2014

Ferri's CLINICAL ADVISOR

5 Books in 1

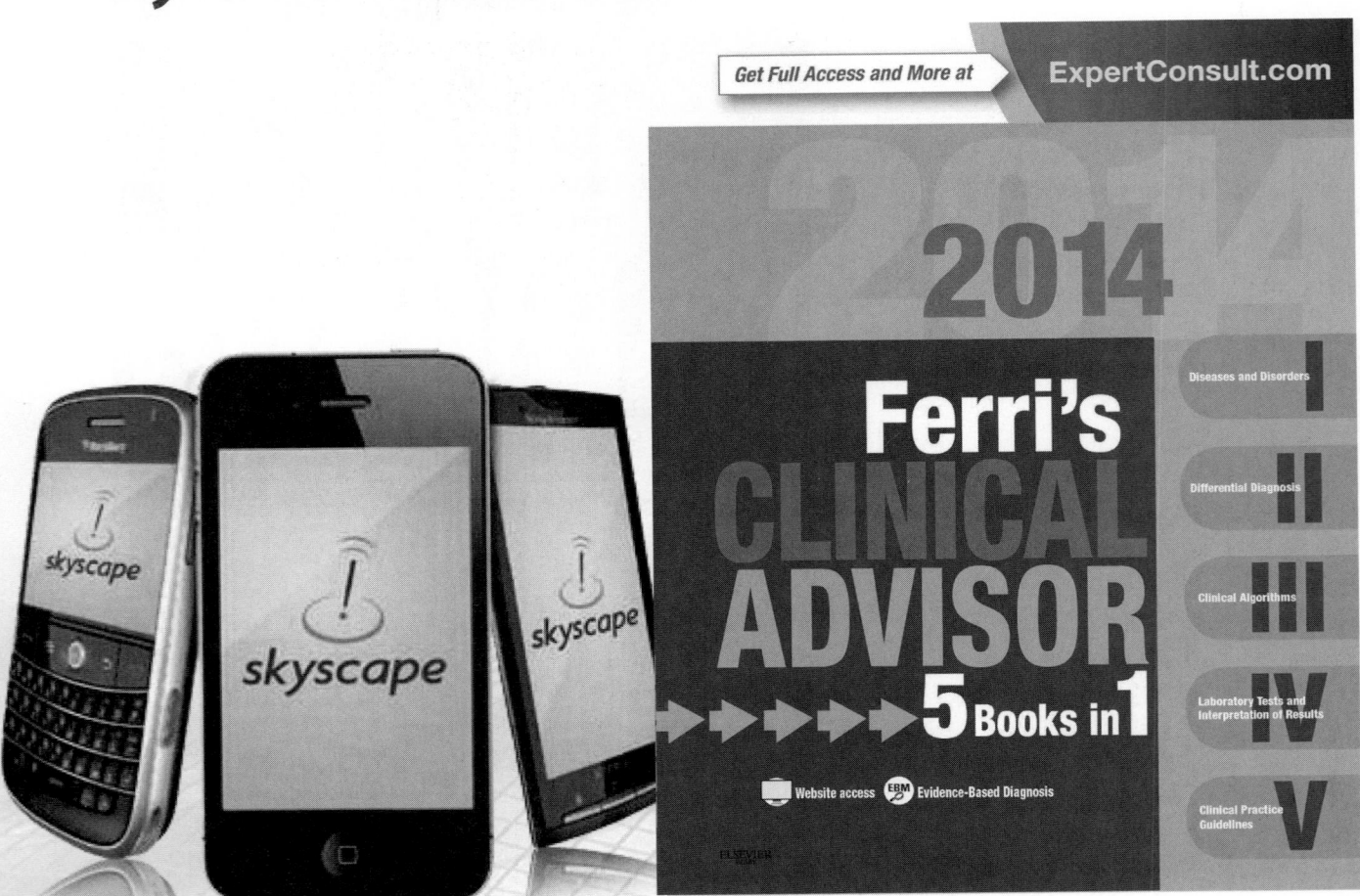

2014

Ferri's CLINICAL ADVISOR

5 Books in 1

FRED F. FERRI, M.D., F.A.C.P.
Clinical Professor
Alpert Medical School
Brown University
Providence, Rhode Island

ELSEVIER
MOSBY

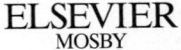

1600 John F. Kennedy Blvd.
Ste 1800
Philadelphia, PA 19103-2899

FERRI'S CLINICAL ADVISOR 2014: 5 BOOKS IN 1

ISBN: 978-0-323-08374-4
ISSN: 1541-4515

Notices

Knowledge and best practice in this field are constantly changing. As new research and experience broaden our
understanding, changes in research methods, professional practices, or medical treatment may become necessary.

Practitioners and researchers must always rely on their own experience and knowledge in evaluating and using
any information, methods, compounds, or experiments described herein. In using such information or methods they
should be mindful of their own safety and the safety of others, including parties for whom they have a professional
responsibility.

With respect to any drug or pharmaceutical products identified, readers are advised to check the most current
information provided (i) on procedures featured or (ii) by the manufacturer of each product to be administered, to
verify the recommended dose or formula, the method and duration of administration, and contraindications. It is the
responsibility of practitioners, relying on their own experience and knowledge of their patients, to make diagnoses,
to determine dosages and the best treatment for each individual patient, and to take all appropriate safety
precautions.

To the fullest extent of the law, neither the Publisher nor the authors, contributors, or editors, assume any liability
for any injury and/or damage to persons or property as a matter of products liability, negligence or otherwise, or
from any use or operation of any methods, products, instructions, or ideas contained in the material herein.

ISBN: 978-0-323-08374-4
ISSN: 1541-4515

Senior Content Strategist: Kate Dimock
Content Development Editor: Angela Rufino
Publishing Services Manager: Patricia Tannian
Senior Project Manager: Kristine Feeherty
Designer: Steven Stave

Printed in the United States of America

Last digit is the print number: 9   8   7   6   5   4   3   2   1

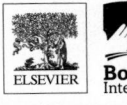

Working together
to grow libraries in
developing countries

www.elsevier.com • www.bookaid.org

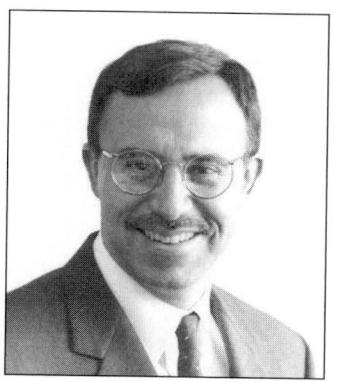

RUBEN ALVERO, M.D.
Director
Assisted Reproductive Technologies
Residency Program Director
Vice Chairman for Education
Department of Obstetrics and
    Gynecology
University of Colorado Denver
Aurora, Colorado
SECTION I

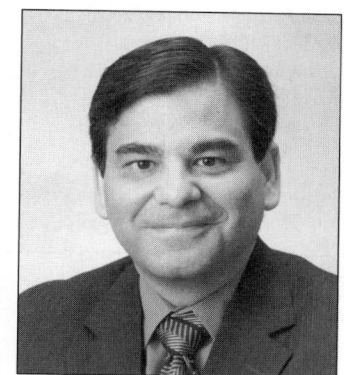

**GLENN G. FORT, M.D.,
M.P.H., F.A.C.P., F.I.D.S.A.**
Clinical Associate Professor of
    Medicine
Alpert Medical School
Brown University
Providence, Rhode Island
Chief
Infectious Diseases
Our Lady of Fatima Hospital
North Providence, Rhode Island
SECTION I

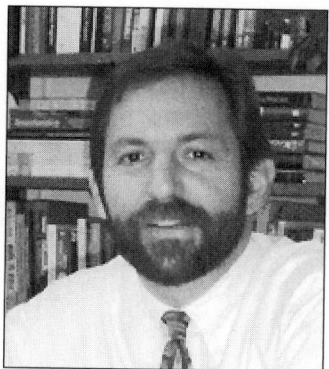

**JEFFREY M. BORKAN,
M.D., Ph.D.**
Professor and Chair
Department of Family Medicine
Memorial Hospital of Rhode Island
Pawtucket, Rhode Island
Alpert Medical School
Brown University
Providence, Rhode Island
SECTION I

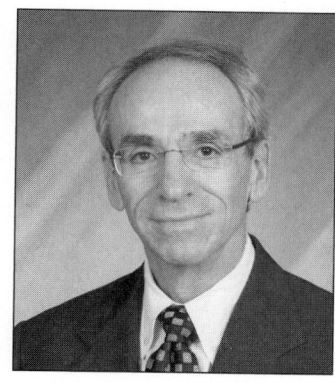

**RICHARD J. GOLDBERG,
M.D., M.S.**
Psychiatrist-in-Chief
Rhode Island Hospital and the
    Miriam Hospital
Professor
Department of Psychiatry and
    Human Behavior
Alpert Medical School
Brown University
Providence, Rhode Island
SECTION I

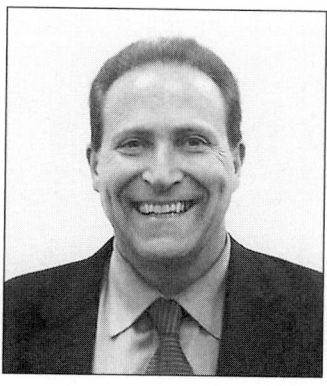

**FRED F. FERRI,
M.D., F.A.C.P.**
Clinical Professor
Alpert Medical School
Brown University
Providence, Rhode Island
SECTIONS I-V

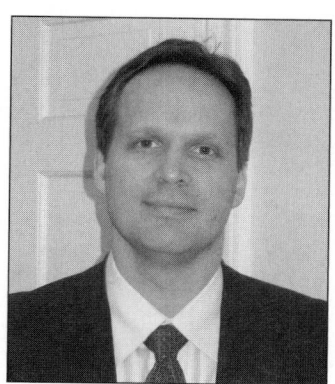

**HARALD ALEXANDER
HALL, M.D.**
Director
Rheumatology Fellowship Program
Roger Williams Medical Center
Assistant Professor of Medicine
Boston University School of
    Medicine
Boston, Massachusetts
SECTION I

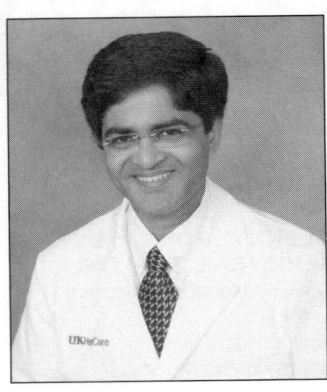

SACHIN KEDAR, M.B.B.S., M.D.
Assistant Professor of Neurology
and Ophthalmology
Director, Neurology Residency
Program
Director, Neuro-ophthalmology
Service
University of Kentucky College of
Medicine
Lexington, Kentucky
SECTION I

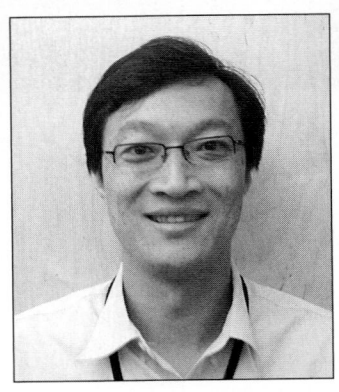

WEN-CHIH WU, M.D., M.P.H.
Associate Professor of Medicine
Alpert Medical School
Brown University
Staff Cardiologist
Providence VA Medical Center
Providence, Rhode Island
SECTION I

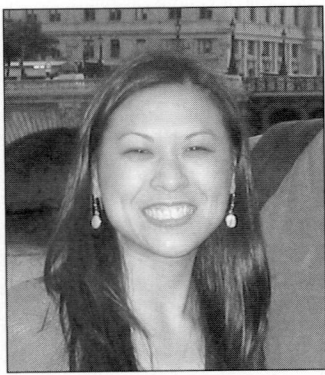

IRIS L. TONG, M.D.
Director, Women's Primary Care
Women's Medicine Collaborative
Assistant Professor
Department of Medicine
Alpert Medical School
Brown University
Providence, Rhode Island
SECTION I

SONYA S. ABDEL-RAZEQ, M.D.
Clinical Assistant Instructor
Department of Obstetrics and Gynecology/Resident Education
State University of New York at Buffalo
Women's and Children's Hospital
Buffalo, New York

ABDULRAHMAN ABDULBAKI, M.D.
Fellow, Cardiology
Louisiana State University and Health Science Center
Shreveport, Louisiana

AKINNIRAN A. ABISOGUN, M.D.
Internal Medicine Resident
Alpert Medical School
Brown University
Providence, Rhode Island

WAFFIYAH AFRIDI, M.D.
Fellow, Rheumatology
Rhode Island Hospital
Alpert Medical School
Brown University
Providence, Rhode Island

MONZR M. AL MALKI, M.D.
Biotherapeutics Development Laboratory
Division of Surgical Research
Boston University School of Medicine
Roger Williams Medical Center
Providence, Rhode Island

TANYA ALI, M.D.
Clinical Assistant Professor of Medicine
Department of Medicine
Alpert Medical School
Brown University
Providence, Rhode Island

PHILIP J. ALIOTTA, M.D., M.S.H.A., F.A.C.S.
Clinical Instructor
Department of Urology
School of Medicine and Biomedical Sciences
State University of New York at Buffalo
Buffalo, New York
Medical Director
Center for Urologic Research of Western New York
Williamsville, New York

RUBEN ALVERO, M.D.
Director, Assisted Reproductive Technologies
Residency Program Director
Vice Chairman for Education
Department of Obstetrics and Gynecology
University of Colorado Denver
Aurora, Colorado

SRIVIDYA ANANDAN, M.D.
Attending Physician
Internal Medicine
Harvard Vanguard Medical Associates
Quincy, Massachusetts

EMILY ANASTASIA, PHARM.D.
PGY-1 Resident
Veterans Affairs Tennessee Valley Healthcare System
Nashville, Tennessee

MEL L. ANDERSON, M.D., F.A.C.P.
Assistant Professor of Medicine
University of Colorado School of Medicine
Denver Veterans Affairs Medical Center
Denver, Colorado

LAURA M. ANDOLINA, M.S., C.G.C.
Clinical Instructor of Pediatrics
State University of New York at Buffalo
School of Medicine and Biomedical Sciences
Buffalo, New York

KATHRYN TAYLOR ANILOWSKI, M.S., P.T., C.L.T.-L.A.N.A.
Instructor
Norton School of Lymphatic Therapy
Director
Kinder Touch Lymphedema Center
Saratoga Springs, New York

ANNGENE G. ANTHONY, M.D., M.P.H., F.A.A.F.P.
Clinical Leader
Zufall Health Center
Morristown, New Jersey

MICHELLE STOZEK ANVAR, M.D.
Assistant Professor (Clinical)
Department of Medicine
Alpert Medical School
Brown University
Providence, Rhode Island

ETSUKO AOKI, M.D., PH.D.
Attending Physician
Department of Hematology
Nagoya Medical Center
Nagoya, Japan

NICOLE APPELLE, M.D., M.P.H.
Assistant Professor of Internal Medicine
University of California, San Francisco
San Francisco, California

GRAYSON ARMSTRONG, B.A.
Medical Student
Alpert Medical School
Brown University
Providence, Rhode Island

WISSAM S. Z. ASFAHANI, M.D.
Department of Neurosurgery
University of Kentucky
Lexington, Kentucky

DANIEL K. ASIEDU, M.D., Ph.D., F.A.C.P.
Clinical Instructor of Medicine
Alpert Medical School
Brown University
Staff Physician
Coastal Medical, Inc.
Providence, Rhode Island

SUDEEP KAUR AULAKH, M.D., C.M., F.R.C.P.C.
Director of Ambulatory Education
Baystate High Street Health Center
Assistant Professor of Medicine
Tufts University School of Medicine
Baystate Medical Center
Springfield, Massachusetts

NUPUR BAHL, M.D.
Endocrine Fellow
Warren Alpert Medical School
Brown University
Rhode Island Hospital
Providence, Rhode Island

CRISOSTOMO R. BALIOG, Jr., M.D.
Assistant Professor
Division of Rheumatology
Department of Internal Medicine
University of South Alabama College of Medicine
Mobile, Alabama

PRIYA BANSAL, M.D., M.P.H.
Physician
Internal Medicine
Miriam Hospital/Rhode Island Hospital
Providence, Rhode Island

ROWLAND P. BARRETT, Ph.D.
Associate Professor of Psychiatry & Human Behavior
Alpert Medical School
Brown University
Providence, Rhode Island

AILIN BARSEGHIAN EL-FARRA, M.D.
Division of Cardiology
University of California, Irvine
Orange, California

VIKRAM BEHERA, M.D.
Clinical Instructor of Medicine
Alpert Medical School
Brown University
Providence, Rhode Island

OMRI BERGER, M.D.
Fellow, Psychiatry and the Law Program
Department of Psychiatry
University of California, San Francisco
San Francisco, California

ARNALDO A. BERGES, M.D.
Rhode Island Hospital
Assistant Clinical Professor
Department of Psychiatry and Human Behavior
Alpert Medical School
Brown University
Providence, Rhode Island

SETH A. BERKOWITZ, M.D.
Division of General Internal Medicine
Department of Medicine
University of California, San Francisco
San Francisco, California

JAYDEEP BHAT, M.D., M.P.H.
Fellow, Gastroenterology
Alpert Medical School
Brown University
Providence, Rhode Island

HARIKRISHNA BHATT, M.D.
Assistant Professor of Medicine (Clinical)
Hallett Center for Diabetes and Endocrinology
Alpert Medical School
Brown University
Providence, Rhode Island

COURTNEY CLARK BILODEAU, M.D.
Attending Physician
Obstetric Medicine/Women's Primary Care
Women's Medicine Collaborative
Providence, Rhode Island

MICHAEL BLUNDIN, M.D.
Pulmonary and Critical Care
Rhode Island Hospital
Providence, Rhode Island

SHEENAGH M. BODKIN, M.D.
Women's Primary Care
Women's Medicine Collaborative
Providence, Rhode Island

NIRALI BORA, M.D.
Assistant Clinical Instructor of Family Medicine
Alpert Medical School
Brown University
Providence, Rhode Island
Memorial Hospital of Rhode Island
Pawtucket, Rhode Island

JEFFREY M. BORKAN, M.D., Ph.D.
Professor and Chair
Department of Family Medicine
Memorial Hospital of Rhode Island
Pawtucket, Rhode Island
Alpert Medical School
Brown University
Providence, Rhode Island

ALEXANDRA BOSKE, M.D.
Chief Resident
Department of Neurology
University of Kentucky
Lexington, Kentucky

LYNN BOWLBY, M.D., F.A.C.P.
Medical Director
Duke Outpatient Clinic (DOC)
Duke Internal Medicine Residency Program
Durham, North Carolina

MARK F. BRADY, M.D., M.P.H.
Department of Emergency Medicine
Yale-New Haven Hospital
New Haven, Connecticut

MANDEEP K. BRAR, M.D.
Clinical Assistant Professor
Department of Obstetrics and Gynecology
State University of New York at Buffalo
Buffalo, New York

ELIZABETH J. BROWN, M.D.
Assistant Clinical Instructor of Family Medicine
Memorial Hospital of Rhode Island
Pawtucket, Rhode Island
Alpert Medical School
Brown University
Providence, Rhode Island

GAVIN BROWN, M.D.
Fellow, Neuromuscular Diseases
Emory University
Atlanta, Georgia

JENNIFER BUCKLEY, M.D.
Assistant Clinical Instructor of Family Medicine
Memorial Hospital of Rhode Island
Pawtucket, Rhode Island
Alpert Medical School
Brown University
Providence, Rhode Island

JONATHAN BURNS, M.A., M.D.
Assistant Clinical Instructor of Family Medicine
Alpert Medical School
Brown University
Providence, Rhode Island

D. BRANDON BURTIS, D.O.
Fellow, Behavioral Neurology
Department of Neurology
College of Medicine
University of Florida
Gainesville, Florida

DOUGLAS BURTT, M.D.
Clinical Assistant Professor of Medicine
Division of Cardiology
Alpert Medical School
Brown University
Providence, Rhode Island

STEVEN BUSSELEN, M.D.
Medical Director
Tri-Town Health Center
Johnston, Rhode Island

CLAUDIA RODRIGUEZ CABRERA, M.D.
Internal Medicine Residency Program Director
Hospital Regional Universitario de Jose Maria Cabral y Baez
Santiago, Dominican Republic

PHILIP A. CHAN, M.D.
Infectious Disease Medicine
Miriam Immunology Clinic
The Miriam Hospital
Providence, Rhode Island

SAURAV CHATTERJEE, M.D.
Fellow, Preventive Cardiology
Providence VA Medical Center
Alpert Medical School
Brown University
Providence, Rhode Island

SUNIT-PREET CHAUDHRY, M.D.
Fellow, Cardiovascular Disease
Alpert Medical School
Brown University
Providence, Rhode Island

VICKY CHENG, M.D.
Assistant Professor of Medicine (Clinical)
Hallett Center for Diabetes and Endocrinology
Alpert Medical School
Brown University
Providence, Rhode Island

GAURAV CHOUDHARY, M.D.
Assistant Professor of Medicine
Alpert Medical School
Brown University
Providence, Rhode Island

STEPHANIE W. CHOW, M.D.
Assistant Clinical Instructor of Family Medicine
Alpert Medical School
Brown University
Providence, Rhode Island

LISA COHEN, PHARM.D.
Associate Professor
Department of Pharmacy Practice
University of Rhode Island
Kingston, Rhode Island
Research Pharmacist
Providence VA Medical Center
Providence, Rhode Island

SCOTT COHEN, M.D.
Fellow, Cardiology
Alpert Medical School
Brown University
Providence, Rhode Island

KAILA COMPTON, M.D., Ph.D.
Attending Psychiatrist
Alta Bates/Herrick Hospital
Berkeley, California

MARIA A. CORIGLIANO, M.D., F.A.C.O.G.
Clinical Assistant Professor
Department of Obstetrics and Gynecology
State University of New York at Buffalo
Buffalo, New York

BRIAN J. COWLES, PHARM.D.
Assistant Professor of Pharmacy
Department of Pharmacy Practice
Albany College of Pharmacy and Health Sciences, Vermont Campus
Colchester, Vermont

DAN A. CRISTESCU, M.D.
Fellow, Rheumatology
Roger Williams Medical Center
Boston University School of Medicine
Providence, Rhode Island

PATRICIA CRISTOFARO, M.D.
Assistant Professor of Medicine
Alpert Medical School
Brown University
Physician
Providence VA Medical Center
Providence, Rhode Island

STEPHANIE A. CURRY, M.D.
Internal Medicine Resident
Roger Williams Medical Center
Boston University School of Medicine
Boston, Massachusetts

ALICIA J. CURTIN, Ph.D., G.N.P.
Assistant Professor
Division of Geriatrics
Alpert Medical School
Brown University
Providence, Rhode Island

CATHERINE D'AVANZATO, M.S.
Department of Psychiatry
Rhode Island Hospital
Providence, Rhode Island

ALI DAHHAN, M.D.
Preventive Cardiology Felloe
Providence VA Medical Center
Alpert Medical School
Brown University
Providence, Rhode Island

KRISTY L. DALRYMPLE, Ph.D.
Assistant Professor (Research)
Department of Psychiatry and Human Behavior
Alpert Medical School
Brown University
Staff Psychologist
Department of Psychiatry
Rhode Island Hospital
Providence, Rhode Island

GEORGE T. DANAKAS, M.D., F.A.C.O.G.
Clinical Assistant Professor
Department of Obstetrics and Gynecology
State University of New York at Buffalo
Buffalo, New York

ALEXANDRA DEGENHARDT, M.D., M.M.Sc.
Director
Multiple Sclerosis Center
New York Methodist Hospital
Brooklyn, New York

JOSEPH A. DIAZ, M.D., M.P.H.
Associate Professor of Medicine
Division of General Internal Medicine
Alpert Medical School
Brown University
Providence, Rhode Island

MICHAEL R. DOBBS, M.D.
Associate Professor of Neurology
Vice-Chair for Clinical Operations
Medical Director
Stroke Care
Chandler Medical Center
University of Kentucky
Lexington, Kentucky

NATHALIA DOOBAY, D.P.M.
Roger Williams Medical Center
Department of Podiatric Surgery
Boston University School of Medicine
Providence, Rhode Island

WILLIAM F. DOTSON II, M.D.
Department of Neurology
Medical Center
University of Kentucky
Lexington, Kentucky

ANDREW DUKER, M.D.
Assistant Professor of Neurology
James J. and Joan A. Gardner Family Center for Parkinson's Disease
  and Movement Disorders
University of Cincinnati
Cincinnati, Ohio

STUART J. EISENDRATH, M.D.
Professor of Clinical Psychiatry
Director of the UCSF Depression Center
Director of Clinical Services
Langley Porter Psychiatric Hospital and Clinics
University of California, San Francisco
San Francisco, California

PAMELA ELLSWORTH, M.D.
Associate Professor of Urology
Alpert Medical School
Brown University
Providence, Rhode Island

HODA ELTOMI, M.D.
Assistant Clinical Instructor of Family Medicine
Memorial Hospital of Rhode Island
Pawtucket, Rhode Island
Alpert Medical School
Brown University
Providence, Rhode Island

MICHAEL ENGELS, M.D.
Internal Medicine Resident
Warren Alpert Medical School
Brown University
Rhode Island Hospital
Providence, Rhode Island

PATRICIO SEBASTIAN ESPINOSA, M.D., M.P.H.
Adjunct Professor of Neurology and Pediatric Neurology
College of Health Sciences
Universidad San Francisco de Quito (USFQ)
Medical Staff
Hospital de los Valles
Cumbayá, Quito, Ecuador
Chairman
International Center of Neurosciences
Quito, Ecuador/New Orleans, Louisiana

VALERIA FABRE, M.D.
Clinical Assistant Instructor of Medicine
Memorial Hospital of Rhode Island
Pawtucket, Rhode Island
Alpert Medical School
Brown University
Providence, Rhode Island

MARK J. FAGAN, M.D.
Director
Medical Primary Care Unit
Rhode Island Hospital
Professor of Medicine
Alpert Medical School
Brown University
Providence, Rhode Island

GIL M. FARKASH, M.D.
Assistant Clinical Professor
School of Medicine
State University of New York at Buffalo
Buffalo, New York

TIMOTHY W. FARRELL, M.D.
Assistant Professor of Medicine (Clinical)
Adjunct Assistant Professor of Family Medicine
Division of Geriatrics
School of Medicine
University of Utah
Salt Lake City, Utah

MITCHELL D. FELDMAN, M.D., M.PHIL.
Professor of Medicine
Director of Faculty Mentoring
Division of General Internal Medicine
University of California, San Francisco
San Francisco, California

FRED F. FERRI, M.D., F.A.C.P.
Clinical Professor
Alpert Medical School
Brown University
Providence, Rhode Island

GLEN FINNEY, M.D.
Assistant Professor
Department of Neurology
College of Medicine
University of Florida
Gainesville, Florida

STACI A. FISCHER, M.D., F.A.C.P., F.I.D.S.A.
Associate Professor of Medicine
Division of Infectious Diseases
Alpert Medical School
Brown University
Director, Graduate Medical Education Lifespan
Director, Transplant Infectious Diseases
Rhode Island Hospital
Providence, Rhode Island

MARLENE FISHMAN, M.P.H., C.I.C.
Director
Nosocomial Infection
St. Joseph Health Services of Rhode Island
North Providence, Rhode Island

ILJIE KIM FITZGERALD, M.D.
Psychiatrist
Veterans Affairs Greater Los Angeles Healthcare Center
Los Angeles, California

TAMARA G. FONG, M.D., PH.D.
Assistant Professor of Neurology
Harvard Medical School
Staff Neurologist
Beth Israel Deaconess Medical Center
Assistant Scientist, Aging Brain Center
Institute for Aging Research, Hebrew SeniorLife
Boston, Massachusetts

MICHELLE FORCIER, M.D., M.P.H.
Associate Professor of Pediatrics
Division of Adolescent Medicine
Alpert Medical School
Brown University
Providence, Rhode Island

PHILIP FORMICA, M.D.
Fellow, Cardiovascular Diseases
Alpert Medical School
Brown University
Providence, Rhode Island

FRANK G. FORT, M.D., F.A.C.S.
Medical Director
Capital Region Vein Centre
Schenectady, New York

GLENN G. FORT, M.D., M.P.H., F.A.C.P., F.I.D.S.A.
Clinical Associate Professor of Medicine
Alpert Medical School
Brown University
Providence, Rhode Island
Chief
Infectious Diseases
Our Lady of Fatima Hospital
North Providence, Rhode Island

DAVID J. FORTUNATO, M.D., F.A.C.C.
Clinical Associate Professor of Medicine
Alpert Medical School
Brown University
Cardiology Section
Providence VA Medical Center
Providence, Rhode Island

JUSTIN F. FRASER, M.D.
Assistant Professor of Cerebrovascular, Endovascular, and Skull Base
    Surgery
Department of Neurological Surgery
University of Kentucky
Lexington, Kentucky

GREGORY K. FRITZ, M.D.
Professor and Director
Division of Child and Adolescent Psychiatry
Interim Vice Chair
Department of Psychiatry and Human Behavior
Alpert Medical School
Brown University
Academic Director
E.P. Bradley Hospital
Associate Chief and Director
Child Psychiatry
Rhode Island Hospital
Hasbro Children's Hospital
Providence, Rhode Island

SAINATH GADDAM, M.D.
Fellow, Preventive Cardiology
Providence VA Medical Center
Alpert Medical School
Brown University
Providence, Rhode Island

ANTHONY GALLO, M.D.
Assistant Clinical Professor of Psychiatry
Alpert Medical School
Brown University
Providence, Rhode Island

PAUL F. GEORGE, M.D.
Assistant Professor of Family Medicine
Alpert Medical School
Brown University
Providence, Rhode Island

NEIL M. GHEEWALA, M.D.
Fellow, Cardiovascular Disease
Alpert Medical School
Brown University
Providence, Rhode Island

CINDY GLEIT, M.D.
Assistant Clinical Instructor
Department of Family Medicine
Alpert Medical School
Brown University
Providence, Rhode Island

RICHARD J. GOLDBERG, M.D., M.S.
Psychiatrist-in-Chief
Rhode Island Hospital and The Miriam Hospital
Professor
Department of Psychiatry and Human Behavior
Alpert Medical School
Brown University
Providence, Rhode Island

ALLA GOLDBURT, M.D.
Assistant Instructor of Family Medicine
Department of Family Medicine
Memorial Hospital of Rhode Island
Pawtucket, Rhode Island

GEETHA GOPALAKRISHNAN, M.D.
Associate Professor of Medicine
Alpert Medical School
Brown University
Providence, Rhode Island

PAUL GORDON, M.D.
Clinical Assistant Professor of Medicine
Division of Cardiology
Alpert Medical School
Brown University
Providence, Rhode Island

NANCY R. GRAFF, M.D.
Associate Clinical Professor
Department of Pediatrics
University of California, San Diego
San Diego, California

JOHN A. GRAY, M.D., Ph.D.
Postdoctoral Fellow
NARSAD Hammerschlag Family Investigator
Department of Cellular and Molecular Pharmacology
University of California, San Francisco
San Francisco, California

ELLIOTT M. GROVES, M.D.
Fellow, Cardiovascular Medicine
University of California, Irvine
Orange, California

STEPHEN L. GRUPKE, M.D., M.S.
Resident
Department of Neurological Surgery
University of Kentucky
Lexington, Kentucky

PAVAN GUPTA, M.D., M.ENG.
Cardiovascular Disease Fellow
Alpert Medical School
Brown University
Providence, Rhode Island

PRIYA SARIN GUPTA, M.D., M.P.H.
Assistant Clinical Instructor of Family Medicine
Alpert School of Medicine
Brown University
Providence, Rhode Island

NAWAZ HACK, M.D.
Department of Neurology
Chandler Medical Center
University of Kentucky
Lexington, Kentucky

WILLIAM O. HAHN, M.D.
Brown Internal Medicine Residency Program
Providence, Rhode Island

HARALD ALEXANDER HALL, M.D.
Director
Rheumatology Fellowship Program
Roger Williams Medical Center
Assistant Professor of Medicine
Boston University School of Medicine
Providence, Rhode Island

SAJEEV HANDA, M.D., S.F.H.M.
Director
Division of Hospital Medicine
Rhode Island Hospital
Clinical Assistant Professor of Medicine
Alpert Medical School
Brown University
Providence, Rhode Island

ERICA HARDY, M.D.
Attending Physician
Obstetric Medicine/Women's Primary Care
Women's Medicine Collaborative
Providence, Rhode Island

TAYLOR HARRISON, M.D.
Assistant Professor of Neurology
Department of Neurology
Emory University
Atlanta, Georgia

DON HAYES, Jr., M.D., M.S.
Associate Professor
The Ohio State University
Nationwide Children's Hospital
Columbus, Ohio

DAWN HOGAN, M.D.
Clinical Assistant Professor of Family Medicine
Alpert Medical School
Brown University
Providence, Rhode Island

N. WILSON HOLLAND, M.D., F.A.C.P.
Assistant Professor of Medicine
Fellowship Director
Department of Medicine
Division of Geriatrics and Gerontology
Emory University School of Medicine
Atlanta Veterans Administration Medical Center
Atlanta, Georgia

SUSIE L. HU, M.D.
Assistant Professor of Medicine
Division of Renal Diseases
Department of Internal Medicine
Alpert Medical School
Brown University
Rhode Island Hospital
Providence, Rhode Island

ANNE L. HUME, PHARM.D.
Professor of Pharmacy
Department of Pharmacy Practice
University of Rhode Island
Kingston, Rhode Island
Adjunct Professor of Family Medicine
Memorial Hospital of Rhode Island
Pawtucket, Rhode Island

HARKAWAL S. HUNDAL, M.D., M.S.
Fellow, Cardiovascular Medicine
University of California, Irvine
Orange, California

SHARLISA HUTSON, M.D.
Pediatric Neurology Resident
Department of Neurology
University of Kentucky
Lexington, Kentucky

RICHARD S. ISAACSON, M.D.
Associate Professor of Clinical Neurology
Vice-Chair of Education
Miller School of Medicine
University of Miami
Miami, Florida

AHMAD M. ISMAIL, M.D.
Academic Hospitalist
Memorial Hospital of Rhode Island
Pawtucket, Rhode Island
Assistant Program Director
Internal Medicine Residency Program
Alpert Medical School
Brown University
Providence, Rhode Island

MATTHEW D. JANKOWICH, M.D.
Staff Physician
Pulmonary and Critical Care Medicine
Providence VA Medical Center
Assistant Professor of Medicine
Alpert Medical School
Brown University
Providence, Rhode Island

NOEL S. C. JAVIER, M.D.
Clinical Assistant Professor of Medicine and Pediatrics
Alpert Medical School
Brown University
Providence, Rhode Island

JENNIFER JEREMIAH, M.D.
Clinical Associate Professor of Medicine
Alpert Medical School
Brown University
Providence, Rhode Island

BREE JOHNSTON, M.D., M.P.H.
Associate Professor of Medicine
Division of Geriatrics
Department of Medicine
Veterans Affairs Medical Center
University of California, San Diego
San Diego, California

KIMBERLY JONES, M.D.
Assistant Professor of Neurology and Pediatrics
University of Kentucky
Lexington, Kentucky

LUCY KALANITHI, M.D.
Postdoctoral Fellow
Stanford University School of Medicine
Stanford, California

SIDDHARTH KAPOOR, M.D.
Assistant Professor of Neurology
University of Kentucky College of Medicine
Lexington, Kentucky

EMILY R. KATZ, M.D.
Director
Child & Adolescent Psychiatry Consultation-Liaison Service
Hasbro Children's Hospital
Rhode Island Hospital
Assistant Professor (Clinical) of Psychiatry and Human Behavior
Alpert Medical School
Brown University
Providence, Rhode Island

ALI KAZIM, M.D.
Clinical Associate Professor
Department of Psychiatry
David Geffen School of Medicine at UCLA
Los Angeles, California
Associate Chief of Mental Health
Sepulveda Veterans Administration Ambulatory Health Care
Sepulveda, California

SACHIN KEDAR, M.B.B.S., M.D.
Assistant Professor of Neurology and Ophthalmology
Director, Neurology Residency Program
Director, Neuro-ophthalmology Service
University of Kentucky College of Medicine
Lexington, Kentucky

BROOKE E. KEELEY, D.P.M.
Roger Williams Medical Center
Department of Podiatric Surgery
Boston University School of Medicine
Providence, Rhode Island

KARA A. KENNEDY FISTER, D.O.
Assistant Professor of Neurology
KY Clinic L-445
Department of Neurology
University of Kentucky College of Medicine
Lexington, Kentucky

BEVIN KENNEY, M.D.
Instructor in Medicine
Harvard University
Cambridge, Massachusetts
Primary Care Internist
Brookside Community Health Center
Jamaica Plain, Massachusetts

WAN J. KIM, M.D.
Department of Obstetrics and Gynecology
Hayward Medical Center
Hayward, California

ROBERT M. KIRCHNER, M.D.
Fellow, Cardiology
Division of Cardiology
Alpert Medical School
Brown University
Providence, Rhode Island

MICHAEL KLEIN, M.D.
Clinical Assistant Professor
Department of Family Medicine
Alpert Medical School
Brown University
Providence, Rhode Island

MELVYN KOBY, M.D.
Associate Clinical Professor of Medicine
Department of Ophthalmology
University of Louisville School of Medicine
Louisville, Kentucky

ROBERT KOHN, M.D.
Professor
Department of Psychiatry and Human Behavior
Director
Geriatric Psychiatry Fellowship Training Program
Brown University
Providence, Rhode Island

ARAVIND RAO KOKKIRALA, M.D.
Clinical Instructor in Medicine
Alpert Medical School
Brown University
Providence, Rhode Island

KRISTINA KRAMER, M.D.
Medical Director
Intensive Care Unit
John Muir Medical Center
Walnut Creek, California

DAVID KURSS, M.D., F.A.C.O.G.
Clinical Assistant Professor
Department of Obstetrics and Gynecology
State University of New York at Buffalo
Buffalo, New York

CINDY LAI, M.D.
Associate Professor of Clinical Medicine
Intersessions Course Director
Site Director
Medicine Clerkships
University of California, San Francisco
San Francisco, California

EDWARD V. LALLY, M.D.
Director
Division of Rheumatology
Rhode Island Hospital
Professor of Medicine
Alpert School of Medicine
Brown University
Providence, Rhode Island

QUANG P. LE, M.D., M.P.H.
Le & Chang Family Urgent Care
Worcester, Massachusetts

KACHIU LEE, B.A.
Medical Student
Department of Dermatology
Feinberg School of Medicine
Northwestern University
Chicago, Illinois

MARGARET LEKANDER DOBSON, M.D.
Assistant Instructor
Department of Family
Alpert Medical School
Brown University
Providence, Rhode Island
Memorial Hospital of Rhode Island
Pawtucket, Rhode Island

ANDRE LEVCHENKO, Ph.D.
Professor of Biomedical Engineering
Johns Hopkins University
Baltimore, Maryland

DONITA DILLON LIGHTNER, M.D.
Assistant Professor of Pediatric Neurology
Department of Neurology
University of Kentucky
Lexington, Kentucky

CUI LI LIN, M.D.
Fellow, Gastroenterology
Division of Gastroenterology
Alpert Medical School
Brown University
Providence, Rhode Island

RICHARD LONG, M.D.
Adjunct Clinical Associate Professor
Department of Family Medicine
Alpert Medical School
Brown University
Providence, Rhode Island
Clinical Associate Professor of Family Medicine
Department of Family Medicine
Boston University School of Medicine
Boston, Massachusetts

ELIZABETH A. LOWENHAUPT, M.D., F.A.A.P.
Instructor
Department of Psychiatry and Human Behavior
Alpert Medical School
Brown University
Providence, Rhode Island

SUSANNA R. MAGEE, M.D., M.P.H.
Assistant Professor
Department of Family Medicine
Alpert Medical School
Brown University
Providence, Rhode Island
Director of Maternal and Child Health
Memorial Hospital of Rhode Island
Pawtucket, Rhode Island

ACHRAF A. MAKKI, M.D., M.Sc.
Resident
Department of Neurology
Emory University
Atlanta, Georgia

ATIZAZUL H. MANSOOR, M.D.
Fellow, Cardiovascular Diseases
Alpert Medical School
Brown University
Providence, Rhode Island

DOUGLAS W. MARTIN, M.D.
Fellow, Pulmonary Diseases and Critical Care
Alpert Medical School
Brown University
Providence, Rhode Island

ELISABETH B. MATSON, D.O.
Rheumatologist
Exeter, New Hampshire

KATE MAVRICH, M.D.
Assistant Professor (Clinical)
Department of Medicine
Alpert Medical School
Brown University
Providence, Rhode Island

ALISON C. MAY, M.D.
Department of Psychiatry
VA Medical Center
Clinical Instructor
University of California, San Francisco
San Francisco, California

MAITREYI MAZUMDAR, M.D., M.P.H.
Assistant Professor of Neurology
Harvard Medical School
Children's Hospital Boston
Department of Neurology
Boston, Massachusetts

JEFFREY C. McCLEAN II, M.D.
Chief of Electrodiagnostic Medicine
Department of Neurology
San Antonio Military Medical Center
San Antonio, Texas

KELLY A. McGARRY, M.D.
Program Director
General Internal Medicine Residency Program
Rhode Island Hospital
Associate Professor of Medicine
Alpert Medical School
Brown University
Providence, Rhode Island

LYNN McNICOLL, M.D., F.R.C.P.C.
Assistant Professor of Medicine (Clinical)
Alpert Medical School
Brown University
Geriatrician
Division of Geriatrics
Rhode Island Hospital
Providence, Rhode Island

LAURA H. McPEAKE, M.D.
Assistant Professor of Emergency Medicine
Brown University Attending Physician of Emergency Medicine
Rhode Island Hospital/Miriam Hospital
Providence, Rhode Island

ERIN MEDLIN, M.D.
Resident
Department of Obstetrics and Gynecology
University of Colorado School of Medicine
Aurora, Colorado

AKANKSHA MEHTA, M.D.
Fellow, Male Reproductive Medicine and Microsurgery
Department of Urology
Weill Cornell Medical College
New York, New York

DANIEL E. MENDEZ-ALLWOOD, M.D.
Fellow, Rheumatology
Roger Williams Medical Center
Boston University School of Medicine
Providence, Rhode Island

LONNIE R. MERCIER, M.D.
Clinical Instructor
Department of Orthopedic Surgery
Creighton University School of Medicine
Omaha, Nebraska

THERESA A. MORGAN, M.PHIL.
Resident in Clinical Psychology
Alpert Medical School
Brown University
Department of Psychiatry
Rhode Island Hospital
Providence, Rhode Island

NADIA MUJAHID, M.D.
Fellow
Department of Geriatrics
Rhode Island Hospital
Alpert Medical School
Brown University
Providence, Rhode Island

VINCENT A. MUKKADA, M.D.
Assistant Professor (Clinical) of Pediatrics
Alpert Medical School
Brown University
Pediatric Gastroenterologist
Hasbro Children's Hospital
Rhode Island Hospital
Providence, Rhode Island

LAURENCE MURPHY, M.D.
Internal Medicine Resident
Warren Alpert Medical School
Brown University
Rhode Island Hospital
Providence, Rhode Island

BILAL H. NAQVI, M.D.
Hematologist/Oncologist
Marshfield Clinic Regional Cancer Center
Eau Claire, Wisconsin

JACK H. NASSAU, PH.D.
Clinical Assistant Professor of Psychiatry and Human Behavior
Alpert Medical School
Brown University
Pediatric Psychologist
Rhode Island Hospital
Hasbro Children's Hospital
Providence, Rhode Island

JUDY NEE, M.D.
Fellow, Gastroenterology
Alpert Medical School
Brown University
Providence, Rhode Island

TAKUMA NEMOTO, M.D.
Research Associate Professor of Surgery
State University of New York at Buffalo
Buffalo, New York

JAMES J. NG, M.D.
Staff Physician
The Vancouver Clinic
Vancouver, Washington

MELISSA NOTHNAGLE, M.D.
Assistant Professor of Family Medicine
Alpert Medical School
Brown University
Providence, Rhode Island

BETH NOWAK, M.D.
Fellow, Geriatric Medicine
Boston Medical Center
Boston, Massachusetts

GAIL M. O'BRIEN, M.D.
Alliance Internal Medicine
Edgartown, Massachusetts

CAROLYN J. O'CONNOR, M.D.
Assistant Clinical Professor
School of Medicine
Yale University
Department of Medicine
St. Mary's Hospital
Waterbury, Connecticut

ALEXANDER B. OLAWAIYE, M.D.
Fellow
Division of Gynecologic Oncology
Vincent Department of Obstetrics, Gynecology and Reproductive Biology
Massachusetts General Hospital
Harvard Medical School
Boston, Massachusetts

MICHAEL K. ONG, M.D., PH.D.
Assistant Professor
UCLA Division of General Internal Medicine/Health Services Research
School of Medicine
University of California, Los Angeles
Los Angeles, California

STEVEN M. OPAL, M.D.
Professor of Medicine
Infectious Disease Division
Alpert Medical School
Brown University
Providence, Rhode Island

JOSEPH R. OWENS, M.D.
Georgetown Neurology
Georgetown, Kentucky

CRISTINA ANTONIO PACHECO, M.D.
Clinical Assistant Professor
Department of Family Medicine
Alpert Medical School
Brown University
Providence, Rhode Island

ROBERTO PACHECO, M.D.
Fellow, Interventional Cardiology
Alpert Medical School
Brown University
Providence, Rhode Island

LISA PAPPAS-TAFFER, M.D.
Dermatologist
University of Pennsylvania Health System
Philadelphia, Pennsylvania

JANICE PATACSIL-TRULL, M.D.
Family Practitioner
Family Medicine Associates of South Attleboro
South Attleboro, Massachusetts

BIRJU B. PATEL, M.D., F.A.C.P.
Assistant Professor of Medicine
Department of Medicine
Division of Geriatrics and Gerontology
Emory University School of Medicine
Atlanta Veterans Administration Medical Center
Atlanta, Georgia

PRANAV M. PATEL, M.D., F.A.C.C., F.S.C.A.I.
Chief (Interim)
Division of Cardiology
Associate Professor of Medicine
University of California, Irvine
Irvine, California

ELENI PATROZOU, M.D.
Clinical Instructor in Medicine
Alpert Medical School
Brown University
Providence, Rhode Island
Attending Physician
Internist-Infectious Diseases Consultant
Hygeia Hospital Greece
Athens, Greece

ALISON PATTERSON, M.D.
Resident in Obstetrics and Gynecology
Department of Obstetrics and Gynecology
University of Colorado
Aurora, Colorado

STEVEN PELIGIAN, D.O.
Medical Director
CODAC Behavioral Healthcare
Providence, Rhode Island

PRANITH PERERA, M.D.
Providence VA Medical Center
Providence, Rhode Island

KIMBERLY PEREZ, M.D.
Assistant Professor
Department of Medicine
Division of Hematology and Oncology
Alpert Medical School
Brown University
Providence, Rhode Island

HEIDI H. PETERSON, M.D.
Clinical Assistant Professor
Department of Family Medicine
Alpert Medical School
Brown University
Providence, Rhode Island
Memorial Hospital of Rhode Island
Pawtucket, Rhode Island

KATHARINE A. PHILLIPS, M.D.
Director
Body Dysmorphic Disorder Program
Director
Research for Adult Psychiatry
Rhode Island Hospital
Professor of Psychiatry and Human Behavior
Alpert Medical School
Brown University
Providence, Rhode Island

PAUL A. PIRRAGLIA, M.D., M.P.H.
Assistant Professor of Medicine
Alpert Medical School
Brown University
Rhode Island Hospital
Providence, Rhode Island

WENDY A. PLANTE, PH.D.
Clinical Assistant Professor of Psychiatry and Human Behavior
Alpert Medical School
Brown University
Pediatric Psychologist
Rhode Island Hospital
Hasbro Children's Research Center
Providence, Rhode Island

ANDREEA POENARIU, M.D.
Assistant Professor
Department of Medicine
Division of Nephrology and Hypertension
University of Florida Health Science Center
Jacksonville, Florida

SHARON S. HARTMAN POLENSEK, M.D., PH.D.
Assistant Professor of Neurology
Center for Dizziness and Balance Disorders
Emory University
Atlanta, Georgia
Chief
Audiology and Speech Pathology
Atlanta VA Medical Center
Decatur, Georgia

SAMUEL H. POON, M.D.
Assistant Director
Rheumatology Fellowship Program
Roger Williams Medical Center
Boston University School of Medicine
Providence, Rhode Island

DONN POSNER, PH.D., C.B.S.M.
Director, Clinical Behavioral Medicine
Sleep Disorders Center of Lifespan Hospitals
Clinical Associate Professor
Alpert Medical School
Brown University
Providence, Rhode Island

ARUNDATHI G. PRASAD, M.D.
Clinical Instructor
Department of Obstetrics and Gynecology/Resident Education
State University of New York at Buffalo
Women's and Children's Hospital
Buffalo, New York

AMANDA PRESSMAN, M.D.
Assistant Professor (Clinical)
Department of Medicine
Alpert Medical School
Brown University
Women's Gastrointestinal Health
Women's Medicine Collaborative
Providence, Rhode Island

MICHAEL PRODROMOU, M.D.
Internal Medicine Resident
Warren Alpert Medical School
Brown University
Rhode Island Hospital
Providence, Rhode Island

KITTICHAI PROMRAT, M.D.
Assistant Professor
Division of Gastroenterology
Department of Medicine
Alpert Medical School
Brown University
Chief
Gastroenterology Section
Providence VA Medical Center
Providence, Rhode Island

SHAHNAZ PUNJANI, M.D.
Fellow, Preventive Cardiology
Providence VA Medical Center
Alpert Medical School
Brown University
Providence, Rhode Island

MATTHEW I. QUESENBERRY, M.D.
Assistant Professor
Hematology/Oncology
Alpert Medical School
Brown University
Rhode Island Hospital
Providence, Rhode Island

RADHIKA A. RAMANAN, M.D., M.P.H.
Assistant Professor of Medicine
University of California, San Francisco
San Francisco, California

WASIM RASHID, M.D.
Director
Geriatric Psychiatry
Rhode Island Hospital
Providence, Rhode Island

JOHN L. REAGAN, M.D.
Fellow, Hematology/Oncology
Rhode Island Hospital/The Miriam Hospital
Alpert Medical School
Brown University
Providence, Rhode Island

RICHARD REGNANTE, M.D.
Division of Cardiovascular Medicine
Alpert Medical School
Brown University
Providence, Rhode Island

VICTOR I. REUS, M.D.
Professor
Department of Psychiatry
School of Medicine
Langley Porter Psychiatric Institute
University of California, San Francisco
San Francisco, California

HARLAN G. RICH, M.D., F.A.C.P., A.F.A.F.
Director of Endoscopy
Rhode Island Hospital
Associate Professor of Medicine
Alpert Medical School
Brown University
Providence, Rhode Island

JESSICA RISSER, M.D., M.P.H.
Third Year Dermatology Resident
Department of Dermatology
Alpert Medical School
Brown University
Providence, Rhode Island

RACHEL ROACH, A.P.R.N.-B.C.
GNP, Teaching Associate
University Medicine Foundation
Division of Geriatrics
Alpert Medical School
Brown University
Providence, Rhode Island

LUTHER K. ROBINSON, M.D.
Associate Professor of Pediatrics
Director
Dysmorphology and Clinical Genetics
State University of New York at Buffalo
Buffalo, New York

DOMINIC RODA, D.P.M.
Podiatry Resident
Roger Williams Medical Center
Boston University School of Medicine
Boston, Massachusetts

JAMISON ROGERS, M.D.
Clinical Assistant Professor
Department of Psychiatry and Human Behavior
Alpert Medical School
Brown University
Providence, Rhode Island
Bradley Hospital
East Providence, Rhode Island

ANISHKA S. ROLLE, M.D.
Fellow, Rheumatology
Roger Williams Medical Center
Boston University School of Medicine
Providence, Rhode Island

JULIE L. ROTH, M.D.
Assistant Professor
Department of Neurology
Alpert Medical School
Brown University
Rhode Island Hospital
Providence, Rhode Island

AMITY RUBEOR, D.O.
Assistant Professor (Clinical)
Department of Family Medicine
Alpert Medical School
Brown University
Providence, Rhode Island

IMMAD SADIQ, M.D.
Clinical Assistant Professor of Medicine
Division of Cardiology
Alpert Medical School
Brown University
Providence, Rhode Island

NUHA R. SAID, M.D.
Rheumatologist
Medical Clinic of North Texas
Denton, Texas

HEMANT K. SATPATHY, M.D.
Fellow
Division of Maternal Fetal Medicine
Department of Obstetrics and Gynecology
Emory University
Atlanta, Georgia

RUBY K. SATPATHY, M.D.
Fellow, Cardiology
Department of Internal Medicine
Creighton University
Omaha, Nebraska

JASON M. SATTERFIELD, Ph.D.
Director
Behavioral Medicine
Associate Professor of Clinical Medicine
University of California, San Francisco
San Francisco, California

SYEDA M. SAYEED, M.D.
Attending Physician
Internal Medicine Department
Coastal Medicine, Inc.
Providence, Rhode Island

HEIDI SCHNEIDER, M.D., M.P.H.
Rheumatologist
Trinity Clinic
Tyler, Texas

PETER J. SELL, D.O.
Assistant Professor
Department of Pediatrics
University of Massachusetts Medical School
Worcester, Massachusetts

CATHERINE SHAFTS, D.O.
Assistant Clinical Instructor
Alpert Medical School
Brown University
Providence, Rhode Island

MADHAVI SHAH, M.D.
Assistant Clinical Instructor
Department of Family Medicine
Alpert Medical School
Brown University
Providence, Rhode Island

GRACE SHIH, M.D.
Assistant Clinical Instructor
Department of Family Medicine
Alpert Medical School
Brown University
Providence, Rhode Island

ASHA SHRESTHA, M.D.
Medical Resident
Memorial Hospital of Rhode Island
Pawtucket, Rhode Island
Alpert School of Medicine
Brown University
Providence, Rhode Island

MARK SIGMAN, M.D.
Professor of Surgery
Division of Urology
Alpert Medical School
Brown University
Providence, Rhode Island

JOANNE M. SILVIA, M.D.
Clinical Assistant Professor
Assistant Professor
Department of Family Medicine
Memorial Hospital of Rhode Island
Pawtucket, Rhode Island
Alpert Medical School
Brown University
Providence, Rhode Island

DIVYA SINGHAL, M.D.
Department of Neurology
University of Kentucky
Lexington, Kentucky

JOHN SLADKY, M.D.
Staff Neurologist
Associate Program Director
Wilford Hall Medical Center
San Antonio, Texas

JEANETTE G. SMITH, M.D.
Assistant Professor of Medicine
Department of Gastroenterology
Alpert Medical School
Brown University
Providence, Rhode Island

U. SHIVRAJ SOHUR, M.D., Ph.D.
Assistant Professor of Neurology
Harvard Medical School
Boston, Massachusetts

DIVJOT SOOCH, M.D.
Department of Family Medicine
Memorial Hospital of Rhode Island
Pawtucket, Rhode Island

PADMAJA SUDHAKAR, M.B.B.S.
Resident
Neurology Department
University of Kentucky College of Medicine
Lexington, Kentucky

HEATHER SUNTER, M.S.
Medical Student
College of Osteopathic Medicine
University of New England
Biddeford, Maine

MARY BETH SUTTER, M.D.
Assistant Instructor of Family Medicine
Alpert Medical School
Brown University
Providence, Rhode Island

ARUN SWAMINATHAN, M.B.B.S.
Resident
Neurology Department
University of Kentucky College of Medicine
Lexington, Kentucky

JULIE ANNE SZUMIGALA, M.D.
Clinical Instructor
Department of Obstetrics and Gynecology
State University of New York at Buffalo
Buffalo, New York

ANGELA M. TABER (PLETTE), M.D.
Assistant Professor of Medicine
Department of Hematology and Oncology
Alpert Medical School
Brown University
Providence, Rhode Island

DOMINICK TAMMARO, M.D.
Associate Director
Categorical Internal Medicine Residency
Co-Director
Medicine-Pediatrics Residency
Division of General Internal Medicine
Rhode Island Hospital
Associate Professor of Medicine
Alpert Medical School
Brown University
Providence, Rhode Island

SARAH TAPYRIK, M.D.
Fellow, Pulmonary Diseases
NYU Department of Pulmonary and Critical Care
New York, New York

SHAMAIL TARIQ, M.D.
Division of Cardiology
University of California, Irvine
Orange, California

TAHIR TELLIOGLU, M.D.
Assistant Professor of Psychiatry and Human Behavior
Alpert Medical School
Brown University
Director
Substance Abuse Division
Department of Psychiatry
Rhode Island Hospital
Providence, Rhode Island

IRIS L. TONG, M.D.
Assistant Professor
Department of Medicine
Alpert Medical School
Brown University
Director, Women's Primary Care
Women's Medicine Collaborative
Providence, Rhode Island

ALEXANDER G. TRUESDELL, M.D.
Fellow, Cardiology
Alpert Medical School
Brown University
Providence, Rhode Island

MARGARET TRYFOROS, M.D.
Assistant Professor of Family Medicine (Clinical)
Department of Family Medicine
Alpert Medical School
Brown University
Providence, Rhode Island
Memorial Hospital of Rhode Island
Pawtucket, Rhode Island

JOSEPH RALPH TUCCI, M.D., F.A.C.P., F.A.C.E.
Professor of Medicine
Boston University School of Medicine
Boston, Massachusetts
Adjunct Professor of Medicine
Alpert Medical School
Brown University
Director
Division of Endocrinology and Metabolism
Roger Williams Medical Center
Providence, Rhode Island

EROBOGHENE E. UBOGU, M.D.
Associate Professor of Neurology
Director
Neuromuscular Immunopathology Research Laboratory
Department of Neurology
Baylor College of Medicine
Houston, Texas

SEAN H. UITERWYK, M.D.
Clinical Assistant Professor
Department of Family Medicine
Alpert Medical School
Brown University
Providence, Rhode Island

NICOLE J. ULLRICH, M.D., PH.D.
Associate Professor
Harvard Medical School
Department of Neurology
Children's Hospital Boston
Boston, Massachusetts

MARISA E. VAN POZNAK, M.D.
Women's Primary Care
Women's Medicine Collaborative
Providence, Rhode Island

JORGE A. VILLAFUERTE, M.D.
Attending Orthopedic Surgeon
VA Medical Center
West Roxbury, Massachusetts

TARA M. WAYT, D.O.
Emergency Medicine Residency Program
University of Connecticut School of Medicine
Farmington, Connecticut
Hartford Hospital
Hartford, Connecticut

ADAM J. WEINBERG, M.D.
Resident
Internal Medicine
Boston University Medical Center
Boston, Massachusetts

DENNIS M. WEPPNER, M.D., F.A.C.O.G.
Associate Professor of Clinical Gynecology/Obstetrics
State University of New York at Buffalo
Clinical Chief
Department of Gynecology/Obstetrics
Millard Fillmore Hospital
Buffalo, New York

JORDAN WHITE, M.D.
Assistant Instructor
Department of Family Medicine
Alpert Medical School
Brown University
Providence, Rhode Island
Memorial Hospital of Rhode Island
Pawtucket, Rhode Island

HILARY B. WHITLACH, M.D.
Chief of Endocrinology
Providence VA Medical Center
Assistant Professor of Medicine
Alpert Medical School
Brown University
Providence, Rhode Island

MATTHEW P. WICKLUND, M.D., F.A.A.N.
Professor
Department of Neurology
Penn State College of Medicine
Hershey, Pennsylvania

CHARLES WOLFF, M.D.
Interim Chief of Geriatrics and Assistant Professor of Clinical Medicine
Department of Family Medicine
Memorial Hospital of Rhode Island
Pawtucket, Rhode Island
Alpert Medical School
Brown University
Providence, Rhode Island

MARIE ELIZABETH WONG, M.D.
Physician
Family Medicine
Baystate Brightwood Health Center
Springfield, Massachusetts

TZU-CHING (TEDDY) WU, M.D., M.P.H.
Assistant Professor of Neurology
University of Texas Medical School at Houston
Director of Telemedicine
Mischer Neuroscience Institute
Houston, Texas

WEN-CHIH WU, M.D., M.P.H.
Staff Cardiologist
Providence VA Medical Center
Associate Professor of Medicine
Alpert Medical School
Brown University
Providence, Rhode Island

WEN Y. (HELENA) WU-CHEN, M.D.
Department of Neurology
Temple University Hospital
Philadelphia, Pennsylvania

BETH J. WUTZ, M.D.
Clinical Assistant Professor of Medicine
Division of Internal Medicine/Pediatrics
Kajeida Health–Buffalo General Hospital
State University of New York at Buffalo
Buffalo, New York

SARAH L. XAVIER, D.O.
Director of Psychiatric Services
Rhode Island Training School
Director
Child & Adolescent Forensic Psychiatry
Rhode Island Hospital
Clinical Assistant Professor of Psychiatry and Human Behavior
Alpert Medical School
Brown University
Providence, Rhode Island

AUGUSTIN G. YIP, M.D., Ph.D.
Clinical Assistant Professor
Butler Hospital
Department of Psychiatry and Human Behavior
Brown University
Providence, Rhode Island

JOHN Q. YOUNG, M.D., M.P.P.
Assistant Professor
Associate Director
Residency Training Program
Department of Psychiatry
School of Medicine
University of California, San Francisco
Associate Director
Adult Psychiatry Clinic
Langley Porter Psychiatric Hospital and Clinics
Associate Editor
AHRB Web M&M
San Francisco, California

CANDICE YUVIENCO, M.D.
Fellow, Rheumatology
Rhode Island Hospital
Alpert School of Medicine
Brown University
Providence, Rhode Island

FARIHA ZAHEER, M.D.
Department of Neurology
University of Kentucky
Lexington, Kentucky

ZHE ZHENG, M.D., Ph.D.
Fellow, Cardiovascular Diseases
Alpert Medical School
Brown University
Providence, Rhode Island

MARK ZIMMERMAN, M.D.
Director
Outpatient Psychiatry
Rhode Island Hospital/The Miriam Hospital
Associate Professor
Department of Psychiatry
Alpert Medical School
Brown University
Providence, Rhode Island

BERNARD ZIMMERMANN, M.D.
Director
Division of Rheumatology
Roger Williams Medical Center
Associate Professor of Medicine
Boston University School of Medicine
Providence, Rhode Island

SCOTT J. ZUCCALA, D.O., F.A.C.O.G.
Staff Physician
Mercy Hospital of Buffalo
Buffalo, New York

RYAN W. ZUZEK, M.D.
Fellow, Clinical Cardiology
Division of Cardiology
Alpert Medical School
Brown University
Providence, Rhode Island

To our families and colleagues.
Their constant support and encouragement made this book a reality. A special thanks to all the readers who have personally commented on the merits of this book and through their suggestions have helped make this product a best-seller in the medical field.

Fred F. Ferri, M.D.
Clinical Professor
Alpert Medical School
Brown University
Providence, Rhode Island

This book is intended to be a clear and concise reference for physicians and allied health professionals. Its user-friendly format was designed to provide a fast and efficient way to identify important clinical information and to offer practical guidance in patient management. The book is divided into five sections and an appendix, each with emphasis on clinical information.

The tremendous success of the previous editions and the enthusiastic comments from numerous colleagues have brought about several positive changes. Each section has been significantly expanded from prior editions, bringing the total number of medical topics covered in this book to more than 1000. Nearly 500 new illustrations and tables have been added to this new edition to enhance recollection of clinically important facts. The use of ICD-9CM codes in all the topics will expedite claims submission and reimbursement.

Section I describes in detail more than 700 medical disorders. Twenty-five new topics have been added to the 2014 edition. Each medical topic in this section is arranged alphabetically, and the material in each topic is presented in outline format for ease of retrieval. Topics with an accompanying algorithm in Section III are identified with an algorithm symbol (ALG). Similarly, if topics also have a Patient Teaching Guide (PTG) available online, this has been noted. Several new PTGs have been added to the 2014 edition. Throughout the text, key quick-access information is consistently highlighted, clinical photographs are used to further illustrate selected medical conditions, and relevant ICD-9CM codes are listed. Most references focus on current peer-reviewed journal articles rather than outdated textbooks and old review articles. Evidence-based medicine data have been added to relevant topics.

Topics in this section use the following structured approach:
1. Basic Information (Definition, Synonyms, ICD-9CM Codes, Epidemiology & Demographics, Physical Findings & Clinical Presentation, Etiology)
2. Diagnosis (Differential Diagnosis, Workup, Laboratory Tests, Imaging Studies)
3. Treatment (Nonpharmacologic Therapy, Acute General Rx, Chronic Rx, Disposition, Referral)
4. Pearls & Considerations (Comments, Suggested Readings)
5. Evidence-Based Data and References

Section II includes the differential diagnosis, etiology, and classification of signs and symptoms. This section has been significantly expanded for the 2014 edition with the addition of 41 new topics. It is a practical section that allows the user investigating a physical complaint or abnormal laboratory value to follow a "workup" leading to a diagnosis. The physician can then easily look up the presumptive diagnosis in Section I for the information specific to that illness.

Section III includes clinical algorithms to guide and expedite the patient's workup and therapy. Twenty-five new algorithms have been added for the 2014 edition. Many physicians describe this section as particularly valuable in today's managed-care environment.

Section IV includes normal laboratory values and interpretation of results of commonly ordered laboratory tests. By providing interpretation of abnormal results, this section facilitates the diagnosis of medical disorders and further adds to the comprehensive, "one-stop" nature of our text.

Section V focuses on preventive medicine. Information in this section includes recommendations for the periodic health examination, screening for major diseases and disorders, patient counseling, and immunization and chemoprophylaxis recommendations.

The **Appendix** has been divided into five major sections. Section I contains extensive information on complementary and alternative medicine (CAM). With the material in this appendix, we hope to lessen the current scarcity of exposure of allopathic and osteopathic physicians to the diversity of CAM therapies. Section II focuses on nutrition with emphasis on dietary supplements, vitamins, and minerals. Section III deals with diagnosis and treatment of acute poisoning. Section IV, available online, contains an extensive section on primary care procedures. Section V contains several patient teaching guides not linked to Section I topics.

As clinicians, we all realize the importance of patient education and the need for clear communication with our patients. Toward that end, practical patient instruction sheets, organized alphabetically and covering the majority of the topics in this book, are available online and can be easily customized and printed from any computer. All of them have been updated, and several new ones have been added to the 2014 edition. They represent a valuable addition to patient care and are useful for improving physician-patient communication, patient satisfaction, and quality of care.

I believe that we have produced a state-of-the-art information system with significant differences from existing texts. It contains five sections and patient education guides that could be sold separately based on their content, yet are available under a single cover, offering the reader a tremendous value. I hope that the *Clinical Advisor*'s user-friendly approach, numerous unique features, and yearly updates will make this book a valuable medical reference, not only to primary care physicians but also to physicians in other specialties, medical students, and allied health professionals.

Fred F. Ferri, M.D., F.A.C.P.

Note: Comments from readers are always appreciated and can be forwarded directly to Dr. Ferri at fred_ferri@brown.edu.

EVALUATION OF EVIDENCE

Ferri's Clinical Advisor evaluates all evidence based on a rating system published by the American Academy of Family Physicians. In order to indicate the strength of the supporting evidence, each summary statement is accorded one of three levels:

LEVEL A

- Systematic reviews of randomized controlled trials, including meta-analyses
- Good-quality randomized controlled trials

LEVEL B

- Good-quality nonrandomized clinical trials
- Systematic reviews not in Level A
- Lower-quality randomized controlled trials not in Level A
- Other types of study: case-control studies, clinical cohort studies, cross-sectional studies, retrospective studies, and uncontrolled studies

LEVEL C

- Evidence-based consensus statements and expert guidelines

SOURCES OF EVIDENCE

Evidence is summarized principally from three critically evaluated, very highly regarded sources:

- **Cochrane Systematic Reviews** are respected throughout the world as one of the most rigorous searches of medical journals for randomized controlled trials. They provide highly structured systematic reviews, with evidence included or excluded on the basis of explicit quality-related criteria, and they often use meta-analyses to increase the power of the findings of numerous studies.
- *Clinical Evidence* is produced by the BMJ Publishing Group. It provides synopses of the best currently available evidence on the treatment and prevention of many clinical conditions, based on searches and appraisals of the available literature.
- **The National Guideline Clearinghouse™** is a comprehensive database of evidence-based clinical practice guidelines and related documents produced by the Agency for Healthcare Research and Quality in partnership with the American Medical Association and the American Association of Health Plans.

In addition, where evidence exists that has not yet been critically reviewed in one of the three sites above, the evidence is summarized briefly, categorized, and fully referenced. Guidelines are also sourced from government and professional bodies.

Contents

SECTION I Diseases and Disorders

PTG indicates that a Patient Teaching Guide is available at www.expertconsult.com.

Additional Topics Available at www.expertconsult.com

SECTION I Figures, Tables, and Boxes Available at www.expertconsult.com

SECTION II   Differential Diagnosis

SECTION III **Clinical Algorithms**

Additional Algorithms Available at www.expertconsult.com

SECTION IV Laboratory Tests and Interpretation of Results

SECTION V Clinical Practice Guidelines

APPENDIX I Complementary and Alternative Medicine

APPENDIX II Nutrition

APPENDIX III Acute Poisoning

2014

Ferri's CLINICAL ADVISOR

5 Books in 1

Diseases and Disorders

BASIC INFORMATION

DEFINITION

Abruptio placentae is the separation of placenta from the uterine wall before delivery of the fetus. There are three classes of abruption based on maternal and fetal status, including an assessment of uterine contractions, quantity of bleeding, fetal heart rate monitoring, and abnormal coagulation studies (fibrinogen, prothrombin time, partial thromboplastin time).

- Grade I: mild vaginal bleeding, uterine irritability, stable vital signs, reassuring fetal heart rate, normal coagulation profile (fibrinogen 450 mg%)
- Grade II: moderate vaginal bleeding, hypertonic uterine contractions, orthostatic blood pressure measurements, unfavorable fetal status, fibrinogen 150 to 250 mg%
- Grade III: severe bleeding (may be concealed), hypertonic uterine contractions, overt signs of hypovolemic shock, fetal death, thrombocytopenia, fibrinogen <150 mg%

SYNONYMS

Premature separation of placenta

ICD-9CM CODES
641.2 Premature separation of placenta

EPIDEMIOLOGY & DEMOGRAPHICS

INCIDENCE (IN U.S.): One in 86 to 206 births; incidence by grade: I = 40%, II = 45%, III = 15%; 80% occur before the onset of labor
RISK FACTORS: Hypertension (greatest association), trauma, polyhydramnios, multifetal gestation, smoking, use of crack cocaine, chorioamnionitis, preterm premature rupture of membranes
RECURRENCE RATE: 5% to 17%, some studies showing a 5- to 10-fold increase in risk; with two prior episodes, 25%

PHYSICAL FINDINGS & CLINICAL PRESENTATION

- Triad of uterine bleeding (concealed or per vagina), hypertonic uterine contractions or signs of preterm labor, and evidence of fetal compromise exists.
- More than 80% of cases have external bleeding; 20% of cases have no bleeding but have indirect evidence of abruption, such as failed tocolysis for preterm labor.
- Tetanic uterine contractions are found in only 17% of cases unless grade II or III abruption.

ETIOLOGY

- Primary etiology: unknown
- Hypertension: found in 40% to 50% of grade III abruptions
- Rapid decompression of uterine cavity, as can occur in polyhydramnios or multifetal gestation
- Blunt external trauma (motor vehicle accident, spousal abuse)

DIAGNOSIS

DIFFERENTIAL DIAGNOSIS

- Placenta previa
- Cervical or vaginal trauma
- Labor
- Cervical cancer
- Rupture of membranes
- The differential diagnosis of vaginal bleeding in pregnancy is described in Section II

WORKUP

- Initial assessment should evaluate for the source of bleeding, ruling out placenta previa that may contraindicate any type of vaginal examination (e.g., pelvic speculum examination).
- Continuous fetal heart monitoring is indicated for all viable gestations (60% incidence of fetal distress in labor); may show early signs of maternal hypovolemia (late decelerations or fetal tachycardia) before overt maternal vital sign changes.
- Actual amount of blood loss is often greater than initially perceived because of the possibility of concealed retroplacental bleeding and apparent "normal" vital signs. The relative hypervolemia of pregnancy initially protects the patient until late in the course of bleeding, when abrupt and sudden cardiovascular collapse can occur.

LABORATORY TESTS

- Baseline hemoglobin and hematocrit help quantify blood loss and establish baseline values for serial comparisons during expectant management.
- Coagulation profile: platelets, fibrinogen, prothrombin, and partial thromboplastin time. Diffuse intravascular coagulation can develop with severe abruption. If fibrinogen is <150 mg%, estimated blood loss is approximately 2000 ml; if fibrinogen is <100 mg%, consider fresh frozen plasma to prevent further bleeding.
- Type and antibody screen is important to identify Rh-negative patients who may need Rh immune globulin.

IMAGING STUDIES

Ultrasound should include fetal presentation and status, amniotic fluid volume, placental location, as well as any evidence of hematoma (retroplacental, subchorionic, or preplacental).

TREATMENT

ACUTE GENERAL Rx

- Stabilization of the mother is the first priority.
- Treatment depends on gestational age of the fetus, severity of the abruption, and maternal status.
- Initial assessment for signs of maternal hemodynamic compromise or hemorrhagic shock; large-bore intravenous access, with crystalloid fluid resuscitation using a replacement of 3 ml lactated Ringer's solution for every 1 ml estimated blood loss.
- Indwelling Foley catheter to monitor urine output and maternal volume status, with a goal of 30 ml/hr urine output.
- Assess fetal status and gestational age by sonogram and continuous fetal heart rate monitoring.
- Because of the unpredictable nature of abruptions, cross-matched blood should be made available during the initial resuscitation period.

CHRONIC Rx

- In the term fetus or when lung maturity has been documented, delivery is indicated.
- In the preterm fetus or a fetus with an immature lung profile, consider betamethasone 12.5 mg IM q24h for two doses and then delivery, depending on the severity of the abruption and the likelihood of fetal complications from preterm birth.
- Cesarean section should be reserved for cases of fetal distress or for standard obstetric indications. While cesarean delivery may be needed to stabilize the fetal and/or maternal status, the mother's coagulation status may complicate the procedure and availability of blood products may be critical.
- In select cases, such as severe prematurity with a stable mother and mild contractions, magnesium sulfate can be used for tocolysis, 6 g IV loading dose then 3 g/hr maintenance, to allow for a course of steroids.

DISPOSITION

Because of the unpredictable nature of abruptions, expectant management should occur only under controlled circumstances and is rarely practiced.

REFERRAL

Abruptio placentae places mother and fetus in a high-risk situation and should be managed by a qualified obstetrician in a facility with capability for neonatal and maternal resuscitation, for supporting a preterm infant if delivery is indicated at an early gestational age, and for performing emergency cesarean sections.

RELATED CONTENT

Premature Labor (Related Key Topic)
Vaginal Bleeding During Pregnancy (Related Key Topic)
Abruptio Placentae (Patient Information)

AUTHOR: **RUBEN ALVERO, M.D.**

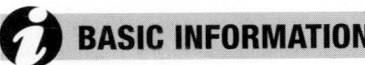 **BASIC INFORMATION**

DEFINITION

A brain abscess is a focal intracerebral infection that can arise as a complication from a bacterial, fungal, or protozoal infection, surgery, or trauma.

ICD-9CM CODES
324.0 Brain abscess

EPIDEMIOLOGY & DEMOGRAPHICS

INCIDENCE: Uncommon (occurs about 2% as commonly as brain tumors)
PEAK INCIDENCE: Preadolescence and middle age (and depends on predisposing condition)
PREDOMINANT AGE: Occurs at any age
PREDOMINANT SEX:
- Men affected more than women (ratio 2:1 to 3:1)

PHYSICAL FINDINGS & CLINICAL PRESENTATION

- Classic triad: fever, headache, and focal neurologic deficit present in less than 50% of cases.
- Clinical presentation is often due to the manifestations of the space-occupying lesion rather than to signs of systemic infection.
- Fever is present in only 32% to 79% of patients.
- Headache is usually localized to the side of the abscess; onset can be gradual or severe; present in an average of 70% to 75% of cases.
- Focal neurologic findings (e.g., seizures, hemiparesis, aphasia, ataxia) depend on the location of the abscess and are seen in 23% to 66% of cases.
- Papilledema is present in 9% to 51% of cases.
- Presence of adjacent infections (dental abscess, otitis media, and sinusitis) may be a clue to the underlying diagnosis and should be sought in any suspected case.
- Time course from symptom onset to presentation ranges from hours in fulminant cases to more than 1 month; 75% present in the first 2 weeks.
- The nonspecific presentation of a brain abscess warrants that clinicians maintain a high index of suspicion. Table 1-1 describes common initial features of brain abscess.

TABLE 1-1 Brain Abscess: Initial Features in 123 Cases

Headache	55%
Disturbed consciousness	48%
Fever	58%
Nuchal rigidity	29%
Nausea, vomiting	32%
Seizures	19%
Visual disturbance	15%
Dysarthria	20%
Hemiparesis	48%
Sepsis	17%

From Goldman L, Schafer AI: *Goldman's Cecil medicine,* ed 24, Philadelphia, 2012, Saunders.

ETIOLOGY

- Brain abscesses are classified based on the likely portal of entry and can arise from:
  Contiguous infection
  Hematogenous spread from a remote site
Likely source of abscess and common organisms involved:
A. Contiguous focus or primary infection (55% of all brain abscesses):
  1. Paranasal sinus: occur in frontal lobe; streptococci (especially microaerophilic and anaerobic streptococci), *Bacteroides, Haemophilus,* and *Fusobacterium* spp.
  2. Otitis media/mastoiditis: occur in temporal lobe and cerebellum; aerobic and anaerobic streptococci, Enterobacteriaceae, *Bacteroides,* and *Pseudomonas* spp.
  3. Dental sepsis: occur in frontal lobe; mixed *Fusobacterium, Bacteroides,* and *Streptococcus* spp. *(especially S. viridans and anaerobic streptococci)*
  4. Penetrating head injury: site of abscess depends on site of wound; *Staphylococcus aureus, aerobic streptococci, Clostridium* spp., Enterobacteriaceae
  5. Postoperative: *Staphylococcus epidermidis* and *S. aureus,* Enterobacteriaceae, and *Pseudomonas aeruginosa*
B. Hematogenous spread from a distant site of infection (25% of all brain abscesses): abscesses most commonly multiple, especially in middle cerebral artery distribution; infecting organisms depend on source.
  1. Congenital heart disease: streptococci, *Haemophilus* spp.
  2. Endocarditis: *S. aureus,* viridans streptococci
  3. Urinary tract: Enterobacteriaceae, Pseudomonadaceae
  4. Intraabdominal: streptococci, Enterobacteriaceae, anaerobes
  5. Lung: streptococci, *Actinomyces* spp., *Fusobacterium* spp.
  6. Immunocompromised host: *Toxoplasma* species, fungi, Enterobacteriaceae, *Nocardia* spp., tuberculosis, listeriosis
C. Cryptogenic (unknown source): 20% of all brain abscesses

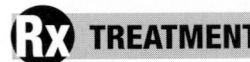 **DIAGNOSIS**

DIFFERENTIAL DIAGNOSIS

- Other parameningeal infections: subdural empyema, epidural abscess, thrombophlebitis of the major dural venous sinuses and cortical veins
- Embolic strokes in patients with bacterial endocarditis
- Mycotic aneurysms with leakage
- Acute hemorrhagic leukoencephalitis
- Parasitic infections: toxoplasmosis, echinococcosis, cysticercosis
- Metastatic or primary brain tumors
- Cerebral infarction
- CNS vasculitis
- Chronic subdural hematoma

WORKUP

Physical examination, laboratory tests, and imaging studies

LABORATORY TESTS

- White blood cell counts are elevated in 60% of patients.
- Erythrocyte sedimentation rate is usually elevated but may be normal.
- Blood cultures are most often negative (10% positive).
- Lumbar puncture is contraindicated in patients with suspected abscess (20% die or experience neurologic decline).
- The yield of Gram stain and culture of material aspirated at time of surgical drainage is very high.

IMAGING STUDIES

- MRI with and without gadolinium is the diagnostic procedure of choice; provides superior detail compared with CT scan (higher sensitivity and specificity than CT scan, but not always immediately available).
- CT scan (Fig. 1-1) with intravenous contrast is still an excellent test (sensitivity 95%-99%).
- Serial CT or MRI scanning is recommended to follow the response to therapy.

Rx TREATMENT

ACUTE GENERAL Rx

- Effective treatment involves a combination of empiric antibiotic therapy and timely excision or aspiration of the abscess.
- If evidence of edema or mass effect, treatment of elevated intracranial pressure is paramount.
  - Hyperventilation of mechanically ventilated patient.
  - Dexamethasone initially in a dosage of 10 mg IV followed by 4 mg IV q6h until symptoms of cerebral edema subside. Steroids should be discontinued as soon as possible.
  - Mannitol 0.25 to 1 g/kg IV over 20 to 30 min q6 to 8h; maximum of 6 g/kg in 24 hr.
- Medical therapy is never a substitute for surgical intervention to relieve increased intracranial pressure. Neurologic deterioration usually mandates surgery.
- Steroids should be limited to patients with severe cerebral edema or midline shift.

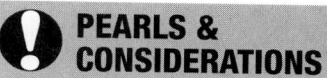

A

I

MEDICAL Rx

If abscess <2.5 cm and patient is neurologically stable and conscious, may start antibiotics and observe. Empiric antibiotic therapy guided by:

- Abscess location
- Suspicion of primary source
- Presence of single or multiple abscesses
- Patient's underlying medical conditions (e.g., HIV, immunocompromised)

Selection of empiric antibiotic therapy:

- Primary infection or contiguous source:
  1. Otitis media/mastoiditis, sinusitis, dental infection: third-generation cephalosporin (cefotaxime 2 g q4h IV or ceftriaxone 2 g q12h IV) plus metronidazole 15 mg/kg IV as a loading dose, then 7.5 mg/kg q8h IV, not to exceed 4 g per day
  2. Dental infection: penicillin G (20 million to 24 million units per day IV in six divided doses) plus mentronidazole (dose as above)
  3. Head trauma: third-generation cephalosporin (cefotaxime 2 g IV q4h or ceftriaxone 2 g IV q12h) plus nafcillin 2 g IV q4h or vancomycin (30 mg/kg IV in two divided doses adjusted for renal function)
  4. Postoperative neurosurgery: vancomycin (dose as above) plus ceftazidime (2 g IV q8h) or cefepime (2 g IV q8h), or meropenem (1 g IV q8h). Replace vancomycin with nafcillin (2g IV q4h) if susceptibility testing reveals methicillin-sensitive *Staphylococcus aureus.*

- Hematogenous spread (congenital heart disease, endocarditis, urinary tract, lung, intraabdominal): vancomycin (empiric therapy, dose as above) or nafcillin (if susceptibility testing reveals methicillin-sensitive *S. aureus,* dose as above) plus metronidazole plus third-generation cephalosporin (cefotaxime 2 g IV q4h or ceftriaxone 2 g IV q12h)

Duration of antibiotic therapy is guided by the clinical course and whether or not the abscess was surgically aspirated or excised. It is usually prolonged. Surgical therapy may be required for clinical failure if the patient is receiving antibiotics alone. Most recommend parenteral treatment for at least 4 to 6 weeks, with repeated neuroimaging to ensure adequate resolution. (Imaging weekly could be considered for first 2 weeks of therapy, then every 2 weeks until resolution.)

SURGICAL Rx

- Two indications for surgical intervention:
  1. Collect specimens for culture and sensitivity
  2. Reduce mass effect
- Stereotactic biopsy or aspirate of the abscess if surgically feasible
- Essential to selection of targeted antimicrobial coverage
- Timing and choice of surgery depends on:
  ○ Primary infection source
  ○ Number and location of the abscesses
  ○ Whether the procedure is diagnostic or therapeutic
  ○ Neurologic status of the patient

DISPOSITION

- Prompt diagnostic consideration, early institution of appropriate antimicrobial therapy, and advanced neuroradiologic imaging have reduced the mortality rate from brain abscesses from 40% to 80% in the preantibiotic era to 10% to 20% at present.
- Morbidity is usually manifest as persistent neurologic sequelae (seizures, intellectual or behavioral impairment, motor deficits).

REFERRAL

Consultation with a neurosurgeon is mandatory.

! PEARLS & CONSIDERATIONS

COMMENTS

- It is important to maintain a high index of suspicion because a brain abscess often presents with nonspecific symptoms.
- Rapid imaging and early institution of appropriate antimicrobial therapy improve patient morbidity and mortality.
- Neurosurgical consultation is mandatory.

PREVENTION

Because brain abscesses arise from either contiguous infections or hematogenously from a remote site, early and appropriate treatment of predisposing infections is paramount to prevent brain abscess.

EBM EVIDENCE

available at www.expertconsult.com

SUGGESTED READINGS

available at www.expertconsult.com

RELATED CONTENT

Brain Abscess (Patient Information)

AUTHORS: **ERICA HARDY, M.D.,** and **KELLY A. MCGARRY, M.D.**

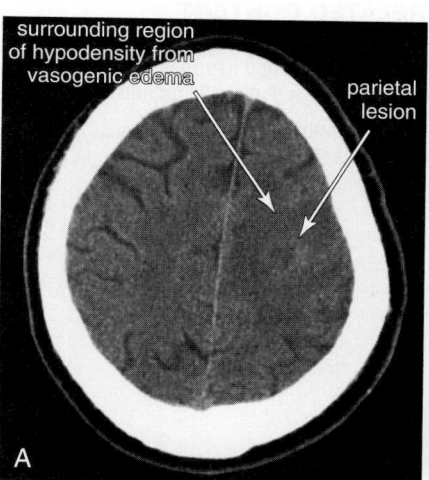
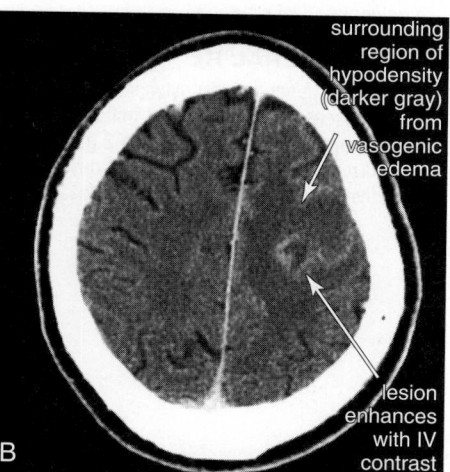
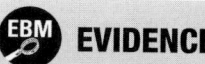

FIGURE 1-1 Brain abscess. This 48-year-old male presented with status epilepticus. Computed tomography (CT) showed a parietal mass, which at brain biopsy was found to be an abscess. Cultures grew mixed gram-positive and gram-negative organisms and anaerobes. The patient was subsequently found to be human immunodeficiency virus positive. **A,** Noncontrast head CT, brain windows. **B,** CT with intravenous (IV) contrast moments later, brain windows. Abscesses and other infectious, inflammatory, or neoplastic lesions typically have surrounding hypodense regions representing vasogenic edema. When IV contrast is administered **(B),** the lesion may enhance peripherally, often referred to as ring enhancement. (From Broder JS: *Diagnostic imaging for the emergency physician,* Philadelphia, 2011, Saunders.)

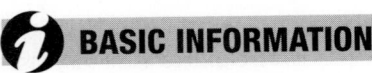

BASIC INFORMATION

DEFINITION

Breast abscess is an acute inflammatory process resulting in the formation of a collection of purulent material in breast tissue. Typically there is painful erythematous mass formation in the breast, occasionally draining through the overlying skin or nipple duct.

SYNONYMS

Subareolar abscess
Lactational or puerperal abscess

ICD-9CM CODES
6.110 Abscess of the breast
675.0 Abscess of the nipple related to childbirth
675.1 Abscess of the breast related to childbirth

EPIDEMIOLOGY & DEMOGRAPHICS

INCIDENCE: 10% to 30% of all breast abscesses are lactational; acute mastitis occurs in 2.5% of nursing mothers, with one in 15 of these women developing abscess. Smoking and diabetes may be risk factors for nonpuerperal mastitis with abscess.

PHYSICAL FINDINGS & CLINICAL PRESENTATION

Painful erythematous induration involving breast and leading to fluctuant abscess

ETIOLOGY

- Lactational abscess: milk stasis and bacterial infection leading to mastitis and then abscess, with *Staphylococcus aureus* the most common causative agent
- Subareolar abscess:
  1. Central ducts involved, with obstructive nipple duct changes leading to bacterial infection
  2. Cultured organisms mixed, including anaerobes, staphylococci, streptococci, and others

DIAGNOSIS

DIFFERENTIAL DIAGNOSIS

- Inflammatory carcinoma
- Advanced carcinoma with erythema, edema, and/or ulceration
- Tuberculous abscess (rare in the United States)
- Hidradenitis of breast skin
- Sebaceous cyst with infection

WORKUP

- Clinical examination sufficient
- If abscess suspected, referral to surgeon for incision, drainage, and biopsy
- If possible abscess suspected, referral for workup required

LABORATORY TESTS

- Perform culture and sensitivity test of abscess contents.
- If mammogram or ultrasound is required but prevented by discomfort, perform after treatment and subsequent resolution of abscess.

TREATMENT

NONPHARMACOLOGIC THERAPY

- Established abscess: incision and drainage
- Biopsy of abscess cavity wall to exclude carcinoma

ACUTE GENERAL Rx

- Antibiotics: generally staphylococci in lactational abscess. Recommended initial antibiotic therapy is nafcillin or oxacillin 2 g q4h IV or cefazolin 1 g q8h IV for 10 to 14 days. Alternative includes vancomycin 1 g IV q12h.

- If acute mastitis is identified and treated early without the development of an abscess, resolution without drainage is possible.
- Subareolar abscess: broad-spectrum antibiotic treatment (e.g., cephalexin 500 mg PO qid or cefazolin 1 g q8h IV for 10 to 14 days for more severe infection) and drainage are needed to control acute phase. If abscess is odoriferous, consider anaerobes as most likely etiology and add metronidazole 500 mg PO/IV tid.

CHRONIC Rx

Further surgical treatment for recurrences or fistula

DISPOSITION

- Lactational abscess: possible to continue breastfeeding without risk of infection to the infant
- Subareolar abscess:
  1. High risk for recurrence or complication of fistula formation
  2. Patient informed and referred to General Surgery for evaluation and treatment

REFERRAL

- If abscess drainage required
- For surgical consultation if subareolar abscess involved

SUGGESTED READINGS

available at www.expertconsult.com

RELATED CONTENT

Breast Cancer (Related Key Topic)
Mastodynia (Related Key Topic)
Breast Abscess (Patient Information)

AUTHORS: **TAKUMA NEMOTO, M.D.,** and **RUBEN ALVERO, M.D.**

BASIC INFORMATION

DEFINITION
Epidural abscess is a suppurative infection of the central nervous system localized between the dura mater and the overlying skull or vertebral column. There are two types of epidural abscess: spinal epidural abscess (SEA) and intracranial epidural abscess (IEA), depending on the location within the central nervous system.

SYNONYMS
Spinal epidural abscess
Intraspinal abscess

ICD-9CM CODES
324.9 Epidural abscess
324.0 Intracranial abscess

EPIDEMIOLOGY & DEMOGRAPHICS
INCIDENCE: Spinal epidural abscess: 2 to 25 patients per 100,000 admissions; spinal epidural abscess is 9 times more common than intracranial abscess
PEAK INCIDENCE: Median age at onset of spinal epidural abscess: 50 years old
PREVALENCE: Greatest between 50 and 70 years of age
PREDOMINANT SEX: More common in men
RISK FACTORS: Bacteremia, secondary to distant infection; epidural catheter placement (0.5% to 3% risk), paraspinal injections of glucocorticoids or for pain management, contiguous bone or soft tissue infection, intravenous drug abuse, diabetes, immunosuppressive therapy, HIV

PHYSICAL FINDINGS & CLINICAL PRESENTATION
- Initially nonspecific, such as fever and malaise
- Classic triad: fever, spinal pain, and neurologic deficits are not common
- More commonly:
  - Localized and significant back pain is present.
  - Nerve root pain is present ("shooting" or "electrical" from involved nerve root).
  - Motor weakness, sensory changes, and even paralysis can occur.
  - Fever may not be a prominent sign.

ETIOLOGY
- Bacteria enter the epidural space most often secondary to hematogenous spread from foci elsewhere in the body (25% to 50% of cases) or by direct extension from nearby infected tissues such as vertebral body or psoas muscle. A local intervention such as injection can also cause infection.
- Hematogenous foci include furuncles, cellulitis, urinary tract infection, pharyngitis, and pneumonia.

- Microbiology:
  - *Staphylococcus aureus,* including methicillin-resistant *S. aureus* (MRSA), accounts for 50% to 90% of cases.
  - Aerobic and anaerobic streptococci account for 8% to 17% of cases.
  - Aerobic gram-negative rods *(Escherichia coli* and *Pseudomonas)* account for 10% to 17% of cases.
  - Coagulase-negative staphylococci can be seen with spinal procedures.

DIAGNOSIS

DIFFERENTIAL DIAGNOSIS
- Disc and degenerative bone disease
- Metastatic tumors
- Vertebral discitis and osteomyelitis

WORKUP
Includes a combination of physical exam with neurologic evaluation, blood work, and radiographic studies

LABORATORY TESTS
- Blood cultures
- Culture of fluid or pus by CT-guided aspiration if possible
- Erythrocyte sedimentation rate and/or C-reactive protein
- CBC with differential

IMAGING STUDIES
- MRI with gadolinium is the diagnostic test of choice and imperative if diagnosis is considered.
- CT is an alternative but not as good as MRI for visualizing spinal cord and epidural space.
- CT myelography can be performed if MRI is not available.

TREATMENT

NONPHARMACOLOGIC THERAPY
- Immediate surgery is required if neurologic deficits occur or the patient worsens with medical therapy.
- CT-guided aspiration of abscess with antimicrobial therapy is an alternative treatment to surgery for patients without neurologic deficits.

ACUTE GENERAL Rx
- Empiric antibiotic regimen should include antibiotics effective against staphylococci (including MRSA), streptococci, and gram-negative rods.
- Examples are vancomycin (30 to 60 mg/kg daily divided in q12h doses adjusted for creatinine clearance *plus* metronidazole (500 mg IV q8h) plus cetriaxone (2 g IV q12h) or ceftazidime (2 g IV q8h) if *Pseudomonas* is suspected.

- If cultures reveal methicillin-sensitive *S. aureus,* use nafcillin 2 g IV q4h

CHRONIC Rx
Antimicrobial therapy tailored to culture results may have to be continued for 4 to 6 weeks depending on whether or not there was surgical or CT-guided drainage. If osteomyelitis is suspected, treat for 6 to 8 weeks.

DISPOSITION
- Mortality rates vary from 5% to 32%. Irreversible paralysis can affect 4% to 22% of patients.
- Complete recovery is more likely if neurologic signs are present less than 24 hours before the start of treatment.
- Final functional capacity may continue to improve for up to 1 year after the end of treatment.

REFERRAL
- Neurosurgery should be involved early when this diagnosis is considered.
- Refer to an interventional radiologist for possible aspiration.
- An infectious diseases evaluation is needed for antimicrobial therapy.

PEARLS & CONSIDERATIONS

COMMENTS
It is important to think of spinal epidural abscess early to permit early treatment and prevent permanent neurologic deficits.

SUGGESTED READINGS
available at www.expertconsult.com

RELATED CONTENT
Abscess, Brain (Related Key Topic)

AUTHOR: **GLENN G. FORT, M.D., M.P.H., F.A.C.P., F.I.D.S.A.**

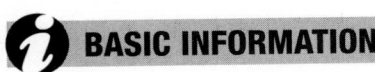

BASIC INFORMATION

DEFINITION
Liver abscess is a necrotic infection of the liver usually classified as pyogenic or amebic.

SYNONYMS
Pyogenic hepatic abscess
Amebic hepatic abscess

ICD-9CM CODES
572.0 Abscess of liver

EPIDEMIOLOGY & DEMOGRAPHICS
INCIDENCE: Incidence of pyogenic liver abscess is 2.3 cases per 100,000 population.
PREVALANCE (WORLDWIDE): Amebic liver abscess is more common than pyogenic liver abscess.
PREVALENCE (IN U.S.): Pyogenic liver abscess is more common than amebic liver abscess.
PREDOMINANT SEX AND AGE: More common in men than women; male/female ratio of 2:1; most common in fourth to sixth decades of life.

PHYSICAL FINDINGS & CLINICAL PRESENTATION
- Fever, chills, and sweats
- Weakness/malaise
- Anorexia with weight loss
- Nausea, vomiting, and diarrhea
- Cough with pleuritic chest pain
- Right upper quadrant abdominal pain
- Hepatomegaly
- Splenomegaly
- Jaundice
- Pleural effusions, rales, and friction rubs may be present
- Most abscesses occur on the right lobe of the liver

ETIOLOGY
- Pyogenic liver abscess is usually polymicrobial (*Klebsiella pneumoniae* [43%], *Escherichia coli* [33%], *Streptococcus* spp. [37%], *Pseudomonas aeruginosa, Proteus* spp., *Bacteroides* spp. [24%], *Fusobacterium* spp., *Actinomyces* spp., gram-positive anaerobes, and *Staphylococcus aureus*).
- Pyogenic liver abscess occurs from:
  1. Biliary disease with cholangitis (accounts for approximately 40% to 60%).
  2. Gallbladder disease with contiguous spread to the liver.
  3. Diverticulitis or appendicitis with spread via the portal circulation.
  4. Hematogenous spread via the hepatic artery, though uncommon; if a solitary organism is isolated, a distant source of hematogenous seeding should be sought.
  5. Penetrating wounds.
  6. Cryptogenic.
  7. Infection by way of portal system (portal pyemia).
  8. No causes found in approximately half of cases.
  9. Incidence increased in patients with diabetes and metastatic cancer.
  10. Table 1-2 summarizes underlying etiology and bacteriology of liver abscesses.
- Amebic hepatic abscess is caused by the parasite *Entamoeba histolytica*. Amebiasis is usually due to fecal-oral contamination and invades the intestinal mucosa, gaining entry into the portal system to reach the liver.

Box 1-1 describes pearls for amebic liver abscesses.

DIAGNOSIS

The diagnosis of liver abscess requires a high index of suspicion after a detailed history and physical examination. Imaging studies and microbiologic, serologic, and percutaneous techniques (e.g., aspiration) confirm the presence of a liver abscess.

DIFFERENTIAL DIAGNOSIS
- Cholangitis
- Cholecystitis
- Diverticulitis

TABLE 1-2 Underlying Etiology and Bacteriology

Etiology	Bacteriology
Biliary, benign	*Escherichia coli* *Klebsiella* spp. *Enterococcus*
Biliary, malignant	*Pseudomonas* spp. Multiply resistant GN aerobes VRE Yeast
Diverticulitis/appendicitis	GN aerobes *Bacteroides fragilis*
Severe cholecystitis	See Biliary, benign *Clostridium perfringens* *Bacteroides* spp.
Subcutaneous abscess	*Staphylococcus* spp. MRSA
Endocarditis	*Enterococcus* spp. *Staphyloccus* spp.
Cryptogenic	Anaerobes

GN, Gram negative.
From Cameron, JL, Cameron AM: *Current surgical therapy,* ed 10, Philadelphia, 2011, Saunders.

- Appendicitis
- Perforated viscus
- Mesentery ischemia
- Pulmonary embolism
- Pancreatitis

WORKUP
- The workup of a liver abscess should focus on differentiating between amebic and pyogenic causes.
- Features suggesting an amebic cause include travel to an endemic area, single abscess rather than multiple abscesses, subacute onset of symptoms, and absence of conditions predisposing to pyogenic liver abscess, as highlighted under "Etiology."
- Laboratory studies are not specific but are useful as adjunctive tests.
- Imaging studies cannot differentiate between the two, and bacteriologic cultures may be sterile in 50% of the cases.

LABORATORY TESTS
- Complete blood count: leukocytosis
- Liver function tests: alkaline phosphatase is most commonly elevated (95% to 100%); aspartate transaminase (AST) and alanine transaminase (ALT) elevated in 50% of cases; elevated bilirubin (28% to 30%); decreased albumin
- Prothrombin time (INR): prolonged (70%)
- Blood cultures: positive in 50% of cases
- Aspiration (50% sterile)
- Stool samples for *E. histolytica* trophozoites (positive in 10% to 15% of amebic liver abscess cases)
- Serologic testing for *E. histolytica* should be done on all patients, but it is important to remember that it does not differentiate acute from old infections.

IMAGING STUDIES
- Ultrasound (80% to 100% sensitivity in detecting abscesses) shows round or oval hypoechogenic mass (Fig. 1-2, *A*).
- CT scan is more sensitive in detecting hepatic abscesses and contiguous organ extension and is the imaging study of choice (Fig. 1-2, *B*).
- Chest x-ray: abnormal in 50% of the cases, may reveal elevated right hemidiaphragm, subdiaphragmatic air-fluid levels, pleural effusions, and consolidating infiltrates.
- Most liver abscesses are single; however, multiple liver abscesses can occur with systemic bacteremia.

BOX 1-1 Pearls for Amebic Liver Abscesses

- Only 10% to 20% of patients with amebic liver abscess have a history of diarrhea.
- Treat the intestinal infection to prevent relapse of amebic liver abscess. Failure to use luminal amebicidal agents after metronidazole in cases of amebic abscess results in a 10% relapse rate.
- Failure to show response to antiamebic medication requires evaluation for polymicrobial infection with bacteria.
- Amebic abscess usually responds clinically to antimicrobial therapy in 3 to 7 days, although imaging takes several months to show resolution.
- Percutaneous drainage is rarely required.

From Cameron, JL, Cameron AM: *Current surgical therapy,* ed 10, Philadelphia, 2011, Saunders.

Rx TREATMENT

NONPHARMACOLOGIC THERAPY

- The management of pyogenic liver abscess differs from that of amebic liver abscess.
- Medical management is the cornerstone of therapy in amebic liver abscess, whereas early intervention in the form of surgical therapy or catheter drainage and parenteral antibiotics is the rule in pyogenic liver abscess.

ACUTE GENERAL Rx

- Percutaneous drainage under CT or ultrasound guidance is essential in the treatment of pyogenic liver abscesses.
- Aspiration of hepatic amebic abscesses is not required unless there is no response to treatment or a pyogenic cause is being considered.
- Empiric broad-spectrum antibiotics are recommended initially until culture results are available. Common choices include:
  1. Metronidazole (500 mg IV q8h) plus ceftriaxone or cefoxitin or levofloxacin.
  2. Metronidazole plus a beta-lactam/beta-lactamase inhibitor, such as piperacillin/tazobactam (4.5 g q6h), ticarcillin-clavulanate (3.1 g q4h), or ampicillin-sulbactam (3 g q6h).

3. Metronidazole plus a carbapenem, such as imipenem (500 mg IV q6h), meropenem (1 g q8h), or ertapenem (1 g daily).
4. In patients with penicillin allergy, clindamycin 600 to 900 mg IV q8h with an aminoglycoside can be considered.
5. Duration of antibiotic treatment is usually 4 to 6 wk with IV antibiotics used for the first 1 to 2 wk or until a favorable clinical response, followed thereafter with oral antibiotics (e.g., metronidazole 500 mg PO q8h plus ciprofloxacin 500 mg PO q12h).
6. Third-generation cephalosporins should not be used as single agents for empiric therapy because of risk of the emergence of beta-lactamase-producing bacteria.

- Antibiotic coverage for amebic liver abscesses includes:
  1. Tissue agent: metronidazole 750 mg PO tid for 10 days
  2. Luminal agent: after therapy with tissue agent treatment with any luminal agent is required even if the stool is negative, such as paromomycin for 10 days or diiodohydroxyquin for 20 days.

CHRONIC Rx

- If fever persists for 2 wk despite percutaneous drainage and antibiotic therapy as outlined under "Acute General Rx," or if there is failure of aspiration or failure of percutaneous drainage, surgery is indicated.

- In patients not responding to intravenous antibiotics and percutaneous drainage, hepatic artery antibiotic infusion can be considered.
- In patients with evidence of metastatic disease that is causing biliary obstruction, a gastroenterology consultation for endoscopic retrograde cholangiopancreatography and stenting should be considered.

DISPOSITION

- Most patients with pyogenic liver abscesses defervesce within 2 wk of treatment with antibiotics and drainage.
- No randomized controlled studies have evaluated the optimal duration of antibiotic therapy for pyogenic liver abscess. Typical duration of antibiotic therapy is at least 4 to 6 wk.
- Pyogenic liver abscess cure rates using percutaneous drainage and antibiotics have been reported to be between 88% and 100%.
- Mortality rate of untreated pyogenic liver abscess is nearly 100%.
- Most patients with amebic liver abscesses defervesce within 4 to 5 days of treatment.
- Amebic liver abscess mortality rate is <1% unless complications occur (see "Comments").
- Follow-up imaging should be used to monitor response to therapy; continue treatment until CT scan shows complete or near-complete resolution of cavity.

REFERRAL

Infectious disease, gastroenterology, interventional radiology, and general surgical consultations are recommended in any patient with hepatic abscess.

! PEARLS AND CONSIDERATIONS

COMMENTS

- Complications of pyogenic and amebic liver abscesses include:
  1. Pleuropulmonary extension, resulting in empyema, abscess, and fistula formation
  2. Peritonitis
  3. Purulent pericarditis
  4. Sepsis
- Amebic liver abscesses complicate amebic colitis in nearly 10% of cases.

SUGGESTED READINGS

available at www.expertconsult.com

RELATED CONTENT

Liver Abscess (Patient Information)

AUTHOR: **TANYA ALI, M.D.**

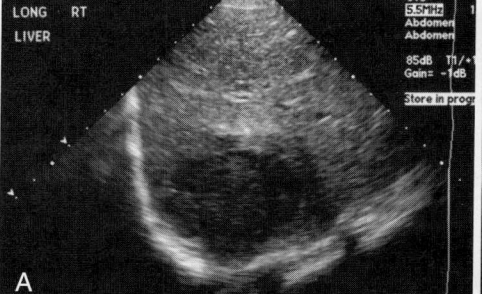
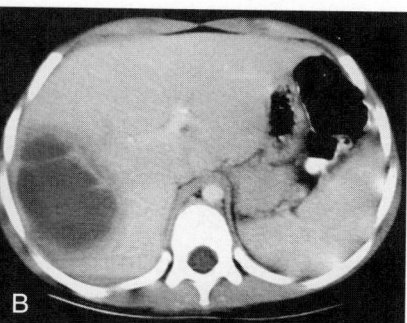

FIGURE 1-2 A, Amebic abscess. Sonogram demonstrates a hypoechogenic mass in the right lobe of the liver with a more hypoechoic surrounding rim. **B,** CT scan demonstrates a low-attenuation mass in the right lobe of the liver with a prominent halo. (From Kuhn JP et al: *Caffrey's pediatric diagnostic imaging,* vol 2, ed 10, Philadelphia, 2004, Mosby.)

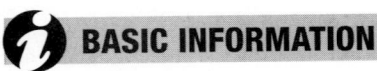

BASIC INFORMATION

DEFINITION
A lung abscess is an infection of the lung parenchyma resulting in a necrotic cavity containing pus.

SYNONYMS
Pulmonary abscess

ICD-9CM CODES
513.0 Abscess of the lung

EPIDEMIOLOGY & DEMOGRAPHICS
INCIDENCE: Has decreased over the last 30 years as a result of antibiotic therapy.
- Lung abscess in patients age 50 and over is associated with primary lung neoplasia in 30% of the cases.
- Lung abscesses commonly coexist with empyemas.

RISK FACTORS (see Table 1-3):
1. Alcohol-related problems
2. Seizure disorders
3. Cerebrovascular disorders with dysphagia
4. Drug abuse
5. Esophageal disorders (e.g., scleroderma, esophageal carcinoma, etc.)
6. Poor oral hygiene
7. Obstructive malignant lung disease
8. Bronchiectasis

PHYSICAL FINDINGS & CLINICAL PRESENTATION
- Symptoms are generally insidious and prolonged, occurring for weeks to months
- Fever, chills, and sweats
- Cough
- Sputum production (purulent with foul odor)
- Pleuritic chest pain
- Hemoptysis
- Dyspnea
- Malaise, fatigue, and weakness
- Tachycardia and tachypnea
- Dullness to percussion, whispered pectoriloquy, and bronchophony
- Amphoric breath sounds (low-pitched sound of air moving across a large open cavity)

ETIOLOGY
- The most important factor predisposing to lung abscess is aspiration.
- Following aspiration as a major predisposing factor is periodontal disease.
- Lung abscess is rare in an edentulous person.
- Approximately 90% of lung abscesses are caused by anaerobic microorganisms (peptostreptococci, microaerophilic streptococci such as *Streptococcus milleri, Bacteroides* species, *Fusobacterium nucleatum, Prevotella*). Pulmonary actinomycosis will also generate lung abscess.
- In most cases anaerobic infection is mixed with aerobic or facultative anaerobic organisms (*S. aureus, E. coli, K. pneumoniae, P. aeruginosa*).
- Parasitic organisms including *Paragonimus westermani* and *Entamoeba histolytica.*
- Fungi including *Aspergillus, Cryptococcus, Histoplasma, Blastomyces,* and *Coccidioides* spp.
- Immunocompromised hosts may become infected with *Aspergillus*, mycobacteria, *Nocardia, Legionella micdadei*, and *Rhodococcus equi.*
- Lung necrosis caused by community strains of MRSA (USA 300 strain) in young adults or adolescents after acute influenza was initially reported in 2002 and can be quite fulminant.

DIAGNOSIS

Lung abscess may be primary or secondary.
- *Primary lung abscess* refers to infection from normal host organisms within the lung (e.g., aspiration, pneumonia).
- Secondary lung abscess results from other preexisting conditions (e.g., endocarditis, underlying lung cancer, pulmonary emboli).

Lung abscess may be acute or chronic.
- Acute lung abscess is present if symptoms are of less than 4 to 6 wk.
- Chronic lung abscess is present if symptoms last longer than 6 wk.

DIFFERENTIAL DIAGNOSIS
The differential diagnosis is similar to that for cavitary lung lesions:
- Bacterial (anaerobic, aerobic, infected bulla, empyema, actinomycosis, tuberculosis)
- Fungal (histoplasmosis, coccidioidomycosis, blastomycosis, aspergillosis, cryptococcosis, zygomycetes)
- Parasitic (amebiasis, echinococcosis)
- Malignancy (primary lung carcinoma, metastatic lung disease, lymphoma, Hodgkin's disease)
- Wegener's granulomatosis, sarcoidosis, endocarditis, and septic pulmonary emboli

WORKUP
- The workup of a patient with lung abscess attempts to elicit a primary or a secondary cause.
- Blood tests are not specific in diagnosing lung abscesses.
- Most diagnoses are made from imaging studies; however, to diagnose a specific cause bacteriologic studies are needed.

LABORATORY TESTS
- CBC with leukocytosis
- Bacteriologic studies
  1. Sputum Gram stain and culture (commonly contaminated by oral flora)
  2. Percutaneous transtracheal aspiration
  3. Percutaneous transthoracic aspiration
  4. Fiberoptic bronchoscopy using bronchial brushings or bronchoalveolar lavage is the most widely used intervention when trying to obtain diagnostic bacteriologic cultures
- Blood cultures on some occasions (<30%) may be positive
- If an empyema is present, obtaining empyema fluid via thoracentesis may isolate the organism

IMAGING STUDIES
- Chest x-ray makes the diagnosis of lung abscess showing the cavitary lesion with an air-fluid level.
- Lung abscesses are most commonly found in the posterior segment of the right upper lobe.
- Chest CT scan can localize and size the lesion and assist in differentiating lung abscesses from other pathologic processes (e.g., tumor, empyema, infected bulla, etc.) (Fig. 1-3).

TREATMENT

NONPHARMACOLOGIC THERAPY
- Oxygen therapy
- Postural drainage
- Respiratory therapy maneuvers

ACUTE GENERAL Rx
Piperacillin/tazobactam 3.375 g IV q6h in aspiration pneumonia with lung abscess
- Ceftriaxone 1 g IV q24h plus metronidazole 1 g IV q12h
- Clindamycin is more effective for anaerobic lung abscess than penicillin alone. Dose: 600 mg IV q8h until improved, then 300 to 600 mg PO q6h.

TABLE 1-3   Risk Factors for Aspiration Pneumonia and Lung Abscess

Increased bacterial inoculum	Periodontal disease, gingivitis, tonsillar or dental abscess, drugs that decrease gastric acidity
Impairment of consciousness	Drugs, alcohol, general anesthesia, metabolic encephalopathy, coma, shock, cerebrovascular accident, cardiopulmonary arrest, seizures, surgery, trauma
Impaired cough and gag reflexes	Vocal cord paralysis, intratracheal anesthesia, endotracheal tube, tracheostomy, myopathy, myelopathy, other neurologic disorders
Impairment of esophageal function	Diverticula, achalasia, strictures, disorders of gastrointestinal motility, neoplasm, tracheoesophageal fistula, pseudobulbar palsy
Emesis	Nasogastric tube, gastric dilation, ileus, intestinal obstruction

From Cohen J, Powderly WG: *Infectious diseases,* ed 2, St Louis, 2004, Mosby.

- Penicillin 1 to 2 million units IV q4h until improvement (afebrile, decreased phelgm production), followed by penicillin VK 500 mg PO q6h for 2 to 3 weeks but often up to 6 to 8 weeks) can be given with metronidazole doses of 7.5 mg/kg IV q6h followed by PO 500 mg bid to qid dosing as an alternative to clindamycin.
- Penicillin should not be used alone because many mouth flora anaerobes now produce penicillinase enzymes. Metronidazole should not be used alone because it is not active against microaerophilic streptococci and some anaerobic cocci.
- Other alternatives are ampicillin/sulbactam and carbapenems such as ertapenem and meropenem.

CHRONIC Rx

- Bronchoscopy to assist with drainage and/or diagnosis is indicated in patients who fail to respond to antibiotics or if there is suspected underlying malignancy.
- Surgery is indicated on rare occasions (<10%) in patients with complications of lung abscess (see "Comments").

DISPOSITION

- More than 95% of patients are cured with the use of antibiotics alone.
- Complications of lung abscesses include:
  1. Empyema
  2. Massive hemoptysis
  3. Pneumothorax
  4. Bronchopleural fistula
- Mortality is low in community-acquired lung abscess (2.5%).
- Hospital-acquired lung abscess carries a high mortality rate (65%).

REFERRAL

If lung abscess is present, consultation with pulmonary and infectious disease specialist is recommended.

⚠ PEARLS & CONSIDERATIONS

COMMENTS

- Complications of lung abscesses include:
  1. Empyema
  2. Bronchopleural fistula

  3. Hepatobronchial fistula
  4. Brain abscess
  5. Bronchiectasis
- Refractory cases are usually the result of:
  1. Large cavity size (>6 cm)
  2. Recurrent aspiration
  3. Thick-walled cavities
  4. Underlying lung carcinoma
  5. Empyema formation
- Necrotizing pneumonia is similar to a lung abscess but differs in size (<2 cm in diameter) and number (usually multiple suppurative cavitary lesions).

SUGGESTED READINGS
available at www.expertconsult.com

RELATED CONTENT
Lung Abscess (Patient Information)

AUTHOR: **GLENN G. FORT, M.D., M.P.H.**

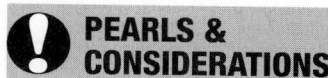
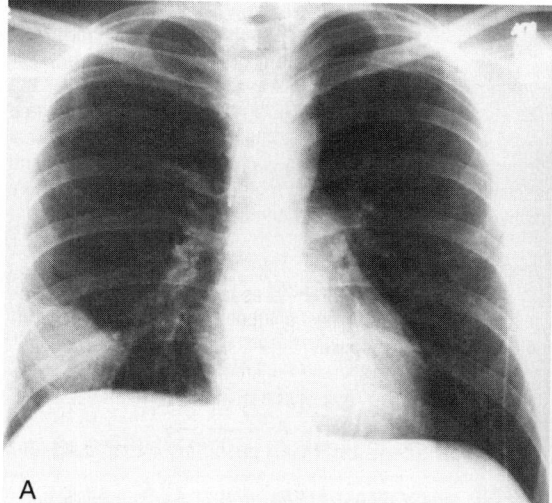
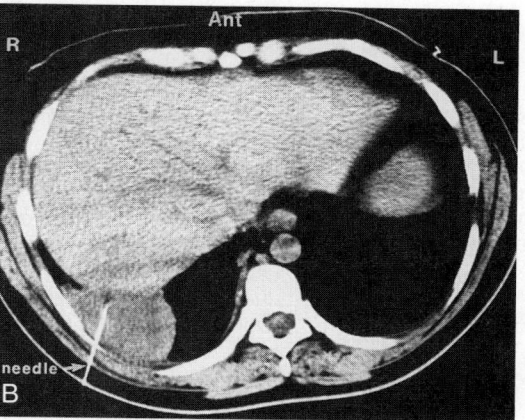

FIGURE 1-3 Lung abscess. On a chest radiograph, a lung abscess may look to be a solid rounded lesion **(A)**, or, if it has a connection with the bronchus, there may be an air-fluid level in a thick-walled cavitary lesion. CT scanning **(B)** can be used to localize the lesion and to place a needle for drainage and aspiration of contents for culture. (From Mettler FA [ed]: *Primary care radiology,* Philadelphia, 2000, Saunders.)

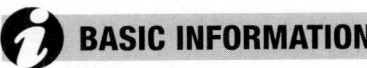

DEFINITION

Pelvic abscess is an acute or chronic infection, most commonly involving the pelvic viscera. Treatment and possible cure require directed therapy that will involve antibiotic therapy and, if medical therapy fails, subsequent surgical therapy. There are four categories based on etiologic factors:

- Ascending infection, spreading from cervix through endometrial cavity to adnexa, forming a tuboovarian complex
- Infection occurring in the puerperium, which spreads to the adnexa from the endometrium or myometrium by a hematogenous or lymphatic route
- Abscess complicating pelvic surgery
- Involvement of the pelvic viscera as a result of spread from contiguous organs, such as appendicitis or diverticulitis

SYNONYMS

Tuboovarian abscess (TOA)
Vaginal cuff abscess

ICD-9CM CODES
614.2 Salpingitis and oophoritis not specified as acute, subacute, or chronic

EPIDEMIOLOGY & DEMOGRAPHICS

INCIDENCE:
- 34% of hospitalized patients with pelvic inflammatory disease
- 1% to 2% of patients undergoing hysterectomy, most with vaginal approach
- Peak incidence third to fourth decade

RISK FACTORS: Same risk factors as for pelvic inflammatory disease, although in 30% to 50% of patients there is no prior history of salpingitis before abscess forms.

PHYSICAL FINDINGS & CLINICAL PRESENTATION

- Abdominal or pelvic pain (90%)
- Fever or chills (50%)
- Abnormal bleeding (21%)
- Vaginal discharge (28%)
- Nausea (26%)
- Up to 60% to 80% present in the absence of fever or leukocytosis; absence of these findings should not exclude diagnosis

ETIOLOGY

- Mixed flora of anaerobes, aerobes, and facultative anaerobes, such as *Escherichia coli*, *Bacteroides fragilis*, *Prevotella* spp., aerobic streptococci, and *Peptococcus* and *Peptostreptococcus* spp.
- *Nesseria gonorrhoeae* and *Chlamydia* are the major etiologic bacteria in cervicitis and salpingitis but are rarely found in abscess cavity cultures.
- In elderly patients consider diverticular disease.

Dx DIAGNOSIS

DIFFERENTIAL DIAGNOSIS

- Pelvic neoplasms, such as ovarian tumors and leiomyomas.
- Inflammatory masses involving adjacent bowel or omentum, such as ruptured appendicitis or diverticulitis.
- Pelvic hematomas, as may occur after cesarean section or hysterectomy.
- Section III describes the diagnostic approach to patients with a pelvic mass; the differential diagnosis of pelvic mass is described in Section II.
- The differential diagnosis of pelvic pain is described in Section II.
- Sonogram or CT scan: commonly used due to associated pain and guarding, resulting in a suboptimal abdominal or pelvic examination, and to characterize anatomic abnormalities such as an adnexal mass.
- Most common cause of preventable death: physician delay in diagnosis.

LABORATORY TESTS

- CBC with differential
- Aerobic as well as anaerobic cultures of cervix, blood, urine, sputum, peritoneal cavity (if entered), and abscess cavity before starting antibiotics
- Pregnancy test in patients of reproductive age

IMAGING STUDIES

- Sonogram: noninvasive, inexpensive study to confirm diagnosis, estimate size of abscess, and monitor response to therapy; sensitivity >90%
- CT scan: used for both diagnosis and therapy (CT-guided drainage) (Fig. E1-4)
  1. Useful where sonogram provides insufficient information, as with intraabdominal abscesses
  2. Success rate with CT-guided abscess drainage: unilocular, 90%; multilocular, 40%

Rx TREATMENT

Major concerns:
1. Desire for future fertility
2. Likelihood of rupture of abscess, with resulting peritonitis, septic shock, and morbid sequelae

ACUTE GENERAL Rx

- Clinical quandary is whether patient requires immediate surgery (uncertain diagnosis or suspicion of rupture) or management with IV antibiotics, reserving surgery for those with inadequate clinical response (e.g., 48 to 72 hr of therapy, with persistent fever or leukocytosis, increasing size of mass, or suspicion of rupture)
- Surgery indicated in poor response to medical therapy. Early surgery may be needed in those with large adnexal masses (>8 cm), or in immunocompromised patients

- Antibiotic combinations:
  1. Clindamycin 900 mg IV q8h or metronidazole 500 mg IV q6-8h plus gentamicin either 5 to 7 mg/kg q24h or 1.5 mg/kg q8h
  2. Alternatives: ampicillin sulbactam 3 g IV q6h or cefoxitin 2 g IV q6h or cefotetan 2 g IV q12h plus doxycycline 100 mg IV q12h
- During medical management, high index of suspicion for acute rupture, such as acute worsening of abdominal pain or new-onset tachycardia and hypotension, mandating immediate surgical intervention after patient stabilization
- Surgical options:
  1. Laparoscopy with drainage and irrigation
  2. Transvaginal colpotomy (abscess must be midline, dissect rectovaginal septum, and be adherent to vaginal fornix)
  3. Laparotomy, including total abdominal hysterectomy with bilateral salpingo-oophorectomy or unilateral salpingo-oophorectomy
  4. Evidence of ruptured tuboovarian abscess is a surgical emergency

DISPOSITION

- Of patients treated with medical therapy, response in 75%, with a 50% pregnancy rate. Pregnancy rate decreases with recurrent episodes.
- No response in 30% to 40%; can be treated with either CT-guided drainage or surgical intervention, keeping in mind that unilateral adnexectomy may give equal chance of cure versus hysterectomy, yet preserve reproductive potential.

REFERRAL

If patient has a tuboovarian abscess, refer to gynecologist.

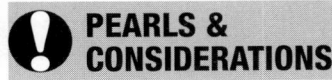 **PEARLS & CONSIDERATIONS**

COMMENTS

If *Actinomyces* species is isolated from culture, treatment with penicillin is required for an extended period (6 wk to 3 mo).

SUGGESTED READINGS
available at www.expertconsult.com

RELATED CONTENT

Pelvic Inflammatory Disease (Related Key Topic)
Pelvic Abscess (Patient Information)

AUTHORS: **SCOTT J. ZUCCALA, D.O.,** and **RUBEN ALVERO, M.D.**

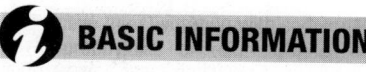

BASIC INFORMATION

DEFINITION

A perirectal abscess is a localized inflammatory process that can be associated with infections of soft tissue and anal glands based on anatomic location. Perianal and perirectal abscesses may be simple or complex, causing suppuration. Infections in these spaces may be classified as superficial perianal or perirectal with involvement in the following anatomic spaces: ischiorectal, intersphincteric, perianal, and supralevator. The Parks classification of anorectal abscess is subdivided into intersphincteric, transsphincteric, suprasphincteric, and extrasphincteric abscess (Fig. 1-5).

SYNONYMS

Rectal abscess
Perianal abscess
Anorectal abscess

ICD-9CM CODES

566 Perirectal abscess

EPIDEMIOLOGY & DEMOGRAPHICS

INCIDENCE (IN U.S.): Commonly encountered
PREDOMINANT SEX: Male > female
PREDOMINANT AGE: All ages
PEAK INCIDENCE: Not seasonal; common
GENETICS: None known

PHYSICAL FINDINGS & CLINICAL PRESENTATION

- Localized perirectal or anal pain—often worsened with movement or straining
- Perirectal erythema or cellulitis
- Perirectal mass by inspection or palpation
- Fever and signs of sepsis with deep abscess
- Urinary retention

ETIOLOGY

- Polymicrobial aerobic and anaerobic bacteria involving one of the anatomic spaces (see "Definition"), often associated with localized trauma

- Microbiology: most bacteria are polymicrobial, mixed enteric and skin flora
- Predominant anaerobic bacteria:
  1. *Bacteroides fragilis*
  2. *Peptostreptococcus* spp.
  3. *Prevotella* spp.
  4. *Porphyromonas* spp.
  5. *Clostridium* spp.
  6. *Fusobacterium* spp.
- Predominant aerobic bacteria:
  1. *Staphylococcus aureus*
  2. *Streptococcus* spp.
  3. *Escherichia coli*
  4. *Enterococcus* spp.

DIAGNOSIS

Many patients will have predisposing underlying conditions including:
- Malignancy or leukemia
- Immune deficiency
- Diabetes mellitus
- Recent surgery
- Steroid therapy

DIFFERENTIAL DIAGNOSIS

- Neutropenic enterocolitis
- Crohn's disease (inflammatory bowel disease)
- Pilonidal disease
- Hidradenitis suppurativa
- Tuberculosis or actinomycosis; Chagas' disease
- Cancerous lesions
- Chronic anal fistula
- Rectovaginal fistula
- Proctitis—often STD-associated, including: syphilis, gonococcal, chlamydia, chancroid, condylomata acuminata
- AIDS-associated: Kaposi's sarcoma, lymphoma, CMV

WORKUP

- Examination of rectal, perirectal/perineal areas
- Rule out necrotic process and crepitance suggesting deep tissue involvement

- Local aerobic and anaerobic culture
- Blood cultures if toxic, febrile, or compromised
- Possible sigmoidoscopy

IMAGING STUDIES

Usually not indicated unless extensive disease abscess but can include CT. One study showed that CT had only a sensitivity of 77% and was particularly poor in detecting a perirectal abscess in immunocompromised patients.

TREATMENT

ACUTE GENERAL Rx

- Incision and drainage of abscess
- Debridement if necrotic tissue
- Rule out need for fistulectomy
- Local wound care—packing
- Sitz baths

Antibiotic treatment: directed toward coverage for mixed skin and enteric flora

OUTPATIENT—ORAL:
- Trimethoprim/sulfamethoxazole DS bid or ciprofloxacin 750 mg bid or levofloxacin 750 mg q24h plus metronidazole 500 mg q6h x 7-10 days
- Amoxicillin/clavulanic acid 875 to 1000 mg 2 tabs bid
- Clindamycin 150 to 300 mg PO q8h ± ciprofloxacin

INPATIENT—INTRAVENOUS:
- Piperacillin/tazobactam 3.375 g IV q6 to 8h
- Ampicillin/sulbactam 1.5 to 3 g IV q6h
- Cefotetan 1 to 2 g IV q8h
- Imipenem or meropenem 500 to 1000 mg IV q8h

DISPOSITION

Follow-up with a general surgeon or infectious disease physician is often warranted.

REFERRAL

- General surgeon or colorectal surgeon for drainage.
- AIDS specialist may be needed for perirectal complications of HIV infection.
- Gastroenterologist follow-up may be warranted in Crohn's disease with perirectal fistula and other complications.

PEARLS & CONSIDERATIONS

Perirectal abscess may be a presenting manifestation of type 2 diabetes mellitus in older adults. Check the blood sugar in patients to exclude the possibility of unrecognized diabetes mellitus.

SUGGESTED READINGS

available at www.expertconsult.com

RELATED CONTENT

Perirectal Abscess (Patient Information)

AUTHOR: **GLENN G. FORT, M.D., M.P.H.**

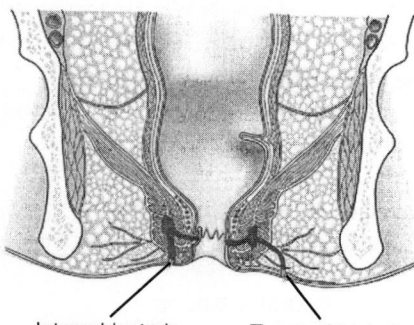
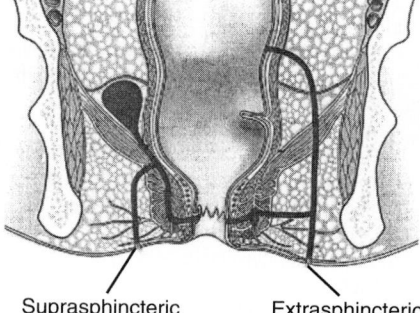

Intersphincteric Transsphincteric Suprasphincteric Extrasphincteric

FIGURE 1-5 Parks classification of anorectal abscess. (From Cameron JL, Cameron AM: *Current surgical therapy*, ed 10, Philadelphia, 2011, Saunders.)

BASIC INFORMATION

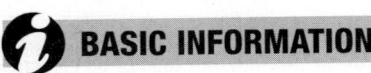

DEFINITION

Peritonsillar abscess is an acute infection located between the capsule of the palatine tonsil and the superior constrictor muscle of the pharynx.

SYNONYMS

Quinsy

ICD-9CM CODES
475.0 Peritonsillar abscess

EPIDEMIOLOGY & DEMOGRAPHICS

INCIDENCE (IN U.S.): 30:100,000/yr for ages 5-59. For adolescents, the incidence is 40:100,000/yr. It is the most common deep infection of the head and neck in children and adolescents, accounting for at least 50% of cases.

PEAK INCIDENCE: Bimodal frequency during the year, with highest occurrence from November to December and April to May.

PREVALENCE: 45,000 cases/yr in the United States

PREDOMINANT SEX: Male > female

PREDOMINANT AGE: Highest incidence is adults aged 20-40 yr.

RISK FACTORS: Smoking, periodontal disease, oropharyngeal or dental infection

PHYSICAL FINDINGS & CLINICAL PRESENTATION

- Sore throat, which may be severe and unilateral
- Dysphagia and odynophagia
- Otalgia on the side of abscess
- Foul-smelling breath
- Facial swelling
- Drooling
- Headache
- Fever
- Trismus
- Hoarseness, muffled voice (also called "hot potato voice")
- Tender submandibular and anterior cervical lymph nodes
- Tonsillar hypertrophy with likely peritonsillar edema
- Contralateral deflection of the uvula
- Stridor

ETIOLOGY

- Peritonsillar abscess is usually a complication of tonsillitis or acute bacterial pharyngitis caused by blockage of salivary ducts. Tonsillitis → peritonsillar cellulitis → peritonsillar abscess
- Group A β-hemolytic *Streptococcus* is the most common bacterial cause, accounting for 15% to 30% of cases in children and 5% to 10% of cases in adults.

- Less common aerobic causes are *Staphylococcus aureus*, *Haemophilus influenzae*, *Neisseria* species.
- The most common anaerobic organism is *Fusobacterium*.

DIAGNOSIS

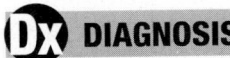

DIFFERENTIAL DIAGNOSIS

- Tonsillitis
- Infectious mononucleosis
- Peritonsillar cellulitis
- Retropharyngeal abscess
- Epiglottitis
- Dental abscess (retromolar)
- Lymphoma
- Ludwig's angina

WORKUP

- Based on history and physical exam
- Consider additional testing if presentation is less clear.

LABORATORY TESTS

- Consider rapid strep antigen testing and/or pharyngeal culture and sensitivity.
- Aspiration of the abscess for culture and sensitivity (see "Treatment" for role of aspiration in tx)

IMAGING STUDIES

- Consider ultrasound, CT scan (Fig. E1-6), or MRI to help differentiate abscess from cellulitis or mass
- Intraoral ultrasound may improve diagnosis and aspiration of peritonsillar abscess compared with visual inspection in adult patients.

TREATMENT

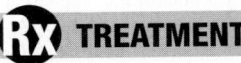

NONPHARMACOLOGIC THERAPY

- Drainage of the abscess by needle aspiration or by surgical incision and drainage

ACUTE GENERAL Rx

- Aspiration or surgical drainage AND antibiotics for 10 to 14 days
- Initial antibiotics should cover group A *Streptococcus* and anaerobes
  Intravenous
  - Piperacillin/tazobactam or ticarcillin/clavulanate. If penicillin allergic, use IV clindamycin (600-900 mg IV q8h).
  - Ampicillin-sulbactam 3 g q6h
  - Penicillin G 10 million units q6h AND metronidazole 500 mg q6h (may use clindamycin 900 mg q8h if penicillin allergic)
  OR oral
  - Amoxicillin-clavulanic acid 875 mg twice daily
  - Penicillin VK 500 mg 4 times daily AND metronidazole 500 mg 4 times daily
  - Clindamycin 600 mg twice daily or 300 mg 4 times daily

- Then appropriate selection of antibiotics should be guided by culture and sensitivity of the organism. Consulting local antimicrobial guidelines for resistance profiles is also advisable for empiric coverage before culture results are available.

CHRONIC Rx

- Tonsillectomy can be considered 3 to 6 mo after diagnosis of peritonsillar abscess with or without the diagnosis of recurrent tonsillitis.
- Though rare, in adults and children with an acute case of peritonsillar abscess and a history of recurrent pharyngitis or previous peritonsillar abscess, a specialist may recommend a *quinsy or hot tonsillectomy,* an immediate removal of the tonsils after starting IV antibiotics.

DISPOSITION

- Successful treatment is defined by symptomatic improvement in sore throat, fever, and/or tonsillar swelling within 24 hr of intervention.
- Treatment failure is defined by lack of symptomatic improvement or worsening despite 24 hr of antimicrobial therapy (with or without surgical drainage).

REFERRAL

- Consider ENT or diagnostic radiology for drainage of abscess.
- Consider ENT for tonsillectomy if criteria are met.

PEARLS & CONSIDERATIONS

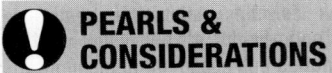

COMMENTS

- Risk for a recurrence is immediate (within 4 days) and long term (2 to 3 yr).
- Most recurrences occur shortly after the initial presentation, suggesting continued infection rather than recurrence.
- Overall recurrence rate is 10% to 15%.

PREVENTION

- Adequate treatment of peritonsillar abscess.
- Up to 30% of patients with peritonsillar abscess meet criteria for tonsillectomy.

PATIENT/FAMILY EDUCATION

Advise family members to call with any trouble breathing, swallowing, or talking.

SUGGESTED READINGS
available at www.expertconsult.com

AUTHORS: **PETER SELL, D.O.,** and **AMITY RUBEOR, D.O.**

BASIC INFORMATION

DEFINITION

Renal abscess and perinephric abscess are a purulent complication of an underlying urinary infection of the ascending tract with an obstructed pyelonephritis. Predisposing factors include diabetes and renal stones. There is lobar necrosis with renal abscess and perirenal fat necrosis in perinephric abscess.

SYNONYMS

Intrarenal abscess
Perinephric abscess

ICD-9CM CODES
590.2 Renal and perinephric abscess

EPIDEMIOLOGY & DEMOGRAPHICS

INCIDENCE: Ranges from 1 to 10 per 10,000 hospital admissions
PREDOMINANT SEX AND AGE: In one study median age was 59.8 years
RISK FACTORS: Diabetes and renal stones

PHYSICAL FINDINGS & CLINICAL PRESENTATION

- Symptoms include fever, flank pain, abdominal pain, and urinary frequency or dysuria
- At times renal abscess can present insidiously in the elderly or persons with diabetes.

ETIOLOGY

These infections may be a complication of a urinary tract infection that ascends to the upper tract, usually due to gram-negative bacteria, or a complication of a bacteremia with hematogenous seeding to the kidney, usually secondary to a *Staphylococcus aureus* infection.

DIAGNOSIS

DIFFERENTIAL DIAGNOSIS

- Acute pyelonephritis with papillary necrosis
- Acute lobar nephronia: acute nonsuppurative renal infection
- Renal cell carcinoma
- Malakoplakia: rare granulomatous inflammatory disease seen with *Escherichia coli* infection
- Emphysematous pyelonephritis: gas formation within the renal parenchyma caused by infection by facultative anaerobes or *Candida* spp.

WORKUP

Combination of laboratory tests and imaging

LABORATORY TESTS

- Blood cultures, urine cultures, urinalysis, and CBC are basic tests.
- Elevated ESR or C-reactive protein may be marker for a deep-seated infection.

IMAGING STUDIES

- Ultrasound may show thick-walled fluid-filled cavity in renal parenchyma. A perinephric abscess is confined to the perinephric space by Gerota's fascia.
- CT with contrast is preferred over ultrasound for the diagnosis (Fig. 1-7).
- MRI and nuclear scans are of limited value.

TREATMENT

Antibiotic therapy and, when necessary, interventional radiology or surgical drainage procedure

NONPHARMACOLOGIC THERAPY

- Therapy for a renal abscess greater than 5 cm in diameter should be percutaneous drainage by CT- or US-guided therapy along with intravenous antibiotics.
- A perinephric abscess should be drained percutaneously with CT or US guidance.
- At times a nephrectomy may be required for severe cases, usually in diabetic patients.

ACUTE GENERAL Rx

A renal abscess less than 5 cm in diameter can be treated successfully with targeted intravenous therapy (92% success rate for abscess 3 to 5 cm in diameter). Antibiotic choices are based

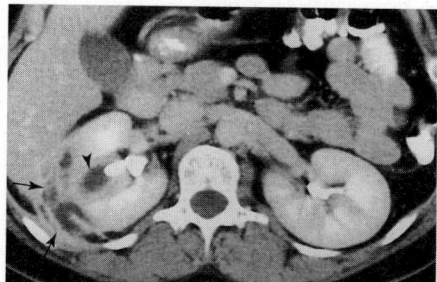

FIGURE 1-7 Renal abscess. Contrast-enhanced CT scan shows an abscess in the medulla of the kidney *(arrowhead)* with penetration and extension into the perinephric space *(arrows)*. (Courtesy L. Towner.)

on culture results but initially should target gram-negative bacteria unless infection is secondary to staphylococcal bacteremia. Empiric antibiotic therapy in geographic areas where fluoroquinolone resistance rates are <10% consists of ciprofloxacin 400 mg IV loading dose. In areas with high fluoroquinolone resistance rates, ceftriaxone 1 g IV is appropriate. If perinephric abscess is associated with staphylococcal bacteremia, give IV nafcillin if methicillin-susceptible *Staphylococcus aureus* (MSSA) or vancomycin 1 g IV q12h if methicillin-resistant *S. aureus*.

CHRONIC Rx

Antibiotic therapy generally continues for 2 to 3 weeks, some of which can be completed with oral therapy.

DISPOSITION

Antibiotics such as trimethoprim-sulfamethoxazole and quinolone antibiotics penetrate well in the kidney and are ideal oral agents for therapy.

REFERRAL

Interventional radiology, urologic surgeon, and infectious diseases consult

PEARLS & CONSIDERATIONS

COMMENTS

This diagnosis should be considered in patients who are being treated for pyelonephritis with appropriate antibiotics and fail to respond clinically after 5 days.

PREVENTION

Early and targeted therapy for urinary tract infections, especially in diabetic patients

SUGGESTED READINGS
available at www.expertconsult.com

RELATED CONTENT

Pyelonephritis (Related Key Topic)
Urinary Tract Infection (Related Key Topic)

AUTHOR: **GLENN G. FORT, M.D., M.P.H.**

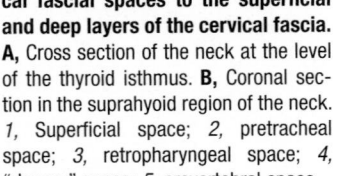
DEFINITION

Retropharyngeal abscess is a soft tissue infection of the throat involving retropharyngeal space. The anatomic boundaries of the retropharyngeal space are the middle layer of the deep cervical fascia (abutting the posterior esophageal wall) anteriorly and the deep layer of the deep cervical fascia posteriorly (Fig. 1-8). These two fasciae fuse inferiorly at the level between the first and second thoracic vertebrae.

ICD-9CM CODES
478.79

EPIDEMIOLOGY & DEMOGRAPHICS

Retropharyngeal abscess occurs most commonly in children between the ages of 2 and 4 yr, analogous to suppurative cervical adenitis. This represents the peak age group for numerous viral upper respiratory tract infections and their attendant complications, acute otitis media and sinusitis. Retropharyngeal space infection is less common in older children and adults because the lymph nodes atrophy by the age of 3 or 4 yr.

PHYSICAL FINDINGS & CLINICAL PRESENTATION

- The onset of a retropharyngeal infection may be insidious, with little more than fever, irritability, drooling, a muffled voice (dysphonia), or possibly nuchal rigidity.
- The acute symptoms relate to pressure and inflammation produced by the abscess on either the airway or the upper digestive tract and pharynx. The patient may have intense dysphagia, drooling, and odynophagia, or there may be some element of respiratory distress from edema and inflammation of the airway (stridor, tachypnea, or both).

- Unwillingness to move the neck because of discomfort is often a prominent presenting feature and should lead to consideration of retropharyngeal abscess if the child is febrile and irritable.
- Extension of the neck is usually affected more than flexion. This causes the patient to hold his or her neck stiffly or to present with torticollis.
- Trismus is unusual.
- On physical examination it may be possible to appreciate midline or unilateral swelling of the posterior pharyngeal wall. The mass may be fluctuant to the examining finger, and care must be taken to avoid rupture of the abscess into the upper airway.

Complications are numerous and could be fatal; these include airway obstruction, septicemia, thrombosis of the internal jugular vein, carotid artery rupture, and acute necrotizing mediastinitis. Aspiration with resultant pneumonia may complicate retropharyngeal abscess if rupture of the abscess occurs and empties into the airway. Infection can spread from one space in the neck to another.

The most dreaded complication is jugular vein suppurative thrombophlebitis (Lemierre's syndrome), in which the vessels of the carotid sheath become infected, leading to bacteremia and metastatic spread of infection to the lungs, brain, and mediastinum.

ETIOLOGY

- The retropharyngeal space comprises two chains of lymph nodes that drain the nasopharynx, adenoids, posterior paranasal sinuses, middle ear, and eustachian tube. Accordingly, suppurative infections in these areas may provide the seeds for infection for retropharyngeal abscess.
- The predominant bacterial species are *Streptococcus pyogenes* (group A *Streptococcus*), *Staphylococcus aureus*, and respiratory anaerobes (including *Fusobacteria, Prevotella,*

and *Veillonella* species). *Haemophilus* species are also occasionally found.
- In young children, infection usually reaches this space by lymphatic spread from a septic focus in the pharynx or sinuses.
- In adults, infection may reach the retropharyngeal space from either local or distant sites. Penetrating trauma (e.g., from chicken bones or after instrumentation) is the usual source of local spread. More distant sources of infection include odontogenic sepsis and peritonsillar abscess (now a rare cause).

DIFFERENTIAL DIAGNOSIS

- Cervical osteomyelitis
- Pott's disease
- Meningitis
- Calcific tendonitis of the long muscle of the neck

IMAGING STUDIES

- A lateral neck film may be helpful in delineating the presence of a retropharyngeal abscess and may demonstrate cervical lordosis; the retropharyngeal space is considered widened and pathologic if it is greater than 7 mm at C2 or 14 mm at C6 (Fig. 1-9).
  - There must be attention to technical issues when performing the study, especially in children. The film should be a perfect lateral, and the child must keep the neck in extension during inspiration to avoid a false thickening of the retropharyngeal space. Crying, particularly in infants, may also cause false thickening of the retropharyngeal space.
- A CT scan of the neck is the best tool to identify abscesses in the retropharyngeal area, but it is not perfect. Both the sensitivity and specificity of the CT scan in predicting the presence of drainable purulent material

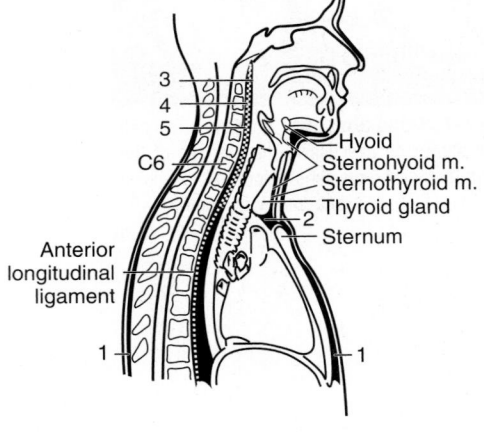

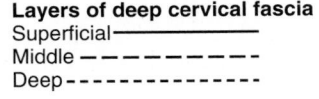

Layers of deep cervical fascia
Superficial ———————
Middle — — — — — — — —
Deep - - - - - - - - - - - - - -

A

FIGURE 1-8 Relation of various cervical fascial spaces to the superficial and deep layers of the cervical fascia. A, Cross section of the neck at the level of the thyroid isthmus. **B,** Coronal section in the suprahyoid region of the neck. *1,* Superficial space; *2,* pretracheal space; *3,* retropharyngeal space; *4,* "danger" space; *5,* prevertebral space.

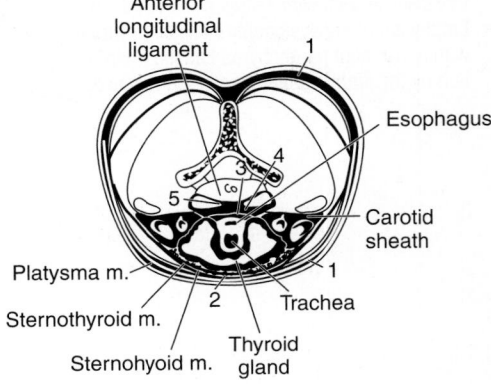

B

are quite variable from study to study, ranging between 68% and 100%.

- The CT scan provides more information than the plain radiograph because it can generally differentiate between retropharyngeal cellulitis and retropharyngeal abscess and can demonstrate extension of the retropharyngeal abscess to contiguous spaces in the neck. Findings on CT common to both cellulitis and abscess are a low-density core, soft tissue swelling, obliterated fat planes, and mass effect. The best differential finding on CT scan is "complete rim enhancement," which is indicative of abscess (Fig. 1-10). The abscess may be seen as a mass impinging on the posterior pharyngeal wall.

- MRI of the neck is more sensitive than CT, and technetium scanning can be helpful in detecting bone involvement. T2-weighted images may identify and localize areas of pus for drainage or aspiration. Gadolinium enhancement is important to accurately define the soft tissue component. Finally, MRI is useful for imaging vascular lesions, such as jugular thrombophlebitis.

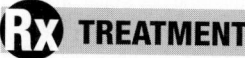 **TREATMENT**

ACUTE GENERAL & CHRONIC Rx

- High-dose penicillin (2 million to 4 million units IV q4h) plus metronidazole (500 mg IV q8h) or ampicillin-sulbactam (50 mg/kg/dose IV q6h) or clindamycin (13 mg/kg/dose IV q8h) are effective antimicrobial selections. Parenteral treatment is maintained until the patient is afebrile and clinically improved. Antibiotics should be adjusted as culture data become available, and oral therapy is continued to complete at least a 14-day course.
- Surgical intervention has historically played a prominent role in the management of retropharyngeal abscess in conjunction with antibiotic therapy. Drainage is indicated when there is a large hypodense area or when a patient has not responded to parenteral therapy alone.
- When the CT does not demonstrate a large hypodense area, a trial of antibiotic therapy without drainage is appropriate. Some investigators also support a trial of IV antibiotic therapy alone when small abscesses are identified by CT scans as long as there is no compromise of the airway.

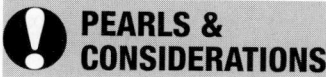 **PEARLS & CONSIDERATIONS**

PREVENTION

The complications of deep neck infection in any space are numerous and potentially fatal. Early diagnosis, with prompt and appropriate management, is key to avoiding these complications.

AUTHOR: **RUBY SATPATHY, M.D.**

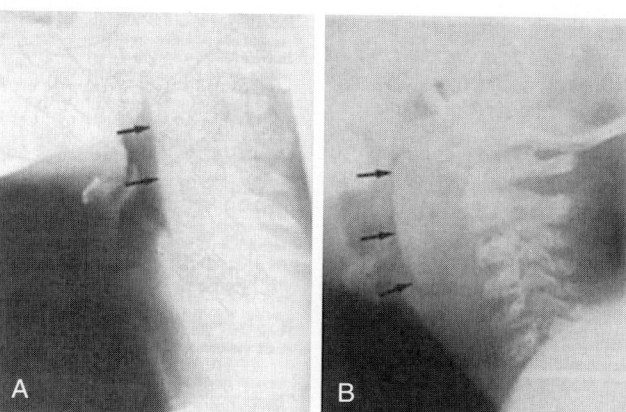

FIGURE 1-9 Lateral radiographs of the neck show normal lateral cervical view **(A)** and expansion of the prevertebral soft tissues by a retropharyngeal abscess **(B)**.

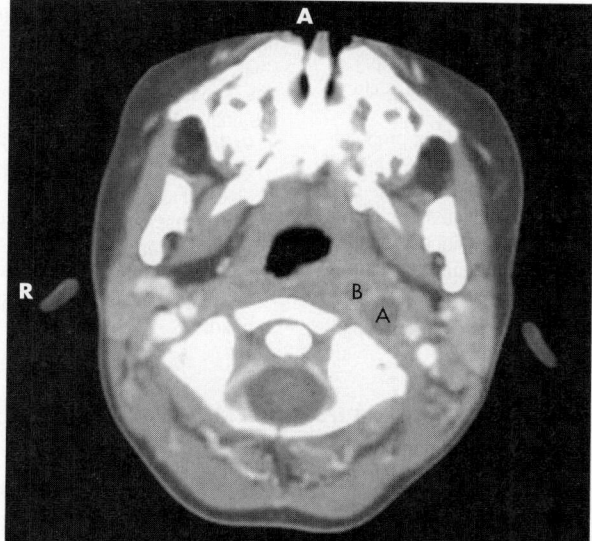

FIGURE 1-10 CT scan of a retropharyngeal abscess (*A* and *B*) demonstrates a low-density core, soft tissue swelling, obliterated fat planes, mass effect, and rim enhancement.

BASIC INFORMATION

DEFINITION

Definition from the Federal Child Abuse Prevention and Treatment Act (CAPTA): any recent act or failure to act on the part of a parent or caretaker that results in death, serious physical or emotional harm, sexual abuse or exploitation of a child; or an act or failure to act which presents an imminent risk of serious harm to a child.

- Neglect: failure to provide for the basic needs of a child
  1. Physical neglect: failure to provide necessary food, shelter, and supervision
  2. Medical neglect: failure to provide necessary medical or mental health care
  3. Educational neglect: failure to meet educational needs
  4. Emotional neglect: failure to attend to emotional needs, exposure to domestic violence
- Physical abuse: physical injury inflicted by a parent or caregiver intentionally or in the course of excessive discipline
- Sexual abuse: sexual act inflicted by parent or caretaker; includes exploitation and pornography
- Emotional/psychological abuse: pattern of behavior of caretaker toward a child that impairs emotional development. This includes verbal abuse, cruelty, and threats. Difficult to prove. Almost always present when other forms of abuse occur.
- Abandonment: child left and parents' whereabouts unknown.
- Substance abuse: includes: prenatal exposure to mother's use of illicit drugs; manufacture of methamphetamine in the presence of a child; selling or giving drugs to a child; use of mood-altering substance by caregivers that impairs their ability to provide care for their child.

SYNONYMS

Child maltreatment syndrome
Physical abuse
Sexual abuse
Battered child syndrome
Shaken baby syndrome
Shaken impact syndrome
Abusive head trauma

ICD-9CM CODES
995.5 Child maltreatment
995.50 Child abuse, unspecified
995.51 Child abuse, emotional or psychological
995.52 Child neglect
995.53 Child abuse, sexual
995.54 Child abuse, physical
995.55 Shaken infant syndrome
995.59 Multiple forms of child abuse or Other Child Abuse and Neglect

EPIDEMIOLOGY & DEMOGRAPHICS

INCIDENCE (IN U.S.): Any reports of incidence are underestimates because many cases are not recognized or reported. The following data are based on Child Protective Services (CPS) state aggregate as reported in Child Maltreatment 2010. In 2010, roughly 695,000 unique children were determined to be victims of abuse or neglect. This is a rate of 9.2 unduplicated victims per 1000 children.

- Types of abuse by percentage (note the total is greater than 100% since children are often victims of more than one type of abuse).
  1. Neglect: 78%
  2. Physical abuse: 17.6%
  3. Sexual abuse: 9.2%
  4. Psychological abuse: 8.1%
  5. Medical neglect: 2.4%
  6. Other: 10.3% (e.g., abandonment, threats of harm, congenital drug addiction)
- For 2010, an estimated 1537 child deaths were caused by abuse or neglect.
  - Overall annual death rate resulting from abuse or neglect is estimated to be 2.07 deaths/100,000 children.
  - More than 32% of these deaths were due to neglect alone; 23% were due exclusively to physical abuse; 41% were due to multiple forms of maltreatment.
  - 80% of these children were <4 yr of age with 48% less than 1 yr old.
  - Most fatalities were directly caused by one or both parents (79%).
  - Many child abuse fatalities are underreported because of misdiagnosis or variations in state definitions and coding.
- 80% of abused children were victimized by one or both of their parents.
- One fifth of adult women report history of molestation or sexual assault as a child or adolescent.

PREDOMINANT SEX: There is a slight predominance of girls as victims. However, boys have a slightly higher child fatality rate than girls.
PREDOMINANT AGE: Youngest children (0 through 3 yr old) have the highest rates of victimization with 34% being younger than the age of 4.
GENETICS: No known genetic factors.

ETIOLOGY

Multiple factors contribute to the incidence. No factor or combination of factors can definitively predict which children will be victimized. Factors contributing to risk of abuse or neglect include the following:
- Parent
  1. Substance abuse
  2. Mental illness
  3. Intellectual impairment
  4. Parental history of being abused as a child
- Child
  1. Low birth weight or prematurity
  2. Chronic physical disability
- Family
  1. Social isolation
  2. Poor parent-child bonding
  3. Stress: unemployment, chronic illness, eviction, arrest, poverty
  4. Domestic violence
- Community/society
  1. Limited transportation
  2. Limited day care
  3. Unsafe neighborhoods
  4. Poverty

DIAGNOSIS

Careful history and physical examination are the most important aspects of the evaluation. Careful documentation of any statements regarding origin of injuries or history of abuse is crucial. Chart and photographic documentation of injuries is also essential. The following are keys to the final diagnosis:
- Patterned bruising (e.g., loop-shaped, square, oval) is indicative of being struck with an object (Fig. 1-11).
- Injury observed is incompatible with the history provided.
- History of injury provided is incompatible with the developmental capabilities of the child.

MARKS from INSTRUMENTS

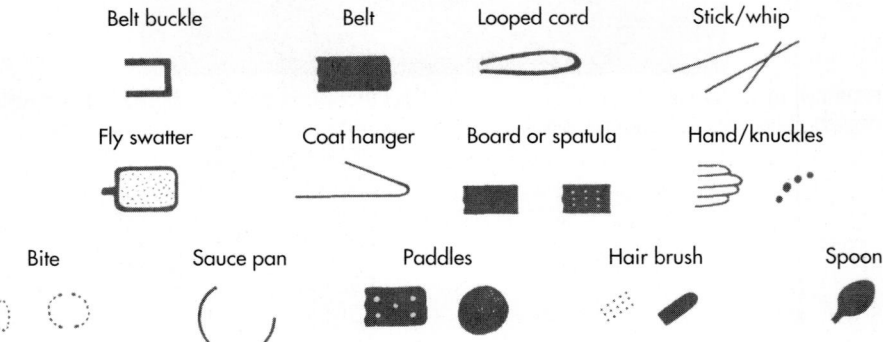

FIGURE 1-11 A variety of instruments may be used to inflict injury on a child. Often the choice of an instrument is a matter of convenience. Marks tend to silhouette or outline the shape of the instrument. The possibility of intentional trauma should prompt a high degree of suspicion when injuries to a child are geometric, paired, mirrored, of various ages or types, or on relatively protected parts of the body. Early recognition of intentional trauma is important to provide therapy and prevent escalation to more serious injury. (From Kliegman RM et al: *Nelson textbook of pediatrics,* ed 19, Philadelphia, 2011, Saunders.)

- Delay in seeking care for a significant injury (e.g., callus formation on a fracture, eschar formation on a burn).
- Bruising is rare in healthy preambulatory infants and warrants further investigation.
- Multiple significant injuries of different ages.
- Infant with clinically significant head trauma attributed to a trivial cause (e.g., a short fall). Often associated with retinal hemorrhages and skeletal fractures, which are indicative of shaken baby syndrome or abusive head trauma.
- Certain fractures in infants without a history of significant trauma (e.g., motor vehicle accident) are characteristic of abuse: metaphyseal, rib, sternum, scapula, vertebral body.
- Inflicted contact burns are indicated by an impression of the burning object: lighter, iron, cigarette (Fig. 1-12).
- Inflicted immersion burns are indicated by "stocking" burns of the feet or "glove" burns of the hands. Stocking burns are often associated with buttocks/perineal burns from immersion of a minor in a flexed position.
- Most sexual abuse victims will have a normal or nonspecific genital examination. A normal genital examination does not mean the child was not abused. History is the most important part of the diagnosis. Forensic interview by a trained professional is recommended, as is an examination by a health care provider experienced in child sexual abuse evaluations for child and adolescent victims of sexual abuse.
- The identification of a sexually transmitted disease in a prepubertal child who is beyond the neonatal period is suggestive of sexual abuse. Reporting and further careful investigation are warranted. Consult current CDC guidelines and a child sexual abuse expert for further guidance.

DIFFERENTIAL DIAGNOSIS

In all categories, accidental injury is the most common entity to be distinguished from abuse. Accidental injuries are most common over bony prominences: forehead, elbows, knees, shins;

soft, fleshy areas are more common for inflicted injury: buttocks, thighs, upper arms. Table 1-4 describes patterns of injury.

BRUISING

- Bleeding disorder (idiopathic thrombocytopenic purpura, hemophilia, leukemia, hemorrhagic disease of the newborn, von Willebrand's disease)
- Connective tissue disorder (Ehlers-Danlos syndrome, vasculitis)
- Pigments (Mongolian spots)
- Dermatitis (phytophotodermatitis, nickel allergy)
- Folk treatment (coining, cupping)

BURNS

- Chemical burn
- Impetigo
- Folk treatment (moxibustion)
- Dermatitis (phytophotodermatitis)

INTRACRANIAL HEMORRHAGE

- Bleeding disorder
- Perinatal trauma (should resolve by 4 wk)
- Arteriovenous malformation rupture
- Glutaric aciduria

FRACTURES

- Osteogenesis imperfecta
- Rickets
- Congenital syphilis
- Very low birth weight (osteopenia of prematurity)

SEXUAL ABUSE

- Normal variants
- Lichen sclerosis et atrophicus
- Congenital abnormalities
- Urethral prolapse
- Hemangioma
- Nonsexually acquired infection (group A *Streptococcus, Shigella*)

WORKUP (Fig. E1-13)

History and physical examination:
- Careful history from all caretakers and child.
- Scene investigation may be necessary.
- Complete physical examination.
- Sexual abuse: forensic interview and magnified examinations by trained professionals are the standard for evaluation and evidence col-

lection. This is especially important to avoid further psychological or physical trauma to the child.

Laboratory tests for physical abuse:
- Tests performed may vary depending on the severity of abuse and clinical presentation of the child.
- CBC with differential and platelets.
- Prothrombin time, activated partial thromboplastin time.
- Consider closure time (PFA-100), von Willebrand panel.
- Alanine aminotransferase, amylase, urinalysis.

Laboratory tests for sexual abuse:
- If within 72 hr of acute sexual assault/abuse, swabs are obtained from the oropharynx, areas of skin exposure (use an alternate light source to ID), genitalia, and rectum to send to the crime lab for DNA and other testing. Also collect samples of foreign hair, blood, saliva, or other tissue if present. A wet mount from cervical/vaginal specimen should be done to look for motile sperm.
- Per current CDC recommendations, adolescent victims of acute assault should have appropriate specimens collected from sites of penetration or attempted penetration for *Neisseria gonorrheae* and *Chlamydia*. Nucleic acid amplification tests (NAATs) may be used and are preferred. In females, wet mount and POC testing or culture of vaginal swab for *T. vaginalis* should also be done. If there is itching, vaginal discharge or malodor present, wet mount for bacterial vaginosis and *Candida* should also be done. Serum should be obtained for HIV, hepatitis B, and syphilis testing acutely. If negative, HIV and syphilis testing should be repeated 6, 12, and 24 wk after the assault.
- Child victims (i.e., prepubertal) should have specimens collected if considered high risk for a sexually transmitted infection (STI) per current CDC recommendations. Cervical specimens are not collected and vaginal specimens must be collected with care by an experienced provider to avoid further trauma to the child. Gonorrhea and *Chlamydia* culture is the gold standard for diagnosis and legal purposes. However, many providers now analyze specimens using urine or vaginal NAAT followed by culture confirmation or 2nd NAAT if any positive results are obtained. Any culture testing positive for *N. gonorrheae* should be confirmed

BURN MARKS

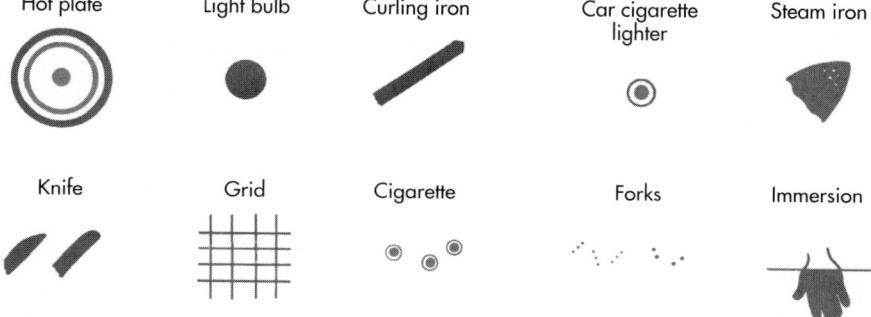

Hot plate   Light bulb   Curling iron   Car cigarette lighter   Steam iron

Knife   Grid   Cigarette   Forks   Immersion

FIGURE 1-12 Marks from heated objects cause burns in a pattern that duplicates that of the object. Familiarity with the common heated objects that are used to traumatize children facilitates recognition of possible intentional injuries. The location of the burn is important in determining its cause. Children tend to explore surfaces with the palmar surface of the hand and rarely touch a heated object repeatedly or for a long time. (From Kliegman RM et al: *Nelson textbook of pediatrics*, ed 19, Philadelphia, 2011, Saunders.)

TABLE 1-4	Patterns of Injury
Accidental	**Nonaccidental**
Unilateral	Bilateral/symmetrical
Isolated injury	Multiple injuries
Amorphous shape	Well-defined shape
Prominent bone areas	Soft tissue areas
Posterior aspect of body	Anterior aspect of body
One age of injury	Multiple ages of injury

From Fuhrman BP et al: *Pediatric critical care*, ed 4, Philadelphia, 2011, Saunders.

by at least two laboratory tests that are based on different principles. Specimens should be collected for gonorrhea and *Chlamydia,* wet mount, and blood for serologic testing (HIV, hepatitis B, syphilis) in the following cases:

1. Child has a past or current symptom of an STI, such as vaginal discharge, genital ulcer, or vaginal pain or currently diagnosed STI
2. Alleged assailant is known to have an STI or be at high risk for an STI
3. A sibling or adult in the same household has a known STI
4. Evidence of ejaculation or of oral, genital, and/or anal penetration is present on the examination
5. Child or parent requests testing

IMAGING STUDIES

Physical abuse:

- Radiographic skeletal survey for all children <2 yr; for 2- to 5-yr-olds, done only for severe abuse. Consider repeat skeletal survey in 2 wk if severe physical injury is present.
- Noncontrast head CT scan or MRI for all children <1 yr; for children >1 yr, clinical judgment should be used.
- Head MRI for children with significant abusive head trauma. This is used as an adjunct a few days after initial head CT.
- Abdominal CT scan if indicated by clinical examination or laboratory evaluation.
- Box E1-2 describes the specificity of radiologic findings for child abuse.

(Rx) TREATMENT

ACUTE GENERAL Rx

- Stabilize and treat acute medical injuries.
- Report to Child Protective Services. HIPAA allows reports for suspected child abuse without parental authorization.
- Early report to law enforcement for suspected physical abuse or sexual abuse to allow scene investigation.
- Disposition, once medically stable, is dependent on CPS. The child cannot be returned home if the environment is not safe.
- Physician should remain available to discuss with investigators. This is often critical to determining the outcome of the case and placement of the child.
- Because follow-up of adolescent sexual assault victims can be difficult, many experts

recommend empiric treatment for STIs: gonorrhea, *Chlamydia, Trichomonas,* and bacterial vaginosis. Pregnancy prophylaxis should also be offered. Hepatitis B immunization should be offered if not previously given. HIV prophylaxis is offered in certain situations depending on local epidemiology and type of assault. Consult local infectious disease experts for current recommendations. Repeat examination should be done in 2 wk for all victims of sexual assault, especially if they declined empiric treatment. If empiric treatment was not done, STI testing should be repeated at the 2-week follow-up visit.

- Empiric treatment of child victims of sexual abuse is generally not recommended. This is especially important if NAATs are used for screening for STIs because confirmation is necessary for any positive results. Careful follow-up within 2 wk and treatment based on culture results are indicated. HIV prophylaxis is offered in certain circumstances according to local epidemiology and risk. Consult with a local infectious disease expert for further recommendations.

CHRONIC Rx

- Often depends on CPS and court-ordered interventions
- Treatment of parental mental illness
- Treatment of parental substance abuse, including requirements for random drug testing
- Instruction for parents in behavior management skills, including appropriate limit setting and discipline
- Anger management classes for parents
- Trauma-focused cognitive-behavioral therapy is an evidence-based practice for victims of sexual abuse and exposure to domestic violence; useful to include nonoffending parent/caregiver
- Ongoing individual and family therapy
  - Parent-child interactive therapy is an evidence-based practice that is used with young children with behavioral problems and parent-child relationship problems
  - Child-parent psychotherapy is an evidence-based practice that is for young children (<5 yr) who have experienced a trauma and their caregivers

- May need long-term placement in foster care before it is safe to return home. In extreme cases of abuse, parental rights may be terminated without offering services.

OUTCOMES

- Victims of chronic abuse and neglect:
  - Have higher rates of mental illness (depression, suicide, posttraumatic stress disorder, eating disorders)
  - Have more cognitive difficulties, often impaired academic performance
  - Are more likely to become aggressive
  - Are more likely as adults to have adverse physical health outcomes (cardiovascular disease, cancer, STDs)
- Victims of abusive head trauma:
  - One third die, one third have severe disability, one third appear normal in the short term.

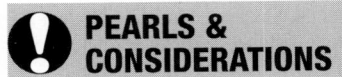

PEARLS & CONSIDERATIONS

PREVENTION

- Home visitation by a specially trained nurse to high-risk families during pregnancy and infancy has shown positive outcomes (Nurse-Family Partnership).
- Anticipatory guidance at health visits to teach normal developmental expectations and appropriate discipline.
- Screening to identify at-risk or abused children.
- Targeted education in the newborn nursery for shaken baby prevention has been shown to be effective.
- Substance abuse prevention and treatment.
- Identification and intervention for domestic violence before children are born.

SUGGESTED READINGS

available at www.expertconsult.com

RELATED CONTENT

Protecting Children from Abuse (Patient Information)

AUTHOR: **NANCY R. GRAFF, M.D.**

BASIC INFORMATION

DEFINITION

Drug abuse is a recurring pattern of harmful use of a substance despite adverse consequences to work, school, relationships, the legal system, or physical health. This may occur concurrently with or independently from *substance dependence,* in which the impairment or distress is more pervasive and often (though not necessarily) includes physical dependence and withdrawal symptoms (Table 1-5).

SYNONYMS

Substance use disorder
Substance abuse
Addiction

ICD-9CM CODES
Defined by specific substance F10-F19
(DSM-IV code is also defined by specific substance 291-292, 303-305)

EPIDEMIOLOGY & DEMOGRAPHICS

INCIDENCE (IN U.S.): Alcohol or drug dependence: 5% to 10% of population
PREVALENCE (IN U.S.): Approximately 15% of patients in primary care practice have an at-risk pattern of drug and/or alcohol use; lifetime prevalence of any alcohol use disorder: 30%; prescription drug misuse is on the rise with 5% past-year prevalence.
PREDOMINANT SEX: Males > females
PREDOMINANT AGE:
- Problematic use of substances may begin in early life (8 to 10 yr).
- Mean age of onset of problem drinking is approximately 25 yr for men and 30 yr for women.

PEAK INCIDENCE: For most substances: age 15 to 30 yr
DURATION OF CONDITION:
- Men: average >20 yr of heavy drinking
- Women: average 15 yr of heavy drinking
- In general, substance use disorders are chronic and relapsing and often progressive

GENETICS: There is evidence of nonspecific genetic factors. Addiction may result in part from underlying, inherited abnormalities in brain structure that impair behavior control and encourage impulsive behavior.

PHYSICAL FINDINGS & CLINICAL PRESENTATION
- Polysubstance use and comorbidity with psychiatric disorders are common.
- History often reveals recurring behavioral problems, such as relationship, work, or legal problems; violence and traumatic injuries; and anxiety, depression, insomnia, and cognitive and memory dysfunction.
- Repeated requests for early refills of controlled substances and obtaining prescriptions from multiple providers should raise concern for prescription drug abuse (Table 1-6).

- Physical findings may include injection marks, nasal lesions or recurrent epistaxis, poor dentition, scars or bruises from falls or trauma, and poor nutritional status; signs/symptoms of intoxication or withdrawal are highly suggestive of substance use disorder.

ETIOLOGY
Several models of addiction have been proposed:
1. Disease model: Addiction is a mental illness, which occurs as a result of the impairment of healthy neurochemical or behavioral processes.
2. Genetic model: Genetic predisposition is often a factor in dependency and certain addictive behaviors.
3. Social model: Person–environment interactions (i.e., socialization, imitation of observable behavior, and the influence of modeling) shape addictive behavior.

DIAGNOSIS

DIFFERENTIAL DIAGNOSIS
- Psychiatric disorders such as depression, mania, psychosis, and anxiety disorders may coexist or occur as a consequence of substance use.
- Rule out seizure disorder and underlying illness.

WORKUP
- A thorough history is crucial for diagnosis.
- The physician's history-taking style and techniques strongly affect patient's willingness to report use and participate in future treatment activities.

TABLE 1-5 Diagnostic Criteria for Dependence and Drug Abuse

Dependence (>3 Needed)	Abuse (>1 for 12 mo)
1. Tolerance	1. Recurrent substance use resulting in failure to fulfill major role obligations at work, school, or home
2. Withdrawal	2. Recurrent substance use in situations in which it is physically hazardous
3. The substance is often taken in larger amounts over a longer period than intended	3. Recurrent substance-related legal problems
4. Any unsuccessful effort or a persistent desire to cut down or control substance use	4. Continued substance use despite having persistent or recurrent social or interpersonal problems caused or exacerbated by the effects of the substance
5. A great deal of time is spent in activities necessary to obtain the substance or recover from its effects	5. Never met criteria for dependence
6. Important social, occupational, or recreational activities given up or reduced because of substance use	
7. Continued substance use despite knowledge of having had persistent or recurrent physical or psychological problems that are likely to be caused or exacerbated by the substance	

Reprinted from Goldman L, Bennett JC (eds): *Cecil textbook of medicine,* ed 22, Philadelphia, 2004, Saunders.

TABLE 1-6 "Red Flags" for Abuse Behavior and Opioid Addiction

Potential Abuse/Addiction Behaviors*

1. Patient displays an overwhelming focus on opioid issues during clinic visits that occupies a significant proportion of the clinic visit and impedes progress with other pain issues or medical problems.
2. Patient has a pattern of early refills (three or more) or escalating drug use in the absence of acute change or progression of his or her medical condition.
3. Patient generates multiple telephone calls or unscheduled visits to request more opioids, early refills, or problems associated with the opioid prescription that often creates a disturbance of the clinic staff.
4. There is a pattern of prescription problems with reports of medications lost, spilled, or stolen.
5. Patient has supplemental sources of opioids from multiple providers, emergency departments, or illegal sources.

Additional "Red Flag" Abuse Behavior

1. Selling prescribed opioid drugs
2. Prescription forgery
3. Stealing another patient's drugs
4. Injecting oral medication
5. Concurrent use of illicit drug
6. Appears intoxicated or oversedated
7. Insists on obtaining a specific opioid medication

*Adapted from Chabal criteria for opioid abuse.
From Hochberg MC et al: *Rheumatology,* ed 5, St Louis, 2011, Mosby.

- A structured, nonjudgmental approach is generally preferable:
  1. Ask about quantity and frequency of alcohol or drug use. For example, the National Institute on Alcohol Abuse and Alcoholism (NIAAA) declares that *problem drinking* is defined as more than 2 drinks per day for men and more than 1 drink per day for women or anyone older than 65 yr.
  2. Use a short screening instrument such as the CAGE questionnaire ("1. Have you ever felt you need to <u>C</u>ut down on your alcohol or drug use? 2. Have people <u>An</u>noyed you by criticizing your alcohol or drugs use? 3. Have you ever felt <u>Guilty</u> about alcohol or drugs use? 4. Have you ever felt you need to drink first thing in the morning [<u>E</u>ye opener] to stop shakiness?").
- Problematic behavior during intoxication or withdrawal is diagnostic.
- Because self-report of substance use and its consequences can be unreliable, obtaining corroborating information, such as from family members, past detoxifications, or drug rehabilitations, is often helpful.
- Adolescent drug abuse detection and treatment is extremely challenging. Stages of adolescent substance use are described in Table 1-7. An assessment for evaluating the seriousness of adolescent drug abuse is described in Table 1-8.

LABORATORY TESTS

- Blood alcohol content (BAC) measured on the breath is practical to define intoxication and provides a rough measure of impairment.
- Obtain toxicology screen in urine or blood samples.
- Biologic markers such as elevated mean corpuscular volume (MCV), γ-glutamyltransferase (GGT), liver function tests (AST and ALT), and carbohydrate deficient transferrin (CDT) may also be used to diagnose and monitor.

IMAGING STUDIES

Not helpful in routine diagnosis and management of substance abuse, but possibly useful in the management of sequelae of substance abuse (e.g., brain imaging to evaluate the alcohol abuse–associated increased risk of subdural hematomas or increased evidence of cerebral atrophy).

Rx TREATMENT

NONPHARMACOLOGIC THERAPY

- First assess readiness for change; if precontemplative or contemplative, counsel about risks of use and benefits of abstinence; a motivational interviewing approach has been shown to be effective.
- Nonpharmacologic strategies have the greatest documented efficacy: advice, feedback, goal setting, problem solving, and additional contacts for further assistance.
- Opiate contracts, prohibiting a patient from getting early refills or obtaining opiates from multiple prescribers, should be considered for all patients with chronic pain receiving opioid painkillers, especially for patients with a history of substance abuse or medication abuse.

- Relapse prevention facilitated by avoidance of trigger stimuli or by uncoupling trigger stimuli from substance ingestion.
- Self-help and support groups such as Alcoholics Anonymous, Narcotics Anonymous, and Al-Anon are helpful in achieving and maintaining sobriety.
- Residential or inpatient treatment programs should be a consideration for any individual with continued or escalating use despite outpatient treatment.

ACUTE GENERAL Rx

- Detoxification is an important first step in substance abuse treatment. Its goals are to facilitate withdrawal and reduce symptoms, initiate abstinence, and refer the patient to ongoing treatment.
- Benzodiazepines are effective in acute alcohol withdrawal for the management of symptoms as well as the prevention of seizures. One strategy is to give the patient a loading dose of a long-acting benzodiazepine (e.g., 20 mg of diazepam) and then continue the benzodiazepine as scheduled while tapering down the dose gradually. An alternative "symptom-driven" strategy is to follow the patient closely with serial assessments, such as the Clinical Institute Withdrawal Assessment for Alcohol (CIWA) scale, and to dose with 1 to 2 mg of lorazepam as needed to treat withdrawal symptoms.
- The prophylactic administration of thiamine and folic acid (first intravenously or intramuscularly followed by supplemental oral doses) in alcohol withdrawal is recommended before starting any carbohydrate-containing fluids or food to prevent Wernicke-Korsakaff syndrome (alcoholic encephalopathy and psychosis). Magnesium appears to be effective in the treatment of alcohol withdrawal–related <u>cardiac arrhythmias</u>, but not other symptoms of alcohol withdrawal. http://en. wikipedia.org/wiki/Cardiac_arrhythmias
- Beta-blockers and clonidine generally should be avoided in alcohol withdrawal; they may mask markers of the severity of the withdrawal (blood pressure and pulse rate).

TABLE 1-7 Stages of Adolescent Substance Abuse

Stage	Description
1	Potential for abuse • Decreased impulse control • Need for immediate gratification • Available drugs, alcohol, inhalants • Need for peer acceptance
2	Experimentation: learning the euphoria • Use of inhalants, tobacco, marijuana, and alcohol with friends • Few, if any, consequences • Use may increase to weekends regularly • Little change in behavior
3	Regular use: seeking the euphoria • Use of other drugs, e.g., stimulants, LSD, sedatives • Behavioral changes and some consequences • Increased frequency of use; use alone • Buying or stealing drugs
4	Regular use: preoccupation with the "high" • Daily use of drugs • Loss of control • Multiple consequences and risk-taking • Estrangement from family and "straight" friends
5	Burnout: use of drugs to feel normal • Polysubstance use/cross-addiction • Guilt, withdrawal, shame, remorse, depression • Physical and mental deterioration • Increased risk-taking, self-destructive, suicidal

From Kliegman RM et al: *Nelson textbook of pediatrics*, ed 19, Philadelphia, 2011, Saunders.

TABLE 1-8 Assessing the Seriousness of Adolescent Drug Abuse

Variable	0	+1	+2
Age (yr)	>15	<15	
Sex	Male	Female	
Family history of drug abuse		Yes	
Setting of drug use	In group		Alone
Affect before drug use	Happy	Always poor	Sad
School performance	Good, improving		Recently poor
Use before driving	None		Yes
History of accidents	None		Yes
Time of week	Weekend	Weekdays	
Time of day		After school	Before or during school
Type of drug	Marijuana, beer, wine	Hallucinogens, amphetamines	Whiskey, opiates, cocaine, barbiturates

Total score: 0-3, less worrisome; 3-8, serious; 8-18, very serious.
From Kliegman RM et al: *Nelson textbook of pediatrics*, ed 19, Philadelphia, 2011, Saunders.

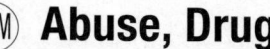
- Unlike withdrawal from alcohol or benzodiazepines, opioid withdrawal is not life threatening.
- Clonidine alleviates the discomfort of opiate withdrawal. Clonidine tablets, 0.1 mg q4-6h as needed, can be used while monitoring patient's blood pressure. Clonidine transdermal patch, 0.1 mg/24 hr, can be used to treat autonomic hyperactivity symptoms; however, it has a very slow onset and may take 2-3 days to achieve therapeutic levels. Antidiarrheals, ibuprofen, and dicyclomine can be used as adjuncts to treat opiate withdrawal symptoms.
- Methadone taper is an effective approach for detoxification in opioid dependence.
- Buprenorphine is a partial μ-opioid receptor agonist that may be used for detoxification and maintenance in treatment of opioid dependence (see dosing in next section).

CHRONIC Rx

- Naltrexone helps reduce craving for alcohol. Naltrexone 50 mg once daily for 12 wk can be a useful adjunct to substance abuse counseling or rehabilitation programs. Randomized treatment studies are equivocal for long-term outcomes. Naltrexone reduces relapse and the intensity or frequency of any drinking that does occur. It can be hepatotoxic and is contraindicated in opiate users. Intramuscular naltrexone (380 mg monthly) may be considered if adherence is an issue.
- Acamprosate also helps reduce craving for alcohol. Acamprosate 666 mg three times daily may be an effective adjunct to counseling. A recent meta-analysis showed overall benefit with increase in the number of abstinent days.
- Disulfiram provokes acetaldehyde accumulation after alcohol ingestion, producing a toxic state manifested by nausea, headache, flushing, and respiratory distress. Studies have shown limited efficacy mostly due to noncompliance.
- Topiramate may be an alternative treatment for alcoholism. In a 12-wk randomized trial topiramate up to 300 mg daily significantly reduced the number of heavy drinking days.
- Methadone maintenance for opiate addiction is effective and involves once-daily dosing of methadone in a controlled setting via methadone clinics.
- Buprenorphine is as effective as low-dose methadone and may be prescribed by physicians who have completed approved training. For induction, initiate 12 to 24 hr after short-acting opioid use and 24 to 48 hr after long-acting opioid use. Use buprenorphine/naloxone tablets in most patients, since buprenorphine-only tablets have risk of abuse. Maximum first-day dosage is 4 to 8 mg of buprenorphine. Titrate buprenorphine dose up to 12 mg on day 2 for signs of withdrawal. Then adjust dosage in frequent outpatient visits (weekly) to minimum needed for maintenance (up to 32 mg daily).
- Naltrexone (oral or injectable) may also be used for maintenance in opioid dependence treatment, though evidence of effectiveness is limited.
- Always combine pharmacotherapy with counseling.
- Treatment of comorbid psychiatric disorders improves outcomes.
- Intervention may be used to break through **denial** of a person with a serious addictive disorder to help the person acknowledge that he or she suffers from a disorder and agree to treatment.

DISPOSITION

- Substance abuse is a chronic relapsing illness, so relapses are best approached as part of the course of the illness, as opposed to as treatment failure.
- The goal of treatment is always abstinence, but success of treatment is measured by return of function, increasing duration between relapses, and prevention of sequelae of use.

REFERRAL

Physicians should refer patients who do not make progress on changing substance use patterns to addiction specialists and/or specialized substance abuse programs. Patients with comorbid psychiatric illness should be referred for mental health care.

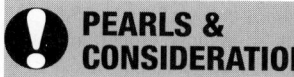 **PEARLS & CONSIDERATIONS**

- Acute withdrawal from alcohol can become life threatening.
- Withdrawal from opioids can resemble a severe case of the flu.
- A brief intervention (providing information and advising the patient to reduce consumption of alcohol) by the primary care doctor has been demonstrated in randomized trials to reduce drinking in at-risk patients.
- Treatment rates for alcohol use disorders remain low despite available effective treatments.

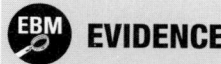 **EVIDENCE**

available at www.expertconsult.com

SUGGESTED READINGS
available at www.expertconsult.com

RELATED CONTENT

Drug Abuse (Patient Information)

AUTHORS: **TAHIR TELLIOGLU, M.D., OMRI BERGER, M.D.,** and **RADHIKA RAMANAN, M.D., M.P.H.**

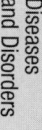
Diseases and Disorders

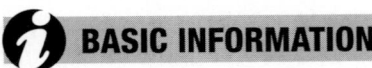

BASIC INFORMATION

DEFINITION

Elder abuse includes abuse commited by someone in a trust relation whether in the community or institutional setting.

- Physical abuse: inflicting physical pain or injury
- Sexual abuse: inflicting nonconsensual sexual activity
- Psychological abuse: inflicting mental anguish, including intimidation, humiliation, or threats
- Financial abuse: improper use of resources, property, or assets without the person's consent
- Neglect: abandonment, failure to fulfill a care-taking obligation, including provision of food, safe shelter, physical health and mental health care, or basic custodial care

SYNONYMS

Battered elder syndrome
Elder mistreatment
Domestic violence in the elderly
Diogenes syndrome

ICD-9CM CODES

995.80 Adult maltreatment, unspecified
995.81 Adult physical abuse
995.82 Adult emotional/psychological abuse
995.83 Adult sexual abuse
995.84 Adult neglect, nutritional
995.85 Other adult abuse and neglect

EPIDEMIOLOGY & DEMOGRAPHICS

INCIDENCE: According to the National Center on Elder Abuse, between 1 and 2 million Americans aged 65 yr and older have been injured, exploited, or mistreated by someone whom they depend on for care.
PEAK INCIDENCE: >75 yr; more recent studies now suggest <75 yr
PREVALENCE:
- 2% to 5% for those older than 65 yr.
- Financial abuse most common form.
- 12-month U.S. prevalence rates: emotional abuse 9.0% and 4.6%; physical abuse 0.2% and 1.6%; sexual abuse 0.6%; neglect 0.5%; and financial abuse 3.5% and 5.2%.
- Family members reported 21% of nursing home residents were neglected on one or more occasion in the past 12 months, and over 24% had been subjected to physical abuse during their entire stay.
- Among caregivers of patients with dementia in the U.K., one half reported behaving abusively at least some of the time, and one third reported "important" levels of abuse. Verbal abuse was common and physical abuse was rare.
- Elder abuse is associated with increased risk of mortality, functional impairment, and greater emotional distress, including depression, anxiety, and posttraumtic stress.
- Adult intimate partner violence perpetrators are significantly more likely to have witnessed intimate partner violence as child than nonperpetrators.

RISK FACTORS (VICTIM):

- Impaired cognition
- Shared living situation and premorbid relationship with abuser
- Social isolation and poor social support
- Mental or physical dependence
- Female
- Low household income
- ADL assistance

RISK FACTORS (PERPETRATOR):

- Substance abuse
- Mental illness, particularly depression
- Dependence on the victim and unemployment
- Being an involuntary caregiver
- History of violence

PHYSICAL FINDINGS & CLINICAL PRESENTATION

- Physical abuse with multiple injuries at various stages with implausible descriptions of their origins.
- Fear, hypervigilance, or withdrawal.
- Evidence of poor nutrition, dehydration, poor hygiene, multiple or neglected pressure ulcers, neglected medical conditions, or evidence of restraint use (bruises around wrists or ankles).
- Toxicologic evidence of unprescribed medications.
- Poor adherence, frequent no-shows, or little contact with health care system.

DIAGNOSIS

DIFFERENTIAL DIAGNOSIS

- Advancing dementia
- Depression, substance misuse, or other psychiatric disorder
- Malnutrition from intrinsic causes
- Conscious nonadherence
- Financial hardship
- Falling

WORKUP

1. Ask direct specific questions such as*:
   - "Has anyone close to you called you names or put you down recently?"
   - "Are you afraid of anyone in your life?"
   - "Are you able to use the telephone anytime you want to?"
   - "Has anyone forced you to do things you didn't want to do?"
   - "Has anyone taken things or money that belong to you without your OK?"
   - "Has anyone close to you tried to hurt you or harm you recently?"
2. Interview patient separately from the suspected abuser.
3. Pelvic examination if sexual abuse suspected.
4. Take photographs of physical injuries as legal evidence.

*University of Maine Center on Aging: Elder abuse screening protocol for physicians: lessons learned from the Maine partners for elder protection pilot project, http://www.umaine.edu/mainecenteronaging/documents/elderabusescreeningmanual.pdf)

LABORATORY TESTS & IMAGING STUDIES

- Toxicology screens and therapeutic drug monitoring are sometimes helpful.
- Other tests and radiology according to presentation.

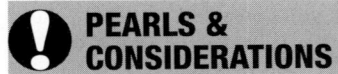 TREATMENT

NONPHARMACOLOGIC THERAPY

- Separate patient and abuser.
- Patient and caregiver may benefit from screening and treatment for substance abuse, mental illness, or cognitive impairment.
- Fig. E1-14 describes a management algorithm for geriatric abuse.

ACUTE GENERAL Rx

As indicated for injury or pain relief

DISPOSITION

If the patient's level of disability does not allow independent living, institutionalization may be required. Guidelines vary at the state and county levels regarding guardianship and conservatorship requirements.

REFERRAL

- For outpatients, report to local adult protective services agency. Reporting is mandatory in most states.
- For nursing home patients, report to regional long-term care ombudsman. Reporting is mandatory under federal law.
- In the U.S., the elder care help line is 1-800-677-1116.
- National Center on Elder Abuse: http://www.ncea.aoa.gov.

PEARLS & CONSIDERATIONS

COMMENTS

Care should be taken in interacting with the alleged abuser so that access to the victim is not lost.

PREVENTION

- Offer social services (e.g., respite care) for stressed caregivers.
- Make financial arrangements and arrange durable power of attorney for health care and finances while patient is still cognitively intact.

PATIENT & FAMILY EDUCATION

National Center on Elder Abuse: http://www.ncea.aoa.gov
JAMA Patient Page: Hildreth CJ et al: JAMA patient page. Elder abuse, *JAMA* 302(5):588, 2009

SUGGESTED READINGS

available at www.expertconsult.com

RELATED CONTENT

Elder Abuse (Patient Information)

AUTHORS: **ROBERT KOHN, M.D.,** and **BREE JOHNSTON, M.D., M.P.H.**

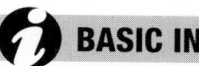

BASIC INFORMATION

DEFINITION

Acetaminophen (APAP) poisoning is a disorder caused by excessive intake of APAP and is manifested by jaundice, nausea, vomiting, and potential death from hepatic necrosis if not treated appropriately.

SYNONYMS

Paracetamol poisoning

ICD-9CM CODES

965.4 Acetaminophen poisoning

EPIDEMIOLOGY & DEMOGRAPHICS

- APAP is one of the most widely prescribed antipyretics and analgesics in the U.S. Potentially toxic ingestions, both intentional and unintentional, exceed 100,000 cases annually in the U.S.
- APAP toxicity has become the number one cause of acute liver failure in the U.S.
- Death rate is approximately one in 1000 persons. Nearly 50% of exposures occur in children ≤6 yr.
- Hepatic necrosis is most likely to occur in people who are chronically malnourished, who regularly abuse alcohol, and who are using other potentially hepatotoxic medications.

PHYSICAL FINDINGS & CLINICAL PRESENTATION

- The physical examination may vary depending on the amount of time since ingestion.
- Phase I (0 to 24 hr): Initial symptoms may be mild or absent and may consist of anorexia, diaphoresis, malaise, nausea, vomiting, and a subclinical rise in transaminase levels.
- Phase II (24 to 72 hr): right upper quadrant pain, vomiting, somnolence, tachycardia, hypotension, and continued increase in transaminases
- Phase III (72 to 96 hr): hepatic necrosis with abdominal pain, jaundice, hepatic encephalopathy, coagulopathy, hypoglycemia, renal failure, fatality from multiorgan failure
- Phase IV (4 days to 3 wk): complete resolution of symptoms and complete resolution of organ failure

ETIOLOGY

- The amount of APAP necessary for hepatic toxicity varies with the patient's body size and hepatic function. It is recommended that APAP intake should not exceed 4 g for adults and 90 mg/kg in children within a 24-hr period.
- Using standardized nomograms calculating the APAP plasma level and the number of hours after ingestion, the clinician can determine potential hepatic toxicity. See the APAP ingestion algorithm (Fig. E1-15).

DIAGNOSIS

DIFFERENTIAL DIAGNOSIS

- Liver disease from alcohol abuse or hepatitis
- Ingestion of other hepatotoxic substances
- Bacterial/viral gastroenteritis

WORKUP

Initial workup is aimed at confirming APAP overdose with plasma APAP level and assessment of hepatic damage. A careful history should elicit the time of APAP ingestion, amount, preparation (e.g., extended release) and possibility co-ingestants (see "Laboratory Tests").

LABORATORY TESTS

- Initial laboratory evaluation should include a STAT plasma APAP level with a second level drawn approximately 4 hr after the initial ingestion. Subsequent levels can be obtained every 2 to 4 hr until the levels stabilize or decline. These levels should be plotted on the Rumack-Matthew nomogram (see acetaminophen ingestion algorithm [Fig. E1-15] to calculate potential hepatic toxicity). The nomogram cannot be used with patients who present >24 hr after ingestion, took extended-release preparations, had chronic ingestions, or when the time of ingestion is unknown.
- Transaminases (AST, ALT), bilirubin level, prothrombin time (INR), blood urea nitrogen, and creatinine should be initially obtained on all patients.
- Serum and urine toxicology screen for other potential toxic substances is also recommended on admission. Screening for infectious hepatitis should also be considered.
- Urine for β-hCG should be obtained from all women of childbearing age.

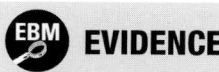 TREATMENT

NONPHARMACOLOGIC THERAPY

Consultation with a Poison Control Center is recommended for patients who have ingested a large amount of APAP and/or other toxic substances. A single toxic dose of APAP usually exceeds 7g or 150 mg/kg in the adult.

ACUTE GENERAL Rx

- Hepatotoxicity is defined as any increase in alanine aminotransferase (ALT) or aspartate aminotransferase (AST) >1000 IU/L, and hepatic failure is hepatotoxicity with hepatic encephalopathy. For those who cannot be risk stratified using the nomogram, the American College of Emergency Physicians recommends that N-acetylcysteine be administered without delay to those >12 yr and >8 hr after ingestion at presentation.
- Administer activated charcoal 1g/kg PO if the patient is seen within 1 hr of ingestion or the clinician suspects polydrug ingestion that delays gastric emptying.
- Determine blood levels 4 hr after ingestion; if in the toxic range, start N-acetylcysteine (NAC) either IV (Acetadote) or PO (Mucomyst). Acetylcysteine IV loading dose is 150 mg/kg ×1 diluted in 200 ml D5W over 15 to 60 min. Maintenance dose is 50 mg/kg diluted in 500 ml D5W over 4 hr, followed by 100 mg/kg diluted in 1000 ml D5W over 16 hr. The dose does not require adjustment for renal or hepatic impairment or for dialysis. Total administration time is 21 hours.
- Oral administration is 140 mg/kg PO as a loading dose, followed after 4 hr by 70 mg/kg PO q4h for a total of 17 doses. N-acetylcysteine therapy should be started within 24 hr of APAP overdose. Total administration time is 72 hours.
- Advantages of IV administration include more reliable absorption, fewer doses, and shorter duration of treatment.
- Monitor APAP level; use graph to plot possible hepatic toxicity. Repeat AST/ALT and APAP levels after 12 to 14 hr of IV acetylcysteine infusion and continue infusion longer than 16 hr if transaminases are elevated, if APAP concentration is measurable, or if coagulopathy exists (INR >1.5-2.0).
- Provide adequate IV hydration (e.g., $D_5\frac{1}{2}NS$ at 150 ml/hr).
- In patients on IV N-acetylcysteine with liver failure, frequent monitoring of vital signs, oxygen saturation by pulse oximetry, AST, and serum creatinine as well as signs of hypoglycemia and infection is essential.
- If APAP level is nontoxic, N-acetylcysteine therapy may be discontinued.

DISPOSITION

Most patients (90%) will recover fully without persisting hepatic abnormalities. Hepatic failure is particularly unusual in children <6 yr.

REFERRAL

Psychiatric referral is recommended after intentional ingestions.

EVIDENCE

available at www.expertconsult.com

SUGGESTED READING

available at www.expertconsult.com

RELATED CONTENT

Acetaminophen Overdose (Patient Information)

AUTHOR: **TARA M. WAYT, D.O.**

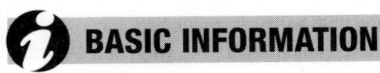

BASIC INFORMATION

DEFINITION

Achalasia is a motility disorder of the esophagus classically characterized by incomplete relaxation of the lower esophageal sphincter (LES) and aperistalsis of esophageal smooth muscle. The result is functional obstruction of the esophagus.

SYNONYMS

Achalasia and cardiospasm
Achalasia (of cardia)
Aperistalsis of esophagus
Megaesophagus
Esophageal achalasia
Esophageal cardiospasm

ICD-9CM CODES
530.0 Achalasia

EPIDEMIOLOGY & DEMOGRAPHICS

- Annual incidence is approximately 0.5 in 100,000 persons.
- Prevalence is <10 per 100,000 persons.
- Although the onset of symptoms may occur at any age, incidence is typically bimodal, 20 to 40 yr, then after 60 yr, with greater incidence in the older group.
- Men and women are affected equally.

PHYSICAL FINDINGS & CLINICAL PRESENTATION

Symptoms:
- Dysphagia (most commonly with both solids and liquids)
- Difficulty belching
- Regurgitation
- Chest pain and/or heartburn
- Globus
- Frequent hiccups
- Vomiting of undigested food
- Symptoms of aspiration such as nocturnal cough; possible dyspnea and pneumonia
- Weight loss
Physical findings:
- Focal lung examination abnormalities and wheezing also possible

ETIOLOGY

- Etiology is poorly understood.
- Loss of myenteric nerve fibers in the LES and smooth muscle portion of the esophagus. This has been associated with lymphocytic and eosinophilic infiltrates and fibrosis in later stages of disease.
- Loss of intrinsic inhibitory neurons in the myenteric plexus, producing nitric oxide synthase, as well as depletion of networks of interstitial cells of Cajal of the LES, leads to incomplete relaxation.
- This motility disorder may be caused by autoimmune degeneration of the esophageal myenteric plexus because association with the HLA class II antigen DQw1 has been noted. Antimyenteric plexus and other antineural autoantibodies have also been described.
- Abnormal immune reactions to neurotropic viruses such as varicella zoster, herpes simplex type 1, and measles viruses have been implicated, but the association has not been confirmed. A host T cell–mediated response may lead to neuronal injury.
- Achalasia is also seen in the rare autosomal recessive disorder Allgrove syndrome (achalasia, alacrima, autonomic disturbance, and acetylcholine insensitivity), which has been linked to a gene mutation on chromosome 12q13. Neurons in this syndrome may be susceptible to oxidative injury.

DIAGNOSIS

DIFFERENTIAL DIAGNOSIS

- Primary achalasia:
  - Idiopathic
- Secondary achalasia:
  - Chagas disease
  - Vagal injury or surgery, including fundoplication
  - Achalasia-like esophageal dilation has been described after laparoscopic gastric banding
- Pseudoachalasia:
  - Esophageal cancer
  - Infiltrating gastric cancer
  - Oat cell and bronchogenic lung cancer
  - Lymphoma

  - Amyloidosis
  - Paraneoplastic syndrome
- Angina
- Bulimia
- Anorexia nervosa
- Gastric bezoar
- Gastritis
- Peptic ulcer disease
- Postvagotomy dysmotility
- Esophageal disease (Table 1-9):
  - Gastroesophageal reflux disease
  - Sarcoidosis
  - Amyloidosis
  - Esophageal stricture
  - Esophageal webs and rings
  - Scleroderma
  - Barrett's esophagus
  - Esophagitis
  - Diffuse esophageal spasm

WORKUP

- Physical examination and laboratory analyses to rule out other causes and assess complications
- Imaging studies, manometry, and endoscopy

LABORATORY TESTS

- Assessment of nutritional status
- Complete blood count, ECG, stress test if diagnosis is in doubt
- Serologic assays for *Trypanosoma cruzi* (Chagas disease) in appropriate individuals

IMAGING STUDIES

Barium swallow with fluoroscopy may demonstrate:
- Uncoordinated or absent esophageal contractions
- An acutely tapered contrast column ("bird's beak"; Fig. 1-16)
- Dilation of the distal (smooth muscle portion) esophagus
- Esophageal air-fluid level with evidence of poor esophageal emptying
Manometry is generally considered to be the "gold standard" test to confirm the diagnosis. In classic achalasia, abnormalities are as follows:
- Low-amplitude disorganized contractions/aperistalsis
- Incomplete or absent LES relaxation after swallow

TABLE 1-9 Esophageal Motor Disorders

	Achalasia	Scleroderma	Diffuse Esophageal Spasm
Symptoms	Dysphagia	Gastroesophageal reflux disease	Substernal chest pain (angina-like)
	Regurgitation of nonacidic material	Dysphagia	Dysphagia with pain
Radiographic appearance	Dilated, fluid-filled esophagus	Aperistaltic esophagus	Simultaneous noncoordinated contractions
	Distal *bird-beak* stricture	Free reflux	
		Peptic stricture	
Manometric findings			
Lower esophageal sphincter	High resting pressure	Low resting pressure	Normal pressure
	Incomplete or abnormal relaxation with swallow		
Body	Low-amplitude, simultaneous contractions after swallowing	Low-amplitude peristaltic contractions or no peristalsis	Some peristalsis
			Diffuse and simultaneous nonperistaltic contractions, occasionally high amplitude

From Andreoli TE et al: *Andreoli and Carpenter's Cecil essentials of medicine*, ed 8, Philadelphia, 2010, Saunders.

- High LES pressure
- A subset of patients with "vigorous achalasia" may have high-amplitude, long-duration, simultaneous esophageal contractions. This term is now felt to be imprecise because of a newer classification of the disease.
- High-resolution manometry (HRM), or high-resolution esophageal pressure topography (HREPT), has recently defined subsets of patients with achalasia who may have different responses to medical or surgical therapies. Unlike classic achalasia (type I), type II achalasia shows panesophageal pressurization to greater than 30 mm Hg with ≥20% of test swallows, and type III achalasia shows spastic lumen-obliterating contractions of the distal esophagus on at least two test with ≥20% of swallows.
- HREPT has also defined an achalasia variant described as esophagogastric junction outflow obstruction.
- Direct visualization by endoscopy should be performed to exclude other causes of dysphagia, including "functional esophagogastric junction obstruction," strictures, secondary causes of achalasia, and pseudoachalasia.

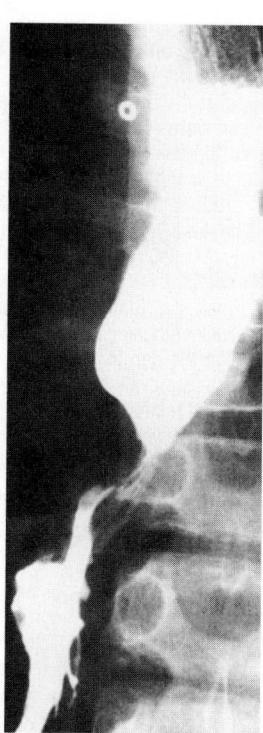

FIGURE 1-16 Classic appearance of achalasia of the esophagus. The dilated esophagus ends in a narrow segment. (From Hoekelman R [ed]: *Primary pediatric care,* ed 3, St Louis, 1997, Mosby.)

Rx TREATMENT

NONPHARMACOLOGIC THERAPY

- The goals of therapy are to decrease LES pressure, relieve symptoms, and prevent progression to a dilated or megaesophagus.
- Pneumatic dilation may benefit 65% to 90% of patients. Multiple sessions may be required, and most protocols use a graded dilation approach, starting with a 30-mm balloon, and repeating if required with a 35-mm or 40-mm balloon. Some studies suggest this may be more effective in women or older patients. Esophageal rupture or perforation is a rare complication (2% to 4%) that may be managed conservatively in some stable patients.
- Surgical: laparoscopic, or now less commonly open, (Heller's) esophagomyotomy is effective (90%). Approximately 35% of patients undergoing surgery will develop reflux disease. As a result, some surgeons will perform a "loose" antireflux repair as part of the surgical procedure. Some studies suggest this may be more effective in men and younger patients. An observational study has suggested that those who have had prior endoscopic treatment before myotomy may not do as well as those who have a primary myotomy.
- Studies suggest that type I and type II patients have better treatment responses to these therapies compared with type III patients.
- A large European study suggested that in experienced hands, patients may expect similar medium-term outcomes from myotomy and balloon dilation. A meta-analysis suggests better long-term durability of myotomy. Balloon dilation may be the more cost-effective treatment.
- Assessment of esophagogastric junction distensibility by an endoscopic functional luminal imaging probe may help to better evaluate the efficacy of treatment.
- Endoscopic submucosal myotomy (POEM [per oral endoscopic myotomy]) has been reported in several series and is being explored as another option for treatment.

GENERAL Rx

- Medications may be useful for short-term symptom relief and in patients with refractory chest pain. They should only be considered in patients unable to receive, or who are scheduled for, more definitive procedures. LES pressure may be lowered by 50% through sublingual use of long-acting nitrates (e.g., isosorbide dinitrate 5 to 20 mg) or calcium channel blockers (e.g., nifedipine 10 to 30 mg). Side effects are common and duration of relief tends to be short. Sildenafil was shown to be effective in a few small, short-term studies, but it is generally not recommended.
- Botulinum toxin injection will benefit up to 85% of patients by inhibiting acetylcholine release from cholinergic nerve endings, but up to half of these patients will require repeat injections by 6 months. A few studies have suggested that repeated injections can lead to fibrosis, which may complicate subsequent attempts at surgical therapy.

! PEARLS & CONSIDERATIONS

COMMENTS

- Medication has a limited role in treatment.
- Botulinum toxin is transiently effective in improving symptoms. Pneumatic dilation and surgical myotomy provide more durable long-term responses and are the treatment of choice for most patients. Botulinum toxin should be considered primarily in patients too elderly or ill to be considered for these other therapies.
- Patients with achalasia may be at long-term risk of squamous cell carcinoma of the esophagus and non–reflux-associated esophagitis. Treated patients may be at long-term risk for reflux esophagitis, Barrett's esophagus, and adenocarcinoma.

EBM EVIDENCE

available at www.expertconsult.com

SUGGESTED READINGS
available at www.expertconsult.com

RELATED CONTENT

AUTHOR: **HARLAN G. RICH, M.D., F.A.C.P., A.F.A.F.**

Diseases and Disorders

DEFINITION

Achilles tendon rupture is a disruption of the continuity of the Achilles tendon that most often results from the combination of mechanical stress and intratendinous degeneration.

ICD-9CM CODES
727.67 Nontraumatic rupture of Achilles tendon

EPIDEMIOLOGY & DEMOGRAPHICS

INCIDENCE: 1 in 10,000/year (third most frequent tendon disruption in the body)
PEAK INCIDENCE: 30 to 39 yr age group
PREDOMINANT AGE: 30 to 55 yr age group
RISK FACTORS: General risk factors include the recreational athlete, advancing age, previous tear or rupture, extreme change in training level, or participation in a new activity. Other risk factors can be categorized into intrinsic and extrinsic.

- **Intrinsic:** Achilles tendinitis/tendinosis, tight musculature, poor vascularity, tibial varum, overpronation, cavus foot, systemic lupus erythematosus, rheumatoid arthritis, gout
- **Extrinsic:** Inadequate training equipment/ training techniques, recent steroid or fluoroquinolone therapy

PHYSICAL FINDINGS & CLINICAL PRESENTATION

The typical patient is a middle-aged man who gives a history of recent physical activity with a sudden push-off, jump, or misstep that causes a snap sensation or audible pop in the back of the leg, followed by the onset of acute pain, swelling, and weakened plantarflexion power. Patients commonly relate feeling as though they were "hit in the back of the leg with a bat." Most often patients have sedentary occupations and indulge occasionally in strenuous activity.

- Depending on the severity of the rupture, initial pain may not be severe.
- Several hours after injury, diffuse pain, swelling, and ecchymosis are usually evident.
- The patient has difficulty walking, with a weakened plantarflexion power and inability to perform a single heel raise on the injured extremity.
- Referred stabbing pain in the posterior leg and ankle from muscle spasm is common.
- A palpable gap within the Achilles tendon, which increases with dorsiflexion of the ankle, is present.

ETIOLOGY

Although a history of direct trauma is uncommon, it may include blunt trauma to the posterior ankle, crushing injury, and laceration. Indirect injury as a cause of rupture is more common. Etiologic factors of indirect injury are of three types: mechanical, vascular, and related to poor tissue quality.

- Mechanical: involves variations of a rapid loading process on an already tensed tendon such as a sudden dorsiflexion of the ankle with the knee extended while an eccentric load is applied
  - ○ Tripping on a curb
  - ○ Lunging for a tennis shot
  - ○ Jumping from a height
- Vascular: factors include the known watershed area located 2 to 6 cm proximal to the insertion, an area of poor blood supply.
- Poor tissue quality: refers to the common notion that prior tendon degeneration is required to weaken the tendon before it is ruptured. This often occurs in the form of repetitive microtrauma from improper training techniques.

![Dx] **DIAGNOSIS**

DIFFERENTIAL DIAGNOSIS

- Achilles tendinopathy
- Retrocalcaneal bursitis
- Ankle sprain
- Calcaneal avulsion fracture
- Partial rupture of gastrocnemius
- Plantaris rupture
- Rupture of Baker's cyst
- Os trigonum syndrome
- Plantaris rupture

WORKUP

Approximately 25% of Achilles tendon ruptures are misdiagnosed initially. A thorough history and physical exam, coupled with high clinical suspicion, can prevent this from happening. The clinical history in most presentations is very specific, and the physical exam is usually diagnostic. Below is a list of specific clinical tests and imaging modalities. Please see section "Physical Findings & Clinical Presentation" for more information.

- Thompson's test: The patient is placed in a prone position with the knees flexed. The examiner squeezes the calf musculature, which should produce plantarflexion of the ankle. If no plantarflexion is obtained, this

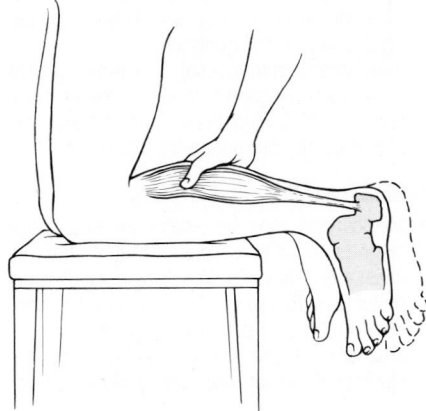

FIGURE 1-17 Thompson's test. Compression of the calf muscles normally produces plantarflexion of the ankle. If the Achilles tendon is ruptured, this reponse is greatly diminished or absent. (From Browner BD et al: *Skeletal trauma: basic science, management, and reconstruction,* ed 3, Philadelphia, 2003, Saunders.)

indicates an Achilles tendon rupture (a positive test). (See Fig. 1-17.)
- Matles' test: The patient is placed in the prone position with the knees flexed to 90 degrees. If the injured foot falls to neutral or a dorsiflexed position, the Achilles tendon is ruptured (a positive test).
- MRI and ultrasound may be useful when clinical suspicion is high, but clinical tests are inconclusive.

![Rx] **TREATMENT**

Controversy exists over conservative versus surgical repair of the ruptured Achilles tendon, but most evidence shows that early treatment has a far better prognosis than later repair. Conservative treatment is associated with a higher re-rupture rate. Surgical repair often facilitates earlier return to full activity. In general, older, more sedentary patients should be treated conservatively and younger athletic patients should receive surgical repair.

- *Conservative treatment:* A long leg cast is applied with the foot in approximately 20 degrees equinovarus, ensuring that the knee is bent during the casting process. The cast is removed at 8 weeks, with gradual reduction in equinovarus with a short leg cast. After removal of the cast, physical therapy should be instituted to regain dorsiflexion of the ankle. This gradual process may take up to 12 weeks. The total conservative rehabilitation period may last 6-9 months.
- *Surgical treatment:* Several surgical techniques exist to repair the ruptured Achilles tendon. Many involve lengthening and flap down methods to bridge the gap in the tendon. Multiple biologic grafts are available that may be used to augment and reinforce the rupture site. After surgery, 10 to 12 weeks of immobilization followed by rehabilitation is recommended.

DISPOSITION

- Conservative care carries a 20%-30% chance of re-rupture.
- Re-rupture rates are very low with surgical repair
- A physical therapist should work closely with the patient in the rehabilitation period regardless of whether surgical or conservative care is used.
- Early treatment, whether conservative or surgical, has far better results than treatment of neglected cases

![EBM] **EVIDENCE**

available at www.expertconsult.com

SUGGESTED READINGS
available at www.expertconsult.com

RELATED CONTENT
Achilles Tendon Rupture (Patient Information)

AUTHOR: **DOMINIC RODA, D.P.M.**

BASIC INFORMATION

DEFINITION

Acne vulgaris is a chronic disorder of the pilosebaceous apparatus caused by abnormal desquamation of follicular epithelium leading to obstruction of the pilosebaceous canal, resulting in inflammation and subsequent formation of papules, pustules, nodules, comedones, and scarring. Acne can be classified by the type of lesion (comedonal, papulopustular, and nodulocystic). The American Academy of Dermatology classification scheme for acne denotes the following three levels:

1. Mild acne: characterized by the presence of comedones (noninflammatory lesions), few papules and pustules (generally <10), but no nodules.
2. Moderate acne: presence of several to many papules and pustules (10 to 40) along with comedones (10 to 40). The presence of >40 papules and pustules along with larger, deeper nodular inflamed lesions (up to five) denotes moderately severe acne (Fig. 1-18).
3. Severe acne (Fig. 1-19): presence of numerous or extensive papules and pustules as well as many nodular lesions.

SYNONYMS

Acne

ICD-9CM CODES
706.1 Acne vulgaris

EPIDEMIOLOGY & DEMOGRAPHICS

- Acne is the most common skin disease in the U.S.
- It is most common in teenagers (highest incidence between ages of 16 and 18 yr).

PHYSICAL FINDINGS & CLINICAL PRESENTATION

- Open comedones (blackheads), closed comedones (whiteheads)
- Greasiness (oily skin)
- Presence of scars from prior acne cysts
- Various stages of development and severity may be present concomitantly
- Common distribution of acne: face, back, and upper chest
- Inflammatory papules, pustules, and ectatic pores

ETIOLOGY

- Overactivity of the sebaceous glands and blockage in the ducts. The obstruction leads to the formation of comedones, which can become inflamed because of overgrowth of *Propionibacterium acnes.*
- Exacerbated by environmental factors (hot, humid, tropical climate), medications (e.g., iodine in cough mixtures, hair greases), industrial exposure to halogenated hydrocarbons.

DIAGNOSIS

DIFFERENTIAL DIAGNOSIS

- Gram-negative folliculitis
- Staphylococcal pyoderma
- Acne rosacea
- Drug eruption
- Sebaceous hyperplasia
- Angiofibromas, basal cell carcinomas, osteoma cutis
- Occupational exposures to oils or grease
- Steroid acne
- Hidradenitis suppurativa
- Perioral dermatitis
- Pseudofolliculitis barbae
- Miliaria
- Seborrheic dermatitis

WORKUP

History and physical examination:
- Inquire about previous treatment
- Careful drug history
- Family history, history of cyclic menstrual flares
- History of use of cosmetics and cleansers
- Oral contraceptive use

LABORATORY TESTS

- Laboratory evaluation is generally not helpful.
- Patients who are candidates for therapy with isotretinoin should have baseline liver enzymes, cholesterol, and triglycerides checked because this medication may result in elevation of lipids and liver enzymes.
- A negative serum pregnancy test or two negative urine pregnancy tests should also be obtained in females 1 wk before initiation of isotretinoin; it is also imperative to maintain effective contraception during and 1 mo after therapy with isotretinoin ends because of its teratogenic effects. Pregnancy status should be rechecked at monthly visits.
- If hyperandrogenism is suspected in female patients, levels of dehydroepiandrosterone sulfate, testosterone (total and free), and androstenedione should be measured. For women with regular menstrual cycles, serum androgen measurements generally are not necessary.

TREATMENT

NONPHARMACOLOGIC THERAPY

Blue light (ClearLight therapy system) can be used for treatment of moderate inflammatory acne vulgaris. Light in the violet/blue range can cause bacterial death by a photoreaction in which porphyrins react with oxygen to generate reactive oxygen species, which damage the cell membranes of *P. acnes.* Treatment usually consists of 15-min exposures twice weekly for 4 wk.

ACUTE GENERAL Rx

Treatment generally varies with the type of lesions (comedones, papules, pustules, cystic lesions) and the severity of acne.

- Comedones (noninflammatory acne) can be treated with retinoids or retinoid analogs. Topical retinoids are comedolytic and work by normalizing follicular keratinization. Commonly available agents are Adapalene (Differin, 0.1% gel or cream, applied once or twice daily), tazarotene (Tazorac 0.1% cream or gel applied daily), tretinoin (Retin-A 0.1% cream or 0.025 gel applied once daily), tretinoin microsphere (Retin-A Micro, 0.1% gel, applied at bedtime). Tretinoin is inactivated by ultraviolet light and oxidized by benzoyl peroxide; therefore it should only be applied at night and not used concomitantly with benzoyl peroxide.
- Tretinoin is pregnancy category C and tazarotene is pregnancy category X. Salicylic acid preparations (e.g., Neutrogena 2% wash) have keratolytic and anti-inflammatory properties and are also useful in the treatment of comedones. Large, open comedones (blackheads) should be expressed.

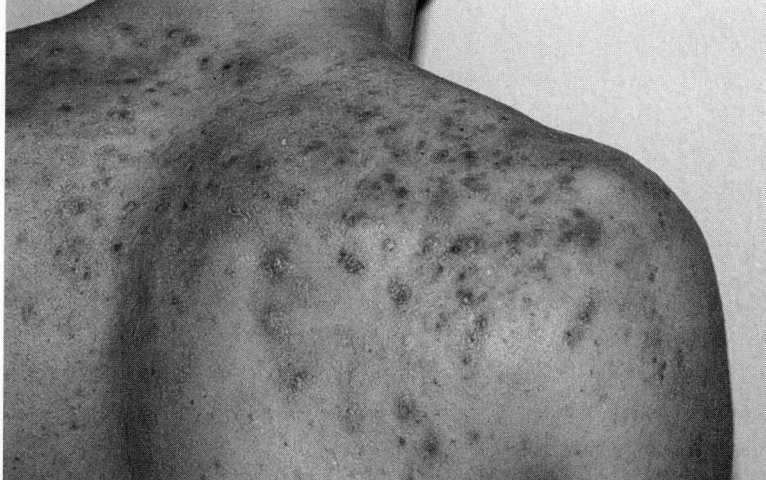

FIGURE 1-18 Acne on back and shoulders. This acne is typically inflammatory and usually needs oral antibiotics or possibly isotretinoin, but the patient may apply topical medication as well. Heat and sweat may aggravate the condition. (From White GM, Cox NH [eds]: *Diseases of the skin*, ed 2, St Louis, 2006, Mosby.)

- Patients should be reevaluated after 4 to 6 wk. Benzoyl peroxide gel (2.5% or 5%) may be added if the comedones become inflamed or form pustules. The most common adverse effects are dryness, erythema, and peeling. Topical antibiotics (erythromycin, clindamycin lotions or pads) can also be used in patients with significant inflammation. They reduce *P. acnes* in the pilosebaceous follicle and have some anti-inflammatory effects. The combination of 5% benzoyl peroxide and 3% erythromycin (Benzamycin) or 1% clindamycin with 5% benzoyl peroxide (BenzaClin) is highly effective in patients who have a mixture of comedonal and inflammatory acne lesions.
- Fixed-dose combinations of clindamycin phosphate 1.2% and tretinoin 0.025% are available (Veltin gel, Ziana) and are more effective than either product used alone; however, they are much more expensive than the individual generic components.
- Pustular acne can be treated with tretinoin and benzoyl peroxide gel applied on alternate evenings; drying agents (sulfacetamide-sulfa lotions [Novacet, Sulfacet]) are also effective when used in combination with benzoyl peroxide; oral antibiotics (doxycycline 100 mg qd or erythromycin 1 g qd given in 2 to 3 divided doses) are effective in patients with moderate to severe pustular acne. Patients not responding well to these antibiotics can be switched to minocycline 50 to 100 mg bid; however, this medication is more expensive.
- Patients with nodular cystic acne can be treated with systemic agents: antibiotics (erythromycin, tetracycline, doxycycline, minocycline), isotretinoin (available on restricted basis), or oral contraceptives. Periodic intralesional triamcinolone (Kenalog) injections by a dermatologist are also effective. The possibility of endocrinopathy should be considered in patients responding poorly to therapy.
- Isotretinoin is indicated for acne resistant to antibiotic therapy and severe acne. It is available only on a restricted basis. Dosage is 0.5 to 1 mg/kg/day in 2 divided doses (maximum of 2 mg/kg/day); duration of therapy is generally 20 wk for a cumulative dose ≥120 mg/kg for severe cystic acne. Before using this medication patients should undergo baseline laboratory evaluation (see "Laboratory Tests"). This drug is absolutely contraindicated during pregnancy because of its teratogenicity. It should be used with caution in patients with history of depression. Physicians, distributors, pharmacies, and patients must register in the iPLEDGE program (http://www.ipledgeprogram.com) before using isotretinoin.
- Azelaic acid is a bacteriostatic dicarboxylic acid used to normalize keratinization and reduce inflammation. It can be used in pregnant women.
- Oral contraceptives reduce androgen levels and therefore sebum production. They represent a useful adjunctive therapy for all types of acne in women and adolescent girls. Commonly used agents are norgestimate/ethinyl estradiol (Ortho Tri-Cyclen) and drosperinone/ethinyl estradiol (Yasmin).

REFERRAL

Referral for intralesional injection and dermabrasion should be considered in patients with severe acne unresponsive to conventional therapy.

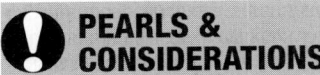

PEARLS & CONSIDERATIONS

- Gram-negative folliculitis should be suspected if inflammatory acne worsens after several months of oral antibiotic therapy.
- Acne may worsen during the first 3 to 4 wk of retinoid therapy before improving.

COMMENTS

Indications for systemic therapy of acne are:
- Painful deep papules or nodules
- Extensive lesions
- Active acne with severe scarring or hyperpigmentation
- Patient's morale

Patients should be educated that in most cases acne can be controlled but not cured and that at least 4 to 6 wk of initial therapy should be required before significant improvement is noted.

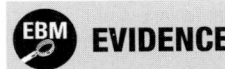 **EVIDENCE**

available at www.expertconsult.com

SUGGESTED READINGS

available at www.expertconsult.com

AUTHOR: **FRED F. FERRI, M.D.**

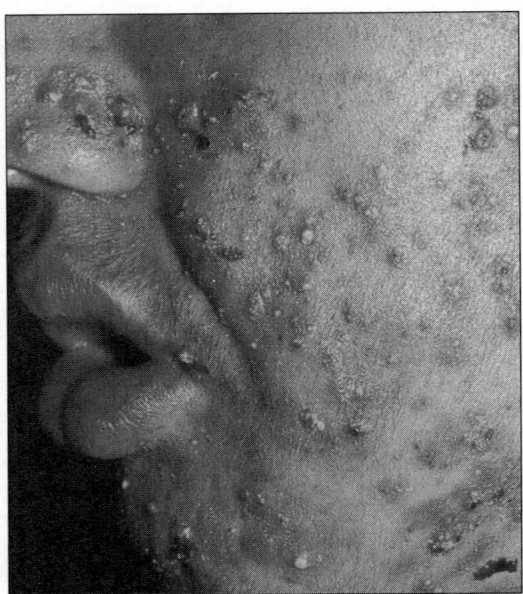

FIGURE 1-19 Severe acne. Acne this severe on presentation should prompt the consideration of early use of isotretinoin. The dose should be low initially to prevent a severe flare. An oral tetracycline or erythromycin may be helpful to calm the acne before isotretinoin. (From White GM, Cox NH [eds]: *Diseases of the skin*, ed 2, St Louis, 2006, Mosby.)

BASIC INFORMATION

DEFINITION

Acoustic neuroma is a benign proliferation of the Schwann cells that cover the vestibular branch of the eighth cranial nerve (CN VIII). Symptoms are commonly a result of compression of the acoustic branch of CN VIII, the facial nerve (CN VII), and the trigeminal nerve (CN V). The glosso-pharyngeal nerve (CN IX) and vagus nerve (CN X) are less commonly involved. In extreme cases compression of the brain stem may lead to ob-struction of cerebrospinal fluid (CSF) outflow and elevated intracranial pressure (ICP).

SYNONYMS

Vestibular schwannoma

ICD-9CM CODES
225.1 Acoustic neuroma

EPIDEMIOLOGY & DEMOGRAPHICS

Annual incidence is approximately one in 80,000 patients per year, with a higher incidence in patients with neurofibromatosis type 2 (NF2). There may be a slight female predominance. The tumor most commonly presents in the fifth and sixth decades.

PHYSICAL FINDINGS & CLINICAL PRESENTATION

- Most frequently unilateral hearing loss and/or tinnitus. Also balance problems, vertigo, fa-cial pain (trigeminal neuralgia) and weak-ness, difficulty swallowing, fullness or pain of the involved ear. Headache may occur.
- With elevated ICP, patients may also have vomiting, fever, and visual changes.
- Hearing loss is the most common presenting complaint and is usually high frequency.

ETIOLOGY

The etiology is incompletely understood, but long-term exposure to acoustic trauma has been impli-cated. Bilateral acoustic neuromas may be inher-ited in an autosomal-dominant manner as part of NF2. This disease is associated with a defect on chromosome 22q1. Childhood exposure to low-dose radiation for benign head and neck conditions may increase risk for acoustic neuromas. There is inconclusive evidence to link chronic exposure to radiofrequency radiation from cellular telephone use and the risk for developing brain tumors.

DIAGNOSIS

DIFFERENTIAL DIAGNOSIS

- Benign positional vertigo
- Ménière's disease
- Trigeminal neuralgia
- Cerebellar disease
- Normal-pressure hydrocephalus
- Presbycusis
- Glomus tumors
- Vertebrobasilar insufficiency
- Ototoxicity from medications
- Other tumors:
  - Meningioma, glioma
  - Facial nerve schwannoma
  - Cavernous hemangioma
  - Metastatic tumors

WORKUP

- A detailed neurologic examination with spe-cial attention to the cranial nerves is crucial.
- Otoscopic evaluation may help rule out other causes of hearing loss.

LABORATORY TESTS

- Audiometry is useful, often showing asymmet-ric, sensorineural, high-frequency hearing loss.
- CSF protein may be elevated.

IMAGING STUDIES

- MRI with gadolinium (Fig. 1-20) is the pre-ferred test. It can detect tumors as small as 2 mm in diameter.
- High-resolution CT scan with and without contrast can detect tumors 1 cm in diameter or larger.
- Treatment decisions should be based on the size of the tumor, rate of growth (older pa-tients tend to have slower growing tumors), degree of neurologic deficit, desire to pre-serve hearing, life expectancy, age of the patient, and surgical risk. A combination of treatments can also be used.

TREATMENT

NONPHARMACOLOGIC THERAPY

- Surgery is the definitive treatment. Choice of approach (middle cranial fossa, translabyrin-thine, or retromastoid suboccipital) may vary depending on the size of the tumor, amount of residual hearing desired, and degree of surgi-cal risk that can be tolerated. Partial resection is sometimes undertaken to minimize the risk of injury to nearby structures. Intraoperative facial nerve monitoring is recommended.

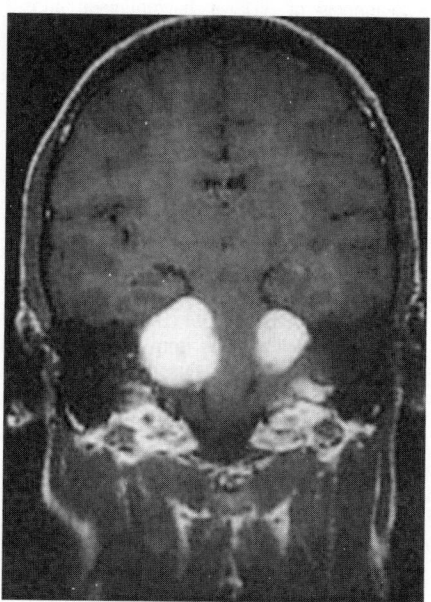

FIGURE 1-20 MR with enhancement shows bilat-eral acoustic neuromas. Coronal view. (From Kanski JJ, Bowling B: *Clinical ophthalmology, a systematic approach,* ed 7, Philadephia, 2011, Saunders.)

- Radiation therapy (stereotactic radiotherapy, stereotactic radiosurgery, or proton beam ra-diotherapy) is useful for tumors <3 cm in di-ameter or for those in whom surgery is not an option. Radiotherapy after partial resection has also been used to minimize complications.
- Age alone is not a contraindication to surgery.

ACUTE GENERAL Rx

Bevacizumab, an antivascular endothelial growth factor (VEGF) monoclonal antibody, has been shown to improve hearing and reduce the volume of growing acoustic neuromas in some neurofibromatosis type 2 patients.

CHRONIC Rx

Observation with MRI every 6 to 12 mo may be appropriate for frail patients with small tumors, but risk of unrecoverable hearing loss may in-crease if surgery is delayed.

DISPOSITION

Hearing can be preserved at near-preoperative levels in more than two thirds of patients with small- to medium-sized tumors. There are no standard posttreatment follow-up recommenda-tions. Therefore, an individualized approach to fol-low-up imaging and audiometry is recommended.

REFERRAL

Prompt referral to an ear-nose-throat specialist or neurosurgeon who is facile with all three surgical approaches is recommended.

PEARLS & CONSIDERATIONS

COMMENTS

- Presents most commonly as unilateral, sen-sorineural hearing loss.
- Treatment outcomes are generally good, with cure rates approaching 90% at 5 years.
- Of those who are managed with observation only, approximately half have continued en-largement and approximately one fifth even-tually have a surgical intervention.

PATIENT/FAMILY EDUCATION

Acoustic Neuroma Association: http://anausa.org.

SUGGESTED READINGS

available at www.expertconsult.com

RELATED CONTENT

Tinnitus (Related Key Topic)
Hearing Loss (Related Key Topic)
Box 3-2 Hearing Loss
Acoustic Neuroma (Patient Information)

AUTHORS: **SRIVIDYA ANANDAN, M.D.,** and **COURTNEY CLARK BILODEAU, M.D.**

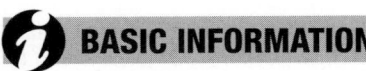

DEFINITION

Acquired immunodeficiency syndrome (AIDS) is a disorder caused by infection with the human immunodeficiency virus (HIV) and marked by progressive deterioration of the cellular immune system, leading to secondary (opportunistic) infections or malignancies.

SYNONYMS

AIDS

ICD-9CM CODES
042 AIDS, unspecified

EPIDEMIOLOGY & DEMOGRAPHICS

INCIDENCE (IN U.S.):
- In the year 2009 the estimated number of persons diagnosed with AIDS was 34,493.
- In the year 2008 the estimated number of deaths of persons with an AIDS diagnosis was 16,605.
- In 2009 about 48% of new AIDS cases were in black/African Americans, almost 20% in Hispanics, and about 27% in white Americans.
- Over 50% of the AIDS cases in 2009 were among gay, bisexual, or other men who have sex with men (MSM).

PREVALENCE (IN U.S.):
- At the end of 2008 the estimated number of persons living with an AIDS diagnosis was 490,696.
- The cumulative number of AIDS diagnoses through 2009 in the U.S. was 1,142,714.

PREDOMINANT SEX: 53% of infections occur in men who have sex with men (MSM).

PREDOMINANT AGE: 80% between ages 20 and 49 yr. In 2009 there were only 13 cases of AIDS under the age of 13 and 846 cases of AIDS over the age of 65.

PEAK INCIDENCE: Ages 20-49

GENETICS:
- Familial disposition: Although there is no proven genetic predisposition, individuals with deletions in the *CCR5* gene are immune from infection with macrophage tropic virus (the predominant virus in sexual transmission).
- Congenital infection:
  1. Transmittable from an infected mother to the fetus in utero in as many as 30% of pregnancies.
  2. No specific congenital malformations associated with infection; low birth weight and spontaneous abortion are possible.
- Neonatal infection: transmission possible to the neonate intrapartum or postpartum through breastfeeding.

PHYSICAL FINDINGS & CLINICAL PRESENTATION

- Nonspecific findings: fever, weight loss, anorexia
- Specific syndromes:

1. Seen in association with opportunistic infection and malignancies, so-called indicator diseases; these include:
   a. Opportunistic infections:
      Disseminated strongyloidiasis
      Disseminated toxoplasmosis, cryptococcosis, histoplasmosis, cytomegalovirus (CMV), herpes simplex, or mycobacterial disease
      Candida esophagitis or bronchopulmonary disease
      Chronic *Cryptosporidia* spp. diarrhea
      Pneumocystis jiroveci pneumonia (PJP)
      Extensive pulmonary and extrapulmonary tuberculosis
      Recurrent bacterial pneumonia
      Progressive multifocal leukoencephalopathy (PML)
   b. AIDS-related neoplasms:
      Kaposi's sarcoma in a person <60 yr of age
      Primary brain lymphoma
      Invasive cervical carcinoma
      High-grade B-cell non-Hodgkin's lymphoma, Burkitt's lymphoma, undifferentiated non-Hodgkin's lymphoma, or immunoblastic lymphoma
2. Most common:
   Respiratory infections (*Pneumocystis jiroveci* [formerly known as *Pneumocystis carinii*] pneumonia, TB, bacterial pneumonia, fungal infection)
   CNS infections (toxoplasmosis, cryptococcal meningitis, TB)
   GI (cryptosporidiosis, isosporiasis, CMV); Sections II and III describe organisms associated with diarrhea in patients with AIDS
   Eye infections (CMV, toxoplasmosis)
   Kaposi's sarcoma (cutaneous or visceral) or lymphoma (nodal or extranodal)
- Possibly asymptomatic
- Diagnosis of AIDS if T-lymphocyte subset analysis demonstrating CD4 cell count <200 or <14% of total lymphocyte in the presence of proven HIV infection even in the absence of other infections
- The various manifestations of HIV infection are described in Section II.

ETIOLOGY

- Caused by infection with HIV-1 or HIV-2
- Transmitted by heterosexual or male homosexual contact, needle-sharing (during IV drug use), transfusion of contaminated blood or blood products, and from infected mother to fetus or neonate as described previously

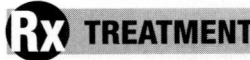

DIFFERENTIAL DIAGNOSIS

- Other wasting illnesses mimicking the nonspecific features of AIDS:
  1. TB
  2. Neoplasms
  3. Disseminated fungal infection
  4. Malabsorption syndromes
  5. Depression

- Other disorders associated with dementia or demyelination producing encephalopathy, myelopathy, or neuropathy

WORKUP

Prompt evaluation of respiratory, CNS, and GI complaints

LABORATORY TESTS

- HIV antibody testing
- T-lymphocyte subset analysis: performed to determine the degree of immunodeficiency
- Viral load assay: to plan long-term antiviral therapy and to follow progression and success of treatment
- CSF examination: for meningitis
- Serologic tests for syphilis, hepatitis B, hepatitis C, and toxoplasmosis
- Genotypic and phenotypic resistance testing: used to assess for primary resistance in naïve patients and secondary resistance in patients failing a regimen
- Eye exam: to evaluate for CMV retinitis in patients with CD4 counts <50 cells/mm^3
- Cryptococcal antigen: part of the evaluation in AIDS patients with CD4 counts <100 cells/mm^3 who have fever, diffuse pneumonia, or symptoms of meningitis
- Evaluation for infection with mycobacterium (TB or MAI) including PPD, sputum cultures, chest radiograph, and blood cultures for acid-fast bacteria, depending on clinical presentation

IMAGING STUDIES

- Cerebral CT for encephalopathy or focal CNS complications (e.g., toxoplasmosis, lymphoma)
- Pulmonary gallium scanning to aid in the diagnosis of *Pneumocystis jiroveci* (*P. carinii*) pneumonia
- Baseline chest radiograph

TREATMENT

NONPHARMACOLOGIC THERAPY

- Maintain adequate caloric intake.
- Encourage good oral hygiene, regular dental care.
- Avoid high-risk behaviors that increase the risk of repeated exposure to HIV and other potential pathogens—safer sexual practices, avoid sharing needles, etc.
- Update vaccines—particularly the pneumococcal and hepatitis B vaccine along with annual influenza vaccines.
- Avoid administration of any live attenuated vaccines that may be a risk to these immunocompromised patients (i.e., MMR, varicella).
- When feasible, avoid activities that might increase risk of exposure to opportunistic infections (i.e., cleaning out a cat litter box [toxoplasmosis], getting scratched by a cat [*Bartonella* infections], exposure to pet reptiles [salmonellosis], traveling to developing countries [cryptosporidiosis, tuberculosis], eating undercooked foods and drinking from unsafe water supplies, etc.).

ACUTE GENERAL Rx

Acute management of opportunistic infections and malignancies is reviewed elsewhere in this text under specific AIDS-related disorders.

CHRONIC Rx

For all HIV-infected patients, particularly those meeting the case definition of AIDS:

- Preventive therapy for *Pneumocystis jiroveci* pneumonia and TB (see specific chapters elsewhere in this text). With the advent of modern antiretroviral therapy many patients have experienced substantial restoration of cellular immune function. It has become clear that preventive therapy for *Pneumocystis jiroveci* and *Mycobacterium avium* complex as well as suppressive therapy for CMV and cryptococcal infection can often be safely withdrawn if the CD4 cell count rises above 200 for at least 6 mo.
- Based on the Department of Health and Human Services (DHHS) Guidelines of 2012, highly active antiretroviral therapy (HAART) should be started regardless of CD4 cell count. Individuals with CD4 cell counts <350 and especially CD4 cell counts <200 should be strongly encouraged to start HAART in a timely fashion.
- HAART usually includes three-drug combinations of:
  1. Nucleoside reverse transcriptase inhibitors (NRTI): tenofovir (TDF), zidovudine (AZT), didanosine (DDI), zalcitabine (DDC), lamivudine (3TC), emtricitabine (FTC), stavudine (D4T), and abacavir (ABC)
  2. Protease inhibitors (PI): saquinavir, amprenavir, indinavir, nelfinavir, agenerase, lopinavir/ritonavir, atazanavir, and darunavir
  3. Nonnucleoside reverse transcriptase inhibitors (NNRTI): nevirapine, delavirdine, efavirenz (EFV), etravirine, and rilpivirine
  4. Integrase inhibitors: raltegravir, elvitegravir, and dolutegravir
  5. Others: maraviroc and enfuvirtide

The protease inhibitor ritonavir should be used in low dose (100 mg) in combination with other protease inhibitors to obtain more sustained drug levels. Usual initial dosing regimens include two NRTIs and an NNRTI (or a PI or raltegravir). Examples of initial regimens recommended by the guidelines:

1. Atripla (EFV/TDF/FTC) in a single combination pill taken once a day
2. Truvada (TDF/FTC) plus either atazanavir (with ritonavir), darunavir (with ritonavir), or raltegravir
3. Truvada (TDF/FTC) may be substituted with either epzicom (ABC/3TC) or combivir (AZT/3TC). Before using ABC, individuals should be tested for the presence of HLA-B*5701 to check for hypersensitivity to this drug.

All these drugs have unique and class-specific side effects and require careful and expert follow-up to achieve optimal antiviral effects, ensure compliance, and maintain efficacy. Antiviral response should be monitored by baseline HIV viral load and CD4 count and repeat measurement at 2 weeks and 4 weeks into treatment and then periodically (every 3 months) to ensure viral suppression.

- An approach to evaluating chronic diarrhea in patients with HIV infection is described in Fig. E1-21, the approach to the acutely ill HIV-infected patient is outlined in Fig. E1-22, and the evaluation of HIV-positive patients with respiratory complaints is described in Figs. E1-23 and E1-24. The approach to a patient with a suspected CNS lesion is described in Figs. E1-25 and E1-26. Fig. E1-27 presents an approach to cardiac dysfunction.
- Genotypic resistance testing is strongly encouraged for all patients initiating treatment and for any patient failing antiretroviral therapy. Poor adherence to therapy, however, often underlies virologic failure.

DISPOSITION

The outlook for AIDS has changed radically since the advent of HAART therapy from an essentially fatal disease to a chronic medical illness compatible with long-term survival and remarkably good quality of life. Patients should be aggressively treated for severe illnesses as outcomes following ICU admissions remain good. This is accomplished through expert and continuous follow-up, use of HAART, and careful detail to compliance to medications and lifestyle modification.

REFERRAL

All patients with AIDS: to a physician knowledgeable and experienced in the management of the disease and its complications

SUGGESTED READINGS

available at www.expertconsult.com

RELATED CONTENT

Acquired Immunodeficiency Syndrome (AIDS) (Patient Information)

AUTHORS: **PHILIP A. CHAN, M.D., M.S.,** and **GLENN G. FORT, M.D., M.P.H.**

A

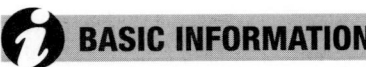

BASIC INFORMATION

DEFINITION

Actinic keratoses (AKs) are common skin lesions usually presenting as multiple, erythematous or yellow-brown, dry, scaly lesions in the middle aged or elderly.

SYNONYMS

Solar keratosis
Senile keratosis
AK

ICD-9CM CODES
702.0 Actinic keratosis

EPIDEMIOLOGY & DEMOGRAPHICS

INCIDENCE: In regions of the northern hemisphere, 11%-25% of adults have a minimum of one AK. In regions closer to the equator, 40%-60% of adults have a minimum of one AK.

PEAK INCIDENCE: The risk of squamous cell carcinoma in patients with AK is 6%-10%. Incidence increases with age, and mortality from non-melanoma skin cancers increases significantly in the sixth decade. The rate of mortality is approximately 0.1% of the incidence rate (Table 1-10).

PREVALENCE:
- In the United States, 58.08 million per year.
- Highest prevalence in those with fair complexions in well-sunlit environments.

- Approximately 60% of predisposed individuals older than 40 years will have one.
- Caucasians' risk increases with age: at age 20-29 prevalence is < 10%; at age 80-89, prevalence is approximately 75%.

PREDOMINANT SEX AND AGE: Males > females, age 65-74. Occurs most in those with fair complexions who burn rather than tan following sun exposure.

GENETICS: There is increased frequency of non-melanoma skin cancers connected to squamous cell cancers with the genetic conditions xeroderma pigmentosum, oculocutaneous albinism, epidermodysplasia verruciformis, dystrophic epidermolysis bullosa, Ferguson-Smith syndrome, and Muir-Torre syndrome.

RISK FACTORS:
- Immunosuppression, exposure to ultraviolet (UV) light, ionizing radiation, arsenic, human papillomavirus, cigarette smoke, chronic ulcers, thermal burns, chronic discoid lupus erythematosus, and nonhealing wounds.
- Lichen planus, lichen sclerosis, linear and classic porokeratosis, and disseminated superficial actinic porokeratosis.
- Age, gender, skin color, mutations in p53 tumor suppressor gene.

PHYSICAL FINDINGS & CLINICAL PRESENTATION

- Typical lesions occur on sun-damaged skin, usually on the face and neck and the dorsal aspects of hands (Fig. 1-29) and forearms.

- Advanced lesions are characterized by a hard, spiky scale (Fig. 1-30) and usually measure 1 cm in diameter or less. Early lesions manifest with redness and minimal scale. With progression, scales become thicker and yellow and may resemble a small squamous cell carcinoma. On examinations, lesions are rough and gritty (Fig. 1-31).
- The surrounding skin frequently shows additional features of sun damage, including atrophy (Fig. 1-32), pigment changes, and telangiectasia.
- Classifications
  - Hypertrophic AK with a cutaneous horn: Biopsy is necessary to distinguish the cutaneous horn from squamous cell carcinoma, seborrheic keratosis, verruca, and trichilemmoma and basal cell carcinoma. Hypertrophic AK has appearance of thick, scaling skin elevations.
  - Lichenoid AK: Most commonly found on the torso and upper extremities. Must be distinguished from BCC due to pink and pearly characteristics.
  - Proliferative AK: Often reappear after treatment and are characterized by a diameter greater than 1 cm. Often occurs in same differential as Bowen's disease or SCC.
  - Spreading pigmented AK: Must be biopsied to distinguish from lentigo maligna–type melanoma in situ as well as solar lentigo.
  - Actinic cheilitis: Characterized by red and sometimes abrasive lesions around the border of the lips and skin.

ETIOLOGY
- Sun exposure, ionizing radiation.
- Arsenic, polycyclic hydrocarbon exposure.

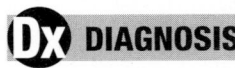

DIAGNOSIS

DIFFERENTIAL DIAGNOSIS
- Heavily pigmented variants may be clinically mistaken for lentigo maligna.
- Basal cell or squamous cell carcinoma.
- Seborrheic keratosis.
- Eczema.
- Bowen disease (intraepithelial carcinoma).
- Wart.
- Lichenoid keratosis.
- Cutaneous lupus.

TABLE 1-10 Incidence Rates Per Year (Per 100,000) of BCC and SCC by Geographic Location

Geographic Location	BCC (Men/Women)	SCC (Men/Women)
Finland	49/45	9/5
Switzerland	52/38	16/8
The Netherlands	53/38	—
United Kingdom	112/54	32/6
New Hampshire	159/87	32/8
Rochester, Minnesota	175/124	63/23
United States	247/150	65/24
Hawaii	576/298	153/92
Nambour, Australia	2074/1579	1035/472

BCC, Basal cell carcinoma; SCC, squamous cell carcinoma.
From Bolognia JL et al (eds): *Dermatology*, ed 2, vol 2, St Louis, 2003, Mosby, p. 1678.

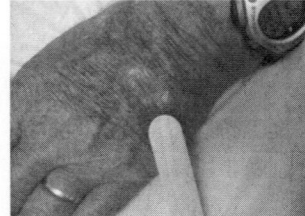

FIGURE 1-29 Several scaly, adherent, yellow-brown lesions on the sun-exposed dorsum of the hand. (From Ferri F et al: *Ferri's fast facts in dermatology*, Philadelphia, 2010, Saunders.)

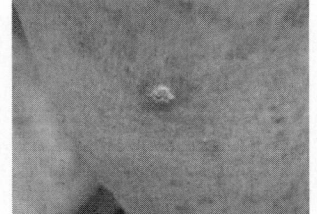

FIGURE 1-30 Scaly, raised lesion on sun-exposed back. Pain was elicited when scraping this lesion. (From Ferri F et al: *Ferri's fast facts in dermatology*, Philadelphia, 2010, Saunders.)

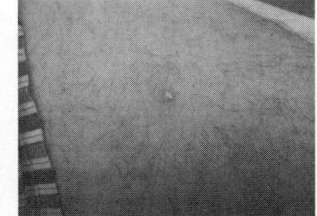

FIGURE 1-31 Raised, rough, gritty actinic keratosis on the anterior thigh of an outdoorsman. (From Ferri F et al: *Ferri's fast facts in dermatology*, Philadelphia, 2010, Saunders.)

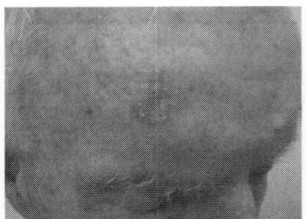

FIGURE 1-32 Actinic keratosis (shown here on a patient's forehead) is often best appreciated by its rough, tactile quality, similar to that of sandpaper. (From Ferri F et al: *Ferri's fast facts in dermatology*, Philadelphia, 2010, Saunders.)

WORKUP

- History, physical, and lesion biopsy. Include risk assessment and family or personal history of skin cancers or previous skin lesions.

LABORATORY TESTS

- Skin biopsy in recurrent lesions or when diagnosis is unclear to rule out squamous cell or basal cell carcinoma.
- Microscopy reveals atypical keratinocytes in the lower epidermis basal layers. They are enlarged and often lack normal polarity. The thickness of the epidermis can be compromised with a distribution of atrophic to hyperplastic. Abnormal keratinocytes can cause parakeratosis of the overlying stratum corneum. Visible signs of an alternating orthohyperkeratosis can overlies the spared epithelium, causing the signature "flag sign." Additionally, there is a distinct margin between normal epidermis and the region of AK at lateral edges. Histologic subtypes are hypertrophic, acantholytic, lichenoid, and bowenoid, which are characterized by a thick stratum corneum, lack of intracellular cohesion, presence of lymphocytic infiltrate in papillary dermis, and either lack of association of adnexal epithelium or full epithelial thickness with pleomorphic kertinocytes, respectively.

 TREATMENT

NONPHARMACOLOGIC THERAPY

- Cryosurgery with liquid nitrogen.
- Carbon dioxide laser.
- Dermabrasion.
- Chemical peel.
- Curettage.
- Excision.
- Photodynamic therapy with aminolevulinic acid and blue light.

ACUTE GENERAL Rx

- Topical 5-fluorouracil bid for 4 weeks.
- Topical diclofenac 3% gel bid for 60-90 days.
- Imiquimod 5% cream bid for 3-4 months.
- Oral retinoids.
- Ingenol mebutate was recently FDA approved for topical treatment of AK. It induces lesion necrosis and activates neutrophils that target residual dysplastic cells. Is available as a gel 0.05%, applied for 2 days with exception of face—or 0.015% for 3 days.

REFERRAL

- To a dermatologist for biopsy of suspicious lesions.

PEARLS & CONSIDERATIONS

COMMENTS

- AKs are of particular importance because they are a sensitive indicator of exposure to UV light and strongly predict the likelihood of developing cutaneous squamous cell carcinoma.
- The cumulative probability of development of invasive squamous cell carcinoma in patients with 10 or more AKs has been estimated at 14% in a 5-year period.
- It is estimated that up to 10% of AKs tend to progress to invasive carcinoma.

PREVENTION

- Avoidance of sun exposure or sunless tanning booths, use of sunscreens.
- Routine self-skin examinations.
- Pharmaceutical prevention:
  - Mild to moderate reduction of AK formation has been documented with the use of topical tretinoin, isotretinoin, and arotinoid methysulfone.
  - Decreased AK development has been documented with the use of high SPF sunscreens.
  - Decreased AK development has been seen in patients with xeroderma pigmentosum who used DNA repair enzymes.
  - Decreased AK formation has been documented in high-risk patients (specifically those with xeroderma pigmentosum, nevoid basal cell carcinoma syndrome, and organ transplantation recipients) with the use of oral retinoids.

SUGGESTED READINGS

available at www.expertconsult.com

AUTHORS: **FRED F. FERRI, M.D.,** and **HEATHER SUNTER, M.S.**

A

Diseases and Disorders

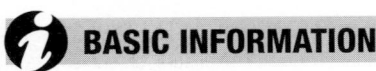

BASIC INFORMATION

DEFINITION

Actinomycosis is an indolent, slowly progressive infection caused by anaerobic or microaerophilic bacteria, mostly from the genus *Actinomyces*, that normally colonize the mouth, vagina, and colon. Actinomycosis is characterized by the formation of painful abscesses, soft tissue infiltration, and draining sinuses.

SYNONYMS

Actinomyces infection
Lumpy jaw

ICD-9CM CODES
039.9 Actinomycosis

EPIDEMIOLOGY & DEMOGRAPHICS

Geographic distribution:
- Actinomycosis is worldwide in distribution.
- Commonly found as normal flora of the oral cavity (within gingival crevices, tonsillar crypts, periodontal pockets, dental plaques, and carious teeth), pharynx, tracheobronchial tree, gastrointestinal tract, and female urogenital tract.

Incidence and prevalence:
- Incidence 1:300,000 in 1970s but now less with better oral hygiene and antibiotic use.
- Males infected more often than females 3:1.
- Can occur at any age but commonly seen in midlife.

PHYSICAL FINDINGS & CLINICAL PRESENTATION

Actinomycosis can affect any organ. Although not typically considered as opportunistic pathogens, *Actinomyces* species capitalize on tissue injury or mucosal breach to invade adjacent structures in the head and neck regions. As a result, dental infections and oromaxillofacial trauma are common antecedent events. Characteristic manifestations include:
- Cervicofacial disease (most common site):
  1. Occurs in the setting of poor dental hygiene, recent dental surgery, or minor oral trauma
  2. Painful soft tissue swelling (Fig. 1-33) commonly seen at the angle of the mandible
  3. Fever, chills, and weight loss
  4. Trismus
  5. Soft tissue facial infection with sinus tract or fistula formation
- Thoracic disease:
  1. Can involve the lungs, pleura, mediastinum, or chest wall.
  2. Presumed secondary to aspiration of *Actinomyces* organisms in patients with poor oral hygiene.
  3. Fever, cough, weight loss, and pleuritic chest pains are common symptoms.
  4. Signs of pneumonia or pleural effusion may be present.
  5. With extension beyond the lungs to mediastinal structures and the chest wall, signs and symptoms of pericarditis, empyema, chest wall sinus drainage, and tracheoesophageal fistula can all occur (Fig. 1-34).
- Abdominal disease:
  1. Occurs most commonly after appendectomy, perforated bowel, diverticulitis, or surgery to the gastrointestinal tract.

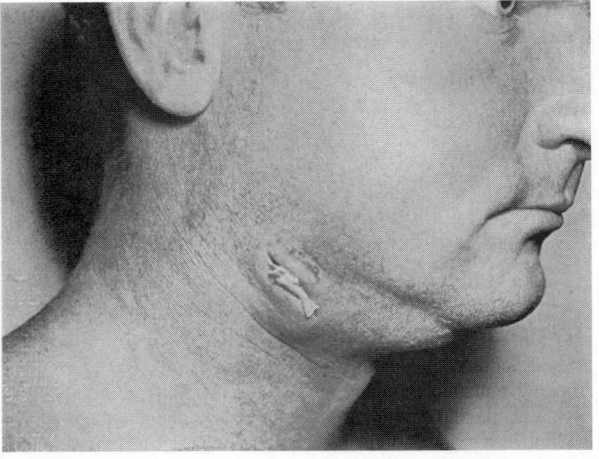

FIGURE 1-33 **Actinomycosis of the jaw, observed at Letterman General Hospital, San Francisco, Calif., in a sergeant who had punctured the floor of his mouth while picking his teeth.** (Office of Medical History, Office of the Surgeon General, U.S. Army; from Goldman L, Schaefer AI: *Goldman's Cecil medicine,* ed 24, Philadelphia, 2012, Saunders.)

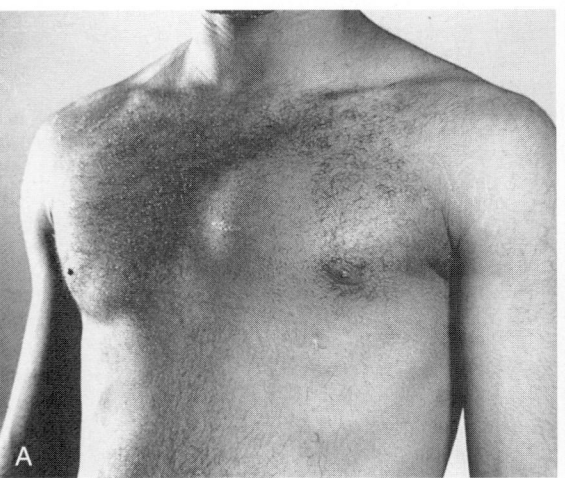 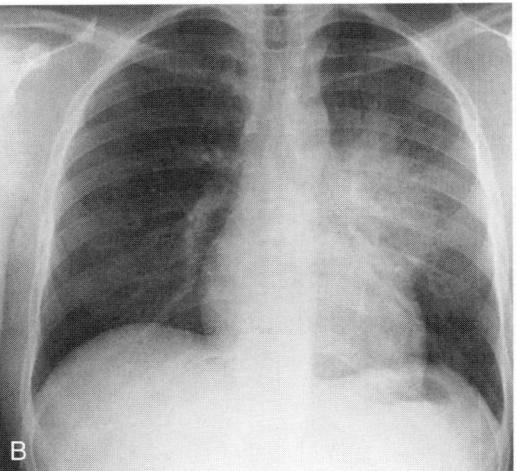

FIGURE 1-34 **Thoracic actinomycosis. A,** Initial presentation with a bulging mass lesion in the chest wall with a central sinus tract. **B,** The chest radiograph with the associated pulmonary infiltrate. (From Gorbach SL: *Infectious diseases,* ed 2, Philadelphia, 1998, Saunders.)

2. Lesions develop most commonly in the ileocecal valve, causing abdominal pain, fever, weight loss, and a palpable mass.
3. Extension may occur to the liver, causing jaundice and abscess formation.
4. Sinus tracts to the abdominal wall can occur.

- Pelvic disease:
  1. Commonly occurs by extension from abdominal disease of the ileocecal valve to the right adnexa (80% of cases).
  2. Endometritis.

ETIOLOGY

- Actinomycosis is most commonly caused by *Actinomyces israelii*. Other causes are *A. naeslundii, A. odontolyticus, A. viscosus,* and *A. meyeri.*
- *Actinomyces* are gram-positive, non–spore-forming, filamentous, anaerobic or micro-aerophilic rods.
- Actinomycosis infections are polymicrobial, usually associated with *Streptococcus, Bacteroides, Eikenella corrodens, Enterococcus,* and *Fusobacterium* spp.
- Infects individuals only after entry into disrupted mucosa or tissue injury.
- Predisposing conditions include diabetes mellitus, malnutrition, and immunosuppression.

DIAGNOSIS

Isolating the bacteria in the proper clinical setting makes the diagnosis of actinomycosis.

DIFFERENTIAL DIAGNOSIS

- Cervicofacial disease: odontogenic abscesses, brachial cleft cyst
- Pulmonary disease: nocardiosis, botryomycosis, chromomycosis, fungal disease of the lung, tuberculosis
- Intestinal disease: intestinal tuberculosis, ameboma, Crohn's disease, colon cancer
- Pelvic disease: chronic pelvic inflammatory disease, Crohn's disease
- CNS disease: other forms of brain abscess, brain tumors, toxoplasmosis, intracranial hematoma

WORKUP

The workup includes obtaining specimens either by aspirating abscesses, excising sinus tracts, or tissue biopsies. All specimens should be set up to culture anaerobic bacteria and held at least 5 to 7 days.

LABORATORY TESTS

- Isolating "sulfur granules" from tissue specimens or draining sinuses confirms the diagnosis of actinomycosis. *Actinomyces* are noted for forming characteristic sulfur granules in infected tissue but not in vitro. The term *sulfur granule* is a misnomer, reflecting only the yellow color of the granule in pus, because the granules are not composed of any sulfur at all.
  1. Sulfur granules are nests of *Actinomyces* species. Sulfur granules may be macroscopic or microscopic.
  2. Sulfur granules are crushed and stained for identification of *Actinomyces* organisms and may take up to 3 wk to grow in culture media.

IMAGING STUDIES

Imaging studies are useful adjunctive tests in localizing the site and spread of infection.
1. Chest x-ray examination
2. CT scan of the head, chest, abdomen, and pelvic areas is useful

TREATMENT

NONPHARMACOLOGIC THERAPY
- Incision and drainage of abscesses
- Excision of sinus tract

ACUTE GENERAL Rx
- Ampicillin 50 mg/kg/day in 3-4 divided doses x 4-6 wk, then Pen VK 2-4 g/day PO x 4-6 wk. In place of ampicillin, can also use penicillin 3-4 million units IV q4h for 4-6 wk.
- In penicillin-allergic patients, erythromycin (500-1000 mg IV q6h), tetracycline or doxycycline (100 mg IV q12h), and clindamycin (900 mg IV q8h) are reasonable alternatives. Other alternatives include cetriaxone, imipenem, and piperacillin/tazobactam.
- Avoid use of metronidazole, aminoglycosides, oxacillin, and cephalexin.

CHRONIC Rx
- Following 4 to 6 wk IV amoxicillin or penicillin, oral penicillin V 500 mg PO qid for 4 to 6 wk. Longer treatment may be necessary in selected cases.
- Other available oral agents are erythromycin, doxycycline, and clindamycin.
- Treatment of associated microorganisms is not needed.

DISPOSITION
- Clinical actinomycosis, if not treated, spreads to contiguous tissues and structures ignoring tissue planes. Hematogenous spread, although possible, is rare.
- Actinomycosis is very sensitive to antibiotics but requires chronic long-term treatment to prevent relapse.

REFERRAL
If the diagnosis of actinomycosis is suspected, consultation with an infectious disease specialist is suggested. General surgical consultation for excision of sinus tracts and abscess incision and drainage is recommended.

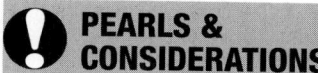

PEARLS & CONSIDERATIONS

COMMENTS
- There is no person-to-person transmission of *Actinomyces.*
- Isolation of the organism in an asymptomatic individual does not mean the person has actinomycosis. Active symptoms must be present to make the diagnosis.
- Pelvic actinomycosis has been associated with use of an intrauterine device (IUD).
- Actinomycosis can also involve the CNS, causing multiple brain abscesses.

SUGGESTED READINGS
available at www.expertconsult.com

AUTHOR: **GLENN G. FORT, M.D., M.P.H.**

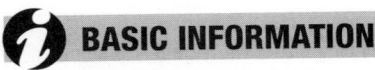

BASIC INFORMATION

DEFINITION

Acute bronchitis is a self-limited inflammation of trachea and bronchi.

SYNONYMS Chest cold

ICD-9CM CODES
466.0 Acute bronchitis

EPIDEMIOLOGY & DEMOGRAPHICS

- Highest incidence in smokers, older adults, and young children and during winter months.
- In the U.S. there are nearly 30 million ambulatory visits annually for cough, leading to more than 12 million diagnoses of "bronchitis."
- Acute lower respiratory tract infection is the most common condition treated in primary care.

PHYSICAL FINDINGS & CLINICAL PRESENTATION

- Cough, usually worse in the morning, often productive; mainly caused by transient bronchial hyperresponsiveness
- Low-grade fever
- Substernal discomfort worsened by coughing
- Postnasal drip, pharyngeal injection
- Rhonchi that may clear after cough, occasional wheezing

ETIOLOGY

- Viral infections are the leading cause of bronchitis (rhinovirus, influenza virus, adenovirus, respiratory syncytial virus)
- Atypical organisms (Mycoplasma, Chlamydia pneumoniae)
- Bacterial infections (Bordetella pertussis, Haemophilus influenzae, Moraxella, Streptococcus pneumoniae)

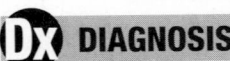 DIAGNOSIS

DIFFERENTIAL DIAGNOSIS

- Pneumonia
- Asthma
- Sinusitis
- Bronchiolitis
- Aspiration
- Cystic fibrosis
- Pharyngitis
- Cough secondary to medications
- Neoplasm (elderly patients)
- Influenza
- Allergic aspergillosis
- Gastroesophageal reflux disease
- Congestive heart failure (in elderly patients)
- Bronchogenic neoplasm

WORKUP

Seldom necessary (e.g., to rule out pneumonia, neoplasm)

LABORATORY TESTS

Laboratory tests are generally not necessary.

IMAGING STUDIES

Chest x-ray examination is usually reserved for patients with suspected pneumonia, influenza, or underlying chronic obstructive pulmonary disease (COPD) and no improvement with therapy.

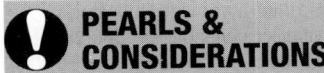 TREATMENT

NONPHARMACOLOGIC THERAPY

- Avoidance of tobacco and other pulmonary irritants
- Increased fluid intake
- Use of vaporizer to increase room humidity

ACUTE GENERAL Rx

- Inhaled bronchodilators (e.g., albuterol, metaproterenol) prn for 1 to 2 wk in patients with wheezing or troublesome cough. Inhaled albuterol has been proven effective in reducing the duration of cough in adults with uncomplicated acute bronchitis.
- Cough suppression with dextromethorphan and guaifenesin is commonly recommended; addition of codeine for cough suppression if cough is severe and is significantly interrupting patient's sleep pattern.
- Use of antibiotics (TMP-SMX, amoxicillin, doxycycline, cefuroxime) for acute bronchitis is generally not indicated; should be considered only in patients with concomitant COPD and purulent sputum or in patients with suspected pertussis. In the few cases of acute bronchitis caused by B. pertussis or atypical bacteria such as C. pneumoniae or Mycoplasma pneumoniae, early use of macrolide antibiotics is reasonable.

- Antibiotics are overused in patients with acute bronchitis (70% to 90% of office visits for acute bronchitis result in treatment with antibiotics); this practice pattern is contributing to increases in resistant organisms.

CHRONIC Rx

Avoidance of tobacco and other pulmonary irritants

DISPOSITION

- Complete recovery within 7 to 10 days in most patients.
- Patients should be informed to expect to have a cough for 10 to 14 days after the visit.

REFERRAL

For pulmonary function testing only in patients with recurrent bronchitis and suspected underlying asthma

PEARLS & CONSIDERATIONS

COMMENTS

- Intervention studies reveal that patient and physician education are effective in reducing the use of antibiotic therapy. No offer or delayed offer of antibiotics for acute uncomplicated lower respiratory tract infection is acceptable, is associated with little difference in symptom resolution, and is likely to reduce antibiotic use and beliefs in the effectiveness of antibiotics.
- It is helpful to refer to acute bronchitis as a "chest cold." Patients should be informed that antibiotics are probably not going to be beneficial and may result in significant side effects.

SUGGESTED READINGS

available at www.expertconsult.com

RELATED CONTENT

Acute Bronchitis (Patient Information)

AUTHOR: **FRED F. FERRI, M.D., F.A.C.P.**

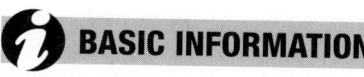

BASIC INFORMATION

DEFINITION

Acute coronary syndrome (ACS) represents a spectrum of clinical disorders that include unstable angina (UA), non–ST-elevation myocardial infarction (NSTEMI), and ST-elevation myocardial infarction (STEMI). Although the severity of disease will vary between the three subsets of ACS, they share a common clinical presentation and pathophysiology. This syndrome is typically caused by atherosclerotic coronary artery disease (CAD). In this spectrum, UA and NSTEMI are represented electrocardiographically by ST-segment depression and T-wave inversion in the appropriate clinical setting (i.e., chest discomfort). NSTEMI would have the addition of positive cardiac biomarkers. STEMI is represented by ST-segment elevation or presumed new left bundle branch block on electrocardiogram (ECG). ACS should be thought of as a continuous spectrum as UA will often progress to a myocardial infarction if left untreated (Table 1-11).

SYNONYMS

Unstable angina
NSTEMI
STEMI
Acute myocardial infarction

ICD-9CM CODES
410.0 Acute myocardial infarction
411.1 Intermediate coronary syndrome

EPIDEMIOLOGY & DEMOGRAPHICS

INCIDENCE: In the United States there are 1.56 million hospitalizations for ACS yearly; 0.89 million are listed as myocardial infarction, and the remainder are UA. Approximately two thirds of myocardial infarctions are listed as NSTEMI, with the remainder being listed as STEMI. The underlying etiology, atherosclerotic CAD, is the number one cause of mortality.

PREDOMINANT SEX AND AGE: In evaluating chest pain, male gender and older age are important clinical factors that can identify ACS as a potential cause. The 2007 overall death rate from cardiovascular disease was 126 per 100,000. The rates were 165.6 per 100,000 for white males, 191.6 per 100,000 for African-American males, 94.2 per 100,000 for white females, and 121.5 per 100,000 for African-American females.

RISK FACTORS: Hypertension, diabetes mellitus, dyslipidemia, tobacco use, family history of premature CAD (CAD in a male first-degree relative younger than 55 years or a female younger than 65 years). Presence of these risk factors causes damage to the vascular endothelium and progression of atherosclerotic coronary artery plaques.

PHYSICAL FINDINGS & CLINICAL PRESENTATION

- Symptoms often, but not always, include chest discomfort described as a pressure that may radiate to the left arm, neck, jaw, or back. Typical angina is substernal in location, brought on by emotional or physical stress, and relieved with rest and/or nitroglycerin.
- Women, diabetics, and the elderly often have an atypical presentation for ACS.
- Angina is considered unstable if it is new onset (<2 months), increasing in frequency (crescendo pattern), or occurring at rest (typically lasting >20 minutes).
- "Anginal equivalents" may include dyspnea, nausea, vomiting, and fatigue.
- ECG for UA and NSTEMI may reveal ST-segment depression and/or T-wave inversion. ECG for definition of STEMI will reveal at least 1-mm ST-segment elevation in two contiguous leads or new left bundle branch block in the appropriate clinical setting.
- Physical exam findings alone are insufficient for the diagnosis of ACS. It is, however, important to assess the patient's hemodynamic stability and volume status. The patient may be diaphoretic and tachycardic. Signs of heart failure may be present, which include elevated jugular venous pressure (JVP), presence of an S3 gallop, and peripheral edema.

ETIOLOGY

Atherosclerotic CAD is the underlying etiology. The hallmark of ACS is the vulnerable atherosclerotic plaque, which typically has a thin fibrous cap and a large lipid core. This vulnerable plaque ultimately ruptures, which leads to platelet activation and aggregation, leading to thrombus formation. STEMI typically results from complete thrombotic occlusion of a coronary artery, whereas UA and NSTEMI often have partial occlusion. Angiographically, it is often the intermediate coronary artery lesions (30% to 50% diameter vessel stenosis) that lead to subtotal or total vessel occlusion in two thirds of STEMI cases.

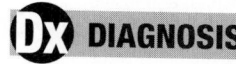

DIAGNOSIS

DIFFERENTIAL DIAGNOSIS

Chest pain mimicking ACS may be the result of various underlying disorders, some of which are also accompanied by ECG changes and/or cardiac biomarker release. Examples include acute pulmonary embolism, acute aortic dissection, pericarditis, myocarditis, costochondritis, pneumonia, tension pneumothorax, perforating ulcer, or Boerhaave syndrome.

WORKUP

Focused history and physical exam, 12-lead ECG, cardiac biomarkers, and chest radiograph (CXR). Initial biomarkers may not be positive. Often serial biomarkers are drawn every 6 to 8 hours for a total of three sets for the purposes of ruling out myocardial infarction (MI), or until peak to determine the severity of an established MI. Echocardiogram may reveal new regional wall motion abnormalities.

LABORATORY TESTS

- Cardiac biomarkers, which include creatine kinase (CK), its MB isoenzyme, myoglobin, and troponin I or T, will be positive in the

TABLE 1-11 Acute Coronary Syndromes

SPECTRUM OF ACUTE CORONARY SYNDROME			
	Unstable Angina	**NSTEMI**	**STEMI**
Chest discomfort	+	+	+
Cardiac biomarkers	−	+	+
ECG changes	TWI and/or ST depression	TWI and/or ST depression	ST elevation or presumed new left bundle branch block
Pathophysiology	Partial/transient thrombotic occlusion	Partial/transient thrombotic occlusion	Complete thrombotic occlusion

NSTEMI, Non–ST-segment elevation myocardial infarction; *STEMI*, ST-segment myocardial infarction; *TWI*, T-wave inversion; *ECG*, electrocardiogram.

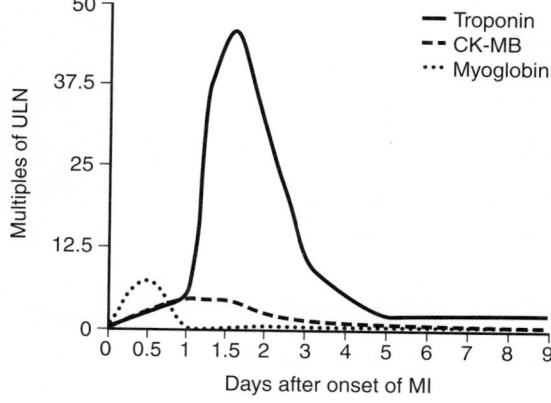

FIGURE 1-35 Timing of release of cardiac biomarkers in ACS. *ULN*, Upper limit of normal; *MI*, myocardial infarction. (Modified from Shapiro BP, Jaffe AS: Cardiac biomarkers. In Murphy JG, Lloyd MA [eds]: *Mayo Clinic cardiology: concise textbook*, ed 3, Rochester, MN: Mayo Clinic Scientific Press and New York, 2007, Informa Healthcare USA, pp 773-780; and Anderson JL et al: *J Am Coll Cardiol* 50:e1-e157, 2007, Fig. 5.)

setting of NSTEMI or STEMI. See Fig. 1-35 for timing of release of each biomarker.

- Testing for B-type natriuretic peptide (BNP) levels may also be helpful in patients with heart failure.
- A complete fasting lipid panel should be obtained during the hospital admission.

IMAGING STUDIES

- CXR to assist in evaluating for volume status and for other possible causes of chest discomfort.
- In patients for whom ECG and cardiac biomarkers are nondiagnostic but the suspicion for ACS is high given the history, an echocardiogram may be helpful to assess left ventricular (LV) function and regional wall motion abnormalities.
- Cardiac stress testing (treadmill ECG, imaging stress studies using echocardiography or nuclear modalities) may further help to diagnose and risk stratify these patients.
- Coronary angiogram/cardiac catheterization will reveal coronary artery luminal irregularities/stenotic lesions.

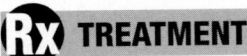 **TREATMENT**

The overall goal for patients with UA and NSTEMI is to relieve myocardial ischemia and to prevent recurrent cardiovascular events. Antithrombotic therapy is needed to reduce thrombus burden, prevent further thrombosis, and improve coronary artery flow. Revascularization is typically needed to prevent further events and improve flow within the coronary artery lumen. For patients with STEMI, the goal is immediate reperfusion therapy, whether it is chemical (i.e., thrombolysis) or mechanical (i.e., percutaneous coronary intervention [PCI]). STEMI patients presenting to a hospital with PCI capability should be treated with primary PCI within 90 minutes of first medical contact (Figs. 1-36 and 1-37). Thrombolytic therapy should not be administered 24 hours after initial diagnosis of STEMI.

NONPHARMACOLOGIC THERAPY

- STEMI is a medical emergency and requires immediate reperfusion therapy; the best outcomes are seen with cardiac catheterization with primary PCI. Guidelines call for a goal door-to-balloon time of ≤90 minutes.
- Patients with UA or NSTEMI should be risk stratified (Fig. E1-38) in conjunction with the cardiology consult service. Risk scores such as the TIMI and GRACE scores can be used to decide between an early invasive strategy and an initial conservative management strategy. Overall, an early invasive strategy is associated with better outcomes and involves cardiac catheterization followed by revascularization with PCI or coronary artery bypass grafting (CABG) within 4 to 24 hours of presentation. An initial conservative strategy involves aggressive medical management and revascularization only if ischemia recurs or is documented on noninvasive testing. This should only be reserved for selected patients with low-risk scores (TIMI score 0-2).
- Bed rest and continuous ECG monitoring is recommended for all ACS patients. Supplemental oxygen should be administered to patients with signs of hypoxia or respiratory distress. Finger pulse oximetry should be utilized to assess arterial oxygen saturation.

ACUTE GENERAL Rx

- All patients with ACS should receive full-dose aspirin for its antiplatelet effects and medical therapy with the statin class of drugs regardless of low-density lipoprotein (LDL) level, unless contraindicated.

- Beta-blocker therapy reduces ischemia by decreasing myocardial oxygen demand and should be initiated within 24 hours of onset of ACS unless signs or symptoms of heart failure are present or arrhythmias preclude its use. Oral administration, titrated to a heart rate of 50-60 beats/min, is preferred. Intravenous beta-blockers should not be administered to STEMI patients who have any of the following:
  1. Signs of heart failure,
  2. Evidence of a low output state,
  3. Increased risk for cardiogenic shock, or
  4. Other relative contraindications to beta-blockade (PR interval >0.24 second, second- or third-degree heart block, active asthma, or reactive airway disease).
- Nitroglycerin is a vasodilator that should be administered to relieve chest discomfort in all ACS patients. It can be administered sublingually at first, followed by intravenous administration if symptoms persist. In the setting of an inferior STEMI, it is wise to rule out a right ventricular (RV) infarct with a right-sided ECG before the administration of nitroglycerin. This is because RV infarcts are preload dependent and nitroglycerin decreases preload through venodilation, which leads to hypotension in this setting. This can be corrected by discontinuing nitroglycerin and starting intravenous fluids. Nitroglycerin provides no mortality benefit in ACS patients.
- Oxygen should be administered to patients with shortness of breath, signs of acute heart failure, cardiogenic shock, or an arterial oxyhemoglobin saturation of less than 94%. The 2011 American College of Cardiology/American Heart Association (ACC/AHA) guidelines recommend against the routine usage of oxygen therapy beyond 6 hours without compelling evidence of benefit.

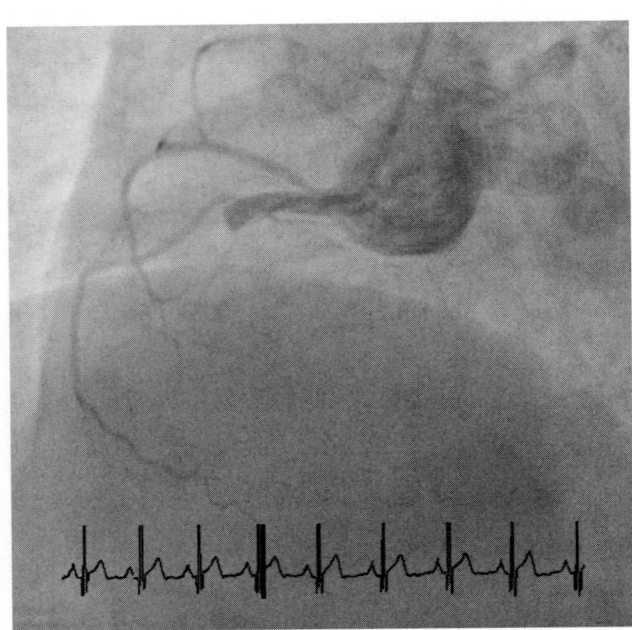

FIGURE 1-36 Right coronary artery totally occluded proximally during STEMI.

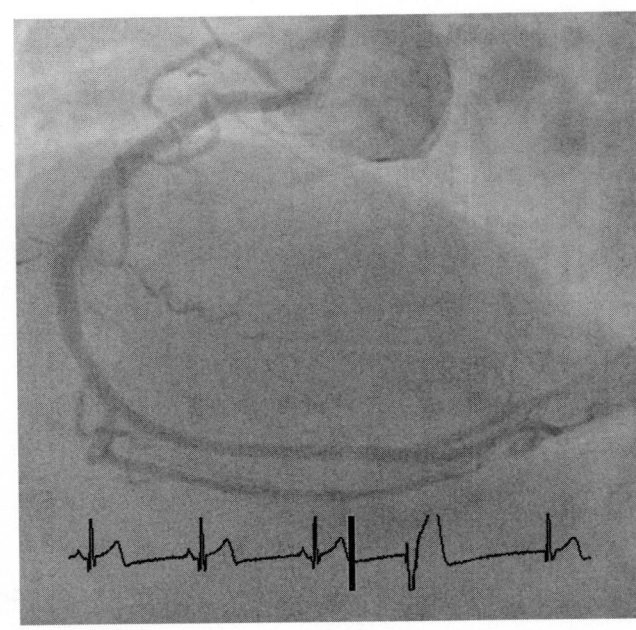

FIGURE 1-37 Right coronary artery after successful percutaneous coronary artery stenting during STEMI.

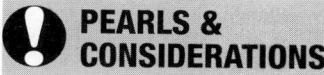

- Calcium channel blockers (nondihydropyridine) may be used in patients with persisting or recurrent symptoms, despite treatment with beta-blockers and nitroglycerin. They work by causing coronary vasodilation and decreasing myocardial oxygen demand. They are useful when beta-blockers are contraindicated and in patients with Prinzmetal variant angina. Calcium channel blockers should not be used in cases of severe LV dysfunction or pulmonary edema.
- Once a diagnosis has been established, morphine is reasonable to relieve chest pain if nitroglycerin is inadequate or contraindicated. Morphine can be used for pain management. Close monitoring of blood pressure and respiratory rate is recommended.
- Patients routinely taking nonsteroidal anti-inflammatory drugs (NSAIDs) (except for aspirin), both nonselective as well as COX-2 selective agents, before STEMI should discontinue those agents at the time of presentation with STEMI because of the increased risks of mortality, reinfarction, hypertension, heart failure, and myocardial rupture associated with their use.
- Angiotensin-converting enzyme (ACE) inhibitors may be added and should be used within 24 hours of onset of ACS in all patients with depressed LV function (ejection fraction [EF] <40%) or pulmonary vascular congestion. Angiotensin receptor blockers (ARBs) should be used in patients who are ACE inhibitor intolerant.
- Antithrombotic therapy is critical in treating the underlying pathophysiology of ACS. This consists of administering antiplatelet and anticoagulant agents.
- Antiplatelet agents inhibit platelet activation and aggregation. Aspirin is a cyclooxygenase inhibitor that blocks platelet aggregation and should be administered to all ACS patients without contraindications at an initial dose of 162 mg to 325 mg. Clopidogrel, prasugrel, and ticagrelor are P2Y12 inhibitors that inhibit platelet activation and aggregation. One should be administered to all ACS patients, with the timing dependent on the clinical scenario and management strategy. A loading dose should be administered, followed by daily dosing. Medication should be chosen by its safety profile specific to the patient. Clopidogrel should be discontinued at least 5 days before CABG, and prasugrel and ticagrelor should be discontinued at least 7 weeks prior. However, prasugrel is not recommended for STEMI patients with stroke

or transient ischemic attack (TIA) or for patients managed with fibrinolysis. Ticagrelor should not be administered to patients with active or intracranial bleeding. Glycoprotein (GP) IIb/IIIa inhibitors (eptifibatide or abciximab) are given intravenously and are effective at blocking the final pathway of platelet aggregation. As a rule, all ACS patients should have two antiplatelet agents.
- Anticoagulant agents should be administered to all ACS patients. Options include either unfractionated heparin (UFH) or low-molecular-weight heparin (LMWH) or direct thrombin inhibitors such as bivalirudin. LMWH is preferred in low-risk NSTEMI/UA. As with antiplatelet agents, the choice of anticoagulant depends on management strategy and institution protocols. For STEMI, fondaparinux can be used for anticoagulation. It has been shown to decrease bleeding complications as compared with either UFH or LMWH. Disadvantages are that it is difficult to monitor. It has a long half-life (15 hours), and thrombosis on catheters has been noted when using only fondaparinux in the cath lab.
- Bivalirudin is a reversible direct thrombin inhibitor and may be considered as an alternative to UFH and GP IIb/IIIa inhibitors in patients with STEMI who are undergoing primary PCI (PPCI). When bivalirudin was compared to UFH plus a glycoprotein inhibitor in patients with STEMI and PPCI, less bleeding and a short- and long-term reduction in cardiac events and overall mortality was observed. With bivalirudin, there is no risk of heparin-induced thrombocytopenia, less bleeding is observed, and no anticoagulant monitoring is needed.

CHRONIC Rx

- Post-ACS medical therapy involves aspirin, statin, beta-blocker, and antiplatelet therapy.
- ACE inhibitors may be added to treat hypertension and should be used in all patients with depressed LV function (EF <40%) or pulmonary vascular congestion. ARBs should be used in patients who are ACE inhibitor intolerant.
- Eplerenone, an aldosterone receptor blocker, should be considered in post-MI patients with LV EF ≤40% and evidence of congestive heart failure.
- Cardiac rehabilitation and a monitored exercise program should be recommended.
- Aggressive risk factor management for secondary prevention of future events is crucial.

REFERRAL

- All ACS patients should be cared for in conjunction with the cardiology consult service.
- When appropriate, referral to a cardiac surgeon may be necessary for CABG.

(!) PEARLS & CONSIDERATIONS

COMMENTS

- ACS is common and a leading cause of mortality in the United States.
- The diagnosis hinges on the basics—history and physical, ECG, biomarkers, and CXR.
- Remember the potentially fatal non-ACS causes of chest discomfort, which include acute pulmonary embolism and acute ascending aortic dissection.
- STEMI patients presenting to a hospital with PCI capability should be treated with primary PCI within 90 minutes of first medical contact.
- STEMI patients presenting to a hospital without PCI capability and who cannot be transferred to a PCI center and undergo PCI within 90 minutes of first medical contact should be treated with fibrinolytic therapy within 30 minutes of hospital presentation unless fibrinolytic therapy is contraindicated.

PREVENTION

- Primary prevention of ACS is based on recognizing the major risk factors for CAD and treating them as appropriate.
- Patients with depressed LV function (ejection fraction <35%) at least 40 days after an acute MI benefit from an implantable cardioverter defibrillator (ICD) for the prevention of sudden cardiac death.

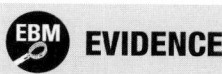 **EVIDENCE**

available at www.expertconsult.com

SUGGESTED READINGS

available at www.expertconsult.com

RELATED CONTENT

Acute Coronary Syndrome (Patient Information)
Angina (Related Key Topic)
Myocardial Infarction (Related Key Topic)

AUTHORS: **SHAMAIL TARIQ, M.D.,** and **PRANAV M. PATEL, M.D., F.A.C.C., F.S.C.A.I.**

A

Diseases and Disorders

I

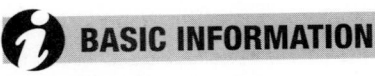

BASIC INFORMATION

DEFINITION

Acute kidney injury (AKI) is the rapid (≤48 hr) impairment in renal function resulting in retention of products in the blood that are normally excreted by the kidneys and thus volume and acid-base dysregulation in the body. Criteria and classifications of AKI are described in Table 1-12.

SYNONYMS

ARF
Acute renal insufficiency syndrome
Acute renal failure
AKI

ICD-9CM CODES
584.9 Acute renal failure, unspecified

EPIDEMIOLOGY & DEMOGRAPHICS

- Incidence of AKI is 3 cases/1000 persons. AKI requiring dialysis develops in five in 100,000 persons annually.
- >10% of intensive care unit patients develop ALL.
- >40% of hospital AKI is iatrogenic.
- The most common cause of AKI in hospitalized patients is intrinsic renal failure caused by acute tubular necrosis (ATN) and prerenal disease.
- AKI occurs in 20% of patients with moderate sepsis and more than 50% of patients with septic shock and positive blood cultures.
- Can occur at any age; however, various underlying causes occur in certain age groups.

PHYSICAL FINDINGS & CLINICAL PRESENTATION

- The physical examination should focus on volume status. The physical findings noted below vary with the duration and rapidity of onset of renal failure.
- Peripheral edema resulting from volume overload, heart failure, liver failure, or nephrotic syndrome
- Skin pallor, ecchymoses
- Arrhythmias due to electrolyte imbalances and acidosis
- Oliguria (i.e., <400 to 500 ml urine/24 hr; however, patients can have nonoliguric renal failure), anuria
- Change in mental status, delirium, lethargy, myoclonus, seizures
- Uremic odor
- Flank pain, fasciculations, muscle cramps
- Tachypnea, tachycardia
- Weakness, anorexia, generalized malaise, nausea
- Pulmonary rales due to volume overload
- Flapping tremors
- Pericardial effusion
- Hypotension or hypertension can occur, suggesting volume depletion and overload, respectively

ETIOLOGY

- Prerenal: inadequate perfusion caused by hypovolemia, congestive heart failure, cirrhosis, sepsis. Sixty percent of community-acquired cases of AKI are from prerenal conditions.
- Postrenal: outlet obstruction from prostatic enlargement, fibrosis, ureteral obstruction (stones), bilateral renal vein occlusion.

Postrenal causes account for 5% to 15% of community-acquired AKI.
- Intrinsic renal: glomerulonephritis, ATN, rhabdomyolysis, systemic hypotension, sepsis, drug toxicity, contrast nephropathy. Contrast-induced nephropathy (increase in serum creatinine >25% within 3 days of intravascular contrast administration in absence of an alternative cause) is the third most common cause of new AKI in hospitalized patients.
- Causes of AKI are described in Table 1-13 and Fig. E1-39.

DIAGNOSIS

DIFFERENTIAL DIAGNOSIS

Refer to "Etiology." Diagnostic tests to distinguish prerenal and renal AKI are described in Table E1-14. A diagnostic approach to patients with suspected AKI is described in Fig. E1-40.

LABORATORY TESTS

- Elevated serum creatinine: the rate of rise is approximately 1 mg/dl/day in complete renal failure.
- Elevated blood urea nitrogen (BUN): BUN/creatinine ratio is >20:1 in prerenal azotemia, postrenal azotemia, and acute glomerulonephritis; it is <20:1 in acute interstitial nephritis and ATN (Table 1-15).
- Electrolytes (potassium, phosphate) are elevated; bicarbonate level, sodium, and calcium are decreased; metabolic acidosis is noted
- Close monitoring of 24-hr urinary volume.
- Complete blood count may reveal anemia because of decreased erythropoietin production, hemoconcentration, hemolysis, or leuckocytosis, suggesting infection.
- Urinalysis may reveal the presence of hematuria (glomerulonephritis), proteinuria (nephrotic syndrome), casts (e.g., granular casts in ATN, red blood cell casts in acute glomerulonephritis, white blood cell casts in acute interstitial nephritis), eosinophiluria (acute interstitial nephritis). However, these urinary findings may be absent in less severe disease.
- Urinary sodium and urinary creatinine should also be obtained to calculate the fractional excretion of sodium (FENa) (FENa = Urine sodium/Plasma sodium × Plasma creatinine/Urine creatinine × 100). FENa is <1 in prerenal failure and >1 in intrinsic renal failure in patients with urine output <400 ml/day. The FENa can be falsely high in patients taking diuretics. It can also be falsely low in several intrinsic renal conditions such as acute glomerulonephritis, contrast-induced nephropathy, and rhabdomyolysis.
- Urinary osmolarity is 250 to 300 mOsm/kg in ATN, <400 mOsm/kg in postrenal azotemia, and >500 mOsm/kg in prerenal azotemia and acute glomerulonephritis (Table 1-16).

TABLE 1-12	RIFLE and AKIN Criteria for Diagnosis of Acute Kidney Injury	
RIFLE CLASSIFICATION		
	GFR Criteria	**Urine Output Criteria**
Risk	S_{Cr} >1.5 × baseline or ΔGFR >25% reduction	UO <0.5 ml/kg/h × 6 h
Injury	S_{Cr} >2.0 × baseline or ΔGFR >50% reduction	UO <0.5 ml/kg/h × 12 h
Failure	S_{Cr} >3.0 × baseline or ΔGFR >75% reduction or S_{Cr} >4.0 mg/dl	UO <0.3 ml/kg/h × 24 h or anuria × 12 h
Loss	Persistent acute kidney injury = Complete loss of function for >4 wk	
ESRD	End-stage renal disease >3 mo	
AKIN CLASSIFICATION		
Stage	**Serum Creatinine Criteria**	**Urine Output Criteria**
1	ΔS_{Cr} ≥0.3 mg/dl (30 μmol/L) or S_{Cr} ≥1.5, ≤2.0 × baseline	UO <0.5 ml/kg/h × 6 h
2	S_{Cr} >2.0, ≤3.0 × baseline	UO <0.5 ml/kg/h × 12 h
3	S_{Cr} >3.0 × baseline or S_{Cr} ≥4.0 mg/dl with an acute rise ≥0.5 mg/dl (50 μmol/L) or on renal replacement therapy	UO <0.3 ml/kg/h × 24 h or anuria × 12 h

AKIN, Acute Kidney Injury Network; *GFR,* glomerular filtration rate; *RIFLE,* risk, injury, failure, loss, ESRD; *SCr,* serum creatinine; *UO,* urinary output.
From Floege J et al: *Comprehensive clinical nephrology,* ed 4, Philadelphia, 2010, Saunders.

TABLE 1-13   Etiologies of Acute Kidney Injury

Prerenal Causes (Decreased Renal Blood Flow)	Intrinsic Renal Causes	Postrenal Causes
Hypovolemia Renal losses (diuretics, osmotic agents, polyuria) Gastrointestinal losses (vomiting, diarrhea) Cutaneous losses (burns, exfoliative syndromes) Hemorrhage Pancreatitis **Decreased Cardiac Output** Congestive heart failure Pulmonary embolism Acute myocardial infarction Severe valvular heart disease Abdominal compartment syndrome Renal artery obstruction (stenosis, embolism, thrombosis, dissection) **Systemic Vasodilation** Sepsis Anaphylaxis Anesthetics Drug overdose **Afferent Arteriolar Vasoconstriction** Hypercalcemia Drugs (NSAIDs, amphotericin B, calcineurin inhibitors, norepinephrine, radiocontrast agents, aminoglycosides) Hepatorenal syndrome Efferent arteriolar vasodilation (angiotensin converting enzyme inhibitors, aldosterone receptor blockers)	**Vascular: Large and Small Vessels** Trauma Renal vein obstruction (thrombosis, ventilation with high-level PEEP, abdominal compartment syndrome) Microangiopathy (thrombotic thrombocytopenic purpura, hemolytic-uremic syndrome, disseminated intravascular coagulation, preeclampsia) Malignant hypertension Scleroderma renal crisis Transplant rejection Atheroembolic disease **Glomerular** Antiglomerular basement membrane disease (Goodpasture syndrome) Antineutrophil cytoplasmic antibody-associated glomerulonephritis (Wegener granulomatosis) Immune complex glomerulonephritis, systemic lupus erythematosus, postinfectious cryoglobulinemia, primary membranoproliferative glomerulonephritis **Tubular** Ischemic Cytotoxic Heme pigment (rhabdomyolysis, intravascular hemolysis) Crystals (tumor lysis syndrome, seizures, ethylene glycol poisoning, vitamin C megadose, acyclovir, indinavir, methotrexate) Drugs (aminoglycosides, lithium, amphotericin B, pentamidine, cisplatin, ifosfamide, radiocontrast agents), synthetic cannabinoid use **Interstitial** Drugs (penicillins, cephalosporins, NSAIDs, proton pump inhibitors, allopurinol, rifampin, indinavir, mesalamine, sulfonamides) Infection (pyelonephritis, viral infection) **Systemic Disease** Sjögren syndrome, sarcoidosis, systemic lupus erythematosus, lymphoma, leukemia, tubulonephritis, uveitis	**Ureteral Obstruction** Calculus Tumor (intrinsic or extrinsic) Fibrosis Ligation during pelvic surgery **Bladder Neck Obstruction** Benign prostatic hypertrophy Prostate cancer Neurogenic bladder Tricyclic antidepressants Ganglionic blockers Bladder tumor Calculus Hemorrhage/clot **Urethral Obstruction** Strictures Tumor Phimosis Renal calcinosis Obstructed urinary catheter, ureteral stent, or ileal conduit Pelvic trauma, retroperitoneal hematoma

NSAIDs, Nonsteroidal anti-inflammatory drugs; *PEEP,* positive end-expiratory pressure.
Modified from Cameron JL, Cameron AM: *Current surgical therapy,* ed 10, Philadelphia, 2011, Saunders.

TABLE 1-15   Serum and Radiographic Abnormalities in Renal Failure

	Prerenal	Postrenal (Acute)	Intrinsic Renal (Acute)	Intrinsic Renal (Chronic)
BUN	↑ 10:1 > Cr	↑ 20-40/day	↑ 20-40/day	Stable; ↑ varies with protein intake
Serum creatinine	N/moderate ↑	↑ 2-4/day	↑ 2-4/day	Stable ↑ (production equals excretion)
Serum potassium	N/moderate ↑	↑ varies with urinary volume	↑↑ (particularly when patient is oliguric) ↑↑↑ with rhabdomyolysis	Normal until end stage, unless tubular dysfunction (type 4 RTA)
Serum phosphate	N/moderate ↑	Moderate ↑	↑	Becomes significantly elevated when serum creatinine surpasses 3 mg/dl
Serum calcium	N	↑↑ with rhabdomyolysis N/-↓ with PO_4^{-3} retention	Poor correlation with duration of renal disease ↓ (poor correlation with duration of renal failure)	Usually ↓
Renal size				
By ultrasonography	N/↑	↑ and dilated calyces	N/↑	↓ and with ↑ echogenicity
FE_{Na}*	<1	<1 → >1	>1†	>1

↑, Increase; ↓, decrease; ↑↑, large increase; ↑↑↑, very high increase; *BUN,* blood urea nitrogen; *Cr,* creatinine; *N,* normal; *Na,* sodium; *P,* plasma; *RTA,* renal tubular acidosis; *U,* urine.

$$*FE_{Na} = \left[\frac{U/P_{Na^+}}{U/P_{Cr}} \times 100 \right]$$ (useful only in oliguric patient).

†May be ≤1 in radiocontrast-induced myoglobinuric acute tubular necrosis and in early sepsis.
From Ferri FF (ed): *Practical guide to the care of the medical patient,* ed 8, St Louis, 2011, Mosby.

- Combined use of cystatin C, a protein that is freely filtered by the glomerulus, and serum creatinine has been shown to improve estimates of GFR in AKI.
- The fractional excretion of urea (FEU) is a useful measure for assessing renal dysfunction in AKI. FEU is calculated as:

$$\frac{\text{Serum creatinine} \times \text{Urinary urea}}{\text{Serum urea} \quad \times \text{Urinary creatinine}}$$

An FEU of less than 35% suggests a prerenal cause of AKI, whereas a value over 50% indicates an intrinsic cause. FEU is more useful than FENa in patients on diuretics.
- Blood cultures for patients suspected of sepsis
- Liver function tests, immunoglobulins, and protein electrophoresis in patients suspected of myeloma
- Decreased complement levels and elevated anti–glomerular basement membrane antibody titers, antineutrophil cytoplasmic antibodies, antinuclear antibodies, cryoglobinemia, and circulating immune complexes are useful diagnostic tools for diagnosing glomerulonephritis or vasculitis.
- Creatinine kinase in patients with suspected rhabdomyolysis.
- Renal biopsy may be indicated in patients with intrinsic renal failure when considering specific therapy; major uses of renal biopsy are differential diagnosis of nephrotic syndrome, separation of lupus vasculitis from other vasculitis and lupus membranous from idiopathic membranous, confirmation of hereditary nephropathies on the basis of the ultrastructure, diagnosis of rapidly progressing glomerulonephritis, separation of allergic interstitial nephritis from ATN, separation of primary glomerulonephritis syndromes.
- Tubular enzymes are studied as biomarkers for renal failure. Among them are proximal renal tubular epithelial antigen (HRTE-1), N-acetyl-beta-glucosaminidase (NAG), alpha-glutathione S-transferase (alpha-GST), gamma-glutamyltranspeptidase (gamma-GT), and lactate dehydrogenase (LDH). The majority of them are released before an increase in serum creatinine; however, they do not provide any clear parameters to differentiate ATN from prerenal failure.
- Alpha1-microglobulin (alpha1-M), beta2-microglobulin (beta2-M), adenosine deaminase binding protein (ABP), retinol binding protein (RBP), urinary cystatin C, and neutrophil gelatinase–associated lipocalin (NGAL) are being further studied for diagnostic evaluation.

IMAGING STUDIES

- ECG is done to evaluate changes especially in hyperkalemia.
- Chest x-ray is useful to evaluate for congestive heart failure and for pulmonary renal syndromes (Goodpasture's syndrome, Wegener's granulomatosis).
- Abdominal x-rays when suspecting renal or ureteric calculi.
- Ultrasound of kidneys is used to evaluate kidney size (useful to distinguish acute from chronic renal failure), evaluate for the presence of obstruction, and evaluate renal vascular status (with Doppler evaluation).
- Computed tomography (CT) with radiocontrast agent administration is usually avoided in AKI; however, unenhanced CT scans are useful for the identification of obstructing ureteral stones.

Rx TREATMENT

NONPHARMACOLOGIC THERAPY

- Stop all nephrotoxic medications.
- Dietary modification to supply adequate calories while minimizing accumulation of toxins; appropriate control of fluid balance. Physicians should recommend a nutrition program with an energy prescription of 120 to 150 KJ/kg/day and restriction of potassium (60 mEq/day), sodium (90 mEq/day), and phosphorus (800 mg/day). Ideal protein supplementation ranges from 0.6 to 1.4 g/kg depending on whether dialysis is required.
- Daily weight.
- Modifications of dosage of renally excreted drugs.

ACUTE GENERAL Rx

- Correction of electrolyte abnormalities
- Loop diuretics in patients with volume overload Specific treatment is variable with etiology of AKI:
- Prerenal: IV volume expansion in hypovolemic patients.
- Intrinsic renal: discontinuation of any potential toxins and treatment of condition causing the renal failure.
- Postrenal: removal of obstruction. Immediate insertion of catheter for lower urinary tract obstruction and nephrostomy or ureteral stents are required in patients with upper urinary tract obstruction.
- IV insulin and glucose for patients with hyperkalemia related ECG changes who could not be admitted to the hospital immediately.
- Intermittent hemodialysis and continuous renal replacement therapy have similar outcomes for patients with AKI.

CHRONIC Rx

- Monitoring of renal function and electrolytes.
- Doses of medications that are renally excreted should be adjusted according to creatinine clearance to prevent further damage to the kidneys.
- Prevention of further insults to the kidneys with proper hydration, especially before contrast studies, and avoidance of nephrotoxic agents. Hydration with sodium bicarbonate (addition of 154 ml of 1000 mEq/L sodium bicarbonate to 846 ml of 5% dextrose in water) before contrast exposure is more

TABLE 1-16 Urinary Abnormalities in Renal Failure

	Prerenal	Postrenal (Acute)	Intrinsic Renal (Acute)	Intrinsic Renal (Chronic)
Urinary volume	↓	Absent-to-wide fluctuation	Oliguric or nonoliguric	1000 ml + until end stage
Urinary creatinine	↑ (U/P Cr ±40)	↓ (U/P Cr ±20)	↓ (U/P Cr <20)	↓ (U/P Cr <20)
Osmolarity	↑ (±400 mOsm/kg)	(<350 mOsm/kg)	(<350 mOsm/kg)	(<350 mOsm/kg)
Degree of proteinuria	Minimum	Absent	Varies with cause of renal failure: Modest with ATN Nephrotic range common with acute glomerulopathies, usually <2 g/24 hr with interstitial disease*	Varies with cause of renal disease (from 1-2 g/day to nephrotic range)
Urinary sediment	Negative, or occasional hyaline cast	Negative or hematuria with stones or papillary necrosis Pyuria with infectious prostatic disease Nephrosis: oval fat bodies	ATN: muddy brown casts Interstitial nephritis: lymphocytes, eosinophils (in stained preparations), and WBC casts RPGN: RBC casts	Broad casts with variable renal "residual" acute findings

↑, Increased; ↓, decreased; *ATN*, acute tubular necrosis; clearance = $\dfrac{\text{urinary concentration} \times \text{urinary volume}}{\text{plasma concentration}}$; *Cr*, creatinine; *RBC*, red blood cell; *RPGN*, rapidly progressive glomerulonephritis; *U/P*, urine/plasma; *WBC*, white blood cell.
*Except nonsteroidal anti-inflammatory drug-induced allergic interstitial nephritis with concomitant "nil disease."
From Ferri FF (ed): *Practical guide to the care of the medical patient*, ed 8, St Louis, 2011, Mosby.

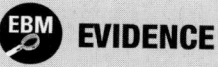
effective than hydration with sodium chloride for prophylaxis of contrast-induced renal failure. Administration of N-acetylcysteine prophylaxis has shown conflicting results regarding its ability to reduce the risk of contrast-induced nephropathy. In high-risk patients having angiography or angioplasty, the RenalGuard System using saline plus N-acetylcysteine and furosemide has been shown to be better than sodium bicarbonate plus N-acetylcysteine for preventing contrast-induced AKI.

- See "Chronic Kidney Disease" entry for indications for initiation of dialysis. Daily hemodialysis is superior to every-other-day hemodialysis in patients with ATN and ARF.

DISPOSITION

- General indications for initiation of dialysis are:
  1. Florid symptoms of uremia (encephalopathy, pericarditis)
  2. Severe volume overload
  3. Severe acid-base imbalance
  4. Significant derangement in electrolyte concentrations (e.g., hyperkalemia, hyponatremia)
- Intermittent hemodialysis and continuous renal replacement therapy have similar outcomes for patients with AKI.
- Renal function recovery (ability to discontinue dialysis) varies from 50% to 75% in survivors of AKI.
- Overall mortality rate in AKI is nearly 50%, varying from 60% in patients with ATN to 35% in patients with prerenal or postrenal AKI.
- The combination of AKI and sepsis is associated with a 70% mortality rate.

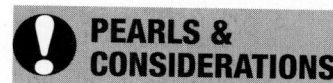

PEARLS & CONSIDERATIONS

- Patients with AKI are susceptible to infections and sepsis.
- Dosing of certain drugs needs to be modified in patients with AKI.

EVIDENCE

available at www.expertconsult.com

SUGGESTED READINGS

available at www.expertconsult.com

RELATED CONTENT

Acute Renal Failure (Patient Information)
Chronic Renal Failure (Patient Information)

AUTHORS: **SYEDA M. SAYEED, M.D.,** and **FRED F. FERRI, M.D.**

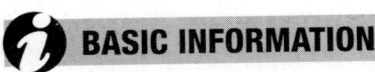

BASIC INFORMATION

DEFINITION

Acute respiratory distress syndrome (ARDS) is a form of noncardiogenic pulmonary edema that results from acute damage to the alveoli. It is characterized by acute diffuse infiltrative lung lesions with resulting interstitial and alveolar edema, severe hypoxemia, and respiratory failure. The cardinal feature of ARDS, refractory hypoxemia, is caused by formation of protein-rich alveolar edema after damage to the integrity of the lung's alveolar-capillary barrier.

The definition of ARDS based on the American–European Consensus Conference (AECC) from 1994 included the following components:
1. The syndrome must present acutely
2. A ratio of Pao_2 to Fio_2 ≤ 200 regardless of the level of positive end expiratory pressure (PEEP)
3. The detection of bilateral pulmonary infiltrates on frontal chest radiograph
4. Absence of congestive heart failure (pulmonary artery wedge pressure [PAWP] ≤ 18 mm Hg or no clinical evidence of elevated left atrial pressure on the basis of chest radiograph or other clinical data)

The Berlin definition of ARDS adopted in 2011 addresses some of the limitations of the AECC definition and establishes the following criteria for ARDS:
- Timing: Within 1 week of a known clinical insult or new or worsening respiratory symptoms
- Chest imaging (chest x-ray or CT scan): Bilateral opacities , not fully explained by effusions, lobar/lung collapse, or nodules
- Origin of edema: Respiratory failure not fully explained by cardiac failure or fluid overload. Need objective assessment (e.g., echocardiography) to exclude hydrostatic edema if no risk factor present
- Oxygenation (if altitude is higher than 1000 m, the correction factor should be calculated as follows: [Pao_2/Fio_2 × {barometric pressure/760}]
1. Mild: 200 mm Hg < Pao_2/Fio_2 ≤ 300 mm Hg with PEEP or CPAP ≥5 cm H_2O (this may be delivered noninvasively in the mild ARDS group)
2. Moderate: 100 mm Hg < Pao_2/Fio_2 ≤ 200 mm Hg with PEEP or CPAP ≥5 cm H_2O
3. Severe; Pao_2/Fio_2 ≤100 mm Hg with PEEP or CPAP ≥5 cm H_2O

SYNONYMS
ARDS
Adult respiratory distress syndrome

ICD-9CM CODES
518.82 Acute respiratory distress syndrome

EPIDEMIOLOGY & DEMOGRAPHICS

- More than 150,000 ARDS cases per year in the U.S. 7.1% of all patients admitted to an ICU and 16.1% of all patients on mechanical ventilation develop ARDS.
- Incidence is 1.5 to 8.3 cases per 100,000 per year.
- Approximately 50% of patients who develop ARDS do so within 24 hours of the inciting event. Mortality rate is 40% to 50%.

PHYSICAL FINDINGS & CLINICAL PRESENTATION

- Signs and symptoms
  1. Dyspnea
  2. Chest discomfort
  3. Cough
  4. Anxiety
- Physical examination
  1. Tachypnea
  2. Tachycardia
  3. Hypertension
  4. Coarse crepitations of both lungs
  5. Fever may be present if infection is the underlying etiology

ETIOLOGY

- Sepsis (>40% of cases)
- Aspiration: near drowning, aspiration of gastric contents (>30% of cases)
- Trauma (>20% of cases)
- Multiple transfusions, blood products
- Drugs (e.g., overdose of morphine, methadone, heroin; reaction to nitrofurantoin)
- Noxious inhalation (e.g., chlorine gas, high O_2 concentration)
- Postresuscitation
- Cardiopulmonary bypass
- Pneumonia
- Burns
- Pancreatitis
- A history of chronic alcohol abuse significantly increases the risk of developing ARDS in critically ill patients
- Table 1-17 describes risk factors associated with development of ARDS.

DIAGNOSIS

DIFFERENTIAL DIAGNOSIS

- Cardiogenic pulmonary edema
- Viral pneumonitis
- Lymphangitic carcinomatosis

WORKUP

The search for an underlying cause should focus on treatable causes (e.g., infections such as sepsis or pneumonia)
- Arterial blood gases (ABGs)
- Hemodynamic monitoring
- Bronchoalveolar lavage (selected patients)

LABORATORY TESTS

- ABGs:
  1. Initially: varying degrees of hypoxemia, generally resistant to supplemental oxygen
  2. Respiratory alkalosis, decreased Pco_2
  3. Widened alveolar-arterial gradient
  4. Hypercapnia as the disease progresses
- Bronchoalveolar lavage:
  1. The most prominent finding is an increased number of polymorphonucleocytes.
  2. The presence of eosinophilia has therapeutic implications because these patients respond to corticosteroids.
- Blood and urine cultures

IMAGING STUDIES

Chest radiograph (Fig. 1-41).
- The initial chest radiograph might be normal in the initial hours after the precipitating event.
- Bilateral interstitial infiltrates are usually seen within 24 hr; they often are more prominent in the bases and periphery.
- "White out" of both lung fields can be seen in advanced stages.
- CT scan of chest: diffuse consolidation with air bronchograms, bullae, pleural effusions. Pneumomediastinum and pneumothoraces may also be present.

TREATMENT

NONPHARMACOLOGIC THERAPY

Treatment of ARDS is supportive.
Hemodynamic monitoring:
- Can be used for the initial evaluation of ARDS (in ruling out cardiogenic pulmonary edema) and its subsequent management. However, a pulmonary catheter is not indicated in the routine management of ARDS and trials have shown that clinical management involving the early use of pulmonary artery catheters in patients with ARDS did not significantly affect mortality and morbidity rates and may result in more complications as compared with a central venous catheter.
- Although no dynamic profile is diagnostic of ARDS, the presence of pulmonary edema, a high cardiac output, and a low pulmonary capillary wedge pressure (PCWP) is characteristic of ARDS.
- It is important to remember that partially treated intravascular volume overload and

TABLE 1-17 Risk Factors Associated with Development of Acute Lung Injury and Acute Respiratory Distress Syndrome

Direct Lung Injury	Indirect Lung Injury
Pneumonia	Sepsis
Aspiration of gastric contents	Multiple trauma
Pulmonary contusion	Cardiopulmonary bypass
Fat, amniotic fluid, or air emboli	Drug overdose
Near-drowning	Acute pancreatitis
Inhalational injury	Transfusion of blood products
Reperfusion pulmonary edema	

From Vincent JL et al: *Textbook of critical care,* ed 6, Philadelphia, 2011, Saunders.

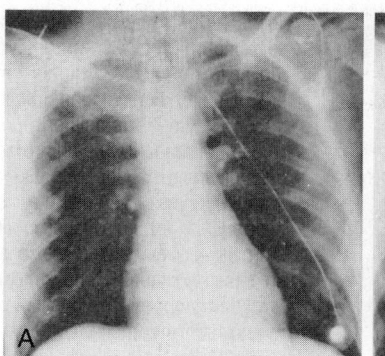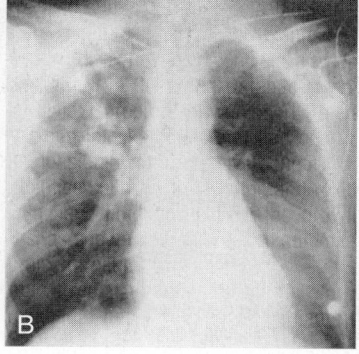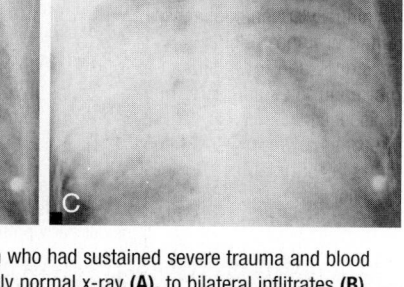

FIGURE 1-41 Acute respiratory distress syndrome. X-ray of a young man who had sustained severe trauma and blood loss in a road traffic accident; the limbs cover a period of 5 days from a relatively normal x-ray **(A)**, to bilateral infiltrates **(B)**, to bilateral "white out"'**(C)**, accompanied by severe hypoxemia. A Swan-Ganz catheter for measurement of pulmonary artery "wedge" pressure (as a reflection of left atrial pressure) can be seen in situ on the x-ray in **C.** The patient died shortly after the last film. (From Souhami RL, Moxham J: *Textbook of medicine,* ed 4, London, 2002, Churchill Livingstone.)

flash pulmonary edema can have the hemodynamic features of ARDS; filling pressures can also be elevated by increased intrathoracic pressures or with fluid administration; cardiac function can be depressed by acidosis, hypoxemia, or other factors associated with sepsis.

Ventilatory support: mechanical ventilation is generally necessary to maintain adequate gas exchange (Fig. E1-42). General recommendations for ventilator settings in ARDS are described in Table 1-18. A low tidal volume and low plateau pressure ventilator strategy are recommended to avoid ventilator-induced injury. Assist-control is generally preferred initially with the following ventilator settings:

- Fio_2 1.0 (until a lower value can be used to achieve adequate oxygenation). When possible, minimize oxygen toxicity by maintaining Fio_2 at <60%.
- Tidal volume: Set initial tidal volume at 6 ml/kg of predicted body weight (PBW = 50.0 + 0.91 [height: 152.4 cm] for men, PBW = 45.5 + 0.91 [height: 152.4 cm] for women). The concept of using PBW is based on the fact that lung size depends most strongly on height and sex; PBW normalizes the tidal volume to lung size. Aim to maintain plateau pressure (Pplat) at <30 mm Hg.
- PEEP 5 cm H_2O or greater (to increase lung volume and keep alveoli open). PEEP should be applied in small increments of 3 to 5 cm H_2O (up to a maximum of 15 cm H_2O) to achieve acceptable arterial saturation (>0.9) with nontoxic Fio_2 values (<0.6) and acceptable airway plateau pressures (>30 to 35 cm H_2O). It is important to remember that an increase in PEEP may lower cardiac output and, despite improvement in Pao_2, may actually have a negative effect on tissue oxygenation (the major determinants of tissue oxygenation are hemoglobin, percent saturation, and cardiac output). The optimal level of PEEP remains unestablished. Although higher levels of PEEP may help prevent life-threatening hypioxemia and be associated with lower

hospital mortality in patients meeting criteria for ARDS, such benefit is unlikely in patients with less severe lung injury and a strategy of treating such patients with high PEEP levels may be harmful.
- Inspiratory flow: 60 L/min.
- Ventilatory rate: high ventilatory rates of 18 to 24 breaths/min are often necessary in patients with ARDS because of their increased physiologic dead space and smaller lung volumes. Patients must be monitored for excessive intrathoracic gas trapping (auto-PEEP or intrinsic PEEP) that can depress cardiac output.
- Sedation: GABA receptor agonists (including propofol and benzodiazepines such as midazolam) have traditionally been the most commonly administered sedative drugs for ICU patients. Recent trials indicate that the alpha-2 agonist dexmedetomidine may have distinct advantages. At comparable sedation levels, dexmedetomidine-treated patients spent less time on ventilator, experienced less delirium, and developed less tachycardia and hypertension. The most notable adverse effect of dexmedetomidine was bradycardia. Preliminary trials involving early administration of the neuromuscular blocking agent cisatracurium in patients with severe ARDS have shown improvement in the adjusted 90-day survival and increase in the time off the ventilator without increase in muscle weakness. However, patients who receive continuous infusions of sedatives generally need to be on mechanical ventilation longer than those who receive intermittent dosing. Paralysis of patients with neuromuscular blockade (NMB) to facilitate controlled ventilation is associated with protracted mechanical ventilation and postparalysis weakness. It should ideally be conducted for a brief period, and limited to patients with severe ARDS. Daily interruption of sedation (daily awakening) in mechanically ventilated patients is safe and is associated with a shorter length of mechanical ventilation.

ACUTE GENERAL Rx

Identify and treat precipitating conditions:
- Blood and urine cultures and trial of antibiotics in presumed sepsis (routine administration of antibiotics in all cases of ARDS is not recommended).
- Prompt repair of bone fractures in patients with major trauma.
- Bowel rest and crystalloid resuscitation in pancreatitis.
- Fluid management: In most patients with ARDS, fluid restriction is associated with better outcomes than a liberal fluid policy. Optimal fluid and hemodynamic management of patients with ARDS should be patient specific; in general, administration of crystalloids is recommended if a downward trend in PCWP is associated with diminished cardiac index, resulting in prerenal azotemia, oliguria, and relative tachycardia. On the other hand, if PCWP increases with little or no change in cardiac index, one should begin diuretic therapy and use low-dose dopamine (2 to 4 μg/kg/min) to maintain natriuresis and support adequate renal flow.
- Positioning the patient: changes in position can improve oxygenation by improving the distribution of perfusion to ventilated lung regions; repositioning (lateral decubitus positioning) should be attempted in patients with hypoxemia that is not responsive to other medical interventions. Placing patients with moderate and severe hypoxemia in a prone position may improve their oxygenation but does not provide significant survival benefit.
- Corticosteroids: routine use of corticosteroids in ARDS is not recommended; corticosteroids may be beneficial in patients with many eosinophils in the bronchoalveolar lavage fluid. Systemic infections should be ruled out or adequately treated before administration of corticosteroids. Use of methylprednisolone has not been shown to increase the rate of infectious complications but is associated with a higher rate of neuromuscular weakness. In addition, starting methylprednisolone

TABLE 1-18   Recommendations for Ventilator Settings in ARDS

Conventional Mechanical Ventilation

Mode		Volume- or pressure-controlled "Airway pressure release ventilation" preferred when preservation of spontaneous ventilation is desired
Tidal volume	6-10 ml/kg	Permissive hypercapnia (increase <5 mm Hg/h) $PaCO_2$ 65-85 mm Hg well tolerated unless increased ICP Arterial pH >7.15
End-inspiratory plateau pressure	<30 cm H_2O	Above this limit, increased risks of barotrauma and air leaks
Positive end-expiratory pressure	10-15 cm H_2O	Lower PEEP levels, if heterogeneous lung injury Higher PEEP levels, if diffuse lung injury Consider early prone positioning (6-12 h)
Respiratory rate	20-60 beats/min	Adjusted to age; higher than normal may limit hypercapnia
Inspiratory/expiratory ratio	1:2 to 1:1	Check for inadvertent PEEP
FiO_2	<60%-80%	Depends on how the diseased lung may be recruited PaO_2 40-60 mm Hg, SpO_2 85%-95%

High-Frequency Oscillatory Ventilation

Amplitude pressure	30-50 cm H_2O	To achieve visible chest vibrations
Mean airway pressure	15-30 cm H_2O	To achieve adequate chest recruitment (7 to 9 ribs)
Respiratory rate	3-10 Hz	Decrease to increase tidal volume (usually not measured)
Inspiratory/expiratory ratio	1:3 to 1:1	1:1 more appropriate in diffuse lung injury
FiO_2	<60%-80%	Depends on whether the lung may be recruited

ICP, Intracranial pressure.
From Fuhrman BP et al: *Pediatric critical care,* ed 4, Philadelphia, 2011, Saunders.

therapy more than 2 wk after the onset of ARDS may increase the risk of death.

- Nutritional support: nutritional support, preferably administered by the enteral route, is necessary to maintain adequate colloid oncotic pressure and intravascular volume. The inclusion of eicosapentaenoic acid from fish oil may be beneficial in improving ventilation requirements and length of stay in patients with ARDS.
- Tracheostomy: tracheostomy is warranted in patients requiring >2 wk of mechanical ventilation; discussion regarding tracheostomy should begin with patient (if alert and oriented) and family members/legal guardian after 5 to 7 days of ventilatory support.
- Some form of deep vein thrombosis prophylaxis is indicated in all patients with ARDS.
- Stress ulcer prophylaxis with sucralfate suspension (by nasogastric tube), or IV proton pump inhibitors or H_2 blockers.
- The use of surfactant remains controversial. Patients who receive surfactant have a greater improvement in gas exchange in the initial 24-hour period than patients who receive standard therapy alone; however, the use of exogenous surfactant does not improve survival.

DISPOSITION

- Patients who survive ARDS are at risk of diminished functional capacity, mental illness, and decreased quality of life. Prognosis for ARDS varies with the underlying cause. Prognosis is worse in patients with chronic liver disease, nonpulmonary organ dysfunction, sepsis, and advanced age.
- Elevated values of dead space fraction ([$Paco_2$ − $Peco_2$]/$Paco_2$; normal is <0.3) is associated with an increased risk of death.
- In ARDS, the percentage of potentially recruitable lung is variable and associated with the response to PEEP.
- Overall mortality rate varies between 32% and 45%. Most deaths are attributable to sepsis or multiorgan dysfunction rather than primary respiratory causes.
- Recent trials have shown that as compared with the current standard of care, a ventilator strategy using esophageal measures to estimate the transpulmonary pressure significantly improves oxygenation and compliance. Further trials will determine if this approach should be widely adapted.
- Strategies for treatment of life-threatening refractory hypoxemia (prone positioning,

inhaled nitric acid, extracorporeal membrane oxygenation (ECMO), high-frequency oscillatory ventilation, recruitment maneuvers) may improve oxygenation, but their impact on mortality remains unproven. Use of ECMO in combination with lung protective ventilation was found to be beneficial as a treatment strategy early in the course of ARDS related to H1N1 infection. Extracorporeal gas exchange may allow the use of low tidal volumes and lower levels of inspired oxygen and use of higher PEEP if desired. ECMO is costly and labor-intensive. The role and proper use of ECMO for patients with ARDS have not been clearly defined. General indications for venovenous ECMO in severe cases of ARDS are:

- ○ Severe hypoxemia (e.g., ratio of PaO_2 to FiO_2 <80 despite the application of high levels of PEEP [typically 15 to 20 cm H_2O]) for at least 6 hr in patients with potentially reversible respiratory failure
- ○ Uncompensated hypercapnia with acidemia (pH <7.15) despite the best accepted standard of care for management with a ventilator
- ○ Excessively high end-inspiratory plateau pressure (>35 to 45 cm H_2O, according to the patient's body size) despite the best accepted standard of care for management with a ventilator

REFERRAL

Surgical referral for tracheostomy (see "Acute General Rx").

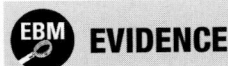 **EVIDENCE**

available at www.expertconsult.com

SUGGESTED READINGS

available at www.expertconsult.com

RELATED CONTENT

Acute Respiratory Distress Syndrome (ARDS) (Patient Information)

AUTHOR: **FRED F. FERRI, M.D.**

BASIC INFORMATION

DEFINITION

The acute cessation of urinary flow; inability to void.

SYNONYMS

Inability to urinate

ICD-9CM CODES
788.20 Retention of urine, unspecified

EPIDEMIOLOGY & DEMOGRAPHICS

INCIDENCE: Can occur in any age group and both sexes. It is the most common urologic emergency.
PEAK INCIDENCE: Males older than age 60. Over a 5-year period, AUR will occur in 10% of men older than 70 and one third of men older than 80.
PREVALENCE: Increased longevity has caused an increase in prevalence.
PREDOMINANT SEX AND AGE: Men older than 60 years.
GENETICS: None known.
RISK FACTORS: Obstructive risk factors include benign prostatic hypertrophy (BPH) and bladder, pelvic, and urethral masses. Acute trauma, surgery, medications (especially over-the-counter [OTC] antihistamines), neurologic disease, and infection can be contributing or precipitating factors, particularly when superimposed on obstructive risk factors.

PHYSICAL FINDINGS & CLINICAL PRESENTATION

- Patients will present with the acute inability to pass urine.
- Pain in the lower abdomen and suprapubic region is typical (this is not typically present with chronic urinary retention due to the more gradual onset).
- The bladder may be palpable on abdominal or rectal exam. There may be tenderness with deep palpation.
- Patients with cognitive deficits may present with restlessness, discomfort, worsened confusion, or delirium but may not be able to give the history of urinary retention.

ETIOLOGY

- Most commonly the result of obstruction from various causes, including BPH and bladder and pelvic masses.
- Nonobstructive causes include medications, surgery, trauma, neurologic disease, and infection.
- Particularly in older patients, the acute presentation may be due to multifactorial causes, with an underlying obstructive risk factor and an acute precipitant.
- In women, AUR may be caused by benign tumors (especially fibroids); malignant tumors of pelvic, urethral, or vaginal origin; postpartum vulvar edema; or labial fusion.
- Infection such as prostatitis, urethritis, and genital herpes and herpes zoster can also cause AUR.

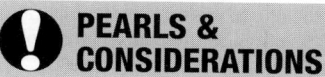 **DIAGNOSIS**

DIFFERENTIAL DIAGNOSIS

- AUR is typically self-evident to the cognitively intact patient, and to the physician. Differential diagnosis focuses on the underlying cause of the problem.

WORKUP

- History should focus on urologic symptoms, including dysuria, hematuria, history of retention, and urologic cancer.
- Review of symptoms (ROS) should include fever, back pain, neurologic symptoms, and rash.
- History should include a complete list of prescribed and OTC medications.
- Rectal exam for masses, fecal impaction, perineal sensation, and sphincter tone.
- Pelvic exam for female patients.
- Neurologic exam to rule out an underlying neurologic cause.

LABORATORY TESTS

- Creatinine level. Note that in acute retention this may not be elevated above baseline.
- Urinalysis and culture (which will be obtained via catheterization).
- BUN, electrolytes
- Prostate-specific antigen (PSA) testing is not helpful in the acute situation, as it is expected to be elevated during an episode of retention.

IMAGING STUDIES

- Imaging may not be necessary when AUR is felt to be due to reversible causes.
- Ultrasound may be valuable, particularly if there is suspicion of a pelvic mass.
- Pelvic computed tomography (CT) scan is done if, on physical exam or ultrasound, masses are found requiring further evaluation.
- Magnetic resonance imaging (MRI) is used when symptoms suggest spinal cord problems.
- Evaluation of bladder function may be considered after initial management, particularly in women with no evidence of anatomic obstruction.

TREATMENT

NONPHARMACOLOGIC THERAPY

- Given that AUR recurs 68% of the time when caused by BPH, consider surgical treatment for this issue. Transurethral resection of the prostate (TURP) should be delayed until at least 30 days after the episode of AUR, to minimize surgical complications.

ACUTE GENERAL Rx

- Prompt bladder decompression and drainage is the initial management of AUR.
- Urethral catheterization should be promptly initiated if the patient has no history of recent genitourinary (GU) surgery.

- If there is a history of recent surgery, suprapubic catheterization is indicated.
- Partial drainage and clamping of catheter is not necessary and may increase the risk of urinary tract infection (UTI).
- Clean intermittent catheterization (CIC) may be considered, although in the acute setting it may be limited by patient acceptance and the time required for teaching this technique. Use of CIC may improve the rate of spontaneous voiding.

CHRONIC Rx

- Consider catheter removal in 2 to 3 days, particularly in patients younger than 65 years old, when the catheterized volume is less than 1 L, and when a precipitating event can be identified.
- Otherwise 1 to 2 weeks of catheterization should be considered before voiding trial.
- Alpha blockers are effective in treatment of the symptoms of BPH and may increase the success of trials of early removal of catheter.
- 5-Alpha reductase inhibitors are not effective for acute management when AUR is caused by BPH, due to slow onset of the decrease of prostate volume.

COMPLEMENTARY & ALTERNATIVE MEDICINE

- None noted.

DISPOSITION

- Patients may be sent home if close follow-up can be assured.
- Hospital admission may be needed, particularly in patients with urosepsis or when retention is due to malignancy or spinal cord compression.

REFERRAL

- To urology, particularly in cases where the underlying cause cannot be addressed acutely or is not self-limited.
- To gynecology when gynecologic masses are the underlying cause of AUR.

PEARLS & CONSIDERATIONS

PREVENTION

Patients with BPH should avoid the use of antihistamines, sedatives, and other medications that can precipitate acute retention.

PATIENT/FAMILY EDUCATION

Education regarding catheter use and care is helpful in patients who are discharged to home.

SUGGESTED READINGS
available at www.expertconsult.com

AUTHOR: **MARGARET TRYFOROS, M.D.**

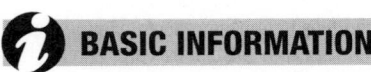

DEFINITION

Addison disease is characterized by inadequate secretion of corticosteroids resulting from partial or complete destruction of the adrenal glands.

SYNONYMS

Primary adrenocortical insufficiency
Adrenal insufficiency

ICD-9CM CODES
255.4 Addison disease

EPIDEMIOLOGY & DEMOGRAPHICS

PREVALENCE: Five cases/100,000 persons
PREDOMINANT SEX: Female/male ratio of 2:1

PHYSICAL FINDINGS & CLINICAL PRESENTATION

- Addison disease may present insidiously with nonspecific symptoms. A high index of suspicion is required for diagnosis. About half of patients may present acutely with adrenal crises.
- Hyperpigmentation of skin (Fig. E1-43) and mucous membranes is a cardinal sign of Addison disease: more prominent in palmar creases, buccal mucosa, pressure points (elbows, knees, knuckles), perianal mucosa, and around areolas of nipples
- Hypotension, postural dizziness
- Generalized weakness, chronic fatigue, malaise, anorexia
- Amenorrhea and loss of axillary hair in females

ETIOLOGY

- Autoimmune destruction of the adrenal glands (80% of cases)
- Tuberculosis (TB) (15% of cases)
- Carcinomatous destruction of the adrenal glands, lymphoma
- Adrenal hemorrhage (anticoagulants, trauma, coagulopathies, pregnancy, sepsis)
- Adrenal infarction (antiphospholipid syndrome, arteritis, thrombosis)
- AIDS (adrenal insufficiency develops in 30% of patients with AIDS, often cytomegalovirus [CMV] adrenalitis)
- Other: sarcoidosis, amyloidosis, hemochromatosis, Wegener's granulomatosis, postoperative, fungal infections (candidiasis, histoplasmosis)

DIAGNOSIS

DIFFERENTIAL DIAGNOSIS

Sepsis, hypovolemic shock, acute abdomen, apathetic hyperthyroidism in the elderly, myopathies, gastrointestinal malignancy, major depression, anorexia nervosa, hemochromatosis, salt-losing nephritis, chronic infection

WORKUP

- If the clinical picture is highly suggestive of adrenocortical insufficiency, the diagnosis can be made with the rapid adrenocorticotropic hormone (ACTH) test (Fig. E1-44):

1. Give 250 mcg ACTH (Sinachten, tetracosatrin) by IV push and measure cortisol levels at 0, 30, and 60 min.
2. An increase in serum cortisol level to peak concentration >500 nmol/L (18 mcg/dl) indicates a normal response. Cortisol level <18 mcg/dl at 30 or 60 min is suggestive of adrenal insufficiency.
3. Measure plasma ACTH. A high ACTH level confirms primary adrenal insufficiency.
- Critical illness-related corticosteroid insufficiency (e.g., in sepsis) is best established with the 1-mcg ACTH stimulation test in which cortisol levels are measured at baseline and 30 min after administration of ACTH. A level <25 mcg/dl (690 nmol/L) or an increment over baseline of <9 mcg (250 nmol/L) represents an inadequate adrenal response.
- Secondary adrenocortical insufficiency (caused by pituitary dysfunction) can be distinguished from primary adrenal insufficiency by the following:
1. Normal or low plasma ACTH level after rapid ACTH
2. Absence of hyperpigmentation
3. No significant impairment of aldosterone secretion (because aldosterone secretion is under control of the renin-angiotensin system)
4. Additional evidence of hypopituitarism (e.g., hypogonadism, hypothyroidism)

LABORATORY TESTS

- Hyponatremia, hyperkalemia
- Decreased glucose
- Increased BUN/creatinine ratio (prerenal azotemia)
- Mild normocytic, normochromic anemia, neutropenia, lymphocytosis, eosinophilia (significant dehydration may mask hyponatremia and anemia), hypercalcemia, metabolic acidosis
- A morning cortisol level >500 mmol/L (18 mcg/dl) generally excludes the diagnosis whereas a level <165 mmol/L (6 mcg/dl) is suggestive of Addison disease and requires further evaluation (see "Workup")
- Useful tests in evaluating the cause of Addison disease are: PPD (rule out TB), adrenal cortex antibodies and 21-hydroxylase antibodies (rule out autoimmune Addison disease), plasma very-long-chain fatty acids (rule out adrenoleukodystrophy)

IMAGING STUDIES

- Chest radiograph may reveal a small heart (Fig. E1-45).
- Abdominal radiograph: adrenal calcifications may be noted if the adrenocortical insufficiency is secondary to TB or fungal infection.
- Abdominal CT scan: small adrenal glands generally indicate either idiopathic atrophy or longstanding TB, whereas enlarged glands are suggestive of early TB or potentially treatable diseases.

TREATMENT

NONPHARMACOLOGIC THERAPY

- Perform periodic monitoring of serum electrolytes, vital signs, and body weight; liberal sodium intake is suggested.
- Periodic measurement of bone density may be helpful in identifying patients at risk for the development of osteoporosis.
- Patients should carry a MedicAlert bracelet and an emergency pack containing hydrocortisone 100-mg ampule, syringe, and needle.
- Patients and partners should be educated on how to give IM injection in case of vomiting or coma.

ACUTE GENERAL Rx

- Addisonian crisis is an acute complication of adrenal insufficiency characterized by circulatory collapse, dehydration, nausea, vomiting, hypoglycemia, and hyperkalemia.
1. Draw plasma cortisol level; do not delay therapy while waiting for confirming laboratory results.
2. Administer hydrocortisone 100 mg IV immediately, followed by 100 to 200 mg of hydrocortisone every 24 hours divided into 3 or 4 doses; if patient shows good clinical response, gradually taper dosage and change to oral maintenance dose (usually prednisone 7.5 mg/day).
3. Provide adequate volume replacement with D_5NS solution until hypotension, dehydration, and hypoglycemia are completely corrected. Large volumes (2 to 3 L) under continuous cardiac monitoring may be necessary in the first 2 to 3 hr to correct the volume deficit and hypoglycemia and to avoid further hyponatremia.
- Identify and correct any precipitating factor (e.g., sepsis, hemorrhage).

CHRONIC Rx

- Give hydrocortisone 15 to 20 mg PO every morning and 5 to 10 mg in late afternoon or prednisone 5 mg in morning and 2.5 mg hs.
- Give oral fludrocortisone 0.05 mg/day to 0.20 mg/day: this mineralocorticoid is necessary if the patient has primary adrenocortical insufficiency. The dose is adjusted based on the serum sodium level and the presence of postural hypotension or marked orthostasis.
- Instruct patients to increase glucocorticoid replacement in times of stress and to receive parenteral glucocorticoids if diarrhea or vomiting occurs. Typical supplementation varies from 25 mg PO qd of hydrocortisone for minor medical and surgical stress to 50 to 100 mg IV hydrocortisone q8h for sepsis-induced hypotension or shock.
- The administration of dehydroepiandrosterone 50 mg PO qd improves well-being and sexuality in women with adrenal insufficiency.

SUGGESTED READINGS
available at www.expertconsult.com

RELATED CONTENT
Addison's Disease (Patient Information)

AUTHOR: **FRED F. FERRI, M.D.**

BASIC INFORMATION

DEFINITION

Moderate drinking has been defined as two standard drinks (e.g., 12 oz of beer) per day and one drink per day for women and persons older than 65 yr. Although not generally included under the alcoholism topic, hazardous or at-risk drinking should also be considered. For men, *at-risk drinking* is defined as more than 14 drinks/wk or more than 4 drinks/occasion. For women, at-risk drinking is defined as approximately half that given for men.

The American Psychiatric Association defines diagnostic criteria for *alcohol withdrawal* as follows:
A. Cessation of (or reduction in) alcohol use that has been heavy and prolonged.
B. Two (or more) of the following, developing within several hours to a few days after criterion A:
   1. Autonomic hyperactivity (e.g., sweating or pulse rate >100 beats/min)
   2. Increased hand tremor
   3. Insomnia
   4. Nausea and vomiting
   5. Transient visual, tactile, or auditory hallucinations or illusions
   6. Psychomotor agitation
   7. Anxiety
   8. Grand mal seizures
C. The symptoms in criterion B cause clinically significant distress or impairment in social, occupational, or other important areas of functioning.

The symptoms are not attributable to a general medical condition and are not better accounted for by another mental disorder.

SYNONYMS

Alcohol abuse
Substance abuse

ICD-9CM CODES
303.9 Alcoholism

EPIDEMIOLOGY & DEMOGRAPHICS

INCIDENCE (IN U.S.):
- The clinical history suggests alcohol problems in 15% to 20% of patients in primary care and hospitalized patients. In the U.S., alcohol abuse generates nearly $223 billion in annual economic costs. An estimated 9% of adults in the U.S. have alcohol dependence.
- 20% achieve abstinence without help; 70% achieve sobriety for 1 yr.

PREVALENCE (IN U.S.): 7% of population ≥18 yr

PREDOMINANT SEX:
- Lifetime risk for males 8% to 10%
- Lifetime risk for females 3% to 5%

PEAK INCIDENCE: 20 to 40 yr. The most common age range for initial treatment of alcohol dependence is 35 to 45 yr. However, the peak period for meeting alcohol dependence criteria is ≥10 years earlier.

GENETICS: More common with a family history of alcoholism and in patients of Irish, Scandinavian, and Native American descent

PHYSICAL FINDINGS & CLINICAL PRESENTATION

- Recurring minor trauma
- Gastrointestinal bleeding from gastritis and/or varices
- Pancreatitis (acute and chronic)
- Liver disease
- Odor of alcohol on breath
- Tremulousness
- Tachycardia
- Peripheral neuropathy
- Recent memory loss

ETIOLOGY

- Social and genetic factors important
- Risk factors:
  1. Broken homes
  2. Unemployment
  3. Divorce
  4. Recurrent depression
  5. Addiction to another substance, including tobacco

DIAGNOSIS

WORKUP

- Several screening tests (CAGE, TWEAK, CRAFFT, AUDIT-C) are available. The four-item CAGE (feeling need to Cut down, Annoyed by criticism, Guilty about drinking, and need for an Eye-opener in the morning) is the most popular screening test in primary care (Fig. E1-46). A positive response should lead to further questioning. The sensitivity of the CAGE ranges from 43% to 94% and its specificity ranges from 70% to 97%. The five-item TWEAK scale (Tolerance, Worry, Eye-openers, Amnesia, [K] cut down) and the TACE questionnaire (Tolerance, Annoyance, Cut down, Eye-opener) are designed to screen pregnant women for alcohol misuse. They detect lower levels of alcohol consumption that may pose risks during pregnancy. The CRAFFT questionnaire (riding in Car with someone who was drinking, using alcohol to Relax, using alcohol while Alone, Forgetfulness, criticism from Friends and Family, Trouble) is useful as a screening tool for adolescents. Its sensitivity is 92% and specificity 64% for alcohol abuse. Single-question screening about alcohol consumption in a day ("When was the last time you had more than X drinks in a day?" [where X = 5 for men and 4 for women]) with the threshold set at "in the past 3 months" is 85% sensitive and 70% specific in men and 82% and 70% in women for unhealthy alcohol use. The 3-question AUDIT-C is a shorter form of the 10-item AUDIT, and the questions center on the quantity and frequency of alcohol use. It asks how often someone has had a drink containing alcohol, how many standard drinks containing alcohol one consumes on a typical day when one is drinking, and how often one has six or more drinks on one occasion. Scoring ranges from 0-4 on each question with a total score range of 0-12. A total score of 3 or higher for women and 4 or higher for men indicates alcohol use disorder and need for further assessment. Its sensitivity ranges from 85% in Hispanic women to 95% in white men.

- Laboratory evaluation (see below).

LABORATORY TESTS

- Lab tests alone do not accurately detect alcohol problems but can help identify medical complications related to alcohol use, such as pancreatitis or cirrhosis.
- Gamma-glutamyltransferase (GGTP), generally elevated
- Liver transaminases (alanine aminotransferase [ALT], aspartate aminotransferase [AST]), often elevated, may be normal or low in advanced liver disease.
- Low albumin level, hypophosphatemia, hypomagnesemia from malnutrition
- Complete blood count (CBC) reveals elevated mean corpuscular volume from toxic effect of alcohol on erythrocyte development in nutritional deficiencies.
- Stool for occult blood may be positive as a result of gastritis or variceal bleeding
- RBC folate, vitamin B_{12} level, vitamin B_6, vitamin B_1 level

IMAGING STUDIES

Indicated only with a history of trauma. CT or ultrasound of abdomen may reveal fatty liver or cirrhosis in advanced stages.

TREATMENT

NONPHARMACOLOGIC THERAPY

- Twelve-step facilitation, cognitive behavioral therapy, and motivational enhancement therapy improve the chances of recovery in patients with alcohol abuse and dependence.
- Depression, if present, should be treated at same time alcohol is withdrawn.

ACUTE GENERAL Rx

Alcohol withdrawal syndrome (AWS) occurs when a person stops ingesting alcohol after prolonged consumption. It can result in four possible clinical patterns depending on the severity of the patient's alcohol abuse and the time from the patient's previous alcohol ingestion. Fig. 1-47 illustrates typical symptoms depending on time course of alcohol withdrawal. Blood ethanol level decreases by ~20 mg/dl/hr (Fig. 1-48) in a normal person. Although discussed separately, these withdrawal states blend together in real life. Table E1-19 summarizes medications for the treatment of alcohol dependence.

1. **Tremulous state** (early alcohol withdrawal, "impending DTs," "shakes," "jitters").
   a. Time interval: usually occurs 6 to 8 hr after the last drink or 12 to 48 hr after reduction of alcohol intake; becomes most pronounced at 24 to 36 hr.
   b. Manifestation: tremors, mild agitation, insomnia, tachycardia; symptoms are relieved by alcohol.
   c. Detoxification can be in the outpatient (ambulatory) or inpatient setting. Candidates for outpatient detoxification should have a reasonable support system (e.g., reliable contact person) who can monitor progress and lack of any significant

comorbid conditions (e.g., suicide risk, seizure disorder, coexisting benzodiazepine dependence, prior unsuccessful outpatient detoxification, pregnancy, cirrhosis) or risk factors for severe withdrawal (age >40 yr, drinking >100 g of ethanol daily [e.g., 1 pint of liquor or eight 12-oz cans of beer, random blood alcohol concentration >200 mg/dl]).

d. Inpatient treatment:
  (1) Admit to medical floor (private room); monitor vital signs q4h; institute seizure precautions; maintain adequate sedation.
  (2) Administer lorazepam as follows:
    (a) Day 1: 2 mg PO q4h while awake and not lethargic.
    (b) Day 2: 1 mg PO q4h while awake and not lethargic.
    (c) Day 3: 0.5 mg PO q4h while awake and not lethargic.
    (d) NOTE: Hold sedation for lethargy or abnormal vital or neurologic signs. The preceding doses are only guidelines; it is best to titrate the dose case by case.
  (3) In patients with mild to moderate withdrawal and without history of seizures, individualized benzodiazepine administration (rather than a fixed-dose regimen) results in lower benzo-

diazepine administration and avoids unnecessary sedation. The Clinical Institute Withdrawal Assessment Scale for Alcohol, Revised (CIWA-Ar) scale can be used to measure the severity of alcohol withdrawal. It consists of 10 items: nausea; tremor; autonomic hyperactivity; anxiety; agitation; tactile, visual, and auditory disturbances; headache; and disorientation. Each item is assigned a score from 0 to 7. For example, in the "agitation" category 0 indicates normal activity, and 7 indicates that the patient constantly thrashes about. For the category of "tremor," 0 indicates that tremor is not present and 7 that tremor is severe, even with arms not extended. The maximum total score is 67. Patients with mild AWS symptoms (CIWA-Ar score <8 to 10 can be monitored on an outpatient basis. Benzodiazepines are recommended in patients with substantial withdrawal symptoms (CIWA-Ar score >12). Patients with CIWA-Ar score of ≥15 should be admitted to detox unit. In-patient treatment is also recommended for patients with history of withdrawal seizures and for those with suicidal ideation and significant comorbidities.

(4) Beta-adrenergic blockers: beta-blockers are useful for controlling blood pressure and tachyarrhythmias. However, they do not prevent progression to more serious symptoms of withdrawal and, if used, should not be administered alone but in conjunction with benzodiazepines. Beta-blockers should be avoided in patients with contraindications to their use (e.g., bronchospasm, bradycardia, or severe congestive heart failure). Centrally acting alpha-adrenergic agonists such as clonidine ameliorate symptoms in patients with mild to moderate withdrawal but do not reduce delirium or seizures.
(5) Vitamin replacement: thiamine 100 mg IV or IM for at least 5 days plus oral multivitamins. The IV administration of glucose can precipitate Wernicke's encephalopathy in alcoholics with thiamine deficiency; therefore thiamine administration should precede IV dextrose.
(6) Hydration PO or IV (high-caloric solution): if IV, glucose with Na^+, K^+, Mg^{2+}, and phosphate replacement prn.
(7) Laboratory studies.
  (a) CBC, platelet count, INR.
  (b) Electrolytes, glucose, blood urea nitrogen, creatinine.
  (c) GGTP, ALT, AST.
  (d) Phosphorus and magnesium.
  (e) Serum vitamin B_{12} and folic acid (if megaloblastic features in blood smear).
(8) Diagnostic imaging: generally not necessary; if subdural hematoma is suspected (evidence of trauma, persistent lethargy), a CT scan should be ordered.
(9) Social rehabilitation: group therapy such as Alcoholics Anonymous; identification and treatment of social and family problems should be initiated during the patient's hospital stay.

2. Alcoholic hallucinosis:
  a. Manifestations: hallucinations usually are auditory, but hallucinations occasionally are visual, tactile, or olfactory; usually there is no clouding of sensorium as in delirium (clinical presentation may be mistaken for an acute schizophrenic episode). Disordered perceptions become most pronounced after 24 to 36 hr of abstinence.
  b. Treatment: same as for DTs (see "withdrawal seizures").
3. Withdrawal seizures ("rum fits"):
  a. Time interval: usually occurs 7 to 30 hr after cessation of drinking, with a peak incidence between 13 and 24 hr.
  b. Manifestations: generalized convulsions with loss of consciousness; focal signs are usually absent; consider further investigation with CT scan of head and electroencephalography if clearly

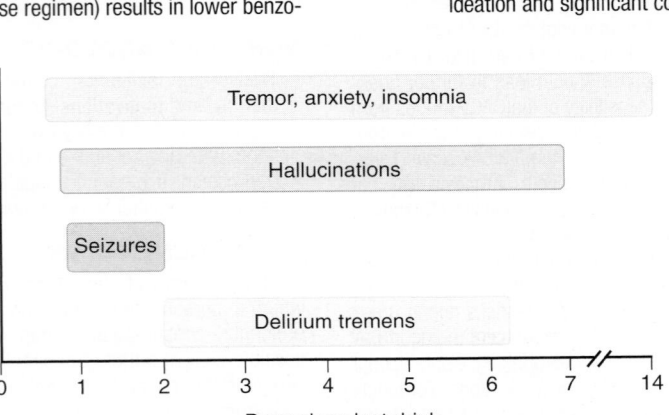

FIGURE 1-47 Time course of alcohol withdrawal. (From Goldman L, Schafer AI: *Goldman's Cecil medicine*, ed 24, Philadelphia, 2012, Saunders.)

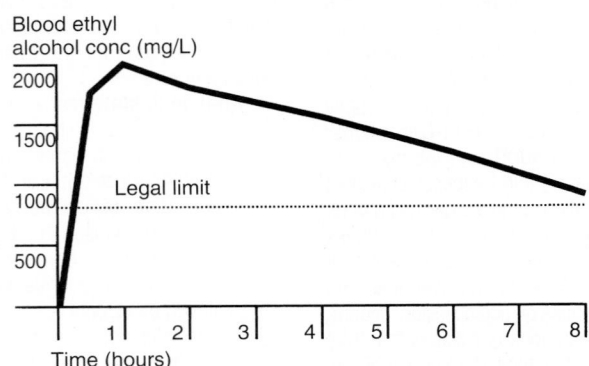

FIGURE 1-48 Blood concentrations after oral administration of ethyl alcohol (2 ml/kg). The concentration declines in a zero-order fashion at an average rate of 190 mg/L each hour. (From Souhami RL, Moxham J: *Textbook of medicine*, ed 4, London, 2002, Churchill Livingstone.)

indicated (e.g., presence of focal neurologic deficits, prolonged postictal confusion state). In addition, in a febrile patient who is having a seizure or altered mental state, a lumbar puncture is necessary.

c. Treatment:

(1) Diazepam 2.5 mg/min IV until seizure is controlled (check for respiratory depression or hypotension) may be beneficial for prolonged seizure activity; IV lorazepam 1 to 2 mg q2h can be used in place of diazepam. Withdrawal seizures generally are self-limited and treatment is not required; the use of phenytoin or other anticonvulsants for short-term treatment of alcohol withdrawal seizures is not recommended.

(2) Thiamine 100 mg IV, followed by IV dextrose, should also be administered.

(3) Electrolyte imbalances (increased Mg^{2+}, decreased K^+, increased or decreased Na^+, decreased PO_4^{3-}) that may exacerbate seizures should be corrected.

4. DTs:

a. Time interval: variable; usually occurs within 1 wk after reduction or cessation of heavy alcohol intake and persists for 1 to 3 days. Peak incidence is 72 hr and 96 hr after the cessation of alcohol consumption.

b. Manifestations: profound confusion, tremors, vivid visual and tactile hallucinations, autonomic hyperactivity; this is the most serious clinical presentation of alcohol withdrawal (mortality rate is approximately 15% in untreated patients).

c. Treatment

(1) Admission to a detoxification unit where patient can be observed closely.

(2) Vital signs q30min (neurologic signs, if necessary).

(3) Use of lateral decubitus or prone position if restraints are necessary

(4) NPO: nasogastric tube for abdominal distention may be necessary but should not be routinely used.

(5) Laboratory studies: same as for early alcohol withdrawal.

(6) Vigorous hydration (4 to 6 L/day): IV with glucose (Na^+, K^+, PO_4^{3-} and Mg^{2+} replacement).

(7) Vitamins: thiamine 100 mg IV qd. The initial dose of thiamine should precede the administration of IV dextrose; multivitamins (may be added to the hydrating solution).

(8) Sedation: control of agitation should be achieved with rapid-acting sedative-hypnotic agents in adequate doses to maintain light somnolence for the duration of delirium.

(a) Initially: lorazepam 2 to 5 mg IM/IV repeated prn.

(b) Maintenance (individualized dosage): chlordiazepoxide, 50 to 100 mg PO q4-6h, lorazepam 2 mg PO q4h, or diazepam 5 to 10 mg PO tid; withhold

doses or decrease subsequent doses if signs of oversedation are apparent.

(c) Midazolam is also effective for managing DTs. Its rapid onset (sedation within 2 to 4 min of IV injection) and short duration of action (approximately 30 min) make it an ideal agent for titration in continuous infusion.

(9) Treatment of seizures (as previously described).

(10) Diagnosis and treatment of concomitant medical, surgical, or psychiatric conditions.

CHRONIC Rx

- See "Referral."
- Pharmacotherapies for alcoholism include:
  ○ Acamprosate is a synthetic compound with a chemical structure similar to the neurotransmitter gamma-aminobutyric acid and the amino acid neuromodulator taurine. Its mechanism of action is not completely understood. It is indicated for the maintenance of abstinence from alcohol in patients with alcohol dependence who are abstinent at treatment initiation. It should be used only as part of a comprehensive psychosocial treatment program. It does not cause a disulfiram-like reaction as a result of ethanol ingestion. Dose is two 333-mg tablets tid. Treatment should be initiated as soon as possible after the period of alcohol withdrawal, when the patient has achieved abstinence, and should be maintained if the patient relapses.
  ○ The long-acting opiate antagonist naltrexone inhibits the rewarding effects of alcohol. The starting dose is 25 mg/day, increased to 50 mg PO qd after 1 wk. An extended-release, once-monthly injection of naltrexone is also available and can be used along with psychosocial support to maintain alcohol abstinence. In patients with opioid dependence, naltrexone can precipitate acute withdrawal syndrome and should not be used at least 7 days from last opioid use. There are no established guidelines on the appropriate length of naltrexone treatment for alcohol dependence. One study recommends at least 3 mo of treatment.
  ○ Disulfiram (Antabuse). Dosage is 500 mg max qd for 1 to 2 wk, then 125 to 500 mg qd. It interferes with the metabolism of alcohol by inhibiting aldehyde dehydrogenase, causing an accumulation of acetaldehyde. It produces unpleasant symptoms (nausea, flushing, elevated blood pressure, headache, weakness) when alcohol is ingested. It is an older drug that is now rarely used.

DISPOSITION

See "Referral."

REFERRAL

- To Alcoholics Anonymous or Adult Children of Alcoholics
- Family members to Al-Anon or Al-A-Teen

- Many cities have Salvation Army Adult Rehabilitation centers; all patients accepted, regardless of ability to pay

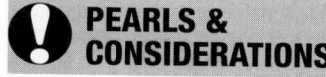
PEARLS & CONSIDERATIONS

COMMENTS

- Relative indications for inpatient alcohol detoxification are as follows: history of DTs or withdrawal seizures, severe withdrawal symptoms, concomitant psychiatric or medical illness, pregnancy, multiple previous detoxifications, recent high levels of alcohol consumption, and lack of reliable support network.
- Detoxification is not a stand-alone treatment but should serve as a bridge to a formal treatment program for alcohol dependence.
- The cure rate for alcoholism is highly disappointing, regardless of the modality. Only those who want to be helped will be helped. An effective strategy for the primary care physician is a prominently displayed sign in the office that states, "If you think you consume too many alcoholic beverages, please discuss it with me." Those who do open up the discussion can be given the facts in a nonjudgmental way and often can be helped. All too often problem drinkers lie on the questionnaire until they face a life-threatening health issue—and even then denial often reigns supreme.
- In a recent clinical trial, patients receiving medical management with naltrexone (100 mg/day), combined behavioral intervention (CBI), or both fared better on drinking outcomes, whereas acamprosate showed no evidence of efficacy, with or without CBI. No combination produced better efficacy than naltrexone or CBI alone in the presence of medical management.

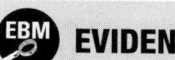
EVIDENCE

available at www.expertconsult.com

SUGGESTED READINGS

available at www.expertconsult.com

RELATED CONTENT

Alcohol Addiction (Patient Information)
Abuse, Drug (Related Key Topic)
AUTHOR: **FRED F. FERRI, M.D.**

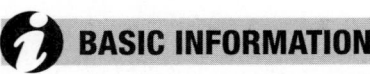

BASIC INFORMATION

DEFINITION

Alopecia is the term used to describe involuntary hair loss, typically on the scalp or beard, but possibly over the entire body. *Nonscarring alopecia* is hair loss without clinically apparent scarring, inflammation, or skin atrophy. *Scarring alopecia* is characterized by hair loss accompanied by tissue destruction in the form of scarring, inflammation, and/or skin atrophy.

SYNONYMS

Hair loss
Balding

ICD-9CM CODES
704.0   Alopecia
704.01   Alopecia Areata
704.02   Telogen Effluvium

EPIDEMIOLOGY & DEMOGRAPHICS

INCIDENCE: Depends on etiology, for example:
- Alopecia areata affects 1% of the U.S. population by age 50 yr.
- Androgenetic alopecia affects females << males but affects up to 40% of females by age 60, increasing after menopause.

GENETICS: Depends on etiology, for example:
- Androgenetic alopecia is autosomal dominant ± polygenic and can be inherited from one or both parents
- Certain scarring alopecias are more predominant in people with coarser hair.

ETIOLOGY

NONSCARRING
- Failure of follicle production
- Hair shaft abnormality
- Pattern hair loss, i.e., androgenetic alopecia
- Hair breakage, i.e., trichotillomania, traction alopecia, cosmetic overprocessing
- Problem with cycling (excess shedding), i.e., telogen effluvium, anagen effluvium, loose anagen syndrome, alopecia areata, syphilis

SCARRING
- Infectious: tinea capitis with inflammation (kerion), bacterial folliculitis as in dissecting folliculitis and folliculitis decalvans
- Neoplasm: alopecia mucinosa in cutaneous T-cell lymphoma or alopecia neoplastica due to metastatic carcinoma (breast cancer)
- Autoimmune: chronic cutaneous lupus erythematosus
- Congenital

CLINICAL FEATURES

HISTORY: A careful history must be taken and should include time course for hair loss, the pattern of hair loss, any recent change in life situation/stresses, any associated medical conditions, new medications, any family history of hair loss, and other skin/nail symptoms.

PHYSICAL EXAMINATION:
- General: patient's emotional response to hair loss
- Hair/skin:
  - Hair thinning/loss
  - May have fine downy hairs also referred to as vellous hairs
  - Skin may show changes consistent with inflammation, infection, and/or atrophy
  - Women may show virilization
  - Exclamation point hairs can be seen in alopecia areata
  - Broken hairs of different length may be seen in traumatic alopecia
  - Hairs that crack or crumble with palpation most often signify shaft damage due to overprocessing

DIAGNOSIS

WORKUP

- Hair pull—no shower for 24 hr, scalp with ~60 hairs is gently pulled, <6 hairs pulled is normal and more is suggestive of telogen effluvium, look for telogen bulbs on recovered hairs
- Punch biopsy—send two punches: one for vertical and one for horizontal sectioning for histopathologic analysis preferably by a dermatopathologist
- Fig. E1-49 describes the evaluation and treatment of alopecia in females.

LABORATORY TESTS

Initiate laboratory studies if not clear based on clinical presentation:
- CBC—rule out Fe deficiency
- Total Fe/ferritin—rule out subclinical Fe deficiency
- TSH—rule out underlying thyroid disease
- ANA—screen for autoimmune disease
- RPR—rule out cutaneous syphilis if history suggestive of increased risk

DIFFERENTIAL DIAGNOSIS

NONSCARRING

- *Telogen effluvium:* This type of alopecia is usually diffuse thinning that follows significant life stress (death of loved one, high fever, severe infection, crash dieting) or change in hormones (postpartum, change in or cessation of oral contraceptives). Patient often presents with a bag of hair that has fallen out. This is caused by a large number of anagen (growing) hairs entering telogen (dying phase) simultaneously. Telogen effluvium is more common in women.
- *Androgenetic alopecia:* Gradual thinning of hair and a trend toward finer hair, which in men has a typical pattern of receding anterior bitemporal hairline resulting in an M-shaped pattern and in women has a typical pattern of thinning along crown with or without frontotemporal thinning. This type of thinning is due to a combination of genetic predisposition and androgenic conversion of hair follicles into vellus-like follicles.
- *Alopecia areata:* Patches of hair loss (Fig. 1-50), typically 2-5 cm in diameter, with normal-appearing skin (including presence of follicular openings) at the base as well as occasional "exclamation point hairs," which are evidence of hair breaking off. Fingernails may show fine pitting. On biopsy, lymphocytes surround the hair bulb "like a swarm of bees," evidence of the autoimmune etiology.
  - AA Universalis (AAU)—generalized loss of body hair
  - AA Totalis (AAT)—complete loss of scalp hair
- *Tinea:* This type of hair loss is evident in round patches, possibly with scarring, erythema, and lymphadenopathy. This is the

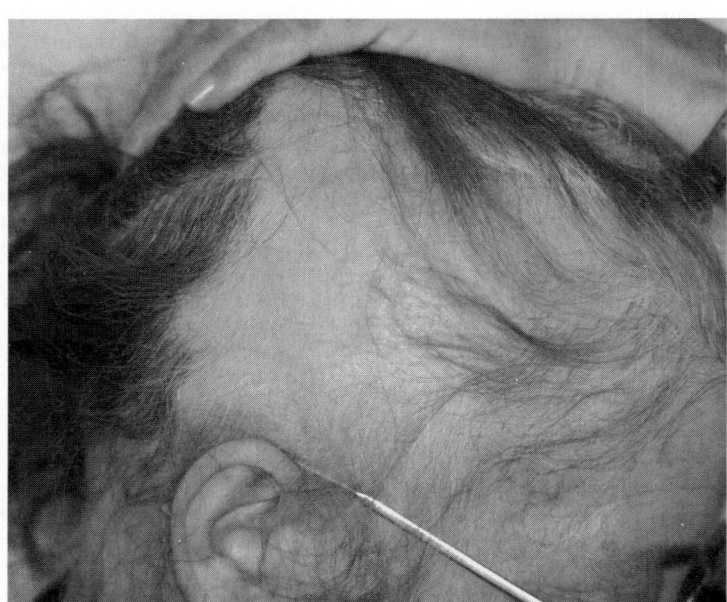

FIGURE 1-50 Alopecia areata: patchy hair loss. The alopecic area is devoid of hairs, and the scalp does not present inflammatory changes. (From Goldman L, Schafer AI: *Goldman's Cecil medicine,* ed 24, Philadelphia, 2012, Saunders.)

more common type of hair loss in children. Diagnosis can be made by scraping the erythematous edge and placing the scraping with KOH under a microscope to check for hyphae. Wood's lamp only fluoresces if tinea is caused by *Microsporum* spp.; however, the more common (in the U.S.) *Trichophyton* spp. does not fluoresce. If a kerion (severe alopecia associated with bogginess) is present, it may cause scarring.

- *Traumatic alopecia:* This type of hair loss is in a pattern consistent with breaking off of hairs due to traction (hair pulling) or chemical agents (hair straightening or permanent). Etiology usually becomes apparent with careful history taking and visualizing the pattern of hair loss. In trichotillomania (Fig. 1-51) the alopecia area has an irregular shape, scalp excoriations may present, and hairs are broken at different lengths.

SCARRING

- *Lichen planus:* The hair loss associated with LP is typically associated with scaling and atrophy of pruritic, painful skin underlying the hair loss. This hair loss is more common in middle-aged women. While there are numerous variations in clinical presentation, the general clinical picture is one of a chronic inflammatory condition of the skin, nails, mucous membranes, and/or hair. The typical skin lesions are flat topped, violaceous lesions with white lines (Wickham's striae), while the typical oral lesions are milky white.
- *Chronic cutaneous (discoid) lupus erthematosus:* This type of hair loss frequently is evident in well-demarcated, erythematous plaques in chronically sun-exposed areas of skin. Lesions exhibit hypopigmentations or hyperpigmentations, atrophy, erythema, and scaling. It may be present concurrently with SLE or be the first presenting symptom of SLE, but in most cases it is a purely cutaneous condition.
- *Tinea with kerion:* A kerion represents an exuberant delayed-type hypersensitivity reaction to the tinea capitis, resulting in one (or many) inflamed boggy plaque(s) on the scalp depending on the severity of the infection.

Rx TREATMENT

- *Telogen effluvium:* Stop insulting stress/medication and in 3-4 months anagen recurs; hair density should be normalized by 12 months. Multiple medications have been shown to be an inciting factor and one should consider stopping them (these include but are not limited to enalapril, colchicine, levodopa, metoprolol, propranolol, oral contraceptives, and lithium). Full regrowth is expected in most cases.
- *Androgenetic alopecia:* For men, the most likely first-line treatment is oral finesteride (type II 5α-reductase inhibitor) which leads to lower levels of dihydrotestosterone. This leads to hair regrowth in about 6 months, but with cessation, hair returns to pattern of loss within 12 months. Topical minoxidil can be useful in partially restoring lost hair in both men and women. In woman with elevated androgens, antiandrogens such as spironolactone, flutamide, and cimetidine may be considered. Other options include surgical intervention with hair transplantation or hair flaps or the use of a hairpiece.
- *Alopecia areata:* Spontaneous remission occurs in patchy AA, but less commonly in AAT or AAU. Glucocorticoids (GCs) are the mainstay of treatment but have little effect on the long-term outcome of hair loss—topical GC for small patches, intralesional injection of high-potency GC, and even systemic steroids can all be temporarily effective but at the cost of glucocorticoid exposure. Induction of allergic contact dermatitis using short-contact anthralin therapy or squaric acid sensitization can be effective but tends to have significant local discomfort, limiting its use. Topical photochemotherapy has shown some beneficial outcomes with alopecia areata. Photochemotherapy to the entire body is effective ~30% of the time.
- *Tinea capitis:* To effectively treat tinea capitis, oral antifungal agents must be used. Griseofulvin is considered the drug of choice in the U.S., and the recommended time course is 6 wk to several months. Other oral agents to consider include terbinafine, itraconazole, fluconazole, or ketaconazole. If there is a kerion (area of boggy, purulent inflammation underlying the area of hair loss), the patient is at increased risk for scarring alopecia due to likely bacterial superinfection and a short course of oral steroids and treatment with an oral antibiotic must be considered.
- *Traumatic alopecia:* First priority is stopping inciting activity/agent, which ideally will lead to gradual resolution of hair loss and hair regrowth.
- *Lichen planus:* Associated hair loss is often permanent; however, for symptomatic control of itching and pain, topical or oral glucocorticoids may be considered.
- *Chronic cutaneous discoid erythematosus:* The best prevention is sun protection, with SPF lotion. Treatment options center around the cautious use of topical or intralesional glucocorticoids. Hydroxychloroquinone and retinoids are also used with caution.

REFERRAL
Dermatology

PATIENT/FAMILY EDUCATION
Alopecia areata: www.naaf.org

SUGGESTED READINGS
available at www.expertconsult.com

AUTHOR: **MARGARET LEKANDER DOBSON, M.D.**

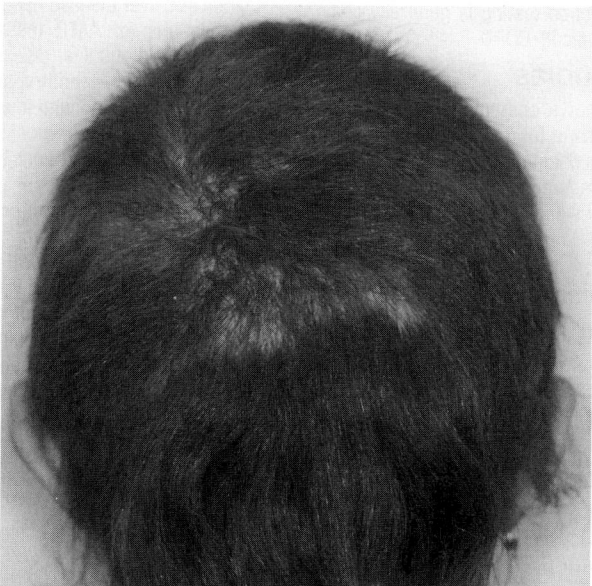

FIGURE 1-51 Trichotillomania: patchy hair loss. The alopecic area has an irregular shape and present hairs are broken at different lengths. Also note scalp excoriations. (From Goldman L, Schafer AI: *Goldman's Cecil medicine,* ed 24, Philadelphia, 2012, Saunders.)

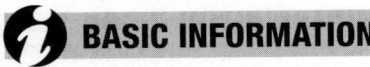

BASIC INFORMATION

DEFINITION

Alpha-1-antitrypsin deficiency is a genetic deficiency of the protease inhibitor alpha-1-antitrypsin that results in a predisposition to pulmonary emphysema and hepatic cirrhosis.

SYNONYMS

AATD

ICD-9CM CODES

277.6 Alpha-1-antitrypsin deficiency

EPIDEMIOLOGY & DEMOGRAPHICS

- Underrecognized by clinicians, but accounts for approximately 2% of chronic obstructive pulmonary disease (COPD) cases in Americans
- Inherited as an autosomal codominant disorder
- Most frequent mutation is in the *SERPINA 1* gene (previously known as *PI* gene)
- Most common alleles are:
  - normal "M" allele (95% frequency in the U.S.)
  - deficient variant "Z" allele (1% to 2%)
  - deficient variant "S" allele (2% to 3%)
- Severe deficiency is most commonly due to homozygotes ZZ
- Risk of COPD is increased with SZ genotype, especially in those who smoke
- Risk of lung disease in heterozygotes (MZ) is uncertain
- One in 10 individuals of European descent carries one of two mutations that may result in partial alpha-1-antitrypsin deficiency

PHYSICAL FINDINGS & CLINICAL PRESENTATION

- Physical findings and clinical presentation are varied and depend on phenotype (see "Etiology")
- Most often affects the lungs but can also involve liver and skin
- Classically associated with early-onset, severe, lower-lobe predominant panacinar emphysema; bronchiectasis may also be seen
- Symptoms are similar to "typical" COPD presentation (dyspnea, cough, sputum production)
- Liver involvement includes neonatal cholestasis, cirrhosis in children and adults, and primary carcinoma of the liver
- Panniculitis is the major dermatologic manifestation

ETIOLOGY

- Degree of alpha-1-antitrypsin deficiency depends on phenotype.
- "MM" represents the normal genotype and is associated with alpha-1-antitrypsin levels in the normal range.
- Mutation most commonly associated with emphysema is Z, with homozygote (ZZ) resulting in approximately 85% deficit in plasma alpha-1-antitrypsin concentrations.
- Development of emphysema is believed to result from an imbalance between the proteolytic enzyme elastase, produced by neutrophils, and alpha-1-antitrypsin, which normally protects lung elastin by inhibiting elastase.
- Deficiency of alpha-1-antitrypsin increases risk of early-onset emphysema, but not all alpha-1-antitrypsin deficient individuals will develop lung disease.
- Smoking increases risk and accelerates onset of COPD.
- Liver disease is caused by pathologic accumulation of alpha-1-antitrypsin in hepatocytes.
- Similar to lung disease, skin involvement is thought to be attributable to unopposed proteolysis in skin.

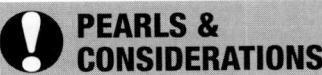

DIAGNOSIS

DIFFERENTIAL DIAGNOSIS

See "COPD."
See "Cirrhosis."

WORKUP

- Suspicion for alpha-1-antitrypsin deficiency usually results from emphysema developing at an early age and with basilar predominance of disease.
- Suspicion for alpha-1-antitrypsin deficiency resulting in liver disease or skin involvement may arise when other more common etiologies are excluded.

LABORATORY TESTS

- Serum level of alpha-1-antitrypsin can confirm or reject suspicion of deficiency.
- Investigate possibility of abnormal alleles with genotyping.
- Pulmonary function testing is generally consistent with "typical" COPD.

IMAGING STUDIES

- Chest x-ray shows characteristic emphysematous changes at lung bases.
- High-resolution chest CT usually confirms the lower-lobe predominant emphysema and may also show significant bronchiectasis.

TREATMENT

NONPHARMACOLOGIC THERAPY

- Avoidance of smoking is paramount.
- Avoidance of other environmental and occupational exposures that may increase risk of COPD.

ACUTE GENERAL Rx

Acute exacerbations of COPD from alpha-1-antitrypsin deficiency are treated in a similar fashion to "typical" COPD exacerbations.

CHRONIC Rx

- The goal of treatment in alpha-1-antitrypsin deficiency is to increase serum alpha-1-antitrypsin levels above a minimum, "protective" threshold.
- Although several therapeutic options are under investigation, IV administration of pooled human alpha-1-antitrypsin is currently the only approved method to raise serum alpha-1-antitrypsin levels. AAT augmentation therapy has been approved by the FDA for patients with AAT deficiency who have COPD. Augmentation therapy is expensive ($93,000 to $125,000/year) and requires lifelong treatment. However, given the cost and a lack of evidence of clinical benefit, a 2010 Cochrane Collaboration review noted that augmentation therapy with alpha-1-antitrypsin cannot be recommended.
- Organ transplantation for patients with end-stage lung or liver disease is also an option.

DISPOSITION

- Prognosis of patients with alpha-1-antitrypsin deficiency will depend on phenotype and level of deficiency.
- Among patients with severe alpha-1-antitrypsin deficiency, the most common underlying causes of death are emphysema (72%) and cirrhosis (10%).

REFERRAL

- Referral to specialists with experience in AAT deficiency is preferred
- Pulmonary and hepatology referrals for advanced lung and liver disease, or if replacement therapy is contemplated (e.g., moderate-severe lung disease)
- Lung and liver transplantation in suitable cases

PEARLS & CONSIDERATIONS

- The liver damage arising from the mutation is not from a deficiency in alpha-1-antitrypsin but from a pathologic accumulation of alpha-1-antitrypsin in hepatocytes.
- Strong association between PI*ZZ phenotypes and liver disease has prompted recommendations for AATD testing in individuals with unexplained liver disease.
- Consider alpha-1-antitrypsin deficiency in patients presenting with lower-lobe predominant emphysema; in most smokers without alpha-1-antitrypsin deficiency, emphysema predominates in the upper lobes.
- Alpha-1-antitrypsin deficiency is believed to be under-recognized.
- The American Thoracic Society and the European Respiratory Society recommend testing for AAT deficiency in all patients with COPD, emphysema, or asthma with irreversible obstruction, whereas the Global Initiative for Chronic Obstructive Lung Disease only recommends testing for those with early-onset COPD (age <45 yr) or a strong family history of COPD.

SUGGESTED READINGS

available at www.expertconsult.com

RELATED CONTENT

Chronic Obstructive Pulmonary Disease (Related Key Topic)
Cirrhosis (Related Key Topic)
Alpha-1-Antitrypsin Deficiency (Patient Information)

AUTHOR: **JOSEPH A. DIAZ, M.D., M.P.H.**

BASIC INFORMATION

DEFINITION

Dementia is a syndrome characterized by progressive loss of previously acquired cognitive skills including memory, language, insight, and judgment. Alzheimer's disease (AD) is believed to account for the majority (50% to 75%) of all cases of dementia.

ICD-9CM CODES
331.0 Alzheimer's disease
290.0 Senile dementia, uncomplicated

EPIDEMIOLOGY & DEMOGRAPHICS

INCIDENCE: Risk doubles every 5 yr after the age of 65; above the age of 85 the incidence is about 8%.

PREVALENCE: Currently an estimated 5.4 million Americans have AD; 6% between the ages of 65 and 74, 44% between 75 and 84, and 46% at 85 years and older.

PREDOMINANT SEX: Female

PHYSICAL FINDINGS & CLINICAL PRESENTATION

- Spouse or other family member, usually not the patient, notes insidious memory impairment.
- Patients have difficulties learning and retaining new information and handling complex tasks (e.g., balancing the checkbook), and have impairments in reasoning, judgment, spatial ability, and orientation (e.g., difficulty driving, getting lost away from home).
- Behavioral changes, such as mood changes and apathy, may accompany memory impairment. In later stages patients may develop agitation and psychosis.
- Atypical presentations include early and severe behavioral changes, focal findings on examination, parkinsonism, hallucinations, falls, or onset of symptoms younger than the age of 65.

DIAGNOSIS

There is no definitive imaging or laboratory test for the diagnosis of AD. Diagnosis is commonly made based on clinical history, a thorough physical and neurologic examination, and use of reliable and valid diagnostic criteria (i.e., DSM-IV or NINDCS-ADRDA) such as the following:

- Loss of memory and one or more additional cognitive abilities (aphasia, apraxia, agnosia, or other disturbance in executive functioning)
- Impairment in social or occupational functioning that represents a decline from a previous level of functioning and results in significant disability
- Deficits that do not occur exclusively during the course of delirium
- Insidious onset and gradual progression of symptoms
- Cognitive loss documented by neuropsychologic tests

- No physical signs, neuroimaging, or laboratory evidence of other diseases that can cause dementia (i.e., metabolic abnormalities, medication or toxin effects, infection, stroke, Parkinson's disease, subdural hematoma, or tumors)

The National Institute on Aging (NIA) and the Alzheimer's Association recommended new diagnostic criteria and guidelines for AD in 2011. These differ from prior DSM-IV or NINDCS-ADRDA criteria in that they now recommend that AD be considered a disease well before the onset of symptoms, they incorporate the use of biomarkers in diagnosis, and they define three distinct stages of AD: (1) *preclinical* AD, in which there is measurable biologic evidence of AD pathology but no symptoms; (2) *mild cognitive impairment* (MCI) due to AD, in which there is mild memory loss but no functional impairment at home or work; and (3) *dementia due to AD*.

DIFFERENTIAL DIAGNOSIS

- Cancer (brain tumor, meningeal neoplasia)
- Infection (AIDS, neurosyphilis, PML)
- Toxic/metabolic (EtOH, hypothyroidism, vitamin B_{12} deficiency, mercury exposure, drug effects)
- Organ failure (dialysis dementia, Wilson's disease)
- Vascular disorder (multiple strokes, severe small vessel changes, chronic vasculitides, or chronic subdural hematoma)
- Depression (pseudodementia)

WORKUP

HISTORY & GENERAL PHYSICAL EXAMINATION:

- Medication lists should always be reviewed for drugs or home remedies that may cause mental status changes.
- Patients should be screened for depression, because it can sometimes mimic dementia but also often occurs as a coexisting condition and should be treated.
- On examination, look for signs of metabolic disturbance, presence of psychiatric features, or focal neurologic deficits.

MENTAL STATUS TESTING: Brief mental status testing can be done easily and quickly in the office. Most commonly used is the Folstein Mini-Mental State Examination (MMSE). An MMSE score <24 (scores range from 0 to 30, with lower scores reflecting poorer performance) suggests cognitive impairment; however, the MMSE is not sensitive enough to detect mild dementia or dementia in patients with high baseline IQ. Scores may be spuriously low in patients with limited education, poor motor function, African American or Hispanic ethnicity, poor language skills, or impaired vision. The MMSE is perhaps most useful to follow AD patients for long-term outcomes.

Mental status testing should include tests that assess the following cognitive functions:
- Orientation: ask the patient to give the day, date, month, year, and place and to name the current president.
- Attention: ask the patient to recite the months of the year forward and in reverse.

- Verbal recall: ask the patient to remember four items; test for recall after a 1- and 5-min delay.
- Language: ask the patient to write and then read a sentence; have the patient name both common and less common objects.
- Visual-spatial: ask the patient to draw a clock and to set the hands of the clock at 11:10.

Patients with AD typically have trouble with verbal recall, plus visual-spatial or language deficits. Attention is usually preserved until the late stages of AD, so consider alternate diagnoses in patients who perform poorly on tests of attention.

LABORATORY TESTS

- CBC
- Serum electrolytes
- Glucose
- BUN/creatinine
- Liver and thyroid function tests
- Serum vitamin B_{12}
- Syphilis serology (RPR), if supported by clinical history
- HIV screening as appropriate
- Lumbar puncture if history or signs of cancer, infectious process, or when the clinical presentation is unusual (i.e., rapid progression of symptoms)
- EEG if there is history of seizures, episodic confusion, rapid clinical decline, or suspicion of Creutzfeldt-Jakob disease
- Measurement of apolipoprotein E genotyping, CSF tau and amyloid, and functional imaging including positron emission tomography (PET) or single proton emission computed tomography (SPECT) are not yet routinely indicated
- Brain biopsy (usually reserved for diagnoses such as prion disease, certain vasculitides)

IMAGING STUDIES

- CT scan or MRI to rule out hydrocephalus and mass lesions, including subdural hematoma
- Florbetapir-PET imaging of the brain correlates with the presence and density of beta-amyloid

TREATMENT

NONPHARMACOLOGIC THERAPY

- Patient safety, including risks associated with impaired driving, wandering behavior, leaving stoves unattended, and accidents, must be addressed with the patient and family early and appropriate measures implemented.
- Wandering, hoarding or hiding objects, repetitive questioning, withdrawal, and social inappropriateness often respond to behavioral therapies.

ACUTE GENERAL Rx

None

CHRONIC Rx

1. Symptomatic treatment of memory disturbance (Table 1-20):
   a. Cholinesterase inhibitors (ChEIs): FDA approved for the treatment of mild to moderate AD. Common side effects

include nausea, diarrhea, and anorexia and may be bothersome enough to require a slower escalation of dosage or switching to another agent.

b. NMDA receptor antagonist: memantine (Namenda)

FDA approved for the treatment of moderate to severe AD. Common side effects include constipation, dizziness, or headache. Memantine is contraindicated in patients with renal insufficiency or history of seizures.

2. Symptomatic treatment of neuropsychiatric and behavioral disturbances (Table 1-21). Depression, agitation, delusions, or hallucinations may respond to medications.

DISPOSITION & REFERRAL

- Patients with complex or atypical presentations or challenging management issues should be referred to a neurologist or another specialist with expertise in dementia.

- Approximately 1 in 8 hospitalized patients with AD who develop delirium will have at least one adverse outcome (e.g., institutionalization, cognitive decline, death) associated with delirium.
- Family education and support may help reduce need for skilled nursing facility, and reduce caregiver stress, depression, and burnout.

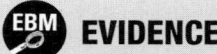

PEARLS & CONSIDERATIONS

The physician should make a thorough search for the treatable causes of dementia. Current American Academy of Neurology practice parameters recommend:

- Treat cognitive symptoms of AD with ChEIs.
- Treat agitation, psychosis, and depression.
- Encourage caregivers to participate in educational programs and support groups.

COMMENTS

- Ginkgo biloba is marketed widely as effective in delaying cognitive impairment; however, trials have shown that it is not effective in reducing the incidence of Alzheimer dementia or dementia overall.
- Higher midlife fitness levels seem to be associated with lower hazards of developing all-cause dementia later in life independent of cerebrovascular disease.
- Lower plasma beta-amyloid 42/40 is associated with greater cognitive decline among elderly persons without dementia over 9 yr, and this association is stronger among those with low measures of cognitive reserve.
- The *APOE* genotype provides information on the risk for AD, but the genotyping of patients raises ethical and emotional concerns. Because the benefits of genetic testing are often modest, and the tests themselves often imprecise in identifying risk, the test is generally discouraged. Recent trials, however, reveal that the disclosure of *APOE* genotyping results to adult children of patients with AD did not result in significant short-term psychological risks. Test-related distress was reduced among those who learned that they were *APOE*4 negative. Persons with high levels of emotional distress before undergoing genetic testing are more likely to have emotional difficulties after disclosure.

For additional information for patients, families, and clinicians, contact the following organizations:

- Alzheimer's Association (www.alz.org; 800-272-3900)
- Alzheimer's Disease Education and Referral Center (http://www.nia.nih.gov/Alzheimers; 800-438-4380)

TABLE 1-20 Symptomatic Treatment of Memory Disturbance

	Initial Dose	Target Dose
Donepezil	5 mg qd for 4-6 weeks	10 mg qd
Rivastigmine	1.5 mg bid with food, increase by 1.5 mg bid weekly	3-6 mg bid
Galantamine	4 mg bid with food, increase by 4 mg bid every 4 weeks	8-12 mg bid
Memantine	5 mg qd, increase by 5 mg weekly	10 mg bid

TABLE 1-21 Treatment of Behavioral and Neuropsychiatric Symptoms

	Initial Dose	Maximum Dose
Atypical Antipsychotics		
Olanzapine	2.5 mg qd to bid, may increase by 2.5 mg as needed	7.5 mg bid
Quetiapine	25 mg bid, may increase by 25 mg every 2 days	250 mg tid
Antidepressants		
Sertraline	25-50 mg qd, may increase by 25 mg every week	200 mg qd
Citalopram	10 mg qd, may increase after 1 week	20 mg qd

EBM EVIDENCE

available at www.expertconsult.com

SUGGESTED READINGS

available at www.expertconsult.com

RELATED CONTENT

AUTHOR: **TAMARA G. FONG, M.D., PH.D.**

BASIC INFORMATION

DEFINITION

Amaurosis fugax is a temporary loss of monocular vision caused by transient retinal ischemia.

ICD-9CM CODES
362.34 Amaurosis fugax

EPIDEMIOLOGY & DEMOGRAPHICS

INCIDENCE (IN U.S.): An uncommon but important presentation of carotid artery disease
PEAK INCIDENCE: ≥55 yr

PHYSICAL FINDINGS & CLINICAL PRESENTATION

- Onset is sudden, typically lasting seconds to minutes, and often accompanied by scotomas such as a shade or curtain being pulled over the front of the eye (usually downward).
- Vision loss can be complete or quadrantic.
- Acute stage: cholesterol emboli may be seen in retinal artery (*Hollenhorst plaque*): carotid bruits or other evidence of generalized atherosclerosis.
- If embolus is cardiac in origin, atrial fibrillation is often present.

ETIOLOGY

- Usually embolic from the internal carotid artery or the heart
- Giant cell arteritis causing inflammation of retinal arteries
- Hyperviscosity syndromes, such as sickle cell disease, which causes ischemia in the vascular territory of the ophthalmic artery
- Hypercoagulability states
- Transient vasospasm often associated with exercise

DIAGNOSIS

DIFFERENTIAL DIAGNOSIS

- Retinal migraine: in contrast to amaurosis, the onset of visual loss develops more slowly, usually over 15 to 20 min.
- Transient visual obscurations occur in the setting of papilledema; intermittent rises in intracranial pressure briefly compromise optic disc perfusion and cause transient visual loss lasting 1 to 2 seconds. The episodes may be binocular. If the visual loss persists at the time of evaluation (i.e., vision has not yet recovered), then the differential diagnosis should be broadened to include:
  ○ Anterior ischemic optic neuropathy: arteritic (classically GCA) or nonarteritic
  ○ Central retinal vein occlusion

WORKUP

- Workup should focus on embolic sources, but GCA should always be considered.

- Careful examination of retina; embolus may be visible and confirm the diagnosis (Fig. 1-52).
- Auscultation of arteries for carotid bruits.
- Examination of all pulses and for temporal artery tenderness.
- Inquire about symptoms of GCA (scalp tenderness, headache, fever, jaw claudication).
- Examine for signs of hemispheric stroke resulting from intracranial aneurysm (contralateral limb and facial weakness or sensory loss, aphasia, etc.).

LABORATORY TESTS

- Complete blood count with erythrocyte sedimentation rate and C-reactive protein.
- Serum chemistries, including lipid profile.
- Cardiac enzymes and ECG.
- Hypercoagulable workup is discretionary based on younger age and history.

IMAGING STUDIES

- Carotid Doppler imaging followed by MR or CT angiography as indicated.
- Transthoracic echocardiography is indicated to screen for embolization in patients with evidence of heart disease and in patients without an evident source for transient neurologic deficit. Transesophageal echocardiography is more sensitive for detecting cardiac sources of embolization (ventricular mural thrombus, atrial appendage, patent foramen ovale, aortic arch).
- MRI of the brain with diffusion-weighted imaging to look for infarcts, especially those presenting with focal neurologic disturbances.

TREATMENT

NONPHARMACOLOGIC THERAPY

- Diet (decrease saturated fatty acids and high-cholesterol foods)
- Exercise
- Cessation of tobacco use

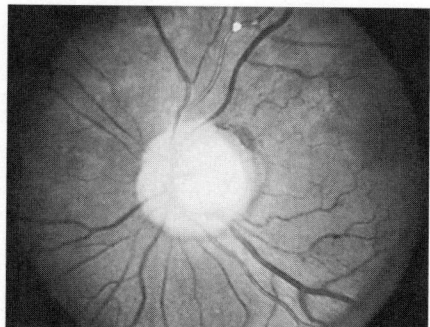

FIGURE 1-52 A cholesterol crystal embolus lodged at an arterial bifurcation. (From Stein JH [ed]: *Internal medicine*, ed 5, St Louis, 1998, Mosby.)

ACUTE GENERAL Rx

- Investigate as an emergency.
- Aspirin if etiology is presumed embolic.
- If GCA is suspected, start prednisone and refer for temporal artery biopsy within 48 hr (see "Giant Cell Arteritis" in Section I).

CHRONIC Rx

- Reduce risks by carotid endarterectomy or carotid stenting if stenosis >70%. Stenting may be performed in high-risk surgical candidates.
- Control hypertension and manage vascular risk factors.
- Antiplatelet therapy.
- Consider starting an HMG-CoA reductase inhibitor.

DISPOSITION

Among patients with >50% carotid stenosis who do not undergo carotid endarterectomy, those who present with transient monocular blindness have an approximate 10% risk of stroke in 3 yr compared with an approximate 20% risk in patients who present with a hemispheric transient ischemic attack (TIA).

REFERRAL

- Recommend referral to a neurologist for evaluation and workup.
- If significant carotid stenosis, consider carotid endarterectomy or carotid stenting for the following:
  1. High-grade (≥70%) stenosis
  2. Multiple TIAs despite medical therapy in the setting of high-grade or ulcerative disease

PEARLS & CONSIDERATIONS

- Cholesterol emboli in retinal arteries on funduscopy confirm the diagnosis.
- Recognize that transient visual loss has multiple other causes.

SUGGESTED READING
available at www.expertconsult.com

RELATED CONTENT

Carotid Stenosis (Related Key Topic)
Giant Cell Arteritis (Related Key Topic)
Transient Ischemic Attack (Related Key Topic)
Amaurosis Fugax (Patient Information)

AUTHOR: **TZU-CHING (TEDDY) WU, M.D.**

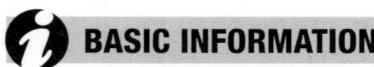

BASIC INFORMATION

DEFINITION

Amblyopia refers to a decrease in vision in one or both eyes in the presence of an otherwise normal ophthalmologic examination. The major types of amblyopia are strabismic, anisometropic (refractive), and combined strabismic and refractive. Less common types are ametropic and deprivation (rare).

SYNONYMS

Deprivation amblyopia
Occlusion amblyopia
Strabismus amblyopia
Refractive amblyopia
Organic or toxic amblyopias
Lazy eye

ICD-9CM CODES
368.00 Amblyopia

EPIDEMIOLOGY & DEMOGRAPHICS

INCIDENCE (IN U.S.): 1% to 5% of the general population. Amblyopia is the leading cause of vision loss in children. It is also the cause of permanent vision loss in 2.9% of adults.
PREVALENCE (IN U.S.): High incidence in premature infants with drug-dependent mothers and in neurologically impaired children. Children with a family history of strabismus or amblyopia are at increased risk.
PREDOMINANT SEX: None
PREDOMINANT AGE: Childhood
PEAK INCIDENCE: Childhood

PHYSICAL FINDINGS & CLINICAL PRESENTATION

Decreased vision using best refraction in the presence of normal corneal, lens, retinal, and optic nerve appearance (Fig. 1-53).

ETIOLOGY

- Visual deprivation
- Strabismus
- Occlusion with patching
- Refractive error organic lesions in the nervous system
- Toxins

DIAGNOSIS

DIFFERENTIAL DIAGNOSIS

- Central nervous system (CNS) disease (brainstem)
- Optic nerve disorders
- Corneal or other eye diseases
- Retinal disorders

WORKUP

- Complete eye examination to find cause of amblyopia or deprivation of vision. Referral to an ophthalmologist is recommended for any child with a visual acuity in either eye of ≤20/40 at age 3 to 5 yr or worse at age ≥6 yr or a two-line difference in acuity between eyes.
- Motility evaluation.

LABORATORY TESTS

Usually none

IMAGING STUDIES

Usually not necessary unless central nervous system (CNS) lesion suspected

TREATMENT

NONPHARMACOLOGIC THERAPY

- Treatment depends on the age of the patient, severity of amblyopia, and compliance with patching or atropine.
- Glasses or prisms to align eyes with minor deviations and improve vision.
- Patching and atropine are both effective. Atropine 1% is used daily for 6 mo; patching is

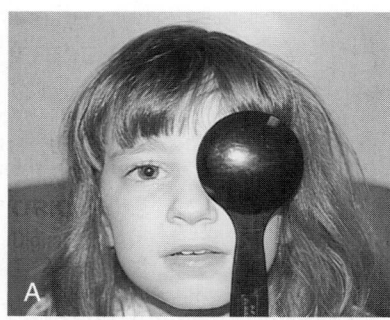
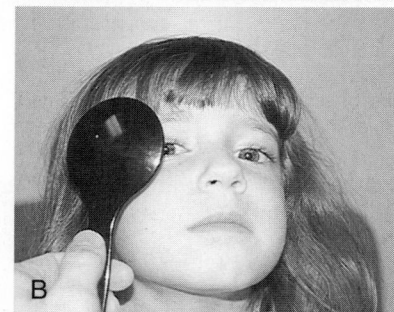

FIGURE 1-53 A, This child happily fixes with her right eye and does not object if the left eye is covered. **B,** When the right eye is covered she moves her head away and tries to remove the cover, demonstrating a fixation preference for the right eye and amblyopia of the left eye. (From Hoekelman R [ed]: *Primary pediatric care,* ed 3, St Louis, 1997, Mosby.)

used 2 to 6 hr/day for 6 mo. Patching may be more effective; 50% get best vision improvement by 16 wk.
- Removal of the cause of the amblyopia if possible.
- Surgery to align the eyes or remove obstruction to vision.

CHRONIC Rx

- Patching or optics, including prisms and atropine, most effective in 3- to 7-yr-olds; although treatment ideally should begin before age 5, a recent trial demonstrated that children may benefit even at an older age.
- Tapering the amount of time a patch is worn each day at the end of treatment reduces the risk of recurrence.

DISPOSITION

Immediate patching, alternating eyes daily

REFERRAL

To ophthalmologist if vision is compromised

PEARLS & CONSIDERATIONS

COMMENTS

- The earlier the referral, the better the outcome. Amblyopia is more responsive to treatment among children younger than 7 years of age. Although the average treatment response is smaller in children 7 to less than 13 years of age, some children show a marked response to treatment.
- The success of therapy is highly dependent on treatment compliance.
- Amblyopia recurs in 25% of children after patching is discontinued.

SUGGESTED READINGS

available at www.expertconsult.com

AUTHOR: **MELVYN KOBY, M.D.**

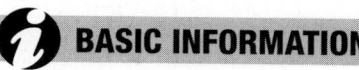 **BASIC INFORMATION**

DEFINITION

Amebiasis is an infection caused by the protozoal parasite *Entamoeba histolytica*. Although primarily an infection of the colon, amebiasis may cause extraintestinal disease, particularly liver abscess.

SYNONYMS

Amebic dysentery (when severe intestinal infection)

ICD-9CM CODES
006.9 Amebiasis

EPIDEMIOLOGY & DEMOGRAPHICS

INCIDENCE (IN U.S.): 1.2 cases per 100,00 U.S. population. Highest in institutionalized patients, and travelers to/immigrants from developing nations.
PREVALENCE (IN U.S.): 4% (80% of infections asymptomatic)
PREDOMINANT SEX:
- Equal sex distribution in general
- Striking male predominance of liver abscess
PREDOMINANT AGE: 2nd through 6th decades
PEAK INCIDENCE: Peaks at age 2 to 3 yr and >40 yr

PHYSICAL FINDINGS & CLINICAL PRESENTATION

- Often nonspecific
- Approximately 20% of cases symptomatic
  1. Diarrhea, which may be bloody
  2. Abdominal and back pain
- Abdominal tenderness in 83% of severe cases
- Fever in 38% of severe cases
- Hepatomegaly, right upper quadrant tenderness, and fever in almost all patients with liver abscess (may be absent in fulminant cases)

ETIOLOGY

- Caused by the protozoal parasite *E. histolytica*. *E. dispar* and *E. moshkovskii* are 10 times more common but nonpathogenic and difficult to distinguish from *E. histolytica*.
- Transmission by the fecal-oral route
- Infection usually localized to the large bowel, particularly the cecum where a localized mass lesion (ameboma) may form
- Extraintestinal infection in which the organism invades the bowel mucosa and gains access to the portal circulation

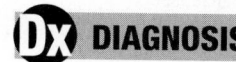 **DIAGNOSIS**

DIFFERENTIAL DIAGNOSIS

- Severe intestinal infection possibly confused with ulcerative colitis or other infectious enterocolitis syndromes, such as those caused by *Shigella*, *Salmonella*, *Campylobacter*, or invasive *Escherichia coli*
- In elderly patients: ischemic bowel possibly producing a similar picture

WORKUP

- Three stool specimens over a period of 7 to 10 days to search for cysts or trophozoites has a sensitivity of 85% to 95%, but microscopy cannot differentiate between the species
- Concentration and staining the specimen with Lugol's iodine or methylene blue to increase the diagnostic yield
- Fecal leukocytes not always present

LABORATORY TESTS

- Fecal ELISA antigen detection is specific for *E. histolytica* (87% percent sensitive) and also useful for diagnosis of liver abscess.
- Mucosal biopsy is occasionally necessary to look for cysts or trophozoites.

- Serum antibody assays specific for *E. histolytica* are available and are particularly sensitive and specific for extraintestinal infection or severe intestinal disease.
- Aspiration of abscess fluid is used to distinguish amebic from bacterial abscesses.

IMAGING STUDIES

Abdominal imaging studies (sonography or CT scan) to diagnose liver abscess

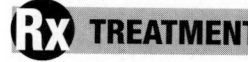 **TREATMENT**

ACUTE GENERAL Rx

- Metronidazole (750 mg PO tid for 10 days) is used in the treatment of mild to severe intestinal infection and amebic liver abscess; it may be administered intravenously when necessary.
- Follow with iodoquinol (650 mg PO tid for 20 days) to eradicate persistent cysts.
- For asymptomatic patients with amebic cysts on stool examination, use iodoquinol or paromomycin (500 mg PO tid for 7 days).
- Avoid antiperistaltic agents in severe intestinal infections to avoid risk of toxic megacolon.
- Liver abscess is generally responsive to medical management but surgical intervention indicated for extension of liver abscess into pericardium or for toxic megacolon.
- Table 1-22 summarizes drug treatment options for amebiasis in adults and children.

DISPOSITION

Host immunity incomplete and reinfection rate high for patients remaining at risk

REFERRAL

- For consultation with infectious diseases specialist for extraintestinal infection or persistent or relapsing intestinal infection
- For surgical consultation:
  1. For toxic megacolon
  2. For impending rupture of or extension of liver abscess into adjacent structures

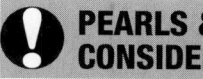 **PEARLS & CONSIDERATIONS**

COMMENTS

- Infection with other intestinal parasites, particularly *Giardia lamblia*, may coexist with amebiasis.
- There is a high prevalence of *E. dispar* in homosexual males, which is nonpathogenic but may be difficult to distinguish from the pathogen *E. histolytica*.

SUGGESTED READINGS

available at www.expertconsult.com

RELATED CONTENT

Amebiasis (Patient Information)

AUTHOR: **GLENN G. FORT, M.D., M.P.H.**

TABLE 1-22 Drug Treatment for Amebiasis

Medication	Adult Dosage (Oral)	Pediatric Dosage (Oral)*
Invasive Disease		
Metronidazole	Colitis or liver abscess: 750 mg tid for 7-10 days	Colitis or liver abscess: 35-50 mg/kg/day in 3 divided doses for 7-10 days
or		
Tinidazole	Colitis: 2 g once daily for 3 days Liver abscess: 2 g once daily for 3-5 days	Colitis: 50 mg/kg/day once daily for 3 days Liver abscess: 50 mg/kg/day once daily for 3-5 days
Followed by:		
Paromomycin (preferred)	500 mg tid for 7 days	25-35 mg/kg/day in 3 divided doses for 7 days
or		
Diloxanide furoate† or	500 mg tid for 10 days	20 mg/kg/day in 3 divided doses for 7 days
Iodoquinol	650 mg tid for 20 days	30-40 mg/kg/day in 3 divided doses for 20 days
Asymptomatic Intestinal Colonization		
Paromomycin (preferred)	As for invasive disease	As for invasive disease
or		
Diloxanide furoate†		
or		
Iodoquinol		

*All pediatric dosages are up to a maximum of the adult dose.
†Not available in the United States.
From Kliegman RM et al: *Nelson textbook of pediatrics*, ed 19, Philadelphia, 2011, Saunders.

A

Diseases and Disorders

I

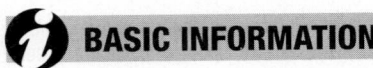

BASIC INFORMATION

DESCRIPTION

Amenorrhea means absence of menstruation. It is classified as either primary or secondary depending on whether the patient has had previous menstrual cycles.

- Primary amenorrhea is defined as the absence of menses by age 16 in the presence of secondary sexual characteristics. However, in the absence of these secondary sexual features by the age of 14 years, one should begin the workup for primary amenorrhea.
- Secondary amenorrhea is the absence of menses for more than six months in a patient who has had previous normal progesterone withdrawal cycles. The duration of amenorrhea required for the diagnosis of secondary amenorrhea varies somewhat depending on the source.

ICD-9CM CODES
626.0 Absence of menstruation

EPIDEMIOLOGY & DEMOGRAPHICS

- Incidence of primary amenorrhea and secondary amenorrhea in the U.S. is <1% and 5% to 7%, respectively.
- There is no racial or ethnic predilection.

ETIOLOGY

- Physiologic amenorrhea
  1. Pregnancy
  2. Lactation
  3. Menopause
- Pathologic amenorrhea (Table 1-23)
  A. Primary amenorrhea
    1. Hypergonadotropic hypogonadism
      a. Turner's syndrome
      b. Pure gonadal dysgenesis
      c. Autoimmune oophoritis
      d. 17,20-desmolase deficiency or 17-hydroxylase deficiency
      e. Galactosemia
    2. Eugonadism
      a. Müllerian agenesis
      b. Transverse vaginal septum
      c. Imperforate hymen
      d. Androgen insensitivity syndrome (AIS) (1%)
      e. 5-alpha reductase deficiency
      f. Polycystic ovarian syndrome (PCOS)
      g. Adult-onset congenital adrenal hyperplasia (CAH)
      h. Cushing's syndrome
      i. Hypothyroidism
    3. Hypogonadotropic hypogonadism
      a. Constitutional delay
      b. Hypothalamic disorders
      c. Pituitary diseases
      d. Other CNS diseases
  B. Secondary amenorrhea
    1. Ovarian diseases
      a. PCOS
      b. Iatrogenic (oophorectomy, S/P radiation)
      c. Premature ovarian failure (POF)
      d. Ovarian tumors
    2. Hypothalamic dysfunction
      a. Functional (eating disorders, exercise, stress)
      b. Congenital GnRH deficiency
      c. Infiltrative diseases (sarcoidosis, histiocytosis, lymphoma)
    3. Pituitary diseases
      a. Hyperprolactinemia (drug induced, hypothyroidism, prolactinoma)
      b. Craniopharyngiomas
      c. Empty sella syndrome
      d. Sheehan's syndrome
      e. S/P radiation
      f. Infiltrative diseases
    4. Asherman's syndrome
    5. Others
       Hypothyroidism, Cushing's syndrome, adult-onset congenital adrenal hyperplasia, drug induced (Lupron Depot, Depo-Provera, progesterone IUD, danazol, etc.), chronic illnesses

PHYSICAL FINDINGS & CLINICAL PRESENTATION

- Turner's syndrome
  - Usually presents with primary amenorrhea unless mosaic
  - Short stature
  - Epicanthic folds
  - Low-set ears
  - High-arched palate
  - Micrognathia
  - Sensorineural hearing loss
  - Otitis media
  - Webbing of the neck
  - Pigmented nevi
  - Square/shield chest
  - Widely spaced nipples
  - Absent breast development
  - Bicuspid aortic valve
  - Coarctation of aorta
  - Cubit valgus
  - Short fourth metacarpal
  - Hyperconvex nails
  - Leg edema
  - Renal abnormalities
  - Autoimmune disorders including thyroiditis
  - Diabetes mellitus
- Pure gonadal dysgenesis
  - Unlike Turner's syndrome has no dysmorphic features
- Müllerian agenesis
  - Sporadic inheritance
  - Primary amenorrhea
  - Normal breast development
  - Normal pubic and axillary hair
  - Normal female external genitalia
  - Absent uterus and upper part of vagina
  - Ovary present
  - Renal and vertebral anomalies
- Transverse vaginal septum and imperforate hymen
  - Primary amenorrhea
  - Progressive cyclic lower abdominal pain
  - Imperforate hymen or transverse vaginal septum on pelvic examination
  - Perirectal fullness from hematocolpos
- Androgen insensitivity syndrome
  - Primary amenorrhea
  - X-linked recessive inheritance
  - Normal breast development
  - Absent pubic and axillary hair
  - Testis may be present in the groin or inguinal canal
  - Uterus and vagina absent
  - No associated renal or vertebral anomalies
- Adult-onset congenital adrenal hyperplasia
  - Commonly seen in Ashkenazi Jewish, Inuit Native American, French Canadian, Mexican population
  - Mimics the presentation of PCOS
  - Features of hyperandrogenism (virilization, hirsutism, acne)
  - Hypertension
- 5-alpha reductase deficiency
  - Primary amenorrhea
  - Undergo striking virilization at puberty
- PCOS
  - Usually presents with secondary amenorrhea and oligomenorrhea
  - Features of hyperandrogenism
  - Obesity (60% to 80% of PCOS patients)
  - Infertility
  - Insulin resistance, predisposition to type II diabetes mellitus
- Cushing's syndrome (rare disorder, prevalence 1/1,000,000)
  - Secondary amenorrhea
  - Features of hyperandrogenism
  - Abnormal fat distribution (dorsocervical fat pad [buffalo hump], spider legs, significant central obesity)
  - Abdominal striae due to weakening of skin integument
  - Easy bruising
  - Hypertension
  - Proximal muscle weakness
- Hypothyroidism
  - Secondary amenorrhea
  - Lethargy
  - Constipation
  - Decreased appetite
  - Weight gain
  - Cold intolerance
  - Hair loss
  - Dry skin
  - Hypotension
  - Bradycardia
- Premature ovarian failure
  - Secondary amenorrhea prior to the age of 40
  - History of oophorectomy or pelvic radiation or chemotherapy
  - Vasomotor symptoms
  - Dry, thin vaginal mucosa without rugosity
- Hyperprolactinemia
  - Usually presents with secondary amenorrhea
  - History of use of drugs such as antipsychotics, oral contraceptive (OC) pills, antidepressants, antihypertensives, H_2 blockers, opioids, etc.
  - Pituitary adenomas may be associated with headache, vomiting, vision changes
  - Galactorrhea
- Sheehan's syndrome
  - History of secondary amenorrhea following postpartum hemorrhage
  - Failure of lactation
  - Other features of hypopituitarism
- Asherman's syndrome
  - History of D&C
  - Secondary amenorrhea

- ○ Recurrent miscarriage/infertility
- Functional hypothalamic disorders
  - ○ Usually presents with secondary amenorrhea
  - ○ History of eating disorders, severe exercise or stress
  - ○ Use of street drugs
- Kallmann's syndrome
  - ○ Usually presents with anosmia, congenital defect of development of both the GnRH neurons and olfactory placode

DX DIAGNOSIS

- First step in the workup of amenorrhea is to rule out pregnancy by serum/urine pregnancy test.
- Diagnostic workup depends on history and physical.
- Primary amenorrhea (Fig. E1-54 and Box E1-3):
  - ○ Pelvic ultrasonography or MRI to detect any anatomic abnormalities of uterus, cervix, ovaries, or vagina. At times examination under anesthesia is needed to assess the pelvic organs.
  - ○ Karyotyping (46,XX in Müllerian agenesis; 46,XY in AIS; 45,XO in Turner's syndrome) is done when uterus is absent or Turner's syndrome is suspected.

- ○ Serum FSH, TSH/FT4, prolactin, estradiol: FSH 40 mIU/ml along with estradiol <20 pg/ml is indicative of ovarian insufficiency.
  Prolactin >200 ng/ml is suggestive of prolactinoma. Lower levels may also be associated with prolactinoma. Threshold levels may vary by laboratory, and providers are advised to become familiar with their institution's normal range.
- ○ Check serum testosterone (male range in AIS; female range in Müllerian agenesis) when uterus is absent or in presence of features of hyperandrogenism.
- ○ 17-alpha hydroxyprogesterone level in presence of features of hyperandrogenism to rule out CAH. In addition to high level of 17 alpha hydroxyprogesterone due to compromised 21-hydroxylase activity, these patients have elevated level of serum progesterone and deoxycorticosterone, hypernatremia, and hypokalemia.
- ○ MRI of head in presence of:
  Primary hypogonadotrophic hypogonadism.
  Hyperprolactinemia.
  Visual field defects.
  Headaches.
  Signs of hypothalamic-pituitary dysfunction.

- Secondary amenorrhea (Fig. E1-55):
  - ○ Serum FSH, TSH/FT4, prolactin, estradiol:
    Low serum FSH with low estradiol indicates secondary (hypogondotropic) hypogonadism.
    High serum FSH with low estradiol suggests primary (hypergonadotropic) hypogonadism.
    Progesterone withdrawal bleeding.
    10 mg medroxyprogesterone is given for 10 days.
    Withdrawal bleeding suggests euestrogenic anovulation in presence of normal end organ (outflow tract) and ovarian function.
  - ○ Estrogen-progesterone withdrawal bleeding:
    In the absence of progesterone withdrawal bleeding, the patients are exposed to 25 to 35 days of estrogen (0.625-2.5 mg Premarin daily) followed by 10 days of medroxyprogesterone.
    Withdrawal bleeding indicates hypogonadism.
    Absence of bleeding indicates defects with end organ (e.g., Asherman's syndrome).
  - ○ Serum LH, testosterone and DHEA-S:

TABLE 1-23 Congenital Anatomic Causes of Primary Amenorrhea with Normal Breast Development*

Diagnosis	Müllerian Agenesis	Androgen Insensitivity (AI)	Transverse Vaginal Septum	Imperforate Hymen
Patients with primary amenorrhea†	15%	1%	3%	1%
Patients with primary amenorrhea and apparent obstruction or absence of vagina†	75%	5%	15%	5%
Chromosomes‡	46,XX	46,XY	46,XX	46,XX
Gonads	Ovaries	Testes	Ovaries	Ovaries
Serum testosterone‡	Normal female level	Normal male level (high)	Normal female level	Normal female level
Vagina	Absent or shallow	Absent or shallow	Obstructed by septum which may be thick or thin, high or low	Obstructed by thin membrane, which may look blue from hematocolpos
Axillary/pubic hair	+	Absent unless AI is incomplete	+	+
Cyclic pain	±	−	+	+
Uterus	Absent or rudimentary	−	+	+
Mass	−	−	+	+
			Can present with acute urinary retention as hematocolpos mass obstructs urethra	Can present with acute urinary retention
Introitus bulges with Valsalva maneuver	−	−	−	+
Associated anomalies	Urinary tract and skeletal	Inguinal hernias; gonadal malignancy in adulthood	Major urinary tract abnormalities in 15%	Possibly some increase in urinary tract abnormalities
Treatment	Vaginal dilation or surgical neovagina	Gonadectomy after age 16-18 yr Vaginal dilation or surgical neovagina	Surgical approach depends on extent and location of septum; may be extensive; should be done as soon as possible	Excision of hymen as soon as possible; diagnostic needle aspiration contraindicated because of risk of infection
Fertility	Advanced reproductive technology required; in vitro fertilization surrogate with uterus to gestate pregnancy	Not fertile	Variable, low septa have a better prognosis than do high septa	Usually fertile

+, Present; −, absent; ±, may be present or absent.
*Cervix not visible on pelvic examination. Short vagina; may be absent or obstructed.
†Data from Reindollar RH, Byrd JR, McDonough PG: Delayed sexual development: a study of 252 patients, *Am J Obstet Gynecol* 140:371, 1981.
‡Sometimes useful in differentiating Müllerian agenesis from androgen insensitivity.
From Kliegman RM et al: *Practical strategies in pediatric diagnosis and therapy,* ed 2, Philadelphia, 2004, Elsevier.

When features of hyperandrogenism seen these tests are ordered.

Serum testosterone >200 ng/ml suggests androgen-producing adrenal or ovarian tumors (high index of suspicion with moderate elevation; threshold value not required in cases of ovarian or adrenal tumors). This level may be mildly elevated in patients with PCOS.

DHEA-S >700 mcg/dl suggests adrenal origin over ovarian (high index of suspicion with moderate elevation; threshold value not required in cases of ovarian or adrenal tumors).

LH/FSH ratio >2 in patient with PCOS.

- Pelvic ultrasound when PCOS or ovarian tumor suspected.
- Abdominal CT when adrenal tumor suspected.
- MRI of head when indicated.
- HSG, sonohysterography, or diagnostic hysteroscopy in patients with suspected Asherman's syndrome.
- Karyotyping is indicated when POF occurs before the age of 30.
- Other tests which are rarely needed:
  Serum transferrin when hemochromatosis is suspected.
  Serum ACE when sarcoidosis is suspected.

TREATMENT

- The treatment of amenorrhea depends on the etiology, as well as the aims of the patient, such as a desire to treat hirsutism or to become pregnant.
- In the absence of pregnancy, withdrawal bleeding may be induced in the majority of patients with amenorrhea using 5 to 10 mg of medroxyprogesterone for 10 days.
- Estrogen replacement along with calcium and vitamin D should be instituted in essentially every patient with hypogonadism to avoid osteoporosis. Women with a uterus require continuous or intermittent progesterone administration to protect against endometrial hyperplasia or cancer. Frequently, it is easiest to prescribe combination OC pills. For most patients, continuation until ~50 years, the usual age of menopause, seems reasonable. Young women in whom secondary sex characteristics have failed to develop fully should be exposed initially to very low dose estrogen (0.3 mg of conjugated equine estrogen or equivalent) given unopposed daily for 6 mo with incremental dose increases at 6-mo intervals until the required maintenance dose is achieved. Cyclic progesterone therapy, 12 to 14 days per month, should be instituted once vaginal bleeding ensues.
- Most patients with anatomic abnormalities will require surgical correction. Creation of a new vagina for patients with Müllerian agenesis is usually delayed until the woman is emotionally mature and ready to participate in the postoperative care required to maintain vaginal patency. However, if adequate correction is impossible, pregnancy will often require a surrogate to carry a gestation. One should not forget to look for the associated urogenital anomalies in these patients and, when present, treat them appropriately.
- In patients with androgen insensitivity syndrome, the incidence of gonadal malignancy is 22%. However, it rarely occurs before the age of 20. Gonadectomy is performed by laparoscopy following breast development and the attainment of adult stature. In the absence of a uterus these individuals only need estrogen replacement without progesterone.
- Women with adult-onset CAH may be treated with low-dose corticosteroids in addition to sex steroids to partially block ACTH stimulation of adrenal function and thereby decrease overproduction of adrenal androgens.
- Patients with POF will need estrogen and progesterone replacement. These patients will require in vitro fertilization using donor oocytes to conceive. These patients have an increased risk of osteoporosis and heart disease. It can also be associated with autoimmune disorders such as hypothyroidism, Addison's disease, and diabetes mellitus. Therefore, fasting blood glucose, TSH, and, if clinically appropriate, morning cortisol should be measured. In the presence of a Y chromosome, removal of gonadal tissue is recommended at the time of diagnosis to avoid gonadal tumors.
- Hypothyroidism should be treated with thyroid replacement.
- Hyperprolactinemia is treated by avoiding the culprit drugs or by giving dopamine agonists, such as bromocriptine or cabergoline. Pituitary adenomas rarely require surgery but may be performed if secondary deficits such as visual changes are observed, when they are resistant to medical therapy, or the lesion is rapidly growing.
- Treatment of hypothalamic amenorrhea depends on the etiology. Patients with eating disorders or who exercise excessively will require behavioral modification and nutritional counseling. Elite athletes may choose not to alter their exercise regimens and will therefore require estrogen treatment and prevention of osteoporosis. When associated with infertility, ovulation induction with clomiphene citrate, exogenous gonadotropins, or pulsatile GnRH therapy should be offered.
- The primary treatment of PCOS is weight loss through diet and exercise. Other treatment options include:
  1. Use of OC pills or cyclic progestational agents to help maintain a normal endometrium.
  2. Insulin-sensitizing agents such as metformin to reduce insulin resistance and improve ovulatory function.
  3. Oral contraceptives and/or spironolactone to treat hyperandrogenism.
  4. Clomiphene citrate to induce ovulation.
- In patients with Asherman's syndrome, hysteroscopic lysis of intrauterine adhesions is followed by administration of long-term exogenous estrogen to stimulate regrowth of endometrial tissue.
- Geneticist consult is given in patients with hereditary causes of amenorrhea.
- Psychiatrist consult is needed in patients with major depression, anorexia nervosa, bulimia nervosa, or other major psychiatric disorders.

COMPLICATIONS

- Osteoporosis
- Endometrial hyperplasia and uterine cancer
- Infertility

PROGNOSIS

Depends on the primary cause of amenorrhea

PATIENT EDUCATION

- Patients with amenorrhea should be reassured that this is, in and of itself, not a concern.
- All women with an intact endometrium should understand the risks of unopposed estrogen action, whether the estrogen is exogenous such as through hormone therapy, or endogenous such as PCOS.
- Hypoestrogenic women should be counseled about the importance of estrogen replacement to protect against bone loss.
- Potential for future childbearing should be discussed.

SUGGESTED READINGS

available at www.expertconsult.com

RELATED CONTENT

Infertility (Related Key Topic)
Pituitary Adenoma (Related Key Topic)
Polycystic Ovary Syndrome (Related Key Topic)
Sheehan's Syndrome (Related Key Topic)
Amenorrhea (Patient Information)

AUTHOR: **HEMANT K. SATPATHY, M.D.**

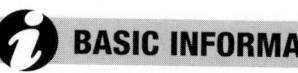

BASIC INFORMATION

The word "amnesia" is derived from the Greek word *amnéstia* meaning "forgetfulness."

DEFINITION

The acquired inability to learn new, or recall previously learned information. The impairment compromises social and occupational functioning. It is caused by an identifiable medical condition or by persisting effects of a substance. Disorder is not caused by delirium or dementia. It may be transient or chronic.

SOME WELL-KNOWN AMNESTIC DISORDERS

Korsakoff syndrome
Transient global amnesia

ICD-9CM CODES
780.9 Amnesia (retrograde); memory disturbance, loss or lack

DSM-IV-TR CODES
294.0 Amnestic disorder due to . . . [indicate the general medical condition]
294.8 Amnestic disorder NOS

EPIDEMIOLOGY & DEMOGRAPHICS

INCIDENCE: Data not available on true incidence or lifetime risk of most amnestic disorders. Transient global amnesia has an incidence in the general population of 23 to 50 per 100,000 population over age 50.
PREDOMINANT AGE: Variable, depending on causative pathology. Transient global amnesia onset usually after age 50 years. Korsakoff syndrome usually presents in patients after the age of 40.

GENETICS: Genetic defect for thiamine metabolism has been described in Korsakoff syndrome.

PHYSICAL FINDINGS & CLINICAL PRESENTATION

HISTORY
- Diagnosis depends on history.
- The inability to learn new or recall previously learned information is the key feature of this disorder.
- The Mini-Mental State Examination is useful. Patients unable to recall events that transpire during the interview but may have a normal digit span and be able to attend to the conversation.
- Neuropsychiatric testing demonstrates specific memory impairments in absence of other cognitive deficits
- Patients are unable to recall events subsequent to the onset of the amnesia.
- Individuals may learn new motor tasks but are unable to recall those learning experiences.
- Amnesia generally is both anterograde and retrograde.
- Commonly, patients are disoriented to time and place. Most lack insight while others may have insight but appear indifferent. Some present with personality change or confabulation.
- Table 1-24 describes memory systems. Clinico-anatomic correlations of memory disorders are described in Table 1-25.

ETIOLOGY (MEDICAL CONDITIONS AND PERSISTENT EFFECTS OF DRUGS)

The etiology can be either medical or due to the persistent effects of a substance/chemical.
- Traumatic brain injury
- Focal tumors or infarction
- Herpes simplex encephalitis
- Cerebral anoxia
- Korsakoff syndrome (thiamine deficiency)
- Carbon monoxide poisoning
- Transient amnesia may arise from concussion, acute intoxication, anesthesia, medications, seizures, transient global amnesia, and electroconvulsive therapy
- Persistent effects of drugs (note that this must not be because of acute effects of intoxication or withdrawl)

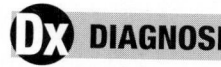

DIAGNOSIS

DIFFERENTIAL DIAGNOSIS
- Dementia
- Delirium
- Major depression
- Minimal cognitive impairment
- Dissociative amnesia
- Memory impairment in substance intoxication or withdrawal
- Malingering
- Factitious disorder

WORKUP
- Complete medical history and mental status testing, with emphasis on identifying underlying medical condition and/or history of drug use
- Neuropsychological testing

LABORATORY TESTS

Tests to determine potential underlying medical condition (e.g., B_{12} levels, TSH, brain imaging).

IMAGING STUDIES
- No specific or diagnostic features of amnestic disorder are detectable on imaging.

TABLE 1-24 Description of Memory Systems

Type of Memory Function	Regional Localization	Learning Efficiency	Time Span until Effective Retrieval	Capacity	Clinical Testing Techniques	Examples in Daily Life
Declarative episodic memory	Hippocampus, medial thalamus	Single exposure	Decades	Very large, with rehearsal and elaboration	Recall of 3-4 words after 5 min	Recall of recent events and conversations
Declarative semantic memory	Temporal-parietal association cortices	Capable of single exposure; enhanced with repetition	Decades	Very large, perhaps limitless	Confrontation naming, general knowledge	Vocabulary, knowledge of life events from remote past
Attention span, "immediate memory"	Primary auditory or visual cortex	Single exposure only	Seconds	Very small: 7 ± 2 digits (auditory)	Digit span	Dialing a telephone number after hearing it or reading it
Working memory	Lateral frontal cortex	Single exposure only	Seconds	Small	Digits backward	Supporting many mental activities, such as mental arithmetic, abstract reasoning
Procedural memory	Basal ganglia, probably association neocortices	Requires extensive training	Decades	Moderate	Experimental laboratory methods only	Retention of motor skills, e.g., riding a bicycle or typing

From Goldman L, Schafer AI: *Goldman's Cecil medicine*, ed 24, Philadelphia, 2012, Saunders.

TABLE 1-25 Clinico-Anatomic Correlations of Memory Disorders

Anatomic Site of Damage	Memory Finding	Other Neurologic and Medical Findings
Frontal lobe	Lateralized deficits in working memory—right: spatial defects, left: verbal defects, impaired recall with spared recognition	Personality change Perseveration Chorea, dystonia Bradykinesia, tremor, rigidity
Basal forebrain	Domain-independent declarative memory deficits	
Ventromedial cortex	Frontal lobe-type declarative memory deficits	Upper visual field defects
Hippocampus and parahippocampal cortex	Bilateral lesions yield global amnesia, unilateral lesions show lateralization of deficits—left: verbal deficits; right: spatial deficits	Myoclonus Depressed level of consciousness Cortical blindness Autonomations
Fornix	Global amnesia	
Mammillary bodies	Declarative memory deficits	Confabulation, ataxia, nystagmus, signs of alcohol withdrawal
Dorsal and medial dorsal nucleus thalamus	Declarative memory deficits	Confabulation
Anterior thalamus	Declarative memory deficits	
Lateral temporal cortex	Deficits in autobiographical memory	

From Goetz CG, Pappert EJ: *Textbook of clinical neurology*, Philadelphia, 1999, Saunders.

- Brain MRI indicates specific atrophy in diencephalic structures in Korsakoff syndrome and in the hippocampus in hypoxic amnesia.
- Neuroradiologic examination with MRI is valuable in the diagnosis of acute Wernicke's encephalopathy.
- Brain MR diffusion-weighted imaging may show hippocampal lesions in transient global amnesia.

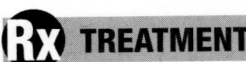 **TREATMENT**

Treatment is as diverse as the medical conditions causing it.

NONPHARMACOLOGIC THERAPY
- Cognitive rehabilitation to promote recovery from brain injury may be helpful.
- Supervised living to ensure appropriate long-term care.

ACUTE GENERAL Rx
Initial treatment directed to the underlying etiology. Generally, transient global amnesia has full remission of symptoms. Korsakoff, on the other hand, is not usually improved significantly, even after administration of thiamine.

CHRONIC Rx
No known effective treatments to reverse or ameliorate memory deficits.

DISPOSITION
Amnesias may be chronic or transient depending upon etiology.

REFERRAL
Refer for neuropsychological testing.

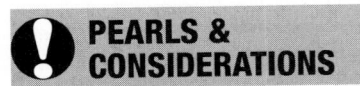 **PEARLS & CONSIDERATIONS**

COMMENTS
In Korsakoff syndrome, anterograde amnesia (disturbance in acquisition of new information) is more prominent than retrograde amnesia (problems remembering old information).

PREVENTION
Cases of amnestic disorder due to trauma are usually not preventable. Refraining from abuse of alcohol and other drugs prevents substance-induced amnestic disorder, and high-dose thiamine has been shown to prevent Korsakoff syndrome.

PATIENT & FAMILY EDUCATION
Respite care and in-home services for family caregivers

SUGGESTED READINGS
available at www.expertconsult.com

AUTHORS: **WASIM RASHID, M.D.,** and **MITCHELL D. FELDMAN, M.D., M.PHIL.**

BASIC INFORMATION

DEFINITION

Amyotrophic lateral sclerosis (ALS) is a progressive, degenerative neuromuscular condition of undetermined etiology affecting corticospinal tracts and anterior horn cells, resulting in dysfunction of both upper motor neurons (UMN) and lower motor neurons (LMN), respectively.

SYNONYMS

Lou Gehrig's disease

ICD-9CM CODES
335.20 Amyotrophic lateral sclerosis

EPIDEMIOLOGY & DEMOGRAPHICS

INCIDENCE:
- 0.5 to 2 cases per 100,000 persons.
- Onset is usually between the ages of 50 and 70 yr.
- Male/female ratio is 2:1.

PREVALENCE: Five in 100,000 persons

PHYSICAL FINDINGS & CLINICAL PRESENTATION

- LMN signs (weakness, hypotonia, wasting, fasciculations, hypoflexia or areflexia).
- UMN signs (loss of fine motor dexterity, spasticity, extensor plantar responses, hyperreflexia, clonus).
- Preservation of extraocular movements, sensation, bowel and bladder function.
- Dysarthria, dysphagia, pseudobulbar affect, frontal lobe dysfunction.
- Respiratory insufficiency typically occurs late in the disease.
- ALS comprises approximately 90% of adult-onset motor neuron diseases. Other presentations of motor neuron disease include progressive muscular atrophy, primary lateral sclerosis, progressive bulbar palsy, progressive pseudobulbar palsy, and ALS-parkinsonism-dementia complex.

ETIOLOGY

- 90% to 95% of all cases are sporadic; of the familial cases, 10% to 20% are associated with a genetic defect in the copper-zinc superoxide dismutase enzyme.

DIAGNOSIS

DIFFERENTIAL DIAGNOSIS

- Multifocal motor neuropathy with conduction block
- Cervical spondylotic myelopathy with polyradiculopathy
- Spinal stenosis with compression of lumbosacral nerve roots
- Chronic inflammatory demyelinating polyneuropathy with central nervous system lesions
- Syringomyelia
- Syringobulbia
- Foramen magnum tumor
- Meningeal carcinomatosis
- Spinal muscular atrophy
- Polyglucosan body disease
- Bulbospinal muscular atrophy (Kennedy disease)
- Monomelic amyotrophy
- ALS-like syndromes have been reported in the setting of lead intoxication, HIV, hyperparathyroidism, hyperthyroidism, lymphoma, and vitamin B_{12} deficiency.

WORKUP

- Electromyography and nerve conduction studies (El Escorial criteria)
- Assessment of respiratory function (forced vital capacity [FVC], negative inspiratory force)

LABORATORY TESTS

- Vitamin B_{12}, thyroid function, parathyroid hormone, HIV may be considered.
- Serum protein and immunofixation electrophoresis.
- DNA studies for SMA or bulbospinal atrophy, hexosaminidase levels in pure LMN syndrome.
- 24-hour urine for heavy metals if indicated.

IMAGING STUDIES

- Craniospinal neuroimaging contingent on clinical scenario
- Modified barium swallow to evaluate aspiration risk

TREATMENT

NONPHARMACOLOGIC THERAPY

- Noninvasive positive-pressure ventilation may improve quality of life and may increase tracheostomy-free survival in patients with respiratory difficulty (defined by orthopnea or FVC 50% of predicted).
- Percutaneous endoscopic gastrostomy (PEG) tube placement improves nutritional intake, promotes weight stabilization, and eases medication administration. Some studies suggest PEG placement may prolong life 1 to 4 mo, particularly when placed before FVC falls to ≤50% of predicted value.
- Nutrition, speech therapy, physical and occupational therapy services.
- Suction device for sialorrhea.
- Communication may be eased with computerized assistive devices.
- Early discussion of living will, resuscitation orders, desire for PEG and tracheostomy, potential long-term care options.
- Encourage contact with local support groups.

ACUTE GENERAL Rx

Riluzole (Rilutek), a glutamate antagonist, is the only FDA-approved medication known to extend tracheostomy-free survival in patients with ALS. Dosage is 50 mg q12h, at least 1 hr before or 2 hr after meals. It is shown to prolong survival by 2 to 3 months. Manufacturer recommends checking alanine aminotransferase (ALT) once a month for 3 months initially, followed by once every 3 months until the first year of therapy is completed. ALT should be checked periodically thereafter.

CHRONIC Rx

- Sialorrhea may respond to either glycopyrrolate or amitriptyline (consider either propranolol or metoprolol if secretions are thick). Botulinum toxin may be effective in medically refractory cases.
- Spasticity may be treated pharmacologically with baclofen, tizanidine, clonazepam.
- Pseudobulbar affect may improve with amitriptyline, sertraline (Zoloft), or dextromethorphan/quinine.

DISPOSITION

- Mean duration of symptoms is 3 to 5 yr.
- Approximately 20% of patients survive >5 yr.

REFERRAL

- Referral to a neurologist experienced in neuromuscular disease is recommended to confirm the diagnosis. One prospective, population-based study suggested improved survival in subjects treated in a multidisciplinary clinic.
- Gastrointestinal referral for PEG placement is recommended while FVC remains >50% to minimize morbidity attributable to risks inherent to the procedure.

PEARLS & CONSIDERATIONS

- Patient-physician communication is an integral and essential part in both the initial diagnosis and subsequent treatment of ALS.
- A multidisciplinary approach to supportive care may lead to an improved level of daily functioning and foster an increased sense of independence.

SUGGESTED READINGS
available at www.expertconsult.com

AUTHOR: **TAYLOR HARRISON, M.D.**

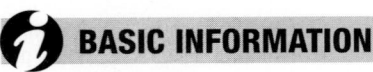

BASIC INFORMATION

DEFINITION

An anaerobic infection is caused by one of a group of bacteria that requires a reduced oxygen tension for growth.

ICD-9CM CODES
See specific condition.

PHYSICAL FINDINGS & CLINICAL PRESENTATION

- May occur at any site, but most are anatomically related to mucosal surfaces
- Should be suspected when there is foul-smelling tissue, soft tissue gas, necrotic tissue, or abscesses
- Head and neck
  1. Odontogenic infections from dental or soft tissue possibly progressing to periapical abscesses, at times extending to bone
  2. Both anaerobic and aerobic pathogens in chronic sinusitis, chronic mastoiditis, peritonsillar abscess, and chronic otitis media
  3. Complications: deep neck space infections, brain abscesses, mediastinitis
  4. Specific examples of anaerobic infections in head and neck:
     a. Ludwig's angina: bilateral infection of sublingual and submandibular spaces that causes swelling of the base of the tongue with potential airway compromise. Usually mixed aerobic and anaerobic flora
     b. Lemierre's syndrome: jugular vein suppurative thrombophlebitis caused by anaerobic bacteria: *Fusobacterium necrophorum*
- Pleuropulmonary
  1. May involve anaerobes present in the oropharynx
  2. Aspiration more common in persons with altered mental status or seizures
  3. Anaerobic bacteria more likely in those with gingivitis or periodontitis
  4. Manifestations: necrotizing pneumonia, empyema, lung abscess
- Intraabdominal
  1. Disruption of intestinal integrity leading to infection involving anaerobic bacteria
  2. Bacteria from colonic neoplasm, perforated appendicitis, diverticulitis, or bowel surgery, causing bacteremia, peritonitis, at times intraabdominal abscesses
  3. Resulting infections usually mixed, containing both anaerobes and aerobes
- Female genital tract
  1. Anaerobes in bacterial vaginosis, salpingitis, endometritis, pelvic abscesses, septic abortion; infections tend to be mixed
  2. Possible pelvic thrombophlebitis when resolving pelvic infection is accompanied by new or persistent fever
- Other anaerobic infections
  1. Skin and soft tissue infection at any site
  2. More commonly associated infections: synergistic gangrene, bite wound infections, infected decubitus ulcers
  3. Clinical significance of anaerobes in diabetic foot infections unclear
  4. Anaerobic bacteremia uncommon with source usually intraabdominal, followed by female genital tract, pleuropulmonary, and head and neck infections
  5. Osteomyelitis especially when associated with decubitus ulcers or vascular insufficiency
  6. Facial bone osteomyelitis from adjacent infections of the teeth or sinuses

ETIOLOGY

- Most commonly endogenous, arising from bacteria that normally line mucosal surfaces
- Disruption of mucosal barriers resulting from various conditions (trauma, ischemia, surgery, perforation), with infection occurring when organisms gain access to normally sterile sites, causing tissue destruction and abscess formation
- Synergy between different anaerobes or between anaerobes and aerobes important
- Examples of anaerobic bacteria include gram-negative bacteria such as *Bacterioides* species, *Fusobacterium* and *Prevotella* species; and gram-positive bacteria such as *Peptostreptococcus, Clostridium* species, and *Actinomyces* species

DIAGNOSIS

DIFFERENTIAL DIAGNOSIS

- Primary differential possibility is an aerobic bacterial infection without the presence of anaerobic bacteria.
- Ischemic necrosis without accompanying anaerobic infection (or "dry" gangrene [noninfected necrosis] vs. "wet" gangrene [infected tissue with anaerobic infection]).

WORKUP

- Specimens submitted for anaerobic culture should be processed within 30 min and may take up to 5 to 7 days to grow
- Large volume of material more likely to have significant growth; swabs less efficient for transporting infected material
- Blood cultures—preferably before antibiotic administration

LABORATORY TESTS

- Elevated WBC count, with extremely high WBC counts sometimes seen with pseudomembranous colitis
- Positive stool *C. difficile* toxin A and B assay
- Increased lactate levels in ischemia or perforation
- Possible positive blood or wound cultures, but failure to grow anaerobes in culture may be common, attributed to inadequate culturing techniques or fastidious organisms

IMAGING STUDIES

- Plain film of an affected area to show gas in tissues, free air resulting from a perforated viscus, or an air/fluid level inside an abscess
- Ultrasound, CT scan, or MRI to reveal abscesses or tissue destruction

TREATMENT

NONPHARMACOLOGIC THERAPY

- Removal of necrotic tissue
- Drainage of abscesses (accomplished by CT scan–guided percutaneous drainage)

ACUTE GENERAL Rx

Oral antibiotics with anaerobic activity: clindamycin, metronidazole, and chloramphenicol
- Broader spectrum of activity with amoxicillin/clavulanate
- Penicillin VK in odontogenic infections
- Oral metronidazole for *C. difficile*–associated diarrhea, with oral vancomycin used for severe, recurrent, or recalcitrant infections
Parenteral antibiotics for more serious illness
- IV clindamycin, metronidazole, and chloramphenicol
- Cephalosporins (anaerobic or mixed infections): cefoxitin and cefotetan
- Extended-spectrum penicillins (e.g., piperacillin) and combination beta-lactamase plus beta-lactamase inhibitor drugs (e.g., clavulanic acid, sulbactam, tazobactam)
  1. Significant anaerobic activity, plus various degrees of broad-spectrum coverage
  2. Include ampicillin/sulbactam, ticarcillin/clavulanate, and piperacillin/tazobactam
- Imipenem or other carbapenems, such as meropenem, doripenem, or ertapenem, which are broad-spectrum agents with extensive anaerobic activity
- Actinomycosis treated with penicillin for 6 to 12 mo
- SMX/TMP and fluoroquinolones are generally ineffective, but some newer quinolones (e.g., moxifloxacin) have inhibitory activity against anaerobes

DISPOSITION

It is essential that all necrotic debris be removed when treating an anaerobic infection or it will recur; follow-up is critically important to ensure resolution of the process.

REFERRAL

Refer to a surgeon if drainage is required; infectious disease consultation may be useful in complicated patients or if treatment regimen is failing or slow to respond.

SUGGESTED READINGS
available at www.expertconsult.com

RELATED CONTENT
Anaerobic Infections (Patient Information)

AUTHOR: **GLENN G. FORT, M.D., M.P.H.**

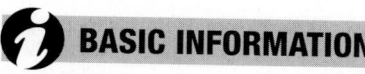

BASIC INFORMATION

DEFINITION

A fissure is a tear in the epithelial lining of the anal canal (i.e., from the dentate line to the anal verge).

SYNONYMS

Anorectal fissure
Anal ulcer

ICD-9CM CODES
565.0 Anal fissure

EPIDEMIOLOGY & DEMOGRAPHICS

PREDOMINANT SEX: Occurs in men more than women. Women are more likely to have anterior fissure than men (10% vs. 1%, respectively). Common in women before and after childbirth.
PREDOMINANT AGE: Can occur at any age. Most common in young and middle-aged adults. Most common cause of rectal bleeding in infants.

PHYSICAL FINDINGS & CLINICAL PRESENTATION

With separation of the buttocks will see a tear in the posterior midline or, less frequently, in the anterior midline (Fig. 1-59)
- Acute anal fissure:
  1. Sharp burning or tearing pain exacerbated by bowel movements
  2. Bright-red blood on toilet paper, a streak of blood on the stool or in the water

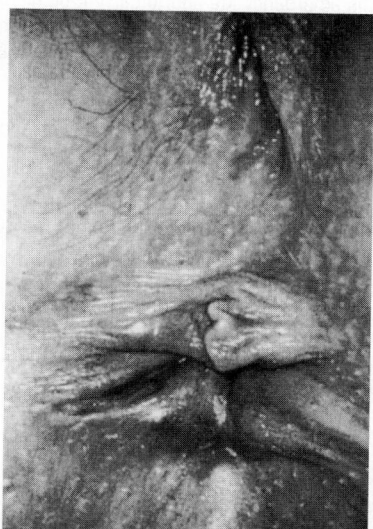

FIGURE 1-59 Lateral anal fissure. (From Seidel HM et al: *Mosby's guide to physical examination*, ed 3, St Louis, 1995, Mosby. Courtesy Gershon Efron, MD, Sinai Hospital of Baltimore.)

- Chronic anal fissure:
  1. Pruritus ani
  2. Pain seldom present
  3. Intermittent bleeding
  4. Sentinel tag at the caudal aspect of the fissure, hypertrophied anal papilla at the proximal end
- Underlying disease possible if the fissure:
  1. Is ectopically located
  2. Extends proximal to the dentate line
  3. Is broad-based or deep
  4. Is especially purulent

ETIOLOGY

- Most initiated after passage of a large, hard stool
- May result from frequent defecation and diarrhea
- Bacterial infections: tuberculosis (TB), syphilis, gonorrhea, chancroid, lymphogranuloma venereum
- Viral infections: herpes simplex virus, cytomegalovirus, human immunodeficiency virus
- Inflammatory bowel disease (IBD): Crohn's disease, ulcerative colitis
- Trauma: surgery (hemorrhoidectomy), foreign bodies, anal intercourse
- Malignancy: carcinoma, lymphoma, Kaposi sarcoma

DIAGNOSIS

DIFFERENTIAL DIAGNOSIS

- Proctalgia fugax
- Thrombosed hemorrhoid

WORKUP

- Digital rectal examination after lubricating the entire anus with anesthetic jelly (i.e., 2% lidocaine) and waiting 5 to 10 min
- Anoscopy
- Proctosigmoidoscopy to exclude inflammatory or neoplastic disease
- Biopsy if doubt exists about the etiology of the condition
- All studies done under adequate anesthesia

IMAGING STUDIES

- Colonoscopy if diagnosis of IBD or malignancy is suspected
- Small-bowel series occasionally obtained for similar reasons

TREATMENT

NONPHARMACOLOGIC THERAPY

- Sitz baths
- High-fiber diet
- Increased oral fluid intake

ACUTE GENERAL Rx

- Bulk-producing agent (e.g., Metamucil) or stool softener

- Local anesthetic jelly (may exacerbate pruritus ani)
- Nitroglycerin ointment (0.4%): apply 1 inch of ointment (equivalent to 1.5 mg of nitroglycerin) intraanally every 12 hours for up to 3 weeks. This medication (Reactiv) is expensive (over $400 for 30-g tube) and can cause headaches. Topical diltiazem (compounded by pharmacist) is also effective and much less expensive.
- Suppositories *not* recommended
- Surgery

CHRONIC Rx

- Surgery: lateral internal anal sphincterotomy. It is a more durable treatment for chronic anal fissure compared with topical nitroglycerin therapy and does not compromise long-term fecal continence
- Topical glyceryl trinitrate ointment
- Injection of botulinum toxin (an injection into each side of the internal anal sphincter) is effective in healing chronic anal fissures in more than 90% of patients

DISPOSITION

Outpatient surgery

REFERRAL

- If fissure does not resolve with conservative therapy in 4 to 6 wk
- If patient prefers surgery for acute fissure
- If patient has chronic fissure

PEARLS & CONSIDERATIONS

COMMENTS

HIV-positive patients should be referred to clinicians who are well versed in the myriad infectious and neoplastic conditions that masquerade as anal ulcers in these patients.

SUGGESTED READINGS

available at www.expertconsult.com

RELATED CONTENT

Anorectal Fistula (Related Key Topic)
Hemorrhoids (Related Key Topic)
Anal Fissure (Patient Information)

AUTHORS: **GEORGE T. DANAKAS, M.D.,** and **RUBEN ALVERO, M.D.**

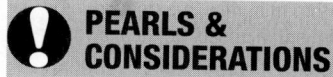

Diseases and Disorders

A

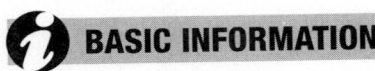

BASIC INFORMATION

DEFINITION

Anaphylaxis is a sudden-onset, life-threatening event characterized by respiratory, cardiovascular, gastrointestinal, and cutaneous manifestations, as well as vasodilatory hemodynamic changes in response to a particular allergen. Anaphylactoid reaction is closely related to anaphylaxis. It is caused by release of mast cells and basophil mediators triggered by non–IgE–mediated events.

SYNONYMS

Anaphylactoid reaction.

ICD-9CM CODES
995.0   Anaphylactic shock
995.60   Anaphylaxis due to food
999.4   Anaphylaxis due to immunization
977.9   Anaphylaxis due to drugs
989.5   Anaphylaxis following stings

EPIDEMIOLOGY & DEMOGRAPHICS

INCIDENCE: The incidence of anaphylaxis in the U.S. is 58.9 cases per 100,000 person-years. Lifetime prevalence is 0.05% to 2%, with a mortality rate of 1%. Anaphylaxis rates are 0.0004% for food, 0.7% to 10% for penicillin, 0.22% to 1% for radiocontrast media, and 0.5% to 5% after insect stings. Annual mortality is 500 to 1000 persons per year in the U.S.

PHYSICAL FINDINGS & CLINICAL PRESENTATION

- Urticaria, pruritus, skin flushing, angioedema
- Dyspnea, cough, wheezing, shortness of breath
- Nausea, vomiting, diarrhea, difficulty swallowing
- Hypotension, tachycardia, weakness, dizziness, malaise, vascular collapse

ETIOLOGY

Anaphylaxis results from sudden systematic release of histamine and other inflammatory mediators from basophils and mast cells. This causes swelling of the mucus membranes and the urticarial rash on the skin. Virtually any substance may induce anaphylaxis.

- Foods and food additives: peanuts, tree nuts, eggs, shellfish, fish, cow's milk, fruits, soy
- Medications: antibiotics, especially penicillins, insulin, allergen extracts, opiates, vaccines, NSAIDs, contrast media, streptokinase
- Bee or wasp sting, snake venom, fire ant venom
- Blood products, plasma, immunoglobulin, cryoprecipitate, whole blood
- Latex

DIAGNOSIS

DIFFERENTIAL DIAGNOSIS

- Endocrine disorders (carcinoid, pheochromocytoma)
- Globus hystericus, anxiety disorder
- Systemic mastocytosis
- Pulmonary embolism, serum sickness, vasovagal reactions
- Severe asthma (the key clinical difference is the abrupt onset of symptoms in anaphylaxis versus a history of progressive worsening of symptoms)
- Septic shock or other form of vasodilatory shock
- Airway foreign body

WORKUP

Workup is aimed at ruling out other conditions that may mimic anaphylaxis (e.g., vasovagal syncope may be differentiated by presence of bradycardia as opposed to tachycardia seen in anaphylaxis; the absence of hypoxemia in arterial blood gas [ABG] analysis may be useful to exclude pulmonary embolism or foreign body aspiration).

LABORATORY TESTS

- Laboratory evaluation is generally not helpful because anaphylaxis is typically diagnosed clinically.
- ABG analysis may be useful to exclude pulmonary embolism, status asthmaticus, and foreign body aspiration.
- Elevated serum and urine histamine levels and serum tryptase levels can be useful for diagnosis of anaphylaxis, but these tests are not commonly available in the emergency setting.

IMAGING STUDIES

Generally not helpful.

- Chest radiography for evaluation of foreign body aspiration or pulmonary pathology is indicated in patients with acute respiratory compromise.
- Consider ECG in all patients with sudden loss of consciousness or reports of chest pains or dyspnea and in any elderly patient. ECG in anaphylaxis usually reveals sinus tachycardia.

TREATMENT

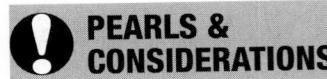

NONPHARMACOLOGIC THERAPY

- Establish and protect airway. Provide supplemental O_2 if indicated.
- IV access should be rapidly established, and IV fluids (i.e., normal saline) should be administered. The patient should be placed supine or in Trendelenburg position if hemodynamically unstable.
- Cardiac monitoring is recommended.

ACUTE GENERAL Rx

- Epinephrine should be rapidly administered as an IM injection at a dose of 0.3 mg of aqueous epinephrine for adults and children >30 kg. Epinephrine 0.15 mg should be given for children <30 kg (1:1000 concentration). Intramuscular administration is preferred because it provides more reliable and quicker rise to effective plasma levels. The dose may be repeated after approximately 5-15 min if symptoms persist.
- Adjunct therapies include H_1 and H_2 receptor antagonists, diphenhydramine 25-50 mg IV or IM, or PO in mild cases, and famotidine 20-40 mg IV, or PO in mild cases. Although useful to improve cutaneous erythema and pruritus, H_1 antagonists are not as effective as epinephrine, since onset of action is 1 to 2 hours and they are not effective in reversing upper airway obstruction or improving hypotension.
- Corticosteroids are not useful in the acute episode because of their slow onset of action; however, they should be administered in most cases to prevent prolonged or recurrent anaphylaxis. Commonly used agents are prednisone, methylprednisolone 40 to 250 mg IV in adults (1 to 2 mg/kg in children), or longer-acting dexamethasone.
- Aerosolized β-agonists (e.g., albuterol, 2.5 mg, repeat prn 20 min) are useful to control bronchospasm.
- Vasopressor therapy with epinephrine (1:10,000), or dopamine is indicated in patients with refractory hypotension after crystalloid resuscitation.

PEARLS & CONSIDERATIONS

COMMENTS

- Patient education regarding the nature of the illness and preventive measures is recommended. A documented history of previous anaphylactic episodes or known anaphylaxis triggers is the most reliable method of identifying individuals at risk.
- Prescription for prefilled epinephrine syringe (EpiPen or EpiPen Jr.) should be given, and the patient should be instructed on the use of this emergency kit, and to carry it on his/her person at all times. School-aged children should keep an additional EpiPen at school with the appropriate staff.
- Patients should also be advised to carry or wear a MedicAlert ID describing substances that have caused anaphylaxis.
- Avoidance of radiologic contrast is also recommended in those who have had a prior reaction. However, pretreatment regimens with methylprednisolone and diphenhydramine exist for those who have had contrast reactions in the past.
- Venom immunotherapy immediately after a sting is effective and recommended for up to 5 yr after the anaphylactic incident.

SUGGESTED READINGS
available at www.expertconsult.com

AUTHOR: **TARA M. WAYT, D.O.**

BASIC INFORMATION

DEFINITION

Aplastic anemia is a bone marrow failure syndrome defined by peripheral blood pancytopenia and hypocellular bone marrow.

SYNONYMS

Refractory anemia
Hypoplastic anemia

ICD-9CM CODES
284.9 Aplastic anemia
284.8 Acquired aplastic anemia
284.0 Congenital aplastic anemia

EPIDEMIOLOGY & DEMOGRAPHICS

INCIDENCE: The annual incidence of aplastic anemia is 2 cases per million.
PREDOMINANT SEX AND AGE: The incidence has two peaks, with most patients presenting between ages 15 and 25 or after 60 yr.

PHYSICAL FINDINGS & CLINICAL PRESENTATION

- Mucosal bleeding, easy bruising, petechiae or heavy menstrual bleeding is seen secondary to thrombocytopenia.
- Fatigue, lassitude, skin pallor, exertional dyspnea, or palpitations are seen secondary to anemia.
- Infection is an uncommon presentation, but neutropenia may lead to fever and sore throat.
- Various physical manifestations like short stature, skeletal or nail changes may be seen in congenital forms of aplastic anemia.

ETIOLOGY

- In most patients with idiopathic aplastic anemia, bone marrow failure results from immunologically mediated, active destruction of blood-forming cells by lymphocytes.
- Mutations in *TERT,* the gene for the RNA component of telomerase, cause short telomerases in congenital aplastic anemia and in some cases of apparently acquired hematopoietic failure. In patients with severe aplastic anemia receiving immunosuppressive therapy, telomere length is unrelated to response but is associated with risk of relapse, clonal evolution, and overall survival.

- Common etiologic factors in acquired aplastic anemia include:
  - Toxins (e.g., benzene, insecticides)
  - Drugs (e.g., felbamate [Felbatol], cimetidine, NSAIDs, antiepileptics, gold salts, chloramphenicol, sulfonamides, trimethadione, quinacrine, phenylbutazone)
  - Ionizing irradiation
  - Infections (e.g., hepatitis C, HIV, Epstein-Barr virus, parvovirus B19)
- Inherited aplastic anemia
  - Fanconi's anemia
  - Reticular dysgenesis
  - Dyskeratosis congenita
  - Nonhematologic syndromes (Down syndrome, etc.)
  - Shwachman-Diamond syndrome
- Pregnancy
- Idiopathic

DIAGNOSIS

DIFFERENTIAL DIAGNOSIS

- Bone marrow infiltration from lymphoma, carcinoma, myelofibrosis
- Severe infection
- Hypoplastic myelodysplastic syndrome or hypoplastic acute myeloid leukemia in adults
- Hypersplenism
- Hairy cell leukemia

WORKUP

- Diagnostic workup (Fig. E1-60) consists primarily of bone marrow aspiration and biopsy, and laboratory evaluation (CBC and examination of blood film).
- Bone marrow examination generally shows paucity or absence of erythropoietic and myelopoietic precursor cells (Fig. E1-61, *B* and *C*); patients with pure red cell aplasia demonstrate only absence of red blood cell (RBC) precursors in the marrow.

LABORATORY TESTS

- CBC reveals pancytopenia (Fig. E1-62, *A*). Macrocytosis and toxic granulation of neutrophils may also be present. Isolated cytopenias may occur in the early stages.
- Reticulocyte count reveals reticulocytopenia.
- Additional initial laboratory evaluation should include Ham test and/or peripheral blood flow cytometry to exclude paroxysmal nocturnal hemoglobinuria and testing for hepatitis C.

IMAGING STUDIES

MRI with spin-echo sequence is helpful in the study of bone marrow disease, and the high fat content of an aplastic marrow can be easily seen on MRI.

TREATMENT

NONPHARMACOLOGIC THERAPY

Discontinue any offending drugs or agents.

ACUTE GENERAL Rx

- Aggressive treatment of neutropenic fevers with parenteral broad-spectrum antibiotics.
- Administer platelet and RBC transfusions as needed; however, it is important to avoid transfusions in patients who are candidates for bone marrow transplantation.
- Fig. E1-63 describes a treatment algorithm for aplastic anemia.

CHRONIC Rx

- Allogenic bone marrow transplantation (ABMT) from a human leukocyte antigen (HLA)–matched sibling donor is curative.
- Patients who do not have a matched sibling can be treated with a matched unrelated transplant, but the mortality rate is higher.
- Immunosuppressive therapy with anti-thymocyte globulin (ATG) is an effective alternate treatment for patients who are not candidates for ABMT.
- Other immunosuppressive agents such as cyclosporin, cyclophosphamide, or corticosteroids also have a role in the treatment of aplastic anemia.
- Androgens such as danazol are effective second-line agents.
- The oral thrombopoietin mimetic eltrombopag can improve hematopoiesis in refractory severe aplastic anemia.

DISPOSITION

- The most recent update of the European Group for Bone Marrow Transplantation long-term survival rate has been reported to be 80%.
- Graft rejection and graft-versus-host disease are the major complications of ABMT.

REFERRAL

Hematology referral is indicated in all patients with aplastic anemia.

SUGGESTED READINGS
available at www.expertconsult.com

RELATED CONTENT
Fig. 3-9 Algorithm for Diagnosis of Anemias

AUTHORS: **BILAL H. NAQVI, M.D.,** and **FRED F. FERRI, M.D.**

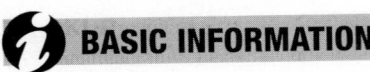

BASIC INFORMATION

DEFINITION

Autoimmune hemolytic anemia (AIHA) is anemia secondary to premature destruction of red blood cells (RBCs) caused by the binding of autoantibodies and/or complement to RBCs. A classification of the hemolytic anemias is described in Table 1-27.

ICD-9CM CODES

283.0 Autoimmune hemolytic anemia

EPIDEMIOLOGY & DEMOGRAPHICS

Predominant sex and age: most common in women <50 yr.

PHYSICAL FINDINGS & CLINICAL PRESENTATION

- Pallor, jaundice.
- Tachycardia with a flow murmur may be present if anemia is pronounced.
- Most common presentation is dyspnea and fatigue.
- Patients with intravascular hemolysis may present with dark urine and back pain.
- The presence of hepatomegaly and/or lymphadenopathy suggests an underlying lymphoproliferative disorder or malignancy; splenomegaly may indicate hypersplenism as a cause of hemolysis.

ETIOLOGY

- Warm antibody mediated: immunoglobulin (Ig) G (often idiopathic or associated with leukemia, lymphoma, thymoma, myeloma, viral infections, and collagen-vascular disease)
- Cold antibody mediated: IgM and complement in majority of cases (often idiopathic; at times associated with infections, lymphoma, or cold agglutinin disease)

TABLE 1-27 Classification of the Hemolytic Anemias

Acquired

Environmental factors
  Antibody: immunohemolytic anemias
  Mechanical trauma: TTP, HUS, heart valve
  Toxins, infectious agents: malaria, etc.

Membrane defects
  Paroxysmal nocturnal hemoglobinuria
  Spur cell anemia

Hereditary spherocytosis, etc.

Congenital

Defects of cell interior
  Hemoglobinopathies: sickle cell, thalassemia
  Enzymopathies: G6PD deficiency, etc.

G6PD, Glucose-6-phosphate dehydrogenase; *HUS*, hemolytic-uremic syndrome; *TTP*, thrombotic thrombocytopenic purpura.
From Goldman L, Schafer AI: *Goldman's Cecil medicine*, ed 24, Philadelphia, 2012, Saunders.

- Drug induced: three major mechanisms:
  1. Antibody directed against Rh complex (e.g., methyldopa)
  2. Antibody directed against RBC-drug complex (hapten induced; e.g., penicillin)
  3. Antibody directed against complex formed by drug and plasma proteins; the drug-plasma protein-antibody complex causes destruction of RBCs (innocent bystander; e.g., quinidine)

DIAGNOSIS

DIFFERENTIAL DIAGNOSIS

- Hemolytic anemia caused by membrane defects (paroxysmal nocturnal hemoglobinuria, spur cell anemia, Wilson disease)
- Non–immune mediated (microangiopathic hemolytic anemia, hypersplenism, cardiac valve prosthesis, giant cavernous hemangiomas, march hemoglobinuria, physical agents, infections, heavy metals, certain drugs [nitrofurantoin, sulfonamides, ribavirin])

WORKUP

Evaluation consists primarily of laboratory evaluation to confirm hemolysis and exclude other causes of the anemia. Although most cases of AIHA are idiopathic, potential causes should always be sought. Section III describes an algorithm for evaluation of suspected hemolytic anemia.

LABORATORY TESTS

- Initial laboratory tests: complete blood count (anemia), reticulocyte count (elevated; Fig. E1-64 describes the evaluation of anemia with elevated reticulocyte count), liver function studies (elevated indirect bilirubin, lactate dehydrogenase), evaluation of peripheral smear (Fig. E1-65), Coombs test (positive direct Coombs test indicates presence of antibodies or complement on the surface of RBCs [Fig. E1-66]; positive indirect Coombs test implies presence of anti-RBC antibodies freely circulating in the patient's serum [Fig. E1-67]), haptoglobin level (decreased)
- IgG antibody and IgM antibody
- Hepatitis serology, antinuclear antibody
- Urinary tests may reveal hemosiderinuria or hemoglobinuria

IMAGING STUDIES

- Chest x-ray
- CT scan of chest and abdomen to rule out lymphoma should be considered

TREATMENT

NONPHARMACOLOGIC THERAPY

- Discontinuation of any potentially offensive drugs
- Plasmapheresis exchange transfusion for severe life-threatening cases only
- Avoid cold exposure in patients with cold antibody

ACUTE GENERAL Rx

- Prednisone 1 to 2 mg/kg/day in divided doses initially in warm antibody AIHA. Corticosteroids are generally ineffective in cold antibody AIHA.
- Splenectomy in patients responding inadequately to corticosteroids when RBC sequestration studies indicate splenic sequestration.
- Immunosuppressive drugs and/or immunoglobulins only after both corticosteroids and splenectomy (unless surgery is contraindicated) have failed to produce an adequate remission.
- Danazol, typically used in conjunction with corticosteroids (may be useful in warm antibody AIHA).
- Immunosuppressive drugs (azathioprine, cyclophosphamide) may be useful in warm antibody AIHA but are indicated only after both corticosteroids and splenectomy (unless surgery is contraindicated) have failed to produce an adequate remission.

DISPOSITION

Prognosis is generally good unless anemia is associated with underlying disorder with a poor prognosis (e.g., leukemia, myeloma).

REFERRAL

- Hematology referral in all cases of AIHA
- Surgical referral for splenectomy in refractory cases

PEARLS & CONSIDERATIONS

COMMENTS

- The direct Coombs test (also known as the direct antiglobulin test) demonstrates the presence of antibodies or complement on the surface of RBCs and is the hallmark of autoimmune hemolysis.
- Warm AIHA is often associated with autoimmune diseases, whereas cold AIHA often follows viral infections (e.g., mononucleosis) and *Mycoplasma pneumoniae* infections.
- HIV can induce both warm and cold AIHA.

SUGGESTED READINGS

available at www.expertconsult.com

RELATED CONTENT

Fig. E3-13 Anemia with reticulocytosis (Algorithm)

AUTHOR: **FRED F. FERRI, M.D.**

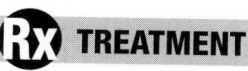

BASIC INFORMATION

DEFINITION

Inflammatory anemia refers to mild to moderately severe anemias (with hemoglobin [Hb] ranging from 7-12 g/dl), associated with chronic infections and inflammatory disorders, and some malignancies. Inflammatory anemia is also commonly referred to as anemia of chronic disease (ACD). may also refer to normal total body iron stores with low circulating iron (<60 mcg/dl).

SYNONYMS

Anemia of chronic disease
Anemia of inflammation
ACD

ICD-9CM CODES

285.21 Anemia in chronic kidney disease
285.22 Anemia in neoplastic disease
285.29 Anemia of other chronic illness
285.3 Antineoplastic chemotherapy induced anemia (effective October 1, 2009)
281.9 Unspecified deficiency anemia

EPIDEMIOLOGY & DEMOGRAPHICS

PREVALENCE: The prevalence rate in the elderly ranges from 8% to 44%, with the greatest prevalence in men 85 yr and older.
- Second-most prevalent anemia after iron deficiency anemia
- Perhaps one third of elderly adults with anemia suffer from anemia of chronic disease, anemia of chronic renal failure, or both
  - 11% of men and 10.2% of women age 65 to 85 yr
  - >20% of adults older than 85 yr

PREDOMINANT SEX AND AGE: Male sex >85 yr of age

RISK FACTORS:
- Chronic inflammatory conditions like autoimmune disorders (e.g., rheumatoid arthritis, systemic lupus erythematosus, vasculitis and sarcoidosis, inflammatory bowel disease [Crohn's disease/ulcerative colitis])
- Neoplasia (both hematologic cancer and solid tumors)
- Renal insufficiency/chronic kidney disease
- Infection (acute/chronic—viral, bacterial, parasitic, and fungal)
- Chronic rejection (graft vs. host disease) after solid-organ transplantation

PHYSICAL FINDINGS & CLINICAL PRESENTATION

Most patients are asymptomatic but may have general findings like skin pallor and conjunctival pallor.

ETIOLOGY

It is caused by several mechanisms (e.g., erythrocyte survival, increased uptake and retention of iron within cells of the reticuloendothelial system, inadequate transfer of iron from the reticuloendothelial system, limited availability of iron from erythroid progenitor cells, iron-restricted erythropoiesis.

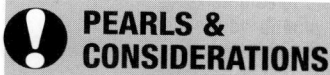

DIAGNOSIS

DIFFERENTIAL DIAGNOSIS

Iron deficiency anemia
Other causes of normocytic anemia
  Red blood cell loss or destruction
    Acute blood loss
    Hypersplenism
    Hemolysis
  Decreased red blood cell production
    Primary causes
      Marrow hypoplasia or aplasia
      Myelopathies
      Myeloproliferative disease
      Pure red blood cell aplasia
    Secondary causes
      Chronic renal failure
      Liver disease
      Endocrine deficiency states
      Sideroblastic anemia

WORKUP

Detailed history and physical examination

LABORATORY TESTS

CBC, reticulocyte count, reticulocyte index and pheripheral smear, serum iron levels, total iron-binding capacity, percentage saturation, and ferritin and erythropoietin level, and sometimes even bone marrow biopsy. Table E1-28 describes laboratory characteristics of inflammatory anemia. Usual findings are as follows:
- Hb levels (typically): 8 to 9.5 g/dl
- Low reticulocyte count (reflecting ineffective erythropoiesis)
- Low serum iron concentration (also low in iron deficiency anemia)
- Low transferrin saturation (also low in iron deficiency anemia)
- Serum ferritin (marker of iron storage) normal or increased (Fig. E1-68).
  - Acute inflammatory states may mimic the hematologic profile of anemia of chronic disease
- Soluble transferrin receptor (sTfR) levels remain within normal limits (they are elevated in iron deficiency anemia)
  - sTfR assays can distinguish iron deficiency anemia from anemia of chronic disease, even in patients with rheumatologic or other inflammatory disorders; enzyme-linked immunosorbent assay (ELISA) testing seems as reliable as bone marrow aspiration
- Erythropoietin level
  - Levels become increased only when Hb <10 g/dl
- Mean corpuscular volume (MCV): 81 to 99 femtoliter (fl)
- Peripheral smear usually reveals hypochromic normocytic RBCs (Fig. E1-69, *A*). Bone marrow shows that erythroid precursors are present in normal numbers (Fig. E1-69, *B*) and iron stores are increased in stromal histiocytes (Fig. E1-70).

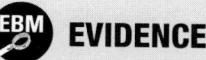

TREATMENT

Treat the underlying disorder/disease.

ACUTE GENERAL Rx

Blood transfusion usually reserved for severe anemia (Hb level <8.0 g/dl) or life-threatening anemia (Hb level <6.5 g/dl), particularly if complicated with ongoing bleeding. Increases survival rates in patients with anemia with myocardial infarction.

CHRONIC Rx

FDA-approved uses of erythropoiesis-stimulating agents epoetin alfa and darbepoetin alfa:
- Treatment of anemia with target Hb level ≤12 g/dl in the following patients:
  - Patients with chronic kidney failure
  - Cancer patients receiving chemotherapy
  - Patients with HIV infection who are taking zidovudine

REFERRAL

Hematology and oncology

PEARLS & CONSIDERATIONS

COMMENTS

The anemia of inflammation, which also includes anemia of critical illness, is a condition that presents similarly to anemia of chronic disease but develops within days of the onset of illness. An anemia similar to anemia of inflammation is seen in some elderly patients in the absence of identifiable chronic disease.

PREVENTION

Consider checking Hb levels or CBC in patients with renal failure, cancer, or other chronic disease for screening purposes.

PATIENT/FAMILY EDUCATION

Am Fam Physician 2000 Nov 15;62(10):2264
http://www.mdconsult.com/das/patient/view/0/10041/32120.html/top (English version)
http://www.mdconsult.com/das/patient/view/0/10041/32121.html/top (Spanish version)

EVIDENCE

available at www.expertconsult.com

SUGGESTED READINGS

available at www.expertconsult.com

AUTHORS: **STEPHANIE W. CHOW, M.D.,** and **NADIA MUJAHID, M.D.**

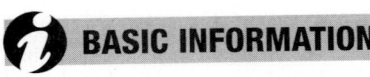

DEFINITION

Anemia is defined as a hemoglobin level 2 standard deviations below normal for age and sex. Iron deficiency anemia is anemia resulting from inadequate iron supplementation or excessive blood loss.

ICD-9CM CODES
280.9 Iron deficiency anemia
648.2 Iron deficiency anemia complicating pregnancy

EPIDEMIOLOGY & DEMOGRAPHICS

- Dietary iron deficiency occurs often in infants as a result of unsupplemented milk diets. It is also commonly seen in women during their reproductive years, as a result of heavy menstrual periods, and during pregnancy (increased demand).
- Iron deficiency is the most common nutritional deficiency worldwide.
- The prevalence of iron deficiency is greatest among toddlers ages 1 to 2 yr (7%) from inadequate intake and female individuals ages 12 to 49 yr (9% to 16%) from menstrual losses.

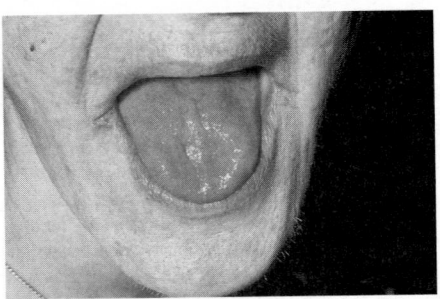

FIGURE 1-71 Iron deficiency. (From White GM, Cox NH [eds]: *Diseases of the skin, a color atlas and text,* ed 2, St. Louis, 2006, Mosby.)

- The prevalence of iron deficiency is 2% in adult men, 9% to 12% in non-Hispanic white women, and 20% in black and Mexican American women.
- GI cancer is diagnosed in 10% of elderly patients with iron deficiency anemia.

PHYSICAL FINDINGS & CLINICAL PRESENTATION

- Most patients have normal examination results.
- Skin pallor and conjunctival pallor may be present.
- Signs and symptoms specific for iron deficiency are koilonychias, pica, pagophagia, blue sclera, glossitis, and angular stomatitis (Fig. 1-71).
- Patients with severe anemia can have palpitations, headache, weakness, dizziness, and easy fatigability.

ETIOLOGY

- Blood loss from GI or menstrual bleeding (genitourinary blood loss less often the cause)
- Dietary iron deficiency (rare in adults)
- Poor iron absorption in patients with gastric or small-bowel surgery
- Repeated phlebotomy
- Increased requirements (e.g., during pregnancy)
- Other: traumatic hemolysis (abnormally functioning cardiac valves), idiopathic pulmonary hemosiderosis (iron sequestration in pulmonary macrophages), paroxysmal nocturnal hemoglobinuria (intravascular hemolysis)
- The most common cause worldwide is hookworm infection

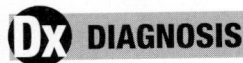 DIAGNOSIS

DIFFERENTIAL DIAGNOSIS

- Anemia of chronic disease
- Sideroblastic anemia
- Thalassemia trait
- Lead poisoning

WORKUP

Diagnostic workup consists primarily of laboratory evaluation. Table 1-29 describes laboratory studies differentiating the most common microcytic anemias. Most patients with iron deficiency anemia are asymptomatic in the early stages. With progressive anemia, the major symptoms are fatigue, dizziness, exertional dyspnea, pagophagia (ice eating), and pica. Patient history may also suggest GI blood loss (melena, hematochezia, hemoptysis).

LABORATORY TESTS

- Laboratory results vary with the stage of deficiency.
- Absent iron marrow stores and decreased serum ferritin are the initial abnormalities.
- Decreased serum iron and increased total iron-binding capacity (TIBC) are the next abnormalities.
- Hypochromic microcytic anemia is present with significant iron deficiency.
- Peripheral smear in patients with iron deficiency generally reveals microcytic hypochromic red blood cells (Fig. 1-72) with a wide area of central pallor, anisocytosis, and poikilocytosis when severe.
- Laboratory abnormalities consistent with iron deficiency are low serum ferritin level, increased RBC distribution width with values generally >15, low mean corpuscular volume, low mean corpuscular hemoglobin, increased TIBC, and low serum iron.
- In patients diagnosed with iron deficiency anemia, a GI workup including an upper endoscopy and colonoscopy is recommended to look for source of iron loss.

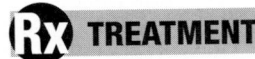 TREATMENT

The goal of therapy is to supply sufficient iron to correct the low hemoglobin and replenish iron stores.

NONPHARMACOLOGIC THERAPY

Patients should be instructed to consume foods that contain large amounts of iron, such as liver, red meat, and legumes.

ACUTE GENERAL Rx

- Treatment consists of ferrous sulfate 325 mg PO daily for at least 6 mo. Doses higher than 325 mg/day are poorly tolerated. Calcium supplements can decrease iron absorption; therefore, these two medications should be staggered.
- Parenteral iron therapy is reserved for patients with poor tolerance, noncompliance with oral preparations, or malabsorption.
- Transfusion of packed RBCs is indicated in patients with severe symptomatic anemia.

CHRONIC Rx

Patients should be instructed to continue their iron supplements for at least 6 mo or longer to correct depleted body iron stores.

TABLE 1-29 Laboratory Studies Differentiating the Most Common Microcytic Anemias

Study	Iron Deficiency Anemia	α or β Thalassemia	Anemia of Chronic Disease
Hemoglobin	Decreased	Decreased	Decreased
MCV	Decreased	Decreased	Normal-decreased
RDW	Increased	Normal	Normal-increased
RBC	Decreased	Normal-increased	Normal-decreased
Serum ferritin	Decreased	Normal	Increased
Total Fe binding capacity	Increased	Normal	Decreased
Transferrin saturation	Decreased	Normal	Decreased
FEP	Increased	Normal	Increased
Transferrin receptor	Increased	Normal	Increased
Reticulocyte hemoglobin concentration	Decreased	Normal	Normal-decreased

Fe, Ferritin; *FEP,* free erythrocyte protoporphyrin; *MCV,* mean corpuscular volume; *RBC,* red blood cell; *RDW,* red cell distribution width.
From Kliegman RM et al: *Nelson textbook of pediatrics,* ed 19, Philadelphia, 2011, Saunders.

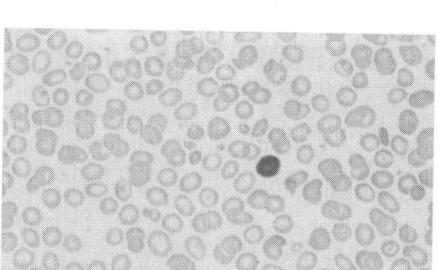

FIGURE 1-72 Iron deficiency anemia. Many of these red blood cells are microcytic (smaller than the nucleus of the normal lymphocyte near the center of the field) and hypochromic (with central areas of pallor that exceed half the diameter of the cells). (From Goldman L, Schafer AI: *Goldman's Cecil medicine,* ed 24, Philadelphia, 2012, Saunders.)

DISPOSITION

- Most patients respond rapidly to iron supplementation with improvement in CBC and general well-being (Table 1-30). GI side effects from oral iron therapy are common and may require decreased dosage to once every other day or to change to parenteral iron.
- A differential diagnosis of microcytic anemia that fails to respond to oral iron is described in Table 1-31.

REFERRAL

GI referral for evaluation of GI malignancy is recommended in all patients with iron deficiency and suspected GI blood loss.

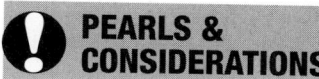 **PEARLS & CONSIDERATIONS**

A

COMMENTS

- Iron deficiency may impair aerobic performance and worsen symptoms in patients with heart failure. Treatment with IV iron in patients with chronic heart failure and iron deficiency has been shown to improve symptoms, quality of life, and functional capacity.
- If the diagnosis of iron deficiency anemia is made, locating the suspected site of iron loss is mandatory.

SUGGESTED READINGS
available at www.expertconsult.com

RELATED CONTENT
Fig. 3-9 Algorithm for diagnosis of anemias
Iron Deficiency Anemia (Patient Information)

AUTHORS: **BILAL H. NAQVI, M.D.,**
and **FRED F. FERRI, M.D.**

Diseases and Disorders

I

TABLE 1-30 Responses to Iron Therapy in Iron-Deficiency Anemia

Time after Iron Administration	Response
12-24 hr	Replacement of intracellular iron enzymes; subjective improvement; decreased irritability; increased appetite
36-48 hr	Initial bone marrow response; erythroid hyperplasia
48-72 hr	Reticulocytosis, peaking at 5–7 days
4-30 days	Increase in hemoglobin level
1-3 mo	Repletion of stores

From Kliegman RM et al: *Nelson textbook of pediatrics,* ed 19, Philadelphia, 2011, Saunders.

TABLE 1-31 Differential Diagnosis of Microcytic Anemia That Fails to Respond to Oral Iron

Poor compliance (true intolerance of iron is uncommon)
Incorrect dose or medication
Malabsorption of administered iron
Ongoing blood loss including gastrointestinal, menstrual, and pulmonary
Concurrent infection or inflammatory disorder inhibiting the response to iron
Concurrent vitamin B_{12} or folate deficiency
Diagnosis other than iron deficiency
- Thalassemias
- Hemoglobin C and E disorders
- Anemia of chronic disease
- Lead poisoning
- Sickle thalassemias, hemoglobin SC disease
- Rare microcytic anemias

From Kliegman RM et al: *Nelson textbook of pediatrics,* ed 19, Philadelphia, 2011, Saunders.

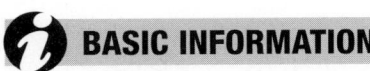

BASIC INFORMATION

DEFINITION
Pernicious anemia (PA) is an autoimmune disease resulting from antibodies against intrinsic factor and gastric parietal cells.

SYNONYMS
Megaloblastic anemia resulting from vitamin B_{12} deficiency

ICD-9CM CODES
281.0 Pernicious anemia

EPIDEMIOLOGY & DEMOGRAPHICS
- Increased incidence in females and older adults (diagnosis is unusual before age 35 yr)
- The overall prevalence of undiagnosed PA after age 60 yr is 1.9%
- Prevalence is highest in women (2.7%), particularly in black women (4.3%)
- Increased incidence of autoimmune disease (e.g., type 1 diabetes mellitus, Graves disease, Addison disease), *Helicobacter pylori* infection

PHYSICAL FINDINGS & CLINICAL PRESENTATION
- Mucosal pallor, glossitis
- Peripheral sensory neuropathy with paresthesias initially and absent reflexes in advanced cases
- Loss of joint position sense, pyramidal or long tract signs
- Possible splenomegaly and mild hepatomegaly
- Generalized weakness and delirium/dementia

ETIOLOGY
- Gastric/antiparietal cell antibodies in >70% of patients; antiintrinsic factor antibodies in >50% of patients
- Atrophic gastric mucosa
- Inborn errors of cobalamin-cofactor synthesis are rare. The cobalamin gene *(cblD)* is localized to human chromosome 2q23.2. Mutations in the gene designated MMADHC (methylmalonic aciduria, cblD type, and homocystinuria) are responsible for the cblD defect in vitamin B_{12} metabolism.
- Fig. E1-73 illustrates the components and mechanism of cobalamin absorption. An etiopathophysiologic classification of cobalamin deficiency is described in Section II.

DIAGNOSIS

DIFFERENTIAL DIAGNOSIS
- Nutritional vitamin B_{12} deficiency
- Malabsorption
- Chronic alcoholism (multifactorial)
- Chronic gastritis related to *H. pylori* infection
- Folic acid deficiency
- Myelodysplasia

WORKUP
- The clinical presentation of PA varies with the stage. Initially, patients may be asymptomatic. In advanced stages patients may have impaired memory, depression, gait disturbances, paresthesias, and reports of generalized weakness.
- Investigation consists primarily of laboratory evaluation.
- Endoscopy and biopsy for atrophic gastritis may be performed in selected cases.
- Diagnosis is crucial because failure to treat may result in irreversible neurologic deficits.

LABORATORY TESTS
- Complete blood count generally reveals macrocytic anemia and leukopenia with hypersegmented neutrophils (Fig. E1-74).
- Mean corpuscular volume (MCV) is generally significantly elevated in the advanced stages.
- Reticulocyte count is low to normal.
- Falsely low serum cobalamin levels can occur in patients with severe folate deficiency, in patients using high doses of ascorbic acid, and when cobalamin levels are measured after nuclear medicine studies (radioactivity interferes with cobalamin radioimmunoassay measurement).
- Falsely high normal levels in patients with cobalamin deficiency can occur in severe liver disease or chronic granulocytic leukemia.
- The absence of anemia or macrocytosis does not exclude the diagnosis of cobalamin deficiency. Anemia is absent in 20% of patients with cobalamin deficiency, and macrocytosis is absent in >30% of patients at the time of diagnosis. It can be blocked by concurrent iron deficiency or anemia of chronic disease and may be masked by thalassemia trait.
- Schilling test is abnormal in part I; part II corrects to normal after administration of intrinsic factor.
- Laboratory tests used for detecting cobalamin deficiency in patients with normal vitamin B_{12} levels include serum and urinary methylmalonic acid level (elevated), total homocysteine level (elevated), intrinsic factor antibody (positive).
- An increased concentration of plasma methylmalonic acid does not predict clinical manifestations of vitamin B_{12} deficiency and should not be used as the only marker for diagnosis of B_{12} deficiency.
- Additional laboratory abnormalities can include elevated lactate dehydrogenase, direct hyperbilirubinemia, and decreased haptoglobin.
- Bone marrow aspirate may show giant C-shaped neutrophil bands and megaloblastic normoblasts (Fig. E1-75).

TREATMENT

NONPHARMACOLOGIC THERAPY
Avoid folic acid supplementation without proper vitamin B_{12} supplementation.

ACUTE GENERAL Rx
Traditional therapy of a cobalamin deficiency consists of IM injections of vitamin B_{12} 1000 mcg/wk for the initial 4 to 6 wk followed by 1000 mcg/mo IM indefinitely. In patients who have no nervous system involvement, intranasal cyanocobalamin may be used in place of IM cyanocobalamin when hematologic parameters have returned to normal range. The initial dose of intranasal cyanocobalamin (Nascobal) is 1 spray (500 mcg) in one nostril once per week. Cost generally exceeds $120/mo. Monitor response and increase dose if serum B_{12} levels decline. Consider return to intramuscular vitamin B_{12} supplementation if decline persists.

CHRONIC Rx
- Parenteral vitamin B_{12} 1000 mcg/mo or intranasal cyanocobalamin 500 mcg/wk (see "Acute General Rx") for the remainder of life.
- Oral cobalamin (1000 to 2000 mcg/day) has been reported as also being effective in mild cases of pernicious anemia because approximately 1% of an oral dose is absorbed by passive diffusion, a pathway that does not require intrinsic factor. Cost for 1 mo of therapy is approximately $5.

DISPOSITION
Anemia generally resolves with appropriate treatment. Neurologic deficits, if present at diagnosis, may be permanent.

REFERRAL
Gastrointestinal referral for endoscopy on diagnosis of PA and surveillance endoscopy every 5 yr to rule out gastric carcinoma.

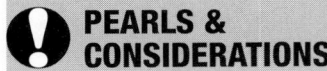

PEARLS & CONSIDERATIONS

COMMENTS
- Patients must understand that therapy is lifelong.
- Self-injection of vitamin B_{12} may be taught in selected patients. Cost of monthly injection is less than $5.

SUGGESTED READING
available at www.expertconsult.com

RELATED CONTENT
Fig. 3-9 Algorithm for diagnosis of anemias Pernicious Anemia (Patient Information)

AUTHOR: **FRED F. FERRI, M.D.**

BASIC INFORMATION

DEFINITION

Sideroblastic anemia is a heterogeneous group of blood disorders whose two distinctive features are ring sideroblasts in the bone marrow (abnormal erythroblasts with excessive iron accumulation in the mitochondria) and impaired heme biosynthesis. They are classified as hereditary, acquired, and reversible.

SYNONYMS

Hereditary sideroblastic anemias
Acquired idiopathic sideroblastic anemia (AISA)
Reversible sideroblastic anemias

ICD-9CM CODES
285.0 Sideroblastic anemia

EPIDEMIOLOGY & DEMOGRAPHICS

- Sex-linked; primarily affects males.
- AISA affects middle-aged and older adults.

PHYSICAL FINDINGS & CLINICAL PRESENTATION

The symptoms for sideroblastic anemia are the same for any anemia and iron overload:
- Fatigue, weakness, palpitations, shortness of breath, headaches, and irritability.
- Physical findings may include pallor, tachycardia, hepatosplenomegaly, S3 gallop, jugular vein distention, and rales.

ETIOLOGY

- The hereditary forms can be X-linked, autosomal dominant or autosomal recessive.
- Acquired forms may be associated with chemotherapy or irradiation.
- Refractory anemia with ringed sideroblast develops as a subtype of myelodysplacia.
- Reversible sideroblastic anemia can be caused by alcohol, isoniazid, pyrazinamide, cycloserine, chloramphenicol, or copper deficiency.

DIAGNOSIS

The principal feature is indolent and progressive, mild, lifelong anemia that goes unnoticed. Symptoms of iron overload may lead to discovery of the underlying disorder. The history and clinical findings, together with typical laboratory findings, usually permit accurate diagnosis of each type of sideroblastic anemia. The molecular defects can be identified in several hereditary forms and in some patients with AISA.

DIFFERENTIAL DIAGNOSIS

- Sideroblastic anemia must be differentiated from other causes of microcytic hypochromic anemia: iron deficiency anemia, thalassemia, anemia of chronic disease, and lead poisoning.
- Tissue iron overload from sideroblastic anemia may act similar to hereditary hemochromatosis with liver cirrhosis, diabetes, congestive heart failure, or cardiac arrhythmias.

WORKUP

Laboratory evaluation: CBC, iron studies, free erythrocyte protoporphyrin level, MRI, bone marrow aspiration, and liver biopsy.

LABORATORY TESTS

- Hypochromic microcytic anemia for the hereditary type and normo- or macrocytic anemia for AISA.
- High serum iron levels, low transferrin along with increased transferrin saturation and high serum ferritin.
- Peripheral smear: dimorphic large and small cells (Fig. E1-76) revealing Pappenheimer bodies or siderocytes when stained for iron.
- Bone marrow shows increased iron stores (Fig. E1-77) and the classic ringed sideroblasts not seen in normal bone marrow tissue (Fig. 1-78). The ringed sideroblasts represent iron storage in the mitochondria of normoblasts.
- In transfusion-dependent anemias, monitoring of ferritin and transferrin saturation levels is recommended despite minimal transfusion needs to avoid iron overload.
- Features of ineffective erythropoiesis like increase in indirect bilirubin concentration, decrease in haptoglobin, increase in LDH, and normal or increase in reticulocyte number is seen.

TREATMENT

Treatment is directed at controlling symptoms of anemia and preventing organ damage from iron overload.

NONPHARMACOLOGIC THERAPY

Avoid alcohol

ACUTE GENERAL Rx

- A trial of pyridoxine (100-200 mg) is indicated for all patients with hereditary sideroblastic anemia.
- 25% to 50% may show full or partial response to pyridoxine.
- Patients who do not respond will need to be treated with blood transfusion.
- Chelation therapy is needed for patients with transfusion-dependant anemia to prevent complications of iron overload.

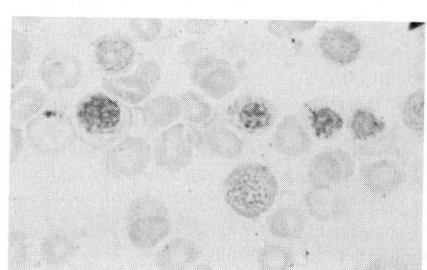

FIGURE 1-78 Prussian blue iron stain of the bone marrow shows ringed sideroblasts. (From Goldman L, Ausiello D [eds]: *Cecil textbook of medicine*, ed 24, Philadelphia, 2012, Saunders.)

- Erythropoietin and granulocyte colony-stimulating factor may show some success in treating MDS-associated refractory anemia with ringed sideroblast.
- Secondary sideroblastic anemia caused by medication can be reversed by withdrawing the medication and administering vitamin B_6 (50 to 200 mg/day).

CHRONIC Rx

- Organ dysfunction resulting from iron overload will require periodic phlebotomy to keep serum ferritin level <300 ng/ml.
- Iron chelating therapy for patients with moderately severe anemia in those who require regular red cell transfusion: deferoxamine continuous infusion or the oral agent deferasirox (EXJADE).
- Splenectomy should be avoided at all costs.

DISPOSITION

In patients with anemia alone, life expectancy is normal. In patients dependent on blood transfusions, morbidity from iron overload can be expected. There are two types of AISA:
1. Pure sideroblastic anemia: with dysplasia confined to the erythroid cell lineage; survival similar to age-matched controls; no incidence of leukemic transformation.
2. Refractory anemia with ringed sideroblasts: dysplastic features involving the red cell lineage, granulopoiesis, and/or megakaryopoiesis; approximately 5% will develop acute leukemia. Erythropoietin and granulocyte colony-stimulating factor therapy do not change survival.

REFERRAL

- Hematology.
- Families with severe forms of hereditary sideroblastic anemia should receive genetic counseling.

PEARLS & CONSIDERATIONS

- Sideroblastic anemia can be thought of as an iron-loading anemia secondary to defective heme synthesis.
- A predisposition to leukemia evolution has not been observed in patients with hereditary forms.
- Symptoms rather than an absolute hemoglobin level or hematocrit should guide transfusion therapy.

COMMENTS

Vitamin B_6, or pyridoxal phosphate, is a required cofactor in heme synthesis, and drugs such as isoniazid, cycloserine, and pyrazinamide can inhibit its function.

SUGGESTED READINGS

available at www.expertconsult.com

RELATED CONTENT

Fig. 3-9 Algorithm for Diagnosis of Anemias

AUTHOR: **BILAL H. NAQVI, M.D.**

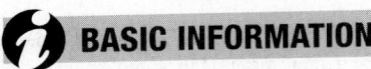

DEFINITION

An abdominal aortic aneurysm (AAA) is a focal dilation of the abdominal aortic artery to at least 1.5 times the diameter measured at the level of the renal arteries, or exceeding the normal diameter of the abdominal aorta by 50%. The normal diameter at the renal arteries is 2 cm (range 1.4-3.0 cm), and a diameter 3 cm or larger is generally considered aneurysmal.

SYNONYMS

AAA

ICD-9CM CODES
441.4 Aneurysm, abdominal (aorta)
441.3 Ruptured abdominal aortic aneurysm

EPIDEMIOLOGY & DEMOGRAPHICS

- Approximately 15,000 deaths/year in the United States are attributed to AAA.
- AAA is predominantly a disease of older adults, affecting men more than women (4:1).
- The prevalence rate ranges from 4% to 9% in men older than age 60.
- Clinically important AAAs ≥4 cm are present in 1% of men ages 55 to 64, and the prevalence rate increases by 2% to 4% per decade thereafter.
- The peak incidence is among men approximately 70 years old.
- The frequency is much higher in smokers than in nonsmokers (8:1), and the risk decreases slowly after smoking cessation.
- AAA is 2 to 4 times more common in first-degree male relatives of known AAA patients.
- Risk factors for AAA are similar to other atherosclerotic cardiovascular diseases; they include age, smoking, male sex, family history, hypertension, hyperlipidemia, and peripheral vascular disease. Aneurysm of other large vessels is also a risk factor for AAA.
- Rupture of the AAA occurs in 1% to 3% of men age 65 or older.
  - Rupture is the 10th leading cause of death in men older than age 55.
  - Mortality from rupture is 70% to 95%.
  - Risk factors for rupture include cardiac or renal transplants, severe obstructive lung disease, uncontrolled blood pressure, female sex, and ongoing tobacco use.
- Risk factors for AAA are similar to other atherosclerotic cardiovascular diseases; they include age, smoking, male sex, family history, hypertension, hyperlipidemia, and peripheral vascular disease. Aneurysm of other large vessels is also a risk factor for AAA.
- The U.S. Preventive Services Task Force recommends one-time screening for AAA by ultrasonography in men ages 65 to 75 who have ever smoked in their lifetime and in those 60 years and older with a history of AAA in a parent or sibling. These populations have been shown to have a higher prevalence of AAA, and selectively screening this group has been shown to decrease AAA-specific mortality.
- Epidemiologic studies have demonstrated a decline in incidence, prevalence, and/or mortality in certain populations.

PHYSICAL FINDINGS & CLINICAL PRESENTATION

- Most aneurysms are asymptomatic and incidentally discovered on imaging studies; however, symptomatic aneurysms are at an increased risk for rupture.
- Physical examination has a sensitivity of 76% for detecting AAAs >5 cm and only 29% for AAAs 3.0-3.9 cm.
- Symptomatic patients may present with abdominal, back, flank, or groin pain.
- A pulsatile epigastric mass that may or may not be tender may be present.
- Abdominal pain radiating to the back, flank, and groin.
- Abdominal bruits can be present in case of renal or visceral arterial stenosis.
- Common iliac arteries can be aneurysmal and palpable in the lower abdominal quadrants. In addition, prominent femoral and popliteal pulses warrant an abdominal ultrasound and lower extremity ultrasound.
- Early satiety, nausea, and vomiting may be caused by compression of adjacent bowel.
- Venous thrombosis or insufficiency may occur from iliocaval venous compression.
- Thromboembolization can cause lower extremity pain and discoloration.
- Ureteral obstruction and hydronephrosis can cause flank and groin pain and lead to obstructive renal failure.
- Rupture classically presents as a triad of abdominal or back pain, hypotension, and a pulsatile abdominal mass in 50% of patients.
- Acute blood loss may lead to myocardial infarction; arteriovenous fistulas may present as heart failure; aortoenteric fistulas may present as hematemesis or melena associated with abdominal and back pain.

ETIOLOGY

- Exact etiology is unknown and is likely multifactorial. AAA formation and rupture may result from elastin and collagen degradation by proteases such as plasmin, matrix metalloproteinases (MMPs), and cathepsin S and K.
- Degenerative:
  - The most common association is atherosclerosis. It is uncertain if atherosclerosis causes or results from AAAs.
  - Tobacco use: >90% of people who develop an AAA have smoked at some point in their life.
- Inherited: Familial clusters are common. High familial prevalence rate is notable in male individuals. The nature of the genetic disorder is unclear but may be linked to alpha-1-antitrypsin deficiency or X-linked mutation. Connective tissue disorders, such as Marfan's syndrome and Ehlers-Danlos syndrome, have also been strongly associated with AAA.
- Inflammatory, arteritis.
- Infection, mycotic: syphilis, *Salmonella.*

NATURAL HISTORY

- The risk of aneurysmal rupture is largely influenced by aneurysm size, rate of expansion, and sex. Other factors associated with increased risk for rupture include continued smoking, uncontrolled hypertension, and increased wall stress.
- AAAs tend to develop in the infrarenal aorta.
- Higher tension in the abdominal aorta (together with histopathologic changes such as accumulation of foam cells, cholesterol crystals, and matrix metalloproteinases) renders the abdominal aortic wall more susceptible to dilation and subsequent rupture.
- The 5-year rupture rate of asymptomatic AAAs is 25% to 40% for aneurysms >5.0 cm, 1% to 7% for AAAs 4.0 to 5.0 cm, and nearly 0% for AAAs <4.0 cm. The rate of rupture of aneurysms that were 4.0-5.5 cm in diameter is four times greater in women compared with men.
- Mortality rate after rupture can be >90% because most patients do not reach the hospital in time for surgical repair. Of those who reach the hospital, the mortality rate is still 50%, compared with the 1% to 4% mortality rate for elective repair of a nonruptured AAA.

Dx DIAGNOSIS

DIFFERENTIAL DIAGNOSIS

Almost 75% of patients with AAA are asymptomatic, and the condition is discovered on routine examination or serendipitously when ordering studies for other symptoms. Diagnosis of AAA should be considered in the differential of the following symptoms: abdominal pain, back pain, and/or pulsatile abdominal mass.

LABORATORY TESTS

Not routinely indicated. For suspected infected or inflammatory aneurysms, WBC, ESR/CRP, and blood cultures can be considered. An elevated D-dimer may indicate a thrombus within the aneurysm.

IMAGING STUDIES (Fig. 1-79)

- Plain radiographs may show the outline of an aneurysm in calcified aortas. This is an insensitive test for diagnosing AAA.

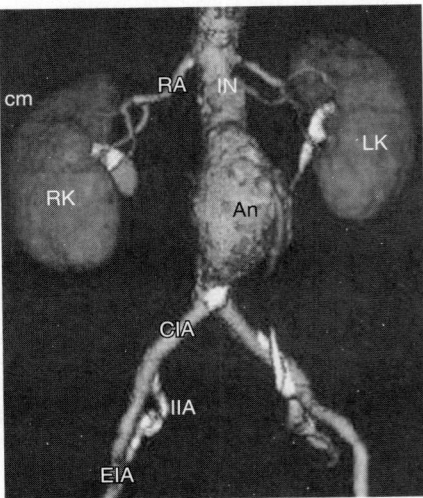

FIGURE 1-79 Three-dimensional CT image illustrates the presence of an infrarenal abdominal aortic aneurysm. *An,* Aneurysm; *CIA,* common iliac artery; *EIA,* external iliac artery; *IIA,* internal iliac artery; *IN,* infrarenal neck; *LK,* left kidney; *RA,* renal artery; *RK,* right kidney. (From Townsend CM et al [eds]: *Sabiston textbook of surgery,* ed 17, Philadelphia, 2004, Saunders.)

- Abdominal ultrasound is nearly 100% accurate in identifying an aneurysm and estimating the size to within 0.3–0.4 cm. It is not accurate in estimating the extension to the renal arteries or the iliac arteries.
- Computed tomography (CT) scan is recommended for preoperative aneurysm imaging and estimates the size of the AAA to within 0.3 mm. There are no false-negative results, and the scan can localize the extent to renal vessels with more precision than ultrasound. CT can also detect the integrity of the wall and exclude rupture.
- Magnetic resonance angiography (MRA) may also be used and is at least as accurate as CT.
- Angiography gives detailed arterial anatomy, localizing the aneurysm relative to the renal and visceral arteries. This is the definitive preoperative study before surgery.

Rx TREATMENT

NONPHARMACOLOGIC THERAPY

- Despite lack of data substantiating reduction in expansion rate through treatment of cardiac risk factors, nonpharmacological treatment continues to focus on risk factor modification (most importantly smoking cessation, diet, and exercise).
- Serial studies have shown that expansion rates are faster in current smokers than in former smokers.
- Definitive treatment depends on the size of the aneurysm (see "Chronic Rx").

ACUTE GENERAL Rx

- AAA repair can be done with open surgical or endovascular aneurysm repair (EVAR). The choice is determined by anatomic considerations, operative risks, and availability of regular patient follow-up for EVAR.
- Emergent open repair has been the traditional method of treatment. That being said, however, several randomized controlled trials had shown fewer perioperative deaths and no increase in morbidity or mortality with endovascular repair. More centers are increasingly using endovascular repair for patients who fit certain anatomic and physiologic criteria. However, in a recent long-term trial among older patients with isolated intact AAA, use of open repair compared with endovascular repair was associated with increased risk of all-cause mortality and AAA-related mortality.

CHRONIC Rx

- Blood pressure and fasting lipids should be monitored and controlled as recommended for patients with atherosclerotic disease. Antihyperlipidemic agents such as the statin family of drugs should be prescribed unless contraindications are present.
- The most commonly used predictor of rupture is the maximum diameter of the AAA.
- Monitoring by ultrasound or CT scan should be performed every 6 to 12 months for patients with AAAs measuring 4.0 to 5.4 cm and every 2 years for those with AAAs measuring <4 cm.
- Long-term beta-blocker therapy has slowed the rate of aortic dilation and decreased the incidence of aortic complications in patients with Marfan's syndrome. Several studies have also suggested that beta-blocker therapy may reduce the rate of expansion and risk of rupture; however, conclusive evidence is lacking. In a Cochrane Database Systematic Review, propranolol was poorly tolerated in all beta-blocker trials and had only minimal, nonsignificant protective benefit.
- Antibiotics such as doxycycline and roxithromycin have potential to limit the growth of AAAs, as shown in small human studies with promising results.
- Surgical repair to eliminate the risk for rupture should be performed for patients with infrarenal or juxtarenal AAA of approximately 5.5 cm. All patients who are symptomatic should undergo repair, regardless of size.
- There is no clear advantage to early repair (open or endovascular) for small AAAs (4.0-5.4 cm).
- Intervention is not recommended for asymptomatic infrarenal or juxtarenal AAAs <5.0 cm in men or <4.5 cm in women.
- Percutaneous, endovascular, stent-anchored grafts placed with the patient under local anesthesia have provided an alternative approach (Fig. 1-80) for patients with favorable anatomy. In patients who have undergone endovascular repair, long-term surveillance is required to assess for endoleak, stent migration, change in aneurysm size, and need for re-intervention.
- Randomized trials have shown that endovascular repair of AAA is associated with a significantly lower operative mortality than open surgical repair but it has increased rates of graft-related complications, increased rates of reintervention, and is more costly. EVAR leads to increased long-term survival among younger patients but not among older patients. There are no differences between endovascular repair and open surgical repair in total mortality or aneurysm-related mortality in the long term.
- Based on current data, less than 1% of endovascular repairs require open conversion and approximately half of all early endoleaks resolve spontaneously within a period of 30 days.
- Endovascular repair in patients who are poor candidates for open repair, as determined by comorbidities, is of uncertain effectiveness.
- In high-risk patients, specifically those with coronary artery disease or those with more than one clinical risk factor based on the American Heart Association (AHA) guidelines, beta-blockers titrated to a goal heart rate of 60 have been shown to decrease incidence of death from cardiac causes or nonfatal myocardial infarctions.
- Patients with chronic obstructive pulmonary disease (COPD) are at higher risk for major clinical complications, particularly if the COPD is suboptimally managed or if it is present in conjunction with cardiac or renal disease. Smoking cessation for 2 months before surgery has also been shown to decrease pulmonary morbidity.
- Renal dysfunction is a strong predictor of mortality, showing up to as high as 41% mortality in those with impaired renal function compared with 6% in those without renal dysfunction.

REFERRAL

- Vascular surgical referral should be made in asymptomatic patients with AAAs that are approximately 4.5 cm.
- In patients with an expansion rate of 0.6-0.8 cm/year, it is reasonable to offer repair, although small studies have shown that using expansion as a criterion for surgical referral is of unclear benefit.
- It is important to optimize any comorbid conditions before surgical referral.

⊘ PEARLS & CONSIDERATIONS

- Repairing AAAs smaller than 5.5 cm has not been shown to improve survival because the risk of rupture is lower than the risk of surgery.

COMMENTS

- Most AAAs are infrarenal.
- Surgical risk is increased in patients with coexisting coronary artery disease, pulmonary disease, or chronic renal failure. Evaluation for ischemia and aggressive perioperative hemodynamic monitoring help identify high-risk patients and decrease postoperative complications.
- It is estimated that AAAs <5 cm expand at a rate of 0.4 cm/year.

SUGGESTED READINGS

available at www.expertconsult.com

RELATED CONTENT

Abdominal Aortic Aneurysm (AAA) (Patient Information)

AUTHORS: **AILIN BARSEGHIAN EL-FARRA, M.D.,** and **PRANAV M. PATEL, M.D., F.A.C.C., F.S.C.A.I.**

FIGURE 1-80 Endovascular abdominal aortic aneurysm repair involves aneurysm exclusion with an endoluminal aortic stent-graft introduced remotely, usually through the femoral artery. An endovascular graft extends from the infrarenal aorta to both common iliac arteries, preserving the flow to the internal iliac arteries. *CIA,* Common iliac artery; *IIA,* internal iliac artery; *IN,* infrarenal aortic neck; *LK,* left kidney; *RK,* right kidney; *SA,* suprarenal aorta. (From Townsend CM et al [eds]: *Sabiston textbook of surgery,* ed 17, Philadelphia, 2004, Saunders.)

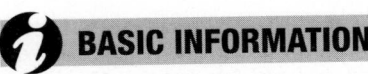

DEFINITION

Angina pectoris is a term used to describe a syndrome, typically characterized by chest discomfort, that is caused by myocardial ischemia (ischemic heart disease [IHD]). This is most commonly related to atheromatous plaque in the coronary arteries; however, myocardial ischemia may occur in the absence of obstructive coronary artery disease (CAD). Any situation that causes an imbalance in myocardial oxygen supply and demand can cause an angina syndrome. Angina can be classified as follows:

1. Chronic (stable IHD [SIHD]):
   - Usually follows a precipitating event (e.g., climbing stairs, sexual intercourse, a heavy meal, emotional stress, cold weather).
   - Generally same severity as previous attacks; relieved by rest or by the customary dose of nitroglycerin.
   - Caused by a fixed coronary artery obstruction secondary to atherosclerosis. The presence of one or more obstructions in major coronary arteries is likely; the severity of stenosis is usually >70%.
2. Unstable (rest or crescendo, acute coronary syndrome):
   - Recent onset.
   - Increasing severity, duration, or frequency of chronic angina.
   - Occurs at rest or with minimal exertion.
3. Prinzmetal's variant:
   - Occurs at rest.
   - Manifests electrocardiographically as episodic ST-segment elevations.
   - Caused by coronary artery spasms with or without superimposed CAD.
   - Patients also more likely to develop ventricular arrhythmias.
4. Microvascular angina (syndrome X):
   - Refers to patients with normal coronary angiograms and no coronary spasm but chest pain resembling angina and positive exercise test.
   - Defective endothelium-dependent dilation in the coronary microcirculation contributing to the altered regulation of myocardial perfusion and the ischemic manifestations in these patients.
   - Patients with chest pain and normal or nonobstructive coronary angiograms are predominantly women, and many have a prognosis that is not as benign as commonly thought (2% risk of death or myocardial infarction [MI] at 30 days of follow-up).
5. Refractory angina:
   - Refers to patients who, despite optimal medical therapy, have both angina and objective evidence of ischemia and are not considered candidates for revascularization.
6. Other:
   - Angina due to aortic stenosis and idiopathic hypertrophic subaortic stenosis, cocaine-induced coronary vasoconstriction.

FUNCTIONAL CLASSIFICATION

It is helpful to grade the severity of stable angina using a grading system. The most commonly adopted is that of the Canadian Cardiovascular Society:

- Class I: Ordinary physical activity, such as walking or climbing stairs, does not cause angina. Angina occurs with strenuous, rapid, or prolonged exertion at work or recreation.
- Class II: Slight limitation of ordinary activity. Angina occurs on walking or climbing stairs rapidly; walking uphill; walking or stair climbing after meals, in cold, in wind, or under emotional stress; or only during the few hours after awakening. Angina occurs on walking more than two level blocks and climbing more than one flight of ordinary stairs at a normal pace and in normal conditions.
- Class III: Marked limitations of ordinary physical activity. Angina occurs on walking one to two level blocks and climbing one flight of stairs in normal conditions and at a normal pace.
- Class IV: Inability to carry on any physical activity without discomfort; anginal symptoms may be present at rest.

ICD-9CM CODES

411.1 Angina, stable
413 Angina pectoris
413.1 Prinzmetal's angina
413.9 Angina, unspecified

EPIDEMIOLOGY & DEMOGRAPHICS

- Angina is most common in middle-aged and elderly men
- Women are usually affected after menopause
- Prevalence of angina pectoris in people older than 30 years of age is >3%
- Within 12 months of initial diagnosis, 10% to 20% of patients with diagnosis of stable angina progress to MI or unstable angina

PHYSICAL FINDINGS & CLINICAL PRESENTATION

- Although there is significant individual variation, most patients report substernal chest pain (pressure, tightness, heaviness, sharp pain, sensation similar to intestinal gas or dysphagia).
- The pain is of short duration (typically <10 minutes); nonpleuritic; and often accompanied by shortness of breath, nausea, diaphoresis, and numbness or pain in the left arm, jaw, or shoulder. Ischemic pain of more than 30 minutes' duration should raise concern for possible myocardial infarction.
- Women are more likely than men to report atypical chest pain or discomfort.
- The elderly and diabetics may report symptoms other than chest pain, such as dyspnea, fatigue, or diaphoresis.

ETIOLOGY

RISK FACTORS:

- Advanced age
- Male sex
- Genetic predisposition
- Smoking (risk is almost double)
- Hypertension (risk is double if systolic blood pressure is >180 mm Hg)
- Hyperlipidemia
- Impaired glucose tolerance or diabetes mellitus
- Obesity (weight >30% over ideal). A higher body mass index during childhood is also associated with an increased risk of coronary heart disease (CHD) in adulthood
- Hypothyroidism
- Left ventricular hypertrophy
- Aortic stenosis or idiopathic subaortic stenosis
- Sedentary lifestyle
- Oral contraceptive use
- Cocaine use (cocaine is used by >5 million Americans regularly and is responsible for >64,000 emergency department [ED] evaluations yearly to rule out myocardial ischemia)
- Metabolic syndrome
- The development of coronary artery calcium is associated with an increased risk of MI
- Long-term use of nonsteroidal anti-inflammatory drugs (NSAIDs) is associated with increased cardiovascular risk
- Exposure to air pollution from traffic (dilute diesel exhaust) promotes myocardial ischemia and is associated with adverse cardiovascular events
- Low serum folate levels. Folate is required for conversion of homocysteine to methionine. Hyperhomocysteinemia has a toxic effect on vascular endothelium and interferes with proliferation of arterial wall smooth muscle cells. Folate deficiencies are associated with an increased risk of fatal CHD
- Elevated homocysteine levels. Elevated plasma homocysteine level is a strong and independent risk factor for CHD events, especially in patients with type 2 diabetes mellitus. Trials lowering homocysteine levels have, however, been disappointing because lowering therapy with folate did not prevent cardiovascular events among patients with coronary disease
- Elevated levels of highly sensitive C-reactive protein (hs-CRP, cardio CRP), suggesting that diseases associated with systemic inflammation can lead to accelerated atherosclerosis
- Depression
- Vasculitis
- Elevated levels of lipoprotein-associated phospholipase A_2
- Elevated fibrinogen levels
- Low level of red blood cell glutathione peroxidase-1 activity
- Radiation therapy

DX DIAGNOSIS

DIFFERENTIAL DIAGNOSIS

Noncardiac pain mimicking angina may be caused by:

- Pulmonary diseases (pulmonary hypertension, pulmonary embolism, pleurisy, pneumothorax, pneumonia)

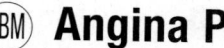
A

- Gastrointestinal disorders (peptic ulcer disease, pancreatitis, esophageal spasm or spontaneous esophageal muscle contraction, esophageal reflux, cholecystitis, cholelithiasis)
- Musculoskeletal conditions (costochondritis, chest wall trauma, cervical arthritis with radiculopathy, muscle strain, myositis)
- Acute aortic dissection
- Herpes zoster
- Anxiety disorder

WORKUP

- In patients with chest pain, the probability of CAD should be estimated on the basis of patient age, sex, cardiovascular risk factors, and pain characteristics
- The most important diagnostic factor is the history. Chest pain or left arm pain or discomfort occurring with exertion and relieved by rest in a patient with cardiovascular risk factors is consistent with a high likelihood of CAD
- In assessing the likelihood of underlying CAD it is helpful to classify the chest pain as typical angina, atypical angina, and or noncardiac chest pain. *Typical angina* will have the following three features: substernal chest discomfort of typical quality and duration, provoked by exertion or emotional stress, and relieved by rest and/or nitroglycerin (NTG). *Atypical angina* will have two of these above three features and *noncardiac chest pain* will have one of these above features
- The physical examination may be completely normal in many patients; however, certain findings may be helpful in the assessment of the patient with suspected stable CAD. Some findings may identify consequences of ischemia or possible causes of the anginal syndrome other than CAD. The presence of hypertension, arcus senilis, xanthelasma, carotid or peripheral bruits, and a prominent S4 are all physical signs that could raise concern for the presence of CAD. A murmur of mitral regurgitation may be a marker of an ischemic cardiomyopathy or transient ischemia. A murmur suggestive of hypertrophic cardiomyopathy or aortic stenosis may suggest a cause of angina other than CAD

LABORATORY TESTS

- Initial laboratory tests in patients with chronic stable angina should include a hemoglobin, fasting glucose, and fasting lipid panel
- Measurement of total cholesterol, low-density lipoprotein cholesterol (LDL-C), high-density lipoprotein cholesterol (HDL-C), and fasting serum triglycerides is recommended for cardiovascular screening. Non–HDL-C and the ratio of total cholesterol to HDL-C and measurements of apolipoprotein fractions (e.g., apolipoprotein B100, apolipoprotein A1) can also be used to estimate cardiovascular risk
- An electrocardiogram should be obtained during pain and when the patient is free of any discomfort. A normal resting electrocardiogram is not unusual in patients with chronic stable angina; in patients who

present with chest pain, 1% to 6% who have an acute MI will have a normal or nondiagnostic electrocardiogram
- Cardio-CRP (hs-CRP): Elevation of cardio-CRP is a relatively moderate predictor of CHD, and it adds prognostic information to that conveyed by the Framingham risk score. However, based on current data, it may be premature to adapt widespread assessment of cardio-CRP

EXERCISE TESTING AND IMAGING STUDIES

- Patients with intermediate likelihood of CAD and angina require further testing for the purpose of diagnosis as well as prognosis. If the patient is physically capable to perform physical exercise, exercise stress testing is useful because of the important prognostic information obtained from exercise performance and the hemodynamic response. The value of further testing is greatest in patients who have an intermediate risk of CAD, as patients in a low-risk or high-risk category are more likely to have a false-positive or false-negative result, respectively. Stress echocardiography or stress testing with myocardial perfusion imaging may be employed when baseline electrocardiographic abnormalities are present that render the electrocardiographic response to exercise uninterpretable. Stress echocardiography has the advantage of higher specificity and a lower cost. Stress radionuclide perfusion imaging has a higher sensitivity, particularly for single-vessel coronary disease, and has a higher technical success rate. When the patient is unable to exercise adequately, pharmacological testing (i.e., dobutamine, adenosine, regadenoson) may be used with these imaging modalities
- A very good predictor of risk for a patient with stable angina is the Duke treadmill score, which incorporates the patient's functional status (METS or time in minutes during the Bruce protocol), ST-segment depression, and an angina index. Patients with favorable Duke scores have a 5-year survival rate of >97%; this is independent of other factors such as coronary anatomy and LV function
- Echocardiography is indicated in patients with systolic murmur suggestive of aortic stenosis, mitral valve prolapse, or hypertrophic cardiomyopathy
- Cardiac computed tomography (CT) is useful for the detection of subclinical CAD in asymptomatic patients with an intermediate Framingham 10-year risk estimate of 10% to 20%. It detects and quantifies coronary calcium and evaluates the lumen and wall of the coronary artery. The calcium score is a strong predictor of incident CHD and provides predictive information beyond that provided by standard risk factors. A coronary artery calcium (CAC) score below 100 indicates low risk, and a score above 300 high risk. Although coronary artery calcium score is a promising tool, CT cost and radiation exposure are limiting factors to recommending widespread routine use of this marker

- Cardiac magnetic resonance imaging (MRI), in addition to its use for diagnosis of arrhythmogenic right ventricular dysplasia, can also be used to assess myocardial perfusion and viability as well as function. Additional studies are needed to determine the cost effectiveness of these studies in patients with ischemic cardiomyopathy
- Although invasive, coronary angiography remains the gold standard for the identification of clinically significant CAD. Angiography is performed to define the location and extent of coronary disease; this is indicated in selected patients who are candidates for coronary artery bypass graft (CABG) surgery or angioplasty

Rx TREATMENT

NONPHARMACOLOGIC THERAPY

- Aggressive modification of preventable risk factors (weight reduction in obese patients, regular aerobic exercise program, correction of folate deficiency, low-cholesterol and low-sodium diet, cessation of tobacco use).
- Diets using nonhydrogenated unsaturated fats as the predominant form of dietary fat, whole grains as the main form of carbohydrates, an abundance of fruits and vegetables, and adequate omega-3 fatty acids are optimal for prevention of CHD.
- Correction of possible aggravating factors (e.g., anemia, hypertension, diabetes mellitus, hyperlipidemia, thyrotoxicosis). Use caution regarding the routine use of blood transfusions to maintain arbitrary hematocrit levels in stable patients with IHD.

PHARMACOLOGIC THERAPY

The major classes of anti-ischemic agents are nitrates, beta-adrenergic blockers, calcium channel blockers, aspirin, and heparin. They can be used alone or in combination.

- Nitrates cause venodilation and relaxation of vascular smooth muscle; the decreased venous return from venodilation decreases diastolic ventricular wall tension (preload) and thereby reduces mechanical activity (and myocardial oxygen consumption) during systole. Relaxation of vascular smooth muscle increases coronary blood flow and reduces systemic pressure. Tolerance to nitrates can be minimized by avoiding sustained blood levels with a daily nitrate-free period (e.g., omission of bedtime dose of oral isosorbide dinitrate or 12 hr on/12 hr off transdermal nitroglycerin therapy). Nitrates are relatively contraindicated in patients with hypertrophic obstructive cardiomyopathy, and should also be avoided in patients with severe aortic stenosis. Nitrates should not be used within 24 hr of sildenafil (Viagra) or vardenafil (Levitra) or within 48 hr of tadalafil (Cialis) because of the potential for hypotension.
- Beta-adrenergic blockers achieve their major antianginal effect by decreasing myocardial oxygen consumption by reducing heart rate

and systolic blood pressure. Absent contraindications, they should be regarded as initial therapy for stable angina for all patients. Their dose should generally be adjusted to reduce the resting heart rate to 50 to 60 beats/min.

- Calcium channel blockers dilate coronary and systemic arteries, increase coronary blood flow, and decrease myocardial oxygen consumption. They play a major role in preventing and terminating myocardial ischemia induced by coronary artery spasm. They are particularly effective in treating microvascular angina. Short-acting calcium channel blockers should be avoided. Calcium channel blockers (particularly nondihydropyridine) should generally also be avoided in patients with CHF secondary to systolic dysfunction due to its negative inotropic effect.
- Use of aspirin reduces cardiovascular mortality and morbidity rates by 20% to 25% among patients with CAD. Initial dose is at least 160 mg/day followed by 81 to 325 mg/day. Aspirin inhibits the enzyme cyclooxygenase and synthesis of thromboxane A_2 and reduces the risk of adverse cardiovascular events by 33% in patients with unstable angina. Patients intolerant to aspirin can be treated with the other antiplatelet agents (see below)
- Clopidogrel is a thienopyridine, which acts by irreversibly blocking the P2Y12 adenosine diphosphate receptor on the platelet surface, thereby interrupting platelet activation and aggregation. Patients are now commonly being tested to see if clopidogrel is effectively inhibiting platelets, although the usefulness of these tests in vivo has not yet demonstrated clinical utility. The hepatic enzyme CYP2C19 is competitively inhibited by most proton pump inhibitors (PPIs), and earlier studies had suggested an increased risk of clopidogel failure, leading to concerns of stent thrombosis. Recent studies have not demonstrated clinically significant increased risk of adverse cardiovascular events due to interference with clopidogrel's efficacy.
- Prasugrel and ticagrelor are newer P2Y12 receptor inhibitors that are more efficacious in platelet inhibition. However, they are associated with an increased risk of bleeding and thus are often used in younger patients and those with lower GI bleeding profiles.
- Use of lipid-lowering drugs is recommended in patients with CAD and in patients with hyperlipidemia refractory to diet and exercise. Among patients who have recently had an acute coronary syndrome, an intensive lipid-lowering statin regimen to reduce LDL cholesterol to <70 mg/dl is a reasonable treatment objective. Statins also decrease the level of the inflammatory marker hs-CRP independently of the magnitude of change in lipid parameters.
- Angiotensin-converting enzyme (ACE) inhibition (e.g., ramipril 10 mg/day) has been shown to be effective in reducing cardiovascular death, MI, and stroke in patients who are at risk for or who had vascular disease (without heart failure). Currently evidence for routine use of ACEs in chronic stable angina is insufficient.
- Ranolazine is indicated for treatment of chronic angina that is inadequately controlled with other antianginals. It represents a new class of drugs known as *metabolic modulators*. Its exact mechanism of action is unknown. It seems to increase the efficiency of energy production in the heart, maintaining cardiac function. Its antianginal and anti-ischemic effects do not depend on reductions in heart rate or blood pressure. It is labeled for use in combination with beta-blockers, amlodipine, or nitrates in patients without an adequate antianginal response to those agents. Side effects include prolongation of QT interval.

REFERRAL

Revascularization (see Table 1-32):

- Revascularization includes either percutaneous coronary intervention (balloon angioplasty and stenting) or CABG.
- CABG surgery is recommended for patients with left main coronary disease, for those with symptomatic three-vessel disease, and for those with left ventricular ejection fraction (LVEF) <40% and critical (>70% stenosis) in all three major coronary arteries. Surgical therapy improves prognosis, particularly in diabetic patients with multivessel disease. Compared with percutaneous coronary intervention (PCI), CABG is more effective in relieving angina and leads to fewer repeated revascularizations but has a higher risk for procedural stroke. Survival to 10 years is similar for both procedures.

Angioplasty and coronary stents (Fig. E1-81):

- PCI should be considered for patients with one- or two-vessel disease that does not involve the main left coronary artery and in whom ventricular function is normal or near normal. PCI has an established place in treating angina but is not superior to intensive medical therapy to prevent MI and death in symptomatic or asymptomatic patients. Patients selected for PCI should also be candidates for CABG. The types of lesions best suited for angioplasty are proximal lesions, noncalcified, concentric, and preferably <5 mm (should not exceed 10 mm). Approximately 80% of patients show immediate benefit after PCI. The development of coronary stents has increased the number of patients who can be treated in the cardiac laboratory. Cardiac stents (Fig. E1-82) are currently used in nearly 95% of all patients with PCI lesions. The rate of restenosis may be reduced by placing a stent electively in primary atheromatous lesions. In patients with symptomatic isolated stenosis of the proximal left anterior descending artery, stenting has advantages over standard coronary angioplasty in that it is associated with

---

TABLE 1-32   Current Recommendations for Myocardial Revascularization in Patients with Chronic Stable Angina

CABG Surgery versus Medical Therapy

Among patients with medically refractory angina pectoris, CABG surgery is indicated for symptom improvement.

Among patients with medically stable angina pectoris, CABG surgery is indicated to prolong life in left main coronary artery disease or three-vessel disease (regardless of left ventricular function) and, possibly, to help symptoms.

CABG surgery may be indicated for prolongation of life if the proximal left anterior descending coronary artery is involved (regardless of the number of diseased vessels).

CABG surgery may reduce the composite end point of death, myocardial infarction, or stroke in diabetic patients with extensive multivessel (two- to three-vessel) coronary artery disease compared with medical therapy.

PCI versus Medical Therapy

For the initial management of patients with stable ischemic heart disease, PCI does not reduce the risk of death, myocardial infarction, or other major cardiovascular events when added to optimal medical therapy.

Among patients with medically refractory angina pectoris, PCI is indicated for symptom improvement.

PCI may be indicated in the presence of severe myocardial ischemia, regardless of symptoms. PCI does not appear to improve survival compared with medical treatment among patients with one- or two-vessel disease.

In the absence of symptoms or myocardial ischemia, PCI is not indicated (merely for the presence of an anatomic stenosis).

PCI versus CABG Surgery

For single-vessel disease, PCI and CABG surgery provide excellent symptom relief, but repeated revascularization procedures are required more frequently after PCI. Intracoronary stenting is preferred to regular PCI, but direct comparison with CABG surgery is limited.

For treated diabetic patients with two- or three-vessel disease, CABG surgery is the treatment of choice.

For nondiabetic patients, multivessel PCI and CABG surgery are acceptable alternatives. The choice of PCI or CABG surgery for initial treatment depends primarily on local expertise and the patient's and physician's preferences.

In general, PCI is preferred for patients at low risk and CABG surgery for patients at high risk.

CABG, Coronary artery bypass graft; *PCI,* percutaneous coronary intervention.
From Goldman L, Schafer AI: *Goldman's Cecil medicine,* ed 24, Philadelphia, 2012, Saunders.

A

both a lower rate of restenosis and a better clinical outcome. The major limitations of stenting are subacute thrombosis, restenosis within the stent, bleeding complications when anticoagulants are used after stenting, and higher cost. The combination of aspirin and clopidogrel (or newer P2Y12 antagonists) is effective in preventing coronary stent thrombosis and the duration of therapy depends on whether bare metal stents (BMS) or drug-eluting stents (DES) are used. Duration of dual antiplatelet therapy can be as short as 4 weeks for BMS, but 12 months of therapy is generally required for DES. This difference in duration is due to the lack of endothelium proliferation in DES initially, which confers a higher risk of stent thrombosis than with BMS. New drug-eluting stents with thin struts releasing Limus-family analogs from durable polymers have lowered the risk of stent thrombosis compared with early-generation stents releasing sirolimus or pallitaxel. Current evidence supports the use of drug-eluting stents in most clinical settings without safety concerns (unless there are contraindications to use of dual antiplatelet therapy). Recent data has shown that extending clopidogrel therapy beyond 6 months after stent placement does not reduce death or ischemic events, and it increases the risk of bleeding complications.

- Other therapies for refractory angina include enhanced external counterpulsation; transcutaneous electrical nerve stimulation; and invasive therapies such as spinal cord stimulation and revascularization. Although some of these therapies may improve symptoms and quality of life, they have not been shown to improve mortality rate.

⚠ PEARLS & CONSIDERATIONS

COMMENTS

- Although nitrate responsiveness is usually an integral part of a diagnostic strategy for chronic stable chest pain, recent reports question its value and conclude that in a general population admitted for chest pain, relief of pain after nitroglycerin treatment does not predict active CAD and should not be used to guide diagnosis in the acute care setting.
- CABG is associated with higher long-term survival rates and lower rates of repeat revascularization than PCI and stenting; however, patients often prefer stenting because it is less invasive, involves a shorter hospital stay, and has a lower in-hospital mortality rate.
- Section III describes an algorithm for the surgical management of ischemic cardiomyopathy.

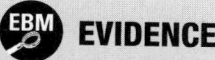

EVIDENCE

available at www.expertconsult.com

SUGGESTED READINGS

available at www.expertconsult.com

RELATED CONTENT

Acute Coronary Syndrome (Related Key Topic)
Angina (Patient Information)

AUTHORS: **NEIL GHEEWALA, M.D.,**
DAVID J. FORTUNATO, M.D., F.A.C.C., and
FRED F. FERRI, M.D.

Diseases and Disorders

I

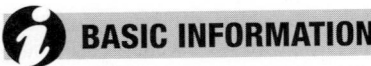
DEFINITION

- The mucocutaneous swelling caused by the release of vasoactive mediators is called urticaria and angioedema.
- Urticaria causes edema of the superficial dermis.
- Angioedema involves the deep layers of the dermis and the subcutaneous tissue.

SYNONYMS

Angioneurotic edema
HAE (hereditary angiodema)

ICD-9CM CODES
995.1 Angioedema (allergic)
277.6 Angioedema (hereditary)

EPIDEMIOLOGY & DEMOGRAPHICS

INCIDENCE: 100 to 3000/100,000 persons (for urticaria and angioedema)
LIFETIME PREVALENCE: Approximately 20% of the population experiences urticaria and/or angioedema at some time during life. The prevalence of hereditary angioedema is 1 case per 50,000 persons.
DEMOGRAPHICS:
Race: Slightly more common among African Americans.
Sex: More occurrences in women than men.
Angioedema commonly occurs after adolescence in the third decade of life.
Angioedema can occur together with urticaria (40%) or alone (20%); the remaining 40% have urticaria alone.

PHYSICAL FINDINGS & CLINICAL PRESENTATION

- Angioedema may be acute or chronic.
  1. Acute angioedema is defined as symptoms lasting 6 wk.
  2. Chronic angioedema is defined as symptoms lasting >6 wk.
- Urticaria is commonly known as "hives" and is:
  1. Pruritic
  2. Palpable and well demarcated
  3. Erythematous
  4. Millimeters to centimeters in size
  5. Multiple in number
  6. Fades within 12 to 24 hr
  7. Reappears at other sites
- Angioedema is characterized by the following:
  1. Nonpruritic
  2. Burning
  3. Not well demarcated
  4. Involves eyelids (Fig. 1-83), lips, tongue, and extremities
  5. Can involve the upper airway, causing respiratory distress
  6. Can involve the gastrointestinal tract, leading to cyclic abdominal pain, nausea, vomiting, and diarrhea
  7. Resolves slowly

ETIOLOGY

- Angioedema, with or without urticaria, is classified as acquired (allergic or idiopathic) or hereditary.
- Angioedema is primarily caused by mast cell activation and degranulation with release of vasoactive mediators (e.g., histamine, serotonin, bradykinins), resulting in postcapillary venule inflammation, vascular leakage, and edema in the deep layers of the dermis and subcutaneous tissue.
- Pathologically, angioedema has both immunologic- and nonimmunologic-mediated mechanisms.
  1. Immunoglobulin E–mediated angioedema may result from antigen exposure (e.g., foods [milk, eggs, peanuts, shellfish, tomatoes, chocolate, sulfites] or drugs [penicillin, aspirin, nonsteroidal anti-inflammatory drugs, phenytoin, sulfonamides, recombinant tissue plasminogen activator]).
  2. Complement-mediated angioedema involving immune complex mechanisms can also lead to mast cell activation that manifests as serum sickness.
  3. Hereditary angioedema is an autosomal-dominant disease caused by a deficiency of or mutation in C1 esterase inhibitor (C1-INH). C1-INH is a protease inhibitor normally present in high concentrations in the plasma. C1-INH serves many functions, one of which is to inhibit plasma kallikrein, a protease that cleaves kininogen and releases bradykinin. Deficient C1-INH activity results in excess concentration of kininogen and the subsequent release of kinin mediators.
  4. Acquired angioedema is usually associated with other diseases, most commonly B-cell lymphoproliferative disorders, but may also result from the formation of autoantibodies directed against C1 inhibitor protein.
  5. Other causes of angioedema include infection (e.g., herpes simplex, hepatitis B, Coxsackie A and B, *Streptococcus, Candida, Ascaris,* and *Strongyloides*), insect bites and stings, stress, physical factors (e.g., cold, exercise, pressure, and vibration), connective tissue diseases (e.g.,

systemic lupus erythematosus, Henoch-Schönlein purpura), and idiopathic causes. Angiotensin-converting enzyme (ACE) inhibitors can increase kinin activity and lead to angioedema.

DIAGNOSIS

A detailed history and physical examination usually establish the diagnosis of angioedema. Extensive laboratory testing is of limited value.

DIFFERENTIAL DIAGNOSIS

- Cellulitis
- Arthropod bite
- Hypothyroidism
- Contact dermatitis
- Atopic dermatitis
- Mastocytosis
- Granulomatous cheilitis
- Bullous pemphigoid
- Urticaria pigmentosa
- Anaphylaxis
- Erythema multiforme
- Epiglottitis
- Peritonsillar abscess

WORKUP

- An extensive workup searching for the cause of angioedema is often unrevealing (90%).
- Workup, including diagnostic blood tests and allergy testing, is performed according to results of the history and physical examination.

LABORATORY TESTS

- Complete blood count, erythrocyte sedimentation rate, and urinalysis are sometimes helpful as part of the initial evaluation.
- Stools for ova and parasites.
- Serology testing.
- C4 levels are usually reduced in acquired and hereditary angioedema (occurring without urticaria). If C4 levels are low, C1-INH levels and activity should be obtained. There are isolated reports of hereditary angioedema with normal C4 levels but reduced C1-INH levels.
- Skin and radioallergosorbent testing may be done if food allergies are suspected.

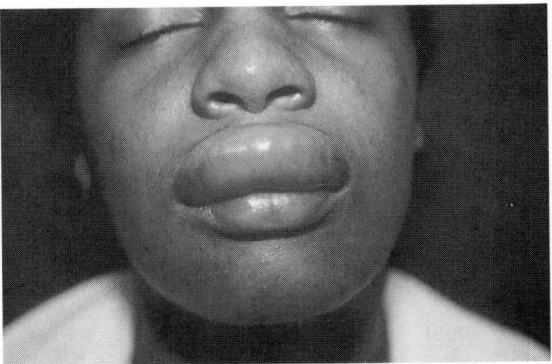

FIGURE 1-83 Angioedema of the upper lip, with severe swelling of deeper tissues. (From Goldstein BG, Goldstein AO: *Practical dermatology,* ed 2, St Louis, 1997, Mosby.)

- Skin biopsy is usually done in patients with chronic angioedema refractory to corticosteroid treatment.

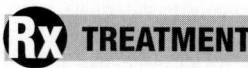 **TREATMENT**

NONPHARMACOLOGIC THERAPY
- Eliminate the offending agent
- Avoid triggering factors (e.g., cold, stress)
- Cold compresses to affected areas

ACUTE GENERAL Rx
- Acute life-threatening angioedema involving the larynx is treated with:
  1. Epinephrine 0.3 mg in a solution of 1:1000 given SC
  2. Diphenhydramine 25 to 50 mg IV or IM
  3. Cimetidine 300 mg IV or ranitidine 50 mg IV
  4. Methylprednisolone 125 mg IV
- Mainstay therapy in nonhereditary angioedema is H$_1$ antihistamines
  1. Diphenhydramine 25 to 50 mg q6h
  2. Chlorpheniramine 4 mg q6h
  3. Hydroxyzine 10 to 25 mg q6h
  4. Cetirizine 5 to 10 mg qd
  5. Loratadine 10 mg qd
  6. Fexofenadine 60 mg qd
- H$_2$ antihistamines can be added to H$_1$ antihistamines
  1. Ranitidine 150 mg bid
  2. Cimetidine 400 mg bid
  3. Famotidine 20 mg bid
- Tricyclic antidepressants
  1. Doxepin 25 to 50 mg qd
- Corticosteroids are rarely required for symptomatic relief of acute angioedema.
- Antihistamines are probably ineffective in acute hereditary angioedema.

- Purified plasma-derived C1-INH replacement therapy is effective and safe in treating acute attacks of hereditary angioedema caused by C1 inhibitor deficiency. Cost is a limiting factor. Available C1 esterase inhibitors are Cinryze and Berinert
- The recombinant protein kallikrein inhibitor ecallantide is also effective for acute attacks of HFA but also very expensive.

CHRONIC Rx
- Chronic angioedema is treated as described under "Acute General Rx."
- Corticosteroids are used more often in chronic nonhereditary angioedema.
- Prednisone 1 mg/kg/day for 5 days and then tapered over a period of weeks.
- Androgens (danazol, stanozolol, oxandrolone, methyltestosterone) and antifibrinolytic agents are used for the treatment of chronic hereditary angioedema, which does not respond to antihistamines or corticosteroids. C1-INH replacement therapy was approved by the FDA in 2008. Available agents are Cinryze and Berinert. Icatibant is a new bradykinin-receptor antagonist in hereditary angioedema currently undergoing trials.

DISPOSITION
- Antihistamines achieve symptomatic relief in more than 80% of patients with nonhereditary acute angioedema.
- In chronic nonhereditary angioedema, corticosteroids are given in addition to antihistamines.
- A small percentage of people will have recurrence of symptoms after steroid treatment.
- Chronic angioedema can last for months and even years.

REFERRAL
Dermatology consultation is recommended in patients with chronic angioedema, hereditary angioedema, and recurring angioedema.

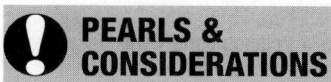 **PEARLS & CONSIDERATIONS**

ACE inhibitors can cause angioedema up to many months after initiation. There are multiple case reports and case series of angiotensin receptor blocker (ARB)–induced angioedema, although the risk is substantially less than that of ACE inhibitors. (Incidence rates per 1000 person-years are 4.38 cases for ACE inhibitors, 1.66 cases for ARBs.) The incidence rate is also very high for the direct renin inhibitor aliskiren (4.67).

COMMENTS
- Identifying a cause for angioedema in patients is often difficult and met with frustration.
- Chronic angioedema, unlike acute angioedema, is rarely caused by an allergic reaction.

SUGGESTED READINGS
available at www.expertconsult.com

RELATED CONTENT
Angioedema (Patient Information)

AUTHOR: **MEL L. ANDERSON, M.D.**

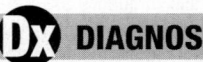
DEFINITION

Ankle fractures involve the lateral, medial, or posterior malleolus of the ankle and may occur either alone or in some combination. Associated ligamentous injuries are included.

CLASSIFICATION

The Danis-Weber (Fig. 1-84) and Lauge-Hensen classifications of ankle fratures are described in Table 1-33.

ICD-9CM CODES
824.8 Ankle fracture (malleolus) (closed)
824.2 Lateral malleolus fracture (fibular)
824.0 Medial malleolus fracture (tibial)

PHYSICAL FINDINGS & CLINICAL PRESENTATION

- Deformity usually depends on extent of displacement
- Pain, tenderness, and hemorrhage at the site of injury
- Gentle palpation of ligamentous structures (especially deltoid ligament) to determine the extent of soft tissue injury
- Evaluation of distal neurovascular status; results recorded

ETIOLOGY

- The ankle depends on its ligamentous and bony support for stability. The joint, or *mortise*, is an inverted U with the dome of the talus fitting into the medial and lateral malleoli. The posterior margin of the tibia is often called the *third* or *posterior malleolus*.

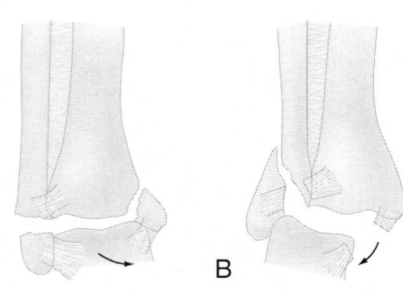

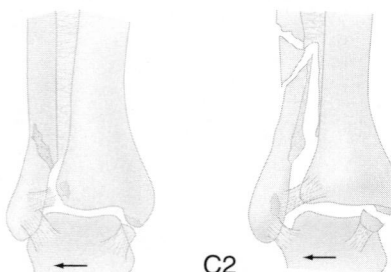

FIGURE 1-84 The Danis-Weber classification of ankle fractures focuses on the location of the fibular fracture in relation to the tibiotalar joint. (From Wilson FC: The pathogenesis and treatment of ankle fractures: classification. In Green WB [ed]: *Instructional course lectures,* ed 39, Easton, PA, 1990, American Academy of Orthopedic Surgeons.)

- Most common ankle fractures are the result of eversion or lateral rotation forces on the talus (in contrast with common sprains, which are usually caused by inversion).

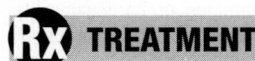
The diagnosis is usually established on the basis of the nature of the injury, the presence of typical findings of bony tenderness with swelling, and abnormal imaging studies.

DIFFERENTIAL DIAGNOSIS

- Ankle sprain
- Avulsion fracture of hindfoot or metatarsal

IMAGING STUDIES

Standard AP and lateral views (Fig. 1-85) accompanied by an AP taken 15 degrees internally rotated. The last view is taken to properly visualize the mortise.

TREATMENT

All fractures: elevation and ice to control swelling for 48 to 72 hr.

ACUTE GENERAL Rx

- Clinical and roentgenographic assessment of the status of the ankle mortise and stability of the injury is mandatory to determine treatment.
- There is potential for displacement if both sides of the joint are significantly injured (e.g., fracture of the lateral malleolus with deltoid ligament injury).
- Deviation of the position of the talus in the mortise could lead to traumatic arthritis.
- If there is no widening of the ankle mortise, many injuries can be safely treated with simple casting without reduction:
  1. Undisplaced or avulsion fractures of either malleolus below the ankle joint line:
     a. Stability of the joint is not compromised and a short leg walking cast or ankle support is sufficient.
     b. Weight bearing is allowed as tolerated.
     c. In 4 to 6 wk, protection may be discontinued.

TABLE 1-33   Classifications and Treatment of Ankle Fractures

	Normal	Abnormal
Talocrural angle—angle formed by parallel line to distal tibial articular surface and line connecting malleolar tips	**8-15 degrees** (or 83 degrees ± 4 degrees if perpendicular used)	> 2-3 degrees difference from contralateral = **fibular shortening**
Medial clear space—distance between lateral border of medial malleolus and lateral border of talus	< **4 mm** and equal to superior clear space	> 4 mm = lateral talar shift and **instability**
Tibiofibular clear space—distance between medial wall of fibula and tibial incisura	< **6 mm** on AP and mortise views	> 6 mm = **syndesmotic disruption (instability)**
Talar tilt—difference between medial and lateral superior clear space measurements	< **2 mm**	> 2 mm = **instability**

Classification:

1. **Danis-Weber**—based on location of fibular fracture
   A. Below syndesmosis
   B. At level of syndesmosis
   C. Above syndesmosis

2. **Lauge-Hansen**—based on position of foot and deforming force
   Supination external rotation—most common
   Supination adduction
   Pronation external rotation
   Pronation abduction

Treatment: Surgical decisions mostly based on stability.

Stable	Unstable
Isolated lateral malleolar fractions if:	**Lateral malleolus fractures** if:
Below syndesmosis	Medial injury/tenderness (bimalleolar equivalent)
No medial ligament injury or talar shift	Talar shift
Displacement < 5 mm	Above syndesmosis
No shortening	Shortened or displaced > 5 mm
Isolated medial malleolus fractures (although 5%-15% nonunion rates have been reported)	**Bimalleolar fractures**
	Trimalleolar fractures (fix posterior if > 25% of articular surface)
	Maisonneuve fractures

From Parvizi J: *High-yield orthopedics,* Philadelphia, 2010, Saunders.

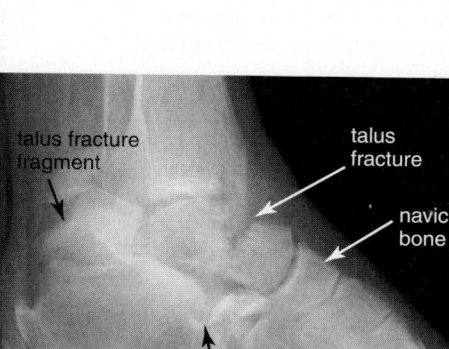

A fibula fracture

depressed talus fracture

B talus fracture fragment

talus fracture

navicular bone

calcaneus fracture

FIGURE 1-85 A, Anterior-posterior view. **B,** Lateral view. A depressed talus fracture is visible. In **B,** this fracture is seen to run through the midbody of the talus. **A** also demonstrates a distal fibula fracture, whereas in **B,** a calcaneal fracture is seen. The patient underwent CT to characterize these fractures further. (From Broder JS: *Diagnostic imaging for the emergency physician,* Philadelphia, 2011, Saunders.)

2. Isolated undisplaced fractures of the medial, lateral, or posterior malleolus:
   a. Usually stable and require only the application of a short leg walking cast with the ankle in the neutral position or fracture cast boot.
   b. Immobilization should be continued for 8 wk.
   c. Fracture line of lateral malleolus may persist roentgenographically for several months, but immobilization beyond 8 wk is usually unnecessary.
   d. Undisplaced bimalleolar fractures are treated with a long leg cast flexed 30 degrees at the knee to prevent motion and displacement of the fracture fragments. In 4 wk, a short leg walking cast may be applied for an additional 4 wk.
3. Isolated fractures of the lateral malleolus that are slightly displaced:
   a. May be treated with casting if no medial injury is present.
   b. A below-knee walking cast is applied with ankle in the neutral position; weight bearing is allowed as tolerated.

   c. Six wk of immobilization is sufficient.
   d. If medial tenderness is present, suggesting deltoid ligament rupture, a carefully molded cast may suffice if weight bearing is not allowed and the patient is followed up closely for signs of instability, especially after swelling recedes. If significant widening of the medial ankle mortise (increase in the "medial clear space") develops as a result of lateral displacement of the talus, referral for possible reduction is indicated.
   e. If signs of instability are already present at initial examination (widening of the medial clear space with medial tenderness), referral is indicated.
4. Undisplaced fracture of the distal fibular epiphysis:
   a. Often diagnosed clinically.
   b. There is tenderness over the epiphyseal plate.
   c. Roentgenographic findings are often negative.
   d. A short leg walking cast or fracture boot is applied for 4 wk.
   e. Growth disturbance is rare.

5. Isolated posterior malleolar fractures involving less than 25% of the joint surface on the lateral roentgenogram:
   Safely treated by applying a short leg walking cast or fracture brace. (Fractures involving >25% of the weight-bearing surface should be referred because of the potential for instability and subsequent traumatic arthritis.)

CHRONIC Rx
- Early motion is encouraged through a home exercise program.
- Protection from reinjury is appropriate for 4 to 6 wk after cast or brace removal.
- Temporary increase in lower extremity swelling that frequently occurs after short leg cast removal may benefit from the use of support hose.

DISPOSITION
Significant factors involved in the development of traumatic arthritis:
- Amount of joint trauma at the time of injury
- Eventual position of the talus in the mortise
Fracture nonunion is uncommon unless displacement is significant.

REFERRAL
Orthopedic consultation for:
- Unstable ankle joint
- Widened ankle mortise
- Posterior malleolar fracture over 25% of joint with incongruity
- Marked displacement of fracture fragment

EBM **EVIDENCE**

available at www.expertconsult.com

SUGGESTED READINGS

available at www.expertconsult.com

RELATED CONTENT
Ankle Fracture (Patient Information)
Ankle Sprain (Related Key Topic)

AUTHOR: **LONNIE R. MERCIER, M.D.**

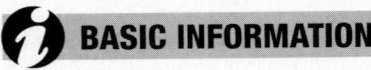

BASIC INFORMATION

DEFINITION

An ankle sprain is an injury to the ligamentous support of the ankle. Most (85%) involve the lateral ligament complex (Fig. 1-86). The anterior inferior tibiofibular (AITF) ligament, deltoid ligament, and interosseous membrane may also be injured. Damage to the tibiofibular syndesmosis is sometimes called a *high sprain* because of pain above the ankle. Lateral ankle sprains classically are graded I, II, or III, representing no, partial, or complete rupture of the lateral ligaments, respectively.

ICD-9CM CODES
845.00 Sprain, ankle or foot

EPIDEMIOLOGY & DEMOGRAPHICS

PREVALENCE: One case/10,000 people each day
PREDOMINANT SEX: Varies according to age and level of physical activity

PHYSICAL FINDINGS & CLINICAL PRESENTATION

- Often a history of a "pop"
- Variable amounts of tenderness and hemorrhage
- Possible abnormal anterior drawer test (pulling the plantar flexed foot forward to determine if there is any abnormal increase in forward movement of the talus in the ankle mortise) (Fig. 1-87)
- Inversion sprains: tender laterally; syndesmotic injuries: area of tenderness is more anterior and proximal
- Evaluation of motor function (Fig. 1-88)

ETIOLOGY

- Lateral injuries usually result from inversion and plantar flexion injuries.
- Eversion and rotational forces may injure the deltoid or AITF ligament or the interosseous membrane.

DIAGNOSIS

DIFFERENTIAL DIAGNOSIS

- Fracture of the ankle or foot, particularly involving the distal fibular growth plate in the immature patient
- Avulsion fracture of the fifth metatarsal base

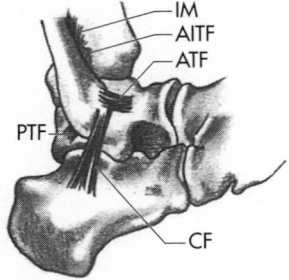

FIGURE 1-86 The lateral ankle ligaments, anterior and posterior talofibular *(ATF, PTF)* and calcaneofibular *(CF)*. Also shown are the anterior inferior tibiofibular ligament *(AITF)* and the beginning of the interosseous membrane *(IM)*. (From Mercier LR [ed]: *Practical orthopaedics,* ed 4, St Louis, 1995, Mosby.)

WORKUP

- History and clinical examination are usually sufficient to establish the diagnosis.
- Plain radiographs are always needed.

IMAGING STUDIES

Roentgenographic evaluation (Fig. 1-89): According to the Ottawa criteria, radiography is indicated if there is pain in the malleolar or midfoot zone, and either bone tenderness over an area of potential fracture or an inability to bear weight for four steps immediately after the injury and in the physician's office.

TREATMENT

ACUTE GENERAL Rx

- The first line of treatment is described by the mnemonic *RICE:*
  - ○ **R**est
  - ○ **I**ce (3 to 7 days)
  - ○ **C**ompression
  - ○ **E**levation
- Pain control with NSAIDs, acetaminophen, mild opioids
- In 48 to 72 hr, active range of motion and weight bearing as tolerated
- Compression, support, and bracing is best achieved with an Air-Stirrup brace combined with an elastic compression wrap, or lace-up support alone.
- In 4 to 5 days, exercise against resistance added
- Possible cast immobilization for some patients who require early independent walking; short leg orthoses also available for the same purpose
- Surgery is rarely recommended, even for grade III sprains; reports of equally satisfactory outcomes with nonsurgical treatment

CHRONIC Rx

- Lateral heel and sole wedge to prevent inversion
- Protective taping or bracing during vigorous activities (Fig. 1-90)
- Strengthening exercises

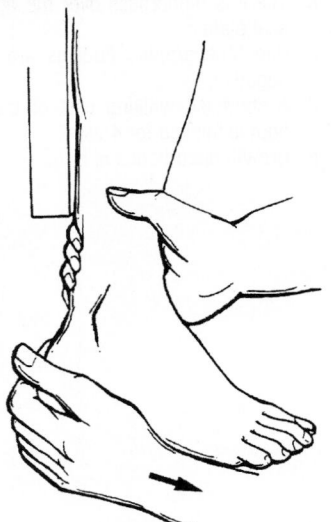

FIGURE 1-87 Anterior drawer test of the ankle (tests the integrity of the anterior talofibular ligament). (From Brinker MR, Miller MD: *Fundamentals of orthopaedics,* Philadelphia, 1999, Saunders.)

DISPOSITION

- Lateral sprains of any severity may cause lingering symptoms for weeks and months.
  1. Some syndesmotic sprains take even longer to heal.
  2. Heterotopic ossification may even develop in the interosseous membrane, but long-term results do not seem to be affected by such ossification.
- Continuing lateral symptoms may require surgical reconstruction, although late traumatic arthritis or long-term instability is rare regardless of treatment.

REFERRAL

For orthopedic consultation for patients who do not respond to conservative treatment. Most ankle sprains resolve in 2-6 wk.

PEARLS & CONSIDERATIONS

COMMENTS

If healing seems delayed (more than 6 wk), the following conditions should be considered:
1. Talar dome fracture
2. Reflex sympathetic dystrophy
3. Chronic tendinitis
4. Peroneal tendon subluxation
5. Other occult fracture
6. Peroneal weakness (poor rehabilitation)
7. A "high" (syndesmotic) sprain
Repeat plain roentgenograms, bone scan, or MRI may be indicated.

EVIDENCE

available at www.expertconsult.com

SUGGESTED READINGS

available at www.expertconsult.com

RELATED CONTENT

Ankle Sprain (Patient Information)
Ankle Fracture (Related Key Topic)

AUTHOR: **LONNIE R. MERCIER, M.D.**

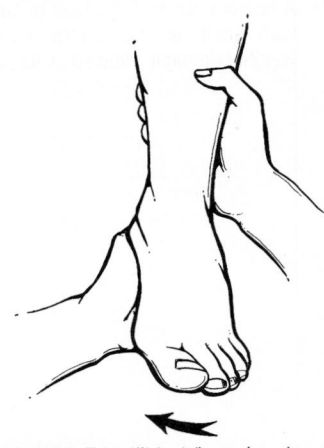

FIGURE 1-88 Talar tilt test (inversion stress) of the ankle (tests the integrity of the anterior talofibular ligament and the calcaneofibular ligament). (From Brinker MR, Miller MD: *Fundamentals of orthopaedics,* Philadelphia, 1999, Saunders.)

Diseases and Disorders

I

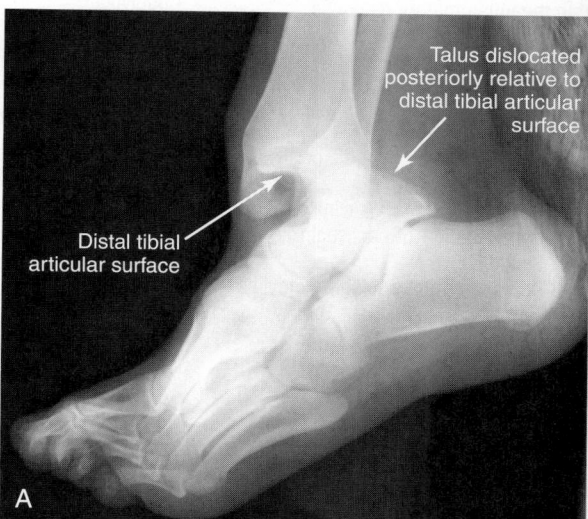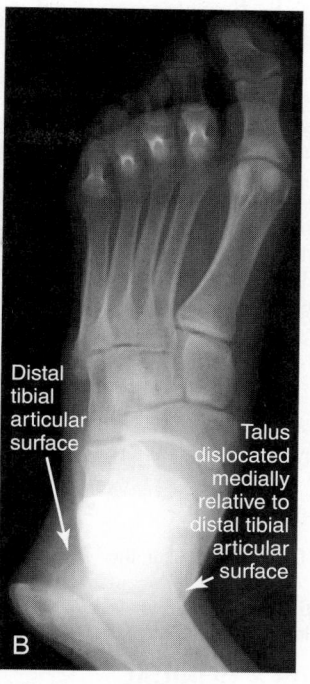

FIGURE 1-89 Tibiotalar dislocation. This 17-year-old male landed on his left ankle after dunking a basketball, sustaining a deformity. His tibiotalar joint is dislocated, with the talus dislocated posteriorly (visible on the lateral view, **A**) and medially (visible on the anterior-posterior view, **B**). No fractures are present in this case, although fractures are commonly associated with this injury because of the amount of force required to dislocate the ankle. This was an open injury, and the patient underwent exploration, irrigation, and debridement with primary closure. (From Broder JS: *Diagnostic imaging for the emergency physician,* Philadelphia, 2011, Saunders.)

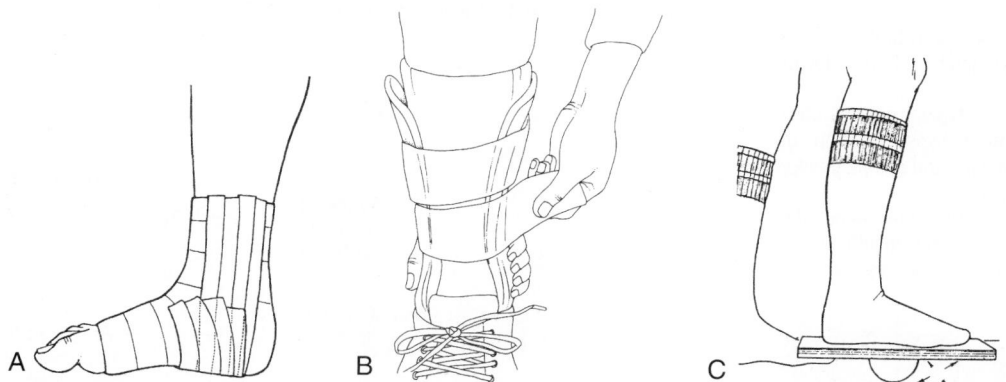

FIGURE 1-90 A, The most effective method of supporting most acute ankle sprains is by using an ACE wrap (BD, Franklin Lakes, NJ) reinforced with 1-inch medial and lateral tape strips. The anterior and posterior aspects of the ankle are left free to allow the patient to flex and extend the ankle. The patient is encouraged to bear weight with crutches. **B,** Diagram of an air splint. Straps are adjusted to heel size, the lower straps are wrapped about the ankle, and the side extensions are centered. The splint is then pressurized and straps adjusted until comfortable support and pressure are attained. **C,** As the ankle pain subsides, about the third to fifth day, balancing exercises can begin to allow the patient to regain ankle proprioception and avoid recurrent instability problems. (From Jardon OM, Mathews MS: Orthopedics. In Rakel RE [ed]: *Textbook of family practice,* ed 5, Philadelphia, 1995, Saunders.)

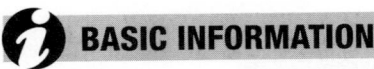

DEFINITION

Ankylosing spondylitis is a type of inflammatory arthritis involving the sacroiliac joints and axial skeleton characterized by ankylosis and enthesitis (inflammation at tendon insertions). It is one of a family of overlapping syndromes called seronegative spondyloarthropathies that includes reactive arthritis (Reiter syndrome), psoriatic spondylitis, and enteropathic arthritis.

SYNONYMS

Marie-Strümpell disease

ICD-9CM CODES
720.0 Ankylosing spondylitis

EPIDEMIOLOGY & DEMOGRAPHICS

PREVALENCE: Between 0.1% and 1% of the population
PREDOMINANT AGE AT ONSET: 15 to 35 yr
PREDOMINANT SEX: Male/female ratio 2 to 3:1

PHYSICAL FINDINGS & CLINICAL PRESENTATION

- Prolonged morning back stiffness of insidious onset lasting more than 3 mo
- Bilateral sacroiliac tenderness (sacroiliitis)
- Limited lumbar spine motion (Fig. 1-91)
- Tenderness at tendon insertion sites, especially the Achilles tendons and plantar fascia
- Loss of chest expansion reflecting rib cage involvement
- Occasionally, peripheral joint arthritis, usually involving the large joints of the lower extremities
- In advanced cases the typical posture consists of compensatory hyperextension of neck, fixed flexion of hips, and compensatory flexion of knees (Fig. 1-92)
- Extraskeletal manifestations may affect the cardiovascular system (aortic insufficiency), lungs (pulmonary fibrosis), and eye (uveitis)

ETIOLOGY

Genetic factors, particularly *HLA-B27*, play an important role in susceptibility to the spondyloarthropathies. Infectious triggers have been implicated in some cases. Tumor necrosis factor is important in the inflammatory response.

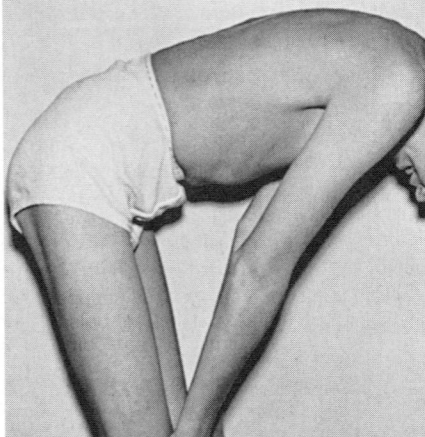

FIGURE 1-91 Loss of lumbodorsal spine mobility in a boy with ankylosing spondylitis. The lower spine remains straight when the patient bends forward. (From Behrman RE: *Nelson textbook of pediatrics,* ed 17, Philadelphia, 2005, Saunders.)

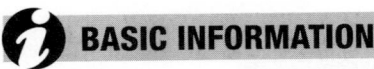 DIAGNOSIS

DIFFERENTIAL DIAGNOSIS

- Diffuse idiopathic skeletal hyperostosis (Forestier disease)
- Noninflammatory back pain (A clinical algorithm for the evaluation of back pain is described in Section III.)
- Table 1-34 compares ankylosing spondylitis and related disorders.

LABORATORY TESTS

- Elevated sedimentation rate, C-reactive protein
- Mild hyperchromic anemia
- Demonstration of inflammatory sacroiliitis by radiography or MRI is essential for diagnosis
- HLA/B27 antigen is not useful in the evaluation of noninflammatory back pain because it is present in up to 8% to 10% of the normal population.

IMAGING STUDIES

- Classic features are those of bilateral sacroiliitis on radiographs of the pelvis
- Vertebral bodies lose anterior concave shape and become square
- With progression, calcification of the annulus fibrosus and paravertebral ligaments develop,

giving rise to the so-called *bamboo spine* and a "trolley track" appearance (Fig. 1-93).
- MRI may be useful in detecting early inflammatory lesions and is especially helpful when the history is suggestive but radiographs are equivocal.

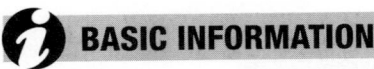 TREATMENT

NONPHARMACOLOGIC THERAPY

- Exercises primarily to maintain on flexibility and aerobic activity are important
- Postural training
  1. Patients must be instructed on spinal extension exercises to avoid fusion in a flexed position
  2. Sleeping should be in the supine position on a firm mattress; pillows should not be placed under the head or knees.

CHRONIC Rx

- NSAIDs: Patients with ankylosing spondylitis should be prescribed full-dose continuous NSAID therapy. There is anecdotal evidence suggesting that indomethacin may be more effective than other NSAIDs, but other NSAIDs are efficacious and may be better tolerated. One study suggested that continuous NSAID therapy may retard the radiographic progression of ankylosing spondylitis.
- Sulfasalazine may be efficacious in some patients, especially for peripheral arthritis
- Tumor necrosis factor (TNF) antagonists such as etanercept, infliximab, and adalimumab have been shown to be very effective for relieving

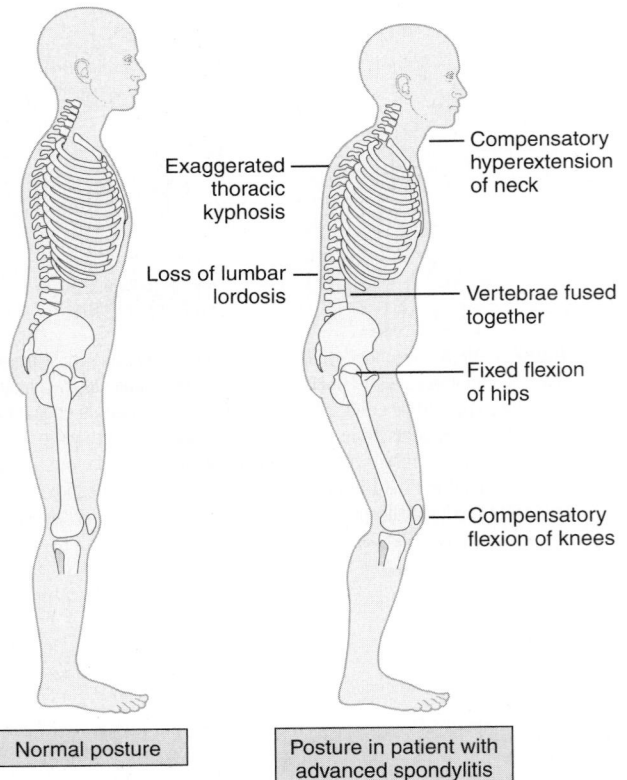

Normal posture

Posture in patient with advanced spondylitis

Exaggerated thoracic kyphosis

Loss of lumbar lordosis

Compensatory hyperextension of neck

Vertebrae fused together

Fixed flexion of hips

Compensatory flexion of knees

FIGURE 1-92 Ankylosing spondylitis. Typical posture in advanced cases compared with normal posture. (From Ballinger A: *Kumar & Clark's essentials of clinical medicine,* ed 6, Edinburgh, 2012, Saunders.)

TABLE 1-34 Comparison of Ankylosing Spondylitis and Related Disorders

Feature	Ankylosing Spondylitis	Psoriatic Arthritis	Reactive Arthritis	Enteropathic Arthropathy
Gender (M:F)	2-3 : 1	1 : 1	8 : 1 (GU) [1 : 1 (GI)]	1 : 1
Age at onset	<40	35-55	20-40	Young adult
Sacroiliitis or spondylitis	100%	~20%	~40%	<20%
Symmetry of sacroiliitis	Symmetric	Asymmetric	Asymmetric	Symmetric
Peripheral arthritis	~25%	95%	90%	15%-20%
Distribution	Axial and lower limbs	Any joint	Lower limbs	Variable
HLA-B27	85%-95%	25%	30%-80%	7%
Uveitis	25%-40%	25%	25%	10%-36%

From Hochberg MC et al: *Rheumatology,* ed 5, St Louis, 2011, Mosby.

symptoms of spinal inflammatory arthritis in numerous controlled studies. Anti-TNF therapy should be recommended for patients whose symptoms are not completely controlled with NSAIDs, and it sometimes results in dramatic improvement in symptoms, range of motion of the spine, and quality of life for these patients.

DISPOSITION
Most patients have a normal life span but many suffer significant disability from loss of spinal mobility

REFERRAL
All patients with seronegative spondyloarthropathy should be referred to a rheumatologist for consideration of anti-TNF therapy

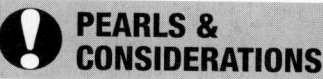 **PEARLS & CONSIDERATIONS**

A family history of seronegative spondyloarthropathy increases the specificity of testing for *HLA-B27.*

SUGGESTED READINGS
available at www.expertconsult.com

RELATED CONTENT
Fig. 3-170 Spondyloarthropathy, diagnosis (Algorithm)
Fig. 3-171 Spondyloarthropathy, treatment (Algorithm)
Ankylosing Spondylitis (Patient Information)

AUTHOR: **BERNARD ZIMMERMANN, M.D.**

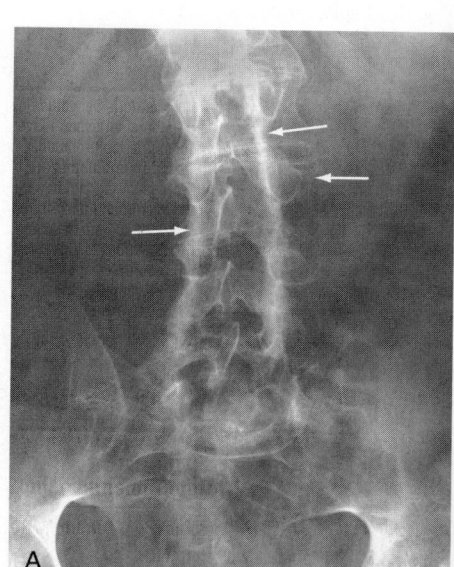
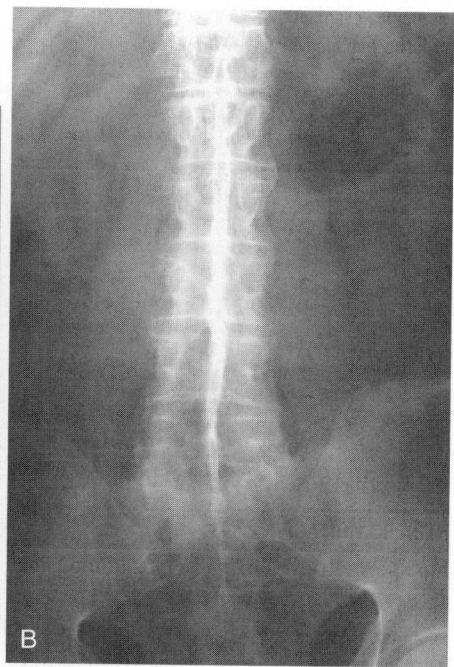

FIGURE 1-93 Ankylosing spondylitis. A, Fusion of the facet joints and ossification of the adjacent soft tissue have produced a "trolley track" appearance *(arrows).* The sacroiliac joints are fused. Syndesmophytes are present. **B,** In another patient, there is a prominent fusion of the interspinous ligaments producing a "saber sheath" appearance. (From Harris ED: *Kelley's textbook of rheumatology,* ed 7, Philadelphia, 2005, Saunders.)

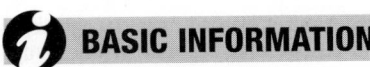

BASIC INFORMATION

DEFINITION

A fistula is an inflammatory tract with a secondary (external) opening in the perianal skin and a primary (internal) opening in the anal canal at the dentate line. It originates in an abscess in the intersphincteric space of the anal canal. Fistulas can be classified as follows:

1. Intersphincteric: fistula track passes within the intersphincteric plane to the perianal skin (most common)
2. Transsphincteric: fistula track passes from the internal opening, through the internal and external sphincter, and into the ischiorectal fossa to the perianal skin (frequent)
3. Suprasphincteric: after passing through the internal sphincter, fistula tract passes above the puborectalis and then tracts downward, lateral to the external sphincter, into the ischiorectal space to the perianal skin (uncommon); if abscess cavity extends cephalad, a supralevator abscess possibly palpable on rectal examination
4. Extrasphincteric: fistula tract passes from the rectum, above the levators, through the levator muscles to the ischiorectal space and perianal skin (rare)

With a horseshoe fistula, the tract passes from one ischiorectal fossa to the other behind the rectum.

SYNONYMS

Fistula-in-ano

ICD-9CM CODES
565.1 Anal fistula

EPIDEMIOLOGY & DEMOGRAPHICS

- Common in all ages
- Occurs equally in men and women
- Associated with constipation
- Pediatric age group: more common in infants; boys more than girls

PHYSICAL FINDINGS & CLINICAL PRESENTATION

- Acute stage: perianal swelling, pain, and fever
- Chronic stage: history of rectal drainage or bleeding; previous abscess with drainage
- Tender external fistulous opening, within 2 to 3 cm of the anal verge, with purulent or serosanguineous drainage on compression; the greater the distance from the anal margin, the greater the probability of a complicated upward extension
- Goodsall's rule:
  1. Location of the internal opening related to the location of the external opening.
  2. With external opening anterior to an imaginary line drawn horizontally across the midpoint of the anus: fistulous tract runs radially into the anal canal.
  3. With opening posterior to the transanal line: tract is usually curvilinear, entering the anal canal in the posterior midline.
  4. Exception to this rule: an external, anterior opening that is >3 cm from the anus. In this case the tract may curve posteriorly and end in the posterior midline.
- If perianal abscess recurs, presence of a fistula is suggested

ETIOLOGY

- Most common: nonspecific cryptoglandular infection (skin or intestinal flora)
- Fistulas more common when intestinal microorganisms are cultured from the anorectal abscess
- Tuberculosis
- Lymphogranuloma venereum
- Actinomycosis
- Inflammatory bowel disease (IBD): Crohn's disease, ulcerative colitis
- Trauma: surgery (episiotomy, prostatectomy), foreign bodies, anal intercourse
- Malignancy: carcinoma, leukemia, lymphoma
- Treatment of malignancy: surgery, radiation

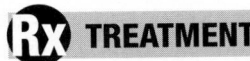

DIAGNOSIS

DIFFERENTIAL DIAGNOSIS

- Hidradenitis suppurativa
- Pilonidal sinus
- Bartholin's gland abscess or sinus
- Infected perianal sebaceous cysts

WORKUP

- Digital rectal examination:
  1. Assess sphincter tone and voluntary squeeze pressure
  2. Determine the presence of an extraluminal mass
  3. Identify an indurated track
  4. Palpate an internal opening or pit
- Gentle probing of external orifice to avoid creating a false tract; 50% do not have clinically detectable opening
- Anoscopy
- Proctosigmoidoscopy to exclude inflammatory or neoplastic disease
- All studies done under adequate anesthesia

LABORATORY TESTS

- Complete blood count
- Rectal biopsy if diagnosis of IBD or malignancy suspected; biopsy of external orifice is useless

IMAGING STUDIES

- Colonoscopy or barium enema if:
  1. Diagnosis of IBD or malignancy is suspected
  2. History of recurrent or multiple fistulas
  3. Patient <25 yr
- Small bowel series: occasionally obtained for reasons similar to above
- Fistulography: unreliable but may be helpful in complicated fistulas

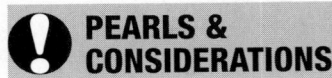

TREATMENT

NONPHARMACOLOGIC THERAPY

Sitz baths

ACUTE GENERAL Rx

- Treatment of choice: surgery
- Broad-spectrum antibiotic given if:
  1. Cellulitis present
  2. Patient is immunocompromised
  3. Valvular heart disease present
  4. Prosthetic devices present
- Stool softener/laxative

CHRONIC Rx

- Surgery
- Surgical goals are as follows:
  1. Cure the fistula
  2. Prevent recurrence
  3. Preserve sphincter function
  4. Minimize healing time
- Methods for the management of anal fistulas: fistulotomy, setons, rectal advancement flaps, colostomy

DISPOSITION

Outpatient surgery

REFERRAL

Refer to a surgeon with expertise in this area

PEARLS & CONSIDERATIONS

COMMENTS

- HIV-positive and diabetic patients with perirectal abscesses/fistulas are true surgical emergencies.
- Risk of septicemia, Fournier's gangrene, and other septic complications make immediate drainage imperative.

SUGGESTED READINGS

available at www.expertconsult.com

RELATED CONTENT

Anal Fissure (Related Key Topic)
Hemorrhoids (Related Key Topic)

AUTHORS: **GEORGE T. DANAKAS, M.D.,** and **RUBEN ALVERO, M.D.**

BASIC INFORMATION

DEFINITION

Anorexia nervosa is a psychiatric disorder characterized by abnormal eating behavior, severe self-induced weight loss, and a specific psychopathology (see "Workup").

ICD-9CM CODES

307.1 Anorexia nervosa

EPIDEMIOLOGY & DEMOGRAPHICS

INCIDENCE/PREVALENCE (IN U.S.):

- Anorexia nervosa occurs in 0.2% to 1.3% of the general population, with an annual incidence of 5 to 10 cases per 100,000 persons.
- Participation in activities that promote thinness (athletics, modeling) is associated with a higher incidence of anorexia nervosa.

PREDOMINANT SEX: Female/male ratio is 9:1. Approximately 0.5% to 1% of women between the ages of 15 and 30 yr have anorexia nervosa.

PREDOMINANT AGE: Adolescence to young adulthood is the predominant age. Mean age of onset is 17 yr. Approximately 0.5% to 1% of college-aged women have anorexia nervosa.

PHYSICAL FINDINGS & CLINICAL PRESENTATION

Eating disorders can affect every organ system. Primary care physicians must be skilled at recognizing this disorder because patients with mild cases usually present with nonspecific symptoms such as asthenia, cold intolerance, lack of energy, or dizziness. Children and adolescents are at particular risk due to their active phase of growth and development. The physical examination may be normal in the early stages or in mild cases. Patients with moderate to severe anorexia have the following physical characteristics:

- Patient is emaciated and bundled in clothing.
- Skin is dry and has excessive growth of lanugo. Skin may also be yellow-tinged from carotenodermia.
- Brittle nails, thinning scalp hair are present.
- Bradycardia, hypotension, hypothermia, and bradypnea are common.
- Female fat distribution pattern is no longer evident.
- Axillary and pubic hair is preserved.
- Peripheral edema may be present.

ETIOLOGY

- Etiology is unknown, but probably multifactorial (sociocultural, psychologic, familial, and genetic factors).
- A history of sexual abuse has been reported in as many as 50% of patients with anorexia nervosa.
- Psychologic factors: anorexics often have an incompletely developed personal identity. They struggle to maintain a sense of control over their environment, they usually have a low self-esteem, and they lack the sense that they are valued and loved for themselves.

DIAGNOSIS

DIFFERENTIAL DIAGNOSIS

- Other eating disorders (see Table 1-35)
- Substance abuse
- Depression with loss of appetite
- Obsessive compulsive disorder
- Schizophrenia
- Conversion disorder
- Occult carcinoma, lymphoma
- Endocrine disorders: Addison disease, diabetes mellitus, hypothyroidism or hyperthyroidism, panhypopituitarism
- Gastrointestinal disorders: celiac disease, Crohn's disease, intestinal parasitosis
- Infectious disorders: AIDS, tuberculosis
- A clinical algorithm for the evaluation of anorexia is described in Section III

WORKUP

- A diagnosis can be made by using the following DSM-IV diagnostic criteria for anorexia nervosa:
  1. Refusal to maintain body weight (BW) at or above a minimally normal weight for age and height (e.g., weight loss leading to maintenance of BW <85% of that expected or failure to make expected weight gain during a period of growth, leading to BW <85% of that expected)
  2. Intense fear of gaining weight or becoming fat, even though underweight
  3. Disturbance in the way in which BW or shape is experienced, undue influence of BW or shape on self-evaluation, or denial of the seriousness of the current low BW
  4. In postmenarchal females, amenorrhea—that is, the absence of at least three consecutive menstrual cycles (A woman is considered to have amenorrhea if her periods occur only after hormone administration, such as estrogen.)

Specify type:

Restricting type: During the current episode of anorexia nervosa, the person has not regu-

TABLE 1-35 Diagnostic Features of Eating Disorders

Anorexia nervosa	Body weight willfully maintained below normal level
	Abnormal perception of body morphology
	Intense fear of weight gain
	Amenorrhea
Bulimia nervosa	Large uncontrolled eating binges at least twice weekly
	Inappropriate compensatory behavior (e.g., vomiting, purging)
Binge eating disorder	Large uncontrolled eating binges at least twice weekly
	No regular inappropriate compensatory disorders
	Marked distress about binges

From Besser CM, Thorner MO: *Comprehensive clinical endocrinology,* ed 3, St Louis, 2002, Mosby.

larly engaged in binge eating or purging behavior (i.e., self-induced vomiting or the misuse of laxatives, diuretics, or enemas).

Binge-eating/purging type: During the current episode of anorexia nervosa, the person has regularly engaged in binge eating or purging behavior (i.e., self-induced vomiting or the misuse of laxatives, diuretics, or enemas).

- The SCOFF questionnaire is a screening tool for eating disorders used in England. It consists of the following five questions:
  1. Do you make yourself *s*ick because you feel full?
  2. Have you lost *c*ontrol over how much you eat?
  3. Have you lost more than *o*ne stone (approximately 6 kg) recently?
  4. Do you believe yourself to be *f*at when others say you are thin?
  5. Does *f*ood dominate your life?
- A positive response to two or more questions has a reported sensitivity of 100% for anorexia and bulimia and an overall specificity of 87.5%.
- In college-aged women a positive response to any of the following screening questions also warrants further evaluation:
  1. How many diets have you been on in the past year?
  2. Do you think you should be dieting?
  3. Are you dissatisfied with your body size?
  4. Does your weight affect the way you think about yourself?
- Baseline ECG should be performed on all patients with anorexia nervosa. Routine monitoring of patients with prolonged QT interval is necessary; sudden death in these patients is often caused by ventricular arrhythmias related to QT interval prolongation.
- A dual-energy x-ray absorptiometry (DEXA) scan to screen for osteopenia should be considered after 6 mo of amenorrhea in patients suspected of anorexia nervosa.

LABORATORY TESTS

- In mild cases, laboratory findings may be completely normal.
- Endocrine abnormalities:
  1. Decreased follicle-stimulating hormone, luteinizing hormone, T_4, T_3, estrogens, urinary 17-OH steroids, estrone, and estradiol
  2. Normal free T_4, thyroid-stimulating hormone
  3. Increased cortisol, growth hormone, rT_3, T_3RU
  4. Absence of cyclic surge of luteinizing hormone
- Leukopenia, thrombocytopenia, anemia, reduced erythrocyte sedimentation rate, reduced complement levels, and reduced CD4 and CD8 cells may be present.
- Metabolic alkalosis, hypocalcemia, hypokalemia, hypomagnesemia, hypercholesterolemia, and hypophosphatemia may be present.
- Increased plasma β-carotene levels are useful to distinguish these patients from others on starvation diets.

TREATMENT

NONPHARMACOLOGIC THERAPY

- A multidisciplinary approach with psychologic, medical, and nutritional support is necessary.
- A goal weight should be set and the patient should be initially monitored at least once a week in the office setting. The target weight is 100% of ideal BW for teenagers and 90% to 100% for older patients.
- Weight gain should be gradual (1 to 3 lb/wk) to prevent gastric dilation. Begin with 800 to 1200 kcal in frequent small meals (to avoid bloating sensation), then increase calories to 1500 to 3000 depending on height and age.
- Add, as necessary, vitamin and mineral supplements.
- In severe cases, total parenteral nutrition must be used (starting at 800 to 1200 kcal/day).
- Electrolyte levels should be strictly monitored.
- Mealtime should be a time for social interaction, not confrontation.
- Postprandially, sedentary activities are recommended. The patient's access to a bathroom should be monitored to prevent purging.

ACUTE GENERAL Rx

- Criteria to decide on the appropriate initial course of treatment for patients with anorexia nervosa are usually based on the presence of complications, percentage of ideal BW, and severity of body image distortion.
- Outpatient treatment is adequate for most patients.
- Indications for hospitalization are described under "Referral" section and summarized in Table 1-36.
- Medically stable patients who are within 85% of ideal BW can be followed up by the primary care physician at 3- or 4-wk intervals, which can be lengthened as the patient improves.
- Pharmacologic treatment generally has no role in anorexia nervosa unless major depression or another psychiatric disorder is present. SSRIs can be used to alleviate the depressed mood and moderate obsessive-compulsive behavior in some individuals.

CHRONIC Rx

- Psychotherapy continued for years and focused specifically on self-image, family and peer interactions, and relapse prevention is an integral part of a successful recovery.
- Family therapy is also recommended, especially in younger patients.

DISPOSITION

- The long-term prognosis is generally poor and marked by recurrent exacerbations. The percentage of patients with anorexia nervosa

TABLE 1-36 Indications for In-Patient Medical Hospitalization of Patients with Anorexia Nervosa

Physical and Laboratory
Heart rate <45 beats/min
Other cardiac rhythm disturbances
Blood pressure <80/50 mm Hg
Postural hypotension resulting in a >10 mm Hg drop or a >20 beats/min increase
Hypokalemia
Hypophosphatemia
Hypoglycemia
Dehydration
Body temperature <97°F
<80% healthy body weight
Hepatic, cardiac, or renal compromise

Psychiatric
Suicidal intent and plan
Very poor motivation to recover (in family and patient)
Preoccupation with ego-syntonic thoughts
Coexisting psychiatric disorders

Miscellaneous
Requires supervision after meals and while using the restroom
Failed day treatment

From Kliegman RM et al: *Nelson textbook of pediatrics,* ed 19, Philadelphia, 2011, Saunders.

who fully recover is modest. Most patients continue to have a distorted body image, disordered eating habits, and psychic difficulties.

- Most patients with anorexia nervosa will recover menses within 6 mo of reaching 90% of their ideal BW. It is important to note that patients with anorexia nervosa can become pregnant despite amenorrhea.
- Mortality rates vary from 5% to 20% and are six times that of peers without anorexia. Frequent causes of death are electrolyte abnormalities, starvation, or suicide.
- Factors that predict improved outcome in patients with eating disorders include early age at diagnosis, brief interval before initiation of treatment, good parent-child relationships, and having other healthy relationships with friends or therapists.
- A prolonged QT interval is a marker for risk of sudden death.

REFERRAL

Hospitalization should be considered in the following situations:
1. Severe dehydration or electrolyte imbalance
2. ECG abnormalities (prolonged QT interval, arrhythmias)
3. Significant physiologic instability (hypotension, orthostatic changes)
4. Intractable vomiting, purging, or bingeing
5. Suicidal thoughts
6. Weight loss exceeding 30% of ideal BW and unresponsiveness to outpatient treatment
7. Rapidly progressing weight loss (>2 lb in a week)
8. Failure to progress in nutritional rehabilitation in outpatient treatment

SUGGESTED READINGS

available at www.expertconsult.com

RELATED CONTENT

Fig. 3-17 Evaluation of anorexia (Algorithm)
Anorexia Nervosa (Patient Information)

AUTHOR: **FRED F. FERRI, M.D.**

BASIC INFORMATION

DEFINITION

Anoxic brain injury is cerebral ischemic injury due to decreased oxygen or blood flow to the brain typically caused by interruption of cardiac circulation or respiratory failure.

SYNONYMS

Hypoxic-ischemic injury

ICD-9CM CODES
348.1 Anoxic brain damage

EPIDEMIOLOGY & DEMOGRAPHICS

INCIDENCE:
- Variable based on diagnostic criteria
- 492,000 out-of-hospital cardiac arrests per year in the U.S.

PREVALENCE:
- Vegetative state varies from 40 to 168 per 1 million population, depending on definition used.
- Recovery is rare after 3 months with life expectancy lasting 2 to 5 years.

RISK FACTORS: Same as risk factors for cardiorespiratory arrest: include HTN, hyperlipidemia, tobacco use, and physical inactivity.

PHYSICAL FINDINGS & CLINICAL PRESENTATION

- Variable depending on degree of insult
- Minimally conscious state: altered consciousness with normal sleep-wake cycles and intermittent interaction with the environment: intermittently follows simple commands, and maintains visual tracking
- Vegetative state: able to maintain normal sleep-wake cycles; there is loss of cognitive awareness and ability to interact with environment
- Coma: pathologic loss of awareness and ability to interact with the environment; loss of sleep-wake cycles
- Brain death: irreversible loss of cortical and brainstem function manifesting as loss of awareness, cranial reflexes, and motor response, isoelectric EEG

ETIOLOGY

- Ischemia (decreased cerebral perfusion): myocardial infarction, hemorrhage, shock
- Hypoxia (decreased oxygenation): drowning, strangulation, aspiration, carbon monoxide poisoning

DIAGNOSIS

DIFFERENTIAL DIAGNOSIS

- Other causes of encephalopathy, including toxic, metabolic, infectious, or neoplastic causes; nonconvulsive status epilepticus; hypothermia

WORKUP

- Neurologic examination (coma examination) to ascertain level of encephalopathy
- Systemic evaluation for causes of cardiorespiratory failure
- Laboratory studies (listed below) to evaluate alternate causes of encephalopathy
- Imaging studies: MRI of brain or CT of head (if MRI cannot be obtained)

LABORATORY TESTS

Urine drug screen, serum metabolic profile, ammonia, complete blood count, coagulation panel, fingerstick glucose, arterial blood gas, blood alcohol panel, serum neuron-specific enolase (if available)

IMAGING STUDIES

- Imaging is usually not revealing within first 24 hr of an anoxic event.
- Head CT without contrast (Fig. 1-94): obtain 24 hr after anoxic event to evaluate for stroke, trauma, or hemorrhage
- MRI of brain (Fig. 1-95): obtain if head CT scan unrevealing; may show cortical necrosis and infarcts of the basal ganglia
- EEG: to assess for nonconvulsive status epilepticus
- SSEP (somatosensory evoked potentials): obtain 48 hr after anoxic event; poor bilateral cortical response is associated with poor prognosis

OTHER STUDIES

- EEG: to assess for nonconvulsive status epilepticus
- Somatosensory evoked potentials (SSEP): obtain 48 hr after anoxic event; poor bilateral cortical response is associated with poor prognosis

TREATMENT

NONPHARMACOLOGIC THERAPY

- Hypothermia: evidence suggests that inducing hypothermia 32°-34° C for 24 hr following anoxic brain injury reduces metabolic need and may improve prognosis for recovery.
- Complications from hypothermia include bradycardia, hemodynamic instability, coagulopathy, infection, hyperglycemia, and hypokalemia.
- Contraindications for hypothermia: active hemorrhage, hemodynamic instability, sepsis, or trauma
- Indication for hypothermia: patients who have been resuscitated from a cardiac arrest with VF/VT as the presenting rhythm
- Hyperbaric oxygen is used in carbon monoxide poisoning.

ACUTE GENERAL Rx

- Supportive care: ABCs, secure airway, cardiopulmonary support in the critical care unit
- Control seizures with antiepileptic medications (may need midazolam or propofol drip if severe uncontrolled seizures).
- Treat myoclonus with clonazepam 8-12 mg daily in divided doses.

CHRONIC Rx

- Maintain adequate nutrition, infection precautions; provide DVT and gastric ulceration prophylaxis.
- Physical, occupational, and speech therapy as indicated per prognosis and patient ability
- May consider withdrawal of treatment per prognosis, family consultation, and respect for autonomy and dignity of the patient

DISPOSITION

Varies per extent of insult from acute rehabilitation to long-term care facility to return to home

REFERRAL

Referral to a neurologist is appropriate for definitive prognostication.

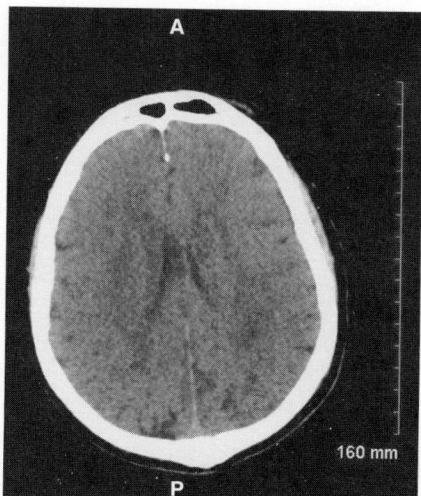

FIGURE 1-94 CT without contrast of a patient 1 day after pulseless electrical activity showing diffuse sulci effacement and loss of gray-white matter differentiation indicating cerebral edema. Diffuse white and gray matter hypodensities are also present. The patient remained comatose and life support was eventually withdrawn.

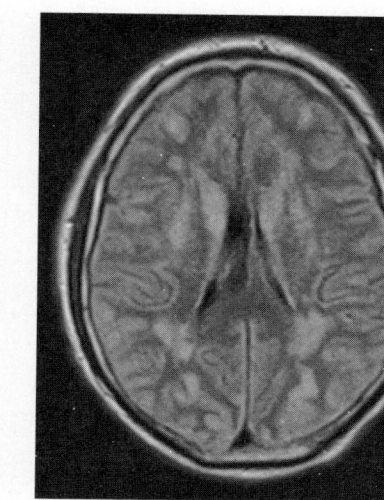

FIGURE 1-95 MRI FLAIR (fluid attenuated inversion recovery) of a patient 1 day after pulseless electrical activity showing bilateral multiple cortical, subcortical, gray and white hyperintensities. The patient remained comatose and life support was eventually withdrawn.

TABLE 1-37 Predictors of Poor Prognosis

Time from Onset of Anoxic Event	Clinical Exam
Initial exam	Pupils do not react to light (reflex absent)
24 hr	Eye movements are not roving conjugate or orienting and motor response is not better than flexor
72 hr	Motor response is not better than flexor
1 wk	Eye movements are not roving conjugate or orienting, no spontaneous eye opening, no following of commands
2 wk	No normal oculocephalic response, no following of commands, no spontaneous eye opening, and eye opening not improved by at least two grades

Composed from data presented in Levy DE et al: Predicting outcome from hypoxic-ischemic coma, *JAMA* 253(10):1420-1426, 1985.

TABLE 1-38 Predictors of Good Prognosis

Time from Onset of Anoxic Event	Clinical Exam
Initial exam	Pupils react to light (reflex present), motor response flexor or extensor, and eye movements spontaneous roving conjugate or orienting
24 hr	Motor response withdrawal or better, and eye opening improved at least 2 grades
72 hr	Motor response withdrawal or better and normal spontaneous eye movements present
1 wk	Follows commands
2 wk	Normal oculocephalic response

Composed from data presented in Levy DE et al: Predicting outcome from hypoxic-ischemic coma, *JAMA* 253(10):1420-1426, 1985.

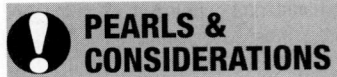

PEARLS & CONSIDERATIONS

COMMENTS
When assessing prognosis, use caution if patient is being treated with anesthetic agents or depressants including anticonvulsants. Refer to Tables 1-37 and 1-38 for indicators of prognosis.

PREVENTION
CPR, risk factor modification, induced hypothermia

PATIENT/FAMILY EDUCATION
Consult with family members regularly and provide accurate assessment of prognosis.

SUGGESTED READINGS
available at www.expertconsult.com

AUTHOR: **ALEXANDRA BOSKE, M.D.**

BASIC INFORMATION

DEFINITION

Antiphospholipid antibody syndrome (APS), the most common acquired thrombophilia, is characterized by clinical features of arterial or venous thrombosis and/or pregnancy morbidity *and* the presence of at least one type of antiphospholipid autoantibody (aPL). aPLs are antibodies directed against serum proteins bound to anionic phospholipids. Autoantibodies bind to antigenic anticoagulants which activate endothelial cells, monocytes, and platelets resulting in complement-mediated thrombosis.

Three types of aPL have been characterized:
- Anticardiolipin antibodies—the most common
- Lupus anticoagulants
- Anti-β_2-glycoprotein-1 antibodies

Primary APS occurs alone; and secondary APS occurs in association with systemic lupus erythematosus (SLE), other rheumatic disorders, or certain infections or medications. APS can affect all organ systems and includes venous and arterial thrombosis, recurrent fetal losses, and thrombocytopenia.

ICD-9CM CODES
795.79 Antiphospholipid antibody syndrome

EPIDEMIOLOGY & DEMOGRAPHICS

PREVALENCE:
- 1% to 5% of healthy individuals have anticardiolipin (aCL) and lupus anticoagulant (LA) antibodies.
- 12% to 30% of patients with SLE have aCL antibodies and 15% to 34% have LA antibodies.

PREDOMINANT AGE: Young to middle-age adults

RISK FACTORS:
- Underlying SLE and collagen-vascular diseases; other autoimmune disorders, including rheumatoid arthritis, Sjögren's syndrome, Behçet's syndrome, and idiopathic thrombocytopenic purpura; AIDS; hypertension (HTN).
- Most individuals are otherwise healthy and have no underlying medical condition.
- Several studies assessing presence of aPL in patients with cardiovascular and cerebrovascular disease have found a higher than expected prevalence of antibody.

GENETICS: Some APS-positive families exist, and human leukocyte antigen (HLA) studies have suggested associations with HLA DR7, DR4, and Dqw7+Drw53.

PHYSICAL FINDINGS & CLINICAL PRESENTATION

No pathognomic findings on examination; abnormal findings consistent with ischemia or infarction.
- Thrombosis:
  - Patients with APS are at risk for both venous and arterial thromboses. Venous thromboses are more common, occurring as the initial manifestation of APS in approximately ~30% of APS patients. Of all patients with venous thrombosis, 5% to −20% have aPL. The most common site for deep vein thrombosis is the calf, but thromboses may also occur in the renal, hepatic, axillary, subclavian, vena cava, and retinal veins. The most common site of arterial thrombosis is the cerebral vessels, followed by the coronary, renal, mesenteric, and bypass arteries. Recurrent thrombosis is common with APS.
- Commonly involved organ systems include:
  - Central nervous system: stroke, transient ischemic attack, migraine, multi-infarct dementia, epilepsy, movement disorders, transverse myelopathy, depression, Guillain-Barré syndrome, and migraine.
  - Pulmonary: pulmonary embolism and infarction; pulmonary hypertension; acute respiratory distress syndrome; intraalveolar pulmonary hemorrhage; a postpartum syndrome characterized by fever, pleuritic chest pain, dyspnea, and patchy infiltrates with pleural effusion on chest radiograph.
  - Cardiology: Libman-Sacks endocarditis, intracardiac thrombosis, coronary artery disease, myocardial infarction.
  - Gastrointestinal: abdominal pain, gastrointestinal bleed secondary to ischemia, splenic or pancreatic infarction, hepatic vein thrombosis, Budd-Chiari syndrome (second most common cause of syndrome).
  - Renal: proteinuria, acute renal failure, hypertension, renal infarct, renal artery or vein thrombosis, postpartum hemolytic-uremic syndrome.
  - Hematology: thrombocytopenia, hemolytic anemia.
  - Endocrine: Addison's disease secondary to adrenal hemorrhage and, less frequently, thrombosis.
  - Cutaneous: livedo reticularis, cutaneous necrosis, skin ulcerations, gangrene of digits (Fig. E1-97).
  - Obstetrics: recurrent spontaneous abortion, premature delivery or fetal growth retardation.
- Catastrophic APS (CAPS) (Table 1-40): CAPS is a rapidly progressive multiorgan thrombotic disease. Approximately 1% of APS is CAPS; approximately ~45% of CAPS do not present as APS initially. A 50% mortality rate

TABLE 1-40 Differential Diagnosis of Catastrophic Antiphospholipid Syndrome (CAPS)

Laboratory Abnormalities	CAPS	TTP	DIC
Microangiopathic hemolytic anemia	−	+	+
Thrombocytopenia	+	+	+
Fibrinogen/FDP	Normal/Normal	Normal/Increased	Decreased/Increased
Anticardiolipin antibody	+	−	−
Lupus anticoagulant	+	−	−

DIC, Disseminated intravascular coagulation; *TTP,* thrombotic thrombocytopenic purpura.

is seen in patients with CAPS. To make the diagnosis of catastrophic APS, four criteria must be satisfied:
1. Evidence of involvement of three or more organs, systems, and/or tissues. The most common symptoms are abdominal pain, dyspnea, neurologic symptoms, chest pain, and skin rash.
2. Development of manifestations simultaneously or in ≤1 week.
3. Confirmation by histopathology of small-vessel occlusion in at least one organ or tissue.
4. Laboratory confirmation of the presence of aPL.

ETIOLOGY
- aPLs react with negatively charged phospholipids.
- Possible mechanisms of thrombosis include effects of aPL on platelet membranes, endothelial cells, and clotting components such as prothrombin, protein C, or protein S.
- Studies have recently shown that prephospholipids are not immunogenic and that a binding protein (β_2-glycoprotein I) may be the key immunogen in the APS.

DIAGNOSIS

DIFFERENTIAL DIAGNOSIS

Other hypercoagulable states (inherited or acquired):
- Inherited: ATIII, protein C and protein, S deficiencies, factor V Leiden, prothrombin gene mutation.
- Acquired: heparin-induced thrombocytopenia, myeloproliferative syndromes, cancer, hyperviscosity.
- Hyperhomocysteinemia.
- Nephrotic syndrome.

WORKUP

Diagnostic criteria of APS include at least one clinical criterion and at least one laboratory criterion. A single clot may not be sufficient, especially with other thrombotic risk factors.
- Clinical:
  1. Venous, arterial, or small vessel thrombosis *or*
  2. Morbidity with pregnancy, defined as:
     - Fetal death at ≥10 weeks' gestation *or*
     - ≥1 premature births before 34 weeks' gestation secondary to eclampsia, preeclampsia, or severe placental insufficiency *or*
     - ≥2 or more unexplained spontaneous abortions at <10 weeks' gestation.
- Laboratory (see Table 1-41):
First steps: screening tests—dilute Russell viper venom time
Initial testing for presence of aPL:
  1. ELISA aCL antibody in medium or high titers *or*
  2. Lupus anticoagulant activity found *or*
  3. Anti-β_2-glycoprotein (GPI)-ELISA antibodies no more than 5 years from the clinical event.
Confirmatory aPL testing: repeat after 12 weeks to confirm persistence of aCL, anti-β2GPI or

LA test. Transient elevations of aCL can occur. Traditional aPL tests include aCL and B2GPI. Newer aPL tests include aps/PT, antiphosphatidyl serine/prothrombin.

LABORATORY TESTS

Diagnostic evaluation of aCL and LA antibodies is indicated in:
- Patient with underlying SLE or collagen-vascular disease with thrombosis.
  - Test patients with SLE without thrombosis regularly.
- Patient with recurrent, familial, or juvenile deep vein thrombosis (DVT) or thrombosis in an unusual location (mesenteric or cerebral).
  - One or more unexplained thrombotic events. Do not test in those at low risk, e.g., the elderly with clot and other risk factors.
  - One or more specific pregnancy events.
  - Unexplained thrombocytopenia.
- Possibly, in patients with lupus or lupuslike disorders in high-risk situations (e.g., surgery, prolonged immobilization, pregnancy).

Abnormal tests include:
- False-positive test for syphilis (RPR/VDRL).
- Lupus anticoagulant activity, demonstrated by prolongation of activated partial thromboplastin time that does not correct with 1:1 mixing study.
- Presence of anticardiolipin antibodies (ELISA for anticardiolipin is the most sensitive and specific test [>80%]).
- Presence of anti-β_2-glycoprotein I antibody.

TREATMENT

ACUTE Rx

Treatment includes use of heparin, low-molecular-weight heparin (LMWH), warfarin, antiplatelet agents, acetylsalicylic acid (aspirin), clopidorgrel, hydroxychloroquine.
- For a patient with positive aPL and venous or arterial thrombosis: Treat as would any other thrombosis.
  - Anticoagulation with heparin or LMWH, then followed by lifelong warfarin treatment, with a target international normalized ratio (INR) of 2.0 to 3.0.
    - There is some evidence to support a higher INR target or the addition of other agents in patients with arterial clots, especially if they have recurrent events while taking warfarin.
- Length of treatment needed is unknown, but possibly is lifelong, as the lifelong recurrence rate is 11% to 29%. Definite APS and thrombosis requires lifelong anticoagulation. Nondiagnostic APL with thrombosis: 3-6 months.
- Unfractionated heparin (UFH) is preferred if quick reversibility is needed.

PRIMARY PREVENTION
- Aspirin is of no benefit for prevention in patients with a prior clot.
- Aspirin may help patients without a history of clot.
- Hydroxychloroquine may be useful in those patients with SLE and aPL.
- Avoid oral contraceptive pills; modifiable risk factors for thrombosis such as smoking and immobility should be addressed.
- For pregnant women with a positive test for aPL antibodies without a history of DVT or pregnancy loss, consider low-dose subcutaneous UFH or LMWH SC, aspirin 81 mg, or surveillance.

SECONDARY PREVENTION
- For pregnant women with previously diagnosed APS:
  - Warfarin should be discontinued in early pregnancy secondary to its teratogenic effects.
  - Aspirin 81 mg, and subcutaneous UFH or LMWH to therapeutic partial thromboplastin time (PTT) or factor Xa levels, respectively.
  - Pregnant patients taking LMWH should be transitioned to unfractionated heparin before delivery due to reversibility.
  - Intravenous immunoglobulin (IVIG), plasmapheresis, hydroxychloroquine, statins, clopidorogrel, dipyridamole, and rituximab have been used when other treatments have failed.
- For pregnant women with a postive test for aPL antibodies and a history of fewer than three spontaneous abortions:
  - Low-dose aspirin at conception, followed by UFH, prophylactically or an intermediate dose at 7 weeks, continuing until 6 weeks' postpartum.
  - A mid-interval PTT should be checked and should be normal or similar to baseline before therapy.
  - LMWH can be used in place of unfractionated heparin and should be titrated to factor Xa levels in the recommended prophylactic range. The combination aspirin (75 mg daily) plus LMWH has been associated with a higher live birth rate when compared with IVIG.

FOR CATASTROPHIC ANTIPHOSPHOLIPID ANTIBODY SYNDROME
- Highest survival rates are achieved with the combination of anticoagulation, corticosteroids, and IVIG or plasma exchange.
- Case reports have shown rituximab to be a successful therapy for patients with life-threatening thrombosis refractory to anticoagulation.

CHRONIC Rx
- Anticoagulation with warfarin therapy.
- Immunosuppressive agents such as corticosteroids and cyclophosphamide are not effective.
- Limited data suggest that hydroxychloroquine may be effective.

DISPOSITION
- APS patients have a 20% to 70% risk for recurrent thrombosis.
- Initial arterial thrombosis tends to be followed by arterial events, and initial venous thrombosis tends to be followed by venous events.
- Catastrophic APS is associated with a high mortality rate, approaching 50%.
- Incidence of developing catastrophic APS is approximately 0.8% among APS patients.

REFERRAL
To hematology or rheumatology and/or obstetric medicine when diagnosis is made.

PEARLS & CONSIDERATIONS

COMMENTS
Cerebral features of SLE may be more related to thrombosis than inflammation and may respond better to anticoagulants than immunosuppression.

TABLE 1-41 Assays Used to Confirm Diagnosis of Antiphospholipid Syndrome

Assay	Methodology
"Criteria" aPL Assays	
aCL	ELISA
Anti-β_2-GPI	ELISA
LAC	Clotting/functional assays
"Noncriteria" aPL Assays	
Assays to detect antibodies to other phospholipids (i.e., phosphatidylserine, phosphatidylinositol, phosphatidic acid, phosphatidylglycerol, phosphatidylethanolamine, phosphatidylcholine)	ELISA
Annexin A5 resistance assay	Clotting/mechanistic assay
Assays to detect antibodies to prothrombin or prothrombin/phosphatidylserine	ELISA
Assays to detect antibodies to clotting proteins (i.e., protein C, protein S)	ELISA

aCL, Anticardiolipin; *aPL,* antiphospholipid antibody; *ELISA,* enzyme-linked immunosorbent assay; *LAC,* lupus anticoagulant.
From Hochberg MC et al: *Rheumatology,* ed 5, St Louis, 2011, Mosby.

PREVENTION

Prophylaxis for asymptomatic patients with positive aPL tests without previous thrombosis:
- No routine prophylaxis is recommended.
- Questionable whether low-dose aspirin is effective.
- Antithrombotic prophylaxis for major surgery, prolonged immobilization, and pregnancy.
- Avoid oral contraceptive pills in women with positive aPL test.

SUGGESTED READINGS

available at www.expertconsult.com

RELATED CONTENT

Hypercoagulable States (Related Key Topic)
Deep Vein Thrombosis (Related Key Topic)
Pulmonary Embolism (Related Key Topic)
Antiphospholipid Antibody Syndrome (Patient Information)

AUTHOR: **LYNN BOWLBY, M.D.**

A

Diseases and Disorders

I

BASIC INFORMATION

DEFINITION

Generalized anxiety disorder (GAD) is most likely to present in combination with other psychiatric and medical conditions. Individuals with GAD commonly present with excessive and disproportionately high levels of anxiety, fear, or worry for most days over at least a 6-mo period. The subjective anxiety must be accompanied by at least three somatic symptoms (e.g., restlessness, irritability, sleep disturbance, muscle tension, difficulty concentrating, or fatigability). GAD cannot be diagnosed if it occurs only in the setting of an active mood disorder, such as depression, or in the setting of another active anxiety disorder, such as PTSD or panic disorder.

SYNONYMS

Anxiety neurosis (former name for a subset of anxiety disorders)
Chronic anxiety
GAD

ICD-9CM CODE
F41.1

DSM-IV CODE
300.02

EPIDEMIOLOGY & DEMOGRAPHICS

INCIDENCE (IN U.S.): 6% to 9% per year in adult primary care clinics
PEAK INCIDENCE: Chronic condition with onset early in life
PREVALENCE (IN U.S.):
- In general population: prevalence of 5% lifetime
- In primary care setting: 3% (the most common anxiety disorder in this setting)

PREDOMINANT SEX: Women are more frequently affected (2:1 ratio) but may present for treatment less often (3:2 female/male).
PREDOMINANT AGE:
- 30% report onset before age 11
- 50% have onset before age 18

GENETICS: Concordance rates in dizygotic twins and monozygotic twins are not different (0% to 5%)

PHYSICAL FINDINGS & CLINICAL PRESENTATION

- Report of being "anxious" all of their lives.
- Excessive worry, usually regarding family, finances, work, or health.
- Sleep disturbance, particularly early insomnia.
- Muscle tension (typically in the muscles of neck and shoulders) or headache.
- Difficulty concentrating.
- Daytime fatigue.
- GI symptoms compatible with IBS (one third of patients).
- Physical symptoms are the usual reason for seeking medical attention.
- Comorbid psychiatric illness (e.g., dysthymia or major depression) and substance abuse (e.g., alcohol abuse) are frequent.

ETIOLOGY

- Hypotheses include models based on neurotransmitters (catecholamines, indolamines) and developmental psychology.
- Prevalence increased with a family history, increase in stress, history of physical or emotional trauma, and medical illness.

DIAGNOSIS

DIFFERENTIAL DIAGNOSIS

- Wide range of psychiatric and medical conditions:
  - Cardiovascular and pulmonary disease, such as cardiac arrhythmias or COPD
  - Hyperthyroidism
  - Substance abuse (e.g., cocaine, amphetamines, and PCP) or withdrawal (e.g., alcohol or benzodiazepines)

WORKUP

- Screening tests may enhance detection. A simple 7-item in-office case finding instrument, the GAD-7, can detect GAD with sensitivity of 89% and specificity of 82%.
- Physical examination: additional laboratory and radiologic workup depend on presenting symptoms.
- Iatrogenic cause should be suspected if anxiety follows recent changes in medication.

TREATMENT

NONPHARMACOLOGIC THERAPY

- Cognitive-behavioral therapy
- Relaxation training
- Biofeedback
- Psychodynamic psychotherapy

PHARMACOLOGIC THERAPY

- SSRIs/SNRIs
- Azapirones (e.g., buspirone)
- Benzodiazepines (less favored)

ACUTE GENERAL Rx

- Acute treatment is rarely indicated because GAD is a chronic condition.
- If patients are in acute distress, the possibility of another cause, including another anxiety disorder such as panic disorder, should be considered.
- Caution in prescribing benzodiazepines because of the propensity for misuse and dependence. If used, the patient should be educated about the options and the risks.

CHRONIC Rx

- SSRIs and SNRIs (e.g., venlafaxine and duloxetine) are effective typical first-line treatment. Particularly useful if comorbid depression present.
- Buspirone can be effective with minimal potential for tolerance or abuse. May be less effective in patients with previous benzodiazepine exposure and may require a high-dose titration.
- Benzodiazepines can be effective under close supervision; however, they have fallen out of favor as a first-line treatment given their potential for functional impairment, abuse, and dependence.
- Sedating antidepressants, such as mirtazapine, may also be useful for initial insomnia secondary to anxious ruminations.

DISPOSITION

- GAD is chronic with periodic exacerbations.
- Treatment is given to reduce level of symptoms. Suicide risk is higher than in the general population.

REFERRAL

- For refractory symptoms.
- For comorbid psychiatric conditions.

SUGGESTED READINGS
available at www.expertconsult.com

RELATED CONTENT
Social Anxiety Disorder (Related Key Topic)
Anxiety (Patient Information)

AUTHOR: **SETH A. BERKOWITZ, M.D.**

BASIC INFORMATION

DEFINITION

Aortic dissection is part of a spectrum of aortic pathologies that include intramural hematomas and penetrating atherosclerotic ulcers. Aortic dissection occurs when blood passes through an intimal tear, separating the intima from the medial layers and creating a false lumen. Intramural hematoma (IMH) occurs when the vasa vasorum ruptures within the medial wall. IMH does not involve an intimal tearing unless a dissection develops. One third of IMH will transform into aortic dissection. Penetrating atherosclerotic ulcers destroy the aortic intima and dissect into the aortic media, resulting in the formation of a pseudoaneurysm. Unlike aortic dissection, penetrating ulcers occur on the basis of extensive atherosclerosis in the aortic intima.

SYNONYMS

Dissecting aortic aneurysm

ICD-9CM CODES
441.00 Aortic dissection
444.01 Aortic dissection, thoracic

EPIDEMIOLOGY & DEMOGRAPHICS

PREDOMINANT SEX AND AGE: Males > females (ratio 3:1), ages 60 to 80 yr; mean, 63 yr
INCIDENCE: Approximately 2000 cases per year; 13th leading cause of death in U.S.
RISK FACTORS:
- Hypertension (found in up to 72% of patients with aortic dissection).
- Age
- Atherosclerosis
- Family history of aortic aneurysms/dissection
- History of cardiac surgery, intraaortic catheterization
- Disorders of collagen (Marfan's syndrome, Ehlers-Danlos syndrome)
- Vascular inflammation (giant cell arteritis, Takayasu arteritis, rheumatoid arthritis, syphilitic aortitis)
- Aortic coarctation, bicuspid aortic valve
- Turner's syndrome
- Cocaine abuse
- Trauma

CLASSIFICATION

Aortic dissection is generally classified according to anatomic location (Fig. 1-98):
- Stanford: type A ascending aorta (proximal), type B descending aorta (distal) (Fig. 1-99)
- DeBakey: type I ascending and descending aorta, type II ascending aorta, type III descending aorta

Aortic dissection can also be classified by acuity of presentation (acute or chronic), based on the time of onset.

PHYSICAL FINDINGS & CLINICAL PRESENTATION

- Sudden onset of severe sharp, tearing, or ripping chest pain
- Anterior chest pain (ascending dissection)
- Back pain, abdominal pain (descending dissection)
- Syncope, congestive heart failure (CHF), malperfusion may occur
- Most present with severe hypertension, 25% with hypotension (systolic blood pressure <100 mm Hg), which can indicate bleeding, cardiac tamponade, or severe aortic regurgitation
- Pulse and blood pressure differentials (>20 mm Hg between arms) in 9% to 30% of cases, caused by partial compression of subclavian arteries
- Aortic regurgitation in 18% to 50% of cases of proximal dissection, often with diastolic decrescendo murmur
- Myocardial ischemia caused by coronary artery occlusion
- Stroke in 5% to 10% of patients
- Horner syndrome
- Vocal cord paralysis/hoarse voice

ETIOLOGY

Aortic dissection shares a common pathway of cystic medial necrosis with abdominal aortic aneurysm formation. Genetics, in addition to other risk factors listed above, contribute to the development of aortic dissection.

DIAGNOSIS

DIFFERENTIAL DIAGNOSIS

- Known as the great imitator: PE, ACS, aortic stenosis/insufficiency, nondissecting aneurysm, pericarditis, cholecystitis, peptic ulcer disease, pancreatitis, musculoskeletal pain
- Acute MI needs to be ruled out.
- Consider aortic dissection in patients with unexplained stroke, chest pain, syncope, acute-onset CHF, abdominal pain, back pain, and malperfusion of extremities or internal organs.

LABORATORY TESTS

- ECG: helpful to rule out MI, although dissection can lead to coronary ischemia
- D-dimer has a 100% negative predictive value but lacks specificity in the setting of acute aortic dissection.
- Three biomarkers with different diagnostic windows can be used in the diagnosis of aortic dissection.
- Smooth muscle myosin heavy chain protein (released from damaged medial smooth muscle) can be used to detect proximal aortic dissections (91% sensitivity and 93%

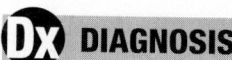

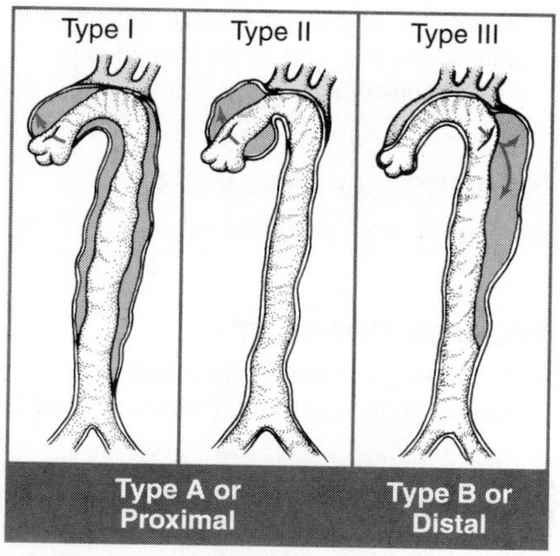

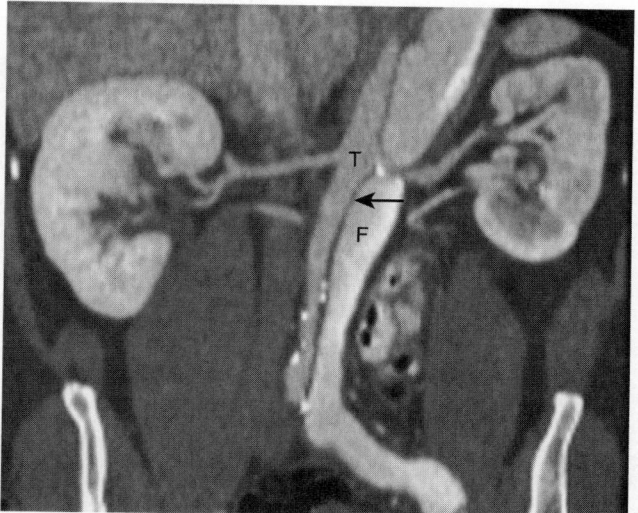

FIGURE 1-98 Classification systems for aortic dissection. (From Isselbacher EM et al: Disease of the aorta. In Braunwald E [ed]: *Heart disease: a textbook of cardiovascular medicine*, ed 5, Philadelphia, 1997, Saunders.)

FIGURE 1-99 Computed tomographic angiogram of the aorta shows type B aortic dissection. The intimal flap *(arrow)* separates the two lumen *(T)* from the false lumen *(F)* and compromises blood flow to the right kidney, causing renal atrophy and cortical thinning. (Image courtesy of Bart Domatch, M.D., Radiology Department, University of Texas Southwestern Medical Center, Dallas, TX; from Andreoli TE et al: *Andreoli and Carpenter's Cecil essentials of medicine*, ed 8, Philadelphia, 2010, Saunders.)

specificity). Myosin heavy chains will peak within 3 hr of dissection and clear within 24 hr of aortic injury.

- CK-BB isoenzyme also peaks within 6 hr of dissection.
- Calponin, a smooth muscle troponin counterpart, increases in aortic dissection with a wider diagnostic window when compared to smooth muscle myosin heavy chain and CK-BB.
- C-reactive protein, fibrinogen, and elastin fragments are under investigation

IMAGING STUDIES (Box E1-4)

- TEE, MRI, multidetector CT are imaging modalities of choice. Sensitivities (98% to 100%) and specificities (95% to 98%) nearly equal in skilled hands. Test of choice depends on clinical circumstances and availability.
- Transesophageal echocardiography (TEE) is study of choice in unstable patients with type A dissection but is operator dependent.
- MRI has high sensitivity and specificity but limited availability; not suitable for unstable patients; contraindicated with pacemakers, metal devices.
- Multidetector CT is considered the gold standard; least operator dependent but involves intravenous contrast. Fig. 1-101 shows a thin-slice CT image of a classic ascending dissection with aneurysmal dilation.
- With medium or high pretest probability, a second diagnostic test should be done if the first is negative.
- Coronary computed tomographic angiography (CTA) may be an alternative and useful diagnostic study when evaluating for pulmonary embolism, acute coronary syndrome, and aortic dissection.
- Aortography rarely done now.
- Chest radiograph may show widened mediastinum (62%) and displacement of aortic intimal calcium (Fig. E1-100).

- Although the diagnostic sensitivity of transthoracic echocardiography is suboptimal, it is useful in assessing potential high-risk features or complications, such as pericardial effusion, and making other potential diagnoses. A negative transthoracic echocardiography, however, does not exclude aortic dissection.

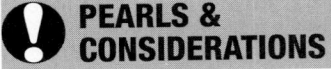 TREATMENT

- Proximal dissections (acute type A) require emergent surgery to prevent rupture or pericardial effusion.
- Distal dissections (Stanford type B) are usually treated medically unless distal organ involvement or impending rutpure occurs.
  - Surgical intervention for distal dissections is reserved for patients who have a complicated course, including occlusion of a major aortic branch, dissection, presence within an aortic aneurysm, and evidence of aortic rupture.

ACUTE GENERAL Rx

- Admit to ICU for monitoring.
- Target SBP 100 to 120 mm Hg or as low as tolerated; heart rate <60 beats/min to reduce aortic wall stress.
- IV beta-blockers are cornerstones of treatment, but multiple medications may be needed.
  - Propanolol 1 mg every 3 to 5 min; metoprolol 5 mg IV every 5 min; or labetalol 20 mg IV, then 20 to 80 mg every 10 min, followed by nitroprusside 0.3 to 10 mg/kg/min.
  - Nitroprusside should not be used without beta-blockade because vasodilation can induce reflex sympathetic stimulation and increased aortic sheer stress.
  - IV calcium channel blockers with negative inotropy may be used if beta-blockers are contraindicated.

- Pain control, often with morphine.
- Endovascular repair is a feasible, less invasive option for type A aortic dissections, but data are limited. Literature has shown favorable short- and mid-term outcomes. However, long-term outcome data are still under investigation.

CHRONIC Rx

- Chronic aortic dissection (>2 wk) managed with aggressive blood pressure control: target <120/80 mm Hg in most patients.
- Target low-density lipoprotein <70 mg/dl.
- Minimize strenuous physical activity.
- Serial imaging of the aorta, usually with contrast CT.
- Endovascular repair in chronic type B dissection should be considered when the aortic diameter exceeds 5.5-6.0 cm, when there is uncontrolled pain or blood pressure, or when there is rapid growth of the dissecting aneurysm (>1 cm per year).

DISPOSITION

- 85% mortality rate within 2 wk if untreated.
- Proximal dissection is a surgical emergency. Time is critical; mortality rate is 1% to 3% per hour.
- Overall, in-hospital mortality rate is 30% with proximal dissections and 10% with distal dissections.

REFERRAL

For ICU management and surgical intervention

! PEARLS & CONSIDERATIONS

- Blood pressure control is essential; beta-blocker is first-line medication.
- Proximal dissection is a surgical emergency.
- Cardiac tamponade is not uncommon in patients with acute type A aortic dissection. Syncope, altered mental status, and a widened mediastinum on chest radiograph on presentation suggest tamponade which warrants urgent operative therapy.
- Surgery for acute type A aortic dissection in patients ≥70 yr can be performed with acceptable outcomes.

SUGGESTED READINGS

available at www.expertconsult.com

RELATED CONTENT

Aortic Dissection (Patient Information)
Abdominal Aortic Aneurysm (Related Key Topic)

AUTHORS: **AHMAD ISMAIL, M.D.,** and **ABDULRAHMAN ABDULBAKI, M.D.**

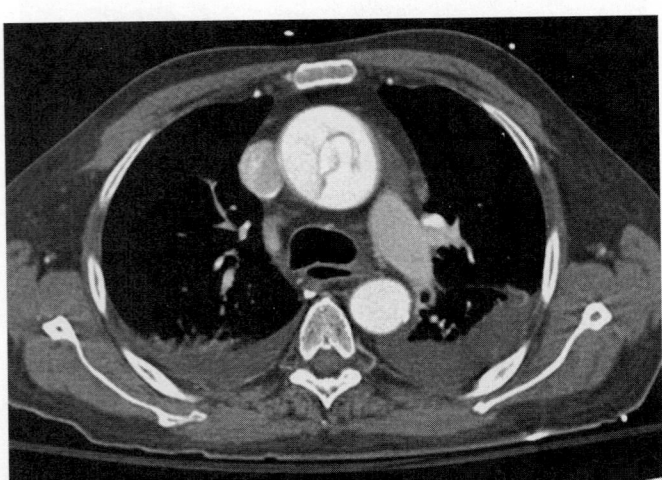

FIGURE 1-101 Thin-slice CT image of a classic ascending dissection with aneurysmal dilation. (From Cameron JL, Cameron AM: *Current surgical therapy,* ed 10, Philadelphia, 2011, Saunders.)

BASIC INFORMATION

DEFINITION

Aortic regurgitation (AR) is retrograde blood flow into the left ventricle from the aorta as a result of an incompetent aortic valve.

SYNONYMS

Aortic insufficiency
AI
AR

ICD-9CM CODES

424.1 Aortic valve disorders

EPIDEMIOLOGY & DEMOGRAPHICS

- Prevalence ranges from 4.9% to 10% and increases with age.
- The most common cause of isolated severe AR is aortic root dilation.
- Infectious endocarditis is the most frequent cause of acute AR.

PHYSICAL FINDINGS & CLINICAL PRESENTATION

The pathophysiology of AR is described in Fig. 1-102. The clinical presentation varies depending on whether aortic insufficiency is acute or chronic. Chronic aortic insufficiency is well tolerated (except when secondary to infective endocarditis), and the patients remain asymptomatic for years. Common manifestations after significant deterioration of left ventricular function are dyspnea on exertion, syncope, chest pain, and congestive heart failure (CHF). Acute aortic insufficiency manifests primarily with hypotension caused by a sudden fall in cardiac output and resultant cardiogenic shock. In addition, a rapid rise in left ventricular diastolic pressure results in a further decrease in coronary blood flow.

Physical findings in chronic aortic insufficiency include the following:
- Widened pulse pressure (markedly increased systolic blood pressure, decreased diastolic blood pressure).
- Findings associated with the widened pulse pressure:
  ○ Bounding pulses, "water hammer" or collapsing pulse (*Corrigan's pulse*), can be palpated at the wrist or on the femoral arteries artery and is caused by rapid rise and sudden collapse of the arterial pressure during late systole.
  ○ Head "bobbing" with each systole (*de Musset's sign*).
  ○ "Pistol shot femorals" (*Traube's sign*) is a term used to describe a loud sound over the femoral artery
  ○ Capillary pulsations (*Quincke's sign*) may occur at the base of the nail beds.

- A to-and-fro Duroziez murmur may be heard over femoral arteries with slight compression.
- Popliteal systolic pressure is increased more than 20 mm Hg over brachial systolic pressure (*Hill's sign*), with a 40 to 60 mm difference representing moderate AR and > 60 mm difference severe AR.
- Other findings associated with AR, which are more of historical than practical interest, include:
  ○ *Mueller's sign*—Systolic pulsations of the uvula.
  ○ *Becker's sign*—Visible pulsations of the retinal arteries and pupils.
  ○ *Mayne's sign*—More than a 15 mm Hg decrease in diastolic blood pressure with arm elevation from the value obtained with the arm in the standard position.
  ○ *Rosenbach's sign*—Systolic pulsations of the liver.
  ○ *Gerhard's sign*—Systolic pulsations of the spleen.
- Cardiac auscultation reveals:
  1. Displacement of cardiac impulse downward and to the patient's left
  2. S_3 heard over the apex
  3. Decrescendo, blowing diastolic murmur heard along left sternal border
  4. Low-pitched apical diastolic rumble (*Austin-Flint murmur*)—the precise etiology of the murmur is uncertain, but it is generally believed to be related to increased velocity of mitral inflow consequent to the AR.
  5. Early systolic ejection sound and systolic ejection murmur.

In patients with acute aortic insufficiency both the wide pulse pressure and the large stroke volume are absent. A short, blowing diastolic murmur may be the only finding on physical examination.

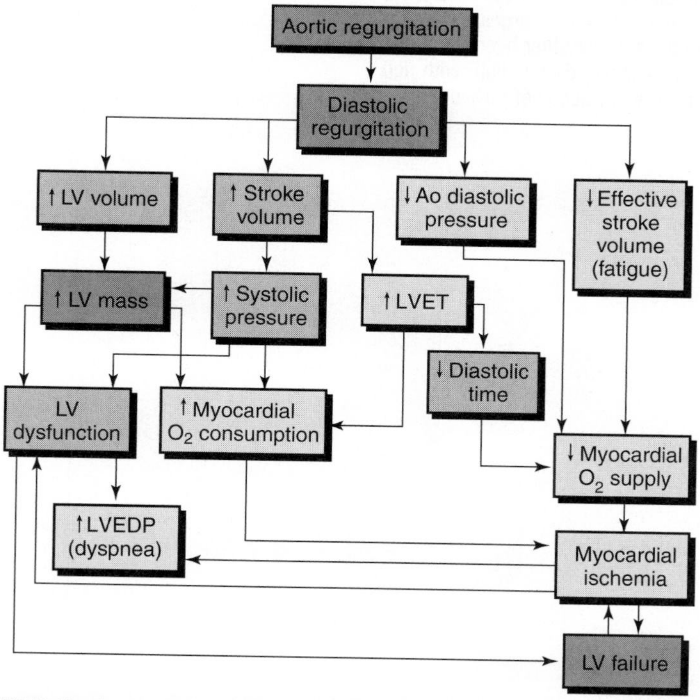

ETIOLOGY

- Leaflet abnormalities:
  ○ Infective endocarditis
  ○ Rheumatic fibrosis (most common cause in developing countries)
  ○ Trauma with valvular rupture
  ○ Congenital bicuspid aortic valve (most common cause in the United States)
  ○ Myxomatous degeneration
  ○ Fenfluramine, dexfenfluramine, pergolide, cabergoline
  ○ Ankylosing spondylitis
- Aortic root or ascending aorta abnormalities:
  ○ Annuloaortic ectasia
  ○ Ehlers-Danlos syndrome
  ○ Marfan's syndrome
  ○ Trauma: ankylosing spondylitis
  ○ Syphilitic aortitis
  ○ Systemic hypertension
  ○ Aortic dissection

DIAGNOSIS

DIFFERENTIAL DIAGNOSIS

- Patent ductus arteriosus, pulmonary regurgitation, and other valvular abnormalities.
- The differential diagnosis of cardiac murmurs is described in Section II.

FIGURE 1-102 **Pathophysiology of aortic regurgitation.** Aortic regurgitation results in an increased left ventricular (*LV*) volume, increased stroke volume, increased aortic (*Ao*) systolic pressure, and decreased effective stroke volume. Increased LV volume results in an increased LV mass, which may lead to LV dysfunction and failure. Increased LV stroke volume increases systolic pressure and prolongation of LV ejection time (*LVET*). Increased LV systolic pressure results in a decrease in diastolic time. Decreased diastolic time (myocardial perfusion time), diastolic aortic pressure, and effective stroke volume reduce myocardial O_1 supply. Increased myocardial O_2 consumption and decreased myocardial O_2 supply produce myocardial ischemia, which further deteriorates LV function. *LVEDP*, LV end-diastolic pressure. (From Boudoulas H, Gravanis MB: Valvular heart disease. In Gravanis MB [ed]: *Cardiovascular disorders: pathogenesis and pathophysiology,* St Louis, 1993, Mosby.)

WORKUP

- Echocardiogram, chest radiograph, electrocardiogram (ECG), and cardiac catheterization (selected patients).
- Medical history and physical examination focused on the following clinical manifestations:
  1. Dyspnea on exertion.
  2. Syncope.
  3. Chest pain.
  4. CHF.

IMAGING STUDIES

- Chest radiography:
  1. Left ventricular hypertrophy (LVH) (chronic AR).
  2. Aortic dilation.
  3. Normal cardiac silhouette with pulmonary edema: possible in patients with acute AR.
- ECG: LVH.
- Echocardiography (Fig. E1-103) is the main imaging modality to diagnose AR and assess left ventricular size and function. Quantification of the severity of regurgitation can be made either qualitatively by Doppler vena contracta width (severe if >0.6 cm) or quantitatively by effective regurgitant orifice area (severe if >0.30 cm^2) and/or regurgitant volume (severe if >60 mL per /beat).
- Cardiac catheterization is indicated in selected patients to assess the degree of left ventricular dysfunction, to assess the degree of AR when echocardiographic parameters are inconclusive, and to determine if there is coexistent coronary artery disease.

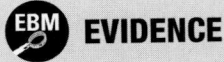 **TREATMENT**

NONPHARMACOLOGIC THERAPY

- Avoidance of competitive sports and heavy weight lifting if the AR is severe.
- Salt restriction.
- In 2007, the American Heart Association (AHA) guidelines for prevention of infectious endocarditis were revised; and routine antibiotic prophylaxis to undergo dental or other invasive procedures is no longer recommended, unless the patient has a prior history of endocarditis.

ACUTE GENERAL Rx

MEDICAL:
- Angiotensin-converting enzyme (ACE) inhibitors, diuretics, and sodium restriction for CHF; nitroprusside in patients with acute AR.
- Short-term vasodilator therapy in patients with severe AR, left ventricular dysfunction, and symptoms of heart failure to improve the hemodynamic profile before surgery.
- Long-term vasodilator therapy with ACE inhibitors or nifedipine in patients who are not candidates for valve replacement, in asymptomatic patients with severe AR and left ventricular dilation but normal left ventricular function.

SURGICAL: Reserved for:
- Symptomatic patients with chronic, severe AR.
- Patients with acute AR (i.e., infective endocarditis) producing left ventricular failure.
- Patients with severe AR undergoing CABG or surgery on the aorta or other heart valves.
- Evidence of systolic dysfunction with left ventricular ejection fraction of 50% or less.

- Asymptomatic patients with severe AR and left ventricular ejection fraction >50%, but with left ventricular dilation:
  1. Echocardiographic end- systolic dimension >55 mm *or*
  2. Echocardiographic end- diastolic dimension >75 mm.

EBM EVIDENCE

available at www.expertconsult.com

SUGGESTED READINGS

available at www.expertconsult.com

RELATED CONTENT

Aortic Insufficiency (Patient Information)

AUTHORS: **PHILIP FORMICA, M.D.,**
DAVID J. FORTUNATO, M.D., F.A.C.C., and
FRED F. FERRI, M.D.

BASIC INFORMATION

DEFINITION

Aortic stenosis (AS) is obstruction to systolic left ventricular outflow across the aortic valve. Symptoms appear when the valve orifice decreases to <1 cm² (normal orifice is 3 to 4 cm²). The stenosis is considered severe when the orifice is <1.0 cm² or the mean pressure gradient is ≥40 mm Hg.

SYNONYMS

Aortic valvular stenosis
AS

ICD-9CM CODES
424.1 Aortic valvular stenosis

EPIDEMIOLOGY & DEMOGRAPHICS

- Aortic stenosis is the most common valve lesion in adults in Western countries.
- Calcific stenosis (most common cause in patients >60 yr) occurs in 75% of patients.

PHYSICAL FINDINGS & CLINICAL PRESENTATION

- Rough, loud, systolic, crescendo-decrescendo murmur best heard at base of heart and radiating into neck vessels; often associated with a thrill or ejection click; may also be heard well at the apex.
- Absence or diminished intensity of the second heart sound (in severe AS).
- Late, slow-rising carotid upstroke with decreased amplitude.
- Strong apical pulse.
- Narrowing of pulse pressure in later stages of AS.
- Some patients with AS experience bleeding into their GI tract or skin. This is caused by an acquired defect in von Willebrand factor. Aortic valve replacement restores normal hemostasis.

ETIOLOGY

- Idiopathic calcification of the aortic valve (most common)
- Progressive stenosis of congenital bicuspid valve (found in 1% to 2% of the population)
- Congenital (major cause of AS in patients <30 yr)
- Rheumatic inflammation of aortic valve is rare as a cause of isolated AS in the U.S.
- Genetic variation in the LPA locus, mediated by Lp(2) levels, is associated with aortic valve calcification across multiple ethnic groups and with incidental clinical aortic stenosis.

DIAGNOSIS

DIFFERENTIAL DIAGNOSIS

- Hypertrophic cardiomyopathy
- Mitral regurgitation
- Ventricular septal defect
- Aortic sclerosis. Aortic stenosis is distinguished from aortic sclerosis by the degree of valve impairment. In aortic sclerosis, the valve leaflets are abnormally thickened but obstruction to outflow is absent or minimal.

WORKUP

- ECG: may demonstrate left ventricular hypertrophy and/or left atrial abnormality (Fig. 1-104).
- Chest radiograph: may demonstrate cardiomegaly. Poststenotic dilation of the ascending aorta may also be evident.
- Laboratory: B-type natriuretic peptide or N-terminal pro-B-type natriuretic peptide (NT-proBNP) correlates with the mean pressure gradient, aortic valve area, and functional status. It is a useful biochemical marker to evaluate severity of AS, monitor disease progression at an early stage, and decide on the optimal time for aortic valve replacement. An increased level of BNP correlates with severity of AS and New York Heart Association functional class.
- Echocardiography (see "Imaging Studies")
- Cardiac catheterization in selected patients (see "Imaging Studies")
- Medical history focusing on symptoms and potential complications:
  1. Angina
  2. Syncope (particularly with exertion)
  3. Congestive heart failure (CHF)
  4. GI bleeding: in patients with associated hemorrhagic telangiectasia (AVM)

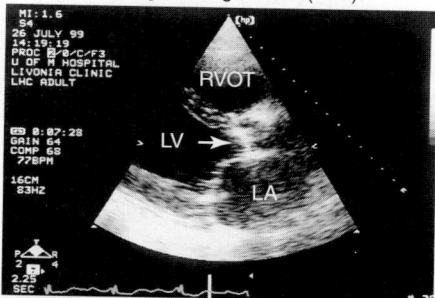
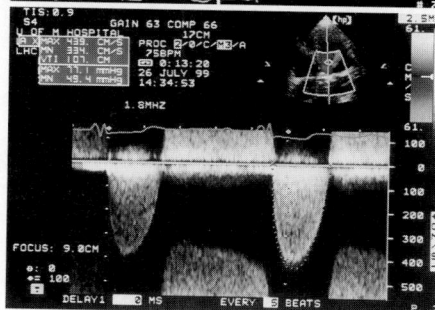

FIGURE 1-104 Echocardiogram recorded in a patient with severe aortic stenosis. The *top panel* is a parasternal long-axis view recorded in systole. Left ventricular function is diminished. The aortic valve is markedly thickened and partially calcified. Its motion is markedly reduced, and in systole it appears that the valve occludes the orifice *(arrow)*. The *lower panel* is a continuous-wave Doppler recorded from the apex of the left ventricle along a line aimed through the stenotic aortic valve. Note the aortic stenosis signal below the zero crossing line. The peak velocity is 430 cm/sec, which corresponds to a maximum gradient of 77 mm Hg and a mean gradient of 49.4 mm Hg. *LA,* left atrium; *LV,* left ventricle; *RVOT,* right ventricular outflow tract. (From Zipes DP et al [eds]: *Braunwald's heart disease,* ed 7, Philadelphia, 2005, Saunders.)

- Figs. E1-105 and E1-106 describe algorithms for evaluation and treatment of AS.

IMAGING STUDIES

- Chest x-ray:
  1. Poststenotic dilation of the ascending aorta
  2. Calcification of aortic cusps
  3. Pulmonary congestion (in advanced stages of AS)
- ECG:
  1. Left ventricular hypertrophy (found in >80% of patients)
  2. ST-T wave changes
  3. Atrial fibrillation: frequent
- Doppler echocardiography: thickening of the left ventricular wall; allows calculation of both aortic valve area and estimation of pressure gradients to determine severity of AS.
- Cardiac catheterization: indicated in symptomatic patients awaiting aortic valve replacement (AVR) in order to detect coexisting coronary artery stenosis that may need bypass at the same time as aortic valve replacement; also indicated in symptomatic patients when noninvasive tests are inconclusive or when there is a discrepancy between noninvasive tests and clinical findings regarding severity of AS as it confirms the diagnosis and the estimates of the severity of the valvular stenosis by directly measuring the gradient across the valve, allowing calculation of the valve area.

TREATMENT

NONPHARMACOLOGIC THERAPY

- Strenuous activity should be avoided in patients with moderate to severe AS
- Sodium restriction if CHF is present

GENERAL Rx
MEDICAL:

- Diuretics and sodium restriction are needed if CHF is present; digoxin and beta-blockers may be useful for rate control if patient has atrial fibrillation.
- ACE inhibitors are relatively contraindicated.
- Statin therapy may be of some benefit in reducing the progression of calcific AS, though further studies are needed.
- In 2007, the AHA guidelines for prevention of infectious endocarditis were revised and routine antibiotic prophylaxis to undergo dental or other invasive procedures is no longer recommended, unless the patient has prior endocarditis.

SURGICAL:

- Valve replacement is the treatment of choice in symptomatic patients because the 5-yr mortality rate after onset of symptoms is extremely high, even with optimal medical therapy. Valve replacement is indicated in symptomatic patients with severe AS, patients with moderate AS undergoing CABG or surgery on the aorta/other heart valves, patients with abnormal blood pressure response (decrease in systolic blood pressure) during exercise, patients with rapidly progressive

stenosis, and in patients with severe AS and left ventricular ejection fraction <50%.

- Percutaneous aortic balloon valvuloplasty serves best as palliative therapy in severely symptomatic patients and as a bridge to surgery in hemodynamically unstable adult patients. It is not an option in patients who are good candidates for surgical valve replacement.
- Percutaneous heart valve replacement is an emerging catheter-based technology that allows for implantation of a prosthetic valve without open heart surgery. Transcatheter aortic-valve replacement (TAVR) has been shown to reduce the death rate in patients with severe AS and coexisting conditions that exclude them as candidates for surgical replacement of the aortic valve. In another randomized trial involving high-risk patients with severe AS who were candidates for surgery, TAVR was found to be noninferior to surgical valve replacement for short-term efficacy with similar all-cause death at 1 yr. The surgical group had double the incidence of new-onset atrial fibrillation and major bleeding, but the TAVR group had a higher rate of paravalvular regurgitation, major stroke, and vascular complications.

DISPOSITION

- The presence of even mild symptoms is an indicator of poor survival for patients with AS. The 5-yr survival rate in adults is 40%.
- The average duration of symptoms before death is angina, 60 mo; syncope, 36 mo; CHF, 24 mo.
- Approximately 75% of patients with symptomatic AS will be dead 3 yr. after onset of symptoms unless the aortic valve is replaced.

REFERRAL

- Surgical referral for valve replacement in symptomatic patients. The risk of aortic valve replacement is greater than any potential benefit for truly asymptomatic patients. There are studies that are examining the presence of moderate or severe valvular calcification, together with a rapid increase in aortic jet velocity and elevated BNP, to identify patients with a very poor prognosis who should be considered for early valve replacement rather than have surgery delayed until symptoms develop.

- Surgical mortality rate for valve replacement is 3% to 5%; however, it varies with patient's age (>8% in patients >75 yr).
- Balloon valvuloplasty is useful in infants and children or poor surgical candidates who do not have calcified valve apparatus; it can be done as an intermediate procedure to stabilize high-risk patients before surgery.

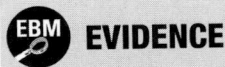

EVIDENCE

available at www.expertconsult.com

SUGGESTED READINGS

available at www.expertconsult.com

RELATED CONTENT

Aortic Stenosis (Patient Information)

AUTHORS: **PHILIP FORMICA, M.D.,**
DAVID J. FORTUNATO, M.D., F.A.C.C., and
FRED F. FERRI, M.D.

BASIC INFORMATION

DEFINITION

Appendicitis is the acute inflammation of the appendix.

ICD-9CM CODES
540.9 Appendicitis
540.0 Appendicitis with generalized peritonitis

EPIDEMIOLOGY & DEMOGRAPHICS

- Appendicitis occurs in 10% of the population, most commonly between the ages of 10 and 30 yr. Median age is 22 years. Lifetime risk is 7%.
- More than 250,000 appendectomies are performed in the U.S. each year.
- It is the most common abdominal surgical emergency.
- Incidence of appendicitis has declined over the past 30 yr.
- Male/female ratio is 3:2 until mid-20s; it equalizes after age 30 yr.

PHYSICAL FINDINGS & CLINICAL PRESENTATION

- In children with abdominal pain, fever is the single most useful sign associated with appendicitis. Vomiting, rectal tenderness, and rebound tenderness along with fever are more indicative of appendicitis in children than in adults.
- Abdominal pain: initially the pain may be epigastric or periumbilical in nearly 50% of patients; it subsequently localizes to the right lower quadrant within 12 to 18 hr. Pain can be found in back or right flank if appendix is retrocecal or in other abdominal locations if there is malrotation of the appendix.
- Pain with right thigh extension *(psoas sign)*, low-grade fever: temperature may be >38° C if there is appendiceal perforation.
- Pain with internal rotation of the flexed right thigh (obturator sign) is present.
- Right lower quadrant (RLQ) pain on palpation of the left lower quadrant (LLQ) *(Rovsing's sign)*: physical examination may reveal right-sided tenderness in patients with pelvic appendix.
- Point of maximum tenderness is in the RLQ *(McBurney's point)*.
- Nausea, vomiting, tachycardia, cutaneous hyperesthesias at the level of T12 can be present.

ETIOLOGY

Obstruction of the appendiceal lumen with subsequent vascular congestion, inflammation, and edema; common causes of obstruction are:

- Fecaliths: 30% to 35% of cases (most common in adults)
- Foreign body: 4% (fruit seeds, pinworms, tapeworms, roundworms, calculi)
- Inflammation: 50% to 60% of cases (submucosal lymphoid hyperplasia [most common etiology in children, teens])
- Neoplasms: 1% (carcinoids, metastatic disease, carcinoma)

DIAGNOSIS

DIFFERENTIAL DIAGNOSIS

- Intestinal: regional cecal enteritis, incarcerated hernia, cecal diverticulitis, intestinal obstruction, perforated ulcer, perforated cecum, Meckel's diverticulitis
- Reproductive: ectopic pregnancy, ovarian cyst, torsion of ovarian cyst, salpingitis, tubo-ovarian abscess, mittelschmerz, endometriosis, seminal vesiculitis
- Renal: renal and ureteral calculi, neoplasms, pyelonephritis
- Vascular: leaking aortic aneurysm
- Psoas abscess
- Trauma
- Cholecystitis
- Mesenteric adenitis

WORKUP

Patients with RLQ pain, nausea, vomiting, anorexia, and RLQ rebound tenderness should undergo prompt clinical and laboratory evaluation. Imaging studies are generally not necessary in typical appendicitis and generally reserved for patients with an equivocal likelihood of appendicitis. They are useful when the diagnosis is uncertain. Laparoscopy may be useful as both a diagnostic and a therapeutic modality.

LABORATORY TESTS

- Complete blood count with differential reveals leukocytosis with a left shift in 90% of patients with appendicitis. Total white blood cell (WBC) count is generally lower than 20,000/mm³. Higher counts may be indicative of perforation. Less than 4% have a normal WBC and differential. A WBC count <10,000/mm³ decreases the likelihood of appendicitis. Low hemoglobin and hematocrit levels in an older patient should raise suspicion for GI tract carcinoma.
- Microscopic hematuria and pyuria may occur in <20% of patients.

IMAGING STUDIES

- Multidetector computed tomography (Fig. 1-107) is a useful test for routine evaluation of suspected appendicitis in adults. CT of the abdomen/pelvis without contrast has a sensitivity of >90% and an accuracy >94% for acute appendicitis. A distended appendix, periappendiceal inflammation, and a thickened appendiceal wall are indicative of appendicitis. Table E1-42 describes CT findings of appendicitis. In children and young adults, exposure to CT radiation is of particular concern. Trials with low-dose CT (116 mGy · cm) have shown that low-dose CT is not inferior to standard-dose CT (521 mGy · cm) with respect to negative (unnecessary) appendectomy rates in young adults with suspected appendicitis.
- Ultrasonography (Fig. E1-108) has a sensitivity of 75% to 90% for the diagnosis of acute appendicitis, although it is highly operator dependent and difficult in patients with large body habitus. Ultrasound is useful, especially in pregnancy and

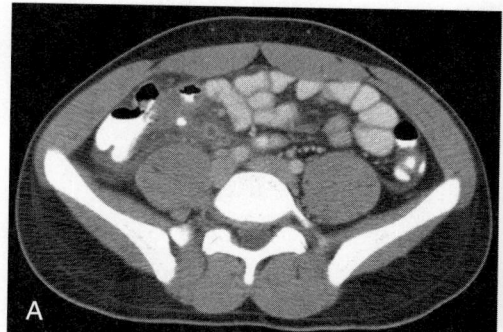
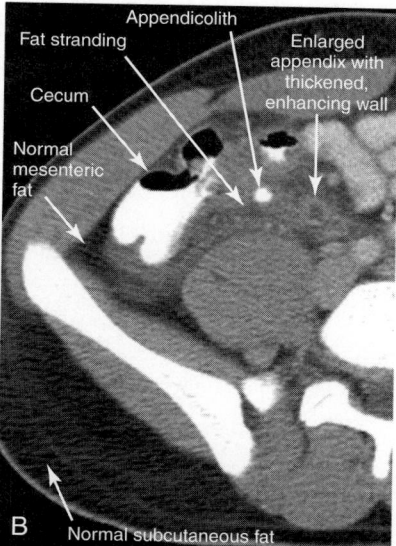

FIGURE 1-107 Appendicitis, CT with IV and oral contrast. This CT demonstrates classic findings of appendicitis in an 18-year-old male with right lower quadrant pain, as seen with CT with IV and oral contrast. Studies suggest that CT without contrast has similar sensitivity and specificity. An enlarged appendix is seen near the cecum as a right lower quadrant tubular structure in short-axis cross section, giving it a circular appearance. The surrounding fat shows stranding, a smoky appearance indicating inflammation (compare with normal mesenteric and subcutaneous fat, which is nearly black). The appendiceal wall shows enhancement, a brightening after administration of IV contrast. This slice also shows an appendicolith, an occasional finding of appendicitis. It does not appear to be within the appendix in this slice, because the appendix bends in and out of the plane of this slice. An appendicolith usually appears as a calcified (white) rounded structure, visible without any contrast. **A,** Axial CT image. **B,** Close-up. (From Broder JS: *Diagnostic imaging for the emergency physician,* Philadelphia, 2011, Saunders.)

in younger women when diagnosis is unclear. Normal ultrasonographic findings should not deter surgery if the history and physical examination are indicative of appendicitis.

- MRI of the abdomen and pelvis can also be used to accurately diagnose acute appendicitis in pregnant patients (100% sensitivity, 93.6% specificity) without exposure to ionizing radiation.

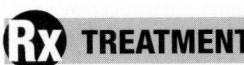
TREATMENT

NONPHARMACOLOGIC THERAPY
- Nothing by mouth
- Do not administer analgesics or antibiotics until the diagnosis is made (may mask signs of peritonitis)

ACUTE GENERAL Rx
- Urgent appendectomy (laparoscopic or open), correction of fluid and electrolyte imbalance with vigorous IV hydration and electrolyte replacement
- IV antibiotic prophylaxis to cover gram-negative bacilli and anaerobes (ampicillin/sulbactam 3 g IV q6h or piperacillin/tazobactam 4.5 g IV q8h in adults)

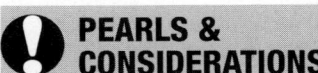
PEARLS & CONSIDERATIONS

COMMENTS
- Perforation is common (20% in adult patients). Indicators of perforation are pain lasting >24 hr, leukocytosis >20,000/mm^3, temperature >102° F, palpable abdominal mass, and peritoneal findings.
- In general, prognosis is excellent. Mortality rate is <1% in young adults without complications; however, it exceeds 10% in elderly patients with ruptured appendix.
- In approximately 20% of patients who undergo exploratory laparotomy because of suspected appendicitis, the appendix is normal.
- Trials comparing antibiotic treatment with emergency appendectomy have shown that amoxicillin plus clavulanic acid is not inferior to emergency appendectomy for acute appendicitis. Researchers have shown that over 60% of patients with uncomplicated appendicitis assigned to the antibiotic group do not need appendectomy. However, the need to remove the appendix in patients with acute appendicitis is so entrenched in the minds of physicians that nonsurgical options are only rarely considered.

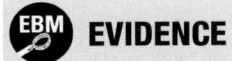
EVIDENCE

available at www.expertconsult.com

SUGGESTED READINGS
available at www.expertconsult.com

RELATED CONTENT
Appendicitis (Patient Information)

AUTHOR: **FRED F. FERRI, M.D.**

BASIC INFORMATION

DEFINITION

Arrhythmogenic right ventricular dysplasia (ARVD) is a disorder characterized by replacement of the normal myocardium by fibrofatty tissue, RV myocyte loss, and RV wall thinning, and represents a kind of cardiomyopathy. It is defined clinically by life-threatening ventricular arrhythmias in otherwise healthy young people.

SYNONYMS

Arrhythmogenic right ventricular cardiomyopathy

ICD-9CM CODES
427.1 Paroxysmal ventricular tachycardia
425.4 Other primary cardiomyopathies
427.89 Other specified cardiac dysrhythmias

ICD-10CM CODES
I47.2 Paroxysmal ventricular tachycardia
I42.8 Other cardiomyopathies
I49.8 Other specified cardiac arrhythmias

EPIDEMIOLOGY & DEMOGRAPHICS

INCIDENCE: ARVD comprises 2% of sudden cardiac arrest cases.
PREVALENCE: 1:5000 persons
PREDOMINANT SEX AND AGE: Men <35 yr old
RISK FACTORS: Family history of ARVD
GENETICS:
- Autosomal dominant with variable penetrance, and polymorphic phenotypic expression
- Desmosomal dysfunction
- 11 subtypes of ARVD are identified based on the involved genes.

PHYSICAL FINDINGS & CLINICAL PRESENTATION

- Suspect when young males present with syncope, sudden cardiac arrest, ventricular tachycardia, premature ventricular beats originating from the right ventricle, or, less commonly, signs and symptoms of right heart failure. Symptoms vary and range from palpitations, dizziness, and syncope to atypical chest pain, dyspnea, and fatigue.
- Cardiac arrest after physical exertion may be the initial presentation.
- Physical examination will be normal in most patients. Widely split S2 is an important diagnostic clue.

ETIOLOGY

ARVD is characterized by progressive replacement of the right ventricular myocardium with fibrofatty tissue

DX DIAGNOSIS

- Diagnosis is made when two major criteria, one major and two minor, or four minor criteria are met.
- See Table 1-43 for diagnostic criteria.

DIFFERENTIAL DIAGNOSIS

- Cardiomyopathy with involvement of the right ventricle
- Uhl's anomaly: rare anomaly that presents mainly in childhood with signs and symptoms and right heart failure. Uhl's anomaly is characterized by a paper thin right ventricle resulting from death of the myocytes throughout the right ventricle
- Idiopathic RV tachycardia
- Left dominant arrhythmogenic cardiomyopathy

WORKUP

- Resting ECG will have diagnostic findings in 50% to 90% of patients with ARVD. These changes include T-wave inversions in anterior precordial leads V_1-V_6, epsilon waves (Fig. 1-109A), and *ventricular tachycardia* (VT) with left bundle branch block pattern.
- Endomyocardial biopsy is the preferred method for diagnosis of ARVD. It has specificity of 92%, but it lacks sensitivity (<20%).
- Electrophysiologic study is important to identify delayed potentials that can lead to tachycardiac events.

TABLE 1-43 Criteria for the Diagnosis of Arrhythmogenic Right Ventricular Dysplasia

Global and/or Regional Dysfunction and Structural Alterations

Major

Severe dilation and reduction of right ventricular ejection fraction with no (or only mild) left ventricular impairment
Localized right ventricular aneurysms
Severe segmental dilation of the right ventricle

Minor

Mild global right ventricular dilation and/or ejection fraction with a normal left ventricle
Mild segmental dilation of the right ventricle
Regional right ventricular hypokinesis

Tissue Characterization of the Walls

Major

Fibrofatty replacement of myocardium on endomyocardial biopsy

ECG Repolarization Abnormalities

Minor

Inverted T waves in the right precordial leads (V_2 and V_3) in patients older than 12 yr and in the absence of right bundle branch block

ECG Depolarization/Conduction Abnormalities

Major

Epsilon waves or localized prolongation (greater than 110 ms) of the QRS complex in right precordial leads (V_1 through V_3)

Minor

Late potentials visible on signal-averaged ECG

Arrhythmias

Minor

Sustained or nonsustained left bundle branch block type VT documented on ECG, Holter monitoring, or during exercise stress testing
Frequent ventricular extrasystoles (more than 1000 per 24 hr on Holter monitoring)

Family History

Major

Familial disease confirmed at autopsy or surgery

Minor

Family history of premature sudden death (younger than 35 yr) caused by suspected ARVD/C
Family history (clinical diagnosis based on present criteria)

The diagnosis of arrhythmogenic right ventricular dysplasia is made if one of the following is met: two major criteria, one major and two minor criteria, or four minor criteria.
ARVD/C, Arrhythmogenic right ventricular dysplasia/cardiomyopathy; *ECG*, electrocardiography; *VT*, ventricular tachycardia.
From Anderson EL: Arrhythmogenic right ventricular dysplasia, *Am Fam Physician* 73[8]:1391-1398, 2006.

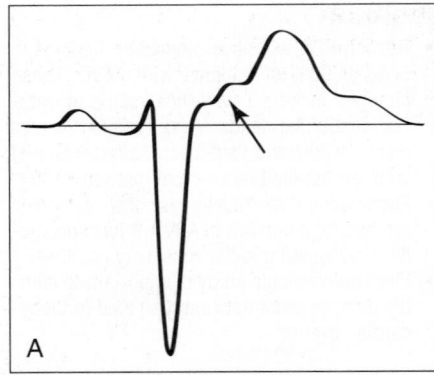

FIGURE 1-109A Epsilon waves are small deflection just beyond the QRS complex. Best visualized in leads V_1-V_3. Any potential in leads V_1-V_3 that exceeds the QRS in leads V6 by more than 25 millisecond should be considered epsilon wave. (From Anderson EL: Arrhythmogenic right ventricular dysplasia, *Am Fam Physician* 73(8):1391-1398, 2006.)

- Routine immunohistochemical analysis of a conventional endomyocardial-biopsy sample appears to be a highly sensitive and specific diagnostic test for arrhythmogenic right ventricular cardiomyopathy.

IMAGING STUDIES
- MRI is a noninvasive method to detect structural changes and regional dysfunction. Cardiac MRI (CMR) is the most sensitive method to detect ARVD, but has high false-positive rates. Cardiac CT angiogram (Fig. 1-109B) will reveal thinning and aneurysmal dilation of the RV anterior wall and outflow tract.
- Echocardiography will show right ventricular dilation with regional wall motion abnormalities that varied with the severity of the disease.
- Other imaging modalities used for evaluation of suspected ARVD include signal averaged ECG, Holter monitor, stress test, and radionuclide ventriculography

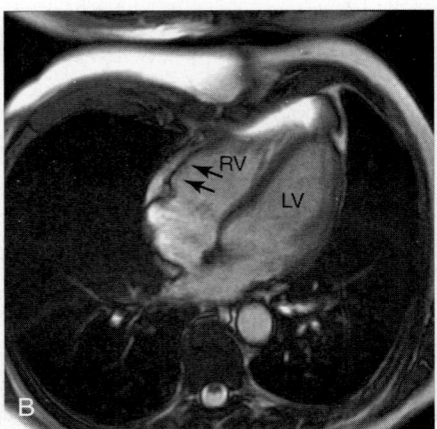
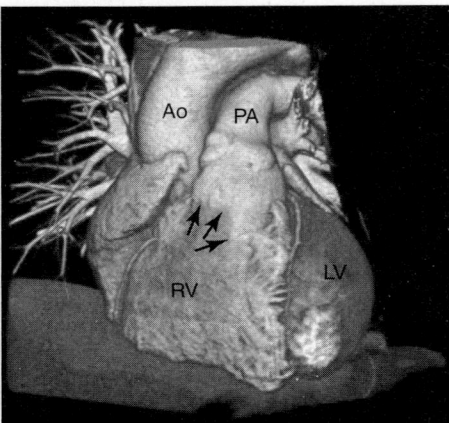
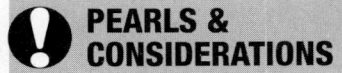

FIGURE 1-109B Right ventricular aneurysm. This cardiac computed tomography angiogram shows thinning and aneurysmal dilation of the RV anterior wall and outflow tract *(arrows)* in a patient with arrhythmogenic right ventricular dysplasia, cardiomyopathy, and ventricular tachycardia. *Ao,* Aorta; *LV,* left ventricle; *PA,* pulmonary artery. (Courtesy of Dr. Nasar Nallamothu, Prairie Cardiovascular Consultants, Springfield, Ill. From Issa Z et al: *Clinical arrhythmology and electrophysiology,* ed 2, Philadelphia, 2012, Saunders.)

Rx TREATMENT

No definitive therapy is available. Treatment goal is to prevent sudden cardiac death.

NONPHARMACOLOGIC THERAPY
- Avoidance of activity that may trigger tachycardia
- Right ventriculotomy
- Cardiac transplantation

ACUTE GENERAL Rx
Intravenous amiodarone has been proved to be effective in terminating VT.

CHRONIC Rx
- Antiarrhythmic therapy with sotalol, amiodarone, propafenone, beta-blocker alone or in combination can be used
- Radiofrequency ablation is used in cases of refractory VT, frequent tachycardia after defibrillator placement, or localized arrhythmia sites
- Implantable cardioverted defibrillators hold promise

REFERRAL
- Early cardiology and electrophysiology referral
- Consider referring for genetic counseling

PEARLS & CONSIDERATIONS

PREVENTION
Test first-degree relatives if there is a positive history of sudden cardiac death or death at an early age.

EDUCATION
Patient handout can be found in *American Family Physician* (American Academy of Family Physicians: Information from your family doctor. Arrhythmogenic right ventricular dysplasia: what you should know. *Am Fam Physician* 73(8):1401, 2006).

SUGGESTED READINGS
available at www.expertconsult.com

AUTHORS: **ABDULRAHMAN ABDULBAKI, M.D.,** and **NADIA MUJAHID, M.D.**

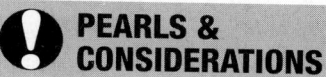

BASIC INFORMATION

DEFINITION

Asbestosis is a slowly progressive diffuse interstitial fibrosis resulting from dose-related inhalation exposure to fibers of asbestos.

ICD-9CM CODES
501 Asbestosis

EPIDEMIOLOGY & DEMOGRAPHICS

- Five to 10 new cases per 100,000 persons per year in U.S.
- Prolonged interval (20 to 30 yr) between exposures to inhaled fibers and clinical manifestations of disease
- Most common in workers involved in the primary extraction of asbestos from rock deposits and in those involved in the fabrication and installation of products containing asbestos (e.g., naval shipyards in World War II; installation of floor tiles, ceiling tiles, acoustic ceiling coverings, wall insulation, and pipe coverings in public buildings)

PHYSICAL FINDINGS & CLINICAL PRESENTATION

- Insidious onset of shortness of breath with exertion is usually the first sign of asbestosis.
- Dyspnea becomes more severe as the disease advances; with time, progressively less exertion is tolerated.
- Cough is frequent and usually paroxysmal, dry, and nonproductive.
- Scant mucoid sputum may accompany the cough in the later stages of the disease.
- Fine end-respiratory crackles (rales, crepitations) are heard more predominantly in the lung bases.
- Digital clubbing, edema, jugular venous distention are present.

ETIOLOGY

Inhalation of asbestos fibers

DIAGNOSIS

DIFFERENTIAL DIAGNOSIS

- Silicosis
- Siderosis, other pneumonoconioses
- Lung cancer
- Atelectasis

WORKUP

Documentation of exposure history, diagnostic imaging, pulmonary function testing

LABORATORY TESTS

- Generally not helpful
- Possible mild elevation of erythrocyte sedimentation rate (ESR), positive antinuclear antibody (ANA) and rheumatoid factor (RF) (these tests are nonspecific and do not correlate with disease severity or activity)
- Pulmonary function testing: decreased vital capacity, decreased total lung capacity, decreased carbon monoxide gas transfer
- Arterial blood gases: hypoxemia, hypercarbia in advanced stages

IMAGING STUDIES

Chest radiograph (Fig. 1-110):
- Small, irregular shadows in lower lung zones.
- Thickened pleura, calcified plaques (present under diaphragm and lateral chest wall).
- CT scan of chest confirms diagnosis. Typical findings on high-resolution CT of the chest include increased interstitial markings found mainly at the bases. As the disease progresses, honeycombing is noted.

TREATMENT

NONPHARMACOLOGIC THERAPY

- Smoking cessation, proper nutrition, exercise program to maximize available lung function
- Home oxygen therapy prn
- Removal of patient from further asbestos fiber exposure

GENERAL Rx

- Prompt identification and treatment of respiratory infections
- Supplemental oxygen on a prn basis

- Annual influenza vaccination, pneumococcal vaccination

DISPOSITION

- There is no specific treatment for asbestosis.
- Death is usually from respiratory failure from cor pulmonale.
- Patients with asbestosis have increased risk for mesotheliomas, lung cancer, and tuberculosis. Recent reports indicate that the risk of asbestos-induced lung cancer may be overestimated.
- Survival in patients after development of mesothelioma is 4 to 6 yr.

REFERRAL

To pulmonologist initially

PEARLS & CONSIDERATIONS

COMMENTS

Patient information on asbestosis can be obtained from the American Lung Association, 1740 Broadway, New York, NY 10019.

SUGGESTED READINGS

available at www.expertconsult.com

RELATED CONTENT

Asbestosis (Patient Information)

AUTHOR: **FRED F. FERRI, M.D.**

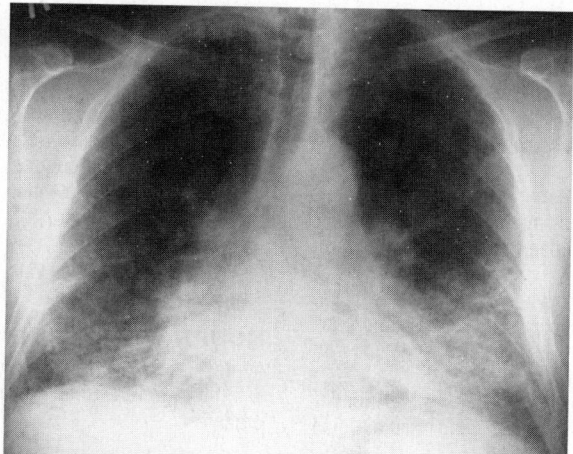

FIGURE 1-110 Asbestosis. Posteroanterior radiograph shows coarse linear opacities at both lung bases obscuring the cardiac borders. (From McLoud TC: *Thoracic radiology: the requisites,* St Louis, 1998, Mosby.)

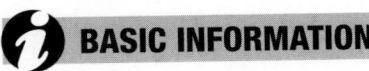

DEFINITION

Ascariasis is a parasitic infection caused by the nematode *Ascaris lumbricoides*. The majority of those infected are asymptomatic; however, clinical disease may arise from pulmonary hypersensitivity, intestinal obstruction, and secondary complications.

SYNONYMS

Round worms
Worms

ICD-9CM CODES
127.0 Ascariasis

EPIDEMIOLOGY & DEMOGRAPHICS

INCIDENCE (IN U.S.):
- Unknown
- Three times the infection rates found in blacks as in whites

PEAK INCIDENCE: Unknown

PREVALENCE (IN U.S.): Estimated at 4 million, the majority of which live in the rural southeastern part of the country; ascariasis is associated with poor sanitation

PREDOMINANT SEX: Both sexes probably equally affected, with a possible slight female preponderance

PREDOMINANT AGE: Most common in children from ages 2 to 10 years old and decreases after age 15; infections tend to cluster in families

NEONATAL INFECTION: Probable transmission, though not specifically studied

PHYSICAL FINDINGS & CLINICAL PRESENTATION

- Occurs approximately 9 to 12 days after ingestion of eggs (corresponding to the larva migration through the lungs)
- Nonproductive cough
- Substernal chest discomfort
- Fever
- In patients with large worm burdens, especially children, intestinal obstruction associated with perforation, volvulus, and intussusception
- Migration of worms into the biliary tree giving clinical appearance of biliary colic and pancreatitis as well as acute appendicitis with movement into that appendage
- Rarely, infection with *A. lumbricoides* producing interstitial nephritis and acute renal failure
- In endemic areas in Asia and Africa, malabsorption of dietary proteins and vitamins as a consequence of chronic worm intestinal carriage; 1 billion people worldwide are infected with this nematode

ETIOLOGY

- Transmission is usually hand to mouth, but eggs may be ingested via transported vegetables grown in contaminated soil.
- Eggs are hatched in the small intestine, with larvae penetrating intestinal mucosa and migrating via the circulation to the lungs.
- Larval forms proceed through the alveoli, ascend the bronchial tree, and return to the intestines after swallowing, where they mature into adult worms.
- Estimated time until the female adult worm begins producing eggs is 2 to 3 mo.
- Eggs are passed out of the intestines with feces and can survive for years in warm, moist, shaded soil.
- Within human host, adult worm lifespan is 1 to 2 yr.

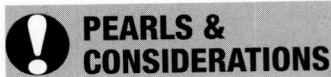 DIAGNOSIS

DIFFERENTIAL DIAGNOSIS

Radiologic manifestations and eosinophilia to be distinguished from drug hypersensitivity and Löffler's syndrome

LABORATORY TESTS

- Examination of the stool for *Ascaris* ova
- Expectoration or fecal passage of adult worm
- Adult male worms: 10 to 30 cm long; adult female worms: larger than male, up to 40 cm
- Eosinophilia: most prominent early in the infection and subsides as the adult worm infestation established in the intestines; usually in 5% to 12% range but can be up to 50%
- Serology: patients develop IgG antibodies, but they cross react with antigens from other helminths and are not protective; thus serology is used more for epidemiologic purposes than for individual diagnosis

IMAGING STUDIES

- Chest x-ray examination to reveal bilateral oval or round infiltrates of varying size (Löffler's syndrome); NOTE: infiltrates are transient and eventually resolve.
- Plain films of the abdomen and contrast studies to reveal worm masses in loops of bowel.
- Ultrasonography and endoscopic retrograde cholangiopancreatography (ERCP) to identify worms in the pancreaticobiliary tract.
- CT scan with oral contrast (Fig. E1-111) can also assist in the detection of GI foreign bodies such as parasites.

Rx TREATMENT

NONPHARMACOLOGIC THERAPY

Aggressive IV hydration, especially in children with fever, severe vomiting, and resultant dehydration

ACUTE GENERAL Rx

- All infected patients, including asymptomatic ones, should be treated
  1. Albendazole: 400 mg PO × 3 days is the first-line agent for intestinal infection with *A. lumbricoides*
  2. Mebendazole 100 mg daily × 3 days
- Cure rate with these agents is 95% to 100%, but they are contraindicated in pregnancy.
- Side effects: GI discomfort, headache, and rarely leukopenia

- Alternative agent or for use in pregnancy: pyrantel pamoate (Antiminth)
  1. Given at a dose of 11 mg/kg PO (maximum dose of 1 g/day)
  2. Considered safe for use in pregnant women
- Other alternative agents:
  1. Ivermectin: 150 to 200 mcg/kg orally once
  2. Nitazoxanide: cure rates in heavy worm burden are only 50% to 80%
  3. Piperazine citrate: no longer first-line agent due to toxicity but still used in cases of intestinal or biliary obstruction, as drug paralyzes the worm, helping its expulsion. Dose: 50 to 75 mg/kg once daily up to maximum of 3.5 g for 2 days.
  4. Levamisole: 2.5 mg/kg once orally is recommended by the WHO as alternative therapy, but not available in the U.S.
- Complete obstruction should be managed surgically

DISPOSITION

Overall prognosis is good. Patients should be reevaluated in 2 to 3 months. Reinfection is common.

REFERRAL

- To gastroenterologist in cases of visualized pancreaticobiliary tract or appendiceal obstruction
- To surgeon in cases of complete obstruction or suspected secondary complication (e.g., perforation or volvulus)

! PEARLS & CONSIDERATIONS

COMMENTS

- Hepatic abscess, containing both viable and dead worms, complicating *Ascaris*-induced biliary duct disease has been documented.
- Given the known transmission of the parasite, routine hand washing with soap and proper disposal of human waste would significantly decrease the prevalence of this disease.
- Other protective measures to avoid ingestion of worm eggs:
  1. Peel or cook food.
  2. Boil drinking water.
  3. Do not place small children directly on soil.

SUGGESTED READINGS
available at www.expertconsult.com

RELATED CONTENT

Ascariasis (Patient Information)

AUTHOR: **GLENN G. FORT, M.D., M.P.H.**

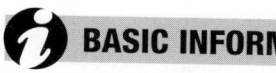

BASIC INFORMATION

DEFINITION

Ascites is the accumulation of excess fluid in the peritoneal cavity, most commonly caused by liver cirrhosis.

SYNONYMS

Fluid in peritoneal cavity
Hydroperitoneum
Hydroperitonia
Hydrops abdominis

ICD-9CM CODES
789.5   Ascites
568.82 Peritoneal effusion (chronic)

EPIDEMIOLOGY & DEMOGRAPHICS

Ascites is the most common complication of cirrhosis. Ascites occurs in 50% of individuals with cirrhosis within 10 yr of diagnosis. Cirrhosis is the cause of 75% of cases of ascites. Other causes include malignancy, heart failure, tuberculosis, pancreatitis, nephrotic syndrome, and Budd-Chiari syndrome.

CLINICAL PRESENTATION

- Important information to elicit within history:
  - Viral hepatitis
  - Alcoholism
  - Increasing abdominal girth
  - Increasing lower extremity edema
  - Intravenous drug use
  - Sexual history (i.e., men who have sex with men)
  - History of transfusions

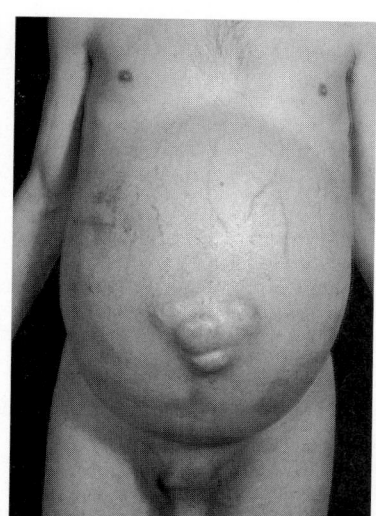

FIGURE 1-112 Ascites in a patient with alcoholic cirrhosis showing distended abdomen; dilated superficial collateral veins; hemorrhagic scratch marks due to pruritus and coagulopathy; umbilical varices; and plaster in left iliac fossa indicating diagnostic paracentesis. (From Forbes A et al [eds]: *Atlas of clinical gastroenterology*, ed 3, Oxford, 2005, Mosby.)

- Important physical exam findings:
  - Bulging flanks
  - Flank dullness to percussion
  - Fluid wave on abdominal exam
  - Lower extremity edema
  - Shifting dullness on abdominal exam
  - Physical signs associated with liver cirrhosis: spider angiomas, jaundice, loss of body hair, Dupuytren's contracture, muscle wasting, bruising, palmar erythema, gynecomastia, testicular atrophy, hemorrhoids, and caput medusae (Fig. 1-112)

ETIOLOGY

Pathophysiology of ascites (Fig. E1-113): increased hepatic resistance to portal flow leads to portal hypertension. The splanchnic vessels respond by increased secretion of nitric oxide, causing splanchnic artery vasodilation. Early in the disease increased plasma volume and increased cardiac output compensate for this vasodilation. However, as disease progresses the effective arterial blood volume decreases, causing sodium and fluid retention through activation of the renin-angiotensin system. The change in capillary pressure causes increased permeability and retention of fluid in the abdomen.

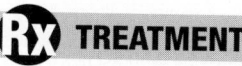

DIAGNOSIS

DIFFERENTIAL DIAGNOSIS

- Chronic parenchymal liver disease, leading to portal hypertension
- Peritoneal carcinomatosis
- Congestive heart failure
- Peritoneal tuberculosis
- Nephrotic syndrome
- Pancreatitis

LABORATORY TESTS

- Initial evaluation should always include:
  - Diagnostic paracentesis (Fig. E1-114). Laboratory tests on this fluid should include a CBC with differential, albumin, total protein, culture and Gram stain. A serum-ascites albumin gradient (SAAG) should be calculated in all patients. If the SAAG is greater than 1.1, the cause of ascites can be attributed to portal hypertension. If SAAG is less than 1.1, a nonportal hypertension etiology of ascites must be sought (see Table 1-44). Optional tests

on paracentesis fluid include amylase, LDH, acid-fast bacilli, and glucose levels.
  - AST, ALT, total and direct bilirubin, albumin, alkaline phosphatase, GGTP
  - CBC, coagulation studies
  - Electrolytes, BUN, creatinine

IMAGING STUDIES

- Abdominal ultrasound (Fig. 1-115) is the most sensitive measure for detecting ascitic fluid; a CT or MRI scan is a viable alternative.
- Endoscopy of the upper GI tract to evaluate for esophageal varices if ascites is secondary to portal hypertension.

TREATMENT

NONPHARMACOLOGIC THERAPY

- Sodium-restricted diet (<2 g/day).
- Fluid restriction to 1 L/day in patients with hyponatremia (sodium <130 mEq/L).

ACUTE GENERAL Rx

- Patients with moderate-volume ascites causing only moderate discomfort may be treated on an outpatient basis with the following diuretic regimen: spironolactone 50 to 200 mg qd or amiloride 5 to 10 mg qd. Add furosemide 20 to 40 mg/day in the first several days of treatment, monitoring renal functions carefully for signs of prerenal azotemia (in patients without edema, goal weight loss is 300 to 500 g/day; in patients with edema it is 800 to 1000 g/day).
- Patients with large-volume ascites causing marked discomfort or decrease in activities of daily living may also be treated as outpatients if there are no complications. There are two options for treatment in these patients: (1) large-volume paracentesis or (2) diuretic therapy until loss of fluid is noted (maximum spironolactone 400 mg qd and furosemide 160 mg qd). No difference in long-term mortality rate was found; however, paracentesis is faster, more effective, and associated with fewer adverse effects.
- Table 1-45 summarizes primary medical therapy and adjunctive medications used to increase the efficacy of primary therapy in the treatment of ascites.

TABLE 1-44 Using the Serum-Ascites Albumin Gradient and the Ascites Total Protein Level to Diagnose the Cause of Ascites

Condition	Serum-Ascites Albumin Gradient*	Ascites Total Protein Level†
Cirrhosis	High	Low
Malignant ascites	Low	High
Cardiac ascites	High	High

*High is greater than 1.1 g/dL; low is less than 1.1 g/dL.
†High is greater than 2.5 g/dL; low is less than 2.5 g/dL.
From Goldman L, Schafer AI: *Goldman's Cecil medicine*, ed 24, Philadelphia, 2012, Saunders.

CHRONIC Rx

5% to 10% of patients with large-volume ascites will be refractory to high-dose diuretic treatment. Treatment strategies include repeated large-volume paracentesis with infusion of albumin every 2 to 4 wk or placement of a transjugular intrahepatic portosystemic shunt (TIPS). A treatment approach to patients with malignant ascites is decribed in Fig. E1-116.

DISPOSITION

Monitor closely for worsening liver function, development of spontaneous bacterial peritonitis (SBP).

REFERRAL

Referral to gastroenterology with ascites

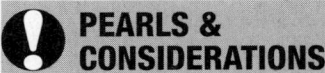

PEARLS & CONSIDERATIONS

COMMENTS

Prevalence of SBP in patients with ascites ranges between 10% and 30%. Presence of at least 250 neutrophils per cubic millimeter of ascitic fluid is diagnostic. Gram negatives such as *E. coli* are the most common isolates. Third-generation cephalosporins are the treatment of choice. By 1 year, 70% of patients have recurrence of SBP and may be prophylaxed with trimethoprim/sulfamethoxazole DS 1 tab PO bid 5 days/wk or ciprofloxacin 750 mg PO once/wk.

PREVENTION

Prevention of liver cirrhosis through avoidance of long-term use of alcohol, immunization against hepatitis A and B, and treatment of hepatitis C

SUGGESTED READINGS

available at www.expertconsult.com

RELATED CONTENT

Ascites (Patient Information)

AUTHORS: **JOANNE M. SILVIA, M.D.,** and **PAUL F. GEORGE, M.D.**

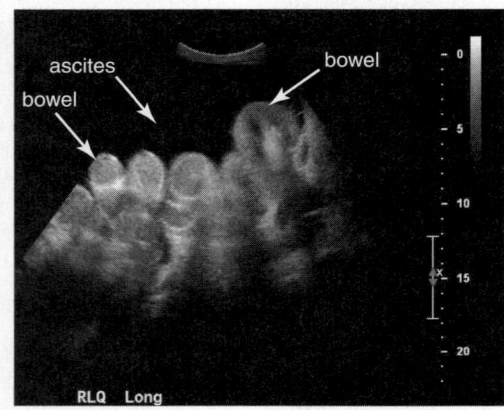

FIGURE 1-115 Ascites, ultrasound. Ultrasound is useful for detection of ascites. Simple fluids such as ascites are excellent sound transmission media, reflecting almost no sound waves. As a consequence, they appear quite hypoechoic *(black)* on ultrasound. This view of the right lower quadrant shows loops of bowel surrounded by fluid. During the ultrasound, the bowel loops would be seen to undergo peristalsis and drift back and forth in the ascitic fluid with patient movement. Ultrasound cannot distinguish the composition of the fluid; ascites, liquid blood, liquid bile, urine, and infectious fluids have a similar appearance, with a few exceptions. Blood may coagulate and form septations within the fluid collection. Infectious fluids also frequently form loculated fluid collections that may be recognized on ultrasound, although the exact composition cannot be determined. (From Broder JS: *Diagnostic imaging for the emergency physician,* Philadelphia, 2011, Saunders.)

TABLE 1-45 Primary Medical Therapy and Adjunctive Medications Used to Increase the Efficacy of Primary Therapy in the Treatment of Ascites

Class	Medication	Dosing	Relevant Action	Notes
Diuretics	Spironolactone	400 mg + qd*	Aldosterone receptor antagonist	Primary therapy
	Furosemide	160 mg + qd*	Inhibits Na-K-2Cl symporter	Primary therapy
	Mannitol	20%*	Osmotic diuresis	Give dose just prior to furosemide and spironolactone
Vasoconstrictors	Octreotide	300 mcg bid*	Splanchnic vasoconstriction, inhibits RAAS	Also used in combination with midodrine to treat hepatorenal syndrome; given for first 5 days following variceal bleeding to decrease recurrence
	Midodrine	7.5 mg tid*	Inhibits RAAS	Also used in combination with octreotide and albumin to treat hepatorenal syndrome
α2-Agonist	Clonidine	0.075 mg bid*	Inhibits sympathetic outflow, inhibits RAAS	Increases sensitivity to spironolactone
Colloid	Albumin	25 g*	Increased oncotic pressure	Also utilized with LVP and in the treatment of hepatorenal syndrome
Aquaretics	None are FDA approved	?	Vasopressin receptor antagonist	May also treat hyponatremia

*The above doses have been derived from various studies and may not be suitable for all patients. Titration is always recommended.
From Cameron JL, Cameron AM: *Current surgical therapy,* ed 10, Philadelphia, 2011, Saunders.

BASIC INFORMATION

DEFINITION

Aspergillosis refers to several forms of a broad range of illnesses caused by infection with *Aspergillus* species.

ICD-9CM CODES
117.3 Aspergillosis
117.3 Aspergillosis with pneumonia
117.3 *Aspergillus* infection *(A. flavus, fumigatus, terreus)*

EPIDEMIOLOGY & DEMOGRAPHICS

INCIDENCE & PREVALENCE:
- *Aspergillus* species are ubiquitous in the environment internationally and occur as a mold found in soil.
- Cause a variety of illness from hypersensitivity pneumonitis to disseminated overwhelming infection in immunosuppressed patients.
- Frequently cultured from hospital wards from unfiltered outside air circulating through open windows as well as water sources.
- Reach the patient by airborne conidia (spores) that are small enough (2.5 to 3 μm) to reach the alveoli on inhalation.
- Can invade the nose, paranasal sinuses, external ear, or traumatized skin.

RISK FACTORS:
- The clinical syndrome depends on the underlying lung architecture, the host's immune response, and the degree of inoculum.
- Incidence of invasive aspergillosis is increasing with advances in the treatment of life-threatening diseases, such as aggressive chemotherapy or bone marrow and organ transplantation. It also can rarely occur in normal hosts, especially associated with influenza A. Liver and lung transplant recipients are at highest risk for pulmonary disease.
- Patients with AIDS and a CD4 count <50/mm³ have an increased susceptibility to invasive aspergillosis.
- Pandemic influenza A (H1N1) infection may predispose immunocompromised patients to invasive aspergillosis.

ETIOLOGY
- *A. fumigatus* is the usual cause.
- *A. flavus* is the second most important species, particularly in invasive disease of immunosuppressed patients and in lesions beginning in the nose and paranasal sinuses. *A. niger* can also cause invasive human infection.

ALLERGIC ASPERGILLOSIS
- Is a hypersensitivity pneumonitis.
- Presents as cough, dyspnea, fever, chills, and malaise typically 4 to 8 hr after exposure.
- Repeated attacks can lead to granulomatous disease and pulmonary fibrosis.

ALLERGIC BRONCHOPULMONARY ASPERGILLOSIS (ABPA):
- Symptoms occur most commonly in atopic individuals during the third and fourth decades of life.

- Hypersensitivity reaction to *Aspergillus* fungal antigens present in the bronchial tree.
- Results from an initial type I (immediate hypersensitivity) and type III reactions (immune complexes).
- Underdiagnosed pulmonary disorder in patients with asthma and cystic fibrosis (reported prevalence in asthmatic patients varies from 6% to 28% and in cystic fibrosis 6% to 25%).

ASPERGILLOMAS ("FUNGUS BALLS"):
- In the absence of invasion or significant immune response, *Aspergillus* can colonize a preexisting cavity, causing pulmonary aspergilloma.
- Forms masses of tangled hyphal elements, fibrin, and mucus.
- Patients typically have a history of chronic lung disease, tuberculosis, sarcoidosis, or emphysema.
- Manifests commonly as hemoptysis.
- Many are asymptomatic.

INVASIVE ASPERGILLOSIS:
- Patients with prolonged and profound granulocytopenia or impaired phagocytic function are predisposed to rapidly progressive *Aspergillus* pneumonia.
- Typically a necrotizing bronchopneumonia, ranging from small areas of infiltrate to intensive bilateral hemorrhagic infarction.
- Most common presentation: unremitting fever and a new pulmonary infiltrate despite broad-spectrum antibiotic therapy in an immunosuppressed patient.
- Dyspnea and nonproductive cough are common; sudden pleuritic pain and tachycardia, sometimes with a pleural rub, may mimic pulmonary embolism; hemoptysis is uncommon.
- Chest radiograph (CXR) may reveal patchy bronchopneumonic, nodular densities, consolidation, or cavitation. High-resolution CT scan is more sensitive and specific than CXR in neutropenic patients.
- Immunocompromised patients: invasive pulmonary *Aspergillus* (IPA) generally is acute and evolves over days to weeks; less commonly, patients with normal or only mild abnormalities of the immune system may develop a more chronic, slowly progressive form of IPA.

EXTRAPULMONARY DISSEMINATION:
- Cerebral infarction from hematogenous dissemination may occur in immunosuppressed individuals.
- Abscess formation from direct extension or invasive disease in the sinuses.
- Esophageal or gastrointestinal ulcerations may occur in the immunosuppressed host.
- Fatal perforation of the viscus or bowel infarction may occur.
- Necrotizing skin ulcers involving the extremities (Fig. 1-117).
- Osteomyelitis.
- Endocarditis in patients who have recently undergone open heart surgery.
- Infection of an implantable cardioverter-defibrillator has been reported.

DIAGNOSIS

DIFFERENTIAL DIAGNOSIS
- Tuberculosis
- Cystic fibrosis
- Carcinoma of the lung
- Eosinophilic pneumonia
- Bronchiectasis
- Sarcoidosis
- Lung abscess

WORKUP
Physical examination and laboratory data

LABORATORY TESTS
ABPA:
- Peripheral blood eosinophilia and an elevated total serum immunoglobulin E (IgE) level.
- Skin test with *Aspergillus* antigenic extract is usually positive but nonspecific.
- *Aspergillus* serum precipitating antibody is present in 70% to 100% of cases.
- Sputum cultures may be positive for *Aspergillus* spp. but are nonspecific.

ASPERGILLOMAS:
- Sputum culture
- Serum precipitating antibody

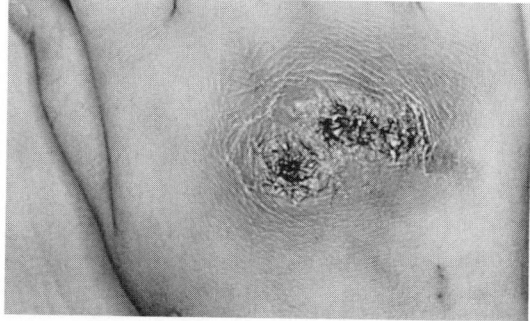

FIGURE 1-117 Cutaneous aspergillosis in a patient with acute leukemia and marked neutropenia. The lesion developed at the site where a steel needle had been left for several days of intravenous infusion. (From Mandell GL [ed]: *Mandell, Douglas, and Bennett's principles and practice of infectious diseases,* ed 6, New York, 2005, Churchill Livingstone.)

Invasive aspergillosis: definitive diagnosis requires the demonstration of tissue invasion (i.e., septate, acute angle branching hyphae) or a positive culture from the tissue obtained by an invasive procedure such as transbronchial biopsy.

- Sputum and nasal cultures: in high-risk patients a positive culture is strongly suggestive of invasive aspergillosis.
- Serology: the *Platelia Aspergillus* ELISA assay detects a circulating fungal antigen, galactomannan, and is used in some centers in neutropenic patients and for those undergoing stem cell transplantation.
- Blood cultures: usually negative.
- Lung biopsy is necessary for definitive diagnosis.
- Biopsy and culture of extrapulmonary lesions.
- Real-time polymerase chain reaction tests are investigational.

IMAGING STUDIES

ABPA:

- CXRs show a variety of abnormalities, from small, patchy, fleeting infiltrates (commonly in the upper lobes) to lobar consolidation or cavitation.
- A majority of patients eventually develop central bronchiectasis.

ASPERGILLOMAS: CXR or CT scans usually show the characteristic intracavity mass partially surrounded by a crescent of air (Fig. 1-118).

INVASIVE ASPERGILLOSIS: CXR and CT scanning may reveal cavity formation.

Ⓡ🆇 TREATMENT

ACUTE GENERAL Rx

ABPA:

- Prednisone (0.5 to 1 mg/kg PO) until the CXR has cleared, followed by alternate-day therapy at 0.5 mg/kg PO (3 to 6 mo).
- If a patient is corticosteroid dependent, prophylaxis for the prevention of *Pneumocystis jiroveci* infection and maintenance of bone mineralization should be considered.

- Bronchodilators and physiotherapy.
- Serial CXR and serum IgE useful in guiding treatment.
- Itraconazole 200 mg PO bid for 4 to 6 mo, then taper over 4 to 6 mo may be considered as a steroid-sparing agent or if steroids are ineffective.

ASPERGILLOMAS:

- Controversial and problematic; the optimal treatment strategy is unknown.
- Up to 10% of aspergillomas may resolve clinically without overt pharmacologic or surgical intervention.
- Observation for asymptomatic patients.
- Surgical resection/arterial embolization for those patients with severe hemoptysis or life-threatening hemorrhage.
- For those patients at risk for marked hemoptysis with inadequate pulmonary reserve, consider itraconazole 200 to 400 mg/day PO.

INVASIVE ASPERGILLOSIS:

- The guidelines of the Infectious Diseases Society of America recommend the use of voriconazole as the primary therapy for invasive aspergillosis. Voriconazole dose is 6 mg/kg IV bid followed by 4 mg/kg IV q12h or 200 mg PO q12h for body weight >40 kg but 100 mg PO q12h for body weight <40 kg.
- Amphotericin B 0.8 to 1.2 mg/kg IV qd to total dose of 2 to 2.5 g; itraconazole 200 to 400 mg/d PO × 1 yr.
- Amphotericin B lipid complex (ABLC) 5 mg/kg IV qd in those intolerant of or refractory to amphotericin B.
- Amphotericin B colloidal dispersion (ABCD) 3 to 6 mg/kg IV qd; stepwise approach in those who have not responded to amphotericin B.
- Liposomal amphotericin B (L-AMB) 3 to 5 mg/kg IV qd; stepwise approach is indicated as empiric therapy for presumed fungal infection in febrile neutropenic patients who are refractory to or intolerant of amphotericin B.
- Itraconazole 200 mg IV bid × 4 doses followed by 200 mg IV qd or 200 mg tid for 4 days, then 200 mg PO bid—first-line ther-

apy if not taking p450 inducers. Levels may be obtained to ensure compliance and adequate absorption. Approved only for salvage therapy in the United States at this time.

- Posaconazole 200 mg PO tid with food or liquid nutritional supplement to enhance absorption is approved in the European Union, but in the United States is approved only for prophylaxis in leukemic neutropenic patients, those with myelodysplasia, or those who have undergone allogeneic hematopoietic stem cell transplantation; ravuconazole is currently under investigation.
- Caspofungin (Candigas) is the first of a new class of antifungals, the echinocandins, approved for the treatment of invasive aspergillosis in patients who do not respond to or are unable to tolerate other antifungal drugs. Starting dose 70 mg IV over 1 hr on day 1, then 50 mg IV qd thereafter (reduce to 35 mg IV qd in cases with moderate hepatic insufficiency). Can switch to oral voriconazole after 2 to 3 wk if the response is favorable. Micafungin 150 mg IV qd is another alternative.
- Because azoles and echinocandins target different cellular sites, combination therapy may have additive activity against *Aspergillus* species. Although still under investigation, some bone marrow transplant units use caspofungin and voriconazole as the preferred initial treatment, especially in patients receiving high-dose corticosteroids.
- Cytokine therapy may offer future treatment options in conjunction with the currently available antifungals.

REFERRAL

To an infectious diseases specialist

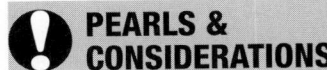

PEARLS & CONSIDERATIONS

- Unlike fluconazole, the potential for drug-drug interactions with voriconazole is high. Azoles may interact with drugs used for chemotherapy by increasing toxicity and/or by reducing efficacy.
- Agitation of hospital buildings by renovations or repairs may increase the incidence of *Aspergillus* infections in immunosuppressed individuals.
- Breakthrough zygomycosis infection may occur with voriconazole treatment.
- *A. terreus* is clinically resistant to amphotericin B.

SUGGESTED READINGS

available at www.expertconsult.com

RELATED CONTENT

Aspergillosis (Patient Information)

AUTHOR: **SAJEEV HANDA, M.D., S.F.H.M.**

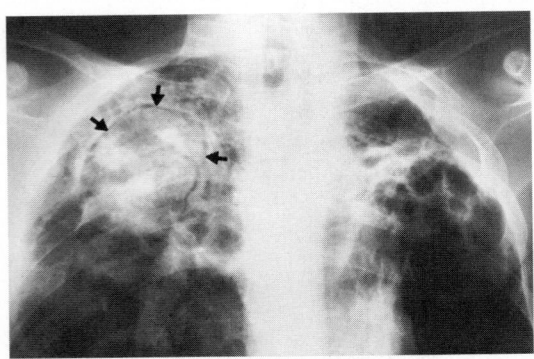

FIGURE 1-118 Fungus ball or mycetoma caused by *Aspergillus*. Coned-down posteroanterior view of the chest of a patient with biapical fibrocavitary tuberculosis accompanied by volume loss. There is a mass in a large right upper-lobe cavity with air dissecting into the cavity producing "air crescents" *(arrows)*. (From McLoud TC: *Thoracic radiology: the requisites*, St Louis, 1998, Mosby.)

BASIC INFORMATION

DEFINITION

The National Asthma Education and Prevention Program (NAEPP) guidelines define asthma as "a chronic inflammatory disease of the airways in which many cells and cellular elements play a role: in particular mast cells, neutrophils, eosinophils, T lymphocytes, macrophages, and epithelial cells. In susceptible individuals, this inflammation causes recurrent episodes of coughing (particularly at night or early in the morning), wheezing, breathlessness, and chest tightness. The episodes are usually associated with widespread but variable airflow obstruction that is reversible either spontaneously or as a result of treatment." *Status asthmaticus* can be defined as a severe continuous bronchospasm.

SYNONYMS

Bronchospasm
Reactive airway disease
Bronchial asthma

ICD-9CM CODES
493.9 Asthma, unspecified
493.1 Intrinsic asthma
493.0 Extrinsic asthma

EPIDEMIOLOGY & DEMOGRAPHICS

- Asthma affects 5% to 12% of the population and accounts for more than 450,000 hospitalizations and nearly 2 million emergency department visits yearly in the U.S.
- It is more common in children (10% of children, 5% of adults).
- 50% to 80% of children with asthma develop symptoms before 5 yr of age. Early childhood risk factors for asthma are described in Table 1-46.
- Overall asthma mortality rate in the U.S. is 20 per 1 million persons.

TABLE 1-46   Early Childhood Risk Factors for Persistent Asthma

Parental asthma
Allergy:
  Atopic dermatitis (eczema)
  Allergic rhinitis
  Food allergy
  Inhalant allergen sensitization
  Food allergen sensitization
Severe lower respiratory tract infection:
  Pneumonia
  Bronchiolitis requiring hospitalization
Wheezing apart from colds
Male gender
Low birthweight
Environmental tobacco smoke exposure
Possible use of acetaminophen (paracetamol)
Exposure to chlorinated swimming pools
Reduced lung function at birth

From Kliegman RM et al: *Nelson textbook of pediatrics,* ed 19, Philadelphia, 2011, Saunders.

- The population of seniors with asthma is increasing rapidly in the U.S. These patients have a high level of morbidity and mortality from their asthma.

PHYSICAL FINDINGS & CLINICAL PRESENTATION

Physical examination varies with the stage and severity of asthma and may reveal only increased inspiratory and expiratory phases of respiration. Physical examination during status asthmaticus may reveal:

- Tachycardia and tachypnea
- Use of accessory respiratory muscles
- Pulsus paradoxus (inspiratory decline in systolic blood pressure >10 mm Hg)
- Wheezing: absence of wheezing (silent chest) or decreased wheezing can indicate worsening obstruction
- Mental status changes: generally secondary to hypoxia and hypercapnia and constitute an indication for urgent intubation
- Paradoxic abdominal and diaphragmatic movement on inspiration (detected by palpation over the upper part of the abdomen in a semirecumbent position): important sign of impending respiratory crisis, indicates diaphragmatic fatigue
- The following abnormalities in vital signs are indicative of severe asthma:
  1. Pulsus paradoxus >18 mm Hg
  2. Respiratory rate >30 breaths/min
  3. Tachycardia with heart rate >120 beats/min

ETIOLOGY

- Symptoms are more commonly due to specific (aeroallergens) or nonspecific (dust, cigarette smoke, fumes, cold air, exercise, etc.) exposures.
- Traditionally, intrinsic asthma was described as occurring in patients who have no history of allergies possibly triggered by upper respiratory infections or psychologic stress and extrinsic asthma (allergic asthma) brought on by exposure to allergens (e.g., dust mites, cat allergen, industrial chemicals).
- Exercise-induced asthma: seen most frequently in adolescents; manifests with bronchospasm after beginning exercise and improves with discontinuation of exercise.
- Drug-induced asthma: often associated with use of NSAIDs, β-blockers, sulfites, and certain foods and beverages.
- There is a strong association of the *ADAM 33* gene with asthma and bronchial hyperresponsiveness.
- Experimental, genetic, and clinical studies support an important role for Th2 immune pathways in the pathogenesis of severe asthma.

DIAGNOSIS

DIFFERENTIAL DIAGNOSIS

- CHF
- COPD
- Pulmonary embolism (in adult and elderly patients)

- Foreign body aspiration (most frequent in younger patients)
- Pneumonia and other upper respiratory infections
- Rhinitis with postnasal drip
- TB
- Hypersensitivity pneumonitis
- Anxiety disorder
- Wegener's granulomatosis
- Diffuse interstitial lung disease

WORKUP

- The clinician should evaluate for environmental causes (e.g., house dust mites, indoor pets) and exposure to other allergens such as tobacco smoke. For symptomatic adults and children aged >5 yr who can perform spirometry, asthma can be diagnosed after a medical history and physical examination documenting an episodic pattern of respiratory symptoms and from spirometry that indicates partially reversible airflow obstruction (>12% increase and 200 ml in forced expiratory volume in 1 sec [FEV_1] after inhaling a short bronchodilator or receiving a short [2 to 3 wk] course of oral corticosteroids). For children aged <5 yr, spirometry is generally not feasible. Young children with asthma symptoms should be treated as having suspected asthma once alternative diagnoses are ruled out.
- The degree of reversibility measured by spirometry correlates with airway obstruction, and patients with a high degree of reversibility have a greater risk of irreversible airflow obstruction in subsequent years.
- Fig. E1-119 describes an algorithm for diagnosing asthma.
- After diagnosis severity of asthma should be classified during the initial assessment before initiating therapy. The following questions from Asthma Control and endorsed by the American Lung Association are important in assessing patients with asthma:
  1. Has your asthma prevented normal activities at home or work?
  2. Have you had shortness of breath in the past 4 wk?
  3. Has your asthma kept you awake at night?
  4. How often have you used your asthma inhaler in the last 4 weeks?
  5. Overall, how have you kept your asthma in control in the last 4 weeks?
- Once therapy is initiated, the emphasis for clinical management is changed to the assessment of asthma control. The level of asthma control should be used to guide decisions either to maintain or adjust therapy.
- Schedule visits at 2- to 6-wk intervals for patients who are just starting therapy or who require a step up in therapy to achieve or regain asthma control. Schedule visits at 1- to 6-mo intervals, after asthma control is achieved, to monitor whether asthma control is maintained. The interval will depend on factors such as the duration of asthma control or the level of treatment required. Consider scheduling visits at 3-mo intervals if step-down therapy is anticipated.

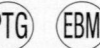
TABLE 1-47 Relative Severity of an Asthmatic Attack as Indicated by PEFR, FEV₁, and MMEFR

Test	Predicted Value (%)	Severity of Asthma
PEFR	>80	
FEV₁	>80	No spirometric abnormalities
MMEFR	>80	
PEFR	>80	
FEV₁	>70	Mild asthma
MMEFR	55-75	
PEFR	>60	
FEV₁	45-70	Moderate asthma
MMEFR	30-50	
PEFR	<50	
FEV₁	<50	Severe asthma
MMEFR	10-30	

FEV₁, Forced expiratory volume in the first second; *MMEFR*, maximal mid-expiratory flow rate; *PEFR*, peak expiratory flow rate.

From Goldman L, Schafer AI: *Goldman's Cecil medicine*, ed 24, Philadelphia, 2012, Saunders.

LABORATORY TESTS

Laboratory tests are usually not necessary and the results can be normal if obtained during a stable period.

- Arterial blood gases (ABGs) can be used during acute bronchospasm in staging the Severity of an asthmatic attack:
  - Mild: decreased Pao_2 and $Paco_2$, increased pH
  - Moderate: decreased Pao_2, normal $Paco_2$, normal pH
  - Severe: marked decreased Pao_2, increased $Paco_2$, and decreased pH
- Complete blood count: leukocytosis with left shift may indicate the existence of bacterial infection.
- Spirometry is recommended at the initial assessment and at least every 1 to 2 yr after treatment is initiated and when the symptoms and peak expiratory flow have stabilized. Spirometry as a monitoring measure may be performed more frequently, if indicated, based on severity of symptoms and the disease's lack of response to treatment.
- Pulmonary function studies: during acute severe bronchospasm, FEV₁ is <1 L and peak expiratory flow rate (PEFR) <80 L/min. Table 1-47 describes the relative severity of an asthma attack as indicated by PEFR, FEV₁ and MMEFR.

IMAGING STUDIES

- Chest x-ray: usually normal, may show evidence of thoracic hyperinflation (e.g., flattening of the diaphragm, increased volume over the retrosternal air space).
- ECG: tachycardia, nonspecific ST-T wave changes are common during an asthma attack; may also show cor pulmonale, right bundle branch block, right axial deviation, counterclockwise rotation.

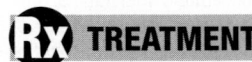

NONPHARMACOLOGIC THERAPY

- Avoidance of triggering factors (e.g., salicylates, sulfites), environmental or occupational triggers
- Encouragement of regular exercise (e.g., swimming)
- Patient education regarding warning signs of an attack and proper use of medications (e.g., correct use of inhalers)

GENERAL Rx

- The 2007 NAEPP guidelines (see Tables 1-48 to 1-56) broadly classify treatment options by age: 0 to 4 yr, 5 to 11 yr, and >12 yr. An approach to home management of acute asthma is described in Fig. E1-120. When asthma symptoms are mild, short-lived, or

TABLE 1-48 Classifying Asthma Severity and Initiating Treatment in Youths ≥12 Yr and Adults (Assessing severity and initiating treatment for patients who are not currently taking long-term control medications)

Components of Severity		Intermittent	CLASSIFICATION OF ASTHMA SEVERITY (≥12 yr) PERSISTENT Mild	Moderate	Severe
Impairment Normal FEV₁/FVC: 8-19 yr 85% 20-39 yr 80% 40-59 yr 75% 60-80 yr 70%	Symptoms	≤2 days/wk	>2 days/wk but not daily	Daily	Throughout the day
	Nighttime awakenings	≤2×/mo	3-4×/mo	>1×/wk but not nightly	Often 7×/wk
	Short-acting beta₂-agonist use for symptom control (not prevention of EIB)	≤2 days/wk	>2 days/wk but not daily, and not more than 1× on any day	Daily	Several times per day
	Interference with normal activity	None	Minor limitation	Some limitation	Extremely limited
	Lung function	Normal FEV₁ between exacerbations			
		FEV₁ >80% predicted	FEV₁ >80% predicted	FEV₁ >60% but <80% predicted	FEV₁ <60% predicted
		FEV₁/FVC normal	FEV₁/FVC normal	FEV₁/FVC reduced 5%	FEV₁/FVC reduced >5%
Risk	Exacerbations requiring oral systemic corticosteroids	0-1 per yr	≥2 per yr ————————————————————————————→		
		←——— Consider severity and interval since last exacerbation. Frequency and severity may fluctuate ———→ over time for patients in any severity category. Relative annual risk of exacerbations may be related to FEV₁.			
Recommended Step for Initiating Therapy		Step 1	Step 2	Step 3	Step 4 or 5 and consider short course of oral systemic corticosteroids
		In 2-6 wk, evaluate level of asthma control that is achieved and adjust therapy accordingly.			

The stepwise approach is meant to assist, not replace, the clinical decision-making required to meet individual patient needs.

Level of severity is determined by assessment of both impairment and risk. Assess impairment domain by patient's/caregiver's recall of previous 2-4 wk and spirometry. Assign severity to the most severe category in which any feature occurs.

At present, there are inadequate data to correspond frequencies of exacerbations with different levels of asthma severity. In general, more frequent and intense exacerbations (e.g., requiring urgent, unscheduled care, hospitalization, or ICU admission) indicate greater underlying disease severity. For treatment purposes, patients who had ≥2 exacerbations requiring oral systemic corticosteroids in the past year may be considered the same as patients who have persistent asthma, even in the absence of impairment levels consistent with persistent asthma.

To access the complete *Expert Panel Report 3: Guidelines for the Diagnosis and Management of Asthma*, go to www.nhlbi.nih.gov/guidelines/asthma/asthgdln.pdf.

EIB, Exercise-induced bronchospasm; *FEV₁*, forced expiratory volume in 1 second; *FVC*, forced vital capacity; *ICU*, intensive care unit.

From National Asthma Education and Prevention Program: *Expert panel report 3: Guidelines for diagnosis and management of asthma*, National Institutes of Health, National Heart, Lung, and Blood Institute, August 2007, NIH publication 08-4051.

infrequent, use of short-acting beta-selective adrenergic agonists (SABAs) administered by inhalation is the most effective therapy for quick relief of asthmatic symptoms. They are recommended for use only as needed for relief of symptoms or before anticipated exposure to known triggers such as exercise. When symptoms become more frequent or more severe, step-up treatment includes use of an inhaled steroid or leukotriene receptor antagonist (LTRA). If symptoms persist, recommendations include use of long-acting beta-agonist (LABA) or LTRA plus inhaled steroid. There are currently several corticosteroid/LABA combination inhalers available (fluticasone/salmeterol [Advair], budesonide/formoterol [Symbicort], mometasone/formoterol [Dulera]). None of these combinations is indicated for the initial treatment of asthma or for acute therapy of asthma symptoms. There is no evidence that one product is more effective than the others. If asthma control remains inadequate, additional treatment consists of inhaled steroid plus LABA plus long-term medication. The ad-

dition of omalizumab, an anti-IgE monoclonal antibody, is indicated for the treatment of moderate and severe persistent asthma refractory to other treatment noted earlier. It is administered subcutaneously every 2 or 4 wk. This medicine is expensive ($10,000 to $30,000/yr). Patients should be closely monitored in the first month because omalizumab can result in allergic reactions (anaphylaxis) in 1 to 2 patients/1000. The NIH guidelines recommend considering omalizumab only after consultation with an asthma specialist.

Treatment of *status asthmaticus* is as follows:
- Oxygen generally started at 2 to 4 L/min by nasal cannula or Venti-Mask at 40% FiO_2; further adjustments are made according to the ABGs.
- Bronchodilators: Initiate treatment with high-dose SABA plus ipratropium bromide administered by means of a nebulizer every 20 min. Use of a metered-dose inhaler with valved holding chamber may be acceptable for patients with mild-to-moderate exacerbations.

- Albuterol nebulizer solution (0.63 mg/3 ml, 1.25 mg/3 ml, 2.5 mg/3 ml, or 5.0 mg/ml): 2.5 to 5 mg every 20 min over the first hr, then 2.5-10 mg every 1-4 hr as needed or 10-15 mg/hr continuously. Other useful medications are levalbuterol nebulizer solution (0.31 mg/3 ml, 0.63 mg/3 ml, 1.25 mg/3 ml), and ipratropium nebulizer solution (0.25/ml [0.025%]).
- Corticosteroids:
  1. Early administration is advised, particularly in patients using steroids at home.
  2. Patients may be started on systemic corticosteroids: methylprednisolone, prednisone, or prednisolone may be used. Dose range is from 40-80 mg/day in one or two divided doses, generally given until peak expiratory flow reaches 70% of predicted value.
  3. Generally for corticosteroid courses < 1 week there is no need to taper the dose
- IV hydration: judicious use is necessary to avoid congestive heart failure in elderly

TABLE 1-49 Assessing Asthma Control and Adjusting Therapy in Youths ≥12 Yr and Adults

Components of Control		CLASSIFICATION OF ASTHMA CONTROL (≥12 yr)		
		Well Controlled	Not Well Controlled	Very Poorly Controlled
Impairment	Symptoms	≤2 days/wk	>2 days/wk	Throughout the day
	Nighttime awakenings	≤2×/mo	1-3×/wk	≥4/wk
	Interference with normal activity	None	Some limitation	Extremely limited
	Short-acting beta₂-agonist use for symptom control (not prevention of EIB)	≤2 days/wk	>2 days/wk	Several times per day
	FEV₁ or peak flow	>80% predicted/personal best	60%-80% predicted/personal best	<60% predicted/personal best
	Validated questionnaires			
	ATAQ	0	1-2	3-4
	ACQ	≤0.75*	≥1.5	N/A
	ACT™	≥20	16-19	≤15
Risk	Exacerbations requiring oral systemic corticosteroids	0-1 per yr	≥2 per yr	
		Consider severity and interval since last exacerbation		
	Progressive loss of lung function	Evaluation requires long-term follow-up care		
	Treatment-related adverse effects	Medication side effects can vary in intensity from none to very troublesome and worrisome. The level of intensity does not correlate to specific levels of control but should be considered in the overall assessment of risk.		
Recommended Action for Treatment		Maintain current step. Regular follow-up every 1-6 mo to maintain control. Consider step down if well controlled for at least 3 mo.	Step up 1 step and Reevaluate in 2-6 wk. For side effects, consider alternative treatment options.	Consider short course of oral systemic corticosteroids. Step up 1-2 steps. Reevaluate in 2 wk. For side effects, consider alternative treatment options.

The stepwise approach is meant to assist, not replace, the clinical decision-making required to meet individual patient needs.
The level of control is based on the most severe impairment or risk category. Assess impairment domain by patient's recall of previous 2-4 wk and by spirometry or peak flow measures. Symptom assessment for longer periods should reflect a global assessment, such as inquiring whether the patient's asthma is better or worse since the last visit.
At present, there are inadequate data to correspond frequencies of exacerbations with different levels of asthma control. In general, more frequent and intense exacerbations (e.g., requiring urgent, unscheduled care, hospitalization, or ICU admission) indicate poorer disease control. For treatment purposes, patients who had ≥2 exacerbations requiring oral systemic corticosteroids in the past year may be considered the same as patients who have not-well-controlled asthma, even in the absence of impairment levels consistent with not-well-controlled asthma.
Validated questionnaires for the impairment domain (the questionnaires do not assess lung function or the risk domain)
 – ATAQ = Asthma Therapy Assessment Questionnaire
 – ACQ = Asthma Control Questionnaire (user package may be obtained at www.qoltech.co.uk or juniper@qoltech.co.uk)
 – ACT = Asthma Control Test™
 – Minimal Important Difference: 1.0 for the ATAQ; 0.5 for the ACQ; not determined for the ACT
Before step up in therapy:
 – Review adherence to medication, inhaler technique, environmental control, and comorbid conditions
 – If an alternative treatment option was used in a step, discontinue and use the preferred treatment for that step
*ACQ values of 0.76-1.4 are indeterminate regarding well-controlled asthma.
EIB, Exercise-induced bronchospasm; *FEV₁*, forced expiratory volume in 1 second; *ICU*, intensive care unit.
The Asthma Control Test is a trademark of QualityMetric Incorporated.
From National Asthma Education and Prevention Program: *Expert panel report 3: Guidelines for diagnosis and management of asthma*, National Institutes of Health, National Heart, Lung, and Blood Institute, August 2007, NIH publication 08-4051.

patients. Aggressive IV hydration is not recommended
- IV antibiotics are indicated when there is suspicion of bacterial infection (e.g., infiltrate on chest radiograph, fever, or leukocytosis).
- Intubation and mechanical ventilation are indicated when previous measures fail to produce significant improvement (Fig. E1-121).
- Discharge home from the emergency department is appropriate if the FEV₁ or PEF after treatment is 70% or greater of the personal best or predicted value and if there is sustained improvement in lung function and symptoms for at least 1 hr.

REFERRAL

Box 1-5 describes indications for referral to an asthma specialist.

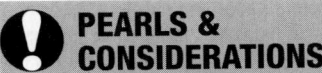

COMMENTS

- The differentiation of asthma from COPD can be challenging. A history of atopy and intermittent, reactive symptoms points toward a diagnosis of asthma, whereas smoking and advanced age are more indicative of COPD. Spirometry is useful in distinguishing asthma from COPD.
- In all asthma patients it is important to treat or prevent comorbid conditions (e.g., rhinosinusitis, vocal cord dysfunction, gastroesophageal reflux disease). However, despite the presumed association between asthma and GERD trials of PPIs in patients with poorly controlled asthma did not reveal any beneficial effects.

- Inhaled low-dose corticosteroids are the single most effective therapy for adult patients with asthma who require more than an occasional use of SABAs to control their asthma.
- Leukotriene modifiers/receptor agonists represent a reasonable alternative in adults unable or unwilling to use corticosteroids; however, these agents are less effective than monotherapy with inhaled corticosteroids.
- Use of LABAs alone without use of a long-term asthma medication, such as an inhaled corticosteroid, is contraindicated. LABAs should also not be used in patients whose asthma is adequately controlled on low- or medium-dose inhaled corticosteroids. Continued use of LABAs may cause down-regulation of the beta-2 receptor with loss of the bronchoprotective effect from from rescue therapy with a SABA.

TABLE 1-50 Stepwise Approach for Managing Asthma in Youths ≥12 Yr and Adults

Intermittent Asthma	Persistent Asthma: Daily Medication Consult with asthma specialist if step 4 care or higher is required. Consider consultation at step 3.

Step 1	Step 2	Step 3	Step 4	Step 5	Step 6	Step up if needed
Preferred: SABA prn	*Preferred:* Low-dose ICS *Alternative:* Cromolyn, LTRA, nedocromil, or theophylline	*Preferred:* Low-dose ICS + LABA OR Medium-dose ICS *Alternative:* Low-dose ICS + either LTRA, theophylline, or zileuton	*Preferred:* Medium-dose ICS + LABA *Alternative:* Medium-dose ICS + either LTRA, theophylline, or zileuton	*Preferred:* High-dose ICS + LABA AND Consider omalizumab for patients who have allergies	*Preferred:* High-dose ICS + LABA + oral corticosteroid AND Consider omalizumab for patients who have allergies	(first, check adherence, environmental control, and comorbid conditions) **Assess control** Step down if possible (and asthma is well controlled at least 3 months)

Each step: Patient education, environmental control, and management of comorbidities
Steps 2-4: Consider subcutaneous allergen immunotherapy for patients who have allergic asthma

Quick-Relief Medication for All Patients
- SABA as needed for symptoms. Intensity of treatment depends on severity of symptoms: up to 3 treatments at 20-minute intervals as needed. Short course of oral systemic corticosteroids may be needed.
- Use of SABA >2 days a week for symptom relief (not prevention of EIB) generally indicates inadequate control and the need to step up treatment.

The stepwise approach is meant to assist, not replace, the clinical decision-making required to meet individual patient needs.
If alternative treatment is used and response is inadequate, discontinue it and use the preferred treatment before stepping up.
Zileuton is a less desirable alternative due to limited studies as adjunctive therapy and the need to monitor liver function. Theophylline requires monitoring of serum concentration levels.
In step 6, before oral systemic corticosteroids are introduced, a trial of high-dose ICS + LABA + either LTRA, theophylline, or zileuton may be considered, although this approach has not been studied in clinical trials.
Steps 1, 2, and 3 preferred therapies are based on Evidence A; step 3 alternative therapy is based on Evidence A for LTRA, Evidence B for theophylline, and Evidence D for zileuton. Step 5 preferred therapy is based on Evidence B. Step 6 preferred therapy is based on (EPR-2 1997) and Evidence B for omalizumab.
Immunotherapy for steps 2-4 is based on Evidence B for house-dust mites, animal danders, and pollens; evidence is weak or lacking for molds and cockroaches. Evidence is strongest for immunotherapy with single allergens. The role of allergy in asthma is greater in children than in adults.
Clinicians who administer immunotherapy or omalizumab should be prepared and equipped to identify and treat anaphylaxis that may occur.
This information is directly abstracted from the 2007 NAEPP *Expert Panel Report 3: Guidelines for the Diagnosis and Management of Asthma* and is not intended to promote or endorse any of the listed products.
To access the complete *Expert Panel Report 3: Guidelines for the Diagnosis and Management of Asthma*, go to www.nhlbi.nih.gov/guidelines/asthma/asthgdln.pdf.
EIB, Exercise-induced bronchospasm; *ICS*, inhaled corticosteroid; *LABA*, inhaled long-acting beta₂-agonist; *LTRA*, leukotriene receptor antagonist; *SABA*, inhaled short-acting beta₂-agonist.
From National Asthma Education and Prevention Program: *Expert panel report 3: Guidelines for diagnosis and management of asthma*, National Institutes of Health, National Heart, Lung, and Blood Institute, August 2007, NIH publication 08-4051.

Diseases and Disorders

TABLE 1-51 Classifying Asthma Severity and Initiating Treatment in Children 5-11 Yr (Assessing severity and initiating treatment in children who are not currently taking long-term control medications)

Components of Severity		Intermittent	Mild	Moderate	Severe
			PERSISTENT		
Impairment	Symptoms	≤2 days/wk	>2 days/wk but not daily	Daily	Throughout the day
	Nighttime awakenings	≤2×/mo	3-4×/mo	>1×/wk but not nightly	Often 7×/wk
	Short-acting beta₂-agonist use for symptom control (not prevention of EIB)	≤2 days/wk	>2 days/wk but not daily	Daily	Several times per day
	Interference with normal activity	None	Minor limitation	Some limitation	Extremely limited
	Lung function	Normal FEV₁ between exacerbations			
		FEV₁ >80% predicted FEV₁/FVC >85%	FEV₁ = >80% predicted FEV₁/FVC >80%	FEV₁ = 60%-80% predicted FEV₁/FVC = 75%-80%	FEV₁ <60% predicted FEV₁/FVC <75%
Risk	Exacerbations requiring oral systemic corticosteroids	0-1 per yr	≥2 per yr		
		←———— Consider severity and interval since last exacerbation. Frequency and severity may fluctuate over time for patients in any severity category. ————→			
		Relative annual risk of exacerbations may be related to FEV₁.			
Recommended Step for Initiating Therapy		Step 1	Step 2	Step 3, medium-dose ICS option	Step 3, medium-dose ICS option, or Step 4
				and consider short course of oral systemic corticosteroids	
		In 2-6 wk, evaluate level of asthma control that is achieved and adjust therapy accordingly.			

The stepwise approach is meant to assist, not replace, the clinical decision-making required to meet individual patient needs.
Level of severity is determined by both impairment and risk. Assess impairment domain by patient's/caregiver's recall of previous 2-4 wk and spirometry. Assign severity to the most severe category in which any feature occurs.
At present, there are inadequate data to correspond frequencies of exacerbations with different levels of asthma severity. In general, more frequent and intense exacerbations (e.g., requiring urgent, unscheduled care, hospitalization, or ICU admission) indicate greater underlying disease severity. For treatment purposes, patients who had ≥2 exacerbations requiring oral systemic corticosteroids in the past year may be considered the same as patients who have persistent asthma, even in the absence of impairment levels consistent with persistent asthma.
EIB, Exercise-induced bronchospasm; *FEV₁,* forced expiratory volume in 1 second; *FVC,* forced vital capacity; *ICU,* intensive care unit.
From National Asthma Education and Prevention Program: *Expert panel report 3: Guidelines for diagnosis and management of asthma,* National Institutes of Health, National Heart, Lung, and Blood Institute, August 2007, NIH publication 08-4051.

TABLE 1-52 Assessing Asthma Control and Adjusting Therapy in Children 5-11 Yr

Components of Control		Well Controlled	Not Well Controlled	Very Poorly Controlled
		CLASSIFICATION OF ASTHMA CONTROL (5-11 yr of age)		
Impairment	Symptoms	≤2 days/wk but not more than once on each day	>2 days/wk or multiple times on ≤2 days/wk	Throughout the day
	Nighttime awakenings	≤1×/mo	≥2×/mo	≥2×/wk
	Interference with normal activity	None	Some limitation	Extremely limited
	Short-acting beta₂-agonist use for symptom control (not prevention of EIB)	≤2 days/wk	>2 days/wk	Several times per day
	Lung function			
	FEV₁ or peak flow	>80% predicted/personal best	60%-80% predicted/personal best	<60% predicted/personal best
	FEV₁/FVC	>80% predicted	75%-80%	<75% predicted
Risk	Exacerbations requiring oral systemic corticosteroids	0-1 per yr	≥2 per yr	
		Consider severity and interval since last exacerbation		
	Reduction in lung growth	Evaluation requires long-term follow-up care		
	Treatment-related adverse effects	Medication side effects can vary in intensity from none to very troublesome and worrisome. The level of intensity does not correlate to specific levels of control but should be considered in the overall assessment of risk.		
Recommended Action for Treatment		Maintain current step. Regular follow-up every 1-6 mo. Consider step down if well controlled for at least 3 mo.	Step up 1 step and Reevaluate in 2-6 wk. For side effects, consider alternative treatment options.	Consider short course of oral systemic corticosteroids. Step up 1-2 steps. Reevaluate in 2 wk. For side effects, consider alternative treatment options.

The stepwise approach is meant to assist, not replace, the clinical decision-making required to meet individual patient needs.
The level of control is based on the most severe impairment or risk category. Assess impairment domain by patient's/caregiver's recall of previous 2-4 wk and by spirometry or peak flow measures. Symptom assessment for longer periods should reflect a global assessment such as inquiring whether the patient's asthma is better or worse since the last visit.
At present, there are inadequate data to correspond frequencies of exacerbations with different levels of asthma control. In general, more frequent and intense exacerbations (e.g., requiring urgent, unscheduled care, hospitalization, or ICU admission) indicate poorer disease control. For treatment purposes, patients who had ≥2 exacerbations requiring oral systemic corticosteroids in the past year may be considered the same as patients who have persistent asthma, even in the absence of impairment levels consistent with persistent asthma.
Before step up in therapy:
– Review adherence to medications, inhaler technique, environmental control, and comorbid conditions.
– If an alternative treatment option was used in a step, discontinue it and use preferred treatment for that step.
EIB, Exercise-induced bronchospasm; *FEV₁,* forced expiratory volume in 1 second; *ICU,* intensive care unit.
From National Asthma Education and Prevention Program: *Expert panel report 3: Guidelines for diagnosis and management of asthma,* National Institutes of Health, National Heart, Lung, and Blood Institute, August 2007, NIH publication 08-4051.

TABLE 1-53 Stepwise Approach for Managing Asthma in Children 5-11 Yr

Intermittent Asthma	Persistent Asthma: Daily Medication
	Consult with asthma specialist if step 4 care or higher is required. Consider consultation at step 3.

Step 1
Preferred:
SABA prn

Step 2
Preferred:
Low-dose ICS

Alternative:
Cromolyn, LTRA, nedocromil, or theophylline

Step 3
Preferred:
Low-dose ICS + either LABA, LTRA, or theophylline

OR

Medium-dose ICS

Step 4
Preferred:
Medium-dose ICS + LABA

Alternative:
Medium-dose ICS + either LTRA or theophylline

Step 5
Preferred:
High-dose ICS + LABA

Alternative:
High-dose ICS + either LTRA or theophylline

Step 6
Preferred:
High-dose ICS + LABA + oral corticosteroid

Alternative:
High-dose ICS + either LTRA or theophylline + oral systemic corticosteroid

Step up if needed
(first, check adherence, inhaler technique, environmental control, and comorbid conditions)

Assess control

Step down if possible

(and asthma is well controlled at least 3 months)

Each step: Patient education, environmental control, and management of comorbidities
Steps 2-4: Consider subcutaneous allergen immunotherapy for patients who have allergic asthma

Quick-Relief Medication for All Patients
• SABA as needed for symptoms. Intensity of treatment depends on severity of symptoms: up to 3 treatments at 20-minute intervals as needed. Short course of oral systemic corticosteroids may be needed.
• Caution: Increasing use of SABA or use >2 days a week for symptom relief (not prevention of EIB) generally indicates inadequate control and the need to step up treatment.

The stepwise approach is meant to assist, not replace, the clinical decision-making required to meet individual patient needs.
If alternative treatment is used and response is inadequate, discontinue it and use the preferred treatment before stepping up.
Theophylline is a less desirable alternative due to the need to monitor serum concentration levels.
Step 1 and step 2 medications are based on Evidence A. Step 3 ICS + adjunctive therapy and ICS are based on Evidence B for efficacy of each treatment and extrapolation from comparator trials in older children and adults–comparator trials are not available for this age group; steps 4-6 are based on expert opinion and extrapolation from studies in older children and adults.
Immunotherapy for steps 2-4 is based on Evidence B for house-dust mites, animal danders, and pollens; evidence is weak or lacking for molds and cockroaches. Evidence is strongest for immunotherapy with single allergens. The role of allergy in asthma is greater in children than in adults. Clinicians who administer immunotherapy should be prepared and equipped to identify and treat anaphylaxis that may occur.
This information is directly abstracted from the 2007 NAEPP *Expert Panel Report 3: Guidelines for the Diagnosis and Management of Asthma* and is not intended to promote or endorse any of the listed products.
ICS, Inhaled corticosteroid; *LABA,* inhaled long-acting beta₂-agonist; *LTRA,* leukotriene receptor antagonist; *SABA,* inhaled short-acting beta₂-agonist.
From National Asthma Education and Prevention Program: *Expert panel report 3: Guidelines for diagnosis and management of asthma,* National Institutes of Health, National Heart, Lung, and Blood Institute, August 2007, NIH publication 08-4051.

BOX 1-5 Possible Indications for Referral to an Asthma Specialist

• Severe, acute asthma that has caused loss of consciousness, hypoxia, respiratory failure, convulsions, or near death
• Poorly controlled asthma as indicated by admission to a hospital, frequent need for emergency care, need for oral corticosteroids, absence from school or work, disruption of sleep, interference with quality of life
• Severe, persistent asthma requiring step 4 care (consider for patients who require step 3 care)
• Patient <3 yr who requires step 3 or 4 care (consider for patient <3 yr who requires step 2 care)
• Requirement for continuous oral corticosteroids or high-dose inhaled corticosteroids or more than two short courses of oral corticosteroids within 1 yr

• Need for additional diagnostic testing such as allergy skin testing, rhinoscopy, provocative challenge, complete pulmonary function testing, bronchoscopy
• Consideration for immunotherapy
• Need for additional education regarding asthma, complications of asthma and treatment of asthma, problems with adherence to management recommendations, or allergen avoidance
• Uncertainty of diagnosis
• Complications of asthma, including sinusitis, nasal polyposis, aspergillosis, severe rhinitis, vocal cord dysfunction, gastroesophageal reflux

Modified from National Asthma Education and Prevention Program, National Heart, Lung, and Blood Institute: *Expert Panel Report 2: guidelines for the diagnosis and management of asthma,* Bethesda, MD, 1997, National Institutes of Health, NIH publication No 97-4051.

TABLE 1-54 Classifying Asthma Severity and Initiating Treatment in Children 0-4 Yr
(Assessing severity and initiating treatment in children who are not currently taking long-term control medications)

Components of Severity		Intermittent	CLASSIFICATION OF ASTHMA SEVERITY (0-4 yr of age)		
			PERSISTENT		
			Mild	Moderate	Severe
Impairment	Symptoms	≤2 days/wk	>2 days/wk but not daily	Daily	Throughout the day
	Nighttime awakenings	0	1-2×/mo	3-4×/mo	>1×/wk
	Short-acting beta₂-agonist use for symptom control (not prevention of EIB)	≤2 days/wk	>2 days/wk but not daily	Daily	Several times per day
	Interference with normal activity	None	Minor limitation	Some limitation	Extremely limited
Risk	Exacerbations requiring oral systemic corticosteroids	0-1 per yr	≥2 exacerbations in 6 mo requiring oral systemic corticosteroids, or ≥4 wheezing episodes/1 yr lasting >1 day AND risk factors for persistent asthma.		
			←————— Consider severity and interval since last exacerbation. —————→ Frequency and severity may fluctuate over time.		
			Exacerbations of any severity may occur in patients in any severity category.		
Recommended Step for Initiating Therapy		Step 1	Step 2	Step 3 and consider short course of oral systemic corticosteroids	
			In 2-6 wk, depending on severity, evaluate level of asthma control that is achieved. If no clear benefit is observed in 4-6 wk, consider adjusting therapy or alternative diagnoses.		

The stepwise approach is meant to assist, not replace, the clinical decision-making required to meet individual patient needs.

Level of severity is determined by assessment of both impairment and risk. Assess impairment domain by patient's/caregiver's recall of previous 2-4 wk. Symptom assessment for longer periods should reflect a global assessment such as inquiring whether the patient's asthma is better or worse since the last visit. Assign severity to the most severe category in which any feature occurs.

At present, there are inadequate data to correspond frequencies of exacerbations with different levels of asthma severity. For treatment purposes, patients who had ≥2 exacerbations requiring oral systemic corticosteroids in the past six months, or ≥4 wheezing episodes in the past year, and who have risk factors for persistent asthma may be considered the same as patients who have persistent asthma, even in the absence of impairment levels consistent with persistent asthma.

To access the complete Expert Panel Report 3: Guidelines for the Diagnosis and Management of Asthma, go to www.nhlbi.nih.gov/guidelines/asthma/asthgdln.pdf.

EIB, Exercise-induced bronchospasm.

From National Asthma Education and Prevention Program: *Expert panel report 3: Guidelines for diagnosis and management of asthma,* National Institutes of Health, National Heart, Lung, and Blood Institute, August 2007, NIH publication 08-4051.

TABLE 1-55 Assessing Asthma Control and Adjusting Therapy in Children 0-4 Yr of Age

Components of Control		CLASSIFICATION OF ASTHMA CONTROL (0-4 yr of age)		
		Well Controlled	Not Well Controlled	Very Poorly Controlled
Impairment	Symptoms	≤2 days/wk	>2 days/wk	Throughout the day
	Nighttime awakenings	≤1×/mo	>1×/mo	>1×/wk
	Interference with normal activity	None	Some limitation	Extremely limited
	Short-acting beta₂-agonist use for symptom control (not prevention of EIB)	≤2 days/wk	>2 days/wk	Several times per day
Risk	Exacerbations requiring oral systemic corticosteroids	0-1 per yr	2-3 per yr	>3 per yr
	Treatment-related adverse effects	Medication side effects can vary in intensity from none to very troublesome and worrisome. The level of intensity does not correlate to specific levels of control but should be considered in the overall assessment of risk.		
Recommended Action for Treatment		Maintain current step. Regular follow-up every 1-6 mo. Consider step down if well controlled for at least 3 mo.	Step up 1 step. Reevaluate in 2-6 wk. If no clear benefit in 4-6 wk, consider alternative diagnoses or adjusting therapy. For side effects, consider alternative treatment options.	Consider short course of oral systemic corticosteroids. Step up 1-2 steps. Reevaluate in 2 wk. If no clear benefit in 4-6 wk, consider alternative diagnoses or adjusting therapy. For side effects, consider alternative treatment options.

The stepwise approach is meant to assist, not replace, the clinical decision-making required to meet individual patient needs.

The level of control is based on the most severe impairment or risk category. Assess impairment domain by caregiver's recall of previous 2-4 wk. Symptom assessment for longer periods should reflect a global assessment such as inquiring whether the patient's asthma is better or worse since the last visit.

At present, there are inadequate data to correspond frequencies of exacerbations with different levels of asthma control. In general, more frequent and intense exacerbations (e.g., requiring urgent, unscheduled care, hospitalization, or ICU admission) indicate poorer disease control. For treatment purposes, patients who had ≥2 exacerbations requiring oral systemic corticosteroids in the past year may be considered the same as patients who have not-well-controlled asthma, even in the absence of impairment levels consistent with not-well-controlled asthma.

Before step up in therapy:

− Review adherence to medications, inhaler technique, and environmental control.

− If an alternative treatment option was used in a step, discontinue it and use preferred treatment for that step.

EIB, Exercise-induced bronchospasm; *ICU,* intensive care unit.

From National Asthma Education and Prevention Program: *Expert panel report 3: Guidelines for diagnosis and management of asthma,* National Institutes of Health, National Heart, Lung, and Blood Institute, August 2007, NIH publication 08-4051.

Diseases and Disorders

A

I

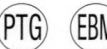

- Patients who remain symptomatic despite inhaled corticosteroids benefit from the addition of LABAs. Trials in patients with poorly controlled asthma despite the use of inhaled glucocorticoids and LABAs have shown that the addition of tiotropium, a long-acting anticholinergic bronchodilator approved for treatment of COPD, increased the time to the first severe exacerbation and provided modest sustained bronchodilation.
- Therapy with with systemic corticosteroids accelerates the resolution of acute asthma and reduces the risk of relapse. There is no evidence that doses >50-100 mg prednisone equivalent are beneficial.
- In patients with allergies and elevated serum immunoglobulin (Ig) E levels, use of anti-IgE therapy is beneficial.
- Bronchial thermoplasty (Alair System) may be used to reduce airway smooth muscle mass and widen the airway in adult patients with severe persistent asthma not well controlled with inhaled corticosteroids and LABAs. It requires the insertion of a catheter via bronchoscopy and use of a radiofrequency controller.
- Biologic modifiers of the Th2 immune pathways (neutralizing monoclonal antibodies, receptor antagonists, soluble receptors) are potential options for the development of new treatments of severe asthma.
- The response to treatment for asthma is characterized by wide individual variability. A functional glucocorticoid-induced transcript 1 gene (GLCCI1) variant is associated with substantial decrements in the response to inhaled glucocorticoids in patients with asthma. Another potential cause of the variability in response to treatment is heterogeneity in the role of interleukin-13 expression in the clinical asthma phenotype. Patients with asthma who have a certain biochemical signature are more likely to respond to an anti–interleukin-13 monoclonal antibody than those without such a signature. Identification of genetic variants can eventually lead to personalized asthma treatment.

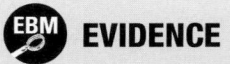 **EVIDENCE**

available at www.expertconsult.com

SUGGESTED READINGS
available at www.expertconsult.com

RELATED CONTENT
Asthma (Patient Information)

AUTHOR: **FRED F. FERRI, M.D.**

TABLE 1-56 Stepwise Approach for Managing Asthma in Children 0-4 Yr

Intermittent Asthma	Persistent Asthma: Daily Medication — Consult with asthma specialist if step 3 care or higher is required. Consider consultation at step 2.

Step 1
Preferred:
SABA prn

Step 2
Preferred:
Low-dose ICS

Alternative:
Cromolyn or montelukast

Step 3
Preferred:
Medium-dose ICS

Step 4
Preferred:
Medium-dose ICS + either LABA or montelukast

Step 5
Preferred:
High-dose ICS + either LABA or montelukast

Step 6
Preferred:
High-dose ICS + either LABA or montelukast

Oral systemic corticosteroid

Step up if needed
(first, check adherence, inhaler technique, and environmental control)

Assess control

Step down if possible

(and asthma is well controlled at least 3 months)

Patient Education and Environmental Control at Each Step

Quick-Relief Medication for All Patients
- SABA as needed for symptoms. Intensity of treatment depends on severity of symptoms.
- With viral respiratory infection: SABA q 4-6 hours up to 24 hours (longer with physician consult). Consider short course of oral systemic corticosteroids if exacerbation is severe or patient has history of previous severe exacerbations.
- Caution: Frequent use of SABA may indicate the need to step up treatment. See text for recommendations on initiating daily long-term-control therapy.

The stepwise approach is meant to assist, not replace, the clinical decision-making required to meet individual patient needs.
If alternative treatment is used and response is inadequate, discontinue it and use the preferred treatment before stepping up.
If clear benefit is not observed within 4-6 wk and patient/family medication technique and adherence are satisfactory, consider adjusting therapy or alternative diagnosis.
Studies on children 0-4 yr are limited. Step 2 preferred therapy is based on Evidence A. All other recommendations are based on expert opinion and extrapolation from studies in other children.
This information is directly abstracted from the 2007 NAEPP *Expert Panel Report 3: Guidelines for the Diagnosis and Management of Asthma* and is not intended to promote or endorse any of the listed products.
ICS, Inhaled corticosteroid; *LABA,* inhaled long-acting beta₂-agonist; *SABA,* inhaled short-acting beta₂-agonist.
From National Asthma Education and Prevention Program: *Expert panel report 3: Guidelines for diagnosis and management of asthma,* National Institutes of Health, National Heart, Lung, and Blood Institute, August 2007, NIH publication 08-4051.

BASIC INFORMATION

DEFINITION

Astrocytoma is a type of neuroepithelial tumor that arises from glial precursor cells (astrocytes, oligodendrocytes, ependymal cells, epithelial cells of the choroid plexus, and others). Astrocytoma arises from astrocytes within the central nervous system (CNS). They are commonly graded by the World Health Organization (WHO) or the Saint Anne–Mayo grading system.

The WHO grades astrocytomas as follows:
- Grade I: pilocytic astrocytoma
- Grade II: low-grade astrocytoma (LGA), fibrillary infiltrating astrocytoma
- Grade III: anaplastic astrocytoma
- Grade IV: glioblastoma multiforme (GBM)
- Grades III and IV are considered high-grade astrocytomas (HGAs) or malignant.

Kernohan system grades astrocytomas based on histologic features: cellularity, mitoses, pleomorphism, vascularity, and necrosis. It has proved to be of prognostic value.
- Grade I: increased cellularity
- Grade II: greater cellularity than grade I plus pleomorphism
- Grade III: greater cellularity and pleomorphism than grade II plus vascular proliferation
- Grade IV: all the above, plus necrosis and pseudopalisading

SYNONYMS

Astroglial neoplasms

ICD-9CM CODES
191.9 Astrocytoma, unspecified site

EPIDEMIOLOGY & DEMOGRAPHICS

- According to SEER registry, the incidence of primary CNS tumor is 2.2 to 8.3/100,000 persons and about 30% of these tumors are astrocytomas.
- Astrocytomas can be found at all ages, with an early peak from birth to 4 yr, followed by a trough between the ages of 15 and 24 yr, and then a steady increase in incidence.
- Male/female ratio is 2:1.
- In adults, glioblastoma is the most common brain tumor.
- In children, astrocytomas are the second most common primary brain tumor and medulloblastoma is the most common.
- Low-grade astrocytomas represent approximately 25% of all CNS gliomas in children.
- Peak age of incidence for juvenile pilocytic astrocytomas is 5 to 14 yr.
- Peak age of incidence for glioblastoma is 45 to 70 yr.

GENETICS:
- Alteration of *p53,* a tumor-suppressor gene encoded by the *TP53* gene on chromosome 17, plays a key role in the development of a large number of adult astrocytomas.
- Genetic abnormalities occur in a stepwise manner with accumulation of multiple abnormalities leading to dedifferentiation and transformation into higher grade.

- Abnormalities of the cell cycle regulatory complex that includes p16, cdk6/cyclinD1, cdk4/cyclinD1, and loss of chromosome 9P that targets the CDKN2A locus is thought to play an important role in progression to grade III astrocytoma.
- Transformation to GBM is the result of multiple mitogenic effects, with deregulation of p16-CDK4D1-pRb pathway being an important component. Loss of chromosome 10, which targets the PTEN tumor-suppressor gene, is also a frequent finding.

PHYSICAL FINDINGS & CLINICAL PRESENTATION

The presenting symptoms of astrocytoma depend, in part, on the location of the lesion and its rate of growth. Astrocytomas classically present with any one or more of the following features:
- Headache (less frequent)
- New-onset partial or generalized seizures (>50%)
- Nausea and vomiting
- Focal neurologic deficit (cranial nerve palsy, hemiplegia, ataxia)
- Change in mental status
- Papilledema (rare)

ETIOLOGY

- The specific etiology of astrocytoma is unknown.
- The only proven risk factor for development of astrocytoma has been significant exposure to ionizing radiation.
- Other risk factors, such as increased exposure to certain chemicals (petroleum, solvents, lead, pesticides and herbicides), have been proposed but not proved.

DIAGNOSIS

A provisional diagnosis of astrocytoma is made on clinical grounds and radiographic imaging studies. Tissue pathology is needed to establish the diagnosis and to grade the astrocytoma.

DIFFERENTIAL DIAGNOSIS

The differential diagnosis is vast and includes any cause of headache, seizures, change in mental status, and focal neurologic deficits.

WORKUP

- A CT scan or MRI of the head makes the diagnosis of an intracranial brain tumor. However, tissue is needed to establish a diagnosis of astrocytoma.
- Stereotactic biopsy under CT or MRI guidance has been shown to be a relatively safe and accurate method for diagnosis of LGA.
- In the presence of mass effect, either clinically or radiologically, craniotomy with open biopsy and tumor debulking is more appropriate than stereotactic biopsy to establish a tissue diagnosis.

LABORATORY TESTS

There are no diagnostic or supportive blood tests for astrocytoma.

IMAGING STUDIES

- MRI (Fig. 1-122) is the diagnostic imaging study of choice. MRI with contrast and magnetic resonance angiography are used to locate the margins of the tumor, distinguish vascular masses from tumors, detect LGAs not seen by CT scan, and provide clear views of the posterior fossa.
- Newer imaging modalities like magnetic resonance spectroscopy, dynamic enhanced MRI, diffusion perfusion MRI, and functional MRI may lead to improved tumor delineation and functional mapping, and provide information to facilitate resection.

TREATMENT

ACUTE GENERAL Rx

- Once a clinical diagnosis is made on imaging and there is evidence of edema, patients should be started on dexamethasone 10 mg intravenously (IV) followed by 4 mg IV q6h.

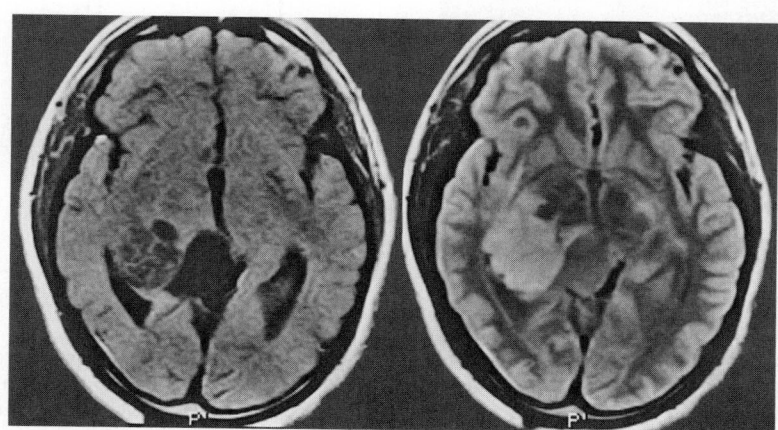

FIGURE 1-122 MR image of a low-grade astrocytoma, demonstrating a hypointense right temporal lesion without contrast enhancement on T1 and hyperintense signal on T2. (From Goetz CG, Pappert EJ: *Textbook of clinical neurology,* Philadelphia, 1999, Saunders.)

A

Diseases and Disorders

I

- If there is increased intracranial pressure and impending herniation, patient should be started on IV mannitol, and mechanical ventilation with hyperventilation should be considered if there is depressed consciousness.
- Surgery remains the initial treatment of almost all astrocytomas, particularly if the tumor is in an anatomically accessible location. Surgery helps in the following ways:
  1. Establishing a pathologic diagnosis and providing information on grade
  2. Debulking the tumor
  3. Alleviating intracranial pressure
- Grade I astrocytomas are usually circumscribed, and complete resection is possible with a high likelihood of long-term remission.
- In grade II astrocytomas, the extent of surgical resection and amount of postoperative residual disease is an important variable for time to first relapse. Randomized trials have shown that postoperative radiotherapy in grade II astrocytoma increases progression-free survival (PFS), but no increase in median survival occurs.
- In grade III and grade IV astrocytomas, gross total resection is the initial treatment of choice. Patients with no residual enhancing tumor have a longer median survival (17.9 vs 12.9 mo; $P < 0.001$) than patients with residual tumor.
- Use of radiation after surgery in high-grade astrocytomas has shown a clear benefit in overall survival.
- In a randomized trial of patients with GBM, radiation with concurrent temozolomide versus radiation alone followed by six cycles of adjuvant temozolomide increases median and overall survival, and this is considered the standard of care for patients with GBM.

CHRONIC Rx

- Attempt at reresection again should be considered in all types of astrocytomas on relapse if possible and in grade I astrocytomas can lead to long-term remissions.
- Radiation therapy can be considered in the relapsed setting in grade II astrocytomas if not given in the adjuvant setting. Chemotherapy has been tried but has no proven role in these tumors.
- Chemotherapy in anaplastic astrocytomas that have relapsed after radiation (Fig. 1-123) does have a role, and the active agents are nitrosourea-based regimen and temozolomide. Grade III anaplastic astrocytomas that have 1p and 19q deletions are especially sensitive to chemotherapy.
- Bevacizumab alone or more commonly in combination with irinotecan is an effective regimen in relapsed GBM, with a response rate of 30% to 50% on the basis of at least two prospective phase II trials.
- Patients presenting with seizures should be treated with anticonvulsants.

DISPOSITION

- Approximately 10% to 35% of astrocytomas (usually grade I pilocytic astrocytomas) are amenable to complete surgical excision and cure. WHO grade I astrocytomas usually do not progress to higher grade tumors.
- Grade II astrocytomas have a median survival of 7.7 yr if they are low risk and 3.2 yr if they are high risk.
- Grade III astrocytomas have a 3-yr survival rate of 55%.
- Median survival for patients with GBM is about 1 yr. Median survival of patients with GBM treated with supportive care is approximately 14 wk. This increases to 20 wk with surgical resection alone, 36 wk with surgery plus x-ray therapy, and 40 to 50 wk with the addition of adjuvant chemotherapy.

REFERRAL

A team of specialty consultations is indicated in patients diagnosed with astrocytoma. A neurosurgeon, radiation oncologist, and neurooncologist are all needed to assist in establishing the diagnosis and to provide immediate and follow-up treatment.

SUGGESTED READINGS

available at www.expertconsult.com

RELATED CONTENT

Astrocytoma (Patient Information)

AUTHOR: **BILAL H. NAQVI, M.D.**

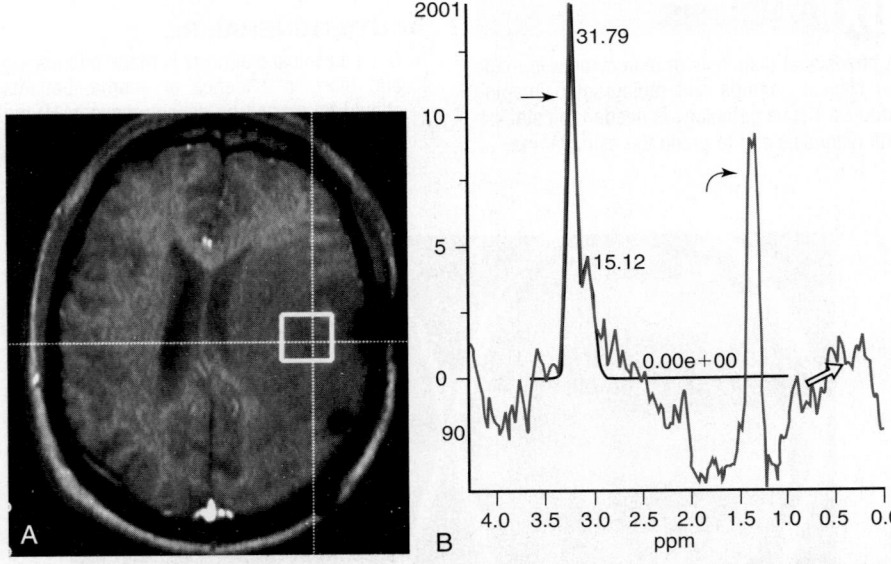

FIGURE 1-123 Recurrent high-grade astrocytoma. Study performed after radiation therapy (not shown) showed increased edema and mass effect; differential diagnosis included recurrent tumor and radiation necrosis. **A,** Axial MRI scan shows volume of tissue *(box)* selected for spectroscopy. **B,** Proton spectroscopy reveals increase in choline peak *(arrow)*, decrease in *N*-acetyl aspartate peak *(curved arrow)*, and appearance of a lactate peak *(open arrow)*. This appearance is consistent with recurrent tumor, which was verified with repeat surgery and biopsy. (From Vincent JL et al: *Textbook of critical care*, ed 6, Philadelphia, 2011, Saunders.)

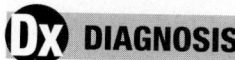

BASIC INFORMATION

DEFINITION

Atelectasis is the collapse of lung volume.

ICD-9CM CODES
518.0 Atelectasis

EPIDEMIOLOGY & DEMOGRAPHICS

- Occurs frequently in patients receiving mechanical ventilation with higher FiO_2
- Dependent regions of the lung are more prone to atelectasis: they are partially compressed, they are not as well ventilated, and there is no spontaneous drainage of secretions with gravity

PHYSICAL FINDINGS & CLINICAL PRESENTATION

- Decreased or absent breath sounds
- Abnormal chest percussion
- Cough, dyspnea, decreased vocal fremitus and vocal resonance
- Diminished chest expansion, tachypnea, tachycardia

ETIOLOGY

- Mechanical ventilation with higher FiO_2
- Chronic bronchitis
- Cystic fibrosis
- Endobronchial neoplasms
- Foreign bodies
- Infections (e.g., TB, histoplasmosis)
- Extrinsic bronchial compression from neoplasms, aneurysms of ascending aorta, enlarged left atrium
- Sarcoidosis
- Silicosis
- Anterior chest wall injury, pneumothorax
- Alveolar injury (e.g., toxic fumes, aspiration of gastric contents)
- Pleural effusion, expanding bullae
- Chest wall deformity (e.g., scoliosis)
- Muscular weaknesses or abnormalities (e.g., neuromuscular disease)
- Mucus plugs from asthma, allergic bronchopulmonary aspergillosis, postoperative state

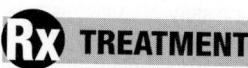

DIAGNOSIS

DIFFERENTIAL DIAGNOSIS

- Neoplasm
- Pneumonia
- Encapsulated pleural effusion
- Abnormalities of brachiocephalic vein and the left pulmonary ligament

WORKUP

- Chest radiograph (Fig. 1-125)
- CT scan and fiberoptic bronchoscopy (selected patients)

IMAGING STUDIES

- Chest radiograph will confirm diagnosis.
- CT scan is useful in patients with suspected endobronchial neoplasm or extrinsic bronchial compression.
- Fiberoptic bronchoscopy (selected patients) is useful for removal of foreign body or evaluation of endobronchial and peribronchial lesions.

TREATMENT

NONPHARMACOLOGIC THERAPY

- Deep breathing, mobilization of the patient
- Incentive spirometry
- Tracheal suctioning
- Humidification
- Chest physiotherapy with percussion and postural drainage

ACUTE GENERAL Rx

- Positive-pressure breathing (continuous positive airway pressure by face mask, positive end-expiratory pressure for patients on mechanical ventilation)
- Use of mucolytic agents (e.g., acetylcysteine [Mucomyst])
- Recombinant human DNase (dornase alpha) in patients with cystic fibrosis
- Bronchodilator therapy in selected patients

CHRONIC Rx

- Chest physiotherapy
- Humidification of inspired air
- Frequent nasotracheal suctioning

DISPOSITION

Prognosis varies with the underlying etiology

REFERRAL

- Bronchoscopy for removal of foreign body or plugs unresponsive to conservative treatment
- Surgical referral for removal of obstructing neoplasms

PEARLS & CONSIDERATIONS

COMMENTS

Patients should be educated that frequent changes of position are helpful in clearing secretions. Sitting the patient upright in a chair is recommended to increase both volume and vital capacity relative to the supine position.

RELATED CONTENT

Atelectasis (Patient Information)

AUTHOR: **FRED F. FERRI, M.D.**

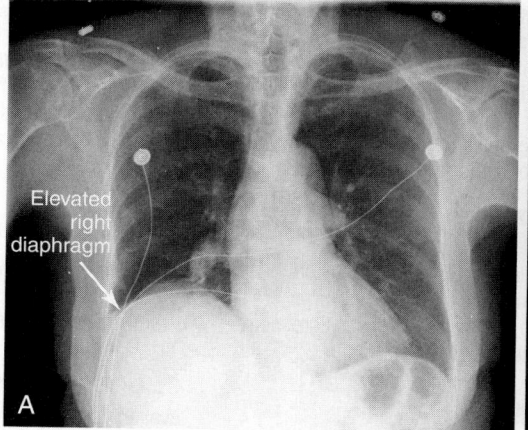
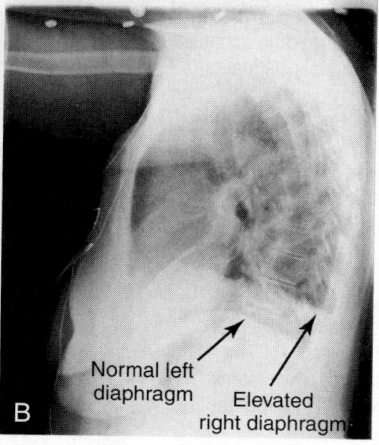

FIGURE 1-125 Atelectasis with elevated diaphragm: an example of volume loss. The right hemidiaphragm in this patient appears elevated on both the posterior-anterior (**A**) and the lateral (**B**) views. Is this the correct interpretation of the x-ray, and if so, what is the cause? Consider the alternative interpretations. A subpulmonic pleural effusion would appear similar, as it would have the same density as liver, heart, and diaphragm and would layer over the diaphragm with the patient upright. This appears less likely in that a meniscus might be seen along the lateral chest wall with a pleural effusion but is not present here. In addition, a pleural effusion occupies space and might be expected to push the heart to the left, whereas in this case the heart may be slightly deviated to the right. Atelectasis of the lower right lung would result in volume loss, pulling the heart and hemidiaphragm into the space normally occupied by lung. This is consistent with the observed features. An infiltrate in this location could explain the x-ray findings but appears less likely for similar reasons to those cited for effusion. Some simple maneuvers could narrow the differential diagnosis. Chest ultrasound, decubitus x-ray views, or CT could identify an effusion. (From Broder JS: *Diagnostic imaging for the emergency physician,* Philadelphia, 2011, Saunders.)

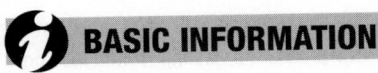

DEFINITION

Atopic dermatitis is a genetically determined eczematous eruption that is pruritic, symmetric, and associated with personal family history of allergic manifestations (atopy).

SYNONYMS

Eczema
Atopic neurodermatitis
Atopic eczema

ICD-9CM CODES
691.8 Atopic dermatitis

EPIDEMIOLOGY & DEMOGRAPHICS

- Incidence is between 5 and 25 cases/1000 persons.
- Highest incidence is among children (10% to 20%). It accounts for 4% of acute care pediatric visits. It affects 1% to 3% of the adult population.
- Onset of disease before age 5 yr in 85% of patients.
- More than 50% of children with generalized atopic dermatitis develop asthma and allergic rhinitis by age 13 yr.
- Concordance in monozygotic twins is 77%.

PHYSICAL FINDINGS & CLINICAL PRESENTATION

- Atopic dermatitis presentation can be subdivided into three phases:
  ○ Acute: vesicular, crusting, weeping eruption
  ○ Subacute: dry, scaly, erythematous papules and plaques
  ○ Chronic: lichenification from repeated scratching
- The lesions are typically on the neck, face, upper trunk, and bends of elbows and knees (symmetric on flexural surfaces of extremities) (Fig. E1-126). Atopic dermatitis lesions are usually discrete but vaguely delineated, scaly, and erythematous.
- There is dryness, thickening of the involved areas, discoloration, blistering, and oozing.
- Papular lesions are frequently found in the antecubital and popliteal fossae.
- In children, red scaling plaques are often confined to the cheeks and the perioral and perinasal areas.
- Inflammation in the flexural areas and lichenified skin is a very common presentation in children.
- Constant scratching may result in areas of hypopigmentation or hyperpigmentation (more common in blacks).
- In adults, redness and scaling in the dorsal aspect of the hands or about the fingers are the most common expression of atopic dermatitis; oozing and crusting may be present.
- Secondary skin infections may be present (*Staphylococcus aureus*, dermatophytosis, herpes simplex).

ETIOLOGY

Unknown; elevated T-lymphocyte activation, defective cell immunity, and B-cell IgE overproduction may play a significant role.

DIAGNOSIS

DIFFERENTIAL DIAGNOSIS

- Scabies
- Psoriasis
- Dermatitis herpetiform
- Contact dermatitis
- Photosensitivity
- Seborrheic dermatitis
- Candidiasis, tinea
- Lichen simplex chronicus
- Other: xerosis, impetigo, Wiskott-Aldrich syndrome, PKU, ichthyosis, HIV dermatitis, non-nummular eczema, histiocytosis X, malignancies (T-cell lymphoma/Mycosis fungoides, Letterer-Siwe disease), graft-versus-host disease, metabolic and nutritional deficiencies (zinc, niacin, pyridoxine deficiencies)

WORKUP

Diagnosis is based on the presence of three of the following major features and three minor features.
MAJOR FEATURES:
- Pruritus
- Personal or family history of atopy: asthma, allergic rhinitis, atopic dermatitis
- Facial and extensor involvement in infants and children
- Flexural lichenification in adults
MINOR FEATURES:
- Elevated IgE
- Eczema-perifollicular accentuation
- Recurrent conjunctivitis
- Ichthyosis
- Nipple dermatitis
- Wool intolerance
- Cutaneous *S. aureus* infections or herpes simplex infections
- Food intolerance
- Hand dermatitis (nonallergic irritant)
- Facial pallor, facial erythema
- Cheilitis
- White dermographism
- Early age of onset (after 2 mo of age)

LABORATORY TESTS

- Lab tests are generally not helpful.
- Elevated IgE levels are found in 80% to 90% of atopic dermatitis.
- Consider skin biopsy only in cases unresponsive to treatment.

TREATMENT

NONPHARMACOLOGIC THERAPY

- Clip nails to decrease abrasion of skin
Avoidance of triggering factors:
- Sudden temperature changes, sweating, low humidity in the winter

- Contact with irritating substance (e.g., wool, cosmetics, some soaps and detergents, tobacco)
- Foods that provoke exacerbations (e.g., eggs, peanuts, fish, soy, wheat, milk)
- Stressful situations
- Allergens and dust
- Excessive hand washing

GENERAL Rx

- Emollients can be used to prevent dryness. Severely affected skin can be optimally hydrated by occlusion in addition to application of emollients.
- Low-potency topical corticosteroids (e.g., 1% to 2.5% hydrocortisone) may be helpful and are generally considered first-line therapy. Use intermediate-potency steroids (e.g., triamcinolone, fluocinolone) for more severe cases and limit potent corticosteroids (e.g., betamethasone, desoximetasone, clobetasol) to severe cases.
- Oral antihistamines (e.g., hydroxyzine, diphenhydramine) are effective in controlling pruritus and inducing sedation, restful sleep, and prevention of scratching during sleep. Doxepin and other tricyclic antidepressants also have antihistamine effect, induce sleep, and reduce pruritus.
- The topical immunomodulators pimecrolimus and tacrolimus are especially useful for treatment of the face and intertriginous sites, where steroid-induced atrophy may occur. However, due to concerns about carcinogenic potential, the FDA recommends limiting their use for short periods in patients who are intolerant or unresponsive to other treatments. Pimecrolimus cream 1% is applied bid and has anti-inflammatory effects secondary to blockage of activated T-cell cytokine production. Tacrolimus ointment (0.03% or 0.1%) applied bid is a macrolide that suppresses humoral and cell-mediated immune responses.
- Oral prednisone, IM triamcinolone, Goeckerman regimen, PUVA are generally reserved for severe cases.
- Cyclosporine, azathioprine, mycophenolate, and interferon gamma are sometimes tried for recalcitrant disease in adults by physicians who specialize in severe inflammatory skin conditions.

DISPOSITION

- Resolution occurs in approximately 70% of patients by adulthood.
- Most patients have a course characterized by remissions and intermittent flares.

SUGGESTED READINGS
available at www.expertconsult.com

RELATED CONTENT
Dermatitis (Patient Information)

AUTHOR: **FRED F. FERRI, M.D.**

BASIC INFORMATION

DEFINITION

Atrial fibrillation (AF) is a supraventricular tachyarrhythmia characterized by uncoordinated atrial activation with resultant deterioration in atrial mechanical function and often times irregular and rapid ventricular conduction. The ventricular rate is dependent on the conduction properties of the atrioventricular node, which can be influenced by vagal/sympathetic tone, medications, or disease of the atrioventricular node.

Multiple classification schemes have been used in the past to characterize AF. The current classification scheme (divided into three major types) used by the ACC/AHA guideline committee is as follows:

- Paroxysmal AF—episodes of AF that terminate spontaneously within 7 days (most episodes last less than 24 hr)
- Persistent AF—episodes of AF that last longer than 7 days and may require either pharmacologic or electrical intervention to terminate
- Permanent AF—AF that has persisted for longer than 1 yr, either because cardioversion has failed or because cardioversion has not been attempted
- In addition to the previous AF categories, which are mainly defined by episode timing and termination, the ACC/AHA/ESC guidelines describe additional AF categories in terms of other characteristics of the patient:
- Lone atrial fibrillation (LAF)—generally refers to AF in younger patients (<60 yr old) who have normal echocardiographic findings
- Nonvalvular AF—absence of rheumatic mitral valve disease, a prosthetic heart valve, or mitral valve repair
- Secondary AF—occurs in the setting of a primary condition that may be the cause of the AF, such as acute myocardial infarction, cardiac surgery, pericarditis, myocarditis, hyperthyroidism, pulmonary embolism, pneumonia, or other acute disease. It is considered separately because AF is less likely to recur once the precipitating condition has resolved.

SYNONYMS

AF
PAFA-fib
A-fib

ICD-9CM CODES
427.31 Atrial fibrillation

EPIDEMIOLOGY & DEMOGRAPHICS

- The prevalence of AF increases with age, from 0.1% in adults ≤55 yr old to 9% of those ≥80 yr old.
- AF affects 2.7 million people in the U.S. AF is uncommon in infants and children and, when present, almost always occurs in association with structural heart disease.
- The incidence of AF is significantly higher in men than in women in all age groups (1.1% versus 0.8%). AF appears to be more common in whites than in blacks, who may have lower awareness of the disease.
- The rate of ischemic stroke in patients with nonrheumatic AF averages 5% a year, which is somewhere between two and seven times the rate of stroke in patients without AF. The risk of stroke is not due solely to AF; it increases substantially in the presence of other cardiovascular diseases. The attributable risk of stroke from AF is estimated to be 1.5% for those aged 50 to 59 yr old, and it approaches 30% for those aged 80 to 89 yr old.

PHYSICAL FINDINGS & CLINICAL PRESENTATION

Clinical presentation is variable:
- Palpitations, dizziness, or lightheadedness
- Fatigue, weakness, or impaired exercise tolerance
- Angina
- Dyspnea
- Some patients are asymptomatic
- Cardiac auscultation revealing irregularly irregular rhythm

ETIOLOGY

- Vascular causes: hypertensive heart disease, increased pulse pressure (calculated as the difference between systolic and diastolic pressure), a reflection of aortic stiffness
- Valvular heart disease
- Pulmonary causes: pulmonary embolism, chronic obstructive pulmonary disease, obstructive sleep apnea, carbon monoxide poisoning
- Structural cardiac disease: pericarditis, myocarditis, cardiomyopathy, congestive heart failure, coronary artery disease, myocardial infarction, congenital heart disease (especially those that lead to atrial enlargement such as atrial septal defect), tachycardia-bradycardia syndrome
- Arrhythmias: atrial tachycardia, Wolff-Parkinson-White syndrome
- Endocrine: thyrotoxicosis, hyperthyroidism or subclinical hyperthyroidism, pheochromocytoma, obesity
- Surgery: both cardiac and noncardiac
- Electrolytes: hypokalemia, hypomagnesemia
- Systemic stress: fever, anemia, hypoxia, sepsis, infections (e.g., pneumonia)
- Medications/toxins: digitalis, adenosine, theophylline, amphetamines, cocaine, antihistamines, alcohol abuse and/or withdrawal, caffeine, steroidal anti-inflammatory drugs (SAIDs), nonsteroidal anti-inflammatory drugs (NSAIDs)
- Frequency of vigorous exercise is associated with an increased risk of developing AF in young men and joggers
- Porphyrias have been associated with autonomic dysfunction and increased risk of AF

DIAGNOSIS

DIFFERENTIAL DIAGNOSIS

- Multifocal atrial tachycardia
- Atrial flutter
- Frequent atrial premature beats
- Atrial tachycardia
- Atrioventricular nodal reentry tachycardia (AVNRT)
- Paroxysmal supraventricular tachycardia
- Wolff-Parkinson-White syndrome

WORKUP

The evaluation of atrial fibrillation involves diagnosis, determination of the etiology, and classification of the arrhythmia. A minimal evaluation includes a history and physical examination, ECG, transthoracic echocardiogram, and case-specific laboratory work to rule out secondary AF.

LABORATORY TESTS

- Thyroid-stimulating hormone, free T_4
- Serum electrolytes
- Toxicity screen
- CBC count (looking for anemia, infection)
- Cardiac enzymes—CK and/or troponin level (to investigate myocardial infarction as a primary or secondary event)
- BNP (to evaluate for CHF)
- D-dimer/CT scan of chest PE protocol (if the patient has risk factors to merit a pulmonary embolism workup)

IMAGING STUDIES

- ECG (Fig. 1-127)
- Absence of P waves
- Fibrillatory or f waves at the isoelectric baseline with varying amplitude, morphology, and intervals
- Irregular ventricular rate
- Echocardiography to rule out structural heart disease (evaluate ventricular size, thickness, and function, atrial size, and valve function)
- Holter monitor: useful only in selected patients to evaluate paroxysmal AF
- Transesophageal echocardiography (TEE): helpful to evaluate for left atrial thrombus (particularly in the LA appendage) to guide cardioversion (if thrombus is seen, cardioversion should be delayed)
- CT and MRI: in patients with a positive D-dimer result, chest CT angiography may be necessary to rule out pulmonary embolus. Three-dimensional imaging technologies (CT scan or MRI) are often helpful to evaluate atrial anatomy if AF ablation is planned
- Six-minute walk test or exercise test: six-minute walk or exercise testing can help assess the adequacy of rate control. Exercise testing can exclude ischemia prior to treatment of patients with class Ic antiarrhythmic drugs and can be used to reproduce exercise-induced AF
- Holter monitor or event recording: useful only in selected patients to establish diagnosis (e.g., paroxysmal AF) and evaluate for rate control

TREATMENT

NONPHARMACOLOGIC THERAPY

- Avoidance of alcohol in patients with suspected excessive alcohol use
- Avoidance of caffeine and nicotine

- Treatment of underlying source/cause, if any found
- The Maze surgical procedure, with its recent modifications creating electrical barriers to the macroreentrant circuits that are believed to underlie AF, is being performed with good results in several medical centers (preservation of sinus rhythm in >95% of patients without the use of long-term antiarrhythmic medication). Success rates are higher in paroxysmal than in persistent or permanent atrial fibrillation. It is important to understand that ablation therapy will not eliminate the need to take anticoagulant drugs. Even after ablation, patients with AF face increased risk of thromboembolic events and most electrophysiologists suggest lifelong anticoagulation. Although catheter-based radiofrequency ablation is no longer considered experimental, it is not the first-line treatment for most patients. Clear indications for catheter ablation remain undefined. In general, surgery is reserved for patients with rapid heart rate refractory to pharmacologic therapy or those who cannot tolerate pharmacologic therapy.
- Pulmonary vein ablation for chronic AF: Sinus rhythm can be maintained long term in the majority of patients with chronic AF by circumferential pulmonary vein ablation, independently of the effects of antiarrhythmic drug therapy, cardioversion, or both. The American College of Cardiology/American Heart Association/European Society of Cardiology (ACC/AHA/ESC) guidelines state that catheter ablation is a reasonable alternative to medical therapy to prevent recurrent AF in symptomatic patients in the absence of significant left atrial enlargement (class 2A recommendation).
- Pulmonary vein isolation is being increasingly used to treat AF in patients with heart failure. Trials have shown that pulmonary vein isolation is superior to AV node ablation with biventricular pacing in patients with heart failure who have drug-refractory AF.

ACUTE GENERAL Rx

New-onset AF:
- If the patient is hemodynamically unstable (hypotension, congestive heart failure or angina), perform synchronized cardioversion after immediate conscious sedation with a rapid short-acting sedative (e.g., midazolam). The likelihood of cardioversion-related clinical thromboembolism is low in patients with AF lasting <48 hr. Patients with AF lasting >2 days have a 5% to 7% risk for clinical thromboembolism if cardioversion is not preceded by several weeks of warfarin therapy. However, if transesophageal echocardiography reveals no atrial thrombus, cardioversion may be performed safely after anticoagulation has been achieved. Anticoagulant therapy should be continued for at least 1 mo after cardioversion to minimize the incidence of adverse thromboembolic events. It can be stopped after 1 mo as long as AF has not recurred.
- If the patient is hemodynamically stable, a rate-control strategy is typically pursued initially.

Treatment options include the following:
1. Diltiazem 0.25 mg/kg (maximum of 25 mg) given intravenously (IV) over 2 min followed by a second dose of 0.35 mg/kg (maximum of 25 mg) 15 min later if the rate is not slowed to <100 beats/min. May then follow with IV infusion 10 mg/hr (range, 5 to 15 mg/hr) to achieve a resting heart rate of <100 beats/min. Onset of action after IV administration is usually within 3 min, with peak effect most often occurring within 10 min. After the ventricular rate is slowed, the patient can be changed to oral diltiazem 60 to 90 mg q4 to 6h.
2. Verapamil 2.5 to 5 mg IV initially, then 5 to 10 mg IV 10 min later if the rate is still not slowed to <100 beats/min. After the ventricular rate is slowed, the patient can be changed to oral verapamil 80 to 120 mg q6 to 8h. Main concern is hypotension with this medication.
3. Esmolol, metoprolol, and atenolol are beta-blockers available in IV preparations that can be used in AF.
4. Digoxin is not a potent atrioventricular nodal blocking agent, has a potential for toxicity and, therefore, cannot be relied on for acute control of the ventricular response, unless the patient is hypotensive or has a low left ventricular systolic function. When used, give 0.5 mg IV loading dose (slow), then 0.25 mg IV 6 hr later. A third dose may be needed after 6 to 8 hr; daily dose varies from 0.125 to 0.25 mg (decrease dosage in patients with renal insufficiency and elderly patients) depending on the heart rate and signs/symptoms of digoxin toxicity.
5. Amiodarone has a class IIa recommendation from the ACC/AHA/ESC for use as a rate-controlling agent for patients who are intolerant of or unresponsive to other agents, such as patients with heart failure who may otherwise not tolerate diltiazem or metoprolol. Caution should be exercised in those who are not receiving anticoagulation because amiodarone can promote cardioversion.
- All atrioventricular nodal blocking agents should be avoided in patients with Wolff-Parkinson-White syndrome and AF because, by blocking the AV node, AF impulses may be transmitted exclusively down the accessory pathway, which can result in ventricular fibrillation. If this happens, the patient will require immediate defibrillation. Procainamide, flecainide, or amiodarone can be used instead.
- In the acute setting, pharmacologic cardioversion is less commonly used than electrical cardioversion. A major disadvantage with pharmacologic cardioversion is the risk of development of ventricular tachycardia and other serious arrhythmias.

CHRONIC Rx

- Long-term management of *paroxysmal* atrial fibrillation is described in Fig. E1-128. A management approach for patients with *persistent* atrial fibrillation is decribed in Fig. E1-129. The long-term management of *permanent* atrial fibrillation is outlined in Fig. E1-130.
- For patients without symptomatic AF, rate-control strategy with calcium channel blockers, beta-blockers, or digoxin is a reasonable option. Race 2 trial indicates that a lenient rate control strategy, with a target resting heart rate of <110 beats/min is noninferior for a composite primary end point that included CV death, heart-failure hospitalization, stroke, and other major events over a median 3-yr follow-up as compared to a strict control strategy, with a target resting heart rate of <80 beats/min and an exercise heart rate of <110 beats/min.
- In patients with symptomatic AF or with difficult to control heart rate, attempt should be made to maintain sinus rhythm with antiarrhythmic agents. Options of antiarrhythmic agents include amiodarone, dronedarone, (paroxysmal atrial fibrillation only), dofetilide, flecainide, propafenone, procainamide, or sotalol. The decision of which strategy to follow should be best made in consultation with cardiology. Use of dronedarone should be avoided in patients with persistent and/or permanent atrial fibrillation due to worsened cardiovascular outcomes, especially in those with concomitant cardiovascular risk factors.
- The decision whether to pursue long-term anticoagulation must be made in light of the patient's risk for a cardioembolic event versus risk for a bleeding event. The CHA2DS2-VASc has largely superseded the CHADS2 scoring system (congestive heart failure, hypertension, diabetes, vascular disease, age 65-74 years, and woman, which are 1 point each, and age ≥75 yr or ischemic stroke, transient ischemic attack, or thromboembolic disease, which are 2 points each if present). Patients with a CHA2DS2-VASc score of 0 are considered low risk, 1 to 2 are considered moderate risk, and ≥2 are considered high risk and would benefit from long-term anticoagulation (e.g., warfarin).
- Anticoagulation with warfarin is generally not recommended in patients with CHADS-VASc score of zero. For patients with CHADS-VASc score of 1 who do not want to undergo anticoagulation, low-dose aspirin is an appropriate alternative in these patients.
- For patients in whom anticoagulation with warfarin is contraindicated, aspirin plus clopidogrel has been shown to be of similar benefit in reducing thromboembolic events as warfarin with a similar bleeding risk.
- Dabigatran is an FDA-approved direct thrombin inhibitor indicated to reduce the risk of stroke and systemic embolism in patients with nonvalvular atrial fibrillation. In the RE-LY trial, 18,113 patients with nonvalvular AF and at least one risk factor for stroke (mean CHADS2 score 2.1) were randomly assigned to receive oral dabigatran at one of two doses (110 or 150 mg) twice daily, or adjusted-dose warfarin. After a median follow-up of 2 yr, the rate of the primary efficacy outcome of stroke (including hemorrhagic stroke) or systemic embolism was 1.54%, 1.11%, and 1.71% per year in the dabigatran 110 mg, dabigatran

150 mg, and warfarin groups, respectively. Dabigatran 110 mg was noninferior compared to adjusted-dose warfarin, whereas dabigatran 150 mg was significantly more effective than warfarin. In patients <75 yr, lower risks of both intracranial and extracranial bleeding were found in both doses of dabigatran compared with warfarin. In patients >75 yr, intracranial bleeding risk is lower, but extracranial bleeding risk is similar or higher with both doses of dabigatran when compared with warfarin. No monitoring is generally required for dabigatran unless risk of renal insufficiency exists where dose adjustment is needed. Disadvantages include twice-daily dosing, the need for consistent timing of doses because its effects wear off quickly compared to warfarin, and association with higher risk of myocardial infarction.

- Factor Xa inhibitors (apixaban, rivaroxaban) are also effective in reducing stroke and systemic embolism in patients with atrial fibrillation. The ARISTOTLE trial in patients at high risk for stroke (mean CHADS2 score 2.1) using apixaban and the ROCKET AF trial using rivaroxaban in patients with CHADS2 score 3.5 showed that these anticoagulants reduce the risk of stroke, systemic embolism, and serious bleeding compared with warfarin.

PROGNOSIS

- AF is associated with a 1.5- to 1.9-fold higher risk of death, which is in part due to the strong association between AF and thromboembolic events.
- Development of AF predicts heart failure and is associated with a worse New York Heart Association Heart Failure classification. AF may also worsen heart failure in individuals who are dependent on the atrial component of the cardiac output.

- AF in the setting of acute myocardial infarction was associated with a 40% increase in mortality compared to patients in sinus rhythm.

DISPOSITION

Factors associated with maintenance of sinus rhythm after cardioversion include:
- Left atrium diameter <60 mm
- Absence of mitral valve disease
- Short duration of AF

REFERRAL

Refer to a cardiologist those patients in whom antiarrhythmic therapy or catheter-based/surgical intervention is being considered.

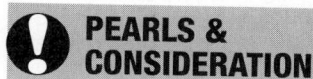 **PEARLS & CONSIDERATIONS**

COMMENTS

The American Academy of Family Physicians and the American College of Physicians provide the following recommendations for the management of newly detected AF:
- Rate control with chronic anticoagulation is the recommended strategy for the majority of asymptomatic patients with chronic AF. Rhythm control has not been shown to be superior to rate control (with chronic anticoagulation) in reducing morbidity and mortality, and may be inferior in some patient subgroups to rate control. Rhythm control is appropriate when based on other special considerations, such as patient symptoms, exercise tolerance, and patient preference.
- Patients with AF should receive chronic anticoagulation, unless they are at low risk for stroke as stated earlier or have specific contraindications.

- For patients with AF, the following drugs are recommended for their demonstrated efficacy in rate control during exercise and while at rest: atenolol, metoprolol, diltiazem, and verapamil (drugs listed alphabetically by class). Digoxin is effective only for rate control at rest and, therefore, should be used only as a second-line agent for rate control in AF.
- For patients who elect to undergo acute cardioversion to achieve sinus rhythm in AF, both direct-current cardioversion and pharmacologic conversion are appropriate options in an otherwise healthy patient.
- Both transesophageal echocardiography with short-term prior anticoagulation followed by early acute cardioversion (in absence of intracardiac thrombus) with postcardioversion anticoagulation vs. delayed cardioversion with preanticoagulation and postanticoagulation are appropriate management strategies for patients who elect to undergo cardioversion.

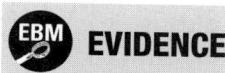 **EVIDENCE**

available at www.expertconsult.com

SUGGESTED READINGS

available at www.expertconsult.com

RELATED CONTENT

Fig. 3-129 Palpitations, dizziness, and/or syncope (Algorithm)
Fig. 3-175 Tachycardia, diagnostic approach (Algorithm)
Atrial Fibrillation (Patient Information)

AUTHORS: **SAURAV CHATTERJEE, M.D., FRED F. FERRI, M.D.,** and **WEN-CHIH WU, M.D., M.P.H.**

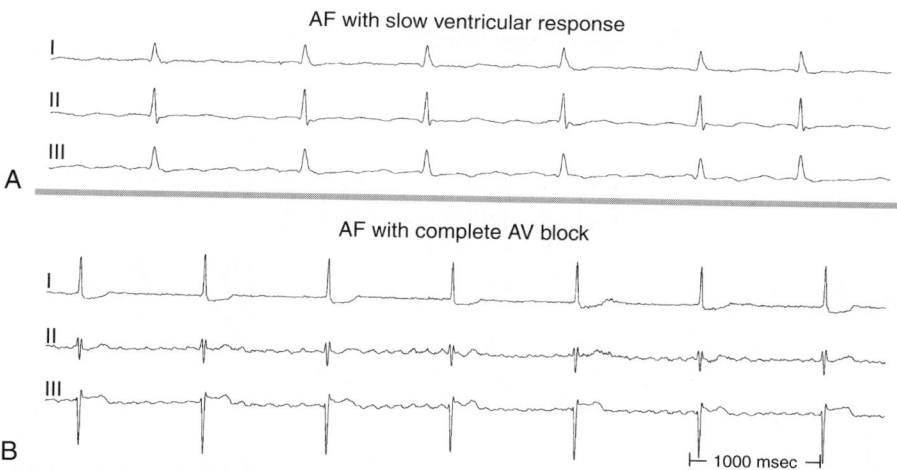

FIGURE 1-127 Atrial fibrillation (AF) with slow ventricular rate. A, The ventricular rhythm is irregular, indicating that it is the result of conducted atrial beats. **B,** The ventricular rhythm is regular, consistent with the presence of complete atrioventricular *(AV)* block and a regular junctional escape rhythm. (From Issa Z et al: *Clinical arrhythmology and electrophysiology,* ed 2, Philadelphia, 2012, Saunders.)

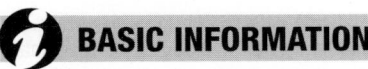

BASIC INFORMATION

DEFINITION
Atrial flutter is characterized by an atrial macro-reentrant circuit (typically in the right atrium) leading to regular atrial depolarizations, typically at a rate of 250 to 350 beats/min. There is typically 2:1 conduction through the atrioventricular node, resulting in heart rates close to 150 beats/min. Higher degrees of atrioventricular (AV) block can occur in patients with AV nodal disease, with increased vagal tone, or when certain drugs such as AV-blocking agents are used. The atrial impulses may be conducted at a constant rate through the atrioventricular node, resulting in a regular rhythm, or the atrial impulses may be conducted at a variable rate, resulting in an irregular rhythm.

ICD-9CM CODES
427.32 Atrial flutter

EPIDEMIOLOGY & DEMOGRAPHICS
- Atrial flutter is the second most common atrial tachyarrhythmia after atrial fibrillation, with an estimated 200,000 new cases annually in the United States.
- Atrial flutter is common during the first week after open-heart surgery.
- Atrial flutter occurs 2.5 times more frequently in men than in women.
- Patients taking antiarrhythmics for chronic suppression of atrial fibrillation may convert to atrial flutter.
- Atrial flutter is typically seen in patients with underlying structural heart disease and is uncommon in children or young adults.

CLASSIFICATION
The Wells classification remains the most commonly used. There are two types of atrial flutter, the common type I and rarer type II. They can only manifest as one type at a time.
TYPE I: Type I atrial flutter, also known as common atrial flutter or typical atrial flutter, has an atrial rate of 240 to 350 beats/min. The reentrant loop circles the right atrium, passing through the cavo-tricuspid isthmus—a body of fibrous tissue in the lower atrium between the inferior vena cava, and the tricuspid valve.

Type I flutter is further divided into two subtypes, known as counterclockwise atrial flutter and clockwise atrial flutter, depending on the direction of the current passing through the loop.
- Counterclockwise atrial flutter (also known as cephalad-directed atrial flutter or typical atrial flutter) is the most common type. The flutter waves are inverted in electrocardiogram (ECG) leads II, III, and aVF.
- Clockwise atrial flutter (atypical): The reentry loop cycles in the opposite direction; thus, the flutter waves are upright in leads II, III, and aVF.

TYPE II: Type II atrial flutter is considered to result from an intraatrial reentrant circuit that is much shorter than type I, at an atrial rate of usually 340 to 440 beats/min. Left atrial flutter type II is common after incomplete left atrial ablation procedures.

Type I is distinguished from type II by:
1. The flutter rate (240-340 beats/min compared to 340-440 beats/min in type II).
2. The observation that type II can change in a "stepwise" manner to type I.
3. The existence of an excitable gap in type I, defined as a period after the wave of depolarization that has recovered its excitability and can be reactivated. After a depolarizing stimulus excites an area of the atrium in type I atrial flutter, it travels slowly in a long pathway with sufficient time for an "excitable gap." In contrast, type II lacks excitable gaps, likely due to short intraatrial reentrant circuits.

PHYSICAL FINDINGS & CLINICAL PRESENTATION
- Palpitations
- Dizziness, lightheadedness, syncope, or near syncope
- Angina
- Congestive heart failure
- Embolic phenomena from intracardiac thrombus

ETIOLOGY
- Rheumatic heart disease
- Congenital heart disease
- Left ventricular dysfunction
- Acute myocardial infarction (rarely)
- Thyrotoxicosis
- Pulmonary embolism
- Mitral valve disease
- Cardiac surgery
- Chronic obstructive pulmonary disease
- Obesity
- Pericarditis
- Pulmonary hypertension
- Atrial flutter can also occur spontaneously or as a result of organization of atrial fibrillation from antiarrhythmic therapy

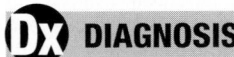

DIAGNOSIS

DIFFERENTIAL DIAGNOSIS
- Atrial fibrillation
- Paroxysmal atrial tachycardia:
  Supraventricular tachycardia, atrioventricular node reentry
  Supraventricular tachycardia, junctional ectopic tachycardia
  Supraventricular tachycardia, Wolff-Parkinson-White syndrome

WORKUP
- ECG
- Laboratory evaluation

LABORATORY TESTS
- Thyroid function studies
- Serum electrolytes

IMAGING STUDIES
- ECG (Fig. 1-131):
  - Absence of P waves.
  - Regular, "sawtooth," or "F" (flutter)" wave pattern in the isoelectric baseline, best seen in leads II, III, and AVF.

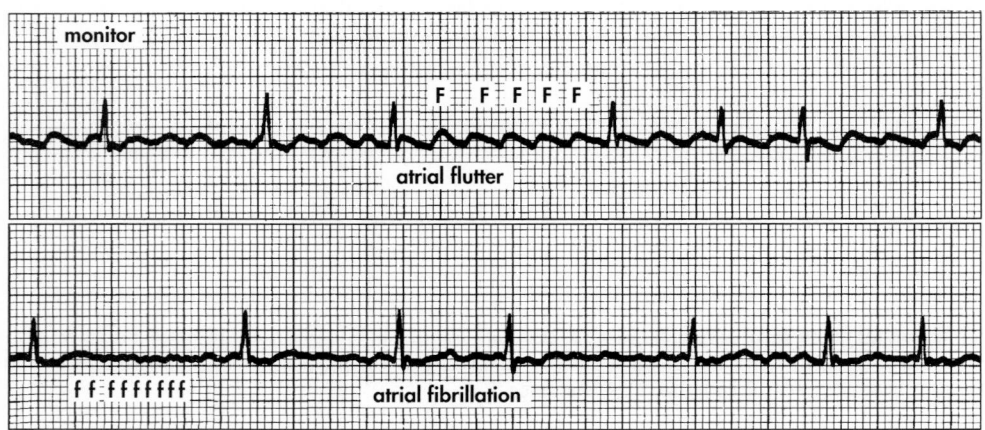

FIGURE 1-131 Atrial flutter and fibrillation. Notice the sawtooth waves with atrial flutter *(F)* and the irregular fibrillatory waves with atrial fibrillation *(f)*. (From Goldberger AL [ed]: *Clinical electrocardiography,* ed 5, St Louis, 1994, Mosby.)

○ There is rarely 1:1 atrioventricular (AV) conduction in atrial flutter (unless pre-excitation is present). Rather, AV conduction is usually in a 2:1, 3:1, or 4:1 fashion, with corresponding usual ventricular rates of 150, 100, or 75 beats/min, respectively (assuming an atrial rate of 300 beats/min).
- Echocardiography to evaluate for structural heart disease (ventricular size, thickness, and function; atrial size, and valve function).
- Transesophageal echocardiography: consider in patients with associated structural or functional heart disease to ascertain the presence of intracardiac thrombi, in the absence of an appropriate duration of anticoagulation.
- Holter monitoring or event recorder to assess for paroxysmal atrial flutter or rate control or to identify the arrhythmia if symptoms are nonspecific or to identify triggering events.
- Electrophysiologic studies: required for a precise diagnosis, for mapping pathway, and for ablation.

Rx TREATMENT

NONPHARMACOLOGIC THERAPY
- Valsalva maneuver or carotid sinus massage usually slows the ventricular rate (increases grade of AV block) and may make flutter waves more evident. Adenosine may be similarly helpful.
- Direct current cardioversion is the treatment of choice for acute management of atrial flutter associated with hemodynamic instability or debilitating symptoms such as angina, congestive heart failure, or poor perfusion. Electrical cardioversion may be successful with energies as low as 25 joules, but since 100 joules is virtually always successful, this may be a reasonable initial shock strength. If the electrical shock results in atrial fibrillation, a second shock at a higher energy level is used to restore normal sinus rhythm. Sedation of a conscious patient is highly recommended before cardioversion is performed. The use of external defibrillators with biphasic waveforms decreases the amount of energy required for cardioversion and improves cardioversion success rate.
- Overdrive pacing in the atrium may also terminate atrial flutter. This method is especially useful in patients who have recently undergone cardiac surgery and still have temporary atrial pacing wires.
- Radiofrequency ablation to interrupt the atrial flutter is highly effective for patients with chronic or recurring atrial flutter and is generally considered first-line therapy in those with recurrent episodes of atrial flutter. It has been shown to improve health-related quality of life. However, there remains an increased risk of subsequent atrial fibrillation and stroke.

ACUTE Rx
- Treatment choices are based on clinical circumstances. If the patient is unstable, proceed directly to electrical cardioversion.
- In the hemodynamically stable patient, proceed with rate control or rhythm control strategy.
- AV blocking agents such as calcium channel blockers, beta-blockers, and digitalis may all be used for rate control. Atrial flutter may spontaneously convert to normal sinus rhythm with this strategy.
- In general, atrial flutter is more difficult to rate-control than atrial fibrillation.
- The rate of recurrence of atrial flutter is difficult to determine because most published data combine atrial flutter with atrial fibrillation. However, the recurrence rate is substantial, perhaps 50% at 1 year.
- Ibutilide is the first-line medication for chemical cardioversion of atrial flutter in patients with normal systolic function and QT intervals. Success rate is approximately 60% to revert atrial flutter to a sinus mechanism and it is more effective than procainamide, sotalol, or amiodarone.

CHRONIC Rx
- Fewer data exist to decide on the choice of rate control versus rhythm control in patients with atrial flutter. There are several options to help maintain sinus rhythm after cardioversion of atrial flutter, such as dofetilide, amiodarone, flecainide, propafenone, or sotalol. The choice of antiarrhythmic therapy is, in part, dictated by the presence or absence of underlying structural heart disease. In patients who have chronic atrial flutter, rate control (to rates as physiologic as possible) can be achieved using AV blocking agents, to prevent occurrence of tachycardia-mediated cardiomyopathy.

- Although data are much less convincing than in atrial fibrillation, current consensus is to treat atrial flutter similar to atrial fibrillation in terms of the risk for thromboembolic events and the need for anticoagulation. In this case, the CHADS2 scoring system (see "Atrial Fibrillation" entry) can be used to risk-stratify patients for their need to stay on long-term anticoagulation.

DISPOSITION
More than 85% of patients convert to regular sinus rhythm after cardioversion with as little as 25 to 50 joules.

REFERRAL
Refer patients who are considered for rhythm control of atrial flutter to cardiologists, especially patients who are candidates for radiofrequency ablation.

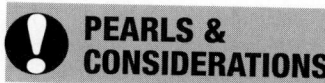 **PEARLS & CONSIDERATIONS**

COMMENTS
- Patients with atrial flutter have a stroke risk at least as high as those with atrial fibrillation and carry a greater risk for subsequent development of atrial fibrillation than in the general population.
- Anticoagulation should be considered for all patients whose CHA2DS2-VASc score is ≥2.
- Anticoagulation with warfarin is generally not recommended in patients with a CHA2DS2-VASc score of zero. For patients with a CHA2DS2-VASc score of 1 who do not want to undergo anticoagulation, low-dose aspirin is an appropriate alternative.

SUGGESTED READINGS
available at www.expertconsult.com

RELATED CONTENT
Fig. 3-129 Palpitations, dizziness, and/or syncope (Algorithm)
Fig. 3-175 Tachycardia, diagnostic approach (Algorithm)
Fig. 3-176 Tachycardia, narrow complex (Algorithm)

AUTHORS: **SAURAV CHATTERJEE, M.D., FRED F. FERRI, M.D.,** and **WEN-CHIH WU, M.D., M.P.H.**

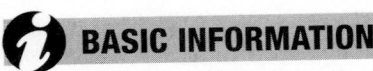

DEFINITION

Atrial myxoma is a benign neoplasm of mesenchymal origin and is the most common primary tumor of the heart.

SYNONYMS

Cardiac myxoma

ICD-9CM CODES
212.7 Benign neoplasm, heart

EPIDEMIOLOGY & DEMOGRAPHICS

- Primary cardiac tumors are extremely rare, with an autopsy frequency of 0.001% to 0.03%. The most frequent cardiac tumors are metastases, occurring 30 times more frequently than primary tumors.
- Myxomas account for 30% to 50% of all primary tumors of the heart.
- 65% of cardiac myxomas occur in females. 4.5% to 10% of cardiac myxomas are familial.
- Average age of incidence of sporadic cases is 30 to 50 yr but can occur at any age.
- Average age of incidence of familial cases is 25 yr.

PHYSICAL FINDINGS & CLINICAL PRESENTATION

Patients with atrial myxomas, when symptomatic, characteristically present in one of three ways:

1. Atrioventricular valve obstruction (e.g., mitral or tricuspid valve): dyspnea, orthopnea, paroxysmal nocturnal dyspnea, edema, dizziness, syncope, elevated jugular venous pressure, widely split loud S_2, secondary pulmonary hypertension, murmurs of regurgitation (holosystolic) or stenosis (rumbles), third heart sound "tumor plop," atrial fibrillation, and sudden death (rarely)
2. Systemic embolization: leading to cerebrovascular accidents, pulmonary embolism, paradoxical embolism
3. Constitutional symptoms: fever, weight loss, arthralgias, Raynaud's phenomenon

ETIOLOGY

- Most cases (90%) of atrial myxomas are sporadic with no known cause
- Carney syndrome, transmitted in an autosomal dominant pattern, accounts for the majority of familial myxomas and as much as 7% of cardiac myxomas. Carney syndrome manifests as cardiac and extracardiac myxomas, pigmented skin discoloration, endocrine hyperactivity, and other tumors.

Dx DIAGNOSIS

DIFFERENTIAL DIAGNOSIS

- Primary valvular diseases: mitral stenosis, mitral regurgitation, tricuspid stenosis, tricuspid regurgitation
- Pulmonary hypertension
- Endocarditis
- Vasculitis
- Atrial thrombus
- Pulmonary embolism
- Cerebrovascular accidents
- Collagen-vascular disease
- Carcinoid heart disease

WORKUP

A high index of suspicion is needed because the clinical manifestations are nonspecific and similar to many common cardiovascular and pulmonary diseases.

LABORATORY TESTS

Although not very specific, the following laboratory findings may be abnormal in patients with atrial myxomas:

- Complete blood count: anemia, polycythemia, thrombocytopenia may occur
- Erythrocyte sedimentation rate, C-reactive protein, and serum immunoglobulins are commonly elevated
- Electrocardiogram: left or right atrial enlargement, atrial fibrillation, premature ventricular depolarizations, or ventricular tachycardia

IMAGING STUDIES

- Echocardiography: initial test of choice in suspected cases of atrial myxoma
- Chest radiograph: about one third of patients have normal findings. Evidence of altered cardiac contour, pulmonary edema, and chamber enlargement may be present.
- Transesophageal echocardiography: is the recommended measure for initial assessment and may better define cardiac masses not clearly visualized by transthoracic echocardiography
- CT: often used for diagnosis; defines tumor extension and evaluates adjacent cardiac structures
- MRI (Fig. 1-132): delineates size, shape, and tissue characteristics, helping distinguish thrombus from tumor

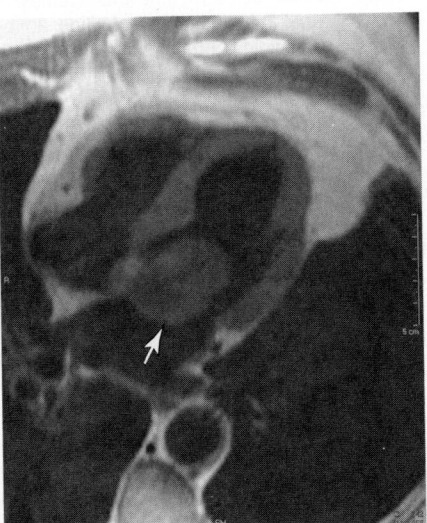

FIGURE 1-132 Diastolic magnetic resonance image of a large left atrial myxoma (arrow) showing that it is attached to the atrial septum and is prolapsing across the mitral valve.
(From Goldman L, Schafer AI: *Goldman's Cecil medicine,* ed 24, Philadelphia, 2012, Saunders.)

- Cardiac catheterization: will show neovascularization in 50% of the cases and may be required to rule out concomitant coronary artery disease in anticipation of surgical excision

Rx TREATMENT

ACUTE GENERAL THERAPY

- Surgical excision is the treatment of choice
- Surgery should be done promptly because systemic embolization and/or sudden death can occur while waiting for the procedure

CHRONIC Rx

Postoperative arrhythmias and conduction abnormalities were present in 26% of patients and can be treated accordingly.

DISPOSITION

- Surgical results have reported a 95% survival rate after a follow-up of 3 yr.
- Careful follow-up is necessary because up to 5% of sporadic cases and 20% of familial cases of atrial myxoma may recur within the first 6 yr after surgery.
- Sudden death in untreated patients may occur in up to 15%, resulting from coronary or systemic embolization or obstruction of the mitral or tricuspid valve.

REFERRAL

- Consultation with a cardiologist is recommended.
- Once the presence of cardiac tumor is confirmed, consultation with a cardiovascular surgeon is needed for prompt surgical excision.

PEARLS & CONSIDERATIONS

- Approximately two thirds of patients present with cardiovascular symptoms, specifically dyspnea, often suggestive of valvular obstruction.
- Nearly one third of patients have evidence of systemic embolization.

COMMENTS

Annual echocardiograms should be performed to monitor for recurrence of atrial myxomas after surgical excision.

SUGGESTED READINGS
available at www.expertconsult.com

RELATED CONTENT
Atrial Myxoma (Patient Information)

AUTHORS: **ABDULRAHMAN ABDULBAKI, M.D., FRED F. FERRI, M.D.,** and **WEN-CHIH WU, M.D., M.P.H.**

BASIC INFORMATION

DEFINITION

Atrial septal defect (ASD) is an abnormal communication within the atrial septum that allows blood flow between the atria. It should be distinguished from patent foramen ovale, which is a persistent patency of the flaplike communication in which the septum primum covering the fossa ovalis overlaps the superior limbic band of the septum secundum. Fig. 1-133 illustrates the physiology of ASD. There are several forms of ASD (Fig. 1-134):

- Primum: This type of ASD occurs when there is failure of fusion of endocardial cushion with the septum primum. The inferior location of the defect on the septum frequently results in involvement of the atrioventricular valves, with resultant cleft anterior mitral leaflet.
- Secundum: The most common form of ASD; it represents a deficiency of the septum primum or a septum secundum, or both. This defect most often occurs in the region of the fossa ovalis.
- Sinus venosus defect: This defect is located at the junction of the right atrium and superior vena cava, and is not a "true ASD" as it does not involve the true atrial septum. In a sinus venosus defect, the wall separating the pulmonary veins and the right atrium is deficient, causing a left-to-right shunt. Most commonly this defect involves the right upper pulmonary vein, which is still connected to the left atrium, but the drainage is anomalous. Less commonly, the right lower pulmonary vein is involved.
- Coronary sinus septal defect (unroofed coronary sinus): This defect results when the wall separating the coronary sinus from the left atrium is deficient, causing a right-to-left shunt. This is not a "true ASD" because it is not a defect in the atrial septum. This defect is often associated with a persistent left superior vena cava.

SYNONYMS

ASD
Interatrial septal defect

ICD-9CM CODES
429.71 Atrial septal defect
745.60 Endocardial cushion defect, unspecified type
745.61 Ostium primum defect
745.5   Ostium secundum type atrial septal defect
745.6   Endocardial cushion defects

EPIDEMIOLOGY & DEMOGRAPHICS

- Secundum, 75%; primum, 15%-20%; sinus venosus, 5%-10%; coronary sinus, <1%
- Incidence is greater in female sex and in patients with Down syndrome
- Accounts for 8% to 10% of congenital heart abnormalities
- Prevalence is 1.6 per 1000 live births

PHYSICAL FINDINGS & CLINICAL PRESENTATION

- Pansystolic murmur best heard at apex secondary to mitral regurgitation (ostium primum defect)
- Wide fixed split of S_2
- Visible and palpable pulmonary artery pulsations
- Ejection systolic flow murmur (pulmonary valve flow murmur)
- Diastolic rumble (atrioventricular valve flow murmur)
- Prominent right ventricular (RV) impulse
- Increased jugular venous pressure (with RV failure)
- Cyanosis and clubbing (severe cases)
- Exertional dyspnea
- Infants with large ASDs: recurrent respiratory infections, heart failure, and failure to thrive
- Patients with small defects: generally asymptomatic

ETIOLOGY

Unknown

DIAGNOSIS

DIFFERENTIAL DIAGNOSIS

- Primary pulmonary hypertension
- Pulmonary stenosis
- Rheumatic heart disease

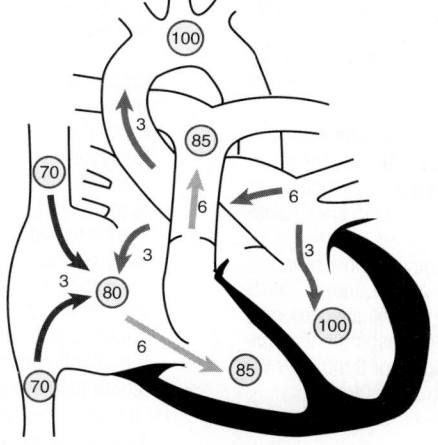

FIGURE 1-133 Physiology of atrial septal defect (ASD). Circled numbers represent oxygen saturation values. The numbers next to the arrows represent volumes of blood flow (in L/min/m²). This illustration shows a hypothetical patient with a pulmonary-to-systemic blood flow ratio (Qp:Qs) of 2:1. Desaturated blood enters the right atrium from the venae cavae at a volume of 3 L/min/m² and mixes with an additional 3 L of fully saturated blood shunting left to right across the ASD; the result is an increase in oxygen saturation in the right atrium. Six liters of blood flow through the tricuspid valve and cause a mid-diastolic flow rumble. Oxygen saturation may be slightly higher in the right ventricle because of incomplete mixing at the atrial level. The full 6 L flows across the right ventricuar outflow tract and causes a systolic ejection flow murmur. Six liters return to the left atrium, with 3 L shunting left to right across the defect and 3 L crossing the mitral valve to be ejected by the left ventricle into the ascending aorta (normal cardiac output). (From Kliegman RM et al: *Nelson textbook of pediatrics*, ed 19, Philadephia, 2011, Saunders.)

FIGURE 1-134 A, Schematic diagram outlining the different types of interatrial shunting that can be encountered. Note that only the central defect is suitable for device closure. **B,** Subcostal right anterior oblique view of a secundum atrial septal defect *(ASD) (asterisk)* that is suitable for device closure. The right panel is a specimen as seen in a similar view, outlining the landmarks of defect. *CS,* Coronary sinus; *IVC,* inferior vena cava; *LA,* left atrium; *RA,* right atrium; *SVC,* superior vena cava. (From Zipes DP et al [eds]: *Braunwauld's heart disease,* ed 7, Philadelphia, 2005, Saunders.)

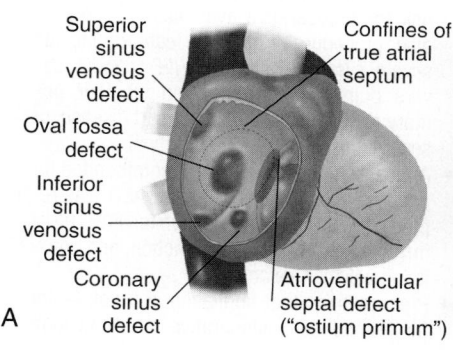
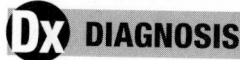
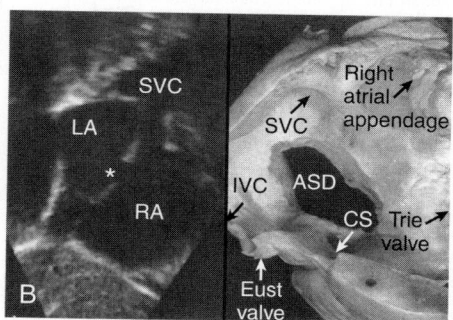

- Mitral valve prolapse
- Cor pulmonale

WORKUP

- ECG:
  - Ostium primum defect: left axis deviation, incomplete or total right bundle branch block, prolongation of PR interval
  - Sinus venosus defect: left axis deviation, abnormal P axis
  - Ostium secundum defect: right axis deviation, incomplete or total right bundle branch block, right atrial enlargement
- Chest x-ray examination
- Echocardiography
- Cardiac catheterization
- Cardiac magnetic resonance imaging (MRI), CT, or both

IMAGING STUDIES

- Chest x-ray: cardiomegaly, right heart enlargement, increased pulmonary vascular pattern
- Echocardiography with saline bubble contrast and Doppler flow studies: may demonstrate the size of the defect, the direction of shunting, presence of anomalous pulmonary return (in sinus venosus ASD), right heart volume overload, and elevated pulmonary artery pressures; transesophageal echocardiography is much more sensitive than transthoracic echocardiography in identifying sinus venosus defects and is preferred by some for the initial diagnostic evaluation
- Cardiac catheterization: not usually a diagnostic necessity; is only useful when the coronary arteries need to be assessed before surgery
- Cardiac MRI and CT: may be useful if echo is not diagnostic; MRI is gold standard for assessing RV size and function, and it can determine whether the right-sided chambers are, in fact, enlarged. MRI is also good to assess pulmonary venous return; cardiac CT can offer similar information

Rx TREATMENT

NONPHARMACOLOGIC THERAPY

- Symptomatic patients should avoid strenuous activity.
- Patients with small shunts (<10 mm) without pulmonary artery hypertension (PAH) and normal RV size are generally asymptomatic and require no medical therapy. Routine assessment of these patients includes symptoms, arrhythmias, and embolic events. A repeat echocardiogram should be obtained every 2 to 3 years to assess RV size and function, and pulmonary pressure.

GENERAL Rx

- Children and infants: Closure of ASD before age 10 yr is indicated if pulmonary to systemic flow ratio is >1.5:1.
- Small ASDs with a diameter of <5 mm and no evidence of RV volume overload do not impact the natural history of the individual

and thus may not require closure unless associated with paradoxical embolism.

- Closure of an ASD either percutaneously or surgically is indicated for right atrial and RV enlargement with or without symptoms.
- A sinus venosus, coronary sinus, or primum ASD should be repaired surgically rather than by percutaneous closure.
- Surgical closure of secundum ASD is reasonable when concomitant surgical repair/replacement of a tricuspid valve is considered or when the anatomy of the defect precludes the use of a percutaneous device.
- Closure of an ASD, either percutaneously or surgically, may be considered in the presence of net left-to-right shunting, pulmonary artery pressure less than two-thirds systemic levels, PVR less than two-thirds systemic vascular resistance, or when responsive to either pulmonary vasodilator therapy or test occlusion of the defect (patients should be treated in conjunction with providers who have expertise in the management of pulmonary hypertensive syndromes).
- Concomitant maze procedure may be considered for intermittent or chronic atrial tachyarrhythmias in adults with ASDs.
- Patients with severe irreversible PAH and no evidence of a left-to-right shunt should not undergo ASD closure.
- Closure of an ASD, either percutaneously or surgically, is reasonable in the presence of:
  - Paradoxical embolism (Class 2a indication)
  - Documented orthodeoxia-platypnea (Class 2a indication)
- Percutaneous catheter device closure is advocated in patients with secundum ASDs (<18 mm in size), with ~95% success rate. A combination of low-dose aspirin and clopidogrel is usually prescribed for 3 mo after the procedure to prevent thrombus formation.

DISPOSITION

- Mortality rate is high in patients with significant ostium primum defect if left untreated, with complications like RV failure, cerebral abscess, and PAH leading to permanent right-to-left shunting (Eisenmenger syndrome).
- Patients with small shunts (<10 mm) have a normal life expectancy.
- Basic preoperative assessment for adult congenital heart disease (ACHD) patients should include systemic arterial oximetry, an ECG, chest radiograph, TTE, and blood tests for full blood count and coagulation screen.
- Intracardiac shunts are considered moderate risk for preoperative evaluation for noncardiac procedure. High-risk features include severe systolic dysfunction (EF <35%), severe pulmonary hypertension whether primary or secondary, cyanotic heart disease, or severe left-side outlet obstruction.
- Annual clinical follow-up is recommended for patients postoperatively if their ASD was repaired as an adult to monitor for PAH, atrial arrhythmias, RV or LV dysfunction, and coexisting valvular lesions.
- Preoperative atrial fibrillation is a risk factor for immediate postoperative and long-term

atrial fibrillation. Patients with a repaired ASD still have an increased risk for development of atrial fibrillation that directly correlates with the age at which the defect is corrected (later correction = greater risk).

  - After closure, anticipated benefits include improved functional status and exercise capacity, improved survival after closure as a child, improved quality of life, prevention of right-heart failure, and prevention of PAH.
  - Potential mid- to long-term complications after ASD closure in adulthood include tachyarrhythmias (atrial fibrillation or atrial flutter), bradyarrhythmias (sinus node dysfunction or heart block), stroke (greater risk in older patients), residual ASDs (small usually close spontaneously, large may be because of patch dehiscence), right-heart failure or pulmonary artery hypertension (risk is inversely related to age at time of closure), mitral valve regurgitation or subaortic stenosis (usually in patients with primum ASDs), device migration/erosion, and pulmonary venous congestion (uncommon).
  - Pregnancy is usually well tolerated in women with ASDs. Follow-up is recommended because of small risk for paradoxical embolus, stroke, arrhythmia, and heart failure. If known, ASDs should be closed before pregnancy if indicated. The sole contraindication to pregnancy in women with an ASD is severe PAH.
  - Scuba diving is generally contraindicated in patients with small ASDs who are medically managed for such risks as paradoxical emboli. In addition, high-altitude climbing should be avoided because it can cause oxygen desaturation from right-to-left shunting in these patients.
- In regard to infective endocarditis prophylaxis for dental procedures,
  - Prophylaxis is not indicated for an ASD.
  - Prophylaxis is indicated for a completely repaired ASD, or any congenital heart disease with prosthetic material during the first 6 mo after the procedure.
  - Prophylaxis is indicated for a repaired ASD, or any congenital heart defect with residual defects at the site or adjacent to the site of a prosthetic patch or prosthetic device (both of which inhibit endothelialization).

The estrogen-containing oral contraceptive pill is not recommended in ACHD patients at risk of thromboembolism, such as those with cyanosis related to an intracardiac shunt, atrial fibrillation, severe PAH, or Fontan repair.

SUGGESTED READINGS

available at www.expertconsult.com

RELATED CONTENT

Atrial Septal Defect (ASD) (Patient Information)

AUTHORS: **SYEDA M. SAYEED, M.D.,**
FRED F. FERRI, M.D., and
WEN-CHIH WU, M.D., M.P.H.

BASIC INFORMATION

DEFINITION

Attention deficit hyperactivity disorder (ADHD) is a chronic disorder of attention and/or hyperactivity-impulsivity. Symptoms must be present before 7 yr of age, last at least 6 mo, and cause functional impairment in multiple settings. The DSM-IV diagnostic criteria for ADHD are described in Table 1-57.

SYNONYMS

Hyperactivity
Hyperkinetic disorder
Attention deficit disorder (ADD)

ICD-9CM CODES
314.00 Attention deficit hyperactivity disorder

EPIDEMIOLOGY & DEMOGRAPHICS

PEAK INCIDENCE: Diagnosis is usually first made in school-aged children (6 to 9 yr).
PREVALENCE: 8% to 10% of school-aged children and 2% to 5% of adults

PREDOMINANT SEX: Among children, male predominance with ratio of 2:1 to 4:1. Among adults, ratio is closer to 1:1 (sex difference may reflect referral bias).
PREDOMINANT AGE: Some symptoms must occur before age 7 yr. Symptoms (especially hyperactivity) tend to diminish with age. Up to 70% continue to meet criteria in adolescence, and an estimated 40% to 65% have some symptoms in adulthood.
GENETICS: Strong polygenetic component. First-degree relatives of ADHD patients have 5 times greater risk of ADHD relative to controls. Studies suggest potential involvement of several genes, including those associated with serotonin and glutamate transporters as well as dopamine metabolism.
RISK FACTORS: Possible environmental and epidemiologic risk factors include in utero tobacco/drug exposure or hypoxia, low birth weight, prematurity, pregnancy, lead exposure (though most children with elevated lead levels do not develop ADHD), head trauma in young children, family dysfunction, low socioeconomic status. Evidence does not support a clear association between dietary factors (e.g., refined sugar, food additives) and ADHD.

PHYSICAL FINDINGS & CLINICAL PRESENTATION

- Three types:
  1. Predominantly inattentive: difficulty organizing, planning, remembering, concentrating, starting/completing tasks; symptoms may not be present during preferred activities.
  2. Predominantly hyperactive-impulsive: edgy/restless, talkative, disruptive/intrusive, disinhibited, impatient.
  3. Combined.
- Usually diagnosed in elementary school when achievement is compromised and behavioral problems are not tolerated. Children with academic underproductivity, problems with peer and family relations, or discipline issues are often referred for evaluation. Of the more than 4 million children in the U.S. who have ADHD, most have comorbid conditions (see below) and nearly half use special education and mental health services.
- Up to 50% may have associated disorders such as psychiatric diagnoses (oppositional defiant disorder, conduct disorder, depression, anxiety), learning disabilities, or substance abuse.
- In adults, hyperactivity is less common, but restlessness, edginess, and difficulty relaxing are often seen. Disorganization and difficulty completing tasks are other common complaints.

TABLE 1-57 DSM-IV Diagnostic Criteria for Attention Deficit Hyperactivity Disorder

A. Either 1 or 2
  1. Six (or more) of the following symptoms of inattention have persisted for ≥6 mo to a degree that is maladaptive and inconsistent with developmental level:
    Inattention
    a. Often fails to give close attention to details or makes careless mistakes in schoolwork, work, or other activities
    b. Often has difficulty sustaining attention in tasks or play activities
    c. Often does not seem to listen when spoken to directly
    d. Often does not follow through on instructions and fails to finish schoolwork, chores, or duties in the workplace (not due to oppositional behavior or failure to understand instructions)
    e. Often has difficulty organizing tasks and activities
    f. Often avoids, dislikes, or is reluctant to engage in tasks that require sustained mental effort (such as schoolwork or homework)
    g. Often loses things necessary for tasks or activities (e.g., toys, school assignments, pencils, books, tools)
    h. Is often easily distracted by extraneous stimuli
    i. Is often forgetful in daily activities
  2. Six (or more) of the following symptoms of hyperactivity-impulsivity have persisted for ≥6 mo to a degree that is maladaptive and inconsistent with developmental level:
    Hyperactivity
    a. Often fidgets with hands or feet or squirms in seat
    b. Often leaves seat in classroom or in other situations in which remaining seated is expected
    c. Often runs about or climbs excessively in situations in which it is inappropriate (in adolescents or adults, may be limited to subjective feelings of restlessness)
    d. Often has difficulty playing or engaging in leisure activities quietly
    e. Is often "on the go" or often acts as if "driven by a motor"
    f. Often talks excessively
    Impulsivity
    g. Often blurts out answers before questions have been completed
    h. Often has difficulty awaiting turn
    i. Often interrupts or intrudes on others (e.g., butts into conversations or games)
B. Some hyperactive-impulsive or inattentive symptoms that caused impairment were present before 7 yr of age
C. Some impairment from the symptoms is present in 2 or more settings (e.g., at school [or work] or at home)
D. There must be clear evidence of clinically significant impairment in social, academic, or occupational functioning
E. Symptoms do not occur exclusively during the course of a pervasive developmental disorder, schizophrenia, or other psychotic disorder, and are not better accounted for by another mental disorder (e.g., mood disorder, anxiety disorder, dissociative disorder, personality disorder)

Code Based on Type

314.01	Attention-deficit/hyperactivity disorder, combined type: if both criteria A1 and A2 are met for the past 6 mo
314.00	Attention-deficit/hyperactivity disorder, predominantly inattentive type: if criterion A1 is met but criterion A2 is not met for the past 6 mo
314.01	Attention-deficit/hyperactivity disorder, predominantly hyperactive-impulsive type: if criterion A2 is met but criterion A1 is not met for the past 6 mo

From American Psychiatric Association: *Diagnostic and statistical manual of mental disorders, fourth edition, text revision,* Washington, DC, 2000, American Psychiatric Association. Copyright 2000 American Psychiatric Association.

ETIOLOGY

Strongest evidence exists for genetic inheritance. Other theories include abnormal metabolism of brain catecholamines, structural brain abnormalities, reduced activation in the basal ganglia and anterior frontal lobe, as well as environmental factors (see earlier).

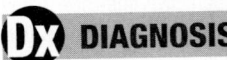 **DIAGNOSIS**

DIFFERENTIAL DIAGNOSIS

- Medical: visual/hearing impairment, seizure disorder, head injury, sleep disorder, medication interactions, mental retardation, developmental delay, thyroid abnormalities, lead toxicity.
- Psychiatric: depression, bipolar disorder, anxiety, obsessive-compulsive disorder, conduct disorder, posttraumatic stress disorder, and substance abuse.
- Psychosocial: mismatch of learning environment with ability, family dysfunction, abuse/neglect.

WORKUP

- Clinical interview should include assessment of symptoms and impact on work/school and relationships; developmental history; personal and family psychiatric history, including substance abuse; social history, including family dysfunction; medical history.
- Physical examination should be performed to investigate medical causes for symptoms, coexisting conditions, and contraindications to treatment. Special focus should be paid to evaluation of dysmorphic features; neurologic examination, including assessment for neurocutaneous findings; and assessment of hearing and vision.
- Information from collateral sources (parents, partners, teachers) is crucial to diagnosis. Many patients will not display symptoms during an office visit and may underreport or overreport symptoms.
- Self-rating scales and standardized symptom-specific questionnaires from collateral sources can help diagnose and assess response to treatment. The use of ADHD-specific rating scales over broadband behavioral scale is associated with improved sensitivity and specificity.
- Laboratory or imaging studies should be undertaken only if indicated by history or physical examination.
- Ancillary testing (e.g., IQ/achievement testing, language evaluation, and mental health assessment) may be indicated based on clinical findings and may require referral.

TREATMENT

NONPHARMACOLOGIC THERAPY

- The majority of studies comparing the efficacy of pharmacologic vs nonpharmacologic interventions demonstrate the superiority of pharmacologic treatments.
- Studies on combined treatments have not shown significant improvements in core ADHD symptoms when behavioral treatments are added to stimulant medications. However, improvements in related areas of concern such as parent-child relations, aggressiveness, teacher-rated social skills, and reaching achievement have been seen in combined treatment groups.
- Prevailing opinion favors a multimodal approach in which nonpharmacologic behavioral therapies including parent-child behavioral therapy and social skills training can be used to target comorbid conditions or behaviors that have not responded to medication.
- Behavioral therapy alone is often considered when symptoms and impairment are mild, if parents are opposed to or patients cannot tolerate medications, or if there is uncertainty or disagreement about the diagnosis (e.g., between parents and teachers).
- Educational interventions are recommended, particularly in the setting of learning disabilities. Children with ADHD are entitled to reasonable educational accommodations under a 504 Plan or the Individuals with Disabilities Education Act.
- Behavioral interventions (e.g., goal setting and rewards systems) show short-term efficacy and are endorsed by most national organizations (e.g., American Academy of Pediatrics, American Medical Association). Time management and organizational skills appear useful. Social skills training may also be useful.
- Psychotherapy such as cognitive therapy, play therapy, or insight-oriented therapy are unlikely to be useful in addressing the core symptoms of ADHD. However, it may be beneficial in treating comorbid psychiatric conditions.
- Elimination diets are not routinely recommended.
- Many support and advocacy groups provide education and other resources (e.g., Children and Adolescents with ADHD, National ADD Association, American Academy of Child and Adolescent Psychiatry).

ACUTE GENERAL Rx

- Most studies on treatment of ADHD are performed in children; limited data available on adults.
- Mainstay of treatment is stimulant medications. Second-line therapies include antidepressants and alpha-agonists.
- Stimulants:
  1. Release or block uptake of dopamine and norepinephrine.
  2. Include short- and long-acting methylphenidate, dextroamphetamine, and dextroamphetamine/amphetamine combinations (mixed amphetamine salts). A methylphenidate patch is available, as is a pro-drug form of dextroamphetamine, lisdexamfetamine (Vyvanse), which is designed to limit the abuse potential.
  3. All stimulants equally effective; however, not all patients improve with stimulants. Patients who do not respond well to one stimulant may respond to another.
  4. Do not cause euphoria or lead to addiction when taken as directed.
  5. Improve cognition, inattention, impulsiveness/hyperactivity, and driving skills. Limited impact on academic performance, learning, and emotional problems.
  6. Side effects are usually mild, reversible, and dose dependent, including anorexia, weight loss, sleep disturbances, increased heart rate and blood pressure, irritability, moodiness, headache, onset or worsening of motor tics, reduction of growth velocity (but not adult height). Do not worsen seizures in patients on adequate anticonvulsant therapy. Rebound of symptoms can occur with withdrawal of medication.
  7. Stimulants have generally been associated with cardiovascular events and death. Patients should be carefully evaluated for cardiovascular disease before beginning therapy and be periodically monitored, including blood pressure checks, while they are treated. However, despite concerns regarding cardiovascular risk, these medications are generally safe. Recent studies have shown that among young and middle-aged adults, current or new use of ADHD medications, compared with nonuse or remote use, is not associated with an increased risk of serious cardiovascular events. Routine, pre-treatment screening with ECGs is not currently recommended by the American Academy of Pediatrics or the American Academy of Child and Adolescent Psychiatry.
- Atomoxetine (Strattera):
  1. Selective norepinephrine reuptake inhibitor.
  2. Generally felt to be less effective than stimulants, but a useful alternative in patients who have not tolerated or responded to stimulants or in the setting of patient or family substance abuse.
  3. Efficacy and safety of use beyond 2 years of treatment have not been studied. There have been reports of behavioral abnormalities and increased suicidality in children and adolescents.
  4. Side effects: gastrointestinal upset, sleep disturbance, decreased appetite, dizziness, sexual side effects in men. Cardiovascular side effects have also been reported.
  5. There have been rare reports of severe liver injury in adults and children.
- Antidepressants (bupropion, imipramine, desipramine, nortriptyline):
  1. May be useful in patients with coexisting psychiatric disorders.
  2. Studies comparing efficacy versus stimulants are inconclusive.
  3. Side effects: arrhythmias, anticholinergic effects, lowering of seizure threshold.
- Alpha-2-adrenergic agonists (clonidine, guanfacine):
  1. Appear to be less effective than stimulants, but may be particularly useful as an adjunctive treatment to stimulants, particularly in patients with a partial stimulant response or who experience side

effects such as sleep disturbance or concurrent symptoms of overarousal, irritability, or aggression.

2. Extended-release formulations of guanfacine (Intuniv) and clonidine (Kapray) have been approved by the FDA for treatment of ADHD in children ages 6 to 17 yr. A transdermal clonidine patch is also available.

3. Potential side effects include sedation, fatigue, headache, bradycardia, hypotension, and depression.

- Use of medications, particularly stimulants (which are monitored under the Controlled Substance Act), requires frequent monitoring.

DISPOSITION

- Although symptoms may change over time, for many patients ADHD represents a chronic condition that requires lifelong management.
- Patients are at higher risk for academic underachievement, lower socioeconomic status, work and relationship difficulties, high-risk behavior, and psychiatric comorbidities.

REFERRAL

- Diagnosis complicated by difficult-to-treat comorbid psychiatric conditions, developmental disorders, or mental retardation
- Lack of adequate response to stimulants/atomoxetine

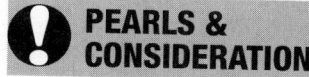
PEARLS & CONSIDERATIONS

- The World Health Organization's Adult Self-Report Scale (ASRS) v1.1 has good sensitivity and adaptability to the primary care setting.
- Among adults with persistent ADHD symptoms treated with medication, trials have shown that the use of cognitive behavioral therapy compared with relaxation with educational support resulted in improved ADHD symptoms, which were maintained at 12 mo.
- ADHD has been associated with criminal behavior in some studies. Data analysis has shown that among patients with ADHD, rates of criminality are lower during periods when they receive ADHD medication.

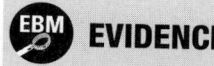
EVIDENCE

available at www.expertconsult.com

SUGGESTED READINGS
available at www.expertconsult.com

RELATED CONTENT
Attention Deficit Hyperactivity Disorder (ADHD) (Patient Information)

AUTHORS: **EMILY R. KATZ, M.D.,** and **MITCHELL D. FELDMAN, M.D., M.PHIL.**

A

Diseases
and Disorders

I

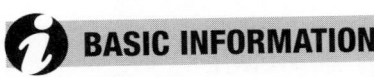 **BASIC INFORMATION**

DEFINITION

Autism spectrum disorders encompass a continuum of developmental disorders characterized by marked social impairment. Table 1-58 describes the DSM-IV-TR diagnostic criteria for autistic disorder. There is usually impairment in several additional domains, integral to social functioning, including language and communication. Stereotypic behavior and sensory issues (i.e., hypersensitivity, hyposensitivity) also are prominent. Onset is typically before age 3 yr. and may be diagnosed as early as 15-18 mo of age. In rare cases, a child may be observed to develop normally to 18-24 mo and be diagnosed with autism at 30-36 mo. The diagnosis of Asperger's syndrome is typically made at a later age with 50% of affected children first diagnosed in kindergarten or 1st grade. DSM-5 criteria will no longer differentiate autism and Asperger's as separate disorders. Instead, an overarching diagnosis of autism spectrum disorder will be applied to both syndromes using severity levels to identify the magnitude of social and behavioral impairment.

SYNONYMS

ASD
Autism
Autistic disorder
Early infantile autism
Childhood autism
Kanner's autism
Asperger disorder
Pervasive developmental disorder

ICD-9CM CODES
F84.0   Autistic disorder

DSM-IV-TR CODES
299.00 Autistic disorder

299.80 Asperger's disorder
299.80 Pervasive developmental disorder NOS

DSM-5 CODE
299.00 Autism spectrum disorder

EPIDEMIOLOGY & DEMOGRAPHICS

INCIDENCE (IN U.S.): Autism spectrum disorder afflicts less than 1% of children in the U.S.
PREVALENCE: 1:88 (1:54 for boys)
PREDOMINANT SEX: Male/female ratio of 2.1 to 6.5:1.0
PREDOMINANT AGE: Lifelong
PEAK INCIDENCE: Before age 3 yr
GENETICS:

- Autism spectrum disorder is highly heritable with a heritability index of .82 to .90.
- De novo mutations account for 10% to 20% of autism spectrum disorder cases. Active research into common biologic mechanisms underlying autism spectrum disorders (including defective synaptic function) has identified chromosomal abnormalities in 6 major genes with as many as 20-30 additional genes in contributory roles, including glutamate-related genes.
- 5% risk rate for siblings of an affected individual, unless fragile X syndrome is determined as the pathway, increasing the risk rate to 50%.
- 70% to 95% concordance for autism spectrum disorder in monozygotic twins and 5% for dizygotic pairs.
- Clinical signs of autism spectrum disorder correlate with abnormal brain development. Overgrowth and neural dysfunction are evidence at young ages and involves an abnormal excess number of neurons in the prefrontal cortex (PFC). This entirely neurobiologic signal of abnormal development has been reported to begin at 9 to 18 months of age.

PHYSICAL FINDINGS & CLINICAL PRESENTATION

- Common triad of marked impairment in social interactions, impaired and atypical verbal and nonverbal communication, and repetitive and usual behavior or play
- Marked impairment in the understanding and use of both verbal and nonverbal communication, including unchanging facial expression and lack of gestures during interactions
- Stereotypic behavior or language (i.e., echolalia, palilalia)
- Perceptual hypersensitivity (i.e., auditory, tactile, olfactory, gustatory) and avoidance of novel stimuli; or perceptual hyposensitivity (e.g., abnormally high threshold for pain)

ETIOLOGY

- Majority of cases are not associated with a comorbid medical condition. However, 2/3 of cases have a comorbid psychiatric feature (ADHD 29%, Anxiety 22%, Bipolar 20%, Depression 20%).
- Significant increase in comorbid seizure disorder (25%) and developmental delay (75%).
- Autism spectrum disorder is sometimes associated with other neurologic conditions (e.g., encephalitis, cytomegalovirus, toxoplasmosis, tuberous sclerosis, phenylketonuria [PKU], fragile X syndrome), suggesting that it also may result from nonspecific neuronal injury.
- Several studies have shown that there is no association between immunizations (specifically MMR vaccine) or thimerosal-containing vaccines (i.e., DPT) and autism spectrum disorder.

TABLE 1-58   DSM-IV-TR Diagnostic Criteria for Autistic Disorder

A. A total of six (or more) items from (1), (2), and (3), with at least two from (1), and one each from (2) and (3):
  1. Qualitative impairment in social interaction, as manifested by at least two of the following:
    a. Marked impairment in the use of multiple nonverbal behaviors such as eye-to-eye gaze, facial expression, body postures, and gestures to regulate social interaction
    b. Failure to develop peer relationships appropriate to developmental level
    c. A lack of spontaneous seeking to share enjoyment, interests, or achievements with other people (e.g., by a lack of showing, bringing, or pointing out objects of interest)
    d. Lack of social or emotional reciprocity
  2. Qualitative impairments in communication as manifested by at least one of the following:
    a. Delay in, or total lack of, the development of spoken language (not accompanied by an attempt to compensate through alternative modes of communication such as gesture or mime)
    b. In individuals with adequate speech, marked impairment in the ability to initiate or sustain a conversation with others
    c. Stereotyped and repetitive use of language or idiosyncratic language
    d. Lack of varied, spontaneous make-believe play or social imitative play appropriate to developmental level
  3. Restricted repetitive and stereotyped patterns of behavior, interests, and activities, as manifested by at least one of the following:
    a. Encompassing preoccupation with one or more stereotyped and restricted patterns of interest that is abnormal either in intensity or focus
    b. Apparently inflexible adherence to specific, nonfunctional routines or rituals
    c. Stereotyped and repetitive motor manners (e.g., hand or finger flapping or twisting, or complex whole-body movements)
    d. Persistent preoccupation with parts of objects
B. Delays or abnormal functioning in at least one of the following areas, with onset prior to age 3 years: (1) social interaction, (2) language as used in social communication, or (3) symbolic or imaginative play.
C. The disturbance is not better accounted for by Rett's Disorder or Childhood Disintegrative Disorder.

From American Psychiatric Association: *Diagnostic and statistical manual of mental disorders*, ed 4, text revision, Washington, DC, 2000, American Psychiatric Association.

- Current research on the Shank family of proteins (SHANK3 [SH3 and multiple ankyrin repeat domains 3]) suggest that the systematic effects of alterations in Shank3 might contribute to the systematic features of autism spectrum disorders found in many patients.

Dx DIAGNOSIS

DIFFERENTIAL DIAGNOSIS

- Rett's syndrome: occurs in females; follows a brief period of normal development (i.e., 12-15 mo; characterized by severe neurodevelopmental regression including head growth deceleration, loss of purposeful use of hands, hyperventilation (risk of aerophagia), and motor incoordination
- Childhood disintegration disorder: normal development until age 4 yr, followed by marked neurodevelopmental and behavioral regression beginning with loss of bladder and bowel control
- Childhood-onset schizophrenia: follows period of normal development
- Asperger's syndrome: lacks the language and cognitive deficits characteristic of autism
- Isolated symptoms of autism spectrum disorder: when occurring in isolation, defined as disorders (i.e., Phelan-Mcdermid syndrome, Aciardi syndrome, selective mutism, expressive language disorder, mixed receptive-expressive language disorder, stereotypic movement disorder, severe-to-profound intellectual disability [aka mental retardation])

WORKUP

- Rule out underlying medical condition including genetic intellectual disability syndromes
- Administer age-appropriate diagnostic instruments based on questionnaires and observation noting scales. Validated autism spectrum disorder–specific screening tools are available for children age ≥18 mo (e.g., Modified Checklist for Autism in Toddlers, Childhood Autism Rating Scale; Autism Diagnostic Observation Scale; Autism Diagnostic Interview-Revised; PDDST-III; Asperger's Syndrome Diagnostic Scale; Gilliam Asperger's Diagnostic Scale) and are being developed for younger children. General developmental screening tools are currently used in children <18 mo.

LABORATORY TESTS

- PKU screen (usually done at birth in the U.S.)
- Lead exposure screening
- Audiology testing for young children with autism spectrum disorders; school-based hearing screening may be sufficient in older children with autism spectrum disorders and without significant language or learning deficits
- Karyotype, microarray analysis, and DNA testing for fragile X syndrome in both boys and girls

IMAGING STUDIES

- EEG to diagnose coexisting seizure disorder if seizure is suspected or if language regression is present (i.e., Landau-Kleffner syndrome)
- Brain MRI if tuberous sclerosis or Aicardi syndrome (callosal agenesis) is suspected

Rx TREATMENT

NONPHARMACOLOGIC THERAPY

- Consistent behavioral training program in both the home and school environments
- A number of programs are currently used; many are based on applied behavioral analysis (ABA), others include Pivotal Response Training (PRT), Floortime, and the Early Start Denver Model for Young Children with Autism.
- Special educational program focused on language and communication skills, social and life skills development
- Highly structured home environment
- Education for families and teachers; the Autism Speaks™ website may be helpful in this regard: http://www.autismspeaks.org/about_us.php

ACUTE GENERAL Rx

- Obsessive or ritualistic behaviors: selective serotonin reuptake inhibitors (SSRIs), atypical antipsychotics, valproic acid
- Aggression, irritability, self-injury: atypical antipsychotic agents (e.g., risperidone), α-agonists, anticonvulsant mood stabilizers, SSRIs, beta-blockers, opiate antagonist (self-injury only)
- Hyperactivity, impulsivity, inattention: stimulants, alpha-agonists, atypical antipsychotics
- Anxiety: SSRIs, buspirone, mirtazapine
- Bipolar, mood lability: valproic acid, carbamazepine, lithium, aripiprazole
- Depression: SSRIs, mirtazapine

CHRONIC Rx

- Extended use of medications used for acute management of comorbid psychiatric disorder.
- Pharmacotherapy is palliative, not curative of autism spectrum disorder

DISPOSITION

- Most children will require some degree of assistance as adults.
- With early diagnosis and proper treatment/support, the prognosis for children without language and intellectual impairment (aka Asperger's syndrome) is fair to very good despite ongoing symptoms.
- Poorer outcomes include a lack of joint attention by age 4 yr, a lack of functional speech by age 5 yr, intellectual disability, seizures, comorbid medical or psychiatric syndromes, and a pervasive lack of social relatedness.
- Best outcomes are associated with early identification and treatment, the development of oral communication skills, and the cognitive and behavioral capacity for inclusion in regular education settings with typically developing peers.

REFERRAL

Assistance may be needed in diagnosis (child psychiatrist, clinical psychologist, geneticist, pediatric neurologist, developmental pediatrician), management (speech language pathologist, occupational therapist), parental teaching (psychiatric social worker), or intervention with the school system (educational advocate, attorney).

! PEARLS & CONSIDERATIONS

- There is no scientific evidence of a relation between childhood vaccination and the development of autism.
- Preliminary evidence suggests that a disproportionate number of children with autism spectrum disorder suffer from sleep difficulties, including obstructive sleep apnea, with sequelae mimicking ADHD.
- The Center for Autism & Developmental Disabilities at Bradley Hospital, an affiliate of the Brown Medical School, is the largest and most comprehensive treatment program in the U.S. for children with autism spectrum disorder and comorbid psychiatric illness (www.bradleyhospital.org).
- University of California Davis M.I.N.D. Institute is devoted to the study of autism (http://www.ucdmc.ucdavis.edu/mindinstitute).

EBM EVIDENCE

available at www.expertconsult.com

SUGGESTED READINGS
available at www.expertconsult.com

RELATED CONTENT

Autism (Patient Information)

AUTHORS: **ROWLAND P. BARRETT, PH.D.,** and **MITCHELL D. FELDMAN, M.D., M.PHIL.**

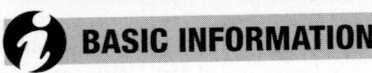

BASIC INFORMATION

DEFINITION
Cerebral arteriovenous malformations (AVMs) are congenital vascular lesions that are characterized by blood flow from high-pressure arterial vessels directly into thin-walled veins without passing through an intervening capillary/venule system (Fig. 1-135A).

SYNONYMS
AVM

ICD-9CM CODES
Q28.2 Arteriovenous malformation of cerebral vessels
I60.8 Ruptured cerebral arteriovenous malformation

EPIDEMIOLOGY & DEMOGRAPHICS
INCIDENCE:
- Detection rates in large prospective studies range from 1.1 to 1.4 per 100.000 person-years.
- Incidence of hemorrhage, the most common and often most clinically dangerous presentation, is estimated to be 2% to 4% per year.

PREVALENCE: Estimated about 1.3 per 100,000
PREDOMINANT SEX AND AGE:
- There is a slight male preponderance, studies of varying populations show 1.04:1 to 1.2:1 M:F ratio.
- Peak age at time of hemorrhage occurrence is about 20 years, but it can occur in younger and older patients.

GENETICS:
- Cerebral AVMs are sporadic in most cases.
- AVMs are present in about 20% of cases of Osler-Weber-Rendu syndrome (also known as hereditary hemorrhagic telangiectasia [HHT]), an autosomal dominant disorder that results in abnormal blood vessel formation in the skin, lungs, liver, brain, and other organs.

RISK FACTORS:
- Male sex and presence of HHT are risk factors for AVM.
- The risk of hemorrhage is increased with prior hemorrhage, presence of a single draining vein, and diffuse nidus morphology.

PHYSICAL FINDINGS & CLINICAL PRESENTATION
- The most common presentation is hemorrhage; symptoms vary based on location and magnitude of hemorrhage.
- Patients may present with seizures or neurologic deficits related to mass effect of the AVM nidus.
- Headache and pulsatile tinnitus may be present.
- In infants, AVM may present as cyanotic heart failure, macrocephaly, or hydrocephalus.
- In nonsymptomatic AVMs a bruit may be auscultated through the scalp or orbit.
- AVMs may also present with associated intracranial aneurysms that occur on distant, unrelated vessels, on a proximal artery that feeds the aneurysm (flow-related aneurysm), or within the AVM nidus itself (intranidal aneurysm). Patients may present with a subarachnoid hemorrhage related to the aneurysm rather than to the AVM.

ETIOLOGY
AVMs are congenital abnormalities caused by failure of formation of a capillary bed between embryonic arterial and venous vascular plexuses during the first trimester of gestation.

DIAGNOSIS

DIFFERENTIAL DIAGNOSIS
The differential diagnosis of cerebral AVMs includes other vascular lesions such as cavernous malformations, dural arteriovenous fistulas, and intracranial aneurysms. Table E1-59 compares vascular malformations, and Table E1-60 describes major differences between hemangiomas and vascular malformations.

LABORATORY TESTS
- CBC and BMP with renal function panel prior to contrast dye administration with CT angiography/cerebral angiogram.
- PT/INR/PTT should be drawn and corrected in the case of bleeding diathesis.

IMAGING STUDIES
- In the acute setting, a CT scan of the head to check for hemorrhage and a CT angiogram of the head for characterization of the lesion may be helpful (although calcification may be present and potentially pose as small acute blood).
- MRI of the brain delineates the nidus and its relationship to surrounding soft tissue structures better than a CT scan; however, in the setting of an acute hemorrhage these details will be obscured.
- Four-vessel cerebral angiogram (arteriogram) is the best study to evaluate AVM. Angiography in multiple projections helps identify the number and location of feeding and draining vessels for treatment planning (Fig. 1-135B). High-resolution images of the nidus may also reveal other irregularities such as aneurysms that often arise given the abnormal histology of the vessel walls and the high-pressure blood flow traversing them.

TREATMENT

Pharmacologic management of seizures with antiepilepsy drugs and of headaches with oral analgesics can provide symptomatic relief.

NONPHARMACOLOGIC THERAPY
- Nonemergent outpatient setting: cerebral angiogram provides characterization of the lesion. Based on angiographic characteristics, the Spetzler-Martin AVM grading system may be used to help guide treatment (Table 1-61). In general, grade 5 AVMs are considered unresectable; they are not treated because the risks of treatment likely outweigh the risk of hemorrhage. Current tools for the treatment of AVMs include surgical resection, radiosurgery, and endovascular embolization (with liquid glues or embolic agents).
- Surgical resection: in low-grade lesions by an experienced neurosurgeon yields a high cure rate (~95% in published studies). Resection should include removal of all of the nidus of the AVM; failure to remove the complete nidus may increase the risk of recurrence. An increasing Spetzler-Martin grading scale increases risk of neurologic complications. Intraoperative imaging techniques such as indocyanine-green in-field angiography and conventional digital subtraction angiography are used to verify complete resection.
- Radiosurgery: alternative definitive treatment for AVMs. Traditionally employed to treat AVMs in eloquent areas such as the brainstem. Sterotactic radiosurgery is increasingly used for higher Spetzler-Martin grade AVM. Reported rates of confirmed radiographic obliteration after AVM radiosurgery range from 47%-90%.
- Endovascular embolization involves transarterial superselective blockage of the AVM. It has become an important adjunctive tool. Currently recommended and approved for use before resection, preoperative embolization can reduce arterial flow and pressure within the AVM, assisting in speed and safety of surgical resection. In addition, embolization may often be used to treat intranidal or flow-related aneurysms in coordination with either resection or radiosurgery. Embolization alone in obliterating an AVM is not routinely recommended.
- Treatment decisions should take into consideration the morbidity associated with the treatment modality versus the risk of future hemorrhage or neurologic deterioration. Disability stemming from intractable seizures or severe headaches may make invasive definitive treatment a more attractive option.

Acute cerebral hemorrhage: In the case of an acute hemorrhage, airway and breathing must be maintained, with intubation if necessary. Acute neurosurgical intervention for clot evacuation may be warranted. Microsurgical resection of the AVM may or may not be feasible in the acute setting and is controversial.

DISPOSITION
Whether the patient is receiving elective treatment of a known lesion or presenting with an acute hemorrhage, the patient should receive care in a progressive or intensive care unit with experience dealing with cerebrovascular disease. Once the patient is stabilized, appropriate rehabilitation should be arranged.

REFERRAL
- Cerebral AVMs should be managed by a qualified neurosurgeon.
- Referral to radiation medicine for adjuvant radiosurgery should be made when indicated.

- Referral to an interventional radiologist for endovascular treatment may be warranted.
- Treatment in a primary stroke center or other specialized center that offers all treatment modalities is recommended.

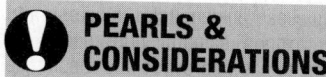

PEARLS & CONSIDERATIONS

COMMENTS

No two AVMs are exactly the same; individualization of treatment decisions is the mainstay. Additionally, many AVMs could be effectively treated through one of several modalities or a combination thereof. Factors such as patient age, overall health status, radiographic characteristics, route of surgical access, and potential morbidities of each treatment modality are vital variables in consideration for treatment.

PATIENT/FAMILY EDUCATION

If a patient with a known AVM suffers from acute-onset neurologic deficits or strokelike symptoms, emergency medical attention is warranted for potential hemorrhage. Presence of AVMs, cerebral or otherwise, in family members should be disclosed to the patient's primary care physician because the presence of a genetic condition predisposing to cerebral AVMs should be considered.

SUGGESTED READINGS

available at www.expertconsult.com

AUTHORS: **STEPHEN L. GRUPKE, M.D.**, and **JUSTIN F. FRASER, M.D.**

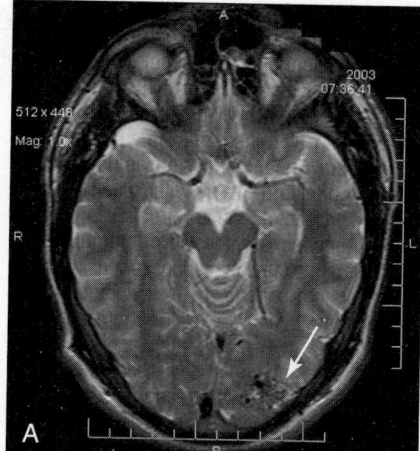
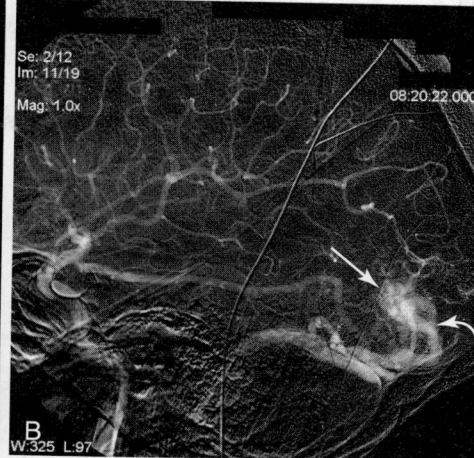
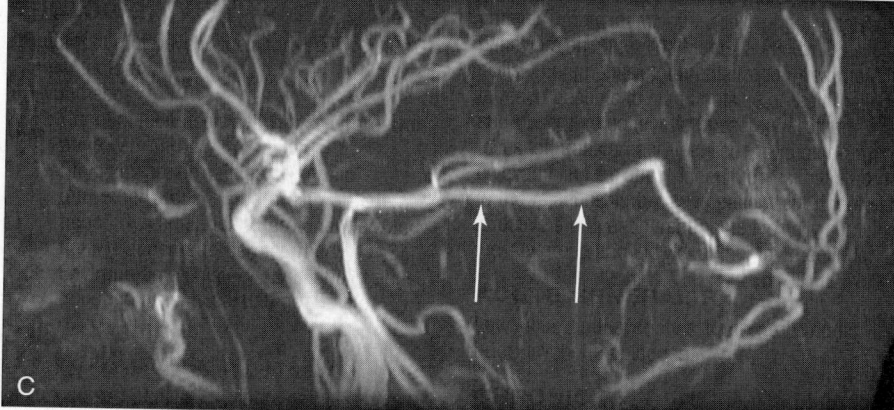

FIGURE 1-135A A 14-year-old child with a left occipital arteriovenous malformation (AVM). A, MRI shows multiple flow voids in the left occipital lobe *(arrow)*. **B,** Lateral view from catheter angiogram confirms the presence of an AVM *(arrow)* and early draining veins *(curved arrow)*. **C,** Lateral maximum intensity projection image from an MR angiogram shows an enlarged posterior cerebral artery branch *(arrows)*, which feeds the tangle of abnormal vessels. (From Fuhrman BP et al: *Pediatric critical care,* ed 4, Philadelphia, 2011, Saunders.)

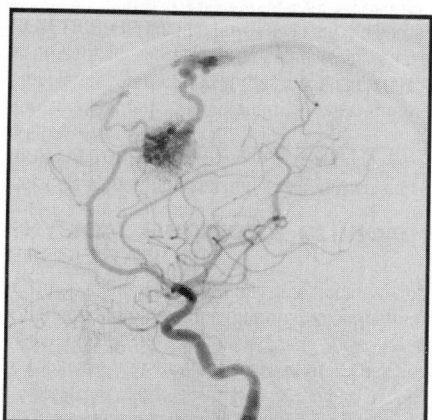

FIGURE 1-135B Arteriovenous malformation of the frontal lobe. The anterior cerebral artery provides primary arterial supply with venous drainage superficially into the superior sagittal sinus.

TABLE 1-61 Spetzler-Martin Arteriovenous Malformation (AVM) Grading Scale*

Characteristic	Points Assigned
AVM Size	
Less than 3 cm	1
3-6 cm	2
Greater than 6 cm	3
Location	
Eloquent	1
Noneloquent	2
Venous Drainage Pattern	
Deep	1
Superficial	0

*The grade is the sum of the points from all three categories. Eloquent brain is defined as sensorimotor, language, or visual cortex, internal capsule, brainstem, diencephalon, cerebellar peduncles, and deep cerebellar nuclei. Venous drainage is considered deep if any of the venous drainage is by deep veins (as opposed to exclusively cortical venous drainage).

From Spetzler RF, Martin NA: A proposed grading system for arteriovenous malformations, *J Neurosurg* 65:476-483, 1986.

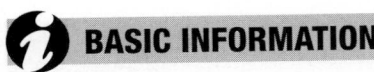

DEFINITION

Avascular necrosis (AVN) is ischemic death of bone due to insufficient blood supply. Osteonecrosis is not a specific disease entity but a final common pathway to several disorders that impair blood supply to the femoral head and other locations.

SYNONYMS

AVN
Osteonecrosis
Aseptic necrosis

ICD-9CM CODES
733.40 Aseptic necrosis
733.43 Aseptic necrosis of femoral condyle
733.42 Aseptic necrosis of femoral head
733.41 Aseptic necrosis of humeral head
733.44 Aseptic necrosis of talus

EPIDEMIOLOGY & DEMOGRAPHICS

- 15,000 new cases per year in the U.S. It is most commonly associated with the hip and accounts for 10% of total hip replacements in the U.S.
- Usually occurs in middle age and is more frequent in males than females
- Associated conditions:
  1. Corticosteroid treatment: 35%
  2. Alcohol abuse: 22%
  3. Idiopathic and other: 43%
  4. Hemoglobinopathies, pancreatitis, chronic renal failure, SLE, chemotherapy, decompression sickness
- Common sites involved
  1. Femoral head
  2. Femoral condyle
  3. Humeral head
  4. Navicular and lunate wrist bones
  5. Talus

PHYSICAL FINDINGS & CLINICAL PRESENTATION

- May be asymptomatic in early stages
- Pain in the involved area exacerbated by movement or weight bearing in later stages
- Decreased range of motion as the disease progresses
- Functional limitation

ETIOLOGY

Final common pathway of conditions that lead to impairment of the blood supply to the involved bone. Trauma disrupting the blood supply is the most common cause of AVN. Arterial factors are considered the most common cause of AVN.
  Stages:
- Stage 0
  - Asymptomatic
  - Normal imaging
  - Histologic findings only (i.e., silent osteonecrosis)

- Stage 1
  - Asymptomatic or symptomatic
  - Normal radiographs and CT scan
  - Abnormal bone scan or MRI
- Stage 2
  - Abnormal radiographs or CT scan, including linear sclerosis, focal bead mineralization, cysts; however, the overall architecture of the involved bone is normal
- Stage 3
  - Early evidence of mechanical bone failure (subchondral fracture), but the overall shape of the bone is still intact
- Stage 4
  - Flattening or collapse of the bone
- Stage 5
  - Joint space narrowing
- Stage 6
  - Extensive joint destruction

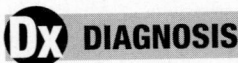 **DIAGNOSIS**

DIFFERENTIAL DIAGNOSIS

- None in late stages
- Early: any condition causing focal musculoskeletal pain, including arthritis, bursitis, tendinitis, myopathy, neoplastic bone and joint diseases, traumatic injuries, pathologic fractures

IMAGING STUDIES (Fig. 1-136)

1. MRI: the most sensitive technology to diagnose early aseptic necrosis. The first sign is a margin of low signal. An inner border of high signal associated with a low-signal line is specific of aseptic necrosis ("double line sign"). Sensitivity is 75% to 100%.
2. Radiography: insensitive early in the course. The earliest changes include diffuse osteopenia, areas of radiolucency with sclerotic border, and linear sclerosis. Later, a subchondral lucency (crescent sign) indicates subchondral fracture. More advanced cases reveal flattening, collapsed bone, and abnormal bone contour. In late disease, osteoarthritic changes are seen.

3. Bone scan:
   - Early: "cold" area.
   - Later: increased radionuclide uptake as a result of remodeling.
   - Sensitivity in early disease is only 70% and specificity is poor.
4. CT scan: may reveal central necrosis and area of collapse before those are visible on radiographs.

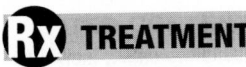 **TREATMENT**

PREVENTION

- Manage etiologic conditions
- Minimize corticosteroid use

NONPHARMACOLOGIC THERAPY

- Core decompression: effectiveness 35% to 95% in early phases
- Bone grafting
- Osteotomies
- Joint replacement

ACUTE GENERAL Rx

- Decrease weight bearing of affected area.
- Pulsing electromagnetic fields applied externally (still experimental).
- Peripheral vasodilators (e.g., dihydroergotamine) (unproven).
- Late-stage AVN is most often treated by total joint arthroplasty.

PROGNOSIS

- When diagnosed at an early stage treatment is appropriate in all cases because 85% to 90% can be expected to progress to a more advanced stage.
- Contralateral joint involvement is common (30% to 70%).

SUGGESTED READINGS
available at www.expertconsult.com

RELATED CONTENT

Avascular Necrosis (Patient Information)

AUTHOR: **FRED F. FERRI, M.D.**

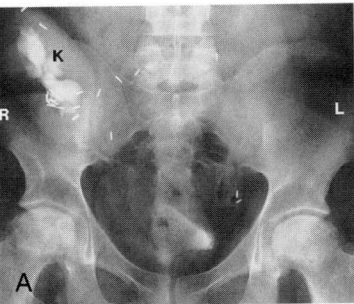
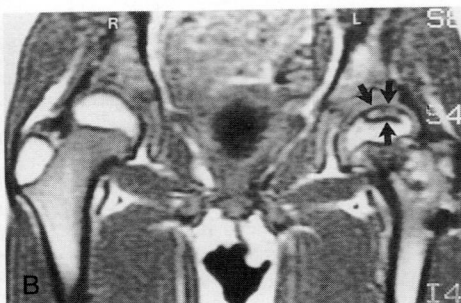

FIGURE 1-136 Aseptic necrosis of the hips. A, Aseptic necrosis can occur from a number of causes, including trauma and steroid use. In this patient, an anteroposterior view of the pelvis shows a transplanted kidney (K) in the right iliac fossa. Use of steroids has caused this patient to have bilateral aseptic necrosis. The femoral heads are somewhat flattened, irregular, and increased in density. **B,** Aseptic necrosis in a different patient is demonstrated on an MRI scan as an area of decreased signal *(arrows)* in the left femoral head. This is the most sensitive method for detection of early aseptic necrosis. (From Mettler FA [ed]: *Primary care radiology,* Philadelphia, 2000, Saunders.)

BASIC INFORMATION

DEFINITION

Babesiosis is a tick-transmitted protozoan disease of animals, caused by intraerythrocytic parasites of the genus *Babesia*. Humans are incidentally infected, resulting in a nonspecific febrile illness. The disease can be severe in immunocompromised hosts.

ICD-9CM CODES
088.82 Babesiosis

EPIDEMIOLOGY & DEMOGRAPHICS

INCIDENCE (IN U.S.): Unknown
PREVALENCE (IN U.S.):
- In areas of high endemicity, seropositivity ranging from 9% (Rhode Island) to 21% (Connecticut)
- Highest number of reported cases in New York

PREDOMINANT SEX: Males (most likely through increased exposure to vectors during recreational or occupational activities)
PREDOMINANT AGE: Severity apparently increasing with age >60 yr
PEAK INCIDENCE: Spring and summer months, May through September
GENETICS: None known
CONGENITAL INFECTION: At least one case of probable vertical transmission
NEONATAL INFECTION: At least two cases of perinatal transmission
BLOOD TRANSFUSION: Many instances

PHYSICAL FINDINGS & CLINICAL PRESENTATION

- Incubation period 1 to 4 wk, or 6 to 9 wk in transfusion-associated disease
- Gradual onset of irregular fever, chills, diaphoresis, headache, myalgia, arthralgia, fatigue, and dark urine
- On physical examination: petechiae, frank or mild hepatosplenomegaly, and jaundice. Most patients have a normal physical exam.
- Infection with *B. divergens* (Europe) producing a more severe illness with a rapid onset of symptoms and increasing parasitemia progressing to massive intravascular hemolysis and renal failure

ETIOLOGY

- Vector: Deer tick, *Ixodes scapularis* (also known as *I. dammini*)
  1. Feeds on rodents during the spring and summer while in its larval and nymphal stages and on deer as an adult
  2. Requires a blood meal to mature to each stage, hence human infection
  3. During the warmer months in endemic areas, humans are readily infected while engaging in outdoor activities
- *B. microti* and *B. divergens* account for most human infections.
- In the U.S., cases caused by *B. microti* are acquired on offshore islands of the northeastern coast, including Nantucket Island, Cape Cod, and Martha's Vineyard in Massachusetts; Block Island in Rhode Island; and Long Island, Fire Island, and Shelter Island in New York; as well as the nearby mainland including Connecticut and New Jersey.
- Sporadic cases reported from California, Georgia, Maryland, Minnesota, Virginia, Wisconsin, and most recently the WA-1 strain from Washington State and the MO-1 strain from Missouri.
- *B. divergens* is implicated in human disease in Europe, where the disease remains rare and predominantly associated with asplenia.
- Majority of cases are asymptomatic.
- May be transmissible by transfusion, through platelets and erythrocytes.
- Mixed infections (*B. microti* and *Borrelia burgdorferi*, the causative agent of Lyme disease) are estimated to occur in 10% (Rhode Island and Connecticut) to 60% (New York) of cases.

DIAGNOSIS

DIFFERENTIAL DIAGNOSIS

- Amebiasis
- Ehrlichiosis
- Hepatic abscess
- Leptospirosis
- Malaria
- Salmonellosis, including typhoid fever
- Acute viral hepatitis
- Hemorrhagic fevers

WORKUP

Should be suspected in any febrile patient living or traveling in an endemic area, irrespective of exposure history to ticks or tick bites, especially if asplenic

LABORATORY TESTS

- The preferred method for diagnosing babesiosis is PCR using whole blood specimens.
- Babesial DNA by polymerase chain reaction (PCR) has comparable sensitivity and specificity to microscopic analysis of thin blood smears. PCR is more sensitive than smears at the onset of infection when parasite load may be minimal.
- Diagnosis achieved serologically by indirect immunofluorescence assay (IFA) is specific for *B. microti*.
  1. Assay is hampered by the inability to distinguish between exposed patients and those who are actively infected.
  2. Titer of ≥1:64 is indicative of seropositivity, whereas one ≥1:256 is considered diagnostic of acute infection.
  3. Immunoglobulin M indirect immunofluorescent-antibody test may be highly sensitive and specific for diagnosis.
- CBC to reveal mild to moderate pancytopenia
- Abnormally elevated serum chemistries, including creatinine, liver function profile, lactate dehydrogenase, and indirect and total bilirubin levels; hepatoglobin is low.
- Urinalysis to reveal proteinuria and hemoglobinuria
- Examination of Giemsa- or Wright-stained thin blood films for intraerythrocytic parasites
  1. In its classic, though infrequently seen, form a "tetrad" or "Maltese cross" composed of four daughter cells attached by cytoplasmic strands is observed (Fig. 1-137).
  2. More commonly, smaller forms composed of a single chromatin dot are eccentrically located within bluish cytoplasm.
  3. Parasitized erythrocytes may be multiply infected but not enlarged.
  4. Extra-erythrocytic forms may be seen.

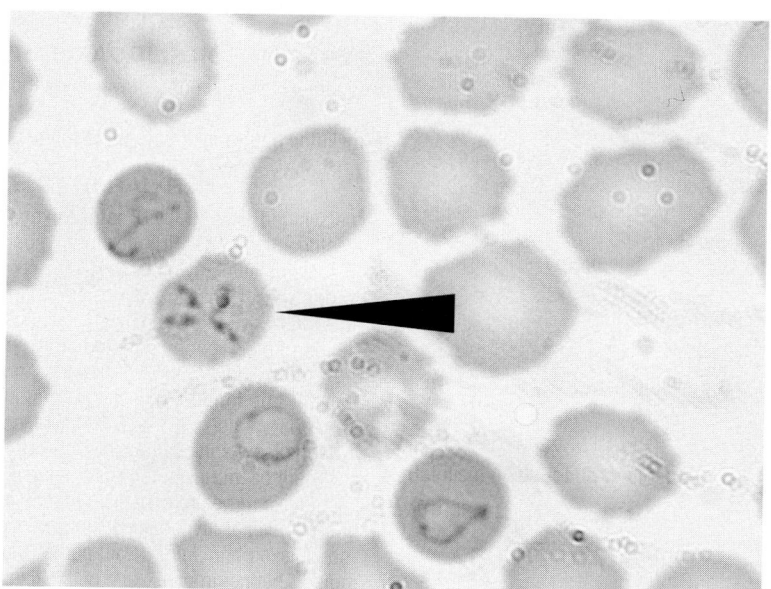

FIGURE 1-137 *Babesia* **spp.** Single and multiple intraerythrocytic parasites can be seen. The *arrow* marks a typical Maltese cross. (From Cohen J, Powderly WG: *Infectious diseases,* ed 2, St Louis, 2004, Mosby.)

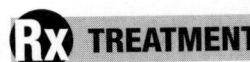

TREATMENT

NONPHARMACOLOGIC THERAPY
Supportive care with adequate hydration

ACUTE GENERAL Rx
- In patients with intact spleens: predominantly asymptomatic or if symptomatic, generally self-limited
- Therapy reserved for the severely ill patient, especially if asplenic, elderly, or immunosuppressed
- Combination of atovaquone 750 mg q12h and azithromycin 500 mg on day 1 and 250 mg per day thereafter for 7 to 10 days appears to be as effective as a regimen of clindamycin and quinine with fewer adverse reactions. This is the preferred regimen for mild disease.
- Combination of quinine sulfate 650 mg PO tid plus clindamycin 600 mg PO tid (600 mg parenterally qid) taken for 7 to 10 days: effective but may not eliminate parasites
- Severely ill patients are hospitalized and treated with clindamycin and quinine
- Exchange transfusions in addition to antimicrobial therapy: successful treatment for severe infections in asplenic patients associated with high levels of *B. microti* or *B. divergens* parasitemia. Exchange transfusion is recommended for patients with >10% parasitemia.
- Relapsed and immunocompromised patients may require a longer duration of therapy.

DISPOSITION
Prognosis is usually good and fatal outcomes are rare.

REFERRAL
- For prompt consultation with an infectious disease specialist if the diagnosis is acutely suspected, especially in the asplenic, elderly, or immunocompromised patient
- For hospitalization for the severely ill patient who may require exchange transfusions in addition to antibiotic therapy

PEARLS & CONSIDERATIONS

COMMENTS
- Prevention of babesiosis in asplenic or immunocompromised hosts is best achieved by avoidance of areas where the vector is endemic, especially May through September.
- If residence or travel in endemic areas is unavoidable, advise patients to perform daily cutaneous self-examination, wear light-colored clothing (to facilitate removal of ticks), tuck pants into socks, and apply tick repellent (diethyltoluamide and dimethylphthalate) to skin or clothing.
- Advise a daily inspection for ticks in family pets (e.g., cats and dogs).
- Infection with *B. divergens,* especially in the asplenic patient, is often fatal.
- Concurrent cases of babesiosis and Lyme disease have been documented—check for combined infection in severely ill patients.
- A combination of clindamycin and quinine has been successfully used to treat babesiosis during the third trimester of pregnancy without incurring apparent adverse effect on the fetus.
- In 2011 the CDC added babesiosis to the list of nationally notifiable diseases.

SUGGESTED READINGS
available at www.expertconsult.com

RELATED CONTENT
Babesiosis (Patient Information)

AUTHOR: **PATRICIA CRISTOFARO, M.D.**

BASIC INFORMATION

DEFINITION

Baker's cyst is a fluid-filled popliteal bursa located along the medial border of the popliteal fossa. It is an extension of the semimembranosus bursa posteriorly (see Fig 1-138).

SYNONYMS

Popliteal synovial cyst

ICD-9CM CODES
727.51 Baker's cyst (knee)

EPIDEMIOLOGY & DEMOGRAPHICS

- Most are asymptomatic and incidentally found on imaging exams.
- Occurs at all ages, most commonly between the ages of 35 and 70, with increasing frequency as one ages.
- Incidence is unknown.
- Between 2% and 6% of all patients believed to have clinical deep venous thrombosis (DVT) have symptomatic Baker's cysts.
- Approximately 5% to 40% of MRIs performed for osteoarthritis or internal derangement reveal popliteal cysts.

PHYSICAL FINDINGS & CLINICAL PRESENTATION

- Pain in the popliteal space
- Knee swelling or stiffness
- Leg edema
- Prominence of the popliteal fossa
- Decreased range of motion of the knee
- Locking of the knee
- Foucher's sign: The cyst becomes hard with knee extension and soft with knee flexion.
- Neuropathic lancinating pains radiating from the knee down the back of the leg
- Pain/discomfort with prolonged standing and hyperflexion of the knee
- Presence of associated DVT

ETIOLOGY

- Believed to represent fluid distention of the bursal sac separating the semimembranous tendon from the medial head of the gastrocnemius.
- May represent a true cyst but more often results from the posterior herniation of a tense

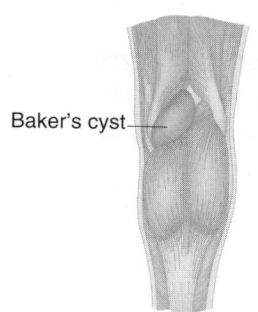

FIGURE 1-138 Baker's cyst is an extension of the semimembranosus bursa posteriorly. This bursa is often connected with a joint cavity. (From Marx J: *Rosen's emergency medicine: concepts and clinical practice,* ed 6, Philadelphia, 2006, Saunders.)

knee effusion. Thus a Baker's cyst usually denotes increased intraarticular pressure from underlying joint disease.
- In children, Baker's cysts are believed to result from trauma and irritation of the knee.
- In adults, Baker's cysts are usually associated with pathologic changes of the knee joint, such as the following:
  - Rheumatoid arthritis (RA)
  - Osteoarthritis of the knee
  - Meniscal tears
  - Patellofemoral chondromalacia
  - Fracture
  - Gout
  - Pseudogout
  - Infection (tuberculosis)

DIAGNOSIS

Baker's cyst frequently mimics DVT and is sometimes referred to as *pseudothrombophlebitis syndrome.*

DIFFERENTIAL DIAGNOSIS

- DVT
- Popliteal artery aneurysm
- Abscess
- Tumor (sarcomas/lymphomas)
- Lymphadenopathy
- Varicosity
- Synovial cysts
- Ganglion cysts

WORKUP

The diagnosis can be made by physical examination alone. However, anyone suspected of having a popliteal cyst should undergo imaging studies to exclude other causes.

LABORATORY TESTS

Blood tests are not specific in the diagnosis of Baker's cysts.

IMAGING STUDIES

- Plain radiographs (AP and lateral views) may show calcification in a solid tumor or in the posterior meniscal area.
- Ultrasound (Fig. 1-139) is safe, portable, cost effective, and excludes other clinically important causes of popliteal fossa pathology, including DVT.
- MRI of the knee identifies coexisting joint pathology (e.g., osteoarthritis, torn meniscus).

TREATMENT

NONPHARMACOLOGIC THERAPY

- Rest
- Strenuous activity avoidance
- Knee immobilization necessary in some cases

ACUTE GENERAL Rx

- NSAIDs can be used to treat Baker's cyst caused by RA, gout, and pseudogout.
- Arthrocentesis with intraarticular injection or injection of the cyst with corticosteroids, triamcinolone acetonide 40 mg, is sometimes tried.

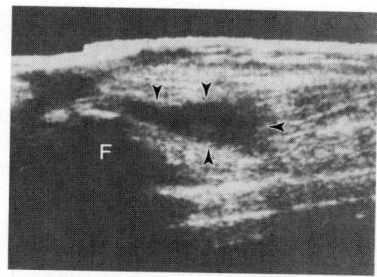

FIGURE 1-139 Sonography of a popliteal cyst. Sagittal sonographic section through the popliteal space in this patient demonstrates a sonolucent fluid collection *(arrowheads)* posterior and inferior to the medial femoral condyle *(F).* (From DeLee D, Drez D [eds]: *DeLee and Drez's orthopaedic sports medicine,* ed 2, Philadelphia, 2003, Saunders.)

CHRONIC Rx

- The majority of Baker's cysts are successfully treated conservatively.
- Surgical procedures addressing the underlying cause include:
  1. Arthroscopic surgery to remove loose cartilaginous fragment
  2. Partial or total meniscectomy
  3. Open excision of the cyst

DISPOSITION

- Baker's cyst may spontaneously resolve without treatment.
- Complications of Baker's cysts include:
  1. Rupture
  2. DVT
  3. Nerve impingement resulting in posterior tibial nerve entrapment, anterior compartment syndrome, or posterior compartment syndrome
  4. Popliteal artery occlusion

REFERRAL

Rheumatology or orthopedics if surgery is contemplated

PEARLS & CONSIDERATIONS

- A Baker's cyst may serve as a protective mechanism for the knee. Intrinsic intraarticular disorders cause joint effusion. The knee effusion is displaced into the Baker's cyst, thus reducing potentially destructive pressure in the joint space.

COMMENTS

Baker's cyst and DVT can coexist. It is imperative to exclude the diagnosis of DVT before discharging the patient.

SUGGESTED READINGS
available at www.expertconsult.com

RELATED CONTENT

Baker Cyst (Patient Information)

AUTHORS: **SUNIT-PREET CHAUDHRY, M.D.,** and **RICHARD REGNANTE, M.D.**

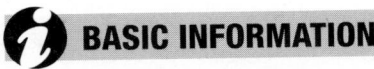

DEFINITION

Balanitis is an inflammation of the superficial tissues of the penile head (glans penis). If the foreskin (prepuce) is involved, it is called *balanoposthitis*.

ICD-9CM CODES
112.2 Balanitis

EPIDEMIOLOGY & DEMOGRAPHICS

INCIDENCE (IN U.S.): More common in uncircumcised males and in diabetic patients
PREVALENCE (IN U.S.): One study reports that 11% of adult men seen in a urology clinic and 3% of male children (mostly uncircumcised) have balanitis.
PREDOMINANT SEX: Almost exclusive to males but can affect clitoris
PEAK INCIDENCE: All ages, especially in sexually active men. It occurs in ¼ of male sex partners of women infected with *Candida*.

PHYSICAL FINDINGS & CLINICAL PRESENTATION

- Itching and tenderness
- Pain, dysuria, and local edema
- Rarely, ulceration and lymph node enlargement
- Severe ulcerations leading to superimposed bacterial infections
- Inability to void: unusual, but a more distressing and serious complication

ETIOLOGY

- Causes include infectious agents, skin disorders, or miscellaneous.
- Infectious diseases: *Candida species (40%)*, *Neiserria gonorrhoeae*, HPV, herpes simplex, *Gardnerella vaginalis*, *Treponema pallidum* (syphilis), HIV, *Trichomonas*, *Staphylococcus aureus*, anaerobic bacteria
- Skin disorders: circinate balanitis **of Reiter's syndrome,** lichen sclerosis
- Miscellaneous: poor hygiene, causing erosion of tissue with erythema and promoting growth of *Candida albicans* (Fig. 1-140), trauma (zippers, urinary catheters), allergic reactions to condoms or medications

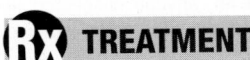 **DIAGNOSIS**

DIFFERENTIAL DIAGNOSIS

- Leukoplakia
- Nummular eczema
- Balanitis xerotica obliterans
- Psoriasis
- Carcinoma of the penis
- Plasma cell balanitis (noninfectious)
- Erythroplasia of Queyrat
- Nodular scabies
- Circinate balanitis (Reiter's syndrome)

WORKUP

- Sexually active males: assessment for evidence of other sexually transmitted diseases
- Biopsy if lesions do not heal

LABORATORY TESTS

- VDRL for syphilis
- Serum glucose to rule out diabetes
- Wet mount for *Trichomonas*
- KOH prep for yeast
- Microbial culture to rule out STD

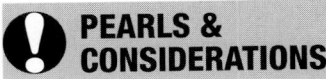 **TREATMENT**

NONPHARMACOLOGIC THERAPY

- Maintenance of meticulous hygiene
- Retraction and bathing of prepuce several times a day
- Warm sitz baths to ease edema and erythema
- Consideration of circumcision, especially when symptoms are severe or recurrent
- With Foley catheters, strict catheter care strongly advised

ACUTE GENERAL Rx

- Metronidazole 2 g PO as a single dose or Fluconazole 150 mg PO × 1 or itraconazole 200 mg PO bid × 1 day
- Clotrimazole 1% cream applied topically twice daily to affected areas
- Bacitracin or Neosporin ointment applied topically 4 times daily
- With more severe bacterial superinfection: cephalexin 500 mg PO qid
- Topical corticosteroids added 4 times daily if dermatitis severe
- Patients with suspected urinary tract infections: trimethoprim-sulfa DS twice daily or ciprofloxacin 500 mg PO bid after obtaining appropriate cultures

DISPOSITION

Balanitis is often self-limited and usually responds to conservative therapy; if it does not improve, consider circinate balanitis of Reiter's syndrome, nodular scabies, and primary skin lesions including skin carcinoma.

PEARLS & CONSIDERATIONS

Don't forget about nodular scabies involving the prepubic area—examine the region carefully for burrows and tracks of *Sarcoptes scabiei*.

REFERRAL

- For surgical evaluation for circumcision if symptoms are recurrent, especially if phimosis or meatitis occurs (NOTE: Severe phimosis with an inability to void may require prompt slit drainage.)
- For biopsy to rule out other diagnosis such as premalignant or malignant lesions if lesions are not healing

SUGGESTED READINGS
available at www.expertconsult.com

RELATED CONTENT
Balanitis (Patient Information)
AUTHOR: **GLENN G. FORT, M.D., M.P.H.**

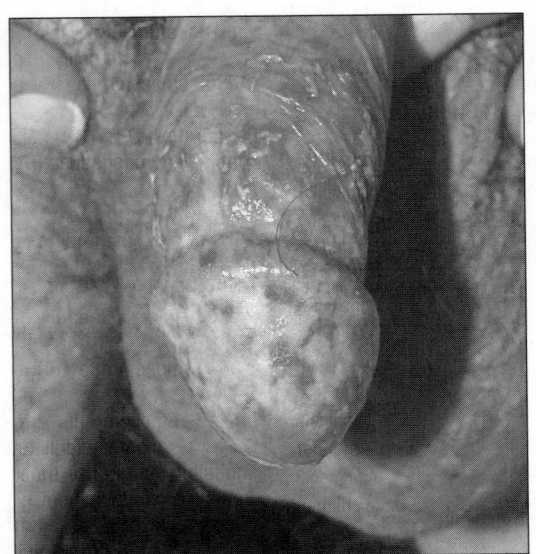

FIGURE 1-140 Candidal balanitis. (From White GM, Cox NH [eds]: *Diseases of the skin: a color atlas and text*, ed 2, St Louis, 2006, Mosby.)

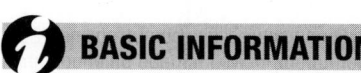

ℹ️ BASIC INFORMATION

DEFINITION

Barrett's esophagus occurs when the squamo-columnar junction is displaced proximal to the gastroesophageal junction and the squamous lining of the lower esophagus is replaced by metaplastic columnar epithelium, which predisposes to the development of esophageal adenocarcinoma. The presence of intestinalized epithelium is still considered essential for the diagnosis. While cardia-type epithelium has been shown to predispose to esophageal cancer, recent data show that the absolute annual risk for esophageal carcinoma in Barrett's esophagus is 0.12%, which is much lower than the assumed risk of 0.5% that is the basis for current surveillance guidelines.

SYNONYMS

Esophagus, Barrett's
Esophagus, columnar-lined
Ulcer, Barrett's

ICD-9CM CODES
530.85 Barrett's esophagus

EPIDEMIOLOGY & DEMOGRAPHICS

- Male/female ratio of 4:1
- Mean age of onset is 40 yr, with a mean age range of diagnosis of 55 to 60 yr
- Occurs more frequently in white and Hispanic individuals than in African American individuals, with a ratio of 10 to 20:1
- Mean prevalence of 5% to 15% in patients undergoing endoscopy (EGD) for symptoms of gastroesophageal reflux disease (GERD)
- Obesity may be an independent risk factor
- Prevalence rate in asymptomatic cohorts ranges from 5% to 25%

PHYSICAL FINDINGS & CLINICAL PRESENTATION

SYMPTOMS:
- Chronic heartburn
- Dysphagia with solid food
- May be an incidental finding on EGD in patients without reflux symptoms
- Less frequent: chest pain, hematemesis, melena
- Patients may be asymptomatic.

PHYSICAL FINDINGS:
- Nonspecific; can be completely normal
- Epigastric tenderness on palpation

ETIOLOGY

- Metaplasia is thought to result from reepithelialization of esophageal tissue injured as a result of chronic GERD.
- Patients with Barrett's esophagus tend to have more severe esophageal motility disturbances (decreased lower esophageal sphincter pressure, ineffective peristalsis) and greater esophageal acid exposure on 24-hour pH monitoring.
- Intraesophageal bile reflux may also play a role in the pathogenesis.

- Familial clustering of GERD and Barrett's esophagus suggests a genetic predisposition, but no gene has yet been identified. Early data suggest that patients who develop Barrett's are genetically predisposed to a severe inflammatory response to GERD.
- Progression from metaplasia to carcinoma is associated with changes in gene structure and expression, including the Caudal-related homeobox family of transcription factors (CDX1 and CDX2) and the tumor suppressors p16 (CDKN2A) and TP53.

Dx DIAGNOSIS

DIFFERENTIAL DIAGNOSIS
- GERD, uncomplicated
- Erosive esophagitis
- Gastritis
- Peptic ulcer disease
- Angina
- Malignancy
- Stricture or Schatzki's ring

WORKUP
- The Practice Parameters Committee of the American College of Gastroenterology (ACG) has suggested that the highest yield for Barrett's esophagus screening is in older (age >50 yr) white men with longstanding heartburn. The American Gastroenterological Association Medical Position Panel gave a weak recommendation for screening patients with multiple risk factors, including age over 50, male sex, white race, chronic GERD, hiatal hernia, elevated body mass index, and intraabdominal distribution of body fat. General population screening is not currently recommended. The benefit of screening in high-risk populations is not established. Although screening has become standard of practice in some communities, the effectiveness of screening using current techniques is controversial because it may not improve mortality rates from adenocarcinoma or be cost-effective.
- EGD with biopsy is necessary for diagnosis.
- Wireless esophageal capsule endoscopy may detect Barrett's, but with a lower sensitivity and specificity than EGD. Imaging studies are nonspecific and insensitive for the diagnosis.
- Diagnosis requires the presence of metaplastic columnar epithelium proximal to the gastroesophageal junction (Fig. 1-141). Longer-segment Barrett's esophagus is more readily diagnosed (Fig. 1-142) At least two expert gastrointestinal pathologists should concur if dysplasia is diagnosed.
- Intestinal metaplasia of the gastric cardia is not Barrett's esophagus and does not have the same risk for malignancy.
- A variety of biomarkers are being evaluated to assist with diagnosis and to better understand progression of disease, prediction of response to therapy, or prognosis.

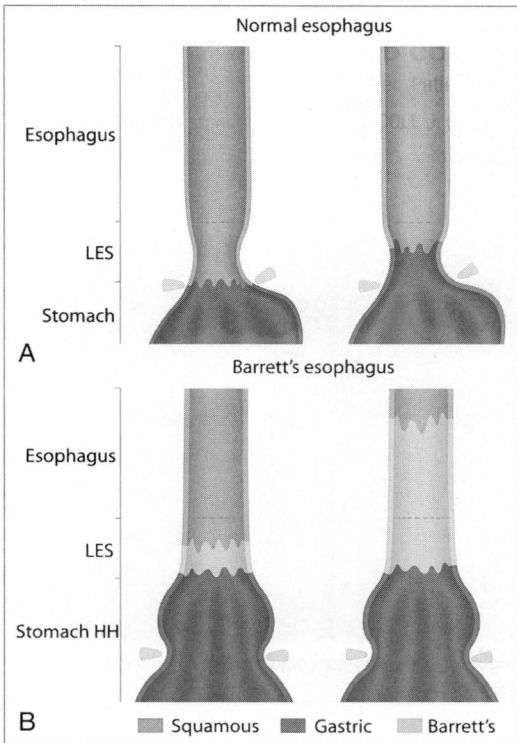

FIGURE 1-141 Anatomic landmarks of the normal LES region (A) and of Barrett's esophagus (B). Note that gastric mucosa is very common and normal in the LES region and that in Barrett's esophagus, the squamocolumnar junction is not only proximally displaced within the tubular esophagus, but that the intervening mucosa is composed of intestinalized Barrett's metaplastic epithelium. *HH,* Hiatial hernia. (From Silverburg SG: *Principles of practice of surgical pathology and cytopathology,* ed 4, New York, 2006, Churchill Livingstone.)

- Screening for *Helicobacter pylori* infection in patients with GERD and Barrett's esophagus is not recommended.

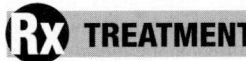 **TREATMENT**

The goal is to control GERD symptoms and maintain healed mucosa.

NONPHARMACOLOGIC THERAPY

Nonpharmacologic therapy includes lifestyle modifications; elevating head of bed; and avoiding chocolate, tobacco, caffeine, mints, and certain drugs (see "Gastroesophageal Reflux Disease").

ACUTE GENERAL Rx

- Proton pump inhibitors are the most effective treatment for GERD. Therapy should be dosed to control symptoms and/or to promote healing of endoscopic signs of disease.
- If patient is asymptomatic and incidentally found to have Barrett's esophagus, medication use may be considered.

CHRONIC Rx

- Chronic acid suppression is often necessary to control symptoms and maintain healing.
- Antireflux surgery may be considered for management of GERD and associated sequelae, but it has not been proven to be superior to medical therapy. Patients continue to require endoscopic surveillance of their esophagus.
- When GERD is controlled by either medical or surgical therapy, ablation of metaplastic epithelium usually leads to replacement by normal squamous epithelium. Because only a minority of patients with Barrett's esophagus progress to high-grade dysplasia or carcinoma, these techniques cannot be currently recommended in patients with Barrett's esophagus without dysplasia.
- Endoscopic eradication therapy may be offered to patients with low-grade dysplasia, but a long-term benefit has not been clearly established.
- Radiofrequency ablation, thermal ablation techniques, or photodynamic therapy, combined with endoscopic mucosal resection of visible mucosal irregularities, are accepted approaches to the treatment of patients with Barrett's esophagus and high-grade dysplasia, in conjunction with aggressive surveillance and eradication of all remaining Barrett's epithelium. Endoscopic therapy is preferred over surgical treatment in properly staged individuals. These therapies may even be considered for patients with focal intramucosal carcinoma, if properly staged (T1SM1 or lower). Cryotherapy is currently being evaluated for the complete eradication of both dysplasia and intestinal metaplasia and reduced risk for disease progression. All these options run the risk for residual or buried metaplasia.
- Surgical resection may be offered for multifocal high-grade dysplasia or carcinoma that has extended into the submucosa. Mortality appears to be lower with experienced surgeons operating in high-volume centers.
- Patients with cardiovascular risk factors may be considered for low-dose aspirin therapy for chemoprevention of esophageal adenocarcinoma.

DISPOSITION

- The relative risk of developing esophageal adenocarcinoma for a patient with Barrett's esophagus, as compared with the general population is 11.3, a substantial drop from the increase by a factor of 30 or 40 estimated in early reports.

- The risk of progression from untreated Barrett's with high-grade dysplasia to esophageal adenocarcinoma ranges from 6% to 19% per year.
- Frequency of monitoring is controversial; no studies have proved that surveillance increases life expectancy; some studies have suggested that close adherence to surveillance protocols is associated with higher rates of dysplasia and cancer detection.
- Patients with Barrett's esophagus should undergo surveillance EGD and systematic four-quadrant biopsy at intervals determined by the presence and grade of dysplasia. All mucosal abnormalities should undergo biopsy. Patients who have had two consecutive EGDs showing no dysplasia should have follow-up every 3 to 5 yr. Patients with low-grade dysplasia should have extensive mucosal sampling within 6 mo and follow-up every 6 to 12 mo. Patients with high-grade dysplasia should have expert confirmation and extensive mucosal sampling. High-grade dysplasia with visible mucosal irregularities should be removed by endoscopic mucosal resection. Consider intensive surveillance every 3 mo. Endoscopic treatment is preferred over intensive surveillance in patients with high-grade dysplasia.
- Patients should be treated aggressively for GERD before surveillance.

REFERRAL

- Consider EGD with biopsy in patients (particularly white men >50 yr old) with multiple risk factors who have not had previous EGD.
- Refer patients with GERD for evaluation if "red flag" symptoms are present (dysphagia, odynophagia, weight loss, vomiting, early satiety, GI bleeding, iron deficiency).
- Refer patients with biopsy-proved Barrett's esophagus for surveillance.
- For those with high-grade dysplasia, refer for ablative therapy with endoscopic mucosal resection if appropriate, followed by intensive surveillance. Esophageal resection may be considered.

SUGGESTED READINGS

available at www.expertconsult.com

RELATED CONTENT

Esophageal Tumors (Related Key Topic)
Barrett's Esophagus (Patient Information)
AUTHOR: **HARLAN G. RICH, M.D., F.A.C.P., A.F.A.F.**

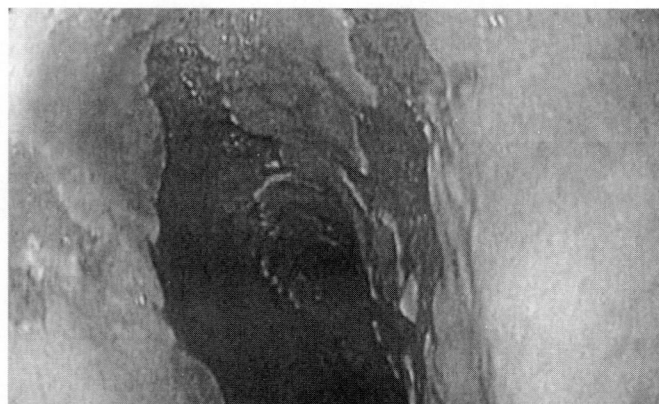

FIGURE 1-142 Long-segment Barrett's esophagus. (From Cameron JL, Cameron AM: *Current surgical therapy,* ed 10, Philadelphia, 2011, Saunders.)

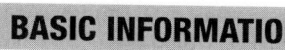

BASIC INFORMATION

DEFINITION

Basal cell carcinoma (BCC) is a malignant tumor of the skin arising from basal cells of the lower epidermis and adnexal structures. It may be classified as one of six types: nodular, superficial, pigmented, cystic, sclerosing or morphreaform, and nevoid. The most common type is nodular (21%); the least common is morpheaform (1%). A mixed pattern is present in approximately 40% of cases. BCC advances by direct expansion and destroys normal tissue.

SYNONYMS

BCC

ICD-9CM CODES

179.9 Basal cell carcinoma, site unspecified
173.3 Basal cell carcinoma, face
173.4 Basal cell carcinoma, neck, scalp
173.5 Basal cell carcinoma, trunk
173.6 Basal cell carcinoma of the limb
173.7 Basal cell carcinoma, lower limb

EPIDEMIOLOGY & DEMOGRAPHICS

- Most common cutaneous neoplasm
- 85% of cases appear on the head and neck region
- Most common site: nose (30%)
- Increased incidence with age >40 yr
- Increased incidence in men
- Risk factors: fair skin, increased sun exposure, use of tanning salons with ultraviolet A or B radiation, history of irradiation (e.g., Hodgkin's disease), personal or family history of skin cancer, impaired immune system

PHYSICAL FINDINGS & CLINICAL PRESENTATION

Variable with the histologic type:
- Nodular: dome-shaped, painless lesion that may become multilobular and frequently ulcerates (rodent ulcer); prominent telangiec-tatic vessels are noted on the surface. Border is translucent, elevated, pearly white (Fig. 1-143). Some nodular BCCs may contain pigmentation, giving an appearance similar to a melanoma.
- Superficial: circumscribed, scaling, black appearance with a thin, raised, pearly-white border (Fig. 1-144); a crust and erosions may be present. Occurs most frequently on the trunk and extremities.
- Morpheaform: flat or slightly raised yellowish or white appearance (similar to localized scleroderma); appearance similar to scars; surface has a waxy consistency.

DIAGNOSIS

DIFFERENTIAL DIAGNOSIS

- Keratoacanthoma
- Melanoma (pigmented BCC)
- Xeroderma pigmentosa
- Basal cell nevus syndrome
- Molluscum contagiosum
- Sebaceous hyperplasia
- Psoriasis

WORKUP

Biopsy to confirm diagnosis

TREATMENT

Variable with tumor size, location, and cell type:
- Excision surgery: preferred method for large tumors with well-defined borders on the legs, cheeks, forehead, and trunk.
- Mohs' micrographic surgery: preferred for lesions in high-risk areas (e.g., nose, eyelid), very large primary tumors, recurrent BCCs, and tumors with poorly defined clinical margins.
- Electrodesiccation and curettage: useful for small (<6 mm) nodular BCCs.
- Cryosurgery with liquid nitrogen: useful in BCCs of the superficial and nodular types with clearly definable margins; no clear advan-tages over the other forms of therapy; generally reserved for uncomplicated tumors.
- Radiation therapy: generally used for BCCs in areas requiring preservation of normal surrounding tissues for cosmetic reasons (e.g., around lips); also useful in patients who cannot tolerate surgical procedures or for large lesions and surgical failures.
- Imiquimod 5% cream can be used for treatment of small, superficial BCCs of the trunk and extremities. Efficacy rate is approximately 80%. Its main advantage is lack of scarring, which must be weighed against higher cure rates with surgical intervention.
- Vismodegib, an orally active hedgehog pathway inhibitor has been FDA approved for metastatic BCC, recurrent basal call carcinoma post-surgery, and locally advanced BCC in patients who are not candidates for surgery or radiation. Dose is 150 mg PO qd. Cost of 1-month supply exceeds $7000.

DISPOSITION

- More than 90% of patients are cured; however, periodic evaluation for at least 5 yr is necessary because of increased risk of recurrence of another BCC (>40% risk within 5 yr of treatment).
- A lesion is considered low risk if it is <1.5 cm in diameter, is nodular or cystic, is not in a difficult-to-treat area (H zone of face), and has not been previously treated.
- Nodular and superficial BCCs are the least aggressive.
- Morpheaform lesions have the highest incidence of positive tumor margins (>30%) and the greatest recurrence rate.

SUGGESTED READING
available at www.expertconsult.com

RELATED CONTENT

Basal Cell Skin Cancer (Patient Information)

AUTHOR: **FRED F. FERRI, M.D.**

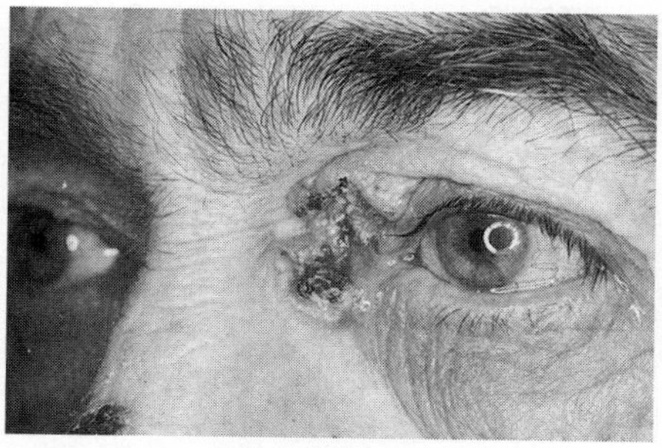

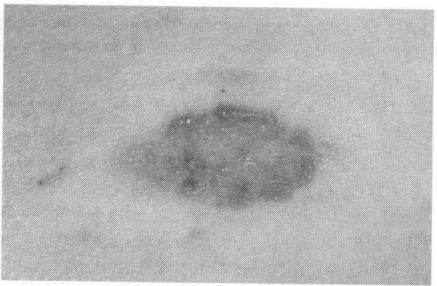

FIGURE 1-143 Basal cell carcinoma. Note rolled translucent border and central ulceration in typical facial location. (From Noble J et al: *Textbook of primary care medicine,* ed 3, St Louis, 2001, Mosby.)

FIGURE 1-144 Superficial variant of basal cell carcinoma. Multiple lesions are common with this variant, often on the trunk. Closer examination shows the typical raised pearly edge. (From White GM, Cox NH [eds]: *Diseases of the skin: a color atlas and text,* ed 2, St Louis, 2006, Mosby.)

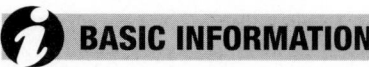

BASIC INFORMATION

DEFINITION

A bedbug's bite is a wound caused by the penetration of the bedbug mouthpiece into the skin as the insect feeds on blood from vessels or extravasated blood from the damaged surrounding tissue. The saliva of the bedbug contains pharmacologically active substances responsible for a spectrum of undesirable skin reactions depending on the individual.

SYNONYMS

Insect bite
Bedbug *Cimex lectularius* bite

ICD-9CM CODES
919.4 Insect bite w/o infection (may also code based on bite location)

EPIDEMIOLOGY & DEMOGRAPHICS

- Traditionally, bedbugs were considered more common in poorer areas, but they are now increasingly found in areas of frequent travel.
- Bedbug infestations may spread among multifamily and institutional facilities with shared walls and are consequently difficult to eradicate.
- Reports of bedbug infestations have increased dramatically in the U.S., as well as worldwide, likely because of the decreased use of pesticides and increased international travel.
- Bedbugs are attracted to carbon dioxide gas and warm bodies.
- Bedbugs do not have a preference for specific age groups, ethnicity, or sex.
- Studies have shown increased sensitivity of cutaneous reaction in previous bite victims.

PHYSICAL FINDINGS AND CLINICAL PRESENTATION

- Firm, purpuric or erythematous macules, urticaria, papules (Fig. E1-145), or bullae may be present. Bites are often inflammatory and pruritic, although bedbug-naive individuals may be asymptomatic to their first bites.
- Bite may have a central hemorrhagic punctum.
- Victim may observe a linear series of three bites ("breakfast, lunch, and dinner").
- As bedbug bites usually do not penetrate clothing, bite distribution is generally on areas of exposed skin. Otherwise, there is no preferential distribution.

ETIOLOGY

- The *Cimex lectularius* species, also known as the common bedbug, feeds on mammals and birds. *Cimex hemipterus* is a tropical species that bites mostly humans, and hybrid species of the two insects exist. Both generally feed nocturnally on the blood of sleeping humans. The adult bedbug is wingless and about 5 to 7 mm in length. It has a modified mouthpart for piercing and sucking that usually leaves a bite mark of papular urticarial presentation to exposed areas of skin. Bedbugs have weak appendages for latching on to their hosts and are not usually transported from person to person.
- The saliva of the bedbug contains nitrophorin that enables vasodilation, an anticoagulant that interferes with production of coagulation factor Xa, a salivary apyrase that inhibits platelet aggregation, and an anesthetic. Consequently, the host often does not feel the bite until the effects have worn off.

DIAGNOSIS

DIFFERENTIAL DIAGNOSIS

Scabies, flea and mite bites, vesicular disorders, delusional parasitosis, dermatitis herpetiformis, pemphigus herpetiformis, ecthyma, drug eruptions

WORKUP

- Workup begins with history and physical for clinical symptoms and environmental findings.
- Victims should carefully scrutinize the bedroom for signs of bedbug infestation. One may encounter fecal smears or flecks of blood on bed linens, inside furniture cracks and crevices, and behind peeling wallpaper. Bedbugs may travel as far as 20 feet for a meal. Densely infested rooms may also have a distinctive, pungent, soda syrup–like odor.

LABORATORY TESTS

- No specific tests recommended except for identification of the insect.
- The histology of bedbug bites is similar to other insect bites. Perivascular infiltrate of lymphocytes, histiocytes, eosinophils, and mast cells are seen within the upper dermis. One may also observe collagen bundles with interstitial eosinophils, dermal edema, and extravasated erythrocytes.

IMAGING STUDIES

None

TREATMENT
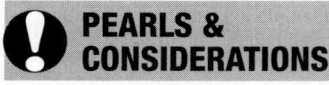

- Treatment of bites is often not necessary. Bites may self-resolve within a week for milder cases and a few weeks for more severe cases.
- Topical glucocorticoids or systemic antihistamines are appropriate in patients with severe pruritus from the bedbug bite.
  - triamcinolone cream 0.1%, apply thin film to affected areas bid
  - chlorpheniramine 4 mg PO at bedtime (adults), 2 mg PO at bedtime (children)
- Insecticides may be effective in eradicating the bedbug, but growing resistance has been seen and multi-insecticide therapy is recommended.
  - Use permethrin spray for clothing and bedsheets or bednets
  - Diethyltoluamide (DEET): Be wary of toxic levels in children when used at high concentrations.
  - Deltamethrin and chlorfenapyr are two common insecticides used.
  - Please consult a pest control professional for safe eradication.

NONPHARMACOLOGIC THERAPY

Vacuuming is effective in removing bedbugs but does not remove the eggs. Wash bedsheets and clothing in hot water with detergent with at least 20 minutes in a dryer. Bedbugs have a high thermal death point of 45° C and also may survive at temperatures as low as 7° C. Coating bedposts with antifriction or adhesive substances such as petrolatum or duct tape may hinder bedbugs from gaining access to the bed.

ACUTE GENERAL Rx

Immunologic response is dependent on immunocompetence and individual sensitivity to the salivary components of the bedbug bite. Often, patients with papular urticaria have IgG antibodies to specific bedbug proteins. IgE antibodies may also mediate bullae formation. Anaphylaxis and death from bites is rare but documented in literature.

DISPOSITION

Patient may resume normal activity and lifestyle. Travelers should inspect their clothing and suitcases before returning home.

BEDBUGS AS POTENTIAL VECTORS

The bedbug has been studied extensively as a potential vector for human pathogens such as HIV and viral hepatitis, as well as many other diseases. To date, there is no evidence of transmission from an infected bedbug to a human.

PEARLS & CONSIDERATIONS

COMMENTS

- Bedbugs are an increasing source of anguish and frustration for humans, and clinicians should evaluate for signs of stress and depression.
- A combination of chemical and physical intervention is often necessary for complete eradication. All hiding areas must be carefully inspected and cleaned. Treatment may include pesticides plus laundering, heat, freezing, and vacuuming.

SUGGESTED READINGS
available at www.expertconsult.com

RELATED CONTENT
Bedbugs (Patient Information)

AUTHOR: **STEPHANIE W. CHOW, M.D.**

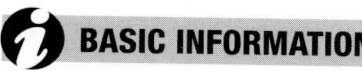

BASIC INFORMATION

DEFINITION

Behçet's disease is a chronic, relapsing, inflammatory disorder characterized by the presence of recurrent oral aphthous ulcers, genital ulcers, uveitis, and skin lesions (Fig. 1-146).

SYNONYMS

Behçet's syndrome

ICD-9CM CODES

136.1 Behçet's syndrome

EPIDEMIOLOGY & DEMOGRAPHICS

PREVALENCE:
- Behçet's disease is observed in two different geographic locations.
  1. One region consists of Eastern Asia, Turkey, and the Mediterranean basin.
     - Prevalence ranges from 13 to 17 cases per 100,000 persons.
     - Turkey has the highest prevalence at up to 300 cases per 100,000 persons.
  2. The second region consists of North America and Northern Europe.
     - Prevalence ranges from 0.5 to 17 cases per 100,000 persons. Germany has the greatest prevalence.
     - Prevalence of Behçet's disease in the U.S. is 6.6 cases per 100,000 persons.
- In these regions, the prevalence of HLA-B51 is greater in patients with Behçet's disease.

PREDOMINANT SEX: Equal sex distribution

GENETICS: No clear pattern of inheritance can be determined. Familial disease was noted in 15% of affected children.

PHYSICAL FINDINGS & CLINICAL PRESENTATION

- Behçet's disease typically affects individuals in the third to fourth decade of life and primarily presents with painful aphthous oral ulcers. The ulcers occur in crops measuring 2 to 12 mm and are found on the mucous membrane of the cheek, gingiva, tongue, pharynx, and soft palate.
- Genital and perianal ulcers are similar to the oral ulcers. They may result in scarring.
- Decreased vision secondary to uveitis, keratitis, and retinal artery occlusion with ischemia may be followed by neovascularization, vitreous hemorrhage and contraction, glaucoma, and retinal detachment. Younger male individuals are at greater risk for ocular involvement.
- Skin findings (41% to 97%) include nodular lesions, which are histologically divided to erythema nodosum–like lesions, pseudofolliculitis, papulopustular lesions, acneiform nodules, or pyoderma gangrenosum–like lesions (cutaneous aphthosis).
- Intermittent, symmetric oligoarthritis (40% to 70%) is the most common; ankylosing spondylitis or arthralgias may occur.
- Central nervous system (CNS; 30% in U.S. and 5% in Turkey) meningeal findings including headache, fever, and stiff neck can occur. Cerebellar ataxia, pseudobulbar palsy, and dementia occur with involvement of the brainstem.
- Vascular involvement (25% to 30%), arterial and venous, of all sizes may cause systemic arterial vasculitis (aneurysms and occlusions), pulmonary artery vasculitis, venous occlusions (including superficial, deep, cerebral, portal, and mesenterial veins), pulmonary embolus, right ventricle thrombosis, and Budd-Chiari syndrome.
- GI involvement is more common in Japanese individuals; ulcerative lesions primarily involve distal ileum and cecum, but any region can be affected. GI lesions tend to perforate or bleed and may recur after surgery.

ETIOLOGY

The etiology of Behçet's disease is unknown. An immune-related vasculitis, a perivascular inflammation, or both are thought to lead to many of the manifestations of Behçet's disease. Multiple triggers for this process have been investigated, including herpes simplex virus infection, streptococcal antigen, and others.

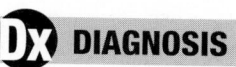 ## DIAGNOSIS

According to the International Study Group for Behçet's Disease, the diagnosis of Behçet's disease is established when oral ulcerations recur at least three times in one 12-mo period plus at least two of the following conditions in the absence of other systemic diseases:
- Recurrent genital ulceration
- Eye lesions
- Skin lesions
- Positive pathergy test (erythematous papules or pustules [>2 mm in diameter] at sterile needle injection sites after 24 to 48 hours)

DIFFERENTIAL DIAGNOSIS

- Inflammatory bowel disease (ulcerative colitis and Crohn's disease)
- Sprue disease
- Herpes simplex infection
- Benign aphthous stomatitis
- Cyclic neutropenia
- Acquired immune deficiency syndrome (AIDS)
- Systemic lupus erythematosus
- Reiter's syndrome
- Ankylosing spondylitis
- Hypereosinophilic syndrome
- Sweet's syndrome
- Lichen planus
- Pemphigoid

WORKUP

The diagnosis of Behçet's disease is a clinical diagnosis. Laboratory tests and x-ray imaging may be helpful in working up the complications of Behçet's disease or excluding other diseases in the differential.

LABORATORY TESTS

No diagnostic laboratory tests for Behçet's disease exist. The measurements of T-cell proliferative response to heat shock protein (HSP) and impaired fibrinolytic activity have been proposed for the diagnosis of Behçet's disease, but the value of testing has not been confirmed.

IMAGING STUDIES

CT scan, MRI, and angiography are useful for detecting CNS and vascular lesions.

B

Diseases and Disorders

I

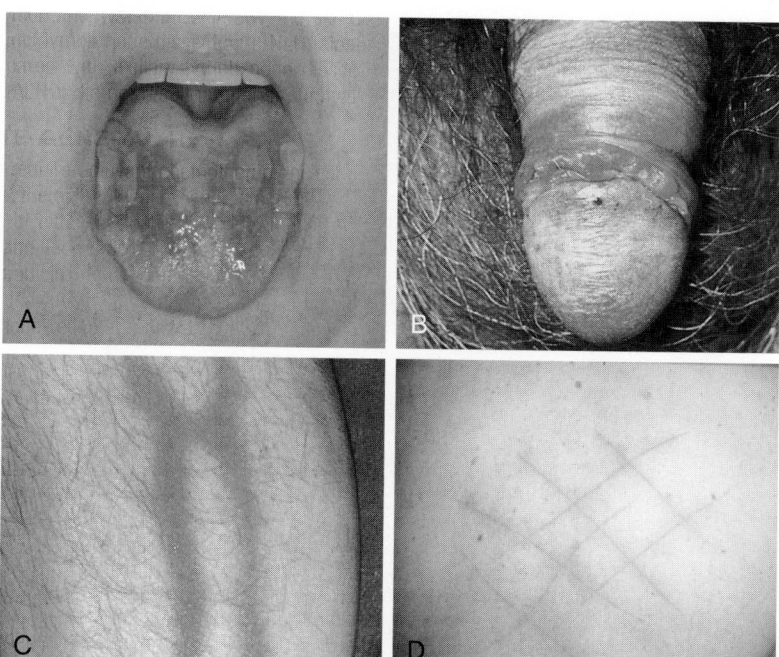

FIGURE 1-146 Behçet's syndrome. A, Major aphthous ulceration; **B,** genital ulceration; **C,** superficial thrombophlebitis; **D,** dermatographia. (**C** courtesy Mir MA: *Atlas of clinical diagnosis,* Philadelphia, 2003, Saunders.) (From Kanski JJ, Bowling B: *Clinical ophthalmology, a systemic approach,* ed 7, Philadelphia, 2010, Saunders.)

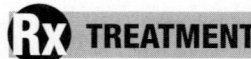 **TREATMENT**

Treatment is directed at the patient's clinical presentation and complications (e.g., mucocutaneous lesions, ocular lesions, arthritis, GI, CNS, or vascular lesions).

NONPHARMACOLOGIC THERAPY

Supportive care and rest during flares, and moderate exercises such as swimming or walking when symptoms improve or disappear

ACUTE GENERAL Rx

- Oral and genital ulcers:
  1. Topical and intralesional corticosteroids (e.g., triamcinolone acetonide ointment applied tid)
  2. Tetracycline tablets 250 mg dissolved in 5 cc water and applied to the ulcer for 2 to 3 min
  3. Colchicine 0.5 to 1.5 mg/day PO
  4. Thalidomide 100 to 300 mg PO daily
  5. Dapsone 100 mg PO daily
  6. Pentoxifylline 300 mg/day PO
  7. Azathioprine 1 to 2.5 mg/kg/day PO
  8. Methotrexate 7.5 to 25 mg/wk PO or intravenously
  9. Interferon alfa-2a and interferon alfa-2b (generally given 3 to 19 million units three times weekly)
- Ocular lesions:
  1. Anterior uveitis is treated by an ophthalmologist with topical corticosteroids (e.g., betamethasone drops 1 to 2 drops tid); topical injection with dexamethasone 1 to 1.5 mg has also been tried

  2. Infliximab 5 mg/kg single dose
  3. Cyclosporine A (5 mg/kg/day) with or without prednisone or azathioprine 1 to 2.5 mg/kg/day PO
- CNS disease:
  1. Chlorambucil 0.1 mg/kg/day is used in the treatment of posterior uveitis, retinal vasculitis, or CNS disease; patients not responding to chlorambucil can be tried on cyclosporine 5 to 7 mg/kg/day.
  2. In CNS vasculitis, cyclophosphamide 2 to 3 mg/kg/day is used. Prednisone can be used as an alternative.
- Arthritis:
  1. NSAIDs (e.g., ibuprofen 400 to 800 mg tid PO or indomethacin 50 to 75 mg/day PO)
  2. Sulfasalazine 1 to 3 g/day PO is an alternative treatment
- GI lesions:
  1. Sulfasalazine 1 to 3 g/day PO
  2. Prednisone 40 to 60 mg/day PO
- Vascular lesions:
  1. Prednisone 40 to 60 mg/day PO
  2. Cytotoxic agents as mentioned previously
  3. Heparin 5000 to 20,000 U/day followed by oral warfarin

CHRONIC Rx

- Chronic therapy is usually continued for approximately 1 yr after remission.
- Surgery may be indicated in patients with complications of bowel perforation, vascular occlusive disease, and aneurysm formation.

DISPOSITION

- The aphthous oral ulcers last 1 to 2 wk, recurring more frequently than genital ulcers.

- 25% of Japanese patients with ocular lesions become blind.
- The disease course is unpredictable.
- The morbidity of Behçet's disease comes primarily from ocular and cutaneous involvement; however, mortality relates primarily to large-size vessel involvement and CNS diseases.

REFERRAL

If the diagnosis of Behçet's disease is suspected, a referral to dermatology, rheumatology, and ophthalmology is indicated because the disease is so rare.

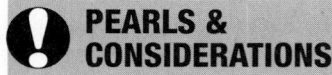 **PEARLS & CONSIDERATIONS**

COMMENTS

- The pathergy test refers to the formation of an erythematous papule or pustule of ≥2 mm after oblique insertion of a sterile 20- or 25-gauge needle into the skin after 24 to 48 hours.
- Because of the rarity of this disease, data from controlled, prospective, randomized clinical trials are lacking.

SUGGESTED READINGS

available at www.expertconsult.com

RELATED CONTENT

Behçet's Syndrome (Patient Information)

AUTHOR: **MONZR M. AL MALKI, M.D.**

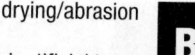

BASIC INFORMATION

DEFINITION
Acute peripheral facial (seventh) nerve palsy

SYNONYMS
Idiopathic facial paralysis

ICD-9CM CODES
351.0

EPIDEMIOLOGY & DEMOGRAPHICS
INCIDENCE: 20-30 cases per 100,000
PEAK INCIDENCE: People >70 yr and pregnant females, especially during the third trimester and/or 1 wk postpartum
PREDOMINANT SEX AND AGE: Sexes are equally affected. Median age is 40 yr.
RISK FACTORS: Diabetes, older age, pregnancy.

PHYSICAL FINDINGS & CLINICAL PRESENTATION
- Dependent on location of facial nerve injury. Onset is usually acute to subacute over hours of unilateral facial paralysis with maximal weakness at 3 wk. One third of patients demonstrate incomplete paralysis, whereas the remaining two thirds have complete paralysis. Recovery is present within the first 6 mo.
- Based on the following criteria: Diffuse facial nerve involvement depicted by paralysis of the facial muscles (Fig. 1-147), along with variable involvement of taste over the anterior two thirds of the tongue or altered secretion of the lacrimal and salivary glands.
  - The degree of involvement is dependent on proximity of facial nerve involvement and involvement of associated branches.

ETIOLOGY
Most cases of Bell's palsy are thought to be secondary to a viral inflammatory/immune mechanism of injury. Herpes simplex virus is thought to be the most common viral pathogen, followed by herpes zoster. Other infectious causes include EBV, CMV, adenovirus, rubella, and mumps.

DIAGNOSIS

DIFFERENTIAL DIAGNOSIS
- Lyme disease: Facial nerve palsy is the most common cranial neuropathy associated with Lyme meningitis. May be unilateral or bilateral.
- HIV
- Ramsay-Hunt syndrome: Facial nerve paralysis associated with ipsilateral zoster oticus
- Parotid gland tumors
- Trauma/temporal bone fracture
- Meningeal processes
  - Infectious: Lyme (mentioned earlier), HIV, syphilis, leprosy, tuberculosis
  - Inflammatory: sarcoid, Sjögren's, Guillain-Barré syndrome
  - Carcinomatous: breast, lung, lymphoma
- Congenital: Mobius syndrome
- Melkerson-Rosenthall syndrome:
- Brainstem stroke: Affecting the nucleus or fascicle of the seventh nerve
- Bell's palsy is a clinical diagnosis.

WORKUP
- Additional workup may be necessary in those patients with complete injury or lack of any recovery or in whom the diagnosis of Bell's palsy is uncertain.

LABORATORY TESTS
Not typically recommended. However, if the diagnosis of Bell's palsy versus facial nerve paralysis from secondary causes is in question (especially if the facial paralysis is bilateral), the following are reasonable:
- Lyme antibody followed by Western blot for positive cases
- ACE level
- Glycosylated hemoglobin
- HIV
- VDRL
- ESR

ELECTRODIAGNOSTIC TESTING
May be performed 2 wk after onset to assess prognosis. Facial motor response remains normal for the first 3 days following injury and then rapidly decreases depending on severity of lesion. Facial motor study may be performed at 10 days and compared to contralateral side. A motor response that is 10% the amplitude of the unaffected side has been defined as a critical value in one study in which recovery was poor when associated with 90% degeneration. EMG can be used to visualize any motor units in the affected muscles that would assess the integrity of the facial nerve.

IMAGING STUDIES
Not usually indicated.
- Brain MRI is indicated in certain cases, such as an upper motor neuron pattern (able to wrinkle forehead) where the temporalis branch of the facial nerve is spared.
- Brain MRI with gadolinium is indicated when other cranial nerve palsies are present or when a meningeal process is suspected.
- CT temporal bone: is indicated in cases of trauma or cases with complete facial paralysis in which the surgeon is considering decompression.

TREATMENT

NONPHARMACOLOGIC THERAPY
- Reassurance that most patients have a full recovery and that the patient did not sustain a stroke.
- Eye patch: To prevent corneal drying/abrasion and subsequent ulceration.
  - Lacrilube to eye at night and artificial tears during the day.

ACUTE GENERAL Rx
- Steroids (based on early findings of inflammation and swelling during decompression studies) and antiviral therapy (predicated on findings of herpes simplex virus in the endoneurial fluid)
  - Two high-quality randomized trials assessed efficacy of early (<72 hr) treatment with glucocorticoids alone, antiviral treatment alone, and combination therapy of Bell's palsy. Glucocorticoid treatment alone was effective, while antiviral therapy showed no benefit when given either alone or with concomitant glucocorticoid therapy.
  - Largest study compared prednisolone (60 mg daily) versus valacyclovir (1000 mg 3 times daily × 7 days) versus combination therapy versus placebo with 72 hr of presentation.
  - At 1-year follow-up, time to recovery was shorter in prednisolone-treated group, while valacyclovir therapy efficacy did not differ from placebo. No added benefit was seen with combination therapy.
- Treatment guidelines, in lieu of above, recommend prednisone 60 to 80 mg/day for 1 wk.
  - Some authors still recommend treatment with valacyclovir (1000 mg 3 times daily for 1 wk) despite lack of clinical evidence.
- Surgical decompression: Not currently recommended.
  - AAN Practice Parameter (2001) concluded there was insufficient evidence to make any recommendation regarding surgical decompression for Bell's palsy.

CHRONIC Rx
Botulinum toxin may be used in cases of hemifacial spasm.

DISPOSITION
- 71% of patients had complete recovery.
- 85% show recovery at 3 wk.
- 13% had slight sequelae.
- 16% had residual weakness, synkinesis, or contracture.
- Prognosis is favorable if recovery is seen within the first 3 wk.
- Recurrence rate is 7%. Average time to recurrence was 10 yr.

REFERRAL
- Neurologist if clinical diagnosis is in question
- Ophthalmologist if concern for corneal abrasion or ulceration

! PEARLS & CONSIDERATIONS

COMMENTS

- Assess wrinkling of forehead (Fig. 1-148). If present on affected side, need to ensure that the facial weakness is not central.
- Assess for other cranial nerve deficits or long-tract signs because brainstem fascicular lesions of the seventh nerve can show peripheral facial pattern of weakness.

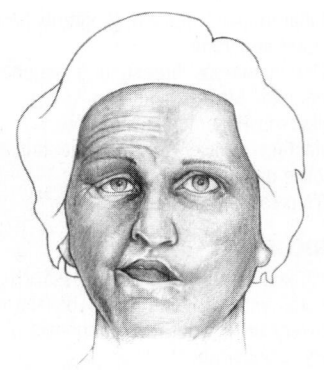

FIGURE 1-148 Bell's palsy. The patient with Bell's palsy (facial nerve palsy) will demonstrate an unwrinkled forehead, widely opened eyes (with weakness of eyelid color), flattening of the nasolabial fold, and a droop of the corner of the mouth. (From Remmel KS et al: *Handbook of symptom-oriented neurology,* ed 3, St Louis, 2002, Mosby.)

SUGGESTED READING

available at www.expertconsult.com

RELATED CONTENT

Bell's Palsy (Facial Palsy) (Patient Information)

AUTHOR: **JOHN SLADKY, M.D.**

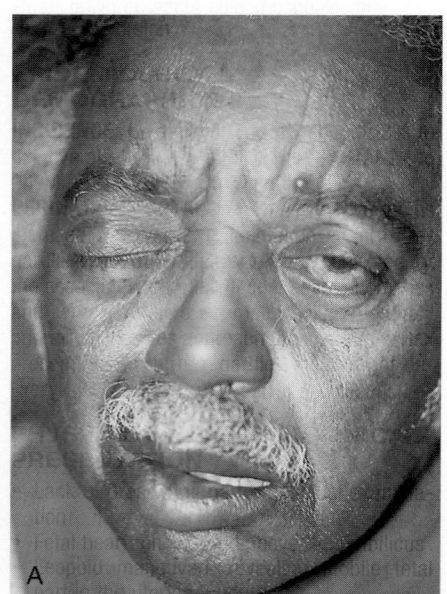

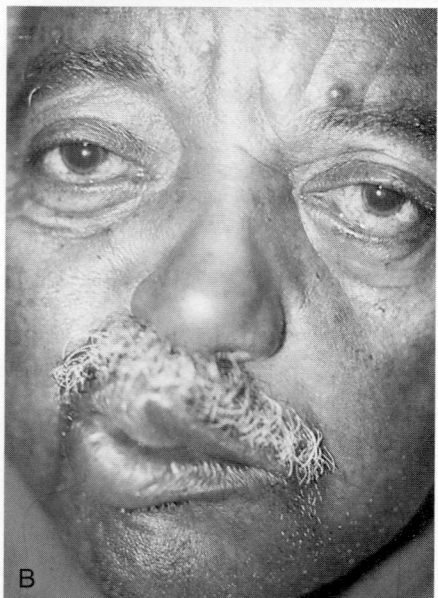

FIGURE 1-147 A patient with a lesion of the facial nerve. A, The patient has difficulty in closing his left eye, and the left corner of his mouth droops. **B,** The latter defect is especially evident when the patient attempts to purse his lips. (From Haines DE: *Fundamental neuroscience for basic and clinical applications,* ed 3, Philadelphia, 2006, Churchill Livingstone.)

BASIC INFORMATION

DEFINITION

Biceps tendonitis is a common cause of anterior shoulder pain characterized by an inflammatory process that involves the long head of the biceps tendon as well as its sheath within the bicipital groove. The tendon involvement can be intra-articular from its attachment to the superior glenoid labrum as it runs across the glenohumeral joint and extra-articular as it runs in the bicipital or intertubercular groove (Fig. 1-149).

SYNONYMS

Bicipital tendonitis
Bicipital tenosynovitis
Biceps tendinosis

ICD-9CM CODES
726.12 Bicipital tenosynovitis

EPIDEMIOLOGY & DEMOGRAPHICS

INCIDENCE: 41% of complete rotator cuff tears have concomitant biceps tendonitis
PREVALENCE: Common but prevalence uncertain
PREDOMINANT AGE: 18 to 35 yr old
RISK FACTORS: Athletes involved in throwing sports, swimming, contact sports, weight lifting, gymnastics, martial arts, repetitive overhead movements among carpenters, electricians, mechanical wheelchair users

PHYSICAL FINDINGS & CLINICAL PRESENTATION
- Pain referred to the anterior shoulder
- Pain that worsens at night

- A history of trauma may or may not be present
- Pain on lifting, pulling, and repetitive overhead reaching
- Most common physical exam finding is tenderness over bicipital groove by palpating the biceps tendon 3 to 6 cm below the anterior acromion and felt most easily in 10 degrees of internal rotation
- Yergason's test—pain on biceps tendon area on resisted supination of pronated forearm with elbow at 90 degrees
- Speed's test—pain on the biceps tendon area on resisted forward flexion of the shoulder with elbows and arms fully supinated and extended

ETIOLOGY
- Primary—of unknown cause and the inflammation is specific to the intertubercular groove without any associated shoulder pathology
- Secondary—associated with other pathologic conditions such as rotator cuff disease, impingement syndrome, SLAP (Superior Labrum from Anterior to Posterior) injuries, presence of spurs or any systemic inflammatory disease involving the shoulders

DX DIAGNOSIS

DIFFERENTIAL DIAGNOSIS
- Impingement syndrome
- Rotator cuff tendonitis
- Subacromial bursitis
- Rotator cuff tears
- SLAP injuries
- Adhesive capsulitis

- Acromioclavicular joint arthritis
- Glenohumeral joint arthritis
- Cervical radiculopathy
- Coracoid impingement
- Brachial plexus neuritis

WORKUP
May proceed to imaging modalities

IMAGING STUDIES
- X-ray plain films are usually normal in primary tendinopathy; special views of the bicipital groove may demonstrate presence of spurs
- Musculoskeletal ultrasound evaluates dynamic movements of the biceps tendon; it is 49% sensitive but 91% to 97% specific; use in both diagnosis and treatment
- CT/MRI Arthrography are early techniques used to reliably identify shoulder pathology
- MRI is a non-invasive way of getting detailed images of the biceps tendon and other shoulder structures such as the superior labrum and rotator cuff structures and identify pathologies that may or may not coexist
- Ultrasound may reveal the presence of effusion in the long head of the biceps tendon sheath (Fig. 1-150)
- Arthroscopy is the gold standard technique for diagnosis and treatment.

Rx TREATMENT

It is often necessary to establish whether the tendonitis is primary or secondary to address certain aspects of the treatment. Initial conservative treatment is usually very successful.

NONPHARMACOLOGIC THERAPY
Ice, rest from overhead physical activities, physical therapy after acute phase

ACUTE GENERAL Rx
Nonsteroidal anti-inflammatory drugs (NSAIDs) are good adjuncts to treatment that expedites the recovery process by decreasing edema, inflammation, and pain.

CHRONIC Rx
- If with persistent pain or severe night symptoms that fail to resolve after 6 to 8 wk of conservative treatment, corticosteroid injections may be considered
- Injection into the tendon sheath, with care not to inject into the biceps tendon, may have good to excellent results; best done under ultrasound guidance
- Subacromial steroid injections can address tendonitis secondary to impingement
- Glenohumeral joint injection delivers the steroids directly to the intra-articular portion of the biceps that is often irritated
- Gradual biceps and rotator cuff strengthening with physical therapy if symptoms have decreased
- Low-power laser therapy has reported beneficial effects but disputes exist

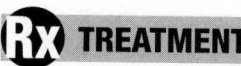

FIGURE 1-149 Anatomic location of the long head of the biceps tendon with surrounding structures of the shoulder. (From Roberts et al: *Clinical procedures in emergency medicine*, ed 5, Philadelphia, 2009, Saunders.)

Site of inflammation
Bursa
Greater tuberosity of the humerus
Biceps tendon
Bicipital groove
Biceps
Lesser tuberosity of the humerus
Scapula

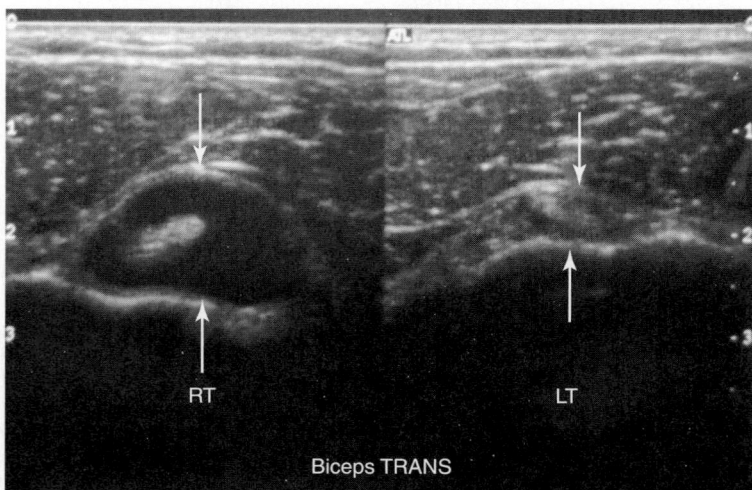

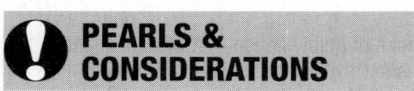

FIGURE 1-150 Ultrasound image of bicipital tendinitis. Transverse image shows large effusion in the long head of biceps tendon sheath. (From Hoechberg MC et al: *Rheumatology,* ed 5, St Louis, 2011, Mosby.)

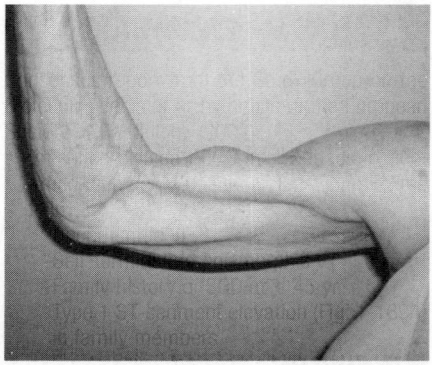

FIGURE 1-151 Popeye deformity after a biceps tendon rupture. (Illustration borrowed from Fernandez et al FIGURE 4, PAGE 7. Seminarios de la Fundación Española de Reumatologia Maniobras exploratorias del hombro doloros martes, 13 jul 2010, Elsevier.)

DISPOSITION

- Usually self-limited with conservative measures
- If pain persists after 3 mo, referral to orthopedic surgery
- Surgical options are tendon debridement, release of constricted synovial sheath, tenodesis, or tenotomy.
- Tenodesis is done by moving the attachment to relieve pressure of the irritated tendon; results in better strength and cosmesis but requires longer rehab; consider for younger, active patients
- Tenotomy consists of cutting the long head of the biceps tendon prior to its intra-articular superior labral insertion; technically simple procedure with short rehabilitation but deformity, weakness, and cramping may occur; consider for older patients
- Can progress to tendon rupture resulting in a "Popeye deformity" (Fig. 1-151)

REFERRAL

- Refer to physical therapy early in the phase of conservative treatment
- Refer to orthopedics if symptoms persist beyond 3 to 4 mo

PEARLS & CONSIDERATIONS

COMMENTS

A complete rotator cuff tear almost always involves the biceps tendon as its intra-articular portion gets exposed to the overlying acromion, which causes further impingement and pain.

PREVENTION

After corticosteroid injection, patient should not return immediately to vigorous physical activities that could potentially progress into a biceps tendon complete tear.

SUGGESTED READINGS

available at www.expertconsult.com

AUTHOR: **CRISOSTOMO R. BALIOG, JR., M.D.**

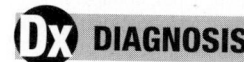

BASIC INFORMATION

DEFINITION

Bipolar disorder is an episodic, recurrent, and frequently progressive condition in which the afflicted individual experiences at least one episode of mania, characterized by at least 1 wk of continuous symptoms of elevated, expansive, or irritable mood, in association with three or four of the following symptoms:
- Decreased need for sleep
- Grandiosity
- Pressured speech
- Subjective or objective flight of ideas
- Distractibility
- Increased level of goal-directed activity
- Problematic behavior

Most individuals with bipolar disorder also experience one or more episodes of major depression over their lifetimes or have symptoms of a depressive episode commingled with those of mania (mixed episode).

SYNONYMS

Manic-depression
Cycloid psychosis

ICD-9CM CODES

296.4-6 Circular manic, circular depressed, circular type mixed

EPIDEMIOLOGY & DEMOGRAPHICS

INCIDENCE: 0.016% to 0.021%
PREVALENCE (IN U.S.): 0.4% to 1.6% (lifetime); bipolar spectrum disorders: 2.8%
PREDOMINANT SEX: Equal distribution among male and female
PREDOMINANT AGE: Lifelong condition with age of onset 14 to 30 yr
PEAK INCIDENCE: Onset in 20s
GENETICS:
- Concordance rates for monozygotic twins: 0.7 to 0.8; for dizygotic twins: 0.2
- Risk of affective disorder in offspring with one affected parent with bipolar disorder: 27% to 29%; with two affected parents: 50% to 74%
- Heritability estimate of 0.85
- No specific causal mutations have been identified. Genome-wide association analyses have suggested a role for *ANK3, CACNA1C, TRANK1,* and a gene at 3p21.1 and implicated ion channelopathies in pathogenesis of bipolar disorder.

PHYSICAL FINDINGS & CLINICAL PRESENTATION

- Mania associated with:
  - Psychomotor activation that is usually goal directed but not necessarily productive
  - Increase in goal-directed activity and excessive involvement in activities leading to unexpected adverse outcomes
  - Elevated, euphoric, and frequently labile mood
  - Decreased need for sleep
  - Flight of ideas with rapid, loud, pressured speech

- Psychosis may occur, with delusions, hallucinations, and formal thought disorder
- Depressive episodes resembling major depressive disorder (see "Depression, Major"); however, atypical features (hypersomnia, weight gain) may be present
- Mixed states, characterized by activation, irritability, and dysphoria, also possible

KEY DIAGNOSTIC CRITERIA DISTINGUISHING BIPOLAR I DISORDER FROM BIPOLAR II DISORDER*:

Manic episode (Bipolar I Disorder)
- Distinct period during which there is an abnormally and persistently elevated, expansive, or irritable mood lasting at least 1 wk (or less if hospitalization is required)
- Must be accompanied by at least three of the following symptoms (four if mood is only irritable): inflated self-esteem or grandiosity, decreased need for sleep, pressured speech, racing thoughts, distractibility, increased involvement in goal-directed activity or psychomotor agitation, excessive involvement in pleasurable activities with a high potential for painful consequences
- Symptoms do not meet criteria for a mixed episode
- Disturbance must be sufficiently severe to cause marked impairment in social or occupational functioning or to require hospitalization, or it is characterized by the presence of psychotic features
- Symptoms not due to direct physiologic effect of medication, general medication condition, or substance abuse

Hypomanic episode (Bipolar II Disorder)
- Distinct period during which there is an abnormally and persistently elevated, expansive, or irritable mood lasting at least 4 days
- Must be accompanied by at least three of the following symptoms (four if mood is only irritable): inflated self-esteem or grandiosity, decreased need for sleep, pressured speech, racing thoughts, distractibility, increased involvement in goal-directed activity or psychomotor agitation, excessive involvement in pleasurable activities with a high potential for painful consequences
- Hypomanic episodes must be clearly different from the person's usual nondepressed mood, and there must be a clear change in functioning that is not characteristic of the person's usual functioning
- Changes in mood and functioning must be observable by others. In contrast to a manic episode, a hypomanic episode is not severe enough to cause marked impairment in social or occupational functioning or to require hospitalization, and there are no psychotic features
- Symptoms not due to direct physiologic effect of medication, general medication condition, or substance abuse

---

*Criteria are from the American Psychiatric Association: *Diagnostic and statistic manual of mental disorders, fourth edition, text revision,* Washington, DC, 2000, American Psychiatric Association.

ETIOLOGY

Hypotheses:
1. Abnormalities of receptor and membrane function, calcium dysregulation
2. Alteration of cAMP, MAP kinase, protein kinase C, arachidonic acid cascade, and glycogen synthase kinase-3 signal transduction pathways; mitochondrial dysfunction
3. Alteration in cell survival pathways, glial and neuronal death and loss of neuroplasticity

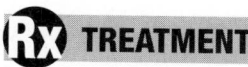

DIAGNOSIS

DIFFERENTIAL DIAGNOSIS

- Secondary manias caused by medical disorders (e.g., hyperthyroidism, AIDS, stroke, Cushing syndrome) or pharmacologic treatment (e.g., steroids, stimulants).
- First onset of mania after age 50 yr suggestive of secondary mania.
- Less severe, and possibly distinct, conditions of bipolar type II and cyclothymia
- Comorbid substance abuse or dependency may confound diagnosis and treatment.
- Presentation can be confused with schizophrenia or paranoid psychosis.

WORKUP

- History
- Physical examination
- Mental status examination
- Mood Disorder Questionnaire (MDQ)

LABORATORY TESTS

Because of high rate of secondary manias, initial evaluation to confirm health of all major organ systems (routine chemistries, complete blood count, urinalysis, sedimentation rate)

IMAGING STUDIES

- Consider brain imaging if late onset or if neurologic examination is abnormal.
- Neuroimaging may show evidence of ventricular enlargement or increased white matter hyperintensities; decrements in right prefrontal and temporal lobe gray matter also reported.

TREATMENT

NONPHARMACOLOGIC THERAPY

- Cognitive-behavioral and family-focused psychoeducational psychotherapy to help patients cope with consequences of the disease, improve adherence with medications, and identify possible environmental triggers
- Bright light therapy in the northern latitudes in individuals exhibiting a seasonal pattern of winter depression
- Lifestyle "regularization"

ACUTE GENERAL Rx

- First-line agents for acute mania: lithium 1500 to 1800 mg/day (0.8 to 1.2 mEq/L), valproate 1000 to 1500 mg/day (50 to 125 ng/ml), carbamazepine 600 to 800 mg/day (4 to 12 micrograms/ml), oxcarbazepine 900 to

2400 mg/day, olanzapine 10 to 20 mg/day, risperidone 2 to 4 mg/day, quetiapine 350 to 800 mg/day, ziprasidone 80 to 120 mg/day, or aripiprazole 10 to 30 mg/day.
- Useful adjuncts to acute treatment: benzodiazepines: lorazepam 1 to 2 mg q4h, clonazepam 1 to 2 mg q4h.
- Traditional antidepressants can induce manic episodes and exacerbate mania in mixed episodes.
- Lamotrigine can have acute antidepressant benefit, but appears more effective in prophylaxis of future episodes.
- Although best evidence data are limited, first-line options for bipolar depression include lithium, quetiapine, lamotrigine, and olanzapine/fluoxetine combination.

CHRONIC Rx
- Goal of long-term treatment: prevention of relapse or episode recurrence
- Best agents for prophylaxis of mania: lithium, valproate, and olanzapine (carbamazepine/oxcarbazepine possibly beneficial)
- Best agents for prophylaxis of depression: lamotrigine and lithium
- Risk/benefit of atypical antipsychotics in maintenance unclear
- Long-term use of antidepressants: frequently destabilizes patient and leads to more frequent relapses; depression outweighs mania as the most debilitating dimension over the life span.

DISPOSITION
- Course is variable.
- More than 90% of patients having a single manic episode are likely to experience others.

- Uncontrolled manic or depressive episodes can lead to additional episodes.
- Lithium shown to specifically decrease suicidal risk.
- Psychosocioeconomic consequences of both mania and depression can be severe and disabling.

REFERRAL
- If use of antidepressant contemplated
- If patient is severely manic, rapid cycling, or suicidal or is in a bipolar, mixed episode

❗ PEARLS & CONSIDERATIONS

COMMENTS
- All patients presenting with depression should be asked about past personal and family history of mania and hypomania; 70% of bipolar patients have previously been misdiagnosed.
- Prompt recognition of the earliest signs of mania in a given individual (e.g., decreased need for sleep, increased rate of speech) allows earlier intervention and a better likelihood of preventing a full episode.
- Bipolar disorder in children frequently manifests as behavioral disinhibition and temper dysregulation, but current consensus indicates that the condition is overdiagnosed in this age group.
- Patients treated with atypical antipsychotic agents should be carefully monitored for development of metabolic syndrome.
- Despite some variation in prevalence, the severity, impact, and patterns of comorbidity

of bipolar disorder are similar in different countries in world health surveys.
- Bipolar disorder often co-occurs with anxiety disorders, and attention deficit hyperactivity disorder (ADHD), making attribution of specific symptoms difficult.
- Patients receiving anticonvulsants or antidepressants should be monitored for a possible increase in suicidal thoughts or behavior.

PATIENT/FAMILY EDUCATION
Information available at www.NMHA.org/ and www.dbsalliance.org/.

SUGGESTED READINGS
available at www.expertconsult.com

RELATED CONTENT
Depression (Related Key Topic)
Bipolar Disorder (Patient Information)
AUTHOR: **VICTOR I. REUS, M.D.**

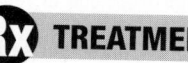

B

Diseases and Disorders

I

BASIC INFORMATION

DEFINITION

Bone cell death in the jaw observed with therapeutic dosages of bisphosphonates (BPs). Osteoclast apoptosis may occur due to the antiresorptive effects of BPs preventing the release of bone regenerative proteins and thus preventing renewal of bone. This results in ischemic tissue loss and exposed bone. BPs are not believed to be toxic to osteoblasts, although evidence suggests some antiangiogenic effects.

Bisphosphonate-related osteonecrosis of the jaw (BRONJ) primarily involves the jawbone due to its higher risk for complications from minor injury and infection when the healing potential or vascular supply is compromised. BPs may accumulate more in bones with higher turnover rates, such as the maxilla and mandible.

SYNONYMS

Bisphosphonate-induced osteonecrosis of the jaw (BIONJ)

ICD-9CM CODES
Not applicable

EPIDEMIOLOGY & DEMOGRAPHICS
INCIDENCE
- The incidence with alendronate has been estimated to be 0.7 per 100,000 persons per year by the original manufacturer.
- The incidence after tooth extraction has ranged from 8.3% to 40% in the medical literature.
  - Incidence at 42 months after tooth extraction has been estimated at 3.9% with oral BPs and 14.8% with IV BPs.
PEAK INCIDENCE: BRONJ has been identified as early as 7 months after the use of IV BPs in patients with cancer, and as early as 13 months in patients with osteoporosis and absence of malignant disease. Incidence may depend on when dentoalveolar surgery occurs.
PREVALENCE
- Prevalence in 2008 estimated at 13.3% of patients with cancer who received an IV BP
- Most prevalent in patients with multiple myeloma or breast cancer vs. other cancers or osteoporosis
PREDOMINANT SEX AND AGE
- Sex not statistically associated with BRONJ
- Age greater than or equal to 65
GENETICS: Single nucleotide polymorphisms (SNPs) have been identified in the *CYP2C8* gene among patients with multiple myeloma and exposure to IV BPs.
RISK FACTORS: The 2009 American Association of Oral and Maxillofacial Surgeons (AAOMS) position paper indicated that dentoalveolar surgery such as tooth extraction or root canal and use of IV BPs are the greatest risk factors for development of BRONJ.
- Patients with cancer exposed to IV BPs who undergo dentoalveolar surgery have an estimated fivefold to 21-fold increased risk for BRONJ than similar patients who do not undergo this surgery.
- IV formulations such as zoledronic acid: risk ratio for developing BRONJ is 14.6 with IV versus oral products. The risk of developing BRONJ with oral forms may increase when duration is greater than 3 years and may be potentiated by concomitant use of chronic corticosteroids.
- Patients with cancer who are exposed to IV BPs have a 2.7- to 4.2-fold increased risk versus similar patients not exposed to IV BPs.
- Longer duration of BP therapy
- Age greater than or equal to 65 with risk ratio estimated to be 200.2 in those exposed to IV BPs vs. similar patients not exposed
- Malignancy
- Chemotherapeutic agents and corticosteroids
- History of periodontal and dental abscesses
- Bacterial infection

PHYSICAL FINDINGS & CLINICAL PRESENTATION
- Exposed bone in the maxilla or mandible, with 65% of cases involving the mandible. Multifocal or bilateral involvement may be present.
- Pain in the maxillofacial region, although one third of lesions may be painless
- Tooth mobility/spontaneous tooth loss
- Mucosal swelling, erythema, ulceration, altered sensation
- Infection

ETIOLOGY
- Exposure to IV or oral BPs

DIAGNOSIS

The AAOMS considers a diagnosis of BRONJ if the following three characteristics are present:
1. Current or previous treatment with a BP
2. Exposed bone in the maxillofacial region persisting for more than 8 weeks
3. No history of radiation therapy to the maxillofacial region

DIFFERENTIAL DIAGNOSIS
- Suppurative osteomyelitis of the jaw (SOJ)
- Osteoradionecrosis of the jaw (ORNJ)
- Alveolar osteitis, gingivitis, periodontitis, dental caries, and temporomandibular joint disorders.

WORKUP
- Treatment history, including medications and radiation therapy
- Past medical history, including malignancy

LABORATORY TESTS
Tissue biopsy should only be performed if metastatic disease is strongly suspected and its detection would change the management of BRONJ. Histopathology of BRONJ shows empty osteocytic lacunae, empty Haversian and Volkmann canals, an absence of inflammatory cells or blood vessels in the marrow space, and absence of extracellular collagenase.

IMAGING STUDIES
Panoramic and periapical radiographs

TREATMENT

Goals of treatment for BRONJ include:
- Control and/or reduce pain.
- Control secondary infection.
- Minimize progression or occurrence of bone necrosis.

NONPHARMACOLOGIC THERAPY
Surgery for BRONJ should be deferred if possible as a surgical margin with viable bone is difficult to obtain. The entire jawbone likely has been exposed to accumulation of BPs, and therefore successful eradication of necrotic bone is often not possible. Those areas of necrosis that consistently irritate soft tissues should undergo debridement as necessary. Hyperbaric oxygen therapy is considered ineffective for preventing progression.

The AAOMS recommends the following surgical strategies based on BRONJ staging:
- Stage 0 (no clinical evidence of necrotic bone): no surgery
- Stage I (exposed and necrotic bone, asymptomatic): no surgery
- Stage II (exposed and necrotic bone with pain and/or infection): superficial debridement
- Stage III (exposed and necrotic bone with pain, infection, **and** one of the following features: necrosis extending beyond alveolar bone, pathologic fracture, extraoral fistula, oral antral or nasal communication, osteolysis extending to mandible of sinus floor): surgical debridement or resection for palliation of infection and pain

ACUTE GENERAL Rx
Both chlorhexidine mouth rinse and antibiotics for 1 to 3 weeks have been found useful for stage reduction.
- Chlorhexidine 0.12% antibacterial mouth rinse daily for Stages I to III
- Oral antibiotics for symptomatic Stage II, and oral or IV antibiotics for Stage III
- Analgesics for Stages II or III

CHRONIC Rx
- Determine whether discontinuation of BPs is appropriate.
  - Evaluate potential benefit of remaining on BP therapy.
  - Patients with cancer may benefit from a reduction in bone pain with use of BPs.
  - BPs have a prolonged half-life, so return to normal osteoclast function and bone turnover may be too gradual.
  - Consider other risks of BPs such as atypical fractures.
- If discontinuing BP therapy, consider other alternative treatments for osteoporosis or bone pain.
- Anecdotal case reports exist for using teriparatide to heal BRONJ.

DISPOSITION

- Patients with involvement of the maxilla appear to have a greater likelihood of repeat surgery.
- Patients on oral BPs may have less severe complications and may have a better response.
- Treatment with antibiotics and chlorhexidine mouth rinse, withdrawal of BPs, and surgical removal of loose sequestra may possibly reduce pain and lesions of osteonecrosis.

REFERRAL

Oral and maxillofacial surgeon

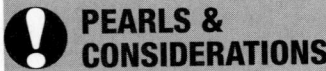

PEARLS & CONSIDERATIONS

COMMENTS

- Patients may be asymptomatic for weeks to years before BRONJ is apparent. Radiographic changes may not be observed until significant disease has developed.
- Tooth extraction may be difficult to avoid in patients at high risk of BRONJ if an underlying bacterial infection is present.

- Patients with cancer are at highest risk as the dosage of BPs are much greater for osteoporosis.
- The most appropriate duration of BPs is unclear, when considering benefits (relief of bone pain in malignancy, prevention of fractures with high morbidity and mortality) vs. serious adverse effects (BRONJ, spontaneous atypical fractures). In September 2011, the FDA asked manufacturers to establish a timeframe for discontinuation.

PREVENTION

- Regular dental hygiene
- Assessment of patients for other risk factors of BRONJ
- Completion of any anticipated dental procedures before beginning BP therapy
- Consideration of appropriateness of oral BP instead of IV forms
- After dentoalveolar surgery, initiation of BPs delayed by 2 to 3 weeks to allow for osseous healing
- Careful monitoring of patients after dentoalveolar surgery
- Examination of mucosa in patients with full or partial dentures
- In asymptomatic patients receiving IV BPs, limiting dental surgery to removal of nonrestorable teeth and avoiding dental implants in patients who also have cancer
- In asymptomatic patients exposed to less than 3 years of oral BPs with concomitant corticosteroids 3 months before dental surgery, consider a drug holiday
- In asymptomatic patients exposed to more than 3 years of oral BPs, consider a drug holiday before dental surgery

PATIENT/FAMILY EDUCATION

- All healthcare providers should be aware of past and current BP use
- Contact a healthcare provider if any of the following are noticed:
  - Presence of exposed bone in the maxillofacial area
  - Persisting pain in the maxillofacial area
  - Signs of infection such as fever, pus, and swelling
- Practice good dental hygiene and keep regular dental appointments

SUGGESTED READINGS

available at www.expertconsult.com

AUTHORS: **CHRISTINE EISENHOWER, PHARM.D.,** and **ANNE L. HUME, PHARM.D.**

BASIC INFORMATION

DEFINITION

A bite wound can be animal or human, accidental or intentional.

ICD-9CM CODES
879.8 Bite wound, unspecified site

EPIDEMIOLOGY & DEMOGRAPHICS

- Bite wounds account for 1% of emergency department visits.
- More than 1 million bites occur in human beings annually in the U.S.
- Dog bites account for 85% to 90% of all bites and result in 10 to 20 fatalities yearly in the U.S.; cat bites account for 10% to 20%. The animal typically is owned by the victim.
- Infection rates are highest for cat bites (30% to 50%), followed by human bites (15% to 30%) and dog bites (5%).
- The extremities are involved in 75% of bites.

PHYSICAL FINDINGS & CLINICAL PRESENTATION

- The appearance of the bite wound is variable (e.g., puncture wound, tear, avulsion).
- Cellulitis, lymphangitis, and focal adenopathy may be present in infected bite wounds.
- Patient may have fever and chills.

ETIOLOGY

- Increased risk of infection: human and cat bites, closed-fist injuries, wounds involving joints, puncture wounds, face and lip bites, bites with skull penetration, bites in immunocompromised hosts
- Most frequent infecting organisms:
  1. *Pasteurella* spp.: responsible for majority of infections within 24 hr of dog (*P. canis*) and cat (*P. multocida, P. septica*) bites
  2. *Capnocytophaga canimorsus* (formerly DF-2 bacillus): a gram-negative organism responsible for late infection, usually after dog bites
  3. Gram-negative organisms (*Pseudomonas, Haemophilus*): often found in human bites
  4. *Streptococcus* spp., *Staphylococcus aureus*
  5. *Eikenella corrodens* in human bites

DIAGNOSIS

DIFFERENTIAL DIAGNOSIS

- Bite from a rabid animal (often the attack is unprovoked)
- Factitious injury

WORKUP

- Determination of the time elapsed since the patient was bitten, status of rabies immunization of the animal, and underlying medical conditions that might predispose the patient to infection (e.g., DM, immunodeficiency)
- Documentation of bite site, notification of appropriate authorities (e.g., police department, animal officer)

LABORATORY TESTS

- Generally not necessary
- Hct if there has been significant blood loss
- Wound cultures (aerobic and anaerobic) if there is evidence of sepsis or victim is immunocompromised; cultures should be obtained before irrigation of the wound but after superficial cleaning

IMAGING STUDIES

Radiographs are indicated when bony penetration is suspected or if there is suspicion of fracture or significant trauma; they are also useful for detecting foreign bodies (when suspected).

TREATMENT

NONPHARMACOLOGIC THERAPY

- Local care with debridement, vigorous cleansing, and saline irrigation of the wound; debridement of devitalized tissue
- High-pressure irrigation to clean bite wound and ensure removal of contaminants (e.g., use saline solution with a 30- to 35-ml syringe equipped with a 20-gauge needle or catheter with tip of syringe placed 2 to 3 cm above the wound)
- Avoid blunt probing of wounds (increased risk of infection)
- If the animal is suspected to be rabid: infiltrate wound edges with 1% procaine hydrochloride, swab wound surface vigorously with cotton swabs and 1% benzalcuronium solution or other soap, and rinse wound with normal saline

ACUTE GENERAL Rx

- Avoid suturing of hand wounds and any wounds that appear infected
- Puncture wounds should be left open
- Give antirabies therapy and tetanus immune globulin (250 to 500 units IM in limb contralateral to toxoid) and toxoid (adult or child older than 5 yr: 0.5 ml DT given IM, child <5 yr 0.5 ml DPT IM) as needed

- Use empiric antibiotic therapy in high-risk wounds (e.g., cat bite, hand bites, face bites, genital area bites, bites with joint or bone penetration, human bites, immunocompromised host): amoxicillin-clavulanate 875 to 1000 mg bid for 7 days or cefuroxime 500 mg bid for 7 days
- In hospitalized patients, IV antibiotics of choice are cefoxitin 1-2 g q6h, ampicillin-sulbactam 1.5-3 g q6h, ticarcillin-clavulanate 3 g q6h, cefoxitin 2 g IV q8h, or ceftriaxone 1-2 g q24h
- Penicillin allergy: animal bite (doxycycline or moxifloxacin or trimethoprim/sulfamethoxazole with either clindamycin or metronidazole); human bite (moxifloxacin plus clindamycin, trimethoprim/sulfamethoxazole plus metronidazole)
- Prophylactic therapy for persons bitten by others with HIV and hepatitis B (see Section V)

DISPOSITION

- Prognosis is favorable with proper treatment.
- Important prognostic factors are type and depth of wound, which compartments are entered, and pathogenicity of inoculated bacteria.
- Punctures that are difficult to irrigate adequately, carnivore bites over vital structures (arteries, nerves, joints), and tissue crushing that cannot be debrided have a worse prognosis.
- In general, human bites have a higher complication and infection rate than do animal bites.
- Nearly 50% of the anaerobic gram-negative bacilli isolated from human bite wounds may be penicillin resistant and beta-lactamase positive.

REFERRAL

- Hospitalization and IV antibiotic therapy for infected human bites; bites with injury to joints, nerves, or tendons; or any animal bites unresponsive to oral therapy.
- Human bites with tendon involvement should go to operating room for washout.
- In the outpatient setting, bite wounds should be reevaluated within 48 hr to assess for signs of infection.

SUGGESTED READING

available at www.expertconsult.com

RELATED CONTENT

Animal and Human Bites (Patient Information)

AUTHOR: **FRED F. FERRI, M.D.**

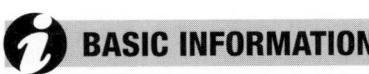

BASIC INFORMATION

DEFINITION

There are two major classes of arthropods: insects and arachnida. This chapter focuses on the class arachnida. Arachnid bites consist of bites caused by:

- Spiders
- Scorpions
- Ticks

ICD-9CM CODES

E905.1 Venomous spiders (black widow spider, brown spider, tarantula)
E905.2 Scorpion
989.5 Bites of venomous snakes, lizards, and spiders; tick paralysis
E906.4 Bite of nonvenomous arthropod; insect bite NOS

EPIDEMIOLOGY & DEMOGRAPHICS

- Spiders—ubiquitous; only three types potentially significantly harmful:
  1. Sydney funnel web spider—Australia
  2. Black widow (Fig. E1-152)—worldwide (excluding Alaska)
  3. Brown recluse (Fig. E1-153)—most common (South Central U.S.)
- Scorpions—various warm climates: Africa, Central South America, Middle East, India; Texas, New Mexico, California, and Nevada in the U.S.
- Ticks—woodlands

PHYSICAL FINDINGS & CLINICAL PRESENTATION

Spiders:
- Sydney funnel web—natracotoxin toxin
  1. Piloerection, muscle spasms leading to tachycardia, hypertension, increased intracranial pressure, coma
- Black widow—females toxic
  1. Initial reaction: local swelling, redness (two fang marks) leading to local piloerection, edema, urticaria, diaphoresis, lymphangitis
  2. Pain in limb leading to rest of body (chest pain, abdominal pain), compartment syndrome
- Brown recluse
  1. Minor sting or burn.
  2. Wound may become pruritic and red with a blanched center with vesicle. Can necrose, especially in fatty areas. Leaves eschar, which sloughs and leaves ulcer; can take months to heal.
  3. Systemic symptoms: headache, fever, chills, gastrointestinal upset, hemolysis, renal tubular necrosis, disseminated intravascular coagulation possible.

Scorpions:
- Sting leading to sympathetic and parasympathetic stimulation: hypertension, bradycardia, vasoconstriction, pulmonary edema, reduced coronary blood flow, priapism, inhibition of insulin

- Also possible: tachycardia, arrhythmia, vasodilation, bronchial relaxation, excessive salivation, vomiting, sweating, bronchoconstriction, pancreatitis.
- Clinically significant scorpion envenomation by *Centruroides sculpturatus* produces a severe neuromotor syndrome and respiratory insufficiency that often requires ICU admission.

Ticks: U.S., Europe, Asia
- Very small (<1 mm). Must be attached >36 hr to transmit disease.
- Lyme disease—most common
  1. Early: erythema migrans in 60% to 80% of cases
  2. 7 to 10 days: mild to moderate constitutional symptoms—disseminated—secondary skin lesions, fever, adenopathy, constitutional symptoms, facial palsy, peripheral neuropathy, lymphocytic meningitis, meningoencephalitis, cardiac manifestations (heart block)
  3. Late: chronic arthritis, dermatitis, neuropathy, keratitis
- Babesiosis (see "Babesiosis")
- Ehrlichiosis/Anaplasmosis (see "Babesiosis" and "Lyme Disease")

DIAGNOSIS

DIFFERENTIAL DIAGNOSIS

- Cellulitis
- Urticaria

Other tick-borne illnesses:
- Babesiosis
- Tick-borne relapsing fever
- Tularemia
- Rocky Mountain spotted fever
- Ehrlichiosis/anaplasmosis
- Colorado tick fever
- Tick paralysis
- Community-acquired cutaneous methicillin-resistant *Staphylococcus aureus*

WORKUP

Physical examination: thorough skin examination may reveal fang marks, attached ticks, black eschar.

TREATMENT

ACUTE GENERAL Rx

Spiders:
- Sydney funnel web
  1. Pressure, immediate immobilization, supportive care, antivenin.
- Black widow
  1. Treatment based on severity of symptoms; bite is rarely fatal.
  2. All should receive oxygen, IV, cardiac monitor, tetanus prophylaxis.
  3. Symptomatic/supportive therapy.
  4. 10% calcium gluconate for muscle cramps (controversial).
  5. Antivenin only for more severe reactions; it carries a risk of anaphylaxis.

  - Dose: one vial in 100 ml 0.9% saline over 20 to 30 min.
  - Skin test before use.
  - Give antihistamines with use.
- Brown recluse
  1. Pain management, tetanus, supportive treatment.
  2. No consensus regarding best treatment; some evidence for hyperbaric oxygen.

Scorpions:
- Fluids, supportive care, species-specific antivenin (equine based, risk of serum sickness) is controversial.
- IV administration of scorpion-specific F(ab')2 antivenom has been reported effective in resolving the clinical syndrome within 4 hours and reducing the need for concomitant sedation with midazolam and reducing the levels of circulating unbound venom.

Ticks:
- Prophylactic: tick >36 hr: single dose of doxycycline 200 mg
- Early localized disease
  1. Treatment of choice in children: amoxicillin for 14 days.
  2. Doxycycline preferred in patients with possible concurrent ehrlichiosis.
  3. Early disseminated: treatment depends on manifestation.
  4. Late disease: may require longer term or IV therapy; controversial for neurologic disease (see "Lyme Disease").

DISPOSITION

- For patients with systemic reactions, send home with emergency epinephrine kit.
- If severe or anaphylactic reaction, admit and observe for 48 hr for cardiac, renal, or neurologic problems.

REFERRAL

For patients with systemic reactions, refer to allergist for immunotherapy; 95% to 98% effective in preventing anaphylaxis.

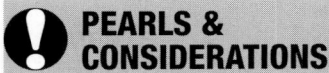

PEARLS & CONSIDERATIONS

Actual spider bites rare, need witnessed bite, patient should bring spider if possible for confirmation. Bites usually occur in settings of unusually close contact with spider. Bedbugs becoming more prevalent, repeated exposure increases severity of reaction.

SUGGESTED READINGS

available at www.expertconsult.com

RELATED CONTENT

Bites and Stings, Insect (Related Key Topic)
Bites and Stings (Patient Information)

AUTHOR: **GAIL M. O'BRIEN, M.D.**

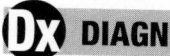

BASIC INFORMATION

DEFINITION

Most stinging insects belong to the Hymenoptera order and include yellow jackets (most common cause of reactions), hornets, bumblebees, sweat bees, wasps, harvester ants, fire ants, and the Africanized honey bee ("killer bee"). Brown recluse spiders, although not insects, are another common cause of bites (see "Bites and Stings, Arachnids"). The usual effect of a sting is intense local pain, some immediate erythema, and often a small area of edema from the injecting venom. Allergic reactions can be either local or generalized, leading to anaphylactic shock. The majority of reactions occur within the first 6 hr after the sting or bite, but a delayed presentation may occur up to 24 hr.

SYNONYMS   Venom allergy

ICD-9CM CODES
989.5 Stings (bees, wasps)
989.5 Bites (fire ant, brown recluse spider)

EPIDEMIOLOGY & DEMOGRAPHICS
PREVALENCE (OF BEE STINGS AND INSECT BITES):
- Unknown.
- Account for 2.3% of ED visits.
- From 0.5% to 3.3% of the population is allergic to the venom of one or more stinging insects.
- Most anaphylactic reactions occur during summer months in those most likely to be exposed, including children, males, outdoor workers.
- Approximately half of fatal reactions occur without prior allergic response.
- Bites by fire ants and brown recluse spiders are less likely to cause systemic disease.

INCIDENCE (IN U.S.): Forty to 100 people die each year from insect sting anaphylaxis; anaphylaxis occurs more often within 10 to 30 min of a sting. Delayed reactions are rare, occurring only in <0.3% of stings.

PHYSICAL FINDINGS & CLINICAL PRESENTATION
Stings:
- Cutaneous: the skin is the most common site of an allergic reaction. Manifestations include flushing, urticaria, pruritus, and angioedema. Local reactions may last several days.
- Respiratory: Symptoms of upper and lower airway obstruction including hoarseness, choking, throat tightness or tingling may progress to stridor, laryngeal edema, laryngospasm, and bronchoconstriction. This is the leading cause of anaphylactic death.
- Cardiovascular: most common reaction is hypotension which can progress to profound hypovolemic shock. Tachycardia and arrhythmia may occur. Myocardial infarction is rare. Cardiac manifestations are the second leading cause of death from anaphylaxis.
- Other symptoms: abdominal pain, nausea, vomiting, and diarrhea.

Fire ant bites:
- Initial wheal and flare response.
- Subsequent development of circularly arrayed blisters within 24 hr.
- Blisters may develop appearance of pustules, but they are not infected.

ETIOLOGY
Stings:
- Most systemic reactions to insect stings are classic immunoglobin E (IgE)–mediated reactions.
- Reactions occur in previously sensitized patients who have produced high titers of IgE antibody to insect venom antigens.
- Sensitization to wasp venom requires only a few stings and can occur after a single sting.
- Sensitization to bee venom occurs mainly in people who have been stung frequently by bees.
Bites:
- Fire ant venom contains proteins toxic to the skin.

 DIAGNOSIS

DIFFERENTIAL DIAGNOSIS
- Stings: cellulitis, bites
- Bites: stings, cellulitis

WORKUP
History is essential for accurate diagnosis including timing of sting or bite and type of insect (bee, wasp, spider, or ant) if known.

LABORATORY TESTS
- Skin test: either skin prick test or intradermal method with fire ant or hymenoptera venom.
- Venom skin tests and occasionally radioallergosorbent tests (RAST) to provide additional information.

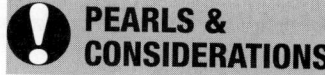 TREATMENT

ACUTE GENERAL Rx
Sting:
- Removal of the stinger most easily performed with a flat tool such as a credit card, followed by cleansing and application of ice.
- Avoid squeezing, which may push venom out of the venom sac and into the tissue.
- Consider treatment with oral antihistamines and nonsteroidal antiinflammatory medications and topical corticosteroids for limited reactions.
- Patients with previous reactions or multiple stings to the mouth or neck should be evaluated in an emergency department.
- Larger swellings may benefit from oral steroids.
- Generalized reactions should be treated with epinephrine. Antihistamines, oxygen, IV corticosteroids, beta-agonists, pressors, and IV fluids may also be beneficial for anaphylaxis.
Bite:
- Supportive care
- Application of ice

- Surveillance for secondary infection

DISPOSITION
Sting:
- Prognosis for a limited reaction is excellent.
- Subsequent anaphylaxis may occur in 35% to 65% of patients stung again.
- There is no evidence that the next sting will necessarily cause a more severe reaction. The reasons for the variable outcome include patient's age, comorbidities, time elapsed since prior exposure, dose of venom injected, and site of sting.
- Watch for secondary cellulitis.
- Patients who have a history of a systemic reaction:
  - Should be educated in avoidance of stinging insects
  - Carry syringes preloaded with epinephrine for self-administration
  - Undergo testing for IgE antibodies to stinging insects
  - Be considered for immunotherapy
  - Consider carrying medical identification for stinging insect hypersensitivity
Bite:
- Prognosis for fire ant bite is excellent.
- Large lesions from brown recluse spider bites may take months to heal.
- Watch for secondary cellulitis.

REFERRAL
- Consider a referral to an allergist for venom immunotherapy (VIT).
- Risk of subsequent anaphylaxis with immunotherapy falls to <3%.
- VIT for 3 to 5 yr induces long-term protection in most patients.

PEARLS & CONSIDERATIONS

Hypersensitivity to stings is common. Reactions range from local nonallergic reaction to venom to life-threatening anaphylaxis. Venom-specific immunotherapy is highly effective in decreasing subsequent anaphylaxis. Although venom immunotherapy is currently indicated only for systemic reactions, investigation is underway to assess efficacy for prevention of large local reactions, which can result in significant morbidity.

SUGGESTED READINGS
available at www.expertconsult.com

RELATED CONTENT
Bites and Stings, Arachnids (Related Key Topic)
Insect Bites (Bites and Stings) (Patient Information)

AUTHOR: **JENNIFER JEREMIAH, M.D.**

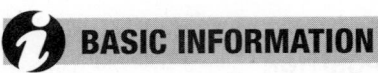

DEFINITION

Injury resulting from snake biting a human.

ICD-9CM CODES
989.5 Venomous poisoning

EPIDEMIOLOGY & DEMOGRAPHICS

- 45,000 snakebites occur annually in the U.S. Of the 4000 to 6000 caused by poisonous snakes, approximately 5 to 12 result in fatality (i.e., <1%-2%). Children, the elderly, and those in whom treatment has been delayed are at highest risk.
- In the U.S., at least one species of poisonous snake (Fig. 1-154) has been identified in every state except Alaska, Hawaii, and Maine.

Table 1-63 summarizes medically important snake families. The Crotalidae family, which includes rattlesnakes, copperheads, and cottonmouths, is responsible for the vast majority of venomous snakebites. The Elapidae family, which includes the coral snake, is less common and does not tend to be aggressive. Coral snake bites account for only 1% of venomous snakebites in the U.S.

PHYSICAL FINDINGS & CLINICAL PRESENTATION

In addition to local tissue injury, envenomation may affect the renal, neurologic, gastrointestinal, vascular, and coagulation systems. Symptoms vary widely depending on type of envenomation. Not all snakebites are poisonous and not all bites lead to envenomation. Species-specific signs and symptoms follow.

CROTALIDAE (PIT VIPERS): Signs and symptoms:
- Pain within 5 min
- Edema within 30 min
- Erythema of site and adjacent tissues/serous or hemorrhagic bullae, ecchymosis, and/or lymphangitis over the ensuing hours (Fig. E1-155)

If no edema or erythema is manifested within 8 hr after a confirmed Crotalid snakebite, it is safe to assume envenomation did not occur. (Roughly 25% of cases do not involve envenomation.) In general, rattlesnake bites are more severe than those of the other snakes in the Crotalid family.

Systemic manifestations may include:
- Mild to moderate manifestations: nausea/vomiting, perioral paresthesias, metallic taste, tingling of fingers or toes (especially with rattlesnake bites), and/or fasciculations (local or generalized)
- Severe manifestations: hypotension (due to increased vascular permeability), mental status change, respiratory distress, tachycardia, acute renal failure, rhabdomyolysis, and coagulopathies including intravascular hemolysis and disseminated intravascular coagulation

ELAPIDAE (CORAL SNAKES): Signs and symptoms:
- Local symptoms are far less pronounced (little or no pain/swelling immediately after the bite).
- Systemic symptoms predominate, but onset may be delayed for up to 12 hr. Examples include:
  - Altered mental status and cranial nerve palsies featuring ptosis, dysphagia, or dysarthria
  - Tremors

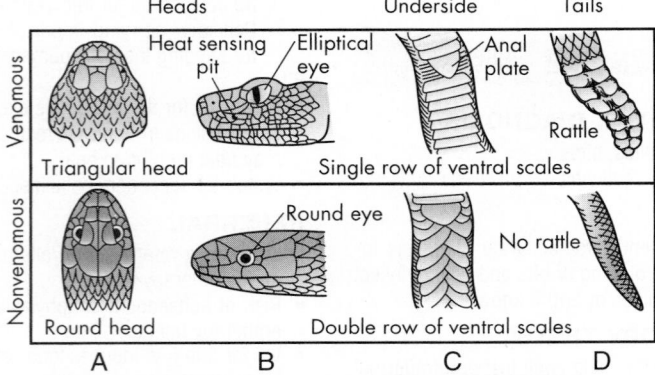

FIGURE 1-154 Comparison of pit vipers and nonvenomous snakes. Rattle in **D** (*top*) applies to rattlesnakes only. (**A** to **D**, From Sullivan JB et al: North American venomous reptile bites. In Auerbach PS [ed]: *Wilderness medicine: management of wilderness and environmental emergencies*, ed 3, p. 684, St Louis, 1995, Mosby.)

TABLE 1-63	Medically Important Snake Families			
Family	**Venomous?**	**Location**	**Examples**	**Toxin Effects/Other Comments**
Colubridae	Some species	Most parts of the world	Garter snakes (*Thamnophis* spp), king snakes and milk snakes (*Lampropeltis* spp)	Largest family of snakes; most are considered harmless to humans; a few species are dangerously toxic (e.g., African boomslang [*Dispholidus typus*])
Boidae	None	Most parts of the world	*Boa* sp, *Python* sp	Constrictors; unsupervised children should not be allowed access to large constrictors
Viperidae				
Subfamily Crotalinae (pit vipers)	All	Americas, Asia	Rattlesnakes (*Crotalus* spp), cottonmouths and copperheads (*Agkistrodon* spp), Lancehead pit vipers (*Bothrops* spp)	Heat-sensing "pit" between each eye and nostril
Subfamily Viperinae (true vipers)	All	Europe, Africa, Middle East, Asia	Puff adder (*Bitis arietans*), Gaboon viper (*Bitis gabonica*)	No heat-sensing pits
Elapidae	All	Americas, Africa, Middle East, Asia	Cobras (*Naja* spp), mambas (*Dendroaspis* spp), kraits (*Bungarus* spp), coral snakes (*Micrurus* spp), and the venomous snakes of Australia	Highly variable venom effects—some largely neurotoxic, others causing severe local tissue damage
Hydrophiidae	All	Warm waters of the Pacific Ocean, Indian Ocean, and Oceania (none in the Atlantic Ocean)	Sea snakes including the pelagic sea snake (*Pelamis platurus*)	Neurotoxins and myotoxins; rarely bite humans unless provoked

From Kliegman RM et al: *Nelson textbook of pediatrics*, ed 19, Philadelphia, 2011, Saunders.

○ If the patient has not responded after 1 hr, repeat the initial dose.

- Relapse may occur in up to two thirds of patients after an initial response. Consequently, it is recommended that three maintenance doses—each consisting of 2 vials—be given at 6, 12, and 18 hr following the patient's initial response to the loading dose.
- The manufacturer of Crofab maintains a 24/7 hotline: 877-377-3784
- Antivenin Crotalidae Polyvalent horse serum is no longer produced but may still be available at some pharmacies. It should be given as follows:
  ○ Progressive local or any systemic symptoms: 5 to 10 vials
  ○ Severe symptoms: 15 vials
  ○ Shock: 20 vials

ANTIVENOM TREATMENT OF ELAPIDAE (CORAL SNAKE) ENVENOMATIONS:

- Production of horse serum–based coral snake antivenom was discontinued in 2006 (horse serum–based antivenoms are being phased out due to much higher risk of hypersensitivity). All stock is expired as of October 31, 2008, except for lot 4030026, which received a 3-yr extension until October 31, 2012, and there has been no update at the time of this submission. After that date, one option will be to seek compassionate release of expired stock in conjunction with your local Poison Control Center. A potent, safe, sheep-based antivenom for elapid bites exists and is being used internationally but is not yet approved in the U.S. Another option is to contact a zoo that cares for exotic snakes and obtain Mexican coral snake or Australian Tiger snake antivenom, although efficacy for North American coral snake envenomation is unproved.
- For confirmed coral snake bites, antivenom should be administered immediately if available.
- If there are no systemic symptoms at the time of administration, start with 3 vials. If symptoms evolve, repeat with 5 vials.
- If systemic symptoms are already present, an initial dose of 6 to 10 vials is recommended.

TREATMENT OF NONNATIVE (EXOTIC) SNAKEBITES:

- For bites by exotic or nonnative snakes, contact a Poison Control Center or your local zoo. (Zoos with exotic snakes are required to maintain a supply of snake-specific antivenom on their premises.)

DISPOSITION

Prognosis is good with prompt evaluation and treatment. All patients who receive antivenom should be monitored in an ICU setting. Patients should be monitored for 18 to 24 hours after initial control of progression of symptoms. If at that time they have no progression of symptoms and labs prior to discharge are normal, patients can be safely discharged home. Give instructions to return for worsening nondependent swelling, abnormal bleeding, or signs of serum sickness and to follow bleeding precautions (no contact sports, elective surgery, etc.) for 2 weeks. Patients who received antivenom need follow-up in 2 to 3 days and in 5 to 7 days to evaluate for delayed hematologic complications and serum sickness.

REFERRAL

Refer to a medical facility with ICU for administration of antivenom. The approach to snakebites should be multidisciplinary and should include medical toxicology or other physican snakebite speacialist, as well as hematology or nephrology consultations if needed. All cases of snake bites should also be reported to Poison Control and the local health department as data are limited.

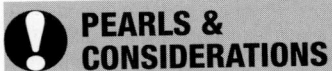

PEARLS & CONSIDERATIONS

OTHER CONSIDERATIONS

- Dosage of antivenom is based on typical envenomation rather than age or weight, so dose is the same for children and adults.
- Pregnancy is not a contraindication to antivenom. The rate of miscarriage is significantly lower in pregnant patients treated with antivenom.
- Immunize against tetanus if no booster within past 5 yr; if never immunized, give immunoglobulin as well as toxoid.
- Manage pain as needed (narcotic preferred to NSAIDs due to theoretical bleeding complications).
- Avoid sedation in Mojave rattlesnake, Eastern diamondback rattlesnake, and coral snake bites as all can have more systemic than local effects.
- Antibiotics rarely needed; reserve for moderate to severe contamination or definite infection; broad-spectrum coverage to include

gram negatives preferred (i.e., ampicillin-sulbactam or quinolone derivatives).

- Antivenom is most effective when given within 4 hr of the bite and least effective if delayed beyond 12 hr. Systemic symptoms (coagulopathy, CNS effects, etc.) respond better to treatment than do local symptoms (erythema/edema, bullae, etc.).
- Although local wound effects can be severe, wound management should not take precedence over antivenom administration. Some studies suggest that even in the case of compartment syndrome, antivenom may be more effective than fasciotomy, although both may be necessary.

COMPLICATIONS

- Allergic reactions were very frequent with horse serum antivenoms.
- Anaphylaxis occurs within 30 min and should be treated by immediately stopping the infusion to manage the symptoms of anaphylaxis, including epinephrine SQ or IM initially and IV if needed, diphenhydramine IV, and hydrocortisone IV. If the anaphylactic symptoms can be managed and the envenomation is severe, the infusion can then be resumed.
- Delayed hematologic complications are common and can manifest up to 4 days post treatment. Most bleeding is self-limited but can rarely be severe.
- Serum sickness occurs 7 to 14 days after antivenom administration and is characterized by fever, rash, arthralgias, and lymphadenopathy. It can be treated with prednisone 60 mg/d PO, tapered over 7 to 10 days.
- Injuries also result from:
  ○ Tourniquet placement, which should be avoided
  ○ Ice application (cryotherapy), which can worsen tissue damage
- National Poison Control hotline: 800-222-1222

SUGGESTED READINGS

available at www.expertconsult.com

AUTHOR: **LAURA H. McPEAKE, M.D.**

ⓘ BASIC INFORMATION

DEFINITION

Bladder cancer is a heterogeneous spectrum of neoplasms ranging from non–life-threatening, low-grade, superficial papillary lesions to high-grade invasive tumors, which often have metastasized at the time of presentation. It is a field change disease in which the entire urothelium from the renal pelvis to the urethra may be susceptible to malignant transformation. The three types of bladder cancer are transitional cell carcinoma (TCCa), squamous cell carcinoma, and adenocarcinoma.

ICD-9CM CODES
Primary:	188.9
Secondary:	198.1
CIS:	233.7
Benign:	223.3
Uncertain behavior:	236.7
Unspecified:	239.4

EPIDEMIOLOGY & DEMOGRAPHICS

Each year over 70,000 new cases are diagnosed and more than 14,000 deaths are attributed to bladder cancer. Overall, bladder cancer is the sixth most prevalent malignancy in the U.S. and the seventh leading cause of solid-cancer–related death.

Until 1990, the incidence of bladder cancer in the U.S. was rising. Since 1990, the incidence of bladder cancer is decreasing at a rate of 0.8% per year (1.2% among men and 0.4% among women).

PREDOMINANT SEX: In males, it is the fourth most common cancer, accounting for 10% of all cancers. In females, it is the eighth most common cancer, accounting for 4% of all cancers.

RISK: The lifetime risk of developing bladder cancer is 2.8% in white males, 0.9% in black males, 1% in white females, and 0.6% in black females.

Smoking:
- Users of "black" tobacco in place of "blond" tobacco have a twofold to threefold increase in developing bladder cancer.
- Smoking risk is based on consumption:
  - A twofold to threefold increase for subjects smoking at least 10 cigarettes per day
  - The risk increases again when the daily consumption rises above 40 to 60 cigarettes per day
- Smokers of low-tar and nicotine cigarettes have a lower risk when compared with higher tar and nicotine cigarettes.
- Those who smoke unfiltered cigarettes have a 50% increased risk of bladder cancer compared with those who smoke filtered cigarettes.
- Pipe smokers have a lower risk of bladder cancer compared with cigarette smokers.
- Cigars, snuff, and chewing tobacco, although implicated in nonurologic cancers, are not believed to influence bladder cancer risk.

Diet:
- Diets rich in beef, pork, and animal fat increase risk of bladder cancer.

- There is no indication that consumption of non-beer alcoholic drinks contributes to bladder cancer development.
- Beer consumption has been linked to bladder cancer development as a result of the presence of nitrosamines in the beer. Nitrosamines have also been implicated in the development of rectal cancer.
- Drinking coffee is not believed to contribute to bladder cancer risk. There is additional evidence that coffee consumption is protective for colorectal cancers, possibly by diminishing fecal transit time.
- Medications: Long-term (>1 yr) use of pioglitazone and rosiglitazone

PEAK INCIDENCE: Incidence increases with age: higher after age 60 yr, uncommon younger than 40 yr.

GENETICS: It is thought to be multifactorial in etiology, involving both genetic and environmental interactions. Overall, approximately 20% to 25% of the male population in the U.S. with bladder cancer is estimated to have the disease as a result of occupational exposure.

DISTRIBUTION: In North America, transitional cell carcinomas comprise 93%, squamous cell carcinomas comprise 6%, and adenocarcinomas account for 1% of bladder cancers.

PATHOGENESIS: Two pathways exist for bladder cancer (TCCa):
1. Papillary superficial disease occasionally leading to invasive cancer (75%)
2. Carcinoma in situ (CIS) and solid invasive cancer with high risk of disease progression (25%)

Two distinct forms of "superficial cancer" exist:
1. T_a: Papillary low-grade tumor with a high rate of recurrence; disease progression occurs in 5%.
2. T_1: Higher grade papillary tumor that infiltrates the lamina propria; often associated with flat CIS that may involve the urothelium diffusely. Disease progression occurs in 30% to 50%.

Subdivided into:
- T_{1a}: Penetration of tumor up to the muscularis mucosa; disease progression in 5.3%
- T_{1b}: Penetration of tumor through the muscularis mucosa; disease progression 53%

Flat CIS:
- Entirely different and separate pathway of cancer development whose mechanism is manifested by dysplasia, which leads to the occurrence of poorly differentiated malignant cells that replace or undermine the normal urothelium and extend along the plane of the bladder wall. It penetrates the basement membrane and lamina propria in 20% to 30% of cases and is associated with the development of solid tumor growth. A defect in chromosome 17p53 occurs in 50% of the cases.

At presentation, 72% of cancers are localized to the bladder, 20% of the cancers extend to the regional lymph nodes, and 3% present with distant metastases. Eighty percent of superficial TCCa recur, with up to 30% progressing to a higher stage or grade. Younger patients most commonly develop low-grade papillary nonin-

vasive TCCa and are less likely to have recurrences when compared with older patients with similar lesions. Involvement of the upper tracts with tumor occurs in 25% to 50% of the cases.

STAGING (BASED ON THE TNM SYSTEM):

T_0	No tumor in specimen
T_{is}	CIS
T_a	Papillary TCCa noninvasive
T_1	Papillary TCCa into lamina propria
T_2	TCCa invasive of superficial muscle
T_{3a}	Invasive of deep muscle
T_{3b}	Invasive of perivesical fat
T_{4a}	Invasive of adjacent pelvic organ
T_{4b}	Invasive of pelvic wall with fixation

Invasive of nodal status:

N_0	No nodal involvement
N_{1-3}	Pelvic nodes
N_4	Nodes above bifurcation
N_x	Unknown

Invasive of metastatic status:

M_0	No distant metastases
M_1	Distant metastases
M_x	Unknown

MOLECULAR EPIDEMIOLOGY: TCCa is usually a field change disease with tumors arising at different times and sites in the urothelium, suggesting a polyclonal etiology of bladder cancer. Bladder cancers have been associated with abnormalities on chromosomes 1, 4, 11, 5, 7, 3, 9, 21, 18, 13, 8; with alterations in suppressor genes *P53*, retinoblastoma gene, and *P16;* and with alterations in oncogenes H-ras and epidermal growth factor receptor.

PHYSICAL FINDINGS & CLINICAL PRESENTATION

- Gross, painless hematuria
- Microhematuria
- Frequency, urgency, occasional dysuria
- With locally invasive to distant metastatic disease, the presentation can include:
  - Abdominal pain
  - Flank pain
  - Lymphedema
  - Renal failure
  - Anorexia
  - Bone pain

ETIOLOGY

Bladder cancer is a potentially preventable disease associated with specific etiologic factors:
- Cigarette smoking is associated with 25% to 65% of cases. The risk of developing a TCCa is two to four times higher in smokers than in nonsmokers, and that risk persists for many years, being equal to nonsmokers only after 12 to 15 yr of smoking abstinence. Smoking tobacco is associated with tumors that are characterized by higher histologic grade, increased tumor stage, increase in the numbers of tumor present, and increased tumor size.
- Occupational exposures: dye workers, textile workers, tire and rubber workers, petroleum workers.
- Chemical exposure: O-toluidine, 2-naphthylamine, benzidine, 4-amino-biphenyl, and nitrosamines.

- Exposure to herpes papilloma virus type 16.

Squamous carcinomas are associated with:
- Schistosomiasis
- Urinary calculi
- Indwelling catheters
- Bladder diverticula

Miscellaneous causes:
- Phenacetin abuse
- Cyclophosphamide
- Pelvic irradiation
- Tuberculosis

Adenocarcinomas are associated with:
- Exstrophy
- Endometriosis
- Neurogenic bladder
- Urachal abnormalities
- As a secondary site for distant metastases from other organs (e.g., colon cancer)

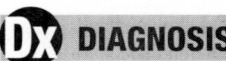 **DIAGNOSIS**

- History and physical examination.
- Urinalysis.
- Cystoscopy with bladder barbotage and biopsy. Fluorescence cystoscopy offers improvement in the detection of flat neoplastic lesions such as carcinoma in situ.
- Transurethral resection of bladder tumor(s).
- There is insufficient evidence to determine whether a decrease in mortality rate from bladder cancer occurs with hematuria testing, urinary cytology, or a variety of other tests on exfoliated urinary cells or other substances.
- In addition to urinary cytology and bladder barbotage, BTA, NMP22, and fibrin degradation products have been approved by the FDA as bladder cancer tumor markers. No marker has general, widespread acceptance because the results are affected by the presence of stents, recent urologic manipulation, stones, infection, bowel interposition, and prostatitis, creating false-positive results.

DIFFERENTIAL DIAGNOSIS
- Urinary tract infection
- Frequency-urgency syndrome
- Interstitial cystitis

- Stone disease
- Endometriosis
- Neurogenic bladder

LABORATORY TESTS
- Urine cytology.
- Urine telomerase: telomerase activity in voided urine or bladder washings determined by the telomeric repeat amplification protocol (TRAP) assay. This test has been reported to accurately detect the presence of bladder tumors in men. It represents a potentially useful noninvasive diagnostic innovation for bladder cancer detection in high-risk groups such as habitual smokers or in symptomatic patients.

RADIOLOGIC TESTS
- IVP, renal ultrasound, retrograde pyelography, CT scan, and MRI.
- One or a combination of studies can be used. In the absence of skeletal symptoms, bone scan is not recommended.

(Rx) **TREATMENT**

NONPHARMACOLOGIC THERAPY
- Initially, transurethral resection of bladder tumor (TURBT) (Fig. 1-156)
- Loop biopsy of the prostatic urethra if high-grade TCCa is suspected
- If superficial disease, follow-up protocol with repeat TURBT and/or the use of intravesical agents is recommended
- For advanced bladder cancer, radical cystectomy with urethrectomy (unless orthotopic diversion is planned) and either ileal loop conduit or orthotopic diversion

BLADDER PRESERVATION APPROACHES: After cystectomy for muscle-invasive disease, 50% or more of the patients will develop metastases. Most patients develop metastases at distant sites, a third relapse locally. Bladder preservation management is offered in individuals who refuse surgery or who might not be suitable radical cystectomy patients. Bladder-sparing protocols include extensive TURBT or partial cystectomy with external-beam or interstitial radiotherapy and systemic chemotherapy.

Radiotherapy as a single treatment modality is not effective. The best predictor of successful bladder preservation is a complete response after the combination of initial TURBT and two cycles of CMV (cisplatin, methotrexate, vinblastine) chemotherapy used with stages T_2 to T_{3a}.

INDICATIONS FOR PARTIAL CYSTECTOMY:
- Tumor within a bladder diverticulum
- Solitary, primary, and muscle-invasive or high-grade lesion of a region of the bladder that allows complete excision with adequate surgical margins
- Inability to adequately resect tumor by TURBT alone because of size or location
- Tumor overlying a ureteral orifice requiring ureteral reimplantation
- Biopsy of a radiation-induced ulceration
- Palliation of severe local symptoms
- Patient refusal of urinary diversion
- Poor-risk patient who is not a diversion candidate

CONTRAINDICATIONS:
- Multiple tumors
- CIS
- Cellular atypia on biopsy
- Prostatic invasion
- Invasion of the trigone
- Inability to achieve adequate surgical margins
- Prior radiotherapy
- Inability to maintain adequate bladder volume after resection
- Evidence of extravesical tumor extension
- Poor surgical risk

ACUTE GENERAL Rx
INDICATIONS FOR INTRAVESICAL CHEMOTHERAPY:
- High-grade tumor
- Tumor size >5 cm
- Tumor multiplicity
- Presence of CIS
- Positive urinary cytologic findings after a resection
- Incomplete tumor resection

Intravesical agents: thiotepa, Adriamycin, mitomycin C, AD-32, BCG, interferon, bropirimine, Epodyl, interleukin-2, and keyhole-limpet hemocyanin. Photodynamic therapy with hematoporphyrin derivatives has also been used.

INDICATIONS FOR CYSTECTOMY:
- Large tumors not amenable to complete TURBT
- High-grade tumor
- Multiple tumors with frequent recurrences
- Diffuse CIS not responsive to intravesical chemotherapy
- Prostatic urethra involvement
- Irritative bladder symptoms with upper tract deterioration
- Muscle-invasive disease
- Disease outside the bladder

SYSTEMIC CHEMOTHERAPY: Used as neoadjuvant and adjuvant therapy for systemic disease. The most effective agents are cisplatin, methotrexate, vinblastine, Adriamycin (MVAC). Other agents include mitoxantrone, vincristine, etoposide (VP16), 5-fluorouracil, ifosfamide, Taxol, gemcitabine, Piritrexim, mitomycin C, and gallium

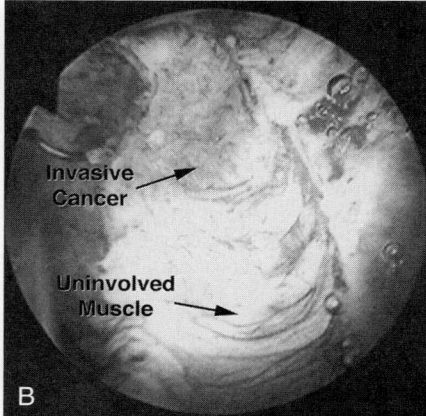

FIGURE 1-156 **A,** Papillary bladder cancer in right lower aspect of photo with resection loop poised to begin transurethral resection. **B,** Demonstration of grossly uninvolved muscularis propria *(bottom)* and cancer grossly invading the bladder wall *(top)*. (From Abeloff MD: *Clinical oncology*, ed 3, Philadelphia, 2004, Churchill Livingstone.)

nitrate. Chemotherapy in combination can provide palliation and modest survival benefit.

RADIOTHERAPY: Conflicting reports suggest that superficial bladder cancer is more sensitive to radiotherapy. Squamous changes within the tumor and secretion of human chorionic gonadotropin by the lesion are associated with poor response to radiotherapy. Only 20% to 30% of patients with invasive bladder cancer can be cured by external-beam radiation therapy alone. It is used in combination with surgery or with systemic agents to treat bladder cancer primarily in patients who are not surgical candidates or who refuse surgery. Trials with synchronous chemotherapy with fluorouracil and mitomycin C combined with radiotherapy have shown significant improved locoregional control of bladder cancer, as compared with radiotherapy alone in patients with muscle-invasive bladder cancer.

CHRONIC Rx

FOLLOW-UP RECOMMENDATIONS FOR SUPERFICIAL BLADDER CANCER:

- Cystoscopy, bladder barbotage, and bimanual examination every 3 mo for 2 yr, then every 6 mo for 2 yr, and annually thereafter.
- Upper tract studies are based on the risk of upper tract tumor development, generally every 2 to 5 yr.

FOLLOW-UP RECOMMENDATIONS FOR ADVANCED DISEASE:

Bladder preservation:

- Cystoscopy, barbotage, bimanual examination, biopsy (when indicated), every 3 mo for 2 yr, then every 6 mo for 2 yr, yearly thereafter
- CT scan of abdomen and pelvis every 6 mo for 2 yr in addition to chest x-ray examination, liver function testing, and serum creatinine

Cystectomy with ileal loop/orthotopic bladder:

- Neobladder endoscopy and IVP yearly
- CT scan of abdomen and pelvis every 6 mo for 2 yr in addition to chest x-ray examination, liver function tests, and serum creatinine
- Loopogram every 6 mo for 2 yr, then annually

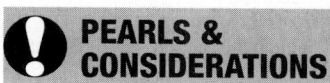

PEARLS & CONSIDERATIONS

COMMENTS

- The most useful prognostic parameters for bladder tumor recurrence and subsequent cancer progression are tumor grade, depth of tumor penetration, multifocal tumors, frequency of recurrence, tumor size, CIS, lymphatic invasion, papillary or solid tumor configuration.
- Box 1-6 describes the American Urological Association Guideline Recommendations for bladder cancer.

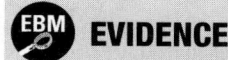

EVIDENCE

available at www.expertconsult.com

SUGGESTED READINGS

available at www.expertconsult.com

RELATED CONTENT

Bladder Cancer (Patient Information)

AUTHORS: **PHILIP J. ALIOTTA, M.D., M.S.H.A.,** and **RUBEN ALVERO, M.D.**

BOX 1-6 American Urological Association Guideline Recommendations

For all index patients:
- Standard: Physicians should discuss with the patient the treatment options and the benefits and harms, including side effects, of intravesical treatment.

For a patient who presents with an abnormal growth on the urothelium but who has not yet been diagnosed with bladder cancer:
- Standard: If the patient does not have an established histologic diagnosis, a biopsy should be obtained for pathologic analysis.
- Standard: Under most circumstances, complete eradication of all visible tumors should be performed.
- Standard: If bladder cancer is confirmed, periodic surveillance cystoscopy should be performed.
- Option: An initial single dose of intravesical chemotherapy may be administered immediately postoperatively.

For a patient with small volume, low-grade Ta bladder cancer:
- Recommendation: An initial single dose of intravesical chemotherapy may be administered immediately postoperatively.

For a patient with multifocal and/or large volume, histologically confirmed, low-grade Ta or a patient with recurrent low-grade Ta bladder cancer:
- Recommendation: An induction course of intravesical therapy with bacillus Calmette-Guérin or mitomycin C is recommended for the treatment of these patients with the goal of preventing or delaying recurrence.
- Option: Maintenance bacillus Calmette-Guérin or mitomycin C may be considered.

For a patient with initial histologically confirmed high-grade Ta, T1, and/or carcinoma in situ bladder cancer:
- Standard: For patients with lamina propria invasion (T1) but without muscularis propria in the specimen, repeat resection should be performed prior to additional intravesical therapy.
- Recommendation: An induction course of bacillus Calmette-Guérin followed by maintenance therapy is recommended for treatment of these patients.
- Option: Cystectomy should be considered for initial therapy in select patients.

For a patient with high-grade Ta, T1, and/or carcinoma in situ bladder cancer that has recurred after prior intravesical therapy:
- Standard: For patients with lamina propria invasion (T1) but without muscularis propria in the specimen, repeat resection should be performed prior to additional intravesical therapy.
- Recommendation: Cystectomy should be considered as a therapeutic alternative for these patients.
- Option: Further intravesical therapy may be considered for these patients.

From the American Urological Association, Guideline Division, http://www.auanet.org.

Diseases and Disorders

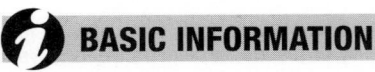

DEFINITION

Blepharitis is a chronic inflammation of the eyelid margins that is often refractory to treatment with infectious and noninfectious etiologies.

SYNONYMS

Eye lid infection or inflammation
Eczema of the eye lids
Dermatoblepharitis
Angular blepharitis

ICD-9CM CODES
373.0 Blepharitis

EPIDEMIOLOGY & DEMOGRAPHICS

- Common in children, particularly those with atopic dermatitis and eczema
- Adults with seborrhea involving the eyelids

PHYSICAL FINDINGS & CLINICAL PRESENTATION

- Common symptoms: red eyes, burning sensation, excessive tearing, blurred vision, pruritic eyelids
- Chronically infected lids are usually diffusely erythematous, with collarettes (fibrin exudate) at the base of the lashes (Fig. 1-159)
- Lid margins thicken over time, with associated loss of eyelashes (madarosis), misdirected growth of lashes (trichiasis), and overflow or inspissation of the meibomian glands.

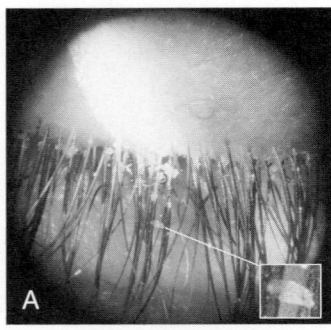
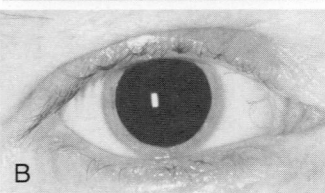

FIGURE 1-159 A, Seborrheic blepharitis. The typical scales (scurf) are translucent and easily removed. **B,** Staphylococcal blepharitis showing the typical lid margin erythema and discharge. (From Palay D [ed]: *Ophthalmology for the primary care physician,* St Louis, 1997, Mosby.)

- Associated conjunctivitis with erythema, edema but no discharge.
- Chalazion: chronic sterile inflammation of an oil gland of the eyelid
- Superficial punctate erosions of the inferior corneal epithelium are common.
- More severe findings, such as corneal pannus, ulcerative keratitis, or lid ectropion, are less common.

ETIOLOGY

Multiple: bacterial and nonbacterial causes
- Staphylococcal infection most common but streptococcal, Moraxella, and other bacterial infections; viral infections (e.g., herpes simplex, herpes zoster, *Molluscum contagiosum*); and a number of ecoparasites, including pediculosis, may cause blepharitis
- Seborrheic dermatitis
- Rosacea
- Dry eye (keratoconjunctivitis sicca): decrease in tear volume
- Meibomian gland dysfunction
- Contact lens intolerance
- Two categories of blepharitis:
  1. Anterior blepharitis, most often associated with staphylococcal infection
  2. Posterior blepharitis, associated with meibomian gland dysfunction and seborrheic dermatitis or rosacea

NOTE: Blepharitis patients have normal skin microflora in greater amounts (mostly *S. epidermidis* and *Propionibacterium acnes*). (*S. aureus* and *S. epidermidis* can be cultured in 10% to 35% and 90% to 95% of healthy persons, respectively.)

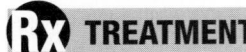 DIAGNOSIS

DIFFERENTIAL DIAGNOSIS
- Keratoconjunctivitis sicca
- Eyelid malignancies
- Herpes simplex blepharitis
- Molluscum contagiosum
- Phthiriasis palpebrarum
- *Phthirus pubis* (pubic lice)
- Demodex folliculorum (transparent mites)
- Allergic blepharitis

WORKUP
Scrapings of the eyelids to show polymorphonuclear leukocytes and gram-positive cocci

LABORATORY TESTS
Eyelid cultures and antibiotic sensitivity testing (usually not done unless patient fails to respond to initial treatment regimen)

TREATMENT

NONPHARMACOLOGIC THERAPY
- Alkaline soaps may be beneficial; alcohol and some detergents remove surface lipids and microflora.
- Hot compresses applied to closed lids for 5 to 10 min: heat loosens debris from lid margins and increases meibomian gland fluidity.
- Firm massage of the lid margins to enhance the flow of secretions from glands, followed by cleansing of the lids with cotton-tipped applicators dipped in a 50:50 mixture of baby shampoo and water.
- Lashes and lid margins scrubbed vigorously while the eyelids are closed, followed by thorough rinsing.
- Following local massage and cleansing, the mainstay of treatment is application of topical antibiotic ointment to the eyelid margins.
  1. Most effective topical antibiotics include bacitracin, erythromycin or 1% azithromycin solution, aminoglycoside and fluoroquinolone ophthalmic ointments.
  2. Ointment is applied 1 to 4 times daily, depending on the severity, for 1 to 2 wk, followed by once daily, at bedtime, for another 4 to 8 wk until all signs of inflammation have disappeared.
- Oral antibiotics: long-term use of doxycycline or tetracycline in a tapering dose may be helpful in severe cases for patients older than 8 years of age.
- Topical glucocorticoids: short-term use in acute exacerbations of blepharitis

For patients with rosacea:
1. Tetracycline 250 mg orally 4 times daily or doxycycline 100 mg orally bid along with local treatment for several months

Recalcitrant cases with antibiotic resistance:
1. Vancomycin eye drops 1%
2. Ciprofloxacin or ofloxacin eye drops

CHRONIC Rx
By definition, this is a chronic condition for which there is frequently no cure.

Some newer agents being evaluated are topical cyclosporine 0.05% eye drops, thermal pulsation systems to break up material in meibomian glands, topical metronidazole and topical tacrolimus, and tear lipid substitutes.

DISPOSITION
This condition may be refractory to treatment.

REFERRAL
To an ophthalmologist if patient fails to respond to local therapy.

SUGGESTED READINGS
available at www.expertconsult.com

AUTHOR: **GLENN G. FORT, M.D., M.P.H.**

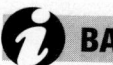

BASIC INFORMATION

DEFINITION

Body dysmorphic disorder (BDD) is a somatoform disorder characterized by preoccupation with one or more perceived defects or flaws in physical appearance that are not observable or appear slight to others, as well as repetitive behaviors (e.g., excessive grooming) in response to the appearance concerns. The preoccupations cause clinically significant distress or impairment in social, occupational, or other important areas of functioning. The appearance preoccupations are not better explained by concerns with body fat or weight in a person who has an eating disorder.

SYNONYMS

Dysmorphophobia

ICD-9CM CODES
300.7

DSM-IV CODES
300.7

EPIDEMIOLOGY & DEMOGRAPHICS

- Affects 1.7% to 2.4% of the general population (in nationwide epidemiologic studies)
- Prevalence among cosmetic surgery patients (in most studies) is 7% to 15%.
- Prevalence among dermatology patients is 9% to 14%.
- Slightly higher prevalence among females
- Onset most commonly in adolescence

PHYSICAL FINDINGS & CLINICAL PRESENTATION

- Excessive preoccupation (obsession) with one or more perceived defects in appearance that are not observable or appear slight to others. Any part of the body may be a focus of concern; skin, hair, and nose concerns are most common. Most patients are preoccupied with multiple body areas.
- The patient usually appears physically normal; if a physical defect is present, it is slight, and the patient's reaction to it is excessive.
- Most patients have poor insight or are delusional (i.e., completely convinced) regarding the accuracy of their belief about the appearance of the perceived defects.
- Over the course of the disorder, all patients engage in repetitive behaviors such as frequent mirror checking, excessive grooming, camouflaging (trying to hide the perceived flaws—e.g., with makeup, a hat, hair), skin picking, reassurance seeking, and repeatedly measuring or feeling the perceived defect. The intent of these behaviors is to check, try

to improve, or be reassured about the appearance of the perceived flaws.
- Nearly all experience impairment in psychosocial functioning and quality of life; impairment is usually substantial.
- Suicidal ideation, suicide attempts, and completed suicide appear common.
- Commonly co-occurring mental disorders are major depressive disorder, substance use disorders, social phobia, obsessive-compulsive disorder (OCD), and personality disorder.

ETIOLOGY

Likely multifactorial, with both genetic and environmental risk factors (e.g., teasing). Neuropsychological and fMRI studies indicate abnormalities in visual processing consisting of excessive focus on details rather than larger configural elements of visual stimuli.

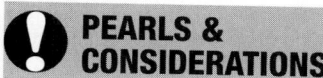

DIAGNOSIS

Psychiatric interview
- Ask:
  1. Are you very worried about your appearance in any way? OR: Are you unhappy with how you look?
  2. Does this concern with your appearance preoccupy you?
  3. How much distress does this concern cause you?
  4. What effect does this concern have on your life?

DIFFERENTIAL DIAGNOSIS

- Often undiagnosed because of patient's reluctance to divulge symptoms due to shame and fear of being misunderstood (e.g., considered vain)
- OCD
- Eating disorder
- Social phobia
- Major depressive disorder

WORKUP

Clinical evaluation focused on BDD symptoms and associated impairment in functioning.

TREATMENT

NONPHARMACOLOGIC THERAPY

- CBT, with a focus on cognitive restructuring, exposure and response prevention; CBT must be specifically tailored to BDD's unique symptoms.
- Do not try to talk patients out of their concern; it is ineffective.
- Avoid cosmetic procedures.

ACUTE GENERAL Rx

Precautions/hospitalization if actively suicidal

CHRONIC Rx

- SRIs are medication of choice; relatively high doses often needed.
- Other agents (e.g., neuroleptics, tricyclic antidepressants other than clomipramine) do not appear as beneficial.
- CBT tailored specifically to BDD is recommended with or without an SRI.
- Support groups if available.

DISPOSITION

- Untreated BDD tends to be chronic and can lead to social isolation; school dropout; major depression; unnecessary surgery, dermatologic treatment, or other cosmetic treatment; and even suicide.
- With correct diagnosis and treatment, a majority improve.

REFERRAL

Refer for psychiatric evaluation and treatment if diagnosis is suspected.

PEARLS & CONSIDERATIONS

- In clinical settings, more than 60% have co-occurring major depressive disorder.
- Reassurance is rarely helpful.
- Patients often have an unrealistic expectation of improvement with plastic surgery, dermatologic treatment, and other cosmetic procedures; these treatments do not appear to be effective.
- All patients should be screened for suicidality.

PATIENT/FAMILY EDUCATION

- Patients and family members usually benefit from psychoeducation.
- Family support and encouragement of appropriate treatment is important.
- Phillips KA: *Understanding Body Dysmorphic Disorder: An Essential Guide.* Oxford University Press, 2009
- http://www.BDDProgram.com (http://www.rhodeislandhospital.org/RIH/Services/MentalHealth/BodyImage/default.htm)
- Body Dysmorphic Disorder Central: http://www.BDDCentral.com

SUGGESTED READINGS

available at www.expertconsult.com

RELATED CONTENT

Obsessive Compulsive Disorder (Related Key Topic)
Body Dysmorphic Disorder (Patient Information)

AUTHOR: **KATHARINE A. PHILLIPS, M.D.**

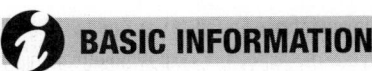

BASIC INFORMATION

DEFINITION

Primary malignant bone tumors are invasive and anaplastic and have the ability to metastasize. Most arise from the marrow (myeloma), but tumors may develop from bone, cartilage, fat, and fibrous tissues. Leukemia and lymphoma are excluded from this discussion.

FIBROSARCOMA AND LIPOSARCOMA: Extremely rare. They are similar to tumors arising in soft tissue.

OSTEOSARCOMA: A rare primary malignant tumor of bone characterized by malignant tumor cells that produce osteoid or bone. Several variants have been described: parosteal sarcoma, periosteal sarcoma, multicentric, and telangiectatic forms.

CHONDROSARCOMA: A malignant cartilage tumor that may develop primarily or secondarily from transformation of a benign osteocartilaginous exostosis or enchondroma.

EWING'S SARCOMA: A malignant tumor of unknown histogenesis.

MULTIPLE MYELOMA: A neoplastic proliferation of plasma cells.

SYNONYMS

Multiple myeloma:
1. Plasma cell myeloma
2. Plasmacytoma

ICD-9CM CODES	
203.0	Multiple myeloma
170.9	Neoplasm, bone (periosteum), primary malignant
M9180/3	Osteosarcoma
N9220/3	Chondrosarcoma
M9260/3	Ewing's sarcoma

EPIDEMIOLOGY & DEMOGRAPHICS

MULTIPLE MYELOMA:
- The most common tumor in bone
- Age at onset: usually >40 yr
- Male/female ratio of 2:1

OSTEOGENIC SARCOMA:
- Average age at onset: 10 to 20 yr
- Males afflicted more often than females
- Parosteal sarcoma in older patients

CHONDROSARCOMA:
- Age at onset: 40 to 60 yr
- Male/female ratio of 2:1

EWING'S SARCOMA: Age at onset: 10 to 15 yr

PHYSICAL FINDINGS & CLINICAL PRESENTATION

MULTIPLE MYELOMA:
- May present as a systemic process or, less commonly, as a "solitary" lesion
- Early manifestations: anorexia, weight loss, and bone pain; majority of cases present initially with back pain that often leads to the detection of a destructive skeletal lesion
- Other organ systems eventually become involved, resulting in more bone pain, anemia, renal insufficiency, and/or bacterial infections, usually as a result of the dysproteinemia typical of this disorder
- Possible secondary amyloidosis, leading to cardiac failure or nephrotic syndrome

OSTEOSARCOMA:
- Most originating in the metaphysis
- 50% to 60% around the knee
- Possible pain and swelling, but otherwise healthy patient
- Osteosarcoma in conjunction with Paget's disease, manifested primarily as a sudden increase in bone pain

CHONDROSARCOMA:
- Tumor most commonly involving the pelvis, upper femur, and shoulder girdle
- Painful swelling

EWING'S SARCOMA:
- Painful soft tissue mass often present
- Possibly increased local heat
- Midshaft of a long bone usually affected (in contrast to other tumors)
- Weight loss, fever, and lethargy

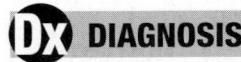

DIAGNOSIS

DIFFERENTIAL DIAGNOSIS
- Osteomyelitis
- Metastatic bone disease

LABORATORY TESTS
- Slightly elevated alkaline phosphatase in osteosarcoma
- In Ewing's sarcoma: reflective of systemic reaction; include anemia, an increase in white blood cell count, and an elevated sedimentation rate
- In multiple myeloma:
  1. Bence Jones protein in the urine
  2. Anemia and elevated sedimentation rate
  3. Characteristic dysproteinemia on serum protein electrophoresis
  4. Diagnostic feature: peak in the electrophoretic pattern suggestive of a monoclonal gammopathy

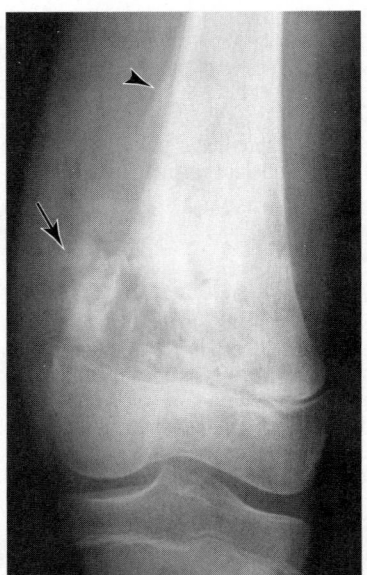

FIGURE 1-160 Conventional central osteosarcoma. AP radiograph of the distal femur showing a classic osteosarcoma with mixed lytic and sclerotic areas, tumor bone formation in the extraosseous mass *(arrow),* and a proximal Codman's triangle *(arrowhead).* (From Adam A et al: *Grainger & Allison's diagnostic radiology,* ed 5, Philadelphia, 2008, Churchill Livingstone.)

5. Rouleaux formation in the peripheral blood smear
6. Often presence of hypercalcemia, but alkaline phosphatase levels usually normal

IMAGING STUDIES
- Classic osteogenic sarcoma penetrates the cortex early in many cases.
  1. A blastic (dense), lytic (lucent), or mixed response may be seen in the affected bone (Fig. 1-160).
  2. An aggressive perpendicular sunburst pattern may be present as a result of periosteal reaction, and peripheral Codman's triangles are often noted.
  3. Margins of the tumor are poorly defined.
- Speckled calcifications in a destructive radiolucent lesion are usually suggestive of chondrosarcoma.
- Ewing's sarcoma is characterized radiographically by mottled, irregular destructive changes with periosteal new bone formation. The latter may be multilayered, producing the typical "onion skin" appearance.
- Typical roentgenographic finding in multiple myeloma is the "punched out" lesion with sharply demarcated edges.
  1. Multiple lesions are usual.
  2. Diffuse osteoporosis may be the only finding in many cases.
  3. Pathologic fractures are common.

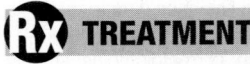

TREATMENT

The evaluation and treatment of malignant bone tumors are complicated. Diagnostic studies and treatment should be supervised by an orthopedic cancer specialist and oncologist.

DISPOSITION
- In the past 20 yr, dramatic improvements have been made in the treatment protocols for osteosarcoma with the use of adjuvant multidrug regimens and limb-sparing surgery.
- Prognosis of multiple myeloma remains poor despite new therapies.
- Prognosis for Ewing's sarcoma has improved with a combination of chemotherapy, local resection, and radiation therapy.
- Chondrosarcomas are not sensitive to chemotherapy or radiation, and prognosis depends on the grade of the tumor and the ability to obtain an adequate resection.

PEARLS & CONSIDERATIONS

Early diagnosis is important because most tumors have not metastasized at the time of initial presentation.

SUGGESTED READINGS
available at www.expertconsult.com

RELATED CONTENT
Fig. E1-548 Multiple myeloma
Fig. E1-551 A current treatment algorithm for multiple myeloma (Algorithm)
Multiple Myeloma (Patient Information)

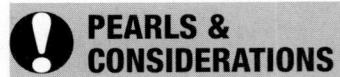

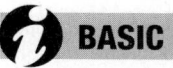 **BASIC INFORMATION**

DEFINITION

Borderline personality disorder (BPD) is characterized by a pervasive pattern of instability in interpersonal relationships, self-image, affect regulation, and impulse control that causes significant subjective distress or impairment of functioning. The individual must meet five or more of the following criteria:

1. Frantic efforts to avoid real or imagined abandonment
2. Unstable and intense personal relationships characterized by alternating between extremes of idealization and devaluation
3. Identity disturbance characterized by an unstable self-image
4. Impulsivity in at least two areas that are potentially self-damaging (e.g., overspending, sex, substance abuse, binge eating, reckless driving)
5. Recurrent suicidal behavior, gestures, threats, or self-mutilating behavior
6. Affective instability due to a marked reactivity of mood
7. Chronic feelings of emptiness
8. Inappropriate, intense anger or difficulty controlling anger
9. Transient, stress-related paranoid ideation or severe dissociative symptoms

ICD-9CM CODES
301.83 Borderline personality

EPIDEMIOLOGY & DEMOGRAPHICS

PREVALENCE: Affects approximately 1% to 2% of the general population and up to 10% of psychiatric outpatients
PREDOMINANT SEX: Female (3:1)
PREDOMINANT AGE: 20s
GENETICS: BPD is five times as likely if disorder is present in a first-degree relative. Increased prevalence of mood disorders and substance abuse disorders also found in first-degree relatives.
RISK FACTORS: Association with childhood physical, sexual, or emotional abuse and/or neglect

PHYSICAL FINDINGS & CLINICAL PRESENTATION

- No specific associated physical findings.
- Mental status examination may reveal affective lability.
- Clinical presentation may reveal the following:
  - A pervasive sense of loneliness and emptiness.
  - Underlying negative affect with dysphoria.
  - High frequency of multiple psychiatric disorders, especially posttraumatic stress disorder (PTSD), mood disorders, attention-deficit/hyperactivity disorder, and substance use disorders. Intense emotions with difficulty returning to emotional baseline.
  - All-or-nothing, either/or cognitive style that is represented by a phenomenon known as "splitting," in which patient sees situations or people as all good or all bad.
  - Difficulty in maintaining commitment to long-term goals; history of numerous stormy relationships and multiple jobs.
  - Reports a high number of sexual partners due to either/both impulsivity and victimization.
  - Reacts with rage, panic, despair to actual or perceived abandonment; may present with suicidality or self-mutilating behavior in response to recent stressor.
  - Attempts to block the experience of pain, which may induce feelings of derealization, depersonalization, changes in consciousness, and/or brief psychotic reactions with delusions and hallucinations.
  - Substance use, gambling, overspending, eating binges, and/or self-mutilation as a way to escape intensely painful affect.
- Some patients may display psychotic symptoms.

ETIOLOGY

- Interaction of psychosocial adversity plus genetic factors
- Hypotheses:
  1. Genetic: increased risk if first-degree relative with BPD.
  2. Biologic: abnormalities in limbic system and other areas of the brain cause emotional dysregulation. Serotonergic functioning appears to be disturbed.
  3. Environmental: history of childhood abuse (most commonly sexual) or neglect.

DIAGNOSIS

DIFFERENTIAL DIAGNOSIS

- Histrionic and narcissistic personality disorders share some common features.
- Dysthymia and other depressive disorders: requires a stability of affective symptoms not seen in BPD.
- Bipolar disorder: mood changes in BPD often triggered by stressors and less sustained than in bipolar disorder. Many patients with BPD are incorrectly diagnosed with bipolar disorder.
- Substance abuse or dependence: often induces impulsive, emotionally labile behavior.
- Posttraumatic stress disorder (PTSD): individuals with BPD often have history of trauma but do not avoid the feared stimulus or reexperience the trauma, as with PTSD.
- Mild cases of schizophrenia may superficially resemble BPD.

WORKUP

- History (helpful to gather collateral information from family and friends)
- Physical examination
- Mental status examination

LABORATORY TESTS

- Toxicology screen; substance use is common and can mimic features of personality disorders.
- Screen for HIV and other sexually transmitted illnesses.

IMAGING STUDIES

Structural and functional MRI demonstrate amygdala hyperactivity, reduced hippocampus and amygdala volume, greater activation within the insula and posterior cingulate cortex, and less activation in regions extending from the amygdala to the cingulate and prefrontal cortex. PET scans reveal reduced metabolism in prefrontal cortex. Recent PET research reveals dysregulation of endogenous opioid function. Imaging is not recommended as part of routine evaluation.

TREATMENT

NONPHARMACOLOGIC THERAPY

Dialectical behavior therapy (DBT), mentalization-based therapy, variations of cognitive behavior therapy (CBT), and transference-focused psychotherapy, a type of psychodynamic therapy, have the most empirical support from randomized trials. The goal of DBT and most CBT variations is to help patients improve mindfulness, control impulsive behaviors and angry outbursts, and develop social skills. The emphasis of mentalization treatment is to teach patients to stand outside of their feelings and observe emotions in oneself and others. The focus of transference-focused psychotherapy is on examining the affect-laden themes that emerge in the relationship between patient and therapist. Effective therapeutic treatments typically combine weekly group and individual therapy meetings.

ACUTE GENERAL Rx

Low-dose antipsychotics to control impulsivity, brief psychotic episodes.

CHRONIC Rx

- Medications have low-to-moderate effectiveness and are most effective in improving symptoms of impulsivity, mood instability, and self-destructive behavior. Effectiveness only studied for the first 3 mo of treatment.
- SSRIs if concurrent mood disorder. Higher doses may be required than for major depression.
- Low-dose antipsychotics.
- Mood stabilizers (lithium, valproate, carbamazepine, topiramate).
- In preliminary studies, omega-3 fatty acids improve irritability.

DISPOSITION

- Course is variable. The most unstable period is typically in early adulthood; the majority achieve greater stability in social/occupational functioning later in life but often continue with difficulty maintaining intimate relationships.
- Clinically salient features such as alcohol/substance use and self-injury may be less common in older adults.
- No evidence of progression to schizophrenia, but there is a high incidence of concurrent major depression and other Axis I disorders.
- Patients with high pre-treatment symptom severity who report a strong therapeutic alliance with their providers report highest treatment benefits.

REFERRAL

- Referral to mental health specialist:
  - For diagnosis and management.
  - Use of pharmacotherapy
  - Patient is severely impaired or suicidal

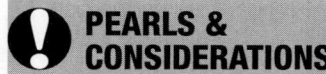

PEARLS & CONSIDERATIONS

COMMENTS

- Consider frequent, brief, scheduled visits for needy, demanding, or somaticizing patients with BPD.
- Validate the patient's feelings while stating the expectation of behavior control.
- Be matter-of-fact; avoid expressing extreme emotions.
- Be alert to the risk of suicide and assess suicide risk often.
- Be alert to the risk of nonsuicidal self-harm, such as cutting
- Convey a demeanor of competence but openly acknowledge minor errors.
- Have a low threshold for seeking psychiatric consultation.
- At the time of this writing, Borderline Personality Disorder type has been recommended for retention in the DSM-5.

PREVENTION

- There are no known ways to prevent BPD (or other personality disorders).
- Suicidality should be actively and consistently monitored.
- Benzodiazepines, narcotic analgesics, and other drugs with potential for dependency should be used rarely and with great caution, due to impaired impulse control and risk of addictive behavior.
- Patients should be asked frequently and in detail about parenting practices. Low frustration tolerance, externalization of blame for psychological distress, and impaired impulse control put children at risk for neglect or abuse.

PATIENT & FAMILY EDUCATION

National Alliance for the Mentally Ill (NAMI; http://www.nami.org) provides patient information, online chat groups, and information on support groups throughout the U.S. for people with BPD and their families.

Additional, local support groups for BPD are common and should be investigated.

SUGGESTED READINGS
available at www.expertconsult.com

RELATED CONTENT

Borderline Personality Disorder (Patient Information)

AUTHORS: **MARK ZIMMERMAN, M.D., THERESA A. MORGAN, M. PHIL,** and **MITCHELL D. FELDMAN, M.D., M.PHIL.**

BASIC INFORMATION

DEFINITION

Botulism is an illness caused by a neurotoxin produced by *Clostridium botulinum*. Five types of disease can occur: foodborne botulism, wound botulism, infant intestinal botulism, adult enteric botulism (which is similar to infant botulism), and inhalational botulism: aerosolized toxin released as an act of bioterrorism. Recent concern has increased about a possible fourth type of disease: inhalational botulism, which does not occur naturally, but may occur as a result of bioterrorism.

SYNONYMS

Clostridium botulinum food poisoning
Botulinum toxin food poisoning
Wound botulism
Infantile botulism

ICD-9CM CODES
005.1 Botulism

EPIDEMIOLOGY & DEMOGRAPHICS

INCIDENCE (IN U.S.): Approximately 24 cases/yr of foodborne illness, 3 cases/yr of wound botulism, and 71 cases/yr of infant botulism

PHYSICAL FINDINGS & CLINICAL PRESENTATION

- Symptoms usually begin 12 to 36 hr following ingestion.
- Severity of illness is related to the quantity of toxin ingested.
- Significant findings:
  1. Cranial nerve palsies, with ocular and bulbar manifestations being most frequent (diplopia, ophthalmoplegia, ptosis, dysphagia, dysarthria, fixed and dilated pupils, and dry mouth)
  2. Usually bilateral nerve involvement that may progress to a descending flaccid paralysis
  3. Typically, absence of sensory findings; sensorium intact
  4. GI symptoms (nausea, vomiting, diarrhea, or cramps)
  5. Usually no fever
- Wound botulism
  1. Occurs mostly in injecting drug users (subcutaneous heroin injection—"skin popping") or with traumatic injury.
  2. Presentation is similar to that of foodborne disease, except for a longer incubation period and the absence of GI symptoms.
  3. Wound infection is not always apparent, but injection sites frequently reveal cellulitis, draining pus, or abscess formation.

ETIOLOGY

- Cause is one of several types of neurotoxins (usually A, B, or E) produced by *C. botulinum*, an anaerobic, gram-positive bacillus. Spore production guarantees survival of the organism in extreme conditions. Botulinum toxin is the most powerful neurotoxin known.

- Disease results from absorption of toxin into the circulation from a mucosal surface or wound. Botulinum toxin does not penetrate intact skin.
- In foodborne variety, disease is caused by ingestion of preformed toxin. Although rapidly inactivated by heat, the toxin can survive the proteolytic environment of the stomach.
- In wound botulism, toxin is elaborated by organisms that contaminate a wound. Most cases reported are from California from injection drug use.
- In infant botulism, toxin is produced by organisms in the GI tract.
- Inhalational botulism has been demonstrated experimentally in primates. This manufactured form results from aerosolized toxin and has been attempted by bioterrorists.

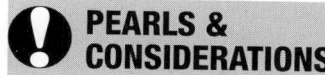

DIAGNOSIS

DIFFERENTIAL DIAGNOSIS

- Myasthenia gravis, Lambert-Eaton myasthenic syndrome
- Guillain-Barré syndrome
- Tick paralysis
- CVA
- Other: polio, heavy metal intoxication, and shellfish poisoning

WORKUP

- Search made for toxin and the organism (see "Laboratory Tests")
- Electrophysiologic studies (e.g., EMG) may aid in the diagnosis

LABORATORY TESTS

- Samples of food and stool are cultured for the organism.
- Food, serum, and stool are sent for toxin assay.

TREATMENT

NONPHARMACOLOGIC THERAPY

- Supportive care with intubation if respiratory failure occurs
- Debridement of the wound in wound botulism

ACUTE GENERAL Rx

- **For non-infants:** Give equine heptavalent botulinum antitoxin (HBAT), which contains antibodies for seven known botulism types (A through G), as early as possible. Once a clinical diagnosis is made, antitoxin should be administered before laboratory confirmation.
  1. The antitoxin is available from the Centers for Disease Control and Prevention (1-404-639-2206 Monday-Friday or 1-404-639-2888 evenings/weekends); it is derived from horse serum, so there is a significant incidence of serum sickness.
  2. Skin testing (conjunctival instillation and observation for 15 min), and possible desensitization, is recommended before treatment.

- Give wound botulism patients penicillin 2 million U IV q4h after antitoxin has been given. Use metronidazole 500 million U IV q8h as alternative for penicillin allergic patients.
- **For infants:** Give human botulinum immunoglobulin (BIG) IV, single dose. Call 1-510-540-2646. Do not use equine antitoxin. Babies with infantile intestinal botulism may benefit from a cathartic to mechanically clear the number of *C. botulinum* vegetative forms and spores residing in the gastrointestinal tract. Avoid antibiotics in infant botulism because antimicrobials may lyse C. botulinum in the gut and increase toxin load.

CHRONIC Rx

- Supportive
- Rehabilitation/physical therapy

DISPOSITION

- Highest mortality in the first case in an outbreak, with subsequent cases receiving rapid treatment
- Complete recovery for most individuals (this may take several weeks in severely affected individuals)

REFERRAL

Immediate for all cases to an ER and an infectious disease consultant

PEARLS & CONSIDERATIONS

COMMENTS

- Routine cooking inactivates the toxin, but spores are resistant to environmental factors. At room temperature, spores can germinate and produce toxin.
- Most outbreaks are associated with home-canned foods, especially vegetables.
- Patients must be closely monitored for progression to respiratory paralysis.
- There is increasing concern over the potential use of botulinum toxin as a biologic weapon, either by the enteric route or by aerosolization.
- Notify public health authorities immediately to alert other health care services of possible additional cases and to initiate investigation into cause and scope of outbreak.
- Recent botulism food recalls have involved carrot juice, cut green beans, and olives.

SUGGESTED READINGS

available at www.expertconsult.com

RELATED CONTENT

Botulism (Patient Information)

AUTHOR: **GLENN G. FORT, M.D., M.P.H.**

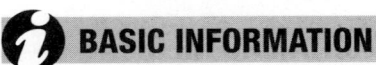

BASIC INFORMATION

DEFINITION

Brain metastases result from a spread of cancers originating in other organs to the brain. Brain metastases are the most common intracranial tumors in adults and account for more than one half of brain tumors.

SYNONYMS

ICD-9CM CODES
198 Secondary neoplasm of other specified sites

EPIDEMIOLOGY & DEMOGRAPHICS
INCIDENCE:
- In the United States, an estimated 98,000 to 170,000 new cases occur each year, which represents 24% to 45% of all cancer patients. The increased incidence is likely due to improved detection and better control of extracerebral disease. The incidence is higher in autopsy series, where 20% of patients with systemic disease have brain metastases.
- The prevalence is thought to be 120,000 to 140,000/yr. Incidence is significantly higher in autopsy series, where 20% of patients with systemic disease have brain metastases.

PREDOMINANT SEX AND AGE:
- In patients with systemic malignancies, brain metastases occur in 10% to 30% of adults and 6% to 10% of children. Of these, about 60% of patients are between the ages of 50 to 70.
- There is no gender predilection.

RISK FACTORS:
- In adults, the most common primary tumors accounting for brain metastases are carcinomas, including lung (16% to 20%), breast (5%), kidney (7% to 10%), and colorectal cancers (1% to 2%), and melanoma (7%).
- In children, the most common primary tumors are sarcomas, neuroblastoma, and germ cell tumors.

PHYSICAL FINDINGS & CLINICAL PRESENTATION
- Brain metastases should be suspected in any cancer patient who develops acute neurologic signs or symptoms. Neurologic symptoms, however, are common in patients with systemic cancer. In an analysis of more than 800 patients with neurologic symptoms, brain metastases were found in only 16%.
- Symptoms:
  - Headache occurs in 40% to 50% of patients with brain metastases. Frequency is higher with metastases located in the posterior fossa, which may result in obstructive hydrocephalus. The headache is accompanied by nausea, vomiting, focal neurologic signs, and postural variation.
  - Focal neurologic signs/symptoms are the presenting symptom in 20% to 40% of patients. Hemiparesis is the most frequent complaint.
  - Cognitive dysfunction, including memory problems and/or mood/personality changes, is the presenting problem in 30% to 45% of patients.
  - The frequency of seizures in patients with metastatic brain tumor is 30% to 40%.
  - Acute stroke secondary to hemorrhage into a metastasis, hypercoagulability, or local vascular invasion accounts for 5% to 10% of patients.

ETIOLOGY
The most common mechanism of metastasis to the brain is by hematogenous spread. The most common location is at the junction of the gray and white matter. The blood vessels decrease in diameter in these regions, which is thought to act like a trap for clumps of tumor cells. Different tumor types have a tendency to metastasize to different regions of the brain. For example, metastases of small cell lung carcinoma are equally distributed in all regions, whereas pelvic (prostate and uterine) and gastrointestinal tumors more commonly metastasize to the posterior fossa.

DIAGNOSIS

DIFFERENTIAL DIAGNOSIS
- Primary brain tumor
- Infection: abscess/fungal disease
- Progressive multifocal leukoencephalopathy
- Demyelinating disease: multiple sclerosis, postinfectious encephalomyelitis
- Cerebral infarction/bleeding
- Effects of treatment, such as radiation necrosis

LABORATORY TESTS
- Routine laboratory studies are not typically helpful.
- Lumbar puncture is generally contraindicated due to increased intracranial pressure and risk of herniation.
- Brain biopsy is necessary in some cases for a definitive diagnosis, particularly in the case of unknown primary tumor.

IMAGING STUDIES
- MRI (Fig. 1-161) with and without contrast is the imaging study of choice. Important features on MRI that suggest brain metastases include: presence of multiple lesions, localization at the junction of the gray and white matter, circumscribed margins, large amounts of vasogenic edema. CT of head with contrast (Fig. 1-162) can be used when MRI is contraindicated.
- MR spectroscopy and PET are useful to delineate tumor from other space-occupying lesions or from radiation necrosis.

- Newer experimental imaging studies, such as receptor-targeted and ligand-based molecular imaging, are on the horizon.
- Patients without a known primary tumor. In about 80% of patients, brain metastases develop after the diagnosis of systemic cancer. In the remaining patients, brain metastases are diagnosed simultaneously or before the primary tumor is found. In patients without a known primary tumor, the lung should be the primary focus of evaluation. Other frequent sites include melanoma, colon cancer, and breast cancer. PET scan may be useful in these patients to help identify the primary tumor or to identify other sites of metastatic disease—these latter sites might also be more amenable to biopsy.

TREATMENT

- Manamagent of patients with brain metastases is influenced by the overall prognosis and may include treatments targeted at the metastases, management and prevention of complications (seizures, edema), and treatment of systemic malignancy, where appropriate.
- In patients considered to have a favorable prognosis, treatment focuses on eradication or control of the brain metastases. Approaches include surgical resection and radiation therapy.
- In patients with poor prognosis, treatment focuses on symptom control.

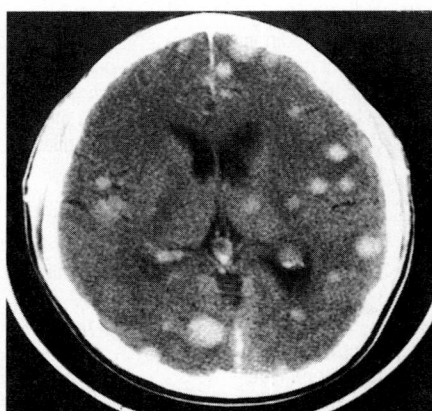

FIGURE 1-162 Intracranial metastatic disease. Axial contrast-enhanced CT scan of head reveals multiple enhancing nodules throughout gray and white matter structures consistent with metastatic disease. (From Vincent JL et al [eds]: *Textbook of critical care,* ed 6, Philadelphia, 2011, Saunders.)

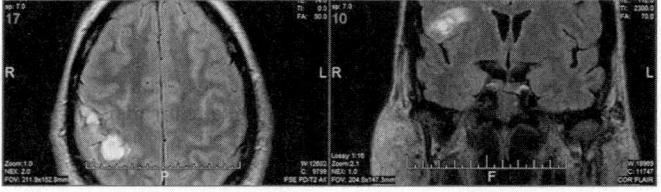

FIGURE 1-161 Brain magnetic resonance imaging (axial and coronal fluid-attenuated inversion recovery sequences) showing hemorrhagic metastatic deposition in the inferior right frontoparietal lobe (lobulated high signal focus) in a 40-year-old woman with metastatic choriocarcinoma to the brain. (From Fielding JR et al: *Gynecologic imaging,* Philadelphia, 2011, Saunders.)

ACUTE GENERAL Rx

- Steroids are used to reduce peritumoral edema and intracranial pressure.
- Antiepileptics are started for patients who present with seizures. Prophylactic treatment for seizure is not necessary in patients with no prior history of seizure.
- Anticoagulants are sometimes used to prevent venous thromboembolic disease.

CHRONIC Rx

- Radiation therapy has become the mainstay of treatment for brain metastases, including whole brain radiation therapy and stereotactic radiosurgery (SRS).
- For highly chemosensitive tumors, chemotherapy has been integrated into the primary management of patients with disseminated disease.
- For other tumors (e.g., small cell and non-small cell lung cancers, breast cancer, melanoma) systemic chemotherapy or molecularly targeted agents may be of palliative value when surgery, whole brain radiation therapy, and SRS have failed or are inappropriate. In most cases, two to three agents in combination and in conjunction with whole brain radiation therapy are used.

DISPOSITION

- The median survival of patients who receive supportive care and are treated with corticosteroids only is approximately 1 to 2 mo.
- Key prognostic factors are performance status, extent of systemic disease, and age. Most favorable outcome is found in patients with Karnofsky performance score >70, age younger than 70 yr, no systemic disease or local control of primary tumor without extracranial metastases, and female gender. In this group, median survival is estimated at 7.1 mo.

REFERRAL

Treatment involves a multispecialty team. Consultations from oncology, neurosurgery, neurology, radiation oncology, psychiatry, and physical therapy are all warranted.

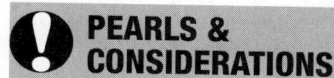

PEARLS & CONSIDERATIONS

COMMENTS

- Brain metastases are the most common intracranial tumors in adults, accounting for more than half of all brain tumors.

- Lung cancer, melanoma, renal cell carcinoma, and breast cancer are the most common primary tumors that metastasize to the brain.
- MRI is the most reliable imaging modality.
- Patient treatment depends upon the overall prognosis.

PATIENT/FAMILY EDUCATION

American Brain Tumor Association (http://www.abta.org)
National Brain Tumor Society (http://www.braintumor.org)

SUGGESTED READINGS

available at www.expertconsult.com

RELATED CONTENT

Brain Cancer (Patient Information)

AUTHOR: **NICOLE J. ULLRICH, M.D., PH.D.**

B

Diseases
and Disorders

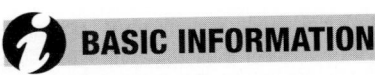

DEFINITION

Brain neoplasms are a diverse group of primary (nonmetastatic) tumors arising from one of many different cell types within the central nervous system (CNS). Specific tumor subtypes and prognosis depend on the tumor cell of origin and pattern of growth. The diffuse low-grade gliomas (LGGs) include World Health Organization Grade II astrocytomas, oligodendrogliomas, and oligoastrocytomas.

SYNONYMS

Low-grade glioma (LGG)
Glioneuronal tumor
Meningioma
Primary brain tumor

ICD-9CM CODES
225.0 Brain neoplasm (benign)
239.2 Brain neoplasm (unspecified)

EPIDEMIOLOGY & DEMOGRAPHICS

INCIDENCE: U.S. incidence rate is approximately 24.6 cases/100,000 persons per yr for all primary brain tumors (Table 1-65). One third of these are considered malignant and the remainder benign or borderline malignant. The incidence rate in children aged 0 to 19 years is lower (48.6/1,000,000 children). Primary brain neoplasms account for ~2% of all cancers, with a disproportionate share of cancer morbidity and mortality. It is the most common cause of cancer death in children up to 15 yr.
PEAK INCIDENCE: Depends on histology, though highest peak at ~age 50 yr
PREDOMINANT SEX AND AGE: Slight male preponderance (8.0 vs. 5.5/100,000 person/yr)
GENETICS: Most primary CNS neoplasms are sporadic; 5% is associated with hereditary syndromes that predispose to neoplasia. The most common of these include:
- Li-Fraumeni syndrome: *p53* mutation on chromosome 17q13, gliomas
- Von Hippel-Lindau: VHL, chromosome 3p25, hemangioblastoma
- Tuberous sclerosis: TSC1/TSC2 (chromosome 9q34/16p13), subependymal giant cell astrocytoma
- Neurofibromatosis type 1: NF1, chromosome 17q11, neurofibroma, optic nerve glioma, low-grade glioma
- Neurofibromatosis type 2: NF2, chromosome 22q12, schwannoma, meningioma, ependymoma
- Retinoblastoma: pRB, chromosome 13q, retinoblastoma
- Gorlin's syndrome: chromosome 9q31, desmoplastic medulloblastoma

RISK FACTORS: Exposure to ionizing radiation has been implicated in meningiomas, gliomas, and nerve sheath tumors. No convincing evidence has shown a link with trauma, occupation, cellular phone use, diet, or electromagnetic fields.

PHYSICAL FINDINGS & CLINICAL PRESENTATION

- In general, the location, size, and rate of growth will determine the symptoms and signs of a brain tumor.
- Headache is common and is the worst symptom in nearly half of all patients. Symptoms of intracranial pressure may also be present, including nausea and vomiting. Headache may be localizing. Papilledema is suggestive of obstructive hydrocephalus.
- Seizures occur in 33% of patients and are among the most common symptoms, particularly with brain metastases and low-grade gliomas. The type of seizure and clinical presentation depends on location. Seizures are more common in low-grade compared with high-grade gliomas. It is thought that patients with seizures typically have smaller tumors at time of diagnosis compared with those with other symptoms, because the onset of seizures prompts an imaging study, leading to an earlier diagnosis.
- Focal neurologic signs and symptoms, including muscle weakness, sensory changes, or visual disturbances are also quite frequent. In addition, cognitive dysfunction, accompanied by changes in memory or personality change, may be recounted, often in retrospect.

ETIOLOGY

Most cases are idiopathic, though specific chromosomal abnormalities have been implicated in some tumor types.

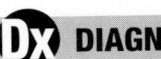 **DIAGNOSIS**

- Diagnosis is typically based on clinical presentation and imaging characteristics.
- Tumors are best seen on MRI; calcifications are sometimes present.
- Benign and low-grade tumors, typically in the glioma family, are heterogeneous. Recent results have implicated molecular pathway alterations in a subset of patients.

LABORATORY

- Ultimately, only histologic examination can provide the exact diagnosis. Information may also be gleaned from additional features such as proliferative index, immunohistochemical stains, and electron microscopy.
- The current classification schema for gliomas is based on pathologic and microscopic criteria. Tumor histology/histologic diagnosis (World Health Organization [WHO] grading system), includes number of mitoses, capillary endothelial proliferation, and necrosis (*Note:* There can be a high degree of morbidity based on tumor location, even with more benign histology.)
- Genetic analysis of tumors is rapidly becoming important for genetic classification, stratification of treatments, and predicting outcome. Different subtypes of gliomas have distinct gene-expression profiles, which can be distinguished from one another and from normal tissue; these differences typically involve pathways of cell proliferation, energy metabolism, and signal transduction. In adults, global expression profiling identified differences in 360 genes between low-grade and high-grade tumors.

DIFFERENTIAL DIAGNOSIS

- Stroke/cerebral hemorrhage
- Abscess/parasitic cyst
- Demyelinating disease: multiple sclerosis, postinfectious encephalomyelitis
- Metastatic tumors
- Primary CNS lymphoma

WORKUP

- Neuroimaging studies and pathologic sampling are the most important diagnostic modalities in evaluation of brain tumors and may be critical for preoperative planning.

IMAGING STUDIES

- MRI with gadolinium enhancement is highly sensitive, though CT scanning is useful if calcification or hemorrhage suspected. MRI permits visualization of the tumor, as well as the relation to the surrounding tissue.

TABLE 1-65 Frequency of Primary CNS Tumors

CHILDREN (0-14 YEARS)		ADULTS (≥15 YEARS)	
Type	Percentage	Type	Percentage
Glioblastoma	20	Glioblastoma	50
Astrocytoma	21	Astrocytoma	10
Ependymoma	7	Ependymoma	2
Oligodendroglioma	1	Oligodendroglioma	3
Medulloblastoma	24	Medulloblastoma	2
Neuroblastoma	3	Neurilemmoma	2
Neurilemmoma	1	Pituitary adenoma	4
Craniopharyngioma	5	Craniopharyngioma	1
Meningioma	5	Meningioma	17
Teratoma	2	Pinealoma	1
Pinealoma	2	Hemangioma	2
Hemangioma	3	Sarcoma	1
Sarcoma	1	Others	5
Others	5	TOTAL	100
TOTAL	100		

From Goetz CG, Pappert EJ: *Textbook of clinical neurology*, Philadelphia, 1999, Saunders.

Enhancing tumor can be distinguished from surrounding edema. Low-grade tumors often present as an infiltrating lesion without mass effect. MRI is superior to CT scanning to evaluate the meninges, subarachnoid space, and posterior fossa, and for defining relation to major intracranial vessels.

- Magnetic resonance spectroscopy is increasingly being used as a diagnostic tool to define metabolic composition of an area of interest and may be useful to contrast areas of tumor progression from radiation necrosis. N-acetylaspartate is often decreased in brain tumors, whereas choline, a component of cell membranes, is increased because of high cellular turnover.
- PET scan is helpful to distinguish neoplastic lesions (with high rate of metabolism) from other lesions such as demyelination or radiation necrosis (with a much lower metabolic rate). Such lesions take up greater amounts of glucose than surrounding tissues or tumors with slower metabolic rates. May be useful to help map functional areas of the brain before surgery or radiation.
- Functional MRI is now used as an adjunct in perioperative planning for patients whose lesion is in vital regions, such as those responsible for speech, language, and motor control.

TREATMENT

NONPHARMACOLOGIC THERAPY

- Maximal surgical removal or debulking is the initial treatment of choice and provides tissue for diagnosis and molecular characterization. Maximal safe resection is often favored with a trend toward improved survival with this approach.
- Biopsy alone is performed if the tumor is located in eloquent regions of brain or is inaccessible; this is essential for histopathologic diagnosis. Biopsy can be performed under CT or MRI guidance using stereotactic localization.
- If the tumor is benign (e.g., meningioma, acoustic neuroma), often no further therapy is required.

ACUTE GENERAL Rx

Antiseizure medications have been used perioperatively and to control seizures resulting from focal lesions. Prophylactic use of anticonvulsants is not typically recommended without clear history of seizures.

CHRONIC Rx

- Chemotherapy (combination or single agent) may be used before, during, or after surgery and radiation therapy. (In children, chemotherapy is often used to delay radiation therapy.) Radiosensitizers may help increase the therapeutic effect of radiation therapy.
- Radiation is useful for certain types of tumors and is often used if there is residual tumor after surgery; conventional radiation uses external beams over a period of weeks, whereas stereotactic radiosurgery delivers a single, high dose of radiation to a well-defined area (usually <1 cm). Long-term effects of radiation therapy include radiation necrosis (particularly of white matter), blood vessel hyalinization, and secondary tumors (usually meningiomas, sarcomas, and malignant astrocytomas).
- Experimental therapies are continually in development and are typically based on molecular characterization of tumors and small molecule blockers of signal transduction cascades. Some of these therapies involve antisense molecules, biologic agents, immunotherapies, or angiogenesis inhibitors. Intratumoral drug infusions and convection-enhanced delivery of novel agents are currently under study.

DISPOSITION

In general, younger age, high performance status, and lower pathologic grade have more favorable prognosis. For all histologic subtypes of brain tumors, pediatric and young adult patients have a better survival rate.

REFERRAL

- All cases warrant evaluation by an oncologist and neurosurgeon.
- Patients should be evaluated for physical and occupational therapy.
- Children should undergo neuropsychologic evaluations and screening for learning disabilities.

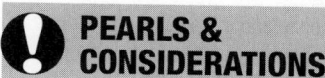 **PEARLS & CONSIDERATIONS**

COMMENTS

In general, younger age, high performance status, and lower pathologic grade have more favorable prognosis. For all histologic subtypes of brain tumors, pediatric and young adult patients have a better survival.

PATIENT/FAMILY EDUCATION

American Brain Tumor Association
National Brain Tumor Society (http://www.braintumor.org)

SUGGESTED READINGS

available at www.expertconsult.com

RELATED CONTENT

Brain Cancer (Patient Information)

AUTHOR: **NICOLE J. ULLRICH, M.D., PH.D.**

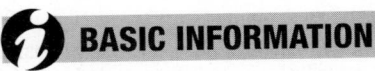

DEFINITION

Brain neoplasms are a diverse group of primary (nonmetastatic) tumors arising from one of the many different cell types within the central nervous system. Malignant brain tumors are defined by histopathologic features and a rapidly progressive pattern of growth. Glioblastoma is the most common primary brain tumor in adults, accounting for 50% to 60% of primary brain tumors.

SYNONYMS

Glioblastoma
GBM

ICD-9CM CODES
191.9

EPIDEMIOLOGY & DEMOGRAPHICS

INCIDENCE: Annual incidence rate of glioblastoma is approximately 2 to 3 cases/100,000 persons in Europe and North America. High-grade/malignant astrocytomas are slightly more common in whites than in blacks, Latinos, and Asians.

PREDOMINANT SEX AND AGE: Glioblastoma is slightly more common in men than women with a male/female ratio of 3:2. Peak incidence is between 45 and 70 yr. Approximately 10% of glioblastomas occur in children.

PEAK INCIDENCE: High-grade gliomas, such as anaplastic astrocytoma and glioblastoma, tend to originate in the fourth to fifth decade of life and beyond.

RISK FACTORS: Prior radiation may increase risk for primary brain tumor. Glioblastomas are more common in individuals who have a heritable cancer predisposition syndrome, such as Li-Fraumeni syndrome and Turcot syndrome.

GENETICS: Malignant progression is associated with inactivation of *PTEN* tumor-suppressor gene and amplification of epidermal growth factor receptor *(EGFR)* gene. Overexpression of *EGFR* gene occurs in 40% to 50% of primary glioblastoma cases. Loss of heterozygosity on chromosome 10q occurs in 60% to 90% of both primary and secondary glioblastoma cases and is associated with poor prognosis. The pathway involving mutations of the tumor-suppressor gene *p53* is typically associated with secondary glioblastoma. Other genetic mutations have also been recognized as potential contributors in the pathogenesis of glioblastoma, including *PTEN* and *MDM2*. Deletion of *NFKBIA* has an effect that is similar to the effect of *EGFR* amplification in the pathogenesis of glioblastoma and is associated with comparatively short survival.

PHYSICAL FINDINGS & CLINICAL PRESENTATION

- In general, the location, size, and rate of growth will determine the symptoms and signs. Clinical history of patients with glioblastoma is typically brief, <3 mo in the majority of patients with primary glioblastoma.

- Most frequent symptoms include:
  - Headache occurs in the majority of cases. The headache can be localizing or may result from increased intracranial pressure.
  - Seizures occur in 30% to 60% depending on tumor location and grade.
  - Symptoms and signs of hydrocephalus and raised intracranial pressure (headache, vomiting, clouding of consciousness, papilledema).
  - Other symptoms seen in 20% or more of patients include memory loss, focal motor weakness, visual changes, language deficits, and cognitive disturbances or memory changes.

ETIOLOGY

- Glioblastomas are classified as primary or secondary. Primary glioblastoma constitutes the majority of cases (60%) in adults older than 50 yr and are considered de novo tumors. Secondary glioblastoma typically involves malignant progression from a lower grade (grade II or III) glioma.

DX DIAGNOSIS

DIFFERENTIAL DIAGNOSIS

- Stroke
- Arteriovenous malformations
- Abscess/parasitic cyst (neurocysticercosis)
- Demyelinating disease: tumefactive multiple sclerosis, postinfectious encephalomyelitis
- Metastatis
- Primary central nervous system lymphoma

LABORATORY TESTS

- Routine laboratory studies are not typically helpful.
- Lumbar puncture is generally contraindicated; cerebrospinal fluid studies do not add much specific additional information for the diagnosis for glioblastoma.
- Ultimately, only a histologic examination can provide the exact diagnosis. Information may also be gleaned from additional features such as proliferative index, immunohistochemical stains, and electron microscopy, as well as molecular markers.

IMAGING STUDIES (Fig. 1-163)

- MRI with and without contrast is the imaging study of choice, though CT scanning is useful if calcification or hemorrhage is suspected. MRI permits visualization of the tumor, as well as the relation to the surrounding tissue. Enhancing tumor can be distinguished from surrounding edema. MRI is superior to CT scanning to evaluate the meninges, subarachnoid space, and posterior fossa, and for defining relation to major intracranial vessels.
- Magnetic resonance spectroscopy (MRS) is increasingly being used as a diagnostic tool to define metabolic composition of an area of interest and may be useful to contrast areas of tumor progression from radiation necrosis. N-acetylaspartate, a marker of neurons, is often decreased in brain tumors, whereas choline, a component of cell membranes, is increased because of high cellular turnover.
- PET scan is helpful to distinguish neoplastic lesions (with high rate of metabolism) from other lesions such as demyelination or radiation necrosis (with a much lower metabolic rate). Such lesions take up greater amounts of glucose than surrounding tissues or tumors with slower metabolic rates. May also aid in preoperative planning to increase diagnostic yield and to help map functional areas of the brain before surgery.
- Functional MRI is now used as an adjunt to in perioperative planning for patients whose lesion is in vital regions (eloquent regions), such as those responsible for speech, language, and motor control.

Rx TREATMENT

- Current standard-of-care therapies include surgery, radiation, and palliative chemotherapy, all of which have significant adverse effects and limited efficacy. Median time to recurrence after standard therapy is 6.9 mo.

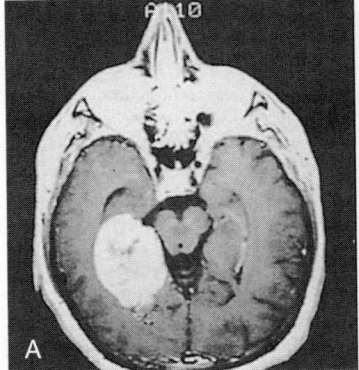
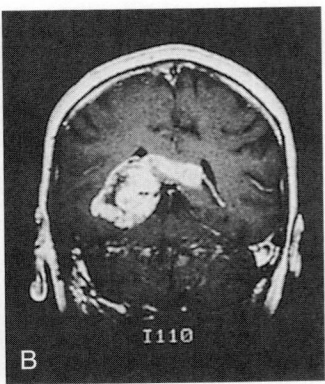

FIGURE 1-163 Glioblastoma multiforme. Axial **(A)** and coronal **(B)** postcontrast enhanced T1-weighted image showing a large homogeneously contrast-enhancing mass in the right medial temporal lobe with extension across the midline. (From Specht N [ed]: *Practical guide to diagnostic imaging*, St Louis, 1998, Mosby.)

B

PHARMACOLOGIC AND NONPHARMACOLOGIC THERAPY

- Maximal surgical removal or debulking is the initial treatment of choice and is the first stage in treatment.
- Biopsy alone is performed if the tumor is located in eloquent regions of brain or is inaccessible; this is essential for histopathologic diagnosis. Biopsy can be performed with CT or MRI guidance using stereotactic localization.
- Radiation therapy is the mainstay of treatment for individuals with glioblastoma and improves local control and overall survival after surgery. Even patients with a gross total resection of tumor have a high recurrence rate.
- Chemotherapy (combination or single agent) may be used before, during, or after surgery and radiation therapy. (In children, chemotherapy is often used to delay radiation therapy.) Radiosensitizers may help increase the therapeutic effect of radiation therapy. Conventional treatment includes radiation in combination with temozolomide.
- Experimental therapies in development are typically based on molecular characterization of tumors and small molecule blockers of signal transduction cascades. Some of these therapies involve antisense molecules, biologic agents, immunotherapies, or angio-genesis inhibitors. Intratumoral drug infusions and convection-enhanced delivery of novel agents are currently under study. In addition, delivery systems such as the use of a vector to permit gene transfer with the goal to selectively kill cancer cells are being investigated.

ACUTE GENERAL Rx

- Steroids are used to reduce edema and may also be used perioperatively or during radiation therapy.
- Antiepileptic medications have been used perioperatively and to control seizures resulting from focal lesions. Prophylactic use of anticonvulsants is not typically recommended without clear history of seizures.

DISPOSITION

- Glioblastoma multiforme is the most aggressive form of primary brain tumor. The important prognostic factors include the extent of resection, patient age, tumor grade/histology, and performance status. In general, younger age, high performance status, and lower pathologic grade have more favorable prognosis. For all histologic subtypes of brain tumors, pediatric and young adult patients have a better survival.
- Terminal events typically result from increased intracranial pressure.

REFERRAL

Treatment should involve a multispecialty team with consultations from oncology, neurosurgery, neurology, radiation oncology, psychiatry, and physical therapy.

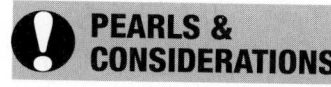 **PEARLS & CONSIDERATIONS**

COMMENTS

Glioblastoma is distinguished pathologically by the presence of vascular proliferation and necrosis.

PATIENT/FAMILY EDUCATION

American Brain Tumor Association
National Brain Tumor Society (http://www. braintumor.org)

SUGGESTED READINGS

available at www.expertconsult.com

RELATED CONTENT

Brain Cancer (Patient Information)

AUTHOR: **NICOLE J. ULLRICH, M.D., PH.D.**

Diseases and Disorders

I

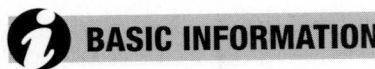

BASIC INFORMATION

DEFINITION
The term *breast cancer* refers to invasive carcinoma of the breast, whether ductal or lobular.

SYNONYMS
Carcinoma of the breast

ICD-9CM CODES
174.9 Malignant neoplasm female breast

EPIDEMIOLOGY & DEMOGRAPHICS
- Nearly exclusively the disease of women, with only 1% of breast cancers in males
- Steady increase in its incidence in the U.S., with 205,000 new patients annually
- Annual mortality of 40,000
- Risk steadily increases with age. Table 1-66 describes risk factors for breast cancer.
- Genetically defined group of women with *BRCA-1* or *BRCA-2* genes identified to carry lifetime risk as high as 85%

PHYSICAL FINDINGS & CLINICAL PRESENTATION
- Increasing number of small breast cancers found by mammograms

TABLE 1-66 Risk Factors for Breast Cancer

Risk Factor	Relative Risk
Any benign breast disease	1.5
Postmenopausal hormone replacement (estrogen with or without progestin)	1.5
Menarche at <12 yr	1.1-1.9
Moderate alcohol intake (two to three drinks/day)	1.1-1.9
Menopause at >55 yr	1.1-1.9
Increased bone density	1.1-1.9
Sedentary lifestyle and lack of exercise	1.1-1.9
Proliferative breast disease without atypia	2
Age at first birth >30 yr or nulliparous	2-4
First-degree relative with breast cancer	2-4
Postmenopausal obesity	2-4
Upper socioeconomic class	2-4
Personal history of endometrial or ovarian cancer	2-4
Significant radiation to chest	2-4
Increased breast density on mammogram	2-4
Older age	>4
Personal history of breast cancer (in situ or invasive)	>4
Proliferative breast disease with atypia	>4
Two first-degree relatives with breast cancer	5
Atypical hyperplasia and first-degree relative with breast cancer	10

From Goldman L, Schafer AI: *Goldman's Cecil medicine*, ed 24, Philadelphia, 2012, Saunders.

- Patients usually completely free of physical findings
- Palpable tumors possibly as small as 1 cm or even smaller
- Size of the mass and its location measured and documented
- Skin and/or nipple retraction and skin edema, erythema, ulcer, satellite nodule
- Nodal enlargement in axilla and supraclavicular areas
- Advanced disease: clinical signs of pleural effusion and/or hepatomegaly
- Rare instances: clear, serous, or bloody discharge only symptom
- Nipple evaluation (see "Paget's Disease of the Breast")

ETIOLOGY
- Precise mechanism of carcinogenesis not understood. Gene expression analysis has altered the way breast cancer is perceived in that it is no longer regarded as a single disease. Estrogen receptor (ER)-positive and ER-negative cancers are clinically distinct diseases.
- Possibly interaction of ovarian estrogen, non-ovarian estrogen, estrogens of exogenous origin with breast tissue of varied carcinogenic susceptibility to develop cancer
- Other known or suspected variables: childbearing, breastfeeding practice, diet, physical activities, body mass, alcohol intake
- Women with *BRCA-1* and *BRCA-2* genes associated with high risk

DX DIAGNOSIS

DIFFERENTIAL DIAGNOSIS
The following nonmalignant breast lesions can simulate breast cancer on both physical and mammogram examinations:

- Fibrocystic changes
- Fibroadenoma
- Hamartoma

WORKUP
- Physical examination:
  1. Mass detected by patient or medical professional: workup required
  2. Negative mammogram: breast cancer not ruled out
  3. Sonogram: to demonstrate mass to be cyst, usually eliminating need for further workup
  4. Screening with both MRI and mammography might rule out cancerous lesions better than mammography alone in women who are known or likely to have an inherited predisposition to breast cancer
- To establish diagnosis:
  1. Positive aspiration cytology on a clinically and mammographically malignant mass—highly accurate but still requires open biopsy confirmation
  2. Stereotactic core needle biopsy diagnosis: Stereotactic- and ultrasonography-guided core-needle biopsy procedures seem to be almost as accurate as open surgical biopsy with lower complication rates. They are reliable with invasive carcinoma identified, but negative or equivocal results require careful evaluation
  3. Atypical hyperplasia or in situ carcinoma found by core needle biopsy: open surgical biopsy confirmation still required
  4. Excisional or incisional biopsy: establishes diagnosis

NOTE: Do not rely on negative mammogram or negative aspiration cytology findings to exclude malignancy. Make appropriate referral. Obtain imaging studies such as bone scan,

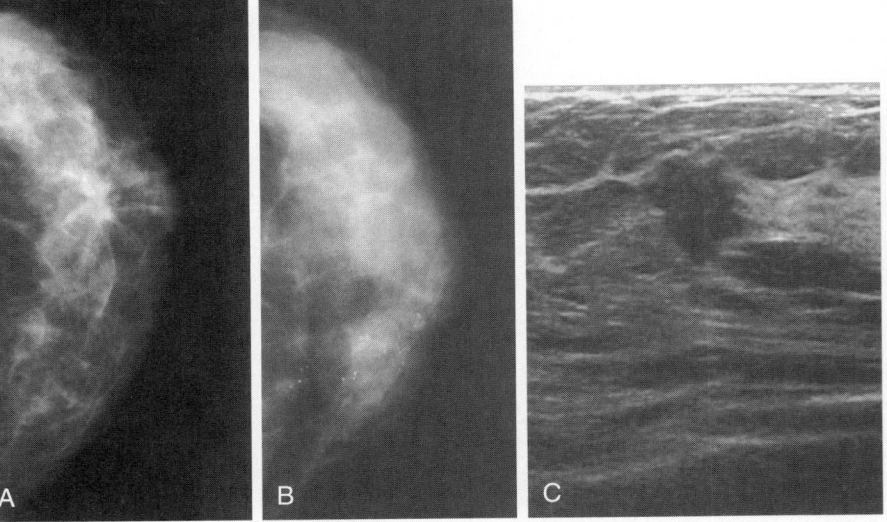

FIGURE 1-164 Mammogram and ultrasound findings of breast disease. A, A stellate mass in the breast. The combination of a density with spiculated borders and distortion of surrounding breast architecture suggests a malignancy. **B,** Clustered microcalcification. Fine, pleomorphic, and linear calcifications that cluster together suggest the diagnosis of ductal carcinoma in situ (DCIS). **C,** An ultrasound image of breast cancer. The mass is solid, containing internal echoes, and displaying an irregular border. Most malignant lesions are taller than they are wide. (From Townsend CM et al [eds]: *Sabiston textbook of surgery*, ed 17, Philadelphia, 2004, Saunders.)

chest x-ray, CT scan of abdomen, or CT scan of liver.
- Breast radiologic evaluation and an algorithm for breast cancer screening and evaluation are described in Section III. The differential diagnosis of breast lumps is described in Section II.

IMAGING STUDIES

Mammograms (Fig. 1-164): 30% to 50% of breast cancers detected by screening mammograms only as a spiculated mass, a mass with or without microcalcifications, or a cluster of microcalcifications. MRI is an excellent modality that is particularly useful in patients with breast implants and when there is a strong family history of breast cancer. MRI is also better than other methods of assessing the response to neoadjuvant chemotherapy and is useful in identifying the primary tumor in patients who present with axillary adenopathy.

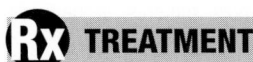 **TREATMENT**

NONPHARMACOLOGIC THERAPY

- Early breast cancer: primarily surgical or surgical and radiotherapeutic. Table 1-67 compares ductal versus lobular carcinoma in situ. Adjuvant treatment guidelines for patients with early-stage invasive breast cancer are described in Table 1-68.
- Choice in 60% to 70% of women between modified mastectomy and breast-conserving treatment, which consists of lumpectomy, axillary staging with sentinel node biopsy or axillary dissection, and breast irradiation
- Recent trials reveal that among patients with limited sentinel lymph nodes (SNL), metastatic breast cancer treated with breast conservation and systematic therapy, the use of sentinel lymph node dissection (SNLD) alone compared with axillary lymph node dissection (ALND) did not result in inferior survival

ACUTE GENERAL Rx

- May require adjuvant chemotherapy or endocrine therapy. Standard chemotherapy consists of either cyclophosphamide, methotrexate, and fluorouracil or cyclophosphamide plus doxorubicin. Endocrine therapy is recommended after chemotherapy in patients with hormone-receptor positive tumors. Adjuvant hormone therapy with anti-estrogen drugs reduces disease recurrence and mortality in these postmenopausal women with breast cancer. Aromatase inhibitors decrease the agonist effect of estrogen by inhibiting estrogen synthesis and have become preferred first-line hormonal treatment agents over the selective estrogen receptor modulator tamoxifen.
- Table 1-69 describes intrinsic molecular subtypes of breast cancer. Molecular targets in clinical breast cancer management are described in Table 1-70. Clinicopathologic considerations for patients with ER-positive and human epidermal growth factor receptor 2 (HER2)-negative disease are summarized in Table 1-71.

TABLE 1-67 Carcinoma in Situ: Lobular Versus Ductal

Feature	Lobular Carcinoma in Situ	Ductal Carcinoma in Situ
Age	Younger	Older
Palpable mass	No	Uncommon
Mammographic appearance	Not detected on mammography	Microcalcifications, mass
Immunophenotype	E-cadherin negative	E-cadherin positive
Usual manifestation	Incidental finding on breast biopsy	Microcalcifications on mammography or breast mass
Bilateral involvement	Common	Uncertain
Risk and site of subsequent breast cancer	25% risk for invasive breast cancer in either breast over remaining lifespan	At site of initial lesion; 0.5% risk/yr of invasive breast cancer in opposite breast
Prevention	Consider tamoxifen or raloxifene	Consider tamoxifen or raloxifene if estrogen-receptor positive
Treatment	Yearly mammography and breast examination	Lumpectomy ± radiation; mastectomy for large or multifocal lesions

From Goldman L, Schafer AI: *Goldman's Cecil medicine*, ed 24, Philadelphia, 2012, Saunders.

TABLE 1-68 Adjuvant Treatment Guidelines for Patients with Early-Stage Invasive Breast Cancer*

Patient Group*	Treatment
Favorable Histology (Tubular or Colloid)	
ER- and/or PR-Positive Breast Cancer	
<1 cm	No adjuvant therapy
1-2.9 cm	Consider adjuvant hormonal therapy[†]
≥3 cm or node-positive	Adjuvant hormonal therapy ± adjuvant chemotherapy[†]
ER- and PR-Negative Breast Cancer	
<1 cm	No adjuvant therapy
1-2.9 cm	Consider adjuvant chemotherapy
≥3 cm or node-positive	Adjuvant chemotherapy
Hormone Receptor-Positive (ER- and/or PR-Positive) Breast Cancer	
Lymph Nodes Negative	
≤0.5 cm	No adjuvant therapy
0.6-1.0 cm well differentiated and no unfavorable features[‡]	Consider adjuvant hormonal therapy
0.6-1.0 cm moderate or poorly differentiated or unfavorable features	Adjuvant hormonal therapy ± adjuvant chemotherapy
>1 cm	Adjuvant hormonal therapy ± adjuvant chemotherapy
Lymph Nodes Positive	
	Adjuvant hormonal therapy + adjuvant chemotherapy
Hormone Receptor-Negative (ER- and PR-Negative) Breast Cancer	
≤0.5 cm	No adjuvant therapy
0.6-1.0 cm	Consider chemotherapy
>1 cm or lymph-node positive	Adjuvant chemotherapy
HER2 Positive	
	Trastuzumab should be added to the suggested treatment above for all node-positive patients; trastuzumab not recommended for tumors ≤1 cm for most node-negative patients; for tumors >1 cm, trastuzumab should be considered for most patients

*Data are insufficient to make chemotherapy recommendations for patients ≥70 yr. Treatment should be individualized for these patients based on life expectancy and comorbidity.
[†]In ER-positive or PR-positive patients, decisions regarding the added value of chemotherapy in addition to hormonal therapy alone can be aided by accurately assessing the added value of chemotherapy in individual patients using a web-based model: www.adjuvantonline.com or Oncotype Dx assay.
[‡]Unfavorable characteristics include high-grade tumor, blood vessel or lymphatic invasion by tumor, and high tumor proliferation rate (high S phase by flow cytometry or high Ki-67 value by immunohistochemistry) or HER2-positive status.
ER, Estrogen receptor; *HER2,* human epidermal growth factor receptor 2; *PR,* progesterone receptor.
Modified from National Comprehensive Cancer Network Guidelines. Available at www.nccn.org.

- Weekly paclitaxel after standard adjuvant chemotherapy with doxorubicin and cyclophosphamide improves disease-free and overall survival in women with breast cancer. However, patients with *HER2*-negative, estrogen-receptor–positive, node-positive breast cancer may gain little benefit from administration of paclitaxel after adjuvant chemotherapy with doxorubicin plus cyclophosphamide.
- Fig. 1-165 illustrates considerations for adjuvant chemotherapy in the management of recurrent and metastatic breast cancer.

- The combination of the aromatase inhibitor anastrozole and fulvestrant is superior to anastrozole alone or sequential anastrozole and fulvestrant for the treatment of HR-positive metastatic breast cancer.
- Trastuzumab emtansine (T-DM1), an antibody-drug conjugate incorporating HER2-targeted antitumor properties of trastuzumab with the cytotoxic activity of the microtubule inhibitor agent DM1, has been shown to significantly prolong progression-free and overall survival with less toxicity than lapatinib plus capecitabine in patients with HER2-positive advanced breast cancer.

CHRONIC Rx
Follow-up required after proper treatment of primary breast cancer includes:
- Periodic clinical evaluations as delineated by medical oncologist or surgeon
- Annual mammograms/MRI
- Other tests as indicated
- Patient instruction in monthly breast self-examination technique

DISPOSITION
- Prognosis after curative therapy: depends on size of tumor, extent of nodal metastasis, and pathologic grade of tumor
  1. Patient with 1-cm tumor with no axillary node metastasis: 10-yr disease-free survival rate of 90%
  2. Patient with 3-cm tumor with metastasis in four nodes: 10-yr disease-free survival rate of 15% if no systemic adjuvant therapy given
  3. Outlook for most patients is between these extremes
- Systemic adjuvant therapy: improves prognosis significantly. Women who take tamoxifen for 10 yr lower their risk of recurrence by 25% and dying of breast cancer by 27% compared with those who took the pills for just 5 yr.
- Isolated tumor cells or micrometastases in regional lymph nodes is associated with a reduced 5-yr rate of disease-free survival among women with favorable early-stage breast cancer who do not receive adjuvant therapy. Survival is improved in patients with isolated tumor cells or micrometastases who received adjuvant therapy.
- Retrospective analyses suggest that occult lymph-node metastases are an important prognostic factor for disease recurrence of survival among patients with breast cancer; however, recent trials indicate that the magnitude of the difference in outcome at 5 yrs is small (1.2 percentage points). These data do not favor a clinical benefit of additional evaluation (including immunohistochemical analysis) of initially negative sentinel nodes in patients with breast cancer.
- The addition of zoledronic acid to adjuvant endocrine therapy improves disease-free survival in premenopausal patients with estrogen-responsive early breast cancer.

REFERRAL
Referral is necessary as soon as breast cancer is suspected.

TABLE 1-69 Intrinsic Molecular Subtypes of Breast Cancer

Type	Characteristics	Markers
Luminal A	Low grade, high ER, 50% of breast cancer	ER+, PR+, HER2−, CK8+, CK18+
Luminal B	Higher grade, lower ER, 10% of breast cancer	ER+, PR+/−, HER2+/−
HER2	High grade, p53 mutations, 5% to 10% of breast cancer	ER−, PR−, HER2+
Basal	High proliferation CK5+, CK14+, CK17+, EGFR+, 30% of breast cancer	ER−, PR−, HER2−

CK, Cytokeratin.
From Cameron JL, Cameron AM: *Current surgical therapy,* ed 10, Philadelphia, 2011, Saunders.

TABLE 1-70 Molecular Targets in Clinical Breast Cancer Management

Target	Drug	Status
ER	Tamoxifen	Survival benefit, adjuvant treatment, and metastatic disease, premenopausal and postmenopausal women
	Aromatase inhibitors (anastrozole, letrozole, exemestane)	Survival benefit, adjuvant and metastatic disease, postmenopausal women
	Fulvestrant	Second-line therapy, metastatic disease in postmenopausal women
HER2	Trastuzumab	Survival benefit, adjuvant and metastatic disease
HER1 + HER2	Lapatinib	Second-line therapy, metastatic disease; phase II adjuvant trials ongoing
HER1 (EGFR)	Gefitinib, erlotinib	Benefit unclear after phase II trials
	Cetuximab	In trial
VEGF	Bevacizumab	Progression-free survival benefit, metastatic disease; phase III adjuvant trials ongoing
PARP1/PARP2	PARP1 inhibitor	Improved PFS, OS in phase II trial, phase III initiated

OS, Overall survival; *PFS,* progression-free survival.
From Cameron JL, Cameron AM: *Current surgical therapy,* ed 10, Philadelphia, 2011, Saunders.

TABLE 1-71 Clinicopathologic Considerations for Patients with ER-Positive, HER2-Negative Disease

Clinicopathologic Features	Consider Adding Chemotherapy	Factors Not Useful for Decision	Consider Endocrine Therapy Only
ER and PR	Lower ER/PR levels		Higher ER/PR levels
Grade	Grade 3	Grade 2	Grade 1
Proliferation	Ki-67 >30%	Ki-67 16% to 30%	Ki-67 ≤15%
Nodes	Node positive (four or more nodes)	Node positive (one to three nodes)	Node negative
Peritumoral vascular invasion	Extensive PVI		Absence of PVI
Tumor size	>5 cm	2.1-5 cm	≤2 cm
Patient preference	Favors using all possible treatments		Favors avoiding side effects of chemotherapy

Adapted from highlights of the St. Gallen consensus panel. From Cameron JL, Cameron AM: *Current surgical therapy,* ed 10, Philadelphia, 2011, Saunders.

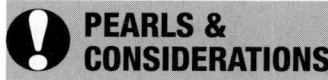

PEARLS & CONSIDERATIONS

Breast cancer in pregnancy and lactation:
1. Frequency in women 40 yr or younger reported to be 15%
2. May carry worse prognosis because disease discovery delayed by engorged and nodular breast changes and/or because disease progression more rapid in pregnancy

3. Survival rates similar to those for nonpregnant early-stage breast cancer patients in same age group
4. Mass usually found by patient or obstetrician
5. Expedient workup recommended, including mammography and sonography
6. Diagnosis to be made without delay
7. Choice of mastectomy or lumpectomy with axillary dissection for treatment
8. Adjuvant chemotherapy delayed until third trimester or after delivery
9. Irradiation to breast after lumpectomy delayed until after delivery

Ductal carcinoma in situ (DCIS, intraductal carcinoma) (see Table 1-67):
1. Discovered by mammogram as cluster of microcalcifications and/or density
2. Presents less often as a palpable mass or nipple discharge
3. Before mammogram screening, DCIS accounted for 1% of all breast cancers
4. Now 15% to 20% or even higher proportion have DCIS
5. Formerly treated with mastectomy, now lumpectomy
6. Cure rates 98% to 99%
7. No axillary dissection required
8. With radiation, breast recurrences reduced
9. Mastectomy possibly required with extensive and/or high-grade DCIS
10. Systemic adjuvant treatment is not indicated

Inflammatory carcinoma:
1. Rare but rapidly progressive and often lethal form of breast cancer
2. Presents as erythematous and edematous breast resembling mastitis
3. Biopsy required, including skin
4. Treatment with combination chemotherapy followed by surgery and radiation therapy
5. Prognosis once dismal, now 5-yr disease-free survival in 50% of patients

COMMENTS
- The U.S. Preventive Services Task Force (USPSTF) now recommends against automatic "routine" screening of younger women (age range 40 to 49). The task force recommends biennial screening mammography for all middle-aged women (age range 50 to 74). It also states that current evidence is insufficient to assess the benefits and harms of screening mammography in older women (aged 75 and older). The task force also discourages women from performing breast self-examination. Several other U.S. organizations, however, still recommend annual screening beginning at age 40. This has created confusion among both physicians and the general public. Physicians should be familiar with the risks and benefits of various competing recommendations in order to better counsel patients.

- Breast radiologic evaluation, evaluation of nipple discharge, and evaluation of palpable mass are described in Section III.
- Exposure of the heart to ionizing radiation during breast cancer radiotherapy increases risk of ischemic heart disease. The increased rate of ischemic heart disease begins within a few years of exposure and continues for at least 20 yr. The increase is proportional to the mean radiation dose to the heart.

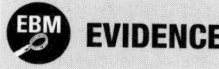 **EVIDENCE**

available at www.expertconsult.com

SUGGESTED READINGS
available at www.expertconsult.com

RELATED CONTENT

AUTHORS: **TAKUMA NEMOTO, M.D.,** and **RUBEN ALVERO, M.D.**

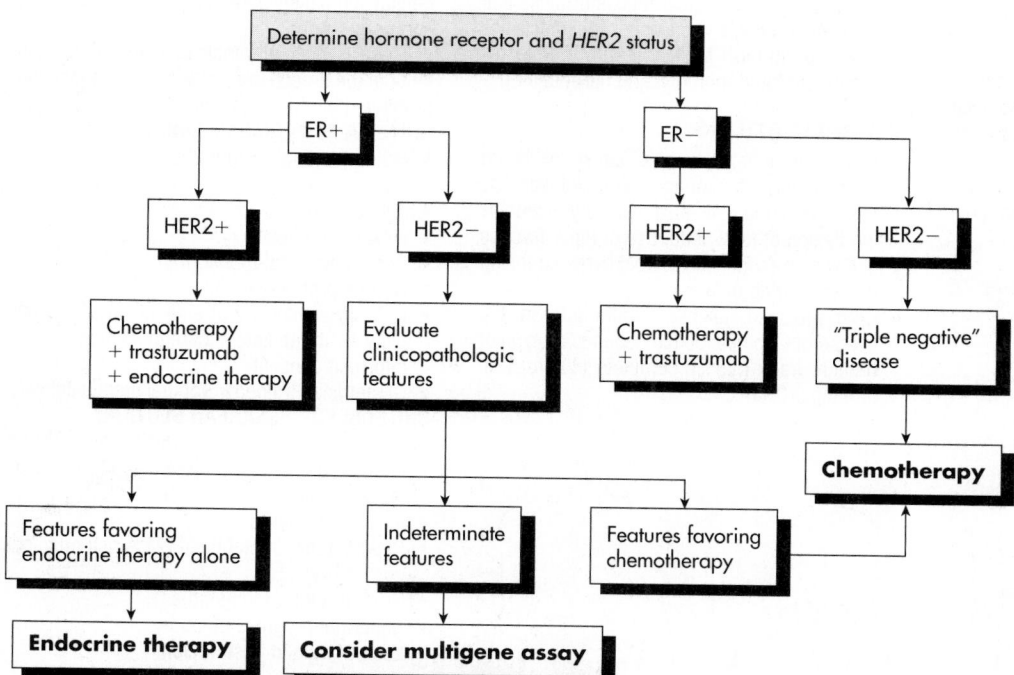

FIGURE 1-165 Management of recurrent and metastatic breast cancer. Considerations for adjuvant chemotherapy. (From Cameron JL, Cameron AM: *Current surgical therapy,* ed 10, Philadelphia, 2011, Saunders.)

B

Diseases and Disorders

I

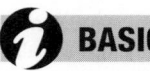

BASIC INFORMATION

DEFINITION

Breech presentation occurs when the fetal longitudinal axis is such that the cephalic pole occupies the uterine fundus (Fig. 1-166). Three types exist with respective percentages at term: frank (48% to 73%, flexed hips, extended knees), complete (4.6% to 11.5%, flexed hips and knees), and footling (12% to 38%, hips extended).

ICD-9CM CODES
652.2 Breech presentation without mention of version

EPIDEMIOLOGY & DEMOGRAPHICS

INCIDENCE: Gestational age dependent: 3% to 4% overall, 14% at 29 to 32 wk, 33% at 21 to 24 wk

PERINATAL MORTALITY: Three to five times increase over vertex presentation at term, regardless of route of delivery. When corrected for the associated increase in congenital anomalies and complications of prematurity, the morbidity and mortality rates approach those of the vertex presentation at term regardless of route of delivery.

PHYSICAL FINDINGS & CLINICAL PRESENTATION

- Lack of presenting part on vaginal examination
- Fetal heart tones heard above the umbilicus
- Leopold maneuvers revealing mobile fetal part in the uterine fundus

ETIOLOGY

- Abnormal placentation (fundal), uterine anomalies (fibroids, septa), pelvic or adnexal masses, alterations in fetal muscular tone, or fetal malformations
- Associated conditions: trisomy 13, 18, 21; Potter syndrome; myotonic dystrophy; prematurity

DIAGNOSIS

DIFFERENTIAL DIAGNOSIS

Vertex, oblique, or transverse lie

WORKUP

- Determine reason for breech presentation, history of uterine anomalies, gestational age, or associated fetal congenital anomalies
- Assess fetal status by continuous fetal heart rate monitoring or ultrasound
- Assess pelvis to determine feasibility of vaginal delivery
- Assess risk for safety of vaginal versus abdominal delivery

IMAGING STUDIES

Ultrasound to evaluate for:
- Fetal anomalies, such as hydrocephalus
- Placental location
- Position of fetal head relative to spine (check for hyperextension)
- Estimated fetal weight (2500 to 3800 g)
- Type of breech (frank, complete, footling)

TREATMENT

ACUTE GENERAL Rx

- Vaginal delivery in selected patients (see "Comments" section): allow maternal expulsive forces to deliver fetus until scapula visible (avoiding traction); with flexion and/or Piper forceps, deliver fetal head
- Perform cesarean section (see "Comments")
- External cephalic version: success 60% to 75% after 37 wk, contraindicated with placental abruption, low-lying placenta, maternal hypertension, previous uterine incision, multiple gestation, nonreassuring fetal status
- Adequate pelvic/cervical relaxation essential for vaginal breech (i.e., need anesthesia in-room during birth [delivery] with uterine relaxants on hand [nitroglycerin, terbutaline])

COMPLICATIONS

- Head entrapment: leading cause of death (with the exception of anomalous fetuses), 88 cases per 1000 deliveries; avoid by maintaining flexion of fetal head, use of Piper forceps or Dührssen's incisions. Avoid hyperextension of head during delivery.
- Cord prolapse: usually occurs late in the course of labor. Incidence depends on type of breech: frank (0.5%), complete (4% to 5%), footling (10%).

- Nuchal arm: arm extended above fetal head, occurs when there is undue traction before delivery of fetal scapulas. Treatment depends on bringing trapped arm across infant's face.

DISPOSITION

If confounding variables are corrected for, such as prematurity and associated congenital anomalies (6.3% of breeches vs. 2.4% in general population), route of delivery plays a less important role in fetal outcome than previously believed. This presupposes that the obstetrician performing the delivery is experienced in breech delivery. As fewer providers perform breech deliveries and experience decreases as seasoned obstetricians retire, fewer new physicians learn the technique of breech delivery.

REFERRAL

An obstetrician trained in delivery of the vaginal breech is a prerequisite for attempting vaginal route, although it must be explained to the patient that with cesarean section certain risks (such as hyperextension of the fetal head with resultant spinal cord injury) may be minimized but not eliminated.

PEARLS & CONSIDERATIONS

COMMENTS

In general, for breech presentation, mortality rate is increased 13-fold and morbidity sevenfold. The main reasons are an increase in congenital anomalies, perinatal hypoxia, birth injury, and prematurity.

There is no contraindication to induction of labor in the breech presentation, and labor is not prohibited in a primigravida.

CRITERIA FOR TRIAL OF LABOR:
- Estimated fetal weight 2000 to 3800 g
- Frank breech
- Adequate pelvis
- Flexed fetal head
- Continuous fetal monitoring
- Normal progress of labor
- Bedside availability of anesthesia and capability for immediate cesarean section
- Informed consent
- Obstetrician trained in vaginal breech delivery

CRITERIA FOR CESAREAN SECTION:
- Estimated fetal weight <1500 g or >4000 g
- Footling presentation (20% risk of cord prolapse, usually late in course of labor)
- Inadequate pelvis
- Hyperextended fetal head (21% risk of spinal cord injury)
- Nonreassuring fetal status
- Abnormal progress of labor
- Lack of trained obstetrician

RELATED CONTENT

Premature Birth (Related Key Topic)
Breech Birth (Patient Information)

AUTHORS: **SCOTT J. ZUCCALA, D.O.,** and **RUBEN ALVERO, M.D.**

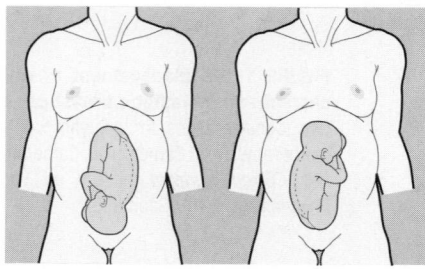
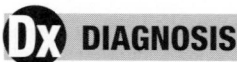

Cephalic 95%   Breech 4%
Longitudinal lie 99%

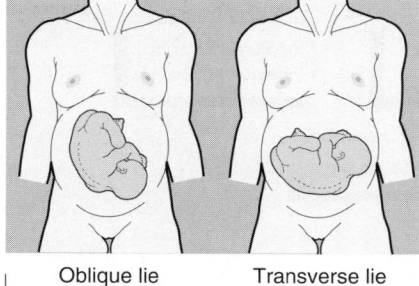
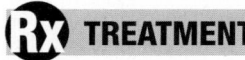

Oblique lie   Transverse lie
1%

FIGURE 1-166 Fetal lie at term. (From Drife J, Magowan B: *Clinical obstetrics and gynecology,* Philadelphia, 2004, Saunders.)

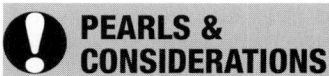

BASIC INFORMATION

DEFINITION

Bronchiectasis is the abnormal dilation and destruction of bronchial walls, which may be congenital or acquired.

ICD-9CM CODES
494.0 Bronchiectasis

EPIDEMIOLOGY & DEMOGRAPHICS

- Cystic fibrosis is responsible for nearly 50% of all cases of bronchiectasis.
- Acquired primary bronchiectasis is uncommon because of rapid diagnosis of pulmonary infections and frequent use of antibiotics.
- Effective childhood immunizations have led to a significant decrease in the incidence of bronchiectasis resulting from pertussis.

PHYSICAL FINDINGS & CLINICAL PRESENTATION

- Moist crackles at lung bases
- Cough with expectoration of large amount of purulent sputum
- Fever, night sweats, generalized malaise, weight loss
- Hemoptysis
- Halitosis, skin pallor
- Clubbing (infrequent)

ETIOLOGY

- Cystic fibrosis
- Lung infections (pneumonia, lung abscess, TB, fungal infections, viral infections)
- Abnormal host defense (panhypogammaglobulinemia, Kartagener's syndrome, AIDS, chemotherapy)

- Localized airway obstruction (congenital structural defects, foreign bodies, neoplasms)
- Inflammation (inflammatory pneumonitis, granulomatous lung disease, allergic aspergillosis)

DIAGNOSIS

DIFFERENTIAL DIAGNOSIS

- TB
- Asthma
- Chronic bronchitis or chronic sinusitis
- Interstitial fibrosis
- Chronic lung abscess
- Foreign body aspiration
- Cystic fibrosis
- Lung carcinoma

LABORATORY TESTS

- Sputum for Gram stain, culture and sensitivity, and acid-fast bacteria
- Complete blood count with differential (leukocytosis with left shift, anemia)
- Serum protein electrophoresis to evaluate for hypogammaglobulinemia
- Antibody test for aspergillosis
- Sweat test in patients with suspected cystic fibrosis

IMAGING STUDIES

- Chest radiograph: hyperinflation, crowded lung markings, small cystic spaces at the base of the lungs.
- High-resolution CT scan of the chest (Fig. 1-167) has become the best tool to detect cystic lesions and exclude underlying obstruction from neoplasm. The CT study should be a noncontrast study with the use of 1- to 1.5-mm window every 1 cm with acquisition time of 1 sec. Typical findings on CT include dilation of airway lumen, lack of tapering of an airway toward periphery, ballooned cysts at the end of bronchus, and varicose constrictions along airways.
- Bronchoscopy may be helpful to evaluate hemoptysis, rule out obstructive lesions, and remove mucus plugs.

TREATMENT

NONPHARMACOLOGIC THERAPY

- Postural drainage (reclining prone on a bed with the head down on the side) and chest percussion with use of inflatable vests or mechanical vibrators applied to the chest may enhance removal of respiratory secretions.
- Adequate hydration.
- Supplemental oxygen for hypoxemia.

ACUTE GENERAL Rx

- Antibiotic therapy is based on the results of sputum, Gram stain, and culture and sensitivity; in patients with inadequate or inconclusive results, empiric therapy with amoxicillin/clavulanate 500 to 875 mg q12h, TMP-SMX q12h, doxycycline 100 mg bid, or cefuroxime 250 mg bid for 10 to 14 days is recommended.
- Bronchodilators are useful in patients with demonstrable airflow obstruction.

CHRONIC Rx

- Avoidance of tobacco
- Maintenance of proper nutrition and hydration
- Prompt identification and treatment of infections
- Pneumococcal vaccination and annual influenza vaccination

DISPOSITION

Prognosis is variable with severity of the disease and underlying etiology of bronchiectasis.

REFERRAL

Surgical referral for partial lung resection in patients with localized severe disease unresponsive to medical therapy or in patients with massive hemoptysis

SUGGESTED READING

available at www.expertconsult.com

RELATED CONTENT

Bronchiectasis (Patient Information)

AUTHOR: **FRED F. FERRI, M.D.**

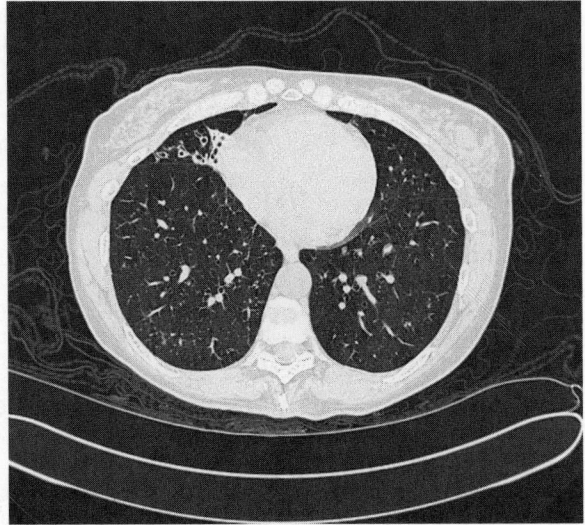

FIGURE 1-167 High-resolution computed tomographic image of nodular bronchiectasis due to nontuberculous mycobacterium infection. (From Goldman L, Schafer AI: *Goldman's Cecil medicine,* ed 24, Philadelphia, 2012, Saunders.)

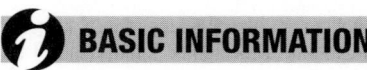

BASIC INFORMATION

DEFINITION

Brugada syndrome (BS) is a genetically determined disease characterized by typical electrocardiographic signs, and it predisposes to sudden cardiac death (SCD) secondary to polymorphic ventricular tachycardia (PVT)/ventricular fibrillation (VF) in the absence of structural heart disease.

ICD-9CM CODES
746.89 Other specified congenital anomalies of heart

EPIDEMIOLOGY & DEMOGRAPHICS

INCIDENCE: The incidence ranges from 1 to 5:10,000 people in Europe and 12:10,000 in Southeast Asia.
PREVALENCE: It comprises 4% of SCD and 20% of SCD in structurally normal hearts.
PREDOMINANT SEX AND AGE: BS is more common in males (80% of patients). Mean age at presentation is 40 to 45.
GENETICS: The disease is autosomal dominant with variable expression.

Cardiac sodium channel gene *SCN5A* mutation accounts for 20% to 25% of clinically confirmed cases of BS. *GPD1-L* (glycerol 3 phosphate dehydrogenase 1–like protein) gene was recently identified and was present in up to 1% of cases. Therefore, the impact of genetic testing is limited but, when available, it is useful to identify silent carriers.

RISK FACTORS:
- First-degree relatives with the disease

PHYSICAL FINDINGS & CLINICAL PRESENTATION

- Physical exam is usually benign.
- Classic ECG finding is a pattern of right bundle branch block (RBBB) with persistent ST elevation of cove-like morphology and T-wave inversion in the anterior leads (V_1-V_3)
- Often an incidental finding diagnosed from a typical ECG pattern
- Palpitations
- Syncope
- Sudden cardiac arrest (SCA)/SCD secondary to rapid PVT that frequently degenerates into VF
- Three ECG patterns were described. Type 1 is the most common and characteristic (Fig. 1-169A).
- Type 1 ECG pattern can be transient and may be provoked (sodium channel blockers, vagal maneuvers, increased alpha-adrenergic tone, beta-blockers, tricyclic or tetracyclic antidepressants, fever, hypokalemia, hyperkalemia, hypercalcemia, and alcohol and cocaine toxicity). Table E1-73 describes drugs used to unmask Brugada ECG pattern.

ETIOLOGY

- Autosomal dominant inheritance with varying prenetration
- Mutations in SCN5A16 gene leading to a loss of function of the cardiac sodium (Na^+) channel by different mechanisms is the most common genotype found among BS patients. Table E1-74 describes the molecular basis of BS.

DIAGNOSIS

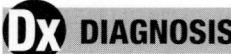

Consensus report from the Study Group on the Molecular Basis of Arrhythmias of the European Society of Cardiology (2002).
- Presence of type I ECG in ≥2 leads in right precordium (V_1-V_3) and at least one of the following:
  - Documented VF
  - Self-terminating polymorphic VT
  - Family history of SCD at <45 yr
  - Type 1 ST-segment elevation (Fig. 1-169A) in family members
  - Electrophysiologic inducibility of VT
  - Unexplained syncope suggestive of a tachyarrhythmia
  - Nocturnal agonal respiration
- Presence of type II or III ECG (Fig. 1-169A) that converts into type I ECG following sodium channel blocker challenge AND one of the features previously described.

DIFFERENTIAL DIAGNOSIS

- Long QT syndrome
- Sudden unexpected nocturnal death syndrome
- Commotio cordis (disruption of heart rhythm as a result of trauma to the precordium)
- Preexcitation syndrome

WORKUP

- Cardiology consult is strongly recommended if BS is suspected.
- Detailed history with emphasis for history of syncope, cardiac arrest, SCD in family
- Two-dimensional echocardiogram
- Electrophysiologic study may be indicated.
- First-degree relatives should obtain ECG and be evaluated for symptoms.

LABORATORY TESTS

No tests are required. Currently, the presence of *SCN5A* mutation is not considered a diagnostic criterion.

IMAGING STUDIES

- Two-dimensional echocardiogram

TREATMENT

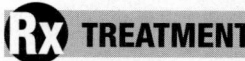

Implantable cardioverter-defibrillator (ICD) implantation reserved for patients with high-risk features; risk stratification of patients becomes the critical step in patient management (Fig. 1-169B).

NONPHARMACOLOGIC THERAPY

ICD is reserved for patients with high-risk features for SCD.

Candidates for ICD are patients who survived SCA or patients who have type 1 ECG pattern in the absence of class IC drug test associated with history of syncope.

Patients with spontaneous type 1 ECG without syncope are considered intermediate risk, and which strategy to follow is less clear.

Patients with a provoked type 1 ECG pattern are considered to be a lower-risk group for SCD.

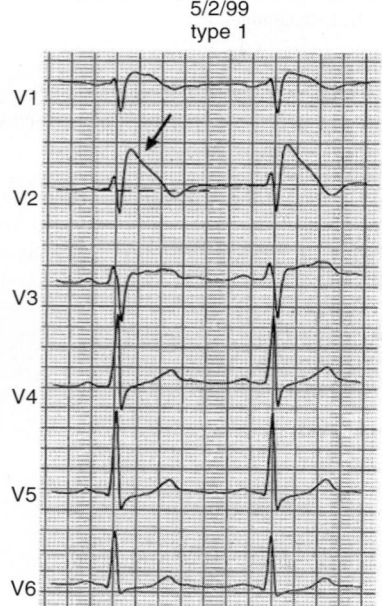

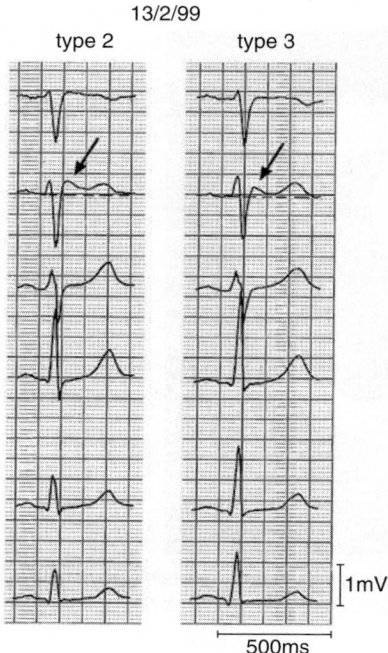

FIGURE 1-169A ECG changes in Brugada syndrome. ST elevation occurs in the anterior precordial leads, leads V_1 and V_2. Type 1 (coved) ECGs with 1 mV of ST elevation have the most prognostic significance. (From Strickberger SA et al: AHA/ACCF scientific statement on the evaluation of syncope, *J Am Coll Cardiol* 47:473-484, 2006.)

ACUTE GENERAL Rx

- Isoproterenol (class IIa) is also used for electrical strom.
- Quinidine (class IIb) is used to treat ventricular tachycardia storm and to reduce the number of ICD shocks.

DISPOSITION

If patient has had recent high-risk symptoms (syncope, SCA/SCD), they should be admitted for an inpatient evaluation. If there are no recent high-risk symptoms, then an outpatient referral to cardiology is reasonable.

REFERRAL

Consultation with cardiology is strongly recommended if BS is suspected.

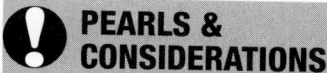

PEARLS & CONSIDERATIONS

COMMENTS

- The clinical manifestations, such as syncope and SCD, are rare in the pediatric group, but fever can acutely predispose to cardiac arrest.

- Increased severity of symptoms are noted in patients in the 3rd to 4th decade of life; mean age at presentation is 40 to 45.
- Cardiac events may occur during sleep, at rest, or after a large meal.
- BS patients should be advised to avoid all drugs that may induce a type 1 ECG pattern and/or be known to trigger ventricular arrhythmias, and avoid unnecessary use of drugs (a drug that is not yet identified as potentially dangerous for these patients does not make its use safe). For up-to-date information on this matter, the following website has been developed: www.brugadadrugs.org.
- Fever may induce the appearance of a type 1 BS ECG pattern and may trigger episodes of PVT/VF in BS patients. In the case of fever, close ECG monitoring is appropriate in combination with lowering of the body temperature.
- The classic ECG changes in BS can be transient and are often provokable.
- Patients with type II ECG, with genetically confirmed diagnosis can still get life-threatening cardiac events.
- The appearance of syncope, seizures, or nocturnal agonal respiration must lead to prompt medical evaluation.

- Family screening of BS in first-degree relatives is strongly recommended.
- All patients must be followed up on a regular basis in order to identify the development of symptoms.
- Genetic testing, when available, is recommended (to support clinical diagnosis).

PREVENTION

Identification of patients with BS, risk stratification, and appropriate screening of family members is paramount to the prevention of SCD.

PATIENT/FAMILY EDUCATION

Immediate family members should be notified and be screened for BS.

SUGGESTED READINGS

available at www.expertconsult.com

AUTHORS: **ABDULRAHMAN ABDULBAKI, M.D.**, and **WEN-CHIH WU, M.D., M.P.H.**

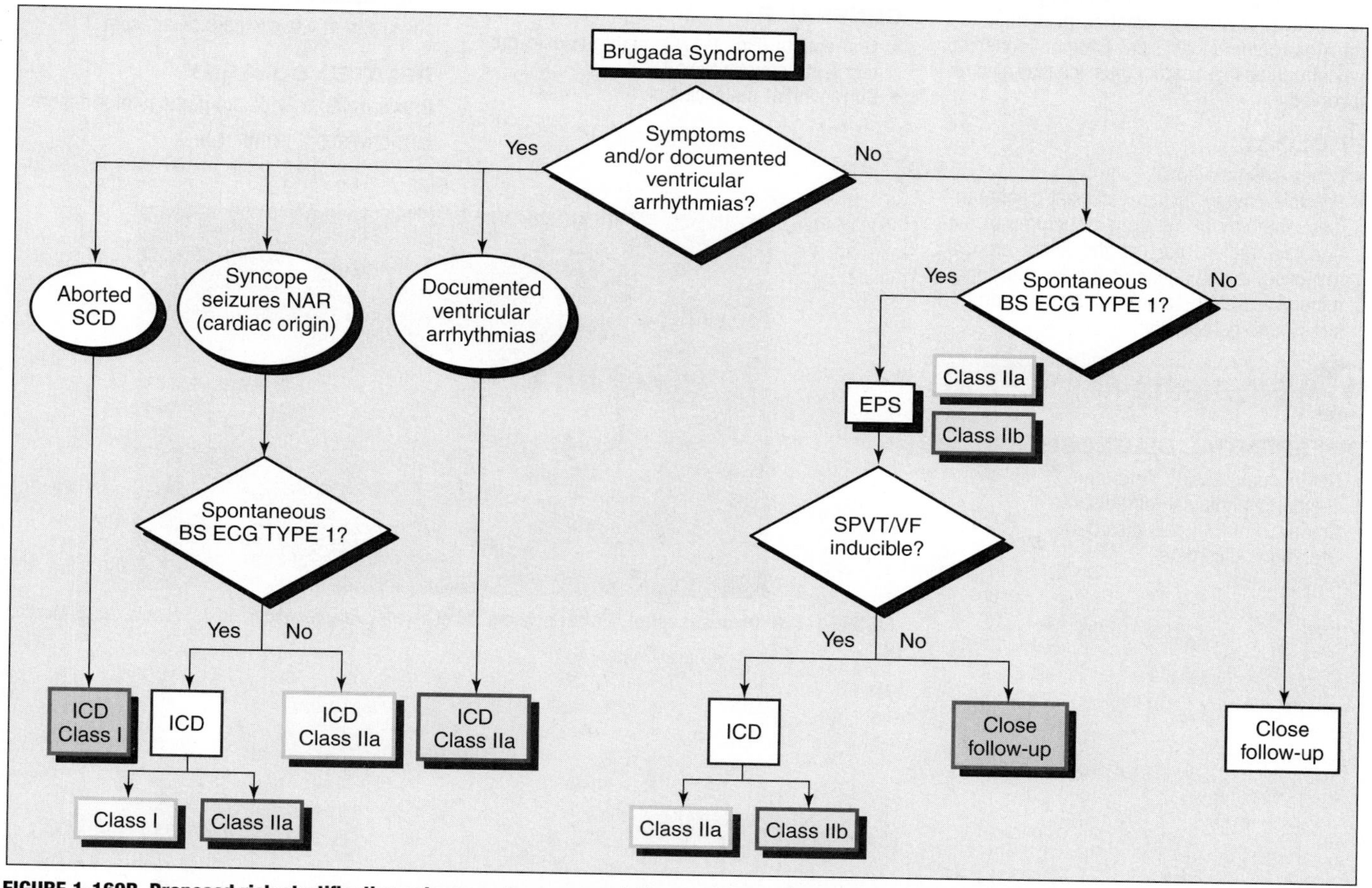

Diseases and Disorders

FIGURE 1-169B Proposed risk stratification scheme and recommendations of ICD in Brugada syndrome patients. *Lightly shaded boxes with dashed lines:* Recommendations from 2nd Consensus on Brugada Syndrome. *Medium shaded boxes with dotted lines:* Recommendations from ACC/AHA/ESC Practice Guidelines for Management of Patients With Ventricular Arrhythmias and the Prevention of Sudden Cardiac Death (2006). *Darkly shaded boxes with dot-dash lines:* Recommendations in Agreement with 2nd Consensus on Brugada Syndrome and Practice Guidelines for Management of Patients With Ventricular Arrhythmias and the Prevention of Sudden Cardiac Death (2006). Recommendation classes: Class I: clear evidence that the treatment/intervention is useful or effective; Class II: conflicting evidence about usefulness or efficacy; Class IIa, weight of evidence in favor of usefulness or efficacy; Class IIb: usefulness or efficacy less well established. *BS,* Brugada syndrome; *EPS,* electrophysiologic study; *ICD,* implantable cardioverter defibrillator; *NAR,* nocturnal agonal respiration; *PVT,* polymorphic ventricular tachycardia; *SCD,* sudden cardiac death; *VF,* ventricular fibrillation. (From Berne P, Brugada J: Brugada syndrome 2012, *Circ J* 76:1563-1571, 2012.)

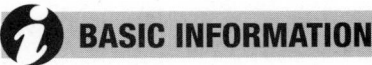

BASIC INFORMATION

DEFINITION

Forcible clenching or grinding of the teeth during sleep or wakefulness, often leading to damage of the teeth.

ICD-9CM CODES
306.8 Bruxism

EPIDEMIOLOGY & DEMOGRAPHICS

- Occurs in 15% of children and 75% of adults
- Familial cases have occasionally been described.
- Bruxism often presents between age 10 and 20 yr but may persist throughout life.
- Nocturnal bruxism is noted most often during stages I and II NREM sleep and REM sleep.

PHYSICAL FINDINGS & CLINICAL PRESENTATION

Complaints of grinding of teeth from a sleep partner or members of the family are common. In many cases the masticatory system will adapt to the phenomenon, but in severe cases nearly every part of the masticatory system may be damaged. Excessive wearing of dentition is the most common physical finding. Tender or hypoatrophied masticatory muscles may also be observed.

ETIOLOGY

- Cause is controversial.
- Possible causes include occlusal discrepancies, anatomy of the bony structures of the orofacial region, part of the sleep arousal response, disturbances of the central dopaminergic system, smoking, alcohol, drugs, stress, and personality.

DIAGNOSIS

DIFFERENTIAL DIAGNOSIS

- Dental compression syndrome
- Temporomandibular joint disorders
- Chronic orofacial pain disorders
- Oral motor disorders
- Malocclusion

WORKUP

- History should have an emphasis on sleep habits, including excessive snoring, pain in the temporal mandibular region, interview with close family members, health habits, personality quirks.
- Physical examination of the teeth and masticatory muscles is mandatory.
- Sleep studies in selected cases may be helpful.

LABORATORY TESTS

None indicated unless a systemic disease is suspected (e.g., infection, autoimmune disorder)

IMAGING STUDIES

X-ray studies of teeth and temporomandibular joints

TREATMENT

NONPHARMACOLOGIC THERAPY

Biofeedback, psychological counseling, and elimination of harmful health habits have been used with limited success.

GENERAL Rx

- Oral splints (Fig. 1-170); nightguard to protect teeth may be useful
- Correction of malocclusion
- Pain management (e.g., gabapentin, ibuprofen)
- Medication to relieve anxiety and improve sleep (e.g., benzodiazepine or trazodone at bedtime)
- Local injections of botulinum toxin into masseter muscles to prevent dental and temporomandibular joint complications

DISPOSITION

Referral to dentist mandatory if damage to teeth evident

PEARLS & CONSIDERATIONS

- Like any poorly understood disease, treatment is often unsatisfactory and subject to quackery.
- Both diurnal and nocturnal bruxism may be associated with various movement and degenerative disorders (e.g., Huntington disease, oromandibular dystonia) and are quite common in children with cerebral palsy and mental retardation.

SUGGESTED READINGS
available at www.expertconsult.com

RELATED CONTENT
Bruxism (Tooth Grinding) (Patient Information)

AUTHOR: **FRED F. FERRI, M.D.**

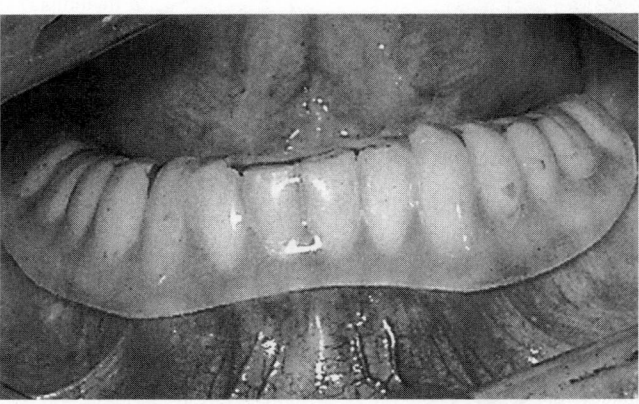

FIGURE 1-170 Occlusal splint. (From Hochberg MC et al [eds]: *Rheumatology*, ed 3, St Louis, 2003, Mosby.)

BASIC INFORMATION

DEFINITION

Budd-Chiari syndrome (BCS) is a rare disease defined by the obstruction of hepatic venous outflow anywhere from the small hepatic veins to the junction of the inferior vena cava (IVC) and the right atrium. Primary BCS is defined by endoluminal obstruction as seen in thromboses or webs. Secondary BCS occurs when the obstruction is caused by compression or invasion by a lesion originating outside the veins (tumor, abscess, cyst, etc.). It can also be a postoperative complication of orthotopic liver transplantation.

SYNONYMS

Hepatic vein thrombosis
Obliterative endophlebitis of the hepatic veins
IVC thrombosis (obliterative hepatocavopathy)

ICD-9CM CODES
453.0 Budd-Chiari syndrome

EPIDEMIOLOGY & DEMOGRAPHICS

INCIDENCE: 1/2.5 million persons per yr
PREDOMINANT SEX: In Western countries, women are more commonly affected (approximately 2/3 of cases)
PREDOMINANT AGE: Presentation is usually in the third and fourth decades of life, with the median age being 35

PHYSICAL FINDINGS & CLINICAL PRESENTATION

Clinical presentation and characteristics vary with geography. In Africa and South Asia, intravascular webs are more often associated with IVC thrombosis with a stronger association with subsequent hepatocellular carcinoma. In the U.S., BCS is more commonly associated with primary myeloproliferative disorders and underlying hypercoagulable states. Underlying factors that contribute to BCS can be identified in ~85% of cases, and multiple causative factors are identified in 50% of cases.

- Clinical manifestations can be caused by complete or partial occlusion of any or all of the three major hepatic veins, or inferior vena cava.
- Variable according to the degree, location, acuity of obstruction, and presence of collateral circulation:
  - Fulminant/acute (20%): severe right upper quadrant abdominal pain, fever, nausea, vomiting, jaundice, hepatomegaly, transudative ascites, marked elevation in serum aminotransferases (ALT >5 times the upper limit of normal), elevation of alkaline phosphatase to 300 to 400 IU/L, decrease in coagulation factors, variceal bleeding, encephalopathy within 8 wk of onset of jaundice; biopsy, if performed, would reveal liver cell loss; early recognition and treatment are essential for survival; a slow decrease in ALT is associated with poor survival.
  - Subacute/chronic (60%): vague abdominal discomfort, gradual progression to caudate lobe hypertrophy with atrophy of the rest of the liver, portal hypertension with or without cirrhosis and its sequelae, transudative ascites, lower extremity edema, esophageal varices, splenomegaly, coagulopathy, hepatorenal syndrome in up to half of patients, hepatopulmonary syndrome in up to 28% of patients, and rarely, encephalopathy
  - Asymptomatic (5% to 20%): usually discovered incidentally by abnormal liver function tests

ETIOLOGY

- Primary myeloproliferative diseases: 20% to 53%
  - Polycythemia vera, responsible for 10% to 40% of cases
  - Essential thrombocythemia and idiopathic myelofibrosis are less common causes
  - JAK2 mutations are implicated in cases of idiopathic BCS (identified in 26% to 59% of cases)
  - Rare but recently reported: idiopathic hypereosinophilia syndrome
- Hypercoagulable states (inherited and acquired): often coexist with other causes, 30% to 65%
  - Factor V Leiden (25%)
  - Factor II gene mutation (5%)
  - Anticardiolipin antibodies (25%)
  - Hyperhomocysteinemia (22%)
  - Paroxysmal nocturnal hemoglobinuria (19%)
- Protein C, protein S, and antithrombin III deficiency are difficult to interpret because the presence of liver disease may confound results.
- Heterozygosity for G20210A prothrombin gene mutation or methylene-tetrahydrofolate reductase (MTHFR) mutation may be seen in BCS
- Pregnancy and oral contraceptive pills (cases reported after <2 wk of use)
- Malignancy (up to 10% of cases, causing external compression or invasions of vascular structures)
  - Most commonly due to hepatocellular carcinoma but also can be due to neoplasms of the kidney, adrenal gland, pancreas, stomach, and sarcomas of the right atrium, inferior vena cava, and hepatic veins
- Rare but reported: sickle cell anemia, infections with liver abscess, hydatid cyst (echinococcosis), schistosomiasis, sarcoidosis, Behçet's disease (<5%), membranous webs of IVC or hepatic veins (more common in Africa and South Asia, can be congenital or acquired secondary to underlying myeloproliferative disorder), abdominal trauma, liver torsion, ulcerative colitis, celiac disease, idiopathic (10% to 20%)

DIAGNOSIS

DIFFERENTIAL DIAGNOSIS

- Hepatitis from ischemia, viral infection, toxin, alcohol
- Cholecystitis
- Hepatic venoocclusive disease (sinusoidal obstruction syndrome)
- Congestive hepatopathy, also known as cardiac cirrhosis, from tricuspid regurgitation, right atrial myxoma, constrictive pericarditis
- Cirrhosis from any etiology

LABORATORY TESTS

- Assessment of liver injury and function: serum aminotransferases, alkaline phosphatase, prothrombin time (PT), albumin, bilirubin
- Exclusion of another form of liver disease: viral hepatitis panel, autoantibodies (antinuclear antibody, anti–smooth muscle antibody, anti-mitochondrial antibody), serum iron, transferrin saturation, ferritin, ceruloplasmin, and α-1 antitrypsin
- Ascites protein content >3.0 g/dl and serum ascites albumin gradient ≥1.1 g/dl are suggestive of transudative ascites from BCS, cardiac or pericardial disease
- Evaluation for underlying myeloproliferative disorder and hypercoagulable state: CBC, bone marrow biopsy, tests for hypercoagulable states (Factor V Leiden, prothrombin gene G20210A mutation, protein C, protein S, and antithrombin deficiencies, antiphospholipid antibodies, hyperhomocysteinemia, paroxysmal nocturnal hemoglobinuria, and MTHFR C677T mutation); protein C, protein S, and antithrombin deficiencies may be difficult to interpret in the setting of liver dysfunction, but levels <20% of normal are suggestive of a true deficiency; thrombophilia screening for the JAK2 V617F mutation may be useful if no other for myeloproliferative disorders/hypercoagulable states identified

IMAGING STUDIES

- Diagnosis of BCS is made by radiographic imaging.
- Ultrasound and color and pulsed Doppler are the first-line tests. Diagnostic sensitivity and specificity are 85% to 90%. Findings include large hepatic vein with an absent flow signal, or with reversed or turbulent flow; large

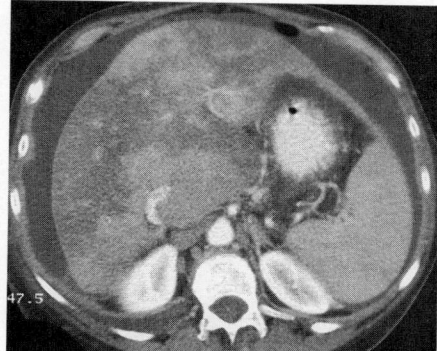

FIGURE 1-171 CT scan of Budd-Chiari syndrome. The appearances are not immediately diagnostic for the nonexpert, and infiltrative disease is sometimes suspected. (From Forbes A et al [eds]: *Atlas of clinical gastroenterology*, ed 3, 2005, Mosby.)

intrahepatic collateral vessels; enlarged, stenotic, thickened or tortuous hepatic veins; and caudate lobe hypertrophy (as the caudate lobe has an alternate blood supply through anastomoses).

- MRI with gadolinium contrast—better than contrast-enhanced CT (Fig. 1-171), with a sensitivity and specificity of approximately 90%—is the second-line test. Findings include obstructed hepatic veins or IVC; large, intrahepatic or subcapsular collaterals; and caudate lobe hypertrophy. Three-dimensional contrast-enhanced magnetic resonance angiography (MRA, see Fig. 1-172) rivals hepatic venography in sensitivity.
- Contrast-enhanced CT may reveal similar findings as Doppler ultrasound, as well as delayed or absent filling of the hepatic veins, parenchymal opacification of the liver, and narrowing of the inferior vena cava.
- CT image reconstruction of vasculature is becoming available.
- Venography: This is not essential for diagnosis; it should be performed when other noninvasive imaging tests are nondiagnostic in the setting of strong clinical suspicion for BCS measurement of pressure gradients can help predict success of percutaneous or surgical shunt intervention and plan surgical intervention. Confirms the pathognomonic web pattern caused by collateral venous flow.
- Liver biopsy: This is not necessary to diagnose BCS but may be helpful in patients with cirrhosis in whom the diagnosis remains uncertain and critical for differentiating from hepatic venoocclusive disease. Findings include hepatic congestion, hepatocyte necrosis and fibrosis in centrilobular areas, and compensatory nodular regenerative hyperplasia with progression to fibrosis and cirrhosis. In advanced BCS, may also see infarction caused by concomitant thrombosis of the intrahepatic, extrahepatic, and portal veins. There are conflicting studies regarding the association of histologic findings and prognosis.

 TREATMENT

NONPHARMACOLOGIC THERAPY

- Goal of therapy is decompression of hepatic congestion.
- In general, therapeutic procedures should be introduced by order of increasing invasiveness based on response/failure to therapy rather than disease severity.
- Hypercoagulable states should be investigated in all patients.

ACUTE GENERAL Rx

- Anticoagulation, first with low-molecular-weight heparin (LMWH), followed by warfarin, even in the absence of an underlying hypercoagulable disorder
- In situ thrombolysis: can be successful when performed in recently thrombosed veins (clot less than 3 to 4 weeks old) that are well defined on venography and do not involve the inferior vena cava; mature clots are nonresponsive to thrombolysis, and bleeding risk is high if portal hypertension has developed
- Balloon angioplasty: complicated by 50% restenosis rate; effective when membranous webs are the etiology
- Stenting: may improve long-term patency rates to 90%, but if placed above the intrahepatic IVC, may complicate future liver transplantation
- Transjugular intrahepatic portosystemic shunt (TIPS) has been increasingly used in recent years; usually performed in patients with no improvement on anticoagulation therapy or when a dilatable lesion cannot be found; TIPS has replaced surgical shunting as the most common invasive therapeutic procedure; recently polytetrafluoroethylene (ePTFE)-coated stents have improved TIPS-patency rates,

especially in patients with underlying hypercoagulable defects.
- Surgical portal systemic shunts: feasibility depends on technical factors, long-term patency of the stent, the extent of liver damage before surgery, as well as on locating a center with well-trained surgeons
- Liver transplant may be indicated in patients with fulminant hepatic failure and in patients who fail to respond to TIPS; 10-year survival reported to range between 69% and 84%.
- Supportive measures

CHRONIC Rx

- Lifelong anticoagulation: Warfarin therapy with a target international normalized ratio of (INR) 2 to 3 lessens, but does not completely prevent, recurrence. This should be continued permanently unless the patient has an adverse event to anticoagulation.
- In patients with an underlying myeloproliferative disorder, treatment with hydroxyurea and aspirin, or anagrelide, may be given instead of traditional anticoagulation.
- Treat liver dysfunction and complications related to portal hypertension, such as ascites (diuretics and low-sodium diet).
- Invasive interventions should be reserved for symptomatic patients who do not improve with medical therapy.
- Manage shunt thrombosis, which is a common complication.
- Liver transplantation is another treatment option; up to 10% recurrence of BCS after transplant has been recognized
- Monitor for development of hepatocellular carcinoma and transformation of myeloproliferative disease in patients with longstanding, well-controlled BCS.

DISPOSITION

Prognosis is variable and depends on multiple factors, including time to recognition and treatment, etiology, acuity, the type of intervention, and the condition of the patient at the time of treatment. Overall mortality rates are decreasing with the use of anticoagulation and early diagnosis of asymptomatic cases. Survival rates have been reported as 77%, 65%, and 57% at 1, 5, and 10 yr from diagnosis. A prognostic index called the *Rotterdam BCS Index* has been described: $1.27 \times$ Encephalopathy $+ 1.04 \times$ Ascites $+ 0.72 \times$ PT $+ 0.004 \times$ Bilirubin. Encephalopathy and ascites are scored as 1 for present or 0 as absent, and PT is scored as greater (1) or less than (0) an INR of 2.3. An index of <1.1 correlates to low risk (5-yr survival rate, 89%), 1.1 to 1.5 with intermediate risk (5-yr survival rate, 74%), and >1.5 with high risk (5-yr survival rate, 42%).

REFERRAL

Fulminant presentations should immediately be referred to a center capable of liver transplantation. All cases benefit from referral to a hepatologist, a hematologist, an interventional radiologist, and a surgeon specializing in hepatobiliary disease.

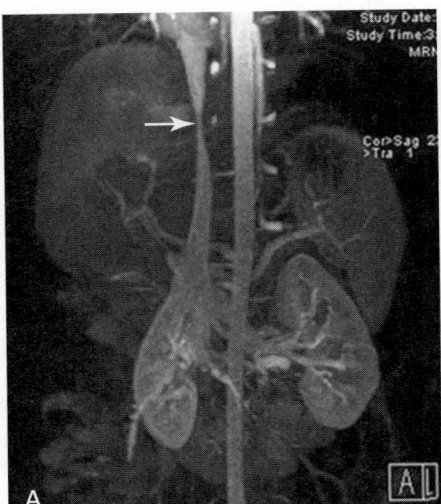
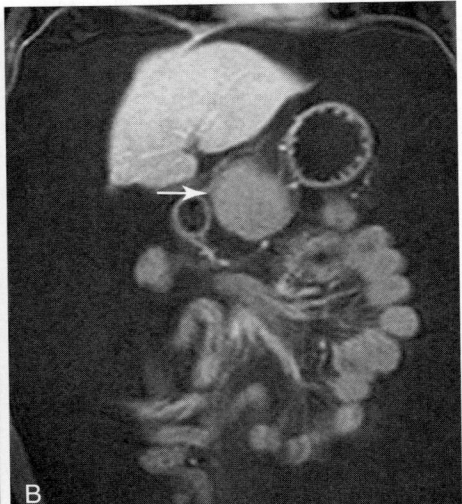

FIGURE 1-172 Magnetic resonance venogram. A, IVC obstruction *(arrow)* at the level of the caudate. **B,** Hypertrophic caudate lobe. (From Cameron JL, Cameron AM: *Current surgical therapy,* ed 10, Philadelphia, 2011, Saunders.)

PEARLS & CONSIDERATIONS

COMMENTS

- Look for one or more underlying causes, especially hypercoagulable or hematologic disorders, and malignancies or space-occupying lesions that may compress or invade the hepatic outflow tract.
- Myeloproliferative disorders are most common.
- Diagnosis relies on imaging, beginning with Doppler ultrasound.
- Treatment with anticoagulation comes first, followed by invasive interventions as needed. Prophylaxis of portal hypertension can reduce the risk of major bleeding associated with anticoagulation therapy.

- Referral for liver transplantation may be necessary.
- Prognosis depends on presence of ascites, encephalopathy, PT, and serum bilirubin levels.

PREVENTION

In the setting of known risk factors, such as a hypercoagulable state or myeloproliferative disorder, any additional risks, such as smoking or oral contraceptive therapy, should be avoided.

SUGGESTED READINGS
available at www.expertconsult.com

RELATED CONTENT
Hypercoagulable States (Related Key Topic)
Budd-Chiari Syndrome (Patient Information)

AUTHORS: **MICHAEL PRODROMOU, M.D.** and **JEANETTE G. SMITH, M.D.**

BASIC INFORMATION

DEFINITION

Bulimia nervosa is a prolonged illness characterized by a specific psychopathology. It is characterized by recurrent episodes of binge eating that are coupled with compensatory behaviors whose intent is to undo the effects of the binge episodes. According to the *Diagnostic and Statistical Manual of Mental Disorders,* 4th edition, Revised (DSM-IV-R), there are 2 main types: ***Purging type:*** During the current episode of bulimia nervosa, the person has regularly engaged in self-induced vomiting or misuse of laxatives, diuretics, or enemas. ***Non-purging type:*** During the current episode of bulimia nervosa, the person has used other inappropriate compensatory behaviors, such as fasting or excessive exercise, but has not regularly engaged in self-induced vomiting or misuse of laxatives, diuretics, or enemas.

ICD-9CM CODES
783.6 Bulimia

EPIDEMIOLOGY & DEMOGRAPHICS

INCIDENCE/PREVALENCE: Affects 1% to 3% of female adolescents and young adults
PREDOMINANT SEX: Female/male ratio of 10:1
PREDOMINANT AGE: Adolescence to young adulthood; mean age of onset: 17 yr

PHYSICAL FINDINGS & CLINICAL PRESENTATION

- Parotid and salivary gland swelling
- Scars on the back of the hand and knuckles (Russell sign) from rubbing against the upper incisors when inducing vomiting
- Eroded enamel, particularly on the lingual surface of the upper teeth; pyorrhea and other gum disorders possible
- Petechial hemorrhages of the cornea, soft palate, or face possibly noted after vomiting
- Loss of gag reflex, well-developed abdominal musculature
- Often no emaciation; normal physical examination possible

ETIOLOGY

- Etiology is unknown but likely multifactorial (sociocultural, psychologic, familial factors).
- Bulimia is much more common in Western societies, where there is a strong cultural pressure to be slender.
- According to the American Psychiatric Association, patients with eating disorders display a broad range of symptoms that occur along a continuum between those of anorexia nervosa and bulimia.

DIAGNOSIS

DIFFERENTIAL DIAGNOSIS

- Schizophrenia
- Gastrointestinal disorders
- Neurologic disorders (seizures, Kleine-Levin syndrome, Klüver-Bucy syndrome)
- Brain neoplasms
- Psychogenic vomiting

WORKUP

- The following questions are useful to screen patients for bulimia:
  1. "Are you satisfied with your eating habits?"
  2. "Do you ever eat in secret?"
- Answering "no" to the first question and/or "yes" to the second question has 100% sensitivity and 90% specificity for bulimia. The SCOFF questionnaire can also be used as a screening tool for eating disorders (see "Anorexia Nervosa").
- A diagnosis can be made using the following DSM-IV diagnostic criteria for bulimia nervosa:
  1. Recurrent episodes of binge eating (rapid consumption of a large amount of food in a discrete period)
  2. A feeling of lack of control over eating behavior during the eating binges
  3. Self-induced vomiting, use of laxatives or diuretics, strict dieting or fasting, or rigorous exercise to prevent weight gain
  4. A minimum of two binge-eating episodes a week for at least 3 mo
  5. Persistent overconcern with body shape and weight
- Table 1-75 describes eating and weight control habits commonly found in children and adolescents with an eating disorder.

LABORATORY TESTS

- Electrolyte abnormalities from vomiting (hypokalemia and metabolic alkalosis) or diarrhea from laxative abuse (hypokalemia and hyperchloremic metabolic acidosis)
- Hyponatremia, hypocalcemia, hypomagnesemia (caused by laxative abuse)
- Elevated cortisol, decreased luteinizing hormone, decreased follicle-stimulating hormone

TREATMENT

NONPHARMACOLOGIC THERAPY

- Cognitive behavioral therapy, particularly interpersonal therapy to control abnormal behaviors
- Use of food diaries, nutritional counseling, and planning meals at least 1 day in advance are useful measures to counter abnormal eating behaviors
- Correction of electrolyte abnormalities

ACUTE GENERAL Rx

- Selective serotonin reuptake inhibitors are generally considered to be the safest medication option in these patients. They are useful in severely depressed patients and in those who do not benefit from cognitive behavioral therapy.
- Prompt recognition and treatment of complications:
  1. Ipecac cardiotoxicity from laxative abuse
  2. Electrolyte abnormalities (see "Laboratory Tests")
  3. Esophagitis and Mallory-Weiss tears; esophageal rupture from repeated vomiting
  4. Aspiration pneumonia and pneumomediastinum
  5. Menstrual irregularities (including amenorrhea)
  6. Gastrointestinal abnormalities: acute gastric dilation, pancreatitis, abdominal pain, constipation

CHRONIC Rx

- Psychotherapy continued for years and focused specifically on self-image and family and peer interactions is an integral part of successful recovery.
- Family therapy is also recommended, especially in younger patients.

DISPOSITION

Course is variable and marked by frequent recurrence of exacerbations.

REFERRAL

- In addition to the primary care physician, the multidisciplinary team should include a dietician, a psychiatrist, and a family therapist.
- Hospitalization should be considered for patients with severe electrolyte abnormalities or those with suicidal thoughts.

PEARLS & CONSIDERATIONS

COMMENTS

- Bulimia has a close association with depression, bipolar disorder, obsessive-compulsive disorder, alcoholism, and substance abuse.
- Bulimia should be considered in all patients (especially adolescents) with unexplained hypokalemia and metabolic alkalosis.

SUGGESTED READINGS

available at www.expertconsult.com

RELATED CONTENT
Bulimia (Patient Information)

AUTHOR: **FRED F. FERRI, M.D.**

TABLE 1-75 Eating and Weight Control Habits Commonly Found in Children and Adolescents with an Eating Disorder

	PROMINENT FEATURES		CLINICAL COMMENTS REGARDING EATING DISORDER HABITS	
Habit	**Anorexia Nervosa**	**Bulimia Nervosa**	**Anorexia Nervosa**	**Bulimia Nervosa**
Overall intake	Inadequate energy (calories), although volume of food and beverages may be high due to very low caloric density of intake due to "diet" and nonfat choices	Variable, but calories normal to high; intake in binges often "forbidden" food or drink that differs from intake at meals	Consistent inadequate caloric intake leading to wasting of the body	Inconsistent balance of intake, exercise and vomiting, but severe caloric restriction is short-lived
Food	Counts and limits calories, especially from fat; emphasis on "healthy food choices" with reduced caloric density Monotonous, limited "good" food choices, often leading to vegetarian or vegan diet Strong feelings of guilt after eating more than planned leads to exercise and renewed dieting	Aware of calories and fat, but less regimented in avoidance than AN Frequent dieting interspersed with overeating, often triggered by depression, isolation, or anger	Obsessive-compulsive attention to nutritional data on food labels and may have "logical" reasons for food choices in highly regimented pattern, such as sports participation or family history of lipid disorder	Choices less structured, with more frequent diets
Beverages	Water or other low- or no-calorie drinks; nonfat milk	Variable, diet soda common; may drink alcohol to excess	Fluids often restricted to avoid weight gain	Fluids ingested to aid vomiting or replace losses
Meals	Consistent schedule and structure to meal plan Reduced or eliminated caloric content, often starting with breakfast, then lunch, then dinner Volume can increase with fresh fruits, vegetables, and salads as primary food sources	Meals less regimented and planned than in AN; more likely impulsive and unregulated, often eliminated following a binge-purge episode	Rigid adherence to "rules" governing eating leads to sense of control, confidence, and mastery	Elimination of a meal following a binge-purge only reinforces the drive for binge later in the day
Snacks	Reduced or eliminated from meal plan	Often avoided in meal plans, but then impulsively eaten	Snack foods removed early because "unhealthy"	Snack "comfort foods" can trigger a binge
Dieting	Initial habit that becomes progressively restrictive, although often appearing superficially "healthy" Beliefs and "rules" about the patient's idiosyncratic nutritional requirements and response to foods are strongly held	Initial dieting gives way to chaotic eating, often interpreted by the patient as evidence of being "weak" or "lazy"	Distinguishing between healthy meal planning with reduced calories and dieting in ED may be difficult	Dieting tends to be impulsive and short-lived, with "diets" often resulting in unintended weight gain
Binge eating	None in restrictive subtype, but an essential feature in binge-purge subtype	Essential feature, often secretive Shame and guilt prominent afterward	Often "subjective" (more than planned but not large)	Relieves emotional distress, may be planned
Exercise	Characteristically obsessive-compulsive, ritualistic, and progressive May excel in dance, long-distance running	Less predictable May be athletic, or may avoid exercise entirely	May be difficult to distinguish active thin vs. ED	Males often use exercise as means of "purging"
Vomiting	Characteristic of binge-purge subtype May chew then spit out, rather than swallow, food as a variant	Most common habit intended to reduce effects of overeating Can occur after meal as well as a binge	Physiologic and emotional instability prominent	Strongly "addictive" and self-punishing, but does not eliminate calories ingested—many still absorbed
Laxatives	If used, generally to relieve constipation in restrictive subtype, but as a cathartic in binge-purge subtype	Second most common habit used to reduce or avoid weight gain, often used in increasing doses for cathartic effect	Physiologic and emotional instability prominent	Strongly "addictive," self-punishing, but ineffective means to reduce weight (calories are absorbed in the small intestine, but laxatives work in the colon)
Diet pills	Very rare, if used; more common in binge-purge subtype	Used to either reduce appetite or increase metabolism	Use of diet pills implies inability to control eating	Control over eating may be sought by any means

AN, Anorexia nervosa; *BN,* bulimia nervosa; *ED,* eating disorder.
From Kliegman RM et al: *Nelson textbook of pediatrics,* ed 19, Philadelphia, 2011, Saunders.

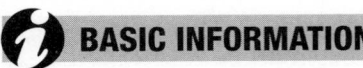

DEFINITION

Bullous pemphigoid is an autoimmune, subepidermal blistering disease commonly seen in the elderly. A related entity is cicatricial pemphigoid, which predominantly affects the mucous membranes.

SYNONYMS

Pemphigoid

ICD-9CM CODES
694.5 Pemphigoid

EPIDEMIOLOGY & DEMOGRAPHICS

- Occurs most commonly in people older than 60 yr, with peak incidence in those aged ≥80 yr
- Incidence is approximately 10 cases per 1 million persons
- No gender or racial predilection
- Most common of the autoimmune bullous dermatoses

PHYSICAL FINDINGS & CLINICAL PRESENTATION

HISTORY:
- Skin lesions typically start as eczematous or urticarial plaques on the extremities and are often very pruritic
- Taut blisters can form within 1 wk to several months

PHYSICAL FINDINGS:
- Anatomic distribution
  1. Flexor surfaces of the arms and legs, groin, axilla, chest, and abdomen; generally spares the head and neck
  2. Rare involvement of mucous membranes
- Lesion configuration
  1. May be localized to the extremities or generalized
  2. Lesions irregularly grouped but may sometimes be serpiginous (Fig. 1-173)
- Lesion morphology
  1. Taut blisters (bullae) measuring 5 mm to 2 cm in diameter filled with clear or bloody fluid on either normal or erythematous skin are characteristic
  2. Heal without scarring but may leave postinflammatory hyperpigmentation

ETIOLOGY

- Autoimmune disease with immunoglobulin (Ig) G and/or C3 complement targeting hemidesmosomal antigens located in the epidermal basement membrane zone
- Drug-induced pemphigoid, although rare, can occur in patients taking penicillamine, furosemide, captopril, penicillin, or sulfasalazine

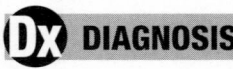 **DIAGNOSIS**

Skin biopsy aids in the diagnosis, and specimens should be sent for routine histochemical staining and direct immunofluorescence.

DIFFERENTIAL DIAGNOSIS

- Cicatricial pemphigoid
- Epidermolysis bullosa acquisita
- Pemphigus
- Linear IgA disease

LABORATORY TESTS

- Histology of lesional skin shows a subepidermal blister with a superficial inflammatory infiltrate, often with numerous eosinophils
- Indirect immunofluorescence detects anti–basement membrane antibodies in 70% of patients with bullous pemphigoid.
- Direct immunofluorescence of perilesional skin shows C3 and IgG linearly arranged along the epidermal basement membrane.
- Approximately half of patients will have a peripheral blood eosinophilia.

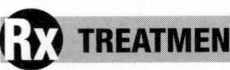 **TREATMENT**

Bullous pemphigoid may be a self-limited disease, but its course may last from months to years. Treatment is based on the degree of disease involvement and the rate of disease progression.

NONPHARMACOLOGIC THERAPY

- Mild soaps with emollients to wet skin after bathing
- Topical antipruritic creams

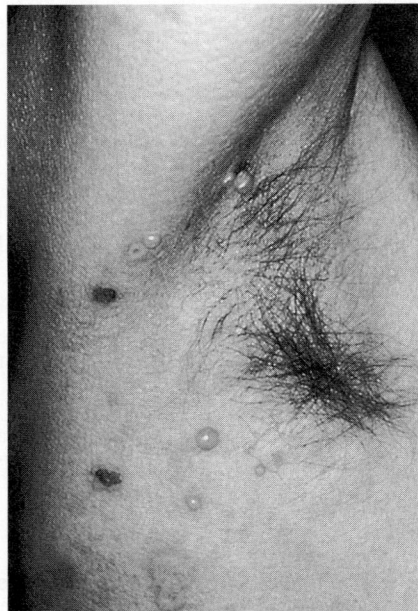

FIGURE 1-173 Bullous pemphigoid. Note intact bullae with erosions in a flexural distribution. (From Goldstein BG, Goldstein AO: *Practical dermatology,* ed 2, St Louis, 1997, Mosby.)

ACUTE GENERAL Rx

Localized disease:
- Potent topical steroids (e.g., clobetasol) until blistering ceases with gradual tapering over several weeks
- Oral antihistamines to control pruritus

Generalized disease:
- Mainstay of therapy is prednisone, usually beginning with a minimal dose of 1 mg/kg/day
- Steroid-sparing agents, such as azathioprine or mycophenolate mofetil, may be started with prednisone or shortly after prednisone therapy is initiated and may be continued once prednisone is discontinued
- Tetracyclines
- Low-dose methotrexate has recently been suggested to be an optimal therapy in the elderly
- Rituximab, a monoclonal antibody to CD20, has been used for treatment-refractory bullous pemphigoid

CHRONIC Rx

- Prednisone combined with steroid-sparing agents with the goal of limiting oral corticosteroid intake
- Other immunosuppressive agents, such as cyclophosphamide or cyclosporine, are occasionally used

DISPOSITION

Mortality rates are estimated at between 10% and 40% after 1 yr. Patients with widespread disease requiring immunosuppressive therapy and with other comorbidities are at highest risk for complications from the disease. Approximately 50% of treated patients experience remission within 2 to 6 yr.

REFERRAL

Dermatology

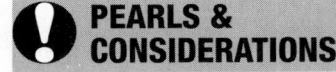 **PEARLS & CONSIDERATIONS**

COMMENTS

- Bullous pemphigoid is mainly a disease of elderly persons and should be suspected in older persons with chronic pruritic eruptions and in those patients who have new-onset taut vesicles and bullae
- Not believed to represent a paraneoplastic process.

SUGGESTED READINGS
available at www.expertconsult.com

RELATED CONTENT
Bullous Pemphigoid (Patient Information)

AUTHORS: **JESSICA RISSER, M.D., M.P.H.,** and **KACHIU LEE, B.A.**

BASIC INFORMATION

DEFINITION

- Cutaneous burns can be classified by type of injury (e.g., thermal vs. chemical), burn depth (e.g., 1st, 2nd, 3rd degree), extent of burn (total burn surface area [TBSA]), and burn severity (e.g., minor vs. major). Types of burn injury include thermal (flames, scalds, hot contactants), chemical, electrical, and radiation burns. This chapter will focus on thermal and electrical burns.
- Burns can affect skin and respiratory, ocular, oral, and genital mucosa.

SYNONYMS

Thermal injury
Chemical injury
Electrical injury
Radiation injury

ICD-9CM CODES
942-949 (by region, % burn)

EPIDEMIOLOGY & DEMOGRAPHICS

PREVALENCE (IN U.S.):

- More than 1.2 million individuals experience burns in the U.S., and burn injuries account for approximately 500,000 emergency department visits, with 9% (45,000) requiring hospitalization, with 0.8% (4,000) resulting in death annually.
- Of thermal injury, scald burn from liquid is most common—followed by flame, flash burn, then contact burn.

PREDOMINANT AGE & SEX:

- Children ages 2-4 years have the greatest frequency of burns (most commonly scald burns), with male adolescent and young adults ages 17-25 with second greatest frequency (most commonly from flammable liquids).

PHYSICAL FINDINGS & CLINICAL PRESENTATION

- It is important to note that burns occur unevenly—often with various depths (Table 1-76).

- 1st-degree (superficial) burns—penetrate epidermis only (minimal barrier loss)
  - Very painful, intact, erythematous skin with minimal to no edema and no blistering.
- 2nd-degree (partial-thickness) burns—epidermis and part of dermis is affected.
  - Moist, very painful skin with edema and blistering/blebs
  - Superficial partial-thickness burns—cherry red with two-point discrimination intact, incredibly painful.
  - Deep partial-thickness burns—mottled white and cherry red; only the sensation of pressure is intact in these areas
- 3rd-degree (full-thickness) burns—entire epidermis and dermis are affected, with destruction of hair follicles and sweat glands.
  - The skin is dry, charred, pale, painless, and leathery. Charred vessels may be visible beneath, little or no pain, and hair pulls out easily.

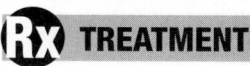 DIAGNOSIS

CLASSIFICATION

- Burns are classified by (1) depth of injury, (2) extent of injury, and (3) severity, according to the American Burn Association.
- Depth of injury (see Table 1-76)
  - Indicates how the wound will heal and whether grafting will be needed
- Extent of TBSA
  - The TBSA is best classified by using age-specific burn charts and the "rule of nines"(Fig. 1-174).
  - For scattered burns, utilizing patient's palm including fingers to equate 1% body surface area can be helpful.
  - TBSA indicates how aggressively the patient will need to be resuscitated
- Severity—determined by burn depth, TBSA, age, location, type of injury, and presence/absence of coexisiting conditions. Severity classification helps triage patients to outpatient, inpatient, or burn unit care (see Table 1-77).
  - Minor burns—outpatient management.

  - Moderate burns—admission to hospital with experience managing burns or burn center referral.
  - Major burns—referral to burn center

LABORATORY STUDIES (MODERATE OR MAJOR BURNS)

- CBC, electrolytes, BUN, creatinine, glucose, liver function tests, venous blood gas, blood coagulation, type and screen in anticipation of blood transfusion
- *If smoke inhalation expected:* serial ABG carboxyhemoglobin, and continuous ECG
- *If electrical burn or if concern for rhabdomyolysis:* urinalysis, urine myoglobin, and CPK levels
- *If severe lactic acidosis:* consider checking cyanide level.

IMAGING STUDIES

- If smoke inhalation suspected: chest radiograph and bronchoscopy
- If high-voltage electrical burn: cardiac monitoring 1st 24 hours

TREATMENT

DIFFERENTIAL DIAGNOSIS

Cultural practices leading to burnlike lesions in distinctive patterns (cupping, coining, moxibustion), cellulitis, Stevens-Johnson syndrome/toxic epidermolytic necrolysis

ACUTE GENERAL Rx

MINOR BURNS (1ST DEGREE BURNS AND 2ND/3RD DEGREE BURNS OF LIMITED TBSA)

- Outpatient management—"6 Cs"
  - Clothing: Remove hot or burned clothing
  - Cooling: Cool (approximately 54° F) for 10-30 minutes (under faucet or compress) to reduce edema/pain by conducting heat away from skin. Not recommended with extensive burns due to theoretical risk of hypothermia and shock. No ice packs.
  - Cleaning: Wash gently with mild alcohol-free soap, then normal saline daily. Remove all old ointment and any loose skin. Blot dry. No evidence supports vigorous

TABLE 1-76   Categorization of Burn by Depth

Burn Type	Histologic Depth	Clinical Presentation	Treatment	Healing Time/Prognosis
1st degree	Epidermis	Erythematous but intact skin, no blisters, pain may range in severity	Topical salves, cold compresses, NSAIDs for pain control	2-5 days with no scarring
Superficial 2nd degree (partial thickness)	Papillary dermis	Erythematous with superficial blisters, intense pain	Topical antimicrobials with gauze dressing or biosynthetic dressing (if widespread), pain control	5-21 days with no grafting
Deep 2nd degree (partial thickness)	Reticular dermis	Erythematous with superficial/deep blisters, range of pain depending on nerve involvement	Same	21-35 days with no infection; if infected, converts to full-thickness burn
3rd degree (full thickness)	Through dermis to subcutaneous tissue. Can involve fascia, muscle and bone.	White or black, possible eschar, may or may not be painful depending on nerve damage	Usually requires grafting, may require resuscitation depending on TBSA affected, pain control	Large areas require grafting, but small areas may heal from the edges after weeks

From Kliegman RM et al: *Nelson textbook of pediatrics,* ed 19, Phildelphia, 2011, Saunders; and Kessides MC, Skelsey MK: Management of acute partial-thickness burns, *Cutis* 86:249-257, 2010.

cleansing with antiseptic solutions. Embedded materials should be removed by copious irrigation using a large-gauge syringe.

○ Chemoprophylaxis: Tetanus immunization (all deep 2nd and 3rd degree burns). Routine skin cultures are NOT recommended except when wound infection suspected, and prophylactic systemic antibiotics are NOT recommended. All 2nd and 3rd degree burns are treated with topical antimicrobial agent. This may include silver sulfadiazine, bacitracin, bismuth-impregnated Vaseline gauze, or silver-impregnated synthetic dressings.

○ Covering: All 2nd and 3rd degree burns should be covered with sterile dressing. If financial resources are limited, instead of gauze can purchase cotton gloves, T-shirts, or similar at discount stores, wash, and reuse.

○ Comfort: Analgesics around the clock are recommended. Tylenol and NSAIDs—alone or in combination with opioids. Additional "rescue" analgesics before dressing changes and physical activity recommended.

Moderate & Major Burns (2nd/3rd degree burns of extensive TBSA)

• Patients with moderate/major burns should be admitted to the hospital or referred to a burn center. Indications for hospitalization for burns are described in Table 1-77.

• Resuscitation (in addition to above)
  ○ Assessment of ABCs: Establish airway and assess breathing (inspect for inhalation injury and intubate for suspected airway edema, often seen 12-24 hr later; O_2; establish circulation (place two large-bore peripheral IV lines, ECG).
  ○ IV fluid resuscitation—Parkland formula (Ringer's lactate at 2-4 ml/kg per % TBSA per 24 hr with half the calculated fluid given in the first 8 hr is an effective modality in severe burns).
  ○ Baseline neurologic and vascular assessment
  ○ Foley catheter and NG tube (20% of patients develop an ileus)—urine output 30 ml/hr

○ Optimize nutritional support: Mayes equations to calculate energy requirements after burn (Box 1-7)

• Frequent reassessment in the first 24-72 hours, as wound depth can change significantly

• The four phases of burn care, with physiologic changes and objectives are described in Table E1-78. Box E1-9 describes the modified Brooke resuscitation formula.

BURN WOUND CARE BY BURN DEPTH Rx

General

• Vigilant wound care with dressings to prevent evaporation and minimize threat of wound colonization and infection of nonintact skin.

• Daily activity necessary to maintain function of burned extremity, decrease pain and swelling, and promote healing

1st-degree burns (skin intact):

• *Dressing:* None required (except to protect from injury); topical antibacterial agents not recommended

• *Other:* Emollients, cool compresses (avoid ice), if pruritic trial of antihistamines

• *Prognosis:* Heals within 1 week without scarring. May heal with pigmentary changes (limit by sunscreen and sun avoidance of area for 1 year).

2nd degree (superficial partial-thickness) burns without adherent exudate or eschar:

• *Blisters:* Sharp debridement of ruptured blisters; leave intact blisters. Quicker healing and reduced infections when intact blisters are not disturbed. Consider unroofing blisters that show no sign of resorption over several weeks, contain cloudy fluid.

• *Dressing:* Topical antimicrobial ointment (bacitracin) or A&D ointment with nonadherent dressing twice a day. Alternate: biosynthetic dressing (alginates, hydrofibers, or foam dressings)—many with silver as antimicrobial (absorb exudates, maintain moist environment, require fewer dressing changes, which reduces pain/anxiety)

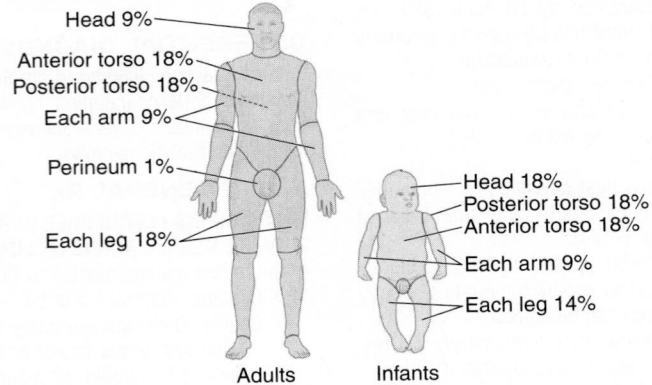

FIGURE 1-174 The "rule of nines" for estimating second-degree and third-degree burns. Because infants have significantly larger heads and smaller legs than do adults, different rules must be used in evaluating these patients. A simple, practical rule is that the palm of the patient's hand, with fingers, equals 1% of the total body area. (From Ferri F: *Practical guide to the care of the medical patient,* ed 8, St Louis, 2010, Mosby.)

TABLE 1-77 Classification of Burns by Severity and Indications for Hospitalization or Burn Center Referral

Criteria	Minor Burn	Moderate Burn	Major Burn
Total body surface area (%)	• All 1st degree burns <10% adults <5% children or elderly • <2% for 3rd degree	• 2nd degree burns 10-20% adults 5-10% in children or elderly • 2-5% 3rd degree	• All 1st degree burns >20% adults >10% children and elderly • >5% 3rd degree
Type of burn injury		• Low-voltage burn • Suspected inhalation injury	• High-voltage burn • Chemical burn, • Known
Location		Circumferential burn	• Clinically significant burn to face, eyes, ears, genitalia, over joints
Coexisting conditions		• Concomitant medical problem predisposing to infection (e.g., diabetes, sickle cell anemia)	• Significant associated injuries (e.g., fracture, other major trauma)
	Outpatient management	Inpatient management—consider referral to burn center*	Referral to burn center

* Per the American Burn Association (ABA), any partial-thickness burn >10% total body surface area, or any factors listed in moderate or major burn category warrant referral to burn center. Additional factors per the ABA include burned children in a hospital without qualified personnel or equipment for the care of children and burn injury in a patient who will require special social, emotional, or rehabilitative intervention (including suspected child abuse).

Modified from Singer AJ, Dagum AB: Current management of acute cutaneous wounds, *N Engl J Med 359* (10):1037-1046, 2008; www.ameriburn.org.

- *Prognosis:* heal with minimal scarring in 10-14 days. May heal with pigmentary changes (limit by sunscreen and sun avoidance of area x 1 year)

2nd degree (deep partial-thickness) burns with adherent exudates; localized 3rd degree burns; cellulitic wounds:

- *Dressing:* silver sulfadiazine 1%: broader spectrum, better penetration of necrotic tissue than bacitracin, but inhibits epithelialization. Must stop use once exudates and eschar have separated from wound. Alternative: enzymatic debrider (e.g., Santyl or Accuzyme)—chemically debrides devitalized tissue without harming healthy tissue.
- *Referral:* Burn specialist for consultation regarding need for excision and grafting.
- *Prognosis:* Deep 2nd degree burns heal with significant scarring, often take 3-4 weeks to heal. If infected, converts to 3rd degree burn. 3rd degree burns typically require skin graft, but small areas may heal from edges after weeks.

DISPOSITION/FOLLOW-UP CARE

- Outpatient: Evaluate next day to assess level of injury, level of pain, and ability to manage dressing changes on own. If insufficient, daily evaluation until complete wound epithelialization recommended. Epithelialization = tiny islands of epithelialization throughout wound. If no epithelialization after 2 weeks, or subsequent evaluation reveals 3rd degree burn, referral to burn surgeon recommended. Box E1-8 describes common complications in burn patients.
- Following re-epithelialization, visits every 4-6 weeks to monitor for hypertrophic scar formation (early referral to burn/scar specialist if occurs).
- Mortality rates higher in patients > 60 yr of age, with burns > 40% TBSA, or with inhalation injury. Long-term risk of developing squamous cell carcinoma of the skin within burn injury. Long-term monitoring necessary.

REFERRAL

Consultation of burn specialist or burn center referral per Table 1-77.

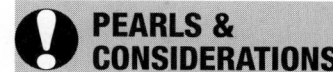 **PEARLS & CONSIDERATIONS**

COMMENTS

- In circumferential skin burns, look for compartment syndrome of limbs (e.g., tightening, progressive deterioration of peripheral motor and sensory exam findings, severe pain, and loss of arterial Doppler signals). Escharotomy may be necessary.
- If child abuse is suspected, social services at the hospital or child protective services must be contacted.

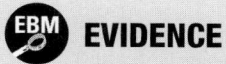 **EVIDENCE**

available at www.expertconsult.com

SUGGESTED READINGS

available at www.expertconsult.com

RELATED CONTENT

Burns (Patient Information)

AUTHOR: **LISA PAPPAS-TAFFER, M.D.**

BOX 1-7 Mayes Equations to Calculate Energy Requirement After a Burn

Mayes equation for a 5- to 10-year-old burn patient with injury <50% TBSA:

818 + 37.4 (weight in kilograms) + 9.3 × % TBSA burn

Mayes equation for a 5.5-year-old patient with a 45% TBSA scald burn weighing 20 kg:

818 + 37.4 (20 kg) + 9.3 × 45% TBSA scald

818 + 748 + 481.5 = 2047.5 calories/day

From Fuhrman BP et al: *Pediatric critical care,* ed 4, Philadelphia, 2011, Saunders.

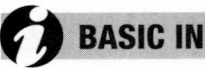 **BASIC INFORMATION**

DEFINITION

Bursitis is an inflammation of a bursa, which is a thin-walled sac lined with synovial tissue. Bursae facilitate movement of tendons and muscles over bony prominences.

SYNONYMS

Student's elbow (olecranon bursitis)
Housemaid's knee (prepatellar bursitis)
Weaver's bottom (ischial gluteal bursitis)
Baker's cyst (gastrocnemius-semimembranosus bursa)

ICD-9CM CODES
726.19 Subacromial bursitis
726.33 Olecranon bursitis
726.5   Ischiogluteal bursitis (hip)
726.5   Iliopsoas bursitis (hip)
726.61 Anserine bursitis
726.5   Trochanteric bursitis
726.65 Prepatellar bursitis
727.51 Baker's cyst
726.79 Retrocalcaneal bursitis

PHYSICAL FINDINGS & CLINICAL PRESENTATION

- Local swelling, tenderness, erythema, warmth over the site of bursa
- Pain with active joint movement greater than passive range of motion or at rest
- Range of motion may be less painful and less restricted in septic bursitis compared with septic arthritis
- Referred pain

ETIOLOGY

- Direct trauma or repetitive injury
- Infection (septic bursitis)—from hematogenous seeding or spread from contiguous infection (*Staphylococcus aureus* >80%)
- Crystal diseases (e.g., gout, pseudogout)
- Systemic inflammatory arthritis (i.e., rheumatoid arthritis [RA])
- Bleeding

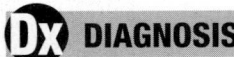 **DIAGNOSIS**

DIFFERENTIAL DIAGNOSIS

- Acute monoarthritis due to septic arthritis or crystal arthritis (gout, pseudogout)
- Tendinitis, tenosynovitis (sometimes occurs with bursitis)
- Cellulitis

WORKUP

- Bursal fluid aspiration: send for Gram stain; culture and sensitivity; cell count; and crystal analysis

IMAGING STUDIES

- Plain radiography can rule out foreign body penetration and other potential or coexisting bone or joint problems such as fracture (Fig. 1-175)
- MRI may aid in defining the extent of soft tissue involvement
- Musculoskeletal ultrasound can aid visualization of superficial and deep bursae, and guide aspiration/injection

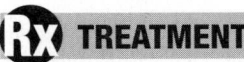 **TREATMENT**

NONPHARMACOLOGIC THERAPY

- Avoidance of direct pressure or repetitive irritation
- Joint protection (e.g., kneeling pads)
- Rest, ice, elevation for acute phase
- Physical therapy

ACUTE GENERAL Rx

- Septic:
  1. Appropriate antibiotic coverage and drainage. If MSSA, use nafcillin or oxacillin 2 g IV q4h or dicloxacillin 500 mg PO qid. If MRSA, use vancomycin 15-20 mg/kg IV q8-12h or linezolid 600 mg PO bid.
  2. Serial aspirations of purulent fluid or surgical drainage may be indicated.

- Nonseptic:
  1. Aspiration of bursal fluid or blood from acute trauma
  2. Nonpharmacologic therapy
  3. Traumatic bursitis may respond well to aspiration and corticosteroid injection.
  4. Crystal-related bursitis: systemic antiinflammatories or injection of corticosteroid

CHRONIC Rx

- Aspiration of fluid, followed by compression dressing to prevent fluid reaccumulation (repeat aspiration may be required)
- Steroid injection into bursa (40 mg triamcinolone mixed with 1-3 ml lidocaine, depending on size of bursa)
- NSAIDs, although steroid injection may be more effective in certain types of bursitis

DISPOSITION

- Nonsurgical treatment is effective in most cases. Surgical drainage may be indicated for loculated bursitis. Recurrent bursitis may require open bursectomy.

REFERRAL

Orthopedic consultation may be needed to assist in treatment of septic bursitis or for excision of chronic enlarged bursa when indicated.

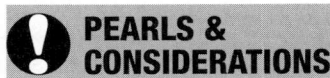 **PEARLS & CONSIDERATIONS**

- Bursae in patients with RA are not usually the sole site of active flare. Therefore, in patients with RA, acute bursitis should be considered septic bursitis until proven otherwise.

COMMENTS

- Scapulothoracic bursitis is underrecognized and undertreated. It results from friction between superomedial angle of scapula and adjacent second and third ribs. Crepitus, snapping, and tenderness are suggestive findings; it can also cause chest wall pain.
- Sterile bursae should not be incised and drained because a chronic draining sinus tract may develop.
- In bursitis caused by infectious or systemic inflammatory disorders, the leukocytosis in bursal fluid may be substantially less intense than the elevations in the joint fluid.
- Patients with crystal-induced bursitis should be investigated for underlying metabolic or hematologic diseases such as hemochromatosis and hyperparathyroidism (for calcium pyrophosphate deposition disease), and for causes of hyperuricemia (for gout).

SUGGESTED READINGS
available at www.expertconsult.com

RELATED CONTENT

Bursitis (Patient Information)
Gout (Related Key Topic)
Pseudogout (Related Key Topic)

AUTHOR: **CANDICE YUVIENCO, M.D.**

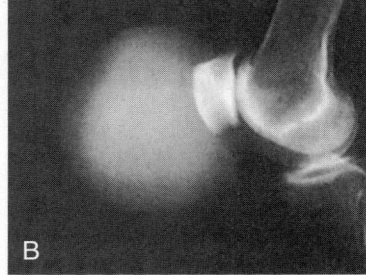

FIGURE 1-175 A, Bursae around the knee. **B,** Markedly swollen prepatellar bursa. (From Scudieri G [ed]: *Sports medicine principles of primary care,* St Louis, 1997, Mosby.)

Suprapatellar bursa

Superficial prepatellar bursa

Deep infrapatellar bursa

Superficial infrapatellar bursa

Pes anserine bursa

A

BASIC INFORMATION

DEFINITION

Infection caused by the species of the genus *Candida*, mainly *Candida albicans*. *Candida* species are ubiquitous. They are the most common fungal pathogens affecting mankind. Cutaneous candidiasis comprises superficial *Candida* infections of the skin and mucosal membranes.

Cutaneous candidiasis can be classified into two subgroups: cutaneous candidiasis syndromes and chronic mucocutaneous syndromes. Cutaneous candidiasis syndromes include:
- Generalized cutaneous candidias
- Intertrigo
- *Candida* folliculitis
- Paronychia/onychomycosis
- Perianal candidiasis
- Erosio interdigitalis blastomycetica
- Balanitis

Chronic mucocutaneous syndromes include:
- Oropharyngeal candidiasis
- Esophageal candidiasis
- Vulvovaginal candidiasis
- GI candidiasis (gastric/intestines/perianal)
- *Candida* cystitis

SYNONYMS

Yeast infection
Candidosis
Moniliasis
Oidiomycosis

ICD-9CM CODES
112 Candidiasis

EPIDEMIOLOGY & DEMOGRAPHICS

- *Candida* species: it is the most common fungal infection in immunocompromised people.
- Most females (75%) experience an episode of vulvovaginal candidiasis in their lifetime.

INCIDENCE: Estimated to be 50 cases per 100,000 persons
PREVALENCE: Colonizes more than 50% of U.S. population
PREDOMINANT SEX AND AGE
- Female > male
- No predominant age, but neonates and the elderly (adults >65 yr) are susceptible to *Candida* colonization and to getting nucocutaneous candidiasis.

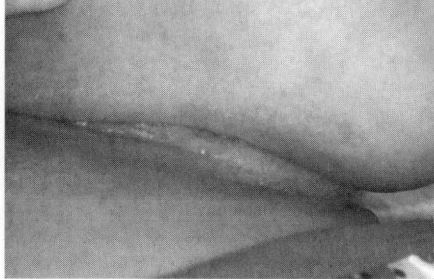

FIGURE 1-176 Intertriginous candidosis of the neck. (From Kliegman RM et al: *Nelson textbook of pediatrics*, ed 19, Philadelphia, 2011, Saunders.)

RISK FACTORS

Risk factors that allow *Candida* infection include:
- Age >65 yr
- Females in the third trimester
- Defects in the mucocutaneous barrier (e.g., wounds, burns, ulcerations)
- Decreased/defective granulocytes/monocytes
- Diseases of white blood cells (e.g., chronic granulomatous disease)
- Complement deficiency
- Certain diseases associated with cell-mediated immunity (e.g., HIV, DM)
- Use of certain medications (e.g., broad-spectrum antibiotics, high doses of steroids)
- Increased skin pH due to panty liners and occlusive attires

Anatomical sites predisposed to *Candida* infection include:
- Axilla
- Beneath the breast, abdominal fold, intertriginous areas
- Periungual creases
- Inguinal creases
- Back and buttocks of bedridden persons

PHYSICAL FINDINGS & CLINICAL PRESENTATION

There are several clinical presentations of cutaneous candidiasis. A few are presented here.
A. Cutaneous candidiasis
  1. Presents as erythematous, sometimes shiny with flakes and fluid lesions at the edge of the redness (satellite pustules). It is itchy and the skin becomes inflamed. Pustules may be present in candidiasis of the scrotal and perineal skin.
B. Gastrointestinal tract candidiasis
  1. Oropharyngeal candidiasis
     - Usually seen in diabetics, after exposure to inhaled steroids or broad-spectrum antibiotics and in immunosuppressed individuals (e.g., patients with a history of HIV infection). Symptoms include:
       ○ White thick patches on the oral mucosa
       ○ Dysphagia, mouth soreness, and pain
       ○ Tongue burning
     - Physical examination shows:
       ○ Erythema of the buccal mucosa
       ○ White patches on buccal cavity surfaces
       ○ Transverse fissuring
  2. Esophageal candidiasis:
     - History of oropharyngeal candidiasis
     - Symptoms include:
       ○ Dysphagia
       ○ Odynophagia
       ○ Epigastric pain
       ○ Retrosternal pain
     - Physical examination shows:
       ○ Affects of mainly the distal one third of the esophagus
       ○ Endoscopy shows areas of the erythema and edema; scattered white patches or ulcers.
  3. Perianal candidiasis
     - Skin maceration
     - Itching

- Frequently extends to the perineum
C. Paronychia/onychomycosis
  - Fungal infection of the nail and surrounding tissues
  - Associated with diabetes mellitus and immersion of hands or feet in water
  - History: pain and redness around and beneath the nail and nail bed
  - Physical exam: inflammation around the toe nail. There may also be nail thickening and discoloration (dystrophic nails). Nail loss may also occur.
D. Respiratory tract candidiasis
  1. Usually seen in hospitalized patients
  2. About 25% of outpatients have their respiratory tract colonized by *Candida* species
     - Genitourinary tract candidiasis
     - Vulvovaginal candidiasis
       ○ It causes itching, curdy white discharge, and occasionally dysuria and dyspareunia.
       ○ On examination the mucosa may be inflamed.
       ○ Painful erythema or itchy penile inflammation may occur in male sexual partners of affected females.
     - *Candida* balanitis
       ○ Usually acquired through sexual contact with a partner who has vulvovaginal candidiasis.
       ○ Symptoms include penile pruritus and white patches on penis.
       ○ Physical exam: dry, erythematous, and scaly patches on penis.
E. Others
  1. Erosio interdigitalis blastomycetica: Denudating/macerating area commonly seen in third web space
  2. *Candida* folliculitis: Pustulous nodules in hairy areas
  3. Intertrigo: This occurs in folds of the skin and creases (Fig. 1-176). It is characterized by erosions, exudation, oozing, and maceration.

ETIOLOGY

The most common cause of cutaneous candidiasis is *Candida albicans*.

DIAGNOSIS

DIFFERENTIAL DIAGNOSIS

Intertrigo

WORKUP

Mucocutaneous and cutaneous candidiasis
- Obtain scrapings from the skin, oral, and vaginal mucosa or nails.
- The presence of hyphae/pseudohyphae or budding yeast cells on wet smear, as well as confirmation by culture, is the recommended procedure to diagnose cutaneous candidiasis.
- KOH smears are helpful.

Respiratory candidiasis
- Sputum Gram stain: shows yeast cells
- Sputum cultures
- Lung biopsy: establishes the diagnosis

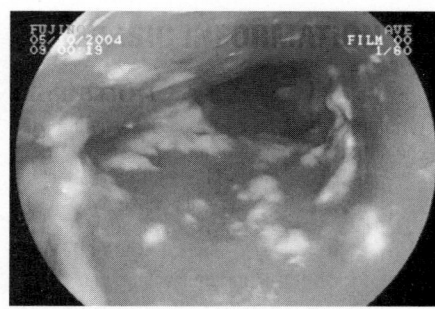

FIGURE 1-177 Endoscopic appearance of esophageal candidiasis. (Courtsey Dr. B. Rembacken, Leeds, U.K.)

Gastrointestinal candidiasis
- Upper endoscopy with or without biopsy (Fig. 1-177)

℞ TREATMENT

PHARMACOLOGIC THERAPY

A. Cutaneous candidiasis
 1. Decrease/prevent moisture in area
 2. Apply antifungal agents (nystatin powder or cream with an azole or ciclopirox [e.g., clotrimazole, econazole, miconazole])

B. Gastrointestinal candidiasis
 1. Oropharyngeal candidiasis
  - Treat with either
   ○ Oral topical antifungal agent (e.g., nystatin swish and swallow)
   OR
   ○ Systemic oral azoles (e.g., fluconazole)
  - In HIV-positive patients, use high doses of fluconazole (100-200 mg PO qd for 7-14 days), itraconazole, or posaconazole.
 2. *Candida* esophagitis
  - Treat with systemic fluconazole for 2 to 3 wk.
  - Treat with IV fluconazole if patient is unable to take oral medication.
C. Genitourinary tract candidiasis
  - Vulvovaginal candidiasis: Treatment options for acute cases include:
   ○ A single dose of oral fluconazole (fluconazole 150 mg PO × 1 dose)
   OR
   ○ Topical antifungal agent
  - For chronic or recurrent cases, treat with fluconazole 150 mg qod × 3 doses and then 150 mg/wk for 6 mo.
D. Chronic mucocutaneous candidiasis
  - Treatment with azoles are effective (e.g., fluconazole 100-400 mg daily).
  - When patient improves, follow with maintenance treatment with same azole for life.

FOLLOW-UP CARE

Mucocutaneous candidiasis
- Patient should be instructed to call or follow up if symptoms persist, recur, or worsen.
- For recurrent infections:
 ○ Check HIV antibodies.
 ○ Check FBS, HbA$_{1c}$.
 ○ Rule out hematologic malignancy or solid organ malignancy.
 ○ Refer to linfectious disease specialist if no etiology is found.

PREVENTION

- Maintaining dry environment (e.g., by wearing cotton underwear)
- Decreased use of antibiotic
- No douching

SUGGESTED READING
available at www.expertconsult.com

RELATED CONTENT

Candidiasis (Patient Information)

AUTHOR: **DANIEL K. ASIEDU, M.D., Ph.D., F.A.C.P.**

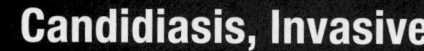

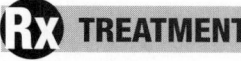 BASIC INFORMATION

DEFINITION

Severe and invasive diseases are caused by *Candida* infection. Invasive candidiasis embodies a variety of diseases including candidemia, disseminated candidiasis, meningitis, and endophthalmitis.

SYNONYMS

Systemic candidiasis

ICD-9CM CODES
112.5 Disseminated candidiasis

EPIDEMIOLOGY & DEMOGRAPHICS

INCIDENCE: Estimated to be 22 to 24 cases per 100,000 persons per year
PREVALENCE: No data available
PREDOMINANT SEX AND AGE: Equal between males and females; all ages are susceptible.
RISK FACTORS: Prolonged hospitalization and ICU stay, use of broad-spectrum antibiotics, prolonged indwelling of catheters (especially central venous catheters), acute and chronic renal failure, surgery requiring general anesthesia, cancer (e.g., solid neoplasms), transplantation (bone marrow or solid organ), recent chemotherapy/radiation therapy, use of immunosuppressive drugs, parenteral alimentation, use of internal prosthetic devices

PHYSICAL FINDINGS & CLINICAL PRESENTATION

1. History
   - Fever unresponsive to broad-spectrum antibiotics
   - History of prolonged indwelling IV catheter
   - A personal history of any of the risk factors listed earlier
2. Physical findings (general)
   - Fever
   - Hypotension
   - Generalized malaise
   - Tachycardia
   - Change in mental status
3. Specific diseases
   - Candidemia
     - *Candida* species are isolated from at least one blood culture.
     - Most common form of invasive candidiasis
     - Physical exam may include fever, macronodular skin lesions, septic shock, *Candida* endophthalmitis.
   - Disseminated candidiasis
     - Seen in patients with neutropenia
     - Associated with multiple deep-organ infections or failure
     - Blood culture negative
     - Fever not responding to broad-spectrum antibiotics
     - Physical exam: discrete erythematous or palpable rash, sepsis/septic shock

- Endophthalmitis
  - Iatrogenic/accidental fungal infection of the eye (exogenous) or hematogenous seeding of the eye (endogenous)
  - Starts as choroidal lesion, progresses to vitreitis and endophthalmitis and eventually blindness
  - Physical exam shows fever. Funduscopic examination shows large and off-white cottonball-like lesions with indistinct borders.
- *Candida* infection of the CNS
  - Exogenous and endogenous forms
  - Commonly found in long-term ICU patient
  - May present as meningitis, mycotic aneurysms, change in mental status
  - Physical examination reveals fever, neck rigidity, confusion, and coma.
- Candidal musculoskeletal infections
  - Previously uncommon; now relatively common probably due to increased frequency of candidemia and disseminated candidiasis
  - Knee and vertebral column (especially lumbosacral vertebral disks and vertebral bodies) are involved.
  - Physical exam is usually unremarkable but may show tenderness over involved area, fever, erythema, bone deformity, weight loss, and sometimes a draining fistulous tract.
- Candidal infections of the heart
  - May present as infective endocarditis, myocarditis, or pericarditis.
  - Physical examination reveals fever, hypotension, tachycardia, new or changing murmur.
- Hepatosplenic candidiasis (chronic systemic candidiasis)
  - Seen in patients with hematologic malignancy and neutropenia; usually develops during recovery from a neutropenic state (normally after undergoing myeloablative chemotherapy)
  - On examination, patients have low-grade fever, right upper quadrant pain, palpable/tender liver, splenomegaly, and rarely jaundice.
- *Candida* peritonitis
  - Associated with GI surgery, peritoneal dialysis
  - Clinical manifestations include fever, chills, abdominal pain; nausea, vomiting, constipation.
  - Physical examination reveals abdominal distention, abdominal pain, absent bowel sounds.
- Other forms of invasive candidiasis
  - *Candida* splenic abscess
  - *Candida* cholecystitis
  - Renal candidiasis

ETIOLOGY

- Several species of *Candida* exist in nature
- Medically significant include:
  - *C. albicans:* together with *C. glabrata*, they account for 70% to 80% of *Candida* in invasive candidiasis.
  - *C. glabrata:* together with *C. albicans*, they account for 70% to 80% of *Candida* in invasive candidiasis.
  - *C. parapsilosis:* associated with indwelling vascular catheters and prosthetic devices
  - *C. tropicalis:* especially in leukemic patients
  - *C. krusei:* resistant to fluconazole and ketoconazole

Dx DIAGNOSIS

DIFFERENTIAL DIAGNOSIS

- Sepsis (bacterial)
- Septic shock
- Cryptococcosis
- Aspergillosis

WORKUP
LABORATORY TESTS
- Laboratory studies are nonspecific.
- High index of suspicion is needed.
- Candidemia/disseminated candidiasis
  - Blood cultures: helpful but low positive yield
  - Serum (1,3) beta-D-glucan detection assay: high specificity and high positive predictive value
- Hepatosplenic candidiasis (focal)
  - Elevated serum alkaline phosphatase

IMAGING STUDIES
- Imaging studies are generally not required or useful.
- Ultrasound is useful for diagnosing hepatosplenic abscess. "Bull's eye or target lesions" are observed in the liver and spleen.
- CT scanning may be used to diagnose hepatosplenic candidiasis, as well as intraabdominal/renal abscesses.
- ECHO is useful to rule in or rule out *Candida* endocarditis.

Rx TREATMENT

- To successfully treat invasive *Candida* infection, it is important to start antifungal medication as early as possible.
- Antifungals available include:
  - Azoles (e.g., fluconazole, posaconazole, itraconazole, voriconazole). They inhibit the synthesis of ergosterol, a fungal cell component.
  - Echinocandins (e.g., caspofungin, micafungin, anidulafungin). These are glucan synthesis inhibitors. Glucan is an important component of fungal cell walls.
  - Polyenes (e.g., amphotericin B, lipid formulation of amphotericin, nystatin). Broad spectrum. Their mechanism of

action is to increase cytoplasmic permeability.

○ Antimetabolites (e.g., flucytosine). Flucytosine is deaminated to 5-fluorouracil in fungal cell. 5-Fluorouracil inhibits RNA and protein synthesis.

TREATMENT PLANS

CANDIDEMIA

- Treatment depends on whether the patient is neutropenic or not.
  ○ Nonneutropenic adult patients: drug of choice is fluconazole; 800 mg as loading dose then 400 mg/day for at least 2 wk after clinical improvement or negative blood culture. Amphotericin B is equally efficacious.
  ○ Neutropenic adult patients: an echinocandin is the drug of choice (e.g., caspofungin 70 mg IV loading dose then 50 mg/day IV or micafungin 100 mg/day IV or anidulafungin 200 mg IV loading dose then 100 mg IV all for at least 2 wk after clear blood culture and after clinical improvement.

DISSEMINATED CANDIDIASIS
Fluconazole is the drug of choice.

DISSEMINATED CANDIDIASIS WITH END-ORGAN INFECTION

- Treatment is the same as for candidemia of nonneutropenic patients. In most cases, therapy is prolonged for at least 4 to 6 wk.
- The echinocandins are the first-line therapy.

OSTEOMYELITIS OR SEPTIC ARTHRITIS

- Fluconazole 400 mg IV or PO *or*
- Lipid-based amphotericin B 3-5 mg/kg qd

ENDOCARDITIS

- Caspofungin 50-150 mg/day or
- Micafungin 100-150 mg/day or
- Anidulafungin 100-200 mg/day

MYOCARDITIS

- Lipid-based amphotericin B 3-5 mg/kg daily *or*
- Fluconazole 400-800 mg daily IV or PO

ESOPHAGITIS

- Fluconazole 200-400 mg/day or
- Caspofungin 50 mg IV daily

PERICARDITIS

- Lipid-based amphotericin B 3-5 mg/kg daily *or*
- Fluconazole 400-800 mg PO qd IV or PO

SURGICAL CARE

Include:

- Drainage
- Removal of any foreign bodies
- Surgical debridement
- Organ-specific care (e.g., valve replacement for endocarditis, splenectomy for splenic abscess, or vitrectomy for fungal endophthalmitis)

DISPOSITION

- Several factors affect prognosis: infection site, degree of immune suppression, and how quickly diagnosis and therapy is initiated
- Overall mortality rate: 30% to 40%

REFERRAL

- Always involve an infectious disease specialist.
- Referral to specialist will depend on the organ involved. For example:
  ○ Endocarditis will require a cardiothoracic surgeon.
  ○ Endophthalmitis will require an ophthalmologist.

FOLLOW-UP CARE

- Prolonged periods, mainly in the hospital, of antifungal treatment may be necessary.
- Closely monitor patients on amphotericin B because of the high incidence of side effects. Check basic metabolic panel, magnesium, and CBC at least twice a week.

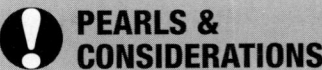

PEARLS & CONSIDERATIONS

PREVENTION

Basic preventative measures are similar to those used for nosocomial infections. This includes:

- Maximizing hand hygiene recommendations:
  ○ Hand washing
  ○ Using alcohol/chlorhexidine solution
- Adhering strictly to recommendations for placement and care of central lines and catheters.
- Judicious use of antimicrobials

PROPHYLAXIS

Antifungal prophylaxis recommended for:

- Solid organ transplant recipients
- Stem cell transplant recipients

PATIENT/FAMILY EDUCATION

- Inform them about the risk factors for invasive candidiasis.
- Inform them of the seriousness of the disease and the associated high morbidity/mortality rates, thus requiring aggressive treatment.
- Side effects and toxicities associated with treatment

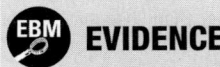 **EVIDENCE**

available at www.expertconsult.com

SUGGESTED READINGS

available at www.expertconsult.com

RELATED CONTENT

Candidiasis (Patient Information)

AUTHOR: **DANIEL K. ASIEDU, M.D., PH.D., F.A.C.P**

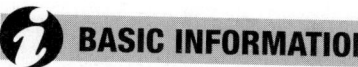 BASIC INFORMATION

DEFINITION

Carbon monoxide (CO) is a colorless, odorless, tasteless, nonirritating gas. When inhaled it produces toxicity by causing cellular hypoxia and damage.

ICD-9CM CODES
986 Carbon monoxide poisoning

EPIDEMIOLOGY & DEMOGRAPHICS

- A leading cause of accidental and intentional poisoning in the U.S.
- CO poisoning is seen more frequently during the fall and winter months in cold climates. Frequently seen after storm-related power outages, mostly due to the use of portable gasoline-powered electrical generators.
- In adults, 20% of CO poisonings occur in occupational settings.

PHYSICAL FINDINGS & CLINICAL PRESENTATION

- Depends on the severity and duration of exposure. The brain and heart are most sensitive to CO poisoning.
- Presentation is often nonspecific and may be mistaken for a flulike illness.
- Severity of poisoning does not correlate with carboxyhemoglobin (COHgb) levels.
- Mild to moderate poisoning may present with headache, malaise, dizziness, nausea, dyspnea, difficulty concentrating, confusion, and blurred vision. Patients may have tachypnea and tachycardia.
- Severe poisoning may present with hypotension, arrhythmias, myocardial ischemia, pulmonary edema, lethargy, ataxia, loss of consciousness, seizure, coma, or rarely, cherry-red skin.
- Delayed neurologic sequelae may develop days to weeks after apparent recovery from acute poisoning. Patients may present with neurologic or psychiatric symptoms (cognitive deficits, memory loss, personality changes, movement disorders, Parkinson's, psychosis, neurologic deficits).

ETIOLOGY

- CO results from the incomplete combustion of carbon-containing compounds. CO poisoning occurs from inhaling smoke from fires, motor vehicle exhaust, or the burning of fuel (oil, wood, coal, natural gas) in poorly functioning or improperly ventilated devices (heating systems, stoves/grills, portable generators, etc.). Methylene chloride (paint stripper) fumes are converted to CO by the liver.
- CO toxicity results from tissue hypoxia and direct CO-mediated damage at the cellular level. This may explain why COHgb levels alone are not predictive of clinical toxicity. The mechanisms of CO toxicity are not completely understood.
- CO impairs oxygen delivery. CO binds hemoglobin with an affinity 250 times greater than oxygen, displacing oxygen from hemoglobin and decreasing the oxygen-carrying capacity of blood. By binding to hemoglobin, CO changes the structure of the hemoglobin molecule and decreases oxygen release to tissue.
- CO also interferes with peripheral oxygen utilization. It binds to other heme-containing proteins including cytochromes and myoglobin. Cellular respiration is depressed by inhibition of the mitochondrial cytochrome oxidase system. By binding to myoglobin, CO decreases its ability to use and store oxygen.
- Neurologic toxicity is not explained by hypoxia alone and is related to the complex intracellular actions of CO. CO precipitates an inflammatory cascade that results in oxidative damage and brain lipid peroxidation.

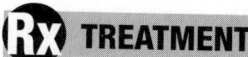 DIAGNOSIS

DIFFERENTIAL DIAGNOSIS

- Viral syndromes
- Cyanide, hydrogen sulfide
- Methemoglobinemia
- Amphetamines and derivatives
- Cocaine, phencyclidine (PCP)
- Cyclic antidepressants
- Phenothiazines
- Theophylline

WORKUP

History (duration and source of CO exposure, loss of consciousness), physical examination (detailed neurologic examination), laboratory and imaging tests

LABORATORY TESTS

- COHgb level (measured by co-oximetry on arterial blood; venous blood may be used to screen large populations exposed to CO: COHgb level >3% in nonsmokers confirms exposure. Table 1-79 describes the half-life of COHgb. Heavy smokers may have baseline levels of up to 10%. Levels may be low if the patient has already received supplemental oxygen or if delay occurs between exposure and testing.
- Direct measurement of arterial oxyhemoglobin (by co-oximetry): Pulse oximetry and arterial blood gas (ABG) may be falsely normal because neither measures oxygen saturation of hemoglobin directly. Pulse oximetry is inaccurate because of the similar absorption characteristics of oxyhemoglobin and COHgb. An ABG is inaccurate because it measures oxygen dissolved in plasma (which is not affected by CO) and then calculates oxygen saturation of hemoglobin.
- Electrolytes, glucose, BUN, creatinine, cardiac biomarkers, ABG (lactic acidosis and rhabdomyolysis may develop), CBC (polycythemia from hypoxia in chronic CO poisoning).
- ECG (ischemia, arrhythmia).
- Pregnancy test (fetus at high risk).
- Consider toxicology screen.

IMAGING STUDIES

- Chest x-ray (noncardiogenic edema)
- Brain CT, MRI if neurologic abnormalities are present

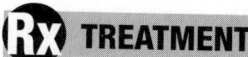 TREATMENT

ACUTE GENERAL Rx

- Remove from site of CO exposure.
- Ensure adequate airway.
- Continuous ECG monitor.
- Fetal monitoring if pregnant.
- 100% oxygen by nonrebreather mask or endotracheal tube (decreases half-life of COHgb from 4 to 6 hr to 60 to 90 min) until COHgb level is <10% and patient is asymptomatic. Fig. 1-178 illustrates the effects of oxygen on the dissociation of CO from carboxyhemoglobin.
- Hyperbaric oxygen (2.5 to 3 atm).
  - Questionable beneficial effect over normobaric oxygen. Disparate findings in various studies: some suggest hyperbaric oxygen treatment reduces the incidence of neurologic sequelae, and others have found it worsens neurologic outcomes compared to normobaric oxygen treatment.
  - Decreases half-life of COHgb to 20 to 30 min; increases amount of oxygen dissolved in plasma. It also reduces CO binding to other heme-containing proteins.
  - Consider for individuals with:
    1. Severe intoxication (COHgb >25%, history of loss of consciousness, neurologic symptoms or signs, cardiovascular compromise, severe metabolic acidosis)
    2. Pregnant women with COHgb >20% or signs of fetal distress. CO elimination is slower in fetus than mother, fetal Hgb has greater affinity for CO than adult Hgb
  - Should be instituted quickly if deemed necessary
- Consider concomitant poisoning with other toxic/irritant gases that may be present in smoke (e.g., cyanide) or thermal injury to airway. Toxic effects of CO and cyanide are synergistic.
- Identify source of exposure and determine if poisoning was accidental.

DISPOSITION

- Patients with mild accidental poisoning can be treated in an ambulatory setting. Those with moderate/severe poisoning or coexisting illness require hospitalization.
- Survivors of severe poisoning are at 14% to 40% risk for neurologic sequelae.
  - Deficits are usually apparent within 3 wk of poisoning but may present months later.

TABLE 1-79   Half-Life of COHb

Oxygen Concentration	Half-Life
21% (room air)	4-5 hr
100% (mask or endotracheal)	60-90 min
100% (hyperbaric molecular oxygen)	20-30 min

From Fuhrman BP et al: *Pediatric critical care*, ed 4, Philadelphia, 2011, Saunders.

- ○ Risk of developing sequelae is greater if patient lost consciousness during acute poisoning and with older age.
- ○ Brain MRI may reveal changes; damage is seen most often in the globus pallidus and deep white matter
- ○ Recovery may occur over months to years.
- CO-mediated cardiac damage is associated with increased long-term mortality rate.
- High risk of fetal demise.

REFERRAL

- American Association of Poison Control Centers: 1-800-222-1222

- Hyperbaric unit; accredited facilities are listed on the Undersea & Hyperbaric Medical Society website (www.uhms.org)
- Psychiatric evaluation if intentional poisoning

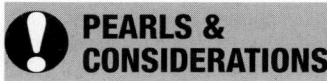

PEARLS & CONSIDERATIONS

- Severity of poisoning and prognosis do not correlate with COHgb levels.
- Neuropsychometric testing is an objective measure of cognitive function but is not universally used.

- Imaging techniques and biomarkers to allow for early prediction of CNS damage are being studied but are not ready for application.
- Pulse oximeter measurement of CO saturation has limited clinical use.
- Contact local Fire Department to assess environment and identify source of CO.

SUGGESTED READINGS

available at www.expertconsult.com

RELATED CONTENT

Carbon Monoxide Poisoning (Patient Information)

AUTHOR: **SUDEEP KAUR AULAKH, M.D.**

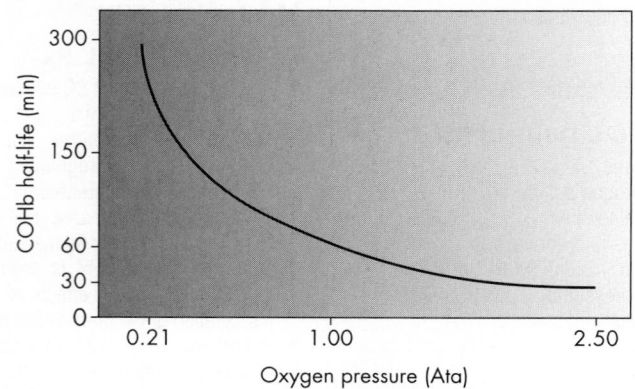

FIGURE 1-178 The effects of oxygen on the dissociation of CO from carboxyhemoglobin (COHb). Oxygen breathing at 1.0 atm decreases the half-life of COHb to 60 min from approximately 300 min, allowing most of the COHb to be removed from the body within 90 min. (From Auerbach P: *Wilderness medicine*, ed 4, St Louis, 2001, Mosby.)

BASIC INFORMATION

DEFINITION

Carcinoid syndrome is a symptom complex characterized by paroxysmal vasomotor disturbances, diarrhea, and bronchospasm. It is caused by the action of amines and peptides (serotonin, bradykinin, histamine) produced by tumors arising from neuroendocrine cells.

SYNONYMS

Flush syndrome
Argentaffinoma syndrome

ICD-9CM CODES
259.2 Carcinoid syndrome

EPIDEMIOLOGY & DEMOGRAPHICS

INCIDENCE:
- Carcinoid tumors are found incidentally in 0.5% to 0.75% of autopsies.
- Carcinoid tumors are principally found in the following organs: appendix (40%); small bowel (20%; 15% in the ileum); rectum (15%); bronchi (12%); esophagus, stomach, and colon (10%); and ovary, biliary tract, and pancreas (3%).
- The incidence of carcinoids is 2.47 to 4.48/100,000, depending on race and sex, and is highest in black men. The overall incidence has increased over the last 30 years due in part to improved diagnostic modalities.
- Carcinoid tumors can be classified as typical or atypical. Atypical carcinoids tend to be more aggressive (higher rate of metastases) and have a worse prognosis than typical carcinoids.

PHYSICAL FINDINGS & CLINICAL PRESENTATION

- Cutaneous flushing (75% to 90%)
  1. The patient usually has red-purple flushes starting in the face, then spreading to the neck and upper trunk.
  2. The flushing episodes last from a few minutes to hours (longer lasting flushes may be associated with bronchial carcinoids).
  3. Flushing may be triggered by emotion, alcohol, or foods or may occur spontaneously.
  4. Dizziness, tachycardia, and hypotension may be associated with the cutaneous flushing.
- Diarrhea (>70%): often associated with abdominal bloating and audible peristaltic rushes
- Intermittent bronchospasm (25%): characterized by severe dyspnea and wheezing
- Facial telangiectasia
- Tricuspid insufficiency, pulmonic stenosis from carcinoid heart lesions

ETIOLOGY

- Carcinoid syndrome is caused by neoplasms originating from neuroendocrine cells.

- Carcinoid tumors do not usually produce the syndrome unless liver metastases are present or the primary tumor does not involve the gastrointestinal tract.

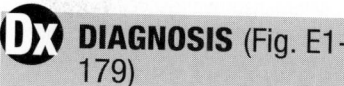 **DIAGNOSIS** (Fig. E1-179)

DIFFERENTIAL DIAGNOSIS

- Flushing: Carcinoid syndrome must be distinguished from idiopathic flushing (IF); patients with IF more often are female, are younger, and have a longer duration of symptoms; palpitations, syncope, and hypotension occur primarily in patients with IF. Additional causes of flushing that need to be ruled out are menopause, medications (niacin, nitrates), alcohol, renal cell carcinoma, medullary cancer of thyroid, VIPoma, mastocytosis, and chronic use of food additives (nitrites, sulfites)
- Diarrhea: IBD, IBS, laxative abuse, infectious colitis
- Bronchospasm: asthma, foreign body, GERD, lung neoplasm

LABORATORY TESTS

- The biochemical marker for carcinoid syndrome is increased 24-hr urinary 5-hydroxyindoleacetic acid, a metabolite of serotonin (5-hydroxytryptamine).
- False elevations can be seen with ingestion of certain foods (bananas, pineapples, eggplant, avocados, walnuts) and certain medications (acetaminophen, caffeine, guaifenesin, reserpine); therefore patients should be on a restricted diet and avoid these medications when the test is ordered.
- Falsely low results can occur with use of alcohol, aspirin, MAO inhibitors, and St. John's wort.
- Liver function studies are an unreliable indicator of liver involvement.

IMAGING STUDIES

- CT scan of chest is useful to detect bronchial carcinoids.
- CT scan of abdomen or a liver and spleen radionuclide scan is useful to detect liver metastases (palpable in >50% of cases).
- Iodine-123–labeled somatostatin can detect carcinoid endocrine tumors with somatostatin receptors.
- Scanning with radiolabeled octreotide (Fig. E1-180) can visualize previously undetected or metastatic lesions.

Rx **TREATMENT**

NONPHARMACOLOGIC THERAPY

Avoidance of ethanol ingestion (may precipitate flushing)

GENERAL Rx

- Surgical resection of the tumor can be curative if the tumor is localized or palliative and results in prolonged asymptomatic periods if metastases are present. Surgical manipulation of the tumor can, however, cause severe vasomotor abnormalities and bronchospasm (carcinoid crisis).
- Percutaneous embolization and ligation of the hepatic artery can decrease the bulk of the tumor in the liver and provide palliative treatment of tumors with hepatic metastases.
- Cytotoxic chemotherapy: combination chemotherapy with 5-fluorouracil and streptozocin can be used in patients with unresectable or recurrent carcinoid tumors; however, it has only limited success.
- Control of clinical manifestations:
  1. Somatostatin analogues (octreotide and lanreotide) are effective for both flushing and diarrhea in most patients. Interferon alfa may be useful as an additive therapy for persistent symptoms despite use of somatostatin analogues; however, data remain inconclusive.
  2. Flushing may be controlled by the combination of H_1- and H_2-receptor antagonists (e.g., diphenhydramine 25 to 50 mg PO q6h and ranitidine 150 mg bid).
  3. Diarrhea may respond to diphenoxylate with atropine (Lomotil).
  4. Bronchospasm can be treated with aminophylline and/or albuterol.
- Nutritional support: supplemental niacin therapy may be useful to prevent pellagra because the tumor uses dietary tryptophan for serotonin synthesis, resulting in a nutritional deficiency in some patients.
- Interferon alfa may be useful as an additive to control symptoms unresponsive to somatostatin analogues.
- Echocardiography and monitoring for right-sided congestive heart failure are recommended for patients with unresectable disease because endocardial fibrosis, involving predominantly the endocardium, chordae, and valves of the right side of the heart, can occur.

DISPOSITION

Carcinoids of the appendix and rectum have a low malignancy potential and rarely produce the clinical syndrome; metastases are also uncommon if the size of the primary lesion is <2 cm in diameter.

RELATED CONTENT

Carcinoid Syndrome (Patient Information)

AUTHOR: **FRED F. FERRI, M.D.**

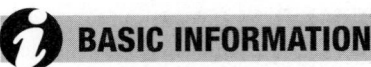

BASIC INFORMATION

DEFINITION

Cardiac tamponade is a life-threatening condition where an accumulation of fluid within the pericardial sac impairs filling of the ventricles during diastole and causes a decline in cardiac output.

ICD-9CM CODES
423.9 Unspecified diseases of the pericardium

PHYSICAL FINDINGS & CLINICAL PRESENTATION

- Chest pain
- Tachypnea/dyspnea
- Beck's triad
  1. Absolute or relative hypotension
  2. Elevated jugular venous pressure (with prominent *x* descent and blunted *y* descent)
  3. Muffled heart sounds
- Tachycardia (except in uremia or hypothyroid patients)
- Pulsus paradoxus (decrease in systolic arterial pressure of 10 mm Hg or more during normal inspiration while in normal sinus rhythm)
- Pericardial friction rub may be present
- Reduced or absent apical cardiac impulse

ETIOLOGY

Acute (rapidly accumulating pericardial effusion leading to cardiac tamponade): does not need a large amount of effusion to cause tamponade
- Penetrating trauma
- Aortic dissection
- Post-infarction myocardial rupture and/or hemorrhagic pericarditis
- Iatrogenic (central line and pacemaker insertions, post–coronary bypass surgery or post–percutaneous coronary intervention)
Subacute or chronic (effusion is usually large):
- Malignancy (e.g., lung, breast, lymphoma)
- Viral pericarditis (e.g., Coxsackie, human immunodeficiency virus)
- Bacterial, fungal, or tuberculous pericarditis
- Uremia
- Hypothyroidism/myxedema (rare)
- Collagen vascular disease (e.g., lupus, rheumatoid arthritis, scleroderma)
- Radiation
- Idiopathic

DIAGNOSIS

Cardiac tamponade is a clinical diagnosis made at the bedside from history and physical examination. The echocardiogram will help confirm or reject the clinical diagnosis. Tamponade can be confirmed invasively by the measurement of elevated intrapericardial pressures with an intrapericardial catheter and right-sided heart catheterization. Typical findings are diastolic equalization of pressures, usually ranging from 15 to 30 mm Hg (diastolic pulmonary artery pressure = right ventricular diastolic pressure = right atrial pressure = intrapericardial pressure) and lowering of the intrapericardial pressure with fluid drainage. Thereafter, the underlying etiology must be determined with specific laboratory work (see "Laboratory Tests" below).

DIFFERENTIAL DIAGNOSIS

Other conditions that can also lead to elevated jugular venous pressure, decreased systemic pressure, and pulsus paradoxus include:
- Chronic obstructive pulmonary disease
- Constrictive pericarditis
- Restrictive cardiomyopathy
- Right ventricular infarction
- Pulmonary embolism
- Chronic biventricular heart failure

LABORATORY TESTS

- Electrolytes, blood urea nitrogen, creatinine, erythrocyte sedimentation rate, thyroid function tests, antinuclear antibody, rheumatoid factor, PPD, blood cultures, viral titers, and pericardial fluid analysis and cultures
- Possible 12-lead ECG findings:
  - Sinus tachycardia
  - PR depression and/or diffuse ST elevations if acute pericarditis is present
  - Electrical alternans (beat to beat alternations in the QRS complex)
  - Low voltage if massive effusion is present. (QRS complex <0.5 mV in the limb leads and <1.0 mV in precordial leads)

IMAGING STUDIES

- Chest radiograph (enlarged cardiac silhouette with clear lung fields) (Fig. 1-181)
- Chest CT (may overestimate size of the effusion) (Fig. 1-182)
- Echocardiogram finding:
  - Pericardial effusion
  - Diastolic collapse of the right atrium (late diastole)
  - Right ventricle (early diastole)
  - Mitral and tricuspid valve inflow variation with respiration
  - Plethoric inferior vena cava
  - Left atrial collapse (high specificity)
- Cardiac catheterization as discussed earlier will see equalization of intracardiac diastolic pressures and increase of right-sided pressures and reduction of left-sided pressures, which subsequently causes pulsus paradoxus

TREATMENT

NONPHARMACOLOGIC THERAPY

- Cardiac tamponade should be treated emergently.
- Avoid drugs that reduce preload (e.g., nitrates, diuretics).
- Large pericardial effusions without hemodynamic compromise (tamponade) can be managed conservatively with careful monitoring, treatment of the underlying cause, clinical follow-up, and frequent serial surveillance echocardiography.

ACUTE GENERAL Rx

- Aggressive intravascular volume expansion (saline or blood)
- Emergency pericardial fluid removal by pericardiocentesis or surgical pericardiotomy by way of the subxiphoid pericardial window
- Pericardiocentesis should be performed under fluoroscopic or echocardiographic guidance when available
- Inotropic or vasopressor support if above measures cannot be performed immediately

CHRONIC Rx

- Depends on etiology.
- Pericardiocentesis with draining catheter: the catheter can be left inside the pericardium to allow continued drainage for 24 to 48 hr. If residual fluid still persists with hemodynamic compromise, surgical drainage should be

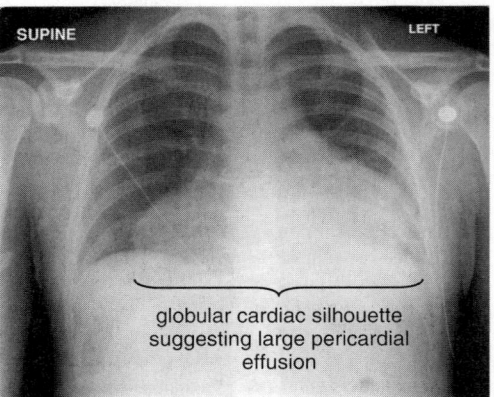

globular cardiac silhouette suggesting large pericardial effusion

FIGURE 1-181 Massive pericardial effusion and tamponade. This 23-year-old male has a history of aortic valve replacement for infective endocarditis. He presented with increased chest pain and dyspnea. His chest x-ray shows a globular cardiac silhouette, suggesting a large pericardial effusion. The lung fields and right costophrenic angle appear clear, although the left costophrenic angle is hidden behind the heart and cannot be assessed. The patient underwent chest computed tomography to evaluate his aorta, as he complained of severe interscapular pain as well (see Fig. 1-182). (From Broder JS: *Diagnostic imaging for the emergency physician,* Philadelphia, 2011, Saunders.)

sought. In the absence of hemodynamic compromise or significant residual fluid, discontinuation of the draining catheter can be done with periodic postprocedure echocardiographic monitoring of reaccumulation (e.g., 24 hr, 7 days, 30 days, 3 mo, 6 mo, 12 mo) depending on the etiology and rate of reaccumulation.

- Other surgical drainage procedures include:
  1. Subxiphoid pericardiotomy drainage
  2. Limited pericardiectomy draining the pericardial fluid into the left hemithorax
  3. Pericardial window
  4. Complete pericardiectomy, especially in patients with effusive-constrictive pericarditis or bacterial pericarditis (see "Pearls & Considerations" below).

DISPOSITION

The prognosis of cardiac tamponade depends on the underlying cause.

REFERRAL

- Emergent cardiology consultation should be made if cardiac tamponade is suspected.
- Cardiothoracic surgery consultation should also be considered if surgical pericardial drainage is indicated.

PEARLS & CONSIDERATIONS

- Cardiac tamponade should always be considered during pulseless electrical activity arrest and may require emergent pericardiocentesis.
- Evaluation for pulsus paradoxus should always be performed during normal respiration because deep inspiration may render a false positive finding.
- Strong consideration should be given to performing early pericardiocentesis in patients who have pericardial effusion associated with bacterial pneumonia or empyema because the incidence of bacterial pericarditis is especially high in this clinical situation and the subsequent development of cardiac tamponade and severe chronic constrictive pericarditis occurs frequently.

COMMENTS

As little as 100 ml of fluid can lead to acute cardiac tamponade, whereas with gradual accumulation, the pericardial sac can hold up to 5 L of fluid before tamponade occurs.

SUGGESTED READINGS
available at www.expertconsult.com

RELATED CONTENT

Cardiac Tamponade (Patient Information)

AUTHORS: **ARAVIND RAO KOKKIRALA, M.D., SCOTT COHEN, M.D., GAURAV CHOUDHARY, M.D.,** and **ROBERTO PACHECO, M.D.**

C

Diseases and Disorders

I

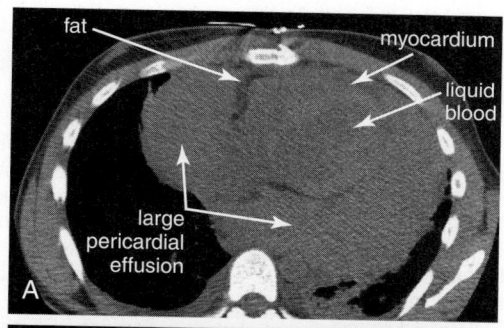
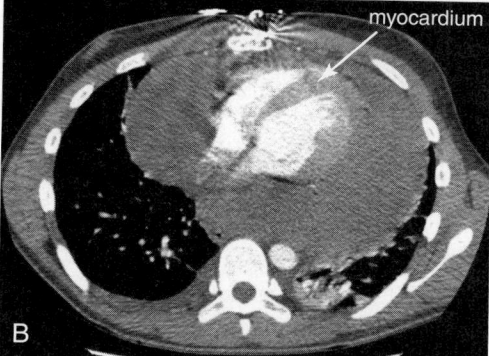

FIGURE 1-182 Massive pericardial effusion. Same patient as Fig. 1-181. The patient underwent chest computed tomography (CT) without **(A)** and then with **(B)** intravenous contrast to evaluate his aorta, which was normal. However, the CT confirmed a massive pericardial effusion surrounding a normal-appearing heart. Without contrast, note that fluid blood within the chambers of the heart has a slightly lower density than the pericardial effusion, which has a density more similar to that of myocardium. When contrast is administered, the ventricular chambers fill completely, and the myocardium enhances and becomes somewhat brighter than the surrounding pericardial effusion. The heart itself is outlined by a thin stripe of fat, which appears nearly black on soft tissue windows. The patient developed hypotension, suggesting cardiac tamponade, and pericardial window was performed for drainage of the effusion. In the operating room, the effusion was found to be coagulated blood. (From Broder JS: *Diagnostic imaging for the emergency physician,* Philadelphia, 2011, Saunders.)

DEFINITION

Cardiomyopathy, chemical-induced (CMc) is the changes of cardiac structure and function caused by chemical compounds, either medically prescribed or not medically prescribed. The common chemicals available in the U.S. include alcohol, cocaine, amphetamine, doxorubicin, 5-fluorouracil (5-FU), zidovudine, and trastuzumab.

SYNONYMS

Alcoholic cardiomyopathy (ACM)
Cocaine-induced CM
Anabolic steroid–induced CM
Anthracycline-induced CM

ICD-10CM CODES
I42.7 Cardiomyopathy due to drug and external agent

EPIDEMIOLOGY & DEMOGRAPHICS

- ACM occurs in about 10% of alcoholics. The prevalence ranges from 23% to 40% of nonischemic cardiomyopathy.
- One study revealed that two thirds of elite U.S. power-lifters admitted to using anabolic steroids to enhance performance.
- In one study of doxorubicin-based chemotherapy, acute cardiotoxicity, including heart failure and arrhythmia, occurred in 3.2% of patients with lymphoma. The incidence was 0.14% at doses less than 400 mg/m^2, 7% at 550 mg/m^2, and as great as 18% at 700 mg/m^2.
- The incidence of 5-FU cardiotoxicity is 1% to 19% in the serial literature.

PREDOMINANT SEX AND AGE: Among ACM cases, men represent more than 80% and have higher mortality. In all races, blacks have higher death rates compared to whites.

GENETICS

- In patients with ACM, deletion (DD) genotype of ACE is more common than insertion (II) and deletion insertion (DI) genotypes.
- Anthracycline-induced cardiomyopathy is linked to an increase in cardiac oxidative stress, via the pathways of mitochondria, nitric oxide synthesis, and nicotinamide adenine dinucleotide phosphate reduced.
- One study suggests that polymorphisms in the carbonyl reductase genes could be related to anthracycline-induced CM.

RISK FACTORS

- The occurrence of chronic anthracycline-induced CM is correlated to cumulative dose (ranging from 7% to 26% of patients who received >550 mg/m^2), age, preexisting heart disease, concomitant chemotherapy, and history of mediastinal radiation therapy. Children are more susceptible to anthracycline-induced CM.
- Continuous infusion of 5-FU has higher risk for cardiotoxicity, compared to bolus regimen.

PHYSICAL FINDINGS & CLINICAL PRESENTATION

The majority of clinical characteristics of CMc are similar to the dilated cardiomyopathy of other etiologies. Symptoms may develop either insidiously or acute in onset.

- The acute anthracycline-induced cardiotoxicity can start at anytime after the first dose and presents with arrhythmias, most commonly supraventricular tachycardia, ventricular dysfunction, and pericardial diseases. The sub-acute and chronic symptoms occur from 3 months after the last dose to 10 years later. Patients usually present with congestive heart failure (CHF). More recently, mortality has improved as a result of medical treatment with ACE inhibitors and beta-blockers.
- Cardiac symptoms after 5-FU treatment include angina (most common), myocardial infarction, arrhythmia, acute pulmonary edema, cardiac arrest, and pericarditis. The mortality of 5-FU–induced cardiotoxicity is 2% to 13%.
- In patients with ACM, the consumption of >90 g/day of alcohol for >5 years generally leads to changes in cardiac structure and function. The presentation of CHF may occur over 15 years of heavy drinking. In the presentation of arrhythmia, atrial fibrillation is most common and ventricular tachycardia is also experienced frequently.
- Patients with cocaine CM may present with adrenergic symptoms (palpitations, pallor, diaphoresis, and anxiety), hypertension, angina, atrial and ventricular arrhythmia, and heart failure.
- Anabolic steroids can cause left ventricular hypertrophy and dilation, and can lead to heart failure, arrhythmia, myocardial infarction, hypertension, and sudden death.

ETIOLOGY

The underlying mechanism of chemotherapy is not well established. Several pathways have been proposed, including an increase in oxidative stress, free radical production, apoptosis, disturbance of DNA, RNA and protein synthesis, and vasospasm. Nutritional deficiency also plays a role in ACM.

DX DIAGNOSIS

DIFFERENTIAL DIAGNOSIS

- Ischemic cardiomyopathy
- Dilated cardiomyopathy, related to valvular disease, hypertension, and causes other than chemicals
- Cirrhotic cardiomyopathy

WORKUP

- The diagnosis is based on the history of chemical exposure and the clinical presentation of heart failure, arrhythmia, and angina pectoris.
- Electrocardiogram (ECG) and serum electrolytes, renal function, and liver function
- Serum troponin and brain natriuretic peptide (BNP) levels
- Transthoracic echocardiogram for the evaluation of heart structure and function
- Rule out the diagnosis of coronary artery disease by coronary angiography.

LABORATORY TESTS

- Serum electrolytes, renal function, liver function, thyroid-stimulating hormone, iron profile, and inflammatory factors
- Serum troponin and BNP (nonspecific)

IMAGING STUDIES

- ECG
  - ST deviation and atrial and ventricular arrhythmia in 5-FU toxicity
  - Anthracycline-induced cardiomyopathy
    - Sinus tachycardia
    - Nonspecific ST-T change
    - Decreased QRS voltage
    - Prolonged QT interval
- Echocardiogram
  - Asymptomatic alcoholics may present with mild left ventricular (LV) hypertrophy, diastolic dysfunction, LV dilation, and decrease in left ventricular ejection fraction (LVEF).
  - Equilibrium radionuclide angiography (ERNA) is highly reproducible with quantitative nature and is the best noninvasive method for monitoring LV systolic function during doxorubicin therapy.
  - Baseline LVEF performed before initiation of doxorubicin treatment of before 100 mg/m^2
  - Subsequent evaluation
    - Baseline LVEF 50% or higher
      - Second study after 250-300 mg/m^2
      - Repeat study after 400 mg/m^2 in patients with known heart disease, hypertension, radiation exposure, ECG findings, or cyclophosphamide therapy; or after 450 mg/m^2 in the absence of risk factors
      - Sequential studies before each dose
      - Doxorubicin therapy should be discontinued if there is a 10% or greater drop in absolute LVEF to a level <50%
    - Baseline LVEF ≤50%
      - Doxorubicin should not be started with baseline LVEF <30%
      - For baseline LVEF of 30% to 50%, perform study with each dose
      - Doxorubicin should be discontinued if there is a 10% or greater drop in absolute LVEF 10% and/or if final LVEF is ≤30%
- Endomyocardial biopsy: used only in research.

RX TREATMENT

NONPHARMACOLOGIC THERAPY

- The noninvasive assessment of LV function before, during, and after anthracycline-containing chemotherapy by means of echocardiograms and ERNA.
- To reduce the risk of anthracycline-induced cardiotoxicity, the lifetime cumulative dosage should be limited to 450 to 500 mg/m^2 in adults.
- Other approaches include the use of infusion other than bolus, liposome encapsulation of

doxorubicin, less cardiotoxic analogs of doxorubicin, and co-administration of dexrazoxane.

- Termination of 5-FU treatment if presenting cardiac symptoms and readministration is not recommended
- In patients with ACM, abstinence can significantly reverse LV systolic dysfunction.

ACUTE GENERAL Rx

- Treat decompensated CHF with diuresis, and vasopressors if low cardiac output.
- For angina in acute cocaine intoxication, benzodiazepines, nitrites, and calcium channel blockers are the first line of therapy. Once myocardial infarction is indicated by ECG and serum troponin, patients should be evaluated by cardiac catheterization.

CHRONIC Rx

- Nitrites, beta-blockers, and calcium channel blockers angina caused by 5-FU

- Dexrazoxane is an ethylenediaminetetraacetic acid–like chelator that acts by binding to iron, which prevents anthracycline cardiotoxicity. American Society of Clinical Oncology 2008 guideline suggests a 10:1 ratio of dexrazoxane to anthracycline, administered 15 to 30 minutes prior to doxorubicin administration. However, the routine use of the drug is not recommended except in the case of a cumulative dose of doxorubicin of 300 mg/m^2 or greater.
- Beta-blocker: In one study, carvedilol preserves LV diastolic function and chamber size after doxorubicin treatment, compared to placebo.
- ACE inhibitor: Enalapril and ramipril can improve myocardial contractility after doxorubicin or epirubicin treatment.
- Thiamine, folic acid, and multivitamins are adjunctive treatment of ACM.

DISPOSITION

Prognosis depends on the dosage of chemicals and the severity of LV dysfunction.

REFERRAL

Closely follow up with cardiologist.

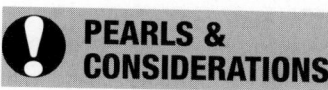

PEARLS & CONSIDERATIONS

Routine follow up is not recommended. Acute cardiotoxicity of chemotherapy is uncommon and not life-threatening. The presentation of chronic toxicity ranges from asymptomatic decline in LVEF to heart failure. The incidence is dose-limited.

SUGGESTED READINGS

available at www.expertconsult.com

AUTHORS: **ZHE ZHENG, M.D., PH.D.,** and **ARAVIND RAO KOKKIRALA, M.D.**

C

Diseases and Disorders

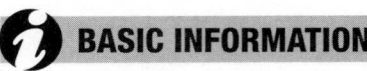

DEFINITION

Dilated cardiomyopathy describes a group of diseases involving the myocardium and characterized by myocardial dysfunction that is not wholly the result of hypertension, coronary atherosclerosis, valvular dysfunction, or congenital or other structural heart disease. As a result, the heart is enlarged and the ventricles are dilated with impaired systolic function.

SYNONYMS

Congestive cardiomyopathy

ICD-9CM CODES
425.4 Other primary cardiomyopathies
425.5 Alcoholic cardiomyopathy
425.8 Cardiomyopathy in other diseases classified elsewhere
425.9 Secondary cardiomyopathy, unspecified

EPIDEMIOLOGY & DEMOGRAPHICS

- The estimated prevalence of dilated cardiomyopathy in the general adult population is approximately 1:2500. The incidence is approximately 4 to 8 per 100,000 persons per yr.
- The incidence of dilated cardiomyopathy is greatest in middle age and among men.
- It is the most common cardiomyopathy and accounts for 25% of cases of congestive heart failure.

PHYSICAL FINDINGS & CLINICAL PRESENTATION

The patient will present the common symptoms of congestive heart failure, which may be of insidious or more sudden onset. The patient may also be asymptomatic and the diagnosis made by the unexpected finding of cardiomegaly on a chest x-ray. The history should focus also on information that could help determine the etiology. Classical signs of heart failure may be absent. When present, findings are indistinguishable from other heart failure syndromes, including:
- Increased jugular venous pressure
- Narrow pulse pressure
- Pulmonary rales, hepatomegaly, peripheral edema
- S3, S4
- Mitral regurgitation, tricuspid regurgitation (less common)

ETIOLOGY

In approximate order of occurrence:
- Idiopathic (often a viral infection that cannot be confirmed)
- Infections (viral [Coxsackie B, adenovirus, parvovirus, HIV], rickettsial, mycobacterial, toxoplasmosis, trichinosis, Chagas' disease)
- Alcoholism (15% to 40% of all cases in Western countries)
- Uncontrolled tachyarrhythmia ("tachycardia-mediated")

- Peripartum (greatest risk from last trimester of pregnancy to 6 mo postpartum)
- Chemotherapeutic (anthracycline, doxorubicin, daunorubicin) or pharmacologic agents (antiretrovirals, phenothiazines)
- Substance abuse (cocaine, heroin, organic solvents "glue-sniffer's heart")
- Postmyocarditis
- Toxins (cobalt, lead, phosphorus, carbon monoxide, mercury)
- Collagen-vascular disease (systemic lupus, rheumatoid arthritis, polyarteritis, dermatomyositis, sarcoidosis)
- Heredofamilial neuromuscular disease (e.g., muscular dystrophy)
- Excess hormones (acromegaly, osteogenesis imperfecta, myxedema, thyrotoxicosis, diabetes)
- Hematologic (e.g., sickle cell anemia, hemochromatosis)
- Stress-induced (i.e., takotsubo or broken heart syndrome)
- TTN truncating mutations (mutations in TTN, the gene encoding the sarcome protein titin) are a common cause of dilated cardiomyopathy, occurring in approximately 25% of familial cases of idopathic dilated cardiomyopathy and in 18% of sporadic cases.

Dx DIAGNOSIS

Dilated cardiomyopathy is a diagnosis of exclusion, made after ruling out other potential causes of myocardial dysfunction.

DIFFERENTIAL DIAGNOSIS

- Coronary atherosclerosis, that is, left ventricular dysfunction secondary to ischemia and/or myocardial infarction
- Valvular dysfunction (especially aortic and mitral regurgitation)
- Other cardiomyopathies (restrictive, hypertrophic)
- Pulmonary disease (embolism, obstructive, restrictive)
- Pericardial abnormalities (constrictive pericarditis, tamponade)
- Hypothyroidism/myxedema

WORKUP

- Medical history: emphasis on symptoms of dyspnea, orthopnea, paroxysmal nocturnal dyspnea, weight gain, palpitations, or signs of systemic and pulmonary embolism
- Physical exam (see "Physical Findings & Clinical Presentation")
- Testing (see "Laboratory Tests" and "Imaging Studies" for more detail): laboratory, chest x-ray, ECG, echocardiogram, cardiac catheterization; myocardial biopsy is not routinely recommended, unless acute myocarditis requiring immunosuppressive therapy is considered (e.g., giant cell myocarditis)

LABORATORY TESTS

- Chemistries/metabolites (deficiencies), renal function tests (renal dysfunction)

- Cardiac biomarkers (elevation of cardiac troponin or BNP)
  - Persistently increased cardiac troponin T levels are a marker of poor outcome in cardiomyopathy patients
- Endocrine (particularly thyroid)
- Iron studies (hemochromatosis, deficiency)
- Rheumatologic and Inflammatory (ANA, ESR, CRP)
- Others as indicated (HIV, Lyme, neurohormonal)

IMAGING STUDIES

Chest x-ray:
- Cardiac silhouette enlargement (particularly left ventricle)
- Pulmonary vascular redistribuition and congestion (Kerley B lines, cephalization of vasculature), pleural effusion (may appear as unilateral, most often on the right side)

ECG:
- ECG findings are typically nonspecific, and sinus tachycardia is usually a reflection of underlying heart failure
- Intraventricular conduction defects and left bundle branch block
- Arrhythmias (atrial fibrillation, premature ventricular or atrial contractions, ventricular tachycardia)

Echocardiogram:
- Low ejection fraction with global hypokinesis
- Four-chamber enlargement (LV enlargement usually predominates)
- Mitral or tricuspid regurgitation (due to incomplete leaflet closure caused by ventricular dilation)

Cardiac catheterization:
- On initial presentation to exclude obstructive epicardial coronary artery disease

Cardiac magnetic resonance imaging (CMRI):
- Particularly if infiltrative or inflammatory etiology suspected

Rx TREATMENT

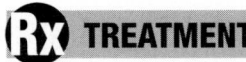

NONPHARMACOLOGIC THERAPY

- Treatment of underlying disease (systemic lupus, alcoholism)
- Dietary sodium restriction (<2 g/day).
- Exercise training has been shown to be associated with reduced risk for hospitalization and death in patients with history of heart failure in limited trials; enrollment in a formal cardiac rehabilitation program may be beneficial in improving patient's functional status

ACUTE GENERAL Rx

- Diuretics are indicated for all patients with current symptoms or history of heart failure and reduced left ventricular ejection fraction (LVEF) with evidence of volume overload (peripheral edema, orthopnea, paroxysmal nocturnal dyspnea).
- ACE inhibitors (and angiotensin receptor blockers) have been shown to have favorable effects on ventricular remodeling in patients with cardiomyopathy and a demonstrable mortality benefit in these patients. Therefore

they are recommended in all patients with reduced LV systolic function, regardless of symptoms, unless specific contraindications exist.

- Beta-blockers (in particular, carvedilol, long-acting metoprolol, and bisoprolol) work by inhibiting the adverse effects of the sympathetic nervous system in patients with ventricular systolic dysfunction, and have likewise shown a mortality benefit in patients with LV systolic dysfunction; unless specifically contraindicated, they should be started once the acute exacerbation has resolved.
- Aldosterone antagonists have shown mortality benefit along with decreased rate of hospitalization for heart failure in patients with symptomatic heart failure and reduced LV systolic function. They should be used following label guidelines and with close monitoring of renal function and potassium.
- Additional medical therapies (direct renin inhibitors, hydralazine/nitrates, digitalis) can be considered in certain patient subpopulations with persistent symptoms on otherwise optimal medical management.
- Patients with associated coronary atherosclerosis (angina, ECG changes, reversible defects on myocardial perfusion imaging)

may benefit from percutaneous or surgical revascularization.

CHRONIC Rx
- As above in "Acute General Rx."

DISPOSITION
- Annual mortality rate is 20% in patients with moderate heart failure, and it exceeds 50% in patients with severe heart failure. Once symptomatic, hospitalizations are frequent and readmission rates are high (>50% at 3 mo). A multispecialty treatment approach (e.g., primary care, cardiology, nutrition, cardiac rehabilitation) is recommended.
- Factors associated with an adverse outcome in dilated cardiomyopathy are described in Table 1-80.

REFERRAL
- Patients with dilated cardiomyopathy are at increased risk for ventricular arrhythmias and sudden cardiac death. Implantation of a cardiac defibrillator for primary prevention of sudden cardiac death can be considered for patients with LVEF <35% on optimal medical therapy regardless of symptom status.

- Patients with LVEF <35%, bundle branch block on ECG (QRS ≥0.12 sec), and persistent heart failure symptoms may benefit from cardiac resynchronization therapy via a biventricular pacemaker.
- Consider heart transplantation for relatively young patients (there is no precise age threshold) free of other significant comorbid conditions who are unresponsive to medical therapy. Dilated cardiomyopathy is the reason for 45% of all heart transplantations in the U.S.

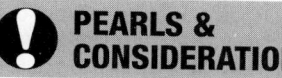 **PEARLS & CONSIDERATIONS**

COMMENTS
- Patients should be encouraged to restrict or eliminate alcohol and reduce sodium intake (<2 g daily).
- Patients may benefit from daily weight checks as a means of early detection of volume overload and decompensated heart failure.
- Vulnerability to cardiomyopathy among chronic alcohol abusers is partially genetic and related to the presence of the ACE DD genotype.
- Idiopathic dilated cardiomyopathy is often familial, and apparently healthy relatives may have latent, early, or undiagnosed disease. Echocardiographic evaluation of family members is recommended.
- Incorporation of sequencing approaches that detect TTN truncations into genetic testing for dilated cardiomyopathy may substantially increase test sensitivity and allow earlier diagnosis of dilated cardiomyopathy.

SUGGESTED READINGS
available at www.expertconsult.com

RELATED CONTENT
Fig. 3-39 Initial approach to classification of cardiomyopathy (Algorithm)
Table 3-2 Profiles of Myocardial Disease
Dilated Cardiomyopathy (Patient Information)

AUTHORS: **ATIZAZUL H. MANSOOR, M.D., DAVID J. FORTUNATO, M.D., F.A.C.C.,** and **FRED F. FERRI, M.D.**

TABLE 1-80 Factors Associated with an Adverse Outcome in Dilated Cardiomyopathy

Clinical	Noninvasive	Invasive
NYHA Class III/IV	Low LV ejection fraction	High LV filling pressures
Increasing age	Marked LV dilation	
Low exercise peak oxygen consumption	Low LV mass	
Marked intraventricular conduction delay	≥Moderate mitral regurgitation	
Complex ventricular arrhythmias	Abnormal diastolic function	
Abnormal signal-averaged ECG	Abnormal contractile reserve	
Evidence of excessive sympathetic stimulation	Right ventricular dilation or dysfunction	
Protodiastolic gallop (S₃)		
Elevated serum BNP		
Elevated uric acid		
Decreased serum sodium		

BNP, Brain natriuretic peptide; ECG, electrocardiogram; LV, left ventricular; NYHA, New York Heart Association.
From Hare JM: The dilated, restrictive, and infiltrative cardiomyopathies. In Bonow RO et al (eds): *Braunwald's heart disease—a textbook of cardiovascular medicine*, ed 9, St Louis, 2011, Saunders.

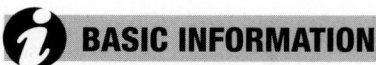

BASIC INFORMATION

DEFINITION

Hypertrophic cardiomyopathy (HCM) is a genetic myocardial disorder characterized by disorganized myocyte architecture and severe thickening (hypertrophy) of the left ventricular wall (>15 mm), without dilation, not explained by another cardiac or systemic disorder. The interventricular septum is the most common site of enlargement, though hypertrophy may involve other focal regions or may be concentric. HCM may result in hemodynamically significant obstruction within the left ventricular outflow tract (LVOT) and/or impairment of the diastolic function of the left ventricle.

SYNONYMS

HCM
Hypertrophic cardiomyopathy
Idiopathic hypertrophic subaortic stenosis (IHSS)
Hypertrophic obstructive cardiomyopathy (HOCM)
Asymmetric septal hypertrophy (ASH)

ICD-9CM CODES
425.1 Hypertrophic obstructive cardiomyopathy
425.4 Other primary cardiomyopathies
746.84 Congenital obstructive anomalies of the heart not elsewhere classified

EPIDEMIOLOGY & DEMOGRAPHICS

- Prevalence in the general population is 1 in 500 (the most common genetically transmitted cardiovascular disease).
- HCM is the most common cause of sudden cardiac death in young athletes (more commonly among blacks).
- There is equal prevalence in men and women (probably underdiagnosed in women).
- It occurs across ethnicities, perhaps underdiagnosed among blacks.
- Mortality rate is approximately 1%/yr, as high as to 2%/yr in children.
- The most common form of the disease is familial (60% to 70% of cases), and it follows an autosomal dominant inheritance pattern with variable expression.
- Spontaneous mutations can also occur, accounting for approximately 20% of cases. It is otherwise indistinguishable from the familial form.
- A variant form seen in the elderly (5% to 10% of cases) has a better prognosis, and it is not typically associated with sudden cardiac death.
- The familial form is usually diagnosed in young patients. It is most often caused by a mutation in one of the contractile protein genes of the cardiac sarcomere. >1400 mutations with variable phenotype and penetrance have been identified thus far.
- Nonsarcomeric genetic mutations that cause storage disease (e.g., Fabry disease) have a very similar clinical presentation.
- Apical HCM is a variant more common among Asians: as many as 41% of Chinese HCM and 15% of Japanese HCM patients. Clinically there is no LVOT obstruction.

PHYSICAL FINDINGS & CLINICAL PRESENTATION

Patients may have subtle symptoms of progressive congestive heart failure (CHF). At time of diagnosis, most patients are asymptomatic, referred and diagnosed based on family history. HCM may be suspected on the basis of abnormalities found on physical examination. Classic findings include:

- Harsh, systolic, crescendo–decrescendo murmur at the left sternal border or apex. The murmur increases with maneuvers that decrease venous return or LV size (Valsalva, standing), and decreases with those that increase venous return or afterload (squatting, hand grip, post-Valsalva release).
- Paradoxic splitting of S2 (if left ventricular obstruction is present).
- S4 may be present.
- Double or triple LV apical impulse ("triple ripple": atrial contraction, early rapid ejection, and late slow ejection).
- Pulsus bisferens (double pulsation on palpation of the carotid pulse).

Increased obstruction can occur with:

- Drugs: digitalis, β-adrenergic stimulators (isoproterenol, dopamine, epinephrine), nitroglycerin, vasodilators, diuretics, alcohol
- Hypovolemia
- Tachycardia
- Valsalva maneuver
- Standing position

Decreased obstruction is seen with:

- Drugs: β-adrenergic blockers, calcium channel blockers, disopyramide, α-adrenergic stimulators
- Volume expansion
- Bradycardia
- Hand-grip exercise
- Squatting position
- Release phase of the Valsalva maneuver

Clinical manifestations are as follows:

- Dyspnea
- Syncope (usually seen with exercise)
- Angina
- Palpitations

ETIOLOGY

- Genetic: Autosomal dominant trait with variable penetrance caused by mutations in multiple genes encoding proteins of the cardiac sarcomere. To date, >1400 mutations have been identified among at least 11 genes.
- Sporadic occurrence.

DIAGNOSIS

DIFFERENTIAL DIAGNOSIS

- Hypertensive heart disease
- Valvular disease, especially aortic stenosis
- Cardiac amyloidosis
- Fabry disease
- Non–sarcomeric protein mutations: gamma 2 regulatory subunit of AMP-activated protein kinase (PRKAG2) mutation
- Lysosome-associated membrane protein 2 (LAMP2) mutation: Danon disease
- Athlete's heart

WORKUP

- Medical history: focus on signs and symptoms of CHF (dyspnea, orthopnea, paroxysmal nocturnal dyspnea), palpitations, any history of syncope or presyncope, chest pain, and family history of sudden death (Fig. E1-183).
- Physical exam: see "Physical Findings & Clinical Presentation."
- Genetic counseling with or without testing.
- ECG is abnormal in 75% to 95% of patients, although there are no pathognomonic findings. Typical findings include:
  ○ LV hypertrophy (abnormally tall R waves in the precordial leads)
  ○ Abnormal Q waves in lateral and inferior leads (Fig. 1-184)
  ○ T wave inversions (associated with the apical hypertrophy predominant variant)
- Echocardiography (Fig. 1-185) is usually diagnostic as the majority of patients have significant LV hypertrophy. (See "Imaging Studies" for details.)
- 24-hour Holter monitor to screen for potentially lethal ventricular arrhythmias (principal

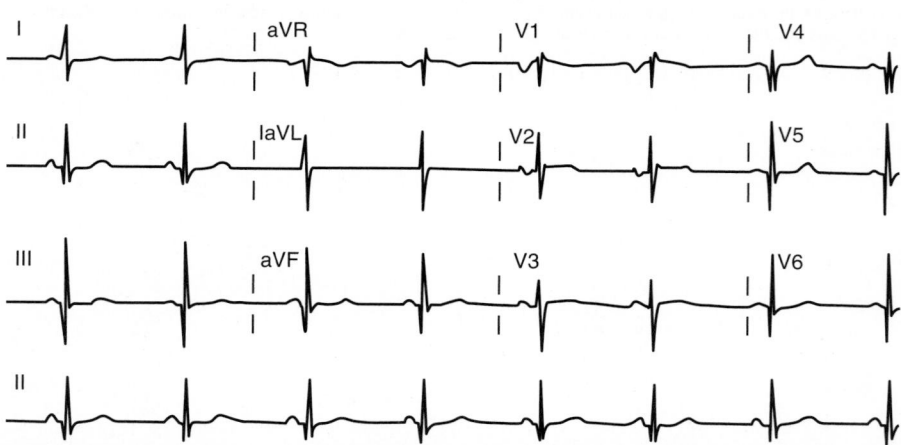

FIGURE 1-184 Surface ECG in a patient with hypertrophic cardiomyopathy. Note the deep narrow Q waves in the inferolateral leads. (From Issa Z et al: *Clinical arrhythmology and electrophysiology*, ed 2, Philadelphia, 2012, Saunders.)

cause of syncope or sudden death in obstructive cardiomyopathy) should be performed at diagnosis and annually afterward as part of routine follow-up regardless of symptoms.
- In the absence of significant LVOT obstruction, exercise testing is indicated at diagnosis and annually afterward to evaluate for symptoms and response to exercise. A drop in systolic blood pressure or failure to augment with exercise is a marker of poor prognosis and it is one of the indicators for referral for myotomy/myomectomy.
- Screening for sarcomere protein gene mutations in family members of patients with HCM can identify a broad subgroup of patients with increased propensity toward long-term impairment of left ventricular function and adverse outcome, irrespective of the myofilament (thick, intermediate, or thin) involvement.

IMAGING STUDIES
- Chest x-ray may be normal or show cardiomegaly.
- Two-dimensional echocardiography is used to establish the diagnosis and assess the severity of obstruction when present. LV wall thickness will usually be >15 mm (although some may be genetically positive but phenotype negative), and most patients (up to 95%) will have asymmetric (ratio of septum thickness to left ventricular wall thickness >1.3:1) LV wall hypertrophy. Symmetric LV hypertrophy is less common. The septum is most often affected, followed by the left ventricular mid-cavity and apex. In addition, 25% to 30% of patients will manifest systolic anterior motion of the anterior leaflet of the mitral valve, causing obstruction of the LVOT and mitral regurgitation. Two-dimensional strain imaging echocardiography is useful for differentiation of HCM and cardiac amyloidosis from other causes of ventricular wall thickening. Up to 80% of HCM patients will also have diastolic dysfunction as evidenced by pulsed mitral valve inflow pattern and tissue Doppler.

- Cardiac MRI may be of diagnostic value when echocardiographic studies are technically inadequate. MRI is also useful in identifying unusual segmental hypertrophy undetectable by standard echocardiography.

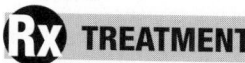 **TREATMENT**

NONPHARMACOLOGIC THERAPY
- Avoid volume depletion: HCM patients experience decrease in stroke volume and consequent increase in left ventricular outflow gradient with exercise. This may lead to hypotension, dizziness, and syncope.
- Exercise restriction: the risk of sudden cardiac death is increased by exercise in HCM patients. Participation in competitive sports and intense physical activity should be avoided. As a part of a healthy lifestyle, low-intensity aerobic exercise is reasonable.
- Advise avoidance of alcohol: alcohol use (even in small amounts) may result in increased obstruction of the left ventricular outflow tract.

GENERAL Rx
- Therapy for HCM is directed at blocking the effect of catecholamines that can exacerbate the dynamic left ventricular outflow tract obstruction and avoiding vasodilator or diuretic agents that can also worsen the obstruction.
- Beta-blockers: The beneficial effects of beta-blockers on symptoms (principally dyspnea and chest pain) and exercise tolerance appear to be largely a result of a decrease in the heart rate with consequent prolongation of diastole and increased passive ventricular filling. By reducing the inotropic response, beta-blockers may also reduce myocardial oxygen demand and decrease the outflow gradient during exercise, when sympathetic tone is increased.
- The nondihydropyridine calcium channel blockers (verapamil, diltiazem) can also decrease left ventricular outflow obstruction through a mechanism similar to beta-blockers. However, they

are mainly second-line agents used in patients who cannot tolerate beta-blockers. They should be used with caution in patients with symptomatic obstruction. Administration in the hospital setting is recommended in these patients.
- Disopyramide is an antiarrhythmic that is also a negative inotrope, resulting in further decrease in outflow gradient. It is sometimes used in combination with beta-blockers.
- Prophylactic antibiotics before dental, GI, and genitourinary procedures are no longer recommended according to the 2007 American Heart Association (AHA) guidelines.
- Avoid use of digitalis, intravenous inotropes, dihydropyridine calcium channel blockers, nitrates, and vasodilators.
- Diuretics, angiotensin-converting enzyme inhibitors, and angiotensin receptor blockers should be used with caution.
- Implantable cardiac defibrillators (ICDs) are a safe and effective therapy in HCM patients prone to ventricular arrhythmias. In their practice guidelines, the major cardiology societies (AHA/ACC/HRS) give a strong recommendation (Class I) for ICD implantation in all patients with HCM who have had an episode of sustained ventricular tachycardia or fibrillation. In addition, they endorse the prophylactic placement of an ICD (Class IIa recommendation) for patients with one or more of the major risk factors for sudden cardiac death (outlined in "Disposition").
- Dual-chamber pacing may provide symptomatic relief, particularly in those who are over 65 yrs of age.
- HCM patients are at an increased risk of atrial fibrillation (AF) as well as systemic thromboembolization. AF is an important source of symptoms, morbidity and mortality and correlates to a worse prognosis. AF therapy should aim for thromboembolic risk mitigation with a vitamin K antagonist (unless contraindicated) and symptom alleviation via rate or rhythm control.

DISPOSITION
HCM is not a static disease. Some adults may experience subtle regression in wall thickness, whereas others (~5% to 10%) paradoxically evolve into an end-stage cardiomyopathy resembling dilated cardiomyopathy, characterized by cavity enlargement, left ventricular wall thinning, and systolic dysfunction. Patients with HCM are at increased risk for sudden death, especially if onset of symptoms began during childhood. Severe left ventricular outflow obstruction at rest is also a strong, independent predictor of severe symptoms of heart failure and death. ICD implantation for primary prevention should be considered if patients (particularly the young) have any of the following:
- A family history of premature death caused by HCM
- Unexplained syncope
- Nonsustained ventricular tachycardia during Holter monitoring
- A marked outflow tract gradient (≥50 mm Hg)
- Substantial hypertrophy (>30 mm)
- Marked left atrial enlargement
- Abnormal blood pressure response during exercise

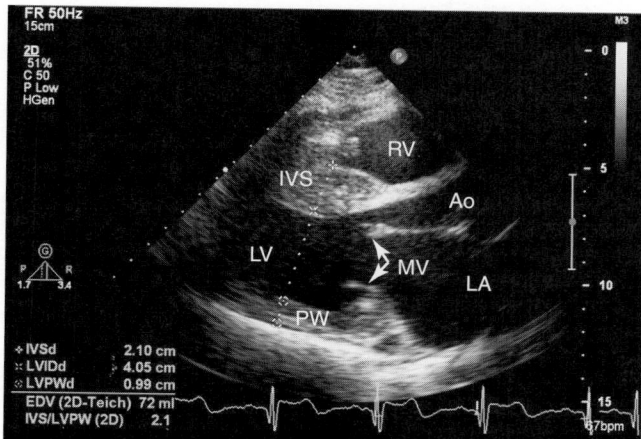

FIGURE 1-185 Echocardiographic appearance of hypertrophic cardiomyopathy. Parasternal long-axis view from a patient with hypertrophic cardiomyopathy demonstrating asymmetrical septal hypertrophy. The interventricular septum (marked by *arrow*) measures 2.1 cm; the posterior wall measures 0.99 cm. *Ao,* Aorta; *IVS,* interventricular septum; *LA,* left atrium; *LV,* left ventricle; *MV,* mitral valve; *PW,* posterior wall; *RV,* right ventricle. (From Issa Z et al: *Clinical arrhythmology and electrophysiology,* ed 2, Philadelphia, 2012, Saunders.)

REFERRAL

- Surgical treatment (myotomy-myectomy involving resection of the basal septum) is reserved for patients who have both a large outflow gradient (≥50 mm Hg) and severe symptoms of heart failure unresponsive to medical therapy. The risk for sudden death from arrhythmias is not altered by surgery. When this operation is performed by experienced surgeons in tertiary referral centers, the operative mortality rate is <2%, and many patients are able to achieve near-normal exercise capacity after surgery.

- As an alternative, nonsurgical reduction of the interventricular septum can be done in patients with HCM refractory to pharmacologic treatment, particularly in those who are not candidates for myomectomy due to high surgical risk. This technique involves the injection of ethanol in a septal perforator branch of the left anterior descending coronary artery, producing a controlled myocardial infarction of the interventricular septum, and thereby reducing septal mass and consequently the left ventricular outflow tract gradient. This method may lead to improvement in both subjective and objective measures of exercise capacity, but results are not as effective as surgery and are associated with a high incidence of heart block, requiring permanent pacing in approximately one fourth of patients and/or recurrence of obstruction and symptoms.

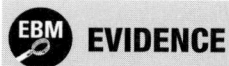

PEARLS & CONSIDERATIONS

COMMENTS

- Clinical screening of first-degree relatives with two-dimensional echocardiography and ECG is indicated. Starting at the age of 12, periodic screening at 12-18 month intervals is recommended for children of patients with HCM. Periodic screening of first-degree adult family members at 5-yr intervals is recommended because hypertrophy may not be detected until the sixth decade of life. Genetic testing is not indicated in relatives of index patients who do not have a definite pathogenic mutation.

- Genetic counseling and screening is recommended in first degree relatives of patients with HCM. Genetic screening of first degree relatives can refine or eliminate the need for periodic clinical screening. At least 11 genes are known to cause HCM, among them: cardiac myosin binding protein-C, beta-myosin heavy chain, troponin T, troponin I, alpha tropomyosin, actin regulatory light chain, and essential light chain. Clinical predictors of positive genotype, such as the presence of ventricular arrhythmias, age at diagnosis, degree of left ventricular wall hypertrophy, and family history of HCM, may aid in patient selection for genetic testing and increase the yield of cardiac sarcomere gene screening.

- The mortality rate in HCM is approximately 1% to 2% per yr.

- About one third of HCM patients will not have a resting or labile outflow gradient (i.e., nonobstructive form of HCM), and lethal ventricular arrhythmias can occur in the absence of obstruction or symptoms.

- Myocardial fibrosis is a hallmark of hypertrophic cardiomyopathy. Biomarkers of collagen metabolism such as serum C-terminal propeptide of type I procollagen (PICP) are significantly higher in mutation carriers without left ventricular hypertrophy and in subjects with overt hypertrophic cardiomyopathy than in controls indicating that a probiotic state precedes the development of hypertrophy of fibrosis identifiable with cardiac MRI.

EBM EVIDENCE

available at www.expertconsult.com

SUGGESTED READINGS

available at www.expertconsult.com

AUTHORS: **ATIZAZUL H. MANSOOR, M.D., DAVID J. FORTUNATO, M.D., F.A.C.C.,** and **FRED F. FERRI, M.D.**

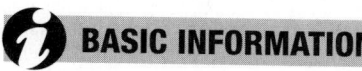

BASIC INFORMATION

DEFINITION

Cardiomyopathy, in general, describes a group of diseases involving the myocardium and characterized by myocardial dysfunction that is not primarily the result of hypertension, coronary atherosclerosis, valvular dysfunction, congenital or other structural heart disease. Restrictive cardiomyopathy is characterized by decreased ventricular compliance, with impaired ventricular filling (of either or both ventricles) and generally normal systolic function.

ICD-9CM CODES
425.4   Other primary cardiomyopathies
425.9   Secondary cardiomyopathy, unspecified
277.39 Restrictive cardiomyopathy secondary to amyloidosis

EPIDEMIOLOGY & DEMOGRAPHICS

- Relatively uncommon cardiomyopathy, accounting for 5% of all primary myocardial diseases
- Most frequently caused by amyloidosis, myocardial fibrosis (following open heart surgery, transplantation or radiation).
- Patients classified as having "idiopathic" restrictive cardiomyopathy may have mutations in the gene for cardiac troponin I, and restrictive cardiomyopathy may represent an overlap with hypertrophic cardiomyopathy in many familial cases.

PHYSICAL FINDINGS & CLINICAL PRESENTATION

Restrictive cardiomyopathy presents with symptoms of progressive left-sided and right-sided heart failure:

- Fatigue, weakness (caused by low output as patients are unable to augment cardiac output by increasing heart rate without compromising ventricular filling).
- Progressively worsening exercise intolerance and dyspnea.
- Anginal chest pain can be seen (particularly in patients with amyloidosis) from myocardial compression of small coronaries.
- Palpitations (atrial fibrillation is common), dizziness or syncope (from orthostasis, heart block, or malignant arrhythmia).
- Edema, ascites, hepatomegaly, distended neck veins (from elevated heart pressures).
- Kussmaul's sign may be present (rise, or failure to fall, of the jugular venous on inspiration).
- On auscultation: murmurs of mitral or tricuspid regurgitation may be heard; an S3 may be present but an S4 almost never is (likely due to infiltration of the atria).
- Apical impulse may be palpable (can help distinguish it from constrictive pericarditis).

ETIOLOGY

Disease may be classified according to pathophysiologic processes:
Infiltrative:
- Amyloidosis (most common overall)
- Sarcoidosis (usually results in a dilated cardiomyopathy with regional wall motion abnormalities)

Noninfiltrative:
- Idiopathic (familial subtypes may have genetic overlap with hypertrophic cardiomyopathy)
- Scleroderma
- Diabetic cardiomyopathy
- Pseudoxanthoma elasticum

Storage diseases:
- Hemochromatosis (unusual as it is commonly associated with a dilated cardiomyopathy)
- Glycogen or other storage diseases (Gaucher, Hurler, Fabry—all rare)

Endomyocardial:
- Endomyocardial fibrosis
- Hypereosinophilic syndrome (Loeffler's)
- Carcinoid heart disease
- Radiation
- Metastatic cancers
- Drug related (anthracyclines, serotonin, ergotamine, busulfan, methysergide)

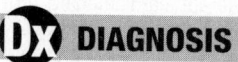 DIAGNOSIS

DIFFERENTIAL DIAGNOSIS

- Constrictive pericarditis (see Table 1-81)
- Valvular dysfunction (especially aortic stenosis)
- Hypertrophic cardiomyopathy
- Hypertension
- Coronary atherosclerosis
- Chronic lung disease

TABLE 1-81   Differentiation between Restrictive Cardiomyopathy and Constrictive Pericarditis

Type of Evaluation	Restrictive Cardiomyopathy	Constrictive Pericarditis
Physical examination	Kussmaul sign present Apical impulse may be prominent Regurgitant murmurs are common	Kussmaul sign may be present Apical impulse usually not palpable Pericardial knock may be present
Electrocardiography	Low QRS voltage (especially in amyloidosis) Pseudoinfarction pattern Bundle branch blocks AV conduction disturbances Atrial fibrillation	Low QRS voltage Repolarization abnormalities
Chest radiography		Calcification of the pericardium may be present
Echocardiography	Marked enlargement of the atria Increased wall thickness (especially in amyloidosis)	Atria usually of normal size Normal wall thickness Pericardial thickening may be seen
Doppler echocardiography	Restrictive mitral inflow (dominant E wave with short deceleration time) No significant variation of transvalvular velocities with respiration (<10%) Reversal of forward flow in hepatic veins during inspiration	Restrictive mitral inflow (dominant E wave with short deceleration time) Increased velocity of RV filling and decreased velocity of LV filling with inspiration; opposite with expiration; variation in velocity exceeds 15% Reversal of forward flow in hepatic veins during expiration
Cardiac catheterization	Prominent atrial x and y descents (w sign) Dip-and-plateau appearance of ventricular diastolic pressure Diastolic pressures increased but not equalized (LV diastolic pressure higher than RV diastolic pressure)	Prominent atrial x and y descents (w sign) Dip-and-plateau appearance of ventricular diastolic pressure Increase and equalization of diastolic pressures Discordance of RV and LV peak systolic pressures (with inspiration, RV systolic pressure increases and LV systolic pressure decreases)
Endomyocardial biopsy	May reveal specific cause of restrictive cardiomyopathy	No specific findings on endomyocardial biopsy Pericardial biopsy may reveal abnormality
Computed tomography, magnetic resonance imaging		Pericardial thickening

AV, Atrioventricular; LV, left ventricular; RV, right ventricular.
From Andreoli TE et al [eds]: Andreoli and Carpenter's Cecil essentials of medicine, ed 8, Philadelphia, 2010, Saunders.

WORKUP

- Blood count (to identify eosinophilia), iron studies, serum renal function studies, chest x-ray, ECG, echocardiogram.
- Cardiac catheterization, magnetic resonance imaging, and computed tomography (selected cases)
- Aspiration biopsy of subcutaneous fat to detect amyloidosis.
- Endomyocardial biopsy if diagnostic confirmation needed.
- Brain natriuretic peptide (BNP) serum levels: there is data suggesting that BNP levels are markedly elevated in restrictive cardiomyopathy but near normal in patients with constrictive pericarditis, despite nearly identical clinical and hemodynamic features.

IMAGING STUDIES

- Chest x-ray:
  - Ranges from normal cardiomediastinal silhouette to moderate cardiomegaly (primarily because of biatrial enlargement).
  - Evidence of heart failure may be present.
  - Presence of pericardial calcification favors alternate diagnosis of constrictive pericarditis.
- ECG:
  - Nonspecific ST-T wave abnormalities are the most common finding. Voltage may be low in infiltrative etiologies such as amyloidosis.
  - Frequent atrial and ventricular ectopy are often present. Atrial fibrillation may be present.
  - High-degree atrioventricular block, intraventricular conduction delay may be seen in advanced cases.
- Echocardiogram (Fig. 1-186):
  - Biatrial enlargement almost always present.
  - Wall thickness depends on etiology, often normal but may be thickened in infiltrative disease such as amyloidosis.
  - Myocardial appearance may be altered (speckled pattern suggestive of infiltration).
  - Ventricular chamber sizes and systolic function are often normal or reduced.
  - Echo Doppler shows evidence of diastolic dysfunction.

- Cardiac catheterization:
  - Characteristic hemodynamic finding is a dip and plateau, or square-root sign in the left ventricular tracing, where deep and rapid decline in ventricular pressure at the onset of diastole is immediately followed by rapid rise and plateau in early diastolic phase. To distinguish restrictive cardiomyopathy from constrictive pericarditis:
    Constrictive pericarditis: Usually involves both ventricles and leads to equalization of diastolic pressures between all four cardiac chambers to within 5 mm Hg.
    Restrictive cardiomyopathy: Impairs the left ventricle more than the right, often with left-sided end-diastolic pressures of 5 mm Hg greater than the right. The presence of increased pulmonary arterial systolic pressures is also suggestive of restrictive disease.
- Cardiac computed tomographic scan may be helpful to identify a thickened and calcified pericardium, consistent with constrictive pericarditis.
- Cardiac magnetic resonance imaging (CMRI) may also be useful to distinguish restrictive cardiomyopathy from constrictive pericarditis (thickness of the pericardium greater than 4 mm in the latter). CMRI is particularly helpful in the diagnosis of the amyloid or sarcoid variants and may have value in other variants as well.

Rx TREATMENT

NONPHARMACOLOGIC THERAPY

Congestive symptoms may respond to dietary sodium restriction (<2 g/day).

ACUTE GENERAL Rx

Treatment of volume overload and heart failure symptoms with diuretic therapy.

CHRONIC Rx

- Treatment involves management of the underlying disease if it exists:
  - Hemochromatosis may respond to repeated phlebotomy to decrease iron deposition in the heart.
  - Sarcoidosis may respond to corticosteroid therapy.

- Primary amyloidosis may respond to antiplasma cell therapy with chemotherapeutics (usually melphalan) and steroids. Autologous bone marrow biopsy, if EF is >40%, may also be indicated.
  - Eosinophilic cardiomyopathy may respond to corticosteroid and cytotoxic drugs.
  - There is no effective therapy for other causes of restrictive cardiomyopathy.
- Overall, the goal of treatment is to reduce symptoms by decreasing filling pressures while preserving cardiac output. Since there is currently no drug available to specifically act on myocardial relaxation, therapy centers on low-dose diuretics to lower the preload.
- Beta-blockers or calcium channel blockers have not been demonstrated to improve symptoms or alter the course of disease.
- ACE inhibitors (or angiotensin receptor blockers [ARBs]) should be avoided in patients with amyloidosis as they are poorly tolerated. Even small doses can trigger profound hypotension (probably due to associated autonomic neuropathy).
- Atrial fibrillation is common and patients with it or with a history of embolization should be anticoagulated. Tachycardia (of any cause) is poorly tolerated and a common cause of decompensation. Rate control is of paramount importance. Cardioversion in case of rapid atrial fibrillation should be considered. Of note, digoxin should be used with caution as it is potentially arrhythmogenic (particularly in patients with amyloidosis).
- Fibrosis of the cardiac conduction system may result in complete heart block presenting as dizziness or syncope (especially in amyloidosis) and pacemaker implantation may be required. The course of restrictive cardiomyopathy is variable and depends on the underlying etiology. Death usually results from heart failure or arrhythmias, and interventions aimed at addressing these are recommended.
  - For the amyloid variant, an implantable cardiac defibrillator offers little prophylactic benefit as the cause of sudden cardiac death is usually electromechanical disassociation.

DISPOSITION

Prognosis varies with the etiology of the cardiomyopathy but is poor overall as disease is rarely detected before advanced stages.

REFERRAL

Cardiac transplantation can be considered in patients with refractory symptoms and idiopathic or familial restrictive cardiomyopathies.

SUGGESTED READINGS

available at www.expertconsult.com

RELATED CONTENT

Fig. 3-39 Initial approach to classification of cardiomyopathy (Algorithm)
Restrictive Cardiomyopathy (Patient Information)

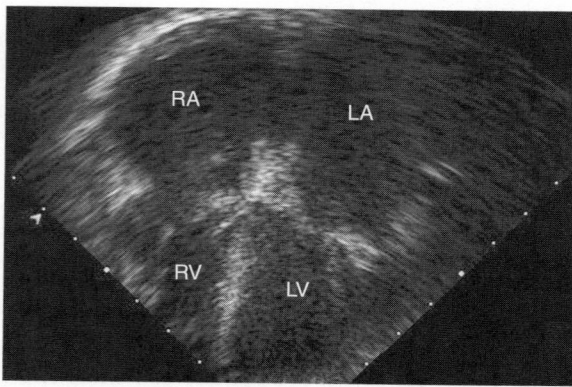

FIGURE 1-186 Echocardiogram of a patient with restrictive cardiomyopathy. The optical four-chamber view shows the markedly enlarged right and left atria, compared to the normal-sized left and right ventricular chambers. *LA,* Left atrium; *LV,* left ventricle; *RA,* right atrium; *RV,* right ventricle. (From Kliegman RM et al: *Nelson textbook of pediatrics,* ed 19, Philadelphia, 2011, Saunders.)

AUTHORS: **ATIZAZUL M. MANSOOR, M.D.,**
DAVID J. FORTUNATO, M.D., F.A.C.C., and
FRED F. FERRI, M.D.

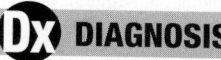

BASIC INFORMATION

DEFINITION

Stress cardiomyopathy (SC) is a syndrome characterized by transient systolic dysfunction and ballooning of the apical and/or mid segments of the left ventricle (LV) that mimics acute myocardial infarction (MI) but in the absence of obstructive (≤70% for the three epicardial coronary vessels or ≤50% for left main) coronary artery disease that can explain the wall motion abnormality. Typically, but not always, it is preceded by severe illness or intense stress.

SYNONYMS

Takotsubo cardiomyopathy (TTC)
Left ventricular apical ballooning syndrome (LVABS)
Broken heart syndrome

ICD-9CM CODES
429.83

EPIDEMIOLOGY & DEMOGRAPHICS

INCIDENCE: Uncertain, although increasingly reported. The recurrence rate is 11.4% over 4 yr after initial presentation.
PREVALENCE: Studies suggest that it comprises 0.7% to 2.5% of cases presenting with acute coronary syndrome (ACS).
PREDOMINANT SEX AND AGE: Postmenopausal women (90%) are predominantly affected.
RISK FACTORS: Frequently, but not always, triggered by severe medical illness or intense emotional or physical stress (death of loved ones, domestic abuse, fierce arguments, financial hardships, etc.)

PHYSICAL FINDINGS & CLINICAL PRESENTATION

Acute substernal chest pain, dyspnea, syncope, shock, electrocardiographic (ECG) changes, or elevated cardiac biomarkers; similar to an acute MI.

ETIOLOGY

Not well understood. Hypotheses include excessive catecholamine release, coronary artery spasm, and/or microvascular disease. Unknown why women are more commonly affected or why the apex and/or mid cavity are affected.

Dx DIAGNOSIS

Mayo Clinic proposed criteria (2008): All 4 criteria required to make diagnosis.
- Transient hypokinesis, akinesis, or dyskinesis in the left ventricular mid segments with or without apical involvement (Fig. 1-187); regional wall motion abnormalities (RWMA) that extend beyond a single epicardial vascular distribution; and frequently, but not always, a stressful trigger.
- Absence of obstructive coronary disease or angiographic evidence of acute plaque rupture.
- New ECG abnormalities (ST-segment elevation and/or T-wave inversion) or modest elevation in cardiac troponins.
- Absence of pheochromocytoma or myocarditis.
- An inverted Takotsubo pattern—mid ventricular ballooning with sparing of the basal and apical segments—atypical variant.
- The RWMA of the right ventricle is present in 30% of patients who tend to develop CHF and who have a poor outcome.

DIFFERENTIAL DIAGNOSIS
- Acute MI
- Cardiac syndrome X
- Prinzmetal's angina
- Myocarditis
- Cocaine abuse

WORK-UP
- This should be suspected in postmenopausal women who present with ACS after intense stress.
- Cardiology consult should be immediately obtained

- Significant CAD should be ruled out as an etiology of the cardiomyoapthy, usually by coronary catheterization.

LABORATORY TESTS
Cardiac biomarkers are often elevated, but typically less than MI

IMAGING STUDIES
- Typically diagnosed in the catheterization lab during left ventriculography, although echocardiography (ECHO) can also show the characteristic apical ballooning. Contrast ECHO is quite useful to exclude apical thrombus. Cardiovascular MRI at the time of initial clinical presentation may provide relevant functional and tissue information that might aid in the establishment of the diagnosis of SC.
- Cardiac magnetic imaging (CMR) features helpful in diagnosis: absence of late gadolinium enhancement (LGE) in contrast to MI and presence of patchy LGE in myocarditis.

COMPLICATIONS
- Approximately 20% include cardiogenic shock, heart failure, arrhythmias, intraventricular thrombus formation (incidence 2.5%), acute clinically significant mitral regurgitation, LV outflow tract (LVOT) obstruction, free wall rupture, and even death. An LV apical thrombus carries a great risk of cerebrovascular accident and distant embolization during the recovery phase.
- Risk score to predict likelihood of acute HF based on three variables: age >70 years, presence of physical stressor, and LV ejection fraction <40%.

Rx TREATMENT

There are no randomized data or established consensus. In most cases, supportive care is sufficient without specific therapy, due to a favorable prognosis. Standard treatment for systolic dysfunction including beta blockers, ACE inhibitors, and diuretics for volume overload. Patients who are in shock should get urgent ECHO to determine presence of LVOT obstruction.

NONPHARMACOLOGIC THERAPY
Patients in shock without significant LVOT obstruction may benefit from an intra-aortic balloon pump (IABP).

ACUTE GENERAL Rx
- Patients who are hemodynamically stable should be started on a beta-blocker, ACE inhibitor, and diuretic if needed.
- Patients who are in shock and with significant LVOT obstruction may benefit from cautious fluid resuscitation (if no significant pulmonary congestion), and use of beta-blockers (can improve hemodynamics by resolution of the obstruction). The use of IABP in this case is controversial due to the potential worsening of LVOT obstruction.

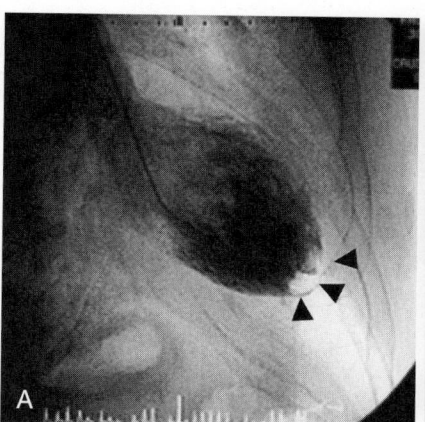
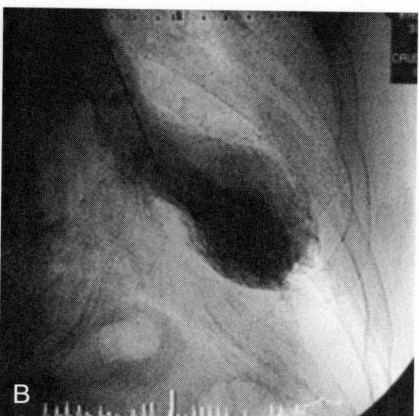

FIGURE 1-187 A and **B,** Left ventriculogram showing apical ballooning characteristic of stress-induced cardiomyopathy. (From Mitsuma W et al: *JACC* 51(1): cover, 2008.)

- Patients with systolic anterior motion (SAM) of the anterior mitral valve leaflet or LVOT obstruction should not be exposed to inotropic agents even if they are in shock.

CHRONIC Rx

- Continued medical therapy and repeat ECHO (in 4 to 6 wk) to ensure normalization of systolic function (most patients normalize by this time).
- Duration of medical therapy is debatable.
- Three months of anticoagulation is suggested if an intraventricular thrombus is detected.

Recently published data could not find the protective effect of beta blockers in preventing the occurrence or recurrence of stress induced cardiomyopathy.

DISPOSITION

Carries a favorable prognosis compared to STEMI or NSTEMI; in-hospital mortality is approximately 2%.

REFERRAL

Follow-up with a cardiologist is suggested.

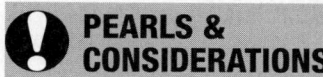 **PEARLS & CONSIDERATIONS**

COMMENTS

The term *takotsubo* is the Japanese name for an octopus trap (*tako-tsubo*), which has a similar shape of the LV in systole during a left ventriculogram (see Fig. 1-187).

PREVENTION

Minimizing stress may reduce incidence but no data to support this.

SUGGESTED READINGS

available at www.expertconsult.com

RELATED CONTENT

Table 3-2 Profiles of Myocardial Disease

AUTHORS: **SHAHNAZ PUNJANI, M.D.**, and **WEN-CHIH WU, M.D., M.P.H.**

BASIC INFORMATION

DEFINITION

Cardiorenal syndrome (CRS) is a pathophysiologic disorder in which acute or chronic dysfunction of the heart or kidneys can induce acute or chronic dysfunction of the other organ. Another definition proposed by the National Heart, Lung, and Blood Institute (NHLBI) is one in which therapy to relieve congestive symptoms of heart failure is limited by further decline in renal function. There are five types of CRS:

Type 1: Acute cardiac dysfunction leading to acute kidney injury

Type 2: Chronic heart failure leading to renal dysfunction

Type 3: Acute kidney injury leading to or resulting in acute cardiac dysfunction

Type 4: Chronic kidney disease (CKD) leading to cardiac dysfunction

Type 5: Systemic conditions that cause both cardiac and renal dysfunction

This section will focus on CRS types 1 and 2.

ICD-9CM CODES
404 Cardiorenal syndrome

EPIDEMIOLOGY & DEMOGRAPHICS
- CKD is present in 20% to 67% of patients with congestive heart failure (CHF).
  - Women, the elderly, whites, and patients with diabetes or systolic blood pressure >160 mm Hg have an increased incidence.
- 20%-30% of patients who are treated for acute or chronic CHF will develop acute kidney injury.
  - In patients with acute CHF, the severity of acute kidney injury is increased with decreased left ventricular systolic function and baseline CKD.

PHYSICAL FINDINGS & CLINICAL PRESENTATION
- Acute/subacute decompensated heart failure (ADHF)
  - Clinical symptoms:
    - Dyspnea with exertion or at rest
    - Orthopnea
    - Paroxysmal nocturnal dyspnea
    - Right upper quadrant pain
  - Vital signs:
    - Sinus tachycardia
    - Elevated respiratory rate
    - Narrow pulse pressure
  - Physical exam findings:
    - Elevated jugular venous pressures in the neck
    - Peripheral edema
    - Third heart sound (S3)
    - Respiratory crackles
    - Abdominal ascites
    - Hepato- and splenomegaly
    - Scrotal edema
- Chronic heart failure
  - Clinical symptoms:
    - Dyspnea
    - Fatigue
    - Anorexia
  - Vital signs:
    - Similar to ADHF, but may not have sinus tachycardia, and may have hypotension
  - Physical exam findings:
    - Similar to ADHF, but may lack respiratory crackles because crackles are more a sign of the rapidity of the collection of fluid within the alveoli rather than the total volume of fluid
- These findings of heart failure will be associated with laboratory findings of kidney disease (discussed later) or in extreme cases physical exam findings of severe kidney disease such as asterixis, uremic frost, or uremic smell.

ETIOLOGY
The etiology of CRS can be divided into four mechanisms:
- Reduced renal perfusion
  - Is a common cause of CRS type 1
- Increased renal venous pressure
  - Can occur secondary to elevated central venous pressure or elevated intraabdominal pressure
- Right ventricular dysfunction
  - May result in increased central venous pressures, which results in increased renal venous pressures
  - May result in poor forward flow
- Neurohormonal
  - Caused by activation of the renin-angiotensin-aldosterone system, antidiuretic hormone, and endothelin-1, which results in systemic vasoconstriction leading to decreased renal perfusion

DIAGNOSIS

DIFFERENTIAL DIAGNOSIS
- Before making the diagnosis of CRS, it is necessary to rule out other causes of renal failure such as:
  - Prerenal causes
    - Volume depletion (overdiuresis, gastrointestinal losses, or vomiting)
    - Fluid overload states besides CHF (cirrhosis, nephrotic syndrome)
  - Intrinsic renal disease
    - Acute tubular necrosis
    - Glomerular disease
      - Nephrotic and nephritic syndromes
  - Postrenal causes
    - Obstruction

WORKUP
- The medical history will be consistent with symptoms of CHF and may include dyspnea, orthopnea, paroxysmal nocturnal dyspnea, edema, increasing abdominal girth, or weight gain. Additionally, laboratory results will show signs of kidney injury.
- Diagnostic workup includes chest radiograph, echocardiogram, renal ultrasound, and laboratory tests (see next section)

LABORATORY TESTS
- Serum creatinine
  - Patients with CRS whose creatinine levels were elevated at least 0.3 to 0.5 mg/dl had an odds ratio of 1.48 for mortality compared with those whose creatinine levels were elevated less than 0.3 mg/dl.
    - If creatinine levels increased by >0.5 mg/dl, the odds ratio of mortality increased to 3.22.
- Estimated glomerular filtration rate (eGFR)
  - Similar results to that of creatinine, but is more accurate for diagnosing elderly patients with less muscle mass
- Blood urea nitrogen
  - Admission levels >43 mg/dl are associated with a higher in-hospital mortality rate in patients with CRS
- Cystatin C
  - Better correlation to GFR than serum creatinine
- Beta natriuretic peptide (BNP)
  - Patients with initial admission values exceeding 480 pg/ml had a 51% chance of death, hospital readmission, or emergency room visit within 6 months compared with patients whose levels were <230 pg/ml.

IMAGING STUDIES
- Chest radiograph
  - May show signs of fluid overload, such as pulmonary edema, pulmonary effusions, or fluid in the fissure
- Echocardiogram
  - Will help to determine if there is underlying systolic or diastolic dysfunction
- Renal ultrasound
  - Can help to distinguish between acute and chronic kidney disease, and can help rule out obstruction as a cause of worsening renal function

TREATMENT

NONPHARMACOLOGIC THERAPY
- Fluid restriction
- Hemodialysis/ultrafiltration
  - Can be used if there is no response to pharmacologic treatment or if the use of pharmacologic agents is limited secondary to hemodynamics or worsening laboratory values
- Left ventricular assist device/cardiac resynchronization therapy (CRT)
  - Can be used to improve forward flow and cardiac dyssynchrony. Use of CRT has been proven to improve ejection fraction by 7%.

ACUTE GENERAL Rx
There is no treatment that directly improves eGFR/creatinine, but an increase in cardiac output can reduce the incidence of the four mechanisms of CRS listed previously.

- Diuretics
  - Fluid off-loading helps patients return to their ideal position on the Frank-Starling curve.
  - Removal of fluid will improve renal perfusion pressure, decrease central venous pressure, and reduce right ventricular dilation.
  - May need high doses to achieve success because of decreased diuretic responsiveness as eGFR decreases
- Inhibitors of the renin-angiotensin-aldosterone system
  - Includes angiotensin converting enzyme (ACE) inhibitors, angiotensin receptor blockers, and aldosterone antagonists
    - Use is limited by worsening renal function
    - Allows for decreasing of diuretic therapy
- Vasodilators
  - Includes nitroglycerin, nitroprusside, and nesiritide
    - Work by increasing renal perfusion pressure
- Ionotropic agents
  - Includes dobutamine, dopamine, and milrinone
  - Are used in treatment of cardiogenic shock and work by improving cardiac output, resulting in better renal perfusion pressures

DISPOSITION

Is based upon improvement of patient's volume status as creatinine levels return to baseline

REFERRAL

Consultation by a cardiologist and nephrologist are recommended.

SUGGESTED READINGS
available at www.expertconsult.com

RELATED CONTENT

Acute Kidney Injury (Related Key Topic)
Heart Failure (Related Key Topic)

AUTHORS: **SUNIT-PREET CHAUDHRY, M.D.,** and **ARAVIND RAO KOKKIRALA, M.D.**

BASIC INFORMATION

DEFINITION

Light-headedness, dizziness, presyncope, or syncope in a patient with carotid sinus hypersensitivity is defined as carotid sinus syndrome (CSS). Carotid sinus hypersensitivity is the exaggerated response to carotid stimulation resulting in bradycardia, hypotension, or both. CSS is often considered a variant of neurocardiogenic syncope.

SYNONYMS

Carotid sinus syncope
CSS
Carotid sinus hypersensitivity

ICD-9CM CODES
337.0 Idiopathic peripheral autonomic neuropathy
780.2 Syncope or collapse

EPIDEMIOLOGY & DEMOGRAPHICS

- Carotid sinus hypersensitivity accounts for 1% of syncopal episodes.
- Carotid sinus hypersensitivity is frequently associated with atherosclerosis and diabetes mellitus.
- Incidence increases with age, with an average age of onset at 61 to 74 yr.
- Men are affected more often than women (2:1).
- CSS is rarely found in patients younger than 50 yr.

PHYSICAL FINDINGS & CLINICAL PRESENTATION

- Usually associated with sudden neck movements or tight-fitting collars
- Usually associated with prodrome of nausea, warmth, pallor, or diaphoresis
- Light-headedness or presyncopal symptoms
- Syncope

Properly performed carotid sinus massage (CSM) at the bedside is diagnostic. European Society of Cardiology recommends carotid sinus massage as part of the exam in patients with syncope of unknown etiology and age over 40. This maneuver can elicit three types of responses in patients with carotid sinus hypersensitivity (see "Diagnosis").

1. CSM should be performed with the patient in the supine and upright position while monitoring the patient's blood pressure by cuff and heart rate by ECG.
2. CSM should be performed on only one carotid artery at a time.
3. Vigorous circular pressure is applied over one carotid artery at the level of the cricoid cartilage for 10 seconds and repeated on the opposite side if no effect is produced.
4. Contraindications to CSM include the presence of carotid artery bruits, documented carotid artery stenosis >70%, history of stroke or transient ischemic attack <3 mo, history of myocardial infarction <6 mo, history of serious ventricular arrhythmia, or prior carotid endarterectomy.
5. Complications of transient visual disturbance or transient paresis occur in <1% of patients.
6. False positive results with carotid sinus massage may be relatively common in the elderly population. Thus alternative explanation for syncope should be investigated prior to attribution of symptoms to carotid sinus hypersensitivity.

ETIOLOGY

- Idiopathic
- Head and neck tumors (e.g., thyroid)
- Significant lymphadenopathy
- Carotid body tumors
- Prior neck surgery

DIAGNOSIS

- The diagnosis of CSS is made when carotid sinus hypersensitivity is demonstrated by CSM and no other cause of syncope is identified.
- CSM can elicit three types of responses diagnostic of carotid sinus hypersensitivity:
  1. Cardioinhibitory type: CSM producing (1) asystole for at least 3 sec in the absence of symptoms or (2) reproduction of symptoms occurring with a decline in heart rate of 30% to 40% or asystole of up to 2 sec in duration. Symptoms should not recur when CSM is repeated after atropine infusion.
  2. Vasodepressor type: CSM producing (1) a decrease in systolic blood pressure of 50 mm Hg in the absence of symptoms or 30 mm Hg in the presence of neurologic symptoms; (2) no evidence of asystole; or (3) neurologic symptoms that persist after infusion of atropine.
  3. Mixed type: CSM producing both types of responses.

DIFFERENTIAL DIAGNOSIS

All causes of syncope

WORKUP

- CSS is a diagnosis of exclusion.
- Exclude other causes of syncope or presyncope: detailed history, physical examination including orthostatic vital signs, ECG. Other tests should be considered depending on the clinical setting.

TREATMENT

NONPHARMACOLOGIC THERAPY

Reassurance and education are important. Avoid applying neck pressure from tight collars, shaving, or rapid head turning.

ACUTE GENERAL Rx

Treatment will vary according to the type of carotid hypersensitivity response and symptoms present (see "Chronic Rx").

CHRONIC Rx

Therapy is divided into three classes: medical, surgical (carotid denervation), and cardiac pacing. Surgical therapy has been largely abandoned except in cases of compressing tumors or masses responsible for CSS.

For infrequent and mildly symptomatic carotid sinus hypersensitivity of either the cardioinhibitory or vasodepressor type, treatment is generally not necessary.

Cardiac pacing: 2008 ACC/AHA/HRS device guidelines recommend pacing in patients with recurrent syncope in spontaneous occurring carotid sinus stimulation, in whom carotid sinus pressure induces ventricular asystole of more than 3 seconds.

Permanent pacing may be considered in patients with recurrent syncope of unexplained origin, and a hypersensitive cardioinhibitory response of 3 seconds or more.

Permanent pacing is not indicated for carotid sinus hypersensitivity with no, or only vague, symptoms.

For symptomatic patients with a vasodepressor response to CSM:

- No medical treatment is proven to be effective
- Drugs, such as vasodilators, that would worsen the response should be discontinued or reduced if feasible
- Sympathomimetics: midodrine 2.5 to 10 mg tid
- Serotonin-specific reuptake inhibitors
- Fludrocortisone
- Elastic knee-high or thigh-high stockings
- Carotid sinus denervation

For symptomatic patients with CSS with a mixed response to CSM:

- Combination of dual-chamber permanent pacemaker and agents used to treat vasodepressor response

DISPOSITION

- Up to 50% of the patients have recurrent symptoms.
- No increased mortality rate in patients with idiopathic CSS compared with the general population.

REFERRAL

Cardiology referral is indicated if cardiac testing, such as tilt-table test, or pacemaker placement is being considered.

Neurology referral is indicated if neurologic causes of syncope are suggested by history or physical examination findings.

PEARLS & CONSIDERATIONS

The most common type of CSS is cardioinhibitory, followed by mixed and vasodepressor responses.

Driving restrictions in the 2009 ESC syncope update and 1996 AHA/NASPE statement are stratified according to whether patients have mild or severe syncope.

Mild syncope is defined as infrequent mild symptoms (usually without syncope), clear precipitating causes (usually standing), warning signs, and infrequent occurrence. For patients with mild sinus hypersensitivity, no driving restrictions are recommended for private or commercial driving.

Severe syncope is classified as severe symptoms (with syncope), without warning and in any position, no clear precipitating causes, and/or frequent occurrence. For patients with severe hypersensitivity, all driving is prohibited. If symptoms are controlled, driving is permitted 1 to 6 months after, based on the modality of treatment.

COMMENTS

Prognosis depends on the underlying cause.

SUGGESTED READINGS
available at www.expertconsult.com

RELATED CONTENT
Fig. E1-799 Syncope (Algorithm)
Box E1-69 Syncope
Fig. 3-88 Hypotension (Algorithm)
Syncope (Patient Information)

AUTHORS: **ABDULRAHMAN ABDULBAKI, M.D.,** and **WEN-CHIH WU, M.D., M.P.H.**

BASIC INFORMATION

DEFINITION

Carotid stenosis is narrowing of the arterial lumen within the carotid artery that is typically a result of atherosclerosis.

SYNONYMS

Atherosclerotic disease of the carotid artery

ICD-9CM CODES
433.1 Carotid stenosis

EPIDEMIOLOGY & DEMOGRAPHICS

INCIDENCE: 2.2 to 8/1000 persons per yr
PREVALENCE: 1.1 to 77/100,000 persons; it is estimated that 5/1000 persons aged 50 to 60 yr and 100/1000 persons >80 yr have carotid stenosis >50%. (*Note:* The incidence of carotid stenosis is unknown as screening is not routine. However, the incidence of transient ischemic attack [TIA], a common presenting symptom of carotid stenosis, is well known.)
PREDOMINANT SEX AND AGE: Male/female ratio of 2:1; more common in whites than African Americans and Asians
PEAK INCIDENCE: Peak incidence is between 50 and 60 yr of age.
GENETICS: Multifactorial; twin studies (monozygous vs. dizygous) suggest a familial influence
RISK FACTORS: Hypertension, dyslipidemia, diabetes mellitus, and smoking are the four major risk factors.

PHYSICAL FINDINGS & CLINICAL PRESENTATION

Patients with carotid stenosis are often asymptomatic, but many have the presence of a carotid bruit or TIA.

- Carotid bruit: In general, the presence of a carotid bruit is a better indicator of generalized atherosclerosis and as such, is a better predictor of ischemic heart disease than future stroke.
- TIA: Carotid stenosis is classically heralded by ipsilateral transient monocular blindness (amaurosis fugax), contralateral numbness or weakness, contralateral homonymous hemianopsia, aphasia, or *syncope (if bilateral disease is present)*.

ETIOLOGY

- Atherosclerosis (most common by far)
- Aneurysm
- Arteritis
- Carotid dissection
- Fibromuscular dysplasia
- Postradiation necrosis
- Vasospasm

DIAGNOSIS

DIFFERENTIAL DIAGNOSIS

Aneurysm, arteritis, and carotid dissection

WORKUP

Systematic history, examination, and diagnostic studies to assess for carotid stenosis and other risk factors of TIA

LABORATORY TESTS

CBC, basic metabolic panel, fasting lipid profile, PT/international normalized ratio, APTT, CRP

IMAGING STUDIES

- Four imaging modalities are available for the evaluation of carotid stenosis (Table 1-82).
- Patients who have neurologic sequelae suggestive of carotid stenosis should be screened via carotid duplex. If carotid stenosis is suspected on carotid duplex, but inconclusive, magnetic resonance angiography, computed tomography angiography, or conventional angiography should be obtained to confirm the degree of stenosis (Fig. 1-188).

TREATMENT

NONPHARMACOLOGIC THERAPY

Carotid endarterectomy (CEA) and carotid angioplasty and stenting (CAS) are available.
CEA—several studies have proved the efficacy of this procedure. The selection of surgical candidates should be guided primarily by the presence or absence of symptoms and the degree of stenosis.

Asymptomatic patients: Four major trials have investigated the benefit of CEA in an asymptomatic patient with carotid stenosis: Carotid Artery Surgery Asymptomatic Narrowing Operation vs Aspirin (CASANOVA), Veterans Affairs Cooperative Study Group, Asymptomatic Carotid Atherosclerosis Study (ACAS), and Asymptomatic Carotid Surgery Trial (ACST). In addition, a meta-analysis was subsequently performed.

Pearls:
  Most studies have shown that a benefit from CEA in asymptomatic patients is not seen until 2 yr after surgery.
  CEA should be considered in asymptomatic patients only if the perioperative risk for stroke and death at the given surgical institution is less than 3%.
  The studies failed to show a benefit in the presence of contralateral carotid occlusion.
Recommendations for asymptomatic patients with carotid stenosis:
  CEA should be considered in patients between the ages of 40 and 75 yr with asymptomatic 60% to 99% stenosis if their life expectancy is greater than 5 yr and the perioperative stroke and mortality rates are <3%. However, medical therapy has improved since early trials comparing medical management and revascularization. Stroke rates have fallen to about 1% in medically treated patients over the past decade, and many experts are favoring intensified medical management rather than revascularization procedures in patients with ACS.

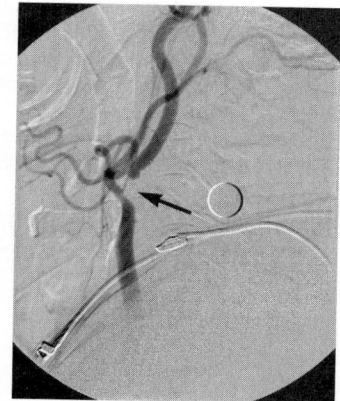

FIGURE 1-188 Conventional angiography demonstrating severe stenosis of the internal carotid artery at the bifurcation.

TABLE 1-82 Imaging Modalities for Carotid Stenosis

Imaging Modality	Benefit	Drawback
Cerebral angiography	• Gold standard • Assesses plaque morphology • Assesses presence of collaterals	• Invasive • High cost • 4% incidence rate of complications • 1% incidence rate of serious complications or death
Carotid duplex	• Sensitive in detecting high-grade stenosis (>70%) • Less invasive • Lower cost	• Can be limited by body habitus • Technician dependent • Overestimates degree of stenosis
Magnetic resonance angiography (MRA)	• Sensitive in detecting high-grade stenosis (>70%) • Less operator dependent	• Overestimates degree of stenosis • Cannot be performed in patients who are critically ill, unable to tolerate supine positioning, have pacemaker or other ferromagnetic hardware, or are claustrophobic* • Expensive • Takes much longer to obtain compared with other modalities
Computed tomography angiography (CTA)	• Sensitive for high-grade stenosis	• Contraindicated in patients with serum creatinine concentration >1.5 mg/dl

*One study revealed that ~17% of patients are unable to tolerate MRA secondary to claustrophobia or are unable to lie still for procedure.

All patients undergoing CEA should be started on aspirin (ASA; 81 or 325 mg daily) before surgery and should be continued indefinitely. Although variations exist among surgeons, ASA is typically continued during the perioperative period.

Symptomatic patients: Two major trials (North American Symptomatic Carotid Endarterectomy Trial [NASCET] and European Carotid Surgery Trial [ECST]) and subsequent pooled analysis have shown the benefit of CEA in patients with symptomatic carotid stenosis.

Pearls:

There is improved outcome in patients with mild stroke or TIA for surgical treatment within 2 wk of the symptomatic event.

Men seem to benefit more when compared with women.

CEA does not appear to be beneficial in women with 50% to 69% stenosis.

Despite increased perioperative risk, patients with contralateral carotid occlusion who undergo CEA have benefit in terms of stroke and death rate when compared with patients undergoing medical management alone.

Recommendations:

CEA is recommended for recently symptomatic patients with 70% to 99% stenosis if their life expectancy is >5 yr and perioperative risk for mortality is <6%. Number needed to treat (NNT) at 5 yr = 6.3.

CEA is beneficial for recently symptomatic men with 50% to 69% stenosis if their life expectancy is >5 yr and perioperative risk of mortality is <6%. NNT at 5 yr = 22.

Medical management is recommended for patients with stenosis <50%.

ASA (81 or 325 mg daily) should be initiated before CEA and continued after surgery.

CAS (stenting) is a less invasive alternative to CEA. Five major studies have compared stenting and CEA (Stent-Protected Angioplasty vs. Carotid Endarterectomy [SPACE], endarterectomy vs. stenting in patients with symptomatic severe carotid stenosis [EVA-3S], Stenting and Angioplasty with Protection in Patients at High Risk for Endarterectomy [SAPPHIRE]), Carotid Revascularization Endarterectomy Versus Stenting [CREST] and the International Carotid Stenting Study [ICSS].

Recommendations:

CAS may be considered for symptomatic patients with >70% carotid stenosis who have either difficult surgical access, intracranial stenosis, or medical risk that increases the risk of surgery (those with severe cardiac or pulmonary disease, contralateral carotid occlusion, prior neck surgery, prior neck irradiation, contralateral laryngeal nerve palsy, recurrent stenosis after prior CEA, age >0 yr).

CAS should be considered only if operators have periprocedural morbidity and mortality rates between 4% and 6%.

ASA should be given before procedure and indefinitely after procedure.

Clopidogrel should be given for 6 mo to 2 yr after stent placement or continued indefinitely depending on individual circumstances.

Risk for CAS:

Minor or major stroke related to hyperperfusion syndrome, periprocedural bradycardia, hypotension, and restenosis. Hyperperfusion syndrome: 1.1%
Restenosis: 0.5% to 2%

Stenting vs. Endarterectomy for Treatment of Carotid Artery Stenosis

The large CREST study, published in 2010, demonstrated no difference in primary outcomes (stroke, myocardial infarction or death in the periprocedural period or ipsilateral stroke within 4 years following randomization).

Results from ICSS, a large, multicenter, international study comparing CEA and CAS, were recently released. This study showed an increased risk of stroke, periprocedural complication, and death in those patients undergoing stenting compared to those undergoing CEA. Additionally, a study on MRI findings following the procedure revealed an increased occurrence of "silent strokes" in those patients undergoing CAS. Long-term follow-up is still ongoing.

Despite the recent reports from ICSS, individual results may depend on factors such as the surgeon's experience and skill, and age of the patient with older patients (>70 yr) possibly doing better with CEA.

Results from SPACE, a multicenter European trial designed to test the hypothesis that CAS is not inferior to CEA, failed to demonstrate a higher incidence of periprocedural complications at 2 yr when CAS was compared to CEA. In addition, the study failed to demonstrate a significant difference in primary outcomes (ipsilateral stroke or death). However, the study failed to demonstrate CAS was noninferior to CEA.

ACUTE GENERAL Rx

- General medical therapy should be aimed at risk factor reduction. As stated earlier, the major risk factors for carotid stenosis are hypertension, diabetes mellitus, dyslipidemia, and smoking (see "Stroke, Secondary Prevention").
- Antiplatelet therapy: Three antiplatelet options are available for patients with carotid stenosis: ASA, ASA plus dipyridamole, and clopidogrel.

DISPOSITION

Disposition and prognosis depend on several variables (Table 1-83): the degree of stenosis, the presence of symptoms, medication compliance, and the type of intervention (if any).

PEARLS & CONSIDERATIONS

There are ongoing studies concerning the best treatment of patients with carotid artery stenosis. Based on the results of these studies, guidelines may change rapidly.

SPECIAL CONSIDERATION

Some studies have shown that in patients with bilateral hemodynamically significant stenosis (>70%), reduction of blood pressure resulted in worse outcome in terms of stroke. These patients would likely be candidates for CEA.

Carotid artery occlusion (100% blockage), for which there is no routine treatment, is being reexamined in the national Carotid Occlusion Surgery Study (http://www.cosstrial.org). Consider referring symptomatic carotid occlusion patients for consideration of this study.

PREVENTION

Prevention of carotid stenosis should be guided at pursuing a healthy lifestyle and management of risk factors for development of atherosclerosis.

PATIENT/FAMILY EDUCATION

Patients should be counseled on pursuing a healthy lifestyle to include exercise and smoking cessation. In addition, patients should take an active role in controlling blood pressure and blood glucose. Further educational materials can be found online at: http://www.strokecenter.org/education.

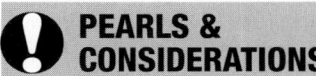 **EVIDENCE**

available at www.expertconsult.com

SUGGESTED READINGS

available at www.expertconsult.com

RELATED CONTENT

Carotid Stenosis (Patient Information)

AUTHOR: **JOSEPH R. OWENS, M.D.**

TABLE 1-83 Carotid Stenosis Management

Degree of Carotid Stenosis	<50%	50%-69%	70%-99%
Asymptomatic	• Medical management	• Men: CEA if stenosis >60% and age <75 yr; otherwise, medical management • Women: medical management	• Men <75 yr: CEA • Women: medical management
Symptomatic	• Medical management	• Men: CEA • Women: medical management	• Men: CEA • Women: CEA

CEA, Carotid endarterectomy.

Diseases and Disorders

I

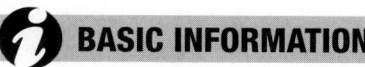
BASIC INFORMATION

DEFINITION

Carpal tunnel syndrome is a compressive neuropathy of the median nerve as it passes under the transverse carpal ligament at the wrist (Fig. E1-189). It is the most common entrapment neuropathy.

ICD-9CM CODES
354.0 Carpal tunnel syndrome

EPIDEMIOLOGY & DEMOGRAPHICS

PREVALENT AGE: 30 to 60 yr
PREVALENT SEX: Females are affected two to five times as often as males.

PHYSICAL FINDINGS & CLINICAL PRESENTATION

- Pain, paresthesia in 1st, 2nd, 3rd, and lateral ½ of 4th fingers, worse at night
- Tinel's sign at wrist (Fig. 1-190): tapping lightly over the median nerve on the volar surface of the wrist produces a tingling sensation radiating from the wrist to the hand
- Phalen's sign (Fig. 1-191): reproduction of symptoms after 1 min of gentle, unforced wrist flexion
- Carpal compression test: direct pressure over the patient's carpal tunnel for 30 sec elicits symptoms
- Findings may be bilateral in up to 65% of patients
- Thenar atrophy in longstanding cases with weakness of thumb abduction and opposition

ETIOLOGY

- Idiopathic in most cases
  - Increased intracarpal tunnel pressure
  - Ischemia, friction, or angulation of median nerve
- Space-occupying lesions in carpal tunnel (tenosynovitis, ganglia, aberrant muscles)
- Can be associated with diabetes, hypothyroidism, pregnancy, connective tissue diseases, acromegaly, amyloidosis
- Repetitive strain or job-related mechanical overuse may be a risk factor
- Crystal-induced rheumatic disorders

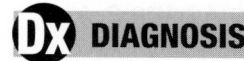
DIAGNOSIS

DIFFERENTIAL DIAGNOSIS

- Cervical radiculopathy
- Chronic tendinitis
- Other arthritides
- Complex regional pain syndrome
- Brachial plexopathy, thoracic outlet syndrome
- Polyneuropathy
- Other entrapment neuropathies
- Traumatic wrist injuries

IMAGING STUDIES

Carpal tunnel syndrome is a clinical diagnosis but imaging may assist workup in uncertain situations. High-resolution ultrasound has been very effective in supporting the diagnosis. Roentgenograms or MRI may be helpful in ruling out other conditions.

ELECTRODIAGNOSTIC STUDIES

Nerve conduction velocity tests demonstrate impaired sensory conduction across the carpal tunnel. Electromyography may show active denervation muscle potentials.

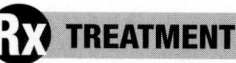
TREATMENT

ACUTE GENERAL Rx

- Activity modification
- Nocturnal wrist splint
- No evidence for effectiveness of NSAIDs
- Corticosteroid injection of carpal canal on ulnar side of palmaris longus tendon proximal to wrist crease: can be done with palpation guidance or under ultrasound guidance
- Low-dose oral corticosteroids can be considered.
- Short-term benefit from ultrasound therapy (physical therapy modality)
- Ergonomic keyboards

DISPOSITION

Clinical course may have remissions and exacerbations. Some may progress from intermittent to persistent sensory complaints (numbness, tingling, paresthesias), then later to develop motor symptoms. In pregnancy, symptoms usually resolve spontaneously weeks after delivery.

REFERRAL

Surgical referral is needed if conservative treatment fails. It is usually reserved for severe symptoms or presence of weakness/thenar atrophy. Surgery (sectioning of transverse carpal ligament) to release pressure on the median nerve is done by open or endoscopic approach, with good long-term results.

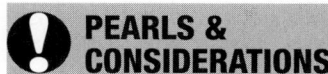
PEARLS & CONSIDERATIONS

- The sensory changes of carpal tunnel syndrome spare the thenar eminence. This distinctive pattern occurs because the palmar sensory cutaneous branch of the median nerve arises proximal to the wrist, passing over, rather than through, the tunnel.
- Role of repetitive hand or wrist use and workplace factors in the development of carpal tunnel syndrome remains controversial.

SUGGESTED READINGS
available at www.expertconsult.com

RELATED CONTENT
Carpal Tunnel Syndrome (Patient Information)

AUTHOR: **CANDICE YUVIENCO, M.D.**

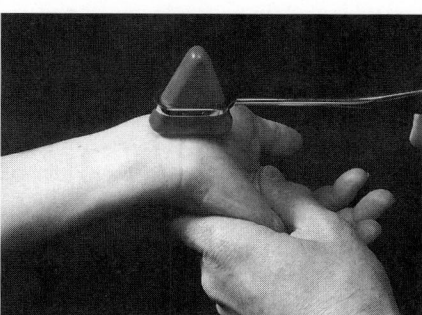

FIGURE 1-190 Tinel's sign. The wrist is held in extension while gentle percussion is performed over and just proximal to the transverse carpal ligament. (From Hochberg MC et al: *Rheumatology,* ed 5, St Louis, 2011, Mosby.)

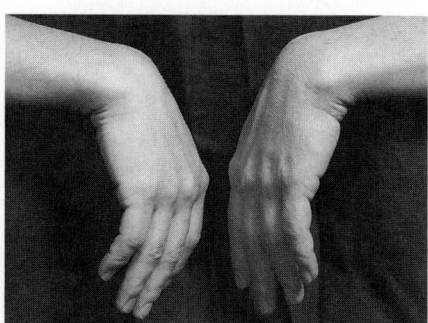

FIGURE 1-191 Phalen's (wrist flexion) test. With the wrists held in unforced flexion for 30 to 60 seconds, a positive test reproduces or worsens the patient's symptoms. (From Hochberg MC et al: *Rheumatology,* ed 5, St Louis, 2011, Mosby.)

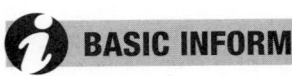 **BASIC INFORMATION**

DEFINITION

Cataracts are the clouding and opacification of the normally clear crystalline lens of the eye. The opacity may occur in the cortex, the nucleus of the lens, or the posterior subcapsular region, but it is usually in a combination of areas.

SYNONYMS

Congenital cataracts (e.g., from rubella)
Metabolic cataracts (e.g., caused by diabetes)
Collagen-vascular disease cataracts (caused by lupus)
Hereditary cataracts
Age-related senile cataracts
Traumatic cataracts
Toxic or drug-induced cataracts (e.g., caused by steroids)
Lenticular opacities

ICD-9CM CODES
366 Cataract

EPIDEMIOLOGY & DEMOGRAPHICS

INCIDENCE (IN U.S.): Most common cause of treatable blindness; cataract removal is the most frequent surgical procedure in patients >65 yr (1.3 million operations per year, with an annual cost of approximately $3 billion). By year 2020 more than 30 million Americans will have cataracts. Of Americans >40 yr, 20.5 million (17.2%) have cataracts. Of these, 5% have had surgery.
PEAK INCIDENCE:
- In early life: congenital and hereditary causes predominant; consider drug related and trauma
- In older age group: senile cataracts (after 40 yr)
PREDOMINANT AGE: Elderly; some stage of cataract development is present in >50% of persons 65 to 74 yr and in 65% of those >75 yr. Lens clouding begins at 39 to 40 yr and then usually progresses either slowly or rapidly depending on individual and health.
GENETICS: Hereditary with syndromes such as galactosemia, homocystinuria, diabetes

PHYSICAL FINDINGS & CLINICAL PRESENTATION
- Cloudiness and opacification of the crystalline lens of the eye (Figs. 1-192 and E1-193)
- Decrease or absence of the red reflex
- Painless decreased visual acuity
- Decreased night vision
- Glare, diplopia

ETIOLOGY
- Heredity
- Trauma
- Toxins
- Age related
- Drug related (e.g., statins)
- Congenital
- Inflammatory
- Diabetes
- Collagen vascular disease

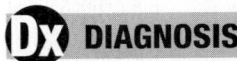 **DIAGNOSIS**

DIFFERENTIAL DIAGNOSIS
- Corneal lesions
- Retinal lesions, detached retina, tumors
- Vitreous disease, chronic inflammation

WORKUP
- Complete eye examination, including slit lamp examination, funduscopic examination, and brightness acuity testing
- Complete physical examination for other underlying causes

LABORATORY TESTS
- Rarely, urinary amino acid screening and central nervous system imaging studies with congenital cataracts
- Fasting glucose in young adults with cataracts
- Diabetes, collagen vascular disease, other metabolic diseases in younger patients
- Genetic and hereditary evaluation

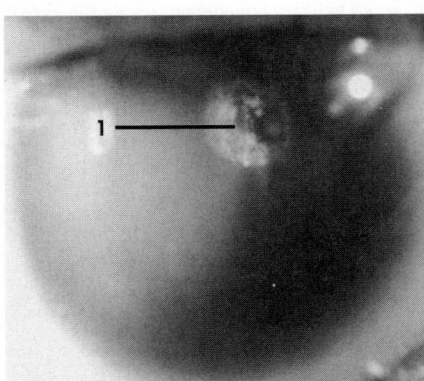

FIGURE 1-192 The central location of a posterior subcapsular cataract *(1)*. (From Palay D [ed]: *Ophthalmology for the primary care physician*, St Louis, 1997, Mosby.)

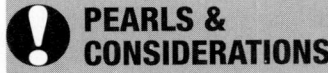 **TREATMENT**

There is no evidence that antioxidants or drugs will slow or treat cataracts.

NONPHARMACOLOGIC THERAPY
- Wait until vision is compromised before doing surgery.
- Surgery is indicated when corrected visual acuity in the affected eye is >20/30 in the absence of other ocular disease; however, surgery may be justified when visual acuity is better in specific situations (especially disabling glare, monocular diplopia). Surgery indicated when vision in one eye is greatly different from the other and affects the patient's life.

ACUTE GENERAL Rx
None necessary except when acute glaucoma or inflammation occurs

CHRONIC Rx
- Change glasses as cataracts develop.
- Myopia is common, and glasses can be adjusted until surgery is contemplated.

DISPOSITION
Refer if sight is compromised or the eye is red or inflamed.

REFERRAL
Refer to ophthalmologist for evaluation for extraction when vision is compromised (see "Nonpharmacologic Therapy").

(!) PEARLS & CONSIDERATIONS

- Patients want to know five things about cataracts:
  1. Chance for vision improvement
  2. When vision will improve
  3. Risk from surgery
  4. Effect of surgery
  5. Types of complications
- Men planning cataract surgery should, if possible, avoid use of alpha blockers until after surgery has been completed. The risk of intraoperative floppy iris syndrome is substantial among men taking tamsulosin, ranging from about 43% to 90%.

SUGGESTED READINGS
available at www.expertconsult.com

RELATED CONTENT
Cataracts (Patient Information)

AUTHORS: **MELVYN KOBY, M.D., FRED F. FERRI, M.D.**

BASIC INFORMATION

DEFINITION

Cat-scratch disease (CSD) is an infectious disease consisting of gradually enlarging regional lymphadenopathy occurring after contact with a feline. Atypical presentations are characterized by a variety of neurologic manifestations as well as granulomatous involvement of the eye, liver, spleen, and bone. The disease is usually self-limiting, and recovery is complete; however, patients with atypical presentations, especially if immunocompromised, may suffer significant morbidity and mortality.

SYNONYMS

Cat-scratch fever
Benign inoculation lymphoreticulosis
Nonbacterial regional lymphadenitis

ICD-9CM CODES
078.3 Cat-scratch disease

EPIDEMIOLOGY & DEMOGRAPHICS

PREVALENCE: Unknown
INCIDENCE (IN U.S.):
- 9 to 10 cases per 100,000 persons per year (22,000 cases per year)
- Majority of reported cases occur in persons <21 yrs

PEAK INCIDENCE: August through January

PHYSICAL FINDINGS & CLINICAL PRESENTATION

- Classic, most common finding: regional lymphadenopathy occurring within 2 wk of a scratch or contact with felines; usually a new kitten in the household
- Tender, swollen lymph nodes most commonly found in the head and neck (Fig. E1-194), followed by the axilla and the epitrochlear, inguinal, and femoral areas
- Erythematous overlying skin, showing signs of suppuration from involved lymph nodes
- On careful examination; evidence of cutaneous inoculation in the form of a nonpruritic, slightly tender pustule or papule
- Fever in most patients
- Malaise and headache in fewer than a third of patients
- Atypical presentations in fewer than 15% of cases
  1. Usually in association with lymphadenopathy and a low-grade or frank fever (>101° F, >38.3° C)
  2. Include granulomatous involvement of the conjunctiva (Parinaud's oculoglandular syndrome) and focal masses in the liver, spleen, and mesenteric nodes
- CNS involvement: neuroretinitis, encephalopathy, encephalitis, transverse myelitis, seizure activity, and coma
- Osteomyelitis in adults and children
- Can be a cause of culture-negative endocarditis
- In HIV-infected and other immunocompromised patients, B. *henselae* is the cause of bacillary angiomatous and peliosis hepatis

ETIOLOGY

- Major cause: *Bartonella henselae,* possibly *Afipia felis* and *Bartonella clarrigeiae*
- Mode of transmission: predominantly by direct inoculation through the scratch, bite, or lick of a cat, especially a kitten
- Also can be transmitted by flea bite (with the flea obtaining the bacteria from a bacteremic cat); rarely after exposure to a dog, probably secondary to flea bites
- Approximately 2 wk after introduction of the bacteria into the host, regional lymphatic tissues displaying granulomatous infiltration associated with gradual hypertrophy
- Possible dissemination to distant sites (e.g., liver, spleen, and bone), usually characterized by focal masses or discrete parenchymal lesions

DIAGNOSIS

DIFFERENTIAL DIAGNOSIS

Granulomas of this syndrome must be differentiated from those associated with:
- Tularemia
- Tuberculosis or other myobacterial infections
- Brucellosis
- Sarcoidosis
- Sporotrichosis or other fungal diseases
- Toxoplasmosis
- Lymphogranuloma venereum
- Benign and malignant tumors such as lymphoma

WORKUP

Diagnosis should be considered in patients who present with a predominant complaint of gradually enlarging regional (focal) lymphadenopathy, often with fever and a recent history of having contact with a cat. A primary ulcer at the site of the cat scratch may or may not be present at the time lymphadenopathy becomes manifest.

LABORATORY TESTS

- Serologies: An IFA or EIA *Bartonella* serology (titer ≥1:64) is diagnostic. A PCR assay on tissue or blood is also available.
- Lymph node biopsy: granulomatous inflammation consistent with CSD.
- Warthin-Starry silver stain on biopsy can identify the bacteria.
- Histopathologically, Warthin-Starry silver stain has been used to identify the bacillus.
- Culture: B. *henselae* is a fastidious, slow-growing, gram-negative rod that requires specific culture techniques for tissue or blood.
- Routine laboratory findings:
  1. Mild leukocytosis or leukopenia
  2. Infrequent eosinophilia
  3. Elevated ESR or CRP
- Abnormalities of bilirubin excretion and elevated hepatic transaminases are usually secondary to hepatic obstruction by granuloma, mass, or lymph node.
- In patients with neurologic manifestations, lumbar puncture usually reveals normal CSF, although there may be a mild pleocytosis and modest elevation in protein.
- CSD skin test is no longer used for clinical purposes.

TREATMENT

NONPHARMACOLOGIC THERAPY

- Warm compresses to the affected nodes
- In cases of encephalitis or coma: supportive care

ACUTE GENERAL Rx

- This disease is typically self-limited and generally resolves within 2 to 6 months. Most studies show no additional benefit from antibiotic therapy.
- It would be prudent to treat severely ill patients, especially if immunocompromised, with antibiotic therapy, because these patients tend to suffer dissemination of infection and increased morbidity.
- *Bartonella* is usually sensitive to a 5-day course of azithromycin, or alternatively tetracycline, sulfa, and the quinolones can be used for 7 to 10 days.
- When the isolate is proven by culture, the patient should receive antibiotic therapy as directed by the obtained susceptibilities.
- Antipyretics and NSAIDs may also be used.

DISPOSITION

Overall prognosis is good.

REFERRAL

- To an appropriate subspecialist to evaluate specific lesions
- For diagnostic aspiration or excision in presence of regional lymphadenopathy, bone lesions, and mesenteric lymph nodes and organs
- To ophthalmologist for ocular granulomas
  1. Usually diagnosed clinically
  2. Rarely require excision

PEARLS & CONSIDERATIONS

COMMENTS

- A presentation of this syndrome, especially in patients with HIV infection or impaired cellular immunity, may be fever of unknown origin.
- Hepatic and splenic granulomas, coronary valve infections may offer few physical clues to diagnosis, emphasizing the need for a complete history.
- CSD should be considered in the differential diagnosis of school-aged children presenting with status epilepticus.
- Chronically immunocompromised patients considering the acquisition of a young feline should be made aware of the possible risk of infection.
- No signs of illness may be apparent in bacteremic kittens.

SUGGESTED READINGS
available at www.expertconsult.com

RELATED CONTENT
Cat-Scratch Disease (Patient Information)

AUTHOR: **GLENN G. FORT, M.D., M.P.H.**

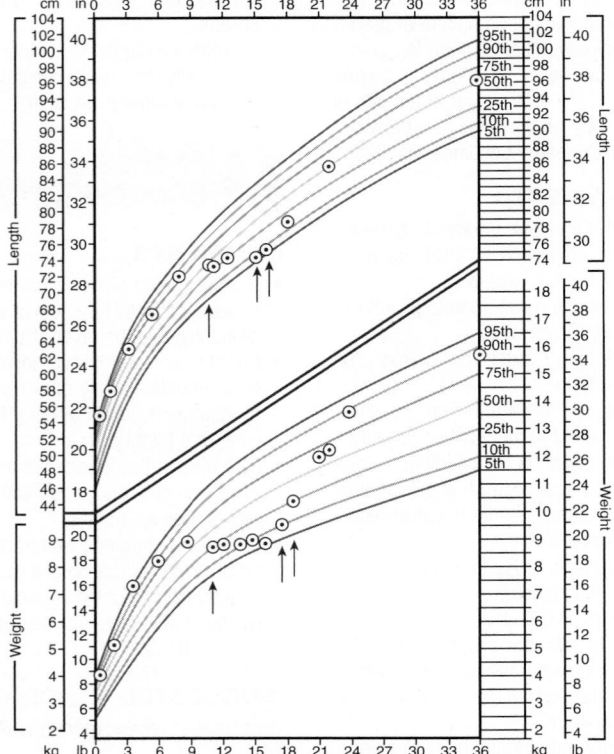

BASIC INFORMATION

DEFINITION

Celiac disease is a chronic autoimmune disease characterized by malabsorption and diarrhea precipitated by ingestion of food products containing gluten. Gluten is a protein complex found in wheat, rye, and barley.

SYNONYMS

Gluten-sensitive enteropathy
Celiac sprue
Nontropical sprue

ICD-9CM CODES
579.0 Celiac disease

EPIDEMIOLOGY & DEMOGRAPHICS

- The prevalence of celiac disease is 1% in the general population in North America and Western Europe and 5% in high-risk groups such as first-degree relatives of persons with the disease. The prevalence of celiac disease in the U.S. has increased fourfold over the past three decades. Worldwide celiac disease affects 0.6% to 1% of the population.
- Incidence is highest during infancy and the first 36 mo of life (after introduction of foods containing gluten), in the third decade (frequently associated with pregnancy and severe anemia during pregnancy), and in the seventh decade.

- There is a slight female predominance.
- The average age of diagnosis is in the fifth decade of life.
- The risk for celiac disease is 5% to 10% in newborn children of parents with the disease and nearly 20% in siblings.
- It is estimated that only 10% to 15% of persons with celiac disease in the U.S. have been diagnosed.

PHYSICAL FINDINGS & CLINICAL PRESENTATION

- Physical examination may be entirely within normal limits.
- Weight loss, dyspepsia, short stature, and failure to thrive may be noted in children and infants (Fig. 1-195).
- Weight loss, fatigue, and diarrhea are common in adults.
- Abdominal pain, nausea, and vomiting are unusual.
- Pallor as a result of iron-deficiency anemia is common.
- Atypical forms of the disease are being increasingly recognized and include osteoporosis, short stature, anemia, infertility, and neurologic problems. Manifestations of calcium deficiency, such as tetany and seizures, are rare and can be exacerbated by coexistent magnesium deficiency.
- Angular cheilitis, aphthous ulcers, atopic dermatitis, and dermatitis herpetiformis are frequently associated with celiac disease.

- Table 1-84 summarizes the clinical spectrum of celiac disease.

ETIOLOGY

- Celiac sprue is considered an autoimmune-type disease, with tissue transglutaminase (tTG) suggested as a major autoantigen. It results from an inappropriate T-cell–mediated immune response against ingested gluten in genetically predisposed individuals who carry either HLA-DQ2 or HLA-DQ8 genes. There is sensitivity to gliadin, a protein fraction of gluten found in wheat, rye, and barley. In patients with celiac disease, immune responses to gliadin fractions promote an inflammatory reaction, mainly in the upper small intestine, manifested by infiltration of the lamina propria and the epithelium with chronic inflammatory cells and villous atrophy.
- Seroconversion to celiac autoimmunity may occur at any time.
- Timing of introduction of gluten into the infant diet is associated with the appearance of celiac disease in children at risk. Children initially exposed to gluten in the first 3 mo of life have a fivefold increased risk. Current recommendations are to delay introduction of gluten into the diet of a genetically susceptible infant until 4 to 6 mo of age while the mother continues to breastfeed.

DIAGNOSIS

Diagnostic criteria for celiac disease require at least four out of five or three out of four if the HLA genotype is not performed:
1. Typical symptoms of celiac disease
2. Positivity of serum celiac disease Ig A class autoantibodies at high titer
3. *HLA-DQ2* or *HLA-DQ8* genotypes

TABLE 1-84 Clinical Spectrum of Celiac Disease

Symptomatic

Frank malabsorption symptoms: chronic diarrhea, failure to thrive, weight loss

Extraintestinal manifestations: anemia, fatigue, hypertransaminasemia, neurologic disorders, short stature, dental enamel defects, arthralgia, aphthous stomatitis

Silent

No apparent symptoms in spite of histologic evidence of villous atrophy

In most cases identified by serologic screening in at-risk groups (see laboratory tests)

Latent

Subjects who have a normal histology, but at some other time, before or after, have shown a gluten-dependent enteropathy

Potential

Subjects with positive celiac disease serology but without evidence of altered jejunal histology

It might or might not be symptomatic

From Kliegman RM et al: *Nelson textbook of pediatrics,* ed 19, Philadelphia, 2011, Saunders.

FIGURE 1-195 Gluten-sensitive enteropathy. Growth curve demonstrates initial normal growth from 0 to 9 mo, followed by onset of poor appetite with intermittent vomiting and diarrhea after initiation of gluten-containing diet *(single arrow).* After biopsy-confirmed diagnosis and treatment with gluten-free diet *(double arrow),* growth improves. (From Kliegman RM et al: *Nelson textbook of pediatrics,* ed 19, Philadelphia, 2011, Saunders.)

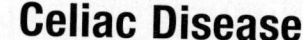

C

4. Celiac enteropathy at the small intestinal biopsy
5. Response to gluten-free diet

DIFFERENTIAL DIAGNOSIS
- Inflammatory bowel disease
- Laxative abuse
- Intestinal parasitic infestations
- Lactose intolerance
- Other: irritable bowel syndrome, tropical sprue, chronic pancreatitis, Zollinger-Ellison syndrome, cystic fibrosis (children), lymphoma, eosinophilic gastroenteritis, short bowel syndrome, Whipple's disease

LABORATORY TESTS
- IgA anti-tTG antibody by enzyme-linked immunosorbent assay (tissue transglutaminase [tTG] test) is the best screening serologic test for celiac disease. IgA antiendomysial antibodies (EMA) test is also a good screening test for celiac disease but is best used as a confirmatory test in cases of borderline positive results. In patients with IgA deficiency, the IgG DPG test (deamidated gliadin peptides) can be used for diagnosis. Screening of close relatives is initially done with PCR testing for HLA DQ2 or HLA DQ8. Thoise that are positive should then have serum tTG IgA screening
- CBC, ferritin level: Iron-deficiency anemia (microcytic anemia, low ferritin level) may be present.
- Celiac disease can lead to malabsorption: Screen for vitamin B_{12} level, folate level, vitamin D level, serum calcium, albumin, magnesium; vitamin B_{12} deficiency, vitamin D deficiency, hypomagnesemia, and hypocalcemia are not uncommon in celiac disease.
- Biopsy of the small bowel, considered the gold standard, has been questioned as a reliable and conclusive test in all cases. It may be reasonable in children with significant elevations of tTG levels (>100 U) to first try a gluten-free diet and consider biopsy in those who do not improve with diet.
- The HLA-DQ2 allele is identified in >90% of patients with celiac disease, and HLA-DQ8 is identified in most of the remaining patients. These genes occur in only 30% to 40% of the general population. Their greatest diagnostic value is in their negative predictive value, making them useful when negative in ruling out the disease.

IMAGING STUDIES
- Consider bone density in newly diagnosed adult patients.
- Capsule endoscopy can be used to evaluate mucosa of the small intestine, especially if future innovations will allow mucosal biopsy.

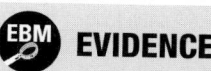 TREATMENT

NONPHARMACOLOGIC THERAPY
Patients should be instructed on a gluten-free diet (avoidance of wheat, rye, and barley). Safe grains (gluten-free) include rice, corn, oats, buckwheat, millet, amaranth, quinoa, sorghum, and teff (an Ethiopian cereal grain). The lowest amount of daily gluten that causes damage to the celiac intestinal mucosa is 10-15 mg/day. One slice of bread contains 1.6 g of gluten.

GENERAL Rx
- Correct nutritional deficiencies with iron, folic acid, calcium, vitamin D, and vitamin B12 as needed.
- Prednisone 20 to 60 mg qd gradually tapered is useful in refractory cases.
- Lifelong gluten-free diet is necessary. A referral to a nutritionist experienced in celiac disease and gluten-free diet is recommended at initial diagnosis.

DISPOSITION
- Prognosis is good with adherence to a gluten-free diet. Rapid improvement is usually seen within a few days of treatment. Healing of the intestinal damage typically occurs within 6-24 mo after initiation of the diet. Lack of response to gluten-free diet occurs in 5% of patients and is due to unintentional ingestion of gluten or presence of coexisting GI disorders such as IBD, lactose or other carbohydrate intolerance, and pancreatic insufficiency.
- Serial antigliadin or antiendomysial antibody tests can be used to monitor the patient's adherence to a gluten-free diet.
- Repeat small-bowel biopsy after treatment generally reveals significant improvement. It is also useful to evaluate for increased risk of small-bowel T-cell lymphoma in these patients, especially untreated patients. Some experts recommend a repeat biopsy only in selected patients who have an unsatisfactory response to a strict gluten-free diet.

⊘ PEARLS & CONSIDERATIONS

COMMENTS
- In close relatives, repeated serum tTG IgA testing may be useful in those with positive HLA DQ2 or HLA DQ8 tests because celiac disease may not manifest until later in life,

and initial negative results do not preclude the possibility of future onset of celiac disease
- Celiac disease should be considered in patients with unexplained metabolic bone disease, osteoporosis, or hypocalcemia, because gastrointestinal symptoms are absent or mild. Clinicians should also consider testing children and young adults for celiac disease if unexplained weight loss, abdominal pain or distention, or chronic diarrhea present.
- Screening for celiac disease is recommended in first-degree relatives. It should also be considered in patients with type 1 diabetes mellitus and in those with certain autoimmune disorders such as primary biliary cirrhosis, primary sclerosing cholangitis, autoimmune hepatitis, IBD, thyroid disease (hypothyroidism occurs in up to 15% of patients with celiac disease), SLE, RA, and Sjogren's syndrome due to increased risk of celiac disease in these populations. Screening persons with Down syndrome or Turner syndrome has also been recommended.
- The prevalence of celiac disease in patients with dyspepsia is twice that of the general population. Screening for celiac disease should be considered in all patients with persistent dyspepsia.
- Patients with celiac disease have an overall risk of cancer that is almost twice that of the general population. The risk of adenocarcinoma of the small intestine is increased manifold compared with the risk in the general population. Celiac disease is also associated with an increased risk for non-Hodgkin's lymphoma, especially of T-cell type and primarily localized in the gut. Lymphoma is 4 to 40 times more common, and death from lymphoma is 11 to 70 times more common in patients with celiac disease.
- Patients with celiac disease who have followed a gluten-free diet for prolonged periods may not experience relapse of symptoms for several months after gluten is reintroduced.

EVIDENCE
available at www.expertconsult.com

SUGGESTED READINGS
available at www.expertconsult.com

RELATED CONTENT
Celiac Disease (Patient Information)
AUTHOR: **FRED F. FERRI, M.D.**

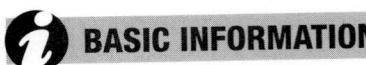

DEFINITION Cellulitis is a superficial inflammatory condition of the skin and underlying tissues characterized by erythema, warmth, and tenderness of the involved area.

SYNONYMS

Erysipelas (cellulitis generally caused by group A β-hemolytic streptococci)
SSSIs (skin and skin structure infections)
ABSSSIs (acute bacterial skin and skin structure infections)

ICD-9CM CODES
682.9 Cellulitis

EPIDEMIOLOGY & DEMOGRAPHICS

- Occurs most frequently in diabetics, immunocompromised hosts, and patients with venous and lymphatic compromise.
- Frequently found near skin breaks (trauma, surgical wounds [surgical site infections develop in 2% to 5% of all surgical procedures], ulcerations, tinea infections). Edema, animal or human bites, subadjacent osteomyelitis, and bacteremia are potential sources of cellulitis.
- Skin and soft-tissue infections (SSTIs) account for more than 14 million outpatient visits in the U.S. each year.

PHYSICAL FINDINGS & CLINICAL PRESENTATION

Variable with the causative organism:
- Erysipelas (Fig. E1-196): superficial-spreading, warm, erythematous lesion distinguished by its indurated and elevated margin; lymphatic involvement and vesicle formation are common.
- Staphylococcal cellulitis: area involved is erythematous, hot, and swollen; differentiated from erysipelas by nonelevated, poorly demarcated margin; local tenderness and regional adenopathy are common; up to 85% of cases occur on the legs and feet.
- *Haemophilus influenzae* cellulitis: area involved is a blue-red/purple-red color; occurs mainly in children; generally involves the face in children and the neck or upper chest in adults.
- *Vibrio vulnificus:* larger hemorrhagic bullae, cellulitis, lymphadenitis, myositis; often found in critically ill patients in septic shock.

ETIOLOGY

- Group A β-hemolytic streptococci (may follow a streptococcal infection of the upper respiratory tract). β-hemolytic streptococci are implicated in most cases of non-traumatic cellulitis.
- Staphylococcal cellulitis: Diabetics, athletes, men who have sex with men, people living in public housing, and incarcerated men are at greater risk for methicillin-resistant *S. aureus* (MRSA) infection. A community-acquired MRSA strain, USA 300, is replacing nosocomial strains of MRSA in hospitals.
- IV drug use: MRSA, *P. aeruginosa.*
- *V. vulnificus:* higher incidence in patients with liver disease (75%) and in immunocompromised hosts (corticosteroid use, diabetes mellitus, leukemia, renal failure). *V. vulnificus*

infection is the leading cause of death related to seafood consumption in the United States.
- *Erysipelothrix rhusiopathiae:* common in people handling poultry, fish, or meat.
- *Aeromonas hydrophila:* generally occurs in contaminated open wounds in fresh water.
- Fungi *(Cryptococcus neoformans):* may be present in immunocompromised granulopenic patients.
- Gram-negative rods *(Serratia, Enterobacter, Proteus, Pseudomonas):* may be present in immunocompromised or granulopenic patients.
- Hot tub exposure: *P. aeruginosa*; fish tank exposure: *Mycobacterium marinum.*
- Bites: Human *(Eikenella corrodens),* dog *(Pasteurella multocida, C. canimorsus),* cat *(P. multocida),* rat *(Streptobacillus moniliformis).*

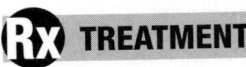 DIAGNOSIS

DIFFERENTIAL DIAGNOSIS

- Necrotizing fasciitis (reddish-purple discoloration of skin, rapid increase in size, woody induration and pale appearance rather than erythema, violaceous bullae, pain out of proportion to appearance, sepsis)
- Deep vein thrombosis
- Peripheral vascular insufficiency
- Paget disease of the breast
- Thrombophlebitis
- Acute gout
- Psoriasis
- *Candida* intertrigo
- Pseudogout
- Osteomyelitis
- Insect bite
- Fixed drug eruption
- Lymphedema
- Contact dermatitis
- Olecranon bursa infection
- Herpetic whitlow, early herpes zoster (before blisters)
- Erythema migrans (Lyme disease)
- Rare: *Vaccinia* vaccination, Kawasaki disease, pyoderma gangrenosum, Sweet syndrome, carcinoma erysipeloides, anaerobic myonecrosis, erythromelalgia, eosinophilic cellulitis (Well's syndrome), familial Mediterranean fever

LABORATORY TESTS

- Gram stain and culture (aerobic and anaerobic):
  1. Aspirated material from:
     a. Advancing edge of cellulitis
     b. Any vesicles
  2. Swab of any drainage material
  3. Punch biopsy (in selected patients)
- Blood cultures in hospitalized patients, in patients who have cellulitis superimposed on lymphedema, in patients with buccal or periorbital cellulitis, and in patients suspected of having a salt-water or fresh-water source of infection. Bacteremia is uncommon in cellulitis (positive blood cultures in only 4% of patients).
- Anti-streptolysin O (ASLO) titer (in suspected streptococcal disease)

Despite the previous measures, the cause of cellulitis remains unidentified in most patients. Patients with recurrent lower-extremity cellulitis should be inspected for tinea pedis. If found it should be treated.

IMAGING STUDIES

CT or MRI in patients with suspected necrotizing fasciitis (deep-seated infection of the subcutaneous tissue that results in the progressive destruction of fascia and fat).

TREATMENT

NONPHARMACOLOGIC THERAPY

Immobilization and elevation of the involved limb. Cool sterile saline dressings to remove purulence from any open lesion. Support stockings in patients with peripheral edema.

ACUTE GENERAL Rx Erysipelas:
- PO: dicloxacillin 500 mg PO q6h
- IV: cefazolin 1 g q6 to 8h or nafcillin 1.0 or 1.5 g IV q4 to 6h

NOTE: Use vancomycin 1 g IV q12h in patients allergic to penicillin.
Staphylococcal cellulitis:
- PO: dicloxacillin 250 to 500 mg qid
- IV: nafcillin 1 to 2 g q4 to 6h
- Cephalosporins (cephalothin, cephalexin, cephradine) also provide adequate antistaphylococcal coverage, except for MRSA.
- Trimethoprim-sulfamethoxazole (160 mg/800 mg 1 PO bid) may be appropriate in mild MRSA infections. Use vancomycin 1.0 to 2.0 g IV qd or linezolid 0.6 g IV q12h in patients allergic to penicillin or cephalosporins and in patients with moderate/severe MRSA. Daptomycin (Cubicin), a cyclic lipopeptide, can be used as an alternative to vancomycin for complicated skin and skin structure infections. Usual dose is 4 mg/kg IV given over 30 min every 24 hr. Telavancin is a new glycopeptide derivative of vancomycin effective for gram-positive skin and skin structure infections, including those caused by MRSA. Tedizolid is an oxazolidinone effective in ABSSSI as an alternative to linezolid. Ceftaroline fosamil (Teflaro) is a new IV cephalosporin also effective against MRSA.

H. influenzae cellulitis:
- PO: cefixime or cefuroxime
- IV: cefuroxime or ceftriaxone

Vibrio vulnificus:
- Doxycycline 100 mg IV bid plus ceftazidime 2 g IV q8h or IV ciprofloxacin 400 mg bid. Mild cases can be treated with oral antibiotics (doxycycline 100 mg bid plus ciprofloxacin 750 mg bid).
- IV support and admission into intensive care unit (mortality rate >50% in septic shock).

E. rhusiopathiae:
- Penicillin

A. hydrophila:
- Aminoglycosides
- Chloramphenicol
- Complicated skin and skin structure infections in hospitalized patients can be treated with daptomycin (Cubicin) 4 mg/kg IV q24h

SUGGESTED READINGS
available at www.expertconsult.com

RELATED CONTENT
Cellulitis (Patient Information)

AUTHOR: **FRED F. FERRI, M.D.**

BASIC INFORMATION

DEFINITION

Cerebral palsy (CP) is a group of disorders of the central nervous system characterized by aberrant control of movement or posture, present since early in life and not the result of a progressive or degenerative disease. Fig. 1-197 provides a classification of CP.

SYNONYMS

Little's disease
Congenital static encephalopathy
Congenital spastic paralysis
CP

ICD-9CM CODES
343 Infantile cerebral palsy
342 Hemiplegia and hemiparesis
344 Quadriplegia and quadriparesiss

EPIDEMIOLOGY & DEMOGRAPHICS

INCIDENCE (IN U.S.): 2 to 2.5 persons per 1000 live births
PREDOMINANT SEX: Males and females affected equally
PREDOMINANT AGE: Diagnosis typically made at 3 to 5 yr

PHYSICAL FINDINGS & CLINICAL PRESENTATION

- Monoplegia, diplegia, quadriplegia, hemiplegia
- Often hypotonic in newborn period, followed by development of hypertonia
- Spasticity
- Athetosis
- Delay in motor milestones
- Hyperreflexia
- Seizures
- Mental retardation in many individuals

ETIOLOGY

Multifactorial, including low birth weight, congenital malformation, asphyxia, multiple gestation, intrauterine exposure to infection, neonatal stroke, hyperbilirubinemia, and maternal thyroid malfunction

DIAGNOSIS

A motor deficit is always present. The usual presenting complaint is that child is not reaching motor milestones at the appropriate age. Medical history establishes that the child is not losing function. This history, combined with a neurologic examination establishing that motor deficit is due to a cerebral abnormality, establishes the diagnosis of CP. Serial examinations may be necessary.

DIFFERENTIAL DIAGNOSIS

Other causes of neonatal hypotonia include muscular dystrophies, spinal muscular atrophy, Down syndrome, and spinal cord injuries.

WORKUP

- Laboratory tests are not necessary to establish the diagnosis.
- Workup is helpful for assessment of recurrence risk, implementation of prevention programs, and medicolegal purposes.

LABORATORY TESTS

- Metabolic and genetic testing should be considered if on follow-up the child has (1) evidence of deterioration or episodes of metabolic decompensation, (2) no etiology determined by neuroimaging, (3) family history of childhood neurologic disorder associated with CP, or (4) developmental malformation on neuroimaging. Hypercoagulability workup should be considered if neuroimaging is suggestive of a remote stroke.
- EEG should be obtained when a child with CP has a history suggestive of seizures.

- Children with CP should be screened for ophthalmologic and hearing impairments, as well as speech and language disorders. Nutrition, growth, and swallowing function should be monitored.

IMAGING STUDIES

- Neuroimaging is recommended if the etiology has not been established previously, for example by perinatal imaging.
- MRI, when available, is preferred to CT scanning because of higher yield in determining an etiology and timing of the insult leading to CP.

TREATMENT

NONPHARMACOLOGIC THERAPY

- Physical therapy, occupational therapy, and speech therapy.
- Orthotics and casting are used to increase musculotendinous length.

ACUTE GENERAL Rx

If present, treatment of seizures

CHRONIC Rx

- Treatment of seizures, as directed by seizure type.
- Medical treatment of spasticity includes baclofen (oral and intrathecal), as well as botulinum toxin A.
- Surgical treatments of spasticity include dorsal rhizotomy, tendon lengthening, and osteotomy.

DISPOSITION

Most children with CP live at home. Those children with severely impaired mobility or other disabilities often live in chronic-care nursing facilities.

REFERRAL

If the child has difficulty with spasticity, physical medicine and rehabilitation referrals are especially helpful.

PEARLS & CONSIDERATIONS

- In full-term infants, there is usually no history of traumatic delivery.
- Compared with delivery at 40 wks' gestation, delivery at 37 or 38 wks or at 42 wks or later was associated with an increased risk of CP.

SUGGESTED READINGS
available at www.expertconsult.com

RELATED CONTENT
Cerebral Palsy (Patient Information)

AUTHOR: **MAITREYI MAZUMDAR, M.D., M.P.H., M.SC.**

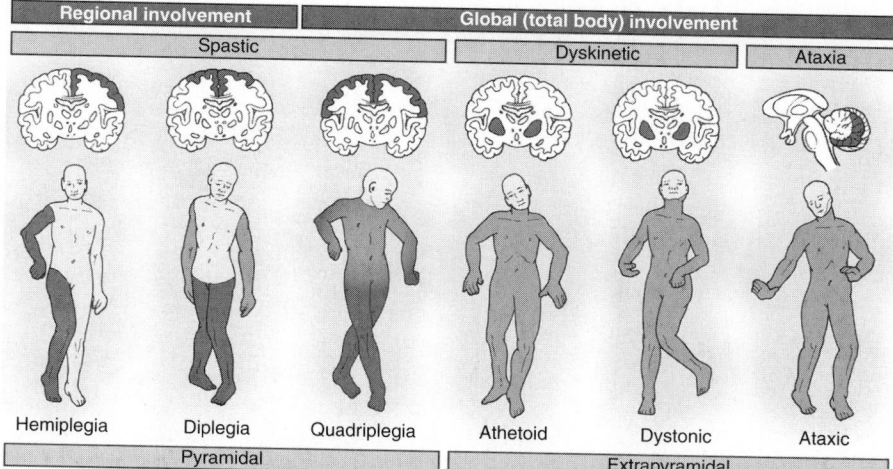

Regional involvement	Global (total body) involvement	
Spastic	Dyskinetic	Ataxia

Hemiplegia	Diplegia	Quadriplegia	Athetoid	Dystonic	Ataxic
Pyramidal			Extrapyramidal		

FIGURE 1-197 Classification of cerebral palsy. Although overlaps in terminology exist, cerebral palsy can be classified according to distribution (regional versus global involvement, hemiplegic, diplegic, quadriplegic), physiologic type (spastic, dyskinetic/dystonic, dyskinetic/athetoid, ataxic), or presumed neurologic substrate (pyramidal, extrapyramidal). (From Canale ST, Beaty JH: *Campbell's operative orthopaedics,* ed 11, Philadelphia, 2007, Mosby.)

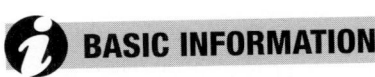

BASIC INFORMATION

DEFINITION
Cerebral vasculitis refers to a group of heterogenous disorders characterized by pathologic inflammation and leukocytoclastic changes in the blood vessel walls.

SYNONYMS
Central nervous system angiitis
Cerebral arteritis

ICD-9CM CODES
437.4 Cerebral arteritis

EPIDEMIOLOGY & DEMOGRAPHICS
INCIDENCE: Average annual incidence rate is 2.4 cases per 1,000,000 person-yr.
PEAK INCIDENCE: Fourth decade of life
PREDOMINANT SEX: Males are affected twice as often as females.
PREDOMINANT AGE: Usual age of presentation is in the third and fourth decades of life, but can present in age ranging from 17 to 70 yr.
GENETICS: Multifactorial
RISK FACTORS: Infections, connective tissue disorders, systemic vasculitis, and substance abuse are the prominent risk factors for secondary cerebral vasculitis.
CLASSIFICATION:
- Primary cerebral vasculitis or primary angiitis of the central nervous system (CNS): involvement of the blood vessels in brain or spinal cord without involvement of blood vessels or organs beyond the CNS.
- Secondary CNS vasculitis (Table 1-85): involvement of the brain or spinal cord blood vessels by a systemic disorder such as systemic vasculitis, connective tissue disorders, infections, malignancy, or substance abuse.

PHYSICAL FINDINGS & CLINICAL PRESENTATION
- Presentation of cerebral vasculitis is diverse and includes the following:
  - Nonspecific symptoms such as weight loss, lethargy, vomiting, headache, and confusion in the early course of the disease.
  - Neurologic manifestations: seen in 80% of patients during course of illness; may mimic multiple sclerosis, with a relapsing and remitting course.
  - Stroke can occur in 40% of the patients; transient ischemic attacks have been reported in 30%-50% of patients.
  - Seizures occur in 25% of patients.
  - Other common presentations include intracerebral hemorrhage (11%) and intracranial space-occupying lesions (15%).
- Secondary vasculitis often presents with stroke-like symptoms. Sjögren's syndrome and Behçet's disease can have varied presentations that mimic multiple sclerosis, seizures, movement disorders, encephalopathy, dementia, and aseptic meningitis.

ETIOLOGY
The exact etiology of primary cerebral vasculitis is unknown. It has been associated with various infectious agents such as herpes zoster, mycoplasma, HIV, and unknown viruses. Amyloid angiopathy has been described with primary cerebral vasculitis.

DIAGNOSIS

DIFFERENTIAL DIAGNOSIS
- Reversible cerebral vasoconstriction syndromes
- Intracranial vessels atherosclerosis
- Cerebral emboli
- Intravascular lymphoma
- Sarcoidosis

TABLE 1-85 Common Causes of Secondary Cerebral Vasculitis and Associated Features

Giant cell arteritis/Takayasu's arteritis	"Pulseless disease," fever, weight loss, syncope, visual field defects
Polyarteritis nodosa	Fever, weight loss, arthralgia, renal failure, myocardial infarction
Churg-Strauss syndrome	Asthma-like features followed by multiple-organ system involvement including GI, skin, kidneys, CNS, heart
Wegener's granulomatosis	Rhinitis, epistaxis, hemoptysis, hematuria, chronic renal failure
Behçet's disease	Oral ulcers, genital ulcers, skin lesions, uveitis, iritis
Systemic lupus erythematosus	Malar rash, oral ulcers, photosensitivity, arthralgia, renal failure, anemia, ANA positive
Rheumatoid arthritis	Arthritis involving hand joints, radiologic evidence of joint erosion, rheumatoid factor positive
Sjögren's syndrome	Dry mouth, dry eyes, involvement of lung, liver, pancreas, joints
Lymphoma	Fever, weight loss, night sweats, lymph node enlargement, hepatosplenomegaly

- Cerebral autosomal dominant arteriopathy with subcortical infarcts and leukoencephalopathy (CADASIL)

WORKUP
- Brain biopsy (usually nondominant temporal lobe tip along with overlying leptomeninges) is the gold standard for diagnosis of cerebral vasculitis.
- Cerebral angiography supports the diagnosis of CNS vasculitis but has low sensitivity and specificity (Fig. 1-198).

LABORATORY TESTS
- Lumbar puncture: may show elevated cerebrospinal fluid opening pressure, elevated protein, lymphocytic pleocytosis, and negative microbial cultures.

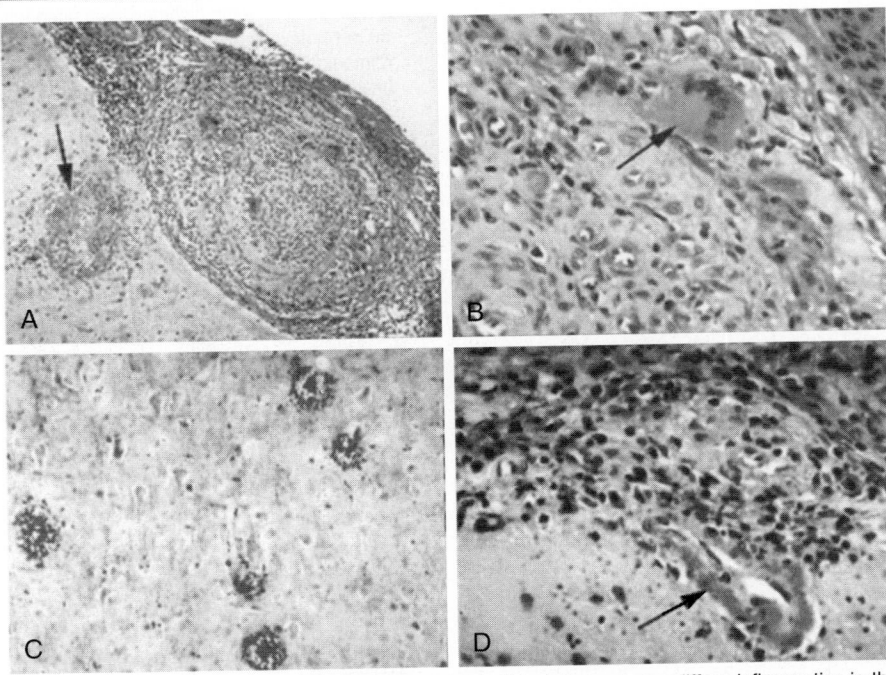

FIGURE 1-198 A, Low-power hematoxylin and eosin stain (10×) demonstrates diffuse inflammation in the leptomeninges with infiltration of lymphocytes, eosinophils, and macrophages with destruction of the vessel wall. **B,** A multinucleated giant cell *(arrow)*. **C,** Multiple neuritic plaques are seen on this silver stain. **D,** Congo red stain demonstrating the presence of amyloid within a vessel wall *(arrow)*. (From Jacobs DA et al: Primary central nervous system angiitis, amyloid angiopathy and Alzheimer's pathology presenting with Balint's syndrome, *Surv Ophthalmol* 49[4]:454-459, 2004.)

- Basic laboratory testing: should include CBC with differential, blood urea nitrogen and serum creatinine, hepatic functions and enzymes, erythrocyte sedimentation rate, RPR (for syphilis), C-reactive protein, and urine analysis.
- Specific serologic tests to evaluate autoimmune causes: ANA, rheumatoid factor, anti–double-stranded DNA, anti SS-A, anti SS-B, anti–neutrophil cytoplasmic antibody (ANCA), complement 3 and 4, cryoglobulins, serum immunoglobulins, and HIV testing.

IMAGING STUDIES

Magnetic resonance imaging (MRI) is the neuroimaging of choice. Abnormal findings are seen in 90% to 100% of the patients. Cerebral cortex, deep white and gray matter changes are commonly reported (Fig. 1-199).

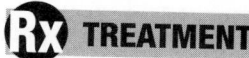

TREATMENT

There are no randomized controlled trials evaluating treatment of cerebral vasculitis. Treatment strategies are similar to other systemic vasculitis.

NONPHARMACOLOGIC THERAPY

Patients with permanent deficits are provided with physical and occupational therapy.

ACUTE GENERAL Rx

- Steroids: For suspected cases, empiric therapy with glucocorticoids is started after exclusion of infectious causes. Intravenous methylprednisolone 1 g daily for 3 days is preferred for patients with severe disease; otherwise, oral prednisone is started at 1 mg/kg/day.

CHRONIC Rx

- Steroids: Oral prednisone is continued at high dose (1 mg/kg/day) for 4 to 6 wk and then tapered over 12 mo.
- Immunosuppressive treatment: cyclophosphamide orally for 3 to 6 months for remission induction. Once stable, milder and relatively safer immunosuppressants such as azathioprine, methotrexate, or mycophenolate are used for 2 to 3 years.

DISPOSITION

Course and prognosis of the disease is variable. It depends on the extent of neurologic involvement, severity of deficits, and response to treatment. Neurologic deficits may resolve acutely, slowly, or not at all. Some patients have symptomatic improvement with resolution of headache or altered mental status. Some have improvement in laboratory values, and others have improved MRI scans.

REFERRAL

- Neurology: referral to neurology is indicated in patients with neurologic deficits of uncertain etiology, younger age, intractable headaches, or uncertain diagnosis.
- Neurosurgical consult for brain biopsy.

PEARLS & CONSIDERATIONS

COMMENTS

- Cerebral vasculitis is a rare disorder that is difficult to diagnose because of variable presentation.
- Early recognition of the clinical symptoms and signs is important to prevent long-term morbidity and mortality.
- Systemic causes should be excluded.
- Patients may need chronic immunosuppressive treatment.

SUGGESTED READINGS

available at www.expertconsult.com

RELATED CONTENT

Vasculitis (Related Key Topic)

AUTHOR: **FARIHA ZAHEER, M.D.**

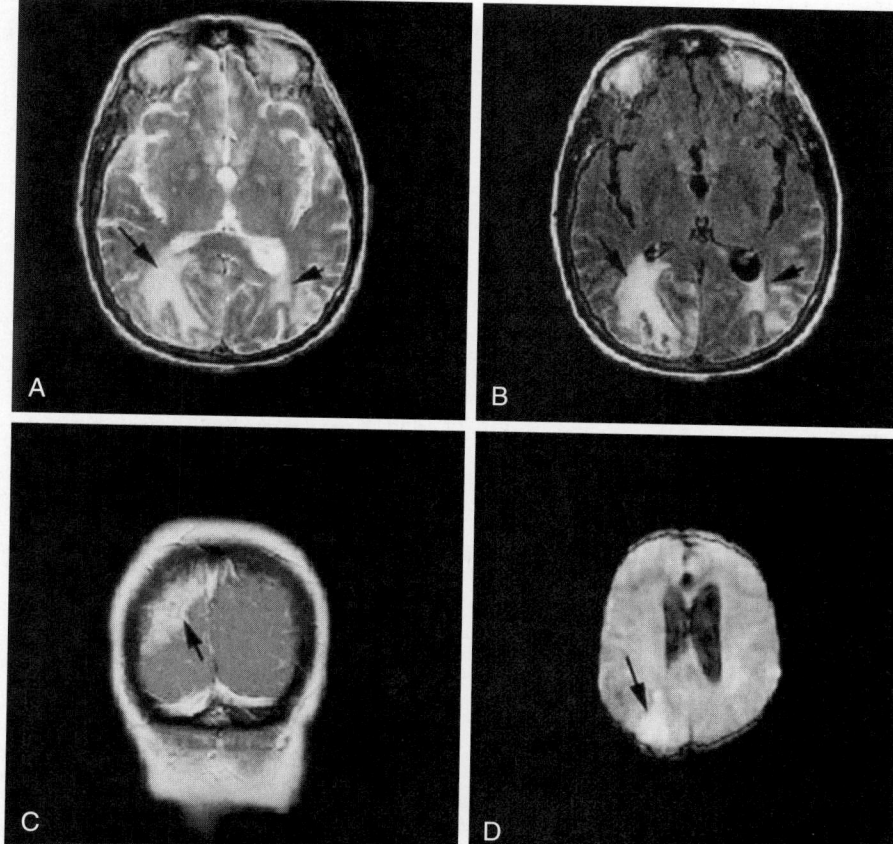

FIGURE 1-199 A, Axial T2-weighted image shows abnormal signal in bilateral parietooccipital lobes, greater on the right than left *(arrows)*. **B,** Axial fluid attenuated inversion recovery image further delineating the extent of bilateral parietooccipital lesions *(arrow)*. **C,** Coronal T1-gadolinium study demonstrating nodular leptomeningeal enhancement in the lesion *(arrow)*. **D,** Diffusion-weighted magnetic resonance imaging shows bright signal in the right parietooccipital region, suggesting ischemic changes *(arrow)*. (From Jacobs DA et al: Primary central nervous system angiitis, amyloid angiopathy and Alzheimer's pathology presenting with Balint's syndrome, *Surv Ophthalmol* 49[4]:454-459, 2004.)

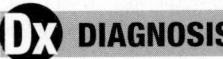 **BASIC INFORMATION**

DEFINITION

Cervical cancer is the penetration of the basement membrane and infiltration of the stroma of the uterine cervix by malignant cells.

ICD-9CM CODES
180 Malignant neoplasm of cervix uteri

EPIDEMIOLOGY & DEMOGRAPHICS

INCIDENCE: There are approximately 15,000 new cases annually, with 4000 to 5000 associated deaths. The U.S. has an age-adjusted mortality rate of 2.6 per 100,000 persons for cervical cancer.
PREDOMINANCE: Higher incidence rates occur in developing countries. Among the U.S. population, Hispanics have a higher incidence than African Americans, who likewise have a higher incidence than whites. Worldwide, cervical cancer is the third most common cancer in women.
RISK FACTORS: Smoking, early age at first intercourse, multiple sexual partners, immunocompromised state, nonbarrier methods of birth control, infection with high-risk human papillomavirus (HPV; types 16 and 18), and multiparity.

PHYSICAL FINDINGS & CLINICAL PRESENTATION

- Unusual vaginal bleeding, particularly postcoital
- Vaginal discharge and/or odor
- Advanced cases may present with lower extremity edema or renal failure
- In early stages there may be little or no obvious cervical lesion; more advanced cases may present with large, bulky, friable lesions encompassing the majority of the vagina

ETIOLOGY

- Infection with high-risk HPV types is a necessary, although not sufficient, cause of almost all cases of cervical cancer. Persistent HPV infection leads to precancerous changes of the cervix, known as cervical intraepithelial neoplasia (CIN). CIN can progress over time to invasive cervical cancer.
- More than 40 HPV types can infect the cervix. Most cases of cervical cancer are believed to be linked to the presence of HPV 16, 18, 45,

and 56 by interaction of E6 oncoprotein on p53 gene product.
- There may be an association with past infection with *Chlamydia trachomatis.*

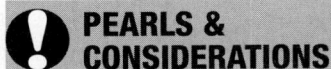 **DIAGNOSIS**

DIFFERENTIAL DIAGNOSIS

- Cervical polyp or prolapsed uterine fibroid
- Preinvasive cervical lesions
- Neoplasia metastatic from a separate primary neoplasia

WORKUP

- Thorough history and physical examination.
- Pelvic examination with careful rectovaginal examination.
- Compared with Pap testing, HPV testing has a greater sensitivity for the detection of CIN. The addition of an HPV test for high-risk types to the Pap test to screen women in their mid-30s for cervical cancer reduces the incidence of grade 2 or 3 CIN or cancer detected by subsequent screening examinations.
- Colposcopy with directed biopsy and endocervical curettage.
- FIGO staging of cervical cancer is described in Table 1-86.

LABORATORY TESTS

- Complete blood count, chemistry profile
- SCC antigen in research setting
- Carcinoembryonic antigen

IMAGING STUDIES

- Chest x-ray
- Depending on stage, may need cystoscopy, sigmoidoscopy or barium enema, CT scan or MRI (Fig. E1-200), lymphangiography
- Intravenous pyelogram

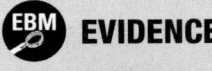 **TREATMENT**

NONPHARMACOLOGIC THERAPY

- FIGO stage IA: cone biopsy or simple hysterectomy
- FIGO stage IB or IIA: type III radical hysterectomy and pelvic lymphadenectomy or pelvic radiation therapy
- Advanced or bulky disease: multimodality therapy (radiation, chemotherapy, and/or surgery); platinum use before radiation therapy

ACUTE GENERAL Rx

Table 1-96 summarizes treatment according to tumor stage. Chemotherapy is cisplatin-based. In advanced cases, cervical cancer may present with massive and acute vaginal bleeding requiring volume and blood replacement, vaginal packing or other hemostatic modalities, and/or high-dose local radiotherapy.

CHRONIC Rx

- Physical examination with Pap smear every 3 mo for 2 yr, every 6 mo during the third to fifth year, and annually thereafter
- Chest x-ray examination annually

DISPOSITION

Five-year survival varies by stage:
- Stage I: 60% to 90%
- Stage II: 40% to 80%
- Stage III: <60%
- Stage IV: <15%
  Early detection by Pap smear is imperative to long-term improvements in survival.

REFERRAL

Gynecologic oncologist for all invasive disease

PEARLS & CONSIDERATIONS

- Gardasil is a vaccine indicated in girls and women age 9-26 yr for the prevention of cervical cancer caused by HPV types 6, 11, 16, and 18. In October 2009 the FDA approved the use of Gardasil for boys and men age 9-26 yr as well.
- Available evidence supports discontinuation of cervical cancer screening among women aged 65 yrs or older who have had adequate screening and are not otherwise at high risk.

EVIDENCE

available at www.expertconsult.com

SUGGESTED READINGS
available at www.expertconsult.com

RELATED CONTENT

Cervical Dysplasia (Related Key Topic)
Cervical Cancer (Patient Information)

AUTHORS: **GIL M. FARKASH, M.D.,** and **RUBEN ALVERO, M.D.**

TABLE 1-86 FIGO Staging of Cervical Cancer

Stage	Invasion	Prognosis 5-yr Survival	Treatment
1$_{A1}$	Depth of invasion up to 3 mm and width up to 7 mm (includes early stromal invasion of up to 1 mm)	84-90% if tumor < 3 cm; 85% will have negative pelvic nodes and 95% of these patients will be 'cured'	Local excision; if margins of a cone clear (i.e., no residual tumor or CIN) then conization is adequate, with no need for pelvic lymphadenectomy
1$_{A2}$	Depth of invasion between 3 and 5 mm (i.e., 3.1-5 mm) and width up to 7 mm		Simple hysterectomy and pelvic lymphadenectomy
1$_{B1}$	Tumor confined to cervix and diameter less than 4 cm	66% if tumor > 3 cm	Radical hysterectomy or radiotherapy
1$_{B2}$	Tumor confined to cervix and diameter more than 4 cm		Radical hysterectomy or radiotherapy
II$_A$	Upper 1/3 vagina	62%	Radical hysterectomy or radiotherapy
II$_B$	Upper 2/3 of vagina plus parametrial disease		Radiotherapy ± chemotherapy
III$_A$	Lower 1/3 vagina	40%	Radiotherapy ± chemotherapy
III$_B$	Pelvic sidewall and/or hydronephrosis		Radiotherapy ± chemotherapy
IV$_A$	Bladder, rectum	15%	Radiotherapy ± chemotherapy
IV$_B$	Beyond pelvis		Radiotherapy ± chemotherapy

From Drife J, Magowan B: *Clinical obstetrics and gynecology,* Philadelphia, 2004, Saunders.

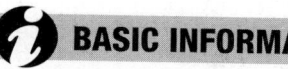

BASIC INFORMATION

DEFINITION

Cervical disk syndromes refer to diseases of the cervical spine resulting from disk disorder, either herniation or degenerative change (spondylosis). When posterior osteophytes compress the anterior spinal cord, lower extremity symptoms may result, a condition called *cervical spondylotic myelopathy*.

ICD-9CM CODES
722.4   Degenerative intervertebral cervical disk
722.71 Degenerative cervical disk with myelopathy

EPIDEMIOLOGY & DEMOGRAPHICS

PREVALENCE: 10% of general adult population (symptoms in 50% of population at some time in their life)
PREDOMINANT SEX: Males and females affected equally
PREDOMINANT AGE: 30 to 60 yr

PHYSICAL FINDINGS & CLINICAL PRESENTATION

- Neck pain, radicular symptoms, or myelopathy, either alone or in combination
- Limited neck movement
- Pain with neck motion, especially extension
- Referred unilateral interscapular pain, resulting in a local trigger point
- Radicular arm pain (usually unilateral), numbness, and tingling possible, most commonly involving the C6 (C5-C6 disk) or C7 (C6-C7 disk) nerve root
- Weakness and reflex changes (C6, biceps; C7, triceps)
- Myelopathy, possibly resulting in gait disturbance, weakness, and even spasticity
- Sensory examination usually not helpful

ETIOLOGY

Unknown

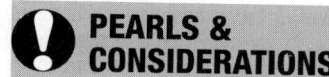

DIAGNOSIS

DIFFERENTIAL DIAGNOSIS

- Rotator cuff tendinitis
- Carpal tunnel syndrome
- Thoracic outlet syndrome
- Brachial neuritis

A differential diagnosis for evaluation of neck pain is described in Section II.

WORKUP

- In most cases, the diagnosis can be established on a clinical basis alone.
- Fig. E1-201 describes an algorithm for a workup of suspected cases.

IMAGING STUDIES

- Plain roentgenograms within the first few weeks
  1. Usually normal in soft disk herniation
  2. With chronic degenerative disk disease, usually loss of height of the disk space, anterior and posterior osteophyte formation, and encroachment on the intervertebral foramen by osteophytes
- Myelography, CT scanning, and MRI indicated in patients whose symptoms do not resolve or when other spinal pathology suspected
- Electrodiagnostic studies to confirm the diagnosis or rule out peripheral nerve disorders

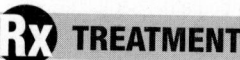

TREATMENT

NONPHARMACOLOGIC THERAPY

- Rest and cervical collar if needed
- Local modalities such as heat
- Physical therapy (Fig. 1-202)
- Avoid extreme range-of-motion exercises in degenerative disk disease

ACUTE GENERAL Rx

- Nonsteroidal anti-inflammatory drugs
- "Muscle relaxants" for their sedative effect
- Analgesics as needed
- Epidural steroid injection for radicular pain

DISPOSITION

- Usually improves with time
- Surgical intervention in <5%

REFERRAL

Orthopedic or neurosurgical consultation for intractable pain or neurologic deficit

PEARLS & CONSIDERATIONS

Myelopathy from cervical spondylosis is the most common cause of acquired spastic paralysis in the adult and is usually progressive. Whether to intervene surgically is a complicated decision in these patients.

COMMENTS

- Pain relief with physical therapy seems anecdotal and short lived; any overall improvement usually parallels what would have probably occurred naturally.
- Sometimes carpal tunnel syndrome and cervical radiculopathy occur together; this is called *double-crush syndrome* and results from nerve compression at two separate levels. Proximal compression may decrease the ability of the nerve to tolerate a second, more distal compression.
- Surgical intervention is indicated primarily for relief of radicular pain caused by nerve root compression or for the treatment of myelopathy; it is generally not helpful when the chief complaint is neck pain alone.
- In many cases of cervical spondylosis with myelopathy, the lower extremity symptoms are much more disabling than the neck symptoms, a situation that can cause some difficulty in determining their etiology.

SUGGESTED READINGS
available at www.expertconsult.com

RELATED CONTENT
Cervical Disc Syndrome (Patient Information)

AUTHOR: **LONNIE R. MERCIER, M.D.**

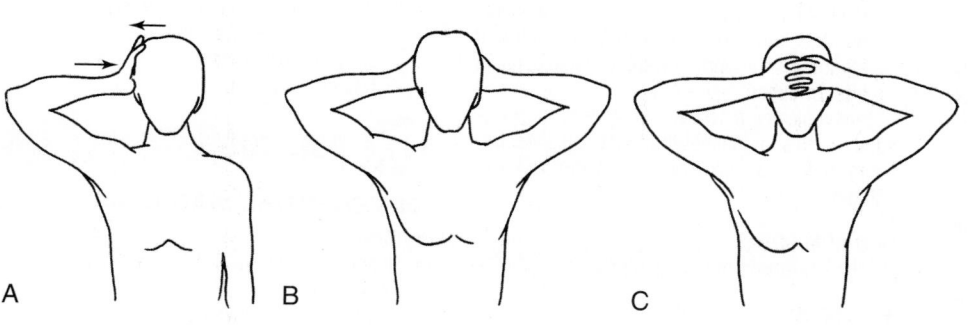

FIGURE 1-202 Isometric neck exercises. A, The hand is placed against the side of the head slightly above the ear, and pressure is gradually increased while resisting with the neck muscles and keeping the head in the same position. The position is held 5 sec, relaxed, and repeated five times. **B,** The exercise is performed on the other side and then from the back and front **(C).** The exercise should be performed three to four times daily. (From Mercier LR [ed]: *Practical orthopedics*, ed 4, St Louis, 1995, Mosby.)

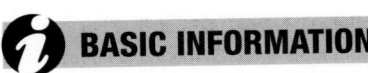

BASIC INFORMATION

DEFINITION

Cervical dysplasia refers to atypical development of immature squamous epithelium that does not penetrate the basement epithelial membrane. Characteristics include increased cellularity, nuclear abnormalities, and increased nuclear:cytoplasmic ratio. A progressive loss of squamous differentiation exists beginning adjacent to the basement membrane and progressing to the most advanced stage (severe dysplasia), which encompasses the complete squamous epithelial layer thickness. The revised 2001 Bethesda System terminology was used in a National Institutes of Health consensus conference, sponsored by the American Society for Colposcopy and Cervical Pathology (ASCCP) and its partner professional organizations in 2006. The conference updated therapeutic options for women based on studies such as the **A**SC-US (atypical squamous cells of undetermined significance)/**L**SIL (low-grade squamous intraepithelial lesions) **T**riage **S**tudy (ALTS) that appeared after revision of the Bethesda classification.

BETHESDA 2001 UPDATED CLASSIFICATION:

The Bethesda 2001 System was the result of a year-long iterative process held to update the original 1991 system and to broaden participation in the consensus process, clarify reporting of abnormalities, and incorporate data that had been collected since the initial system was created.

The reporting system includes the following areas:

Specimen adequacy: The system defines the specimen as either satisfactory for evaluation or unsatisfactory and then specifies the reason for inadequacy if necessary.

General categorization (optional): This serves to triage the specimen into normal finding (negative for intraepithelial lesion or malignancy) or identifies it as an "epithelial abnormality." The descriptions are meant to be mutually exclusive.

Interpretation/result: Makes a distinction between "interpretation" and "diagnosis" of the specimen so that the interpretation may be incorporated into the overall clinical context for the particular patient being evaluated.

Negative for intraepithelial lesion or malignancy: In this screening test, no intraepithelial lesion or malignancy is identified. Non-neoplastic findings such as organisms or reactive cellular findings may be specified but are still considered to be a negative result.

Epithelial cell abnormalities:

Squamous cell:

- Atypical squamous cell (ASC) of undetermined significance (ASC-US) emphasizing the unusual but still possible association with underlying cervical intraepithelial neoplasia (CIN) II/III and extremely rare possibility of squamous cell carcinoma
- ASC cannot exclude high-grade squamous intraepithelial lesion (HSIL) (ASC-H), suggesting a risk for CIN II/III that is intermediate between ASC-US and HSIL
- Low-grade squamous intraepithelial lesion (LSIL) suggests a transient viral infection with a greater likelihood for regression, more likely to encompass human papillomavirus (HPV) infection and CIN I histologically
- HSIL suggestive of a more persistent viral infection and with a greater risk for progressive disease, more likely to encompass CIN II/III and carcinoma in situ (CIS) histologically
- Squamous cell carcinoma

Glandular cell

- Atypical glandular cells (should specify endocervical, endometrial, or not otherwise specified)
- Atypical glandular cell, favor neoplasia (should specify endocervical or not otherwise specified)
- Endocervical adenocarcinoma in situ (AIS)
- Adenocarcinoma

Other: Endometrial cells in a woman ≥40 yr of age. Because menopausal status is sometimes uncertain, age was chosen to discriminate women who might, with the findings of endometrial cells on cytology, warrant further evaluation with endometrial sampling

KEY POINTS:

1. The cytologic distinction of low grade (LSIL) and high grade (HSIL) do not necessarily equate to the histologic classifications CIN I and CIN II/III.
2. The 2006 conference notes that one cytologic abnormality can have different histologic risk in different women and highlights "special populations" such as adolescent and young women, and those women who are pregnant. In young women, spontaneous HPV clearance rates are exceptionally high; therefore, it is worthwhile to defer aggressive evaluative and therapeutic steps to assess whether spontaneous remission has taken place. In pregnant women, colposcopy may be deferred if the patient is at low risk for invasive cancer, and therapy should take place only if there is a strong suspicion for carcinoma.
3. DNA testing for high-risk HPV types is incorporated into the evaluation and treatment algorithms for women with cytologic cervical abnormalities.

Histologically, a two-tiered system is developed in this guideline that distinguishes between the lower risk CIN I and higher risk CIN II/III diagnoses.

ICD-9CM CODES
622.1 Dysplasia of cervix (uteri)

EPIDEMIOLOGY & DEMOGRAPHICS

PREDOMINANT AGE:

- Dysplasia: peak age, 26 yr (3600 cases/100,000 persons)
- CIS: peak age, 32 yr (1100 cases/100,000 persons)
- Invasive cancer: peak age >60 yr (800 cases/100,000 persons)

PEAK INCIDENCE:

- Age 35 yr
- Abnormal Pap smear rate revealing dysplasia approximates 2% to 5% depending on population risk factors and false-negative rate variance
- False-negative rate approaching 40%
- Average age-adjusted incidence of severe dysplasia is 35 cases/100,000 persons

PHYSICAL FINDINGS & CLINICAL PRESENTATION

- Cervical lesions associated with dysplasia often are not visible to the naked eye; therefore, physical findings are best viewed by colposcopy of a 3% acetic acid–prepared cervix.
- Patients evaluated by colposcopy are identified by abnormal cervical cytology screening from Pap smear screening.
- Colposcopic findings:
  1. Leukoplakia (white lesion seen by the unaided eye that may represent condyloma, dysplasia, or cancer)
  2. Acetowhite epithelium with or without associated punctation, mosaicism, abnormal vessels
  3. Abnormal transformation zone (abnormal iodine uptake, "cuffed" gland openings)

ETIOLOGY

- Strongly associated and initiated by oncogenic HPV infection (high-risk HPV types are 16, 18, 31, 33, 35, 45, 51, 52, 56, and 58; low-risk HPV types are 6, 11, 42, 43, and 44)
- Risk factors:
  - HPV
  - Any heterosexual coitus
  - Coitus during puberty (transformation-zone metaplasia peak)
  - Diethylstilbestrol exposure
  - Multiple sexual partners
  - Lack of prior Pap smear screening
  - History of STD
  - Other genital tract neoplasia
  - HIV
  - Tuberculosis
  - Substance abuse
  - "High-risk" male partner (HPV)
  - Low socioeconomic status
  - Early first pregnancy
  - Tobacco use

DIAGNOSIS

DIFFERENTIAL DIAGNOSIS

- Metaplasia
- Hyperkeratosis
- Condyloma
- Microinvasive carcinoma
- Glandular epithelial abnormalities
- Vulvar intraepithelial neoplasm
- Vaginal intraepithelial neoplasm
- Metastatic tumor involvement of the cervix

C

WORKUP

- Periodic history and physical examination (including cytologic screening) depending on age, risk factors, and history of preinvasive cervical lesions
- Consider screening for sexually transmitted disease (gonorrhea, *Chlamydia,* herpes, HIV, HPV)
- Abnormal cytology (HSIL/LSIL, initial ASC/ASC-US/ASC-H in high-risk patients, recurrent in low-risk/postmenopausal patients) and grossly evident suspicious lesions; refer for colposcopy and possible directed biopsy/endocervical cu-rettage (ECC) (examination should include cervix, vagina, vulva, and anus)
- For glandular cell abnormalities (AGCs): refer for colposcopy and possible directed biopsy/ECC, and consider endometrial sampling
- In pregnancy: abnormal cytology followed by colposcopy in the first trimester and at 28 to 32 wk; only high-grade lesions suspect for cancer biopsied; ECC contraindicated

LABORATORY TESTS

- Gonorrhea, Chlamydia to rule out STD
- Pap cytology screening (requires appropriate sampling, preparation, cytologist interpretation, and reporting)
- Colposcopy and directed biopsy, ECC for indications (see "Workup")
- HPV DNA typing if identified abnormal cytology
- As compared with Pap testing, HPV testing has greater sensitivity for the detection of intraepithelial neoplasia

IMAGING STUDIES

- Cervicography
- Computer-enhanced Pap cytology screening (e.g., PAPNET)

MANAGEMENT

Refer to the literature for a more comprehensive approach. The following treatment paradigms give a general outline for care. Where identified below, HPV status refers to oncogenic types (e.g., 16, 18, 31, 33, 35, 45, 51, 52, 56, 58)

- ASC-US: Patients with ASC-US who are HPV negative can repeat cytologic screen in 12 mo. Women who have oncogenic HPV type should have colposcopy performed. Adolescent women should not have HPV testing performed and can be followed with cytologic screen, with colposcopy performed if ASC-US persists after 24 mo or if HSIL is found. Pregnant women can be followed as with nonpregnant women; but if colposcopy is deferred, it can be deferred until at least 6 wk after delivery. Pregnant women should not have endocervical curettage performed.
- ASC-H: Patients with ASC-H should have a colposcopic evaluation.
- LSIL: Colposcopy with endocervical biopsy is recommended for women with LSIL. Adolescent women with LSIL may be followed with cytology at 12 and 24 mo, and referred for colposcopy if they retain a finding of ASC-US or greater. Postmenopausal women may have DNA testing and be referred for colposcopy if

this test is positive for oncogenic HPV type. Pregnant women should have colposcopy, but this procedure may be deferred until the patient is postpartum, particularly if there is no other clinical suspicion for higher grade lesions.
- HSIL: Either colposcopy with endocervical curettage or immediate loop electrosurgical excision procedures (LEEPs) are acceptable with HSIL. If CIN II/III is not found by either method, the patient may be followed colposcopically or a LEEP performed if only colposcopy was initially used. If CIN II/III is identified by adequate colposcopy, a LEEP or ablation may be performed. Adolescent girls in whom CIN II/III is not identified may be observed by colposcopy and cytology at 6-mo intervals up to 24 mo. If CIN II/III persists for 24 mo, then the adolescent girl may be treated by excisional or ablative therapy. Pregnant women should have colposcopy and biopsies performed where CIN II/III or cancer is suspected. Colposcopy should be performed 6 wk or later after delivery when CIN II/III is not found antepartum.
- AGC/AIS: Colposcopy with endocervical biopsy should be performed in these women. In women older than 35 and in women with high risk for endometrial hyperplasia or carcinoma (oligo-ovulation, unscheduled bleeding), an endometrial biopsy should also be performed. Pregnant women should also be colposcoped, but endocervical and endometrial curettings should not be performed during the gestation.

DISPOSITION

- Because of the large number of women in high-risk groups, the prevalence of HPV, and the high false-negative Pap smear rate, routine Pap smear screening should be strongly encouraged for all women, especially those with a history of cervical dysplasia. The addition of an HPV test to the Pap test reduces the incidence of CIN II or III, or cancer detected by subsequent screening.
- Success rates for treatment approach 80% to 90%.
- Detection of persistence of recurrence requires careful follow-up.
- Cervical treatment possibly results in infertility (cervical stenosis or incompetence), which requires careful consideration and discretion for use of LEEP and cone biopsy.
- Appropriate counseling and informed consent are needed when considering any form of management of cervical dysplasia.

REFERRAL

- Patients with abnormal Pap cytology should not be monitored by repeat Pap smear screening.
- Patients with identified abnormal cytology should be evaluated by a skilled colposcopist (defined as documented didactic and preceptorship training, including 50 cases of identified pathology, ongoing colposcopy activity with a minimum of 2 cases/wk, quality-assurance log, and periodic continuing medical education).
- If treatment is required, patient should be referred to a gynecologist or gynecologic

oncologist skilled in the diagnosis and treatment of preinvasive cervical disease.

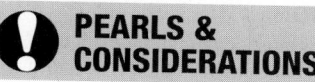

PEARLS & CONSIDERATIONS

COMMENTS

- Testing for human papillomavirus by Hybrid capture 2 DNA test will identify 91% of the small proportion of women with post-treatment residual or recurrent disease, but 30% of all women who are tested will test positive and need colposcopy.
- Gardasil is a vaccine indicated in girls and women aged 9 to 26 yr for the prevention of CIN caused by HPV types 6, 11, 16, and 18. Food and Drug Administration approval for boys and men 9 to 26 yr was given in 2009.
- ACOG cervical cytology screening recommendations are as follows:
  1. Cervical cancer screening should begin at age 21 regardless of age at onset of sexual activity
  2. Cervical cytology screening from age 21 to 29 is recommended every 2 years but should be more frequent in women who are HIV-positive, are immunosuppressed, were exposed in utero to diethylstilbestrol, or have been treated for intraepithelial neoplasia (CIN) 2,3 or cervical cancer. The American Cancer Society, American Society for Colposcopy and Cervical Pathology, American Society for Clinical Pathology, and U.S. Preventive Task Force recommend screening at 3-yr intervals with cytology alone for women age 21-29 yr.
  3. Women age 30 or over who have 3 consecutive negative screens and who do not fit the above criteria for more frequent screening may be tested every 3 years. Co-testing with cervical cytology and high-risk HPV typing is also appropriate; if both tests are negative, re-screening in 3 years is warranted
  4. Cervical cancer screening is unnecessary in women who have undergone hysterectomies for benign disease and who have no histories of CIN
  5. Discontinuation of screening after age 65 or 70 is reasonable in women with 3 or more negative consecutive tests and no cervical abnormalities during the previous decade.
  6. Women with histories of CIN 2, 3, or cancer should undergo annual screening for 20 years after treatment
  7. HPV vaccination does not change these recommendations

SUGGESTED READINGS
available at www.expertconsult.com

RELATED CONTENT
Cervical Cancer (Related Key Topic)
Cervical Polyps (Related Key Topic)
Cervical Dysplasia (Patient Information)

AUTHORS: **DENNIS M. WEPPNER, M.D.,** and **RUBEN ALVERO, M.D.**

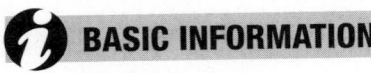

BASIC INFORMATION

DEFINITION

A cervical polyp is a growth protruding from the cervix or endocervical canal. Polyps that arise from the endocervical canal are called *endocervical polyps*. If they arise from the ectocervix, they are called *cervical polyps*.

ICD-9CM CODES
622.7 Mucous polyp of cervix

EPIDEMIOLOGY & DEMOGRAPHICS

Cervical polyps are found in approximately 4% of all gynecologic patients. They most commonly present in perimenopausal and multigravida women between the ages of 30 and 50 yr. Endocervical polyps are more common than cervical polyps and are almost always benign (Fig. 1-203). Malignant degeneration is extremely rare.

PHYSICAL FINDINGS & CLINICAL PRESENTATION

Polyps may be single or multiple and vary in size from being extremely small (a few mm) to large (4 cm). They are soft, smooth, and reddish-purple to cherry-red in color. They bleed easily when touched. Very large polyps can cause some cervical dilation. There may be vaginal discharge associated with cervical polyps if the polyp has become infected.

ETIOLOGY

- Most unknown
- Inflammatory
- Traumatic
- Pregnancy

DIAGNOSIS

DIFFERENTIAL DIAGNOSIS

- Endometrial polyp
- Prolapsed myoma
- Retained products of conception
- Squamous papilloma
- Sarcoma
- Cervical malignancy

WORKUP

Polyps are most commonly asymptomatic and are usually found at the time of annual gynecologic pelvic examination. Polyps are also found in women who present for evaluation of intermenstrual or postcoital bleeding and for profuse vaginal discharge. Polyps are generally painless. Unless a patient has a bleeding abnormality that necessitates evaluation by a physician, polyps would go undiagnosed until the next Pap smear was obtained.

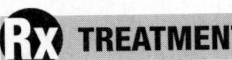 TREATMENT

NONPHARMACOLOGIC THERAPY

Simple surgical excision can be done in the office. The physician should be prepared for bleeding, which can easily be controlled with silver nitrate or Monsel's solution. Most commonly a polyp is excised by grasping it at the stalk with a sponge forceps or similar device and twisting it off. Polyps can also be excised by electrocautery or, in the case of very large polyps, in an outpatient surgical suite. Sexual intercourse and tampon use are to be avoided until the patient's follow-up visit. Douching is not to be performed.

ACUTE GENERAL Rx

Generally no medication is needed.

CHRONIC Rx

Patient is followed up in 2 wk for recheck of the surgical excision site unless there is active bleeding, in which case she would be seen immediately. The cervix should be checked at the patient's routine gynecologic visits.

DISPOSITION

Because these are almost always benign, no further treatment is usually needed. Annual gynecologic examinations should be performed to check for any regrowths.

REFERRAL

To a gynecologist for removal of polyps

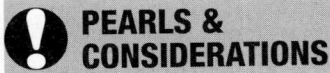 PEARLS & CONSIDERATIONS

COMMENTS

A Pap smear should be obtained before removing the polyp. If an abnormal Pap smear is obtained, it is highly probable that the cause will be the polyp. If a colposcopic evaluation is needed, this should also be performed. During pregnancy the cervix is highly vascularized. If the polyps are stable and benign appearing, they should be observed during the pregnancy and removed only if they cause bleeding.

SUGGESTED READINGS
available at www.expertconsult.com

RELATED CONTENT
Cervical Dysplasia (Related Key Topic)
Cervical Polyps (Patient Information)

AUTHORS: **GEORGE T. DANAKAS, M.D.,** and **RUBEN ALVERO, M.D.**

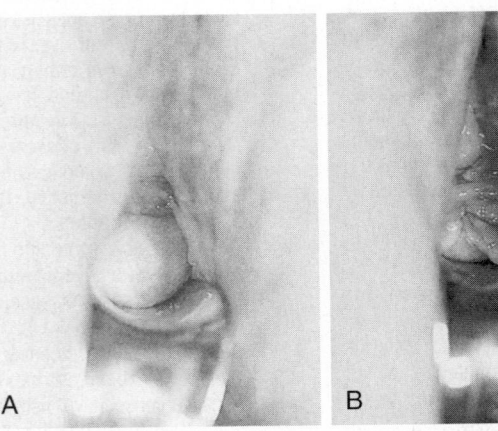
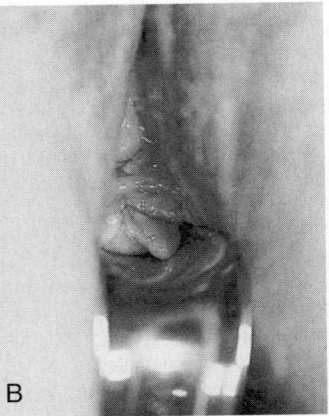

FIGURE 1-203 A, Fibroid polyp protruding through the external cervical os. **B,** Small endocervical polyp. (From Symonds EM, Macpherson MBA: *Color atlas of obstetrics and gynecology,* St Louis, 1994, Mosby.)

BASIC INFORMATION

DEFINITION

Cervicitis is an infection of the cervix. It may result from direct infection of the cervix, or it may be secondary to uterine or vaginal infection.

SYNONYMS

Endocervicitis
Ectocervicitis
Mucopurulent cervicitis

ICD-9CM CODES

616.0   Cervicitis
098.15   Acute gonococcal cervicitis
079.8   *Chlamydia* infection

EPIDEMIOLOGY & DEMOGRAPHICS

Cervicitis accounts for 20% to 25% of patients with abnormal vaginal discharge. It is most common in adolescents, but it can be found in any sexually active woman. Practicing unsafe sex with multiple partners increases the risk of developing cervicitis as well as other sexually transmitted diseases.

PHYSICAL FINDINGS & CLINICAL PRESENTATION

Cervicitis is usually asymptomatic or associated with mild symptoms. Copious purulent or mucopurulent vaginal discharge (Fig. 1-204), pelvic pain, and dyspareunia may be present if cervicitis is severe. The cervix can be erythematous and tender on palpation during bimanual examination. The cervix may also bleed easily when obtaining cultures or a Pap smear. Patients may have postcoital bleeding.

ETIOLOGY

- *Chlamydia trachomatis*
- *Trichomonas*
- *Neisseria gonorrhoeae*
- Herpes simplex
- *Trichomonas vaginalis*
- Human papillomavirus

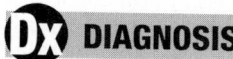

DIAGNOSIS

DIFFERENTIAL DIAGNOSIS

- Carcinoma of the cervix
- Cervical erosion
- Cervical metaplasia

WORKUP

The patient usually presents with a vaginal discharge or history of postcoital bleeding. Otherwise the patient is asymptomatic and diagnosed during routine examination. On examination there is gross visualization of yellow, mucopurulent material on the cotton swab.

LABORATORY TESTS

A finding of leukorrhea (>10 WBC per high-power field on microscopic examination of vaginal fluid) has been associated with chlamydial and gonococcal infection of the cervix. Positive Gram stain is found. Nucleic acid amplification tests (NAAT) should be used for diagnosing *C. trachomatis* and *N. gonorrhoeae* in women with cervicitis; this testing can be performed in either vaginal, cervical, or uterine samples. Use a wet mount to look for trichomonads, but because the sensitivity of microscopy to detect *T. vaginalis* is relatively low (~50%), symptomatic women with cervicitis and negative microscopy for trichomonads should receive further testing with culture. Obtain a Pap smear. HIV testing is recommended in all patients with supposed cervicitis. Although HSV-2 infection has been associated with cervicitis, the utility of specific testing (i.e., culture or serologic testing) for HSV-2 in this setting is unknown.

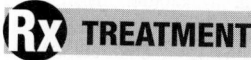

TREATMENT

NONPHARMACOLOGIC THERAPY

- Cervicitis is treated in an outpatient setting. Safe sex should be practiced with the use of condoms.
- Partners should be treated in all cases of infection proven by culture.

ACUTE GENERAL Rx

Because *Chlamydia* and *N. gonorrhoeae* cause 50% of cases of infectious cervicitis, if it is suspected treat without waiting for test results. Administer ceftriaxone 125-mg IM single dose followed by azithromycin 1-g single dose or doxycycline 100 mg PO bid for 7 days. If the patient is pregnant, treat with azithromycin 1-g single dose instead of using doxycycline, which is contraindicated in pregnant or nursing mothers. If *Trichomonas* is the etiologic agent, treat with metronidazole 2-g single dose. For herpes, treat with acyclovir 200 mg PO five times daily for 7 days.

DISPOSITION

Cervicitis responds well to antibiotics. Possible complications to watch for are a subsequent pelvic inflammatory disease (PID) and infertility (found in 5% to 10% of patients with increasing rates with repeat episodes of PID). Repeat cultures should be performed after treatment. Sexual relations can be resumed after negative cultures.

REFERRAL

If subsequent PID develops, consider hospital admission for IV antibiotics.

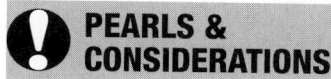

PEARLS & CONSIDERATIONS

COMMENTS

Management of sex partners of women tested for cervicitis should be appropriate for the identified or suspected STD.

SUGGESTED READINGS

available at www.expertconsult.com

RELATED CONTENT

Chlamydia Genital Infections (Related Key Topic)
Gonorrhea (Related Key Topic)
Urethritis, Nongonococcal (Related Key Topic)
Cervicitis (Patient Information)

AUTHORS: **GEORGE T. DANAKAS, M.D.**, and **RUBEN ALVERO, M.D.**

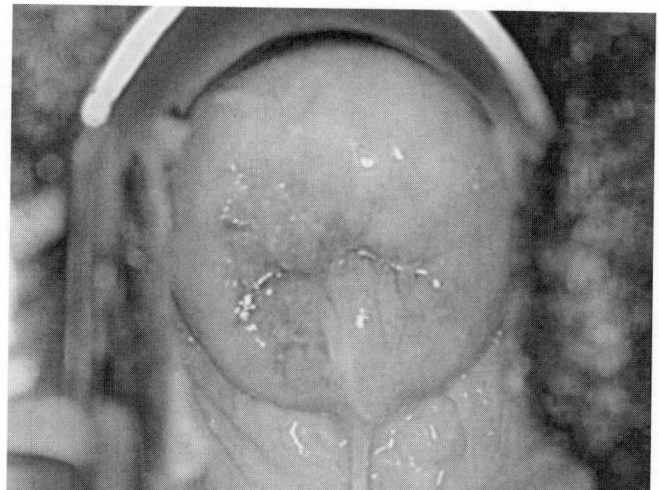

FIGURE 1-204 Colposcopy of a woman with mucopurulent cervicitis and purulent discharge from endocervical os. (Courtesy Dr. David Soper, Richmond, VA. From Mandell GL [ed]: *Mandell, Douglas, and Bennett's principles and practice of infectious diseases*, ed 6, New York, 2005, Churchill Livingstone.)

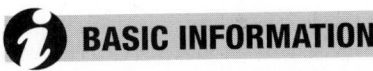

DEFINITION

Chagas' disease is an infection caused by the protozoan parasite *Trypanosoma cruzi*. This is a vector-borne disease transmitted by reduviid bugs from multiple wild and domesticated animal reservoirs. The disease is characterized by an acute nonspecific febrile illness that may be followed, after a variable latency period, by chronic cardiac, GI, and neurologic sequelae. Globally, Chagas' disease affects 8 to 11 million persons.

SYNONYMS

American trypanosomiasis

ICD-9CM CODES
086.2 Chagas' disease

EPIDEMIOLOGY & DEMOGRAPHICS

INCIDENCE (IN U.S.):
- Seven cases of autochthonous transmission in California, Texas, Tennessee, Louisiana
- In the last 2 decades, six cases of laboratory-acquired infection, three cases of transfusion-associated transmission, and nine cases of imported disease reported to the Centers for Disease Control and Prevention (none of the imported cases involving returning tourists)
- Infection has been transmitted by organ transplantation
- Infection has been transmitted congenitally from mother to fetus over more than one generation

PREVALENCE (IN U.S.): Based on regional seroprevalence studies in Hispanic blood donors, it is estimated that between 300,000 and 300,500 persons infected with *T. cruzi* are currently residing in the U.S.

In the Americas, 8 to 10 million people are believed to be infected.

PREDOMINANT SEX: Male = female
PREDOMINANT AGE:
- In highly endemic areas, mean age of acute infection: approximately 4 yr
- Variable age distribution for both types of chronic disease, depending on geography
- Mean age of onset of chronic disease: usually between 35 and 45 yr

PEAK INCIDENCE: Unknown
GENETICS:
Congenital infection: Congenital transmission has been documented with attendant high fetal mortality and morbidity in surviving infants.
Neonatal infection: In rural areas, within substandard housing, transmission is likely to occur.

PHYSICAL FINDINGS & CLINICAL PRESENTATION

- Inflammatory lesion that develops about 1 wk after contamination of a break in the skin with infected insect feces (chagoma)
  1. Area of induration and erythema

2. Usually accompanied by local lymphadenopathy
- Presence of Romaña's sign, which consists of unilateral painless palpebral and periocular edema, when conjunctiva is portal of entry
- Constitutional symptoms of fever, fatigue, and anorexia, along with edema of the face and lower extremities, generalized lymphadenopathy, and mild hepatosplenomegaly after the appearance of local signs of disease
- Myocarditis in a small portion of patients, sometimes with resultant CHF
- Uncommonly, CNS disease, such as meningoencephalitis, which carries a poor prognosis
- Symptoms and signs of disease persisting for weeks to months, followed by spontaneous resolution of the acute illness; patient then in the indeterminate phase of the disease (asymptomatic with attendant subpatent parasitemia and reactive antibodies to *T. cruzi* antigens)
- Chronic disease may become manifest years to decades after the initial infection:
  1. Most common organ involved: heart, followed by GI tract, and to a much lesser extent the CNS
     a. Cardiac involvement takes the form of arrhythmias or cardiomyopathy, but rarely both.
     b. Cardiomyopathy is bilateral but predominantly affects the right ventricle and is often accompanied by apical aneurysms and mural thrombi.
     c. Arrhythmias are a consequence of involvement of the bundle of His and have been implicated as the leading cause of sudden death in adults in highly endemic areas.
     d. Right-sided heart failure, thromboembolization, and rhythm disturbances associated with symptoms of dizziness and syncope are characteristic.
  2. Patients with megaesophagus: dysphagia, odynophagia, chronic cough, and regurgitation, frequently resulting in aspiration pneumonitis

3. Megacolon: abdominal pain and chronic constipation, which, when severe, may lead to obstruction and perforation
4. CNS symptoms: most often secondary to embolization from the heart
5. Varying degrees of peripheral neuropathy

ETIOLOGY

- *T. cruzi*
  1. Found only in the Americas, ranging from the southern U.S. to southern Argentina
  2. Transmitted to humans by various species of bloodsucking reduviid ("kissing") insects, primarily those of the genera *Triatoma, Panstrongylus,* and *Rhodnius*
  3. Usually found in burrows and trees where infected insects transmit the parasite to natural reservoirs (e.g., opossums and armadillos)
  4. Intrusion into enzootic areas for farmland, allowing insects to take up residence in rural dwellings, thus including humans and domestic animals in the cycle of transmission
  5. Initial infection of insects by ingesting blood from animals or humans that have circulating flagellated trypanosomes (trypomastigotes)
  6. Multiplication in the insect midgut as epimastigotes, then differentiation into metacyclic trypomastigotes discharged with the feces during subsequent blood meals (Fig. 1-205)
  7. Transmission to the second mammalian host through contamination of mucous membranes, conjunctivae, or wounds with insect feces containing infected forms
- In the vertebrate host
  1. Movement of parasites into various cell types, intracellular transformation into amastigotes, and thereafter differentiation into trypomastigotes
  2. Following rupture of the cell membrane, parasitic invasion of local tissues or hematogenous spread to distant sites, maintaining a parasitemia infective for vectors
- In addition to insect vectors, *T. cruzi* is transmitted through blood transfusions, transplacentally,

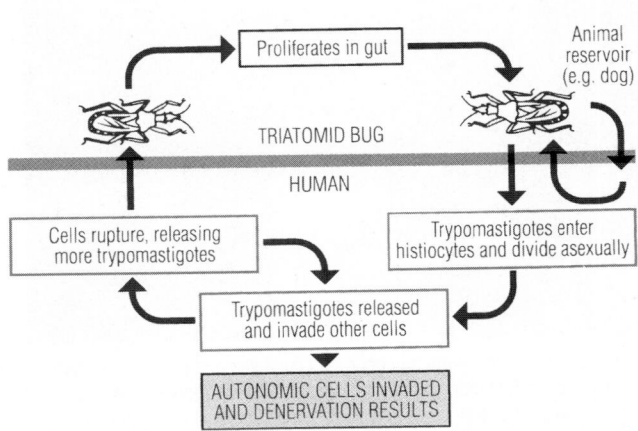

FIGURE 1-205 Lifecycle of *Trypanosoma cruzi*. (From Souhami RL, Mozham J: *Textbook of medicine,* ed 4, London, 2002, Churchill Livingstone.)

and, occasionally, secondary to laboratory accidents or ingestion, including breast milk

- In 2007, voluntary screening was initiated in the U.S. blood supply; it is estimated to cover 75% to 90% of the blood supply.
- Platelet transfusions appear to be more infective than packed red blood cells.

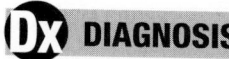 DIAGNOSIS

DIFFERENTIAL DIAGNOSIS

Acute disease
- Early African trypanosomiasis
- New World cutaneous and mucocutaneous leishmaniasis

Chronic disease
- Idiopathic cardiomyopathy
- Idiopathic achalasia
- Congenital or acquired megacolon

WORKUP

Principal considerations in diagnosis:
- A history of residence where transmission is known to occur
- Recent receipt of a blood product while in an endemic area
- Occupational exposure in a laboratory

LABORATORY TESTS

For acute diagnosis:
- Demonstration of *T. cruzi* in wet preparations of blood (Fig. 1-206), buffy coat, or Giemsa-stained smears
- Xenodiagnosis, a technique involving laboratory-reared insect vectors fed on subjects with suspected infection thereafter examined for parasites, and culture of body fluids in liquid media to establish diagnosis
  1. Hampered by the length of time required for completion
  2. Of limited use in clinical decision making with regard to drug therapy
  3. Although xenodiagnosis and broth culture are considered to be more sensitive than microscopic examination of body fluids, sensitivities may not exceed 50%

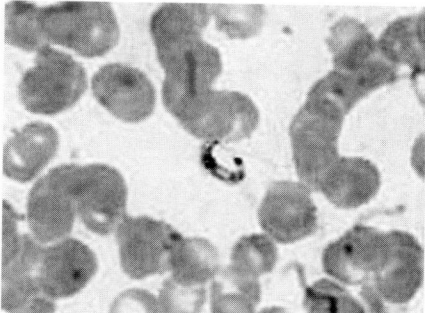

FIGURE 1-206 *T. cruzi* in human blood film. The causative agent occurs in blood films characteristically as short C-shaped or S-shaped trypomastigotes with a prominent kinetoplast. It is otherwise monomorphic *(Giemsa × 950)*. (From Hoffmann R et al: *Hematology: basic principles and practice*, ed 5, Philadelphia, 2009, Churchill Livingstone.)

- Recent advances in serologic testing include immunoblot assay, in situ indirect fluorescent antibody, PCR-based techniques, and an immunochromatographic assay (Chagas Stat Pak)
- Response to treatment in acute, reactivated, or congenital infection can be assessed by quantitative PCR.

For chronic *T. cruzi* infection:
- Traditional serologic tests including: complement fixation (CF), indirect immunofluorescence (IIF), indirect hemagglutination, and enzyme-linked immunosorbent assay (ELISA)
- Serologic tests have variable sensitivity and specificity and frequent false-positive results
- Saliva ELISA may be useful as a screening diagnostic test in epidemiologic studies of chronic trypanosomiasis infection in endemic areas
- Confirmation requires at least two different tests, and if discordant, three tests.

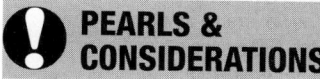 TREATMENT

NONPHARMACOLOGIC THERAPY

- Chronic chagasic heart disease: mainly supportive
- Megaesophagus: symptoms usually amenable to dietary measures or pneumonic dilation of the esophagogastric junction
- Chagasic megacolon: in its early stages responsive to a high-fiber diet, laxatives, and enemas

ACUTE GENERAL Rx

It is now recommended that all patients—acute, indeterminant, and chronic—be treated with antiparasitic therapy. Treatment for individuals older than 50 years requires consideration of risk/benefit as the treatment appears to be more toxic at this age.

A single course of each of the medications below is thought to offer an approximately 50% cure rate. Neither drug is approved by the FDA but both can be obtained free of charge from the FDA and used under investigational protocol. Consultations and requests for drugs can be made to: Parasitic Diseases Public Inquiries Line (770-448-7775), parasites.cdc.gov, www.cdc.gov/parasites/chagas, CDC Drug Service (404-639-3670).

Benznidazole, a nitroimidazole derivative:
- Has demonstrated similar efficacy as nifurtimox in limited trials, is usually better tolerated and is viewed by most experts as first-line treatment
- Recommended oral dosage: 5 to 7 mg/kg/day for 30 to 90 days

Nifurtimox:
- Recommended oral dosage for adults: 8 to 10 mg/kg/day given in 3 to 4 divided daily doses and continued for 90 to 120 days
- Parasitologic cure in approximately 50% of those treated; should be begun as early as possible
- Neither drug can be used during pregnancy.
- Do not use in cases of severe renal or hepatic dysfunction.

- Triazoles offer a new class of therapy. Case reports have had success with posaconazole.

CHRONIC Rx

- In patients with indeterminate phase or chronic disease: Some evidence of benefit in a recent uncontrolled trial with benznidazole in patients with chagasic cardiomyopathy
- In patients exhibiting bradyarrhythmias: pacemakers
- In individuals with congestive heart failure:
  1. Treat with standard modalities for dilated, right-sided, cardiomyopathic disease.
  2. Cardiac transplant is an option for end-stage cardiomyopathy; moreover, reactivation rate found to be low and amenable to therapy without subsequent infection of the allograft.
  3. Myotomy or esophageal resection is reserved for patients with advanced disease.
- In advanced chagasic megacolon associated with chronic fecal impaction, perforation, or, less commonly, volvulus: surgical resection

DISPOSITION

Based on a few prospective studies, most patients infected with *T. cruzi* will not develop symptomatic Chagas' disease.

REFERRAL

- For consultation with an infectious disease specialist or communication with the Centers for Disease Control and Prevention when the disease is acutely suspected
- To a cardiologist for pacemaker implantation for patients with bradyarrhythmias
- To a surgeon for symptomatic disease with chagasic megaesophagus or megacolon

⚠ PEARLS & CONSIDERATIONS

COMMENTS

- All children of an infected mother should be screened for Chagas; household members should also be screened.
- In recipients of solid organ or bone marrow transplants, patients with AIDS, or those receiving chemotherapy, there may be reactivation of indeterminate phase disease.
- Mortality predictors associated with chagasic cardiomyopathy include CHF, QT-interval dispersion, left ventricular (LV) end-systolic dimension, the presence of pathologic Q waves, frequent PVCs, and isolated LAFB on ECG.
- Chagasic esophageal disease has an increased incidence of esophageal malignancy.
- The use of pyrethroid-impregnated curtains may represent an option for the reduction or elimination of Chagas' disease transmission in certain endemic areas.

SUGGESTED READINGS

available at www.expertconsult.com

AUTHOR: **PATRICIA CRISTOFARO, M.D.**

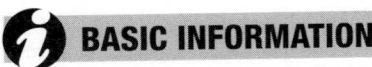

BASIC INFORMATION

DEFINITION

Charcot-Marie-Tooth disease (CMT) is a heterogeneous group of noninflammatory inherited peripheral neuropathies characterized by chronic motor and sensory polyneuropathy. It is the most common inherited neuromuscular disorder (see also "Neuropathy, Hereditary").

SYNONYMS

Peroneal muscular atrophy
Hereditary motor and sensory neuropathy (HMSN)
CMT

ICD-9CM CODES
356.1 Charcot-Marie-Tooth disease, paralysis, or syndrome

EPIDEMIOLOGY & DEMOGRAPHICS

PREVALENCE: 1:2500; CMT type 1 and type 2 are the major divisions with an estimated prevalence of 40 per 100,000
PREDOMINANT AGE: Onset usually 10 to 20 yr, and infants may be symptomatic.
GENETICS: Transmission may be autosomal dominant, autosomal recessive, or X-linked, with some sporadic cases reported. Duplication of *peripheral myelin protein 22* (PMP22) is the most common cause of CMT. CMT is classified into types 1 through 7 and is genetically heterogeneous with at least 43 CMT genes known.

PHYSICAL FINDINGS & CLINICAL PRESENTATION

- Wide variation in clinical presentation, but affected individuals in a family tend to have similar symptoms
- Symmetric, slowly progressive distal motor neuropathy resulting in weakness and atrophy in legs, often progresses to involve hands
- High-arched feet (pes cavus), claw toe deformities (Fig. 1-208), and hammer toes
- Atrophy of the lower legs producing a stork-like appearance (muscle wasting does not involve the upper legs) (Fig. 1-209)
- Nerve enlargement
- Mild to moderate distal sensory loss; uncommonly can have painful paresthesias
- Decreased proprioception and weakness of ankle dorsiflexors often interfere with balance and gait (steppage gait)

- Depressed or absent deep tendon reflexes in many cases
- Hearing loss and hip dysplasia are under-recognized manifestations
- Ambulation usually maintained throughout life
- CMT has been reported to be associated with renal diseases, mostly focal segmental glomerulosclerosis (FSGS)

ETIOLOGY

Genetic abnormalities cause defects in either peripheral nerve myelination, or result in axonal degeneration. Mutations in one of several myelin genes result in defects in myelin structure, maintenance, and formation. Duplication of the PMP22 gene causes CMT1A, the most common type of hereditary motor sensory neuropathy (~40% overall). INF_2 mutations appear to cause many cases of FSGS-associated CMT.

DIAGNOSIS

DIFFERENTIAL DIAGNOSIS

- Other inherited neuropathies
- Acquired peripheral neuropathies such as toxic, metabolic, infectious, endocrine, inflammatory, immune-mediated, and nutritional polyneuropathies

WORKUP

- Clinical diagnosis is based on family history, characteristic presentation, and findings on detailed physical and neurologic examination.
- Electrophysiologic studies are often diagnostic and may help define various subtypes of CMT.
- Occasionally, sural nerve biopsy is helpful in establishing diagnosis.

TREATMENT

ACUTE GENERAL Rx

- Symptomatic and supportive, managed by multidisciplinary team including physical and occupational therapy
- Special shoes with good ankle support, ankle/foot orthoses.
- Some require crutches/cane for gait stability; <5% need wheelchair.
- Daily heel cord stretching exercises and hand grip exercises.
- Musculoskeletal pain may respond to acetaminophen or NSAIDs; neuropathic pain may respond to tricyclic antidepressants or drugs such as carbamazepine or gabapentin.

CHRONIC Rx

Occasionally, orthopedic surgery is required to correct severe pes cavus deformity or hip dysplasia. Avoiding obesity is essential as this makes walking difficult; avoiding potentially neurotoxic medications is also important, particularly *Vinca* alkaloids.

DISPOSITION

- Disability is usually compatible with a long life.
- 10% to 20% of patients are asymptomatic.

REFERRAL

- Orthopedic consultation for bracing and surgical treatment of deformity
- Genetic counseling and family planning

PEARLS & CONSIDERATIONS

COMMENTS

Patient information on CMT disease is available from the Muscular Dystrophy Association, 3300 East Sunrise Drive, Tucson, AZ 85718; (520) 529-2000.

EVIDENCE

available at www.expertconsult.com

SUGGESTED READINGS

available at www.expertconsult.com

RELATED CONTENT

Charcot-Marie-Tooth Disease (Patient Information)

AUTHOR: **CANDICE YUVIENCO, M.D.**

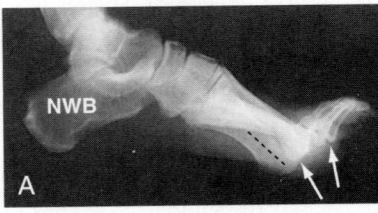
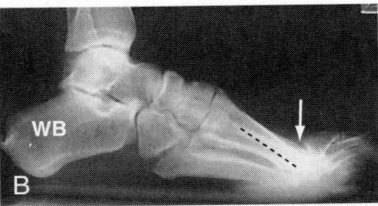

FIGURE 1-208 A, Non–weight-bearing view of cavus and claw toe deformities in a patient with Charcot-Marie-Tooth disease. **B,** On weight-bearing view, plantar flexion of first ray is less noticeable, but clawed hallux remains, indicating fixed extension contracture at first metatarsophalangeal joint. (From Canale ST, Beaty JH: *Campbell's operative orthopedics,* ed 11, Philadelphia, 2007, Mosby.)

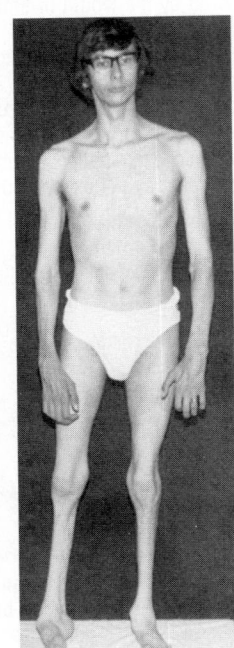

FIGURE 1-209 Patient with Charcot-Marie-Tooth disease showing marked wasting of calf muscles and intrinsic foot muscles. (From Dubowitz V: *Muscle disorders in childhood,* London, 1995, Saunders.)

BASIC INFORMATION

DEFINITION

Charcot's joint was first described by Jean Martin Charcot in reports of patients with tabes dorsalis. It is a chronic progressive condition associated with peripheral neuropathy that commonly results in destruction of the bone and soft tissues at peripheral weight-bearing joints. It is characterized early on by acute inflammation that often leads to joint degeneration, instability from joint dislocation and pathologic fractures, and gross deformities.

SYNONYMS

Neuropathic arthropathy
Charcot osteoarthropathy
Charcot neuroosteoarthropathy

ICD-9CM CODES
094.0 Charcot's arthropathy

EPIDEMIOLOGY & DEMOGRAPHICS
PREVALENCE:
- Estimated as 0.08% to 13% in patients with diabetes mellitus.
- 5 cases per 100 of those with peripheral neuropathy, primarily affecting the foot.
- 20% to 40% of patients with syringomyelia (shoulder, elbow, and wrist are most commonly involved).
- 5% to 10% of patients with tabes dorsalis; usually >60 years old (spine, hip, knee, and ankle are most commonly involved).
- Average age of onset is 50 to 60 years.
- No definite sex predilection, and ethnic variance is unknown.

PHYSICAL FINDINGS & CLINICAL PRESENTATION
- Initial presentation is with a diffusely warm, erythematous, and swollen joint with or without associated pain.
- Pain is typically less than expected based on the severity of clinical and radiographic findings.
- It commonly affects the mid-foot, but the forefoot and hind foot can also be involved.
- Joint instability, osseous debris around the joint, and crepitus may be seen with progressive disease.
- Frank dislocation, fracture, and subsequent bony deformity may occur over time. Additionally, plantar ulcers may affect neuropathic foot joints.

ETIOLOGY

The most common identifiable risk factors for Charcot osteoarthropathy include any condition that causes a peripheral or autonomic neuropathy. Diabetes mellitus with peripheral neuropathy is the most common cause (Fig. 1-210). Less common associations include renal dialysis, syringomyelia, tabes dorsalis, Charcot-Marie-Tooth disease, congenital indifference to pain, chronic alcoholism, poliomyelitis, syphilis, leprosy, familial amyloid neuropathy, spinal or peripheral nerve surgery, and spinal dysraphism. Two theories contribute to the underling processes involved in the disease:

1. Neurotraumatic theory:
   - Impairment or loss of protective joint sensation with continued weight bearing and repetitive stress.
   - Rapid and extensive bone destruction leads to joint subluxation, dislocation, and possible deformity.
   - Chronic inflammation eventually contributes to joint instability and incongruity.
2. Neurovascular theory:
   - Autonomic neuropathy leads to increased blood flow to the affected joints.
   - Enhanced osteoclastic bone resorption contributes to osteopenia and further susceptibility to bone destruction.

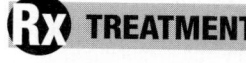

DIAGNOSIS

DIFFERENTIAL DIAGNOSIS
- Osteomyelitis
- Cellulitis
- Inflammatory arthritides, particularly gout
- Deep vein thrombosis
- Infectious arthritis
- Osteoarthritis

WORKUP

Early diagnosis, before radiographic changes are evident, requires a high index of suspicion because the acute phase is characterized by the classical signs of an acute inflammatory process.
- Patients should be tested for an underlying peripheral neuropathy.

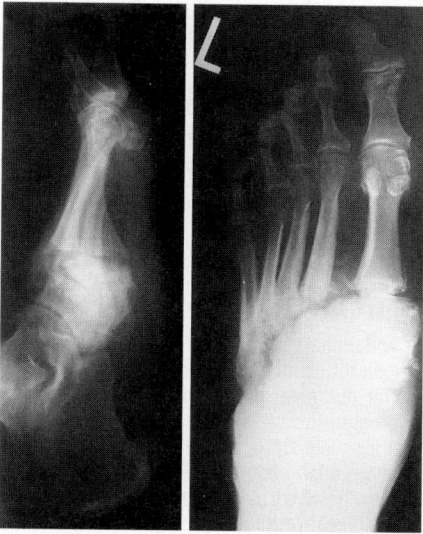

FIGURE 1-210 Diabetes mellitus and neuropathic arthritis. Note lateral displacement of metatarsals *(left)* and fragmentation and osseous debris *(right)*. (From Goldman L, Ausiello D [eds]: *Cecil textbook of medicine,* ed 22, Philadelphia, 2004, Saunders.)

- It may be helpful to diagnose or rule out a previously unrecognized contributing condition or risk factor for the above.

LABORATORY TESTS
- A complete blood count and metabolic panel, while additional testing to determine a possible underlying cause may include vitamin B_{12}, folate, RPR, ALP, and PTH
- In questionable cases, aspiration, sometimes including biopsy, to rule out soft tissue of bone infection

IMAGING STUDIES
Plain roentgenography:
- May reveal variable degrees of destruction and joint disruption. This is usually sufficient to establish the diagnosis in most cases.
- Three radiographic stages correspond to clinical progression of the disease: fragmentation, coalescence, and reconstruction.
- A technetium diphosphate bone scan or MRI can provide more detail when the clinical picture is not too clear.

TREATMENT

ACUTE GENERAL Rx

The cornerstone of therapy involves offloading, which is best achieved with total contact casts (or, alternatively, removable cast walkers) and cessation of weight-bearing activities. The average use of a cast is 12 to 18 wk. In some instances, surgical correction of a joint might be necessary.

PHARMACOLOGIC THERAPY

Antiresorptives such as bisphosphonates and calcitonin have shown improved symptom control and decreased bone turnover markers in controlled trials.

DISPOSITION

Early diagnosis of Charcot's joint is imperative to avoid compromise of bone and joint integrity. In general, it typically takes 1 to 2 yr for complete healing of a Charcot's joint. Once bony changes set in they are very difficult if not impossible to reverse. Timely, appropriate treatment can greatly reduce the risk of irreversible damage and future morbidity.

REFERRAL

Patient should be referred to a high-risk foot clinic.

SUGGESTED READINGS
available at www.expertconsult.com

RELATED CONTENT
Charcot Joint (Patient Information)

AUTHOR: **ANISHKA S. ROLLE, M.D.**

BASIC INFORMATION

DEFINITION

Chemotherapy-induced nausea and vomiting (CINV) refers to adverse effects of drugs used to treat cancer. There are three recognized subtypes: acute-phase CINV, where nausea and vomiting begin minutes to hours after administration of the drug(s); delayed-phase CINV, where symptoms can begin or return 24 hours or more after taking the medication(s); and anticipatory CINV, where nausea and vomiting begin before receiving treatment.

SYNONYMS

Drug-induced nausea and vomiting
Chemotherapy-induced emesis

ICD-9CM CODES

787.01 Nausea with vomiting
787.02 Nausea alone
787.03 Vomiting alone
E933.1 Adverse effect of antineoplastic and immunosuppressive drugs
V58.11-V58.12 Encounter for antineoplastic chemotherapy and immunotherapy

EPIDEMIOLOGY & DEMOGRAPHICS

- The patient's risk for development of nausea and vomiting is most strongly dependent on the drugs used.
- With certain medications, nausea and vomiting will occur in almost 100% of patients. With other drugs, the risk for symptoms can be as low as 10%.
- Symptoms may be dose dependent (the higher the dose, the greater the risk for symptoms).
- CINV is more likely to affect female and younger patients.
- Those patients expecting CINV from medications are more likely to have it (anticipatory emesis).
- Those patients with a history of alcohol consumption are at lower risk.
- Patients with a history of motion sickness are at greater risk.

PHYSICAL FINDINGS & CLINICAL PRESENTATION

- For acute-phase CINV, nausea and vomiting start within minutes to hours after receiving chemotherapy.
- For delayed-phase CINV, nausea and vomiting begin or return 24 hours or more after receiving chemotherapy.
- With anticipatory CINV, symptoms begin before receiving the medication.
- Other symptoms may include anxiety and lightheadedness.
- Physical findings are most commonly elevated pulse and abnormal blood pressure (high if the person is highly anxious, low if the patient is getting dehydrated).

- Symptoms such as diarrhea, fever, headache, and abdominal pain may suggest an etiology of symptoms other than chemotherapy; physical examination findings such as increased blood pressure, abdominal tenderness, or focal neurologic deficits may suggest symptoms caused by cancer progression or other acute illness such as infection.

ETIOLOGY

CINV is probably the result of chemotherapy drugs acting in two places: in the gastrointestinal tract directly and in the vomiting center of the brain. In both areas, nausea and vomiting are mediated by the actions of certain neurotransmitters, with serotonin, dopamine, and neurokinin being the most important.

DIAGNOSIS

DIFFERENTIAL DIAGNOSIS

- The two main considerations are progression of cancer and infection
- Intestinal/gastric: obstruction or partial obstruction of the digestive tract from tumor
- Neurologic: metastases to the brain causing vomiting; infiltration of nerves affecting the digestive tract
- Infectious: acute bacterial, viral, or parasitic infectious of the digestive tract causing symptoms (usually diarrhea will be present)
- Renal: dehydration leading to kidney failure, causing a worsening of nausea and vomiting

WORKUP

No workup is indicated if patient's symptoms and timeframe of nausea and vomiting fit the usual presentation for CINV. If other symptoms or unexpected physical examination findings are present, then other causes need to be ruled out. A combination of blood work and imaging may be helpful.

LABORATORY TESTS

- If the onset of symptoms is not typical for CINV, then blood tests such as a CBC, liver tests, and kidney tests may be indicated.
- Stool studies looking for infections from bacteria or parasites may be ordered if diarrhea is also present.

IMAGING STUDIES

- Abdominal radiographs may be ordered to look for obstruction of the digestive tract but will not give any information about tumor progression.
- Abdominal CT scan will give more detailed information about cancer in the proximity of the digestive tract and whether obstruction of the digestive tract is present.
- Brain CT scan or magnetic resonance imaging (MRI) will give information about possible metastases to the brain.

TREATMENT

- Treatment depends on the likelihood of a given drug or drug regimen to cause CINV and is preventative in nature.
- For those medications with a high probability of causing CINV, a combination of antinausea medications has proved to be highly effective.
- Which combination of drugs is used and for how many days is dependent on the chemotherapy regimen used.
- The most common combination includes a serotonin-receptor antagonist (ondansetron, granisetron, dolasetron, tropisetron, or palonosetron), a corticosteroid (methylprednisolone or dexamethasone), and a neurokinin-1 receptor antagonist (aprepitant).
- Many other drugs are available, such as prochlorperazine, metochlopramide, haloperidol, and marinol, but most are less effective and have greater potential for adverse effects.
- Benzodiazepines (usually lorazepam) may help in patients with high anxiety levels leading to anticipatory CINV.
- Patients with uncontrolled symptoms may require hospitalization for supportive care including intravenous fluids.

NONPHARMACOLOGIC THERAPY

For those patients with a significant anxiety component to their CINV, behavior therapy may help, as may some complementary alternative therapies.

DISPOSITION

Although CINV is one of the most feared complications of cancer therapy, its treatment has been revolutionized in the last 20 years, with most patients achieving adequate symptom control.

PEARLS & CONSIDERATIONS

COMMENTS

- Aggressive attempts to control the acute phase of CINV are the key to symptom control. Prevention of the acute phase has led to much greater control of the delayed phase, which, in turn, has greatly decreased the incidence of anticipatory CINV.
- Prevention of symptoms is much easier to achieve than controlling/treating symptoms once they have begun.

SUGGESTED READINGS
available at www.expertconsult.com

AUTHOR: CHARLES WOLFF, M.D.

BASIC INFORMATION

DEFINITION

Genital infection with *Chlamydia trachomatis* may result in urethritis, epididymitis, cervicitis, and acute salpingitis, but often it is asymptomatic in women (see "Pelvic Inflammatory Disease"). In men, urethritis, mucopurulent discharge, dysuria, and urethral pruritus are noted.

ICD-9CM CODES
597.80 Urethritis
604.0 Epididymitis
616.0 Cervicitis
381.51 Acute salpingitis

EPIDEMIOLOGY & DEMOGRAPHICS

- *Chlamydia trachomatis* is the most common sexually transmitted disease in the U.S. More than 4 million infections occur annually, although the exact number is unknown because reporting is not required in all states. Occurrence is common worldwide and has been increasing steadily over the last 2 decades in the U.S., Canada, Australia, and Europe.
- Most women with endocervical or urethral infections are asymptomatic.
- Up to 45% of cases of gonococcal infection may have concomitant chlamydial infection.
- Infertility or ectopic pregnancy can result as a complication from symptomatic or asymptomatic chronic infections of the endometrium and fallopian tubes.
- Conjunctival and pneumonic infection of the newborn may result from infection in pregnancy.
- In men 15% to 55% of cases are caused by *C. trachomatis*. Complications of nongonococcal urethritis in men infected with *C. trachomatis* include epididymitis and Reiter's syndrome.

PHYSICAL FINDINGS & CLINICAL PRESENTATION

Clinical manifestations may be similar to those of gonorrhea: mucopurulent endocervical discharge, with edema, erythema, and easily induced endocervical bleeding caused by inflammation of endocervical columnar epithelium. Less-frequent manifestations may include bartholinitis, urethral syndrome with dysuria and pyuria, and perihepatitis (Fitz-Hugh–Curtis syndrome).

ETIOLOGY

- *Chlamydia trachomatis*, serotypes D through K
- Obligate, intracellular bacteria

DIAGNOSIS

DIFFERENTIAL DIAGNOSIS

Gonorrhea, nongonococcal urethritis (nonchlamydial etiologies)

WORKUP

Diagnosis based on laboratory demonstration of evidence of infection in intraurethral or endocervical swab by various tests. The intracellular organism is less readily recovered from the discharge.

LABORATORY TESTS

- Cell culture is the reference method for diagnosis (single culture sensitivity 80% to 90%), but it is labor intensive and takes 48 to 96 hr; it is not suited for large screening programs.
- Nonculture methods:
  - NAATs are very sensitive tests for cervical and male urethral specimens and are FDA-approved for use with urine.
  - Direct fluorescent antibody tests
  - Enzyme immunoassay
  - DNA probes
  - Polymerase chain reaction (PCR)
- With the exception of PCR, the other tests are probably less specific than cell culture and may yield false-positive results.
- Because this is an intracellular organism, purulent discharge is not an appropriate specimen. An adequate sample of infected cells must be obtained.
- Ten white blood cells per high-power field.

TREATMENT

ACUTE GENERAL Rx

Nongonococcal urethritis, urethritis, cervicitis, conjunctivitis (except for lymphogranuloma venereum):
- Azithromycin 1 g PO × 1 *or*
- Doxycycline 100 mg PO bid for 7 days
- Alternatives
  1. Erythromycin base 500 mg PO qid for 7 days *or*
  2. Erythromycin ethylsuccinate 800 mg PO qid for 7 days *or*
  3. Ofloxacin 300 mg PO bid for 7 days
  4. Levofloxacin 500 mg PO qd for 7 days

Infection in pregnancy:
- Erythromycin base 500 mg PO qid for 7 days *or*
- Amoxicillin 500 mg PO tid for 7 days
Alternatives:
  1. Erythromycin base 250 mg PO qid for 7 days *or*
  2. Erythromycin ethylsuccinate 800 mg PO qid for 7 days *or*
  3. Erythromycin ethylsuccinate 400 mg PO qid for 14 days *or*
  4. Azithromycin 1 g PO (single dose)
NOTE: Doxycycline and ofloxacin are contraindicated in pregnancy. Safety and efficacy of azithromycin are not established in pregnancy and lactation, although preliminary data indicate that it may be safe and effective. Erythromycin estolate is contraindicated in pregnancy because of drug-related hepatotoxicity.
FOLLOW-UP: Reculture after therapy completion and refer partners for evaluation and treatment.

RECURRENT AND PERSISTENT URETHRITIS:
Retreat noncompliant patients with the above regimens. If patient was initially compliant, recommended regimens: metronidazole 2 g PO in single dose plus erythromycin base 500 mg PO qid for 7 days or erythromycin ethylsuccinate 800 mg PO qid for 7 days.

CLINICAL PEARL

When treating *Chlamydia,* it is best to assume concomitant gonorrhea because co-infection is common. Combination of cetriaxone 125 mg IM single dose plus azithromycin 1 g PO single dose will treat both.

REFERRAL

Refer to infectious disease specialist if persistent infection or gynecologist if salpingitis is suspected.

SUGGESTED READINGS
available at www.expertconsult.com

RELATED CONTENT

Cervicitis (Related Key Topic)
Gonorrhea (Related Key Topic)
Pelvic Inflammatory Disease (Related Key Topic)
Urethritis, Gonococcal (Related Key Topic)
Urethritis, Nongonococcal (Related Key Topic)

AUTHORS: **MARIA A. CORIGLIANO, M.D.,** and **RUBEN ALVERO, M.D.**

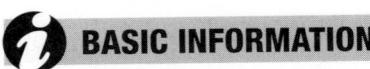

BASIC INFORMATION

DEFINITION

Cholangitis refers to an inflammation and/or infection of the hepatic and common bile ducts associated with obstruction of the common bile duct.

SYNONYMS

Biliary sepsis
Ascending cholangitis
Suppurative cholangitis

ICD-9CM CODES
576.1 Cholangitis

EPIDEMIOLOGY & DEMOGRAPHICS

INCIDENCE (IN U.S.): Complicates approximately 1% of cases of cholelithiasis
PEAK INCIDENCE: Seventh decade
PREVALENCE (IN U.S.): 2 cases/1000 hospital admissions
PREDOMINANT SEX:
- Females, for cholangitis secondary to gallstones
- Males, for cholangitis secondary to malignant obstruction and HIV infection
PREDOMINANT AGE: Seventh decade and older; unusual <50 yr of age

PHYSICAL FINDINGS & CLINICAL PRESENTATION

- Usually acute onset of fever, abdominal pain (RUQ), and jaundice (Charcot's triad)
- All signs and symptoms in only 50% to 85% of patients
- Often, dark coloration of the urine resulting from bilirubinuria
- Complications:
  1. Bacteremia (50%) and septic shock
  2. Hepatic abscess and pancreatitis

ETIOLOGY

Obstruction of the common bile duct causing rapid proliferation of bacteria in the biliary tree
- Most common cause of common bile duct obstruction: stones, usually migrated from the gallbladder
- Other causes: prior biliary tract surgery with secondary stenosis, tumor (usually arising from the pancreas or biliary tree), and parasitic infections from *Ascaris lumbricoides* or *Fasciola hepatica*
- Iatrogenic after contamination of an obstructed biliary tree by endoscopic retrograde cholangiopancreatoscopy (ERCP) or percutaneous transhepatic cholangiography (PTC)
- Primary sclerosing cholangitis (PSC)
- HIV-associated sclerosing cholangitis: associated with infection by CMV, *Cryptosporidium,* Microsporidia, and *Mycobacterium avium* complex

DIAGNOSIS

DIFFERENTIAL DIAGNOSIS

- Biliary colic
- Acute cholecystitis
- Liver abscess
- Peptic ulcer disease (PUD)
- Pancreatitis
- Intestinal obstruction
- Right kidney stone
- Hepatitis
- Pyelonephritis

WORKUP

- Blood cultures
- CBC
- Liver function tests

LABORATORY TESTS

- Usually, elevated WBC count with a predominance of polymorphonuclear forms
- Elevated alkaline phosphatase and bilirubin in chronic obstruction
- Elevated transaminases in acute obstruction
- Positive blood cultures in 50% of cases, typically with enteric gram-negative aerobes (e.g., *E. coli, Klebsiella pneumoniae*), enterococci, or anaerobes

IMAGING STUDIES

- Ultrasound:
  1. Allows visualization of the gallbladder and bile ducts to differentiate extrahepatic obstruction from intrahepatic cholestasis
  2. Insensitive but specific for visualization of common duct stones
- CT scan (Fig. E1-211):
  1. Less accurate for gallstones
  2. More sensitive than ultrasound for visualization of the distal part of the common bile duct
  3. Also allows better definition of neoplasm
- ERCP:
  1. Confirms obstruction and its level
  2. Allows collection of specimens for culture and cytology
  3. Indicated for diagnosis if ultrasound and CT scan are inconclusive
  4. May be indicated in therapy (see "Treatment")

TREATMENT

NONPHARMACOLOGIC THERAPY

Biliary decompression
- May be urgent in severely ill patients or those unresponsive to medical therapy within 12 to 24 hr
- May also be performed semielectively in patients who respond

- Options:
  1. ERCP with or without sphincterotomy or placement of a draining stent
  2. Percutaneous transhepatic biliary drainage for the acutely ill patient who is a poor surgical candidate
  3. Surgical exploration of the common bile duct

ACUTE GENERAL Rx

- Nothing by mouth
- Intravenous hydration
- Broad-spectrum antibiotics directed at gram-negative enteric organisms, anaerobes, and enterococcus such as carbapenems (meropenem: 1 g q8h or imipenem: 500 mg IV q6h if life threatening), piperacillin/tazobactam: 3.375 or 4.5 g IV q6h, or ampicillin-sulbactam, or ticarcillin-clavulanate; if infection is nosocomial, post-ERCP, or the patient is in shock, broaden antibiotic coverage.

CHRONIC Rx

Repeated decompression may be necessary, particularly when obstruction is related to neoplasm.

DISPOSITION

Excellent prognosis if obstruction is amenable to definitive surgical therapy; otherwise relapses are common.

REFERRAL

- To biliary endoscopist if obstruction is from stones or a stent needs to be placed
- To interventional radiologist if external drainage is necessary
- To a general surgeon in all other cases
- To an infectious disease specialist if blood cultures are positive or the patient is in shock or otherwise severely ill

PEARLS & CONSIDERATIONS

- Cholangitis is a life-threatening form of intra-abdominal sepsis, though it may appear to be rather innocuous at its onset.
- Antibiotics alone will not resolve cholangitis in the presence of biliary obstruction because high intrabiliary pressures prevent antibiotic delivery. Decompression and drainage of the biliary tract to alleviate the obstruction with antimicrobial therapy is the therapy of choice.

SUGGESTED READINGS
available at www.expertconsult.com

AUTHOR: **GLENN G. FORT, M.D., M.P.H.**

BASIC INFORMATION

DEFINITION
Cholecystitis is acute or chronic inflammation of the gallbladder generally caused by gallstones (>95% of cases).

SYNONYMS
Gallbladder attack

ICD-9CM CODES
575.0 Acute cholecystitis
574.0 Calculus of the gallbladder with acute cholecystitis
575.1 Cholecystitis without mention of calculus

EPIDEMIOLOGY & DEMOGRAPHICS
- Acute cholecystitis occurs most commonly in women during the fifth and sixth decades. Approximately 120,000 cholecystectomies are performed for acute cholecystitis annually in the U.S.
- The incidence of gallstones is 0.6% in the general population and much higher in certain ethnic groups (>75% of Native Americans by age 60 yr). Most patients with gallstones are asymptomatic. Of such patients, biliary colic develops in 1% to 4% annually.

PHYSICAL FINDINGS & CLINICAL PRESENTATION
- Pain and tenderness in the right hypochondrium or epigastrium; pain possibly radiating to the infrascapular region
- Palpation of the right upper quadrant (RUQ) eliciting marked tenderness and stoppage of inspired breath (Murphy's sign)
- Guarding
- Fever (33%)
- Jaundice (25% to 50% of patients)
- Palpable gallbladder (20% of cases)
- Nausea and vomiting (>70% of patients)
- Fever and chills (>25% of patients)
- Medical history often revealing ingestion of large, fatty meals before onset of pain in the epigastrium and RUQ

ETIOLOGY
- Gallstones (>95% of cases)
- Ischemic damage to the gallbladder, critically ill patient (acalculous cholecystitis)
- Infectious agents, especially in patients with AIDS (cytomegalovirus, *Cryptosporidium*)
- Strictures of the bile duct
- Neoplasms, primary or metastatic
- Risk factors for cholelithiasis include age, obesity, female sex, rapid weight loss, ethnicity/race (Native American), use of contraceptives, pregnancy, diabetes mellitus, hemolysis, total parenteral nutrition, biliary parasites

DIAGNOSIS

DIFFERENTIAL DIAGNOSIS
- Hepatic: hepatitis, abscess, hepatic congestion, neoplasm, trauma
- Biliary: neoplasm, stricture, sphincter of Oddi dysfunction
- Gastric: pelvic ulcer disease, neoplasm, alcoholic gastritis, hiatal hernia, non-ulcer dyspepsia
- Pancreatic: pancreatitis, neoplasm, stone in the pancreatic duct or ampulla
- Renal: calculi, infection, inflammation, neoplasm, ruptured kidney
- Pulmonary: pneumonia, pulmonary infarction, right-sided pleurisy
- Intestinal: retrocecal appendicitis, intestinal obstruction, high fecal impaction, irritable bowel syndrome (IBS), inflammatory bowel disease (IBD)
- Cardiac: myocardial ischemia (particularly involving the inferior wall), pericarditis
- Cutaneous: herpes zoster
- Trauma
- Fitz-Hugh-Curtis syndrome (perihepatitis), ruptured ectopic pregnancy
- Subphrenic abscess
- Dissecting aneurysm
- Nerve root irritation caused by osteoarthritis of the spine

WORKUP
Workup consists of detailed history and physical examination coupled with laboratory evaluation and imaging studies. No single clinical finding or laboratory test is sufficient to establish or exclude cholecystitis without further testing.

LABORATORY TESTS
- Leukocytosis (12,000 to 20,000) is present in >70% of patients.
- Elevated alkaline phosphatase, ALT, AST, bilirubin; bilirubin elevation >4 mg/dl is unusual and suggests presence of choledocholithiasis.
- Elevated amylase may be present (consider pancreatitis if serum amylase elevation exceeds 500 U).

IMAGING STUDIES
- Ultrasound of the gallbladder (Fig. E1-212) is the preferred initial test; it will demonstrate the presence of stones and also dilated gallbladder with thickened wall and surrounding edema in patients with acute cholecystitis.
- Nuclear imaging (HIDA scan) (Fig. E1-213) is useful for diagnosis of cholecystitis when sonogram is inconclusive: sensitivity and specificity exceed 90% for acute cholecystis. This test is only reliable when bilirubin is <5 mg/dl. A positive test result (absence of gallbladder filling within 60 min after the administration of tracer) will demonstrate obstruction of the cystic or common hepatic duct; the test will not demonstrate the presence of stones.
- CT scan of abdomen is useful in cases of suspected abscess, neoplasm, or pancreatitis.
- Plain radiograph of the abdomen generally is not useful because <25% of stones are radiopaque.

TREATMENT

NONPHARMACOLOGIC THERAPY
Provide IV hydration; withhold oral feedings.

ACUTE GENERAL Rx
- Laparoscopic (percutaneous) cholecystectomy (PC) is considered the treatment of choice for most patients. The rate of conversion to open cholecystectomy is higher when laparoscopic cholecystectomy (CCY) is performed for acute cholecystitis rather than for uncomplicated cholelithiasis; conservative management with IV fluids and antibiotics (ampicillin-sulbactam 3 g IV q6h or piperacillin-tazobactam 4.5 g IV q8h) may be justified in some high-risk patients to convert an emergency procedure into an elective one with a lower mortality rate.
- Endoscopic retrograde cholangiopancreatography with sphincterectomy and stone extraction can be performed in conjunction with laparoscopic cholecystectomy for patients with choledochal lithiasis; approximately 7% to 15% of patients with cholelithiasis also have stones in the common bile duct.

DISPOSITION
- Prognosis is good; elective laparoscopic cholecystectomy can be performed as outpatient procedure.
- Hospital stay (when necessary) varies from overnight with laparoscopic cholecystectomy to 4 to 7 days with open cholecystectomy.
- Complication rate is approximately 1% (hemorrhage and bile leak) for laparoscopic cholecystectomy and <0.5% (infection) with open cholecystectomy.

REFERRAL
Surgical referral in all patients with acute cholecystitis

PEARLS & CONSIDERATIONS

COMMENTS
- Patients should be instructed that stones may recur in bile ducts.
- Gallbladder aspiration, in which all fluid visualized by ultrasound is aspirated, represents a nonsurgical treatment when patients who are at high operative risk develop acute cholecystitis. Salvage cholecystectomy is reserved for nonresponders.

SUGGESTED READINGS
available at www.expertconsult.com

RELATED CONTENT
Gallbladder Attack (Cholecystitis) (Patient Information)
Cholelithiasis (Related Key Topic)

AUTHOR: **FRED F. FERRI, M.D.**

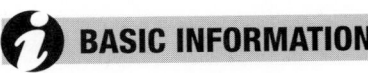

BASIC INFORMATION

DEFINITION

Cholelithiasis is the presence of stones in the gallbladder.

SYNONYMS

Gallstones

ICD-9CM CODES
574.2 Calculus of the gallbladder without mention of cholecystitis
574.0 Calculus of the gallbladder with acute cholecystitis

EPIDEMIOLOGY & DEMOGRAPHICS

- Gallstone disease can be found in 12% of the U.S. population. Of these, 2% to 3% (500,000 to 600,000) are treated with cholecystomies each year.
- Annual medical expenditures for gallbladder surgeries in the U.S. exceed $5 billion.
- Incidence of gallbladder disease increases with age. Highest incidence is in the fifth and sixth decades. Predisposing factors for gallstones are female sex, pregnancy, age >40 yr, family history of gallstones, obesity, ileal disease, oral contraceptives, diabetes mellitus, rapid weight loss, estrogen replacement therapy.
- Patients with gallstones have a 20% chance of developing biliary colic or its complications at the end of a 20-yr period.

PHYSICAL FINDINGS & CLINICAL PRESENTATION

- Physical examination is entirely normal unless patient is having biliary colic; 80% of gallstones are asymptomatic.
- Typical symptoms of obstruction of the cystic duct include intermittent, severe, cramping pain affecting the right upper quadrant.
- Pain occurs mostly at night and may radiate to the back or right shoulder. It can last from a few minutes to several hours.

ETIOLOGY

- 75% of gallstones contain cholesterol and are usually associated with obesity, female sex, and diabetes mellitus; mixed stones are most common (80%); pure cholesterol stones account for only 10% of stones.
- 25% of gallstones are pigment stones (bilirubin, calcium, and variable organic material) associated with hemolysis and cirrhosis. These tend to be black-pigmented stones that are refractory to medical therapy.
- 50% of mixed-type stones are radiopaque.

DIAGNOSIS

DIFFERENTIAL DIAGNOSIS

- Pelvic ulcer disease
- Gastroesophageal reflux disease
- Irritable bowel disease
- Pancreatitis
- Neoplasms
- Nonnuclear dyspepsia
- Inferior wall myocardial infarction
- Hepatic abscess

LABORATORY TESTS

Generally normal unless patient has biliary obstruction (elevated alkaline phosphatase, bilirubin).

IMAGING STUDIES

- Ultrasound of the gallbladder (Fig. E1-214) will detect small stones and biliary sludge (sensitivity, 95%; specificity, 90%); the presence of dilated gallbladder with thickened wall is suggestive of acute cholecystitis.
- Nuclear imaging (HIDA scan) can confirm acute cholecystitis (>90% accuracy) if gallbladder does not visualize within 4 hr of injection and the radioisotope is excreted in the common bile duct.
- Common bile duct stones can be detected noninvasively by magnetic resonance cholangiopancreatography or invasively by endoscopic retrograde cholangiopancreatography (ERCP) and intraoperative cholangiography.

TREATMENT

NONPHARMACOLOGIC THERAPY

Lifestyle changes (avoidance of diets high in polyunsaturated fats, weight loss in obese patients; however, avoid rapid weight loss)

ACUTE GENERAL Rx

- The management of gallstones is affected by the clinical presentation.

TABLE 1-87 Proposed Criteria for Prophylactic Cholecystectomy

Life expectancy >20 years

Calculi >2 cm in diameter

Calculi >3 mm and patent cystic duct

Radiopaque calculi

Gallbladder polyps >15 mm

Nonfunctioning or calcified gallbladder ("porcelain" gallbladder)

Women <60 years

Patients in areas with high prevalence of gallbladder cancer

From Cameron JL, Cameron AM: *Current surgical therapy,* ed 10, Philadelphia, 2011, Saunders.

- Asymptomatic patients do not require therapeutic intervention. Proposed criteria for prophylactic cholecystectomy are described in Table 1-87.
- Surgical intervention is generally the ideal approach for symptomatic patients. Laparoscopic cholecystectomy is generally preferred over open cholecystectomy because of the shorter recovery period and lower mortality rate. Between 5% and 26% of patients undergoing elective laparoscopic cholecystectomy will require conversion to an open procedure. Most common reason is the inability to clearly identify the biliary anatomy.
- Laparoscopic cholecystectomy after endoscopic sphincterectomy is recommended for patients with common bile duct stones and residual gallbladder stones. Where possible, single-stage laparoscopic treatments with removal of duct stones and cholecystectomy during the same procedure are preferable.
- Patients who are not appropriate candidates for surgery because of coexisting illness or patients who refuse surgery can be treated with oral bile salts: ursodiol or chenodiol. Candidates for oral bile salts are patients with cholesterol stones (radiolucent, noncalcified stones), with a diameter of ≤15 mm and having three or fewer stones. Candidates for medical therapy must have a functioning gallbladder and must have absence of calcifications on CT scans.
- Extracorporeal shock wave lithotripsy (ESWL) is another form of medical therapy. It can be used in patients with stone diameter of ≤3 cm and having three or fewer stones.

DISPOSITION

- Recurrence rate after bile acid treatment is approximately 50% in 5 yr. Periodic ultrasound is necessary to assess the effectiveness of treatment.
- After ESWL, stones recur in approximately 20% of patients after 4 yr.
- Patients with at least one gallstone <5 mm in diameter have a greater than fourfold increased risk of presenting with acute biliary pancreatitis. A policy of watchful waiting in such cases is generally unwarranted.
- A potential serious complication of gallstones is acute cholangitis. ERCP and endoscopic sphincterectomy followed by interval laparoscopic cholecystectomy are effective in acute cholangitis.

SUGGESTED READINGS

available at www.expertconsult.com

RELATED CONTENT

Gallstones (Patient Information)
Cholecystitis (Related Key Topic)

AUTHOR: **FRED F. FERRI, M.D.**

BASIC INFORMATION

DEFINITION

Chronic fatigue syndrome (CFS) is characterized by four or more of the following symptoms, present concurrently for at least 6 mo:
- Impaired memory or concentration
- Sore throat
- Tender cervical or axillary lymph nodes
- Muscle pain
- Multijoint pain
- New headaches
- Unrefreshing sleep
- Postexertion malaise for longer than 24 hr

SYNONYMS

Yuppie flu
CFS
Chronic Epstein-Barr syndrome

ICD-9CM CODES
780.7 Chronic fatigue syndrome
300.8 Neurasthenia

EPIDEMIOLOGY & DEMOGRAPHICS

PREVALENCE IN U.S.: 10 to 300 cases per 100,000 persons
PREDOMINANT AGE: Young adulthood and middle age
PREDOMINANT SEX: Females affected more often than males
ECONOMICS: The estimated annual cost of lost productivity exceeds $10 billion.

PHYSICAL FINDINGS & CLINICAL PRESENTATION

- There are no physical findings specific for CFS.
- The physical examination may be useful to identify fibromyalgia and other rheumatologic conditions that may coexist with CFS.

ETIOLOGY

- The etiology of CFS is unknown.
- Some theorize that a viral illness may trigger certain immune responses that lead to the various symptoms. Most patients often report the onset of their symptoms with a flulike illness.
- The presence of numerous psychiatric comorbidities in CFS have led some experts to question the existence of any organic etiology.

DIAGNOSIS

DIFFERENTIAL DIAGNOSIS

- Psychosocial depression, dysthymia, anxiety-related disorders, and other psychiatric diseases
- Infectious diseases (subacute bacterial endocarditis, Lyme disease, fungal diseases, mononucleosis, HIV, chronic hepatitis B or C, tuberculosis (TB), chronic parasitic infections)
- Autoimmune diseases: systemic lupus erythematosus, myasthenia gravis, multiple sclerosis, thyroiditis, rheumatoid arthritis
- Endocrine abnormalities: hypothyroidism, hypopituitarism, adrenal insufficiency, Cushing's syndrome, diabetes mellitus, hyperparathyroidism, pregnancy, reactive hypoglycemia
- Occult malignant disease
- Substance abuse
- Systemic disorders: chronic renal failure, chronic obstructive pulmonary disease, cardiovascular disease, anemia, electrolyte abnormalities, liver disease
- Other: inadequate rest, sleep apnea, narcolepsy, fibromyalgia, sarcoidosis, medications, toxic agent exposure, Wegener's granulomatosis, vitamin deficiency

LABORATORY TESTS

- No specific laboratory tests exist for diagnosing CFS. Initial laboratory tests are useful to exclude other conditions that may mimic or may be associated with CFS.
  1. Screening laboratory tests: CBC, ESR, ALT, total protein, albumin, globulin, alkaline phosphatase, calcium, phosphorus, glucose, BUN, creatinine, electrolytes, TSH, and urinalysis are useful.
  2. Serologic tests for Epstein-Barr virus, *Candida albicans,* human herpesvirus 6, and other studies for immune cellular abnormalities are not useful; these tests are expensive and generally not recommended.
- Other tests may be indicated depending on the history and physical examination (e.g., ANA, RF in patients presenting with joint complaints or abnormalities on physical examination, Lyme titer in areas where Lyme disease is endemic).

IMAGING STUDIES

Generally not recommended unless history and physical examination indicate specific abnormalities (e.g., chest radiography in any patient suspected of TB or sarcoidosis)

TREATMENT

NONPHARMACOLOGIC THERAPY

- Patients should be reassured that the illness is not fatal and that most patients improve over time.
- An initially supervised exercise program to preserve and increase strength is beneficial for most patients and can improve symptoms.
- Cognitive behavioral therapy trials have shown positive effects on fatigue levels, work, depression/anxiety, and social adjustment.

GENERAL Rx

Therapy is generally palliative. The following medications may be helpful; however, evidence is conflicting:
- Antidepressants: The choice of antidepressant varies with the desired side effects. Patients with difficulty sleeping or fibromyalgia-like symptoms may benefit from low-dose tricyclics (doxepin 10 mg hs or amitriptyline 25 mg qhs). When sedation is not desirable, low-dose SSRIs (paroxetine 20 mg qd) often help alleviate fatigue and associated symptoms.
- NSAIDs can be used to relieve muscle and joint pain and headaches.

"Alternative" medications (herbs, multivitamins, nutritional supplements) are very popular with many CFS patients but are generally not very helpful.

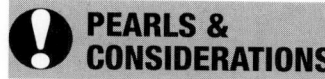

PEARLS & CONSIDERATIONS

COMMENTS

- In CFS the symptoms are serious enough to reduce daily activities by >50% in the absence of any other medically identifiable disorders.
- Moderate to complete recovery at 1 yr occurs in 22% to 60% of patients with CFS.

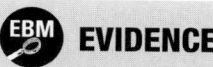

EVIDENCE

available at www.expertconsult.com

SUGGESTED READINGS

available at www.expertconsult.com

RELATED CONTENT

Fig. 3-28 Evaluation of Fatigue (Algorithm)
Chronic Fatigue Syndrome (Patient Information)

AUTHOR: **FRED F. FERRI, M.D.**

BASIC INFORMATION

DEFINITION
Symmetric proximal and distal weakness with associated sensory loss along with reduced or absent reflexes for >2 mo

SYNONYMS
Chronic inflammatory demyelinating polyneuropathy

Chronic inflammatory demyelinating polyradiculoneuropathy

ICD-9CM CODES
357.81 Chronic inflammatory demyelinating polyneuritis

EPIDEMIOLOGY & DEMOGRAPHICS
PREVALENCE: 0.5/100,000 children; 1 to 2/100,000 adults

PREDOMINANT SEX AND AGE: Slightly higher in males

RISK FACTORS: Association with certain systemic medical conditions (see under "Differential Diagnosis" below), but association is unclear

PHYSICAL FINDINGS & CLINICAL PRESENTATION
- Occurrence of symmetrical weakness in both proximal and distal muscles that progressively increases over 2 mo
- Associated with impaired sensation, postural instability, reduced or absent deep tendon reflexes, and variable craniofacial-bulbar involvement

ETIOLOGY
Immune-mediated disorder emerging from interplay of both cell-mediated and humoral immune responses directed against incompletely characterized peripheral nerve antigens. May also be associated with various concurrent illnesses (Table 1-89), although the pathogenetic significance is unclear.

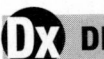 DIAGNOSIS

There is no universal consensus regarding diagnostic criteria for CIDP. The three most widely used are the American Academy of Neurology (AAN), Saperstein, and Inflammatory Neuropathy Cause and Treatment (INCAT) criteria.
- The AAN and INCAT criteria are the least stringent regarding clinical criteria and require motor and sensory function in one limb, whereas the Saperstein criteria are more stringent requiring both symmetrical proximal and distal weakness.
  - Therefore, a patient with DADS (distal acquired demyelinating symmetric neuropathy) could fulfill AAN and INCAT criteria for CIDP.
- All require cerebral spinal fluid analysis to assess for albuminocytologic dissociation.
- Nerve conduction study (NCS): All require some features of demyelination including prolonged distal latencies and F-waves, slowed velocities, and at least one nerve demonstrating partial conduction block (feature of acquired demyelination).
- INCAT criteria do not require a nerve biopsy.
- See Table 1-89 for complete review of differences.

DIFFERENTIAL DIAGNOSIS
- Other demyelinating neuropathies such as:
  - Distal acquired demyelinating symmetric neuropathy (DADS)
  - Multifocal motor neuropathy (MMN)
  - Multifocal acquired demyelinating sensory and motor neuropathy (MADSAM; Lewis-Sumner syndrome)
- Inherited neuropathies: family history, genetic testing, and lack of acquired demyelinating features on NCS will help differentiate it from CIDP

- Metabolic neuropathies: diabetes, uremia
- Paraneoplastic neuropathy: associated with lymphoma or carcinoma
- Neuropathy associated with monoclonal gammopathy: associated with osteosclerotic myeloma, MGUS, and Waldenström's macroglobulinemia.
- Neuropathy associated with infectious diseases: HIV and leprosy
- Neuropathy associated with systemic inflammatory or immune-mediated diseases:
  - Sarcoidosis
  - Amyloidosis
  - Vasculitis: PAN, Behcet's, Sjögren's, cryoglobulinemia, lupus, Castleman's disease, Wegener's, Churg-Strauss
- Toxic neuropathies: ETOH, acrylamide, drugs (platinum-based agents, amiodarone, tacrolimus, perhexilene)

WORKUP
Nerve conduction studies and EMG to assess for demyelinating polyneuropathy with features of acquired demyelination (temporal dispersion and conduction block (Fig. 1-216)

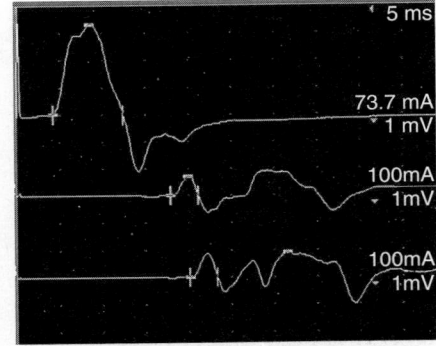

FIGURE 1-216 Conduction block.

TABLE 1-89 Diagnostic Criteria

Feature	American Academy of Neurology (AAN) Criteria	Saperstein Criteria	Inflammatory Neuropathy Cause and Treatment Criteria
Clinical involvement	Motor dysfunction, sensory dysfunction of >1 limb or both	Major: Symmetric proximal and distal weakness; minor: exclusively symmetrical distal weakness or sensory loss	Progressive or relapsing motor and sensory dysfunction of >1 limb
Time course	≥2 mo	≥2 mo	≥2 mo
Reflexes	Reduced or absent	Reduced or absent	Reduced or absent
Electrodiagnostics	Any 3 of the following 4 criteria: partial conduction block of ≥1 motor nerve, reduced velocity of ≥2 motor nerves, prolonged distal latency of ≥2 motor nerves, or prolonged F-waves of ≥2 motor nerves	2 of the 4 AAN electrodiagnostic criteria	Partial conduction block of ≥2 motor nerves and abnormal conduction velocity or distal latency or F-wave latency in 1 other nerve; or, in the absence of partial conduction block, abnormal conduction velocity, distal latency, or F-wave latency in 3 motor nerves; or electrodiagnostic abnormalities indicating demyelination in 2 nerves and histologic evidence of demyelination
CSF analysis	WBC count <10, negative CSF VDRL, and elevated protein (supportive)	Protein >45, WBC <10 (supportive)	CSF recommended but not mandatory
Biopsy findings	Evidence of demyelination and remyelination	Predominant features of demyelination; inflammation (not required)	Not mandatory (except in cases with electrodiagnostic abnormalities in only 2 motor nerves)

LABORATORY TESTS

- CSF analysis to assess for albumin-cytologic dissociation (i.e., elevated protein with normal cell count), along with appropriate laboratory studies to exclude associated conditions.
- Nerve biopsy specimens (rarely done now) also reveal signs of demyelination with variable degrees of inflammation and secondary axonal loss.

IMAGING STUDIES

MRI with/without gadolinium may show enlargement and enhancement of the proximal nerve root segments, respectively (Figs. 1-217 and 1-218)

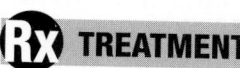 **TREATMENT**

Therapies are directed at blocking the underlying immune processes to arrest demyelination and inflammation and to prevent secondary axonal degeneration. The most widely used forms of immunomodulatory therapy are IV immunoglobulin (IVIg), plasmapheresis/plasma exchange (PE), and corticosteroids. There is no difference in efficacy between these three modalities of treatment. Azathioprine, myocophenylate mofetil, cyclophosphamide, rituximab, and cyclosporine may be used as secondary agents.

NONPHARMACOLOGIC THERAPY

Orthotics/braces for significant distal weakness

ACUTE GENERAL Rx

IVIg 2 g/kg divided over 2 to 5 days; plasmapheresis (5 to 6 exchanges)

CHRONIC Rx

- Oral prednisone (1 mg/kg daily starting dose). Typically changed to every other day after 1 mo or when strength plateaus. Reduce by 10 mg every month until 20 mg every other day. Then reduce by 5 mg/mo. Get tuberculin skin test prior to administration. Treat with calcium and vitamin D; low-sodium/high-protein diet, routine ophthalmologic evaluation for cataract and glaucoma screening, and surveillance for diabetes and GERD symptoms/signs.
- IVIg: 0.4 to 1 g/kg administered monthly. Check baseline IgA level. Check renal function panel and survey for hypercoagulable states and development of headache.
- Mycophenylate mofetil: Start 500 mg bid and increase in 2 to 4 wk to 1 g bid (check CBC, LFTs, and CBC monthly for first 3 mo, then every 3 mo thereafter). May cause GI upset.
- Imuran: Start 25 to 50 mg bid and increase in 4 wk to 100 mg bid (check baseline LFTs and CBC for first 3 mo, then every 3 mo thereafter). Watch for idiosyncratic reaction of fever, GI upset. If occurs, cannot re-challenge patient.
- Cytoxan: Used for severe cases. 1000 mg/m^2 monthly for 6 months (moderate dose) or 50 mg/kg daily × 4 days (high dose).

- Other treatments used (case reports/anecdotal evidence): etanercept, rituximab, tacrolimus, interferon beta-1a.

DISPOSITION

- In one series, 90% of patients with CIDP improved. However, relapse rate was approximately 50%. In Mayo Clinic series, 64% of the patients were either improved or in remission and able to work, 8% were ambulatory but unable to work, 11% were bedridden or wheelchair bound, and 11% died from the disease.
- Patients with CIDP associated with IgM monoclonal gammopathy often respond poorly to treatment.
- Younger age, female gender, and relapsing-remitting course may portend a more favorable prognosis.

REFERRAL

- Neurologist, physical therapy/occupational therapy, orthotics

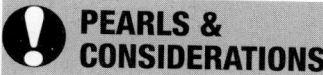 **PEARLS & CONSIDERATIONS**

- Patients are compliant with Imuran treatment if MCV > 100.
- Always place PPD prior to initiation of steroid treatment.
- Consider Bactrim 3 times weekly in patients concomitant with steroids and other immunosuppressant agent for *Pneumocystis* pneumonia prophylaxis (especially in patients with coexisting lung disease).
- NCS: Look for acquired features of demyelination
  - Conduction block
  - Temporal dispersion
- CSF: Albuminocytologic dissociation; high CSF protein with normal cell count.

PATIENT/FAMILY EDUCATION

CIDP is a chronic illness usually characterized by a relapsing-remitting course that typically responds well to treatment. Early referral to a neurologist is important, and education on steroid side effects and mitigating factors is paramount.

SUGGESTED READINGS

available at www.expertconsult.com

AUTHOR: **JOHN SLADKY, M.D.**

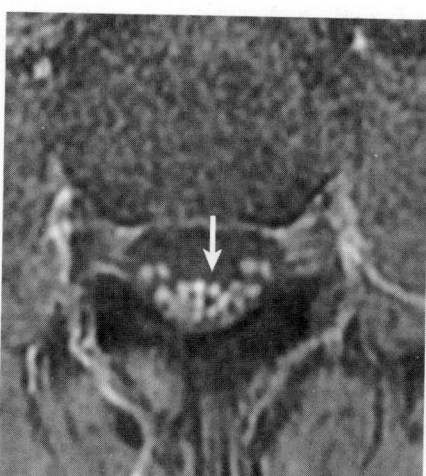

FIGURE 1-217 Contrast-enhanced MRI shows enhancement of nerve roots.

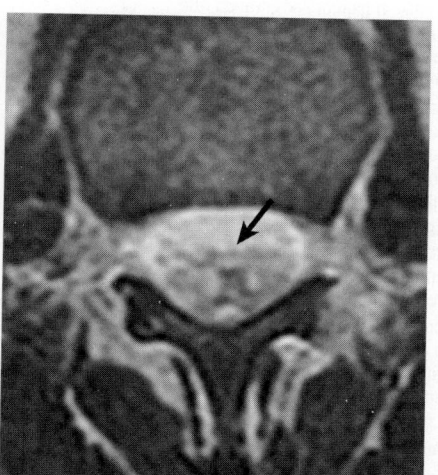

FIGURE 1-218 T2-weighted axial MRI shows enlarged nerve roots.

DEFINITION

Chronic kidney disease (CKD) is a progressive decrease in renal function (glomerular filtration rate [GFR] <60 ml/min for >3 mo) with subsequent accumulation of waste products in the blood, electrolyte abnormalities, and anemia. The mechanisms and manifestations of CKD are summarized in Table 1-90. The National Kidney Foundation Disease Outcomes Quality Initiative defines CKD as follows, regardless of clinical diagnosis (Table 1-91): kidney damage (usually defined as an albumin-creatinine ratio [ACR] ≥30 mg/g) or a glomerular filtration rate (GFR) <60 ml/min per 1.73 m^2 (usually estimated from the serum creatinine level) for at least 3 mo. Table 1-92 describes standardized terminology for stages of chronic renal failure.

Table E1-93 describes the risk, injury, failure, and end-stage kidney disease (RIFLE) classification.

SYNONYMS

CRF
Chronic kidney disease
Chronic renal failure
End-stage renal disease

ICD-9CM CODES
585 Chronic renal failure

EPIDEMIOLOGY & DEMOGRAPHICS

- The prevalence of patients with CKD in the U.S. is approximately 11%.
- The number of patients with end-stage renal disease (ESRD) is increasing at the rate of 7% to 9% per year in the U.S. The increases are partially explained by the increasing prevalence of diabetes mellitus and hypertension, the leading risk factors for CKD. Each year two in 10,000 persons develop end-stage CKD.
- In the U.S., >250,000 people per year receive dialysis treatment for ESRD.
- Although kidney transplantation is considered the best choice for renal replacement therapy, many patients are not eligible for transplantation and more than 100,000 patients start dialysis each year.

PHYSICAL FINDINGS & CLINICAL PRESENTATION

- Skin pallor, ecchymoses.
- Edema, leg cramps, restless legs, peripheral neuropathy.
- Hypertension.
- Emotional lability and depression, decreased mental acuity.
- The clinical presentation varies with the degree of renal failure and its underlying etiology. Common symptoms are generalized fatigue, nausea, anorexia, pruritus (Fig. E1-219), sleep disturbances, smell and taste disturbances, hiccups, and seizures.
- Clinical manifestations of uremic encephalopathy are described in Table 1-90

ETIOLOGY

- Diabetes (37%), hypertension (30%), chronic glomerulonephritis (12%)
- Polycystic kidney disease
- Tubular interstitial nephritis (e.g., drug hypersensitivity, analgesic nephropathy), obstructive nephropathies (e.g., nephrolithiasis, prostatic disease)
- Vascular diseases (renal artery stenosis, hypertensive nephrosclerosis)
- Autoimmune diseases

![Dx] DIAGNOSIS

- CKD is primarily distinguished from acute RF by the duration (progression over several months).

TABLE 1-90 Pathophysiology of Chronic Kidney Disease

Manifestation	Mechanisms
Accumulation of nitrogenous waste products	Decrease in glomerular filtration rate
Acidosis	Decreased ammonia synthesis Impaired bicarbonate reabsorption Decreased net acid excretion
Sodium retention	Excessive renin production Oliguria
Sodium wasting	Solute diuresis Tubular damage
Urinary concentrating defect	Solute diuresis Tubular damage
Hyperkalemia	Decrease in glomerular filtration rate Metabolic acidosis Excessive potassium intake Hyporeninemic hypoaldosteronism
Renal osteodystrophy	Impaired renal production of 1,25-dihydroxycholecalciferol Hyperphosphatemia Hypocalcemia Secondary hyperparathyroidism
Growth retardation	Inadequate caloric intake Renal osteodystrophy Metabolic acidosis Anemia Growth hormone resistance
Anemia	Decreased erythropoietin production Iron deficiency Folate deficiency Vitamin B_{12} deficiency Decreased erythrocyte survival
Bleeding tendency	Defective platelet function
Infection	Defective granulocyte function Impaired cellular immune functions Indwelling dialysis catheters
Neurologic symptoms (fatigue, poor concentration, headache, drowsiness, memory loss, seizures, peripheral neuropathy)	Uremic factor(s) Aluminum toxicity Hypertension
Gastrointestinal symptoms (feeding intolerance, abdominal pain)	Gastroesophageal reflux Decreased gastrointestinal motility
Hypertension	Volume overload Excessive renin production
Hyperlipidemia	Decreased plasma lipoprotein lipase activity
Pericarditis, cardiomyopathy	Uremic factor(s) Hypertension Fluid overload
Glucose intolerance	Tissue insulin resistance

From Kliegman RM et al: *Nelson textbook of pediatrics*, ed 19, Philadelphia, 2011, Saunders.

TABLE 1-91 Criteria for Definition of Chronic Kidney Disease

Kidney damage for ≥3 months, as defined by structural or functional abnormalities of the kidney, with or without decreased GFR, that can lead to decreased GFR, manifest by either:
- Pathologic abnormalities
- Markers of kidney damage, including abnormalities in the composition of blood or urine, or abnormalities in imaging tests
- GFR <60 ml/min/1.73 m^2 for ≥3 months, with or without kidney damage

GFR, Glomerular filtration rate.
From Floege J et al: *Comprehensive clinical nephrology*, ed 4, Philadelphia, 2010, Saunders.

WORKUP

- Laboratory evaluation and imaging studies should be aimed at identifying reversible causes of acute decrements in GFR (e.g., volume depletion, urinary tract obstruction, congestive heart failure [CHF]) superimposed on chronic renal disease.
- Sonographic evaluation of the kidneys reveals smaller kidneys with increased echogenicity in CKD.
- Kidney biopsy: generally not performed in patients with small kidneys or with advanced disease.

LABORATORY TESTS

- Elevated blood urea nitrogen (BUN), creatinine, creatinine clearance. GFR is the best overall indicator of kidney function. It can be estimated by using prediction equations that take into account the serum creatinine level and some or all specific variables (body size, age, sex, race). GFR calculators are available on the National Kidney Foundation website (http://www.kidney.org/kls/professionals/gfr_calculator.cfm).
- Urinalysis: may reveal proteinuria, red blood cell casts.
- Serum chemistry: elevated BUN and creatinine, hyperkalemia, hyperuricemia, hypocalcemia, hyperphosphatemia, hyperglycemia, decreased bicarbonate. Measure urinary protein excretion. The finding of a protein/creatinine ratio of >1000 mg/g suggests the presence of glomerular disease.

- Special studies: serum and urine immuno-electrophoresis (in suspected multiple myeloma), antinuclear antibody (in suspected systemic lupus erythematosus).
- Cystatin C is a cysteine proteinase inhibitor produced by all nucleated cells, freely filtered at the glomerulus but not secreted by tubular cells. Given these characteristics, it may be superior to creatinine concentration both in kidney disease and as a marker of acute kidney injury. It is a better index of kidney function in elderly patients and a better predictor of outcomes than creatinine. The association of cystatin C is stronger than the association of measured GFR with all-cause and cardiovascular mortality in patients with advanced CKD.

IMAGING STUDIES

- Ultrasound of kidneys to measure kidney size and rule out obstruction
- Plain x-rays done for other reasons may reveal extraskeletal calcifications (Fig. E1-220).

CLASSIFICATION

A classification of CKD based on GFR is described in Table 1-94.

 TREATMENT

The management plan for patients with CKD varies according to stage (Table 1-95)

NONPHARMACOLOGIC THERAPY

- Provide adequate nutrition and calories (147 to 168 kJ/kg/day in energy intake, chiefly from carbohydrate and polyunsaturated fats). Table 1-96 describes nutritional recommendations in renal disease. Referral to a dietitian for nutritional therapy for patients with GFR <50 ml/1.73 m² is recommended and is now a covered service by Medicare.
- Restrict sodium (approximately 100 mmol/day), potassium (≤60 mmol/day), and phosphate (<800 mg/day).
- Blood pressure: The optimal blood pressure target in patients with CDK is unclear. Available evidence is inconclusive but does not prove that a blood pressure target of <130/80 mm Hg improves clinical outcomes more than a target of <140/90 mm Hg in adults with CKD. Whether a lower target benefits patients with proteinuria >300 to 1000 mg/dl requires further evaluation.
- Adjust drug doses to correct for prolonged half-lives.
- Restrict fluid if significant edema is present.
- Resistance exercise training can preserve lean body mass, nutritional status, and muscle function in patients with moderate CKD.
- Avoid radiocontrast agents. Hydration with sodium bicarbonate before contrast exposure is more effective than hydration with sodium chloride for prophylaxis of contrast-induced renal failure.
- Smoking cessation.
- Initiate hemodialysis, usually performed in center three times per week, or peritoneal dialysis, usually done by the patient at home (see "General Rx"). Prompt referral to nephrologist is helpful. Late evaluation of patients with chronic renal disease is associated with greater burden and severity of comorbid disease and shorter survival. Suggested criteria for referral to a nephrologist is described in Table 1-97.
- Kidney transplantation in selected patients.

GENERAL Rx

- Angiotensin-converting enzyme (ACE) inhibitors and angiotensin receptor blockers (ARBs) are useful in reducing proteinuria and slowing the progression of chronic renal disease, especially in hypertensive diabetic patients. The combination of ACEi and ARBs should be used only with great caution in patients with CKD due to increased risk of hyperkalemia, hypotension, and worsening renal failure. A systolic blood pressure between 110 and 129 mm Hg may be beneficial in patients with urine protein excretion >1.0 g/day. Systolic blood pressure <110 mm Hg may be associated with a higher risk for kidney disease progression.
- Initiation of dialysis:
  1. Urgent indications: uremic pericarditis, neuropathy, neuromuscular abnormalities, CHF, hyperkalemia, seizures.
  2. Judgmental indications: creatinine clearance 10 to 15 ml/min; progressive

---

TABLE 1-92 Standardized Terminology for Stages of Chronic Kidney Disease

Stage	Description	GFR (ml/min/1.73 m²)
1	Kidney damage with normal or increased GFR	>90
2	Kidney damage with mild decrease in GFR	60-89
3	Moderate decrease in GFR	30-59
4	Severe decrease in GFR	5-29
5	Kidney failure	<15 or on dialysis

GFR, Glomerular filtration rate.
From Kliegman RM et al: *Nelson textbook of pediatrics,* ed 19, Philadelphia, 2011, Saunders.

TABLE 1-94 Classification of Chronic Kidney Disease Based on GFR

CKD Stage	Definition
1	Normal or increased GFR; some evidence of kidney damage reflected by microalbuminuria, proteinuria, and hematuria as well as radiologic or histologic changes
2	Mild decrease in GFR (89-60 ml/min per 1.73 m²) with some evidence of kidney damage reflected by microalbuminuria, proteinuria, and hematuria as well as radiologic or histologic changes
3	GFR 59 to 30 ml/min per 1.73 m²
3A	GFR 59 to 45 ml/min per 1.73 m²
3B	GFR 44-30 ml/min per 1.73 m²
4	GFR 29-15 ml/min per 1.73 m²
5	GFR <15 ml/min per 1.73 m²; when renal replacement therapy in the form of dialysis or transplantation has to be considered to sustain life

GFR, Glomerular filtration rate.
The suffix p to be added to the stage in proteinuric patients (proteinuria >0.5 g/24h)
Classification of CKD based on GFR as proposed by the Kidney Disease Outcomes Quality Initiative (KDOQI) guidelines and modified by NICE in 2008.
From Floege J et al: *Comprehensive clinical nephrology,* ed 4, Philadelphia, 2010, Saunders.

anorexia, weight loss, reversal of sleep pattern, pruritus, uncontrolled fluid gain with hypertension and signs of CHF.

3. General indications for initiation of dialysis are summarized in Table 1-98. Suggested steps for resolving conflict in the shared decision about starting dialysis are described in Fig. E1-221. Recent trials have shown that early initiation of dialysis in patients with stage 5 CKD is not associated with increased survival. Initiation of dialysis when the GFR is 10 to 14 ml/min per 1.73 m² does not enhance survival compared with a strategy of symptom-driven initiation or initiation of dialysis at eGFR <7 ml/min per 173 m².

- Erythropoiesis-stimulating agents epoetin-alpha and darbepoetin-alpha can be used to reduce the need for transfusions in patients with anemia. Anemia should not be fully corrected in patients with CKD. Maintaining a target hemoglobin of 10 g/dl or hematocrit 30% to 33% is satisfactory. Targeting higher hemoglobin levels in CKD may increase risks for stroke, hypertension, and serious cardiovascular events.

- Diuretics for significant fluid overload (loop diuretics are preferred).
- Correction of hypertension to at least 130/85 mm Hg with ACE inhibitors (avoid in patients with significant hyperkalemia), ARBs, and/or nondihydropyridine calcium channel blockers (verapamil, diltiazem) can be used in patients intolerant to ACE inhibitors or when other agents are needed to control blood pressure.
- Correction of electrolyte abnormalities (e.g., calcium chloride, glucose, sodium polystyrene sulfonate for hyperkalemia), sodium

TABLE 1-95 Management Plan for Patients with Chronic Kidney Disease, According to Stage

KDOQI Classification	GFR (ml/min)	Typical Serum Creatinine in 65-kg Subject	Consequences	Actions to Consider
3	30-59	2 mg/dl (170 μmol/L)	Hypertension, secondary hyperparathyroidism	6-monthly eGFR initially 12-monthly eGFR if stable Annual Hb, K, Ca, P Treat hypertension Immunize against hepatitis B
4	15-29	4 mg/dl (350 μmol/L)	*Plus* anemia, hyperphosphatemia	3-monthly eGFR initially 6-monthly eGFR if stable 6-monthly Hb, K, Ca, P, and PTH Start phosphate-restricted diet and phosphate binders Correct vitamin D deficiency Start vitamin D analogue Plan renal replacement therapy, including vascular access
5	<15	8 mg/dl (700 μmol/L)	*Plus* sodium and water retention, anorexia, vomiting, reduced higher mental function	Plan elective start of dialysis or preemptive renal transplant
5	<5	17 mg/dl (1500 μmol/L)	*Plus* pulmonary edema, coma, fits, metabolic acidosis, hyperkalemia, death	Start dialysis or provide palliative care

The table gives a rough guide to the level of serum creatinine corresponding to each stage of CKD in a typical 65-kg subject and shows the approximate timing of the anticipated clinical problems and interventions required as CKD progresses. At each stage, the action plan for the previous CKD stage should be followed if it has not already been initiated.
eGFR, Estimated glomerular filtration rate; *PTH*, parathyroid hormone.
From Floege J et al: *Comprehensive clinical nephrology*, ed 4, Philadelphia, 2010, Saunders.

TABLE 1-96 Nutritional Recommendations in Renal Disease

Daily Intake	Predialysis CRF	Hemodialysis	Peritoneal Dialysis
Protein (g/kg ideal BW) (see KDOQI[24] for estimation of adjusted edema-free body weight)	0.6-1.0 Level depends on the view of the nephrologist 1.0 for nephrotic syndrome	1.1-1.2 This is a broad recommendation as protein intake would be individualized for the patient's nutritional status, serum phosphate levels, and dialysis adequacy	1.0-1.3
Energy (kcal/kg BW)	35 (<60 yr) 30-35 (>60 yr)	35 (<60 yr) 30-35 (>60 yr)	35 including dialysate calories (<60 yr) 30-35 including dialysate calories (>60 yr)
Sodium (mmol)	<100 (more if salt wasting)	<100	<100
Potassium	Reduce if hyperkalemic	Reduce if hyperkalemic	Reduce if hyperkalemic; potassium restriction is generally not required
	If hyperkalemic, advice will take the form of decreasing certain foods (e.g., some fruits and vegetables) and giving information about cooking methods		
Phosphorous	Reduce; level dependent on protein intake Advice will take the form of reducing certain foods (e.g., dairy, offal, some shellfish) and giving information about the timing of binders with high phosphorus meals and snacks		
Calcium	In CKD stages 3-5, total intake of elemental calcium (including dietary calcium) should not exceed 2000 mg/day	Total intake of elemental calcium (including dietary calcium) should not exceed 2000 mg/day	Total intake of elemental calcium (including dietary calcium) should not exceed 2000 mg/day

Recommendations are for typical patients but should always be individualized on the basis of clinical, biochemical, and anthropometric indices.
BW, Body weight; *CKD*, chronic kidney disease; *CRF*, chronic renal failure; *KDOQI*, Kidney Disease Outcomes Quality Initiative.
From Floege J et al: *Comprehensive clinical nephrology*, ed 4, Philadelphia, 2010, Saunders.

TABLE 1-97 Suggested Criteria for Referral of Patients with Chronic Kidney Disease to a Nephrologist

New Diagnosis	Stage 3	Stage 4
eGFR <30 ml/min/per 173 m²	eGFR falling by >4 ml/min per year	eGFR <20 ml/min per 173 m²
Hemoglobin <11 g/dl	eGFR <50 ml/min in patient younger than 50 years	eGFR falling by >4 ml/min per year
K⁺ >6 mmol/L	Hemoglobin <11 g/dl	Hemoglobin <11 g/dl
Ca <2.1 mmol/L	K⁺ >6 mmol/L	K⁺ >6 mmol/L
Pi >1.5 mmol/L	Ca <2.1 mmol/L	Ca <2.1 mmol/L
PTH >3× upper limit normal	Pi >1.5 mmol/L	Pi >1.5 mmol/L
Hematuria		PTH >3× upper limit normal
Urine ACR >30 mg/mmol		
Suspected renovascular disease		

ACR, Albumin to creatinine ratio; *eGFR,* estimated glomerular filtration rate; *PTH,* parathyroid hormone.
Modified from NICE CKD guideline. From Floege J et al: *Comprehensive clinical nephrology,* ed 4, Philadelphia, 2010, Saunders.

TABLE 1-98 When to Initiate Dialysis

Indications for early start on dialysis
- Intractable fluid overload
- Intractable hyperkalemia
- Malnutrition due to uremia
- Uremic neurologic dysfunction
- Uremic serositis
- Functional deterioration otherwise unexplained

Uremic cognitive dysfunction can affect learning
Therefore, home-based self-dialysis may need to start earlier than center-assisted dialysis.

Start of dialysis may be delayed if patient is
asymptomatic, awaiting imminent kidney transplant, awaiting imminent placement of permanent HD or PD access, or, after appropriate education, has chosen conservative therapy.

If start of dialysis is delayed,
patient should be re-evaluated regularly to see if dialysis has become necessary.

Patients who choose PD
should not be required to have HD access placed, but venous sites for possible future HD access in arms should be preserved since HD may be required in the future.
Incremental start on PD may be considered if there is significant residual renal function.

Nephrologists should consider conservative (nondialysis) treatment of kidney failure an integral part of their clinical practice.

HD, hemodialysis; *PD,* peritoneal dialysis.
Modified from NKF KDOQI Clinical Practice Guideline for initiation of dialysis. http://www.kidney.org/professional/Kdoqi/guideline_upHD_PD_VA/pd_rec1.htm. From Floege J et al: *Comprehensive clinical nephrology,* ed 4, Philadelphia, 2010, Saunders.

bicarbonate in patients with severe metabolic acidosis.
- Lipid-lowering agents in patients with dyslipidemia; target low-density lipoprotein cholesterol is <100 mg/dl. Lipid-lowering therapy has been shown to decrease cardiac death and atherosclerosis-mediated cardiovascular events in persons with CKD.
- Control of renal osteodystrophy with calcium supplementation and vitamin D. Starting dose of calcium carbonate is 0.5 g with each meal, increased until the serum phosphorus concentration is normalized (most patients require 5 to 10 g/day). Calcitriol 0.125 to 0.25 mcg/day PO is effective in increasing serum calcium concentration. Paricalcitol, a new vitamin D analogue, has been reported to be more effective than calcitriol in lessening the elevations in serum calcium and phosphorus levels.
- Dietary phosphate restriction effectively reduces serum phosphate levels and is recommended in all patiens with ESRD. For additional management of hyperphosphatemia, calcium-based agents are inexpensive, well tolerated, and should be the first-line phosphate binders for patients undergoing dialysis. Sevelamer and lanthanum are also effective as phosphate binders, but are much more expensive.
- General considerations in the continuing assessment of the CKD patient are described in Table 1-99.
- A sequential approach to the uremic patient with pruritus is described in Fig. E1-222.

DISPOSITION

- Prognosis is influenced by comorbidity of multisystem diseases. Late referral of patients to a nephrologist is associated with higher mortality and morbidity rates and higher costs. Despite recommendations for early referral, up to 64% of patients with CKD are still referred late.
- Lower predialysis serum sodium concentration is associated with an increased risk of death.
- Apolipoprotein E variation predicts CKD progression, independent of diabetes, race, lipid, and nonlipid factors. The e2 allele moderately increases risk of kidney disease progression, whereas allele e4 decreases the risk.
- Kidney transplantation in selected patients improves survival. The 2-yr kidney graft survival rate for living related donor transplantations is >80%, whereas the 2-yr graft survival rate for cadaveric donor transplantation is approximately 70%.
- Principles underlying withdrawal of dialysis are described in Table 1-100.

TABLE 1-99 Continuing Assessment of the Chronic Kidney Disease Patient

Kidney Function

Has kidney function declined?
Has kidney function declined at the predicted rate?
If not, are there exacerbating factors?
Should dialysis be started?
Are there life-threatening complications?
   Pericarditis
   Fluid overload
   Resistant hypertension
   Hyperkalemia
   Uncompensated metabolic acidosis
Should access be created or transplantation planned?

Supportive Treatment

Can salt, potassium, and fluid balance be improved by diet or diuretics?
Is the phosphate controlled?
Is the dose of vitamin D compound appropriate?
Should erythropoietin (EPO) be prescribed?
Are nutritional supplements needed?
Does the patient need counseling?

Questions to be posed in evaluation of the patient.
From Floege J et al: *Comprehensive clinical nephrology,* ed 4, Philadelphia, 2010, Saunders.

TABLE 1-100 Principles Underlying Withdrawal of Dialysis

The ultimate responsibility for the decision rests with the physician, not the relative.
The patient's interests and dignity should be protected at all times.
The process should not be rushed. If there is any doubt about the correctness of the decision, treatment should continue.
There should be an open discussion among the multidisciplinary team to avoid any damaging disagreements.
The psychological needs of the health care team should not be overlooked.
Palliative care must be given in the most appropriate environment, e.g., a hospice or, ideally, the patient's own home.

From Floege J et al: *Comprehensive clinical nephrology,* ed 4, Philadelphia, 2010, Saunders.

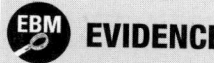 **EVIDENCE**

available at www.expertconsult.com

SUGGESTED READINGS
available at www.expertconsult.com

AUTHOR: **FRED F. FERRI, M.D.**

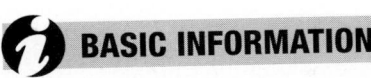

BASIC INFORMATION

DEFINITION

Chronic obstructive pulmonary disease (COPD) is an inflammatory respiratory disease usually caused by exposure to tobacco smoke. It is characterized by the presence of airflow limitation that is not fully reversible. The pathophysiology of COPD is related to chronic airway irritation, mucus production, and pulmonary scarring. Traditionally, COPD was described as encompassing *emphysema*, characterized by loss of lung elasticity and destruction of lung parenchyma with enlargement of air spaces, and *chronic bronchitis*, characterized by obstruction of small airways and productive cough >3 mo for more than 2 successive yr. These terms are no longer included in the formal definition of COPD, although they are still used clinically. Although emphysema and chronic bronchitis are commonly associated with COPD, neither is required to make the diagnosis.

SYNONYMS

COPD
Emphysema
Chronic bronchitis

ICD-9CM CODES
496 COPD
492.8 Emphysema

EPIDEMIOLOGY & DEMOGRAPHICS

- COPD affects more than 5% of adults in the U.S.
- Between 10% and 20% of COPD in the U.S. is due to occupational or other exposure to chemical vapors, irritants, and fumes; 80% to 90% is due to cigarette smoking.
- COPD is the third leading cause of death in the U.S.
- Highest incidence is in males >40 yr.
- 16 million office visits, 500,000 hospitalizations, 120,000 deaths annually, and >$18 billion in direct health care costs annually can be attributed to COPD.
- Patients with COPD living in isolated rural areas of the U.S. are at greater risk for COPD exacerbation-related mortality than those living in urban areas, independent of hospital rurality and volume.

PHYSICAL FINDINGS & CLINICAL PRESENTATION

- Patients with COPD have historically been classically subdivided in two major groups based on their appearance:
  1. *Blue bloaters* are patients with chronic bronchitis; the name is derived from the bluish tinge of the skin (as a result of chronic hypoxemia and hypercapnia) and from the frequent presence of peripheral edema (from cor pulmonale); chronic cough with production of large amounts of sputum is characteristic.
  2. *Pink puffers* are patients with emphysema; they have a cachectic appearance but pink skin color (adequate oxygen saturation); shortness of breath is manifested by pursed-lip breathing and use of accessory muscles of respiration.
- COPD may present with combinations of the following manifestations:
  1. Cyanosis, chronic cough (usually productive but may be intermittent and may be unproductive), tachypnea, tachycardia.
  2. Dyspnea (persistent, progressive), pursed-lip breathing with use of accessory muscles for respiration, decreased breath sounds, wheezing.
  3. Chronic sputum production.
  4. Chest wall abnormalities (hyperinflation, "barrel chest," protruding abdomen).
  5. Flattening of diaphragm.
- Acute exacerbation of COPD is mainly a clinical diagnosis and generally manifests with worsening dyspnea, increase in sputum purulence, and increase in sputum volume. However, respiratory symptom status is not a reliable indicator of the presence of airflow obstruction. Individuals with normal spirometric values may report respiratory symptoms, whereas individuals who have severe to very severe airflow obstruction by spirometry may report no symptoms.

ETIOLOGY

- Tobacco exposure
- Occupational exposure to pulmonary toxins (e.g., dust, noxious gases, vapors, fumes, cadmium, coal, silica). The industries with the highest exposure risk are plastics, leather, rubber, and textiles.
- Atmospheric pollution.
- Alpha-1-antitrypsin deficiency (rare; <1% of COPD patients).

Dx DIAGNOSIS

DIFFERENTIAL DIAGNOSIS

- Congestive heart failure
- Asthma
- Tuberculosis, other respiratory infections
- Bronchiectasis
- Cystic fibrosis
- Neoplasm
- Pulmonary embolism
- Obliterative bronchiolitis
- Diffuse panbronchiolitis
- Sleep apnea, obstructive
- Hypothyroidism <50% predicted

WORKUP

Chest x-ray (seldom diagnostic but useful to exclude alternative diagnosis [CHF, TB]), pulmonary function testing (spirometry), oxygen saturation, blood gases (in selected patients with FEV_1 < 50% predicted or with acute exacerbation). Alpha-1-antitrypsin deficiency screening may be useful in Caucasians with suspected COPD and no clear risk factors.

LABORATORY TESTS

- CBC: generally not helpful, may reveal leukocytosis with left shift during acute exacerbation. Recent trials have shown that eosinophilia in COPD patients predicts response to corticosteroids.
- Sputum may be purulent with bacterial respiratory tract infections. Sputum staining and cultures are usually reserved for cases refractory to antibiotic therapy.
- Arterial blood gases: normocapnia, mild to moderate hypoxemia may be present. ABGs and pulse oximetry are usually used to determine if a patient is a candidate for long-term oxygen therapy or if hypercapnia is present (ABGs).
- Spirometry pulmonary function testing (PFT) with measurement of forced vital capacity (FVC) and forced expiratory volume in 1 s (FEV_1). Spirometry should be obtained to diagnose airflow obstruction in patients with respiratory symptoms. It should not be used to screen for airflow obstruction in individuals without respiratory symptoms. Spirometry reveals that the primary physiologic abnormality in COPD is an accelerated decline in FEV_1 from the normal rate in adults >30 yr of approximately 30 ml/yr to nearly 60 ml/yr. PFT results in COPD reveal abnormal diffusing capacity, increased total lung capacity and/or residual volume, and fixed reduction in FEV_1 in patients with emphysema; normal diffusing capacity and reduced FEV_1 are found in patients with chronic bronchitis. Stage and severity of COPD according to postbronchodilator spirometry are described in Table 1-101. It is important to note that FEV_1 does not correlate well with individual patients' severity of dyspnea, exercise limitations, or health status. Evaluation of patients should also focus on

TABLE 1-101 Stage and Severity of COPD According to Postbronchodilator Spirometry

Stage and Severity	Definition
I: Mild	FEV_1/FVC <0.70, FEV_1 ≥80% of predicted
II: Moderate	FEV_1/FVC <0.70, 50%≤FEV_1 <80% of predicted
III: Severe	FEV_1/FVC <0.70, 30%≤FEV_1 <50% of predicted
IV: Very severe	FEV_1/FVC <0.70, FEV_1 <30% of predicted or FEV_1 <50% of predicted plus chronic respiratory failure

Data from the Global Initiative for Chronic Obstructive Lung Disease. http://www.goldcopd.com.
From Goldman L, Schafer AI: *Goldman's Cecil medicine,* ed 24, Philadelphia, 2012, Saunders.

symptom control and risk for adverse events in addition to FEV₁.

- Patients with COPD can generally be distinguished from asthmatics by their incomplete response to albuterol (change in FEV₁ <200 ml and 12%) and absence of an abnormal bronchoconstrictor response to methacholine or other stimuli. However, nearly 40% of patients with COPD respond to bronchodilators.

IMAGING STUDIES

Chest x-ray:
- Hyperinflation with flattened diaphragm, tenting of the diaphragm at the rib, and increased retrosternal chest space (Fig. 1-223)
- Decreased vascular markings and bullae in patients with emphysema
- Thickened bronchial markings and enlarged right side of the heart in patients with chronic bronchitis

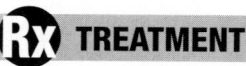 **TREATMENT**

NONPHARMACOLOGIC THERAPY

- Avoidance of tobacco and elimination of air pollutants.
- Supplemental oxygen, usually through a face mask, to ensure oxygen saturation >90% as measured by pulse oximetry. Continuous oxygen therapy should be prescribed for patients with COPD who have arterial partial pressure of oxygen 55 mm Hg or less, or oxygen saturation 88% or less as measured by pulse oximetry.
- Pulmonary clearing: careful nasotracheal suction is indicated only in patients with excessive secretions and an inability to expectorate. Mechanical percussion of the chest as applied by a physical or respiratory therapist is ineffective with acute exacerbations of COPD.
- Pulmonary rehabilitation should be considered in COPD patients who remain symptomatic despite optimal medical management. Medicare will cover up to 36 sessions of pulmonary rehabilitation in COPD patients.
- Weight loss in obese patients.

GENERAL Rx

- Pharmacologic treatment should be administered in a stepwise approach according to the severity of disease and patient's tolerance for specific drugs. Fig. E1-224 describes general management approaches for COPD.
  - Bronchodilators improve symptoms, quality of life, and exercise tolerance, and decrease incidence of exacerbations. Inhaled bronchodilators *may be used* for stable COPD patients with respiratory symptoms and FEV₁ between 60% and 80% of predicted. They are *recommended* for stable COPD patients with respiratory symptoms and FEV₁ <60% of predicted. Recent guidelines from ACP, ACCP, ATS, and ERS recommend that clinicians prescribe monotherapy using either long-acting inhaled anticholinergics or long-acting inhaled beta-agonists for symptomatic patients with COPD and FEV₁ <60% of predicted.

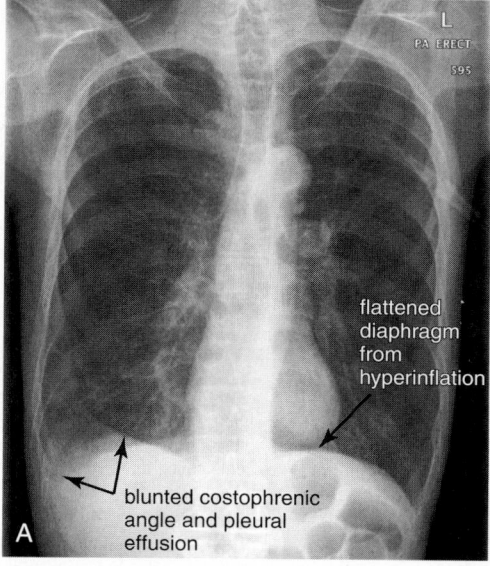 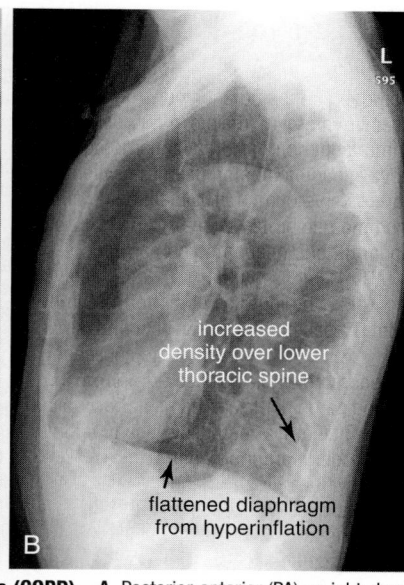

FIGURE 1-223 Chronic obstructive pulmonary disease (COPD). A, Posterior-anterior (PA) upright chest x-ray. **B,** Lateral upright chest x-ray. This 63-year-old man with a history of COPD presented with 2 weeks of worsening cough with yellow sputum and dyspnea. His oxygen saturation was 87% in the emergency room. He has evidence of hyperinflation with flat diaphragms (particularly evident on the lateral x-ray, **B**). The patient also has a blunted right costophrenic angle with an apparent effusion and increased densities in both the right and the left lung base **(A)**. The lateral x-ray also shows increased density overlying the inferior thoracic spine, an abnormal spine sign. (From Broder JS: *Diagnostic imaging for the emergency physician,* Philadelphia, 2011, Saunders.)

Clinicians should base the choice of specific monotherapy on patient preference, cost, and adverse effect profile.
- Short-acting beta-2 agonists (e.g., albuterol metered-dose inhaler 1 to 2 puffs q4 to 6h prn) or short-acting anticholinergic agents (e.g., ipratropium inhaler 2 puffs qid) are acceptable in patients with mild, variable symptoms. Anticholinergics are also effective and are available in combination with albuterol (Combivent). Long-acting inhaled agents are preferred in patients with mild to moderate or continuous symptoms. Tiotropium is an excellent long-acting bronchodilator. It is very effective for long-term, once-a-day use. It has been shown to be superior to salmeterol, an inhaled long-acting beta-agonist (LABA) in patients with moderate to severe COPD; however, recent trials have shown higher hospitalization rates and mortality with tiotropium compared to LABAs. Aclidinium is another orally inhaled long-acting anticholinergic for long-term maintenance treatment of bronchospasm associated with COPD. Unlike tiotropium, which is predominantly renally excreted, it can be used safely in renal impairment.
- Addition of inhaled steroids (fluticasone, budesonide, triamcinolone) is used to reduce exacerbations in patients with moderate to severe COPD. Inhaled steroids are reserved for patients with either ≥2 exacerbations annually or FEV₁ <50% of predicted. The role of inhaled corticosteroids (ICS) in COPD is controversial. Although some trials have demonstrated mild improvement in patients' symptoms and

decreased frequency of exacerbations, most pulmonologists believe that these drugs are ineffective in most patients with COPD but should be considered for patients with moderate to severe airflow limitation who have persistent symptoms despite optimal bronchodilator therapy. ICS therapy does not affect 1-yr all-cause mortality among patients with COPD and is associated with a higher risk of pneumonia.
- Roflumilast is a selective oral PDE4 inhibitor useful to reduce the risk of COPD exacerbations in patients with severe COPD associated with chronic bronchitis and a history of exacerbations. It is not a bronchodilator and is not indicated for the relief of acute bronchospasm.
- Recent guidelines from ACP (American College of Physicians), ACCP (American College of Chest Physicians), ATS (American Thoracic Society), and ERS (European Respiratory Society) suggest that clinicians may administer combination inhaled therapies for symptomatic patients with stable COPD and FEV₁ <60% predicted. They also recommend that clinicians should prescribe pulmonary rehabilitation for symptomatic patients with an FEV₁ <50% predicted and continuous oxygen therapy in patients with COPD who have resting hypoxemia (Pao₂ <55 mm Hg or Spo₂ <88%).
- Acute exacerbation of COPD (increase in sputum volume and purulence, worsening dyspnea) can be treated with:
  - Aerosolized beta-2 agonists (e.g., metaproterenol nebulizer solution 5% 0.3 ml or albuterol nebulized 5% solution 2.5 to 5 mg).

TABLE 1-102 Guideline Recommendations for Hospital Management of COPD Exacerbations

	Global Initiative for Chronic Obstructive Lung Disease*	American Thoracic Society/ European Respiratory Society†	National Institute for Clinical Excellence‡
Date of statement	2010	2004	2010
Diagnostic testing	Chest radiograph, oximetry, ABGs, and ECG. Other testing as warranted by clinical indication.	Chest radiograph, oxygen saturation, ABGs, ECG, sputum Gram stain and culture.	Chest radiograph, ABG, ECG, complete blood count, sputum smear and culture, blood cultures if febrile.
Bronchodilator therapy	Inhaled short-acting β_2-agonist is recommended. Consider ipratropium if inadequate clinical response. Consider theophylline or aminophylline as second-line intravenous therapy.	Inhaled short-acting β_2-agonist and/or ipratropium with spacer or nebulizer, as needed.	Administer inhaled drugs by nebulizer or handheld inhaler. Specific agents and dosing regimens not specified. Consider theophylline if inadequate response to inhaled bronchodilators.
Antibiotics	Recommended if (1) increases in dyspnea, sputum volume, and sputum purulence all are present; (2) increase in sputum purulence along with increase in either dyspnea or sputum volume; or (3) need for assisted ventilation. See original document for complex treatment algorithm.	Base choice on local bacterial resistance patterns. Consider amoxicillin/clavulanate or respiratory fluoroquinolones. If *Pseudomonas* species and/or other Enterobacteriaceae are suspected, consider combination therapy.	Administer only if history of purulent sputum. Initiate with an aminopenicillin, a macrolide, or a tetracycline, taking into account local bacterial resistance patterns. Adjust therapy according to sputum and blood cultures.
Systemic corticosteroids	Daily prednisolone 30-40 mg (or its equivalent) orally for 7-10 days.	Daily prednisone 30-40 mg orally for 10-14 days. Equivalent dose intravenously if unable to tolerate oral intake. Consider inhaled corticosteroids.	Daily prednisolone 30 mg (or its equivalent) orally for 7-14 days.
Supplemental oxygen	Maintain oxygen saturation >90%. Monitor ABGs for hypercapnia and acidosis.	Maintain oxygen saturation >90%. Monitor ABGs for hypercapnia and acidosis.	Maintain oxygen saturation within the individualized target range. Monitor ABGs.
Assisted ventilation	Indications for NPPV include severe dyspnea, acidosis (pH ≤7.35) and/or hypercapnia (PCO$_2$ >45 mm Hg), and respiratory rate >25 breaths/min. Contraindications to NPPV include respiratory arrest, hemodynamic instability, impaired mental status, copious bronchial secretions, and extreme obesity. Intubate if contraindication to NPPV or failure of NPPV (worsening ABGs or clinical status). Consider likelihood of recovery and patient's wishes and expectations before intubation.	Consider with pH <7.35 and PCO$_2$ >45-60 mm Hg and respiratory rate >24 breaths/min. Institute NPPV in a controlled environment, unless there are contraindications (e.g., respiratory arrest, hemodynamic instability, impaired mental status, copious bronchial secretions, and extreme obesity). Intubate if contraindication to NPPV or failure of NPPV (worsening ABGs or clinical status).	NPPV treatment of choice for persistent hypercapnic respiratory failure. Consider functional status, body mass index, home oxygen, comorbidities, prior ICU admissions, age, and FEV$_1$ when assessing suitability for intubation and ventilation.

*Data from http://www.goldcopd.com.
†Data from MacNee W. Standards for the diagnosis and treatment of patients with COPD: a summary of the ATS/ERS position paper. *Eur Respir J* 23:932-946, 2004.
‡Data from http://www.nice.org.uk.
ABGs, Arterial blood gases; *ECG,* electrocardiogram; *ICU,* intensive care unit; *NPPV,* noninvasive positive pressure ventilation.
From Goldman L, Schafer AI: *Goldman's Cecil medicine,* ed 24, Philadelphia, 2012, Saunders.

○ Anticholinergic agents, which have equivalent efficacy to inhaled beta-adrenergic agonists. Inhalant solution of ipratropium bromide 0.5 mg can be administered every 4 to 8 hr.

○ Short courses of systemic corticosteroids have been shown to improve spirometric and clinical outcomes. Treatment failure occurs less often in patients who receive low-dose steroids than in those receiving high-dose parenteral steroids. Oral prednisone 40 mg/day for 10 to 14 days is generally effective. Courses of treatment that are extended for >14 days confer no added benefit and increase the risk of adverse events.

○ Use of noninvasive positive pressure ventilation (NIPPV) decreases the risk of endotracheal intubation and decreases intensive care unit admission rates. Contraindications to its use are uncooperative patient, decreased level of consciousness, hemodynamic instability, inadequate mask fit, and severe respiratory acidosis. Increased airway pressure can be delivered by using inspiratory positive airway pressure, continuous positive airway pressure, or bilevel positive airway pressure, which combines the other modalities. When using NIPPV, the nasal mask is usually tolerated the best; however, patients must be instructed to keep their mouths closed while breathing with the nasal apparatus. Oxygen can be delivered at 10 to 15 L/min and started in spontaneous ventilation mode with an initial expiratory positive airway pressure setting of 3 to 5 cm H$_2$O and an inspiratory positive airway pressure setting of up to 10 cm H$_2$O. Adjustments in these settings should be made in 2-cm H$_2$O increments. It is important to monitor patients with frequent vital signs measurements, arterial blood gases, or pulse oximetry. Intubation and mechanical ventilation may be necessary if previous measures fail to provide improvement.

○ IV aminophylline administration is controversial and generally not recommended. When used in patients with refractory symptoms, serum levels should be closely monitored (keep level 8 to 12 mcg/ml) to minimize risks of tachyarrhythmias.

• Appoximately 50% of COPD exacerbations are caused by bacterial infection. Antibiotics are indicated in suspected respiratory infection (e.g., increased purulence and volume of phlegm).

○ *Haemophilus influenzae* and *Streptococcus pneumoniae* are frequent causes of acute bronchitis.

○ Oral antibiotics of choice are azithromycin, levofloxacin, amoxicillin-clavulanate, trimethoprim-sulfamethoxazole, doxycycline, and cefuroxime.

○ The use of antibiotics is beneficial in exacerbations of COPD presenting with increased dyspnea and sputum purulence (especially if the patient is febrile).

• Guaifenesin may improve cough symptoms and mucus clearance; however, mucolytic medications are generally ineffective. Their benefits may be greatest in patients with more advanced disease.

• Guideline recommendations for hospital management of COPD exacerbations are described in Table 1-102. Indications for invasive mechanical ventilation are described in Box 1-10.

Lung volume reduction surgery has been proposed as a palliative treatment for severe emphysema. Overall it increases the chance of improved exercise capacity but does not

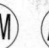

BOX 1-10 Indications for Invasive Mechanical Ventilation

Severe dyspnea, with use of accessory muscles and paradoxical abdominal motion
Respiratory frequency >35 breaths/min
Life-threatening hypoxemia (Pao_2 <40 mm Hg or Pao_2/Fio_2 <200 mm Hg)
Severe acidosis (pH <7.25) and hypercapnia ($Paco_2$ >60 mm Hg)
Respiratory arrest
Somnolence, impaired mental status
Cardiovascular complications (hypotension, shock, heart failure)
Other complications: metabolic abnormalities, sepsis, pneumonia, pulmonary embolism, barotrauma, massive pleural effusion
Noninvasive positive-pressure ventilation failure (or exclusion criteria)

Fio_2, inspired oxygen fraction; Pao_2, partial pressure of carbon dioxide in arterial blood; Pao_2, partial pressure of oxygen in arterial blood.
From Vincent JL et al: *Textbook of critical care,* ed 6, Philadelphia, 2011, Saunders.

---

confer a survival advantage over medical therapy. It is most beneficial in patients with both predominantly upper-lobe emphysema and low baseline exercise capacity.

- In patients with end-stage emphysema who have an FEV_1 <25% of predicted normal value after administration of bronchodilator and additional complications such as severe hypoxemia, hypercapnia, and pulmonary hypertension, single-lung transplantation should be considered a surgical option.
- Trials involving endobronchial valves that allow air to escape from a pulmonary lobe but not to enter it have been done to improve lung function by reducing lobar volume in patients with advanced heterogeneous emphysema. Results have shown modest improvements in lung function, symptoms, and exercise tolerance, but more frequent exacerbations of COPD. Other complications included pneumonia and hemoptysis postimplantation.

DISPOSITION

- After the initial episode of respiratory failure, 5-yr survival is approximately 25%.
- Development of cor pulmonale or hypercapnia and persistent tachycardia are poor prognostic indicators.

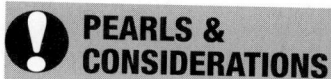

PEARLS & CONSIDERATIONS

COMMENTS

- All patients with COPD should receive pneumococcal vaccine and yearly influenza vaccine.
- Early antibiotic administration is associated with improved outcomes among patients hospitalized for acute exacerbations of COPD regardless of the risk of treatment failure.
- In assessing the severity of COPD, the FEV_1 is limited by the fact that it does not take into account the systemic manifestations of COPD. The BODE index (body mass index, degree of obstruction, dyspnea, and exercise capacity) has been proposed as a multidimensional scale to better assess the morbidity and mortality associated with COPD. It is better than the FEV_1 alone at predicting the risk of death from any cause and from respiratory causes among patients with COPD. In the BODE index, obstruction is measured by FEV_1 and dyspnea is measured by the modified Medical Research Council (MMRC) dyspnea questionnaire in a 6-minute walk test. A score of 0 on the MMRC indicates that the individual is not troubled with breathlessness except with strenuous exercise, 1 indicates shortness of breath when hurrying or walking up a slight hill, and 2 means the individual walks slower than people of the same age due to breathlessness or has to stop for breath when walking at own pace on level ground. A score of 3 means severe dyspnea because the person has to stop for breath after walking approximately 100 meters or after a few minutes on level ground, and a score of 4 indicates very severe dyspnea and is given when the individual is too breathless to leave the house or is breathless when dressing or undressing.

- Pulmonary artery enlargement as determined by a ratio of the diameter of the pulmonary artery to the diameter of the aorta [PA:A ratio] of >1 detected by CT is associated with severe exacerbations of COPD.
- The average person with COPD has one or two acute exacerbations each year. Prophylactic use of macrolide antibiotics (azithromycin 250 mg/day) has been shown to decrease the frequency of exacerbations and improve quality of life among selected patients with COPD; however, it leads to hearing decrements in a small percentage of patients and increased prevalence of macrolide-resistant bacteria colonizing the airway and is therefore not recommended.

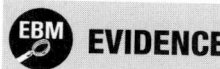

available at www.expertconsult.com

SUGGESTED READINGS
available at www.expertconsult.com

RELATED CONTENT
Chronic Obstructive Pulmonary Disease (Patient Information)

AUTHOR: **FRED F. FERRI, M.D.**

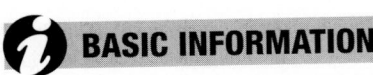

DEFINITION

Churg-Strauss syndrome (CSS) refers to a systemic granulomatous vasculitis accompanied by severe asthma (core clinical feature) and hypereosinophilia. Classification criteria and definition for CSS are described in Table 1-103.

SYNONYMS

Allergic angiitis
Allergic granulomatosis

ICD-9CM CODES
446.4 Angiitis, allergic granulomatous

EPIDEMIOLOGY & DEMOGRAPHICS

- Overall incidence of 2.4 cases per 1 million persons in the U.S. Among asthma patients, the annual incidence of CSS is estimated to average 34.6 per 1 million patients.
- Usually occurs at a mean age of 50 yr but may present as young as 4 yr or in the elderly
- Slight male/female predominance (1.3:1).
- With treatment, 1-year survival is approximately 90% and 5-year survival is 62%.

PHYSICAL FINDINGS & CLINICAL PRESENTATION

The clinical picture of CSS typically consists of three partially overlapping phases, which may or may not be sequential:

1. Prodromal phase:
   - Severe adult-onset asthma, with or without allergic rhinitis, sinusitis, headache, cough, and wheezing
   - Precedes development of systemic vasculitis by several years
2. Eosinophilic/tissue infiltration phase:
   - Peripheral eosinophilia and eosinophilic infiltration of the lungs, myocardium, and gastrointestinal (GI) tract, with or without granulomas
   - Signs and symptoms of cough, fever, anorexia, weight loss, sweats, malaise, nausea, vomiting, abdominal pain, and diarrhea
3. Systemic vasculitic phase:
   - Development of necrotizing vasculitis that is clinically apparent primarily in peripheral nerves, skin, and kidneys
   - Any organ can be affected, with skin involvement present in 50% to 67% of patients

Skin involvement is divided into three categories:

1. Erythematous maculopapules (can resemble erythema multiforme)
2. Hemorrhagic lesions (associated with wheals)
3. Cutaneous and subcutaneous nodules

ETIOLOGY

- Etiology unknown, but believed to be an autoimmune-mediated process
- Triggering factors implicated in CSS include inhaled allergens, vaccinations, infections, and drugs such as macrolides (see "Comments").

DIAGNOSIS

- Clinical findings and biopsy showing eosinophilic vasculitis
- The American College of Rheumatology (ACR) has established the criteria for CSS diagnosis in patients without vasculitis:
  - Asthma
  - Eosinophilia >10% of white blood cell count
  - Mononeuropathy or polyneuropathy
  - Migratory pulmonary infiltrates
  - Paranasal sinus abnormalities
  - Extravascular eosinophils on biopsy

The presence of any four or more of the six criteria yields a sensitivity of 85% and a specificity of 99.7%. For patients with vasculitis, the presence of asthma and eosinophilia was 90% sensitive and 99% specific for CSS.

DIFFERENTIAL DIAGNOSIS

- Polyarteritis nodosa (PAN)
- Wegener's granulomatosis (WG)
- Goodpasture syndrome
- Loeffler syndrome
- Hypereosinophilia syndrome
- Rheumatoid arthritis
- Leukocytoclastic vasculitis

Although similar and at times grouped with patients with PAN or WG, CSS differs in that:

- CSS vasculitis involves small-sized arteries, veins, and venules
- CSS, unlike PAN, predominantly involves the lung. Other organs affected include heart, GI system, central nervous system, kidney, and skin
- Kidney involvement is much less common in CSS than in WG. Pulmonary lesions in WG usually involve the upper respiratory tract rather than the peripheral lung parenchyma in CSS
- CSS shows necrotizing vasculitis along with eosinophilic granulomas

LABORATORY TESTS

- Complete blood count with differential: eosinophilia >10% is an American College of Rheumatology (ACR) diagnostic criterion
- Blood urea nitrogen and creatinine may be mildly elevated, suggesting renal involvement
- Urinalysis may show mild hematuria and proteinuria.
- 24-hour urine for protein; greater than 1 g/day is a poor prognostic factor
- Perinuclear antineutrophilic cytoplasmic antibody (P-ANCA) is found in 13% to 70% of patients. Negative ANCA does not rule out CSS
- Stools may be positive for occult blood (enteric involvement during eosinophilic phase)
- Elevation of aspartate aminotransferase, alanine aminotransferase, and creatine phosphokinase may indicate liver or muscle (skeletal or cardiac) involvement
- Rheumatoid factor and antinuclear antibody may be positive. Erythrocyte sedimentation rate is usually elevated
- Biopsy helps confirm the diagnosis. Surgical lung biopsy is the gold standard. Transbronchial biopsy is rarely helpful. Necrotizing vasculitis and extravascular necrotizing granulomas, usually with eosinophilic infiltrates, are suggestive of CSS. The presence of eosinophils in extravascular tissues is most specific for CSS

IMAGING STUDIES

- Chest radiograph is abnormal in eosinophilic and vasculitic phases: asymmetrical bilateral patchy migratory infiltrates, interstitial lung disease, or nodular infiltrates (Fig. 1-225). Small pleural effusions are found in 29% of cases
- Lung lesions in CSS are noncavitating, as opposed to those in WG
- Paranasal sinus films may reveal sinus opacification, which is an ACR diagnostic criterion
- Angiography is sometimes done in patients with mesenteric ischemia or renal involvement

TABLE 1-103 Classification Criteria and Definition for Churg-Strauss Syndrome

CLASSIFICATION CRITERIA		DEFINITION
Lanham (Requires 2 of 3)	**American College of Rheumatology (Requires 4 of 6)**	**Chapel Hill Consensus Conference**
Asthma	Asthma	Eosinophil-rich and granulomatous inflammation involving the respiratory tract, necrotizing vasculitis affecting small to medium-sized vessels, and associated with asthma and eosinophilia
Eosinophilia (>10% WBC count or >1.5 · 10⁹)	Eosinophilia (>10% total WBC count)	
Systemic vasculitis affecting at least two extrapulmonary sites	Neuropathy (mono or polyneuropathy)	
	Pulmonary infiltrates (migratory or transitory)	
	Paranasal sinus abnormality (pain, tenderness or radiologic abnormality)	
	Extravascular eosinophils (in a biopsy including an artery, arteriole, or venule)	

WBC, White blood cell.
From Hochberg MC et al: *Rheumatology*, ed 5, St Louis, 2011, Mosby.

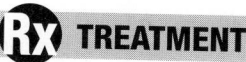 **TREATMENT**

NONPHARMACOLOGIC THERAPY

Oxygen therapy in severe asthmatic exacerbations

PHARMACOLOGIC THERAPY

The following five factors suggest poor prognosis (five-factor score) and determine the aggressiveness of the immune suppressive therapy:
1. Proteinuria >1 g/day
2. Creatinine >1.58 mg/dl
3. Cardiomyopathy
4. GI tract involvement
5. Central nervous system involvement

ACUTE GENERAL Rx

- Corticosteroids are the treatment of choice if no poor prognostic factors are present. Prednisone 1 mg/kg/day is the starting dose and is continued for 6 to 12 wk and then tapered to 10 mg/day at 1 yr as clinical disease resolves. Response to steroids may be dramatic. Patients with extensive disease may require IV corticosteroids.
- A drop in the patient's eosinophil count and the erythrocyte sedimentation rate indicates a response to treatment. ANCA does not reliably correspond with disease activity.

CHRONIC Rx

- In patients with one or more poor prognostic factors, immunosuppressant agents (cyclophosphamide 1 to 2 mg/kg/day) are used with corticosteroids as first-line therapy. Limit duration of cyclophosphamide to a maximum of 6 mo.

- In patients who do not respond to corticosteroid treatment or in CSS relapse, cyclophosphamide therapy is indicated as a second-line therapy.
- Azathioprine (2 mg/kg/day) or high-dose intravenous immunoglobulin has shown benefit in patients with severe disease and in patients unresponsive to corticosteroids.
- Corticosteroids, in combination with interferon-alpha, have also been used in refractory cases but may be difficult to tolerate.
- Patients with persistent symptoms of asthma will require long-term corticosteroids even if vasculitis is no longer present.
- Maintenance therapy using methotrexate (15 to 25 mg/wk) or azathioprine (2 mg/kg/day) is an alternative to cyclophosphamide.

DISPOSITION

- Clinical remission is obtained in more than 90% of patients after treatment. Relapse is common on cessation of therapy (approximately 26%).
- 5-yr survival rate with treatment is between 60% and 90% and decreases to 50% at 7 yr. Asthma generally remains persistent, and ischemic damage to peripheral nerves can be permanent.
- The 5-yr survival rate of untreated CSS is 25%.
- Death usually occurs from progressive refractory vasculitis, myocardial involvement (approximately 50% of deaths), or severe GI involvement (mesenteric ischemia, pancreatitis).

REFERRAL

- A pulmonary referral for diagnosis and management is appropriate.

- Patients should be followed up closely by rheumatology. Patients usually need long-term immunosuppressive medications.

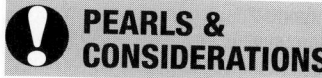 **PEARLS & CONSIDERATIONS**

COMMENTS

- CSS is a rare disease that is less common than other ANCA-associated vasculitides
- CSS is distinguished from other vasculitides by the nearly universal presence of adult-onset asthma that typically precedes all other symptoms. Family history is often negative for allergies or asthma
- Up to 77% of patients in the prodromal phase of CSS require oral steroids for asthma control
- Patients often have constitutional symptoms of weight loss, fever, and malaise before specific organ involvement is clinically evident
- Peripheral nerve involvement from vasculitis of the vasa vasorum commonly manifests as mononeuritis multiplex. Patients may present with sudden foot or wrist drop, along with sensory deficits in the distribution of one or more distal nerves
- Most patients with GI involvement are symptomatic. Gastroenteritis, acute abdomen, cholecystitis, hemorrhage, bowel perforation, and mesenteric ischemia have all been reported in patients with CSS
- Most patients with CSS respond to corticosteroid treatment and do not require cytotoxic therapy
- Symptoms of CSS typically appear as oral corticosteroids are being decreased or discontinued for the treatment of asthma and not triggered by leukotriene receptor-1 antagonists, as previously reported
- Compared to WG, patients more often present with history of atopy, asthma, or allergic rhinitis. When present, eosinophilia in CSS is often >1000 eosinophils/mm^3 compared with WG, where eosinophilia is much milder (<500 eosinophils/mm^3)
- The heart is involved in up to 60% of patients with CSS and represents a major cause of mortality

SUGGESTED READINGS

available at www.expertconsult.com

AUTHORS: **KACHIU LEE, B.A.,** and **JESSICA RISSER, M.D., M.P.H.**

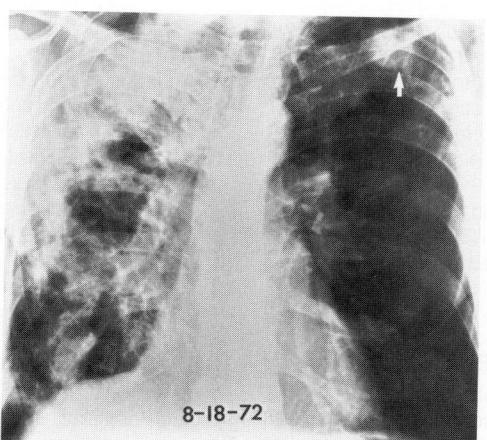

8-18-72

FIGURE 1-225 Allergic angiitis and granulomatosis. Posteroanterior chest radiograph demonstrates peripheral air space consolidation in the right lung and a nodule *(arrow)* in the left upper lobe in this asthmatic patient. (From McLoud TC [ed]: *Thoracic radiology: the requisites,* St Louis, 1998, Mosby.)

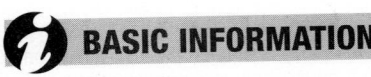

BASIC INFORMATION

DEFINITION

Cirrhosis is defined histologically as the presence of fibrosis and regenerative nodules in the liver. It can be classified as micronodular, macronodular, or mixed; however, each form may be seen in the same patient at different stages of the disease. Cirrhosis manifests clinically with portal hypertension, hepatic encephalopathy, and variceal bleeding.

ICD-9CM CODES
571.5 Cirrhosis of the liver
571.2 Cirrhosis of the liver secondary to
       alcohol

EPIDEMIOLOGY & DEMOGRAPHICS

- Cirrhosis is the eleventh leading cause of death in the U.S. (9 per 100,000 persons annually).
- Alcohol abuse and viral hepatitis are the major causes of cirrhosis in the U.S.

PHYSICAL FINDINGS & CLINICAL PRESENTATION

SKIN: Jaundice, palmar erythema (alcohol abuse), spider angiomata, ecchymosis (thrombocytopenia or coagulation factor deficiency), dilated superficial periumbilical vein (caput medusae), increased pigmentation (hemochromatosis), xanthomas (primary biliary cirrhosis), and needle tracks (viral hepatitis). Cutaneous lesions often accompany cirrhosis and can be found in >40% of people with chronic alcoholism.
EYES: Kayser-Fleischer rings (corneal copper deposition seen in Wilson's disease; best diagnosed with slit lamp examination), scleral icterus
BREATH: Fetor hepaticus (musty odor of breath and urine found in cirrhosis with hepatic failure)
CHEST: Possible gynecomastia in men
ABDOMEN: Tender hepatomegaly (congestive hepatomegaly), small, nodular liver (cirrhosis), palpable, nontender gallbladder (neoplastic extrahepatic biliary obstruction), palpable spleen (portal hypertension), venous hum auscultated over periumbilical veins (portal hypertension), ascites (portal hypertension, hypoalbuminemia)
RECTAL EXAMINATION: Hemorrhoids (portal hypertension), guaiac-positive stools (alcoholic gastritis, bleeding esophageal varices, peptic ulcer disease, bleeding hemorrhoids)
GENITALIA: Testicular atrophy in males (chronic liver disease, hemochromatosis)
EXTREMITIES: Pedal edema (hypoalbuminemia, failure of right side of the heart), arthropathy (hemochromatosis)
NEUROLOGIC: Flapping tremor, asterixis (hepatic encephalopathy), choreoathetosis, dysarthria (Wilson's disease)

ETIOLOGY
- Alcohol abuse
- Secondary biliary cirrhosis, obstruction of the common bile duct (stone, stricture, pancreatitis, neoplasm, sclerosing cholangitis)
- Drugs (e.g., acetaminophen, isoniazid, methotrexate, methyldopa)
- Hepatic congestion (e.g., CHF, constrictive pericarditis, tricuspid insufficiency, thrombosis of the hepatic vein, obstruction of the vena cava)
- Primary biliary cirrhosis
- Hemochromatosis
- Chronic hepatitis B or C
- Wilson's disease
- Alpha-1-antitrypsin deficiency
- Infiltrative diseases (amyloidosis, glycogen storage diseases, hemochromatosis)
- Nutritional: jejunoileal bypass
- Others: parasitic infections (schistosomiasis), idiopathic portal hypertension, congenital hepatic fibrosis, systemic mastocytosis, autoimmune hepatitis, hepatic steatosis, inflammatory bowel disease (IBD)

DIAGNOSIS

WORKUP

In addition to an assessment of liver function, the evaluation of patients with cirrhosis should also include an assessment of renal and circulatory function. Diagnostic workup is aimed primarily at identifying the most likely cause of cirrhosis. The history is extremely important:
- Alcohol abuse: alcoholic liver disease
- History of hepatitis B (chronic active hepatitis, primary hepatic neoplasm, or hepatitis C)
- History of IBD (primary sclerosing cholangitis)
- History of pruritus, hyperlipoproteinemia, and xanthomas in a middle-aged or elderly woman (primary biliary cirrhosis)
- Impotence, diabetes mellitus, hyperpigmentation, arthritis (hemochromatosis)
- Neurologic disturbances (Wilson's disease, hepatolenticular degeneration)
- Family history of "liver disease" (hemochromatosis [positive family history in 25% of patients], alpha-1-antitrypsin deficiency)
- History of recurrent episodes of right upper quadrant pain (biliary tract disease)
- History of blood transfusions, IV drug abuse (hepatitis C)
- History of hepatotoxic drug exposure
- Coexistence of other diseases with immune or autoimmune features (immune thrombocytopenic purpura, myasthenia gravis, thyroiditis, autoimmune hepatitis)

LABORATORY TESTS

- Decreased hemoglobin and hematocrit, elevated mean corpuscular volume, increased blood urea nitrogen (BUN) and creatinine (the BUN may also be "normal" or low if the patient has severely diminished liver function), decreased sodium (dilutional hyponatremia), and decreased potassium (as a result of secondary aldosteronism or urinary losses). Evaluation of renal function should also include measurement of urinary sodium and urinary protein from 24-hr urine collection.
- Decreased glucose in a patient with liver disease, indicating severe liver damage.
- Other laboratory abnormalities:
  - Alcoholic hepatitis and cirrhosis: possible mild elevation of alanine aminotransferase (ALT) and aspartate aminotransferase (AST), usually <500 IU; AST > ALT (ratio > 2:3).
  - Extrahepatic obstruction: possible moderate elevations of ALT and AST to levels <500 IU.
  - Viral, toxic, or ischemic hepatitis: extreme elevations (>500 IU) of ALT and AST.
  - Transaminases may be normal despite significant liver disease in patients with jejunoileal bypass operations or hemochromatosis or after methotrexate administration.
  - Alkaline phosphatase elevation can occur with extrahepatic obstruction, primary biliary cirrhosis, and primary sclerosing cholangitis.
  - Serum lactate dehydrogenase is significantly elevated in metastatic disease of the liver; lesser elevations are seen with hepatitis, cirrhosis, extrahepatic obstruction, and congestive hepatomegaly.
  - Serum gamma-glutamyl transpeptidase is elevated in alcoholic liver disease and may also be elevated with cholestatic disease (primary biliary cirrhosis, primary sclerosing cholangitis).
  - Serum bilirubin may be elevated; urinary bilirubin can be present in hepatitis, hepatocellular jaundice, and biliary obstruction.
  - Serum albumin: significant liver disease results in hypoalbuminemia.
  - Prothrombin time/INR: elevation in patients with liver disease indicates severe liver damage and poor prognosis.
  - Presence of hepatitis B surface antigen implies acute or chronic hepatitis B.
  - Presence of antimitochondrial antibody suggests primary biliary cirrhosis, chronic hepatitis.
  - Elevated serum copper, decreased serum ceruloplasmin, and elevated 24-hr urine may be diagnostic of Wilson's disease.
  - Protein immunoelectrophoresis may reveal decreased α-1 globulins (alpha-1-antitrypsin deficiency), increased IgA (alcoholic cirrhosis), increased IgM (primary biliary cirrhosis), increased IgG (chronic hepatitis, cryptogenic cirrhosis).
  - An elevated serum ferritin and increased transferrin saturation are suggestive of hemochromatosis.
  - An elevated blood ammonia suggests hepatocellular dysfunction; serial values, however, are generally not useful in monitoring patients with hepatic encephalopathy because there is poor correlation between blood ammonia level and degree of hepatic encephalopathy.
  - Serum cholesterol is elevated in cholestatic disorders.
  - Antinuclear antibodies (ANA) may be found in autoimmune hepatitis.
  - Alpha fetoprotein: levels >1000 pg/ml are highly suggestive of primary liver cell carcinoma.

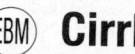
○ Hepatitis C viral testing identifies patients with chronic hepatitis C infection.

○ Elevated level of serum globulin (especially gamma-globulins) and positive ANA test may occur with autoimmune hepatitis.

○ End-stage liver disease is characterized by decreased levels of most procoagulant factors with the notable exceptions of factor VIII and von Willebrand factor, which are elevated.

IMAGING STUDIES

- Ultrasonography is the procedure of choice for detecting gallstones and dilation of common bile ducts. The use of sonography on a periodic basis to screen for hepatocellular carcinoma in patients with cirrhosis has been questioned and should be avoided until additional data are available.
- CT scan is useful for detecting mass lesions in liver and pancreas, assessing hepatic fat content, identifying idiopathic hemochromatosis, diagnosing Budd-Chiari syndrome early, assessing dilation of intrahepatic bile ducts, and detecting varices and splenomegaly.
- MRI can be used to identify hemangiomas.
- Technetium-99m sulfur colloid scanning is rarely used but can be useful for diagnosing cirrhosis (there is a shift of colloid uptake to the spleen and bone marrow), identifying hepatic adenomas (cold defect is noted), and diagnosing Budd-Chiari syndrome (there is increased uptake by the caudate lobe).
- Endoscopic retrograde cholangiopancreatography can be used for diagnosing periampullary carcinoma and common duct stones; it is also useful in diagnosing primary sclerosing cholangitis.
- Percutaneous transhepatic cholangiography is useful when evaluating patients with cholestatic jaundice and dilated intrahepatic ducts by ultrasonography; presence of intrahepatic strictures and focal dilation is suggestive of primary sclerosing cholangitis.
- Percutaneous liver biopsy is useful in evaluating hepatic filling defects; diagnosing hepatocellular disease or hepatomegaly; evaluating persistently abnormal liver function tests; and diagnosing hemachromatosis, primary biliary cirrhosis, Wilson's disease, glycogen storage diseases, chronic hepatitis, autoimmune hepatitis, infiltrative diseases, alcoholic liver disease, drug-induced liver disease, and primary or secondary carcinoma.

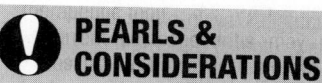 **TREATMENT**

NONPHARMACOLOGIC THERAPY

- Avoid any hepatotoxins (e.g., ethanol, acetaminophen), improve nutritional status
- Transjugular intrahepatic portosystemic shunt (TIPS) in patients with recurrent

variceal hemorrhage despite optical medical therapy (Fig. E1-226). Early use of TIPS is associated with significant reductions in treatment failure and in mortality in patients with cirrhosis who are hospitalized for acute variceal bleeding and are at high risk for treatment failure.

GENERAL Rx

- Beta-blockers with or without nitrates in patients with cirrhosis and variceal hemorrhage.
- Pruritus due to liver disease may be treated with cholestyramine 4 g/day initially. Dose can be increased to 24 g/day as needed
- Remove excess body iron with phlebotomy and deferoxamine in patients with hemochromatosis.
- Remove copper deposits with D-penicillamine in patients with Wilson's disease.
- Long-term ursodiol therapy will slow the progression of primary biliary cirrhosis. It is, however, ineffective in primary sclerosing cholangitis.
- Glucocorticoids (prednisone 20 to 30 mg/day initially or combination therapy or prednisone and azathioprine) is useful in autoimmune hepatitis.
- Liver transplantation may be indicated in otherwise healthy patients (age <65 yr) with sclerosing cholangitis, chronic hepatitis cirrhosis, or primary biliary cirrhosis with prognostic information suggesting <20% chance of survival without transplantation. Contraindications to liver transplantation are AIDS, most metastatic malignancies, active substance abuse, uncontrolled sepsis, and uncontrolled cardiac or pulmonary disease.
- Treatment of complications of portal hypertension (ascites, esophagogastric varices, hepatic encephalopathy, and hepatorenal syndrome; refer to these individual topics in Section I).

DISPOSITION

- Prognosis varies with the etiology of the patient's cirrhosis and whether there is ongoing hepatic injury. Regression of cirrhosis has been demonstrated after antiviral therapy in some patients with chronic hepatitis C. Regression is associated with decreased disease-related morbidity and improved survival. Mortality rate exceeds 80% in patients with hepatorenal syndrome.
- If advanced cirrhosis is present and transplantation is not feasible, survival is 1 to 2 yr.
- Cirrhosis is associated with an increased risk for hepatocellular carcinoma. However, the risk is low (1% 5-year cumulative risk in alcoholic cirrhosis).

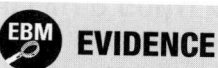 **PEARLS & CONSIDERATIONS**

COMMENTS

- Thrombocytopenia and advanced Child-Pugh cases (Table 1-104) are associated with the presence of varices. These factors are useful to identify cirrhotic patients who benefit most from referral for endoscopic screening for varices.
- A combination of endoscopic and drug therapy reduces overall and variceal rebleeding in cirrhosis more than either therapy alone.
- PPI use, but not H_2RA use, is associated with risk for serious infections in patients with decompensated cirrhosis.

EBM EVIDENCE

available at www.expertconsult.com

SUGGESTED READINGS

available at www.expertconsult.com

AUTHOR: **FRED F. FERRI, M.D.**

TABLE 1-104 Child-Pugh Staging Criteria

CHILD-PUGH SCORE			
Criteria	**1 Point**	**2 Points**	**3 Points**
Total serum bilirubin (mg/dl)	<2	2-3	>3
Serum albumin (g/dl)	>3.5	2.8-3.5	<2.8
INR	<1.70	1.71-2.20	>2.20
Ascites	No ascites	Ascites controlled	Ascites not controlled
Encephalopathy	No encephalopathy	Encephalopathy controlled	Encephalopathy not controlled

INTERPRETATION OF CHILD-PUGH SCORES			
	Points	**Life Expectancy**	**Perioperative Mortality**
Child Class A	5-6	15-20 yr	10%
Child Class B	7-9	Candidate for liver transplant	30%
Child Class C	10-15	1-3 yr	82%

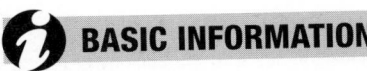

DEFINITION

Primary biliary cirrhosis (PBC) is a chronic, variably progressive cholestatic liver disease most often affecting women and characterized by destruction of the small intrahepatic bile ducts leading to portal inflammation, fibrosis, cirrhosis, and ultimately, liver failure.

SYNONYMS

Biliary cirrhosis
Nonsuppurative destructive cholangitis
Autoimmune cholangiopathy

ICD-9CM CODES
571.6 Biliary cirrhosis
698 Pruritus
780.7 Malaise and Fatigue

EPIDEMIOLOGY & DEMOGRAPHICS

INCIDENCE:
- PBC affects all races and accounts for 0.6% to 2% of deaths from cirrhosis worldwide.
- Annual incidence rates range from 0.7 to 49 cases per million.

PREVALENCE: Prevalence is greatest in the U.K., Scandinavia, Canada, and the U.S., and varies tremendously by geographic areas, ranging from 6.7 to 402 cases per million. Disease burden seems to be increasing, which may be a result of better detection rather than true rise in disease incidence.

PREDOMINANT SEX: Female to male ratio of up to 10:1.

PREDOMINANT AGE: Onset typically occurs between the ages of 30 and 65 yr, and it is uncommon before age 25 yr.

PREDOMINANT RACE: Predominantly Caucasian but can be seen in other races.

GENETICS:
- Although there are no clearly identified genetic factors associated with PBC, there is a clear familial occurrence. Prevalence among first-degree relatives is 5% to 6%, and 1% to 6% of all patients have at least one affected family member. The concordance rate among monozygotic twins is 63%.
- Up to 84% of patients with PBC have at least one other autoimmune disorder, such as thyroiditis, Sjögren's syndrome, rheumatoid arthritis, Raynaud's phenomenon, or scleroderma. A variant form of PBC exists as an overlap syndrome with autoimmune hepatitis (AIH).
- PBC is closely associated with a greater risk of hepatocellular carcinoma as well as an overall greater risk of cancer.

ETIOLOGY

- Although the cause of PBC remains unknown, it is believed to require both a genetic susceptibility as well as an environmental trigger, ultimately leading to the modification of mitochondrial proteins triggering a persistent T lymphocyte–mediated attack on intralobular bile duct epithelial cells.
- PBC is associated with the DRB1*08 family of alleles, but there is a great deal of variation among ethnicities.
- Possible environmental triggers include cigarette smoking, urinary tract infections, reproductive hormone replacement, nail polish, and toxic waste sites (particularly exposure to halogenated hydrocarbons), as well as xenobiotics in animal models of PBC.
- Recent studies have identified a group of autoantigens collectively known as the "M2 subtype" of autoantigens that play a major role in the early pathogenesis of PBC. These are peptides within the mitochondrial membrane that share structural homology. The enzyme complex subunit (PDC-E2) is one of the key autoantigens in this group. Patients with PBC have a tenfold increased concentration of cytotoxic CD8$^+$ lymphocytes recognizing this peptide in their livers compared with their blood, and most antimitochondrial antibodies (AMAs), which are the serologic hallmark of this disease, react to the PDC-E2 subunit. In addition, bile duct epithelial cells handle PDC-E2 in a unique way that exposes them to immune-mediated attack by PDC-E2–oriented cytotoxic T cells. Future therapies may be specific immunomodulation directed at these peptides.
- In addition to the T lymphocyte–mediated direct destruction of small bile ducts, secondary damage to hepatocytes results from the chronic accumulation of bile acids.

PHYSICAL FINDINGS & CLINICAL PRESENTATION

Clinical stages:
- Asymptomatic
- Symptomatic
- Cirrhotic
- Hepatic failure

Symptoms:
- 50% to 60% of patients may be asymptomatic; 40% to 100% of these patients will develop symptoms, and nearly 25% of symptomatic patients at diagnosis will progress to liver failure within 10 yr without treatment.
- Fatigue (78% of patients) and pruritus (20% to 70% of patients) are the usual presenting symptoms.
- Pruritus is worse at night, under constricting, coarse garments; in association with dry skin; and in hot, humid weather. The cause is unknown; it is no longer believed to be a result of the retention of bile acids in skin. Pruritus may first occur during pregnancy but is distinguished from pruritus of pregnancy because it persists into the postpartum period and beyond.
- Other common symptoms include jaundice, unexplained right upper quadrant pain (10%), manifestations of portal hypertension, sicca symptoms, and scleroderma-like lesions.
- Musculoskeletal complaints caused by inflammatory arthropathy in 40% to 70% of patients: 5% to 10% experience development of chronic rheumatoid arthritis and 10% experience development of "arthritis of PBC."
- Steatorrhea may be seen in advanced disease.

Physical:
- Variable: Results depend on stage of disease at time of presentation; patients at the early stage may be completely unaffected.
- Excoriations may be present.
- Hepatomegaly (70%) and splenomegaly (initially 35%) may be present in more advanced disease.
- Xanthomas and jaundice appear in advanced disease. Kayser-Fleischer rings are rare and result from copper retention. Hyperpigmentation of the skin due to melanin deposition may be present.
- Late physical findings mirror those of cirrhosis: spider nevi, temporal and proximal limb wasting, ascites, and edema.

DIAGNOSIS

The diagnosis of PBC can be established when two of the following three criteria are met.
- Positive serum AMA, titer >1:40
- Biochemical evidence of cholestasis (mainly alkaline phosphatase elevation)
- Characteristic liver histology: nonsuppurative destructive cholangitis and destruction of interlobular bile ducts

DIFFERENTIAL DIAGNOSIS

- Drug-induced cholestasis
- PBC-AIH overlap syndrome: reported in almost 10% of adults with AIH or PBC; transition from stable PBC to AIH and vice versa also seen
- Other etiologies of chronic liver disease and cirrhosis, such as alcoholic cirrhosis, chronic viral hepatitis, primary sclerosing cholangitis, AIH, sarcoidosis, chemical/toxin-induced cirrhosis, other hereditary or familial disorders (e.g., cystic fibrosis, α-1-antitrypsin deficiency)
- Biliary obstruction

WORKUP

History, physical examination, laboratory evaluation, liver biopsy

LABORATORY TESTS

- AMAs found in 95% of patients with PBC and are 98% specific.
- Antinuclear antibodies (ANAs) and AMAs found in approximately 50% of patients. In approximately 5% of patients, AMAs are absent or present only in low titer (AMA-negative PBC). Nearly all of these patients have ANA or AMAs, or both.
- Cholestatic pattern of liver biochemical markers, that is, markedly increased alkaline phosphatase (of hepatic origin).
- γ-Glutamyl transpeptidase is increased.
- Serum IgM levels are increased (lower in AMA-negative PBC).
- Bilirubin level is normal early; increases with disease progression (direct and indirect) in 60% of patients. Increased serum bilirubin level is a poor prognostic sign.

- Aminotransferase level may be normal and, if increased, is rarely more than five times the upper limit of normal.
- Markedly increased serum lipids in more than 50% of patients. Total cholesterol may exceed 1000 mg/dl. No increased risk for death from atherosclerosis seen, possibly because of high levels of LP-X, an antiatherogenic low-density lipoprotein particle, very-high-density lipoprotein levels, and low serum levels of lipoprotein(a).
- Percutaneous liver biopsy confirms or rules out the diagnosis, allows staging, but is not essential in order to initiate medical therapy in patients with typical liver chemistry and positive AMA test.
- Histology is not uniform, so histologic stage is based on the most advanced lesion present.
  - Stage I: Lymphocytic infiltration of the epithelial cells of the small bile ducts with granuloma-like lesions, limited to portal triads (bridging fibrosis)
  - Stage II: Extension of inflammatory cells to periportal parenchyma, invasion by foamy macrophages, and development of biliary piecemeal necrosis
  - Stage III: Fibrous septa link portal triads
  - Stage IV: Frank cirrhosis; hyaline deposits and accumulation of stainable copper are also seen

IMAGING STUDIES

If history, physical examination, blood tests, and liver biopsy are all consistent with PBC, neither imaging nor cholangiography is necessary.

PROGNOSIS

- Median survival was 10 yr but may be getting longer with earlier diagnosis and initiation of treatment.
- Mean time of progression from stage I or II disease to cirrhosis with no medical treatment is 4 to 6 yr.
- Neither presence nor total titer level of AMAs predicts survival, disease progression, or response to therapy.
- Prognostic laboratory measures: Serum bilirubin is most important.
- Response to ursodiol therapy can be prognostic: Patients with a decrease in alkaline phosphatase level of at least 40% or to the reference range after 1 yr of treatment with ursodeoxycholic acid (UDCA) may have a prognosis similar to an age-matched healthy population. Similarly, the Mayo Risk score, a predictor of short-term survival probability (http://www.mayoclinic.org/gi-rst/mayomodel1.html), can also reliably predict life expectancy when calculated after 6 mo of ursodiol therapy.
- Poorer prognosis exists with jaundice, advanced histologic stage, advanced age, edema, coagulopathy, and ascites.

Rx TREATMENT

- Treatment is according to the clinical stage of the disease.
- Asymptomatic stage: Follow bilirubin every 3 mo. Once liver function test results become abnormal, begin UDCA at 13 to 15 mg/kg/day in a twice-daily divided dose regardless of histologic stage. Side effects may include weight gain of approximately 5 lbs during the first 1 to 2 yr and, less commonly, thinning of hair and loose stools. Watch for interactions with cholestyramine and other bile-acid sequestrants, as well as antacids, which may interfere with UDCA absorption. Efficacy is best if started during stage I or II disease but should be started at any stage of disease. Lifelong therapy is currently recommended, but benefits are still observed if therapy is interrupted and restarted.
- Treatment also includes treatment of associated conditions such as pruritus, osteoporosis, increased low-density lipoprotein level, and any eventual complications of cirrhosis.
- 20% of patients will not respond to medical therapy and will proceed to liver transplantation, which is the only definitive treatment for this disease.

ACUTE GENERAL Rx

- Symptomatic stage: Goals of treatment are resolution of pruritus, decrease of alkaline phosphatase levels, and delay of progression to liver failure.
- Ursodiol can significantly improve bilirubin and alkaline phosphatase levels, prolong survival without liver transplantation, and delay progression of liver fibrosis and development of portal hypertension.
- The addition of colchicine, methotrexate, or benzafibrate has not been found to be of benefit to mortality or time to liver transplantation in controlled trials.
- Prednisone, azathioprine, penicillamine, and cyclosporine are no longer used because of limited efficacy and significant toxicity.
- For the pruritus of PBC, cholestyramine resin (4 g/dose; maximum, 16 g/day) reduces pruritus in most patients but must be given at least 2 to 4 hr apart from ursodiol to avoid reducing the efficacy of that drug. Antihistamines at bedtime help nighttime symptoms. Rifampin (150 to 300 mg bid) or oral opiate antagonists such as naltrexone (50 mg daily) can be used for pruritus refractory to bile acid sequestrants. Intractable pruritus can be an indication for liver transplantation.

CHRONIC Rx

- Liver function tests should be checked every 3 to 6 mo.
- Management of sicca syndrome: Artificial tears can be used initially for dry eyes. Saliva substitutes can be used for xerostomia and dysphagia; pilocarpine or cevimeline for refractory cases. Moisturizers can be given for vaginal dryness.
- Treatment/Prevention of osteopenia/osteoporosis: Patients with PBC should be provided 1000 to 1500 mg calcium and 1000 IU of vitamin D daily in the diet and as supplements if needed. Bone densitometry should be done every 2 to 4 yr. Alendronate (70 mg weekly) should be considered if patients are osteopenic in the absence of acid reflux or known varices.

- Hyperlipidemia is common in patients with cholestatic liver disease. Statins are safe in patients who may need treatment even if liver chemistry is abnormal.
- Vitamin A, K, and E deficiencies can be clinically important in advanced cases and respond to oral replacement.
- Upper endoscopy to assess for varices should be done every 2 to 3 yr in patients with cirrhosis or Mayo risk score >4.1. Nonselective beta-blockers or endoscopic banding can be considered for prevention of variceal hemorrhage.
- Regular screening for hepatocellular carcinoma with ultrasound and α-fetoprotein every 6 to 12 mo is recommended for patients with cirrhosis.
- Liver transplantation is the only effective treatment for patients with liver failure. Indications for transplantation include hepatic decompensation (ascites, encephalopathy, jaundice), hepatocellular carcinoma fulfilling Milan criteria (see "Hepatocellular Carcinoma"), and intractable pruritus.
- The outcome of liver transplantation for patients with PBC is more favorable than that of nearly all other liver disease categories. The survival rates are 85% to 90% and 80% to 85% at 1 and 5 yr, respectively. Although recurrent disease may develop in 20% to 25% of patients after liver transplantation over 10 yr, patient and graft survival is usually not affected.

DISPOSITION

Definitive treatment requires liver transplantation; survival is 7 to 16 yr depending on symptoms at time of diagnosis.

REFERRAL

Gastroenterology and/or hepatology for treatment, evaluation for liver transplantation, and management of portal hypertension

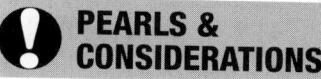 **PEARLS & CONSIDERATIONS**

- AMA is the serologic hallmark of PBC.
- The prototypical patient with PBC is a middle-aged, Caucasian woman reporting fatigue and pruritus.
- Ursodiol should be started as soon as liver biochemical markers begin to increase and is most effective when started early in the course of the disease.
- Associated illnesses must be detected and treated.
- Liver transplantation is the only effective treatment for PBC with end-stage liver failure.

SUGGESTED READINGS

available at www.expertconsult.com

RELATED CONTENT

Primary Biliary Cirrhosis (PBC) (Patient Information)

AUTHORS: **MICHAEL ENGELS, M.D.**, and **JEANETTE SMITH, M.D.**

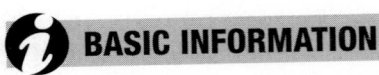

BASIC INFORMATION

DEFINITION

Claudication refers to reproducible discomfort of muscles brought on by exertion and relieved with rest. This disorder results from an imbalance between supply and demand of blood flow that fails to satisfy ongoing metabolic requirements. This intermittent vascular claudication is most common in the calves and lower extremities but it can also affect the upper extremities.

SYNONYMS

Intermittent claudication

ICD-9CM CODES
443.9   Peripheral vascular disease, unspecified
440.21 Intermittent claudication due to atherosclerosis

EPIDEMIOLOGY & DEMOGRAPHICS

- The prevalence of peripheral arterial disease (PAD) is approximately 12% to 21% of Americans ≥65 yr old and affects about 10 million Americans.
- The risk factors associated with development of PAD are similar to coronary atherosclerosis. Increasing age, cigarette smoking, hypertension, diabetes mellitus, and dyslipidemia are significant risk factors. Nontraditional risk factors include race/ethnicity, with African American patients being at higher risk. In addition, chronic renal disease, metabolic syndrome, and patients with elevated levels of C-reactive protein, lipoprotein(a), and homocysteine increase risk.
- There is a strong correlation among peripheral artery disease, carotid artery stenosis, and cardiovascular disease.
- In a 2011 update, the American College of Cardiology/American Heart Association (ACC/AHA) guidelines suggested the following distribution of clinical presentation of PAD in patients >50 yr of age:
  - Asymptomatic: 20% to 50%
  - Atypical leg pain: 40% to 50%
  - Classic claudication: 10% to 35%
  - Critical limb ischemia: 1% to 2%

PHYSICAL FINDINGS & CLINICAL PRESENTATION

- The severity of symptoms varies with degree of stenoses, collateral blood supply, and exertional demand.
- Classic symptoms include exertional calf pain, causing patient to stop exertion and pain resolves within 10 min of rest. Claudication can present in the buttock and hip, thigh, calf, or foot, with one or more of the following depending on the level and degree of stenosis:
  - Diminished or absent pedal pulses, with cool skin temperature
  - Bruit over the distal aorta, iliac, or femoral arteries

- Pallor of the distal extremities on elevation
- Rubor with prolonged capillary refill on dependency
- Trophic changes, including hair/nail loss and muscle atrophy
- Nonhealing ulcers, necrotic tissue, and gangrene
- Weakness, numbness, or heaviness in the lower extremities
- True vascular claudication must be distinguished from "pseudoclaudication" caused by severe venous obstructive disease, chronic compartment syndrome, lumbar disease and spinal stenosis, osteoarthritis, and inflammatory muscle diseases. The characteristic features of pseudoclaudication that distinguish it from claudication are summarized in Table 1-105.
- Location of pain usually corresponds to analogous anatomy:
  - Buttock and hip: aortoiliac disease
  - Thigh: aortoiliac or common femoral artery
  - Upper two thirds of calf: superficial femoral artery
  - Lower one third of calf: popliteal artery
  - Foot: tibial or peroneal artery
- Asymptomatic PAD is typically diagnosed by screening studies or incidentally on physical exam. Symptoms of intermittent claudication classically start distally within a muscle group (below the stenosis) and then ascend with continued activity. Rest pain that occurs with leg elevation and is relieved paradoxically by walking may suggest severe PAD (the effects of gravity increase arterial perfusion of muscle groups). Critical PAD may present as tissue ulceration and gangrene.

ETIOLOGY

The primary cause of claudication is peripheral atherosclerosis, resulting in inability to supply enough blood to meet the metabolic demand of limb muscles.

Dx DIAGNOSIS

DIFFERENTIAL DIAGNOSIS

- Spinal stenosis (neurogenic or pseudoclaudication)
- Musculoskeletal disorders: arthritis or myositis
- Degenerative osteoarthritic joint disease, predominantly of the lumbar spine and hips

- Compartment or popliteal artery entrapment syndrome
- Peripheral neuropathy
- Atheromatous embolization and deep venous thrombosis
- Vasculitis: thromboangiitis obliterans, Takayasu, or giant cell arteritis

WORKUP

History and physical findings suggest the diagnosis of claudication. Noninvasive studies help confirm the diagnosis.

- Measurement of resting ankle–brachial index (ABI) should be performed in all patients at risk for PAD and repeated at least once every 5 yr. These patients include:
  - Patients ≥18 yr old with walking impairment, claudication, or lower extremity non-healing wounds
  - Asymptomatic patients 50 to 69 yr old with a history of smoking or diabetes
  - All patients ≥70 yr old.
- An ABI is the ratio of highest ankle systolic pressure to the highest brachial systolic pressure of either arm. A normal ABI is 1.00 to 1.40. A low ABI has been shown to be an independent predictor of mortality.
- The severity of PAD is based on the resting ABI. ABI correlates with the severity of perfusion deficit but does not define the level of obstructive disease. It is classified as follows:
  - Borderline: ABI at rest 0.91 to 0.99
  - Mild: ABI at rest 0.71 to 0.90
  - Moderate: ABI at rest 0.41 to 0.70
  - Severe: ABI at rest <0.40
- Segmental systolic pressures are measured from thigh, calf, ankle, metatarsal, and toes. Normally, there should be <20 mm Hg difference in pressures between adjacent segments. If the gradient is >20 mm Hg, significant narrowing is suspected in the intervening segment.
- Both ABI and segmental pressures can be taken before and after exercise (1 to 2 mi/hr, 5 min, or symptom-limited) to quantify severity of symptoms objectively. An ABI that decreases by at least 15% following exercise indicates significant PAD.
- ABI >1.3 may represent significant PAD. In such cases, measuring a toe–brachial index can increase the sensitivity of testing, as highly calcified arteries are not compressible and may have a normal or increased ABI.

TABLE 1-105 Characteristic Features of Pseudoclaudication That Distinguish It from Claudication

	Claudication	Pseudoclaudication
Characteristics	Cramping, tightness, fatigue	Similar to claudication and numbness
Location of discomfort	Lower extremity involving buttock, hip, thigh, calf, foot	Similar to claudication
Induced by exercise	Yes	Variable
Reproducible with distance walked	Consistent	Variable
Occurs with standing	No	Yes
Actions which provide relief	Stand	Sit
Time to relief	<5 min	≤30 min

C

A toe–brachial index <0.7 is considered abnormal.

IMAGING STUDIES

- Duplex ultrasound can be used to assess occlusion location, length, and patency of the distal arterial system or prior vein grafts. Ultrasound is a great noninvasive modality for surveillance monitoring after revascularization.
- In patients with prior infrainguinal bypass grafts, the long-term patency should be evaluated at regular intervals using a duplex ultrasound. The 2011 ACC guidelines recommends routine surveillance using a duplex ultrasound at approximately 3, 6, and 12 mo and then yearly after graft placement.
- Magnetic resonance angiography (MRA) and spiral CT angiography are effective for imaging of the aorta and peripheral lower extremity arteries above the knee. MRA has almost replaced catheter-based angiography, with 90% sensitivity and 97% specificity in identification of hemodynamically significant stenoses in the lower extremities.
- MRA and CT angiography are useful to delineate the anatomy and help plan percutaneous and surgical revascularization.
- Angiography (Fig. 1-227) remains the gold standard for diagnosing peripheral arterial occlusion, especially below the knee, and before revascularization.

(Rx) TREATMENT

NONPHARMACOLOGIC THERAPY

- Smoking cessation is vital.
- Aggressive risk factor modification for hypertension, dyslipidemia, and diabetes mellitus, including diet and weight loss counseling, is recommended.

- Walking 30 to 60 min/day, at least 3 times per week at approximately 2 mi/hr to near-maximal pain for 6 mo is recommended.
- New prospective data point to intermittent pneumatic compression as a promising adjunctive therapy.

ACUTE GENERAL Rx

Revascularization by endovascular or surgical approach is usually reserved for patients with symptoms refractory to medical therapy or impending ischemic limb loss.

CHRONIC Rx

- Aspirin 75 to 325 mg daily; thienopyridines (clopidogrel and ticlodipine) can be considered as alternatives, especially for those intolerant of aspirin. There is no current data to support combination treatment (CHARISMA trial).
- Hydroxymethyl glutaryl (HMG) coenzyme-A reductase inhibitor (statin) medication is indicated for all patients with PAD.
  - LDL cholesterol level of less than 100 mg/dl is recommended.
  - Patients with concomitant high risk for ischemic events should be treated to a goal LDL cholesterol level of less than 70 mg/dl.
- Antihypertensive therapy with beta-adrenergic blocking drugs and/or ACE inhibitors should be administered to all hypertensive patients with PAD to reduce the risk of MI, stroke, congestive heart failure, and cardiovascular death.
  - In non-diabetics, the target blood pressure is <140 mm Hg systolic over 90 mm Hg diastolic.
  - In diabetics or patients with chronic renal disease, the target blood pressure is <130 mm Hg systolic over 80 mm Hg diastolic.

- Cilostazol 100 mg bid may be used in conjunction with aspirin or clopidogrel. It has been shown to increase walking distance by 50% to 67% in symptomatic patients.
- Pentoxifylline 400 mg three times per day may be considered as second-line alternative therapy to cilostazol to improve walking. However, the clinical effectiveness of pentoxifylline as therapy for claudication is not well established.
- Individuals with intermittent claudication who are offered the option of endovascular or surgical therapies should:
  - Be provided information regarding supervised claudication exercise therapy and pharmacotherapy
  - Receive comprehensive risk factor modification and antiplatelet therapy
  - Have a significant disability, either being unable to perform normal work or having serious impairment of other activities important to the patient
  - Have lower extremity PAD lesion anatomy such that the revascularization procedure would have low risk and a high probability of initial and long-term success
- Revascularization is indicated in patients with refractory rest pain or claudication that limits their lifestyle, results in non-healing ulcers or gangrene, or in a select group of patients with functional disability. Common procedures include:
  - Aorto-iliofemoral reconstruction or bypass or infrainguinal bypass (e.g., femoropopliteal, femorotibial).
  - Angioplasty, often with stenting, is used primarily on short, discrete stenotic lesions in the iliac or femoropopliteal arteries
  - Endovascular intervention is recommended as the preferred revascularization for iliac and femoropopliteal arterial lesions.
  - Stenting is effective primary therapy for common iliac artery and external iliac artery stenosis and occlusions; however, it is not recommended in the femoral, popliteal, or tibial arteries.

COMPLEMENTARY & ALTERNATIVE MEDICINE

- A meta-analysis found that over 12 to 24 wk, *Ginkgo biloba* increased pain-free walking distance by 34 m compared with placebo, although the benefit is not well established according to ACC/AHA guidelines.
- Naftidrofuryl, a serotonin receptor inhibitor, available in Europe, has shown some efficacy in improving claudication symptoms.
- Estrogen replacement therapy, propionyl-L-carnitine, L-arginine, oral vasodilators, prostaglandins, and chelation therapy are ineffective in the treatment of intermittent claudication.

DISPOSITION

- Intermittent claudication progressing to an ischemic leg or limb loss is unusual, especially if maintaining conservative treatments of risk factor modification, exercise, and smoking cessation.

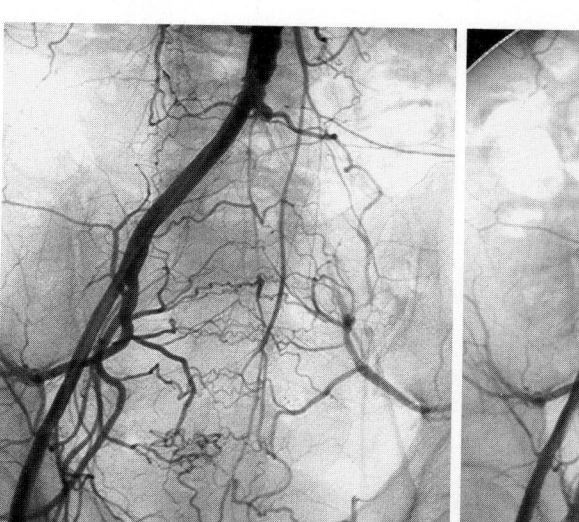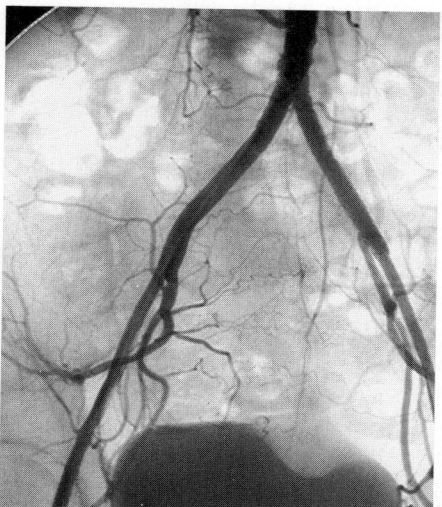

FIGURE 1-227 Angiogram of the distal abdominal aorta and iliac arteries demonstrates an occluded left common iliac artery with extensive collateral circulation from contralateral internal iliac artery *(left panel),* which resolved after successful stent implantation *(right panel).* (Images courtesy of Bart Domatch, MD, Radiology Department, University of Texas Southwestern Medical Center, Dallas, Texas. From Andreoli TE et al: *Andreoli and Carpenter's Cecil essentials of medicine,* ed 8, Philadelphia, 2010, Saunders.)

- The 5-yr risk for development of ischemic ulceration in patients treated for diabetes and with ABI <0.5 was 30% compared with only 5% in patients with neither characteristic.

REFERRAL

Consultation with physicians specializing in vascular medicine is recommended in the patient with threatened limb loss, rest pain, non-healing ulcers, functional disability from pain, and gangrene.

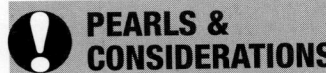

PEARLS & CONSIDERATIONS

- Approximately 70% of patients with peripheral vascular disease will have concomitant coronary artery disease.
- Beta-blockers may worsen claudication symptoms in some patients, although their underuse is associated with excess cardiovascular death. Patients with intermittent claudication are less likely to receive beta-blocker therapy after an initial myocardial infarction. Those who did not receive this treatment have at least a significant threefold higher mortality.
- Patients with peripheral vascular disease may benefit from secondary cardiovascular prevention with clopidogrel versus aspirin more so than other high-risk patients (CAPRIE trial).

COMMENTS

- Claudication is a marker for generalized atherosclerosis. This group of patients has a higher risk of death from cardiovascular events than from limb loss. Patients with claudication experience diminished overall quality of life similar to patients with diagnosed coronary or cerebrovascular disease.
- The ABI is more closely associated with leg function in persons with peripheral arterial disease than is intermittent claudication or other leg symptoms.

SUGGESTED READINGS
available at www.expertconsult.com

RELATED CONTENT

Claudication (Patient Information)

AUTHORS: **SHAMAIL TARIQ, M.D.,** and **PRANAV M. PATEL, M.D., F.A.C.C., F.S.C.A.I.**

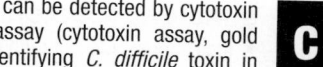

BASIC INFORMATION

DEFINITION *Clostridium difficile* infection (CDI) is the occurrence of diarrhea and bowel inflammation associated with antibiotic use. CDI can manifest clinically in several forms ranging from fulminant diarrhea and leukocytosis associated with pseudomembranous colitis, mild to severe acute diarrhea, short-term colonization seen typically in health care facilities, and recurrent CDI with 60 days after initial treatment occurring in 20% to 30% of cases.

SYNONYMS

Antibiotic-induced colitis
Pseudomembranous colitis
CDI

ICD-9CM CODES
008.45 *Clostridium difficile*,
    pseudomembranous colitis

EPIDEMIOLOGY & DEMOGRAPHICS

- Cephalosporins are the most frequent offending agent in pseudomembranous colitis because of their high rates of use.
- The antibiotic with the highest incidence is clindamycin (10% incidence of pseudomembranous colitis with its use).
- Since 1996, the incidence of CDI has more than doubled. Severity of CDI has also increased due to the emergence of an epidemic virulent strain (NAP1/BI/027). CDI is the most common infectious cause of healthcare-associated diarrhea in adults and is responsible for approximately 3 million cases of diarrhea and colitis in the U.S. every year.

PHYSICAL FINDINGS & CLINICAL PRESENTATION

- Abdominal tenderness (generalized or lower abdominal)
- Fever
- In patients with prolonged diarrhea, poor skin turgor, dry mucous membranes, and other signs of dehydration may be present

ETIOLOGY

The NAP1 strain is predominant among patients with *C. difficile* infection, whereas asymptomatic patients are more likely to be colonized with other strains. Risk factors for *C. difficile* (the major identifiable agent of antibiotic-induced diarrhea and colitis):

- Administration of antibiotics: can occur with any antibiotic, but occurs most frequently with clindamycin, ampicillin, cephalosporins, and fluoroquinolone
- Prolonged hospitalization
- Advanced age
- Abdominal surgery
- Underlying disease (malignancy, renal failure, debilitated status)
- Hospitalized, tube-fed patients are at risk for *C. difficile*–associated diarrhea. Clinicians should consider testing for *C. difficile* in tube-fed patients with diarrhea unrelated to the feeding solution.
- PPI and H$_2$ blocker therapy increases risk of CDI and recurrent CDI. Risk is 1.7-fold higher with PPIs.

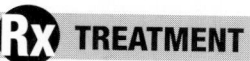

DIAGNOSIS

The clinical signs of CDI generally include diarrhea, fever, and abdominal cramps after use of antibiotics.

DIFFERENTIAL DIAGNOSIS

- Gastrointestinal bacterial infections (e.g., *Salmonella, Shigella, Campylobacter, Yersinia*)
- Enteric parasites (e.g., *Cryptosporidium, Entamoeba histolytica*)
- Inflammatory bowel disease
- Celiac sprue
- Irritable bowel syndrome
- Ischemic colitis
- Antibiotic intolerance

WORKUP

- All patients with diarrhea accompanied by current or recent antibiotic use should be tested for *C. difficile* (see later discussion). Testing and treatment for CDI is not recommended in asymptomatic individuals.
- Sigmoidoscopy (without cleansing enema) may be necessary when the clinical and laboratory diagnosis is inconclusive and the diarrhea persists.
- In antibiotic-induced pseudomembranous colitis, the sigmoidoscopy often reveals raised white-yellow exudative plaques adherent to the colonic mucosa (Fig. 1-228).

LABORATORY TESTS

- Stool test for *C. difficile* toxin: enzyme-linked immunosorbent assay for *C. difficile* toxins A and B. The latter is used most widely in the clinical setting. It has a sensitivity of 85% and a specificity of 100%.

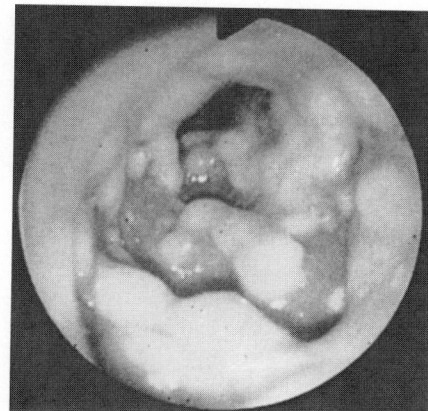

FIGURE 1-228 Pseudomembranous plaques seen with colonoscopy in a patient with *Clostridium difficile*–associated pseudomembranous colitis. (From Gorbach SL: *Infectious diseases*, ed 2, Philadelphia, 1998, Saunders.)

- *C. difficile* toxin can be detected by cytotoxin tissue-culture assay (cytotoxin assay, gold standard for identifying *C. difficile* toxin in stool specimen). This test is difficult to perform and results are not available for 24 to 48 hr.
- Fecal leukocytes (assessed by microscopy or lactoferrin assay) are generally present in stool samples.
- Complete blood count usually reveals leukocytosis. A sudden increase in white blood cells to >30,000/mm^3 may be indicative of fulminant colitis.

IMAGING STUDIES

Abdominal film (flat plate and upright) is useful in patients with abdominal pain or evidence of obstruction on physical examination.

TREATMENT

NONPHARMACOLOGIC THERAPY

- Discontinue offending antibiotic.
- Fluid hydration and correction of electrolyte abnormalities
- Probiotics to restore natural defense mechanisms may be useful as adjuvant therapy; however, evidence is limited.
- Fecal microbiota transplantation is an excellent treatment modality for recurrent CDI. Trials have shown that it is more effective than vancomycin and may become standard treatment for recurrent CDI.

ACUTE GENERAL Rx

- Metronidazole 500 mg PO qid for 10 to 14 days.
- Vancomycin 125 mg PO qid for 10 to 14 days in cases resistant to metronidazole. However, vancomycin may be considered as first-line therapy in hospitalized patients who are seriously ill.
- When parenteral therapy is necessary (e.g., patient with paralytic ileus), IV metronidazole 500 mg qid can be used. It can also be supplemented with vancomycin 500 mg by nasogastric tube with intermittent clamping or retention enema.
- IV tigecycline (a broad-spectrum antibiotic used for skin or soft-tissue infection) can be used as adjunctive or alternative therapy for severe refractory *C. difficile* toxin infection.
- The addition of monoclonal antibodies against *C. difficile* toxins to antibiotic agents has been shown to reduce the recurrence of *C. difficile* infection.
- Fidaxomicin, a newer antibiotic, has shown non-inferiority to vancomycin and a lower rate of CDI recurrence.
- Fecal transplantation: When standard treatment has failed, intestinal microbiota transplantation (IMT) is an effective alternative therapy (eradication rate is 94%). It involves infusing intestinal microorganisms (in a suspension of healthy donor stool) into the intestine of a sick patient via enema, gastroscope /colonoscope, or nasojejunal tube to restore the microbiota.

C

Diseases and Disorders

I

SURGICAL MANAGEMENT OF CDI

- Indications: CDI unresponsive to medical therapy, fulminant colitis
- Clinical features: colonic distention, severe abdominal pain/tenderness, systemic inflammatory response syndrome. Diarrhea may be absent because of ileus.
- Surgical approaches:
  - Traditional (subtotal or total colectomy), high mortality (50%)
  - Colon-sparing (loop ileostomy with intraoperative colonic lavage using warmed polyethylene glycol solution via the ileostomy and instillations of postoperative vancomycin flushes via the ileostomy); lower mortality compared to traditional approach

CHRONIC Rx

Judicious future use of antibiotics to prevent recurrences (e.g., avoid prolonged antibiotic therapy)

DISPOSITION

- Most patients recover completely with appropriate therapy. Fever resolves within 48 hr and diarrhea within 4 to 5 days. Overall mortality rate is 1% to 2.5% but exceeds 10% in untreated patients. CDI recurrence after an initial episode is 20% to 25% regardless of initial treatment with metronidazole or vancomycin. Each recurrence increases risk of repeat episodes (65% chance of recurrence after 3 CDI episodes). Recurrent CDI usually represents relapse rather than reinfection, no matter how long between episodes. Recurrent episodes are best treated with a prolonged course of oral vancomycin tapered off over several weeks to months.
- Hospital-acquired CDI is independently associated with an increased risk of in-hospital death.

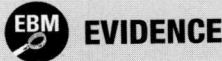

EVIDENCE

available at www.expertconsult.com

SUGGESTED READINGS

available at www.expertconsult.com

RELATED CONTENT

Pseudomembranous Colitis (Patient Information)

AUTHOR: **FRED F. FERRI, M.D.**

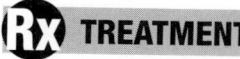 BASIC INFORMATION

DEFINITION

Cocaine is an alkaloid derived from the coca plant *Erythroxylum coca,* native to South America, which contains approximately 0.5% to 1% cocaine. The drug produces physiologic and behavioral effects when administered orally, intranasally, intravenously, or by inhalation after smoking. Cocaine has potent pharmacologic effects on dopamine, norepinephrine, and serotonin neurons in the central nervous system (CNS) involving alteration and blockade of cellular membrane transport and prevention of reuptake. Cocaine's second action involves the blockage of voltage-gated sodium ion membrane channels, which is responsible for its anesthetic effect. The mechanisms by which cocaine may induce myocardial ischemia or infarction are described in Fig. 1-229.

SYNONYMS

Cocaine hydrochloride: topical solution (FDA approved as a topical anesthetic)

Freebase: aqueous solution of cocaine hydrochloride converted to a more volatile base state by the addition of alkali, thereby extracting the cocaine base in a residue or precipitate

Crack: potent, purified smokable form; produces effects similar to those of intravenous administration

Street names include Bernice, Bernies, C, Cadillac or Champagne of drugs, Carrie, Cecil, Charlie, Coke, Dust, Dynamite, Flake, Gin, Girl, Gold dust, Green gold, Jet, Powder, Star dust, Paradise, Pimp's drug, Snowflake, Stardust, White girl

Liquid lady = alcohol + cocaine

Speedball = heroin + cocaine

Street measures: hit (2 to 200 mg), snort, line, dose, spoon (approximately 1 g)

ICD-9CM CODES
304.2 Cocainism

EPIDEMIOLOGY & DEMOGRAPHICS

- The 1993 National Household Survey on Drug Abuse estimated that 4.5 million Americans used cocaine in 1992, with 1.3 million reporting use at least monthly. By 1998 this had not significantly changed.
- Between 1993 and 1994, intravenous cocaine and heroin abusers accounted for a major new group of persons with HIV in several metropolitan areas.
- In 1999 an estimated 25 million Americans admitted that they used cocaine at least once—3.7 million the previous year and 1.5 million currently. It is the most frequent cause of drug-related death reported by medical examiners and is increasing more sharply in women than in men.
- The 2010 National Survey on Drug Use and Health indicates that there were 1 million individuals aged 12 yr. or older who had dependence or abuse of cocaine in the preceding year. This compares with 1.1 million in 2009, 1.4 million in 2008, and 1.6 million in 2007.

PHYSICAL FINDINGS & CLINICAL PRESENTATION

PHASE I:
- CNS: euphoria, agitation, headache, vertigo, twitching, bruxism, unintentional tremor
- Nausea, vomiting, fever, hypertension, tachycardia

PHASE II:
- CNS: lethargy, hyperreactive deep tendon reflexes, seizures (status epilepticus)
- Sympathetic overdrive: tachycardia, hypertension, hyperthermia
- Incontinence

PHASE III:
- CNS: flaccid paralysis, coma, fixed dilated pupils, loss of reflexes
- Pulmonary edema
- Cardiopulmonary arrest

Psychologic dependence manifests with habituation, paranoia, and hallucinations (cocaine "bugs"):

CNS: Cerebral ischemia and infarction, cerebral arterial spasm, cerebral vasculitis, cerebral vascular thrombosis, subarachnoid hemorrhage, intraparenchymal hemorrhage, seizures, cerebral atrophy, movement disorders, and hyperthermia

Cardiac: Acute myocardial ischemia and infarction, arrhythmias and sudden death, dilated cardiomyopathy and myocarditis, infective endocarditis, aortic rupture, acceleration of coronary atherosclerosis

Pulmonary: Inhalation injuries (secondary to smoking crack cocaine): cartilage and nasal septal perforation, oropharyngeal ulcers; immunologically mediated diseases: hypersensitivity pneumonitis, bronchiolitis obliterans; pulmonary vascular lesions and hemorrhage, pulmonary infarction, pulmonary edema secondary to left ventricular failure, pneumomediastinum, and pneumothorax

Gastrointestinal: Gastroduodenal ulceration and perforation; intestinal infarction or perforation, colitis

Renal: Acute renal failure secondary to rhabdomyolysis and myoglobinuria; renal infarction; focal segmental glomerulosclerosis

Obstetric: Placental abruption, low infant weight, prematurity, microcephaly

Psychiatric: Anxiety, depression, paranoia, delirium, psychosis, suicide

ETIOLOGY

Cocaine may be absorbed through different routes with varying degrees of speed:
- Nasal insufflation/snorting: 2.5 min
- Smoking: <30 sec
- Oral: 2 to 5 min
- Mucosal: <20 min
- Intravenous injection: <30 sec

DX DIAGNOSIS

DIFFERENTIAL DIAGNOSIS
- Methamphetamine ("speed") abuse
- Methylenedioxyamphetamine ("ecstasy") abuse
- Cathione ("khat") abuse
- Lysergic acid diethylamide (LSD) abuse

WORKUP
Physical examination and laboratory evaluation

LABORATORY TESTS
- Toxicology screen (urine): cocaine is metabolized within 2 hr by the liver to major metabolites, benzoylecgonine and ecgonine methyl ester, which are excreted in the urine. Metabolites can be identified in urine within 5 min of IV use and up to 48 hr after oral ingestion.
- Blood: CBC, electrolytes, glucose, BUN, creatinine, calcium.
- Arterial blood gas analysis.
- ECG.
- Serum creatinine kinase and troponin concentration.

Rx TREATMENT

There is no specific antidote and, at present, no drug therapy is uniquely effective in treating cocaine abuse and dependence. In addition, adulterants, contaminants, and other drugs may be admixed with street cocaine. Amantadine may provide effective treatment for cocaine-dependent patients with severe cocaine withdrawal symptoms, as well as the other dopamine agonist bromocriptine (1.5 mg PO tid), which may alleviate some of the symptoms of craving associated with acute cocaine withdrawal.

ACUTE GENERAL Rx

Acute cocaine toxicity requires following advanced poisoning treatment and life support. A suspected "body packer" should have an abdominal radiograph to detect the continued presence of cocaine-containing condoms in the intestinal tract. If present, gentle catharsis with charcoal and mineral oil should be performed with ICU admission and monitoring.

SPECIFIC TREATMENT

INHALATION: Wash nasal passages

AGITATION:
- Check STAT glucose
- Diazepam 15 to 20 mg PO or 2 to 10 mg IM or IV for severe agitation

HYPERTHERMIA:
- Check rectal temperature, creatine kinase, electrolytes
- Monitor with continuous rectal probe; bring temperature down to 101° F within 30 to 45 min

RHABDOMYOLYSIS:
- Vigorous hydration with urine output at least 2 ml/kg

- Mannitol or bicarbonate for rhabdomyolysis resistant to hydration

SEIZURE MANAGEMENT (STATUS EPILEPTICUS):
- Diazepam 5 to 10 mg IV over 2 to 3 min; may be repeated every 10 to 15 min.
- Lorazepam 2 to 3 mg IV over 2 to 3 min; may be repeated.
- Phenytoin loading dose 15 to 18 mg/kg IV at a rate not to exceed 25 to 50 mg/min under cardiac monitoring.
- Phenobarbital loading dose 10 to 15 mg/kg IV at a rate of 25 mg/min; an additional 5 mg/kg may be given in 30 to 45 min if seizures are not controlled.
- For refractory seizures, consider:
  1. Pancuronium 0.1 mg/kg IV
  2. Halothane general anesthesia
  3. Both require EEG monitoring to determine brain seizure activity.

HYPERTENSION: Cocaine-induced hypertension usually responds to benzodiazepines. If this fails:

- Consider arterial line for continuous blood pressure monitoring
- Avoid the use of calcium channel blockers because they may potentiate the incidence of seizures and death, especially in body packers.
- The use of beta-blockers may exacerbate cocaine-induced vasoconstriction.
- Phentolamine (unopposed adrenergic effects) or nitroglycerin may be required.
- If diastolic pressure >120 mm Hg: hydralazine hydrochloride 25 mg IM or IV; may repeat q1h.
- If hypertension is uncontrolled or hypertensive encephalopathy is present: sodium nitroprusside initially at 0.5 μg/kg/min not to exceed 10 μg/kg/min.

CHEST PAIN:
- Chest radiograph, ECG, cardiac enzymes.
- Benzodiazepines for agitation.
- Acetylsalicylic acid and nitroglycerin for ischemic pain. (Aspirin is contraindicated if dissection is suspected.)

- Percutaneous transluminal coronary angioplasty possibly better than thrombolysis for cocaine-associated myocardial infarction.
- Phentolamine will reverse cocaine-induced vasoconstriction and may be administered 5 to 10 mg every 5 to 10 minutes.
- The use of beta-adrenergic blockers remains controversial because of the unopposed alpha-adrenergic effects of cocaine.
- If beta-blockers are to be used, this should be preceded by administration of phentolamine to prevent unopposed alpha adrenergic stimulation. Many authors recommend not using beta-blockers until the cocaine has been systemically eliminated.

VENTRICULAR ARRHYTHMIAS (CONSIDERATIONS):
- Antiarrhythmic agents should be used with caution during the early period after cocaine exposure as a result of their proarrhythmic and proconvulsant effects.
- Lidocaine 1.5 mg/kg IV bolus followed by IV infusion (controversial: may be proarrhythmic and proconvulsant).
- Termination of ventricular arrhythmias may be resistant to lidocaine and even cardioversion.
- $NaHCO_3^-$ is under investigation in cocaine-mediated conduction abnormalities and rhythm disturbances.
- In a cardiac arrest situation secondary to cocaine toxicity, vasopressin offers a theoretical advantage over epinephrine.

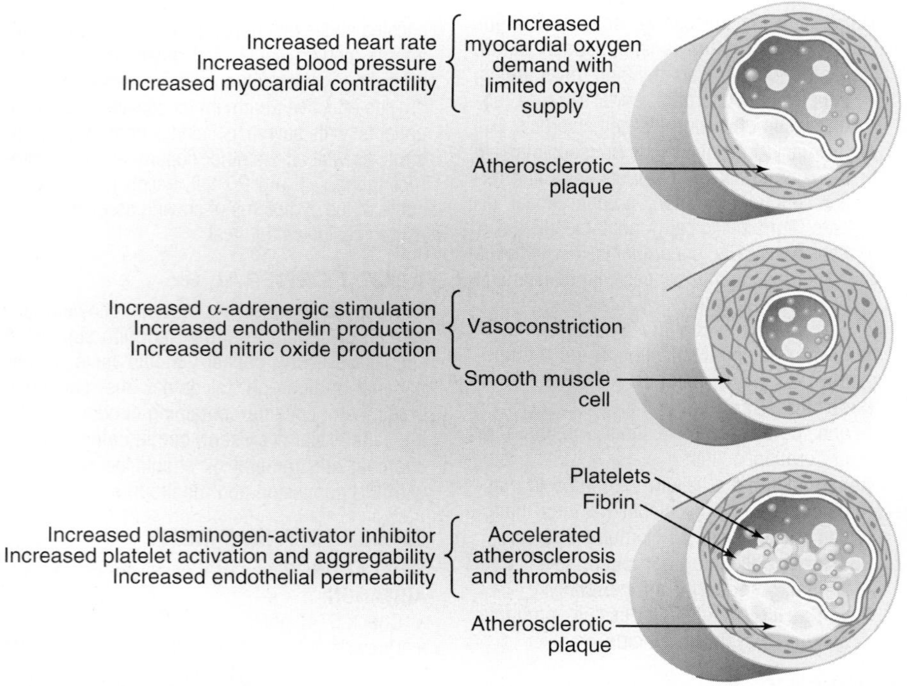

DISPOSITION

Although many patients who use cocaine may not require treatment because of the short half-life of the drug, others may require specific treatment for possible cocaine-related complications.

REFERRAL

Consider psychotherapy or behavioral therapy once stable.

PEARLS & CONSIDERATIONS

- Cocaine-induced vasoconstriction may be exacerbated by the use of selective and non-selective beta-adrenergic blocking agents.
- The use of lidocaine in treating ventricular arrhythmias may precipitate seizures and further arrhythmias.

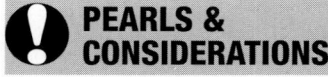
FIGURE 1-229 The mechanisms by which cocaine may induce myocardial ischemia or infarction. Cocaine may cause increase in the determinants of myocardial oxygen demand when oxygen supply is limited *(top)*, when intense vasoconstriction of the coronary arteries occurs *(middle)*, or when accelerated atherosclerosis and thrombosis are present *(bottom)*. (From Andreoli TE et al: *Andreoli and Carpenter's Cecil essentials of medicine,* ed 8, Philadelphia, 2010, Saunders.)

Labels in figure:
- Increased heart rate / Increased blood pressure / Increased myocardial contractility → Increased myocardial oxygen demand with limited oxygen supply
- Atherosclerotic plaque
- Increased α-adrenergic stimulation / Increased endothelin production / Increased nitric oxide production → Vasoconstriction
- Smooth muscle cell
- Platelets / Fibrin
- Increased plasminogen-activator inhibitor / Increased platelet activation and aggregability / Increased endothelial permeability → Accelerated atherosclerosis and thrombosis
- Atherosclerotic plaque

SUGGESTED READINGS

available at www.expertconsult.com

RELATED CONTENT

Abuse, Drug (Related Key Topic)
Cocaine Abuse and Dependence (Patient Information)
Drug Abuse (Patient Information)

AUTHOR: **SAJEEV HANDA, M.D., S.F.H.M.**

BASIC INFORMATION

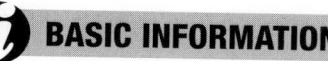

DEFINITION

Coccidioidomycosis is an infectious disease caused by inhaling the spores of the fungus *Coccidioides immitis*. Clinical syndromes range from subclinical pulmonary disease to pneumonia and disseminated disease mostly in immunocompromised hosts. Most cases occur in the southwest part of the U.S.

SYNONYMS

San Joaquin Valley fever

ICD-9CM CODES
114.0 *Coccidioides* pneumonia
114.1 Cutaneous or extrapulmonary (primary) coccidioidomycosis
114.3 Disseminated or prostate coccidioidomycosis
114.5 Pulmonary coccidioidomycosis
114.2 Coccidioidal meningitis
114.4 Chronic coccidioidomycosis

EPIDEMIOLOGY & DEMOGRAPHICS

INCIDENCE (IN U.S.): Estimated annual infection rate 150,000 persons, predominantly in southwest U.S. and appears to be rising due to increased population and construction in the area.
PEAK INCIDENCE: Seasonal in endemic areas with the higest risk being in the dry season after a rainy season as the mold lies a few inches below desert surface in soil and can become aerosolized.
PREVALENCE: 28.65 cases per 1 million population in the southwest U.S. in 2002 based on patients requiring hospital admission.
PREDOMINANT SEX: Males, between the ages of 25 and 55 yr
Clinical disease more severe in older children and adults

PHYSICAL FINDINGS & CLINICAL PRESENTATION

- The clinical manifestations vary widely according to the host, the severity of the illness, and location of dissemination.
- Asymptomatic infections or illness consistent with a nonspecific upper respiratory tract infection in at least 60%.
- Symptoms of primary infection—cough, malaise, fever, chills, night sweats, anorexia, weakness, and arthralgias (desert rheumatism)—in remaining 40% within 3 wk of exposure.
- Erythema nodosum and erythema multiforme more common in women.
- Scattered rales and dullness on percussion.
- Spontaneous improvement within 2 wk of illness, with complete recovery usual.
- Pulmonary nodules and cavities in <10% of those patients with primary infection; half of these patients asymptomatic.
- In a small portion of these patients: a progressive pneumonitis, often with a fatal outcome.

- Immunocompromised or diabetic patients may progress to chronic pulmonary disease.
- Over many years, granulomas rupture, leading to new cavity formation and continued fibrosis, often accompanied by hemoptysis.
- Disseminated or extrapulmonary disease in approximately 0.5% of acutely infected patients.
  1. Early signs of probable dissemination: fever, malaise, hilar adenopathy, and elevated ESR persisting in the setting of primary infection.
  2. Most organs are susceptible to dissemination, with heart and GI tract generally spared.
- Musculoskeletal involvement: bone lesions often unifocal, ribs, long bones, and vertebral lesions are common.
  1. Joint lesions predominantly unifocal, most commonly involving the ankle and knee, and often accompanying adjacent sites of osteomyelitis.
- Meningeal involvement: headache, fever, weakness, confusion, lethargy, cranial nerve defects, seizures; meningeal signs often minimal or absent.
- Cutaneous involvement: variable lesions—pustules, papules, plaques, nodules, ulcers, abscesses, or verrucous proliferative lesions.
  1. Dissemination and fatal outcomes most common in men, pregnant women, neonates, immunocompromised hosts, and individuals of dark-skinned races, especially those of African, Filipino, Mexican, and Native American ancestry.

ETIOLOGY

- *Coccidioides immitis* is endemic to North and South America.
- In the U.S., endemic areas coincide with the Lower Sonoran Life Zone, with semiarid climate, sparse flora, and alkaline soil in Arizona, California, New Mexico, and Texas.
- Fungus exists in the mycelial phase in soil, having barrel-shaped hyphae (arthroconidia). Arthrospores are aerosolized and deposit in the alveoli, then fungus converts to thick-walled spherule.
- Internal spherical spores (endospores) are released through spherule rupture and mature into new spherules (parasitic cycle).
- Fungus incites a granulomatous reaction in host tissue, usually with caseation necrosis.

DIAGNOSIS

DIFFERENTIAL DIAGNOSIS

- Acute pulmonary coccidioidomycoses:
  1. Community-acquired pneumonias caused by *Mycoplasma* and *Chlamydia*
  2. Granulomatous diseases, such as *Mycobacterium tuberculosis* and sarcoidosis
  3. Other fungal diseases, such as *Blastomyces dermatitidis* and *Histoplasma capsulatum*
- Coccidioidomas: true neoplasms

WORKUP

Suspected in patients with a history of residence or travel in an endemic area, especially during periods favorable to spore dispersion (e.g., dust storms and drought followed by heavy rains)

LABORATORY TESTS

- CBC to reveal eosinophilia, especially with erythema nodosum
- Routine chemistries: usually normal but may reveal hyponatremia
- Elevated serum levels of IgE; associated with progressive disease
- CSF cell counts and chemistry: pleocytosis with mononuclear cell predominance associated with hypoglycorrhachia and elevated protein level
- Definitive diagnosis based on demonstration of the organism by culture from body fluids or tissues
  1. Greatest yield with pus, sputum, synovial fluid, and soft tissue aspirations, varying with the degree of dissemination
  2. Possible positive cultures of blood, gastric aspirate, pleural effusion, peritoneal fluid, and CSF, but less frequently obtained
  3. Lab personnel are at risk of infection by inhalation on opening culture plates so lab should be notified the disease is suspected, but it is not contagious from person to person.
- Serologic evaluations
  1. Latex agglutination and complement fixation
  2. Elevated serum complement-fixing antibody (CFA) titers ≥1:32 strongly correlated with disseminated disease, except with meningitis where lower titers seen
  3. In meningeal disease: CFA detected in CSF except with high serum CFA titers secondary to concurrent extraneural disease
  4. Enzyme-linked immunosorbent assay (ELISA) against a 33-kDa spherule antigen to detect and monitor CNS disease
- PCR
- Skin test: currently not available, and its use was limited as patients with severe disease may be anergic. Skin testing may still have use in epidemiologhic surveys.

IMAGING STUDIES

Chest x-ray:
- Reveals unilateral infiltrates, hilar adenopathy, or pleural effusion in primary infection
- Shows areas of fibrosis containing usually solitary, thin-walled cavities that persist as residua of primary infection
- Possible coccidioidoma, a coinlike lesion representing a healed area of previous pneumonitis

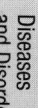

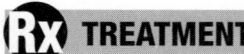 **TREATMENT**

NONPHARMACOLOGIC THERAPY

- Supportive care in mild symptomatic disease
- In patients with extrapulmonary manifestations involving draining skin, joint, and soft tissue infection: local wound care to avoid possible bacterial superinfection

ACUTE GENERAL Rx

- In general, drug therapy is not required for patients with asymptomatic pulmonary disease and most patients with mild symptomatic primary infection.
- Chemotherapy is indicated under the following circumstances:
    1. Severe symptomatic primary infection
    2. High serum CFA titers
    3. Persistent symptoms >6 wk
    4. Prostration
    5. Progressive pulmonary involvement
    6. Pregnancy
    7. Infancy
    8. Debilitation
    9. Concurrent illness (e.g., diabetes, asthma, COPD, malignancy)
    10. Acquired or induced immunosuppression
    11. Racial group with known predisposition for disseminated disease
- Fluconazole
    1. Most commonly, oral therapy with 400 mg/day up to 1.2 g/day appears to be the drug of choice for meningeal and deep-seated mycotic infections.
    2. In patients with AIDS, fluconazole may be considered the drug of choice for initial and maintenance therapy.
    3. All patients with coccidioidal meningitis should continue azole therapy indefinitely.
- Itraconazole
    1. 400 to 600 mg/day achieves 90% response rate in bone, joint, soft tissue, lymphatic, and genitourinary infections.
    2. Itraconazole may be more efficacious than fluconazole in the treatment of skeletal (bone) infections.
- Posaconazole is a new triazole that has recently been approved for use for systemic mycoses such as coccidioidomycosis; its relative efficacy compared to other agents will need additional clinical study.
- For pulmonary infections, treatment with either fluconazole or itraconazole, given for 6 to 12 wk, appears to be equal in efficacy.
- Amphotericin B is the classic therapy for disseminated extraneural disease, dose 0.6 to 1 mg/kg/day, qd for the first week then 0.8 mg/kg every other day, for a total dose of 1 to 2.5 g or until clinical and serologic remission is accomplished.
    1. Local instillation into body cavities such as sinuses, fistulae, and abscesses has been adjunct to therapy.
    2. Liposomal amphotericin B is probably equally effective.

    3. Duration of therapy for extraneural disease is undefined but probably about 1 yr.
- With meningeal disease: fluconazole 400 to 1000 mg PO q24h indefinitely
    1. Intrathecal amphotericin B is the alternate treatment modality, given alone or preceding the use of oral agents.
    2. Begin in doses of 0.01 to 0.025 mg/day, gradually increasing the dose as tolerated, to 0.5 mg/day with the patient in Trendelenburg's position.
    3. If given via Ommaya reservoir, as in ventriculitis, dose may be increased to 1.5 mg/day if tolerated.
    4. Concomitant parenteral therapy with amphotericin B is used for simultaneous extraneural disease as standard doses and with purely meningeal disease in smaller doses, although not strictly indicated.
    5. Intrathecal therapy is usually given three times a week for at least 3 mo, then discontinued or gradually tapered until once every 6 wk through 1 yr of therapy.
    6. Patients need routine monitoring of CSF, CFA, cell count, and chemistries for at least 2 yr following cessation of therapy.
- For osteomyelitis, soft tissue closed-space infections, and pulmonary fibrocavitary disease: surgical debridement, drainage, or resection, respectively, in addition to oral azole therapy or parenteral administration of amphotericin B.

CHRONIC Rx

For chronically immunocompromised patients, lifelong therapy with oral azoles or amphotericin B

DISPOSITION

- Prognosis for primary symptomatic infection is good.

TABLE 1-106 Risk Factors for Poor Outcome in Young Patients with Active Coccidioidomycosis

Primary Infections

Severe, prolonged (≥6 wk), or progressive infection

Risk Factors for Extrapulmonary Dissemination

Primary or acquired cellular immune dysfunction (including patients receiving tumor necrosis factor inhibitors)

Neonates, infants, the elderly

Male sex (adult)

Filipino, African, Native American, or Latin American ethnicity

Late-stage pregnancy and early postpartum period

Standardized complement fixation antibody titer >1:16 or increasing titer with persisting symptoms

Blood group B

HLA class II allele-DRBI*1301

From Kliegman RM et al: *Nelson textbook of pediatrics,* ed 19, Philadelphia, 2011, Saunders.

- Immunocompromised patients are most likely to have disseminated disease and higher morbidity and mortality.
- Risk factors for poor outcome in patients with active coccidioidomycosis are described in Table 1-106.

REFERRAL

- To surgeon for the evaluation of chronic hemoptysis, enlarging cavitary lesions despite chemotherapy and intrapleural rupture, osteomyelitis, and other synovial or soft tissue closed space infections
- For neurosurgical consultation in patients with meningeal disease to establish the delivery route of intrathecal drug therapy

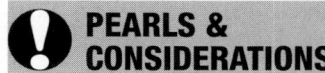 **PEARLS & CONSIDERATIONS**

COMMENTS

- Although coccidioidomycosis is a great imitator, a diagnosis will become apparent if a high degree of suspicion is maintained and appropriate testing (serologic testing, cultures, and histology) is performed.
- Infected body fluids contained within a closed moist environment (e.g., sputum in a specimen cup) provide the opportunity for the fungus to revert to its hyphal form whereby spores may be made airborne on opening of the container. This is a biohazard for laboratory personnel. Purulent drainage into a cast, allowing conversion of fungus to the saprophytic phase, has been responsible for acute disease when the cast was opened and the spores were unintentionally made airborne.
- Patients with a remote history of exposure, especially if immunosuppressed by medication or disease, may reactivate primary disease and suffer rapid dissemination.
- Although cardiac disease is rare, constrictive pericarditis in the setting of disseminated coccidioidomycosis has been documented and is potentially fatal.
- Organ transplant recipients may develop disease if the transplant donor has unrecognized active coccidioidomycosis at the time of death.

SUGGESTED READINGS

available at www.expertconsult.com

RELATED CONTENT

Coccidioidomycosis (Patient Information)

AUTHOR: **GLENN G. FORT, M.D., M.P.H.**

C

I

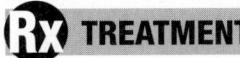 **BASIC INFORMATION**

DEFINITION

Cogan's syndrome is an autoimmune inner ear disorder that is temporally associated with interstitial keratitis and is thought to be the result of an underlying systemic vasculitis.

SYNONYMS

Cogan syndrome

ICD-9CM CODES
370.52 Cogan's syndrome

EPIDEMIOLOGY & DEMOGRAPHICS

INCIDENCE: No population studies are available for incidence calculation. More than 100 cases have been described in the literature.
PREVALENCE: No population studies are available for prevalence analysis.
PREDOMINANT SEX: No gender preference.
PREDOMINANT AGE: Median age of onset is 25 yrs.
GENETICS: Unknown.
RISK FACTORS: None.

PHYSICAL FINDINGS & CLINICAL PRESENTATION (Table 1-107)

- Clinical hallmarks: Cogan's syndrome is characterized by an acute or subacute or recurrent onset of inner ear loss of function resembling Meniere's disease (tinnitus, vertigo, and gradual hearing loss). The resultant hearing loss typically is bilateral. This is temporally related to the onset of a nonsyphilitic keratitis manifested as pain, redness, and blurry vision in the affected eye. Keratitis and cochleovestibular symptoms should occur within 2 yrs of each other.

TABLE 1-107 Systemic Manifestations of Cogan's Syndrome

Manifestations	Percentage of Cases (%)
Fever	25
Fatigue	20
Arthralgias/myalgias	15
Arthritis	15
Weight loss	15
Abdominal pain	10
Gastrointestinal bleeding	10
Lymphadenopathy	10
Hepatomegaly	10
Splenomegaly	10
Central nervous system findings	5
Pleuritis	5
Rash	5
Peripheral nervous system findings	<5
Polychondritis	<5

From Hochberg MC et al: *Rheumatology*, ed 4, St Louis, 2008, Mosby.

Systemic vasculitis features are marked by large vessel vasculitis and can occur in up to 10% of patients. This leads to aortic regurgitation. Medium vessel vasculitis resembling polyarteritis nodosa to small vessel vasculitis manifestations are possible.
- Constitutional: fever, headache, weight loss, malaise
- Ocular: redness, pain, and blurred vision as a result of interstitial keratitis (72% to 100%). Scleritis or episcleritis (23%).
- Hearing/Vestibular: hearing loss to deafness, usually bilateral (100%), vertigo (90%), tinnitus (80%). Imbalance with associated nausea, vomiting.
- Cardiovascular: aortitis (aortic aneurysm, aortic insufficiency)
- Musculoskeletal: arthralgia, arthritis, myalgia
- Gastrointestinal: abdominal pain (13% to 16%)
- Renal: hematuria (7%), glomerulonephritis (3%)
- Dermatologic: cutaneous nodules, rash

ETIOLOGY

The exact etiology of Cogan's syndrome is unknown. It is an autoimmune disease, which is supported by the binding of autoantibodies from patients with Cogan's syndrome to the cochlea in mice in passive transfer studies. Infection is thought to be a trigger for Cogan's syndrome. Some HLA loci, including HLA-B17, HLA-A9, HLA-Bw35, and HLA-Cw4, correlate with the disorder.

DX **DIAGNOSIS**

DIFFERENTIAL DIAGNOSIS
- Infectious diseases
  - Syphilis
  - Tuberculosis, Lyme disease, chlamydia, leprosy, brucellosis, mumps, EBV, herpes zoster, and herpes simplex; rubeola should be considered in the differential for interstitial keratitis
- Rheumatology
  - ANCA-associated vasculitis: granulomatosis with polyangiitis (Wegener's granulomatosis)
  - Takayasu's arteritis
  - Giant cell arteritis
  - Rheumatoid arthritis with vasculitis
  - Polyarteritis nodosa
  - Behçet's disease
  - Sarcoidosis
- Neurology
  - Susac syndrome
- Neoplastic
  - Lymphoma (CNS)
- Miscellaneous
  - Vogt-Koyanagi-Harada syndrome

LABORATORY TESTS
- Inflammatory markers are often elevated, including the erythrocyte sedimentation rate (ESR) and C-reactive protein.
- Complete blood cell count with differential; may show leukocytosis.

- ANCA serology test to exclude ANCA-associated vasculitis.
- Serologic test result should be negative for syphilis.

IMAGING STUDIES
- MRI with gadolinium of the brain to rule out noninner ear causes for acute or subacute hearing loss and vestibular dysfunction. Brain MRI can range from normal to gadolinium enhancement of the vestibular-cochlear structures.
- Magnetic resonance angiography (MRA) of the aorta and its proximal branches may be used to assess for vascular inflammation. This can be supportive of large vessel vasculitis.

Rx **TREATMENT**

NONPHARMACOLOGIC THERAPY
- Cochlear implant

ACUTE GENERAL Rx
- Treatment guidelines are based on grade C (fair evidence from ancillary studies) recommendations.
- Eye symptoms: Topical corticosteroids, mydriatics may be considered.
- Fluconazole Vestibuloauditory symptoms: Oral prednisone 1 to 2 mg/kg/day is recommended.
- Vasculitis symptoms: Oral prednisone 1 to 2 mg/kg/day is recommended. Oral or intravenous cyclophosphamide should be considered for life-threatening features.

CHRONIC Rx
- Methotrexate or azathioprine may be considered as steroid-sparing agent.

DISPOSITION
- Ocular outcomes are good.
- Hearing loss may occur in up to 50% of cases.

REFERRAL
- Refer to ophthalmologist for complete ocular examination, including slit-lamp examination.
- Refer to rheumatologist for all patients with suspected disease.
- Refer to audiologist for complete hearing assessment.
- Refer to otolaryngologist for confirmation of sensorineural hearing loss.

SUGGESTED READINGS
available at www.expertconsult.com

AUTHOR: **SAMUEL H. POON, M.D.**

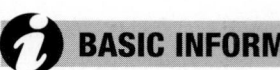 **BASIC INFORMATION**

DEFINITION

Colorectal cancer (CRC) is a neoplasm arising from the luminal surface of the large bowel; locations include descending colon (40% to 42%), rectosigmoid and rectum (30% to 33%), cecum and ascending colon (25% to 30%), and transverse colon (10% to 13%).

ICD-9CM CODES
154.0 Colorectal cancer

EPIDEMIOLOGY & DEMOGRAPHICS

- CRC is the second leading cause of cancer deaths in the U.S. (>160,000 new cases and >55,000 deaths/yr).
- Peak incidence is in the seventh decade of life. The lifetime risk for development of CRC is 1 in 17, with 90% of cases occurring after age 50 yr.
- 50% of rectal cancers are within reach of the examiner's finger, and 50% of colon cancers are within reach of the flexible sigmoidoscope.
- CRC accounts for 14% of all cases of cancer (excluding skin malignancies) and 14% of all yearly cancer deaths.
- Risk factors:
  - Hereditary polyposis syndromes
    Familial polyposis (high risk)
    Gardner's syndrome (high risk)
    Turcot's syndrome (high risk)
    Peutz-Jeghers syndrome (low to moderate risk)
  - Inflammatory bowel disease (IBD), both ulcerative colitis and Crohn's disease
  - Family history of "cancer family syndrome"
  - Heredofamilial breast cancer and colon carcinoma
  - History of previous colorectal carcinoma
  - Women undergoing irradiation for gynecologic cancer
  - First-degree relatives with colorectal carcinoma
  - Age >40 yr
  - Possible dietary factors (diet high in fat or meat, beer drinking, reduced vegetable consumption); prolonged high consumption of red and processed meat may increase the risk for cancer of the large intestine
  - Hereditary nonpolyposis colon cancer (HNPCC): autosomal dominant disorder characterized by early age of onset (mean age, 44 yr) and right-sided or proximal colon cancers, synchronous and metachronous colon cancers, mucinous and poorly differentiated colon cancers; accounts for 1% to 5% of all cases of CRC
  - Previous endometrial or ovarian cancer, particularly when diagnosed at an early age

PHYSICAL FINDINGS & CLINICAL PRESENTATION

- Physical examination may be completely unremarkable.
- Digital rectal examination can detect approximately 50% of rectal cancers.
- Palpable abdominal masses may indicate metastasis or complications of colorectal carcinoma (abscess, intussusception, volvulus).
- Abdominal distention and tenderness are suggestive of colonic obstruction.
- Hepatomegaly may be indicative of hepatic metastasis.

ETIOLOGY

CRC can arise through two mutational pathways: microsatellite instability or chromosomal instability. Germline genetic mutations are the basis of inherited colon cancer syndromes; an accumulation of somatic mutations in a cell is the basis of sporadic colon cancer.

Dx DIAGNOSIS

DIFFERENTIAL DIAGNOSIS

- Diverticular disease
- Strictures
- IBD
- Infectious or inflammatory lesions
- Adhesions
- Arteriovenous malformations
- Metastatic carcinoma (prostate, sarcoma)
- Extrinsic masses (cysts, abscesses)

WORKUP

The clinical presentation of colorectal malignancies is initially vague and nonspecific (weight loss, anorexia, malaise). It is useful to divide colon cancer symptoms into those usually associated with the right side of the colon and those commonly associated with the left side of the colon because the clinical presentation varies with the location of the carcinoma.

- Right side of colon:
  - Anemia (iron deficiency from chronic blood loss).
  - Dull, vague, and uncharacteristic abdominal pain may be present, or patient may be completely asymptomatic.
  - Rectal bleeding is often missed because blood is mixed with feces.
  - Obstruction and constipation are unusual because of large lumen and more liquid stools.
- Left side of colon:
  - Change in bowel habits (constipation, diarrhea, tenesmus, pencil-thin stools).
  - Rectal bleeding (bright red blood coating the surface of the stool).
  - Intestinal obstruction is frequent because of small lumen.

Early diagnosis of patients with surgically curable disease (Dukes A/B) is necessary because survival time is directly related to the stage of the carcinoma at the time of diagnosis. Appropriate screening recommendations are discussed in Section V.

CLASSIFICATION AND STAGING

Dukes and UICC classification for CRC:
- A. Confined to the mucosa-submucosa (stage I)
- B. Invasion of muscularis propria (stage II)
- C. Local node involvement (stage III)
- D. Distant metastasis (stage IV)

TNM Classification:

Stage	TNM Classification
I	T1-2, N0, M0
IIA	T3, N0, M0
IIB	T4, N0, M0
IIIA	T1-2, N1, M0
IIIB	T3-4, N1, M0
IIIC	T(any), N2, M0
IV	T(any), N(any), M1

LABORATORY TESTS

- Positive fecal occult blood test (FOBT): Many primary care physicians use single digital FOBT as their primary screening test for CRC. Single FOBT has low specificity for detecting human hemoglobin, is a poor screening method for CRC (sensitivity, 4.9%), and is inappropriate as the only test because negative results do not decrease the odds of advanced neoplasia. The American College of Gastroenterology recommends fecal immunochemical test as a replacement for guaiac-based FOBT for CRC detection. Annual Hemoccult SENSA and fecal DNA testing every 3 yr are alternative cancer detection tests.
- Microcytic anemia on CBC may be indicative of chronic blood loss.
- Increased plasma carcinoembryonic antigen (CEA) level: CEA should not be used as a screening test for CRC because it can be increased in patients with many other conditions (smoking, IBD, alcoholic liver disease). A normal CEA result does not exclude the diagnosis of CRC.
- Liver function tests should be ordered.

IMAGING STUDIES

- Colonoscopy with biopsy (primary assessment tool): The American College of Physicians (ACP) recommends that patients should be offered a colonoscopy beginning at age 50 yr and repeated every 10 yr in average-risk patients. Screening is recommended in African Americans beginning at 45 yr of age. Persons with only one first-degree relative with CRC or advanced adenomas diagnosed at 60 yr or older may be screened as at average risk. A family history of small tubular adenomas in first-degree relatives is not considered to increase the risk for CRC. The U.S. Preventive Services Task Force guidelines state that screening should not be routinely recommended in persons older than 75 yr, and it should not be recommended at all in persons older than 85 yr. If persons between the ages of 75 and 85 yr have never undergone screening, the decision about screening should be individualized according to health status. The ACP recommends that clinicians stop screening for colorectal cancer in adults over age 75 yr or in adults with a life expectancy of <10 yr. Table 1-108 describes CRC screening and surveillance recommendations.

- Computed tomography colonoscopy (CTC) virtual colonoscopy (VC) uses helical (spiral) CT scanning to generate a two- or three-dimensional virtual colorectal image. CTC does not require sedation; but, like optical colonoscopy, it requires some bowel preparation (either bowel cathartics or ingestion of iodinated contrast medium with meals during the 48 hr before CT) and air insufflation. It also involves substantial exposure to radiation. In addition, patients with lesions detected by VC will require traditional colonoscopy. Compared with colonoscopy, CTC sensitivity for detection of polyps >10 mm ranges from 70% to 96%, and specificity ranges from 72% to 96%. CTC has replaced double-contrast barium enema as the radiographic screening alternative when patients decline colonoscopy.
- Capsule endoscopy allows visualization of the colonic mucosa but is not recommended as a screening procedure because its sensitivity for detecting colonic lesions is low compared with colonoscopy.
- CT scanning of the abdomen, pelvis, and chest assists in preoperative staging.
- PET scanning can display functional information and is accurate in the detection of CRC and its distant metastases. Combined PET/CT scanners are increasingly more available, and are useful to detect and characterize malignant lesions. Colonography composed of a combined modality of PET and CT is a newer diagnostic modality that can provide whole-body tumor staging in a single session.

 TREATMENT

GENERAL Rx

- Surgical resection: 70% of CRCs are resectable for cure at presentation; 45% of patients are cured by primary resection. Stage I and II tumors are curable by surgical resection, and up to 73% of cases of stage III can be cured by surgery combined with adjuvant chemotherapy.
- The backbone of chemotherapy treatment of CRC is fluorouracil (FU). Leucovorin (folinic acid) enhances the effect of FU and is given concomitantly. Adjuvant chemotherapy with combination of 5-FU and levamisole substantially increases cure rates for patients with stage III colon cancer and should be considered standard treatment for all such patients and selected patients with high-risk stage II colon cancer (adherence of tumor to an adjacent organ, bowel perforation, or obstruction).
- Radiation therapy is a useful adjunct to FU and leucovorin therapy for stage II or III rectal cancers.
- When given as adjuvant therapy after a complete resection in stage III disease, FU increases overall 5-yr survival rate from 51% to 64%. The use of adjuvant FU in stage II disease (no involvement of regional nodes) is controversial because 5-yr overall survival is 80% for treated or untreated patients, and the addition of FU only increases the probability of a 5-yr disease-free interval from 72% to 76%. For patients with standard-risk stage III tumors (e.g., involvement of one to three

regional lymph nodes), both FU alone and FU with oxaliplatin (Eloxatin, an inhibitor of DNA synthesis) are reasonable choices. In general, reversible peripheral neuropathy is the main side effect of FU plus oxaliplatin. The oral fluoropyrimidine capecitabine (Xeloda) is a prodrug that undergoes enzymatic conversion to FU. It is an effective alternative to IV FU as adjuvant treatment for stage III colon cancer because it has a lower incidence of mouth sores and bone marrow suppression. It does, however, have an increased incidence of palmar-plantar erythrodysesthesia (hand-foot syndrome).
- Irinotecan (Camptosar), a potent inhibitor of topoisomerase I, a nuclear enzyme involved in the unwinding of DNA during replication, can be used to treat metastatic CRC refractory to other drugs, including 5-FU; it may offer a few months of palliation but is expensive and is associated with significant toxicity.
- Oxaliplatin (Eloxatin), a third-generation platinum derivative, can be used in combination with FU and leucovorin (FL) for patients with metastatic CRC whose disease has recurred or progressed despite treatment with FL plus irinotecan. FL plus oxaliplatin should be considered for high-risk patients with stage III cancers (e.g., more than three involved regional nodes [N2] or tumor invasion beyond the serosa [T4 lesion]).
- Laboratory studies have identified molecular sites in tumor tissue that may serve as specific targets for treatment by using epidermal growth factor receptor (EGFR) antagonists and angiogenesis inhibitors. The monoclonal antibodies cetuximab (Erbitux), panitumumab (Vectibix), and bevacizumab (Avastatin) have been approved by the FDA for advanced CRC. Bevacizumab is an angiogenesis inhibitor that binds and inhibits the activity of human vascular endothelial growth factor. Cetuximab and panitumumab are EGFR blockers that inhibit the growth and survival of tumor cells that overexpress EGFR. Cetuximab has synergism with irinotecan, and its addition to irinotecan in patients with advanced disease resistant to irinotecan increases the response rate from 10% when cetuximab is used alone to 22% with combination of cetuximab and irinotecan. The addition of bevacizumab to FL in patients with advanced CRC has been reported to increase the response rate from 17% to 40%. Severe dermatologic toxicity can occur with both cetuximab and panitumumab.
- The liver is generally the initial and most common site of CRC metastases. Resection of metastases limited to the liver is curative in more than 30% of selected patients. In patients who undergo resection of liver metastases, postoperative treatment with a combination of hepatic arterial infusion of floxuridine and IV FU improves the outcome at 2 yr. Trials comparing hepatic resection (HR) and radiofrequency ablation (RFA) in the treatment of solitary colorectal liver metastases reveal that HR has better outcome; however, in tumors <3 cm, RFA can be

TABLE 1-108 Colorectal Cancer (CRC) Screening and Surveillance Recommendations

Indication	Recommendations
Average risk	Beginning at age 50 yr: Colonoscopy every 10 yr; Computed tomographic colonography every 5 yr; Flexible sigmoidoscopy every 5 yr; Double-contrast barium enema every 5 yr (Stool blood testing annually or stool DNA testing acceptable but not preferred)
One or two first-degree relatives with CRC at any age or adenoma at age < 60 yr	Colonoscopy every 5 yr beginning at age 40 yr, or 10 yr younger than earliest diagnosis, whichever comes first
Hereditary nonpolyposis CRC	Genetic counseling and screening†; Colonoscopy every 1 to 2 years beginning at age 25 yr and then yearly after age 40 yr‡
Familial adenomatous polyposis and variants	Genetic counseling and testing†; Flexible sigmoidoscopy yearly beginning at puberty‡
Personal history of CRC	Colonoscopy within 1 yr of curative resection; repeat at 3 yr and then every 5 yr if normal
Personal history of colorectal adenoma	Colonoscopy every 3 to 5 yr after removal of all index polyps
Inflammatory bowel disease	Colonoscopy every 1 to 2 yr beginning after 8 yr of pancolitis or after 15 yr if only left-sided disease

*Recommendations proposed by the American Cancer Society and U.S. Multi-Society Task Force on Colorectal Cancer; recommendations for average-risk patients also endorsed by the American College of Radiology.
†Whenever possible, affected relatives should be tested first because of potential false-negative results.
‡Screening recommendation for individuals with positive or indeterminate tests as well as for those who refuse genetic testing.
From Andreoli TE et al: *Andreoli and Carpenter's Cecil essentials of medicine*, ed 8, Philadelphia, 2010, Saunders.

recommended in patients who are not surgical candidates due to comorbidities or when the liver met is poorly localized anatomically.

CHRONIC Rx

Follow-up is indicated with:

- Physician visits with a focus on the clinical and disease-related history, directed physical examination guided by this history, coordination of follow-up, and counseling every 3 to 6 mo for the first 3 yr, then decreased frequency thereafter for 2 yr
- Colonoscopy yearly for the initial 2 yr, then every 3 yr
- Baseline CEA level can be obtained; if elevated, it can be used after surgery as a measure of completeness of tumor resection or to monitor tumor recurrence. If used to monitor tumor recurrence, CEA should be obtained every 3 to 6 mo for up to 5 yr. The role of CEA for monitoring patients with resected colon cancer has been questioned because of the small number of cures attributed to CEA monitoring despite the substantial cost in dollars and physical and emotional stress associated with monitoring.

DISPOSITION

The 5-yr survival rate varies with the stage of the carcinoma:

- Dukes:
  - Dukes A 5-yr survival rate >80%
  - Dukes B 5-yr survival rate 60%
  - Dukes C 5-yr survival rate 20%
  - Dukes D 5-yr survival rate 3%
- TNM classification:

Stage	TNM Classification	5-yr Survival Rate
I	T1-2, N0, M0	>90%
IIA	T3, N0, M0	60-85%
IIB	T4, N0, M0	60-85%
IIIA	T1-2, N1, M0	25-65%
IIIB	T3-4, N1, M0	25-65%
IIIC	T(any), N2, M0	25-65%
IV	T(any), N(any), M1	5-7%

- Overall 5-yr disease-free survival rate has increased from 50% to 63% during the past two decades.
- High-frequency microsatellite instability in CRC is independently predictive of a relatively favorable outcome and reduces the likelihood of metastases.
- In patients with Dukes C (stage III) CRC, there is improved 5-yr survival among women treated with adjuvant chemotherapy (53%

with chemotherapy vs. 33% without) and among patients with right-sided tumors treated with adjuvant chemotherapy.
- Retention of 19q alleles in microsatellite-stable cancers and mutation of the gene for the type I receptor for tumor growth factor B1 in cancers with high levels of microsatellite instability point to a favorable outcome after adjuvant chemotherapy with FU-based regimens for stage II colon cancer.
- Expression patterns of microRNA are systemically altered in colon adenocarcinomas. High miR-21 expression is associated with poor survival and poor therapeutic outcome.
- Guanylyl cyclase 2 C (GUCY2C) has been identified as a marker expressed by colorectal tumors that could reveal occult metastases in lymph nodes. Expression of GUCY2C in histologically negative lymph nodes appears to be independently associated with time to recurrence and disease-free survival in patients with lymph nodes free of tumor cells by histopathology (pNO) in CRC.
- The optimal timing from surgery to initiation of adjuvant chemotherapy is unknown. Meta-analysis of available literature suggests that longer time to adjuvant chemotherapy is associated with worse survival rates among patients with resected CRC.
- Regular aspirin use after the diagnosis of CRC has been reported to be associated with lower risk for CRC-specific and overall mortality, especially among individuals with tumors that overexpress cyclooxygenase-2. All aspirin doses starting with 75 mg daily had similar effects on CRC incidence and mortality.

REFERRAL

- Surgical referral for resection
- Oncology referral for adjuvant chemotherapy in selected patients
- Radiation oncology referral for patients with stage II or III rectal cancers

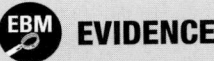

PEARLS & CONSIDERATIONS

COMMENTS

- Metastases of tumor cells to regional lymph nodes is the single most important prognostic factor in patients with colon cancer.
- Decreased fat intake to 30% of total energy intake, increased fiber, and fruit and vegetable

consumption may reduce CRC risk. Recent literature reports, however, do not support a protective effect from dietary fiber against CRC in women.
- Chemoprophylaxis with aspirin (81 mg/day) reduces the incidence of colorectal adenomas in persons at risk.
- Statins inhibit the growth of colon cancer lines. Use of statins is associated with a 47% relative reduction in the risk for CRC. Additional trials are necessary to investigate the overall benefits of statins in preventing CRC.
- The National Cancer Institute has published consensus guidelines for universal screening for HNPCC in patients with newly diagnosed CRC. Tumors in mutation carriers of HNPCC typically exhibit microsatellite instability, a characteristic phenotype caused by expansion or contraction of short nucleotide repeat sequences. These guidelines (Bethesda Guidelines) are useful for selective patients for microsatellite instability testing. Screening patients with newly diagnosed CRC for HNPCC is cost effective, especially if the benefits to their immediate relatives are considered.
- Expression of guanylyl cyclase C mRNA in lymph nodes is associated with recurrence of CRC in patients with stage II disease. Analysis of guanylyl cyclase mRNA expression by reverse transcription polymerase chain reaction may be useful for CRC staging.
- The use of either annual or biennial FOBT significantly reduces the incidence of CRC.
- The detection of mutations in the *APC* gene from stool samples is a promising new modality for early detection of colorectal neoplasms.
- KRAS mutations are consistently associated with reduced overall and progression-free survival and increased treatment failure.

RELATED CONTENT
Colon Cancer (Patient Information)

AUTHOR: **FRED F. FERRI, M.D.**

ℹ️ BASIC INFORMATION

DEFINITION

Compartment syndrome is a condition that occurs when elevated pressure within a limited space compromises the circulation, with increased risk of irreversible damage to its contents and their function. Acute compartment syndrome is a surgical emergency.

SYNONYMS

None

ICD-10CM CODES
958.90 Compartment syndrome unspecified
958.90 Compartment syndrome, not otherwise specified

EPIDEMIOLOGY & DEMOGRAPHICS

- Occurs most commonly after acute trauma, especially with long bone fractures, comprising 75% of cases.
- It usually occurs in persons <35 yr.
- Incidence is higher in males.
- It can occur in other parts, such as the foot, thigh, gluteal region, and abdomen.
- Supracondylar fractures in children can commonly lead to compartment syndrome.
- 6%-9% of open tibial fractures are complicated by compartment syndrome.

RISK FACTORS: It is seen in all races and ethnicities.

PATHOPHYSIOLOGY

Compartment syndrome occurs when the blood flow is less than the tissue metabolic demands, causing tissue injury. It occurs when the intracompartment pressure increases limiting venous outflow with rising venous pressure, resulting in compromise of the local circulation and tissue hypoxia with decreased arteriovenous pressure gradient. Venous congestion additionally leads to tissue edema and interstitial pressure, and the compartment pressure continues to increase. Compartment pressure able to cause the condition ranges between 10 and 30 mm Hg of diastolic pressure.

Different conditions are known to cause compartment syndrome:

- Conditions that limit compartment volume, such as when patients have fracture casts, when sedated or comatose patients lie on a limb for a prolonged period, and when patients have tight dressings that are applied externally
- Conditions that cause increased compartment content, such as bleeding from vascular injury or diathesis, fractures or finger injuries, reperfusion after ischemic injury such as embolectomy and arterial bypass grafting, and thermal or electrical burn injuries
- Other injuries, such as extravasation of IV fluids, injection of recreational drugs, and snake bites.

PHYSICAL FINDINGS & CLINICAL PRESENTATION

Signs and symptoms are usually apparent but can be unreliable and can lead to delayed diagnosis. Acute compartment syndrome can worsen within hours; therefore serial examination is important in a patient with suspected compartment syndrome. Patients with tense painful limbs are considered to have acute compartment syndrome; however, diagnosis is confirmed with the assessment of elevated compartment pressure. Clinical signs and symptoms include the following:

- Pain disproportional to injury (the earliest sign)
- Constant deep pain and pain that is referred to the compartment on passive stretching of the muscles of the affected compartment (Fig. 1-231A)
- Reduced sense of touch or sensation (hypesthesia) within the territory of the nerve passing the compartment (in acute anterior compartment syndrome, the patient may have hypesthesia in the territory of the first webspace)
- Tense and swollen compartment (Figs. 1-231B and 1-231C)
- Muscle weakness
- Paresis (late finding) that suggests permanent muscle damage
- Capillary refill can be slow but normal.
- Peripheral pulses that are normally palpable even in severe conditions
- Tingling and numbness in the affected limb. Hypesthesia or paresthesia should be evaluated with pinprick, light touch, and two-point discrimination tests.

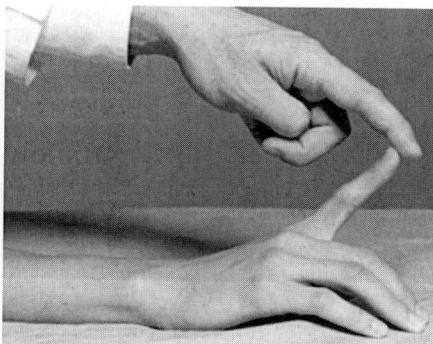

FIGURE 1-231A Passive extension of the digit causes pain referred to the compartment. (From Browner BD et al [eds]: *Skeletal trauma,* ed 4, Philadelphia, 2009, Saunders.)

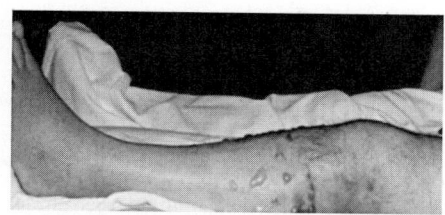

FIGURE 1-231B Acute compartment syndrome of the leg. (From Browner BD et al [eds]: *Skeletal trauma,* ed 4, Philadelphia, 2009, Saunders.)

🅳🅷 DIAGNOSIS

Diagnosis is based on clinical signs and symptoms along with compartment pressure. Compartment pressure testing may be unnecessary if the diagnosis is clinically obvious.

DIFFERENTIAL DIAGNOSIS

- Muscle strains
- Cellulitis
- Gangrene
- Peripheral vascular injury
- Necrotizing fasciitis
- Stress fractures
- Deep vein thrombosis and thrombophlebitis
- Tendinitis
- Muscle contusion
- Tarsal tunnel syndrome
- Posterior ankle syndrome
- Popliteal artery impingement
- Claudication
- Tumor
- Venous insufficiency

LABORATORY TESTS

Diagnosis is based on clinical findings and the measurement of compartment pressures. Laboratory values are not useful in the diagnosis of compartment syndrome. Laboratory studies are important, though, for other diagnoses or associated conditions.

- CBC with differential for evaluation of infection

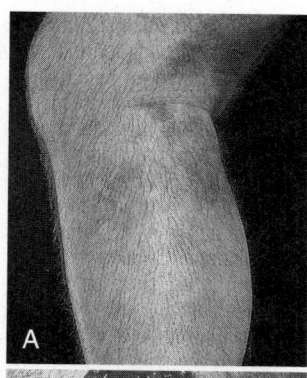

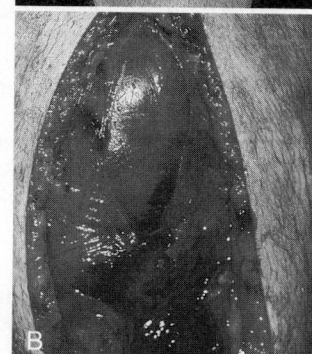

FIGURE 1-231C A, Severe calf swelling due to anterior and posterior compartment syndromes after ischemia-reperfusion. **B,** Appearance after emergency fasciotomy. Note edematous muscle and hematoma. (Courtesy Michael J. Allen, FRCS, Leicester, UK. From Floege J et al: *Comprehensive clinical nephrology,* ed 4, Philadelphia, 2010, Saunders.)

- Creatine phosphokinase levels, which can rise as muscle injury develops
- Metabolic panel for the assessment of electrolytes and renal function
- Coagulation profile for bleeding diathesis
- Urinalysis for rhabdomyolysis
- Urine and serum myoglobin levels

IMAGING STUDIES

- Direct intracompartment pressure measurement can be done by handheld manometer, wick or slit catheter technique, and simple needle manometer system. Compartment syndrome is diagnosed when the difference between diastolic blood pressure and compartment pressure (Δ pressure) is ≤ 30 mm Hg.
- Ultrasonography can be used to rule out deep vein thrombosis, or Doppler ultrasonography can be used to evaluate blood flow to the extremity. Arteriography, though, should be used to evaluate the adequate blood flow through a compartment.
- Near-infrared spectroscopy and technetium-99m methoxyisobutylisonitrile scintigraphy can also be used.
- Radiography can be used on the affected limb for fracture or foreign body evaluation.

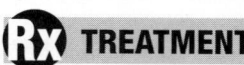 **TREATMENT**

Treatment goal is to keep intracompartment pressure low and prevent tissue injury (Fig. 1-231D).

NONPHARMACOLOGIC THERAPY

- Immediate relieving of all external pressure on the affected compartment
- Removal of casts, splints, and dressings
- Placing limb at heart level to avoid decreased or increased blood flow

ACUTE GENERAL RX

- Analgesics for pain
- Hyperbaric oxygen
- Hypotension can worsen tissue ischemia and thus should be treated with IV isotonic saline.
- Fasciotomy of the affected compartment is indicated if there has been >6 hr of limb ischemia, or immediate decompression should be performed when the compartment pressure > 30-35 mm Hg.
- When compartment pressures are trending downward, it is often safe to hold fasciotomy emergently, provided the Δ pressure is also improving.

CHRONIC RX

- Aftercare of fasciotomy wound: Wound is inspected after 48 hours and dead tissue is removed.
- Wounds are left open, requiring later skin grafting or delayed wound closure.
- Opsite sheet and boot lace techniques are also used for closing fasciotomy wounds.
- Concomitant fractured bones should also be stabilized with plating, external fixation, or intramedullary nailing.

DISPOSITION

With early diagnosis and treatment, the prognosis is excellent for recovery of the muscles and nerves inside the compartment. The following conditions can be prevented:
- Permanent nerve damage/paralysis
- Muscle contracture
- Gangrene
- Amputation
- Muscle necrosis
- Fracture nonunion
- Rhabdomyolysis that leads to renal failure
- Compartment syndrome that can occur in open fractures
- Permanent nerve injury, which can occur after 12-24 hr of compression; mortality rates in patients who need fasciotomy is $\approx 15\%$.

REFERRAL

Patients with suspected compartment syndrome should be referred promptly to orthopaedic and general surgery.

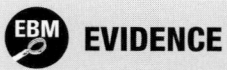 **PEARLS & CONSIDERATIONS**

- Universal precautions and aseptic measures are necessary for patients undergoing fasciotomy because the risk of local and systemic infection is high with the procedure.

- Invasive monitoring techniques should be undertaken with adequate analgesia so that patient immobility is ensured while the pressure is measured.
- Injection of local anesthetics into the compartment can increase the pressure and pain and therefore should be avoided.
- Patients with fracture casts should be informed about the risks of swelling, and patients should also be encouraged to wear appropriate equipment while playing sports.
- A history of coagulation disorders and the use of anticoagulants should be mentioned in a patient's medical history.

EBM EVIDENCE

available at www.expertconsult.com

SUGGESTED READINGS

available at www.expertconsult.com

AUTHOR: **SYEDA M. SAYEED, M.D.**

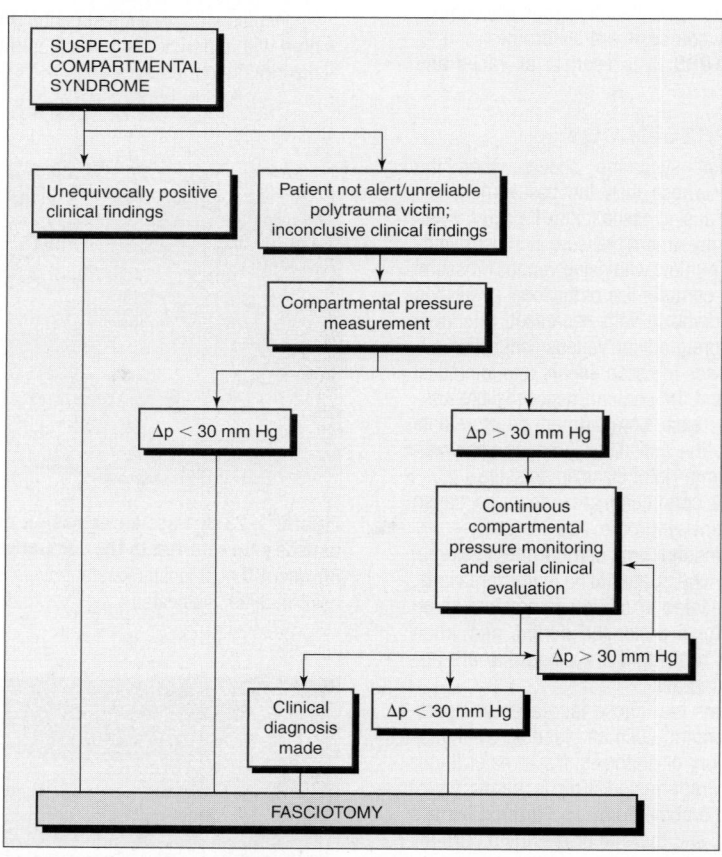

FIGURE 1-231D Algorithm for management for a patient with suspected compartment syndrome. Δp is defined as the difference between the diastolic pressure and the measured compartment pressure in mm Hg as documented by McQueen and Court-Brown. (From Browner BD et al [eds]: *Skeletal trauma*, ed 4, Philadelphia, 2009, Saunders.)

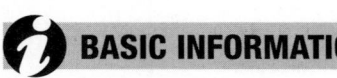

BASIC INFORMATION

DEFINITION

Complex regional pain syndrome (CRPS) is a pain disorder characterized by constant and intense limb pain associated with vasomotor and neurosensory abnormalities, skin changes, and demineralization of bone. CRPS has been divided into type I, in which there is usually an initiating noxious event but no distinct nerve lesion, and type II, in which a definable (usually traumatic) nerve lesion exists. CRPS type I generally correlates with the syndrome formerly known as reflex sympathetic dystrophy (RSD) and CRPS type II equates with what was previously termed causalgia. The term *shoulder-hand syndrome* has been used to describe CRPS in the setting of myocardial infarction or ischemia.

SYNONYMS

Reflex sympathetic dystrophy

ICD-9CM CODES
337.20 Dystrophy, sympathetic (posttraumatic) (reflex)

EPIDEMIOLOGY & DEMOGRAPHICS

The incidence and prevalence of CRPS are not known. It occurs in adults and children. Common situations in which CRPS is seen include extremity trauma, burns, stroke, and orthopedic and podiatric procedures. Immobilization of the limb often precedes the development of symptoms. CRPS in the setting of myocardial infarction seems to be decreasing, presumably due to early mobilization and more effective pain control.

PHYSICAL FINDINGS & CLINICAL PRESENTATION

CRPS is divided into three stages:
1. Acute stage (occurring within hours to days after the injury).
   - Burning or aching pain occurring over the injured extremity.
   - Hyperalgesia (exaggerated response to nociceptive stimuli).
   - Edema.
   - Dysthermia.
   - Increased hair and nail growth.
2. Dystrophic stage (3-6 months after injury).
   - Burning pain radiating both distally and proximally from the site of injury.
   - Brawny edema (Fig. E1-232).
   - Hyperhidrosis.
   - Hypothermia and cyanosis.
   - Muscle tremors and spasms.
   - Increased muscle tone and reflexes.
3. Atrophic stage (6 months after injury).
   - Spread of pain proximally.
   - Alllodynia (pain response to stimuli that are not normally painful).
   - Cold, pale, cyanotic skin.
   - Tropic skin changes with subcutaneous atrophy.
   - Contractures.

ETIOLOGY

The exact pathogenetic mechanisms underlying CRPS have not been fully elucidated, but most theories include the formation of an abnormal reflex arc in the sympathetic nervous system that is modulated by cortical centers to produce peripheral vascular disturbances. Persistent pain in the peripheral nervous system is modulated by inflammatory neuropeptides including substance P, which has been shown to be elevated in the serum of patients with CRPS-I. Increased concentrations of tumor necrosis factor and IL-6 have been demonstrated in the skin of patients with CRPS-I, and immune abnormalities such as reduced numbers of CD8-positive T lymphocytes have also been seen.

DIAGNOSIS

Criteria proposed for the diagnosis of CRPS type I include:
- An initiating noxious event, spontaneous pain or alloying/hyperalgesia disproportionate to the inciting event.
- Evidence of edema, skin blood flow, or sweating abnormality in the region of the pain.
- Absence of other conditions that could explain the symptoms.

Tests such as nuclear medicine bone scanning, nerve conduction testing, and plain radiographs are often indicated to confirm the diagnosis and rule out other possibilities.

DIFFERENTIAL DIAGNOSIS

The differential diagnosis includes nerve entrapment syndromes such as cervical radiculopathy, myofascial pain syndromes, and fibromyalgia.

WORKUP

- Bone scintigraphy (Fig. E1-233) shows decreased perfusion of the affected areas if done soon after the onset of symptoms. If done after 6 weeks of symptoms, bone scan may show increased uptake in the region of the peripheral joints of the involved extremity.
- Electrophysiologic testing is useful to identify nerve injury in patients with type II CRPS.
- Plain radiographs show diffuse patchy osteopenia.
- Skin temperature measurements can be used as a diagnostic test.
- Autonomic testing, although not commonly done, has been proposed.
  1. Measuring resting sweat output.
  2. Measuring resting skin temperature.
  3. Quantitative sudomotor axon reflex test.

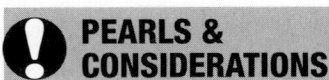

TREATMENT

Treatment of CRPS is largely empiric, based mostly on anecdotal reports, extrapolation from drug trials for other painful conditions, and clinical experience. Therapy should be tailored to stage of disease progression and severity of symptoms.

NONPHARMACOLOGIC THERAPY

- Physical therapy.
- Patient education.

PHARMACOLOGIC THERAPY

Suggested regimens:
Stage 1
  Tricyclic antidepressants (amitryptaline 25-150 mg or doxepin 5-20 mg).
  Prednisone 1 mg/kg for 2 weeks, then taper by 10 mg every 2 weeks.
  Alendronate 70 mg PO weekly.
Stage II
  Topical capsaicin.
  Gabapentin 300 mg tid.
  Regional nerve blocks.
Stage III
  Sympathetic ganglion blocks.
  Refer to multidisciplinary pain center.
NOTE: High-dose vitamin C may decrease the incidence of CRPS following wrist fracture and foot and ankle surgery or trauma.

DISPOSITION

Spontaneous remission can occur after several weeks to months.

REFERRAL

Cases in which the diagnosis is not clear or there is suboptimal response to therapy should promptly be referred to a multidisciplinary pain clinic.

PEARLS & CONSIDERATIONS

COMMENTS

- CRPS is a common clinical entity without clear definition, pathophysiologic features, or treatment.
- Early mobilization in high-risk situations is important for prevention of CRPS.
- Prompt diagnosis and aggressive physical and pharmacologic therapy may prevent progression to chronic, intractable pain.

SUGGESTED READINGS

available at www.expertconsult.com

AUTHOR: **BERNARD ZIMMERMANN, M.D.**

C

Diseases and Disorders

I

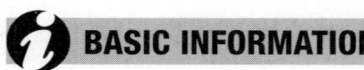

BASIC INFORMATION

DEFINITION

- Complex pathophysiologic process affecting the brain, induced by traumatic biomechanical forces. It may be caused by a direct blow to the head, face, neck, or elsewhere on the body with an "impulsive" force transmitted to the head.
- Concussion typically results in the rapid onset of short-lived impairment of neurologic function that resolves spontaneously. It may result in neuropathologic changes, but the acute clinical symptoms largely reflect a functional disturbance rather than a structural injury.
- Concussion results in a graded set of clinical syndromes that may or may not involve loss of consciousness. Table 1-109 describes a grading scale for concussion. Resolution of the clinical symptoms typically follows a sequential course. It is typically associated with grossly normal structural neuroimaging studies.

SYNONYMS

Sports-related mild traumatic brain injury (mTBI)

ICD-9CM CODES

850.0 Concussion (no loss of consciousness)
850.11 Concussion (loss of consciousness of ≤30 min)
850.9 Concussion unspecified

EPIDEMIOLOGY & DEMOGRAPHICS

INCIDENCE: 1.6 million to 3.8 million sports and recreation related concussions occur each year in the United States.

PREVALENCE: Each year, U.S. emergency departments treat an estimated 135,000 sports- and recreation-related TBIs, including concussions, among children ages 5 to 18.

PREDOMINANT SEX AND AGE: Children and teens are more likely to get a concussion and take longer to recover than adults.

RISK FACTORS: High-impact sports and recreation; six times more likely in organized sports than leisure physical activity.

PHYSICAL FINDINGS & CLINICAL PRESENTATION

See Table 1-110.

ETIOLOGY

- Concussion occurs when rotational or angular acceleration forces are applied to the brain, resulting in shear strain of the underlying neural elements.
- This may be associated with a blow to the skull; however, direct impact to the head is not required.

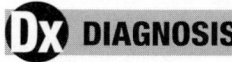 DIAGNOSIS

DIFFERENTIAL DIAGNOSIS

See "Postconcussive Syndrome"

TABLE 1-110 Symptoms and Signs of Concussion

Mental Status Changes

Amnesia
Confusion
Disorientation
Easily distracted
Excessive drowsiness
Feeling dinged, stunned, or foggy
Impaired level of consciousness
Inappropriate play behaviors
Poor concentration and attention
Seeing stars or flashing lights
Slow to answer questions or to follow directions

Physical or Somatic

Ataxia or loss of balance
Blurry vision
Decreased performance or playing ability
Dizziness
Double vision
Fatigue
Headache
Lightheadedness
Nausea, vomiting
Poor coordination
Ringing in the ears
Seizures
Slurred, incoherent speech
Vacant stare/glassy-eyed
Vertigo

Behavior or Psychosomatic

Emotional lability
Irritability
Low frustration tolerance
Personality changes
Nervousness, anxiety
Sadness, depressed mood

From Patel DR et al: Sports related concussions in adolescents, *Pediatr Clin N Am* 57:652, 2010.

WORKUP

- Sideline assessment:
  - No athlete with a suspected concussion should return to play that day.
  - Neurologic assessment using a standardized tool, such as
    SCAT2 (Sport Concussion Assessment Tool)
    SAC (Standardized Assessment of Concussion)
  - Monitor for deterioration; no athlete should be left alone
- Neurocognitive testing:
  - Computer-based programs, such as ImPACT, ANAM, CogSport
  - Neuropsychiatric testing administered by a neuropsychologist
- Gait/balance testing with a tool such as the Balance Error Scoring System (BESS)
- When used in combination, symptom assessment, balance assessment, and neurocognitive testing provide a sensitivity of >90% for the identification of concussion.

IMAGING STUDIES

- CT imaging is indicated in any athlete with a Glasgow Coma Scale score of ≤15 or a rapidly changing neurologic exam.
- Neuroimaging using PECARN guidelines
- Brain MRI is recommended for persons with grade 2 and 3 concussions who have persistent abnormalities on examination or symptoms lasting longer than 1 week.

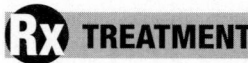 TREATMENT

ACUTE GENERAL Rx

- Removal from game
- Physical rest
  - No return to play until asymptomatic for 24 hr
  - Follow return-to-play guidelines (Table 1-111)
- Cognitive rest to limit symptoms
  - Modifications at school
  - Modifications at home/recreation
  - Encourage sleep

CHRONIC Rx

See "Postconcussive Syndrome"

DISPOSITION

See Table 1-111. Table 1-112 summarizes the American Academy of Neurology recommendations on diagnosis and management of concussion

REFERRAL

Sports-medicine physician, neuropsychology or concussion center

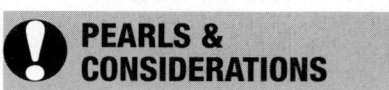 PEARLS & CONSIDERATIONS

PREVENTION

- Preparticipation evaluations for all athletes

TABLE 1-109 Grading Scales for Concussion

Scale	GRADE OF CONCUSSION		
	I	II	III
Colorado	Confusion; no LOC; PTA <30 min	LOC <5 min; confusion; PTA >30 min	LOC >5 min; PTA >24 hr
Cantu	PTA <30 min; no LOC	LOC <5 min; PTA 30 min to 24 hr	LOC >5 min; PTA >24 hr
AAN	Transient confusion; symptoms <15 min; no LOC	No LOC; transient confusion; symptoms >15 min	Any LOC

AAN, American Academy of Neurology; *LOC,* loss of consciousness; *PTA,* posttraumatic amnesia.
From Vincent JL et al: *Textbook of critical care,* ed 6, Philadelphia, 2011, Saunders.

TABLE 1-111 Graduated Return to Play Protocol

Rehabilitation Stage	Functional Exercise at Each Stage of Rehabilitation	Objective of Each Stage
1. No activity	Complete physical and cognitive rest	Recovery
2. Light aerobic exercise	Walking, swimming, or stationary cycling, keeping intensity <70% maximum predicted heart rate. No resistance training	Increase heart rate
3. Sport-specific exercise	Skating drills in ice hockey, running drills in soccer. No head impact activities	Add movement
4. Noncontact training drills	Progression to more complex training drills, e.g., passing drills in football and ice hockey. May start progressive resistance training	Exercise, coordination, and cognitive load
5. Full contact practice	After medical clearance, participate in normal training activities	Restore confidence and assess functional skills by coaching staff
6. Return to play	Normal game play	

From Putukian M: The acute symptoms of sports-related concussion: diagnosis and on-field management, *Clin Sports Med* 30(58), 2011.

TABLE 1-112 American Academy of Neurology: Diagnosis and Management of Concussion

Grade 1 (Mild)*	Grade 2 (Moderate)†	Grade 3 (Severe)‡
Remove from duty/work/play	Remove from duty for the rest of the day	Take to the emergency department
Examine immediately and at 5-min intervals	Examine frequently for signs of CNS deterioration	Neurologic evaluation, including appropriate neuroimaging
	Physician's neurologic examination as soon as possible (within 24 hr)	
May return to duty/work if clear within 15 min	Return to duty after 1 full asymptomatic week (after being cleared by the physician)	Consider hospital admission

Grade of Concussion	Return to Play/Work
Grade 1 (first)	15 min
Grade 1 (second)	1 wk
Grade 2 (first)	1 wk
Grade 2 (second)	2 wk
Grade 3 (first) (brief loss of consciousness)	1 wk
Grade 3 (first) (long loss of consciousness)	2 wk
Grade 3 (second)	1 mo
Grade 3 (third)	Consult a neurologist

*Mild: transient confusion, no loss of consciousness, symptoms associated with concussion (such as amnesia) or mental status changes lasting less than 15 min.
†Moderate: transient confusion, no loss of consciousness, symptoms lasting longer than 15 min.
‡Severe: any loss of consciousness.
From Goldman L, Schafer AI: *Goldman's Cecil medicine,* ed 24, Philadelphia, 2012, Saunders.

- Preparticipation neurocognitive and balance testing to establish a baseline
- There is currently no evidence to support the use of concussion prevention head bands or mouth guards

PATIENT/FAMILY EDUCATION
Centers for Disease Control and Prevention: http://www.cdc.gov/concussion/support.html.

SUGGESTED READINGS
available at www.expertconsult.com

AUTHORS: **PETER J. SELL, D.O.,** and **AMITY RUBEOR, D.O.**

C

Diseases and Disorders

I

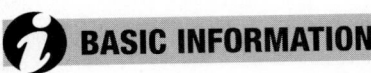

BASIC INFORMATION

DEFINITION

Conduct disorder (CD) is a repetitive and persistent pattern of behaviors in which either the basic rights of others are violated and/or major age-appropriate societal rules are violated. Classified under the DSM-IV-TR category "disorders usually first diagnosed in infancy, childhood or adolescence," and more specifically considered a "disruptive behavior disorder."

ICD-9CM CODES
312.81 Conduct disorder, childhood onset type
312.82 Conduct disorder, adolescent onset type
312 Disturbance of conduct, not elsewhere classified

EPIDEMIOLOGY & DEMOGRAPHICS

INCIDENCE: 1% (12-mo span, National Comorbidity Survey-Replication [NCS-R])
PREVALENCE: Approximately 1% to 16%; NCS-R: 9%. Disruptive behavior disorders are considered the most common reason for referral of children to mental health providers. There is wide variation in documented prevalence rates when subgroups are considered (i.e., gender, age, neighborhood, acts of physical aggression, acts of rule breaking). Subtypes characterized by rule violations, deceit, and theft are more prevalent than subtypes characterized by aggression.
PREDOMINANT SEX: More common in males (4:1 preadolescence and 2:1 postadolescence). It is unclear if CD females are underrepresented, as diagnostic criteria were validated on male samples. Nonconfrontational aggression and promiscuity are examples of possible gender-specific criteria that, at this time, have unknown predictive validity.
PREDOMINANT AGE: Most common onset in early adolescence. Median age of onset is 11 yr.
GENETICS: Meta-analyses of twin and adoption studies report a heritability estimate of approximately 50%.
RISK FACTORS: Factors associated with illness onset include parental criminality, hostile parenting, perinatal complications, low IQ, impulsivity, and overcrowded neighborhoods. Factors associated with poor prognosis include early onset, more severe behaviors, and comorbid attention deficit hyperactivity disorder (ADHD) and/or substance abuse.

PHYSICAL FINDINGS & CLINICAL PRESENTATION

- The DSM-IV-TR lists 15 possible behavioral manifestations of CD, grouped into four categories: aggression to people and animals, destruction of property, deceitfulness or theft, and serious violations of rules. Three of the 15 behaviors are required to have occurred in the last 12 mo, and one behavior must have occurred in the last 6 mo.
- Specifiers describe the age of onset and the severity of the disorder.

- CD represents a heterogeneous group with respect to presentation, etiology, severity, and course.
- Symptom severity often progresses over time with age (i.e., lying and truancy to sexual assault and robbery).
- Aggressive youth are more likely to interpret as negative or hostile the intent of neutral others and are more likely to believe that conflict can be adequately resolved via aggression.
- Poor frustration tolerance, irritability, temper outbursts, and recklessness are often associated with CD.
- Slow resting heart rate associated with underarousal of the autonomic nervous system is the most replicated of all biologic markers for conduct problems.

ETIOLOGY

Estimated population variance in antisocial behavior accounted for by:
- Genes: 50%
- Environmental factors shared among family members: 20%
- Environmental factors unshared among family members: 20% to 30%

DIAGNOSIS

DIFFERENTIAL DIAGNOSIS

- Oppositional defiant disorder
- ADHD
- Mood disorder
- Adjustment disorder
- Substance abuse, dependence, intoxication, or withdrawal
- Post-traumatic stress disorder
- Antisocial personality disorder (for those >18 yr)
- Adaptive behavior or subcultural delinquency

WORKUP

Diagnosis is made based on history, including individual and family interviews as well as collateral data from additional sources (e.g., parents, teachers, other medical providers, therapist).

LABORATORY TESTS

Consider urine toxicology for possible substance use comorbidity.

TREATMENT

Initial treatment of CD should include psychosocial and environmental interventions aimed at decreasing the frequency and severity of delinquent behaviors. If the interventions listed here are not effective, or if serious concerns exist regarding safety or impairment in functioning, pharmacologic interventions targeting specific symptoms (e.g., aggression) or comorbid disorders (e.g., ADHD, anxiety disorders, or mood disorders) may help. There are currently no medications approved by the FDA for the treatment of CD.

NONPHARMACOLOGIC THERAPY

- Parent management training
- Cognitive problem-solving skills training (including elements of social skills, conflict resolution, anger management, impulse control, and vocational training)

- Multisystemic therapy
- Social skills training
- Individual psychotherapy
- Family psychotherapy
- Higher levels of care such as a hospital or acute residential setting may be required for stabilization if acute safety concerns develop in the context of CD, such as severe aggression.
- Legal involvement and/or out-of-home-placements may be necessary to monitor safety of both the patient and the community.

PHARMACOLOGIC THERAPY

Medication may be considered as an adjunct to behavioral treatment or in cases where comorbidity is a factor. There is some evidence for symptom improvement with trials of several classes of psychotropic medications—including stimulants, mood stabilizers, atypical antipsychotics, antidepressants, and alpha-2 agonists such as clonidine—all of which seem to target aggressive symptoms in particular; medication, however, should never be used alone or as first-line treatment for CD.

DISPOSITION

- Approximately half of those with early onset of CD persist with antisocial behaviors into adulthood. There is no reliable way to predict which 50% will persist.
- Approximately half of those with early onset of CD do not develop antisocial personality disorder in adulthood. This subgroup appears to become depressed, anxious, and socially isolated adults.
- Approximately 85% of those with adolescent onset of CD do not demonstrate lifetime persistent violence, convictions, and incarcerations. However, adult prognosis may often include substance abuse and crimes that go largely undetected.

PEARLS & CONSIDERATIONS

COMMENTS

- Expect 30% treatment noncompliance rate.
- Due to the high rate of comorbidity of substance abuse and depression, educate youth who are treated with SSRIs regarding serotonin syndrome and other commonly abused serotonergic substances such as ecstasy, dextromethorphan, cocaine, and stimulants.

PATIENT/FAMILY EDUCATION

Conduct Disorder Resource Center: A Guide for Families by the American Academy of Child and Adolescent Psychiatry (http://www.aacap.org/cs/ConductDisorder.ResourceCenter)
American Academy of Pediatrics: HealthyChildren.org (http://www.healthychildren.org/English/health-issues/conditions/emotional-problems/Pages/Disruptive-Behavior-Disorders.aspx)

SUGGESTED READINGS
available at www.expertconsult.com

AUTHORS: **ELIZABETH A. LOWENHAUPT, M.D.,** and **SARAH L. XAVIER, D.O.**

BASIC INFORMATION

DEFINITION

Condyloma acuminatum is a sexually transmitted viral disease of the vulva, vagina, and cervix caused by the human papillomavirus (HPV). 90% of genital warts are caused by HPV 6 or 11.

SYNONYMS

Genital warts
Venereal warts
Anogenital warts

ICD-9CM CODES
078.11 Condyloma acuminatum

EPIDEMIOLOGY & DEMOGRAPHICS

- Seen mostly in young adults, with a mean age of onset of 16 to 25 yr
- A sexually transmitted disease spread by skin-to-skin contact
- Highly contagious, with 25% to 65% of sexual partners developing it
- Virus shed from both macroscopic and microscopic lesions
- Average incubation time is 2 mo (range, 1 to 8 mo)
- Predisposing conditions: diabetes, pregnancy, local trauma, and immunosuppression (e.g., transplant recipients, those with HIV infection)

PHYSICAL FINDINGS & CLINICAL PRESENTATION

- Usually found in genital area but can be present elsewhere
- Lesions usually in similar positions on both sides of perineum
- Initial lesions pedunculated, soft papules about 2 to 3 mm in diameter, 10 to 20 mm long; may occur as single papule or in clusters
- Size of lesions varies from pinhead to large cauliflower-like masses (Fig. E1-234)
- Usually asymptomatic, but if infected can cause pain, odor, or bleeding
- Vulvar condyloma more common than vaginal and cervical
- Four morphologic types: condylomatous, keratotic, papular, and flat warts
- Intra-anal warts are observed predominantly in persons who have had receptive anal intercourse.

ETIOLOGY

- HPV DNA types 6 and 11 usually found in exophytic warts and have no malignant potential
- HPV types 16 and 18 usually found in flat warts and are associated with increased risk of malignancy

- Recurrence associated with persisting viral infection of adjacent normal skin in 25% to 50% of cases

DIAGNOSIS

DIFFERENTIAL DIAGNOSIS

- Abnormal anatomic variants or skin tags around labia minora and introitus
- Dysplastic warts

WORKUP

- Colposcopic examination of lower genital tract from cervix to perianal skin with 3% to 5% acetic acid
- Biopsy of vulvar lesions that lack the classic appearance of warts and that become ulcerated or do not respond to treatment
- Biopsy of flat, white, or ulcerated cervical lesions

LABORATORY TESTS

- Pap smear
- Cervical cultures for *Neisseria gonorrhoeae* and *Chlamydia*
- Serologic test for syphilis
- HIV testing offered
- Wet mount for trichomoniasis, *Candida albicans,* and *Gardnerella vaginalis*
- Testing for diabetes (blood glucose)

TREATMENT

NONPHARMACOLOGIC THERAPY

- Keep genital area dry and clean.
- If present, keep diabetes well controlled.
- Advise use of condoms to prevent spread of infection to sexual partner.

ACUTE GENERAL Rx

Factors that influence selection of treatment include wart size, wart number, anatomic site of wart, wart morphology, patient preference, cost of treatment, convenience, adverse effects, and provider experience.
Keratolytic agents:

- Podophyllin (Podofilox 0.5% solution or gel)
  - Acts by poisoning mitotic spindle and causing intense vasospasm
  - Applied directly to lesion weekly and washed off in 6 hr
  - Used in minimal vulvar or anal disease
  - Applied cautiously to nonkeratinized epithelial surfaces
  - Contraindicated in pregnancy
  - Discontinued if lesions do not disappear in 6 wk; switch to other treatment
- Sinecatechin 15% ointment
  - Applied tid (0.5 cm strand of ointment to each wart)
  - Should not be continued longer than 16 wk

- Trichloroacetic acid (30% to 80% solution)
  - Acts by precipitation of surface proteins
  - Applied twice monthly to lesion
  - Indicated for vulvar, anal, and vaginal lesions; can be used for cervical lesions
  - Less painful and irritating to normal tissue than podophyllin
- Fluorouracil
  - Causes necrosis and sloughing of growing tissue
  - Can be used intravaginally or for vulvar, anal, or urethral lesions
  - Better tolerated; 3 g (two thirds of vaginal applicator) applied weekly for 12 wk
  - Possible vaginal ulceration and erythema
  - Patient's vagina examined after four to six applications
  - 80% cure rate

Physical agents:
- Cryotherapy with liquid nitrogen or cryoprobe
  - Can be used weekly for 3 to 6 wk
  - 62% to 79% success rate
  - Not suitable for large warts
- Laser therapy
  - Done by physician with necessary expertise and equipment
  - Painful; requires anesthesia
- Electrocautery or excision
  - For recurrent, very large lesions
  - Local anesthesia needed

Immunotherapy:
- Interferon
  - Injected intralesionally at a dose of 3 million U/m^2 three times weekly for 8 wk
  - Side effects: fever, chills, malaise, headache
- Imiquimod 5% cream at hs, 3× wk up to 16 wk increases wart clearance after 3 mo
- Interferon, topical: increases wart clearance at 4 wk

DISPOSITION

- Follow-up exam every 6 to 12 mo, as needed.
- Correct and consistent male condom use might lower the chances of giving or getting genital HPV, but such use is not fully protective because HPV can infect areas that are not covered by a condom.

SUGGESTED READING
available at www.expertconsult.com

RELATED CONTENT

Chancroid (Related Key Topic)
Lymphogranuloma Venereum (Related Key Topic)
Syphilis (Related Key Topic)
Genital Warts (Patient Information)

AUTHORS: **GEORGE T. DANAKAS, M.D.,** and **RUBEN ALVERO, M.D.**

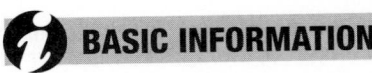

BASIC INFORMATION

DEFINITION

The term *conjunctivitis* refers to an inflammation of the conjunctiva resulting from a variety of causes, including allergies and bacterial, viral, and chlamydial infections.

SYNONYMS

"Red eye"
Pink eye
Acute conjunctivitis
Subacute conjunctivitis
Chronic conjunctivitis
Purulent conjunctivitis
Pseudomembranous conjunctivitis
Papillary conjunctivitis
Follicular conjunctivitis
Newborn conjunctivitis

ICD-9CM CODES
372.30 Conjunctivitis, unspecified

EPIDEMIOLOGY & DEMOGRAPHICS

INCIDENCE (IN U.S.): 1.6% to 12% in *newborns*
PREVALENCE (IN U.S.):
- Allergic conjunctivitis (Fig. E1-236), the most common form of ocular allergy, is usually associated with allergic rhinitis and may be seasonal or perennial.
- Bacterial or viral conjunctivitis is often seasonal and can be extremely contagious.

PREDOMINANT AGE: Occurs at *any* age. Most cases in adults are due to viral infection. Children are more prone to develop bacterial conjunctivitis than viral forms.
PEAK INCIDENCE: More common in the fall, when *viral* infections and pollens increase

PHYSICAL FINDINGS & CLINICAL PRESENTATION

- Infection and chemosis of conjunctivae with discharge. Gluing of the eyelids and no itching is more indicative of a bacterial cause (Fig. 1-237).

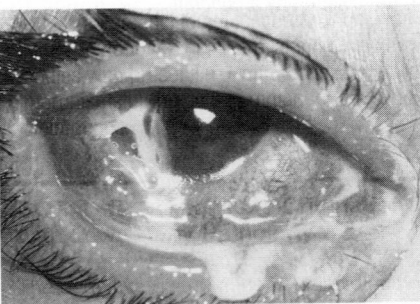

FIGURE 1-237 Bacterial conjunctivitis. Purulent discharge and conjunctiva hyperemia suggest bacterial conjunctivitis. Viral conjunctivitis produces watery discharge, foreign body sensation, preauricular lymphadenopathy, and conjunctival follicles seen on slit lamp examination. (Reproduced with permission from the American Academy of Ophthalmology.) (From Goldman L, Schafer AI: *Goldman's Cecil medicine*, ed 24, Philadelphia, 2012, Saunders.)

- Cornea is clear or can be involved.
- Vision is often normal but can be blurred.

ETIOLOGY

- Bacterial: *Haemophilus influenzae*, *Streptococcus pneumoniae*, and *Moraxella catarrhalis* in children; *Staphylococcus* species in adults. Gram-negative infections are more common in contact lens wearers. Gonococcal ophthalmia neonatorum is caused by *Neisseria gonorrhoeae* acquired by exposure of the neonatal conjunctivae to infected cervicovaginal secretions during delivery.
- Viral.
- Chlamydial.
- Allergic.
- Traumatic.

DIAGNOSIS

DIFFERENTIAL DIAGNOSIS

- Acute glaucoma
- Corneal lesions
- Acute iritis
- Episcleritis
- Scleritis
- Uveitis
- Canalicular obstruction

WORKUP

- History and physical examination
- Reports of itching, pain, and visual changes

LABORATORY TESTS

Cultures are useful if not *successfully* treated with antibiotics; initial culture is usually not necessary.

TREATMENT

NONPHARMACOLOGIC THERAPY

- Warm compresses if infective conjunctivitis.
- Cold compresses if irritative or allergic conjunctivitis.
- Contact lenses should be taken out until an infection is completely resolved. Nondisposable lenses should be cleaned thoroughly as recommended by the manufacturer, and a new lens case should be used. Disposable contact lenses should be thrown away.

ACUTE GENERAL Rx

- Antibiotic drops (e.g., levofloxacin, ofloxacin, ciprofloxacin, tobramycin, gentamicin ophthalmic solution, 1 or 2 drops q2 to 4h) are indicated for suspected bacterial conjunctivitis.
- Caution: be careful with ophthalmic corticosteroid treatment and avoid unless sure of diagnosis; corticosteroids can exacerbate infections and have been associated with increased intraocular pressure and cataract formation.
- An oral antihistamine (cetirizine, loratadine, desloratadine, or fexofenadine) is effective in relieving itching.
- Mast cell stabilizers (e.g., cromolyn [4%, 1 to 2 drops q4 to 6h], lodoxamide [0.1%, 1 to

2 drops qid]) are effective for allergic conjunctivitis. Others include Elestat, Optivar, and Patanol.
- Bepotastine, alcaftadine, azelastine, epinastine, and ketotifen are H1-antihistamines effective for topical treatment of itching associated with allergic conjunctivitis. The topical NSAID ketorolac (0.5%, 1 drop qd) is also useful in allergic conjunctivitis. Table E1-114 describes topical ophthalmic medications for allergic conjunctivitis.
- Antihistamine/decongestant combinations such as pheniramine/naphazoline (Visine A), available over the counter, are more effective than either agent alone but have a short duration and can result in rebound vasodilatation with prolonged use. Others include Naphcon-A, Albacon-A, and Opcon-A.

CHRONIC Rx

- Depends on cause.
- If allergic, nonsteroidals such as Voltaren, Acular, and Xibrom ophthalmic solution; mast cell stabilizers such as Elestat, Alocril, Patanol, and Zaditor are useful for improving ocular itching in patients with allergic conjunctivitis.
- If an infection, use antibiotic drops (see "Acute General Rx").
- Dry eyes need artificial tears (Restasis) or lacrimal duct plugs when indicated.

DISPOSITION

Follow carefully for the first 2 wk to ensure secondary complications do not occur. Otitis media can develop in 25% of children with *Haemophilus influenzae* conjunctivitis. Bacterial keratitis occurs in 30/1000 contact lens wearers.

REFERRAL

To ophthalmologist if symptoms are refractory to initial treatment. Indications for urgent referral are severe eye pain or headache, photophobia, decreased vision, and contact lens use.

PEARLS & CONSIDERATIONS

COMMENTS

- Red eyes are not simply conjunctivitis when the patient has significant pain or loss of sight. However, it is usually safe to treat pain-free eyes and the normal-seeing red eye with lid hygiene and topical treatment.
- Use caution with patients wearing soft contact lenses, infants, and the elderly.
- Do not use steroids indiscriminately; use only when the diagnosis is certain.
- Bacterial conjunctivitis is generally self-limiting. Over 60% of persons will improve with placebo within 2 to 5 days.

RELATED CONTENT

Conjunctivitis (Patient Information)

AUTHORS: **MELVYN KOBY, M.D.,** and **FRED F. FERRI, M.D.**

BASIC INFORMATION

DEFINITION

Contact dermatitis is an acute or chronic skin inflammation, usually eczematous dermatitis resulting from exposure to substances in the environment. It can be subdivided into "irritant" contact dermatitis (nonimmunologic physical and chemical alteration of the epidermis) and "allergic" contact dermatitis (delayed hypersensitivity reaction).

SYNONYMS

Irritant contact dermatitis
Allergic contact dermatitis

ICD-9CM CODES
692 Contact dermatitis and other eczema

EPIDEMIOLOGY & DEMOGRAPHICS

- 20% of all cases of dermatitis in children are caused by allergic contact dermatitis.
- Rhus dermatitis (poison ivy, poison oak, and poison sumac) is responsible for most cases of contact dermatitis.
- Frequent causes of irritant contact dermatitis are soaps, detergents, and organic solvents.
- Chemical irritants (e.g., cutting fluids used in machining, solvents) account for most cases of irritant contact dermatitis. Occupational skin diseases are second only to traumatic injuries as the most common types of occupational disease.

PHYSICAL FINDINGS & CLINICAL PRESENTATION

Clinical presentation varies with the responsible agent and affected area of skin.

IRRITANT CONTACT DERMATITIS:
- Mild exposure may result in dryness, erythema, and fissuring of the affected area (e.g., hand involvement in irritant dermatitis caused by exposure to soap (Fig. E1-238), genital area involvement in irritant dermatitis caused by prolonged exposure to wet diapers).
- Eczematous inflammation may result from chronic exposure.

ALLERGIC CONTACT DERMATITIS:
- Poison ivy dermatitis can present with vesicles and blisters; linear lesions (as a result of dragging of the resins over the surface of the skin by scratching) are a classic presentation.
- The pattern of lesions is asymmetric; itching, burning, and stinging may be present.
- The involved areas are erythematous, warm to touch, swollen, and may be confused with cellulitis.

ETIOLOGY
- Irritant contact dermatitis: cement (construction workers), rubber, ragweed, malathion (farmers), orange and lemon peels (chefs, bartenders), hair tints, shampoos (beauticians), rubber gloves (medical, surgical personnel)
- Allergic contact dermatitis: poison ivy, poison oak, poison sumac, rubber (shoe dermatitis), nickel (jewelry), balsam of Peru (hand and face dermatitis), neomycin, formaldehyde (cosmetics)

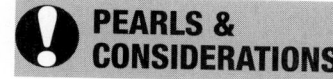

DIAGNOSIS

DIFFERENTIAL DIAGNOSIS
- Impetigo
- Lichen simplex chronicus
- Atopic dermatitis
- Nummular eczema, dyshidrotic eczema
- Seborrheic dermatitis
- Inverse psoriasis, palmoplantar psoriasis
- Scabies
- Tinea pedis

WORKUP
- Medical history: gradual onset versus rapid onset, number of exposures, clinical presentation, occupational history.
- Physical examination: contact dermatitis in the neck may be caused by necklaces, perfumes (Fig. E1-239), after-shave lotion. Involvement of the axillae is often secondary to deodorants, clothing. Face involvement can occur with cosmetics, airborne allergens, aftershave lotion.

LABORATORY TESTS
- Patch testing has a sensitivity and specificity of 70% to 80%. It is useful to confirm the diagnosis of contact dermatitis; it is indicated only when inflammation persists despite appropriate topical therapy and avoidance of suspected causative agent; patch testing should not be used for irritant contact dermatitis because this is a nonimmunologic-mediated inflammatory reaction.
- Dermoscopy and microscopy when suspecting scabies and mites.
- A potassium hydroxide (KOH) preparation may be useful if suspecting tinea or *Candida* infection.

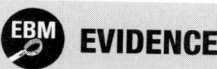

TREATMENT

NONPHARMACOLOGIC THERAPY
Avoidance of suspected allergens

ACUTE GENERAL Rx
- Removal of the irritant substance by washing the skin with plain water or mild soap within 15 min of exposure is helpful in patients with poison ivy, poison oak, or poison sumac dermatitis.
- Cold or cool water compresses for 20 to 30 min 5 to 6 times a day for the initial 72 hr are effective during the acute blistering stage.
- Topical steroids (clobetasol 0.05%, triamcinolone 0.1%) are effective for acute localized allergic contact dermatitis lesions. Lower potency topical steroids are preferred on face, anogenital regions and flexural surfaces to minimize risk of skin atrophy. Oral corticosteroids (e.g., prednisone 20 mg bid for 6 to 10 days) are generally reserved for severe, widespread dermatitis.
- IM steroids (e.g., Kenalog) are used for severe reactions and in patients requiring oral corticosteroids but unable to tolerate PO.
- Oral antihistamines (e.g., hydroxyzine 25 mg q6h) will control pruritus, especially at night; calamine lotion is also useful for pruritus; however, it can lead to excessive drying.
- Colloidal oatmeal (Aveeno) baths can also provide symptomatic relief.
- Patients with mild to moderate erythema may respond to topical steroid gels or creams.
- Patients with shoe allergy should change their socks at least once a day; use of aluminum chloride hexahydrate in a 20% solution (Drysol) qhs will also help control perspiration.
- Use hypoallergenic surgical gloves in patients with rubber and surgical glove allergy.

DISPOSITION
Allergic contact dermatitis generally resolves within 2 to 4 wk if reexposure to allergen is prevented.

REFERRAL
For patch testing in selected patients, see "Laboratory Tests."

PEARLS & CONSIDERATIONS

COMMENTS
Commercially available corticosteroid dose packs should be avoided, because they generally provide an inadequate amount of medication.

EVIDENCE

available at www.expertconsult.com

SUGGESTED READING
available at www.expertconsult.com

AUTHOR: FRED F. FERRI, M.D.

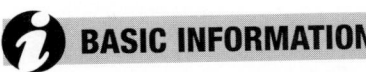

BASIC INFORMATION

DEFINITION

Contraception refers to the various modalities that a sexually active couple use to prevent pregnancy. These options can be either medical or nonmedical and used by men or women or both. An algorithm for helping couples select a contraceptive method is described in Fig. E1-240. The options are as follows:

- No contraception (unprotected intercourse): failure rate 85% both typical use and perfect use
- Abstinence
  - 12.4% of unmarried men
  - 13.2% of unmarried women
  - More frequently practiced before age 17 yr
  - No intercourse experienced by 13% of women ages 30 to 34 yr
  - Failure rate 0%
- Withdrawal
  - Used in only 2% of sexually active women
  - Failure rate with perfect use, 4%; with typical use, 19%
- Rhythm method (natural family planning)
  - Failure rate with perfect use, 1% to 9%; with typical use, 20%
  - Symptothermal type: mucus method and ovulation pain combined with basal body temperature
  - Ovulation (Billings' method): takes into account mucus quality
  - Basal body temperature method: uses biphasic temperature chart
  - Lactation amenorrhea method: effective in fully breastfeeding women, especially 70 to 100 days after delivery; depends on number of feedings per day
- Barriers
  - Diaphragm and cervical cap: failure rate 5% to 9% in nulliparous women, 20% in multiparous women
  - Female condom: failure rate with perfect use, 5.1%; with typical use, 12.4%; FDA labeling states 25% failure rate
  - Male condom: failure rate with perfect use, 3%; with typical use, 12%
  - Spermicides (aerosols, foam, jellies, creams, tabs): failure rate with perfect use, 3%; with typical use, 21%
- Oral contraceptives (Fig. E1-241)
  - Failure rate with perfect use, <1%; with typical use, 3%
  - Come in combinations of estrogen/progestin or as progestin only
- Hormonal implants and injectables
  - Implanon (etonogestrel) implant 2-yr cumulative pregnancy rate 0.05%. Nexplanon is essentially the same as Implanon but with a barium sulfate core for easier radiologic detection and a preloaded applicator to facilitate insertion.
  - Depo-Provera: failure rate 0.3% in first year of use
  - Lunelle failure rate 0.2% in first year
  - Nestorone-releasing single implant: not yet available

- Jadelle implant: Succesor to the Norplant implant, which has been discontinued in the U.S. The Jadelle implant is not available in the U.S.
- Mini pill (progesterone only pill)
  - Failure rate with typical use, 1.1% to 13.2%
  - With perfect use, 5 pregnancies per 1000 women
- Emergency postcoital contraception
  - Decreases pregnancy rate by 75% with women treated immediately postcoitally
  - Involves dedicated hormonal (Plan B, which contains levonorgestrel) use or intrauterine device (IUD) insertion
- IUD (available over the counter in some states)
  - Progestasert: failure rate with perfect use, 2%; with typical use, 3%
  - Copper T (30-A): failure rate with perfect use, 0.8%; with typical use, 3%
  - Levonorgestrel Intrauterine System (Mirena)
    - 1-yr failure rate, 1%
    - 5-yr cumulative failure rate, 0.71 per 100 women
- Female sterilization (tubal ligation): failure rate with perfect use, 0.2%; with typical use, 3%
- Male sterilization (vasectomy): failure rate of 0.1% in first year
- Vaginal ring (Nuva ring): failure rate pearl index 0.77
- Contraceptive patch (Ortho Evra): failure rate 0.4% to 0.7%

SYNONYMS

Birth control
Family planning

ICD-9CM CODES
V25.01 Oral contraceptives
V25.02 Other contraceptive measures
V25.09 Family planning
V25.1   IUD
V25.2   Sterilization

DIAGNOSIS

WORKUP

- Thorough medical history
- Thorough surgical history
- Obstetric history (fertility desired?)
- Gynecologic history, including:
  - History of previous sexually transmitted diseases
  - Number of partners
  - Previous difficulties with contraception
  - Frequency of intercourse
- Family history

LABORATORY TESTS

- Pap smear
- Cultures, aerobic and *Chlamydia*
- Pregnancy test if suspected pregnancy
- Lipid profile if family history of premature vascular event

TREATMENT

NONPHARMACOLOGIC THERAPY

- Male condoms
  - 95% latex (rubber), 5% skin or natural membrane
  - Proper use: place on an erect penis and leave ½-inch empty space at the tip of the condom; use with non–oil-based lubricants
  - Effectiveness increased when used with spermicides
- Female condoms
  - Composed of polyurethane, with one end open and one end closed
  - Proper use: place closed end over cervix, open end hanging out of vagina to cover penis and scrotum
  - Highly effective against HIV
- Spermicides
  - Types: nonoxynol, octoxynol
  - Forms: jellies, creams, foams, suppositories, tablets, soluble films
  - Proper use: put in immediately before intercourse; may be used with other barrier methods
- Diaphragm and cervical cap
  - Must be fitted by practitioner, used with contraceptive gels, and refitted with weight gain or loss of 4.5 kg. Must also be refit after pregnancy.
  - Diaphragm sizes: 50 to 105 mm; cervical cap sizes 26, 28, and 30 mm
  - The correct fit allows the woman to remain ambulatory without feeling the device
  - Proper use of diaphragm: put in immediately before intercourse and keep in for 6 hr after intercourse; must not remain in the vagina for longer than 24 hr
  - Proper use of cervical cap: fit over the cervix exactly; must not remain in place for longer than 48 hr
- Lactation amenorrhea method
  - Depends on number of feedings per day; effective as birth control for 6 mo if 15 or more feedings, lasting 10 min each, are accomplished daily. If woman meets criteria (e.g., breastfeeding only source of infant feeding) 0.5%-2.0% failure rate in the first 6 months after delivery.
  - Not a common practice in the U.S.
- Withdrawal
  - Withdrawal of the penis from the vagina before ejaculation
  - Depends on self-control
- Rhythm method
  - Depends on awareness of physiology of male and female reproductive tracts
  - Sperm viable in vagina for 2 to 7 days
  - Ovum life span 24 hr
- Sterilization
  - Male:
    - Vasectomy to interrupt vas deferens and block passage of sperm to seminal ejaculate

- Scalpel and nonscalpel techniques available
- More easily performed procedure than female sterilization and does not require general anesthesia
○ Female:
- Leading method of birth control in U.S. in women older than 30 yr
- Interrupts fallopian tubes, blocking passage of ovum proximally and sperm distally through tube
- Several types; modified Pomeroy done during cesarean section or interval laparoscopic using clips (Filshie, Hulka) or banding
- Essure-tubal occlusion through hysteroscopic placement of micro-inserts into the fallopian tubes.

ACUTE GENERAL Rx

- Combination oral contraceptives
○ Taken daily for 21 days, pill-free interval of 7 days
○ Less than 50 mcg ethynyl estradiol in most common combination oral contraceptives; progestins most commonly used in combination pills are norethindrone, levonorgestrel, norgestrel, norethindrone acetate, ethynodiol diacetate, norgestimate, or desogestrel; triphasic combination oral contraceptives (give varying doses of progestin and estrogens throughout cycle); monophasic oral contraceptives: offer same dose of progestin and estrogen throughout cycle, taken daily at same time; estrophasic pill (constant progesterone with variation of estrogen throughout the cycle)
○ If pill taken with antibiotics, efficacy affected by inadequate gastrointestinal absorption in most cases; only rifampin truly reduces pill's effectiveness
○ Increased body weight decreases effectiveness
- Mini pill
○ Progestin only; taken without a break
○ Causes much irregular bleeding because of the lack of estrogen effect on the lining of the uterus
- Hormonal implants and injectables
○ Implanon/Nexplanon
- Single etonogestrol-secreting device that is inserted underneath the skin
- Among the most effective contraceptive available
- Approved by FDA in 2006 and effective over 3-yr period

○ Depo-Provera
- Medroxyprogesterone acetate given every 3 mo in IM injection form
- Major side effect: irregular bleeding
- Fertility return possibly delayed up to 1 year or longer after last injection
○ Lunelle: monthly injectable administered intramuscularly. Contains 0.5 ml aqueous, 5 mg estradiol cypionate and 25 mg medroxyprogesterone acetate
- Postcoital contraception
○ Done on emergency basis, usually as a result of noncompliance with birth control or failure of birth control (e.g., condom breakage) at the time of ovulation
○ Methods:
- Hormonal methods
- Levonorgestrel is available either as two 0.75 mg tablets taken 12 hr apart (next choice) or as a 1.5 mg tablet taken once (Plan B, one step). It is indicated for emergency contraception to be used within 72 hr after unexpected intercourse. It can be obtained OTC by women ≥15 yr of age and by prescription by younger patients
- Ulipristal (ELLA) is a progesterone-receptor agonist/antagonist available by prescription only. It is a 30-mg, single-dose tablet and can be taken up to 5 days after unexpected intercourse
- Copper IUD insertion within 5 days of coitus
- IUD
○ Device inserted into uterus to prevent sperm and ovum from uniting in fallopian tube
○ Types available in the U.S.:
- ParaGard (Copper T/30-A): a polyethylene T wrapped with a fine copper wire effective for 10 yr
- Mirena Levonorgestrel Intrauterine System: a T-shaped system with a chamber that contains levonorgestrel. Releases 20 mcg/day; is effective for 5 yr
- Vaginal ring (NuvaRing)
○ Provides daily dose of 120 mcg of etonogestrel and 15 mcg ethinyl estradiol
○ Stays in vagina 3 wk and is removed the fourth for a contraceptive-free interval analogous to the placebo pills in oral contraceptive pills
○ Increased body weight decreases effectiveness

- Contraceptive patch (Ortho-Evra)
○ Provides low daily dose of steroids
○ Releases a progestin and estrogen (ethinyl estradiol)
○ Patch size 20 cm²
○ Each patch contains 6 mg norelgestromin and delivers an estimated continuous systemic dose of 150 mcg of norelgestromin and 20 mcg of ethinyl estradiol; common dose 250 mcg/day progestin and 25 mcg/day estrogen
○ Worn 3 out of 4 wk
○ Increased body weight decreases effectiveness
○ Concern for increased risk of thromboembolic events

CHRONIC Rx

- With all the previously mentioned types of birth control, patient is followed up at least yearly, or as necessary, if problems arise.
- Full history, physical examination, and Pap smear, including cultures when needed, are performed yearly.
- Patients with medical problems are followed up approximately every 6 mo when taking hormonal therapy.

DISPOSITION

- Follow yearly or more frequently according to patient's side effects.
- Tailor birth control to patient according to different needs or side effects present at different times in life. Effective counseling also requires an understanding of a woman's preference and medical risks, benefits, side effects, and contraindications of each contraceptive method.

COMMENTS

- With hormonal contraception, if neurologic or cardiac symptoms arise, stop method immediately, evaluate, and refer to internist when appropriate.
- The effectiveness of long-actiing reversible contraception (IUDs and implants) is superior to that of contraceptive pills, patch, or ring and is not altered in adolescents and young women.

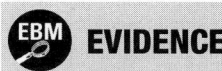 **EVIDENCE**

available at www.expertconsult.com

SUGGESTED READINGS
available at www.expertconsult.com

RELATED CONTENT
Contraception (Patient Information)

AUTHORS: **MARIA A. CORIGLIANO, M.D.,** and **RUBEN ALVERO, M.D.**

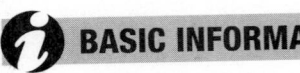

BASIC INFORMATION

DEFINITION

Conversion disorder is a diagnosis of exclusion that presents with neurologic symptoms that cannot be explained by medical evaluation or a culturally sanctioned behavior or experience. The symptom or deficit is not intentionally produced, distinguishing conversion disorder from factitious disorder or malingering. Conversion disorder is usually characterized by a single symptom that is sporadic, such as paralysis, blindness, numbness, or the inability to speak. Symptoms are preceded by a psychological conflict or stressor that may or may not be remembered and may have happened recently or in the distant past. The conversion symptom is presumed to express and manage the psychological distress, or "convert" the distress into a physical symptom. There is no well validated neurobiologic model for conversion disorder, but advances in neuroscience and neuroimaging may reveal new etiologies in the future.

SYNONYMS

Dissociative conversion
Hysterical neurosis
Medically unexplained symptom
Psychogenic, nonorganic, or functional symptoms

ICD-10CM CODES
Dissociative (Conversion) Disorders

EPIDEMIOLOGY & DEMOGRAPHICS

- Incidence estimated at 5 to 10/100,000 in general population, 20 to 100/100,000 in hospital inpatients
- All ages, including early childhood
- Associated with axis I (depression more than anxiety) and axis II disorders (most commonly histrionic, passive dependent, and passive aggressive)

PHYSICAL FINDINGS & CLINICAL PRESENTATION

- Presents with a motor symptom (e.g., paralysis, aphonia, difficulty swallowing), a sensory symptom (loss of sensation, double vision, blindness, deafness), a psychogenic seizure, or "mixed" (symptoms from more than one category).
- Symptoms tend to occur in isolation (compared with multisystem involvement in somatization disorder).
- The symptoms or signs persist whether the patient is observed or unobserved, though are typically worse when the patient is attentive to them.
- May last from hours to years and tends to be sporadic.
- May occur in the context of documented medical illness (e.g., a patient with epileptic seizure may also have psychogenic seizure).
- May have comorbid axis I or axis II disorders, commonly depression, panic attacks, generalized anxiety, and PTSD.

ETIOLOGY

- Complex interplay of neurologic and psychologic factors is not well-understood.
- Presumed to be preceded by psychological conflict or stressor that is completely or partially unconscious.
- Functional brain imaging studies suggest alterations in processing of sensory and motor signals.

DIAGNOSIS

DIFFERENTIAL DIAGNOSIS

Broad differential diagnosis depending on presenting signs and symptoms, including multiple sclerosis, CNS neoplasm, myasthenia gravis, Guillain-Barré syndrome, amyotrophic lateral sclerosis, Parkinson's disease, seizure disorder, systemic lupus erythematosus, spinal cord compression, intracerebral infarct, drug-induced dystonia, and HIV.

WORKUP

Thorough history and physical examination, including careful neurologic examination

LABORATORY TESTS

- No gold standard diagnostic tests exist; no single finding is pathognomonic.
- Laboratory tests or procedures may be needed to rule out other etiologies (e.g., EEG for seizures, EMG for lower motor neuron paralysis, optokinetic drum test in blindness).

IMAGING STUDIES

As indicated by presenting signs and symptoms

TREATMENT

NONPHARMACOLOGIC THERAPY

- No good evidence exists demonstrating the efficacy of any treatment.
- Cognitive behavioral therapy is often the treatment of choice, although evidence is mixed.
- A long tradition of psychodynamic therapy exists but has not been validated by controlled trials.
- Treatment success has been associated with a caring, long-term relationship between patient and physician and a safe, nonconfrontational approach, with the exception of psychogenic seizure for which empathic confrontation and acceptance of disease is advocated as a foundation of treatment.
- Physical and occupational therapy can help "retrain" the patient in normal behaviors and is important for maintaining strength and function in extended cases of paralysis.
- Studies have shown no additional benefit to hypnosis, although case records describe successful treatment with hypnosis.

ACUTE GENERAL Rx

- Antidepressants may be helpful for underlying mood or anxiety disorders.

- Longstanding symptoms may require inpatient treatment.

CHRONIC Rx

See "Nonpharmacologic Therapy" and "Acute General Rx."

DISPOSITION

Long-term follow-up essential for recurrent conversion symptoms and underlying mood disorders.

REFERRAL

To rule out other psychiatric disorders and for psychotherapy.

PEARLS & CONSIDERATIONS

COMMENTS

- Three modifications have been proposed for the diagnostic criteria in DSM-5: the removal of the requirements that the clinician establish that 1) the patient is not feigning or 2) that there is an associated psychological stressor, as both of these can be difficult and sometimes impossible to demonstrate; 3) the importance of positive neurologic evidence, such as the absence of seizure activity on EEG or Hoover's sign for motor weakness.
- Good prognostic factors: sudden onset, presence of psychological stressors at onset, short duration between diagnosis and treatment, high level of intelligence, absence of other psychiatric or medical disorders.
- Poor prognostic factors: severe disability, long duration of symptoms, age >40 yr at onset, and convulsions or paralysis as presenting symptoms.
- Differentiation between conversion, somatization, dissociative, factitious, and malingering disorders, as well as organic versus functional etiologies, may be challenging.
- Studies show an association between sexual trauma and conversion symptoms, although evidence does not support causality because of confounding and methodologic factors.
- Although not well demonstrated, some argue that conversion and somatized symptoms are more prevalent in cultures without an articulated concept of affective disorder or in which mental illness is highly stigmatized.

SUGGESTED READINGS
available at www.expertconsult.com

RELATED CONTENT
Conversion Disorder (Patient Information)

AUTHOR: **KAILA COMPTON, M.D., PH.D.**

BASIC INFORMATION

DEFINITION

Cor pulmonale is an alteration in the structure and function of the right ventricle (RV) from pulmonary hypertension caused by diseases of the upper or lower airways, lungs, or pulmonary vasculature. It is a state of cardiopulmonary dysfunction that may result from multiple etiologies rather than a specific disease state. Right-sided heart failure resulting from primary disease of the left heart and congenital heart disease are not considered in this disorder.

SYNONYMS

Acute cor pulmonale
Chronic cor pulmonale

ICD-9CM CODES
415.0 Cor pulmonale, acute
416.9 Cor pulmonale, chronic

ETIOLOGY

Most conditions that cause cor pulmonale are chronic. Acute cor pulmonale is often life threatening but transient. For example, acute pulmonary embolus may present with acute cor pulmonale, cardiogenic shock, or death, but if the patient survives the initial event, then the RV often recovers and cor pulmonale is no longer existent after several weeks.

In general, cor pulmonale occurs as a result of the inability of the RV to adapt to increased afterload in the pulmonary circuit, resulting in either acute or chronic right ventricular failure depending on the time course of the elevation in pulmonary vascular resistance. Mechanisms leading to pulmonary hypertension and thus predisposing to the development of cor pulmonale include:
- Pulmonary vasoconstriction leading to increased RV afterload, often resulting from conditions causing alveolar hypoxia and/or respiratory acidosis (e.g., high altitude/hypobaric hypoxia, obstructive sleep apnea/obesity-hypoventilation syndrome, chronic obstructive pulmonary disease). In pulmonary arterial hypertension (PAH), pulmonary vasoconstriction may occur in the absence of a primary cause of hypoxemia, due to imbalances between vasoconstrictor and vasodilator expression in the pulmonary circulation.
- Anatomic reduction or remodeling of the pulmonary vascular bed leading to increased RV afterload (e.g., emphysema, interstitial lung disease, pulmonary emboli, pulmonary arterial hypertension)
- Increased blood viscosity leading to increased RV afterload (e.g., polycythemia related to chronic hypoxemia, polycythemia vera, Waldenström's macroglobulinemia)

PHYSICAL FINDINGS & CLINICAL PRESENTATION

No symptoms are specific for cor pulmonale. Typically, the symptoms depend on the underlying disease process. The symptoms are most often a result of right ventricular failure:

- Dyspnea, fatigue, chest pain, or syncope with exertion (from pulmonary hypertension, RV ischemia, and impaired cardiac output)
- Right upper quadrant abdominal pain and anorexia (from passive hepatic congestion)
- Hoarseness (caused by compression of the left recurrent laryngeal nerve by dilation of the main pulmonary artery; known as *Ortner's syndrome*)
- Signs of right ventricular failure: jugular venous distention, peripheral edema, hepatic congestion, ascites, and a right ventricular third heart sound
- Signs of associated tricuspid regurgitation: holosystolic murmur heard best along the left parasternal border (augments during inspiration), prominent V-wave on jugular venous pulse, and pulsatile hepatomegaly (in severe tricuspid regurgitation)
- Pulmonary hypertension will increase the intensity of the pulmonic component of S2, which may be narrowly split
- Rarely, cough and hemoptysis

DIAGNOSIS

WORKUP

Search for an underlying pulmonary process resulting in pulmonary hypertension:
- Left ventricular dysfunction should be excluded in initial assessment.
- Worldwide, chronic mountain sickness is an important cause of cor pulmonale.
- 80% to 90% of cor pulmonale cases not related to high altitude are attributable to chronic obstructive pulmonary disease (COPD).
- Consideration of obstructive sleep apnea, chronic thromboembolic disease, pulmonary arterial hypertension, and musculoskeletal disease should be given in the absence of parenchymal lung disease.

LABORATORY TESTS
- Complete blood count may show erythrocytosis from chronic hypoxia.
- Arterial blood gas levels confirm hypoxemia and acidosis or hypercapnia.
- BNP may be elevated from RV dilation.
- Pulmonary function tests.

IMAGING STUDIES
- Chest radiograph may show underlying pulmonary disease and evidence of pulmonary hypertension (e.g., enlargement of the pulmonary arteries or right atrium and right ventricular dilation) (Fig. 1-242).
- ECG may reveal right ventricular hypertrophy, right atrial enlargement (P-pulmonale), right-axis deviation, or incomplete/complete right bundle branch block.
- Echocardiogram to detect right ventricular enlargement and/or hypertrophy and estimate pulmonary artery pressure.
- Radionuclide ventriculography to measure right ventricular ejection fraction, which may be reduced.
- Cardiac MRI can accurately measure right ventricular dimensions and function.
- Right-sided heart catheterization measures pulmonary artery pressures and pulmonary vascular resistance. It can also determine response to oxygen or vasodilators. Importantly, right heart catheterization allows assessment of pulmonary capillary wedge pressure, allowing right heart failure from pulmonary venous hypertension due to left heart disease to be ruled out.

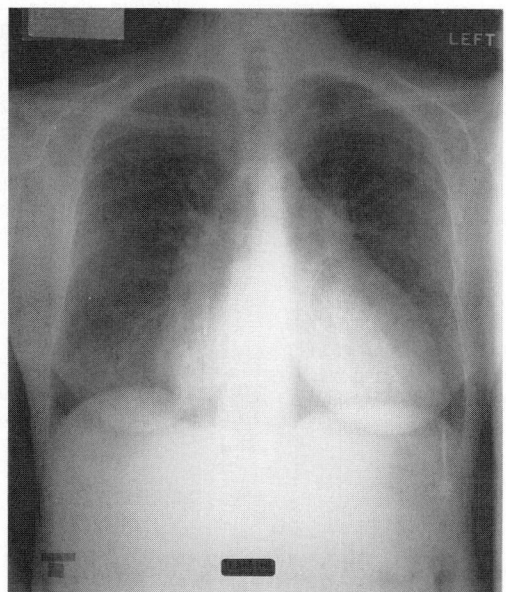

FIGURE 1-242 Chest radiography in a patient with severe intrinsic pulmonary vascular disease demonstrating enlargement of the main pulmonary artery, right ventricle, and right atrium. (From Crawford MH et al [eds]: *Cardiology*, ed 2, St Louis, 2004, Mosby.)

- Chest CT can assess for pulmonary parenchymal disease and embolus in the pulmonary vasculature.

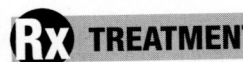 **TREATMENT**

The treatment of cor pulmonale is directed toward the underlying etiology while also reversing hypoxemia, improving right ventricular contractility, decreasing pulmonary artery vascular resistance, and improving pulmonary hypertension

NONPHARMACOLOGIC THERAPY

- Supplemental oxygen to correct hypoxemia is an important management step in the treatment of cor pulmonale related to hypoxemia. Goal O_2 sat of more than 90% is reasonable.
- Continuous positive airway pressure is used in patients with obstructive sleep apnea.
- Sodium and fluid restriction in setting of edema from RV failure
- Phlebotomy is reserved as adjunctive therapy in patients with polycythemia (hematocrit >55%) who have acute decompensation of cor pulmonale or remain polycythemic despite long-term oxygen therapy. Phlebotomy has been shown to decrease mean pulmonary artery pressure and pulmonary vascular resistance.

ACUTE GENERAL Rx

- Pulmonary embolism is the most common cause of acute cor pulmonale (see "Pulmonary Embolism"). The treatment is anticoagulation, hemodynamic support, and consideration of thrombolytics. Cathether-based thrombectomy or surgical embolectomy are potential salvage therapies in patients who cannot receive anticoagulation or thrombolysis, or whose condition continues to deteriorate despite thrombolytics and anticoagulation.
- Acute cor pulmonale may also be seen in cases of acute respiratory distress syndrome (ARDS), related to hypercapnea/acidosis, hypoxic pulmonary vasoconstriction, and the effects of mechanical ventilation. The treatment is supportive care for ARDS with low tidal volume ventilation. Extracorporeal membrane oxygen support (ECMO) while awaiting lung recovery from ARDS may also be helpful in maintaining blood oxygenation. Venoarterial ECMO can provide hemodynamic support as well as blood oxygenation.
- In patients with preexisting cor pulmonale, acute pulmonary illnesses or hypoxia can increase pulmonary hypertension and worsen right ventricular function. The underlying exacerbating conditions should be treated.

- Careful attention to fluid balance is important in the management of acute decompensated right heart failure. Both overhydration and overdiuresis should be avoided, with careful monitoring of intake and output, electrolytes and creatinine, and hemodynamics.
- Intravenous inotropes may be employed to support right heart contractility in decompensated right heart failure.
- In acutely decompensated right heart failure due to pulmonary arterial hypertension, IV prostanoid medications are the treatment of choice. Oral pulmonary vasodilators may also be added to the IV prostanoids, but should not be initiated as monotherapy in patients with advanced right heart failure from PAH. Atrial septostomy is a salvage option for patients with ongoing decompensated right heart failure from PAH despite pulmonary vasodilators. Such patients should undergo rapid assessment for possible transplantation.

CHRONIC Rx

- Long-term oxygen supplementation improves survival in hypoxemic patients with COPD.
- Right ventricular volume overload should be treated with diuretics (e.g., furosemide). However, excessive diuresis can reduce right ventricular filling and decrease cardiac output.
- Theophylline and sympathomimetic amines may improve diaphragmatic excursion, myocardial contraction, and pulmonary artery vasodilation, but can cause toxicity and arrhythmias.
- Digoxin may be employed as an oral inotropic agent to improve right heart contractility.
- Selective oral or parenteral pulmonary vasodilators to combat pulmonary hypertension should not be administered empirically in the absence of a right-sided heart catheterization and have not been proven to be of specific benefit in pulmonary hypertension related to hypoxemia or parenchymal lung disease. However, such agents have been shown to be beneficial in the treatment of idiopathic PAH, PAH related to connective tissue disease, and PAH due to congential heart disease. Pulmonary vasodilators are sometimes considered in other forms of PAH when primary disease management strategies have failed to improve right heart failure.
- Pulmonary thrombendarterectomy may be curative in the special case of cor pulmonale due to chronic thromboembolic pulmonary hypertension.
- Lung transplantation or heart-lung transplantation should be considered in the setting of cor pulmonale from lung diseases or from pulmonary vascular disease.

DISPOSITION

Patients with cor pulmonale should have regular assessment of their functional class (e.g., NYHA or WHO functional class); worse functional class indicates a poorer prognosis. High right atrial pressure and impaired cardiac output are also markers of increased mortality in RV failure from PAH. The presence of hyponatremia and elevated BNP levels are adverse indicators in PAH, as is low systemic blood pressure. Six-minute walk testing can be helpful in assessing exercise tolerance and is used for prognostication in PAH and COPD.

REFERRAL

Patients with pulmonary disease who have progressed to cor pulmonale should be followed up by a pulmonologist.

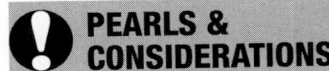 **PEARLS & CONSIDERATIONS**

- There is no differential diagnosis, but rather an evaluation of the patient to identify the underlying cause.
- Prognosis and treatment are related to the underlying cause, whereas the presence of cor pulmonale is merely a marker of the underlying disease severity.

COMMENTS

There is increasing interest in selective pulmonary vasodilators to improve right ventricular heart function in patients with cor pulmonale outside of the setting of idiopathic PAH, PAH related to connective tissue disease, and PAH related to congenital heart disease. However, more data on the safety and efficacy of these agents, especially in the setting of hypoxemic lung disease, is needed.

The importance of maintaining or improving right heart function, rather than solely lowering pulmonary pressures, is becoming increasingly apparent in the therapeutic management of patients with pulmonary hypertension and right heart failure.

SUGGESTED READINGS

available at www.expertconsult.com

AUTHORS: **MATTHEW D. JANKOWICH, M.D.,** and **GAURAV CHOUDHARY, M.D.**

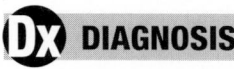

BASIC INFORMATION

DEFINITION

A corneal abrasion is a loss of surface epithelial tissue of the cornea caused by trauma.

SYNONYMS

Corneal erosion
Corneal contusion

ICD-9CM CODES

918.1 Corneal abrasion

EPIDEMIOLOGY & DEMOGRAPHICS

INCIDENCE (IN U.S.): A universal problem. Corneal abrasions comprise 8% of all eye presentations in primary care.
PEAK INCIDENCE: Childhood through active adulthood and older and debilitated patients
PREDOMINANT AGE: Any age

PHYSICAL FINDINGS & CLINICAL PRESENTATION

- Haziness of the cornea
- Disruption of the corneal surface (Fig. 1-243)
- Redness and infection of the conjunctiva
- Pain
- Light sensitivity
- Tearing
- Gritty feeling
- Pain on opening or closing eyes
- Sensation of a foreign body

ETIOLOGY

- Trauma (direct mechanical event)
- Foreign body
- Contact lenses
- Chemical or flash burns

DIAGNOSIS

DIFFERENTIAL DIAGNOSIS

- Acute-angle glaucoma
- Herpes ulcers and other corneal ulcers

- Foreign body in the cornea (be certain it is not a keratitis)
- Infective keratitis

WORKUP

- Fluorescein staining, slit lamp evaluation. After fluorescein staining of the cornea, an abrasion will appear yellow under normal light and green in cobalt blue light.
- Assessment of visual acuity. Vision loss of more than 20/40 requires referral.
- Intraocular pressure
- Rule out corneal laceration
- Rule out other eye pathology. Inspect anterior chamber for blood (hyphema) or pus (hypopyon). If present, refer immediately to ophthalmologist.
- Examine for foreign bodies and remove them if present.
- Confirm rod reflex to rule out significant global injury.

TREATMENT

NONPHARMACOLOGIC THERAPY

- Patching is controversial (see below) and not recommended because it does not improve pain and can delay healing.
- Bandage.
- Contact lenses.
- Warm compresses.
- Pressure dressing is controversial. Although eye patching traditionally has been recommended in the treatment of corneal abrasions, several studies show that patching does not help and may hinder healing.
- Removal of any foreign particles if present.

ACUTE GENERAL Rx

- Topical antibiotics such as 10% sulfacetamide or ofloxacin 0.3% solution 2 drops qid are commonly prescribed to prevent bacterial superinfection, but evidence for their use is lacking. Antipseudomonal topical antibiotics are, however, recommended for contact lens–related abrasions.

- Pressure patching of eye with eyelid closed is no longer recommended because it can result in decreased oxygen delivery, increased moisture, and a higher chance of infection.
- Cycloplegics such as 5% homatropine are often prescribed to relieve ciliary muscle spasm; however, their benefit has been questioned and they are no longer routinely recommended.
- Topical nonsteroidal anti-inflammatory drugs (NSAIDs) (e.g., diclofenac 0.1% or ketorolac 0.5%) 1 drop qid may be used for pain relief.
- Oral NSAIDs may be used for severe pain.

DISPOSITION

Follow-up in 24 hr and then every 3 days until abrasion has cleared and vision has returned to normal. Less frequent follow-up is appropriate for abrasions ≤4 mm or for uncomplicated abrasions.

REFERRAL

To ophthalmologist if patient has no relief within 24 hr or for patients with deep eye injuries, foreign bodies that cannot be removed, or suspected recurrent corneal erosion.

PEARLS & CONSIDERATIONS

COMMENTS

- Never give the patient topical anesthetic to use at home because these can cause decomposition of the cornea and permanent damage.
- Most corneal abrasions heal in 24 to 48 hr and rarely progress to corneal erosion or infection.

SUGGESTED READINGS

available at www.expertconsult.com

RELATED CONTENT

Fig. E3-45 Approach to the patient with corneal disorders (Algorithm)
Corneal Foreign Body or Abrasion (Patient Information)

AUTHOR: **MELVYN KOBY, M.D., and FRED F. FERRI, M.D.**

Diseases and Disorders

I

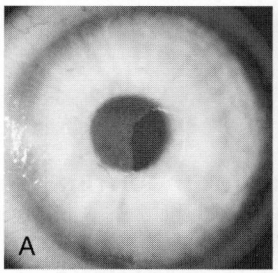
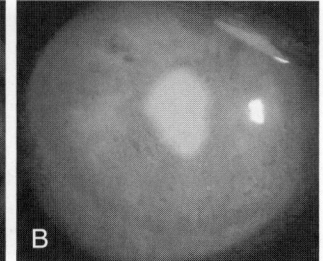

FIGURE 1-243 Corneal epithelial abrasion. A, Epithelial defect without fluorescein highlighting the defect. An irregularity in the otherwise smooth corneal surface is the key to identifying the defect if no fluorescein is available. **B,** Classic fluorescein staining of an epithelial defect. (From Palay D [ed]: *Ophthalmology for the primary care physician,* St Louis, 1997, Mosby.)

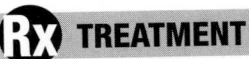

BASIC INFORMATION

DEFINITION

Corneal ulceration refers to the disruption of the corneal surface and/or deeper layers caused by trauma, contact lenses infection, degeneration, or other means.

SYNONYMS

Infectious keratitis with ulceration
Bacterial keratitis with ulceration
Viral keratitis with ulceration
Fungal keratitis with ulceration

ICD-9CM CODES
370.0 Corneal ulcer NOS

EPIDEMIOLOGY & DEMOGRAPHICS

INCIDENCE (IN U.S.): Four to six cases per month seen by an average general ophthalmologist
PREVALENCE (IN U.S.): Common
PREDOMINANT SEX: Either
PREDOMINANT AGE: All ages

PHYSICAL FINDINGS & CLINICAL PRESENTATION

- Localized, well-demarcated, infiltrative lesion with corresponding focal ulcer (Fig. 1-244) or oval, yellow-white stromal suppuration with thick mucopurulent exudate and edema. Usually red, angry-looking eye with infiltration in surrounding area of cornea.
- Eye possibly painful, with conjunctival edema and infection.
- Sterile neurotrophic ulcers with tissue breakdown and no pain.

ETIOLOGY

- Complication of contact lens wear, trauma, or diseases such as herpes simplex keratitis or keratoconjunctivitis sicca. Often associated with collagen vascular disease and severe exophthalmus and thyroid disease.
- Viral causes often contagious.

DIAGNOSIS

DIFFERENTIAL DIAGNOSIS

- *Pseudomonas* and pneumococcus and other bacterial infection—virulent
- *Moraxella, Staphylococcus,* α-*Streptococcus* infection—less virulent
- Herpes simplex infection or disease caused by other viruses
- Contact lens ulcers differ

WORKUP

- Fluorescein staining, slit lamp
- Appearance often typical

- Differentiate carefully with contact lens wearers
- Note previous eye surgery or laser vision correction

LABORATORY TESTS

Microscopic examination and culture of scrapings

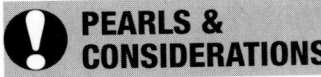

TREATMENT

NONPHARMACOLOGIC THERAPY

- Warm compresses
- Bandage contact lenses
- Patching
- Stop contact lens wearing
- Remove eyelid crusting

ACUTE GENERAL Rx

- An ophthalmic emergency
- Intense antibiotic and antiviral therapy
- Nonsteroidal antiinflammatory drugs
- Viroptic/Zymar
- Bacterial infection: subconjunctival cefazolin or gentamicin (topical Zymar, Vigomax, etc.)
- Fungal infection: hospitalization and topical application of antifungal agents
- Herpes: Viroptic and oral therapy

DISPOSITION

Ideally treated by an ophthalmologist if the patient does not rapidly respond to antibiotics (within 24 hr)

PEARLS & CONSIDERATIONS

- Always stop contact lens wearing.
- Always refer ulcers to ophthalmologist.
- Never treat with topical anesthetics or steroids.

COMMENTS

Do not use topical steroids because herpes, fungal, or other ulcers may be aggravated, leading to perforation of the cornea. Antibiotics may delay response and result in overgrowth of nonbacterial (fungal and amoebic) pathogens.

SUGGESTED READINGS
available at www.expertconsult.com

RELATED CONTENT
Fig. E3-45 Approach to the patient with corneal disorders (Algorithm)

AUTHOR: **MELVYN KOBY, M.D.**

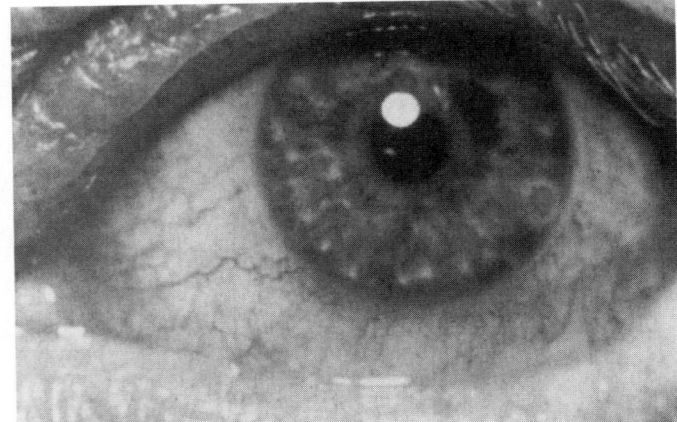

FIGURE 1-244 Peripherally located corneal ulcer. (From Marx JA [ed]: *Rosen's emergency medicine,* ed 5, St Louis, 2002, Mosby.)

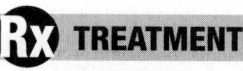

BASIC INFORMATION

DEFINITION

Clinical condition characterized by pain and tenderness at costochondral or chondrosternal joints of the anterior chest wall without swelling or induration, usually at multiple levels.

SYNONYMS

Anterior chest wall syndrome
Chest wall pain syndrome
Costosternal syndrome
Parasternal chondrodynia

ICD-9CM CODES
733.6 Costochondritis

EPIDEMIOLOGY & DEMOGRAPHICS

PREVALENCE: Fairly common, comprises approximately 28% of undifferentiated noncardiac chest pain patients.
PREDOMINANT SEX: Women > men
PREDOMINANT AGE: >40 years of age

PHYSICAL FINDINGS & CLINICAL PRESENTATION

SYMPTOMS:
- Anterior chest wall pain, usually described as sharp, aching, or pressure-like. Pain is usually aggravated by coughing, sneezing, deep inspiration, or any chest-wall movement.
- In children, especially teenagers, may present as sudden episode of sharp chest pain, with feeling that they cannot take deep breath, but actually improves with deep breathing.
- May radiate to arms and shoulders mimicking cardiac pain.

SIGNS:
- Reproducible tenderness of costochondral (second through fifth) or costosternal junction without localized swelling.
- Pain on crossed-chest adduction of arm and backward extension of arm from 90 degrees of abduction signifies pain of musculoskeletal origin.

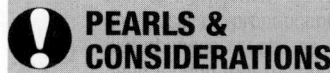

DIAGNOSIS

DIFFERENTIAL DIAGNOSIS

- Cardiac pain: primary concern; ischemic chest pain, acute pericarditis, aortic dissection
- Gastrointestinal: gastroesophageal reflux disease
- Pulmonary embolism, pneumonia, pneumothorax
- Musculoskeletal (Table 1-115): Tietze's syndrome, cervical or thoracic spine disease, fibromyalgia, arthritis
- Involvement of ribs by trauma, infections (*Candida albicans*) or neoplasms (breast cancer, prostate cancer, sarcoma, plasma cell cytoma)
- Psychiatric: panic attack

WORKUP

- A diagnosis of exclusion for chest pain after ruling out more serious conditions including cardiac chest pain. Key to diagnosis are detailed history, a meticulous physical examination and a few rationally selected diagnostic studies. Usefulness of nuclear scanning with technetium99 scintigraphy, gallium, or bone scanning to assist diagnosis of costochondritis is not clear.

TREATMENT

ACUTE GENERAL Rx

- Often self-limiting, so reassurance is important.
- Symptomatic treatment includes local application of heat, minimize activities that aggravate symptoms, stretching exercises for chest-wall muscles, and nonsteroidal anti-inflammatory drugs or acetaminophen.
- Refractory cases can be treated with local injections of combined lidocaine and corticosteroid (may be a useful diagnostic and therapeutic tool).
- Recurrent costochondritis may respond to sulfasalazine; however, there are no clinical trials on pharmacologic therapy for costochondritis.

PEARLS & CONSIDERATIONS

Presence of costochondritis in a patient with chest pain does not exclude more serious problems including cardiac pain.

SUGGESTED READINGS
available at www.expertconsult.com

RELATED CONTENT
Costochondritis (Patient Information)

AUTHOR: **ASHA SHRESTHA, M.D.**

TABLE 1-115 Musculoskeletal Chest Pain

Disorder	Clinical Features	Comments
Tietze's syndrome	Painful swelling of usually 2nd or 3rd costochondral junctions.	Less common than costochondritis; commonly affects young people of either sex. Exact cause is unknown, but a traumatic pathogenesis has been associated. The disease course is mostly self-limited.
Costochondritis	Pain and tenderness at the costochondral or chondrosternal junctions without a notable swelling. The 2nd-5th costal cartilages are most commonly involved.	Certain maneuvers like "crowing rooster" maneuver (extension of the cervical spine and traction on the posteriorly extended arm) and traction on the adducted arm with head rotated to ipsilateral side may reproduce the pain.
Slipping rib syndrome	Pain at the lower costal cartilages, associated with increased mobility of the anterior end of a costal cartilage. Most commonly affects 10th rib and occasionally 8th and 9th ribs.	Maneuver such as hooking the fingers under the anterior costal margin and pulling the rib cage anteriorly may produce a palpable click of the cartilages slipping over one another
Cervical, thoracic disc disease	Referred regional pain from affected areas. Often aggravated by spine motion and may be accompanied by radicular pain into arm if cervical origin or along intercostal nerve if thoracic origin. Symptoms reproduced by Spurling's maneuver (steady pressure to head causing increased axial loading on the nerve root).	May mimic chest disease if spinal complaints are minimal and referred or radicular symptoms predominate.
Fibromyalgia	Widespread pain with other multiple peripheral tender points. Symptoms often change in location.	Female/male ratio of 9:1. Prevalent age 30-50 yr. Frequently associated with tension headache, irritable bowel syndrome, and psychiatric symptoms.
Sternoclavicular or manubriosternal joint involvement in osteoarthritis, rheumatoid arthritis, ankylosing spondylitis, psoriatic arthritis, and infection	Dull, aching local pain with tenderness. Occasional bony joint enlargement with soft tissue swelling. Pain may radiate to anterior chest wall mimicking pain of cardiopulmonary origin.	Crepitus may rarely be present.

C

Diseases
and Disorders

I

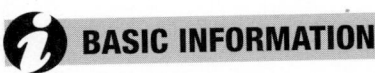

DEFINITION

Craniopharyngiomas are tumors arising from squamous cell remnants of Rathke's pouch, located in the infundibulum or upper anterior hypophysis.

SYNONYMS

Subset of nonadenomatous pituitary tumors

ICD-9CM CODES
237.0 Craniopharyngioma

EPIDEMIOLOGY & DEMOGRAPHICS

PEAK INCIDENCE: Occurs at all ages; peak during the first 2 decades of life, with a second small peak occurring in the sixth decade.
PREDOMINANT SEX:
- Both sexes are usually equally affected.
- Craniopharyngiomas are the most common nonglial tumors in children and account for 3% to 5% of all pediatric brain tumors.

PHYSICAL FINDINGS & CLINICAL PRESENTATION

- The typical onset is insidious and a 1- to 2-year history of slowly progressive symptoms is common.
- Presenting symptoms are usually related to the effects of a sella turcica mass. Approximately 75% of patients report headache and have visual disturbances.
- The usual visual defect is bitemporal hemianopsia. Optic nerve involvement with decreased visual acuity and scotomas and homonymous hemianopsia from optic tract involvement may also occur.
- Other symptoms include mental changes, nausea, vomiting, somnolence, or symptoms of pituitary failure. In adults, sexual dysfunction is the most common endocrine complaint, with impotence in men and primary or secondary amenorrhea in women. Diabetes insipidus is found in 25% of cases. In children, craniopharyngiomas may present with dwarfism.
- More than 70% of children at the time of diagnosis present with growth hormone deficiency, obstructive hydrocephalus, short-term memory deficits, and psychomotor slowing.

ETIOLOGY

Craniopharyngiomas are believed to arise from nests of squamous epithelial cells that are commonly found in the suprasellar area surrounding the pars tuberalis of the adult pituitary.

DX DIAGNOSIS

DIFFERENTIAL DIAGNOSIS

- Pituitary adenoma
- Empty sella syndrome
- Pituitary failure of any cause
- Primary brain tumors (e.g., meningiomas, astrocytomas)
- Metastatic brain tumors
- Other brain tumors
- Cerebral aneurysm

LABORATORY TESTS

- Hypothyroidism (low FT_4, FT_3 with high thyroid-stimulating hormone).
- Hypercortisolism (low cortisol) with low adrenocorticotropic hormone.
- Low sex hormones (testosterone, estriol) with low follicle-stimulating hormone and luteinizing hormone.
- Diabetes insipidus (hypernatremia, low urine osmolarity, high plasma osmolarity).
- Prolactin may be normal or slightly elevated.
- Pituitary stimulation tests may be required in some cases.

IMAGING STUDIES

- Visual field testing for bitemporal hemianopsia.
- Skull film.
  - Enlarged or eroded sella turcica (50%)
  - Suprasellar calcification (50%)
- MRI (Fig. 1-245) or head CT. MRI features include a multicystic and solid enhancing suprasellar mass. Hydrocephalus may also be present if the mass is large. CT usually reveals intratumoral calcifications.

RX TREATMENT

GENERAL Rx

- Surgical resection (curative or palliative).
  - Transsphenoidal surgery for small intrasellar tumors
  - Subfrontal craniotomy for most patients

- Postoperative radiation.
- Intralesional ^{32}P irradiation or bleomycin for unresectable tumors. Long-term complications of radiation include secondary malignancies, optic neuropathy, and vascular injury.

PROGNOSIS

- Operative mortality rate: 3% to 16% (higher with large tumors).
- Postoperative recurrence rate: 30% of cases after total resection and 57% of cases after subtotal resection.
- 5-yr and 10-yr survival: 88% and 76%, respectively, with surgery and radiation.
- The most important factors that correlate with prognosis are the extent of resection and postoperative radiation.

RELATED CONTENT

Craniopharyngioma (Patient Information)

AUTHOR: **FRED F. FERRI, M.D.**

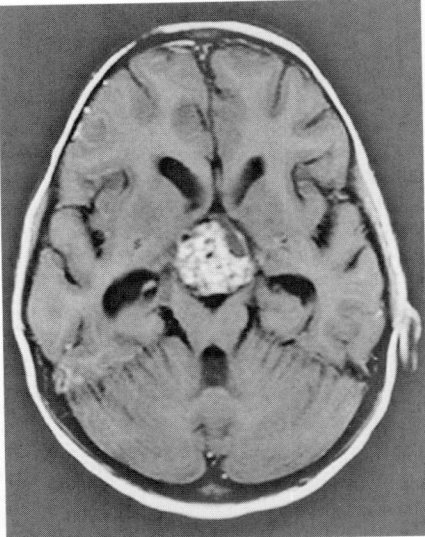

FIGURE 1-245 MRI scan of a craniopharyngioma, demonstrating a cystic contrast-enhancing mass in the suprasellar area extending upward and compressing the hypothalamus. (From Goetz CG: *Textbook of clinical neurology,* Philadelphia, 1999, Saunders.)

BASIC INFORMATION

DEFINITION

Creutzfeldt-Jakob disease (CJD) is a progressive, fatal, dementing neurologic illness caused by an infectious protein agent known as a *prion*.

SYNONYMS

Transmissible spongiform encephalopathy
Mad cow disease
Prion disease
Bovine spongiform encephalopathy

ICD-9CM CODES

046.1 Creutzfeldt-Jakob disease

EPIDEMIOLOGY & DEMOGRAPHICS

- Incidence of one per 1 million population per year
- Peak age 60 yr (range, 16 to 82 yr)—sporadic cases are seen in an older population while the variant subtype is commonly seen in younger patients
- 5% to 10% familial, remaining cases are sporadic; iatrogenic cases (corneal transplants, dura mater allograft, human pituitary extract, blood or blood product transfusion, reused medical equipment such as EEG depth electrodes) are very rare—about 1%; variant CJD is caused by ingestion of meat from cows with prion disease
- Normal prion protein (PRNP) gene found on human chromosome 20
- Methionine and valine distribution on codon 129 of the PRNP determines the six clinical phenotypes of CJD

PHYSICAL FINDINGS & CLINICAL PRESENTATION

- Cognitive deficits: Patients present with cognitive deficits (dementing illness—memory loss, behavioral abnormalities, higher cortical function impairment), usually a subacute progressive encephalopathy or dementia. Other manifestations include prodromal symptoms such as fatigue, depression, weight loss, and disorders of sleep and appetite in about one third of patients. Early stages are characterized by confusion with hallucinations, delusions, and agitative behavior.
- More than 80% will have myoclonus—generalized and exaggerated by startle.
- Pyramidal tract signs (weakness), cerebellar signs (clumsiness), and extrapyramidal signs (parkinsonian features) are seen in more than 50% of the cases.
- Less common features include cortical visual abnormalities, abnormal eye movements, vestibular dysfunction, sensory disturbances, autonomic dysfunction, lower motor neuron signs, and seizures.

ETIOLOGY

Small proteinaceous infectious particle (prion). Noninfectious prion protein (PrP) is a cellular protein found on the surfaces of neurons. Normal function is not known. Protein is converted to protease-resistant and infectious agent by infectious prion protein.

DIAGNOSIS

- Definite CJD: Neuropathologically confirmed spongiform encephalopathy in a case of progressive dementia.
- Probable CJD: History of rapidly progressive dementia (<2 yr) with typical EEG and with at least two of the following clinical features: myoclonus, visual or cerebellar dysfunction, pyramidal or extrapyramidal features, akinetic mutism.
- Possible CJD: Same as probable CJD without EEG findings.

DIFFERENTIAL DIAGNOSIS

- Other dementias (Alzheimer's disease, frontotemporal dementia, Lewy body dementia, and vascular dementia)
- Infectious (viral, HIV, fungal, TB, Whipple's disease)
- Inflammatory/Autoimmune (CNS vasculitis, Hashimoto's encephalopathy, SSPE)
- Metabolic (vitamin deficiency, endocrine)
- Cancers (CNS lymphoma, gliomatosis cerebri, paraneoplastic)

A clinical algorithm for the evaluation of dementia is described in Section III, "Dementia."

WORKUP

- Evaluate for treatable causes of dementia (see "Alzheimer's Disease").
- Brain biopsy is gold standard for diagnosis, but it is usually not performed because there is no treatment or cure.
- Lumbar puncture with spinal fluid analysis for presence of 14-3-3 protein or human prion protein (PrP^{Sc}).
- Recent guidelines issued by the American Academy of Neurology states that clinicians should order assays for 14-3-3 in patients with rapidly progressive dementia, strong suspicion of sporadic CJD and an uncertain diagnosis (pretest probability 20% to 90%). The test has a high false positive and false negative rate due to its presence in other chronic noninflammatory dementing diseases.

LABORATORY TESTS

- Presence of periodic sharp wave complexes on EEG in cases of rapidly progressive dementia has a sensitivity of 67% and a specificity of 86%.
- In cases of probable or possible CJD, presence of the 14,3,3 protein in CSF has a 95% positive predictive value with its absence having a 92% negative predictive value. Test for presence of human prion protein (PrP^{Sc}) in CSF has been reported to be 83% sensitive and 100% specific. Repeated testing for 14.3.3 protein increases the probability of a positive result. Enolase and neopterin in CSF are the other nonspecific markers that may have adjunct diagnostic value.

IMAGING STUDIES

MRI scan can show areas of restricted diffusion in the basal ganglia and cerebral cortex. MRI diffusion-weighted imaging has a sensitivity of 92.3% and a specificity of 93.8% only in cases of rapidly progressive dementia. T2-weighted imaging may also show subtle hyperintensities in the lenticular nuclei in about 82% of cases.

TREATMENT

NONPHARMACOLOGIC THERAPY

Full-time caregiver and/or nursing home. Social work can be helpful with end-of-life discussions, family counseling, and optimizing appropriate home services. Proper disposal of medical equipment and avoidance of organ transplants from these patients prevent transmission of the disease.

ACUTE GENERAL Rx

No known therapy

CHRONIC Rx

No known therapy

DISPOSITION

The disease is fatal. Mean duration of illness is 8 mo (range, 1 to 130 mo). One in 7 survives to 1 yr, and 1 in 30 survives to 2 yr. Better survival found in younger age at onset of disease and female gender. Increased survival may be falsely reported due to coexisting dementias such as Alzheimer's with earlier onset of dementia than CJD.

REFERRAL

- Neurology for evaluation of any rapidly progressive dementia
- Social work

PEARLS & CONSIDERATIONS

COMMENTS

- Related diseases in human beings: kuru, fatal familial insomnia, Gerstmann-Sträussler-Scheinker syndrome, new-variant CJD.
- Related diseases in animals: scrapie, bovine spongiform encephalopathy (mad cow disease).

EVIDENCE

available at www.expertconsult.com

SUGGESTED READINGS

available at www.expertconsult.com

AUTHOR: ARUN SWAMINATHAN, M.B.B.S., and SACHIN KEDAR, M.B.B.S., M.D.

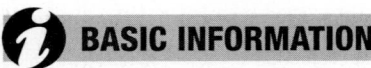

BASIC INFORMATION

DEFINITION

Crohn's disease is an inflammatory disease of the bowel of unknown etiology, most commonly involving the terminal ileum and manifesting primarily with diarrhea, abdominal pain, fatigue, and weight loss.

SYNONYMS

Regional enteritis
Inflammatory bowel disease (IBD)

ICD-9CM CODES
555.9 Crohn's disease, unspecified site
555.0 Crohn's disease, small intestine
555.1 Crohn's disease involving large intestine

EPIDEMIOLOGY & DEMOGRAPHICS

PREVALENCE:
- One case per 1000 persons; most common in whites and Jews
- Crohn's disease affects approximately 380,000 to 480,000 persons in the U.S.
- Incidence: bimodal with a peak in the third decade of life and another in the fifth decade

PHYSICAL FINDINGS & CLINICAL PRESENTATION

- Abdominal tenderness, mass, or distention
- Chronic or nocturnal diarrhea
- Weight loss, fever, night sweats
- Hyperactive bowel sounds in patients with partial obstruction, bloody diarrhea
- Delayed growth and failure of normal development in children
- Perianal and rectal abscesses, multiple sinuses and scarring (Fig. E1-246), mouth ulcers, cobblestone appearance of oral mucosa (Fig. E1-247) and atrophic glossitis
- Extraintestinal manifestations: joint swelling and tenderness, hepatosplenomegaly, erythema nodosum, clubbing, tenderness to palpation of the sacroiliac joints

- Symptoms may be intermittent with varying periods of remission

ETIOLOGY

Unknown. Pathophysiologically, Crohn's disease involves an immune system dysfunction.

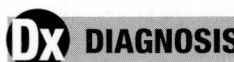

DIAGNOSIS

DIFFERENTIAL DIAGNOSIS

- Ulcerative colitis (see Table 1-116)
- Infectious diseases (tuberculosis, *Yersinia, Salmonella, Shigella, Campylobacter*)
- Parasitic infections (amebic infection)
- Pseudomembranous colitis
- Ischemic colitis in elderly patients
- Lymphoma
- Colon carcinoma
- Diverticulitis
- Radiation enteritis
- Collagenous colitis
- Fungal infections *(Histoplasma, Actinomyces)*
- Gay bowel syndrome (in homosexual patient)
- Carcinoid tumors
- Celiac sprue
- Mesenteric adenitis

LABORATORY TESTS

- Decreased hemoglobin and hematocrit from chronic blood loss, effect of inflammation on bone marrow, and malabsorption of vitamin B_{12}
- Hypokalemia, hypomagnesemia, hypocalcemia, and low albumin in patients with chronic diarrhea
- Vitamin B12 and folate deficiency
- Elevated erythrocyte sedimentation rate
- Positive anti–*Saccharomyces cerevisiae* antibodies
- Elevated INR (due to vitamin K malabsorption)
- Fecal calprotectin has been reported as useful in screening of patients with suspected IBD. Based on a pretest probability of 32% in adults, an abnormal calprotectin test results increases the posttest probability to 91%, and a normal result reduces the probability of

IBD to 3%. False elevations may occur with other gastrointestinal diseases such as bacterial, viral, and protozoal causes of infective diarrhea

ENDOSCOPIC EVALUATION

Endoscopic features of Crohn's disease include asymmetric and discontinued disease, deep longitudinal fissures, cobblestone appearance, and presence of strictures. Crypt distortion and inflammation are also present. Granulomas may be present.

IMAGING STUDIES

- Barium imaging studies are essentially outdated examinations. When performed, they reveal deep ulcerations (often longitudinal and transverse) and segmental lesions (skip lesions, strictures, fistulas, cobblestone appearance of mucosa caused by submucosal inflammation); "thumbprinting" is common, and "string sign" in terminal ileum may be noted. Although the diagnosis may be suggested by radiographic studies, it should be confirmed by endoscopy and biopsy when possible.
- CT of abdomen may show thickening of the terminal ileum (Fig. 1-248) and is helpful in identifying abscesses and other complications.
- Magnetic resonance enterography (MRe) is superior to other imaging modalities in its ability to distinguish active from chronic fibrotic disease. It is, however, more expensive.
- In 5% to 10% of patients with IBD, a clear distinction between ulcerative colitis and Crohn's disease cannot be made. In general, Crohn's disease can be distinguished from ulcerative colitis by the presence of transmural involvement and the frequent presence of noncaseating granulomas and lymphoid aggregates on biopsy.

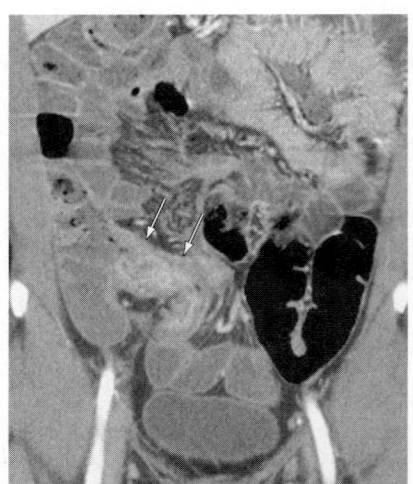

FIGURE 1-248 Coronal reformat from a contrast-enhanced computed tomographic scan shows thickening in the terminal ileum with enhancement *(arrows)* suggestive of Crohn's disease. (From Fielding JR et al: *Gynecologic imaging*, Philadelphia, 2011, Saunders.)

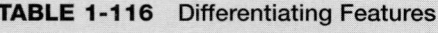

TABLE 1-116 Differentiating Features

	Ulcerative Colitis	Crohn's Disease
Site of involvement	Only involves colon Rectum almost always involved	Any area of the gastrointestinal tract Rectum usually spared
Pattern of involvement	Continuous	Skip lesions
Diarrhea	Bloody	Usually nonbloody
Severe abdominal pain	Rare	Frequent
Perianal disease	No	In 30% of patients
Fistula	No	Yes
Endoscopic findings	Erythematous and friable Superficial ulceration	Aphthoid and deep ulcers Cobblestoning
Radiologic findings	Tubular appearance resulting from loss of haustral folds	String sign of terminal ileum RLQ mass, fistulas, abscesses
Histologic features	Mucosa only Crypt abscesses	Transmural Crypt abscesses, granulomas (about 30%)
Smoking	Protective	Worsens course
Serology	p-ANCA more common	ASCA more common

ASCA, Anti–*Saccharomyces cerevisiae* antibodies; *p-ANCA,* perinuclear antineutrophil cytoplasmic antibody; *RLQ,* right lower quadrant.
From Andreoli TE et al: *Andreoli and Carpenter's Cecil essentials of medicine,* ed 8, Philadelphia, 2010, Saunders.

C

Diseases and Disorders

I

TREATMENT

The medical management of Crohn's disease is based on disease activity. According to Hanauer and Sanborn, disease activity can be defined as follows:

- Mild to moderate disease: The patient is ambulatory and able to take oral alimentation. There is no dehydration, high fever, abdominal tenderness, painful mass, obstruction, or weight loss of >10%.
- Moderate to severe disease: Either the patient has not responded to treatment for mild to moderate disease or has more pronounced symptoms, including fever, significant weight loss, abdominal pain or tenderness, intermittent nausea and vomiting, or significant anemia.
- Severe fulminant disease: Either the patient has persistent symptoms despite outpatient steroid therapy or has high fever, persistent vomiting, evidence of intestinal obstruction, rebound tenderness, cachexia, or evidence of an abscess.
- Remission: The patient is asymptomatic or without inflammatory sequelae, including patients responding to acute medical intervention.

NONPHARMACOLOGIC THERAPY

- Nutritional supplementation is needed in patients with advanced disease. Total parenteral nutrition may be necessary in selected patients.
- Low-residue diet is necessary when obstructive symptoms are present.
- If diarrhea is prominent, increased dietary fiber and decreased fat in the diet are sometimes helpful.
- Psychotherapy is useful for situational adjustment crises. A trusting and mutually understanding relationship and referral to self-help groups are very important because of the chronicity of the disease and the relatively young age of the patients.
- Avoid oral feedings during acute exacerbation to decrease colonic activity: a low-roughage diet may be helpful in early relapse.

ACUTE GENERAL Rx

- Traditionally, initial treatment consists of 5-aminosalicylate drugs (sulfasalazine, olsalazine, balsalazide, mesalamine: oral or rectal). Sulfasalazine, 500 mg PO qid initially,

increased qd or qod by 1 g until therapeutic dosages of 4 to 6 g/day are achieved, is often initially used. Individuals with sulfa allergies should avoid sulfasalazine. Folate supplementation is recommended because sulfasalazine inhibits folate absorption. Oral salicylates, such as mesalamine (Asacol, Rowasa), are as effective as sulfasalazine and better tolerated and have become preferred agents despite their higher cost.
- Corticosteroids have been the mainstay for treating moderate to severe active Crohn's disease. Prednisone 40 to 60 mg/day is useful for acute exacerbation. Steroids are usually tapered over approximately 2 to 3 mo. Some patients require a low dose for a prolonged period of maintenance.
- Steroid analogues are locally active corticosteroids that target specific areas of inflammation in the gastrointestinal tract. Budesonide is available as a controlled-release formulation and is approved for mild to moderate active Crohn's disease involving the ileum and/or ascending colon. The adult dose is 9 mg qd for a maximum of 8 wk.
- Immunosuppressants such as azathioprine 150 mg/day, methotrexate, or cyclosporine can be used for severe, progressive disease. In patients with Crohn's disease who enter remission after treatment with methotrexate, a low dose of methotrexate maintains remission.
- Metronidazole 500 mg qid may be useful for colonic fistulas and treatment of mild to moderate active Crohn's disease. Ciprofloxacin 1 g qd has also been found to be effective in decreasing disease activity.
- TNF inhibitors: Infliximab, a chimeric monoclonal antibody targeting tumor necrosis factor-α, is effective in the treatment of enterocutaneous fistulas. This medication can induce clinical improvement in 80% of patients with Crohn's disease refractory to other agents. It can be used in combination with other medications such as azathioprine in patients with severe Crohn's disease. A PPD test should be done before using this medication. Adalimumab and certolizumab are other TNF inhibitors also effective in inducing remissions and may be useful in adult patients with Crohn's disease who cannot tolerate infliximab or have symptoms despite receiving infliximab therapy.
- Natalizumab, a selective adhesion-molecule inhibitor, has been reported to be effective in

increasing the rate of remission and response in patients with active Crohn's disease. It is effective for patients in whom anti-TNF therapy has been unsuccessful. Recent trials with pegylated antibody fragments in patients with moderate to severe Crohn's disease involving certolizumab pegol revealed a modest improvement in response rates but no significant improvement in remission rates.
- Hydrocortisone enema bid or tid is useful for proctitis.
- Most patients who have anemia associated with Crohn's disease respond to iron supplementation. Erythropoietin is useful in patients with anemia refractory to treatment with iron and vitamins.

CHRONIC Rx

- Monitor disease activity with symptom review and laboratory evaluation (complete blood count and sedimentation rate)
- Liver tests and vitamin B_{12} levels monitored on a yearly basis

DISPOSITION

One tenth of patients have prolonged remission, three quarters have a chronic intermittent disease course, and one eighth have an unremitting course.

REFERRAL

- Surgical referral is needed for complications such as abscess formation, obstruction, fistulas, toxic megacolon, refractory disease, or severe hemorrhage. Approximately 40% to 50% of patients will require some type of bowel surgery within the first 5 years of Crohn's disease. A conservative surgical approach is necessary because surgery is not curative. Multiple surgeries may also result in short bowel syndrome.

EBM EVIDENCE

available at www.expertconsult.com

SUGGESTED READINGS
available at www.expertconsult.com

RELATED CONTENT
Crohn's Disease (Patient Information)

AUTHOR: **FRED F. FERRI, M.D.**

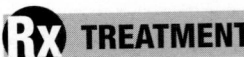

BASIC INFORMATION

DEFINITION

Cryoglobulins are serum immunoglobulins that precipitate when cooled and redissolve when heated. A classification of cryoglobulins is described in Table E1-117. Cryoglobulinemia is a clinical syndrome that results from systemic inflammation caused by cryoglobulin-containing immune complexes. Mixed cryoglobulinemia is a vasculitis of small and medium-sized arteries and veins due to the deposition of complexes of antigen, cryoglobulin, and complement in the vessel walls.

SYNONYMS

Cryoglobulinemic vasculitis
Cryoproteinemia
Mixed cryoglobulinemia
Essential cryoglobulinemia

ICD-9CM CODES
273.2 Cryoglobulinemia, cryoglobulinemic vasculitis (CV), mixed cryoglobulinemia (MC)

EPIDEMIOLOGY & DEMOGRAPHICS

PREVALENCE:
- Prevalence of mixed cryoglobulinemia is approximately 1:100,000
- More than 50% of patients with HCV are found to have mixed cryoglobulinemia
- Three types: I (monoclonal), II (IgM monoclonal and IgG polyclonal), and III (polyclonal)

PREDOMINANT SEX AND AGE: Female:male ratio of 3:1

PREDOMINANT AGE: Mean age reported is 42 to 52 yr

RISK FACTORS: Hepatitis C virus (HCV) infection, connective tissue disorders, lymphoproliferative disorders

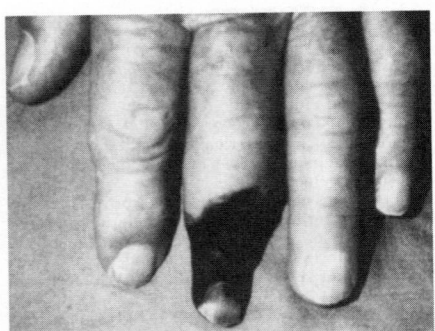

FIGURE 1-249 Cryoglobulinemia. (From Hoffman R et al: *Hematology, basic principles and practice*, ed 5, New York, 2009, Churchill Livingstone.)

PHYSICAL FINDINGS & CLINICAL PRESENTATION

- **Meltzer triad** of purpura, arthralgias/myalgia, and weakness
- Other symptoms include dyspnea, cough, numbness, abdominal pain, acrocyanosis
- Hypertension, hepatosplenomegaly, Raynaud's phenomenon, and in severe cases, distal necrosis and ulcerations of lower limbs (Fig. 1-249)

ETIOLOGY

- Intravascular deposition of cryoglobulins leads to ischemic insults in territory supplied by vasa nervorum
- Necrotizing vasculitis caused by cryoglobulin precipitation
- Infections: HCV, mycosis fungoides, HBV, Epstein-Barr virus, cytomegalovirus, *Treponema pallidum, Mycobacterium leprae,* and in post-streptococcal glomerulonephritis
- Lymphoproliferative disorders: chronic lymphocytic leukemia, Waldenström's macroglobulinemia, multiple myeloma
- Connective tissue disorders: rheumatoid arthritis, systemic lupus erythematosus (SLE), scleroderma, Sjögren's syndrome, vasculitis
- Renal diseases including proliferative glomerulonephritis

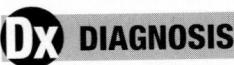 DIAGNOSIS

DIFFERENTIAL DIAGNOSIS

Antiphospholipid syndrome, SLE, lupus, Churg-Strauss syndrome, cirrhosis, glomerulonephritis, Goodpasture syndrome, hemolytic uremic syndrome, hepatitis, lymphoma, sarcoidosis, Waldenström's hypergammaglobulinemia

WORKUP

History and physical examination; laboratory tests; imaging tests depending on patients' presentations

LABORATORY TESTS

- Serum cryoglobulins, rheumatoid factor, serum complement, hepatitis C titers, urinalysis, CBC, ALT, AST, BUN, creatinine
- Electromyogram/nerve conduction studies may demonstrate axonal changes and distal muscle denervation
- Sural nerve and skin biopsy

IMAGING STUDIES

Chest x-ray for pulmonary involvement, CT to study for malignancy, and angiography for vasculitis

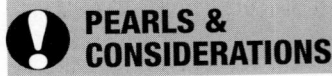 TREATMENT

- Immunosuppressive therapies such as corticosteroids are the mainstay treatment for mixed cryoglobulinemia.
- In patients with HCV, IFN-α can be added. The treatment of HCV-related mixed cryoglobulinemia is difficult due to the multifactorial origin and polymorphism of the syndrome. Therapy is aimed at eradicating the HCV infection, suppressing B-cell clonal expansion and cryoglobulin production and ameliorating symptoms
- Combination of pegylated IFN-α with ribavirin results in 77% remission.
- Variable success rate with plasma exchange, intravenous immunoglobulin, and anti-CD20 (rituximab) treatments

NONPHARMACOLOGIC THERAPY

Avoidance of cold exposure

ACUTE GENERAL Rx

NSAIDs in those with general fatigue and arthralgia; see "Treatment" for further management

DISPOSITION

Overall prognosis is worse with concomitant renal disease. Mean survival rate is ~50% at 10 yr.

REFERRAL

Consider referring to a nephrologist if there is renal involvement; hematologist in those with lymphoproliferative disorders; gastroenterologist/hepatologist in hepatitis; rheumatologist in connective tissue disease cases; and consider clinical immunologist in severe cases.

PEARLS & CONSIDERATIONS

COMMENTS

Always look for underlying causes for cryoglobulinemia.

PREVENTION

Avoidance of cold exposure, avoidance of late complications

PATIENT/FAMILY EDUCATION

Inform patients about early signs/symptoms of cryoglobulinemia so that treatments can be rendered before the development of complications.

SUGGESTED READINGS
available at www.expertconsult.com

AUTHOR: **QUANG P. LE, M.D., M.P.H.**

BASIC INFORMATION

DEFINITION

Cryptococcosis is an infection caused by the fungal organism *Cryptococcus neoformans*.

SYNONYMS

C. neoformans var. *neoformans* infection
C. neoformans var. *gatti* infection
C. neoformans var. *grubii* infection

ICD-9CM CODES
117.5 Cryptococcosis

EPIDEMIOLOGY & DEMOGRAPHICS

INCIDENCE (IN U.S.)
- 0.8 cases/million persons/year
- 6% to 7% in HIV-infected persons with AIDS

PEAK INCIDENCE: 20 to 40 yr (parallel to AIDS epidemic)

PREDOMINANT SEX: Equal sex distribution when corrected for HIV status

PREDOMINANT AGE: Less than 2 yr of age; 20 to 40 yr of age

NEONATAL INFECTION: Very uncommon

PHYSICAL FINDINGS & CLINICAL PRESENTATION

- More than 90% present with meningitis; almost all have fever and headache.
- Meningismus, photophobia, mental status changes are seen in approximately 25%.
- Increased intracranial pressure.
- Most common infections outside the CNS:
  1. In the lungs (fever, cough, dyspnea)
  2. In the skin (cellulitis, papular eruption)
  3. In the lymph nodes (lymphadenitis)
  4. Potential involvement of virtually any organ

ETIOLOGY

- Caused by the fungal organism *C. neoformans*

There are 3 varieties of *Cryptococcus spp.* and 4 capsular serotypes: Serotype A is *Cryptococcus neoformans* var. *grubii* and Serotype D is known as *Cryptococcus neoformans* var. *neoformans*. Both cause disease primarily in immunocompromised patients. Serotype B and C are known as *C. neoformans* var. *gatti*. This organism causes disease primarily in normal hosts.

- Infection originates by inhalation into the respiratory tract followed by dissemination to the CNS in most cases, usually without recognizable lung involvement
- Almost always in the setting of AIDS or other disorders of cellular immune function
- Neutropenia alone poses a much lower risk of significant cryptococcal infection

DIAGNOSIS

DIFFERENTIAL DIAGNOSIS

- Subacute meningitis (caused by *Listeria monocytogenes*, *Mycobacterium tuberculosis*, *Histoplasma capsulatum*, viruses)

- Intracranial mass lesion (neoplasms, toxoplasmosis, TB)
- Pulmonary involvement confused with *Pneumocystis jiroveci* pneumonia when diffuse or confused with TB or bacterial pneumonia when focal or involving the pleura
- Skin lesions confused with bacterial cellulitis or molluscum contagiosum

WORKUP

- Lumbar puncture to exclude cryptococcal meningitis.
- CT scan of the head when focal lesion or increased intracranial pressure is suspected.
- Biopsy of enlarged lymph nodes and skin lesions if feasible.

LABORATORY TESTS

- Culture and India ink stain (60% to 80% sensitive in culture-proven cases [Fig. 1-250]) examination of the CSF in all cases when CNS involvement is suspected
- Blood and serum cryptococcal antigen assay (>90% sensitivity and specificity)
- Culture and histologic examination of biopsy material

IMAGING STUDIES

- CT scan or MRI of the head if focal neurologic involvement is suspected
- Chest x-ray examination to exclude pulmonary involvement

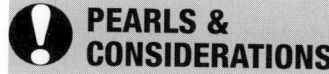 TREATMENT

ACUTE GENERAL Rx

- Induction therapy for CNS disease (meningitis) is initiated with IV amphotericin B (0.5 to 0.8 mg/kg/day) with flucytosine 37.5 mg/kg PO q6h until afebrile and cultures negative (≈6 wk), then stop amphotericin B/flucytosine and start fluconazole 200 mg PO q24h or fluconazole 400 mg PO q24h for 8-10 wk or longer (up to 2 yr) to reduce relapse rate.
- Alternative: IV fluconazole for initial therapy in patients unable to tolerate amphotericin B.

- If symptomatic increased intracranial pressure, consider multiple therapeutic lumbar taps or intraventricular shunt.

CHRONIC Rx

- Fluconazole (200 to 400 mg PO qd) is highly effective in preventing a relapse in HIV-infected patients; development of resistance may occur. Itraconazole is an alternative agent.
- Immune reconstitution syndrome following the institution of HAART can cause transient worsening of meningitis and necessitate the use of a short course of corticosteroids.

DISPOSITION

Without maintenance therapy, relapse rate is >50% among AIDS patients.

REFERRAL

- For consultation with infectious diseases specialist in all cases
- For neurologic consultation if level of consciousness is depressed or focal lesion is present

PEARLS & CONSIDERATIONS

Cryptococcal meningitis can be remarkably insidious in nonimmunocompromised patients.

COMMENTS

Cryptococcosis is considered an AIDS-defining infection; thus all patients should be HIV tested.

SUGGESTED READINGS
available at www.expertconsult.com

RELATED CONTENT
Cryptococcosis (Patient Information)

AUTHORS: **PHILIP A. CHAN, M.D., M.S.**, and **GLENN G. FORT, M.D., M.P.H.**

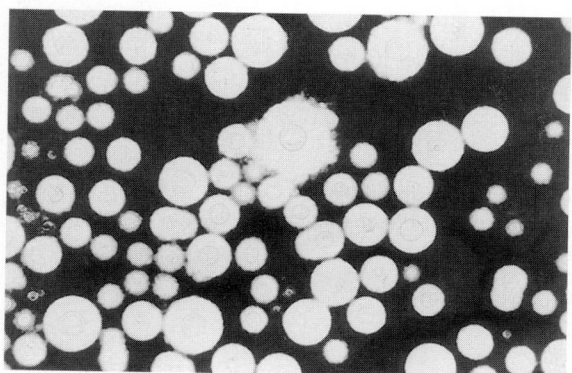

FIGURE 1-250 India ink preparation of cerebrospinal fluid revealing encapsulated cryptococci. Note the large capsules surrounding the smaller organisms. (From Andreoli TE [ed]: *Cecil essentials of medicine*, ed 4, Philadelphia, 1997, Saunders.)

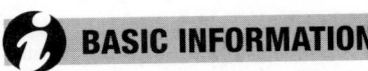

DEFINITION

The intracellular protozoan parasite *Cryptosporidium parvum* is associated with gastrointestinal disease and diarrhea, especially in AIDS patients or immunocompromised hosts. It is also associated with sporadic infections and waterborne outbreaks in immunocompetent hosts.

Other species, including *C. hominis, C. felis, C. muris,* and *C. meleagridis,* are now described to be pathogens as well.

SYNONYMS

Cryptosporidiosis

ICD-9CM CODES

007.4 Cryptosporidia infection

EPIDEMIOLOGY & DEMOGRAPHICS

INCIDENCE (IN U.S.):
- Approximately 2% in industrial countries, 5% to 10% in developing countries
- 10% to 20% of HIV patients in U.S. may excrete cyst

PREVALENCE: Worldwide, especially third world countries; associated with poor hygiene as a waterborne pathogen

PREDOMINANT SEX: Male = female

TRANSMISSION:
- Person to person (daycare, family members)
- Animal to person (pets, farm animals)
- Environmental (water-associated outbreaks, including travel associated with swimming in or drinking contaminated water or eating contaminated food)
- May be significant pathogen causing diarrhea in AIDS

PHYSICAL FINDINGS & CLINICAL PRESENTATION

- Spectrum of illness ranging from asymptomatic to severe enteritis
- Usually limited to gastrointestinal tract
- Diarrhea, severe abdominal pain (2 to 28 days)
- Impaired digestion, dehydration
- Fever, malaise, fatigue, nausea, vomiting
- Pneumonia if aspirated

ETIOLOGY

Cryptosporidium hominis, C. parvum, C. felis, C. muris, C. meleagridis

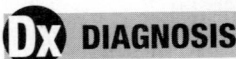
DIAGNOSIS

Clinical presentation of acute gastrointestinal illness, especially associated with HIV or with travel and waterborne outbreaks.

DIFFERENTIAL DIAGNOSIS

- *Campylobacter*
- *Clostridium difficile*
- *Entamoeba histolytica*
- *Giardia lamblia*
- *Salmonella*
- *Shigella*
- Microsporidia
- Cytomegalovirus
- *Mycobacterium avium*

Disease may cause cholecystitis, reactive arthritis, hepatitis, pancreatitis, pneumonia in immunocompromised or HIV-infected patients.

WORKUP

- Stool evaluation looking for characteristic oocyst by modified acid-fast stain (Fig. 1-252).
- Direct immunofluorescence using monoclonal antibodies is the gold standard for stool exams.

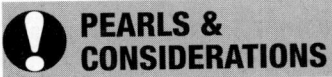
TREATMENT

- May be self-limited in normal host over several weeks. Antidiarrhea agents Pepto-Bismol, Kaopectate, or loperamide may give symptomatic relief.
- Pharmacologic treatment with antibiotics has been largely unsatisfactory in AIDS patients. Antiviral therapy is the treatment of choice to restore the immune system. Oocyst excretion reduction has been shown with nitazoxanide 500 mg PO bid for 3 days in immunocompetent patients. If treatment fails, consider a trial of paromomycin, metronidazole, or trimethoprim/sulfamethoxazole. However, these medications have not been approved for treatment of *Cryptosporidium*.
- Nitazoxanide elixir has been approved for the treatment of cryptosporidiosis in children ages 1 to 11 yr.
- Biliary cryptosporidiosis can be treated with antiretroviral therapy in the HIV setting.

DISPOSITION

- A self-limited disease in immunocompetent patients with complete recovery over 2 to 3 weeks.
- Chronic arthralgia, headache, malaise, and weakness may persist after cryptosporidial infection even in immunologically normal people.
- If severe and prolonged disease (>30 days), testing for HIV and other immunocompromised states is appropriate along with a referral to an infectious disease specialist or gastroenterologist.

REFERRAL

- To an infectious disease specialist if symptoms persist and if HIV infection is found
- To a gastroenterologist if chronic malabsorption, or biliary or pancreatic complications occur

PEARLS & CONSIDERATIONS

- Chronic cryptosporidiosis (>30 days of diarrhea from *Cryptosporidium* spp. infection) in a patient with HIV is an AIDS-qualifying opportunistic infection.
- *Cryptosporidium hominis* has a limited host range (humans), whereas *Cryptosporidium parvum* has a wide host range including humans, horses, cattle, other domesticated animals, and wild animals; both species present a similar illness in humans.

SUGGESTED READINGS

available at www.expertconsult.com

AUTHORS: **PHILIP A. CHAN, M.D., M.S.,** and **GLENN G. FORT, M.D., M.P.H.**

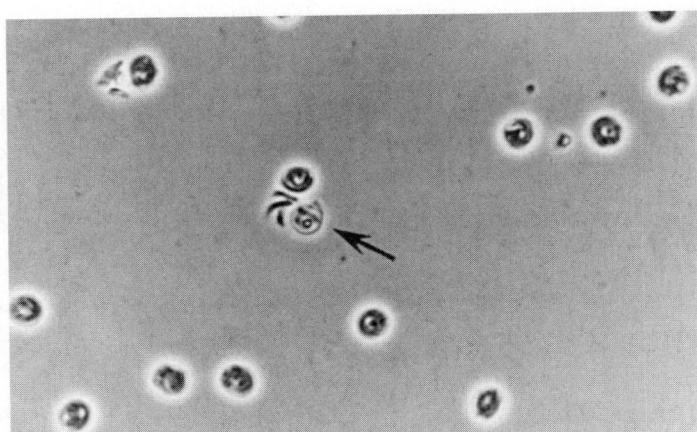

FIGURE 1-252 Human stool-derived *Cryptosporidium* oocysts. Excysting oocyst *(arrow)* is releasing three of its four sporozoites. (Phase-control microscopy ×630.) (From Gorbach SL: *Infectious diseases,* ed 2, Philadelphia, 1998, Saunders.)

BASIC INFORMATION

DEFINITION

Cubital Tunnel Syndrome is a compression neuropathy of the ulnar nerve as it traverses the cubital tunnel at the elbow (Fig. 1-253). It is the second most common entrapment neuropathy of the upper extremity.

ICD-9CM CODES
354.2 Cubital tunnel syndrome

EPIDEMIOLOGY & DEMOGRAPHICS

Males and females equally affected

PHYSICAL FINDINGS & CLINICAL PRESENTATION

- Paresthesias, numbness along distribution of ulnar nerve (little finger and medial half of ring finger); pain is less common
- Positive Tinel's sign at elbow over the ulnar groove—highest negative predictive value
- Positive elbow flexion test (flexion of elbow with wrist extended for 30 sec may reproduce symptoms)
- Pressure provocation test (direct pressure over cubital tunnel for 60 sec elicits symptoms)
- "Scratch collapse" test—positive if temporary loss of external rotation resistance after examiner scratches over the compressed ulnar nerve; due to allodynia
- Signs of old trauma or elbow instability (valgus stress)
- Ulnar nerve may be subluxable over medial epicondyle with elbow motion
- Weakness/atrophy of intrinsic musculature of hand in longstanding cases (Fig. 1-254)
- "Intrinsic minus" or claw hand; due to paralysis of lumbricals and interossei (clawing usually worse in ring and small fingers)

- Masse's sign—hand appears flattened due to hypothenar muscle paralysis
- Wartenberg's sign—due to weakness of interossei: weak adduction of small finger
- Froment's sign—compensation by thumb flexor (flexor pollicis longus, median-nerve innervated) for diminished thumb pinch strength (paralysis of adductor pollicis, which is innervated by ulnar nerve)

ETIOLOGY

- Previous trauma, fractures
- Chronic pressure over ulnar groove from occupational stress, unusual elbow positioning
- Cubitus valgus deformity
- Subluxation of ulnar nerve
- Repeated stretching during throwing motion
- Elbow synovitis, osteophytes
- Local muscular hypertrophy
- Increased cubital tunnel pressure, particularly in elbow flexion
- Symptoms develop due to local nerve ischemia

DIAGNOSIS

DIFFERENTIAL DIAGNOSIS

- Tardy ulnar palsy
- Medial epicondylitis
- Other peripheral neuropathies
- Carpal tunnel syndrome
- Cervical radiculopathy
- Ulnar nerve compression at wrist (Guyon's canal)

WORKUP

Diagnosis can usually be established clinically. Provocative tests have either inadequate or inconsistent sensitivity and specificity. These tests are operator dependent and may have substantial inter-rater variation.

IMAGING STUDIES

- Routine roentgenograms may be helpful in ruling out other conditions.

- Electrodiagnostic studies: nerve conduction tests and electromyography are useful to confirm the clinical diagnosis and can help localize site of compression.
- High-resolution ultrasound may be a valuable adjunct to diagnosis.
- On ultrasound, there was strong correlation found between greater ulnar nerve cross-sectional area at the elbow and presence of cubital tunnel syndrome, using electrodiagnostic criteria as the reference standard.

TREATMENT

ACUTE GENERAL Rx

- Activity modification, avoiding prolonged/repetitive flexion
- Elbow pads to relieve pressure, splints limiting flexion
- Physical therapy

DISPOSITION

- There is tendency toward spontaneous recovery with mild/moderate or intermittent symptoms if provocative causes are avoided.
- If muscle atrophy has developed, recovery of strength may be incomplete despite treatment.

REFERRAL

Surgical referral needed in cases of failed medical management. Patients with constant symptoms or muscle atrophy usually require surgical treatment.

PEARLS & CONSIDERATIONS

Patients with cubital tunnel syndrome are 4 times more likely to present with atrophy than those with carpal tunnel syndrome. Surgical decompression has been shown to be successful and may be adequate in most cases. More recently, endoscopic decompression techniques have been described. Ulnar nerve transposition and medial epicondylectomy are other surgical options.

SUGGESTED READINGS
available at www.expertconsult.com

RELATED CONTENT
Cubital Tunnel Syndrome (Patient Information)

AUTHOR: **CANDICE YUVIENCO, M.D.**

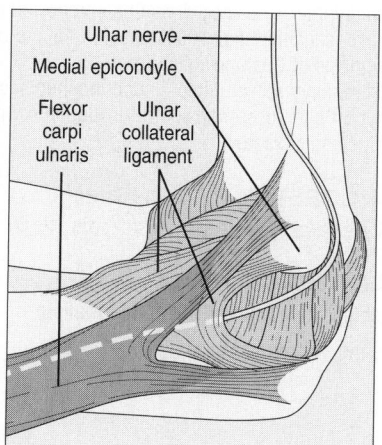

FIGURE 1-253 The cubital tunnel. The fibro-osseous canal is formed by the medial epicondyle, ulnar collateral ligament, and flexor carpi ulnaris muscle. Elbow flexion decreases the volume of the channel. (From Hochberg MC et al: *Rheumatology*, ed 5, St Louis, 2011, Mosby.)

Labels: Ulnar nerve; Medial epicondyle; Flexor carpi ulnaris; Ulnar collateral ligament

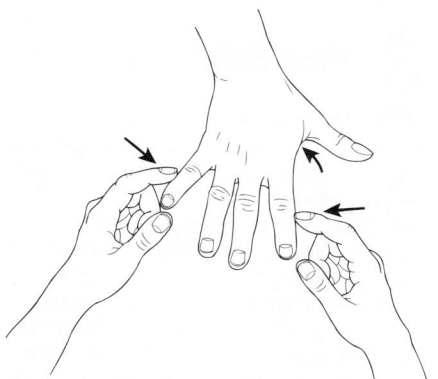

FIGURE 1-254 Testing for intrinsic (ulnar) motor weakness (fanning the fingers against resistance). Always look for atrophy of the first dorsal interosseus *(curved arrow)* when ulnar nerve lesions are suspected. (From Mercier LR: *Practical orthopedics*, ed 5, St Louis, 2000, Mosby.)

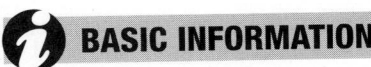

BASIC INFORMATION

DEFINITION

- Cushing's syndrome is the occurrence of clinical abnormalities associated with glucocorticoid excess as a result of exaggerated adrenal cortisol production or long-term glucocorticoid therapy.
- Cushing's disease is Cushing's syndrome caused by pituitary adrenocorticotropic hormone (ACTH) excess.

ICD-9CM CODES
255.0 Cushing's disease or syndrome

PHYSICAL FINDINGS & CLINICAL PRESENTATION

- Hypertension
- Central obesity with rounding of the facies (moon facies); thin extremities
- Hirsutism, menstrual irregularities, hypogonadism
- Skin fragility, ecchymoses, red-purple abdominal striae (Fig. E1-255), acne, poor wound healing, hair loss, facial plethora, hyperpigmentation (with ACTH excess)
- Psychosis, emotional lability, paranoia
- Muscle wasting with proximal myopathy

NOTE: The previous characteristics are not commonly present in Cushing's syndrome caused by ectopic ACTH production. Many of these tumors secrete a biologically inactive ACTH that does not activate adrenal steroid synthesis. These patients may have only weight loss and weakness.

ETIOLOGY

- Iatrogenic from long-term glucocorticoid therapy (common)
- Pituitary ACTH excess (Cushing's disease; 60%)
- Adrenal neoplasms (30%)
- Ectopic ACTH production (neoplasms of lung, pancreas, kidney, thyroid, thymus; 10%)

DIAGNOSIS

DIFFERENTIAL DIAGNOSIS

- Alcoholic pseudo-Cushing's syndrome (endogenous cortisol overproduction)
- Obesity associated with diabetes mellitus
- Adrenogenital syndrome

WORKUP

- In patients with a clinical diagnosis of Cushing's syndrome the initial screening test is the overnight dexamethasone suppression test (Fig. E1-256):
  1. Dexamethasone 1 mg PO given at 11 PM
  2. Plasma cortisol level measured 9 hr later (8 AM)
  3. Plasma cortisol level <5 mcg/100 ml excludes Cushing's syndrome
- Serial measurements (two or three consecutive measurements) of 24-hr urinary free cortisol and creatinine (to ensure adequacy of collection) are undertaken if overnight dexamethasone test is suggestive of Cushing's syndrome. Persistent elevated cortisol excretion (>300 mcg/24 hr) indicates Cushing's syndrome.
- The low-dose (2 mg) dexamethasone suppression test is useful to exclude pseudo-Cushing's syndrome if the previous results are equivocal. Corticotropic-releasing hormone (CRH) stimulation after low-dose dexamethasone administration (dexamethasone-CRH test) is also used to distinguish patients with suspected Cushing's syndrome from those who have mildly elevated urinary free cortisol level and equivocal findings.
- The high-dose (8 mg) dexamethasone test and measurement of ACTH by radioimmunoassay are useful to determine the etiology of Cushing's syndrome.
  1. ACTH undetectable or decreased and lack of suppression indicate adrenal cause of Cushing's syndrome.
  2. ACTH normal or increased and lack of suppression indicate ectopic ACTH production.
  3. ACTH normal or increased and partial suppression suggest pituitary excess (Cushing's disease).

Bilateral inferior petrosal sinus sampling (BIPSS) can be used to distinguish pituitary Cushing's disease from the ectopic ACTH syndrome.

LABORATORY TESTS

- Hypokalemia, hypochloremia, metabolic alkalosis, hyperglycemia, hypercholesterolemia
- Increased 24-hr urinary free cortisol (>100 mcg/24 hr)

IMAGING STUDIES

- CT scan or MRI of adrenal glands in suspected adrenal Cushing's syndrome
- MRI of pituitary gland with gadolinium is the preferred procedure for localizing a pituitary edema in suspected pituitary Cushing's syndrome
- Additional imaging studies to localize neoplasms of the lung, pancreas, kidney, thyroid, or thymus in patients with ectopic ACTH production

TREATMENT

GENERAL Rx

The definitive treatment of Cushing's syndrome is surgical removal of the tumor causing excessive production of cortisol:

- Pituitary adenoma: transsphenoidal microadenomectomy is the therapy of choice in adults. Pituitary irradiation is reserved for patients not cured by transsphenoidal surgery. In children, pituitary irradiation may be considered as initial therapy because 85% of children are cured by radiation. Stereotactic radiotherapy (photon knife or gamma knife) is effective and exposes the surrounding neuronal tissues to less irradiation than conventional radiotherapy. Total bilateral adrenalectomy is reserved for patients not cured by transsphenoidal surgery or pituitary irradiation.
- Adrenal neoplasm:
  1. Surgical resection of the affected adrenal
  2. Glucocorticoid replacement for approximately 9 to 12 mo after the surgery to allow time for the contralateral adrenal gland to recover from its prolonged suppression
  3. In nonsurgical candidates, suppression of adrenal steroid production can be accomplished with ketoconazole. Mifepristone, an antiprogestin, can also be used for control of hyperglycemia secondary to hypercortisolism in adults with endogenous Cushing's syndrome. It should be avoided in women who are or who could become pregnant.
- Bilateral micronodular or macronodular adrenal hyperplasia: bilateral total adrenalectomy
- Ectopic ACTH:
  1. Surgical resection of the ACTH-secreting neoplasm
  2. Control of cortisol excess with metyrapone, aminoglutethimide, mifepristone, or ketoconazole
  3. Control of the mineralocorticoid effects of cortisol and 11-deoxycorticosteroid with spironolactone
  4. Bilateral adrenalectomy: a rational approach to patients with indolent, unresectable tumors

DISPOSITION

Prognosis is favorable in patients with surgically amenable disease.

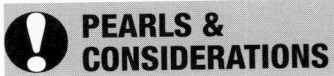

PEARLS & CONSIDERATIONS

COMMENTS

- A single midnight serum cortisol level (normal diurnal variation leads to a nadir around midnight) >7.5 mcg/dl has been reported as 96% sensitive and 100% specific for the diagnosis of Cushing's syndrome.
- Screening for multiple endocrine neoplasia type I should be considered in patients with Cushing's disease.

SUGGESTED READING
available at www.expertconsult.com

RELATED CONTENT
Cushing's Syndrome (Patient Information)

AUTHOR: **FRED F. FERRI, M.D.**

BASIC INFORMATION

DEFINITION
Cystic fibrosis (CF) is an autosomal recessive disorder characterized by dysfunction of exocrine glands.

ICD-9CM CODES
277.0 Cystic fibrosis

EPIDEMIOLOGY & DEMOGRAPHICS
- CF is the most common fatal hereditary disorder of whites in the U.S. (one case per 2500 whites) and second most common life-shortening childhood-onset inherited disorder in the U.S., behind sickle cell disease.
- Median age at diagnosis is 5.3 mo. Median survival is 30 yr.
- Carrier screening is associated with a decrease in incidence of CF.

PHYSICAL FINDINGS & CLINICAL PRESENTATION
- Failure to thrive in children
- Increased anterior/posterior chest diameter
- Basilar crackles and hyperresonance to percussion
- Digital clubbing
- Chronic cough
- Abdominal distention
- Greasy, smelly feces

ETIOLOGY
Chromosome 7 gene mutation (*CFTR* gene) resulting in abnormalities in chloride transport and water flux across the surface of epithelial cells; the abnormal secretions cause obstruction of glands and ducts in various organs and subsequent damage to exocrine tissue (recurrent pneumonia, atelectasis, bronchiectasis, diabetes mellitus, biliary cirrhosis, cholelithiasis, intestinal obstruction, increased risk of gastrointestinal malignancies).

TABLE 1-119 Diagnostic Criteria for Cystic Fibrosis (CF)

Presence of typical clinical features (respiratory, gastrointestinal, or genitourinary)
OR
A history of CF in a sibling
OR
A positive newborn screening test
PLUS
Laboratory evidence for CFTR (CF transmembrane regulator) dysfunction:
  Two elevated sweat chloride concentrations obtained on separate days
  OR
  Identification of two CF mutations
  OR
  An abnormal nasal potential difference measurement

From Kliegman RM et al: *Nelson textbook of pediatrics,* ed 19, Philadelphia, 2011, Saunders.

DIAGNOSIS

DIFFERENTIAL DIAGNOSIS
- Immunodeficiency states
- Celiac disease
- Asthma
- Recurrent pneumonia

WORKUP
A diagnosis of CF requires a positive quantitative pilocarpine iontophoresis test with one or more phenotypic features consistent with CF (e.g., chronic suppurative obstructive lung disease, pancreatic insufficiency) or documented CF in a sibling or first cousin. Table 1-119 describes diagnostic criteria for CF. Conditions suggesting the diagnosis of CF in adults and recommended diagnostic studies are described in Table 1-120.

LABORATORY TESTS
- Pilocarpine iontophoresis (sweat test): diagnostic of CF in children if sweat chloride is >60 mmol/L (>80 mmol/L in adults) on two separate tests on consecutive days. Repeat testing may be necessary because not all infants have sufficient quantities of sweat for reliable testing. Table 1-121 describes conditions associated with false-positive and false-negative sweat test results.
- DNA testing may be useful for confirming the diagnosis and providing genetic information for family members.
- Sputum culture and sensitivity and Gram stain (frequent bacterial infections with *Staphylococcus aureus, Pseudomonas aeruginosa* [most common virulent respiratory pathogen], *Haemophilus influenzae*). Bronchoalveolar lavage (BAL) is used at times to aid in the early diagnosis of pulmonary infection in non-expectorating patients. However, evidence for its

TABLE 1-120 Approach to Diagnosis of Cystic Fibrosis in Adult Patients

Conditions Suggesting the Diagnosis of Cystic Fibrosis in Adults
Recurrent pancreatitis
Male infertility
Chronic sinusitis
Nasal polyposis
Nontuberculous mycobacterial infection
Allergic bronchopulmonary mycosis
Bronchiectasis

Recommended Diagnostic Studies
Sweat electrolyte determination
Extended CFTR mutation analysis
Nasal potential difference
High-resolution CT scan to identify bronchiectasis
CT scan of sinuses for polyposis
Sputum induction or bronchoalveolar lavage to identify bacterial and fungal pathogens

CFTR, Cystic fibrosis transmembrane conductance regulator; *CT,* computed tomography.
From Goldman L, Schafer AI: *Goldman's Cecil medicine,* ed 24, Philadelphia, 2012, Saunders.

clinical benefit is lacking. Trials have shown that among infants diagnosed with CF, BAL-directed therapy did not result in a lower prevalence of *P. aeruginosa* infection or lower total CF-CT score when compared with standard therapy at age 5 years.
- Low albumin level, increased 72-hr fecal fat excretion.
- Pulse oximetry or arterial blood gases: hypoxemia.
- Pulmonary function studies: decreased total lung capacity, forced vital capacity, pulmonary diffusing capacity.

IMAGING STUDIES
- Chest x-ray (Fig. 1-258): may reveal focal atelectasis, peribronchial cuffing, bronchiectasis, increased interstitial markings, hyperinflation
- High-resolution chest CT scan: bronchial wall thickening, cystic lesions, ring shadows (bronchiectasis)

TREATMENT

NONPHARMACOLOGIC THERAPY
- Postural drainage and chest percussion

TABLE 1-121 Conditions Associated with False-Positive and False-Negative Sweat Test Results

With False-Positive Results
Eczema (atopic dermatitis)
Ectodermal dysplasia
Malnutrition/failure to thrive/deprivation
Anorexia nervosa
Congenital adrenal hyperplasia
Adrenal insufficiency
Glucose-6-phosphatase deficiency
Mauriac syndrome
Fucosidosis
Familial hypoparathyroidism
Hypothyroidism
Nephrogenic diabetes insipidus
Pseudohypoaldosteronism
Klinefelter syndrome
Familial cholestasis syndrome
Autonomic dysfunction
Prostaglandin E infusions
Munchausen syndrome by proxy

With False-Negative Results
Dilution
Malnutrition
Edema
Insufficient sweat quantity
Hyponatremia
Cystic fibrosis transmembrane conductance regulator (CFTR) mutations with preserved sweat duct function

From Kliegman RM et al: *Nelson textbook of pediatrics,* ed 19, Philadelphia, 2011, Saunders.

- Encouragement of regular exercise and proper nutrition
- Psychosocial evaluation and counseling of patient and family members

ACUTE GENERAL Rx

- Antibiotic therapy based on results of Gram stain and culture and sensitivity of sputum (PO quinolones for *Pseudomonas,* cephalosporins for *S. aureus,* IV aminoglycosides [tobramycin] plus ceftazidime or ticarcillin for life-threatening *Pseudomonas* infections). Inhaled antibiotics (aztreonam or tobramycin) can also be used and can achieve high airway concentration with lower systemic side effects. Macrolides are also active against *Pseudomonas aeruginosa.* For *S. aureus* infection, use oxacillin or nafcillin 2 g IV p4h if MSSA; if dealing with MRSA, use IV vancomycin 1 g q12h. A recent study using azithromycin maintenance in children with CF for 6 mo found less use of additional antibiotics and improvement in some aspects of pulmonary function. Additional studies may be necessary to determine if azithromycin should be used as a primary therapy or rescue treatment.
- Bronchodilators for patients with airflow obstruction.
- Long-term pancreatic enzyme replacement.
- Alternate-day prednisone (2 mg/kg) possibly beneficial in children with CF (decreased hospitalization rate, improved pulmonary function); routine use of corticosteroids not rec-ommended in adults; among children with CF who have received alternate-day treatment with prednisone, boys, but not girls, have persistent growth impairment after treatment is discontinued.
- Proper nutrition and vitamin supplementation.
- Recombinant human deoxyribonuclease (DNase [Dornase alpha]) 2.5 mg qd or bid given by aerosol for patients with viscid sputum. It lowers the viscosity of sputum. It is useful to improve mucociliary clearance by liquefying difficult-to-clear pulmonary secretions. It is, however, very expensive (annual cost to the pharmacist is >$10,000); most beneficial in patients with forced vital capacity values >40% of predicted. Its cost can be decreased by using alternate-day rhDNase therapy.
- Intermittent administration of inhaled tobramycin has been reported beneficial in CF.
- Newer treatment modalities involve increasing the activity of CF transmembrane conductance regulator (CFTR) protein. Ivacaftor (a CFTR potentiator) is FDA approved for oral treatment of CF in patients 6 years and older with the G551D mutation (5% of patients with CF). It can decrease the frequency of pulmonary exacerbations and improve lung function. Dose is 150 mg PO BID. Cost is more than $250,000/year.
- Treatment of impaired glucose tolerance and diabetes mellitus.

CHRONIC Rx

Pneumococcal and influenza vaccination

DISPOSITION

- More than 50% of children with CF live beyond age 20 yr. During the past 2 decades, survival among patients with late-stage CF has lengthened substantially. This is believed due to increased use of NBH DNase.
- Lung transplantation is the only definitive treatment; 3-yr survival after transplantation exceeds 50%.
- Obstructive azoospermia is present in >98% of postpubertal males.
- The SERPINA Z allele is a risk factor for liver disease in CF. Patients that carry the Z allele are at a greater risk of developing severe liver disease with portal hypertension.

REFERRAL

- For lung transplantation in selected patients. Indications for lung transplantation are FEV$_1$ <30% of predicted, rapidly progressive respiratory deterioration, increasing number of hospital admissions, massive hemoptysis, recurrent pneumothorax, arterial partial pressure of oxygen <55 mm Hg, arterial partial pressure of carbon dioxide >50 mm Hg, multiresistant organisms, wasting. Young female patients should be referred earlier because of overall poor prognosis.
- For screening of family members with DNA analysis.

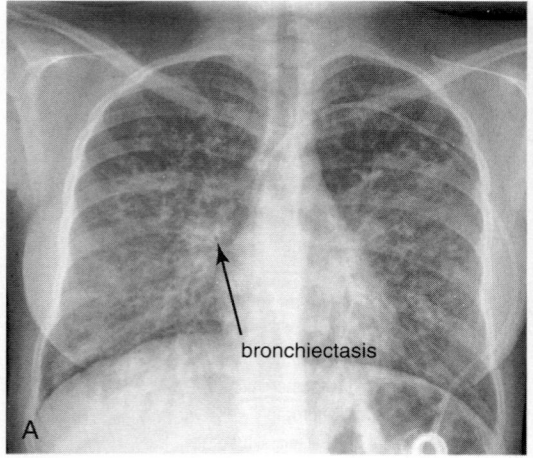
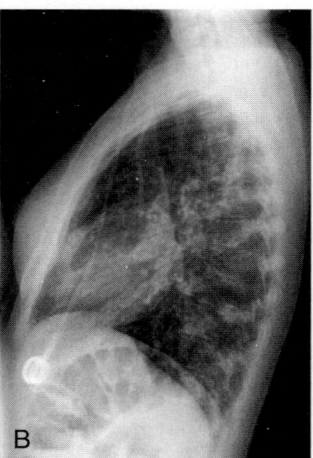
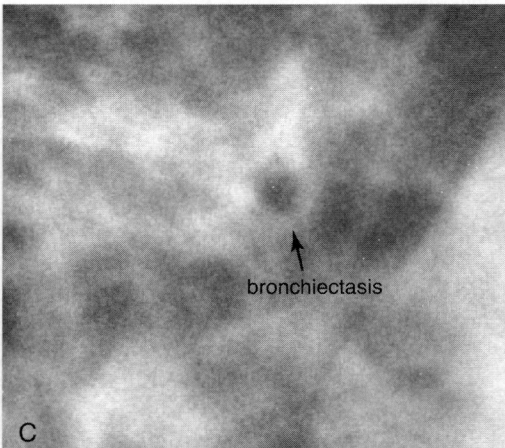

FIGURE 1-258 Cystic fibrosis. Cystic fibrosis is aptly named. Chest x-ray findings include increased interstitial density of fibrosis and cystic changes of lung parenchyma similar to chronic obstructive pulmonary disease. Bronchiectasis (dilation of bronchi, potentially erodmg into bronchial arteries and presenting with hemoptysis) may be visible on chest x-ray as large and thickened bronchioles particularly when viewed in short axis (when bronchioles are oriented perpendicular to the frontal plane). This l5-year-old with cystic fibrosis presented with cough and dyspnea. Does she have pneumonia? Comparison with prior x-rays showed no changes. **A,** Posterior-anterior chest x-ray. **B,** Lateral chest x-ray. **C,** Close-up from **A** showing bronchiectasis. (From Broder JS: *Diagnostic imaging for the emergency physician,* Philadelphia, 2011, Saunders.)

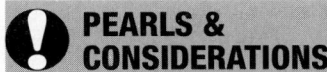

PEARLS & CONSIDERATIONS

COMMENTS

- Clinicians should think of CF in any patient with bronchiectasis plus any of the following: male infertility, recurrent idiopathic pancreatitis, recurrent nasal polyposis.
- Genetic testing for CF should be offered to adults with a positive family history of CF, couples currently planning a pregnancy, and couples seeking prenatal care.
- Inhalation of hypertonic saline (5 mL of 7% sodium chloride qid) has been reported to produce a sustained acceleration of mucus clearance and improved lung function.
- The prevalence of MRSA in the respiratory tract of individuals with CF has increased dramatically over the past decade and is associated with worse survival.

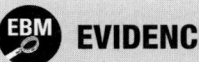 **EVIDENCE**

available at www.expertconsult.com

SUGGESTED READINGS

available at www.expertconsult.com

RELATED CONTENT

Cystic Fibrosis (Patient Information)
Bronchiectasis (Related Key Topic)

AUTHOR: **FRED F. FERRI, M.D.**

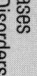

Diseases and Disorders

BASIC INFORMATION

DEFINITION
Cysticercosis is an infection caused by the tissue deposition of larval forms of the pork tapeworm *Taenia solium*. *T. solium* cysts, or cysticerci, may accumulate in any human tissue, including the eyes, spinal cord, skin, muscle, heart, and brain. Central nervous system (CNS) involvement is common and is known as neurocysticercosis. Humans most commonly acquire cysticercosis from human tapeworm carriers, or via ingestion of larval cysts in infected pork or soil tapeworm eggs in contaminated water. Larvae in the gastrointestinal tract migrate hematogenously to tissues, where they encyst, forming cysticerci.

SYNONYMS
Cysticerciasis
Taeniasis
Pork tapeworm

ICD-9CM CODES
123.1 Cysticercosis

EPIDEMIOLOGY & DEMOGRAPHICS
- *T. solium* infection is worldwide in distribution. Tapeworm infection and cysticercosis are endemic in developing countries where pigs are raised as a food source.
- Serologic studies from endemic areas of Latin America have demonstrated seroprevalences of 4% to 24% in native populations.
- Neurocysticercosis is the most common cause of acquired epilepsy worldwide and has become an important parasitic disease in the U.S., especially in states with large immigrant populations from countries where the disease is endemic.

PHYSICAL FINDINGS & CLINICAL PRESENTATION
- After ingestion of *T. solium* eggs or cysts, human beings may remain asymptomatic for years.
- The symptoms vary and depend on the location of cysticerci. Cysticerci in muscles and skin may form "cold" nodules, which are usually asymptomatic but may calcify and be seen on radiographs.
- Neurocysticercosis, or the presence of cysts within the brain parenchyma, is usually asymptomatic. Symptoms stem from inflammation associated with the degeneration of cysts.
- Seizures are the most common manifestation of neurocysticercosis, occurring in 70% to 90% of symptomatic cases. Headache is also common.
- Inflammation around degenerating cysts may result in focal encephalitis, vasculitis, chronic meningitis, and cranial nerve palsies.
- In 10% to 20% of cases of neurocysticercosis, cysts lodge within the ventricular system and result in obstructive hydrocephalus, causing acute intracranial hypertension. Symptoms are caused by the presence of the parasite itself, ependymal inflammation, and/or fibrosis, each of which block the circulation of cerebrospinal fluid (CSF). Death may occur from progressive hydrocephalus, cerebral edema, or intractable seizures.
- Ocular cysticercosis occurs in less than 5% of infections and is generally asymptomatic. Inflammation in response to degenerating cysticerci may result in chorioretinitis, vasculitis, or retinal detachment, threatening vision.

ETIOLOGY
- *T. solium* has a complex two-host life cycle.
- Human beings are the only definitive host and harbor the adult worm in the intestine (taeniasis). However, both human beings and pigs can serve as intermediate hosts and harbor the larvae or cysticerci.

DIAGNOSIS

DIFFERENTIAL DIAGNOSIS
- Idiopathic epilepsy
- Migraine
- CNS vasculitis
- Primary neoplasia of CNS
- Chronic CNS infections, including toxoplasmosis, coccidioidomycosis, tuberculosis, and cryptococcosis
- Brain abscess
- CNS involvement with sarcoidosis or systemic lupus erythematosus

WORKUP
Comprehensive clinical history: obtain information on current and previous travel and residence, including geographic area, sanitary conditions, and dietary habits, most importantly consumption of undercooked pork.

LABORATORY TESTS
- Definitive diagnosis is based on the histopathologic demonstration of cysticerci in the tissue involved.
- Peripheral eosinophilia is usually absent.
- Stool examination for ova and proglottids of *T. solium* is insensitive and not specific for the diagnosis of cysticercosis.
- CSF examination may demonstrate pleocytosis, with lymphocytic or eosinophilic predominance, low glucose, and elevated protein with neurocysticercosis. However, CSF is normal in most cases.
- Serologic testing is supportive of a suspected diagnosis of cysticercosis. An enzyme-linked immunoelectrotransfer blot (EITB) assay is the test of choice for detecting anticysticercal antibodies and can be performed on serum or CSF. This assay uses purified glycoprotein antigens and has higher sensitivity (98%) and specificity (100%) than other enzyme-linked antibody (e.g., ELISA) tests. However, the diagnostic performance of the EITB can vary in different patient populations depending on the activity of the cysts and number of lesions. Single calcified lesions are more likely to be associated with a false-negative assay result, with 38% of patients with a single brain lesion testing negative in one study. Antibodies detected by EITB can persist for years after successful therapy limiting the usefulness of this assay in following patients after treatment. In endemic regions, the test is useful in ruling out disease but is positive in a significant proportion of exposed individuals without disease.
- Antigen detection tests are also being developed. The antigen-detecting ELISA performs better for CSF samples than for serum samples, but for both specimen types it is less sensitive than the EITB assay. The antigen-detecting ELISA seems to correlate better with viable and nonviable cysts. Furthermore, high antigen levels suggest the presence of subarachnoid neurocysticercosis. This method may be particularly useful in monitoring patients following therapy. Parasite antigen levels usually fall within 3 months of successful treatment.
- More recently, amplification of *T. solium* DNA, with the method of polymerase chain reaction, has been achieved (sensitivity 96.7%).

IMAGING STUDIES
- Plain radiographs of the extremities may reveal calcified cysts in patients with soft tissue or muscle involvement.
- For diagnosis of neurocysticercosis, CT and MRI are most commonly used.
- Brain CT (Fig. 1-259) has a sensitivity and specificity of 95% and can identify living cysticerci, which appear as hypodense lesions, as well as degenerating cysts, which appear as isodense or hyperdense lesions with surrounding edema. CT is the best method for detecting calcification associated with prior infection, which suggests inactivity.
- Brain MRI is the most accurate technique to assess the extent of infection, location, and evolutionary stage of the parasites. MRI provides detailed images of living and degenerating cysts, perilesional edema, as well as small cysts or those located in the ventricles, brainstem, and cerebellum.

TREATMENT

ACUTE GENERAL Rx
Asymptomatic cysticercosis:
- There is no evidence that administering antiparasitic therapy is beneficial.

Symptomatic neurocysticercosis:
- Treatment decisions in neurocysticercosis should be individualized. Initial measures should focus on the symptomatic management before considering antiparasitic therapy when appropriate.
- Patients with active lesions, with evidence of surrounding edema and/or inflammation, generally warrant treatment with antiparasitics, corticosteroids, and anticonvulsants.
  - Anticonvulsant therapy:
    Patients who have seizures or are considered at risk for recurrent seizures based on imaging should be treated with anticonvulsants.
  - Antiparasitic therapy:
    Pharmacologic therapy is indicated in the treatment of symptomatic patients with multiple viable brain parenchymal cysticerci. However, despite treatment, only

C

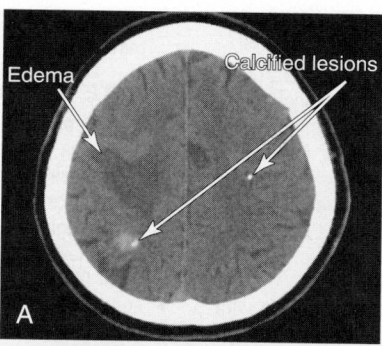

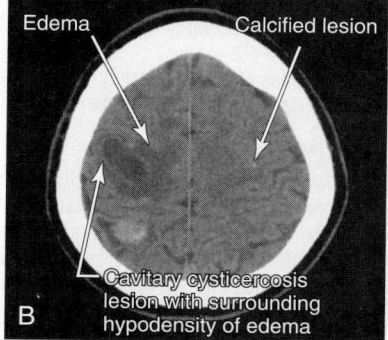
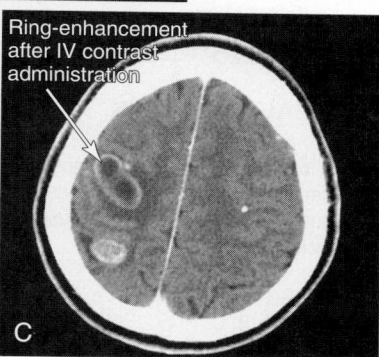

FIGURE 1-259 Neurocysticercosis. This 40-year-old Bolivian male presented with left-hand weakness. **A-B,** Noncontrast head CT, brain windows. **C,** CT with contrast moments later—compare this with image **B.** a slice through the same level of the brain before contrast administration. Hypodense lesions are present, with surrounding hypodensity *(dark gray)* representing edema. Scattered calcifications are also seen, which are a common feature of old neurocysticercosis lesions. Administration of IV contrast leads to ring enhancement, a feature of many infectious and inflammatory conditions, including neurocysticercosis, brain abscess, and toxoplasmosis. (From Broder JS: *Diagnostic imaging for the emergency physician,* Philadelphia, 2011, Saunders.)

CHRONIC Rx

- A recently published study suggests that prolonged antiparasitic therapy does not improve outcomes in patients with neurocysticercosis and seizures. Antiparasitic therapy, in fact, delayed calcification of lesions. Antiepileptic medications may need to be continued indefinitely.
- Rare patients with neurocysticercosis develop chronic or recurrent perilesional inflammation, requiring long-term, high-dose steroid therapy. Methotrexate has been reported to be of use as a steroid-sparing agent in this setting.

DISPOSITION

- In seizure-free, stable neurocysticercosis, outpatient management is appropriate.
- Patients with seizures should be restricted from driving.

REFERRAL

- Infectious diseases consultation
- Neurology consultation in patients with seizures
- Neurosurgical consultation if extraparenchymal neurocysticercosis or obstructive hydrocephalus is present

PREVENTION

- Eradication of taeniasis/cysticercosis is possible with implementation of meat inspection, improvement of pig husbandry, and improvement of socioeconomic conditions in endemic areas.
- A porcine vaccine against *T. solium* has been developed and successfully implemented in Peru, Mexico, and Australia.
- There is currently no human vaccine to prevent tapeworm infection or cysticercosis.

PATIENT & FAMILY EDUCATION

- Pork should be inspected for the presence of cysticerci, which are visible in raw meat.
- Pork must be well cooked.
- Proper disposal of human excreta and handwashing are of utmost importance to break the transmission cycle in households.

SUGGESTED READINGS
available at www.expertconsult.com

RELATED CONTENT
Cysticercosis (Patient Information)

AUTHORS: **ELENI PATROZOU, M.D.,**
and **STACI A. FISCHER, M.D.**

30% to 50% of lesions resolve within 6 months.

Calcified cysticerci are inactive and do not warrant antiparasitic treatment.

Antiparasitic therapy is often unnecessary in patients with single cysts, which are usually self-limited and resolve within 6 months.

○ Cysticidal therapy:

Antiparasitic therapy hastens the disappearance of cysts and should initially be given in conjunction with corticosteroids to control the inflammation associated with dying organisms.

Patients with viable parenchymal or subarachnoid cysts should be treated with albendazole 15 mg/kg/day PO divided BID for 7 days or praziquantel 50 mg/kg/day divided TID for 28 days. Albendazole is preferred since praziquantel management is more complicated due to an interaction with corticosteroids. Patients should be medicated with prednisolone 2 mg/kg/day or 0.15 mg/kg/day oral dexamethasone, either concurrent with albendazole, or starting albendazole on the third day of corticosteroids. Antiparasitics should be used cautiously in patients with massive cysticercal infection of the brain parenchyma (≥50 cysts) or cysticercal encephalitis. These patients should be managed initially with corticosteroids, and perhaps mannitol, to control intracranial hypertension. Once the inflammation and the edema have resolved by MRI, antiparasitics can be administered.

Praziquantel may cause drug interactions with other agents metabolized by the cytochrome p450 systems, including phenytoin and phenobarbital. Furthermore, praziquantel serum levels are decreased by concomitant use of corticosteroids.

Albendazole has no significant drug interactions with anticonvulsants.

Albendazole is considered to be the drug of choice due to slightly better efficacy, greater availability and lower cost.

The combined use of albendazole and praziquantel for neurocysticercosis has been reported.

○ Surgical therapy:

Surgery may be indicated in patients with obstructive hydrocephalus or giant cysts with associated intracranial hypertension.

Minimally invasive neurosurgery (neuroendoscopy) for cyst removal and ventricular shunt formation has greatly improved the management of intraventricular neurocysticercosis.

Extraparenchymal cysticercosis, including ocular, subarachnoid, and intraventricular disease, carries a poor prognosis and requires a more aggressive approach. When feasible, complete surgical excision of lesions remains the definitive therapy.

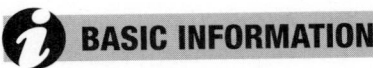
BASIC INFORMATION

DEFINITION

Infection with cytomegalovirus (CMV), a herpes virus, is common in the general population, with multiple mechanisms for transmission, often during childhood and adolescence. CMV is associated with pregnancy and can be a congenital disease. CMV is also associated with immunocompromised states and may be life threatening.

SYNONYMS

CMV
Heterophil-negative mononucleosis
Cytomegalic inclusion disease virus

ICD-9CM CODES
078.5 CMV infection
771.1 Congenital or perinatal CMV infection
V01.7 Exposure to CMV

EPIDEMIOLOGY & DEMOGRAPHICS

- Seroprevalence is widespread: 40% to 100% antibody positivity in adults.
- Increased infection develops perinatally, in day care exposure, and then during reproductive age, related to sexual activity.

ROUTES OF TRANSMISSION

- Blood transfusions
- Sexually (STDs) via uterus, cervix, and semen
- Perinatally via breast milk
- Transplant of organs—bone marrow, kidneys, liver, heart, or lung

PHYSICAL FINDINGS & CLINICAL PRESENTATION

CHILDREN: Congenital—25% of infected children with symptoms if congenital:
- Petechial rash
- Jaundice and/or hepatosplenomegaly
- Lethargy
- Respiratory distress
- CNS involvement, seizures
Postnatal acquisition:
- CMV mononucleosis
- Pharyngitis, croup, bronchitis, pneumonia
HEALTHY ADULTS:
Common
- May be asymptomatic
- CMV mononucleosis similar to EBV mononucleosis
- Fever—lasting 9 to 30 days—mean of 19 days
Less common
- Exudative pharyngitis
- Lymphadenopathy, hepatitis, splenomegaly
- Interstitial pneumonia (rare)
- Nonspecific rash
- Thrombocytopenia/hemolytic anemia
Rare
- Guillain-Barré syndrome
- Meningoencephalitis
- Myocarditis

IMMUNOSUPPRESSED PATIENTS:
- Febrile mononucleosis
- GI ulcerations, hepatitis, pneumonitis, retinitis, encephalopathy, meningoencephalopathy
- HIV associated—dementia, demyelination, retinitis, acalculous cholecystitis, adrenalitis, diarrhea, enterocolitis, esophagitis
- Diabetes associated with pancreatitis
- Adrenalitis associated with HIV

ETIOLOGY

CMV infection can remain latent, reactive with immunosuppression.

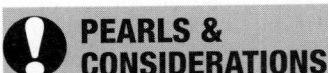
DIAGNOSIS

DIFFERENTIAL DIAGNOSIS

Congenital:
- Acute viral, bacterial, parasitic infections including other congenitally transmitted agents (toxoplasmosis, rubella, syphilis, pertussis, croup, bronchitis)
Acquired:
- EBV mononucleosis
- Viral hepatitis—A, B, C
- Cryptosporidiosis
- Toxoplasmosis
- *Mycobacterium avium* infections
- Human herpesvirus 6
- Acute HIV infection

WORKUP

- Laboratory confirmation combined with clinical findings often with leukopenia, thrombocytopenia, lymphocytosis
- Serology:
  1. Detection of CMV-IgM antibodies suggests recent infection. CMV-IgG antibodies usually appear 2 to 3 weeks after infection.
  2. Molecular amplification tests: options include PCR assays on plasma, leukocytes and whole blood, nucleic acid sequence based amplification (NASBA), and Hybrid Capture System CMV DNA test. These tests are used in immunocompromised patients, AIDS and transplant patients.
- Cultures: using human fibroblast cultures of blood, CSF, urine, BAL, and biopsy specimens but can take 1 to 6 weeks
- Funduscopic—necrotic patches with white granular component of retina
- Biopsy—"owl's eye" inclusion bodies on tissue sample

IMAGING STUDIES

- Chest radiograph—if pneumonitis suspected, consider bronchoscopy
- Endoscopy—if GI involvement
- CT scan/MRI—if CNS involvement

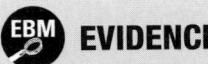
TREATMENT

NONPHARMACOLOGIC THERAPY

- Strict hand washing and standard precautions limit CMV transmission in health care facilities.
- Highly active antiretroviral therapy (HAART) in patients with CD4 count <50/mm^3 for the goal of CD4 >100/mm^3 for a 3- to 6-mo period

ACUTE GENERAL Rx

For compromised hosts with CMV retinitis or pneumonitis:
- Ganciclovir 5 mg/kg q12h IV x 14 to 21 days, then valganciclovir: 900 mg PO q24h or alternative regimen
- Ganciclovir intraocular implant plus valganciclovir 900 mg PO q24h or alternative regimen
- Foscarnet 90 mg/kg q12h x 14 to 21 days, then 90 mg to 120 mg/kg IV q24h or alternative regimen
- Cidofovir 5 mg/kg IV q day x 14 days, then 5 mg/kg IV q 2 weeks
- Fomivirsen-salvage therapy for CMV retinitis 300 µg injected into vitreous

DISPOSITION

- CMV infection in patients who are immunocompromised (especially those with AIDS, bone marrow and solid organ transplant recipients, and disorders of cell-mediated immune function) will need expert, long-term follow-up by an infectious disease specialist or immunologist familiar with the care of such patients.
- CMV mononucleosis, hepatitis, pharyngitis, etc. in immunologically normal hosts are usually self-limiting infections requiring no special follow-up plans.

REFERRAL

- To an ophthalmologist if CMV retinitis is present
- To an infectious disease specialist or AIDS specialist for patients who are HIV-positive with CMV disease
- To a cellular immunologist or transplant specialist in the case of CMV infection in a transplant recipient
- To a pediatric infectious disease specialist for congenital CMV infection

PEARLS & CONSIDERATIONS

CMV is ubiquitous in the environment and is asymptomatically shed by latently infected persons with CMV infection, making it difficult to protect patients who are immunocompromised from acquiring this infection.

EVIDENCE

available at www.expertconsult.com

SUGGESTED READINGS
available at www.expertconsult.com

AUTHOR: **GLENN G. FORT, M.D.**

BASIC INFORMATION

DEFINITION

Venous thromboembolism is any thromboembolic event occurring within the venous system. Deep vein thrombosis (DVT) is the development of thrombi in the deep veins of the extremities or pelvis.

SYNONYMS

DVT
Venous thromboembolism (VTE) (VTE includes DVT and pulmonary embolism [PE])
Deep venous thrombosis

ICD-9CM CODES
451.1   Thrombosis of deep vessels of lower extremities
451.83   Thrombosis of deep veins of upper extremities
541.9   Deep vein thrombosis of unspecified site

EPIDEMIOLOGY & DEMOGRAPHICS

- Annual incidence in urban population is 1.6 cases/1000 persons.
- The risk of recurrent thromboembolism is higher among men than women.
- About 5% to 15% of persons with untreated DVT die from pulmonary embolism.

PHYSICAL FINDINGS & CLINICAL PRESENTATION

- Pain and swelling of the affected extremity
- In lower extremity DVT: leg pain on dorsiflexion of the foot (*Homans' sign*)
- Physical examination may be unremarkable in early DVT

ETIOLOGY

The etiology is often multifactorial (prolonged stasis, coagulation abnormalities, vessel wall trauma). The following are risk factors for DVT:
- Prolonged immobilization (>3 days)
- Postoperative state
- Trauma to pelvis and lower extremities for lower extremity DVT; central line placement for upper extremity DVT
- Birth control pills, high-dose estrogen therapy; conjugated equine estrogen but not esterified estrogen is associated with increased risk of DVT; estrogen plus progestin is associated with doubling the risk of venous thrombosis. The use of bevacizumab is also significantly associated with an increased risk of developing DVT in cancer patients receiving this drug.
- Visceral cancer (lung, pancreas, alimentary tract, genitourinary tract)
- Age >60 yr
- History of thromboembolic disease
- Hematologic disorders (e.g., factor V Leiden mutation [FVL], antithrombin III deficiency, protein C deficiency, protein S deficiency, heparin cofactor II deficiency, sticky platelet syndrome, G20210A prothrombin mutation, lupus anticoagulant, dysfibrinogenemias,

anticardiolipin antibody, hyperhomocystinemia, concurrent homocystinuria, high levels of factors VIII, XI, and single nucleotide polymorphisms [SNPs] such as CYP4V2)
- Pregnancy and early puerperium
- Obesity (BMI >30)
- Congestive heart failure
- Surgery, fracture, or injury involving lower leg or pelvis
- Plaster cast immobilization
- Surgery requiring >30 min of anesthesia
- Gynecologic surgery (particularly gynecologic cancer surgery)
- Recent travel (within 2 wk, lasting ≥2 hr). Every 2 hr spent traveling increases VTE risk by 18%.
- Smoking and abdominal obesity
- Central venous catheter or pacemaker insertion
- Superficial vein thrombosis (10% risk of DVT within 3 mo), varicose veins
- Collagen vascular disease
- Nephrotic syndrome
- Myeloproliferative disorders
- Long-term exposure to particulate air pollution is also associated with altered coagulation function and DVT risk.

DIAGNOSIS

DIFFERENTIAL DIAGNOSIS

- Postphlebitic syndrome
- Superficial thrombophlebitis
- Ruptured Baker's cyst
- Cellulitis, lymphangitis, Achilles tendinitis
- Hematoma
- Muscle or soft tissue injury, stress fracture
- Varicose veins, lymphedema
- Arterial insufficiency
- Abscess
- Claudication
- Venous stasis

WORKUP

- The clinical diagnosis of DVT is inaccurate. Pain, tenderness, swelling, or color changes are not specific for DVT.

- Clinical prediction rules can be used to establish pretest probability of DVT. The Wells prediction rules for DVT and for pulmonary embolism are described in Box 1-11. These rules perform better in younger patients without a history of DVT and in those without comorbidities. In younger patients without associated comorbidities and a low pretest probability using Wells criteria and a negative high-sensitivity D-dimer test, the diagnosis of DVT can be reasonably excluded.
- Compression ultrasonography (CUS) is preferred as the initial study to diagnose DVT in patients with intermediate to high pretest probability (Fig. E1-260). An initial negative test limited to the proximal leg should be repeated after 5 days (if the clinical suspicion of DVT persists) to exclude DVT that is propagating proximally from the calf. Comprehensive ultrasonography (whole-leg CUS) is a more extensive test that examines the deep veins from the inguinal ligament to the level of the malleolus. Literature reports indicate that it may be safe to withhold anticoagulation after negative results on comprehensive duplex ultrasonography in nonpregnant patients with a suspected first episode of symptomatic DVT of the leg.

LABORATORY TESTS

- Laboratory tests are not specific for DVT. Baseline prothrombin time (INR), partial thromboplastin time, and platelet count should be obtained on all patients before starting anticoagulation. D-dimer testing is sensitive but not specific for DVT. A negative result (D-dimer <0.5 mcg/ml) can exclude the diagnosis, but a positive result (≥0.5 mcg/ml) mandates additional testing with venous ultrasonography.
- Use of D-dimer assay by ELISA is useful in the management of suspected DVT. The combination of a normal D-dimer study on presentation together with a normal compression venous ultrasound is useful to exclude DVT and generally eliminate the need to do repeat ultrasound at 5 to 7 days. Recent trials indicate that DVT can be ruled out in patients who

---

BOX 1-11 Wells Prediction Rule for Diagnosing Deep Venous Thrombosis: Clinical Evaluation Table for Predicting Pretest Probability of Deep Venous Thrombosis*

Clinical Characteristic	Score
Active cancer (treatment ongoing, within previous 6 mo, or palliative)	1
Paralysis, paresis, or recent plaster immobilization of the lower extremities	1
Recently bedridden >3 days or major surgery within 12 wk requiring general or regional anesthesia	1
Localized tenderness along the distribution of the deep venous system	1
Entire leg swollen	1
Calf swelling 3 cm larger than asymptomatic side (measured 10 cm below tibial tuberosity)	1
Pitting edema confined to the symptomatic leg	1
Collateral superficial veins (nonvaricose)	1
Alternative diagnosis at least as likely as deep venous thrombosis	−2

*Clinical probability: low, ≤0; intermediate, 1-2; high, ≥3. In patients with symptoms in both legs, the more symptomatic leg is used.

Reprinted from Wells PS et al: Value assessment of pretest probability of deep-vein thrombosis in clinical management, *Lancet* 351:1795-1798, 1997.

are clinically unlikely to have DVT and who have a negative D-dimer test. Compressive ultrasonography can be safely omitted in such patients. Fig. E1-261 is an algorithm for the diagnosis DVT.

- Laboratory evaluation of young patients with DVT, patients with recurrent thrombosis without obvious causes, and those with a family history of thrombosis should include protein S (both total and free PS), protein C, fibrinogen, antithrombin III level, lupus anticoagulant, anticardiolipin antibodies, anti-β2 glycoprotein1, factor V Leiden, factor VIII, factor IX, and fasting plasma homocysteine levels. HIT antibody may also be useful in the correct context (heparin exposure and abrupt onset of unexplained decrease in platelet count, whether thrombocytopenic or not). It is important to remember that the lupus anticoagulant assay and antithrombin, protein C, protein S, and dysfibrinogenemia testing cannot be properly interpreted if the patient is already on warfarin, whereas anticardiolipin antibody test, prothrombin G20210A factor VII:C, factor V Leiden, and PT polymorphism can be performed when the patient is on warfarin.

IMAGING STUDIES

- Compression ultrasonography (CUS) is generally preferred as the initial study because it is noninvasive and can be repeated serially (useful to monitor suspected acute DVT); it offers good sensitivity for detecting proximal vein thrombosis (in the popliteal or femoral vein) (see Fig. E1-260). Its disadvantages are poor visualization of deep iliac and pelvic veins and poor sensitivity in isolated or nonocclusive calf vein thrombi. Whole-leg compression ultrasound can generally exclude proximal and distal DVT in a single evaluation. Withholding anticoagulation following a single negative whole-leg CUS is associated with a relatively low risk of venous thromboembolism (3.5% of inpatients will develop DVT) during a 3-mo follow-up.
- Contrast venography is the gold standard for evaluation of DVT of the lower extremity. It is, however, invasive and painful. Additional disadvantages are the increased risk of phlebitis, new thrombosis, renal failure, and hypersensitivity reaction to contrast media; it also gives poor visualization of the deep femoral vein in the thigh and the internal iliac vein and its tributaries.
- Magnetic resonance direct thrombus imaging (MRDTI) is an accurate noninvasive test for diagnosis of DVT. It is particularly useful in suspected DVT patients with leg casts, which prevent CUS and in pregnant patients with positive D-dimer and negative CUS (Fig. E1-262). Current limitations are its cost and lack of widespread availability.

(Rx) TREATMENT

NONPHARMACOLOGIC THERAPY

- Gradual resumption of normal activity. Immobility promotes stasis and propagation of

DVT. Patients should get up and walk as tolerated. The theoretical risk that ambulation may dislodge thrombi in the legs, precipitating PE, is unfounded.
- Patient education on anticoagulant therapy and associated risks.

ACUTE GENERAL Rx

- Low-molecular-weight heparin (LMWH) for 4 to 7 days followed by warfarin therapy. Recommended dose of enoxaparin is 1 mg/kg q12h SC and continued for a minimum of 5 days and until a therapeutic INR (2 to 3) has been achieved with warfarin. Once-daily fondaparinux, a synthetic analog of heparin, is also as effective and safe as twice-daily enoxaparin in the initial treatment of patients with symptomatic DVT. Warfarin therapy should be initiated when appropriate (usually within 72 hr of initiation of heparin). Long-term LMWH may be preferable to warfarin in patients with cancer or those whose INR is difficult to control. Other possible alternatives to warfarin may include dabigatran, a direct oral thrombin inhibitor recently FDA approved for anticoagulation in non-valvular atrial fibrillation. It is as effective as warfarin but does not require laboratory monitoring. Recent trials have also shown that rivaroxaban or apixaban, oral factor Xa inhibitors, are safe and effective alternatives to standard acute DVT therapy. They are noninferior to warfarin, do not require periodic lab monitoring, and have a relatively low bleeding risk. They may eventually become preferred agents for extended treatment of venous thromboembolism.
- Outpatient treatment of DVT is appropriate for patients without prior DVT, thrombophilic conditions, or substantial comorbidity, but not for those who are pregnant or likely not to adhere to therapy.
- Exclusions from outpatient treatment of DVT include patients with potential high complication risk (e.g., hemoglobin <7, platelet count <75,000, guaiac-positive stool, recent cerebrovascular accident or noncutaneous surgery, noncompliance).
- Compression stockings are effective in reducing the incidence of postthrombotic syndrome and should be used starting within 1 mo of proximal DVT and continued for at least 1 yr after diagnosis.
- Insertion of an inferior vena cava filter to prevent pulmonary embolism is recommended in patients with contraindications to anticoagulation (e.g., hemorrhagic stroke, active internal bleeding, pregnancy), HIT in a patient with an active VTE/PE, recurrent PE despite adequate anticoagulant therapy, emergent surgery in patient with DVT, presence of free-floating iliofemoral thrombus, lower IVC thrombosis (incipient embolization), and chronic pulmonary (thromboembolic) hypertension with limited pulmonary reserve.
- Thrombolytic therapy (streptokinase) can be used in rare cases (unless contraindicated) in patients with extensive iliofemoral venous thrombosis and a low risk of bleeding. There

are concerns about hemorrhagic complications related to the large doses of thrombolytics required in systemic thrombolysis for DVT (2% to 10% risk of major hemorrhagic complications).
- Other treatment modalities for DVT include surgical thombectomy and catheter-directed thrombolysis (CDT). Thromboreduction by surgical thrombectomy is effective but invasive and expensive. CDT is also invasive, carries a bleeding risk and will require ICU admission.

CHRONIC Rx

- Conventional-intensity warfarin therapy is more effective than low-intensity warfarin therapy for the long-term prevention of recurrent DVT. The low-intensity warfarin regimen does not reduce the risk of clinically important bleeding.
- The optimal duration of anticoagulant therapy varies with the cause of DVT and the patient's risk factors. The risk of recurrence is low if VTE is provoked by surgery, intermediate if provoked by a nonsurgical risk factor, and high if unprovoked. These risks should determine whether patients with VTE should undergo short-term vs. indefinite treatment.
- Therapy for 3 mo is generally satisfactory in patients with reversible risk factors (low-risk group). A high D-dimer level measured after 3 mo of anticoagulation in patients with unprovoked DVT should favor a longer duration of therapy.
- Anticoagulation for 6 mo is recommended for patients with idiopathic venous thrombosis or medical risk factors for DVT (intermediate-risk group). About 20% of patients with unprovoked venous thromboembolism have a recurrence within 2 yr after the withdrawal of oral anticoagulant therapy. Use of daily low-dose aspirin after discontinuation of anticoagulant treatment has been shown in recent trials to reduce the risk of DVT recurrence with no apparent increase in the risk of major bleeding. Additional trials are currently under way to determine the role of aspirin use to prevent recurrent DVT in clinical practice.
- Indefinite anticoagulation is necessary in patients with DVT associated with active cancer; long-term anticoagulation is also indicated in patients with inherited thrombophilia (e.g., deficiency of antithrombin III, protein C or S antibody), high factor VIII levels, antiphospholipid antibody, and those with recurrent episodes of idiopathic DVT (high-risk group). Long-term anticoagulation should also be considered in the presence of comorbidities such as paroxysmal nocturnal hemoglobinuria (PNH), SLE (especially with nephrotic syndrome), some myeloproliferative disorders, IBD, and Cushing's syndrome.
- Measurement of D-dimer after withdrawal of oral anticoagulation may be useful to estimate the risk of recurrence. In patients with a first unprovoked DVT, positive D-dimer test results after cessation of anticoagulation predict recurrence, regardless of test timing or pt's age. Patients with a first spontaneous DVT and a D-dimer level <250 mg/ml after

withdrawal of oral anticoagulation have a low risk of DVT recurrence. Recent trials show that in patients who have completed at least 3 mo of anticoagulation for a first episode of unprovoked DVT and after approximately 2 yr of follow-up, a negative D-dimer result was associated with a 3.5% annual risk of recurrent disease, whereas a positive D-dimer result was associated with an 8.9% annual risk for recurrence. Hence, elevated D-dimer levels would be an indication for prolonged therapy (for 1 or 2 more yr at a minimum).

- The presence of residual thrombosis on ultrasonography when warfarin therapy is discontinued is also associated with an increased risk for subsequent recurrent DVT; a recent trial showed that tailoring the duration of anticoagulation on the basis of the persistence of residual thrombi on ultrasonography may reduce the rate of recurrent DVT. Additional trials are needed before this approach can be adapted for all patients.

- Patients with DVT and pulmonary embolism are at high risk of recurrence whenever anticoagulation is discontinued; therefore, many experts recommend prolonged anticoagulation in this population group, especially if other risk factors for recurrence are present.

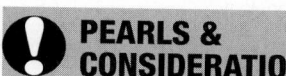

PEARLS & CONSIDERATIONS

COMMENTS

- When using heparin, there is a risk of heparin-induced thrombocytopenia (HIT) (with unfractionated more so than with LMWH). Platelet count should be obtained initially and repeated every 3 days while on heparin.

- Prophylaxis of DVT is recommended in all patients at risk (e.g., low-molecular-weight heparin [enoxaparin 30 mg SC bid] after major trauma, post surgery of hip and knee; enoxaparin 40 mg SC qd post-abdominal surgery in patients with moderate to high DVT risk; gradient elastic stockings alone or in combination with intermittent pneumatic compression [IPC] boots following neurosurgery). Graduated compression stockings (GCSs) are effective for preventing air-travel-related DVT and in reducing the risk of DVT in patients hospitalized for conditions other than stroke. The type of GCSs is also important because proximal DVT occurs more often in patients with stroke who wear below-knee stockings than in those who wear high-length stockings.

- Fondaparinux, a synthetic analog of heparin, can also be used for prevention of DVT after hip fracture surgery, hip replacement, or knee replacement. Initial dose is 2.5 mg SC given 6 to 8 hr postoperatively and continued daily. Its bleeding risk is similar to enoxaparin; however, it is more effective in preventing DVT.

- Desirudin is an injectable direct thrombin inhibitor available for prevention of DVT after selective hip arthroplasty. Unlike unfractionated heparin and LMWH, desirudin does not cause HIT.

- Rivaroxaban, 10 mg PO qd is the first oral, selective inhibitor of factor Xa approved by the FDA for prophylaxis of DVT in patients undergoing knee or hip replacement surgery. Recent trials have also shown that another oral Xa inhibitor, apixaban, is more effective and as safe as enoxaparin for DVT prophylaxis after hip replacement.

- The risk of recurrent venous thromboembolism in heterozygous carriers of factor V Leiden and a first spontaneous venous thromboembolism is similar to that of noncarriers of factor V Leiden; therefore, heterozygous patients should receive secondary thromboprophylaxis for a similar length of time as patients without factor V Leiden.

- Approximately 20% to 50% of patients with DVT develop postthrombotic syndrome characterized by leg edema, pain, venous ectasia, skin induration, and ulceration. Patients with extensive DVT and those with more severe postthrombotic manifestations 1 month after DVT have poorer long-term outcomes.

- Exercise following DVT is reasonable because it improves flexibility of the affected leg and does not increase symptoms in patients with postthrombotic syndrome.

- Previously undiagnosed cancer is frequent in patients with newly diagnosed DVT. A cancer screening strategy should be considered in all patients with unprovoked venous thromboembolism.

- *UPPER EXTREMITY DVT:* It is less common than lower extremity DVT and is seen more frequently in patients requiring central venous catheters or wires. It confers risk for mortality, recurrent thromboembolic events, and postthrombotic syndrome similar to that of lower extremity DVT. It is classified as primary upper extremity DVT (*Paget-Schroetter syndrome*) defined as a thrombus in the axillary and subclavian veins in absence of identifiable thrombosis risk factors. It accounts for 20% of upper extremity DVT cases and may be due to an underlying anatomic abnormality at the thoracic outlet in combination with local hypercoagulability due to venous stretching or perivascular fibrosis from recurrent venous compression. Secondary upper extremity DVT is defined as any DVT related to a predisposing factor (e.g., insertion of central venous catheter, wires, or other devices, malignancy). In patients with secondary upper extremity DVT removal of the catheter is not routinely recommended but is warranted if there is a catheter malfunction or infection, if anticoagulation therapy is contraindicated or has failed, or if the catheter is no longer needed. Anticoagulation therapy in upper extremity DVT consists of use of vitamin K antagonists except in patients with cancer, for whom low-molecular-weight heparin is preferred. Optimal duration of anticoagulation treatment in upper extremity DVT is 3 to 6 mo (including in those in whom a central catheter has been removed)

- *REVERSAL OF ANTICOAGULATION:* Vitamin K (1 mg PO or 2 mg IV) can be used to reverse elevated INR (3 to 6) when elective or urgent procedures are needed. The administration of vitamin K can take more than 24 hr to fully restore vitamin K dependent coagulation factors II, VII, IX, and X. The American College of Chest Physicians recommends the following guidelines for managing elevated INRs or bleeding in patients receiving vitamin A antagonist therapy:
  - INR 5 to <9 and no significant bleeding: omit dose and give vitamin K (1 to 2.5 mg orally). Monitor the next day and use additional vitamin K if necessary.
  - INR >9 and no significant bleeding: hold vitamin K antagonist, give 5 to 10 mg orally of vitamin K. Monitor the next day and use additional vitamin K if necessary. Resume therapy at lower dose when INR therapeutic.
  - Serious bleeding at any elevation of INR: hold vitamin K antagonist and supplement with prothrombin complex concentrates (PCC). Give vitamin K (10 mg by slow IV infusion over 30 min to reduce the risk of anaphylaxis). Vitamin K1 can be repeated every 12 hr. PCC composition in the U.S. (3-factor PCC) includes clotting factors II, IX, and X but minimal amounts of factor VII (unlike PCC products available outside of the U.S. [4-factor PCC], which have a significant amount of factor VII). In order to replace the low factor VII some clinicians in the U.S. will also give fresh frozen plasma (FFP) in addition to vitamin K and PCC in patients with life-threatening warfarin-related bleeding.

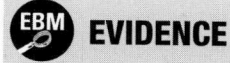

EVIDENCE

available at www.expertconsult.com

SUGGESTED READINGS
available at www.expertconsult.com

RELATED CONTENT

Deep Vein Thrombosis (DVT) (Patient Information)
Hypercoagulable State (Related Key Topic)
Antiphospholipid Antibody Syndrome (Related Key Topic)
Pulmonary Embolism (Related Key Topic)

AUTHOR: **FRED F. FERRI, M.D.**

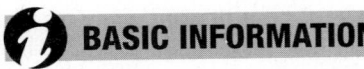

BASIC INFORMATION

DEFINITION

Pubertal delay refers to delayed development and maturation of the reproductive system. The diagnostic criterion is a delay of more than 2 standard deviations from the mean age of pubertal onset.

SYNONYMS

Pubertal delay

ICD-9CM CODES

259.0 Delay in sexual development and puberty, not elsewhere classified

EPIDEMIOLOGY & DEMOGRAPHICS

PREVALENCE: 2.5% of healthy adolescents have a diagnosis of pubertal delay using the statistical diagnostic criteria

GENETICS: Constitutional delay of puberty often runs in families. Pubertal delay occurs with some congenital syndromes, such as Prader-Willi syndrome and Noonan syndrome, and in patients with enzyme defects in sex steroid synthesis, as well as others.

PHYSICAL FINDINGS & CLINICAL PRESENTATION

Puberty is clinically delayed for girls if there is no evidence of breast development by 13 yr of age, absence of menarche by age 16 yr, or absence of menarche within 5 yr of pubertal onset. Puberty is clinically delayed for boys if there is no evidence of testicular enlargement by 14 yr of age, or >5 yr between start and completion of growth of genitalia.

ETIOLOGY

Puberty begins with increased pulsatile secretion of gonadotropin-releasing hormone (GnRH) from the hypothalamus, increased pituitary responsiveness to GnRH, secretion of gonadotropins, gonadal maturation, and increasing production of sex steroids. Increased concentration of sex steroids induces the development of secondary sexual characteristics, acceleration of growth, and fertility. Numerous causes can lead to pubertal delay, including chronic disease, normal variation, congenital syndromes, or other factors.

DIAGNOSIS

DIFFERENTIAL DIAGNOSIS

Normal or low serum gonadotropins
- Constitutional delay
- Hypothalamic dysfunction
  - Malnutrition or eating disorder
  - Strenuous exercise
  - Chronic illness
  - Severe obesity
  - Central nervous system tumors
- Hypopituitarism
  - Panhypopituitarism
  - Isolated gonadotropin deficiency
  - Kallmann syndrome (associated with anosmia)

- Hypothyroidism
- Hyperprolactinemia
  - Pituitary adenoma
  - Drug-associated (cannabis, cocaine)

Increased serum gonadotropins
- Turner's syndrome (gonadal dysgenesis)
- Klinefelter syndrome
- Bilateral gonadal failure
  - Primary testicular failure
  - Anorchia
  - Premature ovarian failure
  - Resistant ovary syndrome
  - Irradiation, cytotoxic therapy
  - Trauma
  - Infections (e.g., mumps, orchitis)

Other conditions
- Prader-Willi syndrome
- Noonan syndrome
- Androgen resistance
- Steroidogenic enzyme defects

WORKUP

- Given the extensive differential diagnosis for pubertal delay, a systematic and focused approach is necessary. A careful history, including family history and social history, can identify eating and exercise habits, chronic illnesses, and parental history of pubertal delay. Fig. E1- 263 is an algorithm for the evaluation of patients with delayed puberty.
- Growth measurement should include height and weight, a growth chart to assess rate of growth, and calculation of the sex-adjusted midparental height that represents the statistically most probable adult height for the child.
  - For boys, add 2.5 inches (6.5 cm) from the mean of the parents' heights. For girls, subtract 2.5 inches (6.5 cm) from the mean of the parents' heights.
  - Physical exam can reveal signs of sexual maturation, stigmata of congenital syndromes, and nutritional status. Include neurologic exam (visual fields, ophthalmologic), thyroid, chest, heart, abdomen, and Tanner staging.

LABORATORY TESTS

- Serum gonadotropin levels (luteinizing hormone, follicle-stimulating hormone) can help distinguish disorders of congenital or acquired gonadal failure from other causes. By bone age 10 to 12 yr gonadal failure produces elevated levels of serum gonadotropins. If levels are low or normal, constitutional delay is the most frequent diagnosis.
- Chromosomal analysis if there is a suspicion of gonadal dysgenesis or Klinefelter syndrome.
- Screening studies include complete blood count, erythrocyte sedimentation rate, serum prolactin, serum thyroid-stimulating hormone.
- Endocrinologist may do further studies such as IGF-1 to screen for growth hormone disorders and GnRH stimulation testing.

IMAGING STUDIES

Consider bone age (left hand and wrist film), which is delayed in constitutional delay and GnRH deficiency; consider MRI of the head to evaluate for tumors of pituitary or hypothalamus

and absence of olfactory bulb and tract, which occurs in Kallmann syndrome (absence of GnRH); and pelvic ultrasound, which can be helpful in detecting intraabdominal testes and to evaluate müllerian anatomy.

TREATMENT

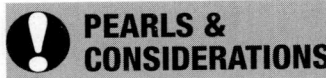

- Treat underlying cause if it is identified.
- Constitutional delay can be managed with reassurance that the delay will have no effect on final adult height or development. Short-term hormonal therapy can be used to hasten puberty if the delay is causing severe psychosocial difficulties. Monthly testosterone injections may be used for boys who have begun pubertal development.
- Short stature in puberty may be dealt with through pharmacologic interventions, though definitive data on some medications are lacking and long-term safety issues require further study.
- Gonadotropin deficiency or hypogonadism may require lifelong sex steroid replacement.
- Psychosocial evaluation, support, and treatment as needed.

REFERRAL

Pediatric endocrinology

PEARLS & CONSIDERATIONS

COMMENTS

- Constitutional delay is the most common cause of pubertal delay and is often associated with a positive family history in parents and/or siblings, but other causes, such as Turner syndrome and systemic disorders, should be excluded.
- Bone age demonstrates more clearly than chronologic age how far an individual has progressed toward maturity and predicts the potential for further growth.
- No studies reliably distinguish constitutional delay from gonadotropin deficiency.

PATIENT & FAMILY EDUCATION

- The Magic Foundation, a support group for patients and their families (http://www.magicfoundation.org)
- The American Academy of Family Physicians (http://www.aafp.org)
- American Academy of Pediatrics (http://www.aap.org)
- Pediatric Endocrine Society (http://www.lwpes.org)

SUGGESTED READINGS

available at www.expertconsult.com

RELATED CONTENT

Delayed Puberty (Patient Information)

AUTHOR: **NIRALI BORA, M.D.**

BASIC INFORMATION

DEFINITION

The key to delirium is that it has an acute/subacute onset. The American Psychiatric Association's *Diagnostic and Statistical Manual*, 4th edition (DSM-IV) defines delirium as:

- Disturbance of consciousness (i.e., reduced clarity of awareness about the environment) with reduced ability to focus, sustain, or shift attention.
- A change in cognition (e.g., memory deficit, disorientation, language disturbance) or development of a perceptual disturbance that is not better accounted for by a preexisting, established, or evolving dementia.
- The disturbance develops over a short period of time (usually hours to days) and tends to fluctuate during the course of a day.

Three main theories prevail regarding pathophysiology of delirium:

- Neuroinflammation, with increased permeability of the blood-brain barrier
- Acetylcholine deficiency
- Other neurotransmitter imbalances, including excesses of norepinephrine, serotonin (which may actually exert a beneficial effect on the stress of illness), and, most important, dopamine

SYNONYMS

Acute confusional state
Acute brain syndrome
Toxic or metabolic encephalopathy

ICD-9CM CODES
780.09 Delirium

EPIDEMIOLOGY & DEMOGRAPHICS

Currently classified into hyperactive, hypoactive, and mixed subtypes. Although hypoactive is more common (20% to 86% prevalence vs. 6% to 31% for hyperactive), it is often overlooked and seems to portend a worse prognosis. Any age, race, or gender can be affected. Pediatric delirium is often missed but remains important because delirium is associated with longer hospital stays, decreased cognitive performance, and increased mortality. Risk factors include extremes of age, severe pain, illicit substance use, surgery, dementia, and kidney or liver failure (Tables E1-122 and E1-123).

PHYSICAL FINDINGS & CLINICAL PRESENTATION

- Pay particular attention to reversible causes for delirium.
- Start with a careful history, especially including the time course of the symptoms. Symptoms may differ both among and within one patient. Thus history from various caregivers may conflict because delirium implies a mental status that is frequently in flux. Symptoms may include poor attention, sleepiness, agitation, or psychosis. Take notice of new medications, recent surgeries or illnesses, and treatments.
- Next perform a physical examination focusing on signs of infection, dehydration, or chronic disease that may be exacerbated. Vital signs are key. Consider using the Mini-Mental Status Exam or the Montreal Cognitive Assessment.
- An algorithm for the evaluation of patients with delirium is presented in Fig. E1-264, and Fig. E1-265 describes an algorithm for evaluation of mental status changes in an older patient.

ETIOLOGY

Can be multifactorial; often falls into one of the following categories:

- Drugs: benzodiazepines are the worst offenders, but also remember narcotics, anticholinergics, beta-blockers, steroids, nonsteroidal anti-inflammatory drugs, digoxin, cimetidine, among others
- Infection or inflammation: any, including abdominal processes
- Metabolic: kidney or liver failure, thyroid, adrenal or glucose dysregulation, anemia, vitamin deficiency
- Stress: surgery, sleep problems, pain, fever, hypoxia, anesthesia, environmental changes, fecal or urinary retention
- Fluids, electrolytes, nutrition (FEN): dysregulation of calcium, magnesium, potassium, or sodium; dehydration; volume overload; altered pH

Dx DIAGNOSIS

DIFFERENTIAL DIAGNOSIS

- Psychosis
- Dementia
- Depression or mania

Remember, delirium may coexist with any of the above!

LABORATORY TESTS

- Complete blood count, blood urea nitrogen, creatinine, and electrolytes
- Toxicology screen, liver function tests, ammonia
- Thyroid function tests, vitamin B_{12}, and folate levels
- Rapid plasma reagin for syphilis, blood, urine, and spinal culture
- Arterial blood gas measurement

IMAGING STUDIES

- Consider head CT (to look for bleed, trauma, tumor, atrophy, dementia, stroke)
- Chest radiograph (to look for tumor, infection)

Rx TREATMENT

NONPHARMACOLOGIC THERAPY

- The most important consideration is to keep the patient safe by using a variety of methods, including frequent reorientation.
- A quiet, restful, simplified environment with cues to time and location such as clock or calendar are helpful, as well as consistent staff providing both personal and medical care. If possible, encourage familiar family members and friends to keep the patient company.
- Physical restraints if necessary to ensure safety.

ACUTE GENERAL Rx

- Reverse any treatable cause.
- Haloperidol can be used with caution to control agitation, with doses ranging from 0.25 to 2 mg IM/IV twice daily, repeating the dose every 20 to 30 min until patient has calmed and using lower doses for the elderly.
- Risperidone 0.5 mg twice daily (off-label use, non-FDA approved) can also be used with caution with a slow increase to desired dose, not to exceed 1.0 to 2.0 mg.
- Avoid benzodiazepines and meperidine.

CHRONIC Rx

Delirium is not a chronic condition; if assessing a more long-term mental status change, consider other diagnoses.

DISPOSITION

Requires frequent monitoring often necessitating hospital level of care to ensure safety and assess etiology.

REFERRAL

Consider neurologic or psychiatric consultation if not improved in several days or in complicated cases.

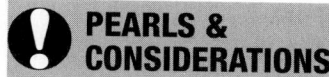 PEARLS & CONSIDERATIONS

COMMENTS

Although benzodiazepines are frequently used in hospitalized patients for sedation and are the mainstay of therapy for alcohol withdrawal, they must be used with caution in the elderly because they can have a paradoxical effect on agitation.

PREVENTION

- Avoid polypharmacy as much as possible.
- Optimize chronic medical conditions.
- Provide frequent reorientation and a soothing environment for high-risk patients (e.g., lights on during the day, off at night; open curtains during the day so patient can see the weather).
- In patients over 70 without dementia, regular exercise has been associated with lower risk for developing delirium, and early return to physical activity can improve outcomes in ill patients.

PATIENT & FAMILY EDUCATION

Inform about the above preventive techniques, especially polypharmacy risks.

SUGGESTED READINGS
available at www.expertconsult.com

RELATED CONTENT

Delirium Tremens (Related Key Topic)

AUTHOR: **CRISTINA ANTONIO PACHECO, M.D.**

BASIC INFORMATION

DEFINITION

Delirium tremens is overactivity of the central nervous system after cessation of alcohol intake. The time interval is variable; it usually occurs within 1 wk after reduction or cessation of heavy alcohol intake and persists for 1 to 3 days.

SYNONYMS

Alcohol withdrawal syndrome
DTs
Alcoholic delirium

ICD-9CM CODES
291.00 Alcohol withdrawal delirium

EPIDEMIOLOGY & DEMOGRAPHICS

INCIDENCE (IN U.S.): Up to 500,000 cases annually
PEAK INCIDENCE: 30 yr and older
PREDOMINANT SEX: Male
PEAK AGE: Teenage years and older
GENETICS: More common with patients who have relatives who are alcoholics

PHYSICAL FINDINGS & CLINICAL PRESENTATION

- Initially: anxiety, insomnia, tremulousness
- Early: tachycardia, sweating, anorexia, agitation, headache, gastrointestinal distress
- Late: seizures, visual hallucinations, delirium

ETIOLOGY

Alcoholism

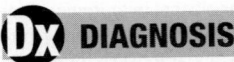

DIAGNOSIS

DIFFERENTIAL DIAGNOSIS

- Coexisting illness
- Trauma
- Drug use

WORKUP

- Frequent rating of symptoms (hallucinations, tremor, sweating, agitation, orientation).
- The Clinical Institute Withdrawal Assessment-Alcohol (CIWA-A) scale can be used to measure the severity of alcohol withdrawal. It consists of the 10 following items:
  1. Nausea
  2. Tremor
  3. Autonomic hyperactivity
  4. Anxiety
  5. Agitation
  6. Tactile disturbances
  7. Visual disturbances
  8. Auditory disturbances
  9. Headache
  10. Disorientation

The maximum score is 67.

LABORATORY TESTS

- Electrolytes (including magnesium, phosphate)
- Close monitoring of glucose levels
- Drug screen (blood and urine)

IMAGING STUDIES

CT scan of head if there is a history of head trauma.

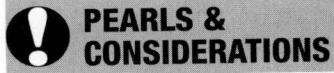

TREATMENT

NONPHARMACOLOGIC THERAPY

Refer to drug rehabilitation program after patient recovers.

ACUTE GENERAL Rx

- Admission to a detoxification unit where patient can be observed closely.
- Vital signs q30min initially (neurologic signs, if necessary).
- Use of lateral decubitus or prone position if restraints are necessary.
- Nothing by mouth: nasogastric tube for abdominal distention may be necessary but should not be routinely used.
- Vigorous hydration (4 to 6 L/day): IV with glucose (Na^+, K^+, PO_4^{-3}, and Mg^{2+} replacement). Use with caution in patients with CHF.
- Vitamins: thiamine 100 mg IV qd. The initial dose of thiamine should precede the administration of IV dextrose; multivitamins (may be added to the hydrating solution).
- Sedation:
  - Initially: lorazepam 2 to 5 mg IM/IV repeated prn
  - Maintenance (individualized dosage): chlordiazepoxide, 50 to 100 mg PO q4 to 6h, lorazepam 2 mg PO q4h, or diazepam 5 to 10 mg PO tid; withhold doses or decrease subsequent doses if signs of oversedation are apparent.
  - Midazolam is also effective for managing DTs. Its rapid onset (sedation within 2 to 4 min of IV injection) and short duration of action (approximately 30 min) make it an ideal agent for titration in continuous infusion.
- Treatment of seizures: diazepam 2.5 mg/min IV until seizure is controlled (check for respiratory depression or hypotension) may be beneficial for prolonged seizure activity; IV lorazepam 1 to 2 mg q2h can be used in place of diazepam. In general, withdrawal seizures are self-limited and treatment is not required; the use of phenytoin or other anticonvulsants for short-term treatment of alcohol withdrawal seizures is not recommended.
- Diagnosis and treatment of concomitant medical, surgical, or psychiatric conditions.

CHRONIC Rx

Alcoholics Anonymous has the best record in breaking addiction, but the results are still disappointing.

DISPOSITION

Refer to drug rehabilitation program.

REFERRAL

If cardiac arrhythmias are prominent or respiratory distress develops

PEARLS & CONSIDERATIONS

COMMENTS

This is a potentially lethal disease if not carefully treated. Mortality rate is 15% in untreated patients.

SUGGESTED READING

available at www.expertconsult.com

RELATED CONTENT

Alcoholism (Related Key Topic)
Delirium Tremens (Patient Information)
Delirium (Related Key Topic)

AUTHOR: **FRED F. FERRI, M.D.**

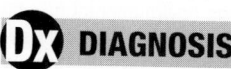

BASIC INFORMATION

DEFINITION

A fixed belief characterized by a person's preoccupation that his or her skin is infested by insects, worms, or other living organisms.

SYNONYMS

Morgellon's disease

ICD-9CM CODES
297.10 Paranoia—delusional disorders, delusional disorder

ICD-10CM CODES
F22 Delusional disorders

EPIDEMIOLOGY & DEMOGRAPHICS

INCIDENCE: Unknown
PEAK INCIDENCE: Occurs more often later in life
PREVALENCE: Unknown
PREDOMINANT SEX AND AGE: For patients less than age 50, the male/female ratio is 1:1; for patients older than 50, females predominate by a ratio of 3:1
GENETICS: Unknown
RISK FACTORS: None known

PHYSICAL FINDINGS & CLINICAL PRESENTATION

- Patients complain of living organisms infesting their skin, sometimes including mucosal tissues.
- Patients have often been to specialists, including dermatologists, allergists, and infectious disease specialists.
- Patients may bring in samples of skin or hair, stating that they have looked at tissue under a microscope and have seen organisms. These samples are often brought in a matchbox ("matchbox sign") or wrapped in plastic wrap ("Saran sign").
- Skin may show areas of excoriation.

ETIOLOGY

Unknown: Thought to be mediated through dopaminergic pathways in the brain given the known etiology of other psychotic disorders and the ability of cocaine use to create symptoms of formication (see below).

DIAGNOSIS

DIFFERENTIAL DIAGNOSIS

- Primary psychiatric disorders include formication, in which patients experience crawling and biting sensations on their skin, although they are not delusional about the cause.

- Neuropsychiatrically, B_{12} deficiency, diabetic neuropathy, cardiovascular disease, multiple sclerosis, and brain lesions can all cause similar delusions.
- Other medical causes that deserve workup include primary skin lesions, systemic diseases that may present with skin lesions, and disorders of infestation.

WORKUP

- Skin biopsy may exclude dermatitis herpetiformis (although many patients have already been to their primary care doctor and dermatologist and have had a skin biopsy done, likely many times).
- Mineral oil preparation may exclude scabies, and a microscopic examination may exclude louse infestation.
- Thorough history is likely to yield the very fixed nature of the belief and an unwillingness to come to terms with the lack of findings on the exam.

LABORATORY TESTS

- Pruritus workup: iron studies, LFTs, CBC, UA, TSH, Chem 7, Folate, B_{12}
- Lumbar puncture (especially when multiple sclerosis is highly suspected)
- CRP (especially when an infectious etiology is suspected)
- Urine toxicology screen to evaluate substance use

IMAGING STUDIES

- Head CT, without contrast
- MRI

TREATMENT

- Antipsychotics have been shown to lead to full to partial remission in 60% to 100% of cases.
- Classically, Orap was the treatment of choice, although it has been associated with QTc prolongation.
- Multiple studies describe the use of second-generation antipsychotics, but these have been shown to cause weight gain and metabolic syndrome.
- Numerous antipsychotics have a black box warning about the risk of sudden death in the elderly and must be administered carefully for patients who have issues with QTc.
- Given all of these issues, a careful risk/benefit analysis is needed, including the assistance of family members of elderly patients.

NONPHARMACOLOGIC THERAPY

- Given the fixed nature of the belief, patients often refuse referral to a mental health specialist.

- A treatment (e.g., Permethrin) should not be recommended "just in case" because it may reinforce the patient's belief.
- Repeat visits with medical providers may be helpful to provide assurance and prevent harm from further workup.

ACUTE GENERAL Rx

Antipsychotics (Table 1-124)

COMPLEMENTARY & ALTERNATIVE MEDICINE

There is no evidence on the use of complementary or alternative medicine for this disorder.

REFERRAL

Referral to an outpatient psychiatrist may be helpful, but patients are often resistant.

PREVENTION

No preventive measures have been identified.

PATIENT/FAMILY EDUCATION

Psychoeducation may be helpful for the patient and family, although resistance from the patient can be expected.

SUGGESTED READINGS
available at www.expertconsult.com

RELATED CONTENT

Schizophrenia (Related Key Topic)
Alcoholism (Related Key Topic)
Cocaine Overdose (Related Key Topic)
Delirium (Related Key Topic)

AUTHOR: **ANTHONY GALLO, M.D.**

TABLE 1-124 Antipsychotics

Antipsychotic Drug	Dosage
Haloperidol	0.5-10 mg PO bid
Pimozide	2-12 mg PO qam
Perphenazine	4-16 mg PO tid
Olanzapine	2.5-10 mg PO bid
Aripiprazole	2.5-20 mg PO qam
Quetiapine	12.5-200 mg PO bid
Ziprasidone	20-80 mg PO bid
Risperidone	0.5-3 mg PO bid

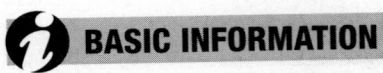

BASIC INFORMATION

DEFINITION

A neurodegenerative disease characterized by dementia concurrent with or preceding parkinsonian symptoms typically by 1 yr with other core features including fluctuations in attention and alertness and recurrent visual hallucinations. Diagnostic criteria for dementia syndrome associated with Lewy body pathology are described in Box 1-12. The disease characteristically responds to cholinesterase inhibitors, is relatively unresponsive to L-dopa, and is very sensitive to neuroleptics.

SYNONYMS

Lewy body dementia
Diffuse Lewy body disease
Lewy body type senile dementia
Cortical Lewy body disease

ICD-9CM CODES
Lewy bodies
331.82 [294.11] with behavioral disturbance
331.82 [294.10] without behavioral disturbance

EPIDEMIOLOGY & DEMOGRAPHICS

INCIDENCE: Accounts for 10% to 22% of all dementias.
PEAK INCIDENCE: Affects individuals in their sixth decade or older.
PREVALENCE: Estimated 0.7% of individuals older than age 65.
PREDOMINANT SEX AND AGE:
- Sex: Male predominance
- Mean age of onset: 75 yr. On average, 10 yr greater for dementia with Lewy bodies (DLB) than Parkinson's disease (PD).

GENETICS:
- Most cases are sporadic with a discordance among monozygotic twins, which suggests that environment or other epigenetics play a major role in the incidence of DLB.
- Multiplication of alpha-synuclein gene (SNCA) has been reported in families with DLB.
- Other factors include glucocerebrosidase genetic mutations, high prevalence of Lewy bodies with presenilin-1 mutations, and polymorphisms of the coding region for the synuclein genes.

RISK FACTORS:
- Male sex
- Advanced age

PHYSICAL FINDINGS & CLINICAL PRESENTATION

- Importance of recognizing DLB relates to its pharmacologic management, including responsiveness to cholinesterase inhibitors, sensitivity to side effects of neuroleptics, and relative unresponsiveness to L-dopa.
- Insidious onset of dementia with core features of fluctuations in cognition, recurrent visual hallucinations, and extrapyramidal motor symptoms, along with other features either suggestive or supportive of the clinical diagnosis. Refer to "Revised Criteria for the Clinical Diagnosis of Dementia with Lewy Bodies" (McKeith I et al, *Neurology*, 2005).
- Detailed neuropsychological assessment demonstrates a characteristic profile of impairments in visuoperceptual, attentional, and executive functions, which reflects a combination of cortical and subcortical damage.

ETIOLOGY

- SNCA is a protein normally found at the synapse with a role in vesicle production. In its insoluble form, SNCA aggregates into Lewy bodies found at the cortical and subcortical levels.
- Lewy bodies are round, eosinophilic, intracytoplasmic inclusions in the nuclei of neurons.
- Cortical Lewy bodies are found in deep cortical layers of the anterior frontal and temporal lobes, the cingulate gyrus, and insula.
- As in PD, Lewy bodies aggregate in the following structures: substantia nigra, locus coeruleus, raphe nuclei, nucleus basalis of Meynert, and brain stem nuclei.

DIAGNOSIS

DIFFERENTIAL DIAGNOSIS

- Similar to Parkinson's disease with dementia, including fluctuation in neuropsychological function, neuropsychiatric features, and extrapyramidal motor features
- Diagnosis of DLB when dementia occurs before or concurrently with extrapyramidal features—arbitrarily set as the "1-yr rule" vs. Parkinson's disease with dementia, which occurs after 1 yr

- Dementia: Alzheimer's disease (AD), vascular dementia
- Parkinsonian features: progressive supranuclear palsy, multisystem atrophy, corticobasal degeneration
- Rapidly progressive form: Creutzfeldt-Jakob disease. Lack of cerebellar signs may help distinguish DLB from classic CJD (but not variant form of CJD)
- Psychiatric features: late-onset psychosis or depression with psychotic features
- Hallucinations with fluctuations in consciousness: temporal lobe epilepsy (TLE)

WORKUP

- Lumbar puncture to rule out underlying chronic infections. Protein 14-3-3 may be present in both DLB and CJD.
- EEG to rule out potential TLE. However, either DLB or TLE may show nonspecific slowing or periodic complexes.

LABORATORY TESTS

- Rule out other potential reversible causes for dementia including:
  - Hormonal dysregulation: thyroid stimulating hormone, free thyroxine
  - Vitamin deficiency: thiamine, cyanocobalamin, folate
  - Vascular risk factors: lipid profile, Hgb A_{1c}, homocysteine, syphilis (FTA-ABS), or ApoE genetype

IMAGING STUDIES

- MRI typically shows a relative preservation of the hippocampi and medial temporal lobe volumes (as found in AD) but generalized atrophy and white matter changes.
- Functional imaging including single photon emission computed tomography (SPECT) demonstrates hypoperfusion of the occipital region.

TREATMENT

Patient and caregiver education on benefits, side effects, and limitations of treatment is very important. Based on the preference of the patient and caregiver, a fine balance between psychosis and Parkinsonism features confounds the treatment choices.

NONPHARMACOLOGIC THERAPY

- Social interaction and environmental novelty may improve cognitive dysfunction and psychiatric features often exacerbated by low levels of arousal and attention.
- Behavioral methods, such as avoiding previously exposed environmental triggers known to cause anxiety, agitation, or aggression.
- Physical therapy, mobility aids, and daily exercise.

ACUTE GENERAL Rx

Neuroleptic for disabling, persistent psychotic features despite initiation of a cholinesterase inhibitor. A very low dose of an atypical antipsychotic (quetiapine 12.5 mg daily) may be started after patient/caregiver education regarding the sensitivity to neuroleptics.

BOX 1-12 Diagnostic Criteria for the Dementia Syndrome Associated with Lewy Body Pathology

The cognitive disturbance is of insidious onset and is progressive, based on evidence from the history or serial cognitive examination
The presence of at least two of the following:
   Parkinsonism (rigidity, resting tremor, bradykinesia, postural instability, parkinsonian gait disorder)
   Prominent, fully formed visual hallucinations
   Substantial fluctuations in alertness or cognition
   Rapid eye movement sleep behavior disorder
   Severe worsening of parkinsonism by antipsychotic drugs
The disturbance is not better accounted for by a systemic disease or another brain disease

From Goldman L, Schafer AI: *Goldman's Cecil medicine*, ed 24, Philadelphia, 2012, Saunders.

CHRONIC Rx

- Cholinesterase inhibitors for cognitive and behavioral symptoms. Rivastigmine (6 to 12 mg per day orally or 9.5 mg per day by transdermal patch) has shown in RCT a significant reduction in anxiety, delusions, and hallucinations, as well as significantly improved performance on neuropsychological testing.
- Antiparkinson medications for disabling parkinsonian features. L-Dopa is reported to be more effective with fewer side effects than dopamine agonists. Begin at a low dose of L-dopa (25/100 mg tid), and slowly titrate over several weeks as tolerated and according to response.
- Selective serotonin reuptake inhibitors are commonly used for depression.
- If REM sleep disorder remains disabling (or patient has not responded to an atypical antipsychotic initiated for psychosis), a trial of low-dose clonazepam (0.25 to 0.5 mg) or melatonin (3 mg) at bedtime remains an option.
- Orthostatic hypotension may be aided by nonpharmacologic therapy, such as supportive stockings, or pharmacologically by midodrine and/or fludrocortisone.
- Memantine demonstrated an improvement in clinical global measure and remains well-tolerated but may worsen hallucinations or delusions.
- Avoid anticholinergics (including tricyclic antidepressants) and benzodiazepines.

DISPOSITION

- Survival resembles the progression of AD, but a minority of cases may have a rapid disease course.
- Progression in cognitive decline, similar to AD, by an approximate 10% per year on cognitive testing.

REFERRAL

DLB requires a multidisciplinary approach including the general practitioner, neurologist, neuropsychologist, and/or neuropsychiatrist.

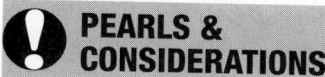

PEARLS & CONSIDERATIONS

COMMENTS

- Clinical presentation helps differentiate DLB from AD. AD presents with early signs of anterograde episodic memory loss without the benefit of recognition on neuropsychological testing due to cortical atrophy at the medial temporal lobe region.
- Vascular dementia may also present with evidence of frontal-subcortical features but typically without the core features listed in the criteria above.

- Bed partners may report that individuals with DLB "act out their dreams," sometimes violently, leading to sleeping in separate beds. A history of REM sleep behavior may precede the diagnosis by many years.

PATIENT/FAMILY EDUCATION

- Visual hallucinations (VH) typically consist of innocuous, well-formed, detailed images of animate figures. Unless VH lead to a potential threat to self or others, avoid antipsychotics due to the sensitivity of neuroleptics. Family/friends are often more alarmed by the VH than the patient with DLB.
- Apathy is a common clinical feature of DLB and mimics changes in mood, including depression, or excessive daytime somnolence. These features are often noticed by family/friends.

SUGGESTED READINGS

available at www.expertconsult.com

AUTHORS: **D. BRANDON BURTIS, D.O.,** and **GLEN FINNEY, M.D.**

Diseases and Disorders

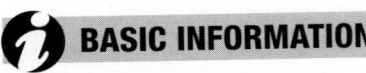

BASIC INFORMATION

DEFINITION

Dependent personality disorder (DPD) is characterized by a pervasive and excessive need to be taken care of that leads to submissive and clinging behavior and fears of separation. DPD begins by early adulthood and causes significant distress or impairment in multiple domains of functioning. Individuals must meet five or more of the following criteria:

1. Difficulty making routine decisions without an excessive amount of advice and reassurance from others.
2. Need others to assume responsibility for most major areas of their life.
3. Difficulty expressing disagreement with others because of fear of loss of support or approval.
4. Difficulty initiating or completing projects on own because of a lack of self-confidence in abilities rather than lack of motivation or energy.
5. Excessive attempts to obtain nurturance and support from others.
6. Feel uncomfortable or helpless when alone because of exaggerated fears of being unable to care for self.
7. Urgently seek another relationship when a close relationship ends.
8. Unrealistically preoccupied with being left to take care of self.

SYNONYMS

None

ICD-9CM CODES

301.6

EPIDEMIOLOGY & DEMOGRAPHICS

PREVALENCE: 0.5% in general population. Dependent traits, as opposed to the disorder itself, are among the most frequently reported in outpatient mental health clinics.
PREDOMINANT SEX: Female (2:1) in clinical settings.

CLINICAL PRESENTATION

- Early onset and chronic course. Impairment is frequently mild.
- On interview, will defer excessively to partner or parent.
- Indecision in routine decisions.
- Depend on a parent or spouse to decide where they should live, work, and recreate and who they should befriend.
- Need for others to function for them goes beyond age-appropriate and situation-appropriate requests for assistance.
- Will agree with objectionable opinions, submit to unreasonable requests, and not express appropriate anger or disappointment for fear of alienating the person without whom they believe they cannot function.
- Convinced that they are not capable of independent function and present themselves as inept.
- Often do not develop independent living skills, perpetuating their dependency.
- Social relations tend to be limited to those few people on whom the person depends.

ETIOLOGY

Chronic physical illness or separation anxiety disorder may predispose for DPD.

DIAGNOSIS

DIFFERENTIAL DIAGNOSIS

- Dependency and personality changes arising as a consequence of an Axis I disorder.
- Dependency arising as a consequence of a general medical condition.
- Most common comorbid Axis I conditions are major depressive and other mood disorders, anxiety disorders, including social phobia, and adjustment disorder.
- Most common comorbid personality disorders are histrionic, avoidant, and borderline. Each of these disorders is characterized by dependent features. DPD is distinguished by its predominantly submissive, reactive, and clinging behavior.

WORKUP

- History: collateral information is essential to establishing the presence of longstanding interpersonal pattern in multiple domains of the patient's life.
- Physical examination.
- Mental status examination.

LABORATORY TESTS

Tests necessary to rule out medical causes of personality changes

IMAGING STUDIES

Tests necessary to rule out medical causes of personality changes

TREATMENT

NONPHARMACOLOGIC THERAPY

- Cognitive-behavioral and psychodynamic psychotherapy to diminish and better contain anxiety and to help patients develop sense of self as competent and requisite assertiveness skills
- Psychodynamic psychotherapy to help develop improved self-concept and interpersonal functioning

ACUTE GENERAL Rx

Benzodiazepines to control highly anxious states

CHRONIC Rx

Selective serotonin reuptake inhibitors (SSRIs) and selective serotonin-norepinephrine reuptake inhibitors (SNRIs) for comorbid depression, social phobia, other anxiety disorders, and agoraphobia

DISPOSITION

- Chronic course; severity is variable
- Impairments often mild
- At increased risk for major depression, social phobia, and other anxiety disorders, including panic and agoraphobia

REFERRAL

- If pharmacotherapy or psychotherapy is contemplated
- If patient's functioning is impaired

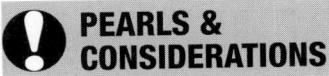

PEARLS & CONSIDERATIONS

COMMENTS

- DPD patients fear illness will lead to abandonment by others.
- This fear of simultaneous helplessness and abandonment intensifies neediness and may lead to dramatic demands for urgent medical attention.
- When physicians do not respond as wanted, angry outbursts may ensue.
- Medical care can also become a means by which dependency needs are met. As a result, some of these patients may unconsciously or consciously prolong their illness for primary gain.
- Physicians often react to the extreme neediness with avoidance or overengagement, leading to burnout.
- Management guidelines:
  1. Overall strategy is to provide reassurance and allay fear of abandonment.
  2. Specific strategies include scheduling frequent visits, noncontingent care (i.e., scheduling visits regardless of whether ill or not).
  3. Establish firm and realistic limits to availability as early as possible in treatment.
  4. Enlist other members of health care team for support.
  5. Encourage patient to develop additional "outside" support systems.

SUGGESTED READINGS

available at www.expertconsult.com

AUTHOR: **JOHN Q. YOUNG, M.D., M.P.P.**

BASIC INFORMATION

DEFINITION

Major depression is an episodic, frequently recurring syndrome. The diagnosis requires that five of nine criteria be present for 2 wk. One of these nine criteria must be either a persistent depressed mood or pervasive anhedonia (loss of interest or pleasure in all, or almost all, usual interests or activities). Other symptoms include sleep disturbance (insomnia or hypersomnia), appetite loss/gain or weight loss/gain, fatigue, psychomotor retardation or agitation, difficulty concentrating or indecisiveness, feelings of guilt or worthlessness, and recurrent thoughts of death or suicidal ideation.

SYNONYMS

Unipolar affective disorder
Clinical depression
Melancholia
Manic-depressive illness, depressed type
Depressive episode

ICD-9CM CODES
296.2
296.3
311

EPIDEMIOLOGY & DEMOGRAPHICS

LIFETIME RISK (IN U.S.): 10% of men, 20% of women
PREVALENCE (IN U.S.): Point prevalence in a community sample is 3% of men, 4.5% to 9.3% of women, and 1% of children. Prevalence of 20% to 40% in patients with comorbid medical conditions.
PREDOMINANT SEX: Female/male ratio 2:1
PREDOMINANT AGE: 25 to 44 yr; 5% of adolescents
PEAK INCIDENCE: 30 to 40 yr; 13% of postpartum women
GENETICS:
- Clear evidence of familial predominance
- Prevalence is 2 to 3 times greater among first-degree relatives.
- Concordance among monozygotic twins approximately 50%
- No established pattern of inheritance

PHYSICAL FINDINGS & CLINICAL PRESENTATION

- Clinical evaluation facilitated by organizing the major symptoms into four hallmarks: (1) depressed mood, (2) anhedonia, (3) physical symptoms (sleep disturbance, appetite problem, fatigue, psychomotor changes), and (4) psychologic symptoms (difficulty concentrating or indecisiveness, guilt or worthlessness, and suicidal ideation).
- A stressful life event, typically a serious loss, may trigger a depressive episode; however, the presence or absence of identifiable precipitants is irrelevant to the diagnosis.
- Patients often present with somatic complaints such as pain, fatigue, insomnia, dizziness, headache, or gastrointestinal problems.

- May be associated with mood-congruent delusional thinking (paranoid and melancholic themes).
- May be associated with active or passive suicidal ideation.
- Serious misconduct may appear in adolescents.
- May be misdiagnosed in elderly patients, with signs and symptoms attributed to normal aging.

ETIOLOGY

- A heterogeneous group of disorders probably arising from various etiologies.
- Genetic and environmental experiences, and their interaction, each contribute.
- Significant psychosocial stressors, especially loss, often trigger depression, particularly for first episodes.
- Numerous biologic correlates have been identified, though none is considered causative or diagnostic. Genes that influence the production and reuptake of serotonin, norepinephrine, and dopamine, as well as nerve cell growth in brain regions underlying memory and emotional processing, are of greatest interest. Abnormalities in brain regions underlying emotion regulation and reward processing, as well as irregularities in cortisol responding, appear to play a role.
- Cognitive risk factors include a pessimistic style of explaining negative events, a tendency to ruminate, and biases in processing emotional information and events.

DIAGNOSIS

DIFFERENTIAL DIAGNOSIS

- Anxiety disorders (e.g., social phobia, PTSD, obsessive compulsive disorder), substance abuse, and personality disorders often present with depressive symptoms.
- Important to determine if a depressive episode is part of major depression or part of bipolar disorder.
- Important to distinguish from adjustment disorder. Depression in the context of a stressful life event is diagnosed as major depressive disorder if the symptom criteria are met and adjustment disorder if the symptom criteria are not met. There is no evidence that medication is effective for adjustment disorder.
- Approximately 10% to 15% of depression caused by general medical illnesses, such as

Alzheimer's disease, Parkinson's disease, stroke, end-stage renal failure, cardiac disease, HIV infection, and cancer.
- Some medical conditions present as depression (e.g., hypothyroidism, hyperthyroidism or neurosyphilis).
- Premenstrual dysphoric disorder.
- In elderly, depression often coexists with dementia.

WORKUP

- Careful medical history is required
- Physical examination reveals no specific diagnostic signs of depression
- Mental status examination
- Self-report scales can assist in screening.
- Commonly used validated screening tools include the 15-item Geriatric Depression Scale in the elderly and the Patient Health Questionnaire (PHQ)-2 and PHQ-9. The PHQ-2 has a 97% sensitivity and 67% specificity in adults. If it is positive for depression, the PHQ-9 should be administered. The PHQ-9 has a 61% sensitivity and 94% specificity for depression in adults.

LABORATORY TESTS

- No laboratory studies are diagnostic.
- The following can assist in ruling out other confounding issues:
  1. Routine blood chemistry evaluation
  2. CBC with differential
  3. Thyroid function studies
  4. Vitamin B_{12} levels

IMAGING STUDIES

With unusual presentations (e.g., associated with new-onset severe headache, focal neurologic signs, a cognitive or sensory disturbance), the following may be performed:
- EEG (diffuse slowing indicates metabolic encephalopathy)
- Anatomic brain imaging (CT scan or MRI)

TREATMENT
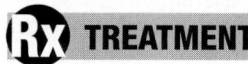

NONPHARMACOLOGIC THERAPY

- Good evidence that cognitive-behavioral therapy is as effective as antidepressant medication in achieving significant reduction or remission (Table 1-125).
- Problem solving and interpersonal psychotherapies have efficacy rates of 50% to 60%.

TABLE 1-125   Treatments of Depression

Name of Psychotherapy	Approach
Cognitive psychotherapy	Identify and correct negativistic patterns of thinking.
Interpersonal psychotherapy	Identify and work through role transitions or interpersonal losses, conflicts, or deficits.
Problem-solving therapy	Identify and prioritize situational problems; plan and implement strategies to deal with top-priority problems.
Psychodynamic psychotherapy	Use therapeutic relationship to maximize use of the healthiest defense mechanisms and coping strategies.

From Goldman L et al: *Goldman's Cecil medicine,* ed 24, Philadelphia, 2012, Saunders.

- "New wave" cognitive-behavioral therapies (e.g., acceptance and commitment therapy, mindfulness-based CBT) have demonstrated efficacy, but as of yet it is unknown whether they are superior to traditional CBT.
- By 12 wk, psychotherapy and medication approaches are equally effective.
- Patients with severe symptoms should generally not be treated by psychotherapy alone.
- Evidence, although mixed, that combined psychotherapy and medication may be more effective than either treatment alone.
- Factors, including history of childhood maltreatment, presence of precipitant stressful life events, and depression severity, may affect treatment response and risk of recurrence.

ACUTE GENERAL Rx

- Concurrent medical or psychiatric illnesses, history of prior response, cost, and side effects should be considered when selecting initial treatment. Fig. E1-270 describes guidelines for the treatment of depression in the primary care setting.
- Antidepressants are helpful in approximately 60% to 70% of cases, though sustained remission rates are lower.
- Selective serotonin reuptake inhibitors (SSRIs) generally are first-line.
- According to the STAR-D trial, approximately 30% achieve remission with the first prescribed medication after 3 months of treatment. Another 25% to 30% respond to treatment, but do not achieve remission. Treatment-refractory patients should be switched to another SSRI or to another class of medication, offered adjunctive medication such as bupropion, or referred for evidence-based counseling. Approximately 25% more patients will achieve remission with this secondary intervention.
- Response to antidepressants for many patients is seen as early as 2 wk, and among patients showing little to no response, the odds of later response decrease the longer patients remain unimproved.
- To date no benefit has been shown with combining antidepressants. Also no clear advantage has been identified for switching medications within vs. across different classes, or to switching vs. augmentation.
- Therapy should be continued for 4 to 9 mo after the full remission of symptoms.
- Electroconvulsive therapy is the most effective means available for the treatment of severe, refractory depression. Transcranial magnetic stimulation has also shown evidence of efficacy though effects are modest and to date electroconvulsive therapy showed superior efficacy.
- Antipsychotic medication should be added for psychotic depression. Antipsychotic medication has also been shown to be helpful in augmenting antidepressants for nonpsychotic depression.

CHRONIC Rx

Long-term treatment, in some cases, lifelong recommended for multiple depressive episodes, an episode duration longer than 2 yr, a severe episode or significant suicidality, or a strong family history of severe depression or bipolar disorder.

DISPOSITION

- Major depression is often a relapsing and remitting illness.
- Physical symptoms predict a favorable response to biologic intervention.
- Additional episodes experienced by >50% after one episode, with each additional episode linked to increased risk for subsequent episodes.
- Without treatment, episodes last an average of 6 to 12 mo; risk of recurrence higher without treatment.
- For many depressed individuals, subthreshold residual symptoms are present between episodes and define the majority of an individual's course of depression. Such symptoms may lead to impairment and warrant prolonged treatment.

REFERRAL

- If treatment refractory
- If patient suicidal or psychotic
- For suspected bipolar depression

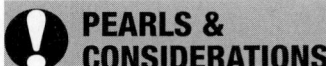

PEARLS & CONSIDERATIONS

COMMENTS

- All threats of suicide should be taken very seriously. Clinicians can use the mnemonic SAL: Is the method specific? Is it available? Is it lethal?
- Rule out bipolar affective disorder before initiating antidepressant medication.
- Many patients and families reluctant to acknowledge depression because of stigma.
- A two-question screener is as effective as longer instruments. A positive answer to either question warrants a full assessment.
  1. Over the past 2 weeks, have you ever felt down, depressed, or hopeless?
  2. Over the past 2 weeks, have you felt little interest or pleasure in doing things?
- Depression screening programs without treatment programs are unlikely to improve depression outcomes.
- Strict monitoring of patients who initiate antidepressant therapy is necessary both for safety and to ensure optimal treatment. Use of self-report scales to measure symptom severity are helpful in monitoring outcome.

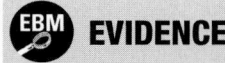 **EVIDENCE**

available at www.expertconsult.com

SUGGESTED READINGS

available at www.expertconsult.com

RELATED CONTENT

Bipolar Disorder (Related Key Topic)
Depression (Patient Information)

AUTHORS: **MARK ZIMMERMAN, M.D., CATHERINE D'AVANZATO, M.S.,** and **MITCHELL D. FELDMAN, M.D.**

BASIC INFORMATION

DEFINITION

De Quervain's tenosynovitis refers to a painful inflammatory process of the first dorsal retinacular compartment containing the tendons of the abductor pollicis longus and extensor pollicis brevis.

SYNONYMS

Stenosing tenosynovitis of the radial styloid process
Stenosing tenovaginitis of the first dorsal compartment
De Quervain's disease
De Quervain's tendonitis
De Quervain's stenosinig tenosynovitis
Tendinosis

ICD-9CM CODES
727.04 Radial styloid tenosynovitis, de Quervain disease
727.0 Synovitis and tenosynovitis
727.05 Other tenosynovitis of hand and wrist

EPIDEMIOLOGY & DEMOGRAPHICS

- More common in women than in men (10:1)
- Usually occurs between the ages of 30 and 50
- Associated with rheumatoid arthritis (RA)
- Can be seen in new mothers or daycare providers due to holding the babies with an outstretched thumb
- Seen more frequently in certain occupations involving repetitive wrist motion (e.g., clerical, assembly, and manual labor)

PHYSICAL FINDINGS & CLINICAL PRESENTATION

- Pain over the styloid process of the radius with grasping and isometric thumb abduction
- Swelling on the radial styloid
- Tenderness in the anatomic snuffbox
- Positive Finkelstein's test (Fig. 1-271)
- Crepitance
- Numbness of the dorsum of the thumb is rarely noticed.
- Absence of local heat on examination

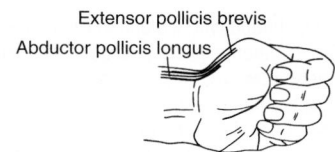
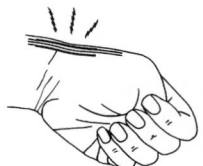

Extensor pollicis brevis
Abductor pollicis longus

FIGURE 1-271 Finkelstein's test is positive in de Quervain's stenosing synovitis. Ulnar flexion of the wrist produces pain over the dorsal compartment containing the extensor pollicis brevis and abductor pollicis longus. (From Noble J [ed]: *Textbook of primary care medicine,* ed 2, St Louis, 1996, Mosby.)

ETIOLOGY

- The cause is usually repetitive use or overuse of the hand and thumb involving pinching with the thumb while moving wrist in radial and ulnar directions causing thickening of the fibrous tendon sheath (e.g., typing, writing, nailing, golfing, fly-fishing, etc.).
- Acute trauma to the first extensor dorsal compartment can also lead to tenosynovitis.
- It can also occur in inflammatory joint conditions like RA and conditions causing calcium apatite deposition.

DIAGNOSIS

- The diagnosis of de Quervain's tenosynovitis is based on the clinical triad of:
  1. Tenderness over the radial styloid
  2. Swelling over the first dorsal retinacular compartment
  3. Pain on ulnar movement of the wrist with the thumb adducted and flexed (Finkelstein's test; see Fig. 1-271).
- Consideration can be given to injecting 1.5 ml of 1% Xylocaine into the tenosynovial sac, and if all three physical signs resolve, the diagnosis is confirmed, allowing for differentiation from carpometacarpal (CMC) osteoarthritis (OA).
- Finkelstein maneuver can also be present in first CMC joint OA; therefore it should also be evaluated if this test is positive.

DIFFERENTIAL DIAGNOSIS

- Carpal tunnel syndrome
- Arthritis (e.g., degenerative OA or RA)
- Gout
- Infiltrative tenosynovitis
- Radiculopathy
- Compression neuropathy (e.g., superficial branch of the radial nerve "bracelet syndrome")
- Ganglia
- Infection (e.g., tuberculosis, bacterial)
- Scaphoid fracture
- Intersection syndrome

LABORATORY TESTS

- ESR is usually normal in patients with de Quervain's tenosynovitis.
- Arthrocentesis can be used to rule out gout (crystals) and infection (Gram stain and culture of aspirate).

IMAGING STUDIES

- Imaging of the wrist and thumb is not necessary unless a fracture or arthritis is suspected.

TREATMENT

NONPHARMACOLOGIC THERAPY

- Rest
- Avoiding repetitive movements of the hand or thumb
- Splinting (thumb spica)
- Icing (4-6 times day for 15 minutes)
- Physiotherapy

ACUTE GENERAL Rx

- Corticosteroid injection using 20 to 40 mg triamcinolone acetonide and 1% Xylocaine is effective in relieving pain.
- NSAIDs (ibuprofen 800 mg tid or naproxen 500 mg bid)
- Topical hydrocortisone on the radial styloid for mild conditions

CHRONIC Rx

- Once signs of active inflammation have resolved after 3-4 wk, gentle stretching exercises involving abductor and extensor tendons usually help recovery.
- Surgical release is generally reserved for patients not responding to NSAIDs and corticosteroid injection therapy.

DISPOSITION

- ~90% of patients have relief of symptoms with either single or multiple steroid injections.
- Rarely, steroid injection use can cause infection and tendon rupture.
- If left untreated, can lead to fibrosis and decrease in mobility (stenosing tenosynovitis).
- Surgical control of symptoms achieved in 90% of referred cases
- Complications of surgery include:
  1. Radial nerve damage
  2. Paresthesia (~10%)
  3. Neuroma
  4. Scarring
- Recovery rates are higher with early treatment to ~80% after 6 wk but <40% after 4 yr.

REFERRAL

Rheumatologist or orthopedist

PEARLS & CONSIDERATIONS

- Steroid injection is generally recommended after failure of conservative treatment for 2-6 wk.
- Pain relief is usually noted within 48 hr with patient becoming asymptomatic by the first or second week after corticosteroid injection.
- If there is no improvement by 6 wk post second corticosteroid injection, referral to an orthopedic hand surgeon is recommended.
- Without treatment it will not improve and can get worse.
- Condition can recur if triggering activity continues.

SUGGESTED READINGS

available at www.expertconsult.com

RELATED CONTENT

De Quervain's Tenosynovitis (Patient Information)

AUTHOR: **SYEDA M. SAYEED, M.D.**

BASIC INFORMATION

DEFINITION

Dermatitis herpetiformis (DH) is an autoimmune blistering disease that is considered to be a cutaneous manifestation of celiac disease (CD). It is associated with gluten-sensitive enteropathy in nearly all cases, although only 20% of patients have gastrointestinal symptoms. Approximately 25% of patients with CD will have DH.

SYNONYMS

Duhring diease

ICD-9CM CODES
694.0 Dermatitis herpetiformis

EPIDEMIOLOGY & DEMOGRAPHICS

PREVALENCE (IN U.S.): 11.2 cases per 100,000 persons; prevalence for CD is one in 133 adults
PREDOMINANT SEX: Male predominance (2:1); however, female predominance in children
PREDOMINANT AGE: Fourth decade of life, but can occur at any age
PREDOMINANT RACE: Most common in Caucasians of Northern European ancestry
GENETICS: Both CD and DH have a strong genetic component. Eleven percent of patients with DH have a first-degree relative with either DH or CD. Specific HLA genes (involved in processing gliadin antigen in genetically susceptible individuals) have also been shown to predispose to developing DH (HLA-DQ2 in 90%, DQ8 in the remaining 10%). However, less than 50% of genetic predisposition is attributed to HLA genes.

PHYSICAL FINDINGS & CLINICAL PRESENTATION

- Classically, small fragile clusters ("herpetiform" vesicles) distributed symmetrically on extensor surfaces (elbows, knees, scalp, back, and buttocks) (Fig. 1-272). However, due to intense pruritus, pin-point erosions and excoriations are often the most prominent findings on examination, with intact vesicles rare.
- Spontaneous improvement with cyclic exacerbations is common.
- Celiac-type enamel defects to permanent teeth, oral vesicles, or palmoplantar purpura have been reported as potential associated findings.

PATHOGENESIS

CD and DH are both autoimmune-mediated by IgA class autoantibodies. Dietary gluten is central to the pathogenesis in both. It is hypothesized that gluten byproduct, gliadin, complexes with tissue transglutaminase (tTG) in the gut, binding as an antigen to HLA-DQ2 on T-cells, creating an immune response. Anti-tTG IgA antibodies (i.e., anti-endomysial antibodies) in the blood result. However, unlike CD, patients with DH also have high-affinity antibodies against epidermal transglutaminase (eTG) and antigenetic cross-reactivity has been suggested.

DIAGNOSIS

Physical examination and routine histopathology are often suggestive of DH; however, direct immunofluorescence (DIF) of a perilesional skin biopsy has pathognomonic findings and is the gold standard for diagnosis.

DIFFERENTIAL DIAGNOSIS

- Clinically and histologically, the differential diagnosis includes linear IgA dermatosis, bullous pemphigoid, and bullous lupus—can be differentiated by DIF on perilesional skin biopsy
- Other clinical diagnoses to consider:
  - Scabies (check for interdigital burrows, involvement of genitalia)
  - Arthropod bite (popular urticaria over exposed areas)
  - Eczematous dermatitis (ill-defined, weeping erythematous plaques)
  - Herpes simplex or zoster infection (painful, not symmetric)
  - Generalized pruritus (no blister history)

WORKUP, LABORATORY TESTS

- Evaluation for gastrointestinal symptoms, family history of DH or CD, and pruritus should be sought in patients with suspected DH
- **Lesional skin biopsy:** will demonstrate a neutrophil-rich subepidermal bulla and rule out many conditions.
- **DIF of normal-appearing perilesional skin biopsy:** will demonstrate pathognomonic IgA deposits localized to the dermal papillae and dermal-epidermal junction in a granular pattern.
- Checking for circulating antibodies in the blood (anti-gliadin, anti-endomysial, or anti-reticulin IgA antibodies) is not recommended as part of the diagnostic workup for DH. However, they can be helpful in confirming the diagnosis of DH in cases where linear IgA cannot be excluded on DIF.

TREATMENT

A gluten-free diet (GFD) and dapsone are considered first-line therapy, and are often started in conjunction.

- GFD improves symptoms of both GI and skin disease, with GI responding quicker (skin responds after 2 months).
- Dapsone results in improvement of skin manifestations within days but does not treat GI manifestations. Dapsone is often tapered over time, while lifelong gluten avoidance is often necessary.
- A recent small study demonstrated that a GFD alone was comparable to a gluten-free diet plus dapsone in the treatment of DH; hence GFD is an essential component in the treatment of DH.

NONPHARMACOLOGIC THERAPY

- First line: GFD
  - Avoid barley, rye, wheat (rice, corn, and oats okay)
  - Consultation with a dietitian recommended
  - Most patients need to follow diet indefinitely; however, cases of spontaneous remission have been reported.
- Second line: elemental diet (controversial)
  - Can consider elemental diet (avoidance of whole proteins) in those patients who do not adequately respond to a strict GFD; however, data are limited.

ACUTE GENERAL Rx

- First line: dapsone
  - Initial dose 25-50 mg PO daily with gradual increase to an average maintenance dose of 0.5-1 mg/kg daily (often maintenance dose of 100 mg daily).
  - Clinical monitoring weekly is recommended to optimize dose (optimal dose is when 1-2 new lesions/wk)

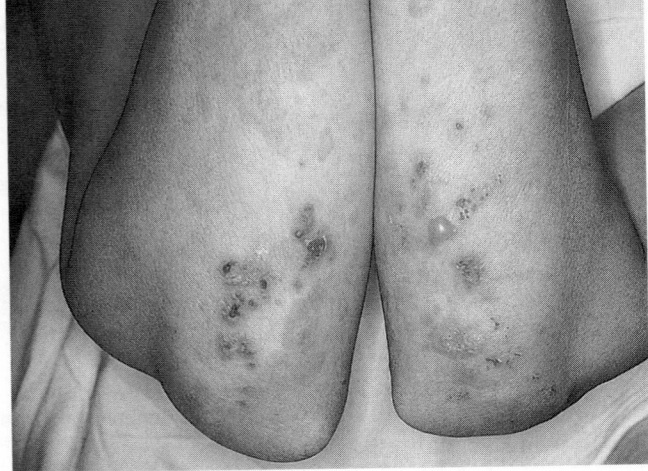

FIGURE 1-272 Dermatitis herpetiformis is an immunologically mediated blistering disease. There is a strong association of dermatitis herpetiformis with HLA-B8, DR3. Gluten-sensitive enteropathy is a common associated finding. The lesions are grouped (herpetiform) and extremely pruritic. (From Callen JP [ed]: *Color atlas of dermatology,* ed 2, Philadelphia, 2000, Saunders.)

○ Caution: dapsone may produce hemolysis (expecially if G6PD deficiency), agranulocytosis, methemoglobinemia, systemic drug hypersensitivity reaction (DRESS), and a peripheral neuropathy.

○ Baseline labs: CBC, LFTs, G6PD levels. After the initiation of therapy, monitor CBC every week x1 month, then every other week x2 months, monthly x4 months, then every 3-4 months. Monitor LFTs every 3-4 months.

- Second-line alternatives
  ○ Sulfapyridine (500-1500 mg/day) or sulfasalazine (500-1000 mg bid) may be substituted in cases of dapsone intolerance.
  ○ Reported efficacy in uncontrolled studies and case reports have suggested efficacy with tetracyclines, nicotinamide, cyclosporine, colchicine, and heparin
- Symptomatic relief for pruritus
  ○ Potent and superpotent topical corticosteroids (atrophy with prolonged use, limit to 14 days per month), antihistamines at bedtime, sarna lotion

CHRONIC Rx

- As DH is considered to represent the cutaneous manifestations of CD, lifelong avoidance of gluten is typically recommended. Information about educational resources, such as national and local support groups, should be provided (www.celiac.org).
- Patients with DH and CD have an increased risk of developing Hashimoto's thyroiditis, non-Hodgkin lymphoma, and GI lymphomas. An increased incidence of other autoimmune disorders (type 1 diabetes mellitus, pernicious anemia, Addison's disease, vitiligo, systemic lupus erythematosus, rheumatoid arthritis, and Sjögren's syndrome) and osteoporosis have also been reported.

○ Screening for thyroid disease (TSH, antithyroid peroxidase antibody titers) is typically recommended

○ Screening for autoimmune connective tissue diseases should be considered if suspicious signs or symptoms

○ Routine screening for GI lymphomas is controversial

REFERRAL

- Dermatologist for skin biopsy and management of cutaneous disease
- Gastroenterology for evaluation of CD
- Nutritionist to educate patients about gluten-free diet
- National support groups (www.celiac.org) and local support groups

! PEARLS & CONSIDERATIONS

- Classic areas involved are those that are exposed if in a "fetal position."
- Lesions may be worsened by iodides and certain NSAIDs; systemic steroids ineffective.
- Location of biopsies is important! False-negative DIF can result if biopsies are taken from lesional skin (should be taken from normal-appearing skin adjacent to lesion) as diagnostic IgA deposits are usually destroyed by the blistering process.
- GFD results in reduced IgA in skin on DIF (with eventual disappearance) and reduced anti-endomysial antibodies in the blood. Hence, serologies (e.g., anti-endomysial antibodies) can be used to monitor degree of compliance to dietary gluten restriction.
- Some studies have suggested a possible protective effect of GFD against intestinal lymphoma. First-degree relatives do not appear to be at increased risk for GI or systemic lymphomas in the absence of DH or CD.

SUGGESTED READINGS

available at www.expertconsult.com

RELATED CONTENT

Celiac Disease (Related Key Topic)
Celiac Disease (Patient Information)

AUTHORS: **LISA PAPPAS-TAFFER, M.D.,** and **IRIS TONG, M.D.**

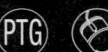
 BASIC INFORMATION

DEFINITION

Diabetes insipidus is a polyuric disorder resulting from insufficient production of antidiuretic hormone (ADH) (pituitary [neurogenic] diabetes insipidus) or unresponsiveness of the renal tubules to ADH (nephrogenic diabetes insipidus).

ICD-9CM CODES
253.5 Diabetes insipidus

EPIDEMIOLOGY & DEMOGRAPHICS

GENETICS:
- Nephrogenic diabetes insipidus can be inherited as a sex-linked recessive trait.
- There is also a rare autosomal-dominant form of neurogenic diabetes insipidus.

PHYSICAL FINDINGS & CLINICAL PRESENTATION
- Polyuria: urinary volumes ranging from 2.5 to 6 L/day
- Polydipsia (predilection for cold or iced drinks)
- Neurologic manifestations (seizures, headaches, visual field defects)
- Evidence of volume contractions

NOTE: The physical findings and clinical manifestations are generally not evident until vasopressin secretory capacity is reduced to <20% of normal.

ETIOLOGY

Neurogenic diabetes insipidus:
- Idiopathic
- Neoplasms of brain or pituitary fossa (craniopharyngiomas, metastatic neoplasms from breast or lung)
- Posttherapeutic neurosurgical procedures (e.g., hypophysectomy)
- Head trauma (e.g., basal skull fracture)
- Granulomatous disorders (sarcoidosis or tuberculosis)
- Histiocytosis (Hand-Schüller-Christian disease, eosinophilic granuloma)
- Familial (autosomal dominant); some cases autosomal recessive
- Other: interventricular hemorrhage, aneurysms, meningitis, postencephalitis, multiple sclerosis, Guillain-Barré syndrome

Nephrogenic diabetes insipidus:
- Drugs: lithium, aminoglycosides, antivirals amphotericin B, demeclocycline, methoxyflurane anesthesia
- Familial: X-linked
- Metabolic: hypercalcemia or hypokalemia
- Other: sarcoidosis, amyloidosis, pyelonephritis, polycystic disease, sickle cell disease, postobstructive, low-protein diets (protein malnourishment)

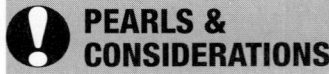 **DIAGNOSIS**

DIFFERENTIAL DIAGNOSIS
- Diabetes mellitus, nephropathies
- Primary polydipsia, medications (e.g., chlorpromazine)
- Osmotic diuresis (glucose, mannitol, anticholinergics)
- Psychogenic polydipsia, electrolyte disturbances

WORKUP
- The diagnostic workup is aimed at showing that polyuria is caused by the inability to concentrate urine and determining whether the problem is the result of decreased ADH or insensitivity to ADH. This is done with the water deprivation test (Table E1-126):
  - After baseline measurement of weight, ADH, plasma sodium, and urine and plasma osmolarity, the patient is deprived of fluids under strict medical supervision.
  - Frequent (q2h) monitoring of plasma and urine osmolarity follows.
  - The test is generally terminated when plasma osmolarity is >295 mOsm/kg or the patient loses ≥3.5% of initial body weight.
  - Diabetes insipidus is confirmed if the plasma osmolarity is >295 mOsm/kg and the urine osmolarity is <500 mOsm/kg.
  - To distinguish nephrogenic from neurogenic diabetes insipidus, the patient is given 5 U of vasopressin (ADH) and the change in urine osmolarity is measured. A significant increase (>50%) in urine osmolarity after administration of ADH is indicative of neurogenic diabetes insipidus.
- A diagnostic algorithm for diabetes insipidus is described in Fig. E1-273.

LABORATORY TESTS
- Decreased urinary specific gravity (≤1.005)
- Decreased urinary osmolarity (usually <200 mOsm/kg) even in the presence of high serum osmolality
- Hypernatremia, increased plasma osmolarity, hypercalcemia, hypokalemia

IMAGING STUDIES
MRI of the brain if neurogenic diabetes insipidus is confirmed

TREATMENT

NONPHARMACOLOGIC THERAPY
- Patient education regarding control of fluid balance and prevention of dehydration with adequate fluid intake or IV D_5W
- Daily weight

ACUTE GENERAL Rx
Therapy varies with the degree and type of diabetes insipidus (Table E1-127).
- Neurogenic diabetes insipidus:
  - Desmopressin acetate (DDAVP) 20-40 mcg qd intranasally in 1-3 divided doses or in tablet form 0.1-1.2 mg. Usual oral dose is 0.1 to 1.2 mg/day in 2-3 divided doses. Desmopressin is also available in injectable form given as 2-4 mcg/day SC or IV in 2 divided doses.
  - Vasopressin tannate in oil: 2.5 to 5 U IM q24 to 72h; useful for long-term management because of its long half-life.
  - In mild cases of neurogenic diabetes insipidus, polyuria may be controlled with HCTZ 50 mg qd (decreases urine volume by increasing proximal tubular reabsorption of glomerular infiltrate).
- Nephrogenic diabetes insipidus:
  - Removal of the underlying cause. However, prolonged lithium therapy can lead to irreversible nephrogenic diabetes insipidus even after lithium therapy is withdrawn.
  - Amiloride 5 mg/day for lithium-related disease
  - Low-sodium diet and chlorothiazide to induce mild sodium depletion

CHRONIC Rx
Patients should be aware of the danger of dehydration and the need for liberal water intake.

REFERRAL
Endocrinology consultation for diagnostic testing

! PEARLS & CONSIDERATIONS

COMMENTS
- Patients should be instructed to wear a medical identification tag or bracelet identifying their medical illness.
- In central diabetes insipidus, the use of DDAVP has become the standard of care. Extensive clinical experience has shown it to be both safe and effective in the treatment of this disorder.
- The treatment of nephrogenic diabetes insipidus is more complicated than the central form, and opinion varies among experts in the field. Consultation with a specialist is always recommended in this setting.

SUGGESTED READING
available at www.expertconsult.com

RELATED CONTENT
Diabetes Insipidus (Patient Information)

AUTHOR: **FRED F. FERRI, M.D.**

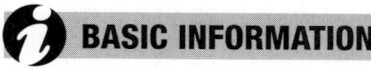

BASIC INFORMATION

DEFINITION

- Diabetes mellitus (DM) refers to a syndrome of hyperglycemia resulting from many different causes (see "Etiology"). It is broadly classified into type 1 and type 2 DM. The terms "insulin-dependent" and "non–insulin-dependent" diabetes are obsolete because when a person with type 2 diabetes needs insulin, he or she remains labeled as type 2 and is not reclassified as type 1. Table 1-128 provides a general comparison of the two types of DM.
- The American Diabetes Association (ADA) defines DM as follows:
  - A fasting plasma glucose (FPG) ≥126 mg/dl, which should be confirmed with repeat testing on a different day. Fasting is defined as no caloric intake for at least 8 hr.
  - Symptoms of hyperglycemia and a casual (random) plasma glucose ≥200 mg/dl. Classic symptoms of hyperglycemia include polyuria, polydipsia, and unexplained weight loss.
  - An oral glucose tolerance test (OGTT) with a plasma glucose ≥200 mg/dl 2 hr after a 75 g (100 g for pregnant women) glucose load.
  - A hemoglobin A_{1c} (HbA1c) value ≥6.5%.
- Individuals with glucose levels higher than normal but not high enough to meet the criteria for diagnosis of DM are considered to have "prediabetes," the diagnosis of which is made as follows:
  - A fasting plasma glucose 100 to 125 mg/dl; this is referred to as impaired fasting glucose.
  - After OGTT, a 2-hr plasma glucose 140 to 199; this is referred to as impaired glucose tolerance.
  - A hemoglobin A_{1c} value 5.7% to 6.4%.

- Table 1-129 describes diagnostic categories for DM and at-risk states.

SYNONYMS

IDDM (insulin-dependent diabetes mellitus)
NIDDM (non–insulin-dependent diabetes mellitus)
Type 1 diabetes mellitus (insulin-dependent diabetes mellitus)
Type 2 diabetes mellitus (non–insulin-dependent diabetes mellitus)

ICD-9CM CODES

250.0 Diabetes mellitus (NIDDM)
250.1 Insulin-dependent diabetes mellitus without complication (IDDM)

EPIDEMIOLOGY & DEMOGRAPHICS

- DM affects 9% to 10% of the U.S. population. Prevalence rates vary considerably by race/ethnicity.
- Incidence rate increases with age, varying from 2% in persons age 20 to 44 yr to 18% in persons 65 to 74 yr. Type 2 DM can have a long presymptomatic phase, leading to a 4- to 7-yr delay in diagnosis.
- Diabetes accounts for 8% of all legal blindness in the United States and is the leading cause of end-stage renal disease (ESRD).
- Patients with diabetes are 2-4 times more likely than nondiabetic patients to experience development of cardiovascular disease.

PHYSICAL FINDINGS & CLINICAL PRESENTATION

1. Physical examination varies with the presence of complications and may be normal in early stages
2. Diabetic retinopathy:
   a. Nonproliferative (background diabetic retinopathy):
      (1) Initially: microaneurysms, capillary dilation, waxy or hard exudates, dot and flame hemorrhages, atrioventricular shunts
      (2) Advanced stage: microinfarcts with cotton wool exudates, macular edema
   b. Proliferative retinopathy: characterized by formation of new vessels, vitreous hemorrhages, fibrous scarring, and retinal detachment
3. Cataracts and glaucoma occur with increased frequency in patients with diabetes
4. Diabetic neuropathy
   a. Distal sensorimotor polyneuropathy
      (1) Symptoms include paresthesia, hyperesthesia, or burning pain involving bilateral distal extremities, in a "stocking-glove" distribution. This can progress to motor weakness and ataxia.
      (2) Physical examination may reveal decreased pinprick sensation, sensation to light touch, vibration sense, and loss of proprioception. Motor disturbances such as decreased deep tendon reflexes and atrophy of interossei muscles can also be seen.
   b. Autonomic neuropathy:
      (1) GI disturbances: esophageal motility abnormalities, gastroparesis, diarrhea (usually nocturnal)
      (2) Genitourinary (GU) disturbances: neurogenic bladder (hesitancy, weak stream, and dribbling), impotence
      (3) Cardiovascular (CV) disturbances: orthostatic hypotension, tachycardia, decreased heart rate variability (HRV). Decreased heart rate variability is associated with increased cardiac mortality, independent of ejection fraction.

TABLE 1-128 General Comparison of the Two Types of Diabetes Mellitus

	Type 1	Type 2
Previous terminology	Insulin-dependent diabetes mellitus (IDDM), type I, juvenile-onset diabetes	Non–insulin-dependent diabetes mellitus, type II, adult-onset diabetes
Age of onset	Usually <30 yr, particularly childhood and adolescence, but any age	Usually >40 yr, but any age
Genetic predisposition	Moderate; environmental factors required for expression; 35%-50% concordance in monozygotic twins; several candidate genes proposed	Strong; 60%-90% concordance in monozygotic twins; many candidate genes proposed; some genes identified in maturity-onset diabetes of the young
Human leukocyte antigen associations	Linkage to DQA and DQB, influenced by DRB (3 and 4) (DR2 protective)	None known
Other associations	Autoimmune; Graves' disease, Hashimoto's thyroiditis, vitiligo, Addison's disease, pernicious anemia	Heterogenous group, ongoing subclassification based on identification of specific pathogenic processes and genetic defects
Precipitating and risk factors	Largely unknown; microbial, chemical, dietary, other	Age, obesity (central), sedentary lifestyle, previous gestational diabetes
Findings at diagnosis	85%-90% of patients have one and usually more autoantibodies to ICA512/IA-2/IA-2β, GAD$_{65}$, insulin (IAA)	Possibly complications (microvascular and macrovascular) caused by significant preceding asymptomatic period
Endogenous insulin levels	Low or absent	Usually present (relative deficiency), early hyperinsulinemia
Insulin resistance	Only with hyperglycemia	Mostly present
Prolonged fast	Hyperglycemia, ketoacidosis	Euglycemia
Stress, withdrawal of insulin	Ketoacidosis	Nonketotic hyperglycemia, occasionally ketoacidosis

GAD, Glutamic acid decarboxylase; IA-2/IA-2β, tyrosine phosphatases; IAA, insulin autoantibodies; ICA, islet cell antibody; ICA512, islet cell autoantigen 512 (fragment of IA-2).
From Andreoli TE (ed): *Cecil essentials of medicine*, ed 6, Philadelphia, 2005, Saunders.

c. Polyradiculopathy: painful weakness and atrophy in the distribution of ≥1 contiguous nerve roots.
d. Mononeuropathy involving cranial nerves III, IV, or VI or peripheral nerves can also occur.
5. Diabetic nephropathy: pedal edema, pallor, weakness, uremic appearance
6. Foot ulcers: occur in 15% of individuals with diabetes (annual incidence rate 2%) and are the leading causes of hospitalization; they are usually secondary to a combination of factors, including peripheral vascular insufficiency, repeated trauma (unrecognized because of sensory loss), and superimposed infection.
   a. Patient symptoms are usually less than would be expected from clinical findings, due to loss of sensation related to peripheral neuropathy.
   b. Comprehensive foot exams include visual inspection, assessment of pedal pulses, and assessment of protective sensation using a 10-g monofilament to test sensation.
   c. Prevention of foot ulcers in an individual with diabetes includes strict glucose control, patient education, prescription footwear, intensive podiatric care, and evaluation for surgical interventions
7. Neuropathic arthropathy (Charcot's joints): bone or joint deformities from repeated trauma (secondary to peripheral neuropathy; Fig. 1-274).
8. Necrobiosis lipoidica diabeticorum: plaquelike reddened areas with a central area that fades to white-yellow found on the anterior surfaces of the legs (Fig. 1-275); in these areas, the skin becomes very thin and can ulcerate easily.

ETIOLOGY
IDIOPATHIC DIABETES:
Type 1 DM: results from beta-cell destruction, usually leading to absolute insulin deficiency
- Hereditary factors:
  1. Islet cell antibodies (found in 90% of patients within the first yr of diagnosis)
  2. Higher incidence of human leukocyte antigen (HLA) types DR3, DR4
  3. 50% concordance rate in identical twins
- Environmental factors: viral infection (possibly Coxsackie virus, mumps virus)
Type 2 DM: results from insulin resistance and a progressive defect in insulin secretion.

- Hereditary factors: 90% concordance rate in identical twins
- Environmental factor: obesity, sedentary lifestyle, high carbohydrate content in food
DIABETES SECONDARY TO OTHER FACTORS:
- Hormonal excess: Cushing's syndrome, acromegaly, glucagonoma, pheochromocytoma
- Drugs: glucocorticoids, diuretics, oral contraceptives
- Insulin receptor unavailability (with or without circulating antibodies)
- Pancreatic disease: pancreatitis, pancreatectomy, hemochromatosis, cystic fibrosis
- Genetic syndromes: maturity onset diabetes of the young (MODY, monogenetic diabetes accounting for 2% to 5% of diabetes), familial hyperlipidemias, myotonic dystrophy, lipoatrophy
- Gestational diabetes (GDM): diabetes diagnosed during pregnancy that is due to pregnancy-related insulin resistance

DIAGNOSIS
DIFFERENTIAL DIAGNOSIS
- Diabetes insipidus
- Stress hyperglycemia
- Diabetes secondary to hormonal excess, drugs, pancreatic disease

LABORATORY TESTS
- Diagnosis of DM is made on the basis of the following tests:
  1. Fasting glucose ≥126 mg/dl on two occasions
  2. Non-FPG ≥200 mg/dl and symptoms of DM
  3. OGTT (75-g glucose load for nonpregnant individuals) with 2-hr value >200 mg/dl
  4. Glycosylated hemoglobin (HbA1c) ≥6.5%
- Screening for prediabetes and diabetes in asymptomatic patients (see Table 1-130):
  1. Should be considered in adults of any age who are overweight or obese (body mass index [BMI] >25 kg/m²) and who have one or more additional risk factors for diabetes.

TABLE 1-129 Diagnostic Categories*: Diabetes Mellitus and At-Risk States

Fasting Plasma Glucose Level	<140 mg/dl	140-199 mg/dl	≥200 mg/dl
<100 mg/dl	Normal	IGT†	DM
100-125 mg/dl	IFG†	IGT† and IFG†	DM
≥126 mg/dl	DM	DM	DM
HbA1c Level	**<5.7%**	**5.7-6.4%**	**≥6.5%**
	Normal	High-risk†	DM

*These diagnostic categories are based on the combined fasting plasma glucose level and a 2-hour, 75-g oral glucose tolerance test (OGTT) result. Note that a confirmed random plasma glucose level of 200 mg/dl or higher in the appropriate clinical setting is diagnostic of diabetes and precludes the need for further testing.
†May be referred to as prediabetes.
DM, Diabetes mellitus; IFG, impaired fasting glucose; IGT, impaired glucose tolerance.
From Goldman L, Schafer AI: Goldman's Cecil medicine, ed 24, Philadelphia, 2012, Saunders.

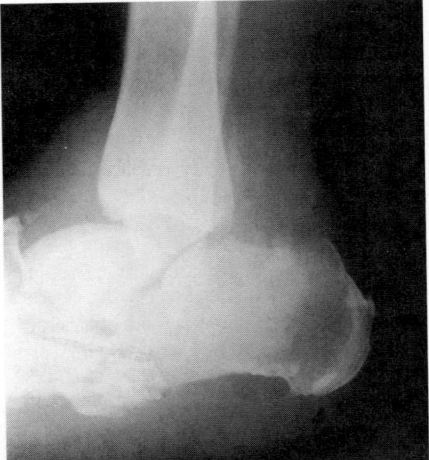

FIGURE 1-274 Diabetic neuropathy of the hindfoot. Destruction of the joint with collapse and fragmentation. (From Hochberg MC et al [eds]: Rheumatology, ed 3, St Louis, 2003, Mosby.)

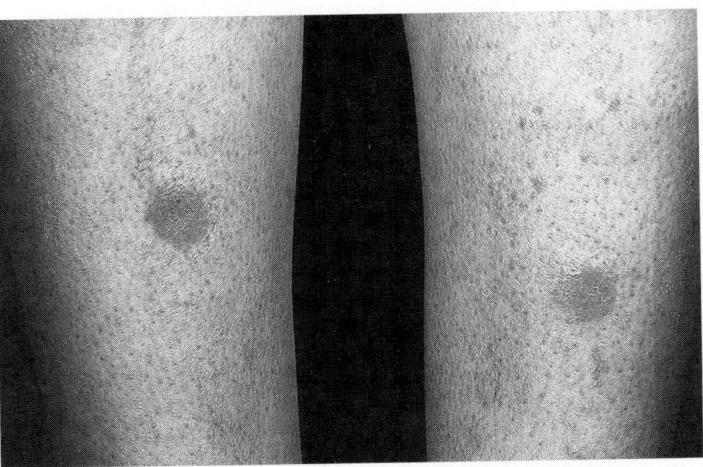

FIGURE 1-275 Necrobiosis lipoidica: symmetrical early lesions with erythema. (Courtesy of the Institute of Dermatology; from McKee PH et al [eds]: Pathology of the skin with clinical correlations, ed 3, St Louis, 2005, Mosby.)

D

Diseases
and Disorders

I

2. In those who are without these risk factors, testing should begin at age 45 yr.
3. If screen is normal, repeat testing should be carried out at least at 3-yr intervals.
• Detection and diagnosis of gestational diabetes mellitus (GDM)
  1. Screen for GDM using risk factor analysis and use of an OGTT. Pregnant women who are not known to have diabetes should be screened for gestational diabetes at 24 to 48 weeks' gestation with a 75-g oral glucose tolerance test. A diagnosis of GDM is made if any of the following levels of plasma glucose are exceeded: ≥92 mg/dl (5.1 mmol/L) when fasting, ≥80 mg/dl (10 mmol/L) at 1 hour, or ≥153 mg/dl (8.5 mmol/L) at 2 hours.
  2. Women with GDM should be screened for diabetes 6 to 12 wk postpartum and should be followed with subsequent screening for the development of diabetes or prediabetes at least every 3 yr

• Screening for diabetic nephropathy (Fig. 1-276)
  1. Screening should be done at diagnosis and then yearly for type 2 diabetes and 5 yr after diagnosis then yearly in type 2 diabetics.
  2. Screening can be performed using a albumin:creatinine ratio (microalbumin) in a random spot urine collection or by measurement of a 24-hour urine collection for albumin, and creatinine clearance. The urine albumin to creatinine ratio (ACR) is independently associated with mortality at all levels of estimated glomerular filtration rate (eGFR) in older adults with diabetes.
  3. The diagnosis of microalbuminuria (ACR 30-299 mg/24 hr) should be based on 2 to 3 elevated levels within a 3- to 6-mo period because there is a marked variability in day-to-day albumin excretion. Patients with overt macroalbuminuria (>300 mg albumin/24 hr or albumin: creatinine ratio >300) should be followed by urine protein:creatinine ratio.
• A fasting serum lipid panel, serum creatinine, and electrolytes should be obtained yearly on all adult patients with diabetes.
• Self-monitoring of blood glucose (SMBG) is crucial for assessing the effectiveness of the management plan. The frequency and timing of SMBG varies with the needs and goals of each patient. In most patients with type 1 DM and pregnant women taking insulin, SMBG is recommended at least 3 times/day. In patients with type 2 DM not on insulin, recommendations are unclear for SMBG, but testing once or twice/day is acceptable in most patients.

TABLE 1-130 Criteria for Diabetes Screening in Asymptomatic Individuals

1. Testing should be considered in all adults who are overweight (BMI >25 kg/m²*) and have additional risk factors:
   • Physical inactivity
   • A first-degree relative with diabetes
   • High-risk ethnic population (e.g., African American, Hispanic American, Native American, Asian American, Pacific Islander)
   • Delivered a baby weighing more than 9 lb or diagnosed with gestational diabetes mellitus
   • Systemic hypertension (blood pressure >140/90 mm Hg or on antihypertensive therapy)
   • High-density lipoprotein cholesterol level <35 mg/dl or triglyceride level >250 mg/dl
   • Polycystic ovary syndrome
   • Hemoglobin A_{1c} ≥5.7%, impaired glucose tolerance or impaired fasting glucose on prior testing
   • Other clinical conditions associated with insulin resistance (e.g., severe obesity, acanthosis nigricans)
   • History of cardiovascular disease
2. If none of the above criteria are present, screening for diabetes should begin at age 45 yr.
3. If the results are normal, screening should be repeated at least every 3 yr. Depending on initial results and risk status, more frequent testing may need to be considered.

*In some ethnic groups, such as Asians, at-risk body mass index (BMI) may be lower.
Modified from American Diabetes Association, Diagnosis and classification of diabetes mellitus *Diabetes Care* 33(Suppl. 1):S14, 2010. Borrowed from Goldman L, Schafer AI: *Goldman's Cecil medicine*, ed 24, Philadelphia, 2012, Saunders.

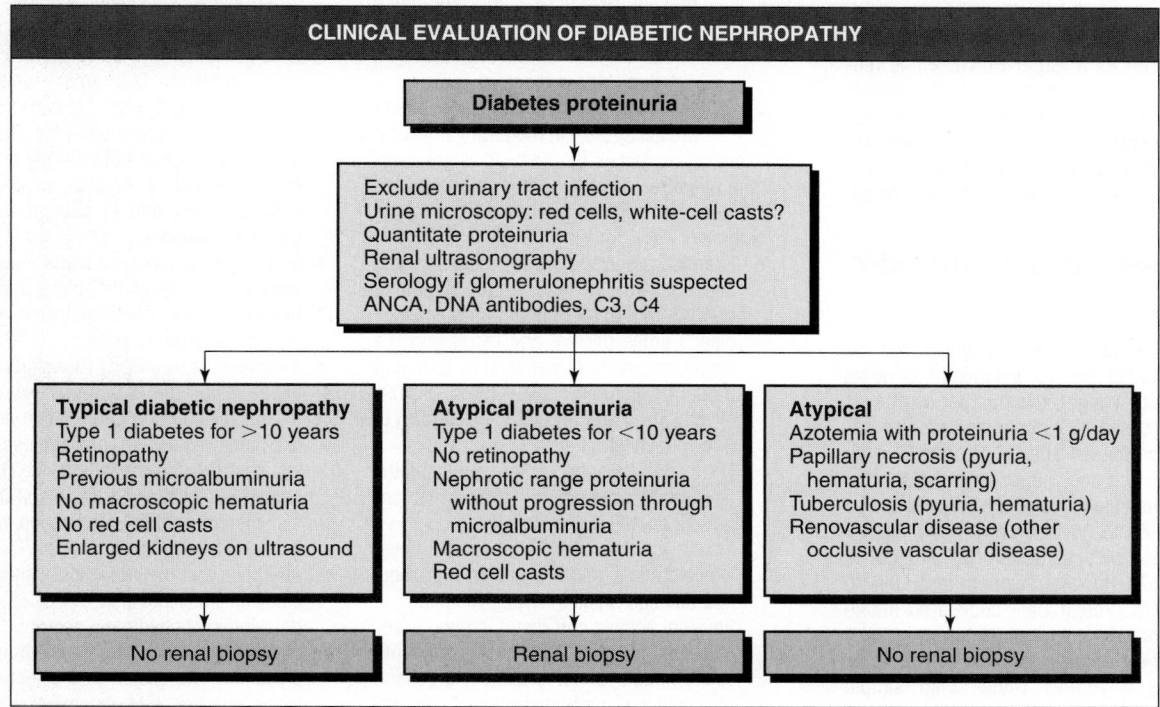

FIGURE 1-276 Clinical evaluation of diabetic renal disease. *ANCA,* Antineutrophil cytoplasmic antibody. (From Floege J et al: *Comprehensive clinical nephrology,* ed 4, Philadelphia, 2010, Saunders.)

- Screening for thyroid dysfunction (TSH level), Vitamin B_{12} deficiency, and celiac disease should be considered in type 1 diabetes due to the increased frequency of other autoimmune diseases in these individuals.

Rx TREATMENT

- Type 1 diabetes requires immediate initiation of insulin therapy.
- The ADA and European Association for the Study of Diabetes recommend lifestyle intervention (diet and exercise) and metformin initiation (unless contraindication such as renal failure) at the time of diagnosis of type 2 diabetes. Therapy should then be augmented with additional agents (including early initiation of insulin therapy) to achieve adequate glycemic control.
- In Type 1 diabetes, intensive glycemic control (HbA1c <7) has been shown in randomized controlled trials (RCT) to reduce the risk of microvascular (neuropathy, retinopathy, nephropathy) and macrovascular (cardiovascular events) complications.
- In Type 2 diabetes, intensive glycemic control (HbA1c <7) has been shown in RCT to reduce the risk of microvascular complications. While intensive glucose control reduced the risk of some cardiovascular disease outcomes (such as nonfatal MI), it did not reduce the risk of cardiovascular death or all cause mortality and increased the risk of severe hypoglycemia.
- It is important to remember that tight glycemic control may burden patients with complex treatment programs, hypoglycemia, weight gain, and costs. Clinicians should individualize HbA1c targets so that they are reasonable and reflect patients' personal and clinical contexts and their informed values and preferences A target HbA1c <7 is reasonable for motivated new diabetic patients with long life expectancies, whereas less stringent controls (HbA1c 7.5 or higher) may be reasonable in elderly patients with limited life expectancy and elevated risk of hypoglycemia.

NONPHARMACOLOGIC THERAPY

1. Diet
   a. Calories
      (1) The patient with diabetes can be started on 15 calories/lb of ideal body weight; this number can be increased to 20 calories/lb for an active person and 25 calories/lb if the patient does heavy physical labor.
      (2) The calories should be distributed as 45% to 65% carbohydrates, <30% fat, with saturated fat limited to <7% of total calories, and 10% to 30% protein. Daily cholesterol intake should not exceed 300 mg.
      (3) The emphasis should be on complex carbohydrates rather than simple and refined starches, and on polyunsaturated instead of saturated fats in a ratio of 2:1.
   b. Seven food groups
      (1) The exchange diet of the ADA includes bread or starches, meat or proteins, vegetables, fruits, fats, milk, and free foods (e.g., black tea, sugar-free gelatin).
      (2) The name of each exchange is meant to be all-inclusive (e.g., cereal, muffins, spaghetti, potatoes, rice are in the bread group; meats, fish, eggs, cheese, peanut butter are in the protein group).
      (3) The glycemic index compares the increase in blood sugar after the ingestion of simple sugars and complex carbohydrates with the increase that occurs after the absorption of glucose; equal amounts of starches do not give the same increase in plasma glucose (pasta equal in calories to a baked potato causes less of an increase than the potato); thus, it is helpful to know the glycemic index of a particular food product.
      (4) Fiber: Insoluble fiber (bran, celery) and soluble globular fiber (pectin in fruit) delay glucose absorption and attenuate the postprandial serum glucose peak; they also appear to reduce the increased triglyceride level often present in patients with uncontrolled diabetes. A diet high in fiber should be emphasized (20 to 35 g/day of soluble and insoluble fiber).
   c. Other principles
      (1) Modest sodium restriction to 2400 to 3000 mg/day. If hypertension is present, restrict to <2400 mg/day; if nephropathy and hypertension are present, restrict to <2000 mg/day.
      (2) Moderation of alcohol intake recommended (≤2 drinks/day in men, ≤1 drink/day in women).
      (3) Non-nutritive artificial sweeteners are acceptable in moderate amounts.
2. Exercise: increases the cellular glucose uptake by increasing the number of insulin receptors. The following points must be considered:
   a. Exercise program must be individualized and built up slowly. Consider beginning with 15 min of low-impact aerobic exercise 3 times per wk and increasing the frequency and duration to 30 to 45 min of moderate aerobic activity (50% to 70% of maximum age predicted heart rate) to 3 to 5 days/wk.
      (1) In the absence of contraindications, resistance training three times per wk should be encouraged.
   b. Insulin is more rapidly absorbed when injected into a limb that is then exercised, and this can result in hypoglycemia.
   c. Physical activity can result in hypoglycemia if medication dose or carbohydrate consumption is not modified. Ingestion of additional carbohydrates is recommended if pre-exercise glucose levels are <100 mg/dl.

3. Weight loss: to ideal body weight if the patient is overweight. Recent trials have shown that although weight loss has many positive health benefits for people with type 2 DM, such as slower decline in mobility, it does not reduce the number of cardiovascular events.
4. Screening for nephropathy, neuropathy, and retinopathy: annual serum creatinine and urine albumin excretion; initial comprehensive eye examination and at least annually thereafter
5. Diabetes self-management education: could also address psychosocial issues
6. Self-monitoring of blood glucose should occur three to four times per day for patients using multiple insulin injections or on insulin pump therapy
7. Perform HbA1c at least two times a year in patients who are meeting treatment goals and who have stable glycemic control
   ○ HbA1c quarterly in patients whose therapy has changed or who are not meeting glycemic goals
   ○ The HbA1c goal for nonpregnant adults in general is <7%
   ○ In the elderly, those with comorbidities, or those at risk for complications from hypoglycemia, a more moderate glycemic target (HbA1c 7-8) may be appropriate

GENERAL Rx

- When the previous measures fail to normalize the serum glucose, oral hypoglycemic agents should be added to the regimen in type 2 DM. Table 1-131 describes commonly used oral hypoglycemic agents.
- The primary mechanism of metformin is to decrease hepatic glucose production and improve insulin sensitivity. Because metformin does not produce hypoglycemia when used as a monotherapy, it is preferred initially for most patients. Metformin reduces mean HbA1c level by 1.1 %. It is contraindicated in patients with severe renal insufficiency with an estimated glomerular filtrate rate <30 ml/min, heart failure, or other clinical states of hypoperfusion, and in patients with significant liver disease.
- Sulfonylureas increase insulin secretion and work best when given before meals. All sulfonylureas are contraindicated in patients who are allergic to sulfa.
- Sitagliptin, saxagliptin, vildagliptin, and linagliptin inhibit the enzyme DPP-4, responsible for inactivation and degradation of glucagon-like peptide-1 (GLP-1) and glucose-dependent insulinotropic polypeptide (GIP). These drugs, known as "gliptins," raise blood incretin levels, thereby inhibiting glucagon release and lowering blood glucose levels.
- Acarbose and miglitol inhibit pancreatic amylase and small intestinal glucosidases, thereby delaying carbohydrate absorption in the gut and reducing associated post-prandial hyperglycemia. The major side effects are flatulence, diarrhea, and abdominal cramps.
- Exenatide and liraglutide are glucagon-like peptide-1 (GLP-1) agonists. They are incretin

TABLE 1-131 Non-Insulin Antidiabetic Agents

	Sulfonylureas	Biguanides	α-Glucosidase Inhibitors	Thiazolidine-diones	Meglitinides	Dipeptidyl Peptidase-4 Inhibitors	Incretin Mimetics	Amylin Analogue
Generic name	Glimepiride, glyburide, glipizide	Metformin	Acarbose, miglitol	Pioglitazone	Repaglinide, nateglinide	Sitagliptin, linagliptin, saxagliptin	Exenatide, liraglutide	Pramlintide
Mode of action	↑↑ Pancreatic insulin secretion chronically	↓↓HGP; ↓ peripheral IR; ↓ intestinal glucose absorption	Delays PP digestion of carbohydrates and absorption of glucose	↓↓ Peripheral IR; ↑↑ glucose disposal; ↓ HGP	↑↑ Pancreatic insulin secretion acutely	Potentiate insulin synthesis and release	Mimics incretin action by increasing glucose-dependent insulin secretion	Amylinomimetic agent; modulates gastric emptying, prevents postprandial glucagon secretion, and promotes satiety
Preferred patient type	Type 2 DM	Overweight, IR, fasting hyperglycemia, dyslipidemia	PP hyperglycemia	Overweight, IR, dyslipidemia, renal dysfunction	PP hyperglycemia	Type 2 DM	DM type 2 as monotherapy or adjunct, overweight	As an adjunct type 1 and type 2 DM

Therapeutic Effects

	Sulfonylureas	Biguanides	α-Glucosidase Inhibitors	Thiazolidine-diones	Meglitinides	Dipeptidyl Peptidase-4 Inhibitors	Incretin Mimetics	Amylin Analogue
↓ HBA$_{1c}$* (%) decrease	1-2	1-2	0.5-1	0.8-1	1-2	0.5	0.7-0.9	With the start of pramlintide, reduce preprandial, rapid acting or short acting insulin dosages by 50%
↓ FPG* (mg/dl) decrease	50-70	50-80	15-30	25-50	40-80			
↓ PPG* (mg/dl) decrease	~90	80	40-50	—	30			
Insulin levels	↑	—	—	—	↑			
Weight	↑	—/↓	—	—/↑	↑		↓	↓
Lipids	—	↓ LDL ↓↓ TG		↑ Large "fluffy" LDL ↓↓ TG ↑ HDL	—			
Side effects	Hypoglycemia	Diarrhea, lactic acidosis	Abdominal pain, flatulence, diarrhea	Heart failure; edema	Hypoglycemia (low-risk)		Hypoglycemia, nausea, vomiting, diarrhea, headache, pancreatitis	Severe hypoglycemia, abdominal pains, loss of appetite, nausea, vomiting, headache, cough
Dose(s)/day	1-2	1-3	1-3	1-2	+−2		Injectable exenatide (Byetta, Bydureon) bid weekly Injectable liraglutide qd (Victoza)	Type 1 initial: 15 mcg SUBQ prior to major meals; maintenance: titrate 15-mcg increments to 30-60 mcg; type 2 initial 60 mcg SUBQ immediately prior to major meals; maintenance, 120 mcg SUBQ as tolerated
Maximum daily dose	Glimepiride 8 mg, glyburide 20 mg, glipizide 40 mg	2550 mg	150 mg (<60-kg bw), 300 mg (>60-kg bw or above)	45 mg for pioglitazone	16 mg (repaglinide), 360 mg (nateglinide)	Sitagliptin 100 mg; saxagliptin 5 mg; linagliptin 5 mg	10 mcg SUBQ twice a day	Type 1: 60 mcg as tolerated; type 2: 120 mcg as tolerated
Renal impairment	Glipizide preferred—no adjustment needed	Can be used in creatinine clearance > 30 ml/min	Can be used when serum creatinine < 2 mg/dl	No dose adjustment needed	Repaglinide: CrCl 20-40 ml/min: start lower at 0.5 mg, avoid if CrCl < 20 ml/min; nateglinide: no adjustment needed	50% of the dose when CrCl < 50 ml/min, no dose adjustment for linagliptin	No dose adjustment needed	No dose adjustment needed when CrCl > 20 ml/min, not studied < 20 ml/min
Optimal administration time	~30 min premeal	After meal	With first bite of meal	With meal (breakfast)	Preferably <15 (0-30 min) pre-meals (omit if no meal)		Within 30-60 min period before meals twice a day	Immediately prior to major meals
Main site of metabolism/ excretion	Hepatic/renal, fecal	Not metabolized/renal	Only 2% absorbed/fecal	Hepatic/fecal	Hepatic/fecal		Renal	Renal

*Values combined from numerous studies; values are also dose dependent.

↑, Increased; ↓, decreased; —, unchanged; *bw*, body weight; *FPG*, fasting plasma glucose; *HDL*, high-density lipoprotein; *HGP*, hepatic glucose production; *IR*, insulin resistance; *LDL*, low-density lipoprotein; *PP*, postprandial; *PPG*, postprandial plasma glucose; *TG*, triglyceride.

Modified from Andreoli TE (ed): *Cecil essentials of medicine*, ed 6, Philadelphia, 2005, Saunders.

mimetics that stimulate release of insulin from pancreatic beta cells and can be used as adjunctive therapy for patients with type 2 DM. GLP-1 agonists are not indicated in type 1 DM and are contraindicated in patients with severe renal impairment.

- Pramlintide is a synthetic analog of human amylin, which is synthesized by pancreatic beta cells and cosecreted with insulin in response to food intake. It suppresses glucagon secretion and slows stomach emptying and can be used as an adjunctive treatment for patients with type 1 or type 2 DM who inject insulin at mealtime. Nausea is its major side effect.
- Thiazolidinediones (pioglitazone and rosiglitazone) increase insulin sensitivity and have been used in the therapy of type 2 diabetes. Serum transaminase levels should be obtained before starting therapy and monitored periodically. Thiazolidinediones, in general, result in moderate weight gain and increase the risk for heart failure and osteoporosis/fractures. Rosiglitazone has an FDA black box warning for heart failure exacerbations and myocardial ischemia. Pioglitazone and rosiglitazone cause increased incidence of bladder cancer.
- Combination therapy of various hypoglycemic agents is commonly used when monotherapy results in inadequate glycemic control.
- Insulin is indicated for the treatment of all type 1 DM and for type 2 DM patients whose condition cannot be adequately controlled with diet and oral agents. The American College of Endocrinology and the American Association of Clinical Endocrinologists recommend initiation of insulin therapy in patients with type 2 diabetes and an initial HbA1c level >9%, or if the diabetes is uncontrolled despite optimal oral glycemic therapy. Insulin therapy may be initiated as augmentation, starting at 0.3 unit/kg, or as replacement, starting at 0.6 to 1.0 unit/kg. Table 1-132 describes commonly used types of insulin.
  1. The risks of insulin therapy include weight gain, hypoglycemia, and in rare cases, allergic or cutaneous reactions.
  2. Replacement insulin therapy should mimic normal release patterns.
     a. Approximately 50% to 60% of daily insulin can be given as a long-acting insulin (NPH, ultralente, glargine, detemir) injected once or twice daily
     b. The remaining 40% to 50% can be short-acting (regular) or rapid-acting (lispro, aspart, glulysine) to cover mealtime carbohydrates and correct increased current glucose levels.
- Continuous subcutaneous insulin infusion (CSII, or insulin pump) provides comparable or slightly better control than multiple daily injections. It should be considered for diabetes presenting in childhood or adolescence and during pregnancy. The guidelines for insulin pump therapy from the American Association of Diabetes Educators include "frequent and unpredictable fluctuations in blood glucose" and "patient perceptions that diabetes management impedes the pursuit of personal or professional goals."
- Low-dose aspirin (ASA; 81 mg/day) has been proven to lower the risk of subsequent myocardial infarction, stroke, or vascular death in secondary prevention studies. The ADA recommends low-dose aspirin for primary prevention in diabetic patients with one additional cardiovascular risk factor, including age older than 40 yr, cigarette smoking, hypertension, obesity, albuminuria, hyperlipidemia, and family history of coronary artery disease.
- Measure fasting lipid profile at least annually in adults with low-risk lipid values (low-density lipoprotein [LDL] cholesterol <100 mg/dl, high-density lipoprotein [HDL] cholesterol >50 mg/dl, and triglycerides <150 mg/dl).
  1. All patients with diabetes older than 40 yr with one or more additional risk factors for cardiovascular disease should be on statin therapy together with lifestyle modification regardless of baseline lipid levels.
  2. The primary goal is an LDL cholesterol level <100 mg/dl without overt coronary-artery disease (CAD), and in patients with overt CAD, a goal of <70 mg/dl.
  3. In patients for whom target goals cannot be easily reached on maximal tolerated therapy, an alternative therapeutic goal should be the reduction in LDL of ~30% to 40% from baseline.
- Aggressive antihypertensive therapy is recommended to keep systolic blood pressure (BP) <130 and diastolic BP <80 mm Hg. Use of angiotensin-converting enzyme (ACE) inhibitors or angiotensin receptor blockers (ARBs) to decrease albuminuria and for prevention of progression of kidney disease should be considered regardless of presence of hypertension.
- Bariatric surgery should be considered in adults with BMI >35 kg/m² and type 2 diabetes, especially if the diabetes is difficult to control with lifestyle and pharmacologic therapy.
- Treat hypoglycemia in a conscious person with glucose tab or gel 15 to 20 g, and intramuscular injection of glucagon if unconscious. Patient and family members should be instructed on the administration of glucagon for individuals at significant risk for severe hypoglycemia.

DISPOSITION

- Diabetic retinopathy occurs in ~15% of patients with diabetes after 15 yr of diagnosis and increases 1%/yr after diagnosis. Retinal laser photocoagulation and vitrectomy are effective treatment modalities. Prevention is best accomplished by strict glucose and BP control. Early blockade of the renin-angiotensin system has been shown to slow progression of retinopathy in patients with type 1 diabetes.
- The frequency of neuropathy in patients with type 2 diabetes approaches 70% to 80%. It can be subdivided into sensorimotor neuropathy and autonomic neuropathy. Duloxetine, a selective serotonin and norepinephrine reuptake inhibitor, is effective and FDA approved for relief of diabetic peripheral neuropathy. Pregabalin and gabapentin (900 to 3600 mg/day) are also effective for the symptomatic treatment of peripheral

TABLE 1-132 Types of Insulin[a]

Preparation	Brand	Onset (hr)[b]	Peak (hr)	Duration (hr)[c]	Route
Insulin Aspart	NovoLog[d]	<0.25	1-3	3-5	SC, IV, CSII
Insulin Aspart Protamine/ Insulin Aspart	NovoLog Mix 70/30[d]	<0.25	1-4	24	SC
Insulin Detemir	Levemir[e]	1	None	24	SC
Insulin Glargine	Lantus[d]	1.1	None	≥24	SC
Insulin Glulisine	Apidra[d]	≤0.25	1	2-4	SC, IV
Insulin Lispro	Humalog[d]	<0.25	1	3.5-4.5	SC
Insulin Lispro Protamine/ Insulin Lispro	Humalog Mix 75/25[d]	≤0.25	0.5-1.5	24	SC
	Humalog Mix 50/50[d]	≤0.25	1	16	SC
Insulin Injection Regular (R)	Humulin R[f]	0.5	2-4	6-8	SC, IM, IV
	Novolin N[e]	0.5	2.5-5	8	SC, IM, IV
Insulin Isophane Suspension (NPH)/Regular Insulin (R)	Humulin 70/30[f]	0.5	2-12	24	SC
	Humulin 50/50[f]	0.5	3-5	24	SC
	Novolin 70/30[e]	0.5	2-12	24	SC
Insulin Isophane Suspension (NPH)	Humulin N[f]	1-2	6-12	18-24	SC
	Novolin N[e]	1.5	4-12	24	SC

[a]Injectable insulins listed are available in a concentration of 100 U/ml; Humulin R, in a concentration of 500 U/ml for SC injection. SC injection only is available by prescription from Lilly for insulin-resistant patients who are hospitalized or in need of medical supervision.
[b]Onset for injectable formulations is always for the subcutaneous (SC) route. All times are approximate.
[c]Maximum effect occurs between these times; actual effect may last longer.
[d]Recombinant human insulin analogue (using *E. coli*).
[e]Recombinant (using *S. cerevisiae*).
[f]Recombinant (using *E. coli*).
CSII, Continuous subcutaneous infusion; *IM,* intramuscularly; *IV,* intravenously.

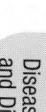

neuropathic pain. Topical capsaicin, 5% lidocaine transdermal patches, amitriptyline, and carbamazepine are also modestly effective.

- Diabetic gastroparesis is most often seen in patients who have had diabetes for at least 10 yr and typically have retinopathy, neuropathy, and nephropathy. Major manifestations are postprandial fullness, nausea, vomiting, and bloating. Pharmacologic therapy involves prokinetic agents (metoclopramide). Endoscopic injection of botulinum toxin into the pylorus and gastric electrical stimulation (using f electrodes placed laparoscopically in the muscle wall of the stomach antrum and connected to a neurostimulator) represent newer approaches to nonpharmacologic therapy.

- Nephropathy: The first sign of renal involvement in patients with DM is most often microalbuminuria, which is classified as incipient nephropathy. Before the current period of intensive glycemic control and blood pressure with ACE inhibitors and angiotensin receptor blockade, it was suggested that 25% to 45% of diabetic patients would develop clinically evident renal disease (proteinuria) and 4% to 17% would progress to end-stage renal disease. In the current era of intensive glycemic and blood pressure control and ACE/ARB use, clinically evident diabetic nephropathy has declined to 9% and end-stage renal disease 2% to 7%.

- Infections are generally more common in patients with diabetes because of multiple factors, such as impaired leukocyte function, decreased tissue perfusion secondary to vascular disease, repeated trauma because of loss of sensation, and urinary retention secondary to neuropathy.

- Prevention/delay of type 2 diabetes: Patients with prediabetes should achieve weight loss of 5% to 10% of body weight and increase physical activity to at least 150 min/wk of moderate activity such as walking. Metformin therapy may be considered in those at high risk, especially if they have hyperglycemia (HbA1c ≥6) despite lifestyle interventions.

REFERRAL

- Patients with diabetes should be advised to have annual ophthalmologic examinations. In type 1 DM, ophthalmologic visits should begin within 3 to 5 yr of diagnosis, whereas type 2 DM patients should be seen from disease onset.
- Podiatric care can significantly reduce the rate of foot infections and amputations in patients with DM. Noninfected neuropathic foot ulcers require debridement and reduction of pressure.
- Nephrology consultation in all cases of proteinuria, hyperkalemia, uncontrolled BP, and when GFR has decreased to <30 ml/min/1.73 m².

PEARLS & CONSIDERATIONS

COMMENTS

- Because normalization of serum glucose level is the ultimate goal, every patient with diabetes should measure his or her blood glucose with commercially available glucometers unless contraindicated by senility or blindness.
- Underinsured children and those with psychiatric illness are at greater risk for acute complications in type 1 DM and require frequent monitoring and aggressive risk management with diet, exercise, and periodic laboratory evaluation.
- Significant sustained weight loss using bariatric surgery has been reported as effective in achieving remission of type 2 diabetes in morbidly obese patients. Bariatric surgery may be considered for adults with BMI >35 μg/m² and type 2 DM, especially if diabetes or associated comorbidities are difficult to control with lifestyle and pharmacologic therapy.
- Cigarette smoking predicts incident type 2 diabetes. For a smoker at risk for diabetes, smoking cessation should be coupled with strategies for diabetes prevention and early detection.
- Glycemic control in hospitalized patients: The American College of Physicans (ACP) recommends against using intensive insulin therapy to strictly control blood glucose in nonsurgical intensive care unit (SICU)/medical intensive care unit (MICU) in patients with or without DM. The ACP recommends a target blood glucose level of 140 to 200 mg/dl if insulin therapy is used.
- Statin medication use in postmenopausal women has been reported to be associated with an increased risk for DM.

SUGGESTED READINGS
available at www.expertconsult.com

RELATED CONTENT

Diabetic Ketoacidosis (Related Key Topic)
Diabetic Polyneuropathy (Related Key Topic)
Diabetic Retinopathy (Related Key Topic)
Gestational Diabetes Mellitus (Related Key Topic)
Hyperosmolar Nonketotic State (Related Key Topic)
Diabetes Mellitus Type 1 (Patient Information)
Diabetes Mellitus Type 2 (Patient Information)

AUTHORS: **HILARY B. WHITLATCH, M.D., SAINATH GADDAM, M.D.,** and **FRED F. FERRI, M.D.**

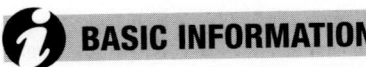

DEFINITION

Diabetic ketoacidosis (DKA) is a life-threatening complication of diabetes mellitus resulting from absolute insulin deficiency or insulin resistance with relative insulin deficiency. It is characterized by the presence of an anion gap metabolic acidosis, ketonemia, and hyperglycemia. Patients often present with severe dehydration and altered sensorium.

SYNONYMS

DKA

ICD-9CM CODES
250.1 Diabetic ketoacidosis

EPIDEMIOLOGY & DEMOGRAPHICS

INCIDENCE/PREVALENCE: 6 episodes per 10,000 individuals with diabetes; it accounts for 8% to 29% of all hospital admissions of patients with diabetes
PREDOMINANT AGE: 36% in persons younger than age 30, 27% in persons 30 to 60 years of age, 23% in persons 51 to 70 years of age, and 14% occurring in persons older than 70 years.

PHYSICAL FINDINGS & CLINICAL PRESENTATION

- Evidence of dehydration (tachycardia, hypotension, dry mucous membranes, sunken eyeballs, poor skin turgor)
- Altered mental status
- Tachypnea with air hunger (Kussmaul's respiration)
- Fruity breath odor (caused by acetone)
- Lipemia retinalis in some patients
- Possible evidence of precipitating factors (infected wound, pneumonia)
- Abdominal tenderness in some patients

ETIOLOGY

- Metabolic decompensation in individuals with diabetes is frequently precipitated by an infectious process (up to 40%).
- Poor compliance with insulin therapy and severe medical illness (e.g., pancreatitis, cardiovascular events) are other common causes.
- There is a subgroup of type 2 diabetics who have ketosis-prone diabetes. These persons are often black or Latino, overweight, middle aged, males with a family history of diabetes or newly diagnosed diabetes. This subgroup represents 20% to 50% of persons with DKA.
- Cocaine abuse has been reported as a risk factor for DKA in adult and teenage patients, particularly in patients with multiple admissions.
- Lack of education of primary caregiver (mother, sibling), as well as deficiencies in proper monitoring of blood glucose, correct administration of insulin, supervision of insulin pump maintenance, and monitoring of diabetic caloric restraints are causes of recurrent episodes of DKA.

DIFFERENTIAL DIAGNOSIS

- Hyperosmolar nonketotic state
- Alcoholic ketoacidosis
- Uremic acidosis
- Metabolic acidosis caused by methyl alcohol or ethylene glycol
- Salicylate poisoning

WORKUP

- Laboratory evaluation (see "Laboratory Tests") to confirm diagnosis and evaluate precipitating factors
- Identification of "trigger," such as infection (blood cultures, urine cultures, chest radiographs), pancreatitis (pancreatic enzymes), or myocardial ischemia (ECG, cardiac enzymes)

LABORATORY TESTS

- Glucose level demonstrates severe hyperglycemia (serum glucose generally >250 mg/dl)
- Arterial blood gases demonstrate metabolic acidosis: arterial pH usually <7.30 with P_{CO_2} <40 mm Hg
- Serum ketonemia (β-hydroxybutyrate >300 μmol/L), ketonuria, and glycosuria
- Serum electrolytes:
  1. Serum bicarbonate is usually <15 mEq/L.
  2. Serum potassium (K^+) may be low, normal, or elevated. There is always significant total body potassium depletion regardless of the initial potassium level.
  3. Serum sodium is usually decreased as a result of hyperglycemia, dehydration, and lipemia. Assume 1.6-mEq/L decrease in extracellular sodium for each 100-mg/dl increase in glucose concentration.
  4. Calculate the anion gap (AG):

     $$AG = Na^+ - (Cl^- + HCO^-_3)$$

     In DKA, the anion gap is increased (>12) because of high levels of ketones.
  5. Mixed metabolic disturbances demonstrating anion gap metabolic acidosis overlapping with metabolic alkalosis may be present; this is common in patients with DKA with persistent vomiting.
- CBC with differential, urinalysis, and urine and blood cultures to rule out infectious precipitating factor
- Serum calcium, magnesium, and phosphorus; the plasma phosphate and magnesium levels may be significantly depressed and should be rechecked within 12 hr because they may decrease further with correction of DKA
- Blood urea nitrogen and creatinine generally reveal significant dehydration and acute kidney injury.
- A pregnancy test should be performed in all female patients of child-bearing years who present with DKA.
- Amylase, lipase, and liver enzymes should be checked in patients with abdominal pain.

IMAGING STUDIES

- Chest radiographs are helpful to rule out pneumonia. The initial chest film may be negative if the patient has significant dehydration. Repeat chest x-ray after 24 hr if pulmonary infection is strongly suspected.
- Additional imaging, such as CT scanning or abdominal ultrasound, should be considered in the presence of physical exam findings, such as abdominal tenderness.

NONPHARMACOLOGIC THERAPY

- Monitor mental status, vital signs, and urine output hourly until improved, then monitor every 2 to 4 hours.
- Fingersticks should be checked every 1 to 2 hours while patient is on an insulin drip.
- Basic metabolic panel should be checked every 2 to 4 hours to monitor for anion gap closure (see "Acute General Rx").

ACUTE GENERAL Rx (Fig. E1-277)

Fluid replacement (usual deficit is 6 to 8 L)

1. Do not delay fluid replacement until laboratory results have been received. Fluid deficits are typically 100 ml/kg of body weight. The total fluid administered should not exceed 4 L/m²/24 hours for fear of causing cerebral edema (CE). One rule of thumb is to deliver fluids (deficit and maintenance) over a period of 48 hours if serum osmolality is >360 mOsm/L.
2. The initial fluid replacement should be with 0.9% normal saline (NS) to expand vascular volume and ensure blood pressure stabilization and organ perfusion. In patients with severe hypernatremia (serum sodium >160 mEq/L), 0.45% normal saline infusion can be used. Careful monitoring for fluid overload is necessary in elderly patients and those with a history of congestive heart failure.
3. The rate of fluid replacement varies with the age of the patient and the presence of significant cardiac or renal disease.
   - The usual rate of infusion is 1 L of 0.9% NS over the first hour, followed by 15 ml/kg/hr 0.9% NS during the second hour. Then change to 0.45% NS at 15 ml/kg/hr to replenish free water.
   - Switch to dextrose D5 0.45% NS when serum glucose is <250 to prevent hypoglycemia and introduce additional glucose substrate (necessary to suppress lipolysis and ketogenesis).

Insulin administration:

1. The patient should be given an initial loading IV bolus of 0.1 U/kg regular insulin followed by a constant infusion at a rate of 0.1 U/kg/hour. Insulin replacement should generally not be started until serum potassium is >3.3 mEq/L to prevent life-threatening hypokalemia.
2. Monitor serum glucose every 1 to 2 hr while patient is on insulin drip, then every 2 to 4 hr.
3. The goal is to decrease serum glucose level by 80 mg/dl/hour (after an initial decline

because of rehydration); if the serum glucose level is not decreasing at the expected rate, double the rate of insulin infusion.

4. When the serum glucose level approaches 250 mg/dl, decrease the rate of insulin infusion to 2 to 3 U/hour and continue this rate until the patient has received adequate fluid replacement, HCO_3^- is close to normal, and ketones have cleared. After target glucose levels are achieved, it usually takes 5 to 7 hr for ketosis to clear. Young children and adolescents have greater levels of human growth hormone, resulting in a prolonged time lag for plasma glucose to reach above levels. Patients with infection and fever have higher metabolic requirements and may need 15% to 20% more insulin than the usual starting dose.

5. Prior to stopping the IV insulin infusion, administer an SC dose of insulin (dose varies with the patient's demonstrated insulin sensitivity). Short (regular) or rapid-acting (aspart, lispro, glulisine) insulins should be administered SC 1 to 2 hr before stopping IV insulin infusion. Intermediate (NPH) or long-acting (glargine, detemir) insulins should be administered 2 to 4 hr before stopping IV insulin infusion.

6. In individuals with newly diagnosed diabetes, the total daily insulin dose to maintain metabolic control ranges from 0.5 to 0.8 U/kg/day. Approximately half of this dose should be given as intermediate or long-acting insulin, and half of this dose should be given as mealtime or prandial insulin, provided the patient is eating.

Electrolyte replacement:
- Potassium replacement: the average total potassium loss in DKA is 300 to 500 mEq.
- K^+ can be supplemented as chloride- and phosphate-containing solutions.
  1. The rate of replacement varies with the patient's serum potassium level, degree of acidosis (decreased pH, increased potassium level), and renal function (potassium replacement should be used with caution in patients with renal failure).
  2. As a rule of thumb, potassium replacement can be guided by presenting serum K level. If K is <3.3, give KCl 20 to 30 mEq/L of intravenous fluid (IVF) until K is >3.3. If K is 3.3 to 5.3, give KCl at 10 to 30 mEq/L IVF to maintain a K of >4. If K is >5.3, hold potassium supplementation until K is <5.3.
  3. Monitor serum potassium level hourly for the first 2 hours, then monitor q2 to 4h.
- Phosphate replacement: If the serum PO_4 is <1.5 mEq/L, give 2.5 mg/kg IV over 6 hours of elemental phosphate. Routine replacement

of phosphate (in the absence of laboratory evidence of significant hypophosphatemia) is not indicated. Rapid IV phosphate administration can cause hypocalcemia.
- Magnesium replacement: Replacement is indicated only in the presence of significant hypomagnesemia or refractory hypokalemia/hypocalcemia.

Bicarbonate therapy:
- Routine use of bicarbonate in DKA is contraindicated because it can worsen hypokalemia and can cause cerebral edema. Bicarbonate therapy should be considered only if the arterial pH is <6.9 and HCO_3^- is <5.
- In these patients, 44 to 88 mEq sodium bicarbonate can be added to 1 L of 0.45% NS q2-4h until pH increases to >7.
- Use of bicarbonate therapy is particularly dangerous in the pediatric population. Children with DKA are at increased risk for cerebral edema. Bicarbonate therapy in children with DKA should be limited to those with severe circulatory failure and a high risk for cardiac decompensation resulting from profound acidosis.

PREVENTION
- Provide information/education for teachers, parents, school staff, and caregivers on how to recognize children with undiagnosed diabetes.
- Review sick day management; increase home blood glucose monitoring, education on how to measure urinary or fingerstick ketones, compliance with insulin; and maintain adequate hydration and nutrition.

DISPOSITION
- Average mortality rate in DKA is 5% to 10%.
- In children <10 yr, DKA causes 70% of diabetes-related deaths.
- Cerebral edema (CE) occurs in 1% of episodes of DKA in children and is associated with a mortality rate of 40% to 90%.

REFERRAL
In general, patients with DKA should be admitted to the intensive care unit on an insulin drip. Alert patients who are able to take fluids orally and have mild DKA occasionally can be treated with short-acting insulin analogues under observation and sent home. The American Diabetes Association admission guidelines are a plasma glucose level >250 mg/dl with arterial pH <7.30, serum bicarbonate level <15 mEq/L, and a moderate or greater level of ketones in the serum or urine.

PEARLS & CONSIDERATIONS

COMMENTS
- Although DKA occurs more commonly in type 1 diabetes mellitus, a significant proportion (>20%) occurs in patients with type 2 diabetes, particularly under conditions of extreme stress, severe infection or surgery, and marked hyperglycemia (results in glucose toxicity).
- 30% to 40% of DKA admissions involve patients with newly diagnosed diabetes.
- Potential complications of DKA therapy include hypoglycemia, cerebral edema, cardiac arrhythmias, shock, myocardial infarction, and acute pancreatitis.
- Risk factors for cerebral edema include age <5 yr, high initial BUN, hyperventilation to a $Paco_2$ of <22 mm Hg, and presenting arterial pH of <7.00. It presents 4 to 8 hours after start of rehydration therapy. Presentation may be abrupt with sudden severe headache, vomiting, sudden hypertension, and obtunded sensorium. First management response to CE is to elevate head of the patient to 30-degree angle, IV mannitol, intubation and hyperventilation, and, finally, cutting back of the maintenance fluid to 75%.
- Underinsured children and those with psychiatric illness are at greater risk for DKA.
- Subcutaneous administration of rapid-acting insulin analogues may be reasonable alternatives to IV regular insulin infusion for treating uncomplicated DKA.
- DKA can occur with blood glucose <350 mg/dl in the setting of poor oral intake or pregnancy.
- Ketones can be positive in starvation or with heavy alcohol intake; DKA can coexist with other causes of metabolic acidosis such as lactic acidosis.

SUGGESTED READINGS
available at www.expertconsult.com

RELATED CONTENT
Diabetes Mellitus (Related Key Topic)
Hyperosmolar Nonketotic State (Related Key Topic)

AUTHORS: **HILARY B. WHITLATCH, M.D., SAINATH GADDAM, M.D.**, and **FRED F. FERRI, M.D.**

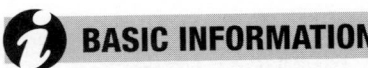

BASIC INFORMATION

DEFINITION

Diabetic polyneuropathy is a term used to encompass the various forms of peripheral nerve dysfunction that occur in the setting of diabetes. The most common form of diabetic polyneuropathy is distal symmetric polyneuropathy (DSPN), which is a length-dependent process typically characterized by numbness, tingling, and occasionally, pain that begins in the feet and slowly progresses more proximally. Besides DSPN, in which distal sensory nerves are predominantly involved, diabetes is also associated with autonomic neuropathies, as well as focal or multifocal neuropathies that can lead to proximal and asymmetric presentations.

SYNONYMS

Chronic distal symmetric polyneuropathy
Diabetic peripheral neuropathy

ICD-9CM CODES
250.6 Diabetes with neurological manifestations
357.2 Polyneuropathy in diabetes

EPIDEMIOLOGY & DEMOGRAPHICS

PREVALENCE: The true prevalence of diabetic polyneuropathy in its varying forms is unknown, but it is the most common cause of peripheral neuropathy in developed countries. As many as 66% of individuals with diabetes may have some form of neuropathy.
RISK FACTORS: Patients with poor glycemic control and patients with diabetic nephropathy or retinopathy are at increased risk.

PHYSICAL FINDINGS & CLINICAL PRESENTATION

DSPN:
- Patients most commonly experience numbness and tingling, but may also experience feelings of tightness or a sensation of heat or cold.
- Pain is not uncommon, is often worst at night, and can be burning, aching, shooting, or lancinating in nature.
- These symptoms begin in the feet and may slowly ascend over months to years. Symptoms in the hands do not generally occur until symptoms in the lower extremities have reached the level of the knees. In more severe cases, the symptoms can spread to the trunk and head.
- Neurologic examination reveals early loss of small-fiber modalities resulting in decreased pinprick and temperature sensation with later involvement of large-fiber modalities leading to a reduction in vibratory and proprioceptive sensation. Ankle reflexes are usually reduced or absent, and more proximal reflexes may also become involved as the neuropathy progresses. Strength is usually normal, but there can be some motor involvement leading to mild weakness and atrophy

which is usually limited to intrinsic foot muscles and ankle dorsiflexors.

OTHER DIABETIC NEUROPATHIES

Autonomic neuropathy (Fig. E1-278):
- Some form of autonomic dysfunction may be present in up to half of diabetic individuals and usually occurs along with a DSPN.
- Symptoms are usually mild and may include difficulty adjusting to changes in light or dryness of the eyes or mouth.
- Gastrointestinal symptoms are common and can include early satiety, bloating, vomiting, constipation, or diarrhea.
- Cardiovascular complications include cardiac arrhythmias and postural hypotension.
- Patients may also have symptoms related to dysfunction of the genitourinary (erectile dysfunction and incontinence) or thermoregulatory (excessive or reduced sweating, intolerance of cold or heat) systems.

Regional diabetic polyneuropathy:
- In contrast to DSPN, the regional diabetic polyneuropathies tend to be subacute in onset, predominantly proximal, and asymmetric or unilateral.
- These usually occur in individuals who also have a DSPN
- The most common presentation is the diabetic lumbosacral radiculoplexus neuropathy, which is also known as *diabetic amyotrophy* or *Bruns-Garland syndrome*. Patients usually report acute or subacute onset of severe pain involving the lower back, hip, and thigh. Weakness and atrophy of the affected leg progresses over the course of days to weeks, often predominantly in the anterior thigh. There may also be numbness, tingling, and significant weight loss. Although the initial onset is typically unilateral, asymmetric involvement of the other leg commonly occurs within weeks or months. Progression of weakness usually plateaus within several months, followed by some degree of gradual improvement that can take 2 to 3 yr. The degree of improvement is variable, and many individuals have significant, chronic pain, weakness, or sensory loss.
- Less commonly, involvement of several thoracic nerve roots may cause a thoracoabdominal neuropathy, resulting in pain and numbness in the chest, back, or abdomen. The symptoms are usually in a dermatomal distribution but may mimic more common causes of pain in these areas. There may also be associated weakness of the abdominal muscles.
- The cervical roots and brachial plexus are not usually involved.

Focal diabetic neuropathy:
- These also tend to occur in patients who also have DSPN.
- Diabetic patients are at increased risk for common limb mononeuropathies, particularly median neuropathy at the wrist and ulnar neuropathy at the elbow, but other nerves (femoral, sciatic, or peroneal) may be involved as well.

- A diabetic cranial mononeuropathy usually presents acutely and unilaterally, with or without pain. The examination findings should be limited to dysfunction of a single cranial nerve, usually cranial nerve III, VI, VII, or, less frequently, IV. There is typically significant improvement or complete resolution within several months.

ETIOLOGY

The etiology is unknown but most likely involves a complex interaction of metabolic derangements and microvascular insults that occur in the setting of diabetes.

DIAGNOSIS

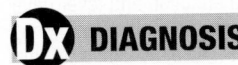

DIFFERENTIAL DIAGNOSIS

Although diabetes is the leading cause of peripheral neuropathy in developed countries, there are many other causes.

WORKUP

- A thorough history and neurologic examination are essential to confirm features consistent with a diabetic polyneuropathy and exclude other features that would suggest alternative diagnoses.
- For some patients, neuropathy may be the presenting feature of previously undiagnosed diabetes.
- Electrodiagnostic evaluation to include nerve conduction studies and electromyography can be helpful in confirming the presence, extent, and severity of a neuropathy.
- Patients with DSPN typically have a reduction of amplitudes and slowing of conduction velocities involving sensory and possibly motor nerves in a length-dependent and symmetric fashion.
- Electromyographic examination of distal muscles may reveal fibrillation potentials, positive sharp waves, and large motor unit action potentials, suggestive of denervation and reinnervation.
- Skin biopsy and nerve biopsy are not necessary in the vast majority of cases.

LABORATORY TESTS

- Fasting blood sugar, hemoglobin A_{1c}, and oral glucose tolerance test should all be considered in patients with peripheral neuropathy without a known history of diabetes.
- A focused laboratory evaluation for other common or potentially treatable causes of neuropathy is also indicated: complete blood cell count, complete metabolic panel to include electrolytes and liver function tests, erythrocyte sedimentation rate, vitamin B_{12} and folate levels, thyroid function tests, serum protein electrophoresis and immunofixation electrophoresis.
- Additional laboratory tests can be considered based on history or exam findings that may suggest other underlying diagnoses: antinuclear antibodies, extractable nuclear antigens, and rheumatoid factor.

IMAGING STUDIES

Imaging is not necessary unless there is concern for an alternate or coexisting process based on the history and examination.

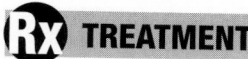 TREATMENT

CHRONIC Rx

- The primary treatment for diabetic polyneuropathy is effective glycemic control as this may improve or at least slow progression of the neuropathy.
- Another aspect of treatment is the symptomatic management of pain and paresthesias. The American Academy of Neurology, the American Association of Neuromuscular and Electrodiagnostic Medicine, and the American Academy of Physical Medicine and Rehabilitation have developed an evidence-based guideline for the treatment of painful diabetic neuropathy. Pregabalin, an anticonvulsant, is the only agent in the guideline that has been established as effective for painful diabetic neuropathy. Other probably effective agents are listed below:
  - Topical agents: Lidocaine 5% patch can be applied to painful areas for 12 hours a day, capsaicin 0.075% applied qid.
  - Anticonvulsants: gabapentin (100 to 1200 mg tid) and pregabalin (50 to 100 mg tid)
  - Antidepressants: amitriptyline (10 to 100 mg qhs), nortriptyline (25 to 150 mg qhs), duloxetine (60 to 120 mg daily), and venlafaxine (75 to 225 mg/day). The American Academy of Neurology, the American Association of Neuromuscular and Electrodiagnostic Medicine, and the American Academy of Physical Medicine and Rehabilitation have developed an evidence-based guideline for the treatment of painful diabetic neuropathy. Pregabalin, an anticonvulsant, is the only agent in the Other probably effective agents are listed below:
  - Tramadol (50 mg qid as needed) can be a useful adjunctive analgesic

DISPOSITION

The distal sensory loss of diabetic polyneuropathy places patients at increased risk of trauma to the extremities with the potential for ulceration and infection which could ultimately necessitate amputation.

REFERRAL

- A neurologist can assist in the diagnosis and management of diabetic polyneuropathy.
- Patients with diabetic polyneuropathy should also be evaluated at least annually by a podiatrist and ophthalmologist

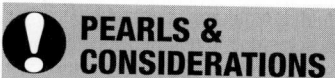 PEARLS & CONSIDERATIONS

COMMENTS

- For many patients, a DSPN or other form of diabetic neuropathy may be the initial presentation of previously undiagnosed diabetes.
- In addition to regular visits with podiatry, patients with diabetic polyneuropathy should be educated on aggressive foot hygiene and the importance of examining their own feet

PATIENT/FAMILY EDUCATION

Website: http://www.mayoclinic.com/health/diabetic-neuropathy/DS01045

SUGGESTED READINGS

available at www.expertconsult.com

AUTHOR: **JEFFREY C. MCCLEAN II, M.D.**

D

Diseases and Disorders

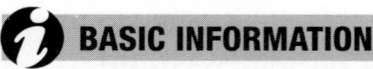

BASIC INFORMATION

DEFINITION

Diabetic retinopathy is an eye abnormality of the retina associated with diabetes and consisting of microaneurysms, punctate hemorrhages, white and yellow exudates, flame hemorrhages, and neovascular vessel growth and can ultimately end in blindness. Diabetic retinopathy can be classified into two stages: nonproliferative and proliferative (Fig. 1-279 and Table 1-133).

SYNONYMS

Nonproliferative diabetic retinopathy (NPDR)
Proliferative (advanced) diabetic retinopathy (PDR)
Diabetic retinopathy (DR)

ICD-9CM CODES
250.5   Diabetes with ophthalmic manifestations
362.1   Retinopathy, diabetic, background
362.02 Retinopathy, diabetic, proliferative

EPIDEMIOLOGY & DEMOGRAPHICS

INCIDENCE (IN U.S.):
- Affects 11 million persons. Approximately 40% of patients with diabetes who are over age 40 have retinopathy, including 8.2% who have vision-threatening retinopathy
- A leading cause of blindness in the U.S. between the ages of 20 and 74 yr
- There are 12,000 to 24,000 new cases of diabetic retinopathy-induced blindness each year in the U.S.
- 5000 new cases annually

PEAK INCIDENCE: Begins 10 yr after onset of diabetes

PREVALENCE (IN U.S.): Prevalence of retinopathy increases with duration of diabetes. Found in 18% of people diagnosed with diabetes for 3- to 4-yr duration and in up to 80% of diabetics with a diagnosis of ≥15 yr.

PREDOMINANT SEX: Males and females affected equally

PREDOMINANT AGE: ≥30 yr

GENETICS: Type 1 diabetes: 80% have retinopathy before 30 yr, with 30% having vision-threatening retinopathy.

PHYSICAL FINDINGS & CLINICAL PRESENTATION (Fig. E1-280)
- Microaneurysms
- Hemorrhages
- Exudates
- Macular edema
- Neovascularization
- Retinal detachment
- Hemorrhages in the vitreous
- In early cases, patient may not report a visual disturbance

ETIOLOGY

Vascular endothelial growth factor and erythropoietin have been identified as factors involved in angiogenesis in proliferative diabetic retinopathy. Risk factors for diabetic retinopathy are duration of diabetes, hyperglycemia/glycated hemoglobin value, hypertension, hyperlipidemia, pregnancy, and nephropathy or renal disease.

DIAGNOSIS

DIFFERENTIAL DIAGNOSIS
- Retinal examination: look for background retinopathy, microaneurysms, exudate, macular edema, retinal hemorrhage, proliferative neovascular growth on surface of retina
- Retinal inflammatory diseases
- Tumor
- Trauma
- Arteriosclerotic vascular disease
- Hypertension
- Vein or artery occlusion

WORKUP
- Fluorescein angiogram
- Frequent retinal examinations

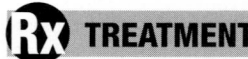 TREATMENT

NONPHARMACOLOGIC THERAPY
- Tight glycemic control remains the cornerstone in the primary prevention of diabetic retinopathy
- Laser treatment when indicated
- Laser treatment with proliferative disease or macular edema
- Photocoagulation of neovascular areas
- Exercise, diet, sugar and lipids control can slow progression of background retinopathy but have no effect on proliferative retinopathy. Trials have shown that glycemic control and combination treatment of dyslipidemia, but not intensive blood-pressure control, reduce the rate of diabetic retinopathy. Intensive glycemic therapy (vs. standard therapy) lowers the incidence of progressive retinopathy (7.3% vs. 10.4%) but not vision loss (16.3% vs. 16.7%) and can result in excess mortality (ACCORD trial)

ACUTE GENERAL Rx
- Laser therapy: pan-retinal and focal retinal laser photocoagulation reduces the risk of visual loss in patients with severe diabetic retinopathy and macular edema
- Vitrectomy
- Repair of retinal detachment
- Medical control of disease and complications and associated diseases (e.g., hypertension)

CHRONIC Rx
- Repeated laser treatments may be necessary
- Diet and exercise; good medical control of disease

DISPOSITION
- Retinal examination should be performed on all routine medical visits. Referral if abnormality seen.
- Routine annual eye examination in all patients with diabetes.
- Prognosis is improved with early diagnosis and treatment.

REFERRAL

Refer to ophthalmologist immediately on finding retinal abnormality to institute early treatment.

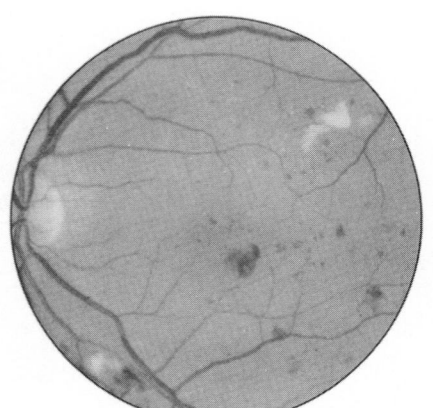
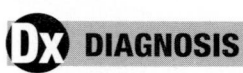
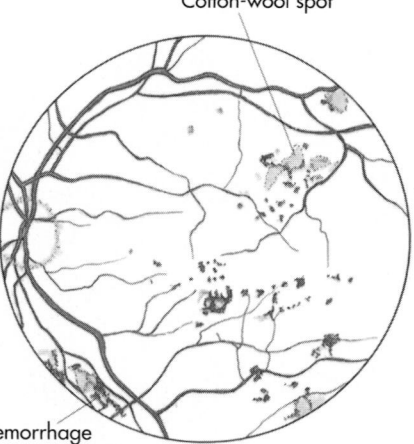

FIGURE 1-279 Background diabetic retinopathy. Note flame-shaped and dot-blot hemorrhages, cotton-wool spots, and microaneurysms. (From Barkaukas VH et al: *Health and physical assessment,* ed 2, St Louis, 1998, Mosby.)

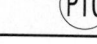

TABLE 1-133 Abbreviated Early Treatment Diabetic Retinopathy Study Classification of Diabetic Retinopathy

Category/Description	Management
Nonproliferative Diabetic Retinopathy (NPDR)	
No DR	Review in 12 mo
Very mild Microaneurysms only	Review most patients in 12 mo
Mild Any or all of: microaneurysms, retinal hemorrhages, exudates, cotton wool spots, up to the level of moderate NPDR. No IRMA or significant beading	Review range 6-12 mo, depending on severity of signs, stability, systemic factors, and patient's personal circumstances
Moderate • Severe retinal hemorrhages (more than ETDRS standard photograph 2A: about 20 medium-large per quadrant) in 1-3 quadrants *or* mild intraretinal microvascular abnormalities (IRMA) • Significant venous beading can be present in no more than 1 quadrant • Cotton-wool spots commonly present	Review in approximately 6 mo PDR in up to 26%, high-risk PDR in up to 8% within a yr
Severe The 4-2-1 rule; one or more of: • Severe hemorrhages in all 4 quadrants • Significant venous beading in 2 or more quadrants • Moderate IRMA in 1 or more quadrants	Review in 4 mo PDR in up to 50%, high-risk PDR in up to 15% within a yr
Very severe Two or more of the criteria for severe	Review in 2-3 mo High-risk PDR in up to 45% within a yr
Proliferative Diabetic Retinopathy (PDR)	
Mild-moderate New vessels on the disc (NVD) or new vessels elsewhere (NVE), but extent insufficient to meet the high-risk criteria	Treatment considered according to severity of signs, stability, systemic factors, and patient's personal circumstances such as reliability of attendance for review. If not treated, review in up to 2 mo
High-risk • New vessels on the disc (NVD) greater than ETDRS standard photograph 10A (about disc area) • Any NVD with vitreous or preretinal hemorrhage • NVE greater than disc area with vitreous or preretinal hemorrhage (or hemorrhage with presumed obscured NVD/E)	Treatment advised—see text Should be performed immediately when possible, and certainly same day if symptomatic presentation with good retinal view

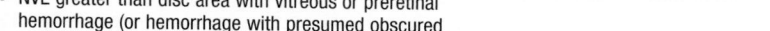

From Kanski JJ, Bowling B: *Clinical ophthalmology, a systematic approach,* ed 7, Philadelphia, 2010, Saunders.

PEARLS & CONSIDERATIONS

COMMENTS
- Early laser treatment of severe, nonproliferative, and proliferative retinopathy may minimize complications and visual loss.
- Retinopathy is an independent risk marker for cardiovascular disease in patients with type 2 DM.

SUGGESTED READINGS
available at www.expertconsult.com

RELATED CONTENT
Retinopathy, Diabetic (Patient Information)
Diabetes Mellitus (Related Key Topic)

AUTHORS: **MELVYN KOBY, M.D.,** and **FRED F. FERRI, M.D.**

Diseases and Disorders

D

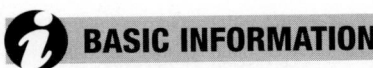

BASIC INFORMATION

DEFINITION

Discoid lupus erythematosus (DLE) refers to a chronic inflammatory autoimmune skin disorder that can lead to significant disfiguration and scarring. It can be associated with systemic lupus erythematosus (SLE).

SYNONYMS

Chronic cutaneous lupus erythematosus (CLE)

ICD-9CM CODES
695.4 Lupus erythematosus
erythematosus (discoid)
Erythematosus (discoid), not
disseminated

EPIDEMIOLOGY & DEMOGRAPHICS

- Slightly more common in African Americans than in Asians or whites
- CLE is two to three times more likely in women than in men
- Approximately 5% to 10% of patients presenting with DLE will develop SLE; those with widespread, numerous lesions are more likely to progress

PHYSICAL FINDINGS & CLINICAL PRESENTATION

General:
- Early lesions: single or multiple erythematous or violaceous, discrete papules or plaques with scale, often extending into dilated hair follicles (Fig. 1-283)
- Older lesions: peripheral hyperpigmentation with scarring, central depigmentation (Fig. E1-284), and telangiectasia
Anatomic distribution:
- Commonly involves the scalp, face, ears, and extensor surface of the arms
- Mucosal and nail involvement is also possible
Lesion configuration:
- Irregularly grouped, confluent and disfiguring plaques
Lesion morphology:
- Plaque lesions with scale

- Follicular plugging
- Atrophy
- Irreversible, scarring alopecia (34%)
- May be associated with other clinical findings of SLE (e.g., oral ulcers, arthritis, pleuritis, pericarditis)

ETIOLOGY

Unknown, but thought to be an autoimmune-mediated disorder

DIAGNOSIS

Clinical findings and skin biopsy are used to establish the diagnosis of DLE

DIFFERENTIAL DIAGNOSIS

Psoriasis, lichen planus or lichen planopilaris, dermatophyte infections, photosensitivity eruption, sarcoidosis, subacute CLE, rosacea, dermatomyositis, cutaneous T-cell lymphoma

LABORATORY TESTS

- Complete blood count is usually normal in isolated DLE, but a small percentage of patients may show low-grade anemia
- Blood urea nitrogen and creatinine are normal in isolated DLE
- Erythrocyte sedimentation rate is elevated in active disease
- Urinalysis may show proteinuria
- Antinuclear antibody positive in 30% to 40% of patients with isolated DLE
- Anti-Ro (SS-A) autoantibodies are present in 1% to 3% of patients
- dsDNA antibodies are uncommon
- Complement levels may be low in rare instances
- Histology of skin reveals hyperkeratosis with follicular plugging, a thickened basement membrane, and a perivascular, interstitial, and appendageal lymphocytic infiltrate

TREATMENT

NONPHARMACOLOGIC THERAPY

Avoid sun exposure by using protective clothing and a broad-spectrum sunscreen of SPF >30

ACUTE GENERAL Rx

1. Topical steroids: intermediate- to high-potency steroids are needed; use caution when applying to the face
2. Intralesional steroids: triamcinolone acetonide 2.5 to 5.0 mg/ml with 1% Xylocaine
3. Topical calcineurin inhibitors: pimecrolimus 1% cream and tacrolimus 0.1% ointment
4. Antimalarial drugs are first-line systemic therapy for cutaneous lupus: hydroxychloroquine sulfate 400 mg PO qd
5. Avoid use of systemic glucocorticoids in patients with isolated DLE because of risks of side effects

CHRONIC Rx

1. Chloroquine 250 to 500 mg PO qd
2. Additional options are methotrexate, mycophenolate mofetil, and cyclosporine.
3. Thalidomide 100 to 300 mg PO before sleep, with water, and >1 hr after meals for refractory CLE
4. Azathioprine 1 mg/kg/day PO for 6 to 8 wk, increase by 5 mg/kg q4 wk until response is seen or dose reaches 2.5 mg/kg/day
5. Dapsone: 100 mg/day

DISPOSITION

If untreated, DLE can lead to significant and permanent atrophy and scarring of the skin.

REFERRAL

Dermatology, rheumatology

PEARLS & CONSIDERATIONS

- Cutaneous lesions account for four of the 11 criteria in the diagnosis of SLE (e.g., malar rash, discoid rash, photosensitivity, and oral ulcers).
- Rarely, patients with DLE may develop nonmelanoma skin cancer in areas of disease.

SUGGESTED READINGS
available at www.expertconsult.com

RELATED CONTENT

Discoid Lupus Erythematosus (Patient Information)

AUTHORS: **KACHIU LEE, B.A.**, and **JESSICA RISSER, M.D., M.P.H.**

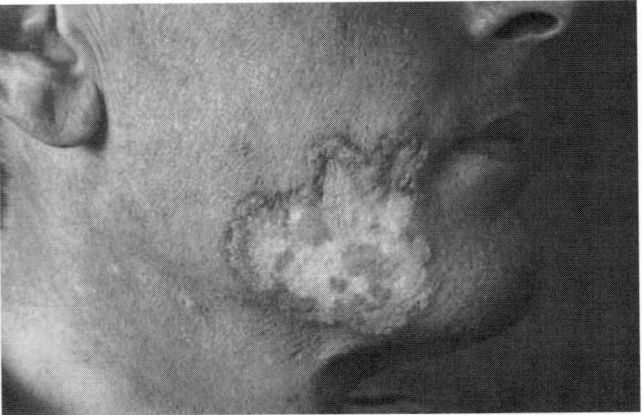

FIGURE 1-283 Classic discoid lupus erythematosus of the face. Note central scarring and erythematous hyperkeratotic borders. (From Hochberg MC et al: *Rheumatology*, ed 5, St Louis, 2011, Mosby.)

BASIC INFORMATION

DEFINITION

Disseminated intravascular coagulation (DIC) is an acquired thromboembolic disorder characterized by generalized activation of the clotting mechanism, which results in the intravascular formation of fibrin and ultimately thrombotic occlusion of small and midsize vessels.

SYNONYMS

Consumptive coagulopathy
DIC
Defibrination syndrome

ICD-9CM CODES
286.6 Disseminated intravascular
  coagulation

EPIDEMIOLOGY & DEMOGRAPHICS

More than 50% of cases are associated with gram-negative sepsis or other septicemic infections.

PHYSICAL FINDINGS & CLINICAL PRESENTATION

- Wound site bleeding, epistaxis, gingival bleeding, hemorrhagic bullae
- Petechiae, ecchymosis, purpura (Fig. E1-285)
- Dyspnea, localized rales, delirium
- Oliguria, anuria, gastrointestinal bleeding, metrorrhagia

ETIOLOGY

- Infections (e.g., gram-negative sepsis, Rocky Mountain spotted fever, malaria, viral or fungal infection)
- Obstetric complications (e.g., dead fetus, amniotic fluid embolism, toxemia, abruptio placentae, septic abortion, eclampsia, placenta previa, uterine atony)
- Tissue trauma (e.g., burns, hypothermia rewarming)
- Neoplasms (e.g., adenocarcinomas [gastrointestinal, prostate, lung, breast], acute promyelocytic leukemia)
- Quinine, cocaine-induced rhabdomyolysis
- Liver failure
- Acute pancreatitis
- Transfusion reactions
- Respiratory distress syndrome
- Toxins (snake bites, amphetamine overdose)
- Other: systemic lupus erythematosus (SLE), vasculitis, aneurysms, polyarteritis, cavernous hemangiomas
- Box E1-14 describes underlying conditions associated with DIC.

DIAGNOSIS

DIFFERENTIAL DIAGNOSIS

- Hepatic necrosis: normal or elevated factor VIII concentrations
- Vitamin K deficiency: normal platelet count
- Hemolytic uremic syndrome
- Thrombotic thrombocytopenic purpura
- Renal failure, SLE, sickle cell crisis, dysfibrinogenemias
- HELLP syndrome (**h**emolysis, **e**levated **l**iver function tests, and **l**ow **p**latelets)
- Fig. E1-286 describes an algorithm for the differential diagnosis of deep vein thrombosis.

WORKUP

Diagnostic workup includes laboratory screening to confirm the diagnosis and exclude conditions noted in the differential diagnosis (Figs. E1-286 and E1-287). Workup is also aimed at distinguishing DIC progression (acute vs. chronic), chief manifestations (thrombotic or hemorrhagic), and extent (localized or systemic). The International Society on Thrombosis and Haemostasis scoring system for DIC is described in Box E1-15.

LABORATORY TESTS

- Peripheral blood smear generally shows red blood cell fragments (schistocytes) and low platelet count.
- Coagulation factors are consumed at a rate in excess of the capacity of the liver to synthesize them, and platelets are consumed in excess of the capacity of the bone marrow megakaryocytes to release them. Diagnostic characteristics of DIC are decreased fibrinogen level; thrombocytopenia; and increased prothrombin time (PT), partial thromboplastin time (PTT), TT, fibrin split products, and D-dimer.
- Coagulopathy secondary to DIC must be differentiated from that secondary to liver disease or vitamin K deficiency.
  1. Vitamin K deficiency manifests with prolonged PT and normal PTT, TT, platelet, and fibrinogen level; PTT may be elevated in severe cases.
  2. Patients with liver disease have abnormal PT and PTT; TT and fibrinogen are usually normal unless severe disease is present; platelets are usually normal unless splenomegaly is present.
  3. Factors V and VIII are low in DIC, but they are normal in liver disease with coagulopathy.

IMAGING STUDIES

Imaging studies are generally not useful. Chest radiographs may be helpful to exclude infectious processes in patients with pulmonary symptoms such as dyspnea, cough, or hemoptysis.

TREATMENT

NONPHARMACOLOGIC THERAPY

No specific precautions regarding activity level are necessary unless thrombocytopenia is severe.

ACUTE GENERAL Rx

- Correct and eliminate underlying cause (e.g., antimicrobial therapy for infection, removal of necrotic bowel, evacuation of uterus in obstetric emergencies).
- Give replacement therapy with fresh frozen plasma (FFP) and platelets in patients with significant hemorrhage:
  1. FFP 10 to 15 ml/kg can be given with a goal of normalizing international normalized ratio.
  2. Platelet transfusions are given when platelet count is <10,000 (or higher if major bleeding is present).
  3. Cryoprecipitate 1 U/5 kg is reserved for hypofibrinogen states.
  4. Antithrombin III treatment may be considered as a supportive therapeutic option in patients with severe DIC. Its modest results and substantial cost are limiting factors.
- Heparin therapy at a dose lower than that used in venous thrombosis (300 to 500 U/hr) may be useful in selected cases to increase neutralization of thrombin (e.g., DIC associated with acute promyelocytic leukemia, purpura fulminans, acral ischemia).

CHRONIC Rx

Follow-up management includes coagulation screening to assess factor replacement therapy. Laboratory abnormalities generally correct with treatment of the underlying disorder. Long-term laboratory monitoring is not required.

DISPOSITION

Mortality rate in severe DIC exceeds 75%. Death generally results from progression of the underlying disease and complications such as acute renal failure, intracerebral hematoma, shock, or cardiac tamponade.

REFERRAL

Hematology consultation is recommended in all cases of DIC.

PEARLS & CONSIDERATIONS

COMMENTS

The treatment of chronic DIC is controversial. Low-dose SC heparin and/or combination antiplatelet agents such as aspirin and dipyridamole may be useful.

RELATED CONTENT

Disseminated Intravascular Coagulation (Patient Information)

AUTHOR: **FRED F. FERRI, M.D.**

BASIC INFORMATION

DEFINITION

- Colonic diverticula are herniations of mucosa and submucosa through the muscularis. They are generally found along the colon's mesenteric border at the site where the vasa recta penetrates the muscle wall (anatomic weak point).
- *Diverticulosis* is the asymptomatic presence of multiple colonic diverticula.
- *Diverticulitis* is an inflammatory process or localized perforation of diverticulum.

ICD-9CM CODES
562.10 Diverticulosis of colon
562.11 Diverticulitis of colon

EPIDEMIOLOGY & DEMOGRAPHICS

- Incidence of diverticulosis in the general population is 35% to 50%.
- Diverticulosis is more common in Western countries, affecting >30% of people >40 yr and >50% of people >70 yr.

PHYSICAL FINDINGS & CLINICAL PRESENTATION

- Physical examination in patients with diverticulosis is generally normal.
- Painful diverticular disease can present with left lower quadrant (LLQ) pain, often relieved by defecation; location of pain may be anywhere in the lower abdomen because of the redundancy of the sigmoid colon.
- Diverticulitis can cause muscle spasm, guarding, and rebound tenderness predominantly affecting the LLQ.

ETIOLOGY

Diverticular disease is believed to be secondary to low intake of dietary fiber.

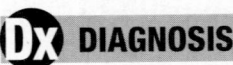 DIAGNOSIS

DIFFERENTIAL DIAGNOSIS

- Irritable bowel syndrome
- IBD
- Carcinoma of colon
- Endometriosis
- Ischemic colitis
- Infections (pseudomembranous colitis, appendicitis, pyelonephritis, PID)
- Lactose intolerance

LABORATORY TESTS

- WBC count in diverticulitis reveals leukocytosis with left shift.
- Microcytic anemia can be present in patients with chronic bleeding from diverticular disease. MCV may be elevated in acute bleeding secondary to reticulocytosis.

PROCEDURES: Colonoscopy should be avoided during acute diverticulitis due to the risk of perforation. It can generally be performed after 6 wk to rule out the presence of cancer and IBD.

IMAGING STUDIES

- A CT scan of the abdomen (Fig. E1-288) is recommended as the initial radiologic examination to diagnose acute diverticulitis; It can also diagnose diverticulosis (Fig. E1-289). It has a sensitivity of 93% to 97% and a specificity approaching 100% for diverticulitis. Typical findings are thickening of the bowel wall, fistulas, or abscess formation. CT may also reveal other disease processes (e.g., appendicitis, tubo-ovarian abscess, Crohn's disease) accounting for lower abdominal pain
- Evaluation of suspected diverticular bleeding:
  1. Arteriography if the bleeding is faster than 1 ml/min (advantage: the possible infusion of vasopressin directly into the arteries supplying the bleeding, as well as selective arterial embolization; disadvantages: its cost and invasive nature)
  2. Technetium-99m sulfa colloid
  3. Technetium-99m labeled RBC (can detect bleeding rates as low as 0.12 to 5 ml/min)

TREATMENT

NONPHARMACOLOGIC THERAPY

- Increase in dietary fiber intake and regular exercise to improve bowel function. However, recent studies have challenged the common view that fiber intake protects against diverticulosis
- NPO and IV hydration in severe diverticulitis; NG suction if ileus or small bowel obstruction is present

ACUTE GENERAL Rx

TREATMENT OF DIVERTICULITIS:

- Mild case: broad-spectrum PO antibiotics (e.g., Ciprofloxacin 750 mg bid or levofloxacin 750 mg bid or trimethoprim/sulfamethoxazole DS bid to cover aerobic component of colonic flora and metronidazole 500 mg q6h for anaerobes) and liquid diet for 7 to 10 days
- Severe case: NPO and aggressive IV antibiotic therapy
  a. Ampicillin-sulbactam 3 g IV q6h *or*
  b. Piperacillin-tazobactam 4.5 g IV q8h *or*
  c. Ciprofloxacin 400 mg IV q12h plus metronidazole 500 mg IV q6h *or*
  d. Ticarcillin-clavulanate 3.1 g IV q6h
- Life-threatening case: Imipenem 500 mg IV q6h *or* meropenem 1 g IV q8h
- Surgical treatment consisting of resection of involved areas and reanastomosis (if feasible); otherwise a diverting colostomy with reanastomosis performed when infection has been controlled; surgery should be considered in patients with:
  1. Repeated episodes of diverticulitis (two or more)
  2. Poor response to appropriate medical therapy (failure of conservative management)
  3. Abscess or fistula formation
  4. Obstruction

  5. Peritonitis
  6. Immunocompromised patients, first episode in young patient (<40 yr old)
  7. Inability to exclude carcinoma (10% to 20% of patients diagnosed with diverticulosis on clinical grounds are subsequently found to have carcinoma of the colon)

DIVERTICULAR HEMORRHAGE:

1. Bleeding is painless and stops spontaneously in the majority of patients (60%); it is usually caused by erosion of a blood vessel by a fecalith present within the diverticular sac.
2. Medical therapy consists of blood replacement and correction of volume and any clotting abnormalities.
3. Colonoscopic treatment with epinephrine injections, bipolar coagulation, or both may prevent recurrent bleeding and decrease the need for surgery.
4. Surgical resection is necessary if bleeding does not stop spontaneously after administration of 4 to 5 U of PRBCs or recurs with severity within a few days; if attempts at localization are unsuccessful, total abdominal colectomy with ileoproctostomy may be indicated (high incidence of rebleeding if segmental resection is performed without adequate localization).

CHRONIC Rx

Asymptomatic patients with diverticulosis can be treated with a high-fiber diet or fiber supplements.

DISPOSITION

- Most patients with diverticulitis respond well to antibiotic management and bowel rest. Up to 30% of patients with diverticulitis will eventually require surgical management.
- Diverticular bleeding can recur in 15% to 20% of patients within 5 yr.

REFERRAL

GI referral for colonoscopy. Surgical referral when considering resection.

SUGGESTED READINGS
available at www.expertconsult.com

RELATED CONTENT
Diverticulitis (Patient Information)
Diverticulosis (Patient Information)

AUTHOR: **FRED F. FERRI, M.D.**

BASIC INFORMATION

DEFINITION

Down syndrome is a disorder characterized by mental retardation and multiple organ defects and is caused by a chromosomal abnormality (trisomy 21).

SYNONYMS

Trisomy 21

ICD-9CM CODES
758.0 Down Syndrome

EPIDEMIOLOGY & DEMOGRAPHICS

INCIDENCE (IN U.S.): 1 in 800 births
PEAK INCIDENCE: Newborn
PREVALENCE (IN U.S.): 300,000 persons
PREDOMINANT SEX: Male/female ratio of 1.3:1.0
PREDOMINANT AGE: Newborn to early adulthood
GENETICS: Nondisjunction causing trisomy 21

PHYSICAL FINDINGS & CLINICAL PRESENTATION

(Fig. 1-290)
- Microcephaly
- Flattening of occiput and face
- Upward slant to eyes with epicanthal folds
- Brushfield spots in iris
- Broad, stocky neck
- Small feet, hands, digits
- Single palmar crease
- Hypotonia

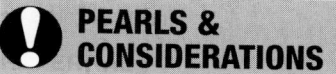

FIGURE 1-290 Down syndrome. Note depressed nasal bridge, epicanthal folds, mongoloid slant of eyes, low-set ears, and large tongue. (From Zitelli BJ, Davis HW: *Atlas of pediatric physical diagnosis,* ed 3, St Louis, 1997, Mosby.)

- Short stature
- Associated with congenital heart disease, malformations of the GI tract, cataracts, hypothyroidism, hip dysplasia, obstructive sleep apnea, and myeloproliferative disorders
- About half of children with Down syndrome are born with congenital heart disease, with the most common lesions being atrial septal defect and ventricular septal defect
- Persistent primary congenital hypothyroidism is found in 1 in 141 newborns with Down syndrome, as compared with 1 in 4000 in the general population
- Ophthalmologic disorders increase in frequency with age; >80% of children aged 5 to 12 yr have disorders that need monitoring or intervention, such as refractive errors, strabismus, or cataracts
- Renal and urinary tract abnormalities

ETIOLOGY

Nondisjunction of chromosome 21

DIAGNOSIS

- The American College of Obstetrics and Gynecology recommends offering fetal chromosomal screening to all pregnant women regardless of age due to improvements in noninvasive screening methods.
- Combined use of serum screening and fetal ultrasound testing for thickened nuchal fold has 85% detection rate with 5% false-positive results. Second-trimester serum screening in combination with maternal age is improved with use of multiple serum markers
- Prenatal cytogenic diagnosis by amniocentesis or chorionic villus sampling
- Postnatal chromosomal karyotype

DIFFERENTIAL DIAGNOSIS

- Congenital hypothyroidism
- Other chromosomal abnormalities

WORKUP

Postnatal chromosomal karyotype

TREATMENT

- Thyroid screen at birth, at age 6 mo, and yearly thereafter
- Echocardiogram in all newborns and cardiac assessment of adolescents for development of mitral valve prolapse
- Treatment consists of vigilant monitoring for comorbid states, such as obesity, hypothyroidism, leukemia, hearing loss, and valvular heart disease
- Prevention of obesity with low-calorie, high-fiber diet
- Auditory brain stem responses in all newborns and aggressive testing for hearing loss in children with chronic otitis media
- Ophthalmologic assessment by age 6 mo for congenital cataracts and annual examinations for monitoring of refractive errors and strabismus
- Regular dental care

- Pelvic examination of women who are sexually active or who have menstrual problems
- Dermatologic issues such as folliculitis can become problematic in adolescents, and require topical antibiotics and careful attention to hygiene

DISPOSITION

Most children with Down syndrome live at home. As these individuals reach adulthood, those with higher functioning sometimes live in supervised settings away from their families.

REFERRAL

Down syndrome clinics use a preventive checklist to anticipate many clinical challenges.

PEARLS & CONSIDERATIONS

COMMENTS

- Screening for atlantoaxial subluxation is controversial.
- Most patients experience neuropathologic changes typical of Alzheimer's disease. Presenting symptoms include seizures, focal neurologic signs, and apathy. If Alzheimer's disease is suspected, screen for treatable diseases such as depression or hypothyroidism.
- This syndrome accounts for approximately one third of moderate-to-severe cases of mental retardation.
- Individuals with Down syndrome have a wide range of function, but all will have decrease in intelligence quotient (IQ) in first decade of life.
- Deficiency of language production relative to other areas of development often causes substantial impairment.
- Individuals with Down syndrome have more behavioral and psychiatric problems than other children, but fewer than other individuals with mental retardation.
- Though increased maternal age is a risk factor, most children with Down syndrome are born to women younger than 35 yr.

SUGGESTED READINGS
available at www.expertconsult.com

RELATED CONTENT
Down Syndrome (Trisomy, Mongolism) (Patient Information)

AUTHOR: **MAITREYI MAZUMDAR, M.D., M.P.H.**

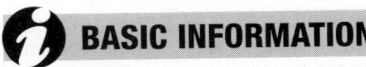

BASIC INFORMATION

DEFINITION

Dumping syndrome refers to a constellation of postprandial symptoms resulting from rapid delivery of hypertonic stomach contents into the small bowel that is most often caused by gastric surgery, such as procedures for peptic ulcer disease and gastric bypass.

SYNONYMS

Postgastrectomy syndrome
Rapid gastric emptying

ICD-9CM CODES
564.2 Postgastric surgery syndromes

EPIDEMIOLOGY & DEMOGRAPHICS

Incidence is 10% of all patients having gastric surgery.
- Vagotomy and pyloroplasty (8.5% to 20%)
- Vagotomy and antrectomy (4% to 27%)
- Subtotal gastrectomy (10% to 40%)
- Parietal cell vagotomy (3% to 5%)
- Gastric bypass surgeries (up to 50%)
- Males and females are affected equally

PHYSICAL FINDINGS & CLINICAL PRESENTATION

1. Early dumping syndrome: symptoms start within 1 hr after eating food:
   - No symptoms in fasting state
   - Nausea, vomiting, and belching
   - Epigastric fullness, cramping, and diarrhea
   - Dizziness, flushing, diaphoresis, and syncope
   - Palpitations and tachycardia
2. Late dumping syndrome: symptoms occurring 1 to 3 hr after eating:
   - Diaphoresis
   - Irritability
   - Difficulty in concentration
   - Tremulousness

ETIOLOGY

Dumping syndrome occurs almost exclusively in patients who have had gastric surgery.
- Systemic symptoms in early dumping syndrome are thought to be partially due to hypovolemia caused by rapid shifts of fluid from the intravascular space into the lumen of the bowel.
- Increase in vasoactive substances related to rapid gastric emptying is thought to play a role in dumping syndrome.
- Late dumping symptoms are thought to be due to reactive hypoglycemia.

DIAGNOSIS

A detailed clinical history and evidence of prior gastric surgery are necessary for the diagnosis.

DIFFERENTIAL DIAGNOSIS

- Pancreatic insufficiency
- Inflammatory bowel disease
- Afferent loop syndromes
- Bile acid reflux after surgery
- Bowel obstruction
- Gastroenteric fistula

WORKUP

Diagnosis is typically made on clinical grounds. In certain clinical settings, where patients exhibit symptoms with no prior history of gastric surgery, oral glucose challenge and imaging studies may be pursued and aid in establishing the diagnosis.

LABORATORY TESTS

Oral glucose challenge test:
- After overnight fasting, oral intake of 50 g of glucose is followed by serial measurements of heart rate, serum glucose, and hydrogen breath test every 15 to 30 min for 3 to 6 hrs. A 30-min hematocrit can also be taken.
- An increase in the heart rate >12 beats/min and a rise in hydrogen breath excretion have a sensitivity of 94% and specificity >92%. An increase of >3% in the 30-min hematocrit is also suggestive of a positive test. A nadir blood glucose <3.3 mmol/L (<59 mg/dl) was present in 75% of late dumpers.

IMAGING STUDIES

- Upper GI series properly defines anatomy.
- Scintigraphic imaging documents rapid gastric emptying and may be useful in patients with dumping syndrome and no prior history of gastric surgery.

TREATMENT

NONPHARMACOLOGIC THERAPY

- Diet modification
  1. Divide caloric intake over six small meals
  2. Limit fluid intake with meals (try to avoid fluids 30 min before meals and following meals)
  3. Decrease carbohydrate intake and avoid simple sugars
  4. Increase/supplement dietary fibers
  5. Avoid milk/milk products

ACUTE GENERAL Rx

- Acarbose 50 mg PO daily can be tried if dietary modification does not help.
- Octreotide 25 to 50 μg SC 30 min before meals is effective in relieving symptoms of dumping syndrome.
- Pectin and guar have been used to increase viscosity of intraluminal contents and relieve symptoms from rapid emptying and absorption.

CHRONIC Rx

- Surgery is considered in patients with severe symptoms refractory to the above-mentioned dietary and acute general treatment.
- Surgical procedures include: reconstruction of the pylorus, converting Billroth II to a Billroth I anastomosis, and a Roux-en-Y reconstruction.
- In severe cases, can consider depot long-acting-release octreotide, given as 10 mg intramuscularly every 4 wks for symptom relief.

DISPOSITION

- Dumping syndrome improves with time. Approximately 1% to 2% of patients will continue to have significant symptoms several months after surgery.
- Dietary modification effectively treats the majority of patients.

REFERRAL

- A gastrointestinal specialist consult is recommended in patients suspected of having dumping syndrome.
- If medical management is unsuccessful, a general surgical consultation is warranted.

PEARLS & CONSIDERATIONS

COMMENTS

- The majority of patients usually manifest with early dumping symptoms or a combination of early and late symptoms. Few have late dumping symptoms alone.
- Octreotide has an inhibitory effect on the release of insulin and other vasoactive substances released by the gut. It also works by decreasing gastric emptying.

SUGGESTED READINGS
available at www.expertconsult.com

AUTHOR: **MARK F. BRADY, M.D., M.P.H., M.M.S.**

BASIC INFORMATION

DEFINITION

Dupuytren's contracture is a disease of the palmar fascia characterized by nodular fibroblastic proliferation that often results in progressive contractures of the fascia and flexion deformity of the fingers.

Dupuytren's diathesis is a more aggressive presentation of the disease. Risk factors include >40 yr, strong family history, bilateral involvement, and ectopic manifestations like plantar and penile fibromatosis.

ICD-9CM CODES
728.6 Dupuytren's contracture

EPIDEMIOLOGY & DEMOGRAPHICS

PREVALENCE: Varies depending on ethnicity. The disorder is more common in Scandinavians; some Northern Europeans have a 25% prevalence after the age of 60.
PREVALENT SEX: Male/female ratio of 3.5 to 9:1, becomes 1:1 after age 80 yr.
PREVALENT AGE: 40 to 60 yr
RISK FACTORS: Age >40 yr, positive family history, diabetes mellitus, alcoholism, smoking, HIV infection
GENETICS: Aberrations in genes encoding proteins in the Wnt-signaling pathways are believed to be implicated in the process of fibromatosis in Dupuytren's disease

PHYSICAL FINDINGS & CLINICAL PRESENTATION

- Usually asymptomatic
- Most common complaints: deformity and interference with the use of the hand by the flexed, contracted fingers (Fig. 1-291)
- Process usually begins on the ulnar side of the hand, often starting at the ring finger; other fingers can be involved
- Isolated, painless nodules that eventually harden and mature into a longitudinal cord that extends into the finger
- Later stages: fibrous cord begins to contract and pull the finger into flexion
- Skin pitting, atrophic grooves
- Tabletop test of Hueston: place hand and fingers prone on a table. Test is positive if hand won't go flat (Fig. E1-292). Surgery is generally not indicated if test is negative
- A staging classification for Dupuytren's contracture is described in Table 1-134.

ETIOLOGY
Unknown.

DIAGNOSIS

DIFFERENTIAL DIAGNOSIS
- Soft tissue tumor
- Tendon cyst

WORKUP
The typical case is easily diagnosed clinically. Plain radiographs may be useful to rule out bony abnormalities.

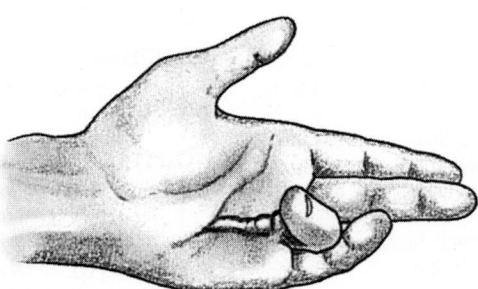

FIGURE 1-291 Dupuytren's contracture. A flexion deformity of the finger is present, with nodular thickening of the fascia to the ring finger.

TREATMENT

- Avoidance of repetitive hand trauma; measures include the use of gloves and damping tape to widen grips.
- Stretching exercises.
- Radiotherapy.
- Enzymatic fasciotomy by *Clostridium histolyticum* collegenase injection: collagenase *C. histolyticum* is the first FDA-approved, nonsurgical treatment option for adult Dupuytren's contracture patients with a palpable cord that is highly effective and well tolerated.
- Surgery is usually performed when the metacarpophalangeal joint contracture exceeds 30 degrees or when the proximal interphalangeal joint has any degree of contracture. Another indication for surgery is if there is neurovascular damage of the finger.
- Surgery may consist of closed fasciotomy, limited fasciotomy, regional fasciotomy, extensive fasciectomy, and dermofasciectomy. Percutaneous needle aponeurotomy performed in the office represents an alternative to surgery.

DISPOSITION
Rate of development is variable.

REFERRAL
Evaluation by hand or plastic surgeon if joint contracture begins to develop or for excision of rare nodule that is painful (at any stage)

PEARLS & CONSIDERATIONS

COMMENTS
- Dupuytren's contracture develops earlier and more often in certain families.
- Approximately 5% of patients develop a similar condition elsewhere, such as Peyronie's disease or Ledderhose disease (involvement of the plantar fascia).
- Tender knuckle pads (*Garrod's knuckle pad*) over the dorsal aspect of the PIP joints may also be present.
- Individuals with these additional findings are considered to have Dupuytren's diathesis, and their disease is generally more severe and recurrent.

SUGGESTED READINGS
available at www.expertconsult.com

RELATED CONTENT
Dupuytren's Contracture (Patient Information)

AUTHOR: **DANIEL E. MENDEZ-ALLWOOD, M.D.**

TABLE 1-134 Staging Classification for Dupuytren's Contracture (Woodruff, 1998)

Stage	Description	Management
1	Early palmar disease with no contracture	Leave alone
2	One finger involved, with only metacarpophalangeal joint contracture	Surgery
3	One finger—metacarpophalangeal joint + proximal interphalangeal joint	Surgery difficult
4	Stage 3 + more than one finger involved	Surgery prolonged and only partly successful
5	Finger-in-palm deformity	Consider amputation

From Parvizi J: *High-yield orthopedics,* Philadelphia, 2010, Saunders.

BASIC INFORMATION

DEFINITION

Dysfunctional uterine bleeding (DUB) describes abnormal uterine bleeding in the absence of disease in the pelvis, pregnancy, or medical illness. Parameters of normal menstrual function are described in Box 1-16. Specific types of abnormal bleeding include the following:

- Hypermenorrhea: excessive bleeding amount during normal duration of regular menstrual cycles
- Hypomenorrhea: decreased bleeding amount in regular menstrual cycles
- Menorrhagia: regular normal intervals, excessive flow and duration
- Metrorrhagia: irregular intervals, excessive flow and duration
- Menometrorrhagia: irregular or excessive bleeding during menstruation and between periods
- Oligomenorrhea: intervals >35 days
- Polymenorrhea: intervals <21 days

These terms, while commonly used in practice, increasingly are felt to be confusing. In fact, The FIGO Menstrual Disorders Working Group has been working since 2009 to eliminate many of the confusing and overlapping terms and create simpler definitions that can be intuitively understood by medical professionals and lay people alike. The term *dysfunctional uterine bleeding* was initially used in 1935 but has never been clearly defined and has been used as both a diagnosis and a symptom. It is generally understood to be a term of exclusion when no other cause of bleeding has been established. FIGO recommends that the three diagnoses (disturbances of molecular control of menses, HPO axis abnormalities, and disorders of hemostasis) be grouped under the nonstructural causes of abnormal uterine bleeding. However, these new FIGO terms have not yet made their way into common usage. In addition, the ICD-9 codes have not been updated to reflect this new usage.

SYNONYMS

DUB

ICD-9CM CODES

626	Disorders of menstruation and other abnormal bleeding from female genital tract
626.2	Hypermenorrhea
626.1	Hypomenorrhea
626.2	Menorrhagia
626.6	Metrorrhagia
626.2	Menometrorrhagia
626.1	Oligomenorrhea
626.2	Polymenorrhea

EPIDEMIOLOGY & DEMOGRAPHICS

- Most cases of DUB occur in postmenarchal and perimenopausal age groups.
- During reproductive age, <20% of abnormal bleeding results from anovulatory DUB.

PHYSICAL FINDINGS & CLINICAL PRESENTATION

- A clinical diagnosis of exclusion
- Thorough physical and pelvic examination to exclude the other causes of abnormal bleeding
  1. Includes thyroid, breast, liver, presence or absence of ecchymotic lesions
  2. Patient possibly obese and hirsute (polycystic ovarian disease)
  3. No evidence of any vulvar, vaginal, cervical lesions, uterine (fibroid) or ovarian tumor, urethral caruncle, urethral diverticula, hemorrhoids, anal fissure, colorectal lesions
  4. Bimanual pelvic examination: normal-sized or slightly enlarged uterus

ETIOLOGY

- 90% is caused by anovulation.
- 10% is ovulatory in origin; can be caused by dysfunction of corpus luteum or midcycle bleeding.
- Section II describes the various causes of abnormal uterine bleeding.

DIAGNOSIS

DIFFERENTIAL DIAGNOSIS

- Pregnancy-related cause
- Anatomic uterine causes:
  1. Leiomyomas
  2. Adenomyosis
  3. Polyps
  4. Endometrial hyperplasia
  5. Cancer
  6. Sexually transmitted diseases
  7. Intrauterine contraceptive devices
- Anatomic nonuterine causes:
  1. Cervical neoplasia, cervicitis
  2. Vaginal neoplasia, adhesions, trauma, foreign body, atrophic vaginitis, infections, condyloma
  3. Vulvar trauma, infections, neoplasia, condyloma, dystrophy, varices
  4. Urinary tract: urethral caruncle, diverticulum, hematuria
  5. Gastrointestinal tract: hemorrhoids, anal fissure, colorectal lesions
- Systemic diseases:
  1. Exogenous hormone intake
  2. Coagulopathies: von Willebrand's disease, thrombocytopenia, hepatic failure
  3. Endocrinopathies: thyroid disorder, hypothyroidism and hyperthyroidism, diabetes mellitus
  4. Renal diseases
- Section II describes a differential diagnosis of vaginal bleeding abnormalities.

BOX 1-16 Parameters of Normal Menstrual Function

Cycle interval (days)	21-35
Duration of flow (days)	2-8
Blood loss/cycle (ml)	30-80

From Carlson KJ et al: *Primary care of women,* ed 2, St Louis, 2002, Mosby.

WORKUP

- A detailed history and thorough physical examination, including a pelvic examination to exclude causes mentioned above.
- Clinical algorithms for the evaluation of vaginal bleeding are described in Section III, "Bleeding, Vaginal."

LABORATORY TESTS

- Complete blood count with platelets; possible iron-deficiency anemia or thrombocytopenia
- Prothrombin; partial thromboplastin and bleeding time if coagulopathy is suspected
- Serum human chorionic gonadotropin
- Chemistry profile, including liver function tests
- Thyroid profile
- Stool testing for occult blood
- Urinalysis for hematuria
- Pap smear
- Cultures for gonorrhea and *Chlamydia*
- Serum gonadotropins and prolactin
- Serum androgens
- Endometrial biopsy in women >35 yr or earlier if longstanding history of anovulatory bleeding
- Hysterogram and hysteroscopy
- Von Willebrand's panel, particularly in perimenarchal women

IMAGING STUDIES

- Pelvic ultrasound, including measurement of endometrial thickness
- Fluid contrast ultrasound (also called saline sonogram, sonohysterogram, hydrosonogram, and various other names)

TREATMENT

NONPHARMACOLOGIC THERAPY

Increase iron intake in the form of pills and in a diet rich in iron.

ACUTE GENERAL Rx

- Progestational agents (see Box 1-17)
  1. Progesterone in oil, 100 to 200 mg
  2. Medroxyprogesterone acetate, 20 to 40 mg qd for 15 days
  3. Megestrol acetate, 40 to 120 mg daily in divided doses for 15 days
  4. Oral contraceptives: any oral contraceptive pill, 1 tablet qid for 5 to 7 days,

BOX 1-17 Equivalent Daily Doses of Oral Progestins for the Treatment of Dysfunctional Uterine Bleeding

Medroxyprogesterone acetate (Provera, Cycrin)	10 mg
Micronized progesterone (Prometrium)	400 mg
Norgestrel (Ovrette)	150 µg
Norethindrone acetate (Micronor, Nor-QD)	0.7-1.0 mg

From Carlson KJ et al: *Primary care of women,* ed 2, St Louis, 2002, Mosby.

followed by 1 tablet low-dose estrogen qd for 21 days; causes withdrawal bleeding; should then be on cyclical Provera or continue on oral contraceptives
- Estrogens
  1. Conjugated estrogen (Premarin) 25 mg IV q4h until bleeding is under control (in cases of severe or life-threatening bleeding); maximum three doses
  2. For prolonged bleeding that is not life threatening: Premarin 1.25 mg (Estrace 2 mg) q4h for 24 hr, followed by Provera to bring on withdrawal bleeding; then sequential regimen of estrogen and progestin (Premarin 1.25 mg qd for 24 days, Provera 10 mg for last 10 days) or oral contraceptives
- Surgical treatment
  1. Dilation and curettage (D&C) and hysteroscopy
  2. Endometrial ablation
  3. Hysterectomy

CHRONIC Rx

- Progestational agents
  ○ Medroxyprogesterone acetate 10 mg qd for 12 days, then cyclically to induce monthly withdrawal bleeding
  ○ Norethindrone 2.5 to 10 mg qd for 12 days

○ Depo-Provera 150 mg IM and then 150 mg every 3 mo
○ Oral contraceptives, 1 tablet qd
○ Levonorgestrel-releasing intrauterine device (Mirena, currently has an FDA indication for heavy menstrual bleeding in women who use an IUD for contraception)
- Clomiphene citrate: patients with anovulatory bleeding who want to become pregnant
- Others
  ○ Antiprostaglandins
  ○ Danazol (rarely used due to side-effect profile)
  ○ Gonadotropin-releasing hormone analogs (GnRH)
  ○ Human menopausal gonadotropin (HMG) (desire pregnancy)
  ○ Tranexamic acid (Lysteda) is an antifibrinolytic agent recently FDA approved for cyclic heavy menstrual bleeding. Dosage in normal renal function is 3900 mg daily (650-mg tablets, 2 tablets tid) for up to 5 days during menses
- Surgical treatment
  1. D&C and hysteroscopy
  2. Endometrial ablation
  3. Hysterectomy

DISPOSITION

Cyclical treatment on birth control pills or Provera for several cycles, then discontinue pill and watch patient for onset of regular menses

REFERRAL

To gynecologist in case of failure of treatment

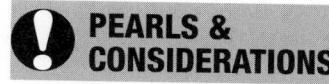 **PEARLS & CONSIDERATIONS**

COMMENTS

- Table 1-135 describes management options for DUB.
- Patient education material may be obtained from the American College of Obstetricians and Gynecologists, 409 12th Street SW, Washington, DC 20024-2188; phone 202-638-5577.

SUGGESTED READING

available at www.expertconsult.com

RELATED CONTENT

Endometrial Cancer (Related Key Topic)
Uterine Fibroids (Related Key Topic)
Fig. 3-28 Evaluation of ovulatory bleeding (Algorithm)
Fig. 3-29 Evaluation of anovulatory bleeding (Algorithm)
Dysfunctional Uterine Bleeding (Patient Information)

AUTHORS: **MANDEEP K. BRAR, M.D.**, and **RUBEN ALVERO, M.D.**

TABLE 1-135	Management of Dysfunctional Uterine Bleeding (DUB)	
Bleeding Pattern	**Cause**	**Treatment**
Ovulatory DUB		
Heavy menstrual bleeding	Imbalance in endometrial prostacyclins and prostaglandins	Nonsteroidal anti-inflammatory drugs Combination oral contraceptive pill Progestin intrauterine device Endometrial ablation
Midcycle spotting	Periovulatory estrogen decline	None
Delayed menses	Persistent corpus luteum	None (rule out pregnancy)
Anovulatory DUB		
Irregular menses	Unopposed estrogen stimulation of endometrium	Combination oral contraceptive pill Cyclic progestins Endometrial ablation
Postmenopausal bleeding	Endometrial atrophy	Hormone replacement therapy Endometrial ablation

From Carlson KJ, Eisenstat SA et al: *Primary care of women,* ed 2, St Louis, 2002, Mosby.

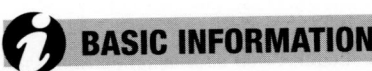

BASIC INFORMATION

DEFINITION

Dysmenorrhea is pain with menstruation, usually cramping and usually centered in the lower abdomen. It is defined as *primary dysmenorrhea* when there is no associated organic pathology and *secondary dysmenorrhea* when there is demonstrable organic pathology.

SYNONYMS

Menstrual cramps
Painful periods

ICD-9CM CODES
625.3 Dysmenorrhea

EPIDEMIOLOGY & DEMOGRAPHICS

- Approximately 50% of menstruating women are affected by dysmenorrhea, with approximately 10% of them having severe dysmenorrhea with incapacitation for 1 to 3 days/mo.
- Dysmenorrhea is most common in the age group from 20 to 24 yr, and primary dysmenorrhea usually appears within 6 to 12 mo after menarche.
- Dysmenorrhea is more common in women who have menarche at an earlier age, and in those with a longer duration of menstruation.

PHYSICAL FINDINGS & CLINICAL PRESENTATION

- Sharp, crampy, midline, lower abdominal pain without a lower quadrant or adnexal component but possible radiation to the lower back and upper thighs
- Unremarkable pelvic examination in non-menstruating patient
- Accompanying symptoms: nausea, vomiting, headaches, anxiety, fatigue, diarrhea, fainting, and abdominal bloating
- Cramps usually lasting <24 hr and seldom lasting >2 to 3 days
- Secondary dysmenorrhea: dyspareunia is a common complaint, and bimanual pelvic-abdominal examination may demonstrate uterine or adnexal tenderness, fixed uterine retroflexion, uterosacral nodularity, a pelvic mass, or an enlarged, irregular uterus

ETIOLOGY

Prostaglandin $F_{2\alpha}$ is the agent responsible for dysmenorrhea. It stimulates uterine contractions and cervical stenosis (narrowing) and increases vasopressin release. Behavior and psychological factors have also been implicated in the etiology of primary dysmenorrhea. Primary dysmenorrhea only occurs in ovulatory cycles. Secondary dysmenorrhea is usually caused by endometriosis, adenomyosis, leiomyomas and, less commonly, chronic salpingitis, intrauterine device (IUD) use, or congenital or acquired outflow tract obstruction, including cervical stenosis.

DIAGNOSIS

DIFFERENTIAL DIAGNOSIS

- Adenomyosis
- Adhesions
- Allen-Masters syndrome
- Cervical structures or stenosis
- Congenital malformation of müllerian system
- Ectopic pregnancy
- Endometriosis, endometritis
- Imperforate hymen
- IUD use
- Leiomyomas
- Ovarian cysts
- Pelvic congestion syndrome, pelvic inflammatory disease
- Polyps
- Transverse vaginal septum

WORKUP

- Primary dysmenorrhea: characteristic history, physical examination normal with the absence of an identifiable cause of pelvic pain
- Secondary dysmenorrhea: history of onset generally >2 yr after menarche; physical examination may reveal uterine irregularity, cul-de-sac tenderness, or nodularity or pelvic masses

LABORATORY TESTS

- No specific tests diagnostic for dysmenorrhea
- Elevated white blood cell count in the presence of infection
- Human chorionic gonadotropin to rule out ectopic pregnancy

IMAGING STUDIES

- Ultrasound scan of the pelvis to evaluate the presence of leiomyomas, ovarian cysts, or ectopic pregnancy
- Hysterosalpingogram or saline ultrasonography to assess the uterine cavity to rule out endometrial polyps or submucosal or intraluminal leiomyomas

TREATMENT

NONPHARMACOLOGIC THERAPY

- Applying heat to the lower abdomen with hot compresses, heating pads, or hot water bottles seems to offer some relief.
- Other reassurance that this is a treatable condition.

ACUTE GENERAL Rx

- Nonsteroidal anti-inflammatory drugs such as ibuprofen 400 to 600 mg q4 to 6h or naproxen sodium 500 mg q12h, mefenamic acid 500 mg initial dose followed by 250 mg q6h prn
- Oral contraceptives may be effective at reducing pain in women with primary dysmenorrhea
- Nifedipine 30 mg qd in difficult cases of dysmenorrhea
- Vitamin E supplements may reduce pain compared to placebo
- Magnesium supplements have been found likely to be beneficial
- Thiamine supplements may reduce pain
- The Chinese herbal remedy toki-shakuyaku-san may be effective in reducing pain. However, few studies have been of good quality
- Secondary dysmenorrhea: treatment directed to the specific underlying condition; surgery may be indicated if pathology is found on physical examination or by imaging

CHRONIC Rx

Acupuncture and transcutaneous electrical nerve stimulation may be tried. In cases in which medical therapy has not worked, laparoscopy or other surgical treatments should be considered depending on the secondary cause of the dysmenorrhea.

DISPOSITION

The majority of patients are satisfactorily treated with good outcomes. Possible chronic complications with primary dysmenorrhea that has not been adequately treated can lead to anxiety and depression. With certain causes of secondary dysmenorrhea, infertility can become a problem.

REFERRAL

If a secondary cause of dysmenorrhea is revealed, refer to the appropriate specialist for further medical or surgical treatment (e.g., gynecologist, pain management center).

RELATED CONTENT

Dyspareunia (Related Key Topic)
Endometriosis (Related Key Topic)
Premenstrual Syndrome (Related Key Topic)
Dysmenorrhea (Patient Information)

AUTHORS: **GEORGE T. DANAKAS, M.D.,** and **RUBEN ALVERO, M.D.**

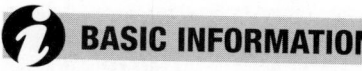 BASIC INFORMATION

DEFINITION

Persistent and/or recurrent pain associated with sexual intercourse

SYNONYMS

Painful intercourse

ICD-9CM CODES

625.0   Pain associated with female genital organs

302.76 Sexual deviations and disorders with functional dyspareunia, psychogenic dyspareunia

EPIDEMIOLOGY & DEMOGRAPHICS

PREVALENCE: 7% to 60% depending on definition

PREDOMINANT SEX: Female

AT-RISK POPULATION: No consistent findings regarding:

- Age
- Parity
- Educational status
- Race
- Income
- Marital status

RISK FACTORS:

Lower:

- Frequency of intercourse
- Levels of desire and arousal
- Orgasmic response
- Physical and emotional satisfaction
- General happiness

HISTORICAL FACTORS:

- Pain parameters
  1. Character
  2. Location (Introital, middle, deep)
  3. Onset
  4. Duration
  5. Timing
  6. Chronicity
  7. Cyclicity
  8. Recurrence
- Gynecologic history
  1. History of sexually transmitted disease
  2. History of herpes simplex virus (HSV) or human papillomavirus (HPV)
  3. Other sexual dysfunctions
  4. Prior abdominal or gynecologic surgery
  5. Prior pelvic or abdominal radiation
  6. History of endometriosis, fibroids
  7. History of genital or uterine prolapse
  8. History of gynecologic infection
  9. History of pelvic pain
  10. History of menopausal symptoms
  11. Sexual misinformation
- Obstetric history
  1. Lacerations
  2. Episiotomy
- General medical causes
  1. History of chronic diseases
  2. Gastrointestinal or genitourinary symptoms
  3. Medications
  4. History of psychological disorders
  5. History of dermatologic condition
  6. Religious beliefs
  7. Generalized anxiety

PHYSICAL FINDINGS & CLINICAL PRESENTATION

- Primary versus secondary dyspareunia
  1. Latter with history of pain-free coitus
- Visual inspection of lower genital tract
  1. Discoloration
  2. Ulcerations
  3. Discharge
  4. Prolapse
  5. Dysplastic changes
  6. Infestations
- Physical examination
  1. Sensitivity to light touch
  2. Tenderness to palpation
  3. Genital prolapse
     a. Uterus
     b. Bladder
     c. Cervix
     d. Vagina
     e. Adnexa
     f. Rectum
     g. Bowel
  4. Ridges, septum
  5. Levator muscle tone
  6. Evidence of previous surgery
  7. Vaginal length, depth, caliber constrictions

ETIOLOGY

- Pathology or alteration or reduction of genital-associated tissue
- Psychosocial factors
- Marital or relationship discord
- History of sexual abuse

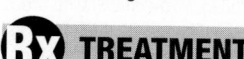 DIAGNOSIS

DIFFERENTIAL DIAGNOSIS

- Congenital deformities (septa/agenesis)
- Imperforate hymen
- Menopausal changes
- Atrophic tissue
- Impaired lubrication
- Psychogenic
- Vaginismus
- Inadequate foreplay
- Endometriosis
- Levator ani myalgia
- Chronic pelvic pain
- Previous surgery (posterior colporrhaphy, perineorrhaphy)
  1. Alteration in vaginal length, depth, caliber
  2. Adhesions
- Infectious
  1. HPV
  2. HSV
  3. Candidiasis
  4. *Tinea cruris*
  5. Acute or chronic salpingitis or endometritis
- Pelvic carcinoma
- Previous radiation
- Adnexal attachment or tubal prolapse
- Pelvic tumor
- Uterine prolapse, malposition, enlargement, or retroversion
- Genital prolapse
- Cystocele, rectocele, enterocele
- Urethral or bladder pathology
- Pelvic congestion
- Vulvar vestibulitis
- Postcoital cystitis
- Broad ligament pathology
- Neuroma at the site of previous episiotomy
- Previous sexual abuse
- Vulvodynia
- Contact or allergic dermatitis
- Vitamin A, B, or C deficiency
- Equestrian dyspareunia
- Interstitial cystitis
- Pudendal neuralgia
- Myofascial pain syndrome
- Rectal pathology
- Structural abnormalities or alterations
  1. Muscle
  2. Bone
  3. Ligament

WORKUP

- History and physical examination are key
- If needed:
  1. Colposcopy
  2. Cystoscopy
  3. Consider laparoscopy for unexplained deep dyspareunia

LABORATORY TESTS

- Erythrocyte sedimentation rate
- White blood cell count
- Wet mount
- Cultures
  1. Cervical
     a. Gonorrhea
     b. *Chlamydia*
  2. Vaginal
  3. Lesions
  4. Urine
- Vulva, vaginal, or cervical biopsy
- Pap smear
- HSV antibodies
- Gonadotropin levels

IMAGING STUDIES

Pelvic or abdominal ultrasonography. Transvaginal ultrasonography provides for greater resolution of uterus and ovaries due to proximity to pelvic organs. MRI when diagnosis is unclear with other diagnostic modalities (Fig. 1-293).

RX TREATMENT

NONPHARMACOLOGIC THERAPY

- Patient education
- Discontinue exacerbating activity and irritants
- Lubrication with coitus
- Coital position changes: female superior position
- Warm or cool soaks
- Reassurance to patient of nonmalignant condition

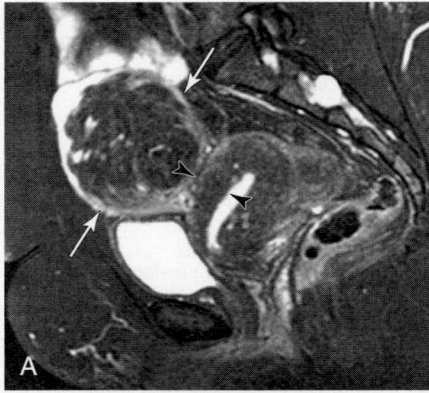

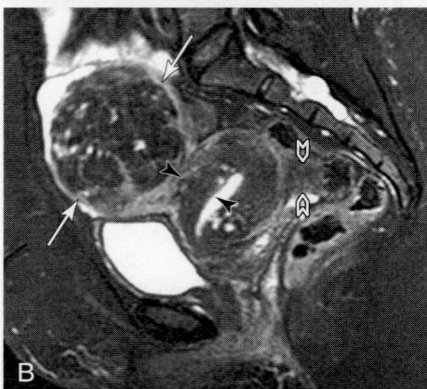

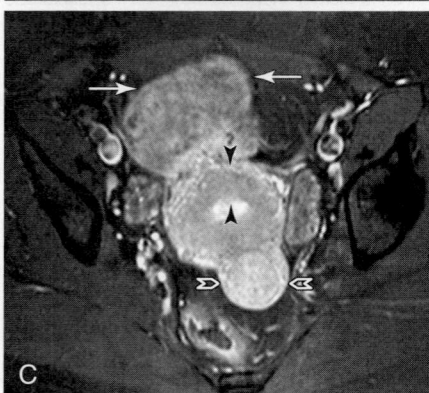

FIGURE 1-293 Adenomyosis and leiomyomata in a 41-year-old woman with pelvic pain, irregular menses, menorrhagia, and dyspareunia. A and B, Sagittal T2-weighted fat-suppressed images show a large anterior subserosal fibroid with mixed but predominately low signal *(arrows),* and a smaller posterior subserosal fibroid with low to intermediate signal *(chevrons).* There is also widening of the junctional zone *(black arrowheads)* with areas of increased T2 signal, indicative of adenomyosis. **C,** Axial three-dimensional gradient echo postcontrast image with fat suppression shows enhancement of the leiomyomata *(white arrowheads and chevrons)* and the thickened junctional zone *(black arrowheads).* (From Fielding JR et al: *Gynecologic imaging,* Philadelphia, 2011, Saunders.)

- Psychosocial interventions
  1. Systemic desensitization techniques
  2. Behavior modification
- Vaginal dilators
- Vaginal muscle exercises and relaxation techniques
- Excision of pathologic tissue
- Surgical correction of altered, reduced, or deformed tissues

ACUTE GENERAL Rx

- Topical lidocaine
- Corticosteroids
- Antiinfective agents
- Trigger point injections
- Massage
- Acupuncture
- Transcutaneous electrical nerve stimulation
- Stress reduction techniques
- Safe sexual practices
- Hormonal replacement therapy
- Antiviral agents
- Intralesional interferon
- Mild analgesics
- Antidepressants

CHRONIC Rx

All the previous plus:

- Set supportive visits as needed
- Oral contraceptives
- Regular sexual activity
- Balanced diet
- Vitamin supplementation
- Proper hygiene

DISPOSITION

Most patients will have a reduction and/or resolution of their symptoms by using the appropriate therapeutic approaches.

REFERRAL

As with other chronic pain conditions, a multidisciplinary approach using the expertise of psychologists, dermatologists, gynecologic surgeons, infectious disease specialists, or urologists is helpful.

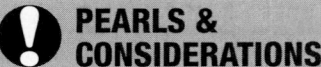

PEARLS & CONSIDERATIONS

- Dyspareunia is a symptom complex resulting from a multitude of etiologies, some of which act simultaneously.
- Uncovering the etiology of dyspareunia is predominantly based on a comprehensive history and physical examination.
- The differential diagnoses can be sorted into superficial, intermediate, and deep dyspareunia categories.
- As with the physical evaluation of any painful condition, attempt—by precise touching (moistened cotton swab), palpation, or applied pressure—to reproduce the patient's chief complaint.
- Performing a one-finger pelvic examination without concurrent abdominal palpation allows a more precise assessment of the source of genital pain.
- Individualize therapy.
- Initiate and maintain an honest diagnosis and compassionate demeanor with the patient and her partner.
- Be open minded, approachable, nonjudgmental, and diligent in your search for a solution to help these often silently suffering patients.

SUGGESTED READINGS

available at www.expertconsult.com

RELATED CONTENT

Dysmenorrhea (Related Key Topic)
Endometriosis (Related Key Topic)

AUTHORS: **DAVID I. KURSS, M.D.,** and **RUBEN ALVERO, M.D.**

BASIC INFORMATION

DEFINITION

Nonulcerative dyspepsia is a term used to describe signs and symptoms of persistent or recurrent dyspepsia centered in the upper abdomen that have no obvious cause or evidence of organic disease

SYNONYMS

Functional dyspepsia
Idiopathic dyspepsia

ICD-9CM CODES
536.8 Nonulcerative dyspepsia

EPIDEMIOLOGY & DEMOGRAPHICS

- Annual prevalence of dyspepsia approximately 25% of population.
- Dyspepsia, gastroesophageal reflux disease, peptic ulcer disease (PUD) account for 2% to 5% of all primary care visits.

PHYSICAL FINDINGS & CLINICAL PRESENTATION

An international committee of clinical investigators, sponsored by the American Gastroenterological Association (AGA), developed the Rome III criteria in 2006 to define Functional Dyspepsia (nonulcerative dyspepsia) for both research purposes and clinical practice:

Diagnostic criteria* must include:
One or more of the following:
  a. Bothersome postprandial fullness
  b. Early satiation
  c. Epigastric pain
  d. Epigastric burning
AND
No evidence of structural disease (including at upper endoscopy) that is likely to explain the symptoms

ETIOLOGY

The etiology and pathophysiology are still unclear but research is focused on the following factors:
- Abnormalities of gastric motor function—especially in delayed gastric emptying, antral hypomotility, the relationship between low fasting gastric volumes and faster gastric emptying, and lower gastric compliance
- Visceral hypersensitivity
- *Helicobacter pylori* infection
- Psychosocial factors—associated with anxiety and depression

RISK FACTORS

Risk factors include excessive amounts of caffeine, alcohol, or smoking or taking steroids, NSAIDs, or certain other medications, and living in a high *H. pylori* prevalence area.

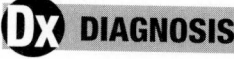 **DIAGNOSIS**

DIFFERENTIAL DIAGNOSIS

Made from the exclusion of other causes of dyspepsia

*Criteria need to be fulfilled for the last months with symptom onset at least 6 mo prior to diagnosis.

Other possible etiologies for dyspepsia:
- PUD
- Gastroesophageal reflux
- Gastric/esophageal/all abdominal cancers
- Biliary tract disease
- Gastroparesis
- Pancreatitis
- Medications (i.e., NSAIDs, erythromycin, steroids)
- Infiltrative diseases of the stomach (i.e., Crohn's or sarcoidosis)
- Metabolic disturbances (i.e., hypercalcemia or hyperkalemia)
- Ischemic bowel disease
- Systemic disorders (i.e., diabetes, thyroid disorders, or connective tissue diseases)

WORKUP

The American Gastroenterological Association and the Maastricht III and IV European consensus reports have similar recommendations.
- The pattern of symptoms overlaps considerably for all types of dyspepsia; therefore, the history and physical should focus on finding specific symptoms that help exclude other causes of dyspepsia.
- The AGA guidelines recommend that patients 55 yr of age or younger without alarm features should receive *H. pylori* testing and treatment, followed by acid suppression if symptoms remain. The European Guidelines IV also recommend an *H. pylori* test-and-treat approach for uninvestigated dyspepsia in populations in whom *H. pylori* prevalence is high (≥20%), subject to local cost/benefit considerations. Test-and-treat is not considered applicable to patients with alarm symptoms or older patients (age to be determined locally according to cancer risk), and further workup such as endoscopy should be considered. In areas with low *H. pylori* prevalence, either a test-and-treat or an acid-suppression strategy may be appropriate.

ENDOSCOPY:
- AGA Guidelines recommend endoscopy for patients older than 55 yr and for younger patients with alarm features (e.g., weight loss, progressive dysphagia, recurrent vomiting, evidence of gastrointestinal bleeding, or family history of cancer) presenting with new-onset dyspepsia. Biopsy specimens should be obtained during endoscopy for *H. pylori* and eradication therapy offered to those who are infected since this may reduce the risk of subsequent PUD and gastric malignancy
- It should be noted that the value of alarm features in younger patients is controversial and endoscopy may add little in younger patients who continue to have symptoms.

LABORATORY TESTS

H. pylori testing. Laboratory methods include certain validated serologic tests, monoclonal stool antigen, or urea breath test.
Other lab testing as appropriate.

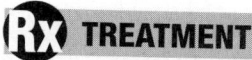 **TREATMENT**

NONPHARMACOLOGIC THERAPY

Treatment modalities may be controversial and disappointing. Goal should be to help patients reduce risk or exacerbating factors, accept, diminish, and cope with symptoms rather than seek to totally eliminate them. The Maastricht IV guidelines note that *H. pylori* eradication may be better than any other treatment for dyspepsia, yet it produces long-term relief of dyspepsia in only 1 of every 12 patients.

ACUTE GENERAL Rx

PHARMACOLOGIC THERAPY: Treatment may depend on the predominant symptoms. Possible approaches, based on predominant symptoms, may include the following:

Predominant Symptom	Possible Etiology	Medication Recommended
Nausea	Motility dysfunction	Prokinetic agent
Bloating	Motility dysfunction	Simethicone and/or prokinetic agent
Pain	Mucosal disease or *H. pylori* infection	Antibiotic trial
Somatic complaints	Psychosocial	Psychotropic medication trial

Medication categories:
- Antacids (i.e., aluminum hydroxide, calcium carbonate)
- Gas-reducing agents, such as those containing simethicone
- H_2-receptor antagonists (i.e., cimetidine)
- Proton pump inhibitors (PPIs) (i.e., omeprazole)
- Prokinetic agents (i.e., metoclopramide)
- Antidepressants (i.e., selective serotonin receptor inhibitors)
- *H. pylori* therapy/antibiotic therapy (various antibiotic regimens, usually + PPI)

CHRONIC Rx

Controversy currently exists around the long-term use of PPIs.

COMPLEMENTARY & ALTERNATIVE THERAPIES

Peppermint and caraway oil may be helpful, as well as acupuncture; however, no definitive trials have been performed.

REFERRAL

- Referral to gastroenterology if patient with alarming symptoms (such as GI bleeding, dysphagia, odynophagia, unexplained anemia, change in appetite, and weight loss) or when endoscopy is indicated—although controversy exists about the workup of younger patients.
- Referral to cardiology if cardiac etiology suspected.

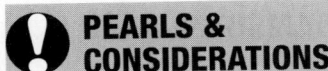

PEARLS & CONSIDERATIONS

PREVENTION
Avoid excessive amounts of caffeine, alcohol, smoking, or long-term use of steroids and NSAIDs.

PATIENT AND FAMILY EDUCATION
http://www.mayoclinic.com/health/stomach-pain/DS00524

SUGGESTED READINGS
available at www.expertconsult.com

RELATED CONTENT
Fig. 3-58 Approach to the patient with dyspepsia (Algorithm)

AUTHOR: **JEFFREY BORKAN, M.D., PH.D.**

BASIC INFORMATION

DEFINITION

The term "dysphagia" is derived from the Greek words *dys* (with difficulty) and *phagia* (to eat). It is characterized by abnormal transfer of food from mouth to the stomach, which may involve the oral, pharyngeal, or esophageal stages of swallowing.

ICD-9CM CODES
782.2 Dysphagia

EPIDEMIOLOGY & DEMOGRAPHICS

- This is seen in 10% of individuals above the age of 50 yr. Its prevalence increases with advancing age.
- Nearly 12% of hospitalized patients have symptoms of dysphagia.
- Up to 30% to 60% of nursing home patients have some form of dysphagia.
- Special populations, including patients with head injury, stroke, or Parkinson's disease, have 30% to 50% prevalence of oropharyngeal dysphagia.

ETIOLOGY
- Oropharyngeal
  1. Neuromuscular causes
     - Stroke
     - Parkinson's disease
     - Multiple sclerosis
     - Myasthenia gravis
     - Amyotrophic lateral sclerosis
     - CNS tumors
     - Muscular dystrophy
     - Thyroid dysfunction
     - Polymyositis and dermatomyositis
     - Sarcoidosis
     - Cerebral palsy
     - Head trauma
     - Metabolic encephalopathy
     - Dementia
     - Bell's palsy
  2. Structural causes
     - Oropharyngeal tumors
     - Zenker's diverticulum
     - Infection of pharynx or neck (mucositis from *Candida,* herpes, and CMV)
     - Thyromegaly
     - Prior surgery or radiotherapy
     - Osteophytes and other spinal disorders
     - Proximal esophageal webs
     - Congenital anomalies (e.g., cleft palate)
     - Poor dentition
- Esophageal
  1. Neuromuscular disorders
     - Achalasia
     - Diffuse esophageal spasm
     - Nutcracker esophagus
     - Hypertensive lower esophageal sphincter
     - Ineffective esophageal motility
     - Scleroderma
     - Reflex-associated dysmotility

  2. Structural disorder
     - Peptic stricture
     - Esophageal rings and webs
     - Diverticuli
     - Carcinoma and benign tumors
     - Foreign bodies
     - Vascular compression
     - Mediastinal masses
     - Spinal osteophytes
     - Mucosal injury (from pills, infection, gastroesophageal reflux disease [GERD], etc.)

PATHOGENESIS

The inability to swallow is caused either by a problem in strength or coordination of the muscles required to move material from the mouth to stomach or by a fixed obstruction somewhere between the mouth and the stomach.

CLINICAL FEATURES
Oropharyngeal dysphagia
- Problem arises within 2 seconds of initiating the voluntary phase of swallowing.
- Typical symptoms include drooling, spillage of food, postnasal regurgitation, difficulty in initiation of swallowing, sialorrhea, sensation of food stuck in the neck, coughing or choking during swallowing, the need to swallow repeatedly to clear food or fluid from the pharynx, dysphonia, nasal speech, hoarseness of voice, and dysarthria.
- A thorough physical examination including that of the nervous system, oral cavity, and the head/neck is very important in patients with oropharyngeal dysphagia.

Esophageal dysphagia
- Problem usually arises several seconds after swallowing.
- Patients often complain of food being stuck in lower substernal area.
- Dysphagia to solids suggests mechanical obstruction.
- Neuromuscular causes result in dysphagia to both solids and liquids. Particularly, patients with achalasia tend to drink a lot of fluids while eating or apply maneuvers such as straightening the back, raising their arms over their heads, or standing to increase intraesophageal pressure to facilitate the emptying of food into the stomach.
- Oftentimes, ingestion of very cold or very hot foods precipitates the dysphagia associated with neuromuscular disorder.
- Delayed regurgitation of food, heartburn, and chest pain are usually present.
- Weight loss is usually associated with malignancy or achalasia.
- Symptoms are intermittent in patients with esophageal dysphagia from benign causes of structural obstruction or diffuse esophageal spasm. However, it is progressive in patients with peptic stricture, esophageal carcinoma, scleroderma, and achalasia.
- In patients with structural obstruction, when the luminal diameter is more than 18 to 20 mm, they are rarely symptomatic, whereas those with a diameter of less than 13 mm are nearly always symptomatic.

- These patients with esophageal dysphagia usually do not have any characteristic physical findings.

DIAGNOSIS

Laboratory evaluation
- CBC
- Thyroid studies
- Nutritional assessment by checking serum protein and albumin levels
- Other studies based on specific clinical conditions

Special studies
- Oropharyngeal dysphagia
  1. Videofluoroscopy is the first test often ordered in evaluation of patients with oropharyngeal dysphagia
  2. Double contrast modified barium swallow study (Fig. 1-294)
  3. Fiberoptic flexible nasopharyngeal laryngoscopy is mandatory in all cases when a structural lesion, particularly malignancy, is suspected.
  4. Pharyngeal and upper esophageal manometry (Fig. 1-295) is occasionally of value to predict which patients will have a favorable outcome from cricopharyngeal myotomy or dilation.
  5. Radiography of head and neck when indicated
- Esophageal dysphagia
  1. Barium esophagography should precede upper endoscopies to identify patients at

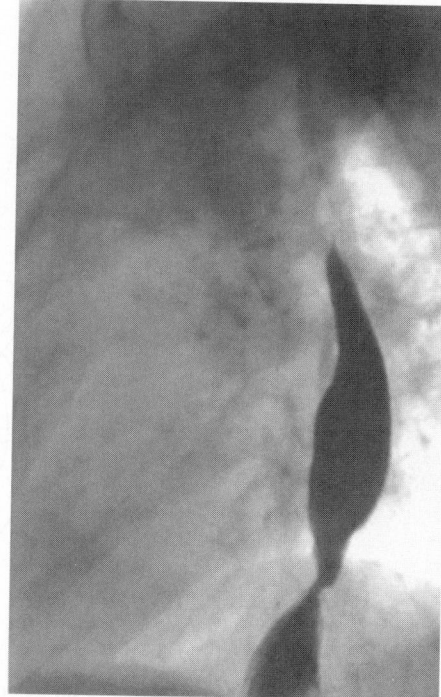

FIGURE 1-294 Barium swallow demonstrating a benign peptic stricture in a patient with gastroesophageal reflux disease and dysphagia. (From Talley NJ, Martin C: *Clinical gastroenterology: a practical problem-based approach,* ed 2, Sydney, 2006, Churchill Livingstone.)

risk from potential perforation with an endoscopy and to help plan fluoroscopically guided dilation. It is often the first step in evaluating patients with dysphagia, especially if an obstructive lesion is suspected.

2. EGD
3. Esophageal manometry is indicated if no abnormality is identified by barium study or EGD.
4. Esophageal pH monitoring in patients with suspected reflux disease
5. Endoscopic ultrasonography
6. Radiograph, CT, and MRI of chest

DIFFERENTIAL DIAGNOSIS
(Fig. E1-296)
- Globus pharyngeus
- Odynophagia
- Phagophobia
- GERD

 TREATMENT

- Treatment should be approached with the help of specialists of multiple disciplines (ENT, head and neck surgeon, radiologist, speech pathologist, physical therapist, dietitian, gastroenterologist, physical medicine and rehabilitation specialist, dentist, neurologist, etc.).
- Goal of therapy is airway protection and maintenance of nutrition.
- Alteration of food consistency, volume, and delivery rate plays a major role.
- The goal of direct therapy is to change swallowing physiology with medical treatment of primary disease, maxillofacial prosthesis, and cricopharyngeal myotomy
- Indirect therapies include exercise programs for tongue coordination and chewing under the guidance of a speech therapist.
- Maintenance of oral feeding often requires compensatory techniques such as chin-tuck position, rotation of head to the affected side, tilting of head to the strong side, and lying on one's back or on one's side during swallowing.
- Some of the voluntary maneuvers applied include supraglottic swallow, effortful swallow, Mendelson maneuver, Shaker exercise, and the Heimlich maneuver.
- Placement of nasogastric tube, jejunostomy tube, or percutaneous endoscopic gastrotomy (PEG) tube is considered for enteral feeding when other measures fail and the patient remains at significant risk for aspiration or nutrition becomes compromised.
- Treatment of associated GERD should not be forgotten.
- Surgery for chronic aspiration may involve tracheostomy, medialization, laryngeal suspension, laryngeal closure, and/or laryngotracheal separation-diversion.
- Other measures include esophageal dilation removal of foreign body, esophageal resection, chemotherapy, radiotherapy, endoscopic ablation of tumor, phodynamic therapy, esophageal prosthesis/stents, diverticulectomy, intrasphincteric injection of botulinum toxin, surgical myotomy, and others. Smooth muscle relaxants such as nitrates and calcium channel blockers have been used to effectively treat patients with diffuse esophageal spasm and nutcracker esophagus.
- Several scales have been suggested to determine patients' functional outcome. One of them is the "Swallowing Rating Scale."

COMPLICATIONS
- Dehydration
- Malnutrition
- Aspiration pneumonia
- Airway obstruction
- Death resulting from pulmonary complications

PROGNOSIS
- Depends on the etiology.
- Nursing home patients with oropharyngeal dysphagia and a history of aspiration have an approximately 45% mortality rate over 1 yr.
- All patients, especially the elderly, should take their medications with a full glass of water while in upright position well before bedtime.
- Dysphagia should be considered an alarm symptom, indicating the need for immediate evaluation.

PATIENT EDUCATION
Elderly patients with dysphagia should not attribute their symptoms to aging.

EBM EVIDENCE

available at www.expertconsult.com

SUGGESTED READINGS

available at www.expertconsult.com

RELATED CONTENT
Esophageal Tumors (Related Key Topic)
Gastroesophageal Reflux Disease (Related Key Topic)
Dyspepsia, Nonulcerative (Related Key Topic)

AUTHOR: **HEMANT K. SATPATHY, M.D.**

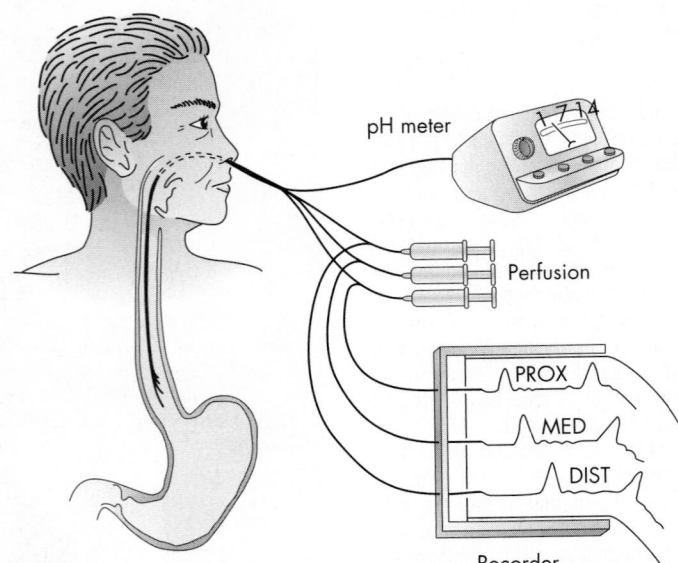
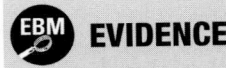

FIGURE 1-295 Combined manometric-pH recording system used in the evaluation of esophageal function. The triple-lumen perfused recording catheter measures intraluminal pressures from three levels in the esophagus. Measurements are made in terms of centimeters from the nostrils to the proximal opening of the recording catheter *(PROX)*. The medial catheter *(MED)* records pressures 5 cm distal to the proximal opening and the distal catheter *(DIST)* 5 cm below this. The intraesophageal pH electrode is used to document gastroesophageal reflux. (From Townsend CM et al: *Sabiston textbook of surgery*, ed 17, Philadelphia, 2004, Saunders.)

BASIC INFORMATION

DEFINITION

Dystonia refers to a group of disorders characterized by involuntary muscle contractions (sustained or spasmodic) that lead to abnormal body movements or postures. Dystonia can be generalized or focal, of early (<20 yr) or late onset, and primary or secondary.

SYNONYMS

Blepharospasm
Oromandibular (orofacial) dystonia
Spasmodic (limb or axial) dystonia
Torticollis
Writer's cramp

ICD-10CM CODES
G24   Dystonia
G24.1 Idiopathic familial dystonia
G24.0 Drug induced dystonia
G24.3 Spasmodic torticollis

EPIDEMIOLOGY & DEMOGRAPHICS

PREVALENCE: Estimated at one in 3000 persons.
PREDOMINANT SEX: Cervical dystonia has a 3:2 female preponderance.
PREDOMINANT AGE:
- Onset of focal cervical dystonia is usually in the fifth decade.
- Hereditary forms may have an onset in childhood or adulthood and tend to be more severe.
GENETICS: Autosomal-dominant, autosomal-recessive, and X-linked forms of dystonia have been identified. Ashkenazi Jews are particularly susceptible to primary early-onset dystonia.

CLINICAL PRESENTATION

Focal dystonias produce abnormal sustained muscle contractions in a single region of the body:
- Neck (**torticollis**): most commonly affected site with a tendency for the head to turn to one side
- Eyelids (**blepharospasm**): involuntary closure of the eyelids that leads to excessive eye blinking, sometimes with persistent eye closure and functional blindness
- Mouth (**oromandibular dystonia**): involuntary contraction of muscles of the mouth, tongue, or face
- Hand (**writer's cramp**) (Fig. 1-297)
Generalized dystonia affects multiple areas of the body and can lead to marked joint deformities.
- Isolated foot dystonia is very rare and may suggest an underlying parkinsonian disorder or brain structural abnormality

ETIOLOGY

- Exact pathophysiology of primary dystonia is unknown but believed to involve abnormalities of basal ganglia. Specifically, reduced and abnormal patterns of neuronal activity in the basal ganglia result in disinhibition of the motor thalamus and cortex, leading to abnormal movement.
- Fifteen hereditary forms have been described, including the severe progressive form, dystonia musculorum deformans.
- Secondary dystonia results from central nervous system (CNS) disease of the basal ganglia (stroke, demyelination, hypoxia, trauma), Huntington's disease, Wilson's disease, Parkinson syndromes, and lysosomal storage diseases.
- Acute dystonia can occur with drugs that block dopamine receptors, such as phenothiazines or butyrophenones.
- Tardive dyskinesia can result from long-term treatment with antiemetics (e.g., phenothiazines), antipsychotics (e.g., haloperidol), levodopa, anticonvulsants, or ergots.

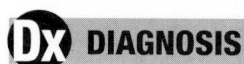

DIAGNOSIS

DIFFERENTIAL DIAGNOSIS
- Parkinson's disease
- Progressive supranuclear palsy
- Wilson's disease
- Huntington's disease
- Drug effects

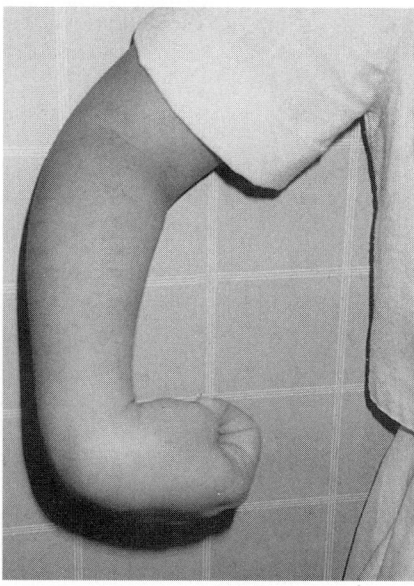

FIGURE 1-297 Focal dystonia of the distal right arm. (From Goldman L, Ausiello D [eds]: *Cecil textbook of medicine,* ed 22, Philadelphia, 2004, Saunders.)

- Table 1-136 describes selected causes of primary and secondary dystonia in childhood

WORKUP
History (family history, birth history, trauma, medication use), physical examination

LABORATORY TESTS
- Usually not helpful for diagnosis
- Serum ceruloplasmin if Wilson's disease is suspected

IMAGING STUDIES
- Primary dystonias are generally not associated with structural CNS abnormalities. CT scan or MRI of brain if a CNS lesion is suspected as a cause of secondary dystonia.
- Electrophysiologic testing can provide diagnostic support for the diagnosis.

TREATMENT

NONPHARMACOLOGIC THERAPY
- Heat, massage, physical therapy to relieve pain
- Splints to prevent contractures

ACUTE GENERAL Rx
For acute dystonic reactions to phenothiazines/butyrophenones, use diphenhydramine 50 mg IV or benztropine 2 mg IV.

CHRONIC Rx
- Pharmacologic treatment is often ineffective.
- Slowly withdraw offending agents.
- Diazepam, baclofen, or carbamazepine may be helpful.
- Intrathecal baclofen is most useful for spastic or truncal dystonia.
- Trihexyphenidyl or benztropine may be helpful in up to 50% of tardive dystonias.
- For generalized dystonia, a trial of carbidopa/levodopa may be beneficial and diagnostic of dopa-responsive dystonia (DYT5).
- Injections of botulinum toxin into the affected muscles is the standard treatment for focal dystonias. Both type A and type B toxins produced by *Clostridium botulinum* block cholinergic transmission at the neuromuscular junction by inhibiting release of acetylcholine. There are currently several botulinum toxins (Botox, Dysport, Xeomin, Myobloc) FDA approved for cervical dystonia. Botox and Xeomin are also FDA approved for blepharospasm.
- Surgical procedures, including denervation, myectomy, rhizotomy, thalamotomy (pallidotomy), or functional stereotactic surgery, may be helpful for severe, refractory cases.
- Deep brain stimulation is becoming more promising, especially for refractory primary generalized dystonias.

DISPOSITION

Spontaneous remission of focal cervical dystonia can occur, but dystonia is generally progressive and pharmacologic therapy is often ineffective.

REFERRAL

Neurology and/or neurosurgery for severe or refractory cases.
Physical therapy for maintaining flexibility.

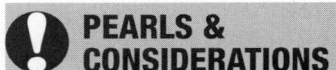

PEARLS & CONSIDERATIONS

COMMENTS

- Avoid triggers/exacerbating factors.
- Early physical therapy and splinting to prevent contractures.

- Consider botulism injections or deep brain stimulation surgery for severe or refractory dystonia, and for focal dystonias.

SUGGESTED READINGS

available at www.expertconsult.com

AUTHORS: **LYNN MCNICOLL, M.D., F.R.C.P.C.,** and **JULIE L. ROTH, M.D.**

TABLE 1-136 Selected Causes of Primary and Secondary Dystonia in Childhood

Diagnosis	Additional Clinical Features	Diagnosis	Additional Clinical Features
Aicardi-Goutieres syndrome	Encephalopathy, developmental regression; Acquired microcephaly; Sterile pyrexias; Lesions on the digits, ears (chilblain); Epilepsy; CT: calcification of the basal ganglia	Leigh syndrome	Motor delays, weakness, hypotonia; Ataxia, tremor; Elevated lactate; MRI: bilateral symmetric hyperintense lesions in the basal ganglia or thalamus
Alternating hemiplegia of childhood	Episodic hemiplegia/quadriplegia; Abnormal ocular movements; Autonomic symptoms; Epilepsy; Global developmental impairment; Environmental triggers for spells	Lesch-Nyhan syndrome (X-linked)	Male; Self-injurious behavior; Hypotonia; Oromandibular dystonia, inspiratory stridor; Oculomotor apraxia; Cognitive impairment; Elevated uric acid
Aromatic amino acid decarboxylase deficiency (AADC)	Developmental delay; Oculogyric crises; Autonomic dysfunction; Hypotonia	Myoclonus dystonia	Myoclonus; Head, upper limb involvement
ARX gene mutation (X-linked)	Male; Cognitive impairment; Infantile spasms, epilepsy; Brain malformation	Niemann-Pick type C	Hepatosplenomegaly; Hypotonia; Supranuclear gaze palsy; Ataxia, dysarthria; Epilepsy; Psychiatric symptoms
Benign paroxysmal torticollis of infancy	Episodic; Cervical dystonia only; Family history of migraine	Neuroacanthocytosis	Oromandibular and lingual dystonia
Complex regional pain syndrome	Lower limb involvement; Prominent pain	Neurodegeneration with brain iron accumulation	Cognitive impairment; Retinal pigmentary degeneration, optic atrophy
Dopa-responsive dystonia (DRD)	Diurnal variation	Rapid onset dystonia parkinsonism (DYT12)	Acute onset; Distribution face>arm>leg; Prominent bulbar signs
Drug-induced dystonia		Rett syndrome	Female; Developmental regression following a period of normal development; Stereotypic hand movements; Acquired microcephaly; Epilepsy
Dystonia-deafness optic neuropathy syndrome	Sensorineural hearing loss in early childhood; Psychosis; Optic atrophy in adolescence		
DYT1 dystonia	Lower limb onset followed by generalization		
Glutaric aciduria type 1	Macrocephaly; Encephalopathic crises; MRI: striatal necrosis	Spinocerebellar ataxia 17 (SCA17)	Ataxia; Dementia, psychiatric symptoms; Parkinsonism
GM1 gangliosidosis type 3	Short stature, skeletal dysplasia; Orofacial dystonia; Speech/swallowing disturbance; Parkinsonism; MRI: putaminal hyperintensity	Tics	Stereotyped movements; Premonitory urge, suppressible
Huntington disease (HD)	Parkinsonism; Epilepsy; Family history of HD	Tyrosine hydroxylase deficiency	Infantile encephalopathy, hypotonia; Oculogyric crises, ptosis; Autonomic symptoms; Less diurnal fluctuation than DRD
Kernicterus	Jaundice in infancy; Hearing loss; Impaired upgaze; Enamel dysplasia; MRI: hyperintense lesions in the globus pallidus		

From Kliegman RM et al: *Nelson textbook of pediatrics,* ed 19, Philadelphia, 2011, Saunders.

BASIC INFORMATION

DEFINITION

Echinococcosis is a chronic infection caused by the larval stage of several animal cestodes (tapeworms) of the genus *Echinococcus*.

SYNONYMS

Hydatid disease

ICD-9CM CODES

122.9 *Echinococcus* infection

EPIDEMIOLOGY & DEMOGRAPHICS

INCIDENCE (IN U.S.): Seen primarily in immigrants.
PEAK INCIDENCE: Presumed to be acquired in childhood or early adulthood in most cases.
PREVALENCE (IN U.S.): See Incidence
PREDOMINANT SEX: Male = female
PREDOMINANT AGE: 0 to 50 yr of age

PHYSICAL FINDINGS & CLINICAL PRESENTATION

- Signs of an enlarging mass lesion in a visceral site such as the liver, lungs, kidneys, bone, or CNS
- Occasional cyst rupture causing allergic manifestations such as urticaria, angioedema, or anaphylaxis that bring the patient to medical attention
- Incidental discovery of cysts by abdominal or thoracic imaging studies performed for other reasons

ETIOLOGY

- Four species of *Echinococcus*: *E. granulosus*, *E. multilocularis*, *E. oligarthrus*, and *E. vogeli*.
  1. *E. granulosus* is the cause of cystic hydatid disease.
  2. *E. multilocularis* and *E. vogeli* are the causes of alveolar and polycystic disease.
- The disease is transmitted to humans by infected canines (domestic or wild dogs, wolves, foxes) and seen most commonly in livestock-producing areas of the Middle East, Africa, Australia, New Zealand, Europe, and the Americas, including the southwestern U.S.
- Eggs are present in the feces of infected canines; human infection occurs by ingestion of viable eggs in contaminated food.
- It is common in many areas of the world, especially the Middle East.

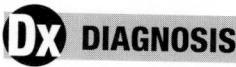 DIAGNOSIS

DIFFERENTIAL DIAGNOSIS

- Cystic neoplasms (see Table 1-137)
- Abscess (amebic or bacterial)
- Congenital polycystic disease

WORKUP

- Antibody assay
- Imaging study (CT scan [Fig. 1-298], ultrasonography)

- Classification (Fig. 1-299): Table 1-138 describes the World Health Organization Informal Working Group on Echinococcosis classification of hepatic echinococcal cysts.
- Histologic examination of cyst or contents obtained by aspiration or resection (if possible) to confirm diagnosis

LABORATORY TESTS

Antibody assays (ELISA, latex agglutination, and Western blot): >90% sensitive and specific for liver cysts, but less accurate for cysts in other sites. A PCR assay is now available for problematic cases.

IMAGING STUDIES

Ultrasonography and/or CT scan:
- Both are extremely sensitive for the detection of cysts, especially in the liver.
- Both lack specificity and are inadequate to establish the diagnosis of echinococcosis with certainty.

TREATMENT

ACUTE GENERAL Rx

- Albendazole 400 mg PO bid followed by percutaneous aspiration-injection-reaspiration (PAIR) for uncomplicated larval cysts. It consists of puncture (P) and needle aspirate (A) of cyst content followed by inspiration (I) of hypertonic saline (15%-30%) or absolute alcohol, waiting 20 to 30 minutes, then reaspirating (R) with final irrigation. Albendazole is continued for 28 days. Cure rate is 96%.
- Surgical resection: cure rate 90%

DISPOSITION

- Long-term follow-up is necessary following surgical or medical therapy because of the potential for late relapse.
- Antibody assays and imaging studies are repeated every 6 to 12 mo for several years following successful surgical or medical therapy.

TABLE 1-137 Hepatic Cyst Disease: Differential Features on Imaging Studies

Characteristics	Hydatid Cyst	Congenital Cyst	Cystadenoma
Configuration	Cyst within cyst	Single or multiple ± septations	Single ± septations
Wall character	Thick, uniform ± calcification	Thin, uniform	Mural nodules
Cyst contents	Daughter cysts Hydatid sand	Low density	Low density

From Cameron JL, Cameron AM: *Current surgical therapy*, ed 10, Philadelphia, 2011, Saunders.

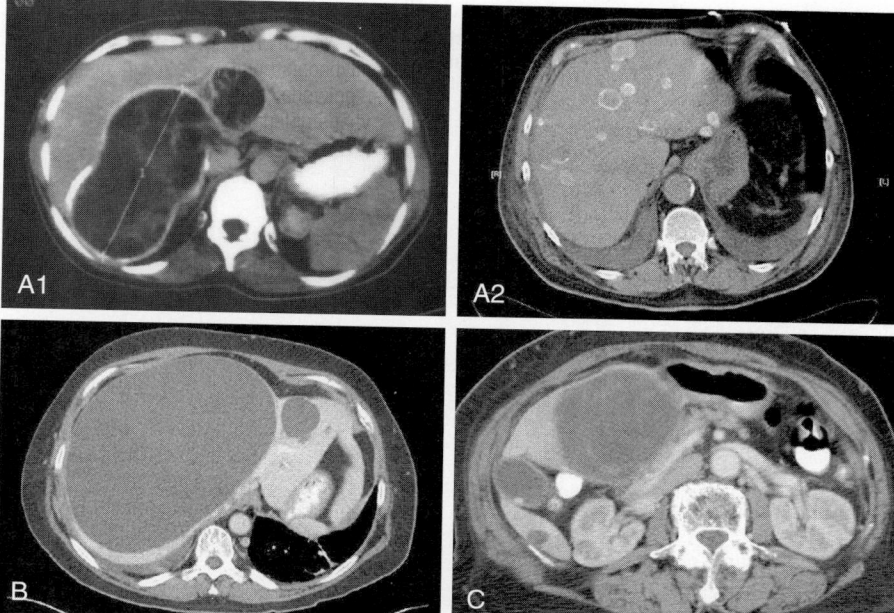

FIGURE 1-298 A comparison of computed tomography scans. A, Hepatic echinococcal cysts. **B,** Congenital cyst. **C,** Cystadenoma. For echinococcal cyst. **A1** demonstrates a single cyst with calcification and daughter cyst caused by *E. granulosa*. **A2** shows multiple small cysts characteristic of *E. multilocularis* infection. (Courtesy Barbara M. Kadell, MD, Professor of Radiology, David Geffen School of Medicine at University of California, Los Angeles. From Cameron JL, Cameron AM: *Current surgical therapy*, ed 10, Philadelphia, 2011, Saunders.)

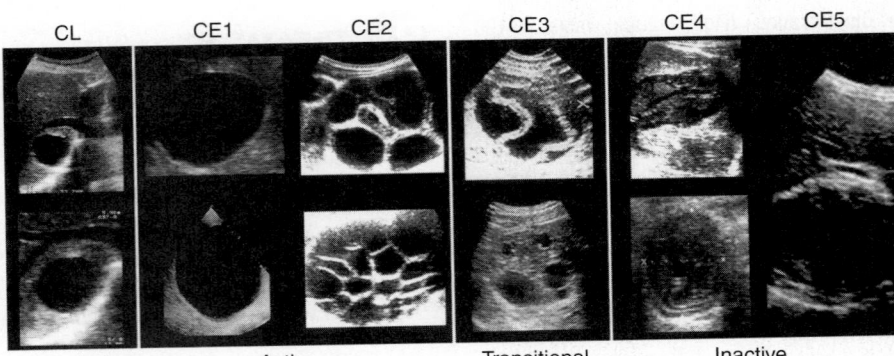

Cystic lesion   Active   Transitional   Inactive

FIGURE 1-299 WHO Informal Working Group on Echinococcosis standardized ultrasound classification of cystic echinococcosis. CL lesions are cystic lesions lacking a distinct wall and may have other diagnoses. CE1 lesions are cystic lesions with a visible wall that may demonstrate protoscolices ("hydatid sand"). CE2 lesions include internal septation. CE3 lesions may be detached from the wall or have daughter cysts with internal thickening. CE4 lesions are heterogeneous lesions with degeneration. CE5 lesions show thick calcification. (From Goldman L, Schafer AI: *Goldman's Cecil medicine*, ed 24, Philadelphia, 2012, Saunders.)

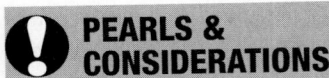

REFERRAL

All patients for evaluation for possible surgical resection of cysts versus PAIR

⚠ PEARLS & CONSIDERATIONS

COMMENTS

Cyst resection, if indicated, should be performed by surgeons experienced with this procedure.

SUGGESTED READINGS

available at www.expertconsult.com

RELATED CONTENT

Echinococcosis (Patient Information)

AUTHOR: **GLENN G. FORT, M.D., M.P.H.**

TABLE 1-138   WHO-IWGE Classification of Hepatic Echinococcal Cysts

Type of Cyst	Status	Ultrasound Features	Remarks
CL	Active	Signs not pathognomonic, unilocular, no cyst wall	Usually early stage, not fertile; differential diagnosis necessary
CE 1	Active	Cyst wall, hydatid sand	Usually fertile
CE 2	Active	Multivesicular, cyst wall, rosette-like	Usually fertile
CE 3	Transitional	Detached laminated membrane, "water lily" sign, less round, decreased intracystic pressure	Starting to degenerate, may produce daughter cyst
CE 4	Inactive	Heterogeneous hypoechogenic or hyperechogenic degenerative contents; no daughter cyst	Usually no living protoscolices; differential diagnosis necessary
CE 5	Inactive	Thick, calcified wall, calcification partial to complete; not pathognomonic but highly suggestive of diagnosis	Usually no living protoscolices

WHO-IWGE, World Health Organization Informal Working Group on Echinococcosis.
From Cameron JL, Cameron AM: *Current surgical therapy,* ed 10, Philadelphia, 2011, Saunders.

BASIC INFORMATION

DEFINITION

Eclampsia is the occurrence of seizures or coma in a woman with preeclampsia, occurring at >20 wk of gestation or <48 hr postpartum. Atypical eclampsia occurs at <20 wk of gestation or as much as 14 days postpartum.

SYNONYMS

Toxemia
Seizures of pregnancy

ICD-9CM CODES
642.6 Eclampsia

EPIDEMIOLOGY & DEMOGRAPHICS

INCIDENCE: One case per 150 to 3000 pregnancies; 2% to 4% of those with preeclampsia
GENETICS: Increased incidence with a first-degree relative (sister or mother) having had eclampsia
RISK FACTORS: Multifetal gestation (3.6% in twin gestation), molar pregnancy, nonimmune hydrops fetalis, uncontrolled hypertension, preexisting hypertension, renal disease

PHYSICAL FINDINGS & CLINICAL PRESENTATION

- Seizure begins as facial twitching, then spreads to generalized clonicotonic state, with cessation of respiration followed by a postictal period of amnesia, agitation, and confusion.
- 40% have severe hypertension, 40% have mild to moderate hypertension, and 20% are normotensive.
- Generalized edema with rapid weight gain (>2 lb/wk) may be one of the earliest signs of eclampsia.
- Persistent occipital headache and hyperreflexia with clonus occur in 80% of patients with eclampsia; epigastric pain occurs in 20% of these patients.

ETIOLOGY

- Exact etiology unknown.
- Common pathway relates to abnormalities in autoregulation of cerebral blood flow. This may involve transient vasospasm, ischemia, cerebral hemorrhage, and edema occurring by a mechanism involving hypertensive encephalopathy, decreased colloid osmotic pressure, and prostaglandin imbalance.

DIAGNOSIS

DIFFERENTIAL DIAGNOSIS

- Preexisting seizure disorder
- Metabolic abnormalities (hypoglycemia, hyponatremia, hypocalcemia)
- Substance abuse
- Head trauma, infection (meningitis, encephalitis)
- Intracerebral bleeding or thrombosis
- Amniotic fluid embolism
- Space-occupying brain lesions or neoplasms
- Pseudoseizure

WORKUP

- Rule out other causes of seizures during pregnancy.
- Atypical presentations such as prolonged postictal state; status epilepticus; gestational age <20 wk or >48 hr postpartum; or signs of meningitis, substance abuse, or severe uncontrolled hypertension should prompt a search for other seizure etiologies.

LABORATORY TESTS

- Proteinuria: severe (49%), mild to moderate (29%), absent (22%)
- HCT: elevated as a result of hemoconcentration
- Platelet count: decreased; LFTs elevated in HELLP syndrome (hemolysis, elevated liver enzymes, and low platelet count)
- BUN and creatinine: elevated with renal involvement
- Serum electrolytes, glucose, calcium, toxicology profile: rule out other causes of seizures
- Hyperuricemia: >6.9 mg/dl found in 70% of eclamptics
- ABG: maternal acidemia and hypoxia

IMAGING STUDIES

- CT scan or MRI indicated in atypical presentation, suspected intracerebral bleeding, or focal neurologic deficit
- There are abnormal findings, including cerebral edema, hemorrhage, and infarction, in 50% of patients.

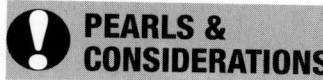 TREATMENT

NONPHARMACOLOGIC THERAPY

- Airway protection (risk of aspiration)
- Supportive care during acute event

ACUTE GENERAL Rx

- Maintain airway, adequate oxygenation, and IV access.
- Fetal resuscitation, involving maternal oxygenation, left lateral positioning, and continuous fetal heart rate monitoring, is needed.
- Magnesium sulfate is the drug of choice. Give magnesium sulfate 6 g IV load over 20 min, then 3 g/hr maintenance, for recurrent seizure prophylaxis. If repeated convulsions, may give an additional 2 g IV over 3 to 5 min. Approximately 10% to 15% of patients will have a second seizure after initial loading dose. Check magnesium level 1 hr after loading dose, then q6h (therapeutic range 4 to 6 mg/dl). Antidote for toxicity is calcium gluconate 10 ml of 10% solution. Phenytoin has been used as an alternative in patients in whom magnesium sulfate is contraindicated (renal insufficiency, heart block, myasthenia gravis, hypoparathyroidism).
- Give sodium amobarbital 250 mg IV over 3 min for persistent seizures.
- Treat blood pressure if >160 mm Hg/110 mm Hg with labetalol 20- to 40-mg IV bolus, hydralazine 10 mg IV, or nifedipine 10 to 20 mg sublingual q20min.
- Evaluate patient for delivery.

CHRONIC Rx

- The first priority is stabilization of the mother in terms of adequate oxygenation, hemodynamics, and laboratory abnormalities, such as associated coagulopathies.
- Cervical status and gestational age should be assessed. If unfavorable cervix and <30 wk of gestation, consider C-section; otherwise consider induction.
- Controlled epidural is the anesthesia of choice for labor or C-section.
- Avoid general anesthesia in uncontrolled hypertension to minimize risk of catastrophic cerebral events.

DISPOSITION

The maternal mortality rate for eclampsia averages 5% to 6%. Morbidity rate is 25%, including placental abruption (10%), maternal apnea with fetal asphyxia, aspiration pneumonia, pulmonary edema (4%), renal failure, cardiopulmonary arrest, and coma.

REFERRAL

Because of the potential for serious permanent maternal and fetal sequelae, all cases should be managed by a team approach of obstetrician, neonatologist, and intensivist.

PEARLS & CONSIDERATIONS

COMMENTS

- Eclampsia antepartum, 50%; intrapartum, 20%; and postpartum, 30%.
- Postseizure there is an associated period of fetal bradycardia from 1 to 9 min; if there is evidence of fetal compromise beyond that time, consider alternative etiologies such as placental abruption (23% incidence).

SUGGESTED READINGS

available at www.expertconsult.com

RELATED CONTENT

Fatty Liver of Pregnancy, Acute (Related Key Topic)
HELLP Syndrome (Related Key Topic)
Preeclampsia (Related Key Topic)
Eclampsia (Patient Information)

AUTHORS: **SCOTT J. ZUCCALA, D.O.,** and **RUBEN ALVERO, M.D.**

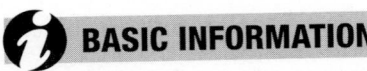

BASIC INFORMATION

DEFINITION

An ectopic pregnancy (EP) occurs when a fertilized ovum implants outside the endometrial lining of the uterus.

SYNONYMS

Abdominal pregnancy (0.03% to 1%)
Cervical pregnancy (0.5%)
Interstitial pregnancy (1% to 2%)
Ovarian pregnancy (1%)
Tubal pregnancy (97%)

ICD-9CM CODES
633 Ectopic pregnancy

EPIDEMIOLOGY & DEMOGRAPHICS

- 1% to 2% of pregnancies
- 13% of maternal deaths

PREVALENCE (IN U.S.): Increasing number of EPs; 17,800 reported cases in 1970 and currently over 100,000 reported cases/year.

RISK FACTORS: Previous salpingitis, previous EP, previous tubal ligation, previous tuboplasty, intrauterine device use, progestin-only pill, assisted reproductive techniques

PHYSICAL FINDINGS & CLINICAL PRESENTATION

- Abdominal tenderness: 95%
- Adnexal tenderness: 87% to 99%
- Peritoneal signs: 71% to 76%
- Adnexal mass: 33% to 53%
- Enlarged uterus: 6% to 30%
- Shock: 2% to 17%
- Amenorrhea or abnormal vaginal bleeding: 75%
- Shoulder pain: 10%
- Tissue passage: 6% to 7%

ETIOLOGY

- Anatomic obstruction to zygote passage
- Abnormalities in tubal motility
- Transperitoneal migration of the zygote

DIAGNOSIS

DIFFERENTIAL DIAGNOSIS

- Corpus luteum cyst
- Rupture or torsion of ovarian cyst
- Threatened or incomplete abortion
- Pelvic inflammatory disease
- Appendicitis
- Gastroenteritis
- Dysfunctional uterine bleeding
- Degenerating uterine fibroids
- Endometriosis

WORKUP

1. The classic presentation of EP includes the triad of abnormal vaginal bleeding, pelvic pain, and an adnexal mass. Fig. E1-300 describes a diagnostic approach to suspected EP. Fig. 1-301 *(top)* describes potential sites of ectopic implantations. Consider in all women with abdominopelvic pain and a positive pregnancy test
2. Transvaginal ultrasound
3. Quantitative serum human chorionic gonadotropin level
4. Laparoscopy in equivocal situations and possibly for treatment

LABORATORY TESTS

- Quantitative human chorionic gonadotropin (QhCG): if normal intrauterine pregnancy (IUP), 85% have doubling time of 2 days. If abnormal

Sites of Ectopic Implantations

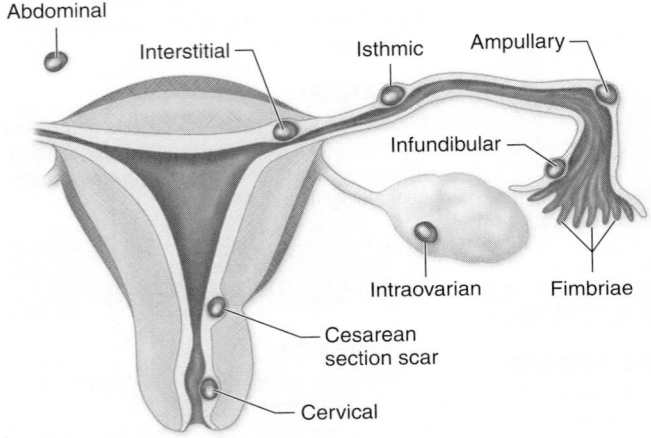

FIGURE 1-301 *Top,* Schematic drawing depicting implantation sites of ectopic pregnancies. **A** and **B,** Heterotopic pregnancy. This pregnant patient presented with vaginal bleeding at 5 to 6 wk of gestational age. **A,** Transverse transvaginal ultrasound (TVUS) image of the uterus reveals an intrauterine gestational sac containing a yolk sac. Note small subchorionic hemorrhage *(arrows),* most likely accounting for the vaginal bleeding. **B,** Sagittal TVUS image of the right adnexa reveals an echogenic tubal ring *(arrow)* clearly separate from the right ovary *(OV),* which was surgically confirmed to be an ectopic pregnancy. (From Fielding JR et al: *Gynecologic imaging,* Philadelphia, 2011, Saunders.)

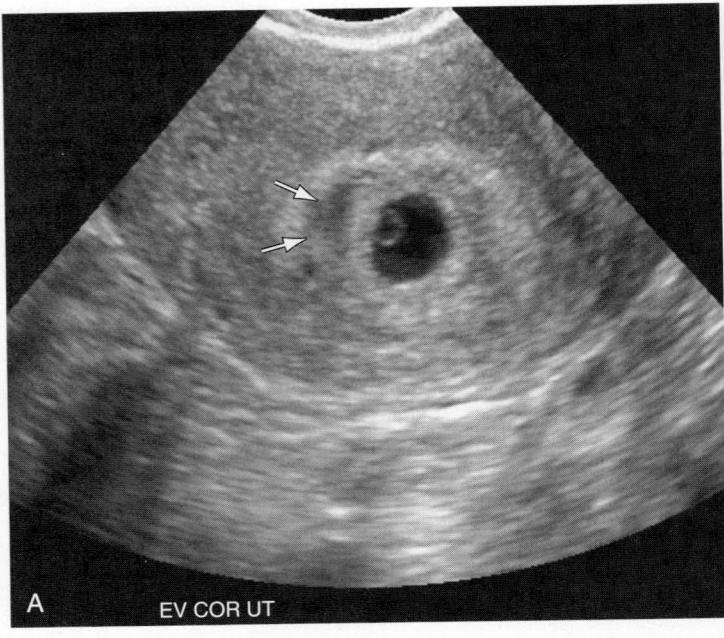

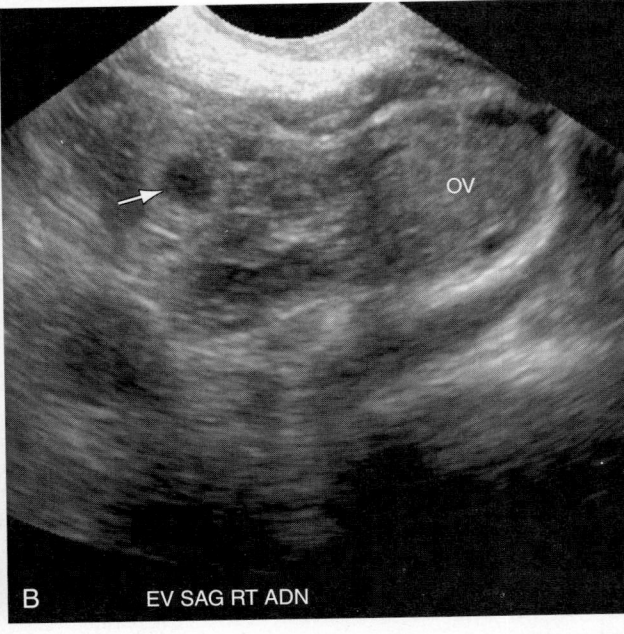

gestation, will show <66% increase of QhCG within 2 days. However, 13% of ectopic pregnancies have a normal doubling time.

- Progesterone: decreased production in EP; <5 ng/ml strongly predictive of abnormal pregnancy. If >25 ng/ml, strongly predictive of normal IUP.
- Dropping hematocrit associated with tubal rupture, resolving EP, or abnormal intrauterine pregnancy.
- Leukocytosis.

IMAGING STUDIES

- Ultrasound: presence of an IUP makes EP extremely unlikely. However, if the patient used assisted reproductive technologies, a heterotopic pregnancy (a pregnancy in the uterus as well as in the fallopian tube) is much more likely to occur (Fig. 1-301, *A* and *B*). A repeat ultrasonographic examination 2 to 7 days after presentation may identify the location of a pregnancy that was not identified on initial ultrasonographic examination.
- If QhCG >6000 mIU/ml, should see IUP on abdominal scan; QhCG >1500 mIU/ml for transvaginal scan. Since transvaginal ultrasonography is overwhelmingly the preferred modality for imaging, the latter value is clearly the discriminatory threshold that is used in diagnosis.
- Findings on ultrasound in EP include:
  1. Empty uterus
  2. Adnexal mass
  3. Cul-de-sac fluid
  4. Fetal sac in tube
  5. Fetal cardiac activity in adnexa

(Rx) TREATMENT

NONPHARMACOLOGIC THERAPY

Surgery can be performed by laparoscopy if patient is stable or, rarely, by laparotomy if patient is very unstable. Salpingiosis is the direct injection of chemotherapy into the EP by laparoscopy, transvaginal ultrasound, or hysteroscopy.

- Conservative surgery, salpingostomy or segmental resection, depends on tubal location and size of EP.
- Salpingectomy should be considered in the following circumstances:
  1. Ruptured tube
  2. Future fertility not desired
  3. Recurrent EP in the same tube
  4. Uncontrolled hemorrhage

ACUTE GENERAL Rx

- If the patient is stable and compliant, consider medical management with methotrexate. Patient should not have contraindications to methotrexate such as hepatic or renal disease, thrombocytopenia, leukopenia, or significant anemia. There should be no evidence of hemoperitoneum on transvaginal ultrasound. EP should be <3.5 cm mass with QhCG <6,000 to 15,000 mIU/ml, but these are relative contraindications. Presence of cardiac activity in the fetus is also a relative contraindication to methotrexate.
- Most common regimen is methotrexate 50 mg/m^2 of body surface area. May require second dose or surgical intervention if QhCG increases or plateaus (<15% drop) when comparing values from the fourth through seventh day after treatment (day 1 is the day

that methotrexate is given). Absolute contraindications to methotrexate include breast feeding, preexisting blood dyscrasias, known sensitivity to methotrexate, active pulmonary disease, chronic liver disease, alcoholism, laboratory evidence of immunodeficiency, renal disease, and peptic ulcer disease.

CHRONIC Rx

Persistent EP results from residual trophoblastic tissue or secondary implantation after conservative surgery. There is a 5% incidence of persistent EP with conservative treatment.

DISPOSITION

If diagnosed and treated early (before rupture), prognosis is excellent for good recovery. Monitor QhCG weekly until negative. Use reliable contraception until hCG is negative. With subsequent pregnancies, follow QhCG and perform early ultrasound to confirm IUP. There is a 12% recurrence rate for EP.

REFERRAL

Should obtain gynecologic consultation if EP is suspected.

SUGGESTED READINGS
available at www.expertconsult.com

RELATED CONTENT

Spontaneous Miscarriage (Related Key Topic)
Vaginal Bleeding during Pregnancy (Related Key Topic)
Ectopic Pregnancy (Patient Information)

AUTHORS: **GEORGE T. DANAKAS, M.D.,** and **RUBEN ALVERO, M.D.**

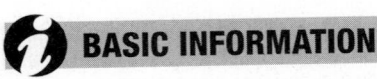

BASIC INFORMATION

DEFINITION

Ehlers-Danlos syndrome (EDS) refers to a group of inherited, clinically variable, and genetically heterogeneous connective tissue disorders. EDS is characterized by skin hyperextensibility, skin fragility, joint laxity, and joint hyperextensibility.

ICD-9CM CODES
756.83 Ehlers-Danlos syndrome

EPIDEMIOLOGY & DEMOGRAPHICS

- The prevalence of EDS is estimated to be approximately one in 5000 births, although it is somewhat higher in African Americans.
- There are several distinct forms of EDS (see Table 1-139).
- Classic and hypermobility EDS are most prevalent. Classic EDS accounts for approximately 80% of reported cases.
- Vascular EDS is the most dangerous because it is associated with spontaneous rupture of medium and large arteries and hollow organs, especially the large intestine and uterus; occurs in 4% of patients with EDS. Vascular events typically occur between the third and fifth decade.
- In most cases, transmission is autosomal dominant except for some unclassified forms of EDS (previously known as type V and type IX, which are x-linked; type X is autosomal recessive).

PHYSICAL FINDINGS & CLINICAL PRESENTATION

- Classic (previously types I and II): patients have moderate-to-severe skin hyperelasticity (easy scarring and bruising ("cigarette-paper scars"); smooth, velvety skin and subcutaneous spheroids (small, firm, cystlike nodules) along shins or forearms, hyperextensibility ("Gorlin's sign": ability to touch tip of tongue to nose, and joint hypermobility (Fig. 1-302) and dislocation; patients have complications such as hernias, pelvic organ prolapsed, premature arthritis, and cervical insufficiency
- Hypermobility (type III): most frequent form, causing recurrent joint dislocations, often leaving a patient unable to walk; chronic limb/joint pain is a prominent feature; skin involvement is less prominent

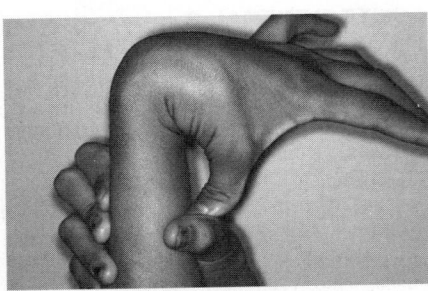

FIGURE 1-302 Joint hyperextensibility in classic Ehlers-Danlos syndrome. (From Kliegman RM et al: *Nelson textbook of pediatrics*, ed 19, Philadelphia, 2011, Saunders.)

- Vascular (type IV): cardinal features include distinctive facial features (pinched nose, thin lips, tight skin, hollow cheeks, lobeless ears), acrogeria, thin, translucent skin, excessive bruising, and most importantly, rupture of vessels and viscera including arterial, intestinal, and uterine walls; spontaneous rupture of organs occurs in the sigmoid colon, spleen, liver, and uterus; facial features are often not prominent in children, and vascular EDS is usually not diagnosed until adulthood
- Kyphoscoliotic (type VI): rare; characterized by marked muscular hypotonia, osteopenia, joint hypermobility, progressive scoliosis, ocular fragility and possible globe rupture, mitral valve prolapse, and aortic dilation
- Arthrochalasia (types VIIA and VIIB): prominent joint hypermobility with subluxations, congenital hip dislocation, skin hyperextensibility, and tissue fragility
- Dermatosparaxis (type VIIC): severe skin fragility with decreased elasticity, bruising, hernias
- Unclassified types: type V—X-linked recessive, similar to classic EDS with skin fragility but less joint hypermobility and bruising; type IX—classic characteristics; type VIII—classic characteristics and severe periodontal disease; type X—mild classic characteristics, mitral valve prolapse; type XI—joint instability

ETIOLOGY

- Defects of collagen in extracellular matrices of multiple tissues (skin, tendons, blood vessels, and viscera) underlie all forms of EDS.

TABLE 1-139 Types of Ehlers-Danlos Syndrome

Type	Name	Genetics	Etiology	Clinical Features
EDS I	Gravis	AD	30% of cases caused by null allele	Soft skin with scars for *COL5A1* or *COL5A2* Hypermobile joints Easy bruising
EDS II	Mitis	AD	30% of cases caused by null allele for *COL5A1* or *COL5A2*	Less severe form of type I EDS
EDS III	Hypermobile	AD	Unknown	Soft skin without scars Marked mobility of large and small joints
EDS IV	Vascular	AD (AR)	Defects of type III collagen	Translucent skin Marked bruising Ruptured arteries, uterus, bowel Normal joint mobility
EDS V	X-linked	XL	Unknown	Similar to EDS II
EDS VI	Ocular-scoliotic	AR		Skin soft and extensible
	VIA—decreased lysyl hydroxylase case type		Defects in lysyl hydroxylase	Scoliosis Ocular fragility
	VIB—decreased lysyl hydroxylase case type		Unknown	Hypermobile joints
EDS VII	Arthrochalasis multiplex congenita			
	VIIA—α1(I) type	AD	α1(I) DE6	Congenital hip dislocation
	VIIB—α2(I) type	AD	α2(I) DE6	Hypermobile joints
	VIIC—enzyme deficiency	AR	Deficient procollagen N-proteinase	Skin soft without scars
EDS VIII	Periodontitis type	AD	Unknown	Generalized periodontitis Skin soft and extensible Easy bruising Hypermobile joints
EDS X	Fibronectin	AR	Fibronectin	Mild joint hypermobility Easy bruising Abnormal platelet aggregation

AD, Autosomal dominant; *AR*, autosomal recessive.
From Hochberg MC et al: *Rheumatology*, ed 5, St Louis, 2011, Mosby.

- Classic EDS is associated with defects in type V collagen, corresponding to mutations of *COL5A* genes.
- Vascular EDS involves a deficiency in type III collagen, and several studies suggest that mutations of gene *COL3A1* lead to this deficiency.
- Arthrochalasia EDS results from a defect in type I collagen, caused by mutations in the *COL1A1* and *COL1A2* genes.

DIAGNOSIS

Diagnosis is based solely on clinical criteria. It is important to identify patients with vascular EDS because of the grave consequences of the disease.

- Clinical criteria for vascular EDS: two of four major diagnostic criteria establish the diagnosis; ≥1 minor criterion supports but is not sufficient to establish the diagnosis.
- Major criteria:
  1. Easy bruising
  2. Arterial, intestinal, or uterine fragility
  3. Thin, translucent skin
  4. Characteristic facial features (thin, delicate, and pinched nose, hollow cheeks, prominent staring eyes): occur in <30% of patients with vascular EDS
- Minor criteria:
  ○ Small joint hypermobility
  ○ Skin hyperextensibility
  ○ Spontaneous pneumothorax/hemothorax
  ○ Tendon or muscle rupture
  ○ Early-onset varicose veins
  ○ Carotid-cavernous fistula
  ○ Talipes equinovarus (clubfoot)

DIFFERENTIAL DIAGNOSIS

- Marfan's syndrome
- Osteogenesis imperfecta

- Autosomal dominant cutis laxa
- Familial joint hypermobility

WORKUP

Diagnosis is based solely on clinical criteria.

LABORATORY TESTS

- Biochemical and gene testing for known molecular defects recommended to confirm the diagnosis in vascular EDS.
- Plain radiographs may reveal calcified nodules along the shin or forearms corresponding to the subcutaneous spheroids.
- Echocardiogram can identify mitral valve prolapse and aortic dilation.

TREATMENT

- All patients should receive genetic counseling about the mode of inheritance of their EDS.
- Management of most skin and joint problems should be conservative and preventive. Joint hypermobility and pain in EDS usually does not require surgical intervention. Physical therapy to strengthen muscles is helpful. Surgical repair and tightening of joint ligaments can be performed, but ligaments frequently will not hold sutures. Surgical intervention should be considered on an individual basis.
- For patients with vascular EDS:
  ○ Special surgical care is required because of increased tissue friability.
  ○ Patients should be advised to avoid contact sports.
  ○ Elevated blood pressure should be aggressively treated with beta-blockers, given the risk of arterial dissection.

DISPOSITION

Prognosis varies according to type of EDS. For vascular EDS:

- 25% will have a complication by age 25 yr; >80% will have a complication by age 40 yr.
- Most vascular complications consist of arterial dissections.
- Vascular events typically occur between the third and fifth decade.
- Median age of survival is 48 years. Most deaths are related to arterial rupture.

REFERRAL

Referral to dermatology for skin biopsy to confirm diagnosis of vascular EDS and to cardiology, orthopedic surgery, general surgery, and physical therapy as needed.

PEARLS & CONSIDERATIONS

- Women with vascular EDS should be counseled about the risk of uterine, intestinal, and arterial rupture.
  ○ Pregnancy is associated with up to a 25% mortality rate; however, successful childbirth is possible.
  ○ There is a 50% chance that the child will be affected.
- Family members of patients with EDS should be recommended for evaluation for EDS and genetic testing/counseling.

SUGGESTED READINGS
available at www.expertconsult.com

RELATED CONTENT
Ehlers-Danlos Syndrome (Patient Information)

AUTHORS: **AHMAD ISMAIL, M.D.**, and **IRIS TONG, M.D.**

E

Diseases and Disorders

I

BASIC INFORMATION

DEFINITION

Human monocytic ehrlichiosis (HME) and human granulocytic anaplasmosis (HGA) are tick-borne rickettsial diseases. HGA was formerly known as human granulocytic ehrlichiosis (HGE). Table 1-140 describes the agent, vector, and geographic prevalence of these diseases.

SYNONYMS

Human granulocytic ehrlichiosis (HGE)
Ehrlichiosis
Human monocytic ehrlichiosis (HME)
Human granulocytic anaplasmosis (HGA)
Anaplasmosis
Ehrlichia phagocytophila
Anaplasma phagocytophilum

ICD-9CM CODES

082.8 Other tick-borne rickettsiosis

EPIDEMIOLOGY & DEMOGRAPHICS

INCIDENCE (IN U.S.): Highest overall incidence in Rhode Island (36.5 per 1 million), New York, New Jersey, Connecticut, Wisconsin, Minnesota, and northern California; >3000 cases identified in the United States since 2006.
PREDOMINANT SEX: Males outnumber females by 2 to 1.
PREDOMINANT AGE: Most severe disease 50 to 70 yr
PEAK INCIDENCE: Occurs throughout the year, with peak incidence between May and July and again in November.

PHYSICAL FINDINGS & CLINICAL PRESENTATION

- Most common initial symptoms
  1. Fever
  2. Chills, rigor
  3. Headache
  4. Myalgia
- Subsequent symptoms
  1. Anorexia, nausea
  2. Arthralgia
  3. Cough
  4. Confusion (meningoencephalitis in 20% of patients with HME)
  5. Abdominal pain
  6. Rash (erythematous to pustular) <30% in HME, uncommon in HGA
- Complications
  1. Hepatitis
  2. Interstitial pneumonitis; acute respiratory distress syndrome
  3. Renal and respiratory failure
  4. Demyelinating polyneuropathy
  5. Toxic shock–like syndrome
  6. Life-threatening opportunistic infections

ETIOLOGY

- The causative agents are *Ehrlichia chaffeensis* and *Anaplasma phagocytophilum*
- Vector
  1. Almost certainly tick-borne, recently confirmed to be rarely transmitted by infected blood (including nosocomial infection).
  2. Transmitted by *Ixodes scapularis* in the northeastern states and *Amblyomma americanum* in the south central, southeastern, and mid-Atlantic states.
  3. Tick exposure reported in >90% of patients, with ~60% reporting tick bite.
- Mammalian host: deer, horses, dogs, white-footed mice, cattle, sheep, goats, bison
- Host inflammatory and immune responses define final spectrum of disease beyond granulocytes, including hepatitis, interstitial pneumonitis, and nephritis with mild azotemia
- Between 6% and 21% of patients with HGE also have serologic evidence of other *Ixodes* spp. tick-borne diseases: Lyme disease or babesiosis
- Recovery is usual outcome; fatality rate of HGE is <1%
- ICU care required: 7%

DIAGNOSIS

DIFFERENTIAL DIAGNOSIS

- Rocky Mountain spotted fever, Colorado tick fever, Q fever, relapsing fever
- Babesiosis
- Leptospirosis
- Lyme disease
- Tularemia
- Typhoid fever, paratyphoid fever
- Brucellosis
- Viral hepatitis
- Meningococcemia
- Infectious mononucleosis
- Hematologic malignancy

WORKUP

- Acute blood samples for Giemsa-stained smears
- CBC (leukopenia, thrombocytopenia), liver function (elevated), BUN/creatinine
- Acute serum samples for serology . Antibodies are seldom detected at time of acute infection (they usually appear 2-4 weeks following clinical illness).
- Chest radiograph examination
- Bone marrow rarely needed

LABORATORY TESTS

- Polymerase chain reaction (PCR) to facilitate early diagnosis: detection of *Ehrlichia* DNA in blood or CSF by PCR
- Giemsa-stained smear demonstrating morulae of the organism within granulocytes (sensitivity 20% to 75%) (Fig. 1-303)
- CBC: progressive leukopenia and thrombocytopenia with nadir near day 7
- C-reactive protein concentration is generally elevated
- Liver function tests (LFTs): increase in hepatic transaminases, lactate dehydrogenase, and alkaline phosphatase
- Elevated plasma creatinine concentration may be seen
- Serologic titer (IFA) >80 or fourfold increase in titer to *E. equi* antigen
- Culture on the first 7 days of illness; not readily available in most clinical laboratories

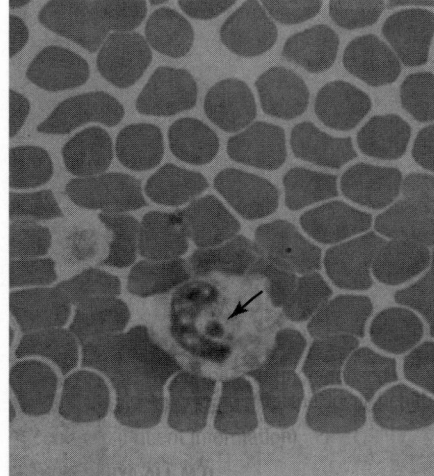

FIGURE 1-303 White blood cells infected with the agent of human granulacytic ehrlichiosis (*Anaplasma phagocytophilum*). (Courtesy Dr. Daniel Caplivski, Division of Infectious Diseases, Mount Sinai School of Medicine.)

TABLE 1-140 Ehrlichioses and Anaplasmoses

Disease	Agent	Vector	Geographic Repartition
American monocytic ehrlichiosis	*Ehrlichia chaffeensis*	*Amblyomma americanum*	South central, southeastern, mid-Atlantic coastal states
Human granulocytic ehrlichiosis	*Anaplasma phagocytophilum*	*Ixodes ricinus*	Europe, China
		Ixodes scapularis	Northeast, upper Midwest, northern California
E. ewingii	*Ehrlichia ewingii*	*Amblyomma americanum*	South central, southeastern, mid-Atlantic coastal states
Japanese monocytic ehrlichiosis	*Neorickettsia sennetsu*	Helminth of the gray mullet?	Japan
E. canis	*Ehrlichia canis*	*Rhipicephalus sanguineus*	Venezuela

From Goldman L, Schafer AI: *Goldman's Cecil medicine*, ed 24, Philadelphia, 2012, Saunders.

IMAGING STUDIES

- Chest radiograph examination to show interstitial pneumonitis (unusual)
- MRI of the brain

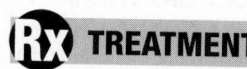 **TREATMENT**

ACUTE GENERAL Rx

- Immediate therapy to limit extent of acute illness and complication
- Doxycycline: 100 mg twice a day for 7 to 14 days is therapy of choice for adults and children >8 yr (4 mg/kg/day in 2 divided doses).
- Rifampin: 300 mg twice a day for 7 to 10 days can be used in pregnancy and for children <8 yr at 10 mg/kg twice per day
- Most patients defervesce within 24 to 48 hr given appropriate treatment.

PROGNOSIS

Poor prognostic indicators include:
- Advanced age
- Concomitant chronic illness (such as diabetes mellitus, collagen-vascular disease)
- Lack of diagnosis recognition
- Delayed onset of specific antibiotic therapy
- Concomitant HIV or organ transplant status

DISPOSITION

- Repeat CBC every 2 to 4 wk until normal.
- A new pathogenic *Ehrlichia* species, close relative of *E. muris* has been identified in Minnesota and Wisconsin. Organism-specific PCR and serologic testing can be used for identification.

REFERRAL

For consultation with infectious diseases specialist in suspected cases

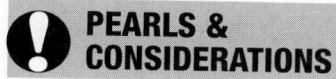 **PEARLS & CONSIDERATIONS**

COMMENTS

- Duration of time tick must be attached to produce illness as few as 4 hr
- Delay in antibiotic treatment results in poorer outcome. Antibiotic treatment should be initiated as soon as infection is suspected.

SUGGESTED READINGS

available at www.expertconsult.com

RELATED CONTENT

Anaplasmosis (Patient Information)

AUTHOR: **PATRICIA CRISTOFARO, M.D.**

E

Diseases and Disorders

I

BASIC INFORMATION

DEFINITION

Clinically significant disorders of ejaculation include failure of emission, retrograde ejaculation, premature ejaculation, delayed ejaculation, painful ejaculation, hematospermia, and anorgasmia. Failure of emission occurs when semen is not propulsed into the urethra during orgasm, resulting in a dry ejaculate. Retrograde ejaculation is a backward flow of semen into the bladder. Premature ejaculation exists when there is an inability to delay ejaculation such that ejaculation occurs sooner than desired, either before or shortly after penetration, causing distress to either one or both partners. Hematospermia is the appearance of blood in the ejaculate. Anorgasmia is the inability to achieve orgasm in a timely manner.

SYNONYMS

Ejaculatory dysfunction
Retarded or delayed ejaculation
Early or rapid ejaculation
Inhibited ejaculation
Anejaculation

ICD-9CM CODES
608.82 Hematospermia
608.87 Ejaculation, retrograde
608.89 Painful ejaculation
306.59 Ejaculation, psychogenic
302.75 Ejaculation, premature
302.74 Orgasm inhibited male (psychosexual)

EPIDEMIOLOGY & DEMOGRAPHICS

Men with ejaculatory dysfunction of any type usually indicate higher levels of relationship stress, sexual dissatisfaction, anxiety about sexual performance, and general health issues, compared to sexually functional men. Premature ejaculation is the most prevalent male sexual complaint, affecting 20% to 30% of men and may be primary (lifelong) or acquired. Retarded or delayed ejaculation is the least common, least studied, and least understood of the male sexual dysfunctions.

CLINICAL PRESENTATION

- Failure of emission: no ejaculate is produced during orgasm. Physical findings may reveal nervous system dysfunction (e.g., spinal cord injury); may present with infertility (e.g., ejaculatory duct obstruction).
- Retrograde ejaculation: little or no ejaculate is expelled out of the urethra at orgasm. Patients may report cloudy postcoital urine. Physical examination is usually normal; may present with infertility.
- Premature ejaculation: ejaculation occurs sooner than desired, either before or shortly after penetration. Physical examination is normal. Sexual and psychological history may be revealing. Up to 30% of patients may report concomitant erectile dysfunction.
- Painful ejaculation: perineal, scrotal, or testicular pain during or shortly after ejaculation.

Physical examination may demonstrate pain on examination of external genitalia, or with digital rectal examination; may present with infertility.
- Hematospermia: reddish-brown ejaculate, usually painless. Physical findings usually unremarkable; not associated with malignancy.
- Anorgasmia: patient is not able to achieve orgasm despite appropriate stimulation.

ETIOLOGY

- Retrograde ejaculation may be caused by anatomic abnormalities of the bladder neck, or nerve injury affecting the bladder neck sphincter.
- Either retrograde ejaculation or failure of emission may result from functional abnormalities, such as spinal cord injury, diabetes mellitus, retroperitoneal surgery, transurethral prostate surgery, urethral strictures, alpha-blocker therapy, antipsychotics, multiple sclerosis, and peripheral neuropathy.
- The etiology of premature ejaculation is complex and multifactorial, and includes genetic, behavioral, and psychologic contributions.
- Causes of painful ejaculation may be infectious (e.g., epididymo-orchitis, urethritis, prostatitis), obstructive (e.g., vasectomy, prostatectomy, hernia repair), or psychologic.
- Hematospermia may be idiopathic, secondary to prolonged abstinence, or due to infection or inflammation of the genitourinary tract.
- Anorgasmia may be caused by spinal cord injury, psychologic factors, dysfunctional sexual techniques, or medications, particularly serotonin re-uptake inhibitors.

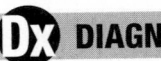 **DIAGNOSIS**

DIFFERENTIAL DIAGNOSIS

- Erectile dysfunction
- Low seminal fluid volume attributable to hypogonadism or ejaculatory duct obstruction
  - Inflammatory disorders of the genitourinary tract
  - Hypoactive sexual desire

LABORATORY TESTS

- In the setting of a dry or low-volume ejaculate, post-ejaculate urine should be evaluated for the presence of spermatozoa, in order to differentiate failure of emission from retrograde ejaculation.
- Hematuria, in the setting of hematospermia or painful ejaculation, may signal an underlying inflammatory disorder or a malignancy and should prompt a complete evaluation.
- A fasting blood glucose may be considered if diabetes is suspected as a cause of lack of emission or retrograde ejaculation.
- Urinalysis, urine culture, and screening for sexually transmitted diseases, when indicated, can rule out an infectious etiology of painful ejaculation.

IMAGING STUDIES

Transrectal ultrasonography can rule out ejaculatory duct obstruction or absence of the seminal vesicles.

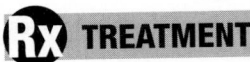 **TREATMENT**

NONPHARMACOLOGIC THERAPY

- Retrograde ejaculation and failure of emission do not require treatment unless fertility is desired.
- In the setting of retrograde ejaculation, viable sperm can be recovered from the post-ejaculate urine and used for intrauterine insemination or in vitro fertilization.
- Premature ejaculation can improve with psychotherapy and behavioral interventions (e.g., "coronal squeeze" or "start-and-stop" technique) and effective partner communication. These approaches may be more effective when combined with pharmacologic therapy.
- Idiopathic hematospermia may be followed expectantly and is usually self-limited to 10 to 15 ejaculations.
- Anorgasmia caused by serotonin reuptake inhibitors usually improves with withdrawal of the medication. Sexual therapy and counseling can improve anorgasmia caused by dysfunctional sexual techniques or psychologic issues. Vibratory or electrical stimulation of emission is helpful in selected cases.

ACUTE GENERAL Rx

- Retrograde ejaculation: pharmacologic therapy is only effective in patients without an anatomic disturbance of the bladder neck. Sympathomimetic medications (phenylpropanolamine, ephedrine, pseudoephedrine) and imipramine may be useful in converting retrograde ejaculation to antegrade ejaculation.
- Failure of emission: may be converted to retrograde ejaculation by oral sympathomimetic therapy, as listed above.
- Premature ejaculation: selective serotonin reuptake inhibitors (SSRI) (sertraline, fluoxetine) and the tricyclic antidepressant clomipramine can successfully delay ejaculation when taken daily. Recent research has focused on dapoxetine, a short-acting SSRI, which has shown promise as an "on-demand" treatment for premature ejaculation. Topical anesthetics such as lidocaine cream and topical sprays have also been used, with variable success. The use of phosphodiesterase inhibitors (PDE5i) (sildenafil, vardenafil, tadalafil) with SSRIs may be beneficial in men with concomitant erectile dysfunction and premature ejaculation.
- Antimicrobial treatment (if indicated), NSAIDs, and muscle relaxants may help decrease discomfort associated with painful ejaculation.
- The use of the pharmacologic therapies listed above for the treatment of various disorders of ejaculation is strictly off label and does not carry FDA approval.

SURGICAL THERAPY

There is no role for surgery for the majority of ejaculatory disorders. Rarely, painful ejaculation due to obstructive causes may show improvement with surgical intervention (e.g., vasectomy reversal).

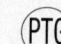
DISPOSITION

Prognosis varies with etiology. Ejaculatory dysfunction attributable to sexual techniques or psychologic issues can improve with psychotherapy. Pharmacologic treatment is helpful in treating premature, retrograde, or painful ejaculation.

REFERRAL

All fertility issues and suspected anatomic problems should be referred to a urologist. Professional psychotherapy should be considered for appropriate patients.

SUGGESTED READINGS

available at www.expertconsult.com

RELATED CONTENT

Erectile Dysfunction (Related Key Topic)
Erectile Dysfunction (Patient Information)

AUTHORS: **AKANKSHA MEHTA, M.D.,**
and **MARK SIGMAN, M.D.**

E

Diseases
and Disorders

I

BASIC INFORMATION

DEFINITION

Premature ejaculation is a persistent or recurrent problem in which a male experiences orgasm or ejaculation in the early phases of sexual contact and before he and his partner wish it. Other definitions have emphasized elapsed time after intromission (with durations of 30 sec to several min), number of thrusts, or rate of partner satisfaction. However, no absolute measure is applicable to the diverse numbers of men with this problem.

SYNONYMS

Rapid ejaculation
Early ejaculation
Inadequate ejaculatory control

ICD-9CM CODES
F52.4 Premature ejaculation

DSM-IV CODES
302.75 Premature ejaculation

EPIDEMIOLOGY & DEMOGRAPHICS

PEAK INCIDENCE: Adolescence and young adulthood
PREVALENCE (IN U.S.):
- 7% to 40% of adult men, most with no underlying physical condition
- Often present more or less since start of sexual life
- Most prevalent sexual disorder in men; more common than low libido and erectile dysfunction

PREDOMINANT AGE: None defined
GENETICS: No identifiable genetic factors

PHYSICAL FINDINGS & CLINICAL PRESENTATION

- Complaint of ejaculation before, upon, or shortly after penetration
- Frequently associated with anxiety either specific to sexual activity or more generalized anxiety disorder
- Premature ejaculation caused by a medical condition frequently associated with low desire and/or erectile insufficiency

ETIOLOGY

- Increasingly believed to be a neurobiologic phenomenon particularly related to serotonergic pathway
- Different theoretical frameworks emphasize anxiety related to performance or personal interactions, behavioral concepts of learned expectations related to early experience, or heightened penile sensitivity

- Organic factors are contributory in some individuals (e.g., abdominal or pelvic trauma or surgery, neuropathies, or urologic pathology such as prostatic urethritis)
- Biologic causes include penile hypersensitivity, hyperexcitable ejaculatory reflex, increased sexual arousability, possible endocrinopathy, a genetic predisposition, and central 5-hydroxytryptamine receptor dysfunction

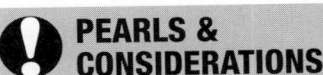 **DIAGNOSIS**

DIFFERENTIAL DIAGNOSIS

- In young adolescents, premature ejaculation may be normally experienced as a consequence of heightened excitation.
- Distinguish comorbid erectile dysfunction, which may influence management.

WORKUP

- History with a specific emphasis on sexual activities and beliefs
- Factors to be assessed include patient's subjective evaluation, degree of sexual satisfaction, sense of control, and personal or interpersonal distress related to ejaculation
- Collateral information from sexual partner when possible
- Additional history regarding surgery, trauma, and neurologic symptoms
- History of prescribed and recreational drugs (e.g., antidepressants, alcohol, opiates)

LABORATORY TESTS

Urinalysis and urine culture after prostatic massage to rule out prostatic infection

IMAGING STUDIES

None routinely indicated

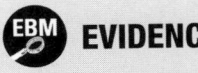 **TREATMENT**

NONPHARMACOLOGIC THERAPY

- Behavioral and psychotherapeutic interventions: strongly guided by a specific theoretical framework; inadequate data to suggest the superiority of any particular approach.
- Use of condoms may reduce penile sensitivity, prolonging erection.
- Use of Masters and Johnson's "pause-squeeze" technique (in which 4 sec of moderate pressure is applied to the frenulum to reduce ejaculatory urge) or "stop-start" technique may be helpful for some patients.

ACUTE GENERAL Rx

- Topical anesthetic, such as lidocaine-prilocaine cream and topical eutectic mixture for PE (TEMPE) aerosol spray (not available in the U.S.), increases ejaculatory latency if

applied <20 min before intercourse. Side effects include mild discomfort and burning for some patients. Use with condom to avoid numbness for partner.
- Daily selective serotonin reuptake inhibitors (SSRIs), such as paroxetine (most potent) or sertraline, delay ejaculation. May take several weeks for response to occur. Clomipramine (tricyclic antidepressant) has also been found to delay ejaculation. Discontinuation of daily SSRIs often leads to recurrence of premature ejaculation. Dapoxetine is a short-acting, on-demand agent that delays ejaculation (available in Europe but not available in the U.S.).
- Sildenafil or vardenafil may be useful in delaying ejaculation, especially in premature ejaculation with comorbid erectile dysfunction.

DISPOSITION

There is gradual improvement with age, but it is frequently a chronic, lifelong problem with few spontaneous remissions.

REFERRAL

Behavioral sex therapy or psychotherapy may be helpful; if recurrent prostate infection, referral to urology is indicated.

PEARLS & CONSIDERATIONS

Various psychological risk factors are cited for premature ejaculation, including lack of sexual experience, infrequent sexual intercourse, fear, anxiety, social phobia, relationship problems, and a lack of sexual education.

Treatment should emphasize partner communication, behavioral technique, and topical anesthetics/condoms as first-line treatment. If these treatments are ineffective and PE is causing significant distress, consider SSRIs and PDE5 inhibitors.

EBM EVIDENCE

available at www.expertconsult.com

SUGGESTED READINGS
available at www.expertconsult.com

RELATED CONTENT
Premature Ejaculation (Patient Information)

AUTHOR: **NICOLE APPELLE, M.D, M.P.H.**

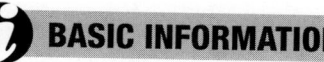 BASIC INFORMATION

DEFINITION

Injuries or wounds that occur as a result of contact with an electrical current.

ICD-9CM CODES
994.8 Electrical shock, nonfatal

EPIDEMIOLOGY & DEMOGRAPHICS

- Causes approximately 1000 deaths annually, with two thirds occurring in persons between ages 15 and 40 yr.
- Most electrical injuries in children occur at home (e.g., oral burns from electrical appliances).
- Most electrical injuries in adults are occupationally related. It ranks fifth as a cause of occupational death.
- Accounts for 4% to 6.5% of all admissions to burn units.
- Lightning strikes kill on average 100 people annually.
  - Eight of every 10 lightning strike victims are male; 75% of lightning deaths in the U.S. occur in the South and Midwest.
  - 25% of lightning deaths are work related.
- Electronic weapons (stun gun and Taser) are capable of causing fatal cardiac arrhythmias.

PHYSICAL FINDINGS & CLINICAL PRESENTATION

- Cognitive changes: depending on the extent of injury, the patient may be unconscious, seizing, or confused and unable to present a history
- Extensive skin burns (>10% of the body surface)
  1. Located over the entry and exit sites (Fig. 1-304)
  2. Most common entry sites are the hands and skull
  3. Most common exit sites are the heels
  4. "Kissing burns" over the flexor creases
  5. Oral burns are common in children; bleeding from the labial artery may present 7 to 10 days after the injury
  6. Charring at the contact site (Fig. 1-305)
- Asystole or ventricular fibrillation may be the initial cardiac rhythm
- Bone fractures and periosteal burns
- Compartment syndrome from severe muscle tissue damage
- Headaches, memory disturbances
- Weakness and paresthesias
- Otologic injury, conductive hearing loss from tympanic membrane rupture or ossicular disruption
- Rhabdomyolysis and myoglobin-induced acute tubular necrosis
- Vascular injury from coagulation of small vessels or compartment syndrome

ETIOLOGY

- Electricity causes tissue injury by converting electrical energy into heat or by blunt trauma

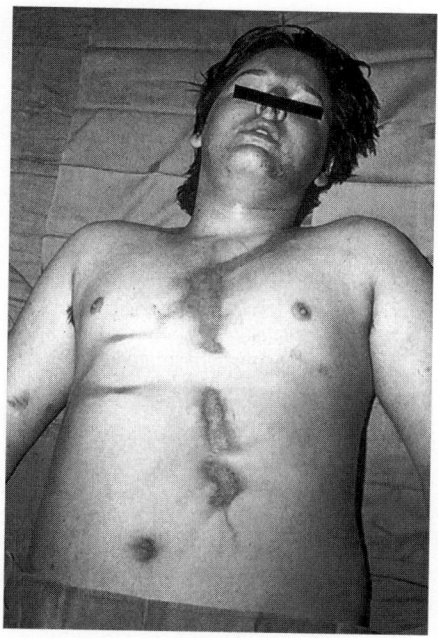

FIGURE 1-304 The arborescent current markings on the face, neck, and anterior trunk of this young patient, which are characteristic of lightning injury, healed without the need for grafting. Note the focal lesions on the right arm, indicating the spread of the current that produced the marks on the right anterolateral aspect of the chest wall. (From Goldman L, Schafer AI: *Goldman's Cecil medicine,* ed 24, Philadelphia, 2012, Saunders.)

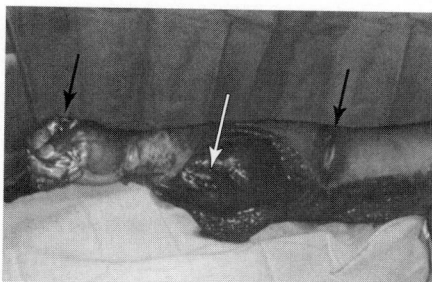

FIGURE 1-305 Charring at the contact site in the first web space and at the site of arcing in the antecubital space *(black arrows)* of a victim of electric injury. The fixed flexion deformity of the thumb and other digits is characteristic of severe high-voltage injury to the hand and forearm. The severity of the injury is indicated by the marked edema of the forearm muscles, bulging above the cut edges of the fasciotomy incision, and by the patchy dark discoloration of the muscles of the arm and the forearm, particularly the deeper muscle exposed in the central portion of the forearm incision *(white arrow).* (From Goldman L, Schafer AI: *Goldman's Cecil medicine,* ed 24, Philadelphia, 2012, Saunders.)

from being thrown from the electrical source or from continuous muscle contraction (tetany).
- The effects of electricity are determined by seven factors: type of current, amount of current, pathway of current, duration, area of contact, resistance of the body, and voltage.

- Tissue damage is greater with higher voltage and longer duration of contact.
- Direct current (DC) contact causes a single muscle contraction, throwing the patient away from the source. Alternating current (AC) contact precipitates a tetanic contraction, not allowing the patient to withdraw from the source and prolonging the duration of contact. AC contact is more ominous than DC contact.
- Electrical injuries are arbitrarily divided into high-voltage (>1000 volts) and low-voltage (<1000 volts) burns. Low-voltage burns involve almost exclusively either the hands or oral cavity. High-voltage injuries have a wide variety of systemic manifestations.
- The entry and exit path of the electrical current determines which tissues are affected.

Dx DIAGNOSIS

WORKUP

Physical examination may not reveal the extent of damage that has occurred. Detailed testing to determine the extent of internal organ damage is indicated. In lightning injuries, male victims may have scrotal (on the undersurface of the scrotum) and penile burns, which may often be overlooked. Hemorrhage behind the eardrum with or without perforation is not uncommon. An otoscopic examination is indicated in all lightning strike victims.

LABORATORY TESTS

- Complete blood count
- Blood chemistry profile including electrolytes
- Blood urea nitrogen and creatinine
- Arterial blood gas analysis
- Myoglobin
- Creatinine kinase with isoenzyme fractionation
- Urinalysis, including screening for myoglobinuria
- Liver function tests
- Type and cross-match
- ECG

IMAGING STUDIES

- Radiographs: any suspicious area for bone fractures
- CT scan of the head and cervical spine in patients with suspected head injury, coma, or neurologic deficit

Rx TREATMENT

NONPHARMACOLOGIC THERAPY

- At the scene: ensure the electrical power source of injury is turned off before approaching patients.
- Basic and advanced cardiac life support with cervical spine precautions. Prolonged cardiopulmonary resuscitation should be undertaken regardless of the initial cardiac rhythm.
- Cardiac monitoring.
- Oxygen.
- Tetanus prophylaxis.

ACUTE GENERAL Rx

- IV fluids to maintain urine output of 50 to 100 ml/hr (IV hydration should be reassessed with central nervous system expert in patients at risk of developing cerebral edema).
- Alkalinization of the urine (sodium bicarbonate 50 mEq in 1 L of normal saline) in patients with or at risk of myoglobinuria.
- Furosemide 20 to 40 mg PO or IV and/or mannitol 12.5 g/kg/hr may be used to force diuresis.
- Seizures are treated in the standard fashion.
- Treat burns with sulfadiazine silver dressings.

CHRONIC Rx

- Hospitalization is indicated in patients with high-voltage injuries, extensive burns, central nervous system symptoms, myonecrosis (creatine kinase level more than twice normal, high serum myoglobin levels, or myoglobinuria), new cardiac arrhythmia or ECG changes, or any internal organ damage.
- Ophthalmology consultation at the follow-up to screen for cataract formation (occurs within 1 to 24 mo of a high-voltage electrical injury in 5% to 20% of patients).

DISPOSITION

- Patients with severe burns should be transferred to the regional burn center.
- Complications of electrical injuries include:
  1. Infection
  2. Renal failure from rhabdomyolysis
  3. Seizure disorder
  4. Fasciotomies
  5. Amputation
- Delayed neurologic damage may present as ascending paralysis, amyotrophic lateral sclerosis, or transverse myelitis weeks to years after the injury.
- Vascular damage may also present in a delayed fashion.

REFERRAL

- Referrals to general surgery, burn surgery, trauma surgery, orthopedic surgery, and/or critical care specialists as appropriate in any patient that meets hospitalization criteria. Ophthalmology and ear-nose-throat specialist referral may be indicated.
- Plastic surgery is recommended in children with oral burns.

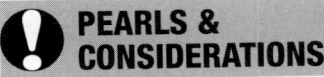

PEARLS & CONSIDERATIONS

COMMENTS

- The size of external skin burns can often underestimate the degree of internal injury.
- Lightning Strike and Electric Shock Survivors International is a support group that serves people from around the world who have sustained an electric injury (http://www.lightning-strike.org).
- Home safety education provided one to one in a clinical setting or at home, especially with the provision of safety equipment, is effective in increasing the range of safety practices.

SUGGESTED READINGS

available at www.expertconsult.com

RELATED CONTENT

Electrical Injury (Patient Information)

AUTHORS: **ROBERT M. KIRCHNER, M.D.,** and **PAUL GORDON, M.D.**

BASIC INFORMATION

DEFINITION

Emergency contraception (EC) can prevent pregnancy soon after unprotected intercourse, sexual assault, or failure or improper use of a birth control method. EC reduces the risk of pregnancy when used up to 120 hr (5 days) after unprotected sex but is more effective if used earlier.

MECHANISM: The primary mechanism of all EC pills is inhibition or delay of ovulation. Emergency insertion of the copper IUD may prevent fertilization or implantation.

EFFECTIVENESS: Levonorgestrel prevents an estimated 89% of unexpected pregnancies after unprotected intercourse. Ulipristal acetate is as effective as, if not more effective than, levonorgestrel up to 72 hr after unprotected sex and more effective than levonorgestrel from 72 to 120 hr. Combined hormonal EC prevents 74% and the copper IUD prevents 99% of unexpected pregnancies. EC pills may be less effective in obese women. Addition of a COX-2 inhibitor (meloxicam 15 mg) to levonorgestrel EC may increase its efficacy.

SYNONYMS

Morning-after pill, postcoital contraception

ICD-9CM CODES
V25.03 Emergency contraceptive counseling and treatment
V25.09 Family planning

EPIDEMIOLOGY & DEMOGRAPHICS

Approximately 49% of all pregnancies and more than 82% of teen pregnancies in the U.S. are unintended. An estimated 1.7 million unintended pregnancies could be prevented annually if EC use were widespread.

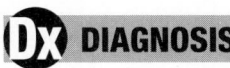 **DIAGNOSIS**

LABORATORY TESTS

- If there is doubt about whether a patient is already pregnant from intercourse that occurred more than 2 wk previously, a pregnancy test may be helpful. However, there is no need for a pregnancy test before administering EC pills. Delays in administration of the medication will reduce its efficacy. The medication in EC pills will not harm an established pregnancy.
- A pregnancy test should be done before insertion of a copper IUD.

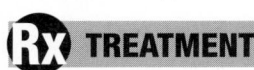 **TREATMENT**

ACUTE GENERAL Rx

- Administer EC as soon as possible after unprotected intercourse. All forms of EC reduce the risk of pregnancy when used up to 120 hr (5 days) after unprotected intercourse but are more effective if used earlier.

- Emergency contraceptive pills (see Table 1-141)
  1. Levonorgestrel (Next Choice, Plan B One-Step)
     - Total dose 1.5 mg levonorgestrel
     - A single dose is equally effective and causes no more side effects than two divided doses.
     - Indicated for use up to 72 hr after unprotected intercourse, although research supports efficacy up to 120 hr.
     - Available "behind the counter" without a prescription if age ≥17. Some Medicaid plans cover generic forms with a prescription.
  2. Ulipristal acetate (Ella)
     - Single dose 30 mg ulipristal acetate, a progesterone-receptor modulator
     - Indicated for use up to 120 hr after unprotected intercourse.
     - More expensive than levonorgestrel EC. Prescription is required.
  3. Combined estrogen/progestin contraceptive pills:
     - Two doses, 12 hr apart, of 100 to 120 mcg ethinyl estradiol and 0.5 to 0.6 mg levonorgestrel (or 1.0 to 1.2 mg norgestrel) per dose.
     - See Table 1-141 for dosing.
     - Prescription is required.
- Side effects:
  - Combined estrogen-progestin EC will cause nausea in 50% of women and vomiting in 20%. Levonorgestrel and ulipristal are associated with a much lower incidence of side effects. Side effects resolve within 1 to 2 days. Anti-nausea medication such as meclizine 25 mg orally is recommended 1 hr before taking combined estrogen-progestin EC.
- Contraindications:
  - Few contraindications to EC exist other than hypersensitivity to the product. EC pills will not affect an established pregnancy.
  - There are no other evidence-based medical contraindications to the use of EC pills. The benefits of EC in preventing pregnancy generally outweigh the theoretical risks for women with contraindications to long-term use of combined hormonal contraception, such as thromboembolic

TABLE 1-141   Emergency Contraceptive Pills Available in the United States

EMERGENCY CONTRACEPTION PILLS		
Brand	**Dose**	**Dose**
Next Choice[1]	2 pills	1.5 mg levonorgestrel
Plan B One-Step	1 pill	1.5 mg levonorgestrel
Ella	1 pill	30 mg ulipristal acetate

COMBINED ORAL CONTRACEPTIVE PILLS FOR EMERGENCY CONTRACEPTION[2]				
Brand	**First Dose**	**Second Dose (12 hours later)**	**Ethinyl Estradiol per Dose (mcg)**	**Levonorgestrel per Dose (mg)**
Aviane	5 orange pills	5 orange pills	100	0.50
Cryselle	4 white pills	4 white pills	120	0.60
Enpresse	4 orange pills	4 orange pills	120	0.50
Jolessa	4 pink pills	4 pink pills	120	0.60
Lessina	5 pink pills	5 pink pills	100	0.50
Levora	4 white pills	4 white pills	120	0.60
Lo/Ovral	4 white pills	4 white pills	120	0.60
LoSeasonique	5 orange pills	5 orange pills	100	0.50
Low-Ogestrel	4 white pills	4 white pills	120	0.60
Lutera	5 white pills	5 white pills	100	0.50
Lybrel	6 yellow pills	6 yellow pills	120	0.54
Nordette	4 light-orange pills	4 light-orange pills	120	0.60
Ogestrel	2 white pills	2 white pills	100	0.50
Portia	4 pink pills	4 pink pills	120	0.60
Quasense	4 white pills	4 white pills	120	0.60
Seasonale	4 pink pills	4 pink pills	120	0.60
Seasonique	4 light-blue-green pills	4 light-blue-green pills	120	0.60
Sronyx	5 white pills	5 white pills	100	0.50
Trivora	4 pink pills	4 pink pills	120	0.50

[1]Package instructions for Plan B and Next Choice recommend 1 pill per dose, 12 hours apart, but research shows similar efficacy and side effects with taking both pills at the same time.
[2]For combined oral contraceptive pills as emergency contraception, take two doses, 12 hours apart. The FDA has declared these products safe for use as emergency contraception.

disease, smoking after age 35, heart disease, or liver disease. Levonorgestrel or ulipristal EC may be preferable to estrogen containing EC for women with any of these conditions or who are breastfeeding. EC is not indicated for breastfeeding women <6 weeks postpartum as ovulation is extremely unlikely.

- Copper IUD for EC
  - ○ Emergency insertion of the copper IUD is the most effective option for EC and can be used up to 5 days after unprotected intercourse.
  - ○ This option may be preferable for women who desire effective long-term contraception and have no contraindications to IUD insertion.
  - ○ A pregnancy test should be done before IUD insertion.

CHRONIC Rx

Because EC pills are less effective than other forms of contraception, they are not recommended as an ongoing method of contraception. The copper IUD is highly effective for EC and can be kept in place to prevent pregnancy for 10 yr.

DISPOSITION

After using EC, most women will have their menses within 3 days of the expected onset date. If a woman's next expected menses are delayed by more than 1 wk, a pregnancy test should be done.

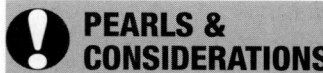

PEARLS & CONSIDERATIONS

COMMENTS

- All forms of EC reduce the risk of pregnancy up to 120 hr (5 days) after unprotected intercourse.
- A pregnancy test is not necessary before administering EC pills because the medicines will not harm an existing pregnancy.
- Advanced prescription of EC pills at routine visits may increase timely use of EC and does not decrease the use of more reliable means of contraception.
- Men and women ≥17 can purchase levonorgestrel EC (Next Choice, Plan B One-Step) without a prescription.
- Copper IUD is the most effective form of EC and is the only method that provides users with long-term contraception.

PREVENTION

- Patients should begin an effective method of birth control immediately after using EC. Hormonal contraceptives can be started the day after EC is administered. A backup method should be used for 7 days.
- EC should be offered to all women after sexual assault.

PATIENT & FAMILY EDUCATION

- EC website: http://www.not-2-late.com

SUGGESTED READINGS

available at www.expertconsult.com

RELATED CONTENT

Fig. E1-240 Helping couples select a contraceptive method (Algorithm)
Fig. E1-241 Contraceptive use (Algorithm)

AUTHORS: **MELISSA NOTHNAGLE, M.D., M.SC.,** and **JENNIFER BUCKLEY, M.D.**

BASIC INFORMATION

DEFINITION
An accumulation of pus in the pleural space, most often caused by bacterial infection.

SYNONYMS
Infected pleuritis
Infected pleural effusion
Purulent pleural effusion

ICD-9CM CODES
510.9 Empyema, lung

EPIDEMIOLOGY & DEMOGRAPHICS
- Empyema is most commonly a complication of bacterial pneumonia, especially in association with pneumococcal or anaerobic infection (40% to 60% of cases of empyema)
- Occur as a complication of thoracic surgery (<20% of cases)
- Penetrating chest trauma (4% to 10% of cases)
- Bronchopleural fistulae resulting from malignancy or lung biopsy

PHYSICAL FINDINGS & CLINICAL PRESENTATION
- May be abrupt or chronic and insidious depending on the etiologic agent and host factors.
- Typically presents as progressive pleuritic chest pain, persistent fever, and other sustained signs and symptoms of infection.
- In anaerobic empyema, particularly that caused by the actinomycetes, the clinical picture is dominated by systemic symptoms and signs: weight loss, malaise, and low grade fever.
- A slowly enlarging chest wall mass.
- As a complication of thoracic trauma or surgery, empyema typically results from contamination of blood within the pleural space several days following the event.
- The physical findings of empyema are those of pleural effusion. Decreased breath sounds and dullness to percussion over the involved part of the thorax is typical. Systemic signs include fever, tachycardia, leukocytosis, and warmth and erythema over the involved area.

ETIOLOGY
Infection of the lung parenchyma spreading to pleural space caused by
- *Streptococcus pneumoniae*
- *Haemophilus influenzae*
- *Staphylococcus aureus*
- *Legionella* species
- *Mycobacterium tuberculosis*
- *Actinomyces* spp.
- A variety of oral anaerobic bacteria have been cultured in 36% to 37% of empyemas: *Bacteroides fragilis*, *Prevotella* species, *Fusobacterium nucleatum*, and *Peptostreptococcus* are the most common

DIAGNOSIS

DIFFERENTIAL DIAGNOSIS
- Uninfected parapneumonic effusion
- Congestive heart failure
- Malignancy involving the pleura
- Tuberculous pleurisy
- Collagen vascular disease (particularly rheumatoid lung and systemic lupus erythematosus)

LABORATORY TESTS
- Complete blood count; arterial blood gas.
- Blood cultures.
- Pleural fluid analysis in empyema has the characteristics of an exudate with a ratio of pleural fluid to serum protein >0.5 or pleural fluid to serum LDH >0.6. Characteristically, empyema fluid is grossly purulent with visible organisms on Gram stain with glucose <50 mg/dl and pH <7. These findings justify immediate drainage by chest tube or surgery because of the high risk of loculation and progressive systemic infection.

IMAGING STUDIES
- Chest x-ray (Fig. 1-306, *A*)
- Lateral decubitus view to establish the presence of free fluid in the pleural space
- Computed tomography (Fig. 1-306, *B*) to establish the presence of fluid loculation, underlying mass lesions, and other intrathoracic pathology

TREATMENT

NONPHARMACOLOGIC THERAPY
Prompt drainage by thoracostomy (chest tube) or open thoracotomy. Video-assisted thoracoscopic surgery (VATS) has greatly improved surgical management of empyemas.

ACUTE GENERAL Rx
- Maintenance of drainage until infection controlled.
- Antibiotics directed at suspected or proven bacterial or fungal pathogens. Initial regimens include cefotaxime or ceftriaxone for suspected *S. pneumoniae* or group A *Streptococcus*, nafcillin or oxacillin for suspected methicillin-sensitive *S. aureus*, vancomycin or linezolid for suspected MRSA, ceftriaxone for suspected *H. influenzae*, and clindamycin plus ceftriaxone when suspecting anaerobes.
- Thoracoscopy or instillation of thrombolytic agents (streptokinase or urokinase) may be considered in refractory, loculated empyema.

CHRONIC Rx
- If thorough drainage cannot be accomplished, open thoracotomy with pleural decortication may be required.
- Lung function should be monitored following completion of therapy.

DISPOSITION
Hospitalization with supplemental oxygen with ventilatory support if necessary

REFERRAL
Consultation by infectious diseases, pulmonary, or thoracic surgery specialists as needed.

PEARLS & CONSIDERATIONS

COMMENTS
- Empyema caused by actinomycetes may present with erosion through the chest wall and formation of a fistulous tract.
- Nosocomial infection caused by relatively resistant bacterial or fungal pathogens may result in empyema in patients with indwelling thoracostomy tubes.

SUGGESTED READINGS
available at www.expertconsult.com

AUTHOR: **GLENN G. FORT, M.D., M.P.H.**

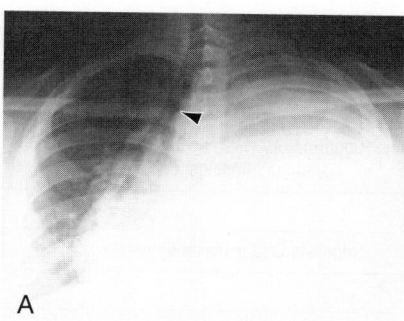
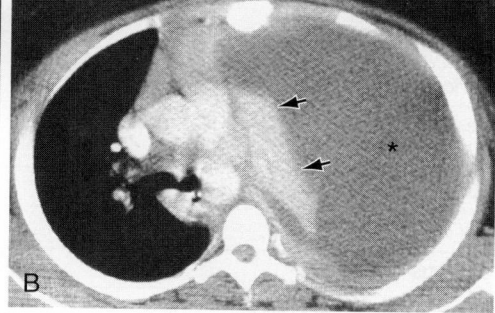

FIGURE 1-306 Empyema and pneumonia in a teenager. A, Chest radiograph shows opacification of the left thorax. Note shift of mediastinum and trachea (arrowhead) to right. **B,** Thoracic CT scan shows massive left pleural effusion *(asterisk)*. Note the compression and atelectasis of the left lung *(arrows)* and shift of the mediastinum to the right. (From Kliegman RM et al: *Nelson textbook of pediatrics*, ed 19, Philadelphia, 2011, Saunders.)

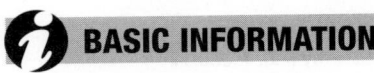

BASIC INFORMATION

DEFINITION

Acute viral encephalitis is an acute febrile syndrome with evidence of meningeal involvement and of derangement of the function of the cerebrum, cerebellum, or brain stem.

SYNONYMS

Arboviral encephalitis
Brain stem encephalitis
Acute necrotizing encephalitis
Rasmussen encephalitis
Encephalitis lethargica

ICD-9CM CODES
049.9 Viral encephalitis, NOS

EPIDEMIOLOGY & DEMOGRAPHICS

INCIDENCE (IN U.S.): About 20,000 cases/yr are reported to the CDC. In 2012 there was an increase in the number of cases of West Nile virus infection in the U.S.
PEAK INCIDENCE: Any age
PREVALENCE (IN U.S.): Unknown
PREDOMINANT SEX: Male = female
PREDOMINANT AGE: Any age
GENETICS: No specific genetic or congenital predisposition

ETIOLOGY

- Can be caused by a host of viruses, with herpes simplex the most common virus identified.
- Arboviruses transmitted by mosquitoes include Eastern equine encephalitis, Western equine encephalitis, St. Louis encephalitis, Venezuelan equine encephalitis, California virus encephalitis, Japanese B encephalitis, Murray Valley and West Nile encephalitis. Tick-borne diseases include Russian spring-summer encephalitis, Powassan encephalitis, and other lesser known agents.
- Also implicated: rabies-causing agents, CMV, Epstein-Barr, varicella-zoster, echo virus, mumps, adenovirus, coxsackie, rubeola, and herpes viruses.
- Meningoencephalitis: acute retroviral infection
- In the U.S., the most commonly identified etiologies are herpes simplex virus, West Nile virus, and the enteroviruses.

PHYSICAL FINDINGS & CLINICAL PRESENTATION

- Initially, fever and evidence of meningeal irritation
- Headache and stiff neck
- Later, development of signs of cortical dysfunction: lethargy, coma, stupor, weakness, seizures, facial weakness, as well as brainstem findings
- Cerebellar findings: ataxia, nystagmus, hypotonia, myoclonus, cranial nerve palsies, and abnormal tendon reflexes
- Patients with rabies: hydrophobia, anxiety, facial numbness, psychosis, coma, or dysarthria
- Rarely, movement disorders, such as chorea, hemiballismus, or dystonia
- Recall of a prodromal viral-like illness (this finding is not at all uniform)

DIAGNOSIS

DIFFERENTIAL DIAGNOSIS

- Bacterial infections: brain abscess, toxic encephalopathies, TB
- Protozoal infections
- Behçet's disease
- Lupus encephalitis
- Sjögren's syndrome
- Multiple sclerosis
- Syphilis
- Cryptococcus
- Toxoplasmosis
- Brucellosis
- Leukemic or lymphomatous meningitis
- Other metastatic tumors
- Lyme disease
- Cat-scratch disease
- Vogt-Koyanagi-Harada syndrome
- Mollaret's meningitis

WORKUP

- Lumbar puncture to reveal pleocytosis, usually lymphocytic, although neutrophils may be seen early on
- Usually, elevated CSF protein
- Normal or low CSF glucose
- In herpes simplex encephalitis: RBCs and xanthochromia
- Selected tests on CSF fluid in viral encephalitis are described in Table 1-142

- EEG changes showing periodic high-voltage sharp waves in the temporal regions and slow wave complexes suggestive of herpes encephalitis (Fig. 1-307).
- CT scan and MRI to reveal edema and hemorrhage in the frontal and temporal lobes
- Temporal lobe involvement suggests herpes simplex encephalitis
- Basal ganglia and thalami are areas involved as generally seen in Eastern equine encephalitis
- With West Nile infection, MRI changes have shown changes in basal ganglia, thalami, mesial temporal structures, brain stem, and cerebellum
- Arboviral infections suspected during outbreaks in specific areas
- Rising titers of neutralizing antibodies from the acute to the convalescent stage demonstrated but often not helpful in the acutely ill patient
- Polymerase chain reaction (PCR) that amplifies DNA from the CSF for herpes simplex encephalitis
- Rarely, brain biopsy to assist in the diagnosis; viral culture of cerebral tissue obtained if biopsy done
- Classic herpetic skin lesions suggestive of herpes encephalitis
- In diagnosing arboviral encephalitis:
  1. Presence of antiviral IgM within the first few days of symptomatic disease; detected and quantified by ELISA
  2. Unusual to recover an arbovirus from the blood or CSF

TABLE 1-142 Selected Tests for Viral Encephalitis

Organism/Syndrome	Test	Comment
West Nile Virus		
West Nile encephalitis	IgM in CSF	Diagnostic of CNS invasive disease or acute flaccid paralysis
Herpes Simplex Virus Type 1		
Herpes simplex encephalitis	PCR in CSF	Sensitive and specific in the acute phase
	CSF–serum antibody ratio	Useful 2 weeks to 3 months after onset
Herpes Simplex Virus Type 2		
Neonatal encephalitis	PCR in CSF	Confirmatory, high sensitivity
Relapsing meningitis	PCR in CSF	Sensitive and specific in first 3 days of illness
Varicella-Zoster Virus		
Meningoencephalitis	PCR in CSF	Confirmatory when used with clinical and spinal fluid findings; sensitivity unclear
Epstein-Barr Virus		
EBV encephalitis	PCR in CSF	Suggests CNS invasion by virus
JC Virus		
Progressive multifocal leukoencephalopathy	PCR in CSF	Diagnostic but incompletely (70%) sensitive
Cytomegalovirus		
CMV ventriculitis	PCR in CSF	Sensitive and specific

CMV, Cytomegalovirus; *CNS,* central nervous system; *CSF,* cerebrospinal fluid; *EBV,* Epstein-Barr virus; *PCR,* polymerase chain reaction.
From Goldman L, Schafer AI: *Goldman's Cecil medicine,* ed 24, Philadelphia, 2011, Saunders.

LABORATORY TESTS

- Aside from the lumbar puncture, most other laboratory studies are nonspecific.
- Skin lesions and urine may be cultured for herpes simplex and CMV.

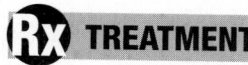 **TREATMENT**

ACUTE GENERAL Rx

- Supportive care, frequent evaluation, and neurologic examination
- Ventilatory assistance for patients who are moribund or at risk for aspiration
- Avoidance of infusion of hypotonic fluids to minimize the risk of hyponatremia
- For patients who develop seizures: anticonvulsant therapy and follow-up in a critical care setting
- For comatose patients:
  1. Aggressive care to avoid decubitus ulcers, contractures, and DVT
  2. Close attention to weights, input/output, and serum electrolytes
- Acyclovir 30 mg/kg/day IV total dose divided in q8 hour intervals for 14 days for herpes simplex encephalitis

- Short courses of corticosteroids to control brain edema and prevent herniation
- In patients with suspected rabies:
  1. Human rabies immune globulin (HRIG) should be given at a dose of 20 U/kg.
  2. Active immunization may be stimulated by rabies vaccine, which is grown on a human diploid cell line (HDCV) and has reduced the number of doses needed to five.
  3. If suspect animal is a dog or cat and can be found, observe closely for 10 days to detect rabid behavior; any significant illness in the animal should promptly initiate humane sacrifice of the animal with the brain submitted to local or state health departments for pathology and immunologic testing for rabies. Any wild animal suspected of rabies should be humanely sacrificed, if possible, and submitted for rabies testing immediately.
  4. If signs are seen, animal should be euthanized and its brain examined for signs of rabies.
- No specific pharmacologic therapy for most other viral pathogens

CHRONIC Rx

Some patients may develop permanent neurologic sequelae; these patients will benefit from intensive rehabilitation programs, including physical, occupational, and speech therapy.

DISPOSITION

- Patients with suspected encephalitis of any cause should generally be admitted for initial diagnostic workup and specific treatment (if available).
- Long-term management of patients with significant neurologic sequelae from encephalitis (e.g., memory defects, depression, difficulty with organization of thoughts, movement disorders) may benefit from rehabilitation services, home care, or nursing home placement.

REFERRAL

- To a neurologist for initial workup and management
- To an infectious disease specialist for diagnostic and therapeutic plan
- To a rehabilitation service for long-term evaluation and convalescent services

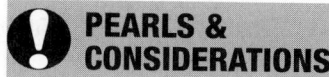 **PEARLS & CONSIDERATIONS**

- West Nile virus encephalitis occurs primarily in elderly patients >65 years of age.
- Rabies may occur months after contact with the rabid animal, and the exposure (especially bat rabies) may have been seemingly insignificant and even inapparent.
- Experimental therapies are worthy of consideration for some forms of viral encephalitis (e.g., immune plasma, ribavirin, interferons), and expert consultation should be obtained early on for possible treatment interventions with promising experimental therapies (e.g., Milwaukee protocol for rabies).

SUGGESTED READINGS
available at www.expertconsult.com

RELATED CONTENT

Rabies (Related Key Topic)
West Nile Virus Infection (Related Key Topic)

AUTHOR: **GLENN G. FORT, M.D., M.P.H.**

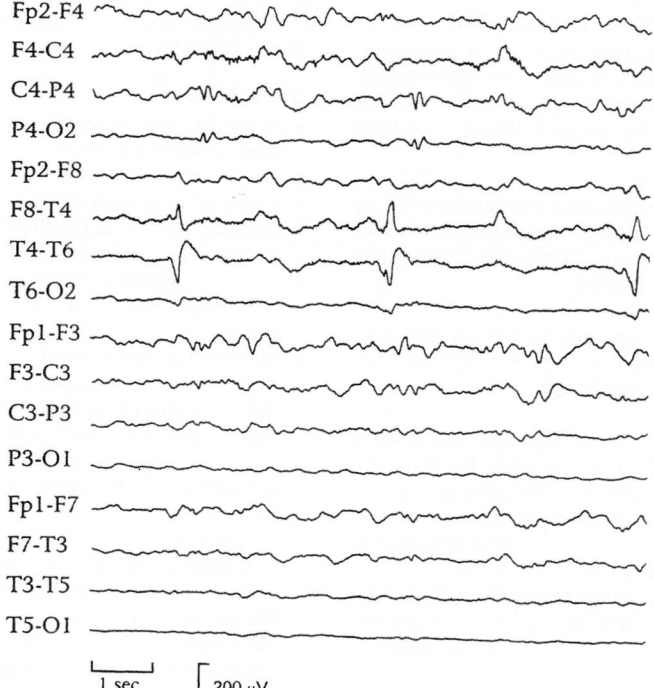

FIGURE 1-307 Repetitive complexes occurring in the right temporal region of a child with herpes simplex encephalitis. (From Goetz CG, Pappert EJ: *Textbook of clinical neurology*, Philadelphia, 1999, Saunders.)

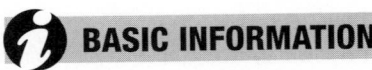

BASIC INFORMATION

DEFINITION

Encephalopathy is a clinical syndrome of global cognitive impairment characterized by impaired arousal, inattention, and disorientation.

SYNONYMS

Delirium, acute confusional state

ICD-9CM CODES
348.3   Encephalopathy, NOS
348.30   Encephalopathy, unspecified
348.31   Encephalopathy, metabolic
348.39   Encephalopathy, other
349.82   Encephalopathy, toxic

EPIDEMIOLOGY & DEMOGRAPHICS

POINT PREVALENCE: 1.1% of adults in the general population >55 yr, 10% to 40% of hospitalized elderly, and 60% of nursing home patients >75 yr; 100,000 to 200,000 cases annually with anoxic encephalopathy
RISK FACTORS: Age, cancer, AIDS, terminal illness, bone marrow transplant, surgery

PHYSICAL FINDINGS & CLINICAL PRESENTATION

- The essential feature of encephalopathy is the patient's inability to maintain a coherent stream of thought or action.
- The history may often suggest a waxing and waning of the level of arousal and general cognitive ability.
- Because toxins and metabolic disturbances are common causes of encephalopathy, the history should focus on exposure to toxins (especially medications) and symptoms suggesting a concurrent illness such as a urinary tract infection or pneumonia.
- Common to all encephalopathies is a fluctuating level of arousal, poor attention, and disorientation.
- Some patients may appear agitated and others lethargic.
- Delusions (fixed false beliefs) and hallucinations are common.
- Asterixis (negative myoclonus) is common.
- Other physical findings may vary depending on the underlying cause of encephalopathy, such as fever, ascites, jaundice, or tachycardia.

ETIOLOGY

The final common pathway of all causes of encephalopathy is widespread, from neuronal dysfunction to structural or functional causes. Many conditions are reversible and carry a good prognosis if treated in a timely manner.
- Organ failure (e.g., hepatic encephalopathy, hypoxia, hypercapnia, uremia)
- Infection: systemic (e.g., urinary tract, pneumonia) or involving the central nervous system (e.g., meningitis, encephalitis)
- Toxin ingestion or withdrawal (e.g., alcohol, medications, recreational drugs)

- Metabolic disturbances: hyperosmolar states, hypernatremia, hyponatremia, hyperglycemia, hypoglycemia, hypercalcemia, hypophosphatemia, acidosis, alkalosis, inborn errors of metabolism
- Endocrinopathy: hyperthyroidism, hypothyroidism, Cushing's syndrome, adrenal insufficiency, pituitary failure
- Neoplasm: tumors of the central nervous system, primary or metastatic; also effect of distant tumors (e.g., paraneoplastic limbic encephalitis)
- Nutritional deficiency, mostly in alcoholics and chronically ill patients, such as vitamin B_1 deficiency (Wernicke's encephalopathy)
- Seizures: postictal state, nonconvulsive status epilepticus, complex partial seizures, absence seizures
- Trauma: concussion, contusion, subdural hematoma, epidural hematoma, diffuse axonal injury
- Vascular: both ischemic and hemorrhagic strokes, vasculitis, venous thrombosis
- Postanoxic encephalopathy
- Other: hypertensive encephalopathy, postoperative status, sleep deprivation

DIAGNOSIS

DIFFERENTIAL DIAGNOSIS

- Dementia: distinguished from encephalopathy by a history of slowly progressive cognitive decline over time (fluctuating cognitive function is rare except in diffuse Lewy body disease).
- Hypersomnia
- Aphasia: distinguished from encephalopathy by virtue of it representing a specific disorder of language rather than a global disturbance of cognitive function.
- Depression
- Psychosis: some overlap with encephalopathy because delusions and hallucinations may be common to both.
- Mania
- Vegetative state from cerebral injury; these patients appear awake (eyes are open) but there is no content to their consciousness.
- Akinetic mutism: these patients do not talk and do not move; there is little fluctuation in their state and there is no asterixis.
- Locked-in syndrome: may be distinguished from encephalopathy by the presence of fixed neurologic deficits (e.g., paralysis of all four limbs).

WORKUP

Electroencephalography is helpful to confirm the presence of encephalopathy (diffuse slowing) and also to exclude nonconvulsive seizures.

LABORATORY TESTS

- General chemistry: electrolytes, glucose, creatinine, ammonia, blood urea nitrogen, transaminases, amylase, lipase
- Arterial blood gases
- Complete blood count
- Drug screen and alcohol level (must order ethylene glycol separately if suspected)

- Lumbar puncture if meningitis, encephalitis, or subarachnoid hemorrhage with negative imaging is suspected
- HIV testing
- Endocrine testing: cortisol level, thyroid function test
- Urinalysis and microscopy

IMAGING STUDIES

- Chest radiograph to rule out pneumonia
- Head CT to rule out bleeding, hydrocephalus, tumors
- Brain MRI with diffusion-weighted images for suspected encephalitis, tumors, and acute strokes
- Magnetic resonance angiography/venography for strokes, arterial dissection, venous thrombosis
- Conventional angiography for central nervous system (CNS) vasculitis and aneurysms

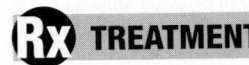 TREATMENT

NONPHARMACOLOGIC THERAPY

The best approach is to treat the underlying toxic or metabolic disturbance. The encephalopathy itself is a symptom of these underlying problems. In general, it is best to avoid treating the symptom of encephalopathy with antipsychotics or sedatives.

GENERAL Rx

- All patients with encephalopathy should have thiamine supplementation.
- Glucose for hypoglycemia
- Antibiotics in cases of infections (choice of an agent with good CNS penetration in cases of primary CNS infections)
- Insulin in hyperglycemic conditions (e.g., diabetic ketoacidosis, hyperosmolar nonketosis, and sepsis)
- The main approach to hepatic encephalopathy is the use of nonabsorbed disaccharides or antibiotics (alone or in combination) to reduce colony counts of ammonia-producing gut flora and to decrease the systemic absorption of ammonia from the intestinal lumen. Lactulose has been used for decades. Probiotics (e.g., 1 capsule containing 112.5 billion viable lyophilized bacteria tid) might also be beneficial in altering gut flora to reduce ammonia production. Rifaximin is a newer agent. It is a minimally absorbed antibiotic useful in both acute hepatic encephalopathy and to maintain remission from recurrent hepatic encephalopathy in patients with chronic liver disease
- Multivitamin, particularly vitamin B_{12}, folate, thiamine replacement when deficiency is suspected
- Anticonvulsants for seizures
- Lorazepam for delirium tremens (alcohol withdrawal)
- Ensure hemodynamic stability (blood pressure and heart rate)

SUGGESTED READINGS
available at www.expertconsult.com

AUTHOR: **ACHRAF A. MAKKI, M.D., M.SC.**

BASIC INFORMATION

DEFINITION/DIAGNOSTIC CRITERIA (*DSM-IV*, 1994)

Encopresis is the voluntary or involuntary passage of stool in inappropriate places, in children over the developmental age of 4 yr. Occurs at least once per month for at least 3 mo and is not due to the effects of a substance (e.g., laxative) or a general medical condition, *except constipation.*

SYNONYMS

Stool incontinence; soiling

ICD-9CM CODES
787.6 Incontinence of feces
307.7 Encopresis

DSM-IV CODES
787.6 Encopresis with constipation and overflow incontinence
307.7 Encopresis without constipation and overflow incontinence

EPIDEMIOLOGY & DEMOGRAPHICS

PEAK INCIDENCE: Preschool age (though also occurs during school age and adolescence)
PREVALANCE (IN U.S.): 1.5% to 7.5% of children 4 to 12 yr old
PREDOMINANT SEX: More often in males (estimates range from 1.9:1 to 9:1)

PHYSICAL FINDINGS & CLINICAL PRESENTATION

- Most children are toilet-trained for stool by age 4. Traditionally, in primary encopresis, fecal continence is never fully established; in secondary encopresis, soiling is preceded by a period of fecal continence. However, definitions of "primary" vs. "secondary" do not reliably correlate with etiology or outcome.
- Constipation and withholding of stool are significant factors in 80% to 90% of cases ("retentive encopresis"). In 10% to 20%, constipation is not a factor ("nonretentive" encopresis).
- When constipation is longstanding, soft or liquid stool may flow around the retained feces, resulting in overflow incontinence. This may occur several times per day and mistakenly be interpreted as diarrhea.
- Children may report a lack of awareness of stool passage when longstanding constipation/impaction has resulted in loss of rectal tone and sensation. Furthermore, some children habituate to the odor.

ETIOLOGY

- Approximately 96% of children have bowel movements between three times daily to once every other day. When bowel movements are less frequent, stool becomes drier and harder and much more uncomfortable or painful to pass. Children may avoid the discomfort or pain by avoiding elimination, resulting in worsening constipation and overflow incontinence.
- Constipation may begin gradually as a result of a decrease in elimination frequency, or more acutely after an illness or changes in diet.
- Toilet training practices that increase anxiety may also play a role in stool retention, the development of constipation, and eventual encopresis.

DIAGNOSIS

DIFFERENTIAL DIAGNOSIS

- Hirschsprung's disease
- Endocrine disease (hypothyroidism)
- Cerebral palsy
- Myelomeningocele
- Pseudoobstruction
- Anorectal lesions (rectal stenosis)
- Malformations
- Trauma
- Rectal prolapse
- Celiac disease
- Hypothyroidism
- Medications

WORKUP

- History: frequency of elimination, character of the stool, associated pain, and presence of enuresis (with which it is frequently associated).
- Evaluate for other developmental or psychiatric problems.
- Physical examination: pay particular attention to the abdomen, anus, rectum, and neurologic examination.

LABORATORY TESTS

- Consider thyroid function tests, celiac screening tests, electrolytes, calcium, urinalysis, and urine culture.
- If concerned about the possibility of Hirschsprung's disease, obtain rectal biopsy.

IMAGING STUDIES

- Abdominal imaging to determine extent of obstruction or megacolon
- Anorectal manometric studies or barium enema can support suspicion of Hirschsprung's disease

TREATMENT

ACUTE GENERAL Rx

- Disimpaction is a necessary first step, by oral or rectal route (or combination).
- For oral disimpaction, polyethylene glycol or high doses of mineral oil are effective (avoid use of mineral oil in patients at risk for aspiration).
- Adding stimulant laxatives such as senna or bisacodyl can sometimes make oral disimpaction more effective.
- For rectal disimpaction, phosphate soda, saline, or mineral oil enemas are effective.
- When medical workup determines that constipation is not present ("nonretentive encopresis"), consider implementing toilet-training routines or referral to behavioral health provider.

CHRONIC Rx

- Prevent recurrence of constipation with oral stool softeners (e.g., polyethylene glycol, sorbital, or lactulose) or stool lubricants (mineral oil).
- In immediate postdisimpaction period (1 mo after acute treatment), stimulant laxatives may be needed because bowel tone remains low; taper use as quickly as possible to avoid dependence.
- Family documentation of stool passage, including location and amount, on a chart or calendar helps inform medication changes and best times for toilet sitting.
- Praise and other small incentives for positive toileting routines and taking medication can help to maintain good bowel habits. Balanced diet and increased fiber intake/supplementation may also help.
- Formal behavioral treatment (education, reinforcement of treatment adherence and exercises to improve anal sphincter control) increases treatment success. Biofeedback to improve sphincter function is advocated by some, with 1-yr results comparable to behavioral treatment. Adjunctive Internet-based interventions that incorporate behavioral therapy and medical management are also beginning to show promise.

DISPOSITION

Encopresis may be self-limited or relatively brief in duration; may require prolonged maintenance therapy. Relapses are common.

REFERRAL

Behavioral family therapy should be considered for patients who do not respond to medical treatment within a few months or who have significant contributing psychiatric or family factors.

PEARLS & CONSIDERATIONS

- It is crucial to educate parents and children about constipation and encopresis and to defuse negative interactions.
- Emphasize that this can require prolonged maintenance therapy and that relapses are common.

SUGGESTED READINGS

available at www.expertconsult.com

RELATED CONTENT

Encopresis (Patient Information)

AUTHORS: **JACK H. NASSAU, PH.D., WENDY A. PLANTE, PH.D.,** and **VINCENT A. MUKKADA, M.D.**

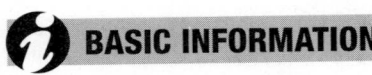

BASIC INFORMATION

DEFINITION

Infective endocarditis is an infection of the endocardial surface of the heart or mural endocardium. Box E1-18 describes the modified Duke criteria for the diagnosis of infective endocarditis.

ACUTE ENDOCARDITIS: Usually caused by *Staphylococcus aureus, Streptococcus pyogenes, Streptococcus pneumoniae,* and *Neisseria* organisms; classic clinical presentation of high fever, positive blood cultures, vascular and immunologic phenomenon

SUBACUTE ENDOCARDITIS: Usually caused by viridans streptococci in the presence of valvular pathology; less toxic, often indolent presentation with lower fevers, night sweats, fatigue

ENDOCARDITIS IN INJECTION DRUG USERS: Often involving *S. aureus* or *Pseudomonas aeruginosa* with variation that may be geographically influenced; tricuspid (Fig. 1-308) or multiple valvular involvement; high mortality rate of 50% to 60%

PROSTHETIC VALVE ENDOCARDITIS (EARLY): Usually caused by *S. aureus* (leading cause of PVE) within 2 mo of valve replacement; other organisms include *S. epidermidis,* gram-negative bacilli, diphtheroids, *Candida* organisms

PROSTHETIC VALVE ENDOCARDITIS (LATE): Typically develops >60 days after valvular replacement; involved organisms similar to early prosthetic valve endocarditis, including viridans streptococci, enterococci, and group D streptococci

NOSOCOMIAL ENDOCARDITIS: Secondary to intravenous catheters, TPN lines, pacemakers; coagulase-negative staphylococci, *S. aureus,* and streptococci most common

Non-HACEK gram-negative bacillus endocarditis is not primarily a disease of injection drug users. More than half of all cases are associated with health care contact

SYNONYMS

Bacterial endocarditis
Subacute bacterial endocarditis (SBE)
Endocarditis

ICD-9CM CODES
421.0   Infective endocarditis
996.61   Prosthetic valve endocarditis

EPIDEMIOLOGY & DEMOGRAPHICS

INCIDENCE (IN U.S.): 5 to 7.9 cases/100,000 persons/yr
PEAK INCIDENCE: Females: often <35 yr old; males: 45 to 65 yr old
NOSOCOMIAL ENDOCARDITIS: 14% to 28% of cases
PREVALENCE (IN U.S.): 0.3 to 3 cases/1000 hospital admissions
PREDOMINANT SEX: Male > female
PREDOMINANT AGE: 45 to 65 yr

PHYSICAL FINDINGS & CLINICAL PRESENTATION

- Clinical manifestations of infective endocarditis are described in Table 1-143.
- Fever may be variable in presentation; may be high, hectic, or absent.
- Fever, chills, fatigue, and rigors occur in 25% to 80% of patients.
- Heart murmur may be absent in right-sided endocarditis.
- Embolic phenomenon with peripheral manifestations is found in 50% of patients.
- Skin manifestations include petechiae, Osler nodes, splinter hemorrhages, Janeway lesions (Fig. E1-309).
- Splenomegaly is more common with subacute course.

ETIOLOGY

Staphylococcal infection is now the leading cause of native or prosthetic valve infection. Variation in incidence may occur that is influenced by the patient's risk for developing infection. Risk factors include hemodialysis (8%), IV drug use (10%), mitral regurgitation (43%), aortic regurgitation (26%), and rheumatic heart disease (3.3%).

ACUTE ENDOCARDITIS:
- *S. aureus*
- *S. lugdunensis*
- *S. pneumoniae*
- Streptococcal species and groups A through G
- *Haemophilus influenzae*

SUBACUTE ENDOCARDITIS:
- Viridans streptococci (alpha-hemolytic)
- *S. bovis*
- Enterococci
- *S. aureus*

ENDOCARDITIS IN INJECTION DRUG USERS:
- *S. aureus*
- *P. aeruginosa*
- *Candida* spp.
- Enterococci

PROSTHETIC VALVE ENDOCARDITIS (EARLY):
- *S. epidermidis*
- *S. aureus*
- Gram-negative bacilli
- Group D streptococci

PROSTHETIC VALVE ENDOCARDITIS (LATE):
- *S. epidermidis*

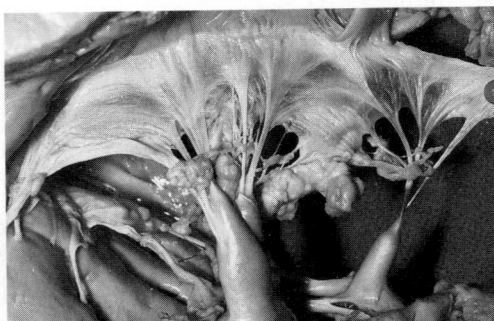

FIGURE 1-308 Tricuspid valve endocarditis. There are large vegetations on the leaflets and the chordae tendineae. (From Crawford MH et al [eds]: *Cardiology,* ed 2, St Louis, 2004, Mosby.)

TABLE 1-143 Clinical Manifestations of Infective Endocarditis Myalgia/Arthralgia

Symptoms	Patients Affected (%)	Signs	Patients (%)
Fever	80	Fever	90
Chills	40	Heart murmur	85
Weakness	40	Changing murmur	5-10
Dyspnea	40	New murmur	3-5
Sweats	25	Embolic phenomenon	>50
Anorexia	25	Skin manifestations	18-50
Weight loss	25	Osler nodes	10-23
Malaise	25	Splinter hemorrhages	15
Cough	25	Petechiae	20-40
Skin lesions	20	Janeway lesion	<10
Stroke	20	Splenomegaly	20-57
Nausea/vomiting	20	Septic complications	20
Headache	20	(e.g., pneumonia, meningitis)	20
Myalgia/arthralgia	15	Mycotic aneurysms	
Edema	15	Clubbing	12-52
Chest pain	15	Retinal lesion	2-10
Abdominal pain and delirium/coma	15	Signs of renal failure	10-25
Delirium/coma	10-15		
Hemoptysis	10		
Back pain	10		

From Mandell GL et al: *Principles and practice of infectious diseases,* ed 6, Philadelphia, 2005, Churchill Livingstone.

- Viridans streptococci
- *S. aureus*
- Enterococci and group D streptococci

NOSOCOMIAL ENDOCARDITIS:

- Coagulase-negative staphylococci
- *S. aureus*
- Streptococci: viridans, group B, enterococcus

HACEK ORGANISMS:

- Fastidious gram-negative bacilli
- *Haemophilus parainfluenzae*
- *Haemophilus aphrophilus*
- *Actinobacillus actinomycetemcomitans*
- *Cardiobacterium hominis*
- *Eikenella corrodens*
- *Kingella kingae*

RISK FACTORS

- Poor dental hygiene
- Long-term hemodialysis
- Diabetes mellitus
- HIV infection
- Mitral valve prolapse

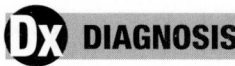 **DIAGNOSIS**

DIFFERENTIAL DIAGNOSIS

- Brain abscess
- FUO
- Pericarditis
- Meningitis
- Rheumatic fever
- Osteomyelitis
- *Salmonella*
- TB
- Bacteremia
- Pericarditis
- Glomerulonephritis

WORKUP

Physical examination to evaluate for the previous physical findings followed by laboratory testing (see "Laboratory Tests"). Fig. E1-310 and Box E1-19 describe a diagnostic evaluation of suspected endocarditis. The modified Duke criteria for diagnosis of endocarditis defines "major criteria" as persistently positive blood cultures of organisms typical of endocarditis or endocardial involvement (new valvular regurgitation or positive echocardiogram). "Minor criteria" is defined as presence of predisposing condition or injection drug use, fever, embolic vascular pneumonia (e.g., glomerulonephritis, rheumatoid factor), or positive blood cultures not meeting major criteria. Definite endocarditis is 2 major criteria or 1 major criteria and 3 minor criteria or 5 minor criteria or presence of organisms by culture or histologic examination of a vegetation.

LABORATORY TESTS

- Blood cultures: three sets in first 24 hr
- More culturing if patient has received prior antibiotic
- CBC (anemia possibly present, subacute)
- WBC (leukocytosis is higher in acute endocarditis)
- ESR and C-reactive protein (elevated)
- Positive rheumatoid factor (subacute endocarditis)
- Proteinuria, hematuria, RBC casts

IMAGING STUDIES

- Echocardiogram: two-dimensional. Transthoracic echocardiography (TTE) is noninvasive and more easily available but has less-than-optimal sensitivity (50%-80%) for endocarditis.
- Transesophageal echocardiography (TEE): more sensitive in detecting vegetations and preferred diagnostic modality. It is especially helpful with prosthetic valves or in detecting perivalvular disease.
- Electrocardiogram: look for cardiac conduction abnormalities, injury pattern, or evidence of pericarditis—any such new findings are suggestive of myocardial abscess

 TREATMENT

Initial IV antibiotic therapy (before culture results) is aimed at the most likely organism.

- **Native valve (no history of IV drugs) empiric therapy awaiting cultures:** Pen G 20 million U IV q24h continuous or divided q4h or ampicillin 12 g IV q24h continuous or divided q4h *plus* nafcillin or oxacillin 2 g IV q4h *plus* gentamicin 1 mg/kg IV q8h; other options are vancomycin 15 mg/kg (assuming CrCl ≥ 80 ml/min) IV q12h *plus* gentamicin 1 mg/kg IM or IV q8h
- **Native valve (IV drug use ± evidence of right-sided endocarditis) empiric therapy:** vancomycin 30-60 mg/kg/day in 2-3 divided doses for trough 15-20 mcg/ml or daptomycin 6 mg/kg IV q24h
- **Native valve (culture positive):** Pen G 12-18 million U/day IV, divided q4h × 2 wk *plus* gentamicin 1 mg/kg q8h IV × 2 wk (target level peak 3 mcg/ml, trough <1 mcg/ml) *or* ceftriaxone 2 g IV q24h × 4 wk
- **Staphylococcal endocarditis (aortic and/or mitral valve)**
  ○ **MSSA:** nafcillin (or oxacillin) 2 g IV q4h × 4-6 wk *or* cefazolin 2 g IV q8h × 4-6 wk *or* vancomycin 15 mg/kg IV q12h (check level if >2 g/day) × 4-6 wk
  ○ **MRSA:** vancomycin 30-60 mg/kg/day 2-3 divided doses with trough conc. 15-20 mcg/ml

- **Patients with prosthetic valves or native valves who are allergic to PCN:** vancomycin (1 g IV q12h × 4 wk) *plus* rifampin 600 mg PO qd *and* gentamicin (1 mg/kg IV q8h × 2 wk), assuming normal renal function in adult patients

Antibiotic therapy after identification of the organism should be guided by susceptibility testing, preferably by formal testing by MIC (minimum inhibitory concentration).

DISPOSITION

- The patient may need outpatient IV antibiotic therapy, and arrangements need to be made to ensure safe vascular access and continuity of care with outpatient IV therapy team.
- Long-term follow-up is essential after therapy has ended; relapse of endocarditis may occur.
- Prophylaxis with antibiotics will be needed before dental procedures as a previous episode of endocarditis increases the risk of recurrent endocarditis associated with transient bacteremia from dental procedures.

REFERRAL

- To an infectious disease specialist
- To a cardiologist or a cardiac surgeon if evidence of heart failure, refractory infection, myocardial abscess, valve disruption, or major embolic events occur.
- The timing and indications for surgical intervention to prevent systemic embolism in infective endocarditis remain controversial. Trials have shown that early surgery in patients with infective endocarditis and large vegetations significantly reduced death and embolic events by decreasing the risk of systemic embolism.

 PEARLS & CONSIDERATIONS

COMMENTS

For endocarditis prophylaxis refer to Section V.

 EVIDENCE

available at www.expertconsult.com

SUGGESTED READINGS

available at www.expertconsult.com

RELATED CONTENT

Endocarditis (Patient Information)

AUTHOR: **GLENN G. FORT, M.D., M.P.H.**

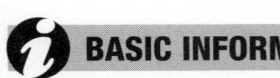 **BASIC INFORMATION**

DEFINITION

Endometrial cancer (EC) is a malignant transformation of endometrial stroma and/or glands typified by irregular nuclear membranes, nuclear atypia, mitotic activity, loss of glandular pattern, and irregular cell size. The two main histologic subcategories of EC, endometrioid and nonendometrioid EC, show unique molecular aberrations and differing clinical behaviors.

SYNONYMS

Uterine cancer (some forms)

ICD-9CM CODES
182 Malignant neoplasm of body of uterus

EPIDEMIOLOGY & DEMOGRAPHICS

INCIDENCE: 21.2 cases per 100,000 persons; approximately 30,000 new cases annually. It is the most common gynecologic malignancy in the U.S.
PREDOMINANCE: Median age at onset: 60 yr; only 5% occur in women <40 yr
RISK FACTORS: Obesity, diabetes, nulliparity, early menarche and late menopause, unopposed estrogen therapy, tamoxifen use, oligoovulation, endometrial atypical hyperplasia, endometrial polyps (malignancy is found in 3.6% of endometrial polyps)

PHYSICAL FINDINGS & CLINICAL PRESENTATION

- Abnormal uterine bleeding or postmenopausal bleeding in 90%
- Pyometra or hematometra
- Abnormal Pap smear

ETIOLOGY

Endogenous or exogenous chronic unopposed estrogen stimulation of the endometrium

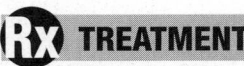 **DIAGNOSIS**

DIFFERENTIAL DIAGNOSIS

- Atypical hyperplasia
- Other genital tract malignancy
- Polyps
- Atrophic vaginitis
- Granuloma cell tumor
- Fibroid uterus

WORKUP

- Complete history and physical examination
- Endometrial biopsy or dilation and curettage
- Assessment of operative risk
- Staging (Table 1-144)

LABORATORY TESTS

- Complete blood count
- Chemistry profile including liver function tests
- Consider CA-125 level

IMAGING STUDIES

- Chest x-ray
- CT scan, and/or pelvic ultrasound (Fig. E1-311)
- Endovaginal ultrasound (Fig. E1-312) in postmenopausal women with vaginal bleeding

 TREATMENT

NONPHARMACOLOGIC THERAPY

- Surgery is the mainstay of treatment, with or without radiation, depending on tumor stage and grade. Laparoscopic surgery for early-stage EC is as safe and effective as laparatomy.
- Surgery generally consists of pelvic washings, total abdominal hysterectomy and bilateral salpingo-oophorectomy, omental biopsy, and selective pelvic and periaortic lymphadenectomy, depending on stage and grade.

- Brachytherapy and/or teletherapy are added in an advanced stage.
- Chemotherapy (cisplatin, Adriamycin) or tamoxifen may also be used.
- Hormonal therapy is an option for some young women with EC who wish to preserve fertility.

ACUTE GENERAL Rx

- A thorough workup should be completed before any therapy for EC.
- Surgery is the treatment of choice.

CHRONIC Rx

- Physical and pelvic examination every 3 mo for 2 yr, then every 6 mo for 2 yr, annually thereafter
- Yearly Pap smear
- Hormone replacement (combination) a consideration in low-risk patients (stage I or early stage II)

DISPOSITION

The majority of cases present early, and the 5-yr survival is generally good:

Stage I	75%-100%
Stage II	65%
Stage III	40%
Stage IV	10%

Some histologic types (clear cell, serous papillary) have worse survival rates.

REFERRAL

Refer to a gynecologic oncologist.

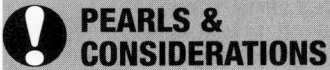 **PEARLS & CONSIDERATIONS**

COMMENTS

- Estrogen replacement therapy after surgery for EC remains controversial. Recent data suggest that it does not increase EC recurrence rates.
- Obesity and sedentary lifestyle put EC survivors at increased risk for health problems. Even moderate activity is associated with better physical functioning in EC survivors.

EBM EVIDENCE

available at www.expertconsult.com

SUGGESTED READINGS
available at www.expertconsult.com

RELATED CONTENT

Dysfunctional Uterine Bleeding (Related Key Topic)
Uterine Malignancy (Related Key Topic)
Endometrial Cancer (Patient Information)

AUTHORS: **GIL M. FARKASH, M.D.,** and **RUBEN ALVERO, M.D.**

TABLE 1-144 FIGO Staging of Endometrial Carcinoma

Stage	Definition	Stage at Presentation	Pelvic Nodes	5-Year Survival
I_A	Tumor limited to the endometrium			
I_B	Growth that has invaded <50% of myometrial thickness	73%	<20%	85%
I_C	Growth that has invaded >50% of myometrial thickness			
II_A	Endocervical glandular involvement only			
II_B	Cervical stroma involved	11%	20%	65%
III_A	Invades sero-serosal surface of uterus, ± adnexa, ± positive washings			
III_B	Vaginal metastases	13%	35%	40%
III_C	Metastases to pelvic or para-aortic nodes			
IV_A	Tumor invasion of bladder and/or bowel			
IV_B	Distant metastases including intra-abdominal and/or inguinal lymph nodes	3%	50%	10%

Histopathology: Degree of Differentiation

Uterine adenocarcinoma should be grouped according to the degree of differentiation as follows:
- G1 – 5% or less of a solid growth pattern
- G2 – 6%-50% of a solid growth pattern
- G3 – More than 50% of a solid growth pattern

From Drife J, Magowan B: *Clinical obstetrics and gynecology*, Philadelphia, 2004, Saunders.

BASIC INFORMATION

DEFINITION

Endometriosis is defined as the presence of functioning endometrial glands and stroma outside the uterine cavity (Fig. 1-313).

ICD-9CM CODES
617.9 Endometriosis

EPIDEMIOLOGY & DEMOGRAPHICS

PREVALENCE:
- Endometriosis affects 10% of reproductive-aged women.
- Women with dysmenorrhea: 40% to 60%
- Subfertile women: 20% to 30%
- Incidence peaks at approximately 40 yr

MOST COMMON AGE AT DIAGNOSIS: 25 to 29 yr

GENETICS:
- Multifactorial inheritance pattern
- 6.9% occurrence rate in first-degree female relatives

PHYSICAL FINDINGS & CLINICAL PRESENTATION

- Classic triad is dysmenorrhea, dyspareunia, and infertility.
- Presence of pelvic pain not correlated with the total area of endometriosis, type of lesion, or volume of disease, but is correlated with the depth of infiltration.
- Other symptoms include abnormal bleeding (premenstrual spotting, menorrhagia), cyclic abdominal pain, intermittent constipation/diarrhea, dyschezia, dysuria, hematuria, and urinary frequency.
- Rare manifestations: catamenial hemothorax, bloody pleural effusion, massive ascites occurring during menses.
- Most severe discomfort is associated with lesions >1 cm in depth.
- Bimanual examination may reveal tender uterosacral ligaments, cul-de-sac nodularity, induration of the rectovaginal septum, fixed retroversion of the uterus, adnexal mass, and generalized or localized tenderness.

ETIOLOGY

- Reflux and direct implantation theory: retrograde menstruation with implantation of viable endometrial cells to surrounding pelvic structures (Sampson's theory)
- Coelomic metaplasia theory: transformation of multipotential cells of the coelomic epithelium into endometrium-like cells
- Vascular dissemination theory: transport of endometrial cells to distant sites by the uterine vascular and lymphatic systems
- Autoimmune disease theory: disorder of immune surveillance allows growth of endometrial implants

DIAGNOSIS

DIFFERENTIAL DIAGNOSIS

- Ectopic pregnancy
- Acute appendicitis
- Chronic appendicitis
- Pelvic inflammatory disease (PID)
- Pelvic adhesions
- Hemorrhagic cyst
- Hernia
- Psychologic disorder
- Irritable bowel syndrome
- Uterine leiomyomata
- Adenomyosis
- Nerve entrapment syndrome
- Scoliosis
- Muscular/skeletal strain
- Interstitial cystitis

WORKUP

- Thorough history and physical examination, including inquiry about physical and emotional abuse. Defining diagnosis of endometriosis can be made only by histology of lesions that have been removed surgically
- Laparoscopy for definitive diagnosis
- Revised American Fertility Society (renamed American Society for Reproductive Medicine) scale to classify endometriosis (since 1985):

Stage I	Minimal
Stage II	Mild
Stage III	Moderate
Stage IV	Severe

LABORATORY TESTS

Cancer antigen 125 (CA125): limited overall value in the diagnosis of endometriosis
- Also elevated in ovarian epithelial neoplasm, myomas, adenomyosis, acute PID, ovarian cysts, pancreatitis, chronic liver disease, menstruation, and pregnancy
- CA125 value >35 U/ml: positive predictive value of 0.58 and a negative predictive value of 0.96 for the presence of endometriosis

IMAGING STUDIES

- Ultrasound: for evaluating adnexal mass; ultrasound characteristics may suggest endometriomas versus other benign or malignant ovarian conditions but persistent solid or cystic-solid ovarian masses require definitive tissue diagnosis with laparoscopy.
- MRI:
  1. Highly accurate in detecting endometriomas
  2. Limited sensitivity in detecting diffuse pelvic endometriosis
- CT scan may show adnexal masses of varying density (Fig. 1-314)

TREATMENT

NONPHARMACOLOGIC THERAPY

Expectant management (observation for 5 to 12 mo) for stage I or stage II endometriosis-associated infertility. Evaluation should take place if the couple meet the diagnostic criteria for infertility.

ACUTE GENERAL Rx

Nonsteroidal anti-inflammatory drugs for symptomatic relief of dysmenorrhea

CHRONIC Rx

PHARMACOLOGIC MANAGEMENT:
Estrogen-progesterone:
- State of "pseudopregnancy" created by continuous (discarding pill pack when placebo pills remaining and starting active pills from new pill pack) use of combination oral contraceptives for minimum of 6 mo and continuing indefinitely
- Breakthrough bleeding treated by administering conjugated estrogens 1.25 mg/day for 2 wk

Progestins:

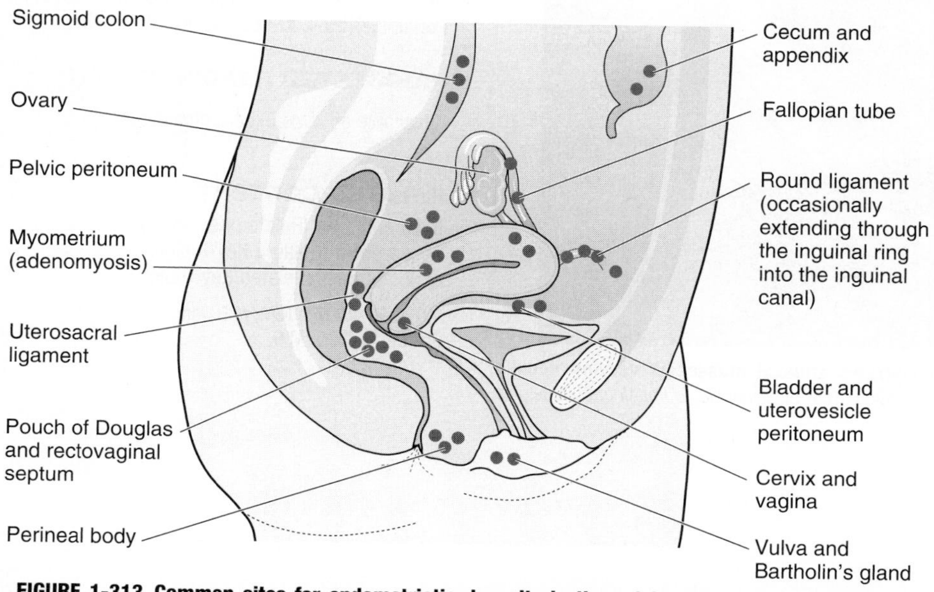

Sigmoid colon
Ovary
Pelvic peritoneum
Myometrium (adenomyosis)
Uterosacral ligament
Pouch of Douglas and rectovaginal septum
Perineal body
Cecum and appendix
Fallopian tube
Round ligament (occasionally extending through the inguinal ring into the inguinal canal)
Bladder and uterovesicle peritoneum
Cervix and vagina
Vulva and Bartholin's gland

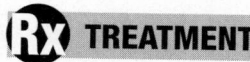

FIGURE 1-313 Common sites for endometriotic deposits in the pelvis. (From Drife J, Magowan B: *Clinical obstetrics and gynecology,* Philadelphia, 2004, Saunders.)

- Medroxyprogesterone acetate 10 to 30 mg PO qd and occasionally up to 100 mg PO qd
- Alternatively, 100 mg IM q2wk for four doses, followed by 200 mg IM monthly for 4 mo
- Breakthrough bleeding treated with ethinyl estradiol (20 mcg/day) or conjugated estrogens (1.25 mg/day) for 1 to 2 wk
- Comparison with danazol: progestins cost less, have a more tolerable side-effect profile, and have comparable efficacy with regard to pain relief and so are often the first-line drug

Gonadotropin-releasing hormone (GnRH) agonists:

- Use usually limited to 6-12 mo due to hypoestrogenic effects such as osteopenia or osteoporosis but can be given longer in certain circumstances, particularly when paired with estrogen add-back therapy. Referral to specialist strongly advised.
- Leuprolide acetate depot 3.75 mg IM monthly or 11.25 mg IM q3mo or nafarelin 200 mcg nasal puffs bid or goserelin 3.6 mg SC monthly
- As effective as danazol for relief of pelvic pain
- Add-back therapy for protection against vasomotor symptoms and bone loss: norethindrone acetate 5 mg PO qd alone or in combination with conjugated estrogen 0.625 mg PO qd
- Add-back therapy allows gonadotropin-releasing hormone (GnRH) agonist use to be extended to 1 yr based on limited studies available

Alternative therapies for inhibition of estrogen action currently under investigation are:

- Aromatase inhibitors: anastrozole, letrozole
- SERM: raloxifene
- Agents enhancing cell-mediated immunity are cytokines (interleukin-12 and interferon-α2b)
- Immunomodulators (loxoribine, levamisole)
- Anti-inflammatory: pentoxifylline

SURGICAL MANAGEMENT:
Conservative:

- Directed at enhancing fertility or treating pain unresponsive to first-line medical treatment
- Usually accomplished through laparoscopy
- Removal or destruction of endometriotic implants by excision, electrocautery, or laser
- Cystectomy for endometrioma; must remove cyst wall to be effective long-term
- Laparoscopic uterosacral nerve ablation for midline pain such as dysmenorrhea or dyspareunia (evidence does not support its use)
- Unless pregnancy is desired, patient is usually started on GnRH agonist therapy or continuous OCP immediately after surgery
- For those desiring pregnancy, surgery alone results in significant increase in fertility

Definitive:

- Directed at relieving endometriosis-associated pain
- Total abdominal hysterectomy with bilateral salpingo-oophorectomy and complete excision or ablation of endometriosis
- Thorough abdominal exploration to ensure removal of all disease
- Must be prepared to manage possible gastrointestinal and urinary tract endometriosis
- 90% effective in pain relief; patient must be counseled that pain relief is not guaranteed

- Estrogen replacement therapy (ERT) to be considered in all women undergoing definitive surgical management; after ERT, recurrence rate is 0% to 5% in women with endometriosis confined to the pelvis but 18% in women with bowel involvement

MANAGEMENT OF ENDOMETRIOSIS-ASSOCIATED INFERTILITY:
Conservative surgery:

- Yields significantly increased pregnancy rate than does expectant management, in part because of correction of mechanical factors such as adhesions

Assisted reproductive technologies:

- Can be used to circumvent unknown mechanism of endometriosis-associated infertility
- Superovulation with clomiphene citrate or human menopausal gonadotropins; clomiphene citrate results in threefold pregnancy rate over either danazol or expectant management
- Further improvement with intrauterine insemination combined with superovulation
- In vitro fertilization if above procedures are unsuccessful

DISPOSITION

Tends to recur unless definitive surgery is performed and should be considered a chronic condition

REFERRAL

To a reproductive endocrinologist for advanced surgical management or infertility management

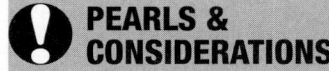

PEARLS & CONSIDERATIONS

COMMENTS

Patient information can be obtained through the following organizations: Endometriosis Association, 8585 North 76th Place, Milwaukee, WI 53223, 414-355-2200 or 800-992-ENDO; Women's Reproductive Health Network, P.O. Box 30167, Portland, OR 97230-9067 or 503-667-7757.

SUGGESTED READINGS

available at www.expertconsult.com

RELATED CONTENT

Dysmenorrhea (Related Key Topic)
Dyspareunia (Related Key Topic)
Endometriosis (Related Key Topic)

AUTHORS: **WAN J. KIM, M.D.,** and **RUBEN ALVERO, M.D.**

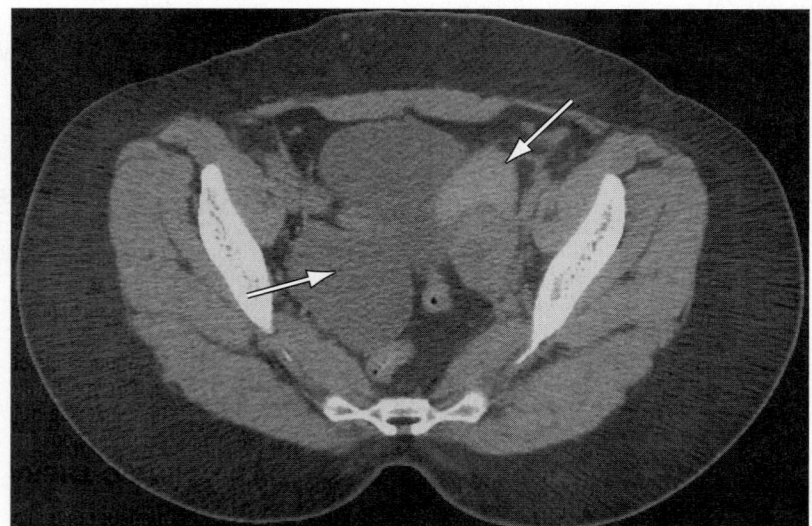

FIGURE 1-314 Computed tomographic scan demonstrates adnexal masses of varying density, subsequently proven to be endometriomas. (From Fielding JR et al: *Gynecologic imaging,* Philadelphia, 2011, Saunders.)

BASIC INFORMATION

DEFINITION
Endometritis is defined as a uterine infection after delivery or abortion.

SYNONYMS
Endomyometritis
Metritis

ICD-9CM CODES
615.9 Endometritis

EPIDEMIOLOGY & DEMOGRAPHICS
- Overall rate of postpartum infection: estimated between 1% and 8%
- Most common genital tract infection after delivery
- Usually presents early in postpartum period; more commonly seen after cesarean section than vaginal delivery; also seen with an incomplete abortion (spontaneous abortion, legal abortion, or illegal abortion)
- More common in preterm deliveries
- Possible after any uterine manipulation in the presence of undiagnosed cervicitis or vaginitis

PHYSICAL FINDINGS & CLINICAL PRESENTATION
- Postpartum oral temperature >37.8° C
- Localized uterine tenderness, purulent or foul lochia; physical examination revealing uterine or parametrial tenderness
- Nonspecific signs and symptoms such as malaise, abdominal pain, chills, and tachycardia

ETIOLOGY
Endometritis is usually associated with multiple organisms: group A or B streptococci, *Staphylococcus aureus* and *Bacteroides* species, *Neisseria gonorrhoeae*, *Chlamydia trachomatis*, enterococci, *Gardnerella vaginalis*, *E. coli*, and *Mycoplasma*.

DIAGNOSIS

DIFFERENTIAL DIAGNOSIS
Causes of postoperative or postprocedural infections

WORKUP
Diagnosis based on symptoms of fever, malaise, abdominal pain, uterine tenderness, and purulent, foul vaginal discharge

LABORATORY TESTS
Complete blood count, blood cultures, and uterine culture

IMAGING STUDIES
Ultrasound (Fig. 1-315) may be useful if retained products are considered a possible source of infection.

TREATMENT

ACUTE GENERAL Rx
Treatment options include doxycycline plus one of the following:
- Cefoxitin
- Ticarcillin-clavulanate
- Ertapenem
- Imipenem-cilastatin
- Meropenem
- Ampicillin-sulbactam
- Piperacillin-tazobactam
- An alternative regimen is clindamycin plus aminoglycoside or ceftriaxone.
- Regimen should be continued for at least 48 hr after substantial clinical improvement. If response is not adequate (Table 1-145), check cultures and treat with appropriate antibiotics.

CHRONIC Rx
Watch for recurrent infection.

DISPOSITION
With appropriate antibiotic therapy, 95% to 98% cure rate

REFERRAL
For patients who do not respond within 48 to 72 hr of appropriate antibiotic therapy, obtain an infectious disease consult or gynecologic consultation.

AUTHORS: **GEORGE T. DANAKAS, M.D.,** and **RUBEN ALVERO, M.D.**

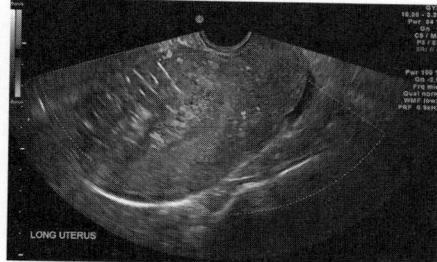

FIGURE 1-315 Endometritis. Patient with uterine tenderness and fever 7 days after classic cesarean section for premature rupture of membranes, chorioamnionitis, and fundic presentation at 27 weeks' gestational age. Sagittal transvaginal ultrasound shows increased vascularity within the endometrium, which can be seen with endometritis. Linear echogenic foci within the anterior myometrium likely represent air and suture material in the vertical uterine incision. Patient's symptoms resolved with antibiotics. (From Fielding JR et al: *Gynecologic imaging*, Philadelphia, 2011, Saunders.)

TABLE 1-145 Identified Causes of Poor Response to Antibiotic Therapy in Patients with Endometritis

Cause	Approximate Prevalence (%)
Infected mass, including abscess, hematoma, septic pelvic thrombophlebitis, pelvic cellulitis, retained placenta	40-50
Resistant organisms, commonly enterococci, in a patient receiving clindamycin-aminoglycoside or a cephalosporin	20
Additional cause, including catheter phlebitis, inadequate dose of antibiotics	10
No cause evident but response to empirical change in antibiotic therapy	20-30

From Gorbach SL: *Infectious diseases*, ed 2, Philadelphia, 1998, Saunders.

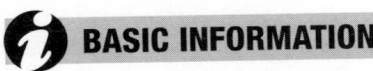

BASIC INFORMATION

DEFINITION

Enuresis refers to the voiding of urine into clothes or in bed that is usually involuntary in individuals who are expected to be continent (>5 yr of age). The diagnosis is made if voiding occurs at least twice a week for 3 mos. Primary enuresis refers to enuresis without a period of continence, whereas secondary enuresis occurs after a period of normal bladder control.

SYNONYMS

Urinary incontinence
Bedwetting

ICD-9CM CODES
788.36 Nocturnal Enuresis

DSM-IV CODES
307.6 Enuresis primary/secondary of nonorganic origin

EPIDEMIOLOGY & DEMOGRAPHICS

PEAK INCIDENCE: Ages 5 to 10 yr
PREVALENCE (IN U.S.):
- Age 5 yr: 7% of males and 3% of females
- Age 10 yr: 3% of males and 2% of females
- Age 18 yr: 1% of males
PREDOMINANT SEX: Twice as many males as females at all ages
PREDOMINANT AGE: By definition, enuresis does not begin before age 5 yr, at which time the prevalence is highest, and decreases steadily thereafter at a rate of approximately 12% to 15% per year.
GENETICS:
- Approximately 75% of children with enuresis have a first-degree relative with enuresis.
- Almost twice as common in monozygotic than dizygotic twins.

PHYSICAL FINDINGS & CLINICAL PRESENTATION

Three enuresis subtypes are defined:
- Nocturnal only: occurs in each sleep stage in proportion to the time spent in the particular stage. May occur during transition from deep sleep to REM.
- Diurnal only: more frequent in girls and rarely after age 9 yr; voiding occurs in early afternoon on school days.
- Combined nocturnal and diurnal; often called complex or complicated enuresis.

ETIOLOGY

- Enuresis often correlates with other maturational delays, particularly language, motor skills, and social development.
- May be related to toilet training issues, stress (secondary enuresis), inability to concentrate urine, altered smooth muscle physiology, or dysfunction of the arousal system.
- Diurnal enuresis associated with a higher rate of urinary tract infections.

DIAGNOSIS

DIFFERENTIAL DIAGNOSIS

- May be associated with encopresis and sleep disorders such as sleep terrors; much less likely to be a primary psychological disorder.
- Organic causes of enuresis include diabetes mellitus, diabetes insipidus, bladder outlet obstruction, small bladder capacity, detrusor instability, urethral valves, meatal stenosis, cerebral palsy, spina bifida, pelvic mass, impacted stool, sedating medications, nocturnal seizures.

WORKUP

- History and physical examination to rule out anatomic abnormalities. Fluid intake and voiding diaries may be useful.
- Children frequently experience shame, so gentleness and care must be exercised when questioning or examining the child.
- Observation of voiding stream is useful.

LABORATORY TESTS

- Urinalysis with specific gravity and urine culture if white cells or nitrites on analysis.
- Serum studies to rule out diabetes, electrolyte abnormalities, or renal dysfunction.

IMAGING STUDIES

- In complicated cases, sleep studies may be useful.
- If an anatomic abnormality suspected, renal ultrasound or intravenous pyelogram is possibly indicated; MRI of the spine if evidence of abnormalities of lower spine or perineum is found on examination.

TREATMENT

NONPHARMACOLOGIC THERAPY

Behavioral treatment:
- Alarm and pad technique: up to 80% cure rate, although 30% relapse.
- Scheduled voiding to reduce the frequency of enuretic episodes.
- Star charts to reward child for dry nights.
- Punishment for enuresis is not effective.

ACUTE GENERAL Rx

- Desmopressin (DDAVP) administered orally (intranasal preparation associated with greater risk for water intoxication and not recommended) at bedtime significantly reduces the incidence of bedwetting.
- Tricyclic antidepressants (imipramine): efficacy supported by randomized control trials. Use with care in children.
- Serotonin reuptake inhibitors: lack of adequate trials is notable.
- Indomethacin suppositories may reduce normal prostaglandin inhibitory effects on antidiuretic hormone.
- Table 1-146 summarizes medications commonly used for treatment of monosymptomatic nocturnal enuresis. Fig. 1-316 describes an algorithm for management of pediatric enuresis and voiding dysfunction.

DISPOSITION

- After age 5 yr, the rate of spontaneous remissions is approximately 12% to 15% per year.
- The disorder usually resolves by adolescence. However, effective treatment spares considerable misery.
- Fewer than 1% will have enuresis as adults.

TABLE 1-146   Medications for Treatment of Monosymptomatic Nocturnal Enuresis

Generic Name (Trade Name)	Dosage Formulation	Dosage Regimen	Mechanisms of Action	Comments
Desmopressin acetate (DDAVP)	Nasal spray pump: 10 µg/0.1 ml spray Tablets: 0.1 mg, 0.2 mg	1 spray (10 µg) per nostril qhs, increasing to 40 µg 0.2 mg PO qhs, increasing up to 0.6 mg	Decreased urine volume Possible effect on sleep arousal through its action as a central nervous system neurotransmitter	Can cause nasal irritation; risk of water intoxication (headache, seizures); hence, restrict fluids 3 hr before the dose
Imipramine hydrochloride (Tofranil)	Tablets: 10 mg, 25 mg, 50 mg; Tofranil PM capsule 75, 100, 125, 150 mg	1.5–2 mg/kg 2 hr before bedtime, not to exceed 2.5 mg/kg or 75 mg max	Anticholinergic effect on bladder Increased resistance of bladder outlet Possible central inhibition of micturition reflex Possible effect on sleep arousal by central noradrenergic facilitation	Can cause sleep disturbance, mood alteration, decreased appetite Risk of cardiac arrhythmia with overdose

Modified from Chandra MM: Enuresis and voiding dysfunction. In Burg FD et al (eds): *Current pediatric therapy*, ed 18, Philadelphia, 2006, Saunders.

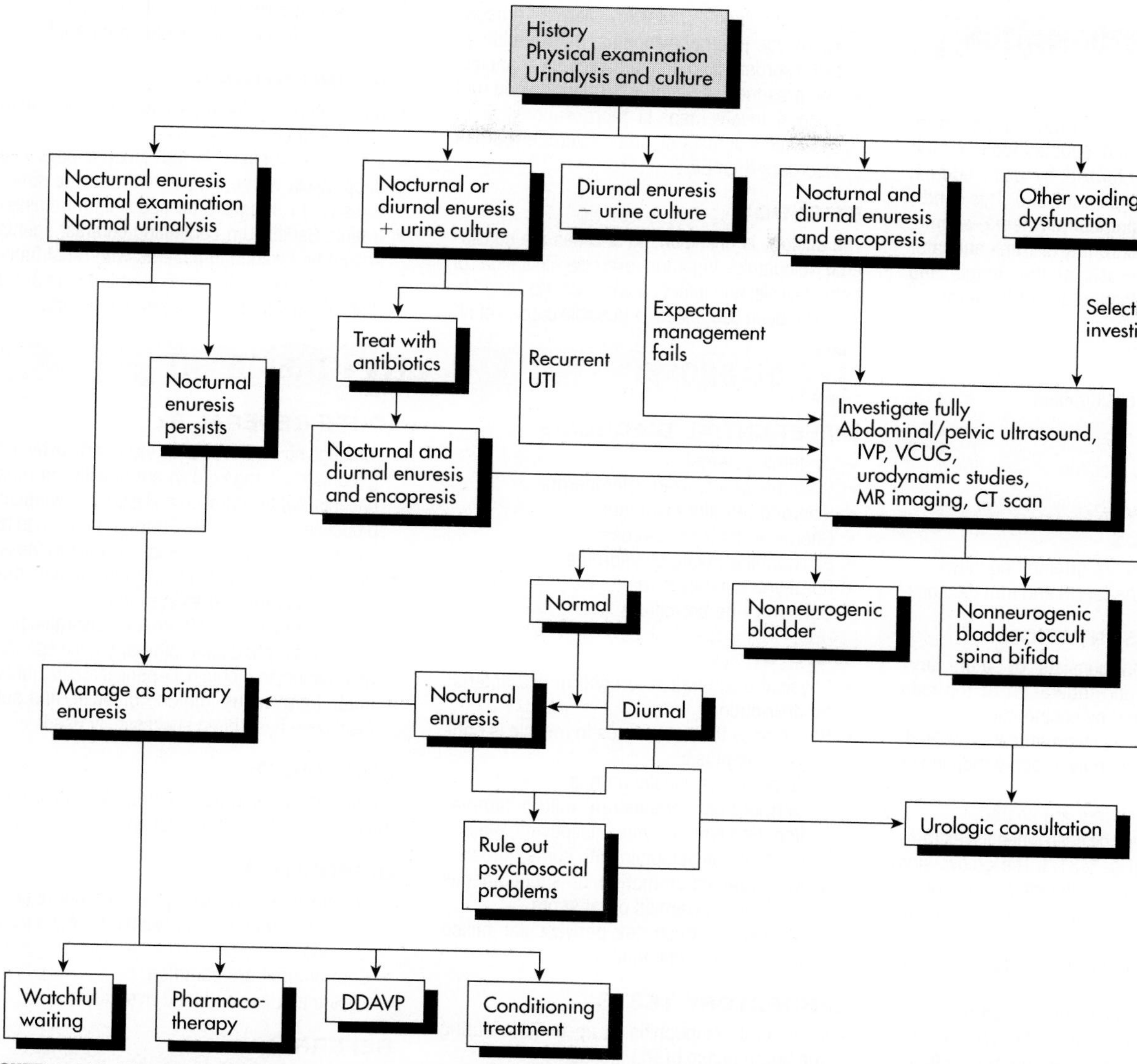

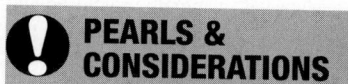

FIGURE 1-316 Algorithm of management of pediatric enuresis and voiding dysfunction. *CT,* Computed tomography; *DDAVP,* desmopressin acetate; *IVP,* intravenous pyelogram; *MR,* magnetic resonance; *UTI,* urinary tract infection; *VCUG,* voiding cystourethrogram. (From Nseyo UO [ed]: *Urology for primary care physicians,* Philadelphia, 1999, Saunders.)

REFERRAL

If coexisting, a psychiatric condition complicates the course of treatment.

PEARLS & CONSIDERATIONS

Illness, hospitalization, and family stressors may precipitate recurrent enuresis after a period of dryness.

PATIENT & FAMILY EDUCATION

Bedwetting: Jasper to the Rescue! video available from Disney Educational Productions (http://dep.disney.go.com/educational/index)

SUGGESTED READINGS

available at www.expertconsult.com

RELATED CONTENT

Bedwetting (Patient Information)

AUTHORS: **GREGORY K. FRITZ, M.D.,** and **MITCHELL D. FELDMAN, M.D., M.PHIL.**

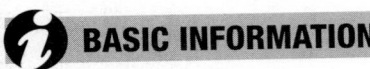

DEFINITION

Eosinophilic fasciitis (EF) is a rare inflammatory disease of the skin and subcutaneous tissue that is initially characterized by pain, edema, and eosinophilia in peripheral blood. This condition starts with symmetrical erythema, edema, and induration of an extremity or trunk and later may progress to sclerosis of the dermis and subcutaneous fascia leading to contractures.

SYNONYMS

Shulman's syndrome
Diffuse fasciitis with eosinophilia

ICD-9CM CODES
728.89 Eosinophilic fasciitis

EPIDEMIOLOGY & DEMOGRAPHICS

- Males and females are affected equally.
- Most common in the fourth and fifth decades.

CLINICAL PRESENTATION

- Initial presentation consists of acute erythema, swelling, and induration of the skin that is accompanied by eosinophilia.
  - Extremities usually symmetrically involved.
  - Upper more commonly affected than lower extremities.
  - Face, hands, and feet are spared.
  - Sunken veins may be seen when the extremity is elevated (Fig. 1-317). The groove sign marks the borders of different muscle groups.
  - Skin may appear deeply rippled (peau d'orange).
- Arthritis was found in 40% of cases in one series.
- Cranial and peripheral neuropathy (carpal tunnel syndrome, mononeuritis multiplex) may occur.
- Myalgia and weakness are common. Inflammatory myositis is uncommon.
- Hematologic abnormalities other than eosinophilia are present in 10% of cases in one

series, including aplastic anemia, amegakaryocytic thrombocytopenia, myeloproliferative disorders, and hematologic malignancies.
- The presence of Raynaud's phenomenon and visceral involvement is more suggestive of systemic sclerosis or other scleroderma-like disorders than EF.

ETIOLOGY

The etiology is unknown. Most cases are considered idiopathic. Vigorous exercise, initiation of hemodialysis, and infection with *Borrelia burgdorferi* have been suggested as possible causes of EF.

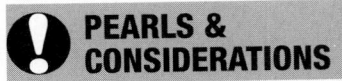

DIAGNOSIS

DIFFERENTIAL DIAGNOSIS

- Systemic sclerosis
- Systemic or localized scleroderma
- Scleroderma-like disorders
- Chemical-induced sclerosis
- Eosinophilia-myalgia syndrome
- Porphyria cutanea tarda
- Chronic Lyme borreliosis

WORKUP

- Physical examination to confirm characteristic distribution.
- Skin biopsy that penetrates to muscle is optimal for diagnosis:
  - Epidermis is usually normal.
  - Dermis may demonstrate mild inflammation with lymphocytes, histiocytes, plasma cells, and eosinophils with some fibrosis.
  - Moderate inflammation of subcutaneous tissue and sclerosis of fat septa.
  - Muscle demonstrates perivascular mixed inflammatory cell infiltrate.

LABORATORY TESTS

- Peripheral eosinophilia in up to 70% during the acute phase of the disease
- Elevated erythrocyte sedimentation rate (29%)
- Hypergammaglobulinemia (35%)
- Creatine kinase is usually normal even in patients with myalgia

- Occasional thrombocytopenia, anemia
- Serum antinuclear antibodies are negative

IMAGING STUDIES

- MRI may be useful in assessing patients with suspected EF.
- Increased T2 signal in the subcutaneous and deep fascia with enhancement of these structures on T1 images after gadolinium administration. Gadolinium-containing contrast agents should be avoided in patients with renal function impairment (GFR <15-30 ml/min) to avoid developing nephrogenic systemic fibrosis.

TREATMENT

ACUTE GENERAL Rx

- Although no controlled trials exist, corticosteroids (prednisone 1 mg/kg/day) are effective in most patients, but the duration and extent of symptom reduction are variable. From 3 to 6 months should be sufficient to assess the effectiveness.
- Hydroxychloroquine is an alternative that may be as effective as steroids.
- In resistant cases, methotrexate, psoralen plus ultraviolet A photochemotherapy, cyclosporine, antithymocyte globulin, D-penicillamine, infliximab, intravenous immune globulin, and sulfasalazine have been successfully used.

CHRONIC Rx

Surgery is sometimes required to reduce contractures and maintain function.

DISPOSITION

- Prognosis is generally good with not uncommon spontaneous regression and response to steroids.
- Contractures are common.
- 10% may develop blood dyscrasias.

REFERRAL

To dermatology for biopsy to make definitive diagnosis. Functional impairment requires surgical evaluation.

PEARLS & CONSIDERATIONS

COMMENTS

- EF is a rare inflammatory disorder of unknown etiology with symmetric painful edema and induration of the arms and legs with peripheral eosinophilia.
- Rapid onset, progression, and good response to systemic corticosteroids are characteristic of the disease.
- Prognosis is usually good.

SUGGESTED READINGS
available at www.expertconsult.com

AUTHOR: ETSUKO AOKI, M.D., PH.D.

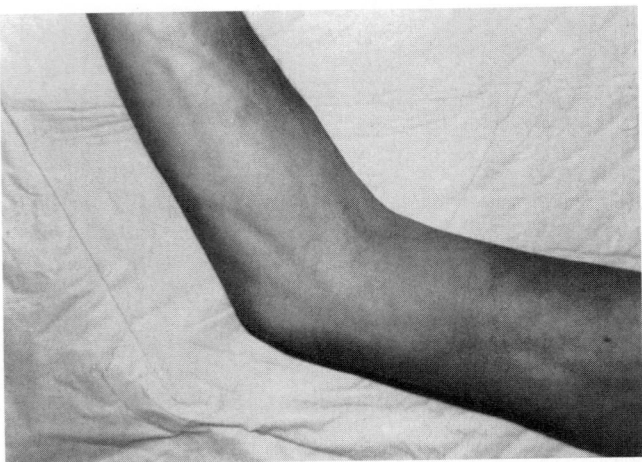

FIGURE 1-317 Eosinophilic fasciitis. This 29-year-old butcher had to stop working because of a generalized painful induration of his skin. Fingers were spared. As he raised his forearms, the collapsed veins appeared as grooves (the "groove sign"), which is pathognomonic of eosinophilic fasciitis. His condition subsided 4 years later, leaving joint contractures. (From Canoso J: *Rheumatology in primary care,* Philadelphia, 1997, Saunders.)

BASIC INFORMATION

DEFINITION

Eosinophilic pneumonias (EPs) are a group of disorders characterized by pulmonary infiltrates, pulmonary parenchymal eosinophilia, and possibly peripheral blood eosinophilia. They manifest by different radiologic and clinical syndromes.

SYNONYMS

Simple pulmonary eosinophilia
Chronic eosinophilic pneumonia
Acute eosinophilic pneumonia
Churg-Strauss syndrome
Idiopathic hypereosinophilic syndrome
Allergic bronchopulmonary aspergillosis
Parasite-induced, fungal-induced, and drug-induced pulmonary eosinophilia

ICD-9CM CODES
518.3 Eosinophilic pneumonia

EPIDEMIOLOGY & DEMOGRAPHICS

Vary depending on the specific cause

PHYSICAL FINDINGS & CLINICAL PRESENTATION

- Fever, cough, and shortness of breath
- Vary depending on the specific cause

ETIOLOGY

SIMPLE PULMONARY EOSINOPHILIA (LÖFFLER'S SYNDROME):

- Transient pulmonary infiltrates
- Symptoms range from asymptomatic to dyspnea and dry cough
- Usually idiopathic
- May be secondary to parasitic infection or drugs (nitrofurantoin, penicillin)
- Remove the offending agent
- If idiopathic and severe symptoms, then give glucocorticoid therapy

IDIOPATHIC ACUTE EP:

- Absence of infection or other cause
- Acute onset of fever, cough, dyspnea (<1 mo); often presents with acute respiratory failure, requiring intensive care
- Erythrocyte sedimentation rate (ESR), C-reactive protein (CRP), and IgE may be elevated but nonspecific
- Bilateral diffuse infiltrates on chest radiograph
- High-resolution CT scan of the chest may demonstrate patchy ground glass with reticular infiltrates; small pleural effusions present in two thirds of cases
- Pleural fluid analysis reveals elevated pH and high eosinophil count
- Hypoxemia (PaO$_2$ <60)
- Lung eosinophilia >25% on bronchoalveolar lavage (BAL)
- Pulmonary function test can demonstrate restrictive dysfunction with reduction in diffusion capacity
- Associations: recent onset of tobacco smoking, World Trade Center dust, Scotchguard

inhalation, tear gas, gasoline, indoor renovation work, multiple medications, firework smoke, cocaine
- Steroids lead to rapid improvement, though there is no consensus about ideal dosing strategy

IDIOPATHIC CHRONIC EP:

- Absence of infection or other cause
- Presentation over weeks to months
- Productive cough, dyspnea, malaise, weight loss, night sweats, and fever (with or without hemoptysis/chest pain)
- Progressive pulmonary infiltrates
- "Photographic negative" pulmonary edema (peripheral alveolar infiltrates) is pathognomonic but only present in 25% of cases; high-resolution CT of the chest may reveal atelectasis, pleural effusions, lymphadenopathy, and septal line thickening
- Blood eosinophilia not always present
- ESR, CRP, platelets, and IgE may be elevated but are nonspecific
- Diagnose by BAL (up to 90% of cases will have 60% eosinophils) or lung biopsy
- Spontaneous remission in 10% of cases
- Treatment with glucocorticoids is rapidly effective
- Relapses are common when glucocorticoids tapered
- Prevalence of patients with asthma

ALLERGIC BRONCHOPULMONARY ASPERGILLOSIS (ABPA):

- Hypersensitivity reaction to *Aspergillus fumigatus*
- Occurs most often in patients with asthma and atopy (up to 13% of the asthma population)

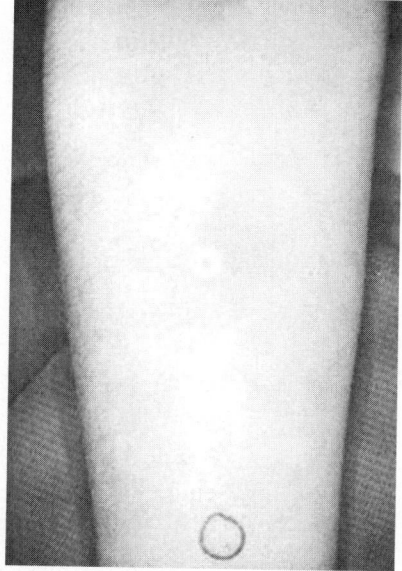

FIGURE 1-318 A positive prick test with *Aspergillus fumigatus* in a patient with allergic bronchopulmonary aspergillosis. The wheal and erythema reaction at 15 min after performing the skin test. (From Fireman P: *Atlas of allergies and immunology*, ed 3, St Louis, 2006, Mosby.)

- Fever, flulike symptoms, myalgias, lassitude, persistent cough and wheezing, hemoptysis, and/or expectoration of brown-black mucous plugs
- A patient with chronic asthma with a component of bronchiectasis and pulmonary infiltrates should be evaluated carefully for ABPA
- Chest radiograph: infiltrates (sometimes migratory) and atelectasis, reflecting endobronchial mucous inspissation ("finger in glove")
- Blood and sputum eosinophilia
- Diagnosis by
  1. *Aspergillus* isolation from multiple sputum samples
  2. Positive skin test to *Aspergillus* (Fig. 1-318)
  3. Elevated serum IgE
  4. *Aspergillus*-specific IgE and IgG
  5. Serum eosinophilia >1000 cells/μL

The disease has been characterized by a staging system:
Patients do not necessarily proceed from one stage to another.

Stage I	Acute phase
Stage II	Remission
Stage III	Exacerbation
Stage IV	Glucocorticoid-dependent ABPA
Stage V	End-stage (fibrotic) ABPA

- Treatment: systemic corticosteroids are the mainstay of treatment. Antifungals may provide additional benefit in modulating airway fungal burden and are recommended for use in patients with relapse or glucocorticoid-dependent disease
- Development of bronchiectasis portends a worse prognosis
- Response to therapy and activity of disease may be monitored by measuring IgE levels, which will decrease by 35% to 50% when a patient is in remission

TROPICAL PULMONARY EOSINOPHILIA:

- Onset of asthma, fever, paroxysmal cough and bronchospasm, marked blood eosinophilia
- Basilar reticulonodular and alveolar infiltrates
- High serum IgE levels
- Presumed etiology: filariasis

PULMONARY VASCULITIS (ALLERGIC GRANULOMATOSIS AND ANGIITIS OR CHURG-STRAUSS SYNDROME):

- Vasculitis and necrotizing granulomatous inflammation that involves many organ systems in the setting of asthma
- Blood eosinophilia and elevated IgE
- Antineutrophilic cytoplasmic antibody may be positive in up to two thirds of patients; antinuclear antibody, rheumatoid factor, and ESR also may be elevated
- Common symptoms include cough, dyspnea, sinusitis, allergic rhinitis; other symptoms depend on other organs involved
- Pulmonary function test may reveal obstructive dysfunction
- Organ and systems involved include lungs, heart (including refractory coronary vasospasm), skin, gastrointestinal, renal, neurologic

HYPEREOSINOPHILIC SYNDROME:

- A disease of persistently elevated eosinophils (>6 mo) with no known cause

- Cardiac problems are the prominent clinical feature with mural thrombi and endocardial/myocardial fibrosis
- Hepatosplenomegaly is common
- Fever, cough, weight loss, wheezing, CNS abnormalities
- May have a myeloproliferative or a lymphocytic etiology
- Diagnosis of exclusion
- Check echocardiogram
- Treat with steroids if symptoms or cardiac abnormalities
- Several potential targets for treatment are currently under investigation, including IL-5, IL5-R, CD2 binding protein, IgE, and IL-4/IL-13 receptor.

DRUG- OR TOXIN-INDUCED EP:

- Can have several different clinical presentations, including simple pulmonary eosinophilia, chronic, or acute
- Symptoms resolve when offending drug is removed
- Described causes of drug/toxin-induced EP: antibiotics, NSAIDs, amiodarone, bleomycin, captopril, gold salts, iodine, methotrexate, venlafaxine, daptomycin, benzbromarone, smoke, illicit drugs, radiation exposure
- BAL to exclude infection or other lung disease
- Laboratory evaluation rarely diagnostic

Dx DIAGNOSIS

- Diagnosis varies depending on specific cause of pneumonia.
- Usually involves chest radiograph, CT, peripheral eosinophil count, BAL, and possibly lung biopsy.

DIFFERENTIAL DIAGNOSIS

- Tuberculosis
- Brucellosis
- Fungal diseases
- Parasitic infection *(Ascaris, Strongyloides)*
- Idiopathic pulmonary fibrosis
- Bronchiolitis obliterans and organizing pneumonia
- Radiation pneumonitis
- Bronchogenic carcinoma
- Hodgkin's disease
- Immunoblastic lymphadenopathy
- Rheumatoid lung disease
- Sarcoidosis

WORKUP

Physical examination, laboratory tests, imaging, bronchoscopy

LABORATORY TESTS

- WBC counts are often normal
- Often blood eosinophilia
- Elevated eosinophil count on BAL

IMAGING STUDIES

Chest radiograph may show a variety of infiltrates depending on the cause of EP. CT demonstrates a more characteristic pattern and distribution of parenchymal opacities than chest radiograph.

Rx TREATMENT

- Varies depending on the cause.
- Remove offending agent or treat with appropriate antibiotic.

- Steroids may be helpful in many cases; doses and length of treatment depend on etiology of symptoms and response to treatment.
- Supportive respiratory care.

DISPOSITION

Prognosis is good if offending agent can be removed or an infectious etiology treated. Glucocorticoids have a good effect, but relapse often recurs with tapering in chronic idiopathic cases.

REFERRAL

To pulmonologist if a BAL or lung biopsy is needed to establish the diagnosis

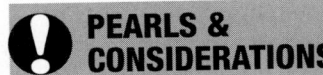 **PEARLS & CONSIDERATIONS**

- History (including travel) and physical examination are most important. Temporal association of eosinophilia and pulmonary abnormalities is an important diagnostic clue.
- Coccidioidomycosis and *Aspergillus* can present as eosinophilic lung disease and are important to recognize because steroid therapy can produce progressive infection.
- *Aspergillus* from respiratory specimens does not always indicate true infection and may be colonization.
- Blood eosinophilia $>1 \times 10^9$ eosinophils/L or BAL $>25\%$ is helpful in narrowing diagnosis.
- Integrating the clinical, radiologic, and pathologic findings facilitates the initial and differential diagnoses of various eosinophilic lung diseases.

SUGGESTED READINGS

available at www.expertconsult.com

RELATED CONTENT

Churg-Strauss Syndrome (Related Key Topic)
Aspergillosis (Related Key Topic)

AUTHOR: **KRISTINA KRAMER, M.D.**

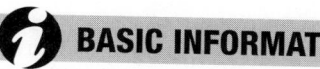

BASIC INFORMATION

DEFINITION

Epicondylitis is inflammation (tendinosis) of the myotendinous junction of the common extensors at the lateral epicondyle or the flexor pronator group at the medial epicondyle of the elbow.

SYNONYMS

Tennis elbow (lateral epicondylitis)
Golfer's elbow (medial epicondylitis)
Elbow tendinosis
Elbow tendinopathy
Epicondylalgia
Elbow tendinitis

ICD-9CM CODES
726.31 Medial epicondylitis
726.32 Lateral epicondylitis
723.4   Radial nerve neuralgia

EPIDEMIOLOGY & DEMOGRAPHICS

PREVALENCE:
- Prevalence is 1% to 3% in the general population.
  - Tennis players who play >2 hr a day have a two to four times greater risk of developing epicondylitis compared with general population.
- The lateral side is involved more often than the medial.

PREVALENT AGE AND SEX:
- Affects women more often than men.
- More common in individuals 40 to 60 years old.

PHYSICAL FINDINGS & CLINICAL PRESENTATION

- Main symptom is of pain in lateral or medial elbow.
  - Pain is typically related to activity.
  - Local tenderness is experienced over the affected epicondyle.
- Pain can be reproduced by administering a forced elbow extension test (Fig. 1-319), offering resistance against wrist extension (Fig. 1-320), or inducing flexion in the affected area.

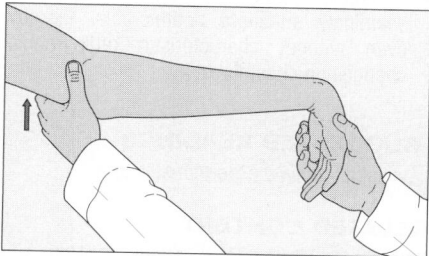

FIGURE 1-319 Forced elbow extension test. (From Hochberg MC et al: *Rheumatology,* ed 5, St Louis, 2011, Mosby.)

ETIOLOGY

- Epicondylitis is thought to be secondary to a chronic tendinosis rather than an acute inflammatory process.
- Overuse likely causes tendinous micro-tears, resulting in inflammation, degeneration, immature repair, and tendinosis.
- Disorganization of normal collagen by invading fibroblasts in association with an immature vascular reparative response and the absence of inflammatory cells is termed angiofibroblastic tendinosis.

DIAGNOSIS

DIFFERENTIAL DIAGNOSIS

- Cervical radiculopathy.
- Intra-articular elbow pathology (osteoarthritis, osteochondritis dissecans, loose body).
- Radial tunnel syndrome (compression of the posterior interosseous nerve).
- Cubital tunnel syndrome (compression of the median nerve).
- Medial collateral ligament instability.
  - Thoracic outlet syndrome.
  - Ulnar neuritis.
  - Valgus extension overload.

IMAGING STUDIES

- Plain radiography is useful to evaluate osteoarthritis, osteochondrosis dissecans, or other bony abnormalities.
- Musculoskeletal (MSK) ultrasonography is not very sensitive; epicondylitis appears as a thickening or thinning of the tendon, as well as decreased echogenecity and poor definition of tendon.
- Magnetic resonance imaging (MRI) is the gold standard in detecting epicondylitis. MRI is the most sensitive test, showing tendon thickening and high T2 signal intensity.

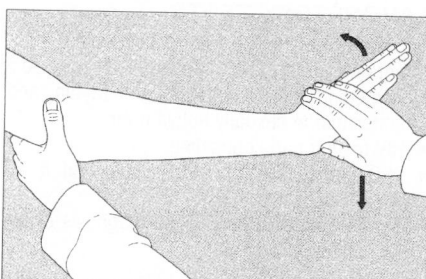

FIGURE 1-320 Resisted wrist extension to test for lateral epicondylitis. The examiner asks the patient to try to extend the wrist but prevents movement by fixing the wrist; this puts tension on the lateral epicondyle without moving the elbow and reproduces the pain of lateral epicondylitis. (From Klippel J et al [eds]: *Primary care rheumatology,* London, 1999, Mosby.)

TREATMENT

- Rest, restricted activities, and proper technique during sports activities.
- Nonsteroidal anti-inflammatory drugs (NSAIDs) can be used topically or orally but usually provide only short-term relief.
- Local steroid/lidocaine injection.
- Counterforce brace/wrist orthoses.
- Acupuncture has been found to be beneficial in some cases.
- Physical therapy and eccentric exercise provides short-term relief.
  - Injection of botulinum toxin A at the myotendinous junction has been found to be helpful in a small randomized-control trial.
- Patients with refractory symptoms after 6 months of nonoperative management may benefit from surgical intervention.

DISPOSITION

- Epicondylitis is self-limited in most cases. Resolution of symptoms may take months to years.
- Prognosis is worse in the following conditions:
  - The dominant hand is involved
  - Patient experiences high physical strain at work
  - Duration of symptoms is more than 3 months
  - Patient experiences severe pain at presentation and concomitant neck pain.

REFERRAL

If symptoms do not respond to injections or a 6-month trial of conservative therapy, surgical referral is appropriate.

SUGGESTED READINGS
available at www.expertconsult.com

RELATED CONTENT

Epicondylitis (Tennis Elbow, Golfer's Elbow) (Patient Information)

AUTHOR: **WAFFIYAH AFRIDI, M.D.**

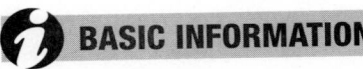

BASIC INFORMATION

DEFINITION

- Epididymitis is an inflammatory reaction of the epididymis caused by either an infectious agent or local trauma. In most cases of acute epididymitis, the testis is also involved (orchitis).
- Epididymitis is considered chronic if lasting ≥6 wk. Chronic epididymitis has been subcategorized into inflammatory chronic epididymitis, obstructive chronic epididymitis, and chronic epididymalgia.

SYNONYMS

Nonspecific bacterial epididymitis
Sexually transmitted epididymitis

ICD-9CM CODES
604 Orchitis and epididymitis

EPIDEMIOLOGY & DEMOGRAPHICS

INCIDENCE (IN U.S.): Cause of >600,000 visits to physicians per year
PEAK INCIDENCE: Sexually active years
PREDOMINANT SEX: Exclusive to males
PREDOMINANT AGE: All ages affected but usually in sexually active men or older males
CONGENITAL: Congenital urologic structural disorders possibly predisposing to infections

PHYSICAL FINDINGS & CLINICAL PRESENTATION

- Tender swelling of the scrotum with erythema, usually unilateral testicular pain and tenderness
- Dysuria and/or urethral discharge
- Fever and signs of systemic illness (less common)
- Pain and redness on scrotal examination
- Hydrocele or even epididymoorchitis, especially late
- Chronic draining scrotal sinuses with a "beadlike" enlargement of the vas deferens in tuberculous disease

ETIOLOGY

- In young, sexually active men (<35 years of age), the most common infectious agents isolated are *N. gonorrhoeae* and *Chlamydia trachomatis.*
- In older men (>35 years of age) or with underlying urologic disease:
  1. Gram-negative aerobic rods are predominant (i.e., *E. coli*).
  2. Similar organisms are found in men following invasive urologic procedures.
  3. Gram-positive cocci are rarely seen in these groups.
  4. Mycobacteria may also be a cause of epididymitis.
- Young, prepubertal boys may present with epididymitis caused by coliform bacteria; almost always a complication of underlying urologic disease such as reflux.
- In AIDS patients, CMV and *Salmonella* epididymitis have been described. CMV may have a negative urine culture. Toxoplasmosis

and *Cryptococcus* should also be considered as a cause of epididymitis in AIDS patients.
- Chronic infectious epididymitis is mostly frequently seen in conditions associated with granulomatous reaction; mycobacterium tuberculosis is the most common granulomatous disease affecting the epididymis.

DIAGNOSIS

DIFFERENTIAL DIAGNOSIS

- Orchitis
- Testicular torsion, trauma, or tumor
- Epididymal cyst
- Hydrocele
- Varicocele
- Spermatocele
- Testicular torsion should be considered in all cases.

WORKUP

- Consideration of a full assessment of the urologic tract in patients with bacterial infection, especially if recurrent
- If discharge is present, cultures and Gram stain smear of urethral exudate. Gram stain will demonstrate ≥5 WBC per oil immersion field.
- In sexually active men: gonococcal cultures of the throat and rectum possibly of value
- If testicular torsion a consideration: radionuclear imaging
- Examination of first void uncentrifuged urine for leukocytes if the urethral Gram stain is negative. Positive leukocyte esterase test on first-void urine or microscopic examination of first-void urine sediment will demonstrate ≥10 WBC per high power field. A culture and Gram-stained smear of this urine specimen should be obtained along with nucleic acid amplification studies (ligase chain reaction [LCR]) from urine samples for gonorrhea and *Chlamydia* spp.
- Imaging with sonogram

LABORATORY TESTS

- Urinalysis and urine culture if dysuria is present or if urinary tract infection is suspected
- Screening test for syphilis, chlamydia, and gonorrhea in sexually active men
- HIV testing and counseling
- PPD placed and chest x-ray viewed if TB suspected (rare cases)
- Rarely, biopsy to assure the diagnosis of tuberculous epididymitis

TREATMENT

ACUTE GENERAL Rx

- Ice packs and scrotal elevation for relief of pain
- Analgesia with acetaminophen with or without codeine or NSAIDs
- Antibiotics to cover suspected pathogens. Empiric therapy is indicated before laboratory test results are available.
- Recommended regimens are ceftriaxone 250 mg IM in a single dose plus doxycycline 100 mg bid for 10 days. For acute epididymitis

most likely caused by enteric organisms, treatment options are levofloxacin 500 mg qd × 10 days or ofloxacin 300 mg bid × 10 days.
- Best treatment for older men with gram-negative bacteriuria: ofloxacin 300 mg PO bid for 10 days or levofloxacin 500 mg PO qd for 10 days
- *Pseudomonas* covered by ciprofloxacin PO or IV or cefepime (2 g IV q12h)
- Consider ampicillin-sulbactam, 3rd-generation cephalosporin, ticarcillin-clavulanate, or piper-acillin-tazobactam in toxic-appearing patients.
- Surgical aspiration of local abscesses or even open surgical drainage
- Diabetics: especially prone to develop more extensive scrotal infections, including Fournier's gangrene
- Reinforcement of compliance with antibiotics to avoid partial treatment

CHRONIC Rx

- Repair of underlying structural defects is considered especially if infections are severe or recur.
- Surgical repair of reflux in young boys should be undertaken promptly and at a young age when possible.
- Sex partners of patient should be referred for evaluation and treatment.

DISPOSITION

Usually self-limited (≤6 wk duration in most cases)

REFERRAL

- If abscess or chronic structural problems suspected
- If another diagnosis, such as testicular torsion, is suspected

PEARLS & CONSIDERATIONS

- Recurrent epididymitis in sexually active men is usually related to failure to simultaneously treat sexual partners for STDs.
- Recurrent epididymitis in non-sexually active men is generally related to structural-anatomic defects in the genitourinary system or relapsing disease from inadequate initial treatment or antimicrobial resistance.
- Tuberculous epididymitis fails to respond to seemingly adequate antimicrobial therapy even without characteristic radiographic changes on chest films.

SUGGESTED READINGS
available at www.expertconsult.com

RELATED CONTENT
Epididymitis (Patient Information)

AUTHORS: **PHILIP A. CHAN, M.D., M.S.,** and **GLENN G. FORT, M.D., M.P.H.**

ⓘ BASIC INFORMATION

DEFINITION
The accumulation of blood in the potential space surrounding the brain, between the dura mater and the inner surface of the skull

SYNONYMS
Extradural hematoma/hemorrhage

ICD-9CM CODES
432.0 Nontraumatic extradural hemorrhage
852.5 Extradural hemorrhage following injury without intracranial wound
852.5 Extradural hemorrhage following injury with open intracranial wound

EPIDEMIOLOGY & DEMOGRAPHICS
INCIDENCE: Exact incidence is unknown; however, it is found in 1% to 4% of traumatic head injury cases and 5% to 15% of autopsy series.
PREDOMINANT SEX AND AGE: Male > female
PEAK INCIDENCE: Peak incidence among adolescents and young adults
GENETICS: There is a role for genetics in spontaneous (nontraumatic) epidural hematoma caused by coagulopathies and vascular malformations.
RISK FACTORS: Head trauma associated with skull fracture

PHYSICAL FINDINGS & CLINICAL PRESENTATION
- History of head trauma is present.
- Transient loss of consciousness, followed by a "lucid interval" in 47% of cases, where the patient is free of any neurologic signs or symptoms. This is followed by clinical deterioration.
- Signs and symptoms vary depending on severity.
- Symptoms: headache, vomiting, drowsiness, confusion, aphasia, seizures, paralysis, and even coma are found.
- Signs: external signs of skull fracture—lacerations, ecchymoses, cerebrospinal fluid (CSF) rhinorrhea or otorrhea are observed.
- Altered mental status, nuchal rigidity, photophobia, focal neurologic deficit—paralysis of one limb, unequal pupils, decerebrate posture, coma—are seen.

ETIOLOGY
- Traumatic: commonly caused by arterial injury (the middle meningeal artery) but may also be injury of the anterior meningeal artery, a dural arteriovenous (AV) fistula at the vertex, or from venous bleeding
- Nontraumatic: caused by an infection/eroding abscess, coagulopathy, hemorrhagic tumors, vascular malformations, postsurgical procedures, and in special populations (e.g., pregnant women, patients receiving hemodialysis)

ⒹⓍ DIAGNOSIS

DIFFERENTIAL DIAGNOSIS
In the setting of head trauma: subdural hematoma, subarachnoid hemorrhage, cerebral contusion, brain laceration, diffuse brain swelling

WORKUP
- Imaging is the mainstay of diagnosis.
- Serial head CT is the test most commonly used due to its simplicity, widespread use, and availability. Typical appearance is a "lens shaped," or "lentiform" hyperdensity (Fig. 1-321). Box 1-20 describes CT findings of epidural hematoma.
- NOTE: Head CT is not conclusive in 8% of cases due to severe anemia, early scanning, and severe hypotension.
- Brain MRI: more sensitive. Indicated in situations in which there is a strong clinical suspicion but no evidence of epidural hematoma on head CT (Fig. 1-322). Preferred in spinal as opposed to intracranial pathology due to higher resolution.

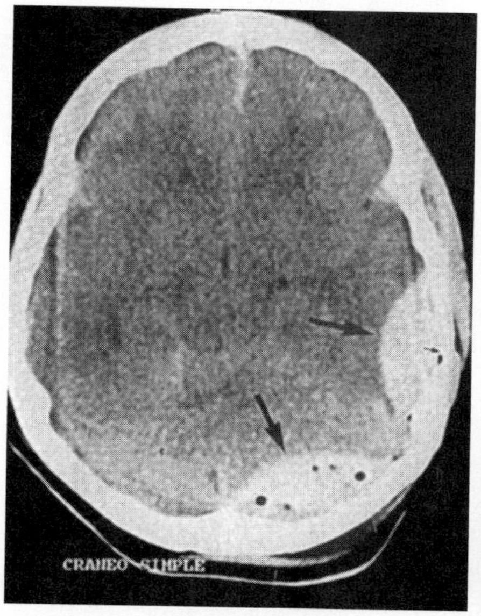

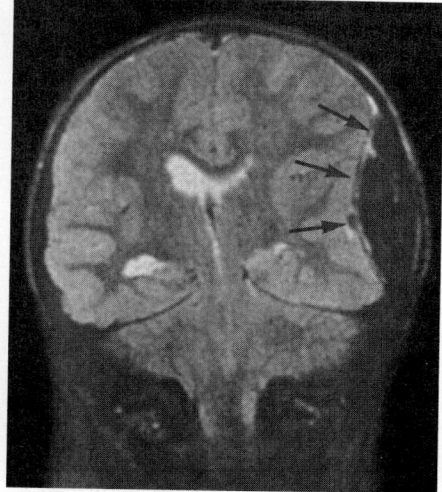

FIGURE 1-321 Head CT showing two epidural hematomas in 23-year-old involved in a motor vehicle accident. Note air bubbles that are a result of linear fracture in the left temporal bone *(short arrow)*.

- Angiography: rarely necessary but may be used to evaluate an underlying vascular lesion.
- NOTE: lumbar puncture (LP) is contraindicated in epidural hematoma due to risk of brain stem herniation.

LABORATORY TESTS
- Laboratory tests are helpful as adjunct to diagnosis but are not the mainstay of diagnosis or treatment.
- CBC may be helpful to evaluate for anemia.
- Other tests: renal functions, electrolytes, liver functions, INR may be helpful depending on the case scenario.

ⓇⓍ TREATMENT

Acute symptomatic epidural hematoma is a neurologic emergency that requires surgical treatment to prevent permanent brain injury.

NONPHARMACOLOGIC THERAPY
- Immediate surgical decompression
- Burr hole evacuation: this involves drilling a hole in the skull to evacuate the hematoma. It is a lifesaving procedure that is indicated if surgical expertise is limited.
- Craniotomy and hematoma evacuation remains the mainstay of treatment. When indicated, identification and ligation of the bleeding vessel.

FIGURE 1-322 Epidural hematoma on MRI. Coronal T2-weighted images show hypointense biconvex extraaxial collection in the left temporal region.

BOX 1-20   CT Findings of Epidural Hematoma

- CT appearance: variable white to gray on brain windows
- Location: peripheral to brain, variable but usually temporal region
- Shape: biconvex disc or lens
- Pearl: does not cross suture lines
- White swirl sign means active bleeding

- Significance: may cause mass effect and herniation
- Look for midline shift
- Look for effacement of ventricles and sulci
- Surgical indications: 15-mm thickness or 5-mm midline shift

From Broder JS: *Diagnostic imaging for the emergency physician*, Philadelphia, 2011, Saunders.

ACUTE GENERAL Rx

- Cardiopulmonary resuscitation and assessment for disability.
- Medical resuscitation maneuvers: head elevation, hyperventilation, monitoring of vital signs and avoidance of hypotension and hyperthermia, sedation if necessary.
- Medications: osmotic diuresis with IV mannitol, cerebrosedating medications, antiepileptics may be used to treat or, in some situations, prevent seizures.
- Reversing anticoagulation should be weighed in terms of advantages versus disadvantages.
- NOTE: glucocorticoid therapy is *not* indicated following head injury and may be related to increased mortality.
- Evaluation for surgery: the best available evidence points toward advantages of decompression procedures. Nonoperative treatment may only be indicated if the patient has no symptoms, no focal neurologic deficit, no coma (Glasgow coma score >8), and epidural hematoma volume is less than 30 ml by CT scan, with clot thickness <15 mm and midline shift of less than 5 mm.
- Nonoperative treatment involves close monitoring, hourly neurologic checks, and serial head CT scans.

CHRONIC Rx

- There is a risk of permanent brain damage whether the disorder is treated or not. Most recovery occurs in the first 6 months with some improvement over 2 years.
- Children recover more quickly.
- Patients should be educated on rehabilitative exercises and to alert medical professionals in the event of new neurologic symptoms.
- Support and encouragement to patient and family should always be provided.

REFERRAL

Clinical nurse practitioners, pastoral care staff, and social workers to help patients and families are also appropriate.

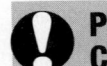 **PEARLS & CONSIDERATIONS**

- Acute symptomatic epidural hematoma is a neurologic emergency.
- Epidural hematoma should be suspected in any patient with a history of blow to the head leading to a period of loss of consciousness.
- Initial resuscitation is extremely important, but surgery is the mainstay of treatment for acute symptomatic epidural hematoma.

PREVENTION

Should be directed toward preventing head trauma: use of appropriate safety equipment (e.g., helmets, hard hats, safe driving, avoiding to dive into unknown depths)

PATIENT/FAMILY EDUCATION

Online head injury support groups are helpful: www.headinjury.com/linktbisup.htm, www.headinjury.com/, www.dailystrength.org/c/Brain-Injury/support-group.

SUGGESTED READINGS

available at www.expertconsult.com

AUTHORS: **JEFFREY BORKAN, M.D., Ph.D.,** and **HODA ELTOMI, M.D.**

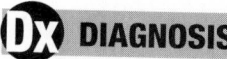

BASIC INFORMATION

DEFINITION

Epiglottitis is a rapidly progressive cellulitis of the epiglottis and adjacent soft tissue structures with the potential to cause abrupt airway obstruction.

SYNONYMS

Supraglottitis
Cherry-red epiglottitis

ICD-9CM CODES
464.30 Epiglottitis

EPIDEMIOLOGY

INCIDENCE (IN U.S.): Highest in young children, 2 to 4 yr
INCIDENCE (IN U.S.): Unknown
PEAK INCIDENCE: Peaks in young boys ages 2 to 4 yr, but it is reported in adults as well
PREDOMINANT SEX: Males

PHYSICAL FINDINGS & CLINICAL PRESENTATION

- Irritability, fever, dysphonia, and dysphagia
- Respiratory distress, with child tending to lean up and forward
- Often, drooling or oral secretions
- Often, presence of tachycardia and tachypnea
- On visualization, edematous and cherry-red epiglottis
- Often, no classic barking cough as seen in croup
- Possibly fulminant course (especially in children), leading to complete airway obstruction

ETIOLOGY

- In children, *Haemophilus influenzae* type b (rare), *Streptococcus pyogenes*, *Streptococcus pneumoniae*, *Staphylococcus aureus* (includes MRSA)
- In adults, group A *Streptococcus, H. influenzae* (can be isolated from blood and/or epiglottis [about 26% of cases])
- Pneumococci, streptococci, and staphylococci are also implicated.
- Role of viruses in epiglottitis unclear.

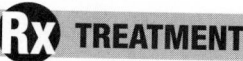

DIAGNOSIS

DIFFERENTIAL DIAGNOSIS

- Croup
- Angioedema
- Retropharyngeal or peritonsillar abscess
- Diphtheria
- Foreign body aspiration
- Lingual tonsillitis

WORKUP

- Cultures of blood and urine
- Lateral neck radiograph to show an enlarged epiglottis, ballooning of the hypopharynx, and normal subglottic structures (Fig. 1-323)
  1. Radiographs are of only moderate sensitivity and specificity and take time to perform.
  2. Visualization of the epiglottis may be safer in adults than in children.
- Cultures of the epiglottis

LABORATORY TESTS

- CBC: may reveal a leukocytosis with a shift to the left
- Chest radiograph examination: may reveal evidence of pneumonia in close to 25% of cases
- Cultures of blood, urine, and the epiglottis, as noted previously

TREATMENT

ACUTE GENERAL Rx

- Maintenance of adequate airway is critical. Fig. E1-324 describes the optimal assessment and management of upper airway obstruction caused by epiglottitis or severe croup. It is crucial to have a tracheostomy set "at bedside."
- Early placement of an endotracheal or nasotracheal tube in a child is advised.
- Closely follow the adult patient, if no signs of airway obstruction, and defer intubation.
- In children, visualization and intubation are best done in the most controlled environment.
- *H. influenzae* in children is much less common in large part due to the HIB vaccine.
Empiric antibiotics:
  ○ **In children:** use cefotaxime 50 mg/kg IV q8h or ceftriaxone 50 mg/kg IV q24h *plus* vancomycin. If penicillin allergy, use levofloxacin 10 mg/kg IV q24h *plus* clindamycin 7.5 mg/kg IV q6h.
  ○ **In adults:** ceftriaxone 2 g IV q24h or cefotaxime *plus vancomycin*
- If possible, obtain cultures before initiating antibiotics.
- If there is an unvaccinated child at home (or in a day care center) who is >4 yr and living with an index case, give close family contacts of the patient (including adults) rifampin 20 mg/kg/day for 4 days (up to 600 mg/day) for prophylaxis.
- Role of epinephrine or corticosteroids in the management of epiglottitis is not firmly established.

DISPOSITION

Invasive *Haemophilus influenzae* infections and epiglottitis are reportable illnesses; this may be particularly important in recognizing an outbreak in a day care center with unvaccinated children.

REFERRAL

- Close cooperation between the pediatrician or internist, anesthesiologist, and otorhinolaryngologist, especially when epiglottis is visualized and when the patient requires endotracheal intubation
- Best managed in a critical care setting or ICU

PEARLS & CONSIDERATIONS

The incidence of epiglottitis has diminished markedly since the introduction of the conjugate vaccine against *H. influenzae* serotype B into routine childhood immunization.

SUGGESTED READINGS
available at www.expertconsult.com

RELATED CONTENT
Epiglottitis (Patient Information)

AUTHOR: **GLENN G. FORT, M.D., M.P.H.**

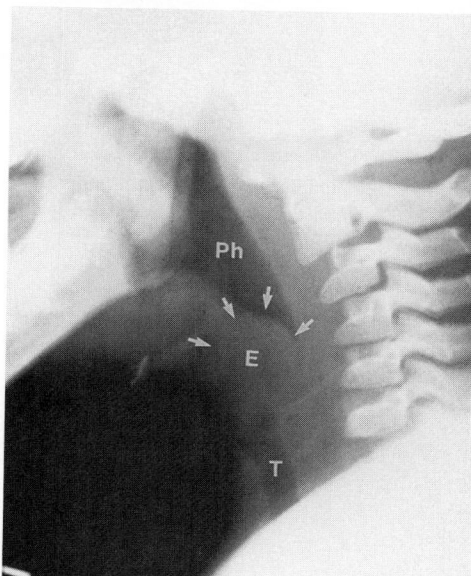

FIGURE 1-323 Epiglottitis. A lateral soft tissue view of the neck shows a ballooned pharynx *(Ph)* with swollen epiglottis *(E)* in the shape of a large thumbprint *(arrows)*. *T*, Trachea. (From Mettler FA [ed]: *Primary care radiology*, Philadelphia, 2000, Saunders.)

BASIC INFORMATION

DEFINITION

Episcleritis is an inflammation of the episclera (Fig. 1-325), the thin layer of vascular elastic tissue between the sclera and conjunctiva.

ICD-9CM CODES

379.0 Scleritis and episcleritis

EPIDEMIOLOGY & DEMOGRAPHICS

INCIDENCE (IN U.S.): Relatively rare in an ophthalmologic practice
PEAK INCIDENCE: Most common in middle and old age
PREDOMINANT SEX: None
PREDOMINANT AGE: 40s

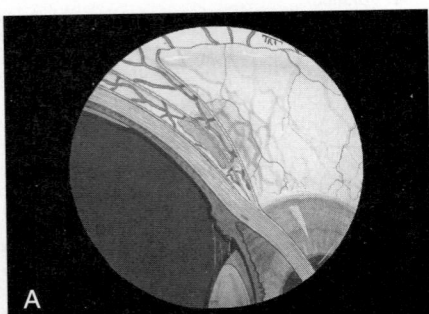

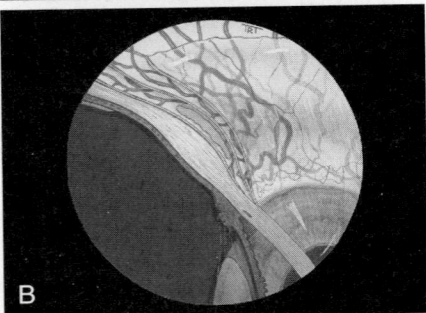

FIGURE 1-325 A, Episcleritis with maximal vascular congestion of the superficial episcleral plexus; **B,** scleritis with scleral thickening and maximal vascular congestion of the deep vascular plexus. (From Kanski JJ, Bowling B: *Clinical ophthalmology, a systematic approach,* ed 7, Philadelphia, 2010, Saunders.)

PHYSICAL FINDINGS & CLINICAL PRESENTATION

- Red, vascular injection of conjunctiva with engorged and enlarged blood vessels beneath the conjunctions (Fig. 1-326)
- Pain in area of inflammation that is usually localized

ETIOLOGY

Associated with collagen-vascular diseases, vasculitis, trauma; often nonspecific

DIAGNOSIS

DIFFERENTIAL DIAGNOSIS

- Acute glaucoma
- Conjunctivitis
- Scleritis
- Subconjunctival hemorrhage
- Congenital or lymphoid masses
- The differential diagnosis of "red eye" is described in Section II

WORKUP

Eye examination, general check-up for collagen-vascular disease or other autoimmune diseases

LABORATORY TESTS

Studies for collagen-vascular disease (e.g., ANA, ESR, RF)

TREATMENT

NONPHARMACOLOGIC THERAPY

Warm compresses

ACUTE GENERAL Rx

- Topical steroids, 1% prednisolone if no glaucoma; nonsteroidal eye drops if there is a tendency for glaucoma
- Nonsteroidal anti-inflammatory drugs (NSAIDs): treat underlying systemic disease

CHRONIC Rx

NSAID eye drops (diclofenac eye drops, ketorolac ophthalmic solution)

DISPOSITION

Close follow-up needed

REFERRAL

To ophthalmologist if patient unresponsive to treatment after a few days

PEARLS & CONSIDERATIONS

COMMENTS

- Often associated with collagen-vascular disease
- Usually related to systemic disease

SUGGESTED READINGS

available at www.expertconsult.com

RELATED CONTENT

Episcleritis (Patient Information)

AUTHOR: **MELVYN KOBY, M.D.**

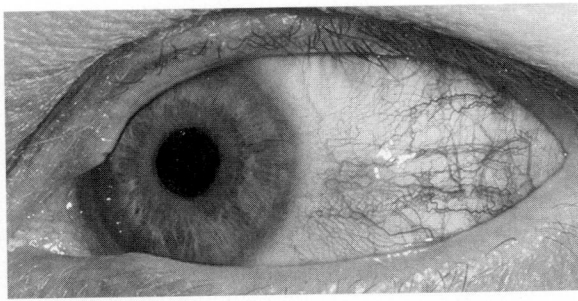

FIGURE 1-326 Nodular episcleritis in a patient with gout. (From Palay D [ed]: *Ophthalmology for the primary care physician,* St Louis, 1997, Mosby.)

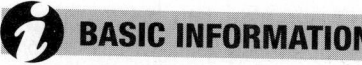

BASIC INFORMATION

DEFINITION

Epistaxis is defined as bleeding from the nose or nasal hemorrhage and is classified as either anterior or posterior.

SYNONYMS

Nosebleed

ICD-9CM CODES
784.7 Epistaxis

EPIDEMIOLOGY & DEMOGRAPHICS

- Epistaxis accounts for one of every 200 emergency department visits in the U.S. annually.
- It increases in frequency after age 20 yr and reaches the highest levels among the elderly population.
- More than 80% of cases of epistaxis are anterior in origin (Little's area) and occur from Kiesselbach's plexus (Fig. 1-327).
- Only 5% of patients with epistaxis have posterior bleeds.

PHYSICAL FINDINGS & CLINICAL PRESENTATION

- Nosebleed
- Hypotension and hemodynamic instability with acute, severe epistaxis

ETIOLOGY

- Approximately 90% of epistaxis events are idiopathic.
- Common identifiable causes are:
  1. Cold, dry environment
  2. Trauma (nose picking, accidents, and physical altercations)
  3. Structural deformities (septal deviations or spurs, chronic perforations)
  4. Inflammatory (rhinosinusitis, nasal polyposis)
  5. Allergies
  6. Foreign bodies in the nasal cavity
  7. Tumors (juvenile angiofibroma)
  8. Irritants
  9. Hypertension
  10. Coagulopathy (hemophilia, von Willebrand's disease, thrombocytopenia)
  11. Osler-Weber-Rendu disease
  12. Renal failure
  13. Drugs: aspirin, nonsteroidal antiinflammatory drugs, warfarin, alcohol, sildenafil, and tadalafil
  14. Blood vessel disorders (connective tissue disease, hereditary hemorrhagic telangiectasia)
  15. Pseudoaneurysm and aneurysm of the internal carotid artery might present as epistaxis

DIAGNOSIS

A good attempt should be made to directly visualize the source of bleeding to confirm the diagnosis and determine the best treatment.

DIFFERENTIAL DIAGNOSIS

Pseudoepistaxis must be ruled out. Common extranasal sites of bleeding that can simulate epistaxis include:
1. Pulmonary hemoptysis
2. Bleeding esophageal varices
3. Tumor bleeding from the pharynx, larynx, or trachea

WORKUP

The workup should include laboratory blood testing to exclude obvious causes. Type and cross in anticipation of transfusion if the bleeding is severe.

LABORATORY TESTS

- Hemoglobin and hematocrit
- Platelet count
- Blood urea nitrogen and creatinine
- Coagulation studies (prothrombin time and partial thromboplastin time)
- Type and crossmatching of blood products

IMAGING STUDIES

Radiographic studies are usually not helpful.

TREATMENT

NONPHARMACOLOGIC THERAPY

- Digital compression or pinching of the lower soft cartilaginous part of the nose for 10 min is the method of choice.
- Use cotton or tissue plug.
- The patient should be sitting and leaning forward, breathing through the mouth, allowing blood to flow out of the nostrils as opposed to bending backward, which would allow the blood to flow down the throat.
- Application of cold compresses to the bridge of the nose to cause a vasoconstrictive effect; the patient may also suck on ice to achieve this effect.

ACUTE GENERAL Rx

Anterior epistaxis:
- Local vasoconstriction is performed by moistening a cotton pledget with either:
  1. 4% lidocaine with 1:1000 epinephrine
  2. 4% lidocaine with 1% phenylephrine (Neo-Synephrine)
  3. 4% lidocaine with 0.05% oxymetazoline (Afrin)
  4. 4% cocaine or cocaine 25% in paraffin base ointment and inserting the pledget into the nasal cavity with bayonet forceps.
- Cauterization with silver nitrate or trichloroacetic acid is performed once hemostasis is achieved.
- Anterior nasal packing is needed when local measures are unsuccessful. Nasal packing is performed under local anesthesia and is done by inserting Vaseline gauze strips in layers from the floor of the nasal cavity to the front entrance of the nasal orifice. Enough pressure is placed to tamponade the epistaxis (Fig. 1-328).
- Other commercially available nasal packing uses sponge packs that expand when exposed to blood or moisture and can be used for anterior epistaxis.

Posterior epistaxis:
- Posterior nasal packing
  1. Commercially available nasal sponge packing can be applied
  2. Rolled gauze technique
- Foley catheter balloon insertion into the nasopharynx can be tried in patients with posterior epistaxis.

Newer agents in the treatment of epistaxis:
- Quick clot hemostatic agent, available OTC. When it comes in contact with blood in and around a wound, it absorbs the smaller water molecules from the blood to promote rapid clotting
- Floseal hemostatic matrix, a combination of human thrombin, gelatin matrix, and calcium

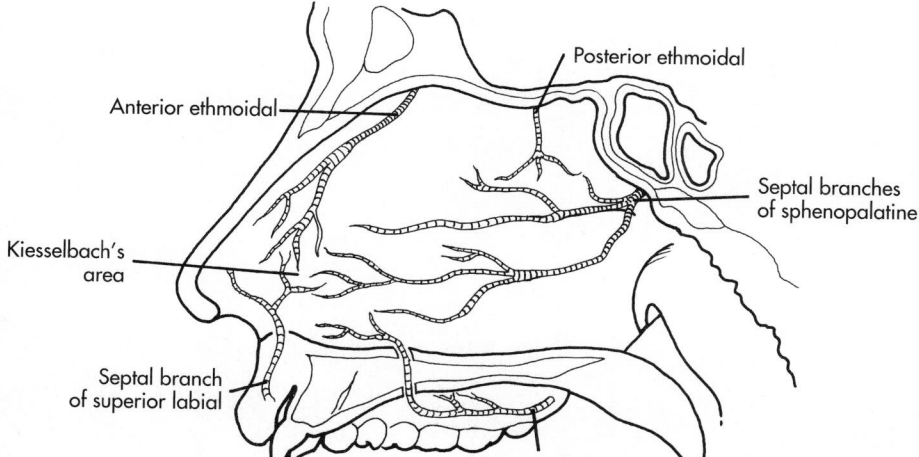

FIGURE 1-327 Kiesselbach's plexus on the anterior septum derives blood supply from the superior labial, descending palatine, and sphenopalatine arteries. (From Noble J: *Primary care medicine*, ed 3, St Louis, 2001, Mosby.)

Labels on figure: Posterior ethmoidal; Anterior ethmoidal; Septal branches of sphenopalatine; Kiesselbach's area; Septal branch of superior labial; Greater palatine

E

Diseases and Disorders

I

chloride, which are mixed together and placed at bleeding site
- Recombinant factor VIIa, generally reserved for uncontrolled epistaxis

CHRONIC Rx
- If acute treatment fails to stop the bleeding or the site of bleeding cannot be located, electrocautery or endoscopic cauterization can be used.
- Electrocautery is performed after suitable anesthesia, such as application of a topical anesthetic followed by local anesthetic injection. Only one side of the nasal septum should be cauterized at a time because perforation can result from bilateral cauterization.
- Arterial ligation or embolization has been used in refractory posterior epistaxis.
- For cases involving irritated or inflamed mucosa, a conservative regimen of triamcinolone 0.025%, Nemdyn, Nasalate, or equivalent cream should be applied once a week, combined with nightly application of a small quantity of petroleum jelly to the septum before bedtime.

DISPOSITION
- Most cases of anterior epistaxis from Kiesselbach's plexus can be stopped by nasal compression and local vasoconstriction or cauterization.
- Nasal packing with gauze or sponge can control 90% of anterior epistaxis.
- Anterior and posterior packs are removed in 2 to 3 days. Hospital admission should be considered in patients who cannot be expected to return for prompt follow-up because prolonged packing increases the risk of pressure necrosis, toxic shock syndrome, sinus infections, and other complications.

- Although rare, epistaxis can lead to death by aspiration of blood, hemodynamic compromise from rapid excessive blood loss, or toxic shock syndrome.

REFERRAL
- If epistaxis cannot be controlled, an ear-nose-throat (ENT) specialist should be called for assistance.
- ENT specialist should be consulted in any patient with posterior epistaxis requiring posterior packing.

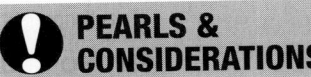

PEARLS & CONSIDERATIONS

COMMENTS
- Silver nitrate cauterization, if done on both sides of the nasal septum, can lead to septal perforation and should be discouraged.
- If anterior nasal packing is done, broad-spectrum antibiotics (e.g., amoxicillin-clavulanate 250 mg PO tid or trimethoprim-sulfamethoxazole 1 tablet PO bid) are used until the anterior packs are removed. Although it is customary to place patients on antibiotics to prevent sinusitis from obstruction, there is no proof that this is effective.
- Complications of nasal packing include:
  1. Aspiration
  2. Dislodged packing
  3. Infection
  4. Nasal trauma

SUGGESTED READINGS
available at www.expertconsult.com

RELATED CONTENT
Noseblleeds (Patient Information)

AUTHOR: **TANYA ALI, M.D.**

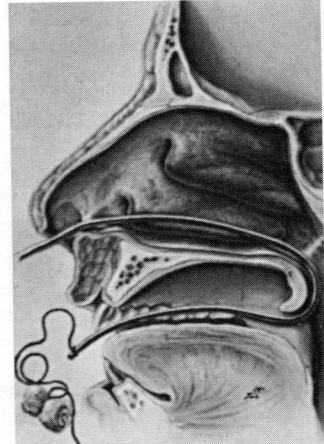
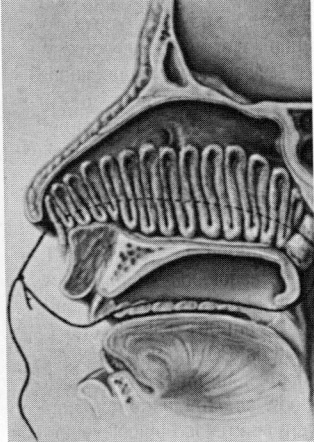

FIGURE 1-328 Packing of the nose for epistaxis with a postnasal pack and an anterior nose pack. (From Boies LR et al: *Fundamentals of otolaryngology: a textbook of ear, nose, and throat diseases,* ed 4, Philadelphia, 1964, Saunders.)

BASIC INFORMATION

DEFINITION

Epstein-Barr virus infection refers to a disease caused by Epstein-Barr virus (EBV), a human herpesvirus.

SYNONYMS

Infectious mononucleosis (IM)
Kissing disease

ICD-9CM CODES
075 Mononucleosis

EPIDEMIOLOGY & DEMOGRAPHICS

INCIDENCE (IN U.S.): 5 cases/100,000 persons per yr of IM
PREDOMINANT SEX: Neither, although peak incidence occurs about 2 yr earlier in women
PREDOMINANT AGE:
- Clinical evidence of IM: occurs most commonly at ages 15 to 24 yr
- EBV infection: occurs earlier in life in lower socioeconomic groups

PHYSICAL FINDINGS & CLINICAL PRESENTATION

- Most EBV infections either are asymptomatic or cause a nonspecific viral illness.
- Incubation period is 1 to 2 mo, possibly followed by a prodrome of anorexia, low-grade fever, malaise, headache, and chills; after several days, clinical triad of pharyngitis, moderate to high fever, and adenopathy may appear, accompanied by fatigue and malaise.
- Pharyngitis is usually the most severe symptom; white or necrotic appearance exudates are common.
- Symmetrical lymphadenopathy is most prominent in the posterior more than anterior cervical region but may be diffuse.
- Splenomegaly (50% of cases) is possible, most commonly during the second week of illness.
- Maculopapular or morbilliform rash is uncommon but will occur in patients who receive ampicillin. Patients may have palatal petechiae, periorbital, or palpebral edema. Mucocutaneous oral hairy leukoplakia (OHL), which is associated with intense EBV replication and the action of EBV-encoded proteins such as latent membrane protein-1, may occur.
- Possible IM presentation: fever and adenopathy without pharyngitis.
- Nausea, vomiting, and anorexia are frequent in patients with IM, probably reflecting mild hepatitis encountered in 90% of infected individuals.
- Although complications such as spleen rupture, airway obstruction, and malignancy may be severe and fatal, they are uncommon and tend to resolve completely.
- Hematologic involvement includes hemolytic or aplastic anemia, thrombocytopenia, thrombotic thrombocytopenic purpura/hemolytic-uremic syndrome, and disseminated intravascular coagulation (DIC). Pneumonia, myocarditis, pancreatitis, mesenteric adenitis, myositis, and glomerulonephritis may occur as well. Nervous system involvement includes Guillain-Barré syndrome, facial nerve palsy, meningoencephalitis, aseptic meningitis, transfer myelitis, peripheral neuritis and optic neuritis.
- IM is usually a self-limited illness. Acute symptoms resolve in 1 to 2 wk, but symptoms of malaise and fatigue often persist for months.
- EBV is related to lymphoproliferative syndromes in transplant recipients and in AIDS patients.
- Increasing evidence showing an association between EBV infection and African Burkitt's, B-cell, T-cell lymphoma, and nasopharyngeal carcinoma. Table E1-147 describes EBV-associated malignancies.

ETIOLOGY

- EBV is a ubiquitous virus.
- Infection during childhood is much less likely to cause significant illness.
- Frequency of IM in late adolescence is attributed to the onset of social contact between the sexes.
- Close personal contact is usually necessary for transmission, although EBV is occasionally transmitted by blood transfusion; transfer via saliva while kissing may be responsible for many cases.

DIAGNOSIS

DIFFERENTIAL DIAGNOSIS

- Heterophile-negative IM caused by cytomegalovirus (CMV)
- Although clinical presentation similar, CMV more frequently follows transfusion
- Bacterial and viral causes of pharyngitis
- Toxoplasmosis
- Acute retroviral syndrome of HIV
- Lymphoma
- Lyme disease

WORKUP

Heterophile antibody and CBC with blood smear. Table E1-148 describes frequently determined EBV-specific antibodies.

LABORATORY TESTS

- Increased WBC common, with a relative lymphocytosis of more than 50% and neutropenia are identified.
- Hallmark of IM: atypical lymphocytes of more than 10% (not pathognomonic) are found.
- Mild thrombocytopenia is present.
- Falling hematocrit signals the possibility of splenic rupture or immune hemolytic anemia.
- Elevated hepatocellular enzymes and cryoglobulins are found in most cases.
- Heterophile antibody:
  - As measured by the monospot test, may be positive at presentation or may appear later in the course of illness.
  - Negative test is repeated in 1 wk if clinical suspicion is high.
  - A positive test has been reported with primary HIV infection.
- Viral capsid antigen (VCA) IgG and IgM are rarely used for diagnosis, but better value in children because heterophile antibody is negative in most of children younger than 8 years.
- PCR DNA for CMV is the test of choice in transplant recipients who develop lymphoproliferative syndromes.

IMAGING STUDIES

Chest radiograph examination:
- May rarely show infiltrates
- Possible elevated left hemidiaphragm with splenic rupture

TREATMENT

NONPHARMACOLOGIC THERAPY

- Supportive including rest
- Splenectomy if rupture occurs
- Transfusions for severe anemia or thrombocytopenia

ACUTE GENERAL Rx

- Pharmacologic therapy is not indicated in uncomplicated illness.
- Avoid aspirin due to the risk of Reye's syndrome.
- Avoid ampicillin and amoxicillin as their use can frequently precipitate a nonallergic rash.
- Use of steroids is suggested in patients who have severe thrombocytopenia, hemolytic anemia, impending airway obstruction resulting from enlarged tonsils, or fulminant liver failure. Prednisone 60 to 80 mg PO qd for 3 days, then tapered over 1 to 2 wk.
- Although it may reduce initial viral shedding, there is little evidence to support the use of antiviral agents such as acyclovir in the management of IM.

CHRONIC Rx

An extremely rare, chronic form of IM with persistent fevers and fatigue has been described and should be differentiated from chronic fatigue syndrome, which is not related to EBV.

DISPOSITION

Eventual resolution of all symptoms

REFERRAL

If more than mild illness

PEARLS & CONSIDERATIONS

COMMENTS

Avoidance of contact sports during the first month of illness because splenic rupture can occur even in the absence of clinically detectable splenomegaly.

SUGGESTED READINGS

available at www.expertconsult.com

RELATED CONTENT

Epstein-Barr Virus Infection (Patient Information)
Mononucleosis (Related Key Topic)

AUTHOR: **MONZR M. AL MALKI, M.D.**

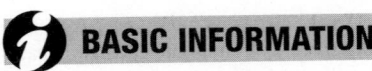

BASIC INFORMATION

DEFINITION

Erectile dysfunction (ED) is the persistent inability to achieve or sustain a penile erection of adequate rigidity to make intercourse possible or satisfactory.

SYNONYMS

ED
Impotence
Male erectile disorder
Sexual dysfunction (a nonspecific term)

ICD-9CM CODES
F52.2 Male erectile disorder

DSM-IV CODES
302.72 Male erectile disorder

EPIDEMIOLOGY & DEMOGRAPHICS

PREVALENCE (IN U.S.):
- Increases with age and presence of vascular comorbidities.
- Approximately 7% in the 20s, 18% in the 50s, 25% in the 60s, 80% in the 80s.

PREDOMINANT SEX: By definition, only in males

PREDOMINANT AGE: Increases with age

RISK FACTORS: Age, coronary artery disease, peripheral vascular disease, hypertension, diabetes mellitus, hypercholesterolemia, prostate surgery, neurologic injury, numerous medications, alcohol, smoking or drug abuse

ETIOLOGY

- Most cases are caused by organic problems related to neurologic, hormonal, or vascular abnormalities or prescription or recreational drugs. In organic ED nocturnal penile tumescence is generally abnormal.
- Psychogenic ED results from mental stress, depression, widower syndrome, and performance anxiety. Characterized by normal nocturnal penile tumescence and otherwise negative test results.
- Vascular disease: History of hypertension (HTN), peripheral vascular disease, ischemic heart disease, diabetes, smoking. In approximately 40% of men >50 yr, the primary cause of ED is related to atherosclerotic disease, diabetes mellitus (DM), neuropathy, or vascular disease.
- Medication side effects: Antihypertensives such as thiazides and clonidine (consider change to ACE inhibitors and calcium channel blockers with lower reported incidence of ED); antiandrogens such as spironolactone, finasteride, ketoconazole; cimetidine; antidepressants such as selective serotonin reuptake inhibitors [SSRIs]; and antipsychotics.
- Alcohol and nicotine use.
- Recreational drugs, including cocaine, heroin, amphetamines, and marijuana. These may increase libido but impair performance.
- Hormonal dysfunction such as testosterone deficiency (decreases libido and erection), hypothyroidism or hyperthyroidism, hyperprolactinemia, and adrenal insufficiency.
- Neurogenic causes including spinal cord lesions, cortical lesions, and peripheral neuropathies.
- Trauma or pelvic surgeries such as radical prostatectomy or cystectomy.

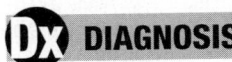

DIAGNOSIS

DIFFERENTIAL DIAGNOSIS

- A useful tool to diagnose/evaluate ED severity is the Sexual Health Inventory for Men.
- Distinguish psychogenic from organic ED.
- Evaluate for underlying etiology of organic ED and comorbid psychiatric condition.

WORKUP

- Clinical history should include time course (abrupt onset may correlate with reversible cause such as medication, psychosocial stress, psychiatric complaint, trauma), cause (psychogenic vs. organic), and change in libido.
- Report of spontaneous nocturnal or morning erections indicate intact neurologic reflexes and penile blood flow.
- Decreased libido may indicate endocrinologic or psychogenic cause.
- If possible, interview partner regarding sexual function.
- Medical and social history should address cardiac disease symptoms and risk factors (HTN, DM, hyperlipidemia, smoking, and substance abuse), pelvic surgery, medications, and mental health.
- Physical examination to check blood pressure, femoral and peripheral pulses, femoral bruits; gynecomastia; neuronal damage (genital sensation, cremasteric reflex); direct penile damage (e.g., plaque formation such as Peyronie's disease); prostate examination; or testicular atrophy and other secondary sexual characteristics.

LABORATORY TESTS

Screen for diabetes mellitus with fasting glucose. Consider lipid panel, thyroid-stimulating hormone, morning serum testosterone (free and total). If decreased testosterone, check prolactin, follicle-stimulating hormone, and luteinizing hormone.

IMAGING STUDIES

Imaging studies are rarely performed except in situations of pelvic trauma or surgery.

OTHER STUDIES

- Nocturnal penile tumescence testing very specific for distinguishing psychogenic versus organic causes.
- Neurogenic etiologies examined by the cremasteric reflex (inner-thigh touch elicits scrotal contraction), the bulbocavernosus reflex, or the pudendal-evoked response.
- Intracorporeal injection of prostaglandin E_1 to distinguish vascular and nonvascular etiologies (erection is achieved in patients with normal vascular systems). If no erection with direct injection of vasoactive substance, consider duplex ultrasound of penile vasculature.

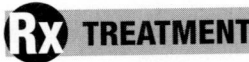

TREATMENT

NONPHARMACOLOGIC THERAPY

- Various psychotherapeutic approaches: cognitive-behavioral therapy preferred; success rates decrease with advancing age and duration of symptoms.
- Psychosexual therapy (sex therapy and couples therapy) is first line for psychogenic ED. Psychosexual therapy may be used as for adjunctive therapy in ED from any cause to address contributing social and relationship issues.
- Mechanical vacuum devices (function by drawing blood into corpus cavernosum) are 70% to 90% effective but are difficult to use.
- Incorporate vascular risk factor reduction including counsel on diet, exercise, smoking cessation, ETOH intake and screening/treatment for HTN, insulin resistance, and hypercholesterolemia as appropriate. Trials have shown that lifestyle modification and pharmacotherapy for cardiovascular risk factors are effective in improving sexual function in men with ED.

ACUTE GENERAL Rx

- First-line treatment: In setting of sexual stimulation, three selective phosphodiesterase type 5 (PDE5) inhibitors prolong nitric oxide–induced vasodilation by increase of intracavernosal cyclic guanosine monophosphate levels. Sildenafil (Viagra) and vardenafil (Levitra, Staxyn) can be taken 30 to 60 min before sexual activity, and both are effective for about 4 hr. Tadalafil (Cialis) can be taken several hours before sexual activity (although 50% respond within 30 min) and lasts up to 36 hr. All three PDE5 inhibitors have similar efficacy and tolerability, but tadalafil has a longer duration of action and is less affected by high-fat meals and alcohol. Counsel patients to avoid high-fat meals and excessive alcohol when taking PDE5 inhibitors, as they may impede effectiveness.
- With PDE5 inhibitors, avoid concomitant use of nitrates (absolute contraindication), drugs that inhibit or induce cytochrome P450 CYP3A4, and drugs that prolong the QT interval. Caution in men on alpha-adrenergic blocker therapy because of concern for hypotension; start the lowest dose of PDE5 inhibitor. Caution in men who have had myocardial infarction in the past 6 mo, resting hypotension or uncontrolled hypertension, unstable angina, positive exercise stress test or poor exercise tolerance. Counsel on side effects of headache, flushing, dyspepsia, nasal congestion, changes in color perception (including blue vision for sildenafil and vardenafil), and priapism (rare). Nonarteritic anterior ischemic optic neuropathy is also a rare association with sildenafil and tadalafil. Consider counseling on safe sexual practices when prescribing PDE5 inhibitors.

- Second-line treatment if PDE5 inhibitors fail: self-injection with intraurethral alprostadil (prostaglandin E_1 [medicated urethral suppository]) applied into meatus of penis before intercourse; or intracavernosal injections of vasodilators (e.g., papaverine or prostaglandin E_1 pellet). Consider combining intraurethral alprostadil with sildenafil. Relatively high success with self-injection, but attrition is high.
- Second-line treatment alternative: vacuum constriction pump; has variable satisfaction rate.

CHRONIC Rx

- Psychosexual therapy is helpful as an adjunctive treatment.
- Psychogenic impotence: PDE5 inhibitors are effective in patients with depression because tissues, nerves, hormones, and vasculature are normal. Full psychologic evaluation is recommended before starting treatment.
- For men not responding to other approaches: surgical implantation of penile prosthesis.
- Testosterone therapy in men with low testosterone (i.e., hypogonadal); evaluate for prostate cancer before prescribing testosterone.
- Aerobic exercise may improve ED along with pharmacologic treatment.

DISPOSITION

- Psychogenic-acquired ED will remit spontaneously in 15% to 30% of cases.
- Lifelong ED is usually a chronic and unremitting condition.
- Situational ED may remit with changes in social environment but usually recurs.

REFERRAL

- Refer if psychotherapy, sex therapy, or invasive organic treatment required
- Refer to urology if PDE5 inhibitors fail or sudden onset occurs after penile trauma

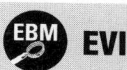 **PEARLS & CONSIDERATIONS**

- ED is commonly evaluated and treated by primary care physician; refer to urologist if oral therapy fails or surgery is required.
- PDE5 inhibitors are treatment of choice for most causes of ED. Main contraindications are nitrate use and decompensated cardiac disease. Caution in patients on alpha-adrenergic blockers and with blood pressures at extreme ends (significant hypotension or hypertension).
- For optimal response, patients should be appropriately informed of proper use, precautions, and adverse effects of PDE5 inhibitors. Try six to eight times at optimal doses before declaring PDE5 inhibitors a failure. Consider switching among the three PDE5 inhibitors if one fails.
- Men with ED are at increased risk of coronary, cerebrovascular, and peripheral vascular diseases. Screen for cardiovascular risk factors in these patients.

EBM **EVIDENCE**

available at www.expertconsult.com

SUGGESTED READINGS

available at www.expertconsult.com

RELATED CONTENT

Erectile Dysfunction (Patient Information)

AUTHORS: **CINDY LAI, M.D.,** and **NICOLE APPELLE, M.D.**

E

Diseases and Disorders

I

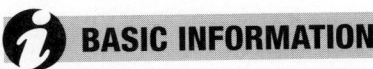 **BASIC INFORMATION**

DEFINITION

Erysipelas is a type of cellulitis caused by infection of the superficial layers of the skin and cutaneous lymphatics. Erysipelas is characterized by redness, induration, and a sharply demarcated, raised border.

SYNONYMS

St. Anthony's fire

ICD-9CM CODES
035 Erysipelas

EPIDEMIOLOGY & DEMOGRAPHICS

PREDOMINANT AGE: Occurs most often in the young or old
RISK FACTORS: Patients with impaired lymphatic or venous drainage (mastectomy, saphenous vein harvesting) and immunocompromised patients. Athlete's foot is a common portal of entry.
RECURRENCE RATE: Relatively common

PHYSICAL FINDINGS & CLINICAL PRESENTATION

- Distinctive red, warm, tender skin lesion with induration and a sharply defined, advancing, raised border (Fig. 1-329).
- Most common sites are lower extremities and face.
- Systemic signs of infection (fever) are often present.
- Vesicles or bullae may develop.
- After several days lesions may appear ecchymotic.
- After 7 to 10 days desquamation of affected area may occur.

ETIOLOGY

- Usually group A β-hemolytic streptococci
- Less often group B, C, or G streptococci
- Rarely *Staphylococcus aureus*

COMPLICATIONS

- Abscess
- Necrotizing fasciitis
- Thrombophlebitis
- Gangrene
- Metastatic infection

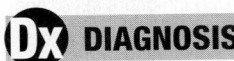 **DIAGNOSIS**

DIFFERENTIAL DIAGNOSIS

- Other types of cellulitis
- Necrotizing fasciitis
- Deep vein thrombosis
- Contact dermatitis
- Erythema migrans (Lyme's disease)
- Insect bite
- Herpes zoster
- Erysipeloid
- Acute gout
- Pseudogout

WORKUP

History, physical examination, and laboratory evaluation

LABORATORY TESTS

Diagnosis is usually made by characteristic clinical setting and appearance.
- Complete blood count and white blood cell count often elevated
- Blood cultures positive in 5% of patients
- Gram stain and culture of any drainage from skin lesions
- Culture of aspirated fluid from leading edge of skin lesion has low yield

IMAGING STUDIES

- Not routinely indicated
- Duplex ultrasound for patients suspected of having deep vein thrombosis
- CT scan or MRI for patients with suspected necrotizing fasciitis

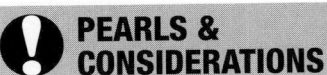 **TREATMENT**

NONPHARMACOLOGIC THERAPY

- Elevation of the affected limb
- Warm compresses

ACUTE GENERAL Rx

Typical erysipelas of extremity in nondiabetic patient:
- PO: penicillin V 500 mg qid
- IV: penicillin G (aqueous) 1 to 2 million units q6h. Use vancomycin 15 mg/kg IV q12h in penicillin-allergic patients.
NOTE: Use azithromycin in patients allergic to penicillin.
Facial erysipelas (include coverage for *Staphylococcus aureus*):
- PO dicloxacillin 500 mg q6h
- IV nafcillin or oxacillin 2 g q4h
- IV vancomycin 1 g q12h
- Daptomycin 4 mg/kg IV q24h
- Linezolid 600 mg IV q12h

DISPOSITION

Prognosis is good with antibiotic treatment but recurrence is common.

REFERRAL

For surgical debridement for patients with necrotizing fasciitis or for drainage of abscess

PEARLS & CONSIDERATIONS

- Consider early surgical referral when necrotizing fasciitis suspected. Consider skin biopsy when not responding to appropriate antibiotics.
- Look for tinea pedis as portal of entry in erysipelas of lower extremities. Treat if present.

SUGGESTED READING
available at www.expertconsult.com

RELATED CONTENT

Cellulitis (Related Key Topic)
Erysipelas (Patient Information)

AUTHORS: **GAIL M. O'BRIEN, M.D.,** and **MARK J. FAGAN, M.D.**

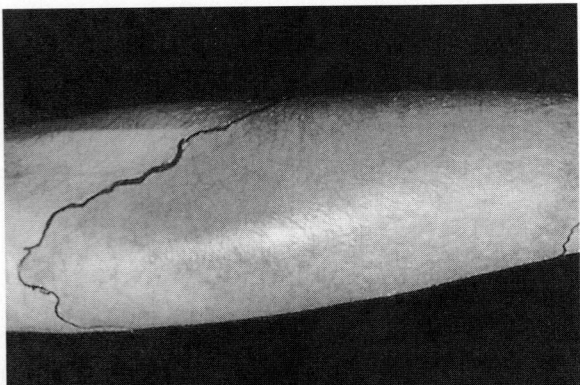

FIGURE 1-329 Erysipelas. Note well-demarcated erythematous plaque on arm. (From Goldstein B [ed]: *Practical dermatology,* ed 2, St Louis, 1997, Mosby. Courtesy Department of Dermatology, University of North Carolina at Chapel Hill.)

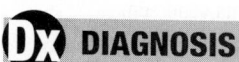 BASIC INFORMATION

DEFINITION

Erythema multiforme is an inflammatory disease characterized by eruption of annular, maculopapular lesions with dark raised, erythematous, or vesiculobullus center surrounded by a pale zone. It is believed to be caused by immune complex formation and subsequent deposition in the skin and mucous membranes. It is considered a hypersensitivity reaction to infection or drugs.

SYNONYMS

EM

ICD-9CM CODES
695.1 Erythema multiforme

EPIDEMIOLOGY & DEMOGRAPHICS

PREDOMINANT AGE: 20 to 40 yr
RISK FACTORS: Often associated with herpes simplex and other infectious agents, drugs, or connective tissue diseases.

PHYSICAL FINDINGS & CLINICAL PRESENTATION

- Prodromal symptoms are mild or absent. Itching or burning at the site of eruption may occur.
- Symmetric skin lesions with a classic "target" appearance (caused by the centrifugal spread of red maculopapules to circumference of 1 to 3 cm with a purpuric, cyanotic, or vesicular center) are present (Fig. 1-330). The papules may enlarge into plaques measuring a few centimeters in diameter with a dark or red central portion. Target lesions may not be apparent for several days.

- Lesions are most common in the back of the hands and feet and extensor aspect of the forearms and legs. Trunk involvement can occur in severe cases.
- Urticarial papules, vesicles, and bullae may also be present and generally indicate a more severe form of the disease.
- Individual lesions heal in 1 to 2 wk without scarring.
- Bullae and erosions may also be present in the oral cavity.

ETIOLOGY

- Immune complex formation and subsequent deposition in the cutaneous microvasculature may play a role in the pathogenesis of erythema multiforme.
- The majority of cases follow outbreaks of herpes simplex virus 1 and 2.
- *Mycoplasma pneumoniae*, fungal infections, medications (bupropion, sulfonamides, penicillins, nonsteroidal anti-inflammatory drugs, barbiturates, phenothiazines, hydantoins).
- In >50% of patients no specific cause is identified.

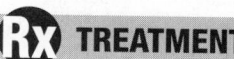 DIAGNOSIS

DIFFERENTIAL DIAGNOSIS

- Chronic urticaria
- Secondary syphilis
- Pityriasis rosea
- Contact dermatitis
- Pemphigus vulgaris
- Lichen planus
- Serum sickness
- Drug eruption
- Granuloma annulare
- Polymorphic light eruption
- Viral exanthem

WORKUP

- Medical history with emphasis on drug ingestion
- Laboratory evaluation in patients with suspected collagen-vascular diseases
- Skin biopsy when diagnosis is unclear

LABORATORY TESTS

- Complete blood count with differential
- Antinuclear antibody
- Serology for *M. pneumoniae*, HSV-1, HSV-2
- Urinalysis

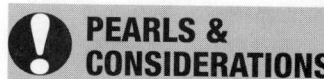 TREATMENT

NONPHARMACOLOGIC THERAPY

- Mild cases generally do not require treatment; lesions resolve spontaneously within 1 mo.
- Potential drug precipitants should be removed.

ACUTE GENERAL Rx

- Treatment of associated diseases (e.g., acyclovir for herpes simplex, erythromycin for *Mycoplasma* infection).
- Prednisone 40 to 80 mg/day for 1 to 3 wk may be tried in patients with many target lesions; however, the role of systemic steroids remains controversial.
- Levamisole, an immunomodulator, may be effective in the treatment of patients with chronic or recurrent oral lesions (dose is 150 mg/day for 3 consecutive days used alone or in combination with prednisone).
- IV immunoglobulins in severe cases.

DISPOSITION

The rash generally evolves over a 2-wk period and resolves within 3 to 4 wk without scarring. A severe bullous form can occur (see entry for "Stevens-Johnson Syndrome").

REFERRAL

Hospital admission in patients with suspected Stevens-Johnson syndrome

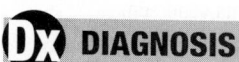 PEARLS & CONSIDERATIONS

COMMENTS

The risk of recurrence of erythema multiforme exceeds 30%. Recurrence may be treated with valacyclovir 500 to 1000 mg/day, famciclovir 125 to 250 mg/day, or acyclovir 400 mg bid. Dapsone, antimalarials, azathioprine, or cyclosporine use is reserved for cases resistant to antivirals.

SUGGESTED READINGS

available at www.expertconsult.com

RELATED CONTENT

Erythema Multiforme (Patient Information)

AUTHOR: **FRED F. FERRI, M.D.**

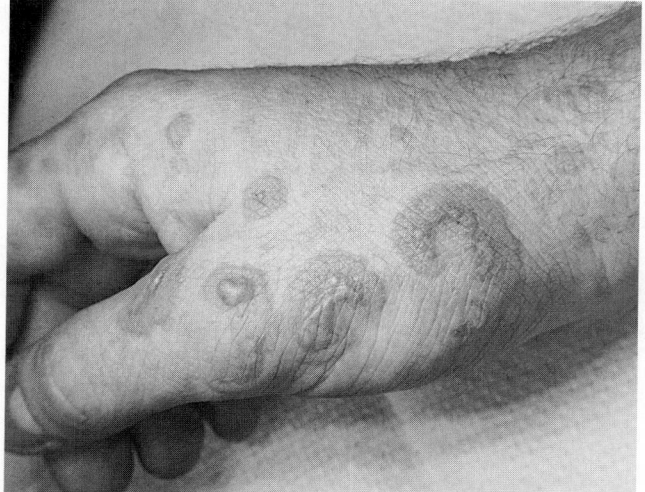

FIGURE 1-330 Iris and arcuate lesions of erythema multiforme. Note erythematous lesions with multiform configurations: target, arcuate, and vesicles. (From Noble J et al: *Textbook of primary care medicine,* ed 2, St Louis, 1995, Mosby.)

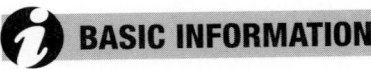

BASIC INFORMATION

DEFINITION

Erythema nodosum (EN) is an acute, tender, erythematous, nodular skin eruption resulting from inflammation of subcutaneous fat, often associated with bruising. It is the most common form of panniculitis.

ICD-9CM CODES
695.2   Erythema nodosum
017.10 Erythema nodosum, tuberculous, NOS

EPIDEMIOLOGY & DEMOGRAPHICS

INCIDENCE: Two to three cases/100,000 persons per yr
PREDOMINANT SEX: Female/male ratio of 3 to 4:1
PREDOMINANT AGE: 25 to 40 yr

PHYSICAL FINDINGS & CLINICAL PRESENTATION

- Acute onset of tender nodules typically located on the shins (Fig. 1-331) and occasionally seen on the thighs and forearms.
- The nodules are usually ⅛ to 1 inch in diameter but can be as large as 4 inches; they begin as light red lesions, then become darker and often ecchymotic. The nodules heal within 8 wk without ulceration.

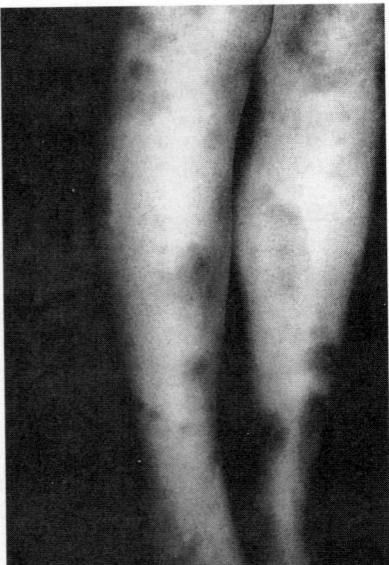

FIGURE 1-331 Erythema nodosum. (From Arndt KA et al: *Cutaneous medicine and surgery, vol 1,* Philadelphia, 1997, Saunders.)

- Associated findings:
  1. Fever
  2. Lymphadenopathy
  3. Arthralgia
  4. Signs of the underlying illness

ETIOLOGY

Cell-mediated hypersensitivity reaction is seen more frequently in persons with human leukocyte antigen (HLA) B8. The lesion results from an exaggerated interaction between an antigen and cell-mediated immune mechanisms leading to granuloma formation. Up to 55% of cases of EN are idiopathic.
Infections:
- Bacteria
  - Streptococcal pharyngitis (28% to 48%)
  - *Salmonella* enteritis
  - *Yersinia* enteritis
  - Psittacosis
  - *Chlamydia pneumoniae* infection
  - *Mycoplasma* pneumonia
  - Meningococcal infection
  - Gonorrhea
  - Syphilis
  - Lymphogranuloma venereum
  - Tularemia
  - Cat-scratch disease
  - Leprosy
  - Tuberculosis
- Fungi
  - Histoplasmosis
  - Coccidioidomycosis
  - Blastomycosis
  - *Trichophyton verrucosum*
- Viruses
  - Cytomegalovirus
  - Hepatitis B
  - Epstein-Barr virus
- Drugs (3% to 10%)
  - Sulfonamides
  - Penicillins
  - Oral contraceptives
  - Gold salts
  - Prazosin
  - Aspirin
  - Bromides
- Sarcoidosis (11% to 25%)
- Inflammatory bowel disease
- Cancer, usually lymphoma
- Ankylosing spondylosis and reactive arthropathies (e.g., associated with inflammatory bowel disease)

DIAGNOSIS

DIFFERENTIAL DIAGNOSIS

- Insect bites
- Posttraumatic ecchymoses
- Vasculitis

- Weber-Christian disease
- Fat necrosis associated with pancreatitis
- Necrobiosis lipoidica
- Scleroderma
- Lupus panniculitis
- Subcutaneous granuloma
- Alpha-1 antitrypsin deficiency

WORKUP

- Physical examination
- Diagnosis of underlying illness by history, physical examination, and laboratory tests as indicated

LABORATORY TESTS

- Erythrocyte sedimentation rate
- Throat culture and antistreptolysin O titer
- PPD
- Others depending on index of suspicion (e.g., stool culture and evaluation for ova and parasites in patients with diarrhea and gastrointestinal symptoms)
- Skin biopsy in doubtful cases:
  1. Early lesion: inflammation and hemorrhage in subcutaneous tissue
  2. Late lesion: giant cells and granulomata

IMAGING STUDIES

Chest radiograph to rule out sarcoidosis and tuberculosis

TREATMENT

- The disease is self-limited and treatment is symptomatic. EN nodules develop in pretibial locations and resolve spontaneously over several weeks without scarring or ulceration.
- Treatment of underlying disorders.
- Avoidance of contact irritation of affected areas.
- Nonsteroidal anti-inflammatory drugs for pain.
- Systemic steroids (prednisone 1 mg/kg of body weight/day, tapered over several days) may be useful in severe cases if underlying risk of sepsis and malignancy have been excluded.

PROGNOSIS

Typical case:
- Pain for 2 wk
- Resolution within 8 wk

SUGGESTED READING
available at www.expertconsult.com

RELATED CONTENT

Erythema Nodosum (Patient Information)

AUTHOR: **FRED F. FERRI, M.D.**

Esophageal Tumors

BASIC INFORMATION

DEFINITION

Esophageal tumors include both benign and malignant neoplasms of the esophageal mucosa and wall. Carcinomas of the esophageal epithelium, both squamous cell and adenocarcinoma, are by far the most common tumors of the esophagus (see Table 1-149). Rare esophageal tumors include both malignant (spindle cell, small cell, sarcoma, lymphoma) and benign neoplasms (leiomyoma, papilloma, and fibrovascular polyps). Approximately 15% of esophageal tumors arise in the proximal esophagus, 50% in the middle third of the esophagus, and 35% in the lower third.

SYNONYMS

Neoplasm of the esophagus
Malignancy of the esophagus

ICD-10CM CODES
C15.X Malignant neoplasm of the esophagus (X defines location)
D00.2 Carcinoma of esophagus, in situ

EPIDEMIOLOGY & DEMOGRAPHICS

INCIDENCE: Varies widely worldwide. It is the eighth most common incident cancer and the seventh leading cause of cancer death worldwide. Rates are increasing every decade and are highest in the Asian esophageal cancer belt, extending from the Caspian Sea to northern China, with certain high-incidence pockets in Finland, Ireland, southeast Africa, and northwest France. Incidence has increased sixfold since 1975. Rates of squamous cell carcinoma are decreasing while rates of esophagus adenocarcinomas are dramatically increasing.

PREVALENCE: In the United States, more than 16,000 new cases and more than 14,000 deaths per year, making it the seventh leading cause of death by cancer among men. The majority are diagnosed at an advanced stage (unresectable or metastatic disease).

RACE, AGE, & SEX PREDOMINANCE: In the United States, squamous cell esophageal cancer is more common among blacks than whites, whereas adenocarcinoma is more common in whites than blacks. The overall male/female ratio is 3 to 4:1; the highest male/female ratio is in the Hispanic population. It usually develops in the seventh and eighth decades and is associated with lower socioeconomic status.

GENETICS: Increasing evidence shows that genetics may play a role by increasing susceptibility to esophageal cancer. One well identified disease condition associated with esophageal cancer is tylosis (focal non-epidermolytic palmoplantar keratoderma), linked to loss of heterozygosity on chromosome 17q. Familiar clustering of Barrett's esophagus and the recent identification of germline mutations in affected sibling pairs support a genetic link to esophageal adenocarcinoma.

CLINICAL PRESENTATION

Symptoms and signs:
- Dysphagia (74%): initially occurs with solid foods and gradually progresses to include semisolids and liquids; latter signs usually indicate incurable disease with tumor involving more than 60% of the esophageal circumference. May be felt as chest pain.
- Unintentional weight loss: usually of short duration. Losing >10% of body mass predicts poor outcome.
- Hoarseness: suggests recurrent laryngeal nerve involvement.
- Odynophagia and halitosis: unusual symptoms.
- Cervical adenopathy: usually involving supraclavicular lymph nodes.
- Dry cough: suggests tracheal involvement.
- Aspiration pneumonia: caused by development of a fistula between the esophagus and trachea.
- Iron deficiency anemia, related to chronic GI blood loss.
- Massive hemoptysis or hematemesis: results from the invasion of vascular structures.
- Advanced disease spreads to lymph nodes, liver, lungs, peritoneum, and pleura.
- Hypercalcemia: associated with squamous cell carcinoma from secretion of a parathyroid-like tumor peptide.

Clinical findings:
- Fifty to sixty percent of patients present with locally advanced, regional, or metastatic disease.

ETIOLOGY

Pathogenesis of esophageal cancers is attributable to chronic recurrent oxidative damage from any of the following etiologic agents, which cause inflammation, and esophagitis, increased cell turnover, and, ultimately, initiation of the carcinogenic process.

ETIOLOGIC AGENTS:
- Excess alcohol consumption is strongly associated with squamous cell esophageal cancer in the United States; hard liquor is associated with a higher incidence than wine or beer.
- Tobacco and alcohol synergistically increase risk for squamous cell cancer.
- Smoking may increase the risk of developing adenocarcinoma, particularly in patients with Barrett's.
- Obesity, hiatal hernia, and low-vitamin, high-fat diet.
- Other ingested carcinogens:
  - Nitrates (converted to nitrites): South Asia, China
  - Smoked opiates: Northern Iran
  - Fungal toxins in pickled vegetables
  - Betel nut chewing
- Mucosal damage:
  - Long-term exposure to extremely hot tea (>70° C)
  - Lye ingestion
- Radiation-induced strictures
- Achalasia: incidence of esophageal cancer is seven times greater in this population
- Host susceptibility as a result of precancerous lesions:
  - Plummer-Vinson syndrome (Paterson-Kelly): glossitis with iron deficiency
  - Congenital hyperkeratosis and pitting of palms and soles (tylosis)
- Chronic GERD leading to Barrett's metaplasia and adenocarcinoma. The annual rate of transformation from Barrett's to adenocarcinoma is 0.5%.
- Human papillomavirus infection (particularly types 16 and 18) has been variably detected in squamous cell carcinoma of the esophagus, sometimes associated with p53 tumor suppressor gene mutations.
- Possible association with celiac sprue or dietary deficiencies of molybdenum, selenium, zinc, vitamin A.
- Questionable relationship with prolonged bisphosphonate use (≥10 prescriptions, or use >3 yr).

DIAGNOSIS

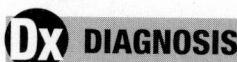

DIFFERENTIAL DIAGNOSIS
- Achalasia
- Scleroderma of the esophagus
- Diffuse esophageal spasm
- Esophageal rings and webs

LABORATORY TESTS

Complete blood cell count, blood chemistry, liver enzymes. No biomarkers are available currently to diagnose, monitor, or predict outcomes.

IMAGING STUDIES

Imaging studies are important not only for diagnosis but for accurate staging (Fig. 1-332):
- Esophagogastroduodenoscopy (EGD) (Fig. E1-333) should be performed initially to visualize smaller tumors, which may be missed by esophagogram, and to allow histopathologic confirmation.
- Endoscopic inspection of the larynx, trachea, and bronchi may identify concomitant cancers of head, neck, and lung ("triple endoscopy").

TABLE 1-149 Classification of Esophageal Cancer

Epithelial

Squamous cell
   Ordinary squamous cell
   Verrucous squamous cell
   Spindle cell (carcinosarcoma)
Adenocarcinoma
   Ordinary
   Adenoacanthoma
   Mucoepidermoid
   Adenoid cystic
Small cell
Melanoma
Choriocarcinoma

Metastatic Disease

Lymphoma
Sarcoma

From Abeloff MD: *Clinical oncology*, ed 3, Philadelphia, 2004, Churchill Livingstone.

- Endoscopic ultrasonogram (EUS) (Fig. E1-333) may be performed for locoregional staging: to determine the depth of tumor invasion and to assess for suspicious lymph nodes.
- Double-contrast esophagogram effectively identifies large esophageal lesions (Fig. 1-334).

  ○ In contrast to benign esophageal leiomyomata, which cause narrowing with preservation of normal mucosal pattern, esophageal carcinomas cause ragged ulcerating mucosal changes in association with deeper infiltration.

- Chest and abdominal CT and/or integrated CT-PET scans can determine tumor spread for preoperative staging.
- Staging laparoscopy may alter treatment plans in 20% to 30% of cases by more accurately staging regional lymph nodes and detecting occult peritoneal metastases.

STAGING
Table 1-150 describes the TNM staging system for cancer of the esophagus from the American Joint Committee on Cancer Criteria.

Rx TREATMENT

ACUTE GENERAL Rx
RESECTION:
- Surgical resection of squamous cell carcinoma and adenocarcinoma of the lower third of the esophagus is indicated for local, resectable disease in the absence of widespread metastasis detected by CT-PET. Gastric pull-through or colonic interposition typically is used to provide luminal continuity.
- Endoscopic mucosal resection may replace radical surgical resection in very early tumors with no lymph node involvement (T stage Tis or T1a), but a recent Cochrane review found no studies comparing endoscopic treatment vs. surgery. This may be performed in conjunction with ablative therapies, including radiofrequency ablation, thermal ablation techniques, or photodynamic therapy.
- Complications of surgery:
  ○ Anatomic fistula (usually with colon interposition, subphrenic abscesses)
  ○ Respiratory complications
  ○ Cardiovascular complications are most common, including MI, CVA, and PE
  ○ Mortality is lower and clinical outcomes are better at high volume hospitals.

RADIATION THERAPY:
- Squamous cell carcinomas are more radiosensitive than adenocarcinoma. Radiation achieves good local control and is generally only used as monotherapy as a palliative modality for obstructive symptoms in unresectable or advanced cancer. It is best used for cervical esophageal tumors.
- Palliative radiation therapy for bone metastasis is also effective.
- Complications of radiation therapy:
  ○ Esophageal stricture, radiation-induced pulmonary fibrosis, and transverse myelitis are the most feared.
  ○ Radiation-induced cardiomyopathy and skin changes are rare.

COMBINATION CHEMOTHERAPY, RADIATION Rx, & SURGICAL Rx:
- Chemotherapy is most often given with concurrent radiation therapy (chemoradiotherapy). Chemotherapy may sensitize tumor cells to the effects of ionizing radiation, improving the tumoricidal effects of treatment. Two-yr survival is improved with chemoradiotherapy (30%) vs. radiotherapy alone (10%). Trials have shown that preoperative chemoradiotherapy improves survival among patients

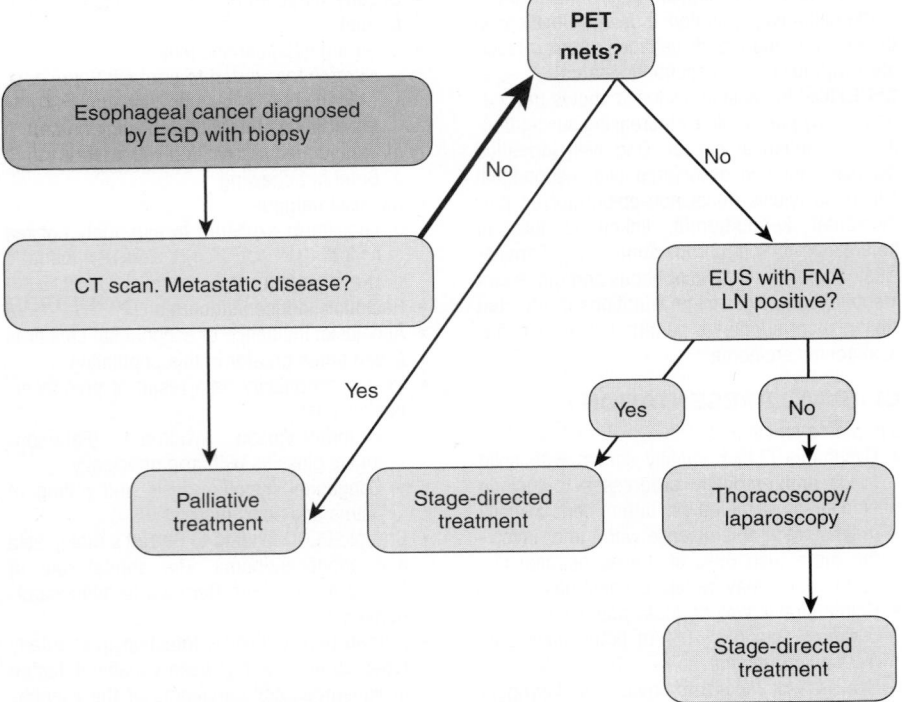

FIGURE 1-332 Algorithm for staging esophageal cancer. *CT,* Computed tomography; *EGD,* esophagogastroduodenoscopy; *mets,* metastases; *PET,* positron emission tomography. (From Cameron JL, Cameron AM: *Current surgical therapy,* ed 10, Philadelphia, 2011, Saunders.)

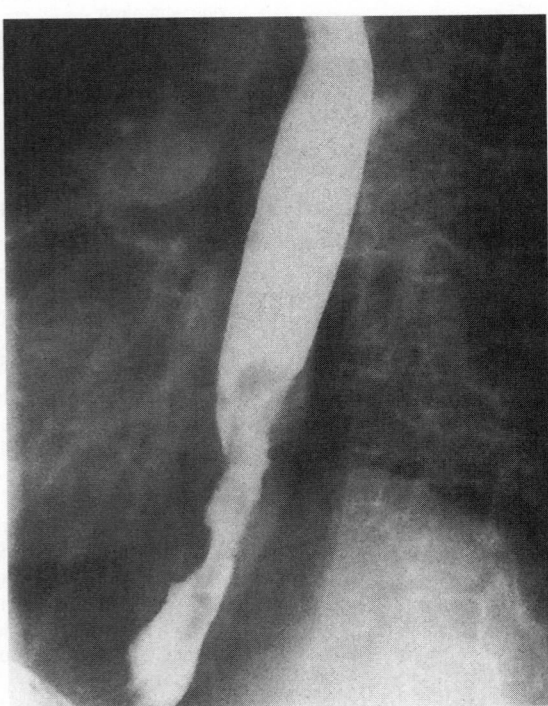

FIGURE 1-334 Barium swallow demonstrating the classic findings in cancer of the distal third of the esophagus. (Reprinted from Noble J [ed]: *Primary care medicine,* ed 2, St Louis, 1996, Mosby.)

with potentially curable esophageal or esoph-agogastric junction cancer.

- Chemoradiotherapy combined with surgery is offered to late Stage I (T2N0 or T3N0), Stage II, and Stage III esophageal cancer patients. Chemoradiotherapy alone may be offered to patients who are not surgical candidates.
- Combination chemotherapy including cisplatin achieved significant tumor reduction in 30% to 60% of patients. Cisplatin is usually given with 5-FU but has also been used in

TABLE 1-150 TNM Staging System for Cancer of the Esophagus (American Joint Committee on Cancer Criteria)

Primary Tumor (T)*	
TX	Primary tumor cannot be assessed
T0	No evidence of primary tumor
Tis	High-grade dysplasia†
T1	Tumor invades lamina propria, muscularis mucosae, or submucosa
T1a	Tumor invades lamina propria or muscularis mucosae
T1b	Tumor invades submucosa
T2	Tumor invades muscularis propria
T3	Tumor invades adventitia
T4	Tumor invades adjacent structures
T4a	Resectable tumor invading pleura, pericardium, or diaphragm
T4b	Unresectable tumor invading other adjacent structures, such as aorta, vertebral body, trachea, etc.

Lymph Node (N)‡	
NX	Regional lymph nodes cannot be assessed
N0	No regional lymph node metastasis
N1	Metastasis in 1-2 regional lymph nodes
N2	Metastasis in 3-6 regional lymph nodes
N3	Metastasis in 7 or more regional lymph nodes

Distant Metastasis (M)	
MX	Metastasis cannot be assessed
M0	No distant metastasis
M1	Distant metastasis

*(1) At least maximal dimension of the tumor must be recorded and (2) multiple tumors require the T(m) suffix.
†High-grade dysplasia includes all noninvasive neoplastic epithelia that was formerly called carcinoma in situ.
‡Number must be recorded for total number of regional nodes sampled and total number of reported nodes with metastasis.
From Goldman L, Schafer AI: *Goldman's Cecil medicine,* ed 24, Philadelphia, 2012, Saunders.

combinations with irinotecan, vinblastine, bleomycin, vindesine, and mitomycin.
- Capecitabine and oxaliplatin are as effective as fluorouracil and cisplatin, respectively, in patients with previously untreated esophagogastric cancer.
- Trastuzumab and Cetuximab, in combination with more traditional chemotherapy, are being studied for a subset of patients with HER-2 overexpressing esophageal adeno-acarcinoma.
- Complications of chemotherapy include mucositis, GI toxicity, myelosuppression, nephrotoxicity; ototoxicity and neurotoxicity occur with cisplatin.
- In several studies, preoperative chemoradiotherapy plus surgery significantly improved local control, reduced recurrence, and reduced mortality compared with surgery alone in patients with resectable esophageal cancer. Trimodal therapy is the preferred treatment for most esophageal cancers.

CHRONIC Rx

Palliative procedures such as repeated endoscopic dilation, endoscopic ablation, endoscopic mucosal resection, photodynamic therapy, brachytherapy, feeding tube insertion, or placement of expandable metal stents or polyvinyl prostheses to bypass tumors have been used for unresectable patients. The morbidity and mortality associated with resection in patients with advanced disease and/or for palliation argues against offering this modality to most of these patients.

DISPOSITION

- Overall 5-yr survival is 13% (37.3% for localized disease, 18.4% for regional disease, and 3.1% for distant disease)
- Endoscopic therapy for highly selected Stage 0 or Stage 1 patients with disease limited to the submucosa may have 5-year survival rates of 60% to 90%.
- Surgery: 5-yr survival rate is 5% to 30%, with higher survival (up to 45% to 50%) in early stage cancers
- Radiation therapy: 5-yr survival rate of 6%-20%
- Combined chemotherapy and radiation therapy: 5-year survival up to 27%
- Combined trimodality: up to 39% 5-year survival rate
- Patients with Stage IV disease receive palliative chemotherapy with a median survival of less than 1 year

REFERRAL

- To gastroenterologist for endoscopy for patients with dysphagia, odynophagia, or unexplained weight loss, or for palliative care
- To medical oncologist for evaluation of preoperative chemotherapy
- To radiation oncologist for palliative therapy if tumor is unresectable or obstruction is present
- To hospice if appropriate

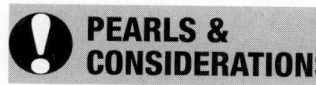 **PEARLS & CONSIDERATIONS**

COMMENTS

More than 50% of patients with esophageal cancer are diagnosed when the disease is metastatic or unresectable.

PREVENTION

- A diet high in fruits, vegetables, and antioxidants may be associated with lower risk of esophageal cancer.
- Avoid tobacco and excessive alcohol use.
- Avoid ingested toxins known to cause esophageal cancers.
- Aspirin may have a chemopreventative role in Barrett's but is only currently recommended for patients with other (e.g., cardiac) indications.
- There is no evidence that vitamins, Chinese herbal regimens, or green tea prevent esophageal cancer.
- Screening the general population is not recommended. If Barrett's esophagus is detected, regularly scheduled surveillance endoscopies are necessary, with consideration for radiofrequency or other ablation therapy if dysplasia is detected.

PATIENT/FAMILY EDUCATION

Provide education and support about the likely prognosis because most esophageal cancers are diagnosed at an advanced stage.

SUGGESTED READINGS

available at www.expertconsult.com

RELATED CONTENT

Barrett's Esophagus (Related Key Topic)
Esophageal Cancer (Patient Information)

AUTHOR: **HARLAN G. RICH, M.D., F.A.C.P., A.F.A.F.**

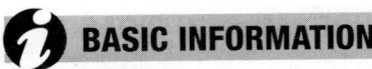

DEFINITION

Esophageal varices are dilated submucosal veins that occur in patients with underlying portal hypertension, function as a shunt between the portal venous and systemic venous circulation, and can result in severe upper GI hemorrhage.

ICD-10CM CODES
85.00 Esophageal varices without bleeding
I85.01 Esophageal varices with bleeding
I85.10 Secondary esophageal varices without bleeding
I85.11 Secondary esophageal varices with bleeding

EPIDEMIOLOGY & DEMOGRAPHICS

INCIDENCE:
- Esophageal varices: 5%-15% per year in patients with cirrhosis
- Hemorrhage:
  - One third of all patients with varices will develop hemorrhage.
  - Variceal hemorrhage occurs in 25%-40% of patients with cirrhosis
  - The risk of bleeding from varices is approximately 15% at 1 year.
  - Survivors of an episode of active bleeding have a 70% risk of recurrent hemorrhage within 1 year.

PREVALENCE: Approximately 50% of patients with cirrhosis have varices at the time of diagnosis.

RISK FACTORS: Cirrhosis, low platelet count and advanced Child-Pugh class, hepatitis C with advanced fibrosis

PHYSICAL FINDINGS & CLINICAL PRESENTATION

- Often asymptomatic until acute upper GI hemorrhage: hematemesis, hypovolemia
- No physical findings specific for esophageal varices
- Stigmata of cirrhosis and portal hypertension may be evident: palmar erythema, telangiectasias, gynecomastia, testicular atrophy, jaundice, caput medusae, lower extremity edema, ascites, splenomegaly, hemorrhoids, asterixis

ETIOLOGY

- Portal hypertension results from obstruction to portal venous outflow, and varices subsequently develop in order to decompress the hypertensive portal vein and return blood to the systemic circulation.
- Varices may appear when portal vein pressures rise above 10-12 mm Hg.
- Cirrhosis is the most common cause of portal hypertension.

DIAGNOSIS

DIFFERENTIAL DIAGNOSIS

- Budd-Chiari syndrome, cirrhosis, portal vein thrombosis, schistosomiasis, Wilson's disease

- Other causes of upper GI bleeding: duodenal or gastric ulcers, gastric cancer, Mallory-Weiss tear

WORKUP

Upper endoscopy, laboratory tests, and imaging

LABORATORY TESTS

- CBC
  - Anemia (blood loss, nutritional deficiencies, alcohol myelosuppression)
  - Thrombocytopenia (hypersplenism, alcohol myelosuppression)
- Renal function panel
  - BUN: often increased in setting of upper GI bleeding
  - Creatinine: often elevated by hypovolemia, monitor for hepatorenal syndrome
  - Sodium: dilutional hyponatremia
- Heme-positive stools
- Type and Crossmatch: in preparation for blood transfusion
- INR/ PT and PTT: coagulation factors produced in liver and may be prolonged in liver disease or impairment
- Liver function tests: ALT/AST may be normal in cirrhotic patients due to longstanding fibrosis; elevated alkaline phosphatase and a direct hyperbilirubinemia may be present if cholestatic liver disease is present
- Serum albumin: severe liver disease results in hypoalbuminemia

IMAGING STUDIES

Invasive:
- Esophagogastroduodenoscopy (EGD) (upper endoscopy):
  - In all patients with cirrhosis, screen for the presence or absence of varices and determine subsequent risk for variceal hemorrhage.
  - In patients with compensated cirrhosis who do not have varices, screening is repeated every 2 to 3 years.
  - In patients with decompensated cirrhosis (ascites, hepatic encephalopathy, variceal hemorrhage, or jaundice), it is repeated every year or at the time of first decompensation.
  - Emergently performed if there is evidence of acute upper GI bleeding to diagnose and treat variceal hemorrhage.
Noninvasive:
- Esophagography with barium can diagnose esophageal varices.
- Capsule endoscopy can also diagnose esophageal varices, although sensitivity is not yet established.

TREATMENT

NONPHARMACOLOGIC THERAPY

- Endoscopic variceal ligation (Fig. 1-335) is an alternative to nonselective beta-blockers for primary prophylaxis against variceal hemorrhage.

- Typically for patients with medium or large varices at highest risk for hemorrhage (Child-Pugh B/C or red wale markings viewed on endoscopy)
- Usually 2-4 sessions
- May not be a permanent solution because varices can recur after initial eradication
- Associated with significant complications, including hemorrhage from banding-induced ulcerations
  - Therefore should be performed by endoscopists with expertise in prophylactic banding
  - First surveillance endoscopy 1-3 months after obliteration, then every 6-12 months indefinitely

ACUTE GENERAL Rx

- Variceal hemorrhage: acute hemodynamic resuscitation with packed red blood cell transfusion, correct coagulopathy and thrombocytopenia, airway protection and intubation as necessary, antibiotics (ceftriaxone or norfloxacin) for SBP prophylaxis, octreotide maintained for 2-5 days in conjunction with endoscopic therapy
- EGD to treat bleeding esophageal varices by esophageal band ligation or sclerotherapy

CHRONIC Rx

Primary prophylaxis:
- Nonselective beta-blockers such as propranolol (20 mg twice daily) and nadolol (40 mg once daily)
  - Increase as tolerated for goal heart rate of approximately 55 beats/min
  - Blocks the adrenergic dilatory tone in mesenteric arterioles, resulting in unopposed alpha-adrenergic mediated vasoconstriction and therefore a decrease in portal inflow
Secondary prophylaxis:
- All patients with compensated cirrhosis who have bled from esophageal varices should receive esophageal band ligation and beta-blockers, unless beta-blockers are contraindicated.
  - Transjugular intrahepatic portosystemic shunt or surgical shunt may be performed if bleeding from esophageal varices continues or recurs despite this dual therapy.
- For patients with decompensated cirrhosis there is evidence, although limited, against the use of prophylactic beta-blockers due to the risk for increased mortality.

REFERRAL

Consultation with a gastroenterologist is recommended in all patients with cirrhosis or portal hypertension in order to screen for esophageal varices.

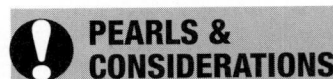 **PEARLS & CONSIDERATIONS**

Besides variceal size, risk factors for variceal hemorrhage include Child-Pugh class B/C or variceal red wale markings on endoscopy.

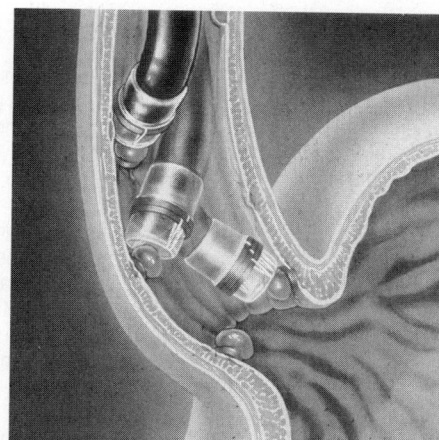

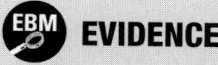

FIGURE 1-335 Esophageal varices. Endoscopic band ligation performed with a multiple-band ligating device. The endoscopist makes circumferential contact between the end of the ligating device and the varix to be ligated. Endoscopic suction draws the varix into the device, after which the elastic band is ejected to ensnare the varix. The ligated tissue sloughs after 3 to 5 days, leaving a shallow ulceration that generally heals within 1 week. (Courtesy Bard Endoscopic Technologies, Billerica, Mass.)

PREVENTION

Treatment of the underling liver disease may help to prevent variceal development. However, treatment with nonselective beta-blockers is not recommended because they do not prevent the development of varices.

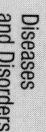

EBM **EVIDENCE**

available at www.expertconsult.com

SUGGESTED READINGS

available at www.expertconsult.com

RELATED CONTENT

Cirrhosis (Related Key Topic)
Portal Hypertension (Related Key Topic)

AUTHOR: **ADAM J. WEINBERG, M.D.**

Diseases and Disorders

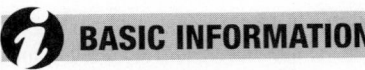

BASIC INFORMATION

DEFINITION

A predominantly postural and action tremor that is bilateral and tends to progress slowly over the years in the absence of other neurologic abnormalities.

SYNONYMS

Benign essential tremor
Familial tremor

ICD-9CM CODES
333.1 Essential tremor

EPIDEMIOLOGY & DEMOGRAPHICS

PREDOMINANT AGE: Can begin at any age, but incidence increases after age 40 yr. Prevalence is 6% to 9% for those >60 yr.
GENETICS: No gender or racial predominance.

PHYSICAL FINDINGS & CLINICAL PRESENTATION

- Patients complain of tremor that is most bothersome when writing or holding something such as a newspaper or trying to drink from a cup. Worsens under emotional distress.
- Tremor, 4 to 12 Hz, bilateral postural and action tremor of the upper extremities. May also affect the head, voice, trunk, and legs. Typically it is the same amplitude throughout the action, such as bringing a cup to the mouth. No other neurologic abnormalities on examination except difficulty with tandem gait. Patients often note improvement with intake of small amounts of alcohol.

ETIOLOGY

Often an inherited disease, autosomal dominant; sporadic cases without a family history are frequently encountered

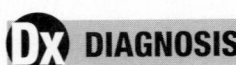

DIAGNOSIS

DIFFERENTIAL DIAGNOSIS

(see Table 1-151)

- Parkinson's disease—tremor is usually asymmetric, especially early on in the disease, and is predominantly a resting tremor. Patients with Parkinson's disease will often also have increased tone, decreased facial expression, slowness of movement, and shuffling gait.
- Cerebellar tremor—an intention tremor that increases at the end of a goal-directed movement (such as finger to nose testing). Other associated neurologic abnormalities include ataxia, dysarthria, and difficulty with tandem gait.
- Drug-induced—there are many drugs that enhance normal, physiologic tremor. These include caffeine, nicotine, lithium, levothyroxine, β-adrenergic bronchodilators, amiodarone, valproate, and SSRIs.
- Wilson's disease—wing-beating tremor that is most pronounced with shoulders abducted, elbows flexed, and fingers pointing towards each other. Usually there are other neurologic abnormalities including dysarthria, dystonia, and Kayser-Fleischer rings on ophthalmologic examination.
- Physiologic tremor

WORKUP

- Essential tremor is a clinical diagnosis
- All imaging studies normal (MRI, CT) and are unnecessary unless there are other associated neurologic abnormalities
- Check TSH (rule out hyperthyroidism)
- In patients younger than 40 yrs with other neurologic abnormalities, send ceruloplasmin, serum Cu, 24-hr urine Cu to rule out Wilson's disease

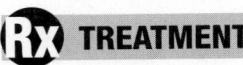

TREATMENT

Treat essential tremor when it is functionally impairing. Treatments are up to 75% effective.

NONPHARMACOLOGIC THERAPY

- Reduction of stress
- Minimize use of caffeine
- Small quantities of alcohol at social functions may be beneficial

ACUTE GENERAL Rx

Propanolol (20 to 40 mg) may be used in preparation for specific event.

CHRONIC Rx

First-line agents:
- Propranolol/Propranolol LA: Usual starting dose is 30 mg. The usual therapeutic dose is 160 to 320 mg. Although not contraindicated, they must be used with caution in those with asthma, depression, cardiac disease, and diabetes.
- Primidone: Usual starting dose is 12.5 to 25 mg qhs. Usual therapeutic dose is between 62.5 and 750 mg daily (assuming side effects are tolerated). Sedation and nausea when first begin medication are biggest side effects.
- Topiramate: 25 mg qhs, may titrate up to about 400 mg

Other agents:
- Gabapentin: 400 mg qhs, usual therapeutic dose is 1200 to 3600 mg
- Alprazolam: 0.75 to 2.75 mg
- Botulinum toxin injected focally may decrease tremor
- Atenonol, sotalol

SURGICAL Rx

Thalamic deep brain stimulation (or possibly thalamotomy) contralateral to side of tremor is reserved for resistant tremor or for patients who do not tolerate drug therapy.

DISPOSITION

Patients should be reassured that the condition is not associated with other neurologic disabilities; however, it can become quite functionally disabling over time.

REFERRAL

This is a condition that usually can be treated by the primary care physician; however, if patient fails first-line therapies then patient should be referred to specialists for other drug trials and other possible surgical options.

PEARLS & CONSIDERATIONS

- Essential tremor is the most common of all movement disorders.
- In addition to motor dysfunction, essential tremor can cause significant psychological impact on patients in social situations.

SUGGESTED READINGS

available at www.expertconsult.com

RELATED CONTENT

Essential Tremor (Patient Information)

AUTHOR: **U. SHIVRAJ SOHUR, M.D., PH.D.**

TABLE 1-151 Overlapping Features of Various Types of Tremor

Feature	Parkinson's Syndrome	Cerebellar Tremor	Essential Tremor
Present at rest	Yes	No	Yes
Increased tone	Yes	No	No
Decreased tone	No	Yes	No
Postural abnormality	Yes	Yes	No
Head involvement	Yes	Yes	Yes
Intentional component	No	Yes	Yes
Incoordination	No	Yes	No

From Remmel KS et al: *Handbook of symptom-oriented neurology,* ed 3, St Louis, 2002, Mosby.

BASIC INFORMATION

DEFINITION

Factitious physical disorder occurs when an individual intentionally strives to create signs or symptoms of disease. The individual may create signs or symptoms by (1) lying, (2) simulating (e.g., putting drops of blood into a urine sample), or (3) actually creating disease (e.g., injecting bacteria or medications). The primary aim is to achieve the patient role, and the individual may seek invasive diagnostic testing, surgery, or treatment. Munchausen's syndrome is the most severe variant of factitious physical disorder and is characterized by exaggerated lying (pseudologia fantastica), sociopathy, geographic wandering from hospital to hospital, and a continuous life of patienthood.

SYNONYMS

Factitious disorder
Munchausen's syndrome (the most severe variant of factitious disorder)
Munchausen by proxy (factitious disorder created in another person, usually a child)
Deliberate disability
Hospital addiction syndrome
Artifactual illness
Peregrinating problem patients
Dermatitis artefacta
Surreptitious illness

ICD-9CM CODES
300.19 Factitious disorder

EPIDEMIOLOGY & DEMOGRAPHICS

INCIDENCE (IN U.S.): Unknown
PEAK INCIDENCE: 30 to 40 yr
PREVALENCE (IN U.S.): Unknown but considerable in specific illnesses. For example, 3.3% of patients with fever of unknown origin have a factitious disorder.
PREDOMINANT SEX: Male/female ratio of 2:1 for Munchausen's syndrome but 1:2 for individuals with non-Munchausen type of factitious physical disorder.
PREDOMINANT AGE: 30 to 40 yr
GENETICS: No genetic predisposition known

PHYSICAL FINDINGS & CLINICAL PRESENTATION

- False complaints or self-inflicted injury or symptoms without clear secondary gain. The intentional aspect of the disorder is often evident, such as injecting bacteria to produce infection or taking medication to produce an abnormality.
- Presentation may be acute and dramatic, but the condition can be a chronic, recurring problem.
- Workup is usually negative for naturally occurring organic etiology.
- Clinical picture is atypical for the natural history of disease (e.g., an infection that does not respond to multiple courses of appropriate antibiotics).

ETIOLOGY

- A history of significant childhood illness; physical or sexual abuse are thought to predispose.
- Personality disorders and psychodynamic factors often play a significant role.

Dx DIAGNOSIS

The diagnosis can be made by (1) direct observation of fabrication, (2) the presence of signs or symptoms that contradict laboratory testing, (3) nonphysiologic response to treatment, (4) the presence of physical evidence of fabrication (e.g., syringes at the bedside), and (5) recurrent patterns of illness exacerbation (e.g., just before discharge) or failure to follow the natural history of disease (e.g., a wound that does not heal for no apparent reason).

DIFFERENTIAL DIAGNOSIS

- Malingering: falsifying an illness for a clear secondary gain (e.g., financial gain or avoidance of unwanted duties).
- Somatoform disorders or hypochondriasis: these disorders are produced unconsciously and are not intentionally produced.
- Self-injurious behavior is common in many other psychiatric conditions; in those conditions the patients confess the intentional self-harm and describe motivating factors. The main intent is the self-harm and not to attain the patient role, as occurs in factitious disorder.
- May also present as Munchausen by proxy, in which a mother (86% of time) or other caregiver induces illness in a child (52% between ages of 3 and 13 yr) for the purpose of obtaining medical attention or some other psychological need. Mothers often have a history of somatoform, factitious, or personality disorder themselves.

WORKUP

- Dictated by the presenting complaints.
- No specific tests for Munchausen's syndrome.
- Diagnosis may be made when the patient is caught in the act of lying or inducing an injury. The diagnosis often rests on organic workup failing to reveal a plausible natural organic disease. The failure of usual, or even extensive, treatment to ameliorate a condition is an important clue.

LABORATORY TESTS

- Laboratory testing often reveals inconsistencies.
- Other laboratory abnormalities may reflect the underlying factitious behavior (e.g., hypokalemia in an individual surreptitiously taking furosemide).

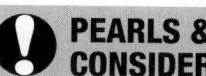 TREATMENT

NONPHARMACOLOGIC THERAPY

Two major approaches:
- Nonpunitive confrontation. Primary physician and psychiatrist conjointly meet with patient and say, "You must be in a lot of distress to be harming yourself as we believe you have been. We would like to help you deal with your distress more adaptively and get you into psychiatric treatment."
- Avoid overt confrontation with patient but provide him or her with a face-saving way to recover. For example, a therapeutic double bind would involve saying, "There are two possibilities here, one is that you have a medical problem that should respond to the next intervention we do, or two, you have a factitious disorder. The outcome will give us the answer."
- Munchausen's syndrome is the most severe variant and may be virtually impossible to treat except to avoid further invasive and iatrogenic disease.

ACUTE GENERAL Rx

Treatment of comorbid psychiatric disorders may be helpful. Treatment with antidepressants or psychotherapy may ameliorate the factitious behavior. Multidisciplinary staff meetings are useful to ventilate feelings and develop cohesive treatment plans.

DISPOSITION

- After being confronted with their behavior, patients may cease factitious behavior, but they more commonly seek other physicians or hospitals, as in the Munchausen variant. Other factitious disorder patients may enter psychotherapy, particularly when they have been given a face-saving approach with avoidance of a humiliating confrontation.
- Extensive medical workups and exploratory surgery are frequent.

REFERRAL

Always obtain psychiatric referral. Risk management attorneys and hospital ethicists may contribute to challenging decision making in these patients.

PEARLS & CONSIDERATIONS

Think of factitious disorders whenever there is an unexplained medical course that continues to repeat despite appropriate treatment, particularly in patients associated with the health care field. There is current consideration of whether factitious disorders should be classified in the upcoming DSM-5 as a subset of somatoform disorders. This possibility is related to the challenge of discriminating whether an illness state is being consciously (factitious) or unconsciously (somatoform) produced. Future research will investigate the utility of this possible change in classification.

SUGGESTED READINGS
available at www.expertconsult.com

RELATED CONTENT
Hypochondriasis (Related Key Topic)

AUTHOR: **STUART J. EISENDRATH, M.D.**

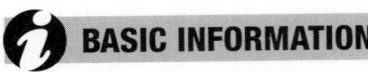

BASIC INFORMATION

DEFINITION

Failure to thrive (FTT) describes a delay in growth and development among children. FTT is a cluster of symptoms rather than a specific disease.

SYNONYMS

Pediatric undernutrition
Faltering growth
Weight faltering
Growth failure

ICD-9CM CODES

263.0	Malnutrition of moderate degree
263.1	Malnutrition of mild degree
263.2	Arrested development following protein-calorie malnutrition
263.8	Other protein-calorie malnutrition
263.9	Unspecified protein-calorie malnutrition
779.34	Failure to thrive in newborn
783.2	Abnormal loss of weight and underweight
783.21	Loss of weight
783.22	Underweight
783.4	Lack of expected normal physiologic development in childhood
783.40	Unspecified lack of normal physiologic development
783.41	Failure to thrive
783.43	Short stature

EPIDEMIOLOGY & DEMOGRAPHICS

INCIDENCE: FTT is a common problem, though its incidence in the community is unclear. A total of 1% to 5% of inpatient pediatric admissions are for evaluation of FTT.
PREDOMINANT SEX AND AGE: FTT most commonly occurs among children ages 6 to 12 months, with 80% presenting before 18 months of age. Most FTT patients present before 3 years of age. Males and females are equally affected.
RISK FACTORS: Poverty is the single greatest risk factor. Nonmedical: poverty, food insecurity, social isolation, neglect, and physical or emotional abuse. Medical: Intrauterine growth restriction (IUGR), prematurity, medical conditions leading to inadequate food intake, food malabsorption, or increased metabolic demand.

PHYSICAL FINDINGS & CLINICAL PRESENTATION

Children have blunted growth in height, weight, head circumference, or any combination of these. Children may have pallid, dry, or cracked skin, sparse hair growth, poorly developed musculature, lack of subcutaneous fat, swollen abdomen, or evidence of vitamin deficiencies.

ETIOLOGY

FTT is the result of inadequate nutrition, which may be due to a wide range of medical or psychosocial causes. FTT can be thought of as stemming from inadequate nutritional intake, malabsorption of nutrients, or increased caloric expenditure, though the actual cause is commonly multifactorial.

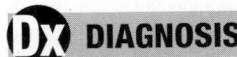

DIAGNOSIS

DIFFERENTIAL DIAGNOSIS

- Inadequate nutritional intake: food insecurity, poor parent knowledge of child's needs, formula dilution, excessive juice, breastfeeding difficulties, neglect, behavioral feeding problem, oromotor dysfunction, developmental delay, emesis, gastroesophageal reflux, volvulus, increased intracranial pressure, genetic disease (trisomy 13, 18, 21), and psychiatric conditions
- Malabsorption: cystic fibrosis, celiac disease, food protein insensitivity or intolerance, and inflammatory bowel disease
- Increased metabolic demand: insulin resistance, congenital infection, other infection, genetic syndrome, hyperthyroidism, chronic disease, and malignancy

WORKUP

- Evaluation should include the child's eating habits, caloric intake, parent-child interactions, psychosocial history, and review of systems.
- Height, weight, and weight-to-length measurements are most sensitive, whereas head circumference and body mass index (BMI) may be useful. Common FTT criteria for children younger than 2 years are below, but clinical judgment should be used because normal causes and biologic variants may exist.
  - Length, weight, or BMI below the 3rd or 5th percentile on more than one consecutive visit
  - Weight that drops below two major percentile lines
  - Weight less than 80% of the ideal weight for age
  - Weight-to-length below the 5th percentile or weight-for-length less than 70% to 79% of the median
  - Weight velocity below the 3rd or 5th percentile
  - Weight less than 70% of the 50th percentile; may require hospitalization
- Obtain caliper measurements of skinfold thickness and midarm muscle circumference.
- A 3-day food diary is helpful, as well as consultation by a nutritionist, to calculate the child's intake of energy, protein, vitamins, and minerals.
- Assess stool frequency, consistency, quantity, as well as fat, blood, or mucus content.
- Routine hospitalization for FTT evaluation is not recommended. Rarely, hospitalization for observed feedings and further workup is warranted.

LABORATORY TESTS

- Laboratory tests have limited utility in screening for FTT unless a specific underlying medical cause is suspected.
- Consider CBC with red blood cell indices, complete chemistry panel, celiac screening, stool examination for fats or reducing substances, or sweat chloride testing. If clinically indicated, thyroid function and growth hormone level can be checked.

IMAGING STUDIES

Imaging tests are not routinely performed but may be warranted depending on underlying medical cause.

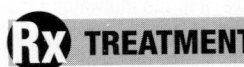

TREATMENT

Identification and management of underlying causes should be implemented. In cases in which there is no underlying medical condition, providing nutrition repletion will, by definition, correct FTT. A multidisciplinary team (including, but not limited to, social workers, occupational/speech therapists, nutritionists/dietitians, nurses, advanced practice nurses, and pediatricians) should be used.

NONPHARMACOLOGIC THERAPY

- Add calorie-dense foods or increase the number of feedings.
- Enteral feeding, percutaneous endoscopic gastrostomy (PEG), and nasogastric feeding tubes can be used to accelerate weight gain, and results should be seen within 2 to 7 days. Caloric intake should be titrated up to goal over 5 to 7 days. Caloric goals by age group: 0 to 6 months: 108 kcal/kg/day, 6 to 12 months: 98 kcal/kg/day, and 1 to 3 years: 102 kcal/kg/day.
- Swift restoration of nutrition can lead to life-threatening refeeding syndrome, where shifts in electrolyte balance (low phosphate, magnesium, potassium), fluid balance (edema), hypoglycemia, and impaired heart function can occur. Calories must therefore be titrated slowly to goal with close monitoring.
- Treat underlying medical conditions, including mental health disorders.
- Assist with family psychosocial stressors.
- Follow up closely, including home nursing visits.
- In cases where economic, psychosocial, or parental issues are suspected and the child's growth is not maintained, state and federal legislation regarding reporting to child protection services must be followed.

ACUTE GENERAL Rx

Multivitamins including iron and zinc

CHRONIC Rx

Nutrient repletion with the goal of accelerated growth should be continued for 4 to 9 months

DISPOSITION

Children with FTT commonly remain small in height and weight. Studies consistently find that children with FTT are more prone to long-term cognitive, learning, and behavioral abnormalities.

REFERRAL

- Indicated based on the cause of FTT
- Hospitalization should be considered in cases of FTT in which a child is less than 70% of predicted weight for length, where outpatient management has failed, when a suspicion of abuse or neglect exists, where signs of traumatic injury are present, or where serious impairment of the child's caregiver is evident.

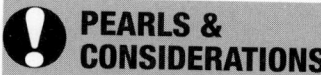

PEARLS & CONSIDERATIONS

COMMENTS

- FTT is a common childhood symptom encountered in the outpatient and inpatient pediatric populations, is caused by undernutrition, and is associated with inadequate nutritional intake, malabsorption, or increased metabolic demand.
- A thorough multidisciplinary approach to assessment, diagnosis, and management should be used to manage nutrient status and any underlying cause(s).
- Child height/length, weight, and weight-for-length measurements with comparison to standard growth curves are useful in the identification of potential cases of FTT.
- FTT treatment should include restoration of nutrition along with treatment of the underlying cause(s), including psychosocial factors.
- Although FTT can usually be managed effectively in the outpatient setting, specific indications for inpatient treatment should be considered.

PREVENTION

Nutritional counseling and anticipatory guidance should be provided at each well-child visit. Enlist dietitians and visiting nurses to provide support to families with children at high risk of FTT.

SUGGESTED READINGS

available at www.expertconsult.com

AUTHOR: **GRAYSON ARMSTRONG, B.A.**

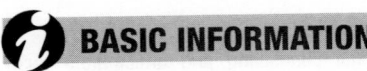

DEFINITION

A fall is an "event which results in a person coming to rest inadvertently on the ground and other than a consequence of the following: loss of consciousness, sudden onset of paralysis, or epileptic seizure" (Kellogg International Work Group, *Danish Medical Bulletin*, 34, 1-24).

SYNONYMS

Syncope
Collapse

ICD-9CM CODES
Accidental fall (E880-E888.9)

EPIDEMIOLOGY & DEMOGRAPHICS

INCIDENCE:
- Falls are the leading cause of accidental death among older adults.
- The incidence of falls among community-dwelling older adults is 30% to 40%.
- The incidence of falls for nursing home and hospitalized older adults is three times the rate of community-dwelling older adults.
- 20% to 30% of older adults who fall suffer significant injury leading to immobility, dependence, and an increased risk of early death.

PREDOMINANT SEX & AGE:
- Fall-related mortality is highest among older white men followed by white women, black men, and black women.
- The incidence rates of falls increase with advancing age.

- Older adults aged 85 years and over are 10 to 15 times more likely to have a fracture compared with those aged 60 to 65 years.

RISK FACTORS: Three groups of risk factors for falls have been identified (Table 1-152):
1. Intrinsic factors inherent in the older adult who falls
2. Extrinsic factors circumstantial to the older adult who falls
3. Situational or the activity in which the older adult is engaged in when a fall occurs

CLINICAL PRESENTATION

- Older adults who fall may present with minor soft tissue injuries, such as lacerations or bruising, hip fracture, or head trauma; however, most falls are not reported unless an injury has occurred.
- If an older adult presents for medical attention for a fall or reports recurrent falls in the past year or difficulties in walking or balance, a multifactorial fall risk assessment should be completed.
- The multifactorial fall risk assessment should include:
  - Focused history: A detailed history of events and circumstances surrounding fall, relevant risk factors including review of medications, acute and chronic medical problems (e.g., osteoporosis, urinary incontinence, and cardiovascular disease).
  - Physical examination
    - Vital signs including orthostatics
    - Cardiovascular examination to look for arrhythmias, carotid bruits, or new murmurs
    - Neurologic examination including vision assessment, evaluation of lower extremity strength, peripheral nerves, proprioception, and testing of cortical, extrapyradmidal, and cerebellar function
    - Gait and balance assessment: "Get up and go test" (Ask patient to stand from a seated position without use of hands, walk 10 feet forward, turn around, and return to chair and sit.)
    - Musculoskeletal exam with attention to joints of lower extremity, feet and footwear.
  - Functional assessment including the older adult's activities of daily living skills, use of adaptive equipment, and fear of falling
  - Environmental assessment of home safety

ETIOLOGY

- Falls are a multifactorial syndrome resulting from the cumulative effects of impaired gait and balance, aging, polypharmacy, depression, cognitive impairment, acute medical illness, or environmental factors (Fig. 1-336).
- Most falls among community-dwelling older adults are due to environmental factors, whereas falls among nursing home residents are a result of confusion, gait impairment, or postural hypotension.

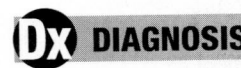 **DIAGNOSIS**

DIFFERENTIAL DIAGNOSIS

Falls are often a nonspecific symptom of an acute illness (such as a urinary tract infection, acute anemia, or pneumonia) or an exacerbation of a chronic disease (chronic heart failure [CHF] or chronic obstructive pulmonary disease [COPD]).

WORKUP

- Older adults presenting with a noninjurious fall need a detailed history and physical exam to identify acute medical illnesses and potential modifiable risk factors. Laboratory and neuroimaging studies may be necessary if the history and physical exam indicate a specific problem. ECG and Holter monitoring may be considered if cardiac arrhythmia is suspected.
- See Fig. 1-336.

LABORATORY TESTS

CBC, blood chemistries, thyroid function, vitamin B_{12} level, vitamin D level, drug levels, and urinalysis depending on physical/historical findings

IMAGING STUDIES

- CT or MRI of the brain or cervical spine films in the presence of neurologic or gait impairment.
- Consider ECG, echocardiography, or Holter monitor if suspicious for structural cardiac abnormality or syncope.

TABLE 1-152 Risk Factors for Falls in the Elderly

Intrinsic

Aging
Age-related decline in vestibular function might lead to increased sway, dizziness, and falls. Aging of the vision system may result in decreased visual acuity, inability to discriminate dark/light, and decreased spatial perception.

Cardiac
Cardiac arrhythmias, carotid sinus hypersensitivity

Neurologic
Parkinson's disease, normal pressure hydrocephalus (NPH), sensory neuropathy, dementia/impaired cognition, cervical myelopathy, senile gait disorder, prior stroke

Musculoskeletal
Lower extremity weakness, deconditioning, arthritis, foot abnormalities (such as bunions, calluses, or nail abnormalities)

Vascular
Vertebrobasilar insufficiency, postural hypotension, postprandial hypotension

Metabolic
Hypoglycemia, hypothyroidism, hyponatremia

Psychiatric
Depression

Extrinsic

Medications
Use of more than four medications may be associated with an increased risk of falls. Medications that may increase fall risk include benzodiazepines, sleeping medications, neuroleptics, antidepressants, anticonvulsants, class I antiarrhythmics, and antihypertensives (Rao, 2005).

Environmental
Inadequate lighting, ill-fitting shoes, slippery floor surfaces, loose rugs, uneven steps

Situational

Tripping over obstacles, carrying heavy items, descending/ascending stairs, rapid turning, reaching overhead, climbing ladders

F

TREATMENT

NONPHARMACOLOGIC THERAPY

- Physical therapy evaluation for gait and balance training, evaluation of appropriate assisted devices (e.g., cane, walker), the use of fall prevention equipment (e.g., low beds, bed alarms), and home safety assessment
- Minimization or discontinuation of certain medications associated with falls (psychotropics)
- Customized exercise program to improve strength, gait, and balance
- Evaluation of proper footwear, hard sole, and low heel height

ACUTE GENERAL Rx

Hospitalization may be necessary for treatment of hip fracture, subdural hematoma, lacerations, or trauma as well as the treatment of underlying cause of the fall such as infection, metabolic disturbances, cardiovascular (e.g., carotid sinus hypersensitivity, vasovagal syndrome, bradyarrhythmias, and tachyarrhythmias) or neurologic abnormality.

CHRONIC Rx

- Screen and treat for osteoporosis as low bone density increases the risk of hip or other fractures.
- Optimize treatment of chronic illnesses such as CHF, COPD, osteoarthritis, Parkinson's disease, dementia, postural hypotension, and visual problems.
- Vitamin D supplementation of at least 800 IU per day. Epidemiological studies reveal that compared to usual care, short-term intervention with oral nutritional supplementation and dietetic counseling significantly decrease falls in malnourished older adults.

COMPLEMENTARY & ALTERNATIVE MEDICINE

T'ai chi has been shown to reduce the risk of falls in community-dwelling study participants.

DISPOSITION

Falls increase the older adult's risk of hospitalization, institutionalization, and mortality.

REFERRAL

- Referral may be appropriate to cardiologist, ophthalmologist, neurologist, or podiatrist depending on the presence of a specific condition.
- Consider referral to physical therapist for gait and balance training, evaluation for assisted device, or strengthening program.

PEARLS & CONSIDERATIONS

COMMENTS

- Fear of falling may lead to restriction of activities, social isolation, and dependence.
- Older adults with four or more risk factors have a 78% chance of falling.
- Mortality from falls has increased by 42% over the past decade.

PREVENTION

The U.S. Preventive Services Task Force recommends exercise or physical therapy and vitamin D supplementation to prevent falls in community-dwelling adults aged 65 or older who are at increased risk for falls. It does not recommend automatically performing an in-depth multifactorial risk assessment in conjunction with comprehensive management of identified risks to prevent falls in community-dwelling adults aged 65 or older because the likelihood of benefit is small. In determining whether this service is appropriate in individual cases, patients and clinicians should consider the balance of benefits and harms on the basis of the circumstances of prior falls, comorbid medical conditions, and patient values.

PATIENT/FAMILY EDUCATION

Providing education and information for the patient and caregiver regarding fall prevention strategies in addition to multifactorial risk reduction strategies

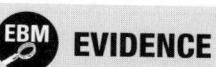 **EVIDENCE**

available at www.expertconsult.com

SUGGESTED READINGS
available at www.expertconsult.com

AUTHORS: **SEAN H. UITERWYK, M.D.,** and **ALICIA J. CURTIN, PH.D., G.N.P.**

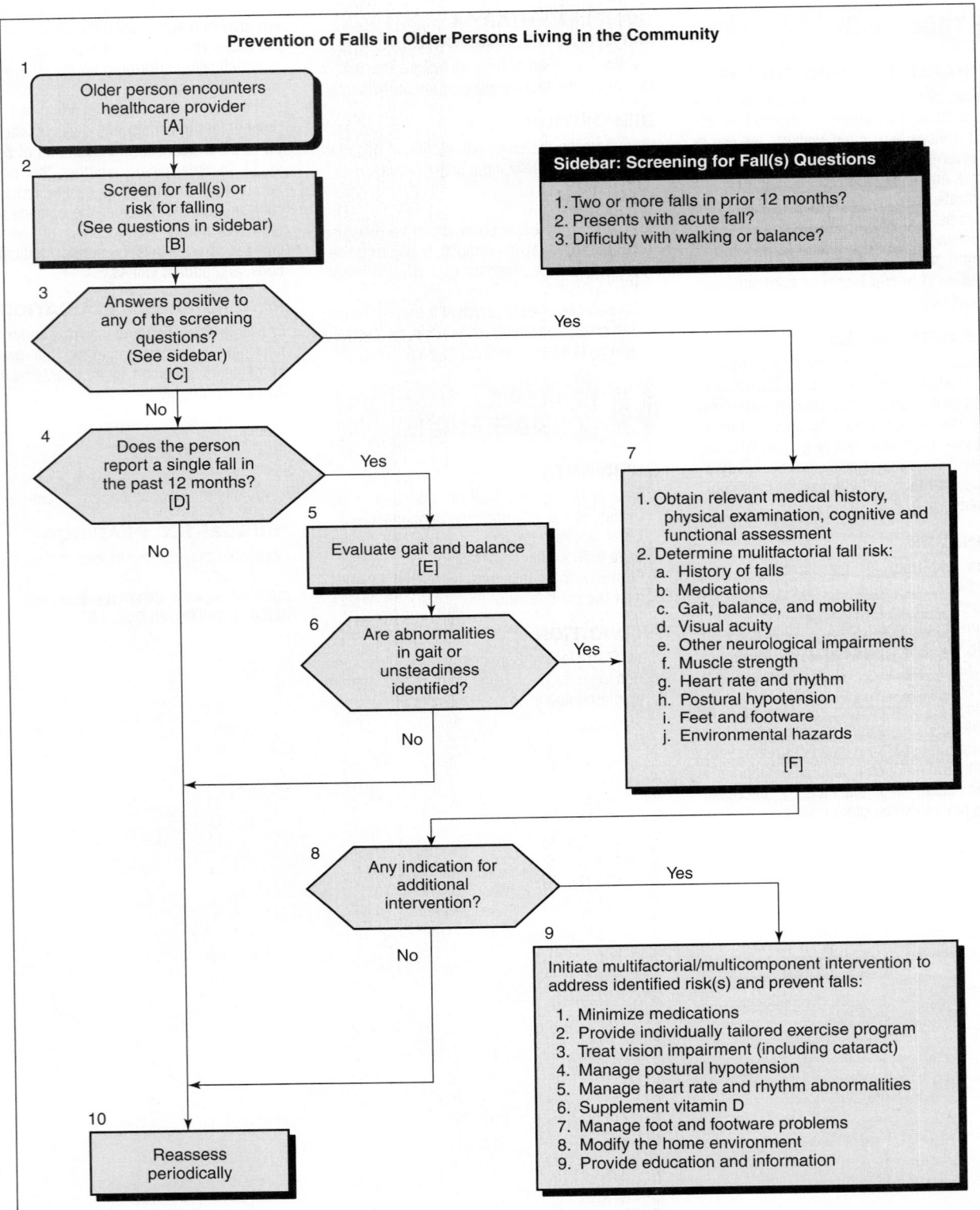

Prevention of Falls in Older Persons Living in the Community

1 — Older person encounters healthcare provider [A]

2 — Screen for fall(s) or risk for falling (See questions in sidebar) [B]

Sidebar: Screening for Fall(s) Questions
1. Two or more falls in prior 12 months?
2. Presents with acute fall?
3. Difficulty with walking or balance?

3 — Answers positive to any of the screening questions? (See sidebar) [C] — Yes / No

4 — Does the person report a single fall in the past 12 months? [D] — Yes / No

5 — Evaluate gait and balance [E]

6 — Are abnormalities in gait or unsteadiness identified? — Yes / No

7 —
1. Obtain relevant medical history, physical examination, cognitive and functional assessment
2. Determine mulitfactorial fall risk:
   a. History of falls
   b. Medications
   c. Gait, balance, and mobility
   d. Visual acuity
   e. Other neurological impairments
   f. Muscle strength
   g. Heart rate and rhythm
   h. Postural hypotension
   i. Feet and footware
   j. Environmental hazards
   [F]

8 — Any indication for additional intervention? — Yes / No

9 — Initiate multifactorial/multicomponent intervention to address identified risk(s) and prevent falls:
1. Minimize medications
2. Provide individually tailored exercise program
3. Treat vision impairment (including cataract)
4. Manage postural hypotension
5. Manage heart rate and rhythm abnormalities
6. Supplement vitamin D
7. Manage foot and footware problems
8. Modify the home environment
9. Provide education and information

10 — Reassess periodically

FIGURE 1-336 Guideline for the prevention of falls in older persons living in the community. (From Panel on Prevention of Falls in Older Persons, American Geriatrics Society and British Geriatrics Society: Summary of the Updated American Geriatrics Society/British Geriatrics Society clinical practice guideline for prevention of falls in older persons, *J Am Geriatr Soc* 59:148-157, 2011.)

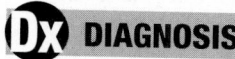

BASIC INFORMATION

DEFINITION

Acute fatty liver of pregnancy (AFLP) is characterized histologically by microvesicular fatty cytoplasmic infiltration of hepatocytes with minimal hepatocellular necrosis.

SYNONYMS

Acute fatty metamorphosis
Acute yellow atrophy

ICD-9CM CODES

646.7 Liver disorders in pregnancy

EPIDEMIOLOGY & DEMOGRAPHICS

INCIDENCE:
- Approximately one in 10,000 pregnancies
- Equal frequencies in all races and at all maternal ages

AVERAGE GESTATIONAL AGE: 37 wk (range 28 to 42 wk)

RISK FACTORS:
- Primiparity
- Multiple gestation
- Male fetus

GENETICS: Some with a familial deficiency of long-chain 3-hydroxyacyl-coenzyme A dehydrogenase (LCHAD)

PHYSICAL FINDINGS & CLINICAL PRESENTATION

- Initial manifestations:
  1. Nausea and vomiting (70%)
  2. Pain in right upper quadrant or epigastrium (50% to 80%)
  3. Malaise and anorexia
- Jaundice often in 1 to 2 wk
- Late manifestations:
  1. Fulminant hepatic failure
  2. Encephalopathy
  3. Renal failure
  4. Pancreatitis
  5. Gastrointestinal and uterine bleeding
  6. Disseminated intravascular coagulation
  7. Seizures
  8. Coma
- Liver:
  1. Usually small
  2. Normal or enlarged in preeclampsia, eclampsia, HELLP syndrome (hemolysis, elevated liver enzymes, and low platelets), and acute hepatitis
  3. Coexistent preeclampsia in up to 46% of patients

ETIOLOGY

- Postulated that inhibition of mitochondrial oxidation of fatty acids may lead to microvesicular fatty infiltration of liver
- Fatty metamorphosis of preeclamptic liver disease believed to be of different etiology

DIAGNOSIS

DIFFERENTIAL DIAGNOSIS

- Acute gastroenteritis
- Preeclampsia or eclampsia with liver involvement
- HELLP syndrome
- Acute viral hepatitis
- Fulminant hepatitis
- Drug-induced hepatitis caused by halothane, phenytoin, methyldopa, isoniazid, hydrochlorothiazide, or tetracycline
- Intrahepatic cholestasis of pregnancy
- Gallbladder disease
- Reye's syndrome
- Hemolytic-uremic syndrome
- Budd-Chiari syndrome
- Systemic lupus erythematosus

WORKUP

- A clinical diagnosis is based predominantly on physical and laboratory findings.
- Most definitive diagnosis is through liver biopsy with oil red O staining and electron microscopy.
- Liver biopsy is reserved for atypical cases only and only after any existing coagulopathy corrected with fresh frozen plasma.

LABORATORY TESTS

Tests to determine the following:
- Hypoglycemia (often profound <60 mg/dl)
- Hyperammonemia
- Elevated aminotransferases (usually <500 U/ml)
- Thrombocytopenia
- Leukocytosis (white blood cell count >15,000)
- Hyperbilirubinemia (usually <10 mg/dl)
- Low albumin
- Hypofibrinogenemia (<300 mg/dl)
- Disseminated intravascular coagulation (DIC) (in 75%)

IMAGING STUDIES

- Ultrasound: best used to rule out other diseases in the differential diagnosis such as gallbladder disease
- CT scan: plays minimal role because of a high false-negative rate

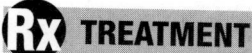

TREATMENT

NONPHARMACOLOGIC THERAPY

- Patient is admitted to intensive care unit for stabilization.
- Fetus is delivered; spontaneous resolution usually follows delivery.
- Mode of delivery is based on obstetric indications and clinical assessment of disease severity.

ACUTE GENERAL Rx

- Decrease in endogenous ammonia through dietary protein restriction; neomycin 6 to 12 g/day PO to decrease presence of ammonia-producing bacteria; magnesium citrate 30 to 50 ml PO or enema to evacuate nitrogenous wastes from colon
- Administration of IV fluids with glucose to keep glucose levels >60 mg/dl
- Coagulopathy corrected with fresh frozen plasma
- Avoidance of drugs metabolized by liver
- Aggressive avoidance and treatment for nosocomial infections; consideration of prophylactic antibiotics
- Monitor closely for development of complications such as hepatic encephalopathy, pulmonary edema, DIC, and respiratory arrest

CHRONIC Rx

Orthotopic liver transplantation is the only treatment for irreversible liver failure.

DISPOSITION

- Before 1980, both maternal and fetal mortality rates were approximately 85%
- Since 1980, both maternal and fetal mortality rates are less than 20%
- Usually rapid return of liver function to normal after delivery
- Minimal risk of recurrence with future pregnancies

REFERRAL

- To tertiary health care facility as soon as diagnosis is suspected.
- Infants of mothers with AFLP should be evaluated for LCHAD deficiency.

SUGGESTED READINGS
available at www.expertconsult.com

RELATED CONTENT
Eclampsia (Related Key Topic)
Preeclampsia (Related Key Topic)

AUTHORS: **ARUNDATHI G. PRASAD, M.D.,** and **RUBEN ALVERO, M.D.**

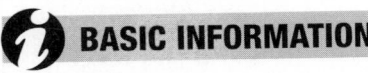

DEFINITION

- The adverse effects of alcohol on the developing human represent a spectrum of structural anomalies and behavioral and neurocognitive disabilities, most accurately termed fetal alcohol spectrum disorder (FASD) (Table 1-153).
- Children at the severe end of the spectrum have been defined as having fetal alcohol syndrome (FAS).

ICD-9CM CODES
760.71 Fetal alcohol syndrome

EPIDEMIOLOGY & DEMOGRAPHICS

- Alcohol is considered to be the most common major teratogen to which the fetus is liable to be exposed.
- 10% report drinking alcohol during pregnancy and 2% to 4% admit to binge drinking.
- FAS represents the most common form of mental retardation in U.S.
- Prevalence is 1-2/1000 live births across U.S.
- Each year 40,000 babies are born with FASD.

RISK FACTORS

- Advanced maternal age (>30 yr)
- High parity
- African-American, Alaskan Natives, and Native Indian race
- Binge drinking >4 drinks per occasion)
- History of prior affected child
- Genetic susceptibility
- Undernutrition
- Low socioeconomic group

PHYSICAL FINDINGS & CLINICAL PRESENTATION

Typical features:
- Growth retardation
  - Prenatal or postnatal
  - Height and/or weight <10%
- Facial dysmorphia
  - Smooth philtrum
  - Thin vermilion border
  - Small palpebral fissure (<10%)
  - Others: epicanthic folds, ptosis of eyelids, flat nasal bridge and midface, upturned nose, railroad track ears, and so forth
- CNS abnormalities
  - Structural
    - Head circumference, 10%
    - Clinically significant brain abnormalities observable through imaging
  - Neurologic
    - Neurologic problems not due to a postnatal insult or fever
  - Functional
    - Intellectual deficit
    - Cognitive or developmental deficits
    - Executive function deficits
    - Motor function delays
    - Problem with attention and hyperactivity
    - Social skills
    - Other problems such as sensory, pragmatic language, and memory

Rare birth defects:
- Cardiac
  - Ventricular septal defect (VSD)
  - Atrial septal defect (ASD)
  - Tetralogy of Fallot
  - Aberrant great vessels
- Skeletal
  - Radioulnar synostosis
  - Hypoplastic nails
  - Clinodactyly
  - Shortened fifth digit
  - Pectus excavatum and carinatum
  - Klippel-Feil syndrome
  - Hemivertebrae
  - Camptodactyly
  - Scoliosis
- Renal
  - Aplastic kidneys
  - Dysplastic kidneys
  - Ureteral duplication
  - Hypoplastic kidneys
  - Hydronephrosis
  - Horseshoe kidneys
- Ocular
  - Strabismus
  - Refractive problems
  - Retinal vascular abnormalities
- Auditory
  - Conductive hearing loss
  - Neurosensory hearing loss
- Others
  - Hockey stick–like palmar crease

ETIOLOGY

- Prenatal damage as a result of chronic alcoholism comes about primarily because of direct action of ethanol or its metabolites (e.g., acetaldehyde) on the fetus.
- The exact damaging mechanism is not clear.
- Although the damaging effect of alcohol is different in the various phases of pregnancy, it is by no means limited to first trimester.
- There is no exact dose-response relationship between the amount of alcohol consumed during the prenatal period and the extent of damage inflicted on the infant.
- An occasional drink during pregnancy carries no risk to the fetus, but no level of drinking is known to be safe during pregnancy.
- The least significant effect recognized at two drinks per day has been slightly smaller birth weight (160 g smaller than average).
- It is not until four to six drinks per day are consumed that additional subtle clinical features are evident.
- Most of the children believed to have FAS have been born to frankly alcoholic mothers whose intake is eight to ten drinks or more per day, and those who engage in binge drinking.
- The risk of serious problem in the offspring of a chronically alcoholic woman has been estimated to be 30% to 50%, the greatest risk being varying degree of mental retardation.

SECONDARY DISABILITIES

- Mental health problems
- Dependent living
- Employment problems
- Disruptive school problems
- Trouble with law
- Confinement
- Inappropriate sexual behavior
- Alcohol or drug problems

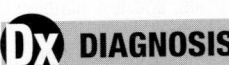 **DIAGNOSIS**

- It is a diagnosis of exclusion.
- Diagnosis is difficult both prenatally and at birth. Unfortunately, most cases are not diagnosed until school age.
- As the characteristic facial features tend to become decreasingly recognizable as the child reaches adolescence, the diagnosis becomes increasingly difficult with advancing age.
- Prenatal exposure to alcohol is not sufficient to warrant a diagnosis. According to the CDC, the diagnosis of FAS requires three specific findings along with the history of prenatal alcohol exposure:

TABLE 1-153 Institute of Medicine's Diagnostic Criteria for Fetal Alcohol–Related Abnormalities

Category 1	
FAS with confirmed maternal alcohol exposure	Presence of classic triad of growth retardation, characteristic facial dysmorphology, and neurodevelopmental abnormalities. This is often defined as full-blown FAS.
Category 2	
FAS without confirmed maternal alcohol exposure	Triad in category 1 is present without confirmed maternal drinking
Category 3	
Partial FAS with confirmed maternal alcohol exposure	Presence of some of the characteristic facial anomalies plus growth retardation or CNS neurodevelopmental abnormalities or behavioral/cognitive abnormalities
Category 4	
FAS with confirmed maternal alcohol exposure and alcohol-related birth defects	These patients will have some congenital anomalies as a result of alcohol toxicity
Category 5	
FAS with confirmed maternal alcohol exposure and alcohol-related neurodevelopmental disorder	There is evidence of CNS neurodevelopmental abnormalities or a complex pattern of behavioral/cognitive abnormalities or both, but not necessarily any obvious physical changes

CNS, Central nervous system; *FAS*, fetal alcohol syndrome.

- Growth restriction (intrauterine or postnatal)
- CNS involvement
- Documentation of all three facial abnormalities (smooth philtrum, thin vermilion border, and short palpebral fissure)
- Imaging recommendation during pregnancy with alcohol exposure:
  - High-risk anatomy scan
  - Serial growth scan
  - Fetal echocardiogram at 22 to 24 weeks' intrauterine pregnancy
- Measurement of the ethyl esters of fatty acids in the meconium and hair of the newborn can substantiate maternal alcohol exposure.
- In school-aged children, the diagnostic process should include a through psychologic evaluation that assesses multiple domains. Also, supplement the observation by obtaining standardized testing through early intervention programs, public schools, and psychologists in private practice.

DIFFERENTIAL DIAGNOSIS

- Other causes of symmetrical growth retardation including intrauterine infection and aneuploidy
- Aneuploidy (T21, T18, T13)
- Syndromes with overlapping features of FAS:
  - Fetal anticonvulsant syndrome
  - Maternal phenylketonuria
  - Toluene embryopathy
  - Velocardiofacial syndrome (deletion 22q11)
  - Williams syndrome
  - Dubowitz syndrome
  - Cornelia de Lange syndrome

(Rx) TREATMENT

- As there is no cure for FAS, we need to emphasize prevention.
- For those women who are planning pregnancy or who have the potential to become pregnant, the U.S. Surgeon General has recommended that the safest course is to avoid alcohol entirely during pregnancy.
- Women of childbearing age who are not pregnant should drink no more than seven alcoholic drinks per week and no more than three drinks on any one occasion.
- Preconception counseling should be offered to women of childbearing age who are at risk for an alcohol-exposed pregnancy.
- Screen all pregnant women for alcohol use.
- The National Institute on Alcohol Abuse and Alcoholism recommends that any woman who reports drinking more than seven drinks per week or more than three drinks on any given day be further assessed for alcohol-related problems.
- The T-ACE (Table 1-154) and TWEAK (Table 1-155) questionnaires are used to identify women drinking enough to potentially damage the fetus. The CAGE questionnaire is less sensitive for screening pregnant women.
- Effective treatment alternatives for women who screen positive for hazardous alcohol use include brief interventions to promote reductions in alcohol use and that facilitate referral to specialized treatment programs.

- Discontinuation or reduction of alcohol consumption at any point in pregnancy may be beneficial.
- The use of alcohol-containing tonics and medications with an alcohol base should be avoided. This applies to medications with an alcohol base, at least when the concentration exceeds 10%.
- Alcoholism is one of the few situations in which pregnancy interruption may be discussed with the patient as it may result in FAS.
- Early diagnosis and appropriate treatment may decrease secondary disabilities and recurrence in future pregnancies.
- A child should be referred for full FAS evaluation when substantial prenatal alcohol use by the mother has been confirmed (more than seven drinks per week, or more than three drinks on multiple occasions, or both).
- If substantial prenatal exposure is known, in the absence of any other positive criteria, the physician should document this exposure and closely monitor the child's ongoing growth and development.
- When information about prenatal exposure is unknown, a child should be referred for full FAS if any of the following conditions are

TABLE 1-154   T-ACE Questions*

T (tolerance)	How many drinks does it take to make you feel high? (3 or more drinks = 2 points)
A (annoyed)	Have people annoyed you by criticizing your drinking? (Yes = 1 point)
C (cut down)	Have you felt you ought to cut down on your drinking? (Yes = 1 point)
E (eye opener)	Have you ever had to drink first thing in the morning to steady your nerves or to get rid of a hangover? (Yes = 1 point)

*A score of 2 or more indicates heavy or problem drinker. Its sensitivity is 70% and specificity is 85%.

TABLE 1-155   TWEAK*

T (tolerance)	How many drinks does it take before you begin to feel the first effects of alcohol? (3 or more drinks = 2 points)
W (worried)	Have close friends or relatives worried about your drinking in the past year? (Yes = 2 points)
E (eye opener)	Do you sometimes take a drink in the morning when you first get up? (Yes = 1 point)
A (amnesia)	Has a friend or family member ever told you about things you said or did while you were drinking that you could not remember? (Yes = 1 point)
K (kut down)	Do you sometimes feel the need to cut down on your drinking? (Yes = 1 point)

*A total of 3 or more points indicates the woman is likely to be a heavy or problem drinker. Its sensitivity is 79% and specificity is 83%.

present: (1) all three dysmorphic facial features (smooth philtrum, thin vermilion border, and small palpebral fissure), (2) one or more of these facial features with growth deficit, (3) one or more facial features with one or more CNS abnormalities, (4) one or more dysmorphic facial features with growth deficit and one or more CNS abnormalities, or (5) any report of concern by a caregiver or parent that a child has or may have FAS.

- Infants and children who are diagnosed with FAS should be evaluated by a physician who is knowledgeable and competent in the evaluation of neurodevelopment and psychosocial problems associated with the diagnosis.
- A multidisciplinary team including a clinical geneticist, developmental pediatrician, mental health professional, social worker, and education specialist is often necessary for management.
- Treatment options include:
  - Medications to help with symptoms
  - Behavior and education therapy
    Friendship training
    Specialized math training
    Executive function training
    Parent-child interaction training
    Parenting and behavior management training
  - Parenting training
    Concentrate on child's strengths and talents
    Accept child's limitations
    Be consistent with everything
    Use concrete language and examples
    Use stable routine that does not change daily
    Keep everything simple
    Be specific (i.e., say exactly what you mean)
    Structure your child's world to provide a foundation for daily living
    Use visualized aids, music, and hands-on activities to help your child learn
    Use positive reinforcement often
    Supervise
    Repeat, repeat, and repeat
  - Emphasis on the following protective factors helps reduce the effects and also assists people with this condition to reach their full potential:
    Diagnosing before 6 yr
    Living in stable nurturing home environment in school years
    Absence of violence
    Involvement in special education and social services
  - Alternative approaches such as biofeedback, auditory training, relaxation therapy, visual imagery, yoga/exercise, acupuncture/acupressure, massage, Reiki, energy healing, animal-assisted therapy, and so forth may play a role.

SUGGESTED READINGS
available at www.expertconsult.com

AUTHOR: **HEMANT SATPATHY, M.D.**

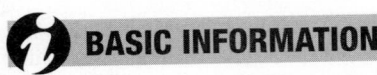

DEFINITION

Fever of undetermined origin (FUO) was defined by Petersdorf and Beeson in 1961 as an illness characterized by temperatures >38.3° C (101° F) on several occasions for >3 wk with no known cause despite extensive workup.

- Persistence for >2 wk separates an FUO from an insignificant viral illness.
- Traditionally, diagnosis was made only after a 1-wk inpatient workup. In contemporary practice, much of the workup is performed as an outpatient.

Table 1-156 provides a summary of definitions and major features of subtypes of FUO.

SYNONYMS

Fever of unknown origin

ICD-9CM CODES
780.6 Pyrexia of undetermined origin

EPIDEMIOLOGY & DEMOGRAPHICS

- The incidence of undiagnosed FUO dropped to <10% in the 1950s but has steadily increased since then.
- True FUOs are uncommon.

CLINICAL PRESENTATION

Fever 38.3° C or (101° F or more) >3 wk

ETIOLOGY

(Most common etiologies italicized)

- Infection (16%)
  - *Abscess: abdominal, pelvic*
  - *Tuberculosis*
  - HIV infection
  - Nosocomial: urinary tract infection, pneumonia, line-related bacteremia, *Clostridium difficile* colitis, sinusitis
  - Bacterial endocarditis (especially caused by difficult-to-isolate organisms)
  - Biliary tract infection
  - Osteomyelitis, vertebral and mandibular
  - Less common infections: Q fever, leptospirosis, psittacosis, tularemia, secondary syphilis, gonococcemia, chronic meningococcemia, Whipple's disease, yersiniosis, fungal infections
- Malignancy (7%): *lymphoma* (especially non-Hodgkin's lymphoma) and *leukemia,* renal cell carcinoma, hepatocellular carcinomas, other tumors metastatic to liver
- Noninfectious inflammatory disease (22%)
  - Adult Still's disease (young to middle-aged patients)
  - Temporal arteritis (elderly patients)
  - Other vasculitis: polyarteritis nodosa, Takayasu's arteritis, Wegener's granulomatosis, mixed cryoglobulinemia
- Other (4%)
  - Drug-induced fever
  - Inflammatory bowel disease
  - Sarcoidosis
  - Pulmonary embolism
  - Alcoholic hepatitis
- No diagnosis (51%)

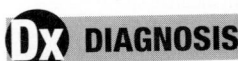

DIFFERENTIAL DIAGNOSIS

Factitious fever

WORKUP

- Accurate history and careful physical examination are essential. Fig. E1-337 describes an approach to the patient with FUO.
- Laboratory tests and imaging dependent on medical history clues and physical findings.
- When in doubt, perform another complete history and physical examination. Examples of subtle physical findings in patients with FUO are described in Table 1-157.

MEDICAL HISTORY CLUES

- Fever duration, tempo; inciting factors
- Rash, myalgia, weight loss, pain
- Sick contacts
- Past medical history: tuberculosis, HIV, malignancies, surgeries
- Medications

TABLE 1-156 Summary of Definitions and Major Features of the Four Subtypes of Fever of Undetermined Origin

Feature	Classic FUO	Health Care–Associated FUO	Immune-Deficient FUO	HIV-Related FUO
Definition	>38.0°C, >3 wk, >2 visits or 1 wk in hospital	≥38.0°C, >1 wk, not present or incubating on admission	≥38.0°C, >1 wk, negative cultures after 48 hr	≥38.0°C, >3 wk for outpatients, >1 wk for inpatients, HIV infection confirmed
Patient location	Community, clinic, or hospital	Acute care hospital	Hospital or clinic	Community, clinic, or hospital
Leading causes	Cancer, infections, inflammatory conditions, undiagnosed, habitual hyperthermia	Health care–associated infections, postoperative complications, drug fever	Majority due to infections, but cause documented in only 40%-60%	HIV (primary infection), typical and atypical mycobacteria, CMV, lymphomas, toxoplasmosis, cryptococcosis, immune reconstitution inflammatory syndrome (IRIS)
History emphasis	Travel, contacts, animal and insect exposure, medications, immunizations, family history, cardiac valve disorder	Operations and procedures, devices, anatomic considerations, drug treatment	Stage of chemotherapy, drugs administered, underlying immunosuppressive disorder	Drugs, exposures, risk factors, travel, contacts, stage of HIV infection
Examination emphasis	Fundi, oropharynx, temporal artery, abdomen, lymph nodes, spleen, joints, skin, nails, genitalia, rectum or prostate, lower limb deep veins	Wounds, drains, devices, sinuses, urine	Skin folds, IV sites, lungs, perianal area	Mouth, sinuses, skin, lymph nodes, eyes, lungs, perianal area
Investigation emphasis	Imaging, biopsies, sedimentation rate, skin tests	Imaging, bacterial cultures	CXR, bacterial cultures	Blood and lymphocyte count; serologic tests; CXR; stool examination; biopsies of lung, bone marrow, and liver for cultures and cytologic tests; brain imaging
Management	Observation, outpatient temperature chart, investigations, avoidance of empirical drug treatments	Depends on situation	Antimicrobial treatment protocols	Antiviral and antimicrobial protocols, vaccines, revision of treatment regimens, good nutrition
Time course of disease	Months	Weeks	Days	Weeks to months
Tempo of investigation	Weeks	Days	Hours	Days to weeks

CMV, Cytomegalovirus; *CXR,* chest radiograph; *FUO,* fever of undetermined origin.
Adapted from Mandell GL, Bennett JE, Dolin R (eds): *Mandell, Douglas, and Bennett's principles and practice of infectious diseases,* ed 7, Philadelphia, 2010, Churchill Livingstone, 2010.
Borrowed from Kliegman RM et al: *Nelson textbook of pediatrics,* ed 19, Philadelphia, 2011, Saunders.

- Family history: tuberculosis, malignancies, familial Mediterranean fever
- Social history: daily routine, rural versus urban, pets and animal contacts, arthropod bites, recent and remote travel, socioeconomic status, occupation, military service, sexual history

PHYSICAL FINDINGS

- HEENT (head, ears, eyes, nose, throat): sinus tenderness, dental abscesses, funduscopic lesions
- Neck: adenopathy, palpable thyroid
- Lungs: auscultate for rales
- Heart: murmur
- Abdomen: organomegaly
- Rectal: prostate tenderness
- Pelvic: cervical motion tenderness, fundal or adnexal masses or pain; inguinal adenopathy
- Extremities: clubbing, splinter hemorrhages; tenderness or fluctuance at IV access site
- Musculoskeletal: joint effusions
- Skin: rashes, wounds

LABORATORY TESTS

- Most FUO workups include:
  - Blood cultures (three sets from different sites)
  - Complete blood count with differential
  - Erythrocyte sedimentation rate or C-reactive protein
  - Urinalysis with microscopic exam and culture
  - Transaminases
  - Serum lactate dehydrogenase
  - PPD testing
- Consider
  - HIV antibody testing
  - Creatinine phosphokinase
  - Rheumatoid factor
  - Serum protein electrophoresis
  - Lumbar puncture
  - Thyroid function testing
  - Stool culture and *C. difficile* assay
  - Biopsy (bone marrow, skin, liver lymph nodes, pleural, etc., based on clinical and laboratory findings)
  - Antinuclear antibody testing

May need to repeat tests at regular intervals until diagnosis is established.

IMAGING STUDIES

- Most workups eventually include chest radiograph and abdominal CT scan.
- Further imaging is based on medical history clues and physical findings.
- FDG-PET is very sensitive to detect anatomic sites of inflammation or malignancy. It may help to identify sites requiring further investigation. Further data are needed to evaluate efficacy.

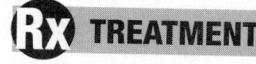 **TREATMENT**

ACUTE GENERAL Rx

Antibiotics and other treatment indicated only after definitive or highly probable diagnosis is established unless patient is neutropenic, severely ill, or septic.

DISPOSITION

In some cases a diagnosis is not made for years. At 5-yr follow-up, mortality rate among patients with undiagnosed FUO was only 3.2% in one study.

REFERRAL

To an infectious disease specialist, hematologist, or rheumatologist if no diagnosis after thoughtful workup

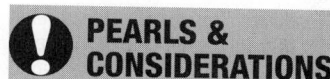 **PEARLS & CONSIDERATIONS**

COMMENTS

Because of improvements in imaging and laboratory tests, fewer cases of FUO are attributed to infectious causes and more are diagnosed as attributable to tumors and collagen-vascular diseases.

SUGGESTED READINGS

available at www.expertconsult.com

RELATED CONTENT

Fever of Undetermined Origin (Patient Information)

AUTHOR: **ETSUKO AOKI, M.D., PH.D.**

TABLE 1-157 Examples of Subtle Physical Findings Having Special Significance in Patients with Fever of Undetermined Origin

Body Site	Physical Finding	Diagnosis
Head	Sinus tenderness	Sinusitis
Temporal artery	Nodules, reduced pulsations	Temporal arteritis
Oropharynx	Ulceration	Disseminated histoplasmosis
	Tender tooth	Periapical abscess
Fundi or conjunctivae	Choroid tubercle	Disseminated granulomatosis*
	Petechiae, Roth's spot	Endocarditis
Thyroid	Enlargement, tenderness	Thyroiditis
Heart	Murmur	Infective or marantic endocarditis
Abdomen	Enlarged iliac crest lymph nodes, splenomegaly	Lymphoma, endocarditis, disseminated granulomatosis*
Rectum	Perirectal fluctuance, tenderness	Abscess
	Prostatic tenderness, fluctuance	Abscess
Genitalia	Testicular nodule	Periarteritis nodosa
	Epididymal nodule	Disseminated granulomatosis
Lower extremities	Deep venous tenderness	Thrombosis or thrombophlebitis
Skin and nails	Petechiae, splinter hemorrhages, subcutaneous nodules, clubbing	Vasculitis, endocarditis

*Includes tuberculosis, histoplasmosis, coccidioidomycosis, sarcoidosis, and syphilis.
From Mandell GL et al (eds): *Mandell, Douglas, and Bennett's principles and practice of infectious diseases*, ed 7, Philadelphia, 2010, Churchill Livingstone, 2010.

F

Diseases and Disorders

I

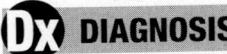

BASIC INFORMATION

DEFINITION

Fibrocystic breast disease (FCD) is a "nondisease" that includes nonmalignant breast lesions such as microcystic and macrocystic changes, fibrosis, ductal or lobular hyperplasia, adenosis, apocrine metaplasia, fibroadenoma, papilloma, papillomatosis, and other changes. Atypical ductal or lobular hyperplasia is associated with a moderate increase in breast cancer risk.

SYNONYMS

Cystic changes
Chronic cystic mastitis
Mammary dysplasia

ICD-9CM CODES
610.0 Solitary cyst of the breast
610.1 Fibrocystic disease of the breast

EPIDEMIOLOGY & DEMOGRAPHICS

- Ubiquitous in premenopausal women after 20 yr of age
- Palpable nodular changes in the breast termed FCD clinically; such changes observable in more than half of adult women aged 20 to 50 yr

PHYSICAL FINDINGS & CLINICAL PRESENTATION

- Tender breasts
- Nodular areas
- Dominant mass
- Thickening
- Nipple discharge
- Can vary with menstrual cycle

ETIOLOGY

- Although it is frequently seen and diagnosed, mechanism of development is not understood.

- Because it is found in the majority of healthy breasts, it is regarded as a nonpathologic process.
- With hormone replacement therapy, the condition may be carried into menopause.

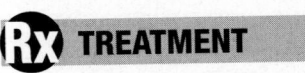

DIAGNOSIS

DIFFERENTIAL DIAGNOSIS

- If presenting as dominant mass or masses, exclude possible carcinoma.
- Carcinoma: detection is difficult with FCD, particularly among premenopausal women.
- If presenting with nipple discharge, differentiate from discharge of possible malignant origin.

WORKUP

- Exclude breast carcinoma if breast mass, thickening, discharge, and/or pain are present.
- Perform biopsy of suspected area for histologic confirmation.

IMAGING STUDIES

Mammography and ultrasound studies required:
- For mammographic changes (suspicious densities, microcalcifications, architectural distortion): careful evaluation, including possibly biopsy to exclude breast cancer
- Ultrasound study: to establish cystic nature of clinical or mammographic mass lesion

TREATMENT

NONPHARMACOLOGIC THERAPY

- Not considered a "disease" and does not require treatment
- Surgical intervention diagnostic to eliminate possibility of breast cancer
- Periodic physician examination to monitor patients with FCD who have pronounced nodular features

- Aspiration for palpable cysts (NOTE: Cysts often recur; repeat aspiration is not always required unless pain is a problem.)

ACUTE GENERAL Rx

The majority of women require no treatment.

CHRONIC Rx

For breast pain:
- Danocrine (Danazol): limited success reported but significant side effect profile of medication
- Bromocriptine or tamoxifen: used less frequently
- Limited caffeine intake: not as successful in controlling pain or nodularity as originally suggested

DISPOSITION

- Careful evaluation to exclude suspicious changes for breast cancer, then reassurance and periodic reevaluation as required
- Regular self-examination, annual physician examination, and annual mammograms for women with atypical ductal or lobular hyperplasia

REFERRAL

- For further evaluation and/or biopsy if there are suspicious changes that may be associated with FCD (including changing of dominant mass or thickening, persistent or spontaneous discharge, suspicious mammographic changes or lesions)
- To alleviate anxiety associated with breast symptoms or changes

RELATED CONTENT

Breast Cancer (Related Key Topic)
Mastodynia (Related Key Topic)
Fibrocystic Breast Changes (Patient Information)

AUTHORS: **TAKUMA NEMOTO, M.D.**, and **RUBEN ALVERO, M.D.**

ℹ BASIC INFORMATION

DEFINITION

Fibromyalgia (FM) is a disorder of pain processing characterized by chronic, widespread pain, a lack of structural pathology, and the presence of pain augmentation. Central features also include fatigue, sleep disturbance, and tenderness.

ICD-9CM CODES
729.0 Rheumatism, unspecified and fibrositis
729.1 Myalgia and myositis, unspecified

EPIDEMIOLOGY & DEMOGRAPHICS

PREVALENCE: 0.5% to 5% worldwide
PREDOMINANT SEX: Female/male ratio of 7:1
PREDOMINANT AGE: 30 to 50 years

PHYSICAL FINDINGS

Tender points (Fig. 1-338) or generalized tenderness

ETIOLOGY

- Unknown. Genetic and environmental factors predispose individuals to FM. Evidence suggests that both the ascending and descending pain pathways operate abnormally, resulting in central amplification of pain signals, analogous to the "volume control setting" being turned up too high. Familial associations of FM provide strongest evidence that reflect both these factors.
- Once predisposed, FM may be precipitated by events such as abuse, injury from motor vehicle accidents, illness including autoimmune disorders, infections, surgical procedures, and psychological stressors.
- Psychosocial and neuroendocrine factors also influence symptom expression.

PATHOGENESIS

- Augmented pain and sensory processing is a hallmark, resulting in diffuse pain, allodynia (pain brought on by normally nonpainful stimuli), and hyperalgesia (more intense and prolonged pain perception)
- Afflicted persons show altered physiologic responses to painful stimulation at spinal and supraspinal levels.
- Brain neuroimaging studies found differences in brain structure, neurochemical concentrations, and functional brain networks in FM compared with control subjects, with increased pain sensitivity demonstrated in these studies.
- Pain augmentation may also result from a loss of tonic inhibition by descending inhibitory pathways from the brain to the spinal cord.

Dx DIAGNOSIS

DIFFERENTIAL DIAGNOSIS

- Presence of any of the disorders mentioned below does not necessarily exclude a diagnosis of FM because it may occur with many conditions
- Other functional somatic or "central sensitivity" syndromes: myofascial pain, chronic fatigue, irritable bowel, headache/migraines, chronic pelvic and bladder pain disorders, and temporomandibular disorder
- Disorders that can mimic FM (thus must be ruled out clinically) include: hypothyroidism, rheumatic diseases (e.g., rheumatoid arthritis, systemic lupus erythematosus, osteoarthritis, inflammatory myopathies), infection
- Mood and anxiety disorders
- Sleep disorders (e.g., sleep apnea, restless leg syndrome)
- Neurologic disorders
- Medications: statin-induced muscle pain, opioid-induced hyperalgesia

WORKUP

- Thorough history, physical examination, and appropriately selected laboratory studies can usually differentiate FM from connective tissue or other systemic diseases.

- Chronic (>3 mo), widespread pain is the hallmark symptom of FM, but fatigue, tenderness, depression/anxiety, nonrestorative sleep, cognitive difficulties, and functional impairment are other key symptoms.
- The 1990 American College of Rheumatology (ACR) FM Classification Criteria was used for clinical studies:
  1. Chronic, widespread pain in all four quadrants of the body and the axial skeleton.
  2. Pain on digital palpation of at least 11 of 18 tender points (see Fig. 1-338).
- The 2010 ACR preliminary diagnostic criteria for FM do not require a tender point examination; it requires the exclusion of other disorders that would otherwise explain the pain.
- A diagnostic screening tool (Fibromyalgia Diagnostic Screen) developed by Arnold and colleagues was found to accurately screen for FM. This tool includes a patient self-reported questionnaire and an abbreviated physical examination with targeted lab tests.

LABORATORY TESTS

- Selective use of laboratory tests complements the history and physical examination in the diagnosis of FM. Testing should be highly focused on the exclusion of FM mimickers or suspected concurrent diseases.
- Complete blood cell count, routine chemistries, thyroid-stimulating hormone (TSH), erythrocyte sedimentation rate (ESR), and C-reactive protein (CRP) are normal in FM.
- Routine testing for antinuclear antibody (ANA) and/or rheumatoid factor should be avoided unless history and physical examination suggest an autoimmune disease.

Rx TREATMENT

GENERAL Rx (Fig. 1-339)

- Strong evidence for: low-dose amitriptyline and cyclobenzaprine, serotonin-norepinephrine reuptake inhibitors (milnacipran and duloxetine), and pregabalin.
- The FDA-approved medications for FM are pregabalin, duloxetine, and milnacipran.
- The only analgesic that has demonstrated efficacy in FM has been tramadol, either alone or in combination with acetaminophen.
- Modest evidence exists for gabapentin and SSRIs.
- No evidence that NSAIDs or corticosteroids are effective in FM.
- Avoid narcotic use. There is concern that opioid use and abuse may aggravate chronic widespread pain.
- Nonpharmacologic: strong evidence to support exercise, cognitive behavioral therapy, and patient education.

DISPOSITION

- The pain and symptoms of FM can wax and wane, vary in physical location and in intensity day to day; many patients continue to have chronic pain and fatigue regardless of therapy.
- Disability rates vary from 9% to 44%.

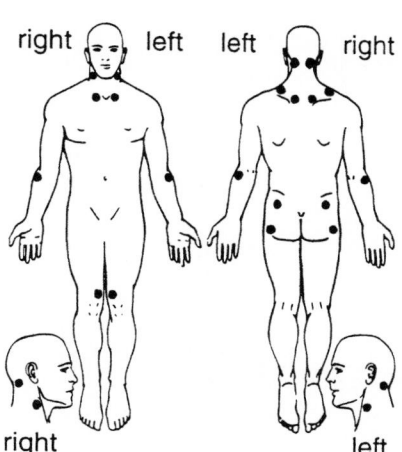

1. Occiput
2. Low cervical
3. Trapezius
4. Supraspinatus
5. Second rib
6. Lateral epicondyle
7. Gluteal
8. Greater trochanter
9. Knees

FIGURE 1-338 The sites of the 18 tender points of the 1990 American College of Rheumatology criteria for the classification of fibromyalgia. (From Conn R: *Current diagnosis,* ed 9, Philadelphia, 1997, Saunders.)

REFERRAL

Referral to rheumatology, mental health professionals, physical therapy, and rehabilitation may be helpful for a multidisciplinary team approach.

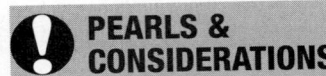

Myofascial pain syndrome may represent a localized form of FM. It is associated with trigger points (rather than tender points as seen in FM). Some patients with myofascial pain syndrome may progress to FM.

COMMENTS

FM occurs frequently in patients with some rheumatic diseases such as rheumatoid arthritis, ankylosing spondylitis, and systemic lupus erythematosus, in which prevalence of FM may reach 20%.

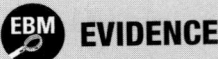 **EVIDENCE**

available at www.expertconsult.com

SUGGESTED READINGS

available at www.expertconsult.com

RELATED CONTENT

Fibromyalgia (Patient Information)

AUTHOR: **CANDICE YUVIENCO, M.D.**

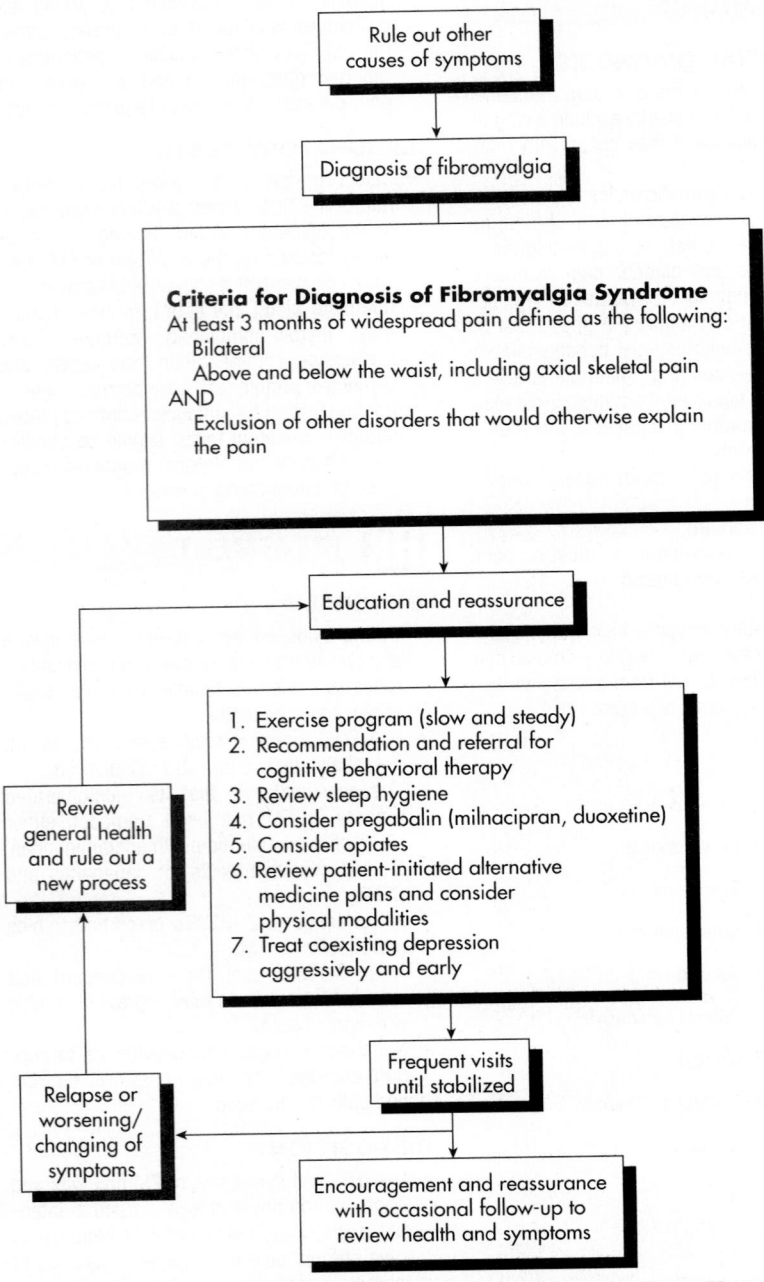

FIGURE 1-339 Treatment algorithm for fibromyalgia. (Modified from Harris ED et al: *Kelley's textbook of rheumatology,* ed 7, Philadelphia, 2005, Saunders.)

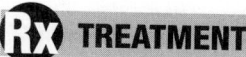 BASIC INFORMATION

DEFINITION

Parvovirus B19 is a nonenveloped DNA virus that causes a spectrum of human disease. Classically, it has been associated with "fifth disease," a viral exanthem of school-aged children historically considered to be the "fifth" in a series of viral exanthems. There is a growing awareness that parvovirus B19 also causes a spectrum of disease in adults, specifically in immunocompromised populations.

SYNONYMS

Erythema infectiosum

ICD-9CM CODES

057.0 Fifth disease (eruptive)

EPIDEMIOLOGY & DEMOGRAPHICS

PEAK INCIDENCE: Late winter and spring, especially April and May
PREDOMINANT AGE: 5 to 18 yr
GENETICS: 50% to 60% of adults have demonstrated protective antibodies to parvovirus B19.

PHYSICAL FINDINGS & CLINICAL PRESENTATION

- Typical bright red, nontender maxillary rash with circumoral pallor over cheeks, producing the classic "slapped cheek" appearance (Fig. 1-340).
- In adults, 90% with erythematous rash, 25% with classic reticular lacy, erythematous, maculopapular rash over trunk and extremities lasting for up to several weeks after the acute episode. May be worsened by heat or sunlight. 60% report pruritus, primarily in lower extremities.

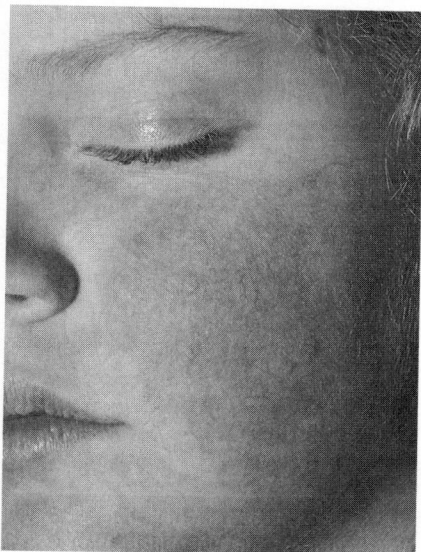

FIGURE 1-340 Fifth disease (erythema infectiosum). Facial erythema "slapped cheek." The red plaque covers the cheek and spares the nasolabial and the circumoral region. (From Habif TP: *Clinical dermatology: a color guide to diagnosis and therapy*, ed 3, St Louis, 1996, Mosby.)

- Polyarthritis and arthralgias are commonly seen in older patients and less commonly in children. Arthritis involves small joints of the extremities in symmetric fashion and typically occurs 1 week after the initial symptoms (5.5 ± 3.2 days).
- Mild fever is seen in up to one third of children, whereas 70% of adults report a fever.

ETIOLOGY

Syndrome caused by parvovirus B19, a single-stranded DNA virus, which has been reclassified in the new genus *Erythrovirus*. Transmission is primarily through droplet exposure to the respiratory tract. As it is heat stable and nonenveloped, parvovirus transmission has been documented through exposure to blood products.

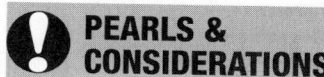 DIAGNOSIS

DIFFERENTIAL DIAGNOSIS

- Juvenile rheumatoid arthritis (Still's disease)
- Rubella, measles (rubeola), and other childhood viral exanthems
- Mononucleosis
- Lyme disease
- Acute HIV infection
- Drug eruption

WORKUP

Diagnosis can be made by typical clinical presentation in well children; laboratory tests required for confirmation in immunosuppressed populations.

LABORATORY TESTS

- Parvovirus B19 IgM
  - An antibody seen in 90% of patients with acute illness. Usually not necessary, as clinical presentation and typical rash are sufficient to establish diagnosis in immunocompetent individuals.
  - Complete blood count (in specific populations at risk for marrow toxicity). Transient aplastic crisis is a syndrome distinct from fifth disease, which may be seen in patients with chronic hematologic illness (described with sickle cell disease, spherocytosis, and other hemolytic processes) or AIDS who are infected with parvovirus B19. There have been recent case reports of patients treated with rituximab who developed aplastic crisis in the setting of parvovirus infection.
    a. Usually self-limited and associated with prodrome of fever and malaise. Lasts for 1 to 2 wk, followed by marrow recovery.
    b. Rash is usually absent.
    c. These patients are highly infective.
- Human chorionic gonadotropin (in women of childbearing age)
  - Infection during early pregnancy may result in fetal death (10%) or severe anemia but is usually asymptomatic and not associated with congenital malformations.
- Quantitative polymerase chain reaction.
- Used for early, rapid diagnosis in immunocompromised patients and to screen plasma products.

TREATMENT

ACUTE GENERAL Rx

- Treatment is supportive only
- Nonsteroidal anti-inflammatory drugs for arthralgias and arthritis
- IV immunoglobulin and transfusion support has anecdotal success reported in patients with immunocompromised state with red cell aplasia.
- Consider immunoglobulin treatment or prophylaxis in pregnancy
- Bone marrow transplantation has been used in individuals with nonresolving aplastic crisis.

DISPOSITION & PROGNOSIS

- Typically self-limited illness lasting 1 to 2 wk.
- Arthritis lasts for weeks. There is some controversy as to whether it can progress to chronic rheumatoid arthritis in adults.
- Pregnant women should avoid contact with patients who have marrow suppression. Maternal parvovirus infection in pregnancy may have a wide range of fetal effects, including hydrops fetalis, and warrants close monitoring of fetal development and health.
- Patients with transient aplastic crisis or chronic parvovirus B19 infection pose a risk for nosocomial spread and, when hospitalized, should be isolated with contact and respiratory precautions.
- Children with fifth disease are not contagious and may attend school and day care.
- Vaccines have not progressed beyond stage I clinical trials.
- Some infected individuals develop aplastic anemia and require bone marrow transplantation.

REFERRAL

- To hematologist if signs of marrow suppression
- To rheumatologist if signs of severe or erosive arthritis

! PEARLS & CONSIDERATIONS

- Generally self-limited disease lasting 1 to 2 wk in immunocompentent individuals
- Symmetric arthritis involving small joints is common in adults, whereas facial rash is common in children
- Can cause aplastic anemia in patients with sickle cell disease, in an immunocompromised state, and after transplantation.

SUGGESTED READINGS

available at www.expertconsult.com

RELATED CONTENT

Fifth Disease (Patient Information)

AUTHORS: **WILLIAM HAHN, M.D.,** and **DOMINICK TAMMARO, M.D.**

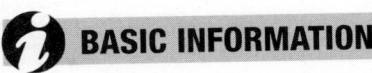

BASIC INFORMATION

DEFINITION

Folliculitis is inflammation of the hair follicle as a result of infection, physical injury, or chemical irritation.

SYNONYMS

Sycosis barbae

ICD-9CM CODES
704.8 Other specified diseases of hair and hair follicles

EPIDEMIOLOGY & DEMOGRAPHICS

PREVALENCE: Staphylococcal folliculitis is the most common form of infectious folliculitis; it occurs most commonly in persons with diabetes.
PREDOMINANT SEX: Sycosis barbae occurs most frequently in men who have commenced shaving.

PHYSICAL FINDINGS & CLINICAL PRESENTATION

- The lesions generally consist of painful yellow pustules surrounded by erythema; a central hair is present in the pustules. Furuncles with pus may be present (Fig. 1-343).
- Patients with sycosis barbae may initially present with small follicular papules or pustules that increase in size with continued shaving; deep follicular pustules may occur surrounded by erythema and swelling; the upper lip is frequently involved.
- "Hot tub" folliculitis occurs within 1 to 4 days after the use of a hot tub with poor chlorination. It is characterized by papules and pustules (Fig. 1-344) with surrounding erythema generally affecting the torso, buttocks, and limbs.

ETIOLOGY

- *Staphylococcus* infection (e.g., sycosis barbae), *Pseudomonas aeruginosa* ("hot tub" folliculitis)
- Gram-negative folliculitis *(Klebsiella, Enterobacter, Proteus)* associated with antibiotic treatment of acne
- Chronic irritation of the hair follicle (use of cocoa butter or coconut oil, chronic irritation from workplace)
- Initial use of systemic corticosteroid therapy (steroid acne), eosinophilic folliculitis (AIDS patients), *Candida albicans* (immunocompromised patients)
- *Pityrosporum orbiculare*

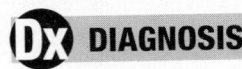

DIAGNOSIS

DIFFERENTIAL DIAGNOSIS

- Pseudofolliculitis barbae (ingrown hairs)
- Acne vulgaris
- Dermatophyte fungal infections
- Keratosis pilaris
- Cutaneous candidiasis
- Superficial fungal infections
- Miliaris

WORKUP

Physical examination and medical history (e.g., use of hot tub: "hot tub" folliculitis; adolescent patients who have started shaving: sycosis barbae; use of occlusive topical steroid therapy: *Staphylococcus* folliculitis).

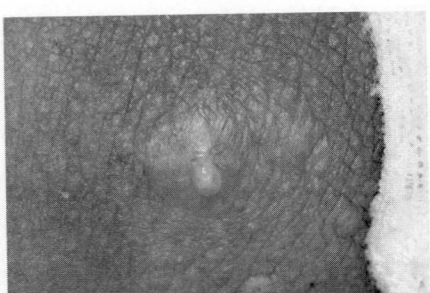

FIGURE 1-343 Rupture and discharge of pus in a furuncle. (From Kliegman RM et al: *Nelson textbook of pediatrics,* ed 19, Philadelphia, 2011, Saunders.)

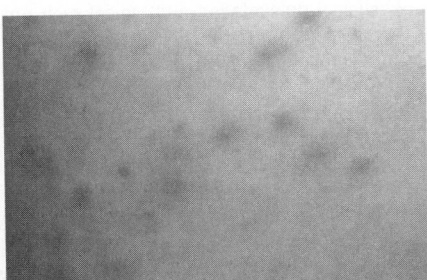

FIGURE 1-344 Papules and pustules in hot tub folliculitis. (From Kliegman RM et al: *Nelson textbook of pediatrics,* ed 19, Philadelphia, 2011, Saunders.)

LABORATORY TESTS

- Generally not necessary.
- Gram stain is useful to identify the infective organisms in infectious folliculitis and to differentiate infectious folliculitis from noninfectious.

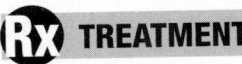 TREATMENT

NONPHARMACOLOGIC THERAPY

- Prevention of chemical or mechanical skin irritation
- Glycemic control in diabetics
- Proper chlorination of hot tubs and spas
- Shaving with a clean razor

ACUTE GENERAL Rx

- Cleansing of the area with chlorhexidine and application of saline compresses to involved area
- Application of 2% mupirocin ointment or 1% Retapamulin ointment for bacterial folliculitis affecting a limited area (e.g., sycosis barbae)
- Treatment of severe cases of *Pseudomonas* folliculitis with ciprofloxacin
- Treatment of *S. aureus* folliculitis with dicloxacillin 250 mg qd for 10 days

CHRONIC Rx

- Chronic nasal or perineal *S. aureus* carriers with frequent folliculitis can be treated with rifampin 300 mg bid for 5 days.
- Mupirocin or Retapamulin ointment applied to nares bid is also effective for nasal carriers.

DISPOSITION

- Most cases of bacterial folliculitis resolve completely with proper treatment.
- Steroid folliculitis responds to discontinuation of steroids.

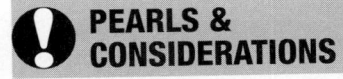 PEARLS & CONSIDERATIONS

COMMENTS

Patients should be instructed in good personal hygiene and avoidance of sharing razors, towels, and washcloths.

RELATED CONTENT

Folliculitis (Patient Information)

AUTHOR: **FRED F. FERRI, M.D.**

BASIC INFORMATION

DEFINITION

Food allergy is an adverse immune response to food proteins. Food allergies are categorized into IgE-mediated or non–IgE-mediated processes.

ICD-9CM CODES
693.1 Food allergy-ICD

EPIDEMIOLOGY & DEMOGRAPHICS

INCIDENCE: Food allergies have a cumulative incidence of 6% to 8% for the first 3 yr of life.
PREVALENCE:
- Food allergies affect 5% to 7% of children and 1% to 3% of adults. 30% of food allergies are self-reported.
- Cow's milk allergy is found in 2.5% of infants. IgE-mediated allergy occurs in 1% of children and non–IgE-mediated allergy occurs in 1.5% of children.
- Egg allergy occurs in 1.5% to 3.2% of children and 1% to 6% of infants have soy allergy.
- There is no predilection for race.
PREDOMINANT SEX: Males are more affected than females among children, and among adults, females are more frequently affected.
GENETICS: Children with parents or close relatives with allergies may have a tendency to become allergic to foods.

PHYSICAL FINDINGS & CLINICAL PRESENTATION

- IgE-mediated reactions: (immediate) pruritus, urticaria or angioedema, atopic dermatitis, GI symptoms, conjunctival injection, sneezing, nasal congestion, rhinorrhea, bronchospasm, and anaphylaxis
- Non–IgE-mediated reactions: food-induced enterocolitis, celiac disease, Crohn's disease, dermatitis herpetiformis, and pulmonary reactions such as Heiner syndrome
- Assess overall nutritional status, growth parameters, and signs of other allergic diseases such as atopic dermatitis, allergic rhinitis, or asthma
- Skin: eczema (dermatitis), angioedema, urticaria
- HEENT: nasal congestion, boggy mucous membranes, lymphoid tissue hypertrophy, postnasal mucous discharge, conjunctival injection

- Oropharyngeal: cobble stoning
- Lungs: stridor or wheezing
- Tachycardia or hypotension may indicate anaphylactic shock

ETIOLOGY

There is insufficient evidence to support the hypothesis that early exposure to food allergens may cause an immature immune system to produce IgE. Eight common foods have been found to be responsible for >90% of food allergies. Food allergies with the greatest likelihood of spontaneous resolution are those involving milk, soy, egg, and wheat. Allergies least likely to resolve spontaneously are peanut, tree nuts, fish, and shellfish.

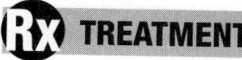 DIAGNOSIS

- Thorough history and physical exam should be performed.
- Differential diagnosis should include toxic reactions (food poisoning), psychological reactions (strongly held beliefs), and carbohydrate malabsorption.
- Skin testing: simple, inexpensive, with excellent sensitivity and negative predictive value. A wheal of 3 mm or greater is considered a positive test. Skin testing if negative can reliably exclude food allergies, but as it has variable specificity and positive predictive value, it does not confirm food allergies when the test is positive. In such cases a food challenge is often necessary.
- In vitro testing: RAST testing: Historically it is less sensitive than skin testing, but sensitivity has improved with cut off points indicating a positive predictive value of 95% for allergies to eggs, milk, peanuts, wheat, and fish. Table 1-158 describes advantages and disadvantages of different allergy testing methods.
- Atopy patch test: used in conjunction with RAST and skin testing in multiallergic children to plan widening the elimination diet.
- Double-blind, placebo-controlled food challenges are the gold standard test for determining food allergies. These need to be done in a supervised and controlled setting.
- In summary, if the history and lab tests are suggestive of specific food allergy, that food should be eliminated from the diet. If reaction involves various food allergens then positive skin tests or specific IgE measurements should be confirmed by double-blind, placebo-controlled food challenges.

DIFFERENTIAL DIAGNOSIS

- Gastrointestinal disorders
- Irritable bowel syndrome
- Carcinoid syndrome
- Giardiasis
- Structural abnormalities like hiatal hernia, pyloric stenosis, Hirschsprung's disease, tracheoesophageal fistula
- Disaccharidase deficiencies: lactase, sucrase-isomaltase complex, glucose-galactose complex
- Pancreatic insufficiency: cystic fibrosis
- Gallbladder disease
- Peptic ulcer disease
- Malignancy
- Metabolic disorders
- Galactosemia
- Phenylketonuria
- Pharmacologic-related conditions
- Gustatory rhinitis
- Auriculotemporal syndrome (facial flush from tart food)

TREATMENT

NONPHARMACOLOGICAL THERAPY

- Elimination diet should be used.
- Formula-fed infants: brief trial of hydrolyzed milk formula as most children with milk allergy induced skin symptoms will respond to the change of formula. Nonresponders may require amino acid–based formula.
- In older children: elimination of one to two suspected foods are appropriate for 2 wk or longer and then reintroducing the foods to determine if symptoms recur.
- Epinephrine and antihistamines should be readily available during food challenges should anaphylactic reactions occur.

ACUTE GENERAL Rx

Antihistamines (both H_1 and H_2 antihistamines), albuterol if wheezing, epinephrine and glucocorticoids in patients with anaphylaxis.

NEW TREATMENTS FOR FOOD ALLERGIES

- Oral and sublingual immunotherapy may play a role in management of food allergies, but this is currently under investigation.
- Recombinant vaccines and other immunomodulatory strategies are under development, although monoclonal anti-IgE antibody has shown benefit in adults with peanut allergy.

TABLE 1-158   Advantages and Disadvantages of Different Allergy Testing Methods

Method	Patient Selection	Clinical Advantages	Clinical Disadvantages
Skin testing	Clinical indication suggesting allergic disease	Rapid (15-30 min) turnaround Sensitive and specific; prick-puncture for aeroallergens, prick-puncture followed by intradermal testing for drugs, sera, and venoms	Patient must not be taking H1-antihistamine agents for 5-7 days Not interpretable in the presence of dermatographism Requires sufficient normal skin to enable testing
In vitro testing	Clinical indication suggesting allergic disease	Antihistamine therapy not contraindicated Dermatographism not a problem Sensitive and specific; equal to prick-puncture skin testing	Requires blood drawn Slow turnaround (7-14 days)

From Goldman L, Schafer AI: Goldman's Cecil medicine, ed 24, Philadelphia, 2012, Saunders.

! PEARLS & CONSIDERATIONS

- Eczema that develops in first 6 to 12 mo of life is usually the first manifestation of atopy.
- Egg allergy or sensitization is the strongest recognized predictor of respiratory allergies in children and asthma in adults.
- Consultation with trained dietitian is critical to avoid potentially adverse nutritional consequences in children with multiple food allergies.
- Skin testing is the preferred method for identifying food-specific IgE. RAST is useful if there is chance of severe food reaction causing risk to the patient.
- American Academy of Pediatrics recommends avoiding influenza vaccine in patients with severe systemic allergic reactions to egg. Skin prick testing using influenza vaccine containing egg is recommended before vaccination in children with egg allergy and asthma. Skin prick testing not required before MMR vaccine in children with egg allergy.

COMMENTS

- Milk allergy usually resolves by age 5. Risk factors for persistence are early cutaneous manifestations following milk ingestion, development of other atopic conditions, and persistence of milk-specific high IgE titers. Soy milk is recommended for these children, keeping in mind that about 15% of these children can develop soy allergy.
- Egg allergy has been thought to resolve in 66% of children by 5 yr of age and in 75% of children by 7 yr of age. Trials have shown that oral immunotherapy can desensitize a high proportion of children with egg allergy and induce sustained unresponsiveness in a clinically significant subset.
- Wheat allergy found to resolve by 5 yr of age and soybean allergy by 2 yr of age.

PREVENTION

- There is conflicting evidence regarding the protective effect of breastfeeding on food allergies.
- There is no evidence to suggest that exclusive breastfeeding for 6 mo or more is superior to exclusive breastfeeding for 4 to 6 mo in terms of developing food allergies.
- In high-risk infants who are not exclusively breast fed, there is limited evidence to suggest that feeding with hydrolyzed formula compared to cow's milk formula reduces allergies.
- Currently, there is no evidence to support the use of prebiotics, probiotics, or synbiotics for the prevention of allergic diseases.
- No current evidence exists to support delaying the introduction of solid foods beyond 4 to 6 mo.

PATIENT/FAMILY EDUCATION

Information can be found on American Academy of Allergy, Asthma and Immunology (www.aaaai.org), the Food Allergy and Anaphylaxis Network (www.foodallergy.org), and the Anaphylaxis Campaign (www.anaphylaxis.org.uk).

REFERRAL

Patients may be referred to an allergy/immunology specialist when the diagnosis is uncertain or if avoidance measures are not successful.

SUGGESTED READINGS
available at www.expertconsult.com

AUTHOR: **DIVJOT SOOCH, M.D.**

ⓘ BASIC INFORMATION

DEFINITION

Food poisoning is an illness caused by ingestion of food contaminated by bacteria and/or bacterial toxins. Table 1-159 describes pathogenic mechanisms in bacterial foodborne disease.

SYNONYMS

Enterotoxin-poisoning
Epidemic vomiting disease

ICD-9CM CODES
See specific illness.

EPIDEMIOLOGY & DEMOGRAPHICS

INCIDENCE (IN U.S.):
- Estimated range of 6 to 8 million cases/yr
- Majority of identifiable causes are bacterial, although more than 250 known diseases can be transmitted through food

PEAK INCIDENCE: Varies with specific organism
- Summer: *Staphylococcus aureus, Salmonella, Shigella* spp.
- Summer and fall: *Clostridium botulinum, Vibrio parahaemolyticus*
- Spring and fall: *Campylobacter jejuni*
- Winter: *Clostridium perfringens, Yersinia enterocolitica*

PREDOMINANT AGE: Varies with specific agent
NEONATAL INFECTION: Rare but severe with *Shigella* and *Salmonella* spp.

PHYSICAL FINDINGS & CLINICAL PRESENTATION

- Any combination of GI symptoms and fever
- Specific organisms suspected on the basis of the incubation period and predominant symptoms (Table E1-160), although a great deal of overlap exists
  1. Short incubation period (1 to 6 hr): involve the ingestion of preformed toxin; noninvasive
     a. *S. aureus:* nausea, profuse vomiting, and abdominal cramps common; diarrhea possible, but fever uncommon; usually resolves within 24 hr; foods implicated in outbreaks include meats, mayonnaise, and cream pastries
     b. *B. cereus:* two forms, a short incubation (emetic) form (characterized by vomiting and abdominal cramps in virtually all patients, diarrhea in one third of patients, fever uncommon) and a long incubation (diarrheal) form; illness usually mild, resolves within 12 hr; unrefrigerated rice most often implicated as vehicle
  2. Moderate incubation period (8 to 16 hr): involves the in vivo production of toxin; noninvasive
     a. *C. perfringens:* severe crampy abdominal pain and watery diarrhea common; fever and vomiting unlikely; symptoms usually resolving within 24 hr; outbreaks invariably related to cooked meat or poultry that is allowed to cool without refrigeration; most cases in the fall and winter months. *C. perfringens* is the third most common cause of foodborne illness in the U.S.
     b. *B. cereus:* diarrheal (or long incubation) form most commonly beginning with diarrhea, abdominal cramps, and occasionally vomiting; fever uncommon; usually resolves within 24 hr; the responsible food is usually fried rice
  3. Long incubation period (>16 hr): some toxin-mediated, some invasive
     a. Toxin-producing organisms include:
        (1) *C. botulinum:* should be considered when a diarrheal illness coincides with or precedes paralysis; severity of illness related to the quantity of toxin ingested; characteristic cranial nerve palsies progressing to a descending paralysis; fever usually absent; usually associated with home-canned foods
        (2) Enterotoxigenic *E. coli* (ETEC): most common cause of travelers' diarrhea; after 1- to 2-day incubation period, abdominal cramps and copious diarrhea occur; vomiting and fever uncommon; usually resolves after 3 to 4 days; vehicle usually unbottled water or contaminated salad or ice
        (3) Enterohemorrhagic *E. coli* (EHEC): can cause severe abdominal cramps and watery diarrhea, which may eventually become bloody; bacteria (strain O157:H7) are noninvasive; no fever; illness may be complicated by hemolytic-uremic syndrome; associated with contaminated beef
        (4) *V. cholerae:* varies from a mild, self-limited illness to life-threatening cholera; diarrhea, nausea, and vomiting, abdominal cramps, and muscle cramps; no fever; severe cases may progress to shock and death within hours of onset; survivors usually have resolution of symptoms in 1 wk; U.S. cases are either imported or result from ingestion of imported food
     b. Invasive organisms include:
        (1) *Salmonella:* associated most often with nontyphoidal strains; incubation period generally 12 to 48 hr; nausea, vomiting, diarrhea, and abdominal cramps typical; fever possible; outbreaks of gastroenteritis related to contaminated poultry, meat, and dairy products
        (2) *Shigella:* asymptomatic infection possible, but some with fever and watery diarrhea that may progress to bloody diarrhea and dysentery; with mild illness, usually self-limited, resolves in a few days; with severe illness, may develop complications; transmission usually from person to person but can occur via contaminated food or water
        (3) *C. jejuni:* the most common foodborne bacterial pathogen; incubation period is about 1 day, then a prodrome of fever, headache, and myalgias; intestinal phase marked by diarrhea associated with fever, malaise, and abdominal pain; diarrhea mild to profuse and bloody; usually resolves in about 7 days, but relapse is possible; associated with undercooked meats and poultry, unpasteurized dairy products, and drinking from freshwater streams
        (4) *Y. enterocolitica* and *Y. pseudotuberculosis:* infrequent causes of enteritis in U.S.; children affected more often than adults; fever, diarrhea, and abdominal pain lasting 1 to 3 wk; some with mesenteric adenitis that mimics acute appendicitis; contaminated food or water is usually responsible
        (5) *V. parahaemolyticus:* In U.S., most outbreaks in coastal states or on

---

TABLE 1-159 Pathogenic Mechanisms in Bacterial Foodborne Disease

Preformed Toxin	Toxin Production in Vivo	Tissue Invasion	Toxin Production and/or Tissue Invasion
Staphylococcus aureus *Bacillus cereus* (short incubation) *Clostridium botulinum*	*Clostridium perfringens* *B. cereus* (long incubation) *C. botulinum* (infant botulism) Enterotoxigenic *Escherichia coli* *Vibrio cholerae* 01 or 0139 *V. cholerae* non-01 Shiga toxin–producing *E. coli*	*Campylobacter jejuni* *Salmonella* *Shigella* Invasive *E. coli*	*Vibrio parahaemolyticus* *Yersinia enterocolitica*

From Mandell GL et al: *Principles and practice of infectious diseases,* ed 6, Philadelphia, 2005, Churchill Livingstone.

cruise ships during the summer months; incubation period usually <1 day, followed by explosive watery diarrhea in the majority of cases; nausea, vomiting, abdominal cramps, and headache also common; fever less common; usually resolves by 1 wk; related to ingestion of seafood

(6) Enteroinvasive *E. coli* (EIEC): a rare cause of disease in the U.S.; high incidence of fever and bloody diarrhea; may resemble bacillary dysentery

(7) *V. vulnificus:* may cause serious, often fatal illness in persons with chronic liver disease; GI symptoms usually absent, but fever, chills, hypotension, and hemorrhagic skin lesions possible; patients with liver disease or at increased risk of developing liver disease should avoid eating raw oysters

ETIOLOGY

Classically categorized as either inflammatory (invasive) or noninflammatory:
- Noninflammatory: *B. cereus, S. aureus, C. botulinum, C. perfringens, V. cholerae,* enterotoxigenic *E. coli* (ETEC), and enterohemorrhagic *E. coli* (EHEC); toxin-producing organisms that are noninvasive; fecal leukocytes are not seen.
- Inflammatory: *Campylobacter,* enteroinvasive *E. coli* (EIEC), *Salmonella, Shigella, V. parahaemolyticus,* and *Yersinia;* cause disease by invasion of intestinal tissue; fecal leukocytes are seen.

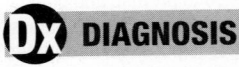 **DIAGNOSIS**

DIFFERENTIAL DIAGNOSIS

Gastroenteritis caused by viruses (Norwalk, Noro, or rotavirus), parasites *(Amoeba histolytica, Giardia lamblia),* or toxins (ciguatoxins, mushrooms, heavy metals)

LABORATORY TESTS

- Test stool for fecal leukocytes to help narrow the differential diagnosis:
  1. Send stool for culture and for ova and parasites.

2. Send stool for *C. difficile* toxin in patients with current or recent antibiotic use.
3. NOTE: Some pathogens are not identified on routine stool culture; laboratory should be advised if *Yersinia, C. botulinum, Vibrio,* or enterohemorrhagic *E. coli* (O157:H7) are suspected.
4. Finding *B. cereus, C. perfringens,* or *E. coli* in stool is of little value, because these may be part of the normal bowel flora.
- If botulism suspected, send food, serum, and stool for toxin assay.
- Blood cultures are needed for all febrile patients.

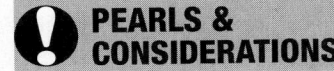 **TREATMENT**

NONPHARMACOLOGIC THERAPY

Adequate rehydration is the mainstay of therapy.

ACUTE GENERAL Rx

- Gastroenteritis caused by the following organisms requires no antimicrobial treatment: *B. cereus, S. aureus, C. perfringens, V. parahaemolyticus, Yersinia,* and enterohemorrhagic and enteroinvasive *E. coli.*
- The usual cause of traveler's diarrhea is enterotoxigenic *E. coli.* Although usually a self-limited illness, antibiotics can shorten the course.
  1. SMX/TMP one DS tab bid for 3 days
  2. Ciprofloxacin 500 mg PO bid for 3 days
- The mainstay of therapy for cholera is fluid replacement. Antibiotics should be given to decrease shedding and duration of illness.
  1. Doxycycline 100 mg PO bid for 3 days
  2. SMX/TMP one DS tab bid for 3 days
- Treatment is not indicated for *Salmonella* gastroenteritis. Patients who are at high risk of developing bacteremia may be treated for 48 to 72 hr (see "Salmonellosis").
- Although shigellosis tends to be a self-limited illness, antibiotics shorten the course of illness and may limit transmission of the illness (see "Shigellosis").

- Those with moderate or severe *Campylobacter* diarrhea may benefit from treatment.
  1. Erythromycin 500 mg PO qid for 5 days
  2. Ciprofloxacin 500 mg PO bid for 5 days
- *V. vulnificus* sepsis should be treated with:
  1. Doxycycline 100 mg IV bid for 2 wk
  2. Ceftazidime 2 g IV q8h for 2 wk
- For suspected botulism, antitoxin should be administered early (see "Botulism").

CHRONIC Rx

Patients with *Salmonella* infections may become carriers and may require treatment (see "Salmonellosis").

DISPOSITION

- Most infections are self-limited and do not require therapy.
- In immunocompromised host or patient with underlying disease, serious complications are possible.
- Postinfectious syndromes are important with some infections:
  1. Reiter's syndrome: *Salmonella, Shigella, Campylobacter, Yersinia* spp.; more common in genetically susceptible host (HLA-B27+)
  2. Guillain-Barré syndrome: *Campylobacter* spp.

REFERRAL

If more than a mild illness

PEARLS & CONSIDERATIONS

COMMENTS

- Grossly underreported and undiagnosed
- All cases to be reported to the local health department

SUGGESTED READINGS

available at www.expertconsult.com

RELATED CONTENT

Bacterial Food Poisoning (Patient Information)
Salmonellosis (Related Key Topic)

AUTHOR: **GLENN G. FORT, M.D., M.P.H.**

ℹ BASIC INFORMATION

DEFINITION

Friedreich's ataxia is the most common neurodegenerative hereditary ataxic disorder, caused by degeneration of dorsal root ganglions, posterior columns, spinocerebellar and corticospinal tracts, and large sensory peripheral neurons.

ICD-9CM CODES
334.0 Friedreich's ataxia

EPIDEMIOLOGY & DEMOGRAPHICS

INCIDENCE (IN U.S.): Estimated at one in 30,000 whites
PEAK INCIDENCE: 8 to 15 yr
PREVALENCE (IN U.S.): Two to four per 100,000. Carrier rate 1:120 to 1:160. Lower prevalence in Asians and people of African descent.
PREDOMINANT SEX: Males and females affected equally
GENETICS: Autosomal recessive; 96% of affected patients are homozygous and 4% are compound heterozygous (two different mutations). Trinucleotide repeat expansion accounts for 94% to 98% of cases, whereas point mutations account for 2% to 6% of cases.

PHYSICAL FINDINGS & CLINICAL PRESENTATION

- Onset of progressive appendicular and gait ataxia, with absent muscle stretch reflexes in the lower extremities.
- With disease progression (within 5 yr): dysarthria, distal loss of position and vibration sense, pyramidal leg weakness, areflexia in all four limbs, and extensor plantar responses.
- Common findings: progressive scoliosis, distal atrophy, pes cavus, and cardiomyopathy (symmetric concentric hypertrophic form in most cases).
- Insulin-requiring diabetes mellitus may occur in 10% of patients, with glucose intolerance occurring in an additional 10% to 20%.

ETIOLOGY

- Genetic: frataxin gene is localized to the centromeric region of chromosome 9q13.
- Normal sequence has six to 27 repeats; abnormal sequence has 120 to 1700 GAA repeats.
- Frataxin deficiency leads to impaired mitochondrial iron homeostasis.

𝖣𝗑 DIAGNOSIS

DIFFERENTIAL DIAGNOSIS

- Charcot-Marie-Tooth disease type 2
- Abetalipoproteinemia
- Severe vitamin E deficiency with malabsorption
- Early-onset cerebellar ataxia with retained reflexes
- Autosomal-dominant cerebellar ataxia (spinocerebellar ataxia)

WORKUP

- Diagnostic criteria include electrophysiologic evidence for a generalized axonal sensory or sensorimotor neuropathy.
- ECG may show widespread T-wave inversion and evidence of left ventricular hypertrophy. ECG abnormalities are present in 65% of patients.
- Sural nerve biopsy shows loss of large myelinated fibers.
- Specific gene testing for the expanded GAA trinucleotide repeat.

LABORATORY TESTS

- Electromyography or nerve conduction study
- ECG and echocardiogram
- Peripheral blood smear for acanthocytes
- Lipid profile
- Two-hour glucose tolerance test
- Vitamin E levels (if necessary)

IMAGING STUDIES

MRI of the spinal cord may demonstrate spinal cord atrophy with essentially normal cerebrum, brainstem, and cerebellum (Fig. 1-345).

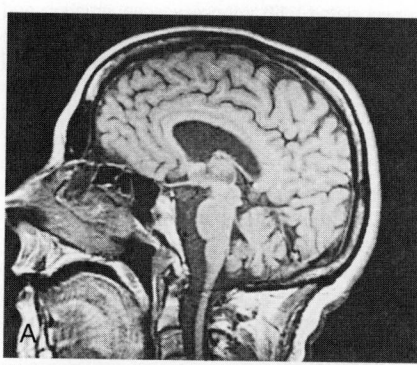
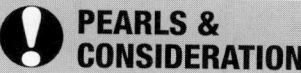
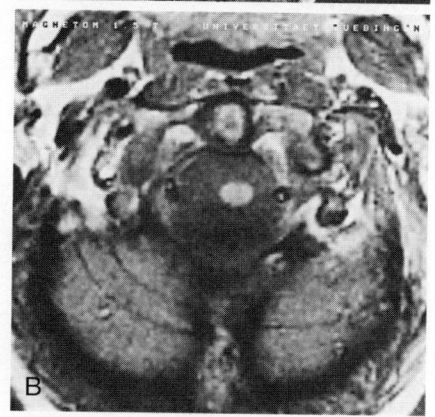

FIGURE 1-345 T1 MRI of the brain (midsagittal section) and spinal cord (axial slice at level of the dens) showing severe shrinkage of the cervical cord, but the cerebellum and brain stem are of normal size. (From Goetz CG: *Textbook of clinical neurology*, Philadelphia, 1999, Saunders.)

℞ TREATMENT

NONPHARMACOLOGIC THERAPY

- Surgical correction of scoliosis and foot deformities in selected patients
- Prosthetic devices as required (e.g., ankle-foot orthosis for foot drop)
- Physical therapy
- Communication devices for patients with severe dysarthria

ACUTE GENERAL Rx

None established.
- An antioxidant, idebenone (short-chain analogue of coenzyme Q10), administered orally at 5 to 20 mg/kg/day with or without vitamin E has demonstrated inconsistent effects on neurologic, cardiac, and psychosocial outcome measures in clinical trials.
- Further research with various antioxidants and iron chelators is ongoing. An open-label pilot study of antioxidants (coenzyme Q10, 400 mg/day, and vitamin E, 2100 U/day) in a small cohort demonstrated slowing in progression of generalized ataxia and kinetic dysfunction and significant improvement in cardiac function with unaltered deterioration in posture, gait, and hand dexterity.

CHRONIC Rx

Chronic management of congestive heart failure is required. Cardiac arrhythmias will warrant pacemaker implantation.

DISPOSITION

- Loss of ambulation typically occurs within 15 yr of symptom onset, and 95% are wheelchair bound by age 45 yr.
- Life expectancy is reduced, particularly if heart disease with or without diabetes mellitus is present.

REFERRAL

- If uncertain about diagnosis
- For genetic counseling (recommended if available)

❗ PEARLS & CONSIDERATIONS

Friedreich's ataxia should be considered in all preadolescent and adolescent children presenting with progressive ataxia. Early recognition of cardiac failure and arrhythmias and institution of appropriate therapy helps prolong survival.

SUGGESTED READINGS
available at www.expertconsult.com

RELATED CONTENT
Friedreich's Ataxia (Patient Information)

AUTHOR: **EROBOGHENE E. UBOGU, M.D.**

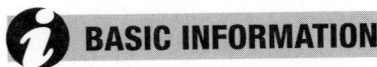

BASIC INFORMATION

DEFINITION

Frostbite represents tissue injury (or death) from freezing and vasoconstriction induced by severe environmental cold exposure.

SYNONYMS

Cold-induced tissue injury

EPIDEMIOLOGY & DEMOGRAPHICS

- Environmental factors include wind chill factor, temperature, duration of exposure, altitude, and degree of wetness. Hands and feet account for 90% of injuries; nose, cheeks, ears, and male genitalia are also more susceptible.
- Host factors include psychiatric illness, neuroleptic and sedative drugs (especially alcohol), immobility, previous frostbite, skin damage, malnutrition, tobacco use, peripheral neuropathy, peripheral vascular disease, diabetes, hypothyroidism, fatigue, and constricting clothing and footwear.

PHYSICAL FINDINGS & CLINICAL PRESENTATION

- Frostbite may be classified into four degrees of injury severity (determined after rewarming) or, more practically, into *superficial* and *deep* groups. This can only be accurately determined after rewarming as initially most frostbite injuries appear similar.
- *Superficial* frostbite involves the skin and subcutaneous tissue. The frozen part is waxy, white (or mottled), and firm but soft and resilient below the surface when gently depressed. After rewarming, there is an initial hyperemia that may be followed by swelling and formation of superficial blisters with clear or milky fluid within 6 to 24 hr (Fig. 1-346). There is no ultimate tissue loss.
- *Deep* frostbite extends into the dermis and may involve muscles, nerves, tendons, or bones. The skin may be hard or wooden, without tissue resilience. Nonblanching cyanosis, hemorrhagic blisters, tissue necrosis

(Fig. 1-347), and gangrene may develop. Affected tissue has a poor prognosis and debridement or amputation is generally required.
- Patients initially feel numbness, prickling, and itching. More severe injury can produce paresthesias and stiffness, with burning or throbbing pain on thawing.

ETIOLOGY

Two mechanisms of tissue injury:
1. Freeze-thaw damage. Intracellular ice crystallization leads to cell membrane lysis and cell death followed by thaw-initiated ischemia-reperfusion injury.
2. Vascular stasis and ischemia. Vessels fluctuate between constriction and dilation (the "hunting response") with associated vascular leak and coagulation; ischemia/infarction ensues from a cascade of inflammatory mediators (prostaglandin F, thromboxane A_2, bradykinins, histamine) that contribute to reperfusion injury and thrombus formation and ultimately lead to destruction of the microcirculation and cell death.

DIAGNOSIS

DIFFERENTIAL DIAGNOSIS

- Frostnip: a superficial nonfreezing cold injury associated with intense vasoconstriction and characterized by frost forming on the surface of the skin. Transient numbness, tingling, and pallor resolve quickly with warming.
- Pernio (chilblains): self-limited, cold-induced vasculitis associated with purple plaques or nodules, often affecting dorsum of hands and feet; seen with prolonged cold exposure to above-freezing temperatures
- Cold immersion (trench foot): caused by ischemic injury resulting from sustained, severe vasoconstriction in appendages exposed to wet cold at temperatures above freezing

WORKUP

- Laboratory work is not indicated unless the patient has systemic hypothermia.
- MRI/MRA or triple-phase bone scanning (with technetium) may be used to predict tissue viability in cases of severe frostbite or when

thrombolysis is being considered. (MRA has the advantage of showing occluded vessels and viability of surrounding tissues.)

TREATMENT (3 PHASES)

1. FIELD MANAGEMENT

- Prioritize treatment of hypothermia (core body temperature <35° C) with systemic and adjunctive rewarming measures if available (e.g., warmed, humidified oxygen, heated IV saline [45° C], and warming blankets) before thawing frostbitten extremities.
- Remove constricting or wet clothing. Pat dry, insulate, splint, and elevate affected areas.
- Avoid thawing if there is any risk of refreezing.
- Never rub or massage the affected area. Avoid dry heat (e.g., fires and heaters)
- Avoid thawing if there is any risk of refreezing and avoid ambulation on thawed lower extremities (unless only distal toes affected).
- Administer pain medication and topical aloe if available.
- Hydrate.

2. REWARMING

- Rapid rewarming is the key objective.
- Immerse affected area in circulating warm water bath with or without a mild antibacterial agent (e.g., chlorhexidene or povidone-iodine) maintained at 37° to 39° C for at least 30 min, until all tissues are thoroughly rewarmed and pliable with a red-purple color. Water should be continually monitored and warmed to the target temperature. Active motion during rewarming is advisable; massage is not.
- Slow thawing is acceptable when this is not possible. For example, relocating to a warm location and warming with adjacent body heat (e.g., axilla or abdomen) from the patient or caregiver.

3. POST-THAW Rx

- Tetanus prophylaxis and topical antibiotics if potentially contaminated skin wound.
- Consider systemic antibiotics for patients with significant trauma or signs of infection.
- Debride broken clear vesicles and avoid disrupting intact blisters (especially hemorrhagic ones) unless they interfere with mobility.
- Topical aloe vera q6h and ibuprofen 400 to 600 mg bid to tid for 1 wk may be beneficial for antiprostaglandin and thromboxane inhibiting effect.
- Thrombolytic therapy. If <24 hr from thawing in a patient with hemorrhagic blisters or loss of Doppler pulses, imaging with MR angiography or technetium triple-phase bone scan (to assess for arterial compromise) followed by intra-arterial or intravenous thrombolytic therapy appears to considerably improve reperfusion and reduce subsequent digit amputation. This should be considered only for deep injuries with potential for significant morbidity (e.g., extending proximally to PIP joints) in a facility with intensive-care monitoring capabilities.

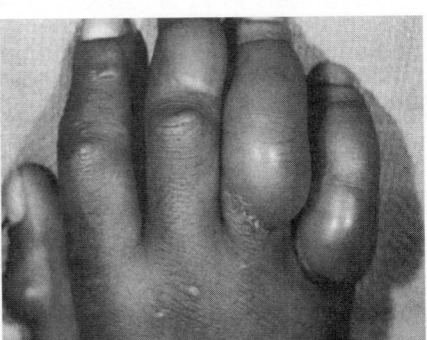

FIGURE 1-346 Large, clear frostbite blisters on the right hand. (From Rosen P [ed]: *Emergency medicine*, ed 4, St Louis, 1998, Mosby.)

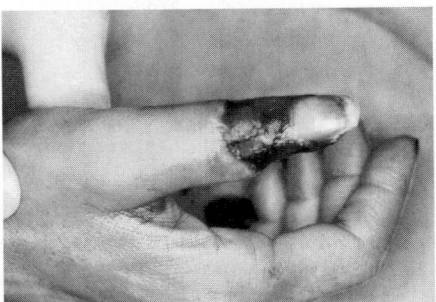

FIGURE 1-347 Third- and fourth-degree frostbite with tissue death. Note demarcation beyond the interphalangeal joint. (From Cameron, JL, Cameron AM: *Current surgical therapy*, ed 10, Philadelphia, 2011, Saunders.)

- If >24 hr from injury imaging with technetium scan or MRA can be used to predict tissue viability and vasodilators (e.g., illoprost infusion daily) may decrease need for subsequent amputation.
- Daily dressing changes with dry, sterile, noncompressive, and nonadherent dressings. Splint and elevate hands and feet to reduce edema and separate digits with cotton gauze. Avoid even slightest abrasion to limit risk of infection.
- Whirlpool hydrotherapy with warm water (38° C) and an antiseptic for 30 min bid until there is a clear demarcation of necrotic tissues or evidence of tissue healing.
- Gentle, progressive physical therapy after edema resolves.
- Keep site warm, and avoid all vasoconstrictors, including nicotine.
- Dextran, vasodilators (e.g., pentoxifylline, nifedipine), and adjunctive heparin with tPA and hyperbaric oxygen are of potential but unproven benefit.

DISPOSITION

A majority of patients have long-term residual symptoms, including neuropathic pain, sensory deficits, hyperhidrosis, secondary Raynaud's disease, edema, hair or nail deformities, and (rarely) arthritis. Treatment with tricyclics, calcium channel blockers, and careful protection from further cold exposure may be helpful.

REFERRAL

- Hospitalize for hypothermia or deep frostbite; a burn unit is best.
- Surgical decisions regarding amputation should be deferred until demarcation of viable tissue is clear (1 to 3 mo) unless refractory pain, sepsis, or gangrene occurs.

SUGGESTED READINGS
available at www.expertconsult.com

RELATED CONTENT
Frostbite (Patient Information)

AUTHOR: **MICHAEL P. JOHNSON, M.D.**

F

Diseases and Disorders

I

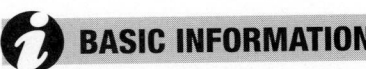

BASIC INFORMATION

DEFINITION

Frozen shoulder is a clinical diagnosis that describes a stiffened glenohumeral (GH) joint accompanied by shoulder pain and restricted passive and active range of motion (ROM) (Fig. 1-348). The condition is categorized as primary when there is no underlying cause and secondary when there is an associated precipitating event or identifiable cause leading to the characteristic shoulder symptomatology.

SYNONYMS

Adhesive capsulitis
Periarthritis
Pericapsulitis
Check-rein shoulder
Bursitis Duplay

ICD-9CM CODES
726.0 Adhesive shoulder capsulitis

EPIDEMIOLOGY & DEMOGRAPHICS

- Prevalence of frozen shoulder is 2% to 5% in the general population. There is a higher incidence of up to 10% to 20% in people with diabetes.
- Predominant sex: Females are affected more often than males.
- Most commonly affects patients 40 to 70 years.

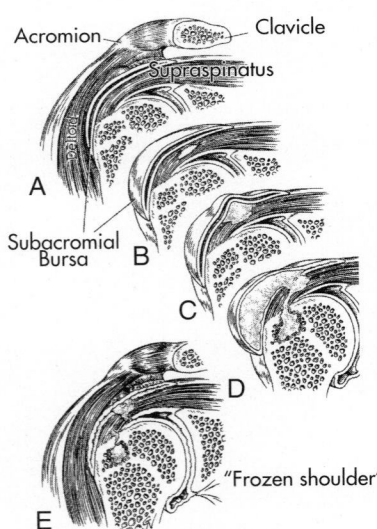

FIGURE 1-348 Sequence of events terminating in frozen shoulder. A, Normal structures of the shoulder. **B,** Supraspinatus tendonitis, sometimes calcific, in the "critical zone." **C,** Spread of inflammation to the tendon sheath and a bulge into the floor of the subacromial bursa. **D,** Rupture into the subacromial bursa and extension of the inflammatory process as an osteitis into the humeral head and greater tuberosity. **E,** Frozen shoulder with involvement of tendons, bursa, capsule, synovium, and muscle with fibrous contracture and markedly diminished volume of the shoulder joint space. (From Noble J [ed]: *Primary care medicine*, ed 2, St Louis, 1996, Mosby.)

PHYSICAL FINDINGS & CLINICAL PRESENTATION

The natural history of frozen shoulder occurs in three phases that usually include full resolution of pain and return of function.
- Painful phase: There is a gradual onset of a painful shoulder, with pain usually worse at night and difficulty lying on the affected side. This may last from weeks to months.
- Frozen phase: Progressive shoulder stiffness may last for 1 yr. In addition to tenderness on palpation of the GH joint, exam findings may include disuse atrophy of the deltoid and supraspinatus, with the arm held in adduction and internal rotation. There is variable loss in the degrees of restricted active and passive shoulder abduction and external rotation.
- Thawing phase: Overall improvement in pain and increase in ROM. This may last for 5-12 mo.

ETIOLOGY

- The pathology of frozen shoulder involves a chronic inflammatory response with fibroblastic proliferation.
- Factors that predispose to increased risk for developing a frozen shoulder include:
  1. Prolonged shoulder immobility from trauma (including fracture of the femoral head and neck), surgery, and overuse injuries.
  2. Systemic diseases (diabetes, thyroid disease, stroke, Parkinson's, cardiovascular disease, and inflammatory disease).
- Fig. 1-348 illustrates the sequence of events terminating in frozen shoulder.

DIAGNOSIS

DIFFERENTIAL DIAGNOSIS

- Trauma: shoulder sprain, dislocation, glenoid labrum tear, rotator cuff tear
- Usage, degenerative, and age-related disorders: GH osteoarthritis, avascular necrosis of the humeral head, rotator cuff tendonopathy
- Mechanical: calcific tendonitis, shoulder impingement or derangement
- Neoplasm: Pancoast tumor
- Cervical spondylosis or other cervical disk disease
- Brachial neuritis
- Milwaukee shoulder

WORKUP

- Laboratory studies only contribute to the diagnosis if an underlying condition such as diabetes, cardiovascular disease, or thyroid disease is suspected.
- Radiographic evaluation should be considered to rule out other pathologic conditions. Nonspecific findings include calcification of the tendons of the rotator cuff.
- MRI might be indicated to further rule out intraarticular pathology. Characteristic MRI findings can include thickening of the coracohumeral ligament and the joint capsule.

TREATMENT

NONPHARMACOLOGIC THERAPY

Patient education is important in prevention and to improve compliance and outcome expectation.

ACUTE GENERAL Rx

- Initial conservative therapy with heat, analgesics (generally NSAIDs), and physical therapy with passive stretching and ROM exercises
- Course of oral corticosteroids
- Local steroid/lidocaine injection into the subacromial space
- Surgical methods include:
  - Shoulder manipulation under anesthesia (rarely needed)
  - Arthroscopic and, rarely, open capsular release when conservative treatment fails

DISPOSITION

- Most patients regain 90% of shoulder motion over time and have improved pain.
- The condition can last from several months to beyond 3 years.
- Recurrence in the same shoulder is rare, although the opposite limb may develop the same symptoms.

REFERRAL

Orthopedic consultation in patients with resistant disease who fail to respond to conservative treatment after 6 mo

PEARLS & CONSIDERATIONS

COMMENTS

- Hallmark symptoms include severe pain, progressive shoulder stiffness, ischemic restricted ROM.
- Frozen shoulder is more common in patients with diabetes, thyroid disease, ischemic cardiovascular disease, and cervical spondylosis.
- Arthroscopic shoulder release has been shown to provide excellent clinical outcome for patients with refractory adhesive capsulitis.

EVIDENCE

available at www.expertconsult.com

SUGGESTED READINGS

available at www.expertconsult.com

RELATED CONTENT

Frozen Shoulder (Patient Information)
Rotator Cuff Syndrome (Related Key Topic)

AUTHOR: **ANISHKA S. ROLLE, M.D.**

BASIC INFORMATION

DEFINITION

Galactorrhea can be defined as inappropriate lactation (in the absence of pregnancy or postpartum state) as a result of nonphysiologic augmentation of prolactin release.

ICD-9CM CODES
611.6 Galactorrhea

PHYSICAL FINDINGS & CLINICAL PRESENTATION

- Milky discharge from nipples (Fig. 1-349) usually occurring bilaterally
- Evidence of chest wall irritation from ill-fitting clothing, herpes zoster, or atopic dermatitis may be present
- Visual field defects (bitemporal hemianopsia) may be present with prolactinomas
- Evidence of acromegaly, Cushing's disease, or hypothyroidism when galactorrhea is caused by these disorders

ETIOLOGY

- Medications (phenothiazines, metoclopramide, selective serotonin reuptake inhibitors, anxiolytics, buspirone, atenolol, valproic acid, conjugated estrogen and medroxyprogesterone, methyldopa, verapamil, H_2 receptor blockers, octreotide, danazol, tricyclic antidepressants, isoniazid, amphetamine, reserpine, opiates, sumatriptan, rimantadine, oral contraceptive formulations); after infancy, galactorrhea is often medication induced
- Breast stimulation (prolonged suckling), sexual intercourse

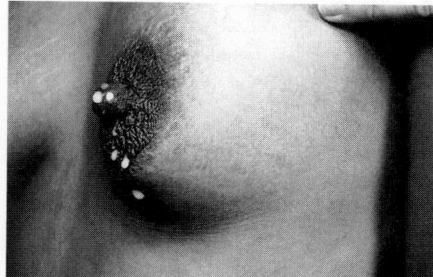

FIGURE 1-349 Galactorrhea. Milk production in a nonpregnant woman resulting from a prolactinoma. (From Haines DE: *Fundamental neuroscience for basic and clinical applications,* ed 3, Philadelphia, 2006, Churchill Livingstone.)

- Pituitary tumors (prolactinomas, craniopharyngiomas)
- Chest wall irritation from ill-fitting clothing, herpes zoster, atopic dermatitis, burns
- Hypothyroidism (diminished feedback inhibition increases thyroid-releasing hormone [TRH], which increases prolactin)
- Increased stress, major trauma
- Chronic renal failure (decreased prolactin clearance)
- Cushing's disease
- Herbs (e.g., fennel, red clover, anise, red raspberry, marshmallow)
- Cannabis
- Spinal cord surgery or injury, or tumors
- Severe gastroesophageal reflux disease, esophagitis (stimulation of thoracic nerves by the cervical and thoracic ganglia)
- Breast surgery
- Idiopathic
- Neonatal ("witch's milk" produced by 2% to 5% of neonates because of precipitous drop in maternal estrogen and progesterone postdelivery)
- Lymphomas, Hodgkin's disease, bronchogenic carcinoma, renal adenocarcinomas
- Sarcoidosis and other infiltrative disorders
- Tuberculosis affecting pituitary gland
- Pituitary stalk resection
- Multiple sclerosis
- Empty sella syndrome
- Acromegaly

DIAGNOSIS

DIFFERENTIAL DIAGNOSIS

- Intraductal papilloma
- Breast cancer
- Paget's disease of breast
- Breast abscess

WORKUP

- Complete history focusing on menstrual irregularity, infertility, previous pregnancies, duration of galactorrhea, medications, visual complaints, fatigue. Age of onset is also significant (e.g., prolactinoma most common between ages 20 and 35 yr; neonatal galactorrhea is usually secondary to transplacental transfer of maternal estrogen)
- Physical examination: hirsutism, acne, obesity, visual field defects, goiter
- Breast examination for presence of nodules, evaluation of discharge (milky versus serosanguineous versus purulent)
- Laboratory testing and imaging studies (see "Laboratory Tests")

LABORATORY TESTS

- Prolactin level (elevated, often >200 ng/ml in prolactinoma)
- Human chorionic gonadotropin level (positive in pregnancy)
- TSH (elevated in hypothyroidism)
- Blood urea nitrogen, creatinine (elevated in renal failure), glucose (elevated in Cushing's syndrome)
- Urinalysis (hematuria in renal cell carcinoma)
- Microscopic examination of nipple discharge (scant cellular material, numerous fat globules)

IMAGING STUDIES

- MRI of brain if prolactin level is elevated, amenorrhea is present, or visual field defects are detected on physical examination.
- High-resolution CT of brain with special coronal cuts through the pituitary region may be helpful in patients with contraindications to MRI; however, it may miss small lesions.

TREATMENT

- Discontinuation of potential offending agents.
- Avoidance of excessive breast stimulation.
- Galactorrhea resulting from prolactinoma can be managed medically or with careful surveillance depending on size and growth of tumor, associated symptoms, and prolactin level. Surgical treatment of prolactinomas is usually reserved for medication failures. Please refer to the topic "Prolactinoma" in Section I for additional information.
- No treatment is necessary for normoprolactinemic patients with idiopathic nonbothersome galactorrhea.
- Normoprolactinemic patients with bothersome galactorrhea may respond to low dose dopamine agonist (e.g., cabergoline 0.5 mg/wk).

REFERRAL

Endocrine and surgical consultation if prolactinoma is detected

SUGGESTED READINGS
available at www.expertconsult.com

RELATED CONTENT
Pituitary Adenoma (Related Key Topic)
Prolactinoma (Related Key Topic)
Galactorrhea (Patient Information)

AUTHOR: **FRED F. FERRI, M.D.**

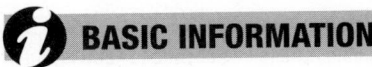

DEFINITION

A fluid-filled sac (cyst) overlying a tendon sheath or joint

SYNONYMS

Ganglion

ICD-9CM CODES
727.43 Ganglion

EPIDEMIOLOGY & DEMOGRAPHICS

- Ganglia are more common in women than men (3:1)
- Can occur at any age, but usually between second and fourth decades of life
- Most common soft tissue tumor of the hand and wrist

PHYSICAL FINDINGS & CLINICAL PRESENTATION

- Most ganglia occur on the dorsum of the wrist (50% to 70%) (Fig. 1-350).
- The volar wrist (18% to 20%) is the next most common site.
- Can also involve the proximal digital flexor tendons and the distal interphalangeal joints.
- Left and right hands are equally affected.
- Ganglia are usually solitary, firm, smooth, round, and fluctuant.
- Pain from mass effect or compression against nearby structure may be present (e.g., median nerve and radial nerve).
- Hand numbness may be present.
- Patient may have hand muscle weakness.
- Ganglia usually develop over a period of months but may arise suddenly.

ETIOLOGY

Ganglia are believed to derive from synovial herniation or expansion from the joint capsule or

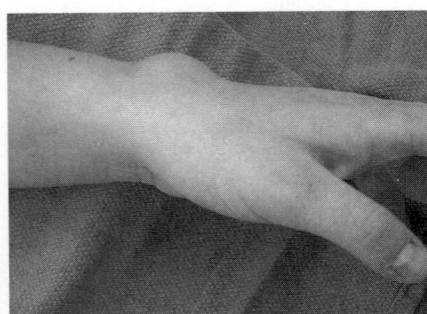

FIGURE 1-350 Dorsal wrist ganglion. (From Hochberg MC et al: *Rheumatology*, ed 5, St Louis, 2011, Mosby.)

tendon sheath. Repetitive movement as an etiology is uncertain, although it may cause enlargement of the lesion or worsen symptoms.

DX DIAGNOSIS

Direct inspection and localization of the cyst often is enough to make the diagnosis of ganglia. Transillumination is an easy method of differentiating ganglia from solid tumors; ganglia transilluminate while solid tumors do not.

DIFFERENTIAL DIAGNOSIS

- Lipoma
- Fibroma
- Epidermoid inclusion cyst
- Osteochondroma
- Hemangioma
- Infection (tuberculosis, fungi, and secondary syphilis)
- Gout
- Rheumatoid nodule
- Radial artery aneurysm

WORKUP

The workup of ganglia usually consists of history, physical examination, and x-ray imaging.

LABORATORY TESTS

Blood tests are not specific in the diagnosis of ganglia.

IMAGING STUDIES

- Radiographs of the hand and wrist are taken to rule out other bone or joint abnormalities.
- Ultrasound studies are helpful in the diagnosis of ganglia by demonstrating smooth cystic walls that may be septated.
- CT scan can be done if the ultrasound is equivocal.
- MRI helps differentiate malignant bone lesions from cystic structures.
- Arthrography may demonstrate a communication between the joint and ganglia (not commonly done).

Rx TREATMENT

Expectant treatment is appropriate if the mass is not painful or interfering with motor function.

NONPHARMACOLOGIC THERAPY

- Attempts to rupture the cyst by sharp blows with a book or with finger compression are not recommended.
- Aspiration, heat, and sclerotherapy have been tried but have met with high recurrence rates (60%).

ACUTE GENERAL Rx

- Aspiration at the base with a large-bore needle (18-gauge) followed by injection of 20 to 40 mg of triamcinolone acetonide can be tried.
- This may be repeated if the ganglia recurs (35% to 40%).

CHRONIC Rx

Total ganglionectomy and repair of the defect after tracing its connection to the tendon sheath is effective and the surgical procedure of choice.

DISPOSITION

- Ganglia spontaneously resolve in approximately 40% to 50% of cases.
- Aspiration with steroid injection is successful in approximately 65% of cases.
- Surgery provides cure in 85% to 95% of the cases.
- Complications of ganglia include:
  1. Carpal tunnel syndrome with pain and muscle atrophy
  2. Radial nerve impingement
  3. Radial artery compression
- Complications of ganglion surgery include:
  1. Infection
  2. Recurrence (5% to 15%), usually from inadequate excision
  3. Reflex sympathetic dystrophy
  4. Scar formation

REFERRAL

It is best to refer patients with symptomatic ganglia to a hand surgeon.

! PEARLS & CONSIDERATIONS

- Dorsal ganglia usually originate from the scapholunate ligament.
- Volar ganglia typically originate between the tendons of the flexor carpi radialis and brachioradialis.

COMMENTS

A ganglion's synovial membrane maintains its secretory function. Aspiration of ganglia often demonstrates a viscous, mucinous, clear fluid containing albumin, globulin, and hyaluronic acid.

SUGGESTED READINGS
available at www.expertconsult.com

RELATED CONTENT

Ganglia (Patient Information)

AUTHORS: **RYAN W. ZUZEK, M.D.,** and **IMMAD SADIQ, M.D.**

BASIC INFORMATION

DEFINITION

Gardner's syndrome is a subset of familial adenomatous polyposis (FAP), with prominent extraintestinal manifestations. It is a highly penetrant autosomal-dominant condition characterized by the following:
- Adenomatous intestinal polyps
- Soft tissue tumors
- Osteomas

SYNONYMS

Familial adenomatous polyposis

ICD-9CM CODES
211.3 Familial adenomatous polyposis

EPIDEMIOLOGY & DEMOGRAPHICS

- FAP occurs in approximately 1 in 10,000 births.
- FAP accounts for <1% of all colorectal cancers.
- Individuals develop hundreds to thousands of adenomatous colorectal polyps.
- Polyps usually present in adolescence.
- 100% lifetime risk for colorectal cancer; most diagnosed by 40 yr of age.
- Gastric, duodenal, periampullary, and small bowel polyps occur but have lower malignant potential.
- Increased risk for other tumors: desmoid (15%), duodenal/periampullary (7%), thyroid (2%), brain (1%), childhood hepatoblastoma (1%), nasopharyngeal angiofibroma, pancreatic (2%), adrenal adenoma (10%), and gastric (1%).

PHYSICAL FINDINGS & CLINICAL PRESENTATION

Phenotypic variability is seen in individuals and families with the same mutation. Soft tissue and bone abnormalities may precede intestinal disease. These findings are reported in at least 20% of individuals with FAP.
- Congenital hypertrophy of the retinal pigment epithelium (CHRPE): benign fundus lesions, usually present at birth
- Dental abnormalities: supernumerary or unerupted teeth
- Soft tissue lesions: epidermal or sebaceous cysts, fibromas, lipomas, desmoid tumors (benign, locally invasive, connective tissue tumors)
- Osteomas (benign bone growths): skull, mandible, long bone
- Anemia, occult blood in stool, bowel obstruction, weight loss

ETIOLOGY

- Caused by mutations of the tumor suppressor gene adenomatous polyposis coli (APC) on chromosome 5q21-q22; more than 700 diseases causing mutations identified. The site of the mutation may explain the prominent extraintestinal lesions found in Gardner's syndrome.
- De novo mutations are responsible for approximately 20% of FAP cases. A subset of these patients have somatic cell mosaicism, which is seen when a new mutation occurs in the APC gene post-fertilization and is present in only a subset of cell types or tissues.

DIAGNOSIS

In individuals with a family history, more than 100 adenomatous colorectal polyps, CHRPE lesions, or genetic testing confirms diagnosis. In those without a family history, more than 100 adenomatous colorectal polyps suggest the diagnosis and genetic testing confirms it. Table 1-161 compares Gardner's syndrome with other polyposis syndromes.

DIFFERENTIAL DIAGNOSIS

- Turcot's syndrome
- Attenuated FAP
- MYH-associated polyposis
- Peutz-Jeghers syndrome
- Juvenile polyposis syndrome
- Hereditary mixed polyposis syndrome
- Hyperplastic polyposis

WORKUP

History, physical examination, laboratory tests, imaging studies

DIAGNOSTIC SCREENING OPTIONS

GENETIC TESTING
NOTE: Genetic counseling should be performed and written informed consent obtained before testing. Refer to a specialized center for counseling and evaluation.
- Should be offered to first-degree relatives of affected individuals (with an identified mutation) at age 10 to 12 yr and clinically suspected individuals.
- Able to identify a mutation in approximately 80% of families. To ensure that the family has a detectable mutation, test an affected family member first.
- If positive in the affected individual, the test can differentiate with 100% accuracy affected and unaffected family members. If negative in the affected individual, screening family members will not be useful in determining disease status.
- If no known family history exists, screening the clinically suspected individual is reasonable. A positive test rules in FAP but a negative test does not rule it out.
- Numerous testing techniques available; may require multiple tests to identify the mutation.

SIGMOIDOSCOPY
- Individuals with a positive genetic test: annual flexible sigmoidoscopy beginning at 10 to 12 yr of age.
- Untested at-risk family members or patients from families with an unidentified APC mutation: annual flexible sigmoidoscopy beginning at 10 to 12 yr until 25 yr of age, then decreasing frequency until age 50 yr, when age-appropriate guidelines may be followed.
- Once adenomatous polyps are detected, patients should undergo colonoscopy and evaluation for colectomy.
- Negative genetic test in patients from families with an identified mutation: average risk screening.

CHRPE: Lesions occur in up to 80% of families and are a reliable indicator of affected status in these families.

TREATMENT

- Prophylactic colectomy or proctocolectomy: timing determined by polyp number, size, and degree of dysplasia.
- Consider celecoxib therapy to reduce polyposis.
- Screening of remaining GI tract and screening for extraintestinal manifestations must continue after colectomy.
  - Annual physical examination: history, examination (including thyroid), and blood tests
  - Upper endoscopy to screen for gastric/duodenal polyps: baseline at age 20 yr (earlier if colon polyps detected) and repeated every 1 to 5 yr based on findings

TABLE 1-161 Comparison of Gardner's Syndrome with Other Polyposis Syndromes

Type	Trait	Gastric	SB	Colon	Histology	GI Malignancy	Extraintestinal
Familial polyposis	AD	<5%	<5%	100%	Adenoma	100%	—
Gardner	AD	5%	5%	100%	Adenoma	100%	Osteoma, others*
Peutz-Jeghers	AD	25%	95%	30%	Hamartoma	Rare	Perioral pigmentation
Juvenile polyposis	AD	—	—	100%	Inflammatory	?	—
Turcot	AR	—	—	100%	Adenoma	100%	Glioma
Cronkhite-Canada	NH	100%	50%	100%	Inflammatory	None	Ectodermal changes
Cowden†	AD	—	—	—	Hamartoma	None	Oral papilloma‡
Ruvalcaba-Myhre†	AD	Yes	Yes	Yes	Hamartoma	None	Macrocephaly, penile macules, mental retardation, SC lipomas

AD, Autosomal dominant; AR, autosomal recessive; GI, gastrointestinal; NH, nonhereditary; SB, small bowel; SC, subcutaneous.
*Soft tissue tumors, sarcomas, ampullary carcinoma, ovarian carcinoma.
†Extremely rare.
‡Gingival hyperplasia, breast cancer, thyroid cancer.
From Weissleder R et al: *Primer of diagnostic imaging*, ed 5, St Louis, 2011, Mosby.

- ○ Some recommend annual thyroid ultrasound
- ○ Other possible cancer sites imaged if symptoms occur or if these cancers have occurred in relatives
- Treat soft tissue lesions and osteomas for symptoms or cosmetic concerns. Treat desmoid tumors if they pose a risk to adjacent structures.

DISPOSITION

- 100% chance of colorectal cancer in untreated individuals. Many other neoplasms occur at higher rates.
- Metastatic colorectal cancer is the leading cause of death (58%), followed by desmoid tumors (11%) and duodenal/periampullary adenocarcinoma (8%).

REFERRAL

- Patients should be managed at centers with expertise in FAP, including a gastroenterologist, medical geneticist, and surgeon.

- Genetic counseling and testing sites can be found at GeneTests (www.ncbi.nlm.nih.gov/sites/GeneTests).

❗ PEARLS & CONSIDERATIONS

- Management should be individualized based on genotype, phenotype, and individual preferences.
- Sulindac (NSAID) and celecoxib (COX-2 inhibitor) cause polyp regression in individuals with FAP. Celecoxib is FDA approved for this indication. Cancer risk remains; neither replaces colon resection for cancer prevention. Small studies suggest combination therapies and dietary supplements may also be effective in reducing polyposis.
- Desmoid tumors frequently occur in the abdomen and are difficult to treat with high rates of recurrence. Growth and recurrence are stimulated by surgery.

- Screen children of affected parents (from infancy to age 10 yr) with alpha-fetoprotein level and liver ultrasound to rule out hepatoblastoma.
- Preimplantation and prenatal genetic testing is available.

SUGGESTED READINGS

available at www.expertconsult.com

RELATED CONTENT

Colorectal Cancer (Related Key Topic)

AUTHOR: **SUDEEP KAUR AULAKH, M.D.**

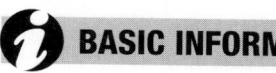

BASIC INFORMATION

DEFINITION

Gastric cancer is an adenocarcinoma arising from the stomach.

SYNONYMS

Stomach cancer
Linitis plastica

ICD-9CM CODES

451 Malignant neoplasm of stomach

EPIDEMIOLOGY & DEMOGRAPHICS

- Annual incidence of gastric cancer in the U.S. is seven cases per 100,000 persons. The incidence is much higher in Japan, with rates as high as 80 cases per 100,000 persons.
- Most gastric cancers arise in the antrum (35%).
- The incidence of distal stomach tumors has greatly declined, whereas that of proximal tumors of the cardia and fundus is on the rise.
- Gastric cancer occurs most commonly in male patients >65 yr (70% of patients are >50 yr).
- Incidence of gastric cancer has been declining over the past 30 yr.
- Male/female ratio is 3:2.
- Familiar diffuse gastric cancer is a disease with autosomal-dominant inheritance in which gastric cancer develops at a young age. Germline truncating mutations in the E-cadherin gene (CDH1) are found in these families.

PHYSICAL FINDINGS & CLINICAL PRESENTATION

- Medical history may reveal complaints of postprandial fullness with significant weight loss (70% to 80%), nausea/emesis (20% to 40%), dysphagia (20%), and dyspepsia, usually unrelieved by antacids; epigastric discomfort, usually lessened by fasting and exacerbated by food intake, is also common.
- Epigastric or abdominal mass (30% to 50%), epigastric pain.
- Skin pallor from anemia.
- Hard, nodular liver: generally indicates metastatic disease to the liver.
- Hemoccult-positive stools.
- Ascites, lymphadenopathy, or pleural effusions: may indicate metastasis.

ETIOLOGY

Risk factors:

- Chronic Helicobacter pylori gastritis. Gastric cancer develops in persons infected with H. pylori but not in uninfected persons. Those with histologic findings of severe gastric atrophy, corpus-predominant gastritis, or intestinal metaplasia are at increased risk. Persons with H. pylori infection and duodenal ulcer are not at risk, whereas those with gastric ulcers, nonulcer dyspepsia, and gastric hyperplastic polyps are. Eradication of H. pylori reduces gastric cancer risk.
- Tobacco abuse, alcohol consumption.
- Food additives (nitrosamines), smoked foods, occupational exposure to heavy metals, rubber, asbestos.
- Chronic atrophic gastritis with intestinal metaplasia, hypertrophic gastritis, and pernicious anemia.

DIAGNOSIS

DIFFERENTIAL DIAGNOSIS

- Gastric lymphoma (5% of gastric malignancies)
- Hypertrophic gastritis
- Peptic ulcer
- Reflux esophagitis

WORKUP

Upper endoscopy with biopsy will confirm diagnosis. Endoscopic ultrasonography in combination with CT scanning and operative lymph node dissection can be used in staging of the tumor. Table 1-162 describes staging systems for gastric carcinoma.

LABORATORY TESTS

- Microcytic anemia
- Hemoccult-positive stools
- Hypoalbuminemia
- Abnormal liver enzymes in patients with metastasis to the liver
- Mutation-specific predictive genetic testing by polymerase chain reaction amplification followed by restriction: enzyme digestion and DNA sequencing for truncating mutations in CDH1 is recommended in families of patients with familiar diffuse cancer because gastric cancer develops in three of every four carriers of a mutant CDH1 gene.

IMAGING STUDIES

Abdominal CT scan to evaluate for metastasis (70% accurate for regional node metastases)

TREATMENT

ACUTE GENERAL Rx

- Gastrectomy with regional lymphadenectomy is performed in patients with curative potential (<30% of patients at time of diagnosis). In patients with operable gastric cancer, a perioperative regimen of epirubicin, cisplatin, and infused fluorouracil decreases tumor size and stage and significantly improves progression-free and overall survival. Postoperative adjuvant chemoradiation therapy using 5-fluorouracil (5-FU) and leucovorin is now the standard of care for resected patients able to tolerate such treatment. Postoperative chemotherapy and radiotherapy, compared with surgical resection alone, can extend the survival rate of patients with gastric cancer in those who are able to complete adjuvant therapy.
- When surgical cure is not possible, palliative resection may prolong duration and quality of life.
- Chemotherapy (5-FU, Adriamycin, and mitomycin C) may provide some palliation; however, it generally does not prolong survival. Chemotherapy with docetaxel, cisplatin, and 5-FU can be used for chemotherapy-naive patients with metastatic or locally recurrent gastric cancer. The addition of trastuzumab to cisplatin plus 5-FU or capecitabine may prolong survival in gastric cancer patients expressing HER2.

DISPOSITION

- 5-yr survival rate of gastric carcinoma is 12% overall.
- 5-yr survival for early gastric cancers (usually detected incidentally with endoscopy in populations where screening is recommended) is >35%.

PEARLS & CONSIDERATIONS

COMMENTS

- Gastrectomy patients will need vitamin B_{12} replacement. They are also at risk for dumping syndrome and should be advised to ingest frequent, small meals.
- Prophylactic gastrectomy should be considered in young, asymptomatic carriers of germ-line truncating CDH1 mutations who belong to families with highly penetrant heredity diffuse gastric cancer.

SUGGESTED READING

available at www.expertconsult.com

RELATED CONTENT

Stomach Cancer (Patient Information)

AUTHOR: FRED F. FERRI, M.D.

TABLE 1-162   Staging Systems for Gastric Carcinoma*

Modified Astler-Coller	TNM	Characteristics
A	TisN0	Nodes negative; lesion limited to mucosa
B1	T1–2N0	Nodes negative; extension of lesion beyond mucosa but still within gastric wall
B2	T3N0	Nodes negative; extension beyond the entire wall (including serosa if present) without adherence to or invasion of surrounding organs or structures
B3	T4N0	Nodes negative; beyond wall with adherence to or invasion of surrounding organs or structures
C1	Tis–2N1–3	Nodes positive; lesion limited to wall
C2	T3N1–3	Nodes positive; extension of lesion through the entire wall (including serosa)
C3	T4N1–3	Nodes positive; beyond wall with adherence to or invasion of surrounding organs or structures

*Comparison of TNM system with a modification of the Astler-Coller rectal system by Gunderson and Sosin.
From Abeloff MD: Clinical oncology, ed 3, Philadelphia, 2004, Elsevier.

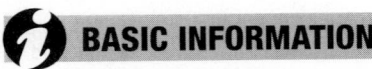

BASIC INFORMATION

DEFINITION

Histologically, *gastritis* refers to inflammation in the stomach. Endoscopically, gastritis refers to a number of abnormal features such as erythema, erosions, and subepithelial hemorrhages. Gastritis can also be subdivided into erosive, nonerosive, and specific types of gastritis with distinctive features both endoscopically and histologically.

SYNONYMS

Erosive gastritis
Hemorrhagic gastritis
Helicobacter pylori gastritis

ICD-9CM CODES
535.5 Gastritis (unless otherwise specified)
535.0 Gastritis, acute
535.3 Alcoholic gastritis
535.1 Atrophic (chronic) gastritis
535.4 Erosive gastritis
535.2 Hypertrophic gastritis

EPIDEMIOLOGY & DEMOGRAPHICS

- Erosive and hemorrhagic gastritis is most commonly seen in patients taking nonsteroidal anti-inflammatory drugs (NSAIDs), alcoholics, and critically ill patients (usually on ventilator support).
- *H. pylori* infection with gastritis is believed to be present in 30% to 50% of the population; however, the majority are asymptomatic.
- The prevalence of *H. pylori* infection increases with age from <10% in whites <40 yr to >50% in patients >50 yr.

PHYSICAL FINDINGS & CLINICAL PRESENTATION

- Patients with gastritis generally present with nonspecific clinical signs and symptoms (e.g., epigastric pain, abdominal tenderness, bloating, anorexia, nausea [with or without vomiting]). Symptoms may be aggravated by eating.
- Epigastric tenderness in acute alcoholic gastritis (may be absent in chronic gastritis).
- Foul-smelling breath.
- Hematemesis ("coffee grounds" emesis).

ETIOLOGY

- Alcohol, NSAIDs, stress (critically ill patients usually on mechanical respiration), hepatic or renal failure, multiorgan failure
- Infection (bacterial, viral)
- Bile reflux, pancreatic enzyme reflux
- Gastric mucosal atrophy, portal hypertension gastropathy
- Irradiation

DIAGNOSIS

DIFFERENTIAL DIAGNOSIS

- Peptic ulcer disease
- Gastroesophageal reflux disease
- Nonulcer dyspepsia
- Gastric lymphoma or carcinoma
- Pancreatitis
- Gastroparesis

WORKUP

Diagnostic workup includes a comprehensive history and endoscopy with biopsy.

LABORATORY TESTS

- *H. pylori* testing by urea breath test, stool antigen test (*H. pylori* stool antigen), endoscopic biopsy, or specific antibody test is recommended.
  1. The urea breath test documents active infection (sensitivity and specificity >90%). A new card test for ^{14}C urea has recently been developed, providing a testing option in primary care settings. It uses a flat breath card read by a small analyzer.
  2. The stool antigen test is an enzymatic immunoassay (ELISA) that identifies *H. pylori* antigen in a stool specimen with a polyclonal anti–*H. pylori* antibody. It is as accurate as the urea breath test for diagnosis of active infection and follow-up evaluation of patients treated for *H. pylori*. A negative result on the stool antigen test 8 wk after completion of therapy identifies patients in whom eradication of *H. pylori* was unsuccessful.
  3. Histologic evaluation of endoscopic biopsy samples is considered by many the gold standard for accurate diagnosis of *H. pylori* infection. However, detection of *H. pylori* depends on the site and number of biopsy samples, the method of staining, and experience of the pathologist.
  4. Serologic testing for antibodies to *H. pylori* is easy and inexpensive; however, the presence of antibodies demonstrates previous but not necessarily current infection. Antibodies to *H. pylori* can remain elevated for months to years after infection has cleared; therefore antibody levels must be interpreted in light of patient's symptoms and other test results (e.g., peptic ulcer disease (PUD) seen on upper gastrointestinal series).
- Vitamin B_{12} level in patients with atrophic gastritis.
- Hematocrit (low if significant bleeding has occurred).

TREATMENT

NONPHARMACOLOGIC THERAPY

- Avoidance of mucosal irritants such as alcohol and NSAIDs
- Lifestyle modifications with avoidance of tobacco and foods that trigger symptoms

ACUTE GENERAL Rx

Eradication of *H. pylori*, when present, can be accomplished with various regimens:
1. Proton pump inhibitor (PPI) bid *plus* amoxicillin 500 mg bid *plus* metronidazole 500 mg for 10 days.
2. PPI bid *plus* clarithromycin 500 mg bid *and* metronidazole 500 mg bid for 10 days. This regimen is useful in those with penicillin allergy.
3. A 1-day quadruple-therapy regimen may be as effective as a 7-day triple-therapy regimen. The 1-day quadruple-therapy regimen consists of two tablets of 262 mg bismuth subsalicylate qd, one 500-mg metronidazole tablet qd, 2 g of amoxicillin suspension qd, and two capsules of 30 mg of lansoprazole.
4. A 5-day treatment with three antibiotics (amoxicillin 1 g bid, clarithromycin 250 mg bid, and metronidazole 400 mg bid) plus either lansoprazole 30 mg bid or ranitidine 300 mg bid is an efficacious, cost-saving option for patients >55 yr with no history of PUD.
5. A combination of levofloxacin 250 mg bid, amoxicillin 1000 mg bid, and a PPI bid for 10 to 14 days can be used as salvage therapy after unsuccessful attempts to eradicate *H. pylori* using other regimens.
   - A 10-day sequential therapy has been reported to be superior to standard triple therapy for eradication of *H. pylori*. It consists of 5 days of treatment with a PPI and one antibiotic (usually amoxicillin) followed by 5-day treatment with the PPI and two other antibiotics (usually clarithromycin and metronidazole).
6. Prophylaxis and treatment of stress gastritis with sucralfate suspension 1 g orally q4-6h, H_2-receptor antagonists, or PPIs in patients on ventilator support.

CHRONIC Rx

- Omeprazole 20 mg/qd in patients receiving long-term NSAIDs
- Avoidance of alcohol, tobacco, and prolonged NSAID or corticosteroid use

DISPOSITION

- Undetectable stool antigen 4 wk after therapy accurately confirms cure of *H. pylori* infection in initially seropositive healthy subjects with reasonable sensitivity.
- Surveillance gastroscopy in patients with atrophic gastritis (increased risk of gastric cancer).

RELATED CONTENT

Gastritis (Patient Information)

AUTHOR: **FRED F. FERRI, M.D.**

BASIC INFORMATION

DEFINITION

Gastroesophageal reflux disease (GERD) is a motility disorder characterized primarily by heartburn and caused by the reflux of gastric contents into the esophagus. A current definition is a condition that develops when the reflux of stomach contents causes at least two heartburn episodes per week and/or complications.

SYNONYMS

Peptic esophagitis
Reflux esophagitis
GERD

ICD-9CM CODES
530.81 Gastroesophageal reflux disease
530.1   Esophagitis
787.1   Heartburn

EPIDEMIOLOGY & DEMOGRAPHICS

- GERD is one of the most prevalent gastrointestinal disorders. It is the most common GI diagnosis recorded during visits to outpatient clinics. From 14% to 20% of adults are affected.
- Nearly 7% of persons in the U.S. have heartburn daily, 20% have it monthly, and 60% have it intermittently. Incidence in pregnant women exceeds 80%.
- Nearly 20% of adults use antacids or over-the-counter H_2 blockers at least once a week for relief of heartburn.

PHYSICAL FINDINGS & CLINICAL PRESENTATION

- Physical examination: generally unremarkable
- Clinical signs and symptoms: heartburn, dysphagia, sour taste, regurgitation of gastric contents into the mouth

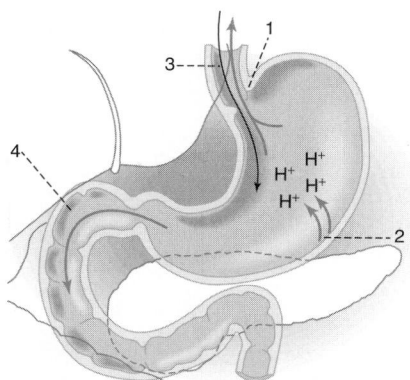

FIGURE 1-351 Pathogenesis of gastroesophageal reflux disease: *(1)* impaired lower esophageal sphincter—low pressures or frequent transient lower esophageal sphincter relaxation; *(2)* hypersecretion of acid; *(3)* decreased acid clearance resulting from impaired peristalsis or abnormal saliva production; *(4)* delayed gastric emptying or duodenogastric reflux of bile salts and pancreatic enzymes. (From Andreoli TE et al: *Andreoli and Carpenter's Cecil essentials of medicine,* ed 8, Philadelphia, 2010, Saunders.)

- Chronic cough and bronchospasm
- Chest pain, laryngitis, early satiety, abdominal fullness, and bloating with belching
- Dental erosions in children

ETIOLOGY

- Incompetent lower esophageal sphincter (LES) (see Fig. 1-351)
- Medications that lower LES pressure (calcium channel blockers, alpha-adrenergic antagonists, nitrates, theophylline, anticholinergics, sedatives, prostaglandins)
- Foods that lower LES pressure (chocolate, yellow onions, peppermint)
- Tobacco abuse, alcohol, coffee
- Pregnancy
- Gastric acid hypersecretion
- Hiatal hernia (controversial) present in >70% of patients with GERD; however, most patients with hiatal hernia are asymptomatic
- Obesity is associated with a statistically significant increase in the risk for GERD symptoms, erosive esophagitis, and esophageal carcinoma

DIAGNOSIS

DIFFERENTIAL DIAGNOSIS

- Peptic ulcer disease
- Unstable angina
- Esophagitis (from infections such as herpes, *Candida*), medication induced (doxycycline, potassium chloride)
- Esophageal spasm (nutcracker esophagus)
- Cancer of esophagus

WORKUP

- Aimed at eliminating the conditions noted in the differential diagnosis and documenting the type and extent of tissue damage. Generally, when symptoms of GERD are typical and the patient responds to therapy, there is no need for further diagnostic tests to verify the diagnosis.
- Upper GI endoscopy is useful to document the type and extent of tissue damage in persistent GERD and to exclude potentially malignant conditions such as Barrett's esophagus. The American College of Physicians recommends endoscopy in the setting of GERD in people with heartburn and alarm symptoms (dysphagia, bleeding, anemia, weight loss, and recurrent vomiting). It is also indicated in people with GERD symptoms that persist despite a therapeutic trial of 4 to 8 weeks of bid PPI therapy in patients with severe erosive esophagus after a 2-month course of PPI therapy to assess healing and rule out Barrettt's esophagus.
- Fig. E1-352 describes an approach to patients with heartburn.

LABORATORY TESTS

- 24-hr esophageal pH monitoring and Bernstein test are sensitive diagnostic tests; however, they are not practical and generally not done. They are useful in patients with atypical manifestations of GERD, such as chest pain or chronic cough.

- Esophageal manometry is indicated in patients with refractory reflux in whom surgical therapy is planned.

IMAGING STUDIES

An upper GI series is useful in patients unwilling to have endoscopy or with medical contraindications to the procedure. It can identify ulcerations and strictures; however, it may miss mucosal abnormalities. Only one third of patients with GERD have radiographic signs of esophagitis on an upper GI series.

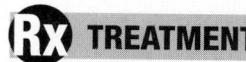 TREATMENT

NONPHARMACOLOGIC THERAPY

- Lifestyle modifications with avoidance of foods (e.g., citrus- and tomato-based products, onions, spicy foods, carbonated beverages, mint, chocolate, fried foods) and drugs that exacerbate reflux (e.g., caffeine, β-blockers, calcium channel blockers, α-adrenergic agonists, theophylline)
- Avoidance of tobacco and alcohol use
- Elevation of head of bed (4 to 8 in) with blocks
- Avoidance of lying down directly after late or large evening meals, consumption of smaller and more frequent meals
- Weight reduction to BMI <25, decreased fat intake
- Avoidance of clothing that is tight around the waist

GENERAL Rx

- Proton pump inhibitors (PPIs) (esomeprazole 40 mg qd, omeprazole 20 mg qd, lansoprazole 30 mg qd, rabeprazole 20 mg qd, or pantoprazole 40 mg qd, or dexlansoprazole 30 mg) are safe, tolerated, and highly effective in most patients (Table 1-163).
- H_2 blockers (nizatidine 300 mg qhs, famotidine 40 mg qhs, ranitidine 300 mg qhs, or cimetidine 800 mg qhs) can be used but are generally much less effective than PPIs.
- Antacids (may be useful for relief of mild symptoms; however, they are generally ineffective in severe cases of reflux).
- Prokinetic agents (metoclopramide) are indicated only when PPIs are not fully effective. They can be used in combination therapy; however, side effects limit their use.
- For refractory cases: surgery with Nissen fundoplication. Potential surgical candidates should have reflux esophagitis documented by esophagogastroduodenoscopy and normal esophageal motility as evaluated by manometry. Surgery generally consists of reduction of hiatal hernia when present and placement of a gastric wrap around the gastroesophageal (GE) junction (fundoplication). Although laparoscopic fundoplication is now widely used, long-term medical therapy is a better choice for most patients who are willing to remain on daily acid-reduction medication. In patients preferring surgical intervention, surgery should not be advised with the expectation that patients with GERD will no longer

need to take antisecretory medications or that the procedure will prevent esophageal cancer among those with GERD and Barrett's esophagus.

- Endoscopic radiofrequency heating of the GE junction (Stretta procedure) is a newer treatment modality for GERD patients unresponsive to traditional therapy. Its mechanism of action remains unclear. Endoscopy gastroplasty (EndoCinch procedure) is also aimed at treating GERD. Initial results appear encouraging; however, long-term studies are needed before recommending these procedures.
- Lifestyle modification must be followed for life because this is generally an irreversible condition.

DISPOSITION

- Recurrence of reflux is common if treatment is discontinued.
- The majority of patients respond well to therapy. In patients with chronic GERD, long-term outcomes are similar between medical therapy with PPIs and anti-reflux surgery. Prolonged use of PPIs is associated with increased risk of fractures of hip, wrist, and spine; increased risk of diarrhea from *Clostridium difficile;* pneumonia; and possible iron deficiency from impaired iron absorption. PPIs also block the effects of clopidogrel by inhibiting cytochrome P450 2C19 isozyme. Therefore all PPIs (other than pantoprazole) should be avoided in patients using clopidogrel. H_2 blockers (e.g., ranitidine) can be used for patients with GERD taking clopidogrel.
- Postsurgical complications occur in nearly 20% of patients (dysphagia, gas, bloating, diarrhea, nausea). Long-term follow-up studies also reveal that within 3 to 5 yr, 52% of patients who had undergone antireflux surgery are taking antireflux medications again.

REFERRAL

- There is a strong and probably causal relation between symptomatic prolonged and untreated GERD, Barrett's esophagus, and esophageal adenocarcinoma. GI referral for upper endoscopy is needed when there are concerns about associated peptic ulcer disease, Barrett's esophagus, or esophageal cancer.

- Patients with Barrett's esophagus should undergo surveillance endoscopy with mucosal biopsy every 2 yr or less because the risk of developing adenocarcinoma of esophagus is at least 30 times greater than that of the general population.
- Testing and treating for *Helicobacter pylori* in patients with GERD has not been shown to improve symptoms.
- All children with dental erosions should be evaluated for GERD.

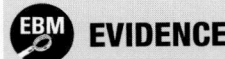

EVIDENCE

available at www.expertconsult.com

SUGGESTED READINGS

available at www.expertconsult.com

RELATED CONTENT

Gastroesophageal Reflux Disease (GERD) (Patient Information)

AUTHOR: **FRED F. FERRI, M.D.**

TABLE 1-163 Drug Therapy for Esophageal Disorders

Agent	Dose
Antacids: Liquid (to Buffer Acid and Increase LESP)	
For example, Mylanta II/Maalox TC (acid-neutralizing capacity, 25 mEq/5 ml)*	15 ml qid 1 hr after meals and at bedtime or as needed
Gaviscon (to Decrease Reflux via a Viscous Mechanical Barrier and Buffer Acid)	
$Al(OH)_3$, $NaHCO_3$, Mg trisilicate, alginic acid	2-4 tablets qid at bedtime or as needed
H_2-Receptor Antagonists (to Decrease Acid Secretion)	
Cimetidine	800 mg bid, 400 mg qid, ≈13 ml bid
Ranitidine	150 mg qid or 10 ml qid; maintenance dose, 150 mg bid, 10 ml bid
Famotidine	20-40 mg bid or 2.5-5 ml bid
Nizatidine	150 mg bid
Proton Pump Inhibitors (to Decrease Acid Secretion and Gastric Volume)†	
Omeprazole	20 mg/day; maintenance dose, 20 mg/day
Lansoprazole	30 mg/day; maintenance dose, 15 mg/day
Pantoprazole	40 mg/day; maintenance dose, 40 mg/day
Rabeprazole	20 mg/day; maintenance dose, 20 mg/day
Esomeprazole	20-40 mg/day; maintenance dose, 20 mg/day
Dexlansoprazole	30-60 mg/day; maintenance dose, 30 mg/day

LESP, Lower esophageal sphinter pressure.

*Patients with reflux are not generally hypersecretors of gastric acid, so the therapeutic doses of antacids are based on their capacity to buffer (normal) basal acid secretion rates of approximately 1 to 7 mEq/hr (mean, 2 mEq/hr) and peak meal-stimulated acid secretion rates of about 10 to 60 mEq/hr (mean, 30 mEq/hr).

†High-dose therapy is a twice-daily administration of the usual daily dose.

From Goldman L, Schafer AI: *Goldman's Cecil medicine,* ed 24, Philadelphia, 2012, Saunders.

BASIC INFORMATION

DEFINITION

Gender dysphoria disorder is a chronic condition resulting when a person's natal or biologic gender (chromosomes, hormones, organs, and secondary sexual characteristics) are incongruent with a person's perceived and asserted core gender identity (innate sense of being male or female). Gender dysphoria implies more than a disconnect or incongruency with physical gender, but a notable discomfort and dislike of one's biologic gender and a desire to be physically different than the gender born into or assigned at birth. Traditional descriptors include transgender or transsexual, male-to-female or female-to-male transgender, or gender queer persons.

Historically, gender and sexuality have been evolving concepts within the psychiatric field. Although discomfort and dislike of one's biologic and anatomic gender and secondary sexual characteristics are a major component of gender dysphoria disorder, newer paradigms embrace a range of gender identity and expression not limited to dysphoria or psychopathology, including gender variance or incongruency, gender nonconformity, transgender, or gender queer. Newer paradigms do not limit gender to a binary or dichotomous place, but contain some potential for movement and fluidity along a spectrum.

SYNONYMS

Gender identity disorder
Gender dysphoria in children, adolescents, adults
Unspecified gender dysphoria
Transgender or transsexual

EPIDEMIOLOGY & DEMOGRAPHICS

DEVELOPMENT & BACKGROUND: Gender development begins as early as 18 months. By age 2 to 4 yr, children understand gender differences and use pronouns such as "him" and "her." Toddlers identify their own gender, and most consider gender a stable personal trait at age 5-6 yr. All children explore and play with gender activities, behaviors, and roles of the opposite gender (called gender play). This stage can last from days to years and does not mean a child is dysphoric or dislikes his or her gender. Many children adopt opposite gender attributes and activities and not want to change to the other gender.

PREDOMINANT AGE

- Gender nonconformity in prepubertal years is more than play; nonconforming prepubertal children exhibit consistent, persistent, and insistent play, dress, attributes, and activities of the other gender. Some of these children, but not all, experience dysphoria and mild to intense discomfort and dislike of their biologic gender. Males with this experience outnumber females by 3:1.
- With puberty, both gender (who you are) and sexuality (attraction, orientation, behaviors,

sexual partner preference) become core developmental tasks of adolescence. At this age, male to female ratio becomes 1:1.
- Incidence may be heavily associated with cultural expectations. It is generally less acceptable to be a feminized boy than a prepubertal girl who is a "tomboy." A peripubertal spike in gender dysphoria also occurs as pubertal females lose their androgenous appearance and begin menses.

PREVALENCE: Overall estimates are between 1 in 10,000 to 1 in 100,000 depending on the study and source. Most believe these numbers vastly underestimate prevalence because they originate from adult surgical or gender specialty clinics.

GENETICS: Although data are emerging about sex hormones, the brain, gender identity, and expression, there is no known single or specific genetic basis for gender dysphoria. The disorder has no specific relationships or associations with parent characteristics, socioeconomic status, or race/ethnicity. There may be a link between autism spectrum disorders and gender nonconformity.

RISK FACTORS: There are no proven risk factors for developing gender dysphoria. However, gender nonconformity may be linked to child abuse, bullying, mental health concerns (e.g., anxiety, depression, suicidality), and substance use. Transgender adult populations have poorer health outcomes, such as depression, anxiety, self-harm and suicide, substance use, underemployment, homelessness, incarceration, and positive HIV status. Poorer health outcomes are explained by using minority stress theory (chronic stress related to stigma and dysphoria) rather than gender variance as a pathology itself.

PHYSICAL FINDINGS & CLINICAL PRESENTATION

Prepubertal children present with consistent, persistent, and insistent interest and expression of other or opposite-gendered activities and behaviors. Boys may be considered more feminine than their same-age peers; they may prefer to wear long hair, nail polish, makeup, girls' jewelry, and clothing. Girls may be considered "tomboys" and reject wearing dresses and skirts, prefer short hair, wear boys' clothing, and participate in traditionally masculine play and activities. During the school-age years, children become sensitive to social expectations and norms. Many gender dysphoric children who do conform in their gender play and expression, however, still experience underlying problems with biology and identity.

Adolescents and adults may present in their natal gender expression as androgenous or as the opposite gender. Many gender dysphoric persons will not present directly with gender dysphoria but present with mood, behavior, or social problems. For many persons, gender dysphoria or the disclosure of gender nonconformity is first elicited as a result of mental health counseling.

For some persons, especially children, social media has provided the initial construct and

terminology to understand and then verbalize their feelings. For many adult persons, disclosing or "coming out" socially as transgender is a deeply personal decision and experience that can have an enormous impact on family, social, and economic relationships.

DIAGNOSIS

- Gender dysphoria is an element of gender identity disorder in the DSM IV. Core components are longstanding discomfort with assigned gender; interference with activities of daily living; and no other illness, physical or psychiatric, that would confuse diagnosis. Future changes in DSM diagnostics are likely. Many argue that focusing on physical or endocrine disorders would be more appropriate and less stigmatizing and allow for improved access to hormonal and surgical therapies.
- Psychiatric evaluations are no longer considered necessary or essential to "diagnose" gender nonconforming persons. Persons may assert a nonconformity identity without severe self-hatred or significant dysphoric presentation. However, persons with severe dysphoria and sequelae from the mismatch in biology with identity usually benefit from participating in therapy, building skills to create successful transition plans, and/or obtaining treatment for comorbid psychiatric concerns. Persons with significant and active psychosis should be evaluated to determine whether gender issues are separate or integrated within the psychotic experience.

WORKUP

- Clinical interview includes assessment of gender experience from childhood until present; desired name, pronoun, and past and current place on the gender spectrum; past and current attempts to feminize or masculinize with clothing, hair, makeup, hormones, and surgeries; future goals of transitioning, gender identity, and expression.
- Review for known comorbidities by asking mental health–specific questions about depression, anxiety, self-harm (cutting and suicidal ideation), psychiatric hospitalization, substance use; sexual attraction and behaviors regarding partners, detailed sexual activities, and risk for sexually transmitted infections and pregnancy; social history, experience of bullying, hate crimes, physical or emotional/verbal abuse, homelessness, joblessness, survival sex, and identified social support systems.
- Ideally, this interview is in the context of interviewing the individual as a person and as a holistic health assessment. Persons with experience in behavioral health and gender issues can perform these interviews. Some patients may benefit from therapy or psychiatric evaluation if they have additional mental health concerns, need support to plan transitioning, and would benefit from self-esteem, social skills, and other protective skill building.
- An initial visit may include a physical examination depending on the patient's goals.

Many gender dysphoric persons are exquisitely uncomfortable with their genitalia and genital examination. This can often be deferred until the patient is more comfortable and familiar with the provider.

- A general physical examination may be performed, but detailed examination of secondary sexual characteristics (breasts, vulva, penis, testicles) often is deferred. Tanner staging genitalia for peripubertal youth interested in puberty "blockers" or cross-gender hormones is important.
- Laboratory studies may include luteinizing hormone, follicle stimulating hormone, testosterone, or estradiol for peripubertal children wanting to start puberty blockers or gonadotropin-releasing hormone (GnRH) analogues. For youth or adults starting GnRH analogues or cross-gender hormones, baseline laboratory values include CBC, liver panel, liver function tests, and testosterone (or estrogen). Screening for sexually transmitted infections (urine, rectal, and oral *Chlamydia* and gonorrhea; syphilis; herpes simplex virus; HIV; hepatitis B and C), and pregnancy is indicated according to sexual practices. Additional preventive care screening and testing may be deferred. Patients should receive typical preventive and screening tests for both biologic gender and asserted gender.
- Ancillary testing may include various psychiatric screening and diagnostic tools for comorbid depression, anxiety, suicidality, substance use, and interpersonal violence.

Rx TREATMENT

Treatment is determined by patient age and development (including Tanner stage) and desired place on the gender spectrum. Moving from biologic gender to asserted gender identity is known as transition. Transition is typically divided into three stages: reversible, partially reversible, and irreversible.

REVERSIBLE TRANSITION

- Taking on clothes, hair, makeup, name, and pronoun of the identified gender. For prepubertal, androgenous children, "social transition" does not require hormones but does require extensive planning for disclosure, social support, and peer- and school-based activities.
- Puberty blockers or GnRH antagonists are reversible and best when used at very early Tanner stage II breast and testicular development. When used in early puberty, blockers stop puberty with regression to prepubertal hormones and secondary sexual characteristics. This often "buys time" for both a child and a family to determine a safe and supportive social transition plan.
- Puberty blockers can be used for patients who are at Tanner stage III or IV according to genital exam but are still androgenous in regards to other secondary sex characteristics, such as voice, facial and body hair, bone, muscle, and fat deposition. Blockers can also

be used to stop penile function or menses, which can be highly distressing to gender dysphoric persons.

- Blockers are completely reversible. If stopped, a person can continue into biologic puberty. Most teens who opt to start blockers continue to create a transition plan and eventually move to cross-gender hormones and puberty in their asserted gender.

PARTIALLY REVERSIBLE TRANSITION

- Cross-gender hormone therapies include testosterone for masculinization and estradiol for feminization. These have many reversible effects on skin changes, fat deposition, and muscle mass. Irreversible effects may include masculine voice changes, areola enlargement with darkening, and clitoromegaly.
- Estradiol creates softer skin, female body fat deposition (hips/thighs), and breast development. It may impair erectile function, which may or may not be desired because some male-to-female persons still want or depend on penile function for both pleasure and/or for sex work. Estradiol is typically administered sublingually but can be taken orally, intramuscularly, or topically. Topical medicines run the risk of undesired feminization (or masculinization) of sex partners or others in close physical contact.
- Testosterone masculinizes by inducing male hair patterns, deepening the voice, and inducing male-pattern fat and muscle deposition (bulk and abdominal girth) and clitoromegaly. It can lead to vaginal atrophy, resulting in dyspareunia for transgender female-to-male persons who use the vagina for sex. Testosterone comes in a variety of vehicles, including subcutaneous, intramuscular, and topical. Testosterone is teratogenic in pregnancy. Both sex hormones should not be used in lieu of contraception, and future fertility cannot be guaranteed. Persons taking testosterone who are having unprotected penile vaginal sex should be counseled and offered birth control in addition to testosterone.
- Consent to what we know and do not know is an important part of beginning the cross-gender hormone process. Current evidence suggests that estrogen or testosterone are not sufficient to act as contraceptives, nor is future fertility guaranteed, for persons who prioritize having biologic children. For male-to-female persons, sperm banking offers future options for biologic children, although at some expense. For female-to-male persons, oocyte banking is extremely expensive and has not yet demonstrated reliable successful outcomes. For many transgender persons, transition to their asserted identity is more important than creating or carrying genetic children. Many transgender persons would prefer to parent or adopt in their identified or asserted gender.

IRREVERSIBLE TRANSITION

Includes mostly surgical options for masculinization (mastectomy, hystero-oophorectomy, and orchi-peniplasty) or feminization (orchiectomy-penectomy with vulvar reconstruction, breast implants, and other cosmetic surgeries). Many

patients opt for partial surgical transition due to expense (surgeries are currently not covered under most insurance plans, or patients are underinsured or uninsured) or function (penile implants are typically not sexually functional). Most common partial surgical options are mastectomy for female-to-male and breast implants for male-to-female. It is important to ask specific goals for surgery because they vary by individual patient.

ADDITIONAL THERAPIES

Anti-androgens such as spironolactone to prevent male-pattern hair growth and vocal coaching for male-to-female. Individual, family, and marital counseling and therapies can be important for dysphoric individuals with comorbid mental health issues. Reparative therapy is *universally* rejected as unethical and harmful by all the national medical and psychological boards and associations. Medications for anxiety, depression, and other mental health concerns may facilitate self-esteem, mood, cognitive function, and social skills building as persons and families negotiate the process of transition. Social support and activity groups may help gender nonconforming persons find community, feel and become less isolated, and improve transition experiences. Support is important to family members who are involved in a patient's transition.

DISPOSITION

- Gender is a physical, emotional, social, and cultural construct across the lifespan that every person experiences. For a gender dysphoric patient or gender nonconforming person, this incongruency may have lifelong implications for physical, emotional, and social well-being.
- Younger patients who begin hormone blockers, are transitioned early both socially and hormonally, and experience puberty in their identified gender may have improved ability to be accepted in their asserted gender, decreased suicidality, and less risk of nonmedical use of street hormones and drugs.
- In addition, evidence suggests that sexual minorities who have early and consistent parental support, despite being gender and sexually nonconforming, have decreased rates of suicide and substance use.
- For persons experiencing some or all of puberty in their biologic but not identified gender, cross-gender hormones and/or gender-affirming surgeries offer the promise of living in their asserted gender. For persons who transition later in life, especially in their 30s and older, physical transition and "passing" are more difficult.
- In addition to minority stress and poorer mental health outcomes, being a visual and visible sexual minority has significant and demonstrated social risks for victimization from hate crimes and interpersonal violence, low socioeconomic status, underemployment, and isolation. Early identification and early transition in a person's identified gender, along with a better likelihood of acceptance, may offer

significant psychosocial benefits to many gender dysphoric persons.
- Regardless of timing of transition, safety is a priority in transition planning and important to consider along the lifespan.

REFERRALS

- Providers who are not comfortable with gender or behavioral assessments may want to refer to medical providers with experience and expertise in gender issues and care. This group may include pediatric, family medicine, medicine-pediatrics, and psychiatry providers. Similarly, there are therapists and social workers with expertise in gender dysphoria assessment and management.

- There are few contraindications to transitioning for most gender dysphoric persons. Active psychosis and inability to consent to care would require further psychiatric evaluation but are extremely rare. For older persons, some medical issues involving cardiac, liver, and thromboembolic risks complicate hormone use and need to be taken into consideration.

PEARLS & CONSIDERATIONS

- Periodic assessment of a person's place on the gender spectrum can begin in toddler age children and can continue into adulthood as a potentially effective way of helping identify and support gender dysphoric persons early.
- Early identification and parental support for gender dysphoric and nonconforming persons may lead to improved mental and physical health outcomes.
- Hormone blockers and cross-gender hormones typically offer far more benefit than risk in the treatment of gender dysphoria when a person desires to transition to the opposite gender.

AUTHOR: **MICHELE FORCIER, M.D., M.P.H.**

G

Diseases
and Disorders

I

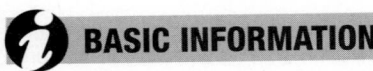

BASIC INFORMATION

DEFINITION

- Glucose intolerance that begins, or is first recognized, during pregnancy. Women are first screened with a 1-hr, nonfasting glucose tolerance test. If the result is >130 mg/dl, a 3-hr glucose tolerance test is ordered. The diagnosis is made if two or more of the glucose values are met or exceeded:
  Fasting: 95 mg/dl
  1-hr: 180 mg/dl
  2-hr: 155 mg/dl
  3-hr: 140 mg/dl
- Pregnant women with diabetes mellitus (DM) (gestational or preexisting) are classified according to White's classification (Table 1-164).
- The International Association of Diabetes in Pregnancy Study Group has recommended a simplified "one-step" approach to screening and diagnosing gestational DM (GDM). It involves a 75-g, 2-hr oral glucose tolerance test. A diagnosis of GDM is made if any of the following levels of plasma glucose are exceeded: ≥92 mg/dl when fasting, ≥180 mg/dl at 1 hr, or ≥153 mg/dl at 2 hr.

SYNONYMS

Gestational diabetes
Sugar of pregnancy
Diet-controlled gestational diabetes (A1)
Insulin-treated gestational diabetes (A2)

ICD-9CM CODES
648.8; if using insulin to treat, add V58.67

EPIDEMIOLOGY & DEMOGRAPHICS

INCIDENCE: Approximately 7% of all pregnancies (may range from 1% to 14% in the U.S. depending on the population studied and the diagnostic tests used)
PREDOMINANT SEX AND AGE: Women of childbearing age
GENETICS: Higher rate in women with family history of GDM or type 2 diabetes; specific HLA alleles (DR3 or DR4) predispose to the development of DM type 1 after delivery

RISK FACTORS

- Obesity
- Family history of GDM or type 2 diabetes
- Glycosuria at first prenatal visit
- Polycystic ovarian syndrome
- Twin gestation
- Hypertension
- Chronic systemic steroid use
- Maternal birth weight >9 lb or <6 lb
- Age >25 y
- Previous infant weighing >9 lb or with shoulder dystocia
- Unexplained perinatal loss or malformation
- Personal history of abnormal glucose tolerance or GDM
- Latin American, Native American, African American, or Asian ethnicity

POTENTIAL RISK FACTORS

- Mixing or applying agricultural pesticides in the first trimester
- Limited physical activity the year before pregnancy
- Prepregnancy diet low in fiber and high in glycemic load

PHYSICAL FINDINGS & CLINICAL PRESENTATION

Suspect GDM if:
- Fetal size greater than dates
- Macrosomia on ultrasound
- Marked maternal obesity or weight gain

ETIOLOGY

- During normal pregnancy there is increased insulin resistance because of placental secretion of diabetogenic hormones in the late second and third trimesters. Pancreatic beta-cell secretion increases to compensate for the increased insulin resistance. GDM occurs when this need cannot be met.
- Insulin resistance is also exacerbated by an increase in maternal adipose deposition, decreased exercise, and increased caloric intake.

DIAGNOSIS

DIFFERENTIAL DIAGNOSIS

Preexisting type 1 or 2 DM not previously diagnosed

WORKUP

- History with focus on personal medical history, prior pregnancy history, and family history
- Routine prenatal examination
- Laboratory evaluation

LABORATORY TESTS

- Screening with 1-hr glucose tolerance test (Nonfasting; 50-g oral glucose load)
  - For screening without risk factors, order at 24 to 28 wk
  - For screening with risk factors, order at first prenatal visit, then repeat at 24 to 28 wk if initial screen was normal. If abnormal at intake, consider possibility of undiagnosed preexisting DM and check hemoglobin A1c.
- If 1-hr test result is abnormal (>130 mg/dl), order 3-hr glucose tolerance test
  - Performed after 3 days of unrestricted diet (carbohydrate load is probably not necessary)
  - Fasting
  - 100-g oral glucose load
- If one fourth of values on 3-hr glucose tolerance test is abnormal, repeat in 1 month and consider beginning a diabetic diet
- The U.S. Preventive Services Task Force (USPSTF) concludes that the evidence is insufficient to recommend for or against routine screening for gestational diabetes. The current evidence is insufficient to assess the balance between the benefits and harms of screening women for GDM either before or after 24 weeks' gestation. Harms of screening include short-term anxiety in some women with positive screening results and inconvenience to many women and medical practices because most positive screening tests are likely false-positives. Until there is better evidence, clinicians should discuss screening for GDM with their patients and make case-by-case decisions. The discussion should include information about the uncertain benefits and harms as well as the frequency and uncertain meaning of a positive screening test result.

IMAGING STUDIES

Ultrasound for fetal size at least once at 36 to 37 wk; more frequently if macrosomia suspected

TREATMENT

NONPHARMACOLOGIC THERAPY

- Glucose monitoring:
  - Four times daily: fasting and 2-hr postprandial
  - Goals: fasting ≤95 mg/dl; 2-hr postprandial ≤120 mg/dl
  - Can also use 1-hr postprandial goal of <140 mg/dl
- Dietary modifications aimed at glycemic control:
  - Follow a low-fat, high-fiber diet; avoid sugar and concentrated sweets; and eat small, frequent meals.

TABLE 1-164 White's Classification for Pregnant Women with Diabetes (Gestational or Preexisting)

Class	Description
A1	DM diagnosed during pregnancy and controlled by diet
A2	DM diagnosed during pregnancy and requiring medication
B	Insulin-requiring DM diagnosed before pregnancy, age >20 yr, lasting <10 yr
C	Insulin-requiring DM, onset at age 10 to 19 yr, with a duration 10 to 19 yr
D	Onset >10 yr or duration >20 yr, or associated with hypertension or background retinopathy
F	DM with renal disease
H	DM with coronary artery disease
R	DM with proliferative retinopathy
T	DM with renal transplant

DM, Diabetes mellitus.

- Nutrition counseling for diet that adequately meets the needs of pregnancy but restricts carbohydrates to 35% to 40% of daily calories.
- For women with a body mass index >30, restrict calories to 25 kcal/kg actual weight per day.
- Regular moderate exercise

PHARMACOLOGIC Rx

Begin if >20% of glucose values are elevated after trial of diet control:
- Oral hypoglycemics:
  - Glyburide: begin at 2.5 mg qd and titrate up to a maximum of 20 mg qd (10 mg bid). Increase dose as needed by 2.5 to 5 mg/wk.
  - Metformin use in pregnancy remains controversial because it crosses the placenta.
- Insulin:
  1. One commonly used regimen:
     - Insulin 0.7 U/kg/day SQ, with two thirds of the total daily dose given in the morning and one third of the total daily dose given in the evening
     - One third of each dose is given as short-acting insulin and the remaining two thirds as NPH insulin
  2. Another option:
     - If fasting values are elevated, use NPH at bedtime with initial dose of 0.2 U/kg
     - If postprandial values are elevated, use rapid-acting insulin before meals with initial dose 1.5 U/10 g carbohydrate at breakfast and 1 U/10 g carbohydrate at lunch and dinner
  3. Long-acting insulin such as Lantus does not have sufficient data to determine whether it crosses the placenta; it may be continued in persons with preexisting diabetes who are well controlled but is not recommended in patients with newly diagnosed GDM
  4. Glyburide and insulin have overall similar rates of clinical effectiveness and fetal safety

ANTENATAL TESTING

Routine blood pressure and urine protein monitoring:
- Class A1: NST/AFI at 40 wk
- Class A2: weekly NST/AFI beginning at 32 wk or when insulin is started
- Poorly controlled diabetes, vascular complications, or hypertension: biweekly NST/AFI beginning at 28 wk and consider admission for initial glycemic control

TIMING AND ROUTE OF DELIVERY

- Class A1 (well controlled): deliver by 41 wk
- Class A2: deliver by 40 wk
- Offer elective cesarean section at 38 wk if estimated fetal weight >4500 g
- Consider delivery by 37 wk if poor control or intrauterine growth retardation after confirmed fetal lung maturity by amniocentesis

INTRAPARTUM MANAGEMENT

- Goal is normoglycemia (80 to 110 mg/dl) using insulin and D5 lactated Ringer's IV fluid
- Monitor glucose hourly
- Preparation for shoulder dystocia
- If on glyburide, discontinue in labor or 12 hr before a scheduled induction

NEONATAL MANAGEMENT

- Check 30- and 60-min glucose
- Watch for signs of hypoglycemia, hypocalcemia, hyperbilirubinemia, and polycythemia

POSTPARTUM MANAGEMENT

- Class A2: check fasting level before discharge; if abnormal, continue checking at home and early follow-up with primary care physician to confirm diagnosis of DM
- 6-wk postpartum visit: screen for diabetes with 2-hr glucose tolerance test or two fasting values
- If no evidence of DM, screen annually for DM and counsel on risk factor modification

REFERRAL

- Nutritionist
- High-risk obstetrician
- Maternal-fetal medicine
- Diabetes educator

COMPLICATIONS

- Maternal: preeclampsia, future type 2 DM or GDM, operative delivery
- Fetal: polyhydramnios, macrosomia, shoulder dystocia, birth trauma, congenital malformations
- Neonatal: hypoglycemia, hypocalcemia, hyperbilirubinemia, polycythemia, perinatal death, future obesity and DM, impaired fine and gross motor functions; increased rates of inattention and hyperactivity

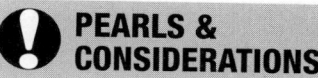

PEARLS & CONSIDERATIONS

Trials have shown that although treatment of mild gestational DM did not significantly reduce the frequency of a composite outcome that included stillbirth or perinatal death and several neonatal complications, it did reduce the risks of fetal overgrowth, shoulder dystocia, cesarean delivery, and hypertensive disorders.

PREVENTION

Regular exercise, maintenance of ideal body weight, and high-fiber low-glycemic diet

PATIENT & FAMILY EDUCATION

Gestational Diabetes Patient Information
American Academy of Family Physicians
http://www.aafp.org/afp/20031101/1775ph.html

American Dietetic Association
Consumer Nutrition Information and Referrals
http://www.eatright.org
Telephone: 800-366-1655

American Diabetes Association: Gestational Diabetes
http://www.diabetes.org
800-DIABETES (800-342-2383)

NOAH: New York Online Access to Health
http://www.noah-health.org

National Institute of Child Health and Human Development
Managing Gestational Diabetes: A Patient's Guide to a Healthy Pregnancy
http://www.nichd.nih.gov/publications/pubs/gest_diabetes/
800-370-2943

Food and Nutrition Information Center
Food Guide Pyramid
http://www.nal.usda.gov.

SUGGESTED READINGS

available at www.expertconsult.com

RELATED CONTENT

Gestational Diabetes (Patient Information)
Diabetes Mellitus (Related Key Topic)

AUTHORS: **JORDAN WHITE, M.D.,**
NIRALI BORA, M.D.,
HEIDI H. PETERSON, M.D., and
SUSANNA R. MAGEE, M.D., M.P.H.

G

Diseases
and Disorders

I

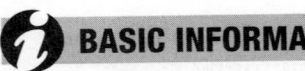

BASIC INFORMATION

DEFINITION

Giant cell arteritis (GCA) is a segmental systemic granulomatous arteritis affecting medium and large arteries in individuals >50 yr. Peak incidence is in patients aged 60 to 80 yr. Inflammation primarily targets extracranial blood vessels, and although the carotid system is usually affected, pathology in the posterior cerebral artery has been reported.

SYNONYMS

Temporal arteritis
Cranial arteritis
GCA
Horton's disease

ICD-9CM CODES

446.5 Temporal arteritis

EPIDEMIOLOGY & DEMOGRAPHICS

INCIDENCE: 17 to 23.3 new cases per 100,000 persons >50 yr
PREVALENCE: 200 cases per 100,000 persons; female/male predominance of twofold to fourfold; more common in Caucasians

PHYSICAL FINDINGS & CLINICAL PRESENTATION

GCA can present with the following clinical manifestations:
- Headache, often associated with marked scalp tenderness—noticed while brushing hair (hair comb allodynia)
- Constitutional symptoms (fever, weight loss, anorexia, fatigue)

TABLE 1-165 Atypical Manifestations of Giant Cell Arteritis

Fever of unknown origin
Respiratory symptoms (especially cough)
Otolaryngeal manifestations
  Glossitis
  Lingual infarction
  Throat pain
  Hearing loss
Large-artery disease
  Aortic aneurysm
  Aortic dissection
  Limb claudication
  Raynaud's phenomenon
Neurologic manifestations
  Peripheral neuropathy
  Transient ischemic attack (TIA) or stroke
  Dementia
  Delerium
Myocardial infarction
Tumorlike lesions
  Breast mass
  Ovarian and uterine mass
Syndrome of inappropriate antidiuretic hormone
  secretion (SIADH)
Microangiopathic hemolytic anemia

From Harris ED et al: *Kelly's textbook of rheumatology*, ed 7, Philadelphia, 2005, Saunders.

- Polymyalgia rheumatica (aching and stiffness of the trunk and proximal muscle groups)
- Visual disturbances (transient or permanent monocular or binocular visual loss)
- Intermittent claudication of jaw and tongue on mastication
- Table 1-165 describes atypical manifestations of GCA.

Important physical findings in GCA:
- Vascular examination: The temporal artery demonstrates tenderness, decreased pulsation, and nodulation (ropy) (Fig. 1-353); diminished or absent pulses in upper extremities may be seen

ETIOLOGY

Vasculitis of unknown etiology

DIAGNOSIS

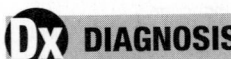

Clinical history and vascular examination remain cornerstones of diagnosis. The American College of Rheumatology has proposed the following criteria for the diagnosis of GCA. Presence of three or more of these criteria in a patient with suspected vasculitis is considered to be diagnostic for GCA.
- Age of onset of symptoms >50 yr
- New-onset of or new type of localized headache
- Temporal artery abnormalities including tenderness or decreased pulsation
- Westergren erythrocyte sedimentation rate (ESR) elevated (typically >50 mm/hr)
- Temporal artery biopsy with vasculitis and mononuclear cell infiltrate or granulomatous changes

DIFFERENTIAL DIAGNOSIS

- Other vasculitic syndromes
- Nonarteritic anterior ischemic optic neuropathy (AION)
- Primary amyloidosis
- Transient ischemic attack, stroke
- Infections
- Occult neoplasm, multiple myeloma

LABORATORY TESTS

- ESR elevated although up to 22.5% of patients with GCA have normal ESR before treatment.
- C-reactive protein is typically included in laboratory investigation; it may have greater sensitivity than ESR.
- Mild to moderate normochromic normocytic anemia, elevated platelet count.

IMAGING STUDIES

- Color duplex ultrasonography of temporal artery produces three characteristic features—periluminal "halo" over the temporal artery involved, segmental arterial stenosis, and arterial luminal occlusion in severe cases. Clinical utility is not felt to be superior to clinical examination with biopsy.
- Contrasted MRI of temporal artery may be performed in patients with contraindications to surgical biopsy of the superficial temporal artery, although the clinical utility remains limited once treatment is started.

TREATMENT

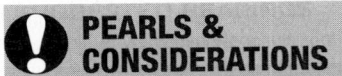

ACUTE GENERAL Rx

- If there is clinical suspicion of GCA, treatment should be initiated without waiting for results of laboratory or imaging studies.
- IV methylprednisolone (250 to 1000 mg qd for 3 to 5 days) is indicated in patients with severe clinical manifestations such as visual loss from ischemic optic neuropathy. IV steroids may have additional benefits over oral steroids in the acute phase.
- Oral prednisone (1 mg/kg/day). High-dose oral regimen should be continued at least until symptoms resolve and ESR returns to normal. Prednisone treatment may last up to 2 yr and is tapered over several weeks to months.
- Corticosteroids are the treatment of choice. There is no evidence for the role of steroid-sparing agents. Methotrexate may be considered as an adjunct treatment.

DISPOSITION

With steroid therapy there is a dramatic improvement of systemic symptoms but not vision in patients with ischemic optic neuropathy. In one study only 4% of eyes improved in both visual acuity and central visual field.

REFERRAL

- Surgical referral for biopsy of temporal artery
- Ophthalmology referral in patients with visual disturbances and after initiation of corticosteroid therapy
- Rheumatology referral for long-term immunosuppressive treatment management

PEARLS & CONSIDERATIONS

- Treatment of GCA should be started if there is clinical suspicion of the disease.
- Temporal artery biopsy should be performed as soon as possible but within 2 weeks of initiating treatment with steroids.
- Treatment should not be withheld pending temporal artery biopsy.

COMMENTS

- The relation between polymyalgia rheumatica and GCA is unclear, but the two frequently coexist. They are considered to be different points along the gradient or spectrum of the same disease.
- Clinical picture rather than ESR should be the prime yardstick for continuing prednisone therapy. A rising ESR in a clinically asymptomatic patient with normal hematocrit should raise suspicion for alternate explanations (e.g., infections, neoplasms).
- GCA is associated with a markedly increased risk for the development of aortic aneurysm, which is often a late complication and may cause death. Annual chest radiograph in chronic CGA patients has been suggested, as well as emergent chest CT or MRI for clinical suspicion—reduction aortoplasty has been often undertaken to treat these aneurysms.

SUGGESTED READINGS
available at www.expertconsult.com

RELATED CONTENT

Giant Cell Arteritis (Patient Information)

AUTHORS: **ARUN SWAMINATHAN, M.B.B.S.,**
and **SACHIN KEDAR, M.B.B.S., M.D.**

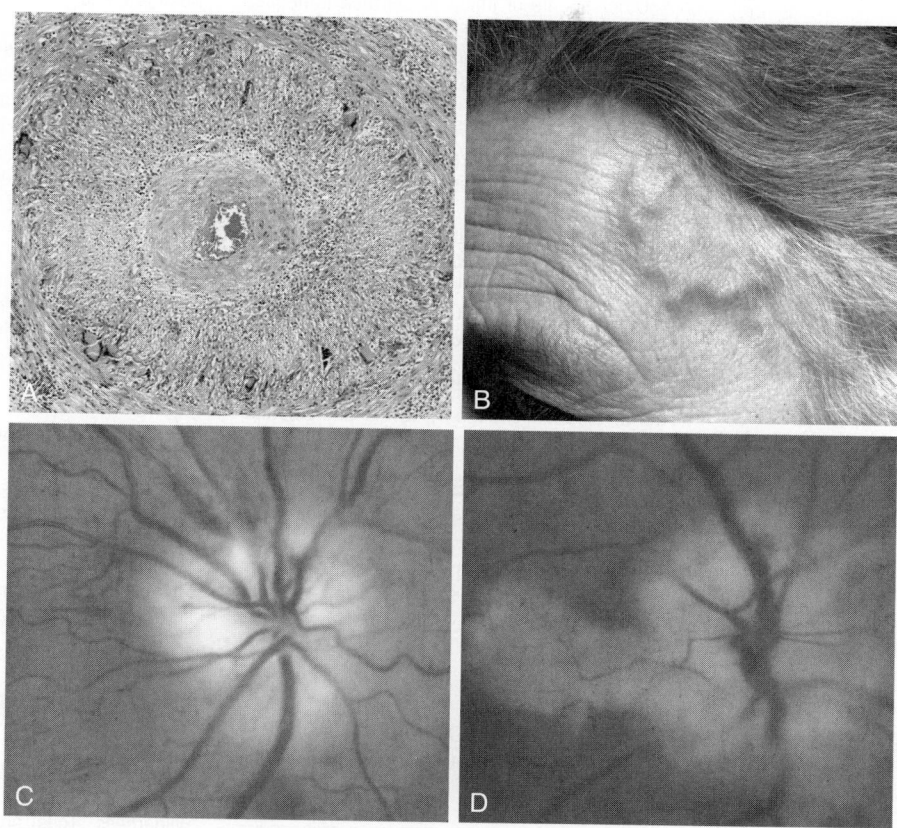

FIGURE 1-353 **Giant cell arteritis. A,** Histology shows transmural granulomatous inflammation, disruption of the internal elastic lamina, proliferation of the intima, and gross narrowing of the lumen. **B,** The superficial temporal artery is pulseless, nodular, and thickened. **C,** Ischemic optic neuropathy. **D,** Ischemic optic neuropathy and cilioretinal artery occlusion. (From Kanski JJ, Bowling B: *Clinical ophthalmology, a systematic approach,* ed 7, Philadelphia, 2010, Saunders.)

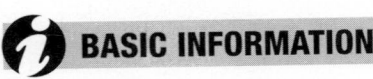

BASIC INFORMATION

DEFINITION

Giardiasis is an intestinal and/or biliary tract infection caused by the protozoal parasite *Giardia lamblia*. The organism is a widespread zoonotic parasite and frequently contaminates fresh water sources worldwide.

SYNONYMS

Giardiasis
Giardia duodenalis
Giardia intestinalis

ICD-9CM CODES
007.1 Giardiasis

EPIDEMIOLOGY & DEMOGRAPHICS

INCIDENCE (IN U.S.):
- Exact incidence unknown
- Frequently occurs as water-borne outbreaks

PREVALENCE (IN U.S.): 4%
PREDOMINANT SEX: Male = female
PREDOMINANT AGE:
- Preschool children, especially if in day care
- 20 to 40 yr of age, especially among sexually active homosexual men

PEAK INCIDENCE:
- Varies with risk factors, outbreaks, but peak onset from early summer through early fall
- All age groups affected

GENETICS: Familial disposition: Patients with common variable immunodeficiency or X-linked agammaglobulinemia are at increased risk of infection.

PHYSICAL FINDINGS & CLINICAL PRESENTATION

- More than 70% with one or more intestinal symptoms (diarrhea, flatulence, cramps, bloating, nausea). Table 1-166 summarizes clinical signs and symptoms of giardiasis
- Fever in <30%
- Chronic diarrhea, malabsorption, and weight loss
- GI bleeding is unusual
- Continuous or intermittent symptoms, lasting for weeks
- Of infected patients, 20% to 25% are asymptomatic

ETIOLOGY

Infection is acquired by ingestion of viable cysts of the organism, typically in contaminated water or by fecal-oral contact.

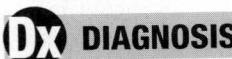

DIAGNOSIS

DIFFERENTIAL DIAGNOSIS

- Other agents of infective diarrhea (amebae, *Salmonella* sp., *Shigella* sp., *Staphylococcus aureus*, *Cryptosporidium*, etc.)
- Noninfectious causes of malabsorption

WORKUP

- Stool specimen (three specimens yield 90% sensitivity) or duodenal aspirate for microscopic examination to establish diagnosis and exclude other pathogens
- Immunoassays for *Giardia* sp. Antigens in stool samples are now routinely used in most clinical laboratories. These assays are 85% to 98% sensitive and 90% to 100% specific.

LABORATORY TESTS

Serum albumin, vitamin B_{12} levels, and stool fat test to exclude malabsorption

IMAGING STUDIES

- Not necessary unless biliary obstruction is suspected
- In detection of organism, possible interference by barium in stool from radiographic studies

TABLE 1-166 Clinical Signs and Symptoms of Giardiasis

Symptom	Frequency (%)
Diarrhea	64-100
Malaise, weakness	72-97
Abdominal distention	42-97
Flatulence	35-97
Abdominal cramps	44-81
Nausea	14-79
Foul-smelling, greasy stools	15-79
Anorexia	41-73
Weight loss	53-73
Vomiting	14-35
Fever	0-28
Constipation	0-27

From Kliegman RM et al: *Nelson textbook of pediatrics*, ed 19, Philadelphia, 2011, Saunders.

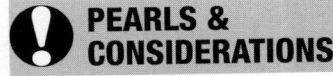

TREATMENT

NONPHARMACOLOGIC THERAPY

Avoidance of milk products to reduce symptoms of transient lactase deficiency that occur in many patients

ACUTE GENERAL Rx

Adult and pediatric:
- Metronidazole 250 mg PO three times daily for 5 to 7 days is considered the drug of choice in the United States. Pediatric dose: 5 mg/kg tid × 7 days (metronidazole should be avoided in pregnancy).
- Tinidazole: 2 g single dose (50 mg/kg in children) is a congener of metronidazole
- Nitazoxanide: aged 12 to 47 mo: 100 mg bid × 3 days. Aged 4 to 11 yr: 200 mg bid × 3 days
- Albendazole 400 mg PO qd x 5 days
- Paromomycin 25 to 35 mg/kg/day in three doses for 5 to 10 days
- Can be used in pregnancy

CHRONIC Rx

May require retreatment.

DISPOSITION

Reinfection is possible.

REFERRAL

For evaluation by gastroenterologist if malabsorption and persistent weight loss

PEARLS & CONSIDERATIONS

COMMENTS

Travelers to endemic areas (developing world, wilderness areas) should be cautioned to boil drinking water or use water purification tablets.

SUGGESTED READINGS

available at www.expertconsult.com

RELATED CONTENT

Giardiasis (Patient Information)

AUTHOR: **GLENN G. FORT, M.D., M.P.H.**

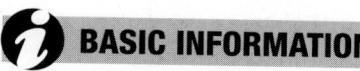

BASIC INFORMATION

DEFINITION

Gilbert's disease is an autosomal-dominant disease characterized by indirect hyperbilirubinemia caused by impaired glucuronyl transferase activity.

SYNONYMS

Gilbert's syndrome

ICD-9CM CODES

277.4 Gilbert's syndrome

EPIDEMIOLOGY & DEMOGRAPHICS

INCIDENCE (IN U.S.): Probable autosomal-dominant disease affecting >5% of the U.S. population
PREDOMINANT SEX: Male/female ratio of 3:1
GENETICS: Most common hereditary hyperbilirubinemia (genotypic prevalence 12%)

PHYSICAL FINDINGS & CLINICAL PRESENTATION

- No abnormalities on physical examination other than mild jaundice when bilirubin exceeds 3 mg/dl.
- A family history of unconjugated hyperbilirubinemia may be present.

ETIOLOGY

- Decreased elimination of bilirubin in bile is caused by inadequate conjugation of bilirubin.
- Alcohol consumption and starvation diet can increase bilirubin level.
- The pathogenesis of Gilbert's syndrome has been linked to a reduction in the bilirubin UGT-1 gene (HUG-Brl) transcription, resulting from a mutation in the promoter region.

DIAGNOSIS

DIFFERENTIAL DIAGNOSIS

- Hemolytic anemia
- Liver disease (chronic hepatitis, cirrhosis)
- Crigler-Najjar syndrome

WORKUP

- Most patients are diagnosed during or after adolescence, when isolated hyperbilirubinemia is detected as an incidental finding on routine biochemical testing.
- Laboratory evaluation to exclude hemolysis and liver diseases as a cause of the elevated bilirubin level (Table 1-167).

LABORATORY TESTS

Elevated indirect (unconjugated) bilirubin (rarely exceeds 5 mg/dl)

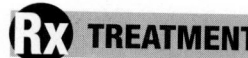

TREATMENT

ACUTE GENERAL Rx

Treatment is generally unnecessary. Phenobarbital (if clinical jaundice is present) can rapidly decrease serum indirect bilirubin level.

DISPOSITION

Prognosis is excellent. Treatment is generally unnecessary.

REFERRAL

Referral is generally not necessary.

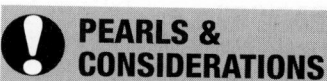

PEARLS & CONSIDERATIONS

COMMENTS

- Patients should be reassured about the benign nature of their condition.
- Fasting for 2 days or significant dehydration may raise the bilirubin level and result in the clinical recognition of jaundice.

AUTHOR: **FRED F. FERRI, M.D.**

TABLE 1-167 Characteristic Patterns of Liver Function Tests

Disorder	Bilirubin	Alkaline Phosphatase	AST	ALT	Prothrombin Time	Albumin
Gilbert's syndrome (abnormal bilirubin metabolism)	↑	NL	NL	NL	NL	NL
Bile duct obstruction (pancreatic cancer)	↑↑↑	↑↑↑	↑	↑	↑-↑↑	NL
Acute hepatocellular damage (toxic, viral hepatitis)	↑-↑↑↑	↑-↑↑	↑↑↑	↑↑↑	NL-↑↑↑	NL-↓↓
Cirrhosis	NL-↑	NL-↑	NL-↑	NL-↑	NL-↑↑	NL-↓↓

ALT, Alanine aminotransferase; AST, aspartate aminotransferase; NL, normal; ↑, increase; ↓, decrease (arrows indicate extent of change: ↑-↑↑↑, slight to large).
From Andreoli TE (ed): Cecil essentials of medicine, ed 6, Philadelphia, 2005, Saunders.

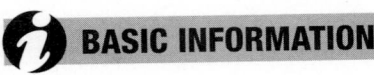

DEFINITION

Inflammation of the gums covering the maxilla and mandible

SYNONYMS

None

ICD-9CM CODES
523.1 Chronic gingivitis
523.01 Acute gingivitis

EPIDEMIOLOGY & DEMOGRAPHICS

Gingivitis generally occurs in adults.

PHYSICAL FINDINGS & CLINICAL PRESENTATION

- Inflammation is usually painless. Red velvety gingiva may be present (Fig. 1-354).
- Bleeding may occur with minor trauma such as brushing teeth.
- A bluish discoloration of the gums and halitosis are sometimes present.
- Subgingival plaque may be seen on close examination, and in time, there is detachment of soft tissue from the tooth surface.
- Longstanding infection may lead to destructive periodontal disease, which may involve teeth and bones.
- A dramatic form of gingivitis called acute ulcerative necrotizing gingivitis (ANUG or "trench mouth") can occur. This is manifested by acute, painful inflammation of the gingivae, with bleeding, ulceration, and halitosis. At times this is accompanied by fever and lymphadenopathy.
- Linear gingival erythema ("HIV gingivitis") presents as a brightly inflamed band of marginal gingiva. It may be painful, with easy bleeding and rapid destruction.
- Severe periodontitis can occur in patients with diabetes mellitus or HIV infection and in primary HIV infection (acute retroviral syndrome).

- Pregnancy may be associated with an acute form of gingivitis. Gingivae become inflamed and hypertrophic; this is likely the result of hormonal shifts.

ETIOLOGY

- A variety of organisms may be found in the environment of plaque. Anaerobes play a predominant role in periodontal disease.
- Improper hygiene and poorly fitting dentures may contribute to the development of gingivitis.
- Excessive use of tobacco and alcohol may predispose individuals to gingival disease.
- In patients with HIV infection, gram-negative anaerobes, enteric organisms, and yeast predominate.
- Appropriate oral hygiene, such as flossing and tooth brushing, can prevent the accumulation of bacterial plaque; once dense plaque is present, adequate hygiene becomes more difficult.

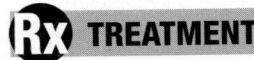 **DIAGNOSIS**

DIFFERENTIAL DIAGNOSIS

Gingival hyperplasia, which may be caused by long-term use of phenytoin or nifedipine

WORKUP

Oral examination

LABORATORY TESTS

Elevated serum glucose in diabetics

IMAGING STUDIES

Radiographs of the teeth and facial bones may reveal extension of infection to these structures.

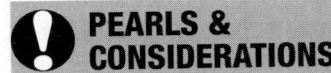 **TREATMENT**

NONPHARMACOLOGIC THERAPY

Removal of plaque, and at times, debridement of soft tissue

ACUTE GENERAL Rx

- Penicillin VK, 500 mg PO qid for 1 to 2 wk or
- Clindamycin, 300 mg PO qid for 1 to 2 wk
- For linear gingival erythema, chlorhexidine gluconate rinses and nystatin rinses or troches may be used

CHRONIC Rx

Extensive or recurrent infection may require periodic evaluation and debridement.

DISPOSITION

Continued inflammation can eventually lead to destruction of teeth and bone.

REFERRAL

Patients should be referred to a dentist or periodontist.

! PEARLS & CONSIDERATIONS

COMMENTS

- Presence of periodontal disease is associated with an increased incidence of anaerobic pleuropulmonary infections.
- Existing data support the recommendation to change a toothbrush every 3 mo. Worn brushes seem to be less effective in plaque reduction.

SUGGESTED READINGS
available at www.expertconsult.com

RELATED CONTENT

Gingivitis (Patient Information)
Gingivitis, Necrotizing Ulcerative (Related Key Topic)

AUTHOR: **GLENN G. FORT, M.D., M.P.H.**

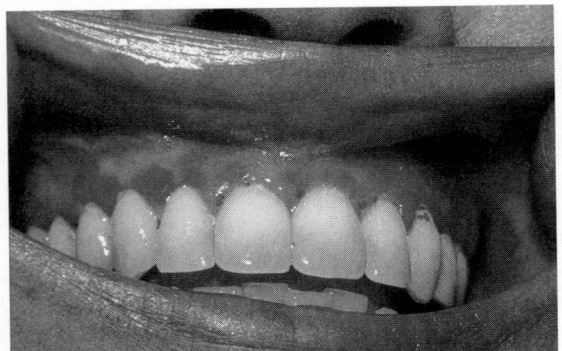

FIGURE 1-354 Gingivitis in a patient with cicatricial pemphigoid. This pattern of periodontal, chronic, red, velvety gingivitis is very suggestive of this disorder but may occur in other blistering diseases. (From White GM, Cox NH [eds]: *Diseases of the skin, a color atlas and text,* ed 2, St Louis, 2006, Mosby.)

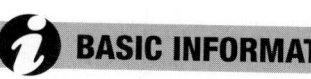

BASIC INFORMATION

DEFINITION

Glaucoma is a chronic degenerative optic neuropathy in which the neuro-retinal rim of the optic nerve becomes progressively thinner, thereby enlarging the optic-nerve cup. The classification of glaucomas is based on the appearance of the iridocorneal angle (open angle vs. closed angle) and is further subdivided into primary and secondary types. Primary open-angle glaucoma can occur with or without elevated intraocular pressure. Normal tension glaucoma refers to primary open-angle glaucoma without elevated intraocular pressure.

SYNONYMS

Chronic simple glaucoma
Primary open-angle glaucoma (POAG)
Open-angle glaucoma
Chronic open-angle glaucoma

ICD-9CM CODES
365.1 Open-angle glaucoma

EPIDEMIOLOGY & DEMOGRAPHICS

INCIDENCE (IN U.S.): Third most common cause of vision loss (75% to 95% of all forms of glaucoma are open angle)
PEAK INCIDENCE:
- Increases after age 40 yr
- Three million cases expected by 2020 because of the rapid increase in aging population
PREVALENCE (IN U.S.):
- Overall prevalence in U.S. population aged >40 yr is estimated to be 1.86%, with 1.57 million white and 398,000 black patients affected.
- 150,000 patients have bilateral blindness.
- Disease occurs in 2% of people >40 yr.
- Prevalence is higher in diabetics, those with high myopia, and older persons.
- More common in blacks (three times the age-adjusted prevalence than whites).
PREDOMINANT AGE:
- Persons >50 yr
- Can occur in 30s and 40s
GENETICS:
- Four to six times higher incidence in blacks than whites
- No clear-cut hereditary patterns but a strong hereditary tendency

PHYSICAL FINDINGS & CLINICAL PRESENTATION

- High intraocular pressures and large optic nerve cup (Ocular Hypertension Treatment Study results very important)
- Corneal edema causes vision loss and blurring
- Abnormal visual fields
- Open-angle gonioscopy
- Red eye
- Restricted vision and field

ETIOLOGY

- Uncertain hereditary tendency
- Topical steroids
- Trauma
- Inflammatory
- High-dose oral corticosteroids taken for prolonged periods

DIAGNOSIS

DIFFERENTIAL DIAGNOSIS

- Other optic neuropathies
- Secondary glaucoma from inflammation and steroid therapy
- Red eye differential
- Trauma
- Contact lens injury

WORKUP

- Intraocular pressure
- Slit lamp examination
- Visual fields
- Gonioscopy
- Nerve fiber analysis (e.g., GDx analyzer, Zeiss, Jena, Germany)
- Corneal thickness—very important in prognosis

LABORATORY TESTS

Blood sugar

IMAGING STUDIES

- Optic nerve photography—stereo photographs
- Visual field testing
- Laser scan of nerve fiber layer, OCT, HRT

TREATMENT

ACUTE GENERAL Rx

- β-blockers (e.g., Timolol) qd to bid depending on individual response to drug
- Carbonic anhydrase inhibitors (e.g., Diamox 250 mg qid or 500 mg bid)
- Prostaglandin analogs (latanoprost, bimatoprost, travopost, tafluprost) commonly used as first-line treatment. They lower intraocular pressure by 25%-30% by increasing uveoscleral outflow
- Alpha-2 agonists and cholinergic agonists
- Hyperosmotic agents (mannitol) in acute treatment (IV)
- Laser trabeculoplasty (SLT) as needed

CHRONIC Rx

- At least biannual checks of intraocular pressure and adjustment of medication
- Poor control = frequent examinations; good control = drugs
- Trabeculectomy
- Filter valves

DISPOSITION

Must be followed by ophthalmologist

REFERRAL

Immediately to ophthalmologist

PEARLS & CONSIDERATIONS

COMMENTS

- Glaucoma is a serious blinding disease that must be monitored professionally by an ophthalmologist. It is mostly asymptomatic until late in the disease when visual problems arise. Even in developed countries half of glaucoma cases are undiagnosed.
- Vision loss from glaucoma cannot be recovered. Early diagnosis and treatment may minimize visual loss.
- Glaucoma is not solely caused by increased intraocular pressure because approximately 20% of patients with glaucoma have normal intraocular pressure. However, high pressure is definitely a risk factor to be considered. Potential sites of increased resistance to aqueous flow are described in Fig. 1-355.

SUGGESTED READINGS

available at www.expertconsult.com

RELATED CONTENT

Glaucoma (Patient Information)

AUTHOR: **MELVYN KOBY, M.D.**

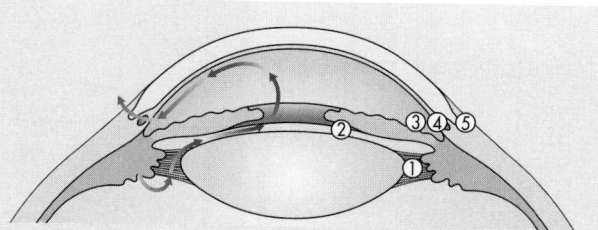

1 Ciliary body processes (when ciliary body swollen by congestion), fibrin debris, vitreous face against the lens equator
2 Pupillary block by anterior position of lens or swollen lens
3 Pretrabecular by neovascular or cellular membranes
4 Trabecular by abnormal accumulation of extracellular matrix
5 Post-trabecular by increased episcleral venous pressure

FIGURE 1-355 Potential sites of increased resistance to aqueous flow. (From Yanoff M, Duker JS: *Ophthalmology*, ed 2, St Louis, 2004, Mosby.)

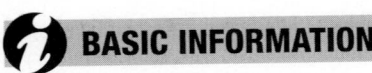

BASIC INFORMATION

DEFINITION

Primary angle-closure glaucoma occurs when elevated intraocular pressure is associated with closure of the filtration angle or obstruction in the circulating pathway of the aqueous humor.

SYNONYMS

Acute glaucoma, angle-closure glaucoma (ACG)
Pupillary block glaucoma
Narrow-angle glaucoma
Angle-closure glaucoma

ICD-9CM CODES
365.2 Primary angle-closure glaucoma (PACG)

EPIDEMIOLOGY & DEMOGRAPHICS

INCIDENCE (IN U.S.):
- 2% to 8% of all patients with glaucoma
- Higher incidence among those with hyperopia, small eyes, dense cataracts, shallow anterior chambers

PEAK INCIDENCE: Greater >50 yr; high association with hypopia, cataracts, and eye trauma
PREDOMINANT SEX: Females are affected more often than males
PREDOMINANT AGE: 50 to 60 yr
GENETICS: High family history

PHYSICAL FINDINGS & CLINICAL PRESENTATION

- Although angle-closure glaucoma can present with an acute painful crisis associated with blurred vision, more than 75% of patients present with an asymptomatic course with progressive loss of the visual field (similar to that in patients with primary open-angle glaucoma)
- Hazy cornea
- Narrow angle (Fig. 1-356)
- Red eyes
- Pain may be present
- Injection of conjunctiva
- Shallow anterior chamber
- Thick cataract
- Old trauma
- Chronic eye infections

ETIOLOGY

- Narrow angles with acute closure: blockage of circulatory path of the aqueous humor causing increase in interior ocular pressure. ACG occurs more commonly in eyes with shorter axial length, shallower anterior chamber, and a relatively larger lens
- Secondary angle-closure glaucoma resulting from neovascularization of iris, iris tumors, pharmacology, lens induced, iris scarring, trauma, chronic inflammation with scarring, malignant glaucoma with aqueous misdirection

DIAGNOSIS

DIFFERENTIAL DIAGNOSIS

- Open-angle glaucoma: Angle-closure glaucoma is distinguished from open-angle glaucoma by the closure of the angle between the iris and cornea, obstructing outflow of aqueous humor
- High pressure
- Optic nerve cupping
- Field loss
- Shallow chamber
- Open-angle glaucoma
- Conjunctivitis
- Corneal disease, keratitis
- Uveitis
- Scleritis
- Allergies
- Contact lens wearing with irritation

WORKUP

- Intraocular pressure
- Gonioscopy
- Slit lamp examination
- Visual field examination
- GDx examination (laser scan of nerve fiber layer), OCT
- Optic nerve evaluation
- Anterior chamber depth
- Cataract evaluation
- High hyperopia

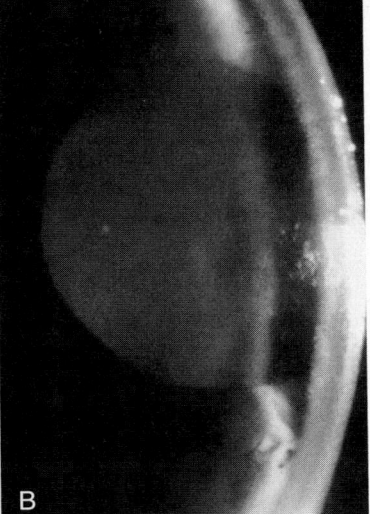

LABORATORY TESTS

- Blood sugar and complete blood count (if diabetes or inflammatory disease is suspected)
- Visual field
- GDx nerve fiber analysis, OCT, Heidelberg retinal tomography

IMAGING STUDIES

- Fundus photography
- Fluorescein angiography for neurovascular disease

TREATMENT

The goal of treatment is to acutely lower pressure on the eye and keep it down.

NONPHARMACOLOGIC THERAPY

Laser iridotomy early in disease process

ACUTE GENERAL Rx

- IV mannitol
- Pilocarpine
- β-blockers
- Diamox
- Laser iridotomy
- Anterior chamber paracentesis (as emergency treatment)

CHRONIC Rx

- Iridotomy
- Trabeculectomy
- Filter valves
- Other laser procedures

DISPOSITION

Refer to ophthalmologist immediately.

REFERRAL

This is an emergency; refer immediately to an ophthalmologist.

PEARLS & CONSIDERATIONS

COMMENTS

- Do not use antihistamines or vasodilators with narrow-angle glaucoma.
- After iridotomy, the majority of patients will be totally cured and will need no further medication and have no visual loss.
- Lower socioeconomic status and higher levels of social deprivation are risk factors for delayed detection and probable worse outcomes in glaucoma.
- Glaucoma is undiagnosed in 9 out of 10 affected people worldwide and is undiagnosed in 50% of those in developed countries.

EVIDENCE

available at www.expertconsult.com

SUGGESTED READINGS

available at www.expertconsult.com

RELATED CONTENT

Glaucoma (Patient Information)

AUTHOR: **MELVYN KOBY, M.D.**

FIGURE 1-356 Acute angle-closure glaucoma. A, Acutely elevated pressure produces an inflamed eye with corneal edema (note fragmented light reflex) and a mid-dilated pupil. **B,** Slit lamp examination shows a very shallow central anterior chamber (space between cornea and iris) and no peripheral chamber. (From Palay D [ed]: *Ophthalmology for the primary care physician,* St Louis, 1997, Mosby.)

BASIC INFORMATION

DEFINITION

Glenohumeral dislocation (Fig. 1-357) is complete separation or displacement of the humeral head from the glenoid surface (partial separation is termed *subluxation*). Most often the cause is traumatic, and the humeral head dislocates anteriorly and inferiorly. This may cause a tear of the glenoid labrum (the Bankart lesion). Less commonly the head dislocates posteriorly.

Rarely, multidirectional instability may be present in which dislocation or subluxation, often bilateral, may occur in multiple directions, usually the result of excessive joint laxity and generally without trauma.

ICD-9CM CODES
831.01 Anterior
831.02 Posterior
831.03 Inferior
718.31 Recurrent
718.81 Instability

PHYSICAL FINDINGS & CLINICAL PRESENTATION

Traumatic:
- The arm is held in external rotation with anterior dislocation and internal rotation with posterior dislocation.
- Little movement is possible without pain.
- The acromion may appear more prominent, and there is absence of the normal "fullness" beneath the acromion.
- The status of the axillary nerve must always be checked (sensation to the mid-deltoid should be assessed).

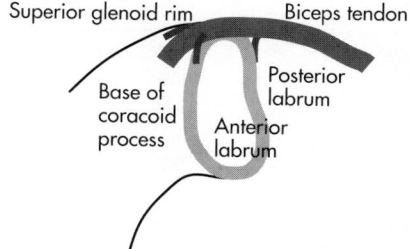

FIGURE 1-357 Glenohumeral dislocation. (From Weisslederer R et al: *Primer of diagnostic imaging,* St Louis, 2007, Mosby.)

Superior glenoid rim — Biceps tendon
Base of coracoid process — Posterior labrum — Anterior labrum

- The apprehension test may become positive if anterior instability persists (pain and apprehension that the shoulder will dislocate when the relaxed arm is manually placed in the "throwing position" of external rotation and abduction).
- Recurrent episodes of anterior dislocation may occur with minor movement, such as putting on a coat or turning off a light.

Multidirectional:
- Often difficult to diagnose, especially if only subluxation occurs.
- Recurrent episodes of giving out and weakness, often bilateral and without trauma.
- Sulcus sign is often positive (the arms are pulled downward with the patient standing; a sulcus [indentation] will form between the acromion and humeral head, indicating excessive inferior movement of the head).
- Other signs of generalized joint laxity may be present, such as joint hyperextensibility and the ability of the patient to touch the thumb against the flexor aspect of the forearm.

ETIOLOGY

- Trauma
- Generalized joint laxity (multidirectional)
- Seizures (posterior dislocations)

DIAGNOSIS

DIFFERENTIAL DIAGNOSIS

- Rotator cuff rupture
- Frozen shoulder (posterior dislocation)
- Suprascapular nerve paralysis
- Anterior instability

IMAGING STUDIES

- Acute shoulder injury: true anteroposterior roentgenogram plus lateral view of the glenohumeral joint, either transaxillary or transcapsular
- MRI: to determine soft tissue status, especially the presence of Bankart lesion or rotator cuff tear; may be indicated after a second episode of dislocation

TREATMENT

- Reduction of the acute dislocation by gentle straight traction in the relaxed patient followed by light immobilization

- Gentle limited range-of-motion exercises as pain subsides followed by strengthening exercises at 2 wk

DISPOSITION

- Recurrence of anterior dislocation is common in the young; these patients may have to avoid the arm position associated with dislocation (external rotation with abduction).
- Primary dislocations in patients >40 yr are not generally complicated by recurrence but may result in shoulder stiffness and associated rotator cuff injuries.
- There is an almost 100% recurrence after the third dislocation.

REFERRAL

Surgical reconstruction may be required in the recurrent dislocator.

PEARLS & CONSIDERATIONS

COMMENTS

- It is important to know if there was an injury involved in the first episode and if a radiograph was taken to determine direction of the dislocation.
- Up to 50% of posterior dislocations are missed by the first examiner, usually the result of an inadequate lateral radiograph of the glenohumeral joint.
- "Voluntary" posterior dislocators should always be treated nonsurgically.
- Sports activities may be resumed when there is pain-free full flexibility and normal strength.
- Multidirectional instabilities are usually treated nonsurgically with strengthening exercises.
- Dislocations in either direction are occasionally overlooked. If the injury is over 2 to 4 weeks old, enough tissue healing will have occurred to make closed reduction fail. Open reduction or arthroplasty will then be needed in the young. Older patients may improve with therapeutic exercises, and the resultant disability is often acceptable.

SUGGESTED READINGS

available at www.expertconsult.com

AUTHOR: **LONNIE R. MERCIER, M.D.**

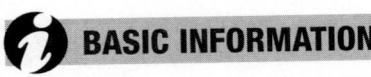

DEFINITION

Acute glomerulonephritis is an immunologically mediated inflammation primarily involving the glomerulus that can result in damage to the basement membrane, mesangium, or capillary endothelium.

SYNONYMS

Postinfectious glomerulonephritis
Acute nephritic syndrome

ICD-9CM CODES

583.9 Glomerulonephritis, acute

EPIDEMIOLOGY & DEMOGRAPHICS

- More than 50% of cases involve children <13 yr.
- Glomerulonephritis is the most common cause of chronic renal failure (25%).
- Immunoglobulin A (IgA) nephropathy glomerulonephritis (Berger's disease) is the most common glomerulonephritis worldwide.

PHYSICAL FINDINGS & CLINICAL PRESENTATION

- Edema (peripheral, periorbital, or pulmonary)
- Joint pains, oral ulcers, malar rash (frequently seen with lupus nephritis)
- Dark urine
- Hypertension

- Findings of palpable purpura in patients with Henoch-Schönlein purpura
- Heart murmurs may indicate endocarditis
- Impetigo, skin pallor, tenderness in the abdomen and/or back, pharyngeal erythema may be present

ETIOLOGY

Acute glomerulonephritis may be caused by primary renal disease or a systemic disease. A number of pathogenic processes (e.g., antibody deposition, cell-mediated immune mechanisms, complement activation, hemodynamic alterations) have been implicated in the pathogenesis of glomerular inflammation. Medical disorders generally associated with glomerulonephritis are:
- Group A beta-hemolytic *Streptococcus* infection (other infectious etiologies including endocarditis and visceral abscess)
- Collagen-vascular diseases (systemic lupus erythematosus [SLE])
- Vasculitis (Wegener's granulomatosis, polyarteritis nodosa)
- Idiopathic glomerulonephritis (membranoproliferative, idiopathic, crescentic, IgA nephropathy)
- Goodpasture's syndrome
- Other cryoglobulinemia (Henoch-Schönlein purpura)
- Drug-induced (gold, penicillamine)

Table 1-168 summarizes primary renal diseases that present as acute glomerulonephritis. Diseases associated with rapidly progressive glomerulonephritis and pertinent laboratory findings are described in Table 1-169.

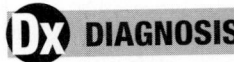

DIFFERENTIAL DIAGNOSIS

- Cirrhosis with edema and ascites
- Congestive heart failure
- Acute interstitial nephritis
- Severe hypertension
- Hemolytic-uremic syndrome
- SLE, diabetes mellitus, amyloidosis, preeclampsia, sclerodermal renal crisis

WORKUP

Initial evaluation of suspected glomerulonephritis consists of laboratory testing.

LABORATORY TESTS

- Urinalysis (hematuria [dysmorphic erythrocytes and red cell casts], proteinuria)
- Serum creatinine (to estimate glomerular filtration rate [GFR]), blood urea nitrogen
- 24-hr urine for protein excretion and creatinine clearance (to document degree of renal dysfunction and amount of proteinuria). Proteinuria in acute glomerulonephritis typically ranges from 500 mg/day to 3 g/day, but nephrotic-range proteinuria (>3.5 g/day) may be present.
- Streptococcal tests (Streptozyme), antistreptolysin O (ASO) quantitative titer (highest in 3 to 5 wk); ASO titer, however, is not related to severity of renal disease, duration, or prognosis.
- Additional useful tests depending on the history: anti-DNA antibodies (rule out SLE), CH_{50} level (if elevated, obtain C_3, C_4 levels), triglycerides, cryoglobulins, hepatitis B and C

TABLE 1-168 Summary of Primary Renal Diseases that Manifest as Acute Glomerulonephritis

Diseases	Poststreptococcal Glomerulonephritis	IgA Nephropathy	Goodpasture Syndrome	Idiopathic Rapidly Progressive Glomerulonephritis
Clinical Manifestations				
Age and sex	All ages, mean 7 yr, 2:1 male	10–35 yr, 2:1 male	15–30 yr, 6:1 male	Adults, 2:1 male
Acute nephritic syndrome	90%	50%	90%	90%
Asymptomatic hematuria	Occasionally	50%	Rare	Rare
Nephrotic syndrome	10–20%	Rare	Rare	10–20%
Hypertension	70%	30–50%	Rare	25%
Acute renal failure	50% (transient)	Very rare	50%	60%
Other	Latent period of 1–3 wk	Follows viral syndromes	Pulmonary hemorrhage; iron deficiency anemia	None
Laboratory findings	↑ ASO titers (70%) Positive streptozyme (95%) ↓ C3–C9; normal C1, C4	↑ Serum IgA (50%) IgA in dermal capillaries	Positive anti-GBM antibody	Positive ANCA in some
Immunogenetics	HLA-B12, D "EN" (9)*	HLA-Bw 35, DR4 (4)*	HLA-DR2 (16)*	None established
Renal Pathology				
Light microscopy	Diffuse proliferation	Focal proliferation	Focal → diffuse proliferation with crescents	Crescentic GN
Immunofluorescence	Granular IgG, C3	Diffuse mesangial IgA	Linear IgG, C3	No immune deposits
Electron microscopy	Subepithelial humps	Mesangial deposits	No deposits	No deposits
Prognosis	95% resolve spontaneously 5% RPGN or slowly progressive	Slow progression in 25–50%	75% stabilize or improve if treated early	75% stabilize or improve if treated early
Treatment	Supportive	Uncertain (options include steroids, fish oil, and ACE inhibitors)	Plasma exchange, steroids, cyclophosphamide	Steroid pulse therapy

*Relative risk.
ACE, Angiotensin-converting enzyme; *ANCA*, antineutrophil cytoplasmic antibody; *ASO*, anti–streptolysin O; *GBM*, glomerular basement membrane; *GN*, glomerulonephritis; *HLA*, human leukocyte antigen; *Ig*, immunoglobulin; *RPGN*, idiopathic rapidly progressive glomerulonephritis.
From Kliegman RM et al: *Practical strategies in pediatric diagnosis and therapy*, ed 2, Philadelphia, 2004, Saunders.

TABLE 1-169 Diseases Associated with Rapidly Progressive Glomerulonephritis and Pertinent Laboratory Studies

Disease	Studies
Renal Limited	
IgA nephropathy	
Postinfectious glomerulonephritis	Low complement, streptococcal serologies, bacterial cultures
ANCA-associated glomerulonephritis (pauci-immune glomerulonephritis)	ANCA titers
Anti-GBM disease (Goodpasture's syndrome)	Anti-GBM antibodies
Systemic Disorders	
Lupus nephritis	Low complement, ANA, dsDNA antibodies
ANCA-associated small-vessel vasculitis	ANCA titers
Anti-GBM disease	Anti-GBM antibodies
Henoch-Schönlein purpura	None
Cryoglobulinemic vasculitis	Low complement, cryoglobulins, hepatitis C serologies

ANCA, Antineutrophil cytoplasmic antibody; *ANA,* antinuclear antibodies; *dsDNA,* double-stranded DNA; *GBM,* glomerular basement membrane; *IgA,* immunoglobulin A.
From Vincent JL et al: *Textbook of critical care,* ed 6, Philadelphia, 2011, Saunders.

TABLE 1-170 Antigens Identified in Glomerulonephritis

Poststreptococcal GN	Streptococcal pyrogenic exotoxin B, plasmin receptor
Anti-GBM disease	α3 type IV collagen (likely induced by molecular mimicry)
IgA nephropathy	Possibly no antigen but rather polymerized polyclonal IgA (?superantigen driven)
Membranous nephropathy	Phospholipase A_2 receptor (idiopathic), neutral endopeptidase in podocyte (congenital), HBeAg (hepatitis associated)
Staphylococcus aureus–associated GN	*Staphylococcus* superantigens induce polyclonal response; not necessarily antigen in glomeruli
Membranoproliferative GN	HCV and HBsAg in hepatitis-associated MPGN
ANCA-associated vasculitis	Proteinase 3 (c-ANCA) and myeloperoxidase (p-ANCA) in neutrophils; antibodies to lysosome-associated membrane protein 2 on endothelial cells (likely induced by molecular mimicry to fimbriated bacterial antigens)

ANCA, Antineutrophil cytoplasmic antibody; *GBM,* glomerular basement membrane; *GN,* glomerulonephritis; *HBeAg,* hepatitis B virus early antigen; *HBsAg,* hepatitis B surface antigen; *HCV,* hepatitis C virus; *IgA,* immuoglobulin A; *MPGN,* membranoproliferative glomerulonephritis.
From Floege J et al: *Comprehensive clinical nephrology,* ed 4, Philadelphia, 2010, Saunders.

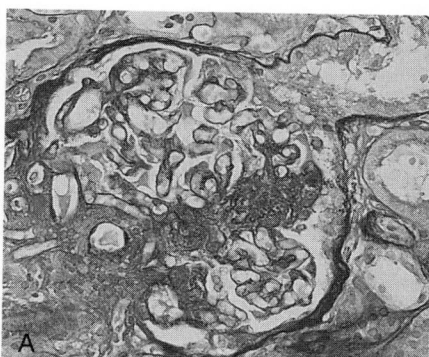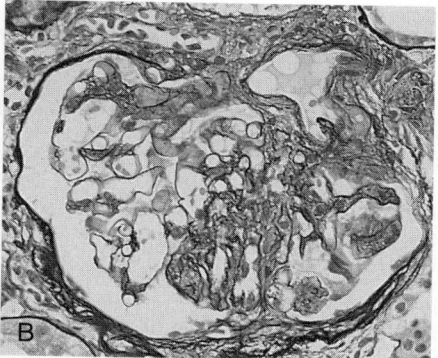

FIGURE 1-358 Light microscopic appearances in focal segmental glomerulosclerosis. Segmental scars with capsular adhesions in otherwise normal glomeruli. A, Periodic acid-Schiff, ×300. **B,** Methenamine silver stain, ×300. (Courtesy Dr. D. Davies. From Johnson RJ, Feehally J: *Comprehensive clinical nephrology,* ed 2, St Louis, 2000, Mosby.)

serologies, antineutrophil cytoplasmic antibody (ANCA), c-ANCA (in suspected cases of Wegener's granulomatosis), p-ANCA found in pauciimmune (lack of immune deposits) idiopathic rapidly progressive glomerulonephritis with or without systemic vasculitis, and antiglomerular basement membrane (type alpha[3] IV collagen) antibodies.
- Hematocrit (decrease in glomerulonephritis) and platelet count (thrombocytopenia in cases of lupus nephritis).
- Anti–glomerular basement membrane antibody (in Goodpasture's syndrome).
- Blood cultures are indicated in all febrile patients.
- Antigens identified in glomerulonephritis are described in Table 1-170.

IMAGING STUDIES
- Chest x-ray: pulmonary congestion, Wegener's granulomatosis, and Goodpasture's syndrome.
- Renal ultrasound if GFR is depressed to evaluate renal size and determine extent of fibrosis. A kidney size of <9 cm is suggestive of extensive scarring and low likelihood of reversibility.
- Echocardiogram in patients with new cardiac murmurs or positive blood cultures to rule out endocarditis and pericardial effusion.
- Renal biopsy and light (Fig. 1-358), electron, and immunofluorescent microscopy to confirm diagnosis.
- Kidney biopsy: generally reveals a granular pattern in poststreptococcal glomerulonephritis and a linear pattern in Goodpasture's syndrome; absence of immune deposits suggests vasculitis. Renal biopsy, although helpful to define the etiology of glomerulonephritis, is not usually essential. It is useful to determine the degree of inflammation and fibrosis. It is also especially important for patients with rapidly progressive glomerulonephritis, in whom prompt diagnosis and treatment are essential.
- Immunofluorescence: generally reveals C_3. Negative immunofluorescence suggests Wegener's granulomatosis, idiopathic crescentic glomerulonephritis, or polyarteritis nodosa.
- Angiography or biopsy of other affected organs if systemic vasculitis is suspected.

Rx TREATMENT

NONPHARMACOLOGIC THERAPY
- Avoidance of salt if edema or hypertension is present
- Low-protein intake (approximately 0.5 g/kg/day) in patients with renal failure
- Fluid restriction in patients with significant edema
- Avoidance of high-potassium foods

ACUTE GENERAL Rx

- Correction of electrolyte abnormalities (hypocalcemia, hyperkalemia) and acidosis (if present)
- Treatment of streptococcal infection with penicillin (or erythromycin in penicillin-allergic patients)
- Furosemide in patients with significant hypertension and/or edema; hydralazine or nifedipine in patients with hypertension
- Immunosuppressive treatment in patients with heavy proteinuria or rapidly decreasing GFR (high-dose steroids, cyclosporin A, cyclophosphamide); corticosteroids generally not useful in poststreptococcal glomerulonephritis
- Fish oil (n-3 fatty acids) 12 g/day; may prevent or slow loss of renal function in patients with IgA nephropathy
- Plasma exchange therapy and immunosuppressive drugs (prednisone and cyclophosphamide); effective in Goodpasture's syndrome
- Short-term therapy with IV cyclophosphamide followed by maintenance therapy with mycophenolate mofetil or azathioprine. Oral mycophenolate mofetil is also effective in induction therapy in patients with lupus nephritis
- Mycophenolate mofetil appears superior to azathioprine in maintaining a renal response to treatment and in preventing relapse in patients with lupus nephritis who responded to induction therapy
- Table 1-171 summarizes suggested management of membranoproliferative glomerulonephritis

CHRONIC Rx

- Frequent monitoring of urinalysis, serum creatinine, and blood pressure in the initial 12 mo
- Monitoring for onset of hypertensive retinopathy, encephalopathy
- Aggressive treatment of infections, particularly streptococcal infections
- Dosage adjustment of all renally excreted medications

DISPOSITION

- Prognosis is generally related to histology, with excellent prognosis in patients with minimal change in glomerulonephritis and focal segmental proliferative glomerulonephritis. Between 25% and 30% of patients with mesangial IgA disease and membranous glomerulonephritis generally progress to chronic renal failure; >70% of patients with mesangial capillary glomerulonephritis will develop chronic renal failure.
- In general, prognosis is worse in patients with heavy proteinuria, severe hypertension, and significant elevations of creatinine.
- Recovery of renal function occurs within 8 to 12 wk in 95% of patients with poststreptococcal glomerulonephritis.

REFERRAL

- Nephrology consultation. The urgency for referral depends on the GFR. Urgent consultation is recommended if GFR is significantly abnormal or rapidly deteriorating or if the patient has systemic symptoms.
- Surgical referral for biopsy in selected cases.

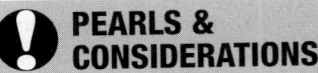

PEARLS & CONSIDERATIONS

COMMENTS

- Anticoagulation to prevent deep vein thrombosis should be considered in patients with a low level of physical activity.
- Monitoring of lipids and aggressive treatment of hyperlipidemias are recommended.
- Close monitoring of side effects of immunosuppressive drugs and complications of corticosteroids is necessary.

SUGGESTED READINGS

available at www.expertconsult.com

RELATED CONTENT

Glomerulonephritis (Patient Information)
Acute Kidney Injury (Related Key Topic)

AUTHOR: **FRED F. FERRI, M.D.**

TABLE 1-171 Suggested Management of Membranoproliferative Glomerulonephritis

Type	Treatment
All types	Supportive therapy following the recommendations discussed in text
Idiopathic MPGN in children	Non-nephrotic proteinuria, normal renal function: follow with 3-month visits Normal renal function and moderate proteinuria (>3 g/day): prednisone 40 mg/m² on alternate days for 3 months Nephrotic or impaired renal function: prednisone 40 mg/m² on alternate days (80 mg maximum) for 2 years, tapering to 20 mg on alternate days for 3-10 years
Idiopathic MPGN in adults	Non-nephrotic, normal renal function: follow with 3-month visits Nephrotic or impaired renal function: 6-month course of corticosteroid with/without cytotoxic agents (cyclophosphamide) or other drugs used: cyclosporine, tacrolimus, mycophenolate mofetil Rapidly progressive renal failure with diffuse crescents: treat as for idiopathic rapidly progressive glomerulonephritis In the presence of chronic renal failure or nephrotic proteinuria: angiotensin-converting enzyme inhibitors
MPGN associated with hepatitis C virus or cryoglobulinemia	Non-nephrotic, normal renal function: treat with interferon alpha based on severity of liver disease (diagnosed by biopsy) Nephrotic syndrome, reduced renal function, or signs of cryoglobulinemia: pegylated interferon alfa-2b (1 μg/kg weekly) and ribavirin (15 mg/kg/day) for 12 months, followed by a short-term course of low-dose corticosteroids; if relapse occurs, consider high-dose interferon alfa (10 million U daily for 2 weeks, then every other day for 6 more weeks) Rapidly progressive renal failure or severe symptoms of vasculitis (heart failure, pulmonary disease): methylprednisolone 1 g daily for 3 days, followed by oral prednisone 60 mg/daily with slow taper during 2-3 months Cyclophosphamide (2 mg/kg/day with adjustment for renal function) and cryofiltration may be added as adjunctive therapy; when the prednisone is reduced to 20 mg/day and the cyclophosphamide is discontinued, add interferon alfa MPGN in the renal or liver transplant recipient: consider course of oral ribavirin (0.6-1 g/day)

MPGN, Membranoproliferative glomerulonephritis.
From Floege J et al: *Comprehensive clinical nephrology,* ed 4, Philadelphia, 2010, Saunders.

ℹ️ BASIC INFORMATION

DEFINITION

Glossitis is an inflammation of the tongue that can lead to loss of filiform papillae.

ICD-9CM CODES
529.0 Glossitis

EPIDEMIOLOGY & DEMOGRAPHICS

Glossitis is seen more frequently in patients of lower socioeconomic status, malnourished patients, alcoholics, smokers, elderly patients, immunocompromised patients, and patients with dentures.

PHYSICAL FINDINGS & CLINICAL PRESENTATION

- The appearance of the tongue varies depending on the etiology of the glossitis (Fig. 1-359). Loss of filiform papillae results in a red, smooth-surfaced tongue.
- The tongue may appear pale in patients with significant anemia.
- Pain and swelling of the tongue may be present when glossitis is associated with infections, trauma, or lichen planus.
- Ulcerations may be present in patients with herpetic glossitis, pemphigus, or streptococcal infection.
- Excessive use of mouthwash may result in a "hairy" appearance of the tongue (Fig. 1-360)

ETIOLOGY

- Nutritional deficiencies (vitamin E, riboflavin, niacin, vitamin B_{12}, iron)
- Infections (viral, candidiasis, tuberculosis, syphilis)
- Trauma (generally caused by poorly fitting dentures)

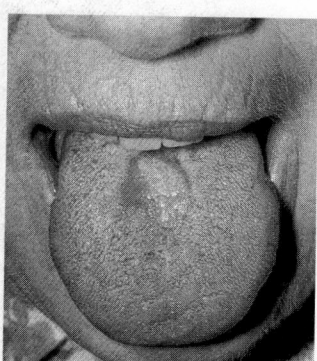

FIGURE 1-359 Median rhomboid glossitis. (From White GM, Cox NH [eds]: *Diseases of the skin, a color atlas and text,* ed 2, St Louis, 2006, Mosby.)

- Irritation of the tongue from toothpaste, medications, alcohol, tobacco, citrus
- Lichen planus, pemphigus vulgaris, erythema multiforme
- Neoplasms

💊 DIAGNOSIS

DIFFERENTIAL DIAGNOSIS

- Infections
- Use of chemical irritants
- Neoplasms
- Skin disorders (e.g., Behçet's syndrome, erythema multiforme)

WORKUP

- Laboratory evaluation to exclude infectious processes, vitamin deficiencies, and systemic disorders
- Biopsy of lesion only when there is no response to treatment

LABORATORY TESTS

- Complete blood count: decreased hemoglobin and hematocrit, low mean corpuscular volume (MCV) (iron-deficiency anemia), elevated MCV (vitamin B_{12} deficiency)
- Vitamin B_{12} level
- 10% KOH scrapings in patients with white patches suspect for candidiasis

℞ TREATMENT

NONPHARMACOLOGIC THERAPY

Avoidance of primary irritants such as hot foods, spices, tobacco, and alcohol

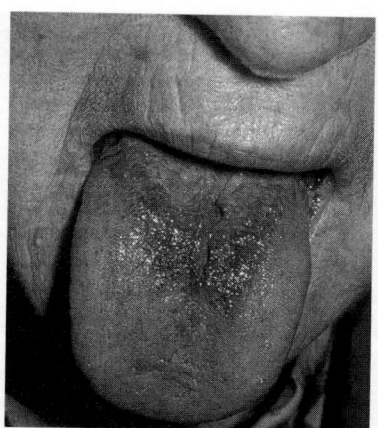

FIGURE 1-360 Black hairy tongue. (From White GM, Cox NH [eds]: *Diseases of the skin, a color atlas and text,* ed 2, St Louis, 2006, Mosby.)

ACUTE GENERAL Rx

Treatment varies with the etiology of the glossitis.

- Malnutrition with avitaminosis: multivitamins
- Candidiasis: fluconazole 200 mg on day 1, then 100 mg/day for at least 2 wk or nystatin 400,000 U suspension qid for 10 days or 200,000 pastilles dissolved slowly in the mouth four to five times qd for 10 to 14 days
- Painful oral lesions: rinsing of the mouth with 2% lidocaine viscous, 1 to 2 tablespoons q4h prn; triamcinolone 0.1% applied to painful ulcers prn for symptomatic relief

CHRONIC Rx

- Lifestyle changes with elimination of tobacco, alcohol, and other primary irritants
- Dental evaluation for correction of ill-fitting dentures
- Correction of associated metabolic abnormalities such as hyperglycemia from diabetes mellitus

DISPOSITION

Most patients experience prompt improvement with identification and treatment of the cause of the glossitis.

REFERRAL

Surgical referral for biopsy of solitary lesions unresponsive to treatment to rule out neoplasm

❗ PEARLS & CONSIDERATIONS

COMMENTS

If the primary cause of glossitis is not identified or cannot be corrected, enteric nutritional replacement therapy should be considered in malnourished patients.

RELATED CONTENT

Glossitis (Patient Information)

AUTHOR: **FRED F. FERRI, M.D.**

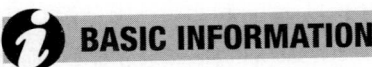

DEFINITION

Gonorrhea is a sexually transmitted bacterial infection with a predilection for columnar and transitional epithelial cells. It commonly manifests as urethritis, cervicitis, or salpingitis. Infection may be asymptomatic. It differs between males and females in course, severity, and ease of recognition.

SYNONYMS

Gonococcal urethritis
Gonococcal vulvovaginitis
Gonococcal cervicitis
Gonococcal bartholinitis
Clap
GC

ICD-9CM CODES

098 Gonococcal infections

EPIDEMIOLOGY & DEMOGRAPHICS

- The disease is common worldwide, affects both sexes and all ages, especially younger adults; highest incidence is in inner-city areas, with an estimated 700,000 new cases annually.
- Asymptomatic anterior urethral carriage may occur in 12% to 50% of cases in men.
- Asymptomatic in 50% to 80% of cases in women. Most common dissemination by mucosal passage to fallopian tubes, resulting in pelvic inflammatory disease (PID) in 10% to 15% of infected women. Hematogenous spread may result in septic arthritis and skin lesions. Conjunctivitis rarely occurs but may result in blindness if not rapidly treated. Infection can occur in both men and women in oropharynx and anorectally.
- 700,000 new infections per year (second most commonly reported bacterial STD).

PHYSICAL FINDINGS & CLINICAL PRESENTATION

- Males: purulent discharge from anterior urethra (Fig. 1-361). with dysuria appearing 2 to 7 days after infecting exposure. May have

rectal infection causing pruritus, tenesmus, and discharge or may be asymptomatic.
- Females: initial urethritis or cervicitis may occur a few days after exposure, frequently mild. In approximately 20% of cases uterine invasion occurs after menstrual period with signs and symptoms of endometritis, salpingitis, or pelvic peritonitis. The patient may have purulent discharge or inflamed Skene's or Bartholin's glands.
- Classic presentation of acute gonococcal PID is fever, abdominal and adnexal tenderness, and often absence of purulent discharge. Physical examination may be normal if asymptomatic. Disseminated gonococcal infection may manifest with various skin lesions (Fig. 1-362).

ETIOLOGY

- *Neisseria gonorrhoeae* is the gonococcus. Plasmids coding for β-lactamase render some strains resistant to penicillin or tetracycline. There is an increasing frequency of chromosomally mediated resistance to penicillin, tetracycline, fluoroquinolones, and cefoxitin. In the Far East, high-level resistance to spectinomycin is endemic.
- There are a rising number of cases of quinolone-resistant *N. gonorrhoeae* worldwide, with the expected number to rise in the U.S. from importation.
- Men who have sex with men are vulnerable to the emerging threat of antimicrobial-resistant *N. gonorrhoeae*.

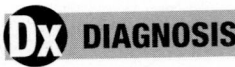

DIFFERENTIAL DIAGNOSIS

- Nongonococcal urethritis (NGU)
- Nongonococcal mucopurulent cervicitis
- *Chlamydia trachomatis*

WORKUP

- Diagnosis depends on bacteriologic investigation.
- Gram-negative intracellular diplococci are diagnostic in male urethral smears (Fig. 1-363). There is a false-negative rate of 60% to 70% in female cervical or urethral smears. Culture, nucleic acid hybridization tests, and nucleic acid amplification tests (NAATs) are available for the detection of genitourinary infection with *N. gonorrhoeae*. Culture and nucleic acid hybridization tests require female endocervical or male urethral swab specimen. NAATs allow testing of the widest variety of specimen types including endocervical swabs, vaginal swabs, urethral swabs (men), and urine (from both men and women).

LABORATORY TESTS

- Gonorrhea culture on Thayer-Martin medium (organism is fastidious; requires aerobic conditions with increased carbon dioxide atmosphere; incubate ASAP). Culture has a sensitivity of 95% or more for urethral specimens from men with symptomatic urethritis and 80% to 90% for endocervical infection in women.
- NAATs: These tests have largely replaced culture in many settings where persons are

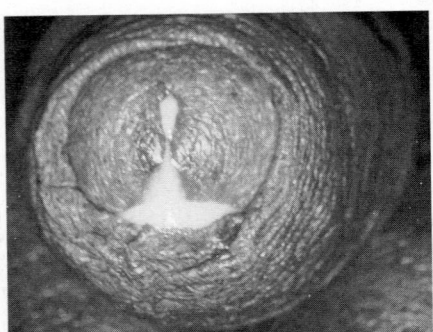

FIGURE 1-361 Purulent urethral discharge from a man with gonococcal urethritis. (From Mandell GL et al: *Principles and practice of infectious diseases,* ed 6, Philadelphia, 2005, Churchill Livingstone.)

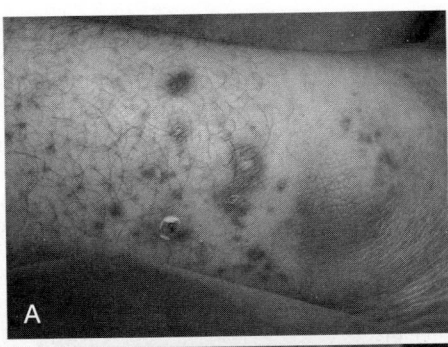
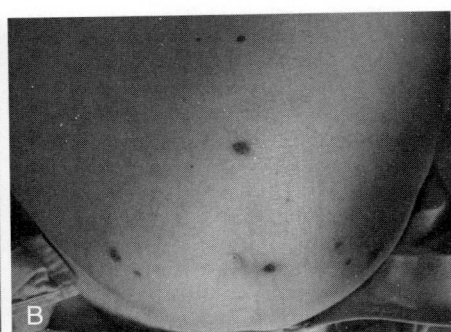
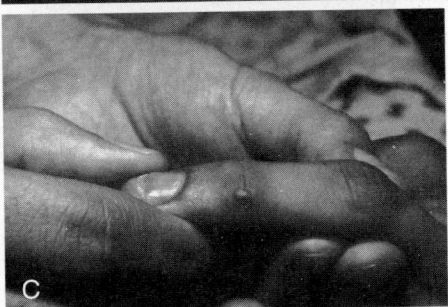

FIGURE 1-362 Disseminated gonococcal infection: skin lesions. A, Macules, papules, and pustules over an ankle. B, Hemorrhagic papules localized in trunk. C, Hemorrhagic vessel over a distal interphalangeal joint. (C Courtesy of Dr. Peter Schlessinger. From Hochberg MC et al: *Rheumatology,* ed 5, St Louis, 2011, Mosby.)

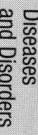

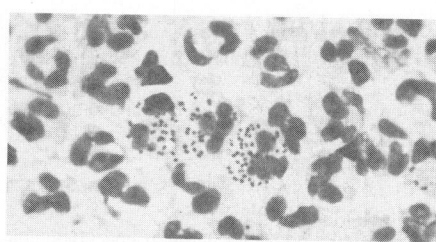

FIGURE 1-363 *Neisseria gonorrhoeae.* Gram stain of urethral exudate in gonorrhea, showing intracellular gram-negative reniform diplococci. (Courtesy of Dr S.E. Thompson. From Hochberg MC et al: *Rheumatology,* ed 5, St Louis, 2011, Mosby.)

screened for asymptomatic genital infection. They are not more sensitive than culture for detecting *N. gonorrhoeae* in cervical or urethral specimen; however, they have specificities >99% and retain sensitivity when used to test voided urine or self-collected vaginal swabs.
- Nonamplified DNA probe tests are less sensitive than culture or NAATs and are not useful in the diagnosis of rectal or pharyngeal infection or for testing urine; however, they are inexpensive, readily available and offered in many laboratories in combination assays for *C. trachomatis.*
- Concomitant serologic testing for syphilis on all patients
- Concomitant *Chlamydia* testing on all patients
- Offer of HIV testing and counseling to all patients

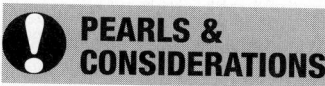

Rx TREATMENT

ACUTE GENERAL Rx
Uncomplicated infections of the cervix, urethra, and rectum:
- Ceftriaxone 250 mg IM × 1 dose *plus* azithromycin 1 g PO single dose *or* doxycycline 100 mg PO bid for 7 days

Alternative regimens:
- Cefixime 400 mg PO x 1 dose *plus* azithromycin 1 g orally single dose *or* doxycycline 100 mg PO bid for 7 days *plus* test of cure in 1 wk
- If the patient has severe cephalosporin allergy, then azithromycin 2 g PO single dose *plus* test of cure in 1 wk

Uncomplicated gonococcal infections of the pharynx:
- Ceftriaxone 250 mg IM x 1 dose *plus* azithromycin 1 g PO single dose *or* doxycycline 100 mg PO bid for 7 days

DISPOSITION
- Pregnant patients require test of cure (as do those treated with regimens other than ceftriaxone/doxycycline); reculture 4 to 7 days after treatment.
- To reduce development of drug resistance, the CDC has recently modified guidelines and recommends reculture of patients who show continued symptoms despite treatment. These patients should be tested with a culture-based gonorrhea test that can detect antibiotic resistance.
- All sexual partners should be identified, examined, tested, and receive presumptive treatment.

REFERRAL
PID requiring hospitalization, disseminated gonococcal infection

PEARLS & CONSIDERATIONS

COMMENTS
- This is a reportable disease.
- The proportion of gonorrhea cases in heterosexual men who are fluoroquinolone resistant (QRNG) has reached 6.7%, an elevenfold increase from 0.6% in 2001. Fluoroquinolone antibiotics are no longer recommended to treat gonorrhea in the U.S.
- The use of azithromycin as the second antimicrobial is preferred over doxycycline due to the high prevalence of tetracycline resistance.

SUGGESTED READINGS
available at www.expertconsult.com

RELATED CONTENT
Cervicitis (Related Key Topic)
Chlamydia Genital Infections (Related Key Topic)
Pelvic Inflammatory Disease (Related Key Topic)
Gonorrhea (Patient Information)

AUTHORS: **MARIA A. CORIGLIANO, M.D.,** and **RUBEN ALVERO, M.D.**

G

Diseases and Disorders

I

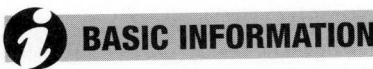

DEFINITION

Goodpasture's syndrome is an antiglomerular basement membrane antibody involving the lung and kidney. It is characterized by idiopathic recurrence of alveolar hemorrhage and rapidly progressive glomerulonephritis. It can also be defined by the triad of glomerulonephritis, pulmonary hemorrhage, and antibody to basement membrane antigens.

ICD-9CM CODES
446.2 Goodpasture's syndrome

EPIDEMIOLOGY & DEMOGRAPHICS

- Goodpasture's syndrome affects predominantly young, white, male smokers.
- Male/female ratio is 6:1.
- Goodpasture's syndrome accounts for 5% of all cases of rapidly progressive glomerulonephritis.
- 80% of patients are HLA-BR2 positive.

PHYSICAL FINDINGS & CLINICAL PRESENTATION

- Dyspnea, cough, hemoptysis
- Skin pallor, fever, arthralgias (may be mild or absent at the time of initial presentation)

ETIOLOGY

Presence of glomerular basement membranes (GBM) antibody deposition in kidneys and lungs with subsequent pulmonary hemorrhage and glomerulonephritis. In the kidneys circulating antibodies bind to the non-collagenous-1 (NC1) domain of type IV collagen in the GBM.

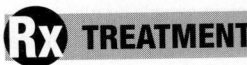 **DIAGNOSIS**

DIFFERENTIAL DIAGNOSIS

- Wegener's granulomatosis
- Systemic lupus erythematosus
- Systemic necrotizing vasculitis
- Idiopathic rapidly progressive glomerulonephritis
- Drug-induced renal pulmonary disease (e.g., penicillamine)

WORKUP

Laboratory evaluation, diagnostic imaging, immunofluorescence studies of renal biopsy

LABORATORY TESTS

- Presence of circulating serum anti-GBM antibodies
- Absence of circulating immunocomplexes, antineutrophils, cytoplasmic antibodies, and cryoglobulins
- Urinalysis revealing microscopic hematuria and proteinuria
- Elevated blood urea nitrogen and creatinine from rapidly progressive glomerulonephritis
- Immunofluorescence studies of renal biopsy material: linear deposits of anti-GBM antibody, often accompanied by C3 deposition
- Anemia from iron deficiency (from blood loss and iron sequestration in the lungs)

IMAGING STUDIES

Chest radiograph: fluffy alveolar infiltrates, evidence of pulmonary hemorrhage (Fig. 1-364)

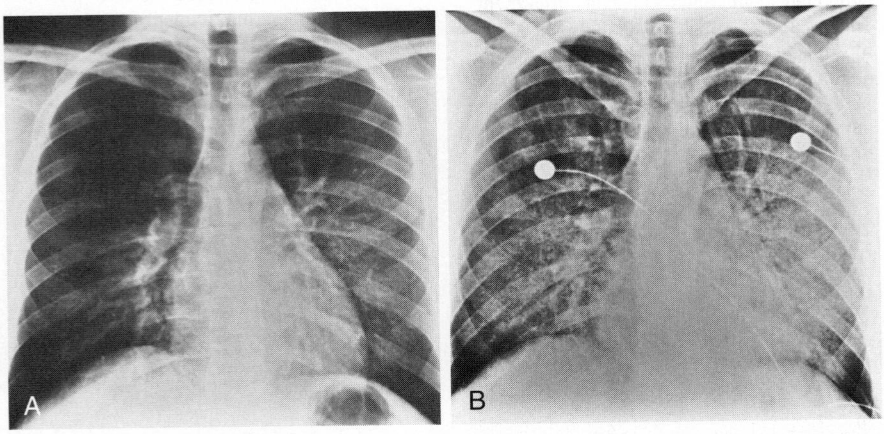

TREATMENT

ACUTE GENERAL Rx

- Combined use of plasmapheresis using albumin replacement for 1-2 wk with immusuppressive therapy with prednisone (1 mg/kg/day) and cyclophosphamide (2 mg/kg/day)
- Dialysis support in patients with renal failure
- Factors influencing decision to treat or not to treat aggressively in Goodpasture's disease are described in Table 1-172

DISPOSITION

Life-threatening pulmonary hemorrhage and irreversible glomerular damage are the major causes of death.

REFERRAL

- Referral for renal biopsy to guide the management
- Consideration for renal transplantation in patients with end-stage renal failure

SUGGESTED READINGS
available at www.expertconsult.com

RELATED CONTENT
Goodpasture's Syndrome (Patient Information)

AUTHOR: **FRED F. FERRI, M.D.**

FIGURE 1-364 Goodpasture's syndrome. Posteroanterior chest radiographs several days apart demonstrate consolidation in the left lung **(A),** which progressed to diffuse alveolar disease (consolidation) **(B).** (From McLoud TC [ed]: *Thoracic radiology: the requisites,* St Louis, 1998, Mosby.)

TABLE 1-172 Factors Influencing Decision to Treat or Not to Treat Aggressively in Goodpasture's Disease

	Factors Favoring Aggressive Treatment	Factors Against Aggressive Treatment
Pulmonary hemorrhage	Present	Absent
Oliguria	Absent	Present
Creatinine	<5.5 mg/dl (approximately 500 μmol/L)	>5.5-6.5 mg/dl (approximately 500-600 μmol/L) and ANCA negative Severe damage on kidney biopsy No desire for early kidney transplantation
Other factors	Creatinine >5.5-6.5 mg/dl (approximately 500-600 μmol/L) *but* Rapid and recent progression ANCA positive Glomerular damage less severe than expected Crescents recent, nonfibrous Early renal transplantation desired	
Associated disease	Absent	Unusually high risk from immunosuppression

ANCA, Antineutrophil cytoplasmic antibody.
From Floege J et al: *Comprehensive clinical nephrology,* ed 4, Philadelphia, 2010, Saunders.

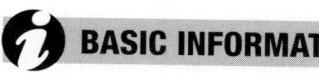

BASIC INFORMATION

DEFINITION

Gout is a term used to refer to a group of disease states caused by tissue deposition of monosodium urate due to prolonged hyperuricemia. Clinical manifestations of gout include acute arthritis, soft tissue inflammation, chronic tophus formation, gouty nephropathy, and nephrolithiasis. Untreated hyperuricemia in patients with gout may lead to chronic destructive deforming arthritis

> **ICD-9CM CODES**
> 274.00 Gouty arthritis
> 274.01 Acute gout
> 274.02 Chronic gout
> 274.03 Gout with tophus

EPIDEMIOLOGY & DEMOGRAPHICS

PREVALENCE: 5 cases per 1000 persons in the United States. Incidence is rising.
PREDOMINANT SEX: Male/female ratio ~4:1
PREDOMINANT AGE: 30 to 50 yr in men. Older than 60 yr in women

ETIOLOGY

- Hyperuricemia and gout develop from excessive uric acid production, a decrease in the renal excretion of uric acid, or both.
- Primary hyperuricemia results from an inborn error of metabolism and may be attributed to several biochemical defects.
- Secondary hyperuricemia may develop as a complication of acquired disorders (e.g., leukemia) or as a result of the use of certain drugs (e.g., diuretics). Consumption of alcohol, especially beer, increases the risk of gout, and fructose-rich beverage intake is associated with hyperuricemia. Lead toxicity can lead to gouty arthritis. Blood lead levels in the range currently considered acceptable are associated with increased prevalence of gout and hyperuricemia.
- Individuals with hyperuricemia who are predisposed with genetic factors develop clinical gout.

PHYSICAL FINDINGS & CLINICAL PRESENTATION

ACUTE GOUT:
- Rapid onset of pain and swelling and erythema of a distal joint and/or periarticular soft tissue. Table 1-173 summarizes key components of gout flares

> **TABLE 1-173** Key Components of Gout Flares
>
> - Marked tenderness and swelling of affected joint
> - Acute onset with maximum pain in 4-12 hr
> - Recurrent pattern of similar attacks
> - Marked impairment of physical function
> - Resolution of symptoms within 3-14 days
>
> From Hochberg MC et al: *Rheumatology,* ed 5, St Louis, 2011, Mosby.

- May present as monoarthritis of any joint. Acute gout of the first metatarsophalangeal (MTP) joint (Fig. 1-365) is known as *podagra*
- 10% to 15% of attacks are polyarticular
- Spontaneous resolution occurs over days to weeks

CHRONIC TOPHACEOUS GOUT (Fig. 1-366)
- Insidious onset of painless arthritis and soft tissue swelling
- Distal small joints characteristic
- May be confused with nodal osteoarthritis

DIAGNOSIS

DIFFERENTIAL DIAGNOSIS OF ACUTE GOUT

- Infectious arthritis
- Cellulitis
- Pseudogout

DIFFERENTIAL DIAGNOSIS OF CHRONIC GOUT

- Osteoarthritis (especially nodal OA in women)
- Rheumatoid arthritis
- Psoriatic arthritis
Section II describes the differential diagnosis of acute monoarticular and oligoarticular arthritis.

WORKUP

Arthrocentesis and examination of synovial fluid (Fig. E1-367 and Box E1-21)

LABORATORY TESTS

- Uric acid: All patients with gout are hyperuricemic at some time, but during an acute attack the serum uric acid may be normal or low.

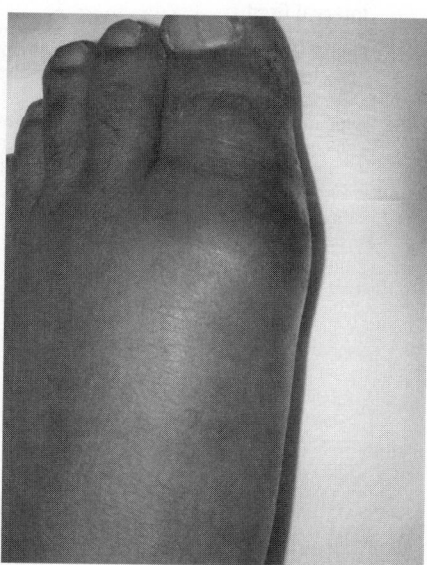

FIGURE 1-365 Podagra or acute gout of the first metatarsophalangeal (MTP) joint is shown. The hyperintense erythema with a dusky hue is characteristic. The area of inflammation usually extends beyond the area of the involved joint. (From Hochberg MC et al: *Rheumatology,* ed 5, St Louis, 2011, Mosby.)

- Synovial aspirate: usually cloudy and markedly inflammatory in nature. Urate crystals in fluid are needle-shaped and strongly negatively birefringent under polarized microscopy.
- CBC: mild leukocytosis often present
- Inflammatory markers: ESR and CRP often elevated

IMAGING STUDIES

- Plain radiography for diagnosis and evaluation.
- No typical findings in early gouty arthritis but late disease is associated with characteristic punched-out marginal erosions and overhanging edges

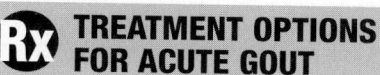

TREATMENT OPTIONS FOR ACUTE GOUT

- Nonsteroidal anti-inflammatory medication (see Table 1-174)
  - Indomethacin 75 mg bid
  - Ibuprofen 800 mg tid
  - Naproxen 500 mg bid
- Low-dose colchicine (less toxic and as effective as traditional high-dose colchicine): 1.2 mg colchicine PO, followed by 0.6 mg PO 1 hr later.
- Intra-articular corticosteroid injection (treatment of choice for monoarticular large joint attack): Triamcinolone hexacetomide 40 mg or equivalent for knee
- Systemic corticosteroid therapy: Prednisone 40 mg PO for 3 days, then taper over 10 days (effective and safe, but evidence is lacking)

NONPHARMACOLOGIC THERAPY

Lifestyle and dietary modification may be effective in highly motivated patients. Should be attempted only in patients with modestly elevated uric acid, as dietary modification can only lower uric acid 1 mg%. Discontinuation of diuretic therapy may help.

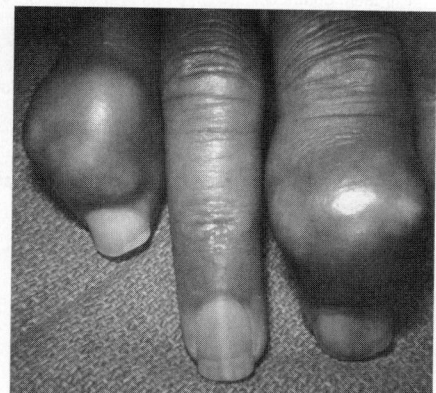

FIGURE 1-366 Large tophi involving the distal interphalangeal joints are commonly seen in gouty patients with preexisting Heberden's nodes. This is particularly characteristic of late-onset gout. (From Hochberg MC et al: *Rheumatology,* ed 5, St Louis, 2011, Mosby.)

PHARMACOLOGIC TREATMENT OF SYMPTOMATIC HYPERURICEMIA

ALLOPURINOL: Allopurinol is very effective and safe when used properly. Correct dosing and patient compliance are essential elements in the prevention of erosive and tophaceous gout. Patients with renal insufficiency are at increased risk for allopurinol hypersensitivity, which is manifest as fever, rash, and hepatitis occurring most commonly in the first 3 mo of therapy. The rash may progress to life-threatening toxic epidermal necrolysis is not recognized early.

Therapy with allopurinol should be initiated several weeks after the acute attack has resolved. The initial dose should be low (≤100 mg/day depending on creatinine clearance) in patients with renal insufficiency and those with very high uric acid levels. The serum uric acid should be reevaluated after 4-6 wk of therapy, and the allopurinol dose adjusted to reduce the serum uric acid to less than 6 mg%. The most common therapeutic dosage of allopurinol is 300 mg/day, but dose may be increased by 50-100 mg every two to three weeks until the target serum uric acid level is achieved. There is evidence that increasing allopurinol doses in patients with renal insufficiency does not result in significant adverse events. Some authors have reported using doses as high as 800 mg daily without excess toxicity.

FEBUXOSTAT: Novel xanthine oxidase inhibitor that has been shown to be more potent than allopurinol 300 mg daily for reducing serum uric acid. The chemical structure of febuxostat is different from allopurinol, making cross-reactive allergy unlikely. The metabolism of febuxostat is primarily hepatic, which obviates the need for dose adjustments due to renal insufficiency. Some cases of hepatic toxicity have been reported, and it is recommended that liver function tests be monitored periodically. Febuxostat has not been tested in patients with severe renal failure.

The primary indication for febuxostat is demonstrated allergy to allopurinol. The cost of febuxostat may be as much as 40 times that of allopurinol.

BENEMID and SULFINPYRAZONE: These uricosuric agents may only be used in patients with good renal function and urinary uric acid less than 600 mg in a 24-hr collection. Compliance is poor due to necessity of taking drugs more often than once daily

PEGLOTICASE: Intravenous pegylated uricase was approved by the FDA in 2010 for treatment of severe refractory tophaceous gout. It is a pegylated recombinant mammalian uricase that rapidly degrades urate when given intravenously. Use is limited by very high cost and significant toxicities including frequent gout flares and anaphylaxis.

PATIENT/FAMILY EDUCATION

It is essential that patients, families, physicians, and other members of the health care team appreciate the importance of compliance with a daily allopurinol regimen if recurrent flares and progression to chronic arthritis and tophi are to be avoided. Allopurinol should be discontinued only for symptoms suggesting the hypersensitivity syndrome. It should be continued during flares, medical illnesses, and surgical procedures.

REFERRAL

- Rheumatologist if diagnosis is not clear or therapy is complicated
- Podiatrist for management of pedal complications

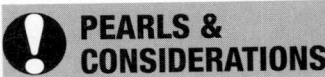

PEARLS & CONSIDERATIONS

Do not stop allopurinol during hospitalizations, surgery, or acute attacks unless there is evidence of drug allergy.

SUGGESTED READINGS

available at www.expertconsult.com

RELATED CONTENT

Gout (Patient Information)

AUTHOR: **BERNARD ZIMMERMANN, M.D.**

TABLE 1-174 Treatment of Gout

Acute Gout	Interval Gout	Treatment of Hyperuricemia
NSAIDs (preferred): Indomethacin 50 mg qid or ibuprofen 800 mg tid (or other NSAID in full doses). Contraindicated in patients with renal insufficiency and gastrointestinal disorders.	**Colchicine, oral:** 0.6-1.2 mg/day as prophylaxis against recurrent attacks. **NSAIDs may also be used for prophylaxis.**	**Colchicine, oral:** 0.6-1.2 mg/day for 4-6 wk before initiating hypouricemic therapy and for several months afterward to prevent recurrent attacks during initiation of hypouricemic therapy.
Or	**Hypouricemic agent:** Indicated for patients with recurrent attacks despite prophylaxis, severe hyperuricemia, presence of tophi, urolithiasis, or gouty arthritis	*And*
Colchicine, oral: 1.2 mg followed by a second dose of 0.6 mg 1 hr later. Contraindicated in patients with renal insufficiency and gastrointestinal disorders	**Other:** Weight loss, reduce alcohol (especially beer), diet low in seafood, red meat, organ meat, and fructose	**Allopurinol:** Initial dose 100 mg/day in patients with renal insufficiency or very high uric acid levels. Increase dose as needed to attain uric acid less than 6 mg/dl.
Or		*Or*
Intra-articular steroids (Treatment of choice for large joint monoarthritis): Triamcinolone 40 mg or equivalent for knee		**Uricosuric agent** (Use only in patients with good renal function and <600 mg uric acid in a 24-hr collection): probenecid, 0.5-1 g bid, or sulfinpyrazone 100 mg tid or qid
Or		**Other:** Consider febuxostat for patients allergic to allopurinol. Pegloticase may be useful for selected patients with severe tophaceous gout.
Systemic steroid therapy (for patients in whom NSAIDs and colchicine are contraindicated)		
Prednisone 30-50 mg PO daily or in divided doses. May use lower dose in diabetic or postsurgical patients.		

NSAIDs, Nonsteroidal anti-inflammatory drugs.

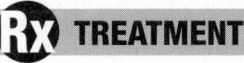
G

Diseases and Disorders

I

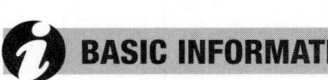 **BASIC INFORMATION**

DEFINITION

Granuloma annulare (GA) is a chronic, usually self-limited, inflammatory disorder of the dermis that classically presents as arciform to annular plaques located on the extremities.

SYNONYMS

Pseudorheumatoid nodule—subcutaneous granuloma annulare
GA

ICD-9CM CODES
695.89 Granuloma annulare

EPIDEMIOLOGY & DEMOGRAPHICS

- Most common in children and young adults; most cases of localized GA are diagnosed in patients <30 yr
- Female predominance (2:1)
- Disseminated form associated with diabetes mellitus
- Recurrent in 40% of affected individuals
- A generalized form of GA can occur in up to 15% of patients

PHYSICAL FINDINGS & CLINICAL PRESENTATION

- The four main clinical variants of GA are localized (75%), disseminated (>10 lesions), subcutaneous (occurring primarily in children aged 2 to 5 yr), and perforating (rare form manifesting with 1- to 4-mm papules with a central crust).
- Localized GA starts as a small ring of colored skin or pale erythematous papules.
- Lesions coalesce and evolve into annular plaques over several weeks.
- Plaques undergo central involution and increase in diameter over several months (0.5 to 5 cm) (Fig. 1-368).
- Most frequently found on the lateral and dorsal surfaces of the hands and feet.
- Most lesions resolve spontaneously after several months.
- The generalized form of GA is characterized by hundreds to thousands of small, flesh-colored papules in a symmetric distribution on the trunk and extremities.
- Deep dermal (subcutaneous GA) presents as large, painless, skin-colored nodules that are frequently mistaken for rheumatoid nodules.

ETIOLOGY

Unknown, but may be related to vasculitis, trauma, monocyte activation, or delayed hypersensitivity.

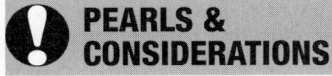 **DIAGNOSIS**

DIFFERENTIAL DIAGNOSIS

- Tinea corporis
- Lichen planus
- Necrobiosis lipoidica diabeticorum
- Sarcoidosis
- Rheumatoid nodules
- Late secondary or tertiary syphilis
- Arcuate and annular plaques of mycosis fungoides
- Papular GA can simulate insect bites, secondary syphilis, xanthoma
- Annular elastolytic giant cell granuloma

WORKUP

- Diagnosis based on clinical appearance and presentation
- Biopsy when diagnosis is unclear

LABORATORY TESTS

- No laboratory tests will help confirm the diagnosis.

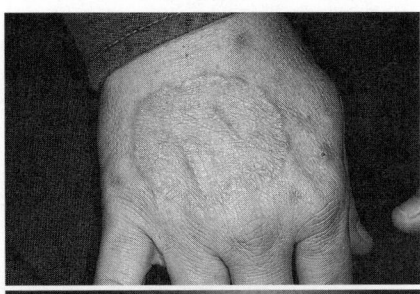
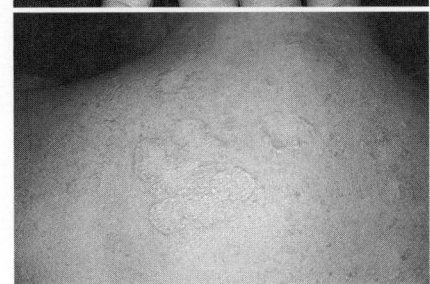

FIGURE 1-368 Granuloma annulare. (From Callen JP [ed]: *Color atlas of dermatology,* ed 2, Philadelphia, 2000, Saunders.)

- Biopsy shows focal degeneration of collagen and elastic fibers, mucin deposition, and perivascular and interstitial lymphohistiocytic infiltrate in the upper and middle dermis.

Rx TREATMENT

NONPHARMACOLOGIC THERAPY

Reassurance, given the self-limited and benign nature of GA

CHRONIC Rx

High-potency topical corticosteroids with or without occlusion and intralesional steroid injection into elevated border with triamcinolone 2.5 to 10 mg/ml are useful first-line local therapies.

- Cryosurgery, psoralen ultraviolet-A (UVA) range or UVA-1 therapy, and carbon dioxide laser treatment can also be used.
- Systemic agents (e.g., niacinamide, hydroxychloroquine, chloroquine, cyclosporine, dapsone) are generally reserved for severe cases. Recent case reports indicate positive outcomes with tacrolimus and pimecrolimus and the tumor necrosis factor infliximab.

DISPOSITION

Most lesions resolve spontaneously within 2 yr.

REFERRAL

Dermatology referral recommended for symptomatic, disseminated disease

! PEARLS & CONSIDERATIONS

COMMENTS

GA has been described as a paraneoplastic granulomatous reaction to Hodgkin's disease, non-Hodgkin's lymphoma, solid organ tumors, and mycosis fungoides.

SUGGESTED READING
available at www.expertconsult.com

RELATED CONTENT

Granuloma Annulare (Patient Information)

AUTHOR: **FRED F. FERRI, M.D.**

BASIC INFORMATION

DEFINITION
Granulomatosis with polyangiitis (**Wegener's granulomatosis**) is a multisystem disease generally consisting of the classic triad of:
1. Necrotizing granulomatous lesions in the upper or lower respiratory tract
2. Generalized focal necrotizing vasculitis involving both arteries and veins
3. Focal glomerulonephritis of the kidneys
   "Limited forms" of the disease can also occur and may evolve into the classic triad; granulomatosis with polyangiitis can be classified using the "ELK" classification, which identifies the three major sites of involvement: *E,* ears, nose, and throat or respiratory tract; *L,* lungs; *K,* kidneys.

SYNONYMS
Wegener's granulomatosis

ICD-9CM CODES
446.4 Wegener's granulomatosis

EPIDEMIOLOGY & DEMOGRAPHICS
INCIDENCE: 3/100,000 persons, equal in men and women
MEAN AGE AT ONSET: 41 yr

PHYSICAL FINDINGS & CLINICAL PRESENTATION
- Clinical manifestations often vary with the stage of the disease and degree of organ involvement. 90% of patients present with symptoms involving the upper or lower airways or both.
- Frequent manifestations are:
  1. Upper respiratory tract: chronic sinusitis, chronic otitis media, mastoiditis, nasal crusting, obstruction and epistaxis, nasal septal perforation, nasal lacrimal duct stenosis, saddle nose deformities (resulting from cartilage destruction) (Fig. 1-370)
  2. Lung: hemoptysis, multiple nodules, diffuse alveolar pattern
  3. Kidney: renal insufficiency, glomerulonephritis
  4. Skin: necrotizing skin lesions
  5. Nervous system: mononeuritis multiplex, cranial nerve involvement
  6. Joints: monarthritis or polyarthritis (nondeforming), usually affecting large joints
  7. Mouth: chronic ulcerative lesions of the oral mucosa, "mulberry" gingivitis
  8. Eye: proptosis, uveitis, episcleritis, retinal and optic nerve vasculitis

ETIOLOGY
Unknown

DIAGNOSIS

DIFFERENTIAL DIAGNOSIS
- Other granulomatous lung diseases (e.g., sarcoidosis, lymphomatoid granulomatosis, Churg-Strauss syndrome, necrotizing sarcoid granulomatosis, bronchocentric granulomatosis, sarcoidosis); the differential diagnosis of granulomatous lung disease is described in Section II
- Neoplasms (especially lymphoproliferative disease)
- Goodpasture's syndrome
- Bacterial or fungal sinusitis
- Midline granuloma
- Viral infections
- Other causes of glomerulonephritis (e.g., poststreptococcal nephritis)

WORKUP
- Granulomatosis with polyangiitis should be suspected in anyone presenting with sinus disease that does not respond to conventional treatment, pulmonary hemorrhage, glomerulonephritis, mononeuritis multiplex resulting in wrist or foot drop, progressive migratory arthralgias or arthritis, and unexplained multisystem disease.
- Chest x-ray, laboratory evaluation, PFTs, and tissue biopsy.

LABORATORY TESTS
- Positive test for cytoplasmic pattern of ANCA (c-ANCA).
- Anemia, leukocytosis.
- Urinalysis: may reveal hematuria, RBC casts, and proteinuria.
- Elevated serum creatinine, decreased creatinine clearance.
- Increased ESR, positive rheumatoid factor, and elevated C-reactive protein may be found.

IMAGING STUDIES
- Chest x-ray: may reveal bilateral multiple nodules, cavitated mass lesions, pleural effusion (20%). Up to one third of patients without pulmonary signs or symptoms have an abnormal chest x-ray (Fig. 1-371).
- Computed tomography (Fig. 1-372)
- PFTs: useful in detecting stenosis of the airways.
- Biopsy of one or more affected organs should be attempted; the most reliable source for tissue diagnosis is the lung. Lesions in the nasopharynx (if present) can be easily biopsied but biopsy is positive in only 20%. Biopsy of radiographically abnormal pulmonary parenchyma provides the highest yield (>90%).

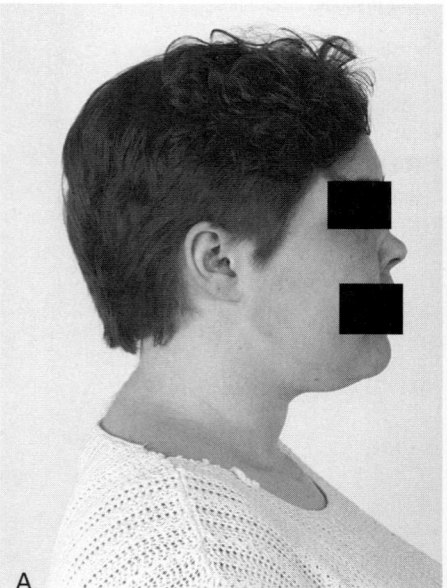
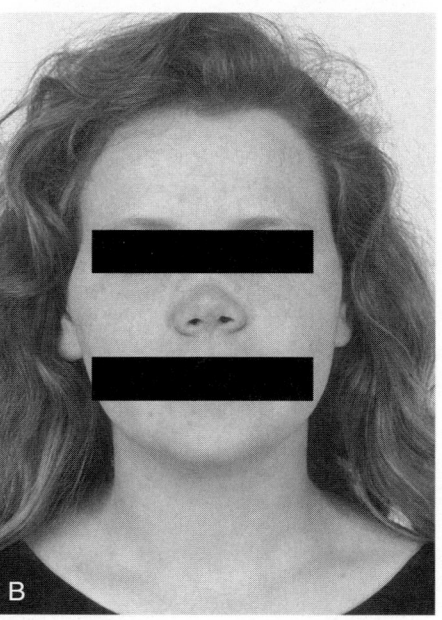

FIGURE 1-370 A and **B,** Saddle nose deformity resulting from collapse of the nasal cartilage in Wegener's granulomatosis. (From Hochberg MC et al: *Rheumatology,* ed 5, St Louis, 2011, Mosby.)

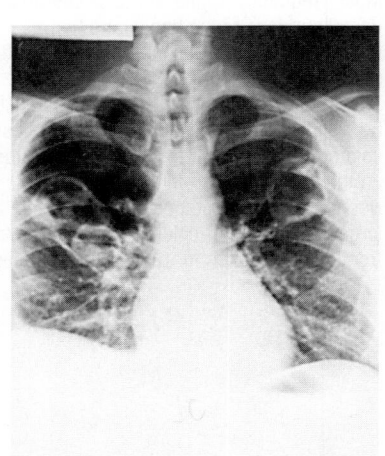

FIGURE 1-371 Chest radiograph shows multiple cavitary pulmonary nodules in patient with Wegener's granulomatosis. (From Weinberg SE et al: *Principles of pulmonary medicine,* ed 5, Philadelphia, 2008, Saunders.)

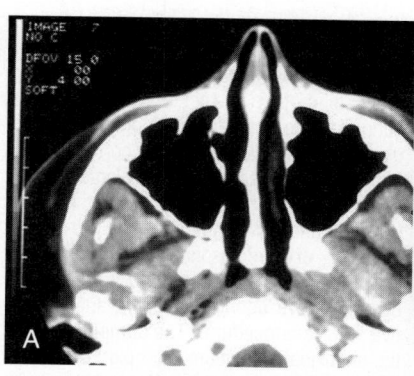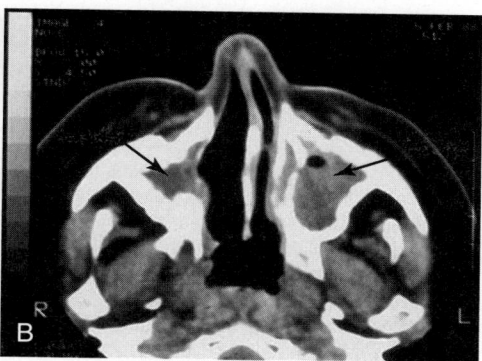

FIGURE 1-372 Computed tomography (CT) scans of the sinuses. A, Normal maxillary sinuses in a recently diagnosed Wegener's granulomatosis (WG) patient. **B,** Sinus CT scan of a patient with long-standing WG: nasal septal deviation to the left, destruction of the medial walls of the right maxillary sinus, opacification of both sinuses with soft tissue densities *(arrows),* and neo-ossification of all maxillary bony structures due to chronic inflammation. (From Hochberg MC et al: *Rheumatology,* ed 5, St Louis, 2011, Mosby.)

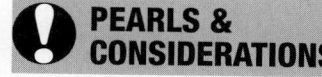 **TREATMENT**

NONPHARMACOLOGIC THERAPY
- Ensure proper airway drainage.
- Give nutritional counseling.

ACUTE GENERAL Rx
- Prednisone 60 to 80 mg/day and cyclophosphamide 2 mg/kg are generally effective and are used to control clinical manifestations; once the disease comes under control, prednisone is tapered and cyclophosphamide is continued. Other potentially useful agents in patients intolerant to cyclophosphamide are rituximab, methotrexate, azathioprine, and mycophenolate mofetil. Recent trials involving rituximab show that it is not inferior to daily cyclophosphamide treatment for induction of remission in severe ANCA-associated vasculitis and may be superior in relapsing disease.
- TMP-SMX therapy may represent a useful alternative in patients with lesions limited to the upper or lower respiratory tracts in absence of vasculitis or nephritis. Treatment with TMP-SMX (160 mg/800 mg bid) also reduces the incidence of relapses in patients with granulomatosis with polyangiitis in remission. It is also useful in preventing *Pneumocystis jirovecii* pneumonia, which occurs in 10% of patients receiving induction therapy. When used for prophylaxis, dose of TMP-SMX (160 mg/800 mg) is 1 tablet three times/wk.

DISPOSITION
Five-year survival with aggressive treatment is approximately 80%; without treatment 2-yr survival is <20%.

REFERRAL
Surgical referral for biopsy

(!) PEARLS & CONSIDERATIONS

COMMENTS
- Methotrexate (20 mg/wk) represents an alternative to cyclophosphamide in patients who do not have immediately life-threatening disease.
- C-ANCA levels should not dictate changes in therapy, because they correlate erratically with disease activity.
- The incidence of venous thrombotic events in granulomatosis with polyangiitis is significantly higher than the general population. Clinicians should maintain a heightened awareness of the risks of venous thrombosis and a lower threshold for evaluating patients for possible DVT or pulmonary embolism.

SUGGESTED READINGS
available at www.expertconsult.com

RELATED CONTENT
Wegener's Granulomatosis (Patient Information)

AUTHOR: **FRED F. FERRI, M.D.**

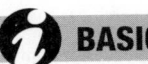 **BASIC INFORMATION**

DEFINITION

Graves' disease is a hypermetabolic state caused by circulating IgG antibodies that bind to and activate the G-protein–coupled thyrotropin receptor. This activation stimulates follicular hypertrophy and hyperplasia, causing thyroid enlargement as well as increases in thyroid hormone production. It is characterized by thyrotoxicosis, diffuse goiter, and infiltrative ophthalmopathy (edema and inflammation of the extraocular muscles and an increase in orbital connective tissue and fat); infiltrative dermopathy characterized by lymphocytic infiltration of the dermis; accumulation of glycosaminoglycans; and occasionally edema.

SYNONYMS

Thyrotoxicosis

ICD-9CM CODES
242.0 Toxic diffuse goiter

EPIDEMIOLOGY & DEMOGRAPHICS

INCIDENCE/PREVALENCE: Hyperthyroidism affects 2% of women and 0.2% of men in their lifetimes. More than 80% of these cases are caused by Graves' disease.
PREDOMINANT AGE: Peak incidence is between 40 and 60 yr.
GENETICS: Increased prevalence of HLA-B8 and HLA-DR3 in whites with Graves' disease. Concordance rate is 20% among monozygotic twins.

PHYSICAL FINDINGS & CLINICAL PRESENTATION

- Tachycardia, palpitations, tremor, hyperreflexia
- Goiter, exophthalmos (50% of patients), lid retraction, lid lag
- Nervousness, weight loss, heat intolerance, atrial fibrillation
- Increased sweating, brittle nails, clubbing of fingers
- Localized dermopathy (1% to 2% of patients) is most frequent over the anterolateral aspects of the skin but can be found at other sites (especially after trauma)
- Men may have gynecomastia, reduced libido, and erectile dysfunction. Women often have irregular menses

ETIOLOGY

Autoimmune etiology: the activity of the thyroid gland is stimulated by the action of T cells, which induce specific B cells to synthesize antibodies against thyroid-stimulating hormone (TSH) receptors in the follicular cell membrane.

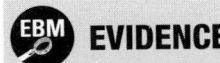 **DIAGNOSIS**

DIFFERENTIAL DIAGNOSIS

- Anxiety disorder
- Premenopausal state
- Thyroiditis
- Other causes of hyperthyroidism (e.g., toxic multinodular goiter, toxic adenoma)
- Other: metastatic neoplasm, diabetes mellitus, pheochromocytoma

WORKUP

The diagnostic workup includes a detailed medical history followed by laboratory and imaging studies and ECG. Patients often present with anxiety, heat intolerance, menstrual dysfunction, increased appetite, and weight loss. Elderly patients can have an atypical presentation (apathetic hyperparathyroidism). For additional information, refer to the topic "Hyperthyroidism."

LABORATORY TESTS

- Increased free thyroxine (T_4) and free triiodothyronine (T_3)
- Decreased TSH
- Presence of thyroid-stimulating immunoglobulin or thyrotropin-receptor antibodies (useful in selected patients to differentiate Graves' disease from toxic nodular goiter)

IMAGING STUDIES

- 24-hr radioactive iodine uptake (RAIU): increased homogeneous uptake
- CT or MRI of the orbits is useful if there is uncertainty about the cause of ophthalmopathy

TREATMENT

NONPHARMACOLOGIC THERAPY

- Patient education and discussion of therapeutic options
- Smoking cessation: smoking is associated with an increased risk of progression of Graves' ophthalmopathy.

ACUTE GENERAL Rx

- Antithyroid drugs (ATDs) to inhibit thyroid hormone synthesis or peripheral conversion of T_4 to T_3:
  1. Methimazole or propylthiouracil (PTU) are available. Methimazole is generally preferred because it has a longer half-life, allowing for once-daily dosing. PTU is preferred during pregnancy.
  2. Side effects: skin rash (3% to 5%), arthralgias, myalgias, granulocytopenia (0.5%); rare side effects: aplastic anemia, hepatic necrosis (PTU), cholestatic jaundice.
- Radioactive iodine (RAI):
  1. Treatment of choice for patients >21 yr and younger patients who have not achieved remission after 1 yr of ATD therapy
  2. Contraindicated during pregnancy and lactation
- Surgery: near-total thyroidectomy is rarely performed. Indications: obstructing goiters despite RAI and ATD therapy, patients who refuse RAI and cannot be adequately managed with ATDs, and pregnant women inadequately managed with ATDs.
- Adjunctive therapy: Beta-adrenergic receptor blockers (e.g., atenolol 25 to 100 mg/day) to alleviate the β-adrenergic symptoms of hyperthyroidism (tachycardia, tremor); contraindicated in patients with bronchospasm.
- Graves' ophthalmopathy: methylcellulose eye drops to protect against excessive dryness, sunglasses to decrease photophobia, intraocular and systemic high-dose corticosteroids for severe exophthalmos. Worsening of ophthalmopathy after RAI therapy is often transient and can be prevented by the administration of prednisone. Other treatment options include antiinflammatory and immunosuppressive agents, radiation, and corrective surgical procedures. The administration of the antioxidant selenium (100 µg PO bid) has been recently reported as effective in improving quality of life, reducing ocular involvement, and slowing progression of the disease in patients with mild Graves' orbitopathy. Its mechanism of action is believed to be an effect on the oxygen free radicals and cytokines that play a pathogenic role in Graves' orbitopathy.

CHRONIC Rx

Patients undergoing treatment with ATDs should be seen every 1 to 3 mo until euthyroidism is achieved and every 3 to 4 mo while they are receiving ATDs.

DISPOSITION

- ATDs induce sustained remission in <60% of cases.
- The incidence of hypothyroidism after RAI is >50% within the first year and 2% per year thereafter.
- Complications of surgery include hypothyroidism (28% to 43% after 10 yr), hypoparathyroidism, and vocal cord paralysis (1%).
- Successful treatment of hyperthyroidism requires lifelong monitoring for the onset of hypothyroidism or the recurrence of thyrotoxicosis.
- RAI therapy is followed by the appearance or worsening of ophthalmopathy more often than is therapy with methimazole, particularly in patients who are cigarette smokers. It can be prevented with the administration of prednisone 0.5 mg/kg body weight per day starting 2 to 3 days after RAI, continued for 1 mo, then tapered off over 2 mo.
- Mild to moderate ophthalmopathy often improves spontaneously. Severe cases can be treated with high-dose glucocorticoids, orbital irradiation, or both. Orbital decompression may be used in patients with optic neuropathy and exophthalmos (see "Hyperthyroidism").

EVIDENCE

available at www.expertconsult.com

SUGGESTED READINGS

available at www.expertconsult.com

RELATED CONTENT

Graves' Disease (Patient Information)
Hyperthyroidism (Related Key Topic)

AUTHOR: **FRED F. FERRI, M.D.**

BASIC INFORMATION

DEFINITION

Guillain-Barré syndrome (GBS) is an acute immune-mediated polyradiculoneuropathy (affects nerve roots and peripheral nerves), with predominant motor involvement. It is the most common cause of acute flaccid paralysis in the Western hemisphere and probably worldwide. By definition, maximal clinical weakness occurs within 4 wk of disease onset.

SYNONYMS

AIDP (acute inflammatory demyelinating polyradiculoneuropathy)
Acute polyneuropathy
Ascending paralysis
Postinfectious polyneuritis

ICD-9CM CODES
357.0 Guillain-Barré syndrome

EPIDEMIOLOGY & DEMOGRAPHICS
INCIDENCE:
- 0.6 to 1.9 cases/100,000 persons annually without geographic variation. Incidence increases with age. A slight peak in incidence occurs between late adolescence and early adulthood. A slight male preponderance (1.25:1) also exists.
- GBS consists of several clinical variants based on the pattern of clinical involvement and electrophysiologic findings. These include:
  - AIDP (most common form in Europe and North America)
  - Acute motor axonal neuropathy (AMAN; most prevalent form in China and Japan)
  - Acute motor and sensory axonal neuropathy (AMSAN; has more severe sensory involvement and is associated with more severe clinical course and poorer prognosis)
  - Miller Fisher syndrome (MFS; triad of ophthalmoplegia, ataxia, and areflexia)
  - Acute pandysautonomia (rapid onset of parasympathetic and sympathetic failure without motor or sensory involvement)
  - Regional variants (e.g., pharyngeal-cervical-brachial GBS, pure ataxic GBS)

PREDISPOSING FACTORS: Viral (HIV, CMV, EBV, influenza) and bacterial (*Campylobacter jejuni, Mycoplasma pneumoniae*) infections; systemic illness (Hodgkin's lymphoma, immunizations). Major antecedents of GBS are described in Box 1-22.

PHYSICAL FINDINGS & CLINICAL PRESENTATION
- Symmetric weakness starts in either distal or proximal appendicular muscles with ascending or descending progression, respectively; difficulty in ambulating, getting up from a chair, or climbing stairs.
- Depressed or absent reflexes bilaterally.
- Minimal to moderate glove and stocking paresthesias/dysesthesia/anesthesia or back pain.
- Pain (caused by involvement of posterior nerve roots) may be prominent.
- Autonomic abnormalities (brady- or tachyarrhythmias, hypo- or hypertension).
- Respiratory insufficiency (caused by weakness of bulbar/intercostal muscles).
- Facial paresis, ophthalmoparesis, dysphagia (secondary to cranial nerve involvement).

ETIOLOGY
- Unknown
- Preceding infectious illness 1 to 4 wk before disease onset in 66% of patients
- Humoral and cell-mediated immune attack of peripheral nerve myelin, Schwann cells; sometimes with primary axonal involvement

DIAGNOSIS

DIFFERENTIAL DIAGNOSIS
- Toxic peripheral neuropathies: heavy metal poisoning (lead, thallium, arsenic), medications (vincristine, disulfiram), organophosphate poisoning, hexacarbon (glue sniffer's neuropathy)
- Nontoxic peripheral neuropathies: acute intermittent porphyria, fulminant vasculitic polyneuropathy, infectious (poliomyelitis, diphtheria, Lyme disease, West Nile virus); tick paralysis
- Neuromuscular junction disorders: myasthenia gravis, botulism, snake envenomations
- Myopathies such as polymyositis, acute necrotizing myopathies caused by drugs
- Metabolic derangements such as hypermagnesemia, hypokalemia, hypophosphatemia
- Acute CNS disorders such as basilar artery thrombosis with brain stem infarction, brain stem encephalomyelitis, transverse myelitis, or spinal cord compression
- Hysterical paralysis or malingering

WORKUP
1. Exclude other causes based on clinical history, examination, and laboratory tests.
2. Lumbar puncture (may be normal in the first 1 to 2 wk of the illness).
   Typical findings include elevated CSF protein with few mononuclear leukocytes (albuminocytologic dissociation) in 80% to 90% of patients. Elevated CSF cell counts is an expected feature in cases associated with HIV seroconversion.
3. EMG/NCS: may be normal in the first 10 to 14 days of the disease. The earliest electrodiagnostic abnormality is prolongation or absence of H-reflexes. EMG/NCS evidence of demyelination (prolonged distal latency, conduction velocity slowing, conduction block, temporal dispersion, and prolonged F-waves) in two or more motor nerves confirms diagnosis of AIDP in the appropriate clinical context.

LABORATORY TESTS
- CBC may reveal early leukocytosis with left shift. Electrolytes are tested to exclude metabolic causes.
- Heavy metal testing, urine porphyria screen, creatine kinase, HIV titers, neuroimaging of the brain and spinal cord if diagnosis uncertain. Nerve root enhancement may be seen on MRI of the lumbosacral spine.
- Antibodies against ganglioside GQ1b may be present in up to 90% of patients with MFS. IgG antibodies against ganglioside GM1 may be associated with AMAN. There are no antiganglioside antibodies commonly associated with AIDP.
- In equivocal cases (especially if peripheral nerve vasculitis is a concern), nerve biopsy may aid in confirming a diagnosis of GBS. Sensory nerve biopsy demonstrates segmental demyelination with infiltration of monocytes and T cells into the endoneurium. Axonal loss is commonly seen in sensory nerve biopsy specimens in GBS.

TREATMENT

NONPHARMACOLOGIC THERAPY
- Close monitoring of respiratory function (frequent measurements of vital capacity, negative inspiratory force, and pulmonary toilet), because respiratory failure is the major complication in GBS
- Frequent repositioning of patient to minimize formation of pressure sores

---

BOX 1-22   Major Antecedents of Guillain-Barré Syndrome

Frequent
Upper respiratory tract infections
Campylobacter jejuni enteritis
Cytomegalovirus infection
Epstein-Barr virus infection
Hepatitis A infection
Hepatitis B infection
Hepatitis C infection
HIV infection

Infrequent
Mycoplasma pneumoniae infection
Haemophilus influenzae infection
Leptospira icterohaemorrhagiae infection
Salmonellosis

Rabies vaccine
Tetanus toxoid
Bacille Calmette-Guérin immunization
Sarcoidosis
Systemic lupus erythematosus
Lymphoma
Trauma
Surgery

Questionable
Hepatitis B vaccine
Influenza vaccine
Hyperthermia
Epidural anesthesia

- Prevention of thromboembolism with anti-thrombotic stockings and SC heparin (5000 U q12h) in nonambulatory patients
- Emotional support and social counseling

ACUTE GENERAL Rx

- Infusion of IV immunoglobulins (IVIG; 0.4 g/kg/day for 5 days). Always check serum IgA levels before infusion to prevent anaphylaxis in rare deficient patients.
- Early therapeutic plasma exchange (TPE or plasmapheresis: 200 to 250 ml/kg over five sessions every other day), started within 7 days of onset of symptoms, is beneficial in reducing the need for mechanical ventilation in patients with rapidly progressive disease and results in improved rate of recovery. It is contraindicated in patients with cardiovascular disease (recent MI, unstable angina), active sepsis, and autonomic dysfunction.
- There is no proven benefit from combining IVIG and plasma exchange.
- Mechanical ventilation may be needed if FVC is <12 to 15 ml/kg, vital capacity is rapidly decreasing or is <1000 ml, negative inspiratory force <20 cm H_2O, PaO_2 is <70, the patient is having significant difficulty clearing secretions or is aspirating.

CHRONIC Rx

- Ventilatory support may be necessary in up to 30% of patients. Adequate fluid/electrolyte support and nutrition are necessary, especially in patients with dysautonomia or bulbar dysfunction.
- Aggressive nursing care to prevent decubitus, infections, fecal impactions, and pressure nerve palsies.
- Monitoring and treatment of autonomic dysfunction (bradyarrhythmias or tachyarrhythmias, orthostatic hypotension, systemic hypertension, altered sweating).

- Treatment of back pain and dysesthesia with low-dose tricyclics, gabapentin, and so on. Opiate narcotics can be used cautiously in the short term but may compound dysautonomia.
- Stress ulcer prevention in patients receiving ventilator support.
- Physical and occupational therapy rehabilitation, including supportive devices.

DISPOSITION

- Mortality is approximately 5% to 10% worldwide. Causes of death include cardiac arrest, pulmonary embolism, and fulminant infections. A recent study showed 62% complete motor recovery, 14% mild weakness, 9% moderate weakness, 4% bed-bound or ventilated, and 8% dead at 1 yr. Another study suggested that about 33% of patients were free from sensory symptoms at 1 yr, with residual sensory loss present in the lower extremities in 67% and 36% in the upper extremities. About 32% had to change their work, 30% were unable to function at home as well as they could before the disease, and 52% had to alter their leisure activities 1 yr after GBS onset. Excessive fatigue is a common complaint in patients during the recovery phase of GBS. This may be treated with exercise therapy (e.g., bicycle exercise training).
- Predictors for poor recovery (inability to walk independently at 1 yr): age >60 yr, preceding diarrheal illness, recent CMV infection, fulminant or rapidly progressing course, ventilatory dependence, reduced motor amplitudes (<20% normal), or inexcitable nerves on NCS. Outcomes may also be influenced by complications of medical therapy.
- GBS is typically a monophasic illness. Recurrence may occur in <5% of patients following full recovery.

REFERRAL

Tracheostomy may be necessary in patients with prolonged ventilatory support. Percutaneous endoscopic gastrostomy may be temporarily required.

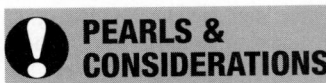

PEARLS & CONSIDERATIONS

- GBS is the most common cause of acute flaccid paralysis.
- Close monitoring of ventilatory function with respiratory mechanics (FVC and NIF) is of paramount importance in all patients with suspected GBS.
- Corticosteroids are of no benefit in the treatment of GBS and may even delay recovery.

COMMENTS

Patient education information may be obtained from the GBS/CIDP Foundation International, The Holly Building, 104 1/2 Forrest Avenue, Narberth, PA 19072; phone: (610) 667-0131; fax: (610) 667-7036; toll-free: (866) 224-3301; E-mail: info@gbs-cidp.org

SUGGESTED READINGS

available at www.expertconsult.com

RELATED CONTENT

Guillain-Barré Syndrome (Patient Information)

AUTHOR: **EROBOGHENE E. UBOGU, M.D.**

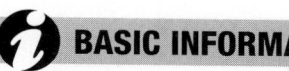

BASIC INFORMATION

DEFINITION

Gynecomastia is a benign enlargement of male breast, resulting from proliferation of glandular breast tissue.

ICD-9CM CODES
611.1 Gynecomastia

EPIDEMIOLOGY

- Most common reason for male breast evaluation.
- Seen in patients of all age groups.
- 60% to 90% of infants have transient gynecomastia due to high estrogenic state of pregnancy.
- Prevalence during adolescence ranges from 4% to 69%. It results from transient increase of estradiol concentration at the onset of puberty.
- Higher incidence in body builders due to use of anabolic steroids.
- 24% to 65% of older men have gynecomastia. It is secondary to decreased testosterone production with advanced age, increased peripheral conversion of testosterone to estrogen, and at times from side effects of medications.

PATHOPHYSIOLOGY

Altered estrogen-androgen balance, in favor of estrogen.

ETIOLOGY

Physiologic
  Infancy
  Puberty
  Persistent pubertal gynecomastia seen in 25% of cases
  Elderly
Pathologic
  Idiopathic (25%)
  Increased estrogen production or action
    Testicular tumors (3%)
    Chronic liver disease
    Malnutrition
    Hyperthyroidism
    Adrenal tumors
    Familial gynecomastia
  Decreased testosterone production or action (10%)
    Testicular trauma
    Testicular torsion

Viral orchitis
Congenital anorchia
Renal failure (1%)
Hyperthyroidism (1.5%)
Malnutrition
Androgen insensitivity syndrome
Five-alpha reductase deficiency
Pituitary tumors
Kallmann syndrome
Klinefelter's syndrome
Medications (10% to 25%)
  Estrogen, gonadotropins, clomiphene, phenytoin, ketoconazole, metronidazole, metoclopramide, alkylating agents, busulfan, methotrexate, cisplatin, cimetidine, ranitidine, omeprazole, flutamide, finasteride, etomidate, HAART therapy, INH, tricyclic antidepressants, phenothiazines, diazepam, haloperidol, calcium channel blocker, ACE inhibitors, spironolactone, digoxin, amiodarone, methyldopa, alcohol, marijuana, heroin, methadone, amphetamine, anabolic steroids

CLINICAL FEATURES

- Although gynecomastia is usually bilateral, it could be unilateral.
- Characterized by concentric rubbery to firm disk of tissue, which is often mobile and located directly beneath the areola.
- Pain is usually not severe. Varying degree of tenderness and nipple sensitivity are more common than pain, usually in the first 6 mo.

DIAGNOSIS

- Good history and physical examination including review of all medications the patient is taking is helpful.
- Mammogram is recommended for suspected breast cancer.
- Serum concentration of hCG, LH, testosterone, and estradiol should be measured, preferably in the morning, unless the cause is clearly apparent. There is no uniformity of opinion regarding what biochemical evaluation, if any, should be performed in patients with asymptomatic gynecomastia (Fig. E1-373).

DIFFERENTIAL DIAGNOSIS

- Breast cancer
  - Mass is usually firm to hard
  - Unilateral
  - Eccentric in location

  - Could be associated with nipple discharge and retraction, lymphadenopathy, and skin dimpling
- Pseudogynecomastia or lipomastia
  - Characterized by fat deposition without glandular proliferation
  - Seen in obese men
  - Bilateral
  - Remain unchanged over time

TREATMENT

- Observation is recommended for most patients with physiologic gynecomastia. They often regress spontaneously. Reassurance and follow-up examination in 3 to 6 mo usually suffice.
- Treat the underlying cause, and stop the offending medications.
- Treatment is most effective in the early stages (first 6 mo). Medical therapy often fails when given for longstanding (>12 mo) cases because of the presence of fibrosis.
- Potential indications of early therapy include severe breast enlargement, pain, tenderness, and psychological embarrassment. Consider giving tamoxifen 10 mg orally twice a day to these patients for up to 3 mo. It is not FDA-approved for this purpose. It results in regression of gynecomastia in approximately 80% of patients and, of which, only 60% had complete regression. As far as breast symptoms, such as pain and tenderness, some improvement is usually seen within a month of therapy.
- Surgery is offered for symptomatic gynecomastia that does not respond to medical therapy. However, for adolescents, surgery is deferred until puberty is completed. The different surgical options include subcutaneous mastectomy, ultrasound-guided liposuction, and suction-assisted lipectomy.
- For prevention of gynecomastia in patients with prostate cancer using antiandrogen therapy, one could offer tamoxifen or radiotherapy.

SUGGESTED READINGS
available at www.expertconsult.com

RELATED CONTENT
Gynecomastia (Patient Information)

AUTHOR: **HEMANT K. SATPATHY, M.D.**

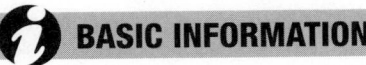

BASIC INFORMATION

DEFINITION

Hand-foot-mouth (HFM) disease is a viral illness characterized by superficial lesions of the oral mucosa and skin of the extremities. HFM is transmitted primarily by respiratory droplet contact in developed countries and feco-oral contact in developing countries. Although children are predominantly affected, adults are also at risk. This disease is usually self-limited and benign, although outbreaks in the Asia Pacific Region have been increasingly complicated by neurological and cardiopulmonary sequelae.

SYNONYMS

Vesicular stomatitis with exanthem
Coxsackie virus infection

ICD-9CM CODES

074.0 Hand-foot-mouth disease

EPIDEMIOLOGY & DEMOGRAPHICS

- Children <5 yr are at the highest risk and have the most severe cases.
- HFM is usually found in children <10 yr.
- HFM is contagious. Close contacts of affected children, including family members and health care workers, are the most commonly affected adults.
- Infection is spread from person to person by direct contact with nasal discharge or stool.
- A person is most contagious during the first week of illness.
- Outbreaks tend to occur during the summer.
- Infection leads to immunity, but a second episode may occur after infection with a different agent.

PHYSICAL FINDINGS & CLINICAL PRESENTATION

Symptoms:
- After a 4- to 6-day incubation period, patients may report odynophagia, sore throat, malaise, and fever (38.3° to 40° C).
- 1 to 2 days later the characteristic oral lesions appear.
- In 75% of cases skin lesions on the extremities accompany these oral manifestations.
- 11% of adults have cutaneous findings.
- Lesions appear over the course of 1 or 2 days.

Physical findings:
- Oral lesions, usually between five and ten, are commonly found on the tongue, buccal mucosa, gingivae, and hard palate.
- Oral lesions initially start as 1- to 3-mm erythematous macules and evolve into gray vesicles on an erythematous base.
- Vesicles are frequently broken by the time of presentation and appear as superficial gray ulcers with surrounding erythema.
- Skin lesions of the hands and feet start as linear erythematous papules (3 to 10 mm in diameter) that evolve into gray vesicles that may be mildly painful (Fig. 1-374). These vesicles are usually intact at presen-

tation and remain so until they desquamate within 2 wk.
- Involvement of the buttocks and perineum is present in 31% of cases.
- In rare cases, encephalitis, meningitis, myocarditis, poliomyelitis-like paralysis, and pulmonary edema may develop. Sporadic acute paralysis and long-term neurologic sequelae have been reported with enterovirus 71.
- Although information is limited, there is no clear evidence that pregnancy outcomes are affected.

ETIOLOGY

- Coxsackie virus group A, type 16, was the first and is the most common viral agent isolated.
- Coxsackie viruses A5, A7, A9, A10, B1, B2, B3, B5, and enterovirus 71 have also been implicated.
- Enterovirus 71 is neurotropic with predilection for the brainstem, leading to more severe cases of the disease. Infection rates have been rising in the Asian Pacific region.
- Epidemics have been reported with coxsackie A16 and enterovirus 71.

DIAGNOSIS

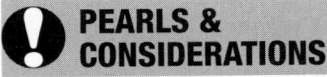

DIFFERENTIAL DIAGNOSIS

- Aphthous stomatitis
- Herpes simplex infection
- Herpangina
- Behçet's disease
- Erythema multiforme
- Pemphigus
- Gonorrhea
- Acute leukemia
- Lymphoma
- Allergic contact dermatitis

WORKUP

The diagnosis is usually made on the basis of history and characteristic physical examination.

LABORATORY TESTS

- Not indicated unless the diagnosis is in doubt.
- Throat culture or stool specimen may be obtained for viral testing but may take from 2 to 4 wk for results.

TREATMENT

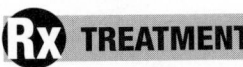

ACUTE GENERAL Rx

- Palliative therapy is given for this usually self-limited disease.
- There are currently no available approved therapies for more severe cases. Antivirals, steroids, and IV immunoglobulin have been tried for enterovirus 71 infections, but these treatments have not been evaluated in randomized, placebo-controlled studies.

DISPOSITION

Prognosis is excellent except in rare cases of central nervous system or cardiac involvement. Most are managed as outpatients.

REFERRAL

Not usually needed

PEARLS & CONSIDERATIONS

- Frequent handwashing, disinfection of contaminated surfaces, and washing of soiled articles of clothing can help reduce transmission.
- HFM has no relation to hoof and mouth disease in cattle.

SUGGESTED READINGS

available at www.expertconsult.com

RELATED CONTENT

Hand, Foot, and Mouth Disease (Patient Information)

AUTHORS: **JAMES J. NG, M.D.,** and **JENNIFER JEREMIAH, M.D.**

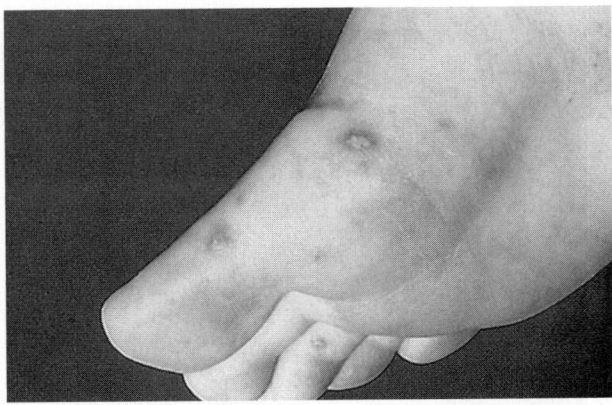

FIGURE 1-374 Hand-foot-mouth disease. Note oval lesions on an erythematous base. (From Goldstein B [ed]: *Practical dermatology,* ed 2, St Louis, 1997, Mosby.)

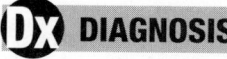

BASIC INFORMATION

DEFINITION

The term *cluster headache* refers to attacks of severe, unilateral pain that is orbital, supraorbital, temporal, or any combination of these sites, lasting 15 to 180 minutes, and occurring from once every other day to eight times a day. The attacks are associated with one or more of the following, all of which are ipsilateral: conjunctival injection, lacrimation, nasal congestion, rhinorrhea, forehead and facial sweating, miosis, ptosis, and eyelid edema. Most patients are restless or agitated during an attack.

SYNONYMS

Ciliary neuralgia
Erythromelalgia of the head
Erythroprosopalgia of Bing
Horton's headache

ICD-9CM CODES
339.00-339.02 Cluster headache

EPIDEMIOLOGY & DEMOGRAPHICS

INCIDENCE: Estimated to occur in 0.05% to 1% of the population
PREDOMINANT SEX: Occurs in males at least five times more commonly than in females
PREDOMINANT AGE: Peak age of onset between 20 and 40 yr
GENETICS: May be inherited (autosomal dominant) in approximately 5% of cases

PHYSICAL FINDINGS & CLINICAL PRESENTATION

- During attack: ipsilateral conjunctival injection, lacrimation, nasal congestion, rhinorrhea, facial sweating, Horner's syndrome.
- In contrast to migraine sufferers, patients are agitated and active during an attack.
- Permanent partial Horner's syndrome in 5% of patients; otherwise examination is normal.

ETIOLOGY

Activation of the posterior hypothalamic gray matter resulting in trigeminal activation coupled with parasympathetic activation. The pathophysiology remains controversial.

DIAGNOSIS

- Severe or very severe unilateral orbital, supraorbital, and/or temporal pain lasting 15 to 180 minutes.

- Frequency of every other day to eight per day; they may cluster seasonally or at a certain time in a patient's life.
- Headache is accompanied by at least one of the following (ipsilateral):
  1. Conjunctival injection and/or lacrimation
  2. Nasal congestion and/or rhinorrhea
  3. Eyelid edema
  4. Forehead and facial sweating
  5. Miosis and/or ptosis
  6. Restlessness or agitation

DIFFERENTIAL DIAGNOSIS

- Migraine
- Trigeminal neuralgia
- Temporal arteritis
- Postherpetic neuralgia
- Venous sinus thrombosis
- Carotid-cavernous fistula or other cavernous sinus lesions
- Other trigeminal autonomic cephalalgias
- Section II describes the differential diagnosis of headaches

WORKUP

Diagnosis is usually established by characteristic history.

IMAGING STUDIES

None, unless history or examination suggests focal neurologic deficit or headaches change in character or are of new onset.

TREATMENT

NONPHARMACOLOGIC THERAPY

Avoidance of alcohol, histamine, nitroglycerin, and tobacco during clusters

ABORTIVE Rx

- Inhalation of 100% oxygen by face mask for 15 min often aborts an attack.
- About 75% of users of triptans (sumatriptan, zolmatriptan) will be pain free within 20 minutes.
- Cafergot, octreotide, intranasal lidocaine, or dihydroergotamine may abort an attack or prevent one if given just before a predictable episode. Acute episode is typically resolved before oral analgesics become effective, although indomethacin and other NSAIDs may also be effective in prolonged attacks.

- Acute episode is typically resolved before oral analgesics become effective, although indomethacin and other NSAIDs may also be effective in prolonged attacks.

PROPHYLAXIS Rx

Various medications have been tried without great success, although good responses may be obtained in up to 50% of cases. Examples include:

- Valproic acid: start at 500 mg/day
- Topiramate: up to 50 mg bid
- Verapamil: up to 480 mg/day as tolerated
- Lithium: 200 mg tid with frequent monitoring and adjustment to maintain therapeutic serum level of 0.4 to 1 mEq/L. Equally effective as verapamil, but with more side effects
- Methysergide: 1 to 2 mg tid; requires familiarity with the potential adverse effects and use of "drug holidays" to decrease risk of fibrosis
- Ergotamine tartrate: 3 to 4 mg/day during clusters
- Prednisone: 60 mg PO qd for 1 wk followed by taper; headaches can return during taper
- There is emerging evidence for benefit of a sphenopalatine ganglion block that may be available at some centers, for treatment and prophylaxis of cluster attacks.

DISPOSITION

Headache-free periods tend to increase with increasing age.

REFERRAL

Refractory cluster headaches may require referral to a headache specialist.

PEARLS & CONSIDERATIONS

COMMENTS

- Cluster headaches are divided into episodic (attacks lasting up to 1 yr with more than 1 mo pain-free periods) and chronic (>1 yr without remission).
- Home oxygen therapy is reasonable for cluster headache sufferers.

SUGGESTED READINGS
available at www.expertconsult.com

RELATED CONTENT
Cluster Headaches (Patient Information)
AUTHOR: **SIDDHARTH KAPOOR, M.D.**

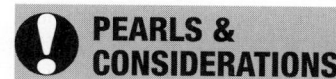

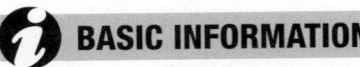
DEFINITION

Migraine headaches are recurrent headaches preceded by a focal neurologic symptom (migraine with aura), occur independently (migraine without aura), or have atypical presentations (migraine variants). The migraine aura typically is characterized by visual or sensory symptoms that develop over a period of 5 to 60 min. If the aura includes motor weakness, the migraine is referred to as hemiplegic. In both migraine with and without aura the headache is typically unilateral, pulsatile, and associated with nausea and vomiting, photophobia, and phonophobia. Migraines that occur ≥15 days every month for ≥3 mo are known as chronic; otherwise, they are referred to as episodic.

ICD-9CM CODES
346 Migraine

EPIDEMIOLOGY & DEMOGRAPHICS

INCIDENCE: Increases from infancy, peaks during the third decade of life, then decreases
PREVALENCE (IN U.S.): Females: 18%; males: 6%. More than 50% of persons affected by migraine headaches report reduced work or school productivity.
PREDOMINANT SEX: Female/male ratio of 3:1
GENETICS:
- Familial predisposition: more than 50% of migraine sufferers have an affected family member
- Autosomal-dominant transmission for some rare migraine variants (familial hemiplegic migraine, cerebral autosomal-dominant arteriopathy with subcortical infarcts and leukoencephalopathy [CADASIL]); familial hemiplegic migraines have been associated with calcium channelopathy, sodium channelopathy, and Na^+/K^+- ATPase dysfunction.

PHYSICAL FINDINGS & CLINICAL PRESENTATION

- Normal between episodes.
- Normal for migraine without aura. Focal motor or sensory abnormalities possible with migraine with aura or migraine variants.
- Common aura types include scintillating scotomata, bright zigzags, homonymous visual disturbance such as paresthesias, speech disturbances, or hemiparesis (familial or sporadic hemiplegic migraine). Other visual phenomena include image distortion or "Alice in Wonderland" effect.

ETIOLOGY

The pathophysiology of migraines is not clearly understood. It is believed that a primary neuronal event results in a trigeminovascular reflex causing neurogenic inflammation. Serotonin, substance P, nitric oxide, and calcitonin gene-related peptide also play a role, but the exact mechanism is unknown. Cortical spreading depression is probably responsible for the aura.

Migraine without aura:
- Five attacks fulfilling criteria
- Headache attacks lasting 4 to 72 hr
- Headache has at least two of the following characteristics:
  1. Unilateral location
  2. Pulsating quality
  3. Moderate or severe pain intensity
  4. Aggravation or causing avoidance of routine physical activity
- At least one of the following during headache:
  1. Nausea and/or vomiting
  2. Photophobia and phonophobia

Migraine with aura:
- At least two attacks
- Aura consisting of at least one of the following, but no motor weakness:
  1. Fully reversible visual symptoms, including positive and/or negative features
  2. Fully reversible sensory symptoms, including positive and/or negative features
- At least two of the following:
  1. Homonymous visual symptoms and/or unilateral sensory symptoms
  2. At least one aura symptom develops gradually over >5 min and/or different aura symptoms occur in succession over >5 min
- A migraine occurring during or within 60 min of the aura

DIFFERENTIAL DIAGNOSIS

- A diagnosis of migraine is possible only after five recurrent episodes.
- The first or the worst headache should always be investigated and the differential includes headaches from all secondary causes.
- Headache red flags can be remembered by the mnemonic SNOOP:
  ○ S: systemic symptoms of fever, weight loss
  ○ S: secondary risk factors of immunosuppression from any cause, cancer
  ○ N: neurologic deficits, altered consciousness
  ○ O: onset is sudden, abrupt, or split second
  ○ O: older, age >50 for new-onset headache should be worked up for giant cell arteritis
  ○ P: previous headache history is different or there is a change to headache
- Section II describes the differential diagnosis of headaches

WORKUP

- In general, no additional investigation is needed with recurrent, typical attacks with usual age of onset, family history, and a normal physical examination.
- If there is an unusual presentation and/or unexpected findings on examination, investigation for other causes is required.

LABORATORY TESTS

Lumbar puncture for history of abrupt-onset headaches and uncertain diagnosis of migraine

IMAGING STUDIES

- Imaging should be done in patients with headaches and an unexplained abnormal finding on the neurologic examination.
- Imaging should be considered in patients with rapidly increasing headache frequency, history of dizziness or incoordination, headache causing wakening from sleep, or headaches worsening with Valsalva maneuver.

Consider the use of a headache log/diary to identify triggers of headaches, record efficacy of treatments, and track history of the headaches.

NONPHARMACOLOGIC THERAPY

- Avoid any identifiable provoking factors: caffeine, tobacco, and alcohol may trigger attacks, as may dietary or other environmental precipitants (less common)
- Avoid stressors in life and minimize variations in daily routine with regular sleep, meals, and exercise
- Relaxation training, behavioral therapy, and biofeedback

ACUTE ANALGESIC Rx

- Many oral agents are ineffective because of poor absorption from migraine-induced gastric stasis. Non-oral route of administration should be selected in patients with severe nausea or vomiting.
- NSAIDs such as ketorolac, combination analgesics, or barbiturates may be used.

ACUTE ABORTIVE Rx

- IV antiemetics (prochlorperazine, metoclopramide, domperidone): Acute dystonic reactions and akathisia are rare side effects. These are generally not used as monotherapy.
- Ergotamine and ergotamine combinations (PO/PR) and dihydroergotamine (DHE 45) (SC, IV, IM, intranasal) have well-documented efficacy against migraines. DHE is usually administered in combination with an antiemetic drug (Table 1-176).
- Triptans (SC, PO, and intranasal) are now considered the drug class of choice for abortive therapy. Meta-analysis suggests that 10 mg rizatriptan, 80 mg eletriptan, and 12.5 mg almotriptan are most effective.
- Early administration improves effectiveness.
- There is an emerging role for the use of IV magnesium 1 g, IV valproate infusions to abort migraine headaches. IV dexamethasone up to 12 mg may be used for headaches lasting more than 72 hours.
- Greater and lesser occipital nerve blocks may also be performed to alleviate pain in the acute setting.

PROPHYLAXIS Rx

- Prophylactic treatment is generally indicated when headaches occur more than once a week or when symptomatic treatments are contraindicated or not effective. They are most effective when initiated during a headache-free period. All prophylaxis should

TABLE 1-176 Abortive and Analgesic Therapy for Migraine*

Drug	Route	Dose
Triptans (Serotonin Agonists)		
Sumatriptan	Subcutaneous	6 mg, repeat in 2 hr (max 2 doses/day)
Sumatriptan	Oral	25 mg, 50 mg, 100 mg, repeat in 2 hr (max 200 mg/day)
Sumatriptan	Nasal spray	5 mg, 20 mg, repeat in 2 hr (max 40 mg/day)
Zolmitriptan	Oral	1.25, 2.5, 5 mg, repeat in 2 hr (max 10 mg/day)
Zolmitriptan	Nasal spray	5 mg, repeat in 2 hr (max 10 mg/day)
Zolmitriptan	Orally disintegrating tab	2.5, 5 mg, repeat in 2 hr (max 10 mg/day)
Naratriptan	Oral	1 mg, 2.5 mg, repeat in 4 hr (max 5 mg/day)
Rizatriptan	Oral	5 mg, 10 mg, repeat in 2 hr (max 30 mg/day)
Almotriptan	Oral	6.25 mg, 12.5 mg, may repeat in 2 hr (max 25 mg/day)
Eletriptan	Oral	20 mg, 40 mg, may repeat in 2 hr (max 80 mg/day)
Frovatriptan	Oral	2.5 mg, may repeat in 2 hr (max 7.5 mg/day); may also be used for mini prophylaxis
Ergotamine Preparations		
Ergotamine and caffeine	Oral	2 tablets, may repeat 1 tab q30 min (max 6/day)
Ergotamine and caffeine	Rectal	1 suppository, repeat in 1 hr (max 2/day)
Ergotamine	Sublingual	1 tablet, repeat in 1 hr (max 2/day)
Dihydroergotamine	Intramuscular Subcutaneous Intravenous Nasal spray	0.5-1.0 mg, repeat twice at 1-hr intervals (max 3 mg/attack)
Sympathomimetics (with or without Barbiturates or Codeine)		
Isometheptene + dichloralphenazone + acetaminophen	Oral	1 to 2 capsules, repeat in 4 hr (max 8/day)
Nonsteroidal Anti-inflammatory Drugs		
Acetaminophen + (should not be used alone)	Oral	2 tablets, repeat in 6 hr (max 8/day aspirin + caffeine)
Naproxen	Oral	550-750 mg, repeat in 1 hr (max 3 times/wk)
Meclofenamate	Oral	100-200 mg, repeat in 1 hr (max 3 times/wk)
Flurbiprofen	Oral	50-100 mg, repeat in 1 hr (max 3 times/wk)
Ibuprofen	Oral	200-300 mg, repeat in 1 hr (max 3 times/wk)
Antiemetics		
Promethazine	Oral Intramuscular	50-125 mg No clear benefit in migraine, may be used
Prochlorperazine	Oral Rectal Intramuscular/IV	1-25 mg 2.5-25 mg (suppository) 5-10 mg, good evidence for strong benefit
Chlorpromazine	Oral Rectal Intravenous	10-25 mg 50-100 mg (suppository) Up to 35 mg, use with monitoring, some evidence for good benefit
Trimethobenzamide	Oral Rectal	250 mg 200 mg
Metoclopramide	Oral Intramuscular Intravenous	5-10 mg 10 mg 5-10 mg
Dimenhydrinate	Oral	50 mg

*For side effects and contraindications consult the manufacturer's drug insert before prescribing any of these drugs.
Modified from Wiederholt WC: *Neurology for non-neurologists,* ed 4, Philadelphia, 2000, Saunders.

be maintained for at least 3 mo before deeming the medication a failure.
- Well-established options for prophylactic treatment include β-blockers (propranolol, timolol, atenolol, metoprolol), tricyclic antidepressants (amitriptyline), and the antiepileptic drugs topiramate and valproic acid.
- Less-established options include calcium channel blockers, selective serotonin reuptake inhibitors, and the antiepileptic drug gabapentin.
- The FDA has recently approved injection of onabotulinum toxin A (Botox) for prevention of headaches in adult patients with chronic migraines (≥15 headache days/mo for ≥3 mo). The recommended total dose is 155 total units administered intramuscularly every 12 wk divided among 31 sites in head and neck area (frontalis, corrugator, procerus, occipitalis, temporalis, trapezius, cervical paraspinal muscle group). A maximum of 195 units is allowed.

DISPOSITION
After age 30 yr, 40% of patients are migraine free.

REFERRAL
To neurologist if uncertain about diagnosis or treatment not effective

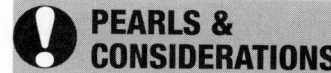

PEARLS & CONSIDERATIONS

- Avoid overuse of narcotics, barbiturates, caffeine, and benzodiazepines because they are habit-forming.
- Long-term use of analgesic medications can result in drug-induced or rebound headaches.

SUGGESTED READINGS
available at www.expertconsult.com

RELATED CONTENT
Migraine Headache (Patient Information)

AUTHOR: **SIDDHARTH KAPOOR, M.D.**

H

Diseases and Disorders

I

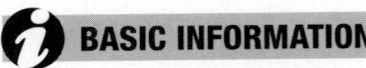

BASIC INFORMATION

DEFINITION

Tension-type headaches (TTH) are recurrent headaches lasting 30 min to 7 days without nausea or vomiting and with at least two of the following characteristics: pressing or tightening quality (nonthrobbing), mild or moderate intensity, bilateral, and not aggravated by routine physical activity.

SYNONYMS

Muscle contraction headache
Tension headache
Stress headache
Essential headache

ICD-9CM CODES

307.81 Tension headache

EPIDEMIOLOGY & DEMOGRAPHICS

INCIDENCE (IN U.S.): Most common type of headache; as high as 70% of all headaches presenting to primary care physician
PEAK INCIDENCE: Occurs at all ages
PREVALENCE (IN U.S.): Males: 63%/yr; females: 86%/yr
PREDOMINANT SEX: Females are affected more often than males

PHYSICAL FINDINGS & CLINICAL PRESENTATION

Pressure or "bandlike" tightness all around the head; may be worse at the vertex. Cervical, paracervical, and trapezius muscle spasm and/or tenderness on palpation may be present. Scalp tenderness or hypersensitivity to pain also occurs. Symptoms suggestive of migraine are usually not present (e.g., throbbing pain, nausea/vomiting, visual complaints, aura). Either one symptom of photo- or phonophobia does not exclude the diagnosis of TTH.

ETIOLOGY

- Unclear; little data to support postulated muscle contraction component. More likely a multifactorial disorder with several possible concurrent pathophysiologic mechanisms.
- No recent data to support the long-standing belief that these headaches arise from stress or other psychological factors. However, components of stress, sleep deprivation, hunger, and eyestrain may exacerbate symptoms. Stress and poor coping mechanisms may initiate and propagate pain (via activation of second messengers in downstream pain substrates). In episodic TTH, peripheral mechanisms are predominant, whereas central mechanisms are involved in chronic TTH.

DIAGNOSIS

DIFFERENTIAL DIAGNOSIS

- Migraine (would expect associated symptoms; see entry "Headache, Migraine")
- Cervical spine disease
- Intracranial mass (may present with focal neurologic signs, seizures, or headache awakening patient from sleep)
- Idiopathic intracranial hypertension (found more often in obese women of childbearing age, may have papilledema, visual loss, or diplopia)
- Rebound headache from overuse of analgesics
- Secondary headache (e.g., temporomandibular joint syndrome, thyrotoxicosis, polycythemia, drug side effects)
- Migraine and TTH may often coexist and may be difficult to differentiate (suggest headache calendar).
- Section II describes the differential diagnosis of headaches.

WORKUP

- Thorough history and physical examination for any new-onset headache
- Neuroimaging should be performed when unexplained neurologic findings are present on examination or in cases of atypical new-onset sudden and severe headaches.

LABORATORY TESTS

- No routine tests
- Erythrocyte sedimentation rate in elderly patients suspected of having temporal arteritis

IMAGING STUDIES

CT scan and/or MRI may be used to exclude intracranial pathology. MRI is better for imaging the posterior fossa. Contrast should be used if mass lesion is suspected.

TREATMENT

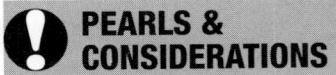

NONPHARMACOLOGIC THERAPY

- Electromyography (EMG) biofeedback has a documented effect, whereas cognitive-behavioral therapy and relaxation training are most likely effective (especially in adolescents and children).
- Physical therapy (including stretching exercises, massage, and ultrasound) and acupuncture may be effective, but there is no robust scientific evidence for efficacy.
- Schultz-type autogenic training (relaxation technique based on passive concentration and body awareness of specific sensations), transcutaneous electrical nerve stimulation, heat

ACUTE GENERAL Rx

Nonnarcotic analgesics (first choice) and combination analgesics containing caffeine (second choice) with limited frequency to prevent drug-induced and/or rebound headache

CHRONIC Rx

- Tricyclic antidepressants (e.g., amitriptyline 10 to 150 mg hs) (first choice); mirtazapine and venlafaxine (second choice); treatment may be limited by side effects.
- Avoid narcotics, limit NSAIDs, consider indomethacin; if related to cervical muscle spasm, may consider trial of muscle relaxants (e.g., Skelaxin 400 to 800 mg tid)
- Botulinum toxin A has been FDA approved for prophylactic treatment of chronic daily headaches. Trials have shown a small-to-modest benefit for chronic headaches but are not associated with fewer tension-type headaches per month.

DISPOSITION

May not respond fully to treatment

REFERRAL

If uncertain about diagnosis or unexplained focal neurologic findings on examination

PEARLS & CONSIDERATIONS

It is imperative to avoid overuse of caffeine- and barbiturate-containing medications because of the risk of rebound headaches.

SUGGESTED READINGS

available at www.expertconsult.com

RELATED CONTENT

Tension Headache (Patient Information)

AUTHOR: **RICHARD S. ISAACSON, M.D.**

BASIC INFORMATION

DEFINITION

Healthcare-associated infections (HAIs) are infections associated with healthcare, generally occurring more than 48 hr after admission to a hospital. Classification criteria are established by the National Healthcare Safety Network.

SYNONYMS

Nosocomial infections

ICD-9CM CODES
008.45 *Clostridium difficile*
041.12 MRSA
482.42 MRSA pneumonia
038.12 MRSA septicemia
998.59 Other postoperative infection
999.31 Bloodstream infection due to central venous catheter
997.31 Ventilator-assisted pneumonia
996.31 Due to urethral [indwelling] catheter

EPIDEMIOLOGY & DEMOGRAPHICS

INCIDENCE (IN U.S.):
- Develop in at least 5% of hospitalized patients; over 1.7 million patients.
- In 2002, HAIs accounted for more than 98,000 deaths.
- In 2002, the annual cost of HAIs in the U.S. was estimated as >$5 billion to $10 billion; adjusts to >$35 billion in 2007 values.
- At least one third of hospital-acquired infections are preventable.
- Leads to increased morbidity and mortality.

PREVALENCE (IN U.S.): 2 million to 4 million cases/yr

PREDOMINANT SEX:
- Overall, approximately equal
- Elderly women: predominantly nosocomial urinary tract infections

PREDOMINANT AGE: Newborns and elderly patients (>60 yr) at highest risk

PEAK INCIDENCE: Varies widely with infection site

RISK FACTORS: Patients with the following conditions can develop HAIs at any age:
- In ICU
- Intubation
- Chronic lung disease
- Renal disease
- Comatose
- Chronic urethral or vascular catheterization
- Malnutrition
- Postoperative state
- Diabetic

PHYSICAL FINDINGS & CLINICAL PRESENTATION

Vary with specific HAIs

ETIOLOGY

- Bacteria (gram-negative bacteria are responsible for >30% of HAIs)
- Fungi
- Viruses

SOURCES AND MODES OF TRANSMISSION:
- Patient's own flora
  - Comprises resistant organisms associated with hospitalization
  - Frequently maintained thereafter by persistent GI colonization
- Unwashed hands of staff
  - Physicians
  - Nurses
- Invasion of protective defenses (intact skin, respiratory cilia, urinary sphincters, and mucosa)
  - IV lines/central lines
  - Catheters
  - Respiratory equipment
  - Surgical wounds
  - Scopes and other imaging devices
- Failure to provide adequate negative pressure, high-volume air flow chambers for airborne infection isolation of patients with TB or disseminated herpes zoster/chickenpox
- Failure to rapidly identify and provide appropriate care (with isolation or precautions) for patients with communicable diseases
- Inanimate environment
  - Clinical equipment should be properly disinfected or sterilized per manufacturer's instructions.
  - High-touch items in patient environment should undergo frequent, thorough disinfection.
- Food
- Fomites
- Personnel attire can become contaminated. Although studies have not yet verified the link between attire contamination and disease transmission, cross-contamination of previously washed hands can occur
- Inattention to safe injection practices leads to outbreaks of hepatitis.
  - Do not administer medications from a syringe to multiple patients even if the needle is changed.
  - Use fluid infusion and administration sets (e.g., IV bags/bottles, tubing, connectors) for one patient only and dispose after each use. Do not use bags or bottles as a common source of supply for multiple patients.
  - Use single-dose vials for parenteral medications whenever possible and do not administer medications from single-dose vials to multiple patients or combine leftover contents for later use.

RISKS AMPLIFIED:
- Use of broad-spectrum antibiotics
  - Select highly resistant bacteria
  - Establish multidrug-resistant bacteria as endemic flora in microenvironments within the hospital
  - Consider antibiotic stewardship programs to reduce these risks
- Highly vulnerable patients with specific risk factors
  - Immunosuppression (as a result of therapy, transplantation, AIDS)
  - Old age
  - Postsurgery
  - Prolonged surgery
  - Chronic lung disease
  - Ventilator dependence
  - Antacid therapy
  - Vascular lines
  - Hyperalimentation
  - ICU stay
  - Recent antibiotic therapy
- Clustering of seriously ill patients
  - Often with wounds or contaminated drainage
  - Intensifying probability of cross-infection

PREVENTION STRATEGIES: Handwashing/hand hygiene between all patient contacts is the single most important method of decreasing HAI:
- Regular soap and water for at least 15 sec
- Chlorhexidine (particularly good for gram-positive organisms like methicillin-resistant *Staphylococcus aureus* [MRSA]), alcohol handrub or other antiseptic for resistant organisms
- Purpose of soap and water handwash
  - Degrease hand surfaces
  - Flushes away oils and associated bacteria, removal of visible dirt or body fluids
- Procedure
  - Lukewarm water
  - Must include all surfaces
  - Special attention to areas between fingers and to the dirtier dominant hand (most people reflexively wash the cleaner, non-dominant hand more vigorously)
- Alcohol handrubs
  - Improve handwashing frequency (less drying to hands, faster, and no need for wash basin and towels for drying)
  - Significantly reduce HAIs
  - Now recommended in essentially all routine healthcare settings
  - Rub hands until dry, approximately 15 sec

METHICILLIN-RESISTANT *STAPHYLOCOCCUS AUREUS* (MRSA)
- Invasive HAIs caused by MRSA decreased 9.4% per year from 2005 through 2008 in the United States.
- Healthcare-associated MRSA strains are typically resistant to many antibiotics, remaining susceptible to vancomycin and trimethoprim/sulfamethoxazole.
- High-risk factors include dialysis, recent stay in acute or long-term care facilities.
- Control measures include hand hygiene, disinfection of equipment, protective attire for isolation, and standard precautions.
- Community-acquired MRSA (CA-MRSA) is associated with soft tissue, presenting as boils, rash, or so-called spider bite, and typically occurs in patients who have no recent healthcare or hospital interaction.
- CA-MRSA often not found in nares.
- CA-MRSA can be sensitive to fluoroquinolones, clindamycin, and/or erythromycin in addition to vancomycin and trimethoprim/sulfamethoxazole.

Refer to Methicillin-Resistant Staphylococcus aureus (MRSA) topic for more information.

VANCOMYCIN-RESISTANT *ENTEROCOCCUS FAECIUM* (VREF):
- The percentage of HAIs caused by VREF increased more than twentyfold between 1989 and 1993, rising from 0% to 9%. By 2005,

VREF, vancomycin-resistant *E. faecalis,* and other vancomycin-resistant species of enterococci had become common and endemic nosocomial pathogens accounting for 15% to 40% of all enterococci isolated in the hospital setting.

- A high percentage of VREF isolated, 80%, are also ampicillin resistant.
- Factors predisposing to VREF colonization or infection include a high percentage of hospital days receiving antibiotic therapy, use of IV, underlying disease, immunosuppression, and abdominal surgery.
- Evidence suggests that the vehicle is the hands of healthcare workers (HCWs).
- Control measures:
  - Aggressive isolation of colonized or infected patients
  - Restraint in using broad-spectrum antibiotics
  - Compliance with hand hygiene best practices

Refer to the topic "Vancomycin-Resistant Enterococcus" for more information.

CLOSTRIDIUM DIFFICILE:
- Causes diarrhea as a result of pseudomembranous colitis.
- Accounts for 15% to 25% of healthcare-associated diarrhea.
- Warrants contact precautions and bleach for disinfection.
- Alcohol-based handrub may not eliminate spores of this organism, so can use soap and water to wash hands at sink.
- Spores can be dispersed in the air or room environment surrounding patients.
- Treatment is tiered based on severity.
- Rising incidence of *C. difficile* infection with emerging strains that have up to twenty-threefold more toxin production.
- Toxin assays vary widely in ability to detect toxin.
- Only unformed stool specimens should be submitted for laboratory *C. difficile* testing.
- Polymerase chain reaction (PCR) and nucleic acid amplification test/loop mediated isothermal DNA amplification (NAAT/LAMP) are more sensitive test methods than enzyme immunoassay (EIA).
- Antibiotics can predispose persons by altering their normal gut flora.
- Can present in healthy patients with no known risk factors.
- Sometimes causes toxic megacolon or fulminant colitis.

NOROVIRUS:
- Patients present with sudden onset of nausea, vomiting, and/or diarrhea.
- Now considered year-round rather than seasonal.
- Disinfection with bleach.
- Often need to isolate exposed persons for average incubation period, such as 3 days, to prevent outbreak.

SURVEILLANCE
- Crucial for early identification of infections. Enables:
  - Immediate intervention
  - Education

- Prospective, concurrent, hospital surveillance:
  - Electronic data mining provides accurate review
  - Feasible with sophisticated computerized data collection and analysis
- Targeted surveillance addresses high-risk procedures and patient populations
- Routine rate calculations and statistical analyses:
  - Use device-specific days, procedure-specific cases, or patient-days as denominators
  - Enhance early recognition of microclusters of infections by body site and by organism
  - Facilitate proper early control of potential outbreaks
- Active surveillance/screening cultures for multi-drug resistant organisms (MDROs); for example, high-risk populations for MRSA

DX DIAGNOSIS

MOST COMMON HAI:
- Urinary tract infections (UTIs) (32%)
- Surgical site and other soft tissue infections (22%)
- Pneumonia (15%) (Fig. 1-375)
- Bloodstream infections (14%)

HEALTHCARE-ASSOCIATED UTIs:
- General associations:
  - Indwelling urinary (e.g., Foley) catheters
  - Inappropriate catheter care (including opening catheter junctions)
  - Female sex
  - Absence of systemic antibiotics
- Physical findings:
  - Fever
  - Dysuria
  - Leukocytosis
  - Pyuria
  - Flank or costovertebral angle tenderness

- Usual organisms:
  - *E. coli*
  - *Candida*
  - *Enterococcus*
  - *Pseudomonas*
  - *Klebsiella*
  - *Enterobacter*
- Sepsis in 1% to 3% of hospital-associated UTIs
- Prevention bundle to eliminate catheter-associated UTIs (CAUTIs):
  - Use meticulous aseptic technique during insertion and daily perineal care
  - Avoid unnecessary urinary catheters; remove promptly
  - Never open the catheter-collection tubing junction (keep system closed)
  - Obtain all specimens using sterile syringe
  - Remove Foley catheters as soon as possible
  - Substitute intermittent catheterization for Foley catheters

HEALTHCARE-ASSOCIATED BLOODSTREAM INFECTIONS:
- General associations:
  - IV lines
  - Arterial lines
  - Central venous pressure (CVP) lines: lead to catheter-associated bloodstream infection (CLABSI)
  - Phlebitis
  - Hyperalimentation
  - Lack of safe injection best practices
- Fever possibly only presenting sign
- Exit site of all vascular lines carefully evaluated for:
  - Erythema
  - Induration
  - Tenderness
  - Purulent drainage

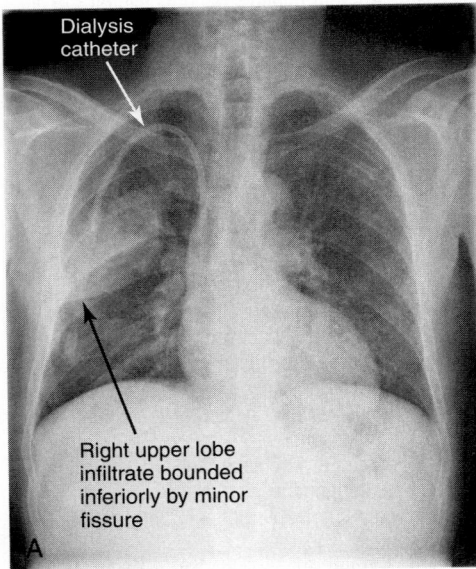 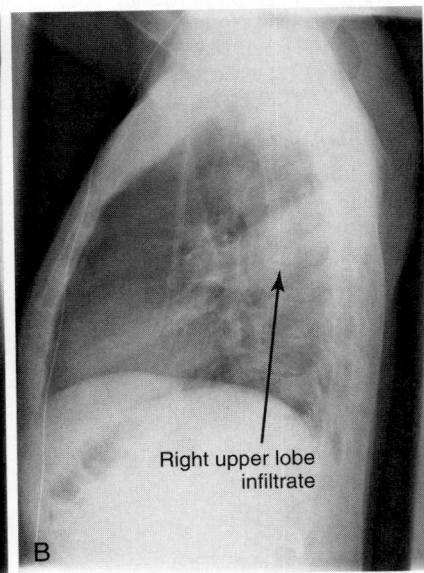

FIGURE 1-375 Healthcare-associated infections: pneumonia in right upper lobe. A, Posteroanterior (PA) chest x-ray. **B,** Lateral chest x-ray. This 46-year-old man with human immunodeficiency virus and end-stage renal disease developed fever to 39.1° C, cough, and right chest pain. **A,** His PA chest x-ray shows a dense infiltrate in the right upper lobe bounded inferiorly by the minor fissure. **B,** On the lateral x-ray, this appears bounded superiorly as well; this boundary identifies this as a right posterior segment upper lobe infiltrate. (From Broder JS: *Diagnostic imaging for the emergency physician,* Philadelphia, 2011, Saunders.)

- Usual organisms for device-associated bacteremia
  - *S. aureus* (including MRSA)
  - *Staphylococcus epidermidis* for long-term IV lines
  - *Enterobacter*
  - *Klebsiella*
  - *Candida* spp.
  - *Pseudomonas aeruginosa* may come from a water source or reflect cutaneous bacteria
- Phlebitis in 1.3 million patients yearly
- Approximately 10,000 annual deaths from IV sepsis
- Prevention bundle to eliminate central line-associated bloodstream infections (CLABSIs):
  - Meticulous sterile technique during central catheter line insertion.
  - Emphasis should be placed on attention to detail, including handwashing, adherence to guidelines for catheter insertion and maintenance, appropriate use of antiseptic solutions such as chlorhexidine (CHG) to prepare the skin before central line insertion.
  - Modified catheter, for example, antiseptic-coated line, may reduce risk for endoluminal colonization and catheter-related sepsis in subclavian lines.
  - Decrease use of routine IVs and encourage PO intake.
  - Avoid using a femoral vein insertion site. Subclavian central line site is associated with lower infection rate than jugular.
  - Bundle to prevent CLABSIs includes hand hygiene, CHG skin prep for insertion of central lines, full barrier protection for insertion of central lines, removal of unnecessary lines, insertion checklist.
  - Consider daily CHG baths in ICUs.

HEALTHCARE-ASSOCIATED PNEUMONIAS:
- More common in ICUs
- General associations:
  - Aspiration
  - Intubation: leads to ventilator-associated events (VAE) or ventilator-associated pneumonia (VAP)
  - Altered consciousness
  - Old age
  - Chronic lung disease
  - Postsurgery
  - Antacids
  - Head of bed not elevated
- Signs of pneumonia common among patients on general wards:
  - Cough
  - Sputum
  - Fever
  - Leukocytosis
  - New infiltrate on chest x-ray examination
- Signs more subtle in ICUs, because many patients have purulent sputum because of chronic intubation
  - Change in sputum character or volume
  - Small changes on chest x-ray examination
- Usual organisms:
  - *S. aureus* (including MRSA)
  - *Pseudomonas aeruginosa*
  - *Enterobacter*
  - *Acinetobacter*
  - *Klebsiella*

- Less common organisms:
  - *Stenotrophomonas* spp.
  - *Legionella, Flavobacterium*
  - Respiratory syncytial virus (infants)
  - Adenovirus
- 1% of hospitalized patients affected
- Mortality rate high (40%)
- Prevention bundle:
  - Use meticulous sterile technique during suctioning and handling airway.
  - Do not routinely change ventilator breathing circuits and components. For heat and moisture exchangers, no more frequently than every 48 hr.
  - Drain respirator tubing without allowing fluid to return to respirator.
  - Wash hands routinely to prevent colonization of patients and transfer of organisms among patients.
  - Use of a bundle to prevent VAEs and VAPs to include: elevate the head of bed, provide deep vein thrombosis (DVT) prophylaxis, provide peptic ulcer disease (PUD) prophylaxis, hold sedation, test for ability to extubate, control glucose, gastric decontamination.
  - Consider oral mouth care with CHG for vented patients in ICUs.

SURGICAL AND HEALTHCARE-ASSOCIATED SOFT TISSUE INFECTIONS:
- Associations:
  - Decubitus ulcers
  - Surgical site risks: contaminated or dirty/infected, the American Society of Anesthesiologists' (ASA) physical status classification of ASA 3 or 4, duration of surgery over national average, usually 3 hr
  - Abdominal surgery
  - Presence of drain
  - Preoperative length of stay
  - Surgeon
  - Presence of other infection
- Physical findings:
  - Decubitus ulcer with fluctuance at margin or under firm eschar
  - Erythema extending >2 cm beyond margin of surgical wound
  - Tenderness
  - Induration
  - Erythema
  - Fluctuance
  - Purulent drainage
  - Dehiscence of sutures
- Usual organisms:
  - *S. aureus* (including MRSA)
  - *Enterococcus*
  - *Enterobacter*
  - *Acinetobacter*
  - *E. coli*
- Prevention:
  - Use careful skin care and frequent, proper positioning of patient to prevent decubitus ulcer.
  - Use meticulous sterile surgical technique.
  - Use properly washed and sterilized instruments, processed in accordance with manufacturer's instructions. Minimize immediate-use steam sterilization (formerly known as flash sterilization).
  - Wash hands to decrease colonization when handling postoperative wound.

- Limit prophylactic antibiotics to 24 hr perioperatively.
- Double-wrap contaminated dressings (hold in gloved hand and evert gloves over dressings) before disposal.
- Surgical Care Improvement Project (SCIP) bundle to include antibiotic prophylaxis selection, receipt of antibiotic within 1 hr prior to surgery, discontinuation of antibiotic within 24 hr of surgery end time, cardiac surgery patients with controlled 6 AM postoperative blood glucose, clip rather than shave prep, postoperative normothermia for colorectal surgery patients, removal of Foley catheter by end of postoperative day 2 (except for urologic, gynecologic, or perineal procedures, or on paralytics, vasopressors/inotropics during ICU stay).
- Preadmission nares MRSA screening often beneficial for open heart and orthopedic implants when time is allowed for decolonization, chlorhexidine showers, and appropriate antibiotic prophylaxis selection.

LABORATORY TESTS
- Appropriate to specific HAI and specific patient's condition
- Cultures generally indicated for proper confirmation of responsible pathogens:
  - Urine
  - Blood
  - Sputum
  - Soft tissue
- Molecular analysis of nosocomial epidemics:
  - Plasmid fingerprinting
  - Restriction endonuclease digestion (plasmid and genomic DNA)
  - Peptide analysis
  - Immunoblotting
  - Ribosomal RNA (rRNA) typing
  - DNA probes
  - Multilocus enzyme electrophoresis
  - Restriction fragment length polymorphism (RFLP)
  - PCR
  - Provide confirmation of point-source or common strains and corroboration of hypotheses reached utilizing classic epidemiology

IMAGING STUDIES
Rarely needed for diagnosis of HAI; helpful for deep surgical site infection.

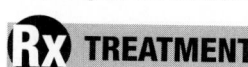 TREATMENT

ACUTE GENERAL Rx
- Appropriate to etiologic organism:
  - Antibiotic
  - Antifungal
  - Antiviral
- Specific therapy determined after careful consideration of resident flora within the microenvironment in which the patient was hospitalized
  - Empiric therapy
  - Frequently difficult to fashion accurately
  - Often undesirable, unless the patient's clinical condition requires urgent treatment

H

Diseases and Disorders

I

- Consultation for expert advice regarding antibiotic selection in view of known epidemiologic risks within the hospital (Hospital Epidemiologist or Infectious Disease Specialist)
- Avoid unnecessary treatment for organisms that are colonizing (no signs or symptoms of infection), but not infecting patients
- Prevention of spread of communicable diseases
  - Isolation or precautions (airborne, droplet, contact isolation precautions, and combinations thereof)
  - Classic schema (strict, respiratory isolation and contact [skin and wound] precautions) have been replaced by more streamlined revised guidelines (airborne, droplet, contact isolation precautions, and combinations thereof)
  - Less careful response to some diseases (e.g., hemorrhagic fevers) inadvertently induced by removal of strict isolation category
  - Universal/standard precautions to protect HCWs against splash or splatter of blood or body fluids
  - Tracking roommates of patients with communicable disease, such as Norovirus or influenza and using precautions during the incubation period
- Universal/standard precautions used for all patients during all anticipated contacts with blood, body fluids, or secretions
  - Gloves
  - Goggles/eye shield
  - Gowns that prevent blood or potentially infectious materials from passing through
- Consider aggressive isolation to restrict spread of multidrug-resistant organisms and their plasmids
  - MRSA
  - VREF
  - MDR-GNRs (multidrug-resistant gram-negative rods) can include extended-spectrum β-lactamases (ESBL), carbapenem-resistant Enterobacteriaceae (CRE), some *Acinetobacter baumanni*. New microbiology interpretive criteria (breakpoints) can result in no longer reporting mechanism of resistance.
  - New Delhi metallo-β-lactamase 1 (NDM-1): these are gram-negative Enterobacteriaceae with a new type of carbapenem-resistance gene.

Refer to the topic "Multidrug-Resistant Gram-Negative Rods (MDR-GNRs)" for more information.

DISPOSITION

The Infection Prevention and Control Service and/or Hospital Epidemiologist should be notified when infectious complications occur in the hospital setting; most, but not all, HAIs are potentially avoidable, and every effort should be taken to minimize the risk of infections associated with healthcare. Nationwide success in achieving and sustaining zero CLABSIs, zero CAUIs, and and zero VAPs warrant widespread use of infection prevention bundles to target zero HAIs.

REFERRAL

- To infection preventionist
- To hospital epidemiologist

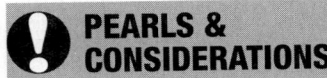

PEARLS & CONSIDERATIONS

COMMENTS

- Sharp and splash injuries to staff are relatively rare, but nearly all are preventable.
  - Nurses incur most injuries.
  - Usual causes:
    1. Needle sticks
    2. Scalpel and surgical needle injuries
    3. Blood splashes
  - Prevention:
    1. Never recap needles.
    2. Dispose of needles only in rigid, impermeable plastic containers.
    3. Clearly announce instrument passes in the operating room and during procedures. Use passing trays.
    4. Use needleless systems for vascular access and connectors whenever possible to limit HCWs' use of sharp medical devices.
    5. Use gloves, mask, and goggles/eye shield if aerosol or splash is likely.
    6. Never leave needles or other sharp items in beds.
    7. Never dispose of sharp items in regular trash bags.
  - Infection Prevention and Control or Employee Health staff should be consulted immediately after exposure to determine need for prophylaxis for hepatitis B or HIV.
  - All clinical staff should be immune to hepatitis B (natural or vaccine).
- Fungi previously considered to be contaminants are now risks for patients with cancer and organ transplantation.
  - *Candida* spp.
    1. *C. guilliermondii*
    2. *C. krusei*
    3. *C. parapsilosis*
    4. *C. tropicalis*
  - *Aspergillus* spp.
  - *Curvularia* spp.
  - *Bipolaris* spp.
  - *Exserohilum* spp.
  - *Alternaria* spp.
  - *Fusarium* spp.
  - *Scopulariopsis* spp.
  - *Pseudallescheria boydii*
  - *Trichosporon beigelii*
  - *Malassezia furfur*
  - *Hansenula* spp.
  - *Microsporum canis*
- Focused, committed efforts by the entire healthcare staff continuously directed toward prevention:
  - Each HAI addressed as an opportunity to improve the organization and delivery of safe patient care
  - Essential for individual staff members to understand that small risks applied to large populations result in a large number of total events (i.e., HAIs)
- Antibiotic stewardship
  - Choose appropriate antibiotic
  - Minimize vancomycin usage
- The Centers for Medicare & Medicaid Services denies inpatient payments for certain HAIs. Total reimbursement is linked to performance (compare HAI outcome to national benchmark).
- The number of surgical-site *S. aureus* infections acquired in the hospital has been reduced by rapid screening and decolonizing of nasal carriers of *S. aureus* on admission.

SUGGESTED READINGS
available at www.expertconsult.com

RELATED CONTENT

Methicillin-Resistant *Staphylococcus aureus* (MRSA) (Related Key Topic)
Multidrug-Resistant Gram-Negative Rods (MDR-GNRs) (Related Key Topic)
Vancomycin-Resistant Enterococcus (VRE) (Related Key Topic)

AUTHORS: **MARLENE FISHMAN, M.P.H., C.I.C.,** and **GLENN G. FORT, M.D., M.P.H.**

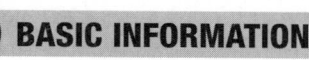 **BASIC INFORMATION**

DEFINITION

Complete heart block (CHB) is the absence of electrical impulse transmission from the atria to the ventricles when atrioventricular (AV) junction is not physiologically refractory.

Atria and ventricles are controlled by independent pacemakers; thus, complete AV block is only one cause of complete AV dissociation. It may be acquired or congenital.

SYNONYMS

Third-degree AV block
CHB
Complete AV block

ICD-9CM CODES
426.0 Complete heart block

EPIDEMIOLOGY & DEMOGRAPHICS

- The prevalence of CHB is 0.04%.
- The prevalence of CHB increases with age.

PHYSICAL FINDINGS & CLINICAL PRESENTATION

Physical examination may be normal. Cannon A waves may appear periodically in jugular vein waveform, and changing intensity of S_1 may occur. Patients may present with the following clinical manifestations:

- Dizziness, palpitations
- Syncope or presyncope (due to reduced cardiac output)
- Fatigue, impaired exercise tolerance
- Mental status changes
- Congestive heart failure
- Angina pectoris
- Some patients may be asymptomatic (e.g., congenital CHB)

ETIOLOGY

- Fibrosis or sclerosis of the conduction system, calcific aortic stenosis
- Acute myocardial infarction—inferior (14%) or anterior (2%) wall of patients, usually within 24 hours
- Drug effect (digitalis, calcium channel blockers, beta-blockers, amiodarone)
- Cardiomyopathy and myocarditis
- Infiltrative processes of the myocardium (amyloidosis, sarcoidosis, sclerodema, tumor)

- Metabolic abnormalities (hyperkalemia, hypoxia, hypothyroidism)
- Lyme carditis, rheumatoid nodules, polymyositis, Chagas' disease
- Neuromuscular disorders (Becker muscular dystrophy, myotonic muscular dystrophy)
- Congenital (birth from mothers with systemic lupus)
- Iatrogenic (cardiac surgery, catheter ablation of arrhythmias, percutaneous coronary intervention). Transcatheter aortic valve implantation (TAVI) is shown to be frequently associated with new conduction abnormalities; patients with preexisting right bundle-branch block are at increased risk of CHB (resolves over time in most patients).

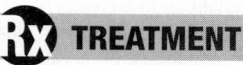 **DIAGNOSIS**

DIFFERENTIAL DIAGNOSIS

The differential diagnosis includes lesser degree of AV block, automatic junctional rhythms, and nonconducted premature atrial contractions.

WORKUP

- Workup such as routine labs, cardiac biomarkers, and cardiac imaging should be dictated by the clinical circumstances.
- ECG: diagnostic of the disease (Figs. 1-376 and 1-377):

- P waves are present with a regular atrial rate that is faster than the ventricular rate.
- P waves are not related to the QRS complexes. The PR intervals are variable.
- RR intervals are regular.
- QRS complexes may be normal with rate of 40 to 60 beats per minute [bpm] (block proximal to His bundle) or wide with a rate of <40 bpm (block distal to His bundle, acquired)—depending on the location of the block in the conduction system.
- Complete AV block can result from block at the level of AV node (congenital CHB), within the His bundle, or distal to it, in the Pukinje system (acquired).

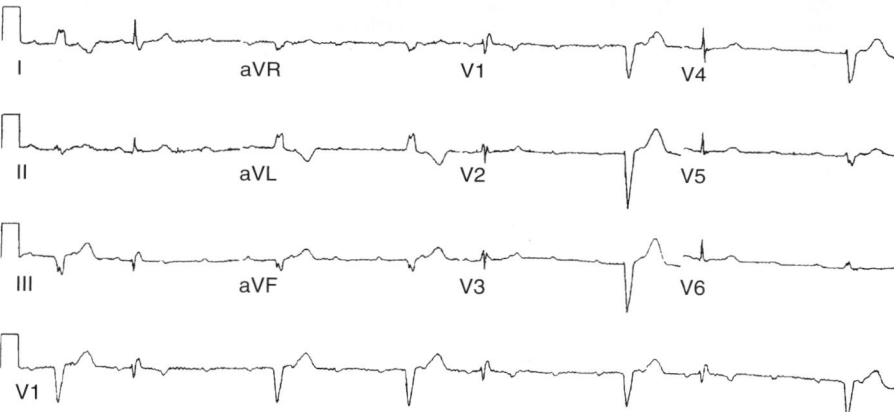 **TREATMENT**

ACUTE GENERAL Rx

- Initial treatment should focus on the hemodynamic stability and symptoms of the patient.
- Consider temporary pacemaker insertion if ventricular escape rate is slow (<40 bpm) and associated with symptoms or hemodynamic compromise.
- CHB as a complication of inferior MI usually only requires temporary pacing; however, a CHB as a result of anterior MI often requires permanent pacing.

FIGURE 1-377 High-grade atrioventricular block. Note that only three P waves conducted to the ventricle in the whole tracing. Conducted P waves were associated with normal PR intervals and right bundle branch block, a finding suggesting infranodal block. All other P waves were blocked, and ventricular escape rhythm with a left bundle branch block pattern is observed. Note that the block is not caused by retrograde concealment in the atrioventricular node or His-Purkinje system from the ventricular escape complexes because the conducted P waves occurred at a short cycle following the escape complexes. (From Issa Z et al: *Clinical arrhythmology and electrophysiology*, ed 2, Philadelphia, 2012, Saunders.)

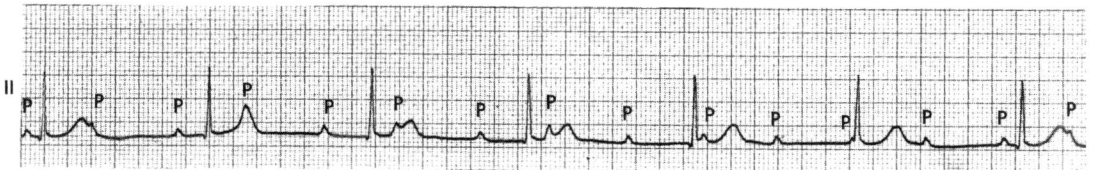

FIGURE 1-376 Third-degree (complete) atrioventricular heart block is characterized by independent atrial (P) and ventricular (QRS) activity. The atrial rate is always faster than the ventricular rate. The PR intervals are completely variable. Some P waves fall on the T wave, distorting its shape. Others may fall in the QRS complex and be "lost." Notice that the QRS complexes are of normal width, indicating that the ventricles are being paced from the atrioventricular junction. (From Goldberger AL [ed]: *Clinical electrocardiography*, ed 5, St Louis, 1994, Mosby.)

Diseases and Disorders

I

- Acquired CHB usually requires pacing, but patients with congenital CHB often have sufficiently rapid escape rhythm to prevent symptoms and avoid permanent pacemaker implantation.
- Withdraw AV-nodal blocking agents if any.
- Short-term therapy (until adequate pacing therapy is established)
  - Vagolytic agents such as atropine may be used to increase the rate of the escape rhythm (for AV nodal level blocks)
  - Catecholamines such as isoproterenol transiently used for a CHB at any site (use with extreme caution or not at all in patients with acute MI).
- Drugs cannot be relied on to increase HR for more than several hours or days without side effects; therefore, temporary or permanent pacemaker insertion is indicated.
- Symptomatic CHB in the absence of a condition that is likely to resolve is an ACC/AHA/HRS Class I indication for permanent pacemaker (PPM) placement.
- Class 1 indications for PPM placement in asymptomatic patients according to the ACC/AHA guidelines include:
  - Patients in sinus rhythm, with documented asystolic pauses greater than or equal to 3.0 sec or an escape rate <40 bpm, or with an escape rhythm that is below the AV node
  - Patients with atrial fibrillation and bradycardia with one or more pauses of at least 5 sec or longer

  - After catheter ablation of the AV junction
  - If cardiomegaly or LV dysfunction is present with ventricular rates of 40 bpm or faster
  - Postoperative CHB that is not expected to resolve
  - When it is associated with neuromuscular diseases, such as Erb dystrophy (limb-girdle muscular dystrophy), Kearns-Sayre syndrome, myotonic muscular dystrophy, and peroneal muscular atrophy
  - CHB present during exercise in the absence of myocardial ischemia
- Therapy is directed toward the underlying etiology if there is a reversible source.
- All patients should be made aware of the high risk of PPM implantation with transcatheter aortic valve implantation (TAVI).

CHRONIC Rx

Patients with PPM need regular follow-up and pacemaker monitoring to ensure proper device functioning.

DISPOSITION

- Mortality is highest in the neonatal period in congenital CHB.
- Prognosis is favorable after insertion of pacemaker and related to the underlying etiology of complete AV block (e.g., myocardial infarction, cardiomyopathy).
- Nonrandomized studies have shown that PPM insertion improves survival in patients with CHB.

REFERRAL

All patients with CHB should be referred to a cardiologist for consideration of temporary and/or PPM implantation.

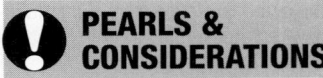

COMMENTS

- Patients should be instructed to avoid activities that may damage the pacemaker (e.g., contact sports).
- Pacemaker manufacturers do not recommend any special restrictions regarding proximity to typical household items.
- The presence of a permanent pacemaker is a strong relative contraindication to MRI.

SUGGESTED READINGS

available at www.expertconsult.com

RELATED CONTENT

Complete Heart Block (Patient Information)

AUTHORS: **SHAHNAZ PUNJANI, M.D.,** **FRED F. FERRI, M.D.,** and **WEN-CHIH WU, M.D., M.P.H.**

BASIC INFORMATION

DEFINITION

Second-degree heart block or second-degree atrioventricular (AV) heart block is characterized by a failure of one or more, but not all, atrial impulses to conduct to the ventricles. The block may be at any level of AV conduction system. When more than one atrial impulse is present for each ventricular complex, the rhythm may be described as a ratio of the number of atrial impulses to the number of ventricular complexes. Electrocardiographically there are three types of second-degree block:

- Mobitz type I (Wenckebach):
  - Characterized by a progressive prolongation of the PR interval prior to a blocked nonconducted beat and a shorter PR interval after that blocked beat; the conducted impulse will generally be narrow. The cycle may repeat periodically, leading to "grouped beating."
  - Site of block is usually AV node (proximal to the His bundle).
- Mobitz type II:
  - High-grade AV block (3:1, 4:1, or greater)
  - Characterized by fixed PR intervals before and after blocked beats and is usually associated with a wide QRS morphology (right bundle branch block [RBBB] or left bundle branch block [LBBB] patterns).
  - Site of block is usually infranodal, especially when QRS is wide.
  - It has a greater propensity for progressing to third-degree AV block.
- Pure 2:1 conduction patterns cannot be reliably classified as Mobitz type I or type II

SYNONYMS

Wenckebach block (Mobitz type I block)
Mobitz type II block

ICD-9CM CODES
426.13 Mobitz type I
426.12 Mobitz type II

EPIDEMIOLOGY & DEMOGRAPHICS

Mobitz type I block is more common and may occur in individuals with heightened vagal tone or as a side effect of medications, such as β-blockers or calcium channel blockers.

PHYSICAL FINDINGS & CLINICAL PRESENTATION

- Patients with Mobitz type I are usually asymptomatic. Sudden loss of consciousness without warning (Adams-Stokes attack) can occur in patients with Mobitz type II; however, it is much more common in patients with complete heart block. Palpitations and feeling of "missing a beat."
- Type I block: there is gradual decrease in the intensity of the first heart sound with widening of the a-c interval in the central venous waveform, ending in a pause, and an a wave not followed by a v wave in the neck along with an irregular pulse.
- Type II block: the first heart sound retains a constant intensity, with intermittent ventricular pauses and a waves not followed by v waves in the neck. There is an irregular pulse for most times with intermittent pauses.

ETIOLOGY

- High vagal tone (young patients, athletes at rest)
- Degenerative changes in the AV conduction system
- Ischemia at the AV nodes (type I with inferior wall myocardial infarction [MI] and type II with anterior way MI)
- Drugs (digitalis, quinidine, procainamide, adenosine, calcium channel blockers [nondihydropyridines], β-blockers)
- Cardiomyopathies, collagen vascular diseases, infiltrative diseases (amyloidosis, sarcoidosis, hematochromatosis)
- Myocarditis/endocarditis (infectious, e.g., Lyme disease, Chagas disease; and noninfectious, e.g., systemic lupus erythematosus)
- Hyperkalemia, hypermagnesemia
- Hypothyroidism
- Prior cardiac valve surgery
- Catheter trauma, catheter ablation for arrhythmias

DIAGNOSIS

DIFFERENTIAL DIAGNOSIS

The ECG easily and reliably distinguishes Mobitz type I from Mobitz type II block and from other conduction abnormalities. It should be distinguished from the less common phenomenon of second-degree sinoatrial node exit block.

Type I AV block with a normal QRS complex tends to be benign and usually does not progress to more advanced forms of AV conduction

within a short period of time. Mobitz type II block often precedes the development of Adams-Stokes syncope, symptoms are frequent, prognosis is compromised, and progression to third-degree AV block is common and sudden. Thus, type II second-degree AV block with a wide QRS typically indicates diffuse conduction system disease.

WORKUP

ECG, ambulatory monitoring (Holter or external loop recorders in selected patients

- Mobitz type I (Fig. 1-378) ECG shows:
  1. Sequential and gradual prolongation of PR interval leading to a nonconducted P wave
  2. Shortened PR interval following the pause as compared to the pre-pause PR interval
  3. Progressive shortening of the R-R interval prior to nonconducted atrial impulse
  4. Usually see "grouped beating" pattern.
- Mobitz type II ECG shows:
  1. Fixed duration of PR interval
  2. Sudden nonconducted P wave
- In 2:1 AV block (Fig. 1-379), it cannot be determined based on the 12-lead ECG whether there is Mobitz type I or type II AV block, although a wide QRS complex is suggestive of Mobitz type II.

TREATMENT

NONPHARMACOLOGIC THERAPY

Elimination of drugs that may induce AV block

ACUTE GENERAL Rx

- Treatment is usually not necessary unless the resting heart rate is <40 beats per min (bpm) while awake.
- If symptomatic (e.g., dizziness), atropine 1 mg (may repeat once after 5 min) may be tried to increase AV conduction; if no response, trial of dobutamine or isoproterenol may be helpful prior to insertion of a pacemaker.
- Atropine
  - Reduces heart block due to hypervagotonia but not due to AV node ischemia
  - Does not increase infranodal conduction (third-degree and second-degree AV block that is below the AV node)
  - Should be used with caution in Mobitz type II AV block due to possible paradoxical decrease in heart rate (as atrial rate increases, AV conduction decreases)
  - Is ineffective in heart transplantation patients

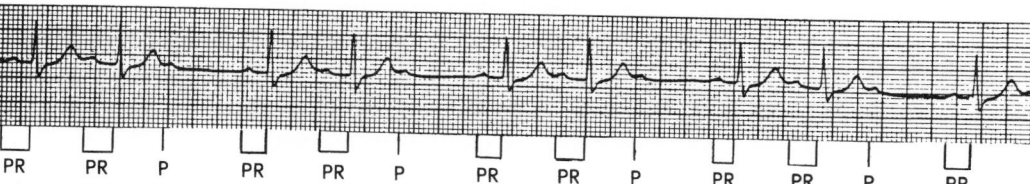

FIGURE 1-378 Wenckebach (Mobitz type I) second-degree atrioventricular block. Notice the progressive increase in PR intervals, with the third P wave in each sequence not followed by a QRS. Wenckebach block produces a characteristically syncopated rhythm with grouping of the QRS complexes (group beating). (From Goldberger AL [ed]: *Clinical electrocardiography*, ed 5, St Louis, 1994, Mosby.)

- If block is the result of drugs (e.g., digitalis), discontinue the drug.
- If associated with anterior wall MI and wide QRS complex, consider insertion of a temporary pacemaker.

ACC/AHA/HRS recommendations for permanent pacemaker (PPM) implantation:

- Second-degree AV block with associated symptomatic bradycardia regardless of the type or site of the block (class I; level of evidence: B).
- Second-degree AV block provoked during exercise in the absence of myocardial ischemia (class I; level of evidence: C).
- Asymptomatic second-degree AV block at intra- or infra-His levels found at electrophysiologic study (class IIa; level of evidence: B).
- First-or second-degree AV block with symptoms similar to those of pacemaker syndrome or hemodynamic compromise (class IIa; level of evidence: B).
- Asymptomatic type II second-degree AV block with narrow QRS. When type II second-degree AV block occurs with a wide QRS, including isolated right bundle-branch block, pacing becomes a class I recommendation; level of evidence: B.
- PPM is not indicated for asymptomatic type I second-degree AV block at supra-His (AV node) level or that which is not known to be intra- or infra-Hisian (class III; level of evidence: C)

DISPOSITION
Prognosis is good with insertion of a pacemaker.

REFERRAL
Referral for pacemaker insertion (see "Acute General Rx")

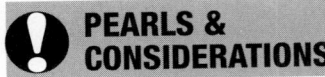

PEARLS & CONSIDERATIONS

COMMENTS
Patients with Mobitz type I should be followed up routinely for potential development of high-grade AV block.

SUGGESTED READINGS
available at www.expertconsult.com

RELATED CONTENT
Second-Degree Heart Block (Patient Information)

AUTHORS: **SHAHNAZ PUNJANI, M.D., FRED F. FERRI, M.D.,** and **WEN-CHIH WU, M.D., M.P.H.**

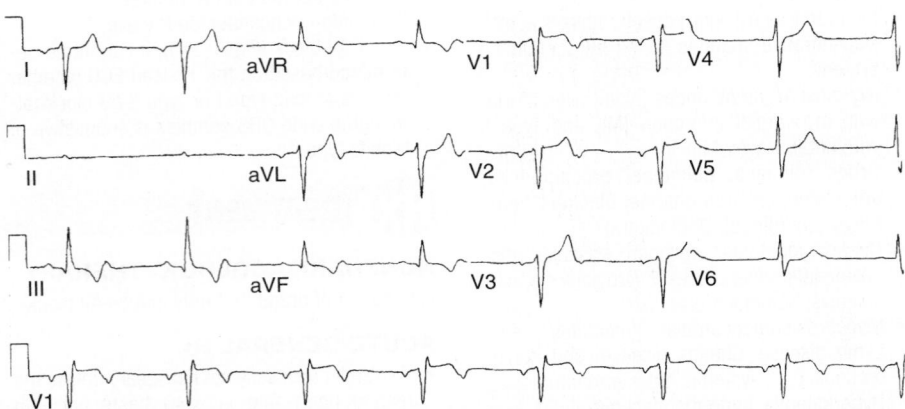

FIGURE 1-379 Second-degree 2:1 atrioventricular block. Notice the short PR interval during conducted complexes and the wide QRS complexes, suggesting block in the His-Purkinje system. (From Issa Z et al: *Clinical arrhythmology and electrophysiology,* ed 2, Philadelphia, 2012, Saunders.)

BASIC INFORMATION

DEFINITION

Heart failure (HF) is a complex clinical syndrome characterized by impaired myocardial performance, resulting in the heart's inability to deliver sufficient oxygenated blood to meet the metabolic demands of peripheral tissues. The pathophysiology of HF is related to progressive activation of the neuroendocrine system to compensate for decreased effective circulating volume, leading to total body volume overload and circulatory insufficiency. Specifically, the renin-angiotensin-aldosterone system (RAAS) is implicated as being activated in HF, leading to volume expansion (sodium retention) and cardiac fibrosis (mediated through angiotensin II). Disordered adrenergic stimulation has also been recognized as a key component of progression of disease. The term "congestive heart failure" (CHF) usually denotes a volume-overloaded status as a result of HF. Given that not all patients have volume overload at the time of the evaluation, "congestive heart failure" should be distinguished from the broader term "heart failure."

CLASSIFICATION: The American College of Cardiology/American Heart Association (ACC/AHA) describes the following four stages of HF. This staging model was designed to emphasize the evolution and progression of HF over a continuum and the preventability of HF in at-risk patients.

Stage A: Patients at high risk (e.g., with hypertension, atherosclerotic disease, diabetes mellitus, metabolic syndrome, cytotoxin, family history) for HF but without structural heart disease or symptoms of HF

Stage B: Patients with structural heart disease (e.g., left ventricular [LV] dysfunction) but without symptoms of HF

Stage C: Patients with structural heart disease with prior or current symptoms of HF

Stage D: Patients with refractory HF requiring specialized interventions

In addition to the ACC/AHA stages described above, the New York Heart Association (NYHA) defines four functional classes of HF designed to describe the symptoms of stage C and D HF. The functional classes are intended to assess the symptoms of HF and may fluctuate with therapy. It should be noted that current guidelines employ the functional classes to aid in determination of appropriate treatment.

I. Asymptomatic or symptomatic only at activity levels that would limit normal individuals

II. Symptomatic with ordinary exertion (e.g., 2 city blocks or 1 flight of stairs in a faster than usual pace)

III. Symptomatic with less than ordinary exertion (e.g., less than 2 city blocks or 1 flight of stairs)

IV. Symptomatic at rest

TERMINOLOGY: HF has been traditionally dichotomized as systolic versus diastolic (see Table 1-177). which has now been replaced with the terms HF with preserved ejection fraction (HFpEF) and HF with reduced ejection fraction (HFREF). Other common classifications include right-sided versus left-sided and high-output versus low-output. Systolic HF or HFREF is defined by the presence of impaired contractility of the LV, as measured by ejection fraction (EF) with clinical signs or symptoms of HF. In contrast, HFpEF or diastolic HF has been described as evidence (clinical) of HF with an EF above 50% and evidence of diastolic dysfunction. The term "HF with preserved EF" is preferred over the term "diastolic HF," given that many of the physiologic derangements in this subset of HF are not solely restricted to diastolic function of the heart. Right-sided HF denotes peripheral signs and symptoms of HF without evidence of pulmonary congestion, as opposed to left HF, which typically manifests with pulmonary congestion and subsequent signs and symptoms of right-sided HF. High-output HF involves signs and symptoms of HF but features an elevated cardiac output unable to meet the abnormally high metabolic demands of peripheral tissues, the result of myriad systemic disorders (e.g., systemic arteriovenous fistulas, hyperthyroidism, anemia). The term "acute decompensated HF" (ADHF) refers to worsening of signs or symptoms of HF due to a wide range of causes. Of note, HF is not equivalent to cardiomyopathy or LV dysfunction. These latter terms describe the possible structural or functional reasons for the development of HF, whereas HF is a clinical syndrome characterized by specific symptoms and signs.

SYNONYMS

HF
Congestive heart failure
CHF
Cardiac failure
Cardiogenic shock
Cardiogenic pulmonary edema

ICD-9CM CODES
428.0 Congestive heart failure

EPIDEMIOLOGY & DEMOGRAPHICS

- Of note, there is variability in the reported demographics of HF due to heterogeneous definitions and classifications of HF.

TABLE 1-177 Systolic versus Diastolic Heart Failure*

Parameters	Systolic (HFREF)	Diastolic (HFpEF)
History		
Coronary artery disease	+++†	++
Hypertension	++	++++
Diabetes	++	++
Valvular heart disease	++++	+
Paroxysmal dyspnea	++	+++
Physical Examination		
Cardiomegaly	+++	+
Soft heart sounds	++++	+
S_3 gallop	+++	+
S_4 gallop	+	+++
Hypertension	++	++++
Mitral regurgitation	+++	+
Rales	++	+
Edema	+++	+
Jugular venous distention	+++	+
Chest Radiograph		
Cardiomegaly	+++	+
Pulmonary congestion	+++	+++
Electrocardiogram		
Left ventricular hypertrophy	++	++++
Q waves	++	+
Low voltage	+++	−
Echocardiogram		
Left ventricular hypertrophy	++	++++
Left ventricular dilation	++	−
Left atrial enlargement	++	++
Reduced ejection fraction	++++	−

*Certain aspects of the history and physical examination, along with clinical measurements, may help to distinguish diastolic from systolic heart failure. For example, patients with hypertensive heart disease and severe left ventricular hypertrophy often experience heart failure because of diastolic dysfunction.
†Plus signs indicate "suggestive" (the number reflects relative weight). Minus signs indicate "not very suggestive."
HFpEF, Heart failure with preserved ejection fraction; HFREF, heart failure with reduced ejection fraction.
From Zipes DP et al (eds): Braunwald's heart disease, ed 7, Philadelphia, 2005, Saunders.

- HF is primarily a condition of the elderly. Approximately 80% of patients hospitalized with HF are older than 65 yr. HF is the most common inpatient diagnosis in the U.S. for patients aged >65 yr.
- In the U.S., 1.1 million hospital discharges and 3.2 million hospitalizations/ambulatory care visits were associated with HF in 2007.
- Prevalence: 5.7 million persons in the U.S. and an estimated 23 million persons worldwide. The risk of development is elevated in African American males. The prevalence of HF is rising, especially in the elderly, particularly due to aging of the population and improved survival from other conditions (e.g., valvular and coronary heart disease).
- In the U.S., more than 550,000 patients annually are diagnosed with HF for the first time. The incidence is higher in the elderly, approaching 1 per 100 persons aged >65 yr per year. Before age 75, the incidence of HF is higher in males but both sexes are equally affected after this age cutoff.
- The estimated (direct and indirect) cost of HF in the U.S. was $39.2 billion in 2010.

PHYSICAL FINDINGS & CLINICAL PRESENTATION

Clinical and physical exam findings with HF vary depending on the severity of disease, precipitant factor, comorbid conditions, and whether the failure symptoms are predominantly right-sided or left-sided.
- Common clinical manifestations are:
  - Dyspnea on exertion, progressively worsening to dyspnea at rest, and caused by increasing pulmonary vascular congestion due to inadequate forward flow and subsequent increased pulmonary venous pressure
  - Orthopnea, caused by increased venous return in the recumbent position and further elevated pulmonary venous pressure
  - Paroxysmal nocturnal dyspnea (PND) resulting from multiple factors including increased venous return in the recumbent position, decreased Pa_{O_2} and decreased adrenergic stimulation of myocardial function during sleep
  - Nocturnal angina resulting from increased myocardial oxygen demand (secondary to increased venous return in the recumbent position causing increased preload) in patients with concomitant coronary artery disease (CAD)
  - *Cheyne-Stokes respiration* (alternating phases of apnea and hyperventilation) caused by prolonged circulation time from lungs to brain as a result of impaired cardiac output
  - Fatigue, lethargy, and decreased functional capacity resulting from low cardiac output and hypoperfusion of peripheral tissues
- Physical examination:
  - Fine pulmonary crackles, wheezes, tachypnea, hypoxia (due to elevated pulmonary pressures). Crackles may be absent in chronic and longstanding high pulmonary venous pressure because it allows for lymphatic drainage in the lungs to increase.

  - Tachycardia and narrowed pulse pressure (due to increased sympathetic tone)
  - S_3 gallop, paradoxical splitting of S_2, jugular venous distention, peripheral edema in dependent tissues, congestive hepatomegaly, ascites, and hepatojugular reflux (due to volume overload)
  - Perioral and peripheral cyanosis, decreased capillary refill, pulsus alternans, and cool extremities (due to decreased cardiac output)
- Six common clinical presentations identified by European Society of Cardiology of Acute Heart Failure Syndromes:
  1. ADHF presenting with hypertension (SBP >160): the hypertension leads to increased afterload causing pulmonary vascular congestion.
  2. Worsening or decompensation of chronic HF
  3. Flash pulmonary edema
  4. Cardiogenic shock
  5. Acute coronary syndrome (ACS) and ADHF
  6. Isolated RV failure

  Each of these scenarios may require different therapies to effectively stabilize and treat the patient.

  Acute precipitants of HF decompensation include noncompliance with salt restriction or medications (most commonly), infection, arrhythmias (e.g., atrial fibrillation), ischemia or infarction, uncontrolled hypertension, new medications (e.g., negative inotropic agents such as calcium channel blockers/antiarrhythmic agents), nonsteroidal anti-inflammatory drugs (NSAIDs), renal dysfunction, toxins (e.g., ethanol and anthracyclines), cardiac surgery, or valvular catastrophe.

ETIOLOGY

LEFT VENTRICULAR FAILURE: The dichotomy of whether HF occurs in the setting of preserved or reduced LV systolic function plays an important role in treatment strategies. Patients with HFpEF may have significant abnormalities in active relaxation and passive stiffness of the LV, renal function, or arterial vasoreactivity.
- Abnormal LV systolic function
  - CAD (acute or chronic ischemia, myocardial infarction [MI], LV aneurysm), which is the most common cause of cardiomyopathy in the U.S., comprising 50%-75% of patients with HF.
  - Increased afterload or pressure overload (severe hypertension, aortic stenosis)
  - Increased preload or volume overload (mitral regurgitation, aortic regurgitation)
  - Cardiomyopathy (dilated cardiomyopathy, dilated phase of hypertrophic cardiomyopathy, ischemic cardiomyopathy)
  - Infectious (Chagas, myocarditis)
  - Infiltrative (amyloidosis, sarcoidosis, hemochromatosis)
  - Toxins (ethanol, cocaine, anthracyclines)
  - Tachycardia induced (e.g., with atrial fibrillation)
- Preserved LV systolic function
  - Impaired relaxation (myocardial ischemia, diabetes mellitus, metabolic syndrome)

  - Tachyarrhythmia (featuring reduced diastolic filling time)
  - Restrictive cardiomyopathy (myocardial stiffness, such as hypereosinophilic syndrome, amyloidosis, hemochromatosis)
  - High cardiac output (thiamine deficiency, anemia, thyrotoxicosis, arteriovenous malformations)
  - Increased afterload (uncontrolled hypertension, aortic stenosis, hypertrophic obstructive cardiomyopathy)
  - Hypervolemia (oliguric renal failure, iatrogenic)

RIGHT VENTRICULAR FAILURE:
- Left-sided HF
- Chronic hypoxemic pulmonary disease
- Valvular heart disease (mitral stenosis or regurgitation)
- Pulmonary embolism
- Primary pulmonary hypertension
- Right-to-left shunts that cause systemic hypoxemia (e.g., large patent foramen ovale and tetralogy of Fallot)
- Left-to-right shunts that cause volume overload (e.g., atrial and ventricular septal defects)
- Bacterial endocarditis (right-sided)
- Right ventricular infarction

DX DIAGNOSIS

DIFFERENTIAL DIAGNOSIS
- COPD, asthma
- Cirrhosis
- Nephrotic syndrome
- Venous insufficiency
- Pulmonary embolism
- ARDS (adult respiratory distress syndrome)
- Pneumonia
- Heroin overdose

WORKUP
- Fig. E1-380 describes the National Institute for Heath and Clinical Excellence recommendation for diagnosis of heart failure.
- Blood work (to diagnose potentially reversible causes, identify comorbidities, and assess disease severity)
  - CBC (to evaluate for anemia, infections), urinalysis, blood urea nitrogen (BUN), creatinine, electrolytes (worsening hyponatremia is a marker of disease severity and is associated with higher mortality rates), liver enzymes (hepatic congestion), thyroid function (especially in the elderly or patients with comorbid atrial fibrillation or known thyroid disease)
  - B-type natriuretic peptide (BNP) is a cardiac neurohormone secreted from the ventricles in response to elevated LV end-diastolic pressure. The sensitivity is low in asymptomatic patients (but elevated BNP levels have been shown to have a negative predictive value up to 90% in symptomatic patients), and BNP elevation generally correlates with severity of disease and parallels closely morbidity and mortality outcome measures.
  - Cardiac biomarkers may be elevated if ischemia is the precipitant factor. However,

slight elevations are very common and may not always be due to obstructive coronary disease. These elevations could be due to subendocardial ischemia (due to increased end-diastolic pressure resulting in decreased perfusion) and necrosis, or cardiomyocyte damage from the inflammatory cytokines or oxidative stress. Impaired renal function is very common, and decreased clearance of the biomarkers can contribute to their elevation. Therefore these elevations should be interpreted in the context of the clinical setting. Despite that, in patients with ADHF, a positive cardiac troponin test (from whatever mechanism) is associated with worse prognosis.

- Screening for dyslipidemia and glucose intolerance, given that CAD remains the predominant cause of HF.
- If hemachromatosis is suspected (specifically in Northern European patients), consider checking a transferrin saturation.
- Consider HIV testing in high-risk patients.
- Electrocardiogram (ECG)
  - Look for signs of prior MI, chamber enlargement, hypertrophy, heart block, arrhythmia, and evidence of pericardial effusion.
  - More than 25% of patients with HF have some form of intraventricular conduction abnormality that is manifest as an increased QRS duration. The most common pattern seen is left bundle-branch block.
- Chest x-ray (Fig. 1-381)
  - Evaluate for pulmonary venous congestion, pulmonary edema, pleural effusion, cardiomegaly, chamber dilation, and Kerley B lines.
- Echocardiography
  - Plays a critical diagnostic role in patients with HF and is useful in assessment of systolic, diastolic, and valvular structure and function
- Exercise stress testing
  - May be useful in evaluating concomitant ischemic etiologies and assessment of degree of disability.
- Cardiac catheterization
  - Useful in selected patients to evaluate intracardiac filling pressures, estimates of valvular areas, presence of intracardiac shunts, coronary artery anatomy, and calculation of hemodynamic properties such as cardiac output, systemic vascular resistance, and pulmonary artery wedge pressure to further guide management.
- Cardiac MRI
  - Useful modality in accurately estimating EF (with less variabiality than conventional 2D echocardiography). MRI is also useful in excluding pericardial disease and is sensitive in identifying infiltrative disease.

RX TREATMENT

NONPHARMACOLOGIC GENERAL MEASURES

- Assess the etiology and severity of disease. Educate the patient and family about the nature of the disorder. Assess the home setting and if patient has social support to ensure compliance, especially for patients with dementia.
- Identify and correct precipitating factors (e.g., increased sodium load, medication noncompliance, ischemia, infections, anemia, thyrotoxicosis) and address lifestyle modification (e.g., smoking and alcohol cessation, weight reduction). Anemia is common in patients with HF; however, treatment with erythropoiesis-stimulating agents (ESAs) such as darbepoetin alfa have not shown improved clinical outcomes in patients with systolic HF and mild-to-moderate anemia and are not recommended.
- Review list of medications and discontinue the ones that can contribute to HF (e.g., NSAIDs, antiarrhythmic drugs, calcium channel blockers, thiazolidinediones)
- Restrict sodium intake: the 2010 Heart Failure Society of America guidelines recommend dietary sodium restriction (2-3 g/day) in all patients with HF and further restriction (<2 g/day) in those with moderate-to-severe HF. Some trials have, however, shown that in patients with systolic HF, low-sodium diets (1.8 g/day) increase mortality and hospital readmission for HF compared with normal-sodium diets (2.8 g/day).
- Restrict fluid intake to <2 L/day in patients with hyponatremia.
- Caloric supplementation should be provided to patients with advanced HF with weight loss and muscle wasting due to cardiac cachexia.
- For patients with coexisting obstructive sleep apnea, continuous positive airway pressure (CPAP) is often recommended after polysomnography, thereby reducing systolic blood pressure and improving LV function.
- Cardiac rehabilitation is unfortunately an underused preventive measure, although it has been shown to reduce morbidity and mortality.
- Pneumococcal vaccination and annual influenza vaccination.

TREATMENT OF ADHF:

- Four phases in treatment of ADHF:
  1st phase: initial stabilization and management
  2nd phase: inpatient hospital care
  3rd phase: early discharge planning and care
  4th phase: early post-discharge care

1st phase: Initial stabilization and management
  Short-term goals: hemodynamic stabilization, stabilization of respiratory status, symptom relief, optimization of tissue perfusion, and recognition of more immediately life-threatening conditions (e.g., arrhythmias, valvular catastrophe, MI, cardiac tamponade). Initial therapy of ADHF is contigent on appropriate determination of clinical scenario.

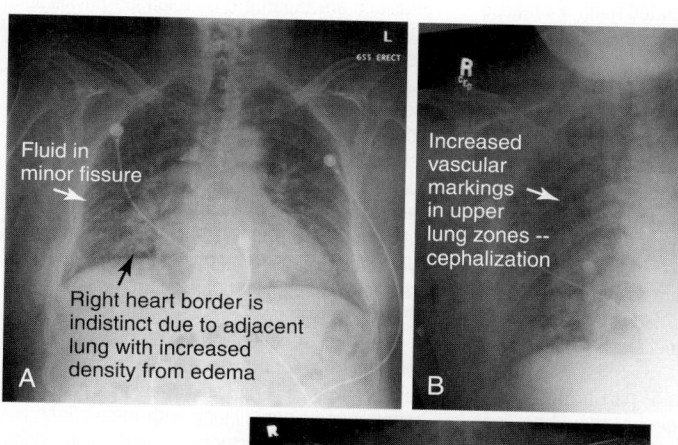

Fluid in minor fissure

Right heart border is indistinct due to adjacent lung with increased density from edema

A

Increased vascular markings in upper lung zones -- cephalization

B

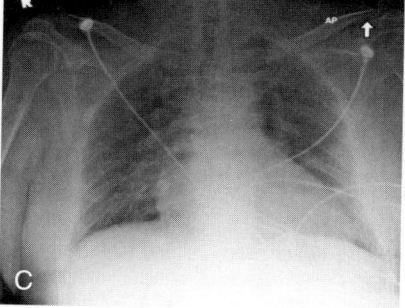

C

FIGURE 1-381 Congestive heart failure. Mild left ventricular hypertrophy with restricted filling, ejection fraction >55%, and no pericardial effusion. This 63-year-old man with coronary artery disease, chronic renal insufficiency, and diastolic heart failure (ejection fraction >55%) presented multiple times for dyspnea (**A, B,** and **C,** first through third clinical presentations). Each of these three radiographs shows signs of moderate pulmonary edema. The diaphragms and costophrenic angles are clear, suggesting no pleural effusion. The right heart border in all three images is indistinct because of interstitial edema in these locations. Portions of the left heart border are also indistinct. The upper lung fields have a hazy appearance indicating mild edema. Fluid is visible in the minor fissure on all three images. Does the similarity of these radiographs mean that edema is not the cause of the patient's dyspnea? No, he simply presented with pulmonary edema on all three occasions. (From Broder JS: *Diagnostic imaging for the emergency physician*, Philadelphia, 2011, Saunders.)

Management as per clinical scenario: (Fig. E1-382)

1. ADHF-associated hypertension: goal is afterload reduction and decrease of systemic hypervolemia. Mode of treatment: diuresis (IV loop diuretics) and vasodilators (acutely nitrates and morphine followed by treatment with ACE inhibitors or angiotensin receptor blockers [ARBs])
2. Worsening or decompensation of chronic HF (HFREF or HFpEF): goal is control of volume status. Treatment is accomplished with vasodilators and diuretics.
3. Flash pulmonary edema: goal is afterload reduction (vasodilators such as nitrates acutely), respiratory status stabilization, and diuresis (IV loop diuretics). May also require careful rate control given that atrial fibrillation or other tachyarrhythmias may decrease cardiac output and result in pulmonary edema.
4. Cardiogenic shock: goal is hemodynamic stabilization. Treatment consists of inotropes + vasopressors ± intraaortic balloon pump ± emergent revascularization if indicated.
5. ACS and ADHF: goal is hemodynamic stabilization + emergent restoration of coronary perfusion. See "Acute Coronary Syndromes."
6. Isolated RV failure: goals are identification of etiology: (1) valvular, (2) pulmonary hypertension, and (3) primary RV failure secondary to ischemia. Treatment: depends on etiology, either corrective surgery vs. treatment of pulmonary hypertension (endothelin antagonists, calcium channel blockers, phosphodiesterase inhibitors) vs. coronary reperfusion therapies.

ACUTE PHARMACOLOGIC TREATMENTS:

- Vasodilators are appropriate in most patients with ADHF (contraindicated in cardiogenic shock and severe aortic stenosis)
  ○ Nitroglycerin (0.4 to 0.8 mg sublingually every 3 to 5 min, or by intravenous infusion starting at 0.2 to 0.4 mcg/kg/min with subsequent up titration) may be administered in the emergency setting until relative hypotension ensues. Nitrates are contraindicated after use of phosphodiesterase inhibitors such as sildenafil due to risk of hypotension.
  ○ Sodium nitroprusside (0.1 to 0.2 mcg/kg/min as an intravenous infusion) is a potent vasodilator with balanced venous and arteriolar effects that usually requires hemodynamic monitoring with an arterial line and may precipitate coronary steal and thiocyanate toxicity (elevated risk in renal failure).
  ○ When given intravenously, loop diuretics have an immediate vasodilator effect that provides clinical relief of symptoms before diuresis begins. Due to gut edema and unpredictable patterns of absorption, oral formulation may become less effective. Therefore intravenous formulation should be used in the acute setting. Studies showed no difference in outcome when using bolus dosing vs. continuous IV infusion. Administration of smaller doses of short-acting loop diuretics multiple times daily is preferable to a single large dose because the kidneys can avidly reabsorb sodium after the initial diuresis. However, if a certain dose is not adequate to force diuresis, the dose, rather than the frequency, should be increased until a single effective dose is reached; more frequent doses can be added as needed. Therefore monitoring of urine output, renal function, and electrolytes is key. The addition of a distal tubule inhibitor such as metolazone 30 min prior to loop diuretic dosing has a synergistic effect and often enhances diuresis because it inhibits sodium reabsorption in the distal segment in the face of increased sodium delivery from the loop. Diuretics should be used with caution in patients with aortic stenosis and are contraindicated in patients with severe hypotension or cardiogenic shock.

- Inotropic agents are used for temporary hemodynamic support, but have not been shown to improve survival. Many of these agents have serious associated adverse events including myocardial necrosis and malignant arrhythmias.
  ○ Dobutamine (starting at 2.5 to 5 mcg/kg/min) can be used for inotropic support but is associated with increased myocardial oxygen demand and cardiac arrhythmias and may result in hypotension from decreased systemic vascular resistance.
  ○ Milrinone (37.5 to 75 mcg/kg loading dose, followed by 0.375 to 0.75 mcg/kg/min) can be used as a vasodilator and inotropic agent, but is associated with increased oxygen demand and cardiac arrhythmias, and may result in hypotension from decreased systemic vascular resistance.
  ○ Levosaminden is a calcium sensitizing drug, which also inhibits potassium channels leading to inotropy. However, this agent is not FDA approved for use in the U.S. Currently, this inotrope has been associated with an elevated risk of malignant arrhythmia and higher mortality.

- Renal replacement therapy (can be used as an alternative to pharmacologic diuresis in ADHF when renal function is significantly compromised).
- ACE inhibitors or ARBs, if part of a patient's chronic medication regimen, should be continued in the absence of hypotension, acute renal failure, or hyperkalemia.
- Beta-blockers, if part of a patient's chronic medication regimen, may be continued or reduced in dosage in mild exacerbations of HF but should be discontinued in patients with hypotension or those requiring inotropic support. Beta-blockers should not be initiated in patients who are not on chronic beta-blocker therapy until euvolemia is achieved unless used for rate control.
- Morphine sulfate can cause venodilation and may be used to reduce patient work of breathing and anxiety, but recent retrospective studies have suggested increased incidence of mechanical ventilation and in-hospital mortality in patients who received morphine.
- If ADHF with preserved EF is suspected, therapy is usually aimed at relief of symptoms and correction of any potential precipitating etiologies (e.g., tachycardia, hypertension, ischemia). Treatment generally involves diuretics to reduce pulmonary congestion with caution not to overdiurese given the need for elevated filling pressures in these patients to ensure adequate stroke volume and cardiac output. Nitrates may be useful in providing symptomatic relief but may precipitate hypotension. Ventricular rate should be controlled in the presence of atrial fibrillation, which, at rapid rates, is poorly tolerated in patients with impaired diastolic filling. Negative inotropic agents such as beta-blockers and calcium channel blockers can be used with caution.
- Nesiritide (recombinant brain natriuretic protein) does not reduce morbidity or mortality (ASCEND-HF trial)

2nd phase: Inpatient hospital care

This phase of treatment includes further diuresis and stabilization of volume status. The patient should be carefully brought to euvolemia with daily volume status and electrolyte monitoring. The patient should also be transitioned to oral diuretics when stabilized. Whilst inpatient, the patient should have his/her medical and device management optimized with the therapies discussed later.

3rd phase: Early discharge planning and care

The patient should be transitioned to oral diuretics and be placed on optimum outpatient maintenance therapy, which will be discussed later. If the patient was on IV inotropic therapy, oral regimens should be adjusted while these infusions are tapered off. Prolonged physiologic effects of these IV inotropic agents after their discontinuation before discharge may mask the inadequate diuretic regimen and intolerance to the vasodilator doses. This can result in readmission, especially with milrinone due to its long half-life that can be further prolonged by the common coexisting impaired renal function. Therefore it may be recommended that patients who received inotropic infusions remain hospitalized for at least 48 hours after inotropic agents are discontinued, and optimize the oral regimen.

4th phase: Early post-discharge care

The patient will require re-evaluation and constant monitoring in order to avoid another episode of ADHF. Emphasis should be placed on importance of compliance with instructions regarding dietary restrictions and daily body weight monitoring. Early follow-up should be scheduled as well as outpatient electrolyte monitoring if required after medication adjustments.

CHRONIC TREATMENT OF HF SECONDARY TO SYSTOLIC DYSFUNCTION:

The goals of HF therapy are clinical improvement followed by stabilizing, slowing, or even reversing deterioration in myocardial function, and ultimately a reduction in risk of morbidity (including hospitalization rates) and mortality.

- ACE inhibitors
  ○ Reduce morbidity and mortality.
  ○ Produce both venous and arterial vasodilation acutely, thereby reducing both preload and afterload.
  ○ Potential mechanism of long-term benefit is attenuation of RAAS activation and decreased myocardial remodeling and fibrosis.
  ○ Used as first-line therapy for asymptomatic LV dysfunction (LVEF <40%) and symptomatic systolic HF (ACC/AHA grades A-D).

- Therapy should be initiated at low doses to prevent hypotension and rapidly titrated to higher doses as tolerated.
- Contraindications to the use of ACE inhibitors are renal insufficiency (creatinine clearance <30 ml/min), bilateral renal artery stenosis, hyperkalemia, hypotension, or adverse reactions (e.g., angioedema).
- ARBs
  - Receptor antagonists to the angiotensin II receptor.
  - Clinical trials have not shown any superiority compared to ACE inhibitors in patients with systolic HF (LVEF <40%).
  - Reserved for patients who are ACE inhibitor intolerant.
  - There are conflictive data on the utility of combination therapy with ARBs and ACE inhibitors in addition to beta-blockers for patients who remain symptomatic in the absence of renal dysfunction, hyperkalemia, and outside the post-MI period.
  - Have a similar contraindication profile to ACE inhibitors.
- Beta-adrenergic blockers (beta-blockers)
  - Reduce morbidity and mortality. Such benefits observed with bisoprolol (CIBIS II trial), metoprolol succinate (MERIT-HF trial), and carvedilol (COPERNICUS trial).
  - Benefit is thought to be conferred by blockade of sympathetic effects of neurohormonal stimulation due to HF.
  - Are considered first-line therapy for symptomatic patients with systolic HF (NYHA class ≥II and LVEF <35%).
  - Only carvedilol, bisoprolol, and metoprolol succinate have been approved for the medical treatment of chronic HF; these agents are generally started in patients judged to be euvolemic and dosage is to be slowly uptitrated as tolerated.
  - Adverse effects include worsening HF (due to negative inotropic effects), fatigue, dizziness, bradycardia, hypotension, and bronchospasm.
- Aldosterone receptor antagonists
  - Reduce morbidity and mortality
  - Indicated in patients with NYHA class III-IV HF, with LVEF <35%, already treated with ACE inhibitors and beta-blockers without significant renal insufficiency or hyperkalemia per 2009 ACC/AHA updated guidelines on the treatment of HF (RALES). Recently, the EMPHASIS-HF trial examined the use of eplerenone in patients with NYHA class II symptoms and left ventricular ejection fraction (LVEF) <35% and demonstrated a mortality benefit compared with current recommended medical therapy. They are also indicated for post-STEMI patients with EF ≤40% who have either symptomatic HF or diabetes mellitus (EPHESUS trial).
  - Spironolactone may cause gynecomastia, galactorrhea, and hyperkalemia (especially in patients with baseline renal insufficiency or type 4 renal tubular acidosis). Eplerenone is associated with less endocrine side effects.

- Diuretics
  - Are used to maintain euvolemia and to improve symptoms as discussed previously.
  - Although data on diuretic efficacy are limited, a meta-analysis of a few small trials found that they were associated with reduction in mortality as well as reduced hospitalization for HF.
  - Of note, loop diuretics with better bioavailability, such as torsemide and bumetanide, may be used in diuretic-resistant patients but are generally more expensive.
- Combination of isosorbide dinitrate and hydralazine
  - Cause venous (nitrates) and arteriolar (hydralazine) vasodilation resulting in decreased preload and afterload.
  - Combination therapy has been shown to confer morbidity and mortality benefit in patients (especially blacks [A-HeFT trial]) with NYHA class III-IV systolic HF (LVEF <40%) already on optimal therapy with a beta-blocker, ACE (or ARB), aldosterone antagonist (if indicated), and diuretics.
  - Adverse effects of nitrates include hypotension, headaches, and tolerance as well as reflex tachycardial and lupuslike syndrome with hydralazine.
- Digoxin
  - Positive inotropic and negative chronotropic drug that works by inhibition of the sodium-potassium transmembrane exchange pump
  - Commonly used in patients with concomitant atrial fibrillation
  - Has been shown to reduce HF-related hospitalizations but does NOT confer any mortality benefit (DIG trial). However, there is evidence suggesting that digoxin may actually have an effect on survival that varies with the serum digoxin level; survival was improved when the level was between 0.5 and 0.8 ng/ml (most often in men) and significantly worsened when it was ≥1.2 ng/ml (most often in women). Digoxin has a very narrow therapeutic range.
  - Caution must be used in patients with abnormal renal function to avoid digoxin toxicity and life-threatening arrhythmia. Avoid hypokalemia because potassium competes with digoxin on the same site of the Na^+-K^+-ATPase pump.
- Cardiac resynchronization therapy (CRT)
  - Improves morbidity and mortality rates in selected patients.
  - The presence of a bundle-branch block or other intraventricular conduction delay (IVCD) can cause ventricular dyssynchrony, which induces regional loading disparities and reduces the efficiency of ventricular contraction, thereby further impairing the systolic function of a failing ventricle.
  - CRT is recommended in patients with advanced HF (NYHA class III-IV despite optimal medical therapy), severe systolic dysfunction (LVEF <35%), and IVCD (QRS duration >120 msec). CRT is NOT indicated in patients whose functional status

and life expectancy are limited predominantly by chronic noncardiac conditions.
- In the appropriate subset of patients, CRT in addition to optimal medical therapy has been shown in numerous clinical trials to improve symptoms by at least one NYHA class, improve 6-min walk distance and quality of life, reduce rate of HF-related hospitalization, and reduce rate of all-cause and cardiovascular mortality.
- Implantable cardioverter-defibrillators (ICDs)
  - Sudden cardiac death (SCD) is a common cause of death in patients with HF in both ischemic and nonischemic cardiomyopathies. Ventricular tachycardia (VT) degenerating into ventricular fibrillation (VF) is the culprit in the majority of patients with SCD, although bradyarrhythmias do also occur with less frequency.
  - In patients with nonischemic cardiomyopathy, primary prevention of SCD with an ICD is appropriate in patients with LVEF <35% and NYHA class II-III HF (and NYHA class IV HF if likelihood of survival is >1 yr). In patients with LVEF <35%, class III-IV HF, and QRS duration >120 msec, a combined biventricular pacemaker and ICD device is indicated. For patients with a history of prior MI (ischemic cardiomyopathy) and LVEF <30% (>40 days post MI and 3 mo post CABG or PCI), regardless of NYHA classification, an ICD is indicated for primary prevention of SCD. In patients who do not meet the above criteria who experience nonsustained VT, the appropriateness of ICD placement is based on electrophysiologic studies.
  - Patients with HF who survive an episode of sudden cardiac arrest or experience sustained VT in the presence of LVEF <35% are at high risk for future arrhythmic events and SCD and obtain a mortality benefit from ICD placement for secondary prevention, with or without adjunctive therapies such as antiarrhythmic drugs, radiofrequency ablation, surgery, or transplant.
- In the absence of an indication (e.g., atrial fibrillation), routine use of anticoagulation is currently not recommended in patients with HF. Even with the increased risk for LV thrombus formation in dilated cardiomyopathy and subsequent thromboembolization, data are conflicting about benefits of antithrombotic (antiplatelet or anticoagulant) therapy for primary prevention to reduce thromboembolic events or mortality in patients with systolic HF who are in sinus rhythm (SOLVD, V-HeFT, SAVE, HELAS, and WASH trials). It may be reasonable to consider anticoagulation for secondary prevention in patients with HF who had a prior thromboembolic event; however, risks and benefits should be carefully assessed.
- Antiplatelet agents are recommended for patients with concomitant CAD.
- Percutaneous coronary intervention (PCI) or surgical revascularization should be considered in patients with HF and significant CAD who are revascularization candidates.

H

Diseases and Disorders

I

- In general, the following sequence of drugs is recommended:
  1. Loop diuretics to provide symptom relief and achieve a euvolemic state.
  2. ACE or ARB started at low doses, then increased to a moderate dose in 1-2 weeks.
  3. Beta-blockers after the patient is stable on ACE/ARB treatment. Start a low dose, then uptitrate to goal based on trial data or maximal dose tolerated. Once achieved, uptitration of ACE or ARB to goal doses can be completed.
- The following drugs can be added in seletected patients in the absence of contraindications:
  - ○ Aldosterone antagonists improve survival in NYHA class II with LVEF <30% or NYHA class III-IV with EF <35%. Kidney function should be stable with eGFR ≥30 ml/min and potassium <5 mEq/L.
  - ○ Combination of hydralazine with a nitrate in patients (particularly blacks) with a reduced EF.
  - ○ Digoxin reduces hospitalizations for HF and controls HR rate in atrial fibrillation. It can also help control symptoms.

CHRONIC TREATMENT OF HF WITH PRESERVED SYSTOLIC FUNCTION:

- To date, there is a relative dearth of clinical trials examining effective chronic treatment strategies in this subset of patients with HF. Current therapies are mainly for symptomatic relief.

- Therapy centers on relief of volume overload with judicious diuretic use, treatment of ischemia via coronary revascularization, heart rate and blood pressure control to prevent acute decompensation, and sodium and fluid restriction to prevent volume overload.
- Surgical options for contributing critical aortic stenosis, constrictive pericarditis, and hypertrophic cardiomyopathy (HCM) should be entertained in appropriate patients.

DISPOSITION

- Annual mortality of systolic HF ranges from 10% in stable patients with mild symptoms to 50% in patients with NYHA class IV disease (a mortality rate rivaling some malignancies). The Seattle Heart Failure Model provides an accurate estimate of 1-, 2-, and 3-year survival before and after different therapies. This model can be useful to assess the need for LV assist device implantation or urgent transplantation. The calculator is available online at http://depts.washington.edu/shfm/.
- Cardiac transplantation has a 5-yr survival rate of ~70% and represents a viable option in selected patients.
- The use of an LV assist device (LVAD) in patients with advanced HF can result in a clinically meaningful survival benefit and improve quality of life in patients who are not candidates for cardiac transplantation. There are two approved uses of LVADs specifically as a bridge to transplant and as destination therapy. There are two major categories of LVAD pulsatile flow devices vs. continuous flow devices. A recent trial (2008) has indicated that continuous flow devices are associated with increased survival as destination therapy as compared to medically managed controls. Interestingly, more recent trials (2010 and 2011) have shown there was no difference in posttransplantation survival between patients who were bridged with continuous-flow VADs vs. no VADs or even between patients bridged with pulsatile vs. continuous-flow VADs.

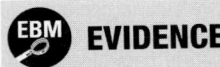 **EVIDENCE**

available at www.expertconsult.com

SUGGESTED READINGS

available at www.expertconsult.com

RELATED CONTENT

Congestive Heart Failure (CHF) (Patient Information)

AUTHORS: **ALI DAHHAN, M.D.,**
FRED F. FERRI, M.D., and
WEN-CHIH WU, M.D., M.P.H.

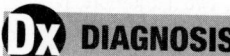

BASIC INFORMATION

DEFINITION

Heat exhaustion and heat stroke are part of a continuum of heat-related illness, and unless factors leading to heat exhaustion are corrected swiftly, affected patients can progress to heat stroke.

- **Heat exhaustion:** an illness resulting from prolonged, heavy activity in a hot environment with subsequent dehydration, electrolyte depletion, and rectal temperature >37.8° C but ≤40° C.
- **Heat stroke:** a life-threatening heat illness characterized by extreme hyperthermia, dehydration, and neurologic manifestations (core temperature >40° C).

SYNONYMS

Heat illness
Hyperthermia

ICD-9CM CODES
992.0 Heat stroke
992.5 Heat exhaustion

EPIDEMIOLOGY & DEMOGRAPHICS

INCIDENCE (IN U.S.): Incidence of heat stroke is approximately 20 cases/100,000 population.
PREDOMINANT AGE: Heat exhaustion and stroke occur more frequently in elderly patients, especially those taking diuretics or medications that impair heat dissipation (e.g., phenothiazines, anticholinergics, antihistamines, beta-blockers). Table 1-178 describes factors predisposing to serious heat illness.

PHYSICAL FINDINGS & CLINICAL PRESENTATION

Heat exhaustion:
- Generalized malaise, weakness, headache, muscle and abdominal cramps, nausea, vomiting, hypotension, tachycardia
- Rectal temperature is usually normal
- Sweating is usually present
Heat stroke:
- Neurologic manifestations (seizures, tremor, hemiplegia, coma, psychosis, other bizarre behavior)
- Evidence of dehydration (poor skin turgor, sunken eyeballs)
- Tachycardia, hyperventilation
- Skin is hot, red, and flushed
- Sweating is often (not always) absent, particularly in elderly patients
- Classic heat stroke generally develops slowly over days and occurs predominantly in older persons and in those with chronic illness. Exertional heat stroke is more common in young, healthy persons, has a more rapid onset, and is associated with higher core temperatures. Table 1-179 compares classic and exertional heat stroke

ETIOLOGY
- Exogenous heat gain (increased ambient temperature)
- Increased heat production (exercise, infection, hyperthyroidism, drugs)
- Impaired heat dissipation (high humidity, heavy clothing, neonatal or elderly patients, drugs [phenothiazines, anticholinergics, antihistamines, butyrophenones, amphetamines, cocaine, alcohol, β-blockers])
- Diuretics, laxatives

DIAGNOSIS

DIFFERENTIAL DIAGNOSIS
- Infections (meningitis, encephalitis, sepsis)
- Head trauma
- Epilepsy
- Thyroid storm
- Acute cocaine intoxication
- Malignant hyperthermia
- Heat exhaustion can be differentiated from heat stroke by the following:
  1. Essentially intact mental function and lack of significant fever in heat exhaustion
  2. Mild or absent increases in creatine phosphokinase (CPK), aspartate aminotransferase (AST), lactate dehydrogenase (LDH), and alanine aminotransferase (ALT) in heat exhaustion

WORKUP
- Heat stroke: comprehensive history, physical examination, and laboratory evaluation
- Heat exhaustion: in most cases, laboratory tests are not necessary for diagnosis

LABORATORY TESTS
Laboratory abnormalities may include the following:
- Elevated BUN, creatinine, hematocrit
- Hyponatremia or hypernatremia, hyperkalemia or hypokalemia
- Elevated LDH, AST, ALT, CPK, bilirubin
- Lactic acidosis, respiratory alkalosis (from hyperventilation)
- Myoglobinuria, hypofibrinogenemia, fibrinolysis, hypocalcemia

TREATMENT

- Treatment of heat exhaustion consists primarily of placing the patient in a cool, shaded area and providing rapid hydration and salt replacement.
  1. Fluid intake should be at least 2 L q4h in patients without history of CHF.
  2. Salt replacement can be accomplished by using one-quarter teaspoon of salt or two 10-grain salt tablets dissolved in 1 L of water.
  3. If IV fluid replacement is necessary, young athletes can be given normal saline IV (3 to 4 L over 6 to 8 hr); in elderly patients, consider using D5½NS IV with the rate titrated to cardiovascular status.
- Patients with heat stroke should undergo rapid cooling.
  1. Remove the patient's clothes and place the patient in a cool and well-ventilated room.
  2. If patient is unconscious, position on his or her side and clear the airway. Protect airway and augment oxygenation (e.g., nasal O_2 at 4 L/min to keep oxygen saturation >90%).
  3. Monitor body temperature every 5 min. Measurement of the patient's core temperature with a rectal probe is recommended. The goal is to reduce the body temperature to 39° C (102.2° F) in 30 to 60 min.
  4. Spray the patient with a cool mist and use fans to enhance airflow over the body (rapid evaporation method).
  5. Immersion of the patient in ice water, stomach lavage with iced saline solution,

TABLE 1-178 Factors Predisposing to Serious Heat Illness

Individual Factors

Lack of acclimatization
Low physical fitness
Excessive body weight
Dehydration
Advanced age
Young age

Health Conditions

Inflammation and fever
Viral infection
Cardiovascular disease
Diabetes mellitus
Gastroenteritis
Rash, sunburn, and previous burns to large areas of skin
Seizures
Thyroid storm
Neuroleptic malignant syndrome
Malignant hyperthermia
Sickle cell trait
Cystic fibrosis
Spinal cord injury

Drugs

Anticholinergic properties (atropine)
Antiepileptic (topiramate)
Antihistamines
Glutethimide (Doriden)
Phenothiazines
Tricyclic antidepressants
Amphetamines, cocaine, "Ecstasy"
Ergogenic stimulants (e.g., ephedrine, ephedra)
Lithium
Diuretics
β-Blockers
Ethanol

Environmental Factors

High temperature
High humidity
Little air motion
Lack of shade
Heat wave
Physical exercise
Heavy clothing
Air pollution (nitrogen dioxide)

From Goldman L, Schafer AI: *Goldman's Cecil medicine,* ed 24, Philadelphia, 2012, Saunders.

H

Diseases and Disorders

I

intravenous administration of cooled fluids, and inhalation of cold air are advisable only when the means for rapid evaporation are not available. Immersion in tepid water (15° C, 59° F) is preferred over ice water immersion to minimize risk of shivering.
6. Use of ice packs on axillae, neck, and groin is controversial because they increase peripheral vasoconstriction and may induce shivering.

7. Antipyretics are ineffective because the hypothalamic set point during heat stroke is normal despite the increased body temperature.
8. Intubate a comatose patient, insert a Foley catheter, and start nasal O_2. Continuous ECG monitoring is recommended.
9. Insert at least two large-bore IV lines and begin IV hydration with NS or Ringer's lactate.

10. Draw initial laboratory studies: electrolytes, complete blood count, blood urea nitrogen, creatinine, AST, ALT, CPK, LDH, glucose, PT (INR), PTT, platelet count, Ca^{2+}, lactic acid, and arterial blood gases.
11. Treat complications as follows:
    a. Hypotension: vigorous hydration with normal saline or Ringer's lactate.
    b. Convulsions: diazepam 5 to 10 mg IV (slowly).
    c. Shivering: chlorpromazine 10 to 50 mg IV.
    d. Acidosis: use bicarbonate judiciously (only in severe acidosis).
12. Observe for evidence of rhabdomyolysis and hepatic, renal, or cardiac failure and treat accordingly.

DISPOSITION

Most patients recover completely within 48 hr. Central nervous system injury is permanent in 20% of cases. Mortality rate can exceed 30% in patients with prolonged and severe hyperthermia. Delayed access to cooling is the leading cause of morbidity and mortality in persons with heat stroke.

SUGGESTED READINGS
available at www.expertconsult.com

RELATED CONTENT
Heat Exhaustion and Heat Stroke (Patient Information)

AUTHOR: **FRED F. FERRI, M.D.**

TABLE 1-179 Comparison of Classic and Exertional Heat Stroke

Patient Characteristics	Classic	Exertional
Age	Young children or elderly	15-55 yr
Health	Chronic illness	Usually healthy
Fever	Unusual	Common
Prevailing weather	Frequent in heat waves	Variable
Activity	Sedentary	Strenuous exercise
Drug use	Diuretics, antidepressants, anticholinergics, phenothiazines	Ergogenic stimulants or cocaine
Sweating	Often absent	Common
Acid-base disturbances	Respiratory alkalosis	Lactic acidosis
Acute renal failure	Uncommon	Common ($\approx$15%)
Rhabdomyolysis	Uncommon	Common ($\approx$25%)
CK	Mildly elevated	Markedly elevated (500-1000 U/L)
ALT, AST	Mildly elevated	Markedly elevated
Hyperkalemia	Uncommon	Common
Hypocalcemia	Uncommon	Common
DIC	Mild	Marked
Hypoglycemia	Uncommon	Common

ALT, Alanine aminotransferase; *AST,* aspartate aminotransferase; *CK,* creatine kinase; *DIC,* disseminated intravascular coagulation.
From Goldman L, Schafer Al: *Goldman's Cecil medicine,* ed 24, Philadelphia, 2012, Saunders.

BASIC INFORMATION

DEFINITION

Infection of the human gastric mucosa with the organism *Helicobacter pylori*, a spiral-shaped gram-negative organism with unique features that allow it to survive in the hostile gastric environment.

SYNONYMS

Previously known as *Campylobacter pylori*

ICD-9CM CODES
041.86 *Helicobacter pylori (H. pylori)*

EPIDEMIOLOGY & DEMOGRAPHICS

H. pylori is the most common chronic bacterial infection in human beings, probably affecting 50% of the earth's population in all age groups and probably 30% to 40% of the U.S. population. In developing nations, infection is acquired at an earlier age and occurs more frequently.

CLINICAL PRESENTATION

- *H. pylori* causes histologic gastritis in all affected individuals. The majority of cases are asymptomatic and unlikely to proceed to serious consequences.
- *H. pylori* is a causative agent in peptic ulcer disease (PUD), gastric adenocarcinoma, and gastric mucosa-associated lymphoid tissue lymphoma, and may be a risk factor for iron-deficiency anemia and chronic idiopathic thrombocytopenic purpura. It may present with the signs and symptoms of these disorders, including abdominal pain, bloating, anorexia, and early satiety. Fig. 1-383 describes association of *H. pylori* infection and disease states.
- "Alarm symptoms" that should prompt more immediate and aggressive workup include weight loss, dysphagia, protracted nausea or vomiting, anemia, melena, and palpable abdominal mass.

ETIOLOGY

- Route of acquisition is unknown but is presumed to be person to person by oral-oral or fecal-oral exposure.
- The majority of cases are acquired in childhood. Socioeconomic status and living conditions in childhood affect risk of acquisition of infection. These factors include housing density, number of siblings, overcrowding, sharing a bed, and lack of running water.
- *H. pylori* does not invade gastroduodenal tissue, but disrupts the mucous layer, causing the underlying mucosa to be more vulnerable to acid peptic damage.
- What differentiates the subset of patients with *H. pylori* who go on to develop ulcers or cancer remains unclear.

DX DIAGNOSIS

DIFFERENTIAL DIAGNOSIS

- Infection with *H. pylori* should be considered in the face of PUD, gastric cancer, gastritis, and gastric MALT lymphoma.
- *H. pylori* should be considered in the differential diagnosis of upper gastrointestinal (GI) tract disease, along with non-ulcer dyspepsia, reflux esophagitis, biliary tract disease, gastroparesis, pancreatitis, and ischemic bowel.

WORKUP

- Workup is indicated in patients with active PUD, a past history of documented peptic ulcer, or gastric MALT lymphoma. The role of routine screening in high-risk populations is not clear. However, numerous studies suggest that *H. pylori* eradication is protective against progression of premalignant lesions. Consider testing for *H. pylori* in patients with idiopathic thrombocytopenic purpura, or with otherwise unexplained iron deficiency anemia. Consider a test-and-treat approach in asymptomatic first-degree relatives of gastric cancer patients.
- Routine identification and treatment of *H. pylori* in cases of non-ulcer dyspepsia, gastroesophageal reflux disease (GERD), nonsteroidal anti-inflammatory drug (NSAID) use, and in asymptomatic individuals in populations at high risk for gastric cancer is considered controversial, although it may be indicated in specific cases. A test-and-treat strategy may be used in patients aged <55 yr with uncomplicated dyspepsia who have no alarm symptoms.
- Results of testing must be interpreted in relation to the individual patient's likelihood of *H. pylori* infection based on demographic risk factors. In the U.S. population, increased probability of infection exists in African Americans, Hispanics/Latinos, immigrants from developing nations, patients with poor socioeconomic status, Native Americans from Alaska, and persons >50 yr.
- Routine screening for *H. pylori* is not indicated in asymptomatic patients who are at low risk of infection.
- Infected patients with nonulcer dyspepsia usually benefit from treatment and should be evaluated for *H. pylori*.

LABORATORY TESTS

- Testing may be invasive or noninvasive depending on the need for endoscopy for other indications. There is no indication for endoscopy solely to diagnose *H. pylori*.
- Tests for *H. pylori* are differentiated as active or passive. Active tests provide direct evidence that *H. pylori* infection is currently present and include urea breath testing and stool antigen testing. Passive testing, which includes all serologic testing for *H. pylori*, gives indirect evidence of its presence by detecting the presence of antibodies to the organism. Serologic testing is limited by its inability to distinguish between active current infection and prior infection that has resolved.
- Tests that use urease as a marker (urea breath and stool antigen tests and biopsy for urease activity) may result in false-negative results in patients taking antibiotics, bismuth, or antisecretory therapy, as well as those with active ulcer bleeding. Patients should be off antibiotics for 4 wk and off protein pump inhibitors for 2 wk before urea breath or stool antigen testing.
- When diagnostic endoscopy is indicated (for suspicion or follow-up of PUD or gastric

FIGURE 1-383 Association of *Helicobacter pylori* colonization and disease states. After *H. pylori* acquisition, virtually all persons develop persistent colonization that lasts for life. Colonization induces tissue responses termed *chronic gastritis*. This process affects gastric physiology, including glandular structure, acid secretion, and antigen processing, which in turn affect disease risk. Colonization with *H. pylori* increases the risk for certain diseases (duodenal ulcer, gastric ulcer, noncardia gastric adenocarcinoma, and B-cell lymphomas) but appears to decrease the risk for gastroesophageal reflux disease and its complications, including Barrett's esophagus, and adenocarcinoma of the esophagus or gastric cardia. (From Mandell GL et al: *Principles and practice of infectious diseases,* ed 7, Philadelphia, 2010, Churchill Livingstone.)

Primary phenomenon: Tissue response (inflammation)

Secondary phenomenon: Atrophic gastritis | Hyperacidity | Antigenic stimulation | ?

Clinical outcome: Noncardia gastric adenocarcinoma | Duodenal ulceration | B-cell lymphoma | Reflux esophagitis and sequelae

Association with H. pylori (odds ratio): 2-8 | 3-6 | 6-20 | 0.2-0.7

MALT), antral biopsy should be tested for urease activity. If urease testing is likely to show a false-negative result because of recent proton pump inhibitor (PPI), bismuth, or antibiotic use or active ulcer bleeding, the sample should undergo histologic examination.

- In cases in which biopsy is not indicated, urea breath testing or stool antigen testing are indicated to evaluate for active infection. The sensitivities and specificities of these two tests are similar (>90%). Urea breath testing is slightly more expensive than stool antigen testing, but both costs are in the modest range. Choice can be made based on patient preference and availability.
- In cases in which biopsy is not indicated, consider using serologic testing as the initial approach. However, in individuals with a low pretest probability of infection, positive results should be confirmed with another testing method.

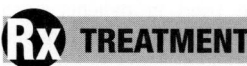

ACUTE GENERAL Rx

- Test only patients whom you intend to treat if positive (see "Workup" above). At this time, the value of eradicating *H. pylori* infection is proven in patients with PUD or gastric MALT lymphoma.
- The optimal antibiotic regimen has not been defined. In addition to efficacy, side effects, cost, and ease of administration must be considered.
- Due to increasing resistance to clarithromycin, decisions regarding appropriate regimens should take into account local rates of clarithromycin resistance.
- The following regimens may be considered for first-line therapy:
  - PPI twice daily, with twice-daily clarithromycin (500 mg) and amoxicillin (1 g) may be used in areas of low clarithromycin resistance.
  - In cases of penicillin allergy, metronidazole (500 mg bid) may be substituted for amoxicillin.
  - PPI twice daily, combined with bismuth four times daily, as well as tetracycline (500 mg qid) and metronidazole (250 mg) four times daily, is now recommended as first-line therapy in areas of high clarithromycin resistance. Sequential therapy, consisting of 5 days of treatment with a PPI and one antibiotic (usually amoxicillin)

followed by 5-day treatment with the PPI and two other antibiotics (usually clarithromycin and metronizadole) may be used in areas of high clarithromycin resistance when bismuth-based therapy is not available.

- Duration of treatment remains controversial. Extending therapy to 10-14 days may improve eradication rates. Use of combination capsules may improve compliance but is likely to be more expensive.
- Prior exposure to a macrolide or metronidazole, for any reason, is associated with increased resistance. A preferable regimen would include medications to which the patient has not been previously exposed.
- Diarrhea and abdominal cramping are commonly observed with many of the regimens. (Probiotics may diminish this effect.) Other side effects may include a metallic taste with metronidazole or clarithromycin, neuropathy, seizures, and disulfiram-like reaction with metronidazole, diarrhea with amoxicillin, photosensitivity with tetracycline, and *Clostridium difficile* infection with any antibiotic exposure. Bismuth may cause black stool and constipation. Tetracycline is contraindicated in pregnant patients.
- 20% of patients may not respond to initial therapy. Optimal retreatment regimens are under investigation. It is important to reinforce compliance. Second-line therapy should be either bismuth-containing quadruple therapy or levofloxacin containing triple therapy (regardless of local clarithromycin resistance patterns). When possible, management of those who do not respond to two courses of therapy should be guided by antimicrobial sensitivity testing.

CHRONIC Rx

- Data do not support routine testing for cure. Accepted indications for confirming eradication include *H. pylori*–associated ulcers, MALT lymphoma, and early gastric cancer. It may be considered in those with persistent dyspepsia despite a test-and-treat management strategy (as well as consideration of other causes for the dyspeptic symptoms).
- Serology does not reliably revert to undetectable levels after treatment and should not be used to determine eradication.
- Active tests (urea breath test and stool antigen testing) are preferable. They are equally accurate in confirming eradication, and either may be used depending on availability and

patient preference. To reduce the likelihood of false-negative results, testing should be performed at least 4 wk after eradication therapy with PPI and antibiotics and at least 2 wk after the cessation of PPI therapy.

DISPOSITION

Consider further evaluation in patients with recurrent symptoms after appropriate treatment.

REFERRAL

- Patients with gastric MALT lymphoma should be followed by a gastroenterologist and oncologist with expertise in the care of lymphoid neoplasms.
- Patients with dyspepsia who have tested positive for *H. pylori* and been treated without resolution should be referred for endoscopy.
- Consider referral for biopsy for culture and sensitivity in patients who have not responded to two attempts at treatment.

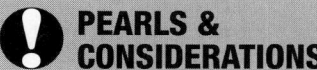

- Whether *H. pylori* eradication reduces the risk of gastric cancer is unclear.
- Outcomes in PUD and gastric MALT lymphoma are improved with treatment of associated *H. pylori* infection.
- Tests that provide direct evidence of active *H. pylori* infection (urea breath and stool antigen testing) are preferred but may result in false-negative results in patients taking antibiotics, bismuth, or antisecretory agents.
- Serologic testing does not differentiate active from prior infection. It may be useful when active tests are not indicated, particularly in high-risk patients.
- Be aware of high-risk populations in low-prevalence settings, including immigrants from Mexico, South America, Southeast Asia, and Eastern Europe.

SUGGESTED READINGS
available at www.expertconsult.com

RELATED CONTENT
Helicobacter pylori Infection (Patient Information)

AUTHOR: **MARGARET TRYFOROS, M.D.**

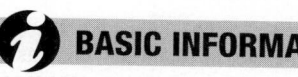

BASIC INFORMATION

DEFINITION

The HELLP syndrome is a serious variant of preeclampsia. HELLP is an acronym for *h*emolysis, *e*levated *l*iver function, and *l*ow *p*latelet count. It is the most frequently encountered microangiopathy of pregnancy. There are three classes of the syndrome based on the degree of maternal thrombocytopenia as a primary indicator of disease severity:

Class 1: Platelets $\leq$ 50,000/mm^3
Class 2: Platelets > 50,000/mm^3 to 100,000/mm^3
Class 3: Platelets > 100,000/mm^3

ICD-9CM CODES
642.50 HELLP, episode of care
642.51 HELLP, delivered
642.52 HELLP, delivered with postpartum complications
642.53 HELLP, antepartum complications
642.54 HELLP, postpartum complications

EPIDEMIOLOGY & DEMOGRAPHICS

- Among women with severe preeclampsia, 6% will manifest with one abnormality suggestive of HELLP syndrome, 12% will develop two abnormalities, and approximately 10% will develop all three.
- The HELLP syndrome, like preeclampsia, is rare before 20 wk of gestation.
- One third of all cases occur postpartum; of these, only 80% are typically diagnosed with preeclampsia before delivery.

RISK FACTORS: Women > 35 yr, white, multiparity
RECURRENCE RATE: 3% to 25%

PHYSICAL FINDINGS & CLINICAL PRESENTATION

- Definitive laboratory criteria remain to be validated prospectively.
- Most commonly used criteria include hemolysis defined by the presence of an abnormal peripheral smear with schistocytes, lactate dehydrogenase (LDH) > 600 U/L, and total bilirubin > 1.2 mg/dl; elevated liver enzymes as serum aspartate aminotransferase (AST) > 70 U/L and LDH > 600 U/L; low platelet count as less than 100,000/mm^3.
- Although many women with HELLP syndrome are asymptomatic, 80% report right upper quadrant pain and 50% to 60% present with excessive weight gain and worsening edema.

ETIOLOGY

As with other microangiopathies, endothelial dysfunction, with resultant activation of the intravascular coagulation cascade, has been proposed as the central pathogenesis of HELLP syndrome.

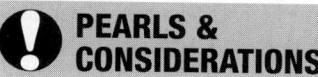

DIAGNOSIS

DIFFERENTIAL DIAGNOSIS

- Appendicitis
- Gallbladder disease
- Peptic ulcer disease
- Enteritis
- Hepatitis
- Pyelonephritis
- Systemic lupus erythematosus
- Thrombotic thrombocytopenic purpura/hemolytic-uremic syndrome
- Acute fatty liver of pregnancy

WORKUP

Because HELLP syndrome is a disease entity based on laboratory values, initial assessment is detailed below.

LABORATORY TESTS

- Initial assessment of suspected HELLP syndrome should include a complete blood count to evaluate platelets, urinalysis, serum creatinine, LDH, uric acid, indirect and total bilirubin levels, and AST/alanine aminotransferase (ALT).
- Tests of prothrombin time, partial thromboplastin time, fibrinogen, and fibrin split products are reserved for women with a platelet count well below 100,000/mm^3.

IMAGING STUDIES

No imaging modalities aid in diagnosis.

TREATMENT

Treatment depends on gestational age of the fetus, severity of condition, and maternal status. Stabilization of the mother is the first priority.

ACUTE GENERAL Rx

- Assess gestational age thoroughly. Fetal status should be monitored with nonstress tests, contraction stress tests, and/or biophysical profile.
- Maternal status should be evaluated by history, physical examination, and laboratory testing.

- Magnesium sulfate is administered for seizure prophylaxis regardless of blood pressure.
- Blood pressure control is achieved with agents such as hydralazine or labetalol.
- Indwelling Foley catheter to monitor maternal volume status and urine output.

CHRONIC Rx

- In pregnancies of 34 wk or with class 1 HELLP syndrome, delivery, either vaginal or abdominal, within 24 hr is the goal.
- In the preterm fetus corticosteroid therapy to enhance fetal lung maturation is indicated.
- Some reports have shown temporary amelioration of HELLP severity with the administration of high-dose steroids measured by increased urine output, improvement in platelet count, and liver function test.
- Judicious use of blood products, especially in those requiring surgery.
- The patient requires intensive observation for 48 hr postpartum; laboratory levels should begin to improve during this time.

DISPOSITION

The natural history of this disorder is a rapidly deteriorating condition requiring close monitoring of maternal and fetal well-being.

REFERRAL

Preterm patients with HELLP syndrome should be stabilized hemodynamically and transferred to a tertiary care center. Term patients can be treated at a local hospital depending on the availability of obstetric, neonatal, and blood banking services.

PEARLS & CONSIDERATIONS

- Not all women with HELLP have hypertension or proteinuria.
- Life-threatening hemorrhage is a rare event in HELLP syndrome. Identifiable risk factors predictive of a major hemorrhage are thrombocytopenia (< 100,000/mm^3), AST > 70 IU/L, and previous gestations.

SUGGESTED READINGS
available at www.expertconsult.com

RELATED CONTENT
Eclampsia (Related Key Topic)
Preeclampsia (Related Key Topic)

AUTHORS: **SONYA S. ABDEL-RAZEQ, M.D.,** and **RUBEN ALVERO, M.D.**

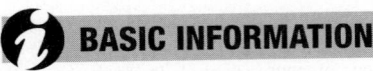

DEFINITION

Hemochromatosis is an autosomal-recessive disorder that disrupts the body's regulation of iron and is characterized by increased accumulation of iron in various organs (adrenals, liver, pancreas, heart, testes, kidneys, pituitary) and eventual dysfunction of these organs if not treated appropriately.

SYNONYMS

Bronze diabetes

ICD-9CM CODES
275.0 Hemochromatosis

EPIDEMIOLOGY & DEMOGRAPHICS

INCIDENCE: In whites, approximately 1 in 385 persons

PREDOMINANT SEX AND AGE:

Generally diagnosed in males in their fifth decade. Diagnosis in females is generally not made until 10 to 20 yr after menopause.

GENETICS:

Most common genetic disorder in North European ancestry. Homozygosity for the *C282Y* mutation is now found in approximately 5 of every 1000 persons of European descent.

PHYSICAL FINDINGS & CLINICAL PRESENTATION

- In earlier stages patients completely asymptomatic and diagnosed due to abnormal laboratory tests
- Hepatic dysfunction leading to hepatomegaly, fibrosis, and eventually cirrhosis
- Arthritis
- Gonadal insufficiency leading to loss of libido and testicular atrophy
- Diabetes mellitus: risk greater in patients with family history
- Iron-induced cardiac disease resulting in cardiomyopathy, heart failure, and arrhythmias
- Skin pigmentation

ETIOLOGY

- The majority of the patients diagnosed with hemochromatosis have mutation in the *HFE* gene and are either homozygous for the *C282Y* mutation (*C282Y/C282Y*) or compound heterozygote for the *C282Y* mutation and either the mutation *H63D* (*C282Y/H63D*) or less commonly the *S65C* (*C282Y/S65C*).
- The remainder of the patients are classified as non–*HFE*-associated hemochromatosis.

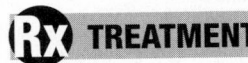 **DIAGNOSIS**

DIFFERENTIAL DIAGNOSIS

- Hereditary anemias with defect of erythropoiesis
- Cirrhosis, chronic liver disease, porphyria cutanea tarda

- Repeated blood transfusions
- African dietary iron overload

WORKUP

Medical history, physical examination, and laboratory evaluation should be focused on affected organ systems (see "Physical Findings & Clinical Presentation"). Fig. 1-384 outlines evaluation for possible hereditary hemochromatosis in an individual with negative family history. Liver biopsy is the gold standard for diagnosis; it reveals iron deposition in hepatocytes, bile ducts, and supporting tissues.

LABORATORY TESTS

- Transferrin saturation is the best screening test. Values >45% are an indication for further testing.
- Elevated serum ferritin is good evidence of iron overload, but other causes like chronic inflammatory conditions, malignancy, and so forth need to be ruled out as ferritin is also an acute phase reactant.
- Genotypical screening for *C282Y* and *H63D* mutation in *HFE* gene should be done in patients with high transferrin saturation, elevated ferritin, or both.

- Liver biopsy (Fig. 1-385) is the gold standard but is not needed in somebody who has a persistently elevated transferrin saturation, elevated ferritin, or both.
- Hepatic iron index can help differentiate between various causes of iron overload.
- Elevated aspartate aminotransferase, alanine aminotransferase, and alkaline phosphatase are seen.
- Hyperglycemia is found.
- Endocrine abnormalities (decreased testosterone, luteinizing hormone, follicle-stimulating hormone) are noted.
- Table 1-180 describes laboratory findings in patients with hereditary hemochromatosis.

IMAGING STUDIES

Routine radiologic imaging is not needed.

Rx TREATMENT

The goal of therapy is the removal of excess iron and maintaining it at a normal or near-normal level.

NONPHARMACOLOGIC THERAPY

Phlebotomy is the treatment of choice.

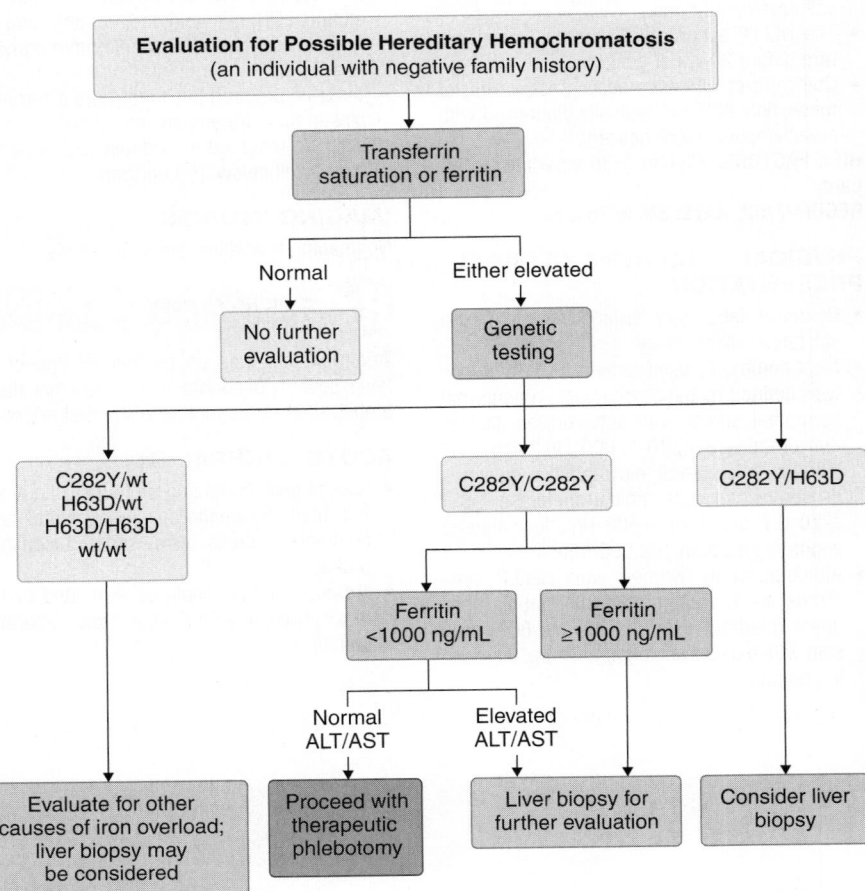

FIGURE 1-384 Algorithm for evaluation of possible hereditary hemochromatosis in a person with a negative family history. *ALT*, Alanine transaminase; *AST*, aspartate transaminase. (From Goldman L, Schafer AI: *Goldman's Cecil medicine*, ed 24, Philadelphia, 2012, Saunders.)

ACUTE GENERAL Rx

- The timing and frequency of phlebotomy needs to be individualized for each patient.
- For patients with heavy iron overload twice weekly phlebotomies should be started. In most patients, weekly phlebotomy is adequate.
- The effectiveness of treatment is monitored by periodic ferritin measurement. The goal is to bring ferritin level below 50 ng/ml.
- Patients with iron overload due to transfusion dependent anemias may not tolerate phlebotomy. For these patients iron chelation may be needed.
- The chelating agent deferoxamine has to be given daily as a 9- to 12-hr IV or SC infusion and compliance is difficult.

- The oral chelating agent deferasirox (Exjade) is effective but should not be used in patients with high-risk myelodysplastic syndrome because it can cause renal impairment, hepatic impairment, or gastrointestinal hemorrhage, which can be fatal.

CHRONIC Rx

After the ferritin has been brought to less than 50 ng/ml phlebotomy is needed on an as needed basis to keep the ferritin at that level.

DISPOSITION

- Serum ferritin measurement is the most useful prognostic indicator of disease severity.
- Prognosis is good if phlebotomy is started early (before onset of cirrhosis or diabetes mellitus); women can have the full phenotypic expression of the disease, including cirrhosis, and should also be aggressively treated.

REFERRAL

For liver biopsy if diagnosis is uncertain

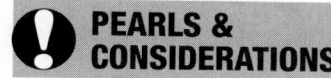 **PEARLS & CONSIDERATIONS**

COMMENTS

- Persons who are homozygous for the HFE gene mutation *C282Y* comprise 85% to 90% of phenotypically affected individuals.
- Patients with hemochromatosis and serum ferritin levels <1000 ng/ml are unlikely to have cirrhosis. Liver biopsy to screen for cirrhosis may be unnecessary in such patients.
- Cirrhotic patients must be periodically monitored (ultrasound or CT scan) because of their increased risk of hepatocellular carcinoma.
- *HFE* gene testing for *C282Y* mutation is a cost-effective method of screening relatives of patients with hereditary hemochromatosis. The American College of Gastroenterology recommends genotyping persons who have abnormal iron screening tests and first-degree relatives of those identified with *C282Y* homozygosity.
- Established cirrhosis, hypogonadism, destructive arthritis, and insulin-dependent diabetes mellitus secondary to hemochromatosis cannot be reversed with repeated phlebotomy, but their progress can be slowed.
- In patients who are heterozygotes for *C282Y* or *H63D* mutation, clinically meaningful iron overload does not develop.
- Screening for hepatocellular carcinoma is reserved for those with hereditary hemochromatosis and cirrhosis.

SUGGESTED READINGS

available at www.expertconsult.com

RELATED CONTENT

Hemochromatosis (Patient Information)

AUTHORS: **BILAL H. NAQVI, M.D.**, and **FRED F. FERRI, M.D.**

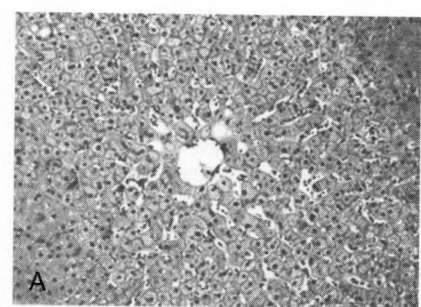
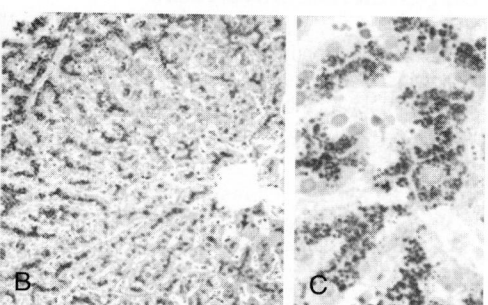

FIGURE 1-385 Hemochromatosis. Liver biopsy sample from a 46-year-old man with homozygous hemochromatosis. Hematoxylin and eosin stain of the liver **(A)** shows intact hepatic architecture. Iron stain **(B, C)** shows marked diffuse iron deposits in the hepatocytes throughout the lobules. A normal liver would show essentially no iron in the hepatocytes. (From Hoffman R et al: *Hematology, basic principles and practice,* ed 5, Philadelphia, 2009, Churchill Livingstone.)

TABLE 1-180   Laboratory Findings in Patients with Hereditary Hemochromatosis

Measurements	Normal Subjects	PATIENTS WITH HEREDITARY HEMOCHROMATOSIS	
		Asymptomatic	Symptomatic
Blood (Fasting)			
Serum iron level (μg/dl)	60-180	150-280	180-300
Serum transferrin level (mg/dl)	220-410	200-280	200-300
Transferrin saturation (%)	20-45	45-100	80-100
Serum ferritin level (ng/ml)			
Men	20-200	150-1000	500-6000
Women	15-150	120-1000	500-6000
Genetic (*HFE* Mutation Analysis)			
C282Y/C282Y	wt/wt‡	C282Y/C282Y	C282Y/C282Y
C282Y/H63D*	wt/wt	C282Y/H63D	C282Y/H63D
Liver			
Hepatic iron concentration			
μg/g dry weight	300-1500	2000-10,000	8000-30,000
μmol/g dry weight	5-27	36-179	140-550
Hepatic iron index†	<1	1 to >1.9	>1.9
Liver histology			
Perls' Prussian blue stain	0, 1+	2+ to 4+	3+, 4+

*Compound heterozygote.
†Calculated by dividing the hepatic iron concentration (in μmol/g dry weight) by the age of the patient (in yr). With the increased use of genetic testing in patients with iron overload, the specificity of the hepatic iron index has diminished.
‡wt/wt: wild type (normal).
From Goldman L, Schafer AI: *Goldman's Cecil medicine,* ed 24, Philadelphia, 2012, Saunders.

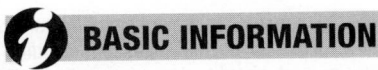

DEFINITION

Hemolytic-uremic syndrome (HUS) refers to an acute syndrome characterized by microangiopathic hemolytic anemia, thrombocytopenia, and severe renal failure.

SYNONYMS

HUS

ICD-9CM CODES
283.11 Hemolytic-uremic syndrome

EPIDEMIOLOGY & DEMOGRAPHICS

- HUS affects mainly children younger than 5 yr with incidence rate of 6.1 cases/100,000.
- Overall incidence is 1 to 2 cases/100,000.
- May be epidemic, most commonly occurring during the summer months in rural populations.
- Most common cause of acute renal failure in children.
- In the U.S., 300 to 700 new cases occur each year.

PHYSICAL FINDINGS & CLINICAL PRESENTATION

- HUS usually preceded by diarrhea in 90% of cases, bloody in 75%
- Abdominal pain, vomiting, and fever
- Neurologic symptoms, principally seizure and somnolence, have been observed in 20% to 25% of cases. Stroke or coma may occur and be associated with significant mortality
- Hypertension
- Hepatomegaly and abnormality in liver function tests
- Anuria or oliguria
- Glucose intolerance and transient diabetes (10%)

ETIOLOGY

Pathologically, it is thought that thrombin generation (probably the result of accelerated thrombogenesis) and inhibition of fibrinolysis lead to renal arteriolar and capillary microthrombi preceding renal injury.
In children:
- *Escherichia coli* serotype O157:H7 is the leading cause of HUS.
- The infection is acquired by eating undercooked red meat, nonpasteurized milk or milk products, water, fruits, or vegetables. A recent large outbreak of the HUS caused by Shiga-toxin–producing *Escherichia coli* O104:H4 in Germany was associated with consumption of contaminated sprouts.
- Other causes of HUS in children and adults are:
  - Drugs (cyclosporine, mitomycin, tacrolimus, ticlopidine, clopidogrel, cisplatin, quinine, penicillin, penicillamine, oral contraceptives, and quinine used to treat muscle cramps) and toxins
  - Infection (*Salmonella, Shigella, Yersinia,* Group A streptococci, *Clostridium difficile, Campylobacter,* coxsackie virus, rubella, influenza virus, Epstein-Barr virus)
  - HIV-associated thrombotic microangiopathy
  - Pneumococcal infection
- Complement disorders involving factors H, I, and membrane cofactors protein have been associated with cases of nondiarrhea-associated HUS (atypical HUS).
- Mutations that impair the function of thrombomodulin occur in about 5% of patients with atypical HUS.
- Table 1-181 describes a classification of HUS.

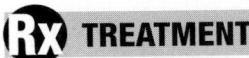

The triad of thrombocytopenia, acute renal failure, and microangiopathic hemolytic anemia establishes the diagnosis of HUS.

DIFFERENTIAL DIAGNOSIS

The differential is vast, including all causes of bloody and nonbloody diarrhea because the GI symptoms usually precede the triad of HUS:
- Thrombotic thrombocytopenic purpura
- Disseminated intravascular coagulation

TABLE 1-181 Classification of Hemolytic-Uremic Syndrome

Infection-induced

Verotoxin-producing *Escherichia coli*

Shiga toxin-producing *Shigella dysentereriae* type 1

Neuraminidase-producing *Streptococcus pneumoniae*

Human immunodeficiency virus

Genetic

Von Willebrand factor-cleaving protease (ADAMTS 13) deficiency

Complement factor H (or related proteins) deficiency or mutation

Membrane cofactor protein (MCP) mutations

Thrombomodulin mutations

Complement factor I mutations

Vitamin B_{12} metabolism defects

Familial autosomal recessive of undefined etiology

Familial autosomal dominant of undefined etiology

Sporadic, recurrent, undefined etiology without diarrhea prodrome

Other Diseases Associated with Microvascular Injury

Systemic lupus erythematosus

Antiphospholipid antibody syndrome

Following bone marrow transplantation

Malignant hypertension

Primary glomerulopathy

HELLP (*h*emolytic anemia, *e*levated *l*iver enzymes, *l*ow *p*latelet count) syndrome

Medication-induced

Calcineurin inhibitors (cyclosporine, tacrolimus)

Cytotoxic, chemotherapy agents (mitomycin C, cisplatin, gemcitabine)

Clopidogrel and ticlopidine

Quinine

From Kliegman RM et al: *Nelson textbook of pediatrics,* ed 19, Philadelphia, 2011, Saunders.

- Prosthetic valve hemolysis
- Malignant hypertension
- Vasculitis
- Catastrophic antiphospholipid syndrome
- Postpartum acute renal failure
- Scleroderma renal crisis

WORKUP

The workup for suspected HUS patients includes blood tests and stool cultures.

LABORATORY TESTS

- Anemia (hemoglobin <8 g/dl) with peripheral smear shows the hallmark microangiopathic hemolytic anemia with schistocytes, burr cells, and helmet cells (Fig. 1-386)
- Thrombocytopenia (platelet counts usually <60,000/mm^3)
- Reticulocyte count high
- LDH level elevated
- Haptoglobin low
- Indirect bilirubin elevated
- Negative Coombs test
- BUN and creatinine elevated
- Urinalysis: proteinuria, microscopic hematuria, and pyuria
- Stool cultures for *E. coli* O157:H7 are positive in more than 90% of cases if obtained during the first week of illness. After the first week, only one third are positive.

IMAGING STUDIES

Imaging studies are not very helpful in the diagnosis of HUS.

The treatment of HUS is primarily supportive.

NONPHARMACOLOGIC THERAPY

- Blood transfusions are used for severe anemia.
- Antibiotics and antimotility agents should be avoided and are not indicated for the treatment of *E. coli* O157:H7.
- Correction of electrolyte abnormalities and fluid management should be performed.

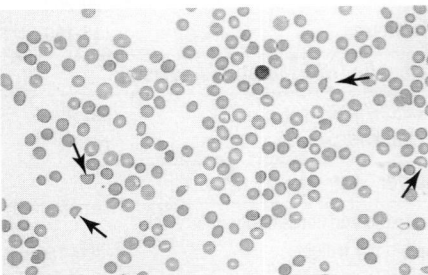

FIGURE 1-386 Hemolytic-uremic syndrome (HUS). Peripheral blood smear from a patient with HUS. The presence of fragmented red blood cells with the appearance of a helmet *(arrows)* is pathognomonic for microangiopathic hemolysis in patients with no evidence of heart valvular disease. (From Floege J et al: *Comprehensive clinical nephrology,* ed 4, Philadelphia, 2010, Saunders.)

- Platelet transfusion is preserved only for patients with HUS who have significant bleed or invasive procedure is required.
- Plasma exchange therapy with immunosuppressive agents has been used in patients with severe CNS involvement. Eculizumab, a monoclonal antibody directed toward complement component C_5, has been approved in adults for treatment of atypical HUS; however, its role remains to be fully defined.
- Tissue-type plasminogen activator (PAI-1) may have a role in improving renal function in recent studies.

ACUTE GENERAL Rx

Hypertension and seizure control

CHRONIC Rx

For anuric or oliguric renal failure, dialysis may be required.

DISPOSITION

- Adults presenting with HUS have a worse prognosis than do children with HUS.
- Mortality rate is less than 5%.

- Morbidity includes:
  - Proteinuria (31%)
  - Renal insufficiency (31%)
  - Hypertension (6%)

REFERRAL

- The local health department should be notified if *E. coli* O157:H7 has been isolated; large food-borne outbreaks have occurred with commercial beef products and asparagus.
- Consultation with hematology and nephrology specialist is recommended for patients with HUS.

⊕ PEARLS & CONSIDERATIONS

COMMENTS

- Children testing positive for the *E. coli* O157:H7 serotype should not return to school or day care facilities until two consecutive stools test negative for the microorganism.
- *E. coli* O157:H7 can be transmitted from person to person; therefore universal precau-

tions and handwashing are recommended in preventing the spread of the infection.
- *E. coli* O111 can also be associated with HUS. In 2008 the largest known U.S. serotype 1 *E. coli* O111 occurred in Oklahoma, causing 341 illnesses. The HUS attack rate in this *E. coli* O111 outbreak was comparable to that for *E. coli* O157-related illness, but most cases occurred among adults. More recently, in May 2011, a large outbreak of diarrhea and HUS caused by an unusual serotype of Shiga-toxin–producing *E. coli* (O104:H4) occurred in Germany, with 908 individuals reported with hemolytic-uremic syndrome, and 34 deaths.

SUGGESTED READINGS

available at www.expertconsult.com

RELATED CONTENT

Hemolytic-Uremic Syndrome (Patient Information)

AUTHORS: **MONZR M. AL MALKI, M.D.,** and **GLENN G. FORT, M.D., M.P.H.**

H

Diseases and Disorders

I

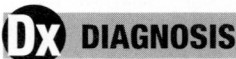

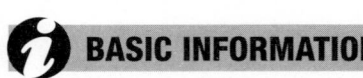 **BASIC INFORMATION**

DEFINITION

Hemophilia is a hereditary bleeding disorder caused by low factor VIII coagulant activity (hemophilia A) or low levels of factor IX coagulant activity (hemophilia B).

SYNONYMS

Hemophilia A: Classic hemophilia, factor VIII deficiency hemophilia

Hemophilia B: Christmas disease, factor IX hemophilia

ICD-9CM CODES
286.0 Hemophilia A
286.1 Hemophilia B

EPIDEMIOLOGY & DEMOGRAPHICS

INCIDENCE/PREVALENCE (IN U.S.): Hemophilia A: 100 cases per 1 million males; hemophilia B: 20 cases per 1 million males. Approximately 400,000 patients have severe hemophilia worldwide.

GENETIC: Both hemophilias have an X-linked recessive pattern of inheritance with only males affected.

PHYSICAL FINDINGS & CLINICAL PRESENTATION

- The clinical features of hemophilia A and B are generally indistinguishable from each other.
- Bleeding is most commonly seen in joints (knees, ankles, elbows), resulting in hot, swollen, painful joints (Fig. 1-387) and subsequent crippling joint deformity. (Fig. E1-388)
- Bleeding can also occur into the muscles and the gastrointestinal tract.
- Compartment syndrome can occur from large hematomas.
- Hematuria may be present.

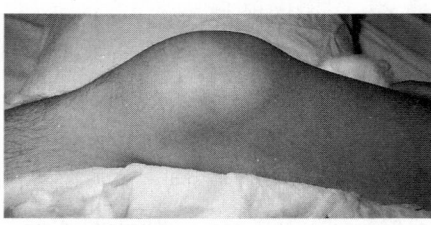

FIGURE 1-387 Acute hemarthrosis of the knee is a common complication of hemophilia. It may be confused with acute infection unless the patient's coagulation disorder is known because the knee is hot, red, swollen, and painful. (From Forbes CD, Jackson WF: *Color atlas and text of clinical medicine,* ed 3, London, 2003, Mosby.)

ETIOLOGY

- Hemophilia A: low factor VIII coagulant (VIII:C) activity; can be classified as mild if factor VIII:C levels are >5%, moderate if levels are 1% to 5%, and severe if levels are <1%.
- Hemophilia B: low levels of factor IX coagulant activity.
- Both disorders are congenital.
- Spontaneous acquisition of factor VIII inhibitors (acquired hemophilia) is rare.

Dx DIAGNOSIS

DIFFERENTIAL DIAGNOSIS

- Other clotting factor deficiencies
- Platelet function disorders
- Vitamin K deficiency

WORKUP

Patients with mild hemophilia bleed only in response to major trauma or surgery and may not be diagnosed until young adulthood. Diagnostic workup includes laboratory evaluation (see "Laboratory Tests").

LABORATORY TESTS

- Partial thromboplastin time (PTT) is prolonged.
- Reduced factor VIII:C level distinguishes hemophilia A from other causes of prolonged PTT.

TABLE 1-182 Treatment of Hemophilia

Type of Hemorrhage	Hemophilia A	Hemophilia B
Hemarthrosis*	50 IU/kg factor VIII concentrate† on day 1; then 20 IU/kg on days 2, 3, 5 until joint function is normal or back to baseline. Consider additional treatment every other day for 7-10 days. Consider prophylaxis.	80-100 IU/kg on day 1; then 40 IU/kg on days 2, 4. Consider additional treatment every other day for 7-10 days. Consider prophylaxis.
Muscle or significant subcutaneous hematoma	50 IU/kg factor VIII concentrate; 20 IU/kg every-other-day treatment may be needed until resolved.	80 IU/kg factor IX concentrate‡; treatment every 2-3 days may be needed until resolved.
Mouth, deciduous tooth, or tooth extraction	20 IU/kg factor VIII concentrate; antifibrinolytic therapy; remove loose deciduous tooth.	40 IU/kg factor IX concentrate‡; antifibrinolytic therapy§; remove loose deciduous tooth.
Epistaxis	Apply pressure for 15-20 min; pack with petrolatum gauze; give antifibrinolytic therapy; 20 IU/kg factor VIII concentrate if this treatment fails.ˡ	Apply pressure for 15-20 min; pack with petrolatum gauze; antifibrinolytic therapy; 30 IU/kg factor IX concentrate‡ if this treatment fails.
Major surgery, life-threatening hemorrhage	50-75 IU/kg factor VIII concentrate, then initiate continuous infusion of 2-4 IU/kg/hr to maintain factor VIII >100 IU/dl for 24 hrˡ then give 2-3 IU/kg/hr continuously for 5-7 days to maintain the level at >50 IU/dl and an additional 5-7 days to maintain the level at >30 IU/dl.¶	120 IU/kg factor IX concentrate‡, then 50-60 IU/kg every 12-24 hr to maintain factor IX at >40 IU/dl for 5-7 days, and then at >30 IU/dl for 7 days.
Iliopsoas hemorrhage	50 IU/kg factor VIII concentrate, then 25 IU/kg every 12 hr until asymptomatic, then 20 IU/kg every other day for a total of 10-14 days.**	120 IU/kg factor IX concentrate‡; then 50-60 IU/kg every 12-24 hr to maintain factor IX at >40 IU/dl until patient is asymptomatic; then 40-50 IU every other day for a total of 10-14 days.**††
Hematuria	Bed rest; 1½ × maintenance fluids; if not controlled in 1-2 days, 20 IU/kg factor VIII concentrate; if not controlled, give prednisone (unless patient is HIV-infected).	Bed rest; 1½ × maintenance fluids; if not controlled in 1-2 days, 40 IU/kg factor IX concentrate‡; if not controlled, give prednisone (unless patient is HIV-infected).
Prophylaxis	20-40 IU/kg factor VIII concentrate every other day to achieve a trough level ≥1%.	30-50 IU/kg factor IX concentrate‡ every 2-3 days to achieve a trough level ≥1%.

*For hip hemarthrosis, orthopedic evaluation for possible aspiration is advisable to prevent avascular necrosis of the femoral head.
†For mild or moderate hemophilia, desmopressin, 0.3 μg/kg, should be used instead of factor VIII concentrate, if the patient is known to respond with a hemostatic level of factor VIII; if repeated doses are given, monitor factor VIII levels for tachyphylaxis.
‡Stated doses apply for recombinant factor IX concentrate; for plasma-derived factor IX concentrate, use 70% of the stated dose.
§Do not give antifibrinolytic therapy until 4-6 hr after a dose of prothrombin complex concentrate.
ˡOver-the-counter coagulation-promoting products may be helpful.
¶Alternatively, give 25 IU/kg every 12 hr to maintain a trough level >50% for 5-7 days followed by 25-30 IU/kg for an additional 5-7 days to maintain trough >25%.
**Repeat radiologic assessment should be performed before discontinuation of therapy.
††If repeated doses of factor IX concentrate are required, use highly purified, specific factor IX concentrate.
Adapted from Montgomery RR et al: Hemophilia and von Willebrand disease. In Nathan DG, Orkin SH (eds): *Nathan and Oski's hematology at infancy and childhood,* ed 5, Philadelphia, 1998, Saunders.

H

Diseases and Disorders

I

- Factor VIII antigen, prothrombin time, fibrinogen level, and bleeding time are normal.
- Factor IX coagulant activity levels are reduced in patients with hemophilia B.
- Coagulation factor activity measurement is useful to correlate with disease severity. Normal range is 50 to 150 U/dl; 5 to 20 U/dl indicates mild disease, 2 to 5 U/dl indicates moderate disease, and <2 U/dl indicates severe disease with spontaneous bleeding episodes.

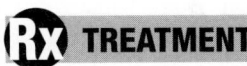 **TREATMENT**

NONPHARMACOLOGIC THERAPY

- Avoidance of contact sports
- Patient education regarding the disease; promotion of exercises such as swimming
- Avoidance of aspirin or other NSAIDs
- Orthopedic evaluation and physical therapy evaluation in patients with joint involvement
- Hepatitis vaccination

ACUTE GENERAL Rx
(see Table 1-182)

Hemophilia A:
- Reversal and prevention of acute bleeding in hemophilia A and B are based on adequate replacement of deficient or missing factor protein.
- The choice of the product for replacement therapy is guided by availability, capacity, concerns, and cost. Recombinant factors cost two to three times as much as plasma-derived factors, and the limited capacity to produce recombinant factors often results in periods of shortage. In the U.S., 60% of patients with severe hemophilia use recombinant products.
- Factor VIII concentrates are effective in controlling spontaneous and traumatic hemorrhage in severe hemophilia. The new recombinant factor VIII is stable without added human serum albumin (decreased risk of transmission of infectious agents).
- Alloantibodies (inhibitors) that neutralize factor VIII clotting function occur in nearly 30% of patients with severe hemophilia A after exposure to factor VIII. In these patients, bypassing agents (anti-inhibitor coagulant complex [AICC] and recombinant activated factor VII [rFVIIa]) can be used to treat bleeding. AICC can also be used prophylactically to decrease the frequency of joint and other bleeding events in patients with severe hemophilia A and factor VIII inhibitors.
- Recombinant activated factor VII is useful to stop spontaneous hemorrhages and prevent excessive bleeding during surgery in 75% of patients with inhibitors. Recommended dose is 90 μg/mg of body weight every 2 to 3 hr for treatment of life-threatening hemorrhage. It is, however, very expensive ($1 per μg).
- Desmopressin acetate 0.3 μg/kg q24h (causes release of factor VIII:C) may be used in preparation for minor surgical procedures in mild hemophiliacs.
- Aminocaproic acid (EACA, Amicar) 4 g PO q4h can be given for persistent bleeding that is unresponsive to factor VIII concentrate or desmopressin.

Hemophilia B:
- Infuse factor IX concentrates. It is important to remember that factor IX concentrates contain other proteins that may increase the risk of thrombosis with recurrent use. Therefore factor IX concentrates must be used only when clearly indicated.
- Daily administration of oral cyclophosphamide and prednisone without empirical factor VIII therapy is an effective and well-tolerated treatment for acquired hemophilia.

CHRONIC Rx
- The aim of chronic treatment is to prevent spontaneous bleeding and excessive bleeding during any surgical intervention.

- Prophylaxis with recombinant factor VIII can prevent joint damage and decrease the frequency of joint and other hemorrhages in young boys with severe hemophilia A. The estimated annual cost for treatment of one patient with recombinant factor VIII is $300,000.
- Implantation of genetically altered fibroblasts that produce factor VIII is safe and well tolerated. This form is feasible in patients with severe hemophilia. Hemophilia will likely be the first common, severe genetic disease to be cured by gene therapy.

DISPOSITION
- Despite the advent of virally safe blood products and blood treatment programs, nearly 70% of hemophiliacs are HIV seropositive. Survival is of normal expectancy in HIV-negative patients with mild disease.
- Intracranial bleeds are the second most common cause of death in hemophiliacs after AIDS. They are fatal in 30% of patients, occur in 10% of patients, and are generally the result of trauma.

SUGGESTED READINGS
available at www.expertconsult.com

RELATED CONTENT
Hemophilia (Patient Information)
AUTHOR: **FRED F. FERRI, M.D.**

BASIC INFORMATION

DEFINITION
Hemoptysis is coughing up of blood originating from the lower respiratory tract, ranging from blood-streaked sputum to gross blood. If greater than 100 to 600 ml in 24 hours, considered massive hemoptysis.

ICD-9CM CODES
786.3 Hemoptysis

EPIDEMIOLOGY & DEMOGRAPHICS
INCIDENCE: Unknown, varies based on underlying pathology
RISK FACTORS: Tobacco smoking predisposes to lung cancer, a common cause of hemoptysis. Systemic processes (rheumatologic, renal hematologic) may contribute to alveolar hemorrhage or vasculitis. Anticoagulation can worsen bleeding.

PHYSICAL FINDINGS & CLINICAL PRESENTATION
- Presentation of hemoptysis is variable and can range from minimal blood-tinged sputum to more than 500 ml of gross blood in 24 hr. Other symptoms depend on the underlying etiology and can include cough, sputum production, fever, shortness of breath, weight loss, night sweats, wheezing, and chest pain.
- There are no specific exam findings, but clues to the etiology may be present, for example, focal wheezing, rhonchi or rales on pulmonary exam, murmur of mitral stenosis on cardiac exam.

ETIOLOGY
- There are many potential causes of hemoptysis including airway disease (bronchitis, bronchiectasis, lung neoplasm), infection (necrotizing pneumonia, lung abscess, tuberculosis, fungal infection), inflammatory diseases (Wegener's granulomatosis, Goodpasture's syndrome, lupus), cardiac disease (mitral stenosis after rheumatic heart disease, congenital heart diseases), and others (pulmonary embolism, cocaine use, foreign body, airway trauma, iatrogenic and cryptogenic).

- In one study of 208 patients, the most common causes of hemoptysis were bronchiectasis, lung cancer, bronchitis, and pneumonia, respectively.

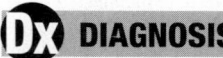 **DIAGNOSIS**

DIFFERENTIAL DIAGNOSIS
- Various potential causes of lower respiratory tract bleeding
  - Airway disease (bronchitis, bronchiectasis, lung neoplasm)
  - Infection (necrotizing pneumonia, lung abscess, tuberculosis, fungal infection)
  - Inflammatory diseases (Wegener's granulomatosis, Goodpasture's syndrome, lupus)
  - Cardiac disease (mitral stenosis after rheumatic heart disease, congenital heart diseases)
  - Pulmonary embolism
  - Cocaine use
  - Foreign body
  - Airway trauma
- Bleeding from upper respiratory tract
- Hematemesis
- Coagulopathy

WORKUP
Complete history and physical exam may suggest a particular etiology; important to ask about duration and quantity of hemoptysis and smoking history.

LABORATORY TESTS
- Complete blood count
- Coagulation profile
- Serum chemistries including creatinine, urinalysis; if abnormal, consider vasculitis serologies (i.e., ANA, ANCA, anti-GBM)
- Arterial blood gas to assess oxygenation
- Sputum for cultures and cytologic studies

IMAGING STUDIES
- Chest x-ray: all patients with hemoptysis should have a chest x-ray but will likely need additional studies to localize site of bleeding.
- Chest CT: chest CT scan combined with flexible bronchoscopy has the highest yield for localizing the site of bleeding.

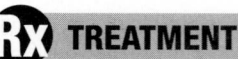 **TREATMENT**

Varies based on underlying etiology and nonmassive versus massive hemoptysis

NONPHARMACOLOGIC THERAPY
Massive hemoptysis:
- Arteriographic embolization of bronchial arteries and/or collateral systemic vessels
- Surgical resection of affected lung

ACUTE GENERAL Rx
Massive hemoptysis:
- Stabilize hemodynamic status and oxygenation.
- Reverse any coagulopathy.
- Bronchoscopy can be used to identify cause of hemoptysis (e.g., neoplasm), as well as to help isolate a side/segment of bleeding.
- If site of bleeding is known, place patient with bleeding lung in dependent position to prevent blood from spilling into nonaffected lung.
- Bronchoscopic lavage with iced saline or topical application of epinephrine can be tried as a temporizing measure.
- Bronchoscopic balloon tamponade of bleeding site can be used as temporizing measure.
- Early consultation with interventional radiology and thoracic surgery for definitive intervention is recommended.
Submassive hemoptysis:
For submassive hemoptysis, identify and treat underlying condition. Referral to pulmonologist or hematologist if indicated.

CHRONIC Rx
For patients requiring anticoagulation or antiplatelet therapy for another disorder, consider risks/benefits of continued anticoagulation or antiplatelet therapy.

DISPOSITION
Generally, patients have a good prognosis after an episode of hemoptysis, but those with massive bleeding and/or malignancy tend to have a poorer prognosis.

SUGGESTED READINGS
available at www.expertconsult.com

RELATED CONTENT
Fig. 3-82 Evaluation of hemoptysis (Algorithm)

AUTHORS: **SARAH TAPYRIK, M.D.,** and **MICHAEL BLUNDIN, M.D.**

BASIC INFORMATION

DEFINITION

A hemorrhoid is a varicose dilation of a vein of the superior or inferior hemorrhoidal plexus, resulting from a persistent increase in venous pressure. External hemorrhoids are below the pectinate line (inferior plexus). Internal hemorrhoids are above the pectinate line (superior plexus).

SYNONYMS

Piles

ICD-9CM CODES
455.6 Hemorrhoids

EPIDEMIOLOGY & DEMOGRAPHICS

Potential for development of symptomatic hemorrhoids in all adults
PREVALENCE: Estimated 50% of the adult population in the United States.
PREDOMINANT SEX: Males and females affected equally

PHYSICAL FINDINGS & CLINICAL PRESENTATION

- Painless bleeding with defecation; bleeding is bright red and staining on toilet paper
- Perianal irritation
- Mucofecal staining of underclothes
- Acute external hemorrhoids: painful, swollen, and often thrombosed (Fig. 1-389)
- Pain on sitting, standing, or defecating (thrombosed hemorrhoid)
- Prolapse (Fig. 1-390)
- Constipation

ETIOLOGY

- Low-fiber, high-fat diet
- Chronic constipation and straining with defecation
- High resting anal sphincter pressures
- Pregnancy
- Obesity
- Rectal surgery (i.e., episiotomy)
- Prolonged sitting
- Anal intercourse

DIAGNOSIS

DIFFERENTIAL DIAGNOSIS

- Fissure
- Abscess
- Anal fistula
- Condylomata acuminata
- Hypertrophied anal papillae
- Rectal prolapse
- Rectal polyp
- Neoplasm (anal cancer, colorectal cancer)
- Inflammatory bowel disease

WORKUP

- Inspection
- Digital rectal examination
- Anoscopy
- Sigmoidoscopy

TREATMENT

NONPHARMACOLOGIC THERAPY

- Avoidance of constipation and straining with defecation
- Avoidance of prolonged sitting on toilet
- High-fiber diet (20 to 30 g/day)

- Increased fluid intake (six to eight glasses of water per day)
- Cleaning with mild soap and water after defecation
- Warm soaks or ice to soothe
- Sitz baths

ACUTE GENERAL Rx

- Fiber supplements to provide bulk (psyllium extracts or mucilloids)
- Medicated compresses with witch hazel
- Topical hydrocortisone (1% to 3% cream or ointment)
- Topical anesthetic spray
- Glycerin suppositories
- Stool softeners
- Surgically remove during first 72 hr after onset

CHRONIC Rx

- Rubber-band ligation
- Injection sclerotherapy
- Photocoagulation
- Cryodestruction
- Hemorrhoidectomy
- Anal dilation
- Laser or cautery hemorrhoidectomy
- Observance for complications: thrombosis, bleeding, infection, anal stenosis or weakness

DISPOSITION

Should resolve, but there is a high rate of recurrence

REFERRAL

To colorectal or general surgeon for any hemorrhoid that does not respond to conservative therapy

PEARLS & CONSIDERATIONS

COMMENTS

- Patients need to understand the importance of a healthy diet, regular exercise, and rectal hygiene.
- Stress the importance of avoiding prolonged sitting and straining on the toilet.
- Stress the need not to defer the urge to defecate.

SUGGESTED READING

available at www.expertconsult.com

RELATED CONTENT

Anal Fissure (Related Key Topic)
Hemorrhoids (Patient Information)

AUTHORS: **MARIA A. CORIGLIANO, M.D.,** and **RUBEN ALVERO, M.D.**

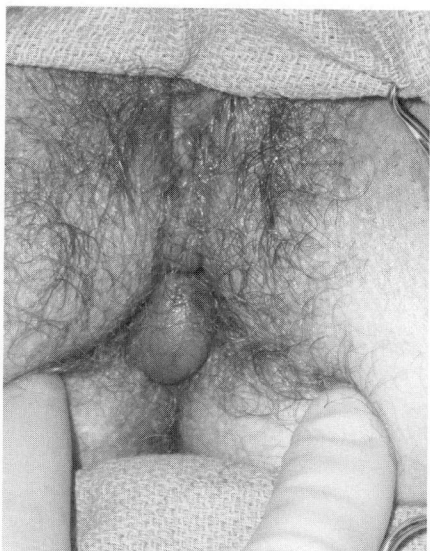

FIGURE 1-389 Thrombosed external hemorrhoid. (From Cameron JL, Cameron AM: *Current surgical therapy,* ed 10, Philadelphia, 2011, Saunders.)

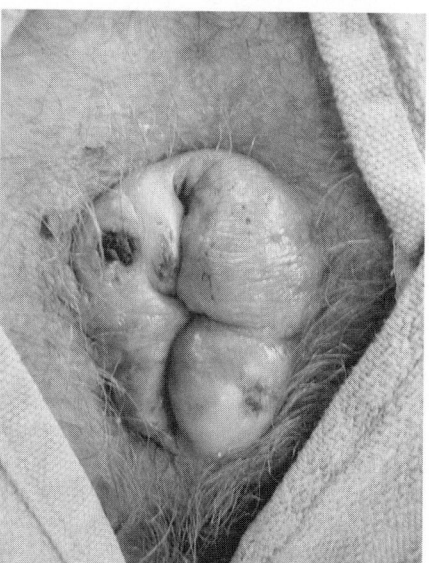

FIGURE 1-390 Prolapsed and thrombosed internal hemorrhoids. (From Cameron JL, Cameron AM: *Current surgical therapy,* ed 10, Philadelphia, 2011, Saunders.)

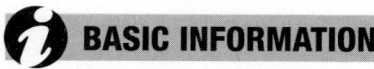

BASIC INFORMATION

DEFINITION

Henoch-Schönlein purpura (HSP) is a systemic, small-vessel, IgA immune complex–mediated leukocytoclastic vasculitis characterized by a tetrad of palpable purpura, abdominal pain, renal disease, and arthritis/arthralgias. It may also present with gastrointestinal (GI) bleeding.

SYNONYMS

Anaphylactoid purpura
Allergic purpura

ICD-9CM CODES
287.0 Henoch-Schönlein purpura

EPIDEMIOLOGY & DEMOGRAPHICS

INCIDENCE: Annual incidence of 20 cases/100,000 population
PEAK INCIDENCE: Majority in spring, rarely in summer
PREVALENCE: Most common vasculitis seen in children and younger age groups; whites and Asians more common than black patients
PREDOMINANT SEX: 2:1 male/female ratio
PREDOMINANT AGE: Seen mostly from ages 4 to 15, although can be seen in older adolescents and young adults

PHYSICAL FINDINGS & CLINICAL PRESENTATION

- Palpable purpura of dependent areas, especially lower extremities and areas subjected to pressure, such as the beltline in adults or buttocks in toddlers.
- Subcutaneous edema.
- Arthralgias and arthritis in 80%. Typically oligoarticular, affecting lower extremity and large joints. Periarticular swelling and tenderness also noted.
- GI symptoms are seen in approximately one third of patients. Common findings are nausea, vomiting, diarrhea, cramping, abdominal pain, hematochezia, and melena. Complications include GI bleeding (20% to 30%), bowel ischemia, intussusception, and bowel perforation.
- Anecdotally may follow upper respiratory infection.
- Renal involvement is seen in as many as 80% of older children, usually within the first month of illness. Fewer than 5% progress to end-stage renal failure, a major cause of morbidity. Renal manifestations may range from isolated hematuria or proteinuria to acute nephropathy with renal insufficiency.

ETIOLOGY

- Presumptive etiology is exposure to a trigger antigen that causes antibody formation.
- Antigen-antibody (immune) complex deposition then occurs in arteriole and capillary walls of skin, renal mesangium, and GI tract. Immunoglobulin (Ig) A deposition is most common.
- Antigen triggers postulated include drugs, foods, immunization, and upper respiratory and other viral illnesses. Group A streptococcal infection is the most common precipitant in children, seen in up to one third of cases. A recent adult case triggered by pantoprazole has also been reported.
- Serologic and pathologic evidence suggests an association between parvovirus B19 and HSP, which may explain observed cases of HSP that do not respond to corticosteroids or other immunosuppressive therapy.
- Case reports describing development of HSP after treatment with immunosuppressive agents (e.g., etanercept) have been published.
- Recent studies suggest an association with the "Mediterranean fever" (MEFV) gene.

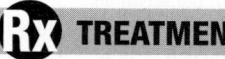

DIAGNOSIS

- Diagnosis is based on the finding of IgA in the affected vessels. Table 1-183 describes common clinical manifestations of HSP.
- Skin manifestations are most common.
- Palpable purpura (see Fig. 1-391) is seen in 70% of adult patients, whereas GI symptoms are more common in children.
- A total of 20% to 54% of children with HSP will have some early renal involvement.
- Skin biopsy shows leukocytoclastic vasculitis. Renal biopsy shows mesangial IgA deposition.
- The presence of two of the following four American College of Rheumatology criteria yields a diagnostic sensitivity of 87.1% and specificity of 87.7%:
  - Palpable purpura unrelated to thrombocytopenia
  - Age <20 yr at onset of first symptoms
  - Bowel angina or ischemia
  - Granulocytic infiltration of arteriole or venule walls on biopsy

DIFFERENTIAL DIAGNOSIS

- Polyarteritis nodosa
- Meningococcemia
- Thrombocytopenic purpura
- Hypersensitivity vasculitis
- Microscopic polyangiitis
- Wegener granulomatosis

WORKUP

History, physical examination, laboratory testing, skin or renal biopsy

LABORATORY TESTS

- Electrolytes, blood urea nitrogen, and creatinine
- Urinalysis
- Complete blood count
- Prothrombin time, fibrinogen, and fibrin degradation products
- Blood cultures

Laboratory abnormalities are not specific for HSP. Leukocytosis and eosinophilia may be seen. IgA levels are elevated in approximately 50% of patients. Glomerulonephritis may be present (microscopic hematuria, proteinuria, and red blood cell casts).

IMAGING STUDIES

Imaging studies are generally not useful in the diagnosis of HSP. Arteriography or magnetic resonance angiography may be helpful in distinguishing from polyarteritis nodosa. Abdominal ultrasound is recommended for patients with severe abdominal pain to detect increased bowel wall thickness, peritoneal fluid, or intussusception.

TREATMENT

- Nonsteroidal anti-inflammatory drugs for arthritis and arthralgias.
- Prednisone 1 mg/kg PO is given if renal or severe GI disease, although clear benefits in renal disease have not been demonstrated according to a recent Cochrane systematic review of pediatric patients.

TABLE 1-183 Clinical Manifestations of Henoch-Schönlein Purpura

	% at Onset	% during Course
Purpura (nl platelet count)	50	100
Subcutaneous edema	10-20	20-50
Arthritis (large joints)	25	60-85
Gastrointestinal	30	85
Renal	?	10-50
Genitourinary (ddx torsion)	?	2-35
Pulmonary (T_LCO)	?	95
Pulmonary hemorrhage	?	Rare, may be fatal
Central nervous system (headache, organic brain syndrome, seizures)	?	Rare, may be fatal

From Hochberg MC et al: *Rheumatology*, ed 5, St Louis, 2011, Mosby.

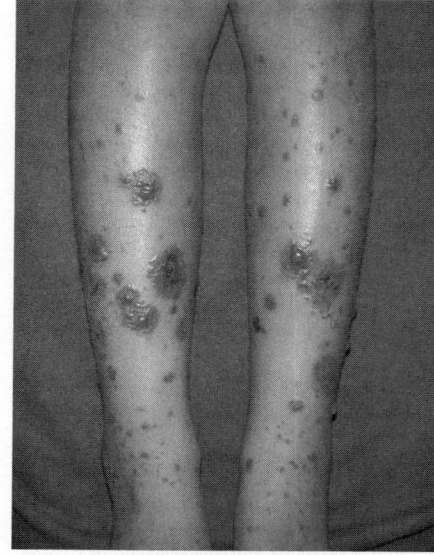

FIGURE 1-391 Extensive palpable purpura over the lower extremities in a 7-yr-old girl with Henoch-Schönlein purpura. (From Hochberg MC et al: *Rheumatology*, ed 5, St Louis, 2011, Mosby.)

- A double-blind, randomized, controlled trial found that early treatment with prednisone reduced abdominal pain and joint symptoms but did not prevent development of renal disease. It was effective in the treatment of renal disease once it was established.
- Corticosteroids and azathioprine may be beneficial if rapidly progressive glomerulonephritis is present. Pulse methylprednisolone therapy has also been proposed in patients with glomerulonephritis, mesenteric vasculitis, or pulmonary involvement. Recent reports describe improvement in rapidly progressive glomerulonephritis and nephrotic-range proteinuria after treatment with mycophenolate mofetil. The combination of cyclosporin A with corticosteroids appears to be effective in inducing remission of nephrotic syndrome in adult patients with HSP nephritis.
- Hospitalization for significant GI or renal involvement.

NONPHARMACOLOGIC THERAPY

Supportive care with pain management, adequate hydration, and nutrition

DISPOSITION & PROGNOSIS

- Prognosis excellent, with spontaneous recovery of most patients within 4 wk.
- Increased age of onset generally correlates with morbidity. While end-stage renal disease (ESRD) occurs in 10% to 30% of adult patients with HSP at 15 years, chronic renal insufficiency is the most common long-term morbidity and affects adults more than children.
- GI complications (mesenteric infarction, perforation, and intussusception).
- Recurrences in up to one third of patients, especially within first 4 to 6 mo after initial episode and most commonly in patients with renal involvement. Recurrences less severe than initial episode.

REFERRAL

Nephrologist or gastroenterologist

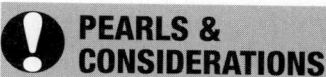

PEARLS & CONSIDERATIONS

- HSP is an IgA-related vasculitis.
- Organ systems involved are skin, joints, GI tract, and kidneys.
- Palpable purpura more common in adults; GI symptoms more common in children.
- Most with spontaneous recovery within 4 wk of onset of symptoms.
- End-stage renal disease occurs in only 5% of patients.
- Steroids and immunosuppressive agents may offer some benefit.

SUGGESTED READINGS

available at www.expertconsult.com

RELATED CONTENT

Henoch-Schönlein Purpura (Patient Information)

AUTHORS: **LAWRENCE MURPHY, M.D.,** and **DOMINICK TAMMARO, M.D.**

H

Diseases and Disorders

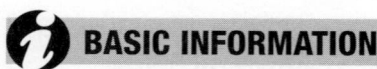

BASIC INFORMATION

DEFINITION

There are two forms of heparin-induced thrombocytopenia (HIT). Type 1 HIT is a mild, transient decrease in platelet count that occurs during the first few days of heparin exposure due to platelet agglutination. This form is benign, and the platelet count will return to normal while heparin is continued. This section will refer to Type 2 HIT, an antibody-mediated thrombocytopenia that is associated with a high risk of developing thrombosis.

SYNONYMS

Type II heparin-induced thrombocytopenia
Heparin-induced thrombocytopenia and thrombosis (HITT)
White clot syndrome
Heparin-associated immune thrombocytopenia

ICD-9CM CODES
289.84 Heparin-induced thrombocytopenia (HIT)

EPIDEMIOLOGY & DEMOGRAPHICS

INCIDENCE: Occurs in 0.2% to 5% of patients exposed to heparin. Unfractionated heparin is associated with a 5 to 10 times higher risk of HIT compared to low-molecular-weight heparin. Initially, there was an overwhelming underdiagnosis of HIT; however, since the introduction of HIT antibody ELISA test, there is a propensity to overdiagnose HIT irrespective of the clinical scenario.
PREDOMINANT SEX AND AGE: Females are at slightly higher risk than males. More common in adults but may also occur in children.
RISK FACTORS: Longer duration of exposure to heparin, type of heparin (unfractionated heparin has a greater risk), type of patient (surgical patients, especially cardiac and orthopedic surgery, are at higher risk than medical patients).

PHYSICAL FINDINGS & CLINICAL PRESENTATION

Suspect in a patient with:
- Exposure to heparin for 4 to 14 days OR who was exposed to heparin in the prior 3 mo
- Unexplained platelet count decrease to 50% below pretreatment baseline
- Onset of thrombocytopenia 5 to 10 days after heparin initiation
- Evidence of acute venous or arterial thrombosis
- Skin lesions/necrosis at heparin injection sites
- Acute anaphylactoid reaction during administration of heparin bolus

ETIOLOGY

Occurs due to the formation of antibodies, directed against heparin in complex with platelet factor 4, which bind to and activate platelets. Activated platelets release platelet factor 4 (leading to more antibody production) and undergo aggregation and premature removal from the circulation (resulting in thrombocytopenia). This platelet activation and antibody formation also can lead to thrombosis. Fig. E1-392 illustrates the mechanism of HIT.

DX DIAGNOSIS

DIFFERENTIAL DIAGNOSIS

Thrombocytopenia due to other causes including:
- Sepsis
- Disseminated intravascular coagulation
- Thrombocytopenic thrombotic purpura
- Hemolytic uremic syndrome
- Drug-induced thrombocytopenia (other than heparin)
- Antiphospholipid antibody syndrome.

WORKUP

HIT is first and foremost a clinical diagnosis. See Table 1-184 for workup based on pretest probability. If the patient has a low pretest probability score, heparin can be safely continued, and there is no need to send for further testing for HIT. If the patient has a moderate to high pretest probability, HIT testing (Table 1-185), imaging studies for lower extremity deep venous thrombosis (also consider imaging of upper extremities if swelling is present or venous catheters are in place), cessation of heparin products, and alternative anticoagulation should all be performed. Patients with intermediate and high pretest probability but no HIT antibodies or intermediate pretest probability and only weakly positive HIT antibodies (based on optical density, see below) can resume heparin use as HIT is unlikely in these scenarios. Patients with high pretest probability and weakly positive antibod-

TABLE 1-184 A Diagnostic and Treatment Approach to Heparin-Induced Thrombocytopenia

Suspicion of HIT based upon the "4 T's"	Score	Pre-test Probability Score Criteria 2	1	0
Thrombocytopenia	☐	nadir 20-100, or >50% platelet fall	nadir 10-19, or 30-50% platelet fall	nadir <10, or <30% platelet fall
Timing of onset of platelet fall	☐	day 5-10, or ≤day 1 with recent heparin*	>day 10 or timing unclear (but fits with HIT)	≤day 1 (no recent heparin)
Thrombosis or other sequelae	☐	proven thrombosis, skin necrosis, or ASR†	progressive, recurrent, or silent thrombosis; erythematous skin lesions	none
OTher cause of platelet fall	☐	none evident	possible	definite
Total Pre-test Probability Score	☐	periodic reassessment as new information can change pre-test probability (e.g., positive blood cultures)		

Total Pre-test Probability Score					
High		**Moderate**		**Low**	
8 | 7 | 6		5 | 4		3 | 2 | 1 | 0	
Stop heparin‡, give alternative non-heparin anticoagulant argatroban¶ or lepirudin# or danaparoid** (or bivalirudin†† or fondaparinux‡‡)		Physician judgment		Continue (LMW) heparin	

Positive test for HIT antibodies ← **HIT Test** → **Negative** test for HIT antibodies
Continue non-heparin anticoagulant until platelet count recovery
Consider continuing or switching back to (LMW) heparin ##

Thrombosis* ← **Imaging studies for lower-limb DVT †††** → **No Thrombosis**
If HIT, continue non-heparin anticoagulant until platelet count recovery, then **cautious coumarin overlap¶¶**
If HIT, consider anticoagulating until platelet count recovery, even if no thrombosis apparent (± coumarin ¶¶)

---

* recent heparin indicates exposure within the past 30 days (2 points) or past 30-100 days (1 point)
† ASR, acute systemic reaction following i.v. heparin bollus (see Table 4)
‡ stop all heparin, including catheter "flushes" and, possibly, heparin-coated catheters
¶ argatroban: approved (U.S., Canada) for isolated HIT and HIT complicated by thrombosis (2 µg/kg/min i.v., adjusted to 1.5-3.0X patient's baseline aPTT or the mean of the laboratory normal range); reduce dose for hepatobiliary compromise: may increase INR more than the other direct thrombin inhibitors, thus requiring care in managing coumarin overlap (see ¶¶ below)
# lepirudin: approved (U.S., Canada, E.U., elsewhere) for treatment of thrombosis complicating HIT (±0.4 mg/kg i.v. bolus, then 0.15 mg/kg/h adjusted to 1.5-2.5X patient's baseline aPTT or mean of the laboratory normal range); used (off-label) also to treat isolated HIT (0.1 mg/kg/h, adjusted by aPTT); to avoid overdosing and anaphylaxis, it may be preferable to omit the bolus, and begin as i.v. infusion (except when facing life- or limb-threatening thrombosis); reduce dose for renal insufficiency
** danaparoid: usual i.v. bolus, 2,250 U (body weight 60-75 kg) followed by infusion (400 U/hr for 4 h, then 300 U/h for 4 h, then 200 U/h, adjusted by anti-factor Xa levels); this therapeutic-dose regimen is appropriate both for isolated HIT and for HIT complicated by thrombosis (though higher than approved dose in some jurisdictions); withdrawn from U.S. market (2002)
†† bivalirudin: no bolus, i.v. infusion 0.15 mg/kg/h adjusted by aPTT; limited experience (off-label)
‡‡ fondaparinux: dosing for HIT not established; limited experience (off-label)
¶¶ delay coumarin pending substantial platelet count recovery (at least >100, preferably >150); begin coumarin in low doses, with at least 4-5 day overlap, stopping alternative anticoagulant when INR therapeutic for 2 days and platelets recovered
depending on physician confidence in the laboratory's ability to rule out HIT antibodies (usually, negative PF4-dependent enzyme-immunoassay and/or washed platelet activation assay performed by an experienced laboratory)
*** some thrombi may require special treatment, e.g., thrombectomy for large limb artery thrombosis
††† routine ultrasound of lower-limb veins recommended, since many HIT patients have subclinical deep-vein thrombosis (DVT)

From Warkentin TE et al: Platelet-endothelial interactions: sepsis, HIT, and antiphospholipid syndrome, *Hematology (Am Soc Hematol Educ Prog)* 497-519, 2003.

ies or intermediate/high pretest probability and moderate to strongly positive antibodies likely have HIT and should be treated as such.

LABORATORY TESTS

In the appropriate clinical setting, testing for HIT antibodies with an enzyme-linked immunosorbent assay, or ELISA, can be useful. This test is very sensitive, but not specific. The majority of patients with positive testing for HIT antibodies will not develop clinical HIT. Thus, HIT antibody testing is more effective for ruling out the diagnosis than confirming the diagnosis of HIT. More recently, use of the HIT Ab optical density as well as the immunoglobulin subtypes of the HIT antibody have entered the diagnostic realm. Higher optical density levels are associated with increased likelihood of a positive functional assay, higher pretest probability score, and increased risk of thrombosis. Weakly positive optical densities (0.4 to 1.0) are only rarely associated with functional assay positivity. In contrast, optical densities greater than 2.0 almost always show heparin-dependent platelet activation. Optical densities are thus defined as weakly positive (0.4-1.0), moderately positive (1.0-2.0), or strongly positive (>2.0). The HIT Ab IgG subtype is the pathologic antibody for HIT. Hence, use of IgG-specific ELISAs increases the test specificity over the polyspecific (IgA/M/G) antibody. Patients with low pretest probability should not have HIT antibody testing performed while all patients with intermediate and high pretest probability of HIT benefit from HIT Ab testing.

The gold standard test for HIT is to measure heparin-dependent platelet activation via the serotonin release assay (14C-SRA). Donor platelets are incubated with radiolabeled serotonin. The platelets internalize the serotonin and are then exposed to the patient's serum and heparin at a therapeutic concentration. If antibodies to the platelet factor 4-heparin complex are present in the patient's serum, the platelets react and released radioactive serotonin is then measured. Availability and turn-around time of this test is dependent on the institution, which can influence the test's clinical utility. Cases where there is intermediate pretest probability but only a weakly positive HIT Ab benefit the most from confirmatory SRA testing. Here, a positive SRA test will argue for HIT while negative SRA tests will suggest absence of HIT.

IMAGING STUDIES

Doppler sonography of the extremities in the correct clinical setting

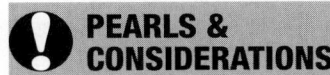

TREATMENT

- For patients with a moderate or high pretest probability, discontinue all heparin exposure. Even if the patient does not have a clinically evident thrombosis, they are at a 50% risk of developing a clot within the subsequent 30 days. Thus, the patient must be started on an alternate anticoagulant.
- Three agents, all direct thrombin inhibitors, are approved for this indication:
  - argatroban (avoid in liver dysfunction)
  - lepirudin (avoid in renal dysfunction)
  - bivalirudin (bivalirudin is approved only for patients with HIT or at risk of HIT who are undergoing PCI).
- These drugs should be continued as a single agent until the platelet count returns to baseline (generally a platelet count of 150×10^9/L but it is important to consider the individual patient's baseline, then warfarin can be added at a maximum dose of 5 mg/day. This overlap therapy should continue until the platelet count has reached a stable plateau, the INR has reached the intended target (remember that argatroban artificially elevates the INR), and after a minimum overlap of 5 days of both the direct thrombin inhibitor and warfarin. The length of treatment is controversial, but most clinicians agree that 1 month of alternate anticoagulation is sufficient in the absence of thrombosis, while 3 to 6 months of treatment is required in the presence of thrombosis.
- There is emerging data showing efficacy and lower bleeding risk in HIT for fondaparinux when compared with the direct thrombin inhibitors. Fondaparinux is a synthetic pentasaccharide that binds antithrombin, causing long-acting inhibition of activated factor X, but not thrombin. It is not FDA approved for HIT, but its use in HIT in pregnancy has been reported. It can initiate the formation of anti-PF4 antibodies, but it does not support platelet activation by the newly formed immune complexes.

NONPHARMACOLOGIC THERAPY

All nonpharmacologic therapies including surgical procedures

REFERRAL

Request a hematology consultation.

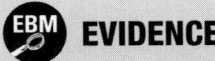

PEARLS & CONSIDERATIONS

COMMENTS

HIT paradoxically causes thrombocytopenia and *clotting*, not bleeding.

PREVENTION

Consider the use of low-molecular-weight heparin (as opposed to unfractionated heparin) as DVT prophylaxis.

(EBM) **EVIDENCE**

available at www.expertconsult.com

SUGGESTED READINGS

available at www.expertconsult.com

AUTHORS: **ANGELA M. TABER (PLETTE), M.D.,** and **JOHN L. REAGAN, M.D.**

TABLE 1-185 Laboratory Assays for Heparin-Induced Thrombocytopenia

Assay	Sensitivity (%)	Specificity (%)	Positive Predictive Value (%)	Negative Predictive Value (%)
Functional assay (e.g., serotonin release assay)	88	≈100	≈100	81
PF4/heparin enzyme immunoassay (ELISA)	95-98	86	93	95

ELISA, Enzyme-linked immunosorbent assay; *PF4*, platelet factor 4.
From Goldman L, Schafer AI: *Goldman's Cecil medicine*, ed 24, Philadelphia, 2012, Saunders.

H

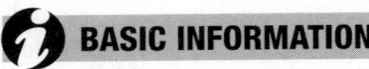
DEFINITION

Hepatic encephalopathy is a neuropsychiatric syndrome occurring in patients with severe impairment of liver function and consequent accumulation of toxic products not metabolized by the liver. It is characterized by gradual impairment of the ability to perform mental tasks and to react to external stimuli. *Minimal hepatic encephalopathy* refers to patients with hepatic cirrhosis and mild cognitive impairment, but no history of overt encephalopathy.

SYNONYMS

Hepatic coma

ICD-9CM CODES
572.2 Hepatic encephalopathy

EPIDEMIOLOGY & DEMOGRAPHICS

INCIDENCE/PREVALENCE: Hepatic encephalopathy occurs in >50% of all cases of cirrhosis.

PHYSICAL FINDINGS & CLINICAL PRESENTATION

Hepatic encephalopathy can be classified by clinical stages described in Table 1-186.

The physical examination in hepatic encephalopathy varies with the stage and may reveal the following abnormalities:

- Skin: jaundice, palmar erythema, spider angiomata, ecchymosis, dilated superficial periumbilical veins (caput medusae) in patients with cirrhosis
- Eyes: scleral icterus, Kayser-Fleischer rings (Wilson's disease)
- Breath: fetor hepaticus
- Chest: gynecomastia in men with chronic liver disease
- Abdomen: ascites, small nodular liver (cirrhosis), tender hepatomegaly (congestive hepatomegaly)
- Rectal examination: hemorrhoids (portal hypertension), guaiac-positive stool (alcoholic gastritis, bleeding esophageal varices, peptic ulcer disease, bleeding hemorrhoids)
- Genitalia: testicular atrophy in males with chronic liver disease
- Extremities: pedal edema from hypoalbuminemia
- Neurologic: flapping tremor (asterixis), obtundation, coma with or without decerebrate posturing

ETIOLOGY

- Precipitating factors in patients with underlying cirrhosis (upper gastrointestinal bleeding, hypokalemia, hypomagnesemia, analgesic and sedative drugs, sepsis, alkalosis, increased dietary protein)
- Acute fulminant viral hepatitis
- Drugs and toxins (e.g., isoniazid, acetaminophen, diclofenac and other NSAIDs, statins, methyldopa, loratadine, propylthiouracil, lisinopril, labetalol, halothane, carbon tetrachloride, erythromycin, nitrofurantoin, troglitazone, herbal products, flavocoxid)
- Reye's syndrome
- Shock and/or sepsis
- Fatty liver of pregnancy
- Metastatic carcinoma, hepatocellular carcinoma
- Other: autoimmune hepatitis, ischemic veno-occlusive disease, sclerosing cholangitis, heat stroke, amebic abscesses

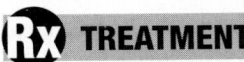
DIFFERENTIAL DIAGNOSIS

- Delirium caused by medications or illicit drugs
- Cerebrovascular accident, subdural hematoma
- Meningitis, encephalitis
- Hypoglycemia
- Uremia
- Cerebral anoxia
- Hypercalcemia
- Metastatic neoplasm to brain
- Alcohol withdrawal syndrome

WORKUP

Hepatic encephalopathy should be considered in any patient with cirrhosis who presents with neuropsychiatric manifestations. Exclude other etiologies with comprehensive history (obtained from patient, relatives, and others), physical examination, and laboratory and imaging studies. A pertinent history should include exposure to hepatitis, ethanol intake, drug history, exposure to toxins, IV drug abuse, measles or influenza with aspirin use (Reye's syndrome), and history of carcinoma (primary or metastatic). Minimal hepatic encephalopathy may not be obvious on clinical examination, but can be detected with neurophysiologic and neuropsychiatric testing.

LABORATORY TESTS

- Alanine aminotransferase, aspartate aminotransferase, bilirubin, alkaline phosphatase, glucose, calcium, electrolytes, blood urea nitrogen, creatinine, albumin
- Complete blood count, platelet count, prothrombin time, partial thromboplastin time
- Serum and urine toxicology screen in suspected medication or illegal drug use
- Blood and urine cultures, urinalysis
- Venous ammonia level
- Arterial blood gases

IMAGING STUDIES

CT scan of the head may be useful in selected patients to exclude other etiologies.

TREATMENT

NONPHARMACOLOGIC THERAPY

- Identification and treatment of precipitating factors
- Restriction of protein intake (30 to 40 g/day) to reduce toxic protein metabolites

---

TABLE 1-187 Management of Fulminant Hepatic Failure

No sedation except for procedures
Minimal handling
Enteric precautions until infection ruled out
Monitor:
- Heart and respiratory rate
- Arterial BP, CVP
- Core/toe temperature
- Neurologic observations
- Gastric pH (>5.0)
- Blood glucose (>4 mmol/L)
- Acid-base
- Electrolytes
- PT, PTT

Fluid balance
- 75% maintenance
- Dextrose 10%-50% (provide 6-10 mg/kg/min)
- Sodium (0.5-1 mmol/L)
- Potassium (2-4 mmol/L)

Maintain circulating volume with colloid/FFP
Coagulation support only if required
Drugs
- Vitamin K
- H_2 antagonist
- Antacids
- Lactulose
- N-acetylcysteine for acetaminophen toxicity
- Broad-spectrum antibiotics
- Antifungals

Nutrition
- Enteral feeding (1-2 g protein/kg/day)
- PN if ventilated

BP, Blood pressure; *CVP,* central venous pressure; *FFP,* fresh frozen plasma; *PN,* parenteral nutrition; *PT,* prothrombin time; *PTT,* partial thromboplastin time.
From Fuhrman BP et al: *Pediatric critical care,* ed 4, Philadelphia, 2011, Saunders.

TABLE 1-186 Clinical Stages of Hepatic Encephalopathy

Stage	Asterixis	EEG Changes	Clinical Manifestations
I (prodrome)	Slight	Minimal	Mild intellectual impairment, disturbed sleep-wake cycle
II (impending)	Easily elicited	Usually generalized	Drowsiness, confusion, coma/inappropriate behavior, disorientation, mood swings
III (stupor)	Present if patient cooperative	Grossly abnormal slowing of rhythm	Drowsy, unresponsive to verbal commands, markedly confused, delirious, hyperreflexia, positive Babinski sign
IV (coma)	Usually absent	Appearance of delta waves, decreased amplitudes	Unconscious, decerebrate or decorticate response to pain present (stage IVA) or absent (stage IVB)

EEG, Electroencephalogram.
From Fuhrman BP et al: *Pediatric critical care,* ed 4, Philadelphia, 2011, Saunders.

ACUTE GENERAL Rx

Table 1-187 summarizes the management of fulminant hepatic failure.

Reduction of colonic ammonia production:

- Lactulose 30 ml of 50% solution qid initially; dose is subsequently adjusted depending on clinical response. Ornithine aspartate 9 g tid is also effective. Lactulose may improve hepatic encephalopathy but may be less effective than antibiotics.
- Neomycin 1 g PO q4 to 6h or given as a 1% retention enema solution (1 g in 100 ml of isotonic saline solution); neomycin should be used with caution in patients with renal insufficiency. Metronidazole 250 mg qid may be as effective as neomycin and is not nephrotoxic; however, long-term use can be associated with neurotoxicity.
- A combination of lactulose and neomycin can be used when either agent is ineffective alone.
- The oral antibiotic rifaximin (550 mg PO bid) is effective in reducing the risk of recurrent hepatic encephalopathy in patients with cirrhosis. It can be taken with lactulose. Rifamaxin has also been shown to be effective in improving psychometric performance and health-related quality of life in patients with minimal hepatic encephalopathy. It is well tolerated but expensive.
- Probiotics (e.g., 1 capsule containing 112.5 billion viable lyophilized bacteria tid) might also be beneficial in altering gut flora to reduce ammonia production.

Treatment of cerebral edema:

- Cerebral edema is often present in patients with acute liver failure, and it accounts for nearly 50% of deaths. Monitoring intracranial pressure by epidural, intraparenchymal, or subdural transducers and treatment of cerebral edema with mannitol (100 to 200 ml of 20% solution [0.3 to 0.4 g/kg of body weight]) given by rapid IV infusion are helpful in selected patients (e.g., potential transplantation patients).
- Dexamethasone and hyperventilation (useful in head injury) are of little value in treating cerebral edema from liver failure.

CHRONIC Rx

- Avoidance of any precipitating factors (e.g., high-protein diet, medications)
- Consideration of liver transplantation in selected patients with progressive or recurrent encephalopathy (Box 1-23). Liver transplantation remains the only curative therapeutic option.

DISPOSITION

Prognosis varies with the underlying etiology of the liver failure and the grade of encephalopathy (generally good for grades 1 or 2; poor for grades 3 or 4).

REFERRAL

The early stages of hepatic encephalopathy can be managed in the outpatient setting, whereas stages 3 or 4 require hospital admission.

PEARLS & CONSIDERATIONS

COMMENTS

- Long-acting benzodiazepines should not be used to treat anxiety and sleep disorders in patients with cirrhosis, as they may precipitate encephalopathy.
- Patients not responding to supportive therapy should be evaluated for liver transplantation.
- Not all patients with cirrhosis develop hepatic encephalopathy. It has been shown that 40% of persons with cirrhosis and minimal hepatic encephalopathy do not develop overt hepatic encephalopathy in long-term follow-up. There are genetic factors associated with development of hepatic encephalopathy in patients with cirrhosis. Genetic analyses have shown that glutaminase TACC and CACC haplotypes are linked to the risk for overt hepatic encephalopathy.

EVIDENCE

available at www.expertconsult.com

SUGGESTED READINGS

available at www.expertconsult.com

RELATED CONTENT

Hepatic Encephalopathy (Patient Information)
Cirrhosis (Related Key Topic)

AUTHOR: **FRED F. FERRI, M.D.**

BOX 1-23 Various Prognostic Criteria Used for Liver Transplantation in Patients with Fulminant Hepatic Failure

King's College Criteria
Acetaminophen overdose:
- Arterial pH <7.3 (irrespective of grade of encephalopathy) or
- PT >100 sec (INR >6.5)
- Serum creatinine >3.4 mg/dl (>300 µmol/L)
- Patients with grade III and IV hepatic encephalopathy
Nonacetaminophen liver injury:
- PT >100 sec (INR >6.5) (irrespective of grade of encephalopathy) or any three of the following variables:
  - Age <10 or >40 years
  - Non-A, non-B hepatitis, halothane hepatitis, idiosyncratic drug reactions
  - Jaundice >7 days before onset of encephalopathy
  - Serum bilirubin 17.4 mg/dl (300 µmol/L)
  - PT >50 sec

Cliché Criteria
Factor V <20% in person <30 years or both of the following:
- Factor V <30% in patients >30 years
- Grade III or IV encephalopathy

Serum Gc Globulin Levels
- Decreasing Gc levels due to dying hepatocytes

Serum α-Fetoprotein Level
- Serial increase from day 1 to day 3 has shown correlation with survival

Liver Biopsy[32]
70% necrosis is discriminant of 90% mortality

Gc, Plasma group-specific component protein; *INR,* international normalized ratio; *PT,* prothrombin time.
From Vincent JL et al: *Textbook of critical care,* ed 6, Philadelphia, 2011, Saunders.

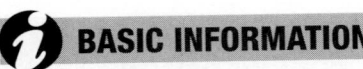

DEFINITION

Hepatitis A is generally an acute self-limiting infection of the liver by an enterically transmitted picornavirus, hepatitis A virus (HAV). Infection may range from asymptomatic to fulminant hepatitis.

SYNONYMS

Infectious hepatitis
Short incubation hepatitis
Type A hepatitis
HAV (hepatitis A virus)

ICD-9CM CODES
070.1 Hepatitis A

EPIDEMIOLOGY & DEMOGRAPHICS

INCIDENCE:
- Hepatitis A occurs worldwide, affecting 1.4 million people annually and accounting for 20% to 40% of cases of viral hepatitis in the United States.
- The seroprevalence increases with age, ranging from 10% in individuals aged <5 yr to 74% in those aged >50 yr.
- In the United States, average disease rate was ~15 cases/100,000 persons/yr prior to routine vaccination of all children in certain states. The incidence after 2005 is about 1 case/100,000.
- The incidence is relatively higher in some regions in the United States, including Arizona, Alaska, California, Idaho, Nevada, New Mexico, Oklahoma, Oregon, South Dakota, and Washington.
- At-risk groups include:
  1. Residents and staff of group homes
  2. Children and employees of day care centers
  3. People who engage in oral-anal contact, regardless of sexual orientation
  4. IV drug abusers
  5. Travel to endemic areas
  6. Areas of overcrowding, poor sanitation, inadequate sewage treatment

PREVALENCE:
- Approximately three fourths of the U.S. population has serologic evidence of prior infection.
- Anti-HAV prevalence has an inverse relation to income and household size.

PREDOMINANT SEX: None, except higher infection rates seen in homosexual males who engage in oral-anal contact.

PREDOMINANT AGE/PEAK INCIDENCE:
- In areas of high rates of hepatitis A, virtually all children are infected while younger than 10 yr, but disease is rare.
- In areas of moderate rates of hepatitis A, disease occurs in late childhood and young adults.
- In areas of low rates of hepatitis A, most cases occur in young adults.

INCUBATION PERIOD: Averages 30 days (15 to 50)

PHYSICAL FINDINGS & CLINICAL PRESENTATION

- Infection with HAV may have acute or sub-acute presentation, icteric or anicteric. Severity of illness seems to increase with age (90% of infection in children aged <5 yr may be subclinical).
- A preicteric, prodromal phase of approximately 1 to 14 days; 15% no apparent prodrome. Symptoms are usually abrupt in onset and may include anorexia, malaise, nausea, vomiting, fever, headache, and abdominal pain.
- Less common symptoms are chills, myalgias, arthralgias, upper respiratory symptoms, constipation, diarrhea, pruritus, urticaria.
- Jaundice occurs in >70% of patients.
- The icteric phase is preceded by dark urine.
- Bilirubinuria is typically followed a few days later by clay-colored stools and icterus.

PHYSICAL EXAMINATION

- Jaundice
- Hepatomegaly
- Splenomegaly
- Cervical lymphadenopathy
- Evanescent rash
- Petechiae
- Cardiac arrhythmias

COMPLICATIONS

- Cholestasis
- Fulminant hepatitis
- Arthritis
- Myocarditis
- Optic neuritis
- Transverse myelitis
- Thrombocytopenic purpura
- Aplastic anemia
- Red cell aplasia
- Henoch-Schönlein purpura
- IgA dominant glomerulonephritis

ETIOLOGY

- Caused by HAV, a 27-nm, nonenveloped, icosahedral, positive-stranded RNA virus.
- Transmission is fecal-oral route, from person to person. Transmission occurs with close contact or with food- or water-borne outbreaks with inadequately purified water or cooked foods. Recent outbreaks have involved green onions and tomatoes.
- Parenteral transmission is considered rare.
- Vertical transmission has also been reported.

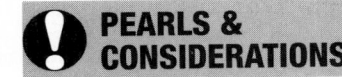 DIAGNOSIS

DIFFERENTIAL DIAGNOSIS

- Other hepatitis virus (B, C, D, E)
- Infectious mononucleosis
- Cytomegalovirus infection
- Herpes simplex virus infection
- Leptospirosis
- Brucellosis
- Drug-induced liver disease
- Ischemic hepatitis
- Autoimmune hepatitis

WORKUP

- IgM antibody specific for HAV
- Liver function tests; ALT and AST elevations are sensitive for liver damage but not specific for HAV
- Elevated ESR
- CBC; may find mild lymphocytosis

LABORATORY TESTS

- DIAGNOSIS confirmed by IgM anti-HAV; it is detectable in almost all infected patients at presentation and remains positive for 3 to 6 mo.
- A fourfold rise in titer of total antibody (IgM and IgG) to HAV confirms acute infection.
- HAV detection in stool and body fluids by electron microscopy.
- HAV RNA detection in stool, body fluids, serum, and liver tissue.
- ALT and AST usually more than 8 times normal in acute infection.
- Bilirubin usually 5 to 15 times normal.
- Alkaline phosphatase minimally elevated but higher level in cholestasis.
- Albumin and prothrombin time are generally normal; if elevated, they may herald hepatic necrosis.
- Fig. 1-393 Illustrates the typical course of hepatis A.

IMAGING STUDIES

- Rarely useful
- Sonogram (fulminant hepatitis)

TREATMENT

- Usually self-limited
- Supportive care
- Those with fulminant hepatitis may require hospitalization and treatment of associated complications
- Activity as tolerated
- Advise to avoid alcohol and hepatotoxic drugs
- Patients with fulminant hepatitis should be assessed for liver transplantation

CHRONIC Rx

No chronic HAV and no chronic carrier state

DISPOSITION

- Follow-up as outpatient
- Most patients recover within 2 months of infection, although 10% to 15% of patients will experience a relapse in the first 6 months.

REFERRAL

- To a hepatologist if severe, fulminant hepatitis develops
- To a transplant surgeon if liver transplant becomes a consideration for fulminant hepatitis and liver failure

PEARLS & CONSIDERATIONS

- All cases of hepatitis A should be reported to the public heath authorities because food-borne or

water-borne outbreaks may occur, and public health efforts (mass vaccination or immuno-globulin therapy) may prevent secondary cases.

- Hepatitis A is a common illness in internationally traveled and developing countries. Pre-travel vaccination is strongly recommended for travelers who are HAV susceptible.

PREVENTION

- Improvement in hygiene and sanitation
- Heating food
- Avoidance of water and foods from endemic area

PASSIVE IMMUNIZATION

- Immunoglobulin provides protection against HAV through passive transfer of antibody.
- Preexposure prophylaxis indicated for people traveling to endemic areas (Ig 0.02 or 0.06 ml/kg given IM) and have not received

or cannot receive the hepatitis A vaccine prior to departure. The lower dose is effective for up to 3 mo, and the higher dose is effective for up to 5 mo.

- Postexposure prophylaxis (Ig 0.02 ml/kg given IM) is indicated for people with recent exposure (within 2 wk) to HAV and who have not been previously vaccinated. In high-risk patients, vaccine may be administered with immunoglobulin.

ACTIVE IMMUNIZATION

- There are several inactivated and attenuated hepatitis vaccines; only the inactivated vaccines are currently available for use and they have been found to be safe and highly immunogenic: HAVRIX or VAQTA. These can be used in adults and children older than 12 mo. They are given as a two-dose regimen 6 mo to 1 yr apart. A combined hepatitis A and

hepatitis B vaccine called TWINRX is also available.

- Protective antibody levels were reached in 94% to 100% of adults 1 mo after the first dose; similar results have been found for children and adolescents.
- Theoretic analyses of antibody levels estimate duration of immunity to be 10 to 20 yr.
- Vaccine should be considered for persons who are at risk: those traveling to or working in endemic areas, homosexual men, illegal drug users, persons with chronic liver disease, children in areas with high rates of hepatitis A infection.
- Beginning in May 2006, the Advisory Committee on Immunization Practices recommended routine hepatitis A vaccination for all children beginning at 12 to 23 mo of age.
- Recent data showed equivalency between use of Ig and hepatitis A vaccine for postexposure prophylaxis in preventing symptomatic hepatitis A in healthy persons 2 to 40 yr of age. The 2007 Advisory Committee guidelines now provide for the use of Ig or the vaccine for this population. Those patients who are immunocompromised, have chronic liver disease, or are less than 1 yr of age should receive Ig.

SUGGESTED READINGS

available at www.expertconsult.com

RELATED CONTENT

Hepatitis A (Patient Information)

AUTHOR: **GLENN G. FORT, M.D., M.P.H.**

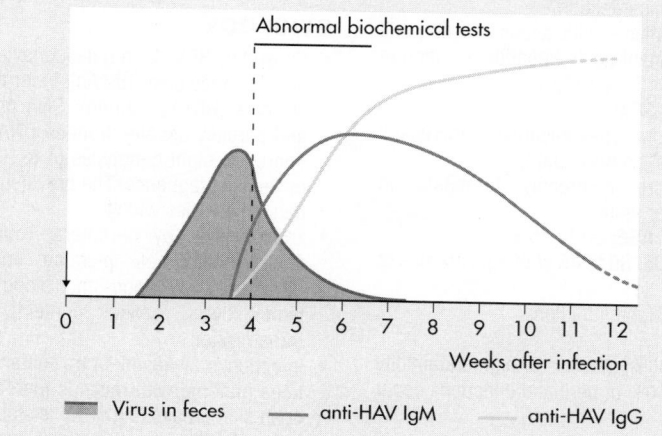

FIGURE 1-393 Course of acute hepatitis A. (From Cohen J, Powderly WG: *Infectious diseases,* ed 2, St Louis, 2004, Mosby.)

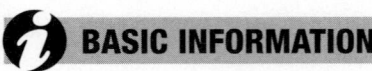

BASIC INFORMATION

DEFINITION

Hepatitis B is an acute infection of the liver parenchymal cells caused by the hepatitis B virus (HBV).

SYNONYMS

Serum hepatitis
Long incubation (30 to 180 days) hepatitis

ICD-9CM CODES
070.3 Hepatitis B

EPIDEMIOLOGY & DEMOGRAPHICS

INCIDENCE (IN U.S.):
- ~200,000 to 300,000 infections annually in the United States.
- Much higher incidence in Europe (~1 million new cases annually) and in areas of high endemicity.
- In U.S., transmission is mainly horizontal (percutaneous and mucous membrane exposure to infectious blood and other body fluids [e.g., sexual transmission, either homosexual or heterosexual]); also from needle sharing among drug abusers; occupational exposure to contaminated blood and blood products; persons receiving transfusions of blood and blood products; and hemodialysis patients.

NOTE: Improved screening of blood and blood products has greatly reduced, although not eliminated, the risk of posttransfusion HBV infection.

- In areas of high endemicity, transmission is largely vertical (perinatal): HBV exists in the blood and body fluids. Perinatal transmission from HBsAg-positive mothers is as high as 90% unless immunoprophylaxis is given.

PREVALENCE (IN U.S.):
- The WHO estimates that 400 million people worldwide (6% of the population) are chronic HBV carriers. North America, Western Europe, and Australia are areas of low prevalence, <2%. In the U.S. an estimated 800,000 to 1.4 million people have chronic HBV infection.
- Africa, Asia, and the Western Pacific region are areas of high prevalence, ≥8%.
- Southern and Eastern Europe have intermediate rates, 2% to 7%.
- Chronically infected persons, those with positive HBsAg for >6 mo, represent the major source of infection.
- As many as 95% of infants and children aged <5, who typically have subclinical acute infection, will become chronic HBV carriers.
- Adults are more likely to have clinically evident acute infection, but only 1% to 5% will develop chronic infection.
- ~0.1% of patients with acute infection will develop fulminant acute hepatitis resulting in death.

PREDOMINANT SEX:
- Predominant in males because of increased IV drug abuse, homosexuality
- Females more commonly terminate in chronic carrier state

PREDOMINANT AGE: 20 to 45 yr
PEAK INCIDENCE: 30 to 45 yr of age, at rates of 5% to 20%
GENETICS: Neonatal infection:
- Rare in U.S.
- High (up to 90%) in areas of high endemicity (only 5% to 10% of perinatal infections occur in utero)

PHYSICAL FINDINGS & CLINICAL PRESENTATION (Fig. 1-394)

- Often nonspecific symptoms
- Profound malaise
- Many asymptomatic cases
- Prodrome:
  1. 15% to 20% serum sickness (urticaria, rash, arthralgia) during early HBsAg
  2. HBsAg-Ab complex disease (polyarteritis nodosa–arthritis, arteritis, glomerulonephritis)
- Hepatomegaly (87%) with right upper quadrant (RUQ) tenderness
  1. Hepatic punch tenderness
  2. Splenomegaly: rare (10% to 15%)
- Jaundice, dark urine, with occasional pruritus
- Variable fever (when present, generally precedes jaundice and rapidly declines following onset of icteric phase)
- Spider angiomata: rare; resolves during recovery
- Rare polyarteritis nodosa, cryoglobulinemia

ETIOLOGY

- Caused by HBV (42-nm hepadnavirus with an outer surface coat [HBsAg], inner nucleocapsid core [HBcAg; HBeAg]; DNA polymerase; and partially double-stranded DNA genome). There are eight genotypes (A to H) based on nucleotide sequence. The prevalence of each genotype varies widely.
- Transmission by parenteral route (needle use, tattooing, ear piercing, acupuncture, transfusion of blood and blood products, hemodialysis, sexual contact), perinatal transmission.
- Infection may result from contact of infectious material with mucous membranes and open skin breaks (e.g., HBV is stable and can be transmitted from toothbrushes, utensils, razors, baby toys, assorted medical equipment [respirators, endoscopes]).
- Oral intake of infectious material may result in infection through breaks in the oral mucosa.
- Food or water are virtually never found to be sources of HBV infection.
- Infection occurs primarily in liver, where necrosis probably results from cytotoxic T-cell response, direct cytopathic effect of HBcAg (core antigen), high-level HBsAg (surface antigen) expression, or coinfection with delta (D) hepatitis virus (RNA delta core within HBsAg envelope).
- Recovery (>90%):
  - Fulminant hepatitis occurring in <1% (especially if coinfected with hepatitis D); 80% fatal
  - Unusual (5%) prolonged acute disease for 4 to 12 mo, with recovery
  - Overall fatality increases with age and viral inoculation (e.g., transfusions)
- Chronic infection (1% to 2%):
  - Persistent carrier state without hepatitis (HBsAg positive)
  - Chronic persistent hepatitis (CPH) (clinically well), or chronic active hepatitis (CAH) (HBsAg positive and HBeAg positive)
  - Cirrhosis

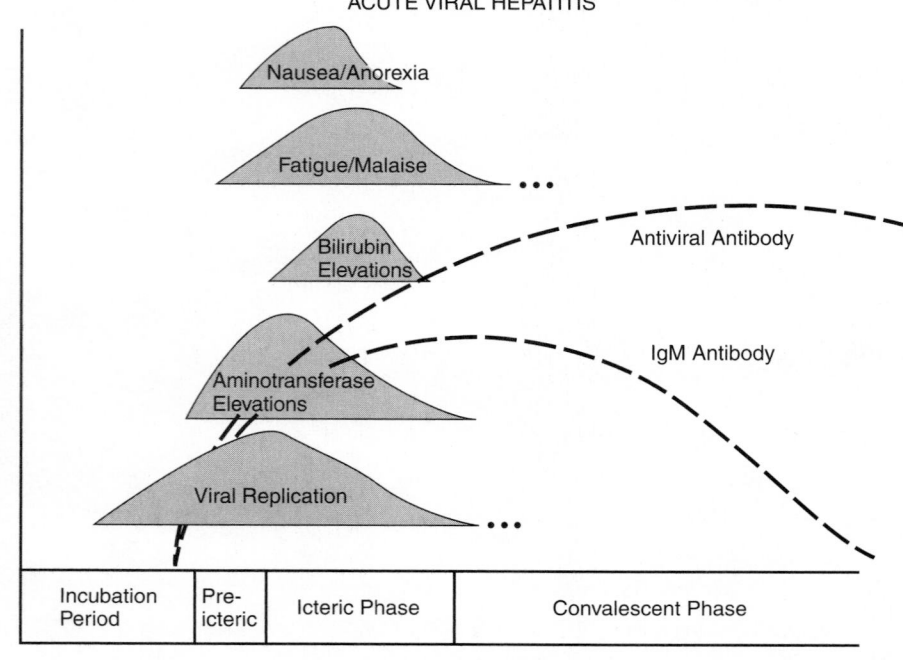

ACUTE VIRAL HEPATITIS

FIGURE 1-394 **The typical course of acute viral hepatitis.** (From Goldman L, Ausiello D [eds]: *Cecil textbook of medicine,* ed 22, Philadelphia, 2004, Saunders.)

- ○ Hepatocellular carcinoma (especially after neonatal infection)
- ○ Chronic infection: more common following low-dose exposure and mild acute hepatitis, with earlier age of infection, in males, and in immunosuppressed patients
- ○ One third to one quarter of chronically infected will develop progressive liver disease (cirrhosis, hepatocellular carcinoma)

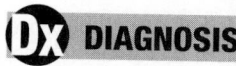 **DIAGNOSIS**

DIFFERENTIAL DIAGNOSIS

- Acute disease confused with other viral hepatitis infections (A, C, D, E)
- Any viral illness producing systemic disease and hepatitis (e.g., yellow fever, EBV, CMV, HIV, rubella, rubeola, coxsackie B, adenovirus, herpes simplex or zoster)
- Nonviral causes of hepatitis (e.g., leptospirosis, toxoplasmosis, alcoholic hepatitis, drug-induced [e.g., acetaminophen, INH], toxic hepatitis [carbon tetrachloride, benzene])

WORKUP

- Acute serum specimen for hepatitis B serology (HBsAg, HBsAb, HBcAb, HBeAg, HBeAb), HBDNA by PCR
- LFTs
- CBC
- Liver biopsy: rarely indicated for diagnosis of fulminant viral hepatitis, chronic hepatitis, cirrhosis, carcinoma

LABORATORY TESTS

- Diagnosis of acute HBV infection is best confirmed by IgM HBcAb in acute or early convalescent serum or by HBDNA by PCR.
  - ○ Generally, IgM present during onset of jaundice
  - ○ Coexisting HBsAg
- HBsAg and IgG-HBcAb during acute jaundice are strongly suggestive of remote HBV infection

and another cause for current illness (Fig. 1-395).
- HBsAb alone is suggestive of immunization response.
- With recovery, HBeAg is rapidly replaced by HBeAb in 2 to 3 mo, and HBsAg is replaced by HBsAb in 5 to 6 mo.
- In chronic HBV hepatitis, HBsAg and HBeAg are persistent without corresponding Ab.
- In chronic carrier state, HBsAg is persistent, but HBeAg is replaced by HBeAb.
- HBcAb develops in all outcomes.
- HBeAg correlation with highest infectivity; appearance of HBeAb heralds recovery.
- LFTs:
  - ○ ALT and AST: usually more than eight times normal (often 1000 U/L) at onset of jaundice (minimal acute ALT/AST rises often followed by chronic hepatitis or hepatocellular carcinoma)
  - ○ Bilirubin: variably elevated in icteric viral hepatitis
  - ○ Alkaline phosphatase: minimally elevated (one to three times normal) acutely
- Albumin and prothrombin time:
  - ○ Generally normal
  - ○ If abnormal, possible harbinger of impending hepatic necrosis (fulminant hepatitis)
- WBC and ESR: generally normal

IMAGING STUDIES

- Rarely useful
- Sonogram to document rapid reduction in liver size during fulminant hepatitis or mass in hepatocellular carcinoma

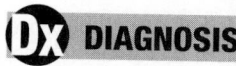 **TREATMENT**

NONPHARMACOLOGIC THERAPY

- Symptomatic treatment as necessary
- Activity as tolerated
- High-calorie diet preferred; often best tolerated in morning

ACUTE GENERAL Rx

- In most cases of acute HBV infection no treatment necessary; >90% of adults will spontaneously clear infection
- Hospitalization advisable for any patient in danger from dehydration caused by poor oral intake, whose PT is prolonged, who has rising bilirubin level >15 to 20 μg/dl, or who has any clinical evidence of hepatic failure
- IV therapy needed (rarely) for hydration during severe vomiting
- Avoid hepatically metabolized drugs
- No therapeutic measures are beneficial
- Steroids not shown helpful

CHRONIC Rx

- The American Association for the Study of Liver Diseases issued guidelines in 2009 for the evaluation and treatment of hepatitis B.
- The aim of therapy in chronic HBV infection is to eradicate the virus.
- The two modalities of therapy available to achieve this goal have been immune modulators (interferon alfa) and antiviral agents in the form of nucleoside analogues (e.g., lamivudine).
- Pegylated interferon alpha (IFN-α) given as a once-a-week SQ injection for 48 wk is a mainstay of therapy and has largely replaced interferon alpha without pegylation, which required daily or thrice weekly injections. Its mechanism of action is to stimulate the immune system to attack HBV-infected hepatocytes, thus inhibiting viral protein synthesis. Dose: 180 μg SQ weekly.
- A 12-mo course of treatment results in a 30% to 40% response with significant reduction of serum HBV DNA, normalization of ALT, and loss of HBeAg. Seroconversion from HBeAg to HBeAb occurs in 15% to 20%.
- Factors that increase the likelihood of response to IFN-α therapy include:
  - ○ Adult onset of infection
  - ○ High baseline ALT

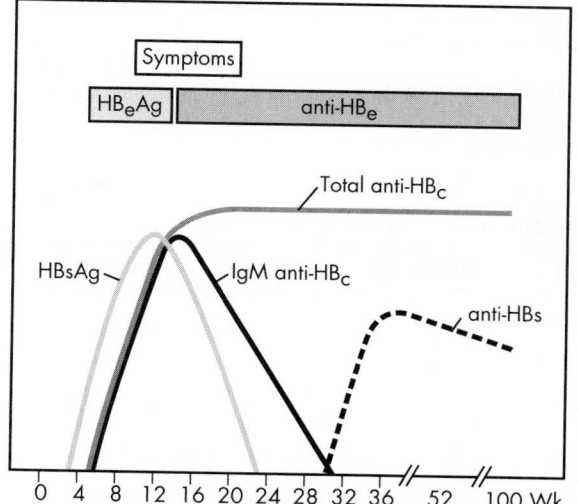
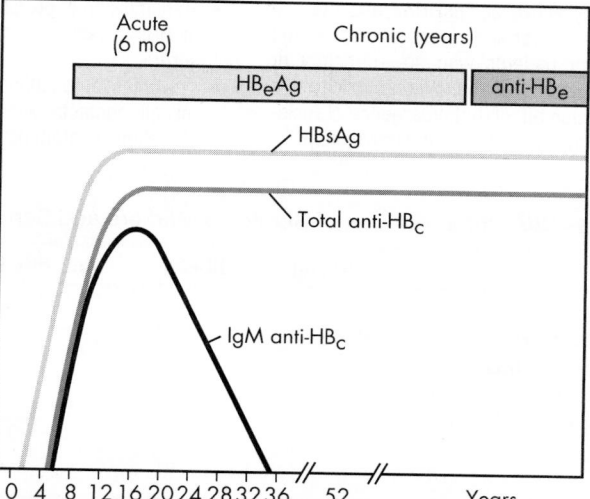

FIGURE 1-395 Typical course of hepatitis B. *Left,* Typical course of acute hepatitis B. *Right,* Chronic hepatitis B. *HBc,* Hepatitis B core; *HBe,* hepatitis B early; *HBsAg,* hepatitis B surface antigen; *IgM,* immunoglobulin M. (From Mandell GL et al: *Principles and practice of infectious diseases,* ed 7, Philadelphia, 2010, Saunders.)

- ○ Low baseline HBV DNA
- ○ Absence of cirrhosis
- ○ Female
- ○ HBeAg positive
- Infrequent relapse after successful completion of therapy.
- 80% of patients who lose HBeAg during therapy lose HBsAg in the decade after therapy.
- >50% of patients who do not seroconvert after initial therapy develop a delayed HBeAg seroconversion months to years after therapy.
- Overall incidence of cirrhosis and hepatocellular carcinoma is decreased in those treated with IFN-α.
- IFN-α is successful only in patients with an active immune response; therefore it is not effective in patients with HIV infection and organ transplant patients.
- Asians respond poorly to IFN-α. Patients with genotype A respond well to IFN-α.
- Treatment with IFN-α in general is not well tolerated: side effects include flulike symptoms, injection-site reactions, rash, weight loss, anxiety, depression, alopecia, thrombocytopenia, granulocytopenia, and thyroid dysfunction.
- Nucleoside analogues block viral replication by inhibiting HBV polymerase.
- Lamivudine was the first nucleoside analogue approved for treatment of chronic HBV infection; it has been shown to rapidly reduce HBV replication and suppress HBV DNA to undetectable levels after a few wk of treatment, and treatment for 1 yr is as effective as IFN-α with respect to loss of HBeAg seroconversion to HBeAb and loss of HBV DNA. The high rate of emergence of resistant HBV strains while on therapy has limited the use of lamivudine as a first-line agent (YMDD variants [tyrosine-methionine-aspartate-aspartate]). Dose: 100 mg orally daily with normal kidney function.
- Adefovir dipivoxil: 10 mg orally daily with normal kidney function is a nucleotide reverse transcriptase inhibitor that also has antiviral activity against HBV. It is a prodrug that is converted to the active drug adefovir. It is highly active against HBV and may be useful as a first-line agent or as salvage therapy for patients who are refractory or intolerant to lamivudine. (Nephrotoxicity is a potential side effect, but emergence of resistant strains is less than with lamivudine.)

- Entecavir is a potent nucleoside agent approved for the treatment of hepatitis B, and it appears to be more effective and to present fewer concerns than lamivudine or adefovir regarding the emergence of resistant strains. Dose: 0.5 mg PO dailiy for nucleoside-naïve patients and 1 mg PO daily for lamiduvine-resistant patients.
- Telbivudine, a thymidine nucleosidase analogue, has demonstrated greater and more consistent HBV DNA suppression than lamivudine or adefovir after 24 wk of treatment but selects for the same resistant strains as lamivudine. Dose: 600 mg PO daily.
- Tenofovir: more potent than adefovir and suppresses lamivudine, telbiduvine, or entecavir resistant strains. In the U.S. it has become a first-line agent. Dose: 300 mg daily with normal kidney function.
- Combination therapy with two or three nucleoside analogues or combination therapy with IFN-α are currently under investigation.
- Liver transplantation (should be considered for fulminant hepatitis).

DISPOSITION
- Follow-up as outpatient
- Acute disease: usually <6 wk
- Rare fatalities (fulminant hepatitis)
- Possible chronic carrier state, cirrhosis, hepatocellular carcinoma

REFERRAL
To infectious disease specialist and gastroenterologist for consultation regarding fulminant hepatitis or prolonged cholestasis, for cases of uncertain etiology, or for treatment of CAH

PEARLS & CONSIDERATIONS

COMMENTS
- Virus and HBsAg in high titers in blood for 1 to 7 wk before jaundice and for a variable time thereafter.
- Transmission is possible during entire period of HBsAg (and especially during HBeAg) in serum.
- Universal precautions should be followed for all contacts with blood or secretions/excretions contaminated with blood.

- Preventing before exposure:
  - ○ Lifestyle changes
  - ○ Meticulous testing of blood supply (although some chronically infected, infectious donors are HBsAg negative)
  - ○ Sterilization via steam or hypochlorite
  - ○ Hepatitis B vaccine for high-risk groups given IM in deltoid to induce HBsAb (response should be confirmed) is protective (>90% effective)
  - ○ Recommendation for universal childhood immunization with doses at birth, 1 mo, and 6 mo
- Prevention after exposure:
  - ○ HBV hyperimmune globulin (HBIG) given immediately after needlestick, within 14 days of sexual exposure, or at birth, followed by HBV vaccination
  - ○ Standard immune globulin: nearly as effective as HBIG
- Preventive therapy with lamivudine for patients who test positive for HBsAg and are undergoing chemotherapy may reduce the risk for HBV reactivation and HBV-associated morbidity and mortality,
- Hepatitis B prophylaxis is described in Section V
- Table 1-188 summarizes interpretation of serologic markers and serum DNA in hepatitis B

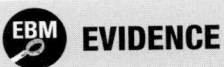

EVIDENCE
available at www.expertconsult.com

SUGGESTED READINGS
available at www.expertconsult.com

RELATED CONTENT
Fig. 3-84 A flow diagram showing the use of specific serologic tests for the diagnosis of acute viral hepatitis in relation to the clinical and epidemiologic setting (Algorithm)
Hepatitis B (Patient Information)

AUTHOR: GLENN G. FORT, M.D., M.P.H.

TABLE 1-188 Interpretation of Serologic Markers and Serum DNA in Hepatitis B

	HBsAg	HBeAg	Anti-HBc IgM	Anti-HBc IgG	Anti-HBs	Anti-HBe	HBV DNA*
Acute hepatitis	+	+/−	+				+
Acute hepatitis, window period			+				
Recovery from acute hepatitis			+	+	+	+/−	
Chronic hepatitis	+	+					+
Chronic hepatitis (precore mutant)	+					+	+
Inactive carrier	+					+/−	
Vaccinated					+		

HBsAg, Hepatitis B surface antigen; *HBeAg*, hepatitis Be antigen; *anti-HBc IgM*, hepatitis B core antibody (IgM type); *anti-HBc IgG*, hepatitis B core antibody (IgG type); *anti-HBs*, hepatitis B surface antibody; *anti-HBe*, hepatitis Be antibody; *HBV DNA*, hepatitis B viral DNA.
*HBV DNA > 10^5 copies/ml.
From Andreoli TE et al: *Andreoli and Carpenter's Cecil essentials of medicine*, ed 8, Philadelphia, 2010, Saunders.

BASIC INFORMATION

DEFINITION

Hepatitis C is an acute liver parenchymal infection caused by hepatitis C virus (HCV).

SYNONYMS

Transfusion-related non-A, non-B hepatitis (incubation period averages 6 wk, intermediate between hepatitis A and B)

ICD-9CM CODES
070.51 Other viral hepatitis

EPIDEMIOLOGY & DEMOGRAPHICS

Hepatitis C infection is the most common chronic blood-borne infection in the U.S. About 3% of baby boomers test positive for the virus. The CDC now recommends testing for hepatits C for anyone born from 1945 to 1965.

INCIDENCE (IN U.S.):
- 150,000 new cases/yr (37,500 symptomatic; 93,000 later chronic liver disease; 30,700 cirrhosis). The incidence of acute HCV has declined substantially over the past 30 yr (from 7.4/100,000 to 0.7/100,000)
- ~9000 of these ultimately die of HCV infection; most common (40%) cause of nonalcoholic liver disease in the United States

PREVALENCE (IN U.S.):
- Overall prevalence of anti-HCV antibody is 1.8% (an estimated 3.9 million persons nationwide)
- Highest prevalence in hemophiliacs transfused before 1987 and users of injection drugs, 72% to 90%. Over past 30 yr, blood transfusion as a risk factor declined from 15% of cases to 1.9%.
- Among low-risk groups, prevalence 0.6%

PREDOMINANT SEX: Slight male predominance
PREDOMINANT AGE: Highest prevalence in 30- to 49-yr age group (65%)

PEAK INCIDENCE:
- 20 to 39 yr of age
- African Americans and whites have similar incidence of acute disease; Hispanics have higher rates
- Prevalence is substantially higher among non-Hispanic blacks than among non-Hispanic whites

GENETICS: Neonatal infection is rare; increased risk with maternal HIV-1 coinfection

PHYSICAL FINDINGS & CLINICAL PRESENTATION

- Symptoms usually develop 7 to 8 wk after infection (range of 2 to 26 wk), but 70% to 80% of cases are subclinical.
- 10% to 20% report acute illness with jaundice and nonspecific symptoms (abdominal pain, anorexia, malaise).
- Fulminant hepatitis may rarely occur during this period.
- After acute infection, 15% to 25% have complete resolution (absence of HCV RNA in serum, normal ALT).
- Progression to chronic infection is common, 50% to 84%. 74% to 86% have persistent viremia; spontaneous clearance of viremia in chronic infection is rare. 60% to 70% of

patients will have persistent or fluctuating ALT levels; 30% to 40% with chronic infection have normal ALT levels.
- 15% to 20% of those with chronic HCV will develop cirrhosis over a period of 20 to 30 yr; in most others, chronic infection leads to hepatitis and varying degrees of fibrosis.
- 0.4% to 2.5% of patients with chronic infection develop hepatocellular carcinoma (HCC).
- 25% of patients with chronic infection continue to have an asymptomatic course with normal LFTs and benign histology.
- In chronic HCV infection, extrahepatic sequelae include a variety of immunologic and lymphoproliferative disorders (e.g., cryoglobulinemia, membranoproliferative glomerulonephritis, and possibly Sjögren's syndrome, autoimmune thyroiditis, polyarteritis nodosa, aplastic anemia, lichen planus, porphyria cutanea tarda, B-cell lymphoma, others).

ETIOLOGY

- Caused by HCV (single-stranded RNA flavivirus).
- Most HCV transmission is parenteral.
- In the United States, advances in screening of blood and blood products in 1990 and 1992 have made transfusion-related HCV infection rare (the risk is estimated to be 0.001% per unit transfused).
- Injecting-drug use accounts for most HCV transmission in the United States (60% of newly acquired cases, 20% to 50% of chronically infected persons).
- Occupational needlestick exposure from an HCV-positive source has a seroconversion rate of 1.8% (range 0% to 7%).
- Nosocomial transmission rates (from surgery and procedures such as colonoscopy and hemodialysis) are extremely low.
- Sexual transmission and maternal-fetal transmission are infrequent (estimated at 5%).
- No identifiable risk in 40% to 50% of community-acquired hepatitis C, but snorting of cocaine by shared use of straw or rolled-up paper has been identified as a risk factor because it causes microscopic bleeding of nasal mucosa.
- HCV infection may stimulate production of cytotoxic T lymphocytes and cytokines (INF-γ), which probably mediate hepatic necrosis.

DIAGNOSIS

DIFFERENTIAL DIAGNOSIS

- Other hepatitis viruses (A, B, D, E)
- Other viral illnesses producing systemic disease (e.g., yellow fever, EBV, CMV, HIV, rubella, rubeola, coxsackie B, adenovirus, HSV, HZV)
- Nonviral hepatitis (e.g., leptospirosis, toxoplasmosis, alcoholic hepatitis, drug-induced hepatitis [acetaminophen, INH], toxic hepatitis)

WORKUP

- Acute hepatitis C antibody
- LFTs; CBC

NOTE: ALT is an easy and inexpensive test to monitor infection and efficacy of therapy. However, ALT levels may fluctuate or even be normal in active or chronic infection and even with

cirrhosis, and ALT may remain elevated even after clearance of viremia.
- Liver biopsy with histologic staging is the gold standard for assessing the degree of disease activity and the likelihood of disease progression, and also to help rule out other causes of liver disease

LABORATORY TESTS

- Diagnosis is often by exclusion, because it takes 6 wk to 12 mo to develop anti-HCV antibody (70% positive by 6 wk, 90% positive by 6 mo).
- Diagnostic tests include serologic assays for antibodies and molecular tests for viral particles.
  - Enzyme immunoassay is the test for anti-HCV antibody:
    The current version can detect antibody within 4 to 10 wk after infection.
    False-negative rate in low-risk populations is 0.5% to 1%.
    False-negatives also occur in immune-compromised persons, HIV-1, renal failure, HCV-associated essential mixed cryoglobulinemia.
    False positives in autoimmune hepatitis, paraproteinemia, and persons with no risk factors.
  - Recombinant immunoblot is used to confirm positive enzyme immunoassays: Recommended only in low-risk settings.
  - Qualitative and quantitative HCV RNA tests using PCR:
    Lower limit of detection is <43 IU/ml
    Used to confirm viremia and to assess response to treatment.
    Qualitative polymerase chain reaction (PCR) useful in patients with negative enzyme immunoassay in whom infection is suspected.
    Quantitative tests use either branched-chain DNA or reverse transcription PCR; the latter is more sensitive.
  - Viral genotyping can distinguish among genotypes 1, 2, 3, and 4, which is helpful in choosing therapy; most of these tests use PCR (genotypes 1, 2, 3, and 4 predominate in the U.S. and Europe [1 is especially common in North America]).
  - LFTs:
    ALT and AST may be elevated to more than eight times normal in acute infection; in chronic infection ALT may be normal or fluctuate.
    Bilirubin may be five to 10 times normal.
    Albumin and prothrombin time generally normal; if abnormal, may be harbinger of impending hepatic necrosis.
  - WBC and erythrocyte sedimentation rate (ESR) are generally normal.

IMAGING STUDIES

Sonogram: rapid liver size reduction during fulminant hepatitis or mass in HCC

TREATMENT

NONPHARMACOLOGIC THERAPY

Activity and diet as tolerated, avoid saw palmetto and green teal leaf herbs

ACUTE GENERAL Rx

- Supportive care
- Avoid hepatically metabolized drugs.
- Specific Rx for acute HCV infection
- Early treatment with interferon-alpha-2b during acute HCV infection prevents chronic infection. The aim is to decrease viral load early in infection and allow the patient's immune system to control viral replication, thus preventing progression to chronic infection. The primary end point was sustained virologic response (SVR), with absence of HCV RNA in serum 24 wk after completion of therapy.
- Further investigations are in progress.

CHRONIC Rx

- Response to therapy is influenced by HCV genotype. Recent advances in treatment now allow for patients with genotypes 1, 2, and 3 to have SVR and cure rates as high as 75% to 80%. Patients with genotype 4 are more difficult to treat and have cure rates of only 45% to 50%.
- Mainstay of therapy currently for patients with genotype 1 is a pegylated interferon-alpha as a weekly SC injection with oral weight-based ribavirin and a protease inhibitor, for a total length of therapy of 12 or 24 wk for most patients. Therapy may go up to 48 wk depending on a history of prior treatment or diagnosis of cirrhosis, and response to therapy measured with viral loads at key intervals during therapy. Two protease inhibitors were approved in 2011: telaprevir and boceprevir.
- For genotypes 2 and 3 treatment consists of a pegylated interferon and ribavirin at a fixed dose of 800 mg daily (400 mg bid) for 24 weeks. This regimen produces SVR rates as high as 75%. For patients with genotype 4, protease inhibitors are not used and therapy extends for 48 weeks with a pegylated interferon and weight-based ribavirin only. This therapy produces SVR rates of about 45% to 50%.
- Pegylated interferons are interferon-alpha with an attached polyethylene glycol (PEG) molecule. The PEG molecule confers a longer half-life and extended therapeutic activity compared with interferon-alpha and reduced dosing to once a week. A third type of interferon, known as consensus interferon, is also available for treatment of hepatitis C, but it is not a long-acting form like the pegylated interferons.
- Two formulations of PEG interferon are available. Peginterferon alpha-2b (PEG INTRON) uses a weight-based dosage in a once-a-week SC Redipen injection. Peginterferon alpha-2a (Pegasys) uses a fixed dosage in a once-a-week premixed syringe, or Redipen, also SC.
- Both PEG interferon-alpha and ribavirin have numerous contraindications (absolute and relative) to use, and may cause a variety of side effects. Interferon-alpha can cause flulike symptoms, thrombocytopenia, granulocytopenia, rash, alopecia, anorexia, psychiatric disturbances, and other side effects. Ribavirin can cause hemolysis, nausea, anemia, nasal congestion, and pruritus. Ribavirin is contraindicated in pregnancy. Patients

should not become pregnant while on therapy and for 6 mo after therapy.
- In patients who fail to respond to interferon-alpha and ribavirin, <10% will respond to retreatment.
- Protease inhibitors:
  - Telaprevir: 750 mg tid taken with a fatty meal is given from the onset of therapy with the pegylated interferon and ribavirin. Telaprevir's side effects include rashes, pruritus, anemia, hemorrhoids, diarrhea, and anorectal discomfort. Severe rash can occur in 4% of patients.
  - Boceprevir: 800 mg tid starts after a lead-in period of 4 wk of the pegylated interferon and ribavirin. The most common side effects of boceprevir include fatigue, anemia, neutropenia, and thrombocytopenia.
  - Use of telaprevir and boceprevir may dramatically improve the cure rates for genotypes 1 and 4 and require only 12 or 24 wk of therapy. They can be used in a cocktail with a pegylated interferon plus ribavirin.
- Combination therapy: Patients with chronic HCV infection who have not had a response to therapy with peginterferon and ribavirin may respond to the addition of multiple direct-acting antiviral agents. Recent trials have shown that the combination of an oral HCV protease and NS5A inhibitor, given for 24 weeks, resulted in an SVR in 36% of these patients.
- Liver transplantation:
  - Hepatitis C is the main indication for liver transplantation in the United States.
  - It is the only option for patients with deteriorating HCV-related cirrhosis and for some patients with HCC.
  - Recurrent infection occurs in almost all patients with progressive fibrosis and cirrhosis; as many as 20% progress to cirrhosis within 5-yr posttransplant.
- Coinfection with HIV:
  - These patients have a poor response to pegylated interferon-alpha and ribavirin if the immune system is depleted, with a low CD4 count as seen in the AIDS category. It is, however, important to treat patients coinfected with HIV and hepatitis C with antiretroviral therapy. Many coinfected patients are stable from their HIV disease, but have significant morbidity and mortality from their hepatitis C.

DISPOSITION

- Recent trials have shown that SVR rates for genotype 1 infection are higher with triple therapy that includes a protease inhibitor than with standard dual therapy.
- SVR after treatment among HCV-infected persons at any stage of fibrosis is associated with reduced HCC.
- Periodic abdominal ultrasonography for HCC screening.
- Recent guidelines recommend against measurement of alpha-fetoprotein (AFP) to screen for HCC in patients with chronic hepatitis C due to lack of sensitivity, specificity, and predictive values.

REFERRAL

- To a hepatologist or infectious disease specialist for treatment for hepatitis C
- To an oncologist if HCC develops. HCC is the fastest rising cause of cancer-related deaths in the United States. This increase is most attributable to an increase in HCV-related HCC.
- To a transplant surgeon for consideration of liver transplant if indicated

⚠ PEARLS & CONSIDERATIONS

- More rapid progression of disease in persons who drink alcohol regularly, persons of advanced age at time of infection, and those coinfected with other viruses (HIV, hepatitis B). All persons with identified HCV infection should receive a brief alcohol screening and intervention as clinically indicated.
- No preventive vaccine available; postexposure Ig provides minimal protection.
- Preventive measures include use of universal precautions, careful screening of blood and blood products, lifestyle changes.
- Major depression is a common (20%-40%) side effect of treatment with interferons. Use of the SSRI escitalopram has been found safe and effective for prevention of interferons-associated depression in these patients.
- Hematologic side effects: use of interferon may result in neutropenia that may require use of Neupogen. Ribavirin may cause sufficient anemia that may require use of Epogen or Procrit or even blood transfusions.
- Eltrombopag is an orally active thrombopoietin-receptor agonist that stimulates thrombopoiesis. It has been reported effective in increasing platelet counts in patients with thrombocytopenia caused by HCV-related cirrhosis.
- Regression of cirrhosis has been demonstrated after antiviral therapy in some patients with chronic hepatitis C. Regression is associated with decreased disease-related morbidity and improved survival.
- The presence of interleukin (IL)-28B and HLA class II are independently associated with spontaneous resolution of HCV infection, and single nucleotide polymorphism IL-28B and DQB1*03:01 may explain approximately 15% of spontaneous resolution of HCV infection.

(EBM) EVIDENCE

available at www.expertconsult.com

SUGGESTED READINGS

available at www.expertconsult.com

RELATED CONTENT

Hepatitis C (Patient Information)

AUTHOR: **GLENN G. FORT, M.D., M.P.H.**

BASIC INFORMATION

DEFINITION

Alcoholic hepatitis is a severe, progressive, inflammatory, and cholestatic liver disease occurring in patients with long-term ethanol abuse.

ICD-9CM CODES
571.1 Acute alcoholic hepatitis

EPIDEMIOLOGY & DEMOGRAPHICS

- Approximately 2 million people in the U.S. (about 1% of the population) are affected by alcoholic liver disease.
- Typical presentation age: 40 to 50 yr. Majority occurs before age 60.

PREVALENCE: Approximately 25% to 30%

PREDOMINANT SEX AND AGE: The majority of patients are males. Males are two times as likely as women to abuse alcohol. However, women develop alcoholic hepatitis after a shorter time and smaller amount of alcoholic exposure than men.

GENETICS: No genetic predilection for any one race. In the U.S., however, there is increased incidence in minority groups.

RISK FACTORS: Drinking multiple alcohol types, drinking alcohol between meal times, poor nutrition, female gender, obesity, Hispanic ethnicity, long-term ingestion of >10 to 20 g/day of alcohol in women and >20 to 40 g/day in men

PHYSICAL FINDINGS & CLINICAL PRESENTATION

Common presenting symptoms include:
- Nausea /vomiting
- Malaise
- Low-grade fever
- Anorexia
- Abdominal distention/pain
- Weight loss
- Complications of liver impairment (GI bleed; confusion, lethargy, ascites)

Findings on physical examination include:
- Fever
- Tachycardia
- Hepatomegaly
- Jaundice
- Splenomegaly
- Asterixis (a flapping tremor)
- Peripheral edema
- Abdominal distention with shifting dullness (ascites)
- Hepatic bruit
- With coexistent cirrhosis look for:
  - Gynecomastia
  - Proximal muscles wasting
  - Spider angiomata
  - Altered hair distribution

DIAGNOSIS

DIFFERENTIAL DIAGNOSIS

- Hepatitis B
- Hepatitis C
- Nonalcoholic steatohepatitis (NASH)
- Chronic pancreatitis
- Drug-induced liver injury
- Hemochromatosis
- Cholangitis

WORK-UP

- A thorough and detailed history is needed.
- Relevant questions may include:
  - When patients started drinking
  - Number of times patient drinks per day
  - How many years of regular/daily drinking
  - Types of alcohol
  - Home or bar drinking?
  - Rehabilitation for drinking?
  - Social problems (e.g., arrest for public intoxication or driving under the influence, marital discord due to alcoholism)

LABORATORY TESTS

- Elevated C-reactive protein
- Electrolyte disorder
- Hypophosphatemia
- Hypomagnesemia
- CBC (may reveal leukocytosis with bandemia or anemia)
- Elevated transaminase (AST >45 U/L but <300 U/L; AST:ALT ratio >1.5)
- S-bilirubin >2 mg/dl
- Increased prothrombin time (PT)
- Decreased gamma glutamyltransferase (GGT)
- Carbohydrate-deficient transferrin (CDT) is a reliable marker for chronic alcoholism
- Screening tests to rule out other conditions include checking:
  - Hepatitis B surface antigen (HBsAg)
  - Anti–hepatic C
  - Ferritin-transferrin saturation
  - Alpha-fetoprotein
  - Alkaline phosphatase

IMAGING STUDIES

Ultrasonography is the preferred imaging study.

LIVER BIOPSY

- Liver biopsy is rarely needed.
- Useful to:
  - Confirm the diagnosis.
  - Evaluate the effect of coexisting disease.
  - Rule out cirrhosis.
  - Exclude other diagnosis (especially other causes of liver diseases).
- Typical finding include:
  - Macrovascular steatosis
  - Hepatocyte injury (ballooning and necrosis)
  - Mallory's bodies (characteristic of alcoholic hepatitis)
  - Perivenular fibrosis
  - Portal and lobular inflammation

TREATMENT

Treatment can be divided into three main components:
1. Lifestyle modifications
2. Nutritional support
3. Pharmacologic therapy

LIFESTYLE MODIFICATIONS

- Abstinence from alcohol (this improves both short- and long-term survival)
- Smoking cessation (to decrease oxidative stress)
- Treatment of substance abuse

NUTRITIONAL SUPPORT

- Good nutrition is an essential part of treatment because many patients with alcoholic hepatitis are usually in a catabolic state.
- Nutritional support includes:
  - Liberal vitamin supplementation (especially thiamine, folic acid, vitamin K)
  - Minerals supplementation (**but not iron**)
  - Calorie counting is essential. A high calorie intake (1.2 to 1.4 times the normal resting intake) may be required.
  - Protein intake of 1.2 to 1.5 g/kg of ideal body weight per day will provide adequate support. **Exception: in patients with severe encephalopathy, protein restriction may be required.**

PHARMACOLOGIC THERAPY

Severe alcoholic hepatitis may require treatment. Severity can be assessed by calculating the Model for End-Stage Liver Disease (MELD) score or Maddrey's Discriminant Function (DF) or the Glasgow score.

- Maddrey's DF = 4.6 × PT in sec prolonged + serum bilirubin (mg/dl)
  - DF >32 indicates significant or severe alcoholic hepatitis (30 day mortality of 50%).
- MELD score can easily be calculated (visit http://www.unos.org/resources/meldpeldcalculator.asp?index=98). This score predicts short-term survival in patients with cirrhosis. A score ≥20 predicts increased short-term mortality.
- Glasgow score: contains four variables (BUN, PT, WBC count, and bilirubin). A score ≥9 indicates increased mortality.

Indications for initiating therapy include:
- DF >30
- MELD >20
- Glasgow score >8
- Hepatic encephalopathy

Patients with severe alcoholic hepatitis may be treated with glucocorticosteroids (prednisolone 40 mg/day for 28 days with a 2-wk taper). Glucocorticosteroids reduce hepatic injury, suppress inflammation, and promote liver regeneration. There are various other treatments, but these are mainly experimental.

LIVER TRANSPLANTATION

- Its role in the management of alcohol hepatitis is unknown.
- Usually reserved for patients with end-stage liver disease.
- Patients with alcoholic hepatitis must be sober for at least 6 mo before they can be eligible for consideration for liver transplantation.

REFERRAL

Severe acute alcoholic hepatitis may require ICU care and referral to different subspecialists:

- GI/hepatology
- Nutritional services
- Nephrology (for acute renal failure, hepatorenal syndrome)
- Neurology (for change in mental status, seizures)
- Infectious disease (for fever/leukocytosis)

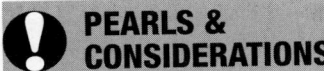

PEARLS & CONSIDERATIONS

COMMENTS

- Referral to substance abuse treatment programs may be helpful.
- Periodic follow-up to monitor patient's response to check BMP and LFTs.

- Encourage alcohol abstinence.
- If patient develops liver cirrhosis, check serum alpha-fetoprotein every 6 mo and liver ultrasound annually to rule out hepatocellular carcinoma.
- Vaccinate patient against hepatitis A and B viruses, pneumococci, and influenza A virus.

SUGGESTED READINGS
available at www.expertconsult.com

RELATED CONTENT
Alcoholic Hepatitis (Patient Information)

AUTHOR: **DANIEL K. ASIEDU, M.D., PH.D., F.A.C.P.**

BASIC INFORMATION

DEFINITION

Autoimmune hepatitis is a chronic inflammatory condition of the liver characterized by elevated serum globulin levels and the presence of circulating autoantibodies. Two types have been described:

- Type 1, or "classic," autoimmune hepatitis is the most predominant form in the U.S. and worldwide (80%); patients are positive for antinuclear antibodies (ANA) and/or anti-smooth muscle antibodies (SMA). Occurs across all age ranges and may be underdiagnosed in the elderly.
- Type 2 is rare in the U.S. and primarily affects young children. Type 2 is characterized by the presence of antibodies to liver/kidney microsomes (anti-LKM-1) or liver cytosol 1.

  This form is generally more advanced at presentation and more difficult to treat.

SYNONYMS

Autoimmune chronic active hepatitis
Chronic active hepatitis
Lupoid hepatitis
Plasma cell hepatitis

ICD-9CM CODES
571.49 Chronic hepatitis

EPIDEMIOLOGY & DEMOGRAPHICS

- Annual incidence (estimated): 1.9 cases per 100,000
- Point prevalence (estimated): 16.9 per 100,000
- Type 1: all age groups; type 2: more common in teenagers and young adults
- Female/male ratio is 3.6:1
- Approximately 100,000 to 200,000 persons affected in the U.S.
- Accounts for 3% to 5.9% of liver transplants in U.S.
- Associated with HLA-DRB1*0301 and HLA-DRB1*0401 alleles

CLINICAL PRESENTATION

- Varies from intermittent asymptomatic elevations of liver enzymes to advanced cirrhosis. Cirrhosis is often the presenting stage. AIH can also present initially as a fulminant hepatitis.
- Symptoms may include fatigue, anorexia, nausea, abdominal pain, pruritus, and arthralgia.
- Autoimmune findings may include arthritis, xerostomia, keratoconjunctivitis, cutaneous vasculitis, and erythema nodosum.
- Patients with advanced disease can show hepatosplenomegaly, ascites, peripheral edema, abnormal bleeding, and jaundice.

ETIOLOGY

- Exact etiology is unknown; liver histology demonstrates cell-mediated immune attack against hepatocytes.
- Presence of a variety of autoantibodies suggests an autoimmune mechanism.
- There are likely two components involved: genetic predisposition and an inciting environmental trigger.
- Potential triggering agents such as viruses (hepatitis A, B, C) or drugs (minocycline, nitrofurantoin) likely possess some homology similar to liver-specific antigens.

DIAGNOSIS

- A simplified diagnostic criteria for routine clinical practice has been developed by the International Autoimmune Hepatitis Group (see Table 1-189).
- Histology: Lymphoplasmacytic infiltrate invading the hepatocyte boundary surrounding the portal triad (limiting plate). Also a periportal infiltrate may be seen (interface hepatitis).

DIFFERENTIAL DIAGNOSIS

- Acute viral hepatitis (A, B, C, D, E, cytomegalovirus, Epstein-Barr, herpes)
- Chronic viral hepatitis (B, C)
- Toxic hepatitis (alcohol, drugs)
- Primary biliary cirrhosis
- Primary sclerosing cholangitis
- Hemochromatosis
- Nonalcoholic steatohepatitis
- SLE
- Wilson's disease
- Alpha-1 antitrypsin deficiency

WORKUP

- History and physical examination with attention to the presence of autoimmune abnormalities such as autoimmune thyroiditis, Graves' disease, inflammatory bowel disease, celiac sprue, and rheumatoid arthritis
- Liver function tests and serum gamma-globulins
- Tests for autoantibodies: ANA, SMA, anti-LKM
- Liver biopsy for establishing diagnosis and disease severity

LABORATORY TESTS

- Aminotransferases generally elevated, may fluctuate
- Bilirubin and alkaline phosphatase moderately elevated or normal
- Elevation of gamma globulin (>2.0 g/dl [20 g/L]) and immunoglobulin G
- Circulating autoantibodies often present:
  1. Rheumatoid factor
  2. ANAs
     a. Present in two thirds of patients
     b. Typical pattern is homogeneous or speckled
     c. Titer does not correlate with the stage, activity, or prognosis
  3. SMAs
     a. Present in 87% of patients
     b. Titer does not correlate with course or prognosis
  4. Anti-LKM antibodies
     a. Typically found in patients who are ANA negative and SMA negative
     b. Characterizes type 2 AIH
     c. Present in pediatric population and up to 20% of adults in Europe; also present in patients with drug-induced hepatitis
  5. Autoantibodies against soluble liver antigen and liver-pancreas antigen (anti-SLA/LP)
     a. Present in 10% to 30% of patients
     b. Associated with higher rate of relapse after corticosteroid therapy
     c. Several studies suggest that patients with anti-SLA/LP have a more severe course
  6. Serum p-ANCA levels are useful for diagnosis of the 10% to 15% of patients with negative SMA, ANA, and low gamma globulin levels.
- Hypoalbuminemia and prolonged prothrombin time with advanced disease
- There is a well-described overlap syndrome with primary biliary cirrhosis (7%), primary sclerosing cholangitis (6%), and autoimmune cholangitis (11%)

IMAGING STUDIES

- Ultrasound of liver and biliary tree to rule out obstruction or hepatic mass
- Cirrhosis secondary to AIH is a risk factor for development of hepatocellular carcinoma (although less so than viral hepatitis). Cirrhotics should get ultrasonography and AFP every 6 months.

TREATMENT

NONPHARMACOLOGIC THERAPY

- Avoid alcohol and hepatotoxic medications.

TABLE 1-189   Simplified Diagnostic Criteria for Autoimmune Hepatitis

Variable	Cutoff	Points	Cutoff	Points
ANA or SMA	≥1:40	1	≥1:80	2
LKM			≥1:40	2
SLA			Positive	2
IgG	≥ULN	1	≥1.1 × ULN	2
Histology	Compatible with AIH	1	Typical of AIH	2
Absence of viral hepatitis			Yes	2

Maximum number of points for all antibodies = 2, total = 8.
Probable AIH ≥6 points, definite AIH ≥7 points.
AIH, Autoimmune hepatitis; *ANA,* antinuclear antibody; *IgG,* immunoglobulin G; *LKM,* liver/kidney microsomes; *SLA,* soluble liver antigen; *SMA,* smooth muscle antibody; *ULN,* upper limit of normal.

- Liver transplantation is an option for end-stage disease or fulminant hepatic failure.

PHARMACOLOGIC THERAPY

- Initial treatment:
  1. Prednisone 60 mg/day PO or combination treatment with prednisone 30 mg/day PO plus azathioprine 50 mg/day PO. A combination of oral budesonide (6 to 9 mg/day) and azathioprine (1 to 2 mg/kg/day) can be used to induce and maintain remission in patients with non-cirrhotic AIH, with a lower rate of steroid-specific side effects.
  2. Combination therapy allows lower prednisone doses and fewer steroid side effects.
  3. Goal of therapy is remission (normalization of gamma-globulin and bilirubin, reduction of aminotransferases to less than twice the upper limit of normal, resolution of symptoms, and improvement in liver histology).
- Indications for treatment:
  1. Serum aminotransferase >10 times the upper limit of normal
  2. Serum aminotransferase more than five times the upper limit of normal, with serum gamma-globulin level twice the upper limit of normal
  3. Histologic features of bridging necrosis or multiacinar necrosis
  4. Incapacitating symptoms such as fatigue and arthralgia
- Evaluation of treatment response:
  1. Goal is the absence of symptoms, resolution of liver function test abnormalities, and histologic improvement. Generally, this is a steroid-responsive condition, but up to 20% do not respond.
  2. Patients whose transaminase levels normalize may continue to have ongoing active hepatitis involving inflammation and fibrosis. 5% to 10% of patients with normal transaminase levels progress to cirrhosis.

3. Histologic improvement may lag behind clinical and laboratory improvement by as much as 6 mo. Because of this, repeat liver biopsy should be considered after normalization of transaminase levels.
4. After initial remission is achieved, one may consider tapering medications. Steroid withdrawal should be done only if liver function tests normalize and histologic quiescence is achieved. About 50% to 86% of patients will relapse after this and require long-term maintenance medications.
5. Complete normalization on biopsy is associated with a 15% to 20% risk of relapse, whereas persistent interface hepatitis is associated with a 90% risk of relapse.

DISPOSITION

- Follow up as outpatient.
- Long-term treatment may be necessary for sustained remission in individuals who continuously relapse and in partial responders.
- Sixty-five percent of patients achieve remission by 18 mo; 80% achieve remission by 3 yr.
- Approximately 10% of patients do not improve with therapy. For these nonresponders, one can try higher dose of combination prednisone/azathioprine. There is limited data pointing toward some success with such agents as cyclosporine and mycophenolate mofetil.
- Patients in whom end-stage liver develops are candidates for liver transplantation. AIH can recur in transplanted livers (18% 5-year probability).

REFERRAL

Patients with advanced cirrhosis or who progress to end-stage liver disease are candidates for liver transplantation and should be referred to appropriate medical centers that provide liver transplantation services.

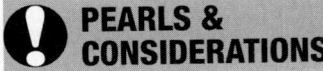

COMMENTS

- ANA and SMA are observed together in 60% of cases. Serum titers >1:40 suggest autoimmune hepatitis.
- A variety of autoimmune conditions can be seen in association with autoimmune hepatitis, including thyroiditis, Graves' disease, ulcerative colitis, rheumatoid arthritis, uveitis, pernicious anemia, Sjögren's syndrome, mixed connective tissue disease, CREST syndrome, and vitiligo.
- Variant forms of autoimmune hepatitis (overlap syndrome) have clinical and serologic findings of autoimmune hepatitis plus features of other forms of chronic liver disease such as primary biliary cirrhosis (PBC) or primary sclerosing cholangitis (PSC).

PREVENTION

None

PATIENT & FAMILY EDUCATION

- American Liver Foundation (ALF): Phone: 800-GO-LIVER (465-4837); Internet: www.liverfoundation.org
- National Digestive Diseases Information clearinghouse: http://digestive.niddk.nih.gov/ddiseases/pubs/autoimmunehep

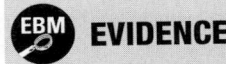 **EVIDENCE**

available at www.expertconsult.com

SUGGESTED READINGS

available at www.expertconsult.com

RELATED CONTENT

Autoimmune Hepatitis (Patient Information)

AUTHORS: **JAYDEEP BHAT, M.D., M.P.H., JUDY NEE, M.D., AMANDA PRESSMAN, M.D.,** and **KITTICHAI PROMRAT, M.D.**

BASIC INFORMATION

DEFINITION

Hepatocellular carcinoma (HCC) is a malignant tumor of the hepatocytes.

SYNONYMS

Hepatoma
HCC

ICD-10CM CODES
C22.0 Liver cell carcinoma
ICD-9CM CODES
155.0 Hepatocellular carcinoma

EPIDEMIOLOGY & DEMOGRAPHICS

Fifth most common cancer worldwide (>500,000 new cases/year) and third most common cause of cancer deaths. Incidence varies worldwide:
- Areas with high rates of hepatitis B and C (Asia, sub-Saharan Africa) have high rates of HCC.
- Males more affected than females, with ratios between 2:1 and 4:1.
- Peak incidence: fifth and sixth decades in Western countries, earlier in areas with perinatal transmission of hepatitis B.
- Incidence rapidly growing in U.S. secondary to chronic hepatitis C infection and obesity leading to nonalcoholic steatohepatitis (NASH).
  - Incidence: during the past two decades, the incidence of HCC in the U.S. has tripled. The greatest proportional increase in cases has been among Hispanics and whites between 45 and 60 years of age
  - Mean age of diagnosis approximately 65 yr
  - HCC is the fastest-rising cause of cancer-related deaths in the United States
- Risk factors:
  - Chronic hepatitis B infection: accounts for 50% of all cases of HCC and virtually all childhood cases
  - Chronic hepatitis C infection: markers of HCV infection are found in 80% to 90% of patients with HCC in Japan, 44% to 66% in Italy, and 30% to 50% in the U.S.
  - Cirrhosis from causes other than viral hepatitis: alcoholic liver disease, nonalcoholic steatohepatitis, primary biliary cirrhosis, hemochromatosis, α1-antitrypsin deficiency, and autoimmune hepatitis
  - Hepatotoxins: alcohol and aflatoxin B1
  - Systemic diseases affecting the liver such as tyrosinemia
  - Obesity and diabetes mellitus

PHYSICAL FINDINGS & CLINICAL PRESENTATION

- One third of patients are asymptomatic. Abdominal pain may be the initial presentation.
- Signs of underlying cirrhosis and portal hypertension are often present.
- Previously compensated cirrhosis with new ascites, encephalopathy, jaundice, or bleeding.
- Paraneoplastic syndromes (hypoglycemia, erythrocytosis, hypercalcemia, severe diarrhea) may be present.

DIAGNOSIS

DIFFERENTIAL DIAGNOSIS

- Metastatic tumor to liver
- Intrahepatic cholangiocarcinoma
- Benign liver tumors such as adenomas, focal nodular hyperplasia, and hemangiomas
- Focal fatty infiltration

WORKUP

- History regarding risk factors
- Physical examination with attention to signs of chronic liver disease
- Laboratory evaluation and imaging studies
- Imaging studies: ultrasound for initial screening; 4-phase multidetector CT scan or dynamic contrast-enhanced MRI for HCC diagnosis

LABORATORY TESTS

- Liver function tests
- α-Fetoprotein levels (AFP) can be elevated in 70% of patients (sensitivity, 40% to 65%; specificity, 80% to 94%). An AFP level of 400 ng/ml or greater is highly suggestive of HCC; however, elevations may not be seen in up to 40% of patients with small HCC lesions (<3 cm).
- Paraneoplastic syndromes associated with HCC may cause hypercalcemia, hypoglycemia, and polycythemia
- Elevated serum HBV DNA level (≥10,000 copies/ml) is a strong risk predictor of HCC independent of HBeAg, serum aminotransferase level, and liver cirrhosis

IMAGING STUDIES

Ultrasound (US), CT scan (Fig. 1-396), or MRI. Ultrasound is most commonly used as a screening test for HCC in high-risk patients every 6 months. The following imaging modalities are recommended based on US findings:
- Hepatic lesion <1 cm needs to be followed with a repeat US every 3 months to ensure the lesion does not change change size. If there is no change in size (remains <1 cm) or

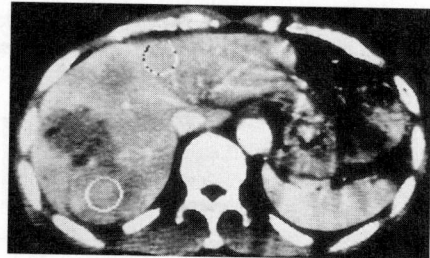

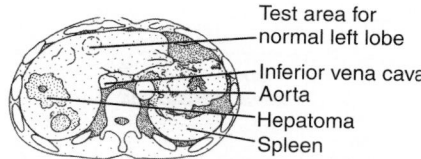

Test area for normal left lobe
Inferior vena cava
Aorta
Hepatoma
Spleen

FIGURE 1-396 Hepatoma. CT scan shows a diffuse lesion in the right lobe of an otherwise normal liver. (From Skarin AT: *Atlas of diagnostic oncology,* ed 3, St Louis, 2003, Mosby.)

characteristics after 24 months, the interval for US surveillance can be increased back to every 6 months
- Hepatic lesion >1 cm needs further imaging to confirm the diagnosis of HCC. Either a 4-phase multidetector CT (MDCT) scan or a dynamic contrast-enhanced MR scan is performed. If the chosen imaging modality shows characteristics typical of HCC (hypervascular in the arterial phase with washout in the portal venous or delayed phase) the diagnosis of HCC is confirmed with no need for additional diagnostic testing or biopsy. If the imaging modality is inconclusive or atypical for HCC then the alternate imaging test must be performed (e.g., if the first modality was MRI then the MDCT scan needs to be performed and vice versa). If the second imaging modality is also inconclusive, a biopsy to confirm diagnosis is recommended.

BIOPSY: Percutaneous biopsy under ultrasound or CT scan is obtained in the event that imaging studies are nondiagnostic or atypical for HCC, or if no cirrhosis is present. Negative biopsy results should be followed and the hepatic nodule reassessed every 3 to 6 months until it is no longer seen, enlarges, or shows diagnostic characteristics.

SCREENING: Screening high-risk patients with US every 6 mo is currently recommended to identify HCC at an early stage. The use of AFP in addition to US is currently under debate; though it does increase detection rate it also increases false-positive results. The use of AFP alone should be discouraged due to limited sensitivity and specificity. Newer tumor markers are currently under investigation, with plasma microRNA expression the most promising. Patients on transplant waiting lists should be regularly screened for HCC because in the U.S. the development of HCC gives increased priority for liver transplantation. Screening for HCC is recommended in the following groups:
- Hepatitis B carriers (HBsAg positive): Asian males >40 yr, Asian females >50 yr, all cirrhotic hepatitis B carriers, family history of HCC and North American blacks/Africans older than age 20 yr
- Cirrhosis (nonhepatitis B): hepatitis C, alcoholic cirrhosis, hemochromatosis, primary biliary cirrhosis, and possibly α1-antitrypsin deficiency, autoimmune hepatitis, and nonalcoholic steatohepatitis

STAGING: According to the Barcelona Clinic Liver Cancer (BCLC) staging classification, treatment is determined according to stage:
- Early stage (A): asymptomatic single tumor 5 cm or 3 nodules, each ≤3 cm (known as Milan criteria)
- Intermediate stage (B): patients with tumors that exceed early criteria but do not yet show cancer-related symptoms, vascular invasion, or metastases
- Advanced stage (C): patients with mild cancer-related symptoms and/or vascular invasion or extrahepatic spread
- End-stage (D): patients with advanced, symptomatic disease

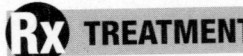 **TREATMENT**

- Fig. 1-397 describes a treatment algorithm for HCC.
- Early stage: curative treatment (surgical resection or liver transplantation). Patients who have a single lesion can be offered surgical resection if they are noncirrhotic or have cirrhosis but still have well-preserved liver function, normal bilirubin, and no significant portal hypertension. Liver transplantation is an effective option for patients with HCC corresponding to the Milan criteria (Table 1-190). Living donor transplantation can be offered for HCC if the waiting time is expected to be long. Local ablation is safe and effective therapy for patients who cannot undergo resection or as a bridge to transplantation. With these options, survival at 5 yr ranges from 50% to 70%.
- Intermediate stage: Transarterial chemoembolization (TACE) is recommended as first-line noncurative therapy for nonsurgical patients with large/multifocal HCC who do not have vascular invasion or extrahepatic spread. Median survival with this option exceeds 2 yr.
- Advanced stage: sorafenib, an oral multikinase inhibitor of the vascular endothelial growth factor receptor (VEGF), the platelet-derived growth factor (PDGF) receptor, and Raf, a serine-threonine kinase, has been shown to improve survival and delay disease progression. The SHARP trial included patients with advanced HCC in Child-Pugh A cirrhosis and showed increased median survival from 7.9 to 10.7 mo.
- End stage: palliative care.

DISPOSITION

- For unresectable tumors, prognosis is poor; 5-yr survival after surgical resection ranges from 30% to 50%.
- In the U.S. the 5-year overall survival rate for HCC is 10% to 12%.

REFERRAL

To gastroenterologist for treatment planning

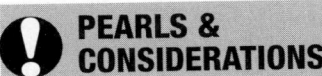 **PEARLS & CONSIDERATIONS**

PREVENTION

- Universal hepatitis B vaccination in children in endemic areas has been shown to decrease the incidence of HCC.
- Treatment of patients with chronic hepatitis B–associated cirrhosis with lamivudine reduces the incidence of HCC. Treatment with entecavir in chronic hepatitis B-HCC can improve hepatic function and MELD score.
- HCC screening is recommended in high-risk patients because curative therapies are available for small and early HCC.
- The expression patterns of microRNAs in liver tissue in patients with HCC differ between men and women. The miR-26 expression status of such patients is associated with survival and response to adjuvant therapy with interferon alfa.

- Several observational studies have suggested that radiofrequency ablation (RFA) may have survival benefits similar to hepatic resection (HR) in cirrhotic patients affected by HCC who are not candidates for liver transplantation.
- Patients diagnosed with HCC with an AFP >1000 are at increased risk for recurrence after transplantation regardless of tumor size.
- Recent trials have shown that among patients with advanced HCC, treatment with sorafenib plus doxorubicin monotherapy resulted in greater median time to progression-free survival. The degree in which this improvement may represent synergism between sorafenib and doxorubicin remains to be defined.
- There are at least 60 new agents, both TKI (tyrosine kinase inhibitors) and monoclonal antibodies, that are being investigated as targeted therapy for advanced HCC in patients who are intolerant or resistant to sorafenib. The future of therapy for advanced HCC will likely lead to the personalized combination of multiple agents to optimize treatment success.

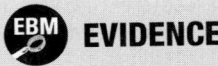 **EVIDENCE**

available at www.expertconsult.com

SUGGESTED READINGS

available at www.expertconsult.com

RELATED CONTENT

Liver Cancer (Patient Information)

AUTHORS: **PRANITH PERERA, M.D.,** and **JEANETTE SMITH, M.D.**

TABLE 1-190 Milan Criteria of Eligibility for Liver Transplantation

Presence of a tumor ≤5 cm in diameter in patients with single hepatocellular carcinomas

or

≤3 tumor nodules, each 3 cm or less in diameter, in patients with multiple tumors

From Cameron JL, Cameron AM: *Current surgical therapy,* ed 10, Philadelphia, 2011, Saunders.

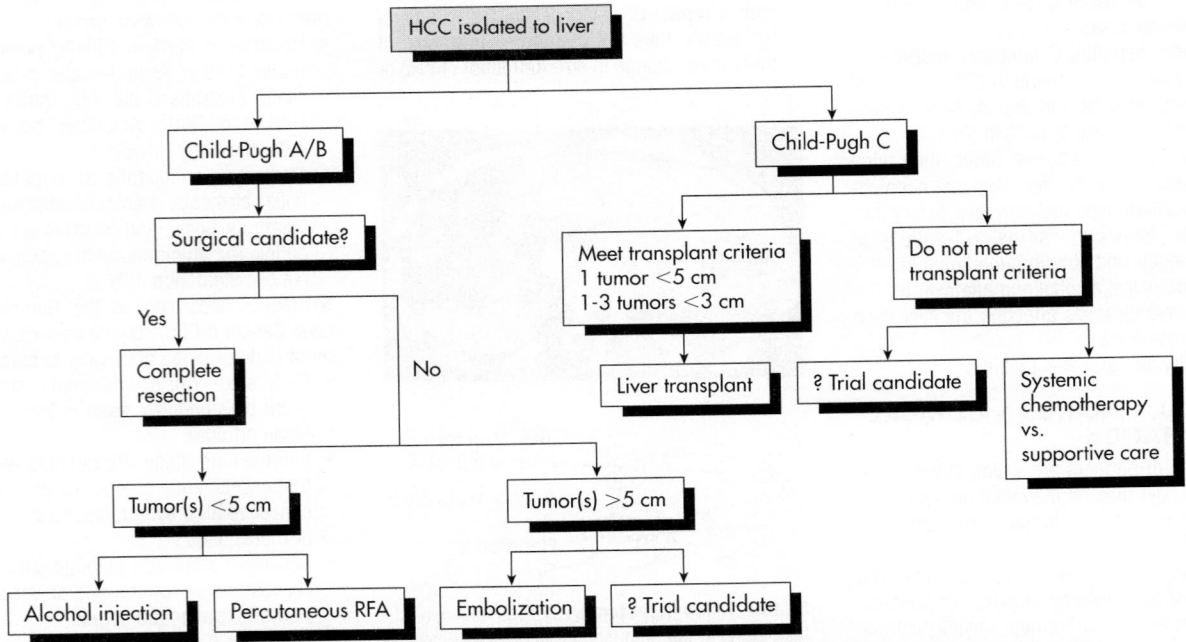

FIGURE 1-397 Treatment algorithm for hepatocellular carcinoma *(HCC).* *RFA,* Radiofrequency ablation. (From Abeloff MD: *Clinical oncology,* ed 3, Philadelphia, 2004, Saunders.)

BASIC INFORMATION

DEFINITION
Hepatopulmonary syndrome (HPS) is characterized by intrapulmonary vascular dilation in the setting of liver disease causing an increased alveolar-arterial (A-a) gradient.

SYNONYMS
HPS

ICD-9CM CODES
417.9 Unspecified disease of pulmonary circulation

EPIDEMIOLOGY & DEMOGRAPHICS
PREVALENCE: Between 5% and 30% of patients with cirrhosis; wide range due to lack of diagnostic criteria
PREDOMINANT SEX AND AGE: There are no data on gender or age prevalence.
RISK FACTORS: Can occur with any degree or etiology of liver disease but is more common in patients with established cirrhosis and portal hypertension. There is no clear relationship between severity of hepatic dysfunction and level of hypoxemia. One recent study suggests that HPS is more common in patients with history of viral hepatitis than in patients with alcoholic cirrhosis.
GENETICS: There are new data suggesting that genes involved in the regulation of angiogenesis are associated with the risk of HPS.

PHYSICAL FINDINGS & CLINICAL PRESENTATION
- Dyspnea
- Platypnea: worsened dyspnea when sitting upright compared to supine position due to further ventilation-perfusion mismatch
- Orthodeoxia: decreased PaO_2 when the patient is sitting upright compared to supine position due to ventilation-perfusion mismatch
- Spider angiomata seen in high number
- Signs of severe hypoxemia (e.g., cyanosis and clubbing of the digits)

ETIOLOGY
Dilation of intrapulmonary arterioles and dilated vascular channels between pulmonary arteries and veins leading to a ventilation-perfusion mismatch and right-to-left shunting (Fig. 1-398). Research shows that nitric oxide plays a role in vasodilation. The relationship of vasodilation to liver disease is unclear. New areas of research include endothelin-1, which is produced by proliferating cholangiocytes, pulmonary angiogenesis, and opiate receptors' influence on NO production.

DIAGNOSIS

DIFFERENTIAL DIAGNOSIS
- Portopulmonary hypertension
- Cavo-pulmonary anastomosis
- Hereditary hemorrhagic telangiectasia (Rendu-Osler-Weber syndrome)
- Chronic lung disease (i.e., COPD or pulmonary fibrosis) with coexisting liver disease

WORKUP
- Diagnosis should be suspected in patients with cirrhosis who develop hypoxemia in absence of other causes (e.g., COPD, thromboembolism).
- Workup includes lab testing and imaging studies (see following), but diagnosis is based on clinical findings.

LABORATORY TESTS
- Arterial blood gas at rest, both supine and erect; PaO_2 <80 mm Hg
- Pulmonary function tests will show nonspecific reduction in DL_{CO}.

IMAGING STUDIES
- The most effective screening tool is transthoracic echocardiogram with bubble study to rule out right-to-left cardiac shunt; microbubble opacification in left atrium shows vasodilation of pulmonary vascular bed.
- Chest x-ray may show nonspecific bibasilar interstitial pattern.
- Scintigraphic perfusion scanning: technetium-99m–labeled albumin found in brain or spleen indicates dilated pulmonary vasculature or cardiac right-to-left shunt.
- Pulmonary angiography rarely used unless there is potential to embolize arteriovenous malformation (AVM).

TREATMENT

Ideal treatment would be targeted against pulmonary vasodilation but no effective medications yet exist. Liver transplantation is the only successful treatment, which leads to improvement in gas exchange or compete resolution in gas exchange in the majority of patients. However, severe hypoxemia with PaO_2 <50 has been associated with a high posttransplant mortality. Some studies have shown benefit of transjugular portosystemic shunting, although it is not currently established treatment. Coil embolization in the setting of pulmonary AVMs is another possible area of treatment.

NONPHARMACOLOGIC THERAPY
Oxygen to correct hypoxemia; PaO_2 will partially correct with administration of supplemental O_2.

ACUTE GENERAL Rx
Correct hypoxemia with supplemental O_2.

CHRONIC Rx
Liver transplantation is only successful treatment.

COMPLEMENTARY & ALTERNATIVE MEDICINE
One study suggested that garlic supplements might decrease A-a gradient in patients with HPS. Studies of diets containing low amount of L-arginine have not shown benefit.

DISPOSITION
The diagnosis of HPS confers a poor prognosis. Patients with HPS have high mortality and shorter median survival than other patients with liver disease, even after adjusting for severity of liver disease. According to one natural history study, compared with patients with similar severity of liver disease and comorbidities whose 5-yr survival was estimated at 63%, those patients with the diagnosis of HPS had a 5-yr survival rate of 23%.

REFERRAL
- Referral to pulmonologist to help in establishing diagnosis
- Referral to a liver transplant center should be considered for patients who would be eligible

PEARLS & CONSIDERATIONS

COMMENTS
Consider the diagnosis of HPS in patients with cirrhosis who present with dyspnea without signs of pulmonary edema from fluid overload.

SUGGESTED READINGS
available at www.expertconsult.com

RELATED CONTENT
Cirrhosis (Related Key Topic)

AUTHOR: **BEVIN KENNEY, M.D.**

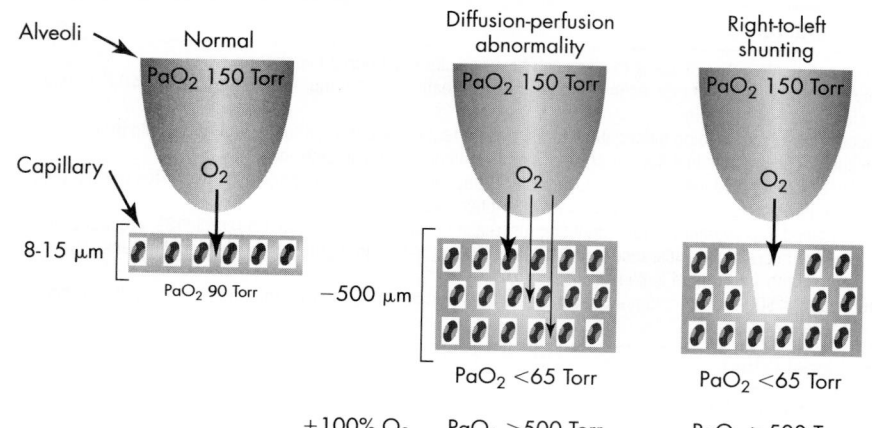

FIGURE 1-398 **Pathophysiology of hypoxemia in hepatopulmonary syndrome.** Abnormal intrapulmonary vascular dilation in combination with increased pulmonary blood flow leads to diffusion-perfusion disturbance and arterial hypoxemia, correctable by oxygen supplementation. Most severe intrapulmonary vascular dilation or formation of arteriovenous malformations causes right-to-left shunting only partially correctable by oxygen administration. (From Hoeper MM et al: Portopulmonary hypertension and hepatopulmonary syndrome, *Lancet* 363:1461, 2004.)

BASIC INFORMATION

DEFINITION

Hepatorenal syndrome (HRS) is a condition of intense renal vasoconstriction (see Fig. 1-399) resulting from loss of renal autoregulation occurring as a complication of severe liver disease. Criteria for HRS are:

1. Serum creatinine concentration >1.5 mg/dl or 24-hr creatinine clearance <40 ml/min
2. Absence of shock, ongoing infection, and fluid loss and no current treatment with nephrotoxic drugs
3. Absence of sustained improvement in renal function (decrease in serum creatinine to <1.5 mg/dl after discontinuation of diuretics and a trial of plasma expansion)
4. Absence of proteinuria (<500 mg/day) or hematuria (<50 red blood cells/high-power field)
5. Absence of ultrasonographic evidence of obstructive uropathy or parenchymal renal disease
6. Urinary sodium concentration <10 mmol/L

Tables 1-191 and 1-192 summarize the classic and the revised diagnostic criteria for HRS.

There are two types of HRS (see Table 1-193):
1. Type 1: progressive impairment in renal function as defined by a doubling of initial serum creatinine >2.5 mg/dl in <2 wk
2. Type 2: stable or slowly progressive impairment of renal function not meeting the above criteria

SYNONYMS

Hepatic nephropathy
Oliguric renal failure of cirrhosis
HRS

ICD-9CM CODES
572.4 Hepatorenal syndrome

EPIDEMIOLOGY & DEMOGRAPHICS

The probability of HRS in patients with cirrhosis is 18% at 1 yr and 39% at 5 yr.

PHYSICAL FINDINGS & CLINICAL PRESENTATION

- Evidence of cirrhosis is usually present: jaundice, spider angiomas, splenomegaly, ascites, fetor hepaticus, pedal edema

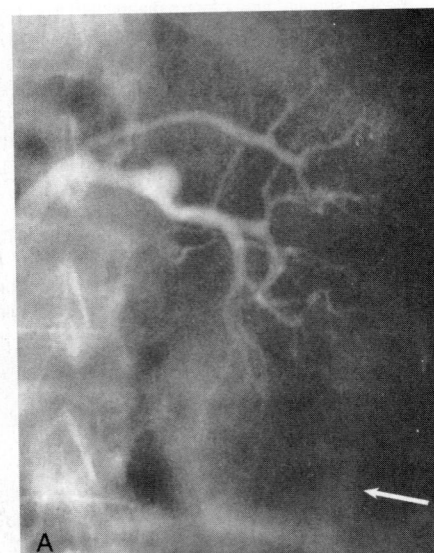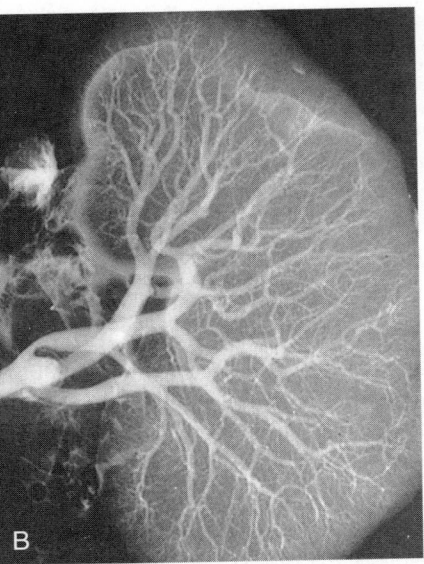

FIGURE 1-399 Hepatorenal syndrome (HRS). A, Renal angiogram (the *arrow* marks the edge of the kidney). **B,** The angiogram carried out in the same kidney at autopsy. Note complete filling of the renal arterial system throughout the vascular bed to the periphery of the cortex. The vascular attenuation and tortuosity seen previously **(A)** are no longer present. The vessels are also histologically normal. This indicates the functional nature of the vascular abnormality in HRS. (From Floege J et al: *Comprehensive clinical nephrology,* ed 4, Philadelphia, 2010, Saunders.)

TABLE 1-191 Diagnostic Criteria for Hepatorenal Syndrome

Major Criteria

Chronic or acute liver disease with advanced hepatic failure and portal hypertension
Low glomerular filtration rate, as indicated by serum creatinine >1.5 mg/dl (135 μmol/L) or 24-hr creatinine clearance <40 ml/min
Absence of shock, ongoing bacterial infection, and current or recent treatment with nephrotoxic drugs
Absence of gastrointestinal fluid losses (repeated vomiting or intense diarrhea)
Absence of renal fluid losses (weight loss >500 g/day for several days in patients with ascites without peripheral edema or 1000 g/day in patients with peripheral edema)
No sustained improvement in renal function (decrease in serum creatinine to 1.5 mg/dl [135 μmol/L] or less or increase in creatinine clearance to 40 ml/min or more) following diuretic withdrawal and expansion of plasma volume with 1.5 liters of isotonic saline
Proteinuria <500 mg/day and no ultrasonographic evidence of obstructive uropathy or parenchymal renal disease

Additional Criteria

Urine volume <500 ml/day
Urine sodium <10 mmol/L
Urine osmolality greater than plasma osmolality
Urine red blood cells <50 per high-power field
Serum sodium concentration <130 mmol/L

From Floege J et al: *Comprehensive clinical nephrology,* ed 4, Philadelphia, 2010, Saunders.

TABLE 1-192 Revised Diagnostic Criteria for Hepatorenal Syndrome

Cirrhosis with ascites
Serum creatinine >1.5 mg/dl (133 μmol/L)
No improvement in serum creatinine (decrease to a level of 1.5 mg/dl) after at least 2 days with diuretic withdrawal and volume expansion with albumin. The recommended dose of albumin is 1 g/kg of body weight per day up to a maximum of 100 g/day.
Absence of shock
No current or recent treatment with nephrotoxic drugs
Absence of parenchymal kidney disease as indicated by proteinuria >500 mg/day, microhaematuria (>50 red blood cells per high-power field) and/or abnormal renal ultrasound

From Floege J et al: *Comprehensive clinical nephrology,* ed 4, Philadelphia, 2010, Saunders.

TABLE 1-193 Definition of Hepatorenal Syndrome Type 1 and Type 2

Type 1 Hepatorenal Syndrome

Doubling of serum creatinine >2.5 mg/dl (220 μmol/L) or a 50% reduction in 24-hr creatinine clearance to <20 ml/min <2 weeks
Frequently follows a precipitating event (e.g., infection)
Median survival without treatment: 2 weeks

Type 2 Hepatorenal Syndrome

Less rapid renal functional deterioration than type 1
Mainly presents with refractory ascites
Median survival without treatment: 4–6 months

From Floege J et al: *Comprehensive clinical nephrology,* ed 4, Philadelphia, 2010, Saunders.

- Hepatic encephalopathy: flapping tremor (asterixis), coma
- Tachycardia and bounding pulse
- Oliguria

ETIOLOGY

An exacerbation of end-stage liver disease, HRS may occur after significant reduction of effective blood volume (e.g., paracentesis, GI bleeding, diuretics) or in the absence of any precipitating factors.

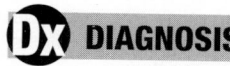 **DIAGNOSIS**

DIFFERENTIAL DIAGNOSIS

- Prerenal azotemia: response to sustained plasma expansion is good (prompt diuresis with volume expansion). Volume challenge (to increase mean arterial pressure) followed by large-volume paracentesis (to increase cardiac output and decrease renal venous pressure) may be useful to distinguish HRS from prerenal azotemia in patients with FENa <1%. In patients with prerenal azotemia, the increase in renal perfusion pressure and renal blood flow will result in prompt diuresis; the volume challenge can be accomplished by giving a solution of 100 g of albumin in 500 ml of isotonic saline.
- Acute tubular necrosis: urinary sodium >30 mEq/L, fractional excretion of sodium (FENa) >1.5%, urinary/plasma creatinine ratio <30, urine/plasma osmolality ratio = 1, urine sediment reveals casts and cellular debris, no significant response to sustained plasma expansion.

WORKUP

Patients with acute azotemia and oliguria in the setting of liver disease should undergo laboratory evaluation to differentiate HRS from acute tubular necrosis and volume challenge to differentiate HRS from prerenal azotemia if FENa <1%.

LABORATORY TESTS

- Obtain serum electrolytes, blood urea nitrogen, creatinine, osmolality, urinalysis, urinary sodium, urinary creatinine, urine osmolality
- Calculate FENa
- In HRS: urinary sodium <10 mEq/L, FENa <1%, urinary plasma creatinine ratio >30, urinary plasma osmolality ratio >1.5, urine sediment unremarkable

IMAGING STUDIES

Renal ultrasound may be indicated if renal obstruction is suspected.

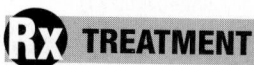 **TREATMENT**

NONPHARMACOLOGIC THERAPY

- Avoidance of precipitating factors.
- Transjugular intrahepatic portosystemic shunts may be effective in selected patients, but data are limited.
- Dialysis with molecular adsorbent recirculating systems remains investigational until more data are available.

ACUTE GENERAL Rx

- The only effective treatment of HRS is liver transplantation; ornipressin is used in some liver units to avoid further deterioration of renal function in patients awaiting liver transplantation. In general, dopamine and prostaglandins are ineffective in treating patients with HRS.
- The best approach to the management of HRS based on its pathogenesis is the administration of vasoconstrictor drugs (terlipressin, norepinephrine, midodrine). Terlipressin may improve renal perfusion by reversing splanchnic vasodilation, which is the hallmark of HRS. Encouraging results were found in a recent study using continuous IV noradrenalin in combination with albumin and furosemide. In this study, reversal of HRS was achieved in 10 of 12 patients.

- Treatment of HRS with vasoconstrictors for 5 to 15 days in attempt to reduce serum creatinine to <1.5 mg/dl is as follows:
  1. Administration of one of the following drugs or drug combinations:
     a. Norepinephrine (0.5 to 3.0 mg/hr IV)
     b. Midodrine (7.5 mg PO tid, increased to 12.5 mg tid if needed) in combination with octreotide (100 micrograms SC tid, increased to tid prn)
     c. Terlipressin (0.2 to 2.0 mg IV q4 to 12h)
  2. Concomitant administration of albumin (1 g/kg IV on day 1, followed by 20 to 40 g daily)

DISPOSITION

Mortality rate exceeds 80%; liver transplantation is the only curative treatment.

REFERRAL

Referral for liver transplantation when indicated (see "Comments")

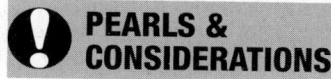 **PEARLS & CONSIDERATIONS**

COMMENTS

Liver transplantation may be indicated in otherwise healthy patients (age preferably <65 yr) with sclerosing cholangitis, chronic hepatitis with cirrhosis, or primary biliary cirrhosis. Contraindications to liver transplantation are AIDS, most metastatic malignancies, active substance abuse, uncontrolled sepsis, and uncontrolled cardiac or pulmonary disease.

SUGGESTED READINGS
available at www.expertconsult.com

RELATED CONTENT
Hepatorenal Syndrome (Patient Information)

AUTHOR: **FRED F. FERRI, M.D.**

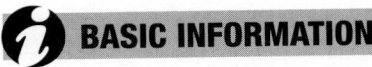

DEFINITION

Herpangina is a self-limited upper respiratory tract infection associated with a characteristic vesicular rash on the soft palate.

SYNONYMS

Vesicular stomatitis
Acute lymphonodular pharyngitis

ICD-9CM CODES
074.0 Herpangina

EPIDEMIOLOGY & DEMOGRAPHICS

INCIDENCE (IN U.S.): Unknown
PEAK INCIDENCE: Summer outbreaks common
PREVALENCE (IN U.S.): Unknown
PREDOMINANT SEX: Male = female
PREDOMINANT AGE: 3 to 10 yr

PHYSICAL FINDINGS & CLINICAL PRESENTATION

- Characterized by ulcerating lesions typically located on the soft palate (Fig. 1-400)
- Usually fewer than six lesions that evolve rapidly from a diffuse pharyngitis to erythematous macules and subsequently to vesicles that are moderately painful
- Fever, vomiting, and headache in the first few days of illness but subsiding spontaneously
- Pharyngeal lesions typical for several more days

ETIOLOGY

- Most cases caused by coxsackie A viruses (A2, A4, A5, A6, A10)
- Occasional cases caused by other enteroviruses (echovirus and enterovirus 71)

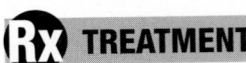 DIAGNOSIS

DIFFERENTIAL DIAGNOSIS

- Herpes simplex
- Bacterial pharyngitis
- Tonsillitis
- Aphthous stomatitis
- Hand-foot-mouth disease

WORKUP

Diagnosis is typically based on characteristic lesions on the soft palate.

LABORATORY TESTS

Viral and bacterial cultures of the pharynx to exclude herpes simplex infection and streptococcal pharyngitis if the diagnosis is in doubt

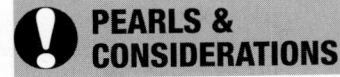 TREATMENT

- Give symptomatic treatment for sore throat: saline gargles and analgesics, and encourage oral fluids.
- No antiviral therapy indicated; avoid antibacterial agents because they are ineffective, increase cost, might result in side effects, and promote antibiotic resistance.

NONPHARMACOLOGIC THERAPY

Analgesic throat lozenges are helpful in some cases.

ACUTE GENERAL Rx

Antipyretics when indicated

CHRONIC Rx

Self-limited infection

DISPOSITION

- Generally, resolution of symptoms within 1 wk
- Persistence of fever or mouth lesions beyond 1 wk suggestive of an alternative diagnosis (see "Differential Diagnosis")

REFERRAL

For consultation with otolaryngologist or infectious disease specialist if the diagnosis is in doubt

PEARLS & CONSIDERATIONS

COMMENTS

Household outbreaks may occur, especially during the summer months.

SUGGESTED READINGS
available at www.expertconsult.com

RELATED CONTENT

Herpangina (Patient Information)

AUTHOR: **GLENN G. FORT, M.D., M.P.H.**

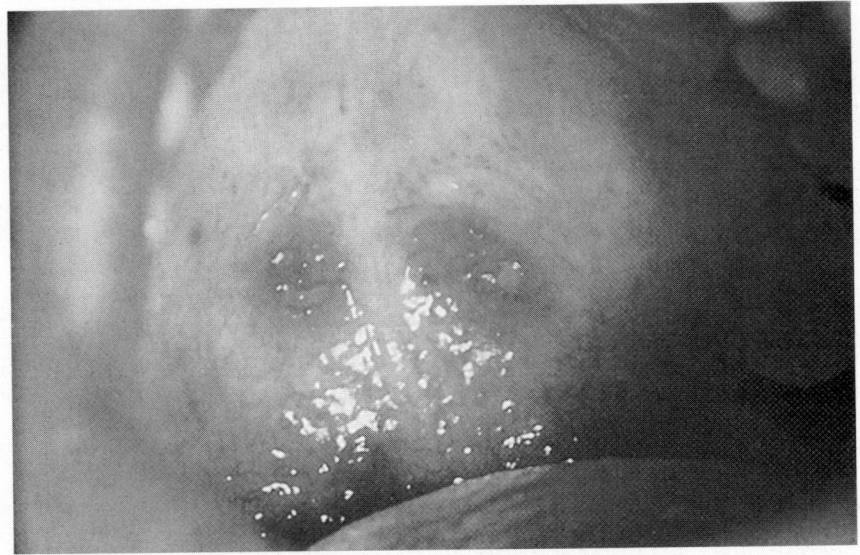

FIGURE 1-400 Herpangina with shallow ulcers in the roof of the mouth. (Courtesy Marshall Guill, M.D. From Goldstein B [ed]: *Practical dermatology,* ed 2, St Louis, 1997, Mosby.)

BASIC INFORMATION

DEFINITION

Herpes simplex is a viral infection caused by the herpes simplex virus (HSV). HSV-1 is associated primarily with oral infections, and HSV-2 causes mainly genital infections. However, either type can infect any site. After the primary infection, the virus enters the nerve endings in the skin directly below the lesions and ascends to the dorsal root ganglia, where it remains in a latent stage until it is reactivated.

SYNONYMS

Genital herpes
Herpes labialis
Herpes gladiatorum
Herpes digitalis

ICD-9CM CODES
054.10 Genital herpes
054.9   Herpes labialis

EPIDEMIOLOGY & DEMOGRAPHICS

- More than 85% of adults have serologic evidence of HSV-1 infection. The seroprevalence of adults with HSV-2 in the U.S. is 25%; however, only approximately 20% of these persons recall having symptoms of HSV infection.
- Most cases of eye or digital herpetic infections are caused by HSV-1.
- Frequency of recurrence of HSV-2 genital herpes is higher than HSV-1 oral labial infection.
- The frequency of recurrence is lowest for oral labial HSV-2 infections.
- The incidence of complications from herpes simplex (e.g., herpes encephalitis) is highest in immunocompromised hosts.
- Male circumcision significantly reduces the incidence of HSV-2.

PHYSICAL FINDINGS & CLINICAL PRESENTATION

Primary infection:
- Symptoms occur from 3 to 7 days after contact (respiratory droplets, direct contact).
- Constitutional symptoms include low-grade fever, headache and myalgias, regional lymphadenopathy, and localized pain.
- Pain, burning, itching, and tingling last several hours.
- Grouped vesicles (Fig. 1-401), usually with surrounding erythema, appear and generally ulcerate or crust within 48 hr.
- The vesicles are uniform in size (differentiating it from herpes zoster vesicles, which vary in size).
- During the acute eruption the patient is uncomfortable; involvement of lips and inside of mouth may make it unpleasant for the patient to eat; urinary retention may complicate involvement of the genital area.
- Lesions generally last from 2 to 6 wk and heal without scarring.
Recurrent infection:
- Generally caused by alteration in the immune system; fatigue, stress, menses, local skin trauma, and exposure to sunlight are contributing factors.
- The prodromal symptoms (fatigue, burning and tingling of the affected area) last 12 to 24 hr.
- A cluster of lesions generally evolves within 24 hr from a macule to a papule and then vesicles surrounded by erythema; the vesicles coalesce and subsequently rupture within 4 days, revealing erosions covered by crusts.
- The crusts are generally shed within 7 to 10 days, revealing a pink surface.
- The most frequent location of the lesions is on the vermilion border of the lips (HSV-1), the penile shaft or glans penis and the labia (HSV-2), buttocks (seen more frequently in women), fingertips (herpetic whitlow), and trunk (may be confused with herpes zoster).
- Rapid onset of diffuse cutaneous herpes simplex (eczema herpeticum) may occur in certain atopic infants and adults. It is a medical emergency, especially in young infants, and should be promptly treated with acyclovir.
- Herpes encephalitis, meningitis, and ocular herpes can occur in patients with immunocompromised status and occasionally in normal hosts.

ETIOLOGY

HSV-1 and HSV-2 are both DNA viruses.

DIAGNOSIS

DIFFERENTIAL DIAGNOSIS

- Impetigo
- Behçet's syndrome
- Coxsackie virus infection
- Syphilis
- Stevens-Johnson syndrome
- Herpangina
- Aphthous stomatitis
- Varicella
- Herpes zoster

WORKUP

Diagnosis is based on clinical presentation. Laboratory evaluation confirms diagnosis.

LABORATORY TESTS

- Direct immunofluorescent antibody slide tests provide a rapid diagnosis.
- Viral culture is the most definitive method for diagnosis; results are generally available in 1 or 2 days. The lesions should be sampled during the vesicular or early ulcerative stage; cervical samples should be taken from the endocervix with a swab.
- Tzanck smear is a readily available test that will demonstrate multinucleated giant cells. However, it is not a highly sensitive test.
- Pap smear will detect HSV-infected cells in cervical tissue from women without symptoms.
- Serologic tests for HSV: immunoglobulin (Ig) G and IgM serum antibodies. Antibodies to HSV occur in 50% to 90% of adults. The presence of IgM or a fourfold or greater rise in IgG titers indicates a recent infection (convalescent sample should be drawn 2 to 3 wk after the acute specimen is drawn).

TREATMENT

- Table 1-194 summarizes antiviral chemotherapy for HSV infection.
- Topical acyclovir, penciclovir, and docosanol are optional treatments for recurrent herpes labialis, but they are less effective than oral treatments.

DISPOSITION

Most patients recover from the initial episode or recurrences without complications; immunocompromised hosts are at risk for complications (e.g., disseminated herpes simplex infection, herpes encephalitis).

REFERRAL

- Hospital admission in patients with herpes encephalitis or herpes meningitis and in immunocompromised hosts with diffuse herpes simplex infection
- Ophthalmology referral in patients with suspected ocular herpes

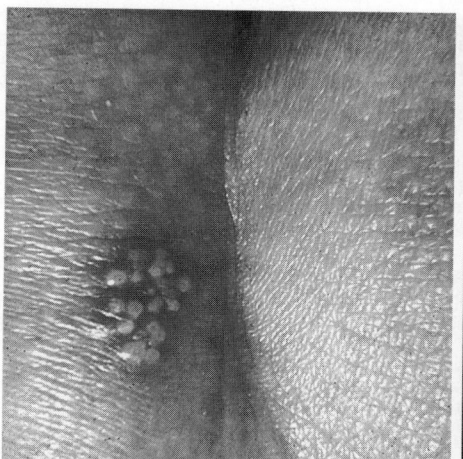
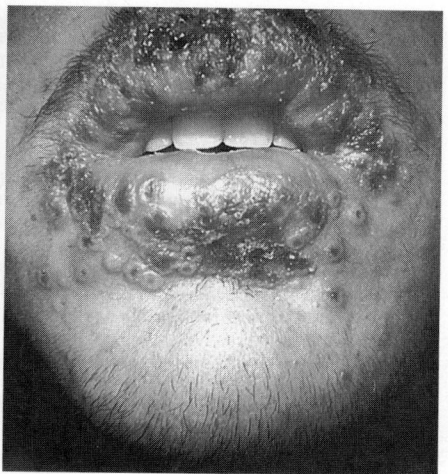

FIGURE 1-401 Herpes simplex. (From Scuderi G [ed]: *Sports medicine: principles of primary care,* St Louis, 1997, Mosby.)

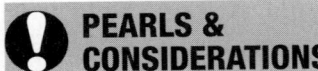 **PEARLS & CONSIDERATIONS**

COMMENTS

- Provide patient education regarding transmission of HSV.
- Condom use offers significant protection against HSV-1 infection in susceptible women.
- Patients should be instructed on the use of condoms for sexual intercourse and on avoiding kissing or sexual intercourse until lesions are crusted.
- Patients should also avoid contact with immunocompromised hosts or neonates while lesions are present.
- Proper handwashing techniques should be explained.

- Patients with herpes gladiatorum (cutaneous herpes in athletes involved in contact sports) should be excluded from participation in active sports until lesions have resolved.
- Many new HSV-2 infections are asymptomatic. Since HSV-2 antibody tests have become commercially available, an increasing number of persons have learned that they have genital herpes through serologic testing. Persons with asymptomatic HSV-2 infection shed virus in the genital tract less frequently than persons with symptomatic infection, but much of the difference is attributable to less frequent genital lesions because generally lesions are accompanied by frequent viral shedding.
- Suppressive treatment of HSV-2 infection lowers the incidence of genital lesions by 70% to 80%, but cuts the rate of HSV-2 transmission to uninfected partners by only 50%.
- Trials involving investigational herpes simplex vaccine have found it to be effective in preventing HSV-1 genital disease and infection, but not in preventing HSV-2 disease or infection.

SUGGESTED READINGS
available at www.expertconsult.com

RELATED CONTENT
Genital Herpes (Patient Information)

AUTHOR: **FRED F. FERRI, M.D.**

TABLE 1-194 Antiviral Chemotherapy for Herpes Simplex Virus Infection

Mucocutaneous HSV Infections
Infections in Immunosuppressed Patients
  Acute symptomatic first or recurrent episodes: IV acyclovir (5 mg/kg q8h) and oral acyclovir (400 mg qid), famciclovir (500 mg PO tid), or valacyclovir (500 mg PO bid) for 7-10 days are effective. Treatment duration may vary from 7-14 days.
  Suppression of reactivation disease: IV acyclovir (5 mg/kg q8h), valacyclovir (500 mg PO bid), or oral acyclovir (400-800 mg three to five times per day) prevents recurrences during the immediate 30-day post-transplantation period. Longer term suppression is often used for persons with continued immunosuppression. In bone marrow and renal transplant recipients, valacyclovir 2 g four times daily is also effective in preventing CMV infection. Valacyclovir 4 g four times daily has been associated with TTP after extended use in HIV-positive persons. In HIV-infected persons, oral famciclovir (500 mg bid) is effective in reducing clinical and subclinical reactivations of HSV-1 and -2.

Genital Herpes
  First episodes: Oral acyclovir (200 mg five times per day or 400 mg tid), oral valacyclovir (1000 mg bid), or famciclovir (250 mg bid) for 10-14 days is effective. IV acyclovir (5 mg/kg q8h for 5 days) is given for severe disease or neurologic complications such as aseptic meningitis.
  Symptomatic recurrent genital herpes: Oral acyclovir (200 mg five times per day for 5 days, 800 mg PO tid for 2 days), valacyclovir (500 mg bid for 3 or 5 days), or famciclovir (125 mg bid for 5 days). All these therapies are effective in shortening lesion duration.
  Suppression of recurrent genital herpes: Oral acyclovir (200-mg capsules bid or tid, 400 mg bid, or 800 mg qd), famciclovir (250 mg bid), or valacyclovir (500 mg or 1000 mg qd or 500 mg bid) prevents symptomatic reactivation. Persons with frequent reactivation (<9 episodes/year) can take 500 mg daily; those with >9 episodes/year should take 1000 mg/daily or 500 mg bid.

Oral-Labial HSV Infections
  First episode: Oral acyclovir (200 mg) is given four or five times per day. Famciclovir (250 mg bid) or valacyclovir (1000 mg bid) has been used clinically.
  Recurrent episodes: Valacyclovir 1000 mg bid for 1 day or 500 mg bid for 3 days is effective in reducing pain and speeding healing. Self-initiated therapy with six times daily topical 1% penciclovir cream is effective in speeding the healing of oral-labial HSV; topical acyclovir cream has also been shown to speed healing.
  Suppression of reactivation of oral-labial HSV: Oral acyclovir (400 mg bid), if started before exposure and continued for the duration of exposure (usually 5-10 days), prevents reactivation of recurrent oral-labial HSV infection associated with severe sun exposure.

Herpetic Whitlow
  Oral acyclovir (200 mg) five times daily for 7-10 days.
HSV Proctitis
  Oral acyclovir (400 mg five times per day) is useful in shortening the course of infection. In immunosuppressed patients or in patients with severe infection, IV acyclovir (5 mg/kg q8h) may be useful.
Herpetic Eye Infections
  In acute keratitis, topical trifluorothymidine, vidarabine, idoxuridine, acyclovir, penciclovir, and interferon are all beneficial. Debridement may be required; topical steroids may worsen disease.
CNS HSV Infections
  HSV encephalitis: Intravenous acyclovir (10 mg/kg q8h; 30 mg/kg per day) for 14-21 days is preferred.
  HSV aseptic meningitis: No studies of systemic antiviral chemotherapy exist. If therapy is to be given, IV acyclovir (15-30 mg/kg/day) should be used.
  Autonomic radiculopathy: No studies are available.
Neonatal HSV infections: Acyclovir (60 mg/kg/day, divided into three doses) is given. The recommended duration of treatment is 21 days. Monitoring for relapse should be undertaken, and some authorities recommend continued suppression with oral acyclovir suspension for 3 to 4 mo.
Visceral HSV Infections
  HSV esophagitis: IV acyclovir (15 mg/kg per day). In some patients with milder forms of immunosuppression, oral therapy with valacyclovir or famciclovir is effective.
  HSV pneumonitis: No controlled studies exist. IV acyclovir (15 mg/kg per day) should be considered.
Disseminated HSV infections: No controlled studies exist. Intravenous acyclovir (10 mg/kg q8h) nevertheless should be tried. No definite evidence indicates that therapy decreases the risk of death.
Erythema multiforme-associated HSV: Anecdotal observations suggest that oral acyclovir (400 mg bid or tid) or valacyclovir (500 mg bid) suppresses erythema multiforme.
Surgical prophylaxis: Several surgical procedures such as laser skin resurfacing, trigeminal nerve root decompression, and lumbar disk surgery have been associated with HSV reactivation. Intravenous acyclovir (3 mg/kg) and oral acyclovir 800 mg bid, valacyclovir 500 mg bid, or famciclovir 250 mg bid is effective in reducing reactivation. Therapy should be initiated 48 hours before surgery and continued for 3 to 7 days.
Infections with acyclovir-resistant HSV: Foscarnet (40 mg/kg IV q8h) should be given until lesions heal. The optimal duration of therapy and the usefulness of its continuation to suppress lesions are unclear. Some patients may benefit from cutaneous application of trifluorothymidine or 5% cidofovir gel.

CMV, Cytomegalovirus; *CNS,* central nervous system; *HIV,* human immunodeficiency virus; *HSV,* herpes simplex virus; *TTP,* thrombotic thrombocytopenic purpura.
From Mandell GL et al: *Principles and practice of infectious diseases,* ed 6, Philadelphia, 2005, Churchill Livingstone.

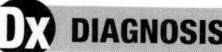

BASIC INFORMATION

DEFINITION

Herpes zoster is a disease caused by reactivation of the varicella-zoster virus. After the primary infection (chickenpox), the virus becomes latent in the dorsal root ganglia and reemerges when there is a weakening of the immune system (as a result of disease or advanced age).

SYNONYMS

Shingles
HZ

ICD-9CM CODES
053.9 Herpes zoster

EPIDEMIOLOGY & DEMOGRAPHICS

- Herpes zoster occurs during the lifetime of 10% to 20% of the population.
- There is an increased incidence in immuno-compromised patients (AIDS, malignancy), the elderly, and children who acquired chickenpox when younger than 2 mo.

PHYSICAL FINDINGS & CLINICAL PRESENTATION

- Pain generally precedes skin manifestation by 3 to 5 days and is generally localized to the dermatome that will be affected by the skin lesions.
- Constitutional symptoms are often present (malaise, fever, headache).
- The initial rash consists of erythematous maculopapules generally affecting one dermatome (thoracic region in majority of cases). Typically the rash does not cross the midline. Some patients (<30%) may have scattered vesicles outside the affected dermatome.
- The initial maculopapules evolve into vesicles and pustules by the third or the fourth day.
- The vesicles have an erythematous base (Fig. E1-402), are cloudy, and have various sizes (a distinguishing characteristic from herpes simplex, in which the vesicles are of uniform size).
- The vesicles subsequently become umbilicated and then form crusts (Fig. E1-403) that generally fall off within 3 wk; scarring may occur.
- Pain during and after the rash is generally significant. Post-herpetic neuralgia occurs after herpes zoster in approximately one third of patients aged 60 years and older and can persist for months or years.
- Secondary bacterial infection with *Staphylococcus aureus* or *Streptococcus pyogenes* may occur.
- Regional lymphadenopathy may occur.
- Herpes zoster may involve the trigeminal nerve (most frequent cranial nerve involved); involvement of the geniculate ganglion can cause facial palsy and a painful ear, with the presence of vesicles on the pinna and external auditory canal (Ramsay Hunt syndrome).

ETIOLOGY

Reactivation of varicella virus (human herpes virus III)

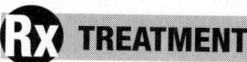

DIAGNOSIS

DIFFERENTIAL DIAGNOSIS

- Rash: herpes simplex and other viral infections
- Pain from herpes zoster: may be confused with acute myocardial infarction, pulmonary embolism, pleuritis, pericarditis, renal colic

LABORATORY TESTS

Laboratory tests are generally not necessary (viral cultures and Tzanck smear will confirm diagnosis in patients with atypical presentation).

TREATMENT

NONPHARMACOLOGIC THERAPY

- Wet compresses (using Burow's solution or cool tap water) applied for 15 to 30 min five to 10 times a day are useful to break vesicles and remove serum and crust.
- Care must be taken to prevent any secondary bacterial infection.

ACUTE GENERAL Rx

- Oral antiviral agents can decrease acute pain, inflammation, and vesicle formation when treatment is begun within 48 hr of onset of rash. Treatment options are:
  1. Valacyclovir 1000 mg tid for 7 days
  2. Famciclovir 500 mg tid for 7 days
  3. Acyclovir 800 mg 5 times daily for 7 to 10 days
- Corticosteroids should be considered in older patients within 72 hr of clinical presentation or if new lesions are still appearing if there are no contraindications. Initial dose is prednisone 40 mg/day decreased by 5 mg/day until finished. When used there is a decrease in the use of analgesics and time to resumption of usual activities, but there is no effect on the incidence and duration of postherpetic neuralgia.
- Immunocompromised patients should be treated with IV acyclovir 500 mg/m² or 10 mg/kg q8h in 1-hr infusions for 7 days, with close monitoring of renal function and adequate hydration; vidarabine (continuous 12-hr infusion of 10 mg/kg/day for 7 days) is also effective for treatment of disseminated herpes zoster in immunocompromised hosts.
- Patients with AIDS and transplant recipients may develop acyclovir-resistant varicella-zoster; these patients can be treated with foscarnet (40 mg/kg IV q8h) continued for at least 10 days or until lesions are completely healed.
- Postherpetic neuralgia (Fig. E1-404)
  - Gabapentin 100 to 600 mg tid is effective in the treatment of pain and sleep interference associated with postherpetic neuralgia. Other effective agents are pregabalin, duloxetine, and tricyclic antidepressants.
  - Lidocaine patch 5% is also effective in relieving postherpetic neuralgia. Patches are applied to intact skin after resolution of blisters and crusts to cover the most painful area for up to 12 hr within a 24-hr period.
  - Capsaicin cream can be useful for treatment of postherpetic neuralgia. It is generally applied 3 to 5 times daily for several weeks after the crusts have fallen off. A topical 8% patch formulation of capsaicin is now available by prescription for postherpetic neuralgia.
  - Sympathetic blocks (stellate ganglion or epidural) with 0.25% bupivacaine and rhizotomy are reserved for severe cases unresponsive to conservative treatment.

DISPOSITION

- The incidence of postherpetic neuralgia (defined as pain that persists more than 30 days after onset of rash) increases with age (30% by age 40 yr, >70% by age 70 yr); antivirals reduce the risk of postherpetic neuralgia.
- Incidence of disseminated herpes zoster is increased in immunocompromised hosts (e.g., 15% to 50% of patients with active Hodgkin's disease).
- Immunocompromised hosts are also more prone to neurologic complications (encephalitis, myelitis, cranial and peripheral nerve palsies, acute retinal necrosis). The mortality rate is 10% to 20% in immunocompromised hosts with disseminated zoster.
- Motor neuropathies occur in 5% of all cases of zoster; complete recovery occurs in >70% of patients.
- Rates of HZ recurrence are more frequently than previously reported and are comparable to rates of first HZ occurrence in immunocompetent individuals.

REFERRAL

- Hospitalization for IV acyclovir in patients with disseminated herpes zoster.
- Patients with herpes zoster ophthalmicus should be referred to an ophthalmologist.
- Vaccination: immunocompetent adults ≥50 yr are appropriate candidates for a single dose of varicella-zoster vaccine (VZV) whether or not they have had a previous episode of herpes zoster. Immunization with VZV (Zostavax) boosts waning immunity in older adults and reduces the severity and duration of pain caused by herpes zoster by 61%. Adults who are VZV seronegative (never had varicella) should be immunized against varicella with two doses of varicella vaccine (Varivax). Despite its efficacy and safety, use of this vaccine remains low (<8% of potential recipients).

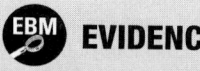

EVIDENCE

available at www.expertconsult.com

SUGGESTED READINGS

available at www.expertconsult.com

RELATED CONTENT

Shingles (Patient Information)

AUTHOR: **FRED F. FERRI, M.D.**

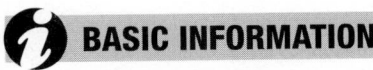

BASIC INFORMATION

DEFINITION

A hiatal hernia is the protrusion of a portion of the stomach into the thoracic cavity through the diaphragmatic esophageal hiatus.

SYNONYMS

Hiatus hernia
Diaphragmatic hernia

ICD-9CM CODES
553.3 Diaphragmatic hernia without obstruction or gangrene
750.6 Congenital hiatal hernia
756.6 Congenital diaphragmatic hernia

EPIDEMIOLOGY & DEMOGRAPHICS

- Found in 50% of patients older than 50 yr.
- Prevalence increases with age.
- More prevalent in Western countries than in Africa and Asia.
- Paraesophageal hiatal hernias are more common in women than in men (4:1).
- Associated with diverticulosis (25%), esophagitis (25%), duodenal ulcers (20%), and gallstones (18%).
- More than 90% of patients with endoscopic documentation of esophagitis have hiatal hernias.

PHYSICAL FINDINGS & CLINICAL PRESENTATION

Most patients are asymptomatic. If symptoms are present, they resemble those of gastroesophageal reflux disease (GERD).

- Heartburn
- Dysphagia
- Regurgitation of gastric contents
- Chest pain
- Postprandial fullness
- GI bleed
- Dyspnea
- Hoarseness
- Wheezing with bowel sounds heard over the left lung base

ETIOLOGY

- The repetitive stretching of the gastroesophageal (GE) junction with swallowing and actions (e.g., vomiting) or states (e.g., obesity, pregnancy) that increase intraabdominal pressure may cause widening of the hiatus, rupture of the phrenoesophageal ligament, and onset of the hernia.
- Hiatal hernias are classified as:
  1. Type I: Sliding (Fig. 1-405, *A*), axial, or concentric hiatal hernia (most common type, 99%). Only the GE junction protrudes into the thoracic cavity and the phrenoesophageal ligament remains intact.
  2. Type II: Paraesophageal or rolling hernia (Fig. 1-405, *B*) (1%). The GE junction stays at the level of the diaphragm, but part of the stomach bulges into the thoracic cavity through a defect in the phrenoesophageal ligament.
  3. Type III: Mixed (rare), a combination of type I and type II.
  4. Type IV: Large defect in hiatus that allows other intraabdominal organs to enter the hernia sac.

DIAGNOSIS

DIFFERENTIAL DIAGNOSIS

- Peptic ulcer disease
- Unstable angina
- Esophagitis (caused by *Candida,* herpes, NSAIDs, etc.)
- Esophageal spasm
- Barrett's esophagus
- Schatzki's ring
- Achalasia
- Zenker's diverticulum
- Esophageal cancer

WORKUP

- Exclude conditions noted in the differential diagnosis and document the presence of a hiatal hernia. Upper endoscopy may also be needed to exclude abnormal metaplasia, dysplasia, or neoplasia.

LABORATORY TESTS

- Blood tests are not specific.
- Esophageal manometry, although not commonly done, can be used in establishing a diagnosis (low sensitivity, but high specificity when compared with endoscopy).

IMAGING STUDIES

- Upper gastrointestinal (UGI) barium contrast swallow series: best defines the anatomic abnormality. Demonstration that the gastric cardia is herniated 2 cm above the hiatus is diagnostic. UGI may also reveal a tortuous esophagus (Fig. 1-406). If endoscopy is performed preoperatively, a barium swallow is generally not necessary.
- UGI endoscopy: documents the presence of a hiatal hernia and also excludes commonly associated findings of esophagitis and Barrett's esophagus (recommended at least once during the workup). Greater than 2 cm of gastric rugal fold seen above the margins of the diaphragmatic crura is diagnostic.
- Abdominal ultrasonography: simple, well tolerated. A transdiaphragmatic esophageal diameter of more than or equal to 18 mm is highly suggestive of the presence of a sliding hiatal hernia.

TREATMENT

NONPHARMACOLOGIC THERAPY

- Lifestyle modifications: avoid foods and drugs that decrease lower-esophageal pressure (e.g., caffeine, chocolate, mint, calcium channel blockers, and anticholinergics)
- Weight loss
- Avoid large quantities of food with meals
- Sleep with the head of the bed elevated 6 inches

ACUTE GENERAL Rx

- Antacids may be useful to relieve mild symptoms.
- H_2 antagonists (e.g., cimetidine 400 mg bid, ranitidine 150 mg bid, or famotidine 20 mg bid).
- If significant GERD is present with documented esophagitis, proton pump inhibitors (e.g., omeprazole 20 mg qd or lansoprazole 30 mg qd) are used. Refractory symptoms may require higher doses (e.g., bid dosing).
- Prokinetic agents (e.g., metoclopramide 10 mg taken 30 min before each meal) can be added to an H_2 antagonist or proton pump inhibitor.

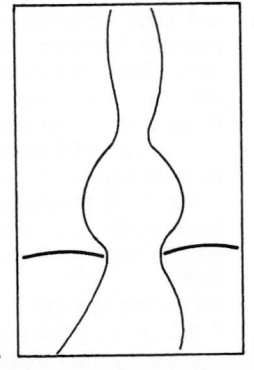
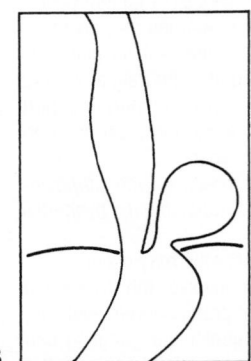

FIGURE 1-405 Types of esophageal hiatal hernia. A, Sliding hiatal hernia, the most common type. **B,** Paraesophageal hiatal hernia. (From Behrman RE: *Nelson textbook of pediatrics,* ed 17, Philadelphia, 2004, Saunders.)

CHRONIC Rx

- When indicated, surgery (laparoscopic or open) can be done in patients with refractory symptoms impairing quality of life, or causing intestinal (e.g., recurrent GI bleeds) or extraintestinal complications (e.g., aspiration pneumonia, asthma, or ear-nose-throat complications).
- Prophylactic surgery is a consideration in all paraesophageal hernias because they have a higher incidence of strangulation.

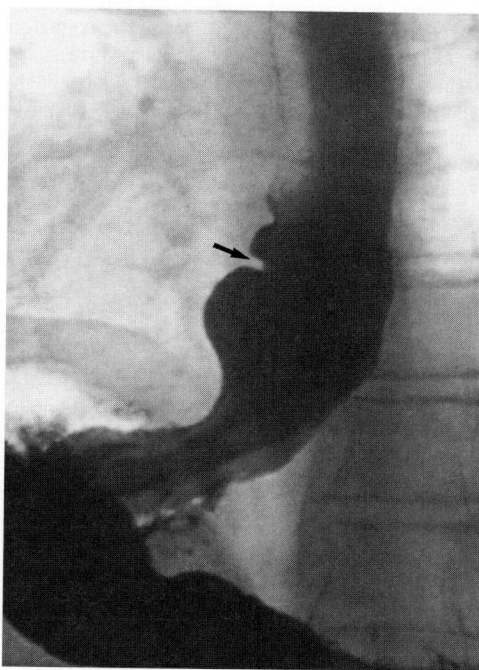

FIGURE 1-406 A sliding hiatal hernia confirmed by the presence of an incisural notch *(arrow)* on the greater curve aspect. (From Grainger RG et al [eds]: *Grainger & Allison's diagnostic radiology,* ed 4, Philadelphia, 2001, Churchill Livingstone.)

DISPOSITION

- More than 90% of patients having GERD symptoms respond well to medical therapy.
- Complications of hiatal hernias are similar to complications occurring in patients with GERD:
  1. Erosive esophagitis
  2. Ulcerative esophagitis
  3. Barrett's esophagus
  4. Peptic stricture
  5. GI hemorrhage
  6. Extraintestinal complications
  7. Lung collapse or heart failure (severe cases)

REFERRAL

Gastroenterologist: for symptoms refractory to conventional therapy (H_2 antagonists, antacids, and proton pump inhibitors) or having complications previously mentioned.

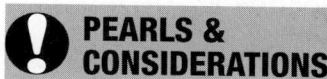 **PEARLS & CONSIDERATIONS**

COMMENTS

- Gastric ulceration and erosions (*Cameron's lesion*) can occur in the paraesophageal hernia pouch and are an uncommon cause of UGI bleeding.
- May cause iron deficiency anemia.
- Gastric volvulus or torsion can also occur and presents as dysphagia and postprandial pain.
- High incidence of esophagitis even after the eradication of *Helicobacter pylori.*
- The appearance of hiatal hernia may resemble a left atrial mass by echocardiography.

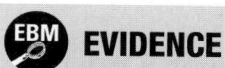 **EVIDENCE**

available at www.expertconsult.com

SUGGESTED READINGS
available at www.expertconsult.com

RELATED CONTENT
Hiatal Hernia (Patient Information)

AUTHOR: **MARK F. BRADY, M.D., M.P.H., M.M.S.**

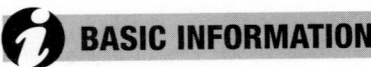

DEFINITION

Hidradenitis suppurativa (HS) is a chronic, relapsing suppurative cutaneous disease affecting skin that bears apocrine glands and manifested by abscesses, fistulating sinus tracts, and chronic infection leading to scarring.

SYNONYMS

Acne inversa
Apocrinitis
Verneuil's disease
Pyoderma fistulas significa
HS

ICD-9CM CODES
705.83 Hidradenitis

EPIDEMIOLOGY & DEMOGRAPHICS

- Onset is postpubertal, with an average age of onset of 23 yr
- An increased frequency is seen in people of African American descent, possibly due to a greater density of apocrine glands; however, this has not been fully studied.

PREVALENCE: Overall prevalence in the United States is ~1% to 2%.
PREDOMINANT SEX: Female to male ratio is 3:1.
RISK FACTORS:
- Obesity
- Family history
- Shorter menstrual cycles and longer duration of menses
- Personal or family history of acne or pilonidal cysts
- Cigarette smoking

PHYSICAL FINDINGS & CLINICAL PRESENTATION

The diagnosis is primarily clinical based on the development of typical lesions in a characteristic distribution, with a relapsing nature.
- Early symptoms include pain, itching, burning, erythema, and hyperhidrosis.
- Typical lesions include:
  - Painful erythematous papules and nodules
  - Painful abscesses and inflamed papules or nodules with foul smelling discharge
  - Dermal contractures and ropelike elevation of the skin
  - Comedones in the apocrine, gland-bearing skin
- Classified into Hurley Stages
  - Stage I: abscesses without sinus tracts or scarring
  - Stage II: multiple abscesses plus sinus tracts and scarring
  - Stage III: diffuse involvement of entire area with abscesses, sinus tracts, and scarring
- The axilla is the most common site (Fig. 1-407).
- Less common sites include inguinal and perineal region, the areola of the breast, and the submammary folds.
- There is a strong tendency toward relapse and recurrence.

- Other characteristics of the disease are:
  - Poor response to conventional antibiotics
  - Often no pathogens from routine cultures of lesions
- The disease is often mistaken for a simple infection and a long delay in diagnosis is common.

ETIOLOGY

- Keratinous materials plug apocrine glands in hair follicles leading to stasis, dilation, rupture, and re-epithelialization of glands.
- Bacteria are trapped and multiply leading to gland rupture with surrounding inflammation and local bacterial infection.
- Over time, repeated nodules and infections cause scarring, which can lead to deep tissue damage and sinus tracts.
- Infectious agents such as *Streptococcus, Staphylococcus,* and *Escherichia coli,* and

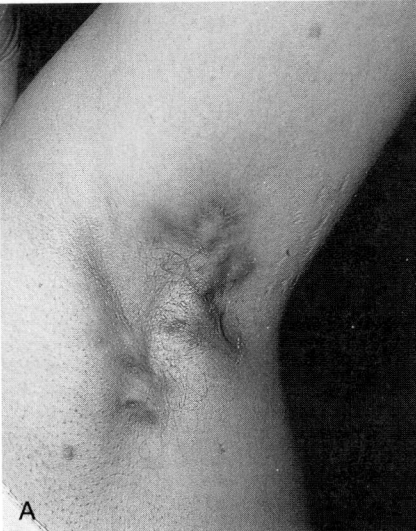

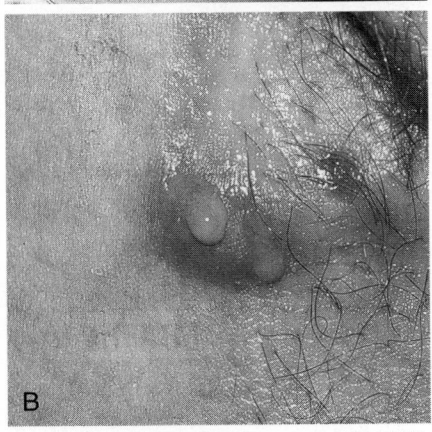

FIGURE 1-407 Hidradenitis suppurativa (HS). A, HS of the axilla. This is the classic appearance with inflammatory nodules and scarred areas. This condition is commonly misdiagnosed as a bacterial infection. **B,** HS of the axilla; a close-up view of the draining pus. When intact, the lesions represent sterile abscesses. Once open, they may become secondarily infected. (From White GM, Cox NH [eds]: *Diseases of the skin: a color atlas and text,* ed 2, St Louis, 2006, Mosby.)

enteric flora have been identified in cultures, but are likely a secondary cause of the disease.
- There is likely some correlation with androgen levels and a genetic component to the disease. About one third of patients report a family history of the disease. Families with an autosomal dominant mode of inheritance have been identified.
- HS has been associated with other endocrine and autoimmune disorders such as diabetes, Cushing's disease, acromegaly, Crohn's disease, and inflammatory arthritis.
- Recent data suggest that the interleukin-12-interleukin-23 pathway and tumor necrosis factor-α (TNF-α) may be involved in the pathogenesis of HS.
- Metabolic syndrome which affects many patients with HS may exacerbate the inflammation associated with HS.

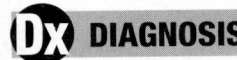

DIFFERENTIAL DIAGNOSIS
- Follicular pyodermas such as folliculitis, furuncles, carbuncles, and pilonidal cysts
- Granuloma inguinale
- Perianal and vulvar manifestations of Crohn's disease
- Actinomycosis
- Lymphogranuloma venereum
- Dermoid, epidermoid, or Bartholin's cysts
- Tuberculous inflammation of the skin
- Lymphadenitis
- Cat-scratch disease
- Tularemia
- Erysipelas

WORKUP
Primarily a clinical diagnosis based on typical lesion (see "Physical Findings & Clinical Presentation")

LABORATORY TESTS
- Patients with acute lesions may have an elevated erythrocyte sedimentation rate or WBC.
- Febrile and toxic appearing patients should have complete blood count, chemistries, and blood cultures.
- Any pus should be sampled for bacterial culture and sensitivity.

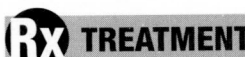

There is no definitive cure for hidradenitis.

NONPHARMACOLOGIC THERAPY
- Avoidance of shaving, depilatory creams, deodorants
- Warm compresses
- Weight loss
- Smoking cessation
- Avoiding tight, synthetic clothing and hot humid climates
- Stress management to reduce flare-ups
- Hydrotherapy
- Incision and drainage of nonpurulent lesions is not recommended due to recurrence

- Benefit seen recently with laser therapy starting at stage I disease
- Radiotherapy and cryotherapy currently under study
- Wide local excision with healing by secondary intention for stage III disease

ACUTE AND CHRONIC Rx

- NSAIDs for inflammation and pain.
- Topical anesthetics and antibacterial soap are useful for stage I (localized) disease.
- Antibiotics never proven to be effective; however, are mainstay of treatment. Can base treatment on the basis of aspirate culture and sensitivities or empirically.
  - Clindamycin is the only topical antibiotic proven to be effective in randomized controlled trial and is appropriate for stage I disease.
  - For oral therapy in stage II: consider clindamycin and rifampin in combination. Cephalosporins, dicloxacillin, erythromycin, minocycline, and tetracycline have also been used.
  - Severe, recurrent disease can require >2 mo of antibiotics.
- Oral contraceptives with low androgenic progesterone for women show mixed effectiveness.

- Isotretinoin has been used with mixed effectiveness.
- Intralesional injections of glucocorticoids may be useful in localized disease.
- Corticosteroids and other immune suppressants such as cyclosporin, infliximab, and etanercept have been used for stage II disease, with mixed results.
- Adalimumab, an anti–tumor necrosis factor-α antibody dosed once per week (40 mg/wk) has been reported effective in alleviating moderate to severe HS.

COMPLICATIONS

- Arthritis secondary to inflammatory injury
- Squamous cell carcinoma
- Scarring and restricted limb mobility
- Lymphedema caused by scarring of lymphatics
- Rectal or urethral fistulas

REFERRAL

- Referral to dermatology during stage I to II disease.
- Referral to a surgeon is indicated for stage III disease.

PEARLS & CONSIDERATIONS

COMMENTS

- Patients with hidradenitis are at risk for severe depression, social isolation, and negatively impacted sexuality as a result of their disease.
- There is an average delay in diagnosis of 12 years and most patients are diagnosed in stage II of the disease (recurrent abscesses with scarring and development of sinus tracts).
- It is important to maximize nonmedical treatment, start medical treatment, and refer to a surgeon early in the disease course to ensure the best quality of life for patients.
- The only definitive treatment for hidradenitis is wide excision of the involved skin.

PATIENT & FAMILY EDUCATION

Handout included in: Shah N: Hidradenitis suppurativa: a treatment challenge, *Am Fam Physician* 72:1547-1552, 1554, 2005.

SUGGESTED READINGS

available at www.expertconsult.com

AUTHOR: **MARY BETH SUTTER, M.D.**

Diseases and Disorders

H

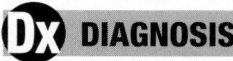 BASIC INFORMATION

DEFINITION

High-altitude sickness refers to a spectrum of illnesses related to hypoxemia occurring during rapid ascension to high altitudes. Common acute syndromes occurring at high altitudes include acute mountain sickness (AMS), high-altitude pulmonary edema (HAPE), and high-altitude cerebral edema (HACE).

SYNONYMS

Altitude sickness
Acute mountain sickness
High-altitude pulmonary edema
High-altitude cerebral edema

ICD-9CM CODES
289   Mountain sickness, acute
993.2 High altitude, effects

EPIDEMIOLOGY & DEMOGRAPHICS

- More than 30 million people are at risk of developing altitude sickness.
- AMS is the most common of the altitude diseases.
  - Approximately 40% to 50% of people ascending to 14,000 ft (4200 m) from lowland living develop AMS.
- HAPE generally arises in people who rapidly ascend to 12,000 to 13,000 ft (3600 to 3900 m); however, it has been reported at altitudes as low as 8000 ft.

- Men are five times more likely to develop HAPE than are women.
- AMS and HACE affect men and women equally.

PHYSICAL FINDINGS & CLINICAL PRESENTATION

AMS
- Occurs within hours to a few days after rapid ascent over 8000 ft (2500 m)
- Headache is the most common symptom
- Dizziness and lightheadedness
- Nausea, vomiting, and loss of appetite
- Fatigue
- Sleep disturbance from an exaggerated hyperventilatory phase of Cheyne-Stokes respiration in response to hypoxemia and alkalosis
- AMS can evolve into HAPE and HACE.

HAPE (Fig. 1-408A)
- Typically occurs 2 to 4 days after ascent over 8000 ft (2500 m).
- Dyspnea
- Dry cough or cough with frothy rust- or pink-tinged sputum
- Chest tightness
- Tachycardia, tachypnea, rales, cyanosis

HACE
- Usually presents several days after AMS
- Confusion, irritability, drowsiness, stupor, hallucinations
- Headache, nausea, vomiting
- Ataxia, paralysis, and seizures
- Coma and death may develop within hours of the first symptoms.

ETIOLOGY

- During ascension to altitudes above sea level, the atmospheric pressure decreases. Although the percentage of oxygen in the air remains the same, the partial pressure of oxygen decreases with increased altitude. This can cause hypoxemia. Fig. 1-408B illustrates the effect of altitude on alveolar PaO_2 and oxygen saturation. Fig. E1-408C describes the pathophysiology of HAPE.
- The body responds to low oxygen partial pressures through a process of acclimatization (see "Comments").

Dx DIAGNOSIS

Made by clinical presentation and physical findings.

DIFFERENTIAL DIAGNOSIS

- Dehydration
- Carbon monoxide poisoning
- Hypothermia
- Infection
- Substance abuse
- Congestive heart failure
- Pulmonary embolism
- Cerebrovascular accident

WORKUP

Typically the diagnosis is self-evident after history and physical examination. Laboratory tests and imaging studies help monitor cardiopulmonary and central nervous system status in patients admitted to the intensive care unit for pulmonary and/or cerebral edema. In patients

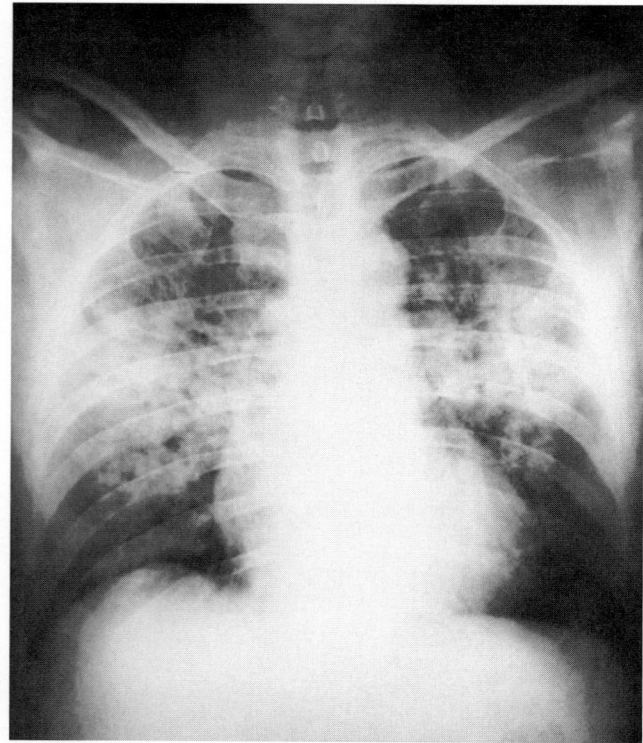

FIGURE 1-408A Chest radiograph showing high-altitude pulmonary edema. (From Strauss RH [ed]: *Sports medicine,* ed 2, Philadelphia, 1991, Saunders.)

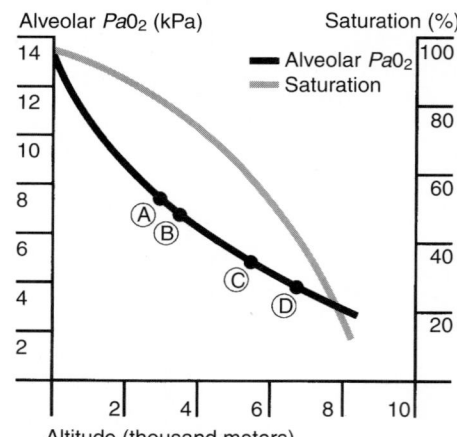

FIGURE 1-408B Effect of altitude on alveolar PaO_2 and oxygen saturation. Because of the steep slope of the oxygen dissociation curve, increasing altitude above 5000 m causes a precipitous fall in saturation. In an unacclimated person, acute change occurs at, *A,* 3000 m (10,000 ft)—slightly impaired memory and judgment, increased heart rate, abdominal cramps and nausea; *B,* 3500 m (12,000 ft)—headache, nausea, diminished visual acuity, and possible pulmonary edema; *C,* 5500 m (18,000 ft)—impaired consciousness after several hours in many people; and *D,* 6750 m (22,000 ft)—loss of consciousness. (From Souhami RL, Moxham J: *Textbook of medicine,* ed 4, London, 2002, Churchill Livingstone.)

with HAPE occurring at lower altitudes (<8000 ft), an evaluation of preexisting pulmonary hypertension or a left-to-right shunt should be considered.

LABORATORY TESTS
Not useful

IMAGING STUDIES
- Chest x-ray showing Kerley B-lines and patchy edema (see Fig. 1-408A)
- CT scan of the head showing diffuse or patchy edema

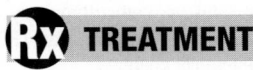 **TREATMENT**

NONPHARMACOLOGIC THERAPY
- Stop the ascent to allow acclimatization or start to descend until symptoms have resolved.
- Oxygen 4 to 6 L/min is used for severe AMS, HAPE, and HACE.
- Portable hyperbaric bags are useful if available at the site.
- Altitude can cause diuresis that may be mediated by enhanced release of atrial natriuretic peptide. When coupled with the increased fluid loss through increased ventilation, there is a higher risk for dehydration, and adequate hydration should be maintained.

ACUTE PHARMACOLOGIC Rx
- Nonsteroidal anti-inflammatory drugs (e.g., ibuprofen 600 mg every 6 hours, beginning 6 hours before ascending) are effective prophylaxis of traditional altitude sickness and in treating headaches in AMS.
- Acetazolamide 125 to 250 mg PO bid has been effective for both prevention and acute therapy in patients with AMS and HAPE.
- Nifedipine 10 mg sublingual followed by long-acting nifedipine 30 mg bid is used for patients with HAPE who cannot descend immediately.
- Dexamethasone 4 mg PO every 6 hr is used in patients with severe AMS, HAPE, or HACE.

CHRONIC Rx
Prevention is the most prudent therapy.
1. Slow, staged ascent to avoid altitude sickness.
2. Start the ascent below 8000 feet.
3. Ascend 1000 feet/day (300 m/day).
4. Spend two nights at the same altitude every 3 days.

5. Sleep at lower heights than the altitude climbed ("climb high, sleep low").
6. Prophylactic therapy with NSAIDs (ibuprofen 600 mg every 6 hours, beginning 6 hours before ascending) or acetazolamide up to 750 mg daily and/or dexamethasone 8 to 16 mg daily decreases the risk of developing AMS (combination may have additive benefit). The drugs should be used until acclimatization occurs.
7. Prophylactic inhalation of a β-adrenergic agonist, salmeterol 125 mcg q12h, or the use of slow-release nifedipine 20 mg bid have both been shown to reduce the risk of HAPE in susceptible individuals.
8. Tadalafil, a long-acting phosphodiesterase inhibitor, has recently been shown to decrease the incidence of HAPE in susceptible individuals.
9. The over-the-counter herbal supplement Ginkgo biloba has gained interest in AMS prophylaxis, primarily because of its low adverse effect profile. However, recent randomized clinical trials have failed to show benefit compared with placebo.

DISPOSITION
- AMS improves over a period of 2 to 3 days.
- HAPE is the most common cause of death among patients with altitude illnesses.
- More than 60% of patients with HAPE will have recurrence of symptoms on subsequent climbs.
- Neurologic deficits may persist for weeks but eventually resolve. If coma occurs, prognosis is poor.

REFERRAL
Cardiology and neurology referrals are made in patients with pulmonary edema and central nervous system findings, respectively.

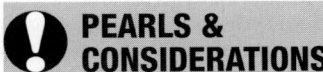 **PEARLS & CONSIDERATIONS**

COMMENTS
- Acclimatization is the process in which an individual who normally resides at low altitude adapts to hypobaric hypoxia to improve tolerance and performance at higher altitude. These mechanisms include:
  1. An increase in respiratory rates and tidal volume. This hyperventilation allows lowering of arterial carbon dioxide to

preserve oxygen delivery, even at extreme altitudes.
  2. An early increase in heart rate and stroke volume to improve oxygen delivery. After 1 wk, both parameters decrease because of diuresis and lower catecholamine levels.
  3. Pulmonary hypertension develops in response to hypoxemia, resulting in improvement of the ventilation-perfusion mismatch but may be maladaptive and lead to the development of HAPE.
  4. Cerebral vasodilation to increase blood flow to the brain.
  5. Rise in hemoglobin and hematocrit. This is a long-term process that takes up to 1 wk to occur in response to the need for improved oxygen delivery.
- Adaptation to altitude is different from acclimatization and refers to physiologic differences in permanent residents at high altitude (e.g., an increased oxygen diffusion capacity).
- Risk factors for the development of altitude sicknesses are:
  1. Rapid ascent
  2. Previous history of altitude sickness
  3. Strenuous exertion on arrival
  4. Obesity
  5. Male gender
- Physical fitness is not protective against high-altitude illness.
- HAPE is characterized by elevated pulmonary pressures, resulting in protein-rich, hemorrhagic exudates into the lung alveoli.
- Both dexamethasone and tadalafil decrease systolic pulmonary artery pressure and may reduce the incidence of HAPE in adults with a history of HAPE. Dexamethasone prophylaxis may also reduce the incidence of AMS in these adults.
- Descent is mandatory for all persons with HACE or HAPE.

SUGGESTED READINGS
available at www.expertconsult.com

RELATED CONTENT
Altitude Sickness (Patient Information)

AUTHORS: **RICHARD REGNANTE, M.D.,** and **PAUL GORDON, M.D.**

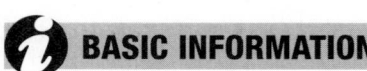
BASIC INFORMATION

DEFINITION

A hip fracture is described as ***intracapsular-femoral neck fracture*** if it occurs between the most distal portion of the articular surface and the most proximal portion of the intertrochanteric region. Location may be subcapital, transcervical, or basicervical. An ***extracapsular-intertrochanteric fracture*** is one with at least one component between the greater and lesser trochanters.

SYNONYMS

Hip fracture
Intracapsular fracture
Subcapital fracture
Extracapsular fracture
Intertrochanteric fracture

ICD-9CM CODES
820.8 Femoral neck fracture
820.2 Peritrochanteric fracture

EPIDEMIOLOGY & DEMOGRAPHICS

PREVALENCE: Lifetime risk in women ~16%
PREDOMINANT SEX: Female/male ratio of 3:1
PREDOMINANT AGE: 90% >60 yr

PHYSICAL FINDINGS & CLINICAL PRESENTATION

- Hip or groin pain
- Affected limb usually shortened and externally rotated in displaced fractures
- Impacted fractures: possibly no deformity and only mild pain with hip motion
- Mild external bruising

RISK FACTORS

- Osteoporosis
- Age >75
- Gait instability, foot deformities, muscular weakness
- Sensory impairment
- Polypharmacy
- Impaired cognition, depression
- Use of alcohol or benzodiazepines
- Orthostatic hypotension
- Environmental hazards at home (e.g., loose rugs, loose cords)

ETIOLOGY

- Trauma
- Age-related bone weakness, usually caused by osteoporosis
- Increased risk of fractures in elderly (decline in muscle function, use of psychotropic medication, etc.)

DIAGNOSIS

DIFFERENTIAL DIAGNOSIS

- OA of hip, RA of hip
- Hip dislocation
- Pathologic fracture
- Lumbar disk syndrome with radicular pain
- Insufficiency fracture of pelvis
- Trochanteric bursitis
- Septic hip joint
- Pelvic fracture
- Lateral femoral cutaneous nerve entrapment (meralgia paresthetica)
- Osteitis deformans (Paget's disease)

WORKUP

Diagnosis is usually obvious based on clinical and radiographic findings (Figs. 1-409 and 1-410). Fig. 1-411 illustrates the Garden classification of femoral neck fractures.

IMAGING STUDIES

- Standard roentgenograms consisting of an anteroposterior view of the pelvis and a cross-table lateral view of the hip to confirm the diagnosis.
- If initial roentgenograms are negative and diagnosis of an occult femoral neck fracture is suspected, hospital admission and further radiographic assessment with either bone scanning or MRI are recommended.
- Bone scanning is sensitive after 48 to 72 hr.

TREATMENT

- Orthopedic consultation
- Surgery indicated in most cases, usually within 24 hr. Treatment depends on type of fracture:
  - Femoral neck, non-displaced, impacted valgus: cannulated screws
  - Displaced: <50 yr, emergent reduction, cannulated screws; >50 yr: hemiarthroplasty, unipolar vs. bipolar or total hip arthroplasty if preexisting degenerative changes
  - Intertrochanteric: stable, two and three parts, dynamic hip screw (DHS) vs. trochanteric

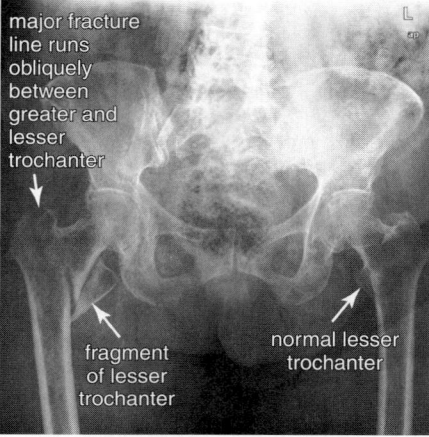

FIGURE 1-409 Intertrochanteric femur fracture: three parts (proximal, distal, and one trochanter). Intertrochanteric femur fractures are common, with the mechanism often being a fall from standing in an elderly patient. The major fracture line usually runs obliquely between the greater and the lesser trochanters. These fractures may have two, three, or four parts classically, although badly comminuted combinations are also possible. Two-part fractures consist of the proximal and distal fragments. Three-part fractures also include a fragment of one trochanter. Four-part fractures include fragments of both trochanters. This 86-year-old female had an unwitnessed fall. She has a typical three-part fracture, with a fragment of the lesser trochanter visible. Note her generalized severe osteopenia. (From Broder JS: *Diagnostic imaging for the emergency physician,* Philadelphia, 2011, Saunders.)

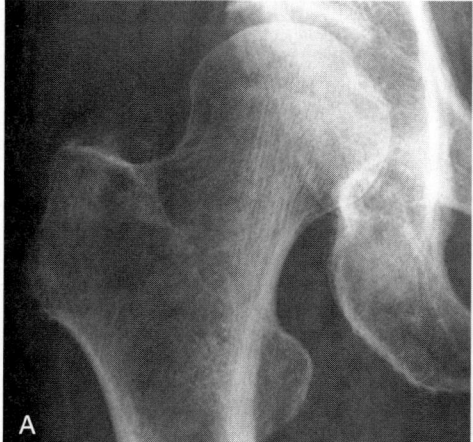 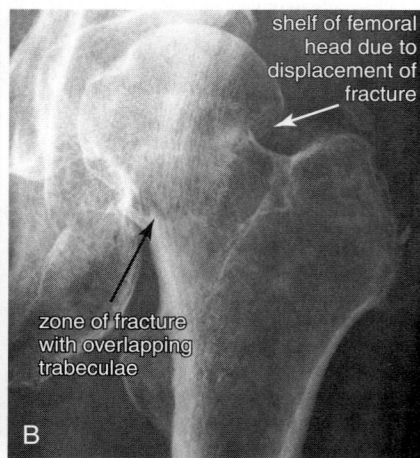

FIGURE 1-410 Femoral neck fracture. This 84-year-old female had an unwitnessed fall. **A,** Normal right hip, osteoporotic. **B,** Left hip, another relatively subtle femoral neck fracture. Note the smudging of the trabeculae of the femoral neck. In addition, the distal fragment has shifted medially, creating an overhanging ledge of the femoral head not seen on the opposite normal side. Some femoral neck fractures are more obvious. (From Broder JS: *Diagnostic imaging for the emergency physician*, Philadelphia, 2011, Saunders.)

H

femoral nail (TFN); unstable, four parts, sub-trochanteric extension, TFN
  - Reverse obliquity: TFN, blade plate, dynamic condylar screw, not DHS
- Deep vein thrombosis prophylaxis (fondaparinux, LMWH, vitamin K antagonist). Mechanical prophylaxis is contraindicated. Prophylaxis is usually continued for 28-35 days post-op
- Pain management: effective pain management is a primary goal in hip fracture. Opioid analgesics have a high incidence of delirium and constipation. Nerve blockade is effective in reducing acute pain after hip fracture
- Prophylactic antibiotics should be initiated before surgery and continued for 24 hours after surgical repair
- Rehabilitation is a major component of hip fracture treatment and should be initiated on the first postoperative day

- Conservative therapy in patients who are not surgical candidates (too ill for surgery, bed- or wheelchair-bound patients before injury)

DISPOSITION

- Surgical mortality after hip fracture repair is 2% to 3%. Older adults have a five- to eight-fold increased risk for all-cause mortality during the first 3 mo after hip fracture. Mortality rate within 1 yr in elderly patients is 25% to 30%. Excess annual mortality persists over time for both women and men, but at any given age, excess annual mortality after hip fracture is higher in men than in women.
- Dementia is a particularly poor prognostic sign.

REFERRAL

For surgical consideration when the diagnosis is made

PEARLS & CONSIDERATIONS

COMMENTS

- Complications: nonunion, avascular necrosis, DVT, infection, delirium, decubitus ulcers, incontinence, persistent pain, loosening of prosthesis
- Intracapsular fractures: occasionally occur in nonambulatory patients
  1. Usually treated nonsurgically, especially in the patient with dementia and limited pain perception
  2. Early bed-to-chair mobilization and vigilant nursing care to avoid skin breakdown
  3. Fracture usually pain free in a short time even if solid bony healing does not occur
- As a result of the increasing life span of the female population, femoral neck fractures are becoming more common. The initial physical examination and roentgenographic studies may be completely negative. Groin pain, sometimes quite severe, may be the only early clue to the diagnosis.
- The rate of hip fracture could be reduced by:
  1. Elimination of environmental hazards (poor lighting, loose rugs)
  2. Regular exercise for balance and strength
  3. Patient education about fall prevention
  4. Medication review to minimize side effects
  5. Prevention and treatment of osteoporosis
- In the U.S., hip fracture rates and subsequent mortality among persons aged 65 yr and older are declining, and comorbidities among patients with hip fractures have increased. Hip fractures are also very expensive ($40,000 in the first year following hip fracture for direct medical costs and $5,000 in subsequent years).
- Fragility (or low-trauma) hip fractures, common in elderly patients with reduced bone density, carry a 1-yr mortality of 26%, while another 58% require long-term care in a nursing facility. Previous fragility hip fracture is associated with a second osteoporotic fracture within the subsequent 5 yr.
- Concurrent prolonged use of proton-pump inhibitors (≥1 yr) is associated with reduced effectiveness of alendronate for preventing hip fractures in older adults.

EBM EVIDENCE

available at www.expertconsult.com

SUGGESTED READINGS

available at www.expertconsult.com

RELATED CONTENT

Hip Fracture (Patient Information)

AUTHOR: **LONNIE R. MERCIER, M.D.**

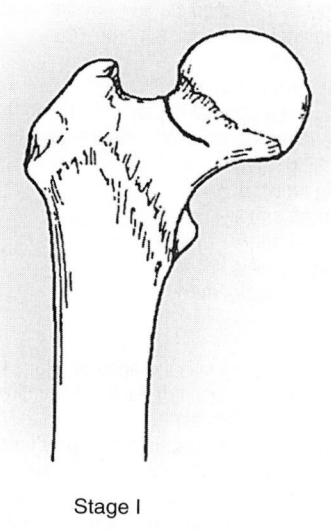

Stage I

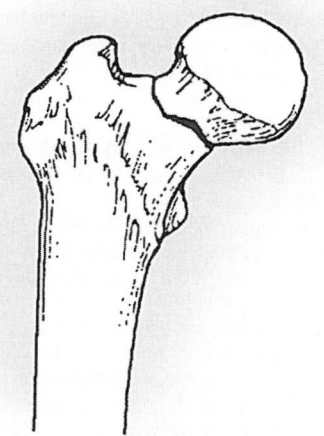

Stage II

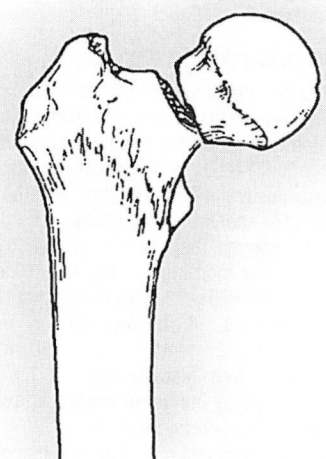

Stage III

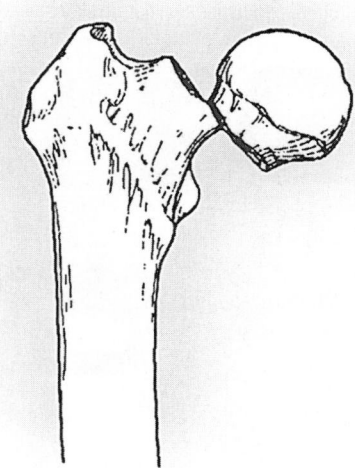

Stage IV

FIGURE 1-411 Garden classification of femoral neck fractures. (From Kyle RF: Fractures of the hip. In Gustilo RB et al [eds]: *Fractures and dislocations,* St Louis, 1993, Mosby.)

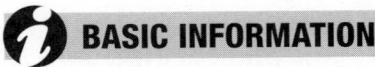

BASIC INFORMATION

DEFINITION

Hirsutism is the development of stiff, pigmented (terminal) facial and body hair (male distribution) in women as a result of excess androgen production.

SYNONYMS

Excessive hair growth

ICD-9CM CODES
704.1 Hirsutism

EPIDEMIOLOGY & DEMOGRAPHICS

- Overall prevalence unknown, estimated 5% to 10% in reproductive age women.
- Race and genetics should be considered. Some distinct ethnic populations have minimal body hair and others (Mediterranean, Middle Eastern, South Asian) have moderate to large amounts of body hair while serum androgen levels are similar.
- Social norms and culture also determine how much body hair is cosmetically acceptable.
- Half of all cases of mild hirsutism do not have hyperandrogenemia. "Patient-important hirsutism" refers to hirsutism causing woman sufficient distress to seek care.
- Incidence and presentation of hirsutism is dependent on underlying cause of androgen excess (see "Differential Diagnosis").

PHYSICAL FINDINGS & CLINICAL PRESENTATION

- Timing of symptoms: abrupt onset, short duration, rapid progression, progressive worsening, more severe signs of virilization, or later age of onset suggest androgen-producing tumor, late-onset congenital adrenal hyperplasia, or Cushing's syndrome. Weight increases may produce increased androgen production.
- Menstrual history: menarche, cycle regularity and symptoms of ovulation, fertility, and contraception use. Anovulatory cycles are the most common underlying cause of androgen excess.
- Medication use history: some drugs cause hirsutism or produce androgenic effects (danazol, phenytoin, valproic acid, androgenic progestins (e.g., norgestrel), cyclosporin, minoxidil, metoclopramide, phenothiazines, methyldopa, diazoxide, penicillamine).
- Family history: known or suspected family history of hirsutism, congenital adrenal hyperplasia, insulin resistance, polycystic ovary syndrome (PCOS), infertility, obesity, menstrual irregularity may be found.
- Physical exam reveals deepening voice, body habitus, increased muscle mass, galactorrhea; abdominal and pelvic exam.
- Associated cutaneous manifestations (Fig. 1-412) are acne, acanthosis nigricans, striae, hair distribution, location and quantity, frontotemporal balding, muscle mass, clitoromegaly.
- Ferriman-Gallwey scale, a simple, pictoral system of scoring nine body areas, is the most common method used to quantify hirsutism. It may be unreliable in non-Caucasian women of other ethnicities.

ETIOLOGY

- Presence of hirsutism indicates androgen excess. Total testosterone may be normal, but free testosterone is elevated.
- Androgens induce vellus hair follicles (soft, unpigmented hair) in sex-specific areas to develop into thicker, more heavily pigmented terminal hairs.
- Anovulatory ovaries are usual source of excess androgens through thecal cell steroidogenesis and conversion of androstenedione to testosterone. The most common cause of hirsutism is polycystic ovary syndrome, which accounts for three out of every four cases.
- Conditions that decrease hepatic production of sex hormone binding globulin (SHBG) decrease protein-bound testosterone and increase free testosterone fraction (e.g., low estrogen, high androgen, and hyperinsulinemic states).
- Late-onset, congenital adrenal hyperplasia enzyme deficiency (most commonly 21-hydroxylase deficiency) produces excess 17 hydroxyprogesterone (17-OHP) and overproduction of androstenedione.
- Rare ovarian tumors primarily derived from Sertoli-Leydig cells, granulosa theca cells, or hilus cells produce excess androgens.
- Rare adrenal tumors produce excess androgens.
- Rare pituitary or hypothalamic tumors produce excess prolactin and can lead to anovulation.

DIAGNOSIS

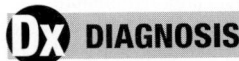

DIFFERENTIAL DIAGNOSIS

- Androgen-independent vellus hair: soft, unpigmented hair that covers entire body
- Hypertrichosis: diffusely increased total body hair (vellus or lanugo-type) not restricted to androgen-dependent areas often an adverse response to a medication or systemic illness (e.g., anorexia nervosa, porphyria)
- PCOS 75%
- Idiopathic 5% to 15%
- Congenital adrenal hyperplasia 1% to 8%
- Insulin resistance syndrome 3% to 4%
- Cushing's syndrome <1%
- Drug induced <1%
- Ovarian tumor <1%
- Adrenal tumor <1%
- Hyperthecosis <1%
- Hyperprolactinemia <1%

WORKUP

- Hirsutism is a clinical diagnosis. Fig. E1-413 describes an algorithm for the evaluation and treatment of hirsutism.
- Management of hirsutism is largely independent of the etiology.
- Workup in selected hirsute women is directed to determine underlying cause of androgen excess.
- See specific conditions for more detailed workup of individual diagnoses.

LABORATORY TESTS

The Endocrine Society Clinical Practice Guideline recommends checking androgen levels in women with moderate or severe hirsutism, sudden onset, rapid progression, or associated menstrual dysfunction, central obesity, clitoromegaly, or acanthosis nigricans.

- Total plasma testosterone or free testosterone: early morning on day 4 to 10 of menstrual cycle to screen for testosterone secreting tumors. If moderately or markedly elevated (total testosterone >150 ng/dl [5.2 nmol/L], free testosterone >2 ng/dl [0.07 nmol/L]) may image adrenals and ovaries for androgen-secreting tumors.

Other laboratory test considerations if appropriate:
- Prolactin: moderately elevated values should prompt imaging of pituitary-hypothalamic region
- 17-OHP (17 α-hydroxyprogesterone): screen for adrenal enzyme deficiencies. Morning value >200 ng/dl in early follicular phase

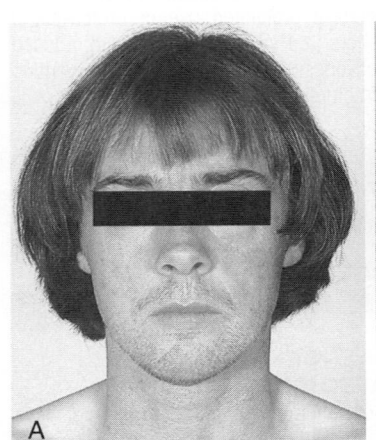
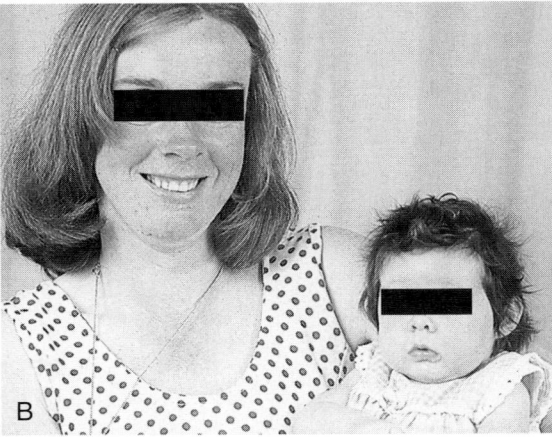

FIGURE 1-412 A patient with an arrhenoblastoma with associated polycystic ovaries before and after treatment. **A,** Before treatment, the patient had marked facial hirsutism. **B,** The patient is shown successfully treated. The tumor was resected and ovulation ensued with clomiphene and human chorionic gonadotropin therapy. (From Besser CM, Thorner MO: *Comprehensive clinical endocrinology*, ed 3, St Louis, 2002, Mosby.)

suggests nonclassic (late onset) congenital adrenal hyperplasia due to 21-hydroxylase deficiency and may be confirmed with high dose (250 mcg) ACTH stimulation test.
- Thyroid-stimulating hormone (TSH): rule out hypothyroidism
- Dehydroepiandrosterone sulfate (DHEA-S): screen for adrenal androgen production as almost entirely produced by adrenals. Levels >700 mcg/dl (13.6 nmol/L) raise suspicion for adrenal androgen-secreting tumor.

Additional laboratory test considerations if appropriate:
- Follicle-stimulating hormone: (FSH): rule out hypoestrogen state (perimenopausal)
- Luteinizing hormone: (LH): typically elevated in PCOS with low or normal FSH
- 24-hour urinary free cortisol: rule out Cushing's syndrome and overproduction of cortisol
- Overnight single-dose dexamethasone suppression test: rule out Cushing's syndrome and adrenal hyperfunction
- Fasting blood sugar (FBS), 2-hr 75-g oral glucose tolerance test, fasting insulin levels: rule out insulin resistance syndrome

IMAGING STUDIES

Imaging study considerations if appropriate:
- Pelvic ultrasound (high resolution, transvaginal): rule out ovarian tumor if total testosterone is elevated
- Abdominal CT/MRI: rule out adrenal tumor if elevated DHEA-S
- Pituitary-hypothalamic region CT/MRI: rule out pituitary tumor if prolactin elevated
- Laparoscopy/laparotomy: rule out small ovarian tumor in cases of elevated testosterone levels without radiologic evidence of adrenal or ovarian pathology

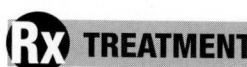 **TREATMENT**

NONPHARMACOLOGIC THERAPY

- Weight reduction: can reduce androgen production indirectly by reducing insulin-stimulated theca cell androgen production and improve menstrual function, and slow hair growth in obese women.
- Cosmetic: temporary.
  - Shaving: does not stimulate hair growth; lasts days, leaves stubble.
  - Epilation: electronic plucking.
  - Bleaching: removes hair pigment. May cause skin irritation.
  - Mechanical waxing/plucking.
  - Depilatories: gels, lotions, or creams that chemically disrupt sulfide bonds of hair causing dissolution of hair shaft. No stubble.
  - Photoepilation (laser and intense pulsed light [IPL]): hair follicles destroyed by wavelengths of light absorbed by melanin. Good for pigmented hair; laser treatment is more effective than shaving, waxing, and electrolysis. It lasts 3 to 6 months as vellus follicles remain and can be converted to terminal pigmented hair under excess androgens.

- Cosmetic: permanent. Electrolysis: destroys individual hair follicles. May be expensive and time consuming.

ACUTE GENERAL Rx
See "Pharmacologic Therapy."

CHRONIC Rx
See "Pharmacologic Therapy."

PHARMACOLOGIC THERAPY

- Usually second-line treatment following non-pharmacologic, physical methods of hair control, and in consideration of patient's co-morbidities and risk factors, patient preferences, area of excess hair amenable to treatment, and access and affordability of treatments.
- Pharmacologic treatments categorized as topical, oral contraceptive pills (OCPs), antiandrogens (potential adverse effects on a developing male fetus, so use with reliable contraception), other treatments directed at specific underlying etiology.
- Topical: Eflornithine topical cream 13.9%: unclear mechanism of action; may inhibit ornithine decarboxylase, retarding hair growth. Temporary cosmetic treatment for facial hair. Applied directly to unwanted facial hair bid with at least 8 hr spaced applications. Does not remove hair, rather slows growth. Slow response over 4 to 8 wk. Hair growth returns upon discontinuation of treatment.
- OCPs: Suppress ovarian steroidogenesis and LH through low-dose estrogen and low androgenic progestational agents. Slow response to treatment. Suppresses new hair growth. Established hair unaffected. Low-dose OCPs with low androgenic progestational agents, for example, desogestrel, norgestimate. Avoid norgestrel and levonorgestrel (higher androgenic progestational agents).
- Antiandrogens: Spironolactone: when OCPs unacceptable or may be added for disappointing results after 6 mo of OCP treatment.
  - Aldosterone-antagonist diuretic inhibits adrenal and ovarian biosynthesis of androgens. May result in ovulation, so consider contraception needs.
  - Slow response usually 6 mo or more.
  - 200 mg PO qd, then decrease to 25 to 50 mg qd maintenance.
  - May cause hyperkalemia.
  - Anovulatory, unopposed estrogen states require progestin management.

REFERRAL

- To endocrinologist if difficulty in determining diagnosis, achieving therapeutic goals, or resistant to first-line therapies. Pre-pubertal and postmenopausal hirsutism is suspicious for neoplastic or secondary endocrine causes and should be referred for further evaluation.
- Consider referral or consultation for following therapies:
  1. Finasteride: antiandrogen, in hair follicle blocks 5α-reductase conversion of testosterone to intranuclearly active 5α-dihydrotestosterone (DHT)

  - Use only with reliable contraception because DHT necessary for normal male fetus urogenital development
  - Not FDA approved for treatment of hirsutism
  - 1 to 5 mg PO qd
  2. Flutamide: inhibits androgen uptake and receptor binding
  - Not recommended by Endocrine Society Clinical Practice Guidelines and not FDA approved for treatment of hirsutism, but used by some European endocrinologists
  - Use only with reliable contraception
  - Reserved for women with severe, resistant hirsutism because of risk of hepatic dysfunction
  - 250 mg PO bid
  3. Cyproterone acetate (not available in U.S.): antiandrogen that competes with DHT for binding androgen receptors. Used as progestin component of OCPs outside U.S.
- Other treatments directed at specific underlying etiology:
  - Metformin/thiazolidinediones: therapy reserved for documented insulin resistant states.
  - GnRH agonists: recommended only in women with severe hyperandrogenemia (e.g., ovarian hyperthecosis) with suboptimal response to combination low-dose estrogen/progestin pills and antiandrogen treatment. Inhibits gonadotropin and consequently ovarian androgen and estrogen secretion.
  - Dexamethasone: adrenal glucocorticoid suppression is reserved for diagnosis of adrenal enzyme deficiency.
  - Total abdominal hysterectomy/bilateral salpingo-oophorectomy reserved for recalcitrant hirsutism in older female with hyperthecosis and undesired fertility.

(!) PEARLS & CONSIDERATIONS

COMMENTS
- Hirsutism is both an endocrine and cosmetic problem for patients.
- Ovulation induction therapy is indicated in women desiring pregnancy.
- Evaluation of incidental adrenal mass is always warranted.

SUGGESTED READINGS
available at www.expertconsult.com

RELATED CONTENT
Hirsutism (Patient Information)

AUTHOR: **RICHARD LONG, M.D.**

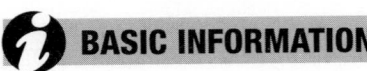

BASIC INFORMATION

DEFINITION

Histoplasmosis is caused by the fungus *Histoplasma capsulatum* and characterized by a primary pulmonary focus with occasional progression to chronic pulmonary histoplasmosis (CPH) or various forms of dissemination. Progressive disseminated histoplasmosis (PDH) may present with a diverse clinical spectrum, including adrenal necrosis, pulmonary and mediastinal fibrosis, and ulcerations of the oropharynx and GI tract. In those patients coinfected with HIV, it is a defining disease for AIDS.

SYNONYMS

North American histoplasmosis
Ohio Valley fever
Vanderbilt disease

ICD-9CM CODES
115.90 Histoplasmosis
115.94 Histoplasmosis with endocarditis
115.91 Histoplasmosis with meningitis
115.93 Histoplasmosis with pericarditis
115.95 Histoplasmosis with pneumonia
115.92 Histoplasmosis with retinitis

EPIDEMIOLOGY & DEMOGRAPHICS

INCIDENCE (IN U.S.):
- Unknown for acute pulmonary disease
- For CPH, estimated at 1/100,000 cases in endemic areas
- For PDH in immunocompetent adults, estimated at 1/2000 cases of histoplasmosis

PREVALENCE: Unknown

PREDOMINANT SEX: Clinically evident disease is most common in males; male/female ratio of 4:1

PREDOMINANT AGE:
- CPH is most often seen in males >50 yr old with an associated history of COPD.
- Presumed ocular histoplasmosis syndrome (POHS) is seen between ages of 20 and 40 yr.

PEAK INCIDENCE: Unknown

PHYSICAL FINDINGS & CLINICAL PRESENTATION

- Conidia are deposited in alveoli then converted to yeast forms where they spread to regional lymph nodes and other organs, especially liver and spleen.
- 1 to 2 wk later, a granulomatous inflammatory response begins to contain the yeast in the form of discrete granulomas.
- Delayed-type hypersensitivity to *Histoplasma* antigens occurs 3 to 6 wk after exposure.
- Clinical disease manifests in various forms, depending on host cellular immunity and inoculum size:
  1. Acute primary pulmonary histoplasmosis
     a. An overwhelming number of patients are asymptomatic.
     b. Most clinically apparent infections manifest by complaints of fever, headache, malaise, pleuritic chest pain, nonproductive cough, and weight loss.
     c. Less than 10%, mainly women, complain of arthralgias, myalgias, and skin manifestations such as erythema multiforme or erythema nodosum.
     d. Acute pericarditis presents in a smaller percentage of patients.
     e. Hepatosplenomegaly is most commonly observed in children.
     f. With particularly heavy exposure, there is severe dyspnea, marked hypoxemia, impending respiratory failure.
     g. Most patients are asymptomatic within 6 wk.
  2. CPH
     a. Presents insidiously with low-grade fever, malaise, weight loss, cough, sometimes with blood-streaked sputum or frank hemoptysis.
     b. Most patients with cavitary lesions present with associated COPD or chronic bronchitis, masking underlying fungal disease.
     c. Tends to worsen preexisting pulmonary disease and further contribute to eventual respiratory insufficiency.
  3. PDH
     a. In both acute and subacute forms, constitutional symptoms of fever, fatigue, malaise, and weight loss are common.
     b. Acute form (seen in infants and children) presents with respiratory symptoms, fever ≥101° F (38.3° C), generalized lymphadenopathy, marked hepatosplenomegaly, and fulminant course resembling septic shock associated with a high fatality rate.
     c. Subacute form is more common in adults and associated with lower temperatures, hepatosplenomegaly, oropharyngeal ulceration, focal organ involvement (including adrenal destruction, endocarditis, chronic meningitis, and intracerebral mass lesions).
     d. Course of subacute form is relentless, with untreated patients dying within 2 yr.
     e. Chronic PDH is found in adults and marked by gradual symptoms of weight loss, weakness, easy fatigability; low-grade fever when present; oropharyngeal ulcerations and hepatomegaly and/or splenomegaly in one third of patients.
     f. Less clinical evidence of focal organ involvement in chronic form than in subacute form.
     g. Natural history of chronic form is protracted and intermittent, spanning months to years.
- Histoplasmoma
  1. A healed area of caseation necrosis surrounded by a fibrous capsule
  2. Usually asymptomatic
- Mediastinal fibrosis
  1. A rare consequence of a fibroblastic process that encases caseating mediastinal lymph nodes producing severe retraction, compression, and distortion of mediastinal structures
  2. Constriction of the bronchi resulting in bronchiectasis, also esophageal stenosis associated with dysphagia, and superior vena cava syndrome
- POHS
  1. Diagnosis characterized by distinct clinical features, including atrophic choroidal scars and maculopathy in patients with histories suggestive of exposure to the fungus (e.g., residence in an endemic area)
  2. Patient complains of distortion or loss of central vision without pain, redness, or photophobia
  3. Usually no evidence of infection except for a positive skin reaction to histoplasmin
- In patients with AIDS
  1. Possible presentation as overwhelming infection similar to acute PDH seen in children
  2. Constitutional symptoms: fever, weight loss, malaise, cough, dyspnea
  3. About 10% with cutaneous maculopapular, erythematous eruptions or purpuric lesions on face, trunk, and extremities
  4. Up to 20% with CNS involvement, manifesting as intracerebral mass lesions, chronic meningitis, or encephalopathy

ETIOLOGY

- *H. capsulatum* is a dimorphic fungus present in temperate zones and river valleys worldwide.
- In the U.S., it is highly endemic in southeastern, mid-Atlantic, and central states.
- Exists as mold at ambient temperature and favors soils enriched with bird or bat droppings.

DIAGNOSIS

DIFFERENTIAL DIAGNOSIS

- Acute pulmonary histoplasmosis
  1. *Mycobacterium tuberculosis*
  2. Community-acquired pneumonias caused by *Mycoplasma* and *Chlamydia*
  3. Other fungal diseases, such as *Blastomyces dermatitidis* and *Coccidioides immitis*
- Chronic cavitary pulmonary histoplasmosis: *M. tuberculosis*
- Histoplasmomas: true neoplasms

WORKUP

- Suspect diagnosis in patients who present with a history of residence or travel in an endemic area, especially if engaged in occupations (e.g., outside construction or street cleaning) or hobbies (e.g., cave exploring) that increase the likelihood of exposure to fungal spores.
- Suspect diagnosis in immunosuppressed patients with remote history of exposure, especially if associated with characteristic calcifications on chest x-ray.

H

Diseases
and Disorders

I

LABORATORY TESTS

- Demonstration of organism on culture from body fluid or tissues to make definitive diagnosis
  1. Especially high yield in patients with AIDS
  2. Characteristic oval yeast cells in neutrophils with Giemsa stain from peripheral smear
  3. Preparations of infected tissue with Gomori's silver methenamine for revealing yeast forms, especially in areas of caseation necrosis
- Serologic tests, including complement-fixing (CF) antibodies and immunodiffusion assays
- Detection of *Histoplasma* antigen in urine: may be influenced by infections with *Blastomyces* and *Coccidioides*
- In PDH
  1. Pancytopenia
  2. Marked elevations in alkaline phosphatase and alanine aminotransferase (ALT) common
- In chronic meningitis (majority of cases)
  1. CSF pleocytosis with either lymphocytes or neutrophils predominating
  2. Elevated CSF protein levels
  3. Hypoglycorrhachia

IMAGING STUDIES

- Chest radiograph examination in acute pulmonary histoplasmosis
  1. Singular or multiple patchy infiltrates, especially in the lower lung fields
  2. Hilar or mediastinal lymphadenopathy with or without pneumonitis
  3. Diffuse nodular or confluent bilateral miliary infiltrates characteristic of heavier exposure
  4. Infrequent pleural effusions, except when associated with pericarditis
- Chest radiograph examination in histoplasmoma: coin lesion displaying central calcification, ranging from 1 to 4 cm in diameter, predominantly located in the subpleural regions
- Chest radiograph examination in CPH:
  1. Upper lobe disease frequently associated with cavities
  2. Preexisting calcifications in the hilum associated with peribronchial streaking extending to the parenchyma
- Chest radiograph examination in acute PDH: hilar adenopathy and/or diffuse nodular infiltrates
- CT scan of adrenals to reveal bilateral enlargement and low-attenuation centers

Rx TREATMENT

NONPHARMACOLOGIC THERAPY

For life-threatening disease seen in acute disseminated disease or infection in patients with AIDS: supportive therapy with IV fluids

ACUTE GENERAL Rx

- No drug therapy is required for asymptomatic pulmonary disease.
- A course of therapy with itraconazole 200 mg PO tid for 3 days, then 200 mg/day PO for 6-12 wk may be beneficial in some patients with acute pulmonary distress. Avoid fluconazole because it is not as active.
- Same therapy appropriate for immunocompetent, mild to moderately symptomatic patients with CPH and subacute and chronic forms of PDH, but duration for 6 to 12 mo.
- Use amphotericin B 0.7 to 1 mg/kg IV for 6 to 12 mo in patients hypersensitive to or intolerant of azole therapy.
- Give amphotericin B for life-threatening disease or continued illness as a result of primary failure or relapse of adequate azole therapy. A lipid formulation of amphotericin B can be used to avoid nephrotoxicity.
  1. For acute pulmonary histoplasmosis associated with acute respiratory distress syndrome (ARDS), acute PDH, and histoplasma meningitis: dose of 0.7 to 1 mg/kg IV q24h
  2. End point of therapy for patient with complicated acute pulmonary disease: total dose of 500 mg
  3. End point for patient with acute PDH: total dose 35 mg/kg or 2.5 g total
  4. For moderately severe or severe acute pulmonary histoplasmosis, add methylprednisolone 0.5-1 mg/kg/day for 1-2 wk to liposomal amphotericin B.
- Chronic cavitary pulmonary histoplasmosis: itraconazole 200 mg PO tid for 3 days, then once or twice daily for at least 12 mo.
- CNS histoplasmosis: liposomal amphotericin B, 5 mg/kg/day for a total of 175 mg/kg over 4-6 wk, then itraconazole 200 mg 2-3×/day for at least 12 mo.
- Endocarditis: surgical treatment with excision of infected valve or graft combined with amphotericin for a total dose of 35 mg/kg or 2.5 g.
- For pericardial disease:
  1. Antifungal therapy: no apparent benefit
  2. Best managed with NSAIDs
- For POHS:
  1. Antifungal therapy: no apparent benefit
  2. May respond to laser therapy

CHRONIC Rx

- In patients with AIDS: lifelong suppressive therapy with either itraconazole, given 200 mg PO qid, or IV amphotericin B at a dose of 50 mg once weekly; a triazole compound posaconazole (400 mg PO bid) may be useful in refractory cases, but clinical experience is limited at this point.
- Prophylaxis in HIV-infected patients with <150 CD4 cells/mm^3: itraconazole 200 mg PO qd

DISPOSITION

For those with chronic or progressive disease, especially if immunocompromised, prognosis is dependent on prompt recognition and timely administration of appropriate antifungal drugs.

REFERRAL

- To an infectious disease specialist in suspected cases of disseminated disease, especially if immunocompromised
- To a pulmonologist for patients with CPH form because of progressive respiratory compromise
- To a thoracic surgeon for decompression procedures for progressive mediastinal fibrosis

! PEARLS & CONSIDERATIONS

- *H. capsulatum*, variety *duboisii*, also known as African histoplasmosis, is restricted to Senegal, Nigeria, Zaire, and Uganda.
- Unlike *H. capsulatum*, pulmonary forms of *duboisii* are not seen, and the disease is limited to the skin, soft tissues, and bone.

COMMENTS

- Patients living in endemic areas, especially if immunocompromised, should take appropriate respiratory precautions when disposing of bird waste from rooftop or home aviaries.
- Appropriate respiratory precautions should also be taken when leisure traveling to areas that act as a natural haven for the fungus, such as bat caves.

SUGGESTED READINGS

available at www.expertconsult.com

RELATED CONTENT

Histoplasmosis (Patient Information)

AUTHOR: **GLENN G. FORT, M.D., M.P.H.**

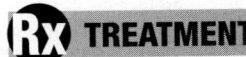

BASIC INFORMATION

DEFINITION

Patients with histrionic personality disorder present with a pervasive pattern of excessive emotionality and attention-seeking behavior that generally begins in early adulthood.

SYNONYMS

Hysterical personality disorder
Psycho-infantile personality disorder
Personality disorder (nonspecific)

ICD-9CM CODES

301.5 Histrionic personality disorder (ICD-9 and DSM IV code)

EPIDEMIOLOGY & DEMOGRAPHICS

PREVALENCE (IN U.S.):
- Diagnosed more often in women (85%); rarely found in men
- Prevalence: 1% to 2%

PREDOMINANT SEX: Female. Cultural factors (e.g., attention-seeking behavior not as acceptable in men) may lead to more common diagnosis in women.

PREDOMINANT AGE: Generally begins in early adulthood

PHYSICAL FINDINGS & CLINICAL PRESENTATION

Features include five or more of the following:
1. Is uncomfortable in situations where he or she is not the center of attention.
2. Interaction with others is often characterized by inappropriate sexually seductive or provocative behavior.
3. Displays rapidly shifting and shallow expression of emotions.
4. Consistently uses physical appearance to draw attention to self.
5. Has a style of speech that is excessively impressionistic and lacking in detail.
6. Shows self-dramatization, theatricality, and exaggerated expression of emotion.
7. Is suggestible (i.e., easily influenced by others or circumstances).
8. Considers relationships to be more intimate than they actually are.

ETIOLOGY

- Unknown
- Hypothesized that childhood events, psychosocial adversity, and genetics are contributory

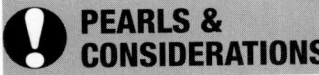

DIAGNOSIS

DIFFERENTIAL DIAGNOSIS

- Narcissistic and borderline personality disorders share common features.
- Other personality disorders (e.g., antisocial personality disorder, dependent personality disorder)
- Personality change attributable to general medical condition
- Symptoms in association with chronic substance abuse

WORKUP

There is no formal test to establish diagnosis.

TREATMENT

NONPHARMACOLOGIC THERAPY

- Long-term individual psychotherapy is treatment of choice.
- No controlled psychotherapy studies
- Unlike other people who have personality disorders, these individuals often seek treatment and exaggerate their symptoms and difficulties in functioning.
- Patients tend to be more emotionally needy and are often reluctant to terminate therapy.

ACUTE GENERAL Rx

- No placebo-controlled trials.
- Care should be given when prescribing medications because of the potential for self-destructive or otherwise harmful behaviors.

DISPOSITION

- Therapeutic approaches should not focus on the long-term personality change, but rather short-term alleviation of specific difficulties and deficits within the person's life.
- Therapeutic approaches that emphasize vague somatic, anxious, or depressive symptoms often fail.
- Patients are likely to be intolerant or drop out of treatment approaches that use delayed gratification.
- Symptoms are moderately stable over adulthood and may remit or decrease in intensity with age.

REFERRAL

Primarily treated by mental health professionals

PEARLS & CONSIDERATIONS

- This disorder is difficult to treat.
- Like most personality disorders, patients present for treatment only when stress or other situational factor within their lives has made their ability to function and cope effectively impossible.
- Suicidality should be assessed on a regular basis, and suicidal threats and self-mutilation should not be ignored or dismissed.
- At the time of this writing, histrionic personality disorder has been recommended for deletion from the DSM-5 (but may be diagnosed by Personality Disorder Trait Specified, Antagonism/attention-seeking).

PATIENT & FAMILY EDUCATION

Group and family therapy approaches are generally not recommended because individuals with this disorder often try to draw attention to themselves and exaggerate every action and reaction.

SUGGESTED READINGS

available at www.expertconsult.com

AUTHORS: **MARK ZIMMERMAN, M.D.,**
THERESA A. MORGAN, M.PHIL., and
MITCHELL D. FELDMAN, M.D., M.PHIL.

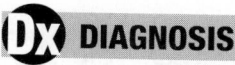

BASIC INFORMATION

- HIV cognitive dysfunction covers a spectrum of disorders ranging from asymptomatic to clinically severe (including AIDS dementia complex or HIV encephalopathy).
- Cognitive, motor, and behavioral abnormalities

SYNONYMS

HIV-associated neurocognitive disorder

ICD-9CM CODES

042 (for diseases related to HIV; no particular code for HIV cognitive dysfunction)

EPIDEMIOLOGY

- Presenting complaint in only 3% of cases
- Incidence: reduced from 60% to 1% since introduction of HIV treatment; however, as more HIV-infected patients live longer, prevalence may be increasing.
- Minor cognitive motor disorders are more common and seen in 20% of patients; not necessarily progressive
- Rarely precedes clinical evidence of HIV infection

CLINICAL FEATURES

- Cognitive changes: forgetfulness, poor attention and concentration, increased difficulty performing complex tasks, slowed psychomotor speed
- Behavioral changes: apathy, lack of initiative, social withdrawal, irritability, occasionally agitation, psychosis or obsessive compulsive disorder
- Motor problems include: clumsiness, unsteady gait, poor balance, tremor, leg weakness
- Progressive/later stages: bedbound, severe dementia, bowel/bladder incontinence

- Subcortical dementia (aphasia, apraxia, agnosia are uncommon)
- Results from inflammation triggered by HIV itself (not related to opportunistic infection) and immune activation of microglia and brain macrophages
- Clinically may resemble Parkinson's disease
- In children: developmental delay, microcephaly, and spasticity are common

RISK FACTORS

- Low CD4 count (less than 200 cells/mm^3)
- High viral load
- Anemia
- Injection drug use
- Hepatitis C
- Female gender
- Older age

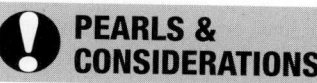

DIAGNOSIS

DIAGNOSTIC EVALUATION

- Diagnosis is based on clinical examination neuropsychometric tests
- MRI head: diffuse, confluent, periventricular white matter lesions on T2 weighted images with normal T1 images
- Lumbar puncture: CSF analysis helps to rule out opportunistic infections. In HIV cognitive dysfunction the CSF may show a nonspecific increase in cell count and protein.
- Potential causes for cognitive impairment that must be ruled out include:
  - Opportunistic infections (toxoplasmosis, CNS lymphoma)
  - Vitamin B_{12} deficiency
  - Substance use
  - Organic affective disorder (such as depression and mania)
  - Side effects of prescribed medications

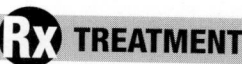

TREATMENT

Early treatment with antiretroviral therapy (ART) leads to clinical improvement.

PEARLS & CONSIDERATIONS

- Initiation of ART can lead to rapid improvement in cognitive function in early stages (untreated, life span is typically 4 to 6 mo)
- Most common presenting complaint in children infected with HIV
- Mini-mental status examination (MMSE): baseline scores in HIV patients are very helpful
- Usually cognitive symptoms precede motor abnormalities
- Four HIV-related opportunistic infections that commonly cause cognitive impairment are: toxoplasmosis, cryptococcal meningitis, progressive multifocal leukoencephalopathy, and CNS lymphoma

REFERRALS

- Upon diagnosis/clinical suspicion for HIV associated cognitive dysfunction, referral to neurology is recommended
- Referral to neuropsychology may be considered

SUGGESTED READINGS

available at www.expertconsult.com

AUTHOR: **DIVYA SINGHAL, M.D.**

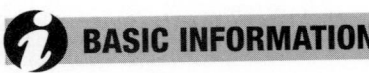

BASIC INFORMATION

DEFINITION

Hodgkin's lymphoma is a malignant disorder of lymphoreticular origin, characterized histologically by the presence of multinucleated giant cells (Reed-Sternberg cells) usually originating from B lymphocytes in germinal centers of lymphoid tissue.

ICD-9CM CODES
201.9 Hodgkin's lymphoma, unspecified
201.4 Hodgkin's lymphoma, lymphocyte predominance
201.5 Hodgkin's lymphoma, nodular sclerosis
201.6 Hodgkin's lymphoma, mixed cellularity
201.7 Hodgkin's lymphoma, lymphocyte depletion

EPIDEMIOLOGY & DEMOGRAPHICS

- There is a bimodal age distribution (15 to 34 yr and >50 yr).
- Concordance for Hodgkin's lymphoma in identical twins suggests that a genetic susceptibility underlies Hodgkin's lymphoma in young adulthood.
- The disease is more common in males (in childhood Hodgkin's lymphoma, >80% occur in males), whites, and higher socioeconomic groups.
- Overall incidence of Hodgkin's lymphoma in the United States is ~4 per 100,000. There are >8000 new cases of Hodgkin's lymphoma diagnosed annually in the United States.

PHYSICAL FINDINGS & CLINICAL PRESENTATION

- Palpable lymphadenopathy that is generally painless is the most common presenting symptom
- Most common site of involvement: neck region
- Fever and night sweats: fever in a cyclical pattern (days or weeks of fever alternating with afebrile periods) is known as Pel-Epstein fever
- Weight loss, generalized malaise
- Persistent, nonproductive cough
- Pain associated with alcohol ingestion often because of heavy eosinophil infiltration of the tumor sites is relatively uncommon
- Pruritus
- Other: superior vena cava syndrome, spinal cord compression (rare), erythema nodosum, ichthyosis

ETIOLOGY

Unknown; evidence implicating Epstein-Barr virus remains controversial.

DIAGNOSIS

DIFFERENTIAL DIAGNOSIS

- Non-Hodgkin's lymphoma
- Sarcoidosis
- Infections (e.g., cytomegalovirus, Epstein-Barr virus, toxoplasmosis, HIV)
- Drug reaction

WORKUP

Diagnosis is confirmed by lymph node biopsy. The World Health Organization classifies Hodgkin's lymphoma into two groups: classical Hodgkin's lymphoma (92% to 97%) and nodular lymphocyte-predominant Hodgkin's lymphoma (3% to 8%). Classic Hodgkin's lymphoma has four main histologic subtypes based on the number of lymphocytes, Reed-Sternberg cells (Fig. 1-415), and the presence of fibrous tissue:
1. Nodular sclerosis (60% to 80%) (Fig. E1-416)
2. Mixed cellularity (15% to 30%) (Fig. E1-417)
3. Lymphocyte predominance (2% to 7%)
4. Lymphocyte depletion (1% to 6%)

Nodular sclerosis occurs mainly in young adulthood, whereas the mixed cellularity type is more prevalent after age 50 yr.

Table 1-196 describes the Cotswolds staging classification.

Proper staging requires the following:
- Detailed history (with documentation of "B symptoms" and physical examination)
- Surgical biopsy
- Laboratory evaluation (complete blood count, erythrocyte sedimentation rate, blood urea nitrogen, creatinine, alkaline phosphatase, liver function tests, albumin, lactate dehydrogenase, uric acid), immunophenotypic markers (see Table 1-197). Gene-expression profiling for tumor-associated macrophages is a new biomarker for risk stratification
- Chest x-ray (posteroanterior and lateral)
- CT scan of chest, abdomen, pelvis, neck
- Positron emission tomography scan (18-FDG PET scan)

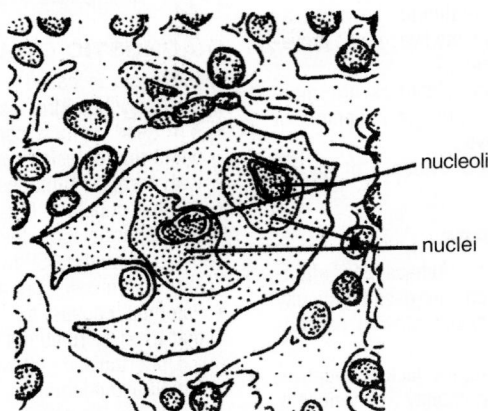

nucleoli

nuclei

FIGURE 1-415 Hodgkin's disease. High-power photomicrograph demonstrates a binucleate Reed-Sternberg cell exhibiting prominent inclusion-like eosinophilic nucleoli, giving it an "owl's eye" appearance. (From Skarin AT: *Atlas of diagnostic oncology,* ed 3, St Louis, 2003, Mosby.)

TABLE 1-196   Cotswolds Staging Classification for Hodgkin's Lymphoma

Classification	Description
Stage I	Involvement of a single lymph node region or lymphoid structure (e.g., spleen, thymus, Waldeyer ring) or involvement of a single extralymphatic site (IE)
Stage II	Involvement of two or more lymph node regions on the same side of the diaphragm (hilar nodes, when involved on both sides, constitute stage II disease); localized contiguous involvement of only one extranodal organ or site and lymph node regions on the same side of the diaphragm (IIE). The number of anatomic regions involved should be indicated by a subscript (e.g., II3)
III1	With or without involvement of splenic, hilar, celiac, or portal nodes
III2	With involvement of paraaortic, iliac, and mesenteric nodes
Stage IV	Diffuse or disseminated involvement of one or more extranodal organs or tissues, with or without associated lymph node involvement Designations applicable to any disease stage
A	No symptoms
B	Fever (temperature, >38° C [100.4° F]), drenching night sweats, unexplained loss of >10% of body weight within the preceding 6 mo
X	Bulky disease (a widening of the mediastinum by more than one third of the presence of a nodal mass with a maximal dimension <10 cm)
E	Involvement of a single extranodal site that is contiguous or proximal to the known nodal site

From Hoffman R et al: *Hematology: basic principles and practice,* ed 5, Philadelphia, 2009, Churchill Livingstone.

TABLE 1-197 Selected Immunophenotypic Markers and Histologic Characteristics of Use in the Differential Diagnosis of Hodgkin's Lymphoma and Other Lymphoid Neoplasms

Marker	Classical HL	Nodular Lymphocyte Predominant HL	TCRBCL	ALCL
CD30	+	–	–	+
CD15	+	–	–	–
CD20	–/+*	+	+	–
CD45	–	+	+	–/+
CD79a	–	+	+	–
ALK	–	–	–	+/–
EMA	–	+	+	+/–
Nodular growth protein	+/–†	+	+	+

+, >90% of cases positive; +/–, majority of cases positive; –/+, minority of cases positive; –, <10% of cases positive; *ALCL*, anaplastic large cell lymphoma; *HL*, Hodgkin's lymphoma; *TCRBCL*, T-cell rich B-cell lymphoma.
*CD20 positivity in classical Hodgkin's lymphoma is quite heterogeneous, with a wide range in brightness of staining.
†In classical Hodgkin's lymphoma, a nodular growth pattern is confined to the nodular sclerosing subtype.
From Abeloff MD: *Clinical oncology*, ed 3, Philadelphia, 2004, Saunders.

BOX 1-24 Recommended Staging Procedures for Hodgkin Lymphoma

The following staging procedures are recommended for the initial workup of Hodgkin lymphoma:
1. Adequate surgical biopsy reviewed by an experienced hematopathologist
2. Core-needle biopsy of bone marrow from the posterior iliac crest; needle or surgical biopsy of any suspicious extranodal (e.g., hepatic, osseous, pulmonary, cutaneous) lesions; and cytologic examination of any effusion
3. Detailed history, with attention to the presence or absence of systemic symptoms, and a careful physical examination, emphasizing node chains, size of the liver and spleen, and inspection of Waldeyer ring
4. Routine laboratory tests: complete blood cell count, erythrocyte sedimentation rate, and liver function tests
5. Chest radiographs (posteroanterior and lateral) with measurement of the mass-to-thoracic ratio
6. Neck, chest, and abdominal CT
7. 18-FDG PET scan

From Hoffman R et al: *Hematology: basic principles and practice*, ed 5, Philadelphia, 2009, Churchill Livingstone.

- Bilateral bone marrow biopsy (selected patients)

Box 1-24 summarizes recommended staging procedures for Hodgkin lymphoma.

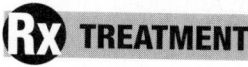 **TREATMENT**

ACUTE GENERAL Rx

The main therapeutic modalities are radiotherapy and chemotherapy; the indication for which one varies with pathologic stage and other factors. In general, chemotherapy plus involved-field radiotherapy can be used as standard treatment for Hodgkin's lymphoma in early stages with favorable prognostic features. In patients with unfavorable features, four courses of chemotherapy plus involved-field radiotherapy should be the standard treatment. Commonly used therapeutic modalities are:

- Stage I and II: radiation therapy alone (involved-field radiotherapy [35 Gy]) unless a large mediastinal mass is present (mediastinal to thoracic ratio ≥1.3); in the latter case, a combination of chemotherapy and radiation therapy is indicated. Various regimens can be used for combination of chemotherapy. Most oncologists prefer the combination

of Adriamycin (doxorubicin), bleomycin, vinblastine, and dacarbazine (ABVD). Table 1-198 describes characteristics of the ABVD regimen. Generally, chemotherapy plus radiation treatment is effective in controlling stage IA or IIA nonbulky lymphoma in a high percentage of patients (>85%), but is associated with late treatment-related deaths. Trials have shown that ABVD therapy alone is associated with a higher rate of overall survival (due to lower rate of death from other causes) when compared with treatment that includes ABVD therapy and subtotal nodal radiation therapy.
- Stage IB or IIB: total nodal irradiation is often used, although chemotherapy is performed in many centers.
- Stage IIIA: treatment is controversial. It varies with the anatomic substage after splenectomy.
  1. III₁A and minimum splenic involvement: radiation therapy alone may be adequate.
  2. III₂ or III₁A with extensive splenic involvement: there is disagreement whether chemotherapy alone or a combination of chemotherapy and radiation therapy is the preferred treatment modality.
  3. IIIB and IVB: the treatment of choice is chemotherapy with or without adjuvant radiotherapy.

TABLE 1-198 Characteristics of the ABVD Regimen

Agents: doxorubicin, bleomycin, vinblastine, dacarbazine
All intravenous, total compliance
80% complete response rate
10% primary refractory disease
60%-65% overall disease-free survival
Most relapses occur within the first 4 yr; however, about 10% of all relapses occur beyond 5 yr
Major side effects are nausea, phlebitis, myelosuppression, less cumulative myelotoxicity than MOPP
No infertility
No leukemia

ABVD, Adriamycin (doxorubicin), bleomycin, vinblastine, dacarbazine; *MOPP,* mechlorethamine, Oncovin (vincristine), procarbazine, prednisone.
From Abeloff MD: *Clinical oncology*, ed 3, Philadelphia, 2004, Saunders.

Recent trials have shown that in patients with early-stage Hodgkin's lymphoma and favorable prognosis, treatment with two cycles of ABVD followed by 20 Gy of involved-field radiation therapy may be as effective as, and less toxic than four cycles of ABVD followed by 30 Gy of involved-field radiation therapy. Long-term effects of this approach need to be fully assessed before it becomes standard of care. BEACOPP, an intensified regimen consisting of bleomycin, etoposide, doxorubicin, cyclophosphamide, vincristine, procarbazine, and prednisone, has been advocated by some as the new standard for treatment of advanced Hodgkin's lymphoma in place of ABVD. Recent trials have shown that treatment with BEACOPP, as compared with ABVD, resulted in better initial tumor control, but the long-term clinical outcome did not differ significantly between the two regimens. In addition, with the use of the escalated BEACOPP regimen, the rate of complications is higher (3% treatment-related death, 20% rate of hospitalization, and 3% rate of secondary leukemia). Thus, if the goal is cure with the least overall toxic effects, it is best to favor ABVD therapy, reserving rescue therapy with high-dose chemotherapy and autologous hematopoietic stem-cell transplantation for patients in whom the primary treatment fails.

- Definitions of treatment groups are described in Table 1-199.
- Recommendations for the primary treatment of Hodgkin's lymphoma outside of clinical trials are described in Table 1-200.

DISPOSITION

- The overall survival at 10 yr is ~60%.
- Cure rates as high as 75% to 80% are now possible with appropriate initial therapy.
- Poor prognostic features (Table 1-201) include presence of B symptoms, advanced age, advanced stage at initial presentation, mixed cellularity and lymphocyte depletion histology, and increased number of tumor-associated macrophages.
- Chemotherapy significantly increases the risk of leukemia.
- The peak in risk of leukemia is seen approximately 5 yr after the initiation of chemotherapy.

H

Diseases and Disorders

I

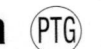
- The risk of leukemia is greater for those who undergo splenectomy and patients with advanced stages of Hodgkin's disease; the risk is unaffected by concomitant radiotherapy.
- Involved-field radiotherapy does not improve the outcome in patients with advanced-stage Hodgkin's lymphoma who have a complete remission after MOPP (mechlorethamine, vincristine, procarbazine, and prednisone)–ABV chemotherapy. Radiotherapy may benefit patients with a partial response after chemotherapy.
- Mediastinal irradiation increases the risk of subsequent death from heart disease caused by sclerosis of the coronary artery from irradiation. Risk increases with high mediastinal doses, minimal protective cardiac blocking, young age at irradiation, and increased duration of follow-up.
- Both chemotherapy and radiation therapy increase the risk of developing secondary solid tumors (Table 1-202).

- Table 1-203 describes potential late complications of Hodgkin's lymphoma treatment and appropriate clinical responses and preventive strategies.

REFERRAL

- To surgery for lymph node biopsy
- Hematology/oncology

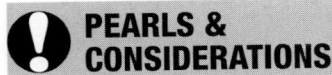

COMMENTS

- Young male patients should consider sperm banking before the initiation of therapy.
- Chemotherapy plus involved-field radiotherapy should be the standard treatment for Hodgkin's disease with favorable prognostic features. In patients with unfavorable features,

four courses of chemotherapy plus involved-field radiotherapy should be the standard of treatment. After failure of ABVD therapy, more than 60% of patients who have had a relapse and about 30% of patients with initially refractory lymphoma can be reliably cured with high-dose chemotherapy and autologous hematopoietic stem-cell transplantation.

SUGGESTED READINGS

available at www.expertconsult.com

RELATED CONTENT

Hodgkin's Lymphoma (Patient Information)

AUTHOR: **FRED F. FERRI, M.D.**

TABLE 1-199 Definition of Treatment Groups According to the EORTC/GELA and GHSG

Treatment Group	EORTC/GELA	GHSG	NCIC/ECOG
Early-stage favorable	CS I-II without risk factors (supradiaphragmatic)	CS I-II without risk factors	Standard risk group: favorable CSD I-II (without risk factors)
Early-stage unfavorable (intermediate)	CS I-II with ≥1 risk factors (supradiaphragmatic)	CS I, CSIIA ≥1 risk factors; CS IIB with C/D but without A/B	Standard risk group: unfavorable CS I-II (at least one risk factor)
Advanced stage	CS III-IV	CS IIB with A/B; CS III-IV	High risk group: CS I or II with bulky disease; intraabdominal disease; CS III, IV
Risk factors (RF)	A large mediastinal mass B age ≥50 yr C elevated ESR* D ≥4 involved regions	A large mediastinal mass B extranodal disease C elevated ESR* D ≥3 involved areas	A ≥ 40 years B not NLPHL or NS histology C ESR ≥ 50 mm/h D ≥ 4 involved nodal regions

*Erythrocyte sedimentation rate (≥50 mm/h without or ≥30 mm/h with B-symptoms).
CS, Clinical stage; *ECOG,* Eastern Cooperative Oncology Group; *EORTC,* European Organization for Research and Treatment of Cancer; *GELA,* Groupe d'Etude des Lymphomes de l'Adulte; *GHSG,* German Hodgkin Study Group; *NCIC,* National Cancer Institute of Canada.
From Hoffman R et al: *Hematology, basic principles and practice,* ed 5, New York, 2009, Churchill Livingstone.

TABLE 1-200 Recommendations for the Primary Treatment of Hodgkin's Lymphoma Outside of Clinical Trials

Group	Stage	Recommendation
Early stages (favorable)	CS I-II A/B, no RFs	2 cycles ABVD; 6 cycles EBVP; *or* VBM ± IF RT (20-30 Gy)
	Early stages (unfavorable, intermediate) CS I-II A/B + RFs	4-6 cycles ABVD; BEACOPP-baseline, Stanford V; *or* MOPP/ABV ± IF RT, 20-30Gy
Advanced stages	CS IIB + RFs, CS III A/B, CS IV A/B	6-8 cycles ABVD; MOPP/ABV; ChlVPP/EVA; BEACOPP-escalated *or* BEACOPP-14 ± RT, 20-30 Gy for residual tumor (PET positive) and/or bulk disease

ABVD regimen, Adriamycin (doxorubicin), vinblastine, bleomycin, and dacarbazine; *BEACOPP-baseline* regimen, bleomycin, etoposide, Adriamycin (doxorubicin), cyclophosphamide, Oncovin (vincristine), procarbazine, and prednisone; *BEACOPP-escalated* regimen, bleomycin, etoposide, Adriamycin (doxorubicin), cyclophosphamide, Oncovin (vincristine), procarbazine, prednisone, and G-CSF; *BEACOPP-14* regimen, bleomycin, etoposide, Adriamycin (doxorubicin), cyclophosphamide, Oncovin (vincristine), procarbazine, prednisone, and G-CSF; *ChlVPP/EVA* regimen, chlorambucil, vinblastine, procarbazine, prednisolone, etoposide, vincristine, Adriamycin (doxorubicin); *CS,* clinical stage; *EBVP* regimen, epirubicin, bleomycin, vinblastine, and prednisone; *IF,* involved field; *MOPP* regimen, mechlorethamine, Oncovin (vincristine), procarbazine, and prednisone; *PET,* positron emission tomography; *RF,* risk factors; *RT,* radiation therapy; *Stanford V* regimen, nitrogen mustard, doxorubicin, vinblastine, bleomycin, vincristine, etoposide, and prednisone; *VBM* regimen, vinblastine, bleomycin, and methotrexate.
From Hoffman R et al: *Hematology, basic principles and practice,* ed 5, New York, 2009, Churchill Livingstone.

TABLE 1-201 Prognostic Factors of Importance in Advanced Hodgkin's Lymphoma*

Gender	male
Age	>45 yr
Stage	IV
Hemoglobin	<105 g/L
White blood cell count	>15 × 10⁹/L
Lymphocyte count	<0.6 × 10⁹/L or <8% of the white cell differential
Serum albumin	<40 g/L

*Identified by the International Prognostic Factors Project on Advanced Hodgkin's Disease.
From Abeloff MD: *Clinical oncology,* ed 3, Philadelphia, 2004, Saunders.

TABLE 1-202 Second Neoplasms Seen with Increased Frequency after Successful Hodgkin's Lymphoma Treatment

Acute myelogenous leukemia/myelodysplasia
Non-Hodgkin's lymphoma
Melanoma
Soft tissue sarcoma
Adenocarcinoma
  Breast
  Thyroid
  Lung
  Stomach and esophagus
Squamous cell carcinoma
  Skin
  Uterine cervix
  Head and neck

From Abeloff MD: *Clinical oncology*, ed 3, Philadelphia, 2004, Saunders.

TABLE 1-203 Potential Late Complications of Hodgkin's Lymphoma Treatment and Appropriate Clinical Responses and Preventive Strategies

Risk/Problem	Incidence/Response
Dental caries	Neck or oropharyngeal irradiation can cause decreased salivation. Patients should have careful dental care follow-up and should make their dentist aware of the previous irradiation.
Hypothyroidism	After external beam irradiation that encompasses the thyroid with doses sufficient to cure Hodgkin's lymphoma, at least 50% of patients will eventually become hypothyroid. All patients whose TSH level becomes elevated should be treated with lifelong thyroxine replacement in doses sufficient to suppress TSH levels to low normal. This is also necessary to assure that the radiation-damaged thyroid is not subjected to long-term stimulation by thyroid-stimulating hormone, which can increase the risk of thyroid neoplasm.
Infertility	ABVD is not known to cause any permanent gonadal toxicity, although oligospermia for 1-2 yr after treatment is common. Direct or scatter radiation to gonadal tissue can cause infertility, amenorrhea, or premature menopause, but this seldom occurs with the current fields used for the treatment of Hodgkin's lymphoma. Thus, with the current chemotherapy regimens and radiation fields used, most patients will not develop these problems. In general, after treatment, women who continue menstruating are fertile, but men require semen analysis to provide a specific answer. High-dose chemoradiotherapy and hematopoietic stem cell transplantation almost always cause permanent infertility in both genders, although some young women occasionally recover fertility.
Impaired immunity to infections	Hodgkin's lymphoma and its treatment can lead to lifelong impairment of full immunity to infection. All patients should be given annual influenza immunization and pneumococcal immunization every 5 years. Patients whose spleen has been irradiated or removed should also be immunized against meningococcal types A and C and *Hemophilus influenza* type B. As for all adults, diphtheria and tetanus immunizations should be kept up-to-date.
Secondary neoplasms	Although uncommon, certain secondary neoplasms occur with increased frequency in patients who have been treated for Hodgkin's lymphoma. These include acute myelogenous leukemia, thyroid, breast, lung, and upper gastrointestinal carcinoma and melanoma and cervical carcinoma in situ. It is appropriate to screen for these neoplasms for the rest of the patient's life because they might have lengthy induction periods.

ABVD, Adriamycin, bleomycin, vinblastine, dacarbazine; *TSH,* thyroid-stimulating hormone.
From Abeloff MD: *Clinical oncology*, ed 3, Philadelphia, 2004, Saunders.

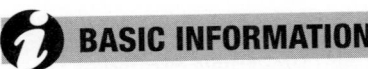

BASIC INFORMATION

DEFINITION

Hookworm is a parasitic infection of the intestine caused by helminths.

SYNONYMS

Ground itch
Ancylostoma duodenale infection
Necator americanus infection

ICD-9CM CODES
126.35 Hookworm

EPIDEMIOLOGY & DEMOGRAPHICS

INCIDENCE (IN U.S.):
- Varies greatly in different areas of the U.S.
- Most common in rural areas of southeastern U.S.
- Poor sanitation and increased rainfall increase incidence

PREVALENCE (IN U.S.): Varies from 10% to 90% in regions where it is found
PREDOMINANT AGE: Schoolchildren

PHYSICAL FINDINGS & CLINICAL PRESENTATION

- Nonspecific abdominal complaints
- Symptoms related to iron deficiency anemia depending on the amount of iron in the diet and worm burden (these organisms consume host's RBCs)
- Fatigue, tachycardia, dyspnea, and high-output failure
- Hypoproteinemia and edema from loss of proteins into the intestinal tract
- Unusual for pulmonary manifestations to occur when the larvae migrate through the lungs
- Skin rash at sites of larval penetration in some individuals without prior exposure

ETIOLOGY

Two species can cause this disease: *N. americanus* and *A. duodenale. N. americanus* is the predominant cause of hookworm in the U.S. They are soil nematodes (geohelminthic infections) that are acquired by skin contact (i.e., bare feet) with contaminated soils in moist, warm climate.
- Infection occurs via penetration of the skin by the larval form, with subsequent migration via the bloodstream to the alveoli, up the respiratory tract, then into the GI tract (Fig. 1-418)
- *Ancylostoma* spp. infection can also occur via the oral route through ingestion of contaminated water supplies
- Sharp mouth parts allow for attachment to intestinal mucosa
- *Ancylostoma* spp. are more likely to cause iron deficiency anemia because they are larger and remove more blood daily from the bowel wall than the other hookworm species, *N. americanus.*

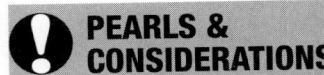

DIAGNOSIS

DIFFERENTIAL DIAGNOSIS

- Strongyloidiasis
- Ascariasis
- Other causes of iron deficiency anemia and malabsorption

WORKUP

Examine stool for hookworm eggs.

LABORATORY TESTS

CBC to show hypochromic, microcytic anemia; possible mild eosinophilia and hypoalbuminemia

IMAGING STUDIES

Chest x-ray examination: occasionally shows opacities

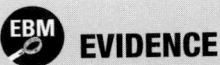

TREATMENT

NONPHARMACOLOGIC THERAPY

- Prevention of disease by not walking barefoot and by improving sanitary conditions
- Vaccines are in development.

ACUTE GENERAL Rx

- Albendazole 400 mg once PO has become preferred treatment.
- Mebendazole 100 mg PO bid for 3 days or as a 500-mg single dose
- Pyrantel pamoate 11 mg/kg (to max dose of 1 g) PO qd × 3 days
- Iron supplementation may be helpful in patients with iron deficiency.

DISPOSITION

Easily treated

REFERRAL

If diagnosis uncertain

PEARLS & CONSIDERATIONS

COMMENTS

- Appropriate disposal of human wastes is important in controlling the disease in areas with a high prevalence of hookworm infestation.
- Wearing shoes will avoid contact with contaminated soils, and the provision of safe water and sanitation for disposing human excreta is important in control of hookworm.

EVIDENCE

available at www.expertconsult.com

SUGGESTED READINGS

available at www.expertconsult.com

RELATED CONTENT

Hookworm Infection (Patient Information)

AUTHOR: **GLENN G. FORT, M.D., M.P.H.**

FIGURE 1-418 Life cycle of intestinal nematodes with a migratory phase through the lungs. Eggs are passed with stools in *Ascaris lumbricoides (A.l.), Necator americanus,* or *Ancylostoma duodenale (A.d.),* or they hatch on their way out in *Strongyloides stercoralis (S.s.).* Ascaris eggs mature in soil, and humans are infected upon ingestion of these eggs. With hookworm and strongyloidiasis, humans are infected via skin penetration by filariform larvae. In all three infections, larvae pass through a migratory phase via the lungs before reaching maturity at their final habitat in the small intestine. (From Mandell GL et al: *Principles and practice of infectious diseases,* ed 7, Philadelphia, 2010, Churchill Livingstone.)

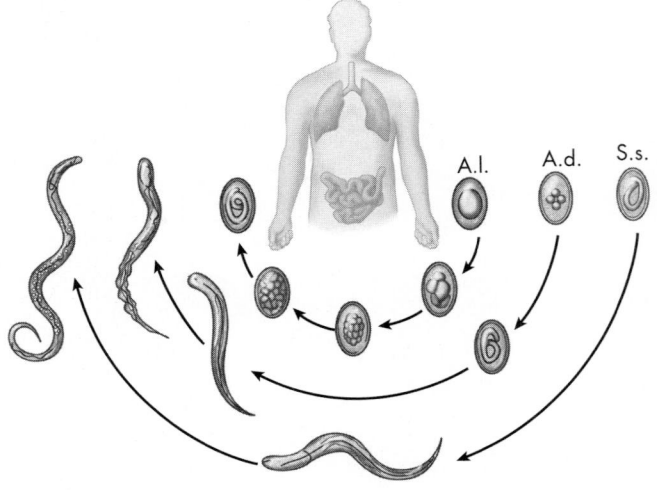

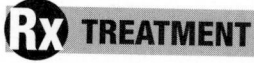

BASIC INFORMATION

DEFINITION

A hordeolum is an acute inflammatory process affecting the eyelid and arising from the meibomian (posterior) or Zeis (anterior) glands. It is most often infectious and usually caused by *Staphylococcus aureus*. When infection involves the meibomian glands, it is called meibomianitis.

SYNONYMS

Stye
Meibomianitis

ICD-9CM CODES
373.11 External hordeolum
373.12 Internal hordeolum

EPIDEMIOLOGY & DEMOGRAPHICS

INCIDENCE (IN U.S.): Unknown
PREVALENCE (IN U.S.): Unknown
PREDOMINANT SEX: No gender predilection
PREDOMINANT AGE: May occur at any age
NEONATAL INFECTION: Rare in the neonatal period
PEAK INCIDENCE: May occur at any age

PHYSICAL FINDINGS & CLINICAL PRESENTATION

- Abrupt onset with pain and erythema of the eyelid
- Localized, tender mass in the eyelid (Fig. 1-419)

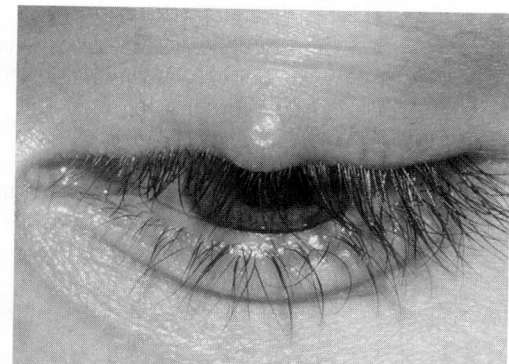

FIGURE 1-419 External stye. (From Palay D [ed]: *Ophthalmology for the primary care physician,* St Louis, 1997, Mosby.)

- May be associated with blepharitis
- External hordeolum: points toward the skin surface of the lid and may spontaneously drain
- Internal hordeolum: can point toward the conjunctival side of the lid and may cause conjunctival inflammation

ETIOLOGY

- 75% to 95% of cases are caused by *S. aureus.*
- Occasional cases are caused by *Streptococcus pneumoniae*, other streptococci, gram-negative enteric organisms, or mixed bacterial flora.

DIAGNOSIS

DIFFERENTIAL DIAGNOSIS

- Eyelid abscess
- Chalazion
- Allergy or contact dermatitis with conjunctival edema
- Acute dacryocystitis
- Herpes simplex infection
- Cellulitis of the eyelid

LABORATORY TESTS

- Generally, none are necessary.
- If incision and drainage are performed, specimens should be sent for bacterial culture.

TREATMENT

NONPHARMACOLOGIC THERAPY

External style (eyelash follicle): Usually responds to warm compresses and will drain spontaneously

ACUTE GENERAL Rx

- Systemic antibiotics generally not necessary
- For internal style, use hot packs *plus* oral dicloxacillin 500 mg qid x 7 days. If suspecting MRSA, use trimethoprim-sulfamethoxazole DS bid in place of dicloxacillin. In patients with hospital-acquired infection, consider linezolid 600 mg PO bid.
- For external style, topical erythromycin ophthalmic ointment applied to the lid margins two to four times daily until resolution may be helpful in some cases.
- Incision and drainage: rarely needed but should be considered for progressive infections

DISPOSITION

- Usually sporadic occurrence
- Possible relapse if resolution is not complete

REFERRAL

- For evaluation by an ophthalmologist if visual acuity or ocular movement is affected or if the diagnosis is in doubt
- For surgical drainage if necessary

PEARLS & CONSIDERATIONS

COMMENTS

Seborrheic dermatitis may coexist with hordeolum.

SUGGESTED READINGS

available at www.expertconsult.com

RELATED CONTENT

Stye (Hordeolum) (Patient Information)

AUTHOR: **GLENN G. FORT, M.D., M.P.H.**

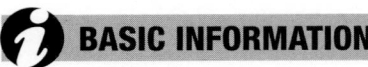

DEFINITION

Horner's syndrome is the clinical triad of ipsilateral ptosis, miosis, and sometimes facial anhidrosis. Disruption of any of the three neurons in the oculosympathetic pathway (central, preganglionic, or postganglionic) can cause Horner's syndrome.

SYNONYMS

Oculosympathetic paresis
Raeder's paratrigeminal syndrome: Horner's syndrome of the postganglionic neuron associated with pain in the trigeminal nerve distribution

ICD-9CM CODES
337.9 Horner's syndrome

EPIDEMIOLOGY & DEMOGRAPHICS

Congenital or acquired

PHYSICAL FINDINGS & CLINICAL PRESENTATION

- Ptosis is usually mild. It results from loss of sympathetic tone to Müller's muscle, which contributes approximately 2 mm of upper eyelid elevation. Weakness of the corresponding muscle in the lower eyelid causes it to elevate slightly. This combination causes narrowing of the palpebral fissure. Levator function of the eyelid is preserved.
- Miosis results from loss of sympathetic innervation to the iris dilator muscle (Fig. 1-420). The affected pupil reacts normally to bright light and accommodation. Anisocoria is greater in dim light.
  - Dilation lag: Horner's pupil dilates more slowly than the normal pupil when lights are dimmed (20 vs. 5 sec) because it dilates passively as a result of relaxation of the iris sphincter.
- Presence of facial anhidrosis is variable and depends on the site of injury. It occurs with lesions affecting central or preganglionic neurons.
- Congenital Horner's syndrome may result in heterochromia. The affected eye has a lighter colored iris.
- Acute cases may also present with conjunctival injection from the loss of sympathetic vasoconstriction.

ETIOLOGY

Disruption of the ipsilateral sympathetic innervation to the eye and face. Lesions can damage any of the three neurons in the oculosympathetic pathway. Central lesions are least common but are usually caused by pathology in the hypothalamus, brainstem, or cervicothoracic spinal cord. Preganglionic lesions are often caused by disease involving the paravertebral cervical spinal cord, lung apex, or anterior neck. Postganglionic lesions are usually seen with disease in the internal carotid artery, skull base, cavernous sinus, or orbital apex. Location is often suggested by the presence of associated findings. Vascular disease and neoplasms must be considered.

Mechanical:
- Syringomyelia
- Trauma
- Tumors: benign, malignant (thyroid, apical lung, mediastinal)
- Lymphadenopathy
- Neurofibromatosis
- Cervical rib

Vascular (ischemia, hemorrhage or arteriovenous malformation):
- Brainstem lesion: commonly occlusion of the posterior inferior cerebellar artery but other arteries may be responsible (vertebral; superior, middle or inferior lateral medullary arteries; superior or anterior inferior cerebellar arteries)
- Carotid artery aneurysm or dissection. Can also be from injury to other major vessels (internal carotid artery, subclavian artery, ascending aorta)
- Cavernous sinus thrombosis
- Cluster headache, migraine

Miscellaneous:
- Idiopathic
- Congenital
- Demyelination (multiple sclerosis)
- Infection (apical tuberculosis, herpes zoster, Lyme disease)
- Myelitis
- Pneumothorax
- Iatrogenic (angiography, internal jugular/subclavian catheter, chest tube, neck or upper thoracic surgery, epidural spinal anesthesia)

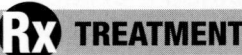 DIAGNOSIS

DIFFERENTIAL DIAGNOSIS

Causes of anisocoria (unequal pupils):
- Normal variant
- Mydriatic use
- Prosthetic eye
- Prior eye surgery
- Unilateral cataract
- Iritis

Causes of ptosis are described in Section II.

WORKUP

History, physical examination, pharmacologic testing, imaging

PHARMACOLOGIC TESTING

- Topical cocaine test: confirms sympathetic denervation (drops dilate normal pupil but not Horner's pupil)
- Topical apraclonidine test: confirms diagnosis (drops reverse anisocoria by causing dilation of Horner's pupil and constriction of normal pupil)
- Topical hydroxyamphetamine test: distinguishes central and preganglionic from postganglionic sympathetic lesions (drops dilate normal pupil and central or preganglionic Horner's pupil, but not postganglionic Horner's pupil)

IMAGING STUDIES

Results of pharmacologic testing as well as accompanying signs and symptoms should guide imaging:
- MRI brain: brainstem (diplopia, vertigo, ataxia); cavernous sinus (eye movement abnormalities, sixth nerve palsy)
- MRI cervical and upper thoracic spinal cord: weakness of extremities, bowel/bladder dysfunction
- MR angiography (or ultrasound, CT angiography): carotid artery dissection (acute Horner's syndrome with face or neck pain)
- CT chest and neck: evaluate lung apex, perivertebral areas, mediastinum if symptoms do not localize to the central nervous system; brachial plexus lesion (arm/hand pain or weakness)

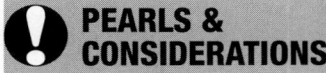 TREATMENT

- Treatment depends on underlying cause.
- Ptosis can be surgically corrected or treated with medication (phenylephrine drops).

DISPOSITION

- Prognosis depends on underlying cause.
- Horner's syndrome is an uncommon presentation for malignancy.
- In one study, 40% of cases were idiopathic.

REFERRAL

Ophthalmologist for pharmacologic testing to confirm diagnosis and localize lesion.

! PEARLS & CONSIDERATIONS

- May be the presentation of a life-threatening condition.
- Anisocoria greater in bright light is likely caused by a defect in parasympathetic innervation, and anisocoria greater in dim light is likely caused by a sympathetic defect.
- Normal variant anisocoria:
  - Occurs in 20% of people
  - Usually <1-mm difference between pupils; more apparent in darkness
  - Pupils are round and display a normal, brisk constriction and dilation response to light

SUGGESTED READINGS
available at www.expertconsult.com

RELATED CONTENT
Lung Neoplasms, Primary (Related Key Topic)
Horner's Syndrome (Patient Information)

AUTHOR: **SUDEEP KAUR AULAKH, M.D.**

FIGURE 1-420 Horner's syndrome. The mild ptosis (1 to 2 mm) and the smaller pupil (in room light) can be seen on the affected right side. (From Palay D [ed]: *Ophthalmology for the primary care physician,* St Louis, 1997, Mosby.)

BASIC INFORMATION

DEFINITION

Hot flashes are sudden onset of intense warmth that begins in the neck or face, or in the chest and progresses to the neck and face; often associated with profuse sweating, anxiety, and palpitations.

ICD-9CM CODES
627.2 Hot flashes

EPIDEMIOLOGY & DEMOGRAPHICS

- Hot flashes affect 75% of postmenopausal women.
- Most hot flashes begin 1 to 2 yr before menopause and resolve after 2 yr.
- 15% of women report duration of hot flashes >15 yr.

PHYSICAL FINDINGS & CLINICAL PRESENTATION

- Profuse sweating and red blotching of skin may be noted during the vasomotor event.
- Palpitations and hyperreflexia may be present during the hot flash.
- Hot flashes typically last 1 to 5 min.
- Each hot flash is associated with increase in temperature, increased pulse rate, and increased blood flow into the hands and face.
- Hot flashes during sleep are common and are referred to as *night sweats*.
- There is considerable variation in the frequency of hot flashes. One third of women report more than 10 flashes per day.

ETIOLOGY

- Dysfunction of central thermoregulatory centers caused by changes in estrogen level at the time of menopause
- Tamoxifen use
- Chemotherapy-induced ovarian failure
- Androgen ablation therapy for prostate carcinoma

DIAGNOSIS

DIFFERENTIAL DIAGNOSIS

- Carcinoid syndrome
- Anxiety disorder
- Idiopathic flushing
- Lymphoma (night sweats)
- Hyperthyroidism
- Hyperhidrosis

WORKUP

Evaluation of hot flashes is aimed at excluding the conditions listed in the differential diagnosis.

LABORATORY TESTS

- Follicle-stimulating hormone (FSH), luteinizing hormone, estradiol level. The serum FSH levels rather than estradiol levels are associated with greater severity of hot flashes in older postmenopausal women, suggesting that nonestrogen feedback systems may be important in modulating the severity of hot flashes. It is not necessary to obtain an FSH to make the diagnosis of menopausal status, however. An amenorrheic woman over age 50 with vasomotor symptoms is assumed to have made the menopausal transition and serum markers of menopause are not required to complete the diagnosis.
- Thyroid-stimulating hormone (TSH).

TREATMENT

NONPHARMACOLOGIC THERAPY

- Behavioral interventions such as relaxation training and paced respiration have been reported effective in reducing symptoms in some women.
- Avoidance of caffeine, alcohol, tobacco, and spicy foods may be beneficial.

GENERAL Rx

- Estrogen replacement therapy reduces hot flashes by 80% to 90%. Estrogen therapy, however, is contraindicated in many women, and others are fearful of its use. Potential risks and side effects should be considered before using estrogen in any patient. When using estrogen, it is best to use low-dose (e.g., Prempro [conjugated equine estrogen 0.45 mg or 0.3 mg plus medroxyprogesterone 1.5 mg]). Femring is an intravaginal ring that is changed every 3 mo and approved to treat vasomotor symptoms in women who have had a hysterectomy. It provides both local and systemic estrogen.
- Megestrol acetate, a progestational agent, is a safer alternative to estrogen in women with a history of receptor-positive breast or uterine cancer and in men receiving androgen ablation therapy for prostate cancer. Usual dose is 20 mg bid.
- The antidepressant venlafaxine has been reported to be 60% effective in reducing hot flashes and represents an alternative treatment modality in women unable or unwilling to use estrogens. Starting dose is 37.5 mg qd, increased as tolerated up to a maximum of 300 mg/day. Other antidepressants such as desvenlafaxine and escitalopram have also been shown to be effective in reducing the number and severity of menopausal hot flashes. A recent trial showed that paroxetine is an effective agent for diminishing hot flashes in men receiving androgen ablation therapy.
- The anticonvulsant gabapentin (300 to 1200 mg/day) represents another nonhormonal alternative in the treatment of hot flashes and can be used alone or in combination with venlafaxine.
- The antihypertensive clonidine is also somewhat effective in reducing the frequency of hot flashes in mild cases. Adverse effects include dry mouth, sedation, and dizziness.
- Vitamin E (800 IU/day) may be effective in patients with mild symptoms that do not interfere with sleep or daily function.
- Soy protein (use of soy extracts that contain plant-derived estrogens [phytoestrogens]) is often used; however, clinical trials have not shown clear efficacy.
- Several classes of herbal remedies are available to patients and are commonly used, generally without significant benefit. Frequently used agents are *Cimicifuga racemosa* (black cohosh, snakeroot, bugbane), *Angelica sinensis,* and evening primrose (evening star). Recent trials using the isopropanolic extract of black cohosh rootstock (Remefemin) did show some improvement in controlling menopausal symptoms. Such alternative medications may be used to treat mild to moderate symptoms, but it is possible that symptomatic improvements may derive in part from a placebo effect.

SUGGESTED READINGS
available at www.expertconsult.com

RELATED CONTENT
Menopause (Related Key Topic)
Hot Flashes (Patient Information)

AUTHOR: **FRED F. FERRI, M.D.**

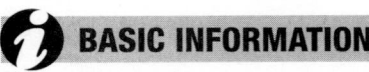

BASIC INFORMATION

DEFINITION

The human immunodeficiency virus, type 1 (HIV) is a retrovirus that is responsible for causing acquired immunodeficiency syndrome (AIDS).

SYNONYMS

AIDS: when a patient with HIV infection meets specific diagnostic criteria (See "Acquired Immunodeficiency Syndrome" in Section I.)

ICD-9CM CODES
042.9 HIV, unspecified

EPIDEMIOLOGY & DEMOGRAPHICS

INCIDENCE (IN U.S.):
- In 2009 there were an estimated 48,100 new HIV infections.
- Greatest incidence is in men who have sex with men (MSM) and minority populations.

PREVALENCE (IN U.S.): Approximately 1.1 million people were living with HIV in the United States at the end of 2006.

PREDOMINANT SEX:
- Adults: males accounted for more than 75% of new infections in 2009.
- Children: male = female

RACIAL DATA:
- In 2009, the rate of new HIV infections in black males was 103.9 new infections per 100,000 vs 15.9 per 100,000 for white men.
- In 2009, the rate of new HIV infections in black females was 39.7 per 100,000 vs 2.6 per 100,000 for white women.
- In 2009, the rate of new HIV infections in Hispanic males was 39.9 per 100,000 vs. 11.8 per 100,000 for Hispanic women.

PEAK INCIDENCE: About half of new infections in 2009 were in patients ages 25 to 44 years. 61% of all new cases were in MSM, 27% were from heterosexual transmission, and 9% from intravenous drug use.

GENETICS:

Familial Disposition:
Individuals with deletions in the *CCR5* gene are immune from infection with macrophage tropic virus (the predominant virus in sexual transmission). Other genetic variants may contribute to rapid progression or long-term control of the virus once infected.

Congenital Infection:
- 80% of childhood cases are caused by peripartum infection, which may occur in utero, during delivery, or after delivery via breastfeeding.
- No specific congenital abnormalities are associated with HIV infection, although risk of spontaneous abortion and low birth weight is greater.

Neonatal Infection:
- May occur during delivery or via breastfeeding
- Typically asymptomatic

PHYSICAL FINDINGS & CLINICAL PRESENTATION

- Signs and symptoms are variable with stage of disease.

- Acute HIV infection (0-3 mo, usually several wk):
  1. May cause a self-limited mononucleosis-like illness in 50% to 80% of individuals characterized by fever, sore throat, lymphadenopathy, headache, and a rash resembling roseola. Individuals may also be asymptomatic.
  2. In a minority of acute cases, aseptic meningitis, Bell's palsy, or peripheral neuropathy may occur.
  3. Rarely, opportunistic infections such as thrush or *Pneumocystis jiroveci* pneumonia (PJP) may occur.
- Chronic HIV infection is usually characterized by a prolonged asymptomatic phase followed by nonspecific symptoms of lymphadenopathy, weight loss, diarrhea, and skin changes including seborrheic dermatitis, localized herpes zoster, and/or fungal infection.
- Advanced disease is characterized by the infections and malignancies associated with AIDS (see specific disorders).
- HIV infection in women may be associated with lower levels of viral load at comparable degrees of immunosuppression when compared with men. Furthermore, women may, on average, have higher CD4 lymphocyte counts at the time of AIDS diagnosis.
- Another special consideration in women infected with HIV is the high incidence of human papillomavirus (HPV) coinfection and the risk for cervical neoplasm that this presents. Even women with normal Pap smears should have this test repeated after 6 months and annually thereafter.
- Coinfection with HIV and hepatitis C is common because of common transmission risk. Patients with HIV and hepatitis C progress faster to cirrhosis. Patients may already have signs of advanced liver disease at the time of diagnosis.

ETIOLOGY

- HIV-1 is a single-stranded RNA retrovirus (Fig. 1-421) that was derived from transmission of a simian immunodeficiency virus (SIV) from chimpanzees in Central Africa; a related virus, HIV-2 was derived from an SIV found in sooty mangabey monkeys from West Africa.
- HIV-1 is the predominant pathogenic retrovirus in human populations; HIV-2 has limited distribution (primarily in West Africa) and tends to be less rapidly immunosuppressive than HIV-1.
- HIV-1 is transmitted by sexual contact, shared needles, blood transfusion, or from mother to child during pregnancy, delivery, or breastfeeding.
- Primary target of infection: CD4 lymphocyte.
- Direct central nervous system (CNS) involvement: manifests as encephalopathy, myelopathy, or neuropathy in advanced cases.

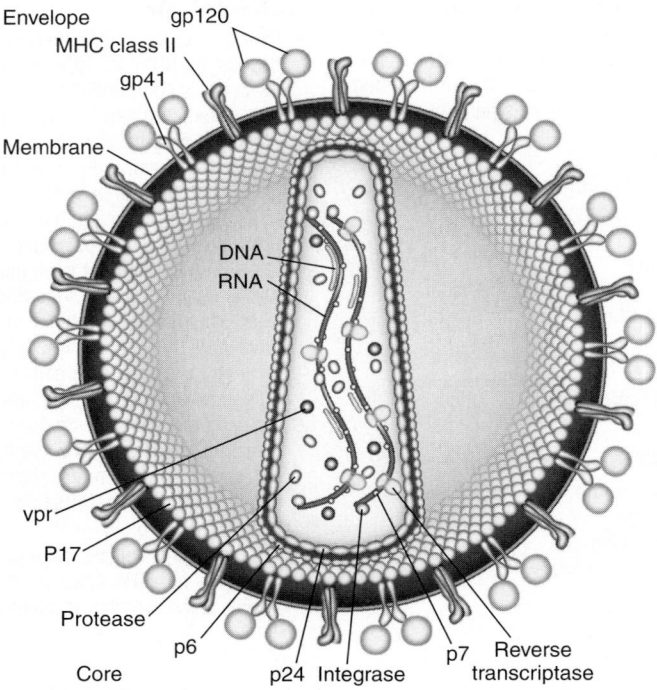

FIGURE 1-421 Structure of the HIV-1 virion. The viral envelope is formed from the host cell membrane, into which the HIV-1 envelope proteins gp41 and gp120 have been inserted and may include several host cell proteins, most significantly the major histocompatibility complex class II proteins. The matrix between the envelope and the core is formed predominantly from gag protein p17. The core contains the viral RNA, closely associated with gag protein p7, in addition to RT and integrase. It has also been proven that virions contain complementary DNA, as shown, synthesized by the RT. The major structural proteins of the core are gag proteins p24 and p6. Also present within the virion are the protease and two cleavage products from the gag precursor protein (p1 and p2, not shown) of undetermined position within the virion is also packaged in the virion and is thought to be localized within the core, as shown. (From Mandell GL et al: *Principles and practice of infectious diseases*, ed 7, Philadelphia, 2010, Saunders.)

- Renal failure, rheumatologic disorders, thrombocytopenia, or cardiac abnormalities may be seen in association with HIV-1.

DIAGNOSIS

DIFFERENTIAL DIAGNOSIS

- Acute HIV infection: mononucleosis or other respiratory viral infections
- Late symptoms: similar to those produced by other wasting illnesses such as neoplasms, tuberculosis (TB), disseminated fungal infection (such as *Candida*), malabsorption, or depression
- HIV-related encephalopathy: confused with Alzheimer's disease or other causes of chronic dementia (cognitive impairment in HIV infection is described in Section II); myelopathy and neuropathy possibly resembling other demyelinating diseases such as multiple sclerosis

WORKUP

Since the debut of HIV/AIDS in the 1980s, diagnosis has been established by testing for antibodies to the virus. An algorithm for HIV detection in patients at risk for HIV infection is described in Fig. E1-422. The CDC is now recommending routine testing for patients in all health care settings unless the patient declines (opt-out screening). This includes routine testing of pregnant women. It is also recommended that separate written consent should no longer be required, although by law this

is being addressed on a state-by-state basis. Generally, all persons aged 13-64 should undergo HIV testing at least once unless the prevalence in the specific population is <0.1%.

- An FDA-approved at-home rapid HIV screening test is now available. It uses swabs of oral fluids from upper and lower gums. A positive test requires confirmatory testing in the office. Negative home tests should be repeated within 3 mo.

LABORATORY TESTS

HIV antibodies are detected by a two-step technique:

- ELISA (enzyme-linked immunosorbent assay), which is a sensitive screening test.
- Confirmation of positive ELISA tests with the more specific Western blot technique.
- ELISA antibody tests will measure HIV-1 and HIV-2 antibodies. The reflex Western blot will only look for HIV-1 proteins. If HIV-2 is suspected (i.e., the individual or sex partners are from Western Africa), a separate HIV-2 Western blot should be ordered.
- Baseline viral resistance testing is recommended for all newly diagnosed patients with HIV to guide choice of antiretroviral therapy (ART).
- The CD4 count and HIV RNA polymerase chain reaction (PCR) should be measured in all patients.
- The CD4 count is a marker of current immune status.

- The HIV RNA PCR (viral load) is predictive of disease progression.
- Rapid serologic tests have been increasingly used and are useful in specific settings: occupational exposures, pregnant women in labor without previous testing, and patients in high seroprevalence areas (for immediate results). Specimens are either blood or saliva and results are given within 20 min. Although sensitivity is high (99.1% to 99.7%), false-positive tests are more common in low seroprevalence populations. Thus, all positive results must be confirmed with standard serology, including Western blot.
- Early during infection (i.e., acute HIV infection), standard antibody tests may be negative ("window period"). The standard for diagnosing HIV during acute HIV infection is by testing for HIV RNA (viral load).

Fig. 1-423 describes the immunologic response to HIV infection.

TREATMENT

NONPHARMACOLOGIC THERAPY
Maintenance of adequate nutrition

ACUTE GENERAL Rx
Acute management of opportunistic infections and malignancies (see AIDS-associated disorders, "*Pneumocystis carinii* (now *P. jirovecii*) Pneumonia," "Cryptococcosis," "Tuberculosis," "Toxoplasmosis" elsewhere in this text.)

CHRONIC Rx
All HIV infected patients should be considered for ART regardless of CD4 cell count. The benefit of ART is well established in preventing progression to AIDS and associated comorbidities. Table 1-204 describes HIV treatment guidelines of the Department of Health and Human Services (DHHS) (www.aidsinfo.nih.gov/guidelines). Other considerations for initiation of antiretroviral therapy are described in Table 1-205. Prophylaxis to prevent first episode of HIV-related opportunistic disease is described in Table 1-206.

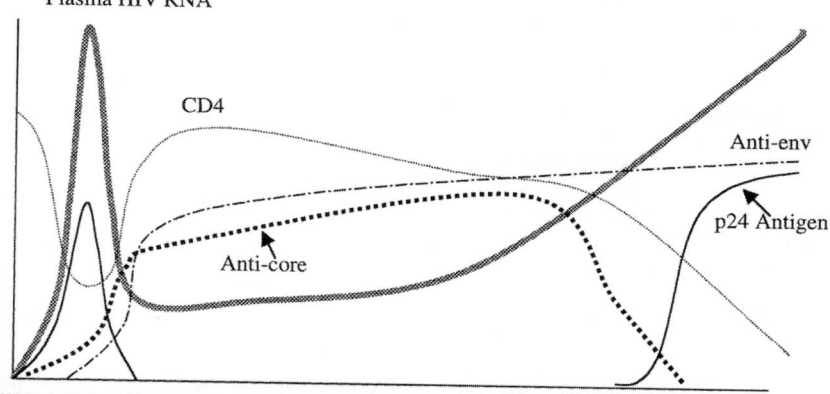

Plasma HIV RNA

FIGURE 1-423 Course of human immunodeficiency virus infection. (From Mandell GL [ed]: *Mandell, Douglas, and Bennett's principles and practice of infectious diseases*, ed 6, New York, 2005, Churchill Livingstone.)

TABLE 1-204 When to Initiate Antiretroviral Therapy (ART) in Treatment-Naïve Patients

ART should be initiated in all patients with a history of an AIDS-defining illness or with a CD4 count of <350 cells/mm³ (AI).
ART is also recommended for patients with CD4 counts between 350 and 500 cells/mm³ (AII).
ART is recommended for patients with CD4 counts greater than 500 cell/mm³ (BIII).
ART should also be initiated, regardless of CD4 count, in patients with the following conditions: HIV-associated nephropathy (HIVAN) and HBV coinfection when treatment of HBV is indicated (AII).
A combination ARV drug regimen is also recommended for pregnant women who are not otherwise on treatment, with the goal to prevent perinatal transmission (AI).
Patients initiating ART should be willing and able to commit to lifelong treatment and should understand the benefits and risks of therapy and the importance of adherence.
Patients may choose to postpone therapy, and providers, on a case-by-case basis, may elect to defer therapy based on clinical and/or psychosocial factors.

Modified from Panel on Antiretroviral Guidelines for Adults and Adolescents. Guidelines for the use of antiretroviral agents in HIV-1–infected adults and adolescents. Department of Health and Human Services. March 27, 2012. http://www.aidsinfo.nih.gov/ContentFiles/AdultandAdolescentGL.pdf.

TABLE 1-205 Conditions Favoring More Rapid Initiation of Antiretroviral Therapy

Pregnancy
AIDS-defining conditions
Acute opportunistic infections
Lower CD4 counts (e.g., <200 cells/mm³)
Rapidly declining CD4 counts (e.g., >100 cells/mm³ decrease per year)
Higher viral loads (e.g., >100,000 copies/ml)
HIV-associated nephropathy
Hepatitis B virus (HBV) coinfection when treatment for HBV is indicated

Modified from Panel on Antiretroviral Guidelines for Adults and Adolescents. Guidelines for the use of antiretroviral agents in HIV-1–infected adults and adolescents. Department of Health and Human Services. March 27, 2012. http://www.aidsinfo.nih.gov/ContentFiles/AdultandAdolescentGL.pdf.

TABLE 1-206 Prophylaxis to Prevent First Episode of HIV-related Opportunistic Disease

Pathogen	Indication	First Choice	Alternative
Pneumocystis jiroveci pneumonia (PJP, previsouly referred to as Pneumocystis carinii, PCP)	CD4$^+$ count <200 cells/mm^3 or oropharyngeal candidiasis CD4$^+$ <14% or history of AIDS-defining illness CD4$^+$ count >200 but <250 cells/mm^3 if monitoring CD4$^+$ count every 1-3 mo is not possible	Trimethoprim-sulfamethoxazole (TMP-SMX) 1 double-strength PO daily; or 1 single-strength daily	TMP-SMX 1 double-strength PO 3 times weekly; or Dapsone 100 mg PO daily or 50 mg PO bid; or Dapsone 50 mg PO daily + pyrimethamine 50 mg PO weekly + leucovorin 25 mg PO weekly; or Aerosolized pentamidine 300 mg via Respirgard II nebulizer every month; or Atovaquone 1500 mg PO daily; or Tovaquone 1500 mg + pyrimethamine 25 mg + leucovorin 10 mg PO daily
Toxoplasma gondii encephalitis	Toxoplasma IgG–positive patients with CD4$^+$ count <100 cells/mm^3 Seronegative patients receiving PCP prophylaxis not active against toxoplasmosis should have Toxoplasma serology retested if CD4$^+$ count declines to <100 cells/mm^3. Prophylaxis should be initiated if seroconversion occurred.	TMP-SMX, 1 double-strength PO daily	TMP-SMX 1 double-strength PO 3 times weekly; or TMP-SMX 1 single-strength PO daily; Dapsone 50 mg PO daily + pyrimethamine 50 mg PO weekly + leucovorin 25 mg PO weekly; or (Dapsone 200 mg + pyrimethamine 75 mg + leucovorin 25 mg) PO weekly; (Atovaquone 1500 mg ± pyrimethamine 25 mg + leucovorin 10 mg) PO daily
Mycobacterium tuberculosis infection (TB) (treatment of latent TB infection or LTBI)	(+) diagnostic test for LTBI, no evidence of active TB, and no prior history of treatment for active or latent TB (−) diagnostic test for LTBI, but close contact with a person with infectious pulmonary TB and no evidence of active TB A history of untreated or inadequately treated healed TB (i.e., old fibrotic lesions) regardless of diagnostic tests for LTBI and no evidence of active TB	Isoniazid (INH) 300 mg PO daily or 900 mg PO twice weekly for 9 mo—both plus pyridoxine 50 mg PO daily; or For persons exposed to drug-resistant TB, selection of drugs after consultation with public health authorities	Rifampin (RIF) 600 mg PO daily × 4 mo; or Rifabutin (RFB) (dose adjusted based on concomitant antiretroviral therapy) × 4 mo
Disseminated Mycobacterium avium complex (MAC) disease	CD4$^+$ count <50 cells/mm^3—after ruling out active MAC infection	Azithromycin 1200 mg PO once weekly; or Clarithromycin 500 mg PO bid; or Azithromycin 600 mg PO twice weekly	RFB 300 mg PO daily (dosage adjustment based on drug-drug interactions with antiretroviral therapy); rule out active TB before starting RFB
Streptococcus pneumoniae infection	CD4$^+$ count >200 cells/mm^3 and no receipt of pneumococcal vaccine in the past 5 yr CD4$^+$ count <200 cells/mm^3—vaccination can be offered In patients who received polysaccharide pneumococcal vaccination (PPV) when CD4$^+$ count <200 cells/mm^3 but has increased to >200 cells/mm^3 in response to antiretroviral therapy	23-valent PPV 0.5 ml IM × 1 Revaccination every 5 yr may be considered	
Influenza A and B virus infection	All HIV-infected patients	Inactivated influenza vaccine 0.5 ml IM annually	
Histoplasma capsulatum infection	CD4$^+$ count ≤150 cells/mm^3 and at high risk because of occupational exposure or live in a community with a hyperendemic rate of histoplasmosis (>10 cases/100 patient-yr)	Itraconazole 200 mg PO daily	
Coccidioidomycosis	Positive IgM or IgG serologic test result in a patient from a disease-endemic area; and CD4$^+$ count <250 cells/mm^3	Fluconazole 400 mg PO daily Itraconazole 200 mg PO bid	
Varicella-zoster virus (VZV) infection	Pre-exposure prevention: Patients with CD4$^+$ count ≥200 cells/mm^3 who have not been vaccinated, have no history of varicella or herpes zoster, or who are seronegative for VZV Note: Routine VZV serologic testing in HIV-infected adults is not recommended. Postexposure—close contact with a person who has active varicella or herpes zoster: For susceptible patients (those who have no history of vaccination or of either condition, or are known to be VZV seronegative)	Pre-exposure prevention: Primary varicella vaccination (Varivax), 2 doses (0.5 ml SC administered 3 mo apart If vaccination results in disease because of vaccine virus, treatment with acyclovir is recommended. Postexposure therapy: Varicella-zoster immune globulin (VariZIG) 125 IU per 10 kg (maximum of 625 IU) IM, administered within 96 hr after exposure to a person with active varicella or herpes zoster Note: As of June 2007, VariZIG can be obtained only under a treatment IND (1-800-843-7477, FFF Enterprises).	VZV-susceptible household contacts of susceptible HIV-infected persons should be vaccinated to prevent potential transmission of VZV to their HIV-infected contacts. Alternative postexposure therapy: Postexposure varicella vaccine (Varivax) 0.5 ml SC × 2 doses, 3 mo apart if CD4$^+$ count >200 cells/mm^3; or Preemptive acyclovir 800 mg PO 5×/day for 5 days These two alternatives have not been studied in the HIV population.

Modified from Centers for Disease Control and Prevention. Guidelines for Prevention and treatment of opportunistic infections in HIV-infected adults and adolescents: Recommendations from CDC, the National Institutes of Health, and the HIV Medicine Association of the Infectious Disease Society of America, *MMWR Morb Mortal Wkly Rep* 58(RR-4), 2009.

Continued on following page

TABLE 1-206 Prophylaxis to Prevent First Episode of HIV-related Opportunistic Disease *(Continued)*

Pathogen	Indication	First Choice	Alternative
Human papillomavirus (HPV) infection	Women aged 11-26 yr. Men aged 11-21 yr	HPV quadrivalent vaccine 0.5 ml IM mo 0, 2, and 6	
Hepatitis A virus (HAV) infection	HAV-susceptible patients with chronic liver disease or who are injection-drug users, or men who have sex with men. Certain specialists might delay vaccination until CD4$^+$ count >200 cells/mm^3.	Hepatitis A vaccine 1 ml IM × 2 doses—at 0 and 6-12 mo IgG antibody response should be assessed 1 mo after vaccination; nonresponders should be revaccinated	
Hepatitis B virus (HBV) infection	All HIV patients without evidence of prior exposure to HBV should be vaccinated with HBV vaccine, including patients with CD4$^+$ count <200 cells/mm^3. *Patients with isolated anti-HBc:* (consider screening for HBV DNA before vaccination to rule out occult chronic HBV infection)	Hepatitis B vaccine IM (Engerix-B 20 μg/ml or Recombivax HB 10 μg/ml) at 0, 1, and 6 mo Anti-HBs should be obtained 1 mo after completion of the vaccine series.	Some experts recommend vaccinating with 40-μg doses of either vaccine.
	Vaccine nonresponders: Defined as anti-HBs <10 IU/ml 1 mo after a vaccination series For patients with low CD4$^+$ count at the time of first vaccination series, certain specialists might delay revaccination until after a sustained increase in CD4$^+$ count with antiretroviral therapy.	Revaccinate with a second vaccine series.	Some experts recommend revaccinating with 40-μg doses of either vaccine.

- Therapy is strongly recommended for all patients with symptomatic established HIV disease regardless of the CD4 count. Symptomatic HIV disease is defined as the presence of any of the following: thrush, vaginal candidiasis, herpes zoster, peripheral neuropathy, bacillary angiomatosis, cervical dysplasia in situ, constitutional symptoms such as fever or diarrhea for more than 1 month, ITP, PID, or listeriosis.
- In asymptomatic individuals, ART is now recommended regardless of CD4 cell counts. The updated recommendations are due to the safety and benefit of newer antivirals in preventing AIDS and decreasing both morbidity and mortality. Earlier treatment may also help reduce transmission of the virus to others due to reductions in viral loads.
- ART generally consists of using a 3-drug regimen to treat HIV-1 infection. Classes of antiretrovirals include:
  1. Nucleoside/nucleotide reverse transcriptase inhibitor (NRTI): zidovudine (AZT), lamivudine (3TC), emtricitabine (FTC), tenofovir (TDF), abacavir (ABC), stavudine (D4T), or didanosine (DDI).
  2. Protease inhibitors (PI): lopinavir/ritonavir, atazanavir, fosamprenavir, darunavir, saquinavir, amprenavir, tipranavir, nelfinavir, and indinavir. These PIs may be "boosted" by ritonavir to increase levels.
  3. Nonnucleoside reverse transcriptase inhibitors (NNRTI): Nevirapine, efavirenz, etravirine, delavirdine, or rilpivirine.
  4. Integrase Inhibitors (II): Raltegravir, elvitegravir, and dolutegravir. Raltegravir is a first-line agent according to the DHHS guidelines.
  5. Fusion Inhibitors: Enfuvirtide (T-20). This drug is administered through subcutaneous injections and is only used as part of a salvage regimen for individuals who have failed multiple other regimens.
  6. CCR5 Inhibitors: Maraviroc. Before using this drug, a viral trophism assay should be

checked to determine if the virus uses the CCR5 co-receptor to infect cells. If the virus uses the CXCR4 co-receptor, this drug will not be effective. Adding a fourth drug to the three-drug regimen does not improve viral suppression or outcomes and is not recommended. Treatment interruptions based upon CD4 responses appear harmful in recent comparative studies versus standard continuous treatment protocols and should be avoided. Antiretroviral regimens for initial therapy are summarized in Table 1-207.
- Usual initial dosing regimen consists of two NRTIs and either a NNRTI, PI, or II. Data support inclusion of lamivudine or emtricitabine as one of the two NRTIs.

Standard NRTIs include:
- Truvada (tenofovir/emtricitabine) 1 tablet once daily.
  ○ Tenofovir: Individuals with underlying renal dysfunction or requiring other nephrotoxic agents may be at increased risk of renal toxicity.
  ○ Epzicom (abacavir/lamivudine) 1 tablet once daily
- Abacavir: association with increased risk of myocardial infarction. Before using this drug, individuals should be checked for having HLA-B*5701. Individuals with this allele are at higher risk of serious hypersentivity reactions and this drug should be avoided.
  ○ Combivir (Zidovudine/lamivudine) 1 tablet twice daily
  ○ Zidovudine: Associated with lipoatrophy and anemia. GI and CNS side effects.

Standard Backbone Regimens include:
- NNRTIs
  ○ Efavirenz 600 mg daily: not recommended for women in the first trimester or those who are contemplating pregnancy. This is considered the preferred agent within the class.
  ○ Nevirapine 200 mg two times a day: avoid with CD4 count >250 in men and >350 in women because of the risk of hepatitis.

The newer agent rilpivirine had higher virologic failures and should be considered an alternative agent.
  ○ Etravirine 200 mg two times a day: This drug is generally used in patients that have failed other regimens. Etravirine retains activity in many patients that have developed resistance against efavirenz and nevirapine.
- PIs (ritonavir boosted)
  ○ Lopinavir/ritonavir (200 mg/50 mg) 2 tablets twice a day (or 4 tablets once a day): most likely to cause diarrhea and has the greatest negative effect on triglyceride levels.
  ○ Atazanavir and ritonavir (300 mg and 100 mg) 2 tablets a day: lower pill burden, but use with caution with acid reducing agents—can alter absorption. This is considered a preferred PI regimen within the DHHS guidelines.
  ○ Fosamprenavir and ritonavir (700 mg and 100 mg) 2 tablets twice a day (or 4 tablets once a day): cannot take fosamprenavir with sulfa allergy.
  ○ Darunavir and ritonavir: 800 mg and 100 mg a day. This is considered a preferred PI regimen within the DHHS guidelines.
  ○ Saquinavir and ritonavir.
- All these drugs have their own unique, as well as class-specific, side effects and require careful follow-up to achieve optimal antiviral effects. Compliance with the drug regimen and tolerance of common side effects are critically important to maintain drug efficacy. Antiviral response should be monitored by baseline HIV viral load and CD4 count and repeat measurement at 2 and 4 wk into treatment and then periodically (every 3 mo) to ensure viral suppression.
- All patients should have genotypic resistance testing upon entry into medical care and before initiation of ART.
- Later, an antiretroviral regimen should be constructed based on past antiretroviral

TABLE 1-207 What Antiretroviral Regimen to Choose for Initial Therapy

Preferred Regimens	Comments
NNRTI-based regimen EFV/TDF/FTC	EFV should not be used during the first trimester of pregnancy or in women trying to conceive or not using effective and consistent contraception.
PI-based regimens (in alphabetical order) ATV/r + TDF/FTC DRV/r (once daily) + TDF/FTC	ATV/r should not be used in patients who are on proton pump inhibitors or other antacids.
Integrase inhibitor-based regimen RAL + TDF/FTC	
Preferred regimen for pregnant women LPV/r (twice daily) + ZDV/3TC	

Alternative Regimens	Comments
NNRTI-based regimens (in alphabetical order) EFV + ABC/3TC RPV/TDF/FTC RPV + ABC/3TC	NVP should not be used in patients with moderate to severe hepatic impairment (Child-Pugh B or C) Should not be used in women with pre-treatment CD4 >250 cells/mm³ or men with CD4 >400 cells/mm³
PI-based regimens (in alphabetical order) ATV/r + ABC/3TC DRV + ABC/3TC FPV/r (once or twice daily) + either ABC/3TC or TDF/FTC LPV/r (once or twice daily) + either [(ABC or ZDV)/3TC] or TDF/FTC	ABC should not be used in patients who test positive for HLA-B*5701 Use with caution in patients with high risk of cardiovascular disease or with pretreatment HIV RNA >100,000 copies/mL Once-daily LPV/r is not recommended in pregnant women.
Integrase inhibitor-based regimens RAL + ABC/3TC	

Acceptable Regimens

EFV + AZT/3TC
NVP + TDF/FTC or ABC/3TC or AZT/3TC
RPV + AZT/3TC
ATV + ABC/3TC or AZT/3TC
ATV/r + AZT/3TC
DRV/r + AZT/3TC
FPV/r + AZT/3TC
LPV/r + AZT/3TC
RAL + AZT/3TC
MVC + AZT/3TC or TDF/FTC or ABC/3TC

3TC, Lamivudine; *ABC,* abacavir; *ATV,* atazanavir; *ddI,* didanosine; *DRV,* darunavir; *EFV,* efavirenz; *FPV,* fosamprenavir; *FTC,* emtricitabine; *INSTI,* integrase strand transfer inhibitor; *LPV,* lopinavir; *MRV,* maraviroc; *NNRTI,* nonnucleoside reverse transcriptase inhibitor; *NRTI,* nucleos(t)ide reverse transcriptase inhibitor; *NVP,* nevirapine; *PI,* protease inhibitor; *r,* low dose ritonavir; *RAL,* raltegravir; *RVP,* rilpivirine; *SQV,* saquinavir; *TDF,* tenofovir; *ZDV,* zidovudine.
The following combinations in the recommended list are available as fixed-dose combination formulations: ABC/3TC, EFV/TDF/FTC, LPV/r, TDF/FTC, RPV/TDF/FTC, and ZDV/3TC.
Modified from Panel on Antiretroviral Guidelines for Adults and Adolescents. Guidelines for the use of antiretroviral agents in HIV-1–infected adults and adolescents. Department of Health and Human Services 1-161, 2012. http://www.aidsinfo.nih.gov/ContentFiles/AdultandAdolescentGL.pdf.

experience and the results of genotypic or phenotypic testing.

- Patients with CD4 lymphocyte count <200/mm³ should be given preventive therapy for PJP (see "*Pneumocystis jirovecii [P. carinii]* Pneumonia").
- Evaluation of chronic diarrhea in patients with HIV is described in Section III, "HIV-Infected Patient, Acutely Ill."
- Criteria for discontinuing and restarting opportunistic infection prophylaxis for adults and adolescents with HIV infection is described in Table 1-208.
- HIV infection in a pregnant woman poses special challenges and considerations. Appropriate and timely ART given to mother and newborn has been shown to dramatically reduce the risk of perinatal transmission of HIV. The goal of therapy is to achieve an undetectable viral load. For HIV-infected pregnant women who are already receiving ART: (1) Continue therapy if suppressing viral replica-

tion, but avoid use of efavirenz in the first trimester (substitution is recommended in the first trimester); (2) If viremia on therapy, genotypic testing is recommended; (3) Nevirapine should be continued, regardless of CD4 count, if there is viral suppression. For HIV-infected pregnant women who have never received ART: (1) Women who require ART for their own health should start on ART in the first trimester. Most antiretrovirals are safe in pregnancy, however, efavirenz should be avoided because of teratogenicity (Class D), DDI and D4T should be avoided (potential of lactic acidosis), and some protease inhibitors may be dose-altered in pregnancy. Nevirapine should not be initiated in an antiretroviral-naive pregnant patient with CD4 counts >250 because of the risk of hepatotoxicity. (2) Women who do not need ART for their own health should also initiate three-drug therapy, but may do so at the end of the first trimester.

(3) Zidovudine (AZT) is recommended as a component of ART.
- Therapy should continue through the baby's birth. Zidovudine is given intravenously at the time of labor, regardless of whether it is an existing component of her three-drug regimen. In women with viral loads persistently >1000 copies/ml despite appropriate ART, cesarean section may further lower risk of transmission. Zidovudine (AZT) should also be given to the newborn for the first 6 weeks of life, and mothers should completely avoid nursing.

DISPOSITION

- Ongoing care consisting of frequent medical evaluations and T-lymphocyte subset analysis (CD4 counts) along with the plasma HIV loads.
- Long-term care focused on providing up-to-date ART and prophylaxis of PJP and other opportunistic infections, as well as early detection of complications (see Section III)
- Ongoing assessment for cardiovascular risk and other primary prevention interventions.
- Screening for hepatitis A, B, and C. Treatment where indicated. Drugs such as tenofovir and lamivudine have activity against both HIV and hepatitis B and may be used in patients with co-infection.
- Vaccinations including hepatitis A and B (when susceptible), Pneumovax, tetanus/diphtheria/pertusis, and influenza.
- Yearly screening for other sexually transmitted infections (*Chlamydia,* gonorrhea, syphilis).
- Consideration of AIDS (lymphomas, HPV) and non-AIDS related (screening for general population, age specific cancers).

REFERRAL

To a physician knowledgeable and experienced in the management of HIV infection and its complications

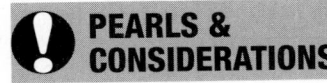

PEARLS & CONSIDERATIONS

COMMENTS

- HIV chemoprophylaxis after occupational exposure is described in Section V.
- A recent analysis of the impact of ART indicates that ART has saved at least 3 million years of life since the introduction into medicine more than 10 years ago.
- In persons with HIV infection, screening for TB needs to include questions about combination of symptoms rather than only inquiring about chronic cough.
- Trials involving antiretroviral chemoprophylaxis before exposure for the prevention of HIV acquisition in MSM have shown that oral tenofovir disoproxil fumarate (FTC-TDF) provides protection against acquisition of HIV infection. Detected blood levels strongly correlated with the prophylactic effect.
- ART in combination with avoidance of breast-feeding and elective cesarean section in women with viremia reduces risk for mother-to-child transmission.

SUGGESTED READINGS
available at www.expertconsult.com

RELATED CONTENT

Fig. E1-21 Diagnostic approach to the patient with chronic diarrhea (patients who are HIV negative) (Algorithm)

Fig. E1-22 Acutely ill HIV-positive patient (Algorithm)

Fig. E1-23 HIV-infected patient with respiratory complaints (Algorithm)

Fig. E1-26 HIV-positive patient with suspected central nervous system infection (Algorithm)

Fig. E1-27 Cardiac dysfunction in HIV-infected patients (Algorithm)

Human Immunodeficiency Virus (HIV) Infection (Patient Information)

AUTHORS: **PHILIP A. CHAN, M.D., M.S.,** and **GLENN G. FORT, M.D., M.P.H.**

TABLE 1-208 Criteria for Discontinuing and Restarting Opportunistic Infection Prophylaxis for Adults and Adolescents with Human Immunodeficiency Virus Infection

Opportunistic Infection	Criteria for Discontinuing Primary Prophylaxis	Criteria for Restarting Primary Prophylaxis	Criteria for Discontinuing Secondary Prophylaxis/ Chronic Maintenance Therapy	Criteria for Restarting Secondary Prophylaxis/ Chronic Maintenance Therapy
Pneumocystis pneumonia (PJP)	CD4$^+$ count >200 cells/mm^3 for >3 mo in response to ART	CD4$^+$ count <200 cells/mm^3	CD4$^+$ count increased from <200 cells/mm^3 to >200 cells/mm^3 for ≥3 mo in response to ART. If PJP is diagnosed when CD4$^+$ count >200 cells/mm^3, prophylaxis should probably be continued for life regardless of CD4$^+$ count rise in response to ART.	CD4$^+$ count <200 cells/mm^3, or if PCP recurred at a CD4$^+$ count >200 cells/mm^3
Toxoplasma gondii encephalitis (TE)	CD4$^+$ count >200 cells/mm^3 for >3 mo in response to ART	CD4$^+$ count <100-200 cells/mm^3	Successfully completed initial therapy, remain asymptomatic of signs and symptoms of TE, and CD4$^+$ count >200 cells/mm^3 for >6 mo in response to ART	CD4$^+$ count <200 cells/mm^3
Microsporidiosis	Not applicable	Not applicable	No signs and symptoms of non-ocular microsporidiosis and CD4$^+$ count >200 cells/mm^3 for >6 mo in response to ART. Patients with ocular microsporidiosis should be on therapy indefinitely regardless of CD4$^+$ count.	No recommendation
Disseminated *Mycobacterium avium* complex (MAC) disease	CD4$^+$ count >100 cells/mm^3 for ≥3 mo in response to ART	CD4$^+$ count <50 cells/mm^3	If fulfill the following criteria: Completed ≥12 mo therapy, and No signs and symptoms of MAC, and Have sustained (≥6 mo) CD4$^+$ count >100 cells/mm^3 in response to ART	CD4$^+$ count <100 cells/mm^3
Bartonellosis	Not applicable	Not applicable	If fulfill the following criteria: Received 3-4 mo of treatment CD4$^+$ count >200 cells/mm^3 for ≥6 mo Certain specialists would discontinue therapy only if *Bartonella* titers have also decreased by fourfold.	No recommendation
Mucosal candidiasis	Not applicable	Not applicable	If used, reasonable to discontinue when CD4$^+$ count >200 cells/mm^3	No recommendation
Cryptococcal meningitis	Not applicable	Not applicable	If fulfill the following criteria: Completed course of initial therapy Remain asymptomatic of cryptococcosis CD4$^+$ count ≥200 cells/mm^3 for >6 mo in response to ART Certain specialists would perform a lumbar puncture to determine if cerebrospinal fluid is culture and antigen negative before stopping therapy.	CD4$^+$ count <200 cells/mm^3
Histoplasma capsulatum infection	If used, CD4$^+$ count >150 cells/mm^3 for 6 mo on ART	For patients at high risk for acquiring histoplasmosis, restart at CD4$^+$ count ≤150 cells/mm^3.	If fulfill the following criteria: Received itraconazole for ≥1 yr Negative blood cultures CD4$^+$ count >150 cells/mm^3 for ≥6 mo in response to ART Serum *Histoplasma* antigen <2 units	CD4$^+$ count ≤150 cells/mm^3
Coccidioidomycosis	If used, CD4$^+$ count ≥250 cells/mm^3 for ≥6 mo	If used, restart at CD4$^+$ count <250 cells/mm^3	**Only for patients with focal coccidioidal pneumonia:** Clinically responded to ≥12 mo of antifungal therapy CD4$^+$ count >250 cells/mm^3 Receiving ART Suppressive therapy should be continued indefinitely, even with increase in CD4$^+$ count on ART for patients with diffuse pulmonary, disseminated, or meningeal diseases.	No recommendation
Cytomegalovirus retinitis	Not applicable	Not applicable	CD4$^+$ count >100 cells/mm^3 for >3-6 mo in response to ART. Therapy should be discontinued only after consultation with an ophthalmologist, taking into account magnitude and duration of CD4$^+$ count increase, anatomic location of the lesions, vision in the contralateral eye, and the feasibility of regular ophthalmologic monitoring. Routine (every 3 mo) ophthalmologic follow-up is recommended for early detection of relapse or immune restoration uveitis.	CD4$^+$ count <100 cells/mm^3
Isospora belli infection	Not applicable	Not applicable	Sustained increase in CD4$^+$ count to >200 cells/mm^3 for >6 mo in response to ART and without evidence of *I. belli* infection	No recommendation

Modified from Centers for Disease Control and Prevention. Guidelines for Prevention and treatment of opportunistic infections in HIV-infected adults and adolescents. Recommendations from CDC, the National Institutes of Health, and the HIV Medicine Association of the Infectious Disease Society of America. *MMWR Morb Mortal Wkly Rep* 58(RR-4), 2009.

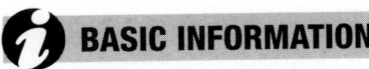

BASIC INFORMATION

DEFINITION

Huntington's disease is an autosomal dominant neurodegenerative disorder characterized by involuntary movements, psychiatric disturbance, and cognitive decline.

SYNONYMS

Huntington's chorea

ICD-9CM CODES
333.4 Huntington's chorea

EPIDEMIOLOGY & DEMOGRAPHICS

PEAK INCIDENCE: Late 30s and 40s, with onsets from ages 2 to 70 yr
PREVALENCE (IN U.S.): 4.1 to 8.4 cases/100,000 persons
PREDOMINANT SEX: Female = male
PREDOMINANT AGE: Adulthood
GENETICS: Autosomal dominant

PHYSICAL FINDINGS & CLINICAL PRESENTATION

- Chorea: irregular, rapid, flowing, nonstereo-typed involuntary movements. When there is a writhing quality, it is referred to as choreoathetosis. Chorea is present early on and tends to decrease in end stages of disease.
- Dancelike, lurching gait, often caused by chorea.
- Westphal variant: cognitive dysfunction, bradykinesia, and rigidity. This variant is more commonly seen in juvenile-onset Huntington's.
- Oculomotor abnormalities are common early on and include increased latency of response and insuppressible eye blinking.
- Psychiatric disorders (can be present early on): depression is commonly seen as well as obsessive-compulsive behaviors and aggression associated with impaired impulse control.

ETIOLOGY

- Trinucleotide repeat disorder
- The responsible gene is the Huntington gene located on chromosome 4. Its function is not known.

DIAGNOSIS

DIFFERENTIAL DIAGNOSIS

- Drug-induced chorea: dopamine, stimulants, anticonvulsants, antidepressants, and oral contraceptives have all been known to cause chorea.
- Sydenham's chorea: decreased incidence with decline of rheumatic fever.
- Benign hereditary chorea: autosomal dominant with onset in childhood. There is no progression of symptoms and no associated dementia or behavioral problems.
- Senile chorea: possibly vascular in origin.
- Wilson's disease: autosomal recessive; tremor, dysarthria, and dystonia are more common presentations than chorea. A total of 95% of patients with neurologic manifestations will have Kayser-Fleischer rings.
- Postinfectious.
- Systemic lupus erythematosus: can be the presenting feature of lupus (rare).
- Chorea gravidarum: presents during first 4 to 5 mo of pregnancy and resolves after delivery.
- Paraneoplastic: seen most commonly in small-cell lung cancer and lymphoma.

WORKUP

Onset of symptoms in an individual with an established family history requires no additional investigation.

LABORATORY TESTS

- Genetic testing for CAG repeats
- If normal, obtain complete blood count with smear, erythrocyte sedimentation rate, electrolytes, serum ceruloplasmin, 24-hr urinary copper excretion, TFTs, antinuclear antibody, liver function tests, HIV, and ASO titer. Consider paraneoplastic markers.

IMAGING STUDIES

CT scan or MRI scan will show atrophy, most notably in the caudate and putamen. The cortex is involved to a lesser extent. A normal scan does not exclude the diagnosis.

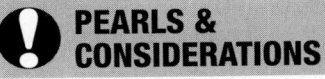

TREATMENT

NONPHARMACOLOGIC THERAPY

- Supportive counseling
- Physical and occupational therapy
- Home health care
- Genetic counseling

CHRONIC Rx

- Chorea does not need to be treated unless it is disabling.
- Tetrabenazine (TBZ) is approved by the FDA for the symptomatic treatment of chorea seen in Huntington's disease. It is a reversible inhibitor of the vesicle monoamine transporter type 2 (VMAT-2). It inhibits primarily dopamine and to a lesser degree serotonin and norepinephrine. Side effects include parkinsonism and severe depression.
- Neuroleptics, typical or atypical, can be used for symptomatic management of neuropsychiatric issues and chorea at low doses (e.g., haloperidol 1 to 10 mg/day).
- Amantadine (up to 300 to 400 mg divided tid).
- Depression with suicidal ideation is common; may improve with tricyclic antidepressants or SSRI

DISPOSITION

Relentless course of variable duration leading to progressive disability and death

REFERRAL

- Should refer to psychiatry and neurology for treatment of mood disorders and movement disorders
- Genetic counseling

PEARLS & CONSIDERATIONS

- Suicide rate is fivefold that of the general population.
- The number of repeats does correlate with age of onset but does not clearly correlate with disease severity. Interpretation of number of repeats is still difficult at this time; therefore it is debatable whether to disclose this information to patients.

SUGGESTED READINGS
available at www.expertconsult.com

RELATED CONTENT

Huntington's Disease (Patient Information)

AUTHOR: **FARIHA ZAHEER, M.D.**

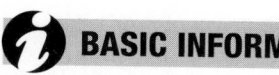

BASIC INFORMATION

DEFINITION

A hydrocele is a fluid collection in a serous scrotal space, usually between the layers of the tunica vaginalis (Fig. 1-424). A hydrocele that fills with fluid from the peritoneum is termed *communicating*. This is distinguished from a *noncommunicating* hydrocele by history of variation in size throughout the day and palpation of a thickened cord above the testicle on the affected side. A communicating hydrocele is a small inguinal hernia in which fluid, but not peritoneal structures, traverses the processus vaginalis. In noncommunicating hydrocele, the processus vaginalis was obliterated during development. An abdominoscrotal hydrocele is a rare variant of a hydrocele in which there is a large, tense hydrocele that extends into the lower abdominal cavity.

ICD-9CM CODES
603.9 Hydrocele

PHYSICAL FINDINGS & CLINICAL PRESENTATION

Symptoms:
- Scrotal enlargement
- Scrotal heaviness or discomfort radiating to the inguinal area
- Back pain

Physical findings:
- Most hydroceles are smooth and nontender. Scrotal distention may make it difficult to palpate the testis, but it is important to palpate the testis because some young men develop a hydrocele in association with a testis tumor
- Transillumination of the scrotum confirms the fluid-filled nature of the mass

ETIOLOGY

Hydroceles may occur as a congenital abnormality in which the processus vaginalis fails to close. In this case an inguinal hernia is virtually always associated with the malformation. Congenital hydroceles are most common in infants (1%-2% of neonates have hydroceles) and children. In adults, hydroceles are more frequently caused by infection, tumor, or trauma. Infection of the epididymis often results in the development of a secondary hydrocele. Tropical infections such as filariasis may produce hydroceles.

DIAGNOSIS

DIFFERENTIAL DIAGNOSIS

- Spermatocele
- Inguinoscrotal hernia
- Testicular tumor
- Varicocele
- Epididymitis

IMAGING STUDIES

Scrotal ultrasound is useful to rule out a testicular tumor as the cause of the hydrocele (Fig. 1-425). The acute development of a hydrocele might be associated with the onset of epididymitis, testicular tumor, trauma, and torsion of a testicular appendage. An ultrasound of the scrotum may provide important diagnostic information.

TREATMENT

- No treatment if asymptomatic and testis is believed to be normal. Most congenital hydroceles resolve by 12 months of age following reabsorption of the hydrocele fluid.
- Surgical repair should be considered if the hydrocele is tense and large. Communicating hydroceles should be repaired in the same manner as an indirect hernia. The indications for repair of a noncommunicating hydrocele include failure to resolve and increase in size to one that is large and tense.
- Surgical correction is similar to a herniorrhaphy: an inguinal incision is made, the spermatic cord is identified, the hydrocele fluid is drained, and a high ligation of the processus vaginalis is performed.

PEARLS & CONSIDERATIONS

- The long-term risk of a communicating hydrocele is the development of an inguinal hernia.
- An inguinal hernia/hydrocele is likely if compression of the fluid-filled mass completely reduces the hydrocele.

SUGGESTED READING
available at www.expertconsult.com

RELATED CONTENT
Hydrocele (Patient Information)

AUTHOR: **FRED F. FERRI, M.D.**

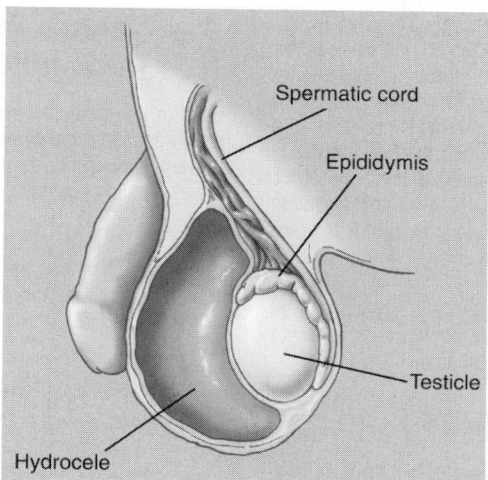

FIGURE 1-424 Schematic representation of the testicle, epididymis, spermatic cord, and a hydrocele. (From Lipshultz LI et al: *Urology and the primary care practitioner,* ed 3, Philadelphia, 2008, Elsevier.)

Spermatic cord
Epididymis
Testicle
Hydrocele

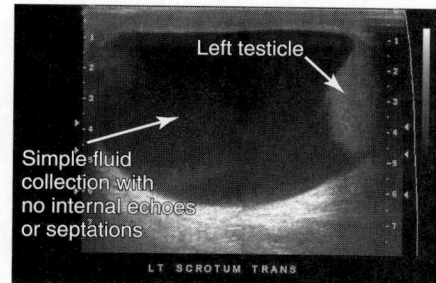

Left testicle
Simple fluid collection with no internal echoes or septations
LT SCROTUM TRANS

FIGURE 1-425 Hydrocele. This patient has a large left hydrocele. The fluid collection has no internal echoes or septations and likely represents serous fluid. Complex fluid collection with internal echoes and septations would be more concerning for infection or blood products. (From Broder JS: *Diagnostic imaging for the emergency physician,* Philadelphia, 2011, Saunders.)

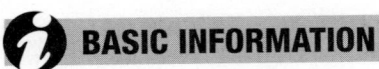

BASIC INFORMATION

DEFINITION

Normal pressure hydrocephalus (NPH) is a syndrome of symptomatic hydrocephalus in the setting of normal cerebrospinal fluid (CSF) pressure. The classic clinical triad of NPH includes gait disturbance, cognitive decline, and incontinence.

SYNONYMS

Occult hydrocephalus
Extraventricular obstructive hydrocephalus
Chronic hydrocephalus

ICD-9CM CODES
331.3 Communicating hydrocephalus

EPIDEMIOLOGY & DEMOGRAPHICS

INCIDENCE: The exact incidence is not known. In one study the incidence was found to be 5.5 per 100,000, but it may account for up to 5% of dementia in the U.S. Hospital discharge data suggest approximately 11,500 new cases diagnosed annually (may be overestimated).
PREDOMINANT SEX: Males = females
PREDOMINANT AGE: NPH is more common with increasing age.

PHYSICAL FINDINGS & CLINICAL PRESENTATION

- Gait difficulty: patients often have difficulty initiating ambulation, and the gait may be broad based and shuffling, with the appearance that the feet are stuck to the floor ("magnetic gait" or "frontal gait disorder").
- Cognitive decline: mental slowing, forgetfulness and inattention typically without agnosia, aphasia, or other cortical disturbances.
- Incontinence: initially may have urinary urgency; incontinence later develops. Fecal incontinence also occasionally occurs.
- Gegenhalten (paratonia) or other frontal lobe signs may be seen.

ETIOLOGY

- Approximately 50% of cases are idiopathic; the remaining cases have a variety of causes, including prior subarachnoid hemorrhage, meningitis, head trauma, or intracranial surgery.
- Symptoms are presumed to result from stretching of sacral motor and limbic fibers that lie near the ventricles as dilation occurs.

DIAGNOSIS

DIFFERENTIAL DIAGNOSIS

- Alzheimer's disease with extrapyramidal features
- Cognitive impairment in the setting of Parkinson's disease or parkinsonism-plus syndromes
- Diffuse Lewy body disease
- Frontotemporal dementia
- Cervical spondylosis with cord compromise in the setting of degenerative dementia
- Multiinfarct dementia
- HIV dementia

WORKUP

- Large-volume lumbar puncture:
  1. Mental status testing and time to walk a prespecified distance (usually 25 feet) are measured, followed by removal of 40 to 50 ml of CSF.
  2. Retest of mental status and timed walking are done later (sometimes at 1 and 4 hr). Patients who have significant improvement in gait or mental status may have a better surgical outcome; those with mild or negative response can have variable outcomes.
  3. Opening and closing pressure are measured; if pressure is elevated, alternative causes must be considered. Higher *normal* pressure may predict a good outcome from CSF shunting.
- Measurement of CSF outflow resistance by an infusion test or CSF pressure monitoring are sometimes used to help predict surgical outcome. External lumbar drainage (ELD) is being used more commonly.

LABORATORY TESTS

CSF should be sent for routine fluid analysis to exclude other pathologies.

IMAGING STUDIES

- CT scan or MRI can be used to document ventriculomegaly. The distinguishing feature of NPH is ventricular enlargement out of proportion to sulcal atrophy (Fig. E1-426).
- MRI has advantages over CT, including better ability to visualize structures in the posterior fossa, visualize transependymal CSF flow (seen as periventricular hyperintensity), and document extent of white matter lesions. On MRI a flow void in the aqueduct and third ventricle ("jet sign"), thinning and elevation of the corpus callosum on sagittal images, and rounding of the frontal horns may be seen.
- Isotope cisternography and dynamic MRI studies have not been shown to be superior in predicting shunt outcome.

TREATMENT

There is no evidence that NPH can be effectively treated with medications.

NONPHARMACOLOGIC THERAPY

Response to ventriculoperitoneal shunting is variable. Some patients (variable depending on series reported) show significant improvement from shunting.

Factors that may predict positive outcome with surgery:
- NPH caused by prior trauma, subarachnoid hemorrhage, or meningitis
- History of mild impairment in cognition <2 yr duration
- Onset of gait abnormality before cognitive decline
- Imaging demonstrates hydrocephalus without sulcal enlargement, including normal-sized sylvian fissures and cortical sulci, and absent or mild white matter lesions.
- Transependymal CSF flow visualized on MRI
- Large-volume tap or ELD produces dramatic but temporary relief of symptoms
- High *normal* opening pressure

Factors that may predict negative outcome with surgery:
- Extensive white matter lesions or diffuse cerebral atrophy on MRI
- Moderate to severe cognitive impairment
- Onset of cognitive impairment before gait disorder
- History of alcohol abuse

ACUTE GENERAL Rx

Shunting in selected patients

DISPOSITION

Symptoms of NPH may progress over time. Prompt diagnosis may improve chances for treatment success.

REFERRAL

To neurologist for initial evaluation, including lumbar puncture, followed by neurosurgeon for shunting in appropriate patients

PEARLS & CONSIDERATIONS

Each of the cardinal symptoms of NPH is commonly seen in the elderly and occurs in multiple disease processes; therefore differential diagnoses should always be considered carefully.

CAUTION

Shunt complications, including subdural or intracerebral hematoma, may occur in 30% to 40% of patients.

SUGGESTED READINGS

available at www.expertconsult.com

RELATED CONTENT

Normal Pressure Hydrocephalus (Patient Information)

AUTHOR: **TAMARA G. FONG, M.D., PH.D.**

BASIC INFORMATION

DEFINITION

Hydronephrosis is dilation of the renal pyelo-calyceal system, most often as a result of impairment of urinary flow.

SYNONYMS

Hydroureter (dilation of ureter, often seen with hydronephrosis when obstruction is in lower urinary tract)
Urinary tract obstruction

ICD-9CM CODES
591 Acquired hydronephrosis
753.2 Congenital hydronephrosis

EPIDEMIOLOGY & DEMOGRAPHICS

Children usually have congenital malformations, whereas adults tend to have acquired defects as etiologies.

CLINICAL PRESENTATION

HISTORY:

- Pain is caused by distention of collecting system or renal capsule and is more related to the rate of onset than the degree of obstruction. It can vary in location from flank to the lower abdomen to the testes/labia. Pain in the flank occurring only on micturition is highly suggestive of vesicoureteral reflux.
- Anuria can occur with total obstruction of urinary flow (bilateral hydronephrosis, or unilateral if only one kidney is present).
- Polyuria or nocturia can occur with chronic (incomplete) obstruction because of deleterious effects on renal concentrating ability (nephrogenic diabetes insipidus).
- Urinary frequency, hesitancy, poor stream, and postvoid dribbling are all symptoms that can occur with obstruction at or below the bladder (e.g., prostatic hyperplasia).
- Chronic urinary infections can either result from chronic urinary obstruction (organisms favoring growth with stasis of urine) or lead to conditions (e.g., urine pH changes) that favor stone formation and subsequent obstruction.

PHYSICAL EXAMINATION:

- Hypertension can be caused by increased renin release in acute or subacute obstruction.
- Fever or costovertebral angle (CVA) tenderness can suggest urinary tract infection.
- Palpate bladder to detect if distention is present.
- Rectal examination to evaluate prostate for size and nodularity and also to check rectal sphincter tone.
- Pelvic examination to assess for vaginal anatomy, pelvic mass, or pelvic inflammatory disease.
- Penile examination to rule out meatal stenosis or phimosis.
- Bladder catheterization to assess postvoid residual volume if urinary tract obstruction is considered. Should rule out postrenal obstruction in unexplained acute renal failure.

ETIOLOGY

MECHANICAL IMPAIRMENTS:

Congenital:
- Ureteropelvic junction narrowing
- Ureterovesical junction narrowing
- Ureterocele
- Retrocaval ureter
- Bladder neck obstruction
- Urethral valve
- Urethral stricture
- Meatal stenosis

Acquired:
- Intrinsic to urinary tract:
  o Calculi
  o Inflammation
  o Trauma
  o Sloughed papillae
  o Ureteral tumor
  o Blood clots
  o Prostatic hypertrophy or cancer
  o Bladder cancer
  o Urethral stricture
  o Phimosis
- Extrinsic to urinary tract:
  o Gravid uterus
  o Retroperitoneal fibrosis or tumor (e.g., lymphoma)
  o Aortic aneurysm
  o Uterine fibroids
  o Trauma (surgical or nonsurgical)
  o Pelvic inflammatory disease
  o Pelvic malignancies (e.g., prostate, colorectal, cervical, uterine, bladder)

FUNCTIONAL IMPAIRMENTS:

- Neurogenic bladder (often with adynamic ureter) can occur with spinal cord disease or diabetic neuropathy.
- Pharmacologic agents such as alpha-adrenergic antagonists and anticholinergic drugs can inhibit bladder emptying.
- Vesicoureteral reflux may occur.
- Pregnancy can cause hydroureter and hydronephrosis (on the right more often than left) as early as the second month. Hormonal effects on ureteral tone combine with mechanical factors.

DIAGNOSIS

DIFFERENTIAL DIAGNOSIS

- Urinary stones
- Neoplastic disease
- Prostatic hypertrophy
- Neurologic disease
- Urinary reflux
- Urinary tract infection
- Medication effects
- Trauma
- Congenital abnormality of urinary tract

LABORATORY TESTS

- Serum blood urea nitrogen and creatinine to assess for renal insufficiency (usually implies bilateral obstruction or unilateral obstruction of a solitary kidney).
- Electrolytes may reveal hypernatremia (if nephrogenic diabetes insipidus), hyperkalemia (from renal failure and effects on tubular function), or distal renal tubular acidosis.
- Urinalysis and examination of sediment may reveal white blood cells, red blood cells, or bacteria in the appropriate setting (e.g., infection, stones), but often the sediment is normal in obstructive renal disease.

IMAGING STUDIES

- Assess kidney and bladder size with ultrasound (Fig. 1-427) as well as contour of collecting system and ureters. Ultrasound is >90% sensitive and specific for hydronephrosis and is noninvasive.
- Abdominal CT scan without IV contrast provides excellent localization of the site of obstruction (Fig. 1-428).
- Once diagnosed, antegrade or retrograde ureterograms can further delineate the point of obstruction.
- Voiding cystourethrogram is helpful in diagnosing vesicoureteral reflux and obstructions of the bladder neck or urethra.

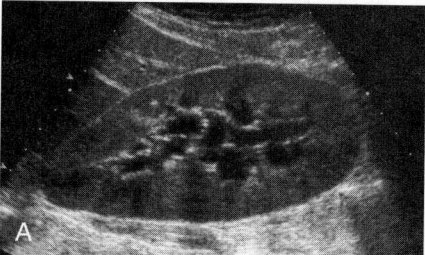
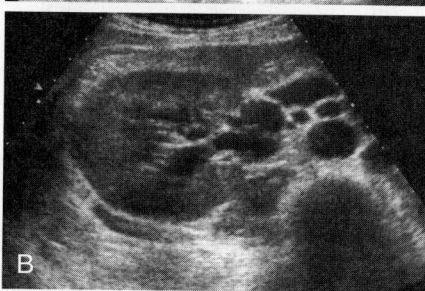
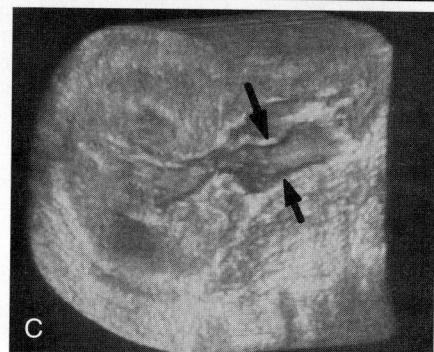

FIGURE 1-427 Renal ultrasound study demonstrating hydronephrosis. A, Sagittal image. B, Transverse image. C, Transverse three-dimensional surface-rendered image; *arrows* indicate the dilated proximal ureter. (From Floege J et al: *Comprehensive clinical nephrology*, ed 4, Philadelphia, 2010, Saunders.)

- Diuretic renogram is sometimes used when there is hydronephrosis without apparent obstruction seen on any of the above studies. A loop diuretic is administered prior to a radionuclide scan. If obstruction is present, there will be slowed transit of the radioisotope during the scan, further dilation of the collecting system, and often reproduction of the patient's symptoms.
- A perfusion pressure flow study should be performed in a symptomatic patient with a negative or equivocal diuretic renogram.

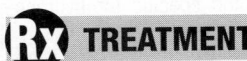

TREATMENT

NONPHARMACOLOGIC THERAPY

- Urgent treatment is required if urinary tract obstruction is associated with urinary tract infection, acute renal failure, or uncontrollable pain.
- Conservative management of calculi with IV fluids, IV antibiotics (if evidence of infection), and aggressive analgesia may be enough to treat acute unilateral urinary tract obstruction depending on the size (90% of stones <5 mm will pass spontaneously).

- Urethral catheter is adequate to relieve most obstructions at or distal to the bladder, but occasionally a suprapubic catheter will be required (e.g., impassable urethral stricture or urethral injury). Neurogenic bladder may require intermittent clean catheterization if frequent voiding and pharmacologic treatments are ineffective.
- Nephrostomy tube can be placed percutaneously to facilitate urinary drainage.
- Extracorporeal shock wave lithotripsy (ESWL) is used to fragment large stones to facilitate spontaneous passage or subsequent extraction. (Note: ESWL is contraindicated in pregnancy.)
- Nephroscopy is performed for extraction of proximal stones under direct visualization.
- Cystoscopy with ureteroscopy is used to remove distal ureteral stones with a loop or basket with or without fragmentation by ultrasonic or laser lithotripsy.
- Ureteral stents can be used for extrinsic and some intrinsic ureteral obstructions.
- Urethral dilation or internal urethrotomy can be used for urethral strictures.
- Nephrectomy or ureteral diversion may be required in severe cases (e.g., malignancy).

- Ureterovesical reimplantation can be used for reflux disease.
- Transurethral retrograde prostatectomy is used for severe obstruction from benign prostatic hypertrophy.
- IV fluid and electrolyte replacement are needed; the patient must be monitored closely during the postobstructive diuresis (usually lasting several days to a week).

ACUTE GENERAL Rx
Antibiotics if indicated

DISPOSITION
Aggressive treatment of infections and early relief of obstruction can usually prevent progressive loss of renal function; however, chronic bilateral obstruction (often from benign prostatic hypertrophy) can lead to chronic renal failure.

REFERRAL
- Urologist consultation early for diagnostic or therapeutic procedures
- Oncologist if a neoplasm is diagnosed
- Gynecologist if pregnancy or female pelvic anatomy is involved

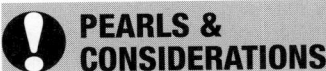

PEARLS & CONSIDERATIONS

COMMENTS
- Not a primary disorder: an underlying etiology should be sought.

PREVENTION
May be achieved through prevention of an underlying potential etiology (e.g., medical or surgical management of benign prostatic hypertrophy before obstruction occurring or medical treatment to avoid formation of renal stones).

SUGGESTED READINGS
available at www.expertconsult.com

RELATED CONTENT
Hydronephrosis (Patient Information)

AUTHORS: **SHEENAGH M. BODKIN, M.D.,** and **PAUL A. PIRRAGLIA, M.D., M.P.H.**

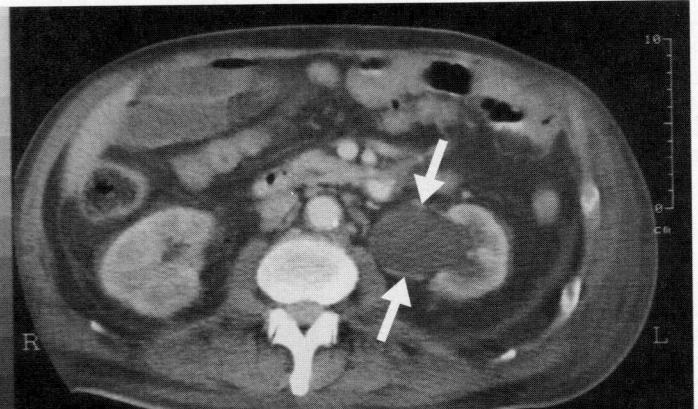

FIGURE 1-428 CT scan of the abdomen showing a grossly hydronephrotic kidney on the left. *Arrows* mark dilated renal pelvis. Dilated loops of small bowel are seen in the right hypochondrium. Sequential sections demonstrated that the ureter was dilated along its length and that there was a pelvic mass, which was responsible for both bowel and left ureteric obstruction. The mass was subsequently shown to be arising from a carcinoma of the colon. (From Johnson RJ, Feehally J: *Comprehensive clinical nephrology,* ed 2, St Louis, 2000, Mosby.)

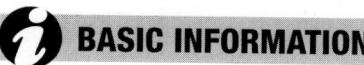

BASIC INFORMATION

DEFINITION

Primary hyperaldosteronism is a clinical syndrome characterized by hypokalemia, hypertension, low plasma renin activity (PRA), and excessive aldosterone secretion.

SYNONYMS

Hyperaldosteronism
Aldosteronism
Primary aldosteronism
Conn's syndrome

ICD-9CM CODES
255.1 Primary aldosteronism

EPIDEMIOLOGY & DEMOGRAPHICS

INCIDENCE: 1% to 2% of patients with hypertension
PREVALENCE: More common in females

PHYSICAL FINDINGS & CLINICAL PRESENTATION

- Generally asymptomatic
- If significant hypokalemia is present, possible muscle cramping, weakness, paresthesias
- Hypertension
- Polyuria, polydipsia

ETIOLOGY

- Aldosterone-producing adenoma (>60%)
- Idiopathic hyperaldosteronism (>30%)
- Glucocorticoid-suppressible hyperaldosteronism (<1%)
- Aldosterone-producing carcinoma (<1%)

DIAGNOSIS

DIFFERENTIAL DIAGNOSIS

- Diuretic use
- Hypokalemia from vomiting, diarrhea
- Renovascular hypertension
- Other endocrine neoplasm (pheochromocytoma, deoxycorticosterone-producing tumor, renin-secreting tumor)

WORKUP

Fig. E1-429 describes a diagnostic approach to patients with suspected primary aldosteronism. CT, MRI, and adrenal vein sampling (AVS) are used to distinguish unilateral from bilateral increased aldosterone secretion. This distinction will dictate treatment options since unilateral primary aldosteronism is treated surgically rather than medically. In patients with hypokalemia and a low PRA, confirming tests for primary hyperaldosteronism include the following:

- 24-hr urine test for aldosterone and potassium levels (potassium >40 mEq and aldosterone >15 mcg).

- Captopril test: administer 25 to 50 mg of captopril (an angiotensin-converting enzyme [ACE] inhibitor) and measure plasma renin and aldosterone levels 1 to 2 hr later. A plasma aldosterone level >15 ng/dl confirms the diagnosis of primary aldosteronism. This test is more expensive and is best reserved for situations in which the 24-hr urine test for aldosterone is ambiguous.
- 24-hr urinary tetrahydroaldosterone (<65 mcg/24 hr) and saline infusion test (plasma aldosterone >10 ng/dl) can also be used in ambiguous cases.
- The renin-aldosterone stimulation test (posture test) is helpful in differentiating idiopathic hyperaldosteronism (IHA) from aldosterone-producing adenoma (APA). Patients with APA have a decrease in aldosterone levels at 4 hr, whereas patients with IHA have an increase in aldosterone levels.
- As a screening test for primary aldosteronism, an elevated plasma aldosterone-renin ratio (ARR), drawn randomly from patients taking hypertensive drugs, is predictive of primary aldosteronism (positive predictive value 100% in a recent study). ARR is calculated by dividing plasma aldosterone (mg/dl) by PRA (mg/ml/hr). ARR >100 is considered elevated.
- Bilateral AVS may be done to localize APA when adrenal CT scan is equivocal. In APA, ipsilateral/contralateral aldosterone level is >10:1, and ipsilateral venous aldosterone concentration is very high (>1000 ng/dl).
- A diagnostic evaluation of hypertensive patients with suspected aldosteronism is described in the online version of Section III.

LABORATORY TESTS

Routine laboratory tests can be suggestive but are not diagnostic of primary aldosteronism. Common abnormalities are:

- Spontaneous hypokalemia or moderately severe hypokalemia while receiving conventional doses of diuretics
- Possible alkalosis and hypernatremia

IMAGING STUDIES

- Adrenal CT scans (with 3-mm cuts) or MRI may be used to localize neoplasm.
- Adrenal scanning with iodocholesterol (NP-59) or 6-beta-iodomethyl-19-norcholesterol after dexamethasone suppression. The uptake of tracer is increased in those with aldosteronoma and absent in those with IHA and adrenal carcinoma.

TREATMENT

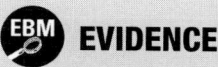

NONPHARMACOLOGIC THERAPY

- Regular monitoring and control of blood pressure

- Low-sodium diet, tobacco avoidance, maintenance of ideal body weight, and regular exercise

ACUTE GENERAL Rx

- Control of blood pressure and hypokalemia with spironolactone, amiloride, or ACE inhibitors
- Surgery (unilateral adrenalectomy) for APA

CHRONIC Rx

Chronic medical therapy with spironolactone, eplerenone, amiloride, or ACE inhibitors to control blood pressure and hypokalemia is necessary in all patients with bilateral IHA.

DISPOSITION

- Unilateral adrenalectomy normalizes hypertension and hypokalemia in 70% of patients with APA after 1 yr. After 5 yr, 50% of patients remain normotensive.
- Experimental animal studies have suggested that long-term exposure to increased aldosterone levels in untreated aldosteronism may result in renal structural damage. However, clinical trials have shown that primary aldosteronism is characterized by partially reversible renal dysfunction in which elevated albuminuria is a marker of a dynamic rather than structural renal defect.

REFERRAL

Surgical referral for unilateral adrenalectomy after confirmation of unilateral APA or carcinoma

PEARLS & CONSIDERATIONS

- Frequent monitoring of blood pressure and electrolytes postoperatively is necessary because normotension after unilateral adrenalectomy may take up to 4 mo.
- Recent investigations regarding serum aldosterone and the incidence of hypertension in nonhypertensive persons indicate that increased aldosterone levels within the physiologic range predispose to the development of hypertension.

EVIDENCE

available at www.expertconsult.com

SUGGESTED READINGS
available at www.expertconsult.com

RELATED CONTENT
Aldosteronism (Patient Information)

AUTHOR: **FRED F. FERRI, M.D.**

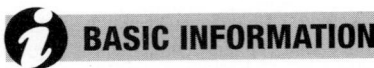

BASIC INFORMATION

DEFINITION

Hypercholesterolemia refers to a blood cholesterol measurement >200 mg/dl. A cholesterol level of 200 to 239 mg/dl is considered borderline high, and a level of >240 mg/dl is considered high.

SYNONYMS

Hypercholesteremia
Dyslipidemia
Type II familial hyperlipoproteinemia

ICD-9CM CODES
272.0 Pure hypercholesterolemia

EPIDEMIOLOGY & DEMOGRAPHICS

- More than half of all U.S. adults have dyslipidemia: 50.4% of men and 50.9% of women.
- Only ~12% of people with high cholesterol are being treated.
- Elevated cholesterol requires drug therapy in ~60 million Americans.
- Incidence of heterozygous familial hypercholesterolemia: ~1:500
- Incidence of homozygous familial hypercholesterolemia: ~1:1 million
- Prevalence of hypercholesterolemia increases with increasing age.
- Familial hypercholesterolemia: autosomal-dominant disorder
- Familial combined hyperlipidemia: possibly an autosomal-dominant disorder
- Multifactorial predilection: apparent in majority of affected individuals

PHYSICAL FINDINGS & CLINICAL PRESENTATION

- A detailed medication history should be performed because some medications may affect lipid levels (e.g., thiazides, corticosteroids, beta-blockers, and estrogens).
- The physical examination should include measurements of BMI and BP, thyroid and liver assessments, and examining peripheral pulses including carotids for bruits.
- Physical findings, particularly in the familial forms may include
  1. Tendon xanthomas
  2. Xanthelasma
  3. Arcus corneae
  4. Arterial bruits (young adulthood)

ETIOLOGY

Primary:
- Genetics
- Obesity
- Dietary intake

Secondary:
- Hypothyroidism
- Diabetes mellitus
- Nephrotic syndrome
- Obstructive liver disease: Hepatoma, extrahepatic biliary obstruction, primary biliary cirrhosis
- Alcohol or tobacco use
- Drugs: Oral contraceptives, progesterone, corticosteroids, thiazide diuretics, β-blockers, androgenic steroids, retinoic acid derivatives

DIAGNOSIS

DIFFERENTIAL DIAGNOSIS

- Always consider underlying secondary causes for the elevated cholesterol.
- Patients with very high LDL cholesterol usually have genetic forms of hypercholesterolemia (see *Hyperlipoproteinemia, Primary*). Early detection of these cases and family testing to identify similarly affected relatives is important.
- Metabolic syndrome:
  1. A constellation of lipid and nonlipid risk factors of a metabolic origin
  2. Diagnosed when three or more of the following are present: abdominal obesity (waist circumference >40 in in men and >35 in in women); fasting triglycerides >150 mg/dl; HDL <40 mg/dl in males and <50 mg/dl in females; systolic BP >130 mmHg and diastolic BP >85 mmHg; fasting glucose >110 mg/dl

WHO SHOULD BE SCREENED:

- The National Cholesterol Education Program Adult Treatment Panel III (NCEP-ATP III) recommends screening of all adults at age 20 yr with fasting lipid profile measurement every 5 yr, regardless of their CHD risk profile.
- The USPSTF supports routine screening for men aged >35 yr and women aged >45 yr by measurement of nonfasting total and HDL cholesterol alone.
- Clinicians should also screen younger adults (men aged 20 to 35 or women aged 20 to 45) who have other risk factors for CVD, family history of premature CHD, or familial lipid disorder or who have evidence of hyperlipidemia on physical examination.
- In 2010, the USPSTF recommended routine screening for overweight and obesity in persons aged <20 yr.
- In 2011, ACC/AHA recommended screening for hypertriglyceridemia by a nonfasting measurement. A nonfasting level of <200 mg/dl is commensurate with an optimal level of <100 mg/dl and no further testing is required. However, a nonfasting level of >200 mg/dl warrants further testing with a fasting lipid profile.

LABORATORY TESTS

- Risk assessment to modify LDL goals (Table 1-209)
- Evaluate for CHD* and CHD equivalents (Table 1-210).

TREATMENT

NONPHARMACOLOGIC THERAPY

- First line of treatment: dietary therapy (use of NCEP-ATP III Therapeutic Lifestyle Change TLC Diet can result in 5% to 15% reduction in LDL cholesterol level).
- Composition of the TLC diet:
  1. Total fat 25% to 30% of total calories
  2. Polyunsaturated fat up to 10% of total calories

*CHD includes history of MI, unstable angina, stable angina, coronary procedures (angioplasty or bypass surgery).

---

  3. Monounsaturated fat up to 20% of total calories
  4. Saturated fats <7% of total calories
  5. Carbohydrate 50% to 60% of total calories
  6. Protein 15% of total calories
  7. No more than 200 mg/day of cholesterol
  8. Fiber 20 to 30 g/day
- Increased physical activity: encourage 20 to 30 min of aerobic exercise three or four times a week
- Weight reduction
- Smoking cessation
- Counseling on CAD risk factors
- Plant-based diets (including stanol-containing margarines, oat bran, and nuts) have shown effectiveness in controlling lipids.

ACUTE GENERAL Rx

No acute treatment needed

CHRONIC Rx

- Elevated LDL cholesterol is the primary target of cholesterol-lowering therapy.
- Risk assessment should be made based on the presence of risk factors (see Table 1-209), CHD and CHD risk equivalents (see Table 1-210) and 10-yr CHD risk using Framingham risk calculator (Table 1-211).
- Drug therapy should be instituted in patients with:
  - LDL >190 and 0-1 risk factor
  - LDL >160 and ≥2 risk factors and <10% 10-yr risk
  - LDL >130 and ≥2 risk factors and 10% to 20% 10-yr risk
  - LDL >100 with CHD, CHD risk equivalents, and >20% 10-yr risk
- Optional goal of LDL cholesterol <70 mg/dl is favored for "very high risk" patients, which includes the presence of established CVD plus multiple major risk factors (especially diabetes), severe and poorly controlled risk factors (especially continued cigarette smoking), multiple

TABLE 1-209 Risk Factors That Modify LDL Goals

1. Cigarette smoking
2. Hypertension (BP ≤140/90 mm Hg or on medications)
3. Low HDL cholesterol (<40 mg/dl)*
4. Family history of premature CHD (<55 yr in first-degree male relative or <65 yr in first-degree female relative)
5. Age (men ≥45 yr, women ≥55 yr)

*HDL cholesterol >60 mg/dl counts as a negative risk factor; its presence removes one risk factor from the total count.

TABLE 1-210 CHD Equivalents

1. Diabetes mellitus
2. Aortic aneurysm
3. Peripheral vascular disease (ABI <0.9)
4. Symptomatic carotid artery disease (stroke, transient ischemic attack)
5. 10-yr risk for coronary artery disease >20% using Framingham risk equation

- risk factors of the metabolic syndrome, and in patients with acute coronary syndromes.
- Non–HDL cholesterol should be secondary target of therapy in patients with elevated triglycerides (>200 mg/dl). The non–HDL cholesterol goal is 30 mg/dl higher than the LDL cholesterol goal.
- Optimal fasting triglyceride level is defined as <100 mg/dl, as a parameter of metabolic health under ACC/AHA guidelines published in 2011.
- Medications that can be used (Table 1-212):
  1. Bile acid sequestrants
  2. Niacin
  3. HMG-CoA reductase inhibitors (statins)
  4. Fibric acids
  5. Ezetimibe
  6. Omega-3 fatty acids
- Bile acid sequestrants are the first-line drugs to lower cholesterol in children and in pregnant women.
- The management of metabolic syndrome includes weight reduction and increased physical activity and treatment of hypertension, elevated triglycerides, and low HDL cholesterol.

- In ten primary prevention clinical trials, statin use resulted in a 30% reduction in coronary events and a 12% reduction in total mortality. Despite their well-known benefits, use of statins is not without potential harms. In addition to risk of serious liver injury and rhabdomyolysis, statin use has been linked to cognitive dysfunction and increased risk of diabetes. Despite the recent addition of these warnings by the FDA, statins remain useful and effective medications.
- Fenofibrates have not been shown to reduce morbidity and mortality in patients.
- The AIM-HIGH trial found no cardiovascular benefit from taking extended-release niacin.

DISPOSITION AND FOLLOW-UP

- The NCEP-ATP III recommends that a 3- to 6-mo trial of lifestyle changes and TLC diet should be completed before initiating treatment.
- It also recommends that 6 weekly reassessments with fasting lipid profiles should be performed once lipid lowering therapy is initiated and further intensification of therapy be considered until goal LDL cholesterol is achieved.

- The American College of Physicians guideline does not recommend routine liver function tests in patients treated with statins.
- Counseling about behavioral lifestyle changes and risk factors for CHD should be provided at every follow-up visit.

REFERRAL Patients with rare lipid disorders, hyperlipoproteinemias, patients resistant to treatment, on complex regimens, and with evidence of disease progression despite treatment should be referred to a lipid specialist.

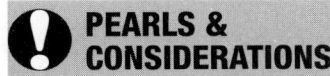
PEARLS & CONSIDERATIONS

COMMENTS

- Nonoptimal levels of LDL and HDL cholesterol during young adulthood are independently associated with coronary atherosclerosis 2 decades later.
- The American Academy of Pediatrics (AAP) guideline (*Pediatrics* 122:198, 2008) recommends consideration toward pharmacologic treatment for children with LDL >190 mg/dl or >160 mg/dl if other risk factors are present.

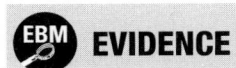
EVIDENCE

available at www.expertconsult.com

SUGGESTED READINGS

available at www.expertconsult.com

RELATED CONTENT

Hyperlipoproteinemia (Related Key Topic)
High Cholesterol (Patient Information)

AUTHOR: **PRIYA BANSAL, M.D., M.P.H.**

TABLE 1-211 Framingham Risk Calculator

Risk Group	Goal LDL Cholesterol (mg/dl)	Initiate Therapeutic Lifestyle Changes	Consider Drug Therapy
High Risk CHD or CHD equivalents (>20% 10-yr risk)	<100 (optional goal <70)	>100	>130 (optional if <100)
Moderately High Risk >2 risk factors (10%-20% 10-yr risk)	<130 (optional goal <100)	>130	>130 (optional if 100-129)
Moderate Risk >2 risk factors (<10% 10-yr risk)	<130	>130	>160
Lower Risk 0-1 risk factor	<160	>160	>190 (optional if 160-189)

TABLE 1-212 Drugs Affecting Lipoprotein Metabolism

Drug Class	Agents and Daily Doses	Lipid/Lipoprotein Effects	Side Effects	Contraindications
HMG-CoA reductase inhibitors (statins)	Lovastatin (10-40 mg) Pravastatin (10-80 mg) Simvastatin (5-80 mg) Fluvastatin (20-40 mg) Atorvastatin (10-80 mg) Rosuvastatin (5-40 mg) Pitavastatin (2-4 mg)	LDL ↓ 20%-60% HDL ↑ 5%-15% TG ↓ 7%-30%	Myalgias, myositis Increased liver enzymes	Active or chronic liver disease Pregnancy Concomitant use of certain drugs*
Bile acid sequestrants	Colestipol (5-20 g) Colesevelam (2.6-3.8 g) Cholestyramine (4-16 g)	LDL ↓ 15%-30% HDL ↑ 3%-5% TG No change or increase	Gastrointestinal distress, constipation, drug interaction, hypertriglyceridemia	TG >300 mg/dl GI motility disorder
Omega-3 fatty acids	Fish oils (4-6 g)	TG ↓ 45% HDL ↑ 13%	Increased bleeding time Nausea	Caution with anticoagulant therapy
Nicotinic acid	Immediate release (niacin) (1.5-3 g) Extended-release (Niaspan) (1-2 g)	LDL ↓ 5%-25% HDL ↑ 15%-35% TG ↓ 20%-50%	Flushing Hyperglycemia Hyperuricemia (or gout) Upper GI distress Hepatotoxicity	Chronic liver disease Severe gout Diabetes Peptic ulcer disease Pregnancy/lactation
Fibric acids	Gemfibrozil (600 mg bid) Fenofibrate (45-145 mg)	LDL ↓ 5%-20% HDL ↑ 10%-20% TG ↓ 20%-50%	Dyspepsia Gallstones Myopathy	Severe renal disease Severe hepatic disease Caution with statins Can worsen LDL cholesterol
Ezetimibe (cholesterol absorption inhibitor)	Ezetimibe (10 mg)	LDL ↓ 18% HDL ↑ 1% TG ↓ 8%	Abdominal pain; myalgias	Liver disease Avoid with resins and fibrates

Modified from The National Cholesterol Education Program, *JAMA* 285:2486, 2001.
*Cyclosporine, macrolide antibiotics, various antifungal agents, and cytochrome P-450 inhibitors (fibrates and niacin should be used with appropriate caution).

H

Diseases and Disorders

I

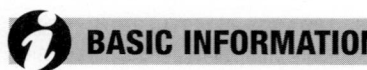 **BASIC INFORMATION**

DEFINITION

Hypercoagulable state is an inherited or acquired condition associated with an increased risk of thrombosis.

SYNONYMS

Thrombophilia

ICD-9CM CODES

289.8 Hypercoagulable state

EPIDEMIOLOGY & DEMOGRAPHICS

INCIDENCE: See Table 1-213.
PREVALENCE, PREDOMINANT SEX, AND AGE: Significant variations in the prevalence rates and thrombotic risks for thrombophilia are reported. This may reflect geographic variation in the prevalence of genetic defects, different populations, or the presence of other unidentified thrombophilic risk factors. When thrombosis occurs, it is often associated with an acquired risk factor (e.g., surgery, pregnancy, oral contraceptive [OC] use). Annual risk of thrombosis is <1%.
GENETICS:
- Most people with a genetic defect will not have thrombotic disease.
- Multiple genetic defects are not uncommon (1% to 2% prevalence in patients with idiopathic venous thromboembolism [VTE]); strong synergistic effect when multiple defects are present. Low risk of recurrent thrombosis in patients with a single genetic defect. Approximately half of patients with unprovoked thrombosis have an identifiable inherited thrombophilia.

RISK FACTORS: Family history of thrombosis, increasing age, tobacco use, immobility, surgery, prior history of DVT, pregnancy, hormone replacement therapy, trauma, connective tissue disease, underlying malignancy, medications (Megace, tamoxifen, birth control pills)

PHYSICAL FINDINGS & CLINICAL PRESENTATION

- Inherited thrombophilia is usually associated with VTE, most commonly deep vein thrombosis (DVT)

- Some acquired thrombophilias are associated with arterial thrombosis. Table E1-214 describes sites of thrombosis according to coagulation defect.
- Pregnancy complications
- Medical conditions associated with increased risk of thrombosis

ETIOLOGY

See Table 1-215A. The differential diagnosis of the patient presenting with thrombosis or thrombotic diathesis is described in Section II. Fig. E1-430 describes components of thrombus formation and actions of various antithrombotic and thrombolytic agents.
- Thrombosis is often a multifactorial process with genetic, environmental, and acquired factors. Table 1-215B describes causes of acquired deficiencies in antithrombin III, protein S, or protein C.
- Thrombotic risk increases with use of OCs or hormone replacement therapy (HRT) and during the pregnancy/postpartum period.
- Adverse pregnancy outcomes may be caused by thrombosis of the uteroplacental circulation.

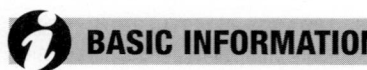 **DIAGNOSIS**

DIFFERENTIAL DIAGNOSIS

INHERITED:
Factor V Leiden (FVL) mutation:
- Autosomal-dominant mutation with low penetrance.
- Causes activated protein C resistance (APCR); 90% of APCR is caused by FVL mutation.
- Most common inherited thrombophilia; accounts for 40% to 50% of cases.
- OC use in heterozygous carriers is associated with an eightfold increased risk of VTE compared with noncarriers and a thirty-fivefold increased risk of VTE compared with noncarriers not using OCs.
- May be associated with cardiovascular disease in select high-risk subgroups.
Prothrombin G20210A mutation:
- Autosomal-dominant mutation with low penetrance.
- OC use in heterozygous carriers is associated with a sixteenfold increased risk of VTE compared with noncarriers not using OCs.

- May be associated with cardiovascular disease in select high-risk subgroups and young patients with ischemic stroke.
Protein C, protein S, antithrombin (AT) deficiency:
- Autosomal-dominant inheritance; many mutations identified for each of these conditions.
- Decreased level (type I deficiency) or abnormal function (type II deficiency).

TABLE 1-215A   Potential Prothrombotic States

Congenital

Deficiency of anticoagulants
  AT-III, protein C or protein S, plasminogen
Resistance to cofactor proteolysis
  Factor V Leiden
High levels of procoagulants
  Prothrombin 20210 mutation
  Elevated factor VIII levels
Damage to endothelium
  Homocysteinemia

Acquired

Obstruction to flow
  Indwelling lines
  Pregnancy
  Polycythemia/dehydration
Immobilization
Injury
  Trauma, surgery, exercise
Inflammation
  IBD, vasculitis, infection, Behçet syndrome
Hypercoagulability
  Pregnancy
  Malignancy
  Antiphospholipid syndrome
  Nephrotic syndrome
  Oral contraceptives
  L-Asparaginase
  Elevated factor VIII levels

Rare Other Entities

Congenital
  Dysfibrinogenemia
Acquired
  Paroxysmal nocturnal hemoglobinuria
  Thrombocythemia
  Vascular grafts

AT-III, Antithrombin III; *IBD*, inflammatory bowel disease.
From Kliegman RM et al: *Nelson textbook of pediatrics,* ed 19, Philadelphia, 2011, Saunders.

TABLE 1-213   Hypercoagulable Conditions

	Prevalence in General Population (%)	Prevalence in Population with Thrombosis (%)	A/V Events	Relative Risk of Thrombosis
FVL mutation	5% of whites; rare in nonwhites	12%-40%	V	Heterozygous: 3-7; homozygous: 80
Prothrombin G20210A mutation	3% of whites; rare in nonwhites	6%-18%	V	3
AT deficiency	0.02%	1%-3%	V	20-50
PC deficiency	0.2%-0.4%	3%-5%	V	7-15
PS deficiency	0.03%-0.1%	1%-5%	V	5-11
Antiphospholipid antibody syndrome	1%-2%	5%-21%	V + A	2-11
Hyperhomocysteinemia	5%-7%	10%	V + A	3
Elevated factor VIII level	11%	25%	V + A	5

A, Arterial; *AT*, antithrombin; *FVL*, factor V Leiden; *PC*, protein C; *PS*, protein S; *V*, venous.

TABLE 1-215B Causes of Acquired Deficiencies in Antithrombin III, Protein C, or Protein S

Antithrombin III	Protein C	Protein S
Neonatal period	Neonatal period	Neonatal period
Pregnancy		Pregnancy
Liver disease	Liver disease	Liver disease
DIC	DIC	DIC
Nephrotic syndrome	Chemotherapy (CMF)	
Major surgery		Inflammatory states
Acute thrombosis	Acute thrombosis	Acute thrombosis
Treatment with:		
Heparin	Warfarin	Warfarin
L-Asparaginase	L-Asparaginase	L-Asparaginase
Estrogens		Estrogens

CMF, Cyclophosphamide, methotrexate, 5-fluorouracil; *DIC,* disseminated intravascular coagulation.
From Hoffman R et al: *Hematology, basic principles and practice,* ed 5, Philadelphia, 2009, Churchill Livingstone.

- First episode of thrombosis is usually in young adults.

Protein C and protein S:
- Homozygous condition is very rare; usually associated with lethal thrombosis in infancy.
- Associated with warfarin-induced skin necrosis, which occurs secondary to depletion of vitamin K–dependent anticoagulant factors sooner than procoagulant factors in the first few days of therapy.

AT deficiency:
- Most thrombogenic of the inherited thrombophilias; 50% lifetime risk of thrombosis.
- Homozygous condition is very rare, probably not compatible with normal fetal development.
- Arterial thrombosis can occur rarely.
- Can cause heparin resistance.

Elevated factor VIII level:
- May be an important risk factor for thrombosis in African-American population.
- Increased risk of recurrent thrombosis.
- Genetic etiology is suspected but not yet identified.

Other possible causes: Non-O blood group, dysfibrinogenemia, elevated thrombin-activatable fibrinolysis inhibitor, elevated factor IX and factor XI levels

ACQUIRED:
Antiphospholipid antibody syndrome (APS):
- Most common cause of acquired thrombophilia.
- Can present as arterial or venous thrombosis, recurrent pregnancy loss, and adverse pregnancy outcomes.
- Thromboembolic events occur in up to 30% of population; high risk of recurrent thrombosis (up to 70% reported).
- See "Antiphospholipid Antibody Syndrome" for more information.

Hyperhomocysteinemia:
- Can be inherited (most commonly an autosomal recessive mutation in methylene tetrahydrofolate reductase gene) but more frequently acquired; folate, vitamin B_6, or vitamin B_{12} deficiency account for two thirds of cases. Other acquired causes include renal disease, hypothyroidism, malignancy, smoking, and certain medications.
- Acquired causes may be associated with VTE and atherosclerotic disease (cardiovascular, cerebrovascular, and peripheral vascular). Inherited causes may be associated with atherosclerotic disease and adverse pregnancy outcomes.

Conditions associated with increased risk of thrombosis:
- Prior thrombosis
- Trauma
- Medical illness: heart failure, respiratory failure, infection, diabetes mellitus, obesity, nephrotic syndrome, inflammatory bowel disease
- Chronic hemolysis–paroxysmal nocturnal hemoglobinuria, sickle cell anemia
- Pregnancy (sixfold increased risk of VTE), postpartum, OC use (fourfold increased risk, higher risk with third-generation OCs), transdermal contraceptive patch, HRT (twofold increased risk), tamoxifen, raloxifene
- Immobilization, travel
- Surgery (especially orthopedic), central venous catheters
- Hyperviscosity syndromes
- Myeloproliferative disorders
- Malignancy: disease or treatment related
- Heparin-induced thrombocytopenia and thrombosis
- Smoking

WORKUP
- History (presence of conditions or use of medications predisposing to thrombosis, family history of thrombosis), physical examination, laboratory tests, imaging studies.
- Age-appropriate cancer screening.
- No consensus exists regarding screening for thrombophilia; little cost-effectiveness or outcomes data are available. Screening laboratory evaluation for patients suspected of having a biologic defect predisposing to thrombosis is described in Box E1-25. Thrombophilia screening is probably overused, as results usually don't change management.
- Thrombophilia screening is not recommended for primary prevention of VTE; some advocate testing prior to OC use or pregnancy in women with a strong family history of thrombosis or thrombophilia.
- Screening not recommended if VTE was associated with an identified risk factor. A possible exception is thrombosis associated with pregnancy, the postpartum period or with OC use.
- Unprovoked VTE:
  ○ Screen individuals for APCR, prothrombin G20210A mutation, protein C, protein S, AT deficiency, and APS if any of the following are present: <50 yr of age at first episode of thrombosis, family history of thrombosis, recurrent thrombosis, thrombosis in unusual anatomic location, life-threatening thrombotic event, warfarin-induced skin necrosis, thrombosis in pregnancy/postpartum/with OC use, or characteristic pregnancy complications.
  ○ Screen all Caucasians <50 yr of age and all women on HRT for APCR, prothrombin G20210A mutation, and APS.
  ○ Screen all others for APS.
- Arterial thrombosis: Screen for APS.
- Note: Routine screening for factor VIII level or hyperhomocysteinemia is not recommended.

TIMING OF WORKUP:
- Ideally >3 wk after discontinuation of anticoagulation (except for APS, which requires prolonged anticoagulation).
- Note: Acute thrombosis, anticoagulation, pregnancy, and many medical conditions can affect the results and must be considered in the timing and interpretation of the workup.

LABORATORY TESTS
- CBC with peripheral smear, electrolytes, calcium, renal and liver function tests, prothrombin time/partial thromboplastin time, prostate-specific antigen (in men aged >50 yr), urinalysis
- Note: Genetic counseling and written informed consent should be obtained before genetic testing. Abnormal nongenetic tests should be repeated after 6 wk to decrease false-positive results.
- APCR: APC-resistance assay (using factor V–deficient plasma) and if positive confirm with genetic test for FVL mutation; use genetic test if lupus anticoagulant present.
- Prothrombin G20210A mutation test.
- AT, protein C, and protein S deficiency: functional assays; if decreased perform antigenic assay to determine type of deficiency. Antigenic assays for protein S should measure free and total levels. In protein C and protein S deficiency, the functional assay may be falsely low in the presence of APCR or elevated factor VIII level and falsely high if lupus anticoagulant is present.
- APS: any of the following found on two occasions at least 12 wk apart: lupus anticoagulant or anticardiolipin antibodies or anti–B_2-glycoprotein-I antibodies.
- Hyperhomocysteinemia: fasting plasma homocysteine level (if normal but suspicion is high, can proceed with methionine loading test and genotyping for methylene tetrahydrofolate reductase).
- Factor VIII level functional assay.

IMAGING STUDIES

Chest radiograph and other tests as appropriate to diagnose thrombosis and rule out associated conditions

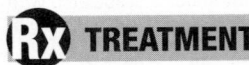 **TREATMENT**

NONPHARMACOLOGIC THERAPY

OC/HRT use and smoking should be avoided.

PROPHYLAXIS

- Prophylactic anticoagulation in high-risk situations.
- Patients with AT deficiency may benefit from antithrombin concentrates in high-risk situations.
- Although homocysteine levels can be lowered with folic acid, vitamin B₆, and vitamin B₁₂ supplements, correcting hyperhomocysteinemia does not decrease risk of thrombosis and routine supplementation is not indicated.
- Vitamin E supplements may decrease risk of VTE in women.
- Pregnancy prophylaxis: timing and intensity of therapy is based on the patient's risk (genetic or acquired defect and clinical history). Women with thrombophilia and recurrent adverse pregnancy outcomes may benefit from prophylaxis with heparin and low-dose aspirin.

ACUTE GENERAL Rx

Initial therapy is the same as for individuals without thrombophilia (exceptions for protein C and AT deficiency).

Venous thrombosis:

- Begin low-molecular-weight heparin (LMWH) and warfarin simultaneously. Continue heparin for at least 5 days and until international normalized ratio (INR) is therapeutic for 2 consecutive days; continue warfarin for at least 3 mo. Aim for INR of 2 to 3. Unfractionated heparin (UH) or fondaparinux (factor Xa inhibitor) may be used as alternatives to LMWH. LMWH is preferred over UH (except in patients with massive pulmonary embolism, increased risk of bleeding or renal failure) because of equivalent or superior effectiveness and a better safety profile.
- Thrombophilia is not associated with a higher risk of recurrent VTE during warfarin therapy, with the exception of cancer patients in whom LMWH for 3 to 6 mo is associated with lower rates of recurrence than warfarin therapy.
- In pregnancy, anticoagulate with heparin throughout pregnancy and for at least 6 wk postpartum. Minimum duration of anticoagulation should be 6 mo. LMWH is preferred over UH. Warfarin may be used postpartum.
- Consider thrombolysis or thrombectomy in patients with massive pulmonary embolism or large proximal lower extremity DVT.

Protein C deficiency:

- Warfarin-induced skin necrosis: Discontinue warfarin, give vitamin K, and start heparin anticoagulation. Consider protein C replacement with protein C concentrate or fresh frozen plasma. Warfarin may be restarted at a low dose (2 mg qd for 3 days and increase by 2 to 3 mg qd until target INR is reached). Continue heparin for at least 5 days and until warfarin-induced anticoagulation is achieved.

AT deficiency:

- AT concentrates may be used if difficulty achieving anticoagulation (heparin resistance), severe thrombosis, or recurrent thrombosis despite adequate anticoagulation.

Arterial thrombosis:

- Anticoagulation and evaluation for thrombolysis or surgery.

CHRONIC Rx

- Optimal duration of anticoagulation remains unknown. Length of therapy may be individualized by assessing the risk of recurrence. Residual thrombosis (on ultrasonography) or elevated D-dimer levels after completion of anticoagulation are associated with an increased risk of recurrence. With these findings, consider prolonging anticoagulation.
- Must consider risk and benefit; risk of major bleeding 2% to 3% annually in general population on anticoagulation but higher in the elderly (7% to 9% per year). Long-term anticoagulation is usually not indicated given the low risk of recurrent thrombosis for most conditions and the bleeding risk associated with anticoagulation.
- Indefinite anticoagulation considered if ≥2 spontaneous thromboses or spontaneous thrombosis associated with any of the following:
  1. Life-threatening thrombosis or thrombosis at an unusual site
  2. More than a single genetic defect
  3. Presence of AT deficiency or APS
- Patients with active cancer may benefit from indefinite anticoagulation.

DISPOSITION

Depends on underlying condition

REFERRAL

Hematology, maternal-fetal medicine, obstetric medicine

PEARLS & CONSIDERATIONS

COMMENTS

- Warfarin therapy effectively reduces the risk of recurrent VTE; when therapy is discontinued VTE risk increases.
- Previous episode of VTE is a major risk factor for recurrence regardless of the presence of

thrombophilia. Risk is greatest in the first 2 yr after thrombosis. ~20% of all patients with unprovoked VTE have recurrence within 5 yr.
- Genetic risk factors for thrombosis in nonwhites remain largely unknown.
- Interpreting workup: many medical conditions cause acquired abnormalities.
  - Acute thrombosis may be associated with lupus anticoagulant, increased anticardiolipin antibodies, and elevated factor VIII levels
  - Heparin therapy: antithrombin levels decrease by up to 30%; can affect lupus anticoagulant testing
  - Warfarin therapy: cannot measure protein C and protein S (levels and function decrease); antithrombin levels may increase; can affect lupus anticoagulant testing
  - Protein C, protein S, and antithrombin levels decrease with acute thrombosis (<2 wk), surgery, liver disease, disseminated intravascular coagulation, and chemotherapy. Protein C level also decreases with severe infection but levels increase with age and hyperlipidemia. Protein S and antithrombin levels also decrease with nephrotic syndrome, pregnancy and estrogen therapy (HRT, OC)
  - APCR is increased with pregnancy, estrogen therapy (HRT, OCs), and certain cancers; elevated factor VIII level and antiphospholipid antibodies can cause APCR

PREVENTION

Risk of postthrombotic syndrome decreases if compression stockings are worn for at least 1 year, starting in the first month after the DVT.

PATIENT & FAMILY EDUCATION

National Blood Clot Alliance
120 White Plains Road, Suite 100
Tarrytown, NY 10591
http://www.stoptheclot.org/contact.htm
National Collaborative Outreach Project of the Blood Clot Outreach Program
at the Hemophilia and Thrombosis Center
University of North Carolina at Chapel Hill
http://www.clotconnect.org/about-clot-connect/about
Factor V Leiden Resources
http://www.fvleiden.org/resources/index.html
APS Foundation of America, Inc.
P. O. Box 801
LaCrosse, WI 54602-0801
http://www.apsfa.org/

SUGGESTED READINGS
available at www.expertconsult.com

RELATED CONTENT

Thrombophilia (Patient Information)

AUTHOR: **SUDEEP KAUR AULAKH, M.D.**

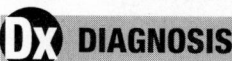

BASIC INFORMATION

DEFINITION

Hyperemesis gravidarum is a severe and persistent form of nausea and vomiting resulting in at least a 5% weight loss, dehydration, ketonuria, and electrolyte imbalance, with typical onset at 4 to 8 wk of pregnancy continuing through 14 to 16 wk of pregnancy.

ICD-9CM CODES
643.0 [0,1,3] Mild hyperemesis gravidarum
643.1 [0,1,3] Hyperemesis gravidarum with metabolic disturbance

EPIDEMIOLOGY & DEMOGRAPHICS

INCIDENCE: 0.5% to 2% of pregnancies
GENETICS: No genetic disposition
RISK FACTORS: Women with increased placental mass, including molar pregnancy or multiple gestation, family history or personal history of hyperemesis gravidarum, prior miscarriage, nulliparity, preexisting diabetes, hyperthyroid disorder, peptic ulceration or other gastrointestinal disorders, depression, and asthma. Female fetus increases the risk by 1.5-fold.

PHYSICAL FINDINGS & CLINICAL PRESENTATION

- Weight loss of more than 5% from pregravid weight
- Symptoms—nausea, vomiting, spitting, enhanced olfactory senses, food and/or fluid intolerance, lethargy
- Signs—dehydration, poor skin turgor, dry mucous membranes, ketonuria, anemia, tachycardia, hypotension
- Complications include inadequate caloric intake, nutritional deficiencies, dehydration, and electrolyte abnormalities including hyponatremia, hypocalcemia, hypokalemia, and in severe cases hypochloremic metabolic acidosis or Wernicke's encephalopathy from thiamine deficiency

ETIOLOGY

Unknown but likely multifactorial. Theories include gestational hyperestrogenemia, gastric dysrhythmias, and hyperthyroidism.

DIAGNOSIS

DIFFERENTIAL DIAGNOSIS

- Gastrointestinal conditions—gastroenteritis, gastroparesis, achalasia, biliary tract disease, hepatitis, intestinal obstruction, peptic ulcer disease, appendicitis
- Genitourinary tract conditions—pyelonephritis, uremia, ovarian torsion, kidney stones, degenerating uterine leiomyoma
- Metabolic disease—diabetic ketoacidosis, porphyria, Addison's disease, hyperthyroidism
- Neurologic conditions—pseudotumor cerebri, vestibular lesions, migraines, tumors of the central nervous system
- Miscellaneous—drug toxicity or intolerance, psychologic
- Pregnancy-related conditions—acute fatty liver of pregnancy, preeclampsia

WORKUP

Diagnosis is one of exclusion. History and physical examination along with laboratory tests to rule out other causes of vomiting should be performed.

LABORATORY TESTS

- Urinalysis may show elevated specific gravity, ketonuria, or proteinuria
- Liver enzymes (elevated but usually <300 U/L)
- Serum bilirubin (<4 mg/dl)
- Serum amylase or lipase (up to 5× greater than normal)
- BMP, may reveal hyponatremia, hypokalemia, low serum urea
- CBC
- Calcium
- TSH and free T4 (transient hyperthyroidism occurs in 2/3 of women with hyperemesis gravidarum; this is biochemical hyperthyroidism that usually resolves by 18 wk gestation; treatment should not be undertaken without evidence of intrinsic thyroid disease)

IMAGING STUDIES

- Ultrasound to evaluate for multiple gestation or molar pregnancy
- Right upper quadrant ultrasound to evaluate for biliary tract disease

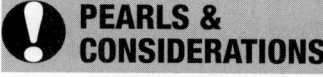 TREATMENT

NONPHARMACOLOGIC THERAPY

- Reassurance and support
- Avoidance of foods and smells that trigger nausea
- Oral ginger root
- Small frequent dry meals
- Eating prior to getting out of bed

ACUTE GENERAL Rx

- Nothing by mouth
- Intravenous fluid and electrolyte replacement with vitamin supplementation
- Thiamine administration prior to giving dextrose to avoid Wernicke's encephalopathy
- Pyridoxine (vitamin B_6)
- Antiemetics, including promethazine, phenothiazines, metoclopramide, and ondansetron, have been shown to be both safe and effective in improving pregnancy outcome
- Restart oral intake gradually no less than 48 hr after vomiting has stopped

CHRONIC Rx

- Nasogastric feedings are useful alternatives in severe cases
- Total parenteral nutrition may be necessary in life threatening cases

COMPLEMENTARY AND ALTERNATIVE MEDICINE

- Supportive psychotherapy
- Acupuncture
- Acupressure with use of a wrist band

DISPOSITION

- Infants born to pregnancies complicated by hyperemesis are more likely to be premature and small for gestational age.
- Lower rates of miscarriage have also been documented when comparing pregnancies complicated by hyperemesis gravidarum vs. controls.

PEARLS & CONSIDERATIONS

COMMENTS

Nausea and vomiting in early pregnancy are associated with psychosocial morbidity.

PREVENTION

Taking a multivitamin at the time of conception

SUGGESTED READINGS

available at www.expertconsult.com

RELATED CONTENT

Hyperemesis Gravidarum (Patient Information)

AUTHOR: **ALISON PATTERSON, M.D.**

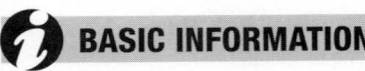

DEFINITION

Hypereosinophilic syndrome (HES) refers to a group of disorders of unknown cause characterized by sustained overproduction of eosinophils, in which eosinophilic infiltration and mediators release cause organ dysfunction.

SYNONYMS

Idiopathic hypereosinophilic syndrome (IHES)

ICD-9CM CODES
288.3 Hypereosinophilic syndrome

EPIDEMIOLOGY & DEMOGRAPHICS

PREDOMINANT SEX: Occurs in men more often than women (9:1)
PREDOMINANT AGE: Usually occurs between the ages of 20 and 50 yr

PHYSICAL FINDINGS & CLINICAL PRESENTATION

- Clinical presentation of HES may vary from an incidental finding of eosinophilia to sudden onset of cardiac or neurologic symptoms.
- Early presentation includes fatigue, cough, breathlessness, muscle pain, angioedema, rash, and fever.
- Cardiac manifestations (58%) include dyspnea, orthopnea, and signs and symptoms of congestive heart failure (CHF). Including three stages: acute necrotic stage secondary to endocardial infiltration of eosinophils; thrombus formation; and fibrotic stage. This may result in a restrictive or dilated cardiomyopathy and/or valvular heart disease.
- Neurologic manifestations (54%) may be of three types:
  1. Thromboembolic (e.g., cardiac emboli or local vascular thrombosis)
  2. CNS dysfunction: confusion, loss of memory, ataxia, upper motor neuron signs, seizures, and behavior changes
  3. Peripheral neuropathy (most common) may be symmetric or asymmetric, sensory or mixed sensory and motor deficits
- Pulmonary manifestations (40%) include a chronic persistent nonproductive cough, shortness of breath, and dyspnea on exertion. Diffuse or focal infiltrate may present in 20% of cases. Complications may include pulmonary fibrosis, CHF, or pulmonary embolus.
- Cutaneous manifestations (56%) usually include eczema, lichenifications, urticaria, angioedema, or erythematous pruritic papules and nodules.
- GI manifestations (23%) include diarrhea, but findings of gastritis, colitis, pancreatitis, cholangitis, and hepatitis can occur.
- Ocular manifestations (23%) are thought to be the result of retinal microemboli.
- Vascular manifestations include venous or arterial thrombosis of unknown mechanism such as femoral artery occlusion, intracranial sinus thrombosis, and digital gangrene.

ETIOLOGY

- The etiology of HES is unknown and is thought of as a composite of many diseases.
- In some cases, a fusion event generating an abnormal and oncogenic tyrosine kinase (FIP1L1-PDGFRA) appears to be causative especially in males.

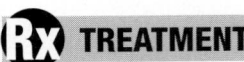 **DIAGNOSIS**

Criteria for the diagnosis of idiopathic HES include:
- Persistent eosinophilia of >1500 eosinophils/mm³ for more than 6 mo
- Exclusion of other conditions causing eosinophilia (Box E1-26)
- Signs and symptoms of organ system dysfunction (e.g., heart, liver, lung).

DIFFERENTIAL DIAGNOSIS

The differential includes all causes of peripheral blood eosinophilia. Parasitic infections, coccidioidomycosis, cat-scratch disease, asthma, Churg-Strauss syndrome, allergic rhinitis, atopic dermatitis, drug-induced eosinophilia, aspergillosis, eosinophilic pneumonia, hypersensitivity pneumonitis, HIV, eosinophilic gastroenteritis, inflammatory bowel disease, leukemias (CML and CMML), systemic mastocytosis with eosinophilia.

WORKUP

The workup of a patient who is suspected of having HES should exclude other causes mentioned in the "Differential Diagnosis" section leading to peripheral eosinophilia.

LABORATORY TESTS

- CBC with differential; often the total WBC ranges from 10,000 to 30,000/mm³ with eosinophilia of 30% to 70%, anemia is present in 50% of the cases, and either thrombocytopenia or thrombocytosis may be noted
- Erythrocyte sedimentation rate (ESR) and rheumatoid factor
- Liver function tests (LFTs), electrolytes, urinalysis, BUN, and creatinine
- HIV assay
- Stools for ova and parasites ×3
- Serologic blood tests for parasitic infections (e.g., *Strongyloides*)
- Total IgE level
- Bone marrow aspirate and biopsy (Fig. E1-431)
- Duodenal aspirate
- ECG
- Tissue biopsies as indicated
- Serum levels of vitamin B_{12}
- Serum levels of tryptase

IMAGING STUDIES

- Chest radiograph may be clear or show infiltrates, effusions, or fibrotic scarring
- CT scan of chest, abdomen, and pelvis
- Echocardiogram (or cardiac MRI for early cardiac involvement) can assess for ventricular function and valvular pathology including regurgitation and thrombi formation

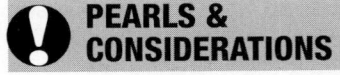 **TREATMENT**

Treatment is initiated only if there is evidence of organ involvement.

NONPHARMACOLOGIC THERAPY

In patients with hypereosinophilia without organ involvement, serial echocardiograms, blood chemistries, and pulmonary function tests are recommended at 6-mo intervals.

ACUTE GENERAL Rx

- In patients with organ involvement without FIP1L1-PDGFRA fusion, initial therapy is with prednisone 1 mg/kg/day or 60 mg/day in adults.
- Patient's symptoms and peripheral eosinophil counts are monitored.
- Doses may be tapered to alternate-day prednisone use in patients whose eosinophil counts have been suppressed.

CHRONIC Rx

- Patients not responding to corticosteroids, hydroxyurea 1 to 2 g/day may be tried.
- Patient with FIP1L1-PDGFRA fusion with or without organ involvement should be started on tyrosine kinase imatinib or dasatinib for resistant cases.
- If the disease continues to progress, vincristine, etoposide, interferon-α, cyclosporine, and leukapheresis are alternative choices.
- Anticoagulation and/or antiplatelet agents are often used in patients with HES.
- If all else fails, bone marrow transplantation may be considered.

DISPOSITION

- Before the use of cardiac imaging (echo) and cardiac surgeries (valve replacement), patients with HES had a poor prognosis with a mean survival of 9 mo and a 3-yr survival of 12%.
- Deaths usually result from CHF, endocarditis, and systemic emboli.
- 5-yr and 15-yr survival rates are 80% and 42%, respectively.

REFERRAL

HES is a rare and complicated disorder requiring a multidisciplinary approach.

PEARLS & CONSIDERATIONS

COMMENTS

There is still much to be learned about HES. The etiology and exact mechanism of organ damage caused by eosinophils remains unknown.

SUGGESTED READINGS
available at www.expertconsult.com

AUTHORS: **MONZR M. AL MALKI, M.D.,** and **GLENN G. FORT, M.D., M.P.H.**

BASIC INFORMATION

DEFINITION

- Primary hyperlipoproteinemia is a group of genetic disorders of the lipid transport proteins in the blood that manifests as abnormally elevated levels of cholesterol, triglycerides, or both in the serum of affected patients.
- Usually defined as total cholesterol, LDL, triglycerides or lipoprotein A levels above 90th percentile or HDL or apo A-1 levels below the 10th percentile for the general population. Table 1-216 describes the ATP III classification for cholesterol.

SYNONYMS

Hyperlipidemia

ICD-9CM CODES
272.4 Hyperlipoproteinemia
272.3 Fredrickson type I
272.0 Fredrickson type IIa
272.2 Fredrickson type IIb, III
272.1 Fredrickson type IV
272.3 Fredrickson type V

EPIDEMIOLOGY & DEMOGRAPHICS

INCIDENCE: The most common types are lipoprotein A excess, hypertriglyceridemia, and combined hyperlipidemia.
- Incidence of heterozygous familial hypercholesterolemia: −1:500.
- Incidence of homozygous familial hypercholesterolemia: −1:1 million.
- Familial hypercholesterolemia: autosomal-dominant disorder.
- Familial combined hyperlipidemia: possibly an autosomal-dominant disorder.
- Multifactorial predilection: apparent in majority of affected individuals.

GENETICS:
- Familial lipoprotein lipase deficiency: autosomal recessive, resulting in an elevation in the plasma chylomicrons and triglycerides
- Familial apoprotein CII deficiency: autosomal recessive, resulting in increased serum chylomicrons, very-low-density lipoprotein (VLDL), and hypertriglyceridemia
- Familial type 3 hyperlipoproteinemia: single-gene defect requiring contributory factors to manifest
- Familial hypercholesterolemia: autosomal-dominant defect of the LDL receptor, resulting in an elevated serum cholesterol level and normal triglycerides
- Familial hypertriglyceridemia: common, autosomal-dominant defect resulting in elevated VLDL and triglycerides
- Multiple lipoprotein–type hyperlipidemia: autosomal dominant, manifesting as isolated hypercholesterolemia, isolated hypertriglyceridemia, or hyperlipidemia
- Polygenic hypercholesterolemia: multifactorial
- Polygenic hyperalphalipoproteinemia: autosomal dominant or polygenic, causing an elevated high-density lipoprotein

- A classification of lipoprotein disorders is described in Table 1-217.

PHYSICAL FINDINGS & CLINICAL PRESENTATION

- Familial lipoprotein lipase deficiency: recurrent bouts of abdominal pain in infancy, eruptive xanthomas, hepatomegaly, splenomegaly, lipemia retinalis
- Familial apoprotein CII deficiency: occasional eruptive xanthomas
- Familial type 3 hyperlipoproteinemia: xanthoma striata palmaris or tuberoeruptive xanthomas, xanthelasmas, arterial bruits at a young age, gangrene of the lower extremities at a young age
- Familial hypercholesterolemia: tendon xanthomas, arcus corneae, xanthelasma
- Familial hypertriglyceridemia: associated obesity; eruptive xanthomas can develop with exacerbations

ETIOLOGY

- Genetic defects causing lipid abnormalities
- Environmental influences including diet, drugs, and alcohol intake

DIAGNOSIS

DIFFERENTIAL DIAGNOSIS

Secondary causes of hyperlipoproteinemias:
- Hypothyroidism
- Diabetes mellitus
- Pancreatitis
- Autoimmune hyperlipoproteinemia
- Nephrotic syndrome

TABLE 1-216 ATP III Classification of LDL, Total, and HDL Cholesterol (mg/dl)

LDL Cholesterol

<100	Optimal
100-129	Near or above optimal
130-159	Borderline high
160-189	High
≥190	Very high

Total Cholesterol

<200	Desirable
200-239	Borderline high
>240	High

HDL Cholesterol

<40	Low
>60	High

From Expert Panel on Detection, Evaluation, and Treatment of High Blood Cholesterol in Adults: Executive Summary of the Third Report of the National Cholesterol Education Program (NCEP) Expert Panel on Detection, Evaluation, and Treatment of High Blood Cholesterol in Adults (Adult Treatment Panel III), *JAMA* 285:2486-2497, 2001.
ATP, Adult treatment panel; *HDL,* high-density lipoprotein; *LDL,* low-density lipoprotein.

- Biliary obstruction

WORKUP

- Family history for premature cardiac disease
- Personal history of recurrent pancreatitis
- Detailed physical examination

LABORATORY TESTS

- Standard lipid profile
- If normal, further testing with measurement of lipoprotein A, apo B, and apo A-1
- Lipoprotein electrophoresis and ultracentrifugation (for phenotypic classification)
- Workup for secondary causes: TSH, fasting glucose, liver function, renal function, urinary protein

TREATMENT

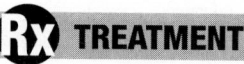

NONPHARMACOLOGIC THERAPY

- Cornerstone of treatment: dietary therapy
  - TLC diet (**t**herapeutic **l**ifestyle **c**hanges): see "Hypercholesterolemia" topic
- Risk factor reduction includes smoking cessation, treatment of hypertension, exercise
- Familial lipoprotein lipase deficiency and familial apoprotein CII deficiency: fat-free diet
- Remainder of cases, except those with polygenic hyperalphalipoproteinemia: fat- and cholesterol-restricted diets
- Interventions to improve adherence are described in Table 1-218

ACUTE GENERAL Rx

No acute treatment needed

CHRONIC Rx

- Familial lipoprotein lipase deficiency, polygenic hyperalphalipoproteinemia, or familial apoprotein CII deficiency: no chronic drug therapy
- Familial type 3 hyperlipoproteinemia: usually responds well to secondary causes being treated and diet therapy; if not, fibric acids may be tried
- Familial hypercholesterolemia: bile acid sequestrants, HMG-CoA reductase inhibitors, or niacin
- Familial hypertriglyceridemia: fibric acids
- Multiple lipoprotein–type hyperlipidemia: drug therapy aimed at the predominant lipid abnormality noted
- Recent data suggest in patients with lipoprotein abnormalities that treatment goals should be based on non-HDL cholesterol rather than LDL cholesterol
- The FDA has approved mipomersen and lomitapide in patients with homozygous familial hypercholesterolemia already taking maximum doses of other lipid-lowering drugs. Both medicines are hepatotoxic and very expensive (>$150,000/yr).

DISPOSITION

- Those with polygenic hyperalphalipoproteinemia: excellent prognosis for longevity
- Those with familial hypercholesterolemia, familial type 3 hypercholesterolemia, or multiple

TABLE 1-217 Classification of Lipoprotein Disorders by Phenotypes, Genotypes, and Corresponding Clinical Manifestations

Phenotype (Frederickson Type)	Genotype	Elevated Cholesterol Type	Genetic Defect	Xanthomas	Other Clinical Manifestations
I (rare)	Familial hyperchylomi-cronemia	Elevated chylomicrons	Familial lipoprotein lipase deficiency, Apo C-II deficiency	Eruptive skin xanthomas	Recurrent abdominal pain, hepatosplenomegaly
IIA	Familial hypercholester-olemia	Elevated LDL	FHC, LDL receptor deficiency	Tendon xanthomas, xanthelasma, tuberous; planar palmar (homozygous)	Premature CAD, arcus corneae, arthritic symptoms
IIB	Familial combined hypercholesterolemia	Elevated LDL and VLDL	Reduced LDL receptor and increased apo B		
III (rare)	Familial dysbetalipopro-teinemia	Elevated IDL	Defective apo E2 synthesis	Tuberous, planar (palmar)	Premature CAD and peripheral vascular disease, male > female, obesity, abnormal glucose tolerance, hyperuricemia, aggravated by hypothyroiditis, good response to therapy
IV	Familial hyperlipemia	Elevated VLDL	Increased VLDL production	None	CAD and peripheral vascular disease, obesity, abnormal glucose tolerance, hyperuricemia, arthritic
V (rare)	Endogenous hypertri-glyceridemia	Elevated VLDL, chylomicrons	Increased VLDL production and reduced LPL	Eruptive	

Apo, Apolipoprotein; *CAD,* coronary artery disease; *FHC,* familial hypercholesterolemia.
Modified from Graber MA: *The family practice handbook,* ed 4, St Louis, 2001, Mosby.

TABLE 1-218 Interventions to Improve Adherence

Focus on the Patient

Simplify medication regimens.
Provide explicit patient instruction and use good counseling techniques to teach the patient how to follow the prescribed treatment.
Encourage the use of prompts to help patients remember treatment regimens.
Use systems to reinforce adherence and maintain contact with the patient.
Encourage the support of family and friends.
Reinforce and reward adherence.
Increase visits for patients unable to achieve treatment goal.
Increase the convenience and access to care.
Involve patients in their care through self-monitoring.

Focus on the Physician and Medical Office

Teach physicians to implement lipid treatment guidelines.
Use reminders to prompt physicians to attend to lipid management.
Identify a patient advocate in the office to help deliver or prompt care.
Use patients to prompt preventive care.
Develop a standardized treatment plan to structure care.
Use feedback from past performance to foster change in future care.
Remind patients of appointments and follow up missed appointments.

Focus on the Health Delivery System

Provide lipid management through a lipid clinic.
Utilize case management by nurses.
Deploy telemedicine.
Utilize the collaborative care of pharmacists.
Execute critical care pathways in hospitals.

From Expert Panel on Detection, Evaluation, and Treatment of High Blood Cholesterol in Adults: Executive Summary of the Third Report of the National Cholesterol Education Program (NCEP) Expert Panel on Detection, Evaluation, and Treatment of High Blood Cholesterol in Adults (Adult Treatment Panel III), *JAMA* 285:2486-2497, 2001.

lipoprotein–type hyperlipidemia: even with aggressive treatment, at high risk for accelerated atherosclerosis and coronary artery disease

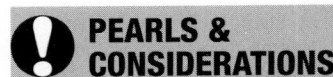
PEARLS & CONSIDERATIONS

COMMENTS
- Patient information is available through the American Heart Association.
- Lipid-lowering drug therapy is recommended for children ≥10 yr whose LDL-C levels remain extremely elevated after 6 mo to 1 yr of dietary modification. Drug therapy also can be considered for children with LDL-C levels of ≥190 mg/dl. Children who may also require treatment are those whose levels are >160 mg/dl and who have ≥2 risk factors for cardiovascular disease or a family history of premature cardiovascular disease.

SUGGESTED READINGS
available at www.expertconsult.com

RELATED CONTENT
Hypercholesterolemia (Related Key Topic)

AUTHOR: **PRIYA BANSAL, M.D., M.P.H.**

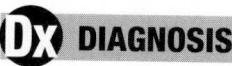

BASIC INFORMATION

DEFINITION

Hyperosmolar hyperglycemic syndrome (HHS) is characterized by severe hyperglycemia, hyperosmolarity, profound dehydration, and altered mental status in the absence of ketosis.

SYNONYMS

Hyperosmolar coma
Nonketotic hyperosmolar syndrome
Hyperosmolar nonketotic state
HHS

ICD-9CM CODES
250.2 Hyperosmolar coma

PHYSICAL FINDINGS & CLINICAL PRESENTATION

- Evidence of extreme dehydration (poor skin turgor, sunken eyeballs, dry mucous membranes)
- Neurologic defects (reversible hemiplegia, focal seizures)
- Orthostatic hypotension, tachycardia
- Evidence of precipitating factors (infection, myocardial ischemia, stroke)
- Suppressed mental status ranging from delirium to obtundation to coma (25% of patients)

ETIOLOGY

- Infections in up to 50% (e.g., pneumonia, urinary tract infection, sepsis)
- New or previously unrecognized diabetes (30%)
- Non-compliance, dose reduction, or recent discontinuation of diabetic medication
- Stress (myocardial infarction, cerebrovascular accident)
- Drugs: diuretics (dehydration), phenytoin, diazoxide (impairs insulin secretion), glucocorticoids, chemotherapeutic agents, calcium channel blockers, total parenteral nutrition, substance abuse (alcohol, cocaine)

DIAGNOSIS

DIFFERENTIAL DIAGNOSIS

- Diabetic ketoacidosis
- The differential diagnosis of coma is described in Section II

LABORATORY TESTS

- Hyperglycemia: serum glucose usually >600 mg/dl, serum/urine ketones absent or "small."
- Hyperosmolarity: serum osmolarity usually >320 mOsm/L.
- Serum sodium: may be low, normal, or high. Because glucose draws fluid from the intracellular space, decreasing the serum sodium, it is necessary to correct sodium for the serum glucose level. The corrected sodium can be obtained by increasing the serum sodium concentration by 1.6 mEq/dl for every 100 mg/dl increase in the serum glucose level over normal.
- Serum potassium: may be low, normal, or high; regardless of the initial serum level, the total body deficit is approximately 5 to 15 mEq/kg.
- Serum bicarbonate: usually >15 mEq/L (average 17 mEq/L).
- Arterial pH: usually >7.3; both serum bicarbonate and arterial pH may be lower if lactic acidosis is present.
- Blood urea nitrogen: generally ranges from 60 to 90 mg/dl due to severe dehydration and pro-renal azotemia.
- Phosphorus: hypophosphatemia (average deficit is 70 to 140 mmol).
- Calcium: hypocalcemia (average deficit is 50 to 100 mEq).
- Magnesium: hypomagnesemia (average deficit is 50 to 100 mEq).
- Complete blood count with differential, urinalysis, and blood and urine cultures should be performed to rule out infectious etiology.
- ECG to rule out a concomitant myocardial infarction.

IMAGING STUDIES

- Chest radiograph is useful to rule out infectious process. The initial radiograph may be negative if the patient has significant dehydration. Repeat chest x-ray after 24 hr of hydration if pulmonary infection is suspected.
- The need for additional imaging, such as CT scans, is determined by biochemical or physical exam findings.

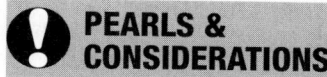

TREATMENT

NONPHARMACOLOGIC THERAPY

- Monitor mental status, vital signs, urine output hourly until improved, then monitor q2-4h.
- Monitor electrolytes, renal function, and glucose level (see "Acute General Rx").

ACUTE GENERAL Rx

- Vigorous fluid replacement: the volume and rate of fluid replacement are determined by renal and cardiac function. Slower infusion rate may be used initially in patients with compromised cardiovascular or renal status. Frequent clinical monitoring of fluid status is essential.
  - During the first hour, infuse 1000 ml of 0.9% normal saline (NS) to expand the intravascular fluid volume.
  - Infuse a second liter of 0.9% NS in the next hour if the patient is persistently hypotensive.
  - Then begin replacing the free fluid deficit with 0.45% NS at 250 to 500 ml/hr. Taper the 0.45% NS to replace the estimated fluid deficit over 24 to 36 hours.
  - When serum glucose reaches 300 mg/dl, change to 5% dextrose with 0.45% NS.
- Correct hyperglycemia: the goal is to decrease plasma glucose by 50 to 100 mg/dl/hr.
  - Vigorous IV hydration will decrease the serum glucose level in most patients by 80 mg/dl/hr. Insulin should not be administered until serum potassium is >3.3 mEq/L to prevent life-threatening hypokalemia.
  - A regular insulin IV bolus (0.1 units/kg of body weight) is followed by an insulin fusion of 0.1 units/kg/hr, adjusted on an hourly basis as needed, until the serum glucose level approaches 300 mg/dl.
  - Before stopping the IV insulin infusion, administer an SC dose of insulin (dose varies with patient's demonstrated insulin sensitivity). Short (regular) or rapid-acting (aspart, lispro, glulisine) insulins should be administered SC 1 to 2 hr before stopping the IV insulin infusion. Intermediate (NPH) or long-acting (glargine, detemir) insulins should be administered SC 2 to 4 hr before stopping IV insulin infusion.
- Total daily insulin doses in insulin-naïve patients range from 0.5 to 0.8 units/kg/day. Approximately half of this dose should be given as intermediate or long-acting insulin, and half of this dose should be given as mealtime or prandial insulin if the patient is eating.
- Replace potassium: monitor potassium every 2 hours until the patient has stabilized. Confirm the patient is not anuric before starting potassium (K) replacement. Rate of K replacement can be based on presenting potassium level. If K is <3.3, give KCl 20 to 30 mEq/L of intravenous fluid (IVF) until K is >3.3. If K is 3.3 to 5.3, give KCl at 10 to 30 mEq/L IVF to maintain a K of >4. If K >5.3, hold potassium supplementation and check K every 2 hours. Continuous telemetry monitoring and hourly measurement of urinary output are recommended.
- Phosphate replacement: replacement can be considered if serum phosphate is <2 mEq/L or there is evidence of phosphate depletion syndrome rhabdomyolysis. In the absence of renal failure, phosphate can be administered at a rate of 0.1 mmol/kg/hr (5 to 10 mmol/hr) to a maximum of 80 to 120 mmol in 24 hr.
- Magnesium replacement, in the absence of renal failure, can be administered IM (0.05 to 0.10 ml/kg of 20% magnesium sulfate) or as IV infusion (4 to 8 ml of 20% magnesium sulfate [0.08 to 0.16 mEq/kg]).
- Individual patients may be appropriate for a trial of oral diabetic therapy as an outpatient after glucose toxicity has completely resolved.

PEARLS & CONSIDERATIONS

COMMENTS

- The typical patient is an elderly or bed-confined diabetic with impaired ability to communicate thirst who is evaluated after an interval of 1 to 2 wk of prolonged osmotic diuresis.
- There is a higher mortality with HHS (5%-20%) than diabetic ketoacidosis (DKA), often due to underlying coexisting comorbities.
  - Risk factors associated with higher mortality include age >70 years, nursing home residency, marked hyperosmolarity or hypernatremia.

SUGGESTED READINGS
available at www.expertconsult.com

RELATED CONTENT
Fig. E1-277 Management of diabetic ketoacidosis (DKA) and hyperglycemic state (HHS) (Algorithm)
Hyponatremia

AUTHORS: **HILARY B. WHITLATCH, M.D.,** **SAINATH GADDAM, M.D.,** and **FRED F. FERRI, M.D.**

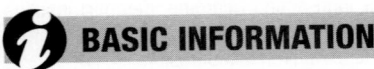

DEFINITION

Hyperparathyroidism is an endocrine disorder caused by excessive secretion of parathyroid hormone (PTH) from the parathyroid glands. Autonomous production of PTH resulting in hypercalcemia defines primary hyperparathyroidism. Secondary hyperparathyroidism occurs when the parathyroid glands appropriately increase PTH production in response to low calcium states. Primary hyperparathyroidism is the focus of this section.

ICD-9CM CODES
252.00 Hyperparathyroidism, unspecified
252.01 Hyperparathyroidism, primary

EPIDEMIOLOGY & DEMOGRAPHICS

INCIDENCE: 4 cases per 100,000 persons per year. Primary hyperparathyroidism is the most common cause of hypercalcemia.
PREVALENCE: 3 cases/1000 persons
PREDOMINANT SEX AND AGE: Most cases occur in women (74%) but the incidence is similar in men and women before 45 years of age. The incidence of primary hyperparathyroidism peaks in the seventh decade.

PHYSICAL FINDINGS & CLINICAL PRESENTATION

The majority of patients with primary hyperparathyroidism are asymptomatic. Diagnosis is usually considered in patients after an incidental discovery of hypercalcemia or during the evaluation for decreased bone mass. The development of symptoms varies with severity and rapidity of disease progression and reflects both the hypercalcemic and hyperparathyroid components of the disease process.
- Cardiovascular: hypertension, shortened QT interval, bradycardia, arrhythmia, valvular calcification, left ventricular hypertrophy, increased mean carotid intima-media thickness.
- GI: anorexia, nausea, vomiting, constipation, abdominal pain, peptic ulcer disease, pancreatitis
- GU: nephrolithiasis, nephrocalcinosis, renal insufficiency, polyuria, nocturia, nephrogenic diabetes insipidus, renal tubular acidosis
- Musculoskeletal: weakness, myopathy, bone pain, osteopenia, osteoporosis, gout, pseudogout, chondrocalcinosis, osteitis fibrosa cystica
- CNS: confusion, anxiety, fatigue, lethargy, obtundation, depression, coma
- Other: hypomagnesemia, hypophosphatemia, pruritus, metastatic calcifications, band keratopathy

ETIOLOGY
- Most cases of primary hyperparathyroidism are sporadic but it can be associated with rare genetic conditions such as multiple endocrine neoplasia (MEN-1 and MEN-2). Pathologic characteristics include adenoma (89%), hyperplasia (10%), or carcinomas (<1%).

- Head and neck irradiation in childhood and long-term lithium therapy are associated with a higher prevalence of primary hyperparathyroidism.

DX DIAGNOSIS

DIFFERENTIAL DIAGNOSIS
- Secondary hyperparathyroidism precipitated by conditions that result in hypocalcemia
  - Medication: loop diuretics
  - Calcium deficiency
  - Vitamin D deficiency
  - Chronic kidney disease (most common)
  - Pseudohypoparathyroidism (PTH resistance)
  - Suppression of bone resorption (due to bisphosphonates)
- Other causes of hypercalcemia include:
  - Medications: thiazide diuretics, lithium therapy
  - Vitamin D intoxication, milk-alkali syndrome
  - Familial hypocalciuric hypercalcemia (FHH)
  - Renal failure (tertiary hyperparathyroidism)
  - Granulomatous disorders (e.g., sarcoidosis)
  - Malignancy (e.g., lung cancer, lymphoma, myeloma, bone metastasis)
  - Prolonged immobilization

WORKUP
- Primary hyperparathyroidism is confirmed with an elevated serum calcium and PTH level.
  - Two measurements of serum calcium are required for the confirmation of hypercalcemia. Total calcium should be corrected for low albumin utilizing the formula: Corrected Calcium = $(0.8 \times [4 - \text{serum albumin}]) + \text{serum calcium}$. If a reliable laboratory is available, an ionized calcium should be considered especially in conditions associated with acid-base disturbances or low albumin states.
  - The serum intact PTH (iPTH) level is the single best test to evaluate the etiology of hypercalcemia. PTH is elevated or in the high normal range (i.e., inappropriately normal for an elevated calcium state) in primary hyperparathyroidism. PTH is decreased in most other conditions associated with elevated calcium.
- Other causes of hypercalcemia should be ruled out. These are typically associated with low PTH levels. Exceptions include lithium use and FHH.
  - Review medication history to determine lithium, thiazide, vitamin D or calcium intake.
  - Check 24-hr urine calcium:creatinine to rule out FHH. Urine calcium is usually low in FHH. PTH can be low, normal, or high in FHH.
  - Consider PTH-related peptide (PTHrP) to evaluate hypercalcemia related to malignancies and vitamin D1,25 to assess hypercalcemia secondary to glaucomatous diseases or lymphomas.

  - Multiple myeloma and bone metastasis can also result in a high calcium state and therefore must be appropriately evaluated.
- Rule out other causes of elevated PTH (i.e., secondary hyperparathyroidism). Serum calcium is typically low or low-normal in secondary hyperparathyroidism.
  - Check calcium and 25 OH-vitamin D to rule out deficiency states.
  - Assess renal function to evaluate for chronic renal failures.

LABORATORY TESTS
- Serum calcium (ionized or corrected calcium): elevated in primary hyperparathyroidism
- Serum phosphorus: low or low normal in primary hyperparathyroidism.
- PTH: elevated or high normal in primary hyperparathyroidism
- 24-hr urine calcium to evaluate risk for renal stones and to exclude FHH.
- Serum creatinine to assess GFR and renal status.
- PTHrP and 1,25 OH-vitamin D levels can be considered to rule out other causes of elevated calcium.
- Evaluation of 25 OH-vitamin D is recommended in all patients with hyperparathyroidism. Vitamin D deficiency can decrease calcium and result in secondary hyperparathyroidism.
- ECG may reveal shortening of the QT interval secondary to severe hypercalcemia (>12 mg/dl)

IMAGING STUDIES
- Neck imaging is not indicated for diagnosis but is useful for localization before planned parathyroidectomy.
- Parathyroid localization with technetium-99m sestamibi can identify potential adenomas.
- Bone mineral density of the spine, hip, and forearm (distal third) is recommended for all patients with hyperparathyroidism in order to assess the risk for osteoporosis and fragility fractures. Cortical bone loss (i.e., forearm or hip) is greater than trabecular bone loss (i.e., spine) in hyperparathyroidism.
- Renal ultrasound can be considered to assess asymptomatic renal stones.
- Plain x-rays may reveal high bone turnover (Fig. 1-432).

RX TREATMENT

Modality of treatment depends on disease progression and which patients are more likely to suffer end-organ effects of hyperparathyroidism or benefit the most from surgery.

NONPHARMACOLOGIC THERAPY
- Surgery is the only definitive treatment for symptomatic primary hyperparathyroidism. Surgery can normalize calcium levels, decrease the risk for kidney stones, improve bone

mineral density and fracture risk, and enhance quality of life measures.

- ○ Indications for parathyroidectomy
  1. All patients younger than 50 yr
  2. Hypercalcemia (Ca >1 mg/dl above upper limit normal)
  3. Creatinine clearance <60 ml/min
  4. Osteoporosis (T-score < −2.5 or prior fragility fracture)
  5. Symptomatic hyperparathyroidism such as history of nephrolithiasis
- ○ Surgical approaches include:
  1. The conventional surgical approach is bilateral neck exploration under general anesthesia. An experienced endocrine surgeon cures >95% of patients undergoing bilateral neck exploration and incurs <1% perioperative mortality. Potential complications include transient and premananent hypocalcemia secondary to hypoparathyroidism and recurrent laryngeal nerve injury.
  2. Minimally invasive parathyroidectomy performed by experienced surgeons is an excellent alternative to conventional surgery. It can be performed under cervical block anesthesia as an outpatient procedure with intraoperative monitoring of PTH before and after re-

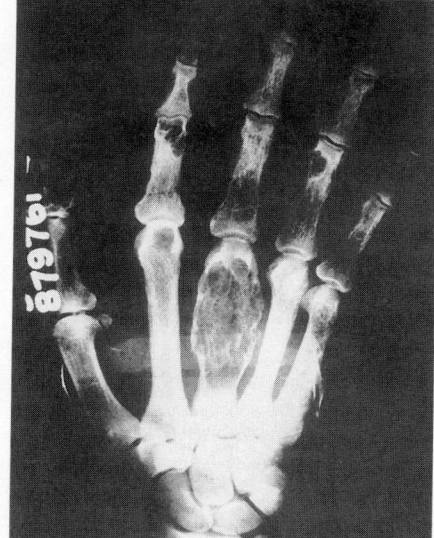

FIGURE 1-432 Radiograph of hand from a patient with severe primary hyperparathyroidism. Note the dramatic remodeling associated with the intense region of high bone turnover in the third metacarpal, in addition to widespread evidence of subperiosteal and trabecular resorption. (Courtesy Fuller Albright Collection, Massachusetts General Hospital. From Larsen PR et al [eds]: *Williams textbook of endocrinology,* ed 10, Philadelphia, 2003, Saunders.)

moval to document the expected fall after abnormal glands are removed.
- Ablation therapy (e.g., ethanol, angiographic, radiofrequency) can be considered in patients who are not surgical candidates. Limited data is available on efficacy and side effects. Repeat abalations may be required if hypercalcemia persists.
- Medical monitoring is recommended for asymptomatic primary hyperparathyroidism. Majority of patients do not manifest disease progression during observation. However, approximately 25% of asymptomatic patients will require surgery over a 10-yr follow-up period.
  - ○ Indications for medical monitoring
    1. Clinically asymptomatic and >50 yr old.
    2. Serum calcium level only mildly elevated (<1 mg/dl above upper limit normal)
    3. GFR > 60 ml/min and no nephrolithiasis or nephrocalcinosis
    4. No evidence of osteoporosis
    5. Medically unfit for surgery or refusing surgery
- Symptoms should be assessed regularly, serum calcium and creatinine should be checked yearly, and bone mineral density may be monitored every 2 yr.
- Medical management
  1. Avoid medications that precipitate hypercalcemia (e.g., thiazide or lithium)
  2. Since inadequate calcium and vitamin D status stimulates PTH, calcium and vitamin D intake should be the same as for patients without hyperparathyroidism (i.e., 1000 mg of elemental calcium and 600-800 IU of vitamin D daily).
  3. Encourage physical activity since immobilization increases bone resorption.
  4. Recommend adequate hydration (at least 2 L) to minimize the risk of nephrolithiasis.

PHARMACOLOGIC THERAPY

For patients who are not surgical candidates, pharmacologic options are available. Indications include symptomatic hyperparathyroidism or osteopenia associated with an increased fracture risk.

- Agents that inhibit bone resorption such as bisphosphonates (e.g., alendronate, pamidronate, zoledronate), improve bone mineral density, and decrease calcium levels in patients with hyperparathyroidism.
- Estrogens, and selective estrogen receptor modulators (e.g., raloxifene) have been shown to increase bone density but have little effect on hypercalcemia.
- Cinacalcet (Sensipar) is an oral calcimimetic agent that activates the calcium sensing receptor in the parathyroid gland. It decreases PTH production and subsequently serum calcium levels, without evidence of a signifi-

cant effect on BMD. Its role in the management of primary hyperparathyroidism is under evaluation. However, it is indicated for the treatment of secondary hyperparathyroidism associated with chronic kidney disease and hypercalcemia associated with parathyroid carcinoma.

ACUTE GENERAL Rx

Severe and/or symptomatic hypercalcemia may require hospitalization especially if serum calcium >12 mg/dl. Acute management of hypercalcemia includes:

- Vigorous hydration with IV normal saline (2-4 L/day). Fluid status must be monitored in patients with cardiac dysfunction or renal insufficiency in order to avoid fluid overload.
- Bisphosphonates can effectively decrease calcium levels. Zoledronate (4 mg IV over 15 min) or pamidronate (60-90 mg IV over 4 hr) are both effective. Onset of action is 24 to 48 hr.
- Calcitonin (4 units/kg IM/SC every 12 hr) may be used with bisphosphonates to achieve a more rapid reduction of calcium levels. Onset of action is within hours.

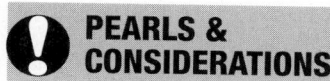 **PEARLS & CONSIDERATIONS**

COMMENTS

- Parathyroidectomy should be considered for all patients with symptomatic hyperparathyroidism. If surgey is contraindicated or not desired, cinacalcet or ablative therapy can be considered.
- Asymptomatic patients can be monitored with serial creatinine, calcium and bone mineral density measurements. Disease progression may result in surgery.
- Most patients can be managed medically by limiting factors that result in hypercalcemia (e.g., dehydration, immobilization, thiazide diuretics) and maintaining normal calcium and vitamin D intake.
- Patients with osteopenia and high fracture risk may require antiresorptive therapy such as bisphosphonates.

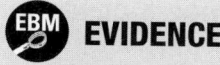 **EVIDENCE**

available at www.expertconsult.com

SUGGESTED READINGS

available at www.expertconsult.com

RELATED CONTENT

Hyperparathyroidism (Patient Information)

AUTHORS: **NUPUR BAHL,** and **GEETHA GOPALAKRISHNAN, M.D.**

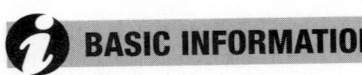

DEFINITION

Hypersensitivity pneumonitis (HP) is a group of immunologically mediated pulmonary diseases, with or without systemic manifestations (e.g., fever, weight loss), caused by the inhalation of an antigen to which the patient is sensitized and hyperresponsive. Sensitization and exposure alone in the absence of symptoms do not define the disease.

SYNONYMS

Extrinsic allergic alveolitis (EAA)
Some specific examples:
- Bird fancier's lung
- Farmer's lung
- Chemical worker's lung
- Humidifier lung
- Hot tub lung
- Sauna taker's lung

ICD-9CM CODES
495.9 Pneumonitis, hypersensitivity

EPIDEMIOLOGY & DEMOGRAPHICS

- Prevalence and incidence of HP vary considerably.
- Depend on definition and methods to establish diagnosis, intensity of exposure, environmental conditions, and genetic risk factors that remain poorly understood.
- More than 300 causative agents have been identified, and the number continues to grow.
- Causative agents in residential and occupational exposures include birds, mold, humidifiers, fountains, steam irons, dry sausage molds, moldy cheese, contaminated wood, wind instruments (e.g., trombone, saxophone), and organic and inorganic chemicals, including metalworking fluids. A large series of patients with HP associated with down pillows, feather duvets, and down-upholstered furniture has been published. Likely several genes are involved that cause an exaggerated lung response to an offending agent. The major histocompatibility complex is the most studied thus far.
- A viral connection has been implicated that may enhance clinical exposure to an offending agent.

PHYSICAL FINDINGS & CLINICAL PRESENTATION

Vary depending on frequency and intensity of antigen exposure.
- Acute: fever, cough, malaise, and dyspnea 4 to 6 hr after an intense exposure, lasting 18 to 24 hr
- Subacute: insidious onset of productive cough, dyspnea on exertion, anorexia, and weight loss, usually from a heavy, sustained exposure
- Chronic: gradually progressive cough, dyspnea, malaise, and weight loss, usually from low-grade or recurrent exposure
- Physical examination: cyanosis and crepitant rales, possible fever

ETIOLOGY

- Numerous environmental agents, often encountered in occupational settings
- Common sources of antigens: "moldy" hay, silage, grain, or vegetables; bird droppings or feathers (including those found commonly in down pillows, blankets, and upholstered furniture); low-molecular-weight chemicals (e.g., isocyanates); pharmaceutical products

DX DIAGNOSIS

- Accurate diagnosis is important for differentiating HP from other interstitial disorders because the prognosis and treatment may differ.
- The clinical syndrome is indistinguishable from an acute respiratory infection without a history of illness occurring within hours of exposure to an antigen.
- Need high index of suspicion.
- Detailed occupational and home exposure history is required.
- Lung biopsy is often necessary for diagnosis.

DIFFERENTIAL DIAGNOSIS

Acute Stages
Acute bronchopulmonary aspergillosis
Pulmonary embolism
Asthma
Aspiration pneumonia
Recurrent pneumonia
Bronchiolitis obliterans–organizing pneumonia
Sarcoidosis
Churg-Strauss syndrome
Wegener granulomatosis

Chronic Stages
Idiopathic pulmonary fibrosis (IPF)
Bronchiectasis
Chronic bronchitis
Nonspecific interstitial pneumonia (NSIP)
Connective tissue–related lung disease

WORKUP

No single radiologic, physiologic, or immunologic test is specific for the diagnosis of HP. HP must be suspected in any patient presenting with cough, dyspnea, fever, and malaise. A thorough history focusing on potential exposures is essential. Table 1-219 describes examples of occupational causes of HP.

Environmental and occupational history questions should ask about grain dusts; animal handling; food processing; cooling towers; fountains; metalworking fluids; symptom improvement away from exposure; pets (particularly birds); hobbies involving chemicals, feathers, or fur; organic dusts; presence of humidifiers, dehumidifiers, or hot tubs/saunas; leaking or flooding indoors; visible fungal growth in living or working environment; feather pillows, bedding, or upholstered furniture.

Major criteria:
- History of symptoms compatible with HP that appear to worsen within hours after antigen exposure
- Confirmation of exposure to the offending agent by history, investigation of the environment, serum precipitin tests to potential agents (often referred to as a "hypersensitivity panel" by many labs), or bronchoalveolar lavage (BAL) antibody
- Compatible changes on chest radiograph or high-resolution CT (HRCT) of the chest
- BAL fluid lymphocytosis (if performed)
- Compatible histologic changes by lung biopsy (if performed): bronchiolocentric interstitial pneumonia, NSIP
- Positive natural challenge (reproduction of symptoms and laboratory abnormalities after exposure to the suspected environment) or controlled inhalation challenge

Minor criteria:
- Basilar crackles

TABLE 1-219 Examples of Occupational Causes of Hypersensitivity Pneumonitis

Occupation	Cause
Farmer	Thermophilic actinomycetes in moldy hay
Metal worker	Contamination of metal-working fluids with microorganisms such as *Mycobacteria immunogens* or fungi
Worker exposed to humidifiers	Contamination with microorganisms such as protozoa or fungi
Sugarcane worker	Moldy sugarcane (bagassosis)
Maple bark stripper	Fungi
Chicken or turkey worker	Avian proteins
Pharmaceutical worker	Penicillin
Food handler	Soybeans
Office worker	Microorganisms contaminating air conditioners or humidifiers
Swimming pool attendant	Fungal contamination in sprays around pool area
Animal worker	Rat proteins
Mushroom worker	Fungi
Wheat farmer or handler	Weevil-infested flour
Greenhouse worker	Fungi
Workers spraying urethane paint or adhesives/sealants (or less often, other workers using diisocyanate)	Methylene diphenyl diisocyanate, hexamethylene diisocyanate, toluene diisocyanates
Chemical worker using plastics, resins, paints	Trimellitic anhydride

From Goldman L, Schafer AI: *Goldman's Cecil medicine*, ed 24, Philadelphia, 2012, Saunders.

- Decreased diffusion capacity
- Arterial hypoxemia (either at rest or with exercise)

LABORATORY TESTS

- Routine laboratory tests do not make the diagnosis, but typically the erythrocyte sedimentation rate, C-reactive protein, lactate dehydrogenase, and leukocyte count are increased; elevated immunoglobulins IgG and IgM are nonspecific; rheumatoid factor (RF) and immune complexes are often positive; peripheral eosinophil count and serum IgE are generally normal.
- Lactate dehydrogenase (LDH) is increased and tends to decrease with improvement.
- Pulmonary function tests: restrictive ventilatory patterns are typically seen. Decreased FEV$_1$, decreased forced vital capacity, decreased total lung capacity, decreased diffusing capacity, and decreased static compliance.
- Arterial blood gases show mild hypoxemia (worsens with exercise).
- A-a gradient shows slight increase.
- Serum precipitin test for IgG antibodies against offending antigen detected in serum. It is sensitive but not specific for HP (asymptomatic patients may have IgG antibodies in serum). HP may also be present without a positive precipitin test.
- Skin testing: unclear if helpful. However, some believe it to be a safe, effective, and rapid procedure in the diagnosis and follow-up of patients with HP. Sensitivity is similar to that of the precipitin test but the specificity is higher.

IMAGING STUDIES

Chest x-ray: nonspecific; may be normal in early stage.
- Acute/subacute: bilateral interstitial and alveolar nodular infiltrates in a patchy or homogeneous distribution. Apices are often spared.
- Chronic: diffuse reticulonodular infiltrates and fibrosis.

High-resolution chest CT scan: no pathognomonic features but demonstrates airspace and interstitial patterns in the acute and subacute stage. The chronic stage reveals honeycombing and bronchiectasis.

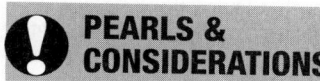 **TREATMENT**

NONPHARMACOLOGIC THERAPY
Early recognition and avoidance of the causative antigen

ACUTE GENERAL Rx
- Glucocorticoids accelerate initial lung recovery but may have no effect long term (from a controlled study in farmer's lung). No prospective, randomized, placebo-controlled trials for other types of HP or subacute and chronic stages.
- Prednisone 0.5 to 1 mg/kg usually over 1 to 2 wk then tapered over 4 wk. Some patients, particularly those with subacute or chronic presentation, may require a longer course of therapy.

DISPOSITION/PROGNOSIS
Prognosis is generally better in patients with acute or subacute HP, and with the finding of NSIP pathologically. Prognosis is worse in those with older age, desaturation during exercise, and findings of severe fibrosis by lung biopsy.
Acute: 4 to 48 hr
- Clinical: fever, chills, cough, hypoxia, malaise
- HRCT: ground-glass infiltrates
- Immunopathology: poorly formed, noncaseating granulomas or mononuclear cell infiltration in a peribronchial distribution, frequently with giant cells
- Prognosis: good
Subacute: weeks to 4 mo
- Clinical: dyspnea, cough, episodic flares
- HRCT: micronodules, air trapping
- Immunopathology: more well-formed, noncaseating granulomas, bronchiolitis, organizing pneumonia, and interstitial fibrosis
- Prognosis: good
Chronic: 4 mo to years
- Clinical: dyspnea, cough, fatigue, weight loss
- HRCT: fibrosis (possible), honeycombing, emphysema
- Immunopathology: granulomatous pneumonitides may be seen in addition to bronchiolitis obliterans (with or without organizing pneumonia) and honeycombing and fibrosis, lymphocytic infiltration, centrilobular and bridging fibrosis, neutrophil-mediated air space destruction, giant cells

REFERRAL
- Bronchoscopy: BAL provides useful supportive data in the diagnosis of HP. Usually reveals intense lymphocytosis (typically T cells >50%) of predominantly CD8+ suppressor cells. In the acute stage neutrophils predominate, but as the disease progresses to chronic form the ratio of CD4+ to CD8+ cells increases. When fibrosis is present the number of neutrophils increases.
- Lung biopsy: the histopathologic features of HP are distinctive but not pathognomonic. Bronchiolitis and interstitial pneumonitis with granuloma formation typically is seen. Variable degrees of interstitial fibrosis are seen in the chronic form. Chronic HP may be difficult to distinguish from IPF or NSIP pathologically.
- Laboratory inhalation challenge: testing to prove a direct relation between a suspected antigen and disease; extract of antigen is inhaled by nebulizer.

PEARLS & CONSIDERATIONS

A clinical prediction rule using six features has high specificity and sensitivity for the diagnosis of acute and subacute HP:
- Exposure to a known offending agent
- Positive specific precipitating antibody
- Recurrent episodes of symptoms
- Inspiratory crackles
- Symptoms occurring 4 to 8 hr after exposure
- Weight loss
HP occurs more frequently in smokers than nonsmokers (likely from an immunosuppressive effect).

SUGGESTED READINGS
available at www.expertconsult.com

RELATED CONTENT
Hypersensitivity Pneumonitis (Patient Information)

AUTHOR: **KRISTINA KRAMER, M.D.**

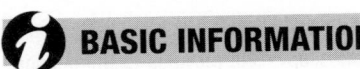 **BASIC INFORMATION**

DEFINITION

Hypersplenism is a syndrome characterized by splenomegaly, cytopenia (one or more of the following: anemia, thrombocytopenia, or leukopenia), and compensatory hyperplastic bone marrow. The cytopenias are correctable with splenectomy.

ICD-9CM CODES
289.4 Hypersplenism

EPIDEMIOLOGY & DEMOGRAPHICS

Most often seen in patients with liver disease, hematologic malignancy, and infection

PHYSICAL FINDINGS & CLINICAL PRESENTATION

- Symptoms depend on the size of the spleen, rate of growth, and underlying disease.
- History: early satiety, abdominal discomfort or fullness, left upper quadrant pleuritic pain (abscess, infarction), episodes of acute left upper quadrant pain (sequestration crisis), referred pain to left shoulder
- Physical examination: splenomegaly (normal spleen not palpable), presence of a rub in left upper quadrant (suggestive of a splenic infarct), stigmata of cytopenias

ETIOLOGY

The spleen is an important component of cellular and humoral immunity. It removes bacteria and other particulates (e.g., opsonized bacteria, antibody-coated cells) from the circulation. It is also responsible for the modification (removal of particles and parasites) and clearance of senescent or poorly deformable red blood cells (RBCs) from the circulation. The spleen is a platelet reservoir, storing 30% of platelet mass. It can become the site of hematopoiesis in certain disease states. The spleen's normal activities are augmented when enlarged.

- Splenomegaly increases the proportion of blood channeled through the red pulp, causing inappropriate splenic pooling of both normal and abnormal blood cells. The size of the spleen determines the amount of cell sequestration. Up to 90% of platelets may be pooled in an enlarged spleen.
- Splenomegaly leads to increased destruction of RBCs. Platelets and white blood cells (WBCs) have about normal survival time even when sequestered and may be available if needed.
- Splenomegaly causes plasma volume expansion, exacerbating cytopenias by dilution.

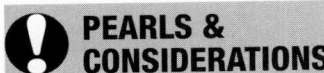 **DIAGNOSIS**

DIFFERENTIAL DIAGNOSIS

Hypersplenism can be caused by splenomegaly of almost any cause.
- Splenic congestion: cirrhosis (portal hypertension); congestive heart failure; portal, splenic, or hepatic vein thrombosis

- Hematologic causes: hemolytic anemia, sickle cell anemia, thalassemia, spherocytosis, elliptocytosis, extramedullary hematopoiesis, following use of granulocyte colony-stimulating factor
- Infections: viral (hepatitis, infectious mononucleosis, cytomegalovirus, HIV/AIDS), bacterial (abscess, endocarditis, tuberculosis, salmonella, brucella, Lyme's disease), parasitic (babesiosis, malaria, leishmaniasis, schistosomiasis, toxoplasmosis), fungal
- Malignancy: acute or chronic leukemia, lymphoma, myeloproliferative diseases (polycythemia vera, essential thrombocythemia, myelofibrosis), metastatic tumors
- Inflammatory diseases: rheumatic fever, rheumatoid arthritis (Felty's syndrome), systemic lupus erythematosus, sarcoid, serum sickness
- Infiltrative diseases: amyloidosis, Gaucher's disease, Niemann-Pick disease, glycogen storage disease
- Anatomic abnormalities: hemangioma, hamartoma

WORKUP

History (including travel), physical examination, laboratory tests, imaging studies

LABORATORY TESTS

- CBC with differential: cytopenia, neutrophilia (infection)
- Peripheral smear: RBC and WBC morphology (abnormal cells may suggest infection, malignancy, bone marrow disease, rheumatologic disease), organisms (bacteria, malaria, babesiosis)
- Bone marrow biopsy: hyperplasia of cytopenic cell lines; hematologic, infiltrative, or infectious disorders
- Tests to diagnose suspected cause of splenomegaly: liver function, hepatitis serology, HIV, rheumatoid factor, antinuclear antibody, tissue biopsy
- Note: red cell mass (^{51}Cr assay) may be used to assess severity of anemia. RBC mass measurement will differentiate true anemia (decrease in RBCs) from dilutional anemia (plasma volume expansion).

IMAGING STUDIES

- Ultrasound: splenic size, presence of cyst or abscess
- CT: estimate volume, obtain structural information: cyst, abscess, tumor, infarct
- MRI: most useful for assessing vascular lesions and infections
- Nuclear medicine: liver-spleen scan: assess anatomy and function; may suggest presence of portal hypertension
- Consider other studies as suggested by history and examination: chest radiograph, echocardiogram

TREATMENT

ACUTE GENERAL Rx

- Treat underlying disease
- Splenectomy is considered if:

1. Indicated for the management of the underlying cause
2. Persistent symptomatic disease (severe cytopenia) not responding to therapy
3. Necessary for diagnosis

Risks:
- Infections (especially encapsulated organisms): risk greatest in the first 2 yr after splenectomy. Mortality rate from sepsis is fiftyfold greater in asplenic patients. Attempts to decrease risk include:
  - Immunization with pneumococcal, meningococcal, and *Haemophilus influenzae* vaccines 3 wk before splenectomy. Revaccination for pneumococcal in 5 yr. Annual influenza vaccination.
  - Prophylactic antibiotics after splenectomy in highest risk patients.
  - Patient education regarding the importance of rapid initiation of antibiotics at the first sign of infection.
- Rapid increase in platelet count may cause thromboembolic complications.
- Possible increased risk of atherosclerotic heart disease.
- Splenectomy should not be performed if the spleen is the main site of hematopoiesis as a result of bone marrow failure (e.g., myelofibrosis).
- Other options include partial splenectomy, partial splenic embolization, radiofrequency ablation, portosystemic shunting (for congestive splenomegaly).

DISPOSITION

- Cytopenias are usually correctable with splenectomy; cell counts return to normal within a few weeks.
- Splenectomy may alleviate portal hypertension.
- Prognosis depends on the underlying disease.

REFERRAL

Hematology

PEARLS & CONSIDERATIONS

- Thrombocytopenia in hypersplenism is usually moderately severe ($>50 \times 10^9$/L) and asymptomatic; severe thrombocytopenia ($<20 \times 10^9$/L) suggests another diagnosis.
- Neutropenia of hypersplenism is rarely symptomatic.

SUGGESTED READINGS
available at www.expertconsult.com

RELATED CONTENT

Felty's Syndrome (Related Key Topic)
Fig. 3-169 Clinical approach to patient with splenomegaly (Algorithm)
Hypersplenism (Patient Information)

AUTHOR: **SUDEEP KAUR AULAKH, M.D.**

BASIC INFORMATION

DEFINITION

The seventh report of Joint National Committee in 2003 on Prevention, Detection, Evaluation, and Treatment of High Blood Pressure (JNC 7) described normal blood pressure (BP) in adults as systolic BP <120 mm Hg and diastolic <80 mm Hg. *Prehypertension* is defined as systolic BP between 120 to 139 mm Hg or diastolic between 80 to 89 mm Hg. *Stage 1 hypertension* (HTN) is systolic BP from 140 to 159 mm Hg or diastolic BP from 90 to 99 mm Hg. *Stage 2 HTN* is systolic BP ≥160 mm Hg or diastolic BP ≥100 mm Hg.

SYNONYMS

Essential hypertension
Idiopathic hypertension
High BP

ICD-9CM CODES
401.1 Essential hypertension (HTN)
401.0-9 with 5th digit 1 Renovascular hypertension
405 Secondary hypertension
642 Hypertension complicating pregnancy
437.2 Hypertensive encephalopathy

EPIDEMIOLOGY & DEMOGRAPHICS

PREVALENCE: Based on NHANES data in 2005 to 2008, between 29% and 31% of U.S. adults have HTN (approximately 65 million) and only 31 million (46%) have it well controlled. There are around 1 billion individuals worldwide who meet the criteria for diagnosis of HTN.
PEAK PREVALENCE: Males and the elderly

PHYSICAL FINDINGS & CLINICAL PRESENTATION

Physical examination may be entirely within normal limits except for the presence of elevated BP. A proper initial physical examination on a hypertensive patient should include the following:
- The BP should be measured with an appropriately sized cuff (bladder of the cuff should cover at least two thirds of the circumference of the arm) and in both arms (the higher of the readings being used).
- The BP should be measured twice on each visit, and separated by at least 1 to 2 min to allow the return of trapped blood.
- Postural BP change should always be recorded in elderly to diagnose postural hypotension. This is assessed by taking BP in supine (after 5-minute rest) and standing (after 2 minutes) positions. A drop of ≥20 mm Hg in systolic, a drop of ≥10 mm Hg diastolic BP, or symptoms of cerebral hypoperfusion is suggestive of postural (orthostatic) hypotension.
- A diagnosis of HTN may be established if the BP is markedly elevated (>180/110 mm Hg) or has evidence of end organ damage; otherwise such a diagnosis should wait until BP is found elevated on at least 3-6 visits, spaced over a period of weeks to months.
- Measure heart rate, height, weight, body mass index, and waist circumference.

- Examine skin for the presence of café-au-lait spots (neurofibromatosis), uremic appearance (renal failure), and violaceous striae (Cushing's syndrome).
- Perform careful funduscopic examination; check for papilledema, retinal exudates, hemorrhages, arterial narrowing, arteriovenous compression.
- Examine neck for carotid bruits, distended neck veins, and enlarged thyroid gland.
- Perform extensive cardiopulmonary examination: check for loud aortic component of S_2, S_4, ventricular lift, murmurs, and arrhythmias.
- Palpate abdomen for renal masses (pheochromocytoma, polycystic kidneys), and auscultate for bruit over the aorta and renal arteries.
- Examine arterial pulses (dilated or absent femoral pulses and BP greater in upper extremities than lower extremities suggest aortic coarctation).
- Look for truncal obesity (Cushing's syndrome) and pedal edema (congestive heart failure [CHF]).
- The clinical evaluation should help to determine if the patient has primary or secondary (possibly reversible) HTN, if there is target organ disease present, and if there are additional cardiovascular risk factors. Table 1-220 provides a guide to evaluation of identifiable causes of HTN. Fig. E1-433 and Box E1-27 describe the investigation of suspected endocrine causes of HTN.

ETIOLOGY

- Essential (primary) HTN (85%)
- Drug induced or drug related (5%)
  1. NSAIDs
  2. Oral contraceptives
  3. Corticosteroids
- Renal HTN (5%)
  1. Renal parenchymal disease (3%)
  2. Renovascular HTN (RVH) (<2%)

- Endocrine (<2%)
  1. Primary aldosteronism (0.5%)
  2. Pheochromocytoma (0.2%)
  3. Cushing's syndrome and long-term steroid therapy (0.2%)
  4. Hyperparathyroidism or thyroid disease (0.2%)
- Coarctation of the aorta (0.2%)

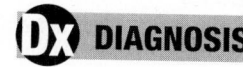

DIAGNOSIS

WORKUP

- The objective for the initial evaluation of HTN is to establish the diagnosis and stage of HTN.
- Gather office and nonoffice BP readings, assess presence of target organ damage (TOD), assess the level of global cardiovascular disease risk and produce a plan for individualized monitoring and therapy.
- ECG, CXR, renal imaging, and tests for plasma aldosterone/plasma renin activity are not routinely recommended at the initial evaluation stage of the patient with newly diagnosed HTN.
- Patient counseling and education should be prominent features of the initial evaluation.
- Pertinent history:
  ○ Age of onset of HTN, previous antihypertensive therapy
  ○ Family history of HTN, stroke, cardiovascular disease
- Diet, salt intake, alcohol, drugs (e.g., oral contraceptives, NSAIDs, decongestants, steroids)
- Occupation, lifestyle, socioeconomic status, psychologic factors
- Other cardiovascular risk factors: hyperlipidemia, obesity, diabetes mellitus

TABLE 1-220 Guide to Evaluation of Identifiable Causes of Hypertension

Suspected Diagnosis	Clinical Clues	Diagnostic Testing
Chronic kidney disease	Estimated GFR <60 ml/min/1.73 m² Urine albumin-to-creatinine ratio ≥30 mg/g	Renal sonography
Renovascular disease	New elevation in serum creatinine, marked elevation in serum creatinine with ACEI or ARB, drug-resistant hypertension, flash pulmonary edema, abdominal, or flank bruit	Renal sonography (atrophic kidney), CT or MR angiography, invasive angiography
Coarctation of the aorta	Arm pulses > leg pulses, arm BP > leg BP, chest bruits, rib notching on chest radiography	MR angiography, TEE, invasive angiography
Primary aldosteronism	Hypokalemia, drug-resistant hypertension	Plasma renin and aldosterone, 24-hr urine aldosterone and potassium after oral salt loading, adrenal vein sampling
Cushing's syndrome	Truncal obesity, wide and blanching purple striae, muscle weakness	1 mg dexamethasone-suppression test, urinary cortisol after dexamethasone, adrenal CT
Pheochromocytoma	Paroxysms of hypertension, palpitations, perspiration, and pallor; diabetes	Plasma metanephrines, 24-hr urinary metanephrines and catecholamines, abdominal CT or MR imaging
Obstructive sleep apnea	Loud snoring, large neck, obesity, somnolence	Polysomography

ACEI, Angiotensin-converting enzyme inhibitor; *ARB,* angiotensin receptor blocker; *BP,* blood pressure; *CT,* computed tomography; *GFR,* glomerular filtration rate; *MR,* magnetic resonance; *TEE,* transesophageal echocardiography.
From Goldman L, Schafer AI: *Goldman's Cecil medicine,* ed 24, Philadelphia, 2012, Saunders.

- Symptoms of secondary HTN:
  1. Headache, palpitations, excessive perspiration (possible pheochromocytoma)
  2. Weakness, polyuria (consider hyperaldosteronism)
  3. Claudication of lower extremities (seen with coarctation of aorta)

LABORATORY TESTS

- Urinalysis with microscopic evaluation, blood urea nitrogen and creatinine, and an albumin/creatinine ratio; for evidence of renal disease. High-serum creatinine is a predictor of cardiovascular risk in essential HTN.
- Nonoffice (home, workplace, 24-hr ambulatory) BP determination to establish the pattern of HTN (sustained, "white coat," or "masked" HTN).
- Serum electrolyte levels: low potassium is suggestive of primary aldosteronism or diuretic use.
- Screening for coexisting diseases that may adversely affect prognosis:
  1. Fasting serum glucose
  2. Serum lipid panel, uric acid, calcium
  3. If pheochromocytoma is suspected: 24-hr urine metanephrines

IMAGING STUDIES

- ECG: check for presence of left ventricular hypertrophy (LVH) with strain pattern.
- Magnetic resonance angiography of the renal arteries in suspected RVH (renal artery stenosis).

Rx TREATMENT

NONPHARMACOLOGIC THERAPY

Lifestyle modifications:
- Weight loss if overweight (target BMI <25).
- Limit alcohol intake to 1 oz of ethanol per day (<2 drinks/day) in men or 0.5 oz (<1 drink/day) in women.
- Regular aerobic exercise (at least 30 min/day on most days).
- Reduce sodium intake to <100 mmol/day (<1.5 g of sodium/day).
- Maintain adequate dietary potassium (>3500 mg/day) intake in patients with normal kidney function.
- Stop smoking.
- The BP reduction seen ranges from 2 to 20 mm Hg, most significant with substantial weight loss and the implementation of the Dietary Approaches to Stop Hypertension (DASH) eating plan, which relies on a diet high in fruits and vegetables, moderate in low-fat dairy products, and low in animal protein but with substantial amount of plant protein from legumes and nuts.

ACUTE GENERAL Rx

According to the JNC 7:
- For patients with prehypertension and no other complications, recommend lifestyle modifications to prevent progression to sustained HTN.
- For patients with prehypertension and diabetes or chronic kidney disease, aggressive

pharmacologic treatment should be undertaken to reduce BP to <130/80 mm Hg.
- Antihypertensive drug therapy should be initiated in patients with stage 1 HTN. Thiazide diuretics are preferred for initial therapy unless there are compelling indications to use other agents for initial therapy. Chlorthalidone has been shown to be more effective than an ACE inhibitor in lowering BP and at least as effective as a calcium blocker or an ACE inhibitor in prevention of cardiovascular events.
- Compelling indications for individual drug classes:
  - CHF due to systolic dysfunction: ACE inhibitors, angiotensin-receptor blockers (ARBs), beta-blockers, diuretics, aldosterone antagonists
  - Post MI: beta-blockers, ACE inhibitors, aldosterone antagonists
  - High cardiovascular risk: beta-blockers, ACE inhibitors, calcium channel blockers (CCBs), diuretics
  - Diabetes: ACE inhibitors, ARBs, CCBs, beta-blockers, diuretics
  - Chronic kidney disease: ACE inhibitors, ARBs
  - Recurrent stroke prevention: ACE inhibitors, diuretics
- A two-drug combination is necessary for most patients with stage 2 HTN. The combination of a diuretic with another agent is preferred unless there is a compelling indication to use other agents.
- When selecting drugs, try to give once per day dosages to improve compliance. Also consider the cost of the medication, metabolic and subjective side effects, and drug-drug interactions.
- The major advantages and limitations of each class of drugs are described as follows:
  1. Diuretics:
     a. Advantages: inexpensive, once-daily dosing. Useful in edematous states, CHF, chronic renal disease, elderly patients (decreased incidence of hip fractures in elderly patients)
     b. Disadvantages: significant adverse metabolic effects, increased risk of cardiac arrhythmias, sexual dysfunction, possible adverse effects on lipids and glucose levels
  2. Beta-blockers:
     a. Advantages: ideal in hypertensive patients with ischemic heart disease or status post MI. Favored in hyperkinetic, young patients (resting tachycardia, wide pulse pressure, hyperdynamic heart) and stable CHF patients.
     b. Disadvantages: adverse effect on quality of life (increased incidence of fatigue, depression, impotence), bronchospasm, hypoglycemia, peripheral vascular disease, adverse effects on lipids, masking of signs and symptoms of hypoglycemia in diabetics.

3. Calcium antagonists:
   a. Advantages: helpful in hypertensive patients with ischemic heart disease. Generally favorable effect on quality of life; can be used in patients with bronchospastic disorders, renal disease, peripheral vascular disease, metabolic disorders, and salt sensitivity. CCBs BP-lowering effect is independent of Na^+ intake.
   b. Disadvantages: diltiazem and verapamil should be avoided in patients with CHF due to systolic dysfunction because of their negative inotropic effects; pedal edema may occur with nifedipine and amlodipine; constipation can be severe in elderly patients receiving verapamil. CCB-related edema is positional in nature, it improves with lying position; additional strategies include switching CCB classes, reducing dosage, giving the medication later in the day, and adding a venodilator (nitrates, an ACE, or an ARB); diuretics may improve edema, but at the expense of a reduction in plasma volume.
4. ACE inhibitors:
   a. Advantages: well tolerated, favorable impact on quality of life; useful in HTN complicated by CHF; helpful in prevention of diabetic renal disease; effective in decreasing LVH.
   b. Disadvantages: cough is a frequent side effect (5% to 20% of patients); hyperkalemia may occur in patients with diabetes or severe renal insufficiency; hypotension may occur in volume-depleted patients; increased risk of renal failure in patients with renal artery stenosis; contraindicated in pregnancy.
5. ARBs:
   a. Advantages: well tolerated, favorable impact on quality of life; useful in patients unable to tolerate ACE inhibitors because of persistent cough and in CHF and diabetic patients; single daily dose. An episode of renal insufficiency with ACE inhibitors does not rule out future therapy with an ARB unless high-grade bilateral renal artery stenosis exists.
   b. Disadvantages: excessive cost; hypotension may occur in volume-depleted patients; hyperkalemia; risk of renal failure in renal artery stenosis; contraindicated in pregnancy.
6. Renin inhibitors: newest class of antihypertensives (Aliskiren):
   a. Advantages: generally well tolerated; once-daily dosing; can be used alone or in combination with other antihypertensive agents (avoid combining with ACEI or ARBs given increase of hyperkalemia)

b. Disadvantages: contraindicated in pregnancy; should not be used in patients with impaired renal function; excessive cost; paucity of cardiovascular outcomes data showing benefit.

7. Alpha-adrenergic blockers:
   a. Advantages: no adverse effect on blood lipids or insulin sensitivity; helpful in benign prostatic hypertrophy.
   b. Disadvantages: postural hypotension, sedation; syncope can be avoided by giving an initial low dose at bedtime.

8. Central alpha-antagonists:
   a. Oral clonidine mainstay of therapy for hypertensive urgencies because of the ease of administration and relative safety.
   b. Transdermal clonidine; useful in management of labile HTN, the hospitalized patient who cannot take medications by mouth, and patients subject to early morning BP surges. At equivalent doses, transdermal clonidine is more apt to precipitate salt and water retention than is the case with oral clonidine.
   c. Dose beyond 0.4 mg causes fatigue, sedation and dry mouth, salt and water retention, and rebound HTN upon abrupt termination of the medication.

9. Combined alpha- and beta-adrenergic receptor blockers:
   a. Labetalol, nebivolol, and carvedilol: Use is reserved to treat complicated hypertensive patient when an antihypertensive effect beyond beta-blockade is sought. IV labetalol is used for hypertensive emergencies. Carvedilol is shown to have less adverse effect on glycemic control than metoprolol and to reduce urinary protein excretion in hypertensive diabetic patients.

TREATMENT OF RENOVASCULAR HYPERTENSION: The therapeutic approach varies with the cause of the RVH (refer to "Renal Artery Stenosis" for additional information).

1. Young patients with fibromuscular dysplasia refractory to medical therapy can be treated with percutaneous transluminal renal angioplasty (PTRA).
2. Medical therapy is advisable in elderly patients with atheromatous RVH; useful agents are:
   a. Beta-blockers: highly effective in patients with elevated plasma renin
   b. ACE inhibitors: highly effective; however, should be avoided in patients with bilateral renal artery stenosis or with a solitary kidney and renal stenosis
   c. Diuretics: often used in combination with ACE inhibitors
3. Surgical revascularization is generally reserved for atheromatous RVH in patients responding poorly to medical therapy (uncontrolled HTN, deteriorating renal function).

HTN DURING PREGNANCY:

1. HTN complicates 5% to 12% of all pregnancies.
2. The American Obstetrical Committee defines BP of 130/80 mm Hg as the upper limit of normal at any time during pregnancy.
3. A rise of 30 mm Hg systolic or 15 mm Hg diastolic is also considered abnormal regardless of the absolute values obtained.
4. Chronic HTN (occurring before pregnancy) must be distinguished from preeclampsia because the risk to mother and fetus is much greater in the latter.
5. Treatment of chronic HTN during pregnancy is as follows:
   a. Initial treatment with conservative measures (proper nutrition, limited physical activity).
   b. When drug therapy is necessary, initiation of methyldopa, hydralazine, labetalol, or atenolol is preferred.

c. ACE inhibitors can cause fetal and neonatal complications; their use should be avoided in pregnancy.
d. The safety of CCBs remains unclear.
e. Diuretics should be used only if there is a specific reason for initiating and maintaining their use (e.g., HTN associated with severe fluid overload or left ventricular dysfunction).

MALIGNANT HTN, HYPERTENSIVE EMERGENCIES, AND HYPERTENSIVE URGENCIES:

Definitions:

1. Malignant HTN is a potentially life-threatening situation caused by elevated BP.
   a. The rate of BP rise is a critical factor.
   b. The clinical manifestations are grade IV hypertensive retinopathy (exudates, hemorrhages, and papilledema); cardiovascular involvement (acute aortic dissection, acute left ventricular failure, acute myocardial infarction; cerebrovascular involvement), encephalopathy, intracerebral hemorrhage; or renal compromise.
   c. Requires immediate BP reduction (not necessarily into normal ranges) to prevent or limit target organ disease.
2. Hypertensive emergencies require rapid (within 1 hr) lowering of BP to prevent end-organ damage.
3. Hypertensive urgencies are significant BP elevations that should be corrected within 24 hr of presentation.

Therapy: The choice of therapeutic agents varies with the cause. IV medications are preferred in hypertensive emergencies.

1. Nitroprusside is the drug of choice in hypertensive encephalopathy, HTN and intracranial bleeding, malignant HTN, HTN and heart failure, dissecting aortic aneurysm (used in combination with propranolol); its onset of action is immediate.

TABLE 1-221 Parenteral Agents for Management of Hypertensive Emergencies

Agent	Dose	Onset of Action	Precautions
Parenteral Vasodilators			
Sodium nitroprusside	0.25-10 mcg/kg/min IV infusion	Immediate	Thiocyanate toxicity with prolonged use
Nitroglycerin	5-100 mcg/min IV infusion	2-5 min	Headache, tachycardia, tolerance
Nicardipine	5-15 mg/hr IV infusion	1-5 min	Protracted hypotension after prolonged use
Fenoldopam mesylate	0.1-0.3 mcg/kg/min IV infusion	1-5 min	Headache, tachycardia, increased intraocular pressure
Hydralazine	5-10 mg as IV bolus or 10-40 mg IM; repeat every 4-6 hr	10 min IV 20 min IM	Unpredictable and excessive falls in blood pressure; tachycardia, angina exacerbation
Enalaprilat	0.625-1.25 mg every 6 hr IV bolus	15-60 min	Unpredictable and excessive falls in blood pressure; acute renal failure in patients with bilateral renal artery stenosis
Parenteral Adrenergic Inhibitors			
Labetalol	20-80 mg as slow IV injection every 10 min, or 0.5-2.0 mg/min IV as infusion	5-10 min	Bronchospasm, heart block, orthostatic hypotension
Metoprolol	5 mg IV every 10 min for three doses	5-10 min	Bronchospasm, heart block, heart failure, exacerbation of cocaine-induced myocardial ischemia
Esmolol	500 mcg/kg IV over 3 min; then 25-100 mg/kg/min as IV infusion	1-5 min	Bronchospasm, heart block, heart failure
Phentolamine	5-10 mg IV bolus every 5-15 min	1-2 min	Tachycardia, orthostatic hypotension

IM, Intramuscular; *IV,* intravenous.
From Andreoli TE et al: *Andreoli and Carpenter's Cecil essentials of medicine,* ed 8, Philadelphia, 2010, Saunders.

2. Fenoldopam is a vasodilator agent useful for the short-term (up to 48 hr) management of severe HTN when rapid but quickly reversible reduction of BP is required. It should be avoided in patients with glaucoma.

3. Other commonly used agents are the IV CCBs nicardipine and clevidipine (useful for urgent treatment of HTN in the intensive care unit or operating room), the beta-blocker esmolol (useful in aortic dissection or postoperative HTN), labetalol (combined β-adrenergic and α-blocker useful in patients with coronary disease), phentolamine (useful for catecholamine-related emergencies), IV nitroglycerin (used in patients with cardiac ischemia and hypertensive crisis), and hydralazine (used for hypertensive emergencies in pregnancy).

4. Table 1-221 describes parenteral agents for management of hypertensive emergencies. *The following are important points to remember when treating hypertensive emergencies:*

   a. Introduce a plan for long-term therapy at the time of the initial emergency treatment.

   b. Agents that reduce arterial pressure can cause the kidney to retain sodium and water; therefore the judicious administration of diuretics should accompany their use.

   c. The initial goal of antihypertensive therapy is not to achieve a normal BP, but rather to gradually reduce the BP; cerebral hypoperfusion may occur if the mean BP is lowered >40% in the initial 24 hr.

ⓘ PEARLS & CONSIDERATIONS

COMMENTS

- For patients with prehypertension, every 20/10 mm Hg increase in BP doubles the risk of cardiovascular events.
- Most patients will require at least two medications for BP control.
- Guidelines now suggest that, if BP is greater than 20/10 mm Hg above goal, therapy should be initiated with two drugs.

- A practical approach to multidrug therapy is use of fixed-dose antihypertensive combinations as an alternative to the sequenced addition of two or three drugs.
- Resistant HTN: HTN is considered resistant if the BP cannot be reduced below target levels in patients who are compliant with an optimal triple-drug regimen that includes a diuretic. Terms *refractory* and *resistant* are used interchangeably. Causes include pseudohypertension, measurement artifact, medication nonadherence, volume overload, and secondary HTN.
  - Pseudohypertension in elderly: hardened and sclerotic artery is not compressible hence falsely elevates BP measurement artifact

TABLE 1-222 Indications for Specialist Referral for Patients with Hypertension

Urgent Treatment Needed

Accelerated hypertension (severe hypertension with grade III-IV retinopathy)

Particularly severe hypertension (>220/120 mm Hg)

Impending complications (e.g., transient ischemic attack, left ventricular failure)

Possible Underlying Cause

Any clue in history or examination of a secondary cause (e.g., hypokalemia with increased or high–normal plasma sodium)

Elevated serum creatinine

Proteinuria or hematuria

Sudden onset or worsening of hypertension

Young age (any hypertension <20 years; needing treatment <30 years)

Therapeutic Problems

Multiple drug intolerances

Multiple drug contraindications

Persistent nonadherence or nonconcordance

Special Situations

Unusual blood pressure variability

Possible white coat hypertension

Hypertension in pregnancy

From Floege J et al: *Comprehensive clinical nephrology,* ed 4, Philadelphia, 2010, Saunders.

- Measurement artifact: BP taken with a small cuff in people with large arm diameter. BP should be taken with the patient in the seated position and the arm supported at heart level, the bladder within the cuff should encircle at least 80% of the arm diameter.

Fig. E1-434 describes an approach to patients with resistant HTN.

- Renal sympathetic denervation is a newer therapeutic option for HTN unresponsive to use of 3 or more antihypertensive agents. Treatment consists of use of a radiofrequency ablation catheter introduced through the femoral artery into the distal segment of the renal artery. Bilateral renal denervation usually requires 4-6 radiofrequency applications in each renal artery to be successful. Mean postprocedure BP drop after 24 months is about 32/14 mm Hg.
- Fig. E1-435 describes an algorithm for evaluation of secondary causes of HTN.
- Barriers to BP control: system issues, provider issues; patient issues, and behavior issues. The rate at which physicians adopt recommended changes based on evidence-based findings can be quite slow and has been properly described as "clinical inertia."
- ACE-ARB combination therapy has gained popularity in the primary care setting, but this practice should be discouraged. Recent studies assessing dual renin-angiotensin-aldosterone system blockade with ACE-ARB combination have not supported the use of this combination.
- Indications for specialist referral for patients with HTN are described in Table 1-222.

SUGGESTED READINGS
available at www.expertconsult.com

RELATED CONTENT
High Blood Pressure
High Blood Pressure–Child (Patient Information)

AUTHORS: **SAINATH GADDAM, M.D.,**
FRED F. FERRI, M.D., and
HILARY B. WHITLATCH, M.D.

BASIC INFORMATION

DEFINITION

Hyperthyroidism is a hypermetabolic state resulting from excess thyroid hormone.

SYNONYMS

Thyrotoxicosis

ICD-9CM CODES
242.9 Hyperthyroidism
242.0 Hyperthyroidism with goiter
242.2 Hyperthyroidism, multinodular
242.3 Hyperthyroidism, uninodular

EPIDEMIOLOGY & DEMOGRAPHICS

INCIDENCE/PREVALENCE:
- Hyperthyroidism affects 2% of women and 0.2% of men in their lifetimes.
- Toxic multinodular goiter usually occurs in women >55 yr and is more common than Graves' disease in the elderly.

PHYSICAL FINDINGS & CLINICAL PRESENTATION

- Patients with hyperthyroidism generally present with tachycardia, tremor, hyperreflexia, anxiety, irritability, emotional lability, panic attacks, heat intolerance, sweating, increased appetite, diarrhea, weight loss, menstrual dysfunction (oligomenorrhea, amenorrhea). Presentation may be different in elderly patients (see below).
- Patients with Graves' disease may present with exophthalmos, lid retraction, and lid lag (Graves' ophthalmopathy). The following signs and symptoms of ophthalmopathy may be present: blurring of vision, photophobia, increased lacrimation, double vision, and deep orbital pressure. Clubbing of fingers associated with periosteal new bone formation in other skeletal areas (Graves' acropachy) and pretibial myxedema may also be noted.
- Clinical signs of hyperthyroidism in the elderly may be masked by manifestations of coexisting disease (e.g., new-onset atrial fibrillation, exacerbation of congestive heart failure).

ETIOLOGY

- Graves' disease (diffuse toxic goiter): 80% to 90% of all cases of hyperthyroidism
- Toxic multinodular goiter (Plummer's disease)
- Toxic adenoma
- Iatrogenic and factitious
- Transient hyperthyroidism (subacute thyroiditis, Hashimoto's thyroiditis)
- Rare causes: hypersecretion of thyroid-stimulating hormone (TSH) (e.g., pituitary neoplasms), struma ovarii, ingestion of large amount of iodine in a patient with preexisting thyroid hyperplasia or adenoma (Jod-Basedow phenomenon), hydatidiform mole, carcinoma of thyroid, amiodarone therapy

DIAGNOSIS

DIFFERENTIAL DIAGNOSIS

- Anxiety disorder
- Pheochromocytoma
- Metastatic neoplasm
- Diabetes mellitus
- Premenopausal state

WORKUP

Suspected hyperthyroidism requires laboratory confirmation and identification of its etiology because treatment varies with cause. A detailed medical history will often provide clues to the diagnosis and etiology of the hyperthyroidism. Fig. E1-436 describes a diagnostic approach to suspected hyperthyroidism.

LABORATORY TESTS

- Elevated free thyroxine (T_4)
- Elevated free triiodothyronine (T_3): generally not necessary for diagnosis
- Low TSH (unless hyperthyroidism is a result of the rare hypersecretion of TSH from a pituitary adenoma)
- Thyroid autoantibodies useful in selected cases to differentiate Graves' disease from toxic multinodular goiter (absent thyroid antibodies)

IMAGING STUDIES

- 24-hr radioactive iodine uptake (RAIU) is useful to distinguish hyperthyroidism from iatrogenic thyroid hormone synthesis (thyrotoxicosis factitia) and from thyroiditis.
- An overactive thyroid shows increased uptake, whereas a normal underactive thyroid (iatrogenic thyroid ingestion, painless or subacute thyroiditis) shows normal or decreased uptake.
- The RAIU results also vary with the etiology of the hyperthyroidism:
  - Graves' disease: increased homogeneous uptake
  - Multinodular goiter: increased heterogeneous uptake
  - Hot nodule: single focus of increased uptake
- RAIU is also generally performed before the therapeutic administration of radioactive iodine to determine the appropriate dose.

TREATMENT

NONPHARMACOLOGIC THERAPY

Patient education regarding thyroid disease and discussion of the therapeutic options. Patients should be informed that radioiodine, antithyroid drugs, and surgery are all reasonable treatment options for hyperthyroidism. It is crucial for the physician to have a detailed discussion with the patient about the benefits and risks relative to lifestyle, patients' values, and coexisting conditions.

ACUTE GENERAL Rx

ANTITHYROID DRUGS (THIONAMIDES): Propylthiouracil (PTU) and methimazole inhibit thyroid hormone synthesis by blocking production of thyroid peroxidase (PTU and methimazole) or inhibit peripheral conversion of T_4 to T_3 (PTU). Methimazole is favored by most endocrinologists. PTU is preferred in pregnant women because methimazole has been associated with aplasia cutis and with choanal and esophageal atresia. Complete blood count and differential should be obtained before their use.

1. Dosage: methimazole 15 to 30 mg/day given as a single dose; PTU 50 to 100 mg PO q8h.
2. Antithyroid drugs can be used as the primary form of treatment or as adjunctive therapy before radioactive therapy or surgery or afterward if the hyperthyroidism recurs.
3. Side effects: skin rash (3% to 5% of patients), arthralgias, myalgias, granulocytopenia (0.5%). Rare side effects are aplastic anemia, hepatic necrosis from PTU, cholestatic jaundice from methimazole.
4. When antithyroid drugs are used as primary therapy, they are usually given for 6 to 18 mo; prolonged therapy may cause hypothyroidism. Monitor thyroid function every 2 mo for 6 mo, then less frequently.
5. The use of antithyroid drugs before radioiodine therapy is best reserved for patients in whom exacerbation of hyperthyroidism after radioactive iodine therapy is hazardous (e.g., elderly patients with coronary artery disease or significant coexisting morbidity). In these patients the antithyroid drug can be stopped 2 days before radioactive iodine therapy, resumed 2 days later, and continued for 4 to 6 wk.

RADIOIODINE THERAPY (RADIOACTIVE IODINE [RAI; ^{131}I]):
1. RAI is the treatment of choice for patients aged >21 yr and younger patients who have not achieved remission after 1 yr of antithyroid drug therapy. RAI is also used in hyperthyroidism caused by toxic adenoma or toxic multinodular goiter.
2. Contraindicated during pregnancy (can cause fetal hypothyroidism) and lactation. Pregnancy should be excluded in women of childbearing age before RAI is administered.
3. A single dose of RAI is effective in inducing a euthyroid state in nearly 80% of patients.
4. There is a high incidence of post-RAI hypothyroidism (>50% within first year and 2%/yr thereafter); these patients should be frequently evaluated for the onset of hypothyroidism (see "Chronic Rx").

SURGICAL THERAPY (SUBTOTAL THYROIDECTOMY):
1. Indicated in obstructing goiters, in any patient who refuses RAI and cannot be adequately managed with antithyroid medications (e.g., patients with toxic adenoma or toxic multinodular goiter), and in pregnant patients who cannot be adequately managed with antithyroid medication or develop side effects to them.
2. Patients should be rendered euthyroid with antithyroid drugs before surgery.
3. Complications of surgery include hypothyroidism (28% to 43% after 10 yr), hypoparathyroidism, and vocal cord paralysis (1%).
4. Hyperthyroidism recurs after surgery in 10% to 15% of patients.

ADJUNCTIVE THERAPY: Propranolol alleviates the beta-adrenergic symptoms of hyperthyroidism; initial dose is 20 to 40 mg PO q6h; dosage is gradually increased until symptoms are controlled. Major contraindications to propranolol are congestive heart failure and bronchospasm. Diagnosis and treatment of thyrotoxic storm is also discussed in Section I.

CHRONIC Rx

- Patients undergoing treatment with antithyroid drugs should be seen every 1 to 3 mo until euthyroidism is achieved and every 3 to 4 mo while they remain on antithyroid therapy. After treatment is stopped, periodic monitoring of thyroid function tests with TSH is recommended every 3 mo for 1 yr, then every 6 mo for 1 yr, then annually.
- Orbital decompression surgery can be used to correct Graves' orbitopathy (Fig. 1-437). The administration of the antioxidant selenium (100 mcg PO bid) has been recently reported as effective in improving quality of life, reducing ocular involvement, and slowing progression of the disease in patients with mild Graves' orbitopathy. Its mechanism of action is believed to be an effect on the oxygen free radicals and cytokines that play a pathogenic role in Graves' orbitopathy.

DISPOSITION

Successful treatment of hyperthyroidism requires lifelong monitoring for the onset of hypothyroidism or the recurrence of thyrotoxicosis.

REFERRAL

- Endocrinology referral is recommended at the time of initial diagnosis and during treatment.
- Surgical referral in selected patients (see "Surgical Therapy").
- Hospitalization of all patients with thyroid storm.

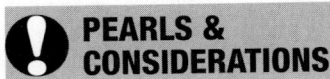

ⓘ PEARLS & CONSIDERATIONS

COMMENTS

- Elderly hyperthyroid patients may have only subtle signs (weight loss, tachycardia, fine skin, brittle nails). This form is known as *apathetic hyperthyroidism* and manifests with lethargy rather than hyperkinetic activity. An enlarged thyroid gland may be absent. Coexisting medical disorders (most commonly cardiac disease) may also mask the symptoms. These patients often have unexplained congestive heart failure, worsening of angina, or new-onset atrial fibrillation resistant to treatment. See the entry "Graves' Disease" for additional information on diagnosis and treatment.
- Subclinical hyperthyroidism is defined as a normal serum-free thyroxine and free triiodothyronine levels with a TSH level suppressed below the normal range and usually undetectable. These patients usually do not present with signs or symptoms of overt hyperthyroidism. Treatment options include observation or a therapeutic trial of low-dose antithyroid agents for 6 mo to attempt to induce remission.
- ***Thyrotoxic periodic paralysis (TPP)*** is a hyperthyroidism-related hypokalemia and muscle-weakening condition resulting from a sudden shift of potassium into cells. Many patients do not have other symptoms of hyperthyroidism. Typical presentation involves an Asian adult male with acute fatigue and muscle weakness initially presenting in the lower extremities. Physical examination reveals decreased deep tendon reflexes, hypertension, and tachycardia. ECG often reveals U waves, high QRS voltage, and first-degree atrioventricular block. Additional laboratory testing reveals normal acid-base state, hypokalemia with low urinary potassium excretion (spot urinary potassium concentration <20 mEq/L from potassium shift into cells), hypophosphatemia, hypophostaturia, and hypercalciuria. Electromyography during attacks shows low-amplitude compound muscle action potential of the tested muscle. Therapy consists of cautious potassium supplementation (increased risk of rebound hyperkalemia). Use of nonselective beta-blockers (e.g., propranolol) to counteract hyperadrenergic activity, which may be causing TPP, may also be useful.

SUGGESTED READINGS

available at www.expertconsult.com

RELATED CONTENT

Hyperthyroidism (Patient Information)
Graves Disease (Related Key Topic)

AUTHOR: **FRED F. FERRI, M.D.**

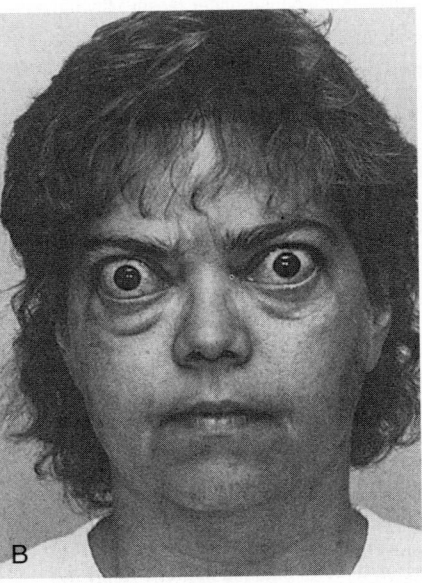

FIGURE 1-437 Characteristic signs of Graves' orbitopathy. A, Subsequently corrected by orbital decompression surgery. **B,** Note the thyroid stare, asymmetry, proptosis, and periorbital edema before correction. (Courtesy Dr. Jack Rootman, University of British Columbia, Vancouver, Canada. From Larsen PR et al [eds]: *Williams textbook of endocrinology,* ed 10, Philadelphia, 2003, Saunders.)

BASIC INFORMATION

DEFINITION

Hypertrophic osteoarthropathy (HOA) is a syndrome of clubbing of the digits, periostosis of long bones, skin changes, and arthritis. Periostosis is usually involved with pain on palpation of the involved area. HOA may be primary or secondary to other underlying disease processes.

SYNONYMS

- Primary hypertrophic osteoarthropathy:
  1. Pachydermoperiostosis
  2. Idiopathic clubbing
  3. Touraine-Solente-Golé syndrome
- Secondary hypertrophic osteoarthropathy
- HOA

ICD-9CM CODES
731.2 Hypertrophic osteoarthropathy

EPIDEMIOLOGY & DEMOGRAPHICS

- Fig. 1-438 provides a classification of HOA.
- Primary HOA is a familial autosomal-dominant disease affecting the age group between 1 and 20 yr and is rare. There is a male/female ratio of 9:1 in occurrence.
- Secondary HOA is more common, typically occurs in adults. 80% to 90% of secondary HOA is associated with non–small cell lung cancer, most frequently adenocarcinoma; other associated illnesses include:

1. Pulmonary: mesothelioma, lung abscesses, bronchiectasis, cystic fibrosis, pulmonary fibrosis, sarcoidosis
2. Gastrointestinal: esophageal carcinoma, biliary atresia, colon cancer, inflammatory bowel disease (Crohn's disease, ulcerative colitis), hepatocellular carcinoma, liver cirrhosis, amebiasis
3. Cardiac: infective endocarditis, right-to-left cardiac shunts, aortic aneurysms
4. Thymoma
5. Hodgkin lymphoma
6. Connective tissue diseases
7. Thyroid acropachy
8. HIV infection
9. POEMS syndrome (polyneuropathy, organomegaly, endocrinopathy, M component, and skin changes)
10. Thalassemia
11. Osteosarcoma
12. Nasopharyngial sarcoma
13. Osteosarcoma
14. Arterial grafts of legs and aortic prosthesis infections

PHYSICAL FINDINGS & CLINICAL PRESENTATION

- Primary HOA typically presents with the insidious onset of clubbing of the hands (Fig. 1-439) and feet, described as "spadelike." Finger clubbing is diagnosed by measurement of the digital index (Fig. 1-440). Other signs and symptoms of HOA include:
  1. Joint pain and swelling
  2. Decreased use of the fingers and hands
  3. Facial changes, coarse facial skin grooves
  4. Thickening of the arms and legs
  5. Oily skin, diaphoresis, gynecomastia, and acne
  6. Thin and shiny appearance of the skin around the nail bed
  7. Nail convexity with nail "floating" sensation within the soft tissue is noticed on palpation of the base of the nail bed
  8. Edema, warmth, and tenderness of the extremities can be seen
- Secondary HOA patients may present with clinical symptoms before the underlying disorder can be detected. Signs and symptoms are similar to the above in addition to findings related to the underlying disease (e.g., bronchogenic carcinoma, infective endocarditis).
- Patients presenting with painful joints prior to developing clubbing can be misdiagnosed as inflammatory arthritis.

ETIOLOGY

The pathogenesis of HOA is not fully understood; current knowledge suggests that HOA results from the activation of one or more growth factors, such as vascular endothelial growth factor (VEGF) and platelet-derived growth factor, that are normally inactivated in the lungs and systemic circulation.

DIAGNOSIS

Diagnosis is primarily clinical; radiographs and bone scans can help confirm the diagnosis.

DIFFERENTIAL DIAGNOSIS

Paget's disease, Reiter's syndrome, psoriatic arthritis, syphilis, osteoarthritis, rheumatoid arthritis, and osteomyelitis.

WORKUP

HOA warrants an investigation into any associated illnesses.

LABORATORY TESTS

- Routine laboratory studies such as blood count, electrolytes, and urine studies are typically normal in primary and secondary HOA.
- Erythrocyte sedimentation rate is elevated in secondary HOA.

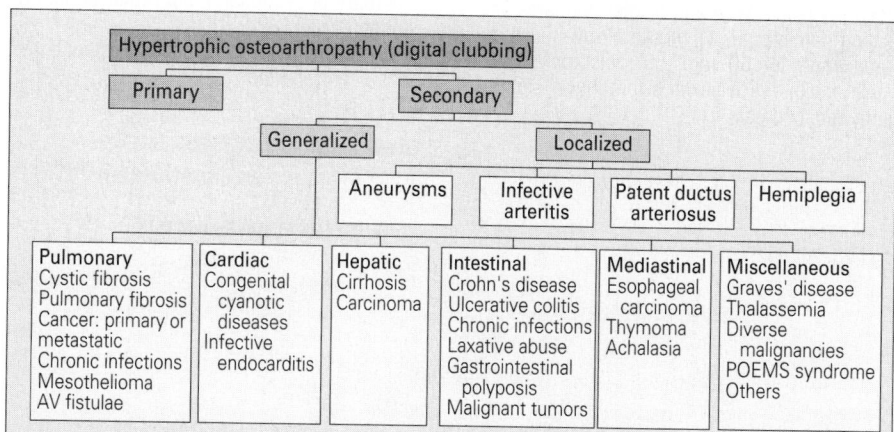

Hypertrophic osteoarthropathy (digital clubbing)					
Primary	Secondary				
	Generalized	Localized			
		Aneurysms	Infective arteritis	Patent ductus arteriosus	Hemiplegia
Pulmonary Cystic fibrosis Pulmonary fibrosis Cancer: primary or metastatic Chronic infections Mesothelioma AV fistulae	Cardiac Congenital cyanotic diseases Infective endocarditis	Hepatic Cirrhosis Carcinoma	Intestinal Crohn's disease Ulcerative colitis Chronic infections Laxative abuse Gastrointestinal polyposis Malignant tumors	Mediastinal Esophageal carcinoma Thymoma Achalasia	Miscellaneous Graves' disease Thalassemia Diverse malignancies POEMS syndrome Others

FIGURE 1-438 Classification of hypertrophic osteoarthropathy. *AV,* Arteriovenous; *POEMS,* polyneuropathy, organomegaly, endocrinopathy, monoclonal proteins, and skin changes. (From Hochberg MC et al: *Rheumatology,* ed 5, St Louis, 2011, Mosby.)

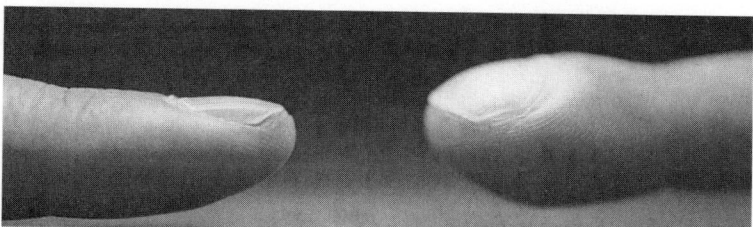

FIGURE 1-439 Clubbing deformity. The finger on the right is clubbed compared with the normal finger shape on the left. (From Hochberg MC et al: *Rheumatology,* ed 5, St Louis, 2011, Mosby.)

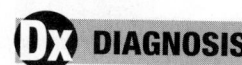
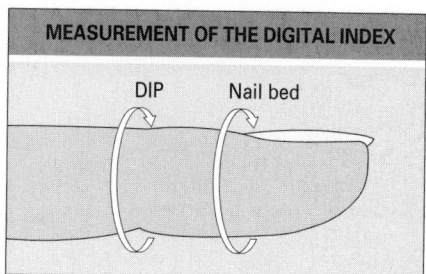

MEASUREMENT OF THE DIGITAL INDEX

DIP   Nail bed

FIGURE 1-440 The digital index. The perimeter of each of the 10 fingers is measured at the nail bed (NB) and at the distal interphalangeal joint (DIP). If the sum of the 10 NB:DIP ratios is more than 10, clubbing is probably present. (From Hochberg MC et al: *Rheumatology,* ed 5, St Louis, 2011, Mosby.)

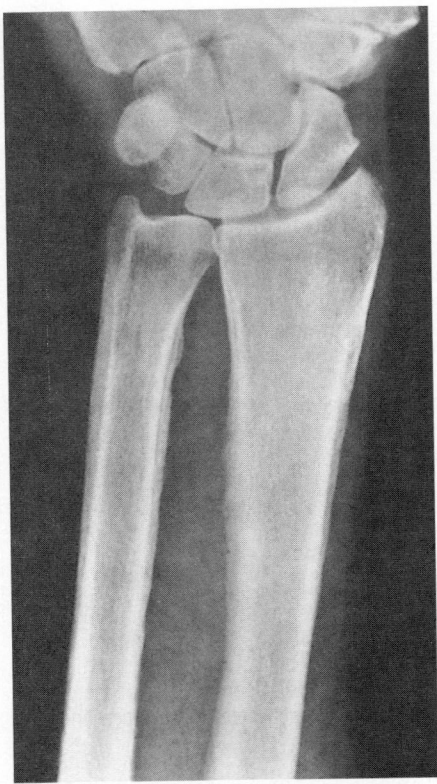

FIGURE 1-441 Hypertrophic osteoarthropathy. Wrist radiograph showing periostosis at the distal ends of the radius and ulna. The coarse, layered appearance is most evident along the diaphyses. The relative sparing of the radial epiphyses is characteristic. (From Hochberg MC et al: *Rheumatology*, ed 5, St Louis, 2011, Mosby.)

- Liver function tests may be abnormal in patients with secondary HOA from gastrointestinal pathology.
- Alkaline phosphatase may be elevated as a result of periostitis of long bones.
- Analysis of the synovial fluid from joint effusions reveals a low white blood cell count with normal viscosity, color, and complement levels.

IMAGING STUDIES

- Radiographs of the long bones show periosteal new bone formation (Fig. 1-441).
- A chest radiograph should be obtained to rule out underlying lung cancer.
- Bone scan with technetium-99m reveals uptake along the long bones, phalanges, and periarticular joint spaces.

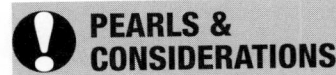 **TREATMENT**

ACUTE GENERAL Rx

- Treatment of primary HOA is symptomatic. Nonsteroidal anti-inflammatory medications such as aspirin, salicylate, ibuprofen, naproxen, or indomethacin can be used.
- Treatment of secondary HOA is to eradicate the underlying disease (e.g., antibiotics for infective endocarditis, surgery for bronchogenic carcinoma). Correction of heart malformation or removal of an underlying tumor is rapidly followed by regression of HOA.

CHRONIC Rx

In patients with secondary HOA refractory to NSAIDs and aspirin, octreotide (100 mcg subcutaneously twice daily) and bisphosphonates, including pamidronate (1 mg/kg intravenously to a maximum of 60 mg) and zoledronic acid, which inhibit VEGF expression, have significantly reduced pain.

Vagotomy has been tried with some success. However, the definitive treatment is to treat the underlying disease.

DISPOSITION

- Patients with primary HOA typically have symptoms of joint pain and swelling for the early part of their life. However, the disease becomes quiescent thereafter.
- Prognosis and disease course in patients with secondary HOA will depend on the underlying cause. The insidious development of clubbing suggests an infectious process, whereas the rapid progression of clubbing may suggest underlying malignancy.

REFERRAL

Referral should be made to rheumatology when the diagnosis of HOA is suspected and the cause remains unclear.

❗ PEARLS & CONSIDERATIONS

Some cases of primary HOA may later be found to be associated with an underlying disease such as patent ductus arteriosus, Crohn's disease, or myelofibrosis, in which case they become secondary.

COMMENTS

- Infections and intrathoracic malignancies are the most common causes of secondary HOA.
- The periostosis and the extent of involvement do not depend on the form of the disease (primary or secondary), but rather on its duration.
- HOA secondary to infection of an arterial graft has been reported.

SUGGESTED READINGS

available at www.expertconsult.com

AUTHOR: **SYEDA M. SAYEED, M.D.**

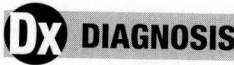
BASIC INFORMATION

DEFINITION

Hyperuricemia may be defined as serum uric acid >7.0 mg/dl in males or >6.0 mg/dl in females. Some persons who are normouricemic by this definition will have levels of uric acid that exceed the limit of solubility of uric acid in tissue. Data from the Framingham study indicates that hyperuricemia increased from 4.8% of the population in the early 1970s to 9.3% in the mid 1980s. Age is an important risk factor in the increasing incidence of hyperuricemia and gout. Women become hyperuricemic at an older age than men due to the uricosuric effect of estrogen. Most people with hyperuricemia are asymptomatic and will remain so; however, 20% of those with serum uric acid >9 mg/dl will develop gout in 5 yr. Hyperuricemia is strongly associated with gout, obesity, diabetes hypertension, and cardiovascular disease but has not been proven to cause any of these conditions.

ASYMPTOMATIC HYPERURICEMIA

Definition: laboratory evidence of elevated serum uric acid without clinical disease known to be caused by hyperuricemia

ETIOLOGY

Overproduction of uric acid accounts for a minority of cases of hyperuricemia. Most cases are due to decreased renal clearance of uric acid and high dietary purine consumption. Fig. 1-442 describes factors affecting urate balance. Table 1-223 describes a classification of hyperuricemia and gout.

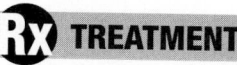
DIAGNOSIS

EVALUATION

The finding of hyperuricemia should prompt a thorough evaluation of potential causes and related diseases. Fig. E1-443 describes the evaluation of patients with hyperuricemia. If there is no clinical evidence of gout, nephrolithiasis, or acute kidney injury, the patient may be said to

TABLE 1-223 Classification of Hyperuricemia and Gout

Impaired Uric Acid Excretion

Primary gout with decreased uric acid clearance
Secondary gout
Clinical conditions
Reduced glomerular filtration rate
Hypertension
Obesity
Systemic acidosis
Familial juvenile hyperuricemic nephropathy
Medullary cystic kidney disease
Lead nephropathy
Drugs
Diuretics
Ethanol
Low-dose salicylates (0.3-3.0 g/day)
Cyclosporine
Tacrolimus
Levodopa

Excessive Urate Production

Primary metabolic disorders
HPRT deficiency
PRPP synthetase overactivity
Glucose-6-phosphatase deficiency
Fructose-1-phosphate aldolase deficiency
Secondary causes
Clinical conditions
Myelo- and lymphoproliferative disorders
Obesity
Psoriasis
Glycogenoses III, V, VII
Drugs and dietary components
Nicotinic acid
Pancreatic extract
Cytotoxic drugs
Red meat, organ meat, shellfish
Alcoholic beverages (especially beer)
Fructose

HPRT, hypoxanthine-guanine phosphoribosyltransferase; PRPP, phosphoribosyl pyrophosphate.
From Goldman L, Schafer AI: *Goldman's Cecil medicine*, ed 24, Philadelphia, 2012, Saunders.

have asymptomatic hyperuricemia. Patients with hyperuricemia should be evaluated for potential causes of elevated uric acid including malignancy, renal insufficiency, toxins, lead toxicity, and dietary indiscretion. If a careful history and physical exam does not reveal an evident cause of persistent hyperuricemia, a 24-hr urine collection for uric acid and creatinine may be considered. Patients with urinary excretion of uric acid >800 mg/24 hr are likely to be overproducers of uric acid and should be investigated more thoroughly for the underlying cause of their hyperuricemia.

LABORATORY TESTS

- CBC with differential
- BUN/creatinine
- Urinalysis
- Lipid profile: Consider 24-hr urine collection

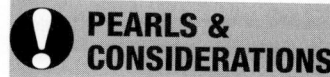
TREATMENT

No specific therapy is indicated for most patients with asymptomatic hyperuricemia. Lifestyle and dietary modification are often advisable.

NONPHARMACOLOGIC THERAPY

- Weight loss
- Reduce alcohol intake, especially beer
- Reduce consumption of foods known to be high in purines such as red meat, organ meat, and high-fructose soft drinks.

PEARLS & CONSIDERATIONS

- Research in progress suggests there may be a causal relationship between hyperuricemia and early hypertension.
- Very high levels of serum uric acid may warrant treatment even if asymptomatic.
- Patient with hyperuricemia and a family history of gout should be followed closely for the development of gouty arthritis.
- Hyperuricemia in patients with gout or presence of tophi (Fig. E1-444) should almost always be treated with urate lowering medication (see "Gout").

SUGGESTED READINGS

available at www.expertconsult.com

RELATED CONTENT

Gout (Related Key Topic)
AUTHOR: **BERNARD ZIMMERMANN, M.D.**

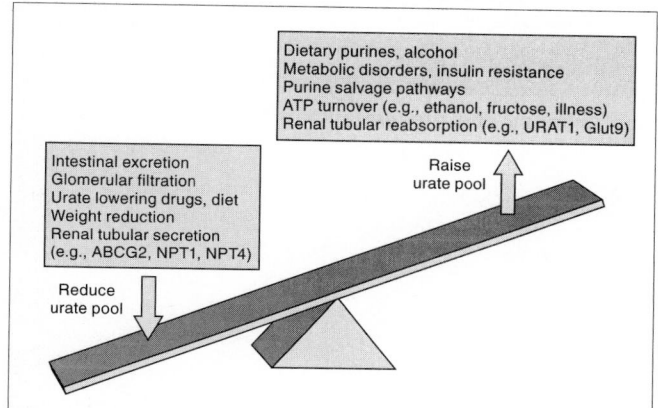

FIGURE 1-442 Factors affecting urate balance. The systemic urate pool and the likelihood of gout are determined by the dynamic balance among dietary purines, endogenous synthesis and recycling, and disposal by the kidney and gut. (From Hochberg MC et al: *Rheumatology*, ed 5, St Louis, 2011, Mosby.)

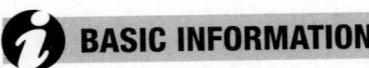

DEFINITION

Hypoaldosteronism is defined as an aldosterone deficiency or impaired aldosterone function.

ICD-9CM CODES
255.4 Hypoadrenalism

EPIDEMIOLOGY & DEMOGRAPHICS

Selective hypoaldosteronism accounts for as many as 10% of cases of unexplained hyperkalemia.

PHYSICAL FINDINGS & CLINICAL PRESENTATION

- Physical examination may be entirely within normal limits.
- Hypertension may be present in some patients.
- Profound muscle weakness and cardiac arrhythmias may be present.

ETIOLOGY

- Hyporeninemic hypoaldosteronism (renin-angiotensin dependent): decreased aldosterone production as a result of decreased renin production; the typical patient has renal disease attributable to various factors (e.g., diabetes mellitus, interstitial nephritis, multiple myeloma).
- Hyperreninemic hypoaldosteronism (renin-angiotensin independent): renin production by the kidneys is intact; the defect is in aldosterone biosynthesis or in the action of angiotensin II. Common causes of this form of hypoaldosteronism are medications (ACE inhibitors, heparin), lead poisoning, aldosterone enzyme defects, and severe illness.

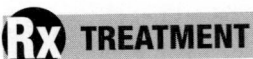

DIFFERENTIAL DIAGNOSIS

Pseudohypoaldosteronism: renal unresponsiveness to aldosterone. In this condition both renin and aldosterone levels are elevated. Pseudohypoaldosteronism can be caused by medications (spironolactone), chronic interstitial nephritis, systemic disorders (systemic lupus erythematosus, amyloidosis), or primary mineralocorticoid resistance.

WORKUP

Measurement of plasma renin activity after 4 hr of upright posture can differentiate hyporeninemic from hyperreninemic causes. Renin levels in the normal or low range identify cases that are renin-angiotensin dependent, whereas high renin levels identify cases that are renin-angiotensin independent. The diagnosis and etiology of hypoaldosteronism can be confirmed with the renin-aldosterone stimulation test:
- Hyporeninemic hypoaldosteronism: low stimulated renin and aldosterone levels
- End-organ refractoriness to aldosterone action: high stimulated renin and aldosterone levels
- Adrenal gland abnormality: high stimulated renin and low aldosterone levels

LABORATORY TESTS

- Increased potassium, normal or decreased sodium
- Hyperchloremic metabolic acidosis (caused by the absence of hydrogen-secreting action of aldosterone)
- Increased BUN and creatinine (secondary to renal disease)
- Hyperglycemia (diabetes mellitus is common in these patients)

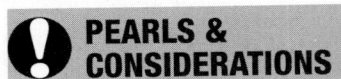

NONPHARMACOLOGIC THERAPY

- Low-potassium diet with liberal sodium intake (at least 4 g of sodium chloride per day)
- Avoidance of ACE inhibitors and potassium-sparing diuretics

ACUTE GENERAL Rx

- Judicious use of fludrocortisone (0.05 to 0.1 mg PO every morning) in patients with aldosterone deficiency associated with deficiency of adrenal glucocorticoid hormones
- Furosemide 20 to 40 mg qd to correct hyperkalemia of hyporeninemic hypoaldosteronism

DISPOSITION

Prognosis varies with the etiology of hypoaldosteronism and presence of associated disorders.

REFERRAL

Endocrinology referral for renin-aldosterone stimulation test

PEARLS & CONSIDERATIONS

COMMENTS

Treatment of pseudohypoaldosteronism is the same as for hypoaldosteronism; however, effect is limited because of impaired renal sensitivity.

AUTHOR: **FRED F. FERRI, M.D.**

BASIC INFORMATION

DEFINITION

Hypochondriasis is the preoccupation with the fear of having, or the idea that one has, a serious undiagnosed disease. The fear is usually based on a misinterpretation of bodily signs or symptoms and persists despite medical reassurance, although the belief does not have the intensity of a delusion. The disorder is defined by clinically significant distress or impairment in social, occupational, or other important areas of functioning and lasts for at least 6 mo. Symptoms that do not rise to the diagnostic criteria of hypochondriasis may be labeled health anxiety.

ICD-9CM CODES
300.7 Hypochondriasis

EPIDEMIOLOGY & DEMOGRAPHICS

PREVALENCE: 1% to 5%, but thought to be higher in primary care outpatient settings, where estimates range from 3% to 10%.
PREDOMINANT SEX: Equal frequency in men and women.
PREDOMINANT AGE: Onset at any age, but most commonly between ages 20 and 30 yr
GENETICS/RISK: No genetic component identified, and neither socioeconomic nor educational factors appear to predispose to this disorder. Patients with hypochondriasis are more likely than the general population to have Axis I disorders, such as generalized anxiety, obsessive-compulsive disorder, and depression, and Axis II personality disorders. Serious childhood illnesses are common in past medical history.

PHYSICAL FINDINGS & CLINICAL PRESENTATION

- Patient may be preoccupied with a specific diagnosis (e.g., malignancy), a physical symptom (e.g., fatigue, headache), or a normal physiologic process (e.g., bowel movements).
- Patient remains preoccupied with concern for a serious medical illness, despite evidence to the contrary.
- Insight (i.e., recognition that the concern about serious illness is excessive or unreasonable) is variable.
- Associated distress and impairment last at least 6 mo.

- Hypochondriacal symptoms often correlate with psychosocial stressors.
- No specific physical examination findings.

ETIOLOGY

Unknown etiology, but psychological theories include disturbance of perception (amplification of normal somatic sensations), cognition (tendency to attribute sensations to a pathologic process), or interpersonal relationships (learning and then reinforcement of the sick role); or variant of another psychiatric condition such as depression.

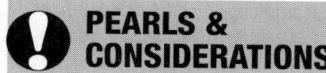

DIAGNOSIS

DIFFERENTIAL DIAGNOSIS

- Underlying medical condition
- Somatization disorder
- Body dysmorphic disorder (restricted to a circumscribed concern about appearance)
- Factitious disorder or malingering
- Generalized anxiety disorder with health concerns is one worry among others
- Major depressive disorder with health concerns occurring only during depressive episodes
- Psychosis, as may occur with depression and schizophrenia

WORKUP

- History, physical examination, and laboratory and imaging tests, as appropriate, to exclude underlying medical condition.
- Symptom measures (e.g., Health Anxiety Inventory, Whiteley Index of Hypochondriasis) may be used for detection and monitoring of severity over time.
- Evaluation for other psychiatric disorders associated with hypochondriasis such as depression and anxiety.

TREATMENT

NONPHARMACOLOGIC THERAPY

- Focus on coping with, rather than eliminating, symptoms.
- Cognitive behavioral therapy (CBT) is the mainstay of treatment, with techniques to alter or restructure maladaptive thinking and behavior. Individual or group CBT, and mindfulness-based approaches, have demonstrated success.

- Brief and regularly scheduled appointments.
- Avoidance of laboratory tests, imaging studies, and diagnostic and surgical procedures unless otherwise indicated.
- Elimination of sources of secondary gain.
- Limit on reading medical texts or websites.
- Benign interventions (e.g., exercise, massage).

CHRONIC Rx

- Antidepressants may be helpful even in patients without features of depression: placebo-controlled trials of fluoxetine and paroxetine suggest benefit.
- Treatment of comorbid psychiatric conditions, if present.

DISPOSITION

Waxing and waning course over decades; recovery rates between 30% and 50%. Positive prognostic factors include acute onset, absence of secondary gain, lack of comorbid psychiatric disorder, and high socioeconomic status.

REFERRAL

Referral for CBT is the mainstay of treatment; referral to a psychiatrist may be needed in the case of comorbid psychiatric condition.

PEARLS & CONSIDERATIONS

- CBT and pharmacotherapy may be helpful treatment modalities for patients open to treatment not directed at the perceived illness.
- The onset of physical symptoms late in life is almost always the result of a medical disorder.

SUGGESTED READINGS
available at www.expertconsult.com

RELATED CONTENT
Somatization Disorder (Related Key Topic)
Hypochondria (Patient Information)

AUTHOR: **LUCY KALANITHI, M.D.**

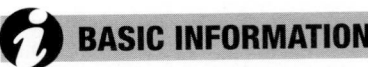

BASIC INFORMATION

DEFINITION

A decrease in parathyroid hormone (PTH) secretion or function results in hypoparathyroidism. In primary hypoparathyroidism, absence or dysfunction of the parathyroid gland results in inadequate PTH secreation and subsequent hypocalcemia and hyperphosphatemia. Impaired function of PTH (i.e., PTH resistance or pseudohypoparathyroidism) can also cause hypocalcemia and hyperphosphatemia but the measured PTH level is elevated in this circumstance. Secondary hypoparathyroidism, a condition in which PTH levels are low in response to hypercalcemic states, is discussed in Section IV (see hypercalcemia discussion in "Calcium" topic).

ICD-9CM CODES
252.1 Hypoparathyroidism

EPIDEMIOLOGY & DEMOGRAPHICS

The incidence and prevalence of primary hypoparathyroidism depends on the etiology of the condition. Postoperative hypoparathyroidism is the most common etiology and occurs in the setting of thyroid or parathyroid surgery. Transient hypoparathyroidism can be as high as 46% postoperatively but permanent dysfunction is less common. Autoimmune disorders are the subsequent most common cause of hypoparathyroidism in adults (female/male ratio of 1.4:1.0). Autoimmune polyglandular syndrome type I is reported to have an incidence worldwide of 1:1,000,000. Typically, patients with this syndrome present in childhood. Other etiologies of hypoparathyroidism are very rare.

PHYSICAL FINDINGS & CLINICAL PRESENTATION

The symptoms of hypoparathyroidism are primarily related to hypocalcemia. The presentation of symptoms varies with the severity and duration of illness.

- Cardiovascular: prolonged QT intervals, QRS and ST segment changes, ventricular arrhythmias
- Musculoskeletal: muscle cramps, laryngospasm, osteomalacia (adults), rickets (children), weakened tooth enamel, osteosclerosis
- CNS: tetany (Chvostek's sign and Trousseau's sign), seizures, paresthesias, visual impairment from cataract formation, altered mental status, papilledema, and basal ganglia calcifications with longstanding disease
- GI: abdominal pain
- Renal: hypercalciuria and nephrolithiasis Other: dry scaly skin, brittle nails, dry hair. In addition to the hypocalcemia-related symptoms, syndromes associated with hypoparathyroidism can have distinct clinical findings.

Conditions associated with hypoparathyroidism include:

- DiGeorge syndrome: dysmorphic facies, cleft palate
- Pseudohypoparathyroidism: short stature, round face, brachydactyly
- Hypoparathyroidism-retardation-dysmorphism syndrome: short stature, microcephaly, microphthalmia, small hands and feet, abnormal teeth
- Hypoparathyroidism-deafness-renal dysplasia syndrome: sensorineural deafness
- Autoimmune polyglandular syndrome type 1: mucocutaneous candidiasis and adrenal insufficiency

ETIOLOGY

There are several etiologies of hypoparathyroidism:

- Developmental defects of the parathyroids
  - Isolated hypoparathyroidism
  - Branchial dysembryogenesis (DiGeorge's syndrome)
  - Hypoparathyroidism-retardation-dysmorphism syndrome
  - Hypoparathyroidism-deafness-renal dysplasia syndrome
  - Mitochondrial dysfunction associated with hypoparathyroidism
- Destruction of the parathyroids
- Postoperative hypoparathyroidism
- Autoimmune polyglandular syndrome type 1
- Radiation to the neck
  - Infiltrative disease (e.g., metastatic carcinoma, Wilson's disease, hemochromatosis, thalassemia, granulomatous disease)
- Functional and secretory defects of the parathyroids
  - Activating mutation of the calcium-sensing receptor alters the set point of the receptor and decreases PTH secretion
  - Activating antibodies to calcium-sensing receptor alters the set point of the receptor and decreases PTH secretion
  - PTH resistance (i.e., target organs unresponsive to PTH action)
  - Pseudohypoparathyroidism: heterogeneous disorder presenting in childhood characterized by hypocalcemia, hyperphosphatemia, and elevated PTH levels
  - Hypermagnesemia and hypomagnesemia

DIAGNOSIS

DIFFERENTIAL DIAGNOSIS

- Secondary hypoparathyroidism as a result of hypercalcemia (discussed in the "Hypercalcemia" section)
- Other conditions associated with hypocalcemia. These conditions are usually associated with an elevated PTH hormone level.

WORKUP

- Serum calcium is usually low and phosphorus is elevated
  - Two measurements of serum calcium are required for the confirmation of hypocalcemia. Total calcium should be corrected for low albumin utilizing the formula: Corrected Calcium = measured calcium + [(4 − albumin) × 0.8]. If a reliable laboratory is available, an ionized calcium should be considered especially in conditions associated with acid-base disturbances or low albumin states.

- Serum phosphorus is usually high normal or elevated in hypoparathyroidism.
- The serum intact PTH (iPTH) level is the single best test to evaluate the etiology of hypocalcemia. PTH is decreased in hypoparathyroidism and elevated in most other conditions associated with low calcium levels. However, PTH is also elevated in disorders associated with impaired PTH function (i.e., pseudohypoparathyroidism).
- Genetic studies as indicated if medical or family history is suggestive.

LABORATORY TESTS

- Total and ionized calcium: low in hypoparathyroidism
- PTH: low in hypoparathyroidism and high in PTH resistance states like pseudohypoparathyroidism
- Phosphorus: high-normal or high in hypoparathyroidism
- Magnesium: both hypomagnesemia and hypermagnesemia can cause hypoparathyroidism
- ECG should be considered in both hypercalcemic and hypocalcemic states. Hypocalcemia associated with prolonged QT interval, rarely ST-segment elevations
- 24-hr urine for calcium to evaluate the risk for renal stones

TREATMENT

NONPHARMACOLOGIC THERAPY

Parathyroid autotransplantation:

Hypoparathyroidism and subsequent hypocalcemia are common problems after neck exploration for total or near-total thyroidectomy or parathyroidectomy. In cases where there is concern for postoperative hypoparathyroidism, parathyroid autotransplantation of one or two parathyroid glands into the forearm or sternocleidomastoid muscle should be performed to prevent postoperative hypoparathyroidism.

PHARMACOLOGIC THERAPY

The mainstay of treatment for primary hypoparathyroidism is pharmacologic therapy with calcium and vitamin D supplementation. The goals of therapy are to control symptoms and minimize complications of therapy. The aim should be to achieve low-normal serum calcium, 24-hr urinary calcium <300 mg/day, and a calcium-phosphorus product <55.

- Vitamin D:
  - There are several vitamin D preparations available on the market but the treatment of choice for patients with primary hypoparathyroidism is calcitriol. It is an active metabolite that does not require hydroxylation in the liver or kidney and therefore bypasses the PTH-mediated 1-α hydroxylation defect that occurs with hypoparathyroidism.
  - Dose of 0.25 to 1 μg once or twice daily is usually required to correct hypocalcemia and improves symptoms. Its maximal effect is seen after 10 hr and it lasts for 2 to 3 days.

- Calcium:
  - Calcium carbonate or calcium citrates are common oral agents used for treatment of hypocalcemia associated with hypoparathyroidism. Calcium carbonate requires an acidic environment for effective absorption, and as a result, it must be taken with food. Its effectiveness is decreased with concomitant use of H_2 blockers or proton pump inhibitors. However, calcium carbonate is cheaper in cost than other calcium supplements and therefore it is first line in the management of hypocalcemia for some patients. The advantage of calcium citrate is that it does not require an acidic environment for effective absorption.
  - Start with a dose of 500 to 1000 mg of elemental calcium tid and adjust the dose for a desired calcium in the low-normal range.
- Magnesium:
  - Hypocalcemia is difficult to correct without normalizing magnesium levels.
  - Magnesium sulfate IV 2 g over 20 min followed by 1 g/hr infusion can be considered in severe deficiency states. Milder deficiencies can be managed with oral magnesium 100 mg tid.
- Thiazide diuretics:
  - Thiazide diuretics decrease urine calcium excretion and decrease kidney stones. They should be considered in individuals with urine calcium >250 mg/day.

- PTH replacement:
  - Preliminary studies involving injectable synthetic human PTH(1-34) and PTH (1-84) have been performed with results showing a decrease in urinary calcium excretion, maintenance of serum calcium in the normal range with reduced requirements for calcium and vitamin D supplementation, and increase in bone density.
  - It is not FDA approved for use in hypoparathyroidism.

ACUTE GENERAL Rx

Severe and/or symptomatic hypocalcemia requires hospitalization. Acute management of hypocalcemia includes:
- Telemetry monitoring for arrhythmias associated with severe hypocalcemia
- IV infusion of calcium gluconate 10 ml of 10% solution to receive a bolus of 90 mg of elemental calcium followed by an infusion of 0.5 to 2 mg/kg/hr until ionized calcium levels are ≥4 mg/dl.

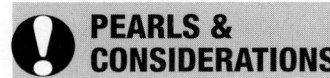

PEARLS & CONSIDERATIONS

COMMENTS

- The mainstay of treatment for primary hypoparathyroidism is calcitriol and calcium supplementation to maintain a goal serum calcium level in the low-normal range. IV calcium should be considered if calcium <7.0 mg/dl. Magnesium levels should be assessed and appropriately replaced in all patients with hypocalcemia. Clinical trials are under way to evaluate the role of recombinant PTH for the treatment of primary hypoparathyroidism.
- In patients undergoing neck exploration, consideration should be given to the parathyroid glands and autotransplantation of one or more parathyroid glands should be considered when appropriate to prevent postoperative hypoparathyroidism.

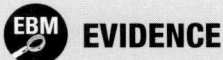

EVIDENCE

available at www.expertconsult.com

SUGGESTED READINGS

available at www.expertconsult.com

RELATED CONTENT

Table 4-9 Laboratory Differential Diagnosis of Hypocalcemia

AUTHORS: **VICKY CHENG, M.D.,** and **GEETHA GOPALAKRISHNAN, M.D.**

TABLE 1-224 Types of Hypoparathyroidism

Type	Calcium	PO₄	PTH	Comments
Hypoparathyroidism	↓	↑	↓	Surgical removal (most common cause)
Pseudohypoparathyroidism	↓	↑	Ø↑	End-organ resistance to parathyroid hormone (hereditary)
Pseudo-pseudohypoparathyroidism	Ø	Ø	Ø	Only skeletal abnormalities (Albright hereditary osteodystrophy)

From Weissleder R et al: *Primer of diagnostic imaging,* ed 5, St Louis, 2011, Mosby.

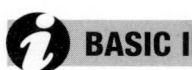 **BASIC INFORMATION**

DEFINITION

Hypopituitarism (from the Latin *pituita,* meaning "phlegm") is the deficiency of one or more of the hormones of the anterior or posterior pituitary gland resulting from diseases of the hypothalamus or pituitary gland. Panhypopituitarism indicates the loss of all the pituitary hormones but is often used in clinical practice to describe patients deficient in growth hormone (GH), gonadotropins, corticotropin, or thyrotropin in whom posterior pituitary function remains intact.

SYNONYMS

Panhypopituitarism
Pituitary insufficiency

ICD-9CM CODES
253.2 Panhypopituitarism

EPIDEMIOLOGY & DEMOGRAPHICS

Incidence of 4.2 cases per 100,000 persons

PHYSICAL FINDINGS & CLINICAL PRESENTATION

Symptoms depend on type of onset, number and severity of hormone deficiencies, their target organs, and age of onset.
- Mass effect of a pituitary tumor can cause headaches and visual disturbances (typically as bitemporal hemianopsia).
- Rhinorrhea.
- Corticotropin deficiency:
  - Fatigue and weakness, no appetite, abdominal pain, nausea, vomiting, failure to thrive in children, and hyponatremia. If the onset is abrupt, hypotension and shock
- Thyrotropin deficiency:
  - Fatigue and weakness, weight gain, cold intolerance, anemia, constipation
  - Bradycardia, hung-up reflexes, pretibial edema, change in voice, and hair loss
- Gonadotropin deficiency:
  - Loss of libido, erectile dysfunction, amenorrhea, hot flashes, dyspareunia, infertility, gynecomastia, decreased muscle mass, and anemia
- GH deficiency:
  - Growth retardation in children
  - Easy fatigue, hypoglycemia
  - Lean mass is reduced and fat mass is increased, leading to obesity
  - Decreased bone mineral density, increased low-density lipoprotein cholesterol, obesity, increased inflammatory cardiovascular markers (interleukin-6 and C-reactive protein)
- Hyperprolactinemia:
  - Galactorrhea, hypogonadism, inability to lactate after delivery
  - Posterior pituitary (vasopressin; antidiuretic hormone [ADH] deficiency): diabetes insipidus with polyuria, polydipsia, nocturia, hypotension, and dehydration

ETIOLOGY
It can be congenital or acquired:
- Congenital: mutations in transcription factors produce multiple hormonal deficiencies. Mutations in genes produce single hormonal deficiency.
- Acquired: the result of destruction of pituitary cells caused by:
  1. Pituitary apoplexy: hemorrhage or infarction of the pituitary gland. Predisposing factors include diabetes mellitus, anticoagulation therapy, head trauma, and radiation therapy. Sheehan's syndrome: postpartum necrosis, a rare complication after pregnancy.
  2. Infiltrative disease, including sarcoidosis, hemachromatosis, histiocytosis X, Wegener's granulomatosis, lymphocytic hypophysitis, and infection of the pituitary (tuberculosis, mycosis, syphilis).
  3. Primary empty sella syndrome: flattening of the pituitary gland caused by extension of the subarachnoid space and filling of cerebrospinal fluid into the sella turcica.
  4. Pituitary tumors: classified by size (microadenomas, <10 mm; macroadenomas, >10 mm) and function. Prolactin-secreting tumors and nonfunctioning tumors account for the majority of pituitary adenomas.
  5. Suprasellar tumors: craniopharyngiomas are the most common.

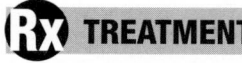 **DIAGNOSIS**

The diagnosis of hypopituitarism is suspected by clinical history and physical findings and is established by blood tests to confirm the presence of hormone deficiency.

DIFFERENTIAL DIAGNOSIS

The differential diagnosis is as outlined under "Etiology."

WORKUP

Includes baseline determination of each anterior pituitary hormone followed by dynamic provocative stimulation tests, radiograph imaging, and formal visual field testing.

LABORATORY TESTS
- Corticotropin deficiency:
  1. The presence of a 9:00 AM cortisol level >20 mcg/dl or <4 mcg/dl usually confirms sufficiency or deficiency, respectively.
  2. Corticotropin stimulation test using 250 mcg of corticotropin given IV and measuring serum cortisol before and 30 and 60 min after administration. A normal response is an increase in serum cortisol level >20 mcg/dl.
  3. With pituitary disease these test results may be indeterminate, and more dynamic testing such as an insulin-tolerance or metyrapone test may be necessary.
- Thyrotropin deficiency:
  1. Thyroid-stimulating hormone (TSH) and free T_4 measurements

  2. Primary hypothyroidism shows elevated TSH with low free T_4. Secondary hypothyroidism shows normal or low TSH with low free T_4 and low T_3 resin uptake.
- Gonadotropin deficiency:
  1. Follicle-stimulating hormone (FSH), luteinizing hormone (LH), estrogen, and testosterone measurements.
  2. In men, hypogonadotropic hypogonadism is seen with low testosterone levels and normal or low FSH and LH levels (ideally measured at 9:00 AM because of diurnal rhythm). Check free testosterone if patient is obese.
  3. In premenopausal women with amenorrhea, low estrogen with normal or low FSH and LH levels is typically seen.
- GH deficiency:
  1. Insulin-induced hypoglycemia stimulation test using 0.1 to 0.15 unit/kg regular insulin given IV and measuring GH 30, 60, and 120 min after administration. A normal response is a GH level >3 mcg/dl. This test is contraindicated in seizure disorder or ischemic heart disease.
  2. Combination of GH-releasing hormone plus arginine is an alternative test, with a diagnostic threshold of 9 mcg/L.
  3. Because the relation between serum insulinlike growth factor (IGF)-1 and GH levels blurs with age, a normal serum IGF-1 does not exclude the diagnosis in older adults.
- Hyperprolactinemia: prolactin levels may be elevated in prolactin-secreting pituitary adenomas.
- Vasopressin deficiency:
  1. Urinalysis shows low specific gravity.
  2. Urine osmolality is low.
  3. Serum osmolality is high.
  4. Fluid deprivation test over 18 hr with inability to concentrate the urine.
  5. Serum vasopressin level is low.
  6. Electrolytes may show hyponatremia and exclude hyperglycemia.

IMAGING STUDIES
- Imaging is the first step in identifying an underlying cause.
- MRI is more sensitive than CT in visualizing the pituitary fossa, sella turcica, optic chiasm, pituitary stalk, and cavernous sinuses. It is also more sensitive in detecting pituitary microadenomas. CT with contrast can be used if MRI is not available.
- Surveillance scan at baseline and 12 mo thereafter depending on protocol and clinical symptoms.

TREATMENT

Threefold: removing underlying cause (surgery or radiation), treating hormonal deficiencies, and addressing any other repercussions from deficiency.

NONPHARMACOLOGIC THERAPY

- IV fluid resuscitation, correction of electrolyte and metabolic abnormalities with potassium bicarbonate, and oxygen therapy.
- Transsphenoidal surgery for tumors causing specific symptoms.
- Radiation or stereotactic radiosurgery ("gamma knife") for medically unresponsive, surgically unresectable tumors and tumors for which other modalities are contraindicated. It is both safe and effective for recurrent or residual pituitary adenomas.

ACUTE GENERAL Rx

Acute situations such as adrenal crisis or myxedema coma can occur in untreated hypopituitarism and should be treated accordingly with IV corticosteroids (e.g., hydrocortisone 100 to 250 mg bolus followed by hydrocortisone 100 mg IV q6h for 24 hr) and levothyroxine (e.g., 5 to 8 mcg/kg IV over 15 min, then 100 mcg IV q24h).

CHRONIC Rx

Treatment is lifelong:

- Adrenocorticotropic hormone (ACTH) deficiency: hydrocortisone 10 mg PO every morning and 5 mg PO every evening or prednisone 5 mg PO every morning and 2.5 mg PO every evening. Dexamethasone or prednisone is often preferred because of longer duration of action.
- LH and FSH deficiency:
  - In men, testosterone enanthate or propionate 200 to 300 mg IM every 2 to 3 wk, or transdermal testosterone scrotal patches can be tried.
  - In women who are not interested in fertility, conjugated estrogen 0.3 to 1.25 mg/day and held the last 5 to 7 days of each month with the addition of medroxyprogesterone 10 mg/day given during days 15 to 25 of the normal menstrual cycle. In those who have secondary hypogonadism and wish to become pregnant, pulsatile gonadotropic-releasing hormone may be of benefit.
- TSH deficiency: levothyroxine 0.05 to 0.15 mg/day.
- GH deficiency:
  - GH replacement in children is universally accepted.

- GH replacement in adults is not generally recommended and requires careful consideration of each individual case. It may have effects on quality of life, body composition, bone density, and cardiovascular risk factors.
- Side effects of replacement includes peripheral edema, arthralgia, and headaches.
- Usual GH dose is between 0.2 and 0.4 mg, determined by the age and gender of a patient and increments of 0.1 mg every 2 to 4 wk until serum IGF-1 is in the upper part of the normal range. Young adults and women taking estrogen require a higher dose.
- ADH deficiency:
  - Desmopressin (DDAVP) 10 to 20 mcg by intranasal spray or 0.05 to 0.1 mg PO bid is used in patients with diabetes insipidus.
  - Vasopressin: 5-10 U given IM or SC q6h.

DISPOSITION

- Hormone replacement therapy is adjusted according to serum hormone monitoring.
- If untreated can lead to adrenal crisis, severe hyponatremia and hypothyroidism, metabolic abnormalities, and death.
- Complications: visual deficit, adrenal crisis, susceptibility to infection and other stressors.
- Prognosis: stable patients have a favorable prognosis with replacement hormone therapy. Patients with acute decompensation are in critical condition with a high mortality rate.

REFERRAL

Consultation with an endocrinologist and neurosurgeon for surgical treatment

(!) PEARLS & CONSIDERATIONS

- All patients sustaining moderate to severe head injury should undergo assessment of anterior pituitary function during the acute phase and at 6 mo.
- IGF-1 can be used as a marker of GH deficiency.
- All tests of GH secretion are more likely to give false-positive results in obese patients.

- The GH axis is the most vulnerable to the effects of radiotherapy; doses as low as 18 Gy in children have caused GH deficiency.
- Sequence of hormonal disruption: GH secretion then gonadotropin secretion. TSH and adrenocorticotropic hormone secretion are somewhat resistant.
- Thyroxine supplementation increases the rate of cortisol metabolism and can lead to adrenal crisis, so corticosteroids should be replaced first.
- All patients receiving glucocorticoid replacement therapy should wear proper identification stating the need for this therapy.
- Stress doses of corticosteroids are indicated before surgery or for any medical emergency (e.g., sepsis, acute myocardial infarction).
- Antidiuretic hormone deficiency may be masked if there is ACTH deficiency with symptoms only appearing when cortisol has been replaced.

COMMENTS

- Mineralocorticoid replacement is not necessary in secondary adrenal insufficiency because the renin-angiotensin-aldosterone system is unaffected by pituitary failure.
- Patients with adult-acquired GH deficiency must meet at least two criteria before replacement therapy: a poor GH response to at least two standard stimuli and hypopituitarism from pituitary or hypothalamic damage. The criteria are different in children in whom GH is required for normal growth.
- Prevention of acute decompensation can be accomplished by reminding patients to increase the dose of hydrocortisone in response to stress.
- Medical therapy should precede surgical therapy.

SUGGESTED READINGS
available at www.expertconsult.com

RELATED CONTENT
Hypopituitarism (Patient Information)

AUTHOR: **SHAHNAZ PUNJANI, M.D.**

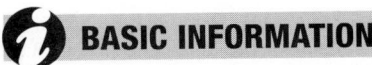

DEFINITION

Hypospadias is a developmental abnormality of the penis characterized by:

- Abnormal ventral opening of the urethral meatus anywhere from the ventral aspect of the glans penis to the perineum
- Ventral curvature of the penis (chordee)
- Dorsal foreskin hood

ICD-9CM CODES
752.61 Hypospadias
752.63 Congenital chordee

EPIDEMIOLOGY & DEMOGRAPHICS

PREVALENCE: One male in 250
GENETICS:

- Pertinent familial aspects of hypospadias include the finding of hypospadias in 6.8% of fathers of affected boys and in 14% of male siblings.
- An 8.5-fold higher rate of hypospadias is reported in monozygotic twins, suggesting insufficient production of human chorionic gonadotropin (hCG) by the single placenta.

PHYSICAL FINDINGS & CLINICAL PRESENTATION

- Genetics: normal karyotypes are seen with glandular hypospadias; abnormal karyotypes are noted in more severe forms of hypospadias
- Cryptorchidism: 8% to 9% occurrence
- Inguinal hernia: 9% to 10% occurrence
- Hydrocele: 9% to 16% occurrence

PENILE CURVATURE (CHORDEE): Three theories:
1. Abnormal development of the urethral plate
2. Abnormal fibrotic mesenchymal tissue at the urethral meatus
3. Corporal disproportion

ETIOLOGY

Multifactorial:
- Endocrine factors:
  1. Abnormal androgen production
  2. Limited androgen sensitivity in the target tissues
  3. Premature cessation of androgenic stimulation as a result of Leydig cell dysfunction
  4. Insufficient testosterone-dihydrotestosterone synthesis as a result of deficient 5-alpha reductase enzyme activity
- Arrested development

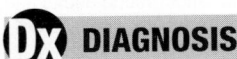 **DIAGNOSIS**

WORKUP

Made by observation and examination (Fig.1-445)

LABORATORY TESTS

Intersex evaluation should be undertaken if there is associated cryptorchidism. The evaluation should include ultrasound; genitographic studies; and chromosomal, gonadal, biochemical, and molecular studies.

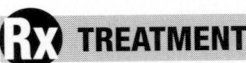 **TREATMENT**

ACUTE GENERAL Rx

DESIGNATION/CLASSIFICATION:
- Anterior: 33%
- Middle: 25%
- Posterior: 41%

SPECIAL CONSIDERATIONS:
- The only reason for operating on any patient with hypospadias is to correct deformities that interfere with the function of urination and procreation.
- Another reason for intervention is cosmetic concern.

- The American Academy of Pediatrics recommends the best time for surgical intervention to be 6 to 12 mo.

HORMONAL MANIPULATION:
- Controversial
- hCG administration is given before repair of proximal hypospadias.
- The effect of hCG administration is decreased hypospadias and chordee severity in all patients, increased vascularity and thickness of the proximal corpus spongiosum.
- Application of topical testosterone increases mean penile circumference and length without any lasting side effects.
- Prepubertal exogenous testosterone does not adversely effect ultimate penile growth.

CHRONIC Rx

SURGICAL PROCEDURES:
- Orthoplasty (correcting penile curvature)
- Urethroplasty
- Meatoplasty
- Glanuloplasty
- Skin coverage

There is no single universally acceptable applicable technique for hypospadias repair.

TYPES OF REPAIR:
- Anterior hypospadias: MAGPI, Thiersch-Duplay urethroplasty, glans approximation procedure, tubularized incised plate (TIP) urethroplasty, Mathieu perimeatal flap, Mustarde technique, megameatus intact prepuce, pyramid procedure
- Midlevel hypospadias: TIP, Mathieu flap, onlay island flap (OIF), King procedure
- Posterior hypospadias:
  1. One-stage repair: OIF, double-onlay preputial flap, pedicled preputial flap, transverse preputial island flap
  2. Two-stage repair: orthoplasty to correct chordee followed 6 mo later or longer by Thiersch-Duplay, bladder and/or buccal mucosal hypospadias repair

COMPLICATIONS OF REPAIR: Hematoma, meatal stenosis, fistula, urethral stricture, urethral diverticulum, wound infection, impaired healing, balanitis xerotica obliterans, penile curvature

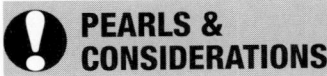 **PEARLS & CONSIDERATIONS**

- Apparent simple isolated hypospadias may be the only visible indication of an underlying abnormality.
- The dorsal hood of redundant foreskin is used in the repair of hypospadias, so the patient with hypospadias and a dorsal hood should not be circumcised.

SUGGESTED READINGS

available at www.expertconsult.com

RELATED CONTENT

Hypospadias (Patient Information)

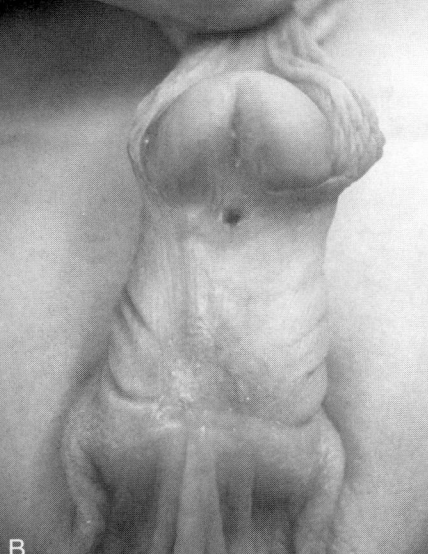

FIGURE 1-445 Varying forms of hypospadias. A, Glanular hypospadias. **B,** Subcoronal hypospadias. Note the dorsal hood of foreskin. (From Kliegman RM et al: *Nelson textbook of pediatrics,* ed 19, Philadelphia, 2011, Saunders.)

AUTHORS: **PHILIP J. ALIOTTA, M.D., M.S.H.A.,** and **RUBEN ALVERO, M.D.**

BASIC INFORMATION

DEFINITION

Hypothermia is a rectal temperature <35° C (95.8° F). Accidental hypothermia is an unintentionally induced decrease in core temperature in the absence of preoptic anterior hypothalamic conditions.

ICD-9CM CODES
991.6 Accidental hypothermia
780.9 Hypothermia not associated with low environmental temperature

EPIDEMIOLOGY & DEMOGRAPHICS

- Hypothermia occurs most frequently in the following groups: alcoholics; learning-impaired; patients with cardiovascular, cerebrovascular, or pituitary disorders; those using sedatives or tranquilizers; and elderly patients.
- ~700 persons in the United States die from hypothermia annually.

PHYSICAL FINDINGS & CLINICAL PRESENTATION

The clinical presentation varies with the severity of hypothermia. Shivering may be absent if body temperature is <33.3° C (92° F) or in patients taking phenothiazines.

Hypothermia may masquerade as cerebrovascular accident, ataxia, or slurred speech, or the patient may appear comatose or clinically dead.

Physiologic stages of hypothermia:
1. Mild hypothermia (32.2° to 35° C [90° to 95° F]): arrhythmias, ataxia
2. Moderate hypothermia (28° to 32.2° C [82.4° to 90° F]):
   a. Progressive decrease of level of consciousness, pulse, cardiac output, and respiration
   b. Fibrillation, dysrhythmias (increased susceptibility to ventricular tachycardia)
   c. Elimination of shivering mechanism for thermogenesis
3. Severe hypothermia (≤28° C [82.4° F]):
   a. Absence of reflexes or response to pain
   b. Decreased cerebral blood flow, decreased CO_2
   c. Increased risk of ventricular fibrillation or asystole

ETIOLOGY

Exposure to cold temperatures for a prolonged period. Contributing factors include:
1. Drugs: ethanol, phenothiazines, sedative-hypnotics
2. Skin disorders: extensive burns, severe psoriasis, exfoliative dermatitis
3. Metabolic disorders: hypopituitarism, hypothyroidism, hypoadrenalism
4. Neurologic abnormalities: stroke, head trauma, acute spinal cord transection, impaired shivering
5. Other: lack of acclimatization, aggressive fluid resuscitation, sepsis, heat stroke treatment

DIAGNOSIS

DIFFERENTIAL DIAGNOSIS

- Cerebrovascular accident
- Myxedema coma
- Drug intoxication
- Hypoglycemia

LABORATORY TESTS

1. Metabolic and respiratory acidosis are usually present.
   a. When blood cools, the arterial pH increases, oxygen tension (Po_2) increases, and the Pco_2 falls:
      (1) pH increases 0.008 U/° F (or 0.015 U/° C), causing a decrease in temperature.
      (2) Pao_2 increases 3.3%/° F, causing a decrease in temperature. Oxygenation considerations during hypothermia are described in Box 1-28.
      (3) $Paco_2$ decreases 2.4%/° F, causing a decrease in temperature.
   b. Blood gas analyzers warm the blood to 37° C, increasing the partial pressure of dissolved gases, resulting in higher oxygen and carbon dioxide levels and a lower pH than the patient's actual values. Correction of arterial blood gases for temperature is unnecessary as a guide to therapy. The use of uncorrected values also permits reference to the standard acid–base nomograms.
2. A decrease in K^+ initially, then an increase in K^+ with increasing hypothermia; extreme hyperkalemia indicates a poor prognosis.
3. Hematocrit increases (caused by hemoconcentration), decreasing leukocytes and platelets (caused by splenic sequestration).
4. Blood viscosity, increased clotting time

IMAGING STUDIES

- Chest x-ray: generally not helpful; may reveal evidence of aspiration (e.g., intoxicated patient with aspiration pneumonia)
- ECG: prolonged PR, QT, and QRS segments, depressed ST segments, inverted T waves, atrioventricular block, and hypothermic J waves (Osborne waves) may appear at 25° to 30° C; characterized by notching of the junction of the QRS complex and ST segments (Fig. 1-446).

TREATMENT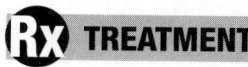

NONPHARMACOLOGIC THERAPY

- Treatment of hypothermia varies with the following:
  1. Degree of hypothermia
  2. Existence of concomitant diseases (e.g., cardiovascular insufficiency)
  3. Patient's age and medical condition (e.g., elderly, debilitated patients vs. young, healthy patients)
- General measures:
  1. Secure an airway before warming all unconscious patients; precede endotracheal intubation with oxygenation (if possible) to minimize the risk of arrhythmias during the procedure.
  2. Peripheral vasoconstriction may impede placement of a peripheral intravenous catheter; consider femoral venous access as an alternative to the jugular or subclavian sites to avoid ventricular stimulation.
  3. A Foley catheter should be inserted, and urinary output should be monitored and maintained >0.5 to 1 ml/kg/hr with intravascular volume replacement.
  4. Box 1-29 summarizes measures for preparing hypothermic patients for transport.

ACUTE GENERAL Rx

- Continuous ECG monitoring of patients is recommended. Ventricular arrhythmias can be treated with bretylium; lidocaine is generally ineffective, and procainamide is associated with an increased incidence of ventricular fibrillation in hypothermic patients.
- Correct severe acidosis and electrolyte abnormalities.
- Hypothyroidism, if present, should be promptly treated (see "Myxedema Coma").
- If clinical evidence suggests adrenal insufficiency, administer IV methylprednisolone.

BOX 1-28   Oxygenation Considerations During Hypothermia

Detrimental Factors
Oxygen consumption increases with rise in temperature; caution if rapid rewarming; shivering also increases demand
Decreased temperature shifts oxyhemoglobin dissociation curve to the left
Ventilation-perfusion mismatch; atelectasis; decreased respiratory minute volume; bronchorrhea; decreased protective airway reflexes
Decreased tissue perfusion from vasoconstriction; increased viscosity
"Functional hemoglobin" concept: capability of hemoglobin to unload oxygen is lowered
Decreased thoracic elasticity and pulmonary compliance

Protective Factors
Reduction of oxygen consumption: 50% at 28° C (82.4° F); 75% at 22° C (71.6° F); 92% at 10° C (50° F)
Increased oxygen solubility in plasma
Decreased pH and increased $Paco_2$ shift oxyhemoglobin dissociation curve to right

From Auerbach P: Wilderness medicine, ed 4, St Louis, 2001, Mosby.

In patients unresponsive to verbal or noxious stimuli or with altered mental status, 100 mg of thiamine, 0.4 mg of naloxone, and 1 ampule of 50% dextrose may be given.

Warm (104° to 113° F [40° to 45° C]), humidified oxygen should also be given if available.

Specific treatment:

1. Mild hypothermia (rectal temperature <32.3° C [90° F]): passive external rewarming is indicated. Place the patient in a warm room (temperature >21° C [69.8° F]), and cover with insulating material after gently removing wet clothing; recommended rewarming rates vary between 0.5° and 20° C/hr but should not exceed 0.55° C/hr in elderly persons.
2. Moderate to severe hypothermia:
   a. Active core rewarming
      (1) Delivery of heat by way of fluids: warm gastrointestinal irrigation (with saline enemas and by nasogastric tube); IV fluids (usually D_5NS without potassium) warmed to 104° to 107.6° F (40° to 42° C), peritoneal dialysis with dialysate heated to 40.5° to 42.5° C.
      (2) Inhalation of heated, humidified oxygen (warmed to 40° C [104° F]) increases core temperature by 1° C (1.8° F) per hr and decreases evaporative heat loss from respiration.
   b. Active external rewarming: immersion in a bath of warm water (40° to 41° C); active external rewarming may produce shock because of excessive peripheral vasodilation. Ideal candidates are previously healthy, young patients with acute immersion hypothermia.
   c. Extracorporeal blood warming with cardiopulmonary bypass appears to be an efficacious rewarming technique in young, otherwise healthy persons.
   d. Patients with cardiac instability and those in cardiac arrest should be transported to a center capable of providing extracorporeal membrane oxygenation (ECMO) unless other conditions (e.g., trauma) require transport to a closer facility.

SUGGESTED READINGS

available at www.expertconsult.com

RELATED CONTENT

Hypothermia (Patient Information)

AUTHOR: **FRED F. FERRI, M.D.**

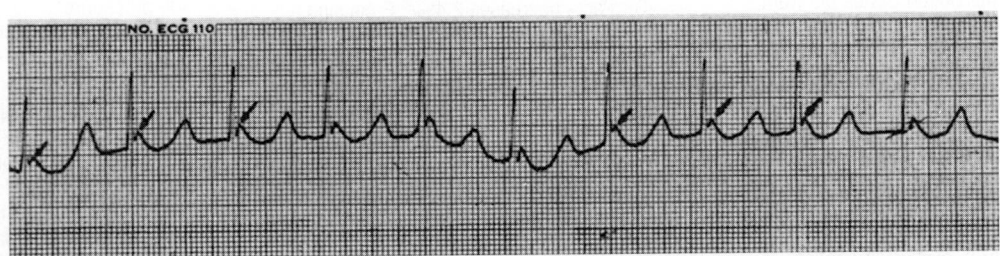

FIGURE 1-446 Hypothermic J waves (Osborne waves) *(arrows)* **in an 80-year-old man with core temperature of 86° F (30° C).** These waves disappeared with rewarming. (From Morse CD, Rial WY: Emergency medicine. In Rakel RE [ed]: *Textbook of family practice*, ed 4, Philadelphia, 1990, Saunders.)

BOX 1-29 Preparing Hypothermic Patients for Transport

1. The patient must be dry. Gently remove or cut off wet clothing and replace it with dry clothing or a dry insulation system. Keep the patient horizontal, and do not allow exertion or massage of the extremities.
2. Stabilize injuries (i.e., the spine; place fractures in the correct anatomic position). Open wounds should be covered before packaging.
3. Initiate intravenous infusions (IVs) if feasible; bags can be placed under the patient's buttocks or in a compressor system. Administer a fluid challenge.
4. Active rewarming should be limited to heated inhalation and truncal heat. Insulate hot water bottles in stockings or mittens and then place them in the patient's axillae and groin.
5. The patient should be wrapped. The wrap starts with a large plastic sheet, on which is placed an insulated sleeping pad. A layer of blankets, a sleeping bag, or bubble wrap insulating material is laid over the sleeping bag; the patient is placed on the insulation; the heating bottles are put in place along with IVs, and the entire package is wrapped layer over layer. The plastic is the final closure. The face should be partially covered, but a tunnel should be created to allow access for breathing and monitoring of the patient.

From Auerbach P: *Wilderness medicine*, ed 4, St Louis, 2001, Mosby.

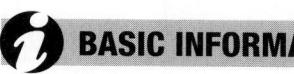 **BASIC INFORMATION**

DEFINITION

Hypothyroidism is a disorder caused by the inadequate secretion of thyroid hormone.

SYNONYMS

Myxedema

ICD-9CM CODES
244	Acquired hypothyroidism
243	Congenital hypothyroidism
244.1	Surgical hypothyroidism
244.3	Iatrogenic hypothyroidism
244.8	Pituitary hypothyroidism
246.1	Sporadic goitrous hypothyroidism

EPIDEMIOLOGY & DEMOGRAPHICS

INCIDENCE/PREVALENCE: 1.5% to 2% of women and 0.2% of men
PREDOMINANT AGE: Incidence of hypothyroidism increases with age; among persons older than 60 yr, 6% of women and 2.5% of men have laboratory evidence of hypothyroidism (thyroid-stimulating hormone [TSH] more than twice normal level).

PHYSICAL FINDINGS & CLINICAL PRESENTATION

- Hypothyroid patients generally present with the following signs and symptoms: fatigue, lethargy, weakness, constipation, weight gain, cold intolerance, muscle weakness, slow speech, slow cerebration with poor memory.
- Skin: dry, coarse, thick, cool, sallow (yellow color caused by carotenemia); nonpitting edema in skin of eyelids and hands (myxedema) secondary to infiltration of subcutaneous tissues by a hydrophilic mucopolysaccharide substance.
- Hair: brittle and coarse; loss of outer third of eyebrows.
- Facies: dulled expression, thickened tongue, thick and slow-moving lips.
- Thyroid gland: may or may not be palpable (depending on the cause of the hypothyroidism).
- Heart sounds: distant, possible pericardial effusion.
- Pulse: bradycardia.
- Neurologic: delayed relaxation phase of the deep tendon reflexes, cerebellar ataxia, hearing impairment, poor memory, peripheral neuropathies with paresthesia.
- Musculoskeletal: carpal tunnel syndrome, muscular stiffness, weakness.

ETIOLOGY

1. Primary hypothyroidism (thyroid gland dysfunction): the cause of >90% of the cases of hypothyroidism
   - Hashimoto's thyroiditis is the most common cause of hypothyroidism after age 8 yr
   - Idiopathic myxedema (nongoitrous form of Hashimoto's thyroiditis)
   - Previous treatment of hyperthyroidism (radioiodine therapy, subtotal thyroidectomy)
   - Subacute thyroiditis
   - Radiation therapy to the neck (usually for malignant disease)
   - Iodine deficiency or excess
   - Drugs (lithium, para-aminosalicylate, sulfonamides, phenylbutazone, amiodarone, thiourea)
   - Congenital (approximately one case per 4000 live births)
   - Prolonged treatment with iodides
2. Secondary hypothyroidism: pituitary dysfunction, postpartum necrosis, neoplasm, infiltrative disease causing deficiency of TSH
3. Tertiary hypothyroidism: hypothalamic disease (granuloma, neoplasm, or irradiation causing deficiency of thyrotropin-releasing hormone)
4. Tissue resistance to thyroid hormone: rare

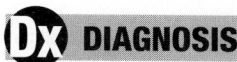 **DIAGNOSIS**

DIFFERENTIAL DIAGNOSIS

- Depression
- Dementia from other causes
- Systemic disorders (e.g., nephrotic syndrome, congestive heart failure, amyloidosis)

LABORATORY TESTS

- Increased TSH (Fig. E1-447): TSH may be normal if patient has secondary or tertiary hypothyroidism, is receiving dopamine or corticosteroids, or the level is obtained after severe illness
- Decreased free T_4
- Other common laboratory abnormalities: hyperlipidemia, hyponatremia, and anemia
- Increased antimicrosomal and antithyroglobulin antibody titers: useful when autoimmune thyroiditis is suspected as the cause of the hypothyroidism

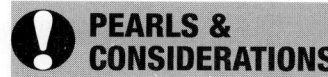 **TREATMENT**

NONPHARMACOLOGIC THERAPY

Patients should be educated regarding hypothyroidism and its possible complications. Patients should also be instructed about the need for lifelong treatment and monitoring of their thyroid abnormality.

ACUTE GENERAL Rx

Start replacement therapy with levothyroxine (L-thyroxine) 25 to 100 μg/day, depending on the patient's age and the severity of the disease. Physiologic combinations of L-thyroxine plus liothyronine do not offer any objective advantage over L-thyroxine alone. The levothyroxine dose may be increased every 6 to 8 wk, depending on the clinical response and serum TSH level. Elderly patients and patients with coronary artery disease should be started with 12.5 to 25 μg/day (higher doses may precipitate angina). The average maintenance dose of levothyroxine is 1.7 μg/kg/day (100 to 150 μg/day in adults). The elderly may require <1 μg/kg/day, whereas children generally require higher doses (up to 3 to 4 μg/kg/day). Pregnant patients also have increased requirements. Estrogen therapy may also increase the need for thyroxine. Women with hypothyroidism should increase their levothyroxine dose by approximately 30% as soon as pregnancy is confirmed. Close monitoring of serum thyrotropin levels and adjustment of levothyroxine dose is recommended throughout pregnancy.

CHRONIC Rx

- Periodic monitoring of TSH level is an essential part of treatment. Patients should be evaluated initially with office visit and TSH levels every 6 to 8 wk until the patient is clinically euthyroid and the TSH level is normalized. The frequency of subsequent visits and TSH measurement can then be decreased to every 6 to 12 mo. Pregnant patients should be checked every trimester.
- For monitoring therapy in patients with central hypothyroidism, measurement of serum free thyroxine (free T_4 level) is appropriate and should be maintained in the upper half of the normal range.

REFERRAL

Admission to the hospital intensive care unit is recommended in all patients with myxedema coma. Additional information on the diagnosis and treatment of this life-threatening complication of hypothyroidism is available under "Myxedema Coma" in Section I.

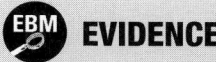 **PEARLS & CONSIDERATIONS**

COMMENTS

Subclinical hypothyroidism occurs in as many as 15% of elderly patients and is characterized by an elevated serum TSH and a normal free T_4 level. Subclinical hypothyroidism is associated with an increased risk of coronary heart disease events and mortality, particularly in those with a TSH concentration of 10 mU/L or greater. Treatment is individualized. In general, replacement therapy is recommended for all patients with serum TSH >10 mU/L and with presence of goiter or thyroid autoantibodies.

EBM **EVIDENCE**

available at www.expertconsult.com

SUGGESTED READINGS

available at www.expertconsult.com

RELATED CONTENT

Hypothyroidism (Patient Information)

AUTHOR: **FRED F. FERRI, M.D.**

BASIC INFORMATION

DESCRIPTION

ID reaction refers to an acute dermatitis developing at cutaneous sites distant from a primary inflammatory focus and is not explained by the inciting primary inflammation.

SYNONYMS

Autoeczematization

ICD-9CM CODES
692.89 Contact dermatitis and other eczema

EPIDEMIOLOGY

- Exact prevalence in U.S. is unknown.
- Seen in all ages.
- Males and females are equally affected.
- No particular race or ethnicity is more vulnerable.

ETIOLOGY

Infection with dermatophytes, mycobacterium, histoplasma, viruses, bacteria, or parasites (e.g., lice)

- Dermatitis such as contact, stasis, or eczematous
- Other causes include retained sutures, ionizing radiation, blunt trauma

PATHOGENESIS

Unknown, but possible explanations include:
1. Abnormal immune recognition of autologous skin antigens
2. Stimulation of normal T cells by altered skin constituents
3. Lowering of the threshold for skin irritation
4. Dissemination of infectious antigen resulting in a secondary response
5. Hematogenous dissemination of cytokines from the primary site of inflammation

CLINICAL FEATURES

- Usually associated with exacerbation of primary dermatitis

- Characteristics of the rash in ID reaction include:
  - Sudden onset of rash appearing within a week or two of primary inflammation
  - The rash could not be identified as a common dermatosis.
  - Lesions are most commonly seen in the side of the fingers. However, ID reaction could be generalized. Particularly in patients with stasis dermatitis, it appears in forearms, thighs, legs, trunk, face (Fig. 1-448), hands, neck, and feet in descending order of frequency.
  - Extremely pruritic
  - Often symmetric in distribution
  - Most of the time it is vesicular.
- It resolves upon treatment of primary inflammation.

DIAGNOSIS

- It is a clinical diagnosis.
- Fungus when suspected could be isolated only from the primary site by using potassium hydroxide or by using fungal culture
- At times skin biopsy is done. The biopsy findings are not pathognomonic for ID reaction. These include spongiotic epidermal vesicles associated with superficial perivascular lymphocytic infiltration of dermis, which may

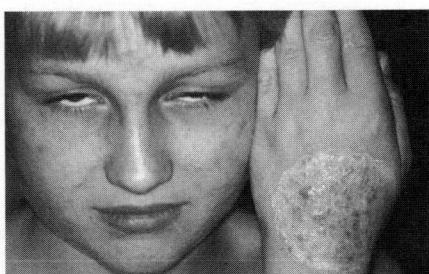

FIGURE 1-448 ID reaction. Papular eruption of the face associated with severe tinea infection of the hand. (From Kliegman RM et al: *Nelson textbook of pediatrics,* ed 19, Philadelphia, 2011, Saunders.)

also contain scattered eosinophils. Most of the lymphocytes in the epidermis are CD3 and CD8 T cells, whereas those in the dermis are primarily CD4 cells.
- Patch testing may be considered to exclude primary or secondary allergic contact dermatitis.

DIFFERENTIAL DIAGNOSIS

- Atopic dermatitis
- Contact dermatitis
- Drug eruptions
- Dyshidrotic eczema
- Folliculitis
- Scabies
- Dermatophytic infection
- Viral exanthema

TREATMENT

- The treatment is best directed toward the inciting cause.
- Medications used for symptomatic treatment of ID reaction include:
  1. Local or systemic steroids
  2. Local or systemic antihistamines
  3. Topical or systemic antibiotics for secondary bacterial infection
  4. Aluminum sulfate or calcium acetate for weeping skin lesions
  5. Rarely, local or systemic macrolactams (e.g., cyclosporine)

COMPLICATIONS

Secondary bacterial infection

PROGNOSIS

It almost always resolves within days when the primary dermatitis is adequately treated.

PATIENT EDUCATION

Treat primary dermatitis promptly.

AUTHOR: **HEMANT K. SATPATHY, M.D.**

BASIC INFORMATION

DEFINITION

Idiopathic intracranial hypertension (IIH) (pseudotumor cerebri) is a syndrome of increased intracranial pressure (ICP) without underlying hydrocephalus or mass lesion and with normal cerebrospinal fluid analysis.

SYNONYMS

Pseudotumor cerebri
IIH
Benign intracranial hypertension

ICD-9CM CODES
348.2 Pseudotumor cerebri

EPIDEMIOLOGY & DEMOGRAPHICS

- Disease of obese women in childbearing age
INCIDENCE:
- General population: 1-2 per 100,000 (including children)
- Women (obese females in reproductive age group): 20 per 100,000
- Men: 0.3 to 1.5 cases per 100,000
- Female/male ratio 9:1
- More than 90% of IIH patients are obese
- Mean age at diagnosis is 30 yr
RISK FACTORS:
- Obesity
- Medications: vitamin A and retinoids (used in treatment of acne and leukemia), chronic oral medications used for acne (tetracycline, minocycline)
- Systemic conditions: chronic kidney disease, polycystic ovarian syndrome, obstructive sleep apnea

PHYSICAL FINDINGS & CLINICAL PRESENTATION

Symptoms:
- Headaches: generalized, throbbing, slowly progressive, worse with straining maneuvers, worse in the morning.
- Transient visual obscuration: a brief blurring of vision or scotomata lasting <30 sec; occurs with postural changes, Valsalva maneuver; may be monocular.
- Double vision: usually due to sixth nerve palsy).
- Pulsatile tinnitus: described as a "whooshing sound" that is synchronous with heartbeat; classic symptom that indicates raised ICP.
- Photopsia: lights, sparkles in the eyes.
- Pain: mainly retro-orbital. Pain may also be located in the shoulders or neck. Could be present without a headache. May be associated with Lhermitte's sign.

Signs:
- Papilledema: seen in virtually all cases; usually bilateral but may be asymmetric
- Sixth nerve palsy: seen in approximately 10% to 20% of patients
- Visual field defects: include enlarged physiologic blind spot, nasal field defects, and constricted visual fields. Ninety percent of patients exhibit some form of visual loss on perimetry.

- Loss of central vision: end result of long-standing and untreated IIH

ETIOLOGY

- The exact etiology remains unknown.
- Proposed pathophysiologic mechanisms underlying the raised ICP include increased brain water content, excess CSF production, reduced CSF absorption, and increased cerebral venous pressure either alone or in combination.
- Another proposed mechanism includes abnormal vitamin A metabolism leading to increased CSF retinol levels and decreased CSF absorption at the arachnoid granulations.

DIAGNOSIS

DIAGNOSTIC CRITERIA
MODIFIED DANDY CRITERIA FOR DIAGNOSIS OF IIH
- Signs and symptoms of raised ICP (listed above)
- Absence of localizing focal neurologic signs (except 6th nerve palsy)
- CSF opening pressure of 25 cm H_2O with normal CSF composition
- Normal neuroimaging studies (MRI brain) including absence of cerebral venous thrombosis; stenosis of transverse sinuses may be seen in IIH without thrombosis.

DIFFERENTIAL DIAGNOSIS

- IIH is a diagnosis of exclusion and criteria listed above have to be satisfied.
- Causes of papilledema include intracranial space-occupying lesions such as tumors, abscesses, hematoma; venous sinus thrombosis; low CSF pressure; carcinomatous meningitis; chronic meningitides such as neurosarcoidosis, CNS lupus, neurosyphilis, cryptococcal meningitis, tuberculous meningitis, and carcinomatous meningitis.

WORKUP

- Neuroimaging studies: MRI of brain with MR venogram; CT head and CT head venogram when MRI of brain cannot be obtained.
- Lumbar puncture: CSF opening pressure (OP) should be obtained in the lateral decubitus position with the legs stretched and patient relaxed. OP exceeding 25 cm H_2O is considered elevated. CSF composition should be normal.
- Ophthalmologic examination: all patients with IIH need an ophthalmologic examination including visual fields at baseline and follow-up visits.

LABORATORY TESTS

CSF analysis shows normal protein, glucose, and cell count.

IMAGING STUDIES

- MRI of the brain to rule out underlying structural lesions
  - Absence of specific causes of raised ICP listed above

  - Empty sella sign often associated with chronic raised ICP but not pathognomonic
- MR or CT venography to exclude cortical venous thrombosis
  - May show transverse sinus stenosis in IIH without thrombosis. Absence of specific causes of raised ICP listed above.
- CT head
  - May show slit-like ventricles

TREATMENT

NONPHARMACOLOGIC THERAPY

- Weight loss in obese patients
- Continuous positive airway pressure if obstructive sleep apnea is suspected

ACUTE GENERAL Rx

- Acetazolamide 250 mg to 4 g per day: reduces CSF production by inhibition of carbonic anhydrase, occasionally causing anorexia and resultant weight loss. Dose can be increased to a maximum of 4 g a day in resistant cases with visual loss.
- Furosemide 40 to 120 mg/day in divided doses: apparent mechanism of action is by reduced sodium transport, leading to decreased total CSF volume.
- Topiramate 100 to 400 mg/day: reported to be effective in treatment of IIH. Weak carbonic anhydrase inhibitor with weight loss as one of its primary side effects.
- Serial lumbar punctures: SHOULD NOT BE CONSIDERED AS STANDARD TREATMENT OF IIH unless used for treatment of IIH during pregnancy. LP should be attempted in patients with severe headaches resistant to medical therapy. Goal is to reduce spinal fluid pressure to allow immediate reduction in headache severity. This treatment should be reserved for the most resistant cases and should be used as a conduit to future surgical intervention. Serial LP should not be used as treatment for IIH with progressive visual loss.

CHRONIC Rx

Surgical intervention is indicated in cases of treatment failure and progressive visual loss.
- Optic nerve fenestration: preferred for patients with visual loss and easily controlled headaches. Proposed mechanism is decompression of the optic nerve. Highly effective; however, has been associated with significant number of failure rates.
- CSF shunting: neurosurgical procedure; performed in patients with significant visual deterioration and difficult-to-control headaches. Provides rapid improvement in symptoms; however, reported to have significant rates of shunt revisions because of shunt malfunction.

DISPOSITION

- IIH is a potentially blinding condition, with severe vision loss in 5%-10% of patients; patients should be co-managed by neurologists and ophthalmologists. Monthly follow-up is essential until visual fields stabilize.
- All patients with IIH should undergo MR or CT venography to rule out the possibility of VST.

REFERRAL

- Neuro-ophthalmologist for serial evaluation of visual fields and fundus photographs
- Nutritionist for weight loss
- General neurologist for the initial workup and eventual treatment of raised ICP

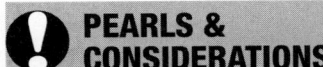

PEARLS & CONSIDERATIONS

COMMENTS

- IIH is a potentially blinding condition.
- IIH is a diagnosis of exclusion.
- IIH is a disease of young obese women.

PREVENTION

Maintenance of ideal body weight is one of the best preventive mechanisms for avoidance of IIH. However, it does occur in patients with normal body weight. In these cases there are no known preventable risk factors.

PATIENT & FAMILY EDUCATION

The combination of weight loss and medical therapy is highly effective in treatment of IIH. Given that most patients with IIH are young and otherwise healthy, high success rates can be accomplished.

SUGGESTED READINGS

available at www.expertconsult.com

RELATED CONTENT

Papilledema (Related Key Topic)
Diplopia (Section II, Differential Diagnosis)
Optic Atrophy (Section II, Differential Diagnosis)
Papilledema (Section II, Differential Diagnosis)

AUTHOR: **SACHIN KEDAR, M.B.B.S, M.D.**

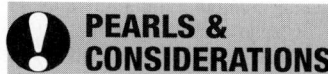

BASIC INFORMATION

DEFINITION

Idiopathic pulmonary fibrosis (IPF) is a specific form of chronic fibrosing interstitial pneumonia with histopathologic characteristics of usual interstitial pneumonia (UIP). Disease characterized by progressive parenchymal scarring and loss of pulmonary function.

SYNONYMS

Cryptogenic fibrosing alveolitis
Usual interstitial pneumonia
Pulmonary fibrosis

ICD-9CM CODES
516.3 Idiopathic pulmonary fibrosis

EPIDEMIOLOGY & DEMOGRAPHICS

- Incidence: 7-16 cases/100,000 persons worldwide. Clinically IPF affects >50,000 people in the U.S.
- Most commonly presents in 5th and 6th decades
- More common in men than women
- Familial forms account for 3% to 25% of cases. Genetic variants: include mutations in surfactant protein C and abnormal telomere shortening.
- No distinct geographic distribution; no clear racial predilection

PHYSICAL FINDINGS & CLINICAL PRESENTATION

- Most present with gradual onset (>6 mo) of exertional dyspnea and nonproductive cough. Progressive dyspnea is usually the most prominent symptom. Cough affects up to 80% of patients with IPF, is frequently disabling, and lacks effective therapy.
- Fine bibasilar inspiratory crackles in >80% of patients, with progression upward as the disease advances.
- Clubbing is found in 25% to 50% of patients.
- Cyanosis and right heart failure (cor pulmonale) may occur late in the disease course.
- Extrapulmonary involvement rarely occurs. Fever and wheezing are rare and suggest alternative diagnosis.

ETIOLOGY

- Unknown
- Cigarette smoking, environmental exposure, and microaspiration have been associated with IPF.
- Aberrant tissue repair and fibrosis are believed to play a greater role in the pathogenesis than generalized inflammation. A number of growth factors have been linked to pulmonary fibrosis (TGF-beta, PDGF, CTGF, FGF, and VEGF).

DIAGNOSIS

DIFFERENTIAL DIAGNOSIS

- Sarcoidosis
- Drug-induced interstitial lung disease
- Pulmonary manifestations of collagen vascular diseases (e.g., rheumatoid arthritis [RA], systemic sclerosis)
- Hypersensitivity pneumonitis (HP)
- Occupational exposures (e.g., asbestos, silica) may cause pneumoconiosis that mimics IPF
- Other idiopathic interstitial pneumonias:
  - Desquamative interstitial pneumonia (DIP)
  - Respiratory bronchitis–interstitial lung disease (RB-ILD)
  - Acute interstitial pneumonia (AIP)
  - Nonspecific interstitial pneumonia (NSIP)
  - Cryptogenic organizing pneumonia (COP)

WORKUP

- Almost all patients have abnormal chest radiograph at presentation, with bilateral reticular opacities most prominent in the periphery and lower lobes. Peripheral honeycombing may be seen.
- High-resolution CT scan shows patchy peripheral reticular abnormalities with intralobular linear opacities, irregular septal thickening, subpleural honeycombing, and ground-glass appearance.
- Pulmonary function testing shows restrictive pattern and reduced carbon monoxide diffusion into the lung.
- Six-minute walk test may show reduced exercise tolerance and/or exertional hypoxia.
- Laboratory abnormalities (nondiagnostic): mild anemia; increases in erythrocyte sedimentation rate, lactate dehydrogenase, C-reactive protein; low titer antinuclear antibody seen in up to 30% of patients.
- There is a limited role for bronchoalveolar lavage either in diagnosis or monitoring IPF.
- Gold standard for diagnosis is lung biopsy (open thoracotomy or video-assisted thoracoscopy). Hallmark features: heterogeneous distribution of parenchymal fibrosis against background of mild inflammation (UIP).
- Lung biopsy is critical to distinguish IPF from diseases with better prognosis and treatment options, especially in patients with any atypical features.

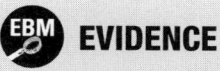

TREATMENT

- No proven treatment for IPF and little evidence to support the routine use of any specific therapy. With the lack of evidence supporting specific therapies in IPF, evaluation for participation in clinical trials of new therapies may be warranted.
- In patients with advanced disease, treatment options include supportive care (pulmonary rehabilitation, supplemental oxygen, influenza and pneumococcal vaccination) and potential lung transplantation.
- Treatment of asymptomatic gastroesophageal reflux may be reasonable given association between pulmonary fibrosis and reflux or microaspiration.
- Lung transplantation is the only therapy shown to prolong survival in IPF. Posttransplant 5-yr survival for IPF patients is approximately 40%. Median survival time is longer after bilateral lung transplantation than single lung transplantation but is associated with more complications during the first year.
- Other treatment options, including pirfenidone, warfarin, and etanercept are not recommended at this time based on prior evidence.
- Acute exacerbation of IPF, defined as worsening dyspnea (<1 mo), the presence of new opacities on radiograph, and the lack of evidence of infection, has an incidence of 10% to 57%. Progressive respiratory failure may require mechanical ventilation. Treatment often includes high-dose corticosteroids and broad-spectrum antibiotics.

DISPOSITION

- Spontaneous remissions do not occur.
- Natural history includes progressive loss of pulmonary function.
- There is an 8 to 14× increased risk of lung cancer.
- Mean survival after the diagnosis of biopsy-confirmed IPF is 2 to 5 yr.
- Respiratory failure is the most common cause of death.

REFERRAL

To pulmonologist for review of abnormal chest imaging and establishing diagnosis

PEARLS & CONSIDERATIONS

- The course is progressive, with a high mortality rate.
- Critical to differentiate IPF from other interstitial lung diseases because prognosis and response to treatment differ.
- There is no proven treatment for IPF. Recent studies have shown an increase in mortality, hospitalizations, and side effects with combination treatment (prednisone/azathioprine/NAC). Novel therapeutic agents targeting aberrant epithelial cell activation and repair may prove beneficial. The tyrosine kinase inhibitor BIBF 1120 at a dose of 150 mg bid has been reported to reduce the decline in lung function, with fewer exacerbations and preserved quality of life as compared to placebo. Trials involving thalidomide, a potent immunomodulary agent, have shown improvement in cough and respiratory quality of life.
- Consider early referral for lung transplant.

EVIDENCE

available at www.expertconsult.com

SUGGESTED READINGS
available at www.expertconsult.com

RELATED CONTENT

Idiopathic Pulmonary Fibrosis (Patient Information)

AUTHORS: **LYNN BOWLBY, M.D.,** and **MICHAEL BLUNDIN, M.D.**

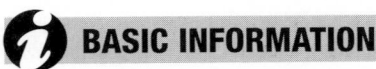

DEFINITION

Immunoglobulin A (IgA) nephropathy is a proliferative glomerulonephritis associated with predominant deposition of IgA in the mesangium.

SYNONYMS

Berger's disease

ICD-9CM CODES
583.81 IgA Nephropathy

EPIDEMIOLOGY & DEMOGRAPHICS

INCIDENCE: It is the most common type of glomerulonephropathy worldwide.
PREVALENCE: Prevalence rate is lower in the U.S. (10% to 15%) compared with Asian countries. Lower rates could be explained by a conservative approach by nephrologists in the U.S., who are reluctant to do renal biopsy in asymptomatic patients with minimal renal abnormalities. In most reports prevalence rates are expressed as a percentage of cases of primary glomerulonephritis or as a percentage of total series of renal biopsies.
PREDOMINANT SEX AND AGE: It is most prevalent in the second and third decades of life with a male/female ratio of 6:1 in the U.S.
GENETICS: Although it is considered a sporadic disease, genetic linkage to locus called *IgAN1* on 6q22 and 6q23 has been shown.
RISK FACTORS: It has a higher association with Asians, whites, and Native Americans and is rarely seen in African Americans.

PHYSICAL FINDINGS & CLINICAL PRESENTATION

- Two common presentations include (1) recurrent macroscopic hematuria often associated with upper respiratory infection and (2) persistent microscopic hematuria.
- Loin pain may be associated with macroscopic hematuria.
- Physical findings are usually unremarkable, except hypertension seen in 20% to 30% of patients with chronic disease and edema in 5% of patients with nephrotic-range proteinuria.
- Mild proteinuria is common.
- Rarely, IgA nephropathy presents as acute renal failure in 5% of patients and chronic renal failure in 10% to 20% of patients.

ETIOLOGY

- Most cases are idiopathic/primary.
- Secondary causes of IgA nephropathy include Henoch-Schönlein purpura; hepatitis B; alcoholic cirrhosis; celiac disease; inflammatory bowel disease; psoriasis; sarcoidosis; cystic fibrosis; cancer of the lungs, larynx, or pancreas; HIV infection; systemic lupus erythematosus; rheumatoid arthritis; diabetic nephropathy; Sjögren's syndrome; and Reiter's syndrome.
- Fig. 1-449 illustrates the pathogenesis of IgA nephropathy.

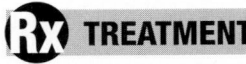 DIAGNOSIS

DIFFERENTIAL DIAGNOSIS

- Henoch-Schönlein purpura
- Hereditary nephritis
- Thin glomerular basement membrane disease
- Lupus nephritis
- Poststreptococcal nephritis
- Secondary causes associated with IgA nephropathy mentioned above

WORKUP

- The diagnosis is suspected on the basis of clinical history and laboratory data but is confirmed by renal biopsy showing IgA deposits in the mesangium.
- Renal biopsy is restricted to patients with sustained proteinuria >1 g/day or worsening renal function.

LABORATORY TESTS

- Urine analysis showing protein, red blood cells and casts, and white blood cells.
- Serum creatinine may be elevated.
- 24-hour urine assay for quantifying proteinuria and to check creatinine clearance.
- Serum IgA is elevated in only 50% of patients and has no clinical utility.

Rx TREATMENT

Although initially considered a benign disease, IgA nephropathy is now recognized as a common cause of renal failure. Currently there is no cure. Table 1-225 summarizes treatment recommendations for IgA nephropathy.

NONPHARMACOLOGIC THERAPY

- Moderate dietary protein restriction
- Discourage smoking

ACUTE AND CHRONIC GENERAL Rx

- Aggressive therapy for hypertension, preferably with angiotensin-converting enzyme (ACE) inhibitors. Goal blood pressure is <125/75 mm Hg in the presence of proteinuria >1 g/day.
- Patients with recurrent gross hematuria or isolated microscopic hematuria, no or minimal proteinuria (<1 g/day), normal blood pressure, and normal kidney function should only be monitored every 6 to 12 mo to assess disease progression.
- If bouts of recurrent macroscopic hematuria are associated with tonsillitis, tonsillectomy may benefit these patients.
- Patients with persistent proteinuria >1 g/day with or without hypertension are treated with ACE inhibitors and/or angiotensin receptor blockers (ARBs). Steroids are reserved for patients with persistent proteinuria >1 g/day despite ACE and/or ARB administration.
- Patients with nephrotic syndrome, preserved kidney function, and minimal change in disease are treated with steroids for 6 mo.
- Patients with severe renal disease or crescentic, rapidly progressive glomerulonephritis in the absence of changes of chronic kidney disease in biopsy are treated with steroid and cyclophosphamide combination for the first 2 mo, followed by steroids and azathioprine for 2 yr for maintenance treatment.

Pathogenesis of IgA nephropathy

Mucosal immune system
Polymeric IgA1 (pIgA1) production↓
IgA1 response to mucosal immunization↓

Bone marrow
pIgA1 production↑
pIgA1 response to systemic immunization↑

Circulation
Monomeric IgA1 (mIgA1)↑
pIgA1↑
IgA rheumatoid factors↑
Abnormal O-glycosylation of IgA↑

Kidney
pIgA1 deposition
± IgG/complement deposition

Liver
Impaired IgA1 clearance

Mesangial cell proliferation

Mesangial matrix↑

Sclerosis

FIGURE 1-449 Pathogenesis of IgA nephropathy. Abnormalities in IgA immunity leading to mesangial IgA deposition and injury. (Modified from Johnson RJ, Feehally J: *Comprehensive clinical nephrology,* ed 2, St Louis, 2000, Mosby.)

- Patients with acute renal failure need renal biopsy to rule out acute tubular necrosis, which needs only supportive therapy, from crescentic IgA nephropathy, which needs aggressive medical management.
- Kidney transplantation is the treatment of choice for end-stage kidney disease. There is no difference in survival in living versus cadaver donors. At present, kidneys with IgA deposits are not used for transplantation.
- Statins are indicated for all IgA nephropathy patients with dyslipidemia, hypertension, and other cardiovascular risks.
- Role of mycophenolate and plasmapheresis is controversial.

COMPLEMENTARY & ALTERNATIVE MEDICINE

Role of fish oil is controversial.

DISPOSITION

- Complete remission occurs in <10% of patients.
- End-stage renal failure develops in 15% to 20% of patients within 10 yr of onset and in 30% to 35% of patients within 20 yr. Prognostic markers at presentation in IgA nephropathy are described in Box 1-30.
- Poor prognostic indicators include (1) male gender, (2) older age, (3) young age at the onset of the disease, (4) absence of episodes of recurrent macroscopic hematuria, (5) hypertension, (6) extent of renal insufficiency, (7) extent of proteinuria, (8) elevated serum uric acid, and (9) certain histologic changes seen in renal biopsy, such as crescents, glomerulosclerosis, and tubulointerstitial fibrosis or atrophy.

REFERRAL

Patients with IgA nephropathy are commonly referred to nephrologists.

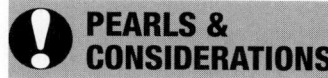

PEARLS & CONSIDERATIONS

COMMENTS

- IgA nephropathy seems to be a kidney-restricted form of Henoch-Schönlein purpura.
- IgA nephropathy is not an entirely benign condition, even when microhematuria is the only clinical presentation.

SUGGESTED READINGS

available at www.expertconsult.com

AUTHOR: **HEMANT K. SATPATHY, M.D.**

TABLE 1-225   Treatment Recommendations for IgA Nephropathy

Recurrent Macroscopic Hematuria (Preserved Renal Function)

Aggressive hydration (no role for antibiotics or tonsillectomy)

Macroscopic Hematuria with Acute Kidney Injury

Renal biopsy mandatory if persistent acute kidney injury (see text)
Acute tubular necrosis: supportive measures only
Crescentic IgA nephropathy
    Induction: Prednisolone 0.5-1 mg/kg/day for up to 8 wk
        Cyclophosphamide 2 mg/kg/day for up to 8 wk
        (no evidence favoring oral or intravenous route—follow local practice)
    Maintenance: Prednisolone in reducing dosage
        Azathioprine 2.5 mg/kg/day

Proteinuria <1 g/24 h (±Microscopic Hematuria)

No specific treatment

Nephrotic Syndrome with Minimal Change on Light Microscopy

Prednisolone 0.5-1 mg/kg/day (children 60 mg/m^2/day) for up to 8 wk, then taper

Non-nephrotic Proteinuria >1 g/24 h (±Microscopic Hematuria)

ACE inhibitor and/or ARB (maximize dosage or combine to achieve target BP and proteinuria <0.5 g/day)
If proteinuria still > 1 g/24 h on maximal supportive therapy and GFR < 70 ml/min, consider fish oil (12 g/daily for 6 mo). If further progression of renal failure, consider prednisolone (40 mg/day decreasing to 10 mg by 2 yr).

Hypertension

ACE inhibitors and ARB are agent of first choice—target BP: 130/80 mm Hg if proteinuria < 1 g/24 h; 125/75 mm Hg if proteinuria > 1 g/24 h

Transplantation

No special measures required

ACE, Angiotensin-converting enzyme; *ARB,* angiotensin receptor blocker; *BP,* blood pressure; *GFR,* glomerular filtration rate.
From Floege J et al: *Comprehensive clinical nephrology,* ed 4, Philadelphia, 2010, Saunders.

BOX 1-30   Prognostic Markers at Presentation in IgA Nephropathy

Clinical	Histopathologic
Poor Prognosis	**Poor Prognosis**
Increasing age	Glomerular sclerosis
Duration of preceding symptoms	Tubular atrophy
Severity of proteinuria	Interstitial fibrosis
Hyperuricemia	Vascular wall thickening
Hypertension	Capillary-loop IgA deposits
Renal impairment	**No Impact on Prognosis**
Good Prognosis	Intensity of IgA deposits
Recurrent macroscopic hematuria	
No Impact on Prognosis	
Gender	
Serum IgA level	

None of the clinical or histopathologic adverse features, except capillary-loop IgA deposits, are specific to IgA nephropathy.
From Feehally J et al: *Comprehensive clinical nephrology,* ed 4, Philadelphia, 2010, Saunders.

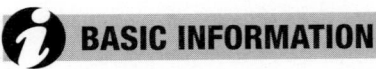

BASIC INFORMATION

DEFINITION

Immune thrombocytopenic purpura (ITP) is an autoimmune disorder in which antibody-coated or immune complex–coated platelets are destroyed prematurely by the reticuloendothelial system, resulting in peripheral thrombocytopenia. In primary ITP the thrombocytopenia is isolated, whereas in secondary ITP the condition is associated with other disorders (e.g., SLE, HIV).

ICD-9CM CODES
287.3 Idiopathic thrombocytopenic purpura (ITP)

EPIDEMIOLOGY & DEMOGRAPHICS

INCIDENCE: Primary ITP incidence is 10 in 100,000 adults, 5 in 100,000 children
PREVALENCE: Five to 10 cases per 100,000 persons
PREDOMINANT SEX: 72% of patients >10 yr are female; in children, males and females are affected equally
PREDOMINANT AGE: Children ages 2 to 4 yr and young women (70% are <40 yr)

PHYSICAL FINDINGS & CLINICAL PRESENTATION

The presentation of ITP is different in children and adults:

- Children generally present with sudden onset of bruising and petechiae from severe thrombocytopenia.
- In adults the presentation is insidious; a history of prolonged purpura may be present; many patients are diagnosed incidentally on the basis of automated laboratory tests that now routinely include platelet counts.
- The physical examination may be entirely normal.
- Patients with severe thrombocytopenia may have petechiae, purpura, epistaxis, or heme-positive stool from gastrointestinal bleeding. Life-threatening bleeding is uncommon and generally confined to patients with platelets <10,000 per cubic mm.
- Splenomegaly is unusual; its presence should alert to the possibility of other etiologies of thrombocytopenia.
- The presence of dysmorphic features (skeletal anomalies, auditory abnormalities) may indicate a congenital disorder as the cause of the thrombocytopenia.

ETIOLOGY

Increased platelet destruction caused by autoantibodies to platelet-membrane antigens. Hundreds of medications can cause thrombocytopenia. Drugs commonly implicated are quinidine, heparin, antibiotics (linezolid, vancomycin, sulfonamides, rifampin), platelet inhibitors (tirofiban, abciximab, eptifibatide), cimetidine, NSAIDs, thiazide diuretics, antirheumatic agents (gold salts, penicillamine), acetaminophen, and chemotherapeutic agents (cyclosporine, fludarabine, oxaliplatin).

DIAGNOSIS

DIFFERENTIAL DIAGNOSIS

- Falsely low platelet count (resulting from EDTA-dependent or cold-dependent agglutinins)
- Viral infections (e.g., HIV, hepatitis C, mononucleosis, rubella)
- Drug-induced (e.g., heparin, quinidine, sulfonamides)
- Hypersplenism resulting from liver disease
- Myelodysplastic and lymphoproliferative disorders
- Pregnancy, hypothyroidism
- SLE, TTP, hemolytic-uremic syndrome
- Congenital thrombocytopenia (e.g., Fanconi's syndrome, May-Hegglin anomaly, Bernard-Soulier syndrome)

LABORATORY TESTS

- Complete blood count, platelet count, and peripheral smear: platelets are decreased but are normal in size or may appear larger than normal (Fig. 1-450). Red blood cells and white blood cells have a normal morphology.
- Additional tests may be ordered to exclude other causes of the thrombocytopenia when clinically indicated (e.g., HIV, ANA, TSH, liver enzymes, bone marrow examination).
- The direct assay for the measurement of platelet-bound antibodies has an estimated positive predictive value of 80% to 83%. A negative test cannot be used to rule out the diagnosis.

IMAGING STUDIES

CT scan of abdomen/pelvis in patients with splenomegaly to exclude other disorders causing thrombocytopenia

TREATMENT

NONPHARMACOLOGIC THERAPY

- Minimize activity to prevent injury or bruising (e.g., contact sports should be avoided).
- Stop any potentially offending drugs (see "Etiology"). Avoid medications that increase the risk of bleeding (e.g., aspirin and other NSAIDs).

ACUTE GENERAL Rx

- Treatment varies with the platelet count, patient's age, and bleeding status (Fig. E1-451).
- Observation and frequent monitoring of platelet count are needed in asymptomatic patients with platelet counts >30,000/mm³.
- Oral prednisone 1 mg/kg/day in a tapering dose generally for 4 to 6 wk is the most common initial regimen. Methylprednisolone 30 mg/kg/day IV infused over a period of 20 to 30 min (maximum dose of 1 g/day for 2 or 3 days) plus IV immunoglobulin (1 g/kg/day for 2 or 3 days) and infusion of platelets should be given to patients with neurologic symptoms, internal bleeding, or those undergoing emergency surgery.

- Prednisone continued until the platelet count is normalized then slowly tapered off is indicated in adults with platelet counts <20,000/mm³ and those who have counts <50,000/mm³ and significant mucous membrane bleeding. Response rates range from 50% to 75%, and most responses occur within the first 3 wk. Oral dexamethasone at a dosage of 40 mg/day for 4 consecutive days has also been reported to induce a high response rate (85%). Continuation of corticosteriods is limited by long-term complications associated with its use (osteoporosis, weight gain, opportunistic infections, emotional lability)
- IV immunoglobulin (0.8-1.0 g/kg) is used in patients who have not responded to corticosteroids and often in pregnant patients. It rapidly increases platelet count in nearly 80% of patients, but its effect is transient. Anti-D immunoglobulin, a pooled IgG product derived from the plasma of Rh(D)-negative donors, is also effective. It can be given only to patients who are Rh(D) positive. Usual dose is 50-75 mcg/kg.
- Rituximab, a monoclonal antibody directed against the CD_{20} antigen, is used as a second-line agent. Usual dose is 375 mg/m² weekly x4 wk.
- Splenectomy is considered second-line treatment and should be considered in adults with platelet count <20,000/mm³ after 6 wk of medical treatment or after 6 mo if more than 10 to 20 mg of prednisone per day is required to maintain a platelet count >30,000/mm³. In children, splenectomy is generally reserved for persistent thrombocytopenia (>1 yr) and clinically significant bleeding. Appropriate immunizations (pneumococcal vaccine in adults and children, *Haemophilus influenzae* vaccine, meningococcal vaccine in children) should be administered before splenectomy.
- Additional second-line agents are thrombopoietin receptor agonists, azathioprine, cyclosporin A, cyclophosphamide, danazol, dapsone, mycophenolate mofetil, and *Vinca* alkaloids. Romiplostim, a recombinant fusion protein, and the oral thrombopoietin-receptor agonist eltrombopag are effective in increasing platelet count in adult patients with chronic ITP refractory to corticosteroids and/or splenectomy. The American Society of Hematology guidelines revised in 2011 recommend the use of thrombopoietin-receptor agonists for adult patients with ITP at risk for bleeding, who have a contraindication to splenectomy, or do not have a response to at least one other therapy.
- Platelet transfusion is needed only in case of life-threatening hemorrhage.
- Third-line therapy for ITP consists of combination chemotherapy and hematopoietic stem cell transplantation.

DISPOSITION

- More than 80% of children have a complete remission within 8 wk.
- In adults, the course of the disease is chronic; only 5% of adults have spontaneous remission.
- The principal cause of death from ITP is intracranial hemorrhage (1% of children, 5% of adults).

SUGGESTED READINGS

available at www.expertconsult.com

RELATED CONTENT

Immune Thrombocytopenic Purpura (Patient Information)

AUTHOR: **FRED F. FERRI, M.D.**

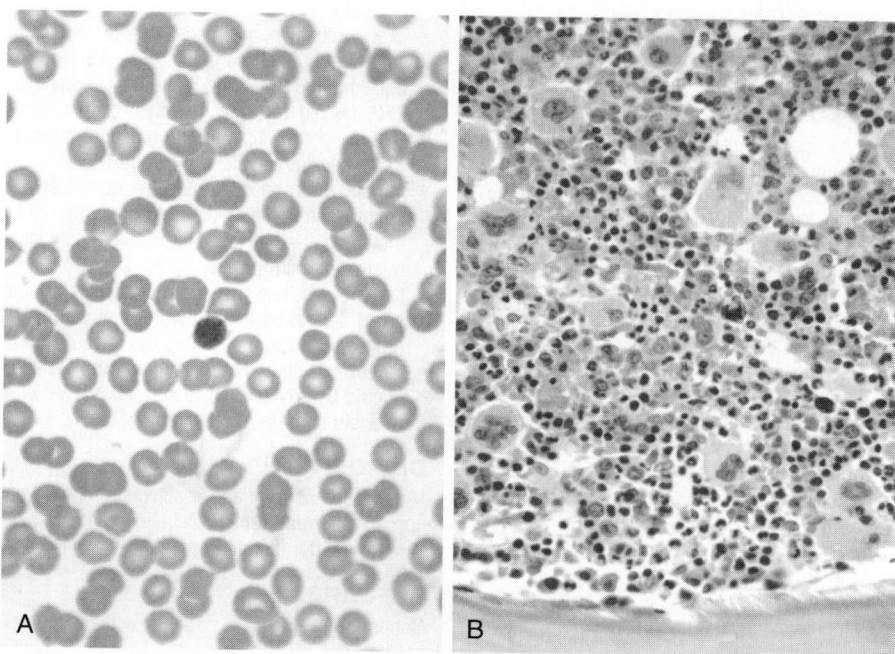

FIGURE 1-450 Immune thrombocytopenic purpura. **A,** Peripheral blood smear of immune thrombocytopenic purpura. A single large platelet is seen at the center. Large platelets reflect early release from the bone marrow. **B,** The bone marrow trephine biopsy section contains increased numbers of megakaryocytes. (From Jaffe ES et al: *Hematopathology,* Philadelphia, 2011, Saunders.)

BASIC INFORMATION

DEFINITION

Impetigo is a superficial skin infection generally caused by *Staphylococcus aureus* and/or *Streptococcus* spp.

Common presentations are bullous impetigo (generally caused by staphylococcal disease) and nonbullous impetigo (from streptococcal infection and possible staphylococcal infection); the bullous form is caused by an epidermolytic toxin produced at the site of infection.

SYNONYMS

Impetigo vulgaris
Pyoderma

ICD-9CM CODES
684 Impetigo

EPIDEMIOLOGY & DEMOGRAPHICS

- Bullous impetigo is most common in infants and children. The nonbullous form is most common in children ages 2 to 5 yr with poor hygiene in warm climates.
- The overall incidence of acute nephritis with impetigo varies between 2% and 5%.

PHYSICAL FINDINGS & CLINICAL PRESENTATION

- Nonbullous impetigo begins as a single red macule or papule that quickly becomes a vesicle. Rupture of the vesicle produces an erosion of which the contents dry to form honey-colored crusts. Multiple lesions with golden yellow crusts and weeping areas are often found on the skin around the nose, mouth (Fig. 1-452), and limbs.

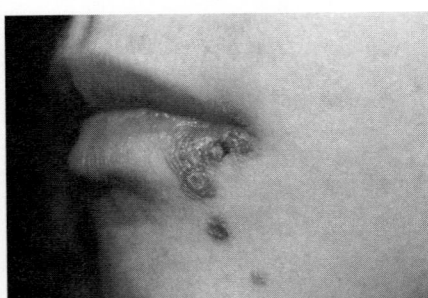

FIGURE 1-452 Multiple crusted and oozing lesions of impetigo. (From Kliegman RM et al: *Nelson textbook of pediatrics*, ed 19, Philadelphia, 2011, Saunders.)

- Bullous impetigo is manifested by the presence of vesicles that enlarge rapidly to form bullae with contents that vary from clear to cloudy. There is subsequent collapse of the center of the bullae; the peripheral areas may retain fluid, and a honey-colored crust may appear in the center. As the lesions enlarge and become contiguous with the others, a scaling border replaces the fluid-filled rim; there is minimal erythema surrounding the lesions.
- Regional lymphadenopathy is most common with nonbullous impetigo.
- Constitutional symptoms are generally absent.

ETIOLOGY

- *S. aureus* coagulase positive is the dominant microorganism.
- *S. pyogenes* (group A β-hemolytic streptococci): M-T serotypes of this organism associated with acute nephritis are 2, 49, 55, 57, and 60.

DIAGNOSIS

DIFFERENTIAL DIAGNOSIS

- Atopic dermatitis
- Herpes simplex infection
- Ecthyma
- Folliculitis
- Eczema
- Insect bites
- Scabies
- Tinea corporis
- Pemphigus vulgaris and bullous pemphigoid
- Chickenpox

WORKUP

Diagnosis is clinical.

LABORATORY TESTS

- Generally not necessary
- Gram stain and culture and sensitivity to confirm the diagnosis when the clinical presentation is unclear
- Sedimentation rate parallel to activity of the disease
- Increased anti-DNAse B and antihyaluronidase
- Urinalysis revealing hematuria with erythrocyte casts and proteinuria in patients with acute nephritis (most frequently occurring in children between ages 2 and 4 yr in the southern part of the U.S.)

TREATMENT

NONPHARMACOLOGIC THERAPY

Remove crusts by soaking with wet cloth compresses (crusts block the penetration of antibacterial creams).

GENERAL Rx

- Application of 2% mupirocin ointment tid for 10 days or retapamulin 1% applied bid for 5 days to the affected area or until all lesions have cleared.
- Oral antibiotics are used in severe cases: commonly used agents are dicloxacillin 250 mg qid for 7 to 10 days, cephalexin 250 mg qid for 7 to 10 days, azithromycin 500 mg on day 1, 250 mg on days 2 through 5, amoxicillin/clavulanate 500 mg q8h.
- Impetigo can be prevented by prompt application of mupirocin or triple-antibiotic ointment (bacitracin, Polysporin, and neomycin) to sites of skin trauma.
- Patients who are carriers of *S. aureus* in their nares should be treated with mupirocin ointment applied to their nares bid for 5 days.
- Fingernails should be kept short, and patients should be advised not to scratch any lesions to avoid spread of infection.

DISPOSITION

Most cases of impetigo resolve promptly with appropriate treatment. Both bullous and nonbullous forms of impetigo heal without scarring.

REFERRAL

Nephrology referral in patients with acute nephritis

PEARLS & CONSIDERATIONS

COMMENTS

- Patients should be instructed on use of antibacterial soaps and avoidance of sharing of towels and washcloths because impetigo is extremely contagious.
- Children attending day care should be removed until 48 to 72 hr after initiation of antibiotic treatment.

RELATED CONTENT

Impetigo (Patient Information)

AUTHOR: **FRED F. FERRI, M.D.**

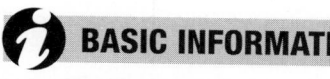 **BASIC INFORMATION**

DEFINITION

Inclusion body myositis (IBM) is the most common myopathy with onset after the age of 50 yr. Although classified among the inflammatory myopathies, its underlying pathophysiology has not yet been delineated.

SYNONYMS

None

ICD-9CM CODES
359.71 Inclusion body myositis

EPIDEMIOLOGY & DEMOGRAPHICS

INCIDENCE: 0.22 to 0.79 cases/100,000 persons; uncommon in Asians and African Americans
PREVALENCE: 0.5 to 7.1 cases/100,000 persons
PREDOMINANT SEX: Male/female ratio 1.3:1
PREDOMINANT AGE: 87% older than 50 yr
PEAK INCIDENCE: Seventh decade
RISK FACTORS: None known
GENETICS: Less than 10% of cases familial

PHYSICAL FINDINGS & CLINICAL PRESENTATION

- Insidious onset of slowly progressive proximal leg and distal arm weakness.
- Time to diagnosis from symptom onset often lags by years to a decade.
- Functional loss of strength in the legs most often precedes arm weakness.
- The cardinal clinical features include early weakness and atrophy of quadriceps muscles (difficulty climbing stairs, arising from chairs, and getting out of cars) along with wrist and finger flexor muscles (difficulty grasping, opening jars and turning doorknobs). Ankle dorsiflexion weakness may also be prominent leading to foot drop and tripping.
- When examining strength, side to side asymmetries are seen in one or more muscle groups in the majority of patients. This stands in contrast to the symmetrical, proximal involvement of polymyositis and most muscular dystrophies.
- Dysphagia and/or mild facial weakness are present in over half of cases. Dysphagia may be the presenting symptom.
- Although sensory symptoms are usually lacking, one third have evidence for peripheral neuropathy on physical examination and/or electrodiagnostic testing.
- 10% to 15% of patients have concomitant autoimmune disorders such as systemic lupus erythematosus, Sjögren's syndrome,

scleroderma, sarcoidosis, or thrombocytopenia. However, different from polymyositis and dermatomyositis, IBM does not portend an increased risk of heart or lung disease nor cancer.

ETIOLOGY

The pathogenesis of IBM is not known. Inflammatory, degenerative, viral and prion etiologies have been postulated, but none substantiated.

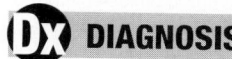 **DIAGNOSIS**

DIFFERENTIAL DIAGNOSIS

- Polymyositis
- Amyotrophic lateral sclerosis
- Late-onset muscular dystrophies
- Acid maltase deficiency

WORKUP

- Thorough neurologic examination with emphasis on the motor exam is important.
- Nerve conduction studies should be performed to exclude other causes and EMG to document a myopathy.
- The diagnosis of definite IBM requires the following features on muscle biopsy: (1) inflammation, (2) inflammatory cells invading healthy muscle fibers, (3) vacuoles, and (4) amyloid deposits by Congo red staining, TDP-43 sarcoplasmic staining, or tubulofilaments on electron microscopy.

LABORATORY TESTS

Creatine kinase level (labs for collagen vascular diseases may be obtained after the diagnosis). A complete blood count and coagulation studies should be drawn in anticipation of the muscle biopsy.

IMAGING STUDIES

MRI may reveal atrophy and signal abnormalities in volar forearm muscle groups and quadriceps atrophy with relative preservation of the rectus femoris muscle.

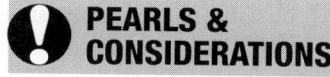 **TREATMENT**

NONPHARMACOLOGIC THERAPY

- Assistive devices for mobility such as canes, walkers, and wheelchairs are the mainstay of therapy.
- Occasionally knee orthoses or ankle-foot orthoses may improve and prolong ambulation.

ACUTE GENERAL Rx

None

CHRONIC Rx

- Experts have not found clinically significant improvement in functional strength with any pharmacologic therapy. Clinical trials of corticosteroids, methotrexate, intravenous immunoglobulin, anti-T lymphocyte globulin, etanercept, interferon β-1a, and oxandrolone have all failed to demonstrate functional improvements in limb strength.
- A short, small trial of a home exercise program demonstrated mild improvements in strength.
- IBM is generally refractory to therapy.

COMPLEMENTARY & ALTERNATIVE MEDICINE

Some patients choose to self-treat with creatine supplementation, coenzyme Q10, or lithium. There is no evidence supporting these treatments.

REFERRAL

- Patients with suspected IBM should be referred to a neurologist with subspecialty expertise in neuromuscular medicine.
- Physical therapy and occupational therapy consultations help the patient optimize ambulation and fine motor tasks, respectively.
- Speech therapy consultations can assist with symptomatic dysphagia.

PROGNOSIS

Life expectancy is not significantly altered in this late-onset, slowly progressive disorder. Some patients require wheelchair use 10 to 20 yr after disease onset.

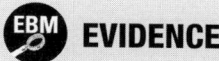 **PEARLS & CONSIDERATIONS**

COMMENTS

A key to diagnosis rests in finding weakness of wrist and/or finger flexors (especially the deep finger flexors at the DIP joints) on examination.

PREVENTION

None known

PATIENT/FAMILY EDUCATION

Patient information and support groups can be found at: www.ninds.nih.gov/disorders/inclusion_body_myositis and http://www.myositis.org.

EBM EVIDENCE

available at www.expertconsult.com

SUGGESTED READINGS
available at www.expertconsult.com

AUTHOR: **MATTHEW P. WICKLUND, M.D.**

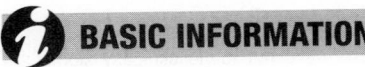

BASIC INFORMATION

DEFINITION

Fecal incontinence is defined as the loss of voluntary bowel control, leading to the inability to hold gas or feces in the rectum.

SYNONYMS

Fecal Incontinence
Anal Incontinence

ICD-9CM CODES

787.6 Incontinence of feces
307.7 Encopresis of non-organic origin

EPIDEMIOLOGY & DEMOGRAPHICS

INCIDENCE: It affects 0.5% to 1.5% of the population younger than age 65 yr but >10% older than age 65. Also more common in institutionalized patients.

PREVALENCE: After age 65: 2.2% of community dwellers, 14% of hospitalized, 54% of nursing-home residents. Prevalence increases with age and body mass index (BMI) in women.

PREDOMINANT SEX AND AGE: More common in females as compared to males

RISK FACTORS:

- History of urinary incontinence (present in 50% of the cases)
- Demented or cognitively impaired individuals
- Age >70 yr
- Presence of neurologic or psychiatric disease
- Poor mobility
- Female sex
- Fecal impaction from chronic constipation

PHYSICAL FINDINGS & CLINICAL PRESENTATION

- On inspection and by performing a digital rectal exam to ascertain the presence of fecal material, prolapsed hemorrhoid, dermatitis, scars, absence of perianal creases, or a gaping anus.
- Also assess for anocutaneous reflex. This can be done by stroking skin in each perianal quadrant (normal response is brisk anal wink).
- Assess the length of the anal sphincter.
- Assess resting and squeezing anal tone.
- Assess for rectal prolapse or excessive perianal descent when patient strains.

ETIOLOGY

- Often multifactorial
- Radiation-induced inflammation and fibrosis
- Rectal inflammation secondary to ulcerative colitis or Crohn's disease
- Neurologic disorders:
  - Status post stroke
  - Dementia
  - Multiple sclerosis
  - Dorsal and spinal cord lesions
- Surgery
  - Anorectal surgery for hemorrhoids, fistula, and fissures
- Medicines
  - Narcotics
  - Antidepressants
  - Antipsychotics
  - Calcium channel blockers
- Number of births and episiotomies in females
- Childhood abuse and adult sexual abuse

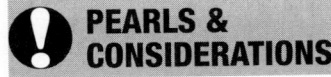

DIAGNOSIS

DIFFERENTIAL DIAGNOSIS

- Fecal encopresis

WORKUP

- Detailed history taking (Fig. E1-453 and Box E1-31) that includes the onset and precipitating events, duration and severity, stool consistency and urgency, and the presence of coexisting problems including urinary incontinence, surgery, or back injury is important.
- Diagnostic workup includes anal manometry, anorectal ultrasound, proctosigmoidoscopy, and anal electromyography (EMG).

IMAGING STUDIES

- Anal endosonography (most widely used and least expensive)
- MRI

TREATMENT

- Loperamide hydrochloride, diphenoxylate/atropine sulfate (mainstay of treatment), estrogen replacement therapy in postmenopausal women (uncontrolled trials)
- Solesta is a tissue bulking agent consisting of dextranomer microspheres and stabilized sodium hyaluronate that can be used for the treatment of fecal incontinence in patients who have failed conservative therapy (fiber therapy, diet, antimotility drugs). It is a gel that is injected in the deep submucosal layer in the proximal part of the high-pressure zone of the anal canal, about 5 mm above the dentate line. It is hypothesized that Solesta may narrow the anal canal and allow for better sphincter control. It should only be used by physicians experienced in anorectal procedures who have successfully completed training and a certification program in Solesta injection procedure.

NONPHARMACOLOGIC THERAPY

- Supportive therapy:
  - Education/counseling/habit training
  - Diet (increase fiber, lactulose, and fructose)
- Biofeedback therapy:
  - Anal sphincter muscle strengthening
  - Rectal sensory conditioning
  - Rectoanal coordination training
- Modified Kegel exercises
- Surgery:
  - Overlapping sphincteroplasty (most common)
  - Anterior repair
  - Artificial bowel sphincter
  - Sacral nerve stimulation
  - Colostomy

REFERRAL

Refer to colorectal surgeon

PEARLS & CONSIDERATIONS

COMMENTS

The shame, embarrassment, and stigma associated with fecal and urinary incontinence pose significant barriers to seeking professional treatment, resulting in many people who suffer from these conditions without help. During routine office visits, ask all patients >70 yr about incontinence.

PREVENTION

- Endoanal ultrasound to detect and repair anal sphincter tears in women with second-degree perineal tears may reduce severe fecal incontinence (mid-level evidence).
- Routine episiotomy is the most easily preventable risk factor for fecal incontinence in females.

PATIENT/FAMILY EDUCATION

Website: www.familydoctor.org/online/famdoc en/home/seniors/common-older/067.html digestive.niddk.nih.gov/ddiseases/pubs/fecal incontinence

SUGGESTED READINGS

available at www.expertconsult.com

AUTHOR: **NADIA MUJAHID, M.D.**

BASIC INFORMATION

DEFINITION

Incontinence is the involuntary loss of urine.

ICD-9CM CODES
788.3	Incontinence
625.6	Stress incontinence
788.33	Mixed stress and urge incontinence
788.32	Male incontinence
788.39	Neurogenic incontinence
307.6	Nonorganic origin

EPIDEMIOLOGY & DEMOGRAPHICS

INCIDENCE/PREVALENCE: In the general population between the ages of 15 and 64 yr, 1.5% to 5% of men and 10% to 25% of women have incontinence. In the nursing home population, 50% of the population has some degree of incontinence. Nearly 20% of children through the mid-teenage years have episodes of urinary incontinence.

CLINICAL, PSYCHOLOGICAL, & SOCIAL IMPACT

Fewer than 50% of the individuals with incontinence living in the community consult health care providers, preferring to suffer silently, turning to home remedies, commercially available absorbent materials, and supportive aids. As their condition worsens, they become depressed, sacrifice their independence, suffer from recurrent urinary tract infection and its sequelae, limit social interaction, refrain from sexual intimacy, and become homebound. In terms of costs, for all ages living in the community, it is estimated that $7 billion is spent for incontinence annually.

MAJOR TYPES OF INCONTINENCE

- **Transient incontinence:** Incontinence occurring as a result or reaction to an acute medical problem affecting the lower urinary tract.

Many of these problems can be reversed with treatment of the underlying problem.
- **Urge incontinence:** Involuntary loss of urine associated with an abrupt and strong desire to void. It is usually associated with involuntary detrusor contractions on urodynamic investigation. In neurologically impaired patients, the involuntary detrusor contraction is referred to as *detrusor hyperreflexia*. In neurologically normal patients the involuntary contraction is called *detrusor instability*.
- **Stress incontinence** (Fig. 1-454): The involuntary loss of urine with physical activities that increase abdominal pressure in the absence of a detrusor contraction or an overdistended bladder. Classification of stress incontinence:
  1. Type 0: Report of incontinence without demonstration of leakage.
  2. Type I: Incontinence in response to stress but with little descent of the bladder neck and urethra.
  3. Type II: Incontinence in response to stress with >2 cm descent of the bladder neck and urethra.
  4. Type III: Bladder neck and urethra wide open without bladder contraction; intrinsic sphincter deficiency; denervation of the urethra. The most common causes include urethral hypermobility and displacement of the bladder neck with exertion, intrinsic sphincter deficiency from failed antiincontinence surgery, prostatectomy, radiation, cord lesions, epispadias, and myelomeningocele.
- **Overflow incontinence:** Loss of urine resulting from overdistention of the bladder with resultant overflow or spilling of the urine. Causes include hypotonic-to-atonic bladder resulting from drug effect, fecal impaction, or neurologic conditions such as diabetes, spinal cord injury, surgery, or vitamin B_{12} deficiency. It is also caused by obstruction at the bladder neck and urethra. In this situation prostatism, prostatic cancer, urethral stenosis, antiincontinence surgery, pelvic prolapse, and

detrusor-sphincter dyssynergia cause the incontinence.
- **Functional incontinence:** Involuntary loss of urine resulting from chronic impairments of physical and/or cognitive functioning. This is a diagnosis of exclusion. It consists of simply not getting to the toilet quickly enough due to significant mobility or cognitive impairment. The condition can sometimes be improved or cured by improving the patient's functional status, treating comorbidities, changing medications, and reducing environmental barriers.
- **Mixed stress and urge incontinence:** See Fig. 1-454.
- **Sensory urgency incontinence:** Involuntary loss of urine as a result of decreased bladder compliance and increased intravesical pressures accompanied by severe urgency and bladder hypersensitivity without detrusor overactivity. This is seen with radiation cystitis, interstitial cystitis, eosinophilic cystitis, myelomeningocele, and radical pelvic surgery. Nephropathy can occur as a complication of this vesicoureteral reflux.
- **Sphincteric incontinence:**
  1. *Urethral hypermobility:* The basic abnormality is a weakness of pelvic floor support. Because of this weakness, during increases in abdominal pressure there is rotational descent of the vesical neck and proximal urethra. If the urethra opens concomitantly, stress urinary incontinence ensues. Urethral hypermobility is often present in women who are not incontinent. Its mere presence is not sufficient evidence to make the diagnosis of sphincteric abnormality unless incontinence is shown.
  2. *Intrinsic sphincter deficiency:* There is an intrinsic malfunction of the sphincter itself. It is characterized by an open vesical neck at rest and a low leak point pressure (<65 cm water). Urethral hypermobility and intrinsic sphincter deficiency may coexist in the same patient. Causes of intrinsic sphincter deficiency are previous pelvic surgery, antiincontinence surgery, urethral diverticulectomy, radical hysterectomy, abdominoperineal resection of the rectum, urethrotomy, Y-V plasty of the vesical neck, myelodysplasia, anterior spinal artery syndrome, lumbosacral disease, aging, and hyperestrogenism.

DIAGNOSIS

HISTORY

- History of present illness, psychosocial factors, congenital disorders, access issues for the physically challenged, neurologic disorders, and disorders pertinent to the urologic tract
- Review of prescription and nonprescription medications
- Voiding diary to assess total voided volume, frequency of micturition, mean volume voided, largest single volume, diurnal distribution, nature and severity of incontinence

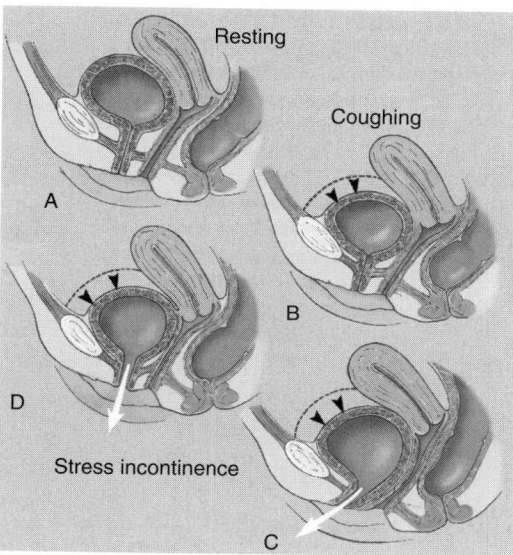

FIGURE 1-454 A, Bladder and urethra in normal position. **B,** Intra-abdominal pressure transmitted to the bladder. **C,** Bladder and urethra in abnormal position with loss of support (hypermobile). **D,** Loss of urethral closure. (From Lipshultz LI et al: *Urology and the primary care practitioner,* ed 3, Philadelphia, 2008, Elsevier.)

Resting

Coughing

Stress incontinence

WORKUP

- Physical examination including general examination, gait of the patient (neuromuscular deficits), estrogen status, vaginal examination to include the periurethral region, evaluation for cystocele, rectocele, and enterocele
- Pelvic floor strength assessment
- Rectal examination to assess sphincter tone and bulbocavernosus reflex
- Neurologic examination
- Postvoid residual check with bladder scan or catheter

LABORATORY TESTS

Urinalysis, urine culture, urine cytology, blood urea nitrogen, creatinine

IMAGING STUDIES

- Radiography: a KUB (kidney, ureter, and bladder) to assess bony skeleton
- CT or intravenous pyelography (IVP) to rule out upper tract abnormalities, developmental anomalies, bladder configuration, and fistula
- Renal ultrasound if dye study is contraindicated

SPECIALIZED STUDIES

Simple cystometrogram, complex urodynamics for leak point pressures and uroflowmetry, endoscopic evaluation, cystogram

TABLE 1-226 Surgical Treatment of Stress Incontinence

Anterior colporrhaphy

Transvaginal needle suspension
  Pereyra
  Stamey
  Gittes
  Raz

Abdominal retropubic urethropexy (suspension)
  Marshall-Marchetti-Krantz
  Burch operation
  Paravaginal repair
  Lapides procedure

Sling procedure
  Pubovaginal (bladder neck) sling
    Autologous
      Rectus abdominis fascia
      Tensor fascia lata
      Anterior vagina wall sling
    Allograft (cadaveric fascia lata fascia)
    Xenograft
      Porcine dermis
      Small intestinal submucosa
    Synthetic mesh (polypropylene)
  Tension-free midurethral sling (polypropylene)
    TVT
    TVT-O
    TOT
    SPARC

Urethral bulking agent
  Bovine collagen
  Carbon-coated zirconium beads
  Ethylene vinyl alcohol copolymer
  Calcium hydroxyapatite

Artificial urinary sphincter

SPARC, Suprapubic arc sling system; *TOT,* trans-obturator tape; *TVT,* tension-free vaginal tape; *TVT-O,* TVT-obturator.
From Lipshultz LI et al: *Urology and the primary care practitioner,* ed 3, Philadelphia, 2008, Elsevier.

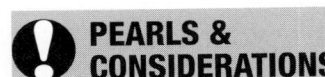 TREATMENT

- Transient incontinence: treatment of underlying medical conditions and behavioral therapy to include habit training and timed voiding
- Urge incontinence: anticholinergic antimuscarinic agents (tolterodine, oxybutynin, trospium chloride, fesoterodine, darifenacin, solifenacin). Anticholinergics bind to muscarinic receptors in the bladder and relax detrusor smooth muscle but can cause dry mouth, constipation, confusion, and cognition abnormalities in the elderly. Other treatment modalities include biofeedback, Kegel exercises, and surgical removal of obstructing or other pathologic lesions. A recent trial comparing oral anticholinergic therapy and onabotulinum toxin A by injection shows similar reductions in the frequency of daily episodes of urgency urinary incontinence. The group receiving onabotulinum toxin A was less likely to have dry mouth and more likely to have complete resolution of urgency urinary incontinence but higher rates of transient urinary retention and urinary tract infections. Mirabegron is a beta-3 adrenergic agonist recently FDA approved for overactive bladder. It is better tolerated than anticholinergic agents but has significant drug interactions and can cause urinary retention.
- Stress incontinence: pelvic floor muscle training (PFMT), Kegel exercises. Duloxetine improves incontinence rates and quality of life but does not cure incontinence. It can be tried if PFMT has been unsuccessful. PFMT is considered first-line therapy for stress incontinence and is also beneficial in mixed urge and stress incontinence.
  - Cystourethropexy (see Table 1-226): Marshall-Marchetti-Krantz procedure, Burch procedure, Raz procedure, Stamey-Raz procedure, Gittes procedure, in situ transvaginal sling, pubovaginal sling with autologous or cadaver graft, laparoscopic Burch procedure, laparoscopic sling, tension-free vaginal tape
  - For intrinsic sphincter deficiency: bulking agents (e.g., collagen), sling, and artificial sphincter
- Overflow incontinence: surgical removal of any obstructing lesions, clean intermittent catheterization, indwelling catheter

TABLE 1-227 Transient Causes of Urinary Incontinence (DIAPPERS)

D	Delirium/confusional state
I	Infection—urinary (symptomatic)
A	Atrophic urethritis/vaginitis
P	Pharmaceuticals (diuretics, etc.)
P	Psychological, especially depression
E	Endocrine (hypercalcemia, hypokalemia, glycosuria)
R	Restricted mobility
S	Stool impaction

From Floege J et al: *Comprehensive clinical nephrology,* ed 4, Philadelphia, 2010, Saunders.

- Functional incontinence: behavioral training to include habit training and timed voiding, incontinence undergarments and pads, external collecting devices, environmental manipulation
- Mixed urgency and stress incontinence: PFMT and use of measures recommended in the management of stress and urge incontinence
- Sensory urgency: bladder relaxants (e.g., anticholinergics, muscle relaxants, and tricyclic antidepressants), behavior therapy to include habit training and timed voiding, cystoscopy and hydrodilation
- Sphincteric deficiency: urethral bulking agents, sling procedure, artificial sphincter, mechanical clamp, external collection devices
- Botox (onabotulinum toxin A injection; Allergan) has been approved for the treatment of urinary incontinence in patients with neurologic conditions (e.g., spinal cord injury) and those with multiple sclerosis who have overactive bladder.

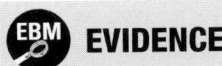 PEARLS & CONSIDERATIONS

COMMENTS

- Overweight and obese women with urinary incontinence have a high prevalence of monthly fecal incontinence (16% found to be associated with low dietary fiber intake after adjustment for other known risk factors for fecal incontinence). Transient causes of urinary incontinence in the elderly are described in Table 1-227.
- Other forms of incontinence:
  - Nocturnal enuresis (ICD-9CM code: 788.3): can be caused by sphincter abnormalities and detrusor overactivity; can occur as idiopathic, neurogenic, and with outlet obstruction
  - Postvoid dribble (ICD-9CM code: 599.2): a postsphincteric collection of urine seen with urethral diverticulum; can be idiopathic
  - Extraurethral incontinence: enterovesical (ICD-9CM codes: 596.1 and 596.2), urethral (ICD-9CM code: 599.1); also known as *fistula*
- Conditions that predispose to surgical failure: advanced age, postmenopausal state, hysterectomy, prior failed incontinence surgery, concurrent detrusor instability, abnormal perineal electromyography, pelvic radiation

EVIDENCE

available at www.expertconsult.com

SUGGESTED READINGS

available at www.expertconsult.com

RELATED CONTENT

Pelvic Organ Prolapse (Related Key Topic)
Urinary Incontinence (Patient Information)

AUTHORS: **PHILIP J. ALIOTTA, M.D., M.S.H.A.,** and **RUBEN ALVERO, M.D.**

BASIC INFORMATION

DEFINITION

Hypotonia typically describes the inability to move or maintain posture against forces that stretch the body, mainly gravity.

SYNONYMS

Floppy infant

ICD-9CM CODES
343.8 Infantile cerebral palsy

EPIDEMIOLOGY & DEMOGRAPHICS

Central causes for hypotonia outweigh peripheral causes 3:1.

PHYSICAL FINDINGS & CLINICAL PRESENTATION

A detailed history and physical exam are the key tools to localizing the lesion, since the cause can be at any level in the neuroaxis, providing an extensive differential.

- Assess tone by observing the fully awake child for body movements, body posture, and signs of decreased in utero movements (hip dislocation, arthrogryposis, plagiocephaly, pectus excavatum).
- When supine, hypotonic infants will lie with their extremities extended and abducted, termed the frog-leg position.
- When pulled gently by the hands from supine toward sitting position, hypotonic infants will have significant head lag and very little resistance to the examiner.
- When held under the arms by the axillae in vertical suspension, hypotonic infants will start to slip through the examiner's hands unlike infants with normal tone.
- If held prone with support under the torso in horizontal suspension, hypotonic infants will fall limply into an "inverted U" position.
- Signs of hypotonia of central origin include abnormal head shape or size, decreased level of consciousness, dysmorphic features, hyperreflexia, seizures, apnea, or abnormal sleep-wake cycles (Table 1-228). Signs of hypotonia of peripheral origin (i.e., a lesion in the motor unit) include an alert and profoundly weak infant with hyporeflexia and atrophic muscles. Tongue fasciculations and intention tremor are seen with anterior horn disease.

- The rest of the neurologic and general exams can provide pertinent clues to specific diagnoses. Cardiac murmurs, skin lesions, hepatosplenomegaly, and so forth help narrow the differential.

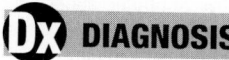 **DIAGNOSIS**

DIFFERENTIAL DIAGNOSIS

Common central causes
- Acquired brain insult
  - Infection
  - Hypoxic encephalopathy
  - Intracranial hemorrhage
- Brain anomalies: neuromigrational disorders
- Genetic disorders
  - Kabuki syndrome
  - Williams syndrome
  - MECP2 duplication syndrome
  - Down syndrome
  - Fragile X syndrome
  - Prader-Willi syndrome
- Congenital syndromes: benign congenital hypotonia

Peripheral causes of hypotonia in infants
- Anterior horn cell disease
  - Spinal muscular atrophy
  - Hypoxic injury
  - Neurogenic arthrogryposis
- Polyneuropathies (motor or sensory)
  - Hereditary motor-sensory neuropathy
  - Charcot-Marie-Tooth disease
  - Guillain-Barré syndrome
  - Congenital hypomyelinating disorder
- Neuromuscular junction disorders
  - Infantile botulism
  - Congenital myasthenia gravis
  - Transient neonatal myasthenia
- Congenital myopathies
  - Central core disease
  - Nemaline rod myopathy
  - Fiber-type disproportion myopathy
  - Multi-minicore disease
  - Myotubular myopathy
- Muscular dystrophies
  - Congenital dystrophinopathy
  - Congenital muscular dystrophy
  - Congenital myotonic dystrophy
- Metabolic disorders
  - Acid maltase deficiency (Pompe's disease)
  - Cerebrohepatorenal syndrome (Zellweger)
  - Cytochrome-c oxidase deficiency

  - Mitochondrial myopathies
  - Neonatal adrenoleukodystrophy

LABORATORY TESTS

- Evaluate neonate for sepsis
- Electrolytes including glucose, creatinine, calcium
- Liver function tests
- Ammonia level
- Creatinine kinase level
- Lactate
- Consider TORCH titers
- Karyotype or specific genetic testing
- Serum amino acids
- Urine organic acids
- Acylcarnitine/carnitine panel
- Very long chain fatty acids
- EMG/nerve conduction velocity (NCV)
- Muscle biopsy

IMAGING STUDIES

MRI with spectroscopy

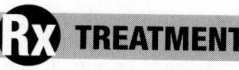 **TREATMENT**

Most of these disorders have no specific treatment.

CHRONIC Rx

- Physical therapy, occupational therapy, and other therapies tailored to the patient's specific needs can provide significant improvement in quality of life and ability to function.
- Respiratory illnesses are common in these children, so vaccinations should be kept up to date.

DISPOSITION

- Long-term outcome varies greatly among different diseases.
- As a general rule, a hypotonic infant that requires mechanical ventilation cannot survive extubation (unless the cause is neonatal myasthenia).

SUGGESTED READINGS
available at www.expertconsult.com

AUTHOR: **KIMBERLY JONES, M.D.**

TABLE 1-228 Localizing Examination Findings

Site of Lesion	Strength	Reflexes	Muscle Mass	Fasciculations
Brain	Normal or slightly impaired	Brisk (low after acute injury)	Normal	None
Anterior horn cell	Weak	Decreased	Significant atrophy	Prominent
Peripheral nerve	Weak	Decreased	Atrophy	None
Neuromuscular junction	Weak	Normal	Normal	None
Muscle	Weak	Decreased or absent	Atrophy or pseudo-hypertrophy	None

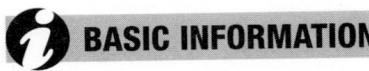

BASIC INFORMATION

DEFINITION

Infertility in a reproductive age couple is the inability to conceive after adequate coital attempts have been made for ≥1 yr. In couples where the female partner is >35 yr of age, an evaluation is justified after 6 mo without successful pregnancy.

SYNONYMS

Sterility

ICD-9CM CODES
628.0 Infertility, female, associated with anovulation
628.2 Infertility, female, of tubal origin
628.9 Infertility, of unspecified origin

EPIDEMIOLOGY & DEMOGRAPHICS

PEAK INCIDENCE: The incidence of infertility increases with increasing age. Subtle decreases in female fertility start as early as age 30. The rate of infertility increases dramatically after age 37 and spontaneous pregnancies become extremely uncommon as women reach the mid-40s. There is also a more subtle but still detectable decrease in male fertility that can also start as early as age 30.

PREVALENCE: One in eight reproductive age couples experience infertility. This prevalence is consistent in all developed countries and there is evidence that it is historically stable.

PREDOMINANT SEX AND AGE: By definition this is a diagnosis of reproductive age couples. Infertility increases with aging in both males and females but more dramatically in women. Male factor is responsible in ~40% of couples and the female factor is responsible in ~40% of couples. The remainder of the cases are either combined male and female or unexplained infertility, meaning a clear cause is not identified.

RISK FACTORS: Aging is among the most common of risk factors, predominantly among females. Women are increasingly deferring pregnancy as a result of careers, which is likely associated with the increasing prevalence in certain sectors of the population. Sexually transmitted disease with *Chlamydia* and gonorrhea is associated with pelvic inflammatory disease, which frequently results in tubal factor infertility. Extremes of weight, especially overweight, are associated with ovulatory dysfunction. Male factor infertility is most commonly idiopathic, although trauma, infection, varicocele, and exposure to environmental toxins may be associated with compromise of semen parameters. Smoking is the most common lifestyle choice that impairs fertility.

PHYSICAL FINDINGS & CLINICAL PRESENTATION
- Age (both partners)
- Previous fertility, particularly if no pregnancy has occurred in another relationship despite absence of contraception (both partners)
- Absence of secondary sexual characteristics (both partners)
- Irregular or absent menstruation (female)
- Hirsutism, acne and alopecia suggestive of hyperandrogenism (female)
- Pelvic exam suggestive of uterine abnormality such as fibroids (female)
- Trauma or torsion of the testes (male)
- Small, firm testes (male)

ETIOLOGY
- Advanced age, especially female
- Pelvic inflammatory disease (results in tubal factor infertility)
- Endometriosis (results in tubal factor infertility)
- Female anatomic (uterine fibroids, polyps, intrauterine adhesions)
- Oligoovulation, most frequently due to polycystic ovarian syndrome (PCOS)
- Idiopathic, both male and female

DIAGNOSIS

DIFFERENTIAL DIAGNOSIS
- Recurrent spontaneous abortion
- Ineffective attempts at natural conception
- Sterility due to previous permanent sterilization procedure

WORKUP
- The components of evaluation depend greatly on whether the female patient is reliably ovulating based on history (regular menses, premenstrual molimina such as breast tenderness) and laboratory testing (midluteal progesterone, basal body temperature testing, urinary LH predictor kits, mid-cycle ovulatory pain [Mittelschmerz], cervical mucus testing). Box E1-32 and Fig. E1-455 describe an approach to infertility diagnosis and management.
- Where the menstrual cycle is important in testing, the first day is defined as the first day of full menstrual flow

- If the female patient does not appear to be ovulating, testing should consist of:
  - ○ TSH
  - ○ Prolactin
  - ○ Total testosterone/free testosterone (to assess for PCOS)
  - ○ Transvaginal pelvic ultrasound to assess for polycystic appearing ovaries
  - ○ 17-Hydroxyprogesterone (to assess for cryptic congenital adrenal hyperplasia)
  - ○ 2-hr glucose tolerance testing (if the patient has PCOS)
  - ○ FSH/LH
  - ○ Lipid panel (if the patient has PCOS, secondary to overlap with metabolic syndrome)
  - ○ Liver function test (if the patient has PCOS, in case treatment with insulin-sensitizing agents indicated)
  - ○ BUN/creatinine (if the patient has PCOS, in case treatment with insulin-sensitizing agents indicated)
  - ○ Semen analysis in the male partner
  - ○ Hysterosalpingogram (especially if the history suggests previous pelvic infection)
- If the female patient appears to be ovulating, testing should consist of:
  - ○ Semen analysis in the male partner
  - ○ Hysterosalpingogram (Fig. 1-456)
  - ○ Mid-luteal progesterone, urinary LH predictor kits (to assess for ovulation)
  - ○ FSH, estradiol, anti-müllerian hormone on day 2 to 3 of menstrual cycle (ovarian reserve testing)
  - ○ Transvaginal pelvic ultrasound to assess for uterine anomalies and antral follicle count as a measure of ovarian reserve

LABORATORY TESTS
- Semen analysis, using Kruger strict morphology after 2 to 3 days of abstinence (male)
- Day 2 or 3 FSH, estradiol, and anti-müllerian hormone as a measure of ovarian reserve (female)

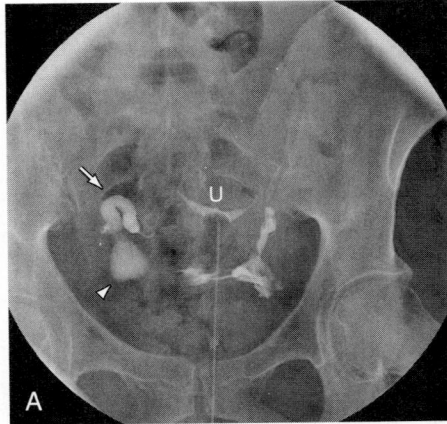
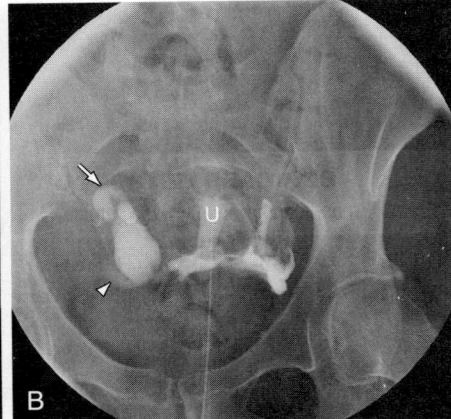

FIGURE 1-456 Hysterosalpingogram spot radiographs early **(A)** and late **(B)** demonstrate a rounded collection of contrast material *(arrowhead)* adjacent to the dilated ampullary portion of the right fallopian tube *(arrow)*, caused by peritubal pelvic adhesions related to previous pelvic inflammatory disease. Normal patient left fallopian tube. *U,* Uterus. (From Fielding JR et al: *Gynecologic imaging,* Philadelphia, 2011, Saunders.)

- Mid-luteal progesterone (ideally 7 days after ovulatory surge)
- Urinary LH ovulatory kits
- See "Workup" for evaluation of couples where the female partner is oligo- or anovulatory

IMAGING STUDIES

- Hysterosalpingogram (between days 6 and 12 of the menstrual cycle)
- Day 2 or 3 transvaginal pelvic ultrasound to assess uterine abnormalities and to count the number of small antral follicles (2 to 9 mm) as a measure of ovarian reserve. If oligo- or anovulatory, to assess for polycystic appearing ovary.

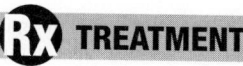 **TREATMENT**

Once the patient presents for evaluation, testing should be completed as quickly as possible, ideally within one menstrual cycle. The couple should follow up with the evaluating provider once all testing is completed and treatment initiated as abnormalities are found.

ACUTE GENERAL Rx

- Mild male factor infertility may be treated with intrauterine insemination but more severe forms will usually require assisted reproductive technologies (ART) with intracytoplasmic sperm injection (ICSI) in the laboratory, where sperm is injected directly into the oocyte.
- Tubal factor infertility may be treated surgically if mild and if the female patient is young and can afford the time to attempt pregnancy over multiple menstrual cycles. If the patient is older or if the tubal pathology is moderate to severe, the patient should use in vitro fertilization (IVF) to achieve pregnancy.
- Oligo- or anovulation should be treated with ovulation induction agents. Women with euestrogenic ovulatory dysfunction can be treated with clomiphene citrate as a first-line agent, using 50 mg in the first cycle attempt and increasing the dose by 50 mg up to a maximum dose of 200 mg if the patient fails to ovulate. Increasingly, aromatase inhibitors such as letrozole or anastrazole are being used both for ovulation induction in anovulatory patients and for superovulation in couples with unexplained infertility. Far less

commonly, ovulatory dysfunction is the result of hypothalamic dysfunction. In these patients, once hypothalamic or pituitary abnormalities are excluded with MRI, ovulation can be achieved using injected gonadotropins.
- Uterine anatomic abnormalities such as submucous fibroids, polyps, or intrauterine adhesions should be corrected if they are identified. Fibroids that do not impact the uterine cavity probably do not interfere with fertility. Removal of intramural or subserosal fibroids is reserved for situations in which these cause excessive vaginal bleeding, pain, or pressure.
- Unexplained infertility can be treated empirically using superovulation with clomiphene citrate or gonadotropins combined with intrauterine insemination with partner's sperm. Most providers recommend using clomiphene citrate with insemination as a first-line superovulatory agent because it is inexpensive. After 3 to 4 such cycles, few pregnancies occur and the couple should be advised to become more aggressive. Controversy exists as to whether gonadotropins with insemination or IVF should be used after clomiphene citrate superovulation induction. There is evidence suggesting that moving to IVF in a *fast-track* fashion shortens the time interval to achieving pregnancy.

COMPLEMENTARY & ALTERNATIVE MEDICINE

Acupuncture is widely used by women being treated for infertility. Limited data suggest some benefit, with possible mechanisms of action including increasing blood flow to the uterus. Patients may additionally benefit from the stress relief that acupuncture provides.

DISPOSITION

- Most couples will achieve a pregnancy, provided that they are willing to use aggressive techniques, including ART such as IVF and gamete donation.
- Adoption can also be used but patients should be aware that this can also be difficult because of limited availability of adoptable children and because of the expense and bureaucratic hurdles.

REFERRAL

Couples should be referred to a reproductive endocrinologist once the complexity of treatment

exceeds the comfort level of the provider, whether a family physician, internist or general gynecologist. Complex ovulation and superovulation induction and ART are usually managed by a board-certified reproductive endocrinologist.

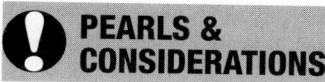 **PEARLS & CONSIDERATIONS**

COMMENTS

- ~1% of all live births in the United States currently are the result of IVF.
- The incidence of heterotopic pregnancy in patients who have undergone IVF is relatively common; identification of a patient with ultrasound-proved intrauterine pregnancy who used ART to conceive should NOT necessarily exclude the possibility of an ectopic gestation.

PREVENTION

- Techniques that reduce the incidence of pelvic inflammatory disease, such as condom use, can reduce pelvic adhesions that are associated with tubal factor infertility.
- Women can be made aware of the fact that delaying pregnancy into the later reproductive years can reduce the chances for successful pregnancy.

PATIENT & FAMILY EDUCATION

Patient support groups such as *Resolve* (www.resolve.org) are available to help couples during evaluation and treatment of infertility, which can be extraordinarily stressful.

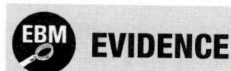 **EVIDENCE**

available at www.expertconsult.com

SUGGESTED READINGS
available at www.expertconsult.com

RELATED CONTENT

Amenorrhea (Related Key Topic)
Pelvic Inflammatory Disease (Related Key Topic)
Polycystic Ovary Syndrome (Related Key Topic)
Infertility (Patient Information)

AUTHOR: **RUBEN ALVERO, M.D.**

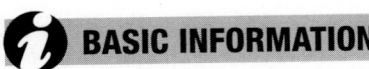

BASIC INFORMATION

DEFINITION

Influenza is an acute febrile illness caused by infection with influenza type A or B virus. Seasonal influenza can include the H1N1 virus. Severe acute respiratory syndrome (SARS) is a similar respiratory illness caused by a coronavirus called SARS-associated coronavirus (SARS-CoV). Table 1-229 compares various viruses. A new novel coronavirus was recognized in two patients in September 2012. This is a very different virus from the SARS agent; the two patients exhibited acute respiratory syndrome, one with renal failure.

SYNONYMS

Flu
Influenza-like illness (ILI)

EPIDEMIOLOGY & DEMOGRAPHICS

PEAK INCIDENCE: Winter outbreaks lasting 5 to 6 wk
PREDOMINANT SEX: Male = female
PREDOMINANT AGE: Attack rates are higher among children than adults, although children are less prone to develop pulmonary complications.
INCIDENCE (IN U.S.): Annual incidence of influenza-related deaths is ~36,000 deaths/yr.

PANDEMICS

DEFINITION: Widespread human community-level outbreaks in ≥two countries in one World Health Organization (WHO) region.
HISTORICAL:
- In the twentieth century, pandemics occurred from H1N1 resulting in 40 to 100 million deaths worldwide in 1918, 70,000 deaths in the United States in 1957 from H2N2, and 36,000 deaths in the United States in 1968 from H3N2.
- H5N1 emerged in Hong Kong in 1997, quickly infecting poultry and birds. More than 400 humans were infected with avian flu (H5N1) by 2009, but transmission from human to human was not efficient.
Novel influenza A virus:
- WHO declared the H1N1 outbreaks a public health emergency in April 2009 and announced a global pandemic in June 2009. The U.S. emergency ended in June 2010, and the WHO declared an end to the global pandemic in August 2010.
- H1N1 is predicted to continue circulation as a seasonal virus for years to come.
- The 2009 H1N1 virus affected more young adults than the elderly.
- In 2009 in the United States, it is estimated that there were 43 million to 88 million cases,

192,000 to 398,000 hospitalizations, and as many as 18,000 deaths from H1N1.
- H3N2 variant virus (H3N2v) normally circulates in swine but sometimes infects humans. Outbreaks occurred in the summer of 2012, mostly associated with exposure to pigs at agricultural fairs. These are not sustained by efficient human-to-human community spread.
- The 2012 H3N2v viruses contain the matrix (M) gene from the 2009 pandemic influenza A (H1N1) virus.
- Influenza A H3N2v clinical presentation is similar to signs and symptoms of uncomplicated seasonal influenza, with vomiting and diarrhea in some pediatric cases. Symptoms can be milder, without fever, lasting 3-5 days.

PHYSICAL FINDINGS & CLINICAL PRESENTATION

- "Classic flu" is characterized by abrupt onset of fever, headache, myalgias, anorexia, and malaise after a 1- to 2-day incubation period.
- Clinical syndromes are similar to those produced by other respiratory viruses, including pharyngitis, common colds, tracheobronchitis, bronchiolitis, and croup.
- Respiratory symptoms such as cough, sore throat, and nasal discharge are usually present at the onset of illness, but systemic symptoms predominate.
- Elderly patients may experience fever, weakness, and confusion without any respiratory complaints.
- Acute deterioration to status asthmaticus may occur in patients with asthma.
- Influenza pneumonia: rapidly progressive cough, dyspnea, and cyanosis may occur after typical flu onset. This may be caused by primary influenza pneumonia or secondary bacterial pneumonia (often pneumococcal or staphylococcal co-infection).
- For influenza A (H3N2v), children younger than 10 years lack immunity. People 65 years and older and those with morbid obesity are at high risk.

ETIOLOGY

- Variation in the surface antigens of the influenza virus, hemagglutinin (HA) and neuraminidase (NA), leading to infection with variants to which immunity is inadequate in the population at risk
- Transmitted by small-particle aerosols and deposited on the respiratory tract epithelium

DIAGNOSIS

DIFFERENTIAL DIAGNOSIS

- Respiratory syncytial virus, adenovirus, parainfluenza virus infection
- Secondary bacterial pneumonia or mixed bacterial-viral pneumonia

WORKUP

- The accuracy of clinical diagnosis of influenza on the basis of symptoms alone is limited because symptoms from illness

caused by other pathogens can overlap considerably with influenza. Diagnostic tests available for influenza include viral cultures, serology, rapid influenza diagnostic tests (RIDTs), reverse transcription-polymerase chain reaction (RT-PCR), and immunofluorescence assays.
- Virus isolation from nasal or throat swab or sputum specimens is the most rapid diagnostic method in the setting of acute illness.
- Specimens are placed into virus transport medium and processed by a reference laboratory.
- For serologic diagnosis:
  1. Paired serum specimens, acute and convalescent, the latter obtained 10 to 20 days later
  2. Fourfold rises or falls in the titer of antibodies (various techniques) considered diagnostic of recent infection
  3. Commercial rapid influenza diagnostic tests (RIDTs) are available. They can detect influenza virus antigens within 15 minutes of testing. Rapid flu test should be collected as early as possible, ideally within 4 days of onset. False negative results are common during the flu season. A negative test result does NOT exclude diagnosis of influenza.
  4. Commercial RIDTs cannot determine if an H3N2 is a variant virus; when suspect H3N2v virus infection, send nasopharyngeal swab or aspirate in viral transport medium to state public health laboratory for rRT-PCR testing using CDC FLU rRT-PCR diagnostic panel assay.

LABORATORY TESTS

Septic syndrome presentation: CBC, ABG analysis, blood cultures

IMAGING STUDIES

- Chest x-ray examination when suspecting viral pneumonia: peribronchial and patchy interstitial infiltrates in multiple lobes with atelectasis. Table 1-229 describes x-ray pulmonary findings based on virus type.
- Possible progression to diffuse interstitial pneumonitis

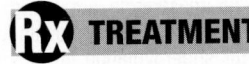

TREATMENT

NONPHARMACOLOGIC THERAPY

- Bed rest
- Hydration

ACUTE GENERAL Rx

- Supportive care: antipyretics; avoid use of aspirin in children because of the association with Reye's syndrome
- Antibiotics if bacterial pneumonia is proved or suspected
- Amantadine is NOT recommended due to resistant isolates.
- Neuraminidase inhibitors block release of virions from infected cells, resulting in shortened duration of symptoms and decrease in complications; effective against both influenza

A and B, including A (H3N2v) for all hospitalized patients, those with severe and progressive illness, and high-risk patients with suspected or confirmed H3N2v.

1. Zanamivir, administered via inhaler:
   For treatment, 10 mg (2 inhalations of 5 mg each) twice daily for 5 days
   For prevention in households, 10 mg (2 inhalations of 5 mg each) once daily for 17 days

2. Oseltamivir, administered orally:
   For treatment, 75 mg PO twice daily for 5 days
   For prevention, 75 mg PO once daily for a minimum of 2 wk in an outbreak setting or 7 days after exposure for an adult

3. Emergency use authorization by the Centers for Disease Control and Prevention (CDC) for intravenous peramivir during the H1N1 pandemic was terminated in June 2010. Intravenous peramivir is still available as an experimental drug.

- Placebo-controlled studies have suggested that antiviral therapy with any of the previously mentioned agents must ideally be initiated within 1 to 2 days of the onset of symptoms and reduces the duration of illness by ~1 day.

- Oseltamivir resistance developed on therapy in individuals with avian flu (H5N1) in Asia, and this is associated with poor outcome.

- Amantadine and rimantadine resistance are documented for novel (H1N1) influenza and H3N2 influenza virus.

- Systemic corticosteroids should not be routinely administered to patients with suspected or confirmed influenza, including H3N2v virus infection, except for patients on chronic corticosteroid therapy for COPD, asthma.

DISPOSITION

Patients are hospitalized if signs of pneumonia are present.

REFERRAL

Infectious disease and/or pulmonary consultation when influenza pneumonia is suspected

PEARLS & CONSIDERATIONS

COMMENTS

- Prevention of influenza in patients at high risk is an important goal of primary care.
- Vaccines reduce the risk of infection and the severity of illness.

1. Antigenic composition of the vaccine is updated annually. The Northern Hemisphere's 2012 to 2013 season vaccine includes one influenza A (H3N2)-like virus, one influenza A (H1N1)-like virus, and one influenza B virus. The influenza A (H1N1) vaccine virus strain is derived from a 2009 pandemic virus. The H3N2 and B vaccine viruses are different from those that were selected for the 2011-2012 vaccine.

2. Revaccination is recommended annually even for those who received the vaccine in the previous season.

3. Seasonal influenza vaccine does not provide protection against the 2012 influenza A (H3N2v) virus.

4. Vaccination should be given at the start of the flu season (September-October) for all persons aged ≥6 mo. Vaccination is particularly important for persons who are at increased risk for severe complications from influenza. When vaccine supply is limited, vaccination efforts should focus on the following groups:
   a. All children aged 6 mo to 4 yr (59 mo).
   b. People 50 years and older
   c. Adults and children with chronic cardiac (except hypertension) or pulmonary (including asthma), renal, hepatic, neurologic, hematologic or metabolic disease (including diabetes mellitus)
   d. Immunocompromised patients (including HIV-infected persons or patients immunosuppressed due to medications)
   e. Women who are or will be pregnant during the influenza season
   f. Children aged 6 mo to 18 yr who are receiving long-term aspirin therapy
   g. Residents of nursing homes and other long-term care facilities
   h. American Indians/Alaska Natives

   i. Persons who are morbidly obese (BMI ≥40)
   j. Health care workers (HCWs)
   k. Household contacts and caregivers of persons in the previous groups

5. Persons with history of egg allergy should be referred to physician with expertise in potential manifestations of egg allergy. Studies with trivalent inactivated vaccine (TIV) indicate successful vaccination when additional safety measures are taken.

6. Vaccination should be delayed for persons with moderate to severe acute febrile illness. Precautions include:
   a. Guillain-Barré syndrome within 6 wk following a previous dose of influenza vaccine
   b. Moderate or severe acute illness with or without fever (for trivalent inactivated influenza vaccine).

7. Contraindication to receiving vaccine is a previous severe allergic reaction to influenza vaccine.

8. Special efforts should be made to vaccinate high-risk patients <65 yr, only 10% to 15% of whom are vaccinated each year.

9. HCW vaccination minimizes transmission to patients and coworkers. States are considering mandated vaccination of HCWs; some states and healthcare facilities promote the wearing of face masks for unvaccinated HCWs during the influenza season.

10. Vaccine efficacy varies by age and by type of circulating virus.

- Alternate vaccine formulations
   1. Intradermal vaccine is available for injection into skin instead of muscle. This uses a smaller needle than the regular flu vaccine and might be preferred by adults aged 18 to 64 yr who do not like shots.
   2. Nasal spray, live-attenuated influenza vaccine (LAIV) is available for nonpregnant, healthy persons aged 2 to 49 yr. Note: give TIV if recipient has egg allergy or asthma or cares for immunosuppressed persons who require a protective environment.
   3. High-dose inactivated vaccine (60 micrograms hemagglutinin each flu strain) is available for persons ≥ 65 yr.

TABLE 1-229 Pulmonary Radiographic Findings Based on Virus Type

Virus	Centrilobular Nodules	Lobar Ground-Glass	Diffuse Ground-Glass	Thickened Interlobular Septa	Consolidation
Influenza	+++	+++	+		+
Epstein-Barr	+	+	+		+
Cytomegalovirus	++	++	++		+
Varicella-zoster	+++	+	+	+	+
Herpes simplex	+	+++	+		+++
Measles	++	+	+		
Hantavirus			+++	+	+
Adenovirus	++	+			++
					+++

From Weissleder R et al: *Primer of diagnostic imaging,* ed 5, St Louis, 2011, Mosby.

4. Thimerosal-free vaccine is available.
5. Quadrivalent LAIV is anticipated for the 2013-2014 influenza season. This will include two influenza B vaccine virus strains.

- Chemoprophylaxis:
1. Table 1-230 describes antiviral agents for influenza. Oseltamivir and zanamivir are recommended in the United States during the influenza season.
2. Consider (after the current circulating strain of influenza has been shown to be sensitive):
   a. For high-risk patients in whom vaccination is contraindicated
   b. When the available vaccine is known not to include the circulating strain
   c. To provide added protection to immunosuppressed patients likely to have a diminished response to vaccination
   d. In the setting of an outbreak, when immediate protection of unvaccinated or recently vaccinated patients is desired

3. Give for 2 wk in the case of late vaccination and for the duration of the flu season in all other patients
4. Treatment should not wait for laboratory confirmation of influenza.
5. Do not give aspirin or aspirin-containing products to children with influenza-like illness due to the risk of Reye's syndrome.

- Other prevention strategies:
1. Hand hygiene, cough etiquette (cover your cough), respiratory hygiene (use of tissues, facemasks for the ill and proper disposal)
2. Personal protective equipment (PPE)—wear gloves and gowns as for universal/standard precautions. Per Centers for Disease Control and Prevention, wear facemask, adhering to Droplet Precautions for 7 days after illness onset or until 24 hr after fever and respiratory symptoms are resolved, whichever is longer. Patient placement in a negative pressure room and N95 respirator for health care workers are recommended when procedures

are conducted that generate respiratory aerosols.
3. Management of ill health care workers—exclude from work until at least 24 hr after they no longer have a fever (without the use of fever-reducing medication). Extended exclusion time period when caring for severely immunocompromised patients.
4. Standard cleaning and disinfection procedures.

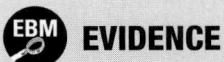 **EVIDENCE**

available at www.expertconsult.com

SUGGESTED READINGS

available at www.expertconsult.com

RELATED CONTENT

Influenza (Flu) (Patient Information)

AUTHORS: **MARLENE FISHMAN, M.P.H., C.I.C.,** and **GLENN G. FORT, M.D., M.P.H.**

TABLE 1-230 Antiviral Agents for Influenza

	Amantadine	Rimantadine	Zanamivir	Oseltamivir
Protein target	M2	M2	Neuraminidase	Neuraminidase
Activity	A only (H1N1 and H3N2 are resistant)	A only (H1N1 and H3N2 are resistant)	A and B	A and B
Side effects	CNS (13%) GI (3%)	GI (6%)	? Bronchospasm	GI (9%)
Metabolism	None	Multiple (hepatic)	None	Hepatic
Excretion	Renal	Renal, + others	Renal	Renal (tubular secretion)
Drug interactions	Antihistamines, anticholinergics	None	None	Probenecid (increased levels of oseltamivir)
Dose adjustments needed	≥65 yr old CrCl <50 ml/min	≥65 yr old CrCl <10 ml/min	None	CrCl <30 ml/min Severe liver dysfunction
Contraindications	Acute-angle glaucoma	Severe liver dysfunction	Underlying airway disease, asthma	
FDA-Approved Indications				
Therapy	Adults and children ≥1 yr old	Adults only	Adults and children ≥7 yr old	Adults and children ≥1 yr old*
Prophylaxis	Yes	Yes	Adults and children >5 yr old	Adults and children ≥13 yr old†

CrCl, Creatinine clearance; *FDA*, U.S. Food and Drug Administration; *GI*, gastrointestinal.
*FDA has authorized treatment of S-OIV (novel H1N1) virus with oseltamivir in children ≥3 mo of age.
†FDA has authorized prophylaxis for S-OIV (novel H1N1) virus with oseltamivir in children ≥1 yr of age.
From Mandell GL et al: *Principles and practice of infectious diseases*, ed 7, Philadelphia, 2010, Churchill Livingstone.

Insomnia

 BASIC INFORMATION

DEFINITION

Insomnia is a disturbance of initiating or maintaining sleep. Restless, nonrestorative sleep may also be described as insomnia. The disturbance occurs despite adequate circumstances and opportunity for sleep and is accompanied by significant distress or impairment in daytime functioning.

SYNONYMS

Sleeplessness

Sleep disorder, sleep disturbance, dyssomnia (NOTE: The terms *sleep disorder, sleep disturbance,* and *dyssomnia* are generic and can refer to disorders of wakefulness [hypersomnia] or sleep-related behavior disorders [parasomnias].)

ICD-9CM CODES
780.52 Insomnia
780.51 Insomnia with sleep apnea
307.41 Insomnia, nonorganic origin
307.42 Insomnia, persistent (primary)
307.41 Insomnia, transient
307.49 Subjective complaint

DSM IV-TR CODES
307.42 Primary insomnia
307.45 Circadian rhythm disorders
780.52 Insomnia due to a general medical condition
291.89, 292.89 Substance-induced insomnia

EPIDEMIOLOGY & DEMOGRAPHICS

INCIDENCE (IN U.S.): 30% to 45% of adults experience insomnia per year.
PREVALENCE (IN U.S.): 1% to 15% of all adults and 25% of older adults develop persistent insomnia.
PREDOMINANT SEX: More common in women.
PREDOMINANT AGE: Transient insomnia can occur at any age; persistent insomnia is more common after age 60 yr.
GENETICS: Can run in families and may be genetically influenced. Circadian rhythm disorders and narcolepsy have been traced to specific genes.

PHYSICAL FINDINGS & CLINICAL PRESENTATION

- Difficulty falling asleep, difficulty staying asleep, early morning awakening, restless or nonrestorative sleep, or difficulty sleeping at desired times.
- Significant distress or impairment in daytime functioning such as fatigue or low energy, sleepiness, cognitive impairments, mood disturbances, or behavioral problems.
- Difficulty occurs despite adequate opportunity for sleep.
- Symptoms may be acute and self-limited, chronic but intermittent, or chronic and frequent.

ETIOLOGY

- Transient insomnia:
  1. Stress
  2. Illness
  3. Travel (across time zones)
  4. Environmental disruptions (noise, heat, cold, poor bedding, bed partners, unfamiliar surroundings, etc.)
- Persistent insomnia:
  1. Mood and anxiety disorders (depression, hypomania/mania, PTSD)
  2. Primary or psychophysiologic insomnia (with or without poor sleep hygiene)
  3. Sleep-related breathing disorders (e.g., obstructive apnea and hypopnea, increased upper airway resistance)
  4. Chronobiologic (also known as circadian rhythm) disorder (delayed sleep phase, advanced sleep phase, shift work, free-running rhythm secondary to blindness)
  5. Drug and alcohol abuse
  6. Restless legs syndrome and periodic leg movements
  7. Neurodegenerative (Alzheimer's disease, Parkinson's disease, etc.)
  8. Medical (pain, GERD, nocturia, orthopnea, medications, etc.)

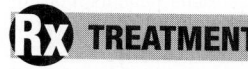 **DIAGNOSIS**

DIFFERENTIAL DIAGNOSIS

Primary or psychophysiologic insomnia is diagnosed when other etiologies (see "Etiology") are ruled out. However, it can be precipitated by a "primary" medical or mental health disorder and continue even after the "primary disorder" has been treated, or as a comorbid condition.

WORKUP

- History (with bed partner interview, if possible)
- Sleep diary for 2 wk (sample sleep diary available at http://www.sleepfoundation.org)
- Wrist actigraphy (detects gross limb movements and can distinguish wake from sleep states) and as an adjunct to a diary—provides some objective verification of the diary data
- Validated sleep-quality rating scale (optional)
  1. Insomnia Severity Index
  2. Pittsburgh Sleep Quality Index
  3. Epworth Sleepiness Scale (see Daytime Sleepiness Test at http://www.sleep foundation.org)

LABORATORY TESTS

- Evaluate for anemia, uremia (for restless legs), thyroid function (if other signs present).
- Polysomnography (in home or in sleep laboratory) is not standard for insomnia but should be reserved for patients whose history suggests specific sleep-related breathing or movement disorders. It is indicated for symptoms suggestive of daytime sleepiness (obstructive sleep apnea, narcolepsy), nonrestorative sleep (periodic leg movements, chronic pain conditions), or sleep behavior suggesting parasomnia (somnambulism, REM sleep behavior).

IMAGING STUDIES

- Not generally helpful for insomnia
- Brain CT or MRI for severe daytime sleepiness or acute onset

Rx TREATMENT

NONPHARMACOLOGIC THERAPY

- Sleep hygiene measures (Box 1-33) as a monotherapy is not very effective. More useful combined with procedures described next.
- Cognitive-behavioral therapy for insomnia (CBT-I) has been shown to reduce time to fall asleep and time awake during the night, can reduce reliance on sleep medications, and has shown lasting effects after treatment has been discontinued.
- The standard components that comprise CBT-I are as follows:
  1. Stimulus Control, which addresses the conditioned cues that create arousal when attempting to sleep by restricting activity in bed to sleep and sex and not permitting sleep effort, worrying, watching TV, reading, etc. in bed
  2. Sleep Restriction, which increases sleep drive by restricting sleep opportunity to the average amount of total sleep time the patient is getting as determined by sleep diary. Sleep time is increased incrementally based on improving sleep efficiency.

BOX 1-33 Sleep Habits (Sleep Hygiene Measures) That May Improve Sleep

1. Reduce caffeine, alcohol, or tobacco late in the day or evening.
2. Avoid heavy meals at night.
3. Increase daytime activity.
4. Increase daytime exposure to natural light.
5. Take warm bath as part of bedtime ritual.
6. Restrict bed to sleep and sex.
7. Get out of bed if not asleep after 30 minutes and return when drowsy.
8. Repeat above if awakened during the night.
9. Maintain regular sleep and wake times.
10. Go to bed with calm mind; resolve arguments or deal with problems earlier in day.

3. Cognitive Therapy, which involves education to address misconceptions and concerns about sleep that serve to increase anxiety

4. Sleep Hygiene, which is aimed at improving sleep habits (e.g., initiating or maintaining exercise, avoiding heavy meals at night, and avoiding or eliminating caffeine, nicotine, and alcohol intake). Environmental factors can also be addressed (e.g., using white noise and/or light attenuating bedroom). Although disruptive to sleep late in the day, caffeine sometimes can prove useful when used judiciously in the morning and early afternoon to combat the increased fatigue and somnolence that are produced early in therapy with sleep restriction and stimulus control.

5. Relaxation Exercises (e.g., progressive muscle relaxation, diaphragmatic breathing) may be considered good adjunctive therapy for insomnia treatment, especially in highly anxious patients, but are not thought to be essential in CBT-I. Mindfulness-based practices have also demonstrated some promise in the treatment of insomnia.

- Insomnia attributable to circadian rhythm disturbances, such as in shift workers, many blind individuals who lack light-dark cycle to synchronize body clock, adolescents and young adults with delayed sleep phase syndrome, and jet lag can be treated with chronobiologic therapies such as chronotherapy, bright light exposure, melatonin, or melatonin agonists.

ACUTE GENERAL Rx

- Benzodiazepine receptor agonists zolpidem 5 mg and zaleplon 5 mg for sleep-onset insomnia, and zolpidem continuous-release formulation 6.25 to 12.5 mg and eszopiclone 1 to 3 mg for maintenance insomnia.
- Benzodiazepine sedative-hypnotics (e.g., temazepam 7.5 to 30 mg, triazolam 0.125 to 0.25 mg).
- A low-dose formulation (6 mg) of the tricyclic antidepressant doxepin, brand name Silenor, is also FDA approved for treatment of insomnia associated with sleep maintenance. This dose retains the hypnotic effect of doxepin without the typical tricyclic effects. A generic 10 mg/ml liquid formulation of doxepin is also available.
- In critical care: lorazepam 0.25 to 0.5 mg PO, SL, or IV as needed for sleep. In patients with acute delirium, haloperidol 0.25 to 0.5 mg IV as needed up to 2 mg/day may be less likely to worsen confusion.
- Melatonin agonist ramelteon 8 mg for sleep-onset insomnia when a mild agent without benzodiazepine side effects is desired.
- Avoid antihistamines except for occasional use.
- Optimize treatment of medical symptoms, especially pain.
- Most prescription and over-the-counter medications carry significant risk of adverse events and drug interactions, especially in the geriatric patient. Preferred pharmacotherapeutic agents in the elderly are zolpidem, zalepton, eszopiclone, and ramelteon.

CHRONIC Rx

- Considerable research supports the efficacy of CBT-I, with acute treatment outcomes equivalent to pharmacotherapy, with better long-term outcomes and maintenance of treatment gains. Three sedative-hypnotics—zolpidem continuous release, eszopiclone, and ramelteon—FDA approved for long-term use.
- Some evidence shows that benzodiazepines and benzodiazepine receptor agonists can be used for chronic insomnia on either intermittent or nightly use with moderate risk of tolerance and dependence but low risk of addiction.
- Sedating antidepressants (e.g., trazodone 25 to 150 mg, mirtazapine 7.5 to 30 mg, amitriptyline 25 to 50 mg, doxepin 10 mg) are in widespread use, with limited data on safety and efficacy. Amitriptyline should be avoided in older adults.
- Sedating antipsychotics (e.g., quetiapine 25 to 200 mg, olanzapine 2.5 to 10 mg at night) considered for severe mood or psychotic disorders associated with insomnia.

COMPLEMENTARY & ALTERNATIVE MEDICINE

Melatonin may shorten sleep-onset latency in some individuals. It may have more use in the treatment of circadian rhythm disorders. Timing of administration in these types of cases requires careful consideration and would not be often administered at bedtime.

DISPOSITION

- Transient insomnia: usually self-limited. May require follow-up if stress-related or illness-related because of risk of depression or persistence.
- Persistent insomnia: Studies have shown that patients who respond well to CBT-I often continue to maintain gains at 1- and 2-yr follow-ups. Insomnia patients may need periodic follow-up to reinforce good sleep hygiene and stimulus control and for reevaluation of pharmacologic therapies. There is now a compelling amount of evidence that insomnia is associated with significant negative mental and health effects over time, and if left untreated can interfere with treatment gains with other "primary disorders" and increase the chance for relapse.

REFERRAL

- A referral to a behavioral medicine specialist may be required for CBT-I or for circadian rhythmn disturbances
- Excessive daytime sleepiness not obviously caused by insomnia (e.g., narcolepsy, sleep-related breathing disorder)
- Nighttime behavior suggestive of a parasomnia (e.g., somnambulism, REM behavior disorder)
- Severe insomnia not responsive to basic interventions

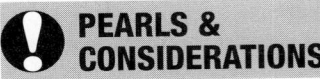

COMMENTS

Early treatment should focus on reducing daytime sleepiness and improving daytime function rather than on trying to achieve the elusive goal of uninterrupted nighttime sleep. CBT-I often results in worse sleep and more fatigue in the short run. Patients often respond to initial worsening of symptoms as a sign of failure; however, they should be encouraged to see this as an important piece of the therapy and to stay the course as new conditioned patterns begin to emerge, sleep efficiency improves, and total sleep time gradually increases.

MODE OF DELIVERY

Access to behavioral sleep medicine specialists can sometimes be limited especially in certain geographic regions. There is now some evidence that the use of Internet based behavioral interventions for insomnia can have modest effect. Such interventions might be best thought of as part of a stepped care model in which this is one level of initial treatment. Patients who fail these attempts should still be encouraged to seek more tailored treatment with a specialist, especially when the insomnia is comorbid with other conditions.

PREVENTION

It is estimated that 50%-70% of individuals demonstrating the syndrome of insomnia (e.g., insomnia symptoms more than 3 days per week for a month along with deleterious daytime sequelae) are still syndromic 1-5 years later. Therefore early intervention with medication or education to prevent the development of maladaptive compensatory behaviors (e.g., napping, sleeping late, avoiding activity) may help to reduce the risk of developing persistent insomnia.

PATIENT & FAMILY EDUCATION

The National Sleep Foundation (http://www.sleepfoundation.org) is a comprehensive resource for health care providers and patients.

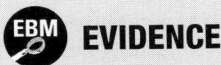 EVIDENCE

available at www.expertconsult.com

SUGGESTED READINGS
available at www.expertconsult.com

RELATED CONTENT
Fig. 3-167 Sleep disorders (Algorithm)
Insomnia (Patient Information)

AUTHORS: **DONN POSNER, PH.D., C.B.S.M.,** and **MITCHELL D. FELDMAN, M.D., M.PHIL.**

BASIC INFORMATION

DEFINITION

Insulinoma is a pancreatic insulin-secreting tumor that leads to inappropriately elevated plasma insulin or proinsulin levels with suppression of hepatic glucose output and subsequent hypoglycemia, especially during periods of fasting.

ICD-9CM CODES
M8151/0 Insulinoma

EPIDEMIOLOGY & DEMOGRAPHICS

INCIDENCE: One case per 250,000 persons annually. 90% of insulinomas are benign.
PREDOMINANT SEX AND AGE: Insulinomas occur in both sexes (approximately 60% in women) and at all ages. In a Mayo Clinic series, the median age at diagnosis was 50 yr in sporadic cases but 23 yr in patients with multiple endocrine neoplasia, type 1 (MEN-1).

PHYSICAL FINDINGS & CLINICAL PRESENTATION

Symptoms typically occur in the morning before breakfast (i.e., fasting hypoglycemia as opposed to reactive hypoglycemia, which is not commonly associated with insulinoma).

Neuroglycopenic Symptoms	%
Various combinations of diplopia, blurred vision, sweating, palpitations, or weakness	85
Confusion or abnormal behavior	80
Unconsciousness or amnesia	53
Grand mal seizures	12
Adrenergic Symptoms	%
Sweating	43
Tremulousness	23
Hunger, nausea	12
Palpitations	10

ETIOLOGY, PATHOLOGY, PATHOPHYSIOLOGY

- Insulinomas are almost always solitary. Malignant insulinomas account for 5% of the total; they tend to be larger (6 cm). Metastases are usually to the liver (47%), regional lymph nodes (30%), or both.
- Insulinomas are evenly distributed in the head, body, and tail of the pancreas; ectopic insulinomas are rare (1% to 3%). Tumor size: 5% are ≤0.5 cm, 34% are 0.5 to 1 cm, 53% are 1 to 5 cm, and 8% are >5 cm.
- Histologic classification includes insulinoma in 86% of patients, adenomatosis in 5% to 15%, nesidioblastosis in 4%, and hyperplasia in 1%. Adenomatosis consists of multiple macroadenomas or microadenomas and occurs especially in patients with MEN-1. Nesidioblastosis is also a diffuse lesion in which islet cells form as buds on ductular structures.

DIAGNOSIS

DIFFERENTIAL DIAGNOSIS (OF FASTING HYPOGLYCEMIA)

Hyperinsulinism:
- Insulinoma
- Nonpancreatic tumors
- Severe congestive heart failure
- Severe renal insufficiency in non-insulin-dependent diabetes

Hepatic enzyme deficiencies or decreased hepatic glucose output (primarily in infants and children):
- Glycogen storage diseases
- Endocrine hypofunction
- Hypopituitarism
- Addison's disease
- Liver failure
- Alcohol abuse
- Malnutrition

Exogenous agents:
- Sulfonylureas, biguanides
- Insulin
- Other drugs (aspirin, pentamidine)

Functional fasting hypoglycemia:
- Autoantibodies to insulin receptor or insulin

LABORATORY TESTS

- An overnight fasting blood sugar level combined with a simultaneous plasma insulin, proinsulin, and/or C peptide level will establish the existence of fasting organic hypoglycemia in 60% of patients. Table 1-231 describes biochemical patterns in patients with various causes of hyperinsulinemic hypoglycemia.
- If single overnight fasting glucose and insulin levels are nondiagnostic, a 72-hr fast is usually done with blood glucose and insulin levels determined at 2- to 4-hr intervals. A total of 75% of patients with insulinoma develop symptoms and a blood sugar level of <40 mg/dl by 24 hr, 92% to 98% develop these by 48 hr, and virtually all patients develop them by 72 hr. The test is considered positive for insulinoma if the plasma insulin/glucose ratio is more than 0.3. If at any point the patient becomes symptomatic, plasma insulin and glucose values should be obtained and IV glucose should be administered.
- The Endocrine Society guidelines for diagnosis of hypoglycemic disorders is based on glucose level <55 mg/dl (<3.1 mmol/L), elevated C-peptide level ≥0.61 ng/ml (≥0.2 nmol/L). Elevated insulin level ≥18 pmol/L, proinsulin level >5 pmol/L, and suppressed β-hydroxy-butyric acid level.
- An "amended" insulin-glucose ratio that accounts for the normal variation in insulin secretion according to prevailing glycemia has been shown to improve diagnostic accuracy of insulinomas. The "amended" insulin-glucose ratio is derived from the simple insulin-glucose ratio by subtracting 30 mg/dl (1.7 mmol/L) from the measured glucose concentrations.

IMAGING STUDIES

- Abdominal CT scan or MRI (Fig. E1-457) detects half to two thirds of insulinomas (abdominal ultrasound is not effective); should be done only after laboratory tests for insulinoma have confirmed the diagnosis
- Intraoperative ultrasound
- Arteriography
- Octreotide scan (Fig. E1-458)

TREATMENT

NONPHARMACOLOGIC THERAPY

- Enucleation of single insulinoma
- Partial pancreatectomy for multiple adenomas

ACUTE GENERAL Rx

- Carbohydrate administration
- Diazoxide directly inhibits insulin release and has an extrapancreatic, hyperglycemic effect that enhances glycogenolysis
- Lanreotide and octreotide (somatostatin analogs)
- Streptozotocin

REFERRAL

To an endocrinologist and then to an endocrine surgeon.

SUGGESTED READINGS

available at www.expertconsult.com

RELATED CONTENT

Fig. E4-16 Diagnostic evaluation of patients with documented hypoglycemia and elevated insulin (Algorithm)

AUTHOR: **FRED F. FERRI, M.D.**

TABLE 1-231 Biochemical Patterns in Patients with Various Causes of Hyperinsulinemic Hypoglycemia

Insulin	C Peptide	Proinsulin	Sulfonylurea	Insulin Antibody	Diagnosis
↑	↓	↓	−	−	Exogenous insulin
↑	↑	↑*	−	−	Insulinoma, congenital hyperinsulinism
↑	↑	↑	+	−	Sulfonylurea
↑	↑†‡	↑†‡	−	+	Insulin autoimmune
±↑	↓	↓	−	−	Insulin receptor autoimmune‡

*> 20% of insulin value.
†Free C peptide and proinsulin ↓.
‡Insulin receptor antibody +.
From Larsen PR et al: *Williams textbook of endocrinology*, ed 10, Philadelphia, 2003, Saunders.

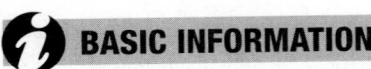

DEFINITION

The International Continence Society defines interstitial cystitis (IC), otherwise known as painful bladder syndrome, as a clinical syndrome consisting of suprapubic pain related to bladder filling and accompanied by other symptoms such as increased daytime and nighttime frequency in the absence of proven infection or other obvious pathology. The American Urological Association defines interstitial cystitis/bladder pain syndrome (IC/BPS) as an unpleasant sensation perceived to be related to the urinary bladder that is associated with lower urinary tract symptoms >6 weeks' duration, in the absence of infection or other unidentifiable causes.

SYNONYMS

Interstitial cystitis/bladder pain syndrome (IC/BPS)
Painful bladder syndrome
Tic douloureux of bladder

ICD-9CM CODES
595.1 Chronic interstitial cystitis

EPIDEMIOLOGY & DEMOGRAPHICS

INCIDENCE: 21 cases per 100,000 women and four cases per 100,000 men annually
PREVALENCE:
- 197 per 100,000 women and 41 per 100,000 men in the U.S.
- Because the disease is substantially underdiagnosed, it may actually affect one in five women and one in 20 men.
- More than 81% of women diagnosed with chronic pelvic pain and up to 84% of men initially diagnosed with chronic prostatitis actually have IC.
- More than 90% of patients diagnosed with overactive bladder who do not respond to anticholinergics are subsequently diagnosed with IC.

PREDOMINANT SEX AND AGE:
- White women constitute 95% of patients with IC.
- Female/male ratio of 5 to 10:1.
- Most prevalent in fourth and fifth decades of life.

PHYSICAL FINDINGS & CLINICAL PRESENTATION

- Urinary urgency, frequency (>8 in daytime), nocturia (>2 at night), and suprapubic pain are the most common symptoms.
- Suprapubic pain is worse with bladder filling or urinating and relieved after emptying.
- Dyspareunia.
- Symptoms lasting longer than 6 mo.
- Intensity of symptoms waxes and wanes.

- Insidious onset and worsens to the final stage within 5 to 15 yr.
- Exercise, stress, sexual activity, ejaculation, certain foods with high potassium and acids (beer, spices, bananas, tomatoes, chocolate, strawberries, artificial sweeteners, oranges, cranberries, caffeine), menstruation, prolonged sitting, and activation of allergies exacerbate the symptoms.
- Often associated with irritable bowel syndrome, migraine, endometriosis, skin sensitivities, multiple drug allergies, other allergies, vulvodynia, fibromyalgia, chronic fatigue syndrome, systemic lupus erythematosus, and mood disorders.
- Dysphoric mood.
- Lower abdominal tenderness.
- Tender prostate in digital rectal examination.
- Levator ani tenderness in female.
- Tenderness of anterior vaginal wall/bladder neck in female.

ETIOLOGY

Unknown

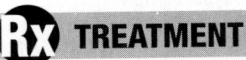 DIAGNOSIS

DIFFERENTIAL DIAGNOSIS

- Chronic pelvic pain
- Overactive bladder
- Recurrent urinary tract infection
- Endometriosis
- Pelvic adhesions
- Vulvar vestibulitis
- Vulvodynia
- Urethral pain syndrome
- Chronic nonbacterial prostatitis
- Frequent vaginitis
- Benign prostatic hyperplasia

WORKUP

- IC can be considered a diagnosis of exclusion when no known cause of painful bladder can be identified.
- There is no definite diagnostic test.
- Validated questionnaires such as Pelvic Pain and Urgency/Frequency scale (PUF), O'Leary-Sant symptoms and problem index, and Wisconsin IC scale. PUF is the most commonly used.
- Voiding diary shows low-volume (<100 ml) and high-frequency voiding pattern.
- National Institute of Diabetes and Diseases of the Kidney diagnostic criteria misses 60% of IC patients and is not clinically used anymore.
- Anesthetic bladder challenge: with this test the symptoms dissipate on instillation of an anesthetic cocktail into the bladder.
- Cystoscopy and hydrodistention under general anesthesia may show terminal hematuria, glomerulation, Hunner's ulcers, and small bladder capacity of less than 350 ml. Cystoscopy and/or urodynamic testing should be considered when the diagnosis is in doubt, but the tests are not necessary to confirm an IC/BPS diagnosis in uncomplicated cases.

- Bladder biopsy is not essential for diagnosis of IC.
- Parson's potassium sensitivity test (PST).
- Urodynamics are unnecessary in diagnosis of IC.

LABORATORY TESTS

- Urine analysis and culture.
- Urine cytology should be performed if microscopic or gross hematuria is present, or with other risk factors such as smoking, age >40 yr, and other bladder cancer risk factors.
- Culture of sexually transmitted diseases if clinically indicated. Nonbacteriuric patients with pyuria should be screened for *Chlamydia*.
- Urine biomarkers (e.g., antiproliferative factor) are promising but not ready for clinical use.

IMAGING STUDIES

CT or ultrasound of abdomen and pelvis may be considered to rule out other pathology.

TREATMENT

- There is no consensus for optimal management.
- There is no cure for this disease.

NONPHARMACOLOGIC THERAPY

- Avoidance of activities associated with flare-ups
- Avoidance of smoking
- Dietary restriction, avoiding common irritants (e.g., coffee, citrus fruits)
- Physical therapy
- Exercise
- Behavioral therapy
- Bladder retraining
- Biofeedback
- Warm sitz bath, ice, heating pad
- Thiele massage (transrectal and transvaginal manual therapy of pelvic floor muscle) in presence of pelvic floor muscle tenderness and spasm
- Hydrodistention only gives temporary relief, so it is not commonly used anymore

ACUTE AND CHRONIC Rx

- A course of empiric antibiotics if not tried yet. Long-term oral antibiotics are not recommended.
- Oral therapy is tried first.
- Pentosan polysulfate sodium (Elmiron) is the only FDA approved and most effective oral therapy.
- Most treatment takes 3 to 6 mo before maximum benefit is seen.
- Adjunct oral therapy includes tricyclic antidepressants (amitriptyline), cimetidine, antihistaminics (hydroxyzine, montelukast), neuroleptics (gabapentin, topiramate), analgesics (NSAIDs, opioid analgesics), and occasionally antimuscarinics.
- Oral therapies can be used in combination.

- Antihistaminics are preferred for patients with an allergy history or those who show mast cells in bladder biopsy.
- Oral prednisone is used in presence of Hunner's ulcers.
- Other drugs rarely used for IC are cyclosporin A, interleukin-10, imatinib, methotrexate, suplatast, misoprostol, and quercetin.
- Growth factor inhibitors, gene therapy, RDP 58, and vitamin B_3 analogue (BXL 628) may represent future therapies.
- Intravesical treatment is used when oral medications fail, for acute flare-ups, or before the oral medications take full effect.
- Dimethyl sulfoxide (DMSO), heparin, lidocaine, hyaluronic acid, capsaicin, botulinum toxin A, chondroitin sulfate, steroids, and Elmiron are drugs used for intravesical treatment.
- DMSO is the only FDA-approved intravesical treatment.
- DMSO is used less often now because of its side effects, specifically a garlic-like odor or taste on breath or skin that lasts 72 hr after treatment.
- Intravesical therapy typically involves mixture of heparin or Elmiron with lidocaine and sodium bicarbonate.
- Silver nitrate and Clorpactin have fallen out of favor.

SURGERY

- Major surgical intervention is not the mainstay of treatment.

- Patients whose condition is extreme and who are miserable may consider surgery if medications fail.
- Sacral neuromodulation (InterStim) is the current preferred surgical intervention.
- Laser ablation, fulguration, or resection is offered when Hunner's ulcers are seen in cystoscopy.
- Augmentation cystoplasty is not recommended.
- Cystourethrectomy with urinary diversion is rarely done.

COMPLEMENTARY & ALTERNATIVE MEDICINE

- Transcutaneous electric nerve stimulation
- Intravaginal electric nerve stimulation
- Acupuncture
- Urinary chelating agents such as Polycitra-K crystals, Urocit-K
- Prelief, an over-the-counter food additive
- Herbal remedies such as Algnot Plus, Cysto-Protek, Cysta-Q, aloe vera

DISPOSITION

- Close follow-up every month for 3 mo and every 3 mo thereafter.
- Voiding diary and symptom questionnaire are helpful to monitor response to treatment.

REFERRAL

- Urologist
- Pain specialist
- Physical therapist

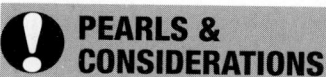

PEARLS & CONSIDERATIONS

COMMENTS

- On average these patients see five physicians and endure irritating voiding symptoms for 5 yr before the disease is identified.
- Besides symptom questionnaire and urine analysis, all other diagnostic tests are optional.
- PST is well tolerated.
- Negative cystoscopy does not rule out IC.

PREVENTION

Early identification and timely intervention improve patient outcome.

PATIENT & FAMILY EDUCATION

- IC support groups
- Interstitial Cystitis Association
- Interstitial Cystitis Network

SUGGESTED READINGS

available at www.expertconsult.com

AUTHOR: **HEMANT K. SATPATHY, M.D.**

Diseases and Disorders

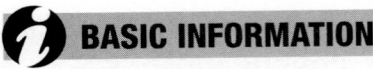

DEFINITION

Diffuse interstitial lung disease (ILD) includes a large group of nonmalignant disorders, which are characterized by diffuse damage to the lung parenchyma via inflammation and fibrosis, and/or granulomatous reaction in interstitial or vascular areas. The term "ILD" can be confusing because in addition to affecting the lung parenchyma, these processes may affect airways, vasculature, and pleura.

SYNONYMS

Interstitial pulmonary disease
ILD
Diffuse parenchymal lung disease (DPLD)

ICD-9CM CODES
136.3 Acute interstitial lung disease
515 Chronic interstitial lung disease

EPIDEMIOLOGY & DEMOGRAPHICS

PREVALENCE: Varies with type of ILD. The most common type of ILD is idiopathic interstitial fibrosis, with a prevalence of 20 cases/100,000 people in the general population, increasing with age to 175 cases/100,000 people aged 75 yr or older.
PREDOMINANT SEX & AGE: Some ILDs are more common in women, such as those resulting from connective tissue disorders. Lymphangiomyomatosis occurs exclusively in postmenopausal women. ILD caused by occupational exposures are more common in men. Generally, ILD occurs in people >50 yr.
RISK FACTORS: Although may be idiopathic, risk factors include history of tobacco abuse; environmental exposures such as to silicone, asbestos, or bird droppings; reactions to drugs such as chemotherapeutic agents, cardiac medications, and some history of connective tissue disease such as rheumatoid arthritis or systemic lupus erythematosus.

PHYSICAL FINDINGS & CLINICAL PRESENTATION

- Shortness of breath (especially with exertion)
- Dyspnea
- Cough (dry)
- Tachypnea
- Bibasilar end-inspiratory dry crackles
- Pulmonary hypertension
- Cyanosis, clubbing

ETIOLOGY

- The hallmark of ILD is restriction caused by decreased lung compliance. The decreased compliance can be the result of a number of factors depending on the type of ILD. Different types of ILD are characterized by three distinct patterns in the alveolar walls:
  1. Inflammatory changes, which are early and potentially reversible
  2. Fibrotic changes
  3. Lung destruction
- Specific changes may be seen:
  - Granulomatous: accumulation of T lymphocytes, macrophages, and epithelioid cells into granulomas in lung parenchyma
  - Inflammation and fibrosis: injury to epithelium causes inflammation; if chronic, inflammation spreads to interstitium and vascular areas

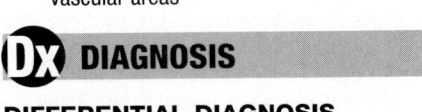
DIAGNOSIS

DIFFERENTIAL DIAGNOSIS

- Congestive heart failure
- Chronic renal failure

WORKUP

- Well-defined patterns in pulmonary function tests are usually consistent with restrictive defect (decreased FRC, RV, and TLC) owing to decreased lung compliance caused by alveolar wall thickening as a result of inflammation and fibrosis. Diffusion capacity is usually reduced also because of inflammation and thickening of alveolar walls, though nonspecific. FEV_1/FVC is usually normal or increased because lung stiffness keeps small airways open, although some conditions (e.g., sarcoidosis) may reduce air flow.
- Bronchoscopy and bronchoalveolar lavage (BAL) may help identify type of ILD. However, their role in defining stage of disease and response to therapy is controversial.
- Biopsy is the most effective method for confirming diagnosis and assessing disease activity.
- Fig. E1-459 describes a diagnostic approach to occupational ILD.

LABORATORY TESTS

- ABGs may be normal or show respiratory alkalosis.
- Blood tests for connective tissue diseases, such as antinuclear antibodies, anti-immunoglobulin antibodies (rheumatoid factors), LDH.
- Serum precipitins confirm exposure if hypersensitivity pneumonitis is suspected.
- Antineutrophil cytoplasmic antibodies or antibasement membrane antibodies if vasculitis is suspected.
- Elevation in angiotensin-converting enzyme level in sarcoidosis.
- ECG and echocardiogram will check for evidence of pulmonary hypertension.

IMAGING STUDIES

- Chest x-ray may be normal but commonly shows a bibasilar reticular pattern.
- High-resolution CT (HRCT) (Fig. 1-460) is the gold standard for evaluating parenchymal opacities seen on chest x-ray; it is also useful for determining potential biopsy sights.
- Echocardiography may be useful to evaluate cardiac function/dilation.

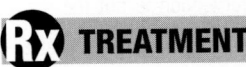
TREATMENT

NONPHARMACOLOGIC THERAPY
Avoidance of tobacco and occupational exposures

ACUTE GENERAL Rx

- Supplemental oxygen in patients with hypoxemia is helpful short and long term.
- Glucocorticoids are the mainstay of therapy, but success rate is low, and some guidelines recommend against use, especially long term. Patients should be reevaluated after this initial course of treatment. If they are stable, steroids may be tapered. If not, the same course may be maintained 4 additional wk. If patient's condition continues to decline, may consider adding second agent (cyclophosphamide, azathioprine).

CHRONIC GENERAL Rx

- Respiratory rehabilitation may be of value.
- Lung transplantation may be considered in appropriate patients in severe stages of the disease.

REFERRAL

- Surgical referral for biopsy
- Pulmonary referral for bronchoscopy and/or BAL

SUGGESTED READINGS
available at www.expertconsult.com

RELATED CONTENT
Interstitial Pulmonary Disease (Patient Information)

AUTHORS: **GRACE SHIH, M.D., CINDY GLEIT, M.D.,** and **JEFFREY BORKAN, M.D., PH.D.**

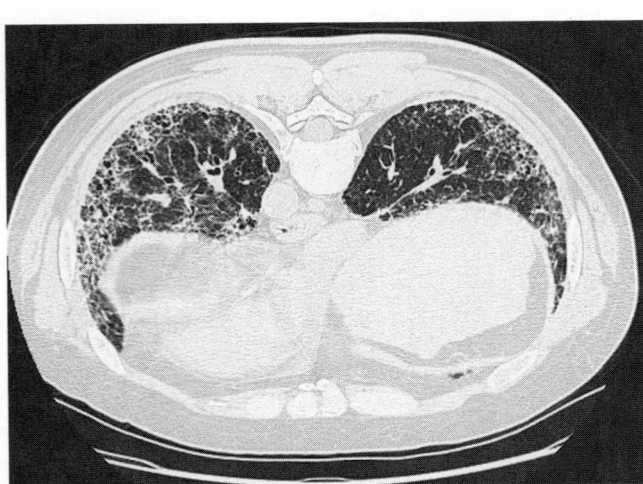
FIGURE 1-460 High-resolution computed tomography scan of the chest shows fibrotic changes in a subpleural distribution with honeycombing consistent with usual interstitial pneumonia. (From Hochberg MC et al: *Rheumatology*, ed 5, St Louis, 2011, Mosby.)

BASIC INFORMATION

DEFINITION

Can be classified into two broad categories:

Acute: Decrease in renal function resulting from immune-mediated injury characterized histopathologically with edema and inflammation of the renal interstitium, classically sparing the glomeruli and blood vessels. Most often drug-induced.

Chronic: Represents a large and diverse group of disorders characterized by interstitial fibrosis with mononuclear leukocyte infiltration and tubular atrophy. It is a final common pathway of many chronic kidney diseases including chronic bacterial infections, obstruction, and high-grade vesicoureteral reflux. Histopathologically seen as atrophy and fibrosis of the renal interstitium.

SYNONYMS

Acute tubulointerstitial nephritis
Contracted kidney
Cirrhosis of the kidney
Granular kidney
Gouty kidney
Renal sclerosis
Chronic productive nephritis without exudation

ICD-9CM CODES

583   Nephritis and nephropathy not specified as acute or chronic
583.7 Nephritis and nephropathy, not specific as acute or chronic, with lesion of renal medullary necrosis
583.8 Nephritis and nephropathy, not specific as acute or chronic, with other specified pathological lesion in kidney
583.9 With unspecified pathological lesions in the kidney

EPIDEMIOLOGY & DEMOGRAPHICS

PREVALENCE: 2% to 3% of all renal biopsies; in cases of acute renal failure, the incidence of acute interstitial nephritis is 7% to 15%.
PREDOMINANT SEX AND AGE: Older patients generally at higher risk given reduced glomerular filtration rates.
PEAK INCIDENCE: Median age at presentation is 65 yr.
GENETICS: Risk of acute interstitial nephritis due to drugs (e.g., NSAIDs, penicillins, sulfa drugs, etc.) increases with volume depletion, underlying kidney disease, age >65 yr, congestive heart failure, and diabetes. Some autoimmune disorders are also risk factors.

PHYSICAL FINDINGS & CLINICAL PRESENTATION

Nonspecific but acutely can present with renal failure, oliguria, hematuria, malaise, mental status changes, rash, nausea, and vomiting. Classic triad of low-grade fever, rash, and arthralgias is present in only 5% of cases of AIN. Chronic interstitial nephritis can be asymptomatic with elevations in BUN or creatinine or the appearance of abnormal urinary sediment.

ETIOLOGY

- Drug-induced (71%) usually hypersensitivity reaction occurring about 15 days after exposure to the drug: antibiotics (penicillins, cephalosporins, sulfonamides), NSAIDs, diuretics, proton pump inhibitors, anticonvulsants
- Infection associated (15%) can be either primary renal infection (acute bacterial pyelonephritis, renal tuberculosis, and fungal nephritis) or complication of systemic infections
  - Bacterial: *Corynebacterium diphtheriae, Legionella,* staphylococci, streptococci, *Yersinia*
  - Viral: Cytomegalovirus, Epstein-Barr virus, hantaviruses, hepatitis C, herpes simplex virus, human immunodeficiency virus, mumps, polyomavirus
  - Other: *Mycobacterium, Mycoplasma, Rickettsia,* syphilis, toxoplasmosis
- Immune disorders: systemic lupus erythematosus, Sjögren's, and Wegener's)
- Neoplastic disorders (multiple myeloma)
- Metabolic diseases (urate nephropathy, hypercalcemic nephropathy, hypokalemic nephropathy, oxalate nephropathy)
- Heavy metals (chronic form)
- Chronic urinary tract obstruction (chronic form)

DIAGNOSIS

DIFFERENTIAL DIAGNOSIS

Any other causes of acute renal failure including acute tubular necrosis, glomerulonephritis, hypertensive nephrosclerosis, prerenal azotemia, obstructive nephropathy, renal vascular disease, and various electrolyte abnormalities

WORKUP

Medical history with focus on recent infection illness or new medication in the presence of acute to chronic onset of kidney failure; evaluation for underlying infection or insult

LABORATORY TESTS

- Urinalysis, urine microscopy (especially eosinophiluria although low sensitivity), serum chemistry profile, complete blood count with differential (eosinophilia occurs in 50% of AIN patients), liver function tests, 24-hr urine specimen collection, consider serum IgE levels
- Renal biopsy is the gold standard for diagnosis but is indicated only when diagnosis is unclear, removal of offending agent does not result in improvement, or steroid initiation is being considered

IMAGING STUDIES

Neither ultrasound nor gallium 67 scan is diagnostic but may be useful for ruling out AIN

TREATMENT

NONPHARMACOLOGIC THERAPY

Largely supportive; removal of offending agent will resolve 60% of all cases.

ACUTE GENERAL Rx

- Correct fluid and electrolyte imbalances, maintain adequate hydration and urine output but avoid volume overload.
- Identify and treat infection as indicated.
- Remove offending drug, substitute as appropriate.
- Avoid medications that impair renal blood flow.
- Initiation of steroids is controversial, but retrospective studies have shown that early steroid treatment may reduce need for chronic dialysis in patients with drug-induced AIN.

CHRONIC Rx

- Limit exposure to known nephrotoxic agents.
- Renally adjust medications as indicated by glomerular filtration rate.
- Tight control of blood pressure, diabetes, and cholesterol to preserve kidney function as needed

DISPOSITION

With acute interstitial nephritis (AIN), 40% of patients will improve in time. Relapse is common with reexposure to offending agents.

REFERRAL

Refer to nephrology with question in diagnosis, multiple comorbidities, with failure to respond to supportive care, or with decision to evaluate for biopsy.

PEARLS & CONSIDERATIONS

COMMENTS

Once known mainly as a complication of streptococcal infection, today acute interstitial nephritis is most often due to drugs; 88% of the time, the drug was started in the past 30 days. Significant fibrosis of the tubules seen in biopsy is the best predictor of transition to chronic interstitial nephritis.

PREVENTION

Use known offending agents with care, especially in the elderly and those with known underlying kidney disease.

SUGGESTED READINGS

available at www.expertconsult.com

RELATED CONTENT

Interstitial Nephritis (Patient Information)

AUTHOR: **ELIZABETH BROWN, M.D.**

BASIC INFORMATION

DEFINITION

Conduction disturbance that occurs at the various levels of the branches in the His-Purkinje system are described as intraventricular conduction defects (IVCDs). Conduction disturbances in the His-Purkinje system can be unifascicular (e.g., right bundle branch block [RBBB]), bifascicular (e.g., left bundle branch block [LBBB]), or nonspecific. The term "nonspecific IVCD" applies to any pattern of intraventricular conduction disturbance that cannot be ascribed to a block in a specific portion of the specialized conduction system such as the LBBB or RBBB. This chapter will focus on the nonspecific type of IVCD. Nonspecific IVCD is defined based on a QRS duration greater than 110 ms in adults, 100 ms or greater in children 4 to 16 yr of age, and 90 ms or greater in children less than 4 yr of age in the electrocardiogram (ECG) and does not satisfy the criteria for either the LBBB or RBBB pattern. The conduction delay causing prolonged QRS is considered to occur beyond the Purkinje's myocardial gates and arises from slowing in cell-to-cell conduction.

SYNONYMS

IVCD
Nonspecific intraventricular conduction disturbance
Unspecified intraventricular conduction disturbance
Intraventricular conduction delay
Intraventicular block

ICD-9CM CODES
426.6 Intraventricular block, NOS

EPIDEMIOLOGY

- Unknown in general population
- The reported prevalence in military aviators was similar to RBBB at 2:1000.

ETIOLOGY

- Any process that affects the intrinsic ventricular conduction system or slows intraventricular conduction can lead to the development of an intraventricular block or conduction delay.
- Nonspecific IVCDs are frequently seen with previous myocardial infarction and scar formation, the use of Class I antiarrhythmic drugs, left ventricular hypertrophy, and hyperkalemia. Etiology can also be unknown in many cases.

PHYSICAL FINDINGS & CLINICAL PRESENTATION

Nonspecific IVCD produces no symptoms and is recognizable only through an ECG.

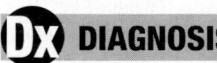 **DIAGNOSIS**

Usually an incidental finding on ECG. Lesions of the ventricular conduction system present as blocks of the bundle branches or fascicles. Ventricular conduction system disturbances can be classified as unifascicular, bifascicular, or trifascicular blocks based on the site of the lesion or lesions.

DIFFERENTIAL DIAGNOSIS

- Unifascicular block
- Bifascicular block
- Wolff-Parkinson-White (WPW) pattern and variants
- LBBB
- RBBB

WORKUP

Workup such as routine labs, cardiac biomarkers, and cardiac imaging should be targeted at the potential known etiologies and dictated by the clinical circumstances.

Clinical correlation is needed to identify associated cardiac problems. If there is a history of heart failure or an abnormal cardiac exam, then an echocardiogram is indicated. If Q waves are present and there is a history of myocardial infarction, then an echocardiogram and/or nuclear stress testing is indicated to determine if further therapy should be given to lessen the possibility of heart failure exacerbation, a future myocardial infarction, and other complications.

If a Class I antiarrhythmic drug like quinidine or flecainide is being taken that relates temporally to the nonspecific IVCD, then increasing the dosage is not indicated. Blood chemistries can be helpful to assess for hyperkalemia.

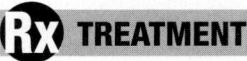 **TREATMENT**

Though cardiac resynchronization therapy has been effective in reducing clinical events in patients with LBBB, a 2012 systematic review of the literature does not support such benefits in patients with wide QRS due to nonspecific IVCD. No specific therapy is needed for IVCD. Patients are usually treated for the underlying heart diseases.

PROGNOSIS

Nonspecific IVCD in an ECG is associated with increased all-cause mortality and a markedly elevated risk of sudden arrhythmic death in a general population. Clinical correlation is needed because prognosis depends on underlying heart disease, if any.

REFERRAL

Refer to a cardiologist if there is a history of heart failure or myocardial infarction, or an abnormal cardiac exam.

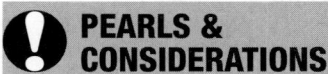 **PEARLS & CONSIDERATIONS**

Nonspecific IVCD can be due to drugs such as Class I antiarrhythmic drugs. Nonspecific IVCD can be a normal variant and is not always associated with cardiac pathology. Clinical correlation (history and physical exam) is needed to identify associated cardiac abnormalities.

SUGGESTED READINGS
available at www.expertconsult.com

AUTHORS: **AKINNIRAN A. ABISOGUN, M.D.,** and **WEN-CHIH WU, M.D., M.P.H.**

BASIC INFORMATION

DEFINITION

Irritable bowel syndrome (IBS) is a chronic functional disorder manifested by alteration in bowel habits and recurrent abdominal pain and bloating. IBS is a symptom complex influenced by a variety of physiologic determinants from gut to brain and back. The ROME III criteria for diagnosis of IBS are:

- Recurrent abdominal pain or discomfort at least 3 days per month in the past 3 mo associated with ≥two of the following:
  - Pain is relieved or improved with defecation.
  - Its onset is associated with a change in the frequency of bowel movement.
  - Its onset is associated with a change in the form or appearance of the stool.
- The criteria must be fulfilled for at least the past 3 mo with symptom onset at least 6 mo before the diagnosis.

SYNONYMS

Irritable colon
Spastic colon
IBS

ICD-9CM CODES
564.1 Irritable bowel syndrome

EPIDEMIOLOGY & DEMOGRAPHICS

- IBS is the most common functional bowel disorder. An estimated 15 million people in the United States have IBS.
- IBS occurs in 20% of the population of industrialized countries and is responsible for >50% of gastrointestinal (GI) referrals. Worldwide adult prevalence is 12%. Incidence increases during adolescence and peaks in third and fourth decades of life.
- Female/male ratio is 2:1. Peak prevalence is from 20 to 39 years of age.
- Nearly 50% of patients have psychiatric abnormalities, with anxiety disorders being most common.

PHYSICAL FINDINGS & CLINICAL PRESENTATION

- The clinical presentation of IBS consists of abdominal pain and abnormalities of defecation, which may include loose stools, usually after meals and in the morning, alternating with episodes of constipation.
- Physical examination is generally normal.
- Nonspecific abdominal tenderness and distention may be present.

ETIOLOGY

- Unknown
- Associated pathophysiology includes altered GI motility, alteration in gut flora, and increased gut sensitivity
- Risk factors: anxiety, depression, personality disorders, history of childhood sexual abuse, and domestic abuse in women

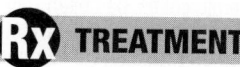

DIAGNOSIS

DIFFERENTIAL DIAGNOSIS

- Inflammatory bowel disease (IBD)
- Diverticulitis
- Colon malignancy
- Endometriosis
- Peptic ulcer disease
- Biliary liver disease
- Chronic pancreatitis
- Constipation caused by medications (opiates, calcium channel blockers, anticholinergics)
- Diarrhea caused by medications (metformin, colchicine, proton pump inhibitors, antacids, antibiotics)
- Small-bowel overgrowth
- Celiac disease
- Parasites
- Lymphoma of GI tract

WORKUP

Diagnostic workup (Fig. E1-461) is aimed primarily at excluding the conditions listed in the differential diagnoses. It is important to identify red flags of other diseases, such as weight loss, rectal bleeding, onset in patients >50 yr, fever, nocturnal pain, and family history of malignancy or IBD. Additional red flags include abnormal examination (e.g., mass, enlarged lymph nodes, stool positive for occult blood, muscle wasting) and abnormal laboratory values (anemia, leukocytosis, abnormal chemistry).

Common clinical criteria for diagnosis of IBS are >3 mo of symptoms, including abdominal pain that is relieved by a bowel movement, or pain accompanied by a change in bowel pattern, and abnormality in bowel movement 25% of the time, characterized by two of the following features:

- Abdominal distention
- Abnormal consistency
- Abnormal defecation (e.g., straining, sense of incomplete evacuation)
- Abnormal frequency
- Mucus with bowel movement

LABORATORY TESTS

- Blood work is generally normal. CBC is reasonable to evaluate for anemia. The presence of anemia should alert to the possibility of a colonic malignancy or IBD.
- Testing of stool for ova and parasites should be considered only in patients with chronic diarrhea. Evaluation of stool for *Clostridium difficile* may be helpful in patients with predominant diarrhea symptoms who have recently taken antibiotics.

IMAGING STUDIES

Imaging studies (e.g., flat and upright abdominal radiograph, small-bowel series, sonogram or CT of abdomen and pelvis) are normal and not necessary for diagnosis.

Lower endoscopy is generally normal except for the presence of some spasms. Colonoscopic imaging should be performed only in persons who have alarm features to rule out organic disease and in persons older than 50 yr to screen for colorectal cancer.

TREATMENT

NONPHARMACOLOGIC THERAPY

- The patient should be encouraged to maintain an adequate fiber intake and to eliminate foods that aggravate symptoms. Avoidance of caffeine, dairy products, fatty foods, and dietary excesses is also helpful.
- Cognitive-behavioral therapy is also recommended, particularly in younger patients because psychosocial stressors are important triggers of IBS. Reassurance and education about trigger avoidance and stress management are important.
- Importance of regular exercise and adequate fluid intake should be stressed.

GENERAL Rx

- The mainstay of treatment of IBS is a high-fiber diet. Fiber is helpful for relief of constipation but not for relief of pain. Because symptoms are chronic, the use of laxatives should generally be avoided.
- Soluble fiber (psyllium) is more effective in symptom relief than insoluble fiber (bran). Fiber supplementation with psyllium 1 tbsp bid or calcium polycarbophil (FiberCon) 2 tablets one to four times daily followed by 8 oz of water may be necessary in some patients.
- Patients should be instructed that there might be some increased bloating on initiation of fiber supplementation, which should resolve within 2 to 3 wk. It is important that patients take these fiber products on a regular basis and not only as needed. Fiber is not effective in patients with diarrhea-predominant IBS and may worsen symptoms in these patients.
- Patients who appear anxious can benefit from use of sedatives or selective serotonin reuptake inhibitors (SSRIs). Tricyclic antidepressants in low doses are also effective in some patients with diarrhea-predominant IBS.
- C-2 chloride channel activators: Lubiprostone (Amitiza) is a chloride channel activator that stimulates chloride-rich intestinal fluid secretion and accelerates small intestine and colonic transmit time. It may be effective in chronic constipation-predominant IBS unresponsive to conventional treatment. Usual dose is 8 to 24 mcg bid with food. Side effects include headache and nausea.
- Linaclotide (Linzess) is a guanylate cyclase-C (GC-C) agonist recently FDA approved for IBS with constipation. It stimulates secretion of chloride and bicarbonate into the intestinal lumen, mainly through activation of the CFTR ion channel, resulting in increased intestinal fluid and accelerated transit. Usual dose for IBS is 290 mcg 30 min before eating. The most common adverse effects are diarrhea, abdominal pain, flatulence, and abdominal distension.

- Loperamide is effective for diarrhea. Alosetron, a serotonin type-3 receptor antagonist previously withdrawn because of severe constipation and ischemic colitis, has been reintroduced with limited availability. It is indicated only for women with severe chronic diarrhea-predominant IBS unresponsive to conventional therapy and not caused by anatomic or metabolic abnormality. Starting dose is 1 mg qd.
- Alterations in gut flora have been identified as potentially contributing to IBS (84% of IBS patients have an abnormal lactulose breath test, suggesting small-intestinal bacterial overgrowth). Rifaximin, a gut-selective antibiotic, has been used in recent trials to eradicate bacterial overgrowth (70% eradication rate). A dose of 400 mg tid for 10 days was reported effective in improving IBS symptoms up to 10 wk after discontinuation of therapy. Until additional evidence is available, use of rifaximin or other antibiotics in IBS should be reserved for patients with proven bacterial overgrowth.
- Antispasmodics-anticholinergics (e.g., dicyclomine, hyoscyamine) are often used, but efficacy data from clinical trials are inconclusive.
- Probiotics: Bifidobacteria and some combinations of probiotics have shown some limited efficacy. Lactobacilli do not appear to be effective for the treatment of IBS. Additional data showing efficacy is needed before probiotics can be endorsed for treatment of IBS.
- Antidepressants: SSRIs are more effective than placebo for relief of global IBS symptoms.

DISPOSITION

More than 60% of patients respond successfully to treatment over the initial 12 mo; however, IBS is a chronic, relapsing condition and requires prolonged therapy.

REFERRAL

GI referral is recommended in patients with rectal bleeding, fever, nocturnal diarrhea, anemia, weight loss, or onset of symptoms >40 yr. Consultation is also necessary if specialized diagnostic procedures such as endoscopy are necessary.

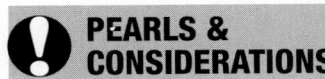

COMMENTS

- Patients should be educated regarding maintenance of a high-fiber diet and elimination of stressors, which can precipitate attacks of IBS. They should be reassured that their condition does not lead to cancer.

- Recent drug efforts (alosetron, tegaserod) are aimed at serotonergic receptors in the gut because most of the serotonin in the body is found in the GI tract and is believed to be involved in the mediation of visceral sensation and motility.
- Cognitive-behavioral therapy is effective in the treatment of patients with IBS and should be considered as part of the armamentarium against this disorder.
- Some patients with IBS but without celiac disease show symptom improvement on a wheat-free diet. A 2- to 3-week trial of wheat avoidance may be reasonable in patients with treatment-resistant IBS.

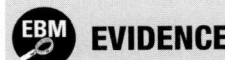 **EVIDENCE**

available at www.expertconsult.com

SUGGESTED READINGS
available at www.expertconsult.com

RELATED CONTENT
Irritable Bowel Syndrome (Patient Information)

AUTHOR: **FRED F. FERRI, M.D.**

BASIC INFORMATION

DEFINITION

Jaundice is a yellowish discoloration of the sclera (Fig. E1-462), skin, and mucous membranes caused by an excessive amount of bilirubin in the bloodstream. Clinically detectable jaundice in adults is a serum bilirubin of 2.5 to 3 mg/dl.

SYNONYMS

Icterus

ICD-9CM CODES
782.4 Jaundice
283.9 Hemolytic jaundice
576.8 Obstructive jaundice

EPIDEMIOLOGY & DEMOGRAPHICS

The major causes of jaundice by age and sex:
- Young adulthood (for either sex): viral hepatitis
- Middle adulthood (for either sex): drug-induced hepatitis and cirrhosis
- Middle-aged and older men: alcoholic liver disease, pancreatic cancer, hepatoma, primary hemochromatosis
- Women: primary biliary cirrhosis, chronic active hepatitis, choledocholithiasis, carcinoma of the gallbladder

PHYSICAL FINDINGS & CLINICAL PRESENTATION

Presentation can vary from an incidental finding to acute and life threatening. History and physical examination give important clues to the underlying condition.
Key history of present illness findings:
- Duration of jaundice
- Associated symptoms: abdominal pain, fever, chills, changes in urine and stool color, anorexia and/or weight loss
Key social history/exposure findings:
- Alcohol use, injection of illicit drugs, use of hepatotoxic medication or herbal products, blood transfusions, unprotected sex, ingestion of shellfish, travel, occupational exposure to toxins
Key past medical history findings:
- Prior abdominal/biliary surgery, prior episodes of jaundice, prior diagnosis of hepatitis B or C
Key physical findings:
- Vital sign abnormalities: fever, hypotension, tachycardia
- Signs of acute disease: abdominal tenderness, splenomegaly, abdominal mass, encephalopathy
- Signs of chronic liver disease: palmar erythema, spider angiomas, bruising, gynecomastia, testicular atrophy, ascites, weight loss, Kayser-Fleischer rings (Wilson's)

ETIOLOGY

Disruption in any of the three phases of bilirubin metabolism can lead to jaundice:
- Prehepatic phase: an increase in heme degradation products from red blood cell catabolism, ineffective erythropoiesis, or breakdown of muscle myoglobin and cytochromes; leads to indirect (unconjugated) hyperbilirubinemia
- Intrahepatic phase: destruction of the hepatocytes or disruption of either of the two separate biochemical processes that conjugate bilirubin in the hepatocyte; may lead to indirect (unconjugated) or direct (conjugated) hyperbilirubinemia
- Posthepatic phase: blockage of the release of water soluble bilirubin from the hepatobiliary system, preventing excretion into the stool or urine or recycling within the gut flora; leads to direct (conjugated) hyperbilirubinemia

DIAGNOSIS

DIFFERENTIAL DIAGNOSIS

Prehepatic causes:
- Consider hemolysis (e.g., sickle cell disease, spherocytosis, G6PD, immune hemolysis), ineffective erythropoiesis (e.g., thalassemia, folate, severe iron deficiency), or large hematoma reabsorption.
Intrahepatic causes:
- If unconjugated hyperbilirubinemia: consider enzyme metabolism disorders, specifically Gilbert's disease, which is common and benign or Crigler-Najjar syndrome, which is rare and severe); drugs that alter the enzymatic pathways such as rifampin, isoniazid, and probenecid.
- If conjugated hyperbilirubinemia: consider intrahepatic cholestasis.
  1. Viruses: hepatitis A, B, and C; Epstein-Barr
  2. Alcohol: alcoholic hepatitis, alcoholic cirrhosis
  3. Autoimmune: primary biliary cirrhosis, primary sclerosing cholangitis
  4. Hepatotoxic drug-induced: acetaminophen (most common), penicillins (specifically Augmentin), chlorpromazine, steroids (estrogenic or anabolic), NSAIDs, some herbals such as kava, ma huang, and off-market weight loss supplements
  5. Hereditary/metabolic: sickle cell disease and other RBC dyscrasias, hemochromatosis, Wilson's disease, Dubin-Johnson and Rotor's syndromes, α-antitrypsin deficiency, glycogen storage disease
  6. Systemic disease: invading liver: sarcoidosis, amyloidosis, tuberculosis, *Mycobacterium avium intracellulare*
  7. Other: cirrhosis, sepsis, total parenteral nutrition, pregnancy, graft-versus-host disease, environmental toxins

Posthepatic causes:
- Intrinsic or extrinsic obstruction of the biliary system
  1. Blockage within hepatobiliary tree: strictures, cholangiocarcinoma, gallbladder cancer, infection (e.g., cytomegalovirus, *Cryptosporidium* in patients with AIDS, parasites)
  2. Blockage outside of hepatobiliary tree: pancreatitis, pancreatic carcinoma, pancreatic pseudocyst
- Pseudojaundice: not related to bilirubin but rather resulting from excessive ingestion of foods containing beta carotene (e.g., carrots, melons, squash)

WORKUP

History, physical examination, and first-line lab tests can often clarify diagnosis. Fig. E1-463 describes a clinical approach to jaundice.

LABORATORY TESTS

First-line tests:
- Serum total and direct bilirubin
- Urinalysis
If serum total bilirubin and direct bilirubin are elevated and urine is positive for bilirubin, consider intrahepatic or posthepatic process:
- Initial evaluation: liver function tests (AST, ALT, GGTP, alkaline phosphatase), CBC, liver synthetic function (albumin, PT, PTT), pancreatic function (amylase, lipase)
- Additional tests if diagnosis unclear:
  1. Screen for hepatitis A, B, and C; if still unclear then consider options 2 to 6 as follow
  2. Other viruses (Epstein-Barr virus, cytomegalovirus)
  3. Autoimmune disorders: antimitochondrial antibody, immunoglobulin (Ig) M (elevated in primary biliary cirrhosis); smooth muscle antibody, antinuclear antibody, IgG (autoimmune chronic active hepatitis); antinuclear cytoplasmic antibody (primary sclerosing cholangitis)
  4. Ceruloplasmin (Wilson's disease)
  5. Alpha-1 antitrypsin deficiency (cirrhosis and emphysema)
  6. Ferritin, Fe saturation (elevated in hemochromatosis)
If serum total bilirubin is elevated but direct bilirubin is normal (unconjugated hyperbilirubinemia) and urine is negative for bilirubin, consider prehepatic or intrahepatic processes.
- Blood smear (abnormal RBC types)
- Diagnosis of exclusion: Gilbert's syndrome
Liver biopsy: essential in diagnosis of chronic hepatitis. Can be used for diagnosis of liver masses but carries a substantial risk.

IMAGING STUDIES

- Abdominal ultrasound: first-line study (Figs. 1-464, 1-465), may be completed bedside, most sensitive for proximal biliary tract disease; presence of dilated ducts hints at an extrahepatic process
- Abdominal CT: often necessary to elucidate more information on liver, pancreas, and distal biliary system
- Endoscopic retrograde cholangiopancreatography: rarely necessary for diagnostics. If needed refer to GI consultant

- Percutaneous transhepatic cholangiography: rarely necessary for diagnostics. If needed refer to GI consultant
- Magnetic resonance cholangiopancreatography: noninvasive visualization of bile and pancreatic ducts; becoming more available. If needed, refer to GI consultant.

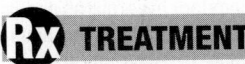 **TREATMENT**

NONPHARMACOLOGIC THERAPY

Depends on underlying cause of the jaundice and clinical stability of the patient. Generally, obstructive causes require surgical treatment, while nonobstructive causes require medical treatment.

ACUTE GENERAL Rx

Acute, life-threatening illness (e.g., cholecystitis or ascending cholangitis) requires prompt diagnosis with basic labs and bedside diagnostics, with early surgical and GI consultation in conjunction with medical management. *N*-Acetylcysteine can be given for acetaminophen overdose.

CHRONIC Rx

Reversible causes must be ruled out first and suspicious medications or ETOH use must be stopped. For intrahepatic disease, consider GI consult for management of hepatitis B or C with interferon, Wilson's disease with penicillamine, hemochromatosis with phlebotomy, etc. Consider surgical consult for resection of pancreatic masses.

Symptomatic pruritus may be treated with cholestyramine for bilirubin binding or with antihistamines to decrease the itch reflex.

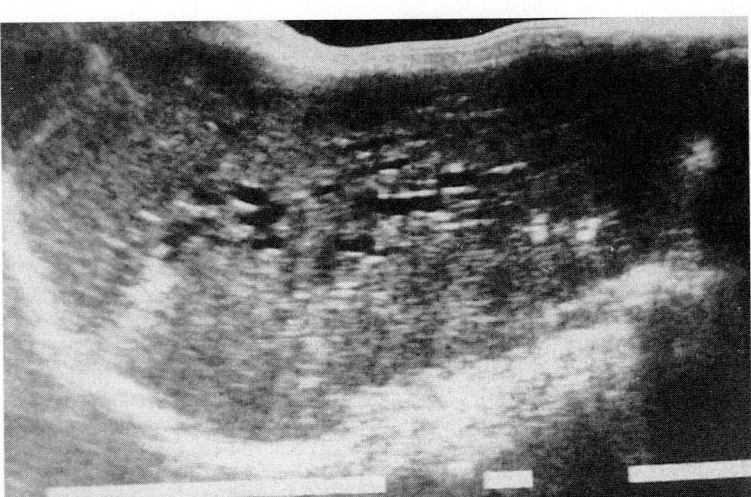

FIGURE 1-464 Ultrasound showing a large calculus in the extrahepatic biliary tree. Dilated bile ducts can be seen to the left. (Courtesy Dr. M.C. Collins. Forbes A et al [eds]: *Atlas of clinical gastroenterology*, ed 3, St Louis, 2005, Mosby.)

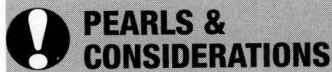

FIGURE 1-465 Schematic representation of ultrasound abnormality seen in Fig. 1-464. (From Forbes A et al [eds]: *Atlas of clinical gastroenterology*, ed 3, St Louis, 2005, Mosby.)

dilated intrahepatic bile ducts

PEARLS & CONSIDERATIONS

COMMENTS

- Heed the warning signs of unstable vital signs to diagnose life-threatening illness; early collaboration with surgical and gastroenterology colleagues is helpful in complex patient care scenarios.
- Careful history and physical examination, basic labs, and prompt bedside imaging frequently lead to accurate diagnosis.
- Very high serum bilirubin (>15 mg/dl) is most likely to be seen in cirrhosis. Watch for hepatorenal syndrome in these patients.

SUGGESTED READINGS

available at www.expertconsult.com

RELATED CONTENT

Jaundice (Patient Information)

AUTHOR: **ALLA GOLDBURT, M.D.**

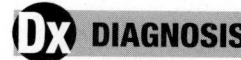

BASIC INFORMATION

DEFINITION

Juvenile idiopathic arthritis (JIA), previously referred to as juvenile rheumatoid arthritis (JRA), is a diverse spectrum of arthritides presenting before 16 yr of age. The arthritis symptoms must be persistent and objective in ≥one joints for at least 6 wk with the exclusion of any other known cause.

SYNONYMS

Still's disease
JIA
Juvenile rheumatoid arthritis

ICD-9CM CODES
714.3 Polyarticular juvenile rheumatoid arthritis, chronic or unspecified

EPIDEMIOLOGY & DEMOGRAPHICS

PREVALENCE (IN U.S.): 57 to 220 per 100,000 children

PHYSICAL FINDINGS & CLINICAL PRESENTATION

JIA is subdivided into seven categories based on the 2001 International League of Associations for Rheumatology (ILAR) classification criteria (subtype characteristics are summarized in Tables 1-232 and E1-233.
Systemic onset JIA
  Arthritis in ≥one joints with or preceded by fever of at least 2 wk duration that is quotidian (once daily) for at least 3 days and associated with at least one of the following: (1) evanescent erythematous rash (Fig. E1-466), (2) generalized lymph node enlargement, (3) hepatomegaly, splenomegaly, or both, and (4) serositis such as pleuritis, pericarditis, or peritonitis.
Oligoarticular JIA (Fig. 1-467)
  Arthritis in one to four joints during a 6-mo period of time. There are two subtypes:
    Persistent: ≤four joints throughout the disease course
    Extended: ≤four joints during the first 6 mo extending to >four joints after 6 mo.
Polyarthritis, rheumatoid factor (RF) negative
  Arthritis involves >six joints during first 6 mo of the disease with negative RF.
Polyarthritis, RF positive
  Arthritis involves >six joints during first 6 mo of the disease with positive RF on at least two tests run 3 mo apart.
  Anti–cyclic citrullinated (CCP) antibodies may also be present
  Most likely to extend beyond childhood and most similar to adult rheumatoid arthritis
Psoriatic arthritis
  Psoriasis and arthritis or psoriasis and ≥two of the following:
    Dactylitis, nail pitting, onycholysis, and psoriasis in a first-degree relative
Enthesitis-related arthritis
  Arthritis and enthesitis or arthritis or enthesitis and ≥two of the following:
    Presence of or a history of SI joint pain, positive HLA-B27, boy aged >6 yr, acute anterior uveitis, or history of ankylosing spondylitis, reactive arthritis, sacroiliitis with inflammatory bowel disease or acute anterior uveitis in a first-degree relative

ETIOLOGY

Idiopathic: Both genetic and environmental triggers thought to play a role.

DIAGNOSIS

DIFFERENTIAL DIAGNOSIS

- Infection: viral or rheumatic fever
- Systemic lupus erythematosus (very rare under age 5)
- Malignancy
- Serum sickness
- Lyme arthritis

LABORATORY TESTS

- Increased erythrocyte sedimentation rate and CRP
- Low-grade anemia
- Leukocytosis
- Rheumatoid factor: rarely demonstrable in the serum of children
- Antinuclear antibodies: often found in children with ocular complications
- If macrophage activation syndrome suspected in patients with systemic JIA: decreased platelets, WBC, and fibrinogen with high ferritin and liver function tests. Bone marrow biopsy is needed to confirm diagnosis.

TABLE 1-232 Overview of the Main Features of the Subtypes of Juvenile Idiopathic Arthritis

ILAR Subtype	Peak Age of Onset (yr)	Female: Male; % of All JIA	Arthritis Pattern	Extra-articular Features	Investigations	Notes on Therapy
Systemic arthritis	2-4	1:1; ~10% of JIA cases	Polyarticular, often knees, wrists, and ankles; also fingers, neck, and hips	Daily fever; evanescent rash; pericarditis; pleuritis	Anemia; WBC ↑↑; ESR ↑↑; CRP ↑↑; ferritin ↑; platelets ↑↑ (normal or ↑ in MAS)	Less responsive to standard treatment with MTX and anti-TNF agents; consider IL-1Ra in resistant cases
Oligoarthritis	<6	4:1; 50%-60% of JIA (but ethnic variation)	Knees ++; ankles, fingers +	Uveitis in ~30%	ANA positive in ;60%; other tests usually normal; may have mildly ↑ ESR/CRP	NSAIDs and intra-articular steroids; occasionally require MTX
Polyarthritis, RF negative	6-7	3:1; 30% of JIA cases	Symmetric or asymmetric; small and large joints; cervical spine; TMJ	Uveitis in ~10%	ANA positive in 40%; RF negative; ESR ↑ or ↑↑; CRP ↑/normal; mild anemia	Standard therapy with MTX and NSAIDs, then if nonresponsive, anti-TNF agents or other biologics
Polyarthritis, RF positive	9-12	9:1; <10% of JIA cases	Aggressive symmetric polyarthritis	Rheumatoid nodules in 10%; low-grade fever	RF positive; ESR ↑↑; CRP ↑/normal; mild anemia	Long-term remission unlikely; early aggressive therapy is warranted
Psoriatic arthritis	7-10	2:1; <10% of JIA cases	Asymmetric arthritis of small or medium sized joints	Uveitis in 10%; psoriasis in 50%	ANA positive in 50%; ESR ↑; CRP ↑/normal; mild anemia	NSAIDs and intra-articular steroids; second-line agents less commonly
Enthesitis-related arthritis	9-12	1:7; 10% of JIA cases	Predominantly lower limb joints affected; sometimes axial skeleton (but less than adult AS)	Acute anterior uveitis; association with reactive arthritis and IBD	80% HLA-B27+	NSAIDs and intra-articular steroids; consider sulfasalazine as alternative to MTX

ANA, Antinuclear antibody; *AS*, ankylosing spondylitis; *CRP*, C-reactive protein; *ESR*, erythrocyte sedimentation rate; *IBD*, inflammatory bowel disease; *ILAR*, International League of Associations for Rheumatology; *IL-1Ra*, interleukin-1 receptor antagonist; *JIA*, juvenile idiopathic arthritis; *MAS*, macrophage activation syndrome; *MTX*, methotrexate; *NSAID*, nonsteroidal anti-inflammatory drug; *RF*, rheumatoid factor; *TMJ*, temporomandibular joint; *TNF*, tumor necrosis factor; *WBC*, white blood cell count.

From Firestein G et al: *Kelley's textbook of rheumatology*, ed 8, Philadelphia, 2008, Saunders.

IMAGING STUDIES

- Roentgenographic findings (Fig. E1-468) are similar to those in adult, with soft tissue swelling and periarticular osteopenia early in the disease.
- Joint destruction (Fig. 1-469) is less frequent.
- Bony erosion and cyst formation may be present as a result of synovial hypertrophy.

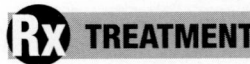

TREATMENT

NONPHARMACOLOGIC THERAPY

Proper management requires close cooperation among primary physician, physical and occupational therapists, pediatric rheumatologist, social workers, and orthopedist.
- Rest
- Physical and occupational therapy
- Patient and family education
- Proper diet and weight maintenance

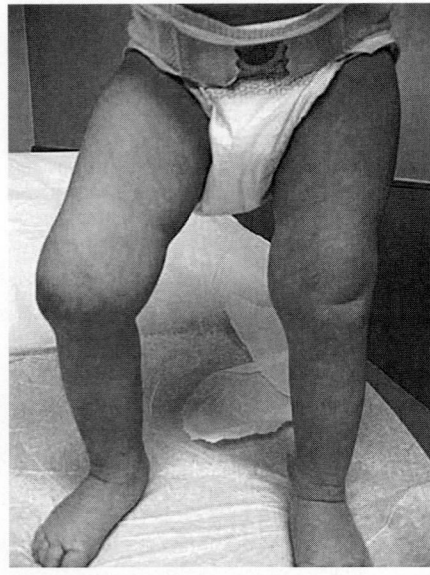

FIGURE 1-467 Oligoarticular juvenile idiopathic arthritis with swelling and flexion contracture of the right knee. (From Kliegman RM et al: *Nelson textbook of pediatrics,* ed 19, Philadelphia, 2011, Saunders.)

ACUTE GENERAL Rx

- NSAIDs
- DMARDs: methotrexate, leflunomide, sulfasalazine
- Patients with polyarticular disease are less likely to respond to methotrexate if they have longer disease duration, positive ANA, higher level of disability, and bilateral wrist arthritis. It may be reasonable to start with anti-TNF therapy first in these cases.
- Axial involvement is also less likely to respond to methotrexate
- Biologics:
  o Tumor necrosis factor blockers such as etanercept and adalimumab
  o T-cell modulator CTLA-4 fusion protein, abatacept, is FDA approved for patients with polyarticular JIA who have not responded to anti-TNF therapy
  o IL-6 (tocilizumab) and IL-1 inhibitors (anakinra, canakinumab) for systemic JIA
- Intra-articular steroids can prevent leg length discrepancies in oligoarticular JIA
- Systemic corticosteroids

DISPOSITION

- Complete remission occurs in the majority of patients and may occur at any age.
- 70% to 85% of children regain normal function.

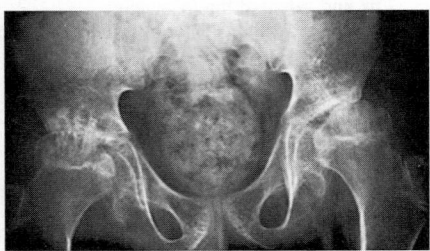

FIGURE 1-469 Severe hip disease in a 13-yr-old boy with active, systemic-onset juvenile idiopathic arthritis. Radiograph shows destruction of the femoral head and acetabula, joint space narrowing, and subluxation of left hip. The patient had received corticosteroids systemically for 9 yr. (From Kliegman RM et al: *Nelson textbook of pediatrics,* ed 19, Philadelphia, 2011, Saunders.)

- Mortality is three- to fourteenfold greater than in the general population of the same age. Macrophage activation syndrome is a life-threatening complication in systemic JIA.
- Oligoarticular JIA patients with positive ANA are at the highest risk for blindness due to chronic iridocyclitis and require frequent ophthalmologic monitoring.
- Systemic and localized growth disturbance can lead to generalized growth failure and leg length discrepancies.
- Arthritis of the temporomandibular joint can lead to jaw malformation.

REFERRAL

- Early rheumatology consultation
- Ophthalmology consultation at diagnosis and regularly thereafter particularly in ANA+, oligoarticular JIA
- Orthopedic consultation for corrective surgery

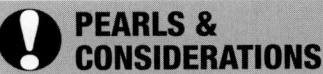

PEARLS & CONSIDERATIONS

COMMENTS

The spontaneous adverse event reports (SERS) in the FDA surveillance system has recently reported a warning for risk of malignancy related to anti-TNF agents in the pediatric population. However, baseline risk of malignancy in children with JIA is unknown and the SERS reporting system has limitations, including incomplete adverse event reporting. Initiation of anti-TNF therapy should be a decision made between families and pediatric rheumatologists.

SUGGESTED READINGS
available at www.expertconsult.com

RELATED CONTENT
Juvenile Rheumatoid Arthritis (JRA) (Patient Information)

AUTHOR: **ELISABETH B. MATSON, D.O.**

BASIC INFORMATION

DEFINITION

Kaposi's sarcoma (KS) is a vascular neoplasm most frequently occurring in AIDS patients. It can be divided into the following four subsets:
1. Classic KS: most frequently found in elderly Eastern European and Mediterranean males. It consists initially of violaceous macules and papules with subsequent development of plaques and red-purple nodules. Growth is slow, and most of the patients die of unrelated causes.
2. Epidemic or AIDS-related KS: most frequently occurs in homosexual men. Lesions are generally multifocal and widespread. Lymphadenopathy may be associated.
3. Endemic KS: usually affects African children and adults. An aggressive lymphadenopathic form affects African children in particular.
4. Immunosuppression-associated, or transplantation-associated, KS: usually associated with chemotherapy.

SYNONYMS

KS

ICD-9CM CODES
173.9 Malignant neoplasm of the skin

EPIDEMIOLOGY & DEMOGRAPHICS

- AIDS-related KS affects >35% of AIDS cases.
- Highest incidence is in homosexual men.

PHYSICAL FINDINGS & CLINICAL PRESENTATION

- AIDS-related KS: multifocal and widespread red-purple (Fig. E1-470) or dark plaques (Fig. E1-471) and/or nodules on cutaneous or mucosal surfaces (Fig. 1-472).
- Generalized lymphadenopathy at the time of diagnosis is present in >50% of patients with AIDS-related KS; the initial lesions have a rust-colored appearance; subsequent progression to red or purple nodules or plaques occurs.
- Most frequently affected areas are the face, trunk, oral cavity, and upper and lower extremities.

ETIOLOGY

A herpesvirus (HHV-8, KS-associated herpesvirus KSHV) has been isolated from patients with most forms of KS and is believed to be the causative agent. It can be transmitted sexually (homosexual or heterosexual activities) and by other forms of nonsexual contact such as maternal-infant transmission (common in African countries).

DIAGNOSIS

DIFFERENTIAL DIAGNOSIS

- Stasis dermatitis
- Pyogenic granuloma
- Capillary hemangiomas
- Granulation tissue
- Postinflammatory hyperpigmentation
- Cutaneous lymphoma
- Melanoma
- Dermatofibroma
- Hematoma
- Prurigo nodularis

The differential diagnosis of cutaneous lesions in patients with HIV infection is described in Section II.

WORKUP

Diagnosis can generally be made on clinical appearance; tissue biopsy will confirm diagnosis.

LABORATORY TESTS

HIV in patients suspected of AIDS

TREATMENT

NONPHARMACOLOGIC THERAPY

Observation is a reasonable option in patients with slowly progressive disease.

GENERAL Rx

- Excisional biopsy often provides adequate treatment for single lesions and resected recurrences in classic KS.
- Liquid nitrogen cryotherapy can result in complete response in 80% of lesions.
- Interlesional chemotherapy with vinblastine is useful for nodular lesions >1 cm in diameter. Intralesional injection of interferon alfa-2b has also been reported as effective and well tolerated.
- Radiation therapy is effective in non-AIDS KS and for large tumor masses that interfere with normal function.

- Systemic therapy with interferon is also effective in AIDS-related KS and is often used in combination with zidovudine.
- Systemic chemotherapy (vinblastine, bleomycin, doxorubicin, and dacarbazine) can be used for rapidly progressive disease and for classic and African endemic KS.
- Sirolimus (rapamycin), an immunosuppressive drug, is effective in inhibiting the progression of dermal KS in kidney transplant recipients.
- Oral etoposide is also effective and has less myelosuppression than vinblastine.
- Paclitaxel is also effective in patients with advanced KS and represents an excellent second-line therapy.
- Thalidomide, retinoids.

DISPOSITION

- Prognosis is poor in AIDS-related KS. Death is often a result of other AIDS-defining illnesses.
- Prognosis is better in African cutaneous KS and classic sarcoma (patients usually die of unrelated causes).

PEARLS & CONSIDERATIONS

COMMENTS

Immunosuppression-associated KS usually regresses with the cessation, reduction, or modification of immunosuppression therapy in most patients. Similarly, in HIV patients KS responds concurrently with the decrease in serum HIV RNA and increase in the CD4 count.

SUGGESTED READING
available at www.expertconsult.com

RELATED CONTENT

Kaposi Sarcoma (Patient Information)

AUTHOR: **FRED F. FERRI, M.D.**

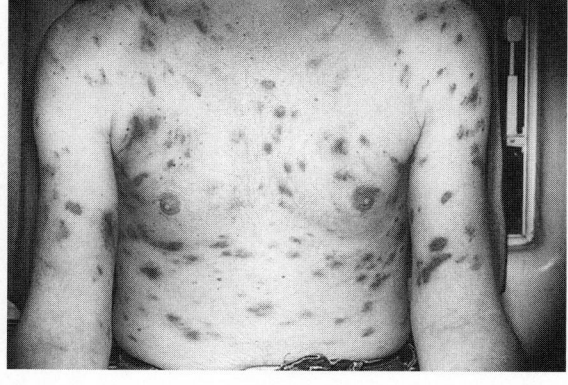

FIGURE 1-472 Kaposi's sarcoma. More advanced lesions. Note widespread hemorrhagic plaques and nodules. (From Noble J [ed]: *Textbook of primary care medicine,* ed 2, St Louis, 1995, Mosby.)

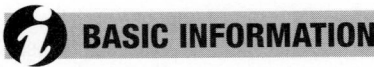

BASIC INFORMATION

DEFINITION

Kawasaki disease (KD) is an acute, febrile vasculitis of small and medium-size blood vessels that predominantly affects children. It is usually a self-limiting condition lasting for an average of 12 days if not treated.

SYNONYMS

Kawasaki syndrome
Mucocutaneous lymph node syndrome
Infantile polyarteritis

ICD-9CM CODES
446.1 Kawasaki disease

EPIDEMIOLOGY & DEMOGRAPHICS

- KD is the leading cause of acquired heart disease in children in developing countries and in the U.S. and Japan.
- Commonly occurs in children <5 yr (80%); peak incidence is in infants aged 9 to 11 mo to 24 mo. Occurrence is rare after late childhood.
- More prevalent in boys than girls (1.5:1).
- The highest incidence is found in Japan (~174 cases/100,000 children).
- Temporal clustering and winter to spring predominance have been observed in KD cases in Japan, supporting an environmental or infectious etiology.
- Incidence of KD in the U.S. is 17 to 18 cases/100,000 children <5 yr.
- Children of Asian descent have the highest incidence of KD compared with those of European or African descent.
- ~4200 new cases are diagnosed each year in the U.S.
- 1% of patients with KD in Japan have a positive family history of KD.
- In the U.S., KD has now surpassed acute rheumatic fever as the leading cause of acquired heart disease in children.

PHYSICAL FINDINGS & CLINICAL PRESENTATION

- The clinical presentations reflect inflammation of small and medium-sized blood vessels. Diagnosis of KD is based on characteristic clinical signs and symptoms and includes fever persisting for >5 days and the presence of at least four of the following five principal features:
  1. Bilateral, painless bulbar conjunctival injection without exudate
  2. Oral mucosal changes: erythema and fissured lips, strawberry tongue (Fig. 1-473, B), diffuse injection of the oropharyngeal mucosae
  3. Polymorphous exanthema (usually in truncal region) (Fig. 1-474, A and B)
  4. Extremity changes: (a) acute: erythema and edema of hands and feet (Fig. 1-473, A); (b) convalescent: membranous desquamation of fingertips
  5. Cervical lymph node enlargement (at least one lymph node >1.5 cm in diameter).
- The fever of KD is mildly responsive to antipyretics and is usually higher than 102.2° F (39° C) and often >104.0° F (40° C). If untreated, it lasts for an average of 12 days.
- The rash of KD can be maculopapular or can take various forms; however, vesicles, bullae, purpura, and petechia are never observed.
- Coronary artery aneurysms can develop in as many as 25% to 30% of untreated children between 1 to 4 weeks of illness. This subset of patients can develop ischemic heart disease, myocardial infarction, and congestive heart failure over time, and, occasionally, death.
- Morbidity and mortality rates are highest if aneurysm diameter is >8 mm.
- Children with KD who are <1 yr or >6 yr are more likely to develop the cardiac sequelae and are least likely to respond to treatment.
- Patients with fever and fewer than four principal symptoms but evidence of coronary artery disease are diagnosed as having atypical or incomplete KD (10%).

- Cervical lymphadenopathy is the most common physical manifestation absent in atypical KD, followed by exanthema and then extremity changes.
- Oral mucosal changes are the most common manifestations of KD affecting approximately 90% of cases (either typical or atypical).
- Patients may also develop sensitivity to light and uveitis along with conjunctival injection.
- On rare occasions aneurysms of peripheral arteries (e.g., axillary) may be seen.
- Redness and induration can be seen at the site of bacille Calmette-Guérin (BCG) inoculation.
- Beau's lines (transverse grooves of the nails), diarrhea, acute myocarditis, cough, rhinorrhea, dyspnea, arthralgia, and myalgia may also be seen.
- Aseptic meningitis can develop in 40% of cases.
- Interstitial nephritis, acute renal failure in rare cases, KD shock syndrome, and macrophage activation syndrome can also occur.

ETIOLOGY

The cause of KD is not known, although evidence suggests an infectious etiology precipitating an immune-mediated reaction in genetically susceptible individuals.

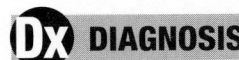 DIAGNOSIS

Diagnosis of KD is made on the basis of clinical features (see "Physical Findings & Clinical Presentation"). The hallmark of KD is fever lasting >5 days. Typically, the clinical signs appear over the course of several days. Laboratory evaluation may be helpful in making the diagnosis in atypical KD. The timely diagnosis and treatment of KD are important in preventing complications.

DIFFERENTIAL DIAGNOSIS

- Scarlet fever
- Stevens-Johnson syndrome
- Drug eruption

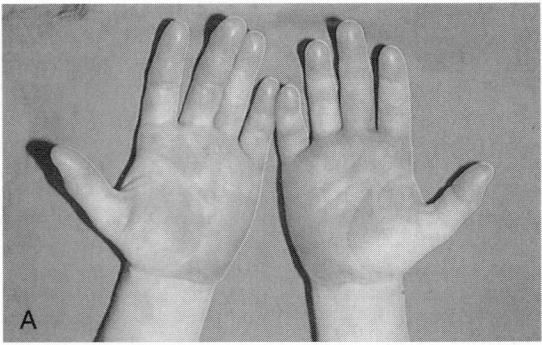 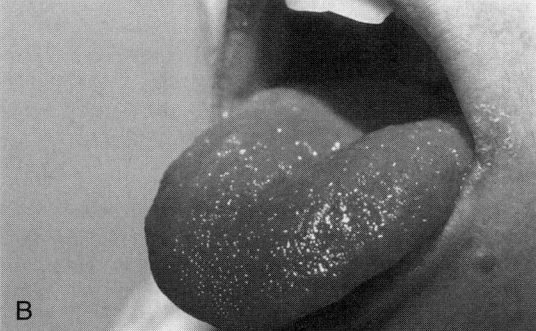

FIGURE 1-473 **A,** Erythema of the hands, to be followed by desquamation. **B,** Strawberry tongue in a patient with Kawasaki disease. (**A** courtesy Department of Dermatology, University of North Carolina at Chapel Hill. In Goldstein B [ed]: *Practical dermatology,* ed 2, St Louis, 1997, Mosby. **B** courtesy Marshall Guill, M.D. In Goldstein B [ed]: *Practical dermatology,* ed 2, St Louis, 1997, Mosby.)

- Henoch-Schönlein purpura
- Toxic shock syndrome
- Measles
- Rocky Mountain spotted fever
- Epstein-Barr virus, adenovirus, echovirus, and enterovirus
- Juvenile rheumatoid arthritis
- Mercury hypersensitivity (acrodynia)
- Leptospirosis

WORKUP

Clinical findings in addition to laboratory and imaging studies are useful in searching for multiorgan system involvement and complications (e.g., cardiac, lung, liver).

LABORATORY TESTS

Inflammatory markers will be increased in KD.
Clinical and laboratory findings observed in patients with this disease are frequently helpful in diagnosis:
- Complete blood count commonly shows a normochromic normocytic anemia, elevated white blood cell count with neutrophil predominance and elevated platelet count, which usually rises by the second week.
- Abnormal liver function tests are found: elevated transaminases (hepatic congestion), elevated bilirubin (gallbladder hydrops), low albumin.
- Elevated erythrocyte sedimentation rate is found (often >40 mm/hr and not uncommonly elevated to levels of >100 mm/hr).
- Hyponatremia is associated with increased risk of coronary aneurysms.

- Elevated C-reactive protein.
- Urinalysis may show sterile pyuria.
- Impaired serum lipid profiles with decreased high-density lipoproteins (HDL) and elevated triglycerides and low-density lipoproteins (LDL) can occur.
- Cerebrospinal fluid (CSF) with increased white cell count without elevated CSF protein is found.

IMAGING STUDIES
- Chest radiograph may reveal pulmonary infiltrates; cardiomegaly may also be present.
- Echocardiogram is recommended at the time of illness, and repeat in 6 wk and 6 mo. Echocardiogram should include careful assessment of the coronary arteries for size and aneurysms, mural or intraluminal thrombi, effusions, valve function, and myocardial function.
- Coronary angiogram, computed tomography angiography, and magnetic resonance angiography can be used to visualize the arterial system and the presence of coronary artery aneurysms. Echocardiography may be able to visualize these aneurysms in infants.
- Intravascular ultrasound can assess for luminal irregularities of the coronary arteries.
- Exercise testing with myocardial perfusion studies can be done to assess for coronary blood flow and the presence of myocardial ischemia.
- ECG changes (arrhythmias, abnormal Q waves, prolonged PR and/or QT intervals, occasionally low voltage, or ST-T wave changes) can be seen.

(Rx) TREATMENT

The goal of treatment of KD in the acute phase is directed at reducing clinical symptoms and reducing inflammation in the systemic and coronary arteries and preventing arterial thrombosis. Long-term therapy in individuals who develop coronary aneurysms is aimed at preventing myocardial ischemia or infarction.

NONPHARMACOLOGIC THERAPY
- Oxygen in selected patients
- Salt restriction in patients with congestive heart failure
- Emollient creams for peeling skin and balms for fissured lips

ACUTE GENERAL Rx
- IV immunoglobulin (IVIG) 2 g/kg over 8 to 12 hr is the treatment of choice in children diagnosed with KD, and ideally should be given within the first 7 to 10 days of the illness.
- Aspirin 80 to 100 mg/kg/day (anti-inflammatory dosing) given in four divided doses until the patient is no longer febrile for 48 hr. Thereafter, aspirin 3 to 5 mg/kg/day (antiplatelet dosing) is continued until laboratory studies (e.g., platelet count, sedimentation rate) return to normal, generally within 6 to 8 wk after disease onset if there are no coronary artery abnormalities or indefinitely if abnormalities are present.
- In patients who do not defervesce within 48 hr or have recrudescent fever after initial IVIG treatment, a second dose of IVIG 2 g/kg IV over 8 to 12 hr should be considered.
- NSAIDs are not effective in the treatment of KD.
- Efficacy of treatment with IVIG along with aspirin is higher than aspirin alone in decreasing risk of coronary artery aneurysms.
- The effect of corticosteroids on coronary artery aneurysms is unclear. Therefore most experts recommend withholding steroids unless fever persists after at least two courses of IVIG. Pulse methyprednisolone at 30 mg/kg daily is given to such patients for 1 to 3 days.
- Other therapies, including urinary trypsin inhibitor (Ulinastatin), pentoxifylline, etanercept, infliximab (monoclonal antibody against tumor necrosis factor-α), plasma exchange, abciximab (platelet glycoprotein IIb/IIIa receptor inhibitor), and immunosuppressive agents (methotrexate, cyclosporine, tacrolimus, anti-thymocyte globulin, cyclophosphamide) have been used, but data are limited on their success.
- Acute coronary thrombosis should be managed with thrombolytic agents under cardiology supervision.
- Most patients with large or giant coronary artery aneurysms (diameter >8 mm) are maintained on aspirin (or clopidogrel) and warfarin to prevent thrombosis within the aneurysm and myocardial infarction.

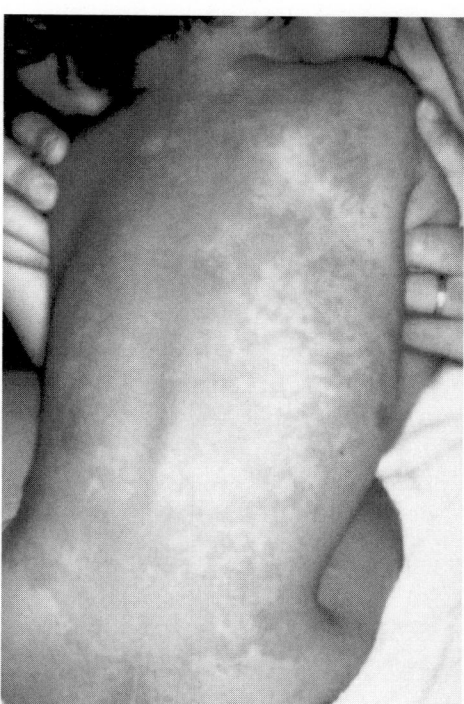 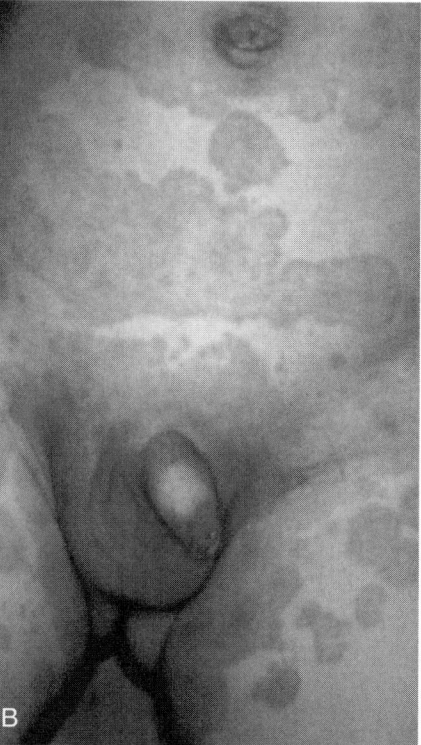

FIGURE 1-474 Clinical manifestations of Kawasaki disease. A and B, Polymorphous exanthema.

CHRONIC Rx

Interventional and surgical procedures can be tried in children who have developed cardiac complications of KD:

- Percutaneous transluminal coronary angioplasty with or without stenting may be performed.
- Coronary bypass graft surgery using the internal mammary artery or the gastroepiploic artery has met with greater patency success than saphenous vein grafts.
- Cardiac transplantation is an option and is indicated in patients with:
  ○ Severe left ventricular failure
  ○ Malignant arrhythmias
  ○ Multivessel coronary artery disease
  For patients with persistent giant (≥8 mm) aneurysms, anticoagulation with warfarin for a goal international normalized ratio of 2.0 to 2.5 should be considered.

DISPOSITION

- Mortality rate of children with KD is 0.5% to 2.8%, usually from coronary aneurysm thrombosis and myocardial infarction.
- Death usually occurs in the third to fourth week of the illness.
- Before the use of IVIG, ~20% of all patients with KD developed coronary artery aneurysms.
- ~ 50% of coronary artery aneurysms return to normal lumen diameter by 1 to 2 yr after onset of illness.
- Treatment with IVIG has reduced the incidence of coronary aneurysms by 80%.
- Aspirin in high dose decreases the coronary artery involvement to <5% from 25%.

- IVIG has also been shown to improve left ventricular function during the acute stages of the disease.
- Risk factors for the development of coronary aneurysms or giant coronary aneurysms 8 mm or greater are:
  ○ Fever lasting >10 days
  ○ Age <1 yr or >6 yr
  ○ Male
  ○ Recurrence of fever
- Recurrence is in about 1% to 3% of cases most commonly within 1 yr of the initial occurrence.
- Aspirin should be discontinued upon exposure to varicella or influenza to decrease the risk of developing Reye's syndrome.

REFERRAL

Multiple specialists may be consulted to assist in the diagnosis of KD, including dermatology, rheumatology, and infectious disease. Cardiology consultation is recommended in any patient with cardiac involvement and in the long-term follow-up of patients with KD.

PEARLS & CONSIDERATIONS

COMMENTS

- KD was first described by Dr. Tomisaku Kawasaki.
- KD is not transmitted from person to person.
- Atypical or incomplete KD can be detected using clinical plus laboratory criteria along with typical findings on echocardiography.
- The mechanism of action of IVIG therapy for KD remains unknown.

- Failure of corticosteroids suggests that the inflammatory response is different compared with other vasculitic conditions.
- Increased risk of atherosclerotic heart disease in adulthood is unclear in patients with history of KD during childhood with normal echocardiographic findings.
- Live vaccine (varicella, measles) administration is suggested to be postponed for 11 mo in children treated with IVIG, since it interferes with vaccine immunogenicity.

PREVENTION

- Without a known etiologic agent for KD, primary prevention is not possible.
- Thrombosis leading to myocardial infarction in a stenotic or aneurysmal coronary artery is the leading cause of death in these children and occurs most often in the first year after illness onset. Therefore serial imaging and stress tests are necessary in patients with significant coronary artery abnormalities (by coronary angiography).

PATIENT & FAMILY EDUCATION

- The Kawasaki Disease Foundation, a nonprofit organization dedicated to KD issues (http://www.kdfoundation.org).
- The American Heart Association has developed guidelines for the diagnosis of KD (http://www.americanheart.org).

SUGGESTED READINGS

available at www.expertconsult.com

RELATED CONTENT

Kawasaki Disease (Patient Information)

AUTHOR: **SYEDA M. SAYEED, M.D.**

ℹ️ BASIC INFORMATION

DESCRIPTION

Keloid may be defined as a benign growth of dense fibrous tissue developing from an abnormal healing response to cutaneous injury, extending beyond the original borders of the wound or inflammatory response (Fig. 1-475).

In 1806, Alibert used the term *cheloide,* derived from the Greek *chele,* or crab's claw, to describe lateral growth of tissue into unaffected skin.

ICD-9CM CODES
701.4 Keloid scar

EPIDEMIOLOGY

- Keloid is seen 5 to 15 times more often in pigmented ethnic groups than in whites.
- Its prevalence is 16% in blacks and Hispanics.
- The highest incidence is seen in the second decade.
- It affects both sexes equally.
- Combined incidence of keloid and hypertrophic scar ranges from 40% to 70% following surgery to up to 91% following burns.

ETIOLOGY

- Wounds from trauma, surgery, or body piercing (Fig. 1-476)
- Burn
- Other injuries such as insect bites, vaccination, folliculitis, or acne
- Rarely can be spontaneous without obvious injury
- Familial predisposition seen in some patients

RISK FACTORS

- Family history of keloids
- Personal history of keloids
- Blacks, Hispanics, and Asians
- Pregnancy

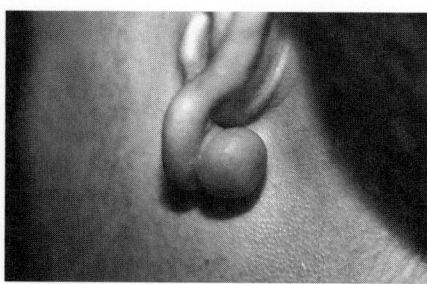

FIGURE 1-475 Keloids. An abnormal reparative reaction to skin injury, keloids are characterized by proliferation of fibroblasts and collagen that extends beyond the margins of the original wound. (From Zitelli BJ, Davis HW: *Atlas of pediatric physical diagnosis,* ed 5, Philadelphia, 2007, Mosby.)

- Puberty
- Patients with blood group A
- Injury over bones

PATHOGENESIS

- Pathophysiology of keloid is not completely understood
- Caused by benign dermal fibroproliferation because of disorder in the regulation of cellularity during the wound healing process

CLINICAL FEATURES

- Keloids usually appear within a few months of the injury, in contrast to the hypertrophic scars, which develop within a few weeks. At times it could take up to a year to appear because the growth is slow.
- Keloids are often symptomatic in the early stages. Common complaints are pruritus, burning, pain, and tenderness.
- Keloids are commonly seen on the shoulders, sternum, upper back, nape of neck, ear lobes, mandibular border, and cheek. Hands and feet are often spared.
- Skin lesions vary from papules to nodules to large tuberous lesions. They have the normal skin color most of the time with well-defined borders. Early on they can appear erythematous, whereas older lesions may be hypo- or hyperpigmented. They can be firm to hard in consistency with smooth surface and are tender to touch. Hair follicles are absent in these keloids.
- Unlike with hypertrophic scar, in keloids the scar extends beyond the margin of the initial wound.

🄳🅇 DIAGNOSIS

- Workup is usually not necessary because it is a clinical diagnosis.
- Biopsy is usually avoided because it may increase the keloid size. When biopsy is done, the histology shows randomly organized large collagen fibers in a dense connective tissue matrix. In fact, both major components of extracellular matrix, collagen and glycosaminoglycans, are increased.

DIFFERENTIAL DIAGNOSIS

- Hypertrophic scar
- Dermatofibroma
- Dermatofibrosarcoma protuberance

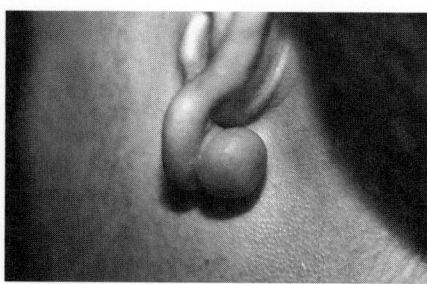

FIGURE 1-476 Keloid of ear lobe after piercing. (From Kliegman RM et al: *Nelson textbook of pediatrics,* Philadelphia, 2011, Saunders.)

- Desmoid tumor
- Foreign body granuloma
- Scar with sarcoidosis
- Lobomycosis

℞ TREATMENT

- There is no universally accepted treatment protocol. Prevention is the best strategy.
- Combination treatment is most effective.
- Surgical excision using cold knife followed by intralesional steroids is the preferred method.
- Treatment outcome is the best when it is initiated shortly after the keloid formation.
- Different treatment options include:
  1. Unlike with hypertrophic scars, **surgery** alone is associated with a 55% to 100% recurrence rate in patients with keloids. Results are significantly better when it is followed by intralesional steroids, radiotherapy, pressure therapy, or silicone application. Both complete and near total excision has been advocated. Few recommend core extirpation. Use of Z-plasties or any wound lengthening techniques is strongly discouraged.
  2. **Intralesional steroid** every 2 to 4 wk is administered either alone or following surgery. Duration of treatment depends on the treatment response. Triamcinolone is the most studied steroid and is used at a concentration of 10 to 40 mg/ml. Higher concentration is used for denser, more calcitrant lesions, and those located in trunks or extremities. It could be used in combination with lidocaine to reduce the discomfort. A 27- to 30-gauge needle is used for its administration. To distribute the suspension evenly, it should be injected while continuously advancing the needle. No more than 20 to 30 mg of the drug is used during each treatment. Liquid nitrogen is applied to the injection briefly for 2 to 4 seconds about 10 to 15 min prior to steroid injection for better dispersal of the steroid and to minimize deposition into surrounding normal tissue. Hypopigmentation, skin atrophy, ulceration, and telangiectasia are the side effects associated with this treatment.
  3. **Cryotherapy** has been used for smaller lesions. When this treatment is chosen, the entire lesion is treated with 2 to 3 freeze-thaw cycles of 30 seconds' duration each. Most lesions need 2 to 10 treatment sessions at 4-wk intervals. Pain and hypopigmentation are the main adverse events.
  4. **Silicone gel sheeting or cushioning** can prevent keloids from recurring after surgery. These are applied as soon as re-epithelialization is achieved and are worn for at least 12 hr/day for 2 to 4 mo.
  5. **Application of pressure** by compression devices has been advocated in the treatment of keloids. These compression treatments include button compression, pressure earrings, pressure gradient garments, ACE bandages, elastic adhesive

K

Diseases and Disorders

I

bandages, compression wraps, Spandex or Elastane bandages, and support bandages. About 24 to 40 mm Hg pressure must be maintained. It must be instituted for long periods (>23 hr/day for 6 to 12 mo) before significant effect can be achieved. Unfortunately, many parts of the body are not amenable to this pressure. Patient discomfort frequently reduces compliance.

6. **Radiation** following surgery can also reduce the recurrence rate. X-rays of 700 to 1500 cGy in fractions over 5 to 6 treatments are the most frequently used treatment. Radiation is usually initiated within 10 days, preferably within 24 hr of surgery. It is avoided in pediatric and pregnant patients. At times brachytherapy with interstitial iridium 192 is used. Most physicians use radiation only for keloids over the extremities. The reported risk of radiation-induced malignancy is theoretical.

7. **5-Fluorouracil** can be used as an individual agent, following surgery, or in combination with intralesional steroids. Weekly injection of 0.5 to 2 ml at a 50 mg/ml concentration of 5-fluorouracil for 12 wk is the recommended dose.

8. Superiority of **laser** use to simple excision currently has not been demonstrated.

9. Topical 5% **imiquimod** cream has some role when used following surgery locally every night for a minimum of 2 mo.

10. Other treatments include Cordran tape, bleomycin, interferon, vitamin A, nitrogen mustard, antihistamines, zinc, tacrolimus, sirolimus, allantoin, botulinum toxin, colchicine, salicylic acid, calcipotriol, NSAIDs, d-penicillamine, relaxin, quercetin, dinoprostone, doxorubicin, ACE inhibitors, hyaluronidase, pentoxifylline, tranilast, mitomycin-C, tamoxifen, silver sulfadiazine, onion extract, vitamin E, intralesional verapamil.

FOLLOW-UP

Because of the high risk of recurrence, a follow-up of at least 12 mo is necessary to fully evaluate the effectiveness of therapy.

PREVENTION

- Avoid nonessential surgery such as body piercing, which carries a high risk for keloid formation.
- LASIK eye surgery and CO_2 laser resurfacing should be avoided in patients with a tendency for keloids.
- Use a laparoscopic approach when surgery is needed.
- Avoid making incisions over joint spaces or over midchest, and ensure that they follow skin creases.
- Handle tissue gently during surgery.
- Ensure good hemostasis intraoperatively.
- Use tension-free primary wound closure.
- Use monofilament, synthetic permanent sutures.
- Use adhesives instead of sutures when possible for closure of wounds.
- Compressive pressure dressing is preferred in high-risk patients following surgery.
- Avoid wound infection.
- Avoid tattoos.
- Aggressively treat inflammatory acnes.

COMPLICATIONS

- Psychological effects secondary to disfigurement.
- Contracture from keloids may result in loss of function if overlying a joint.

PROGNOSIS

- Unlike hypertrophic scars, keloids do not regress with time. However, they may continue to expand in size for decades.
- Regardless of the type of treatment there is a high recurrence rate.
- Keloids never become malignant.

SUGGESTED READINGS
available at www.expertconsult.com

RELATED CONTENT

Keloids (Patient Information)

AUTHOR: **HEMANT K. SAPATHY, M.D.**

BASIC INFORMATION

DEFINITION

Klinefelter's syndrome is a congenital disorder in which a 47,XXY chromosome complement is associated with hypogonadism and infertility.

SYNONYMS

47,XXY Hypogonadism

ICD-9CM CODES
758.7 Klinefelter's syndrome

EPIDEMIOLOGY & DEMOGRAPHICS

INCIDENCE: One in 500 men (most common sex chromosome disorder)
GENETICS: The most common mosaic complement is 46,XY/47,XXY. 47,XXY karyotype 48,XXYY, 48,XXXY, or 49,XXXXY have been reported. The manifestations vary in severity by patient (Table 1-234). This sex chromosome mosaicism is believed to account for the variable presentation. Fertility, although very rare, has been reported in men with Klinefelter's syndrome.

TABLE 1-234 Clinical Features of Klinefelter's Syndrome

Karyotype	47,XXY
Inheritance	Sporadic; associated with advanced maternal age; nondisjunction during first or second meiotic division in either parent (67% maternal, 33% paternal); mitotic nondisjunction
Genitalia	Male
Wolffian duct derivatives	Normal
Müllerian duct derivatives	Absent
Gonads	Small, firm testes; seminiferous tubule dysgenesis; azoospermia; Leydig cell hyperplasia
Habitus	Poor to normal virilization at puberty: gynecomastia; disproportionately long legs
Hormone profile	Testosterone levels variable but usually decreased; increased levels of plasma LH and FSH postpubertally

FSH, Follicle-stimulating hormone; *LH,* luteinizing hormone.
From Larsen PR et al: *Williams textbook of endocrinology,* ed 10, Philadelphia, 2003, Saunders.

PHYSICAL FINDINGS & CLINICAL PRESENTATION

- Classic triad: small firm testes, azoospermia, and gynecomastia
- Prepubertal: small testes; gonadal volume <1.5 ml is a result of loss of germ cells before puberty.
- Postpubertal: gynecomastia (periductal fat growth) with small, firm testes. Exaggerated growth of the lower extremities results in a decreased crown-to-pubis/pubis-to-floor ratio. There are diminished strength, diminished ability to grow a full beard or mustache, and infertility. Decreased intellectual development and antisocial behavior are believed to occur with high frequency.

ETIOLOGY

- Several postulated mechanisms: nondisjunction during meiosis and mitosis and anaphase lag during mitosis or meiosis
- Reason: maternal age
  1. The incidence of Klinefelter's syndrome rises from 0.6% when the maternal age is ≤35 yr to 5.4% when the maternal age is >45 yr.
  2. Of note, the extra X chromosome has a paternal origin as often as a maternal origin.

DIAGNOSIS

- Markedly elevated follicle-stimulating hormone levels.
- Total plasma testosterone levels are decreased in 50% to 60% of patients.
- Free testosterone levels are decreased.
- Plasma estradiol is increased, stimulating the increase in levels of testosterone-binding globulin with resultant decrease in the testosterone/estradiol ratio, which is believed to be the cause of gynecomastia.

LABORATORY TESTS

- Normal to low serum testosterone.
- Increased sex hormone–binding globulin (acts to further suppress any available free testosterone).
- Normal to increased estradiol (a result of augmented peripheral conversion of testosterone to estradiol).
- Testis biopsy shows azoospermia, Leydig cell hyperplasia, hyalinization, and fibrosis of the seminiferous tubules. Mosaics may have focal areas of spermatogenesis and, on rare occasions, a sperm may appear in the ejaculate. The extra X chromosome is the pivotal factor controlling spermatogenesis and also affects neuronal function directly, leading to the behavioral abnormalities related to decreased IQ.

- Buccal smear: one sex chromatin body
- Prepubertal male: Gonadotropin levels are normal.
- Postpubertal male: Gonadotropin levels are elevated even when the testosterone level is normal.
- Disease associations:
  - Malignancies: breast cancer (20 times greater than XY men and 20% the rate of occurrence in women), nonlymphocytic leukemia, lymphomas, marrow dysplastic syndromes, extragonadal germ cell neoplasms
  - Autoimmune disorders: chronic lymphocytic thyroiditis, Takayasu arteritis, taurodontism (enlarged molar teeth), mitral valve prolapse, varicose veins, asthma, bronchitis, osteoporosis, abnormal glucose tolerance testing, diabetes, varicose veins

TREATMENT

- Revolves around three facets of Klinefelter's syndrome:
  1. Hypogonadism: androgen replacement in the form of testosterone
  2. Gynecomastia: cosmetic surgery
  3. Psychosocial problems: androgen therapy and educational support
- After extensive genetic counseling, intracytoplasmic sperm insertion has been used to treat infertility with limited success in mosaic men.

PEARLS & CONSIDERATIONS

COMMENTS

- Androgen therapy should not be used in the case of severe mental retardation.
- Rule out breast and prostate cancer before initiating or continuing androgen therapy.
- Androgen therapy will not improve fertility; it may suppress any spermatogenesis that is taking place within the testes.
- Other causes of primary hypogonadism:
  1. Myotonic muscular dystrophy
  2. Sertoli cell–only syndrome
  3. Kartagener's syndrome
  4. Anorchia
  5. Acquired hypogonadism

SUGGESTED READINGS
available at www.expertconsult.com

RELATED CONTENT
Klinefelter's Syndrome (Patient Information)

AUTHORS: **PHILIP J. ALIOTTA, M.D., M.S.H.A.,** and **RUBEN ALVERO, M.D.**

BASIC INFORMATION

DEFINITION

Labyrinthitis is a peripheral vestibulopathy characterized by acute onset of vertigo usually associated with nausea and vomiting. It may be associated with hearing loss. It may be either serous or purulent.

SYNONYMS

Acute labyrinthitis
Acute vestibular neuronopathy
Vestibular neuronitis
Viral neurolabyrinthitis

ICD-9CM CODES
386.12 Vestibular neuronitis (active and recurrent)
386.3   Labyrinthitis

EPIDEMIOLOGY & DEMOGRAPHICS

INCIDENCE (IN U.S.): Most common cause of prolonged spontaneous vertigo associated with nausea at any age
PREDOMINANT AGE: Any

CLINICAL PRESENTATION

- Vertigo, nausea, and vomiting with onset over several hours.
- Symptoms usually peak within 24 hr, then resolve gradually over several weeks.
- During the first day, the patient usually has difficulty focusing the eyes because of spontaneous nystagmus.
- Usually has benign course, with complete recovery within 1 to 3 mo, although older patients may have intractable dizziness that persists for many months.

PHYSICAL FINDINGS

- Nystagmus
- Nausea
- Vomiting
- Vertigo worsening with head movement
- Abnormal caloric ENG tests
- May have hearing loss in the affected ear
- Normal otoscopic exam typically
- Normal neurologic exam; may have signs of vestibular loss, such as a positive head thrust test

ETIOLOGY

Symptoms often preceded for 1 to 2 wk by a viral-like illness. It may be either bacterial or viral, and be either tympanogenic (i.e., resulting from spread of infection into the inner ear from the middle ear, antrum, or petrous apex), meningogenic, or hematogenic from encephalitis or brain abscess. The round window membrane is considered the most likely pathway of inflammatory mediators from the middle to the inner ear that subsequently give rise to labyrinthitis.

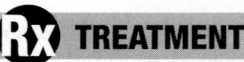

DIAGNOSIS

DIFFERENTIAL DIAGNOSIS

- Acute labyrinthine ischemia (vascular insufficiency)
- Other forms of labyrinthitis (bacterial and syphilitic)
- Labyrinthine fistula
- Benign positional vertigo
- Meniere's syndrome
- Cholesteatoma
- Drug induced
- Eighth nerve tumor
- Head trauma
- Vertebrobasilar stroke

WORKUP

- Otoscopic examination
- Neurologic examination, with close attention to cranial nerves
- Bedside test of vestibular function, that is, head thrust or head heave test
- Audiogram if symptoms accompanied by hearing loss
- Caloric test if presentation is atypical

LABORATORY TESTS

- Routine laboratory tests are generally not helpful.
- If there is a history of significant emesis, check electrolytes, BUN, and creatinine.

IMAGING STUDIES

- Imaging studies are usually not necessary.
- Contrasted MRI may show enhancement of bony labyrinth. MRI of the brain with and without contrast with fine cuts through the internal auditory canal is indicated if there is an abnormal cranial nerve exam or suspicion of eighth nerve tumor.

- Head CT with fine cuts through temporal bones is indicated if there is a history of trauma or suspicion of cholesteatoma.

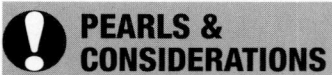

TREATMENT

NONPHARMACOLOGIC THERAPY

- Reassurance.
- Initial bed rest, then encourage increase in activity as tolerated.

ACUTE GENERAL Rx

- Phenergan or other antiemetics are typically effective.
- Vestibular suppressant: meclizine 12.5 to 25 mg qid is often used. Scopolamine patch is also effective.
- Methylprednisolone 100 mg per day for 3 days, with slow taper over 3 wk.
- Valacyclovir has not been shown to be helpful.

CHRONIC Rx

No specific chronic therapy

DISPOSITION

Usually does not require hospital admission unless the patient is unable to tolerate oral intake of liquids.

REFERRAL

- Refer if symptoms persist or neurologic abnormalities are present.
- Consider vestibular rehabilitation, particularly in the elderly.

PEARLS & CONSIDERATIONS

COMMENTS

Labyrinthitis is a term that usually implies peripheral vestibulopathy associated with hearing loss. The term vestibular neuronitis is typically used when hearing is not affected. Despite this technical distinction, many physicians use these terms interchangeably.

SUGGESTED READINGS
available at www.expertconsult.com

RELATED CONTENT
Labyrinthitis (Patient Information)

AUTHOR: **SHARON S. HARTMAN POLENSEK, M.D., PH.D.**

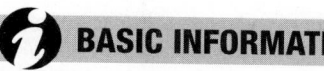

BASIC INFORMATION

DEFINITION

Lactose intolerance is the insufficient concentration of lactase enzyme, leading to fermentation of malabsorbed lactose by intestinal bacteria with subsequent production of intestinal gas and various organic acids, manifesting clinically with diarrhea, abdominal pain, flatulence, or bloating after lactose intolerance. *Lactose malabsorption* occurs when a substantial amount of lactose is not absorbed in the intestine. *Lactase deficiency* is defined as brush-border lactase activity that is markedly reduced relative to the activity observed in infants.

SYNONYMS

Lactase deficiency
Milk intolerance

ICD-9CM CODES

271.3 Lactose intolerance

EPIDEMIOLOGY & DEMOGRAPHICS

Nearly 50 million people in the United States have partial or complete lactose intolerance. There are racial differences, with <25% of white adults being lactose intolerant but >85% of Asian Americans and >60% of African Americans having some form of lactose intolerance.

PHYSICAL FINDINGS & CLINICAL PRESENTATION

- Abdominal tenderness and cramping, bloating, flatulence
- Diarrhea
- Symptoms are directly related to the osmotic pressure of substrate in the colon and occur approximately 2 hr after ingestion of lactose
- Physical examination: may be entirely within normal limits

ETIOLOGY

- Congenital lactase deficiency: common in premature infants; rare in term infants and generally inherited as a chromosomal recessive trait
- Secondary lactose intolerance: usually a result of injury of the intestinal mucosa (Crohn's disease, viral gastroenteritis, AIDS enteropathy, cryptosporidiosis, Whipple's disease, sprue)

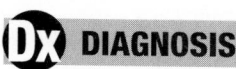

DIAGNOSIS

DIFFERENTIAL DIAGNOSIS

- Inflammatory bowel disease
- Irritable bowel syndrome
- Pancreatic insufficiency
- Nontropical and tropical sprue
- Cystic fibrosis
- Diverticular disease
- Bowel neoplasm
- Laxative abuse
- Celiac disease
- Parasitic disease (e.g., giardiasis)
- Viral or bacterial infections

WORKUP

- The diagnosis can usually be made on the basis of the history and improvement with dietary manipulation.
- Diagnostic workup may include confirming the diagnosis with hydrogen breath test and excluding other conditions listed in the differential diagnosis that may also coexist with lactase deficiency.

LABORATORY TESTS

- Lactose breath hydrogen test: a rise in breath hydrogen >20 ppm within 90 min of ingestion of 50 g of lactose is positive for lactase deficiency. This test is positive in 90% of patients with lactose malabsorption. Common causes of false-negative results are recent use of oral antibiotics or recent high colonic enema.
- The lactose tolerance test is an older and less accurate testing modality (20% rate of false-positive and false-negative results). The patient is administered an oral dose of 1 to 1.5 g of lactose/kg body weight. Serial measurement of blood glucose level on an hourly basis for 3 hr is then performed. The test is considered positive if the patient develops intestinal symptoms and the blood glucose level rises <20 mg/dl above the fasting baseline level.
- Diarrhea associated with lactase deficiency is osmotic in nature with an osmotic gap and a pH <6.5.

IMAGING STUDIES

Imaging studies are generally not indicated. A small bowel series may be useful in patients with significant malabsorption.

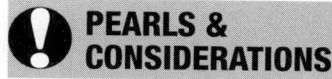

TREATMENT

NONPHARMACOLOGIC THERAPY

Management consists of reducing lactose exposure by avoiding milk and milk-containing products or using milk in which the lactose has been prehydrolized with lactase. A lactose-free diet generally results in prompt resolution of symptoms. Lactose is primarily found in dairy products but may be present as an ingredient or component of common foods and beverages. Possible sources of lactose include breads, candies, cold cuts, dessert mixes, cream soups, bologna, commercial sauces and gravies, chocolate, drink mixes, salad dressings, and medications. Labels should be read carefully to identify sources of lactose.

ACUTE GENERAL Rx

- Addition of lactase enzyme supplement (Lactaid tablets, Dairy Ease) before the ingestion of milk products may prevent symptoms in some patients. However, it is not effective for all lactose-intolerant patients.
- Lactose-intolerant patients must ensure adequate calcium intake. Calcium supplementation is recommended to prevent osteoporosis.

CHRONIC Rx

Patient education regarding foods high in lactose, such as milk, cottage cheese, or ice cream, is recommended.

DISPOSITION

Clinical improvement with restriction or elimination of milk products

REFERRAL

GI referral for endoscopic procedures if concomitant GI disorders are suspected

PEARLS & CONSIDERATIONS

COMMENTS

- There is great variability in signs and symptoms in patients with lactose intolerance depending on the degree of lactase deficiency. Most individuals with presumed lactose malabsorption can tolerate 12 to 15 g of lactose or up to 12 oz of milk daily without symptoms.
- Nondairy synthetic drinks (e.g., Coffee-Mate) and use of rice milk are well tolerated.

SUGGESTED READINGS

available at www.expertconsult.com

RELATED CONTENT

Lactose Intolerance (Patient Information)

AUTHOR: **FRED F. FERRI, M.D.**

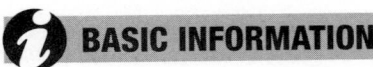

BASIC INFORMATION

DEFINITION

Lambert-Eaton myasthenic syndrome (LEMS) is a disorder of neuromuscular transmission caused by antibodies directed against presynaptic voltage-gated P/Q calcium channels on motor and autonomic nerve terminals. There are two forms: paraneoplastic (most common) and nonparaneoplastic (autoimmune).

SYNONYMS

Eaton-Lambert syndrome

ICD-9CM CODES
199.1 Malignant neoplasm without specification of site, other

EPIDEMIOLOGY & DEMOGRAPHICS

INCIDENCE (IN U.S.): Uncertain; estimated at five cases per 1 million persons annually
PEAK INCIDENCE: Sixth decade
PREVALENCE (IN U.S.): Uncertain; estimated at one per 1,000,000. Up to 3% of small cell lung cancer (SCLC) patients are estimated to develop LEMS.
PREDOMINANT SEX: Male/female ratio of 2:1 in older series. Current series suggest equal frequency between men and women.

PHYSICAL FINDINGS & CLINICAL PRESENTATION

- Weakness with diminished or absent muscle stretch reflexes
- Proximal lower extremity muscles affected most
- Ocular and bulbar muscles less commonly affected
- Transient strength improvement with brief exercise
- Reflexes may be facilitated by repeatedly tapping the tendon or after brief exercise
- Autonomic dysfunction common (dry mouth in 75%, sexual dysfunction, blurred vision, constipation, orthostasis, etc.)

ETIOLOGY

- Antibodies directed against presynaptic voltage-gated P/Q calcium channels are present in most patients (>75% of paraneoplastic and >50% autoimmune cases). The reduction in calcium influx causes a reduction in presynaptic acetylcholine release at motor and autonomic nerve terminals.
- Paraneoplastic forms, usually associated with SCLC, account for 50% to 70% of patients.
- Autoimmune forms, usually in patients with other autoimmune diseases, account for 10% to 30% of patients.

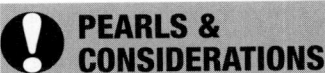

DIAGNOSIS

DIFFERENTIAL DIAGNOSIS

- Myasthenia gravis
- Polymyositis
- Primary myopathies
- Carcinomatous myopathies
- Polymyalgia rheumatica
- Botulism
- Guillain-Barré syndrome

Section II describes the differential diagnosis of muscle weakness.

WORKUP

Confirm diagnosis by characteristic electrodiagnostic (EMG/NCS) findings: reduced motor amplitudes with normal sensory studies; >10% decrement in motor amplitudes on slow repetitive nerve stimulation (RNS) at 2 to 5 Hz, with >100% increment on fast RNS (20 to 50 Hz) or immediately after 10 sec of maximum exercise (postexercise facilitation).

LABORATORY TESTS

Check P/Q calcium channel antibody titers (commercially available).

IMAGING STUDIES

Screen for an underlying malignancy: CT chest, bronchoscopy, or PET scan should be considered. Presentation with LEMS may precede diagnosis of SCLC by up to 5 yr. Chest radiograph or CT of the chest may be required every 6 to 12 mo for SCLC.

TREATMENT

NONPHARMACOLOGIC THERAPY

Symptomatic treatment for autonomic dysfunction.

ACUTE GENERAL Rx

- Anticholinesterase agents (pyridostigmine 30 to 60 mg q4-6h) may yield some improvement.
- Guanidine hydrochloride: start 5 to 10 mg/kg/day up to 30 mg/kg/day in 3-day intervals.
- Plasma exchange (200 to 250 ml/kg over 10 to 14 days) or IV immunoglobulins (2 g/kg divided over 2 to 5 days) often produce significant, temporary improvement.
- Prednisone 1.0 to 1.5 mg/kg/day can be gradually tapered over months to minimal effective dose.

- Azathioprine can be given alone or in combination with prednisone. Give up to 2.5 mg/kg/day. If patient is intolerant, can administer cyclosporine up to 3 mg/kg/day instead.
- 3,4-Diaminopyridine (3,4-DAP) 10 to 20 mg PO qid (maximum of 100 mg/day) may improve muscle strength and reduce autonomic symptoms in up to 85% of patients in uncontrolled series. It is available in Europe and may be available in the U.S. on a compassionate use basis.

CHRONIC Rx

Treat underlying malignancy if present.

DISPOSITION

- Gradually progressive weakness leading to impaired mobility if untreated
- Clinical remission may occur with chronic immunosuppressive therapy in 43% of cases
- Possible substantial improvement with successful treatment of underlying malignancy

REFERRAL

To a neurologist (recommended) because of the infrequency of this disease and risks associated with some treatments. Referral to specialist centers for 3,4-DAP therapy may be warranted in the U.S. Surgical referral for tumor debulking in paraneoplastic forms necessary.

PEARLS & CONSIDERATIONS

COMMENTS

- Prominent autonomic symptoms (dry eyes, dry mouth, impotence, orthostasis) are often the clue to the diagnosis in the appropriate clinical context.
- Many drugs may worsen weakness and should be used only if absolutely necessary. Included are succinylcholine, d-tubocurarine, quinine, quinidine, procainamide, aminoglycoside antibiotics, β-blockers, and calcium channel blockers.

SUGGESTED READINGS

available at www.expertconsult.com

AUTHOR: **EROBOGHENE E. UBOGU, M.D.**

L

Diseases and Disorders

I

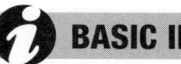 **BASIC INFORMATION**

DEFINITION

Laryngeal carcinoma is cancer of the larynx, including the vocal cords (glottis), supraglottis, and subglottis.

SYNONYMS

Laryngeal cancer
Head and neck cancer (subsite); other sites include oral cavity, pharynx, paranasal sinus, and salivary glands

ICD-9CM CODES
231.0 Carcinoma of larynx

EPIDEMIOLOGY & DEMOGRAPHICS

INCIDENCE: 12,000 new cases per year in the U.S.
PEAK INCIDENCE: Sixth decade
PREDOMINANT SEX: 80% male predominance (current, with past and projected increase in female rates as a result of changing smoking habits)

PHYSICAL FINDINGS & CLINICAL PRESENTATION

- Glottis: Early diagnosis possible because of voice change (hoarseness). Any voice change of more than 2-wk duration should prompt a laryngeal examination.
- Supraglottis:
  1. No early symptom
  2. Cervical lymphadenopathy
  3. Neck pain or ear pain
  4. Discomfort during swallowing
  5. Odynophagia
  6. Later: hoarseness, dysphagia, airway obstruction
- Subglottis: Even more subtle than supraglottic lesion; the same signs occur, only later in the course.

ETIOLOGY

- Smoking (cigarette, cigar, or pipe)
- Alcohol intake/abuse
- Diet and nutritional deficiencies
- Gastroesophageal reflux
- Voice abuse
- Chronic laryngitis
- Exposure to wood dust
- Asbestosis
- Exposure to radiation
- Possible role of human papillomavirus

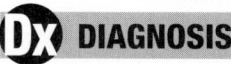 **DIAGNOSIS**

DIFFERENTIAL DIAGNOSIS

- Laryngitis
- Allergic and nonallergic rhinosinusitis
- Gastroesophageal reflux
- Voice abuse leading to hoarseness
- Laryngeal papilloma

- Vocal cord paralysis attributable to a neurologic condition or entrapment of the recurrent laryngeal nerve caused by mediastinal compression
- Tracheomalacia

STAGING:

Supraglottic:
  T_1: Tumor limited to one subsite with normal cord mobility
  T_2: Tumor invades mucosa of more than one subsite (e.g., base of tongue, vallecula, pyriform sinus) without fixation of larynx
  T_3: Tumor limited to larynx with vocal cord fixation or invasion of postcricoid area or preepiglottis
  T_4: Tumor invades thyroid cartilage or extends into soft tissue of the neck, thyroid, or esophagus

Glottic:
  T_1: Tumor limited to vocal cord with normal mobility
  T_{1a}: Tumor limited to one vocal cord
  T_{1b}: Tumor involves both vocal cords
  T_2: Tumor extends to supra- or subglottis or impairs cord mobility
  T_3: Tumor limited to larynx with cord fixation
  T_4: Tumor invades through cartilage or other tissues beyond larynx

Stage grouping:
  Stage I (one anatomic site within the larynx): T_1, N0, M0
  Stage II (one anatomic region within the larynx): T_2, N0, M0
  Stage III (extending beyond one anatomic region but confined to the larynx): T_3, N0, M0
  T_1, T_2, T_3, N1, M0
  Stage IV (distant metastasis): T_4, N0, N1, M0
  Any T, N2, N3, M0
  Any T, any N or M >0

WORKUP

- Laboratory: none
- Endoscopic laryngeal inspection
- After (and only after) diagnosis of the malignancy, imaging with CT or MRI should be undertaken to stage the disease

HISTOLOGIC CLASSIFICATION

Epithelial cancers:
- Squamous cell carcinoma in situ
- Superficially invasive cancer
- Verrucous carcinoma
- Pseudosarcoma
- Anaplastic cancer
- Transitional cell carcinoma
- Lymphoepithelial cancer
- Adenocarcinoma
- Neuroendocrine tumors, including small cell and carcinoid

Sarcomas:
- Metastatic malignancies

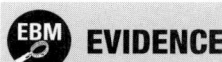 **TREATMENT**

ACUTE GENERAL Rx

- Early stage (T or T_2) has two options:
  1. Conservative surgery (partial laryngectomy) with neck dissection
  2. Primary radiation
- Intermediate stage has four options:
  1. Primary radiation alone
  2. Supraglottic laryngectomy with neck dissection
  3. Supraglottic laryngectomy with postoperative radiation
  4. Chemotherapy with radiation
- Advanced stage:
  1. Chemotherapy and radiation with total laryngectomy reserved for treatment failure

Glottis:
- Carcinoma in situ
  1. Microexcision
  2. Laser vaporization
  3. Radiation
- Early stage (T or T_2) has two options:
  1. Voice conservation surgery
  2. Radiation
- Intermediate stage (T_3)
  1. Combined radiation and chemotherapy (cisplatin and 5-fluorouracil)
  2. Total laryngectomy for treatment failure
- Advanced stage (T_4)
  1. Combined radiation and chemotherapy
  2. Total laryngectomy and neck dissection followed by postoperative radiation in unfavorable lesion or treatment failure

Subglottis:
- Total laryngectomy and approximate neck surgery to excise the tumor, followed by radiation

Unresected cancers:
- Induction chemotherapy and radiation followed by neck dissection in chemosensitive tumors, or by laryngectomy and neck dissection in chemoresistant tumors
- If hypopharyngeal involvement exists: laryngopharyngectomy, neck dissection, and postoperative radiation

DISPOSITION

Supraglottis 5-yr control:
- T_1: 95% to 100%
- T_2: 80% to 90%
- T_3: 65% to 85%
- T_4: 40% to 55%

Glottis 5-yr control:
- T_1: 95% to 100%
- T_2: 50% to 85%
- T_3: 35% to 85%
- T_4: 20% to 65%

EBM **EVIDENCE**

available at www.expertconsult.com

RELATED CONTENT

Laryngeal Cancer (Patient Information)

AUTHOR: **FRED F. FERRI, M.D.**

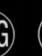

BASIC INFORMATION

DEFINITION
Laryngitis is an acute or chronic inflammation of the laryngeal mucous membranes.

SYNONYMS
Lower respiratory tract infection

ICD-9CM CODES
464.0 Acute laryngitis
476.0 Chronic laryngitis

EPIDEMIOLOGY & DEMOGRAPHICS
It is a common illness in both genders and all age groups, but the diagnosis is imprecise and, therefore, statistics are not readily available with respect to incidence and prevalence.

PHYSICAL FINDINGS & CLINICAL PRESENTATION
ACUTE LARYNGITIS:
- Clinical syndrome characterized by the onset of hoarseness, voice breaks, or episodes of aphonia; may also have accompanying sore throat, cough, nasal congestion, and rhinorrhea
- Usually associated with viral upper respiratory infection
- Larynx with diffuse erythema, edema, and vascular engorgement of the vocal folds, and occasionally mucosal ulceration
- In young children subglottis is often affected, resulting in airway narrowing with marked hoarseness, inspiratory stridor, dyspnea, and restlessness
- Respiratory compromise rare in adults

CHRONIC LARYNGITIS: Characterized by hoarseness or dysphonia persisting for longer than 2 wk

ETIOLOGY
ACUTE LARYNGITIS:
- Most often caused by viruses so treatment consists of supportive measures as outlined in "Nonpharmacologic Therapy" section.
- Studies evaluating the use of antibiotics (erythromycin, penicillin) in acute laryngitis failed to show objective clinical benefit over placebo so they are not routinely recommended. Antibiotics and other antimicrobials may be indicated in cases in which specific treatable pathogens are identified.
- Avoid decongestants because of their drying effect.
- Guaifenesin may be a useful adjunct as a mucolytic agent.

- In gastroesophageal reflux disease (GERD)-associated laryngitis use acid-suppressive therapy (H_2 blockers, proton pump inhibitors) and nocturnal antireflux precautions.

CHRONIC LARYNGITIS:
- Results from any of the following: tuberculosis, usually through bronchogenic spread; leprosy, from nasopharyngeal or oropharyngeal spread; syphilis, in secondary and tertiary stages; rhinoscleroma, extending from the nose and nasopharynx; actinomycosis; cryptococcosis; histoplasmosis; blastomycosis; paracoccidiomycosis; coccidiosis; candidiasis; aspergillosis; sporotrichosis; rhinosporidiosis; parasitic infections including leishmaniasis and *Clinostomum* infection following raw fresh-water fish ingestion.
- Noninfectious causes of both acute and chronic laryngitis include malignancy, voice abuse (singers), GERD, and chemical or environmental irritants such as cigarettes and allergens. Other causes of inflammatory or granulomatous lesions of the larynx include relapsing polychondritis, Wegener's granulomatosis, and sarcoidosis.

DIAGNOSIS

DIFFERENTIAL DIAGNOSIS
- Young children with signs of airway obstruction:
  - Supraglottitis (epiglottitis)
  - Laryngotracheobronchitis
  - Tracheitis
  - Foreign body aspiration
- Adults with persistent hoarseness, consider noninfectious causes of laryngitis as listed previously

WORKUP
- History and physical examination: diagnosis is usually apparent.
- Laryngoscopy for severe or persistent cases.
- Laryngeal cultures should be performed if a cause other than acute viral infection is suspected.
- Imaging not indicated unless there is evidence of airway compromise. Obtain plain radiographs of neck, anteroposterior and lateral views, to differentiate laryngitis from acute laryngotracheobronchitis or supraglottitis.

TREATMENT

NONPHARMACOLOGIC THERAPY
- Rest the voice.
- Use an air humidifier.

- Ensure adequate hydration. Avoid alcohol and caffeine because of diuretic effect.

ACUTE GENERAL Rx
- Antibiotics and other antimicrobials should generally not be used. They are indicated only when a specific pathogen is isolated; commonly employed antibacterial agents are macrolides; clarithromycin 500 mg by mouth bid for 5 to 7 days or azithromycin 500 mg followed by 250 mg once daily for 4 to 5 days if the cause of laryngitis is found to be *Mycoplasma pneumoniae* or *Chlamydiophila pneumoniae* (the new name for what was formerly known as *Chlamydia pneumoniae*).
- Avoid decongestants because of their drying effect.
- Guaifenesin may be a useful adjunct as a mucolytic agent.
- In GERD-associated laryngitis use acid-suppressive therapy (H_2 blockers, proton pump inhibitors) and nocturnal antireflux precautions.

DISPOSITION
Uncomplicated laryngitis is usually benign, with gradual resolution of symptoms.

REFERRAL
- If symptoms persist for >2 wk, refer to otolaryngologist for laryngoscopy.
- Consider referral to gastroenterologist if GERD is suspected.

PEARLS & CONSIDERATIONS

- Most cases of uncomplicated acute laryngitis are viral in origin, and antibacterial agents should not be routinely administered.
- A recent Cochrane analysis found no evidence for the use of empiric antibiotics in adults with laryngitis.
- The most difficult clinical challenge is often convincing patients with acute laryngitis that they do not need and will not benefit from antibacterial agents.

SUGGESTED READINGS
available at www.expertconsult.com

RELATED CONTENT
Laryngitis (Patient Information)

AUTHOR: **GLENN G. FORT, M.D., M.P.H.**

BASIC INFORMATION

DEFINITION

Acute laryngotracheobronchitis is a viral infection of the upper and lower respiratory tract leading to erythema and edema of the tracheal walls and narrowing of the subglottic region.

SYNONYMS

Croup

ICD-9CM CODES
464.4 Croup

EPIDEMIOLOGY & DEMOGRAPHICS

- Croup is primarily a disease of children occurring between the ages of 1 and 6 yr.
- The peak incidence of croup is the second yr of life (50 cases/1000 children).
- Most cases occur in the fall and represent parainfluenza type 1 viral infection.
- Winter outbreaks usually represent infection by influenza A and B viruses.
- Croup accounts for 10% to 15% of lower respiratory tract infections in young children.
- Boys are affected more often than girls.

PHYSICAL FINDINGS & CLINICAL PRESENTATION

Most children with croup present with symptoms of an upper respiratory infection for several days.
- Rhinorrhea
- Cough
- Low-grade fever
- Barking cough that usually occurs at night and awakens the child
- Sore throat
- Stridor
- Apprehension
- Use of accessory muscles of respiration
- Tachypnea
- Tachycardia
- Wheezing

ETIOLOGY

- Parainfluenza viruses (types 1, 2, and 3) are the most common causes of croup in the U.S.
- Influenza A and B, although not common causes of croup, do lead to more severe cases of the disease.
- Adenovirus.
- Respiratory syncytial virus.
- *Mycoplasma pneumoniae* (rare).

DIAGNOSIS

The diagnosis of croup is usually based on the characteristic clinical presentation of a young child between the ages of 1 and 6 yr waking up with a barking cough ("seal's bark") and stridor.

DIFFERENTIAL DIAGNOSIS

- Spasmodic croup
- Epiglottitis
- Bacterial tracheitis
- Angioneurotic edema
- Diphtheria
- Peritonsillar abscess
- Retropharyngeal abscess
- Smoke inhalation
- Foreign body

WORKUP

- The workup of a child with croup is to differentiate viral laryngotracheobronchitis from noninfectious causes of stridor, bacterial tracheitis, and epiglottitis caused by *H. influenzae* (Table E1-235).
- The clinical presentation and plain films of the soft tissues of the neck assist in differentiating viral from nonviral and noninfectious causes.

LABORATORY TESTS

- Laboratory tests are not often used to make the diagnosis of viral tracheobronchitis.
- CBC, viral serology, and tissue cultures can be ordered and may detect the infecting agent in up to 65% of cases.
- Pulse oximetry and ABG determination for patients with tachypnea and respiratory distress.

IMAGING STUDIES

- Plain (AP and lateral) films of the soft tissues of the neck (Fig. E1-477) may show the classic radiographic finding of subglottic stenosis or "steeple" sign.
- CT scan of the soft tissues of the neck may be performed in cases in which the differentiation between croup, epiglottitis, and noninfectious causes is more difficult.
- Direct visualization via laryngoscopy may be useful in some situations under a controlled setting.

TREATMENT

Treatment of croup focuses on airway management.

NONPHARMACOLOGIC THERAPY

- Oxygen
- Cool mist
- Hot steam

ACUTE GENERAL Rx

- 0.25 to 0.75 ml of 2.25% racemic epinephrine every 20 min is used in children with severe respiratory symptoms, rest stridor, and impending intubation.
- Corticosteroids (e.g., dexamethasone 0.6 mg/kg IV or PO, prednisone 2 mg/kg/day) have been shown to be effective.
- Budesonide, a nebulized corticosteroid given at 4 mg, has been shown to improve symptoms in patients with moderate to severe croup.

DISPOSITION

- Croup is usually benign and self-limited, resolving within 3 to 4 days.
- Complications include:
  1. Airway obstruction
  2. Otitis media
  3. Pneumonia
  4. Dehydration

REFERRAL

If intubation is needed (rarely), an emergency consultation with ENT and/or anesthesiology is recommended.

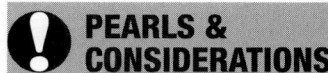

PEARLS & CONSIDERATIONS

COMMENTS

- Most patients with croup can be managed at home (e.g., patients without stridor and in no respiratory distress).
- Hospitalization and observation are required for children with moderate to severe croup (e.g., rest stridor, respiratory distress refractory to the previously mentioned acute treatments).

SUGGESTED READING
available at www.expertconsult.com

RELATED CONTENT

Croup (Patient Information)

AUTHOR: **GLENN G. FORT, M.D., M.P.H.**

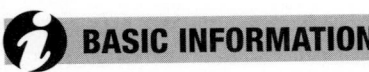

BASIC INFORMATION

DEFINITION

Lead is a potent, pervasive neurotoxicant. Lead poisoning refers to multisystem abnormalities resulting from excessive lead exposure.

SYNONYMS

Plumbism

ICD-9CM CODES
984.0 Lead poisoning

EPIDEMIOLOGY & DEMOGRAPHICS

- Lead poisoning is most common in children ages 1 to 5 yr (17,000 cases/100,000 persons). The highest rates are among blacks, those with low income, and urban children.
- In 1991 the Centers for Disease Control and Prevention (CDC) lowered the definition of a safe blood lead level to <10 mcg/dl of whole blood (a blood lead level of 25 mcg/dl was considered acceptable before 1991).
- It is estimated that >15% of preschoolers in the U.S. have a blood lead level >15 mcg/dl.

PHYSICAL FINDINGS & CLINICAL PRESENTATION

- Findings vary with the degree of toxicity. Examination may be normal in patients with mild toxicity.
- Myalgias, irritability, headache, and general fatigue may be present initially.
- Abdominal cramping, constipation, weight loss, tremor, paresthesias and peripheral neuritis, seizures, and coma may occur with severe toxicity.
- Motor neuropathy is common in children with lead poisoning; learning disorders are also frequent.

ETIOLOGY

Chronic, repeated exposure to paint containing lead, plumbing, storage of batteries, pottery, or lead soldering. Concentration of lead is generally highest in lead-based paint on exterior surfaces. Among interior surfaces, windows are most likely to have the highest lead content.

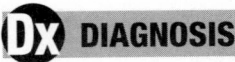

DIAGNOSIS

DIFFERENTIAL DIAGNOSIS

- Polyneuropathies from other sources
- Anxiety disorder, attention deficit disorder
- Malabsorption, acute abdomen
- Iron-deficiency anemia

WORKUP

Laboratory screening: all U.S. children should be considered to be at risk for lead poisoning and should be screened routinely starting at age 1 yr for low-risk children and age 6 mo for high-risk children.

LABORATORY TESTS

- Venous blood lead level: normal level, <5 mcg/dl; levels of 50 to 70 mcg/dl, indicative of moderate toxicity; levels >70 mcg/dl, associated with severe poisoning
- Mild anemia with basophilic stippling on peripheral smear
- Elevated zinc protoporphyrin levels or free erythrocyte protoporphyrin level
- An increased body burden of lead with previous high-level exposure in patients with occupational lead poisoning can be demonstrated by measuring the excretion of lead in urine after premedication with calcium ethylenediamine tetraacetic acid (EDTA) or another chelating agent

IMAGING STUDIES

- Imaging studies are generally not necessary.
- A plain abdominal film can visualize lead particles in the gut.
- "Lead lines" may be noted on x-ray films of long bones.

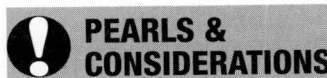

TREATMENT

NONPHARMACOLOGIC THERAPY

- Provide adequate amounts of calcium, iron, zinc, and protein in patient's diet
- Family education on sources of lead exposure and potential adverse health effects

ACUTE GENERAL Rx

- For children with blood levels of 10 to 19 mcg/dl, the CDC recommends nonpharmacologic interventions (see "Nonpharmacologic Therapy").
- For children with blood levels between 20 and 44 mcg/dl, the CDC recommendations include case management by a qualified social worker, clinical management, environmental assessment, and lead hazard control. Chelation therapy should be considered in children with refractory blood lead levels.

Chelation therapy (Table E1-236) is indicated in children with blood lead levels >45 mcg/dl:

- Succimer (DMSA) 10 mg/kg PO q8h for 5 days then q12h for 2 wk can be used in patients with levels between 45 and 70 mcg/dl.
- Edetate calcium disodium (EDTA) and dimercaprol (BAL) are effective in patients with severe toxicity.

- Use of both EDTA and DMSA is indicated in children with blood levels >70 mcg/dl.
- d-Penicillamine (Cuprimine) can also be used for lead poisoning, but it is not FDA approved for this condition.

CHRONIC Rx

- Reduce exposure, remove any potential lead sources.
- Correct iron deficiency and any other nutritional deficiencies.
- Recheck blood lead level 7 to 21 days after chelation therapy.

DISPOSITION

Patients with mild to moderate toxicity generally improve without any residual deficits. The presence of encephalopathy at diagnosis is a poor prognostic sign. Residual neurologic deficits may persist in these patients. Chelation therapy seems to slow the progression of renal insufficiency in patients with mildly elevated body lead burden.

REFERRAL

If exposure to lead is work related, it should be reported to the Office of the United States Occupational Safety and Health Administration (OSHA). Follow-up testing is mandatory in all patients after an abnormal screening blood lead level.

PEARLS & CONSIDERATIONS

COMMENTS

- Even blood lead concentrations as low as 5-10 mcg/dl are inversely associated with children's IQ scores at age 3 and 5 yr.
- Screening of household members of affected individuals is recommended.
- In children with blood lead levels of >45 mg/dl, treatment with succimer does not improve scores on tests of cognition, behavior, or neuropsychological function.
- Lead toxicity may delay growth and pubertal development in girls.
- Low-level environmental lead exposure may accelerate progressive renal insufficiency in patients without diabetes who have chronic renal disease. Repeated chelation therapy may improve renal function and slow the progression of renal failure.

SUGGESTED READINGS
available at www.expertconsult.com

RELATED CONTENT
Lead Poisoning (Patient Information)

AUTHOR: **FRED F. FERRI, M.D.**

BASIC INFORMATION

DEFINITION

Legg-Calvé-Perthes disease (LCPD) is a self-limited disorder of unknown etiology caused by ischemia of the immature femoral head that leads to bone necrosis and variable amounts of collapse during the reparative process. Fig. 1-478 illustrates lateral pillar classification for LCPD.

SYNONYMS

LCPD
Coxa plana
Capital femoral osteochondrosis
Osteonecrosis of the proximal femoral epiphysis

ICD-9CM CODES
732.1 Perthes' disease

EPIDEMIOLOGY & DEMOGRAPHICS

PREVALENCE: One case in 1300 children. More common in Caucasians
INCIDENCE: One in 1200 children, younger than 15 years of age

PREDOMINANT SEX: Male/female ratio of 4:1
PREDOMINANT AGE: 3 to 10 yr

PHYSICAL FINDINGS & CLINICAL PRESENTATION

- Initial symptom: usually a mildly painful limp
- Pain referred down the inner aspect of the thigh to the knee
- Moderate restriction of motion resulting from hip synovitis (abduction and internal rotation are especially limited), decreased range of motion
- Pain at the extremes of movement and tenderness over anterior hip joint
- Condition is bilateral in 10% to 20% of patients

ETIOLOGY

Unknown

DIAGNOSIS

DIFFERENTIAL DIAGNOSIS

- Transient synovitis
- Low-grade septic arthritis
- Juvenile rheumatoid arthritis

WORKUP

Diagnosis is usually based on the physical findings and eventual radiographic findings.

IMAGING STUDIES

- Plain roentgenography to establish the diagnosis
- AP and frog-leg lateral radiographs (Fig. 1-479)
- Technetium bone scanning to help confirm the diagnosis in early cases

TREATMENT

ACUTE GENERAL Rx

- A brief period of bed rest (1 to 3 days) followed by bracing (except in mild cases)
- Bracing possibly required for 2 to 3 yr in small percent of patients
- NSAIDs and non-weight-bearing for pain control
- Range-of-motion physical therapy exercises
- Surgical therapy in refractory cases: tenotomy, various osteotomies

DISPOSITION

- Prognosis depends on age of patient and degree of involvement of the femoral head at onset.
- Young patients (<6 yr) with minimal involvement do well.
- Older patients (>8 yr) often do poorly.
- A few patients eventually develop degenerative arthritis.

REFERRAL

For orthopedic consultation when diagnosis is suspected

PEARLS & CONSIDERATIONS

Both the etiology and the treatment of LCPD remain controversial. Treatment recommendations vary widely and continue to evolve.

COMMENTS

There is great uncertainty regarding treatment and its effect on outcome. Bracing may have no effect whatsoever on the end result.

SUGGESTED READINGS

available at www.expertconsult.com

RELATED CONTENT

Legg-Calvé-Perthes Disease (Patient Information)

AUTHOR: **LONNIE R. MERCIER, M.D.**

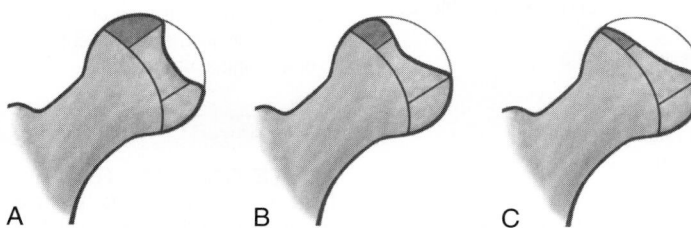

FIGURE 1-478 Lateral pillar classification for Legg-Calvé-Perthes disease. A, There is no involvement of the lateral pillar. **B,** More than 50% of the lateral pillar height is maintained. **C,** Less than 50% of the lateral pillar height is maintained. (From Kliegman RM et al: *Nelson textbook of pediatrics,* ed 19, Philadelphia, 2011, Saunders.)

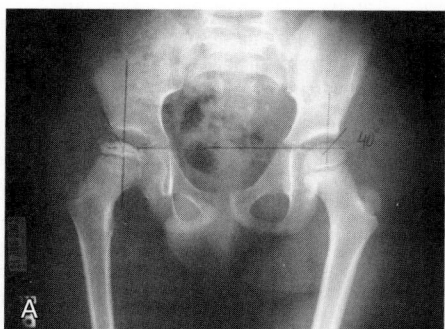
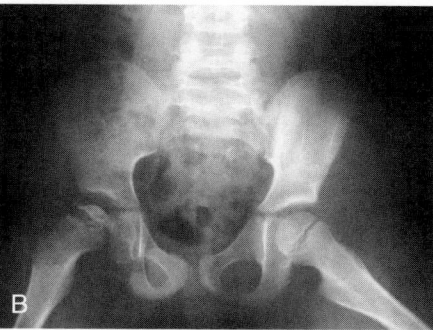

FIGURE 1-479 A, Anteroposterior radiograph of the pelvis shows epiphyseal fragmentation in the right hip, characteristic of the fragmentation phase of Legg-Calvé-Perthes disease. **B,** The frog-leg lateral view demonstrates subchondral fracture, increased density of the femoral head, and some collapse. (From Kliegman RM et al: *Nelson textbook of pediatrics,* ed 19, Philadelphia, 2011, Saunders.)

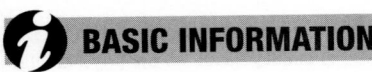

BASIC INFORMATION

DEFINITION

Acute lymphoblastic leukemia (ALL) is a malignancy of B or T lymphoblasts characterized by uncontrolled proliferation of abnormal, immature lymphocytes and their progenitors, ultimately replacing normal bone marrow elements.

SYNONYMS

Lymphoid leukemia
ALL

ICD-9CM CODES
204.0 Acute lymphoblastic leukemia

EPIDEMIOLOGY & DEMOGRAPHICS

- ALL is primarily a disease of children (peak incidence from ages 2 to 10 yr).
- It is diagnosed in 3000 to 4000 persons in the U.S. each year; two thirds are children. It is the most common malignancy of childhood.

PHYSICAL FINDINGS & CLINICAL PRESENTATION

- Skin pallor, purpura, or easy bruising
- Lymphadenopathy or hepatosplenomegaly
- Fever, bone pain, oliguria, weakness, weight loss, mental status changes

ETIOLOGY

- Unknown; increased risk in patients with a previous use of antineoplastic agents (e.g., chemotherapy of non-Hodgkin's lymphoma, Hodgkin's disease, ovarian cancer, myeloma)
- Environmental factors (e.g., ionizing radiation), toxins (e.g., benzene)

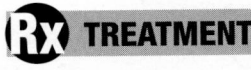

DIAGNOSIS

DIFFERENTIAL DIAGNOSIS

- Acute myeloid leukemia (AML): the distinction between ALL and AML (see Table 1-238) and the classification of the various subtypes are based on the following factors:
  1. Cell morphology
     - Lymphoblasts: a high nucleus/cytoplasmic ratio; cytoplasmic granules are usually not present.
     - Myeloblasts: abundant cytoplasm; cytoplasmic granules (Auer rods) are often present.
  2. Histochemical stains
     - Peroxidase and Sudan black stains: negative in ALL; useful to distinguish nonlymphoid from lymphoid cells.
     - Chloroacetate esterase: a pink cytoplasmic reaction identifies granulocytes; useful to distinguish granulocytes from monocytes in patients with AML.
  3. Cytogenic/molecular markers (Table E1-239)
- Lymphoblastic lymphoma
- Aplastic anemia
- Infectious mononucleosis
- Leukemoid reaction to infection
- Multiple myeloma

WORKUP

- Laboratory evaluation
- Bone marrow examination (with biopsy, cytochemistry, immunophenotyping, and cytogenetics) (Fig. E1-483)
- Lumbar puncture and imaging studies

LABORATORY TESTS

- Complete blood count reveals normochromic, normocytic anemia, thrombocytopenia.
- Peripheral smear will reveal lymphoblasts.
- Initial blood work should also include blood urea nitrogen, creatinine, serum electrolytes, uric acid, and lactate dehydrogenase.
- Special diagnostic tests include immunophenotyping, cytogenetics, and cytochemistry.
- The French, American, British (FAB) Cooperative Study Group has classified ALL into three groups (L1 to L3) on the basis of cell size, cytoplasmic appearance, nucleus shape, and chromatin pattern. The most common form is the L2 type.
- Immunologic classification is made on the basis of expression of surface antigens by blast cells: T lineage and B lineage.

IMAGING STUDIES

- Chest x-ray to evaluate for the presence of mediastinal mass
- CT scan or ultrasound of abdomen/pelvis to assess splenomegaly or leukemic infiltration of abdominal organs

TREATMENT

ACUTE GENERAL Rx

Table 1-240 summarizes the preferred approach to the treatment of adult ALL patients. For younger adults, induction therapy usually consists of an anthracycline, vincristine, L-asparaginase, and a corticosteroid.

DISPOSITION

- Prognosis is generally poorer in adult disease compared with childhood disease (40% adult cure rate versus 80% cure rate in children).
- Five-year leukemia-free survival is <40%.
- The different clinical outcomes associated with the various subtypes of ALL can be attributed primarily to drug sensitivity or resistance of leukemic blasts harboring specific genetic abnormalities. For example, cases of ALL expressing the TEL-AML1 fusion protein are very responsive to intensive chemotherapy with asparaginase, whereas the presence of Philadelphia chromosome (Ph{ΣY}+{/ΣY}), monosomy 5 and 7, and abnormalities of 11q23 are bad prognostic signs in ALL.
- Genetic alteration (deletion) of IKZF1 is associated with a very poor outcome in B-cell-progenitor ALL.
- Outcome of adult ALL patients according to subgroups is summarized in Table 1-241.

REFERRAL

Referral to a hematologist is indicated in all cases of ALL.

TABLE 1-238 Morphologic, Cytochemical, and Biochemical Characteristics Helpful in Distinguishing Acute Lymphoblastic Leukemia from Acute Myelocytic Leukemia

Morphologic Features	ALL	AML
Nuclear/cytoplasmic ratio	High	Low
Nuclear chromatin	Clumped	Spongy
Nucleoli	0-2	2-5
Granules	−	+
Auer rods	−	+/−
Cytoplasm	Blue	Blue-gray
Cytochemical Reaction		
Peroxidase	−	+
Sudan black B	−	+
Periodic acid–Schiff	+/−	−
Naphthyl AS-D chloroacetate esterase	−	+/−
α-Naphthyl acetate esterase	−	+/−
α-Naphthyl butyrate esterase	−	−
Terminal deoxynucleotidyl transferase	+*	−

Table provides information on characteristics that may be useful in differentiating acute lymphoblastic leukemia (ALL) from acute myelocytic leukemia (AML) (see text for details). Wide variation in morphology is encountered in both disease categories. Diagnostic evaluation should include more refined classification of disease according to FAB subtype.

*Terminal deoxynucleotidyl transferase is usually negative in FAB L3 ALL.

From Hoffman R et al: Hematology, basic principles and practice, ed 5, Philadelphia, 2009, Churchill Livingstone.

TABLE 1-240 Preferred Approach to the Treatment of Adult Acute Lymphocytic Leukemia Patients

	Low-Risk ALL	High-Risk ALL	Very High-Risk ALL	Mature B-ALL
Definition	*B-lineage* WBC <30,000/μL Time to CR <4 wk No Pro-B/ t(4;11) *T-lineage* Thy ALL Molecular CR	*B-lineage* WBC >30,000/μL Time to CR >4 wk Pro-B/ t(4;11) *T-lineage* Early T, mature T No molecular CR	Ph/BCR-ABL positive	
Multidrug-induction	Yes	Yes	Yes + imatinib	Short intensive cycles including HDM, fractionated C, HDAC, and other drugs Rituximab
CNS prophylaxis*	Yes	Yes	Yes	Yes
Consolidation (also other combinations)	Alternating cycles, e.g., HDM, HDAC, asparaginase reinduction	One cycle	One cycle + imatinib	6 cycles
SCT in CR1	None	Allogeneic SCT (if matched related or unrelated donor) Autologous SCT After additional (if no donor and negative MRD, consolidation)		None
Maintenance	6-MP/M + intensification for 2-2½ yr		imatinib	None

AC, Cytosine arabinoside; *ALL,* acute lymphocytic leukemia; *CR,* complete remission; *HDM,* high-dose methotrexate; *MRD,* minimal residual disease; *SCT,* stem cell transplantation;*Thy ALL,* thymic ALL.
*Intrathecal therapy with M or triple combination (M, AC, steroid) continued during maintenance therapy; additional CNS irradiation and/or high-dose chemotherapy according to subgroup.
From Hoffman R et al: *Hematology, basic principles and practice,* ed 5, Philadelphia, 2009, Churchill Livingstone.

TABLE 1-241 Outcome of Adult Lymphocytic Leukemia Patients According to Subgroup*

Subgroup	No. of Patients	CR Rate	No. of Patients	LFS
Age				
<30	669	88%	510	42%-60%[‡]
30-59	610	79%	412	33%
≥60	215	58%	141	15%
Subtype				
T-ALL[†]	976	88%	850	40%-60%[‡]
B-Precursor ALL	2366	82%	2036	40%-60%
Pro-B-ALL	987	75%	107	37%-60%[§]
Cytogenetics				
Ph/bcr-abl + (without imatinib)	633	72%	633	21%
Ph/bcr-abl + (with imatinib + Chemo)		90%		50%
WBC				
<30,000/μL	698	81%	746	40%
>30,000/μL	387	75%	409	28%
Time to CR				
<4 wk			1433	44%
>4 wk			253	36%

CR, Complete remission; *LFS,* leukemia-free survival; *MRD,* median remission duration.
*Pooled data from published studies.
[†]Depends on T-ALL subtype.
[‡]Depending on protocol and subtype.
[§]Including allogeneic SCT.
From Hoffman R et al: *Hematology: basic principles and practice,* ed 5, Philadelphia, 2009, Churchill Livingstone.

SUGGESTED READINGS

available at www.expertconsult.com

RELATED CONTENT

Acute Lymphocytic Leukemia (ALL) (Patient Information)

AUTHOR: **FRED F. FERRI, M.D.**

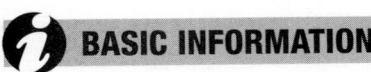

DEFINITION

Acute myelogenous leukemia (AML) is a malignancy of myeloid progenitor cells. It is characterized by uncontrolled proliferation of primitive myeloid cells (blasts), ultimately replacing normal bone marrow elements and frequently resulting in hematopoietic insufficiency (granulocytopenia, thrombocytopenia, or anemia) with or without leukocytosis.

SYNONYMS

Acute nonlymphoblastic leukemia (ANLL)
Acute nonlymphocytic leukemia
Acute myeloid leukemia (AML)

ICD-9CM CODES
205.0 Acute myelogenous leukemia

EPIDEMIOLOGY & DEMOGRAPHICS

- AML usually affects adults (most patients are 30 to 60 yr; median age at presentation is 50 yr).
- Annual incidence is 2 to 4 cases/100,000 persons.

PHYSICAL FINDINGS & CLINICAL PRESENTATION

Patients generally come to medical attention because of the effects of the cytopenias:
- Anemia manifests with weakness or fatigue.
- Thrombocytopenia can manifest with bleeding, petechiae, and ecchymosis.
- Neutropenia can result in infections and fever.
- Physical examination may reveal skin pallor, bruises, petechiae; abdominal examination may reveal hepatosplenomegaly; peripheral lymphadenopathy may also be present.
- Hyperleukocytosis can lead to symptoms of leukostasis, such as ocular and cerebrovascular dysfunction or bleeding.

ETIOLOGY

Risk factors are previous use of antineoplastic agents, chromosomal abnormalities, ionizing radiation, toxins, immunodeficiency states, and chronic myeloproliferative disorders. Congenital disorders or acquired factors predisposing to AML are described in Table 1-242.

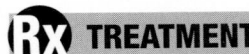 DIAGNOSIS

DIFFERENTIAL DIAGNOSIS

- Acute lymphocytic leukemia
- Leukemoid reaction
- Myelodysplastic syndrome
- Infiltrative diseases of the bone marrow
- Epstein-Barr virus, other viral infection

LABORATORY TESTS

- Complete blood count reveals anemia and thrombocytopenia. Peripheral white blood cell count varies from $<5000/mm^3$ to $>100,000/mm^3$.

- Additional laboratory findings may include elevated lactate dehydrogenase and uric acid levels, decreased fibrinogen, and increased fibrin degradation product as a result of disseminated intravascular coagulation (DIC).
- Cytogenetic abnormalities are common (chromosome 8 is most frequently involved in AML). Table 1-243 describes gene mutations in patients with AML. DNMT3A mutations are highly recurrent in patients with de novo AML with an intermediate-risk cytogenetic profile and are independently associated with a poor outcome.
- The distinction between acute lymphoblastic leukemia (ALL) and AML and the classification of the various subtypes are based on the following factors:
  1. Cell morphology: myeloblasts reveal abundant cytoplasm; cytoplasmic granules are often present (Auer rods).
  2. Histochemical stains:
     - Peroxidase and Sudan black stains are negative in ALL.
     - Chloroacetate esterase: a pink cytoplasmic reaction identifies granulocytes; useful to distinguish granulocytes from monocytes in patients with AML.

TABLE 1-242   Congenital Disorders or Acquired Factors Predisposing to Acute Myeloid Leukemia

Genetic Factors

Down syndrome
Fanconi anemia
Bloom syndrome
Neurofibromatosis type I
Klinefelter syndrome
Turner syndrome

Congenital Bone Marrow Failure Syndromes

Kostmann syndrome
Diamond-Blackfan anemia

Drugs

Benzene
Alkylating agents
Epipodophyllotoxins
Ionizing radiation
Myelodysplastic syndromes

From Hoffman R et al: *Hematology: basic principles and practice*, ed 5, Philadelphia, 2009, Churchill Livingstone.

TABLE 1-243   Gene Mutations in Patients with Acute Myelogenous Leukemia, and Normal Karyotype

Gene Mutation	Frequency (%)	Prognosis
NPM	45-63	Favorable
FLT3	23-33	Adverse
MLL	5-30	Adverse
C/EBP	8-19	Favorable

From Hoffman R et al: *Hematology: basic principles and practice*, ed 5, Philadelphia, 2009, Churchill Livingstone.

- AML is diagnosed by the presence of at least 30% blast cells and positive peroxidase or Sudan black histochemical stain in the bone marrow aspirate.
- The French, American, British (FAB) Cooperative Study Group has classified AML into seven categories (M1 to M7) based on the type and percentage of immature cells. The World Health Organization classification of AML is described in Table 1-244. A summary of diagnostic features of AML in the FAB classification is outline in Table 1-245.
- A stepwise algorithm for diagnosis and classification of AML using cytomorphology, cytochemistry, immunophenotyping, cytogenetics, and molecular genetics is described in Box 1-34 and in Fig. E1-484. Cytogenetic risk categories in AML are described in Table 1-246. Bone marrow findings are described in Fig. E1-485.

IMAGING STUDIES

- Chest x-ray is useful to evaluate for the presence of mediastinal masses.
- CT scan of the abdomen may reveal hepatosplenomegaly or leukemic involvement of other organs.

Rx TREATMENT

ACUTE GENERAL Rx

- Emergency treatment consisting of one or more of the following is indicated in patients with intracerebral leukostasis:
  1. Cranial irradiation
  2. Leukapheresis
  3. Oral hydroxyurea
- Urate nephropathy can be prevented by vigorous hydration and lowering uric acid level with allopurinol and urine alkalinization with acetazolamide.
- Infections must be aggressively treated with broad-spectrum antibiotics.
- Correct significant thrombocytopenia with platelet transfusions.
- Bleeding from DIC is treated with heparin and replacement of clotting factors.
- Intensive induction chemotherapy to destroy a significant number of leukemic cells and achieve remission usually consists of cytarabine and daunorubicin. It is a 7 + 3 regimen consisting of 7 days of continuous IV infusion of cytarabine and 3 days of daunorubicin. With this regimen, the chance of obtaining a complete remission is 65% to 70% with significantly lower rates in older patients (>56 yr old). All-trans retinoic acid is effective for the induction of remission of AML M3 subtype (acute promyelocytic leukemia).
- High-dose cytarabine (ARA-C) (HiDAC) can be used in patients with refractory or relapsed AML. It usually takes 28 to 32 days from the start of therapy to achieve remission. The duration of remission is variable; the median duration of remission in an adult with AML is 1 yr.
- Postremission therapy following complete remission with induction chemotherapy may include either allogeneic bone marrow

transplant (younger patients with donor match) or consolidation chemotherapy.

- Consolidation therapy consists of an aggressive course of chemotherapy with or without radiation shortly after complete remission has been obtained; its purpose is to prolong the remission period or cure. Complications of consolidation therapy are usually attributable to severe bone marrow suppression (anemia, thrombocytopenia, granulocytopenia).
- Goal of therapy is to maintain a state of remission. A postinduction course of high-dose cytarabine can provide equivalent disease-free survival and somewhat better overall survival than autologous marrow transplantation in adults.
- Autologous bone marrow transplantation is indicated in patients <55 yr without a sibling donor. Allogeneic bone marrow transplantation is generally available to <20% of patients; it is usually performed only in patients <40 yr because of higher incidence of graft-versus-host disease with advancing age.

TABLE 1-244 World Health Organization Classification of Acute Myeloid Leukemia

Acute myeloid leukemia with recurrent genetic abnormalities

Acute myeloid leukemia with t(8;21)(q22;q22), (AML1/ETO)

Acute myeloid leukemia with abnormal bone marrow eosinophils and inv(16)(p13;q22) or t(16;16) (p13;q22), (CBFβ/MYH11)

Acute promyelocytic leukemia with t(15;17)(q22;q12), (PML/RARα) and variants

Acute myeloid leukemia with 11q23 (MLL) abnormalities

Acute myeloid leukemia with multilineage dysplasia

Following MDS or MDS/MPD

Without antecedent MDS or MDS/MPD, but with dysplasia in at least 50% of cells in two or more myeloid lineages

Acute myeloid leukemia and myelodysplastic syndromes, therapy related

Alkylating agent/radiation-related type

Topoisomerase II inhibitor-related type (some may be lymphoid)

Others

Acute myeloid leukemia, not otherwise categorized

Classify as:

Acute myeloid leukemia, minimally differentiated

Acute myeloid leukemia without maturation

Acute myeloid leukemia with maturation

Acute myelomonocytic leukemia

Acute monoblastic/acute monocytic leukemia

Acute erythroid leukemia (erythroid/myeloid and pure erythroleukemia)

Acute megakaryoblastic leukemia

Acute basophilic leukemia

Acute panmyelosis with myelofibrosis

Myeloid sarcoma

From Hoffman R et al: *Hematology: basic principles and practice*, ed 5, Philadelphia, 2009, Churchill Livingstone.

DISPOSITION

- Remission can be achieved in nearly 80% of patients <55 yr. Remission rates are highest in children. Patient characteristics relating to duration of remission are described in Table 1-247.
- Allogeneic stem cell transplantation (SCT) after myoablative conditioning is a curative option in younger patients with AML in first complete remission (CR1). However, concerns related to toxicity limit its use. Cure for allogeneic bone marrow transplantation approaches 60%; cure rates with autologous transplantation are lower. Compared with nonallogeneic SCT therapies, allogeneic SCT has significant relapse-free survival (RFS) and overall survival benefit for intermediate- and poor-risk AML but not for good-risk AML in first complete remission.
- Favorable cytogenetics are inv (16) (p13;q22) and t(8;21), t(15;17).
- High expression of an LSC (leukemic stem cell) gene signature is independently associated with adverse outcomes with AML.

BOX 1-34 Stepwise Algorithm for Diagnosis and Classification of Acute Myelogenous Leukemia Using Cytomorphology, Cytochemistry, Immunophenotyping, Cytogenetics, and Molecular Cytogenetics

The criteria are based on Wright-Giemsa–stained blood and marrow smears and biopsy. The percentage of blast cells separates acute myeloid leukemia (AML) from myelodysplastic syndrome (MDS). The World Health Organization (WHO) classification defines AML as greater than 20% blasts in the marrow or blood. The next step is to define the blast population by immunophenotyping and/or immunohistochemistry. The initial evaluation separates AML from ALL. A history of exposure to prior cytoxic chemotherapy or agents associated with AML defines the leukemia as *therapy-related acute myeloid leukemia* (t-AML). The WHO recognizes the unique clinical and biologic features of the therapy-related leukemias (t-AML). This subtype results from prior exposure to cytotoxic chemotherapy and/or radiation therapy. A majority of patients will have clonal cytogenetic abnormalities and now account for more than 40% of all patients with AML. The WHO recognizes two types of t-AML based on the type of prior exposure or treatment: alkylating agent–related AML and topoisomerase II inhibitor–related AML. The WHO classification defines major subgroups of AML that manifest recurring cytogenetic abnormalities. As a group, these AMLs have chromosomal translocations that result in the production of chimeric proteins, which are pivotal in the leukemogenic process. The genetic abnormalities define a specific biology, clinical course, and prognosis and therefore it is important to classify them separately. In this group of patients, the diagnosis is defined by the cytogenetic abnormality independent of the percentage of blasts. There are four recurrent translocations in this group. The diagnosis is defined by the cytogenetic abnormalities and is not dependent on the number of blasts: (a) AML with t(8;21)(q22;q22), (AML1/ETO) (RUNX/CBFA2T1); (b) AML with abnormal bone marrow eosinophils and inv^{16}(p13;q22) or t(16;16)(p13;q22), (CBFB/MYH11); (c) acute promyelocytic leukemia: AML with t(15;17)(q22;q21) (PML/RARA) or t(11;17)(q23;q12) (PLZF/RARA) or t(5;17)(q23;q12)(NPM/RARA), or t(11;17)(q13;q12) (NuMA/RARA); and (d) AML with 11q23 (MLL) abnormalities. If multilineage dysplasia is present, then the leukemia is classified as *acute leukemia with multilineage dysplasia*.

AML with multilineage dysplasia is characterized by the presence of 20% or more blasts in the marrow and dysplasia in at least 50% of the cells of at least two of the three main hemopoietic lines. The leukemia may occur de novo or after a preceding myelodysplastic, myeloproliferative, or overlap myelodysplastic/myeloproliferative syndrome unrelated to prior exposure to chemotherapy. If such a syndrome preceded the development of acute leukemia, the AML is best designated as AML "evolving from a myelodysplastic syndrome." When a leukemia fails to satisfy the cytogenetic, morphologic, or clinical criteria for the newly defined subgroups, it is classified as AML not otherwise categorized. The *not otherwise categorized* designation essentially applies the original FAB classification with some modifications, namely, acute promyelocytic leukemia (M3) is no longer included; a pure erythroleukemia has been distinguished from erythroleukemia, acute erythroid/myeloid type; and acute basophilic leukemia (very rare) has been added, as is a rare entity termed acute panmyelosis with myelofibrosis and the solid tumor myeloid sarcoma.

CD, Cluster designation; *MPO,* myeloperoxidase; *NEC,* nonerythroid cells; *NSE,* nonspecific esterase; *PAS,* periodic acid–Schiff; *SBB,* Sudan black B; *TdT,* terminal deoxynucleotidyl transferase; *TNC,* total nucleated cells.

From Hoffman R et al: *Hematology, basic principles and practice,* ed 5, Philadelphia, 2009, Churchill Livingstone.

TABLE 1-245 Summary of Diagnostic Features of Acute Myeloid Leukemia in the FAB Classification

FAB Subtype (%)	Diagnostic Features
AML-M0 (3%-5%)	≥30% blasts; >3% blasts reactive to MPO, SBB, or NSE; immunophenotyping CD33+, CD13+, may be CD34+, TdT+
AML-M1 (15%-20%)	≥30% blasts; ≥3% blasts reactive to MPO or SBB; <10% of marrow nucleated cells are promyelocytes or more mature neutrophils
AML-M2 (25%-30%)	≥30% blasts; ≥3% blasts reactive for MPO or SBB; ≥10% of marrow nucleated cells are promyelocytes or more mature neutrophils; t(8;21) chromosome abnormality
AML-M3 (10%-15%)	≥30% blasts and abnormal promyelocytes; intense MPO and SBB reactivity; promyelocytes and blasts with multiple Auer rods (faggot cells); t(15;17) cytogenetic abnormality
AML-M4 (20%-30%)	≥30% myeloblasts, monoblasts, and promonocytes; ≥20% monocytic cells in marrow; ≤5 × 10⁹/L monocytic cells in blood: ≥20% neutrophils and precursors in marrow; monocytic cells reactive for NSE; abnormal eosinophils in M4 with associated inv(16) chromosome abnormality
AML-M5a (2%-7%)	≥80% monocytic cells; monoblasts ≥80% of monocytic cells; monoblasts and promonocytes NSE positive; monoblasts usually MPO and SBB negative
AML-M5b (2%-5%)	≥80% monocytic cells; monoblasts ≥80% of monocytic cells; promonocytes predominate; monoblasts and promonocytes NSE positive; promonocytes may have scattered MPO- and SBB-positive granules
AML-M6 (3%-5%)	≥50% erythroid precursors; ≥30% of nonerythroid precursors are myeloblasts; Auer rods may be present in myeloblasts; dysplastic erythroid precursors frequently are PAS positive
AML-M7 (3%-5%)	≥30% blasts; ≥50% cells megakaryoblasts by morphology or electron microscopy; immunophenotyping CD41+, CD61+

AML, Acute myeloid leukemia; *CD,* cluster designation; *FAB,* French-American-British; *MPO,* myeloperoxidase; *NSE,* nonspecific esterase; *PAS,* periodic acid–Schiff; *SBB,* Sudan black B; *TdT,* terminal deoxynucleotidyl transferase.
Percent of all AML.
From Hoffman R et al: *Hematology: basic principles and practice,* ed 5, Philadelphia, 2009, Churchill Livingstone.

TABLE 1-246 Cytogenetic Risk Categories in Acute Myelogenous Leukemia

Category	Abnormality
Favorable	t(8;21),* t(15;17), inv(16) with or without other abnormalities
Intermediate	Normal, +6, +8, +21, +22 −Y, del(9q)
Unfavorable	−5/del(5q), −7/del(7q), abn(3q) t(9;22),t(6;9), abn(11q), 20q or 21q, abn(17p), complex karyotype

*Without deletion 9q or complex karyotype.
From Hoffman R et al: *Hematology: basic principles and practice,* ed 5, Philadelphia, 2009, Churchill Livingstone.

TABLE 1-247 Patient Characteristics Relating to Duration of Remission

Characteristics	Favorable Value
Cytogenetics	t(15;17), t(8;21), inv(16)
Leukocyte count	<100,000/μL⁻¹
Secondary acute myeloid leukemia	Not present
FAB subtype	M1 or M2 with Auer rods, M3 and M4eo
FLT3	Wild-type
Courses to complete remission	1

From Hoffman R et al: *Hematology: basic principles and practice,* ed 5, Philadelphia, 2009, Churchill Livingstone.

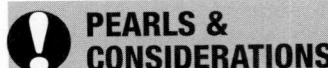

PEARLS & CONSIDERATIONS

- The major complication of chemotherapy is profound marrow depression with pancytopenia lasting 3 to 4 wk. Treatment is aimed at red blood cell and platelet replacement and aggressive monitoring and treatment of suspected infections.
- Low doses of arsenic trioxide can induce complete remission in patients with acute promyelocytic leukemia.

SUGGESTED READINGS
available at www.expertconsult.com

RELATED CONTENT
Acute Myelogenous Leukemia (Patient Information)

AUTHOR: **FRED F. FERRI, M.D.**

BASIC INFORMATION

DEFINITION

Chronic lymphocytic leukemia (CLL) is a lymphoproliferative disorder characterized by proliferation and accumulation of mature-appearing neoplastic lymphocytes.

SYNONYMS

CLL

EPIDEMIOLOGY & DEMOGRAPHICS

- Most frequent form of leukemia in Western countries (10,000 new cases annually in the United States). Incidence rate is 2-6 cases per 100,000 per year, and increases to 13 cases per 100,000 at age 65. It is more common in Caucasians and in those with a family history of CLL or other lymphoid malignancy.
- Generally occurs in elderly patients (70% of diagnoses are made in patients >65 yr of age). Mean age at diagnosis is 65 yr.
- Male/female ratio of 2:1
- CLL accounts for 11% of all hematologic neoplasms.

PHYSICAL FINDINGS & CLINICAL PRESENTATION

- At presentation most patients are asymptomatic. Many cases are diagnosed on the basis of laboratory results obtained after routine physical examination
- Lymphadenopathy, splenomegaly, and hepatomegaly in the majority of patients
- Variable clinical presentation according to stage of the disease
- Some patients come to medical attention because of weakness and fatigue (as a result of anemia) or lymphadenopathy

ETIOLOGY

CLL is a disease derived from antigen-experienced B lymphocytes that differ in the level of immunoglobulin V-gene mutations.

DIAGNOSIS

- Identification of cells bearing the phenotype of CLL in peripheral blood (CD5-positive/CD19-positive)
- Absolute B lymphocyte count in the peripheral blood ≥5000/μL for >3 mo with a preponderant population of morphologically mature-appearing small lymphocytes (Fig. E1-486)
- Demonstration of clonality of circulating B lymphocytes by flow cytometry of peripheral blood
- Table 1-248 describes the evaluation of CLL patients at diagnosis

DIFFERENTIAL DIAGNOSIS

- Hairy cell leukemia
- Adult T-cell lymphoma. Table 1-249 describes major diagnostic features of CLL and small lymphocytic lymphoma (SLL)
- Prolymphocytic leukemia
- Viral infections
- Waldenström's macroglobulinemia

LABORATORY TESTS

- Proliferative lymphocytosis (≥15,000/dl) of well-differentiated lymphocytes is the hallmark of CLL. B-cell clones are early markers for CLL and can be detected in peripheral blood >6 yr before a CLL diagnosis.
- There is monotonous replacement of the bone marrow by small lymphocytes (marrow contains ≥30% of well-differentiated lymphocytes). With the use of cell surface markers for clonality determination, the use of bone marrow aspirate and biopsy has become unnecessary for diagnosis or prognosis.
- Hypogammaglobulinemia and elevated lactate dehydrogenase may be present at the time of diagnosis.
- Anemia or thrombocytopenia, if present, indicates poor prognosis.
- Trisomy-12 is the most common chromosomal abnormality, followed by 14 q+, 13 q, and 11 q; these all indicate a poor prognosis.
- New laboratory techniques (CD 38, fluorescence in situ hybridization) can identify patients with early-stage CLL at higher risk of rapid disease progression. Staining of mononuclear cells by a two-color (fluorescein isothiocyanate/phycoerythrin) flow cytometric assay using antibodies to the chemokine receptors (CXCR1, CXCR2, etc.) can help in the staging and prognosis of patients. Increase in expression of chemokine receptors CXCR4 and CCR7 correlates with advanced Rai stage (stage IV). The presence of V-gene mutations, CD38+, or ZAP-70+ cells also has prognostic relevance. Patients with clones having few or no V-gene mutations or many CD38+ or ZAP-70+ B cells are associated with an aggressive, usually fatal course.
- The percentage of smudge cells (CLL cells ruptured during smear preparation) is associated with mutated IgVH gene status, a favorable prognostic factor. A high percentage of smudge cells on peripheral smear indicates a

---

TABLE 1-248 Evaluation of Chronic Lymphocytic Leukemia (CLL) Patients at Diagnosis

History

B-symptom and fatigue assessment
Infectious history assessment
Occupational assessment for chemical exposure
Familial history of CLL and lymphoproliferative disorders
Preventive interventions for infections and secondary cancers

Physical Exam

Laboratory Assessment

Complete blood count with differential
Morphology assessment of lymphocytes
Chemistry, LFT enzymes, LDH
Flow cytometry assessment to confirm immunophenotype of CLL
Serum immunoglobulins
Serum β2M levels
Interphase cytogenetics for del(17p13.1), del(11q22.3), del(13q14), del(6q21), and trisomy 12
IgVH mutational analysis
Stimulated metaphase karyotype (if available)

Selected Tests Under Certain Circumstances

Direct antiglobulin test (DAT), haptoglobin, reticulocyte count if anemia present
CT scan if unexplained abdominal pain or enlargement present
PET scan and/or biopsy if large nodal mass present
Bone marrow aspirate and biopsy if cytopenias present
Familial counseling if first-degree relative with CLL

Teaching

Varicella zoster identification instruction
Skin cancer identification
Disease education (Leukemia and Lymphoma Society, CLL Topics, ACOR)

From Hoffmann R et al: Hematology: basic principles and practice, ed 5, Philadelphia, 2009, Churchill Livingstone.

TABLE 1-249 Major Diagnostic Features of Chronic Lymphocytic Leukemia (CLL) and Small Lymphocytic Lymphoma (SLL)

CLL

- Absolute mature lymphocytosis of ≥5 × 10⁹/L sustained for at least 3 months
- Monoclonal B cell with mature phenotype, CD5 coexpression, weak CD20, weak surface immunoglobulin, CD23, weak CD22, weak CD11c
- Antigens typically *not* expressed include CD10, FMC7, and CD79b

SLL

- Extramedullary sites of disease predominate
- Diffuse infiltrate of small lymphocytes, proliferation foci
- Monoclonal B cell with mature phenotype similar to CLL

From Jaffe ES et al: Hematopathology, Philadelphia, 2011, Saunders.

longer time to treatment from initial diagnosis and better overall survival in patients with early stage CLL.

STAGING:
Rai et al divided CLL into five clinical stages:
- Stage 0: Characterized by lymphocytosis only (>15,000/mm^3 on peripheral smear, bone marrow aspirate ≥40% lymphocytes). The coexistence of lymphocytosis and other factors increases the clinical stage.
- Stage 1: Lymphadenopathy
- Stage 2: Lymphadenopathy/hepatomegaly
- Stage 3: Anemia (hemoglobin [Hgb] <11 g/mm^3)
- Stage 4: Thrombocytopenia (platelets <100,000/mm^3)

Another well-known staging system developed by Binet divides CLL into three stages:
- Stage A: Hgb >10 g/dl, platelets >100,000/mm^3, and fewer than three areas involved (the cervical, axillary, and inguinal lymph nodes [whether unilaterally or bilaterally]; the spleen; and the liver)
- Stage B: Hgb >10 g/dl, platelets >100,000/mm^3, and three or more areas involved
- Stage C: Hgb <10 g/dl, low platelets (<100,000/mm^3), or both (independent of the areas involved)

IMAGING STUDIES

CT scans at diagnosis for assessment of end-organ involvement are not recommended in diagnostic guidelines. However, CT scan of abdomen may be done to evaluate for hepatomegaly and splenomegaly in patients with poor prognostic features.

Rx TREATMENT

NONPHARMACOLOGIC THERAPY
- Treatment goals are relief of symptoms and prolongation of life.
- Observation is appropriate for patients in Rai stage 0 or Binet stage A.
- There are no survival benefits and a slight trend toward worse survival for patients who have early intervention versus deferred chemotherapy.

ACUTE GENERAL Rx
- Symptomatic patients in Rai stage I or II or Binet stage B: fludarabine-based combination chemotherapy: local irradiation for isolated symptomatic lymphadenopathy and lymph nodes that interfere with vital organs.
- Best response rates are seen when combination chemotherapy and retuximab are used (>70% complete response, median time to disease progression >4 years).
- Rai stages III or IV, Binet stage C: chlorambucil chemotherapy with or without prednisone:
  1. Fludarabine, CAP (**c**yclophosphamide, **A**driamycin, **p**rednisone), or cyclophosphamide, doxorubicin, vincristine, and prednisone (mini-CHOP) can be used in patients who respond poorly to chlorambucil.
  2. Monoclonal antibodies: rituximab, ofatumumab, or alemtuzumab is useful for treatment of patients with CLL refractory to fludarabine.

3. Splenic irradiation can be used in selected patients with advanced disease.
4. Bendamustine, an alkylator in the nitrogen mustard family, is well tolerated and can also be used in some patients with CLL.
5. Combination therapy with fludarabine (F), cyclophosphamide (C), rituximab (R) [FCR] provides additional benefits beyond single-agent therapy. It has shown to improve progression-free and overall survival in patients with CLL who do not have deletion of chromosome 17p and who are considered fit enough for fludarabine-based chemotherapy.
- An algorithm to treatment approach to first relapsed CLL is described in Fig. 1-487.

CHRONIC Rx
Treatment of systemic complications:
- Hypogammaglobulinemia is frequent in CLL and is the chief cause of infections. Immune globulin (250 mg/kg IV every 4 wk) may prevent infections but has no effect on survival rate. Infections should be treated with broad-spectrum antibiotics. Patients should be monitored for opportunistic infections.
- Recombinant hematopoietic cofactors (e.g., granulocyte-macrophage colony stimulating factor and granulocyte colony stimulating factor) may be useful to overcome neutropenia related to treatment.
- Erythropoietin may be useful to treat anemia that is unresponsive to other measures.

DISPOSITION
The patient's prognosis is generally directly related to the clinical stage (e.g., the average survival in patients in Rai stage 0 or Binet stage A is >120 mo, whereas for Rai stage 4 or Binet stage C it is approximately 30 mo). Overall 5-yr survival is 60%. Measurement of ZAP-70 intracellular protein (where available) is also a useful indicator of prognosis.

EBM EVIDENCE

available at www.expertconsult.com

SUGGESTED READINGS

available at www.expertconsult.com

RELATED CONTENT
Chronic Lymphocytic Leukemia (Patient Information)

AUTHOR: **FRED F. FERRI, M.D.**

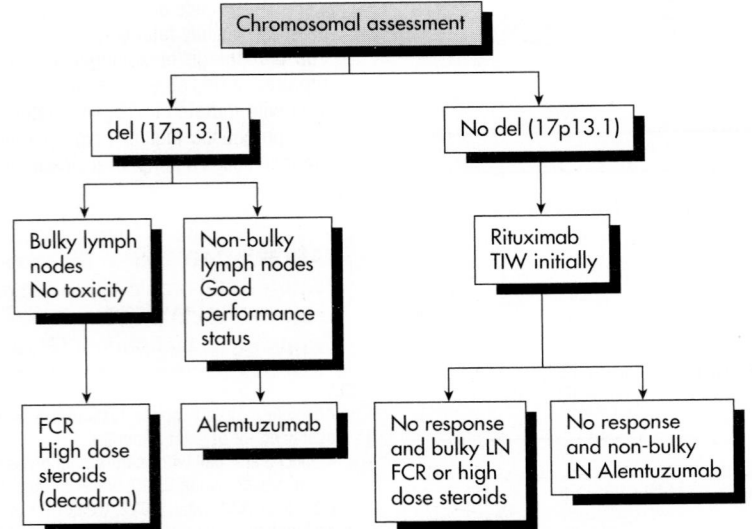

FIGURE 1-487 Algorithm to treatment approach to first relapsed chronic lymphocytic leukemia. (Modified from Hoffman R et al: *Hematology: basic principles and practice*, ed 5, Philadelphia, 2009, Churchill Livingstone.)

BASIC INFORMATION

DEFINITION

Chronic myelogenous leukemia (CML) is a malignant clonal stem disease caused by an acquired somatic mutation that fuses, through chromosomal translocation, the *ABL* and *BCR* genes on chromosomes 9 and 22 and is characterized by abnormal proliferation and accumulation of immature granulocytes. CML manifests with a chronic phase (CP-CML) lasting months to years, followed by an advanced phase (AP-CML) characterized by poor response to therapy, worsening anemia, or decreased platelet count; the second phase then evolves into a terminal phase (acute transformation) that degenerates into acute leukemia (mostly myeloid and approximately 20% lymphoid subtype), characterized by elevated number of blast cells and numerous complications (e.g., sepsis, bleeding).

SYNONYMS

CML
Chronic granulocytic leukemia
Chronic myeloid leukemia

ICD-9CM CODES
201.1 Chronic myelogenous leukemia

EPIDEMIOLOGY & DEMOGRAPHICS

- CML usually affects elderly patients (median age at presentation is 65 yr) and accounts for 15% of adult cases of leukemia
- Incidence is one to two cases per 100,000 people annually

PHYSICAL FINDINGS & CLINICAL PRESENTATION

- The chronic phase usually reveals splenomegaly; hepatomegaly is not infrequent, but lymphadenopathy is highly unusual and generally indicates the accelerated proliferative phase of the disease.
- Common symptoms at the time of diagnosis are weakness or discomfort from an enlarged spleen (abdominal discomfort or pain). Splenomegaly is present in up to 40% of patients at time of diagnosis.
- 40% of patients are asymptomatic, and diagnosis is based solely on an abnormal blood count.

ETIOLOGY

Current evidence strongly implicates the chromosome translocation t(9;22) (q34;q11.2) as the cause of chronic granulocytic leukemia. This translocation is present in >95% of patients. The remaining patients have a complex or variant translocation involving additional chromosomes that have the same end result (fusion of the *BCR* [break point cluster region] gene on chromosome 22 to *ABL* [Ableson leukemia virus] gene on chromosome 9).

DIAGNOSIS

DIFFERENTIAL DIAGNOSIS

- Splenic lymphoma
- Chronic lymphocytic leukemia
- Myelodysplastic syndrome

LABORATORY TESTS

- Elevated white blood cell count (generally >100,000/mm^3) with broad spectrum of granulocytic forms.
- Bone marrow demonstrates hypercellularity with granulocytic hyperplasia, increased ratio of myeloid cells to erythroid cells, and increased number of megakaryocytes (Fig. E1-488). Blasts and promyelocytes constitute <10% of all cells.
- The Philadelphia chromosome results from the reciprocal translocation between the long arms of chromosomes 9 and 22 [Fig. E1-489] and is present in >95% of patients with CML; its presence (Ph^1) is a major prognostic factor because survival rate of patients with Philadelphia chromosome is approximately eight times better than that of those without it. Some believe that Ph^1(+) defines CML and that those who are Ph^1(−) have another disease.
- Leukocyte alkaline phosphatase is markedly decreased (used to distinguish CML from other myeloproliferative disorders).
- Anemia and thrombocytosis are often present.
- Additional laboratory results are elevated vitamin B$_{12}$ levels (caused by increased transcobalamin 1 from granulocytes) and elevated blood histamine levels (because of increased basophils).

IMAGING STUDIES

Chest radiograph and CT scan of abdomen/pelvis

TREATMENT

ACUTE GENERAL Rx

Treatment with a potential to either cure CML or prolong survival should be used during the chronic phase of the disease because it is often futile when administered during the advanced phase. Imatinib mesylate, an oral tyrosine kinase inhibitor, is effective and indicated as first-line treatment for CML myeloid blast crisis, accelerated phase, or CML in its chronic phase. More than 75% of patients have major cytogenetic response (<35% Philadelphia chromosome-positive cells in the marrow), and more than 80% have progression-free survival after 24 mo. Complete hematologic response usually occurs in <1 mo. Nilotinib and dasatinib are newer, more effective agents that also inhibit the activity of the BCR-ABL fusion protein by binding to a particular site and can be used after failure of imatinib and eventually may become first-line agents. Ponatinib is a newer oral tyrosine kinase inhibitor that blocks native and mutated BCR-ABL and has been shown to be highly active in pretreated patients with Ph-positive leukemias with resistance to other tyrosine kinase inhibitors.

- Symptomatic hyperleukocytosis (e.g., central nervous system symptoms) can be treated with leukapheresis and hydroxyurea; allopurinol should be started to prevent urate nephropathy after the rapid lysis of the leukemia cells.
- Allogeneic stem-cell transplantation (SCT) is the only curative treatment for CML in the chronic phase unresponsive to imatinib. In general only 20% of patients are candidates for SCT given the limitations of age or lack of HLA-matched related donors.
  1. It should be considered in "young" patients (increased survival in patients <55 yr) with compatible siblings.
  2. Early transplantation is also important for patient's survival.
- Interferon-alfa is an acceptable alternative in the early chronic phase for patients who do not tolerate tyrosine kinase inhibitors.
- Recent trials have shown that as compared with other treatments, the addition of peginterferon alfa-2a to imatinib therapy resulted in significantly higher rates of molecular response in patients with chronic-phase CML.
- Transplantation of marrow from an HLA-matched, unrelated donor is also now recognized as safe and effective therapy for selected patients with CML.

SUGGESTED READINGS

available at www.expertconsult.com

RELATED CONTENT

Chronic Myelogenous Leukemia (Patient Information)

AUTHOR: **FRED F. FERRI, M.D.**

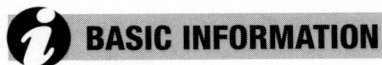
BASIC INFORMATION

DEFINITION

Hairy cell leukemia is a lymphoid neoplasm characterized by the proliferation of mature B cells with prominent cytoplasmic projections (hairs).

SYNONYMS

HCL
Leukemic reticuloendotheliosis

ICD-9CM CODES
202.4 Hairy cell leukemia

EPIDEMIOLOGY & DEMOGRAPHICS

PREVALENCE: Occurs predominantly in men between ages 40 and 60 yr. Approximately 2% of leukemia cases are of the hairy cell type.
PREDOMINANT SEX: Male/female ratio of 4:1

PHYSICAL FINDINGS & CLINICAL PRESENTATION

- Usually, splenomegaly (present in >90% of cases) caused by tumor cell infiltration (Fig. E1-490)
- Pallor, ecchymosis, and evidence of infection if the pancytopenia is severe
- Weakness, lethargy, and fatigue
- Infections (resulting from impaired resistance caused by neutropenia) and easy bruising (caused by thrombocytopenia) also common

TABLE 1-250 Major Diagnostic Features of Hairy Cell Leukemia

Study	Findings
Morphology of hairy cells	Oval or indented nuclei and abundant pale blue cytoplasm Absent or inconspicuous nucleoli Circumferential cell surface "ruffled" projections
Bone marrow biopsy morphology	Diffuse or interstitial bone marrow infiltration, without discrete nodular aggregates Clear cells with "fried egg" or spindled appearance Reticulin fibrosis
Flow cytometry	Clonal B cells expressing *CD103*, *CD25*, and *CD11c* and lacking *CD5* expression
Immunohistochemistry	Positive for DBA.44, TRAP, and ANXA1

From Jaffe ES et al: *Hematopathology,* Philadelphia, 2011, Saunders.

ETIOLOGY

Neoplastic disease of the lymphoreticular system of unknown etiology. A heterozygous mutation in BRAF that results in a BRAF V6000E variant protein has been identified in all patients with hairy cell leukemia

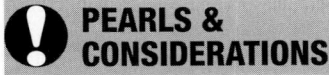
DIAGNOSIS

DIFFERENTIAL DIAGNOSIS

- Other forms of leukemia
- Lymphoma
- Viral syndrome

WORKUP

Comprehensive history, physical examination, and laboratory evaluation to confirm the diagnosis. Table 1-250 describes major diagnostic features of hairy cell leukemia.

LABORATORY TESTS

- Pancytopenia involving erythrocytes, neutrophils, and platelets is common; anemia is usually present and varies from minimal to severe.
- Hairy cells (Fig. 1-491) can account for 5% to 80% of cells in the peripheral blood. The cytoplasmic projections on the cells are redundant plasma membranes.
- Leukemic cells stain positively for tartrate-resistant acid phosphatase stain.
- A bone marrow biopsy (Fig. E1-492) is essential for confirmation and to quantify the degree of hairy cell infiltration. Bone marrow may result in a "dry tap" (because of increased marrow reticulin).

TREATMENT

NONPHARMACOLOGIC THERAPY

Approximately 8% to 10% of patients are asymptomatic and have minimal splenomegaly and minor cytopenia. They are usually detected on routine laboratory evaluation and do not require initial therapy. They should, however,

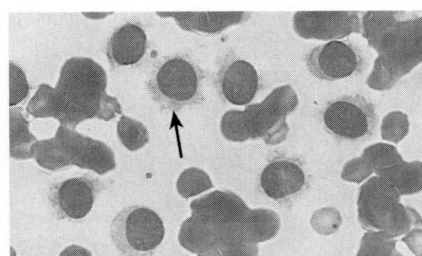

FIGURE 1-491 Hairy cell leukemia. Note the lymphocytes with hairlike cytoplasmic projections surrounding the nucleus. (From Rodak BF: *Diagnostic hematology,* Philadelphia, 1995, Saunders.)

be frequently monitored for progression of disease. Patients require treatment when they have significant cytopenias or occasionally recurrent infections from immunocompromise.

ACUTE GENERAL Rx

- Drugs of choice are the purine analogues 2-chloro-2 deoxyadenosine (cladribine) or 2-deoxycoformycin (DCF, pentostatin). They induce complete remissions in up to 85% of patients and partial responses in 5% to 25%.
- Cladribine may be preferred because it is easy to administer (0.14 mg/kg qd for 7 days), has minimal toxicity, and is able to induce complete durable responses with a single course of therapy.
- The anti-CD 22 recombinant immunotoxin BL 22 can induce complete remission in patients with hairy cell leukemia resistant to treatment with purine analogues.

CHRONIC Rx

- Patients should be monitored with periodic examination and laboratory tests for progression of disease.
- Approximately 40% of patients with HCL eventually relapse. Relapsed patients can be re-treated with purine analogs or the monoclonal CD20 antibody rituximab. If the prior response was <18 months in duration, rituximab may be preferred over retreatment with cladribine.

DISPOSITION

Prognosis has become increasingly favorable with the newer agents. Approximately 90% of patients who are treated have a complete or partial response.

REFERRAL

Hematology consultation is recommended in all patients.

PEARLS & CONSIDERATIONS

COMMENTS

The diagnosis of hairy cell leukemia is occasionally missed and subsequently made by the histopathologist after removal of the spleen for diagnostic purposes.

SUGGESTED READINGS

available at www.expertconsult.com

RELATED CONTENT

Hairy Cell Leukemia (Patient Information)
AUTHOR: **FRED F. FERRI, M.D.**

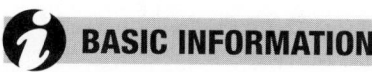

BASIC INFORMATION

DEFINITION

Oral hairy leukoplakia (OHL) is a painless, white, nonremovable, plaquelike lesion typically located on the lateral aspect of the tongue.

ICD-9CM CODES
528.6 Oral hairy leukoplakia

EPIDEMIOLOGY & DEMOGRAPHICS

INCIDENCE AND PREVALENCE: Epstein-Barr virus (EBV) seroprevalence occurs in high incidence in individuals who are HIV seropositive. However, OHL occurs in only 25% of these cases.

RISK FACTORS: OHL is usually found in HIV-seropositive individuals (median CD4 count is 468/μL) but may also be identified in other immunocompromised patients such as transplant recipients (particularly renal) and patients taking steroids. Diagnosing OHL is an indication to institute a workup to evaluate and manage HIV disease.

PHYSICAL FINDINGS & CLINICAL PRESENTATION

- Varying morphology and appearance, which may change daily.
- May be unilateral or bilateral.
- White plaques can be small with fine, vertical corrugations on the lateral margin of the tongue (Fig. 1-493). The plaques from OHL are adherent to the tongue surface (in contrast to candidal plaques, which may be easily scraped off).
- Irregular surface; may have prominent folds or projection, occasionally markedly resembling hairs.
- May spread to cover the entire dorsal surface or spread onto the ventral surface of the tongue where the lesions usually appear flat.

- Rarely, lesions can manifest on the soft palate, buccal mucosa, or posterior oropharynx.
- Usually asymptomatic, but some patients have mouth pain, soreness, or a burning sensation; impaired taste; or difficulty eating; others complain of its unsightly appearance.
- OHL may progress to oral squamous cell carcinoma, which has a poor prognosis.

ETIOLOGY

EBV is implicated in its etiology, and OHL is a result of replication EBV in the epithelium of keratinized cells. OHL differs from most EBV-related diseases in that infection is predominantly lytic rather than latent.

DIAGNOSIS

DIFFERENTIAL DIAGNOSIS

- *Candida albicans*
- Lichen planus
- Idiopathic leukoplakia
- White sponge nevus
- Dysplasia
- Squamous cell carcinoma

WORKUP

Requires physical examination and evaluation of HIV disease

LABORATORY TESTS

The *provisional* diagnosis is clinical and based on:
- Visual inspection
- Inability to scrape the lesion off the tongue with a blade
- Failure to respond to antifungal therapy

The *presumptive* diagnosis requires biopsy and histologic demonstration of:

- Epithelial hyperplasia with hairs
- Absence of inflammatory cell infiltrate

The *definitive* diagnosis requires:
- In situ hybridization of histologic or cytologic specimens revealing EBV DNA *or*
- Electron microscopy of specimens revealing herpes-like particles
- Measurement of the DNA content in cells of oral leukoplakia may be used to predict the risk of oral carcinoma

NOTE: Specimens obtained from lesions may demonstrate hyphae of *Candida albicans,* which may coexist and potentiate EBV-induced OHL.

TREATMENT

NONPHARMACOLOGIC THERAPY

OHL is usually asymptomatic and requires no specific therapy. It may resolve spontaneously and has no known premalignant potential.

ACUTE GENERAL Rx

- Antiretroviral therapy (ART) has considerably changed the frequency of oral lesions caused by opportunistic infections in HIV-seropositive individuals.
- Topical retinoids (0.1% vitamin A) may improve the appearance of OHL-affected oral surfaces through their dekeratinizing and immunomodulation effects; however, they are expensive and prolonged use may result in a burning sensation over the treated area.
- Topical podophyllin resin 25% solution has been reported to induce resolution.
- Surgical excision and cryotherapy may help, but the lesions may recur.
- High-dose acyclovir 800 mg five times per day, valacyclovir 1000 mg tid, famciclovir 500 mg tid, ganciclovir 1000 mg tid, or foscarnet 40 mg/kg IV tid will cause lesions to resolve but only temporarily.

PEARLS & CONSIDERATIONS

- OHL may be the presenting sign of patients infected with HIV who are unaware of their status.
- The incidence has decreased significantly in the era of ART.

SUGGESTED READING

available at www.expertconsult.com

RELATED CONTENT

Epstein-Barr Virus Infection (Related Key Topic)
Human Immunodeficiency Virus (Related Key Topic)
Leukoplakia (Patient Information)

AUTHOR: **SAJEEV HANDA, M.D.**

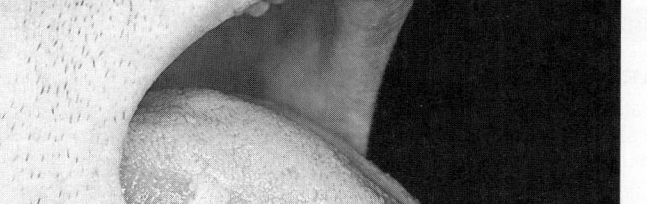

FIGURE 1-493 Oral hairy leukoplakia. Note white verrucoid plaques on the lateral border of the tongue. (From Noble J: *Primary care medicine,* ed 3, St Louis, 2001, Mosby.)

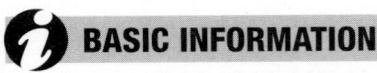

BASIC INFORMATION

DEFINITION

Lichen planus (LP) refers to an idiopathic inflammatory disease manifesting with a papular skin eruption characteristically found over the flexor surfaces of the extremities, genitalia, and mucous membranes.

SYNONYMS

Lichen
Lichen planus et atrophicus
LP

ICD-9CM CODES
697.0 Lichen planus

EPIDEMIOLOGY & DEMOGRAPHICS

INCIDENCE: One in every 100 new patients seen in dermatology clinics in the U.S. is diagnosed with LP
PREVALENCE: 440 cases/100,000 persons
PREDOMINANT SEX: Found equally between males and females (1:1)
PREDOMINANT AGE: Usually found in people between the ages of 30 and 60 yr
PREDISPOSING FACTORS:
1. Associated with other autoimmune disorders (e.g., primary biliary cirrhosis, myasthenia gravis, ulcerative colitis, diabetes)
2. Associated with hepatitis C infection
3. Drug-induced form affects any area of the body surface (e.g., beta-blocker, methyldopa, penicillamine, quinidine, nonsteroidal antiinflammatory drugs, angiotensin-converting enzyme inhibitors, sulfonylurea agents)

PHYSICAL FINDINGS & CLINICAL PRESENTATION

The clinical presentation varies depending on the area involved.
History:
- Usually starts on an extremity and may remain localized or spread to involve other areas over a 1- to 4-mo period
- Pruritic
Physical findings:
- Anatomic distribution:
  1. Flexor surface of wrists, forearms, shins, and upper thighs
  2. Neck and back area
  3. Nails (5%-10% of patients)
  4. Scalp (lichen planopilaris)
  5. Oral mucosa, buccal mucosa, tongue, gingiva, and lips; oral lichen planus can cause extensive dequamative gingivitis
  6. Vulva, penis
Genital mucosa:
- Lesion configuration:
  1. Linear
  2. Annular (more common)
  3. Reticular pattern noted on oral mucosa and genital area
- Lesion morphology:
  1. Papules most common presentation (flat, smooth, shiny) (Fig. 1-494)
  2. Hypertrophic

  3. Follicular
  4. Vesicular
- Color:
  1. Dark red, bluish red, purplish-violaceous color is noted in cutaneous LP.
  2. Individual lesions characteristically have white lines visible (Wickham's striae).
  3. Oral and genital LP has a reticular network of white lines that may be raised or annular in appearance.
- Scalp lesions may result in alopecia.

ETIOLOGY

The cause of LP is unknown. It is believed that LP represents a T-cell–mediated inflammatory disorder.

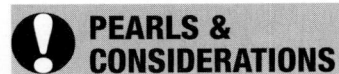

DIAGNOSIS

- Clinical history and physical findings usually establish the diagnosis of LP.
- Skin biopsy (deep shave or punch biopsy of the most developed lesion) can be performed to confirm the diagnosis.

DIFFERENTIAL DIAGNOSIS

Drug eruption, psoriasis, Bowen's disease, leukoplakia, candidiasis, lupus rash, secondary syphilis, seborrheic dermatitis, chronic graft vs. host disease

WORKUP

If the diagnosis is questionable, a skin biopsy is performed.

LABORATORY TESTS

Laboratory tests are not specific for the diagnosis of LP. Lipid panels screening is useful since increases in serum triglycerides and decreases in HDL cholesterol are common in patients with LP.

IMAGING STUDIES

Imaging studies are not helpful in diagnosing LP.

TREATMENT

NONPHARMACOLOGIC THERAPY

- Avoid scratching.
- Use mild soaps and emollients after bathing to prevent dryness.

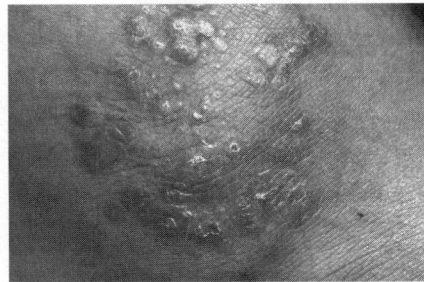

FIGURE 1-494 Flat-topped, purple polygonal papules of the lichen planus. (From Morelli JG: Diseases of the epidermis. In Kliegman RM et al [eds]: *Nelson textbook of pediatrics,* ed 19, Philadelphia, 2011, Saunders.)

ACUTE GENERAL Rx

For cutaneous LP:
- Topical steroids (e.g., triamcinolone acetonide 0.1%, fluocinonide 0.05%, clobetasol propionate 0.05% cream or ointment) with occlusion used twice daily.
- Acitretin 30 mg/day PO for 8 wk.
- Systemic prednisone 30 to 60 mg/day as a starting dose and tapered to 15 to 20 mg/day maintenance for 6 wk.
- Intradermal steroid triamcinolone acetonide 5 mg/ml can be tried for thick hyperkeratotic lesions.
- Hydroxyzine 25 mg PO q6h can be used for pruritus.
- Phototherapy: PUVA or narrow-band ultraviolet B therapy: 2 or 3 times per week, for a total of 12 sessions (i.e., one cycle).
For oral LP:
- Topical steroid fluocinonide in an adhesive base used six times/day for 9 wk.
- Topical calcineurin in steroid-unresponsive cases.
- Topical or systemic retinoids 0.1% retinoic acid in an adhesive base or gel.
- Etretinate 75 mg/day for 2 mo.

CHRONIC Rx

Refer to "Acute General Rx."

DISPOSITION

- Spontaneous remissions of cutaneous LP occur in more than 65% of cases within the first year.
- Spontaneous remission of oral LP usually occurs by 5 yr.
- Approximately 10% to 20% of patients will have recurrence.

REFERRAL

To dermatologist if diagnosis is unclear

PEARLS & CONSIDERATIONS

COMMENTS

- LP can be remembered as purple, planar, pruritic, polygonal, papules, and plaques (six P's).
- Lesions can develop at the site of prior skin injury (Koebner's phenomenon).
- Although there is an increased risk of squamous cell carcinoma in chronic lesions of mucosal LP, transformation to skin cancer is uncommon.

SUGGESTED READINGS

available at www.expertconsult.com

RELATED CONTENT

Lichen Planus (Patient Information)

AUTHOR: **TANYA ALI, M.D.**

BASIC INFORMATION

DEFINITION

Lichen sclerosus is a chronic inflammatory condition of the skin usually affecting the vulva, perianal area, and groin.

ICD-9CM CODES

701.0 Lichen sclerosus

EPIDEMIOLOGY & DEMOGRAPHICS

- Most common in postmenopausal women and men between ages 40 and 60 yr
- More common in females (female/male ratio of 5:1)
- Can occur in children (usually prepubertal girls with involvement of the vulva and perineum)

PHYSICAL FINDINGS & CLINICAL PRESENTATION

- Erythema may be the only initial sign. A characteristic finding is the presence of ivory-white atrophic lesions on the involved area.
- Close inspection of the affected area will reveal the presence of white-to-brown follicular plugs on the surface (dells).
- When the genitals are involved, the white, parchment-like skin assumes an hourglass configuration around the introital and perianal area ("keyhole" distribution; Fig. 1-495). Inflammation, subepithelial hemorrhages, and chronic ulceration may develop.
- Dyspareunia, genital bleeding, and anal bleeding are common.

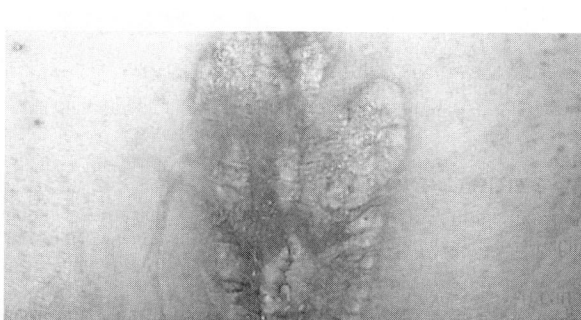

FIGURE 1-495 Lichen sclerosus. Perianal area is thinned and chalk white (keyhole distribution). (Courtesy Department of Dermatology, University of North Carolina at Chapel Hill. From Goldstein BG, Goldstein AO: *Practical dermatology,* ed 2, St Louis, 1997, Mosby.)

ETIOLOGY

Unknown. There may be an autoimmune association and a genetic familial component.

DIAGNOSIS

DIFFERENTIAL DIAGNOSIS

- Localized scleroderma (morphea)
- Cutaneous discoid lupus erythematosus
- Atrophic lichen planus
- Psoriasis

WORKUP

Diagnosis is based on close examination of the lesions for the presence of ivory-white atrophic lesions and typical location.

LABORATORY TESTS

Punch or deep shave biopsy can be used to confirm the diagnosis.

TREATMENT

NONPHARMACOLOGIC THERAPY

Attention to hygiene and elimination of irritants or excessive bathing with harsh soaps

GENERAL Rx

- Application of clobetasol propionate 0.05% topically bid for up to 4 wk is usually effective. Repeat courses of corticosteroids may be necessary because of the chronic nature of this disorder. Continual application of topical steroids may lead to atrophy of the vulva.
- There is no substantial evidence that use of topical sex hormones (e.g., topical testosterone [2%]) is effective in genital lichen sclerosus.
- Lubricants (e.g., Nutraplus cream) are useful to soothe dry tissues.
- Hydroxyzine 25 mg at bedtime is effective in decreasing nocturnal itching.
- Use of intralesional steroids, etretinate, and surgical management is usually reserved for refractory cases.

DISPOSITION

- The disease persists in approximately one third of patients.
- Most prepubertal girls improve spontaneously at menarche.
- Squamous cell carcinoma can develop within the lesions in 3% to 10% of older patients; therefore periodic examination and biopsy of suspicious areas are indicated.

PEARLS & CONSIDERATIONS

COMMENTS

- Prepubertal lichen sclerosus may be confused with sexual abuse in prepubertal girls and may lead to false accusations and investigations.
- Lichen sclerosus of the vulva (kraurosis vulvae) usually occurs after menopause and is generally chronic. It can be painful and interfere with sexual activity.
- Lichen sclerosus of the penis (balanitis xerotica obliterans) is seen more commonly in uncircumcised males. It affects the glans and prepuce and may lead to stricture if it encroaches into the urinary meatus.

SUGGESTED READING

available at www.expertconsult.com

RELATED CONTENT

Lichen Sclerosus (Patient Information)

AUTHOR: **FRED F. FERRI, M.D.**

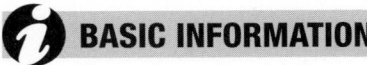

BASIC INFORMATION

DEFINITION

Lichen simplex chronicus is neurodermatitis manifesting with localized areas of thickened scaly skin due to prolonged and severe scratching in patients with no underlying dermatologic condition.

SYNONYMS

Neurodermatitis from rubbing

ICD-9CM CODES

698.3 Lichenification and lichen simplex chronicus

EPIDEMIOLOGY & DEMOGRAPHICS

PEAK INCIDENCE: Between 35 and 50 yr old
PREVALENCE: Increased in patients with underlying anxiety disorders
PREDOMINANT SEX AND AGE:
- Sex: Females > males (2:1)
- Age: Adults over 60

RISK FACTORS: Anxiety disorders, dry skin, insect bites

PHYSICAL FINDINGS & CLINICAL PRESENTATION

- Patients present with profound pruritus and localized scaly plaques with accentuated skin markings said to resemble tree bark (Fig. 1-496).

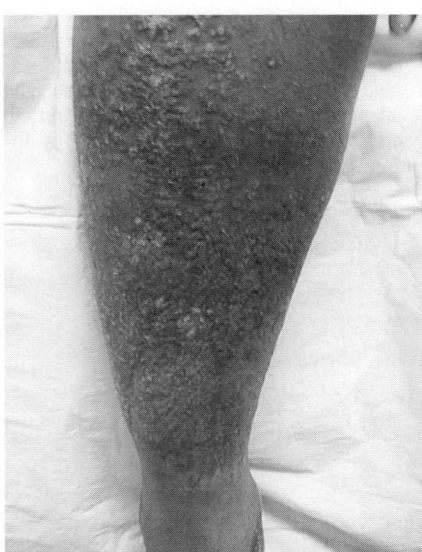

FIGURE 1-496 Lichenified skin of the lower extremity caused by habitual rubbing. The confluence of multiple scaling papules has formed a large plaque of palpably thickened skin. (From Ferri FF et al: *Ferri's fast facts in dermatology,* Philadelphia, 2010, Saunders.)

- Lichenified circumscribed plaques. Trauma from rubbing and scratching accounts for persistence of the plaque.
- Commonly involved areas include hands and wrists (Fig. 1-497), back and sides of neck, anterior tibias, anogenital areas, and ankles.

ETIOLOGY

- Neurodermatitis
- Common triggers are excess dryness of skin, heat, sweat, and psychological stress. It can also accompany other conditions such as the fungal infections candidiasis or tinea cruris, or psoriasis, lichen sclerosus, and neoplasia.
- Other causes include atrophic dermatitis and insect bites. Rare cases have shown links to lithium use, hair dye containing PPD, and long-term exposure to vehicle pollution.

DIAGNOSIS

DIFFERENTIAL DIAGNOSIS

- Lichen planus
- Psoriasis
- Atopic dermatitis
- Insect bite
- Nummular eczema
- Contact dermatitis
- Stasis dermatitis

WORKUP

Patient history and skin examination. Skin biopsy when diagnosis is unclear or persistent symptoms.

LABORATORY TESTS

- Not generally necessary
- Biopsy reveals hyperkeratosis, acanthosis, and mild to moderate lymphohistocytic inflammatory infiltrate with prominent lichenification.

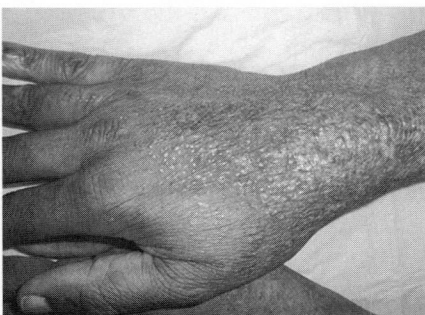

FIGURE 1-497 Longstanding pruritus and scratching resulted in this thickened, hyperpigmented skin on the wrist consisting of numerous 1- to 2-mm papules. This "follicular" pattern is more common in African Americans. (From Ferri FF et al: *Ferri's fast facts in dermatology,* Philadelphia, 2010, Saunders.)

TREATMENT

NONPHARMACOLOGIC THERAPY

- Patient education is essential to break the itch-scratch cycle and facilitate treatment of any underlying dermatitis.
- Psychotherapy

ACUTE GENERAL Rx

- Hydroxyzine 25 mg at bedtime is effective in decreasing nocturnal itching.
- Topical corticosteroids
- Intralesional corticosteroids
- Anxiolytics, SSRIs
- Oral doxepin (an antidepressant and anxiolytic)
- Mirtazapine
- Tropical calcineurin inhibitor for vulvar lichenification

CHRONIC Rx

Constant irritation of the skin must be avoided. Keeping skin moisturized, a covering to prevent scratching, or nail filing may be necessary.

DISPOSITION

Psychological intervention improves recovery. Regular follow-up visits facilitate long-term management.

REFERRAL

Refer to a psychologist for psychological evaluation and consultation, and a dermatologist in resistant cases.

PEARLS & CONSIDERATIONS

- Significant scratching may occur during nocturnal hours.
- The involved area is always at a site that is easily reached for scratching.
- Chronic scratching can also cause keratinocyte necrosis and the development of amyloid in the papillary dermis, called lichen amyloidosis.

COMMENTS

Patients may be at increased risk for scarring of the skin, changes in skin pigmentation, and bacterial and fungal infections of the involved skin.

PREVENTION

Prevent future incidences by continued therapy, stress management, and avoidance of common triggers and accompanying conditions.

SUGGESTED READINGS

available at www.expertconsult.com

AUTHORS: **FRED F. FERRI, M.D.,** and **HEATHER SUNTER, M.S.**

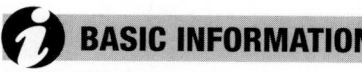

BASIC INFORMATION

DEFINITION

Listeriosis is a systemic infection caused by the gram-positive aerobic bacterium *Listeria monocytogenes*.

SYNONYMS

Listerial infection
Granulomatosis infantisepticum

ICD-9CM CODES
027.0 Listeriosis
771.2 Congenital listeriosis
771.2 Fetal listeriosis
665.4 Suspected fetal damage affecting management of pregnancy

EPIDEMIOLOGY & DEMOGRAPHICS

INCIDENCE (IN U.S.):
- *Listeria* meningitis: about 0.7 cases/100,000 persons (fourth most common cause of community-acquired bacterial meningitis in adults)
- Perinatal listeriosis: 8.6 cases/100,000 persons
- Nonperinatal listeriosis: 3 cases/1 million persons

PREDOMINANT SEX: Pregnant women are more susceptible to *Listeria* bacteremia, accounting for up to one third of reported cases.

PREDOMINANT AGE:
- Pregnant women
- Immunocompromised patients of any age
- Elderly patients are susceptible even in the absence of recognized immunocompromised states

GENETICS:
Congenital infection:
- With transplacental transmission, syndrome termed *granulomatosis infantisepticum* in neonate
- Characterized by disseminated abscesses in multiple organs, skin lesions, and conjunctivitis
- Mortality: 33% to 100%

Neonatal infection:
- Infant becoming ill after 3 days of age; mother invariably asymptomatic
- Clinical picture of sepsis of unknown origin

PHYSICAL FINDINGS & CLINICAL PRESENTATION

Infections in pregnancy
1. More common in third trimester
2. Usually present with fever and chills without localizing symptoms or signs of infection

Meningoencephalitis
1. More common in neonates and immunocompromised patients, but up to 30% of adults have no underlying condition

2. In neonates: poor appetite with or without fever possibly the only presenting signs
3. In adults: presentation often subacute, with low-grade fever and personality change as only signs
4. Focal neurologic signs seen without demonstrable brain abscess on CT scan

Cerebritis/rhombencephalitis
1. Headache and fever may be only presenting complaints
2. Progressive cranial nerve palsies, hemiparesis, seizures, depressed level of consciousness, cerebellar signs, respiratory insufficiency may also be seen

Focal infections
1. Ocular infections (purulent conjunctivitis) and skin lesions (granulomatosis infantisepticum) as a result of inadvertent inoculation by laboratory and veterinary personnel
2. Others: arthritis, prosthetic joint infections, peritonitis, osteomyelitis, organ abscesses, cholecystitis

ETIOLOGY

- Direct invasion of skin and eye has been documented, but mechanism of GI entry is unclear.
- Organism's intracellular life cycle explanatory of:
  1. Importance of cell-mediated immunity in host defense
  2. Increased infection in neonates, pregnant women, and immunocompromised hosts

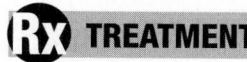

DIAGNOSIS

DIFFERENTIAL DIAGNOSIS

- Meningitis caused by other bacteria, mycobacteria, or fungi
- CNS sarcoidosis
- Brain neoplasm or abscess
- Tuberculous and fungal (especially cryptococcal) meningitis
- Cerebral toxoplasmosis
- Lyme disease
- Sarcoidosis

WORKUP

Dictated by age, end-organ involvement, and immune status

LABORATORY TESTS

- Cultures of blood and other appropriate body fluids
- Variable CSF findings, but neutrophils usually predominate
- Organisms uncommonly seen on Gram stain and may be difficult to identify morphologically
- Monoclonal antibodies, polymerase chain reaction, and DNA probe techniques to detect *Listeria* in foods

IMAGING STUDIES

- If focal cerebral involvement suspected: CT scan or MRI
- MRI most sensitive for evaluation of brainstem and cerebellum

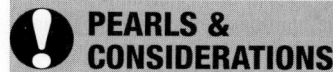

TREATMENT

Empiric therapy should be administered when diagnosis is suspected because overall mortality is 23%.

ACUTE GENERAL Rx

- Drugs of choice:
  1. IV ampicillin 8 to 12 g/day in divided doses
  2. IV penicillin 12 to 24 million U/day in divided doses
- Continuation of therapy for 2 wk
- Alternative (if penicillin allergic): trimethoprim/sulfamethoxazole or vancomycin
- Gentamicin added to provide synergy in meningitis or endocarditis

CHRONIC Rx

Relapses reported, especially in immunocompromised hosts, after 2 wk of therapy.

DISPOSITION

Long-term follow-up of immunodeficiency state

REFERRAL

Infectious disease consultation for all patients

PEARLS & CONSIDERATIONS

COMMENTS

- Foodborne cases have been linked to various products: coleslaw, soft cheeses, unpasteurized milk and milk products, vegetables, undercooked chicken, hot dogs, luncheon meats, refrigerated smoked seafood, and so on.
- Complete decontamination of food products is difficult because *Listeria* is resistant to pasteurization and refrigeration.

SUGGESTED READINGS
available at www.expertconsult.com

RELATED CONTENT
Listeriosis (Patient Information)

AUTHOR: **GLENN G. FORT, M.D., M.P.H.**

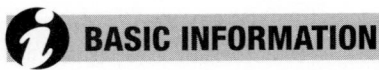

BASIC INFORMATION

DEFINITION

Long QT syndrome (LQTS) is a disorder of myocardial repolarization characterized by a prolongation of rate-corrected QT (QTc) interval on the ECG associated with an increased risk of developing life-threatening ventricular arrhythmias, most commonly torsades de pointes (a specific type of polymorphic ventricular tachycardia), which may lead to ventricular fibrillation and sudden cardiac death (SCD).

SYNONYMS

LQTS
Congenital forms:
  Jervell and Lange-Nielsen syndrome (associated with deafness)
  Romano-Ward syndrome (associated with normal hearing)

ICD-9CM CODES

427.9 Unspecified cardiac dysrhythmia

EPIDEMIOLOGY & DEMOGRAPHICS

- Congenital LQTS is thought to account for more than 3000 deaths per year in the United States.
- Incidence of LQTS is thought to be between 1:2500 and 1:10,000 in the general population, although it has been difficult to estimate due to incomplete penetrance.
- Congenital form associated with deafness is autosomal recessive (Jervell and Lange Nielsen syndrome) and is less common than the autosomal dominant form.
- Congenital form associated with normal hearing (Romano-Ward syndrome) is autosomal dominant. Although inheritance of LQTS is autosomal dominant, female predominance has often been observed and has been attributed to an increased susceptibility to cardiac arrhythmias in women.
- At least 10 different LQTS genes have been identified to date, resulting in at least 10 subtypes.
- LQTS is more common in women than in men.
- Mortality rate is estimated to be about 1% per year.
- Genetic mutations in the congenital LQTS are described in Table 1-251. Common types of LQTS are described in Table 1-252.

PHYSICAL FINDINGS & CLINICAL PRESENTATION

- Many episodes are stress mediated.
- Palpitations, presyncope
- Syncope caused by ventricular tachycardia
- SCD
- Seizure
- Family history of LQTS, but a family history of SCD has not been proved to be a risk factor for SCD in patients with LQTS
- Abnormal ECG (prolonged QT) in asymptomatic relatives of known case
- Prolonged QTc interval on ECG (QTc should be <440 ms in women and <420 ms in men)

ETIOLOGY

- Cardiac repolarization abnormality
- Congenital cause (hundreds of mutations on more than 10 genes have been identified)
- Most of the gene mutations affect function of ion channels leading to prolonged repolarization (i.e., sodium and potassium channels resulting in either increased Na^+ influx or decreased K^+ efflux). These mutations prolong depolarization and predispose the patient to torsades de pointes.
- Acquired causes:
  ○ Drugs: dofetilide, ibutilide, bepridil, quinidine, procainamide, sotalol, amiodarone, ranolazine, disopyramide, phenothiazines and anti-emetic agents (droperidol, domperidone), tricyclic antidepressants, antipsychotics (quetiapine, ziprasidone, iloperidone), citalopram, antihistamines, quinolones, azithromycin, astemizole or cisapride given with ketoconazole or erythromycin,

TABLE 1-251 Genetic Mutations in Congenital Long QT Syndrome

		Location	Gene	Current	Effect
Romano-Ward syndrome (autosomal-dominant inheritance)	LQT1	11p15.5	KvLQT1 (K$^+$ channel)	I$_{Ks}$	↓ Function ↓ Repolarization
	LQT2	7q35-36	HERG (K$^+$ channel)	I$_{Kr}$	↓ Function ↓ Repolarization
	LQT3	3q21-24	SCN5A (Na$^+$ channel)	I$_{Na}$	↑ Function ↑ Depolarization
	LQT4	4q25-27	Unknown	Unknown	Unknown
	LQT5	21q22	KCNE1 (K$^+$ channel, subunit minK)	I$_{Ks}$	↓ Function ↓ Repolarization
Jervell and Lange-Nielsen syndrome (autosomal-recessive inheritance)		11p15.5	KvLQT1 (K$^+$ channel)	I$_{Ks}$	↓ Function ↓ Repolarization
		21q22	KCNE 1 (K$^+$ channel, subunit minK)	I$_{Ks}$	↓ Function ↓ Repolarization

From Crawford MH et al (eds): *Cardiology*, ed 2, St Louis, 2004, Mosby.

TABLE 1-252 Common Types of Long QT (LQT) Syndrome

	LQT1	LQT2	LQT3
Pathophysiology			
Gene	KCNQ1 (K$_v$LQT1)	KCNH2 (HERG)	SCN5A
Protein	K$_v$7.1	K$_v$11.1	Na$_v$1.5
Ionic current	Decreased I$_{Ks}$	Decreased I$_{Kr}$	Increased late I$_{Na}$
Clinical Presentation			
Incidence of cardiac events	63%	46%	18%
Incidence of SCD	4%	4%	4%
Arrhythmia triggers	Emotional/physical stress (swimming, diving)	Emotional stress, arousal (alarm clock, telephone), rest	Sleep/rest
ECG	Broad-based T wave	Low-amplitude, bifid T wave	Long isoelectric ST segment
QT response to exercise	Attenuated QTc shortening and an exaggerated QTc prolongation during early and peak exercise	Normal QT during exercise but with exaggerated QT hysteresis	Supernormal QT shortening
Management			
Exercise restriction	+++	++	?
Response to beta blockers	+++	+++	?
Potassium supplement	+	++	+
Left cervicothoracic sympathectomy	++	++	++
Response to mexiletine	+	+	++

From Issa Z et al: *Clinical arrhythmology and electrophysiology*, ed 2, Philadelphia, 2012, Saunders.

clarithromycin, and antimalarials, particularly among patients with asthma or those using potassium-lowering medications; also common in patients receiving methadone
○ Hypokalemia, hypomagnesemia, hypocalcemia (especially in patients with malabsorption syndrome)
○ Liquid protein diet
○ Central nervous system lesions
○ Mitral valve prolapse
○ Hypothyroidism

Dx DIAGNOSIS

DIFFERENTIAL DIAGNOSIS

See "Syncope." Brugada's syndrome, arrhythmogenic right ventricular dysplasia, and LQTS are major causes of genetic sudden death syndromes (Fig. 1-498).

Diagnostic criteria for the congenital LQTS:
ECG Criteria

QTc >480 ms	3 points
QTc 460-480 ms	2 points
QTc 450-460 ms (males)	1 point
Torsades de pointes	2 points
T-wave alternans	1 point
Notched T wave in 3 leads	1 point
Bradycardia	0.5 point
History	
Syncope with stress	2 points
Syncope without stress	1 point
Congenital deafness	0.5 point
Definite family history of long QT	1 point
Unexplained cardiac death in first-degree relative <30 yr	0.5 point

Total score = 4: definite LQTS; total score = 2 to 3: intermediate probability; total score = 1: low probability.

WORKUP

Cardiology referral is recommended for all cases.

Genetic analysis is an essential step for risk stratification of patients with congenital prolonged QT and is important for identification of potential mutation carriers within the proband family. There is evidence for gene-specific triggers of events and therapeutic efficacy. Molecular screening should become part of the routine clinical management of LQTS.

In relatives of known patients with LQTS or in young patients with syncope:
- Stress test may prolong the QT interval or cause T-wave alternans
- Valsalva maneuver: may prolong the QT interval or cause T-wave alternans
- Prolonged ECG monitoring with various stimulations aimed at increasing catecholamines and assess for QT prolongation (perform in a setting that can provide resuscitation with α- and β-antagonists readily available).
- Epinephrine-induced prolongation of the QT interval (epinephrine infusion QT stress test)
- Genetic analysis
  ○ *LQT1* locus of *KCNQ1* potassium channel gene
  ○ *LQT2* locus of *KCNH2* potassium channel gene
  ○ *LQT3* locus of *SCN5A* sodium channel gene

○ These three variants account for >90% of all genotyped LQTS patients, whereas the remaining genes are responsible for a minority of cases
- Risk stratification for each genetic variant on the basis of gender and QTc: groups are defined on the basis of the probability of the first cardiac event (syncope, cardiac arrest, or sudden death) before the age of 40 years or before therapy. QT interval duration was the strongest predictor of risk for cardiac events; a QTc exceeding 500 ms identifies patients with the highest risk.
  ○ High risk (>50% of cardiac event): QTc ≥ 500 ms and *LQT1* or *LQT2*, or male with *LQT3*
  ○ Moderate risk (30% to 50%): QTc <500 ms in male with *LQT3* or in female with *LQT2 or LQT3*, and female with *LQT3 with QTc ≥ 500 ms*
  ○ Low risk (<30%): QTc <500 ms and *LQT1* or male *LQT2* with QTc < 500 ms
  ○ Prophylactic treatment should be considered in all patients with moderate or high risk for cardiac events based on the above risk stratification scheme (Table 1-253)

Rx TREATMENT

NONPHARMACOLOGIC

- Focuses on exclusion of triggers of life-threatening arrhythmia—there are gene-specific triggers for symptoms:
  ○ *LQT1* patients experience 90% of lethal events under physical and emotional stress. Swimming and diving should be avoided or performed under supervision.
  ○ *LQT2* patients are at highest risk during arousal or emotions, also during sleep and at rest but not at all during exercise; avoid sudden or excessive acoustic stimuli, especially during sleep (e.g., avoid telephone and/or alarm clock in the proximity)—as opposed to *LQT3* patients, in whom 80% of the events occur at rest or while asleep.
- Avoid competitive sports.
- Implantation of an implantable cardioverter-defibrillator (ICD) is recommended according to the ACC/AHA guidelines for patients with a good functional status for more than 1 yr and the following conditions (Table 1-254):
  ○ Survivors of cardiac arrest (class 1)
  ○ Patients with syncope or ventricular tachycardia while receiving β-blockers (class IIa)
  ○ Prophylaxis of SCD with use of β-blocker in patients with characteristics that suggest high risk (such as *LQT2* and *LQT3*, QTc >500 ms) (class IIb)

PHARMACOLOGIC

- With few exceptions (mostly borderline QTc and *LQT1* males older than age 25 to 30 yr), all mutation carriers should be treated because of the risk of SCD during first cardiac event. All symptomatic patients should be treated as well.
- Beta-blockers an initial therapy of choice—there are differential responses to β-blocker

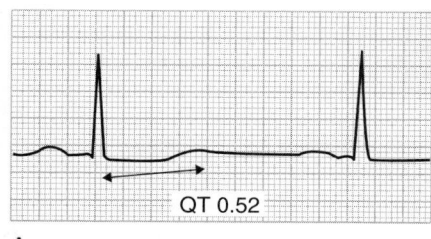

QT 0.52

A

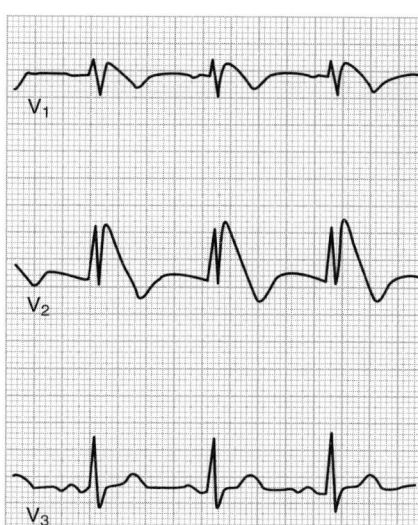

V₁

V₂

V₃

B

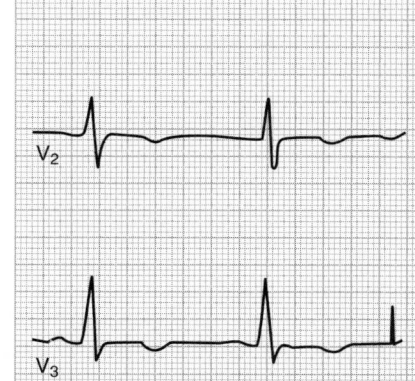

V₁

V₂

V₃

C

FIGURE 1-498 Sinus rhythm electrocardiogram findings in three genetic sudden death syndromes. A, QT prolongation during sinus rhythm in a patient with long QT syndrome. **B,** ST elevation in V₁ and V₂ in a patient with Brugada's syndrome. **C,** T wave inversion in V₁-V₃ in a patient with arrhythmogenic right ventricular dysplasia. (From Goldman L, Schafer AI: *Goldman's Cecil medicine*, ed 24, Philadelphia, 2012, Saunders.)

TABLE 1-253 Cardiac Event Risk Stratification Scheme Based on Genes, Gender, and QTc

Genetic Subtype	QTc <500 ms		QTc >=500 ms	
	Male	Female	Male	Female
LQT1	Low	Low	High	High
LQT2	Low	Intermediate	High	High
LQT3	Intermediate	Intermediate	High	Intermediate

Probability of the first cardiac event (syncope, cardiac arrest, or sudden death) before the age of 40 years or before therapy.
High = >50%, Intermediate = 30%-50%, Low = <30%.

TABLE 1-254 Management of Patients with Long QT Syndrome

Type of Syndrome	Management	Indication
Congenital	Beta-blockers	Asymptomatic patients, symptomatic patients (who do not have bronchospasm)
	Cervicothoracic sympathectomy	Refractory symptoms, especially in pediatric patients
	Cardiac pacing	Refractory symptoms associated with bradycardia, pauses
	Implantable cardioverter-defibrillator	Cardiac arrest, refractory syncope, prophylaxis for moderate- to high-risk patients for cardiac events
Acquired	Elimination of causative drug or condition	All patients
	Magnesium sulfate	Nonsustained ventricular tachycardia, torsades de pointes (even with a normal serum magnesium concentration)
	Administration of potassium (to keep serum K+ >4.5 mEq/L)	Serum K^+ <4.5 mEq/L
	Maneuvers to increase heart rate (cardiac pacing, isoproterenol)	Bradycardia, arrhythmias refractory to magnesium sulfate

K^+, Potassium.
Adapted from Crawford MH et al (eds): *Cardiology*, ed 2, St Louis, 2004, Mosby.

therapy among different genetic variants; especially effective among *LQT1* patients. Studies showed the efficacy of β-blockers with an overall mortality <2% over a mean follow-up exceeding 5 yr.
- From 20% to 30% of patients who continue to have symptoms on a β-blocker, the main options are either left cardiac sympathetic denervation (LCSD) or the prophylactic implantation of an ICD.

- In patients with frequent ICD shocks or in those with high risk for SCD where ICD placement cannot be performed, cardiac pacing and/or LCSD may be indicated.
- In patients with recurrent syncope and/or aborted cardiac arrest despite combined ICD and β-blocker, LCSD as adjunctive therapy.
- Correctable factors including electrolyte disorder—hypokalemia and hypomagnesemia—and avoidance of precipating drugs

that may further prolong the QT interval is mandatory.
- For patients with acquired form and torsades de pointes, IV magnesium and atrial or ventricular pacing are initial choices.
- Table 1-254 summarizes management of patients with LQTS.

PROGNOSIS
In carefully treated patients, mortality is around 0.5% to 1% over 20 years.

The timing and frequency of syncope, QTc prolongation, and gender are predictive of risk for aborted cardiac arrest and SCD during adolescence. Higher risk is present in those with one or two or more episodes of syncope in the last 10 yr compared with those with no syncopal episodes, those with QTc >530 ms, and males aged 10 to 12 yr.

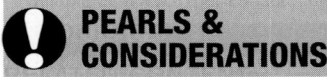

COMMENTS
Family history should be assessed for a history of sudden death and other deaths that may have occurred as manifestations of LQTS (e.g., sudden infant death, drowning, and loss of consciousness while driving).

SUGGESTED READINGS
available at www.expertconsult.com

RELATED CONTENT
Long QT Syndrome (Patient Information)

AUTHORS: **SHAHNAZ PUNJANI, M.D.,**
FRED F. FERRI, M.D., and
WEN-CHIH WU, M.D., M.P.H.

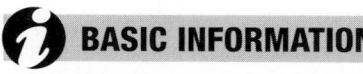

BASIC INFORMATION

DEFINITION

Lumbar disk syndrome includes diseases resulting from disk disorder, either herniation or degenerative change (spondylosis). Massive disk protrusion may rarely lead to paralysis in the lower extremity, a condition termed *cauda equina syndrome.* Gradual narrowing of the spinal canal (lumbar stenosis), usually from spondylosis, may also cause lower extremity symptoms.

SYNONYMS

Lumbago
Sciatica

ICD-9CM CODES
722.10 Lumbar disk displacement
724.02 Lumbar stenosis
344.60 Cauda equina syndrome
721.3 Lumbar spondylosis

EPIDEMIOLOGY & DEMOGRAPHICS

PREVALENCE:
- Variable
- At least one episode in 80% of adults

PREDOMINANT SEX: Approximately equal

PREDOMINANT AGE:
- Herniation: 20 to 40 yr
- Stenosis: >40 to 50 yr
- Disk symptoms: rare <20 yr

PHYSICAL FINDINGS & CLINICAL PRESENTATION

- Overlapping clinical syndromes that may result:
  1. Mild herniation without nerve root compression
  2. Herniation with nerve root compression
  3. Cauda equina syndrome
  4. Chronic degenerative disease with or without leg symptoms
  5. Spinal stenosis
- Low back pain, often worsened by activity or coughing and sneezing
- Local lumbar or lumbosacral tenderness
- Paresthesias, usually unilateral (Fig. E1-499)
- Restricted low back motion
- Increased pain on bending toward affected side
- Weakness and reflex changes (L4—knee jerk and quadriceps, L5—extensor hallucis longus, S1—ankle jerk and toe walking) (Table E1-255)
- Sensory examination usually not helpful
- Lumbar stenosis that possibly produces symptoms (pseudoclaudication), which are often misinterpreted as being vascular. Pseudoclaudication usually recovers quickly with sitting or spine flexion. Vascular disease is unaffected by spine position and is typically associated with atrophic skin changes and diminished pulses.)
- Positive straight leg raising test if nerve root compression is present

ETIOLOGY
Multifactorial

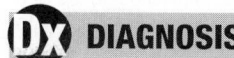

DIAGNOSIS

DIFFERENTIAL DIAGNOSIS

- Soft tissue strain or sprain
- Tumor
- Degenerative arthritis of hip
- Insufficiency fracture of hip or pelvis
  Section II describes the differential diagnosis of common low back pain syndromes. Table E1-256 differentiates the various causes of mechanical low back pain.

WORKUP

In most cases the diagnosis can be established on a clinical basis alone.

IMAGING STUDIES

- Imaging is not warranted for most patients with acute low back pain.
- Plain roentgenograms may be indicated within the first few weeks for persistent pain; they are usually normal in soft disk herniation, but with chronic degenerative disk disease loss of height of the disk space and osteophyte formation can occur.
- MRI (Fig. 1-500) may be indicated in patients whose symptoms do not resolve or when other spinal pathology may be suspected.
- Electrodiagnostic studies may confirm the diagnosis or rule out peripheral nerve disorders.

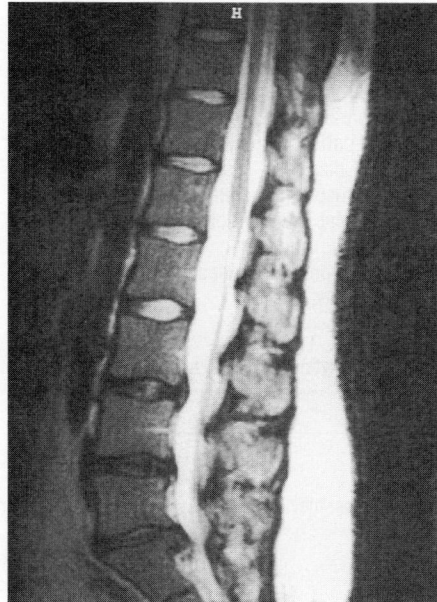

FIGURE 1-500 MRI showing a prolapsed L5/S1 disk. (From Carr A, Hamilton W: *Orthopedics in primary care,* ed 2, Philadelphia, 2005, Saunders.)

TREATMENT

NONPHARMACOLOGIC THERAPY

- Short course (3 to 5 days) of limited physical activity for acute disk herniation with leg pain
- Physical therapy for modalities plus a careful gradual exercise program. Physical therapists generally use the McKenzie method (see http://www.mckenziemdt.org/approach.cfm or http://www.youtube.com/watch?v=bPz9A4TWMCQ) for the treatment of low back pain.
- Lumbosacral corset brace during rehabilitation process in conjunction with exercise program is beneficial only in some cases.
- Percutaneous electrical nerve stimulation may be beneficial in selected patients with chronic back pain.

ACUTE GENERAL Rx

- NSAIDs
- Muscle relaxants for sedative effect
- Analgesics
- Epidural steroid injection for leg symptoms in selected patients

DISPOSITION

- Almost all lumbar disk syndromes improve with time.
- Recurrent episodes usually respond to medical management.
- Recovery from the rare paralytic event is often incomplete.

REFERRAL

- For orthopedic or neurosurgical consultation for intractable pain or significant neurologic deficit
- Emergency referral for cauda equina syndrome

PEARLS & CONSIDERATIONS

Red flags suggesting a more serious condition as a cause of the back pain include:
1. Fever
2. History of malignancy
3. Pain at rest
4. Incontinence
5. Sudden worsening in level of pain
6. Weight loss
7. Significant motor loss, especially if associated with saddle anesthesia

COMMENTS

- Surgery is most consistently helpful when leg pain (not back pain) predominates.
- No substantial benefit has been shown with oral steroids, traction, epidural corticosteroid injections, or lumbar support.

SUGGESTED READINGS

available at www.expertconsult.com

RELATED CONTENT

Lumbar Disc Syndrome (Patient Information)

AUTHOR: **LONNIE R. MERCIER, M.D.**

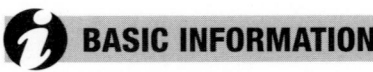

BASIC INFORMATION

DEFINITION

A primary lung neoplasm is a malignancy arising from lung tissue. The World Health Organization distinguishes 12 types of pulmonary neoplasms. The major types are squamous cell carcinoma, adenocarcinoma, small cell carcinoma, and large cell carcinoma. However, the crucial difference in the diagnosis of lung cancer is between small cell lung cancer (SCLC) and non–small cell lung cancer (NSCLC) because the prognosis and therapeutic approach are different.

ADENOCARCINOMA: Represents 35% to 40% of lung carcinomas; frequently located in mid-lung and periphery; initial metastases are to lymphatics; frequently associated with peripheral scars; adenocarcinoma is described as preinvasive, minimally invasive, or invasive

SQUAMOUS CELL (EPIDERMOID): 20% to 30% of lung cancers; central location; metastasis by local invasion; frequent cavitation and obstructive phenomena

SMALL CELL (OAT CELL): 20% of lung carcinomas; central location; metastasis through lymphatics; associated with lesion of the short arm of chromosome 3; high cavitation rate

LARGE CELL: 10% to 15% of lung carcinomas; frequently located in the periphery; metastasis to central nervous system and mediastinum; rapid growth rate with early metastasis

LEPIDIC-PREDOMINANT PATTERN (BRONCHOALVEOLAR): 5% of lung carcinomas; frequently located in the periphery; may be bilateral; initial metastasis through lymphatic, hematogenous, and local invasion; no correlation with cigarette smoking; cavitation rare

SYNONYMS

Lung cancer

ICD-9CM CODES
162.9 Malignant neoplasm of bronchus and lung, unspecified

EPIDEMIOLOGY & DEMOGRAPHICS

- Lung cancer is responsible for >30% of cancer deaths in males and >25% of cancer deaths in females. It has been the most common cancer in the world since 1985 and is the leading cause of cancer-related death.
- Tobacco smoking is implicated in 90% of cases; second-hand smoke is responsible for approximately 20% of cases.
- There are >200,000 new cases of lung cancer yearly in the U.S., most occurring at age >50 yr (<4% in patients <40 yr).
- Among women there has been a 600% increase in incidence of lung cancer during the past 80 years. The rates of death among women with lung cancer in the U.S. are the highest in the world.

PHYSICAL FINDINGS & CLINICAL PRESENTATION

- Weight loss, fatigue, fever, anorexia, dysphagia
- Cough, hemoptysis, dyspnea, wheezing
- Chest, shoulder, and bone pain
- Paraneoplastic syndromes (see Table 1-257):
  - Lambert-Eaton myasthenic syndrome: myopathy involving proximal muscle groups
  - Endocrine manifestations: hypercalcemia, ectopic adrenocorticotropic hormone, syndrome of inappropriate excretion of adrenocorticotropic hormone
  - Neurologic: subacute cerebellar degeneration, peripheral neuropathy, cortical degeneration
  - Musculoskeletal: polymyositis, clubbing, hypertrophic pulmonary osteoarthropathy
  - Hematologic or vascular: migratory thrombophlebitis, marantic thrombosis, anemia, thrombocytosis, or thrombocytopenia
  - Cutaneous: acanthosis nigricans, dermatomyositis
- Pleural effusion (10% of patients), recurrent pneumonias (from obstruction), localized wheezing
- Superior vena cava syndrome:
  - Obstruction of venous return of the superior vena cava is most commonly caused by bronchogenic carcinoma or metastasis to paratracheal nodes.
  - The patient usually reports headache, nausea, dizziness, visual changes, syncope, and respiratory distress.
  - Physical examination reveals distention of thoracic and neck veins, edema of face and upper extremities, facial plethora, and cyanosis.
- Horner's syndrome: constricted pupil, ptosis, facial anhidrosis caused by spinal cord damage between C8 and T1 as a result of a superior sulcus tumor (bronchogenic carcinoma of the extreme lung apex); Pancoast tumor: a superior sulcus tumor associated with ipsilateral Horner's syndrome and shoulder pain

ETIOLOGY

- Tobacco abuse; the chance of developing lung cancer for a 40-pack-year persistent smoker is 20 times that of someone who never smoked
- Environmental agents (e.g., radon) and industrial agents (e.g., ionizing radiation, asbestos, nickel, uranium, vinyl chloride, chromium, arsenic, coal dust)
- Lung cancer susceptibility and risk increased in inherited cancer syndromes caused by germ-line mutations in p53, retinoblastoma, and germ-line mutation in the epidermal growth factor receptor (EGFR) gene; also an association between single-nucleotide polymorphism variation at 15q24-15q25.1 and susceptibility to lung cancer

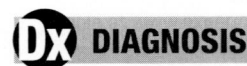

DIAGNOSIS

DIFFERENTIAL DIAGNOSIS

- Pneumonia
- Tuberculosis (TB)
- Metastatic carcinoma to the lung
- Lung abscess
- Granulomatous disease
- Carcinoid tumor
- Mycobacterial and fungal diseases
- Sarcoidosis
- Viral pneumonitis
- Benign lesions that simulate thoracic malignancy:
  - Lobar atelectasis: pneumonia, TB, chronic inflammatory disease, allergic bronchopulmonary aspergillosis
  - Multiple pulmonary nodules: septic emboli, Wegener's granulomatosis, sarcoidosis, rheumatoid nodules, fungal disease, multiple pulmonary atrioventricular fistulas
  - Mediastinal adenopathy: sarcoidosis, lymphoma, primary TB, fungal disease, silicosis, pneumoconiosis, drug-induced (e.g., phenytoin, trimethadione)

TABLE 1-257 Paraneoplastic Syndromes Associated with Bronchogenic Carcinoma

Syndrome	Cell Type	Mechanism
Hypertrophic pulmonary osteoarthropathy and clubbing	All except small cell	Unknown
Hyponatremia	Small cell most common; may be any type	SIADH, ectopic antidiuretic hormone production by tumor
Hypercalcemia	Usually squamous cell	Bone metastases, osteoclast-activating factor, parathyroid hormone–like hormone, prostaglandins
Cushing's syndrome	Usually small cell	Ectopic ACTH production
Lambert-Eaton myasthenic syndrome	Usually small cell	Voltage-sensitive calcium channel antibodies in >75%; affects presynaptic neuronal calcium channel activity
Other neuromyopathic disorders	Small cell most common; may be any type	Antineuronal nuclear antibodies, also known as anti-Hu; others unknown
Thrombophlebitis	All types	Unknown

ACTH, Adrenocorticotropic hormone; *SIADH,* syndrome of inappropriate secretion of antidiuretic hormone.
From Andreoli TE et al: *Andreoli and Carpenter's Cecil essentials of medicine,* ed 8, Philadelphia, 2010, Saunders.

○ Pleural effusion: congestive heart failure, pneumonia with parapneumonic effusion, TB, viral pneumonitis, ascites, pancreatitis, collagen-vascular disease

WORKUP

Workup generally includes chest radiograph, CT scan of chest, positron-emission tomographic (PET) scan, and tissue biopsy. Lab tests should include CBC, serum calcium, and liver chemistry studies. Diagnosis and staging of lung cancer should be performed simultaneously to minimize invasive testing.

LABORATORY TESTS

Obtain tissue diagnosis. Various modalities are available:

- Biopsy of any suspicious lymph nodes (e.g., supraclavicular node)
- Flexible fiberoptic bronchoscopy: brush and biopsy specimens are obtained from any visualized endobronchial lesions
- Transbronchial needle aspiration: done with a special needle passed through the bronchoscope; this technique is useful to sample mediastinal masses or paratracheal lymph nodes
- Transthoracic fine-needle aspiration biopsy with fluoroscopic or CT scan guidance to evaluate peripheral pulmonary nodules
- Mediastinoscopy and anteromedial sternotomy in suspected tumor involvement of the mediastinum
- Pleural biopsy in patients with pleural effusion
- Thoracentesis of pleural effusion and cytologic evaluation of the obtained fluid: may confirm diagnosis

IMAGING STUDIES

- Chest radiograph (Fig. 1-501): The radiographic presentation often varies with the cell type. Pleural effusion, lobar atelectasis, and mediastinal adenopathy can accompany any cell types.
- CT scan of chest (Fig. 1-502) is performed to evaluate mediastinal and pleural extension of suspected lung neoplasms. The chest CT should include liver and adrenal glands (common sites of metastases). CT or MRI of brain should be considered in a patient presenting with neurologic symptoms (e.g., headaches, vision disturbances).
- PET with 18F-fluorodeoxyglucose (18FDG-PET), a metabolic marker of malignant tissue, is superior to CT scan in detecting mediastinal and distant metastases in NSCLC. It is useful for preoperative staging of NSCLC.
- The use of PET-CT for preoperative staging of NSCLC reduces both the total number of thoracotomies and the number of futile thoracotomies but does not affect overall mortality.
- The combination of endoluminal ultrasound (EUS) and endobronchial ultrasound (EBUS) with fine-needle aspiration has been reported to have a 93% sensitivity and 97% specificity for establishing the presence of mediastinal disease in lung cancer patients.

STAGING

After confirmation of diagnosis, patients should undergo staging:

1. The international staging system is the most widely accepted staging system for NSCLC. In this system, stage I (N0 [no lymph node involvement]) and stage II (N1 [spread to ipsilateral bronchopulmonary or hilar lymph nodes]) include localized tumors for which surgical resection is the preferred treatment. Stage III is subdivided into IIIA (potentially resectable) and IIIB. The surgical management of stage IIIA disease (N2 [involvement of ipsilateral mediastinal nodes]) is controversial. Only 20% of N2 disease is considered minimal disease (involvement of only one node) and technically resectable. Stage IV indicates metastatic disease. The pathologic staging system uses a tumor/nodal involvement/metastasis system.

2. In patients with SCLC, a more practical accepted staging system is the one developed by the Veterans Administration Lung Cancer Study Group. This system contains two stages:
   a. Limited-stage disease: confined to the regional lymph nodes and to one hemithorax (excluding pleural surfaces)
   b. Extensive-stage disease: spread beyond the confines of limited-stage disease

3. Pretreatment staging procedures for lung cancer patients, in addition to complete history and physical examination, generally include the following tests:

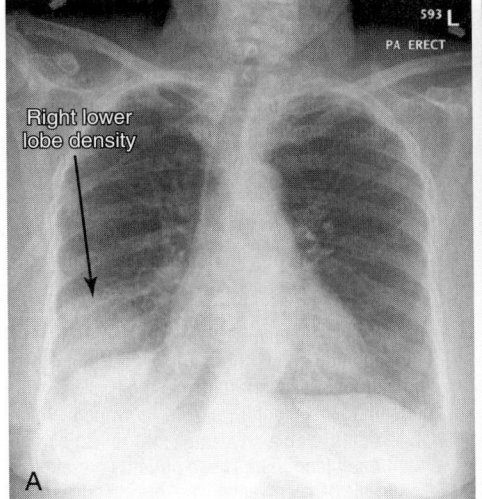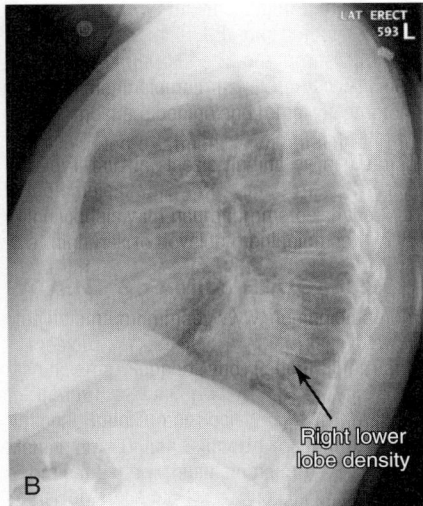

FIGURE 1-501 Lung neoplasm, primary. Lung mass presenting with hemoptysis. **A,** Posterior-anterior (PA) chest x-ray. **B,** Lateral chest x-ray. This 83-year-old female presented with hemoptysis of a quarter-sized clot. Her posterior-anterior chest x-ray shows a rounded right lower lobe density. On the lateral view, this is visible in the retrocardiac space. This density measures 7.6 cm in diameter. Pneumonia, neoplasm, or abscess could have this appearance on chest x-ray. Computed tomography was performed to further delineate the pathology (see Fig. 1-502). (From Broder JS: *Diagnostic imaging for the emergency physician,* Philadelphia, 2011, Saunders.)

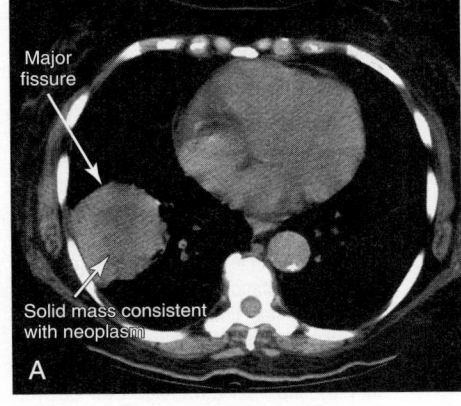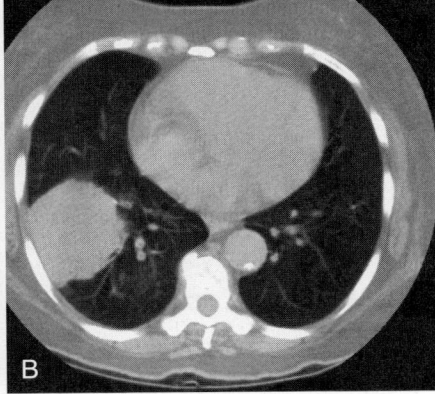

FIGURE 1-502 Lung neoplasm, primary. Lung mass presenting with hemoptysis. Same patient as in Fig. 1-501. Noncontrast computed tomography was performed (contrast was withheld as a consequence of the patient's renal dysfunction) and shows a 6 by 6 cm round lesion abutting the oblique fissure (also called the major fissure) and lateral chest wall. **A,** Soft tissue windows. **B,** Lung windows. On soft tissue windows, the center appears slightly darker, indicating lower density that may represent central necrosis. If IV contrast had been given, an area of necrosis would have failed to enhance. Infection or infarction is technically possible, but a pulmonary neoplasm is the most likely explanation for this lesion. Biopsy showed this to be a moderately differentiated squamous cell carcinoma. (From Broder JS: *Diagnostic imaging for the emergency physician,* Philadelphia, 2011, Saunders.)

a. Chest radiograph (posteroanterior and lateral), ECG
b. Laboratory evaluation: complete blood count, complete metabolic panel, arterial blood gases, pulse oximetry. The identification of molecular signatures of lung cancer to predict prognosis with data from microarray and/or reverse-transcription polymerase chain reaction analysis has been validated in recent trials. A five-gene signature (*DUSP6, MMD, STAT1, ERBB3,* and *LCK*) is closely associated with relapse-free and overall survival among patients with NSCLC. Anaplastic lymphoma kinase (ALK) translocation is found in about 4% to 5% of lung cancers. Detection of mutations in epidermal growth factor receptor (EGFR) in circulating tumor cells from the blood of patients with lung cancer offers the possibility of monitoring changes in epithelial tumor genotypes during the course of treatment
c. Pulmonary function studies
d. CT scan of chest and PET scan: a recent Dutch trial revealed a 51% relative reduction in futile thoracotomies for patients with suspected NSCLC who underwent preoperative assessment with PET with the tracer [18]FDG-PET in addition to conventional workup
e. Mediastinoscopy or anterior mediastinotomy in patients being considered for possible curative lung resection
f. Biopsy of any accessible suspect lesions
g. CT scan of liver and brain; radionuclide scans of bone in all patients with small cell carcinoma of the lung and patients with NSCLC neoplasms suspected of involving these organs
h. Bone marrow aspiration and biopsy only in selected patients with small cell carcinoma of the lung. In the absence of an increased lactate dehydrogenase or cytopenia, routine bone marrow examination not recommended
i. Newer technologies in preoperative staging include endoscopic bronchial ultrasonography and esophageal ultrasonography to guide biopsies; however, cervical mediastinoscopy is criterion standard in preoperative nodal staging (sensitivity >93%, specificity >95%)

Rx TREATMENT

NONPHARMACOLOGIC THERAPY
- Nutritional support
- Avoidance of tobacco and other substances toxic to the lungs
- Supplemental O_2 prn

ACUTE GENERAL Rx
NON–SMALL CELL CARCINOMA:
- Surgical resection is the best hope for cure in patients with operable NSCLC. (stage I or II when the patient is a surgical candidate). Lobectomy is the best standard surgical approach. Lesser resections may be necessary

in patients with marginal pulmonary reserve. Video-assisted thoracic surgery (VATS) is helpful in decreasing morbidity and shortening hospital stay.
1. Surgical resection is indicated in patients with limited disease (not involving mediastinal nodes, ribs, pleura, or distant sites). This represents approximately 15% to 30% of diagnosed cases.
2. Preoperative evaluation includes review of cardiac status (e.g., recent myocardial infarction, major arrhythmias) and evaluation of pulmonary function (to determine if the patient can tolerate any loss of lung tissue). Pneumonectomy is possible if the patient has a preoperative $FEV_1 = 2$ L or if the maximal voluntary ventilation is >50% of predicted capacity. Individuals with FEV_1 >1.5 L are suitable for lobectomy without further evaluation unless there is evidence of interstitial lung disease or undue dyspnea on exertion. In that case, carbon dioxide diffusion in the lung (DLCO) should be measured. If the DLCO is <80% predicted normal, the individual is not clearly operable.
3. Preoperative chemotherapy should be considered in patients with more advanced disease (stage IIIA) who are being considered for surgery because it increases the median survival time in patients with NSCLC compared with the use of surgery alone. Gene expression profiles that predict the risk of recurrence in patients with early stage (IA) NSCLC have been identified. These patients are at high risk of recurrence and may also benefit from adjuvant chemotherapy.
4. Postoperative adjuvant chemotherapy (chemotherapy given after surgical resection of an apparently localized tumor to eradicate occult metastases) with vinorelbine plus cisplatin significantly increases 5-yr survival (69% vs. 54%) in patients with completely resected stage IB or stage II NSCLC and good performance status. Adjuvant chemotherapy is generally indicated for patients with resected stages IIA through IIIA.
- Treatment of unresectable NSCLC:
1. Radiotherapy can be used alone or in combination with chemotherapy; it is used primarily for treatment of central nervous system and skeletal metastases, superior vena cava syndrome, and obstructive atelectasis. Although thoracic radiotherapy is generally considered standard therapy for stage 3 disease, it has limited effect on survival. Palliative radiotherapy should be delayed until symptoms occur because immediate therapy offers no advantage over delayed therapy and results in more adverse events from the radiotherapy. Conventional radiotherapy fails to durably control the primary lung tumor in nearly 70% of patients and 2-yr survival is less than 40%. Stereotactic body radiation (SBRT) uses several highly focused radiation beams to deliver high doses in 15 treatments and appears to be more effective than conventional radiother-

apy, with a survival rate of 55.8% at 3 yr for inoperable early stage lung cancer.
2. Chemotherapy remains the mainstay of treatment for advanced stage IIIB and stage IV NSCLC. (stage I or II when the patient is a surgical candidate). Lobectomy is the best standard surgical approach. Lesser resections may be necessary in patients with marginal pulmonary reserve. Video-assisted thoracic surgery (VATS) is helpful in decreasing morbidity and shortening hospital stay.. A platinum-based treatment is recommended for fit patients, and single agents can be offered in elderly patients and in those with poor performance status. Various combination regimens are available. Current drugs of choice are paclitaxel plus either carboplatin or cisplatin, cisplatin plus vinorelbine, gemcitabine plus cisplatin, and carboplatin or cisplatin plus docetaxel. The overall results are disappointing, and none of the standard regimens for NSCLC is clearly superior to the others. The addition of bevacizumab to paclitaxel plus carboplatin results in significant survival benefit but carries an increased risk of treatment-related death. Gefitinib and erlotinib are oral inhibitors of *EGFR* tyrosine kinase. Activating mutations in the *EGFR* gene confer hypersensitivity to these medications. Sensitivity of lung neoplasms to these agents is seen primarily in tumors with somatic mutations in the tyrosine kinase domain (more common in adenocarcinomas found in patients who never smoked and in Asian patients). Recent trials revealed that gefitinib is superior to carboplatin-paclitaxel as an initial treatment for pulmonary adenocarcinoma among nonsmokers or former smokers in East Asia. In these patients the presence in the tumor of a mutation of the *EGFR* gene was a strong predictor of a better outcome with gefitinib. The National Comprehensive Cancer Network (NCCN) recognizes erlotinib as an option for second- or third-line therapy in patients with advanced NSCLC who have a performance status of 0 to 3. It also recommends erlotinib monotherapy as first line for patients with an EGFR mutation. Erlotinib can also be used as a salvage treatment in this subgroup and as a maintenance agent for patients with stable or responsive disease after first-line platinum-based chemotherapy.Oncogenic fusion genes consisting of EML4 and anaplastic lymphoma kinase (ALK) are present in a subgroup of NSCLCs, representing 4% to 5% of such tumors. The inhibition of ALK in lung tumors with crizotinib, an orally available small-molecule inhibitor of the ALK tyrosine kinase, has resulted in tumor shrinkage and significant prolonged progression-free survival. Crizotinib was recently approved by the FDA for locally advanced or metastatic NSCLC with ALK translocation, which is found in about 5% of lung cancers.
3. The addition of chemotherapy to radiotherapy improves survival in patients with

locally advanced, unresectable NSCLC. The absolute benefit is relatively small, however, and should be balanced against the increased toxicity associated with the addition of chemotherapy.

4. Early initiation of palliative care focusing on management of symptoms, psychosocial support, and assistance with decision making in patients with metastatic NSCLC leads to improved quality of life, longer survival, and less use of aggressive end-of-life care.

SMALL CELL LUNG CANCER:

- Limited-stage disease: standard treatments include thoracic radiotherapy and chemotherapy (cisplatin and etoposide).
- Extensive-stage disease: standard treatments include combination chemotherapy (cisplatin or carboplatin plus etoposide or combination of irinotecan and cisplatin).
- Prophylactic cranial irradiation for patients in complete remission to decrease the risk of central nervous system metastasis.
- Despite high initial response rates, most patients eventually relapse. Topotecan may be an option for these patients.

DISPOSITION

- The 5-yr survival of patients with NSCLC when the disease is resectable is approximately 30%.

- Median survival time in patients with limited-stage disease and SCLC is 15 mo; in patients with extensive stage disease, it is 9 mo. Among patients with metastatic NSCLC, early palliative care results in longer survival and significant improvements in both quality of life and mood.
- Methylation of the promoter region of certain genes (*P16, CDH13, APC,* and *RASSF1A*) in a resected NSCLC specimen is associated with recurrence of the tumor.

PEARLS & CONSIDERATIONS

COMMENTS

- CT screening with use of low-dose computed tomography (LDCT) for detection of lung cancer among persons with a heavy history of smoking increases the percentage of lung cancer cases that are diagnosed in stage 1 and reduces mortality from lung cancer. The National Lung Screening Trial (NLST) showed that lung cancer screening with LDCT resulted in a 20% reduction in mortality from lung cancer. New guidelines from the American College of Chest Physicians, the American Society of Clinical Oncology, and the National Comprehensive Cancer Network recommend annual LDCT for those who are

current or former smokers aged 55-74. However, additional data and risk/benefit evaluation are needed before adaptation of this screening modality in general practice. Controversy also exists on the definition of a positive test result on CT with some proposing a threshold of 7 or 8 mm to define positive results.

- Quitting smoking is the most effective method to reduce risk for lung cancer. Following smoking cessation, the risk of lung cancer remains higher than normal based on duration and quantity of smoking but does not increase further as in a continuing smoker.

SUGGESTED READINGS

available at www.expertconsult.com

RELATED CONTENT

Lung Cancer Diagnosis
Lung Cancer Screening (Patient Information)

AUTHOR: **FRED F. FERRI, M.D.**

L

Diseases and Disorders

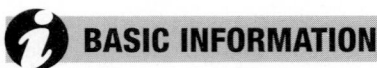

DEFINITION

Lyme disease is a multisystem inflammatory disorder caused by the transmission of a spirochete, *Borrelia burgdorferi*. Lyme disease is spread by the bite of infected *Ixodes* ticks, taking 36 to 48 hr for a tick to feed and transmit the infecting organism *B. burgdorferi* to the host.

SYNONYMS

Bannworth's syndrome (Europe)
Acrodermatitis chronica atrophicans

ICD-9CM CODES
088.8 Lyme disease

EPIDEMIOLOGY & DEMOGRAPHICS

INCIDENCE (IN U.S.): 4.4 cases/100,000 persons; 90% of cases in the U.S. are found in: Massachusetts, Connecticut, Rhode Island, New York, New Jersey, Pennsylvania, Minnesota, Wisconsin, and California.
PEAK INCIDENCE: May to November
PREDOMINANT SEX: Male = female
PREDOMINANT AGE: Median age of 28 yr

PHYSICAL FINDINGS & CLINICAL PRESENTATION

Lyme disease may present in the following stages:
- *Early localized stage (incubation period 3-30 days):* early Lyme disease, erythema migrans (EM); skin rash, often at site of tick bite (the CDC has defined EM rash as an expanding red macule or papule that must reach at least 5 cm in size, with or without central clearing); possible fever, myalgias 3 to 32 days after tick bite
- *Early disseminated stage (incubation period 3-6 weeks):* days to weeks later; multiorgan system involvement, including CNS with aseptic meningitis–type picture or Bell's palsy, joints (arthritis or arthralgias), cardiac including varying degrees of heart block; related to dissemination of spirochete
- *Late stage (incubation period months to years):* mo to yr after tick exposure; affects

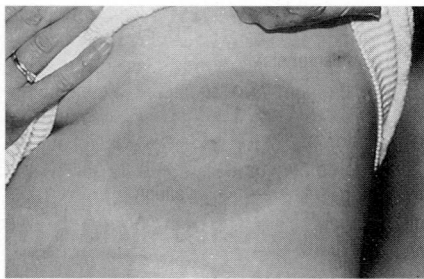

FIGURE 1-503 Erythema migrans. Note expanding erythematous lesion with central clearing on trunk. (Courtesy John Cook, M.D. From Goldstein B [ed]: *Practical dermatology,* ed 2, St Louis, 1997, Mosby.)

central and peripheral nervous system, cardiac, joints

Common presenting signs and symptoms include:
- EM (Fig. 1-503)
- Lymphadenopathy, neck pains, pharyngeal erythema, myalgias, hepatosplenomegaly.
- Patients will complain of malaise, fatigue, lethargy, headache, fever/chills, neck pain, myalgias, back pain.

ETIOLOGY

B. burgdorferi transmitted from bite of an *Ixodes* tick (mostly in the nymph stage, but can also be from adult ticks)

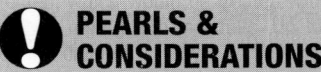 **DIAGNOSIS**

Clinical presentation, exposure to ticks in endemic area, and diagnostic testing for antibody response to *B. burgdorferi*

DIFFERENTIAL DIAGNOSIS

- Chronic fatigue/fibromyalgia
- Acute viral illnesses
- Babesiosis
- Ehrlichiosis

WORKUP

- ELISA testing and if positive or equivocal then followed by a Western blot IgM and IgG. A Western blot IgM assay is positive if 2 of 3 bands present. The Western blot IgG is positive if 5 of 10 bands present.
- Early disease often difficult to diagnose serologically secondary to slow immune response
- Culturing of skin lesions (EM) and polymerase chain reaction (PCR) of skin biopsy and blood to give definitive diagnosis (available only in reference laboratories)

IMAGING STUDIES

- Echocardiogram if conduction abnormalities are present with cardiac involvement
- CT scan, MRI of head for CNS involvement

(Rx) TREATMENT

Early localized Lyme disease:
- Doxycycline 100 mg bid or amoxicillin 500 mg tid for 14 days (doxycycline should be avoided in children >8 yr and pregnant females).
- Alternative treatments: cefuroxime axetil 500 mg bid for 14 to 21 days, azithromycin 500 mg PO for 7 to 10 days but should not be used as a first-line agent.
Early disseminated and late persistent infection:
- 28 days of treatment necessary; doxycycline and ceftriaxone appear equally effective for acute disseminated Lyme disease.
- Arthritis: 28 days of doxycycline or amoxicillin plus probenecid.

- Neurologic involvement requires parenteral antibiotics. Those who fail to respond should be treated with IV ceftriaxone or cefotaxime.
- Ceftriaxone 2 g/day IV for 21 to 28 days; alternative: cefotaxime 2 g q8h IV; alternative: penicillin G 5 million U qid.
- Cardiac involvement: IV ceftriaxone or penicillin plus cardiac monitoring.
- Prolonged treatment with IV or PO antibiotic therapy for up to 90 days did not improve symptoms more than placebo.
Post–Lyme disease syndrome:
- Antibiotics are not indicated.
- Supportive care

DISPOSITION

- The patient often needs careful follow-up and supportive care for the arthralgia-neuritis symptoms.
- Repeat episodes of EM in appropriately treated patients are due to reinfection and not to relapse.

REFERRAL

- To a neurologist if significant neurologic complications (meningitis, myelitis, ophthalmoplegia, Bell's palsy)
- To a cardiologist if the patient develops evidence of cardiac conduction disturbances or pericarditis

(!) PEARLS & CONSIDERATIONS

- The Lyme disease vaccine was taken off the U.S. market in 2002 because of concerns about possible side effects (arthralgia, arthritis) and its infrequent use.
- A physician diagnosis of classic EM in an endemic region of Lyme disease is sufficient to make a definitive diagnosis.
- In some patients with Lyme disease, nonspecific complaints such as headache, fatigue, and arthralgia may persist for months after appropriate (and ultimately successful) antibiotic treatment.
- There is no evidence of current or previous *Borrelia burgdorferi* infection in most patients evaluated at university-based Lyme disease referral centers. Psychiatric comorbidity and other psychological factors are prominent in the presentation and outcome of some patients who inaccurately ascribe longstanding symptoms to "chronic Lyme disease."
- A single dose of 200 mg doxycycline given within 72 hr of *Ixodes* tick bite can prevent development of Lyme disease.

SUGGESTED READINGS
available at www.expertconsult.com

RELATED CONTENT

Lyme Disease (Patient Information)

AUTHOR: **GLENN G. FORT, M.D., M.P.H.**

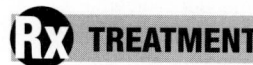

BASIC INFORMATION

DEFINITION

Lymphangitis refers to the inflammation of lymphatic vessels due to infectious or noninfectious causes. Infectious causes include bacteria, mycobacteria, viruses, fungi, and parasites.

SYNONYMS

Nodular lymphangitis
Sporotrichoid lymphangitis

ICD-9CM CODES
457.2 Lymphangitis

EPIDEMIOLOGY & DEMOGRAPHICS

INCIDENCE (IN U.S.): Several hundred cases/yr of sporotrichoid lymphangitis

PHYSICAL FINDINGS & CLINICAL PRESENTATION

ACUTE LYMPHANGITIS:

- Commonly associated with a bacterial cellulitis
- Usually develops after cutaneous inoculation of microorganisms into the lymphatic vessels through a skin wound or as a result of spread from a distal infection
- May or may not recognize site of skin trauma (i.e., laceration, puncture, ulcer)
- In hours to days, distal appearance of erythema, edema, and tenderness, with linear erythematous streaks extending proximally to regional lymph nodes
- Possible lymphadenitis and fever
- Predisposition to group A streptococcal infection of the skin in those with chronic lymphedema and superficial fungal infections (e.g., tinea pedis)

SPOROTRICHOID OR NODULAR LYMPHANGITIS:

- Includes subcutaneous nodules that develop along the path of involved lymphatics
- Most commonly results from inoculation of the skin of the hand
- Usually preceded by well-defined episode of cutaneous inoculation or trauma
- Lesions apparent from one to several wk after inoculation
- Initially, nodular or papular lesion; may ulcerate
- May have frank pus or a serosanguineous discharge

- Systemic complaints uncommon, but infection with certain microorganisms associated with fever, chills, myalgias, and headache

ETIOLOGY

- Acute lymphangitis: usually associated with *Streptococcus pyogenes* (group A streptococcus), but staphylococcal organisms are increasingly recognized as a cause of severe soft tissue infections such as lymphangitis, including community-acquired methicillin-resistant *S. aureus* (CA-MRSA)
- Nodular lymphangitis caused by one of several organisms
  1. *Sporothrix schenckii*
     a. Most common recognized cause in the U.S., usually in the Midwest
     b. Found in soil and plant debris
  2. *Nocardia brasiliensis:* found in soil
  3. *Mycobacterium marinum:* associated with trauma related to water (e.g., aquariums, swimming pools, fish)
  4. *Leishmania brasiliensis*
     a. Protozoal parasite transmitted to humans by sandflies, mostly to travelers in endemic areas
     b. Small endemic focus in Texas
  5. *Francisella tularensis*
     a. Most often in Midwestern states
     b. Associated with contact with infected mammals (e.g., rabbits) or tick bites

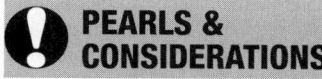

DIAGNOSIS

DIFFERENTIAL DIAGNOSIS

- Nodular lymphangitis
- Insect or snake bites
- Filariasis

WORKUP

- Acute lymphangitis: blood cultures
- Nodular lymphangitis: various stains and cultures of drainage or biopsy specimens of inoculation sites to make definitive diagnosis

LABORATORY TESTS

- WBCs possibly elevated with cellulitis
- Eosinophilia common with helminthic infections

TREATMENT

NONPHARMACOLOGIC THERAPY

Limb elevation

ACUTE GENERAL Rx

- Penicillin possibly sufficient, but 1 wk of dicloxacillin or cephalexin 500 mg PO qid commonly used to ensure antistaphylococcal coverage; if CA-MRSA suspected, then use oral Bactrim DS: one PO bid is the best oral agent and with vancomycin 1 g IV every 12 hr being reserved for patients requiring IV therapy.
- If allergic to penicillin:
  1. Clindamycin 300 mg PO qid for 7 days *or*
  2. Erythromycin 500 mg PO qid for 7 days
  3. Levaquin 500 mg PO daily or moxifloxacin 400 mg PO daily for 7 days
- Nodular lymphangitis: specific therapy directed at etiologic agent.
- For superficial fungal infections: treatment may prevent recurrence of acute lymphangitis.

DISPOSITION

- Acute lymphangitis: usually resolves with therapy
- Recurrent attacks: may lead to chronic lymphedema of limb, rarely resulting in elephantiasis nostras (nonfilarial elephantiasis)
- Nodular lymphangitis: usually responds to appropriate therapy

REFERRAL

- If acute lymphangitis is more than a mild disease or involves the face
- If nodular lymphangitis or filariasis is suspected

PEARLS & CONSIDERATIONS

COMMENTS

- Outside of the U.S., initial episodes of filariasis caused by *Brugia malayi* resemble acute lymphangitis.
- Chronic lymphedema or elephantiasis results from recurrent episodes.

SUGGESTED READINGS
available at www.expertconsult.com

RELATED CONTENT

Lymphangitis (Patient Information)

AUTHOR: **GLENN G. FORT, M.D., M.P.H.**

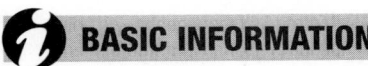

BASIC INFORMATION

DEFINITION

A primary role of the lymphatic system is to transport proteins from the interstitium to the heart. When the transport capacity of the lymphatic system is reduced, proteins accumulate in the interstitium. Accumulated proteins attract water which creates a high protein swelling in the subcutaneous tissues called lymphedema.

SYNONYMS

Elephantiasis

ICD-9CM CODES
457.0   Lymphedema: secondary to breast cancer
457.1   Lymphedema: secondary to all other causes
757   Lymphedema: primary

EPIDEMIOLOGY & DEMOGRAPHICS

PRIMARY LYMPHEDEMA:
- Found in 1.1/100,000 people aged <20 yr
- Females outnumber males 3.5:1.
- Incidence peaks between ages 12 and 16 (puberty)

SECONDARY LYMPHEDEMA: See specific etiology below.

PHYSICAL FINDINGS & CLINICAL PRESENTATION

Lymphedema is a slow onset, progressive disease characterized by an asymmetrical, inflammatory swelling, traveling distal to proximal, that can affect any body part including limbs, trunk, head/neck and genitals (Fig. 1-504). Box 1-35 summarizes lymphedema staging from the International Society of Lymphology.

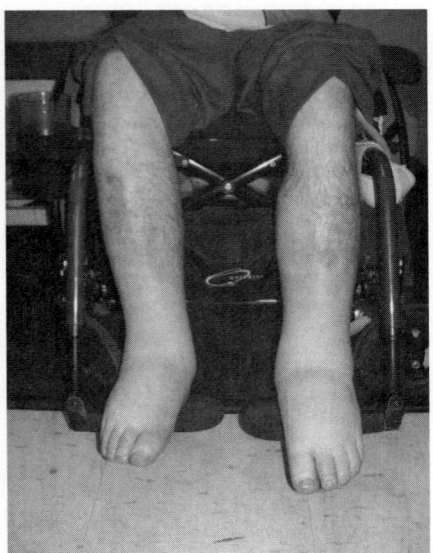

FIGURE 1-504 Lymphedema before treatment.

STAGE 0: LATENCY
- Decreased lymphatic system transport capacity due to primary or secondary etiology
- Subjective complaints of affected body part feeling heavy or achy
- No objective findings, no apparent swelling

STAGE I: REVERSIBLE
- Edema is observable, soft, pitting and reversible with elevation
- No secondary skin changes are present

STAGE II: SPONTANEOUSLY IRREVERSIBLE
- Skin becomes more firm/fibrotic, therefore less pitting
- Edema does not reverse to normal with elevation
- Possibility of infections (cellulitis), wounds or weeping (lymphorrhea)

STAGE III: ELEPHANTIASIS
- Skin becomes very firm/fibrotic, therefore non-pitting
- Evidence of substantial skin changes (e.g., papillomas, lobules, *"peau d' orange"*)

ETIOLOGY

Lymphedema is caused by a reduction in lymphatic system transport and is classified into primary and secondary forms.

PRIMARY LYMPHEDEMA:
- Occurs when the lymphatic system does not maturate properly during fetal development
  1. Aplasia
  2. Hypoplasia
  3. Hyperplasia
- Can be familial, genetic or hereditary
- Lymphedema congenital: symptoms present at birth
- Lymphedema praecox: symptoms onset prior to age of 35 (commonly during puberty)
- Lymphedema tardum: symptoms onset at the age of 35 or after

BOX 1-35   Lymphedema Staging

Stage 0: Latent
- Impaired lymphatic function
- No evident edema; subclinical
- May last months or years before progression

Stage I: Spontaneously Reversible
- Early accumulation of protein-rich fluid
- Pitting edema
- Subsides with elevation

Stage II: Spontaneously Irreversible
- Accumulation of protein-rich fluid
- Pitting edema progresses to fibrosis
- Does not resolve with elevation alone

Stage III: Lymphostatic Elephantiasis
- Nonpitting
- Significant fibrosis
- Trophic skin changes

From International Society of Lymphology: The diagnosis and treatment of peripheral edema: 2009 consensus document of the International Society of Lymphology, *Lymphology* 42(2):51-60, 2009.

SECONDARY LYMPHEDEMA:
- Occurs secondary to a disruption or obstruction of the lymphatic system caused by
  1. Filariasis (#1 cause worldwide)
  2. Lymph node surgery/radiation due to cancer (#1 cause in the United States)
  3. Other: chronic venous insufficiency (CVI), deep vein thrombosis (DVT), infection, surgery/trauma, lipedema and obesity

DIAGNOSIS

- Lymphedema is primarily a clinical diagnosis made on the basis of past medical history and objective findings that distinguish it from other causes of chronic edema
- A Stemmer's sign is often used to identify lymphedema (inability to pick up or pinch a fold of skin at the base of the second toe or finger)
- When physical examination is inconclusive, other available imaging tests can help make the diagnosis (see imaging studies below)

DIFFERENTIAL DIAGNOSIS

Other causes of edema that should be ruled out prior to treatment for lymphedema include cardiac, renal, hepatic, and thyroid dysfunction.

WORKUP

A detailed history and physical examination should help exclude most of the differential diagnoses.

LABORATORY TESTS

- Blood urea nitrogen, creatinine, liver function tests, albumin, urine analysis, and thyroid function tests are obtained to exclude possible systemic causes of edema
- Genetic testing may be practical in defining a specific hereditary syndrome with a discrete gene mutation such as lymphedema distichiasis (*FOXC2*), Milroy's disease (*VEGFR-3*), Meige's disease or Klippel-Trenaunay-Weber syndrome

IMAGING STUDIES

- Lymphoscintigraphy: diagnostic image of choice for lymphedema (if needed)
- Lymphography: phased out in favor of less invasive techniques
- Fluorescent microlymphangiography: primarily used for research purposes
- Magnetic resonance imaging (MRI): primarily used in tumor diagnosis
- Duplex ultrasound: determines venous involvement in the edema
- Computed axial tomography (CAT): distinguishes between fatty tissue and accumulations of protein-rich fluids

TREATMENT

NONPHARMACOLOGIC THERAPY
- Complete decongestive therapy (CDT) is backed by longstanding research and experience as the primary treatment of choice for

lymphedema in both children and adults (Fig. 1-505). It should be delivered by a certified lymphedema therapist (CLT). CDT involves a two-phase treatment program:

- ○ Phase 1—Reduce tissue congestion of affected body part with daily treatments:
  1. Manual lymph drainage
  2. Skin care
  3. Compression wrapping of limb
  4. Decongestive exercises
- ○ Phase 2—Maintain decongestion with Home Maintenance Program:
  1. Daily use of elastic and inelastic compression garments that are properly fitted according to circumference and length to prevent lymphedema from returning
  2. Compression is graduated; most of the compression is distal with decreasing compression in the stocking proximally

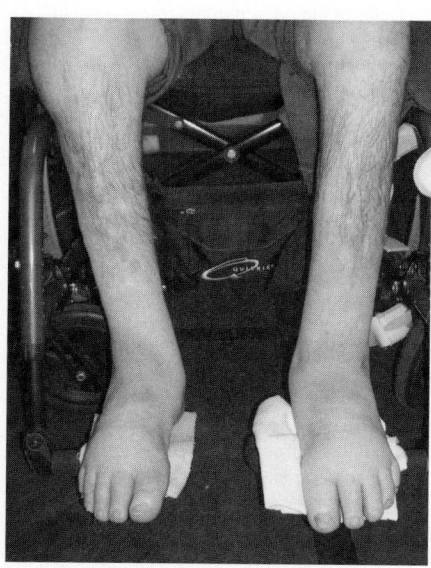

FIGURE 1-505 Lymphedema after treatment.

3. Different knits and compression classes are available for different stages of lymphedema
4. Choices of garments include below the knee stockings, thigh-high stockings, pantyhose, sleeves, bras, and truncal garments

- Massage (or any modality that increases blood flow) can have negative effects on lymphedema by increasing vasodilation. Therefore it is contraindicated on the lymphedematous quadrants
- Compression pumps have not been found to be effective in removing proteins from lymphedematous quadrants
- Nutritional therapy (reducing the amount of proteins ingested) is ineffective in the treatment of lymphedema

PHARMACOLOGIC THERAPY

No drugs have been shown to be beneficial in the treatment of lymphedema. Diuretics, in particular, have not been found to be effective in removing proteins from lymphedematous quadrants and may promote the development of volume depletion.

SURGERY

Surgery for lymphedema has been proven largely unsuccessful and should not be considered prior to CDT. Surgical procedures are divided into two types:

- Physiologic procedures: those performed to improve lymph node drainage (e.g., anastomoses of the lymph system with the venous system, lymph node transplant)
- Excisional or debulking procedures: those performed to excise the subcutaneous tissue (e.g., Charles' procedure, Thompson's procedure, the modified Homans' procedure, and liposuction). Liposuction-circumferential suction-assisted lipectomy represents a newly proposed method to reduce morbidity involved in the traditional excisional techniques

- Lymphedema is a chronic, generally incurable but very manageable condition that requires lifelong care and attention along with psychosocial support
- Children and adolescents (along with parents and adults) should be encouraged to pursue a normal life, participating in school activities and sports (preferably noncontact, such as swimming)
- Infections such as cellulitis should be treated promptly
- If the etiology is filariasis caused by the parasites *Wuchereria bancrofti* or *Brugia malayi*, treatment is diethylcarbamazine citrate 5 mg/kg in divided doses for 3 wk.
- In children with chylous reflux syndromes, a diet low in long-chain triglycerides and high in short- and medium-chain triglycerides has been shown to be of benefit in treatment
- Lymphedema is a slowly progressive disorder that can lead to significant disfigurement of the extremities and other body parts
- Patients with lymphedema commonly manifest psychiatric comorbidities as a result of their disease, such as anxiety, depression, adjustment problems, and difficulty in vocational, domestic, or social domains
- Lymphedema can be complicated by cellulitis or, in rare cases, development of lymphangiosarcomata or other cutaneous malignancies
- Gene therapy to develop new lymphangioles in the affected body parts is a potential clinical remedy in the future

SUGGESTED READINGS

available at www.expertconsult.com

RELATED CONTENT

Lymphedema (Patient Information)

AUTHORS: **FRANK G. FORT, M.D., F.A.C.S.,** and **KATHRYN TAYLOR ANILOWSKI, M.S., P.T., C.L.T.-L.A.N.A.**

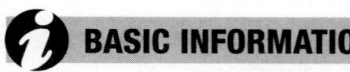

DEFINITION

Non-Hodgkin lymphoma (NHL) is a heterogeneous group of malignancies of the lymphoreticular system.

SYNONYMS

NHL

ICD-9CM CODES
201.9 Lymphoma, non-Hodgkin

EPIDEMIOLOGY & DEMOGRAPHICS

INCIDENCE (IN U.S.): Sixth most common neoplasm (56,000 new cases annually). Incidence increases with age. In patients with HIV, NHL is the second most common tumor (after Kaposi's sarcoma). Diffuse large B-cell lymphoma (DLBCL) is the most common type of HIV-associated lymphoma, accounting for 80% to 90% of cases. Primary CNS lymphoma (PCNSL) accounts for 2% of the cases of lymphoma in patients with HIV infection, but it accounts for 10% of the cases in patients with a diagnosis of AIDS.
PREDOMINANT AGE: Median age at time of diagnosis is 50 yr.

PHYSICAL FINDINGS & CLINICAL PRESENTATION

- Patients often present with asymptomatic lymphadenopathy.
- Approximately one third of NHLs originate extranodally. Involvement of extranodal sites can result in unusual presentations (e.g., gastrointestinal tract involvement can simulate peptic ulcer disease).
- NHL cases associated with HIV occur predominantly in the brain.
- Pruritus, fever, night sweats, and weight loss are less common than in Hodgkin's disease.
- Hepatomegaly and splenomegaly may be present.

Dx DIAGNOSIS

DIFFERENTIAL DIAGNOSIS

- Hodgkin's disease
- Viral infections
- Metastatic carcinoma

A clinical algorithm for evaluation of lymphadenopathy is described in Section III. The differential diagnosis of lymphadenopathy is described in Section II.

WORKUP

Initial laboratory evaluation may reveal only mild anemia and elevated lactate dehydrogenase (LDH) and erythrocyte sedimentation rate (ESR). Proper staging of NHL requires the following:

- A thorough history, physical examination, and adequate biopsy. Laparoscopic lymph node biopsy can be used on an outpatient basis for most patients with intraabdominal lymphoma.
- Routine laboratory evaluation (complete blood count, ESR, urinalysis, LDH, blood urea nitrogen, creatinine, serum calcium, uric acid, liver function tests, serum protein electrophoresis).
- Chest x-ray (posteroanterior and lateral).
- Bone marrow evaluation (aspirate and full bone core biopsy) (Fig. E1-506).
- CT scan of abdomen and pelvis; CT scan of chest if chest x-ray films abnormal.
- Fluorine-18 fluorodeoxyglucose (FDG) positron emission tomography (PET) integrated with CT has emerged as a powerful tool for staging, response evaluation, and posttreatment surveillance in patients with NHL.
- Bone scan (particularly in patients with histiocytic lymphoma).
- Depending on the histopathology (Table E1-258), the results of the above studies and the planned therapy, some other tests may be performed.
- β-2 microglobulin levels should be obtained initially (prognostic value) and serially in patients with low-grade lymphomas (useful to monitor therapeutic response of the tumor).
- Serum interleukin levels have prognostic value in diffuse large cell lymphoma.

CLASSIFICATION: The working formulation of NHL for clinical use subdivides lymphomas into low grade, intermediate grade, high grade, and miscellaneous (Table 1-259).
STAGING: The Ann Arbor staging system with Cotswold modification is described in Table 1-260. Histopathology has greater therapeutic implications in NHL than in Hodgkin's disease. The frequency of indolent lymphomas among all lymphomas is described in Table 1-261. The classification of aggressive lymphomas is described in Table 1-262.

Rx TREATMENT

ACUTE GENERAL Rx

The therapeutic regimen varies with the histologic type and pathologic stage. Following are the commonly used therapeutic modalities:
LOW-GRADE NHL (e.g., NODULAR, POORLY DIFFERENTIATED):

1. Local radiotherapy for symptomatic obstructive adenopathy.
2. Deferment of therapy and careful observation in asymptomatic patients.
3. Single-agent chemotherapy with cyclophosphamide or chlorambucil and glucocorticoids
4. Combination chemotherapy alone or with radiotherapy: generally indicated only when the lymphoma becomes more invasive, with poor response to less aggressive treatment.
5. Monoclonal antibodies directed against B-cell surface antigens can also be used to treat follicular lymphomas resistant to conventional therapy. The anti-CD20 monoclonal antibody rituximab is effective against low-grade NHL in patients who have not received previous treatment. The addition of rituximab to CHOP (CHOP-R) is generally well tolerated.
6. Ibritumomab tiuxetan, an immunoconjugate that combines the linker-chelator tiuxetan with the monoclonal antibody ibritumomab, can be used as part of a two-step regimen for treatment of patients with relapsed or refractory low-grade, follicular, or transformed B-cell NHL refractory to rituximab.
7. New purine analogs (FLAMP, 2CDA) can be used in salvage treatment of refractory lymphomas. They all have activity in follicular lymphomas.
8. Table 1-263 summarizes treatment strategies for indolent lymphomas.

INTERMEDIATE- AND HIGH-GRADE LYMPHOMAS (e.g., DIFFUSE HISTIOCYTIC LYMPHOMA): Combination chemotherapy regimens (e.g., CHOP, PRO-MACE-CYTABOM, MACOP-B, M-BACOD). An anthracycline-containing regimen (such as CHOP) given in standard doses and schedule is generally best for treatment of older patients with advanced stage, aggressive-histology lymphoma who do not have significant comorbid illness.

1. High-dose sequential therapy is superior to standard-dose MACOP-B for patients with diffuse large-cell lymphoma of the B-cell type.
2. Dose-modified chemotherapy should be considered for most HIV-infected patients with lymphoma.
   - Three cycles of CHOP followed by involved-field radiotherapy may be superior to eight cycles of CHOP alone in patients with localized intermediate- and high-grade NHL.
   - High-dose chemotherapy with autologous stem-cell support has been reported to be superior to CHOP in adults with disseminated aggressive lymphoma.
   - The addition of rituximab against CD20 B-cell lymphoma to the CHOP regimen (CHOP-R) increases the complete response rate and prolongs event-free and overall survival in elderly patients with diffuse large B-cell lymphoma without a clinically significant increase in toxicity. Bexxar, a combination of the mononuclear antibody tositumomab and radiolabeled iodine-131, can be used for a single treatment of relapsed follicular NHL in patients who are refractory to rituximab.
   - In patients <61 yr, chemotherapy with three cycles of ACVBP (doxorubicin, cyclophosphamide, vindesine, bleomycin, and prednisone) followed by sequential consolidation has been reported to be superior to three cycles of CHOP plus radiotherapy for treatment of newly diagnosed aggressive lymphoma (diffuse mixed, diffuse large cell, or immunoblastic according to the working formulation).
   - Granulocyte-colony stimulating factor: may be effective in reducing the risk of infection in patients with aggressive lymphoma undergoing chemotherapy.
   - Radioimmunotherapy with (^{131}I) anti-B1 antibody therapy for NHL either by itself or in combination with other treatments represents a new modality in the armamentarium against lymphomas.
   - Treatment with high-dose chemotherapy and autologous bone marrow transplant: compared with conventional chemotherapy, increases event-free and overall survival in

TABLE 1-259 Classification Systems for Grading Lymphomas

Kiel Classification	Working Formulation	Revised European-American Classification
Low-grade malignancy	Low grade	B-cell lymphomas
Lymphocytic, CLL	A. Malignant lymphoma, small lymphocytic	
Lymphocytic, other	Consistent with CLL	B-CLL/SLL
Lymphoplasmacytoid		Lymphoplasmacytoid lymphoma
Centrocytic	B. Malignant lymphoma, follicular, predominantly small cleaved cell	Follicle center lymphomas
		Marginal zone lymphomas (MALT)
Centroblastic/centrocytic		Mantle cell lymphoma
Follicular without sclerosis	Diffuse areas	
Follicular with sclerosis	Sclerosis	
Follicular and diffuse, without sclerosis	C. Malignant lymphoma, follicular mixed, small cleaved and large cell	
Follicular and diffuse, with sclerosis	Diffuse areas	Diffuse large B-cell lymphoma
Diffuse	Sclerosis	Primary mediastinal large B-cell lymphoma
Low-grade malignant lymphoma, unclassified	Intermediate grade	Burkitt's lymphoma
High-grade malignancy	D. Malignant lymphoma, follicular	T-cell lymphomas
Centroblastic	Diffuse areas	
Lymphoblastic, Burkitt's type	E. Malignant lymphoma, diffuse small cleaved cell	
Lymphoblastic, convoluted cell type		T-CLL
Lymphoblastic, other (unclassified) immunoblastic		Mycosis fungoides/Sézary syndrome
High-grade malignant lymphoma, unclassified	F. Malignant lymphoma, diffuse mixed, small and large cell sclerosis	
Malignant lymphoma unclassified (unable to specify high grade or low grade)	G. Malignant lymphoma diffuse	Peripheral T-cell lymphoma, unspecified
Composite lymphoma	Large cell	Angioimmunoblastic T-cell lymphoma
	Cleaved cell	Angiocentric lymphoma
	Noncleaved cell	Intestinal T-cell lymphoma
	Sclerosis	Adult T-cell lymphoma/leukemia
	High grade	Anaplastic large cell lymphoma
	H. Malignant lymphoma large cell, immunoblastic	Precursor T-lymphoid lymphoma/leukemia
	Plasmacytoid	
	Clear cell	
	Polymorphous	
	Epithelioid cell component	
	I. Malignant lymphoma lymphoblastic	
	Convoluted cell	
	Nonconvoluted cell	
	J. Malignant lymphoma small noncleaved cell	
	Burkitt's	
	Follicular areas	

B-CLL, B-cell chronic lymphoid leukemia; *CLL*, chronic lymphocytic leukemia; *MALT*, mucosa-associated lymphoid tumor; *SLL*, lymphoid leukemia; *T-CLL*, T-cell CLL.
From Abeloff MD: *Clinical oncology*, ed 3, New York, 2004, Churchill Livingstone.

TABLE 1-260 Ann Arbor Staging System for Lymphomas

Stage*	Cotswold Modification of Ann Arbor Classification
I	Involvement of a single lymph node region or lymphoid structure
II	Involvement of two or more lymph node regions on the same side of the diaphragm (the mediastinum is considered a single site, whereas the hilar lymph nodes are considered bilaterally); the number of anatomic sites should be indicated by a subscript (e.g., II_3)
III	Involvement of lymph node regions on both sides of the diaphragm: III_1 (with or without involvement of splenic hilar, celiac, or portal nodes) and III_2 (with involvement of para-aortic, iliac, and mesenteric nodes)
IV	Involvement of one or more extranodal sites in addition to a site for which the designation E has been used

*All cases are subclassified to indicate the absence (A) or presence (B) of the systemic symptoms of significant fever (>38.0° C [100.4° F]), night sweats, and unexplained weight loss exceeding 10% of normal body weight within the previous 6 months. The clinical stage (CS) denotes the stage as determined by all diagnostic examinations and a single diagnostic biopsy only. In the Ann Arbor classification, the term pathologic stage (PS) is used if a second biopsy of any kind has been obtained, whether negative or positive. In the Cotswold modification, the PS is determined by laparotomy; X designates bulky disease (widening of the mediastinum by more than one third or the presence of a nodal mass >10 cm), and E designates involvement of a single extranodal site that is contiguous or proximal to the known nodal site.
From Hoffmann R et al: *Hematology: basic principles and practice*, ed 5, Philadelphia, 2009, Churchill Livingstone.

TABLE 1-261 Frequency of Indolent Lymphomas Among All Lymphomas in the World Health Organization Classification

Follicular lymphoma	22.1%
Extranodal marginal zone lymphoma of mucosa-associated lymphoid tissue type	7.6%
Small lymphocytic lymphoma/chronic lymphocytic leukemia	6.7%
Mantle cell	6.0%
Splenic marginal zone lymphoma	1.8%
Lymphoplasmacytic lymphoma	1.2%
Nodal marginal zone B-cell lymphoma (±monocytoid B cells)	1.0%

From Hoffman R et al: *Hematology: basic principles and practice*, ed 5, Philadelphia, 2009, Churchill Livingstone.

TABLE 1-262 Classification of Aggressive Lymphomas

B-cell Neoplasms

Precursor B-cell lymphoma
Precursor B lymphoblastic leukemia/lymphoma
Mature B-cell lymphoma
Mantle cell lymphoma
Diffuse large B-cell lymphoma
Mediastinal (thymic) large B-cell lymphoma
Intravascular large B-cell lymphoma
Primary effusion lymphoma
Burkitt lymphoma/leukemia
B-cell proliferations of uncertain malignant potential
Lymphomatoid granulomatosis
Posttransplant lymphoproliferative disorder, polymorphic

T-cell and NK-cell Neoplasms

Precursor T-cell
Precursor T lymphoblastic leukemia/lymphoma
Blastic NK cell lymphoma
Mature T-cell and NK-cell lymphoma
Adult T-cell leukemia/lymphoma
Extranodal NK/T lymphoma, nasal type
Hepatosplenic T-cell lymphoma
Peripheral T-cell lymphoma, unspecified
Angioimmunoblastic T-cell lymphoma
Anaplastic large cell lymphoma

NK, Natural killer.
From Hoffman R et al: *Hematology: basic principles and practice,* ed 5, Philadelphia, 2009, Churchill Livingstone.

TABLE 1-263 Treatment Strategies for Indolent Lymphomas

Advanced Stage Disease

"Watchful waiting"
Alkylating agents
Purine analogs
Combination chemotherapy
Monoclonal antibodies
  Unconjugated
  Conjugated — radioimmunoconjugates and immunotoxins
Chemotherapy + monoclonal antibodies (chemoimmunotherapy)
High dose chemotherapy plus autologous/allogeneic hematopoietic cell transplantation
Reduced intensity conditioning allogeneic transplantation
Palliative radiotherapy

Localized Disease

Radiotherapy
"Watchful waiting"

From Hoffman R et al: *Hematology: basic principles and practice,* ed 5, Philadelphia, 2009, Churchill Livingstone.

---

patients with chemotherapy-sensitive NHL in relapse.
- An algorithm for the management of NHL in pediatric patients is described in Fig. E1-507. Combination chemotherapy regimens for NHL are described in Table 1-264.

DISPOSITION

- Patients with low-grade lymphoma, despite their long-term survival (6 to 10 yr average), are rarely cured, and the great majority (if not all) eventually die of the lymphoma, whereas patients with a high-grade lymphoma may achieve a cure with aggressive chemotherapy.
- Complete remission occurs in 35% to 50% of patients with intermediate- and high-grade lymphoma. Prognostic factors include the histologic subtype, age of patient, and bulk of disease. Table 1-265 describes the International Prognostic Index for aggressive lymphomas.
- Patients who present with AIDS-related NHL and a low CD4 cell count have a poor prognosis (median duration of survival is 15 to 34 mo). Despite therapeutic advances, the management of HIV-associated lymphomas is challenging due to potential pharmacologic interactions and increased risk of infectious complications. Referral to an HIV oncologist is recommended.

SUGGESTED READINGS

available at www.expertconsult.com

RELATED CONTENT

Non-Hodgkin's Lymphoma (Patient Information)

AUTHOR: **FRED F. FERRI, M.D.**

TABLE 1-264 Combination Chemotherapy Regimens for Non-Hodgkin Lymphoma

Regimen	Dose	Days of Administration	Frequency
CHOP-R			Every 21 days
Cyclophosphamide	750 mg/m² IV	1	
Doxorubicin	50 mg/m² IV	1	
Vincristine	1.4 mg/m² IV*	1	
Prednisone, fixed dose	100 mg PO	1-5	
Rituximab	375 mg/m² IV	1	
CVP-R			Every 21 days
Cyclophosphamide	1000 mg/m² IV	1	
Vincristine	1.4 mg/m² IV*	1	
Prednisone, fixed dose	100 mg PO	1-5	
Rituximab	375 mg/m² IV	1	
FCR			Every 28 days
Fludarabine	25 mg/m² IV	1-3	
Cyclophosphamide	250 mg/m² IV	1-3	
Rituximab	375 mg/m²	1	

*Vincristine dose often capped at 2 mg total.
From Goldman L, Schafer AI: *Goldman's Cecil medicine,* ed 24, Philadelphia, 2012, Saunders.

TABLE 1-265 International Prognostic Index for Aggressive Lymphomas*

Risk Group	IPI Score	CR Rate (%)	5-yr Overall Survival (%)
Low	0, 1	87	73
Low intermediate	2	67	51
High intermediate	3	55	43
High	4, 5	44	26

*One point is given for the presence of each of the following characteristics: age >60 years, elevated serum lactate dehydrogenase level, Eastern Cooperative Oncology Group performance status ≥ 2, Ann Arbor stage III or IV, and more than two extranodal sites.
CR, Complete response; *IPI,* International Prognostic Index.
From Hoffman R et al: *Hematology: basic principles and practice,* ed 5, Philadelphia, 2009, Churchill Livingstone.

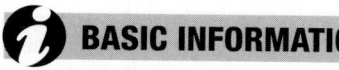 **BASIC INFORMATION**

DEFINITION

Lynch syndrome is a hereditary predisposition to malignancy of the colon that is explained by a germline mutation in a DNA mismatch repair gene.

SYNONYMS

Hereditary nonpolyposis colorectal cancer
Hereditary site-specific colon cancer

ICD-9CM CODES
1539 Lynch syndrome

EPIDEMIOLOGY & DEMOGRAPHICS

The lifetime risk for developing colon cancer in the U.S. is approximately 6%. Of these cases, 2% to 3% may be attributable to Lynch syndrome. The incidence of Lynch syndrome is estimated to be between 1:660 and 1:2000. Lynch syndrome is the most common form of hereditary colon cancer. The average age of diagnosis for Lynch syndrome is 48 years, although diagnosis can occur as early as the 20s or as late as the 70s.

RISK FACTORS: Family history of colon cancer or other hereditary nonpolyposis colorectal cancer (HNPCC)-related cancers such as endometrial (up to 40% of women with Lynch syndrome may develop endometrial cancer), biliary tract, ovarian, stomach, upper urinary tract, or brain.

GENETICS: Autosomal-dominant inheritance pattern

ETIOLOGY

Lynch syndrome is thought to be secondary to germline mutations in DNA mismatch repair genes. The predominant genes involved are *MSH2* and *MLH1,* which are tumor suppressor genes, although other genes have documented involvement *(PMS1, PMS2, MSH6, MLH3).* Mutations in these genes prevent repair of DNA mismatches during DNA replication. This is most prevalent in regions of DNA called microsatellites causing DNA microsatellite instability and leading to an increased risk for malignancy, especially colon cancer. *MSH6* mutations are associated with a markedly lower cancer risk than *MLH1* or *MSH2* mutations.

PHYSICAL FINDINGS & CLINICAL PRESENTATION

- Changes in bowel habits (prolonged constipation)
- Melena
- Hematochezia
- Abdominal pain
- Unexplained weight loss
- Decreased appetite

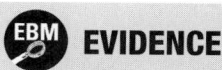 **DIAGNOSIS**

DIFFERENTIAL DIAGNOSIS

- Familial adenomatosis polyposis
- Peutz-Jeghers syndrome
- Juvenile polyposis
- Nonhereditary colorectal cancer
- Gardner syndrome

WORKUP

If an individual presents with numerous adenomatous polyps or has multiple relatives with cancer at a young age, a family history complete with pedigree must be obtained. Clinical diagnosis of the Lynch syndrome can be made with the Amsterdam or Bethesda criteria.

- Revised Amsterdam (II) criteria (must meet all criteria):
  1. HNPCC associated carrier diagnosis in at least three individuals in the family
  2. One of the patients is a first-degree family member of two other patients
  3. Involved patients occur in at least two successive generations with diagnosis of HNPCC
  4. At least one diagnosis in family of HNPCC was made before age 50
  5. The diagnoses are histologically confirmed
  6. Familial adenomatous polyposis is excluded
- Bethesda criteria (must meet all criteria):
  1. Colorectal cancer before age 50
  2. Multiple colorectal cancers or other HNPCC-related cancers such as biliary tract, endometrial, stomach, or ovary
  3. Colorectal cancer with microsatellite instability histology <60 yr of age
  4. Colorectal cancer or HNPCC-related cancer in first-degree relative <50 yr of age
  5. Colorectal cancer or HNPCC-related cancer in at least two first- or second-degree relatives, any age
- If criteria for the Lynch syndrome are not met, no further analysis is necessary (although a genetic syndrome cannot be definitively excluded and genetic referral may be warranted).

LABORATORY TESTS

- If a patient meets criteria for Lynch syndrome, immunohistochemistry can be performed for the presence or absence of mismatch repair genes *MLH1, MSH2, MSH6,* and *PMS2.* Rarely, *MLH3* is identified.
- Microsatellite instability analysis should also be performed if criteria for Lynch syndrome are met.

Rx **TREATMENT**

- If the mutation has been identified in a family member, screening for this mutation can be performed via genetic testing. Informed consent must be obtained after a thorough explanation has been provided to each individual.
- Surveillance using colonoscopy can be performed in individuals who screen positive, while those who screen negative can be discharged. The mismatch repair gene that is mutated guides screening.
- According to the Netherlands Surveillance Protocol, for example, individuals with mutations in *MLH1, MSH2,* or *MSH6* should have colonoscopies every 1 to 2 yr starting at age 20 to 25 yr; urine cytology every 1 to 2 yr starting at age 30 to 35 yr; gastroscopy every 1 to 2 yr starting at age 30 to 35 yr; and, in females, ultrasound of endometrium and CA-125 every 1 to 2 yr starting at age 30 to 35 yr.

REFERRALS

- To gastroenterology for surveillance colonoscopies
- To genetic counselor if patient satisfies Bethesda criteria
- To psychologist as necessary for psychologic support

! **PEARLS & CONSIDERATIONS**

- Prior to genetic testing being instituted, informed consent must be obtained because consequences of this testing include the necessity of lifelong screenings such as colonoscopies.
- The risk of pancreatic cancer is increased in families with Lynch syndrome compared with the U.S. population.

PATIENT & FAMILY EDUCATION

- For information on local genetic counselors, visit the National Society of Genetic Counselors Web site at www.nsgc.org.
- For information on Lynch syndrome, visit www.mayoclinic.com/health/lynch-syndrome/DS00669.

EBM **EVIDENCE**

available at www.expertconsult.com

SUGGESTED READINGS
available at www.expertconsult.com

RELATED CONTENT
Colorectal Cancer (Related Key Topic)

AUTHORS: **PAUL F. GEORGE, M.D.,** and **JOANNE M. SILVIA, M.D.**

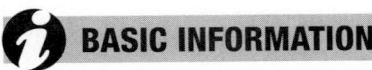

BASIC INFORMATION

DEFINITION

Macular degeneration refers to a group of diseases associated with loss of central vision and damage to the macula. Degenerative changes occur in the pigment, neural, and vascular layers of the macula. Dry macular degeneration is usually ischemic in etiology, and wet macular degeneration is associated with leakage of fluid from blood vessels, usually referred to as *age-related macular degeneration* (AMD).

ICD-9CM CODES
362.5 Degeneration of macula and posterior pole

EPIDEMIOLOGY & DEMOGRAPHICS

INCIDENCE (IN U.S.):
- Leading cause of irreversible blindness in people ≥50 yr in the developed world.
- Increases with age.
- More than 8 million Americans have AMD. The overall prevalence is projected to increase by >50% by 2020.
- About 10% of patients with AMD have the neovascular form manifested by an often rapid decrease in central visual acuity caused by newly developed leaky vessels arising from the choroid towards the subretinal space.

PEAK INCIDENCE:
- Ages 75 to 80 yr
- Dramatically increases in incidence and prevalence with age until ~80% of people ≥75 yr have senile macular degeneration

PREVALENCE (IN U.S.): Varies, but ~5% of people >50 yr have some signs of macular degeneration

PREDOMINANT SEX: Males and females are affected equally (15% of white women >80 yr have severe AMD)

PREDOMINANT AGE: >50 yr

RISK FACTORS:
- Advancing age
- Genetic factors
- Complement factor H, Tyr402His variant
- *LOC387715/ARMS2*, Ala69Ser variant
- History of smoking within past 20 yr
- Dietary factors (low intake of antioxidants and zinc, high fat intake)
- Obesity
- White race

PHYSICAL FINDINGS & CLINICAL PRESENTATION

- Decreased central vision
- Macular hemorrhage, pigmentation, edema, atrophy
- The most common abnormality seen in AMD is the presence of drusen, or yellowish deposits deep to the retina; this may be early in the course of disease
- Choroidal neovascular membrane (CNVM) develops with rapid change in vision

ETIOLOGY

- Subretinal neovascular membrane early
- Pigmentary and vascular changes with exudate, edema, and scar tissue development
- Dry-type atrophy of macular pigment epithelium
- The main mediator of neovascularization in wet AMD is the vascular endothelial growth factor (VEGF). It induces angiogenesis and increases inflammation and vascular permeability

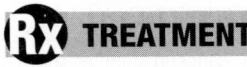

DIAGNOSIS

DIFFERENTIAL DIAGNOSIS
- Diabetic retinopathy (with neovascularization, can mimic CNVM)
- Hypertension
- Histoplasmosis (less common cause of CNVM)
- Trauma with scar

WORKUP
- Complete eye examination, including visual field and fluorescein angiography
- Optical coherence tomography (OCT)

LABORATORY TESTS
Evaluate for diabetes and other metabolic problems as well as vascular diseases

IMAGING STUDIES
- OCT
- Fluorescein angiography

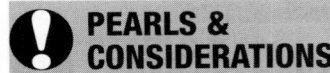

TREATMENT

NONPHARMACOLOGIC THERAPY
- There is no proven treatment for dry AMD.
- Laser treatment to stop progression of disease; photodynamic treatment with verteporfin IV
- Laser (argon) for certain classic membranes (CNVM)
- A high dietary intake of antioxidants, vitamins C and E, and zinc has been reported to substantially reduce the risk of AMD in elderly persons

ACUTE GENERAL Rx
- The introduction of therapies blocking VEGF dramatically changed the management of AMD and it is now standard practice for clinicians to offer intravitreal injections of anti-VEGF agents (ranibizumab, bevacizumab) as first-line treatment for neovascular AMD. Intravitreal administration of ranibizumab, a monoclonal antibody Fab that neutralizes all active forms of VEGF A, has shown to be effective in preventing vision loss and improving mean visual acuity in patients with AMD. It has also been reported to be superior to photodynamic therapy with verteporfin in the treatment of predominantly classic neovascular AMD. Bevacizumab, a monoclonal antibody to VEGF, is also often used off-label as intravitreal therapy. Its cost per intravitreal dose is significantly lower than that of ranibizumab. A major concern regarding anti-VEGF treatment is the potential increased risk of stroke and cardiovascular disease.

- Intravitreous injections of pegaptanib, a more selective anti-VEGF, appear to be less effective therapy in slowing vision loss in neovascular AMD than bevacizumab or ranibizumab. Pegaptanib is administered once every 6 wk by intravitreous injection into one eye.
- Aflibercept, a fusion protein that competes for binding of VEGF, has recently been FDA approved for the treatment of wet (neovascular) AMD. It is injected intravitreally every 8 weeks. It appears to be as effective as ranibizumab and bevacizumab but is more expensive.
- Laser photocoagulation therapy may be useful in patients with extrafoveal lesions but is no longer routinely recommended for wet AMD.

CHRONIC Rx
- Laser phototherapy is not recommended for dry AMD.
- Antioxidants and zinc may slow progression of AMD

DISPOSITION
- Follow closely by ophthalmologist, retinal specialist.
- Most bevacizumab or ranibizumab treatment failures are due to missed follow-up visits. Patients should be reminded repeatedly to call if their vision worsens. There should also be a system in place for calling patients who have been lost to follow-up due to the high risk of recurrent neovascularization and vision loss in these patients.

REFERRAL
- To ophthalmologist early in the course of the disease if vision is to be saved
- Immediate referral if any change in vision

PEARLS & CONSIDERATIONS

COMMENTS
- Sildenafil has no significant effect on macular degeneration.
- Statistically, the vision of only 1 of 10 affected persons can be saved, but the disease is so devastating that vigorous therapy should be considered in all patients.
- Statins plus aspirin may slow progression.
- Vitamins with zinc and antioxidants may slow progression of AMD.
- Quitting smoking significantly reduces the risk of developing AMD.

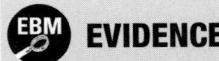

available at www.expertconsult.com

SUGGESTED READING
available at www.expertconsult.com

RELATED CONTENT
Macular Degeneration (Patient Information)

AUTHOR: **MELVYN KOBY, M.D.**, and **FRED F. FERRI, M.D.**

BASIC INFORMATION

DEFINITION

Malaria is a protozoan disease caused by the genus *Plasmodium* and transmitted by female *Anopheles* spp. mosquitoes. It is endemic throughout most of the tropics and is characterized by hectic fever and often presents with classic malarial paroxysm. Five species of genus *Plasmodium* usually infect humans (Table 1-266):

- *P. falciparum*
- *P. vivax*
- *P. malariae*
- *P. ovale*
- *P. knowlesi*

SYNONYMS

Periodic fever
Tertian malaria
Quartan malaria
Tropical splenomegaly

ICD-9CM CODES

084.6 Malaria

EPIDEMIOLOGY & DEMOGRAPHICS

Global:

- ~300 million cases a year in more than 100 countries
- Around 900,000 deaths per year, with more than 80% of the deaths ocurring in children of sub-Saharan Africa
- 3 billion people live in malaria endemic areas

U.S.:

- ~1500 cases reported to the CDC in the United States each year. In the majority of reported cases, U.S. civilians who acquired infection abroad had not adhered to a chemoprophylaxis regimen that was appropriate for the country in which they acquired malaria.
- More than 50% of the reported cases in the U.S. are *P. falciparum*. On average, there are six deaths per year in the United States.

- Most infections limited to:
  1. Immigrant population
  2. Returned travelers or troops from endemic area
- Occasionally, transmission through exposure to infected blood product or shared intravenous needles by users of injection drugs.
- Congenital transmission is possible.
- Local mosquito-borne transmission has been reported.

- Competent mosquito vectors are present.
  1. *A. albimanus* in eastern United States
  2. *A. freeborni* in western United States

Geographic distribution:

- *P. falciparum:* Sub-Saharan Africa, Papua New Guinea, Solomon Islands, Haiti, Indian subcontinent
- *P. vivax:* Central America, South America, North Africa, Middle East, Indian subcontinent
- *P. ovale:* West Africa
- *P. malariae:* worldwide

Parasite life cycle (Fig. 1-508):

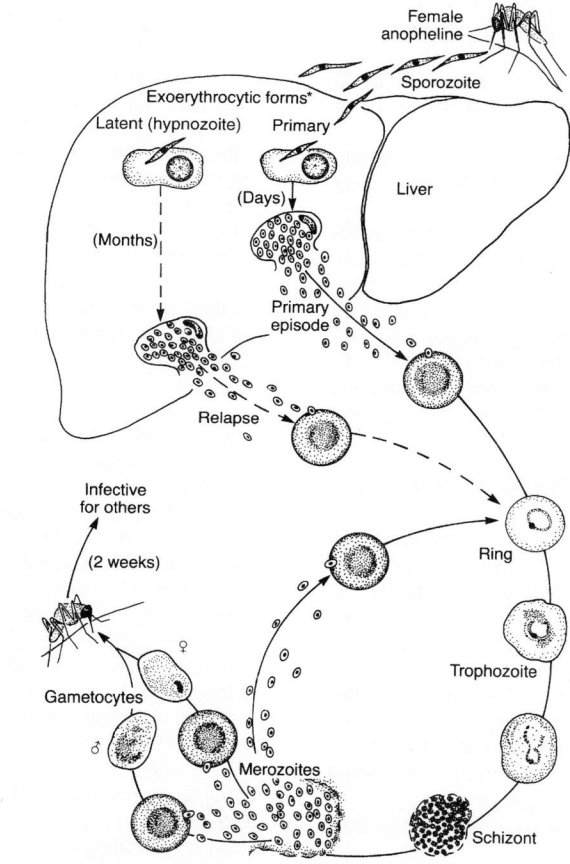

FIGURE 1-508 Life cycle of plasmodia in humans. Exoerythrocytic forms are also called schizonts. (From Gorbach SL: *Infectious diseases,* ed 2, Philadelphia, 1998, Saunders.)

TABLE 1-266 Features of the Five Species of Malaria Known to Cause Disease in Humans

	Plasmodium falciparum	*Plasmodium vivax*	*Plasmodium ovale*	*Plasmodium malariae*	*Plasmodium knowlesi*
Incubation period (days)	6-25	8-27	8-27	16-40	12
Asexual cycle (hours)	48 (tertian)	48 (tertian)	48 (tertian)	72 (quartan)	24 (tertian)
Relapse	No	Yes*	Yes*	No[†]	No
Chloroquine resistance	Yes[‡]	Rare[§]	No	No[‖]	No
Characteristic on thin blood film	Rings predominate, multiply infected RBCs, high parasitemia, rings with thread-like cytoplasm, double nuclei, banana-shaped gametocytes	Enlarged RBCs, Schüffner's dots, trophozoite cytoplasm ameboid, 12-24 merozoites in mature schizont	Oval RBCs with fringed edges, Schüffner's dots, trophozoite cytoplasm compact, 6-16 merozoites in mature schizont	Trophozoite cytoplasm compact (band forms), 6-12 merozoites in mature schizont, RBC unchanged	Similar to *P. malariae*, 8-10 merozoites in mature schizont, often in rosette pattern with central clump of pigment

*Relapses may appear months to years after initial infection due to dormant hypnozoites in the liver.
[†]Although relapse does not occur, *P. malariae* can produce persistent infections that remain below detectable limits in the blood for 20 to 30 years or more.
[‡]*P. falciparum* resistance to sulfadoxine/pyrimethamine, mefloquine, halofantrine, and artemisinin have also been reported in some areas, along with partial resistance to quinine and quinidine.
[§]*P. vivax* resistance to chloroquine now reported in some areas of Southeast Asia, Oceania, and South America.
[‖]Chloroquine-resistant *P. malariae* has also been reported in south Sumatra, Indonesia.
From Vincent JL et al: *Textbook of critical care,* ed 6, Philadelphia, 2011, Saunders.

- Human infection begins when a female anopheline mosquito bites (only female anopheline mosquito takes blood meal) and inoculates plasmodial sporozoites into bloodstream. The bite usually occurs between dusk and dawn.
- The sporozoites then travel to liver and invade to hepatocytes.
- In the hepatocytes, the sporozoites mature to tissue schizont or become dormant hypnozoites.
- The tissue schizonts amplify the infection by producing large number of merozoites (10,000 to 30,000).
- Each merozoite is capable of invading an RBC and can establish the asexual cycle of replication in RBCs.
- Asexual cycles produce and release 24 to 32 merozoites at the end of 48- or 72-hr (*P. malariae*) cycles.
- The hypnozoites are only found in relapsing malaria *P. vivax* or *P. ovale* and may remain dormant for up to 5 yr.
- Eventually some intraerythrocytic parasites develop into gametocytes. Male and female gametocytes are taken up by a female anopheline mosquito with a blood meal where they fertilize in the mosquito gut to produce a diploid zygote that matures to an ookinete; haploid sporozoites are generated that migrate to the salivary gland of the mosquito to infect another human.

PHYSICAL FINDINGS & CLINICAL PRESENTATION

- Fever is the hallmark of malaria, known as malarial paroxysm, initially daily until synchronization of infection after several wk, when fever may occur every other day (tertian) in *P. vivax, P. ovale,* or *P. falciparum* malaria or every third day (quartan) in *P. malariae* malaria. Table 1-267 describes the WHO criteria for severe malaria.
- Classic malarial paroxysm characterized by
  1. Cold stage: abrupt onset of cold feeling associated with rigors, shakes
  2. Hot stage: high fever (~40° C) associated with restlessness
  3. Sweating stage: patient defervesces
- Nonspecific symptoms are
  1. Headache
  2. Cough
  3. Myalgia
  4. Vomiting
  5. Diarrhea
  6. Jaundice
- *P. falciparum:*
  ○ Most pathogenic of the four species.
  ○ Rapidly progresses to high-level parasitemia.
  ○ Important cause of the fatal malaria.
  ○ Classic malarial paroxysm is usually absent.
  ○ Incubation period after exposure is 12 days (range: 9 to 60 days).
  ○ Cytoadherence and resetting of RBCs play central role in pathogenesis.
  ○ The sequestration of RBCs in vital organs leads to fatal complications.
  ○ Cerebral malaria is a feared complication.
  ○ Invades erythrocytes of all ages.
  ○ Lacks hypnozoites (intrahepatic stage), does not relapse.
  ○ Blood smear usually shows ring form only.
  ○ Pigment color is black.
  ○ Banana-shaped gametocytes; if seen in blood, smear is diagnostic.
  ○ Chloroquine resistance is widely present.
- *P. vivax:*
  ○ Known as tertian malaria: fever occurs every other day.
  ○ Duffy blood-group antigen FYA- or FYB-related receptor is needed for attachment to RBC.
  ○ FyFy phenotype (most West African) individuals are resistant to *P. vivax* malaria.
  ○ Incubation period after exposure is 14 days (range: 8 to 27 days).
  ○ Hypnozoites may cause relapse of infection after years.
  ○ Infects mainly reticulocytes.
  ○ Irregularly shaped large rings and trophozoites, enlarged RBCs, and Schüffner's dots are seen in peripheral blood smear (Fig. 1-509).
  ○ Pigment color is yellow-brown.
  ○ *P. vivax* from Papua New Guinea have reduced sensitivity to chloroquine.
  ○ Primaquine is needed to eradicate the hypnozoites.
- *P. ovale:*
  ○ Also known as tertian malaria; fever occurs every other day.
  ○ Occurs mainly in tropical Africa.
  ○ Incubation period after exposure is 14 days (range: 8 to 27 days).
  ○ Hypnozoites may cause relapse of infection.
  ○ Infects mainly reticulocytes.
  ○ Infected RBC is seen as enlarged, oval shape containing large ring or trophozoites with Schüffner's dots.
  ○ Pigment color is dark brown.
  ○ Primaquine needed to eradicate the hypnozoites.
  ○ No chloroquine resistance has been encountered.
- *P. malariae:*
  ○ Known as quartan malaria; fever occurs every third day.
  ○ Common cause of chronic malarial infection.
  ○ May persist for 20 to 30 yr after leaving the endemic area.
  ○ Worldwide distribution.
  ○ Incubation period after exposure is 30 days (range: 16 to 60 days).
  ○ Lacks hypnozoites (intrahepatic stage).
  ○ May persist in blood for many years if treated inadequately.
  ○ Chronic infection may cause soluble immune-complex, resulting in nephritic syndrome.
  ○ Infects mainly mature RBCs.
  ○ Band or rectangular forms of trophozoites are commonly seen in peripheral blood smear.
  ○ Pigment color is brown-black.
- Cerebral malaria:
  ○ Feared complication of *P. falciparum* infection.
  ○ Mortality is ~20%.
  ○ Pathogenesis is poorly understood.
  ○ Ischemia as a result of sequestration of parasites or cytokines induced by parasite toxin(s) is the key debate.
  ○ Seizure and altered mental status leading to coma are cardinal manifestation.
  ○ Hypoglycemia, lactic acidosis, and elevated circulating TNF-α may be present.

TABLE 1-267 World Health Organization Criteria for Severe Malaria, 2000

Impaired consciousness
Prostration
Respiratory distress
Multiple seizures
Jaundice
Hemoglobinuria
Abnormal bleeding
Severe anemia
Circulatory collapse
Pulmonary edema

From Kliegman RM et al: *Nelson textbook of pediatrics,* ed 19, Philadelphia, 2011, Saunders.

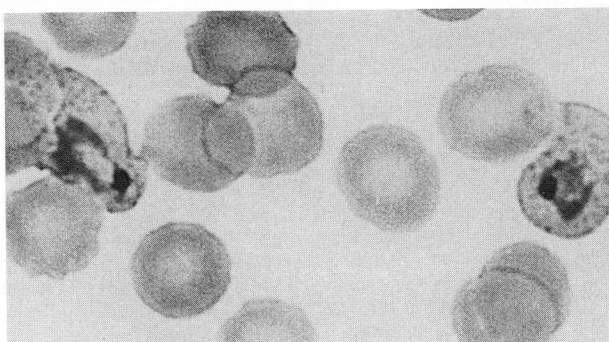

FIGURE 1-509 Giemsa-stained blood smear in *Plasmodium vivax* malaria. Asexual parasites. Note that the parasites are large and ameboid; the infected erythrocytes are the largest cells in the field (because they are reticulocytes), and the erythrocytes contain numerous pink dots (Schüffner's dots) (×2000). (From Klippel JH et al [eds]: *Internal medicine,* ed 5, St Louis, 1998, Mosby.)

Diseases
and Disorders

I

○ CSF studies: no increase of WBC count or protein, raised lactate concentrate, and increased opening pressure, especially in children, may be present.

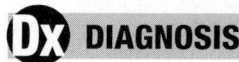

DIAGNOSIS

DIFFERENTIAL DIAGNOSIS

- Typhoid fever
- Dengue fever
- Yellow fever
- Viral hepatitis
- Influenza
- Brucellosis
- UTI
- Leishmaniasis
- Trypanosomiasis
- Rickettsial diseases
- Leptospirosis

WORKUP

- Clinical diagnosis is notoriously inaccurate.
- Demonstration of malarial parasites in blood smear is essential.
- Newer molecular diagnostic techniques (polymerase chain reaction, rapid diagnostic tests) are promising.

LABORATORY TESTS

- The thick and thin blood film is required to identify malarial parasites. A Giemsa-stained film of the patient's peripheral blood should be examined for parasites as soon as possible.
- The thick smears are more sensitive and primarily used to detect the presence of parasites.
- The thin smears are used for species differentiation and parasite density estimation.
- A patient who is suspected of having malaria but who has no parasite seen in blood smears should have blood smears repeated every 12 to 24 hr for 3 consecutive days.

PREPARATION OF BLOOD SMEAR:

- Must be prepared from fresh blood obtained by pricking the fingers.
- The thin smear is fixed in methanol before staining.
- The thick smear is stained unfixed.
- The smear should be stained with a 3% Giemsa solution (pH of 7.2) for 30 to 45 min.
- The parasite density should be estimated by counting the percentage of RBCs infected, not the number of parasites, under an oil immersion lens on thin film.

COMMON ERRORS IN READING MALARIAL SMEARS:

- Platelets overlying an RBC
- Misreading artifacts as parasites
- Concern about missing a positive slide

MOLECULAR DIAGNOSIS OF MALARIA:

- Rapid diagnostic tests (RDT)
  1. Employ immunochromatographic lateral flow technology for antigen detection.
  2. Thus far only one RDT has been FDA approved: BinaxNOW Malaria test kit.
  3. This kit is based on antigens HRP-2 and aldolase.

4. For *P. falciparum:* sensitivity 95% and specificity 94%.
5. For *P. vivax:* sensitivity 69% and specificity 100%.
- Limitations of the BinaxNOW Malaria test:
  1. Not approved for mixed infections
  2. Should not be used for *P. malariae* and *P. ovale* as data are limited
  3. Positive test must be confirmed by microscopy
  4. Negative results require confirmation by thick and thin smears
  5. This test cannot be used to monitor therapy as antigen persists after the elimination of the parasite, causing false positives
- Other diagnostic tests available include:
  1. Tagged monoclonal antibodies for malaria antigen detection
  2. Nucleic acid amplification and detection: PCR can detect parasites down to a level of 1 to 5 parasites per microliter of blood. PCR can detect mixed species infection
  3. Fluorescence microscopy with acridine orange or other staining
  4. Dark field microscopy

TREATMENT

NONPHARMACOLOGIC THERAPY
ANTIMOSQUITO MEASURES:

1. Eradication of mosquito breeding places by chemical spray
2. Use of mosquito nets properly in the endemic areas
3. Use of protective clothing
4. Use of insect spray (permethrin), mosquito coils, or repellents such as diethyltoluamide (DEET). For adults, DEET (30% to 50%) is generally protective for at least 4 hr. For smaller children, use DEET at ≤20% concentration.

ACUTE GENERAL Rx

A definitive diagnosis of malaria is essential for specific antimalarial chemotherapy.

NON-*FALCIPARUM* MALARIA:

- Chloroquine 600 mg base (1000 mg chloroquine phosphate) PO loading dose, 6 hr later 300 mg base (500 mg salt), then 300 mg base (500 mg salt) daily for 2 days.
- In the case of *P. vivax* and *P. ovale,* treatment with primaquine 15 mg daily for 14 days is needed to eradicate the exoerythrocytic forms, especially the hypnozoites responsible for relapses.
- G6PD should be measured before primaquine is given. Primaquine is not recommended for those who are glucose-6-phosphate dehydrogenase deficient, because primaquine can cause hemolysis and even death in G6PD-deficient persons. Normal G6PD levels must be documented before using primaquine for either chemoprophylaxis or treatment.
- Chloroquine-resistant *P. vivax* has been documented; in that case, quinine is given.

FALCIPARUM MALARIA:

- Chloroquine can be used cautiously for *falciparum* malaria acquired in chloroquine-

sensitive areas (chloroquine is more rapidly effective than quinine)
- Mainstay of treatment is oral quinine sulfate 10 mg (salt)/kg (usually 650 mg) q8h for 3 to 7 days + doxycycline 100 mg PO bid both for 7 days for adults. Pediatrics: quinine sulfate: 10 mg/kg PO tid plus clindamycin: 20 mg/kg per day divided in tid dose both for 7 days.
- Atovaquone-proguanil (Malarone): 250 mg atovaquone/100 mg proguanil): 4 adult tabs PO once a day for 3 days with food in adults or for pediatrics: pediatric tablets (62.5 mg atovaquone/25 mg proguanil) are used based on weight:
  5 to 8 kg: 2 pediatric tabs PO once daily for 3 days
  9 to 10 kg: 3 pediatric tabs PO once daily for 3 days
  11 to 20 kg: 1 adult tabs PO once daily for 3 days
  21 to 30 kg: 2 adult tabs PO once daily for 3 days
  31 to 40 kg: 3 adult tabs PO once daily for 3 days
- >40 kg: 4 adult tabs PO once daily for 3 days artemether-lumefantrine (Coartem) tablets: 4 tabs PO (at time zero and 8 hr later) then bid × 2 days for a total of six doses. For pediatrics:
  5 to <15 kg: 1 tablet per dose
  15 to <25 kg: 2 tablets per dose
  25 to <35 kg: 3 tablets per dose
  >35 kg: 4 tablets per dose. The child should receive initial dose based on weight, then followed by second dose 8 hr later, then 1 dose PO bid for following 2 days

ALTERNATIVES:

- Quinine sulfate plus clindamycin 900 mg tid for 7 days in adults, or
- Mefloquine 750 mg PO then 500 mg PO 6 to 12 hr later in adults

NOTE: Parasitemia may paradoxically rise in the first 24 to 36 hr and is not an indication of treatment failure.

SEVERE *FALCIPARUM* MALARIA:

- It is a medical emergency; intensive care is preferred.
- Measurement of blood glucose, lactate, ABG is important.
- IV quinidine gluconate 10 mg salt/kg loading dose (maximum 600 mg) in NS; infuse slowly over 1 to 2 hr, followed by continuous infusion of 0.02 mg/kg/min until patient can swallow.
- Need to monitor ECG for observation of QT interval as can prolong. Also need to monitor blood pressure and glucose to avoid hypoglycemia.
- Alternatively, IV artesunate: 2.4 mg/kg IV first dose then at 12 and 24 hr followed by 2.4 mg/kg once daily. One recent study showed the superiority of parenteral artesuante over parenteral quinine in adults and children who could not take an oral medication.
- Plasmapheresis is an option for parasitemia >30% or in pregnant women and in elderly with severe malaria.

NOTE: WHO recommends IV artesunate as the treatment of choice for severe malaria in adults and children in area of low transmission. Data

on children in high-transmission regions are limited, and WHO recommends treatment with artesunate, artemether, or quinine.

MULTIDRUG-RESISTANT MALARIA:
- Mefloquine 1250 mg as a single dose, or
- Halofantrine 500 mg every 6 hr for 3 doses, repeat same course after 1 wk
- Combination therapy usually preferred

DISPOSITION
RISK FACTORS FOR FATAL MALARIA:
- Failure to take chemoprophylaxis
- Delay in seeking medical care
- Misdiagnosis

COMPLICATIONS OF MALARIA:
- Anemia
- Acidosis
- Hypoglycemia
- Respiratory distress
- DIC
- Blackwater fever
- Renal failure
- Shock

REFERRAL
- To an infectious disease specialist or travel medicine expert for severe malaria complications
- To an intensive care specialist if severe cerebral malaria or other major organ failure develops
- All malaria cases are mandated to be reported to local and state health departments by health care providers or laboratory staff

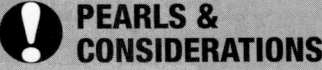 **PEARLS & CONSIDERATIONS**

HOST RESPONSE:
- The specific immune response to malaria confers protection from high-level parasitemia and disease, but not from infection.
- Asymptomatic parasitemia without illness (premunition) is common among adults in endemic areas.
- Immunity is specific for both the species and the strain of infecting malarial parasites.
- Immunity to all strains is never achieved.

- Normal spleen function is an important host factor because of immunologic as well as filtering functions of the spleen.
- Both humoral and cellular immunity is necessary for protection.
- Polyclonal increase in serum level of IgG, IgM, and IgA occurs in immune individuals.
- Antibody to antigenically variant protein PfEMP1 is important for protection in case of *P. falciparum* malaria.
- Passively transferred IgG from immune individuals has been shown to be protective.
- Maternal antibody confers relative protection of infants from severe disease.
- Genetic disorders (sickle cell disease, thalassemia, and G6PD deficiency) confer protection from death because parasites are unable to grow efficiently in low-oxygen tensions, thus preventing high-level parasitemias.
- Individuals deficient of Duffy factor in RBCs are resistant to infection by *P. vivax.*
- Nonspecific defense mechanisms, such as cytokines (TNF-α, IL-1, -6, -8), also play an important role in protection, causing fever (temperatures of 40° C damage mature parasites) and other pathologic effects.

PREVENTION OF MALARIA: Medications are available for the prophylaxis of malaria and will vary depending on level of chloroquine resistance in a given area.

***Areas free of chloroquine-resistant* Falciparum *malaria:*
Chloroquine 300 mg base (500 mg chloroquine phosphate) PO/wk. Start 1 wk prior to arrival in malaria area, then weekly while there and for 4 wk on leaving malaria area. Pediatric dose: 8.3 mg/kg (5 mg/kg base). Alternatives for adults include atovaquone-proguanil (Malarone): 1 adult tablet per day starting 1 to 2 days prior to arriving in malaria area, then daily while there and then for 7 days daily on leaving malaria area. For children, atovaquone-proguanil pediatric tablets based on weight:
- 11 to 20 kg 1 pediatric tablet
- 21 to 30 kg 2 pediatric tablets
- 31 to 40 kg 3 pediatric tablets
- >40 kg 1 adult tablet

***Areas with chloroquine-resistant* Falciparum *malaria:*
- Atovaquone-proguanil (Malarone): dosing as above
- Mefloquine 250 mg (228 mg base) PO/wk, starting 1 wk before arriving in malaria area, weekly while there and then weekly for 4 wk on return. In children, mefloquine dose is based on weight:
  - <15 kg 5 mg/kg
  - 15 to 19 kg ¼ adult dose
  - 20 to 30 kg ½ adult dose
  - 31 to 45 kg ¾ adult dose
  - >45 kg adult dose
- Doxycycline 100 mg PO/day for adults and children aged >8. Start 1 to 2 days before travel, daily while in malaria area, and then daily for 4 wk on return.

SPECIAL CONSIDERATIONS:
- Long-term visitors or travelers
- Children aged <12 yr
- Immunocompromised host
- Pregnant women: chloroquine and mefloquine are safe in pregnancy but not atovaquone-proguanil. Avoid doxycycline and primaquine.

VACCINATION:
- No effective and safe vaccine available yet
- A live, attenuated, whole sporozoite vaccine shown to work
- A synthetic peptide (SPf66) vaccine proved ineffective
- New DNA-based vaccines are in development

MALARIA INFORMATION:
- CDC Travelers' Health Hotline (877) 394–8747; CDC Travelers' Health Fax (888) 232–3299
- CDC Malaria Epidemiology (770) 488–7788; internet: www.cdc.gov

SUGGESTED READINGS
available at www.expertconsult.com

RELATED CONTENT
Malaria (Patient Information)
AUTHOR: **GLENN G. FORT, M.D., M.P.H.**

BASIC INFORMATION

DEFINITION

Malignant hyperthermia is a life-threatening subclinical myopathy that is often triggered by volatile anesthetics or succinylcholine and results in skeletal muscle rigidity and rising temperature. Initial signs may include masseter spasm and rising end-tidal carbon dioxide. There have been case reports of malignant hyperthermia associated with ondansetron and endosulfan poisoning.

SYNONYMS

Malignant hyperthermia of anesthesia
Malignant hyperpyrexia
MH

ICD-9CM CODES
995.86 Malignant hyperthermia of anesthesia

EPIDEMIOLOGY & DEMOGRAPHICS

INCIDENCE: Between 1/200 and 1/250,000. A study by Larach et al demonstrates a mortality rate of 1.4%.
PEAK INCIDENCE: Children account for >50% of cases, but any age may be affected
PREVALENCE: Difficult to determine because of great variations in both penetrance of gene and severity of illness
PREDOMINANT AGE AND SEX: Children, and men more often than women
GENETICS: MH is a heritable disorder of skeletal muscle calcium homeostasis. More than 70% of cases are autosomal dominant, mostly involving a mutation of the ryanodine receptor.
RISK FACTORS: Known family history of malignant hyperthermia or significant problems with general anesthesia. Muscular build increases risk of dying fourteenfold and the risk of cardiac arrest nineteenfold. Northern Europeans seem more affected. There may be a relationship between exertional heat illness/rhabdomyolysis and MH.

PHYSICAL FINDINGS & CLINICAL PRESENTATION

- Within minutes to hours after anesthetic is given, patient develops muscle rigidity (especially masseter spasm), hyperthermia (up to 45° C), tachycardia that may progress to other dysrhythmias, and hypotension. Skin initially reddens but then becomes cyanotic and mottled. There is also increased carbon dioxide production.
- Rhabdomyolysis, acute renal failure, and disseminated intravascular coagulation may soon follow.
- Box 1-36 summarizes positive findings consistent with malignant hyperthermia.

ETIOLOGY

- In contrast to fever, in which elevated core temperature is related to hypothalamus set point adjustment by cytokines, malignant hyperthermia results from overproduction of heat via skeletal muscle metabolism in the context of a normal hypothalamic set point.
- In genetically susceptible individuals, administration of anesthetic agents results in release of calcium from the sarcoplasmic reticulum of skeletal muscles, causing muscle rigidity and hypermetabolism. This results in significant heat production that overwhelms the body's normal ability to dissipate heat.

DIAGNOSIS

DIFFERENTIAL DIAGNOSIS

- Neuroleptic malignant syndrome
- Fever
- Heat stroke
- Thyrotoxicosis
- Pheochromocytoma
- Central nervous system infection or space-occupying lesion
- MDMA (Ecstasy), cocaine, alcohol withdrawal, or amphetamine use
- Serotonin syndrome
- Adverse reaction to monoamine oxidase inhibitor or anticholinergic drug
- Strychnine poisoning
- Delerium tremens
- Sepsis associated with renal and respiratory failure
- Drug withdrawal
- Rhabdomyolysis
- Blood transfusion reaction

WORKUP

Based on history, it is usually easy to distinguish malignant hyperthermia from other causes of hyperthermia. A thorough history, especially including medications and any illicit substances, is important. Consider lumbar puncture to rule out infection.

LABORATORY TESTS

- If the cause of hyperthermia is uncertain, a complete blood count, thyroid function studies, toxicology screen, and urine vanillylmandelic acid (VMA) may be useful.
- Once diagnosis is established, it is important to follow electrolytes (especially potassium, calcium, and phosphorus), creatinine, blood urea nitrogen, liver transaminases, and creatinine kinase.
- Prothrombin time and partial thromboplastin time should be followed to evaluate for disseminated intravascular coagulation.
- Testing for susceptibility to MH can involve genetic testing or an in vitro muscle contracture test (involving a muscle biopsy and exposing the tissue to halothane and caffeine).

IMAGING STUDIES

CT scan to assess for space-occupying lesion if diagnosis is uncertain

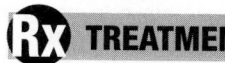

TREATMENT

The most important measures for treatment include stopping the anesthetic agents and substituting propofol if necessary, starting dantrolene, physical cooling, and preventing sequelae. Antipyretics are not useful because the hypothalamic set point is not altered by cytokines.

NONPHARMACOLOGIC THERAPY

- Cooling by ice bath, ice packs in the groin and axillae, cool spray with fans, or cooling blankets. In severe instances extracorporeal partial bypass or iced peritoneal lavage may be used. Stop cooling when core temperature reaches 38° C to prevent overcooling.
- Careful monitoring of cardiovascular and respiratory status with constant core temperature measurements. Hyperventilation may be helpful.

ACUTE GENERAL Rx (see Box 1-37)

- Dantrolene is the mainstay of treatment, starting with a bolus of 5 mg/kg IV, which should be repeated every 5 min until symptoms abate or a maximum of 10 to 20 mg/kg

---

BOX 1-36   Positive Findings Consistent with Malignant Hyperthermia (MH)

History of recent exposure to trigger agent, including volatile anesthetic agents or succinylcholine
Family or personal history of MH susceptibility
Total body rigidity
Masseter spasm
Inappropriately elevated (38.8° C) or rapidly increasing temperature (>1.5° C over 5 min)
Inappropriate tachypnea
Profuse sweating
Mottled, cyanotic skin
Dark urine, urine dipstick testing shows a positive result from blood without red cells in the sediment and no hemolysis
Unexplained, excessive bleeding
Unexplained ventricular tachycardia or fibrillation
Inappropriate hypercarbia (venous $Paco_2$ >65 mm Hg, arterial $Paco_2$ >55 mm Hg) if the patient is receiving positive-pressure ventilation or is spontaneously breathing with greater than normal minute ventilation
Arterial base excess more negative than −8 mEq/L
Arterial pH <7.25
Potassium concentration >6 mEq/L
Creatine kinase >10,000 IU/L

From Fuhrman BP et al: *Pediatric critical care*, ed 4, Philadelphia, 2011, Saunders.

is reached. Then 24 hr of 10 mg/kg/day IV should be given.

- Beta-blockers or lidocaine may be useful for dysrhythmias, but verapamil should be avoided as its use with dantrolene has been shown to depress cardiac function.
- Sodium bicarbonate may be necessary to reverse acidosis.
- Aggressive hydration with forced diuresis and urine alkalinization should be instituted as treatment for rhabdomyolysis.

CHRONIC Rx

This is an acute illness.

COMPLEMENTARY & ALTERNATIVE MEDICINE

None

DISPOSITION

Patient will likely need intensive monitoring for at least 24 hours, necessitating an intensive care unit bed.

REFERRAL

Anesthesia consultants will likely already be involved. Consider cardiac, renal, or hematologic consult if sequelae are significant.

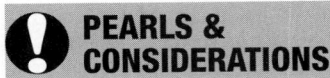 **PEARLS & CONSIDERATIONS**

COMMENTS

Malignant hyperthermia is a life-threatening condition that requires prompt recognition of the signs and symptoms to minimize illness and end-organ damage.

PREVENTION

- Careful family or personal history of significant adverse effects with general anesthesia is an important tip-off.
- Prophylactic dantrolene therapy is no longer recommended in susceptible individuals.

PATIENT & FAMILY EDUCATION

Because family history is so important in this illness, it is important for patients and families to be aware of a history of problems with general anesthesia.

SUGGESTED READINGS

available at www.expertconsult.com

AUTHOR: **CRISTINA ANTONIO PACHECO, M.D.**

BOX 1-37   Management of an Acute Malignant Hyperthermia Episode in the Intensive Care Unit

1. Administer high-flow 100% oxygen via a nonrebreathing mask, and consider endotracheal intubation.
2. For ventilated patients, administer an FiO_2 of 1.0 and increase minute ventilation to control $PaCO_2$.
3. Administer dantrolene (2.5 mg/kg intravenously) over 10 min, and repeat until acidosis and muscle rigidity have resolved. Repeat dantrolene (1 mg/kg) every 6 hr.
4. Initiate cooling with ice packs in the axillae and groin; decrease room temperature; use hypothermia blankets, iced intravenous saline solution (10 mL/kg over 10 min, repeated as needed), and lavage body cavities with cold saline solution if temperature is greater than 39° C. Stop cooling when core temperature falls to 38° C.
5. Correct metabolic acidosis with sodium bicarbonate (1-2 mEq/kg initially), and give subsequent doses based on base excess and body weight.
6. Administer calcium chloride (10 mg/kg) or calcium gluconate (100-200 mg/kg) to cardiotoxicity associated with hyperkalemia.
7. Give regular insulin (0.1 U/kg) and glucose (0.3-0.5 g/kg) to correct hyperkalemia.
8. Administer lidocaine (1 mg/kg) to treat ventricular arrhythmias. Consider amiodarone (5 mg/kg IV) for refractory, stable ventricular tachycardia. Do not delay defibrillation or cardiopulmonary resuscitation if indicated by cardiovascular instability.
9. Maintain urine output of 2 ml/kg/hr with aggressive cold fluid administration, furosemide (0.5-1 mg/kg), and additional mannitol (0.25-0.3 g/kg) if needed.
10. Consider quantitative end-tidal CO_2 monitoring.
11. Monitor core temperature (pulmonary artery, esophageal temperature probe, rectal probe).
12. Place arterial catheter for invasive blood pressure monitoring and frequent blood sampling. Consider central venous catheter and/or pulmonary artery catheter if indicated by cardiovascular instability.
13. Repeat venous blood gas and electrolytes analysis until these normalize. Repeat CK at least every 6 hr while the patient is in ICU and then daily until CK returns to normal. Assess glucose, clotting function, and hepatic and renal functions, and treat symptomatically. Repeat lactic acid measurement after each dantrolene administration.
14. Consider hemodialysis if indicated.
15. Consider intensive care monitoring for at least 24 hr after MH episode or after recrudescence of MH.
16. Refer the patient for muscle caffeine-halothane contracture testing and consider exam of *RYR1*. Pursue a pathologic diagnosis for other occult myopathies.

CK, Creatine kinase; *ICU,* intensive care unit; *MH,* malignant hyperthermia.
From Fuhrman BP et al: *Pediatric critical care,* ed 4, Philadelphia, 2011, Saunders.

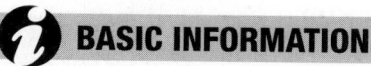
BASIC INFORMATION

DEFINITION

A Mallory-Weiss tear (MWT) is a longitudinal mucosal laceration in the region of the gastroesophageal junction.

SYNONYMS

Mallory-Weiss syndrome

ICD-9CM CODES
530.7   Gastroesophageal laceration-hemorrhage syndrome
530.82 Esophageal hemorrhage

EPIDEMIOLOGY & DEMOGRAPHICS

- Accounts for 5% to 15% of cases of upper gastrointestinal (GI) bleeding
- Reported from early childhood to old age; the majority of patients are age 40 to 60 yr
- More common in males
- Alcohol use is present in 30% to 60%

PHYSICAL FINDINGS & CLINICAL PRESENTATION

- Vomiting, retching, or vigorous coughing will often, but not always, precede hematemesis.
- Patients may be clinically stable or present with tachycardia, hypotension, melena, or hematochezia.
- Bleeding may be self-limited or severe.
- Tears may be seen in association with other upper GI tract lesions, including hiatus hernia (present in as many as 90% of patients), ulcers, and esophageal varices, particularly in alcoholics.

ETIOLOGY

- An acute increase in intraabdominal pressure is transmitted to the esophagus, resulting in mucosal laceration.
- Vomiting may be associated with alcohol use, ketoacidosis, ulcer disease, uremia, pancreatitis, cholecystitis, pregnancy (in particular associated with hyperemesis gravidarum), myocardial infarction, or the postoperative period.
- Tears may be iatrogenic, related to routine endoscopy (especially in struggling or retching patients), enteroscopy, esophageal dilation, lower esophageal pneumatic disruption therapy for achalasia, endoscopic submucosal dissection, transesophageal echocardiography, or in association with polyethylene glycol electrolyte colonic lavage preparation.

DIAGNOSIS

DIFFERENTIAL DIAGNOSIS

- Esophageal or gastric varices
- Esophagitis or esophageal ulcers (peptic or pill-induced)
- Gastric erosions
- Gastric or duodenal ulcer
- Dieulafoy lesion
- Arteriovenous malformations
- Neoplasms (usually gastric)
- Boerhaave's syndrome

WORKUP

Endoscopy is the diagnostic method of choice.

LABORATORY TESTS

- Complete blood count, prothrombin time, partial thromboplastin time
- Electrolytes, blood urea nitrogen, creatinine, liver function tests, pregnancy test, tests to evaluate for predisposing conditions

IMAGING STUDIES

Upper GI series is usually not sensitive. Patients with concurrent chest pain, dyspnea, shock, or physical examination findings of crepitus or pleural effusion should have a chest radiograph or CT to exclude Boerhaave's syndrome.

TREATMENT

NONPHARMACOLOGIC THERAPY

- Supportive care
- Avoidance of aspirin, nonsteroidal anti-inflammatory drugs, and anticoagulants

ACUTE GENERAL Rx

- Patients with active bleeding or hemodynamic instability require large-bore IVs, fluid resuscitation, and transfusion of blood products (red blood cells, fresh frozen plasma, and platelets) as appropriate.
- Nasogastric decompression and antiemetics may be considered.
- Endoscopic therapy for patients with active or ongoing hemorrhage (Fig. 1-510). Therapeutic modalities include electrocoagulation, injection (e.g., 1:10,000 epinephrine, polidocanol), sclerotherapy (for bleeding associated with esophageal varices), band ligation, or endoscopic hemoclips (therapies may be used alone or in combination) (Fig. E1-511).
- Arterial embolization in patients with active bleeding who are poor surgical candidates.
- Laparotomy, with gastrotomy and oversewing of the tear, is required in a small percentage of patients with uncontrolled bleeding.

CHRONIC Rx

- Healing will usually occur without specific therapy.
- H_2 blockers or proton pump inhibitors may be given to help facilitate healing but should not be used long term unless appropriate indications are present.

DISPOSITION

- Prognosis is good, with spontaneous cessation of bleeding in upwards of 90% of patients. Endoscopic features can guide treatment.
- Delayed rebleeding is described in patients with high-risk stigmata (shock at initial presentation, spurting or oozing at initial endoscopy).
- Death has been reported in 3% to 12%, often in association with severe bleeding and underlying comorbid conditions such as advanced age, coagulopathy, elevated transaminases, thrombocytopenia, alcohol use, presentation with a very low hemoglobin level or melena, and multisystem organ failure.

REFERRAL

- Gastrointestinal referral for endoscopy
- Surgical referral for bleeding unresponsive to endoscopic treatment or in the setting of co-existent perforation

PEARLS & CONSIDERATIONS

Conditions predisposing to retching or vomiting should be identified and treated at presentation.

SUGGESTED READINGS

available at www.expertconsult.com

RELATED CONTENT

Mallory-Weiss Tear (Patient Information)

AUTHOR: **HARLAN G. RICH, M.D., F.A.C.P., A.F.A.F.**

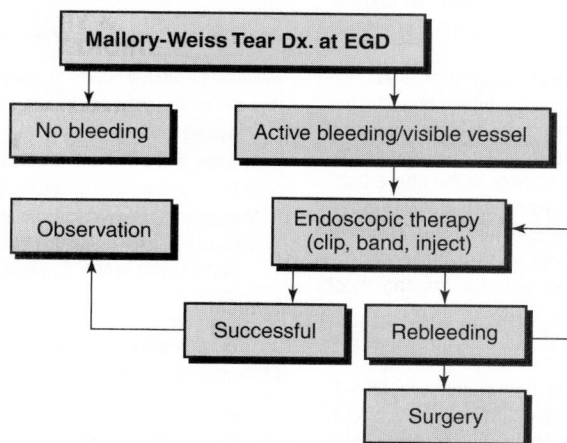

FIGURE 1-510 Treatment algorithm for Mallory-Weiss tear. *EGD,* Esophagogastroduodenoscopy. (From Cameron JL, Cameron AM: *Current surgical therapy,* ed 10, Philadelphia, 2011, Saunders.)

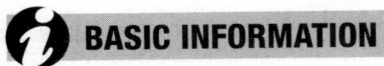

BASIC INFORMATION

DEFINITION

Marfan's syndrome is an inherited disorder of connective tissue involving the skeleton, cardiovascular system, eyes, lungs, and central nervous system.

ICD-9CM CODES
759.82 Marfan's syndrome

EPIDEMIOLOGY & DEMOGRAPHICS

PREVALENCE:
- One case per 10,000 persons.
- Both sexes are affected equally by this autosomal-dominant syndrome.
- Approximately 30% of cases are a new mutation.

PHYSICAL FINDINGS & CLINICAL PRESENTATION

Diagnostic criteria for Marfan's syndrome (Table 1-268):
- Skeleton: joint hypermobility, tall stature (Fig. 1-512, A), pectus excavatum, reduced thoracic kyphosis, scoliosis, arachnodactyly (Fig. 1-512, B), dolichostenomelia, pectus carinatum, and erosion of the lumbosacral vertebrae from dural ectasia*
- Eye: myopia, retinal detachment, elongated globe, ectopia lentis*
- Cardiovascular: mitral valve prolapse, endocarditis, arrhythmia, dilated mitral annulus, mitral regurgitation, tricuspid valve prolapse, aortic regurgitation, aortic dissection,* dilation of the aortic root*
- Pulmonary: apical blebs, spontaneous pneumothorax
- Skin and integument: inguinal hernias, incisional hernias, striae atrophicae
- Central nervous system: attention deficit disorder, hyperactivity, verbal-performance discrepancy, dural ectasia, anterior pelvic meningocele*

If the family history is positive for a close relative clearly affected by Marfan's syndrome, manifestations should be present in the skeleton and one of the other organ systems and the diagnosis confirmed by linkage analysis or mutation detection.

If the family history is negative or unknown, the patient should have manifestations in the skeleton, the cardiovascular system, and one other system and at least one of the manifestations indicated by an asterisk in the above lists.

Manifestations are listed within each organ system in increasing specificity for Marfan's syndrome; although none is completely specific, those indicated by an asterisk are the most specific.

ETIOLOGY

Mutations in the gene that encodes fibrillin-1, the major constituent of microfibrils, which form the frame for elastic fibers. All the manifestations of Marfan's syndrome can be explained by the defective microfibrils.

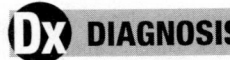

DIAGNOSIS

DIFFERENTIAL DIAGNOSIS

Each of the clinical manifestations of the syndrome may have other causes; however, if the diagnostic criteria are met, the diagnosis is made.

WORKUP

- Echocardiography to establish:
  1. Mitral valve prolapse
  2. Mitral regurgitation
  3. Tricuspid valve prolapse
  4. Aortic regurgitation
  5. Dilation of the aortic root
- Chest radiograph (Fig. 1-513)

TABLE 1-268 Diagnostic Criteria for Marfan's Syndrome

In the absence of a family history of MFS, a diagnosis can be reached in 1 of 4 scenarios:
1. Aortic diameter at Sinuses of Valsalva Z-score ≥2 AND Ectopia Lentis = MFS*
2. Aortic diameter at Sinuses of Valsalva Z-score ≥2 AND FBN1 mutation = MFS
3. Aortic diameter at Sinuses of Valsalva Z-score ≥2 AND Systemic Score ≥7 = MFS*
4. Ectopia Lentis AND FBN1 mutation known to associate with aortic aneurysm = MFS

In the absence of a family history of MFS, alternative diagnoses to MFS include:
1. Ectopia Lentis ± Systemic Score AND FBN1 mutation not known to associate with aortic aneurysm or no FBN1 mutation = Ectopia Lentis syndrome
2. Aortic diameter at Sinuses of Valsalva Z-score <2 AND Systemic Score 2:5 (with at least one skeletal feature) without Ectopia Lentis = MASS phenotype
3. Mitral Valve Prolapse AND Aortic diameter at Sinuses of Valsalva Z-score <2 AND Systemic Score <5 without Ectopia Lentis = Mitral Valve Prolapse syndrome

In the presence of a family history of MFS, a diagnosis can be reached in 1 of 3 scenarios:
1. Ectopia Lentis AND Family History of MFS = MFS
2. Systemic Score ≥7 AND Family History of MFS = MFS*
3. Aortic diameter at Sinuses of Valsalva Z-score ≥2 if older than 20 yr or ≥3 if younger than 20 yr AND Family History of MFS = MFS*

Scoring of Systemic Features (in points)[†]

Wrist AND thumb sign = 3 (wrist OR thumb sign = 1)

Pectus carinatum deformity = 2 (pectus excavatum or chest asymmetry = 1)

Hindfoot deformity = 2 (plain pes planus = 1)

Pneumothorax = 2

Dural ectasia = 2

Protrusio acetabuli = 2

Reduced US/LS AND increased arm/height AND no severe scoliosis = 1

Scoliosis or thoracolumbar kyphosis = 1

Reduced elbow extension = 1

Facial features (3/5) = 1 (dolichocephaly, enophthalmos, downslanting palpebral fissures, malar hypoplasia, retrognathia)

Skin striae = 1

Myopia >3 diopters = 1

Mitral valve prolapse (all types) = 1

Criteria for Causal FBN1 Mutation

Mutation previously shown to segregate in a Marfan family

Any one of the following de novo mutations (with proven paternity and absence of disease in parents):

Nonsense mutation

In-frame and out-of-frame deletion/insertion

Splice site mutations affecting canonical splice sequence or shown to alter splicing on mRNA/cDNA level

Missense mutation affecting/creating cysteine residues

Missense mutation affecting conserved residues of the EGF consensus sequence [(D/N)X(D/N)(E/Q)Xm(D/N) Xn(Y/F), with m and n representing variable number of residues; D, aspartic acid; N, asparagine; E, glutamic acid; Q, glutamine; Y, tyrosine; F, phenylalanine]

Other missense mutations: segregation in family, if possible, + absence in 400 ethnically matched control chromosomes; if no family history, absence in 400 ethnically matched control chromosomes

Linkage of haplotype for n≥6 meioses to the FBN1 locus

MFS, Marfan's syndrome; US/LS, upper segment/lower segment ratio.
*Without discriminating features of Shprintzen-Goldberg syndrome, Loeys-Dietz syndrome, or Ehlers-Danlos syndrome and after TGFBR1/2, collagen biochemistry, COL3A1 testing if indicated. Other conditions/genes will emerge with time.
†Maximum total: 20 points; score ≥7 indicates systemic involvement.
From Loeys BL et al: The revised Ghent nosology for the Marfan syndrome, J Med Genet 47:476-485, 2010.

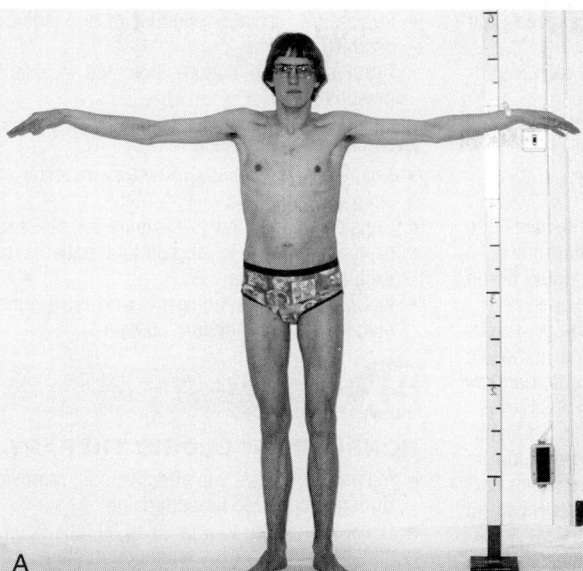

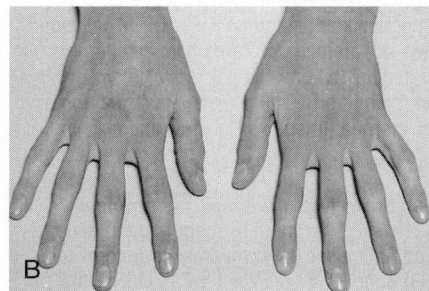

FIGURE 1-512 A, Long limbs compared with the trunk. **B,** Arachnodactyly. (From Kanski JJ, Bowling B: *Clinical ophthalmology, a system approach,* ed 7, Philadelphia, 2010, Saunders.)

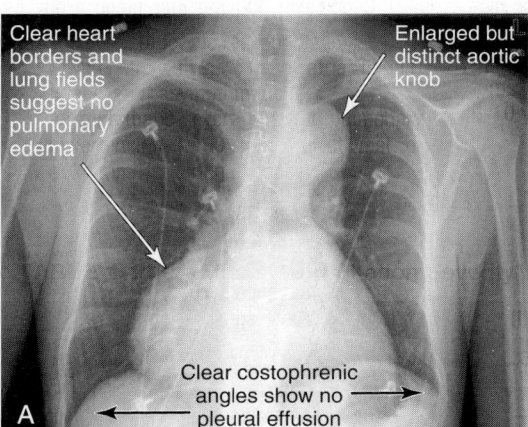

Clear heart borders and lung fields suggest no pulmonary edema

Enlarged but distinct aortic knob

Clear costophrenic angles show no pleural effusion

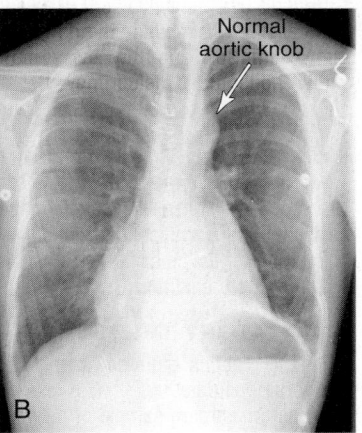

Normal aortic knob

FIGURE 1-513 Cardiomegaly and thoracic aneurysm in Marfan's syndrome. This 24-year-old patient with Marfan's syndrome presented with dyspnea (**A**). The heart appears markedly dilated, as do the aortic root and arch. Ejection fraction was estimated at 10% by magnetic resonance imaging. No effusion was seen despite the globular heart shape. This is a dilated cardiomyopathy. Lung fields, heart borders, and hemidiaphragms appear clear and without evidence of pulmonary edema. **B,** The same patient 3 years earlier. Compare the heart size and aortic contour before progression of disease. Sternotomy wires are visible from a previous mitral valve repair. (From Broder JS: *Diagnostic imaging for the emergency physician,* Philadelphia, 2011, Saunders.)

M

Diseases and Disorders

I

- Transesophageal echocardiography, chest CT scan, chest MRI, or aortography for suspected aortic dissection
- Chest radiograph for pulmonary apical bullae
- Ophthalmologic examination by ophthalmologist

(Rx) TREATMENT

- Regular cardiac and aorta monitoring by physical examination and echocardiography.
- Endocarditis prophylaxis.
- Restriction of contact sports, weight lifting, and overexertion.
- Beta-blockers are commonly prescribed to slow the rate of aortic root dilation. Patients with Marfan's syndrome and associated aneurysm should be receiving beta-blockers unless there is a contraindication to their use. Recent reports indicate that use of angiotensin receptor blockers significantly also slowed the rate of progressive aortic root dilation independent of hemodynamic effects.
- Early use of angiotensin-converting enzyme inhibitors in young patients with Marfan's syndrome and valvular regurgitation should be considered.
- Genetic counseling.
- Monitor aorta during pregnancy because of the increased risk of dissection.

SUGGESTED READINGS
available at www.expertconsult.com

RELATED CONTENT
Marfan's Syndrome (Patient Information)

AUTHOR: **FRED F. FERRI, M.D.**

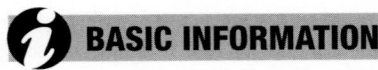

BASIC INFORMATION

DEFINITION

Mastitis is local painful inflammation of the breast that may or may not be accompanied by infection, flulike symptoms, and abscess formation.

ICD-9CM CODES
611.0 Inflammatory disease of the breast
675.1 Postpartum abscess of the breast
675.2 Postpartum nonpurulent mastitis

EPIDEMIOLOGY & DEMOGRAPHICS

- In lactating mothers, mastitis typically occurs in the first 3 mo postpartum (74% to 95% of cases)
- When severe, mastitis can lead to a breast abscess (5% to 11%) or septicemia
- In nonlactating women of childbearing age it often presents as granulomatous mastitis (GM)
- In older nonlactating women it is called periductal mastitis (PM) and is caused by inflamed milk ducts near the nipple
- Mastitis can also occur in early infancy, when breast hypertrophy from maternal hormonal stimulation can lead to infection

PREVALENCE: 9.5% to 33% depending on definition and postpartum timeline
PREDOMINANT SEX: Females
RISK FACTORS:
- Previous mastitis
- Cracked, fissured, or sore nipples
- Primiparity and infant attachment difficulties
- Cleft lip or palate or short frenulum in infant
- Milk stasis and missed feedings
- Poor maternal nutrition
- Using antifungal nipple cream (presumably for nipple thrush) in the same week
- Tight clothing or bras
- Use of manual breast pump
- Diabetes
- Use of steroids
- Lumpectomy with radiation
- Breast implants
- Nipple piercings

PHYSICAL FINDINGS & CLINICAL PRESENTATION

- Warmth, redness, tenderness in breast
- Unilateral or bilateral
- Malaise, myalgias, fevers, chills
- Pain with nursing
- Decreased milk output

- Area of breast is hard, wedge shaped, and swollen
- In PM, breast mass near nipple with retraction or discharge
- In GM, enlarged axillary lymph nodes or sinus tract formation

ETIOLOGY

- Milk stasis and irritation of the milk ducts due to local immune response to milk proteins.
- Bacterial infection of subcutaneous tissue due to breaks in skin.
- The most common organism is *S. aureus* and, less commonly, group A beta-hemolytic streptococci, *S. pneumoniae, E. coli, Candida albicans,* and *M. tuberculosis.*
- GM from inflammation with epithelioid histiocytes and multinucleated giant cells can be caused by etiologies like tuberculosis, sarcoidosis, foreign body reaction, parasitic and mycotic infections, or idiopathic (IGM).
- Mastitis in neonates is caused by infections with *S. aureus* or gram-negative enteric bacteria.

DIAGNOSIS

DIFFERENTIAL DIAGNOSIS

- Engorgement, plugged duct (see Table 1-269)
- Breast abscess
- Inflammatory or other breast cancer (3% of women diagnosed with breast cancer are lactating)
- Mastitis as a symptom of hyperprolactinemia or galactorrhea
- GM can be a manifestation of systemic disease including sarcoidosis, Wegener granulomatosis, giant cell arteritis, polyarteritis nodosa, TB, syphilis

WORKUP

- History of signs and symptoms and clinical exam including thorough breast exam with assessment for axillary nodes and nipple discharge are sufficient to make diagnosis
- Recurrent mastitis should include workup for underlying breast disease

LABORATORY TESTS

- Simple mastitis requires no milk culture or laboratory studies
- Obtain midstream sample of milk for culture for antibiotic sensitivities in refractory mastitis or in MRSA-suspected cases
- CBC and blood cultures in toxic-appearing patients

- In abscess formation, culture of drainage or aspirate fluid
- Gram stain and culture indicated in infant mastitis

IMAGING STUDIES

- Not necessary unless refractory mastitis or abscess suspected
- Consider ultrasound to evaluate for abscess or mammogram in appropriate patients to exclude carcinoma
- In GM, use of mammogram and ultrasound guided FNA are standard studies

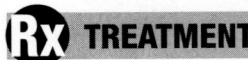

TREATMENT

NONPHARMACOLOGIC THERAPY

- Mainstay of therapy is effective milk removal through continued breastfeeding
- Consider referral to a certified lactation consultant to improve breastfeeding technique
- Warm compresses, increased fluid intake, good nutrition, and rest
- In abscess formation, surgical drainage or needle aspiration is necessary, followed by antibiotic therapy based on sensitivities of culture

ACUTE GENERAL Rx

- NSAIDs and analgesics (e.g., acetaminophen, ibuprofen)
- No MRSA:
  - Dicloxacillin 500 mg four times daily for 10 to 14 days
  - Cephalexin 500 mg four times a day for 10 to 14 days
  - Inpatient nafcillin or oxacillin 2 g IV q4h
- If MRSA suspected:
  - Trimethoprim/sulfamethoxazole 160 mg/800 mg twice daily for 10 to 14 days, should not be used when breastfeeding healthy infants aged <2 mo or compromised infants
  - Clindamycin 300 mg four times daily for 10 to 14 days (for penicillin allergy, MRSA coverage)
  - Inpatient: vancomycin 1 g IV q12h
- Oxytocin nasal spray if letdown reflex disturbed
- Consider treatment for candidal infection if bilateral symptoms and infant with thrush
- Mastitis in early infancy should be treated with parenteral antibiotics based on results of Gram stain

CHRONIC Rx

- Systemic corticosteroids or wide surgical resection in GM.
- No evidence proving benefit of prophylactic antibiotics to prevent mastitis

COMPLEMENTARY & ALTERNATIVE MEDICINE

- Complementary therapies have not been assessed in prospective studies: *Belladonna, Phytolacca, Chamomilla,* sulfur, and *Bellis perennis*
- Several strains of lactobacilli have shown promise as probiotic agents that might be

TABLE 1-269 Comparison of Findings of Engorgement, Plugged Duct, and Mastitis

Characteristics	Engorgement	Plugged Duct	Mastitis
Onset	Gradual, immediately	Gradual, after feedings	Sudden, after 10 days postpartum
Site	Bilateral	Unilateral	Usually unilateral
Swelling and heat	Generalized	May shift/little or no heat	Localized red, hot, and swollen
Body temperature	<38.4° C	<38.4° C	>38.4° C
Systemic symptoms	Feels well	Feels well	Flulike symptoms

From Lawrence RA, Lawrence RM: *Breastfeeding: a guide for the medical profession,* ed 5, St Louis, 1999, Mosby.

useful in treating mastitis. *L. fermentum* and *L. salivarius* have been found to be an effective alternative to antibiotics in recent trials on treatment of infectious mastitis during lactation. These intriguing results should be replicated before this approach is adopted widely.

REFERRAL

Referral to a surgeon for severe PM or significant abscess that does not resolve with conservative measures

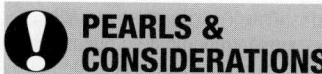

PEARLS & CONSIDERATIONS

COMMENTS

- One quarter of breastfeeding mothers with one episode of mastitis will stop breastfeeding.
- Increasing incidence of MRSA mastitis.
- In reassessing refractory mastitis, the most important consideration is the possibility of cancer.
- Mastitis can be a manifestation of systemic disease.
- Mastitis is a risk factor for vertical transmission of infections including increased transmission of retroviruses (especially HIV-1), CMV, measles, hepatitis B and C.
- GM mimics breast cancer both clinically and radiologically (>50% of reported cases are initially mistaken for carcinoma). This includes fine needle aspiration, which is sometimes interpreted as malignant.
- All infants of mothers with diagnosis of mastitis should receive parenteral antibiotics.

PATIENT & FAMILY EDUCATION

La Leche League International (website: http://www.llli.org),
International Lactation Consultant Association (website: http://www.ilca.org)

SUGGESTED READINGS

available at www.expertconsult.com

AUTHORS: **MARY BETH SUTTER, M.D.,** and **ANDREI LEVCHENKO, M.D.**

M

Diseases and Disorders

I

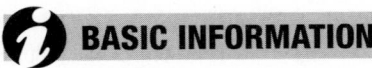

BASIC INFORMATION

DEFINITION
- Pain in the breast
- Usually cyclic condition but may be noncyclic or extramammary

SYNONYMS
Mastalgia

ICD-9CM CODES
611.71 Mastodynia

EPIDEMIOLOGY & DEMOGRAPHICS
- Mastodynia affects up to 70% of women at some time in their reproductive lives.
- Severe cyclic mastodynia lasting more than 5 days/mo and of sufficient intensity to interfere with sexual, physical, social, and work-related activities is reported among 30% of premenopausal women.
- Underlying fear of breast cancer is the reason most of these women seek medical consultation.
- One tenth of women with mastodynia require pain-relieving therapy.

PHYSICAL FINDINGS & CLINICAL PRESENTATION
- Usually the breasts are normal bilaterally
- Full, tender breasts
- Generalized breast nodularity without discrete lumps
- Chest wall tenderness: extramammary breast pain
- Distinguishing mammary from extramammary pain can be difficult
- With the patient lying on her side so that the breast tissue falls away from the chest wall, tenderness can then be reproduced by direct pressure over the offending site
- Cyclic mastodynia presents in the luteal phase of the menstrual cycle
- Women with cyclic mastodynia tend to have abdominal bloating, leg swelling, and other symptoms of premenstrual syndrome
- Noncyclic mastodynia, on the other hand, is unrelated to the menstrual cycle
- Extramammary breast pain simulates noncyclic mastodynia

ETIOLOGY
- Hormonal imbalance
- Abnormal lipid metabolism
- Premenstrual syndrome (20%)
- Fibrocystic breast disease
- Emotional abuse and anxiety
- Excessive caffeine intake
- Breast cancer (10%)
- Tietze syndrome (idiopathic costochondritis)

DIAGNOSIS

DIFFERENTIAL DIAGNOSIS
- See "Etiology."
- The majority of women with mastodynia have no underlying abnormality.

- Breast fullness and tenderness associated with hormonal changes fluctuate with the menstrual cycle.
- Similarly, breast nodularity, which may or may not be the result of fibrocystic breast disease, also fluctuates with the menstrual cycle.
- Discrete breast lumps need full evaluation to rule out malignancy.
- Tietze syndrome is usually unilateral and may be associated with chest wall swelling.

LABORATORY TESTS
Although hormonal imbalance and abnormal lipid metabolism have been implicated in the etiopathogenesis of mastodynia, there is no good evidence to support any consistent pattern of serum hormonal or lipid profile in women with mastodynia. These tests are therefore not recommended.

IMAGING STUDIES
- Mammography should be part of the baseline investigation if the woman is >35 yr.
- Ultrasound can be performed as needed; it is particularly helpful in the assessment of cystic breast lesions.
- In women <35 yr, imaging investigations are not helpful unless a lump has been palpated clinically.
- There are no radiologic features associated with mastodynia: rather, radiologic investigations are performed to exclude the rare presence of a subclinical carcinoma.

TREATMENT

NONPHARMACOLOGIC THERAPY
- 85% of the women with mastodynia can be reassured after full clinical evaluation.
- The remaining 15% require some form of therapy in addition to reassurance.
- A firm, supportive brassiere designed for postpartum use is particularly helpful if mastodynia is associated with breast swelling.
- Follow a low-fat, high-carbohydrate diet.
- Reduce caffeine intake.

ACUTE GENERAL Rx
- Evening primrose oil, which contains gamma-linolenic acid, has been shown to have some effectiveness and is an acceptable treatment for mastodynia.
- Topical NSAID preparations may confer some benefit and can be prescribed for these women.
- Hormonal therapy is the mainstay of treatment.
- Danazol is the only drug approved by the FDA for the treatment of mastodynia. Danazol has some androgenic and peripheral antiestrogenic effects. Its efficacy is well established, with significant relief of mastodynia in 70% to 93% of cases.
  - Widespread use of danazol is limited because of its adverse side effects. These include menstrual irregularities, depression, acne, hirsutism, and, in severe cases,

voice deepening. Women taking danazol should be advised to use effective nonhormonal contraception because of the drug's potential adverse effects on the fetus.
- The side effects of danazol can be significantly reduced by using a low dose (100 mg daily) and confining treatment to 2 wk preceding menstruation.
- Tamoxifen, a synthetic antiestrogen, has also been shown to be effective in the treatment of mastodynia. Although effective in relieving symptoms, its use is extremely limited because of side effects. When used, it should be at a low dosage of 10 mg/day and duration should be limited to 6 mo at a time. In the U.S. this agent is not approved for use in women with mastodynia.
- Bromocriptine is a dopamine-receptor agonist whose primary action is inhibition of prolactin release. It has been used extensively in the treatment of severe cyclic mastodynia and is effective. Again, side effects such as headache and lightheadedness have limited its use.
- Lisuride maleate was recently found to be effective by one study.
- Other hormonal agents that have been reported to be effective in small studies cannot be recommended. Either they have unacceptable side effect profiles or their efficacy is not established. These agents include gestrinone, gonadotropin-releasing hormone analogues, progesterone, and hormone replacement therapy.

CHRONIC Rx
- Longstanding cases of mastodynia can be managed with intermittent low-dose danazol therapy to limit side effects. In between these courses of hormone, nonpharmacologic and nonhormonal therapy can be used.
- Severe, unremitting mastodynia that does not respond to medical treatment may require mastectomy; this is rare.

DISPOSITION
- Cyclic mastodynia resolves spontaneously in 20% to 30% of women.
- Up to 60% of women may develop recurrent symptoms 2 yr after treatment.
- Noncyclic mastodynia responds poorly to treatment but may resolve spontaneously in up to 50% of women.

SUGGESTED READINGS
available at www.expertconsult.com

RELATED CONTENT
Abscess, Breast (Related Key Topic)
Fibrocystic Breast Disease (Related Key Topic)
Breast Pain (Patient Information)

AUTHORS: **ALEXANDER B. OLAWAIYE, M.D.,** and **RUBEN ALVERO, M.D.**

BASIC INFORMATION
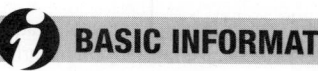

DEFINITION

Mastoiditis is inflammation of the mastoid process and air cells, a complication of otitis media.

SYNONYMS

Mastoid abscess

ICD-9CM CODES
383.00 Mastoiditis, acute or subacute
383.1   Mastoiditis, chronic

EPIDEMIOLOGY & DEMOGRAPHICS

INCIDENCE (IN U.S.): Since the introduction of antibiotic therapy and use of broad-spectrum antibiotics, there has been a marked decline in the incidence of acute mastoiditis.
PREDOMINANT SEX: More common in males
PREDOMINANT AGE: 2 mo to 18 yr
PEAK INCIDENCE: Early childhood

PHYSICAL FINDINGS & CLINICAL PRESENTATION

- Acute mastoiditis is usually a complication of acute otitis media.
- Most common presenting symptom is pain and tenderness in the postauricular region.
- Other signs or symptoms include:
  1. Fever
  2. Postauricular erythema and edema
  3. Protrusion of the pinna inferiorly and anteriorly
  4. Tympanic membrane usually intact with signs of acute otitis media
- Complications of acute mastoiditis include:
  1. Subperiosteal abscess (most common complication)
  2. Hearing loss
  3. Facial nerve palsy
  4. Labyrinthitis
  5. Intracranial complications such as hydrocephalus, meningitis, encephalitis, intracranial abscess, and lateral sinus thrombosis
- Chronic mastoiditis is characterized by chronic otorrhea and chronic tympanic membrane perforation.

ETIOLOGY

- Continuity exists between the middle air space and the mastoid cavity.
- Initial hyperemia and edema of the mucosal lining of the air cells results in accumulation of purulent exudate.
- Dissolution of calcium from bony septa and osteoclastic activity in the inflamed periosteum lead to bone necrosis and coalescence of air cells.
- Most common bacterial isolates are:
  1. *Streptococcus pneumoniae*
  2. *Streptococcus pyogenes*
  3. *Haemophilus influenzae*
  4. *Moraxella catarrhalis*
  5. *Staphylococcus aureus*
- Often, there are multiple organisms in chronic mastoiditis, with predominance of anaerobes and gram-negative bacteria.
- *Mycobacterium tuberculosis*, nontuberculous mycobacteria, *Aspergillus,* and *Rhodococcus equi* have been reported in cases of mastoiditis in severely immunocompromised individuals.

DIAGNOSIS

DIFFERENTIAL DIAGNOSIS

- Children
  1. Rhabdomyosarcoma
  2. Histiocytosis X
  3. Leukemia
  4. Kawasaki syndrome
- Adults
  1. Fulminant otitis externa
  2. Histiocytosis X
  3. Metastatic disease

WORKUP

A thorough history and physical examination are important in establishing diagnosis.

LABORATORY TESTS

- Fluid for Gram stain and culture may be obtained by myringotomy.
- If there is a perforation in the tympanic membrane with drainage, cultures of this may be taken after carefully cleaning the external canal.

IMAGING STUDIES

- Plain x-rays of the mastoid region may demonstrate clouding or opacification in areas of pneumatization.
- CT scan (Fig. E1-514) can demonstrate early involvement of bone (mastoiditis with bone destruction).
- MRI is more sensitive than CT scan in evaluating soft-tissue involvement and is useful in conjunction with CT scan to investigate other complications of mastoiditis.

TREATMENT

NONPHARMACOLOGIC THERAPY

Myringotomy, if the ear is not already draining

ACUTE GENERAL Rx

- Initiated with IV antibiotics directed against the common organisms *S. pneumoniae* and *H. influenzae.* Useful agents are amoxicillin/clavulanate, ceftriaxone, and cefotaxime. If the disease in the mastoid has had a prolonged course, coverage for *S. aureus* with gram-negative enteric bacilli may be considered for initial therapy until results of cultures become available. Add vancomycin or nafcillin/oxacillin if culture is positive for *S. aureus.*
- Antibiotics continued until all signs of mastoiditis have resolved
- Directed against enteric gram-negative organisms and anaerobes in chronic mastoiditis
- Indications for mastoidectomy:
  1. Failure to improve after 72 hr of therapy
  2. Persistent fever
  3. Imminent or overt signs of intracranial complications
  4. Evidence of a subperiosteal abscess in the mastoid bone

DISPOSITION

Proceed with mastoidectomy when medical therapy fails.

REFERRAL

- To otorhinolaryngologist:
  1. If diagnosis is in doubt
  2. If aural complications present
  3. To evaluate for surgical intervention
- To neurosurgeon if intratemporal or intracranial extension of infection suspected
  1. Aural complications: bone destruction, subperiosteal abscess, petrositis, facial paralysis, labyrinthitis
  2. Intracranial complications: extradural abscess, lateral sinus thrombophlebitis or thrombosis, subdural abscess, meningitis, brain abscess, otitic hydrocephalus

PEARLS & CONSIDERATIONS
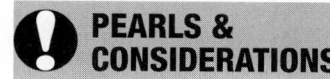

Mastoiditis is particularly difficult to eradicate because the mastoid air cells are poorly vascularized and difficult to drain.

SUGGESTED READINGS

available at www.expertconsult.com

RELATED CONTENT

Mastoiditis (Patient Information)

AUTHOR: **GLENN G. FORT, M.D., M.P.H.**

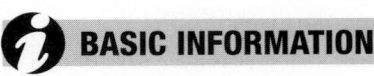

BASIC INFORMATION

DEFINITION

Meckel diverticulum is an ileal diverticulum located 100 cm proximal to the cecum. It results from failure of the omphalomesenteric duct to obliterate completely (as it should by the eighth week of gestation).

SYNONYMS

MD

ICD-9CM CODES
751.0 Meckel diverticulum

EPIDEMIOLOGY & DEMOGRAPHICS

- Meckel diverticulum, based on autopsy studies and intraoperative evidence, occurs in 0.3% to 4% of the population and is the most prevalent congenital anomaly of the gastrointestinal (GI) tract. Complications occur more frequently in males.
- Most patients who develop symptoms are <10 yr.
- The lifetime risk of complications developing in a case of Meckel diverticulum is 4%.
- In adults, complications (small bowel obstruction [25% to 40%], diverticulitis [20%]) are usually attributable to factors other than heterotopic mucosa.
- Tumors have rarely been reported in symptomatic Meckel diverticulum, with carcinoid being the most common type.

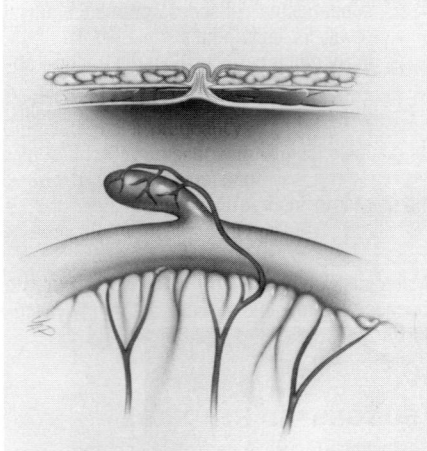

FIGURE 1-518 Typical Meckel diverticulum located on the antimesenteric border. (From Kliegman RM et al: *Nelson textbook of pediatrics,* ed 19, Philadelphia, 2011, Saunders.)

PHYSICAL FINDINGS & CLINICAL PRESENTATION

- Painless lower GI bleeding (4%)
- Intestinal obstruction caused by intussusception, volvulus, herniation, or entrapment of a loop of bowel through a defect in the diverticular mesentery (6%)
- Meckel's diverticulitis mimics acute appendicitis (5%)

20 min.

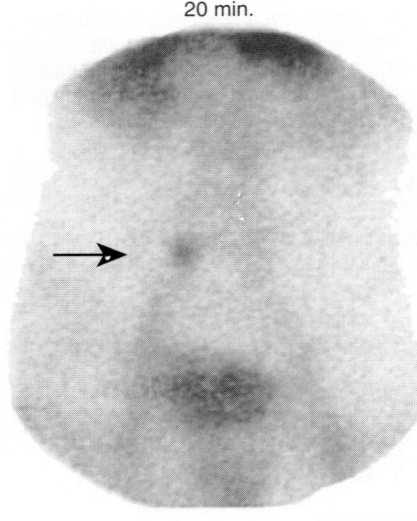

25 min.

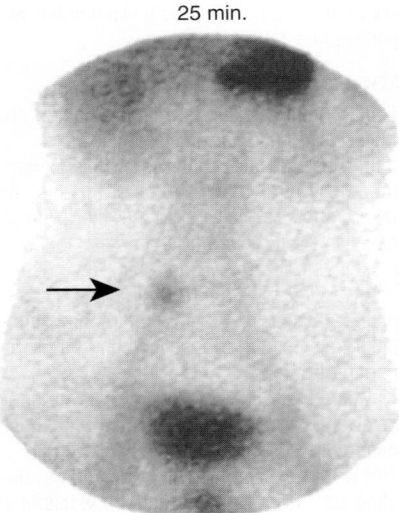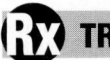

FIGURE 1-519 Meckel scan demonstrating accumulation in the stomach superior bladder (inferior) and in the acid-secreting mucosa of a Meckel diverticulum. (From Kliegman RM et al: *Nelson textbook of pediatrics,* ed 19, Philadelphia, 2011, Saunders.)

- Rare primary tumor arising from diverticulum (carcinoid, sarcoma, leiomyoma, adenocarcinoma)
- Asymptomatic (80% to 95%)

ETIOLOGY & PATHOGENESIS

- As a remnant of the omphalomesenteric duct, Meckel diverticulum contains all layers of the intestinal wall and has its own mesentery and blood supply (branch of the superior mesenteric artery) (Fig. 1-518).
- The majority of complicated cases of Meckel diverticulum contain ectopic mucosa (75% gastric, 15% pancreatic). It causes ulceration and bleeding of ileal mucosa adjacent to the acidic ectopic gastric secretions. Alkaline secretions of ectopic pancreatic tissue can also cause ulcerations.

DIAGNOSIS

DIFFERENTIAL DIAGNOSIS

- Appendicitis
- Crohn's disease
- All causes of lower GI bleeding (polyp, colon cancer, arteriovenous malformation, diverticulosis, hemorrhoids)

WORKUP

- Diagnosis is often made intraoperatively when the preoperative diagnosis is appendicitis.
- Preoperative detection of symptomatic Meckel diverticulum requires a high index of suspicion.
- Meckel scan: In the case of GI bleeding of unknown source, a technetium scan will identify Meckel diverticulum (sensitivity: 85% in children, 62% in adults; specificity: 95% in children, 9% in adults) (Fig. 1-519).
- In patients with suspected small-bowel obstruction, intussusception, or diverticulitis, a CT scan of the abdomen and pelvis is helpful.

TREATMENT

- Surgical resection in symptomatic patients.
- There is controversy regarding the need to remove an incidentally found diverticulum, with most surgeons arguing in favor of resection.

SUGGESTED READINGS
available at www.expertconsult.com

RELATED CONTENT
Meckel Diverticulum (Patient Information)

AUTHOR: **FRED F. FERRI, M.D.**

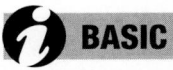 BASIC INFORMATION

DEFINITION

Meigs' syndrome is characterized by the presence of a benign solid ovarian tumor associated with ascites and predominantly right hydrothorax that disappear after tumor removal.

ICD-9CM CODES
620.2 Ovarian mass (unspecified)
220.0 Benign ovarian lesion
789.5 Ascites
511.9 Pleural effusion

EPIDEMIOLOGY & DEMOGRAPHICS

- Occurs in <1% of ovarian fibromas (associated with approximately 0.004% of ovarian tumors)
- Most frequently encountered during middle age (average age, approximately 48 yr)

PHYSICAL FINDINGS & CLINICAL PRESENTATION

- Asymptomatic pelvic mass on bimanual examination
- Intermittent pelvic pain (intermittent torsion)
- Acute pelvic tenderness
- Acute abdominal tenderness
- Abdominal pelvic mass
- Abdominal bloating
- Fluid wave
- Shifting dullness
- "Puddle sign"
- Hyperresonance or flatness to chest percussion, absence of tactile and vocal fremitus
- Absent or loud bronchial breath sounds, rales, mediastinal displacement, tracheal shift
- Weight loss and emaciation

ETIOLOGY

- Not specifically known
- Usually associated with "edematous" fibromas (or other benign ovarian solid tumor) in excess of 10 cm
- Plausible that large fibroma with narrow stalk has inadequate lymphatic drainage; when coupled with intermittent torsion, results in backflow transudation into the peritoneal cavity; accumulated peritoneal ascites then pass to the right pleural cavity by the lymphatics (overloaded thoracic duct) or abdominal pleural commutation (i.e., foramen of Bochdalek)

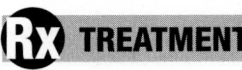 DIAGNOSIS

DIFFERENTIAL DIAGNOSIS

- Abdominal ovarian malignancy
- Various gynecologic disorders:
  1. Uterus; endometrial tumor, sarcoma, leiomyoma ("pseudo-Meigs' syndrome")
  2. Fallopian tube: hydrosalpinx, granulomatous salpingitis, fallopian tube malignancy
  3. Ovary: benign, serous, mucinous, endometrioid, clear cell, Brenner tumor, granulosa, stromal, dysgerminoma, fibroma, metastatic tumor
- Nongynecologic (gastrointestinal tract or genitourinary tract tumor or pathology) causes of pelvic mass
  1. Ascites
  2. Portal vein obstruction
  3. Inferior vena cava obstruction
  4. Hypoproteinemia
  5. Thoracic duct obstruction
  6. Tuberculosis
  7. Amyloidosis
  8. Pancreatitis
  9. Neoplasm
  10. Ovarian hyperstimulation
  11. Pleural effusion
  12. Congestive heart failure
  13. Malignancy
  14. Collagen-vascular disease
  15. Pancreatitis
  16. Cirrhosis

WORKUP

- Clinical condition characterized by ovarian mass, ascites, and predominantly right-sided pleural effusion (the pleural effusion can also be left-sided in a small number of cases)
- Ovarian malignancy and the other causes (see "Differential Diagnosis") of pelvic mass, ascites, and pleural effusion to be considered
- History of early satiety, weight loss with increased abdominal girth, bloating, intermittent abdominal pain, dyspnea, nonproductive cough

LABORATORY TESTS

- Complete blood count to rule out inflammatory process
- Tumor markers (CA-125, hCG, AFP, CEA) to evaluate malignancy
- Chemical and liver function testing profile to evaluate metabolic or hepatic involvement
- Arterial blood gases if respiratory compromise

IMAGING STUDIES

- Pelvic sonography (color-flow Doppler evaluation of adnexal mass) initially to evaluate pelvic pathology (CT scan or MRI to further delineate neoplastic lesions [Fig. E1-520])
- Chest x-ray

RX TREATMENT

NONPHARMACOLOGIC THERAPY

- Informed consent and proper preparation of patient for possible staging laparotomy (total abdominal hysterectomy and bilateral salpingo-oophorectomy, omentectomy, possible bowel resection, pelvic/periaortic lymphadenectomy)
- Bowel prep if considering pelvic malignancy

ACUTE GENERAL Rx

Depending on clinical presentation, size of pelvic mass, amount of ascites, and pleural effusion:

- If pelvic mass <10 cm with minimal ascites/pleural effusion: consider diagnostic laparoscopy (possible exploratory laparotomy) and salpingo-oophorectomy with removal of ovarian fibroma (tumor).
- If pelvic mass >10 cm with moderate/large amount ascites/pleural effusion: consider pleurocentesis if respiratory compromise (cytology: AFB) and exploratory laparotomy with salpingo-oophorectomy and removal of ovarian fibroma (tumor).
- Treat pelvic malignancy, gastrointestinal or genitourinary tumor as indicated.

CHRONIC Rx

- Resolution of ascites and right-sided pleural effusion after removal of ovarian fibroma
- No long-term follow-up for benign ovarian fibroma

DISPOSITION

Excellent progress and complete survival are expected.

REFERRAL

To gynecologist or gynecologic oncologist for evaluation and treatment, especially if malignancy considered or encountered

SUGGESTED READINGS
available at www.expertconsult.com

RELATED CONTENT

Ovarian Cancer (Related Key Topic)

AUTHORS: **DENNIS M. WEPPNER, M.D.,** and **RUBEN ALVERO, M.D.**

BASIC INFORMATION

DEFINITION

Melanoma is a skin neoplasm arising from the malignant degeneration of melanocytes. It is classically subdivided in four types:
1. Superficial spreading melanoma (70%) (Fig. 1-521, *A*)
2. Nodular melanoma (15% to 20%) (Fig. 1-521, *B*)
3. Lentigo maligna melanoma (5% to 10%)
4. Acral lentiginous melanoma (7% to 10%)

SYNONYMS

Malignant melanoma
Cutaneous malignant melanoma
CMM

ICD-9CM CODES
172.9 Melanoma of the skin, site unspecified

EPIDEMIOLOGY & DEMOGRAPHICS

- Annual incidence of melanoma is 13 cases per 100,000 persons. By 2015 the estimated lifetime risk of the development of cutaneous melanoma will be 1 in 50.
- Melanoma has doubled to tripled in incidence over the past 25 yr.
- Melanoma is the most common cancer among women ages 20 to 29 yr.
- Melanoma is much more common in whites (17.2/100,000 white men) than in African Americans (1 in 100,000 African American men). Increased risk of developing melanomas is found in patients with fair skin, red hair, light eyes, abundance of freckles, atypical moles or large amount of moles (>50). A personal history of non-melanoma skin cancer or a family history of melanoma also increases the risk.
- Lifetime risk of cutaneous melanoma for white Americans is 1 in 90. White men >50 yr old are the most likely to have rapidly growing melanomas.
- Melanoma is the leading cause of death from skin disease. Although melanoma represents less than 10% of all skin-cancer diagnoses,

at least 70% of deaths that are related to skin cancer are attributed to melanoma.
- Median age at diagnosis is 53 yr.
- Superficial spreading melanoma occurs most often in young adults on sun-exposed areas.
- Acral lentiginous melanoma is most often found in Asian Americans and African Americans and is not related to sun exposure.
- Death rate for white men with melanoma is 3 per 100,000.
- 8% to 10% of melanomas arise in people with a family history of the disease.

PHYSICAL FINDINGS & CLINICAL PRESENTATION

Variable depending on the subtype of melanoma:
- Superficial spreading melanoma is most often found on the lower legs, arms, and upper back. It may have a combination of many colors or may be uniformly brown or black.
- Nodular melanoma can be found anywhere on the body, but it most frequently occurs on the trunk on sun-exposed areas. It has a dark-brown or red-brown appearance and can be dome shaped or pedunculated. Lesions are frequently misdiagnosed because they may resemble a blood blister or hemangioma and may also be amelanotic.
- Lentigo maligna melanoma is generally found in older adults in areas continually exposed to the sun and frequently arising from lentigo maligna (Hutchinson's freckle) or melanoma in situ. It might have a complex pattern and variable shape; color is more uniform than in superficial spreading melanoma.
- Acral lentiginous melanoma frequently occurs on soles, subungual mucous membranes, and palms (sole of the foot is the most prevalent site). Unlike other types of melanoma, it has a similar incidence in all ethnic groups.
- The warning signs that the lesion may be a melanoma can be summarized with the ABCDE mnemonic:
  A: Asymmetry (e.g., lesion is bisected and halves are not identical)
  B: Border irregularity (uneven, ragged border)
  C: Color variegation (presence of various shades of pigmentation)

D: Diameter enlargement (>6 mm)
E: Evolving (mole changing in size, shape, or color, or mole that differs visibly from surrounding moles ["ugly duckling" sign]) (Fig. 1-522)

ETIOLOGY

- Ultraviolet light is the most important cause of malignant melanoma.
- There is a modest increase in melanoma risk in patients with small nondysplastic nevi and a much greater risk in those with dysplastic lesions.
- The *CDKN2A* gene, residing at the *9p21* locus, is often deleted in people with familial melanoma.
- A mutated signal transduction molecule v-raf murine sarcoma viral oncogene homolog B$_1$ (BRAF) has been identified in about 50% of patients with metastatic melanoma.

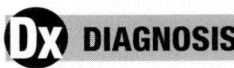

DIAGNOSIS

DIFFERENTIAL DIAGNOSIS

- Dysplastic nevi
- Solar lentigo
- Vascular lesions
- Blue nevus
- Basal cell carcinoma
- Seborrheic keratosis

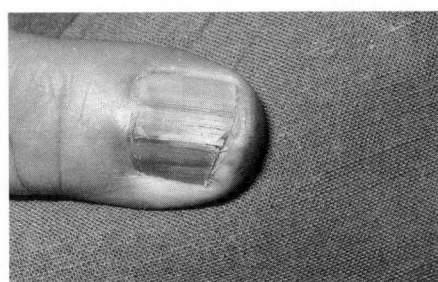

FIGURE 1-522 Subungual melanoma with Hutchinson sign (pigment spreading from under the nail to involve the adjacent skin, usually of the proximal or lateral nail fold). These lesions are thought to emanate from the nail matrix. (From White GM, Cox NH [eds]: *Diseases of the skin, a color atlas and text,* ed 2, St Louis, 2006, Mosby.)

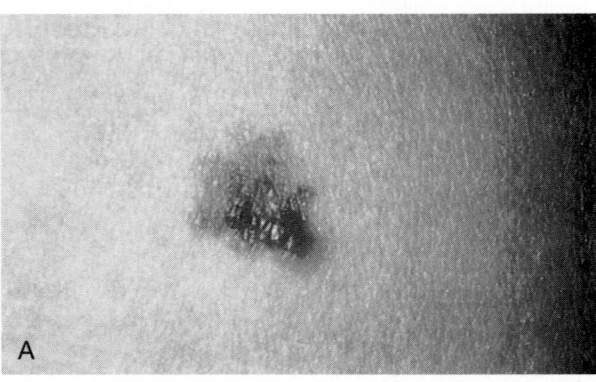

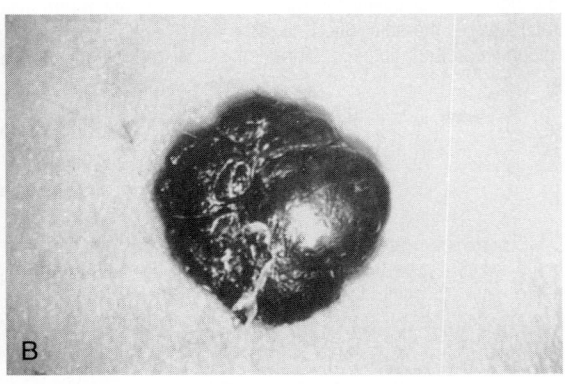

FIGURE 1-521 A, Superficial spreading melanoma. **B,** Nodular melanoma. (From Abeloff MD [ed]: *Clinical oncology,* ed 3, New York, 2004, Churchill Livingstone.)

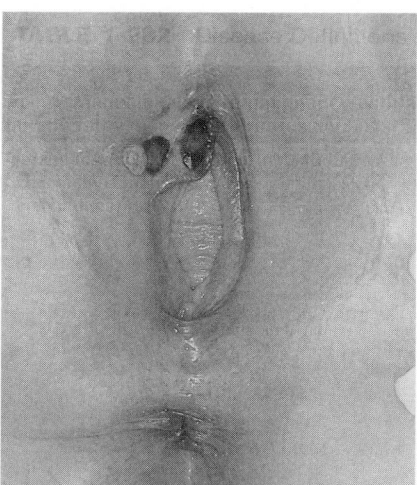

FIGURE 1-523 Melanoma of the vulva. Benign nevi, vulva melanosis, and melanoma may occur in the vulvar region. Any suspicious pigmented lesion should be biopsied. The patient here is 75 years old. (Courtesy Paul Koonings, M.D. From White GM, Cox NH [eds]: *Diseases of the skin, a color atlas and text,* ed 2, St Louis, 2006, Mosby.)

WORKUP

- Dermoscopy (use of an instrument that shines polarized light on skin surfaces and magnifies skin lesions) can increase the accuracy in diagnosing melanoma by 10% to 27%.
- Any suspicious lesion (Fig. 1-523) should be biopsied. Perform excisional biopsy with elliptical excision that includes 1 to 2 mm of normal skin surrounding the lesion and extends to the subcutaneous tissue; incisional punch biopsy is sometimes necessary in surgically sensitive areas (e.g., digits, nose). It is essential that the size of the specimen be adequate to determine the histologic depth of penetration, which is known as the Breslow depth.
- Sentinel lymph node excision (SLNE) is probably the most important diagnostic and potentially therapeutic procedure for patients with melanoma. It should be considered in patients with intermediate (1 to 4 mm) melanomas or high-risk skin tumors to obtain information regarding a patient's subclinical lymph node status with minimal morbidity. The National Comprehensive Cancer Network (NCCN) recommends that sentinel-node biopsy be discussed with and offered to patients classified as stage IB or stage II, and should be considered for patients with stage IA melanoma and "adverse" features that might portend a higher risk of sentinel node involvement (e.g., Clark level IV or V, tumor thickness of 0.75 mm or more, lymphovascular invasion, positive deep margins). Sentinel lymph node biopsy involves the use of radiologic lymphoscintigraphy to map lymphatic drainage from the site of the primary melanoma to the first sentinel lymph node in the region. When properly performed, if the sentinel node is negative the remaining lymph nodes in the region will not have metastases in more than 98% of cases. If the sentinel nodes are negative, no addi-

tional regional surgery is recommended. The staging of intermediate thickness (1.2 to 3.5 mm) primary melanomas, according to the results of sentinel node biopsy, provides important prognostic information and identifies patients with nodal metastases whose survival can be prolonged by immediate lymphadenectomy. SPECT/CT is helpful in detecting micrometastatic melanoma. Among patients with clinically lymph node-negative melanoma, the use of SPECT/CT-aided SLNE compared with SNLE alone is associated with a higher frequency of metastatic involvement and a higher rate of disease-free survival.

- The staging system for melanoma adapted by the American Joint Committee on Cancer (AJCC) is as follows:

T*	Thickness of primary tumor
Tis	In situ
T1	≤1.0 mm
T2	1.01-2.0 mm
T3	2.01-4.0 mm
T4†	>4.0 mm
N†	Number of positive lymph nodes
N0	0
N1	1
N2	2 or 3
N3	≥4 (or combination of in-transit metastases, satellite lesions, or an ulcerated primary lesion with any number of nodes)
M	Metastases
M0	0
M1	Distant subcutaneous or lymph node metastases
M2	Lung metastases
M3	All other visceral or any distant metastases or an elevated lactate dehydrogenase level not attributable to another cause

Clinical Stage	
0	(T0N0M0)
IA	(T1aN0M0)
IB	(T1bN0M0) (T2aN0M0)
IIA	(T2bN0M0) (T3aN0M0)
IIB	(T3bN0M0) (T4aN0M0)
IIC	(T4bN0M0)
IIIA	(T1-T4aN1bM0)
IIIB	(T1-T4aN2bM0)
IIIC	(AnyT, N2c, M0) (Any T, N3, M0)
IV	(Any T, Any N, >M1)

*a, Without ulceration; b, with ulceration.
†a, Micrometastasis; b, macrometastases; c, in-transit metastases with metastatic lymph nodes.

LABORATORY TESTS

The pathology report should indicate the following:
- Tumor thickness (Breslow microstage).
- Tumor depth: the depth of invasion is the most important histologic prognostic parameter in evaluating the primary tumor.
- Mitotic rate: tabulated as mitoses per square millimeter in the dermal part of the tumor in which most mitoses are identified.
- Radial growth rates versus vertical growth rate: radial growth phase describes the growth of melanoma within the epidermis and along the dermal-epidermal junction.

- Tumor infiltrating lymphocytes have a strong predictive value in vertical growth phase melanomas and are defined as brisk, nonbrisk, or absent.
- Histologic regression: characterized by the absence of melanoma in the epidermis and dermis flanked on one or both sides by melanoma.
- Reverse-transcription polymerase chain reaction assay for tyrosine messenger RNA is a useful marker for the presence of melanoma cells. It is performed on sentinel lymph node biopsy and is useful for detection of submicroscopic metastases.
- Identification of somatic mutations in the gene encoding the serine-threonine protein kinase B-RAF (*BRAF*). This mutation is found in approximately 50% of melanomas.

Rx TREATMENT

- Initial excision of the melanoma
- Reexcision of the involved area after histologic diagnosis:
  1. The margins of reexcision depend on the Breslow depth. For melanoma in situ with Breslow depth ≤2.0 mm, recommended surgical margin is 1 cm. If Breslow depth is >2.0 mm, margin should be 2 cm. For melanoma in situ, margin should be 5 mm.
  2. Low-risk or intermediate-risk tumors require excision of 1 to 3 cm.
  3. Melanomas of moderate thickness (0.9 to 2.0 mm) can be excised safely with 2-cm margins.
  4. A 1-cm margin of excision for melanoma with a poor prognosis (as defined by a tumor thickness ≥2 mm) is associated with a significantly greater risk of regional recurrence than is a 3-cm margin, but with a similar overall survival rate. Randomized clinical trials have also shown that radical surgery with 2 cm excision margins did not differ from that with 4 cm margins for survival in patients with cutaneous melanoma >2 mm thick.
- Lymph node dissection: recommended in all patients with enlarged lymph nodes. Lymph node evaluation is important in patients with melanoma 1 mm in depth because it determines the overall prognosis and need for therapeutic lymph node dissection or adjuvant treatment.
  1. Elective lymph node dissection remains controversial.
  2. It is indicated with positive sentinel node. It may be considered in those with a primary melanoma between 1 and 4 mm thick (especially in patients <60 yr).
- Adjuvant therapy with interferon alfa-2b (intron A) in patients with metastatic melanoma is approved by the FDA for AJCC stages IIb and III melanoma; however, its statistical benefit remains unclear. Peginterferon alfa-2b (which has a longer duration of action and can be given once a week compared to 3-5 times/week for standard interferon) has now also been FDA approved for adjuvant treatment of node-positive melanoma after surgical resection.

- Dacarbazine and interleukin-2 can be used in metastatic melanoma. Results are generally poor, with median survival time in patients with distant metastatic melanoma approximately 6 mo.
- Recent attention has focused on combinations of dacarbazine and cisplatin with interleukin-2 and interferon-alfa (biochemotherapy). Novel therapeutics involve cancer vaccines and use of granulocyte-macrophage colony-stimulating factor and angiogenesis inhibitors. Preliminary trials involving the stimulation of immune response with vaccines using high-dose interleukin-2 plus the gp100:209-217 (210 M) peptide vaccine in patients with advanced melanoma have shown increased survival. Trials with ipilimumab, an agent that blocks cytotoxic T-lymphocyte–associated antigen 4 to potentiate an antitumor T-cell response, have shown improved overall survival in patients with previously treated metastatic melanoma. Ipilimumab when used with dacarbazine also showed improved overall survival in patients with previously untreated metastatic melanoma.

- In patients that carry the V600E *BRAF* mutation, trials involving treatment with vemurafenib (PLX4032), an oral inhibitor of mutated *BRAF*, have shown complete or partial tumor regression in the majority of patients with metastatic melanoma and improved rates of overall and progression-free survival in patients with previously untreated melanoma. The oral selective MEK inhibitor trametinib has also shown improved rates of progression-free and overall survival among patients who had metastatic melanoma with a BRAF V600E or V600K mutation.
- Some melanomas harbor activating mutations and amplification of the type III transmembrane receptor tyrosine kinase KIT. In these patients with advanced melanomas harboring KIT alterations, treatment with imatinib mesylate results in significant clinical responses in a subset of patients.
- Patients with a history of melanoma should be followed up with skin examinations every 6 mo or sooner if patient detects any new lesions; the assessments usually consist of medical history, physical examination, laboratory values, and chest radiograph.

DISPOSITION

- Prognosis varies with the stage of the melanoma. The 5-yr survival related to thickness is as follows: <0.76 mm, 99% survival; 0.6 to 1.49 mm, 85%; 1.5 to 2.49 mm, 84%; 2.5 to 3.9 mm, 70%; >4 mm, 44%.
- The 5-yr survival in patients with distant metastasis is <10%.
- Treatment of advanced disease consists (in addition to surgical excision and lymph node dissection) of chemotherapy, immunotherapy, and radiation therapy.

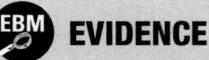 **EVIDENCE**

available at www.expertconsult.com

SUGGESTED READINGS
available at www.expertconsult.com

RELATED CONTENT

Melanoma (Patient Information)

AUTHOR: **FRED F. FERRI, M.D.**

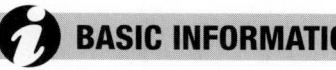

BASIC INFORMATION

DEFINITION

Meniere's disease is a syndrome characterized by recurrent vertigo with fluctuating hearing loss, tinnitus, and fullness in the ear.

SYNONYMS

Endolymphatic hydrops
Lermoyez's syndrome
Idiopathic endolymphatic hydrops

ICD-9CM CODES

386.01 Meniere's disease, cochleovestibular (active)

EPIDEMIOLOGY & DEMOGRAPHICS

INCIDENCE (IN U.S.): 100 cases/100,000 persons
PREVALENCE (IN U.S.): 15 cases/100,000 persons
PREDOMINANT SEX: Male = female
PEAK INCIDENCE: 20 to 50 yr

PHYSICAL FINDINGS & CLINICAL PRESENTATION

- Hearing may be unilaterally decreased.
- Pallor, sweating, and nausea may occur during a severe attack.
- Usually the patient develops a sensation of fullness and pressure along with decreased hearing and tinnitus in a single ear.
- The patient typically experiences severe vertigo, which peaks within minutes, then slowly subsides over hours.
- May see spontaneous nystagmus on examination.
- Persistent sense of disequilibrium for days is typical after an acute episode
- May have vestibulopathy demonstrable with a positive head thrust test.

ETIOLOGY

- Unknown; viral and autoimmune causes have been suggested.
- Associated with endolymphatic hydrops.

DIAGNOSIS

Proposed criteria by the American Academy of Otolaryngology-Head and Neck Surgery (AAO-HNS) for diagnosis of Meniere's disease include the following four features, of which (1) and at least one of (2), (3), or (4) must be present:
1. Two spontaneous episodes of vertigo lasting 20 min or longer without loss of consciousness
2. Hearing loss that is usually, but not always, fluctuating
3. Tinnitus in the ear, which may fluctuate
4. Aural fullness in the ear, which may fluctuate

DIFFERENTIAL DIAGNOSIS

- Acoustic neuroma
- Migrainous vertigo
- Multiple sclerosis
- Autoimmune inner ear syndrome
- Otitis media
- Vertebrobasilar disease
- Labyrinthitis

WORKUP

- Electronystagmography may show peripheral vestibular deficit.
- Electrocochleography and glycerol test used by some otoneurologists and ENT specialists.

LABORATORY TESTS

Audiogram may show sensorineural hearing loss, with lower frequencies primarily affected.

IMAGING STUDIES

MRI to rule out acoustic neuroma, especially if cerebellar or CNS dysfunction is present

TREATMENT

NONPHARMACOLOGIC THERAPY

Limit activity during attacks

ACUTE GENERAL Rx

- Prochlorperazine 5 to 10 mg PO q6h or 25 mg PO bid
- Promethazine 12.5 to 25 mg PO q4 to 6h
- Diazepam 5 to 10 mg IV/PO for acute attack
- Meclizine 25 mg q6h
- Scopolamine patch

CHRONIC Rx

- Diuretics such as hydrochlorothiazide or acetazolamide, salt restriction, and avoidance of caffeine are traditional.
- For refractory cases, surgical interventions.

DISPOSITION

- Patients are usually followed by an otoneurologist or ENT specialist.
- Usual course of disease consists of alternating attacks and remissions.
- Majority of patients can be managed medically. Of patients, 10% to 30% will undergo surgical intervention for persistent incapacitating vertigo.

REFERRAL

To an otolaryngologist for surgical intervention if attacks persist despite medical therapy

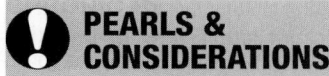

PEARLS & CONSIDERATIONS

COMMENTS

- There are many variations of the classical clinical picture. The essential features for diagnosis are episodic vertigo and sensorineural hearing loss audiometrically documented on at least one occasion.
- In one third of patients, both ears are eventually involved.
- There is some evidence that Meniere's disease and migraines may be pathophysiologically linked.

SUGGESTED READINGS

available at www.expertconsult.com

RELATED CONTENT

Meniere's Disease (Patient Information)

AUTHOR: **SHARON S. HARTMAN POLENSEK, M.D., PH.D.**

DEFINITION

Meningiomas are generally slow-growing tumors arising from arachnoid cells of the arachnoid villi; 90% are benign.

ICD-9CM CODES
225.2 Cerebral meninges

EPIDEMIOLOGY & DEMOGRAPHICS

INCIDENCE: 6/100,000 persons/yr; account for about one third of primary intracranial tumors and are the second most common brain tumor in adults; often underreported.

PREDOMINANT SEX AND AGE: Female/male ratio of almost 3:1 in the brain and up to 6:1 in the spinal cord; male > female in childhood and male = female among African Americans

PEAK INCIDENCE: Males: sixth decade, females: seventh decade, incidence increases with age; rare in childhood

RISK FACTORS: Ionizing radiation results in increased incidence and a shorter latency period. Neurofibromatosis type 2 (NF2) is an autosomal dominant genetic disorder that predisposes to multiple intracranial tumors. Approximately half of all individuals with NF2 have meningiomas, most of which are intracranial. Studies have suggested a link between hormonal factors and development of meningioma. At present, there is no conclusive evidence to support a causal relationship with cell phone usage and subsequent development of meningioma.

GENETICS: Meningiomas may be isolated or found in associated with other genetic diseases, such as neurofibromatosis type 2 and familial meningioma. Approximately half of meningiomas have allelic losses involving of the NF2 and DAL-1 genes. Allelic losses of chromosomes 1p, 2p, 6q, 9q, 10q, 14q, 17p, and 18q may be associated with histologic progression.

PHYSICAL FINDINGS & CLINICAL PRESENTATION

- Neurologic symptoms vary with location and size (see Table 1-270); meningiomas can

TABLE 1-270 Locations and Presentations of Meningiomas

Location	Presenting Manifestation
Parasagittal	Urinary incontinence, dementia, gradual paraparesis, seizures
Lateral convexity	Variable depending on structures compressed, including slow hemiparesis, speech abnormalities
Olfactory groove	Anosmia, visual disturbance, dementia, Foster-Kennedy syndrome
Suprasellar	Hormonal failure, bitemporal hemianopia, optic atrophy
Sphenoid ridge	Extraocular nerve paresis, exostoses, proptosis, seizures

From Goetz CG, Pappert EJ: *Textbook of clinical neurology,* Philadelphia, 1999, Saunders.

arise from the dura at any site, although most commonly occur within the skull and at sites of dural reflection, such as the cerebral convexities and the falx. Other less common locations include the sphenoid wing, olfactory groove, and optic nerve sheath. Focal symptoms depend on the site of origin and the time course of growth.

- Most common presentation is with a focal or generalized seizure or gradually worsening neurologic deficit. Seizures are present preoperatively in 30% to 40%.
- Typically are slow growing and asymptomatic; discovered incidentally on a neuroimaging study or at autopsy.

ETIOLOGY

- Meningiomas are thought to arise from a multistep progression of genetic changes.
- Mutations of the NF2 gene on chromosome 22 are found in patients with neurofibromatosis type 2 and >50% of sporadic meningiomas. This gene is thought to act as a tumor suppressor gene; the protein product, merlin, is also involved in cytoskeletal organization.
- DAL-1 is another tumor suppressor gene, located on chromosome 18p, that has been identified in a subset of the approximately 40% of sporadic meningiomas with neither the NF2 gene mutations nor allelic loss of chromosome 22q.
- Cranial radiation may be responsible for some cases following an appropriate latency period from 10 to 20 yr. Meningiomas that result from radiation are generally more aggressive.
- The link with steroid hormones and their receptors is suggested by the increase in growth rate and/or development of meningiomas during pregnancy and increased incidence in women who use postmenopausal hormones or in association with breast carcinomas.

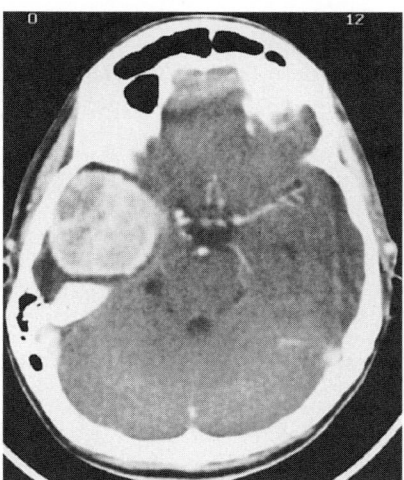

FIGURE 1-524 Contrast-enhanced CT scan demonstrates a large contrast-enhancing right sphenoid wing meningioma. (From Specht N [ed]: *Practical guide to diagnostic imaging,* St Louis, 1998, Mosby.)

DIFFERENTIAL DIAGNOSIS

Other well-circumscribed intracranial tumors that involve the dura or subdural space.
- Acoustic schwannoma (typically at the pontocerebellar junction)
- Ependymoma, lipoma, and metastases within the spinal cord
- Metastatic disease from lymphoma/adenocarcinoma, inflammatory disease such as sarcoidosis and Wegener's granulomatosis, or infections such as tuberculosis

WORKUP

Imaging studies with CT or MRI, followed by surgical removal with histologic confirmation

LABORATORY TESTS

According to the World Health Organization (WHO) classification, there are nine benign histologic variants (account for 90% of all meningiomas) and four variants associated with increased recurrence and rates of metastasis. Ninety percent of meningiomas are classified as benign meningiomas or WHO grade I.

IMAGING STUDIES

- Cranial CT scanning or MRI can detect and determine the extent of meningiomas (Fig. 1-524). CT can show hyperostosis and/or intratumoral calcifications. MRI (Fig. 1-525) is the imaging modality of choice to demonstrate the dural origin of the tumor in most cases, with the characteristic "tail" sign.
- On nonenhanced scans, meningiomas typically are isodense to slightly hyperdense to brain and are homogeneous in appearance.

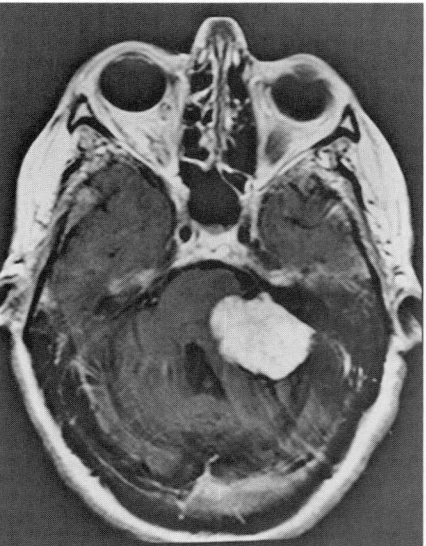

FIGURE 1-525 MRI picture of a posterior fossa meningioma, demonstrated an extra-axial homogeneously contrast-enhanced mass arising from the tentorium and compressing the cerebellar hemisphere. (From Goetz CG, Pappert EJ: *Textbook of clinical neurology,* Philadelphia, 1999, Saunders.)

Meningiomas show homogeneous enhancement; gadolinium can facilitate imaging of smaller additional lesions that are missed on unenhanced images.

- Indistinct margins, marked edema, mushroomlike projections from tumor, brain parenchymal infiltration, and heterogeneous enhancement are suggestive of more aggressive behavior.
- PET scan may help in predicting the aggressiveness of the tumor and the potential for recurrence, but it is not used routinely.

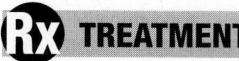 **TREATMENT**

Primary management depends on signs or symptoms, age of patient, and location and size of tumor. Observation may be appropriate if tumors are discovered incidentally and/or if growth is indolent and unlikely to cause symptoms.

PHARMACOLOGIC THERAPY

- Although a variety of chemotherapeutic agents have been studied, such as hydroxyurea, there is no established effective systemic therapy.
- Inhibition of hormone receptors, such as progesterone, estrogen, and androgen, has failed to demonstrate clinical benefit.
- Treatment with molecularly targeted approaches, such as angiogenesis inhibition, is currently under way.

NONPHARMACOLOGIC THERAPY

- The mainstay of treatment for meningiomas remains surgical removal. Complete resection is usually attempted, when feasible. After total excision, recurrence rates of 0% to 20% have been observed, while 20% to 50% of patients recur within 5 yr of a subtotal resection.

- Active surveillance to monitor for tumor recurrence is important.
- Radiation therapy is the only validated form of adjuvant therapy and may be beneficial in patients with incomplete resections or inoperable tumors. Stereotactic radiosurgery can provide local control with more limited toxicity.

ACUTE GENERAL Rx

- For lesions that cause significant mass effect, steroids are sometimes used to decrease brain edema.
- Anticonvulsants are used if the patient presents with seizures.

CHRONIC Rx

- Prophylactic use of anticonvulsants is not recommended in patients without a history of seizures.
- There is limited data on the efficacy of traditional chemotherapy, and the evidence is largely anecdotal. The most extensively evaluated agents are hydroxyurea, mifepristone (RU486), and interferon alfa-2b. Recently, somatostatin analogs have been evaluated in multicenter clinical trials.

DISPOSITION

- Estimated surgical mortality is 7%. Significant morbidity and mortality can be observed in meningiomas with otherwise favorable pathology secondary to unfavorable location (e.g., skull base).
- Long-term outcome varies, based on pathology, tumor grade, location, and completeness of resection.
- Most incidentally discovered meningiomas remain asymptomatic and have a slow rate of growth. Calcified tumors may be less likely to progress than noncalcified ones.

- Meningiomas may recur after surgical resection. In addition, some tumors show histologic progression to a higher grade. Features suggesting increased rate of recurrence include multiple allelic chromosomal losses, local brain invasion, high rate of mitosis, and highly anaplastic features.

REFERRAL

- Neurosurgical consultation for all cases
- Neurology, radiation oncology, and oncology depending on presence of other sequelae and in setting of recurrence

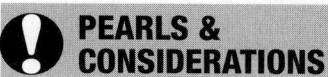 **PEARLS & CONSIDERATIONS**

COMMENTS

- Many meningiomas are discovered incidentally; most are benign and remain asymptomatic.
- "Dural tail" is classic finding on neuroimaging studies.
- Individuals with neurofibromatosis type 2 are at high risk to develop meningiomas.

PATIENT & FAMILY EDUCATION

Meningioma mommas: www.meningiomamommas.org

Meningioma Support and Patient Information Group

National Brain Tumor Society

Meningioma Online Support Group: http://www.brainstrust.org/meningioma.htm

SUGGESTED READINGS
available at www.expertconsult.com

RELATED CONTENT

Meningioma (Patient Information)

AUTHOR: **NICOLE J. ULLRICH, M.D., PH.D.**

Diseases and Disorders

M

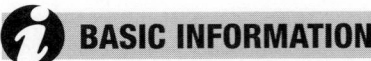
DEFINITION

Bacterial meningitis is an inflammation of meninges with increased intracranial pressure, and pleocytosis or increased WBCs in cerebrospinal fluid (CSF) secondary to bacteria in the pia-subarachnoid space and ventricles, leading to neurologic sequelae and abnormalities.

SYNONYMS Spinal meningitis

ICD-9CM CODES
320 Bacterial meningitis

EPIDEMIOLOGY & DEMOGRAPHICS

INCIDENCE (IN U.S.): 1.3 to 2.0 cases/100,000 persons; 1.2 million cases per year in the world; 135,000 deaths annually worldwide. The rate of bacterial meningitis declined by 55% in the U.S. in the early 1990s with the introduction of the *Haemophilus influenzae* type b (Hib) vaccine.
PREDOMINANT SEX: Male = female
PREDOMINANT AGE: All ages, neonate to geriatric

PHYSICAL FINDINGS & CLINICAL PRESENTATION

- Fever
- Headache
- Neck stiffness, nuchal rigidity, meningismus
- Altered mental state, lethargy
- Vomiting, nausea
- Photophobia
- Seizures
- Coma; lethargy, stupor
- Rash: petechial associated with meningococcal infection (Fig. E1-526)
- Myalgia
- Cranial nerve abnormality (unilateral)
- Papilledema
- Dilated, nonreactive pupil(s)
- Posturing: decorticate/decerebrate
- Physical examination findings of Kernig's sign and Brudzinski's sign in adults with meningitis are often not helpful in determining meningeal inflammation

ETIOLOGY

Neisseria meningitidis is now more common than *Haemophilus influenzae* as a cause of bacterial meningitis in children as well as adults. *H. influenzae* is the cause of >30% of cases of meningitis (usually in infants and children <6 yr of age). It is associated with sinusitis, otitis media.

- Neonates: group B streptococci, *Escherichia coli*, *Listeria monocytogenes*, *Klebsiella* sp.
- Infants: 1 to 23 mo
  1. *S. pneumoniae*
  2. *N. meningitidis*
  3. *S. agalactiae* (group B streptococci)
  4. *H. influenzae*
  5. *E. coli*
- Ages 2 to 50 yr
  1. *N. meningitidis*
  2. *S. pneumoniae*
- >50 yr of age
  1. *S. pneumoniae*
  2. *N. meningitidis*
  3. *L. monocytogenes*
  4. Aerobic gram-negative bacilli

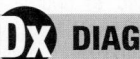 **DIAGNOSIS**

Diagnostic approach is based on patient presentation and physical examination (Fig. 1-528). Lumbar puncture should be performed as soon as possible. Key elements to diagnosis are CSF evaluation (Fig. E1-527) and CT scan or MRI if the patient is in a coma or has focal neurologic deficits, pupillary abnormalities, or papilledema.

DIFFERENTIAL DIAGNOSIS

- Endocarditis, bacteremia
- Intracranial tumor
- Lyme disease
- Brain abscess
- Partially treated bacterial meningitis
- Medications
- SLE
- Seizures
- Acute mononucleosis
- Other infectious meningitides
- Neuroleptic malignant syndrome
- Subdural empyema
- Rocky Mountain spotted fever

WORKUP

CSF examination:
- Opening pressure >100 to 200 mm Hg
- WBC usually >1.0 x 10^8/L
- Neutrophilic predominance: >80%
- Gram stain of CSF: positive in 60% to 90% of patients
- CSF protein: >50 mg/dl
- CSF glucose: <40 mg/dl
- Culture: positive in 65% to 90% of cases
- CSF bacterial antigen: 50% to 100% sensitivity
- E-test for susceptibility of pneumococcal isolates

LABORATORY TESTS

Blood culturing, WBC with differential, and CSF examination (see "Workup")

IMAGING STUDIES

- CT scan or MRI of head: necessary with increased intracranial pressure, coma, neurologic deficits
- Sinus CT: if sinusitis suspected

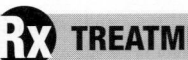 **TREATMENT**

Empiric therapy is necessary with IV antibiotic treatment if patient has purulent CSF fluid at time of lumbar puncture, is asplenic, or has signs of DIC/sepsis pending Gram stain and culture results. Try to obtain blood and CSF cultures before starting antimicrobial therapy, but do not delay therapy if obtaining them is not possible. Therapy after Gram stain pending cultures is recommended for the following:
1. Neonates: ampicillin *plus* cefotaxime
2. 1-23 months: vancomycin *plus* third-generation cephalosporin
3. 2-50 months: vancomycin *plus* third-generation cephalosporin
4. >50 years old: vancomycin *plus* ampicillin *plus* third-generation cephalosporin
5. Immunocompromised patients: vancomycin *plus* ampicillin *plus* either cefepime or meropenem
   - Table E1-271 describes common pathogens of bacterial meningitis and their empiric treatment based on age.
   - Table E1-272 describes specific antibiotic treatments.
   - Corticosteroids: dexamethasone 0.15 mg/kg q6h for first 4 days of therapy should be used for most adults with bacterial meningitis. Decreased mortality and neurologic sequelae are seen with adjunct therapy.
   - Dexamethasone also benefits children with Hib or pneumococcal meningitis and should be given within the first 2 days of illness.

DISPOSITION

Bacterial meningitis is a reportable disease that needs to be reported to local health authorities. Droplet precautions should be used for first 24 hr of therapy for suspected or confirmed *N. meningitidis* infection.

REFERRAL

- To a neurologist if persistent neurologic sequelae develop after bacterial meningitis
- To an infectious disease consultant if a patient has recurrent bacterial meningitis; such patients deserve a workup for an anatomic (CSF dural leak) or immunologic defect (complement defect, hyposplenism, immunoglobulin deficiency)

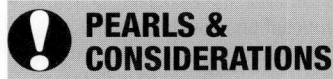 **PEARLS & CONSIDERATIONS**

COMMENTS

- Nosocomial bacterial meningitis may result from invasive procedures (e.g., placement of ventricular catheters, lumbar puncture,

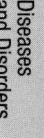

craniotomy, spinal anesthesia). Treatment of this different spectrum of microorganisms requires empirical antimicrobial therapy with vancomycin plus cefepime, ceftazidime, or meropenem. In cases of basilar skull fracture, effective empirical antimicrobial therapy consists of vancomycin plus a third-generation cephalosporin.

- Prevention of meningitis can be achieved through chemoprophylaxis of close contacts (household members and anyone exposed to oral secretions).

- Effective medications are rifampin 10 mg/kg PO bid for 2 days or ceftriaxone 250 mg IM single dose in patients older than age 12; 125 mg IM if age 12 or younger.
- Ciprofloxacin 500 mg for prevention of *Neisseria* meningitis can be given to patients older than 18 yr who cannot tolerate rifampin to eradicate pharyngeal colonization.
- Menactra: a protein-conjugate vaccine against serogroup A, C, Y, W-135 capsular polysaccharides is available for adults (up to 55 yr) and children older than 2 yr.

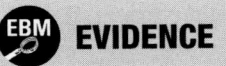 **EVIDENCE**

available at www.expertconsult.com

SUGGESTED READINGS

available at www.expertconsult.com

RELATED CONTENT

Meningitis (Patient Information)

AUTHOR: **GLENN G. FORT, M.D., M.P.H.**

M

Diseases
and Disorders

I

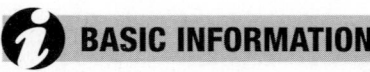

BASIC INFORMATION

DEFINITION
Viral meningitis is an acute febrile illness with signs and symptoms of meningeal irritation, usually with a lymphocytic pleocytosis of the cerebrospinal fluid (CSF) and negative CSF bacterial stains and cultures.

SYNONYMS
Aseptic meningitis

ICD-9CM CODES
047.8 Meningitis, aseptic

EPIDEMIOLOGY & DEMOGRAPHICS (Table 1-273)
INCIDENCE (IN U.S.): 11 cases/100,000 persons
PREDOMINANT SEX: Male = female
GENETICS: Those with abnormal humoral immunity and agammaglobulinemia have associated difficulty with viral clearance.

PHYSICAL FINDINGS & CLINICAL PRESENTATION
- Fever
- Headache
- Nuchal rigidity
- Photophobia
- Myalgias
- Vomiting
- Rash

ETIOLOGY
- Enterovirus: 85% to 95% of all cases
- Parechoviruses
- Mumps virus
- Measles
- Arboviruses from mosquitoes: EEE, West Nile, St Louis
- Herpes: HSV-1, HSV-2, VZV, HHV-6, and HHV-7
- Acute HIV
- Lymphocytic choriomeningitis virus
- Adenovirus
- CMV and EBV
- Other arthropod-borne viruses: Powassan virus
- Influenza A and B virus

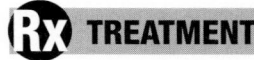

DIAGNOSIS

The diagnostic approach is similar to that for bacterial meningitis (see "Meningitis, Bacterial"); the foremost need is to rule out bacterial meningitis with CSF evaluation. Presentation may be similar to that of meningitis with bacterial involvement.

DIFFERENTIAL DIAGNOSIS
- Bacterial meningitis
- Meningitis secondary to Lyme disease, TB, syphilis, amebiasis, leptospirosis
- Rickettsial illnesses: Rocky Mountain spotted fever
- Migraine headache
- Medications
- SLE
- Acute mononucleosis/Epstein-Barr virus
- Seizures
- Carcinomatous meningitis

WORKUP
CSF examination:
- Usually shows pleocytosis
- Lymphocytic predominance (neutrophils in early stages)
- Opening pressure: 200 to 250 mm Hg
- WBC: 100 to 1000 mm^3
- Increased CSF protein
- Decreased or normal CSF glucose
- Negative Gram stain, cultures, CIE, latex agglutination
- Viral cultures or serologic testing may be diagnostic
- Polymerase chain reaction for HSV, West Nile, or enterovirus (which could shorten duration of antibiotic treatment and hospitalization if bacterial meningitis was suspected)

LABORATORY TESTS
CBC with differential, blood culturing, and CSF examination (see "Workup")

IMAGING STUDIES
CT scan or MRI: if cerebral edema, focal neurologic findings develop

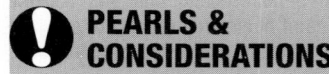

TREATMENT

No specific antiviral therapy for most viruses. Treatment is supportive unless HSV is detected, which would be treated with IV acyclovir: 10 mg/kg q8h in adults. Up to 20 mg/kg q8h in children <12 yr.

DISPOSITION
Viral meningitis is almost always an uncomplicated illness that will resolve; however, relapsing headache, myalgia, and weakness may occur for 2 to 3 wk after onset of symptoms.

PEARLS & CONSIDERATIONS

- Enteroviruses are the most common cause of viral meningitis and are transmitted by fecal-oral and less commonly by the respiratory route.
- Herpes simplex type 2 (HSV-2) causes both primary and recurrent lymphocytic meningitis. HSV-2 meningitis presents most often without a history of genital herpes, recurrent meningitis, or genital symptoms.

SUGGESTED READINGS
available at www.expertconsult.com

RELATED CONTENT
Meningitis (Patient Information)

AUTHOR: **GLENN G. FORT, M.D., M.P.H.**

TABLE 1-273 Epidemiology of Acute Viral Meningitis

		EPIDEMIOLOGIC FACTORS*		
Season	Patient's Age (yr)	Patient's Sex	Risk Factor	Suggested Viral Agent
Summer-fall	Infant	—	Infected mother	Coxsackievirus B
	1-15	—	Swimming pools, closed communities	Enteroviruses
			Geographic area: California, southeastern United States	California serogroup virus
Winter	1-15	—	School exposure	Varicella virus, measles virus
		Male/female 3:1		Mumps virus
	16-21	—	College exposure	Measles virus
		Male/female 3:1		Mumps virus
		—		Epstein-Barr virus (mononucleosis)
	Any	—	Mice, rats, hamsters	Lymphocytic choriomeningitis virus
	Adults	—	Varicella-zoster	Varicella-zoster virus
Any	Any	—	Immunocompromise	Adenovirus
		—	Acquired immunodeficiency syndrome	Human immunodeficiency virus

*Epidemiologic factors are suggestive but should not be used to exclude diagnoses in individual cases.
From Gorbach SI: *Infectious diseases,* ed 2, Philadelphia, 1998, Saunders.

BASIC INFORMATION

DEFINITION

Menopause is the permanent cessation of menstrual periods for 1 yr after age 40 yr or permanent cessation of ovulation after lost ovarian activity. It is the reproductive stage of life marked by waxing and waning estrogen levels followed by decreasing ovarian function. Premature ovarian failure (recently also referred to as Premature Ovarian Insufficiency) and no menstrual periods may also occur because of depletion of ovarian follicles before the age of 40 yr.

SYNONYMS

Change of life
Climacteric ovarian failure

ICD-9CM CODES
627   Premenopausal menorrhagia
627.2   Menopausal or female climacteric states
627.4   States associated with artificial menopause
716.3   Climacteric arthritis

EPIDEMIOLOGY & DEMOGRAPHICS

- Average age of menopause in the United States is 51 yr.
- Age at which menopause occurs is primarily genetically determined.
- Smokers experience menopause an average of 1.5 yr earlier than nonsmokers.
- More than one third of a woman's life will be spent after menopause.
- Onset of perimenopause is usually in a woman's mid- to late-40s.
- ~4000 women each day begin menopause.

PHYSICAL FINDINGS & CLINICAL PRESENTATION

- Atrophic vaginitis, which can cause burning, itching, bleeding, dyspareunia
- Either complete cessation of menses or a period of irregular cycles and diminished or heavier bleeding
- Osteoporosis
- Psychological dysfunction:
  1. Anxiety
  2. Depression
  3. Insomnia
  4. Nervousness
  5. Irritability
  6. Inability to concentrate
- Sexual changes, decreased libido, dyspareunia
- Urinary incontinence
- Vasomotor symptoms (hot flashes, flushes), night sweats, cardiovascular disease, coronary artery disease, atherosclerosis, headaches, tiredness, and lethargy. A recent study from the University of Pennsylvania noted that the median duration of moderate-to-severe hot flashes is 10.2 yr but that the length of hot flashes was largely dictated by how early these began in the perimenopause.

ETIOLOGY

- The most common etiology: physiologic, caused by depleted granulosa and theca cells that fail to react to endogenous gonadotropins, producing less estrogen; decreased negative feedback in the hypothalamic pituitary access, increased follicle-stimulating hormone (FSH), and increased luteinizing hormone (LH), which leads to stromal cells that continue to produce androgens as a result of the LH stimulation
- Surgical castration
- Family history of early menopause, cigarette smoking, blindness, abnormal chromosomal karyotype (Turner's syndrome, gonadal dysgenesis), precocious puberty, and left-handedness

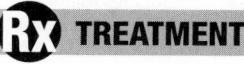

DIAGNOSIS

DIFFERENTIAL DIAGNOSIS

- Asherman's syndrome
- Hypothalamic dysfunction
- Hypothyroidism
- Pituitary tumors
- Adrenal abnormalities
- Ovarian abnormalities
- Polycystic ovarian syndrome
- Pregnancy
- Ovarian neoplasm
- Tuberculosis of the endometrium

WORKUP

- If the clinical picture is highly suggestive of menopause, estrogen can be prescribed. If all symptoms resolve, then diagnosis has essentially been made. Before estrogen is prescribed, a complete history and physical examination are needed. If a patient has estrogen-dependent malignancy, unexplained abnormal uterine bleeding, history of thrombophlebitis, or acute liver disease, estrogen therapy is contraindicated.
- Progesterone challenge test: medroxyprogesterone 10 to 20 mg PO or progesterone 100 mg IM to induce withdrawal bleeding. If no withdrawal bleeding is obtained, a hypoestrogenic state is assumed to be present.
- Physical examination, height, weight, blood pressure, breast examination, and pelvic examination are needed.
- Assess risk for coronary artery disease, osteoporosis, cigarette smoking, personal history, history of breast cancer, liver disease, active coagulation disorder, or any unexplained vaginal bleeding.

LABORATORY TESTS

- FSH, LH, and estrogen levels: markedly elevated FSH and markedly depressed estrogen level constitute laboratory diagnosis of ovarian failure; LH only if polycystic ovarian disease is to be ruled out in a younger patient. It is not necessary to obtain an FSH if the patient fulfills the clinical criteria for menopause. Similarly, since estradiol levels vary during the menstrual cycle, estradiol levels are rarely necessary or informative

- TSH to rule out thyroid dysfunction and prolactin level if patient has symptoms of galactorrhea and if suspicion of pituitary adenoma exists
- A general chemistry profile to check for any systemic diseases
- Pap smear, endometrial biopsy, or dilation and curettage in patients who have had irregular periods or intermenstrual or postmenopausal bleeding
- Mammogram

IMAGING STUDIES

- CT scan or MRI of sella if pituitary tumor is suspected
- Bone density studies if high-risk condition for osteoporosis exists
- Pelvic ultrasound to check endometrial stripe

TREATMENT

NONPHARMACOLOGIC THERAPY

- A balanced diet: low in fat, with total fat intake being <30% of calories; total calories sufficient to maintain body weight or produce weight loss if that is needed
- Avoidance of smoking and excessive alcohol or caffeine intake
- Exercise: weight-bearing exercise for osteoporosis prevention
- Kegel exercises for strengthening the pelvic floor
- Adequate calcium intake: 1500 mg qd is necessary to maintain zero calcium balance in postmenopausal women
- Change in the ambient temperature (may ameliorate hot flashes and reduce night sweats)
- Vitamin E
- Avoidance of caffeine, alcohol, and spicy foods if they trigger hot flashes
- Vaginal lubricants to help with the dyspareunia attributable to vaginal dryness (e.g., Replens, K-Y Jelly, or Gyne-Moistrin cream)

ACUTE GENERAL Rx

Estrogen replacement in symptomatic patients can be done in a variety of forms, including oral estrogen and transdermal estrogen patch. The lowest effective dose should be prescribed.
- Examples of oral estrogen include:
  1. Conjugated estrogens: start with 0.3 mg qd and increase to 1.25 mg qd depending on symptoms.
  2. Estradiol: start with 0.5 mg qd and increase to 2 mg qd.
  3. Esterified estrogens: start with 0.3 to 1.25 mg qd.
  4. Estropipate: start with 0.625 to 2.5 mg qd.
  5. Esterified estrogen/testosterone combination: give 1.25 mg and methyltestosterone 2.5 mg (Estratest) and esterified estrogen 0.625 mg and methyltestosterone 1.25 mg (Estratest HS [half-strength]). May improve sexual enjoyment and libido.
- If the patient has had a hysterectomy for benign disease, estrogen alone is sufficient. However, if she still has her uterus, progestin

should be added for its protective effect against endometrial cancer. Progestins can be prescribed as continual daily dose or cyclic fashion. Most commonly prescribed progestins include medroxyprogesterone acetate 2.5 mg, 5 mg, and 10 mg; Prometrium 100 mg, 200 mg, and 400 mg; and Aygestin 5 mg. Continuous hormone replacement therapy is preferred because after time the patient should be amenorrheic. Patients should be counseled that they may experience some irregular spotting for the first 6 to 9 mo after starting the hormone replacement therapy. Cyclic therapy will cause withdrawal bleeding.

- Combination oral preparations Femhrt, Prefest, Prempro, Activella, Premphase are commonly used. However, the U.S. Preventive Services Task Force recommends against the use of combined estrogen and progestin for the prevention of chronic conditions in post-menopausal women.
- Transdermal patches can be either estradiol (Estraderm, Vivelle, FemPatch) 0.025 to 0.1 mg applied twice weekly or Climara 0.025 to 0.1 mg used once a week. With these preparations, progesterone should be used in a similar fashion. Apply CombiPatch twice weekly (combination estrogen and progesterone) or Climara Pro once per week (one patch).
- Vaginal creams can be used; these should be reserved for local therapy of atrophic vaginitis. Systemic absorption does occur; however, blood levels are unpredictable. Usual dose 0.5 to 2 g intravaginally daily, cyclically 3 wk on 1 wk off. When symptoms improve, once to twice weekly is adequate maintenance.
- Vagifem estradiol vaginal tablets. Initial dosage: one Vagifem tablet, inserted vaginally, qd for 2 wk. Maintenance dose: one Vagifem tablet, inserted vaginally, twice weekly.
- Femring vaginal ring delivering the equivalent of 0.5 mg/day inserted every 3 mo or Estring 0.0075 mg/day.
- EstroGel 0.06% (estradiol gel) One Pump (1.25 g/day) applied to one arm from wrist to shoulder.
- The FDA contraindications to menopause hormone therapy include the following diseases and disorders: active liver disease; current, past, or suspected breast cancer; active or recent anterior thrombembolic dis-

ease (angina, myocardial infarction); known or suspected estrogen-sensitive malignant conditions; known hypersensitivity to the active substance of the therapy or to any of the excipients; porphyria cutanea tarda; previous idiopathic or current venous thromboembolism; undiagnosed genital bleeding; untreated hypertension; untreated endometrial hyperplasia.

- For women in whom estrogen is contraindicated or for those who do not wish to take estrogen, the following regimens can be used:
  1. Serotonin reuptake inhibitors
  2. Depo-Provera 150 mg IM every month (may be helpful in alleviating hot flashes)
  3. Clonidine 0.05 to 0.15 mg PO qd (questionable efficacy) or transdermal clonidine patch
  4. Bellergal-S (questionable efficacy)
- Tibolone significantly improves vasomotor symptoms, libido, and vaginal lubrication.

CHRONIC Rx

Hormone replacement therapy should be used only for the short term unless benefits outweigh the risks of long-term use. As a result of the results of the Women's Health Initiative (WHI), the FDA has instituted a "black box" warning on postmenopausal hormone replacement products suggesting that the lowest dose should be used for the shortest period of time. This necessitates a considered and nuanced counseling session with patients contemplating hormone replacement prior to the initiation of therapy and then on a periodic basis after that, usually at least a yearly basis.

DISPOSITION

If treated, the patient should have resolution of her symptoms and reduced incidence of osteoporosis. Lifelong medical supervision is necessary to monitor adequacy of treatment and prevention of complications. This should include annual Pap smears, pelvic examinations, breast examinations, mammography, and endometrial sampling of any type of abnormal bleeding. If untreated, the vasomotor symptoms will eventually disappear; however, this may take several years in a small percentage of women. Some women who are in their 80s have experienced hot flashes. Urogenital atrophy will continue to worsen. Osteoporosis and coronary artery disease risks will increase with every passing year.

REFERRAL

Most menopausal women are managed by their gynecologists. However, this condition can be managed adequately by the patient's primary care physician who has an interest in treating menopausal women.

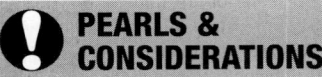

PEARLS & CONSIDERATIONS

COMMENTS

- Short-term risks of hormone replacement therapy (HRT) include an eighteenfold increased rise for cholecystitis, three-and-a-half-fold risk of a thrombocardiac event in the first year, and possible increased risk of stroke and myocardial infarction.
- Results of the WHI study found that for every 10,000 women taking HRT (combination of both estrogen and progesterone) for 1 yr (10,000 person-yr), seven more would have coronary events, eight would have more strokes, eight would have more pulmonary emboli, and eight would have earlier breast cancer than would 10,000 women taking placebo. Benefits of HRT were six fewer cases of colorectal cancer and five fewer hip fractures per 10,000 women.
- HRT should not be initiated or continued for the primary or secondary prevention of coronary heart disease.
- Estrogen-replacement therapy or HRT should only be prescribed for patients with sufficient menopausal symptoms that impact the patient's quality of life.

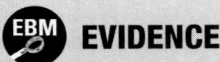 **EVIDENCE**

available at www.expertconsult.com

SUGGESTED READINGS

available at www.expertconsult.com

RELATED CONTENT

AUTHORS: **GEORGE T. DANAKAS, M.D.,** and **RUBEN ALVERO, M.D.**

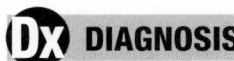

BASIC INFORMATION

DEFINITION

Menorrhagia is menstrual blood loss greater than 80 mL.

Metrorrhagia is bleeding between menses.

Polymenorrhea is bleeding that occurs more often than every 21 days.

Oligmenorrhea is bleeding less than every 35 days.

The new FIGO classification of abnormal uterine bleeding further defines abnormal bleeding by etiology. The acronym PALM-COEIN (polyp, adenomyosis, leiomyoma, malignancy or hyperplasia, coagulaopathy, ovulatory dysfunction, endometrial, iatrogenic, or not yet classified) is now used to define abnormal uterine bleeding.

SYNONYMS

Abnormal uterine bleeding
Menometrorrhagia
Dysfunctional uterine bleeding

ICD-9CM CODES
626.2 Menorrhagia

EPIDEMIOLOGY & DEMOGRAPHICS

PREVALENCE: 30% of women in their lifetime; 5% of medical visits for women

PREDOMINANT SEX AND AGE: Female; peak in adolescence and perimenopausal periods

GENETICS: Von Willebrand disease; hereditary platelet dysfunction disorders; 20% of women at any age have underlying bleeding disorder

RISK FACTORS: genetic predisposition, anticoagulation treatment, obesity

PHYSICAL FINDINGS & CLINICAL PRESENTATION

- History: age, age of menarche or menopause, menstrual bleeding patterns, severity of bleeding, pain, underlying medical conditions, surgical history, use of medications, signs and symptoms of hemostatic disorder including history of heavy bleeding since menarche, postpartum hemorrhage, surgery related bleeding, bleeding from dental work, easy bruising, epistaxis, and frequent gum bleeding, family history of bleeding disorder
- Physical exam: general findings including excessive weight, signs of polycystic ovarian syndrome (PCOS) (hirsutism and acne), signs of thyroid disease (nodule), signs of insulin resistance (acanthosis nigricans), signs of bleeding disorder including petechiae, ecchymoses, pallor, swollen joints, pelvic examination including external, speculum, and bimanual exam

ETIOLOGY

- Pregnancy/miscarriage
- Endometrial polyps
- Adenomyosis

- Uterine leiomyoma
- Endometrial hyperplasia or carcinoma
- Coagulopathy, inherited or acquired
- Ovulatory dysfunction, most likely PCOS
- Endometrial
- Iatrogenic

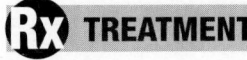

DIAGNOSIS

DIFFERENTIAL DIAGNOSIS

Pregnancy, STD, PCOS, thyroid dysfunction, anovulation due to immature hypothalamic-pituitary-ovarian axis, perimenopausal transition, uterine pathology including endometrial hyperplasia or carcinoma, leiomyoma, adenomyosis, or endometrial polyp, von Willebrand's disease, platelet dysfunction disorder, iatrogenic due to medications including oral contraceptives or anticoagulants (warfarin)

WORKUP

- History
- Physical exam to evaluate for uterine pathology
- Laboratory, pathology, and imaging studies to determine etiology

LABORATORY TESTS

- Pregnancy test
- CBC with platelets to assess for anemia or platelet dysfunction
- TSH to assess for hypothyroidism or hyperthyroidism
- Chlamydia trachomatis testing if high risk for evaluation of pelvic infection
- Evaluation for cyclic menses
- Prothrombin time and partial thromboplastin time
- Testing for von Willebrand disease if clinically suspected (von Willebrand–ristocetin cofactor activity, von Willebrand factor antigen, and factor VIII)
- Endometrial sampling by endometrial biopsy or hysteroscopic sampling for women >45 yr or <45 yr with history of unopposed estrogen (PCOS, obesity), failed medical management, or persistent abnormal bleeding

IMAGING STUDIES

- Transvaginal ultrasound if abnormal exam or persistent symptoms
- Sonohysterography or hysteroscopy if ultrasound not adequate or suspicion for endometrial polyp or submucosal leiomyoma
- Transabdominal ultrasound in adolescents may be considered
- MRI not indicated initially

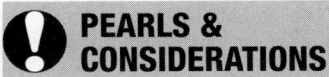 TREATMENT

NONPHARMACOLOGIC THERAPY

- Dilation and curettage
- Uterine artery embolization
- Hysteroscopic resection of uterine pathology including endometrial polyps and submucosal leiomyoma

- Endometrial ablation
- Hysterectomy

ACUTE GENERAL Rx

- Progestin
- Oral contraceptive pills
- Conjugated estrogens
- Surgical management if indicated including dilation and curettage, uterine artery embolization, or hysterectomy
- Hospitalization to maintain hemostasis and administer blood transfusion if severe menorrhagia

CHRONIC Rx

- Oral contraceptive pills
- Levonorgestrel intrauterine device
- Gonadotropin-releasing hormone agonist (goserelin)
- Nonsteroidal anti-inflammatory drugs
- Tranexamic acid, aminocaproic acid
- Danazol (significant side-effect profile requires justification for use)
- Surgery for anatomic causes including resection of leiomyoma and hysterectomy
- Endometrial ablation if completed childbearing

COMPLEMENTARY & ALTERNATIVE MEDICINE

None

REFERRAL

- If concern for uterine pathology as etiology for menorrhagia, referral to a gynecologist for surgical management indicated
- If endometrial sampling reveals endometrial hyperplasia (especially complex or atypical) or malignancy, referral to a gynecologic oncologist is indicated

 PEARLS & CONSIDERATIONS

PREVENTION

Weight reduction

EBM EVIDENCE

available at www.expertconsult.com

SUGGESTED READINGS

available at www.expertconsult.com

RELATED CONTENT

Dysfunctional Uterine Bleeding (Related Topic)

AUTHOR: **ERIN MEDLIN, M.D.**

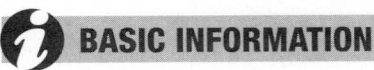

BASIC INFORMATION

DEFINITION

Acute mesenteric lymphadenitis is a syndrome of acute right lower quadrant abdominal pain associated with mesenteric lymph node enlargement and a normal appendix.

ICD-9CM CODES
289.2 Mesenteric adenitis

EPIDEMIOLOGY & DEMOGRAPHICS
• Incidence unknown
• Affects mostly children (<18 yr) with no sex preference
• When *Yersinia* enterocolitis is the cause, boys are more frequently involved

PHYSICAL FINDINGS & CLINICAL PRESENTATION
• Abdominal pain of variable severity (mild ache to severe colic) beginning in upper abdomen or right lower quadrant; eventually localizes in the right side but not in a precise location (unlike appendicitis)
• In *Yersinia* infection outbreaks (see Table E1-274), symptoms include abdominal pain (84%), diarrhea (78%), fever (43%), anorexia (22%), nausea (13%), and vomiting (8%)

• Physical findings:
  ○ Other lymphadenopathy (20% of cases)
  ○ Right lower quadrant tenderness (site of maximal tenderness may vary from one examination to the next)
  ○ Guarding (rare)
  ○ Mild fever

ETIOLOGY & PATHOGENESIS
• Reactive hyperplasia of lymph nodes that drain the ileocecal region, similar to that seen in inflammatory or allergic conditions. One study reported that approximately two thirds of cases are secondary (reactive) and one third are primary (no demonstrable associated inflammatory process).
• *Yersinia enterocolitica, Y. pseudotuberculosis, Salmonella* species, *Escherichia coli*, and streptococci have been implicated in mesenteric adenitis. Clinical manifestations of yersiniosis are described in Table E1-275.

DIAGNOSIS

In general, the diagnosis is made on exploration of the abdomen of a patient suspected of having acute appendicitis. On examination the appendix appears normal, and enlarged mesenteric lymph nodes are noted. Excision of an enlarged lymph node with culture and nodal histology may provide information regarding the etiology but is not routinely used.

DIFFERENTIAL DIAGNOSIS
• Acute appendicitis (5% to 10% of patients admitted to hospitals with a diagnosis of appendicitis are discharged with a diagnosis of mesenteric adenitis)
• Crohn's disease
Section II describes the differential diagnosis of right lower quadrant abdominal pain.

LABORATORY TESTS
• Complete blood count may show leukocytosis
• Abdominal sonography and CT scan with IV and oral contrast (Fig. 1-530). may be useful
• Laparotomy if appendicitis is suspected

PROGNOSIS
Recurrent bouts are common; therefore if laparotomy is performed and a normal appendix is found, it should be removed.

SUGGESTED READING
available at www.expertconsult.com

AUTHOR: **FRED F. FERRI, M.D.**

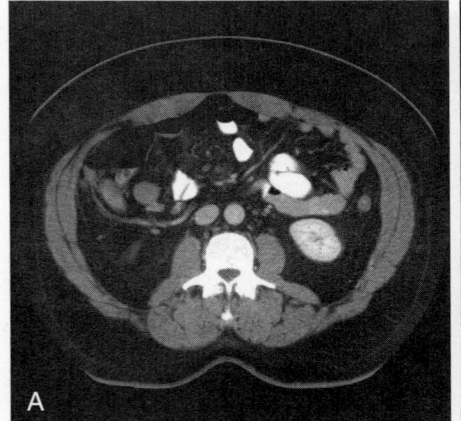
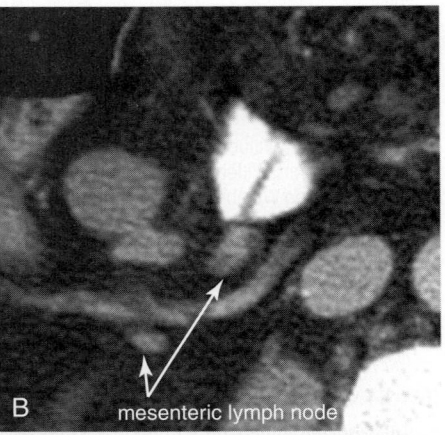
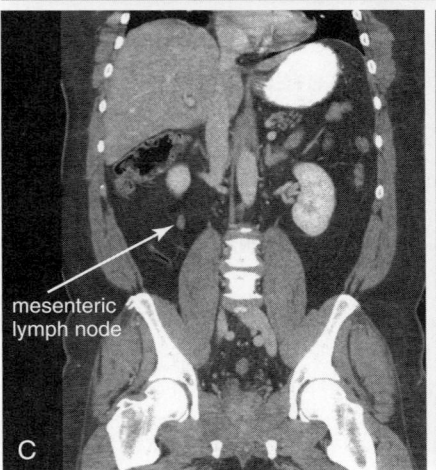
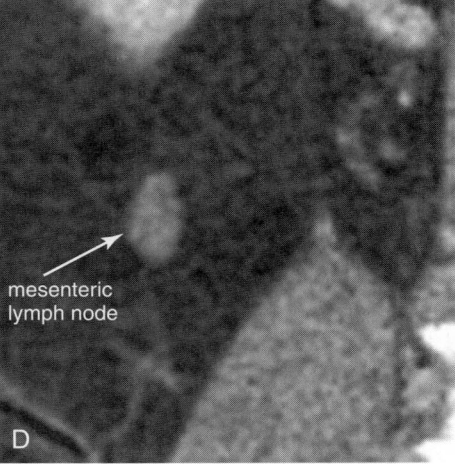

FIGURE 1-530 Mesenteric adenitis, CT with IV and oral contrast, soft-tissue window. Mesenteric adenitis can mimic appendicitis in its clinical presentation. Enlarged lymph nodes are visible on CT. Lymph nodes have soft-tissue density and appear as discrete, rounded structures. On a single image they may appear similar to blood vessels or to the appendix, but on inspection of adjacent images it becomes clear that lymph nodes are rounded, not tubular like a blood vessel or the appendix. **A,** Axial image. **B,** Close-up from **A. C,** Coronal reconstruction. **D,** Close-up from **C.** (From Broder JS: *Diagnostic imaging for the emergency physician,* Philadelphia, 2011, Saunders.)

BASIC INFORMATION

DEFINITION

Acute mesenteric ischemia (AMI) is the sudden onset of intestinal hypoperfusion to all or part of the small bowel caused by emboli, arterial or venous thrombosis (Fig. 1-531), or vasoconstriction from low-flow states.

ICD-9CM CODES
ICD-557.1 Mesenteric vascular insufficiency

EPIDEMIOLOGY & DEMOGRAPHICS

INCIDENCE:
- AMI accounts for 0.1% of hospital admissions.
- The incidence appears to be increasing, likely due to increased awareness among clinicians and aging of the population. The mortality rate is 60% to 85%.
- Improved intensive care, and longer survival of sicker patients, has allowed mesenteric ischemia to occur more frequently as a complication of the initial illnesses.

PREDOMINANT SEX AND AGE:
- AMI caused by arterial embolism or thrombosis occurs more frequently in the elderly.
- AMI from mesenteric venous thrombosis often presents in younger age groups.

GENETICS: No specific genetic predisposition but may be related to underlying factors such as cardiac disease, atherosclerosis, and hypercoagulable states.

RISK FACTORS:
- Advanced age, atherosclerosis, low cardiac output (especially atrial fibrillation), severe cardiac valvular disease, intraabdominal malignancy.
- In the subgroup of cases caused by venous thrombosis, risk factors include hypercoagulable states, portal hypertension, abdominal infection, blunt trauma, pancreatitis, and portal malignancy.
- Additional risk factors for AMI caused by non-occlusive mesenteric ischemia include recent cardiac surgery, dialysis, and cocaine use.
- AMI may occur rarely in patients with no identifiable risk factors.

PHYSICAL FINDINGS & CLINICAL PRESENTATION
- The classic presentation is rapid onset of severe periumbilical pain out of proportion to physical examination findings.

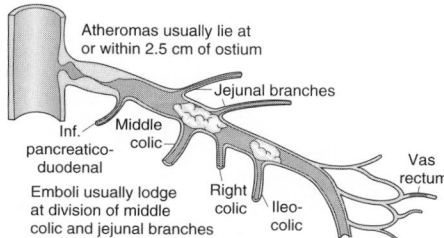

FIGURE 1-531 Typical location of superior mesenteric artery obstruction in patients with embolic and thrombotic occlusion. (From Donaldson MC: Mesenteric vascular disease. In Braunwald S, Creager MA [eds]: *Atlas of heart diseases*, St Louis, 1996, Mosby.)

- Nausea and vomiting are commonly associated.
- Initial abdominal examination may be normal, with no rebound or guarding, or may include minimal distention or stool positive for occult blood.
- Later in the course the patient may present with gross distention, absence of bowel sounds, and peritoneal signs. In the elderly, mental status changes may occur.

ETIOLOGY

The pathophysiologic mechanisms that cause AMI include:
- Mesenteric arterial embolism: typically from the left atrium, left ventricle, or cardiac valves. The superior mesenteric artery is most commonly affected.
- Mesenteric arterial thrombosis: often in patients with prior progressive atherosclerotic stenoses, with superimposed abdominal trauma or infection.
- Mesenteric venous thrombosis may occur in the setting of hypercoagulable states (acquired or inherited), blunt trauma, abdominal infection, portal hypertension, pancreatitis, and portal malignancy.
- Nonocclusive mesenteric ischemia is caused by reduced intestinal perfusion, such as may be seen in a patient with an acute cardiovascular disease process being treated with drugs that reduce intestinal perfusion, or with use of ergot, cocaine, or amphetamines.

DIAGNOSIS

DIFFERENTIAL DIAGNOSIS
Initially include other causes of abdominal pain of acute onset, including perforated peptic ulcer and early appendicitis. Ultimately, the varied causes of peritonitis.

WORKUP
- Early diagnosis is key. Treatment success is related to the duration of symptoms before diagnosis.
- Consider early laparotomy for diagnosis in cases with a high index of suspicion when angiography is not available.

LABORATORY TESTS
- Laboratory test results are nonspecific, especially early in the course. Elevated lactic acid, leukocytosis, acidosis, and elevated hematocrit from hemoconcentration can occur later in the course, often after progression to bowel necrosis has occurred, hence are not useful for early diagnosis.
- When a hypercoagulable state is suspected, workup may include proteins C and S, antithrombin III, and factor V Leiden. This will likely not affect the diagnosis of AMI but may help guide long-term therapy.
- D-dimer testing has been reported to be useful for the early diagnosis of AMI but is very nonspecific.

IMAGING STUDIES
- Biphasic contrast-enhanced CT is the preferred diagnostic mode. It is more easily available and has similar sensitivity to angiography.
- With strong clinical suspicion, workup should proceed directly to angiography without delay for CT scan (Fig. 1-532) or other testing. If angiography cannot be done emergently, diagnositic laparotomy should not be delayed.
- Plain films are normal 25% of the time in the early stages. Suggestive findings may include ileus, bowel wall thickening, or intramural gas. Intraluminal barium should not be used as it is rarely helpful in making a positive diagnosis and will interfere with angiographic studies.
- Doppler ultrasound evaluation of intestinal blood flow is often limited by the presence of air-filled loops of bowel and is not an appropriate part of the diagnostic workup if AMI is the leading working diagnosis.
- Plain CT findings also are commonly nonspecific and more often found late in the course. Portal venous gas or intramural gas may be seen after the development of gangrene; in many cases, even at that advanced stage CT findings remain nonspecific. The use of IV contrast material may affect interpretation of subsequent angiography.
- CT scanning is more useful in cases of mesenteric vein thrombosis causing AMI, with sensitivity approaching 90%. It has also been found useful in monitoring the progress of patients with superior mesenteric venous thrombosis who are treated nonsurgically.

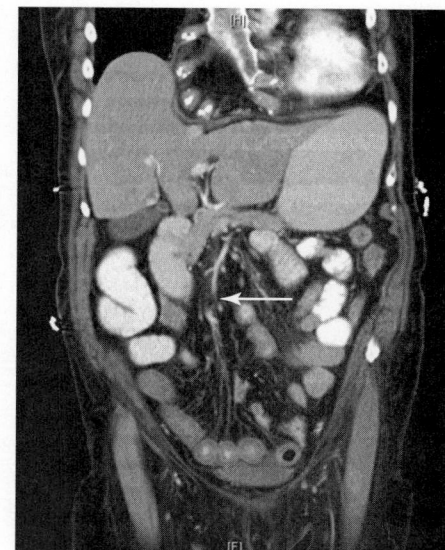

FIGURE 1-532 Mesenteric ischemia, acute. CT after administration of oral and intravenous contrast in patient with embolism to superior mesenteric artery and ischemia of small bowel and right colon. *Arrow* points to embolus in superior mesenteric artery. (From Vincent JL et al: *Textbook of critical care*, ed 6, Philadelphia, 2011, Saunders.)

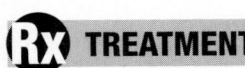 **TREATMENT**

- The goal of treatment is to restore blood flow as rapidly as possible to ischemic bowel before the occurrence of infarction.
- Treatment varies depending on etiology.

ACUTE GENERAL Rx

- Initial management should include hemodynamic monitoring and support, correction of acidosis, administration of broad-spectrum antibiotics, and gastric decompression by nasogastric tube.
- Vasoconstricting agents should be avoided.
- Systemic anticoagulation may be started. Optimal timing of initiation is unclear.

NONPHARMACOLOGIC THERAPY

- Signs of peritonitis mandate early laparotomy and resection of infarcted bowel.
- When workup is positive for major superior mesenteric artery (SMA) embolus, embolectomy is considered standard treatment in the absence of peritoneal signs. Depending on the location and degree of occlusion of the embolus, surgical revascularization, intraarterial infusion of thrombolytics or vasodilators, or systemic anticoagulation may be considered.
- In cases of SMA thrombosis, emergency surgical revascularization is the treatment of choice; stent placement may be a viable alternative.

- Angiography is needed to diagnose nonocclusive mesenteric ischemia before infarct and should be followed up by intraarterial vasodilator infusion. This approach has been shown to significantly reduce mortality rate in this situation.
- In patients with mesenteric vein thrombosis, treatment depends on the presence or absence of peritoneal signs. Laparotomy and resection of infarcted bowel is indicated in more advanced cases. If there are no peritoneal signs, immediate anticoagulant therapy with heparin, and ultimately warfarin, may be adequate treatment.
- Percutaneous treatment with lytic therapy, balloon angioplasty, or stenting may be limited by the frequent presence of nonviable bowel, which would require laparotomy despite success with the percutaneous treatment.

CHRONIC Rx

In the subgroup of patients with mesenteric venous thrombosis, prevention of further thrombosis is indicated. The optimal duration of anticoagulation is unclear.

DISPOSITION

- Prognosis is best in AMI due to mesenteric venous thrombosis and after surgical treatment for acute arterial embolism. It remains poor in cases of arterial thrombosis and nonocclusive ischemia.
- With delayed diagnosis, intestinal infarction—resulting in perforation or gangrenous bowel, sepsis, shock, and death—is typical.

REFERRAL

- Early surgical consultation should be considered. There should be no delay with peritoneal signs.
- If diagnostic angiography is unavailable, surgery may be warranted for diagnostic purposes.

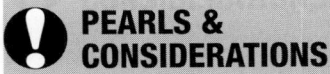 **PEARLS & CONSIDERATIONS**

COMMENTS

- The diagnosis of AMI should be considered in any patient with acute onset of abdominal pain out of proportion to physical findings, particularly in at-risk patients.
- Early diagnosis, before intestinal infarction occurs, is critical and correlates with improved survival rates.
- In a recent case series, the primary location of the ischemic colitis was in the right, transverse, left, and distal colon in 25%, 10%, 33%, and 25% of cases, respectively; 7% were pancolonic.

PREVENTION

Prevention of the underlying factors, most notably atherosclerotic disease

SUGGESTED READINGS

available at www.expertconsult.com

RELATED CONTENT

Mesenteric Venous Thrombosis (Related Key Topic)

AUTHOR: **MARGARET TRYFOROS, M.D.**

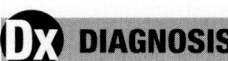

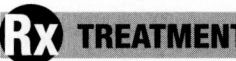

BASIC INFORMATION

DEFINITION

Mesenteric venous thrombosis (MVT) is a thrombotic occlusion of the mesenteric venous system involving major trunks or smaller branches and leading to intestinal infarction in its acute form.

ICD-9CM CODES
557.0 Mesenteric venous thrombosis

EPIDEMIOLOGY & DEMOGRAPHICS

Between 5% and 15% of patients with acute mesenteric infarction have MVT. MVT is slightly more common in men than women. The typical age of occurrence is 50 to 60 yr.

PHYSICAL FINDINGS & CLINICAL PRESENTATION

Acute MVT:
- Symptoms: abdominal pain in 90% of patients, typically out of proportion to the physical findings. Nausea and vomiting occur in 50% and gastrointestinal (GI) bleeding occurs in 50% (occult) and 15% (gross).
- Physical findings:
  - Early: abdominal tenderness, decreased bowel sounds, abdominal distention
  - Later: guarding and rebound tenderness, fever, septic shock

Subacute MVT:
- Symptoms: nonspecific abdominal pain for weeks or months
- Physical findings: none

Chronic MVT:
- Symptoms: upper GI hemorrhage from bleeding varices
- Physical findings: none other than signs of blood loss if significant

ETIOLOGY & PATHOGENESIS

Hypercoagulable states:
- Peripheral deep venous thrombosis
- Neoplasms
- Antithrombin III, protein C, protein S deficiencies
- Lupus anticoagulant (antiphospholipid antibody)
- Oral contraceptive use, pregnancy
- Polycythemia vera
- Thrombocytosis
- Paroxysmal nocturnal hemoglobinuria

Portal hypertension:
- Cirrhosis

Inflammation:
- Pancreatitis
- Peritonitis (e.g., appendicitis, diverticulitis, perforated viscus)
- Inflammatory bowel disease
- Pelvic or intraabdominal abscess
- Intraabdominal cancer

Postoperative state or trauma:
- Blunt abdominal trauma
- Postoperative states (abdominal surgery)
  Thrombosis may begin in small mesenteric branches (e.g., in hypercoagulable states) and propagate to the major venous mesenteric trunks or begin in large veins (e.g., in cirrhosis, intraabdominal cancer, surgery) and extend distally. If collateral drainage is inadequate, the intestine becomes congested, edematous, cyanotic, and hemorrhagic and eventually may infarct.

DIAGNOSIS

DIFFERENTIAL DIAGNOSIS

All other causes of abdominal pain (e.g., peritonitis, intestinal obstruction, pancreatitis, peptic ulcer disease, gastritis, inflammatory bowel disease, perforated viscus). Also to be considered in the differential diagnosis of GI hemorrhage.

WORKUP

Laboratory tests and imaging studies

LABORATORY TESTS
- Complete blood count: leukocytosis
- Electrolytes: metabolic acidosis (lactic) indicates bowel infarction
- Elevated amylase
- Tests for hypercoagulable status

IMAGING STUDIES
- Abdominal plain radiograph: ileus, ascites, bowel dilation, bowel wall thickening, loop separation, thumbprinting
- Abdominal CT scan (diagnostic in 90%): bowel wall thickening, venous dilation, venous thrombus
- Arteriography if CT scan is not diagnostic
- Diagnosis occasionally made by laparotomy

TREATMENT

- Anticoagulation or thrombolytic therapy
- Laparotomy if intestinal infarction is suspected
- Short ischemic segment: resection
- Long ischemic segment:
  1. Nonviable: resection or close
  2. Viable: intraarterial papaverine and/or thrombectomy followed by "second look" intervention
- Treatment of chronic MVT is the same as for portal hypertension

PROGNOSIS
- Mortality rate of acute MVT: 20% to 50%
- Recurrence rate: 15% to 25%

SUGGESTED READINGS
available at www.expertconsult.com

AUTHOR: **FRED F. FERRI, M.D.**

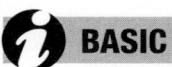

BASIC INFORMATION

DEFINITION

Malignant mesothelioma is a neoplasm that originates from the mesothelial surfaces of the pleural cavities (80%) or peritoneal cavities (20%).There are three major histologic subtypes: epithelial (most common), sarcomatous, and mixed (epithelial/sarcomatous).

ICD-9CM CODES
199.1 Malignant mesothelioma, site NOS

EPIDEMIOLOGY & DEMOGRAPHICS

- Associated with asbestos exposure (all fiber types)
- More than 3000 new cases diagnosed in the United States annually
- More common in men as a result of asbestos exposure in the workplace
- Right-sided involvement is more common
- Incidence of mesothelioma increases with age; median age at presentation is >60 yr
- More than 8 million persons in the United States are currently at risk for mesothelioma because of prior asbestos exposure

PHYSICAL FINDINGS & CLINICAL PRESENTATION

- Dyspnea
- Nonpleuritic chest pain
- Fever, weight loss, sweats, fatigue, loss of appetite
- Dysphagia, superior vena cava syndrome, Horner's syndrome in advanced stages
- Auscultation may reveal unilateral loss of breath sounds
- Dullness on percussion may be present

ETIOLOGY

- Asbestos exposure (>70% of patients)
- Other reported potentially causal factors include prior radiation therapy and extravasated Thorotrast, zeolite, and erionite fibers

DIAGNOSIS

DIFFERENTIAL DIAGNOSIS

Metastatic adenocarcinomas (from lung, breast, ovary, kidney, stomach, prostate)

WORKUP

- Staging evaluation (Fig. E1-533) includes complete history (including occupational history), physical examination, and testing to determine potential operability (CT, bone scan, pulmonary function tests [PFTs])
- Thoracoscopy, pleuroscopy, and open-lung biopsy are useful in obtaining adequate tissue samples for diagnosis
- Pulmonary function tests
- Staging: the International Union Against Cancer (UICC) staging uses the TNM categories to organize mesothelioma in stages I to IV in a manner similar to that used for non–small cell lung cancer

LABORATORY TESTS

- Diagnostic thoracentesis is generally insufficient for diagnosis because pleural effusions may only reveal atypical mesothelial cells.
- Immunohistochemistry is useful to distinguish adenocarcinoma from epithelial malignant mesothelioma (mesotheliomas are generally carcinoembryonic antigen negative and cytokeratin positive).
- Thrombocytosis and anemia may be found on initial laboratory evaluation.
- Fibulin-3 may be useful as a blood and effusion biomarker for pleural mesothelioma. Recent data reveal that plasma fibulin-3 levels can distinguish healthy persons with exposure to asbestos from patients with mesothelioma. In conjunction with effusion fibulin-3 levels, plasma fibulin-3 levels can further differentiate mesothelioma effusions from other malignant and benign effusions.
- Serum osteopontin levels (when available) can also be used to distinguish persons with exposure to asbestos who do not have cancer from those with exposure to asbestos who have pleural mesothelioma.

IMAGING STUDIES

- Chest radiographs may reveal pleural plaques (Fig. 1-534) or calcifications in the diaphragm.
- CT scans of the chest and abdomen and bone scan are used to assess the extent of disease.

TREATMENT

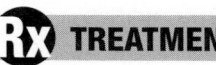

GENERAL Rx

- Operable patient (epithelial type, no positive nodes, confined to pleura, adequate PFTs): the two surgical techniques for therapeutic intervention are decortication (pleurectomy) and extrapleural pneumonectomy. Postoperative chemotherapy with cisplatin, doxorubicin, and cyclophosphamide and subsequent

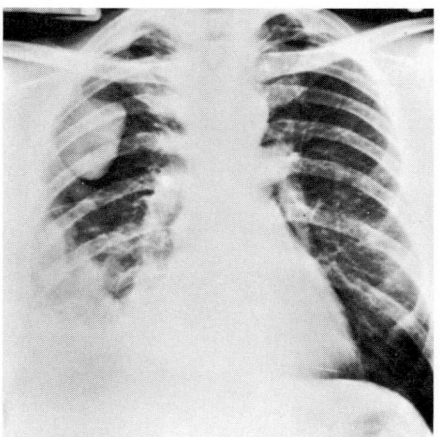

FIGURE 1-534 Chest radiograph of patient with mesothelioma. Note several lobulated, pleural-based masses in right hemithorax accompanied by right pleural effusion. (From Weinberg SE et al: *Principles of pulmonary medicine,* ed 5, Philadelphia, 2008, Saunders.)

external-beam radiation are used in some centers with limited success.
- Inoperable patient (disease too extensive, sarcomatous or mixed histology type, poor PFTs): supportive care with or without radiation therapy for symptoms or supportive care plus chemotherapy. Combined modality therapies (surgery, radiation therapy, chemotherapy, and biologics) have also been used to reduce both local and distant recurrences. The combination of pemetrexed (an antimetabolite that inhibits enzymes involved in folate metabolism) and cisplatin is used for chemotherapy of unresectable malignant pleural mesothelioma.
- Intrapleural instillation of cisplatin or biologics (e.g., interferons, interleukin-2) is generally limited to very early disease because it can only penetrate a very limited depth of the tumor and there is a propensity of the pleural space to become progressively obliterated with advancing disease.
- The role of radiation therapy in the treatment of mesotheliomas remains uncertain. It is often used for palliation of local pain despite lack of trials to prove its utility.
- Obliteration of the pleural space (pleurodesis) with instillation of tetracycline, bleomycin, or biologic substances such as *Cryptosporidium parvum* into the pleural cavity is often attempted in the treatment of recurrent symptomatic pleural effusions.

DISPOSITION

Median survival is from 6.7 to 21 mo for patients undergoing pleurectomy and ranges from 4 to 21 mo for extrapleural pneumonectomy. Survival is better for patients with the epithelial form.

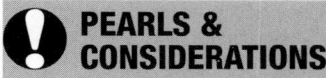

PEARLS & CONSIDERATIONS

COMMENTS

Patients with early disease should be referred to treatment centers specializing in mesothelioma treatment before attempts are made to obliterate the pleural space with pleurodesis.

SUGGESTED READINGS
available at www.expertconsult.com

RELATED CONTENT

Mesothelioma (Patient Information)
Mesenteric Ischemia, Acute (Related Key Topic)

AUTHOR: **FRED F. FERRI, M.D.**

BASIC INFORMATION

DEFINITION

Hyperglycemia, dyslipidemia, abdominal obesity, and hypertension are critical components of metabolic syndrome. Over the years, many definitions of the syndrome have been proposed and debated (see Table 1-276). In 2009, a consensus statement from several organizations including the International Diabetes Federation (IDF) and American Heart Association defined "metabolic syndrome" as the presence of any three of the following criteria:

- Abdominal waist circumference >94 cm (37 in) in men and >80 cm (31 in) in women (the use of population- and country-specific definitions is suggested; however, until better data are available, IDF recommends using these cutoffs)
- Serum hypertriglyceridemia ≥150 mg/dl (1.7 mmol/L) or drug treatment for elevated triglycerides
- Serum high-density lipoprotein (HDL) cholesterol <40 mg/dl (1 mmol/L) in men and <50 mg/dl (1.3 mmol/L) in women or drug treatment for low HDL-C
- Blood pressure ≥130/85 mm Hg or drug treatment for elevated blood pressure
- Fasting glucose ≥100 mg/dl (5.6 mmol/L) or drug treatment for elevated blood glucose

SYNONYMS

Syndrome X
Insulin resistance syndrome
Obesity dyslipidemia syndrome

ICD-9CM CODES
277.7 Metabolic syndrome

EPIDEMIOLOGY & DEMOGRAPHICS

- Affects 22% of U.S. adults.
- Prevalence increases with age, affecting more than 40% of individuals >60 yr.
- Increasing prevalence among women, especially in the African American and Mexican American populations.

TABLE 1-276 Common Definitions for Metabolic Syndrome

Criterion	NCEP ATP III (3 or more criteria)
Abdominal obesity	Waist circumferance
Men	>40 inches (>102 cm)
Women	>35 inches (>88 cm)
Hypertriglyceridemia	>150 mg/dl (≥1.7 mmol/l)
Low HDL	
Men	<40 mg/dl (<1.03 mmol/l)
Women	<50 mg/dl (<1.30 mmol/l)
Hypertension	≥130/85 mm Hg or on anti-hypertensive medication
Impaired fasting glucose or diabetes	>100 mg/dl (5.6 mmol/l) or taking insulin or hypoglycemic medication

From Floege J et al: *Comprehensive clinical nephrology,* ed 4, Philadelphia, 2010, Saunders.

- Prevalence increases with weight. Metabolic syndrome is noted in 5% of normal weight, 22% of overweight, and 60% of obese individuals.
- Other risk factors include low socioeconomic status, lack of physical activity, high carbohydrate diet, no alcohol intake, smoking, genetic predisposition, use of atypical antipsychotics, and postmenopausal status.

CLINICAL PRESENTATION

- Obesity, hypertension, dyslipidemia, and hyperglycemia as defined.
  - Blood pressure: ≥130/85 mm Hg
  - Abdominal obesity with waist circumference: >94 cm (37 in) in men and >80 cm (31 in) in women
  - Triglycerides: ≥150 mg/dl (1.7 mmol/L)
  - HDL: <40 mg/dl (1 mmol/L) in men and <50 mg/dl (1.3 mmol/L) in women
  - High fasting glucose: ≥100 mg/dl (5.6 mmol/L)
- Patients with the metabolic syndrome are at twice the risk of developing cardiovascular disease and have a sevenfold increase in risk for type 2 diabetes and a 1.5-fold increase in all-cause mortality compared to patients without the syndrome. Other complications include cognitive decline in the elderly, fatty liver disease, polycystic ovary syndrome, obstructive sleep apnea, gout, and chronic kidney disease.
- Focus history on symptoms of diabetes and its complications, obesity and its complications, coronary artery disease (angina), and polycystic ovary syndrome.
- Complete physical examination, including height, weight, waist circumference, and blood pressure.

ETIOLOGY

- Genetic and environmental factors associated with obesity increase the risk of developing metabolic syndrome.
- Abdominal obesity is associated with insulin resistance and hyperinsulinemia.
- Insulin resistance results in ineffective glucose and fatty acid utilization leading to type 2 diabetes mellitus.
- Hyperinsulinemia and inflammatory markers/cytokines play an important role in development of abnormal lipid profile, hypertension, and vascular endothelial dysfunction, which can lead to the development of atherosclerotic cardiovascular disease.

DX DIAGNOSIS

DIFFERENTIAL DIAGNOSIS

- Other causes of weight gain or obesity (Cushing's syndrome, hypothyroidism)
- Other causes of hyperlipidemia (familial hyperlipidemia, hypothyroidism)
- Other causes of hypertension (Cushing's syndrome, hyperaldosteronism)
- Other forms of diabetes (type 1)

LABORATORY TESTS

- Fasting lipid profile (total cholesterol, low-density lipoprotein [LDL] cholesterol, HDL cholesterol, and triglycerides)
- Fasting glucose

Rx TREATMENT

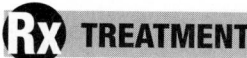

NONPHARMACOLOGIC THERAPY

- Lifestyle modification:
  - Dietary modifications aimed at weight loss
  - Physical activity of moderate intensity (i.e., brisk walking): 30 min daily
  - Smoking cessation
- Consider bariatric surgery in the management of obesity:
  - Body mass index (BMI) ≥40 kg/m² in patients who have not responded to diet and exercise (with or without drug therapy)
  - Individuals with BMI >35 kg/m² and comorbidities (hypertension, impaired glucose tolerance, diabetes mellitus, dyslipidemia, sleep apnea) are also potential surgical candidates.

ACUTE GENERAL Rx

- Treat obesity (see "Obesity"): Pharmacologic treatment: consider orlistat and other approved agents in patients who have not responded to diet and exercise if BMI >30 kg/m² or a BMI of 27 to 30 kg/m² with comorbid conditions. Drug therapy still needs to be in conjunction with diet and exercise.
- Treat hypertension (see "Hypertension"): Systolic blood pressures >130/80 mm Hg: consider angiotensin-converting enzyme inhibitors or angiotensin II receptor blocker as first-line therapy.
- Treat hyperlipidemia:
  - Serum LDL cholesterol of <100 mg/dl (2.6 mmol/L) is recommended for secondary prevention (i.e., coronary artery disease [CAD] or CAD equivalent such as diabetes); however, recent studies suggest greater benefit with a more aggressive goal of <70 mg/dl (2.1 mmol/L). For primary prevention, an LDL goal <130 mg/dl (3.4 mmol/L) is recommended for individuals with more than two coronary heart disease risk factors. HMG-CoA reductase inhibitors (statins) can be used as first-line agents.
  - Patients with high triglycerides (>200 mg/dl) may benefit from fibric acid derivatives to achieve secondary non-HDL cholesterol target (LDL goal + 30).
- Treat diabetes:
  - Goal HgA1C < 7.0% Aspirin should be started in patients with metabolic syndrome and an intermediate or elevated Framingham cardiovascular risk, if there are no contraindications.
  - Metformin as first-line therapy to improve insulin sensitivity
- Treat cardiovascular risk factors:
  - Consider aspirin. Aspirin should be started in patients with metabolic syndrome and an intermediate or elevated Framingham cardiovascular risk, if there are no contraindications.

○ Risk can be lowered with weight loss, exercise, smoking cessation, blood pressure control, diabetes management, and treatment of hyperlipidemia.

CHRONIC Rx

- Encourage lifestyle modification as above.
- Pharmacologic and surgical management to maintain therapeutic goals described above.

DISPOSITION

Weight loss can prevent disease progression. Appropriate treatment of obesity, hypertension, hyperlipidemia, and diabetes can improve morbidity and mortality rates.

REFERRAL

- To nutritionist for dietary counseling
- To weight loss and exercise programs
- To endocrinologist if difficulty reaching therapeutic goals
- To bariatric surgeon if patient meets surgical criteria (as noted previously)

! PEARLS & CONSIDERATIONS

PREVENTION

- Weight loss is essential for the prevention and treatment of metabolic syndrome.
- Recommend dietary modifications and moderate physical activity.
- Consider pharmacologic and surgical options in select individuals (as above).

PATIENT & FAMILY EDUCATION

- Weight reduction programs, including Weight Watchers, Curves, etc.
- American Diabetes Association: http://www.diabetes.org
- Polycystic Ovarian Syndrome Association: http://www.pcosupport.org
- The Hormone Foundation: http://www.hormone.org

SUGGESTED READINGS

available at www.expertconsult.com

RELATED CONTENT

Obesity (Related Key Topic)
Fig. E1-593 Endocrine evaluation of obesity (Algorithm)
Metabolic Syndrome (Patient Information)

AUTHORS: **HARIKRISHNA BHATT, M.D.,** and **GEETHA GOPALAKRISHNAN, M.D.**

BASIC INFORMATION

DEFINITION

The diagnosis of metatarsalgia includes multiple etiologies of pain involving the plantar aspect of the lesser metatarsal heads or metatarsophalangeal joints (Fig. 1-535).

ICD-9CM CODES
726.7 Metatarsalgia

PHYSICAL FINDINGS & CLINICAL PRESENTATION

- Pain beneath any or all of metatarsal heads 2, 3, 4, and 5
- Pain on metatarsophalangeal joint range of motion
- Often associated with hammertoe deformity and gastrocnemius/soleus equinus
- May include predislocation syndrome
- Common with bunion deformity
- Often obesity, recent weight gain, or increased/change in type of activity

ETIOLOGY

- Primary structural/functional factors, all yielding increased submetatarsal pressure:
  - Structural: sagittal plane (cavus foot, ankle equinus, pseudoequinus, elongated lesser metatarsal[s] relative to the optimal metatarsal parabola) or frontal plane (relative fixed dorsiflexion or plantarflexion of adjacent metatarsals)
  - Functional causes yielding transferred pressure (from hypermobile first or fifth rays) or friction (secondary to compensation for transverse plane deformities or lack of sufficient rearfoot mobility).
- Local factors: decreased shock absorption due to hammertoe deformity, predislocation syndrome, translocation of the plantar fat pad, plantar fat pad atrophy.
- Trauma: rupture of plantar plate, metatarsophalangeal joint capsule, or any associated tendon
- Degenerative joint diseases (osteoarthritis, rheumatoid arthritis, psoriatic arthritis, etc.)

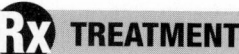

DIAGNOSIS

DIFFERENTIAL DIAGNOSIS

- Interdigital neuroma, most commonly third interspace (Morton's)
- Metatarsal traumatic fracture or stress fracture
- Foreign body, infection/abscess
- Freiberg's infraction, usually of second metatarsal head, frequently in teenage females

- Secondary systemic findings: rheumatoid nodules, gout
- Neoplasms: ganglion cyst, bone tumor
- Skin: verrucous plantaris, intractable plantar keratoma, tinea pedis, etc.
- Neuropathy or peripheral vascular disease

LABORATORY TESTS

As necessary if suspicion of a systemic cause of joint arthritis/destruction

IMAGING STUDIES

- X-rays: rule out fracture, tumor, avascular necrosis, arthritic process/joint disease.
- MRI: evaluate for any plantar plate injury, capsular injury, tendon rupture, or neuroma.
- Bone scan: if stress fracture suspected (may take 2 wk to show up on x-ray).

TREATMENT

- Silicone padding provides symptomatic relief, works well for fat pad atrophy.
- Moleskin or padding will reduce frictional forces without adding bulk for long-term use.
- Custom orthotics with proximal metatarsal pad or submetatarsal cutout to offload.
- Heel lift or shoes with short heel or wedge are effective when equinus is etiology.
- Rocker-bottom to prevent motion in severe or high-risk diabetic patients
- Nonsteroidal anti-inflammatory drugs
- Intraarticular injection if indicated, based on underlying etiology
- **Caution with injection:** risk of plantar plate ruptures; use only if absolutely indicated!

DISPOSITION

Varies depending on etiology

REFERRAL

To podiatric or foot/ankle orthopedic surgeon for biomechanical exam/orthotic management or surgical consultation

SUGGESTED READINGS
available at www.expertconsult.com

RELATED CONTENT
Metatarsalgia (Patient Information)

AUTHOR: **BROOKE E. KEELEY, D.P.M.**

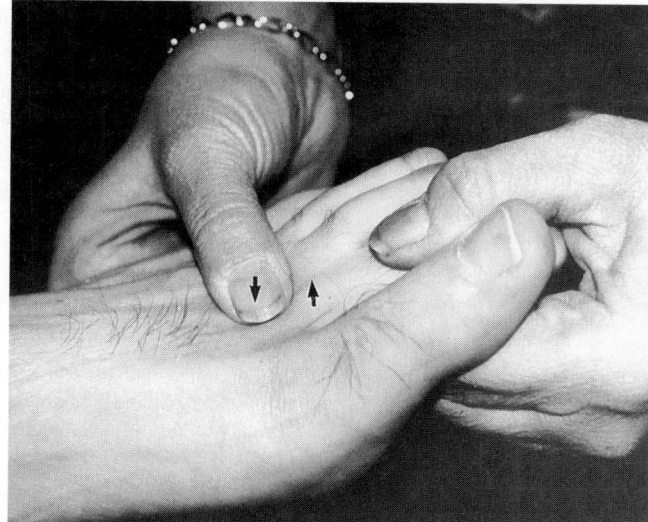

FIGURE 1-535 Vertical stress test for metatarsophalangeal stability. One of the examiner's hands stabilizes the metatarsal head while the other grasps the proximal phalanx. Examiner attempts to displace the proximal phalanx dorsally. A positive test result is the ability to displace dorsally while reproducing symptoms. (From Scuderi G [ed]: *Sports medicine: principles of primary care,* St Louis, 1997, Mosby.)

M

Diseases and Disorders

I

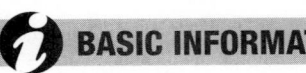

BASIC INFORMATION

DEFINITION

An accidental or intentional ingestion of 1 g/kg of methanol or ethylene glycol is considered lethal, although even small amounts can be toxic. Inhalation and dermal exposures rarely cause toxicity.

SYNONYMS

Antifreeze and moonshine overdose

EPIDEMIOLOGY & DEMOGRAPHICS

INCIDENCE: In 2009, the American Association of Poison Control Centers reported 4852 and 1883 single-exposure cases of ethylene glycol and methanol poisoning, respectively. Most cases reported are in adults older than 19 yr and predominantly males. Accidental exposure is common in children, while alcoholism, polysubstance abuse, depression, and suicide are seen in adults.

PHYSICAL FINDINGS & CLINICAL PRESENTATION

- Historical data crucial for determining dose, duration, source of exposure, and concomitant ingestion of other alcohols/toxins
- Initial symptoms like nausea, vomiting, and inebriation, and late symptoms like coma, convulsions, respiratory failure, and cardiogenic shock are common to both methanol and ethylene glycol toxicity
- Visual symptoms ranging from blurry or snowy vision to complete visual loss and findings of papillary edema, afferent pupillary defect, retinal hyperemia, and parkinsonian-like syndrome are indicative of methanol poisoning
- Abdominal pain, oliguria, hematuria, calcium oxalate crystalluria, tetany, and acute kidney injury suggest ethylene glycol toxicity

ETIOLOGY

- Toxicity of these alcohols is related to its metabolites rather than the parent compound
- Sequential metabolism by alcohol and aldehyde dehydrogenase converts methanol to formic acid and ethylene glycol to glycolic acid and oxalate, resulting in toxicity
- While methanol metabolites primarily cause retinal injury, ethylene glycol metabolites cause renal tubular injury and calcium oxalate stones

DIAGNOSIS

DIFFERENTIAL DIAGNOSIS

- Other causes of anion gap metabolic acidosis include lactic acidosis, diabetic/alcoholic ketoacidosis, renal failure, toluene, and salicylate intoxication

- Elevated plasma osmolal gap can also be seen in ethyl alcohol or isopropyl alcohol ingestion and other serious illnesses like septic shock

WORKUP

- Diagnosis depends on history, clinical presentation, and laboratory abnormalities
- Anion gap metabolic acidosis (AG >12 mEq/L) with elevated plasma osmolal gap (>10 mOsm/L) in an appropriate clinical setting should raise the suspicion for methanol or ethylene glycol ingestion.
- While those with ethylene glycol ingestion may have fewer toxicities and may present without acidosis, anion gap, or symptoms, the osmolar gap will remain elevated.
- Acute kidney injury, hypocalcemia with prolonged QT interval, and calcium oxalate crystalluria can been seen due to ethylene glycol toxicity
- Serum methanol and ethylene glycol levels are elevated in respective ingestions
- Wood's lamp fluorescence uses ultraviolet light to detect fluorescein contained in ethylene glycol preparations but lacks sensitivity as not all preparations contain fluorescein and also lacks specificity due to high rate of false positivity

LABORATORY TESTS

- Anion gap determination: electrolytes, albumin
- Osmolal gap determination: measured and calculated serum osmolality (sodium, BUN, glucose, ± ethanol)
- Arterial blood gas analysis, lactate, calcium, and creatinine kinase
- Creatinine, urine analysis to assess kidney function, tubular injury, and calcium oxalate crystals
- ECG to assess QT interval
- Toxicology screen and quantification: acetaminophen, salicylate, ethyl alcohol, methanol, ethylene glycol, and isopropyl alcohol

TREATMENT

High index of suspicion and immediate recognition with early treatment remain crucial to reduce mortality. Box 1-38 describes common commercial products that may contain ethylene glycol.

BOX 1-38 Common Commercial Products That May Contain Ethylene Glycol

Paints and lacquers
Polishes and detergents
Inks
Cosmetics
Hydraulic brake fluids
Solar collector fluids
Car wash fluids

Data from Kruse JA: Methanol, ethylene glycol, and related intoxications. In Carlson RW, Geheb MA (eds): *Principles and practice of medical intensive care,* Philadelphia, 1993, Saunders.

NONPHARMACOLOGIC THERAPY

- Securing patient's airway, breathing, and circulation and advanced cardiac life support measures instituted as indicated.
- Gastric decontamination (charcoal and/or gastric lavage) is of limited use unless done within 1 hr of ingestion as alcohols are rapidly absorbed.

ACUTE GENERAL Rx

- Volume expansion with isotonic fluids facilitates urinary excretion of the toxins.
- Management of methanol and ethylene glycol poisoning includes preventing formation of toxic metabolites, correcting the acidosis with isotonic sodium bicarbonate solution, and removing toxins such as acidic metabolites by alkalinizing the urine.
- Ethanol, as a competitive substrate, and fomepizole, a competitive inhibitor of alcohol dehydrogenase, prevent the formation of toxic metabolites of ethylene glycol and methanol. Fomepizole is preferred over ethanol given its erratic pharmacokinetics and complications associated with ethanol use.
- Treatment with medications and/or hemodialysis is continued until the methanol or ethylene glycol concentration is < 20 mg/dl.
- Ethanol:
  - Target ethanol concentration is 100-200 mg/dl requiring close monitoring
  - Loading dose: 800 mg/kg in a 10% vol/vol solution of D5W which will raise serum ethanol by 100 mg/dl
  - Maintenance dose: infusion of 80-160 mg/kg/hr based on the levels
- Fomepizole: preferred antidote
- Indications for fomepizole use:
  - Plasma concentration of methanol or ethylene glycol >20 mg/dl OR
  - Documented ingestion with an osmolal gap >10 mOsm/L OR
  - Suspected ingestion with at least three of the following criteria:
  - Arterial pH <7.3
  - Serum bicarbonate <20 mEq/L
  - Osmolal gap >10 mOsm/L
- Urinary oxalate crystals in the case of ethylene glycol toxicity
- Fomepizole dosing:
  - Loading dose: 15 mg/kg
  - Maintenance dose: 10 mg/kg every 12 hr for 4 doses then 15 mg/kg/every 12 hr (if blood levels do not reach goal by 48 hr). The plasma fomepizole concentration that is required to inhibit alcohol dehydrogenase is approximately 0.8 mcg/ml (10 mmol/L).
  - During hemodialysis: Add 1 to 1.5 mg/kg per hr
- Hemodialysis:
  - It should be considered in patients with significant metabolic acidosis (pH <7.25-7.30), renal failure, visual abnormalities, electrolyte imbalances refractory to pharmacologic treatments, hemodynamic instability, and serum concentrations >50 mg/dl.
- Duration of hemodialysis can be estimated using the formula: Time (hr) = $-V \ln(5/A)/0.06\ k$, where V is the Watson estimate of

total body water (in liters); A is the initial alcohol concentration (in mmol/L); and k is 80% of the manufacturer's specified urea clearance (in ml/min). Average duration of dialysis in studies was 8.4 ± 3.2 hr.

ADJUNCTIVE Rx

- Sodium bicarbonate is indicated if the serum pH falls below 7.3 as acidosis promotes penetration of toxic metabolites into end organ tissues.
- In cases of ethylene glycol poisoning, thiamine and pyridoxine may decrease oxalic acid formation and shift metabolism to less toxic metabolites.
- Folinic acid at doses of 1 mg/kg given intravenously every 4 to 6 hr may be used to increase the metabolism of formic acid in methanol overdose.
- Correct electrolyte imbalance.

DISPOSITION

Transfer to a hospital with intensive care and hemodialysis capability should be considered early in the patient's course.

REFERRAL

- Regional poison center (toxicologist) and nephrology recommended to avoid treatment delays
- Ophthalmology for patients with visual symptoms
- Psychiatry if depression and suicidal ideation
- Detoxification centers

PROGNOSIS

- Coma or seizures at presentation and prolonged severe acidosis correlated with increased mortality

 PEARLS & CONSIDERATIONS

- The metabolites of methanol and ethylene glycol cause clinical toxicity rather than the agents themselves.
- Complaints of visual blurring, central scotomata, and blindness suggest methanol poisoning.
- Calcium oxalate crystalluria, oliguria, and hematuria suggest ethylene glycol poisoning.

- Profound anion gap metabolic acidosis with elevated plasma osmolal gap is the vital clue to diagnosis in an appropriate clinical setting.
- Fomepizole is favored over ethanol due to complications associated with ethanol use.
- Emergent hemodialysis is indicated in the setting of end organ damage and severe metabolic acidosis.

 EVIDENCE

available at www.expertconsult.com

SUGGESTED READINGS

available at www.expertconsult.com

RELATED CONTENT

Fig. 3-142 Algorithm for the management of acute poisoning (Algorithm)

AUTHORS: **ANDREEA POENARIU, M.D.,** and **SUSIE L. HU, M.D.**

M

Diseases and Disorders

I

BASIC INFORMATION

DEFINITION

Methicillin-resistant *Staphylococcus aureus* (MRSA) is a common bacterial pathogen with resistance to many antibiotics. It is defined as a *S. aureus* that shows a minimum inhibitory concentration (MIC) of greater than or equal to 4 mcg/ml to oxacillin. There are now two types of MRSA:
- HA-MRSA: hospital-acquired MRSA, usually multidrug resistant
- CA-MRSA: community-acquired MRSA; an emerging pathogen, usually acquired outside of the hospital setting; resistance may differ from HA-MRSA and is generally susceptible to more antibiotics than HA-MRSA

SYNONYMS

Multidrug-resistant *Staphylococcus aureus*
Oxacillin-resistant *Staphylococcus aureus*

ICD-9CM CODES
041.12 Methicillin-resistant *Staphylococcus aureus* in conditions classified elsewhere and of unspecified site

EPIDEMIOLOGY & DEMOGRAPHICS

INCIDENCE: 1:3000
PEAK INCIDENCE: Occurs year round; may peak during summer and fall months for CA-MRSA
PREVALENCE: The national rate of MRSA colonization or infection is 46.3 per 10,000 inpatients. Hospital prevalence rate of MRSA is as high as 60% in hospitals, which means that 60% of *S. aureus* strains in that hospital will be MRSA.
PREDOMINANT SEX AND AGE: All ages and both sexes
GENETICS: NA
RISK FACTORS:
- HA-MRSA: hospitalization; invasive medical device; residing in long-term nursing facility
- CA-MRSA: initially seen in young men engaged in athletic activities and in gyms, prisons, military barracks, etc., but has now spread to the entire age spectrum including neonates and the elderly.

PHYSICAL FINDINGS & CLINICAL PRESENTATION

- CA-MRSA: can present with skin infection, associated with opening in the skin; red bump, pustule, or boil; erythema, swelling; edema, often fluctuant and very painful
- HA-MRSA: bacteremia; infection associated with intravenous device
  - Catheters: pneumonia
  - Skin: cellulitis
  - Bone: osteomyelitis
  - Endocarditis
  - Abscesses: skin or organ
  - Pneumonia: nosocomial

ETIOLOGY

- CA-MRSA: the most prevalent strain in the US on pulse field electrophoresis (PFGE) is called USA 300
  - CA-MRSA: common cause of skin and soft tissue infections in the emergency room. It can, however, also cause necrotizing pneumonia, sepsis, osteomyelitis, etc.
  - Virulence factors particular to CA-MRSA: Panton-Valentine leukocidin (PVL) toxin, alpha-hemolysin toxin, phenol soluble modulins, etc., that enhance ability to cause infection
- HA-MRSA: most strains on PFGE are USA 100 or USA 200 and tend to have multidrug resistance. Patients with HA-MRSA infection have higher mortality and morbidity than patients with a methicillin-sensitive *S. aureus* (MSSA) infection.

DIAGNOSIS

DIFFERENTIAL DIAGNOSIS

- Skin: spider bite (many patients with CA-MRSA feel as if they were bitten by a spider)
- Cellulitis: other organism(s) such as streptococci and methicillin-sensitive *S. aureus* (MSSA)
- Pneumonia: not due to MRSA
- Bacteria: not due to MRSA

WORKUP

- Culture of wound, abscess, blood, sputum; rule out colonization; culture of nares or axillae

LABORATORY TESTS

- See above.
- PFGE: usually done only for epidemiologic or outbreak purposes.

IMAGING STUDIES

- Radiographs or computed tomography scan of suspected organ
- Echocardiogram if endocarditis suspected

TREATMENT

- CA-MRSA: oral antibiotics that may be effective include trimethoprim-sulfamethoxazole, doxycycline, minocycline, or clindamycin; linezolid is another option but very expensive.
- HA-MRSA: intravenous antibiotics, vancomycin, linezolid, daptomycin, tigecycline

NONPHARMACOLOGIC THERAPY

Abscess surgically drained

ACUTE GENERAL Rx

- Trimethoprim-sulfamethoxazole, one double-strength tablet PO bid, is useful in cases of CA-MRSA since 95% of community-acquired MRSA strains are susceptible to it in vitro. Other agents that can be used for CA-MRSA include:
  1. Clindamycin: 300 to 450 mg q6-8h also inhibits toxin production. If strain tests

sensitive to clindamycin but resistant to erythromycin, then a D test must be done to ensure there will not be inducible resistance while on therapy with the clindamycin.
  2. Doxycycline: 100 mg PO q12h and minocycline also have some activity against MRSA.
  3. Rifampin: never used alone but can be used with one of the other oral agents
- Vancomycin 15-20 mg/kg IV q8 to 12h is the mainstay of parenteral therapy for MRSA infections. There is an increasing concern of MRSA strains developing tolerance to vancomycin, requiring higher doses to achieve eradication. True vancomycin resistant strains (MIC ≥32 mg/L) remain rare. Vancomycin trough levels of at least 15 to 20 mcg/ml are recommended to treat MRSA infections.
- Linezolid 600 mg PO or IV bid is a synthetic oxazolidinone FDA-approved for MRSA skin and soft tissue infections and pneumonia. It has been shown to be more effective than vancomycin for MRSA pneumonia. However, its cost is more than 10 times as much as vancomycin.
- Daptomycin: 4 mg/kg/day to 6 mg/kg/day IV is approved for skin and soft tissue infections, bacteremia and right sided endocarditis but should not be used for pneumonia as is inactivated by pulmonary surfactant.
- Tigecycline: 100 mg IV load, then 50 mg IV q12h, is approved for MRSA skin and soft tissue infections and intraabdominal abscess.
- Ceftaroline is a fifth-generation cephalosporin, also effective against MRSA but only skin and soft tissue infections, not pneumonia: 600 mg IV q12h.

CHRONIC Rx

- Patients with MRSA colonization may have reexposure or may be unable to eradicate colonized state.
- Oral agents used to attempt eradication of colonization are rifampin, tetracycline, and minocycline.

COMPLEMENTARY & ALTERNATIVE MEDICINE

- Mupirocin ointment may be administered to the nares to attempt to decolonize; it can also be applied to infected skin sites.
- Chlorhexidine 2% or 4% wash may be used to lower skin burden of colonization.

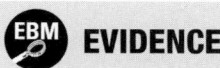 **EVIDENCE**

available at www.expertconsult.com

SUGGESTED READINGS
available at www.expertconsult.com

AUTHOR: **GLENN G. FORT, M.D., M.P.H.**

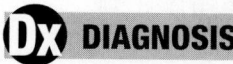 **BASIC INFORMATION**

DEFINITION

Significant cognitive impairment in the absence of dementia with preserved activities of daily living (ADLs). Mild cognitive impairment (MCI) can also be thought of as an intermediate state between normal cognitive function and dementia.

SYNONYMS

Minimal dementia
Isolated short-term memory loss
Cognitive impairment not dementia (CIND)
Predementia
Dementia prodrome

ICD-9CM CODES
331.83 Mild cognitive impairment, so stated
ICD-10CM CODES
F06.7

EPIDEMIOLOGY & DEMOGRAPHICS

INCIDENCE:
- 12 to 15 cases per 1000 person-yr age ≥65
- 51 to 77 cases per 1000 person-yr age ≥75

PEAK INCIDENCE: In the elderly
PREVALENCE: 15% to 25% in those older than age 70.
PREDOMINANT SEX AND AGE: Male, age ≥75
GENETICS: *APOE4* genotype
- Various pathways result in amyloid accumulation and deposition.

RISK FACTORS: Male sex, age, lower socioeconomic status, lower educational level

CLINICAL PRESENTATION

- Subjective memory problems, preferably corroborated by another person.
- Preserved functional status (ADLs).
- Normal general thinking and reasoning skills.
- Subtypes of MCI include amnestic (mainly involves memory loss) vs. nonamnestic with involvement of other cognitive domains (single domain vs. multiple domains).
- Domains affected in MCI include memory, visuospatial skills, language, attention, and executive function.

ETIOLOGY

Neurodegenerative, vascular, traumatic, depression, or due to underlying medical condition

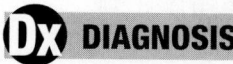 **DIAGNOSIS**

DIFFERENTIAL DIAGNOSIS

- Delirium
- Dementia
- Depression
- "Reversible" cognitive impairment:
  - Medication related (anticholinergics)
  - Hypothyroidism
  - Vitamin B$_{12}$ deficiency
- Reversible CNS conditions
  - Subdural hematoma
  - Normal pressure hydrocephalus
  - Metastatic disease

WORKUP

History

- Focus on cognitive deficits and impairment.
- Review all medications that may impact cognition (i.e., anticholinergics).
- Rule out depression and delirium.
- Perform functional assessment.

Physical exam
- Check blood pressure
- Neurologic exam to rule out reversible CNS causes of cognitive impairment

Cognitive function testing:
Brief mental status testing using MMSE (Mini-Mental Status Exam), MOCA (Montreal Cognitive Assessment), or SLUMS (Saint Louis University Mental Status) for office screening followed by neuropsychological testing if appropriate for specific deficits in cognitive domains.

LABORATORY TESTS

- Complete blood count
- Comprehensive metabolic profile
- TSH
- Vitamin B$_{12}$
- Lipids
- Vitamin D level

IMAGING STUDIES

- CT imaging can detect most reversible CNS conditions leading to cognitive impairment.
- MRI further evaluates vascular, infectious, neoplastic, and inflammatory conditions.

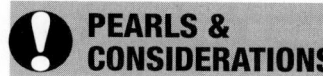 **TREATMENT**

- There is insufficient evidence to recommend use of cholinesterase inhibitors (Table 1-277) for MCI. They are not approved for treating MCI, have shown little efficacy in altering progression to dementia, and can have significant side effects.
- Consider treatment with these medications only if memory complaints appear to be affecting day-to-day quality of life in individual patients or in amnestic subtypes of MCI.

NONPHARMACOLOGIC THERAPY

- Role of cognitive rehabilitation to target specific deficits
- Caregiver education and counseling
- Physical and mental exercises to maintain cognition should be recommended

COMPLEMENTARY & ALTERNATIVE MEDICINE

No clear indications for antioxidants, and studies in humans are inconclusive.

DISPOSITION

- Progression to Alzheimer's at the rate of 5% to 15% per year

- Risk factors for progression to dementia include presence of vascular risk factors, significant cognitive impairment, depression, and presence of extrapyramidal signs.
- Mortality of those with MCI is twice that of those without MCI.
- Two- to threefold increase in risk of nursing home placement in those with MCI.

REFERRAL

Consider referral to a memory specialist if more than just memory is involved or for further evaluation of specific deficits.

(!) PEARLS & CONSIDERATIONS

COMMENTS

Patients with MCI usually report short-term memory concerns such as misplacing things, not remembering names of people, word-finding difficulties, forgetting day-to-day tasks, not being able to read a book, or not being able to follow a conversation.

MCI becomes clinically relevant when quality of life is affected such as problems making financial decisions and problems with personal day-to-day interactions.

Depression should be ruled out prior to making a diagnosis of MCI since it is highly prevalent in the elderly.

Anticholinergic medication use should be evaluated carefully prior to making a diagnosis of MCI.

PREVENTION

Patients with MCI should be counseled on strategies to prevent progression to dementia. They should remain physically and mentally active, have a well-balanced diet, continue activities that are socially engaging, reduce stress in their lives, and aggressively pursue treatment of vascular risk factors.

PATIENT & FAMILY EDUCATION

- Patients with MCI typically have poor retention and rapid loss of newly learned information.
- For additional information for patients, families, and clinicians: Alzheimer's Association (www.alzheimers.org)

SUGGESTED READINGS
available at www.expertconsult.com

AUTHORS: **BIRJU B. PATEL, M.D., F.A.C.P.,** and **N. WILSON HOLLAND, M.D., F.A.C.P.**

TABLE 1-277 Characteristics and Properties of Cholinesterase Inhibitors

Drug Name	Starting Dose	Maintenance Dose	Serum Half-life	Taken with Food?	Elimination
Donepezil	5 mg	10 mg	70 hr	+/−	Hepatic
Rivastigmine pill	1.5 mg bid	6 mg bid	2-8 hr	+	Hepatic
Rivastigmine patch	4.6 mg/24 hr	9.5 mg/24 hr	N/A	N/A	Hepatic
Galantamine	4 mg bid or 8 mg SA daily	12 mg bid or 24 mg SA daily	6-8 hr	+	Hepatic and renal

Adapted from *Physicians' desk reference*, ed 62, Montvale, NJ, 2008, Thomson PDR.

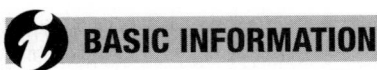

DEFINITION

Mitral regurgitation (MR) is retrograde blood flow into the left atrium resulting from an incompetent mitral valve. This condition can lead to left ventricular (LV) failure as well as increased left atrial and pulmonary pressures, with consequent right heart failure.

SYNONYMS

Mitral insufficiency

ICD-9CM CODES
424.0 Mitral regurgitation

EPIDEMIOLOGY & DEMOGRAPHICS

The incidence of MR has increased over the past 30 yr; however, this may be due to increasing availability of echocardiography and MR diagnosis rather than any real increase in the prevalence of this condition.

PHYSICAL FINDINGS & CLINICAL PRESENTATION

- Holosystolic, high-pitched, "blowing" murmur at apex with radiation to base, left axilla, or back; there is a poor correlation between the intensity of the systolic murmur and the degree of regurgitation. However, an early diastolic to mid-diastolic rumble (pseudo-mitral stenosis) suggests severe MR.
- The murmur of acute MR (e.g., from papillary muscle rupture) can be very soft or inaudible due to a large regurgitant volume entering a noncompliant left atrium, leading to an acute rise in left atrial pressure and thus lack of significant gradient for an audible murmur.
- Hyperdynamic apex, sometimes with palpable LV lift and apical thrill.
- Many patients with mild to moderate MR will remain asymptomatic and without evidence of hemodynamic compromise for years.
- Symptomatic patients with MR generally present with the following:
  ○ Symptoms suggestive of heart failure (fatigue, dyspnea, orthopnea, paroxysmal nocturnal dyspnea, edema)
  ○ Hemoptysis (caused by pulmonary hypertension)
  ○ Atrial fibrillation

ETIOLOGY

- Idiopathic myxomatous degeneration of the mitral valve, mitral valve prolapse (most common cause of MR in industrialized countries)
- Papillary muscle dysfunction or rupture (typically as a result of an inferior wall myocardial infarction)
- Ruptured chordae tendineae
- Infective endocarditis
- Calcified mitral valve annulus
- LV dilation (e.g., secondary to dilated cardiomyopathy)
- Rheumatic valvulitis (may be combined with mitral stenosis; common in Third World countries)

- Hypertrophic cardiomyopathy
- Systemic lupus erythematosus (Libman-Sacks endocarditis)
- Drugs: fenfluramine, dexfenfluramine, pergolide, cabergoline

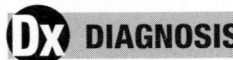

DIFFERENTIAL DIAGNOSIS

- Hypertrophic cardiomyopathy
- Tricuspid regurgitation
- Aortic stenosis
- Aortic sclerosis
- Ventricular septal defect
- Atrial septal defect

WORKUP

- Diagnostic workup consists of echocardiography, ECG, and chest radiograph; cardiac catheterization sometimes needed to confirm severity of the disease.
- Recent studies suggest that in patients with severe asymptomatic MR and normal LV function, elevations of brain natriuretic peptide (BNP) >105 pg/ml have an independent and additive prognostic value that may identify patients at high risk and aid in the selection of patients for early surgery.

IMAGING STUDIES

- Echocardiography (Fig. 1-536): dilated left atrium, hyperdynamic left ventricle (erratic motion of the leaflet is seen in patients with ruptured chordae tendineae); color flow Doppler will show evidence of MR. The most important aspect of the echocardiographic examination is the quantification of the severity of MR (Table 1-279), LV systolic performance, and estimated right ventricular (RV) systolic pressure.
- Chest x-ray:
  ○ Left atrial enlargement, LV enlargement
  ○ Possible pulmonary congestion, although most often normal
- ECG:
  ○ Left atrial enlargement
  ○ LV hypertrophy
  ○ Atrial fibrillation
- Cardiac catheterization: to confirm severity of MR, or to rule out presence of coronary artery disease in patients being evaluated for surgical replacement

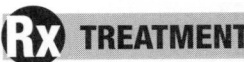

NONPHARMACOLOGIC THERAPY

Salt restriction

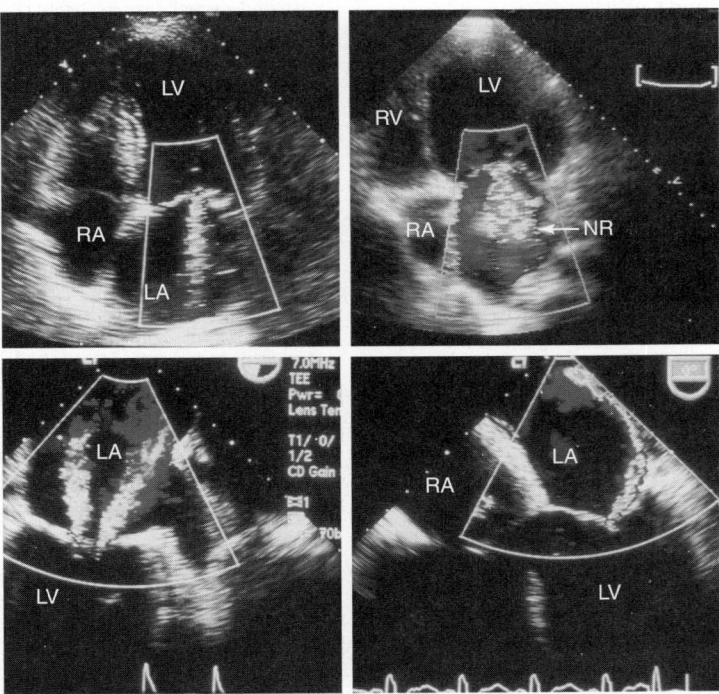

FIGURE 1-536 Mitral regurgitation. Four panels depicting varying degrees of mitral regurgitation; the two *top panels* are apical four-chamber transthoracic views showing, on the *left,* mild mitral regurgitation and, on the *right,* moderate to severe mitral regurgitation. On the *left,* note the relatively narrow jet directed from the tips of the mitral valve toward the posterior left atrial wall. On the right, note the larger jet, filling approximately 40 percent of the left atrial cavity. The two *bottom panels* are transesophageal echocardiograms. On the *left,* note the mitral regurgitation occurring in two discrete jets and, on the *right,* the highly eccentric jet, which courses along the extreme lateral wall of the left atrium. *LA,* Left atrium; *LV,* left ventricle; *RA,* right atrium; *RV,* right ventricle. (From Zipes DP et al [eds]: *Braunwald's heart disease,* ed 7, Philadelphia, 2005, Saunders.)

ACUTE GENERAL Rx

- Medical: medical therapy is primarily directed toward treatment of the source or its complications (e.g., atrial fibrillation, ischemic heart disease, infective endocarditis, and heart failure).
  - The utility of afterload reduction (to decrease the regurgitant fraction and to increase cardiac output) depends upon the etiology of MR and the administration of afterload reducers. In acute MR, intravenous nitroprusside has shown some utility. Long-term use of oral afterload reducers (e.g., ACE inhibitors or angiotensin receptor blockers [ARBs]) has shown mixed results in small studies but may be given if another indication for their use exists (hypertension, LV dysfunction, diabetes).
  - Control ventricular response only if atrial fibrillation with rapid ventricular response is present.
  - Anticoagulants if atrial fibrillation occurs.
- Surgery: surgery is the only definitive treatment for MR. Transesophageal echocardiography allows accurate assessment of the feasibility of valve repair and is indicated before surgical intervention. The timing of surgical repair varies. In general, surgery is indicated in:
  - Acute severe MR
  - Symptomatic patients with severe MR despite optimal medical therapy
  - Asymptomatic patients with severe MR but with evidence of declining LV function (EF <60%) or progressive dilation (LV at end-systole >40 mm)
- In addition, surgery is reasonable in:
  - Severe MR with new onset atrial fibrillation, even if asymptomatic
  - Asymptomatic severe MR with pulmonary hypertension (≥50 mm Hg at rest or ≥60 mm Hg during exercise)

- Finally, mitral valve repair, as opposed to replacement, is recommended in the following two instances:
  - Symptomatic severe MR with severe LV dysfunction or dilatation (LVEF <30% or LV at end-systole >55 mm, respectively) in whom LV dysfunction is not the primary cause for the MR (as opposed to the other way around)
  - Asymptomatic severe MR with preserved LVEF (>60%) and size (<40 mm in end-systole) in whom the likelihood of successful repair without residual MR is >90%
- Quantitative grading of MR is a powerful predictor of the clinical outcome of asymptomatic MR. In general, patients with regurgitant orifice areas of ≥40 mm^2 should be considered for prompt surgery, whereas those with orifices between 20 and 39 mm^2 can be followed closely
- Percutaneous mitral valve repair methods are currently being investigated. Early data has not demonstrated as significant efficacy in MR reduction compared to surgical replacement; however, it has been shown to improve NYHA functional class and quality of life measures.

DISPOSITION

Prognosis is generally good unless there is significant impairment of left ventricular function or significantly elevated pulmonary artery pressures. Most patients remain asymptomatic for many years (average interval from diagnosis to onset of symptoms is 16 yr). In patients with chronic severe MR, MR is commonly progressive, with onset of other symptoms or left ventricular dysfunction within 6-10 yr.

REFERRAL

- Surgical referral in selected patients (see "Acute General Rx"). Emergency surgery is usually necessary in patients with acute MR caused by ruptured papillary muscle or chordae tendineae after myocardial infarction.
- Mitral valve repair can also be accomplished with an investigational procedure that involves the percutaneous implantation of a clip that grasps and approximates the edges of the mitral leaflets at the origin of the regurgitant jet. Preliminary data reveals that although percutaneous repair is less effective at reducing MR than conventional surgery, the procedure is associated with superior safety and similar improvements in clinical outcomes.

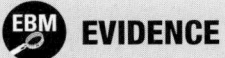 **PEARLS & CONSIDERATIONS**

COMMENTS

- Patients should be counseled regarding weight reduction (if obese), avoidance of tobacco, and maintenance of normal (nonstrenuous) activities.
- In 2007, the AHA guidelines for prevention of infectious endocarditis were revised and routine antibiotic prophylaxis to undergo dental or other invasive procedures is no longer recommended, unless the patient has prior endocarditis.

EBM **EVIDENCE**

available at www.expertconsult.com

SUGGESTED READINGS
available at www.expertconsult.com

RELATED CONTENT
Mitral Regurgitation (Patient Information)

AUTHORS: **NEIL M. GHEEWALA, M.D., DAVID J. FORTUNATO, M.D., F.A.C.C.,** and **FRED F. FERRI, M.D.**

TABLE 1-279 **Mitral Regurgitation Severity***

	(Mild)	II	III	IV (Severe)
MR = jet (%LA)	<15	15-30	35-50	>50
Spectral Doppler	Faint	—	—	Dense
Vena contracta	<3 mm	—	—	>6 mm
Pulmonary vein flow	S > D	—	—	Systolic reversed
RV (ml)	<30	30-44	45-59	≥60
ERO (cm^2)	<0.2	0.2-0.29	0.3-0.39	≥0.40
PISA	Small	—	—	Large

D, Antegrade flow in diastole; ERO, effective regurgitant orifice; %LA, percentage of left atrial area encompassed by the MR jet with color flow Doppler; MR, mitral regurgitation; PISA, proximal isovelocity surface area; RV, regurgitant volume; S, antegrade flow in systole.
*For some parameters, the observation is valid at the extremes of MR severity and there may be marked overlap in intermediate (grades II, III) MR. In these instances, no value is presented.
From Zipes DP et al (eds): *Braunwald's heart disease,* ed 7, Philadelphia, 2005, Saunders.

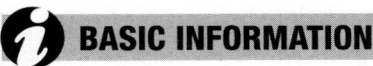

DEFINITION

Mitral stenosis is a narrowing of the mitral valve orifice that prevents proper opening during diastole. Due to thickening of the leaflets there is restricted movement. The cross section of a normal orifice measures 4 to 6 cm^2. Symptoms usually develop with exercise when the orifice measures <2.5 cm^2, and symptoms may develop at rest when the orifice is <1.5 cm^2.

SYNONYMS

MS

ICD-9CM CODES
394.0 Mitral stenosis

EPIDEMIOLOGY & DEMOGRAPHICS

- The predominant cause of mitral stenosis is rheumatic heart disease; however, the occurrence of mitral valve stenosis has decreased worldwide over the past 30 yr (particularly in developed countries) as a result of declining incidence of rheumatic fever.
- The incidence of MS is higher in women (2:1 female-to-male ratio).

PHYSICAL FINDINGS & CLINICAL PRESENTATION

- Dyspnea is the most common symptom along with fatigue and decreased exercise capacity. These occur secondary to an inability to increase cardiac output and elevated pulmonary capillary pressures.
- "Mitral facies" which are pinkish-purple patches on the cheek due to low cardiac output and vasoconstriction, usually indicate severe MS.
- Paroxysmal nocturnal dyspnea (PND) and orthopnea secondary to elevated left atrial pressure may occur.
- Acute pulmonary edema may occur after an increase in flow across the mitral valve secondary to an increase in cardiac output or heart rate (exertion, tachyarrhythmias, fever, anemia).
- Pulmonary hypertension can lead to right ventricular (RV) dysfunction and signs and symptoms of right heart failure (hepatomegaly, pulsatile liver, peripheral edema, ascites).
- Hemoptysis can be present secondary to pulmonary capillary vessel rupture or pulmonary vascular congestion.
- Systemic embolic events are caused by left atrial thrombi. These are associated with atrial fibrillation 80% of the time.
- Chest pain can be caused by RV pressure overload and/or concomitant coronary artery disease in up to 15% of patients.
- Irregularly irregular pulse caused by atrial fibrillation.
- Signs of left and subsequently right heart failure.
- Loud first heart sound (S_1) caused by delayed valve closure and rapid rising left ventricular (LV) pressure.
- A low-pitched rumbling diastolic murmur heard best at the apex. The intensity of the murmur is not related to the severity of the stenosis, but the duration is holodiastolic in severe MS.
- An opening snap (OS) caused by tensing of the valve leaflets after the cusps have opened completely. The OS follows S_2 by 0.03 to 0.14 sec, and the shorter the S_2-OS interval, the more severe the MS, due to higher left atrial pressures.
- Prominent A wave on the venous pulse of patients in normal sinus rhythm.
- A diastolic thrill may be palpable at the apex, especially with the patient in the left lateral recumbent position.
- An RV lift may be palpable at the left sternal border secondary to RV hypertrophy and pulmonary hypertension.
- An accentuated P_2 and/or a soft, early diastolic decrescendo murmur *(Graham Steell murmur)* caused by pulmonary regurgitation may be present in patients with pulmonary hypertension.
- Hoarseness due to the enlargement of the left atrium compressing the recurrent laryngeal nerve.

ETIOLOGY

- Rheumatic fever (RF) is the predominant cause of MS. RF causes thickening of the leaflet edges, commissure fusion, and chordal shortening and fusion.
- Congenital defect (parachute valve) has the usual two mitral leaflets, but the chordae, instead of diverging to insert into two papillary muscles, converge into one major papillary muscle, which allows little mobility of the leaflets, cor triatriatum in which there is a thin membrane which obstructs the pulmonary vein flow and simulates mitral stenosis.
- Rare causes are severe mitral annular calcification, endomyocardial fibroelastosis, malignant carcinoid syndrome, systemic lupus erythematosus, Whipple disease, Fabry disease, and rheumatoid arthritis.
- Medications: methysergide

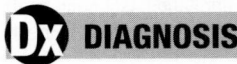

DIFFERENTIAL DIAGNOSIS

- Left atrial myxoma
- Ball valve thrombus
- Other valvular abnormalities (e.g., tricuspid stenosis, mitral regurgitation)
- Atrial septal defect

WORKUP

Physical examination and echocardiography

IMAGING STUDIES

- Echocardiography (Fig. 1-537):
  - Two-dimensional echocardiogram can measure valve area by direct planimetry or calculate it by the Doppler pressure half-time method (this may be inaccurate in patients with concomitant diastolic dysfunction or aortic insufficiency and in patients who have recently undergone mitral valvuloplasty) or the continuity equation. The transmitral gradient can also be calculated. A mean gradient of >10 mm Hg indicates severe MS.
  - Echocardiography will also show a markedly diminished E-to-F slope of the anterior mitral valve leaflet during diastole; there is also fusion of the commissures, resulting in "doming" of the leaflets during diastole.
  - Grading of leaflet thickness, mobility, calcification, and subvalvular thickening; involvement with a score of 0 to 4 for each characteristic can predict hemodynamic results and outcome of balloon mitral valvuloplasty (a low score of less than 8 is favorable for balloon valvuloplasty and a high score is unfavorable).

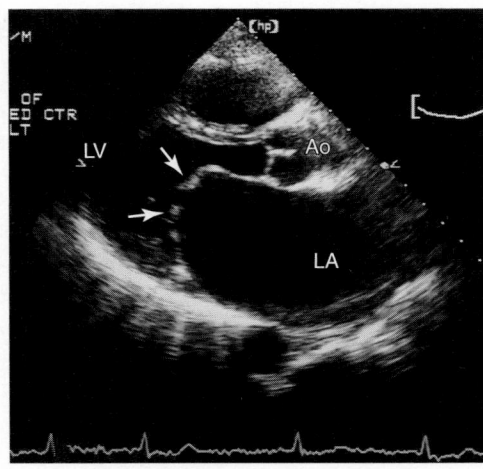

FIGURE 1-537 Mitral stenosis. Parasternal long-axis view of a patient with mitral stenosis and a pliable noncalcified mitral valve leaflet. Note the "doming" motion of the mitral valve leaflets *(arrows)*. Valves with these morphologic features are excellent candidates for percutaneous balloon valvotomy. *Ao,* Aorta; *LA,* left atrium; *LV,* left ventricle. (From Zipes DP et al [eds]: *Braunwald's heart disease,* ed 7, Philadelphia, 2005, Saunders.)

- Doppler echocardiography can be used to assess for pulmonary hypertension and to give an estimate of the pulmonary artery pressure.
- Chest radiograph:
  - Straightening of the left cardiac border caused by dilated left atrium
  - Left atrial enlargement on lateral chest radiograph
  - Prominence of pulmonary arteries
  - Possible pulmonary congestion and edema (Kerley B lines)
- ECG:
  - RV hypertrophy; right axis deviation caused by pulmonary hypertension
  - Left atrial enlargement (broad, notched P waves and duration >0.12 sec in lead II)
  - Atrial fibrillation
- Cardiac catheterization:
  - Allows the measurement of pulmonary artery pressure and transmitral pressure gradients at rest or with exercise (supine biking or raising weights with arms while lying supine).
  - Allows the measurement of transmitral flow and calculation of the valve area.
  - Is not routinely recommended for the evaluation of MS but is useful when the echocardiographic findings are nondiagnostic or discrepant with the clinical scenario.

Rx TREATMENT

NONPHARMACOLOGIC THERAPY

Decrease level of activity in symptomatic patients and salt restriction if pulmonary congestion is present.

ACUTE GENERAL Rx

- Medical:
  - Anticoagulation for the prevention of systemic embolic events in patients with MS and:
    1. Atrial fibrillation
    2. Prior embolic event
    3. Documented left atrial thrombus
    4. Severe left atrial enlargement and spontaneous echo contrast indicating stagnant blood flow (class 2b indication)
  - Ventricular rate control (to increase diastolic filling period) with beta- blockers, calcium channel blockers, or digitalis and aggressive treatment of tachyarrhythmias.
  - Treat congestive heart failure with diuretics and sodium restriction.
  - Antibiotic prophylaxis to prevent recurrent rheumatic fever is usually not indicated unless presence of high-risk features such as prior endocarditis, prosthetic heart valves, valvulopathy of the transplanted heart, and certain cases of cyanotic congenital heart disease.
- Table 1-280 summarizes approaches to mechanical relief of mitral stenosis.
- Percutaneous balloon mitral valvotomy (BMV) is the therapy of choice for symptomatic patients with moderate to severe MS (valve area ≤1.5 cm^2) with a favorable valve score, minimal or no mitral regurgitation and no left atrial thrombus. Balloon valvotomy is also indicated in asymptomatic patients with moderate to severe MS that has resulted in

pulmonary artery pressures of 50 mm Hg at rest or 60 mm Hg with exercise. Percutaneous BMV is also considered the procedure of choice in pregnant women with rheumatic MS and in NYHA class 3 to 4 and/or unresponsive to adequate medical treatment. In addition, it is a reasonable option for patients who are at high risk for surgery even when their valve morphology is not ideal (class 2a indication).
- Surgical intervention is indicated for patients with moderate to severe symptomatic MS when BMV is not available or is contraindicated or the valve is calcified and the surgical risk is acceptable. The surgical approaches include closed mitral valvotomy, open valvotomy and repair (preferred) and mitral valve replacement.

DISPOSITION

- Prognosis is generally good except in patients with chronic pulmonary hypertension.
- Operative mortality rates for mitral valve replacement are 1% to 5% at most institutions.

RELATED CONTENT

Mitral Stenosis (Patient Information)

AUTHORS: **ARAVIND RAO KOKKIRALA, M.D., SCOTT COHEN, M.D.,** and **FRED F. FERRI, M.D.**

TABLE 1-280 Approaches to Mechanical Relief of Mitral Stenosis

Approach	Advantages	Disadvantages
Closed surgical valvotomy	Inexpensive Relatively simple Good hemodynamic results in selected patients Good long-term outcome	No direct visualization of valve Only feasible with flexible, noncalcified valves Contraindicated if MR >2+ Surgical procedure with general anesthesia
Open surgical valvotomy	Visualization of valve allows directed valvotomy Concurrent annuloplasty for MR is feasible	Best results with flexible, noncalcified valves Surgical procedure with general anesthesia
Valve replacement	Feasible in all patients regardless of extent of valve calcification or severity of MR	Surgical procedure with general anesthesia Effect of loss of annular-papillary muscle continuity on LV function Prosthetic valve Chronic anticoagulation
Balloon mitral valvotomy	Percutaneous approach Local anesthesia Good hemodynamic results in selected patients Good long-term outcome	No direct visualization of valve Only feasible with flexible, noncalcified valves Contraindicated if MR >2+

LV, Left ventricular; *MR,* mitral regurgitation.
From Otto CM: *Valvular heart disease,* ed 2, Philadelphia, 2004, Saunders.

BASIC INFORMATION

DEFINITION

Mitral valve prolapse (MVP) is the bulging of one or both of the mitral valve leaflets into the left atrium during systole. MVP syndrome refers to a constellation of MVP and associated symptoms (e.g., autonomic dysfunction, palpitations) or other physical abnormalities (e.g., pectus excavatum).

SYNONYMS

MVP
Mitral click murmur syndrome
Barlow's syndrome

ICD-9CM CODES
424.0 Mitral valve disorders
394.9 Other and unspecified mitral valve diseases

EPIDEMIOLOGY & DEMOGRAPHICS

- MVP can be found by two-dimensional echocardiogram in 1% to 4% of the general population (females more often than males).
- Increased incidence is seen with autoimmune thyroid disorders, Ehlers-Danlos syndrome, Marfan's syndrome, pseudoxanthoma elasticum, pectus excavatum, anorexia nervosa, and bulimia.
- Compared to men, women with MVP have less posterior prolapse (22% vs. 31%), less flail (2% vs. 8%), more leaflet thickening (32% vs. 28%), and less frequent severe regurgitation (10% vs. 23%).
- Although MVP is more common in women than men, men more often develop severe regurgitation requiring surgical intervention.

PHYSICAL FINDINGS & CLINICAL PRESENTATION

- Usually, young female patient with narrow anteroposterior chest diameter, low body weight, low blood pressure
- Mid to late systolic click, heard best at the apex
- Crescendo mid to late systolic murmur, may have a "honking" quality
- Timing of click within the cardiac cycle varies with loading conditions within the left ventricle (i.e., may occur earlier with standing or Valsalva and later with squatting or expiration)
- Most patients with MVP are asymptomatic; symptoms (if present) consist primarily of chest pain, palpitations, and anxiety
- Neurologic abnormalities (e.g., transient ischemic attack [TIA] or stroke) are rare
- Patients may also complain of anxiety, fatigue, and dyspnea

ETIOLOGY

- Myxomatous degeneration of connective tissue within mitral valve, usually involving multiple leaflet segments. In contrast, fibroelastic deficiency of single leaflet segment develops in elderly patients.
- Congenital deformity of mitral valve and supportive structures
- Secondary to other disorders of connective tissue such as Ehlers-Danlos, Marfan, or pseudoxanthoma elasticum; association with other connective tissue disorders suggests MVP result of defective embryogenesis in cells of mesenchymal origin

DIAGNOSIS

DIFFERENTIAL DIAGNOSIS

- Other valvular abnormalities (especially mitral regurgitation [MR])
- Anxiety/panic disorders
- Pulmonary embolism
- Atypical chest pain

WORKUP

- Medical history and physical examination, with increased suspicion in patients with other findings of connective tissue disorder.
- Workup consists primarily of echocardiography in patients with a systolic click or murmur on careful auscultation.
- ECG is most often normal but may show nonspecific ST-T wave changes, prolonged QT interval, or prominent Q waves.

IMAGING STUDIES

Echocardiography (Fig. E1-538) shows one or more leaflets prolapsing at least 2 mm into the left atrium during systole. Mitral leaflets may be thickened (>5 mm). MR may or may not be present, and sometimes it is only present during exertion. If moderate or severe MR is present, findings of dilated left atrium, LV dilation and/or dysfunction, and elevated estimated RV systolic pressures may also be present. There is an increased incidence of secundum-type atrial septal defects (ASDs) in patients with MVP, which may also be identified with echocardiography.

TREATMENT

NONPHARMACOLOGIC THERAPY

Avoidance of stimulants (e.g., caffeine, nicotine) in patients with palpitations. Sometimes, reassurance is sufficient to reduce the severity of symptoms in many patients.

ACUTE GENERAL Rx

β-blockers may be tried in symptomatic patients (e.g., palpitations, chest pain); they decrease the heart rate and contractility, thus potentially decreasing the stretch on the prolapsing valve leaflets.

CHRONIC Rx

Monitoring for complications:
- Bacterial endocarditis (risk is three to eight times that of the general population)
- TIA or stroke caused by embolic phenomena (from fibrin and platelet thrombi) in patients with thickened leaflets; risk in young patients is <0.05% per year; if present aspirin (75-325 mg) is indicated for secondary prevention
- Cardiac arrhythmias (the vast majority are supraventricular and benign)
- Sudden death (rare occurrence, most often caused by ventricular arrhythmias associated with other structural heart disease)
- MR (most common complication of MVP, on rare occasion may occur acutely due to rupture of chordae tendineae)

DISPOSITION

The incidence of complications of MVP is very low (<1% per year) and generally associated with an increase in mitral leaflet thickness to >5 mm; young patients (age <45 yr) with absence of mitral systolic murmur or MR on Doppler echocardiography are at low risk for any complications.

REFERRAL

Surgical referral may be necessary in patients who develop progressive MR with surgical indications as per guidelines for valvular heart disease (see MR topic).

PEARLS & CONSIDERATIONS

COMMENTS

- Recent studies suggest that the prevalence of MVP and its propensity to cause symptoms and serious complications have been overestimated in the past.
- Asymptomatic patients with MVP and mild or no MR can be evaluated clinically every 3 to 5 yr. High-risk patients (those with symptoms, arrhythmias, or significant regurgitation) should undergo a follow-up examination once a year.
- In 2007, the AHA guidelines for prevention of infectious endocarditis were revised and prophylactic antibiotics are no longer recommended for patients with MVP without previous endocarditis.

SUGGESTED READINGS

available at www.expertconsult.com

RELATED CONTENT

Mitral Valve Prolapse (Patient Information)

AUTHORS: **ZHE ZHENG, M.D., PH.D., DAVID J. FORTUNATO, M.D., F.A.C.C.,** and **FRED F. FERRI, M.D.**

ⓘ BASIC INFORMATION

DEFINITION

An overlap syndrome with clinical features seen in systemic lupus erythematosus (SLE), polymyositis (PM), and systemic sclerosis (Scl) in association with high titer of anti U1-RNP antibodies, especially to the 68-70 kD epitope. Not all clinical features are present initially, and it usually takes several years before enough overlapping features are present to be confident that mixed connective tissue disease (MCTD) is the most likely diagnosis. Because of the nonspecific signs and symptoms at presentation, most of the patients may be initially classified as having undifferentiated connective tissue disease.

SYNONYMS

MCTD

ICD-9CM CODES
710.9 Diffuse connective tissue disease NOS

EPIDEMIOLOGY & DEMOGRAPHICS

PREVALENCE: Variable by population.
PREDOMINANT SEX: Female/male ratio of 10:1
PREDOMINANT AGE: Age at onset generally in the second or third decade

PHYSICAL FINDINGS & CLINICAL PRESENTATION

- General: exertional dyspnea, malaise, fatigue, fever
- Joints: arthalgias are an early symptom that can evolve to arthritis resembling RA but without severe erosions. Sausage-shaped fingers (Fig. 1-539)
- Skin and mucosas: Raynaud's phenomenon is an early finding. Malar rash, discoid plaques, oral or genital ulcers, sicca symptoms, subcutaneous nodules, abnormal nail fold capillaries can be seen
- Muscle: myalgias, inflammatory myopathy
- Lung: interstitial lung disease leading to pulmonary fibrosis
- Heart: pulmonary hypertension, pericardial effusion (most frequent cardiac manifestation), pericarditis
- Hematopoietic: anemia of chronic disease, lymphopenia, thrombocytopenia
- Gastrointestinal tract: altered motility, mesenteric vasculitis, pancreatitis, hepatitis
- Kidney: membranous glomerulonephritis, diffuse proliferative glomerulonephritis; kidney involvement is uncommon
- Nervous system: trigeminal neuropathy, headache, aseptic meningitis

ETIOLOGY

Autoimmune disorder

ⓓ DIAGNOSIS

DIFFERENTIAL DIAGNOSIS

Other connective tissue disorders (SLE, progressive Scl, PM, infection, malignancy)

WORKUP (Table 1-281)

Alarcon-Segovia: Serologic criterion accompanied by three or more clinical criteria, one of which must be synovitis or myositis (sensitivity 81.3%, specificity 86.2%).

Kahn: Serologic criterion accompanied by Raynaud's phenomenon and at least two of the three remaining clinical criteria.

LABORATORY TESTS

- Positive antinuclear antibody (ANA) speckled pattern >1:1000 to 1:10,000
- U1-RNP antibodies especially to the 68-70 kD antigen (high titers)
- SLE-specific autoantibodies are generally absent.
- Rheumatoid factor positive (50% to 70%)

℞ TREATMENT

- Considered to be a steroid-responsive disease
- Aimed at the specific features of the overlap syndrome
- Arthralgias, arthritis, fatigue, myalgias usually respond to NSAIDs, antimalarials, and/or steroids. Immunosuppressive medications such as methotrexate and azathioprine can also be used
- Keeping warm, avoiding beta- blockers, stopping smoking, and dihydropiridine calcium channel blockers can be used for Raynaud's
- Pulmonary hypertension and lung disease: Therapies include steroids, cyclophosphamide, low-dose aspirin, anticoagulation, ACE inhibitors, endothelin receptor antagonist, IV prostacyclin, cyclic GMP phosphodiesterase type 5 inhibitors like sildenafil, tadalafil, and mycophenolate mofetil.
- Calcium, vitamin D, and bisphosphonates are used for bone health

DISPOSITION

- Patients with high titers of U1-RNP antibodies have low prevalence of serious renal disease and life-threatening neurologic disorders.
- Disease-related mortality is usually related to pulmonary hypertension and its cardiac sequelae.

REFERRAL

Rheumatology consultation for clarification and assistance in treatment

⚠ PEARLS & CONSIDERATIONS

COMMENTS

Pulmonary arterial hypertension (PAH) is diagnosed by cardiac catheterization. It is the main disease-related cause of death. Early detection of PAH and aggressive treatment may improve prognosis.

SUGGESTED READINGS
available at www.expertconsult.com

RELATED CONTENT
Rheumatoid Arthritis (Related Key Topic)
Scleroderma (Systemic Sclerosis) (Related Key Topic)
Systemic Lupus Erythematosus (Related Key Topic)

AUTHOR: **DANIEL E. MENDEZ-ALLWOOD, M.D.**

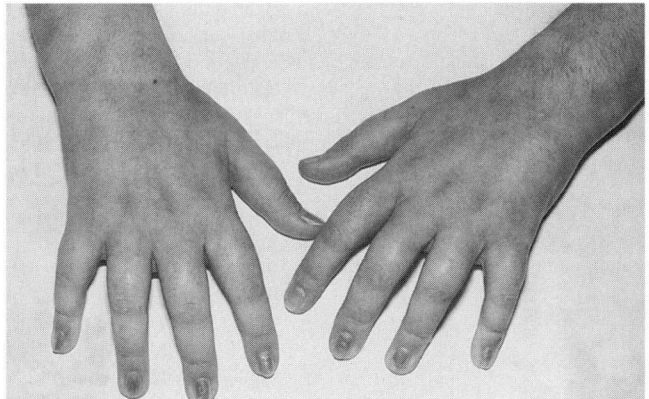

FIGURE 1-539 Sausage-shaped fingers in a patient with mixed connective tissue disease. An identical appearance may be found in patients with early scleroderma and eosinophilic fasciitis. (From Hochberg MC et al: *Rheumatology*, ed 5, St Louis, 2011, Mosby.)

TABLE 1-281 Diagnostic Criteria by Alarcon-Segovia and Kahn

	Alarcon-Segovia Criteria	Kahn Criteria
Serology	Anti-RNP at hemagglutination titer of ≥1:1600	High-titer anti-RNP corresponding to a speckled ANA of ≥1:1200
Clinical	Swollen hands Synovitis Myositis Raynaud's phenomenon Acrosclerosis	Swollen fingers Synovitis Myositis Raynaud's phenomenon

BASIC INFORMATION

DEFINITION

Molar pregnancy is a premalignant gestational disorder. Molar pregnancies are classified as complete or partial based on morphologic and pathologic examination. Both complete and partial molar pregnancies have an abnormal placenta with enlargement and swelling of the chorionic villi and hyperplasia of the villous trophoblastic cells. Most molar pregnancies are complete and are characterized by generalized hydropic villous changes with no fetal tissue. Partial moles are characterized by a mixture of large hydropic villi and normal placental tissue and often have fetal tissue present. The risk of malignant sequelae (gestational trophoblastic neoplasia) for a complete mole is 18% to 29% and for a partial mole is 0% to 11%.

SYNONYMS

Hydatidiform mole
Gestational trophoblastic disease

ICD-9CM CODES
630 Hydatidiform mole

EPIDEMIOLOGY & DEMOGRAPHICS

INCIDENCE: 0.57 to 2/1000 pregnancies with wide regional variation
PREDOMINANT SEX AND AGE: Females of reproductive age, highest rates at extremes of reproductive ages
RISK FACTORS: Extremes of reproductive age (<21 and >40 yr), previous molar pregnancy, history of spontaneous abortion

PHYSICAL FINDINGS & CLINICAL PRESENTATION

Complete molar pregnancy:
- 80% to 90% present with vaginal bleeding at 6 to 16 wk gestational age
- 28% with uterine enlargement greater than expected for gestational age

- 8% with hyperemesis gravidarum
- 1% with gestational hypertension in the first or second trimester
- 15% with bilateral theca lutein cysts
- 15% will have a beta hCG >100,000
Partial molar pregnancy
- 90% present with an incomplete or missed abortion
- 75% present with vaginal bleeding
- <10% will have a beta hCG of >100,000

ETIOLOGY

Complete molar pregnancy
- Fertilization of an oocyte with absent or inactive maternal chromosomes and duplication of paternal chromosomes (90% are 46, XX) or fertilization of an empty oocyte with 2 sperm (46, XY or XX)
- Uniform villous enlargement and no development of a fetus
Partial molar pregnancy
- Fertilization of a normal oocyte with 2 sperm (usually 69, XXY)
- Focal villous edema with identifiable fetus

DIAGNOSIS

DIFFERENTIAL DIAGNOSIS

Complete mole, partial mole, ectopic pregnancy, abortion (incomplete or spontaneous), normal intrauterine pregnancy

WORKUP

- Pelvic exam to evaluate for uterine size and bleeding
- Blood pressure to assess for gestational hypertension or preeclampsia (systolic blood pressure >140 or diastolic blood pressure >90)

LABORATORY TESTS

- Quantitative beta human chorionic growth hormone (beta hCG); significantly elevated levels >100,000 will raise suspicion for molar pregnancy

- Complete blood count (CBC) to assess for acute anemia from vaginal bleeding
- Comprehensive metabolic panel to evaluate for renal or liver disease
- TSH to evaluate for hyperthyroidism
- Urinalysis for proteinuria to evaluate for preeclampsia
- Type and screen to evaluate Rh and to prepare for surgery

IMAGING STUDIES

- Pelvic ultrasound (Fig. 1-540)
  ○ Complete molar pregnancy will show diffuse vesicular changes with no evidence of fetal tissue and may show theca lutein cysts
  ○ Partial molar pregnancy will show focal cystic changes in the placenta and fetal tissue may be present
- Baseline chest x-ray to use for comparison if malignant trophoblastic disease develops

TREATMENT

NONPHARMACOLOGIC THERAPY

Surgical uterine evacuation with dilatation and curettage (D&C)

ACUTE GENERAL Rx

D&C, Rh immune globulin if Rh negative

CHRONIC Rx & DISPOSITION

If pathology results are consistent with complete or partial mole, patients must be followed to evaluate for trophoblastic neoplasia. 15% to 20% of complete moles and 1% to 5% of partial moles will develop into trophoblastic neoplasia. Quantitative beta hCG should be followed weekly until three consecutive results show normal levels. After that, check quantitative beta hCG every 3 mo for a total of 6 mo. Patients should remain on reliable contraception during this time to prevent confusion from a rising beta hCG in the case of a new pregnancy.

REFERRAL

- If there is concern for a molar pregnancy, the patient should be managed by a gynecologist for uterine evacuation and follow-up.
- If there is a plateau or rise of the beta hCG during follow-up, the patient should be referred to a gynecologic oncologist for treatment with chemotherapy.

SUGGESTED READINGS
available at www.expertconsult.com

RELATED CONTENT
Spontaneous Miscarriage (Related Key Topic)
Vaginal Bleeding During Pregnancy (Related Key Topic)

AUTHOR: **LAUREN ROTH, M.D.**

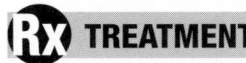

FIGURE 1-540 Endovaginal ultrasound of the theca lutein cyst with early molar pregnancy. Note enlarged anechoic cystic spaces within the ovary *(arrows)*. (From Fielding JR et al: *Gynecology imaging*, Philadelphia, 2011, Saunders.)

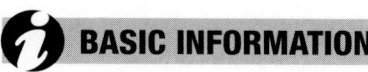

BASIC INFORMATION

DEFINITION

Molluscum contagiosum is a viral infection characterized by discrete skin lesions with central umbilication.

SYNONYMS

MC

ICD-9CM CODES

078.0 Molluscum contagiosum

EPIDEMIOLOGY & DEMOGRAPHICS

- Molluscum contagiosum spreads by autoinoculation, scratching, or touching a lesion.
- It usually occurs in young children. It is also common in sexually active adults and patients with HIV infection.
- Incubation period varies between 4 and 8 wk.
- Spontaneous resolution in immunocompetent patients can occur after several months.

PHYSICAL FINDINGS & CLINICAL PRESENTATION

- The individual lesion appears initially as a small (2-3 mm), flesh-colored, firm, smooth-surfaced papule with subsequent central umbilication. Lesions are frequently grouped (Fig. 1-541). The size of each lesion generally varies from 2 to 6 mm in diameter.
- Typical distribution in children involves the face, extremities, and trunk. Mucous membranes are spared.
- Distribution in adults generally involves pubic and genital areas.
- Erythema and scaling at the periphery of the lesions may be present as a result of scratching or hypersensitivity reaction.
- Lesions are not present on the palms and soles.

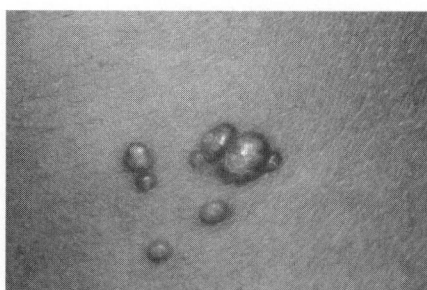

FIGURE 1-541 Grouped molluscum. (From Kliegman RM et al: *Nelson textbook of pediatrics,* ed 19, Philadelphia, 2011, Saunders.)

ETIOLOGY

Viral infection of epithelial cells caused by a poxvirus, molluscum contagiosum

 # DIAGNOSIS

Diagnosis is usually established by the clinical appearance of the lesions (distribution and central umbilication). A magnifying lens can be used to observe the central umbilication. If necessary, the diagnosis can be confirmed by removing a typical lesion with a curette and examining the content on a slide after adding potassium hydroxide and gentle heating. Staining with toluidine blue will identify viral inclusions.

DIFFERENTIAL DIAGNOSIS

- Verruca plana (flat warts): no central umbilication, not dome shaped, irregular surface, can involve palms and soles
- Herpes simplex: lesions become rapidly umbilicated
- Varicella: blisters and vesicles are present
- Folliculitis: no central umbilication, presence of hair piercing the pustule or papule
- Cutaneous cryptococcosis in AIDS patients: budding yeasts will be present on cytologic examination of the lesions
- Basal cell carcinoma: multiple lesions are absent
- Cellulitis

WORKUP

Careful examination of the papules

LABORATORY TESTS

Generally not indicated in children. Screening for other sexually transmitted diseases is recommended in all cases of genital molluscum contagiosum.

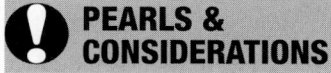 # TREATMENT

GENERAL THERAPY

- Therapy is individualized depending on number of lesions, immune status, and patient's age and preference.
- Observation for spontaneous resolution is reasonable in patients with few, small, nonirritated, and nonspreading lesions. Genital lesions should be treated in all sexually active patients.
- Liquid nitrogen cryotherapy

- Carbon dioxide laser
- Curettage after pretreatment of the area with combination prilocaine 2.5% with lidocaine 2.5% cream (EMLA) for anesthesia is useful for treatment of a few lesions. Curettage should be avoided in cosmetically sensitive areas because scarring may develop.
- Treatments with liquid nitrogen therapy in combination with curettage are effective in older patients who do not object to some discomfort.
- Application of cantharidin 0.7% to individual lesions covered with clear tape will result in blistering over 24 hr and possible clearing without scarring. This medication should be avoided on facial lesions.
- Other treatment measures include use of imiquimod cream or tretinoin 0.025% gel or 0.1% cream at bedtime, daily use of salicylic acid (Occlusal) at bedtime, and use of laser therapy.
- Trichloroacetic acid peel generally repeated every 2 wk for several weeks is useful in immunocompromised patients with extensive lesions.

DISPOSITION

Most patients respond well to the therapeutic modalities listed previously. Spontaneous resolution can occur after 6 to 9 mo in some immunocompetent patients.

REFERRAL

To dermatology when diagnosis is in doubt or in patients with extensive lesions

PEARLS & CONSIDERATIONS

COMMENTS

Genital molluscum contagiosum in children may be indicative of sexual abuse.

RELATED CONTENT

Molluscum Contagiosum (Patient Information)

AUTHOR: **FRED F. FERRI, M.D.**

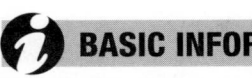
BASIC INFORMATION

DEFINITION

Monoclonal gammopathy of undetermined significance (MGUS) is defined by the presence of a monoclonal protein in persons with no features of multiple myeloma or other malignant gammopathies (Table 1-282). Patients with MGUS have a serum monoclonal protein concentration <3 g/dl, <10% plasma cells on the bone marrow, and no clinical manifestations related to the monoclonal gammopathy.

SYNONYMS

Non-IgM MGUS
IgM MGUS
Light chain MGUS

ICD-9CM CODES
273.1 Monoclonal Gammopathy

EPIDEMIOLOGY & DEMOGRAPHICS

INCIDENCE: The annual incidence of MGUS in men is 120 per 100,000 population at age 50 yr and increases to 530 per 100,000 at age 80 yr. The rates for women are 60 per 100,000 at 50 yr and 370 per 100,000 at 80 yr.
PREVALENCE: Prevalence is higher in blacks than in whites
PREDOMINANT SEX AND AGE: Median age of diagnosis is about 70 yr. Prevalence is higher in men than in women.
RISK FACTORS: Race (African American), older age, male sex, exposure to pesticides and family history of MGUS or multiple myeloma

PHYSICAL FINDINGS & CLINICAL PRESENTATION

- MGUS typically detected after a routine blood test reveals an elevated total protein concentration
- Asymptomatic
- Physical exam is normal

ETIOLOGY

- Unknown mechanism
- Characterized by a rearrangement of immunoglobulin genes that results in the production of a monoclonal protein

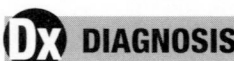
DIAGNOSIS

DIFFERENTIAL DIAGNOSIS

Smoldering myeloma (Table E1-283)
Multiple myeloma
Waldenström's gammaglobulinemia
Secondary monoclonal gammopathies
- Chronic liver disease
- Rheumatologic diseases
- Chronic myelomonocytic leukemia
- Chronic neutrophilic leukemia
- Lichen myxedematosus
Pyoderma gangrenosum

LABORATORY TESTS

Protein studies:
- Serum protein electrophoresis (Fig. 1-542)
  - IgG most common, followed by IgM and IgA
- 24-hour urine protein excretion and urine electrophoresis
- Serum and urine immunofixation
- Determination of serum free light chain ratio (kappa and lambda free light chains)
Hemoglobin
Serum calcium and creatinine
Examination of the bone marrow aspirate

IMAGING STUDIES

- Skeletal survey
- Bone mineral density resting at baseline (MGUS is associated with increased risk of osteoporosis)

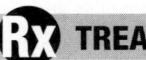
TREATMENT

No formal guidelines for follow-up
Reevaluation annually with:
- Total serum protein–serum electrophoresis
- 24-hour urine protein excretion
- Hemoglobin
- Serum creatinine and calcium
MGUS with low-risk features (IgG type, monoclonal protein <1.5 g/dl and normal light chain ratio) does not need follow-up.

DISPOSITION

- Risk of myeloma at 25 yr is 30%.
- Annual risk of transformation to myeloma is 1% per year after diagnosis.
- Predictors of progression:
  - IgA or IgM monoclonal spike
  - >1.5 g/dl monoclonal protein
  - Abnormal free light chain ratio

REFERRAL

To hematologist/oncologist for evaluation

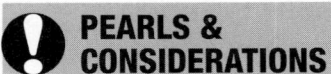
PEARLS & CONSIDERATIONS

- Approximately 55% of 70-yr-old patients diagnosed as having MGUS have had the condition for more than 10 yr.
- Most patients with MGUS should be monitored every 6 to 12 mo for signs and symptoms of progression.
- There is no indicated treatment.

SUGGESTED READINGS

available at www.expertconsult.com

AUTHOR: **KIMBERLY PEREZ, M.D.**

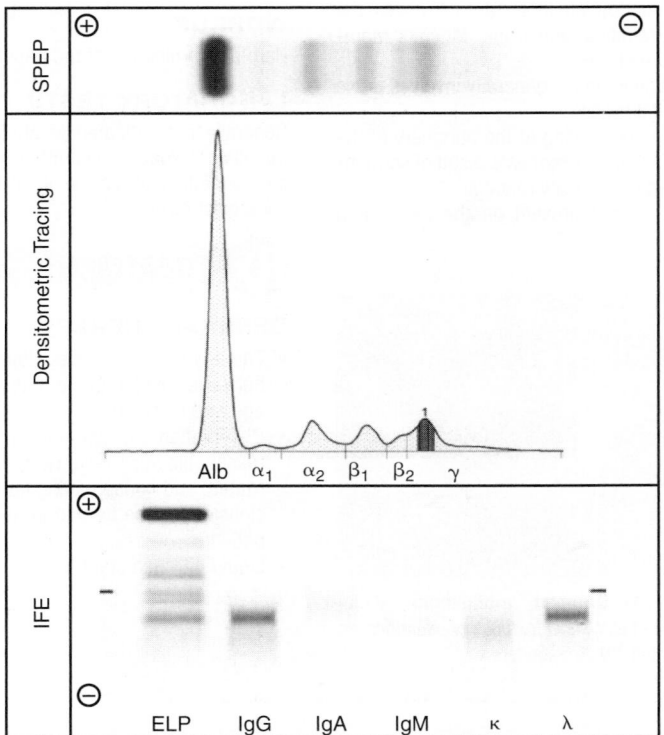

FIGURE 1-542 Serum electrophoresis from a 73-year-old man with monoclonal gammopathy of undetermined significance. The patient has no clinical, hematologic, or imaging evidence of a plasma cell dyscrasia, except for a persistent, modest (0.4 g/dl), single M protein peak on the densitometric tracing *(shaded area, middle panel)* of the serum protein electrophoresis pattern *(SPEP)*. The M protein was identified by immunofixation electrophoresis *(IFE)* as IgGλ, located in the β_2 region of the electrophoresis *(ELP)* pattern. (Courtesy Drs. Frank H. Wians Jr. and Dennis C. Wooten, Department of Pathology, University of Texas Southwestern Medical Center, Dallas. From Jaffe ES et al: *Hematopathology*, Philadelphia, 2011, Saunders.)

TABLE 1-282 Disease Definitions for the Monoclonal Gammopathies: MGUS and Related Disorders

Type of Monoclonal Gammopathy	Premalignancy with a Low Risk of Progression (1%-2% per year)	Premalignancy with a High Risk of Progression (10% per year)	Malignancy

IgG and IgA (non-IgM) monoclonal gammopathies*	**Non-IgM MGUS**
	All 3 criteria must be met:
	• Serum monoclonal protein <3 g/dl
	• Clonal bone marrow plasma cells <10%, and
	• Absence of end-organ damage such as hypercalcemia, renal insufficiency, anemia, and bone lesions (CRAB) that can be attributed to the plasma cell proliferative disorder
		Smoldering multiple myeloma
		Both criteria must be met:
		• Serum monoclonal protein (IgG or IgA) ≥3 g/dl and/or clonal bone marrow plasma cells ≥10%, and
		• Absence of end-organ damage such as lytic bone lesions, anemia, hypercalcemia, or renal failure that can be attributed to a plasma cell proliferative disorder
			Multiple myeloma
			All 3 criteria must be met except as noted:
			• Clonal bone marrow plasma cells ≥10%
			• Presence of serum and/or urinary monoclonal protein (except in patients with true nonsecretory multiple myeloma), and
			• Evidence of end-organ damage that can be attributed to the underlying plasma cell proliferative disorder, specifically
			  ○ Hypercalcemia: serum calcium >11.5 mg/dL or
			  ○ Renal insufficiency: serum creatinine >2 mg/dL or estimated creatinine clearance <40 mL/min
			  ○ Anemia: normochromic, normocytic with a hemoglobin value of >2 g/dL below the lower limit of normal or a hemoglobin value <10 g/dL
			  ○ Bone lesions: lytic lesions or severe osteopenia attributed to a plasma cell proliferative disorder or pathologic fractures

IgM monoclonal gammopathies	**IgM MGUS†** All 3 criteria must be met: • Serum monoclonal protein <3 g/dl • Clonal bone marrow lymphoplasmacytic cells <10%, and • Absence of end-organ damage such as anemia, constitutional symptoms, hyperviscosity, lymphadenopathy, or hepatosplenomegaly that can be attributed to the underlying lymphoproliferative disorder	**Smoldering Waldenström macroglobulinemia** Both criteria must be met: • Serum IgM monoclonal protein ≥3 g/dl and/or bone marrow lymphoplasmacytic infiltration ≥10%, and • No evidence of anemia, constitutional symptoms, hyperviscosity, lymphadenopathy, or hepatosplenomegaly that can be attributed to the underlying lymphoproliferative disorder	**Waldenström macroglobulinemia** All criteria must be met: • IgM monoclonal gammopathy (regardless of the size of the M-protein), and • ≥10% bone marrow lymphoplasmacytic infiltration (usually intertrabecular) by small lymphocytes that exhibit plasmacytoid or plasma cell differentiation and a typical immunophenotype (eg, surface IgM+, CD5+/−, CD10−, CD19+, CD20+, CD23−) that satisfactorily excludes other lymphoproliferative disorders including chronic lymphocytic leukemia and mantle cell lymphoma • Evidence of anemia, constitutional symptoms, hyperviscosity, lymphadenopathy, or hepatosplenomegaly that can be attributed to the underlying lymphoproliferative disorder. **IgM myeloma** All criteria must be met: • Symptomatic monoclonal plasma cell proliferative disorder characterized by a serum IgM monoclonal protein regardless of size • Presence of 10% plasma cells on bone marrow biopsy • Presence of lytic bone lesions related to the underlying plasma cell disorder and/or translocation t(11;14) on fluorescence in situ hybridization.
Light-chain monoclonal gammopathies	**Light-chain MGUS** All criteria must be met: • Abnormal FLC ratio (<0.26 or >1.65) • Increased level of the appropriate involved light-chain (increased kappa FLC in patients with ratio >1.65 and increased lambda FLC in patients with ratio <0.26) • No immunoglobulin heavy-chain expression on immunofixation • Clonal bone marrow plasma cells <10%, and • Absence of end-organ damage such as hypercalcemia, renal insufficiency, anemia, and bone lesions (CRAB) that can be attributed to the plasma cell proliferative disorder	**Idiopathic Bence Jones proteinuria** All criteria must be met: • Urinary monoclonal protein on urine protein electrophoresis ≥500 mg/24 h and/or clonal bone marrow plasma cells ≥10% • No immunoglobulin heavy-chain expression on immunofixation • Absence of end-organ damage such as hypercalcemia, renal insufficiency, anemia, and bone lesions (CRAB) that can be attributed to the plasma cell proliferative disorder	**Light-chain multiple myeloma†** • Same as multiple myeloma except no evidence of immunoglobulin heavy-chain expression

FLC, Free light chain; *MGUS*, monoclonal gammopathy of undetermined significance.
*Occasionally patients with IgD and IgE monoclonal gammopathies have been described and will be considered to be part of this category as well.
†Note that conventionally IgM MGUS is considered a subtype of MGUS, and similarly light-chain multiple myeloma is considered as a subtype of multiple myeloma. Unless specifically distinguished, when the terms MGUS and multiple myeloma are used in general, they include IgM MGUS and light-chain multiple myeloma, respectively.
From Rajkumar SV et al: Advances in the diagnosis, classification, risk stratification, and management of monoclonal gammopathy of undetermined significance: implications for recategorizing disease entities in the presence of evolving scientific evidence, *Mayo Clin Proc* 85(10):945-948, 2010.

M

Diseases
and Disorders

I

BASIC INFORMATION

DEFINITION

Mononucleosis is a symptomatic infection caused by Epstein-Barr virus (EBV) and characterized by fever, tonsillar pharyngitis, and lymphadenopathy.

SYNONYMS

Infectious mononucleosis (IM)

ICD-9CM CODES
075 Infectious mononucleosis

EPIDEMIOLOGY & DEMOGRAPHICS

INCIDENCE (IN U.S.): 500 cases/100,000 persons/yr
PREDOMINANT SEX: Incidence is the same, but occurs earlier in females.
PREDOMINANT AGE: Most common between the ages of 15 and 24 yr.

PHYSICAL FINDINGS & CLINICAL PRESENTATION

- Following an incubation period of 1 to 2 mo, a prodrome may occur, with fever, chills, malaise, and anorexia for several days. This is followed by the classic triad, which includes pharyngitis, fever, and adenopathy. Although fatigue and malaise may be prominent, pharyngitis is usually the most severe symptom. Exudates are common.
- Lymphadenopathy is most prominent in the cervical region but may be diffuse.
- Splenomegaly may occur, most commonly during the second wk of illness.
- Rash is uncommon but will occur in nearly all patients who receive ampicillin.
- At times, IM can present as fever and adenopathy without pharyngitis. Although complications may be severe, they are uncommon and tend to resolve completely. Involvement of the hematologic, pulmonary, cardiac, or nervous system may occur; splenic rupture is rare. IM is usually a self-limited illness, but symptoms of malaise and fatigue may last months before resolving.

ETIOLOGY

The cause of IM is primary infection with EBV. Primary infection during childhood causes few or no symptoms. Infection during childhood is more common in lower socioeconomic groups. The frequency of IM in late adolescence is attributed to the onset of social contact between the sexes. Close personal contact is usually necessary for transmission. Transfer via saliva while kissing may be responsible for many cases. Virus can persist in oropharynx of patients with IM for up to 18 mo. Transmission may also occur sexually as EBV can be isolated in cervical epithelial cells and male seminal fluid and can also be transmitted by blood transfusion.

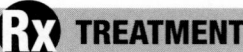 DIAGNOSIS

DIFFERENTIAL DIAGNOSIS

- Heterophile-negative IM caused by cytomegalovirus (CMV); although clinical presentation may be similar, CMV more frequently follows transfusion
- Bacterial and viral causes of pharyngitis
- Toxoplasmosis
- Acute retroviral syndrome of HIV, lymphoma

WORKUP

Initial testing consists of heterophile antibody (monospot) and CBC with differential. Fig. E1-543 illustrates a diagnostic algorithm for EBV infection and IM.

LABORATORY TESTS

- Increased WBC is common, with a relative lymphocytosis and neutropenia. Atypical lymphocytes (Fig. E1-544) are the hallmark of IM, but are not pathognomonic. Mild thrombocytopenia is common. A falling hematocrit may signal splenic rupture or severe immune-mediated hemolytic anemia. Elevated hepatocellular enzymes and cryoglobulins occur in most cases. Heterophile antibody, as measured by the monospot test, may be positive at presentation, or may appear later in the course of illness. A negative test should be repeated if clinical suspicion is high. If this test remains negative for 8 wk, other causes of IM are likely. The monospot usually remains positive for 3 to 6 mo, but can last for 1 yr.
- A positive test has been reported with primary HIV infection.
- In addition to the heterophile antibody, virus-specific antibodies may result in response to IM. Determination of these EBV-specific antibodies is rarely necessary to diagnose IM, although early diagnosis in monospot negative cases may be made by isolating IgM to the viral capsid antigen, which is usually positive during the acute illness.

IMAGING STUDIES

Chest x-ray may rarely show infiltrates. An elevated left hemidiaphragm may occur in cases of splenic rupture.

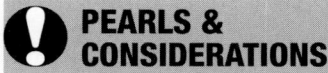 TREATMENT

NONPHARMACOLOGIC THERAPY

- Supportive rest is advocated by some, but effect on outcome is not clear.
- Splenectomy if rupture occurs; transfusions for severe anemia or thrombocytopenia

ACUTE GENERAL Rx

- Pharmacologic therapy is not indicated in uncomplicated illness.
- The use of steroids (Fig. E1-545) is suggested in patients who have severe thrombocytopenia or hemolytic anemia, or impending airway obstruction as a result of enlarged tonsils. Prednisone, 60 to 80 mg PO qid for 3 days, then tapered over 1 to 2 wk. There is no role for antiviral agents such as acyclovir in the management of IM.

CHRONIC Rx

A rare, chronic form of IM with persistent organ infection and inflammation has been described. This should not be confused with chronic fatigue syndrome, which is unrelated to EBV.

DISPOSITION

Eventual resolution of all symptoms is the rule.

REFERRAL

More than mild illness

PEARLS & CONSIDERATIONS

COMMENTS

- Contact sports should be avoided during the first month of illness, because splenic rupture can occur, even in the absence of clinically detectable splenomegaly.
- Between 30% and 75% of college freshmen are seronegative for EBV. Each year nearly 20% of susceptible persons become infected and up to 50% of these persons develop IM.

SUGGESTED READINGS
available at www.expertconsult.com

RELATED CONTENT
Mononucleosis (Patient Information)

AUTHOR: **GLENN G. FORT, M.D., M.P.H.**

BASIC INFORMATION

DEFINITION

Morton's neuroma is an entrapment neuropathy involving one of the common plantar digital nerves of the foot. This condition manifests as pain in the plantar aspect of the forefoot, often localized between the metatarsal heads.

SYNONYMS

Morton metatarsalgia
Morton toe
Interdigital neuroma
Plantar neuroma
Metatarsal neuralgia

ICD-9CM CODES

355.6 Morton's neuroma

EPIDEMIOLOGY & DEMOGRAPHICS

- Morton's neuroma affects one of the common plantar digital nerves located at any of the four interspaces of the foot (Fig. 1-546).
  - It most commonly affects the third common plantar digital proper nerve, located in the third interspace.
  - It occurs most frequently in patients who wear tight-fitting, high-heeled shoes.
- Morton's neuroma is usually unilateral.
- The condition occurs most frequently in women.
- It usually presents between the fourth and sixth decade of life.

PHYSICAL FINDINGS & CLINICAL PRESENTATION

- Patients with Morton's neuroma will present complaining of pain to the plantar aspect of the foot, typically localized between the metatarsal heads of the affected interspace.
- The pain may be described as stabbing, burning, tingling, or "electric" and may radiate to the digits.
- The pain is exacerbated by the use of tight-fitting shoes. The typical indication of a Morton's neuroma is the patient's desire to remove shoes and rub the forefoot.

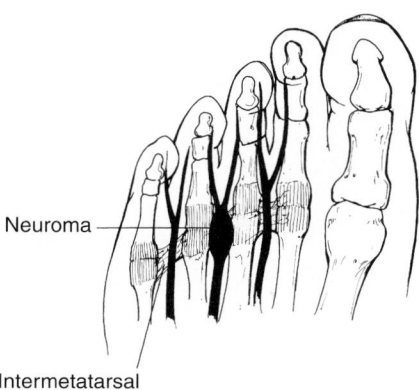

Neuroma

Intermetatarsal ligament

FIGURE 1-546 Interdigital neuroma, plantar view. (From DeLee D, Drez D [eds]: *DeLee and Drez's orthopaedic sports medicine*, ed 2, Philadelphia, 2003, Saunders.)

- The pain can often be recreated by applying pressure at the plantar aspect of the interspace, starting just proximal to the metatarsal heads and proceeding distally.
- Mulder's sign: Compression of the forefoot at the level of the metatarsophalangeal joints, combined with plantar pressure at the affected interspace, elicits a palpable "click."

ETIOLOGY

- Morton's neuroma is considered to be an entrapment neuropathy of the affected common digital plantar nerve. The etiology remains obscure.
- The common plantar digital nerves are branches of the medial plantar nerve, coursing distally to supply the digits of the foot, passing just beneath the deep transverse intermetatarsal ligament. The third common plantar nerve is often supplied by a communicating branch of the lateral plantar nerve (see Fig. 1-546). This anatomic variation results in a thicker nerve that is more prone to trauma, a reason often cited to explain the prevalence of Morton's neuroma in the third common plantar digital nerve.
- The deep transverse intermetatarsal ligament may also be implicated in the cause of a neuroma. If it is thickened or has aberrant bands, it may cause compression of the affected nerve.
- Soft tissue masses, such as a plantar lipoma, may also cause compression of the nerve against the ligament, leading to the formation of a neuroma.
- Histologic examination of resected Morton's neuroma exhibits increased neural width, demyelination, intraneural fibrosis, and thickened endoneural capillaries.

DIAGNOSIS

The diagnosis of Morton's neuroma is primarily a clinical diagnosis. Laboratory tests and imaging modalities are generally not necessary for diagnosis.

DIFFERENTIAL DIAGNOSIS

- Peripheral neuropathy
- Tarsal tunnel syndrome
- Metatarsal stress fracture
- Freiberg's infraction
- Metatarsophalangeal joint capsulitis
- Osteoarthritis
- Rheumatoid arthritis

WORKUP

Exclude other causes mentioned in "Differential Diagnosis".

LABORATORY TESTS

There is no specific laboratory study that can be used to diagnose Morton's neuroma.

IMAGING STUDIES

- Weight-bearing radiographs may be performed to exclude other pathologic conditions.
- MRI may be used to detect and localize a neuroma. The mass is best visualized on a T1-weighted image.
  - MRI is best for patients with recurrent neuromas and atypical symptoms.

- Ultrasound imaging can be used to visualize a neuroma. It will typically present as a hypoechoic mass.

TREATMENT

NONPHARMACOLOGIC THERAPY

- Altering footwear is the first line of treatment.
- Wide shoes with a low heel are recommended.
- A metatarsal pad may also provide relief, as it splays the metatarsal heads, thereby decreasing the pressure on the neuroma.
- If adequate relief is noted with the above, then orthotics may also be considered.

ACUTE GENERAL Rx

- If conservative measures are unsuccessful, other treatment options include serial injections with corticosteroids or a sclerosing agent. The sclerosing solution is commonly composed of bupivacaine and ethyl alcohol.
- Nonsteroidal anti-inflammatory agents may also provide relief.

CHRONIC Rx

- If conservative treatment fails to provide a resolution to symptoms, then surgical intervention should be considered.
- Surgical excision of the neuroma is performed in an operating room under monitored anesthesia care.
- Possible complications of surgery include hematoma formation, numbness, infection, and recurrent neuroma.

DISPOSITION

- Following surgery, patients are often placed on a partial weight-bearing status to the affected foot. Sutures are removed 2 to 3 weeks following the initial surgery. Patients generally return to their previous activity level in 4 to 6 weeks.
- Should a neuroma recur, a second surgical procedure may be performed.

REFERRAL

If surgery is being considered, a consultation with either a podiatrist or a foot and ankle specialized orthopedic surgeon is indicated.

PEARLS & CONSIDERATIONS

COMMENTS

- Dr. Thomas G. Morton is given credit for describing this disorder in 1876.
- Morton's neuroma may occur in any of the four interspaces of the foot but most commonly affects the third interspace.
- If conservative treatment and serial injections fail, surgery should be considered for the excision of the neuroma.

SUGGESTED READINGS

available at www.expertconsult.com

RELATED CONTENT

Morton's Neuroma (Patient Information)

AUTHOR: **NATHALIA DOOBAY, D.P.M.**

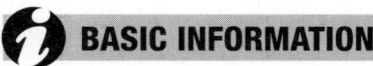 **BASIC INFORMATION**

DEFINITION

Motion sickness is a clinical syndrome associated with motion or perception of motion. Patients with motion sickness suffer perspiration, nausea, vomiting, increased salivation, and generalized malaise in response to movement.

SYNONYMS

Physiologic vertigo

ICD-9CM CODES
994.6 Motion sickness

EPIDEMIOLOGY & DEMOGRAPHICS

INCIDENCE (IN U.S.): Common
PEAK INCIDENCE: Any age
PREVALENCE (IN U.S.): Common
PREDOMINANT SEX: Male = female
PREDOMINANT AGE: Any age
GENETICS: Not known to be genetic

PHYSICAL FINDINGS & CLINICAL PRESENTATION

- Vomiting
- Sweating
- Pallor

ETIOLOGY

- Motion (e.g., amusement rides, rides in automobiles or planes)
- Exacerbated by anxiety, fumes (e.g., industrial pollutants), visual stimuli

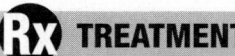 **DIAGNOSIS**

DIFFERENTIAL DIAGNOSIS

- Acute labyrinthitis
- Gastroenteritis
- Metabolic disorders
- Viral syndrome

WORKUP

None necessary in routine case

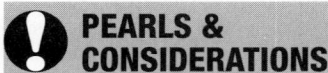 **TREATMENT**

NONPHARMACOLOGIC THERAPY

- Fixate on far object
- Cease motion
- Avoid reading
- Avoid alcohol

ACUTE GENERAL Rx

- Scopolamine patch is most effective. It should be applied to a hairless area behind the ear every 3 days prn. It should be applied >4 hr before antiemetic effect is required.
- Over-the-counter oral preparations (e.g., Dramamine) are less effective.
- Meclizine 12.5 to 25 mg q6h may be effective.

CHRONIC Rx

- Rarely chronic
- Symptoms generally resolve completely with cessation of motion exposure.

DISPOSITION

Follow-up is not needed.

REFERRAL

If another diagnosis is suspected (e.g., purulent ear, fever, cranial nerve abnormalities)

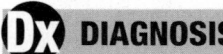 **PEARLS & CONSIDERATIONS**

COMMENTS

- Many patients with migraine report having had severe motion sickness as a child.
- Improved ventilation, avoidance of large meals before travel, semirecumbent sitting, and avoidance of reading while in motion will minimize the risk of motion sickness.

SUGGESTED READINGS

available at www.expertconsult.com

RELATED CONTENT

Motion Sickness (Patient Information)

AUTHOR: **FRED F. FERRI, M.D.**

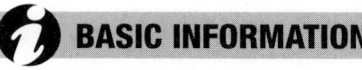

BASIC INFORMATION

DEFINITION

Mucormycosis is a fungal infection by Zygomycetes fungi and includes species in the order Mucorales (*Rhizopus* sp., *Rhizomucor*, *Cunninghamella*, *Apophysomyces*, *Saksenaea*, *Absidia*, *Syncephalastrum*, *Cokeromyces*, *Mortierella*) and in the order Entomophthorales (*Conidiobolus* and *Basidiobolus*).

ICD-9CM CODES
117.7 Mucormycosis

EPIDEMIOLOGY & DEMOGRAPHICS

- These fungi are ubiquitous in nature and can be found in soil and decaying vegetation. Infection is seen in association with underlying conditions, including diabetes mellitus especially with ketoacidosis, hematologic malignancies, stem cell or solid organ transplants, severe burns or trauma, treatment with deferoxamine or iron overload states, steroid treatment, immunodeficiency states (e.g., AIDS), injection drug use, and malnutrition. Immunocompetent hosts may become infected in tropical climates.
- The fungus gains entry to the body most commonly through the respiratory tract. The spores are deposited in the nasal turbinates and may be inhaled into the pulmonary alveoli. In cases of cutaneous mucormycosis, the spores are introduced directly into the skin lesion.
- After a tornado with winds >200 mph struck Joplin, Missouri, in May 2011, there were 13 confirmed cases of mucormycosis *(Apophysomyces trapeziformis),* including five deaths. While two patients had diabetes, none were immunocompromised. It was felt that the fungus entered through wounds sustained during the tornado. Wooden splinters were found in four patients.

PHYSICAL FINDINGS & CLINICAL PRESENTATION

- Rhinocerebral-rhinoorbital-paranasal syndrome may present with fever, facial and orbital pain, headache, diplopia, loss of vision, facial or orbital cellulitis, facial anesthesia, cranial nerve dysfunction, black nasal discharge, epistaxis, and seizure. Physical findings in this situation include proptosis; chemosis; nasal, palatal, or pharyngeal necrotic ulcerations; and retinal infarction. Thrombosis of the cavernous sinus or internal carotid artery may occur. This form of mucormycosis is found most commonly in diabetics, primarily in the presence of acidosis, and in patients with leukemia and neutropenia.
- Pulmonary mucormycosis can present with pneumonia, lung abscess, pulmonary infarction, pleurisy, pleural effusion, hemoptysis, chills, and fever. This form of mucormycosis is found most commonly in immunocompromised neutropenic hosts after chemotherapy for hematologic malignancies.
- Gastrointestinal zygomycosis presents with abdominal pain, diarrhea, gastrointestinal hemorrhage, ulcers, peritonitis, and bowel infarction. This form of mucormycosis is found most commonly in patients with extreme malnutrition and is believed to arise from ingestion of spores of the fungi.
- Cutaneous zygomycosis presents as nodular lesions (hematogenous seeding) or a wound infection. It primarily involves the epidermis and dermis after use of occlusive dressings that have not been properly sterilized.
- Cardiac mucormycosis is a form of endocarditis.
- Septic arthritis and osteomyelitis
- Brain abscess occurs most often from extension of the fungus from the nose or paranasal sinuses through adjacent bones in severely debilitated patients.
- Disseminated zygomycosis (rare but uniformly fatal)
- Physical findings depend on the location of the infection.

ETIOLOGY & PATHOGENESIS

The cause of mucormycosis is infection by a fungus of the Zygomycetes class (see "Definition"). Normal host defenses include leukocytes and pulmonary macrophages. Quantitative (e.g., neutropenia) or qualitative (e.g., diabetes mellitus or steroid treatment) disruption in the host defenses predisposes the patient to infection.

DIAGNOSIS

The hallmark of mucormycosis is infarction and necrosis of host tissues that result from invasion of the vasculature by the fungal elements. Black eschars and discharges should be closely evaluated. Diagnosis depends on the demonstration of the organism in the tissue of a biopsy specimen.

DIFFERENTIAL DIAGNOSIS

- Infection of the sites described previously by other organisms (bacterial [including tuberculosis and leprosy], viral, fungal, or protozoan)
- Noninfectious tissue necrosis (e.g., neoplasia, vasculitis, degenerative) of the sites described previously

WORKUP

- Biopsy of infected tissue with direct-light microscopy examination establishes the diagnosis within minutes of the biopsy in the case of nasopharyngeal infection. Fungal hyphae are broad (5- to 15-micron diameter) and irregularly branched and have rare septations, in contrast to molds such as *Aspergillus,* which are narrower, have regular branching, and have many septations.
- Bronchoalveolar lavage or bronchoscopy with biopsy for smear, culture, and histologic examination
- Radiographs and other imaging studies such as CT of symptomatic sites may be required before infection is suspected and tissue specimens are obtained.

TREATMENT

Aggressive correction of underlying disease (e.g., hyperglycemia, high steroid doses, use of immunosuppressive drugs) should be undertaken.

Standard therapy consists of aggressive surgical debridement of involved tissues and antifungal therapy. For invasive mucormycosis recommended treatment is with a lipid formulation of amphotericin B that allows higher doses with less nephrotoxicity. The start dose is 5 mg/kg of liposomal amphotericin B or amphotericin B lipid complex. Doses as high as 10 mg/kg have also been used.

Traditional amphotericin B given IV at a daily dose of 1.0 to 1.5 mg/kg infused over 2 to 4 hr daily for a total of 1 to 4 g can also still be used, but are associated with significant nephrotoxicity and adverse reactions such as fever, chills, myalgias, vomiting, and electrolyte disturbances.

- Other antifungals do not appear to be effective except possibly posaconazole, which may serve as an oral step-down therapy after amphotericin B at a dose of 400 mg bid with a fatty meal.
- Some studies suggest that caspofungin with amphotericin B may be synergistic for *Rhizopus oryzae* infections only.
- The role of colony-stimulating factors remains unclear, beyond that of increasing the neutrophil count in patients with neutropenia.
- Hyperbaric oxygen has been used in some patients but its utility in therapy is still not clear.

PROGNOSIS

- Sinus infection with no underlying disease: 75% survival
- Sinus infection with diabetes: 60% survival
- Sinus infection with renal disease: 25% survival
- Surgery may increase survival by 5% to 20%.
- Early diagnosis improves survival as well as control of the underlying condition.

SUGGESTED READINGS
available at www.expertconsult.com

AUTHOR: **GLENN G. FORT, M.D., M.P.H.**

BASIC INFORMATION

DEFINITION

These are gram-negative bacteria that are resistant to at least one antimicrobial in three or more antimicrobial classes (antipseudomonal penicillins, third-generation cephalosporins, fluoroquinolones, carbapenems, and aminoglycosides).

SYNONYMS

CRE: carbapenam-resistant Enterobacteriaceae
ESBL: extended-spectrum beta-lactamases
MDR-GNB: multidrug-resistant gram-negative bacilli
MDRO: multidrug-resistant organisms
NDM-1: New Delhi metallo-beta-lactamase-1

ICD-9CM CODES
V09.9 Infection with drug-resistant microorganisms, unspecified
V09.1 Infection with microorganisms resistant to cephalosporins and other beta-lactam antibiotics

EPIDEMIOLOGY & DEMOGRAPHICS

INCIDENCE: There is an increasing incidence of these bacteria in hospitals and long-term care facilities in the U.S. and around the world. ESBL bacteria were first discovered in Europe in 1984 and in the U.S. in 1988. CRE bacteria were first described in the late 1990s in the U.S. The NDM-1 bacteria were first noted in 2009 in Sweden in a patient from India.
PREDOMINANT SEX AND AGE: These bacteria can be seen in any age group. They may be more frequent in women due to increased risk of urinary tract sepsis.
RISK FACTORS: In general, these bacteria are more common in hospitals and long-term care facilities, but they are spread nosocomially through patient care and thus are now entering the community, where the incidence is also increasing. Specific risk factors include:
- Length of stay in the hospital
- Length of ICU stay
- Use of central line catheters
- Abdominal surgery
- Presence of gastrostomy or jejunostomy tube
- Prior administration of any antibiotic
- Prior residence in a long-term care facility
- Presence of indwelling urinary catheter

ETIOLOGY

- Several different classes of MDR-GNRs exist based on their resistance mechanism.
  1. ESBL: These bacteria contain enzymes that break open the beta-lactam ring of penicillins, cephalosporins, and aztreonam and thus inactivate antibiotics from those classes. Enzymes conferring resistance include:
     ○ TEM beta-lactamases
     ○ SHV beta-lactamases
     ○ CTX-M beta lactamases
     ○ OXA beta-lactamases

These enzymes are plasmid-mediated and thus can spread from one gram-negative bacteria to another, causing outbreaks in a single institution.
  2. CRE: Enzymes conferring resistance include:
     ○ Class A beta-lactamases: encoded on chromosomes or plasmids (e.g., *Klebsiella pneumoniae* carbapenamase [KPC], which has caused outbreaks in hospitals around the world)
     ○ Class B: metallo-beta-lactamases (e.g., New Delhi metallo-beta-lactamase-1). Encoded on a mobile plasmid that can spread to other gram-negative bacteria.
     ○ Class C and Class D beta-lactamases
- *Stenotrophomonas maltophilia*: MDR-GNR that acts as an opportunistic pathogen among mostly hospitalized patients with high morbidity and mortality. It has intrinsic or acquired resistance mechanisms to multiple antibiotic classes and has the ability to adhere to foreign materials and form a biofilm, which escapes host defenses.
- *Acinetobacter* sp. (e.g., *Acinetobacter baumannii*): strains have emerged that are resistant to all commercially available antibiotics. These bacteria have the capability to acquire diverse mechanisms of resistance including:
  ○ AmpC beta-lactamases
  ○ Beta-lactamases: serine and metallo-beta-lactamases

CLINICAL PRESENTATION

All these resistant bacteria have the capability of causing diverse infections, including
- Pneumonia
- Bacteremia
- Urinary tract sepsis
- Central line–associated infections
- Ventilator-associated pneumonia (VAP)
- Surgical site infections
  VAP from *A. baumannii* now accounts for 8.4% of GNR pneumonias in the ICU.

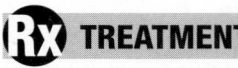

DIAGNOSIS

DIFFERENTIAL DIAGNOSIS

Other gram-negative rods such as:
- *Pseudomonas aeruginosa*
- *Klebsiella pneumoniae* that are not ESBL or CRE by resistance pattern
- *Morganella morgani*
- *Providencia, Proteus* sp., *Serratia*

WORKUP

Detection of ESBL and CRE bacteria can pose problems for the clinical microbiology laboratory:
1. To detect ESBL bacteria: automated systems such as Vitek use disk diffusion or broth dilution techniques, or double disk test or E-test strip with clavulanate
2. To detect CRE: modified Hodge test to detect carbapenamase-producing bacteria
3. In 2010, testing guidelines with respect to susceptibility involving several beta-lactam antibiotics were changed to better identify these bacteria via automated systems.

LABORATORY TESTS

Clinical testing is the same in infections from these resistant organisms as with nonresistant organisms:
- Cultures of any wounds, blood, sputum, urine, catheter tips
- CBC, liver function tests, urinalysis

IMAGING STUDIES

Studies depend on the clinical presentation but are similar to those for nonresistant bacteria causing infections.

TREATMENT

Because of multidrug resistance, only a few reliable antibiotics are available to treat these infections.
1. ESBL bacteria: carbapenem antibiotics such as imipenem, meropenem, ertapenem, or the cephalosporin cefoxitin or tigecycline.
2. CRE bacteria: selection of antibiotic will depend on testing but tigecycline may be used clinically. Other alternatives include:
   ○ IV colistin
   ○ *Stenotrophomonas maltophilia:* only available agents are Bactrim (drug of choice), levaquin, and minocycline
   ○ *A. baumannii:* will depend on susceptibility testing, but ampicillin-sulbactam, imipenem or meropenem, or tigecycline can be used for MDR strains. For pan-resistant strains, IV colistin ± rifampin can be used. Inhaled colistin can be used for pneumonia patients.

DISPOSITION

Morbidity and mortality can be quite high with infections from these MDR bacteria.
1. Nosocomial *Acinetobacter* pneumonia carries a mortality rate of 35% to 70%.
2. *Stenotrophomonas* infections carry a mortality rate of 21% to 69%.
3. ESBL infections carry a mortality rate of 3.7% despite therapy with carbapenem antibiotics.

REFERRAL

- Infectious diseases specialist for selection of best antibiotic choice and follow-up
- Microbiologist for specialized testing and interpretation of results
- Pulmonary specialist for severe forms of pneumonia
- Infection control officer to help prevent spread of these bacteria in an institution

SUGGESTED READINGS
available at www.expertconsult.com

AUTHOR: **GLENN G. FORT, M.D., M.P.H.**

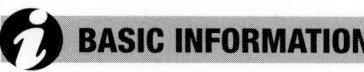 **BASIC INFORMATION**

DEFINITION

Multifocal atrial tachycardia (MAT) is a supraventricular, moderately rapid arrhythmia (rate 100 to 140 beats/min) with P waves having at least three or more different morphologies and irregular P-P intervals. An isoelectric baseline further differentiates MAT from atrial fibrillation or atrial flutter.

SYNONYMS

Chaotic atrial rhythm
Chronic atrial tachycardia
Repetitive multifocal paroxysmal atrial tachycardia
The term *wandering pacemaker* is used for a similar arrhythmia associated with a normal or slow heart rate (<100 beats/min).

ICD-9CM CODES

427.89 Multifocal atrial tachycardia

EPIDEMIOLOGY & DEMOGRAPHICS

Estimated prevalence in hospitalized patients of 0.05% to 0.32%. Average age is 70s. Usually associated with underlying pulmonary disease with right atrial electromechanical delay. Chronic obstructive pulmonary disease (COPD) is present in approximately 55% of patients with MAT.

PHYSICAL FINDINGS & CLINICAL PRESENTATION

Symptoms:
- Palpitation
- Lightheadedness
- Syncope
- Symptoms of the underlying pulmonary disease
- Physical findings associated with the underlying pulmonary disease

ETIOLOGY

- Exact mechanism unknown
- Exacerbated by underlying pulmonary disease (COPD, hypoxia, pulmonary embolism, pneumonia), cardiac disease, hypercarbia, acidosis, electrolyte disturbances, digitalis toxicity

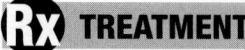 **DIAGNOSIS**

DIFFERENTIAL DIAGNOSIS

- Atrial fibrillation
- Atrial flutter
- Sinus tachycardia
- Paroxysmal atrial tachycardia
- Extrasystole

WORKUP

- ECG (Fig. 1-547)
- Chest x-ray
- Pulmonary function tests
- Electrolytes
- Arterial blood gases
- Digoxin level (if patient on digoxin)

Rx **TREATMENT**

- Correction and/or improvement in the underlying pulmonary or metabolic dysfunction if possible
- Electrolyte repletion, especially magnesium and potassium
- Calcium channel blockers
- β-blockers are typically contraindicated by obstructive lung disease or acute heart failure
- If the arrhythmia is asymptomatic, it can be left untreated
- Direct current cardioversion is ineffective
- No significant role for antiarrhythmics
- No role for radiofrequency ablation

SUGGESTED READINGS

available at www.expertconsult.com

RELATED CONTENT

Fig. 3-129 Algorithm for evaluating patients with symptoms of palpitation, dizziness, or syncope (Algorithm)
Fig. 3-175 Stepwise approach to the diagnosis of type of tachycardia based on 12-lead electrocardiogram during the episode (Algorithm)
Fig. 3-176 Evaluation and management of narrow complex tachycardia (Algorithm)

AUTHORS: **SAURAV CHATTERJEE, M.D.,**
FRED F. FERRI, M.D., and
WEN-CHIH WU, M.D., M.P.H.

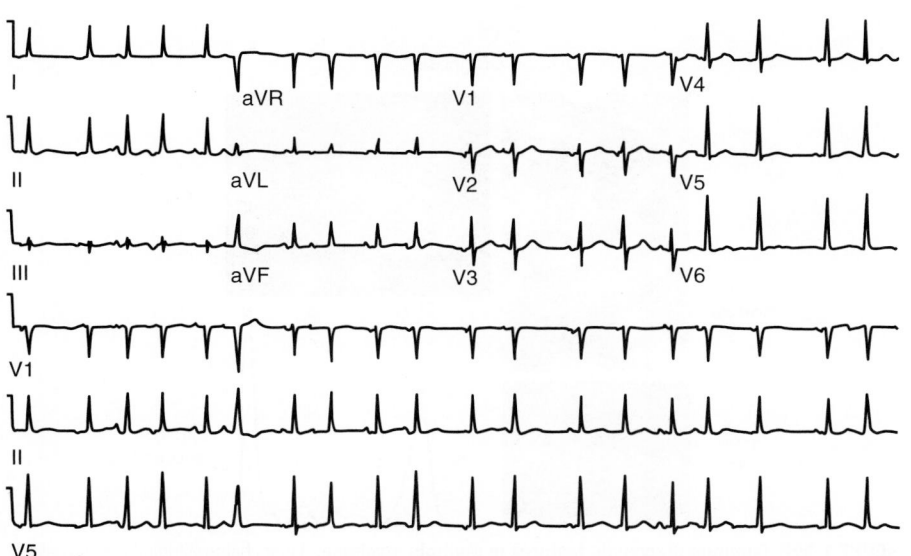

FIGURE 1-547 Surface ECG of multifocal atrial tachycardia. Note the varying morphology of the P waves and the PR intervals. (From Issa Z et al: *Clinical arrhythmology and electrophysiology,* ed 2, Philadelphia, 2012, Saunders.)

BASIC INFORMATION

DEFINITION

Multiple myeloma is a malignancy of plasma cells characterized by clonal proliferation of malignant plasma cells in the bone marrow, monoclonal protein in the blood or urine, and associated organ dysfunction. Diagnostic criteria require the following:

1. Presence of ≥10% plasma cells on examination of the bone marrow (or biopsy of a tissue with monoclonal plasma cells).
2. Monoclonal protein in the serum or urine. Occasional patients without detectable monoclonal protein are considered to have nonsecretory myeloma.
3. Evidence of end-organ damage (*c*alcium elevation, *r*enal insufficiency, *a*nemia, or *b*one lesions [CRAB]).

ICD-9CM CODES
203.0 Multiple myeloma

EPIDEMIOLOGY & DEMOGRAPHICS

ANNUAL INCIDENCE: Five cases/100,000 persons (blacks affected twice as frequently as whites, males more than females); multiple myeloma accounts for 10% of all hematologic cancers. It is the most common primary bone malignancy. More than 20,000 new cases are diagnosed annually in the United States.

PREDOMINANT AGE: Peak incidence is in the seventh decade at a median age of 70 yr.

PHYSICAL FINDINGS & CLINICAL PRESENTATION

The patient usually comes to medical attention because of one or more of the following:

- Bone pain (58%) (back, thorax) or pathologic fractures (30%) caused by osteolytic lesions
- Fatigue (32%) or weakness because of anemia from bone marrow infiltration with plasma cells
- Recurrent infections as a result of impaired neutrophil function and deficiency of normal immunoglobulins
- Nausea and vomiting caused by constipation and uremia
- Delirium resulting from hypercalcemia
- Neurologic complications, such as spinal cord or nerve root compression, blurred vision from hyperviscosity
- Pallor and generalized weakness from anemia
- Purpura, epistaxis from thrombocytopenia
- Evidence of infections from impaired immune system
- Paresthesias (5%), weight loss (24%)
- Swelling on ribs, vertebrae, and other bones

DIAGNOSIS

DIFFERENTIAL DIAGNOSIS (Fig. E1-548)

- Metastatic carcinoma
- Lymphoma (B-cell non-Hodgkin lymphoma)
- Bone neoplasms (e.g., sarcoma)

- Monoclonal gammopathy of undetermined significance
- Primary amyloidosis
- Chronic lymphocytic leukemia
- Waldenström's macroglobulinemia

LABORATORY TESTS

- Normochromic, normocytic anemia; rouleaux formation on peripheral smear (Fig. E1-549)
- Hypercalcemia is present in 15% of patients at diagnosis.
- Elevated blood urea nitrogen, creatinine, uric acid, and total protein
- Urine protein immunoelectrophoresis: proteinuria from overproduction and secretion of free monoclonal kappa or lambda chains (Bence Jones protein)
- Serum protein immunoelectrophoresis: tall homogeneous monoclonal spike (M spike) on protein immunoelectrophoresis in approximately 75% of patients (Fig. 1-550); decreased levels of normal immunoglobulins (Ig)
  1. The increased immunoglobulins are generally IgG (75%) and IgA (15%).
  2. Approximately 17% of patients have a flat level of immunoglobulins but increased light chains in the urine by electrophoresis.
  3. A small percentage (<2%) of patients have nonsecreting myeloma (no increase in immunoglobulins and no light chains in the urine) but have other evidence of the disease (e.g., positive bone marrow examination).
- Reduced ion gap from the positive charge of the M proteins and the frequent presence of hyponatremia in myeloma patients
- Hyponatremia, serum hyperviscosity (more common with production of IgA)
- Bone marrow examination: usually demonstrates nests or sheets of plasma cells, which comprise >30% of the bone marrow; ≥10% are immature
- Serum beta-2 microglobulin has little diagnostic value; it is useful for prognosis be-

cause levels >8 mg/L indicate high tumor mass and aggressive disease.
- Elevated serum levels of lactate dehydrogenase at the time of diagnosis define a subgroup of myeloma patients with very poor prognosis.
- Increased interleukin-6 in serum during active stage of myeloma
- The production of DKK1, an inhibitor of osteoblast differentiation, by myeloma cells is associated with the presence of lytic bone lesions in patients with multiple myeloma.
- Nearly all patients with myeloma present with abnormal chromosomes identified by fluorescence in situ hybridization (FISH). The Mayo Clinic Stratification of Myeloma, for purposes of therapy, identifies high-risk patients (<25% of patients at diagnosis) as those who have any of the following: FISH deletion 17p, FISH translocation 4;14, FISH translocation 14;16, cytogenetic deletion 13q, cytogenetic hypodiploidy, or plasma cell labeling index ≥3%.

IMAGING STUDIES

Radiograph films of painful areas may demonstrate punched-out lytic lesions or osteoporosis (Fig. 1-550). MRI is the preferred technique for suspected spinal compression or soft tissue plasmacytomas. Bone scans are not useful because lesions are not blastic. PET and MRI scans are emerging as useful tools to detect early bone involvement or extramedullary disease.

STAGING

Table 1-284 describes a historical multiple myeloma staging system. With use of newer tumor biology factors (see "Disposition") that can affect prognosis, along with tumor burden described in Table 1-284 and patient-related factors, it is possible to classify patients in three risk groups (high, intermediate, and standard).

Diagnosis

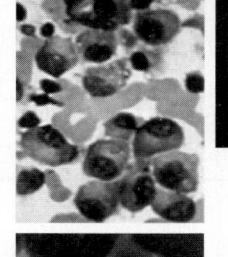
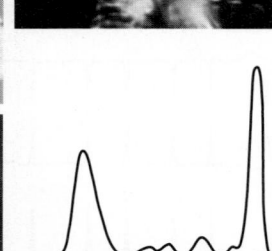

Bone marrow

X-ray

Electrophoresis

FIGURE 1-550 Common diagnostic features in multiple myeloma. Light chain-restricted plasma cells in a bone marrow aspirate; multiple lytic lesions in a skull radiograph; large monoclonal spike in the γ-globulin area in serum electrophoresis. (From Hoffman R et al: *Hematology, basic principles and practice,* ed 5, Philadelphia, 2009, Churchill Livingstone.)

TABLE 1-284 Myeloma Staging System

Stage	Criteria
I	All of the following: 1. Hemoglobin >10 g/dl 2. Serum calcium <12 mg/dl 3. Normal bone radiograph or solitary lesion 4. Low M-component production a. IgG level <5 g/dl b. IgA level <3 g/dl c. Urine light chain <4 g/24 hr
II	Fitting neither I nor III
III	One or more of the following: 1. Hemoglobin <8.5 g/dl 2. Serum calcium >12 mg/dl 3. Advanced lytic bone lesions 4. High M-component production a. IgG level >7 g/dl b. IgA level >5 g/dl c. Urine light chains >12 g/24 hr

Subclassification:
A Serum creatinine <2 mg/dl
B Serum creatinine <2 mg/dl

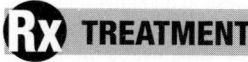 **TREATMENT**

NONPHARMACOLOGIC THERAPY

Prevention of renal failure with adequate hydration and avoidance of nephrotoxic agents and dye contrast studies

ACUTE GENERAL Rx

- Treatment strategy is mainly related to age and comorbidities. It is crucial to identify transplant-eligible patients (Fig. E1-551).
  1. Initiation of induction therapy with thalidomide, lenalidomide, or bortezomib plus autologous stem cell transplant (ASCT) for patients <70 yr who do not have substantial heart, lung, renal, or liver dysfunction.
  2. ASCT with a reduced-intensity conditioning regimen should be considered in older patients or those with coexisting conditions.
  3. Conventional therapy combined with thalidomide, lenalidomide, or bortezomib should be administered in patients >70 yr.
- Induction therapy in patients ineligible for transplantation (old age, coexisting conditions, poor physical conditions) includes the following chemotherapeutic agents:
  1. Thalidomide in combination with melphalan and prednisone.

  2. Melphalan, bortezomib, and prednisone
  3. Bortezomib-thalidominde-prednisone
  4. Melphalan-prednisone-lenalidomide (MPR-R)
  5. Lenalidomide and low-dose dexamethasone
- Therapy for relapsed and refractory myeloma:
  1. If the relapse occurs more than 6 mo after conventional therapy is stopped, the initial chemotherapy regimen can be reinstituted.
  2. Consider autologous stem cell transplantation as salvage therapy in patients who had stem cells cryopreserved early in the course of the disease.
- ~15% of patients with newly diagnosed multiple myeloma are recognized incidentally and present without significant symptoms (asymptomatic MM, formerly known as smoldering myeloma). The rate of progression of smoldering myeloma to symptomatic disease is 10% per year for the initial 5 yr, decreasing to 5% for the next 5 yr, and decreasing further to 1.5% per year thereafter. Observation alone is reasonable in these patients because no survival advantage has been demonstrated by treating them.

CHRONIC Rx

- Promptly diagnose and treat infections. Common bacterial agents are *Streptococcus pneumoniae* and *Haemophilus influenzae*. Prophylactic therapy against *Pneumocystis jirovecii* with trimethoprim-sulfamethoxazole must be considered in patients receiving chemotherapy and high-dose corticosteroid regimens. Vaccinate against *S. pneumoniae*, influenza, and *H. influenzae*.
- Control hypercalcemia with IV fluids and corticosteroids. Monthly infusions of the bisphosphonate pamidronate provide significant protection against skeletal complications and improve the quality of life of patients with advanced multiple myeloma. Zoledronic acid at doses of 2 mg and 4 mg in patients with osteolytic lesions has been shown to be as effective as pamidronate in terms of reducing the need for radiation to bone, increasing bone mineral density, and decreasing bone resorption. It can be infused over 15 min for treatment of hypercalcemia of malignancy. Bisphosphonates (pamidronate, zoledronate, and ibandronate) also appear to have an antitumor effect.
- Control pain with analgesics; radiation therapy to treat painful bone lesions or cord

compression. Perform surgical stabilization of pathologic fractures. Consider vertebroplasty or kyphoplasty for selected vertebral lesions.
- Treat anemia with erythropoietin.
- Aggressive treatment of reversible causes of renal failure such as dehydration, hypercalcemia, and hyperuricemia.

DISPOSITION

- In patients presenting at an age <60 yr, the 10-year survival is approximately 30%. The median length of survival after diagnosis is now 8 yr. Prognosis is better in asymptomatic patients with indolent or smoldering myeloma. Median survival time is approximately 10 yr in persons with no lytic bone lesions and a serum myeloma protein concentration <3 g/dl. Adverse outcome is associated with increased levels of beta-2 microglobulin, low levels of serum albumin, circulating plasma cells, plasmablastic features in bone marrow, increased plasma cell labeling index, complete deletion of chromosome 13 or its long arm, t (4;14) or t (14;16) translocation, and increased density of bone marrow microvessels. In general any chromosomal abnormality that is detected on standard cytogenetic analysis is associated with a worse outcome than that associated with a normal karyotype.
- Compared with a single autologous stem cell transplantation, double transplantation (two successive autologous stem cell transplantations) improves survival among patients with myeloma, especially those who do not have a very good partial response after undergoing one transplantation.
- Recent trials reveal that among patients with newly diagnosed myeloma, survival in recipients of a hematopoietic stem cell autograft followed by a stem cell allograft from an HLA-identical sibling is superior to that in recipients of tandem stem cell autografts.

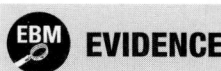 **EVIDENCE**

available at www.expertconsult.com

SUGGESTED READINGS
available at www.expertconsult.com

RELATED CONTENT
Multiple Myeloma (Patient Information)

AUTHOR: **FRED F. FERRI, M.D.**

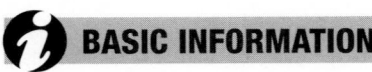

BASIC INFORMATION

DEFINITION

Multiple sclerosis (MS) is a chronic autoimmune demyelinating disease of the central nervous system (CNS) characterized by clinical attacks correlated with lesions separated in time and space. A clinical attack or relapse is the subacute onset of neurologic dysfunction that lasts for a minimum of 24 hr.

Subtypes include:
- Relapsing-remitting MS (RRMS) (most common): relapses followed by complete or near-complete recovery, 50% to 85% of which later transition to secondary progressive MS
- Secondary progressive MS (SPMS): progression of disability with few or no relapses
- Primary progressive MS (PPMS) (<5%): progression from the onset
- Progressive relapsing MS (PRMS): seen in 10% to 15%

Rare MS variants include:
- Marburg's disease (malignant MS): MRI reveals a tumorlike lesion with significant edema in one cerebral hemisphere. Pathology shows severe inflammation with necrosis: typically acute onset with a fulminant course, leading to coma or death.
- Balo's concentric sclerosis: Neuroimaging and pathology show alternating rings of myelination and demyelination—typically more fulminant progression than classic MS.
- Schilder's diffuse sclerosis: childhood onset with one to two large symmetric lesions
- Relapsing optic neuritis

SYNONYMS

MS
Disseminated sclerosis

ICD-9CM CODES
340 Multiple sclerosis

EPIDEMIOLOGY & DEMOGRAPHICS

PEAK INCIDENCE: 20 to 40 yr in two thirds of patients; remaining cases of MS usually before age 20 yr (0.3% to 0.4% occur in first decade). Overall mean age of onset is 37.5 yr.
PREVALENCE: MS is more common in people raised in northern latitudes and in certain genetic clusters. Prevalence per 10^5 varies from 6 to 14 in southern United States and southern Europe to 30 to 80 in Canada, northern United States and northern Europe; 16 to 30 in Middle Eastern Arabs and 30 to 38 in Israeli Jews; and less than 10 in Asia, Central America, and most of Africa. MS affects approximately 400,000 people in the U.S. and 2.5 million people worldwide.
PREDOMINANT SEX & AGE: Female/male ratio is 2 to 3:1. MS is most commonly a disease of young adults.
GENETICS: Frequency of MS in dizygotic twins and siblings is 3% to 5% and 20% to 40% in monozygotic twins. Most common associations include human leukocyte antigen classes I and II (DRB1*1501, DQA1*0102, DQB1*0602),

(DRB1*0405-DQA1*0301-DQB1*0302 in Mediterranean population), T-cell receptor-beta, CTLA4, and ICAM1.

PHYSICAL FINDINGS & CLINICAL PRESENTATION

- Common: both vague and nonspecific complaints such as fatigue, blurred vision, diplopia, vertigo, falls, hemiparesis, paraparesis, monoparesis, numbness, paresthesias, ataxia, cognitive deficits, depression, sexual dysfunction, and urinary dysfunction
- Visual abnormalities: horizontal nystagmus, visual field defects, *Marcus Gunn pupil* (i.e., relative afferent papillary defect—normal direct and consensual light reflexes; however, when swinging flashlight from one eye to the other, direct light causes dilatation of pupil of affected eye), *internuclear ophthalmoplegia* (paresis of the adducting eye on conjugate lateral gaze with horizontal nystagmus of the abducting eye [Fig. 1-552])
- Corticospinal tract(s) involvement: leads to upper motor neuron signs such as spasticity, hyperreflexia, clonus, extensor plantar responses, and UMN pattern of weakness (shoulder abduction, elbow, hand and finger

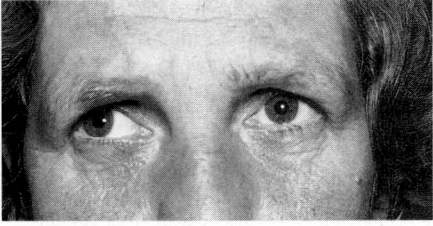

FIGURE 1-552 Internuclear ophthalmoplegia may be an initial feature of brain stem involvement in multiple sclerosis. On lateral gaze to the right, adduction of the left eye is incomplete. On convergence, eye movement was normal. The lesion is in the left medial longitudinal bundle, between the nucleus in the pons and the third nerve nucleus on the opposite side. (From Forbes CD, Jackson WF. *Color atlas and text of clinical medicine,* ed 3, London, 2003, Mosby.)

extension, hip and knee flexion, foot dorsiflexion)
- Sensory loss: numbness and tingling may or may not follow anatomic distribution, dermatomal loss of pain and temperature, loss of vibration (common) and position sense, and a thoracic band of sensory loss
- Ataxia: intention tremor, heel-to-shin ataxia, inability to tandem gait
- Bladder dysfunction: detrusor hyperreflexia (urge incontinence), flaccidity (neurogenic bladder), and dyssynergia (bladder contracts against a closed sphincter)
- *Lhermitte's sign:* flexion of the neck elicits an electrical sensation extending down the spine and occasionally into the extremities
- *Uhthoff's phenomenon:* transient worsening of preexisting symptoms with small increases in body temperature (during exercise or exposure to warm environments)

ETIOLOGY

Remains unknown but likely multifactorial with evidence for autoimmunity (autoreactive T and B cells) and genetics. It is believed that an interaction between multiple genes influencing the immune system and environmental factors (such as certain viruses [e.g., Epstein-Barr virus and human herpes virus 6], low vitamin D level, smoking, and sun exposure) are important factors.

DIAGNOSIS

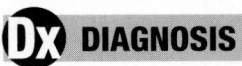

- MS: based on revised 2005 McDonald criteria (Table 1-285)
- RRMS: at least two relapses—two clinical lesions distinctly separated in space and time *or* one clinical lesion plus paraclinical testing (Table 1-285)
- PPMS: insidious progression of disability with a positive CSF and either dissemination in both space and time *or* ongoing progression for at least 1 yr

TABLE 1-285 Summary of Revised 2005-2010 McDonald Criteria for Diagnosis of Multiple Sclerosis

Clinical Attacks	Clinical Lesions	Paraclinical Testing Needed
2	2	None
2	1	MRI dissemination in space *or* two lesions on MRI consistent with multiple sclerosis plus positive CSF
1	2	MRI dissemination in time
1	1	MRI dissemination in space *or* two MRI lesions consistent with multiple sclerosis and positive CSF, *and* MRI dissemination in time

Evidence of clinical lesions by physical examination or evoked potentials.
Diagnosis of PPMS: 1 year evidence of disease progression and 2 of the following:
(1) Evidence for dissemination in space, (2) Evidence for dissemination in time, or (3) Positive CSF
CSF, Cerebrospinal fluid; *MRI,* magnetic resonance imaging; *MRI dissemination in space,* by either (1) one or more T2 lesions in 2 of the 4 typical areas for MS lesions – periventricular, juxtacortical, infratentorial or spinal cord, or (2) await further clinical attack implicating a distinctly separate CNS region; *MRI dissemination in time,* a new enhancing lesion at least 3 mo or a new nonenhancing lesion at least 6 mo after the initial attack; *positive CSF,* positive oligoclonal bands or elevated immunoglobulin G index.
Modified from Degenhardt A: *Ferri's clinical advisor,* ed 11, St Louis, 2011, Mosby. Incorporates 2010 Revisions to Diagnostic criteria of MS (for details, please see original article: Polman CH et al: Diagnostic criteria for multiple sclerosis: 2010 revisions to McDonald's criteria, *Ann Neurol* 69[2]:292-302, 2011).

M

DIFFERENTIAL DIAGNOSIS

- Autoimmune: acute disseminated encephalomyelitis (ADEM), postvaccination encephalomyelitis
- Degenerative: subacute combined degeneration of the cord (vitamin B_{12} deficiency), amyotrophic lateral sclerosis
- Infections: Lyme disease, neurosyphilis, HIV, tropical spastic paraparesis, progressive multifocal leukoencephalopathy, Whipple's disease
- Inflammatory: systemic lupus erythematosus, vasculitis, sarcoidosis, Sjögren's disease, Behçet's disease, celiac disease
- Inherited metabolic disorders: leukodystrophies
- Mitochondrial: Leber's hereditary optic neuropathy, mitochondrial encephalopathy, lactic acidosis, and strokelike episodes (MELAS)
- Neoplasms: CNS lymphoma, metastases
- Vascular: subcortical infarcts, Binswanger's disease

WORKUP

- Lumbar puncture may be considered for cases that are atypical or do not satisfy the diagnostic criteria for MS. Typical CSF abnormalities include increased protein (less than 100 mg/dl), mild elevation of mononuclear white blood cells, and increased IgG synthesis rate. An elevated CSF immunoglobulin (Ig) G index and positive oligoclonal bands are seen in 70% and 90%, respectively, of clinically definite MS. (Serum MS profile needs to be sent to lab simultaneously with CSF MS profile.) False-positive results with IgG index and rarely with positive OCBs (at least two CSF OCBs with polyclonal or negative serum) can be seen in CNS infections (SSPE, neurosyphilis), inflammation (vasculitis), and CNS lymphoma. CSF myelin basic protein is typically elevated following an acute exacerbation.

- Serum: complete blood count (CBC), erythrocyte sedimentation rate, CHEM 7, liver function tests (LFTs), antinuclear antibody, vitamin B_{12}.
- Consider: anti–SS-A antibody, anti–SS-B antibody, neuromyelitis optica IgG antibody, Lyme titer, angiotensin-converting enzyme, TSH, free T_4, anti–thyroglobulin antibody, very-long-chain fatty acids, arylsulfatase A, and possibly heavy metal screen (urine) in select cases.
- Consider evoked potentials (visual, somatosensory and brain stem auditory evoked response). Demyelination causes slow conduction velocities. Visual evoked potentials reveal prolongation of P100.

IMAGING STUDIES

Head imaging (MRI) is strongly recommended. Fig. 1-553 illustrates imaging features of MS. MRI of the head with gadolinium is the modality of choice (Fig. 1-554). MRI of the cervical spine can be helpful. MRI helps to assess disease load, acute lesions, and atrophy. A normal MRI of the brain does not conclusively exclude MS.

Rx TREATMENT

NONPHARMACOLOGIC THERAPY

Patient education regarding disease characteristics, treatment options, and prognosis. Advise patients to schedule intermittent rest periods on a daily basis and avoid exposure to heat as much as possible. Provide encouragement regarding improved quality of life with new disease-modifying drug options.

Recommend physical therapy for spasticity/disability.

ACUTE GENERAL Rx

Relapses: high-dose IV methylprednisolone (3 to 5 days of 1 g/day; alternative dose is 15 mg/kg/day), often followed by a 7- to 10-day prednisone taper. High-dose corticosteroids typically do not alter the long-term course of disease.

CHRONIC Rx

- **Disease-modifying therapy:** includes interferon beta-1a (IM Avonex, SC Rebif), interferon beta-1b (SC Betaseron), and glatiramer acetate (SC Copaxone). Interferons require routine CBC and LFT checks (initially in 1 mo, q3mo thereafter) and occasionally thyroid-stimulating hormone. None needed with glatiramer acetate. Interferons can frequently cause flulike symptoms.
- Two medications approved as oral disease modifying agents:
  1. Fingolimod, a sphingosine-1-phosphate receptor modulator, was approved as the first oral disease-modifying agent in September 2010. Common side effects: liver toxicity, bradycardia with first dose only (requiring cardiac monitoring for at least 6 to 8 hr after administration of first dose), pancytopenia.
  2. Teriflunomide, reversible inhibitor of pyrimidine synthesis, resulting in cytostatic effect on proliferation of B- and T-lymphocytes, was approved by FDA as the second oral disease-modifying agent in MS in September 2012. Common side effects: diarrhea, abnormal liver function tests, nausea and hair loss; pregnancy category X.

Use of either oral agent is reasonable in those who cannot tolerate or do not benefit from alternative disease-modifying therapies, and in those who have had one or more relapses or new white matter lesions on MRI within the past year.

- Dalfampridine (Ampyra) is a potassium channel blocker recently approved to improve walking speed in patients with MS.
- Cytotoxic: methotrexate or azathioprine is occasionally used in RRMS or PPMS. Consider cyclophosphamide or mitoxantrone (causes

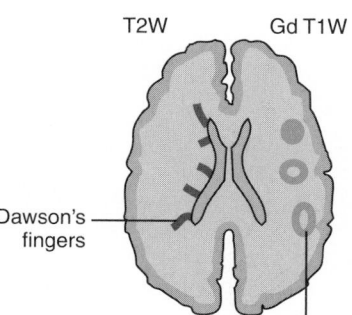

FIGURE 1-553 Imaging features. MRI appearance of plaques.

- Plaques are most commonly multiple. To support the diagnosis of multiple sclerosis, at least three plaques of >5 mm should be present.
- Average size range: 0.5 to 3 cm
- Contrast enhancement may be homogeneous, ringlike, or patchy.
- Inactive plaques do not enhance.
- Bright signal intensity on T2W and PDW images

(From Weisslederer R et al: *Primer of diagnostic imaging,* ed 5, St Louis, 2011, Mosby.)

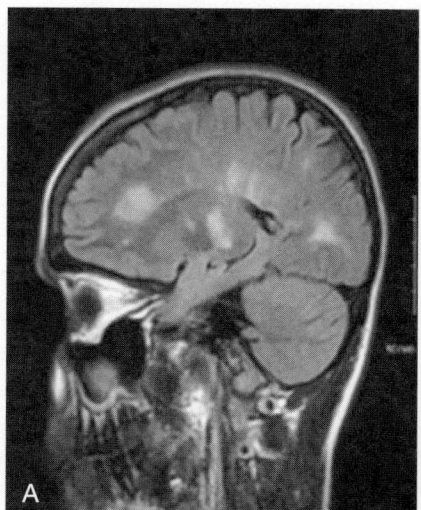
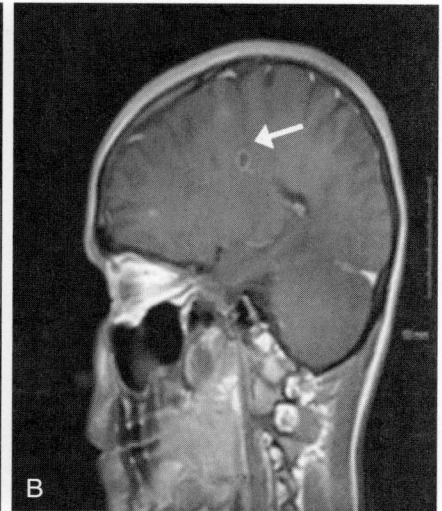

FIGURE 1-554 Multiple sclerosis. A, Sagittal FLAIR image magnetic resonance scan shows multiple lesions in corpus callosum (periventricular and perpendicular to corpus callosum, known as "Dawson's fingers") along with lesions in right frontal, occipital lobes. **B,** Gadolinium-enhanced scan shows one enhancing lesion *(arrow).*

dose-dependent cardiotoxicity) for frequent relapses with significant disability progression and for early SPMS. Emerging agents (currently in phase 2 or 3 of clinical trials) with long-term immunosuppressive effects include cladribine, alemtuzumab, daclizumab, laquinimod, and teriflunomide.

- Monoclonal antibodies: natalizumab (Tysabri) is approved for treatment of RRMS in the form of monthly infusions. It has been associated with an increased risk of developing progressive multifocal leukoencephalopathy (rare and fatal brain infection). Patients taking natalizumab must enter into a registry for monitoring.
- Spasticity: onabotulinum toxin type A injection is FDA approved as first-line therapy for upper limb spasticity. Baclofen, tizanidine, dantrolene, diazepam, lorazepam, and intrathecal baclofen are other alternatives.
- Pain: carbamazepine, gabapentin, or amitriptyline.
- Spastic bladder: oxybutynin, tolterodine, or propantheline. Prazosin for spastic sphincter.
- Fatigue: consider amantadine 100 mg bid, modafinil (most effective for somnolence), or fluoxetine.
- Tremor: clonazepam, carbamazepine, propranolol, or gabapentin. Wrist splints may be helpful.
- Depression: selective serotonin receptor inhibitors or tricyclic antidepressants.

DISPOSITION
Most patients have complete or near-complete recovery weeks to months after a relapse. Typically, two flares occur in RRMS patient per year (75% will have at least one flare). Although the rate of disease progression is highly variable, 50% to 75% of patients progress from RRMS to SPMS.

REFERRAL
- Referral to neurology on diagnosis is highly recommended.
- Consider referrals for physical therapy and occupational therapy to prevent/minimize disability. Consider referral to urology if postvoid residual by bladder scan is more than 100 ml.
- Referral to MS specialist should be strongly considered in case of poor response to therapy, possibility of cytotoxic treatment, and/or concern regarding accuracy of diagnosis.

PEARLS & CONSIDERATIONS

- Clinically isolated syndrome (CIS): patient with an isolated demyelinating event such as optic neuritis with no prior history of neurologic symptoms. If brain MRI is completely normal, there is 20% to 25% chance of subsequent MS. If there are two or more T2 hyperintensities on neuroimaging, there is a 70% to 90% chance of subsequent MS.
- Pseudorelapses may occur with heat, fever, or infections (urinary tract infections common in patients with MS).
- In an African American patient with clinical suspicion for MS, strongly consider possibility of neurosarcoidosis and order CXR, CSF angiotensin-converting enzyme level, and perhaps noncontrast chest CT.

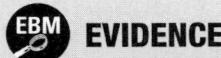 **EVIDENCE**

available at www.expertconsult.com

SUGGESTED READINGS
available at www.expertconsult.com

RELATED CONTENT
Multiple Sclerosis (Patient Information)

AUTHOR: **DIVYA SINGHAL, M.D.**

BASIC INFORMATION

DEFINITION

Mumps is an acute generalized viral infection that is usually characterized by nonsuppurative swelling and tenderness of one or both parotid glands. It is caused by mumps virus, a paramyxovirus and member of the paramyxoviridae family.

SYNONYMS

Viral parotitis
Parotitis

ICD-9CM CODES
072.9 Mumps

EPIDEMIOLOGY & DEMOGRAPHICS

INCIDENCE (IN U.S.):
- About 1600 infections/yr. Sporadic outbreaks occur
- More than 150,000 cases/yr before licensure of mumps vaccine in 1967

PREDOMINANT SEX: Males = females

PREDOMINANT AGE: 75% of disease in teenage years

PEAK INCIDENCE: Late winter and early spring months

GENETICS:
Congenital infection:
- First-trimester infection is associated with excessive fetal deaths.
- Second- and third-trimester infection is not associated with increased fetal mortality.

Neonatal infection:
- Uncommon
- Uncommon in infants <1 yr because of passive immunity conferred by placental transfer of maternal antibody

PHYSICAL FINDINGS & CLINICAL PRESENTATION

- Prodromal period: includes low-grade fever, malaise, anorexia, and headache
- Parotid swelling (Fig. 1-555) and tenderness; often the first signs of infection:
  1. Progresses over 2 to 3 days, then opposite side may become involved
  2. Unilateral parotitis in 25% of cases
  3. Considerable pain with parotid swelling, causing trismus and difficulty with mastication and pronunciation
  4. Pain exacerbated by eating or drinking citrus and other acidic foods
  5. Possible fever with parotid swelling, ranging up to 40° C
  6. Parotid swelling, usually resolving within 1 wk
- CNS involvement:
  1. May occur from 1 wk before to 2 wk after the onset of parotitis or even in its absence
  2. Meningitis:
     a. Occurs in 1% to 10% of patients with mumps parotitis
     b. Occurs three times more often in males than females
     c. Symptoms: headache, fever, nuchal rigidity, and vomiting
     d. Full recovery with no sequelae
  3. Encephalitis:
     a. May develop early, as a result of direct viral invasion of neurons, or late, around the second wk after onset of parotitis, and is a postinfectious demyelinating process.
     b. Mumps accounted for only 0.5% of viral meningitis.
     c. Symptoms: fever, alterations in the level of consciousness, possible seizures, paresis or paralysis, and aphasia. Fever can be quite high (40° to 41° C).
     d. Cerebellitis and hydrocephalus are serious complications of mumps encephalitis.
     e. May result in permanent sequelae or death.
  4. Other rare neurologic complications: include cerebellar ataxia, transverse myelitis, Guillain-Barré syndrome, and facial palsy.
- Epididymoorchitis:
  1. Most common extrasalivary gland complication of mumps in adult men
  2. Occurs in 38% of postpubertal males who have mumps
  3. Most often unilateral but is bilateral in 30% of males who develop this complication
  4. May precede development of parotitis and may be only manifestation of mumps
  5. Two thirds of cases develop during first week of parotitis
  6. Symptoms:
     a. Severe pain, swelling, and tenderness of the testes and scrotal erythema
     b. Fever and chills
  7. Some degree of testicular atrophy in 50% of cases, mo to yr later
  8. Sterility from bilateral orchitis is rare
- Involvement of pancreas and ovaries:
  1. Pancreas: abdominal pain, fever, and vomiting
  2. Ovaries: oophoritis
     a. Occurs in 5% of postpubertal women with mumps
     b. Symptoms include fever, nausea, vomiting, and lower abdominal pain
     c. May rarely result in decreased fertility and premature menopause
- Transient renal impairment: common and manifested by hematura and polyuria
- Joint involvement:
  1. Migratory polyarthritis is most frequent
  2. Infrequently affects adults with mumps
  3. Occurs rarely in children
  4. Self-limited, with complete resolution
- Deafness:
  1. Most often unilateral, involving high frequencies; may rarely cause bilateral involvement
  2. Most patients recover
  3. Permanent unilateral deafness reported in 1 in 20,000 cases
  4. Labyrinthitis and end lymphatic hydrops also reported
- Myocardial involvement:
  1. Uncommon
  2. Rarely causes progressive and fulminant fatal myocarditis with dilated cardiomyopathy
  3. Refractory arrhythmia and congestive heart failure
  4. Coronary artery involvement
- Eye involvement:
  1. Corneal endothelitis following mumps parotitis

ETIOLOGY

- Virus is spread via direct contact, droplet nuclei, fomites, or oral or nasal secretions.
- Patients are contagious from 48 hr before to 9 days after parotid swelling.

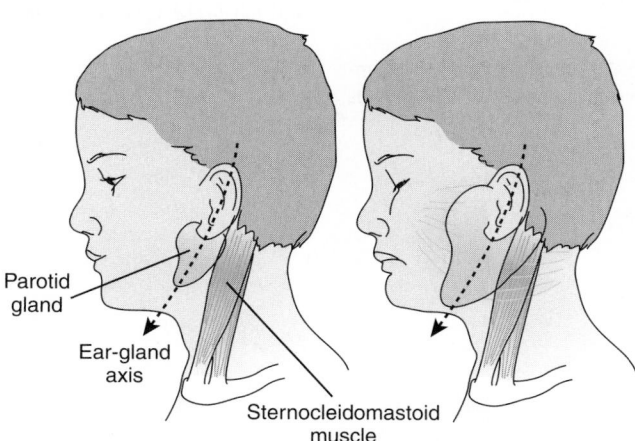

FIGURE 1-555 Schematic drawing of a parotid gland infected with mumps (right) compared with a normal gland (left). An imaginary line bisecting the long axis of the ear divides the parotid gland into two equal parts. These anatomic relationships are not altered in the enlarged gland. An enlarged cervical lymph node is usually posterior to the imaginary line. (From Mumps [epidemic parotitis]. In Krugman S et al [eds]: *Infectious diseases in children*, ed 6, St Louis, 1977, Mosby.)

Parotid gland
Ear-gland axis
Sternocleidomastoid muscle

M

Diseases and Disorders

I

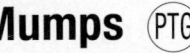

DIAGNOSIS

DIFFERENTIAL DIAGNOSIS

- Other viruses that may cause acute parotitis:
  1. Parainfluenza types 1 and 3
  2. Coxsackie viruses
  3. Influenza A
  4. Cytomegalovirus
- Suppurative parotitis:
  1. Most often caused by *Staphylococcus aureus*
  2. May be differentiated from mumps
     a. Extreme indurations, tenderness and erythema overlying the gland
     b. Ability to express pus from Stensen's duct or massage of parotid
- Other conditions that may occur with parotid enlargement or swelling:
  1. Sjögren's syndrome
  2. Leukemia
  3. Diabetes mellitus
  4. Uremia
  5. Malnutrition
  6. Cirrhosis
- Drugs that cause parotid swelling:
  1. Phenothiazines
  2. Phenylbutazone
  3. Thiouracil
  4. Iodides
- Conditions that cause unilateral swelling:
  1. Tumors
  2. Cysts
  3. Stones causing obstruction
  4. Strictures causing obstruction

WORKUP

- Diagnosis based on history of exposure and physical finding of parotid tenderness with mild to moderate constitutional symptoms.
- Diagnosis is confirmed by a variety of serologic tests or isolation of the virus.

LABORATORY TESTS

- Diagnosis is confirmed by a positive IgM mumps antibody or by fourfold rise between acute and convalescent sera by CF, ELISA, or neutralization tests. A polymerase chain reaction (PCR) assay is also available.
- Virus can be isolated from the saliva, usually from 2 to 3 days before to 4 to 5 days after the onset of parotitis.
- Virus can be cultured from CSF in patients with meningitis during the first 3 days of meningeal findings. More rapid confirmation of mumps in the CSF is IgM antibody capture immunoassay and nested PCR assay.
- Virus can be detected in urine during the first 2 wk of infection.
- WBC:
  1. May be normal or possible mild leukopenia with a relative lymphocytosis
  2. Leukocytosis with left shift with extra–salivary gland involvement, such as meningitis, orchitis, or pancreatitis
- Serum amylase:
  1. Elevated in the presence of parotitis
  2. May remain elevated for 2 to 3 wk
  3. May be differentiated from mumps and parotids by isoenzyme analysis or serum pancreatic lipase
- Mumps meningitis:
  1. CSF WBCs from 10 to 2000 WBC/mm^3 with a predominance of lymphocytes
  2. In 20% to 25% of patients, predominance of polymorphonuclear cells
  3. CSF protein normal or mildly elevated
  4. CSF glucose low, <40 mg/dl, in 6% to 30% of patients

TREATMENT

NONPHARMACOLOGIC THERAPY

- Supportive treatment
- Adequate hydration and nutrition

ACUTE GENERAL Rx

- Analgesics and antipyretics to relieve pain and fever
- Narcotic analgesics, along with bed rest, ice packs, and a testicular bridge, to relieve pain associated with mumps orchitis
- IV fluids for patients with frequent vomiting associated with mumps pancreatitis or meningitis

DISPOSITION

Most patients recover without incident.

REFERRAL

- To a neurologist if significant neurologic complications develop during or following mumps (myelitis, encephalitis, cranial nerve involvement, cerebellar ataxia, etc.)
- To a cardiologist if viral perimyocarditis develops
- To a urologist if orchitis develops

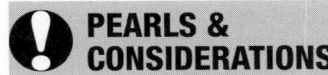

PEARLS & CONSIDERATIONS

COMMENTS

Prevention:
- Attenuated live mumps virus vaccine has been available since 1967.
  1. Usually given in combination with measles and rubella vaccines
  2. Should be given at 15 mo of age, and again at 5 to 12 yr
  3. Seroconversion in about 100% of infants given the vaccine
  4. Contraindicated in pregnant women and immunocompromised patients
  5. Patients with asymptomatic HIV infection and patients with symptomatic HIV infection, in the absence of severe immunosuppression, can safely receive mumps, measles, and rubella (MMR) vaccine
  6. Adverse events of vaccination include local pain, indurations, thrombocytopenic purpura, Guillain-Barré syndrome, and cerebellar ataxia
- The CDC and American Academy of Pediatrics (AAP) recommend that patients with mumps stay home from work or school for 5 days after onset of clinical symptoms.
- Because virus may be shed before the onset of parotid swelling, isolation possibly not of great value in limiting spread of infection. Use droplet precautions as per CDC and AAP.

SUGGESTED READINGS

available at www.expertconsult.com

RELATED CONTENT

Mumps (Patient Information)

AUTHOR: **GLENN G. FORT, M.D., M.P.H.**

BASIC INFORMATION

DEFINITION

Muscular dystrophy (MD) refers to a heterogeneous group of inherited disorders resulting in characteristic patterns of muscle weakness, some with cardiac involvement. Only disorders with childhood or adult onset are considered here (i.e., excluding congenital myopathies).

ICD-9CM CODES
359   Muscular dystrophies and other myopathies
359.1 Hereditary progressive muscular dystrophy

EPIDEMIOLOGY & DEMOGRAPHICS

INCIDENCE:
- Most common childhood MD is Duchenne's muscular dystrophy (DMD) with an incidence of 1/3500 male births.
- Most common adult MD is myotonic dystrophy with an incidence as high as 1/8000.

GENETICS:
- **Dystrophinopathies:** X-linked recessive defect in dystrophin gene resulting in either absence (DMD) or reduced/defective (Becker's MD [BMD]) dystrophin (Fig. 1-556)
- **Myotonic Dystrophy:** Autosomal dominant (AD) CTG trinucleotide repeat (see "Myotonia")
- **Limb-Girdle Muscular Dystrophy:** Autosomal recessive, also autosomal dominant forms with deficiency identified in multiple proteins (sarcoglycan, calpain, dysferlin, telethonin, lamin A/C, myotilin, and caveolin-3)
- **Emery-Dreifuss Muscular Dystrophy:** X-linked recessive defect in nuclear protein emerin or AR defect in inner nuclear lamina proteins lamin A/C

- **Facioscapulohumeral Muscular Dystrophy:** AD; genetic mutation causes deletion of 3.3 kb repeat
- **Oculopharyngeal Muscular Dystrophy:** AD GCG trinucleotide repeat resulting in deficient mRNA transfer from nucleus

PHYSICAL FINDINGS & CLINICAL PRESENTATION

- **Dystrophinopathies:** Proximal arm and leg weakness with hypertrophic calf muscles (Fig. 1-557), delayed motor milestones, cognitive impairment, cardiac involvement, progressive course resulting in respiratory complications and respiratory failure
  - DMD (Fig. 1-558) onset at 2 to 3 yr old, typically wheelchair-bound by 12 yr
  - BMD onset at 5 to 15 yr old, ambulatory beyond age 15
- **Myotonic Dystrophy:** Variable age of onset and severity manifesting as predominately distal weakness with long face, percussion and grip myotonia, temporalis and masseter wasting, ptosis, hypersomnolence, cognitive impairment, and cardiac conduction defects. May be associated with frontal balding, cataracts, impaired glucose tolerance, and male infertility.
- **Limb-Girdle MD:** Phenotypically and genetically heterogenous characterized by proximal hip and shoulder girdle weakness, some genotypes featuring cardiac involvement
- **Emery-Dreifuss MD:** Early adulthood onset with predominately humeroperoneal weakness, early contractures, and cardiac dysfunction
- **Facioscapulohumeral MD:** Onset typically in late childhood or adolescence with weakness mostly in face and shoulder girdle musculature and possible later, mild involvement of lower extremities

- **Oculopharyngeal MD:** Symptom onset typically in mid-adult life with ptosis, dysphagia, dysarthria, and proximal muscle weakness

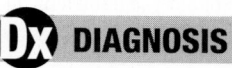 **DIAGNOSIS**

DIFFERENTIAL DIAGNOSIS

Myasthenia gravis, inflammatory myopathy, metabolic myopathy, endocrine myopathy, toxic myopathy, mitochondrial myopathy

WORKUP

- CK
- ECG, Holter monitor, echocardiography
- EMG
- Muscle biopsy with immunohistochemistry useful for diagnosis of dystrophinopathies and limb-girdle MD

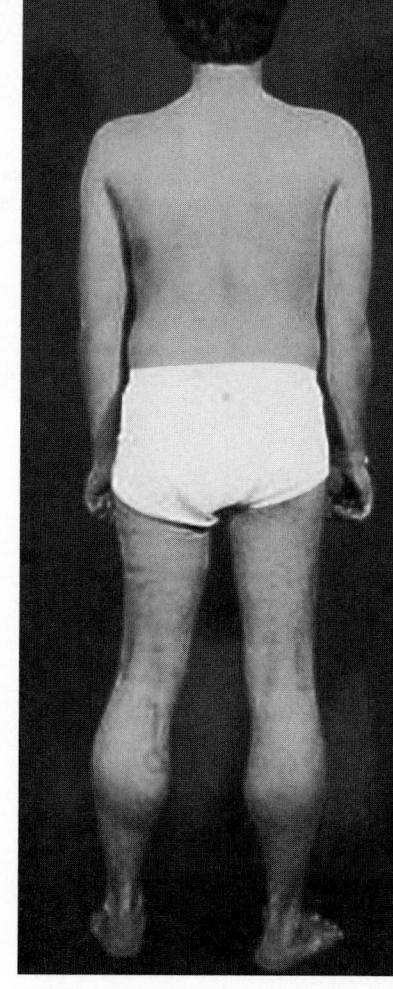

FIGURE 1-557 Becker muscular dystrophy in a 24-year-old male. There is dystrophy of the shoulder girdle and calf pseudohypertrophy. (Courtesy Dr. R. Pascuzzi. From Libby PL et al: *Braunwald's heart disease: a textbook of cardiovascular medicine,* ed 8, Philadelphia, 2007, Saunders.)

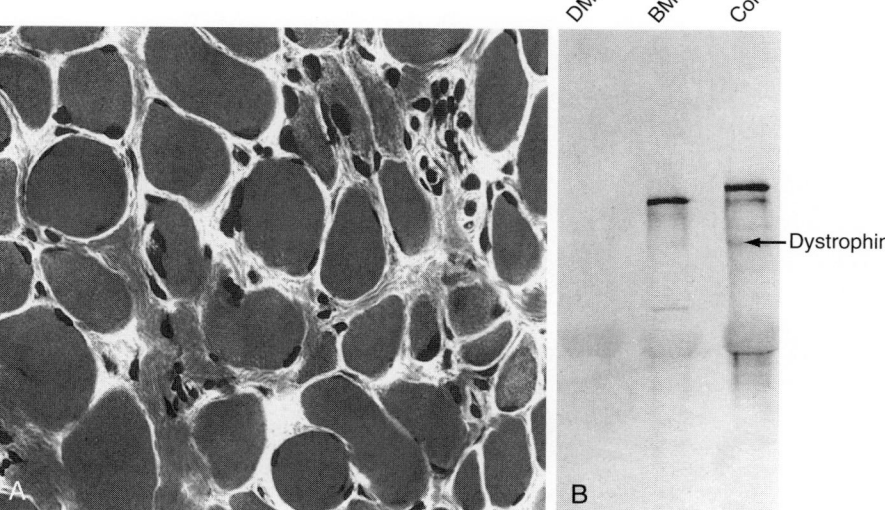

FIGURE 1-556 A, Duchenne muscular dystrophy showing variation in muscle fiber size, increased endomysial connective tissue, and regenerating fibers. **B,** Western blot showing absence of dystrophin in DMD and altered dystrophin size in Becker muscular dystrophy (BMD) compared with control (Con). (Courtesy Dr. L. Kunkel, Children's Hospital, Boston. From Kumar V et al: *Robbins and Cotran pathologic basis of disease,* ed 7, Philadelphia, 2005, Saunders.)

- DNA analysis helpful if clinical suspicion is for myotonic, Emery-Dreifuss, facioscapulo-humeral, and oculopharyngeal MDs
- Assessment of respiratory parameters, including forced vital capacity (FVC)

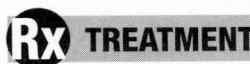 TREATMENT

NONPHARMACOLOGIC THERAPY
- Genetic counseling
- Physical, occupational, respiratory, speech therapy as symptoms dictate

- Screening for sleep-disordered breathing with overnight polysomnogram (PSG) if clinically indicated
- Pacemaker placement may be necessary if cardiac conduction defect present

ACUTE GENERAL Rx
Prednisone may modestly prolong ambulation in DMD. A dose of 0.75 mg/kg/day may improve muscle strength and function over 6 months to 2 years. These short-term benefits must be weighed against the side effects of long-term steroid therapy.

CHRONIC Rx
Vigilance to avoid cardiac and respiratory complications, joint contractures

DISPOSITION
Variable course, because severity of phenotype is contingent upon both diagnosis and genotype

REFERRAL
- Surgical referral for correction of scoliosis or contractures may be necessary
- Assessment and follow-up in an MD specialty clinic

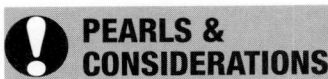 **PEARLS & CONSIDERATIONS**

Formal evaluation by anesthetist is recommended before any operation with general anesthesia in patients with dystrophinopathy.

SUGGESTED READINGS
available at www.expertconsult.com

RELATED CONTENT
Muscular Dystrophy (Patient Information)

AUTHOR: **TAYLOR HARRISON, M.D.**

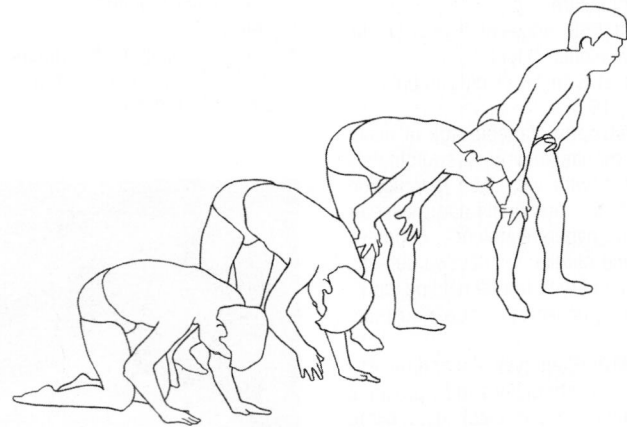

FIGURE 1-558 In Duchenne's muscular dystrophy, the patient will get up from the floor with Gower's maneuver. The boy will "walk up" his body with his hands as he arises. (From Remmel KS et al: *Handbook of symptom-oriented neurology,* ed 3, St Louis, 2002, Mosby.)

BASIC INFORMATION

DEFINITION

Mushroom poisoning is intoxication resulting from ingestion of poisonous mushrooms.

ICD-9CM CODES
988.1 Mushroom poisoning

EPIDEMIOLOGY & DEMOGRAPHICS

- 5% of all mushrooms are poisonous. Distinction between poisonous and edible mushrooms may be difficult even by experienced persons.

- Common poisonous species include *Amanita*, *Russula*, *Gyromitra*, and *Omphalotus*.

PHYSICAL FINDINGS & CLINICAL PRESENTATION (Table 1-286)

- *Russula* causes confusion, delirium, visual disturbance, tachycardia, and diarrhea within a few hours of ingestion. Prognosis: spontaneous recovery (mortality rate <1%).
- *Amanita* (Fig. 1-559) and *Gyromitra* intoxication begins with symptoms of gastroenteritis (nausea, vomiting, diarrhea, abdominal cramps) approximately 10 hr after ingestion. *Amanita* then causes cardiomyopathy and hepatic and renal failure. *Gyromitra* produces jaundice and seizures. Both mushrooms are associated with a 50% mortality rate.
- *Omphalotus* causes symptoms of gastroenteritis that subside spontaneously within 24 hr.

ETIOLOGY

- *Amanita* contains cytotoxic substances and isoxazoles that are gamma-aminobutyric acid neurotransmitter analogs.
- *Gyromitra* contains a pyridoxine antagonist that disrupts the gastrointestinal mucosa and causes hemolysis.
- *Russula* contains a cholinergic substance.

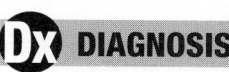

DIAGNOSIS

DIFFERENTIAL DIAGNOSIS

- Food poisoning
- Overdose of prescription or illegal drug
- Other intoxications
- See topic on specific organ failure (e.g., renal or hepatic failure) for differential diagnosis of those conditions

WORKUP

- History
- Inspection and identification of suspected mushrooms
- Mushroom or gastric content analysis (by thin-layer chromatography or radioimmunoassay)

TREATMENT

- Gastric lavage
- Repeated administration of activated charcoal
- Penicillin G or silibinin can be used for *Amanita* mushroom intoxication. Silibinin interferes with hepatic uptake of alpha-amanitin. IV silibinin is not currently available in the U.S. Where available, it is given at a rate of 5 mg/kg IV over 1 hour, followed by 20 mg/kg/day. An oral form of silibinin is available in health food stores as an extract from milk thistle called silymarin. Dose is 1 g PO qid. IV benzyl penicillin reduces hepatocyte uptake of amatoxin.
- Supportive care as needed (may require respiratory assistance, hemodialysis, or emergency liver transplantation)

AUTHOR: **FRED F. FERRI, M.D.**

TABLE 1-286 Mushroom Poisoning Syndromes

Syndrome	Incubation Period (hr)	Species	Toxin
Confusion, restlessness, visual disturbances, lethargy	2	*Amanita muscaria* *Amanita pantherina*	Ibotenic acid, muscimol
Parasympathetic activity	2	*Inocybe* spp. *Clitocybe* spp.	Muscarine
Hallucinations	2	*Psilocybe* spp. *Panacolus* spp.	Psilocybin Psilocin
Disulfiram	2	*Coprinus atramentarius*	Disulfiram-like substances
Gastroenteritis	2	Many	Unknown
Hepatorenal failure	6-24	*Amanita phalloides* *Amanita virosa* *Amanita verna* *Galerina autumnalis* *Galerina marginata* *Galerina venenata*	Amatoxins Phallotoxins
Hepatic failure	6-24	*Gyromitra* spp.	Gyromitrin

From Gorbach SL: *Infectious diseases*, ed 2, Philadelphia, 1998, Saunders.

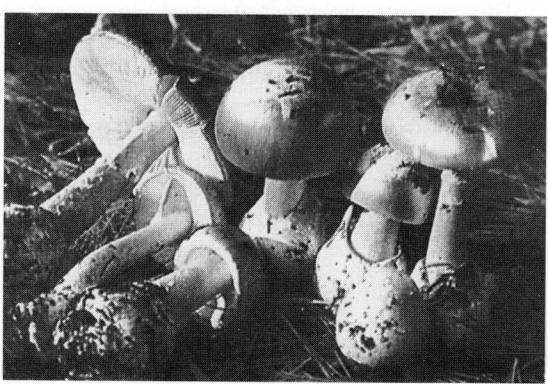

FIGURE 1-559 Death cap *(Amanita phalloides).* (From Auerbach P: *Wilderness medicine*, ed 4, St Louis, 2001, Mosby.)

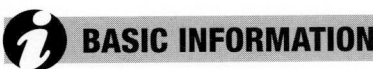

DEFINITION

Myasthenia gravis (MG) is an autoimmune disorder that affects postsynaptic neuromuscular transmission classically mediated by antibodies directed against the nicotinic acetylcholine receptor (AChR) of the neuromuscular junction, resulting in a decrease in functional postsynaptic ACh receptors and consequent weakness.

ICD-9CM CODES
358.0 Myasthenia gravis

EPIDEMIOLOGY & DEMOGRAPHICS

INCIDENCE (IN U.S.): Two to five cases annually per 1 million persons
PEAK INCIDENCE: Female, second to third decades; male, sixth to seventh decades
PREVALENCE (IN U.S.): One per 20,000 persons
PREDOMINANT SEX: Females are affected more often than males (3:2) in adults; they are equally affected in the elderly
GENETICS: Increased frequency of HLA-B8, DR3

PHYSICAL FINDINGS & CLINICAL PRESENTATION

- The hallmark of MG is fluctuating weakness worsened with exercise and improved with rest.
- Generalized weakness involving proximal muscles, diaphragm, and neck extensors is common.
- Weakness is confined to eyelids and extraocular muscles in approximately 15% of patients.
- Bulbar symptoms of ptosis, diplopia, dysarthria, and dysphagia are common.
- Reflexes, sensation, and coordination are normal.

ETIOLOGY

Antibody-mediated decrease in nicotinic AChR in the postsynaptic neuromuscular junction resulting in defective neuromuscular transmission and subsequent muscle weakness and fatigue

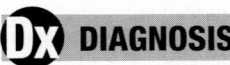 DIAGNOSIS

DIFFERENTIAL DIAGNOSIS

Lambert-Eaton myasthenic syndrome, botulism, medication-induced myasthenia, chronic progressive external ophthalmoplegia, congenital myasthenic syndromes, thyroid disease, basilar meningitis, intracranial mass lesion with cranial neuropathy, Miller-Fisher variant of Guillain-Barré syndrome

WORKUP

- Edrophonium (Tensilon) test (Fig. E1-560): useful in MG patients with ocular symptoms. Cardiac monitoring and atropine ready at the bedside are essential. Patients with MG may also have a positive ice test (Fig. E1-561).
- Repetitive nerve stimulation: successive stimulation shows decrement of muscle action potential in clinically weak muscle; may be negative in up to 50%.
- Single-fiber electromyography: highly sensitive; abnormal in up to 95% of patients.
- Serum AChR antibodies found in up to 80% of patients.
- A subset of patients with seronegative MG may have muscle-specific tyrosine kinase MuSK antibodies.

ADDITIONAL TESTS

- Spirometry to document pulmonary function
- CT scan of anterior chest to look for thymoma or residual thymic tissue
- Thyroid-stimulating hormone, free T_4 to rule out thyroid disease

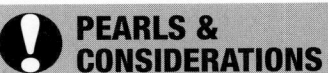 TREATMENT

NONPHARMACOLOGIC THERAPY

- Patient education to facilitate recognition of worsening symptoms and impress need for medical evaluation at onset of clinical deterioration
- Avoidance of selected drugs known to provoke exacerbations of MG (beta-blockers, aminoglycoside and quinolone antibiotics, class I antiarrhythmics)
- Prompt treatment of infections, diet modification, and speech evaluation with dysphagia

ACUTE GENERAL Rx

- Symptomatic treatment with acetylcholinesterase inhibitors:
  1. Pyridostigmine 30 to 60 mg PO q4 to 6h initially; onset of effects is 30 min, duration 4 hr
- Immunosuppressive treatment with corticosteroids, azathioprine, cyclosporine for long-term disease-modifying therapy

1. Prednisone initiated at 15 to 20 mg qd titrate by 5-mg increments to effect or dose of 1 mg/kg/day with improvement in 2 to 4 wk and maximal response by 3 to 6 mo
2. Azathioprine initiated at 50 mg qd titrated to 2 to 3 mg/kg/day with clinical effect in 6 to 12 mo
3. Cyclosporine initiated at 5 mg/kg/day with clinical effect within 1 to 2 mo
- Plasmapheresis and IV immunoglobulin are short-term options for immunotherapy during an exacerbation.
- Mechanical ventilation is lifesaving in setting of a myasthenic crisis. Consider elective intubation if forced vital capacity <15 ml/kg, maximal expiratory pressure <40 cm H_2O, or negative inspiratory pressure <25 cm H_2O.

SURGICAL Rx

- In thymomatous MG, thymectomy is indicated in all patients.
- For nonthymomatous autoimmune MG, thymectomy is an option in select patients, typically <40 yr.

DISPOSITION

Course of disease is highly variable.

REFERRAL

Surgical referral for thymectomy in selected cases (see "Surgical Rx")

PEARLS & CONSIDERATIONS

- Sustained upward or lateral gaze and arm abduction for 120 sec may be necessary to elicit subtle signs on examination.
- Myasthenic patients can worsen rapidly and warrant close, careful observation during an exacerbation.

SUGGESTED READINGS

available at www.expertconsult.com

RELATED CONTENT

Myasthenia Gravis (Patient Information)

AUTHOR: **TAYLOR HARRISON, M.D.**

BASIC INFORMATION

DEFINITION

Mycosis fungoides refers to a T-cell lymphoproliferative disorder with characteristic cutaneous skin lesions and the potential to disseminate into lymph nodes and viscera.

SYNONYMS

Cutaneous T-cell lymphoma

ICD-9CM CODES

202.1 Mycosis fungoides

EPIDEMIOLOGY & DEMOGRAPHICS

- Incidence of mycosis fungoides is four cases per 1 million persons.
- ~1000 new cases are diagnosed annually in the United States.
- More commonly affects males than females (2:1).
- Affects blacks more often than whites (2:1).
- Usually found in males ages 40 to 60.

PHYSICAL FINDINGS & CLINICAL PRESENTATION

Mycosis fungoides characteristically progresses through three phases:

- A *premycotic phase* featuring scaly, erythematous patches that can last from months to years. During this stage the diagnosis can only be suspected because the histopathologic features are not definitive for mycosis fungoides. Lesions are pruritic and can appear anywhere but are usually found in sun-shielded areas. Parapsoriasis in plaques, poikilodermatous parapsoriasis, parapsoria-

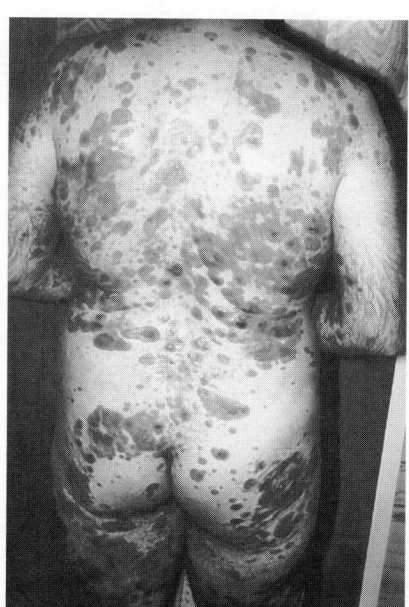

FIGURE 1-562 Cutaneous T-cell lymphoma (mycosis fungoides). Note patch, plaque, and tumor stages. (From Noble J [ed]: *Textbook of primary care medicine*, ed 2, St Louis, 1996, Mosby.)

sis lichenoides, and variegata are skin lesions suspicious of representing premycotic cutaneous T-cell lymphoma.

- The *infiltrative plaque phase* features raised, indurated erythematous palpable plaques that are pruritic and may be associated with alopecia.
  - Stage IA disease is defined as a patch or plaque skin disease involving <10% of the skin surface area and with absence of blood involvement or with low blood tumor burden (<5% of atypical T cells [Sézary cells] in the peripheral blood).
  - Stage IB disease (Fig. 1-562) is defined as a patch or plaque skin disease involving ≥10% of the skin surface area (Fig. E1-563) with absence of blood involvement or low blood tumor burden (<5% Sézary cells).
- The *tumor phase* is characterized by large, lumpy nodules arising from a premycotic patch, plaque, or unaffected skin and represents systemic infiltration and spreading. The tumors can be pruritic and large (>10 cm) and ulceration can occur.
  - Stage IIA and stage IIB diseases are defined by the presence of tumors with or without clinically abnormal peripheral lymph nodes with absence of blood involvement or low blood tumor burden. In approximately 5% of cases of mycosis fungoides, the presentation may be a diffuse, painful, pruritic erythroderma with Sézary cells in the peripheral blood (known as Sézary syndrome) (Fig. E1-564).
  - Stage III disease is defined by the presence of generalized erythroderma from the spread of cancer cells through the skin but not yet to the lymph nodes.
- Lymphadenopathy can occur during the plaque or tumor stages and may be regional or diffuse.
  - Stage IVA disease is defined by a lymph node biopsy showing large clusters of atypical cells, more than six cells, or total effacement by atypical cells.
- Infiltration of the liver, spleen, lungs, bone marrow, kidney, stomach, and brain can occur.
  - Stage IVB disease is defined by the presence of visceral involvement.

ETIOLOGY

The specific cause of mycosis fungoides is not known. Infection with the retrovirus HTLV-1 has been suspected, given the association of individuals infected with HTLV-1 and those with T-cell leukemia. Other considerations listed but unsubstantiated include environmental toxins (e.g., tobacco, pesticides, herbicides, and solvents) and genetic predisposition.

DIAGNOSIS

The diagnosis of mycosis fungoides is established by skin biopsy. This may be difficult to differentiate from other skin lesions in the early phases of the disease (e.g., premycotic patch or early plaque lesions); therefore the diagnosis can only be suspected.

DIFFERENTIAL DIAGNOSIS

- Contact dermatitis
- Atopic dermatitis
- Nummular dermatitis
- Parapsoriases
- Superficial fungal infections
- Drug eruptions
- Psoriasis
- Photodermatitis
- Alopecia mucinosa
- Lymphomatoid papulosis

WORKUP

Any patient who is suspected of having mycosis fungoides should have a staging workup. Prognosis in patients with mycosis fungoides depends on the type of skin lesions and the extent of disease. The workup should focus on:

1. Complete physical examination:
   - The type of skin lesion and the extent of skin involvement of the body (e.g., skin involvement is >10% or <10% of the skin surface)
   - Identification of palpable lymph node (especially those >1.5 cm in largest diameter)
   - Identification of organomegaly (e.g., lungs, liver)
2. Skin biopsy:
   - Biopsy of the most indurated area
   - Immunophenotyping
   - Evaluation for clonality
3. Blood test:
   - Complete blood count with differential, liver function tests, lactate dehydrogenase, chemistry
   - T-cell receptor gene rearrangement
   - Determination of Sézary cell count and/or flow cytometry
4. Radiologic tests
   - Depending on the stage of the disease, chest radiograph; ultrasound; and CT scan of the chest, abdomen, and pelvis alone, with or without fluorodeoxyglucose positron emission tomography scan
5. Lymph node biopsy
   - Excisional biopsy
   - Biopsy of the largest lymph node
   - If multiple nodes enlarged, order of preference is cervical, axillary, and inguinal areas
   - Histopathology, flow cytometry, T-cell receptor gene rearrangement

TREATMENT

Treatment is guided according to the stage of disease. A treatment algorithm is described in Fig. E1-565.

NONPHARMACOLOGIC THERAPY

- For dry, cracking skin, emollients (e.g., lanolin and petrolatum) are applied bid.
- Moisturizing lotion (e.g., ammonium lactate) applied bid.
- Topical antibiotics (e.g., bacitracin) are used on ulcerative tumors.

ACUTE GENERAL Rx

- Treatment of patients with stage IA limited patch or plaque phase includes:
  - Topical agents such as cotriosteroids and rtinoids are used when cutaneous symptoms develop.
  - Psoralen ultraviolet A (PUVA) light therapy where 0.6 mg/kg of 8-methoxypsoralen is ingested 1 to 2 hr before exposure of the skin to UVA light (320 to 400 nm). This is done three times per wk and tapered to twice per wk until all the lesions have cleared. This is typically continued for 6 mo with a 90% complete remission rate.
- Treatment of patients with stage IB and IIA disease is similar to stage IA, with topical corticosteroids and retinoids or PUVA.
  - Total skin electron beam therapy is considered in patients with thick plaques.
  - Interferon-alpha 5 million units SQ three times weekly can be considered in patients with stage IB or IIA disease.

- Retinoids in combination with PUVA are used in refractory cases. Isotretinoin 1 mg/kg per day or acitretin 25 to 50 mg per day is the standard dosing.
- Treatment of patients with stage IIB disease with generalized tumor and plaque disease:
  - Total skin electron beam therapy in doses of 3000 to 3600 cGy given over 8 to 10 wk followed by adjuvant therapy with topical mustard can be used.
- Patients with advanced disease may receive combination chemotherapy (CHOP). Allogeneic HSCT should also be considered and may be curative in patients. Alemtuzumab has been reported effective in patients with organ involvement.

CHRONIC Rx

- In patients developing diffuse erythroderma, stage III disease (e.g., Sézary syndrome, extracorporeal photophoresis), 8-methoxypsoralen is ingested and peripheral blood is exposed to UVA through a membrane filter.

- In stage IV disease, interferon and other systemic chemotherapeutic agents (e.g., methotrexate, cyclophosphamide, doxorubicin, vincristine, prednisone) and alemtuzumab are considered.

DISPOSITION

- The patients with limited patch or plaque disease have excellent prognosis with long-term life expectancy that is similar to an age-, sex-, and race-matched control population.
- The patients with generalized patch or plaque without evidence of extracutaneous involvement have a median survival of greater than 11 yr.
- The patients with cutaneous tumor and generalized erythroderma without extracutaneous involvement have a median survival of 3 to 4.6 yr.
- The patients with extracutaneous disease at presentation involving either lymph node or viscera have median survival of 13 mo.

REFERRAL

Any patient with suspected mycosis fungoides should be referred to a dermatologist for definitive diagnosis and initial therapy. Oncology consultation is also indicated in patients with more advanced disease.

PEARLS & CONSIDERATIONS

A TNM staging classification of mycosis fungoides has been in use for guiding therapy since 1979. The International Society for Cutaneous Lymphomas (ISCL) and the Cutaneous Lymphoma Task Force of the European Organization of Research and Treatment of Cancer (EORTC) recommended revisions to the TNM classification and staging system of cutaneous T-cell lymphoma in 2007. Table 1-287 compares EORTC and WHO classifications of primary cutaneous lymphoma.

COMMENTS

Mycosis fungoides is thought to represent one class of the spectrum of cutaneous T-cell lymphomas.

SUGGESTED READINGS

available at www.expertconsult.com

AUTHOR: **TANYA ALI, M.D.**

TABLE 1-287 Comparison of EORTC and WHO Classifications of Primary Cutaneous Lymphoma

EORTC Classification	WHO Classification
Cutaneous T-Cell Lymphoma	
Indolent clinical behavior	Mycosis fungoides
Mycosis fungoides variants	Mycosis fungoides variants
Follicular mycosis fungoides	Follicular mycosis fungoides
Pagetoid reticulosis	Pagetoid reticulosis
CTCL, large cell, CD30$^+$	Primary cutaneous CD30$^+$ ALCA (CD30$^+$ lymphoproliferative disease, including lymphomatoid papulosis)
Lymphomatoid papulosis	
Aggressive clinical behavior	Sézary syndrome
Sézary syndrome	Peripheral T-cell lymphoma, unspecified (most); extranodal NK/T-cell lymphoma, nasal type
CTCL, large cell, CD30$^-$	
Provisional entities	
CTCL, pleomorphic, small/medium sized	
Subcutaneous panniculitis-like T-cell lymphoma	Subcutaneous panniculitis-like T-cell lymphoma
Cutaneous B-Cell Lymphoma	
Indolent clinical behavior	Extranodal marginal zone B-cell lymphoma
Primary cutaneous immunocytoma (marginal zone B-cell lymphoma)	
Follicle center cell lymphoma (any grade)	
Intermediate clinical behavior	
Primary cutaneous large B-cell	
Lymphoma of the leg	
Provisional Entities	
Primary cutaneous plasmacytoma	Plasmacytoma
Intravascular large B-cell lymphoma	Diffuse large B-cell lymphoma (intravascular)

ALCL, Anaplastic large cell lymphoma; *CTCL,* cutaneous T-cell lymphoma; *EORTC,* European Organization for the Research and Treatment of Cancer; *NK,* natural killer; *WHO,* World Health Organization.
From Hoffman R et al: *Hematology: basic principles and practice,* ed 5, Philadelphia, 2009, Churchill Livingstone.

BASIC INFORMATION

DEFINITION

Myelodysplastic syndrome (MDS) is a group of acquired clonal disorders affecting the hemopoietic stem cells and characterized by cytopenias with hypercellular bone marrow and various morphologic abnormalities in the hemopoietic cell lines. MDS shows abnormal (dysplastic) hemopoietic maturation. Marrow cellularity is increased, reflecting an effective hematopoiesis, but inadequate maturation results in peripheral cytopenias.

CLASSIFICATION

- Myelodysplasia encompasses several heterogenous syndromes. The French-American-British (FAB) classification of MDSs is based on the proportion of immature blast cells in the blood and marrow and on the presence or absence of ringed sideroblasts or peripheral monocytosis (Table 1-288). It includes refractory anemia, refractory anemia with ringed sideroblasts, refractory anemia with excess blasts, chronic myelomonocytic leukemia, and refractory anemia with excess blasts in transformation.
- In 1999 the World Health Organization modified the FAB by incorporating newer morphologic insights and cytogenetic findings. It includes the disease subtypes refractory anemia, refractory anemia with ringed sideroblasts, refractory cytopenia with multilineage dysplasia, refractory cytopenia with multilineage dysplasia and ringed sideroblasts, refractory anemia with excessive blasts (1, 2), unclassified MDS, and MDS associated with isolated del(5q).

SYNONYMS

MDS
Preleukemia
Dysmyelopoietic syndrome

ICD-9CM CODES
238.7 Myelodysplastic syndrome

EPIDEMIOLOGY & DEMOGRAPHICS

INCIDENCE (IN U.S.): Approximately 82 cases/100,000 persons per yr. An estimated 7000 to 12,000 new cases are diagnosed annually in the U.S.
PREDOMINANT AGE: More common in elderly patients; median age, >65 yr

PHYSICAL FINDINGS & CLINICAL PRESENTATION

- Splenomegaly, skin pallor, mucosal bleeding, and ecchymosis may be present.
- Patients often present with fatigue.
- Fever, infection, and dyspnea are common.

ETIOLOGY

Unknown. However, exposure to radiation, chemotherapeutic agents, benzene, or other organic compounds is associated with myelodysplasia. Table 1-289 describes predisposing factors and epidemiologic associations of patients with MDS. Recently targeted resequencing of the gene encoding RNA splicing factor 3B, subunit 1 (SF3B1) has shown that mutations in SF3B1 implicate abnormalities of messenger RNA splicing in the pathogenesis of MDS.

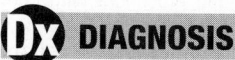 **DIAGNOSIS**

DIFFERENTIAL DIAGNOSIS

- Hereditary dysplasias (e.g., Fanconi's anemia, Diamond-Blackfan syndrome)
- Vitamin B_{12}/folate deficiency
- Exposure to toxins (drugs, alcohol, chemotherapy)
- Renal failure
- Irradiation
- Autoimmune disease
- Infections (tuberculosis, viral infections)
- Paroxysmal nocturnal hemoglobinuria

TABLE 1-288 French-American-British Classification Criteria

Subtype	Abbreviation	Peripheral Blood	Bone Marrow
Refractory anemia	RA	Blasts <1%	Blasts <5%
Refractory anemia with ringed sideroblasts	RARS	Blasts <1%	Blasts <5%, and >15% ringed sideroblasts
Refractory anemia with excess blasts	RAEB	Blasts <5%	Blasts 5%-20%
Refractory anemia with excess blasts in transformation	RAEB-T	Blasts >5%	Blasts 20%-30% or Auer rods
Chronic myelomonocytic leukemia	CMML	Monocytes $>1 \times 10^9$/L	Any of the above
Acute myelogenous leukemia	AML	Blasts >30%	

From Hoffmann R et al: *Hematology, basic principles and practice*, ed 5, Philadelphia, 2009, Churchill Livingstone.

TABLE 1-289 Predisposing Factors and Epidemiologic Associations of Patients with Myelodysplastic Syndrome

Heritable

Constitutional Genetic Disorders

Trisomy 8 mosaicism
Familial monosomy 7
Down syndrome (trisomy 21)
Neurofibromatosis 1
Germ cell tumors [embryonal dysgenesis del(12p)]

Congenital Neutropenia

Kostmann syndrome
Shwachman-Diamond syndrome

DNA Repair Deficiencies

Fanconi anemia
Ataxia-telangiectasia
Bloom syndrome
Xeroderma pigmentosum
Pharmacogenomic polymorphisms (GSTq1-null)

Acquired

Senescence

Mutagen Exposure

Alkylator therapy (chlorambucil, cyclophosphamide, melphalan, N-mustards)
Topoisomerase II inhibitors (anthracyclines)
β Emitters (32p)
Autologous stem cell transplantation
Environmental/occupational (benzene)
Tobacco
Aplastic anemia
Paroxysmal nocturnal hemoglobinuria

From Hoffman R et al: *Hematology, basic principles and practice*, ed 5, Philadelphia, 2009, Churchill Livingstone.

WORKUP

Diagnostic workup (Fig. E1-566) includes laboratory evaluation (Table E1-290) and bone marrow examination (Fig. E1-567). Cytogenetic analysis (Box E1-39) by conventional metaphase karyotyping should be performed in patients with MDS. Physical examination, medical history, and laboratory tests aiding in diagnosis of MDS are described in Table 1-291.

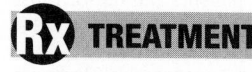 **TREATMENT**

NONPHARMACOLOGIC THERAPY

Red blood cell transfusions in patients with severe symptomatic anemia

ACUTE GENERAL Rx

- Erythropoietin (10,000 to 40,000 U/wk) in patient with symptomatic anemia.
- DNA methyltransferase inhibitors: Azacitidine (Vidaza), a pyrimidine nucleoside analog of cytidine, has been shown to improve the quality of life for patients with MDS and probably prolong survival. Decitabine (Dacogen), another nucleoside analog, has also been FDA approved for patients with MDS. These agents may also be useful in preventing the transition of MDS to AML.
- Immunomodulators: Lenalidomide (Revlimid), a novel analogue of thalidomide, has demonstrated hematologic activity in patients with low-rise MDS who have no response to erythropoietin or who are unlikely to benefit from conventional therapy. Lenalidomide can also reduce transfusion requirements and reverse cytologic and cytogenetic abnormalities in patients who have MDS with the 5q31 deletion.

- Allogeneic stem cell transplantation should be considered in patients ≤60 yr because this is the established procedure with cure potential (Fig. E1-568).
- Results of chemotherapy are generally disappointing. Combination chemotherapy regimens (e.g., cytarabine plus doxorubicin) generally induce a complete response in only a minority of patients, and the average duration of response is <1 yr.
- The role of myeloid growth factors (granulocyte colony-stimulating factor [G-CSF], granulocyte-macrophage CSF) and immunotherapy is undefined. In a recent trial, 34% of patients treated with antithymocyte globulin (40 mg/kg for 4 days) became transfusion independent. Response was also associated with a statistically significantly longer survival.

CHRONIC Rx

Monitor for infections, bleeding, and complications of anemia. Supportive measures include blood transfusions and erythropoietin for anemia and antibiotics to treat opportunistic infections. Iron overload from frequent transfusions may require iron chelation therapy.

DISPOSITION

- Cure rates in young patients with allogeneic bone marrow transplantation approach 30% to 50%.
- The risk of transformation to acute myelogenous leukemia varies with the percentage of blasts in the bone marrow.
- Advanced age, male sex, and deletion of chromosomes 5 and 7 are associated with a poor prognosis.
- The 1997 International Prognostic Scoring System uses the following three elements for staging: (1) the proportion of myeloblasts in the patient's marrow, (2) the number of blood cell lineage deficits, and (3) the type of chromosomal abnormality present (e.g., poor risk includes abnormalities of chromosome 7; good risk includes clonal loss of the Y chromosome). According to the International Myelodysplastic Syndrome Risk Analysis Workshop, the most important variables in disease outcome are the specific cytogenetic abnormalities, the percentage of blasts in the bone marrow, and the number of hematopoietic lineages involved in the cytopenias.

REFERRAL

Hematology referral in all patients with MDS

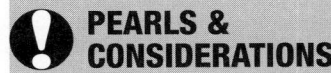

PEARLS & CONSIDERATIONS

COMMENTS

- Somatic point mutations in TP53, EZH2, ETV6, RUNX1, and ASXL1 are predictors of poor overall survival in patients with MDS independent of established risk factors. Patients with cytogenetic abnormalities associated with poor prognosis should be considered for aggressive treatment with high-dose chemotherapy and stem cell transplantation.
- Many younger patients who respond to immunosuppressive therapy with drugs such as antithymocyte globulin and cyclosporine have clonal expansions of cytotoxic CD8+ T cells that suppress normal hematopoiesis, as well as expansion of CD4+ helper T-cell subsets that promote and sustain autoimmunity.
- Nearly 50% of the deaths that result from MDS are the result of cytopenia associated with bone marrow failure.

SUGGESTED READINGS
available at www.expertconsult.com

RELATED CONTENT
Myelodysplastic Syndrome (Patient Information)

AUTHOR: **FRED F. FERRI, M.D.**

TABLE 1-291 Physical Examination, Medical History, and Laboratory Tests Aiding in Diagnosis of Myelodysplastic Syndrome

Medical History

Duration of symptoms
History of blood disease
History of exposure to occupational toxins or cytotoxic agents
Medication history
Alcohol intake
Comorbid conditions

Physical Examination

Pallor
Petechiae
Purpura
Bruising
Tachypnea
Signs of infection
Splenomegaly

Laboratory Testing

Complete blood count with a manual differential
Reticulocyte count
Vitamin B_{12} and folate levels
Consider methylmalonic acid and red blood cell folate levels
Iron, total iron-binding capacity, and ferritin level
Thyroid-stimulating hormone level
Lactate dehydrogenase
Antinuclear antibody
Coombs test and haptoglobin
Serum erythropoietin level
Human leukocyte antigen (histocompatibility antigens) typing in appropriate patients
Paroxysmal nocturnal hemoglobinuria screen

Bone Marrow Testing

Hematopathology
  Percentage of blasts on 200 cell aspirate differential
  Presence or absence of Auer rods
  Percentage of cellularity of bone marrow biopsy
  Iron stain on aspirate (ringed sideroblasts)
  Iron stain on biopsy (storage)
  Dysplastic features (% and number of dysplastic lineages)
Cytogenetics (karyotype of 20 metaphase cells)
Fluorescent in situ hybridization
Flow cytometry (not useful for quantitation)

From Hoffman R et al: *Hematology, basic principles and practice*, ed 5, Philadelphia, 2009, Churchill Livingstone.

BASIC INFORMATION

DEFINITION

Primary myelofibrosis (PMF) is a clonal stem cell disorder characterized by chronic myeloproliferation, atypical megakaryocytic hyperplasia, bone marrow fibrosis (Fig. 1-569A) and extramedullary hematopoiesis in the spleen. PMF is a myeloproliferative neoplasm; however, it does not include patients who present with myelofibrosis with an associated antecedent diagnosis.

ICD-9CM CODES
238.76 Primary myelofibrosis

EPIDEMIOLOGY & DEMOGRAPHICS

INCIDENCE (IN U.S.): ~0.21 per 100,000

PREDOMINANT SEX AND AGE:
- No sex association
- Median age of diagnosis is ~67 years of age

PHYSICAL FINDINGS & CLINICAL PRESENTATION
- Fatigue
- Symptoms related to splenomegaly: abdominal fullness, early satiety
- Acute left upper quadrant pain with the development of spontaneous splenic infarction
- Due to extramedullary hematopoiesis: hepatomegaly and portal hypertension, lymphadenopathy, ascites, or pleural effusions
- Infection
- Skeletal changes
- Leukemic transformation
  - Incidence 3.9% to 20%
  - Within the first 10 yr of diagnosis

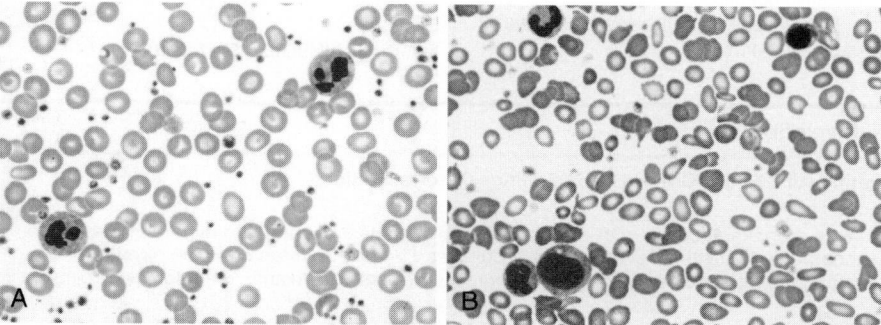
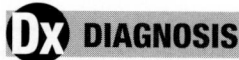

FIGURE 1-569A Blood smears from prefibrotic and fibrotic stages of primary myelofibrosis. **A,** This smear from the prefibrotic stage shows neutrophilia and thrombocytosis but minimal red cell changes. **B,** This smear from the fibrotic stage shows leukoerythroblastosis with marked red cell abnormalities, including many teardrop forms. (From Jaffe ES et al: *Hematopathology,* Philadelphia, 2011, Saunders.)

BOX 1-40 World Health Organization Classification of Myeloid Malignancies and Operational Subcategorization of Myeloproliferative Neoplasms

1. Acute myeloid leukemia and related precursor neoplasms
2. Myelodysplastic syndromes (MDS)
3. Myeloproliferative neoplasms (MPN)
   a. Classic MPN
      i. Chronic myelogenous leukemia (CML), BCR-ABL1 positive
      ii. Polycythemia vera (PV)
         (1) Chronic phase PV
         (2) Post-PV MF
         (3) Blast phase PV
      iii. Essential thrombocythemia (ET)
         (1) Chronic phase ET
         (2) Post-ET MF
         (3) Blast phase ET
      iv. Primary myelofibrosis (PMF)
         (1) Chronic phase PMF
         (2) Blast phase PMF
   b. Nonclassic MPN
      i. Chronic neutrophilic leukemia
      ii. Chronic eosinophilic leukemia, not otherwise specified
      iii. Mastocytosis
      iv. Myeloproliferative neoplasm, unclassifiable (MPN-U)
4. MDS/MPN
5. Myeloid and lymphoid neoplasms with eosinophilia and abnormalities of PDGFRA,*PDGFRB, *FGFR1*

*Genetic rearrangements involving platelet-derived growth factor receptor α/β (PDGFRA/PDGFRB) or fibroblast growth factor receptor 1 (FGFR1).
From Tefferi A: How I treat myelofibrosis, *Blood* 117:3494-3504, 2011.

- >20% blasts in the bone marrow or extramedullary leukemic deposits
- Thrombohemorrhagic events

ETIOLOGY
- Clonal disorder of multipotent hematopoietic progenitors arising from the hematopoietic stem cell compartment
- Single mutation in Janus family of cytoplasmic nonreceptor tyrosine kinase (JAK)–2, which is a guanine-to-thymine mutation resulting in a substitution of valine to phenylalanine codon 617 within the pseudokinase domain (JH2) of JAK2 (JAK2V617F)
- JAK2 mutation results in autoinhibition and constitutive JAK2 activity
- Present in 40% to 50% of PMF patients
- Alternative alleles: somatic mutations at codon 515 of the thrombopoietin receptor gene MPL (three different substitutions—W515L (leucine), W515K (lysine), or W515A (alanine)—present in 10% of JAK2V617F-negative patients

DIAGNOSIS

DIFFERENTIAL DIAGNOSIS
- Myelofibrosis in the setting of preexisting PV or ET (MPN)
- Chronic myelogenous leukemia
- Myelodysplastic syndrome with marrow fibrosis
- Acute myelofibrosis of acute megakaryocytic leukemia
- Marrow fibrosis associated with hairy cell leukemia, lymphoma, and multiple myeloma
- Nonhematologic disorders with bone marrow fibrosis: solid tumor metastases to the bone marrow, autoimmune disorders, and secondary hyperparathyroidism with vitamin D deficiency

WORKUP
- WHO criteria for PMF (3 major, 2 minor; Boxes 1-40 and 1-41)
- Major criteria:
  - Presence of megakaryocytic proliferation and atypia, usually accompanied by reticulin and/or collagen fibrosis, or, in the absence of significant reticulin fibrosis, the megakaryocyte changes must be accompanied by an increased bone marrow cellularity characterized by granulocytic proliferation and often decreased erythropoiesis
  - *Not* polycythemia vera, chronic myelogenous leukemia, myelodysplastic syndrome or other myeloid neoplasm
  - Demonstration of JAK2V617F or other clonal marker (MPLW515K/L), or, in the absence of a clonal marker, no evidence of bone marrow fibrosis due to underlying inflammatory or other neoplastic diseases
- Minor criteria:
  - Leukoerythroblastosis: nucleated red blood cells, granulocyte precursors, and teardrop-shaped erythrocytes
  - Increase in serum lactate dehydrogenase level

- ○ Anemia
- ○ Palpable splenomegaly

LABORATORY TESTS

- Anemia (hemoglobin <10g/dl)
- Platelet count and white blood cell count vary widely
- Peripheral blood smear: nucleated red blood cells, granulocyte precursors, and teardrop-shaped erythrocytes (leukoerythroblastosis)
- Bone marrow is fibrotic, megakaryocytic dysplasia
- Presence of JAK2V617F mutation

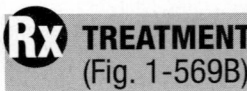 TREATMENT
(Fig. 1-569B)

Risk factors are based on Dynamic International Prognostic Scoring System plus (DIPSS-plus).
- Age >65 years
- Hemoglobin <10 g/dl

- Leukocyte count >25 × 10⁹/L
- Circulating blasts >1%
- Presence of constitutional symptoms
- Red cell transfusion need
- Platelet <100 × 10⁹/L
- Unfavorable karyotype (complex or presence of +8, −7/7q−, i(17q), inv(3), −5/5q−, 12p−, or 11q23 rearrangement)

Scoring: low (0 risk factors); intermediate 1 (1 risk factor); intermediate 2 (2 or 3 risk factors), and high (>4 risk factors)

LOW AND INTERMEDIATE 1 RISK

- Conventional drug therapy if symptomatic:
  - ○ Erythropoiesis stimulating agent
  - ○ Corticosteroids
  - ○ Androgens
  - ○ Danazol
  - ○ Thalidomide
  - ○ Lenalidomide

INTERMEDIATE 2 AND HIGH RISK

- Palliative options:
  - ○ Conventional drug therapy (see above)
  - ○ Splenectomy

- ○ Radiotherapy
- ○ Experimental drug therapy
- Curative options:
  - ○ Allogeneic stem cell transplant

DISPOSITION

Median survival between 3.5 and 5 years based on above DIPSS-plus scoring system

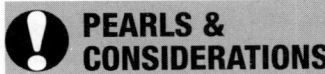 PEARLS & CONSIDERATIONS

- PMF is a clonal stem cell disorder.
- Significant proportion of PMF patients have JAK2V617F or MPL mutations.
- The only curative treatment is autologous stem cell transplant.

SUGGESTED READINGS

available at www.expertconsult.com

AUTHOR: **KIMBERLY PEREZ, M.D.**

BOX 1-41 Diagnostic Criteria for Primary Myelofibrosis

WHO Diagnostic Criteria for PMF Requires Meeting All 3 Major Criteria and ≥2 Minor Criteria Outlined

Major Criteria
1. Megakaryocyte proliferation, including small-to-large megakaryocytes, with aberrant nuclear/cytoplasmic ratio and hyperchromatic and irregularly folded nuclei and dense clustering accompanied by either reticulin and/or collagen fibrosis, or in the absence of reticulin fibrosis (i.e., prefibrotic PMF), the megakaryocyte changes must be accompanied by increased marrow cellularity, granulocytic proliferation, and often decreased erythropoiesis
2. Not meeting WHO criteria for chronic myelogenous leukemia, polycythemia vera, myelodysplastic syndromes, or other myeloid neoplasm
3. Demonstration of JAK2V617F or other clonal marker or no evidence of reactive marrow fibrosis

Minor Criteria
1. Leukoerythroblastosis
2. Increased serum lactate dehydrogenase
3. Anemia
4. Palpable splenomegaly

International Working Group for Myeloproliferative Neoplasms Research and Treatment Criteria for Post–Polycythemia Vera/Essential Thrombocythemia (post-PV/ET) Myelofibrosis Requires Meeting Both Major Criteria and ≥2 Minor Criteria

Major Criteria
1. Documentation of a previous diagnosis of PV or ET as defined by the WHO criteria
2. Bone marrow fibrosis grade 2-3 (on 0-3 scale) or grade 3-4 (on 0-4 scale)*

Minor Criteria
1. A leukoerythroblastic peripheral blood picture (for both PV and ET)
2. Increasing splenomegaly defined as either an increase in palpable splenomegaly of ≥5 cm (distance of the tip of the spleen from the left costal margin) or the appearance of a newly palpable splenomegaly (for both PV and ET)
3. Development of ≥1 of 3 constitutional symptoms: >10% weight loss in 6 months, night sweats, unexplained fever (>37.5° C) (for both PV and ET)
4. Anemia or sustained loss of requirement for phlebotomy in the absence of cytoreductive therapy (for PV)
5. Anemia and a decrease of hemoglobin level ≥2 g/dl from baseline (for ET)
6. Increased serum lactate dehydrogenase (for ET)

*Grade 2-3 according to the European classification: diffuse, often coarse fiber network with no evidence of collagenization (negative trichrome stain) or diffuse, coarse fiber network with areas of collagenization (positive trichrome stain). Grade 3-4 according to the standard classification: diffuse and dense increase in reticulin with extensive intersections, occasionally with only focal bundles of collagen and/or focal osteosclerosis or diffuse and dense increase in reticulin with extensive intersections with coarse bundles of collagen, often associated with significant osteosclerosis.
From Tefferi A: How I treat myelofibrosis, *Blood* 117:3494-3504, 2011.

MYELOFIBROSIS TREATMENT ALGORITHM

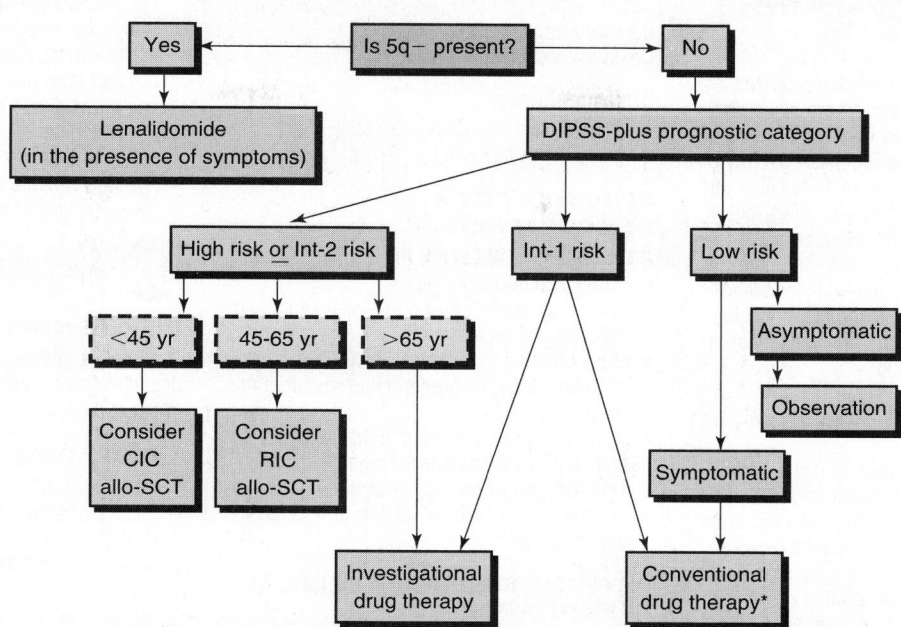

FIGURE 1-569B Risk-adapted therapy in primary myelofibrosis. *Conventional drug therapy includes erythropoiesis-stimulating agents, androgens, danazol, corticosteroids, thalidomide, lenalidomide, hydroxyurea, and cladribine. *allo-SCT,* allogeneic stem cell transplantation; *DIPSS-plus,* Dynamic International Prognostic Scoring System plus prognostic model for primary myelofibrosis; *CIC,* conventional-intensity conditioning; *Int,* intermediate; *RIC,* reduced-intensity conditioning. (From Tefferi A: How I treat myelofibrosis, *Blood* 117(13):3494-3504, 2011.)

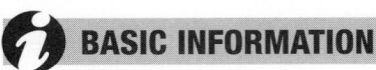

BASIC INFORMATION

DEFINITION

Myocardial infarction (MI) is characterized by myocardial necrosis resulting from an insufficient supply of oxygenated blood to an area of the heart. According to the European Society of Cardiology/American College of Cardiology, either one of the following criteria for acute evolving or recent MI satisfies the diagnosis:

- Typical rise and gradual fall (troponin) or more rapid rise and fall (creatine kinase–MB fraction [CK-MB]) of biochemical markers suggestive of myocardial necrosis with at least one of the following:
  1. Ischemic symptoms
  2. Development of pathologic Q waves on ECG
  3. ECG changes indicative of ischemia (ST-segment elevation or depression)
  4. Imaging evidence of new loss of viable myocardium or a new regional wall motion abnormality
- Pathologic findings of acute MI

MI may be classified as ST-segment elevation MI (STEMI) and non–ST-segment elevation MI [NSTEMI]) depending on the ECG findings on MI presentation. This entry discusses STEMI. For a discussion of NSTEMI, see "Acute Coronary Syndromes."

The *European Heart Journal* and the *Journal of the American College of Cardiology* published a new definition of acute MI that includes subtypes of acute MI, imaging tests supporting the diagnosis, and biomarker thresholds after percutaneous coronary intervention (PCI) or coronary artery bypass grafting (CABG).

- Type 1: Spontaneous MI related to ischemia due to a primary coronary event such as plaque erosion and/or rupture, fissuring, or dissection
- Type 2: MI secondary to ischemia due to either increased oxygen demand or decreased supply (e.g., coronary artery spasm, coronary embolism, anemia, arrhythmias, hypertension, or hypotension)
- Type 3: Sudden unexpected cardiac death, including cardiac arrest, often with symptoms suggestive of myocardial ischemia, accompanied by presumably new ST elevation, new left bundle branch block, or evidence of fresh thrombus in a coronary artery by angiography and/or at autopsy, but death occurring before blood samples could be obtained or at a time before the appearance of cardiac biomarkers in the blood
- Type 4a: MI associated with percutaneous coronary intervention
- Type 4b: MI associated with stent thrombosis as documented by angiography or at autopsy
- Type 5: MI associated with coronary artery bypass grafting

SYNONYMS

MI
Myocardial infarction
Non–ST elevation MI
ST-elevation MI
Heart attack

Acute myocardial infarction
AMI
Coronary thrombosis
Coronary occlusion

ICD-9CM CODES
410.9 Acute myocardial infarction, unspecified site

EPIDEMIOLOGY & DEMOGRAPHICS

INCIDENCE/PREVALENCE (IN U.S.):
- >500:100,000 persons
- >Approximately 800,000 MIs annually; 500,000 will recur
- More prominent in males between the ages of 40 and 65 yr; no predominant sex after age 65 yr
- Women experience more lethal and severe first acute MIs than men regardless of comorbidity, previous angina, or age
- At least one fourth of all MIs are clinically unrecognized

PHYSICAL FINDINGS & CLINICAL PRESENTATION

Clinical presentation:
- Crushing substernal chest pain usually lasting >30 min.
- Pain is unrelieved by rest or sublingual nitroglycerin or is rapidly recurring.
- Pain radiates to the left or right arm, neck, jaw, back, shoulders, or abdomen and is not pleuritic in character.
- Pain may be associated with dyspnea, diaphoresis, nausea, or vomiting.
- There is no pain in ~20% of infarctions (usually in diabetic or elderly patients).

Physical findings:
- Skin may be diaphoretic, with pallor (because of decreased oxygen).
- Rales may be present at the bases of lungs (indicative of heart failure [HF]).
- Cardiac auscultation may reveal an apical systolic murmur caused by mitral regurgitation from papillary muscle dysfunction; S_3 or S_4 may also be present.
- Physical examination may be completely normal.

ETIOLOGY

- Coronary atherosclerosis and plaque rupture
- Coronary artery spasm
- Coronary embolism (caused by infective endocarditis, rheumatic heart disease, intracavitary thrombus)
- Periarteritis and other coronary artery inflammatory diseases
- Dissection into coronary arteries (aneurysmal or iatrogenic)
- Calcium supplementation may promote vascular calcification. Studies have shown that calcium supplementation (but not dietary calcium intake) is associated with elevated risk for MI.
- MI with normal coronaries: more frequent in younger patients and cocaine addicts. The risk of acute MI is increased by a factor of 24 during the 60 min after the use of cocaine in

persons who are otherwise at relatively low risk. Most patients with cocaine-related MI are young, nonwhite, male cigarette smokers without other risk factors for coronary heart disease who have a history of repeated cocaine use. Blood and urine toxicology screen for cocaine is recommended in all young patients who present with acute MI.
- Hypercoagulable states, increased blood viscosity (polycythemia vera)

DIAGNOSIS

DIFFERENTIAL DIAGNOSIS

The various causes of myocardial ischemia are described along with the differential diagnosis of chest pain.

LABORATORY TESTS

- ECG (Fig. 1-570): common ECG findings suggestive of acute myocardial ischemia include inverted T waves ≥1 mm deep and/or ST-segment depression ≥1 mm in two contiguous leads. The presence of pathologic Q waves (Fig. 1-571) indicates an area of infarction that usually develops hours to days after presentation. The joint ESC/ACCF/AHA committee for the definition of MI established definition for the diagnosis of ST-elevation MI, which is considered to be present when there is ST-segment elevation in two contiguous leads, ≥0.20 mm for men and ≥1.5 mm for women, or ≥1 mm in other leads. ST-segment elevation is measured at 0.08 sec after the J point (the junction between the end of the QRS and the beginning of the ST segment). ECG findings alone, without laboratory results, are sufficient to diagnose STEMI; therefore treatment should not be delayed until biomarkers are available.
- Cardiac troponin levels: Cardiac-specific troponin T (cTnT) and cardiac-specific troponin I (cTnI) are generally indicative of myocardial injury with increases in serum levels of >99th percentile of a normal reference population. Detection of a rise and fall pattern of the measurements is essential to the diagnosis of AMI. The rise may occur relatively early after muscle damage (3-12 hr), peak at 24-48 hr, and may be present for several days after MI (up to 7 days for cTnI and up to 10 to 14 days for cTnT). cTnT or cTnI tests can be falsely positive in patients with renal failure. Recently, highly sensitive troponin assays (hs-cTnI, hs-cTnT) have also been developed to facilitate an early diagnosis of AMI. Most patients can be diagnosed with AMI within the first 2-3 hours of presentation. However, an initial negative high-sensitivity troponin at the time of presentation is not sensitive enough to completely rule out AMI. MI can be excluded in most patients by 6 hours of presentation, but guidelines suggest serial samples be obtained if there is a high degree of suspicion to definitively rule out MI.
- CK-MB isoenzyme is also a useful marker for MI if troponin levels are not available. It is released in the circulation in amounts that

correlate with the size of the infarct. An increased CK-MB value for the diagnosis of MI is defined as a measurement above the 99th percentile of the upper reference limit. Troponin, however, is the preferred marker for the diagnosis of myocardial necrosis because of its increased sensitivity and specificity as compared to CK-MB. This preference was recommended by the 2007 Joint ESC/ACCF/ AHA Task Force for the Definition of Myocardial Infarction. Because troponins need 7-14 days to be cleared by the kidneys, they are not sensitive enough to detect a recurrent MI within days from the initial MI. Therefore CK-MB isoenzyme can be useful in such circumstances.

IMAGING STUDIES
- Chest radiograph is useful to evaluate for pulmonary congestion and exclude other causes of chest pain.

- Echocardiography can evaluate wall motion abnormalities and identify mural thrombus or acute mitral regurgitation, which can occur acutely after MI.

RISK ASSESSMENT
Several risk assessment models are available. The Thrombolysis in Myocardial Infarction (TIMI) risk score for STEMI uses the following variables: age ≥65 yr; a history of diabetes,

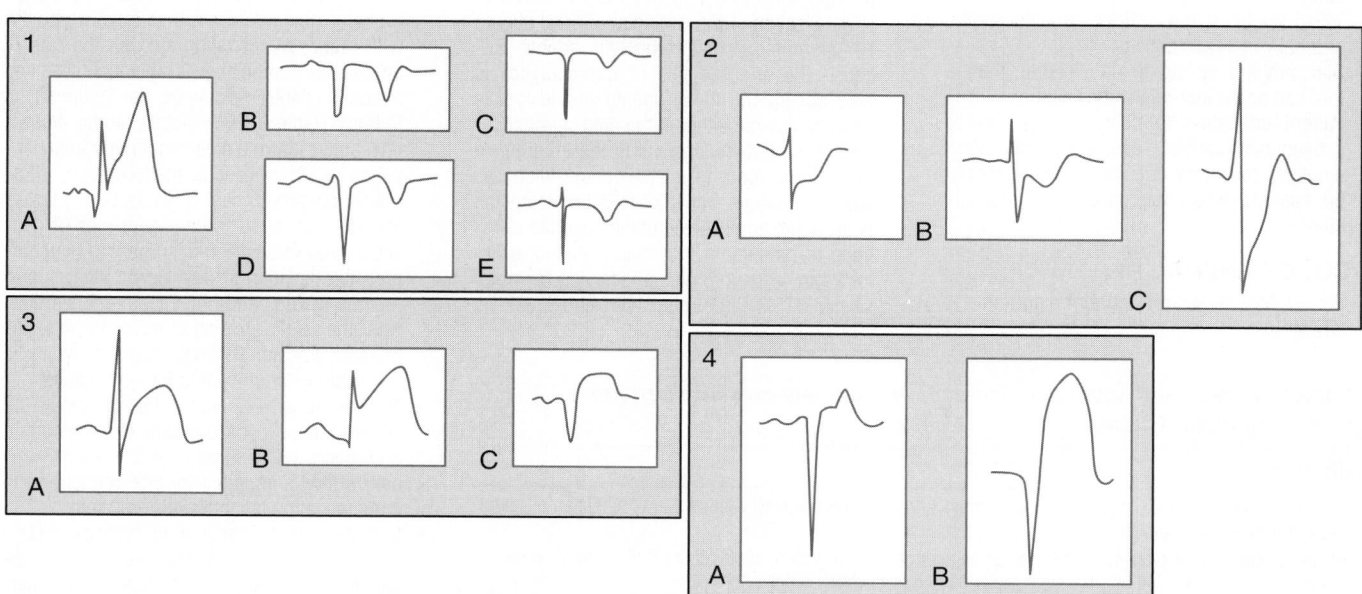

FIGURE 1-570 Electrocardiographic findings of acute myocardial infarction (AMI). 1, T-wave abnormalities of AMI. *A,* Prominent "hyperacute" T wave. *B-E,* T-wave inversions of non-ST-segment elevation MI (NSTEMI). **2,** ST-segment depression. *A,* Flat. *B,* Downsloping. *C,* Upsloping. **3,** ST-segment elevation. *A,* Convex ST-segment elevation. *B,* Obliquely straight ST-segment elevation. *C,* Convex ST-segment elevation. **4,** Pathologic Q waves. *A,* Pathologic Q wave of completed myocardial infarction. *B,* Simultaneous ST-segment elevation with pathologic Q wave 2 hours into the course of ST-segment elevation MI (STEMI). (From Vincent JL et al: *Textbook of critical care,* ed 6, Philadelphia, 2011, Saunders.)

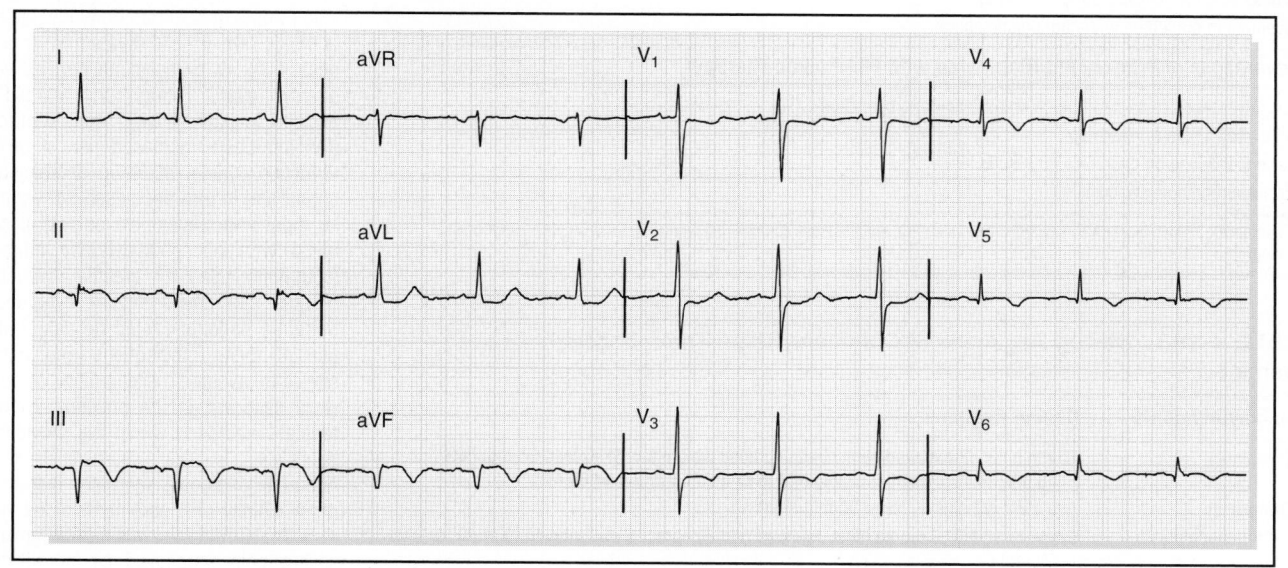

FIGURE 1-571 Evolving inferoposterolateral infarction. Note the prominent Q waves in leads II, III, and aVL, along with ST elevation and T-wave inversion in these leads, as well as V₃ through V₆. ST depression in I, aVL, V₁, and V₂ is consistent with a reciprocal change. Relatively tall R waves are also present in V₁ and V₂. (From Zipes DP et al [eds]: *Braunwald's heart disease,* ed 7, Philadelphia, 2005, Saunders.)

hypertension, or angina; systolic blood pressure <100 mm Hg; heart rate >100 beats/min; Killip class (discussed below) ≥2; weight >67 kg; anterior ST elevation or left bundle branch block; and time to treatment >4 hr. The higher the score, the higher the 30-day mortality rate.

Rx TREATMENT

NONPHARMACOLOGIC THERAPY

- Limit patient's activity: bed rest for the initial 12 to 24 hr; if the patient remains stable, gradually increase activity.
- Diet: nothing by mouth until stable, then a low-salt and a low-cholesterol diet.
- Patient education to decrease the risk of subsequent cardiac events (proper diet, smoking cessation, regular exercise) should be initiated when the patient is medically stable.

ACUTE GENERAL Rx

- Fig. E1-572 shows a treatment algorithm for STEMI.

- Prompt myocardial reperfusion in STEMI can be accomplished with PCI or fibrinolytic therapy. Indications for primary angioplasty and comparison with fibrinolytic therapy are described in Table 1-292. If readily available without delay, PCI is superior to thrombolytic therapy and is the standard of care. It is effective and generally results in more favorable outcomes than thrombolytic therapy.
- Thrombolytic therapy (Table 1-293): in STEMI, if the duration of pain has been <12 hr and primary angioplasty is not readily available, recanalization of the occluded arteries should be attempted with thrombolytic agents. Because the effectiveness of thrombolytics is time dependent, these agents should ideally be administered either in the field or within 30 min of the patient's arrival in the emergency department (door-to-needle time). When tissue plasminogen activator (t-PA) or reteplase is used, heparin is given to increase the likelihood of patency in the infarct-related artery for 24 to 48 hr. In patients receiving fibrinolysis for STEMI, treatment with enoxaparin is

superior to treatment with unfractionated heparin for 48 hr but is associated with an increase in major bleeding episodes. In patients receiving streptokinase or APSAC, heparin after thrombolysis is not indicated because it does not offer any additional benefit and can result in increased bleeding complications. Tenecteplase and reteplase are comparable with accelerated infusion recombinant t-PA in terms of efficacy and safety but are more convenient because they are administered by bolus injection. Lanoplase and heparin bolus plus infusion are as effective as tPA with regard to mortality rate, but the rate of intracranial hemorrhage is significantly higher. Absolute contraindications to thrombolytic therapy (Table 1-294) include aortic dissection, active internal bleeding, intracranial neoplasm or arteriovenous malformation, intracranial surgery in past 6 mo, ischemic stroke in past 1 yr, head trauma with loss of consciousness in past 6 mo, surgery in noncompressible location in past 6 wk, alteration in mental status, and infectious endocarditis. After the administration of thrombolytics, immediate transfer to a PCI-capable facility is advisable without waiting for lytic results.

- Transfer to a PCI-capable facility should be sought if door-to-balloon time (from arrival to emergency department until the culprit coronary artery is engaged for intervention in the catheterization laboratory) is <90 min.
- Until the catheterization team is ready or fibrinolytics are administered, medical therapy should be initiated immediately in the emergency department. This includes:
  - Nasal oxygen: administer at 2-4 L/min
  - Nitrates: increase oxygen supply by reducing coronary vasospasm and decrease oxygen consumption by reducing ventricular preload. Sublingual nitroglycerin (0.4 mg) can be administered immediately on suspicion of MI (unless systolic blood pressure is <90 mm Hg or ≤30 mm Hg below baseline or heart rate is <50 beats/min or >100 beats/min); IV nitroglycerin can be subsequently used. Nitroglycerin should be avoided in patients with right ventricular (RV) infarction (increased risk of preload reduction, which results in decreased RV output and in turn decreased left ventricular input and subsequent output). If combined with phosphodiesterase inhibitors (commonly used for erectile dysfunction), nitrates can cause severe hypotension; therefore patients should be asked about use of these medications and nitrates should be avoided if sildenafil or vardenafil were used within the previous 25 hr or tadalafil was used within the previous 48 hours.
  - Adequate analgesia: morphine sulfate 2-4 mg IV initially with increments of 2-8 mg IV at 5- to 10-min intervals can be given for severe pain unrelieved by nitroglycerin. Morphine can reduce the catecholamine surge caused by anxiety and pain, which in turn can reduce the increased cardiac workload and oxygen demand, leading to

TABLE 1-292 Indications for Primary Angioplasty and Comparison with Fibrinolytic Therapy

Indications

Alternative recanalization strategy for ST segment elevation or LBBB acute MI within 12 hr of symptom onset (or >12 hr if symptoms persist)

Cardiogenic shock developing within 36 hr of ST segment elevation/Q wave acute MI or LBBB acute MI in patients <75 yr old who can be revascularized within 18 hr of shock onset

Recommended only at centers performing >200 PCI/yr with backup cardiac surgery and for operators performing >75 PCI/yr

Advantages of Primary PCI

Higher initial recanalization rates

Reduced risk of intracerebral hemorrhage

Less residual stenosis; less recurrent ischemia or infarction

Usefulness when fibrinolysis contraindicated

Improvement in outcomes with cardiogenic shock

Disadvantages of Primary PCI (Compared with Fibrinolytic Therapy)

Access, advantages restricted to high-volume centers, operators

Longer average time to treatment

Greater dependence on operators for results

Higher system complexity, costs

LBBB, Left bundle branch block; *MI,* myocardial infarction; *PCI,* percutaneous coronary intervention (includes balloon angioplasty, stenting).
From Goldman L, Schafer AI: *Goldman's Cecil medicine,* ed 24, Philadelphia, 2012, Saunders.

TABLE 1-293 Dosing Regimens of Commonly Used Thrombolytic Agents

Thrombolytic Agents	Dosing Regimen
t-PA (alteplase)	15 mg bolus IV, followed by 0.75 mg/kg body weight (not to exceed 50 mg) over 30 min, followed by 0.5 mg/kg (not to exceed 35 mg) over 60 min
r-PA (reteplase)	Two 10-U IV boluses, given 30 min apart
TNK–t-PA (tenecteplase)	Single bolus IV 0.5 mg/kg (dose rounded to the nearest 5 mg, ranging from 30 to 50 mg)
Streptokinase	1.5 million U IV over 60 min

IV, Intravenous; *PA,* plasminogen activator; *r-PA,* reteplase plasminogen activator; *TNK–t-PA,* tenecteplase tissue plasminogen activator; *U,* units.
From Andreoli TE et al: *Andreoli and Carpenter's Cecil essentials of medicine,* ed 8, Philadelphia, 2010, Saunders.

decreased ischemia. Hypotension from morphine can be treated with careful IV hydration with saline solution. If sinus bradycardia accompanies hypotension, use atropine (0.5 to 1.0 mg IV q5min prn to a total dose of 2.5 mg). Respiratory depression caused by morphine can be reversed with naloxone 0.8 mg.
- Aspirin 162-325 mg PO should be crushed and swallowed to enhance drug absorption and delivery. Depending on the clinical and ECG findings, if the patient is suspected to have a coronary anatomy that needs CABG rather than PCI, thienopyridine (clopidogrel) should be avoided because it increases the perioperative bleeding risk; otherwise, surgery is deferred for 7 days. However, if the coronary artery disease is likely to benefit from PCI alone, then a loading dose of thienopyridine 300-600 mg PO should be given as early as possible or by the time of PCI, or prasugel 60 mg as early as possible and no later than 1 hour after PCI.
- Beta-adrenergic blocking agents should generally be given to all patients. Before using beta-blockers, some of the contraindications and side effects (e.g., exacerbation of asthma, central nervous system effects, hypotension, bradycardia) must be carefully assessed. Beta-blockers are useful to reduce myocardial oxygen consumption and prevent tachyarrhythmias. Early IV beta blockage (in the initial 24 hr) followed by institution of an oral maintenance regimen is also effective in reducing recurrent infarction and ischemia. Frequently used agents are metoprolol (IV 5 mg q2min for 3 doses, then PO 25-50 mg q6h, given 15 min after last IV dose, continued for 48 hr; maintenance dosage is 50-100 mg bid) or atenolol (IV 5 mg over 5 min, repeat in 10 min if initial dose is well tolerated, then start PO dose

10 min after the last IV dose; PO 50 mg qd, increasing to 100 mg as tolerated).
- STEMI is due to plaque rupture, which exposes the underlying collagen. With the destruction of the smooth vascular endothelial layer, platelets are activated and the coagulation cascade is initiated. Therefore anticoagulation therapy is important. IV unfractionated heparin or bivalirudin, or subcutaneous enoxaparin or fondaparinux can be used. In patients at high risk of bleeding, use of bivalirudin is reasonable. Anticoagulatin therapy is usually continued for 48 hours after administration of lytic therapy unless streptokinase or APSAC is used.
- Neither facilitation of PCI with reteplase plus abciximab nor facilitation with abciximab alone significantly improves the clinical outcomes compared with abciximab given at the time of PCI in patients with STEMI. In patients with acute MI, treatment with drug-eluting stents is associated with decreased 2-yr mortality rates and a reduction in the need for repeat revascularization procedures compared with treatment with bare-metal stents.

CHRONIC Rx
- Discharge medications in all patients with MI (unless contraindicated) should include antiischemic medications (e.g., nitroglycerin, beta-blocker), lipid-lowering agents, and antiplatelet therapy (aspirin and/or clopidogrel).
- Aspirin 162-325 mg PO can be decreased to 81 mg (baby dose) PO after 30 days, but should be continued indefinitely unless not tolerated (e.g., GI bleed). Clopidogrel 75 mg PO qd can be combined with aspirin and should be continued without interruption for 30 days after bare-metal stent placement or

for 12 months after drug-eluting stent placement and can be discontinued after completion of duration; however, aspirin should be continued indefinitely. Combining clopidogrel with aspirin reduces risk for in-stent restenosis. If there is an elective surgical intervention pending, it is recommended to defer the surgery until completion of the full course of clopidogrel.
- Angiotensin-converting enzyme inhibitors (ACEIs) should be started within the first 24 hours of STEMI, especially if patients have anterior infarction, pulmonary congestion, or LV EF <40%, in the absence of hypotension. They reduce LV dysfunction and dilation and slow the progression to HF during and after acute MI. IV formulations of ACEIs should not be given within the first 24 hours of STEMI due to risk of hypotension. Angiotensin receptor blockers (ARBs) offer no advantage over ACEIs and should be considered only in patients who are intolerant to ACEIs.
  - Commonly used ACEIs are ramipril 2.5 mg PO qd, captopril 12.5 mg PO bid, enalapril 2.5 mg PO bid, and lisinopril 2.5-5 mg PO qd initially, with subsequent titration as needed. Ramipril is associated with a lower mortality rate than most ACEIs.
  - ACEIs may be stopped in patients without complications and no evidence of LV dysfunction after 6 to 8 weeks.
  - ACEIs should be continued indefinitely in patients with impaired LV function (EF <40%) or clinical HF.
- Long-term aldosterone antagonist therapy should be prescribed for post-STEMI patients without significant renal dysfunction (creatinine ≤2.5 mg/dl in men and ≤2.0 mg/dl in women) or hyperkalemia who are already taking an ACEI and have LV EF <40% with symptomatic HF or diabetes.
- Statins should be started as early as possible in all patients with STEMI regardless of lipid panel, not only for their lipid-lowering effects, but also their anti-inflammatory properties (JUPITER trial), which can stabilize the ruptured plaque. Atorvastatin 80 mg qd can be used (PROVE IT-TIMI 22 and MIRACL trials). Lipid panel should be checked during the first 24 hr of hospital course and the intensive therapy can be stepped down if appropriate. Goal LDL cholesterol is <70 mg/dl. Consider addition of fenofibrate or niacin if triglycerides are significantly elevated. Recent data showed no improvement in outcome with increasing HDL cholesterol therapy using niacin; therefore its use to decrease HDL cholesterol is questionable.
- Evaluation of post-MI patients:
  - Submaximal exercise (low-level) treadmill test (can be done 1 to 3 wk after MI) in stable patients who did not undergo cardiac catheterization or noninvasive stress imaging.
    1. Useful to assess the patient's functional capacity and formulate an at-home exercise program
    2. Helpful to determine the patient's prognosis

TABLE 1-294 Contraindications to Thrombolytic Therapy in Acute Myocardial Infarction

Absolute

Suspected aortic dissection
Active bleeding*
Any prior cerebral hemorrhage
Intracranial neoplasm
Cerebral aneurysm or arteriovenous malformation
Ischemic cerebrovascular accident within 3 mo

Relative

Bleeding diathesis, coagulopathy, or anticoagulant use
Major surgery within 3 wk
Puncture of a noncompressible vessel, internal bleeding, or head or major body trauma within previous 2 wk
Nonhemorrhagic stroke or gastrointestinal hemorrhage within 6 mo
Proliferative retinopathy
Active peptic ulcer disease
History of chronic, severe, poorly controlled hypertension
Severe uncontrolled hypertension on presentation (systolic blood pressure >180 mm Hg or diastolic blood pressure >110 mm Hg)
Traumatic or prolonged (>10 min) cardiopulmonary resuscitation
Pregnancy

*Does not include menstrual bleeding.
From Andreoli TE et al: *Andreoli and Carpenter's Cecil essentials of medicine*, ed 8, Philadelphia, 2010, Saunders.

○ Radionuclide angiography or two-dimensional echocardiography:
  1. To evaluate LV ejection fraction
  2. To evaluate ventricular size and segmental wall motion
  3. Echocardiography to rule out presence of mural thrombi in patients suspected of having an extensive infarction (more common with anterior wall MI); contrast echocardiography is added if mural thrombosis is suspected

○ Primary prevention of sudden cardiac death: Forty days after MI, patients with LV ejection fraction <40% and nonsustained ventricular tachycardia may be candidates for programmed electrical stimulation studies and implanted defibrillator, depending on the results of these studies. Patients with LV ejection fraction ≤35% and NYHA class II or III heart failure, or LV ejection fraction ≤30% with documented prior MI should be considered for implanted defibrillator if the life expectancy is >1 yr.

DISPOSITION

The prognosis after MI depends on multiple factors:

- New bundle branch block, Mobitz II second-degree block, and third-degree heart block adversely affect outcome.
- Size of infarct: the larger it is, the higher the post-MI mortality rate. Significant myocardial stunning with subsequent improvement of ventricular function occurs in most patients after anterior MI. A lower level of creatine kinase, an estimate of the extent of necrosis, is independently predictive of recovery of function.
- Site of infarct: inferior wall MI carries a better prognosis than anterior wall MI; however, patients with inferior wall MI and right ventricular involvement have a high risk for arrhythmic complications and cardiogenic shock.

- Ejection fraction after MI: the lower the LV ejection fraction, the higher the mortality rate after MI. The risk of death is highest in the first 30 days after MI among patients with LV dysfunction, HF, or both.
- Presence of post-MI angina indicates a high mortality rate.
- Performance on low-level exercise test: the presence of ST-segment changes during the test is a predictor of high mortality rate during the first year.
- Presence of pericarditis during the acute phase of MI increases mortality: rate at 1 yr.
- Type A behavior (competitive drive, ambitiousness, hostility) is associated with a lower mortality rate after symptomatic MI.
- The Killip classification is an independent predictor of all-cause 30-day mortality: acute MI
  ○ Killip class I includes individuals with no clinical signs of HF. Mortality rate is 6%.
  ○ Killip class II includes individuals with rales or crackles in the lungs, S_3 gallop, and elevated jugular venous pressure. Mortality rate is 17%.
  ○ Killip class III describes individuals with frank acute pulmonary edema. Mortality rate is 38%.
  ○ Killip class IV describes individuals in cardiogenic shock or hypotension (measured as systolic blood pressure <90 mm Hg) and evidence of peripheral vasoconstriction (oliguria, cyanosis, or sweating). Mortality rate is 67%.
- Self-reported moderate alcohol consumption in the year before acute MI is associated with reduced 1-yr mortality rate.
- Discharge medication in patients with MI should include lipid-lowering agents. Statins may also lower vascular inflammation and damage by mechanisms other than reduction of low-density lipoprotein cholesterol. Early initiation of statin treatment in patients with acute MI is associated with reduced 1-yr mortality rate.

- Additional poor prognostic factors include cigarette smoking, history of hypertension or prior MI, presence of ST-segment depression in acute MI, older age, diabetes mellitus, and female sex (especially women >50 yr).
- Renal disease, even mild, as assessed by the estimated glomerular filtration rate, is a major risk factor for cardiovascular complications after MI.
- Although black patients with MI have worse outcomes than white patients, these differences did not persist after adjustment for patient factors and site of care.

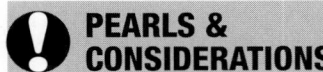

PEARLS & CONSIDERATIONS

COMMENTS

- Approximately 1.5 million patients undergo PCI in the United States each year. Depending on local practices and the diagnostic criteria used, 5% to 30% of these patients have evidence of a periprocedural MI.
- The 12-lead ECG has low sensitivity for the detection of MI if the culprit lesion is in the left circumflex artery (LCX). If the initial 12-lead ECG is not diagnostic and high clinical suspicion for acute coronary syndrome exists, it is reasonable to obtain additional posterior chest leads (V_7 to V_9) to detect LCX occlusion.

SUGGESTED READINGS

available at www.expertconsult.com

RELATED CONTENT

Acute Coronary Syndrome (Related Key Topic)
Angina (Related Key Topic)
Heart Attack (Patient Information)

AUTHORS: **ALI DAHHAN, M.D., FRED F. FERRI, M.D.,** and **GAURAV CHOUDHARY, M.D.**

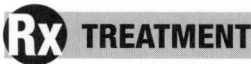

BASIC INFORMATION

DEFINITION

Myocarditis is an inflammatory condition of the myocardium.

ICD-9CM CODES
429.0   Myocarditis, nonspecific
391.2   Myocarditis, rheumatic
422.91 Myocarditis, viral (except Coxsackie)
074.23 Myocarditis, Coxsackie
422.92 Myocarditis, bacterial

EPIDEMIOLOGY & DEMOGRAPHICS

- The incidence of focal myocarditis reported at autopsy is 1% to 7% in asymptomatic patients and ≥50% in patients infected with HIV.
- Myocarditis is a major cause of sudden unexpected death (15% to 20% of cases) in adults <40 yr.

PHYSICAL FINDINGS & CLINICAL PRESENTATION

- Persistent tachycardia out of proportion to fever
- Faint S_1, S_4 sound on auscultation
- Murmur of mitral regurgitation
- Pericardial friction rub if associated with pericarditis
- Clinical features can be variable due to etiology and severity of myocarditis.
- Signs of biventricular failure (hypotension, hepatomegaly, peripheral edema, distention of neck veins, S_3)
- Patients may present with a history of recent flulike syndrome (fever, arthralgias, malaise); children often have a more fulminant presentation. Difficulty breathing is the most common presentation of pediatric myocarditis.
- Most common presentations are dyspnea (72% of patients), chest pain (32%), arrhythmias (sinus tachycardia, atrial and ventricular premature contractions) (18%).
- Acute coronary syndrome, which can occur due to local coronary spasm, and inflammation
- Sudden cardiac death due to VT/VF

ETIOLOGY

- Infection
  1. Viral (adenovirus, parvovirus B19, HCV, Coxsackie B virus, cytomegalovirus, echovirus, poliovirus, mumps, HIV, Epstein-Barr virus)
  2. Bacterial (*Staphylococcus aureus, Clostridium perfringens,* diphtheria, and any severe bacterial infection)
  3. *Mycoplasma*
  4. Mycotic (*Candida, Mucor, Aspergillus*)
  5. Parasitic (*Trypanosoma cruzi*—most common worldwide, *Trichinella, Echinococcus,* amoeba, *Toxoplasma*)
  6. *Rickettsia rickettsii*
  7. Spirochetal (*Borrelia burgdorferi*–Lyme carditis)
- Rheumatic fever

- Drugs (e.g., cocaine, emetine, doxorubicin, sulfonamides, isoniazid, methyldopa, amphotericin B, tetracycline, phenylbutazone, lithium, 5-fluorouracil, phenothiazines, interferon-alfa, tricyclic antidepressants, cyclophosphamides)
- Toxins (carbon monoxide, ethanol, diphtheria toxin, lead, arsenicals)
- Systemic and collagen-vascular disease (systemic lupus erythematosus, scleroderma, sarcoidosis, and Kawasaki syndrome)
- Radiation
- Postpartum status

DIAGNOSIS

DIFFERENTIAL DIAGNOSIS

- Cardiomyopathy
- Acute myocardial infarction
- Valvulopathies
  The differential diagnosis of chest pain is described in Section II.

WORKUP

- Medical history: the clinical presentation of myocarditis is nonspecific and can consist of fatigue, palpitations, dyspnea, precordial discomfort, and myalgias.
- Diagnostic workup includes chest x-ray examination, ECG, laboratory evaluation, echocardiogram, cardiac catheterization, and endomyocardial biopsy (in selected patients on the basis of the likelihood of finding specific treatable disorders such as giant cell myocarditis).

LABORATORY TESTS

- Elevated cardiac troponin T is suggestive of myocarditis in patients with clinically suspected myocarditis. Troponin I specificity is 89%; sensitivity is 34%. A normal level does not rule out the diagnosis.
- Increased creatine kinase (with elevated MB fraction, lactate dehydrogenase), and aspartate aminotransferase from myocardial necrosis.
- Increased erythrocyte sedimentation rate (nonspecific but may be of value in following the progress of the disease and the response to therapy).
- Increased white blood cell count (increased eosinophils if parasitic infection).
- Viral titers (acute and convalescent).
- Cold agglutinin titer, antistreptolysin O titer, blood cultures.
- Lyme disease antibody titer.

IMAGING STUDIES

- Chest radiograph: enlargement of cardiac silhouette
- ECG: sinus tachycardia with nonspecific ST-T wave changes; interventricular conduction defects and bundle branch block may be present
  1. Lyme disease and diphtheria cause all degrees of heart block.
  2. Changes of acute myocardial infarction can occur with focal necrosis.

- Echocardiogram:
  1. Dilated and hypokinetic chambers
  2. Segmental wall motion abnormalities
  3. Abnormal tissue Doppler signal
- Cardiac catheterization and angiography:
  1. To rule out coronary artery disease and valvular disease.
  2. A right ventricular endomyocardial biopsy can confirm the diagnosis, although a negative biopsy result does not exclude myocarditis. Recent studies have shown that myocardial biopsy may be unnecessary because immunosuppression therapy based on biopsy results is generally ineffective.
- Cardiac MRI (Fig. 1-573):
  1. Can be used to detect edema ratio
  2. Focal or global myocardial enhancement in relation to the skeletal muscle
  3. Late gadolinium enhancement (LGE)
  4. Any combination of two of the above has a sensitivity and specificity of 76% and 96%, respectively.
  5. Some viral pathogens have focal involvement of the myocardium. Parvovirus B19 involves the subepicardial lateral wall of the left ventricle. Human herpes simplex virus 6 and parvovirus B19 involve the septum, and also present with heart failure.

TREATMENT

NONPHARMACOLOGIC THERAPY

- Supportive care is the first line of therapy for patients with myocarditis.
- Restrict physical activity (to decrease cardiac work). Bed rest is advisable during viremia.

ACUTE GENERAL Rx

- Treat underlying cause (e.g., use specific antibiotics for bacterial infection).
- Treat congestive heart failure (CHF) with diuretics, angiotensin-converting enzyme inhibitors, and salt restriction. A beta-blocker may be added once clinical stability has been achieved. Digoxin should be used with caution and only at low doses.
- Antiarrhythmics if needed for ventricular arrhythmias.
- Provide anticoagulation to prevent thromboembolism in atrial fibrillation, severe left ventricular dysfunction with an EF <20%, and in patients with segmental wall motion.
- Inotropes or mechanical assist devices if severe heart failure or cardiovascular collapse is present.
- Corticosteroid use is contraindicated in early infectious myocarditis; it may be justified in only selected patients with intractable CHF, severe systemic toxicity, and severe life-threatening arrhythmias.
- Immunosuppressive drugs (prednisone with cyclosporine or azathioprine) do not have any significant effect on the prognosis of myocarditis and should not be used in the routine

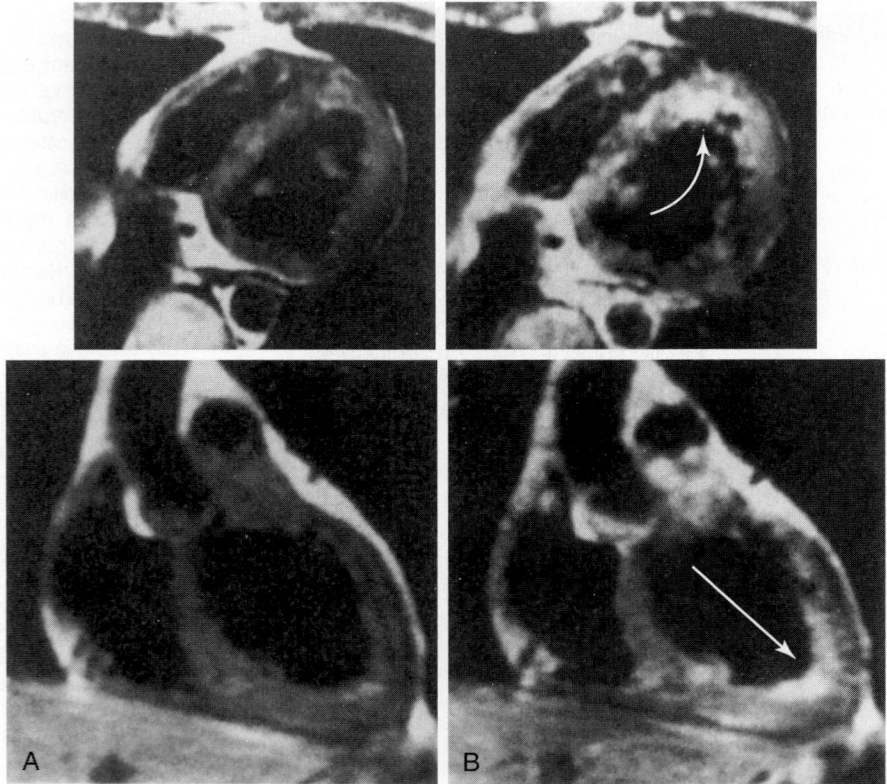

FIGURE 1-573 A, Precontrast T1-weighted transaxial *(upper)* and coronal *(lower)* magnetic resonance images through the left ventricle in a patient with myocarditis. **B,** Postcontrast magnetic resonance images at the same levels after contrast injection. Note enhancement of the myocardial signal in the septum and apical region *(arrows)*. (From Zipes DP et al [eds]: *Braunwald's heart disease*, ed 7, Philadelphia, 2005, Saunders.)

treatment of patients with myocarditis. Immunosuppression may have a role in the treatment of myocarditis from systemic autoimmune disease (e.g., lupus, scleroderma) and in patients with idiopathic giant cell myocarditis.

- There may be a role for immunosuppressive drugs in chronic inflammation; these have been shown to improve LVEF and NYHA functional status.

DISPOSITION

Nearly 50% of patients with myocarditis will die within 5 yr of diagnosis. Prognosis is best for patients with fulminant lymphocytic myocarditis (severe hemodynamic compromise, rapid onset of symptoms, or high fever). These patients tend to have complete recovery with total resolution of myocarditis on repeat biopsy.

REFERRAL

Consider heart transplant if patient develops intractable CHF.

SUGGESTED READINGS
available at www.expertconsult.com

RELATED CONTENT

Myocarditis (Patient Information)

AUTHORS: **ARAVIND RAO KOKKIRALA, M.D., SCOTT COHEN, M.D., FRED F. FERRI, M.D.,** and **GAURAV CHOUDHARY, M.D.**

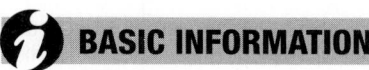 BASIC INFORMATION

DEFINITION

Myoclonus is defined as sudden, brief, jerky, "shocklike" involuntary movements that can involve the muscles of the extremities, face, or trunk. Positive myoclonus is caused by muscle contraction, whereas negative myoclonus is caused by inhibition of active (such as postural) muscles. Myoclonus is a symptom that can be seen in a number of different neurologic disorders.

ICD-9CM CODES
333.2 Myoclonus

EPIDEMIOLOGY & DEMOGRAPHICS

INCIDENCE: 1.3/100,000 persons
PREVALENCE: 8.6/100,000 persons
PREDOMINANT SEX AND AGE: No gender preference; age at onset varies by the etiology of the myoclonus.
GENETICS: Varies by etiology, can be hereditary or sporadic

PHYSICAL FINDINGS & CLINICAL PRESENTATION

- Clinically, myoclonus can be classified by its distribution: focal (only one body part involved), multifocal, segmental (spread to adjacent body parts), axial (muscles innervated by one or several spinal levels), or generalized. It can be stimulus-induced or occur at rest.
- Myoclonus can be seen with involvement or lesions of the cerebral cortex, brain stem, spinal cord, or peripheral nerve. The location of the lesion may not always influence the characteristics of the myoclonus.
- Negative myoclonus is typically seen in postural muscles of the legs, causing a "bobbing" while walking. Asterixis is another form of negative myoclonus.

ETIOLOGY

- The causes of myoclonus are numerous and can be grouped into the categories of physiologic, essential, epileptic, and symptomatic.
- Physiologic myoclonus ranges from sleep (hypnic) jerks to exercise-induced myoclonus and can be seen in normal subjects.
- Essential myoclonus occurs in the absence of other neurologic symptoms and is usually autosomal dominant. When dystonia is present, it is called myoclonus-dystonia.

The myoclonus is often responsive to alcohol in this condition.
- In epileptic myoclonus, seizures dominate the clinical picture. Syndromes include infantile spasms and juvenile myoclonic epilepsy among others.
- Symptomatic or secondary myoclonus comprises myoclonus in the setting of an underlying neurologic disorder or other precipitant. The number of secondary causes prevents giving a full list, but common etiologies include neurodegenerative diseases (Alzheimer's, atypical forms of parkinsonism), CNS infections (Creutzfeldt-Jakob disease, viral encephalitis), metabolic derangements (uremia, hepatic failure), drug-induced (selective serotonin reuptake inhibitors [SSRIs], tricyclics, lithium), and posthypoxic etiologies.

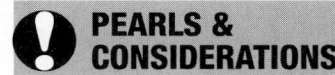 DIAGNOSIS

DIFFERENTIAL DIAGNOSIS

- Tremor: a rhythmic oscillation around a point; slower than myoclonus
- Tic: complex patterned movements that can be suppressed voluntarily for a short time unlike myoclonus, which is simple jerks that are persistent
- Dystonia: patterned contractions of agonist/antagonist muscles causing twisting or pulling; slower than myoclonus
- Chorea: typically slower, writhing, patterned movements
- Psychogenic myoclonus: variable in duration and location, distractible, or entrainable

LABORATORY TESTS

- Evaluate for metabolic precipitants (renal and hepatic function, Mg, Ca, thyroid studies)
- Toxicology screen
- Lumbar puncture if encephalitis is suspected
- Electroencephalography (EEG) to evaluate for epileptic myoclonus

IMAGING STUDIES

MRI of the brain can evaluate for a seizure focus if the myoclonus is epileptic. Creutzfeldt-Jakob disease can show diffusion weighted abnormalities in the striatum and cortex.

TREATMENT

NONPHARMACOLOGIC THERAPY

- Treatment should be directed toward correcting the underlying cause if it is reversible (e.g., hepatic or renal failure).

- Carefully remove or decrease potentially causative medications.

ACUTE GENERAL Rx

For acute treatment of epileptic myoclonus, antiepileptic drugs such as valproic acid, levetiracetam, or clonazepam are helpful.

CHRONIC Rx

- Clonazepam, valproic acid, levetiracetam are typically used for all forms of myoclonus, and often combinations of several medications seem to be more effective.
- If dystonia is present (myoclonus-dystonia), a trial of levodopa is worthwhile although only rarely responsive. Anticholinergics may also help dystonia. Botulinum toxin injections are used for focal dystonias.
- Peripheral focal myoclonus can also be helped by botulinum toxin injections.

DISPOSITION

The ultimate prognosis depends on the etiology of the myoclonus.

REFERRAL

Referral to a general neurologist or movement disorders center is appropriate.

! PEARLS & CONSIDERATIONS

COMMENTS

- When myoclonus is seen with parkinsonism, atypical forms of parkinsonism should be high on the differential such as dementia with Lewy bodies, corticobasal degeneration, and multiple system atrophy. Myoclonus is only rarely seen in idiopathic Parkinson's disease.
- Symptomatic palatal myoclonus is a specific syndrome that is often associated with a focal brain-stem lesion. In essential palatal myoclonus (no lesion), ear "clicking" is an additional symptom, which is not seen in the symptomatic form.

SUGGESTED READINGS
available at www.expertconsult.com

AUTHOR: **ANDREW DUKER, M.D.**

BASIC INFORMATION

DEFINITION

Inflammatory myopathies are idiopathic diseases of muscle characterized clinically by muscle weakness and pathologically by inflammation and muscle fiber breakdown. The three most common are dermatomyositis (DM), polymyositis (PM), and inclusion body myositis (IBM). See separate topic on "Inclusion Body Myositis" for details regarding the latter.

SYNONYMS

Idiopathic inflammatory myopathies
Myositis syndromes
Polymyositis
Dermatomyositis

ICD-9CM CODES
710.3 Dermatomyositis
710.4 Polymyositis

EPIDEMIOLOGY & DEMOGRAPHICS

DM:
- Occurs in children and in adults (bimodal age peak)
- Average age at diagnosis is 40 in adults. Age range in children: 5 to 14 yr
- More common in females than in males (2:1)
- Incidence 1:100,000
- Prevalence 1 to 10 cases/million in adults and 1 to 3.2 cases/million in children
- Up to one third of patients older than 50 with DM have an associated malignancy

PM:
- Occurs mostly in adults, very rare in children
- Average age at diagnosis >20 yr
- More common in females
- Least common inflammatory myopathy
- Exact incidence unknown

PHYSICAL FINDINGS & CLINICAL PRESENTATION

DM and PM:
- Most patients have a subacute onset over weeks to months.
- Pattern is typically symmetric proximal muscle weakness involving the proximal limbs (shoulder and pelvic girdles).
- Weakness of neck flexion and extension is common.
- Difficulty getting up from a chair, climbing stairs, reaching for objects above head, or combing hair.
- Distal muscle and ocular involvement is uncommon.
- Sensation is preserved.
- Reflexes may be preserved or diminished.
- Dysphagia and dysphonia result from involvement of striated muscle of the pharynx and proximal esophagus.
- Esophageal dysmotility is common in DM.
- Respiratory failure from associated pulmonary fibrosis.
- Cardiac conduction abnormalities can be seen with DM.

- Systemic autoimmune disease occurs frequently in PM, and rarely in DM.
- Skin findings in DM:
  - Heliotrope rash on the upper eyelids (Fig. 1-574)
  - Erythematous rash on the face (see Fig. 1-574)
  - May also involve the back and shoulders (shawl sign), neck and chest (V-shape), knees (Fig. 1-575), and elbows
  - Photosensitivity
  - Gottron's papules (violaceous papules overlying dorsal interphalangeal or metacarpophalangeal areas, elbow or knee joints—Fig. 1-576)
  - Nail cracking, thickening, and irregularity (Fig. 1-577) with periungual telangiectasia (see Fig. 1-576)
  - Mechanic's hand: fissured, hyperpigmented, scaly, and hyperkeratotic; also associated with increased risk of interstitial lung disease

ETIOLOGY

DM: complex, immune-mediated microangiopathy. Adaptive immune response via humorally mediated complement attack
PM: unknown:
- Cell-mediated immune major histocompatibility-I (MHC-1) process directed against muscle fibers is likely, given biopsy features.

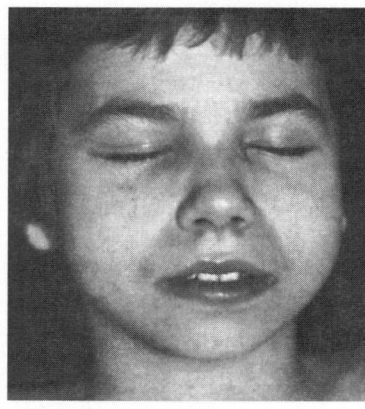

FIGURE 1-574 The facial rash of juvenile dermatomyositis. There is erythema over the bridge of the nose and malar areas, with violaceous (heliotropic) discoloration of the upper eyelids. (From Behrman RE: *Nelson textbook of pediatrics,* ed 17, Philadelphia, 2004, Saunders.)

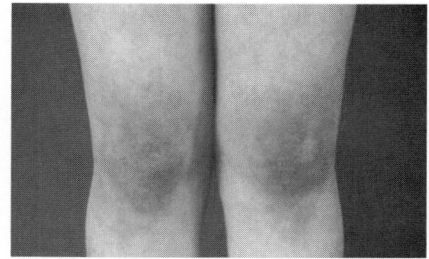

FIGURE 1-575 Violaceous plaques on the knees in a patient with dermatomyositis (Gottron sign). (From Hochberg MC et al: *Rheumatology,* ed 5, St Louis, 2011, Mosby.)

- A viral etiology has been proposed secondary to the presence of autoantibodies to histidyl transferase, anti-Jo-1, and signal recognition particle.

Dx **DIAGNOSIS**

- Myopathic pattern of muscle weakness
- Characteristic rash in DM
- EMG shows myopathic (small-amplitude, short-duration, polyphasic) motor potentials with early recruitment
- Majority of patients have "irritable" features (fibrillations and positive sharp waves) on EMG
- See "Laboratory Tests."
- Biopsy is required for diagnosis and should confirm inflammation before treatment is started: myopathic features (variation in fiber size, fiber splitting, fatty replacement of muscle tissue, and increased endomysial connective tissue) should be seen in addition to the following:
  - DM: perifascicular atrophy, MAC deposition along capillaries
  - PM: endomysial infiltrates composed of CD8+ T cells and macrophages invading nonnecrotic muscle fibers that express MHC-I antigen

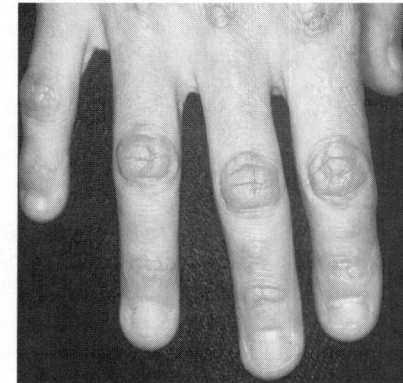

FIGURE 1-576 Dermatomyositis (Gottron's papules). Note erythematous papules over joints and periungual telangiectasias. (From Noble J [ed]: *Textbook of primary care medicine,* ed 2, St Louis, 1996, Mosby.)

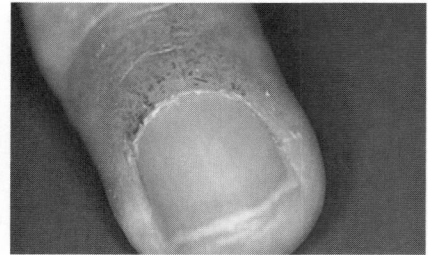

FIGURE 1-577 Enlarged nailfold capillaries in a patient with dermatomyositis. (From Hochberg MC et al: *Rheumatology,* ed 5, St Louis, 2011, Mosby.)

M

DIFFERENTIAL DIAGNOSIS

- IBM
- Muscular dystrophies
- Amyloid myoneuropathy
- Amyotrophic lateral sclerosis
- Myasthenia gravis
- Eaton-Lambert syndrome
- Drug-induced myopathies (e.g., quinidine, NSAIDs, penicillamine, HMG CoA-reductase inhibitors)
- Diabetic amyotrophy
- Guillain-Barré syndrome
- Hyperthyroidism or hypothyroidism
- Lichen planus
- Amyopathic DM (rash without weakness)
- DM sine rash (weakness with characteristic biopsy, but no rash)
- Systemic lupus erythematosus (SLE)
- Contact atopic or seborrheic dermatitis
- Psoriasis

LABORATORY TESTS

- Creatine kinase (CK) is the most sensitive muscle enzyme test for muscle breakdown. It should be checked at onset, and serially monitored several times during treatment.
- CK is typically elevated (5-50x normal) in active PM.
- CK may be normal or only slightly elevated in DM.
- Aldolase, AST, ALT, alkaline phosphatase, and LDH may be elevated.
- Anti-Jo-1 antibodies are seen in myositis with associated interstitial lung disease but are not specific for either DM or PM.
- Electrolytes, thyroid-stimulating hormone (TSH), Ca, and Mg should be evaluated to exclude other causes of weakness.
- Check ECG for cardiac involvement.

IMAGING STUDIES

- Chest x-ray is used to rule out pulmonary involvement. If suspicious for pulmonary interstitial disease, a high-resolution CT scan of the chest may be helpful.
- Video fluoroscopy or barium swallow study to look for upper esophageal dysfunction in patients with dysphagia and DM.

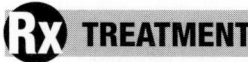 **TREATMENT**

Goal: maintain function, minimize disease/iatrogenic sequelae

NONPHARMACOLOGIC THERAPY

- Sun-blocking agents with SPF 15 or greater for skin protection in patients with DM
- Physical therapy beneficial for gait training and increasing muscle tone and strength
- Occupational therapy assists with activities of daily living
- Speech therapy to monitor patients with swallowing dysfunction

ACUTE GENERAL Rx

- Corticosteroids are the mainstay of therapy. Start prednisone 1 to 2 mg/kg per day, up to a maximum dose of 100 mg/day. Continue until muscle strength improves or muscle enzymes have normalized for at least 4 wk. Begin tapering by 10 mg/mo until 60 mg/day, then slowly taper by 5 mg/mo. Consider every-other-day prednisone treatment at same dose (may decrease side effects).
- Consider IV immunoglobulin (IVIG) if patient fails to improve on prednisone, or muscle enzymes begin rising when tapering off prednisone. See "Chronic Rx" for specific dosage.
- Hydroxychloroquine can be used to treat the cutaneous lesions of DM.

CHRONIC Rx

- Chronic prednisone therapy may be needed for years, but other immunosuppressive ("steroid-sparing") agents may be added early to decrease long-term steroid side effects.
- Azathioprine 2 to 3 mg/kg per day tapered to 1 mg/kg per day once steroid is tapered to 15 mg/day. Reduce dosage monthly by 25-mg intervals. Maintenance dosage is 50 mg/day.
- Methotrexate 7.5 to 10 mg PO/wk, increased by 2.5 mg/wk to total of 25 mg/wk; consider IM dosing if PO is ineffective.
- IV immunoglobulin 2 g/kg total dose over 2 to 5 days.
- IV cyclophosphamide 1 g/M^2 monthly for 6 mo is preferred to oral dosing for refractory cases. However, oral dosing of cyclophosphamide is 1 to 3 mg/kg per day PO or 2 to 4 mg/kg per day in conjunction with prednisone.
- Cyclosporin A: initial dose 2.0 to 2.5 mg/kg bid; long-term maintenance is lowest effective dose.
- Mycophenolate mofetil 500 mg PO bid, titrate to 1500 mg PO bid over 1 to 2 mo.
- Hydroxychloroquine 200 mg PO daily; monitor for visual changes.

DISPOSITION

- 30% to 40% of patients achieve clinical remission with treatment.
- In patients with residual weakness, deficits typically remain stable over long-term follow-up.
- 10% experience recurrent disease.
- Serum CK often returns to normal before symptoms improve.
- During exacerbations, enzymes may rise before clinical symptoms appear.
- Poor prognostic indicators include delay in diagnosis, older age, recalcitrant disease, malignancy, interstitial pulmonary fibrosis, dysphagia, leukocytosis, fever, and anorexia.
- Infection, malignancy, and cardiac and pulmonary dysfunction are the most common causes of death.
- With early treatment, 5- and 8-yr survival rates of 80% and 73%, respectively, have been reported.

REFERRAL

Neurology or rheumatology referral should be made to help establish the diagnosis and implement treatment.

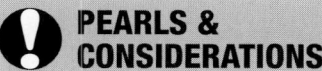 **PEARLS & CONSIDERATIONS**

- Do not implement treatment before muscle biopsy.
- When assessing response to treatment, clinical muscle strength is more important than muscle enzyme tests.
- The concern for malignancies (ovary, lung, breast, GI) associated with DM is legitimate and merits screening in patients older than age 40 at time of diagnosis and every 2 to 3 yr thereafter.
- There does not appear to be any association between juvenile DM and malignancy.
- Overlap syndrome refers to patients with DM who also meet criteria for a connective tissue disorder (e.g., rheumatoid arthritis, scleroderma, SLE).
- In any patient taking steroids, closely monitor for:
  - Diabetes or glucose intolerance (2-hour oral glucose tolerance test)
  - Osteopenia/osteoporosis (DEXA scan q6mo)
  - Cataracts (yearly ophthalmologic appointment)
  - Hypertension
  - Psychiatric side effects including depression or psychosis
  - Poor sleep
  - Peptic ulcer disease (prescribe H$_2$ antagonist or proton pump inhibitor)
- Clinical and immune response features can be used for categorizing heterogeneous myositis syndromes and mutually exclusive and stable phenotypes and are useful for predicting clinical signs and symptoms, associated environmental and genetic risk factors, and responses to therapy and prognosis.

RELATED CONTENT

Dermatomyositis and Polymyositis (Patient Information)

AUTHOR: **GAVIN BROWN, M.D.**

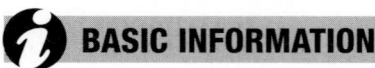

BASIC INFORMATION

DEFINITION

Myotonia is a type of muscular dystrophy in which relaxation of a muscle after contraction is delayed or prolonged. The most common type of muscular dystrophy with myotonia is myotonic dystrophy.

SYNONYMS

Myotonic dystrophy

ICD-9CM CODES
359.2   Myotonic disorders
728.85 Muscle spasm

EPIDEMIOLOGY & DEMOGRAPHICS

- Three to five cases/100,000 persons
- Genetic disorder inherited as an autosomal-dominant illness
- Symptoms usually manifest during adolescence or early adulthood. Cases of infantile myotonic dystrophy have been described.

PHYSICAL FINDINGS & CLINICAL PRESENTATION

- Usual first symptom is distal extremity weakness sometimes associated with muscle stiffness, cramps, or difficulty relaxing grasp.
- Weakness spreads to eventually involve all muscle groups. Flexor neck muscle weakness and masseter and temporal wasting are often prominent features, as is dysarthria.
- Percussion of a muscle produces a slow contraction followed by prolonged relaxation. The myotonic reflex is best tested by percussing the thenar muscles and observing a slow flexion followed by slow relaxation of the thumb.
- As the disease progresses, generalized weakness becomes more pronounced and myotonia becomes less evident.
- Extramuscular involvement:
  o Mental retardation of variable severity (may be absent)
  o Frontal baldness (Fig. 1-578)
  o Cataracts
  o Diabetes mellitus
  o Hypogonadism
  o Adrenal failure
  o Cardiomyopathy
- Infantile myotonic dystrophy presents as neonatal extreme hypotonia with "shark mouth" deformity (upper lip forming an inverted V).

ETIOLOGY & PATHOGENESIS

Genetic disorder encoded on chromosome 19 leading to sustained firing of the muscle membrane, causing prolonged muscle contraction. Myotonic dystrophy 1 (the more common form) is caused by an expanded CTG repeat within the noncoding 3′ untranslated region of the myotonic dystrophy protein kinase *(DMPK)* gene. The less common form (myotonic dystrophy 2) is caused by an expanded CCTG repeat in the first intron of the zinc finger protein 9 *(ZNF9)* gene.

DIAGNOSIS

DIFFERENTIAL DIAGNOSIS

The disease is limited to muscles and causes hypertrophy and stiffness after rest. Muscle function normalizes with exercise. There is no weakness. Symptoms are exacerbated by exposure to cold.
- Myotonia congenita (Thomsen's disease)
- May be autosomal dominant or recessive (two distinct varieties)
- Paramyotonia congenita (autosomal-dominant disease): weakness and stiffness of facial muscles and distal upper extremities, especially or exclusively on cold exposure
- Muscular dystrophies
- Inflammatory myopathies (polymyositis)
- Metabolic muscle diseases
- Myasthenic syndromes
- Motor neuron disease

WORKUP

- History and physical examination usually sufficient

- Muscle enzymes usually abnormal (creatine phosphokinase, aldolase, aspartate aminotransferase)
- Electromyography: typical myotonic "dive bomber" bursts
- Muscle biopsy: type I fiber atrophy, ring fibers, increased central nucleation

TREATMENT

- Phenytoin
- Quinine
- Quinidine
- Procainamide
- Acetazolamide
- Genetic counseling
- Assistive devices, orthotics

DISPOSITION

In myotonic dystrophy, death is usually caused by the wasting of skeletal muscle and defects in cardiac function.

REFERRAL

To neurologist

SUGGESTED READINGS
available at www.expertconsult.com

AUTHOR: **FRED F. FERRI, M.D.**

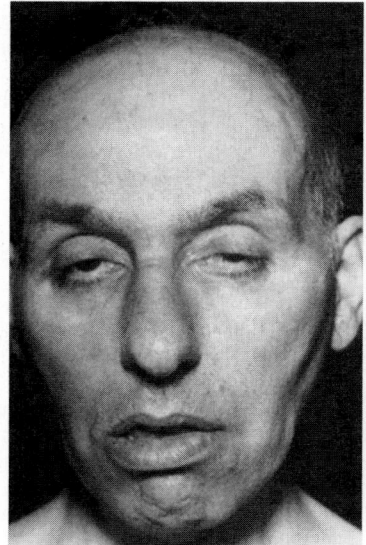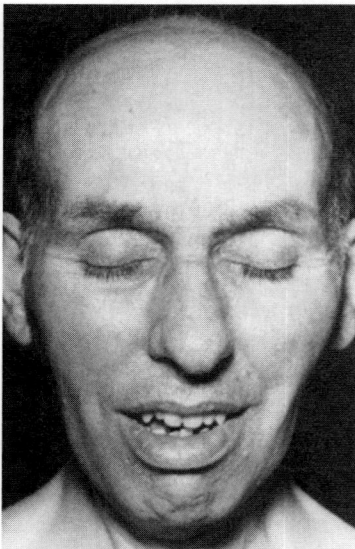

FIGURE 1-578 Myotonic dystrophy with typical myopathic facies, frontal balding, and sunken cheeks. (From Dubowitz V: *Muscle disorders in childhood,* London, 1995, Saunders.)

BASIC INFORMATION

DEFINITION

Myxedema coma is a life-threatening complication of hypothyroidism characterized by profound lethargy or coma and usually accompanied by hypothermia.

ICD-9CM CODES
244.8 Myxedema, pituitary
244.1 Myxedema, primary

PHYSICAL FINDINGS & CLINICAL PRESENTATION

- Mental obtuntation, profound lethargy or coma
- Hypothermia (rectal temperature <35° C [95° F]); often missed by using ordinary thermometers graduated only to 34.5° C or because the mercury is not shaken below 36° C
- Bradycardia, hypotension (attributable to circulatory collapse)
- Delayed relaxation phase of deep tendon reflexes, areflexia
- Myxedema facies (Fig. 1-579)
- Alopecia, macroglossia, ptosis, periorbital edema, nonpitting edema, doughy skin
- Bladder dystonia and distention
- Pleural, pericardial, and peritoneal effusions

ETIOLOGY

Decompensation of hypothyroidism from:
- Sepsis
- Exposure to cold weather
- Central nervous system depressants (sedatives, narcotics, antidepressants)
- Trauma, surgery
- Stroke, congestive heart failure, burns
- Intravascular volume contraction (GI blood loss, diuretic use)

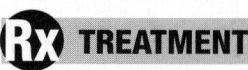

DIAGNOSIS

DIFFERENTIAL DIAGNOSIS

- Severe depression, primary psychosis
- Drug overdose
- Cerebrovascular accident, liver failure, renal failure
- Hypoglycemia, CO_2 narcosis, encephalitis

WORKUP

Diagnosis of hypothyroidism and exclusion of contributing factors (e.g., sepsis, cerebrovascular accident) with laboratory and radiographic studies (see "Laboratory Tests")

LABORATORY TESTS

- Markedly increased thyroid-stimulating hormone (if primary hypothyroidism), decreased serum free T_4
- Complete blood count with differential, urine and blood cultures to rule out infectious process
- Electrolytes, blood urea nitrogen, creatinine, liver function tests, calcium, glucose
- Arterial blood gases to rule out hypoxemia and carbon dioxide retention
- Cortisol level to rule out adrenal insufficiency
- Elevated CPK
- Hyperlipidemia

IMAGING STUDIES

- CT scan of head in suspected cerebrovascular accident
- Chest x-ray to rule out infectious process

TREATMENT

NONPHARMACOLOGIC THERAPY

- Prevent further heat loss; cover the patient but avoid external rewarming because it may produce vascular collapse.

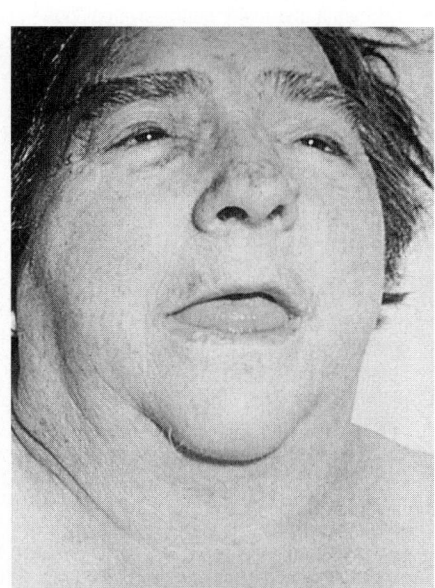

FIGURE 1-579 Myxedema facies. Note dull, puffy, yellowed skin; coarse, sparse hair; temporal loss of eyebrows; periorbital edema; prominent tongue. (Courtesy Paul W. Ladenson, M.D., The Johns Hopkins University and Hospital, Baltimore. In Seidel HM [ed]: *Mosby's guide to physical examination,* ed 5, St Louis, 2004, Mosby.)

- Support respiratory function; intubation and mechanical ventilation may be required.
- Monitor patient in the intensive care unit.

ACUTE GENERAL Rx

- Give levothyroxine 5 to 8 mcg/kg (300 to 500 mcg) IV infused over 15 min, then 100 mcg IV q24h.
- Glucocorticoids should also be administered until coexistent adrenal insufficiency can be ruled out. Hydrocortisone hemisuccinate 100 mg IV bolus is initially given, followed by 100 mg IV q8h until initial plasma cortisol level is confirmed normal.
- IV hydration with D_5NS is used to correct hypotension and hypoglycemia (if present); avoid overhydration and possible water intoxication because clearance of free water is impaired in these patients.
- Rule out and treat precipitating factors (e.g., antibiotics in suspected sepsis).

CHRONIC Rx

Refer to "Hypothyroidism" in Section I.

DISPOSITION

Mortality rate in myxedema coma is 20% to 50%.

REFERRAL

Endocrinology consultation

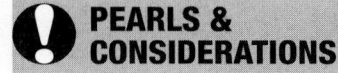

PEARLS & CONSIDERATIONS

COMMENTS

If the diagnosis is suspected, initiate treatment immediately without waiting for confirming laboratory results.

RELATED CONTENT

Hypothyroidism (Related Key Topic)
Hypothyroidism (Patient Information)

AUTHOR: **FRED F. FERRI, M.D.**

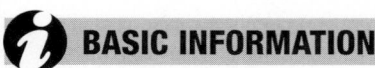

BASIC INFORMATION

DEFINITION

Narcissistic personality disorder (NPD) is characterized by a pattern of grandiosity, need for admiration, and lack of empathy that begins by early adulthood and causes significant distress or impairment in multiple domains of functioning. The individual must meet five or more of the following criteria:

1. Grandiose sense of self-importance. For example, the person may exaggerate achievements and talents or expect recognition as superior without commensurate achievements.
2. Preoccupied with fantasies of unlimited success, power, brilliance, beauty, or ideal love.
3. Views self as "special" and unique and should only associate with other special or highly regarded people and institutions.
4. Requires excessive admiration.
5. Sense of entitlement. For example, unreasonable expectations of especially favorable treatment or automatic compliance with his or her expectations.
6. Interpersonally exploitative.
7. Lacks empathy—unwilling to recognize or identify with the feelings or needs of others.
8. Often envious of others or believes others envious of him or her.
9. Shows arrogant or haughty behaviors.

SYNONYMS

None

ICD-9CM CODES

301.81 Narcissistic personality disorder

EPIDEMIOLOGY & DEMOGRAPHICS

PREVALENCE: Less than 1% of the general population; estimates range from 2% to 16% in the clinical population
PREDOMINANT SEX: More commonly diagnosed in males (up to 3:1)
PREDOMINANT AGE: 20s and 30s

CLINICAL PRESENTATION

- Patients have an underlying sense of inferiority and inadequacy.
- May be related to the failure of parents or parental surrogates to impart a sense of self-worth.
- To avoid these beliefs and their associated painful effects, patients seek to convince self and others that they are special, the best, or unusually talented.
- Astutely aware of status, pecking order.
- Vulnerability in self-esteem makes these patients exquisitely sensitive to criticism, defeat, or perceived weakness, which in turn can lead to feeling humiliated, degraded, and empty.

- These patients react to perceived slights with either more intense grandiosity and admiration seeking or with disdain and rage. Either approach seeks to bolster their sense of self often by devaluing or criticizing the other person.
- Experiences of self-deflation lead to social withdrawal or depressed mood or to feigned humility that protects grandiosity.
- Interpersonal relationships are typically shallow and limited.
- Although ambition and confidence may lead to high achievement, vocational functioning may be disrupted by intolerance for criticism.

ETIOLOGY

- Limited knowledge about role of genetic loading and neurobiologic vulnerability.
- Prevailing hypotheses focus on impaired development of self as "worthy" because of insufficient affirmation and warmth from parents.

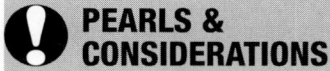

DIAGNOSIS

DIFFERENTIAL DIAGNOSIS

- Mania and hypomania
- Dysthymia and major depressive episode
- Substance-induced euphoria, especially cocaine abuse
- Histrionic, borderline, antisocial, and paranoid personality disorders share common features and are often comorbid
- Personality changes from a general medical condition, including central nervous system processes in the frontal-temporal regions of the brain

WORKUP

- History: collateral information essential to establishing presence of longstanding interpersonal pattern in multiple domains of the patient's life
- Physical examination
- Mental status examination

LABORATORY TESTS

Tests necessary to rule out medical causes of personality changes

IMAGING STUDIES

Those necessary to rule out medical causes of personality changes

TREATMENT

NONPHARMACOLOGIC THERAPY

- Cognitive-behavioral therapy to help patients control rage, manage perceived criticism, and develop social skills

- Psychodynamic psychotherapy to help develop improved self-concept, affect tolerance, and interpersonal functioning

ACUTE GENERAL Rx

Benzodiazepines or low-dose antipsychotics to control rage

CHRONIC Rx

- Selective serotonin reuptake inhibitors for impulsivity or comorbid depression
- Mood stabilizers if comorbid bipolar or to improve impulse control

DISPOSITION

- Severity is variable and course is chronic. The majority of patients obtain greater functioning in fifth decade and beyond when pessimism replaces grandiosity. Often lifelong difficulty maintaining intimate relationships.
- At increased risk for major depressive disorder and substance abuse or dependence (especially cocaine).

REFERRAL

If pharmacotherapy is contemplated

PEARLS & CONSIDERATIONS

COMMENTS

- Illness threatens these patients' image of superiority.
- To defend against this threat, patients may minimize symptoms or deny presence of illness.
- Patients will commonly demand special treatment from senior and well-known physicians.
- Patients may devalue, criticize, or question the behavior or credentials of the treating physician.
- Management guidelines:
  1. Be respectful and nonconfrontational.
  2. Help patient use self-perceived talents in service of treatment.
  3. Do not personalize patient's devaluation, but understand their criticalness as an attempt to manage their own intense insecurity.
  4. Appeal to the patient's narcissism. In other words, agree with the patient that he or she is "entitled" to appropriate care.

SUGGESTED READINGS

available at www.expertconsult.com

RELATED CONTENT

Narcissistic Personality Disorder (Patient Information)

AUTHOR: **JOHN Q. YOUNG, M.D., M.P.P.**

BASIC INFORMATION

DEFINITION

Narcolepsy is a chronic neurologic sleep disorder characterized by excessive daytime sleepiness and dysregulation of rapid eye movement (REM) sleep. It is the second most common cause of disabling daytime sleepiness after obstructive sleep apnea. Symptoms of REM sleep dysregulation include cataplexy, sleep paralysis, and hallucinations during transition between wake and sleep. Difficulty sleeping with either frequent awakenings or disrupted sleep may also occur.

SYNONYMS

Hypersomnia of central origin
Narcolepsy with cataplexy
Narcolepsy-cataplexy syndrome
Narcolepsy with hypocretin deficiency
Gelineau syndrome

ICD-9CM CODES
347.00 Narcolepsy without cataplexy
347.01 Narcolepsy with cataplexy

EPIDEMIOLOGY & DEMOGRAPHICS

INCIDENCE: 0.74/100,000 persons/yr
PREVALENCE: 5 to 50/100,000 people
PREDOMINANT SEX: Males and females are equally affected.
AGE OF ONSET: Peak 15 to 30 yr (range, 10-55 yr)
GENETICS:
- Associated with human leukocyte antigen (HLA) subtypes, specifically, *DQB1*0602,* which is present in 95% of patients with cataplexy and 96% of patients with hypocretin deficiency.
- Risk of narcolepsy increases 20 to 40 times if a family member is affected.
- Monozygotic twin concordance rate is 17% to 36%, thus indicating an incomplete penetrance and suggesting an environmental factor in the disease process.

RISK FACTORS: Anesthesia, head injury, history of meningitis or encephalitis, family history of narcolepsy, tumor, vascular malformations, stroke, and obesity.

PHYSICAL FINDINGS & CLINICAL PRESENTATION

- Overwhelming urge to sleep with chronic hypersomnia may occur during the day.
- Cataplexy occurs in 60% to 100% of patients with narcolepsy and is reported as a partial or complete loss of voluntary muscle control with preserved consciousness that is precipitated by a strong emotion, more commonly with laughter. This is the most specific symptom and is considered pathognomonic for narcolepsy.
- Hypnagogic (wake to sleep) or hypnopompic (sleep to wake) hallucinations have been reported in 60% to 80% of patients with narcolepsy.
- Sleep paralysis, defined as loss of muscle tone during the transition between sleep and wakefulness, occurs in 60% to 80% of patients with narcolepsy. It may occur with hallucinations and can be interrupted by sensory stimuli.
- Only about one third of patients will have all four symptoms: chronic daytime sleepiness, cataplexy, hypnagogic hallucinations, and sleep paralysis.
- Fragmented sleep is seen in 60% to 80% of narcolepsy patients and can often be mistaken for insomnia or other intrinsic sleep disorder.
- Other symptoms that have been reported in narcolepsy include automatic behavior or semipurposeful movements in 40% of patients and memory disturbance in 50% of patients.

ETIOLOGY

The loss of hypocretin/orexin signaling, genetic factors, and rare brain lesions are presently identified factors in the development of narcolepsy.
HYPOCRETIN/OREXIN:
- Loss of hypocretin-1 and hypocretin-2 (also known as orexin-A and orexin-B) producing neurons in the lateral hypothalamus.
- Human cerebrospinal fluid (CSF) levels of hypocretin-1 are low to undetectable in narcoleptics with cataplexy.
- Narcolepsy without cataplexy may have a different cause because CSF hypocretin levels are usually normal in these patients, so there may be a completely separate mechanism in these patients, or it may result from less extensive loss of hypocretin neurons or impaired signaling.

SECONDARY ETIOLOGIES:
- Tumors, vascular malformations, and strokes have all been reported to cause secondary narcolepsy.
- Direct injury to the hypocretin neurons or their projections is the most likely cause of secondary narcolepsy due to central nervous system lesions.
- Narcolepsy has been reported in genetic syndromes, including Prader-Willi syndrome and Niemann-Pick disease type C, as well as paraneoplastic syndromes.

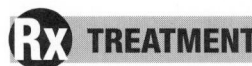

DIAGNOSIS

DIFFERENTIAL DIAGNOSIS

Excessive daytime somnolence:
- Autism
- Autosomal dominant cerebellar ataxia, deafness, and narcolepsy
- Behaviorally induced insufficient sleep syndrome
- Central or obstructive sleep apnea (sleep-disordered breathing)
- Circadian rhythm disorder
- Depression
- Diencephalic lesions
- Drug or alcohol abuse
- Hypothyroidism
- Idiopathic hypersomnia with long or short sleep time
- Inadequate sleep hygiene
- Insufficient sleep
- Increased intracranial pressure
- Insomnia
- Kleine-Levin syndrome
- Medication effect
- Menstrual-related hypersomnia
- Posttraumatic narcolepsy
- Seizures
- Sleep fragmentation (multiple causes)

Cataplexy:
- Seizures
- Periodic paralysis
- Cardiovascular insufficiency
- Psychogenic (multiple causes)
- Lesions of the hypothalamus or brain stem

WORKUP

- Narcolepsy is often diagnosed by clinical history. The Epworth Sleepiness Scale is very useful in determining the degree of excessive daytime sleepiness (Table 1-295).
- The diagnosis of narcolepsy can be made if there is a clear history of cataplexy in the setting of excessive daytime somnolence, without need for further diagnostic testing. Sleep laboratory testing or possibly laboratory testing is required if these symptoms do not exist.
- The medical history should include questions regarding severity of daytime hypersomnia while also evaluating for sleep-disordered breathing, transient muscle weakness triggered by emotion, hallucinations while falling asleep or upon awakening, and inability to move after awakening. The clinical evaluation should also address symptoms of seizures and paraneoplastic disorders while also asking about previous stroke or genetic disorders. A detailed family history is imperative. Hypothalamic dysfunction such as unexplained weight gain, endocrine abnormalities, circadian dysrhythmias, and autonomic nervous system problems may provide useful insight.
- A thorough examination including a detailed neurologic examination should be performed.
- Nocturnal polysomnography followed by a multiple sleep latency test (MSLT) remains to be the gold standard for the diagnosis of narcolepsy. A drug screen should also be performed to rule out pharmacologic modulations of sleep.

LABORATORY TESTS

HLA subtyping and CSF hypocretin/orexin levels may be attempted in suspected cases of narcolepsy. CSF hypocretin/orexin analysis is primarily a research tool. CSF hypocretin levels below 110 pg/ml are indicative of narcolepsy, but high CSF hypocretin levels do not exclude the diagnosis.

TREATMENT

NONPHARMACOLOGIC THERAPY

Avoidance of over-the-counter drugs and illicit drugs, optimal sleep hygiene and scheduled daily naps, and psychosocial support can be used for symptoms of excessive daytime somnolence. However, nonpharmacologic therapy is typically not sufficient for treatment of narcolepsy alone but is often used as adjunct therapy with medications.

PHARMACOLOGIC THERAPY

For excessive daytime somnolence:

- Sodium oxybate (Xyrem): a central nervous system depressant that can be used for the treatment of cataplexy and REM-related symptoms
- Modafinil (Provigil) 200 to 600 mg PO every morning or divided bid
- Armodafinil (Nuvigil) 150 or 250 mg PO as a single dose in the morning
- Methylphenidate (Ritalin) 5 to 15 mg PO bid to tid
- Methylphenidate SR (Concerta) 18 to 54 mg PO every morning or divided bid
- Dextroamphetamine (Dexedrine) 10 to 60 mg PO qd
- Eldepryl (Selegiline HCl) 5 mg PO bid

For cataplexy:

- Sodium oxybate (Xyrem): a central nervous system depressant that can be used for the treatment of cataplexy and REM-related symptoms
- Fluoxetine (Prozac) 20 mg PO qd initially
- Sertraline (Zoloft) 25 mg PO qd initially
- Venlafaxine (Effexor) 25 mg PO qd initially
- Clomipramine (Anafranil) 25 mg/day initially
- Protriptyline (Vivactil) 5 mg tid initially
- Imipramine (Tofranil) 25 to 50 mg/day initially
- Desipramine (Norpramin) 10 mg bid initially

DISPOSITION

This is a chronic sleep disorder that may worsen for the first few years and then persist for life.

REFERRAL

Because of the complexity of this disorder and its ever-changing management and treatment, patients should be referred to centers or programs with highly trained sleep specialists with expertise caring for these patients, especially if sodium oxybate (Xyrem) therapy is needed.

 PEARLS & CONSIDERATIONS

Many narcoleptics report the onset of symptoms beginning in childhood to early adulthood with a long delay of actual diagnosis on the order of 10 to 15 yr. Typically, excessive daytime sleepiness is the initial symptom followed by REM dysregulation (e.g., cataplexy, sleep paralysis, hypnagogic hallucinations). Patients with narcolepsy also have higher than expected incidence of other sleep disorders, including obstructive sleep apnea, periodic limb movements of sleep, and REM sleep behavior disorder.

COMMENTS

Narcolepsy is a rare disorder that is underdiagnosed. Cataplexy is specific for narcolepsy, but other symptoms of REM dysregulation, including sleep paralysis and hypnagogic or hypnopompic hallucinations, can occur even in normal patients. Sleep-onset REM or REM periods on an MSLT may occur as a result of sleep deprivation or withdrawal from REM-suppressing drugs.

SUGGESTED READINGS
available at www.expertconsult.com

RELATED CONTENT
Narcolepsy (Patient Information)

AUTHOR: **DON HAYES, JR., M.D.**

TABLE 1-295 Epworth Sleepiness Scale

How likely are you to doze off or fall asleep in the following situations, in contrast to just feeling tired? This refers to your usual way of life in recent time. Even if you have not done some of these things recently, try to work out how they would have affected you. Use the following scale to choose the most appropriate number for each situation.

0 = would never doze	
1 = slight chance of dozing	
2 = moderate chance of dozing	
3 = high chance of dozing	

Situation	Chance of Dozing
Sitting and reading	
Watching TV	
Sitting and inactive in a public place (theater or meeting)	
As a passenger in a car for an hour without a break	
Lying down to rest in the afternoon when circumstances permit	
Sitting and talking to someone	
Sitting quietly after lunch (without alcohol)	
In a car, while stopped for a few minutes in traffic	
TOTAL	

From Johns MW: A new method for measuring daytime sleepiness: the Epworth Sleepiness Scale, *Sleep* 14:540-545, 1991.

BASIC INFORMATION

DEFINITION

Necrotizing fasciitis is a rapidly spreading bacterial infection of the deep fascia, with associated inflammation, leading to necrosis of subcutaneous tissue planes. This infection can occur in wounds from trauma or surgical wounds or can be spontaneous or idiopathic. There are two clinical types, both of which carry a high rate of morbidity and mortality.

SYNONYMS

Soft tissue gangrene
Flesh eating bacteria
Fournier's gangrene
Hemolytic streptococcal gangrene

ICD-9CM CODES
728.86 Necrotizing fasciitis

EPIDEMIOLOGY & DEMOGRAPHICS

PREDOMINANT SEX: Male > female
PREDOMINANT AGE: 6-50 yr; rare in children
EPIDEMIOLOGY: Invasive group A *Streptococcus* infection occurs at a rate of 3.5 cases per 100,000 persons, with a case fatality rate of around 24%.

PHYSICAL FINDINGS & CLINICAL PRESENTATION

CLINICAL TYPES OF NECROTIZING FASCIITIS
- Type I necrotizing fasciitis: at least one anaerobic species is isolated in conjunction with one or more facultative anaerobic species, such as streptococci (not group A), *and* members of the Enterobacteriaceae:
  - Anaerobic bacteria, most commonly *Bacteroides* or *Peptostreptococcus* spp.
  - Enterobacteriaceae: *Escherichia coli, Klebsiella* spp., *Proteus* spp., *Enterobacter* spp.
  - Usually associated with diabetes or peripheral vascular disease
  - Example of type I: Fournier's gangrene of the perineum
- Type II necrotizing fasciitis: Group A *Streptococcus* is isolated alone or in combination with other bacteria, most likely *Staphylococcus aureus.* Also known as hemolytic streptococcal gangrene
  - Example of type II: Invasive group A *Streptococcus*, associated with virulence factors type 1 and type 3 M protein

EXAMPLES OF NECROTIZING FASCIITIS
- Fournier's gangrene: Aggressive type I infection of the perineum usually caused by penetration of the gastrointestinal or urethral mucosa by enteric organisms. Can rapidly spread to involve the scrotum, penis, and abdominal wall or gluteal muscles, causing gangrene.

- Clostridial cellulitis: Caused by *Clostridium perfringens* associated by local trauma or surgery and crepitus caused by gas production; generally noted in the skin, with deeper tissues generally spared.

PHYSICAL FINDINGS

Minor skin trauma, toxic-appearing patient:
- Open skin wound
- Severe pain at injury or surgical site
- Fever, confusion, weakness, diarrhea
- Early skin erythema, quickly spreading in hours to days
- Skin redness changes to purple discoloration
- Gangrenous skin changes may develop
- Loosening of skin and subcutaneous skin in association with deep fascial necrosis (Fig. 1-580)
- Muscle involvement, thrombosis of blood vessels, and myonecrosis may develop
- Bullae and gas formation at site

ETIOLOGY
- Polymicrobial: mixture of anaerobes and aerobic enteric gram-negative rods
- Group A streptococci *(S. pyogenes)*
- *S. aureus*
- *C. perfringens*
- *Bacteroides fragilis*
- *Vibrio vulnificus*
- Methicillin-resistant *S. aureus* (MRSA), especially community-acquired MRSA

DIAGNOSIS

DIFFERENTIAL DIAGNOSIS
- Cellulitis
- Pyomyositis
- Gas gangrene

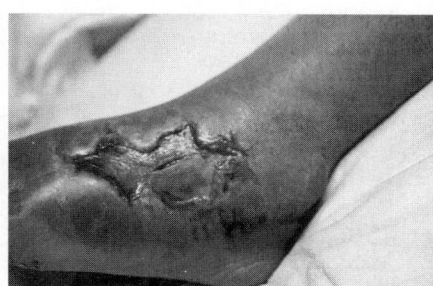

FIGURE 1-580 Necrotizing fasciitis. The so-called flesh-eating bacteria, group A β-hemolytic *Streptococcus,* can cause significant tissue destruction rapidly. This 32-year-old woman had pain, erythema, and swelling of the foot followed by necrotic ulceration over a week. There was no history of trauma. (Courtesy Roger Bitar, MD. From White GM, Cox NH [eds]: *Diseases of the skin, a color atlas and text,* ed 2, St Louis, 2006, Mosby.)

- A classification of necrotizing skin, soft-tissue, and muscle infections is described in Table 1-296.

WORKUP
- Diagnosis of necrotizing fasciitis generally requires incision and probing. In patients with necrotizing fasciitis, there is no resistance to probing subcut and there is fascial plane involvement.
- Laboratory tests:
  - Complete blood cell count (CBC) with differential
  - Cultures of skin, soft tissue, or debrided tissue, aerobically and anaerobically. Blood cultures are positive in 60% of patients with type II infections and 20% with type I infections.
- Imaging:
  - Radiographs show subcutaneous gas in fascial planes (Fig. 1-581).
  - Computed tomography (CT)/magnetic resonance imaging (MRI) may be helpful because they can detect gas in the tissues.

TREATMENT

- Aggressive surgical debridement of involved necrotic tissues is essential as soon as possible to reduce mortality.
- Fasciotomies of extremities may be necessary.
- Empiric antibiotic treatment:
  - Type I: Piperacillin/tazobactam; carbapenems such as imipenem, meropenem, or doripenem; and third-generation cephalosporin + metronidazole or aminoglycoside + clindamycin are reasonable choices pending cultures. It is important to always have anaerobic coverage.
  - Type II: For group A *Streptococcus,* give intravenous (IV) penicillin G, 4 million U q4h in patients who weigh more than 60 kg with clindamycin, 600-900 mg IV q8h.
  - Clindamycin has the added effect of suppressing toxin production. If community associated-MRSA is suspected, add vancomycin.
- Intravenous gammaglobulin, 2 g/kg, neutralizes circulating streptococcal toxins and has been shown beneficial in severe forms of invasive group A streptococcal infections.
- Hyperbaric oxygen evaluation as an adjunct to surgery and IV antibiotics.

SUGGESTED READINGS
available at www.expertconsult.com

AUTHOR: **GLENN G. FORT, M.D., M.P.H.**

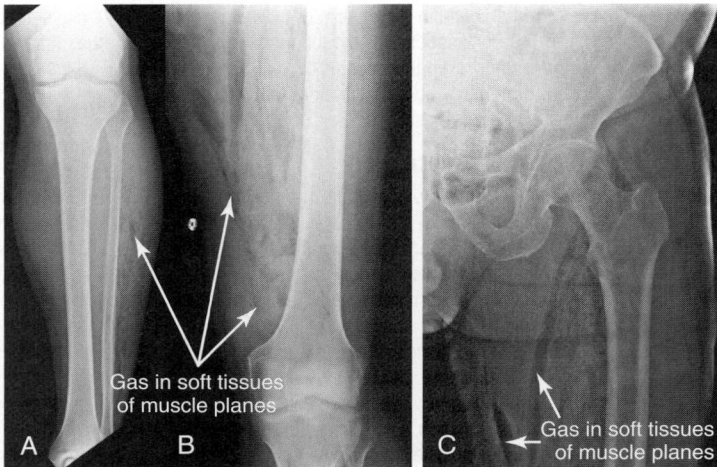

FIGURE 1-581 Necrotizing fasciitis. This 71-year-old man with aplastic anemia presented with fevers to 38.9° C, leg weakness, and extreme leg pain. Initially, the patient was thought to have neuropathic pain and weakness, possibly indicating spinal disease such as epidural abscess. He rapidly developed crepitus of his legs. Radiographs of the patient's legs were obtained, followed by noncontrast CT. **A,** Anterior-posterior (AP) tibia and fibula. **B,** AP femur. **C,** AP hip. Air is seen dissecting in muscle planes of the legs. On radiograph, air appears black. Given the wide distribution of air, a focal abscess is unlikely, and necrotizing fasciitis with gas-producing organisms should be suspected. (From Broder JS: *Diagnostic imaging for the emergency physician,* Philadelphia, 2011, Saunders.)

TABLE 1-296 Classification of Necrotizing Skin, Soft-Tissue, and Muscle Infections

Disease	Bacteriology	Comments
Necrotizing Cellulitis		
Clostridial cellulitis	*Clostridium perfringens*	Local trauma, recent surgery; fascial/deep muscle spared
Nonclostridial cellulitis	Mixed: *Escherichia coli, Enterobacter, Peptostreptococcus* spp., *Bacteroides fragilis*	Diabetes mellitus predisposes; produces foul odor
Meleney's synergistic gangrene	*Staphylococcus aureus,* microaerophilic streptococci	Rare infection; postoperative; slowly expanding, indolent, ulceration in superficial fascia
Synergistic necrotizing cellulitis	Mixed aerobic and anaerobic, including *B. fragilis, Peptostreptococcus* spp.	Diabetes mellitus predisposes; variant of necrotizing fasciitis type I; involves skin, muscle, fat, and fascia
Necrotizing Fasciitis		
Type I	Mixed aerobic and anaerobic; staphylococci, *B. fragilis, E. coli,* group A streptococci, *Peptostreptococcus* spp., *Prevotella, Porphyromonas* spp., *Clostridium* spp.	Usually requires a breach in the mucous membrane layer either through surgery or penetrating injuries or from chronic medical conditions such as diabetes, peripheral vascular disease, malignancy, and anal fissures
Type II	Group A streptococci	Increasing in frequency and severity since 1985; very high mortality; often begins at site of nonpenetrating minor trauma such as a bruise or muscle strain but often no identified precursor
		Predisposing factors: blunt/penetrating trauma, varicella (chickenpox), intravenous drug abuse, surgical procedures, childbirth, nonsteroidal anti-inflammatory drug use
Myonecrosis		
Clostridial myonecrosis	*Clostridium* spp.	Predisposing factors: deep/penetrating injury, bowel and biliary tract surgery, improperly performed abortion and retained placenta, prolonged rupture of the membranes, and intrauterine fetal demise or missed abortion in postpartum patients. Recurrent gas gangrene occurs at sites of previous gas gangrene.
Streptococcal myonecrosis	Streptococci	
Special Type of Necrotizing Soft-Tissue Infection		
Fournier's gangrene	Polymicrobial, with *E. coli* the predominant aerobe and *Bacteroides* the predominant anaerobe. Other microflora: *Proteus, Staphylococcus, Enterococcus,* aerobic and anaerobic *Streptococcus, Pseudomonas, Klebsiella,* and *Clostridium*	Necrosis of the scrotum or perineum that starts with scrotal pain and erythema and rapidly spreads onto anterior abdominal wall and gluteal muscle. It is more often seen in diabetics and can be associated with trauma.

From Vincent JL et al: *Textbook of critical care,* ed 6, Philadelphia, 2011, Saunders.

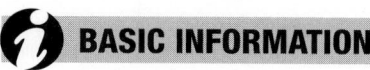

BASIC INFORMATION

DEFINITION

Nephroblastoma is a malignant renal tumor derived from primitive metanephric blastoma. Most tumors are unicentric, but some are multifocal in one or both kidneys. Associated anomalies may be present.

SYNONYMS

Wilms' tumor

ICD-9CM CODES
189.0 Nephroblastoma

EPIDEMIOLOGY & DEMOGRAPHICS

- Pediatric malignancy mean presentation is at 41.5 mo in boys and 46.9 mo in girls.
- Slightly more frequent in girls
- Incidence rate is 7.9 cases per year per 1 million white children <15 yr (a little over 500 new cases annually in the U.S.); the incidence is double in black children.
- Associated syndromes (Table 1-297):
  1. Cryptorchidism
  2. Hypospadias
  3. Hemihypertrophy with or without the Beckwith-Wiedeman syndrome, aniridia
  4. Denys-Drash syndrome (nephroblastoma, pseudohermaphroditism, glomerulonephritis)
  5. WAGR syndrome (**W**ilms' tumor, **a**niridia, **g**enitourinary malformations, and mental **r**etardation)
- Familial nephroblastoma occurs in 1.5% (with younger age at diagnosis and more frequent multifocal tumors).

PHYSICAL FINDINGS & CLINICAL PRESENTATION

- Nephroblastoma often is discovered when a parent notices a mass while bathing or dressing a child, most commonly a child who is approximately age 3 yr, or during a routine physical examination. The mass is unilateral, firm, and nontender and below the costal margin.
- Abdominal swelling and/or pain
- Nausea
- Vomiting
- Constipation
- Loss of appetite
- Fever of unknown origin
- Night sweats
- Hematuria (less common than in adult renal malignancies)

- Malaise
- High blood pressure that is triggered when the tumor obstructs the renal artery
- Varicocele
- Signs of associated syndromes

ETIOLOGY & PATHOGENESIS

- Three cell types: blastomal, stromal, and epithelial may be present. Structural diversity is characteristic.
- Anaplasia is evidenced by the presence of gigantic polyploid nuclei. The term *focal anaplasia* is used to describe such findings when it is confined within the primary tumor in the kidney.
- Staging:
  Stage I: Tumor limited to the kidney whose capsule is intact. The tumor is completely excised.
  Stage II: Tumor extends beyond the kidney but is completely excised. No peritoneal involvement.
  Stage III: Residual tumor confined to the abdomen after surgery. No hematogenous metastases.
  Stage IV: Hematogenous metastases present.
  Stage V: Bilateral renal involvement at time of initial diagnosis.

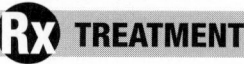

DIAGNOSIS

DIFFERENTIAL DIAGNOSIS

- Other renal malignancies
  1. Hypernephroma
  2. Transitional cell carcinoma
  3. Lymphoma
  4. Clear cell sarcoma
  5. Rhabdoid tumor of the kidney

- Renal cyst
- Other intraabdominal or retroperitoneal tumors

LABORATORY TESTS

- Complete blood count
- Transaminases (alanine aminotransferase, aspartate aminotransferase)
- Alkaline phosphatase
- Blood urea nitrogen and creatinine
- Serum calcium
- Urinalysis

IMAGING STUDIES

- Renal ultrasound to confirm existence of a solid mass in a kidney
- Abdominal CT scan with contrast
- Chest radiograph or CT scan

TREATMENT

- Surgical resection and surgical staging:
  1. Stages I and II: surgery followed by chemotherapy
  2. Stages III and IV: surgery followed by radiation and chemotherapy
- Chemotherapeutic agents used in the treatment of nephroblastoma include vincristine, dactinomycin, and doxorubicin

PROGNOSIS

- Stage I: 95% survival
- Stage II: 91% survival
- Stage III: 91% survival
- Stage IV: 81% survival
- Prognosis is better for patients <2 yr

AUTHOR: **FRED F. FERRI, M.D.**

TABLE 1-297 Syndromes associated with Wilms' Tumor

Syndrome	Clinical Characteristics	Genetic Anomalies
Wilms' tumor, aniridia, genitourinary abnormalities, and mental retardation (WAGR syndrome)	Aniridia, genitourinary abnormalities, mental retardation	Del 11p13 (*WT1* and *PAX6*)
Denys-Drash syndrome	Early-onset renal failure with renal mesangial sclerosis, male pseudohermaphroditism	*WT1* missense mutation
Beckwith-Wiedemann syndrome (BWS)	Organomegaly (liver, kidney, adrenal, pancreas) macroglossia, omphalocele, hemihypertrophy	Unilateral paternal disomy, duplication of 11p15.5 loss of imprinting, mutation of *p57KIP57* Del 11p15.5 *IGF2* and *H19* imprinting control region

From Kliegman RM et al: *Nelson textbook of pediatrics*, ed 19, Philadelphia, 2011, Saunders.

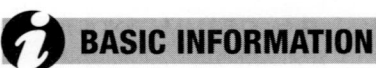

BASIC INFORMATION

DEFINITION

Nephrotic syndrome is characterized by high urine protein excretion (>3.5 g/1.73 m³/24 hr), peripheral edema, and metabolic abnormalities (hypoalbuminemia, hypercholesterolemia). Table 1-298 describes definitions of terms used in idiopathic nephrotic syndrome in adults and children. Fig. 1-582 illustrates the mechanism of nephrotic edema.

ICD-9CM CODES
581.9 Nephrotic syndrome

EPIDEMIOLOGY & DEMOGRAPHICS

- Nephrotic syndrome occurs predominantly in children ages 2 to 6 yr (2 new cases/100,000 persons/yr) and in adults of all ages (3 to 4 new cases/100,000 persons/yr).
- Membranous glomerulonephritis is the most common cause of nephrotic syndrome.

PHYSICAL FINDINGS & CLINICAL PRESENTATION

- Peripheral edema, eyelid edema (Fig. 1-583)
- Ascites, anasarca
- Hypertension
- Pleural effusion
- Typically patients present with severe peripheral edema, exertional dyspnea, and abdominal fullness secondary to ascites. There is a significant amount of weight gain in most patients.

ETIOLOGY

- Idiopathic (may be secondary to the following glomerular diseases: minimal change disease [nil disease, lipoid nephrosis], focal segmental glomerular sclerosis (20% of cases of nephrotic syndrome), membranous nephropathy, membranoproliferative glomerular nephropathy). PLA 2 R is a major antigen in the majority of patients with idiopathic membranous nephropathy. An

---

TABLE 1-298   Nephrotic Syndrome (NS): Definitions

| Term | NS DEFINITIONS | |
	Adult	Pediatric
Relapse	Proteinuria ≥3.5 g/day occurring after complete remission has been obtained for >1 mo	Albu-stix 3+ or proteinuria >40 mg/m/h occurring on 3 days within 1 wk
Frequently relapsing	2+ relapses within 6 mo	2+ relapses within 6 mo
Complete remission	Reduction of proteinuria to ≤0.20 g/day and serum albumin >35 g/L	<4 mg/m/h on at least 3 occasions within 7 days serum albumin >35 g/L
Partial remission	Reduction of proteinuria to between 0.21 g/day and 3.4 g/day ± decrease in proteinuria of ≥50% from baseline	Disappearance of edema. Increase in serum albumin >35 g/L and persisting proteinuria >4 mg/m/h or >100 mg/m/day
Steroid-resistant	Persistence of proteinuria despite prednisone therapy 1 mg/kg/day × 4 mo	Persistence of proteinuria despite prednisone therapy 60 mg/m × 4 wk*
Steroid-dependent—NS recurs when stop or decrease treatment	Two consecutive relapses occurring during therapy or within 14 days of completing steroid therapy	Two relapses of proteinuria within 14 days after stopping or during alternate day steroid therapy

Definition of terms used in idiopathic nephrotic syndrome in adults and children. The definitions were generated by a consensus of the International Society for Kidney Diseases in and the German Pediatric Nephrology Society.
*Or persistence of proteinuria despite prednisone therapy 60 mg m⁻² × 4 weeks and three methylprednisolone pulses.
From Floege J et al: *Comprehensive clinical nephrology,* ed 4, Philadelphia, 2010, Saunders.

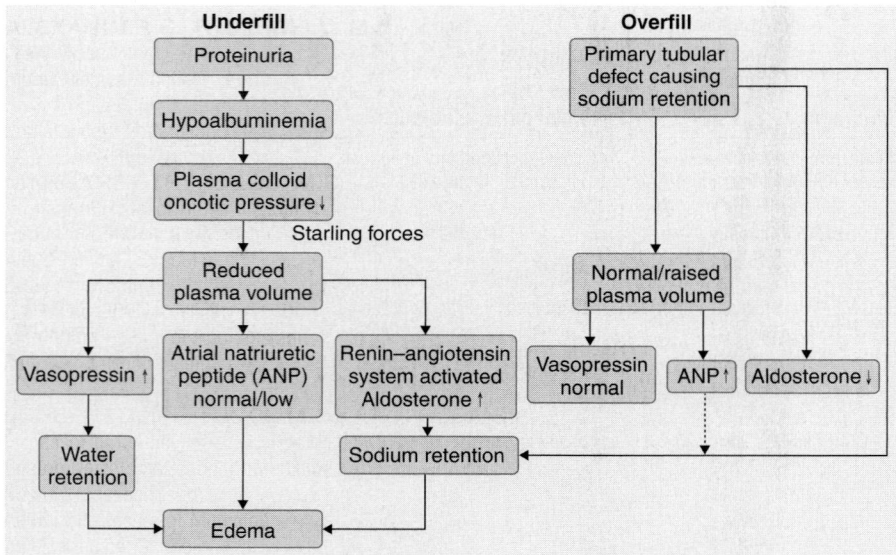

FIGURE 1-582 Mechanisms of nephrotic edema. The kidney is relatively resistant to ANP in this setting, so ANP has little effect in countering sodium retention. (From Floege J et al: *Comprehensive clinical nephrology,* ed 4, Philadelphia, 2010, Saunders.)

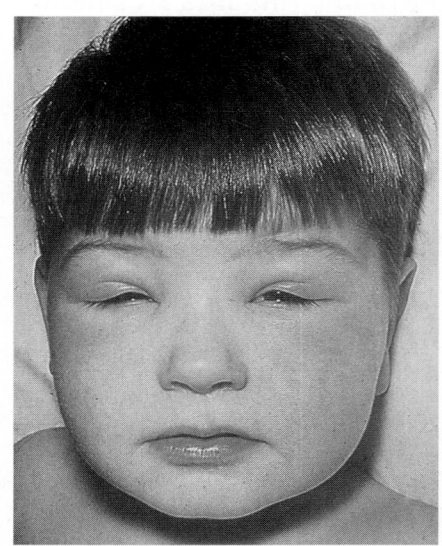

FIGURE 1-583 Nephrotic edema. Periorbital edema in the early morning in a nephrotic child. The edema resolves during the day under the influence of gravity. (From Floege J et al: *Comprehensive clinical nephrology,* ed 4, Philadelphia, 2010, Saunders.)

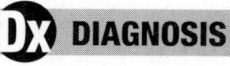

HLA-DQA$_1$ allele on chromosome 6p21 is most closely associated with idiopathic membranous nephropathy in persons of white ancestry. This allele may facilitate an autoimmune response against targets such as variants of PLA 2 R1.

- Associated with systemic diseases (diabetes mellitus, systemic lupus erythematosus [SLE], amyloidosis). Amyloidosis and dysproteinemias should be considered in patients >40 yr.
- Majority of children with nephrotic syndrome have minimal change disease (this form also

associated with allergy, nonsteroidals, and Hodgkin's disease).
- Focal glomerular disease: can be associated with HIV infection, heroin abuse. A more severe form of nephrotic syndrome associated with rapid progression to end-stage renal failure within months can also occur in HIV seropositive patients and is known as "collapsing glomerulopathy."
- Membranous nephropathy: can occur with Hodgkin's lymphoma, carcinomas, SLE, gold therapy

- Membranoproliferative glomerulonephropathy: often associated with upper respiratory infections

DX DIAGNOSIS

DIFFERENTIAL DIAGNOSIS

- Other edema states (CHF, cirrhosis)
- Primary renal disease (e.g., focal glomerulonephritis, membranoproliferative glomerulonephritis [MPGN]). The differentiation between nephrotic syndrome and nephritic syndrome is described in Table 1-299. Table 1-300 summarizes primary renal diseases that present as idiopathic nephrotic syndrome.
- Carcinoma, infections
- Malignant hypertension
- Polyarteritis nodosa
- Serum sickness
- Toxemia of pregnancy

WORKUP

Diagnostic workup consists of family history and history of drug use or toxin exposure and laboratory evaluation. Renal biopsy is generally performed in individuals with persistent proteinuria in whom the etiology of the proteinuria is unclear.

TABLE 1-299 Differentiation between Nephrotic Syndrome and Nephritic Syndrome

Typical Features	Nephrotic	Nephritic
Onset	Insidious	Abrupt
Edema	++++	++
Blood pressure	Normal	Raised
Jugular venous pressure	Normal/low	Raised
Proteinuria	++++	++
Hematuria	May/may not occur	+++
Red-cell casts	Absent	Present
Serum albumin	Low	Normal/slightly reduced

From Johnson RJ, Feehally J: *Comprehensive clinical nephrology,* ed 2, St Louis, 2000, Mosby.

TABLE 1-300 Summary of Primary Renal Diseases That Present as Idiopathic Nephrotic Syndrome

	Minimal-Change Nephropathy Syndrome	Focal Segmental Sclerosis	Membranous Nephrotic	MEMBRANOPROLIFERATIVE GLOMERULONEPHRITIS	
				Type I	Type II
Frequency*					
Children	75%	10%	<5%	10%	10%
Adults	15%	15%	50%	10%	10%
Clinical Manifestations					
Age (yr)	2-6	2-10	40-50	5-15	5-15
Sex	2:1 female	1.3:1 female	2:1 male	Male-female	Male-female
Nephrotic syndrome	100%	90%	80%	60%	60%
Asymptomatic proteinuria	0	10%	20%	40%	40%
Hematuria	10%-20%	60%-80%	60%	80%	80%
Hypertension	10%	20% early	Infrequent	35%	35%
Rate of progression to renal failure	Does not progress	10 years	50% in 10-20 yr	10-20 yr	5-15 yr
Associated conditions	Allergy? Hodgkin's disease, usually none	None			
Laboratory Findings	Manifestations of nephrotic syndrome	Manifestations of nephrotic syndrome	Renal vein thrombosis, cancer, SLE, hepatitis B	None	Partial lipodystrophy
	↑ BUN in 15%-30%	↑ BUN in 20%-40%	Manifestations of nephrotic syndrome	Low C1, C4, C3-C9	Normal C1, C4, low C3-C9
Immunogenetics	HLA-B8, B12 (3.5)[†]	Not established	HLA-DRW3 (12–32)[†]	Not established	C3 nephritic factor
Renal Pathology					Not established
Light microscopy	Normal	Focal	Thickened	Thickened	Lobulation
Immunofluorescence	Negative	IgM	Fine	Granular	C3 only
Electron microscopy	Foot process fusion	Foot	Subepithelial	Mesangial	Dense deposits
Response of Steroids	90%	15%-20%	May slow progression	Not established	Not established

*Approximate frequency as a cause of idiopathic nephrotic syndrome. About 10% of adult nephrotic syndrome is due to various diseases that usually present with acute glomerulonephritis.
[†]Relative risk.
↑, Elevated; *BUN,* blood urea nitrogen; *C,* complement; *GBM,* glomerular basement membrane; *hepatitis B,* hepatitis B virus; *HLA,* human leukocyte antigen; *Ig,* immunoglobulin; *SLE,* systemic lupus erythematosus.
Modified from Goldman L, Ausiello D (eds): *Cecil textbook of medicine,* ed 22, Philadelphia, 2004, Saunders.

LABORATORY TESTS

- Urinalysis reveals proteinuria. The presence of hematuria, cellular casts, and pyuria is suggestive of nephritic syndrome. Oval fat bodies (tubular epithelial cells with cholesterol esters) are also found in the urine in patients with nephrotic syndrome.
- 24-hr urine protein excretion is >3.5 g/1.73 m^3/24 hr.
- Abnormalities of blood chemistries include serum albumin <3 g/dl, decreased total protein, elevated serum cholesterol, glucose, azotemia.
- Additional tests in patients with nephrotic syndromes depending on the history and physical examination are ANA, serum and urine immunoelectrophoresis, C3, C4, CH-50, LDH, liver enzymes, alkaline phosphatase, hepatitis B and C screening, and HIV.

IMAGING STUDIES

- Ultrasound of kidneys
- Chest x-ray

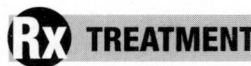 **TREATMENT**

NONPHARMACOLOGIC THERAPY

- Bed rest as tolerated, avoidance of nephrotoxic drugs, low-fat diet, fluid restriction in hyponatremic patients; normal protein intake unless urinary protein loss exceeds 10 g/24 hr (some patients may require additional dietary protein to prevent negative nitrogen balance and significant protein malnutrition)
- Improved urinary protein excretion and serum lipid changes have been observed with a low-fat soy protein diet providing 0.7 g of protein/kg/day. However, because of increased risk of malnutrition, many nephrologists recommend normal protein intake.
- Strict sodium restriction to help manage peripheral edema
- Close monitoring of patients for development of peripheral venous thrombosis and renal vein thrombosis because of hypercoagulable state secondary to loss of antithrombin III and other proteins involved in the clotting mechanism

ACUTE GENERAL Rx

- Furosemide is useful for severe edema (Fig. 1-584).
- Use of ACE inhibitors to reduce proteinuria is generally indicated even in normotensive patients.
- Anticoagulant therapy should be administered as long as patients have nephrotic proteinuria, an albumin level <20 g/L, or both.

The mainstay of therapy is treatment of the underlying disorder:

- Minimal change disease generally responds to prednisone 1 mg/kg/day. Relapses can occur when steroids are discontinued. In these individuals, cyclophosphamide and chlorambucil may be useful.
- Focal segmental glomerulosclerosis: children—empiric therapy with prednisone (60 mg/square meter of BSA) for 4-6 wk because 80% will have glucocorticoid-responsive minimal change disease. Adults receive RAS blockade (ACE inhibitors, ARBs) and dietary sodium restriction. Some genetic forms may respond to empiric therapy with calcineurin inhibitors.
- Membranous glomerulonephritis: prednisone 2 mg/kg/day may be useful in inducing remission. Cytotoxic agents can be added if there is poor response to prednisone.
- MPGN: most patients are treated with steroid therapy and antiplatelet drugs. Despite treatment, the majority of patients will progress to end-stage renal disease within 5 yr.

CHRONIC Rx

- Patients should be monitored for azotemia and should be aggressively treated for hypertension and hyperlipidemia. Furosemide is useful for severe edema. Anticoagulants may be necessary for thromboembolic events. Prophylactic anticoagulation should be considered in patients with membranous glomerulonephritis.
- Oral vitamin D is useful in the treatment of hypocalcemia (because of vitamin D loss).

REFERRAL

Nephrology consultation is recommended in all cases of nephrotic syndrome.

SUGGESTED READINGS

available at www.expertconsult.com

RELATED CONTENT

Nephrotic Syndrome (Patient Information)

AUTHOR: **FRED F. FERRI, M.D.**

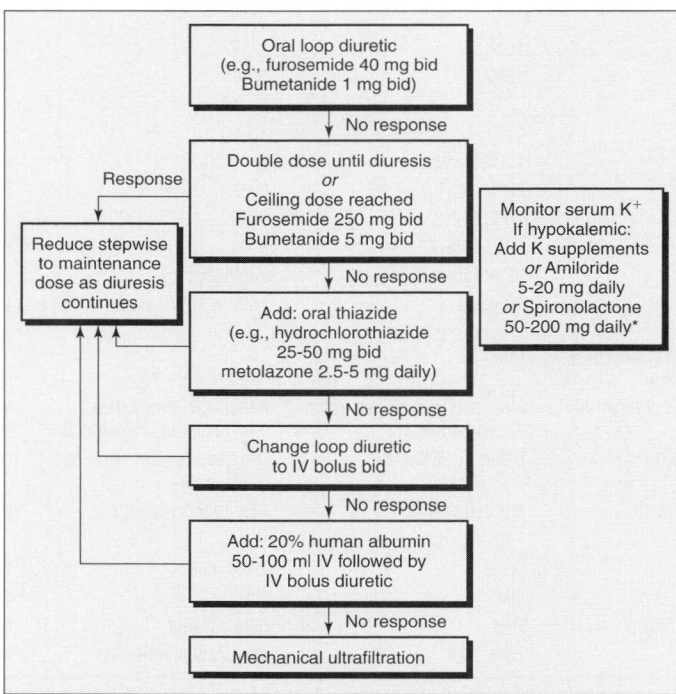

FIGURE 1-584 Management of edema in nephrotic syndrome. Edema is often diuretic resistant, but the response is not predictable. Therefore, stepwise escalation of therapy is appropriate until diuresis occurs. Even when there is anasarca, diuresis should not proceed faster than 2 kg/day in adults to minimize the risk of clinically significant hypovolemia. Mechanical ultrafiltration is rarely required for nephrotic edema unless there is associated renal insufficiency. *Spironolactone is less effective in nephrotic syndrome than in cirrhosis and is often poorly tolerated because of gastrointestinal side effects. Spironolactone should be used with great caution if the glomerular filtration rate is very low. (From Floege J et al: *Comprehensive clinical nephrology,* ed 4, Philadelphia, 2010, Saunders.)

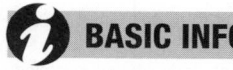

BASIC INFORMATION

DEFINITION

Neuroblastomas are tumors of postganglionic sympathetic neurons that typically originate in the adrenal medulla or the sympathetic chain/ganglion. Often present at birth, but not diagnosed until later, when the child shows symptoms of the disease. They are almost exclusively a disease of childhood.

ICD-9CM CODES
194.0 Neuroblastoma, unspecified site

EPIDEMIOLOGY & DEMOGRAPHICS

INCIDENCE (IN U.S.): 8%-10% of all solid tumors of childhood (third most common childhood cancer, after leukemia and brain tumors); 1/10,000 children <15 yr.
PREDOMINANT SEX: Male/female ratio of 1:1.3
PEAK AGE: Early childhood. Mean age of onset is 18 mo; 33% onset by 1 year; 75% onset by 5 year; 97% by 10 year. In rare cases, neuroblastoma can be discovered by fetal ultrasound.
GENETICS: Chromosomal deletions (loss of heterozygosity) found in nearly half of tumors, most commonly localized to chromosomes 1p, 11q, and 14q. Deletion of 1p36 (leading to amplification and overexpression of *N-MYC* protooncogene) associated with poor prognosis. There is a small subset with an autosomal dominant pattern of inheritance. Somatic recurrent mutations (ATRX gene) in tumors from patients with stage 4 neuroblastoma correlate with age at diagnosis and telomere length in children and young adults.

PHYSICAL FINDINGS & CLINICAL PRESENTATION

- Neuroblastomas can arise anywhere along the sympathetic nervous system. The most common primary site is the adrenal gland (40%), followed by a mass in the abdomen (25%), thorax (15%), neck (5%), and pelvis (5%). In approximately 1% of cases a primary site cannot be identified. Between 70% to 80% of children have regional lymph node involvement or distant metastases to bone marrow, cortical bone, orbits, liver, and skin at time of presentation.
- Spinal cord/paraspinal: can present with localized back pain, signs of compression—paraplegia, stool/urine retention, scoliosis
- Abdominal mass, pain, or constipation
- Horner's syndrome (ptosis, miosis, anhidrosis)
- Thoracic: difficulty breathing, dysphagia, infections, chronic cough
- Secondary symptoms referable to metastatic disease: fatigue, chronic pain (typically bony pain), pancytopenia, periorbital ecchymosis, proptosis, anorexia, weight loss, unexplained fever, multiple subcutaneous bluish nodules, irritability
- Paraneoplastic syndromes: opsoclonus-myoclonus syndrome (OMS) is described as "dancing eyes, dancing feet," which manifest as myoclonic jerks and chaotic eye movements

in all directions. This may be initial presentation before tumor diagnosis; present in 1% to 3% of patients with neuroblastoma; of all patients with opsoclonus-myoclonus, approximately 50% have an underlying neuroblastoma. Patients who present with this syndrome must be evaluated for neuroblastoma; when present, the neuroblastoma often has more favorable biologic features.
- Progressive cerebellar ataxia.
- Abnormal secretion of vasoactive intestinal peptide by the tumor, leading to distention of the abdomen and secretory diarrhea.

DIAGNOSIS

WORKUP
- Careful general physical examination to look for mass
- Biopsy and resection of tumor when possible

LABORATORY TESTS
- Complete blood count, coagulation studies, erythrocyte sedimentation rate.
- 24-hour urine for catecholamines: homovanillic acid (HVA) and vanillylmandelic acid (VMA) are secreted by up to 90% of tumors.
- Nonspecific serum markers such as neuron-specific enolase, lactate dehydrogenase, and ferritin.
- Bone marrow biopsy and aspirate: karyotype, DNA index, *N-MYC* copy number.
- Minimum criteria for diagnosis is based on one of the following: (1) unequivocal pathologic diagnosis made from tumor tissue or (2) combination of bone marrow aspirate with unequivocal tumor cells and increased levels of serum or urinary catecholamine metabolites, as described above.
- Genetic/biologic variables have been studied in children with neuroblastoma, in particular the histology, aneuploidy of tumor DNA, and amplification of the *N-MYC* oncogene within tumor tissue, because treatment decisions may be based on these factors.
  ○ Hyperdiploid DNA is associated with favorable prognosis, especially in infants.
  ○ *N-MYC* amplification is associated with poor prognosis, regardless of patient age, likely due to association with deletion of chromosome 1p and gain of chromosome 17q.
  ○ Other biologic factors studied include profile of GABAergic receptors, expression of neurotrophin receptors, level of telomerase RNA and serum ferritin and lactate dehydrogenase.

IMAGING STUDIES
- Chest x-ray, abdominal plain film, skeletal survey, abdominal and renal/bladder ultrasound
- CT scan or MRI of the chest and abdomen to provide information about regional lymph nodes, vessel invasion, and distant metastases (Fig. 1-585)
- Body scan with ^{131}I-MIBG (meta-iodobenzylguanidine), which is taken up by neuroblasts

and is sensitive to metastases in the bone and soft tissue
- Bone scan with Tc-99 MDP to visualize lytic bone lesions and metastases
- Urine catecholamines: elevated in 90% to 95% of patients with neuroblastomas
- STAGING (International Neuroblastoma Staging System)
  I.   Confined to single organ
  IIA. Localized tumor with incomplete gross resection; lymph nodes negative
  IIB. Localized tumor with incomplete gross resection; ipsilateral lymph nodes positive
  III. Extension across midline, with or without lymph node involvement
  IV.   Distant metastases to lymph nodes, bone, bone marrow, liver, skin
  IVs. Localized primary tumor with dissemination limited to skin, liver, or bone marrow; limited to infants

DIFFERENTIAL DIAGNOSIS
- Other small, round, blue-cell childhood tumors, such as lymphoma, rhabdomyosarcoma, soft tissue sarcoma, and primitive neuroectodermal tumors (PNETs)
- Wilms' tumor. Table 1-301 describes features distinguishing between Wilms' tumor and neuroblastoma.
- Hepatoblastoma

TREATMENT

- Assure patient and family that there is hope for recovery with aggressive treatment.

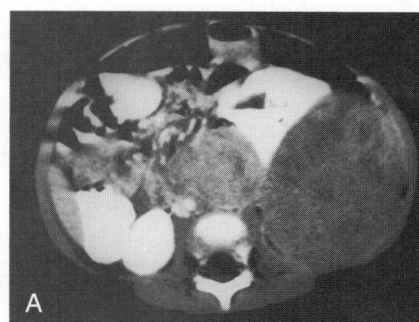

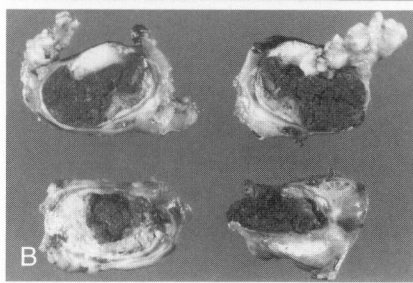

FIGURE 1-585 Computed tomographic scan **(A)** shows adrenal neuroblastoma at diagnosis. Serial sections through adrenal neuroblastoma **(B)** shows tumor with large areas of diffuse hemorrhage and calcification. (From Abeloff MD [ed]: *Clinical oncology,* ed 3, Philadelphia, 2004, Saunders.)

- Overall, treatment will be determined by several factors, including age at diagnosis, stage of disease, site of primary tumor and metastases, and tumor histology.
- Surgery: particularly for low-risk tumors.
- Radiation therapy may be tried for unresectable tumors or tumors that are not responsive to chemotherapy.
- Multiagent chemotherapy is mainstay of treatment (e.g., cisplatinum, etoposide, Adriamycin, cyclophosphamide, carboplatin).
- Autologous bone marrow transplantation following aggressive chemotherapy for stage IV disease or patients who are at highest risk based on presence of disseminated disease or unfavorable markers such as *N-MYC* amplification.
- Novel therapies include immunotherapy using monoclonal antibodies and vaccines that attempt to initiate an immune reaction against the disease and targeting of tumor cells with drugs that induce apoptosis or have antiangiogenic effect. Immunotherapy with ch14.18, a monoclonal antibody against the tumor-associated disialoganglioside GD2, has activity against neuroblastoma. Recent trials have shown that immunotherapy with ch14.18, GM-CSF, and interleukin-2 is associated with a significantly improved outcome as compared with standard therapy in patients with high-risk neuroblastoma.
- Adrenocorticotropic hormone (ACTH) treatment is thought to be effective for patients with opsoclonus/myoclonus syndrome.

DISPOSITION

- Overall survival is >40%. Children under the age of 1 yr have a cure rate as high as 90%.
- Approximately 70% of patients with neuroblastoma have metastases at diagnoses.
- Prognosis is related to age at time of diagnosis, clinical stage, and regional lymph node involvement. Children with localized disease and infants <1 year at diagnosis and favorable disease characteristics have better prognosis whereas poorer prognosis is noted in older children with stage IV disease (20% survival compared with >95% in stage I), age >1 year at diagnosis, increased number of *N-MYC* copies, adrenal tumor, and chronic 1p deletion.
- Children treated for neuroblastoma may be at risk for second malignancies, including renal cell carcinoma.

REFERRAL

Multidisciplinary oncology team with experience in treating cancers of childhood and adolescence.

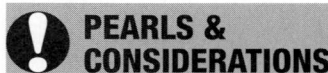

PEARLS & CONSIDERATIONS

- Neuroblastoma is predominantly a tumor of early childhood that originates in the sites where the sympathetic nervous system tissue is present.

- Symptoms occur due to tumor mass or bone pain from metastases.
- Children can present with classic paraneoplastic neurologic symptoms, including cerebellar ataxia and opsoclonus/myoclonus.
- Recent trials have shown a very high rate of survival among patients with intermediate-risk neuroblastoma with biologically based treatment assignment involving a substantially reduced duration of chemotherapy and reduced doses of chemotherapeutic agents as compared with regimens used in earlier trials. These data provide support for further reduction in chemotherapy with more refined risk stratifications.
- Despite recent advances, 50% to 60% of patients with high-risk neuroblastoma have a relapse and currently there are no salvage treatment regimens known to be curative.

SUGGESTED READINGS
available at www.expertconsult.com

RELATED CONTENT
Neuroblastoma (Patient Information)

AUTHOR: **NICOLE J. ULLRICH, M.D., PH.D.**

TABLE 1-301 Features Distinguishing Between Wilms' Tumor and Neuroblastoma

Feature	Wilms' Tumor	Neuroblastoma
Age	2-3 years	<2 years
Origin	Kidney	Retroperitoneal neural crest
Renal mass effect	Intrinsic mass effect	External compression
Laterality	10% bilateral	Almost always
Calcification	<15%	85%-95%
Vessel involvement	Renal vein invasion in 5%-10%	Frequent encasement

From Weissleder R et al: *Primer of diagnostic imaging,* ed 5, St Louis, 2011, Mosby.

BASIC INFORMATION

DEFINITION

Neurofibromatosis (NF) is an autosomal-dominant disorder affecting bone, the nervous system, soft tissue, and skin. There are three major subtypes of NF disorders: NF type 1 (NF1), NF type 2 (NF2), and schwannomatosis. Schwannomatosis has only recently been recognized as a distinct disorder; currently very little is known about it.

SYNONYMS

NF1: von Recklinghausen disease, peripheral NF
NF2: bilateral acoustic neurofibromatosis, central NF

ICD-9CM CODES
237.70 Neurofibromatosis, unspecified
237.71 Type 1, von Recklinghausen's
237.72 Type 2, acoustic

EPIDEMIOLOGY & DEMOGRAPHICS

- Incidence of NF1 (one case/3000 live births), NF2 (one case/25,000 live births).
- Prevalence of NF1 (one case/5000 persons), NF2 (one case/210,000 persons).
- NF1 and NF2 are autosomal dominant; approximately 50% of cases have no family history.
- The two disorders affect approximately 100,000 people in the U.S.
- Affects males and females equally.
- NF1 may be associated with optic gliomas, astrocytomas, spinal neurofibromas, pheochromocytomas, and chronic myeloid leukemia.
- NF2 may be associated with meningiomas, spinal schwannomas, and cataracts.
- For schwannomatosis, the incidence is one per 30,000 persons, and the disease is mostly sporadic in nature.

PHYSICAL FINDINGS & CLINICAL PRESENTATION

- Common features of NF1 include:
  1. Café-au-lait macules (100% of children by age 2 yr)
     a. Hyperpigmented skin lesions (Fig. E1-586) occurring anywhere on the body except the face, palms, and soles
     b. Appear early in life and increase in size and number during puberty
     c. Are focal or diffuse
  2. Axillary and inguinal freckling (70%)
  3. Multiple neurofibromas (Figs. 1-587 and 1-588) can be soft or firm; three subtypes:
     a. Cutaneous: circumscribed, not specific for NF1
     b. Subcutaneous: circumscribed, not specific for NF1
     c. Plexiform: noncircumscribed, thick and irregular; can cause disfigurement of supportive structures and specific for NF1

  4. Lisch nodule (small hamartoma of the iris) found in >90% of adult cases.
  5. Visual defects possibly related to optic gliomas (2% to 5%).
  6. Neurodevelopment problems such as learning disability and mental retardation (30% to 40%).
  7. Skeletal disorders, including long bone dysplasia, pseudoarthrosis, scoliosis, short stature, and decreased bone mineral density.
- Common features of NF2 include:
  1. Hearing loss and tinnitus related to bilateral acoustic neuromas (>90% of adults)
  2. Cataracts (81%)
  3. Headache
  4. Unsteady gait
  5. Cutaneous and subcutaneous neurofibromas but fewer than in NF1
  6. Café-au-lait macules (1%)
- Common features of schwannomatosis include painful multiple schwannomas of the spinal, peripheral, or cranial nerves *except* the vestibular nerve.

ETIOLOGY

- NF1 is caused by DNA mutations located on the long arm of chromosome 17 responsible for encoding the protein neurofibromin.
- NF2 is caused by DNA mutations located in the middle of the long arm of chromosome 22 responsible for encoding the protein merlin, which is a potent inhibitor of glioma growth.
- Both proteins are speculated to act as tumor suppressors.

- The etiology of schwannomatosis remains unclear; however, biallelic NF2 mutations are found in the schwannomas but nowhere else, suggesting that they are secondary mutations.

DIAGNOSIS

- NF1 is diagnosed if the person has two or more of the following features:
  1. Six or more café-au-lait macules >5 mm in prepubertal patients and >15 mm in postpubertal patients
  2. Two or more neurofibromas of any type or one plexiform neurofibroma
  3. Axillary or inguinal freckling
  4. Optic glioma
  5. Two or more Lisch nodules (iris hamartomas)
  6. Sphenoid wing dysplasia or cortical thinning of long bones, with or without pseudoarthrosis
  7. A first-degree relative (parent, sibling, or child) with NF1 based on the previous criteria
- NF2 is diagnosed if the person has either of the following two criteria:
  1. Bilateral eighth nerve masses seen by appropriate imaging studies (e.g., CT, MRI)
  2. A first-degree relative with NF2 and either a unilateral eighth nerve mass or two of the following: neurofibroma, meningioma, glioma, schwannoma, or juvenile posterior subcapsular lenticular opacity

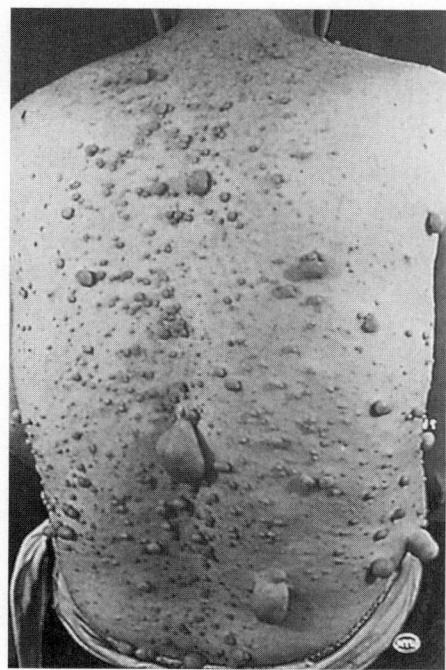

FIGURE 1-587 Nodules. Solid, large (>1 cm), deep-seated mass in dermal or subcutaneous tissues. These nodules are neurofibromas in a patient with neurofibromatosis. (From Goldman L, Ausiello D [eds]: *Cecil textbook of medicine,* ed 22, Philadelphia, 2004, Saunders.)

- Schwannomatosis is diagnosed in an individual >30 yr having either of the following two criteria:
  1. Two nonintradermal schwannomas, no vestibular tumor found on MRI scan, no NF2 mutation
  2. One nonvestibular schwannoma and a first-degree relative fitting the above criteria

DIFFERENTIAL DIAGNOSIS

- Abdominal NF
- Myxoid lipoma
- Nodular fasciitis
- Fibrous histiocytoma
- Segmental NF

WORKUP

The diagnosis of NF is usually self-evident. Workup is dictated by clinical symptoms in NF1 and usually includes MRI evaluation of the head and spine in NF2 and schwannomatosis. In fact, if NF2 is suspected but no vestibular nerve schwannomas are found, the diagnosis points to schwannomatosis.

LABORATORY TESTS

- Genetic testing is possible in individuals who desire prenatal diagnosis for NF1. There is no single standard test and multiple tests are required. Results can only tell if an individual is affected but cannot predict the severity of the disease due to variable expression.
- In NF2, linkage analysis testing provides a >99% certainty the individual has NF2.

IMAGING STUDIES

- MRI with gadolinium is the imaging study of choice in both NF1 and NF2 patients. MRI increases detection of optic gliomas, tumors of the spine, acoustic neuromas, and "bright spots" believed to represent hamartomas.
- MRI of the spine is recommended in all patients diagnosed with NF2 to exclude intramedullary tumors.

OTHER TESTS

- Wood lamp examination may be useful in patients with very pale skin for visualizing café-au-lait spots.
- Slit-lamp examination is recommended for children >6 yr to confirm the presence of Lisch nodules and subcapsular opacity.

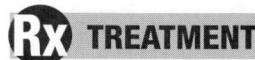

TREATMENT

Treatment is directed primarily at symptoms and complications of NF1 and NF2. As for schwannomatosis, resection should be reserved for tumors that are symptomatic or threaten to cause spinal cord compression.

NONPHARMACOLOGIC THERAPY

- Counseling addressing prognosis and genetic, psychological, and social issues
- Hearing testing and speech pathology evaluation

ACUTE GENERAL Rx

- Surgery is usually not done on skin tumors unless cosmetically requested or if suspicion of malignant transformation exists.
- Surgery may be indicated for spinal or cranial neurofibromas, gliomas, or meningiomas.
- Acoustic neuromas can be treated by surgical excision.

CHRONIC Rx

- Radiation may be indicated in optic nerve gliomas and patients whose central nervous system tumors show radiographic progression.
- Stereotactic radiosurgery with a gamma knife may be an alternative approach to surgery for acoustic neuromas.

DISPOSITION

- Prognosis varies according to the severity of involvement.
- There is no cure for NF.

REFERRAL

A multidisciplinary team of consultants is needed in patients with NF, including neurosurgeon, otolaryngologist, dermatologist, neurologist, audiologist, speech pathologist, geneticist, and neuropsychologist.

PEARLS & CONSIDERATIONS

- Friedrich Daniel von Recklinghausen first reported his cases in 1882, although there had been similar accounts dating back to the 1600s.
- The first report in the literature of NF2 was by Wishart in 1822.
- A high SPRED1 mutation detection rate has been identified in NF1 mutation-negative families with an autosomal dominant phenotype of CALMs with or without freckling and no other NF1 features.

COMMENTS

For additional information and patient resources, refer to the National Neurofibromatosis Foundation (www.nf.org) or Neurofibromatosis Inc. (www.nfinc.org).

SUGGESTED READINGS

available at www.expertconsult.com

RELATED CONTENT

Neurofibromatosis Type 1 (Patient Information)

AUTHORS: **MARK F. BRADY, M.D., M.P.H.,** and **WEN Y. WU-CHEN, M.D.**

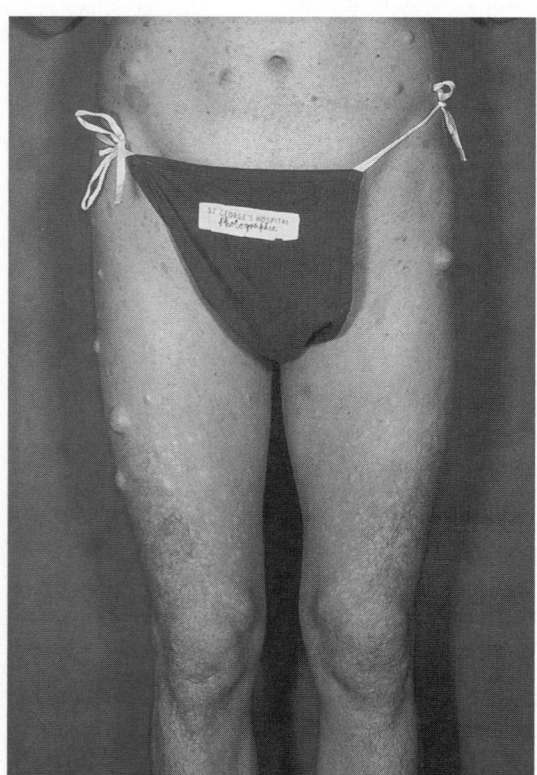

FIGURE 1-588 Type 1 neurofibromatosis: widespread cutaneous neurofibromata are a prominent feature of the classical variant. (Courtesy of R.A. Marsden, M.D., St George's Hospital, London. From McKee PH, Calonje E, Granter SR [eds]: *Pathology of the skin with clinical correlations,* ed 3, St Louis, 2005, Mosby.)

BASIC INFORMATION

DEFINITION

Neuroleptic malignant syndrome (NMS) is a disorder characterized by hyperthermia, muscular rigidity, autonomic dysfunction, and depressed/fluctuating levels of arousal that evolve over 24 to 72 hr. This occurs as an idiosyncratic adverse reaction most commonly to dopamine-receptor antagonists (especially the D2/4 receptor) or sudden withdrawal from a dopaminergic agent or agonist, such as antiparkinsonian medications.

SYNONYMS

None

ICD-9CM CODES
333.92 Neuroleptic malignant syndrome

EPIDEMIOLOGY & DEMOGRAPHICS

INCIDENCE (IN U.S.): 0.07% to 0.15% annual incidence in psychiatric population.
PREDOMINANT SEX: More than two thirds of patients are male.
PREDOMINANT AGE: Young and middle-aged adults
PREDISPOSING FACTORS:
- High-potency dopamine antagonists
- Long-acting depot preparations or multiple agents

PHYSICAL FINDINGS & CLINICAL PRESENTATION

- Syndrome typically begins abruptly while the patient is taking therapeutic (not toxic) dosages of neuroleptics and reaches maximum severity within 72 hr.
- Muscle rigidity (hypertonia, cogwheeling, or "lead pipe" rigidity)
- Hyperthermia (38.6° to 42.3° C, usually <40° C)
- Autonomic symptoms: diaphoresis, sialorrhea, skin pallor, urinary incontinence
- Tachycardia, tachypnea
- Labile blood pressure (hypertension or postural hypotension)
- Agitation, catatonia, fluctuating consciousness, obtundation

ETIOLOGY

- Unknown: Impaired thermoregulation in hypothalamus and limbic cortex may occur as a result of relative lack of dopamine activity (central dopamine-blockade hypothesis: most accepted).
- Neuroleptic drugs have different potencies for inducing NMS:
  1. Typical neuroleptics: high potency, haloperidol; medium potency, chlorpromazine, fluphenazine; low potency, levomepromazine, loxapine
  2. Atypical neuroleptics: low potency, risperidone, olanzapine, clozapine, quetiapine

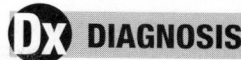

DIAGNOSIS

DIFFERENTIAL DIAGNOSIS

- Heatstroke, drug-induced states and overdose (Ecstasy abuse, phencyclidine), thyrotoxicosis, pheochromocytoma, serotonin syndrome
- Malignant hyperthermia, catatonia, acute psychosis with agitation
- CNS or systemic infections, including sepsis

WORKUP

Careful drug history

LABORATORY TESTS

- Elevated creatine phosphokinase (CPK) (sensitivity 0.71)
- Urinary myoglobin
- Leukocytosis, usually 10,000 to 40,000/mm^3
- Electrolytes and renal function
- Blood gases
- Drug levels

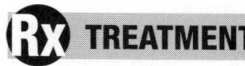

TREATMENT

NONPHARMACOLOGIC THERAPY

- Stop all neuroleptic drugs and reinstitute any recently discontinued dopaminergic agonists.
- Respiratory support; nutritional support in cases with dysphagia or comatose.
- Careful fluid balance monitoring with adequate hydration (intravenous in severe cases).
- Active cooling (cooling blanket and antipyretics).
- Skilled nursing care is necessary to prevent decubitus ulcers in bed-confined patients.

ACUTE GENERAL Rx

- Bromocriptine, a dopamine receptor agonist, is the mainstay of therapy for patients with NMS. Initial doses of 2.5 to 10 mg are given IV q8h and are increased by 5 mg/day until clinical improvement is seen. The drug should be continued for at least 10 days after the syndrome has been controlled and then tapered slowly.
- Dantrolene therapy can inhibit the excessive muscle contractions that generate myoglobinemia. Initially, patients can be given 0.25 mg/kg IV q6-12h, followed by a maintenance dose up to 3 mg/kg/day. After 2 to 3 days, patients may be given the drug orally (25 to 600 mg/day in divided doses). Oral dantrolene therapy (50 to 600 mg/day) may be continued for several days afterward.
- Amantadine, an NMDA receptor antagonist with possible dopaminergic properties, administered orally at doses of 100 to 200 mg PO bid, has also been shown to reduce mortality in comparison to supportive therapy alone.
- IV benzodiazepines (e.g., diazepam 2 to 10 mg, with total daily dose of 10 to 60 mg) to relax muscles and control agitation.
- Electroconvulsive therapy with neuromuscular blockage in pharmacologically refractory cases. Succinylcholine should not be used because it may cause hyperkalemia and cardiac arrhythmias in patients with rhabdomyolysis or dysautonomia.

CHRONIC Rx

- Respiratory care, nutritional support, and physical therapy may be required in more severe cases.
- Appropriate therapy would be required in patients with persistent neuropsychiatric sequelae of NMS (e.g., antidepressants for depression, cognitive behavioral therapy for cognitive deficits, rehabilitation for contractures).

DISPOSITION

- Mortality rate is currently 5% to 10% despite therapeutic measures. Serious sequelae may occur in a further 20%. Complete recovery occurs in >70% of patients. Causes of death include cardiac arrhythmias, myocardial infarction, renal failure secondary to rhabdomyolysis, seizures, pulmonary edema, and bronchopneumonia.
- Factors adversely affecting mortality are development of renal failure and core temperature >104° F (40° C).
- Late neuropsychiatric sequelae.
- Monitor closely for future complications of pharmacologic therapy.

REFERRAL

If the patient's condition is critical, it is preferable to treat the patient in a medical/neurologic ICU.

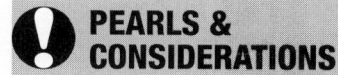

PEARLS & CONSIDERATIONS

COMMENTS

Early detection and diagnosis lead to a more favorable outcome. Refer to recent consensus diagnostic criteria as a guide. Treatment is a medical emergency.

SUGGESTED READINGS
available at www.expertconsult.com

AUTHOR: **EROBOGHENE E. UBOGU, M.D.**

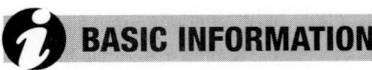

BASIC INFORMATION

DEFINITION

Neuropathic pain is not itself a disease, but rather a symptom that is associated with multiple different diseases. Thus it is not enough to define its presence without searching for a cause. It is defined as the sensation derived from the abnormal discharges of impaired or injured neural structures in either the peripheral or central nervous system. Descriptors include:

- Hyperesthesia: heightened sensitivity to non-painful stimuli (e.g., light touch)
- Hyperalgesia: heightened sensitivity to painful stimuli (e.g., pinprick), or reduced threshold to feel pain
- Allodynia: pain provoked by a stimulus that is not normally painful

SYNONYMS

Neuralgia

ICD-9CM CODES

782.0 Numbness, paresthesias
729.1 Myositis/myalgia, not otherwise specified
729.2 Neuralgia, neuritis, or radiculitis, not otherwise specified

EPIDEMIOLOGY & DEMOGRAPHICS

- Estimates of the prevalence of neuropathic pain in the general population range from 1.6% to 8.2%.
- Demographics vary widely depending on etiology, for example:
  - Postherpetic neuralgia: affects elderly, pain seen in almost 100% of cases
  - AIDS: 30% of patients affected
  - Diabetes mellitus: 20% to 24% affected (prevalence rates vary, increasing with longer disease duration)
  - Fabry disease: affects mostly children, pain in 81% to 90% of patients

PHYSICAL FINDINGS & CLINICAL PRESENATION

- History: localize the disease with questions
  - Quality (description) of neuropathic pain: burning, hot or cold, "icy hot," "pins and needles," stinging, lancinating, sharp, shooting
  - Distribution of symptoms may aid in localization (i.e., "stocking-glove" symptoms in generalized neuropathy, numbness in a peripheral nerve territory in focal neuropathy)
  - Generalized small fiber neuropathy: dysesthesias without numbness common, but many etiologies (e.g., diabetes) cause both small and large fiber dysfunction
  - Large fiber neuropathy (LFPN): coexisting numbness, hyporeflexia, or weakness may be seen, usually worse distally
  - Nerve root: coexisting neck or low back pain that radiates along a specific dermatome; most common cause is structural compression
  - Spinal cord symptoms: coexisting spasticity, bowel or bladder involvement, sensory level
  - Prior history of thalamic stroke in central thalamic pain syndrome (Dejerine-Roussy syndrome)
  - Family history may suggest a genetic cause
- Examination: see Fig. 1-589 and Table 1-302. Table 1-303 describes joint involvement in neuropathic arthropathy. Fig. E1-590 illustrates a diagnostic approach to neuropathic pain.

ETIOLOGY & LABORATORY EVALUATION (Table 1-304)

- Metabolic: diabetes mellitus; malnutrition and alcoholism; vitamin B_{12} deficiency; thiamine deficiency; porphyria; Fabry's disease
- Inflammatory: immune vasculitides (lupus, Sjögren's syndrome, polyarteritis nodosa, etc.), acute inflammatory demyelinating polyneuropathy (classically presents with ascending weakness and numbness, although pain is also a common feature), chronic inflammatory demyelinating polyneuropathy, sarcoid, multiple sclerosis
- Infiltrative: amyloidosis, paraproteinemias (e.g., monoclonal gammopathy of uncertain significance [MGUS])
- Infectious: postviral (brachial neuritis), HIV/AIDS, HSV, varicella-zoster virus (VZV; postherpetic neuralgia), Lyme disease, leprosy (thickened nerves and skin lesions), syphilis
- Neoplastic and paraneoplastic-carcinomatous infiltration of nerve/nerve root, anti-Hu
- Drugs/toxins: history of exposure to alcohol, chemotherapeutic agents (paclitaxel, vincristine), isoniazid, metronidazole, or heavy metals (thallium, arsenic)

DIAGNOSIS

LABORATORY TESTS

- Fasting blood glucose (FBG)
- 2-hour oral glucose tolerance test (OGTT)
- Vitamin B_1 level
- If B_{12} level normal: serum methylmalonic acid and homocysteine levels
- Serum erythrocyte sedimentation rate (ESR), ANA, SS-A and SS-B, c-ANCA, p-ANCA
- RPR or FTA-ABS
- Serum ACE level (sarcoid)
- HIV antibody
- SPEP, UPEP, immunofixation
- Urine and stool protoporphyrins, if porphyria is suspected clinically
- Hu antibody: can be seen in both small cell and non–small cell lung cancers, may be positive without evidence of lung cancer
- Lumbar puncture: protein elevation, oligoclonal bands, CSF/serum IgG index, herpes simplex virus (HSV), VZV, Lyme polymerase chain reaction (PCR), VDRL

ELECTROPHYSIOLOGY STUDIES

- Electrophysiologic testing (electromyography with nerve conduction studies): may be normal in small fiber neuropathies or CNS lesion, but is often abnormal in large fiber neuropathies
- Quantitative sensory testing: abnormal in small and large fiber neuropathy
- Evoked potentials (only if suspicion for spinal cord lesion)

PATHOLOGY STUDIES

- Nerve biopsy is occasionally useful in selected cases, particularly when vasculitis, sarcoid, or amyloid neuropathy are in the differential.
- Skin biopsy for intraepidermal nerve fiber (IENF) density may be useful for small fiber neuropathy when other studies are normal.
- Rectal or abdominal fat pad biopsy may show amyloid deposition in systemic amyloidosis.

IMAGING STUDIES

- MRI (with and without contrast):
  - Of the brain to exclude thalamic pathology if symptoms and signs are consistent with thalamic lesion
  - Of the spinal cord and nerve roots to exclude structural, inflammatory, neoplastic, or infectious causes
  - Of the lumbar spine to evaluate for arachnoiditis
- If MRI cannot be performed, consider:
  - CT of the brain for thalamic pathology
  - CT myelography of the spinal cord to evaluate for structural/neoplastic disease, but only if clinical signs of spinal or nerve root compromise are present

TREATMENT

NONPHARMACOLOGIC THERAPY

- Counseling should be initiated at the beginning of therapy to address psychologic issues exacerbating physiologic pain

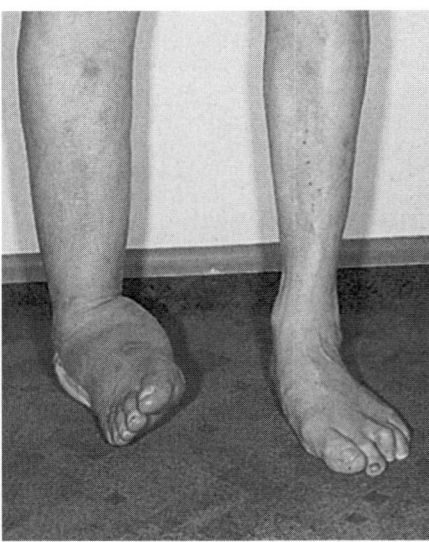

FIGURE 1-589 Neuropathic ankle. Marked instability of the subtalar and midtarsal joints is seen with collapse on weight bearing. (From Hochberg MC et al: *Rheumatology,* ed 5, St Louis, 2011, Mosby.)

- Physical therapy: especially in cases of chronic neck and low back pain

ACUTE GENERAL Rx

- Antidepressants:
  - Tricyclic antidepressants (TCAs): nortriptyline preferred over amitriptyline (fewer anticholinergic side effects with nortriptyline). Begin 25 mg PO qd in adults, or 10 mg qd in elderly. Increase dose by 25 mg every week as tolerated until usual maximal effective dose of 150 mg/day.
  - Paroxetine: begin 10 mg PO qd, increase by 10 mg/wk to a max dose of 60 mg qd.
  - Duloxetine: begin 30 mg daily, increase to 60 to 120 mg daily. Duloxetine is effective in diabetic neuropathy, post-herpetic neuropathy, and chemotherapy-induced painful peripheral neuropathy.
- Antiepileptics:
  - Gabapentin: begin 300 mg PO qd, advance to 300 mg PO tid by the end of the first week. Effective dose: higher than 1600 mg/day. Max dose: 1500 mg PO tid.
  - Carbamazepine: for trigeminal neuralgia. Begin 400 mg PO bid, increase to tid if necessary. Side effects and drug levels help to determine optimal dosing. Risk of aplastic anemia and hyponatremia (monitor CBC and chemistries).
  - Oxcarbazepine: better tolerated than carbamazepine. Start 150 mg PO bid and gradually increase to a maximal dose of 600 mg bid.
  - Lamotrigine: begin 25 mg PO bid, increase slowly (by 100 mg biweekly) until maximum effective dose of 200 to 300 mg PO bid. Risk: Stevens-Johnson syndrome.
  - Pregabalin: begin 50 mg PO tid, increase slowly to 100 to 200 mg PO tid.
- Analgesics:
  - Tramadol: 150 mg/day (50 mg tid), increase by 50 mg/wk, max 200 to 400 mg/day.
  - Morphine (oral): 15 to 30 mg q8h, max 90 to 360 mg/day.
  - Oxycodone: 20 mg q12h, increase by 10 mg/wk, max 40 to 160 mg/day.
  - Fentanyl patch: 25 to 100 mcg transdermally q3 days.
- Topical anesthetics:
  - 5% lidocaine patch, apply to area of pain, max three patches every 12 hr.
  - Capsaicin is inconsistent in its ability to relieve pain and may exacerbate it. Use not recommended.
- Procedural/surgical: this option is considered mostly when the patient suffers from pain secondary to spinal cord or cauda equina injury. Studies are limited and benefit is not completely established. Procedures should be considered only when all other therapeutic modalities have failed. In addition, the patient should be cautioned that surgical procedures may not result in pain relief and may be associated with significant morbidity and even mortality.
  - Dorsal root rhizotomy
  - Nerve blocks
  - Spinal cord stimulator

DISPOSITION

Prognosis depends on multiple factors, including:
- Etiology of pain
- Treatment of any underlying condition
- Initiation of appropriate (often multiple) therapeutic modalities
- Patient compliance with prescribed regimen
Most care is accomplished in the outpatient setting, except when surgery is required.

REFERRAL

- Pain clinic
- Neurology
- Psychiatry
- Psychology
- Physiatry
- Anesthesiology (nerve blocks)
- Neurosurgery if considering surgical management

TABLE 1-302 Examination

Exam Finding	Localization
Pinprick/temperature loss alone	Small fibers only
Pinprick/temperature loss + vibratory/proprioceptive loss	Small and large fibers
Sensory loss and motor dysfunction worse distally than proximal	Large fiber neuropathy
Sensory loss and motor dysfunction along single nerve distribution	Single nerve
Sensory loss and motor dysfunction along multiple single nerves	Multiple mononeuropathies (i.e., mononeuropathy multiplex)
Motor and sensory loss involving multiple nerves belonging to specific region of brachial or lumbar plexus	Plexopathy
Sensory loss along dermatome with multiple myotomal muscles affected	Nerve root lesion
Asymmetric sensory loss without weakness and pseudoathetosis	Dorsal root ganglion
Vibratory/proprioceptive loss without pinprick/temperature loss	Dorsal column dysfunction (from compressive lesion, B_{12} deficiency, or tabes dorsalis from neurosyphilis)
Sensory level with weakness below the level of lesion and long tract signs (spasticity/Babinski's sign)	Spinal cord lesion
Hemisensory hyperalgesia	Contralateral thalamus

TABLE 1-303 Joint Involvement in Neuropathic Arthropathy

Disease	Site of Involvement
Diabetes mellitus	Midtarsal, metatarsophalangeal, tarsometatarsal
Syringomyelia	Shoulder, elbow, wrist
Amyloidosis	Knee, ankle
Congenital sensory neuropathy	Knee, ankle, intertarsal, metatarsophalangeal
Tabes dorsalis	Knee, hip, ankle
Leprosy	Tarsal, tarsometatarsal

From Hochberg MC et al: *Rheumatology,* ed 5, St Louis, 2011, Mosby.

(!) PEARLS & CONSIDERATIONS

- Factitious disorder and malingering frequently manifest with pain complaints. These are diagnoses of exclusion, and require negative evaluation for organic etiologies before diagnosis is made.
- Peripheral neuropathy in diabetics increases the risk of foot ulceration by sevenfold. Abnormal results in monofilament testing and vibratory perception (alone or in combination with the appearance of the feet, ulceration, and ankle reflexes) are the most helpful sign for the detection of LFPN.

TABLE 1-304 Clinical Presentation and Laboratory Findings

Neuropathy Type	Predisposition	Examination Findings	EMG/NCS	Laboratory Analysis
Idiopathic small fiber PN	Age >50	Strength: normal Reflexes: normal Pos/Vib: normal Pain/Temp: decreased distally	Normal	Serum studies: normal Skin biopsy: abnormal Sudomotor studies: abnormal
Diabetic PN	Longstanding disease Family history	Strength normal to reduced, sensation reduced distally	Abnormal	Abnormal glucose tolerance High fasting glucose
Inherited PN	Family history	Pes cavus, hammer toes, reduced reflexes, sensation reduced distally	Abnormal	Genetic studies may be abnormal, other studies normal
Familial amyloid PN	Family history	Pain/temp loss Reduced reflexes Orthostasis	Abnormal if large fibers affected; also carpal tunnel syndrome	Transthyretin genetic study
Acquired amyloid PN	Monoclonal gammopathy	Pain/temp loss Reduced reflexes Orthostasis	Abnormal if large fibers affected; also carpal tunnel syndrome	SPEP, UPEP, immunofixation abnormal
Fabry's disease	Age Renal failure Strokes	Normal; possible reduced pain/temp sensation	Normal	α-Galactosidase levels in cultured fibroblasts
PN + mixed connective tissue disease	History of lupus, rheumatoid arthritis, Sjögren's syndrome	Reduced reflexes and distal sensation	Abnormal	ANA, RF, SS-A/SS-B may be abnormal
Peripheral nerve vasculitis	Asymmetric disease	Multiple peripheral nerves involved	Abnormal	ANA, RF, SS-A/SS-B, ANCA, cryoglobulins may be abnormal
Paraneoplastic neuropathy	Lung cancer risk factors, chemical exposures	Asymmetric sensory loss, pseudoathetosis, relatively preserved strength	Abnormal	Anti-Hu
Sarcoidosis	Pulmonary sarcoid	Multiple mononeuropathies	Abnormal	Abnormal biopsy, elevated serum ACE, CXR abnormal
Arsenic	Pesticides, copper smelting	Reduced reflexes and distal sensation	Abnormal	Elevated arsenic in plasma, urine, and hair
HIV	Promiscuity, unprotected sex, IV drug abuse, blood transfusion	Variable, but most often reduced reflexes and distal sensation	Abnormal if large fibers involved	HIV antibody

ACE, Angiotensin-converting enzyme; *ANA,* antibody to nuclear antigens; *ANCA,* antineutrophil cytoplasmic antibodies; *CXR,* chest x-ray; *EMG,* electromyography; *HbA1C,* glycosylated hemoglobin; *HIV,* human immunodeficiency virus; *IV,* intravenous; *NCS,* nerve conduction studies; *PN,* polyneuropathy; *Pos,* position sensation; *RF,* rheumatoid factor; *SPEP,* serum protein electrophoresis; *SS-A,* Sjögren syndrome A; *SS-B,* Sjögren syndrome B; *Temp,* temperature sensation; *UPEP,* urine protein electrophoresis; *Vib,* vibration sensation.
Adapted from Mendell JR, Sahenk Z: Painful sensory neuropathy, *N Engl J Med* 348(13):1243, 2003.

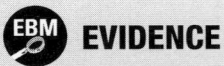 **EVIDENCE**

available at www.expertconsult.com

SUGGESTED READINGS
available at www.expertconsult.com

AUTHOR: **GAVIN BROWN, M.D.**

BASIC INFORMATION

DEFINITION

Any disorder affecting the peripheral nervous system, including nerve roots, plexuses, and individual peripheral nerves, that has a genetic basis of inheritance and has been or is capable of being transmitted along generations.

There are many different types of hereditary peripheral neuropathies, including Dejerine-Sottas disease, inherited metabolic neuropathies, hereditary sensory and autonomic neuropathies (HSANs), and hereditary motor neuropathies. Most disorders are diagnosed in infancy or childhood; as such, adult clinicians rarely see these patients. For this reason, this chapter discusses only the hereditary motor and sensory neuropathies that an adult clinician might encounter.

SYNONYMS

Charcot-Marie-Tooth (CMT) disease, a.k.a. hereditary motor-sensory neuropathy (HMSN)
Hereditary neuropathy with liability to pressure-sensitive palsies (HNPP)

ICD-9CM CODES
CMT: 356.1
HNPP: 689

EPIDEMIOLOGY & DEMOGRAPHICS

All CMT: approximately 30 per 100,000
- CMT type 1 (demyelinating pathophysiology): 1 in 2500
- CMT type 2 (axonal pathophysiology): 7 in 1000
- CMT type 4 and CMT-X: rare (either axonal or demyelinating pathophysiology)
HNPP: 2 to 5 per 100,000

PHYSICAL FINDINGS & CLINICAL PRESENTATION

CMT: Highly variable
- Age at onset earlier for CMT-1 than CMT-2, but both may present from childhood to old age.
- Severely affected patients have severe distal weakness and muscle atrophy with hand (prominently affecting interossei) and foot deformities (pes cavus, high arched feet, hammer toes).
- Mildly affected patients may have only foot deformity (pes cavus) with little or no weakness/sensory loss.
- Legs can be affected greater than arms, and patients will complain of gait abnormalities (steppage), which cause them to trip and fall.
- Sensory complaints (paresthesias, numbness, dysesthesia) are uncommon despite physical findings of impaired sensation.
- Decreased or absent reflexes.
- Some patients may have postural tremor of the upper limbs.

HNPP (a.k.a. tomaculous neuropathy):
- Age at onset is commonly adolescence.
- Disorder is characterized by recurrent entrapment of peripheral nerves with accompanying signs and symptoms (paresthesias and/or weakness in anatomic distributions). Most common are:
  1. Median nerve at the wrist (carpal tunnel syndrome)
  2. Ulnar nerve at the elbow (cubital tunnel syndrome)
  3. Painless brachial plexopathies
  4. Lateral femoral cutaneous nerve (meralgia paresthetica)
  5. Peroneal nerve at the fibular head
- May be associated with a generalized polyneuropathy.

ETIOLOGY

CMT: more than 30 subgroups have been identified and have various chromosomal abnormalities.
- Most common mutation is PMP-22 duplication, giving rise to CMT 1A demyelinating phenotype.
- Other mutations include P0 (demyelinating) and neurofilament light chain mutations (demyelinating or axonal phenotype)—see the following.
- Updated information may be available at http://www.neuro.wustl.edu/neuromuscular.
HNPP: deletion of chromosome 17p11.2–12.

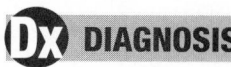

DIAGNOSIS

DIFFERENTIAL DIAGNOSIS

CMT: other genetic, metabolic, and multisystem disorders including:
- Spinocerebellar ataxias
- Friedreich's ataxia
- Leukodystrophies
- Refsum's disease (elevated serum phytanic acid)
- Distal spinal muscular atrophies and distal myopathies, which can present with pes cavus and other foot deformities
- Chronic inflammatory demyelinating polyneuropathy (CIDP)
HNPP:
- Hereditary neuralgic amyotrophy (HNA), which typically is painful rather than painless. In addition, in HNA, there is no evidence of generalized polyneuropathy.
- Multifocal motor neuropathy with conduction block (MMNCB)—autoimmune-mediated pure motor neuropathy
- Neuropathy associated with renal failure
- Lead neuropathy
- Neuropathy relating to paraproteinemia (demyelinating pathophysiology)

EVALUATION

CMT
- History of gradual onset symptoms is important to distinguish CMT from other forms of neuropathy.

- Detailed family history with *pedigree* is essential. Consider examination of multiple family members.
- History should evaluate for potential heavy metal exposure.
- History of dysesthesias is uncommon and should prompt search for acquired neuropathy or other inherited neuropathies (e.g., Fabry's disease).
HNPP: genetic testing after identification of multiple entrapment neuropathies on EMG and nerve conduction studies

LABORATORY TESTS

- Neurophysiology: electromyography (EMG) and nerve conduction studies (NCSs) must be done first to determine type of pathophysiology: demyelinating or axonal. This will guide genetic testing.
- NCSs in CMT-1 will reveal demyelinating physiology characterized by very slow conduction velocities (around 15 to 30 m/s) with prolonged distal latencies. Inherited demyelinating disorders can be distinguished from acquired demyelinating disorders (e.g., chronic inflammatory demyelinating polyneuropathy or CIDP) by the presence of conduction block in the latter.
- In HNPP, diffusely prolonged distal latencies with superimposed entrapment neuropathies at common sites will be seen on NCSs.
- EMG will reveal reinnervation characterized by long-duration, large-amplitude, polyphasic motor unit potentials (MUPs) with decreased MUP recruitment.
- Genetic tests are available for some CMT subtypes:
  1. CMT-1A: chromosome 17p11-PMP-22 duplication
  2. CMT-1B: chromosome 1q22-P0 mutation
  3. CMT-2E: chromosome 8p21-neurofilament light chain (NF-L) point mutation
  4. CMT-X: connexin 32 mutations
  5. HNPP: chromosome 17p11 deletion, which includes the PMP-22 gene
- Serum and 24-hour urine levels of heavy metals (arsenic, lead, etc.)
- SPEP, UPEP, immunofixation (for paraprotein).
- Anti-GM1 antibody (positive in ~50% of patients with MMNCB).
- Lumbar puncture may reveal elevated CSF protein in CIDP.
- Peripheral nerve biopsy:
  1. Demyelination with "onion bulb formation." Tomaculae, or focal thickening of myelin sheaths, seen in HNPP
  2. Generally not indicated unless diagnosis is uncertain

IMAGING STUDIES

- Spine plain films: for evaluation of scoliosis.
- MRI: indicated if dissociative sensory loss (dorsal column dysfunction with intact spinothalamic tract function) or if upper motor neuron findings (spasticity, Babinski's sign, clonus, increased tendon reflexes) are present.

- Exclusion of involvement of brain or spinal cord compressive lesions causing arm or leg weakness.
- Some inherited peripheral demyelinating disorders (i.e., CMT-X) are associated with intracerebral white matter abnormalities on MRI.
- Exclusion of structural, infectious, or inflammatory nerve root pathology.

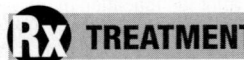 **TREATMENT**

There is no known cure for any of these disorders. Management is supportive.

NONPHARMACOLOGIC THERAPY

- Physical therapy (PT) and occupational therapy (OT) to provide assistance with gait and coordination.
- PT and OT might provide walking aid such as ankle foot orthosis (AFO), cane, walker, or wheelchair depending on the severity of the neuropathy.
- Wrist splints for superimposed carpal tunnel syndrome.
- Elbow pads (Heelbo Pads) to cushion the ulnar nerve at the elbow.
- Heel-cord strengthening.
- Stretching exercises.
- Analgesics for pain associated with foot deformity.
- Surgical correction of foot deformities by orthopedic surgeons if indicated.

Vincristine may worsen existing neuropathy (important for oncologist to know if patient develops cancer requiring chemotherapy).

SURGICAL TREATMENT

- Patients with HNPP should probably not undergo surgical decompression of the median nerve at the wrist or the ulnar nerve at the elbow; these nerves are sensitive to manipulation. Poor results have been reported with ulnar nerve transposition.
- Anesthesiologists should be aware of HNPP diagnosis in patients undergoing surgery to prevent compression neuropathies from occurring during surgical procedures.

GENETIC COUNSELING

Must be routinely done for patient and family when diagnosis is established. Many aspects of the patient and family's life are affected, including:

- Future progeny of patient and/or patient's parents or children
- Psychosocial aspects including social functioning, marriage, employment
- Financial needs
- Medical and life insurability

PROGNOSIS

- CMT: slowly progressive, and patients often remain ambulatory until late in life. Life expectancy is normal. Patients with respiratory involvement (i.e., phrenic nerve involvement with diaphragm paresis) may have shorter life expectancy.
- HNPP: benign prognosis.

DISPOSITION

Outpatient care. Routine follow-up appointments should be done initially every 6 mo, and then every 1 to 2 yr.

REFERRAL

- Neurology and/or neuromuscular disease specialist
- Podiatry for recurrent foot problems, including appropriate arches

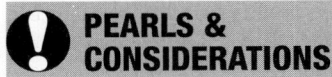 **PEARLS & CONSIDERATIONS**

PATIENT & FAMILY EDUCATION

Patients can benefit from use of Muscular Dystrophy Association (MDA) resources.

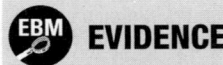 **EVIDENCE**

available at www.expertconsult.com

SUGGESTED READINGS

available at www.expertconsult.com

RELATED CONTENT

Fig. E1-590 Neuropathic pain, diagnostic approach (Algorithm)

Charcot-Marie-Tooth Disease (Related Key Topic)

AUTHOR: **GAVIN BROWN, M.D.**

BASIC INFORMATION

DEFINITION

Nocardiosis is an infection caused by aerobic actinomycetes found in soil and characterized by lung, soft tissue, or central nervous system (CNS) involvement.

SYNONYMS

Mycetoma
Nocardia

ICD-9CM CODES
039 Actinomycotic infections
039.9 Nocardiosis NOS, of unspecified site

EPIDEMIOLOGY & DEMOGRAPHICS

- *Nocardia* species are found worldwide in the soil.
- Nocardiosis is found most commonly in patients who are immunocompromised (e.g., those receiving steroids or immunosuppressive therapy; those with lymphoma, leukemia, or lung cancer; transplant recipients; and those with pulmonary infections).
- Other underlying conditions associated with nocardiosis are pemphigus vulgaris, Whipple's disease, Goodpasture's syndrome, Cushing's disease, cirrhosis, ulcerative colitis, and rheumatoid arthritis.
- Use of steroids is an independent risk factor for developing nocardiosis.
- Between 500 and 1000 new cases are diagnosed each year in the U.S.
- Approximately 2% of patients with AIDS develop nocardiosis.
- Occurs more commonly in men than in women (2:1).
- Adults are affected more often than children.

PHYSICAL FINDINGS & CLINICAL PRESENTATION

- Inhalation of *Nocardia* organisms is the most common mode of entry, and pneumonia is the most common presentation, with 75% manifesting with fever, chills, dyspnea, and a productive cough (Fig. 1-591).
  1. Presentation can be acute, subacute, or chronic.
  2. Nocardiosis should be suspected if soft tissue abscesses or CNS tumors or abscesses form in conjunction with the pulmonary infection.
  3. Pulmonary infection may spread into the pericardium, mediastinum, and superior vena cava.
- Cutaneous disease usually occurs by direct inoculation of the organism as a result of skin puncture by a thorn or splinter, surgery, IV catheter use, or animal scratches or bites manifesting in:
  1. Cellulitis
  2. Lymphocutaneous nodules appearing along lymphatic sites draining the infected puncture wound
  3. Mycetoma (Madura foot), a chronic deep nodular infection usually involving the hands or feet that can cause skin breakdown or fistula formation and that spreads along the fascial planes to infect surrounding skin, subcutaneous tissue, and bone

- The CNS is infected in approximately one third of all cases. Brain abscess is the most common pathologic finding.
- Dissemination of nocardiosis may infect other tissues and organs, including the kidney, heart, skin, and bone.

ETIOLOGY

- The most common *Nocardia* species leading to infection in human beings are:
  1. *N. asteroides* (causing more than 80% of the cases of pulmonary nocardiosis)
  2. *N. brasiliensis* (most common cause of mycetoma)
  3. *N. otitidiscaviarum*
- *N. asteroides* has two subgroups:
  1. *N. farcinica*
  2. *N. nova*

DIAGNOSIS

The diagnosis of nocardiosis requires a high index of suspicion in the proper clinical setting and is confirmed by bacteriologic staining and growth of the organism in culture.

DIFFERENTIAL DIAGNOSIS

There are no pathognomonic findings separating nocardiosis pneumonia from other infectious etiologies of the lung. Diagnoses presenting in a similar manner and often confused for nocardiosis include:
1. Tuberculosis
2. Lung abscess
3. Lung tumor
4. Other causes of pneumonia
5. Actinomycosis
6. Mycosis
7. Cellulitis
8. Coccidioidomycosis
9. Histoplasmosis
10. Aspergillosis
11. Kaposi's sarcoma

WORKUP

All patients with suspected nocardiosis need laboratory identification of the microorganism by obtaining sputum in the case of pneumonia, cultures of the infected skin lesions in mycetoma or lymphocutaneous disease, or the sampling of any purulent material (e.g., brain abscess, lung abscess, or pleural effusion).

LABORATORY TESTS

- Blood tests are not very sensitive in the diagnosis of nocardiosis.
- Gram stain shows gram-positive beaded filaments with multiple branches (Fig. 1-592).
- Gomori methenamine silver staining may detect the organism.
- *Nocardia* species are acid-fast on a modified Ziehl-Neelsen stain.
- *Nocardia* are slow-growing organisms; colony growth in cultures may take up to 2 to 3 wk.

IMAGING STUDIES

- Chest radiograph may demonstrate infiltrates, densities, nodules, cavitary masses, or multiple abscesses.
- CT scan of the brain is indicated in the appropriate clinical setting to exclude CNS brain abscesses.

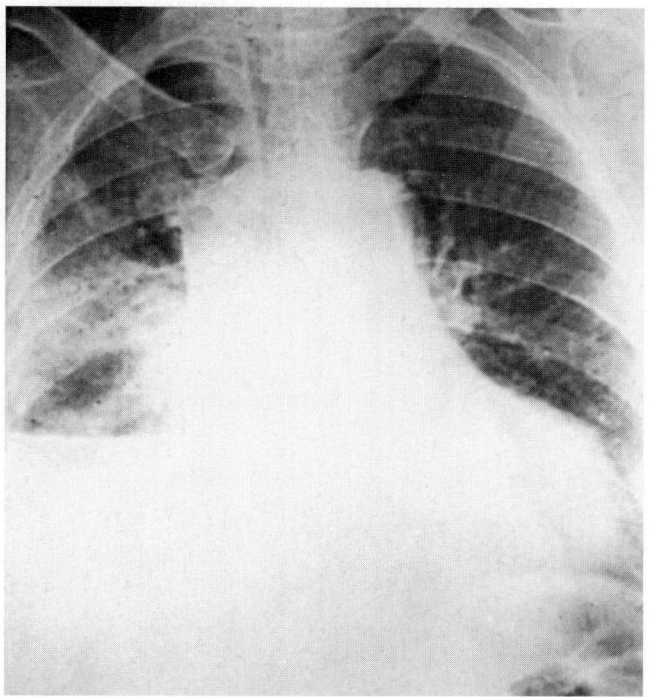

FIGURE 1-591 Right lower lobe *Nocardia* pneumonia in a kidney transplant recipient. (From Gorbach SL: *Infectious diseases*, ed 2, Philadelphia, 1998, Saunders.)

Rx TREATMENT

NONPHARMACOLOGIC THERAPY

- Supportive therapy with oxygen in patients with pneumonia
- Chest physiotherapy
- For any abscess formation, surgical drainage is indicated (e.g., skin, lung, or brain)

ACUTE GENERAL Rx

- There are no prospective, randomized trials to date highlighting the most effective treatment of nocardiosis. Culture and sensitivity should always be done on the specimen.
- For cutaneous infection, trimethoprim-sulfamethoxazole (TMX-SMX) 5 mg/kg of the trimethoprim component divided in 2 doses
- *Nocardia* pneumonia: TMX-SMX 15 mg/kg/day IV/PO in 2-4 divided doses *plus* imipenem 500 mg IV q6h for 3-4 weeks, then TMX-SMX 10 mg/kg/day in 2-4 divided doses for 3 months if immunocompetent or 6 months if immunocompromised. An alternate regimen consists of imipenem 500 mg IV q6h *plus* amikacin 7.5 mg/kg IV q12h for 3-4 weeks, then PO TMX-SMX.

- In patients with CNS disease, TMX-SMX 15 mg/kg/day of TMP and 75 mg/kg/day of SMX IV/PO divided in 2-4 doses *plus* imipenem 500 mg q6h IV. If multiorgan involvement, add amikacin 7.5 mg/kg q12h. Measure peak sulfonamide levels; target is 100-150 mcg/ml 2 hours post dose. An alterative regimen consists of linezolid 600 mg IV or PO q12h *plus* meropenem 2 g q8h.
- Sulfonamide-resistant disease: following two-drug regimens is recommended: imipenem (500 mg IV q6h), and amikacin (7.5 mg/kg IV q12h).
- Alternative drug treatment includes:
  1. Third-generation cephalosporin
  2. Minocycline 100 to 200 mg bid
  3. Extended-spectrum fluoroquinolones (moxifloxacin)
  4. Linezolid (use of linezolid >4 wk is associated with hematologic toxicity)
  5. Tigecycline
  6. Dapsone

CHRONIC Rx

- Although the optimal duration of therapy has not been determined, long-term therapy is generally recommended for all infections caused by *Nocardia*.

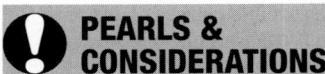

FIGURE 1-592 *Nocardia* pneumonia. Thin, branching, irregularly staining gram-positive bacilli course through necrotic pulmonary tissue (Brown-Hopps Gram, ×1000). (From Silverberg SG et al [eds]: *Silverberg's principles and practice of surgical pathology and cytopathology,* ed 4, Philadelphia, 2006, Churchill Livingstone.)

- Patients with cellulitis and lymphocutaneous syndrome are treated for 2 to 4 mo depending on whether there is bone involvement.
- Mycetomas are best treated with antibiotics for 6 to 12 mo but may require surgical drainage.
- Pulmonary and systemic nocardiosis excluding the CNS is treated for at least 6 mo in immunocompromised hosts.
- CNS involvement is treated with drainage and antibiotics for 12 mo.
- All immunosuppressed patients should receive 12 mo of antibiotic therapy.

DISPOSITION

- Patients with pulmonary nocardiosis have a mortality rate of 15% to 30%.
- CNS involvement carries a >40% mortality rate.
- Isolated skin lesions have a low mortality rate.

REFERRAL

Whenever the diagnosis of nocardiosis is suspected, consultation with infectious disease is indicated. Pulmonary evaluation and assistance may be needed in pulmonary nocardiosis. Neurosurgery consultation is indicated in patients with single or multiple brain abscesses.

! PEARLS & CONSIDERATIONS

- Nocardiosis does not spread from animal to animal.
- Nocardiosis is not transmitted from person to person.
- Nocardiosis is distinguished by its ability to disseminate to any organ and its tendency to relapse despite appropriate antibiotic therapy.

COMMENTS

Tuberculosis and nocardiosis may coexist in the same patient.

SUGGESTED READINGS

available at www.expertconsult.com

RELATED CONTENT

Nocardiosis (Patient Information)

AUTHOR: **TANYA ALI, M.D.**

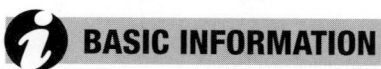

BASIC INFORMATION

DEFINITION

Nonalcoholic fatty liver disease (NAFLD) is a spectrum of diseases based on histiopathologic findings and representing a morphologic rather than a clinical diagnosis. It is liver disease occurring in patients who do not abuse alcohol and manifesting histologically by mononuclear cells and/or polymorphonuclear cells, hepatocyte ballooning, and spotty necrosis. Nonalcoholic steatohepatitis (NASH) is a subset of NAFLD. A diagnosis of NAFLD is contingent on the following factors:

1. Alcohol consumption in amounts less than those considered hepatotoxic
2. Absence of serologic evidence of other hepatic diseases or disorders
3. Liver biopsy showing predominant macrovesicular steatosis or steatohepatitis

SYNONYMS

Nonalcoholic steatohepatitis (NASH)
NAFLD
Fatty liver hepatitis
Diabetes hepatitis
Alcohol-like liver disease
Laënnec's disease

ICD-9CM CODES
571.8 Fatty liver

EPIDEMIOLOGY & DEMOGRAPHICS

- NAFLD affects 10% to 24% of the general population.
- Increased prevalence in obese persons (57% to 74%), type 2 diabetes mellitus, and hyperlipidemia (primarily hypertriglyceridemia)
- Most common cause of abnormal liver test results in adults in the United States (accounts for up to 90% of cases of asymptomatic ALT elevations)
- 30 million obese adults have steatosis; 8.6 million may have steatohepatitis.
- There is a 3:1 female-to-male predominance.

PHYSICAL FINDINGS & CLINICAL PRESENTATION

- Most patients are asymptomatic.
- Patients may report a sensation of fullness or discomfort on the right side of the upper abdomen.
- Nonspecific complaints of fatigue or malaise may be reported.
- Hepatomegaly is generally the only positive finding on physical examination.
- Acanthosis nigricans may be found in children.

ETIOLOGY

- Insulin resistance is the most reproducible factor in the development of NAFLD. High baseline and continuously increasing fasting insulin levels are independent determinants for future development of NFLD.
- Risk factors are obesity (especially truncal obesity), diabetes mellitus, hyperlipidemia.

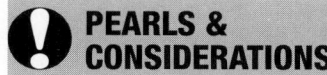

DIAGNOSIS

DIFFERENTIAL DIAGNOSIS

- Alcohol-induced liver disease (a daily alcohol intake of 20 g in females and 30 g in males [three 12-oz beers or 12 oz of wine] may be enough to cause alcohol-induced liver disease)
- Viral hepatitis
- Autoimmune hepatitis
- Toxin- or drug-induced liver disease

WORKUP

Diagnosis is usually suspected on the basis of hepatomegaly, asymptomatic elevations of transaminases, or "fatty liver" on sonogram of abdomen in obese patients with little or no alcohol use. Liver biopsy will confirm diagnosis and provide prognostic information. It should be considered in patients with suspected advanced liver fibrosis (presence of obesity or type 2 diabetes, AST/ALT ratio 1, age 45 yr).

LABORATORY TESTS

- Elevated ALT, AST: AST/ALT ratio is usually <1, but can increase as fibrosis advances
- Negative serology for infectious hepatitis; generally normal GGTP and serum alkaline phosphatase
- Hyperlipidemia (primarily hypertriglyceridemia) may be present.
- Elevated glucose levels may be present.
- Prolonged prothrombin time, hypoalbuminuria, and elevated bilirubin may be present in advanced stages.
- Elevated serum ferritin and increased transferrin saturation may be found in up to 10% of patients; however, hepatic iron index and hepatic iron level are normal.
- Liver biopsy may show a wide spectrum of liver damage, ranging from simple steatosis to advanced fibrosis and cirrhosis.

IMAGING STUDIES

- Ultrasound generally reveals diffuse increase in echogenicity as compared with that of the kidneys; CT scan reveals diffuse low-density hepatic parenchyma.
- Occasionally patients may have focal rather than diffuse steatosis, which may be misinterpreted as a liver mass on ultrasound or CT; use of MRI in these cases will identify focal fatty infiltration.

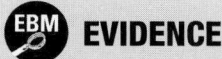

TREATMENT

NONPHARMACOLOGIC THERAPY

- Weight reduction in all obese patients. The American Gastroenterological Association recommends that the initial target weight loss be 10% of baseline weight at a rate of 1 to 2 lb (0.45 to 0.90 kg) per week.
- Increase physical activity.
- Alcohol has a deleterious effect on NAFLD and should be avoided.

GENERAL Rx

- No medications have been proved to directly improve liver damage from NAFLD.
- Medications to control hyperlipidemia (e.g., fenofibrates for elevated triglycerides) and hyperglycemia (e.g., metformin) can lead to improvement in abnormal liver test results.
- Pioglitazone therapy (30 mg/day) and vitamin E (800 IU/day) provide modest benefits in NASH.

DISPOSITION

- Patients with pure steatosis on liver biopsy generally have a relatively benign course.
- The presence of steatohepatitis or advanced fibrosis on liver biopsy is associated with a worse prognosis.

REFERRAL

- Liver transplantation should be considered in patients with decompensated, end-stage disease; however, in these patients there may be a recurrence of NAFLD post transplantation.

PEARLS & CONSIDERATIONS

COMMENTS

- NAFLD is closely associated with metabolic disorders, even in nonobese, nondiabetic subjects. It can be considered an early predictor of metabolic disorders, particularly in the normal-weight population. The presence of metabolic syndrome is a strong predictor of NAFLD.
- NAFLD is associated with an increased risk of incident cardiovascular disease that is independent of the risk conferred by traditional risk factors and components of the metabolic syndrome.

EVIDENCE

available at www.expertconsult.com

SUGGESTED READINGS

available at www.expertconsult.com

RELATED CONTENT

Fatty Liver (Patient Information)

AUTHOR: **FRED F. FERRI, M.D.**

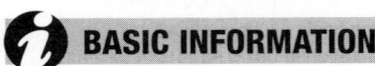 **BASIC INFORMATION**

DEFINITION

Obesity refers to having an excess amount of body fat in relation to lean body mass, or a body mass index (BMI) of $\geq$30 kg/m². Overweight is defined as BMI of 25 to 29.9 kg/m² and morbid obesity refers to adults with a BMI $\geq$40 kg/m². BMI is used as a surrogate measure of obesity. These conditions result from an imbalance between energy intake and expenditure.

ICD-9CM CODES
278.0 Obesity

EPIDEMIOLOGY & DEMOGRAPHICS

- The World Health Organization first recognized obesity as a worldwide epidemic in 1997. As of 2005, 1.6 billion adults worldwide were classified as overweight, 400 million of whom were obese. It is predicted that the combination of overweight and obesity will soon eclipse public health issues such as malnutrition and infectious diseases as the most significant cause of poor health.
- Based on U.S. National Health and Nutrition Examination (NHANES) data from 2009-2010, the prevalence of obesity in the U.S. was 35.7%. By 2015, it is estimated that two in every five adults and one in every four children in the U.S. will be obese.
- The present cost of obesity in the U.S. population is estimated at $100 billion annually.
- For persons with a BMI $\geq$30 kg/m², all-cause mortality is increased by 50% to 100% above that of persons with BMI in the range of 20 to 25 kg/m².
- Obesity is an independent risk factor for cardiovascular disease (CVD) and CVD risks associated with obesity have also been documented in children.
- Obese individuals are at increased risk of morbidity and death from type 2 diabetes, hypertension, coronary heart disease (CHD), cancer (particularly colon, prostate, and breast cancer), sleep apnea, degenerative joint disease, thromboembolic disorders, digestive tract diseases (gallstones), and dermatologic disorders.
- Significant morbidity and risk of death are projected to begin in young adulthood, resulting in more than 100,000 excess cases of CHD by 2035, even with the most modest projection of future obesity.
- Obesity in adolescence is significantly associated with increased risk of incident severe obesity in adulthood, with variations by sex and race/ethnicity. Overweight or obese adults who were obese as children have increased risk of type 2 DM, dyslipidemia, hypertension, and carotid artery atherosclerosis.
- Obesity is a major preventable cause of death and disability in the United States (the other is tobacco).
- Extensive data indicate that weight loss can reverse or arrest the harmful effects of obesity.

PHYSICAL FINDINGS & CLINICAL PRESENTATION

- Physical examination should assess the degree and distribution of body fat and signs of secondary causes of obesity.
- Increased waist circumference is apparent. Excess abdominal fat is clinically defined as a waist circumference >40 inches (>102 cm) in men and >35 inches (>88 cm) in women (in Asian men and women, >36 inches and >33 inches, respectively).
- Symptoms associated with hypertension, coronary artery disease (CAD), and diabetes (e.g., polyuria, polydipsia, acanthosis nigricans, retinopathy, and neuropathy) may be present.
- Obesity is associated with cardiac hypertrophy, diastolic dysfunction, and decreased aortic compliance, which are independent predictors of cardiovascular risk.
- Joint pain and swelling are associated with degenerative joint disease secondary to obesity.
- The physical exam and ECG often underestimate the presence and extent of cardiac dysfunction in obese patients. Jugular venous distention and hepatojugular reflux may not be seen and heart sounds are frequently distant. Obesity is associated with changes in the ECG, including a reduction in voltage and nonspecific ST-T changes that may interfere with diagnosis of left ventricular hypertrophy (LVH) or CAD.
- A large quantity of fluid is present in the interstitial space of adipose tissue, as the interstitial space is ~10% of the tissue wet weight. This excess fluid in this compartment if redistributed into the circulation, can have negative repercussions in obese individuals with heart failure. Obese individuals have higher cardiac output and a lower total peripheral resistance than do lean individuals, and obesity is associated with persistence of elevated cardiac filling pressure during exercise.
- Obesity predisposes to heart failure through several different mechanisms: increased total blood volume, increased cardiac output, LVH, left ventricular diastolic dysfunction, and adipositas cordis (excessive epicardial fat and fatty infiltration of the myocardium).

ETIOLOGY

- The pathophysiology of obesity is complex and poorly understood, but includes social, nutritional, physiologic, psychological, and genetic factors.
- Environmental factors such as a sedentary lifestyle and chronic ingestion of excess calories can cause obesity.
- Obesity may be related to genetic factors, which are thought to be polygenic. Genetic studies with adopted children have demonstrated that they have similar BMIs to their biologic parents but not their adoptive parents. Twin studies also demonstrate a genetic influence on BMI.

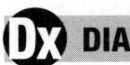 **DIAGNOSIS**

- BMI will establish the diagnosis of obesity. BMI is a measure of an adult's weight in relation to his or her height—more specifically, the adult's weight in kilograms divided by the square of his or her height—and is closely correlated with total body fat content.
- BMI values can categorize patients into three classes of obesity:
  - Class I (mild): BMI of 30.0 to 34.9 kg/m²
  - Class II (moderate): BMI of 35.0 to 39.9 kg/m²
  - Class III (severe): BMI of $\geq$40 kg/m²
- Although BMI is commonly used to define obesity, it is not a highly accurate indicator of body fat composition in children, who are undergoing rapid changes in height, or in bodybuilders or athletes who have large amounts of muscle tissue.
- Waist circumference or waist-hip ratio is indicative of visceral adipose tissue/intraabdominal fat, which may be more deleterious than overall overweight or obesity.

DIFFERENTIAL DIAGNOSIS

It is important to evaluate obese patients for secondary medical causes of obesity. Hypothalamic disorders, hypothyroidism, Cushing's syndrome, insulinoma, depression, and drugs (corticosteroids, antidepressants, second-generation antipsychotics, and HIV protease inhibitors) can cause obesity. In children, certain genetic conditions, such as Prader-Willi syndrome, are associated with obesity.

WORKUP

History should be obtained regarding weight change, family history of obesity, and eating and exercise behavior. Assessment for eating disorders and depression should be made. Attention should be directed to the use of nutritional supplements, over-the-counter medications, hormones, diuretics, and laxatives. The workup of an obese patient typically requires laboratory work to assess for risks and complications as well as to rule out underlying causative medical conditions. Fig. E1-593 describes the evaluation of patients with suspected endocrine cause of obesity.

LABORATORY TESTS

- Obese patients should be assessed for medical consequences of their obesity by screening for metabolic syndrome. This includes measurement of fasting lipid profile, blood pressure, and waist circumference, and screening for diabetes or prediabetes (oral glucose tolerance test, fasting glucose, or hemoglobin A1C).
- In the proper clinical setting, thyroid function studies and dexamethasone suppression testing will exclude hypothyroidism and Cushing's syndrome as underlying causes of obesity. If insulinoma is suspected, the patient will need to undergo a 72-hour fast to confirm hypoglycemia with inappropriate insulin secretion.

IMAGING STUDIES

- Several methods are available for determining or calculating total body fat but offer no significant advantage over the BMI. These include measurement of total body water, total body potassium, bioelectrical impedance, and dual-energy x-ray absorptiometry.
- Buoyancy testing is an accurate method for determining total body fat composition.

OTHER STUDIES

Obesity increases the risk of obstructive sleep apnea, which, in turn, increases the risks of hypertension, cardiac arrhythmias, CVD, stroke, and heart failure. Therefore one should have a low threshold to screen obese patients for obstructive sleep apnea via sleep study/polysomnography.

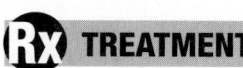 **TREATMENT**

The National Heart, Lung, and Blood Institute (NHLBI) developed guidelines for selecting treatment strategies for overweight and obese patients based on BMI and comorbidities. They recommend a combination of dietary management, physical activity management, and behavior therapy for anyone with a BMI ≥25 or with a high-risk waist circumference and two or more obesity-associated comorbidities. Pharmacotherapy should be considered for patients with a BMI ≥30 or ≥27 with comorbidities.

Surgery is indicated for patients with a BMI ≥35 with comorbidities and for any patient with a BMI ≥40 (Table 1-305).

NONPHARMACOLOGIC THERAPY

- The cornerstones for weight management and reduction are calorie restriction, exercise, and behavioral modification.
- The NHLBI guidelines recommend an initial diet to produce a calorie deficit of 500 to 1000 kcal/day. This has been shown to reduce total body weight by an average of 8% over 3 to 12 mo.
- These guidelines recommend the use of a food diary to focus on dietary substitutes.
- Thirty minutes of moderate-intensity activity on 5 or more days of the week results in health benefits for obese individuals. Moreover, several studies indicate that 60 to 80 min of moderate to vigorous physical activity may provide additional benefit.
- Increased physical activity without caloric restriction (minimal or no weight loss) can reduce abdominal (visceral) adipose tissue and improve insulin resistance.
- The key features of the standard behavioral modification program include goal setting, self-monitoring, stimulus control (modification of one's environment to enhance behaviors that will support weight management), cognitive restructuring (increased awareness of perceptions of oneself and one's weight), and prevention of relapse (weight regain).
- Mammalian sleep is closely integrated with the regulation of energy balance. Trials have shown that the amount of human sleep contributes to the maintenance of fat-free body mass at times of decreased energy intake. Lack of sufficient sleep may compromise the efficacy of typical dietary interventions for weight loss and related metabolic risk reduction.

ACUTE GENERAL Rx

- According to the NHLBI *Guidelines on the Identification, Evaluation, and Treatment of Overweight and Obesity in Adults* and the U.S. Food and Drug Administration (FDA), pharmacotherapy is indicated for:
  - Obese patients with a BMI ≥30
  - Overweight patients with a BMI of ≥27 and concomitant obesity-related risk factors or diseases, such as hypertension, diabetes, or dyslipidemia

- Pharmacologic treatment options include:
  - Gastrointestinal lipase inhibitors: Orlistat is the only drug available for long-term treatment of obesity. It blocks the digestion and absorption of ingested dietary fat. It is a reversible inhibitor of pancreatic, gastric, and carboxyl ester lipases and phospholipase A2, which are required for the hydrolysis of dietary fat in the gastrointestinal tract. Side effects include flatulence, fecal incontinence, cramps, and oily spotting. There can also be impairment of absorption of vitamin A, E, and beta-carotene. Oxalate-associated acute kidney injury and rare severe liver injury have also been reported.
  - C Serotonin agonists: Lorcaserin is a selective serotonin agonist that acts centrally to reduce appetite, aiding weight loss. Adverse effects include headache, upper respiratory infections, dizziness, and nausea. While there is little evidence of serotonin-associated cardiac valvular disease (as seen with nonselective serotonergic agonists fenfluramine and dexfenfluramine), long-term data is currently limited.
  - Sympathomimetic medications: Phentermine and diethylpropion are currently approved for short-term treatment of obesity. They reduce food intake by causing early satiety. Side effects include increased blood pressure and increased pulse. They are Schedule IV drugs with a potential for abuse. Other sympathomimetic drugs that have been removed from the market due to concerns about cardiovascular safety are sibutramine, phenylpropanolamine, and ephedrine.
  - Antidepressants: While not FDA-approved for treatment of obesity alone, bupropion and fluoxetine are antidepressants that have been associated with modest weight loss.
  - Antiepileptic drugs: Zonisamide and topiramate (also used in migraine therapy) have been associated with weight loss in clinical trials but are not currently FDA-approved for treatment of obesity alone.
  - Diabetes drugs: While not FDA-approved for treatment of obesity alone, metformin, pramlintide (synthetic human amylin), and glucagon-like polypeptide-1 agonists (exenatide, liraglutide) have been associated with weight loss in the treatment of individuals with diabetes. Weight loss was also reported in a trial of liraglutide in patients without diabetes.

CHRONIC Rx

- According to the NHLBI guidelines, surgical intervention is an option for selected patients with clinically severe obesity (a BMI ≥40 or a BMI ≥35 with comorbid conditions), when patients are at high risk for obesity-associated morbidity or death, and when less invasive methods of weight loss have failed.
- Bariatric surgery for weight loss falls into one of three general categories:

TABLE 1-305 Weight-Loss Treatment Guidelines from the National Heart, Lung, and Blood Institute*

| Treatment | BMI | | | | |
	25.0-26.9	27.0-29.9	30.0-34.9	35.0-39.9	>40.0
Diet, physical activity, behavioral therapy, or all three	Yes	Yes	Yes	Yes	Yes
Pharmacotherapy†		In patients with obesity-related diseases	Yes	Yes	Yes
Surgery‡				In patients with obesity-related diseases	Yes

*Data are from www.nhlbi.nih.gov/guidelines/obesity/ob_home.htm. These guidelines are generally consistent with those from the American Heart Association, the American Medical Association, the American Diabetic Association, the Obesity Society (Practical Guide), the American Diabetes Association, the American Academy of Family Physicians, the American College of Sports Medicine, and the American Cancer Society. *BMI* denotes body mass index, calculated as the weight in kilograms divided by the square of the height in meters.

†Pharmacotherapy should be considered only in patients who are not able to achieve adequate weight loss with available conventional lifestyle modifications and who have no absolute contraindications for drug therapy.

‡Bariatric surgery should be considered only in patients who are unable to lose weight with available conventional therapy and who have no absolute contraindications for surgery.

- ○ Restrictive surgeries limit the amount of food the stomach can hold and slow the rate of gastric emptying. These include vertical banded gastroplasty and laparoscopic adjustable silicone gastric banding (lap banding).
- ○ Malabsorptive surgeries reduce nutrient absorption by shortening length of small intestine. These include jejunoileal bypass and the duodenal switch operation (DS).
- ○ Restrictive malabsorptive bypass procedures combine the elements of gastric restriction and selective malabsorption. These include Roux-en-Y gastric bypass (considered the gold standard because of its high level of effectiveness and durability) and biliopancreatic diversion.
- Compared with usual care, bariatric surgery is associated with reduced number of cardiovascular deaths and lower incidence of cardiovascular events in obese adults. A study on bariatric surgery patients demonstrated a significant reduction in long-term cardiovascular events. Ten-year follow-up estimated relative risk reductions ranging from 18% to 79% according to the Framingham risk score and 8% to 62% with the PROCAM risk score.
- Liposuction is removal of fat by aspiration after injection of physiologic saline. This technique reduces the subcutaneous fat but has failed to improve insulin sensitivity or risk factors for CHD.

DISPOSITION

- The incidence of venous thromboembolism in the upper tertile of BMI was 2.42 times that of the lowest BMI tertile. Obese patients have a higher incidence of postoperative thromboembolic events when undergoing noncardiac surgery.
- Perioperative obesity (>140% ideal body weight) may increase morbidity and mortality rates after heart transplantation.
- Weight stable obese subjects have an increased risk of arrhythmias and sudden death even in the absence of cardiac dysfunction.
- Obesity and the cardiac autonomic nervous system are intrinsically related. A 10% increase in body weight is associated with a decline in parasympathetic tone accompanied by a rise in mean heart rate. Conversely, a 10% weight loss in severely obese patients is associated with significant improvement in autonomic nervous system cardiac modulation, including decreased heart rate and increased heart rate variability.
- Postmortem Determinants of Atherosclerosis in Youth (PDAY) study data provided convincing evidence that obesity in adolescents and young adults accelerates the progression of atherosclerosis decades before the appearance of clinical manifestations.

- Obesity accelerates the progression of native coronary atherosclerosis and after coronary artery bypass grafting.
- In older adults, obesity is associated with protection against hip fracture, but this protective effect on bone status does not offset the extensive array of potential adverse effects on conditions common in the older population.

REFERRAL

- Obesity is commonly seen in the primary care setting. If pharmacologic therapy is considered, consultation with physicians specializing in obesity and experienced with the use of the drug is recommended. In addition, consultation with nutritionists and behavioral therapists is helpful. A consultation with general surgery is indicated in patients being considered for surgical intervention.
- Recent trials have shown that among adolescents, use of gastric banding compared with lifestyle intervention results in a greater percentage achieving a loss of 50% of excess weight corrected for age. There were associated benefits to health and quality of life.

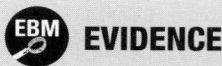

PEARLS & CONSIDERATIONS

COMMENTS

- Enhanced weight-loss counseling helps about one third of obese patients achieve long-term, clinically meaningful weight loss.
- The NHLBI launched the Obesity Education Initiative in January 1991. The overall purpose of the initiative is to help reduce the prevalence of overweight along with the prevalence of physical inactivity to reduce the risk of CHD and overall morbidity and mortality rates from CHD.
- The American Medical Association, in association with the Robert Wood Johnson Foundation and the U.S. Department of Health and Human Services, produced a primer for the assessment and management of adult obesity. The primer consists of 10 booklets that offer practical recommendations for addressing adult obesity in the primary care setting and is available for free at: http://www.ama-assn.org/ama/pub/physician-resources.
- Recent research indicates that brown adipose tissue represents a natural target for the modulation of energy expenditure. The presence of brown adipose tissue in humans may be quantified with the use of ^{18}F-FDG PET-CT. The amount of brown adipose tissue is inversely correlated with BMI, suggesting a potential role of brown adipose tissue in adult human metabolism.
- Obesity, glucose intolerance, and hypertension in childhood are strongly associated with

increased rates of premature death from endogenous causes in this population.
- Recent trials have shown that among persons living in a controlled setting, calories alone account for the increase in fat. Protein affected energy expenditure and storage of lean body mass, but not body fat storage.

PREVENTION

- Prevention of overweight and obesity involves both increasing physical activity and dietary modification to reduce caloric intake.
- There is compelling evidence that prevention of weight regain in formerly obese individuals requires 60 to 90 min of moderate intensity activity or lesser amounts of vigorous intensity activity.
- Moderate intensity activity of approximately 45 to 60 min per day, or 1.7 physical activity level (PAL), is required to prevent the transition to overweight or obesity. For children, even more activity time is recommended.
- Clinicians can help guide patients to develop personalized eating plans and help them recognize the contributions of fat, concentrated carbohydrates, and large portion sizes.
- Clinicians must work with patients to modify other risk factors such as tobacco use, high glycemic intake, and elevated blood pressure to prevent the long-term chronic disease sequelae of obesity.
- Regular screening of body weight and BMI measurements at routine office visits can help identify early weight gain.

PATIENT & FAMILY EDUCATION

Information can be obtained on the American Obesity Association website (http://www.obesity.org) and the American Medical Association website (http://www.ama-assn.org).

EBM EVIDENCE

available at www.expertconsult.com

SUGGESTED READINGS

available at www.expertconsult.com

RELATED CONTENT

Fig. 3-190 Weight gain (Algorithm)
Obesity, Female (Patient Information)
Obesity, Male (Patient Information)

AUTHORS: **HILARY B. WHITLACH, M.D.,**
SAINATH GADDAM, M.D., and
FRED F. FERRI, M.D.

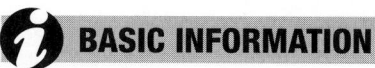 BASIC INFORMATION

DEFINITION

Obsessive-compulsive disorder (OCD) is characterized by recurrent obsessions (intrusive and unwanted thoughts, urges, or images) and/or compulsions (behaviors or mental acts performed in response to obsessions, or according to rules that must be applied rigidly) that are time-consuming (e.g., >1 hr/day) or cause marked impairment or distress. The symptoms are usually perceived as excessive and unreasonable.

SYNONYMS

OCD

ICD-9CM CODES
F42.8 Obsessive-compulsive disorder
(DSM-IV 300.3)

EPIDEMIOLOGY & DEMOGRAPHICS

PEAK INCIDENCE: Mean age at onset is 19.6 yr.
LIFETIME PREVALENCE (IN U.S.): 2.5% of adults
PREDOMINANT SEX: Approximately equal distribution between sexes
PREDOMINANT AGE:
- Modal age of onset for females is between 20 and 29 yr.
- Modal age of onset for males is between 6 and 15 yr.

DISEASE COURSE:
- Condition is chronic with waxing and waning pattern.
- Symptoms typically worsen with stress.
- 15% show progressive deterioration, whereas 5% show an episodic course with little impairment between episodes.

GENETICS:
- There is no clear genetic pattern.
- Rate of concordance is higher in monozygotic (33%) compared with dizygotic (7%) twins.
- Rate of disorder is also higher in first-degree relatives of individuals with OCD and Tourette's disorder than in the general population.

PHYSICAL FINDINGS & CLINICAL PRESENTATION

- Persistent and recurrent intrusive and ego-dystonic obsessive ideas, thoughts, urges, or images that are perceived as alien and beyond one's control.
- Frequent experiencing of obsessions related to contamination (e.g., when using the telephone), excessive doubt (e.g., was the door locked?), organization (the need for a particular order), violent impulses (e.g., to yell obscenities in church), or intrusive sexual imagery.
- Compulsive behaviors (e.g., repeated hand washing, checking, rearranging) or mental rituals (e.g., counting, repeating phrases) meant to temporarily ameliorate anxiety caused by obsessions.
- Obsessions and compulsions almost always accompanied by high anxiety and subjective distress. Both are usually seen as excessive and unreasonable.

ETIOLOGY

- Strong evidence of neurobiologic etiology.
- OCD onset may be temporally associated with infectious illness of CNS (e.g., Von Economo's encephalitis, Sydenham's chorea).
- OCD may follow head trauma or other premorbid neurologic condition, including birth hypoxia and Tourette's syndrome.
- Serotonergic pathways believed important in some ritualistic instinctual behaviors, with dysfunction of these pathways possibly giving rise to OCD.

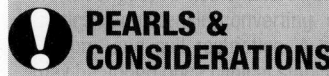 DIAGNOSIS

DIFFERENTIAL DIAGNOSIS

- Obsessive-compulsive personality disorder (OCPD) is a maladaptive personality style defined by excessive rigidity, need for order and control, preoccupation with details, and excessive perfectionism. Unlike OCD, OCPD is ego-syntonic.
- Other psychiatric disorders in which obsessive or intrusive thoughts occur (e.g., body dysmorphic disorder, eating disorders, hypochondriasis, phobias, posttraumatic stress disorder).
- Impulse control disorders (e.g., trichotillomania, pathologic gambling, compulsive shopping, kleptomania, paraphilias/sexual compulsions).
- Neurologic disorders with repetitive behaviors (e.g., Tourette's syndrome, Sydenham's chorea, torticollis, autism).
- Delusions or psychosis, which may be mistaken for obsessive thoughts; unlike OCD, these individuals do not believe their obsessions are unreal and may likely meet criteria for another psychotic spectrum disorder that fully accounts for the obsessions (e.g., schizophrenia).

WORKUP

- Careful history leading to diagnosis
- Neurologic examination to rule out concomitant Tourette's or other tic disorder
- In adolescents and children: psychological testing to reveal learning disabilities

LABORATORY TESTS

No specific tests are indicated.

IMAGING STUDIES

No specific studies are indicated.

Rx TREATMENT

NONPHARMACOLOGIC THERAPY

- Treatment will help ~50% of patients achieve partial remission within the first 6 mo.
- Cognitive-behavioral therapy (CBT), especially exposure/response prevention, is successful in up to 70% of patients, but nearly 25% drop out of treatment because of the initial anxiety the exposures create. Best results are found for contamination obsessions and washing compulsions.

ACUTE GENERAL Rx

Clonazepam may be helpful in patients with extreme anxiety.

CHRONIC Rx

- Antidepressants with serotonin reuptake blockade, including clomipramine, fluvoxamine, fluoxetine, paroxetine, sertraline, citalopram and escitalopram, venlafaxine, and duloxetine; optimal dosages are typically at the high end of the prescription range. Risk/benefit/alternatives discussion is crucial (e.g., dose-related risk of QT interval prolongation with clomipramine and citalopram).
- Most improve with treatment, but few become symptom-free. No response in 15% of patients.
- Likely indefinite treatment. Relapse is common if medications are discontinued.
- Recent studies suggest that combination CBT and pharmacotherapy yields superior outcomes. More severe symptoms warrant combination therapy.
- Patients who do not respond to first-line treatments and those with comorbid psychosis and/or tic disorders may benefit from augmentation with a first- or second-generation antipsychotic medication (e.g., haloperidol, olanzapine, risperidone).
- Surgical intervention (e.g., cingulotomy, deep brain stimulation) is an option for the most extreme, refractory cases.

DISPOSITION

- Most mild to moderate cases can be managed on a regular outpatient basis. Treatment should typically start with SSRI monotherapy with regular follow-up to assess treatment response and side-effect management. Dose should be increased to maximum tolerated.
- Patient and family education may help improve medical adherence and support.

REFERRAL

- If differentiation from other psychiatric conditions, particularly delusional disorder, is not clear
- Refractory illness (treatment resistance) and/or if patient requests CBT

! PEARLS & CONSIDERATIONS

Patients with OCD typically have insight regarding the irrationality of their obsessions and compulsions but lack the ability to control them. This may cause intense shame and avoidance of medical care unless patient education and support are provided. Screen for OCD, especially among patients who present with "depression" or "anxiety."

SUGGESTED READINGS

available at www.expertconsult.com

RELATED CONTENT

Obsessive-Compulsive Disorder (OCD) (Patient Information)

AUTHORS: **AGUSTIN G. YIP, M.D., PH.D.,** **JASON M. SATTERFIELD, PH.D.,** and **MITCHELL D. FELDMAN, M.D., M.PHIL.**

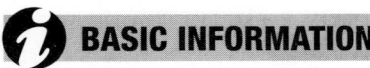

BASIC INFORMATION

DEFINITION

The term *ocular foreign body* refers to a foreign body on the surface of the corneal epithelium.

ICD-9CM CODES
930 Foreign body in external eye

EPIDEMIOLOGY & DEMOGRAPHICS

INCIDENCE (IN U.S.): Universal, with a predominance in active people
PEAK INCIDENCE: Childhood through active adult years
PREDOMINANT SEX: Perhaps slightly more common in men
PREDOMINANT AGE: Childhood through active adult years

PHYSICAL FINDINGS & CLINICAL PRESENTATION

- Pain is most common symptom.
- Causes of most common foreign bodies:
  - Grinding (Fig. 1-594)
  - Drilling
  - Auto repair
  - Working beneath cars
  - Airborne particles, such as blown by fans

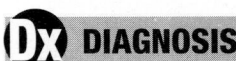 DIAGNOSIS

DIFFERENTIAL DIAGNOSIS

- History of corneal foreign body seen
- Hemorrhage, loss of vision
- Distorted anterior chamber, soft eye
- Corneal abrasion
- Corneal ulceration or laceration
- Glaucoma
- Herpes ulcers
- Infection
- Other keratitis
- Intraocular foreign body

WORKUP

- Fluorescein stain, slit-lamp examination if no foreign body is found
- Ultrasound examination
- Plain radiographs

LABORATORY TESTS

Intraocular pressure to make certain that eye has not been penetrated

IMAGING STUDIES

Occasionally, MRI of the orbits to identify foreign bodies not found by other means. Do not perform MRI if suspect metallic foreign body. Plain radiographs and ultrasound are sufficient.

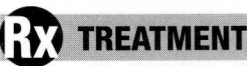 TREATMENT

NONPHARMACOLOGIC THERAPY

- Remove foreign body
- Treat infection
- Repair eye if ruptured
- Treat corneal abrasion or injury

ACUTE GENERAL Rx

- Saline irrigation
- Removal of foreign body with moist cotton-tipped applicator after instillation of topical anesthetic drops
- Use burr or more aggressive treatment if needed
- Cycloplegics, antibiotics, and pressure dressing after removal of foreign body
- Repair corneal laceration or damaged eye

DISPOSITION

If symptoms persist 24 hr after examination, refer to an ophthalmologist.

REFERRAL

To ophthalmology within 24 hr if patient not completely comfortable

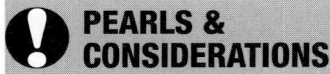 PEARLS & CONSIDERATIONS

COMMENTS

- Make sure foreign body is not intraocular (inside eye).
- Alkaline or acidic chemical foreign bodies can be dangerous; pH test must be performed if either of these is suspected (for all chemical foreign bodies).

SUGGESTED READINGS
available at www.expertconsult.com

RELATED CONTENT

Corneal Foreign Body (Patient Information)

AUTHOR: **MELVYN KOBY, M.D.**

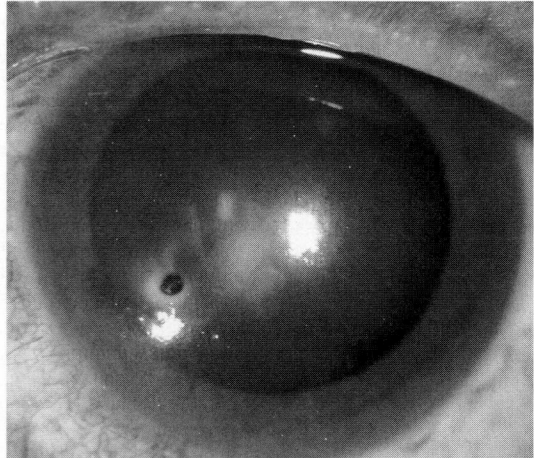

FIGURE 1-594 A small iron foreign body may be seen on external examination. (Courtesy Department of Dermatology, University of North Carolina at Chapel Hill. In Goldstein GB, Goldstein AO: *Practical dermatology,* ed 2, St Louis, 1997, Mosby.)

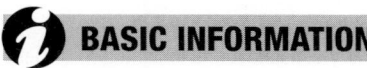

BASIC INFORMATION

DEFINITION

Onychomycosis is defined as a persistent fungal infection affecting the toenails and fingernails.

SYNONYMS

Tinea unguium
Ringworm of the nails

ICD-9CM CODES

110.1 Onychomycosis

EPIDEMIOLOGY & DEMOGRAPHICS

- Onychomycosis is most commonly found in people between the ages of 40 and 60 yr.
- Onychomycosis rarely occurs before puberty.
- Incidence: 20 to 100 cases/1000 population.
- Toenail infection is 4 to 6 times more common than fingernail infection.

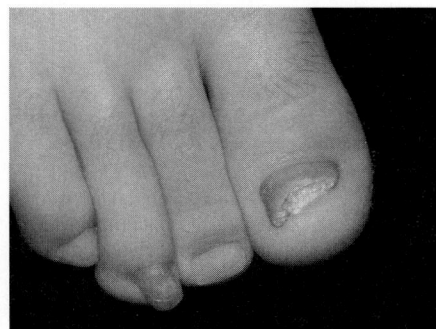

FIGURE 1-595 Distal subungual onychomycosis in a 5-year-old. Note how heavily infected nails occur adjacent to totally normal nails. Cutting back the big toe's nail plate has revealed the friable subungual debris. This material is the most desirable for culture. (From White GM, Cox NH [eds]: *Diseases of the skin, a color atlas and text,* ed 2, St Louis, 2006, Mosby.)

- Onychomycosis affects men more often than women.
- Occurs more frequently in patients with diabetes, peripheral vascular disease, and any conditions resulting in the suppression of the immune system.
- Occlusive footwear, physical exercise followed by communal showering, and incompletely drying the feet predispose the individual to developing onychomycosis.

PHYSICAL FINDINGS & CLINICAL PRESENTATION

- Onychomycosis causes nails to become thick, brittle, hard, distorted, and discolored (yellow to brown color) (Fig. 1-595). Eventually, the nail may loosen, separate from the nail bed, and fall off (Fig. 1-596).
- Onychomycosis is frequently associated with tinea pedis (athlete's foot).

ETIOLOGY

- The most common causes of onychomycosis are dermatophyte, yeast, and nondermatophyte molds.
- The dermatophyte *Trichophyton rubrum* accounts for 80% of all nail infections caused by fungus.
- *Trichophyton interdigitale* and *Trichophyton mentagrophytes* are other fungi causing onychomycosis.
- The yeast *Candida albicans* is responsible for 5% of the cases of onychomycosis.
- Nondermatophyte molds *Scopulariopsis brevicaulis* and *Aspergillus niger,* although rare, can also cause onychomycosis.
- Onychomycosis is classified according to the clinical pattern of nail bed involvement. The main types are:
  1. Distal and lateral subungual onychomycosis (DLSO)
  2. Superficial onychomycosis
  3. Proximal subungual onychomycosis

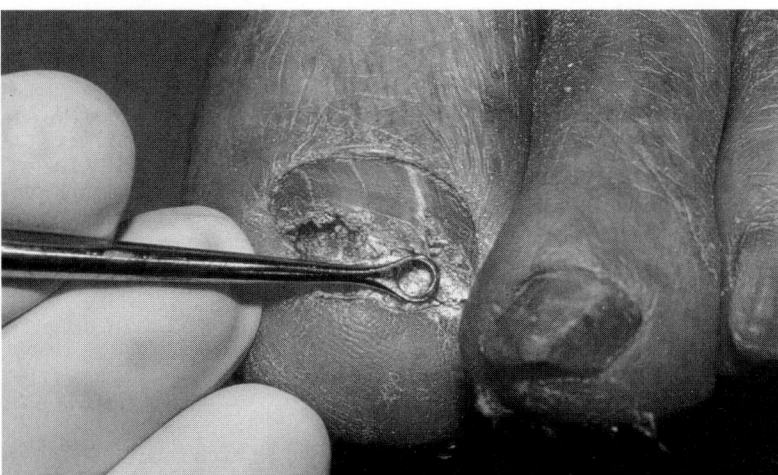

FIGURE 1-596 Collection of nail for culture. The subungual debris is the most valuable material for culture. After the nail is cut back, a curette may be used. Clippings of the nail may be added to the culture. (From White GM, Cox NH [eds]: *Diseases of the skin, a color atlas and text,* ed 2, St Louis, 2006, Mosby.)

  4. Endonyx onychomycosis
  5. Total dystrophic onychomycosis

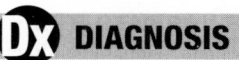

DIAGNOSIS

The diagnosis of onychomycosis is based on the clinical nail findings and confirmed by direct microscopy and culture.

DIFFERENTIAL DIAGNOSIS

- Psoriasis
- Contact dermatitis
- Lichen planus
- Subungual keratosis
- Paronychia
- Infection (e.g., *Pseudomonas*)
- Trauma
- Peripheral vascular disease
- Yellow nail syndrome

WORKUP

The workup of suspected onychomycosis is directed at confirming the diagnosis of onychomycosis by visualizing hyphae under the microscope by KOH prep or by culturing the organism. Although the standard for the diagnosis of fungal nail disease is a positive result on microscopic examination and culture of nail clippings with subungal debris or from surface debris in superficial white onychomycosis, treatment is often prescribed in absence of confirmatory findings.

LABORATORY TESTS

- KOH prep: specificity is high but sensitivity is variable
- Fungal cultures on Sabouraud medium: culture may take 4 to 6 wk
- Dermatophyte test medium (DTM): an alternative to Sabouraud's that takes only 3 to 7 days and can be done in office setting. A color change indicates dermatophyte growth.
- Nail plate biopsy with periodic acid–Schiff (PAS) stain
- Blood tests are not specific in the diagnosis of onychomycosis and therefore not useful

IMAGING STUDIES

- Imaging studies are not very specific in making the diagnosis of onychomycosis and not useful.
- If an infection is present and osteomyelitis is a consideration, an x-ray of the specific area and a bone scan may help establish the diagnosis.

CLASSIFICATION

- The Onychomycosis Severity Index (OSI) is a new classification system for grading the severity of onychomycosis.
- The OSI score is obtained by multiplying the score for the area of involvement (range, 0-5) by the score for the proximity of the disease to the matrix (range, 1-5). Ten points are added for the presence of a longitudinal streak or a patch (dermatophytoma) or for >2 mm of subungual hyperkeratosis.
- Mild onychomycosis corresponds to a score of 1-5; moderate to a score of 6-15; severe to a score of 16-35.

O

Diseases and Disorders

I

Rx TREATMENT

NONPHARMACOLOGIC THERAPY

- Surgical removal of the nail plate is a treatment option; however, the relapse rate is high.
- Prevention of reinfection by wearing properly fitted shoes, avoiding public showers, and keeping feet and nails clean and dry.

ACUTE GENERAL Rx

- Topical antifungal creams are used for early superficial nail infections.
  1. Miconazole 2% cream applied over the nail plate bid
  2. Clotrimazole 1% cream bid
  3. Ciclopirox: topical antifungal nail lacquer can be used for moderate onychomycosis that spares the lunula. Success rate <10%
  4. Amorolfine: nail lacquer for infecton that spares lunula but is not available in the U.S.
- Oral agents.
  1. Terbinafine
     a. For toenails: 250 mg/day for 3 mo
     b. For fingernails: 250 mg/day for 6 wk
  2. Itraconazole
     a. For toenails: 200 mg PO daily for 3 mo
     b. For fingernails: 200 mg PO daily for 6 wk
  3. Fluconazole: not as effective as terbinafine or itraconazole
     a. For toenails: 150 to 300 mg once weekly for 18 to 26 wk
     b. For fingernails: 150 to 300 mg once weekly for 12 to 16 wk

- All oral agents used for onychomycosis require periodic monitoring of liver function blood tests. Patients should be advised to watch for symptoms of drug-induced hepatitis (anorexia, fatigue, nausea, right upper quadrant pain) while taking these oral antifungal agents. They should stop their medication and contact their physician immediately if symptoms occur.
- Itraconazole is contraindicated in patients taking cisapride, astemizole, triazolam, midazolam, and terfenadine. Statins should be discontinued during itraconazole therapy. Itraconazole requires gastric acidity for absorption; patients should be advised not to take oral antacids, H_2 blockers, or proton pump inhibitors while taking itraconazole.
- Fluconazole is contraindicated in patients taking cisapride and terfenadine.
- Oral antifungal agents should not be initiated during pregnancy.
- Short-pulse laser therapy is fungicidal and is a newer treatment modality for onychomycosis. Most patients will require 2-4 treatments, each lasting 15-30 minutes. Laser therapy is useful in patients with contraindications to oral agents. It is, however, expensive ($250-$1,000 per treatment) and not covered by most insurance plans.

DISPOSITION

- Spontaneous remission of onychomycosis is rare.
- A disease-free toenail is reported to occur in approximately 25% to 50% of patients treated with the oral antifungal agents mentioned previously.

REFERRAL

- Podiatry consultation is indicated in diabetic patients for proper instruction in foot care, footwear, and nail debridement or surgical removal of the toenail.
- Dermatology consultation is indicated in patients refractory to treatment or if another diagnosis is considered (e.g., psoriasis).

! PEARLS & CONSIDERATIONS

COMMENTS

- The growth of fungus on an infected nail typically begins at the end of the nail and spreads under the nail plate to infect the nail bed as well.
- Carefully consider the informational insert regarding drug-drug interactions and contraindications before initiating oral antifungal agents.

SUGGESTED READINGS

available at www.expertconsult.com

RELATED CONTENT

Ringworm (Patient Information)
AUTHOR: **GLENN G. FORT, M.D., M.P.H.**

BASIC INFORMATION

DEFINITION

- Opioid addiction/dependence is defined as a cluster of cognitive, behavioral, and physiologic symptoms in which the individual continues use of opiates despite significant opiate-induced problems. Opiate dependence is a chronic, relapsing disorder characterized by repeated self-administration that usually results in opiate tolerance, withdrawal, and compulsive drug use. Tolerance is the need to increase dose to achieve the same effect. Dependence may occur with or without the physiologic symptoms of tolerance and withdrawal.
- There are four stages of addiction:
  1. Stage I, acute drug effects: rewarding effects of drug result from neurobiologic changes in response to the acute drug use. Duration varies from hours to days.
  2. Stage II, transformation to addiction: associated with changes in neuronal function that accumulate with repeated administration and diminish over days or weeks after discontinuation of drug use.
  3. Stage III, relapse after extended periods of abstinence: precipitated by an incubation of cue-induced craving (people, places, and things as triggers) and priming (relapse precipitated by drug exposure).
  4. Stage IV, end-stage addiction: vulnerability to relapse endures for years and results from prolonged changes at the cellular level.
- Pseudoaddiction: undertreatment of pain resulting in "opiate-seeking" behaviors such as "doctor shopping" and multiple emergency department visits. These behaviors disappear with adequate treatment of pain.

SYNONYMS

Opiate addiction
Opiate abuse
Narcotic addiction
Narcotic abuse

ICD-9CM CODES
304.7X/304.8X Opioid dependence

EPIDEMIOLOGY & DEMOGRAPHICS

INCIDENCE: There are 980,000 opiate addicts in the U.S.; less than one third are in treatment.

PREVALENCE:
- Approximately 6 million persons age ≥12 yr used psychotherapeutic drugs for nonmedical purposes in 2004, which represents 2.5% of the population. Most of them reported abusing opiate pain relievers.
- In 2004, 2.4 million persons age ≥12 yr initiated nonmedical use of prescription pain relievers, surpassing for the first time those who initiated abuse of marijuana (2.1 million).
- Opiate addiction is becoming an adolescent disease. Among twelfth-graders, in 2005,

9.5% reported past-year nonmedical use of oxycodone (Vicodin) and 5.5% reported past-year nonmedical use of oxycodone slow-release tablets (OxyContin).
- The percentage of eighth-, tenth-, and twelfth-graders who have used heroin has more than doubled since the late 1990s. This increase has largely been attributed to decreased price and increased purity in the last decade.

PREDOMINANT SEX: Males abuse opiates more commonly than females, with a male/female ratio of 3:1 for heroin and 1.5:1 for prescription opiates.

PEAK INCIDENCE: The majority of new abusers of opiates are <26 yr.

RISK FACTORS:
- Family history
- Prior history of addiction
- Psychiatric disorders

GENETICS:
- Genetic epidemiologic studies suggest a high degree of heritable vulnerability for opiate dependence.
- Gene polymorphism for dopamine receptor/transporters, opioid receptors, serotonin receptors/transporters, proenkephalin, and catechol-*O*-methyltransferase all appear to be associated with vulnerability to opiate dependence. Future interventions for opiate dependence may include medications identified through genetic research.

PHYSICAL FINDINGS & CLINICAL PRESENTATION

- Physical examination is often noncontributory.
- Small-sized pupils may be the only observable sign of use because only mild tolerance develops for miosis.
- Scars or tracks from chronic IV use may be visible over the veins of the arms, hands, ankles, neck, and breasts.
- Inflamed nasal mucosa or respiratory wheezing may be apparent in patients who are snorting heroin or OxyContin.
- Patients in withdrawal may have more dramatic findings such as tachycardia, hypertension, fever, piloerection (goose flesh), mydriasis, lacrimation, central nervous system (CNS) arousal, irritability, and repeated yawning. In patients with sympathetic overactivity and panic attacks, use of CNS stimulants, such as amphetamines or cocaine, should also be ruled out.
- Although gastrointestinal symptoms of nausea, vomiting, and abdominal pain are common in opiate withdrawal, other causes such as gastroenteritis, pancreatitis, peptic ulcer disease, and intestinal obstruction need to be ruled out.
- The history may provide relevant information in making the diagnosis. Significant findings may include:
  1. A long history of opiate self-administration, typically by the IV or intranasal route but sometimes through smoking as well.
  2. Polysubstance use. Intoxication by drugs other than narcotics (e.g., benzodiazepines,

barbiturates) should be ruled out in unconscious patients.
  3. A high incidence of non-opiate-related psychiatric disorders (>80%).
  4. History of problems at work, school, or relationships associated with drug use.
  5. History of legal problems associated with drug use, such as arrest for possession, robbery, or prostitution.
  6. History of interpersonal violence (as perpetrator or victim).
  7. History of physical problems such as skin infections, phlebitis, endocarditis, or liver diseases attributable to acetaminophen toxicity (Vicodin/Percocet) or viral hepatitis. Hepatitis C is the most prevalent blood-borne pathogen. It is present in approximately 90% of opiate-dependent people and is often spread by sharing IV drug paraphernalia or snorting devices. There is also a higher incidence of HIV infection.

ETIOLOGY

Opioid dependence is a biopsychosocial disorder. Pharmacologic, social, genetic, and psychodynamic factors interact to influence abusive behaviors. Pharmacologic factors are especially prominent in opiate addiction because these drugs are strong reinforcing agents because of their euphoric effects and their ability to reduce anxiety and increase self-esteem and the patient's subjective feelings of improved ability to cope with daily challenges.

DIAGNOSIS

DIFFERENTIAL DIAGNOSIS

- Psychiatric disorders (e.g., anxiety, depression, bipolar disorder).
- Acute medical illness (e.g., hypoglycemia, seizure disorder, sepsis, renal or hepatic insufficiency) may mimic opiate withdrawal symptoms.

WORKUP

- The history is the most important part of the workup.
- Observation of opiate withdrawal is indicative of opiate addiction.
- Observation of purposeful behaviors such as complaints and manipulations directed at getting more drugs and anxiety during withdrawal is suggestive of opiate addiction.
- Screen blood and urine for opiate metabolites.
- Screen for communicable diseases: HIV, hepatitis B and hepatitis C, tuberculosis.
- Screen for endocarditis in patients with newly diagnosed murmurs.

LABORATORY TESTS

- Urine and serum toxicology screen
- Complete blood count
- Chemistries (alanine aminotransferase, aspartate aminotransferase, serum creatinine): elevated liver function test (LFT) results may

be from viral hepatitis or acetaminophen toxicity
- Hepatitis screen: if hepatitis C antibody positive, follow up with hepatitis C polymerase chain reaction (viral load) even in patients with normal LFTs
- HIV
- PPD

IMAGING STUDIES

Generally not helpful in routine diagnosis and treatment. Consider echocardiography in patients with heart murmurs and liver sonography or CT scan in patients with elevated LFTs or who are positive for hepatitis C or B (increased risk of hepatocellular carcinoma).

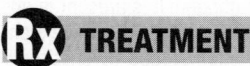 **TREATMENT**

NONPHARMACOLOGIC THERAPY

- Brief counseling interventions during a visit with their primary care physician or OB/GYN have proved efficacious in motivating patients for treatment.
- Therapeutic communities (residential).
- 12-step or other self-help groups (e.g., Alcoholics Anonymous, Narcotics Anonymous).
- Relapse prevention (counseling).

ACUTE Rx

- Medical withdrawal (not overdosed).
- Short- (30 days) or long-term (30 to 180 days) protocols.
- Buprenorphine (opioid partial agonist) or methadone (opioid agonist) is initiated in tapering doses.
- Clonidine 0.1 mg bid to tid can be used to minimize autonomic symptoms (sweating) and craving.
- Nonsteroidal anti-inflammatory drugs for body and muscle aches.
- The anticholinergic dicyclomine can be used to minimize gastrointestinal hyperactivity.
- Nonbenzodiazepine hypnotics, low-dose atypical antipsychotics (e.g., quetiapine), or low-dose tricyclic antidepressants are effective for promoting adequate sleep.

CHRONIC Rx

Opioid antagonist treatment:
- Naltrexone: does not stabilize neuronal circuitry like partial or full opioid agonists and generally results in poor outcomes, much like Antabuse for alcohol.
- Opioid partial agonist therapy: buprenorphine.
- Opioid agonist therapy: methadone.

NOTE: Buprenorphine and methadone are both metabolized by the cytochrome P450 3a4 and 2d6 I isoenzyme pathways. Prescribers should be aware of multiple possible drug interactions.

PATIENT SELECTION FOR BUPRENORPHINE OR METHADONE

- Appropriate patients for buprenorphine office-based treatment:
  - Patients interested (highly motivated) in treatment
  - Have no major contraindications (see following)
  - Can be expected to be reasonably compliant with treatment
  - Understand the benefits and risks of buprenorphine treatment
  - Willing to follow safety precautions
- Less likely to be appropriate for office-based treatment:
  - Have comorbid dependence on benzodiazepines or other CNS depressants (including ethylene alcohol)
  - Have significant untreated psychiatric comorbidities
  - Have active or chronic suicidal or homicidal ideation or attempts
  - Have multiple previous treatments with frequent relapses
  - Have poor response to previous treatment with buprenorphine
  - Have significant medical complications (e.g., hepatic insufficiency, bacterial endocarditis, active tuberculosis)
- Methadone maintenance: narcotic treatment program (clinic setting) indications
- Evidence of opiate addiction >1 yr
- Two failed previous treatment attempts
- Patients not appropriate for office-based treatment
- Eligible without active "use" if prior methadone maintenance patient within previous 2 mo
- Pregnancy

DISPOSITION

- Opioid addiction is a chronic, relapsing disease.
- High rate of relapse after "detox."
- Relapse potential after medically supervised withdrawal from methadone:
  - 90% after 1 yr stable in treatment
  - 80% after 3 yr stable in treatment
  - 70% after 5 yr stable in treatment

REFERRAL

Refer to addiction medicine specialist or narcotic treatment program when the neurobiologic disease of opioid addiction is identified.

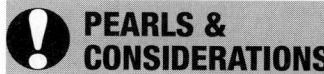 **PEARLS & CONSIDERATIONS**

COMMENTS

- Methadone maintenance is the gold standard for the pregnant opiate-addicted patient re-

gardless of the duration of the addiction or prior treatment attempts. Detoxification is contraindicated during pregnancy.
- Breastfeeding is encouraged in mothers on methadone maintenance. The American Academy of Pediatrics statement regarding "Transfer of Drugs and Other Chemicals into Human Milk" has placed methadone into the "usually compatible with breastfeeding" group based on the assumption that maternal urine is monitored to detect use of illicit drugs. The U.S. Department of Health and Human Services also recommends that mothers on methadone be encouraged to breastfeed.
- When a physician identifies a patient as a "drug seeker," it is imperative that the physician avoid abruptly stopping the opiate prescription because this will often result in the patient's buying the drugs illegally. These patients should be counseled and referred for treatment.
- Patients on methadone or buprenorphine who have pain resulting from an acute injury will need pain medication in addition to their daily dose of methadone or buprenorphine. They will require higher than usual doses of pain medications because of opiate receptor blockade attributable to their methadone or buprenorphine use.
- Opiate-dependent patients have a lower pain threshold resulting from hyperalgesia caused by the long-term use of opiates.

PREVENTION

Education is the hallmark of prevention.
- School drug prevention education programs.
- Educate children about their family medical history, including diseases of addiction.
- Address childhood psychiatric disorders to prevent self-medicating.

PATIENT & FAMILY EDUCATION

- Stigma of addictions and treatment often interferes with good treatment.
- Family needs to be educated so they can support the patient's efforts.
- Encourage family meeting with addiction specialist, counselor.
- Recommend support groups for family members.

SUGGESTED READINGS
available at www.expertconsult.com

RELATED CONTENT
Drug Abuse (Patient Information)

AUTHOR: **STEVEN PELIGIAN, D.O.**

BASIC INFORMATION

DEFINITION

Oppositional defiant disorder (ODD) is an ongoing pattern of uncooperative, defiant, and hostile behavior toward authority figures that is not developmentally appropriate, lasts more than 6 months, and leads to impairment in social, academic, or occupational functioning for a child or adolescent.

SYNONYMS

ODD

ICD-9CM CODES

313.81 Oppositional defiant disorder

EPIDEMIOLOGY & DEMOGRAPHICS

PEAK INCIDENCE:
- Usually diagnosed in school-aged children (roughly ages 6-12)

PREVALENCE:
- Ranges from 1% to 16% based on source (community prevalence)

PREDOMINANT SEX AND AGE:
- Males more than females
- Highest diagnosis in prepubertal children
- Usually present by age 8

GENETICS:
- Some evidence for genetic factors, but studies are not usually specific to ODD (e.g., studies also include conduct disorder or more generally refer to aggressive or delinquent behaviors) and include potential confounding factors (e.g., difficult to distinguish between genetic and environmental contribution)

RISK FACTORS:
- Male gender, low socioeconomic status
- The following risk factors have been identified more generally for development of disruptive behavior disorders or aggression:
  - Family history (especially parental) of aggressive or criminal behaviors
  - Parental substance abuse
  - Prenatal or early childhood exposure to toxins (e.g., lead)
  - Perinatal complications
  - Head injuries
  - Cognitive impairment
  - Learning disabilities
  - History of abuse or witnessed domestic violence
  - Overall family instability

PHYSICAL FINDINGS & CLINICAL PRESENTATION

DSM-IV criteria are met when four or more of the following symptoms are present for at least 6 months:
- Frequent temper tantrums
- Excessive arguing with adults
- Often questioning rules
- Active defiance and refusal to comply with adult requests and rules
- Deliberate attempts to annoy or upset people
- Blaming others for his or her mistakes or misbehavior
- Often touchy or easily annoyed by others
- Frequent anger and resentment
- Mean and hateful talking when upset
- Spiteful attitude and revenge-seeking

Symptoms usually occur in more than one setting (e.g., home, school) and cause significant impairment in social, academic, and/or occupational functioning. Symptoms may not occur only during an active, untreated mood episode or in the context of conduct disorder.

ETIOLOGY

Multiple hypothetical models have been developed for disruptive behavior disorders and antisocial behaviors in general, including a few focused specifically on ODD that address the complex interaction between various predisposing and protective factors. These models identify some biologic factors (including genetic, structural, toxin exposure, etc.), some child functional factors (including cognitive, social, and neuropsychological deficits), and broad psychosocial factors that focus on parenting styles (including history of physical abuse), peer involvement, and other environmental factors.

DIAGNOSIS

DIFFERENTIAL DIAGNOSIS

- Child abuse or neglect
- Learning disorder or other deficits in executive functioning
- Mental retardation
- Language disorder
- Attention-deficit/hyperactivity disorder
- Conduct disorder
- Mood disorder (bipolar disorder or depression)
- Parent-child relational problem

WORKUP

- Diagnosis is made based on history, including individual and family interviews as well as collateral data from additional sources (parents, teachers, other medical providers, therapist, etc.).

LABORATORY TESTS

- None indicated

IMAGING STUDIES

- None indicated

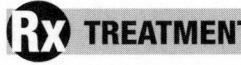 TREATMENT

Initial treatment of ODD should include psychosocial interventions aimed at changing the maladaptive patterns of interaction between the child or adolescent and his or her family and environment. If the interventions listed here are not effective, or if serious concerns exist regarding safety or impairment in functioning, pharmacologic interventions targeting specific symptoms (such as aggression) or comorbid disorders (such as ADHD, anxiety disorders, or mood disorders) may help. There are currently no medications approved by the FDA for the treatment of ODD.

NONPHARMACOLOGIC THERAPY

- Parent management training
- Cognitive problem-solving skills training
- Social skills training
- Individual psychotherapy
- Family psychotherapy

ACUTE GENERAL Rx

- Medication may be considered as an adjunct to behavioral treatment or in cases where comorbidity is a factor. There is some evidence for symptom improvement with trials of stimulants, mood stabilizers, or atypical antipsychotics, but medication should never be used alone or as first-line treatment for ODD.
- Higher levels of care such as a hospital or acute residential setting may be required for stabilization if acute safety concerns develop in the context of ODD, such as severe aggression.

COMPLEMENTARY & ALTERNATIVE MEDICINE

No evidence-based treatments are available.

DISPOSITION

Most patients with ODD can be managed in an outpatient setting with either standard or intensive, home-based support; treatment should always be provided in the least restrictive setting possible. Hospitalization is sometimes necessary for crisis management only; consideration of different levels of care, including day treatment, therapeutic school settings, or residential facilities, may be appropriate for more severe cases or in situations where the family is not willing or able to participate adequately in the outpatient regimen.

REFERRAL

Consider referral to a mental health provider specializing in the treatment of children, adolescents, and families (including potentially a child and adolescent psychiatrist) if the patient and family are not responding to basic parenting interventions or are demonstrating significant safety concerns or other evidence of impairment in functioning at home, in school, or in the community.

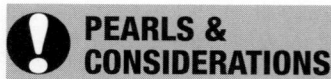

PEARLS & CONSIDERATIONS

COMMENTS

- Involvement of the family and school is crucial in the management of patients with this disorder.
- Polypharmacy (the prescribing of multiple medications simultaneously) to target the more complicated symptoms of this disorder should be implemented with great caution and only after discrete trials of therapeutic interventions and single medication agents have failed.
- Standardized assessment tools used to identify ADHD, disruptive behavior disorders, and general child and adolescent psychopathology may be helpful in confirming the diagnosis of ODD and/or monitoring progress throughout treatment.

- ODD symptoms are independently associated with increased externalizing symptoms, internalizing symptoms, delinquent behaviors, and social and academic functioning.
- One-time, intensive interventions are not considered effective treatment options (including boot camps, shock incarceration) and may carry additional risks.
- When ODD coexists with attention deficit/hyperactivity disorder, stimulant therapy can reduce the symptoms of both disorders.

PREVENTION

Most effective prevention strategies include both individualized treatment and universal interventions that incorporate a parent-directed component as one of the primary elements. They also may incorporate social-cognitive skills training, academic skills training, proactive classroom management and teacher training, and group therapy. These may take place in schools, clinics, and other community-based settings in addition to targeted clinical work.

PATIENT & FAMILY EDUCATION

ODD: A Guide for Families by the American Academy of Child and Adolescent Psychiatry (http://www.aacap.org/cs/ODD.ResourceCenter)
American Academy of Pediatrics: HealthyChildren.org (http://www.healthychildren.org/English/health-issues/conditions/emotional-problems/Pages/Disruptive-Behavior-Disorders.aspx)

SUGGESTED READINGS

available at www.expertconsult.com

RELATED CONTENT

Attention Deficit/Hyperactivity Disorder (Related Key Topic)
Conduct Disorder (Related Key Topic)

AUTHOR: **ELIZABETH A. LOWENHAUPT, M.D.**

BASIC INFORMATION

DEFINITION

- *Optic atrophy* refers to the degeneration of the axons of the optic nerve.
- It is a symptom rather than a disease.

SYNONYMS

Unilateral/bilateral optic atrophy

ICD-9CM CODES
377.10 Atrophy, optic nerve

EPIDEMIOLOGY & DEMOGRAPHICS

PREDOMINANT SEX: Unilateral optic atrophy in women is most commonly multiple sclerosis (MS); may also occur after head injury (more commonly in men)
PREDOMINANT AGE: 21 to 40 yr
PEAK INCIDENCE: Varies depending on cause

PHYSICAL FINDINGS & CLINICAL PRESENTATION

- Asymmetry of disc color is often first subtle finding.
- Temporal part of optic disc is pale initially (Fig. 1-597); later the entire disc becomes pale/white.
- Optic disc pallor occurs 4 to 6 wk after optic nerve injury.

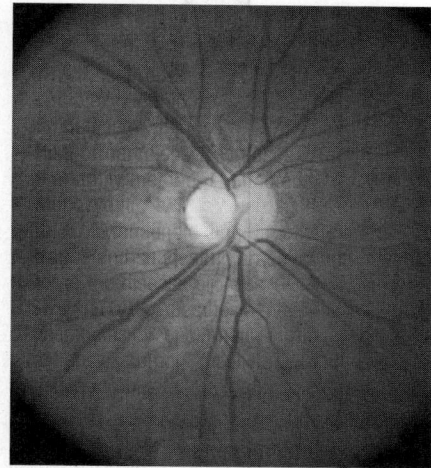

FIGURE 1-597 Optic atrophy. Patient's right eye shows atrophy. (Courtesy John W. Payne, M.D., The Wilmer Ophthalmological Institute, The Johns Hopkins University and Hospital, Baltimore. From Seidel HM [ed]: *Mosby's guide to physical examination,* ed 4, St Louis, 1999, Mosby.)

- Unilateral lesion produces a relative afferent pupillary defect (RAPD): swing flashlight eye to eye; abnormal pupil dilates to direct light.
- Decreased visual acuity, blurred vision, visual field deficits (e.g., central scotoma), abnormal color vision (e.g., red desaturation).

ETIOLOGY

- Optic neuritis—MS, sarcoidosis, infections (syphilis, CMV, HIV, Lyme disease)
- Vascular—ischemic optic neuropathy, central retinal artery occlusion, temporal arteritis
- Compression—glaucoma, pituitary tumor, meningioma, thyroid eye disease
- Hereditary—Leber's hereditary optic neuropathy
- Nutritional, toxic, and metabolic—amiodarone, isoniazid, B_{12} deficiency, tobacco, alcohol
- Trauma

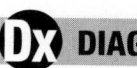

DIAGNOSIS

DIFFERENTIAL DIAGNOSIS

- Nutritional, toxic, and hereditary causes are usually bilateral.
- Unilateral optic atrophy in a young person is more commonly MS.
- Postviral atrophy may be seen in childhood.

WORKUP

- Depends on suspected cause/clinical presentation. History including age of onset, risk factors, acuity of onset of symptoms, trauma, presence of pain, family history, toxic/nutritional factors, and other associated neurologic findings should be considered.
- Visual field testing may help identify cause (e.g., centrocecal field defects may occur with nutritional/toxic causes), but specificity is low.
- To differentiate between optic nerve and macular disease an Amsler chart and/or visual evoked responses may be helpful.
- If high clinical suspicion for MS, consider MRI of brain with contrast, evoked potentials, and LP with oligoclonal bands.
- Measure intraocular pressure (glaucoma).

LABORATORY TESTS

- Depends on suspected cause: none for trauma, tumor, or MS
- Serum B_{12}
- Autoimmune diseases: ESR, ANA, ACE

IMAGING STUDIES

- MRI of the brain with contrast, fat suppression, and special (thin) cuts through orbits is necessary to identify compressive lesions in all patients with unexplained optic atrophy; especially important in patients with positive predictive factors for abnormal imaging (e.g., young age, progression, bilateral findings).
- If sarcoid is suspected, order chest x-ray.

TREATMENT

ACUTE GENERAL Rx

Treat the underlying cause—discontinue identifiable toxins, use B_{12} replacement, neurosurgical intervention is necessary if tumor is found; consider IV steroids if there is evidence for active demyelinating disease.

CHRONIC Rx

The optic nerve does not regenerate, although symptoms often improve.

DISPOSITION

- Visual loss usually occurs over weeks to months.
- Appointment with neurologist or ophthalmologist

REFERRAL

If tumor or demyelinating lesions are found or if etiology is unknown

PEARLS & CONSIDERATIONS

COMMENTS

- An experienced clinician should be able to identify pale optic discs and an RAPD.
- Pupillary dilation with mydriatic agents (e.g., pilocarpine) may be necessary to optimize funduscopic examination.
- Patient education material can be obtained from the National Eye Institute, Department of Health and Human Services, 9000 Rockville Pike, Bethesda, MD 20892.

SUGGESTED READINGS
available at www.expertconsult.com

AUTHOR: **RICHARD S. ISAACSON, M.D.**

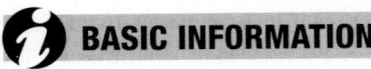

DEFINITION

Optic neuritis is an inflammation of the optic nerve resulting in impaired visual function.

SYNONYMS

Optic papillitis
Retrobulbar neuritis

ICD-9CM CODES
377.3 Optic neuritis

EPIDEMIOLOGY & DEMOGRAPHICS

INCIDENCE (IN U.S.): 1 to 5/100,000 person(s) per year; rates vary according to incidence of multiple sclerosis (MS)
PREVALENCE (IN U.S.): Common in patients with MS
PREDOMINANT SEX: Female/male ratio: 1.8:1
PEAK INCIDENCE: 20 to 49 yr, mean 30
GENETICS: Unknown. If due to MS, it is more common in patients with certain HLA blood types and in monozygotic twins of affected siblings. See topic "Multiple Sclerosis."

PHYSICAL FINDINGS & CLINICAL PRESENTATION

- Presents with acute or subacute (days) visual loss, often accompanied by periocular pain that worsens with eye movements.
- **Marcus Gunn pupil** (relative afferent pupillary defect [RAPD]): direct and consensual response is normal; however, when flashlight is swung from eye to eye, the affected eye's pupil dilates to direct light.
- Decreased visual acuity
- Unilateral visual field abnormalities—often a central scotoma (Fig. E1-598)
- Color desaturation; red is most often affected
- Normal orbit and fundus; occasionally there is disc edema acutely (Fig. 1-599), uveitis, or periphlebitis.
- May have movement or light-induced phosphenes (flashes of light lasting 1 to 2 sec).
- Uhthoff's phenomenon (benign exercise–or heat-induced deterioration of vision) is seen

in some. Vision may also worsen in bright sunlight.
- Over time the optic disc may atrophy and become pale.

ETIOLOGY

An inflammatory response associated with an infection, autoimmune disease (such as MS or neuromyelitis optica), or, rarely, a mitochondrial disorder

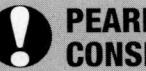 DIAGNOSIS

Consistent clinical presentation and exclusion of alternate ocular pathology, infection, and CNS mass lesions. Classic triad includes loss of vision, pain, and dyschromatopsia. 70% unilateral and 30% bilateral.

DIFFERENTIAL DIAGNOSIS

- Inflammatory: MS, neuromyelitis optica (NMO), sarcoidosis, lupus, Sjögren's, Behçet's, postinfectious, postvaccination, neuroretinitis, acute disseminated encephalomyelitis, paraneoplastic, autoimmune optic neuropathy (with retinopathy is ARRONS)
- Infectious: syphilis, TB, Lyme disease, *Bartonella*, HIV, CMV, herpes, helminths, chickenpox. Q fever, periorbital infections, *Toxocara* sp.
- Ischemic: giant cell arteritis, anterior and posterior ischemic optic neuropathies, diabetic papillopathy, branch or central retinal artery or vein occlusion
- Mitochondrial: Leber's hereditary optic neuropathy
- Mass lesion: pituitary tumor, aneurysm, meningioma, glioma, metastases, sinus mucocele
- Ocular: optic drusen, retinal detachment, vitreous hemorrhage, uveitis, posterior scleritis, neuroretinitis, maculopathies, and retinopathies
- Drugs, toxins, and nutritional: toxins (arsenic, tobacco, etc.), medications (amiodarone, cyclosporine, etc.), and vitamin deficiencies (B_{12}, B_1, B_6, niacin).
- Other: acute papilledema, retinal migraine, factitious visual loss

WORKUP

A thorough neurologic examination; recommend dilated ophthalmoscopy

LABORATORY TESTS

- Recommend CBC, ANA, ACE, ESR.
- Consider HIV Ab, Lyme titer, RPR, other inflammatory or infectious causes.
- Bilateral or recurrent ON:NMO IgG; paraneoplastic CRMP-5-IgG

IMAGING STUDIES

MRI of the brain and orbits (thin section fat-suppressed T_2-weighted) with gadolinium to look for compressive and infiltrative causes. Often enhancement of the optic nerve is seen. The risk to develop MS should be assessed.

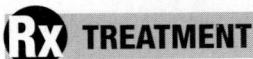 TREATMENT

NONPHARMACOLOGIC THERAPY

Assure patient that in most cases there is near complete recovery of vision.

ACUTE GENERAL Rx

Treat if the visual loss is severe or if there is an abnormal MRI (higher risk of MS). Treatment is with methylprednisolone (MP) 250 mg IV every 6 hr for 3 days followed by an oral prednisone taper of 11 days. MP 1 g IV every day for 3 days followed by an oral MP taper is an alternative.

CHRONIC Rx

None, unless at high risk to develop MS. See topic "Multiple Sclerosis."

DISPOSITION

Most often vision is worst at the end of week 1, followed by recovery over several months. In the Optic Neuritis Treatment Trial (ONTT), 90% had 20/40 or better vision at 1 yr and 3% had 20/200 or worse. Of initial 20/200 or worse cases, only 5% remained in that group at 6 mo.

REFERRAL

- To neurologist if patient has other neurologic signs; urgently needed if proptosis or ophthalmoplegia present
- To ophthalmologist when atypical features or slowly progressive, and urgently when other ocular pathology is present
- To ophthalmologist if vision worsens or does not improve after several wk, pain is severe or persistent, or vision deteriorates as steroids are tapered

 PEARLS & CONSIDERATIONS

- Bilateral optic neuritis suggests a systemic inflammatory disorder, infection, NMO, or paraneoplastic but can also occur in MS.
- Acute bilateral loss of vision with a severe headache or diplopia should raise concern for pituitary apoplexy.

EBM EVIDENCE

available at www.expertconsult.com

SUGGESTED READINGS
available at www.expertconsult.com

RELATED CONTENT

Multiple Sclerosis (Related Key Topic)

AUTHOR: **ALEXANDRA DEGENHARDT, M.D.**

FIGURE 1-599 A case of optic neuritis. The optic disc edema seen here is often not present. Note the otherwise normal fundus. (Courtesy of J. Barton, M.D., Beth Israel Deaconess Medical Center, Boston.)

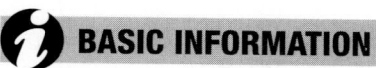

BASIC INFORMATION

DEFINITION

Oral cancer is malignant cell formation in the oral cavity and may occur as a primary lesion initiating in any of the oral tissues, by metastasis from a distant site of origin, or by extension from a neighboring anatomic structure such as the nasal cavity or the maxillary sinus.

SYNONYMS

Oral cancer
Oropharyngeal cancer

ICD-9CM CODES
140.0-149.0 Code varies with specific
anatomic structure

EPIDEMIOLOGY & DEMOGRAPHICS

INCIDENCE & PREVALENCE: Oral and pharyngeal cancer is the sixth most common cancer in the world. An estimated half a million cases are diagnosed annually around the globe and the rates have been rising, particularly in young people. In 2011, oropharyngeal squamous cell carcinoma (OP-SCCA) affected >12,000 new patients, with the most common sites being the tonsillar fossa and base of the tongue. In the U.S., the incidence of OP-SCCA linked to alcohol and tobacco use has been declining, whereas those linked to human papillomavirus (HPV), primarily HPV type 16, is on the increase. In Asian countries where chewing betel nut is customary, oral cancer accounts for up to 40% of cancers in some regions (Ayaz, 2011). Squamous cell carcinoma is the most common malignancy that occurs in the oral cavity. Minor salivary gland cancers, lymphomas, and sarcomas are less common.

PREDOMINANT SEX & AGE:
- Predominantly male, middle aged
- Black males have a higher early incidence in the 50- to 60-yr age group, but with increasing age, white men predominate.

GENETICS: There is no specific genetic factor or translocation, but the human papillomavirus (HPV)–induced oral squamous cell cancer typically seen in younger populations is associated with loss of p53 tumor suppressor due to inactivation by E6 protein from the virus.

RISK FACTORS:
- Tobacco
- HPV infection (primarily types 16 and 18)
- Alcohol
- Immune deficiency
- Syphilis
- Radiation
- Vitamin A deficiency
- Betel nut consumption

PHYSICAL FINDINGS & CLINICAL PRESENTATION

- Often starts as a tiny, unnoticed white or red spot or sore anywhere in the mouth.

- Most lesions begin on the tongue or buccal mucosa.
- Clinically, oral cancer can present as:
  ○ Erythroplakia (flat red patch)
    Can mimic inflammatory or traumatic lesions.
  ○ Leukoplakia (white patch; Fig. 1-600)
  ○ Raised lesion
  ○ Ulcerated lesion
  ○ White warty lesion
- The borders of the oral cavity can be defined as from the skin-vermilion junction of the lips to the junction of the hard and soft palate above and to the line of the circumvallate papilla of the tongue below. The lateral boundary between the oral cavity and oropharynx consists of the anterior tonsillar pillars and glossotonsillar folds.
- Oral cavity cancer can present on the lip, floor of the mouth, oral tongue (anterior two thirds of the tongue), lower alveolar ridge, upper alveolar ridge, retromolar trigone (retromolar gingiva), hard palate, and buccal mucosa.
- Oral cavity tumors often present with local invasion, tissue destruction, and lymph node metastases.
- Oral cancers rarely have distant metastases at the time of presentation, although this may vary depending on the length of time until presentation.

DIAGNOSIS

DIFFERENTIAL DIAGNOSIS

- Traumatic ulcerative granuloma with stromal eosinophilia, especially on the tongue
- Deep fungal infections
- Chancre of early syphilis and gumma of tertiary syphilis
- Chronic ulcer

WORKUP

- Primary workup includes biopsy of the presenting lesion.
- Pretreatment evaluation: Tumor size, the extent of invasion, and the presence or absence of regional lymph node metastases are critical for planning treatment.
- Workup includes staging the cancer: The tumor-node-metastasis (TNM) staging system of the American Joint Committee on Cancer (AJCC) and the International Union for Cancer Control (UICC) is used to classify lip and oral cavity carcinoma.
- By definition, patients with early (stage I and II) disease have tumors <4 cm in greatest dimension without deep invasion into surrounding structures and have no evidence of lymph node involvement.
- Oral cavity cancers tend to invade bone and soft tissue early in their natural history. Therefore, pretreatment imaging studies, such as magnetic resonance imaging (MRI) and computed tomography (CT), are required

in addition to a thorough inspection and palpation of the oral cavity.

LABORATORY TESTS

Send biopsy specimen to oral and maxillofacial pathology, head and neck pathology, or general pathology.

IMAGING STUDIES

Consider MRI or CT based on the extent of clinical presentation.

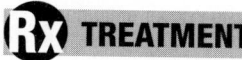

TREATMENT

- Surgery vs. radiation therapy:
  ○ Both primary surgery and definitive radiation therapy are options for patients with oral cavity cancer.
  ○ Outcomes with primary surgery and definitive radiation therapy appear to be similar based on retrospective studies, but the two modes of treatment have not been compared in randomized controlled trials.
- Surgery is generally favored because it is typically associated with less morbidity than radiation therapy. Surgical therapy traditionally involved wide-exposure approaches (mandibulotomy, transpharyngeal access). Newer surgical techniques allow tumor resection through the mouth. Recently, transoral robotic surgery (TORS) has been developed to improve access to oropharyngeal squamous cell carcinomas with excellent oncologic outcomes.
  ○ Acute surgical complications can include infection, bleeding, aspiration, wound breakdown, fistula, and flap loss.
  ○ Surgical procedures can cause functional deficits in speech and swallowing, but these adverse effects can be minimized by appropriate reconstruction.
- Definitive radiation therapy is reserved for patients who cannot tolerate surgery or for whom surgical resection would result in particularly severe functional impairment.
  ○ Radiation therapy can include external beam radiation and brachytherapy.
  ○ Radiation therapy side effects include mucositis, skin reaction, loss of taste, dysphagia, and xerostomia.
  ○ Late complications can include skin and soft tissue atrophy and fibrosis, osteoradionecrosis, and trismus.
- Close margins, typically defined as <5 mm, are associated with a worse prognosis.
- Adjuvant chemotherapy may also be an option in treatment regimen.

DISPOSITION

- Prognosis depends on the stage and extent of cancer.
- Tumor HPV status is a strong and independent prognostic factor for survival among patients with oropharyngeal cancer.

REFERRAL

Refer to oral and maxillofacial or ear, nose, and throat surgeon.

PEARLS & CONSIDERATIONS

COMMENTS

- Oral and pharyngeal cancer is the sixth most common cancer globally.
- Biopsy is the key for diagnosis.
- Posttreatment surveillance is important.

PREVENTION

- Encourage patients to stop smoking.
- Examine oral cavities at annual checkups and work up suspicious lesions.

PATIENT & FAMILY EDUCATION

http://globocan.iarc.fr/factsheets/populations/factsheet.asp?uno=900.

EBM EVIDENCE

available at www.expertconsult.com

SUGGESTED READINGS

available at www.expertconsult.com

RELATED CONTENT

Mouth Cancer (Patient Information)

AUTHOR: **PRIYA SARIN GUPTA, M.D., M.P.H.**

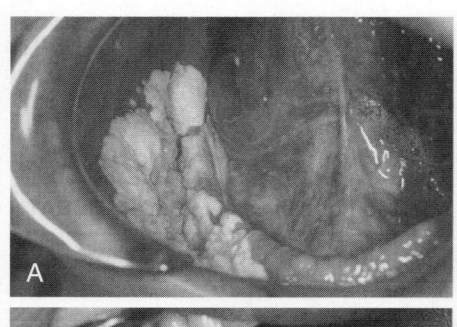
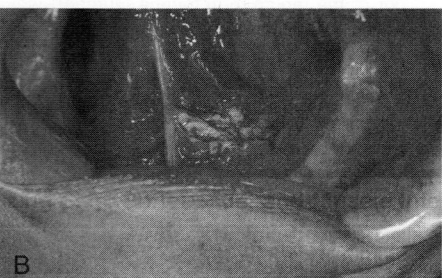
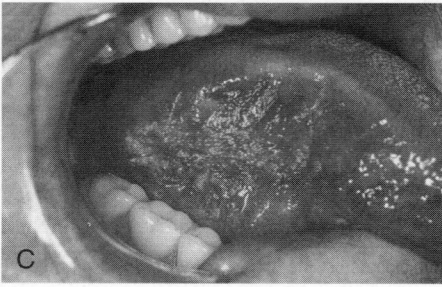

FIGURE 1-600 Squamous cell carcinoma of the oral mucosa. A, Leukoplakia. **B,** Invasive carcinoma of the floor of the mouth. **C,** Invasive carcinoma of the tongue. (Courtesy G. Putnam. In White GM, Cox NH [eds]: *Diseases of the skin: a color atlas and text,* ed 2, St Louis, 2006, Mosby.)

BASIC INFORMATION

DEFINITION

Orchitis is an inflammatory process (usually infectious) involving the testicles. Infection may be viral or bacterial and can be associated with infection of other male sex organs (prostate, epididymis, or bladder) or lower urogenital tract or sexually transmitted diseases often via hematogenous spread. Common causes are:

- Viral: mumps—20% postpubertal; coxsackie B virus
- Bacterial: pyogenic via spread from involving epididymis; bacteria include *Escherichia coli, Klebsiella pneumoniae, P. aeruginosa, Staphylococcus, Streptococcus* or *Rickettsia, Brucella* spp.
- Other:
  - Viral—HIV-associated, CMV
  - Fungi
    1. Cryptococcosis
    2. Histoplasmosis
    3. *Candida*
    4. Blastomycosis
    5. Syphilis
  - *Mycobacterium tuberculosis* and *M. leprae*
  - Parasitic causes: toxoplasmosis, filiariasis, schistosomiasis
- Table E1-306 describes a classification of epididymitis and orchitis based on etiology.

SYNONYMS

Epididymoorchitis
Testicular infection
Testicular inflammation

ICD-9CM CODES
0.72   Mumps
098.13   Acute gonococcal orchitis
095.8   Syphilitic orchitis
016.50   Tuberculous orchitis, unspecified

EPIDEMIOLOGY & DEMOGRAPHICS

PREDOMINANT SEX: Male
PREDOMINANT ORGANISM: The leading cause of viral orchitis is mumps. The mumps virus rarely causes orchitis in prepubertal males but involves one or both testicles in nearly 30% of postpubertal males.

PHYSICAL FINDINGS & CLINICAL PRESENTATION

- Testicular pain, unilateral or bilateral swelling
- May have associated epididymitis, prostatitis, fever, scrotal edema, erythema, cellulitis
- Inguinal lymphadenopathy
- Acute hydrocele (bacterial)
- Rare development: abscess formation, pyocele of scrotum, testicular infarction
- Spermatic cord tenderness may be present
- Granulomatous

DIAGNOSIS

Clinical presentation as described previously with possible history of acute viral illness or concomitant epididymitis.

DIFFERENTIAL DIAGNOSIS

- Epididymoorchitis-gonococcal
- Autoimmune disease
- Vasculitis
- Epididymyosis
- Mumps, with or without parotitis
- Neoplasm
- Hematoma
- Spermatic cord torsion

LABORATORY TESTS

- CBC with differential
- Urinalysis
- Viral titer—mumps
- Urine culture
- Ultrasound of testicle to rule out abscess

IMAGING STUDIES

Ultrasound if abscess suspected (Fig. 1-601)

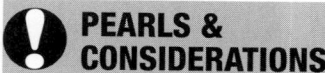

TREATMENT

- Dependent on cause
- Viral (mumps): observation; bed rest, ice packs, analgesics, and a scrotal sling for support may provide some relief of discomfort that accompanies mumps orchitis
- Bacterial: empiric antibiotic treatment with parenteral antibiotic treatment until pathogen identified: ceftriaxone (250 mg IM once) plus doxycycline (100 mg PO bid for 10 days), in men <35 yr old to cover *Neisseria gonorrhoeae* and Chlamydia trachomatis. In homosexual men or men >35 yr old: levofloxacin 500-750 mg IV/PO qd for 10-14 days *or* ampicillin-sulbactam *or* third-generation cephalosporin or ticarcillin-clavulanate.
- Surgery for abscess, pyogenic process

DISPOSITION

Follow-up for evidence of recurrence, hypogonadism, and infertility may be needed with bilateral orchitis.

REFERRAL

- To a urologist if surgical drainage is needed
- To an endocrinologist if hypogonadism develops
- To a fertility specialist if infertility develops

PEARLS & CONSIDERATIONS

Consider tuberculous orchitis if symptoms fail to respond to standard antibacterial therapy, even in the absence of chest radiographic evidence of pulmonary tuberculosis.

SUGGESTED READINGS

available at www.expertconsult.com

RELATED CONTENT

Orchitis (Patient Information)
Epididymitis (Related Key Topic)

AUTHOR: **GLENN G. FORT, M.D., M.P.H.**

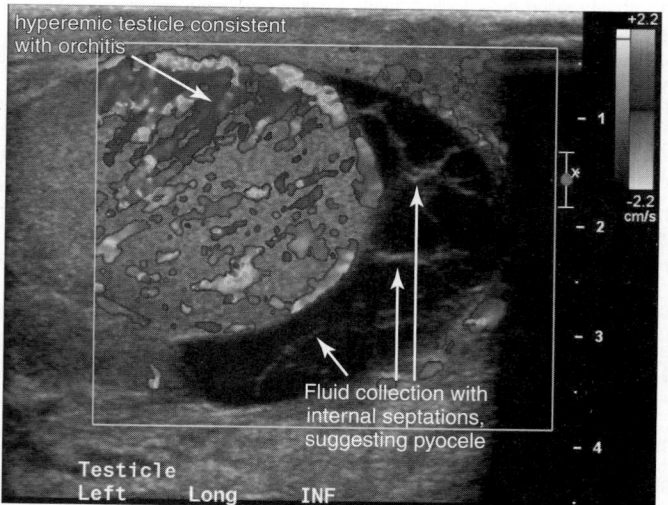

FIGURE 1-601 Orchitis with pyocele: testicular ultrasound. The left testicle is markedly hyperemic on color Doppler ultrasound compared with the right testicle (not shown), consistent with orchitis. There is complex fluid collection with internal septations and internal echoes that is predominantly located inferior to the testicle and raises concern for a pyocele. Simple hydroceles are homogenously black without internal echoes. Fluid collections with internal structure are more likely to represent infection or blood products, whereas simple fluid is more likely serous. (From Broder JS: *Diagnostic imaging for the emergency physician,* Philadelphia, 2011, Saunders.)

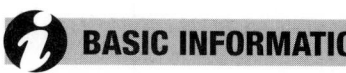

BASIC INFORMATION

DEFINITION

Orthostatic hypotension (OH) is defined as the presence of at least one of the following: a decrease in systolic blood pressure by ≥20 mm Hg or a decrease in diastolic blood pressure by ≥10 mm Hg within 3 min of standing. It is a physical sign that requires further investigation to discern its underlying etiology.

SYNONYMS

Postural hypotension

ICD-9CM CODES
458.0 Orthostatic hypotension

EPIDEMIOLOGY & DEMOGRAPHICS

- The incidence of OH is increased in older people and in those with diseases associated with autonomic dysfunction (e.g., Parkinson disease, diabetes mellitus).
- OH may cause up to 30% of all syncopal events in the elderly, and OH is associated with an increased risk of heart failure among those aged 45 to 55 yr and an increased risk of cardiovascular disease and all-cause mortality among those aged 55 yr and older.

PHYSICAL FINDINGS & CLINICAL PRESENTATION

- Symptoms may include dizziness, lightheadedness, syncope, visual and auditory disturbances, weakness, diaphoresis, pallor, and nausea. OH may also be asymptomatic, especially in older hypertensive patients.
- Associated with increased autonomic activity during meals (from increased splanchnic blood flow), exercise, and hot weather.
- Supine and nocturnal hypertension in patients with OH may indicate an underlying autonomic dysfunction.

ETIOLOGY

- The assumption of an upright posture results in the pooling of approximately 500 ml of blood in the lower extremities due to gravity and decreased venous return, decreased cardiac output, and decreased arterial pressure. The consequent increase in sympathetic tone due to increased carotid baroreceptor activity causes arterial and venous constriction as well as positive inotropic and chronotropic effects, thereby limiting the fall in upright blood pressure. Peripheral vasoconstriction is also mediated by increased activity of the renin-angiotensin system and decreased activity of atrial natriuretic factor.
- Impairment of the baroreceptor reflex, as in central or peripheral autonomic dysfunction and aging, may cause OH because decreased blood pressure cannot be counteracted by the aforementioned regulatory mechanisms.

DIAGNOSIS

DIFFERENTIAL DIAGNOSIS

Common:
- Medications: antihypertensives, antidepressants (tricyclics), antipsychotics (phenothiazines), alcohol, narcotics, barbiturates, insulin, nitrates, PDE-5 inhibitors, alpha-adrenergic antagonists
- Reduced intravascular volume (hemorrhage, dehydration, hyperglycemia, hypoalbuminemia)
- Postprandial effect (especially in the elderly)
- Vasovagal syncope
- Deconditioning
- Central autonomic dysfunction (Parkinson's disease)
- Peripheral autonomic dysfunction (diabetes mellitus, Guillain-Barré syndrome)

Uncommon:
- Central autonomic dysfunction (Shy-Drager syndrome)
- Postganglionic autonomic dysfunction: impaired norepinephrine release
- Autoimmune autonomic dysfunction: nicotinic acetylcholine receptor autoantibodies
- Paraneoplastic autonomic dysfunction: anti-Hu antibodies (in small-cell lung cancer)
- Postural tachycardia syndrome (POTS): usually occurs in young women; an abnormally large increase in heart rate is observed in the upright position caused by increased venous pooling from autonomic dysfunction of the lower extremities, but blood pressure is not affected because of an excess of plasma norepinephrine
- Impaired cardiac output (myocardial infarction, aortic stenosis, arrhythmias)
- Cerebrovascular accident
- Adrenal insufficiency
- Deconditioning
- Carotid sinus hypersensitivity
- Anxiety, panic attacks
- Seizures
- Sepsis
- Idiopathic

WORKUP

- Measure supine blood pressure after the patient has been resting comfortably, stand for 3 min, then measure upright blood pressure. The blood pressure cuff must be held at the level of the right atrium; holding the cuff below this level will result in a 5 to 10 mm Hg underestimation of blood pressure.
- Thorough neurologic examination should be performed.
- Rule out treatable causes (e.g., medications, volume depletion).
- Table 1-307 describes a grading of orthostatic intolerance.

LABORATORY TESTS

- Hemoglobin and hematocrit
- Consider when treatable causes of OH have been ruled out:
  ○ Blood pressure and heart rate monitoring with a tilt table test
  ○ Plasma norepinephrine measurements (to distinguish postganglionic from preganglionic autonomic dysfunction)
  ○ Other methods, which use the Valsalva maneuver or measure sweating as indirect means of evaluating the autonomic nervous system

IMAGING STUDIES

None

TABLE 1-307 Grading of Orthostatic Intolerance

Grade	Symptom Frequency	Activities of Daily Living in the Upright Posture	Standing Time (on Most Occasions)	Orthostatic Blood Pressure
I	Infrequent orthostatic symptoms developing only under conditions of increased stress*	Unrestricted	>15 min	May or may not be abnormal
II	Intermittent orthostatic symptoms occurring at least weekly	Some limitation	>5 min	Some changes in cardiovascular indexes (e.g., oscillations or decrease in pulse pressure by >50%)
III	Frequent orthostatic symptoms occurring on most occasions	Marked limitation	>1 min	Orthostatic hypotension is present >50% of the time, recorded on different days
IV	Orthostatic symptoms are consistently present	Incapacitated and unable to stand without presyncope or syncope developing	<1 min	Orthostatic hypotension is severe and consistently present

*Conditions that increase orthostatic stress include dehydration, deconditioning from prolonged bed rest, physical exertion, heat stress, and medications that lower blood pressure or impair adrenergic function.

Modified from Low PA, Singer W: Update on management of neurogenic orthostatic hypotension, *Lancet Neurol* 7:451-458, 2008.

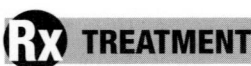 **TREATMENT**

NONPHARMACOLOGIC THERAPY

- Patient education (leg crossing, prolonged sitting before first standing in the morning, avoid excessive straining and hot baths)
- High-salt diet (e.g., bouillon cubes); caution if history of heart failure
- Liberal fluid intake
- Take needed antihypertensive medications at different times of the day
- Raise the head of the bed at night
- Compression stockings (to include splanchnic circulation)
- Multiple low-carbohydrate meals to avoid postprandial OH
- Avoid large carbohydrate loads and excess alcohol consumption

ACUTE GENERAL Rx

- Correction of volume status
- Review medication list and attempt to eliminate those potentially contributing to OH

CHRONIC Rx

- Fludrocortisone: 0.1 mg/day (may combine with an alpha-1 agonist to lower the dose of each); monitor for electrolyte disturbances and supine hypertension

- Midodrine (alpha-1 agonist): 10 mg three times a day; monitor for supine hypertension
- Erythropoietin (consider if anemic)
- Caffeine (for postprandial hypotension)

OTHER TREATMENTS

- Pyridostigmine (enhances renal sodium reabsorption): 0.2 to 0.6 mg/day (not FDA approved for this indication)
- Octreotide: 300 to 600 mg/day (not FDA-approved for this indication)
- Indomethacin (prostaglandin inhibitor)
- DDAVP (experimental)

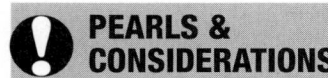 **PEARLS & CONSIDERATIONS**

COMMENTS

- The presence of OH should always trigger a search for an underlying etiology.
- OH is diagnosed by observing changes in blood pressure, not heart rate.
- Volume depletion should cause an increased heart rate on standing; a lack of heart rate response in this setting suggests autonomic dysfunction.
- Pharmacotherapy with mineralocorticoids may require concomitant potassium replenishment and monitoring for hypertension.

- Evidence to support the efficacy of pharmacologic interventions to treat OH, including midodrine, is limited.
- The etiology of OH is often multifactorial in older patients, but increased susceptibility to volume depletion due to decreased baroreceptor reflexes frequently contributes.
- Evidence suggests that nursing home residents with more stringent SBP control (<140 mm Hg) have a lower risk of OH than nursing home residents with less stringent SBP control.
- The physical examination of patients with dizziness, gait disturbance, and/or falls should include an assessment for OH.
- Because OH may be asymptomatic, physical examination of those at risk must include assessment of blood pressure in both the supine and upright positions.

SUGGESTED READINGS

available at www.expertconsult.com

AUTHOR: **TIMOTHY W. FARRELL, M.D.**

O

Diseases and Disorders

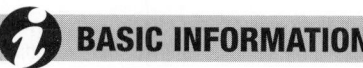

DEFINITION

Osgood-Schlatter disease is painful swelling of the growing tibial tuberosity in growing adolescents.

ICD-9CM CODES
732.4 Osgood-Schlatter disease

EPIDEMIOLOGY & DEMOGRAPHICS

PREVALENCE: 4 cases/100 adolescents
PREDOMINANT SEX: Male/female ratio of 3:1
PREDOMINANT AGE: Males: age 12-15 yr, females: age 8-12 yr

PHYSICAL FINDINGS & CLINICAL PRESENTATION

- Gradual onset of pain and swelling of the tibial tubercle
- Worsening of pain after athletic activity
- Reproduction of pain with resisted knee extension

ETIOLOGY

- Repetitive microtrauma and avulsion of the developing ossification center of the tibial tuberosity
- Anatomic variants such as patella alta

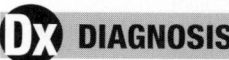 **DIAGNOSIS**

DIFFERENTIAL DIAGNOSIS

- Stress fracture of the proximal tibia
- Hoffa disease
- Sinding-Larsen-Johansson syndrome
- Patellar tendinitis

WORKUP

- The diagnosis of Osgood-Schlatter disease is generally made on clinical grounds.
- Imaging is generally indicated to exclude fracture or bony tumors.

IMAGING STUDIES

- Lateral x-rays may show separation and fragmentation of the upper tibial epiphysis (Fig. 1-602).
- Musculoskeletal ultrasound can also be used and may be helpful in evaluating soft tissue, tendons, and noncalcified cartilage.

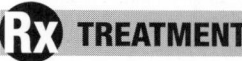 **TREATMENT**

NONPHARMACOLOGIC THERAPY

- Activity modification with increased periods of rest
- Physical therapy

ACUTE GENERAL Rx

- Ice, especially after exercise
- Nonsteroidal anti-inflammatory drugs
- Quadriceps stretching exercises

DISPOSITION

- Condition usually heals when the epiphysis closes.
- 90% of patients respond to conservative treatment.
- Recent studies have shown promising results with the use of hyperosmolar dextrose injections in recalcitrant disease
- Surgery is rarely needed in the treatment of Osgood-Schlatter disease but can be used for relief of persistent symptoms in which patients have separated ossicles or an abnormally ossified tibial tuberosity.

REFERRAL

Orthopedic consultation is recommended when symptoms persist more than 6 to 8 weeks with conservative treatment.

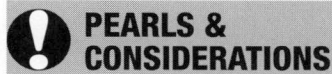 **PEARLS & CONSIDERATIONS**

COMMENTS

Larsen-Johansson disease is a similar disorder. While the diagnosis of Osgood-Schlatter disease is clinical, imaging should be performed to rule out infection, fracture, and malignancy as causes of unilateral anterior knee pain in adolescents.

SUGGESTED READINGS
available at www.expertconsult.com

RELATED CONTENT
Osgood-Schlatter Disease (Patient Information)

AUTHOR: **AMY L. LUNDHOLM, D.O.**

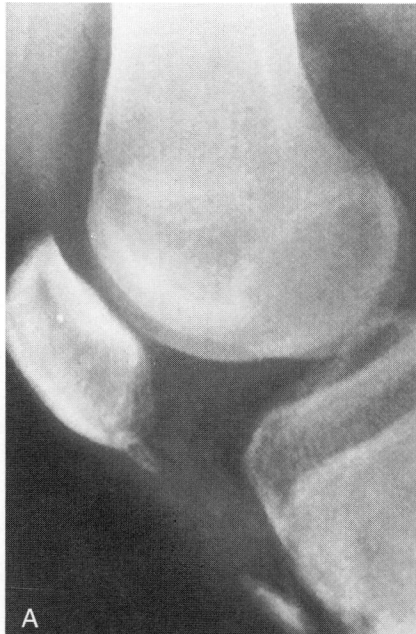
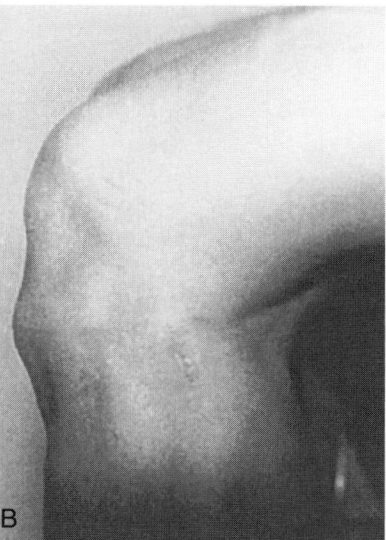

FIGURE 1-602 A, Radiograph of Osgood-Schlatter disease demonstrating thickening of patella tendon, fragmentation of the tibial tubercle, and soft tissue swelling. **B,** Clinical picture of bony prominence anteriorly at the tibial tubercle. (From Scuderi G [ed]: *Sports medicine: principles of primary care,* St Louis, 1997, Mosby.)

BASIC INFORMATION

DEFINITION

Osteoarthritis (OA) is a progressive disease of the joint representing failed repair of joint damage that results from intraarticular stresses that may be initiated by abnormalities in articular cartilage, subchondral bone, ligaments, menisci (when present), periarticular muscles, peripheral nerves, or synovium. This ultimately results in the breakdown of cartilage and bone, leading to symptoms of pain, stiffness, and functional disability. As a disease, it is aptly defined as structural abnormalities visualized on plain radiographs and MRI (magnetic resonance imaging), while as an illness, it encompasses a symptom complex of pain, aching, discomfort, stiffness, fatigue, and sleep disturbance that results in functional limitation, physical disability, and reduced health-related quality of life.

SYNONYMS

Degenerative joint disease
Osteoarthrosis
Arthrosis

ICD-9CM CODES
715.0 Osteoarthrosis and allied disorders

EPIDEMIOLOGY & DEMOGRAPHICS

PREVALENCE: 2% to 6% of general population
PREDOMINANT SEX: Females slightly more than males in a 2:1 ratio
PREDOMINANT AGE: >50 yr
GENETICS: 39% to 65% heritability rate in twin studies of women who have generalized OA, concordance rate of 0.64 in monozygotic twins.
RISK FACTORS: Nonmodifiable are age, female gender, hormonal status, geographic, genetic, and presence of congenital or developmental conditions. Modifiable risk factors such as obesity, smoking, high bone density, nutritional deficiencies such as vitamin D deficiency, and presence of crystal arthropathies such as gout. Local factors are trauma during physical activities, type of occupation, muscle strength, anatomic malalignment of the lower extremities, as well as biomechanical factors such as knee laxity, leg length discrepancy, and proprioceptive deficits.

PHYSICAL FINDINGS & CLINICAL PRESENTATION

- Similar symptoms in most forms: stiffness, pain, crepitus
- Joint tenderness, swelling
- Decreased range of motion
- Crepitus with motion
- Bouchard's nodes: bony enlargement on the proximal interphalangeal (PIP) joints of the hand
- Heberden's nodes: bony enlargement of the distal interphalangeal (DIP) joints of the hand (Fig. 1-604)
- Pain with range of motion

ETIOLOGY

- Primary or idiopathic OA can be mono-, oligo-, or polyarticular.
- Secondary OA is due to an identifiable condition such as trauma, type of occupation, developmental, mechanical, metabolic, and inflammatory conditions.

DIAGNOSIS

DIFFERENTIAL DIAGNOSIS

- Bursitis, tendinitis
- Inflammatory arthritides
- Infectious arthritis
- Crystal arthropathies such as gout and pseudogout
- Rheumatoid arthritis (Fig. 1-605)

WORKUP

- No diagnostic test exists for degenerative joint disease.

- Laboratory evaluation is normal.
- Rheumatoid factor, erythrocyte sedimentation rate, complete blood count, and antinuclear antibody tests may be required if inflammatory component is suggested by history.
- Arthrocentesis of swollen joints: synovial fluid examination is generally normal or noninflammatory in character.

IMAGING STUDIES

- Plain x-ray of the involved joints is the first step and usually of high diagnostic value.
- Roentgenographic evaluation (Fig. 1-606) reveals:
  1. Joint space narrowing
  2. Subchondral sclerosis
  3. New bone formation in the form of osteophytes
- MRI can detect other sources of pain such as synovial thickening, effusions, bone marrow edema, bony attrition, and periarticular lesions.

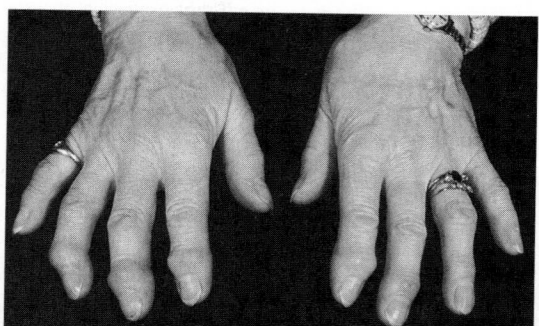

FIGURE 1-604 Osteoarthritis of the distal interphalangeal (DIP) joints. This patient has the typical clinical findings of advanced osteoarthritis of the DIP joints, including large, firm swellings (Heberden's nodes), some of which are tender and red because of associated inflammation of the periarticular tissues and the joint. (From Klippel J et al [eds]: *Primary care rheumatology,* London, 1999, Mosby.)

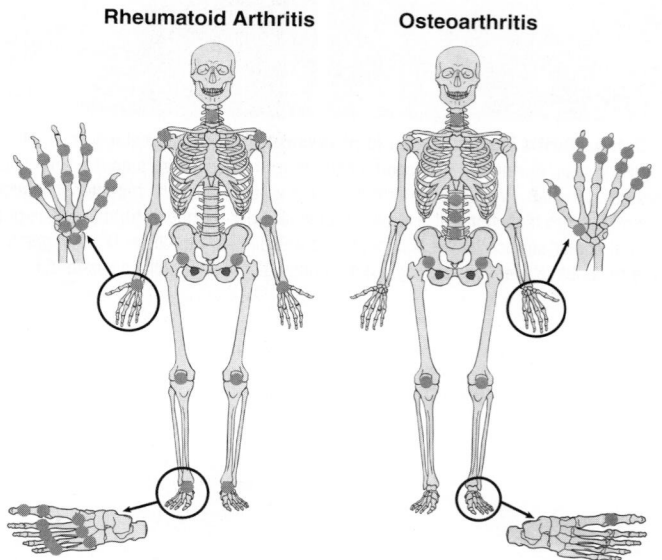

FIGURE 1-605 Distribution of involved joints in the two most common forms of arthritis: rheumatoid arthritis and osteoarthritis. *Shaded circles* are shown over the involved joint areas. (From Goldman L, Schafer AI: *Goldman's Cecil medicine,* ed 24, Philadelphia, 2012, Saunders.)

- Musculoskeletal ultrasound (MSKUS) is emerging as an alternative, fast, and inexpensive modality to identify joint damage, presence of osteophytes, effusions and non-inflammatory synovial proliferation identified using Doppler studies. This is otherwise operator-dependent.

Rx TREATMENT

- Optimal use of both pharmacologic and nonpharmacologic measures. Fig. E1-607 describes an algorithm for the management of OA.
- Education and reassurance

NONPHARMACOLOGIC THERAPY
HAND OA
- Joint protection techniques
- Assistive devices
- Thermal modalities
- Trapeziometacarpal splints

HIP AND KNEE OA
- Aerobic, aquatic, and resistance exercises
- Weight loss for overweight patients
- Medial wedge insoles for valgus knee
- Subtalar strapped lateral insoles for varus knees
- Patellar taping
- Manual therapy
- Assistive devices such as canes or walkers
- Thermal agents
- Tai chi

ACUTE GENERAL Rx/ PHARMACOLOGIC Rx
- Rest and ice
- Acetaminophen recommended for mild to moderate pain
- May add weak opioids such as tramadol
- Oral and topical NSAIDs. Capsaicin may be used.
- Arthrocentesis of the acutely swollen joint followed by intraarticular steroid injection
- Duloxetine, tramadol if above initial treatment fails
- Opioid analgesics recommended only for severe pain unresponsive to other treatment modalities
- Chronic physical therapy for gentle assisted strengthening exercises
- If considering NSAID as long term, evaluate for risk factors such as age, GI bleed, and cardiovascular (CV) risks. Topical rather than oral NSAIDs are preferred for patients age 75 and older.
- If with risk for GI bleed (age >60 yr), may add PPI or use COX-2 inhibitors
- If with CV risks, consider using naproxen. Ibuprofen may render aspirin ineffective as a cardioprotective agent by interfering with the aspirin-binding site on platelets.
- Nutritional supplements (glucosamine and chondroitin) are unproven
- Use of intraarticular hyaluronan injection is controversial. A recent trial in patients with knee OA found viscosupplementation associated with a small and clinically irrelevant benefit and an increased risk for serious adverse events.

DISPOSITION
Progression is not always inevitable, and the prognosis is variable depending on the site and extent of the disease.

REFERRAL
Surgical consultation for patients not responding to nonpharmacologic and pharmacologic management

! PEARLS & CONSIDERATIONS

COMMENTS
Surgical intervention is generally helpful in degenerative joint disease. Arthroplasty, arthrodesis, and realignment osteotomy are the most common procedures performed. Arthroscopic debridement (of the knee) appears to be of questionable value. In patients needing hip arthroplasty, resurfacing hip arthroplasty (in which the femoral head is resurfaced with a cap and the neck is preserved) is increasingly popular among younger patients because it results in more hip movement and allows total hip arthroplasty later in the patient's life if necessary.

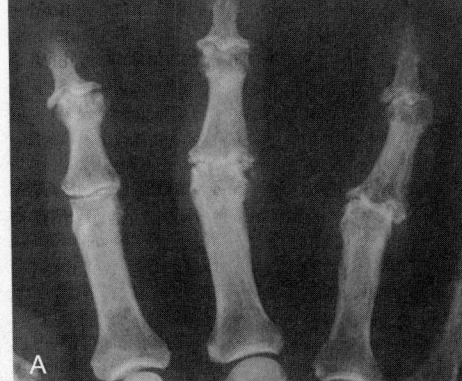
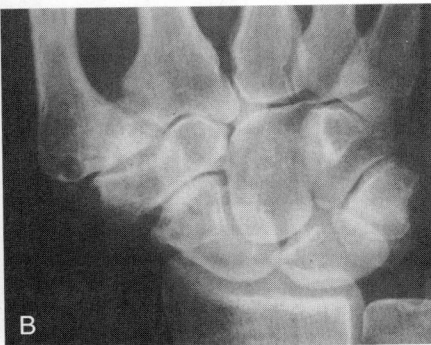

FIGURE 1-606 Osteoarthritis (degenerative joint disease). A, Primary osteoarthritis of the fingers with characteristic cartilage loss, deviations, and spurs of the proximal (Bouchard's nodes) and distal (Heberden's nodes) interphalangeal joints. **B,** Primary osteoarthritis of the carpus showing characteristic involvement of the radial side with cartilage loss, subchondral sclerosis, and small spur formation from the base of the first metacarpal to the distal articular surface of the scaphoid. (From Grainger RG, Allison D: *Grainger & Allison's diagnostic radiology, a textbook of medical imaging,* ed 4, London, 2001, Churchill Livingstone.)

EBM EVIDENCE

available at www.expertconsult.com

SUGGESTED READINGS
available at www.expertconsult.com

RELATED CONTENT
Osteoarthritis (Patient Information)

AUTHOR: **CRISOSTOMO R. BALIOG, JR, M.D.**

BASIC INFORMATION

DEFINITION

Osteochondritis dissecans (OCD) refers to a localized necrosis of the bone with detachment of the overlying subchondral bone and cartilage. The suffix "-itis" is a misnomer, as the disease does not involve inflammation.

SYNONYMS

Osteochondrosis
Avascular necrosis (AVN), aseptic necrosis, ischemic necrosis—AVN and OCD have the same pathophysiology; AVN is a more generic term, whereas OCD is used specifically when a detached fragment of bone and/or cartilage is seen on imaging.

ICD-9CM CODE
732.7 Osteochondritis dissecans

ETIOLOGY & PATHOPHYSIOLOGY

- While the cause remains unknown, predisposing factors have been identified, including genetic predisposition, repetitive microtrauma, and single trauma followed by bone ischemia. The sequence of events likely entails bone injury, hypovascularization with defective repair, bone necrosis with structural collapse, and detachment of the overlying subchondral bone and cartilage.
- OCD is seen more often in children and adolescents and is more commonly associated with repetitive trauma and sports.

EPIDEMIOLOGY & DEMOGRAPHICS

PREVALENCE: 2 cases/10,000 persons
PREDOMINANT SEX: Male/female ratio of 3:1
PREDOMINANT AGE: Typically between 10 and 20 years of age

CLINICAL PRESENTATION & PHYSICAL FINDINGS

- OCD most commonly affects the knee (75%) followed by the elbow (6%) and the ankle (4%); the other joints are affected in 15% of cases.
- Early lesions cause nonspecific pain with activity.

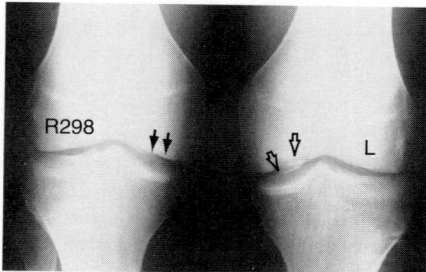

FIGURE 1-608 Bilateral, asymmetrical osteochondritis dissecans with a healed right lesion *(black arrows)* and an unhealed, unstable left lesion *(open arrows)* in a 17-year-old tennis player. (From DeLee D, Drez D [eds]: *DeLee and Drez's orthopaedic sports medicine,* ed 2, Philadelphia, 2003, Saunders.)

- As the disease progresses, stiffness and intermittent swelling occurs.
- Range of motion is usually intact in the knees.
- If a loose fragment becomes detached, it can cause locking or catching.
- Physical exam reveals tenderness at the site of the lesion; crepitus may also be present.
- When the knee is involved, a positive Wilson sign can sometimes be found (pain with knee extension and internal rotation); antalgic gait and limp can occur in chronic cases.
- Rare asymptomatic cases have been reported.

DIAGNOSIS

DIFFERENTIAL DIAGNOSIS

- Knee: torn meniscus, patellofemoral syndrome, medial plica syndrome, stress fracture
- Elbow: Panner's disease, Little League elbow, epicondyle fracture, epicondilitis
- Talus: ankle sprain, os trigonum tarsal coalition

IMAGING STUDIES

- X-rays including "tunnel views" are the initial test of choice.
- Early, small lesions can look normal or show only increased subchondral bone density.
- The defining lesion of OCD is seen on x-ray as a subchondral bone fragment surrounded by a radiolucent, crescent-shaped line (Fig. 1-608).
- MRI (Fig. 1-609) is the most sensitive test (91%) and is useful to identify OCD in symptomatic patients with normal x-rays.
- Contrast is used to evaluate blood supply to the affected fragment, evaluating stability.

TREATMENT

ACUTE GENERAL Rx

- Conservative management: usually indicated in juvenile OCD without an intraarticular for-

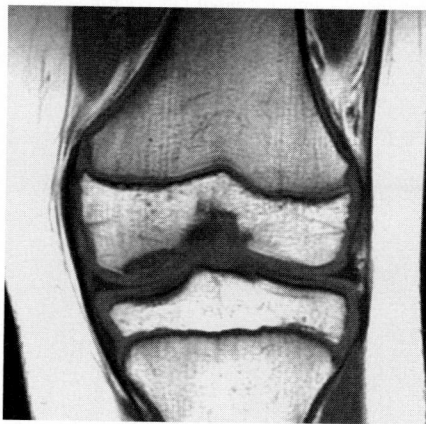

FIGURE 1-609 Osteochondritis dissecans (OCD). A coronal MRI of an OCD lesion of the medial femoral condyle. (From Frontera WR: *Clinical sports medicine: medical management and rehabilitation,* Philadelphia, 2006, Saunders.)

eign body and for adult patients who have a small, stable fragment
- Non–weight bearing and immobilization for 4-6 wk; physical therapy once healing starts
- Surgery: indicated for juvenile OCD with a loose body and in cases that fail to improve after 4-6 mo of conservative management; also indicated in adults with OCD

DISPOSITION & PROGNOSIS

- Office follow-ups are initially frequent, every 2 wk.
- X-ray changes should be monitored every 6 wk while immobilized.
- Once bone healing has been seen on x-rays, follow-ups can be spaced every 3 mo.
- Return to activity can be attempted once the patient is pain free and has an intact active full range of motion; it usually takes from 3 to 6 mo.
- Once complete healing occurs, joint function usually returns to normal.
- Complete healing is frequent in skeletally immature children with small lesions (95%), but in adults with larger lesions complete healing is less common (50%).

REFERRAL

- Orthopedic consultation is helpful in most symptomatic children and adults with OCD for staging and management options.
- Surgical options include arthroscopic drilling, fixation with Kirschner wires, special screws, and chondrocyte transplantation.

PEARLS & CONSIDERATIONS

COMMENTS

- Although inflammation is suggested by the name, it has not been shown to be of significance in this disorder. *Osteochondral lesion* or *osteochondrosis dissecans* may be more appropriate terms to describe these disorders.
- Repetitive trauma with ischemic necrosis is the most likely cause.
- The condition is often bilateral, especially in the knee, which could suggest the possibility of an endocrine or genetic basis.
- This condition should always be considered in the patient whose "sprained ankle" does not improve over the usual course of treatment.

SUGGESTED READINGS
available at www.expertconsult.com

RELATED CONTENT
Osteochondritis Dissecans (Patient Information)
AUTHOR: **DAN CRISTESCU, M.D.**

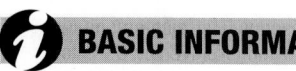

BASIC INFORMATION

DEFINITION

Osteomyelitis is an acute or chronic infection of the bone secondary to the hematogenous or contiguous source of infection or direct traumatic inoculation, which is usually bacterial.

SYNONYMS

Bone infection

ICD-9CM CODES
730.1 Chronic osteomyelitis
730.2 Acute or subacute osteomyelitis

EPIDEMIOLOGY & DEMOGRAPHICS

PREDOMINANT SEX: Male > female
PREDOMINANT AGE: All ages

PHYSICAL FINDINGS & CLINICAL PRESENTATION

HEMATOGENOUS OSTEOMYELITIS:
- Usually occurs in tibia/fibula (children)
- Localized inflammation: often secondary to trauma with accompanying hematoma or cellulitis
- Abrupt fever
- Lethargy
- Irritability
- Pain in involved bone

VERTEBRAL OSTEOMYELITIS:
- Usually hematogenous
- Fever: 50%
- Localized pain/tenderness. Back pain is the most common initial symptom (86% of cases)
- Neurologic defects: motor/sensory (sensory loss, weakness, radiculopathy)

CONTIGUOUS OSTEOMYELITIS:
- Direct inoculation
- Associated with trauma, fractures, surgical fixation
- Chronic infection of skin/soft tissue
- Fever, drainage from surgical site

CHRONIC OSTEOMYELITIS:
- Bone pain
- Sinus tract drainage, nonhealing ulcer
- Chronic low-grade fever
- Chronic localized pain

ETIOLOGY

- *Staphylococcus aureus*
- *S. aureus* (methicillin-resistant)
- *Pseudomonas aeruginosa*
- Enterobacteriaceae
- *Streptococcus pyogenes*
- *Enterococcus*
- Mycobacteria
- Fungi
- Coagulase-negative staphylococci
- *Salmonella* (in sickle cell disease)

DIAGNOSIS

DIFFERENTIAL DIAGNOSIS

- Gaucher's disease
- Bone infarction
- Charcot's joint
- Fracture

WORKUP

- ESR, C-reactive protein
- Blood culturing
- Bone culture. A culture of a biopsy specimen has a significantly higher overall diagnostic yield than does a blood culture. Bone samples should be cultured for aerobic and anaerobic bacteria and for fungi
- Pathologic evaluation of bone biopsy for acute/chronic changes consistent with necrosis or acute inflammation
- PCR analysis of specimens obtained by means of biopsy or puncture may be useful for organisms that are difficult to identify (anaerobic bacteria, *Bartonella* sp., *Kingella kingae*); however, broad-range PCR has suboptimal sensitivity and specificity due to contamination and may not provide sufficient information on the susceptibility of the microorganisms to antibiotics

IMAGING STUDIES

- Bone radiograph examination: initial study but not sensitive in early osteomyelitis as may not show changes for as much as 2 wk
- MRI (Fig. 1-610): most accurate imaging study. CT only if patient has contraindication to MRI
- Triple-phase technetium-99m bone scan (Fig. 1-611). Typically positive within a few days after onset of symptoms but accuracy is lower than that of MRI
- Gallium scan (Ga-67) scintigraphy with single-photon emission CT (SPECT) has higher accuracy than bone scan but is less sensitive for detection of epidural abscess in vertebral osteomyelitis
- Indium-111–labeled leukocyte scintigraphy scan; low sensitivity (<20%) for vertebral osteomyelitis
- Positron-emission tomography (PET) scanning with ^{18}F-fluorodeoxyglucose has high accuracy (similar to MRI) and is useful in patients with metallic implants

TREATMENT

- Surgical debridement in biopsy-positive cases will guide direction for antibiotic therapy. This will vary with type of osteomyelitis. Duration of therapy is usually 6 wk for acute osteomyelitis; chronic osteomyelitis may need a longer course of medication
- *S. aureus:* cefazolin IV, nafcillin IV, vancomycin IV (in patient allergic to penicillin)
- *S. aureus* (methicillin resistant): vancomycin IV, linezolid, daptomycin, or tigecycline
- *Streptococcus* spp.: ceftriaxone, IV penicillin G in sensitive species

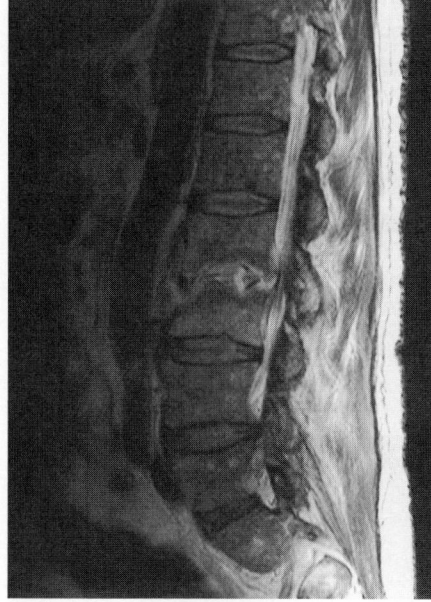

FIGURE 1-610 T1-weighted magnetic resonance images show an abnormal signal in the disk between L2 & L3 with associated vertebral osteomyelitis. A fluid collection is located in the posterior part of L2 and L3 resulting in the evaluation of the posterior ligament. A computed tomography–guided aspirate grew *Staphylococcus aureus*. (From Mandell GL et al: *Principles and practice of infectious diseases*, ed 7, Philadelphia, 2010, Saunders.)

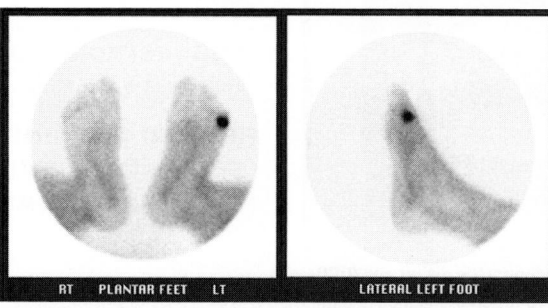

FIGURE 1-611 Osteomyelitis. Intense accumulation of Tc-99m WBCs in proximal phalanx of fifth digit of left foot at 4 hr after injection. (From Specht N [ed]: *Practical guide to diagnostic imaging*, St Louis, 1998, Mosby.)

- *P. aeruginosa:* cefepime plus ciprofloxacin, piperacillin/tazobactam plus ciprofloxacin, or imipenem/cilastatin plus aminoglycoside
- Enterobacteriaceae quinolone-susceptible: fluoroquinolone or ceftriaxone
- Enterobacteriaceae quinolone-resistant: carbapenem (such as imipenem, meropenem, or doripenem)
- Anaerobes: clindamycin, ticarcillin clavulanate, cefotetan, or metronidazole
- Table 1-308 summarizes antimicrobial therapy for selected microorganisms in osteomyelitis
- Hyperbaric oxygen therapy: may be useful in chronic osteomyelitis
- Surgical debridement of all devitalized bone and tissue
- Immobilization of affected bone (plaster, traction) if bone is unstable

DISPOSITION

Acute hematogenous osteomyelitis usually resolves without recurrence or long-term complications, but contiguous focus osteomyelitis, bone infections from open fractures, or osteomyelitis frequently recurs.

REFERRAL

- To an orthopedic surgeon if chronic osteomyelitis with need for bone debridement, bone grafting, or stabilization of infected tissue adjacent to a bone fracture
- To an infectious disease specialist for appropriate treatment for difficult-to-treat or recalcitrant infections
- To a hyperbaric oxygen chamber service for nonhealing, chronic osteomyelitis

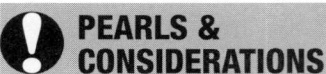 **PEARLS & CONSIDERATIONS**

Chronic osteomyelitis is one of the most challenging infections to treat; the high failure rate is a consequence of poor vascular supply, nondistensible bone tissue, and limited penetration of bone tissue.

SUGGESTED READINGS

available at www.expertconsult.com

RELATED CONTENT

Osteomyelitis (Patient Information)

AUTHOR: **GLENN G. FORT, M.D., M.P.H.**

TABLE 1-308 Antimicrobial Therapy for Selected Microorganisms in Osteomyelitis or Septic Arthritis in Adults

Microorganism	First Choice*	Alternative Choice
Methicillin/oxacillin/nafcillin-sensitive staphylococci	Nafcillin sodium or oxacillin sodium 1.5-2 g IV q4-6h for 4-6 wk *or* cefazolin 1-2 g IV q8h	Vancomycin 15 mg/kg IV q12h for 4-6 wk
Methicillin/oxacillin/nafcillin-resistant staphylococci (MRSA)	Vancomycin† 15 mg/kg IV q12h *or* daptomycin 6 mg/kg IV q24h	Linezolid 600 mg PO/IV q12h *or* levofloxacin† 500-750 mg PO/IV daily
Penicillin-sensitive streptococci	Aqueous penicillin G 20×10^6 U/24 hr IV either continuously or in six equally divided daily doses *or* ceftriaxone 1-2 g IV q24h *or* cefazolin 1-2 g IV q8h	Vancomycin 15 mg/kg IV q12h
Enterococci	Aqueous crystalline penicillin G 20×10^6 U/24 hr IV either continuously or in six equally divided daily doses *or* ampicillin sodium 12 g/24 hr IV either continuously or in six equally divided daily doses; the addition of gentamicin sulfate 1 mg/kg IV or IM q8h for 1-2 wk is *optional*	Vancomycin† 15 mg/kg IV q12h; the addition of gentamicin sulfate 1 mg/kg IV or IM q8h for 1-2 wk is *optional*
Enterobacteriaceae, quinolone resistant	Ticarcillin clavulanate, 3.1 g IV q4h or piperacillin/tazobactam, 3.375 g IV q6h	Ceftriaxone 1-2 g IV q24h
Pseudomonas aeruginosa	Cefepime 2 g IV q12h plus ciprofloxacin 400 mg IV q8-12h	Imipenem/cilastatin 1 g IV q8h, plus aminoglycoside

*Antimicrobial selection should be based on in vitro sensitivity data, as well as allergies, intolerances, and drug interactions in individual patients.
†Doses shown are based on normal renal and hepatic function and may need to be adjusted or serum levels monitored (vancomycin).
MRSA, Methicillin-resistant *Staphylococcus aureus.*
Adapted from Berbari EF et al: Osteomyelitis. In Mandell GL et al (eds): *Mandell, Douglas, and Bennett's principles and practice of infectious diseases,* ed 7, Philadelphia, 2010, Churchill Livingstone.

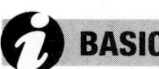

DEFINITION

Osteoporosis is characterized by a progressive decrease in bone mass that results in increased bone fragility and a higher fracture risk. The various types are as follows:

PRIMARY OSTEOPOROSIS: Affects 80% of women and 60% of men with osteoporosis.
- Idiopathic osteoporosis: unknown pathogenesis; may occur in children and young adults
- Type I osteoporosis: may occur in postmenopausal women (ages 51 to 75); characterized by accelerated and disproportionate trabecular bone loss and associated with vertebral body and distal forearm fractures (estrogen withdrawal effect)
- Type II osteoporosis (involutional): occurs in both men and women aged >70 yr; characterized by both trabecular and cortical bone loss and associated with fractures of the proximal humerus and tibia, femoral neck, and pelvis

SECONDARY OSTEOPOROSIS: Affects 20% of women and 40% of men with osteoporosis; osteoporosis that exists as a common feature of another disease process, heritable disorder of connective tissue, or drug side effect (see "Differential Diagnosis")

ICD-9CM CODES
733.0 Osteoporosis

EPIDEMIOLOGY & DEMOGRAPHICS

PREVALENCE (IN U.S.):
- ~25 million men and women
- Twice as common in women
- Results in 1.5 million fractures annually (70% women)
- Osteoporosis-related fractures in 50% of women and 20% of men aged >65 yr
- Results: institutionalization, death, and costs in excess of $10 billion annually

RISK FACTORS:
- Age: each decade after 40 yr associated with a fivefold increased risk
- Genetics:
  1. Ethnicity (white/Asian are affected more often than blacks, with Polynesians affected the least)
  2. Gender (females affected more often than males)
  3. Family history (hip fracture in first-degree relative)
- Environmental factors: poor nutrition, calcium deficiency, physical inactivity, medication (chronic corticosteroid use [>3 mo], PPIs, aromatase inhibitors, anticonvulsants, anticoagulants, SSRIs), tobacco use, alcohol use (>3 drinks/day), traumatic injury, high caffeine intake
- Chronic disease states: estrogen deficiency, androgen deficiency, hyperthyroidism, inflammatory bowel disease, diabetes mellitus, hypercortisolism, cirrhosis, malabsorption, gastrectomy, multiple myeloma

PHYSICAL FINDINGS & CLINICAL PRESENTATION

- Most commonly silent with no signs and symptoms
- Insidious and progressive development of dorsal kyphosis *(dowager's hump),* loss of height, and skeletal pain typically associated with fracture; other physical findings related to other conditions with associated increased risk for osteoporosis (see "Risk Factors")

ETIOLOGY

- Primary osteoporosis: multifactorial, resulting from a combination of factors including nutrition, peak bone mass, genetics, level of physical activity, age of menopause (spontaneous vs. surgical), and estrogen status
- Secondary osteoporosis: associated decrease in bone mass resulting from an identified cause, including endocrinopathies, hypogonadism, hyperthyroidism, hyperparathyroidism, Cushing's syndrome, hyperprolactinemia, acromegaly, diabetes mellitus, gastrointestinal disease, malabsorption, primary biliary cirrhosis, gastrectomy, malnutrition (including anorexia nervosa), and medications (corticosteroids, PPIs, rosiglitazone, pioglitazone)

Dx DIAGNOSIS

DIFFERENTIAL DIAGNOSIS

- Malignancy (multiple myeloma, lymphoma, leukemia, metastatic carcinoma)
- Primary hyperparathyroidism
- Osteomalacia
- Paget's disease
- Osteogenesis imperfecta: types I, III, and IV (see also "Epidemiology & Demographics" and "Etiology")

WORKUP

- History and physical examination (20% of women with type I osteoporosis have associated secondary cause), with appropriate evaluation for identified risk factors and secondary causes
- Diagnosis of osteoporosis made by bone mineral density (BMD) determination (BMD should ideally evaluate the hip, spine, and wrist)
  ○ Dual-energy x-ray absorptiometry (DEXA) is the gold standard for screening and monitoring changes in BMD due to excellent precision, widespread availability, low cost, and minimal radiation exposure
- Recommendations as to when to repeat bone density testing should be based on initial T scores. Data from the Study of Osteoporotic Fractures indicates that in women with normal bone density or mild osteopenia, repeat testing might not be necessary for another 10-15 yr. For women with moderate osteopenia, a screening interval of 3-5 yr may be appropriate. Annual testing may be indicated for women with advanced osteopenia.

LABORATORY TESTS

- Biochemical profile to evaluate renal and hepatic function, primary hyperparathyroidism, and malnutrition
- CBC: for nutritional status and myeloma
- TSH to rule out the presence of hyperthyroidism
- Vitamin D level. Consideration of 24-hr urine collection for calcium (excess skeletal loss, vitamin D malabsorption/deficiency), creatinine, sodium, and free cortisol (to detect occult Cushing's disease); no need to measure calcitropic hormones (parathyroid hormone, calcitriol, calcitonin) unless specifically indicated
- Biochemical markers of bone remodeling; may be useful to predict rate of bone loss and/or follow therapy response; specific biochemical markers followed (e.g., 3-mo interval) to document normalization as a response to therapy
  1. High-turnover osteoporosis: high levels of resorption markers (lysyl pyridinoline, deoxy lysyl pyridinoline, n-telopeptide of collagen cross-links, C-telopeptide of collagen cross-links) and formation markers (osteocalcin, bone-specific alkaline phosphatase, carboxy-terminal extension peptide of type I procollagen); accelerated bone loss responding best to antiresorptive therapy
  2. Low-normal-turnover osteoporosis: normal or low levels of the markers of resorption and formation (see "high turnover osteoporosis" listed previously); no accelerated bone loss; responds best to drugs that enhance bone formation

IMAGING STUDIES

- BMD determination (see "Workup") should be performed on all women with determined risk factors and/or associated secondary causes; criteria for diagnosis of osteoporosis based on measurement of bone density and T score equivalent cut points are summarized in Table 1-309 and Fig. E1-612.
  1. Normal: BMD <1 SD of the young adult reference mean
  2. Osteopenia: BMD 1 to 2.5 SD below the young adult reference mean
  3. Osteoporosis: BMD >2.5 SD below the young adult reference mean
- For patient undergoing treatment: annual BMD to follow response to therapy
- X-ray exam of appropriate part of skeleton to evaluate clinical osteoporotic fracture only

Rx TREATMENT

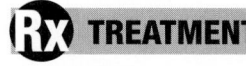

NONPHARMACOLOGIC THERAPY

Prevention:
- Identification and minimization of risk factors
- Appropriate diagnosis and treatment of secondary causes
- Behavioral modification: proper nutrition (dietary calcium >800 mg/day, vitamin D 400 to 800 U/day), physical activity, fracture prevention strategies

ACUTE GENERAL Rx

- Vitamin D supplement: 800 to 1000 IU/day for all adults age 50 and older
- Calcium supplement: 1200 to 1500 mg/day
- Oral bisphosphonates (ibandronate, alendronate, risendronate): they decrease bone resorption by attenuating osteoclast activity. They are first-line therapy for the treatment of most patients with osteoporosis, with proven efficacy to reduce fracture risk. Ibandronate is given 150 mg once monthly, swallowed whole with 8 oz water on empty stomach, with no oral intake for at least 60 min. Do not lie down for 60 min after dose. Alendronate is given 70 mg once weekly on awakening, with 8 oz water on empty stomach, with no oral intake for at least 30 min. Use 70-mg dose for treatment of postmenopausal osteoporosis and a 35-mg tablet for the prevention of osteoporosis in postmenopausal women. Risedronate is given 35 mg once weekly or 75 mg taken on 2 consecutive days per month on awakening, with 8 oz water on empty stomach, with no oral intake for at least 30 min.
- Synthetic salmon calcitonin: 100 U/day SC or 200 U/day intranasally. It decreases bone resorption by attenuating osteoclast activity.
- Raloxifene: 60 mg qd. Selective estrogen-receptor moderator, it has suppressive effects on osteoclast and bone resorption.
- Zoledronic acid: a bisphosphonate given by IV infusion over at least 15 min, 5 mg once/year
- Teriparatide is a recombinant human parathyroid hormone used for postmenopausal women with osteoporosis who are at high risk for fracture. It is also used in men with primary or hypogonadal osteoporosis who are at high risk of fracture. It is administered by injection 20 mcg qd SQ into the thigh or abdominal wall. Use for >2 yr not recommended. It stimulates bone formation and reduces the risk of fracture but may increase the risk of stroke in older women with osteoporosis.
- Denosumab is a human monoclonal antibody that decreases bone resorption by inhibiting the formation and activity of osteoclasts. It was recently approved for treatment of postmenopausal osteoporosis. Dosage is 60 mg subcutaneously every 6 months. Cost of 1 yr of therapy is approximately $2000.
- Other FDA-approved drugs (without osteoporosis indication) used to treat osteoporosis:
  1. Calcitriol
  2. Etidronate
  3. Thiazide
- Estrogen (conjugated equine estrogen or equivalent): 0.3 to 0.625 mg/day
- Progestin: continuous (e.g., 2.5 mg medroxyprogesterone acetate/day or equivalent) or cyclic (e.g., 10 mg medroxyprogesterone acetate days 16 to 25 each mo or equivalent) co-administered in nonhysterectomized women
- Combination estrogen/alendronate or estrogen-progestin/alendronate may be considered in individualized patients on hormone replacement therapy with identified osteoporosis. BMD baseline obtained before onset of therapy and at 1 yr; decrease of 2% or greater results in dosage adjustment or medication change.
- A recent trial on the effects of lasofoxifene on the risk of fractures showed that in postmenopausal women with osteoporosis, lasofoxifene (0.5 mg/day) decreased risk of vertebral and nonvertebral fractures. It also lowered the risk of ER-positive breast cancer, coronary heart disease, and stroke but it increased the risk of venous thromboembolic events.
- Baseline biochemical markers of remodeling baseline considered; identified high-turnover osteoporosis patients rescreened at 3 mo to document marker return to normal

CHRONIC Rx

- Lifelong disorder requiring lifelong attention to behavior modification issues (nutrition, physical activity, fracture prevention strategies) and compliance with pharmacologic intervention. There is little evidence to guide physicians about long-term bisphosphonate therapy. Evidence is accumulating that the risk of atypical fracture of the femur increases after 5 years of bisphosphonate use. It is reasonable to stop bisphosphonates at 3 to 5 yr in women at the lowest risk (T score better than −2.5 and no fractures) and then monitor patients with markers of bone turnover. Continued treatment may be advisable in those at highest risk.
- Continuing need to eliminate high-risk factors when possible and to diagnose and optimally manage secondary causes of osteoporosis

DISPOSITION

Goal for diagnosis and treatment: identification of women at risk; initiation of preventive measures for all women lifelong; institution of treatment modalities that will result in a decrease in fracture risk; and reduction of morbidity, mortality, and unnecessary institutionalization, thereby improving quality of independent life and productivity.

REFERRAL

- To reproductive endocrinologist, medical endocrinologist, gynecologist, or rheumatologist if unfamiliar with diagnosis and management of osteoporosis
- If multidisciplinary management is required, to other specialties depending on presence of acute fracture and/or secondary associated disorders

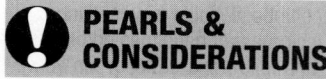 **PEARLS & CONSIDERATIONS**

COMMENTS

- Osteonecrosis of the jaw is a known complication of high-dose IV bisphosphonate therapy for cancer; however, there is considerable debate on whether low-dose bisphosphonates used for osteoporosis can also cause this disorder. Evidence for this is inconclusive.
- Long-term use (>10 yr) of bisphosphonates has been reported to increase risk of atypical subtrochanteric or femoral shaft fractures in several uncontrolled case series. A prodrome of thigh pain, lack of trauma prior to the procedure, and specific radiologic characteristics have been reported. The evidence remains inconclusive. Patients can be reassured that short or intermediate use of bisphosphonates does not increase the risk of atypical femoral fractures. Current strategies should include considering a 12-mo interruption in therapy after 5 yr in patients who are clinically stable and considering teriparatide treatment in individuals who experience an atypical fracture while receiving bisphosphonate therapy.
- Increased risk of esophageal cancer and atrial fibrillation have been reported as possible adverse effects of bisphosphonate therapy.

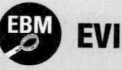 **EVIDENCE**

available at www.expertconsult.com

SUGGESTED READINGS

available at www.expertconsult.com

RELATED CONTENT

Osteoporosis (Patient Information)

AUTHORS: **DENNIS M. WEPPNER, M.D.,** and **RUBEN ALVERO, M.D.**

TABLE 1-309 1994 WHO Criteria for the Diagnosis of Osteoporosis Based on the Measurement of Bone Density and T Score Equivalent Cut Points

Diagnostic Category	Standard Deviations Below the Young-Adult Mean	T Score
Normal	≤1 SD	Equal to or better than −1
Osteopenia (low bone mass)	Between 1 and 2.5 SD	Between −1 and −2.5
Osteoporosis	≥2.5 SD	Equal to or poorer than −2.5
Severe (established) osteoporosis	≥2.5 SD + a fragility fracture	Equal to or poorer than −2.5 + a fragility fracture

From Hochberg MC et al: *Rheumatology*, ed 5, St Louis, 2011, Mosby.

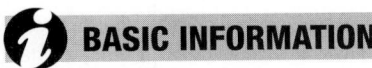

BASIC INFORMATION

DEFINITION

Otitis externa is a term encompassing a variety of conditions causing inflammation and/or infection of the external auditory canal (and/or auricle and tympanic membrane). There are six subgroups of otitis externa:
1. Acute localized otitis externa (furunculosis)
2. Acute diffuse bacterial otitis externa (swimmer's ear)
3. Chronic otitis externa
4. Eczematous otitis externa
5. Fungal otitis externa (otomycosis)
6. Invasive or necrotizing (malignant) otitis externa (Fig. 1-613)

SYNONYMS

See "Definition."

ICD-9CM CODES
38.10 Otitis externa

EPIDEMIOLOGY & DEMOGRAPHICS

INCIDENCE (IN U.S.):
- Among the most common disorders
- Affects 3% to 10% of patients seeking otologic care

PREVALENCE (IN U.S.):
- Diffuse otitis externa (swimmer's ear) is most often seen in swimmers and in hot, humid climates, conditions that lead to water retention in the ear canal.
- Necrotizing otitis externa is more common in elderly, diabetics, and immunocompromised patients.

PREDOMINANT SEX: None

PREDOMINANT AGE:
- Occurs at all ages
- Necrotizing otitis externa: typically occurs in elderly: mean age >65 yr

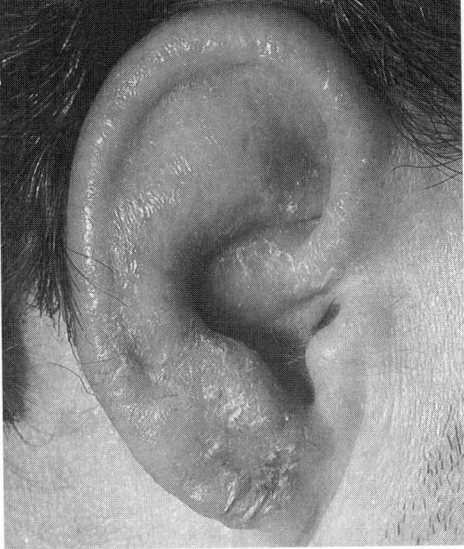

FIGURE 1-613 Malignant external otitis. Severe infection of the ear has occurred after months of chronic inflammation of the pinna. (From Habif TP: *Clinical dermatology: a color guide to diagnosis and therapy,* ed 3, St Louis, 1996, Mosby.)

PHYSICAL FINDINGS & CLINICAL PRESENTATION

The two most common symptoms are otalgia, ranging from pruritus to severe pain exacerbated by motion (e.g., chewing), and otorrhea. Patients may also experience aural fullness and hearing loss as a result of swelling with occlusion of the canal. More intense symptoms may occur with bacterial otitis externa, with or without fever, and lymphadenopathy (anterior to tragus). There are also findings unique to the various forms of the infection:
- Acute localized otitis externa (furunculosis):
  1. Occurs from infected hair follicles, usually in the outer third of the ear canal, forming pustules and furuncles
  2. Furuncles are superficial and pointing or deep and diffuse
- Impetigo:
  1. In contrast to furunculosis, this is a superficial spreading infection of the ear canal that may also involve the concha and the auricle
  2. Begins as a small blister that ruptures, releasing straw-colored fluid that dries as a golden crust
- Erysipelas:
  1. Caused by group A *Streptococcus*
  2. May involve the concha and canal
  3. May involve the dermis and deeper tissues
  4. Area of cellulitis, often with severe pain
  5. Fever, chills, malaise
  6. Regional adenopathy
- Eczematous otitis externa:
  1. Stems from a variety of dermatologic problems that can involve the external auditory canal
  2. Severe itching, erythema, scaling, crusting, and fissuring possible
- Acute diffuse otitis externa (swimmer's ear):
  1. Begins with itching and a feeling of pressure and fullness in the ear that becomes increasingly tender and painful
  2. Mild erythema and edema of the external auditory canal, which may cause narrowing and occlusion of the canal, leading to hearing loss
  3. Minimal serous secretions, which may become profuse and purulent
  4. Tympanic membrane may appear dull and infected
  5. Usually absence of systemic symptoms such as fever, chills
- Otomycosis:
  1. Chronic superficial infection of the ear canal and tympanic membrane
  2. In primary fungal infection, major symptom is intense itching
  3. In secondary infection (fungal infection superimposed on bacterial infection), major symptom is pain
  4. Fungal growth of variety of colors
- Chronic otitis externa:
  1. Dry and atrophic canal
  2. Typically lack of cerumen
  3. Itching, often severe, and mild discomfort rather than pain
  4. Occasionally mucopurulent discharge
  5. With time, thickening of the walls of the canal, causing narrowing of the lumen
- Necrotizing otitis externa (also known as malignant otitis externa). Typically seen in older patients with diabetes or in patients who are immunocompromised.
  1. Redness, swelling, and tenderness of the ear canal
  2. Classic finding of granulation tissue on the floor of the canal and the bone–cartilage junction
  3. Small ulceration of necrotic soft tissue at bone–cartilage junction
  4. Most common symptoms: pain (often severe) and otorrhea
  5. Lessening of purulent drainage as infection advances
  6. Facial nerve palsy often the first and only cranial nerve defect
  7. Possible involvement of other cranial nerves

ETIOLOGY
- Acute localized otitis externa: *Staphylococcus aureus*
- Impetigo:
  1. *S. aureus* including MRSA
  2. *Streptococcus pyogenes*
- Erysipelas: *S. pyogenes*
- Eczematous otitis externa:
  1. Seborrheic dermatitis
  2. Atopic dermatitis
  3. Psoriasis
  4. Neurodermatitis
  5. Lupus erythematosus
- Acute diffuse otitis externa:
  1. Swimming
  2. Hot, humid climates
  3. Tightly fitting hearing aids
  4. Use of ear plugs
  5. *Pseudomonas aeruginosa*
  6. *S. aureus* including MRSA

- Otomycosis:
  1. Prolonged use of topical antibiotics and steroid preparations
  2. *Aspergillus* (80% to 90%)
  3. *Candida*
- Chronic otitis externa: persistent low-grade infection and inflammation
- Necrotizing otitis externa (NOE):
  1. Complication of persistent otitis externa
  2. Extends through Santorini's fissures, small apertures at the bone-cartilage junction of the canal, into the mastoid and along the base of the skull
  3. *P. aeruginosa*

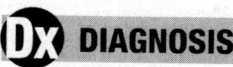

DIFFERENTIAL DIAGNOSIS

- Acute otitis media
- Bullous myringitis
- Mastoiditis
- Foreign bodies
- Neoplasms
- Contact dermatitis
- Eczema
- Ramsey-Hunt syndrome
- Seborrhea
- Otomycosis
- Referred pain

WORKUP

Thorough history and physical examination

LABORATORY TESTS

- Cultures from the canal are usually not necessary unless the condition does not respond to treatment.
- Leukocyte count normal or mildly elevated.
- Erythrocyte sedimentation rate is often quite elevated in malignant otitis externa.

IMAGING STUDIES

- CT scan is the best technique for defining bone involvement and extent of disease in malignant otitis externa.
- MRI is slightly more sensitive in evaluation of soft tissue changes.
- Gallium scans are more specific than bone scans in diagnosing NOE.
- Follow-up scans are helpful in determining efficacy of treatment.

NOTE: Expert opinion supports history and physical examination as the best means of diagnosis. Persistent pain that is constant and severe should raise the question of NOE (particularly in the elderly, diabetics, and immunocompromised patients).

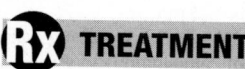

NONPHARMACOLOGIC THERAPY

- Cleansing and debridement of the ear canal with cotton swabs and hydrogen peroxide or other antiseptic solution allows a more thorough examination of the ear.
- If the canal lumen is edematous and too narrow to allow adequate cleansing, a cotton

wick or gauze strip inserted into the canal serves as a conduit for topical medications to be drawn into the canal. Usually remove wick after 2 days.
- Local heat is useful in treating deep furunculosis.
- Incision and drainage is indicated in treatment of superficial pointing furunculosis.

ACUTE GENERAL Rx

Topical medications:
- An acidifying agent such as 2% acetic acid (Vosol) inhibits growth of bacteria and fungi
- Topical antibiotics (in the form of otic or ophthalmic solutions) or antifungals, often in combination with an acidifying agent and a steroid preparation
- The following are some of the available preparations:
  1. Neomycin otic solutions and suspensions:
     a. With polymyxin-B-hydrocortisone (Corticosporin)
     b. With hydrocortisone-thonzonium (Coly-Mycin S)
  2. Polymyxin-B-hydrocortisone (Otobiotic)
  3. Quinolone otic solutions:
     a. Ofloxacin 0.3% solution (Floxin Otic)
     b. Ciprofloxacin 0.3% with hydrocortisone (Cipro HC)
  4. Quinolone ophthalmic solutions:
     a. Ofloxacin 0.3% (Ocuflox)
     b. Ciprofloxacin 0.3% (Ciloxan)
  5. Aminoglycoside ophthalmic solutions:
     a. Gentamicin sulfate 0.3% (Garamycin)
     b. Tobramycin sulfate 0.3% (Tobrex)
     c. Tobramycin 0.3% and dexamethasone 0.1% (TobraDex)
  6. Chloramphenicol 0.5% otic solution or 0.25% ophthalmic solution (Chloromycetin)
  7. Gentian violet (methylrosaniline chloride 1%, 2%)
  8. Antifungals:
     a. Amphotericin B 3% (Fungizone lotion)
     b. Clotrimazole 1% solution (Lotrimin)
     c. Tolnaftate 1% (Tinactin)
- Topical preparations should be applied qid (bid for quinolones, antifungals), generally for 3 days after cessation of symptoms (average 10 to 14 days total)

Systemic antibiotics:
- Reserved for when the infection has spread beyond the ear canal
- Treatment usually for 10 days with ciprofloxacin 750 mg q12h or ofloxacin 400 mg q12h, or with antistaphylococcal agent (e.g., dicloxacillin or cephalexin 500 mg q6h). Use Bactrim when MRSA suspected or cultured at one DS twice a day instead of cephalexin or dicloxacillin. For malignant otitis externa (due to *Pseudomonas aeruginosa* in >90% of cases), effective agents are imipenem-cilastatin 0.5 g IV q6h or ciprofloxacin 400 mg IV q12h or 750 mg PO q12h or cefepime 2 g q12h.

Treatment for NOE:
- Requires prolonged therapy up to 3 mo; whether to use oral parenteral therapy based on clinical judgment

- Oral quinolones, ciprofloxacin 750 mg q12h or ofloxacin 400 mg q12h may be appropriate initial therapy or used to shorten the course of IV therapy
- Intravenous antipseudomonals with or without aminoglycosides are also appropriate
- Local debridement

Pain control:
- May require NSAIDs or opioids
- Topical corticosteroids to reduce swelling and inflammation

CHRONIC Rx

- Patients prone to recurrent infections should try to identify and avoid precipitants to infection.
- Swimmers should try tight-fitting ear plugs or tight-fitting bathing caps and remove all excess water from the ears after swimming.
- Treat underlying systemic diseases and dermatologic conditions that predispose to infection.

DISPOSITION

Inadequate treatment of otitis externa may lead to NOE and mastoiditis.

REFERRAL

To an otolaryngologist:
- NOE
- Treatment failure
- Severe pain

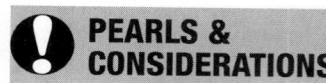

Otitis externa varies in severity from a mild irritation of the external acoustic canal (swimmer's ear) that resolves spontaneously by simply removing the offending agent (stay out of fresh water or wear ear plugs) to a life-threatening infection with the risk of intracranial extension, gram-negative bacterial meningitis, and severe neurologic impairment with multiple cranial neuropathy. Do not miss severe malignant otitis externa in patients who are diabetic or immuno-compromised.

SUGGESTED READINGS
available at www.expertconsult.com

RELATED CONTENT
Otitis Externa (Patient Information)

AUTHOR: **GLENN G. FORT, M.D., M.P.H.**

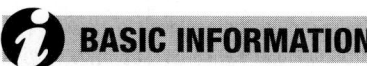

BASIC INFORMATION

DEFINITION

Otitis media is the presence of fluid in the middle ear accompanied by signs and symptoms of infection.

SYNONYMS

Acute suppurative otitis media
Purulent otitis media
Acute otitis media
AOM

ICD-9CM CODES
382.9   Acute or chronic otitis media
381.00 Acute non-suppurative otitis media

EPIDEMIOLOGY & DEMOGRAPHICS

INCIDENCE (IN U.S.):
- Affects patients of all ages but is largely a disease of infants and young children.
- Occurs once in approximately 75% of all children.
- Occurs three or more times in one third of all children by age 3 yr.
- In 2000, costs associated with otitis media were approximately $5 billion, with 40% of the costs occurring from patients ages 1-3
- From 1995 to 2006, 80% of children diagnosed with otitis media received an antibiotic at initial visit.

PEAK INCIDENCE:
- Between 6 and 36 mo
- Second peak between ages 4 and 6 yr
- Fall, winter, early spring

PREDOMINANT SEX: Males

PREDOMINANT AGE:
- 47% to 60% of all children have their first episode of otitis media during their first year of life and 60% to 70% by their fourth birthday.
- Incidence of infection declines with age; seen infrequently in adults.

GENETICS:
Familial disposition:
- Native Americans
- Eskimos
- Australian aborigines
- Those with a strong family history
Congenital infection: high incidence in children born with cleft palates and other craniofacial abnormalities

PHYSICAL FINDINGS & CLINICAL PRESENTATION

- Fluid in the middle ear along with signs and symptoms of local inflammation (Figs. 1-614 and 1-615).
  1. Erythema with diminished light reflex
- Erythema of the tympanic membrane without other abnormalities is not a diagnostic criterion for acute otitis media (AOM) because it may occur with any inflammation of the upper respiratory tract, crying, or nose blowing.

- As infection progresses, middle ear exudation occurs (exudative phase); the exudate rapidly changes from serous to purulent (suppurative phase).
  1. Retraction and poor motility of the tympanic membrane, which then becomes bulging and convex
- At any time during the suppurative phase the tympanic membrane may rupture, releasing the middle ear contents.
- Symptoms:
  1. Otalgia, ranging from slight discomfort to severe, spreading to the temporal region
  2. Ear stuffiness and hearing loss may precede or follow otalgia
  3. Otorrhea
  4. Vertigo, nystagmus, tinnitus, fever, lethargy, irritability, nausea, vomiting, anorexia
- After an episode of AOM:
  1. Persistence of effusion for weeks or months (called secretory, serous, or nonsuppurative otitis media)
  2. Fever and otalgia usually absent
  3. Hearing loss possible (10 to 50 dB, with predominant involvement of the low frequencies)

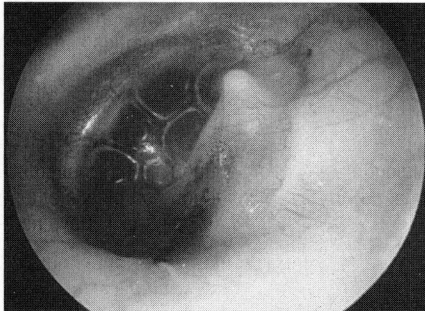

FIGURE 1-614 Otitis media with effusion of left ear. Retracted eardrum, prominent short process of malleus, and air bubbles seen anteriorly through the tympanic membrane. (From Behrman RE: *Nelson textbook of pediatrics,* ed 16, Philadelphia, 1996, Saunders.)

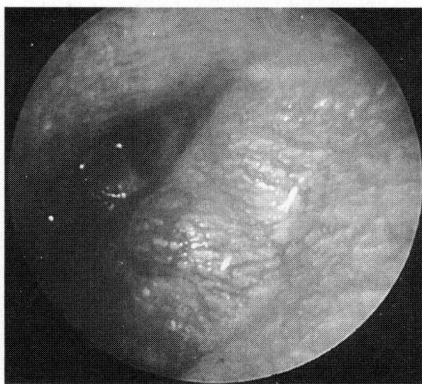

FIGURE 1-615 Acute left otitis media. (From Behrman RE: *Nelson textbook of pediatrics,* ed 16, Philadelphia, 1996, Saunders.)

ETIOLOGY

- Most common etiologic factor is an upper respiratory tract infection (often viral), which causes inflammation and obstruction of the eustachian tube. Bacterial colonization of the nasopharynx in conjunction with eustachian tube dysfunction leads to infection.
- May occasionally develop as a result of hematogenous spread or by direct invasion from the nasopharynx.
- Most common bacterial pathogens:
  1. *Streptococcus pneumoniae* causes 40% to 50% of cases and is the least likely of the major pathogens to resolve without treatment
  2. *Haemophilus influenzae* causes 20% to 30% of cases
  3. *Moraxella catarrhalis* causes 10% to 15% of cases
  4. Of increasing importance, infection caused by penicillin-nonsusceptible *S. pneumoniae* (MIC >0.1 μg/ml), ranging from 8% to 34%. About 50% of PNSSP isolates are penicillin-intermediate (MIC 0.1 to 2.0 μg/ml)
- Viral pathogens:
  1. Respiratory syncytial virus
  2. Rhinovirus
  3. Adenovirus
  4. Influenza
- Others:
  1. *Mycoplasma pneumoniae*
  2. *Chlamydia trachomatis*

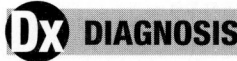 DIAGNOSIS

DIFFERENTIAL DIAGNOSIS

- Otitis externa
- Referred pain
  1. Mouth
  2. Nasopharynx
  3. Tonsils
  4. Other parts of the upper respiratory tract
- Section II describes the differential diagnosis of earache

WORKUP

Thorough otoscopic examination. Adequate visualization of the tympanic membrane requires removal of cerumen and debris.

- Tympanometry
  1. Measures compliance of the tympanic membrane and middle ear pressure
  2. Detects the presence of fluid
- Acoustic reflectometry
  1. Measures sound waves reflected from the middle ear
  2. Useful in infants >3 mo
  3. Increased reflected sound correlated with the presence of effusion

LABORATORY TESTS

- Tympanocentesis
  1. Not necessary in most cases because the microbiology of middle ear effusions has been shown to be quite consistent

Otitis Media 815

O

Diseases and Disorders

I

2. May be indicated in:
   a. Highly toxic patients
   b. Patients who do not respond to treatment in 48 to 72 hr
   c. Immunocompromised patients
- Cultures of the nasopharynx: sensitive but not specific
- Blood counts: usually show a leukocytosis with polymorphonuclear elevation
- Plain mastoid radiographs: generally not indicated; will reveal haziness in the periantral cells that may extend to entire mastoid
- CT or MRI may be indicated if serious complications suspected (meningitis, brain abscess)

Rx TREATMENT

ACUTE GENERAL Rx

Hydration, avoidance of irritants (e.g., tobacco smoke), nasal systemic decongestants, cool mist humidifier
Antimicrobials:

NOTE: Most uncomplicated cases of AOM resolve spontaneously, without complications. Studies have demonstrated limited therapeutic benefit from antibiotic therapy. Watchful waiting is appropriate for children who look well, can be comforted with supportive care, and are old enough to easily evaluate. However, when opting to use antibiotic therapy:

- Amoxicillin remains the drug of choice for first-line treatment of uncomplicated AOM despite increasing prevalence of drug-resistant *S. pneumoniae.*
- Treatment failure is defined by lack of clinical improvement of signs or symptoms after 3 days of therapy.
- With treatment failure, in the absence of an identified etiologic pathogen, therapy should be redirected to cover:
  1. Drug-resistant *S. pneumoniae*
  2. β-lactamase–producing strains of *H. influenzae* and *M. catarrhalis*
- Agents fulfilling these criteria include amoxicillin/clavulanate, second-generation cephalosporins (e.g., cefuroxime axetil, cefaclor), and ceftriaxone (given IM). Cefaclor, cefixime, loracarbef, and ceftibuten are active against *H. influenzae* and *M. catarrhalis* but less active against pneumococci, especially drug-resistant strains, than the agents listed previously.

- TMP/SMX and macrolides have been used as first- and second-line agents, but pneumococcal resistance to these agents is rising (up to 25% resistance to TMP/SMX and up to 10% resistance to erythromycin).
- Cross-resistance between these drugs and the β-lactams exists; therefore patients who do not respond to amoxicillin are more likely to have infections resistant to TMP/SMX and macrolides.
- Newer fluoroquinolones (levofloxacin, moxifloxacin) have enhanced activity against pneumococci compared with older agents (ciprofloxacin, ofloxacin) but are not indicated under the age of 18 due to concerns about the effect on bones, tendons, and joints.
- Treatment should be modified according to cultures and sensitivities.
- Generally treatment course is 10 to 14 days.
- Follow up approximately 4 wk after discontinuation of therapy to verify resolution of all symptoms, return to normal otoscopic findings, and restoration of normal hearing.

NOTE: Effusions may persist for 2 to 6 wk or longer in many cases of adequately treated otitis media.

SURGICAL Rx

- No evidence to support the routine of myringotomy, but in severe cases it provides prompt pain relief and accelerates resolution of infection.
- Purulent secretions retained in the middle ear lead to increased pressure that may lead to spread of infection to contiguous areas. Myringotomy to decompress the middle ear is necessary to avoid complications.
- Complications include mastoiditis, facial nerve paralysis, labyrinthitis, meningitis, and brain abscess.
- Other procedures used for drainage of the middle ear include insertion of a ventilation tube and/or simple mastoidectomy.

CHRONIC Rx

- Myringotomy and tympanostomy tube placement for persistent middle ear effusion unresponsive to medical therapy for ≥3 mo if bilateral or ≥6 mo if unilateral.
- Adenoidectomy, with or without tonsillectomy, often advocated for treatment of recurrent otitis media, although indications for this procedure are controversial.

- Long-term complications include tympanic membrane perforations, cholesteatoma, tympanosclerosis, ossicular necrosis, toxic or suppurative labyrinthitis, and intracranial suppuration.

DISPOSITION

Patients can be treated at home as outpatients with the rare exception of patients with evidence of local suppurative complications (e.g., meningitis, acute mastoiditis, brain abscess, cavernous sinus, or lateral vein thrombosis).

REFERRAL

- To otorhinolaryngologist if:
  1. Medical treatment failure
  2. Diagnosis uncertain: adults with one or more episodes of otitis media should be referred for ear-nose-throat evaluation to rule out underlying process (e.g., malignancy)
  3. Any of the above-mentioned acute and chronic complications

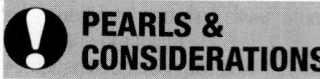 **PEARLS & CONSIDERATIONS**

COMMENTS

- Otoscopic findings are critical for accurate AOM diagnosis. AOM microbiology has changed with use of pneumococcal conjugate vaccine (PCV7). Antibiotics are modestly more effective than no treatment but cause adverse effects in 4% to 10% of children. Most antibiotics have comparable clinical success.

Prevention:
- Multiple component conjugate vaccines hold promise for decreasing recurrent episodes of AOM
- Breastfeed and bottle-feed infants in an upright position
- Avoidance of irritants (e.g., tobacco smoke)

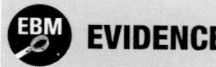 **EVIDENCE**

available at www.expertconsult.com

SUGGESTED READINGS
available at www.expertconsult.com

AUTHOR: **GLENN G. FORT, M.D., M.P.H.**

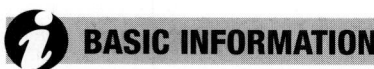

BASIC INFORMATION

DEFINITION

Ovarian tumors can be benign, requiring operative intervention but not recurring or metastasizing; malignant, recurring, metastasizing, and having decreased survival; or borderline, having a small risk of recurrence or metastases but generally having a good prognosis.

SYNONYMS

Epithelial ovarian cancer
Germ cell tumor
Sex cord stromal tumor
Ovarian tumor of low malignant potential

ICD-9CM CODES
183.0 Malignant neoplasm of ovary

EPIDEMIOLOGY & DEMOGRAPHICS

INCIDENCE: 12.9 to 15.1 cases/100,000 persons; ~25,000 new cases annually
PREVALENCE: Median age of 61 yr; peaks at age 75 to 79 yr (54/100,000)
RISK FACTORS: Low parity, delayed childbearing, use of talc on the perineum (unlikely), high-fat diet, fertility drugs (unlikely), Lynch II syndrome (nonpolyposis colon cancer, endometrial cancer, breast cancer, and ovarian cancer clusters in first- and second-degree relatives), breast-ovarian familial cancer syndrome, site-specific familial ovarian cancer.
GENETICS: The greatest risk factors of ovarian cancer are a family history and associated genetic syndromes. Familial susceptibility has been shown with the *BRCA1* gene located on 17q12 to 21. This correlates with breast-ovarian cancer syndrome.

PHYSICAL FINDINGS & CLINICAL PRESENTATION

- 60% present with advanced disease
- Abdominal fullness, early satiety, dyspepsia
- Pelvic pain, back pain, constipation
- Pelvic or abdominal mass
- Lymphadenopathy (inguinal)
- Sister Mary Joseph nodule (umbilical mass)

ETIOLOGY

- Can be inherited as site-specific familial ovarian cancer (two or more first-degree relatives have ovarian cancer)
- Breast-ovarian cancer syndrome (clusters of breast and ovarian cancer among first- and second-degree relatives)
- Lynch syndrome
- No family history and unknown etiology in the majority of ovarian cancer cases

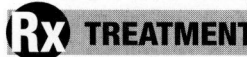

DIAGNOSIS

DIFFERENTIAL DIAGNOSIS

- Primary peritoneal cancer mesothelioma
- Benign ovarian tumor
- Functional ovarian cyst
- Endometriosis
- Ovarian torsion
- Pelvic kidney
- Pedunculated uterine fibroid
- Primary cancer from breast, gastrointestinal tract, or other pelvic organ metastasized to the ovary

WORKUP

- Definitive diagnosis made at laparotomy; epithelial ovarian cancer most common type of ovarian cancer
- Careful physical and history, including family history
- Exclusion of nongynecologic etiologies
- Observation of small cystic masses in premenopausal women for regression for 2 mo
- FIGO classification of ovarian carcinoma is described in Table 1-311.

LABORATORY TESTS

- Complete blood count
- Chemistry profile
- CA-125 or lysophosphatidic acid level. Use of these tests for annual screening is controversial. Only about 50% of early-stage ovarian cancers will be associated with elevated CA-

125. Additionally, false elevations may occur with uterine leiomyoma, endometriosis, pregnancy, and intraabdominal infections. The PLCO cancer screening trial revealed that annual screening based on CA-125 and vaginal ultrasound is ineffective and diagnostic follow-up of false positives resulted in 15% serious complication rate.
- Consider: human chorionic gonadotropin, inhibin, alpha-fetoprotein, neuron-specific enolase, and lactate dehydrogenase in patients at risk for germ cell tumors.
- A panel of 3 serum biomarkers (apolipoprotein A-1 [ApoA-1], transthyretin [TTR], and transferrin [TF]) has been reported useful in distinguishing normal samples from early-stage ovarian cancer with a sensitivity of 84% and normal samples from late-stage ovarian cancer with a sensitivity of 97%.

IMAGING STUDIES

- Ultrasound
- Chest x-ray
- Mammogram
- CT scan to help evaluate extent of disease (Fig. 1-617)
- Other studies (MRI, intravenous pyelogram, etc.) as clinically indicated

TREATMENT

NONPHARMACOLOGIC THERAPY

Virtually all cases of ovarian cancer involve surgical exploration. This includes:
- Abdominal cytology
- Total abdominal hysterectomy and bilateral salpingo-oophorectomy (except in early stages in which fertility preservation is an issue)
- Omentectomy
- Diaphragm sampling
- Selective lymphadenectomy (pelvic and para-aortic nodes)
- Primary cytoreduction with a goal of residual tumor diameter <2 cm
- Bowel surgery, splenectomy if needed to obtain optimal (<2 cm) cytoreduction

---

TABLE 1-311 FIGO Classification of Ovarian Carcinoma

Stage I	Growth limited to the ovaries:
	Stage IA: Growth limited to one ovary, no ascites and no tumor present on the external surface; capsule intact
	Stage IB: Growth limited to both ovaries, no ascites and no tumor present on the external surface; capsule intact
	Stage IC: Stage 1A or 1B where there is tumor on the surface of either ovary; or with ruptured capsules or with ascites containing malignant cells or positive peritoneal washings
Stage II	Growth involving one or both ovaries with pelvic extension:
	Stage IIA: Extension and/or metastases to the uterus and tubes
	Stage IIB: Extension to other pelvic tissues
	Stage IIC: Stage IIA or IIB with tumor on the surface of either ovary or positive peritoneal washings or malignant ascites
Stage III	Growth involving one or both ovaries with peritoneal implants outside the pelvis or positive retroperitoneal or inguinal lymph nodes:
	Stage IIIA: Microscopic seeding of abdominal peritoneal surfaces
	Stage IIIB: Macroscopic disease outside the pelvis less than 2 cm in diameter
	Stage IIIC: Abdominal implants greater than 2 cm and/or positive nodes
Stage IV	Growth involving one or both ovaries with distant metastases including parenchymal (but not superficial) liver metastases and pleural effusions containing malignant cells

From Symonds EM, Symonds IM: *Essential obstetrics and gynaecology*, ed 4, London, 2004, Churchill Livingstone.

- Conventional treatment includes surgical de-bulking (cytoreduction) followed by chemotherapy. However, patients with low-grade, well-differentiated stage I ovarian cancer do not benefit from adjuvant chemotherapy.

ACUTE GENERAL Rx

- Optimal cytoreduction is generally followed by chemotherapy (except in some early-stage disease).
- Cisplatin-based combination chemotherapy is used for stage II or greater, 6-mo treatment. Compared with IV paclitaxel plus cisplatin, IV paclitaxel plus intraperitoneal cis-platin and paclitaxel improves survival rates in patients with optimally debulked stage III ovarian cancer.
- Chemotherapy regimens continue to change as research continues. Bevacizumab, a humanized antivascular endothelial growth factor monoclonal antibody, has been shown to be effective in improving progression-free survival in women with ovarian cancer. Trials using bevacizumab during and up to 10 months after carboplatin and paclitaxel chemotherapy have shown prolongation of the median progression-free survival by about 4 months in patients with advanced epithelial ovarian cancer. Olaparib, an oral polymerase inhibitor, has shown antitumor activity in pa-tients with high-grade serous ovarian cancer with or without BRCA1 and BRCA2 germline mutations. Trials have shown that olaparib as maintenance treatment significantly improved progression-free survival among patients with platinum-sensitive, relapsed high-grade serous ovarian cancer.
- Second-look surgery when chemotherapy is complete generally is no longer recommended because this procedure has not been shown to improve survival.
- Recent trials have shown that neoadjuvant chemotherapy followed by interval debulking surgery is not inferior to debulking surgery followed by chemotherapy as a treatment option for patients with bulky stage IIIC or IV ovarian carcinoma. Complete resection of all macroscopic disease, whether performed as primary treatment or after neoadjuvant chemotherapy, remains the objective whenever cytoreductive surgery is performed.

CHRONIC Rx

- If CA-125 elevated, may have recurrent disease
- Physical and pelvic examinations every 3 mo for 2 yr, every 4 mo during third year, then every 6 mo
- CA-125 every visit
- Yearly Pap smear

DISPOSITION

- Overall 5-yr survival rates remain low because of the preponderance of late-stage disease:
  - Stage I and II: 80% to 100%
  - Stage III: 15% to 20%
  - Stage IV: 5%
- Younger patients (<50 yr) in all stages have a considerably better 5-yr survival than older patients (40% vs. 15%).
- Among women with high-grade serous ovarian cancer, BRCA2 mutation, but not BRCA1 deficiency, is associated with improved survival, improved chemotherapy response, and genome instability compared with BRCA wild-type.
- Among patients with invasive epithelial ovarian cancer (EOC), having a germline mutation in BRCA1 or BRCA2 is associated with improved 5-yr overall survival. BRCA2 carriers have the best prognosis.

COMMENTS

- The U.S. Preventive Services Task Force has concluded that current evidence does not show any mortality benefit to routine screening for ovarian cancer with transvaginal ultrasonography or single-threshold serum CA-125 testing and that the harms of such screening are at least moderate.
- Patients at high risk for developing ovarian cancer (BRCA1/BRCA2 gene mutation, hereditary nonpolyposis colorectal cancer syndrome) should consider prophylactic salpingo-oophorectomy after childbearing is complete. If surgery is declined, the National Comprehensive Cancer Network guidelines recommend intensive surveillance with pelvic and abdominal sonogram and serum CA-125 every 6 mo starting at age 35 or 10 yr earlier than cancer diagnosis in family member.

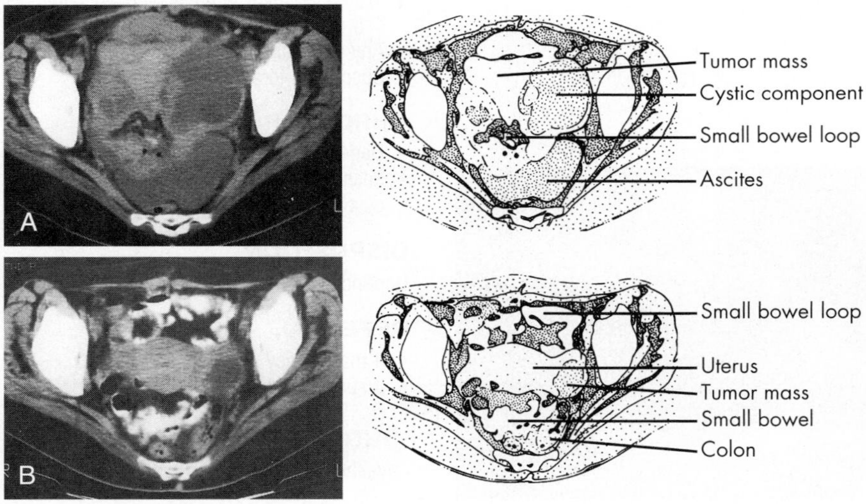

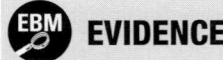

EVIDENCE

available at www.expertconsult.com

SUGGESTED READINGS

available at www.expertconsult.com

RELATED CONTENT

Ovarian Neoplasm, Benign (Related Key Topic)
Ovarian Cancer (Patient Information)

AUTHORS: **GIL M. FARKASH, M.D.,** and **RUBEN ALVERO, M.D.**

Tumor mass
Cystic component
Small bowel loop
Ascites

Small bowel loop
Uterus
Tumor mass
Small bowel
Colon

FIGURE 1-617 Response to chemotherapy. A 51-year-old woman presented with a rapid increase in abdominal girth. **A,** On CT scan, she was found to have a 12 × 8 cm ovarian mass with a cystic component; peritoneal involvement was extensive and 6 L of ascites was removed. Pathologic examination showed a poorly differentiated tumor. The tumor was not resectable, and she was treated with combination chemotherapy. After one cycle of therapy, her abdomen returned to normal size. **B,** A CT scan reveals only a small residual ovarian mass. Surgery after four cycles of chemotherapy showed no gross or microscopic tumor. She received four more cycles of chemotherapy but relapsed 1 year later with abdominal metastases. (From Skarin AT: *Atlas of diagnostic oncology,* ed 3, St Louis, 2003, Mosby.)

Diseases and Disorders

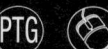
ℹ BASIC INFORMATION

DEFINITION

Benign ovarian neoplasms are often clinically indistinguishable from their malignant counterparts. Therefore all persistent adnexal masses must be considered malignant until proven otherwise. Nonneoplastic tumors include:

- Germinal inclusion cyst
- Follicle cyst
- Corpus luteum cyst
- Pregnancy luteoma
- Theca lutein cysts
- Sclerocystic ovaries
- Endometrioma

Neoplastic tumors derived from coelomic epithelium include:

- Cystic tumors: serous cystadenoma, mucinous cystadenoma, mixed forms
- Tumors with stromal overgrowth: fibroma, adenofibroma, Brenner tumor

Tumors derived from germ cells are dermoids (benign cystic teratomas).

ICD-9CM CODES
220 Benign neoplasm of ovary

EPIDEMIOLOGY & DEMOGRAPHICS

- Reproductive years:
  1. Most common benign ovarian neoplasms: serous cystadenoma and benign cystic teratoma
  2. Most common adnexal mass: functional cyst
- Risk of malignancy increases after age 40 yr.
- Infants: adnexal masses are usually follicular cysts attributable to maternal hormone stimulation that regress during first few months of life.
- Childhood:
  1. Adnexal masses are rare
  2. 8% malignant
  3. Almost always dysgerminomas or teratomas (germ cell origin)
  4. Frequency of malignancy inversely correlated with age
- Adolescence:
  1. Most common adnexal mass is a functional cyst.
  2. Most common neoplastic ovarian tumor is a benign cystic teratoma.
  3. Solid/cystic adnexal tumors are rare and almost always dysgerminomas or malignant teratomas.

PHYSICAL FINDINGS & CLINICAL PRESENTATION

- Usually asymptomatic
- Pelvic pain or pressure
- Dyspareunia
- Abdominal pain ranging from mild to severe peritoneal irritation
- Increasing abdominal girth or distention
- Adnexal mass of pelvic examination
- Children: abdominal or rectal mass

ETIOLOGY

- Physiologic
- Endometriosis
- Unknown

Dx DIAGNOSIS

DIFFERENTIAL DIAGNOSIS

- Ovarian torsion
- Malignancy: ovary, fallopian tube, colon
- Uterine fibroid
- Diverticular abscess, diverticulitis
- Appendiceal abscess, appendicitis (especially in children)
- Tubo-ovarian abscess
- Paraovarian cyst
- Distended bladder
- Pelvic kidney
- Ectopic pregnancy
- Retroperitoneal cyst or neoplasm

WORKUP

- Complete history and physical examination
- Pelvic or rectovaginal examination to reveal firm, irregular, mobile mass
- Laparoscopy or laparotomy to establish diagnosis

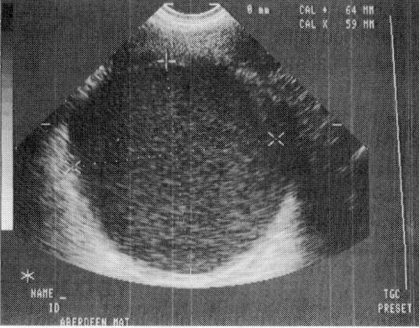

FIGURE 1-618 Ultrasonogram, which reveals a cyst 6.5 cm across, which was found at laparotomy to be an endometrioma, full of altered blood: the so-called chocolate cyst. This may cause cyclical or chronic pelvic pain. (From Greer IA et al: *Mosby's color atlas and text of obstetrics and gynecology*, London, 2000, Harcourt.)

LABORATORY TESTS

- Pregnancy test
- Serum tumor markers:
  1. Cancer antigen 125 (CA-125)
  2. Alpha-fetoprotein (endodermal sinus tumor, immature teratoma)
  3. Beta-human chorionic gonadotropin
  4. Lactate dehydrogenase (dysgerminoma)

IMAGING STUDIES

Ultrasound (Fig. 1-618):

- May differentiate adnexal mass from other pelvic masses
- Features that increase risk of malignancy include solid component, papillae, multiple septations or solitary thick septa, ascites, matted bowel, bilaterality, irregular borders
- CT scan with contrast
- Colonoscopy or barium enema, if symptomatic

Rx TREATMENT

NONPHARMACOLOGIC THERAPY

Repeat pelvic examination for premenopausal women in 4 to 6 wk

ACUTE GENERAL Rx

Indications for surgery:

- Postmenopausal or premenarcheal palpable adnexal mass
- Adnexal mass with suspicious ultrasound features
- Premenopausal woman with persistent cyst >5 cm
- Any adnexal mass >10 cm
- Suspected torsion or rupture

CHRONIC Rx

- Depends on diagnosis
- Possible suppression of formation of new cysts by oral contraceptives

DISPOSITION

Depends on diagnosis

REFERRAL

- If malignancy suspected
- If surgery required

SUGGESTED READINGS
available at www.expertconsult.com

RELATED CONTENT
Ovarian Cysts (Patient Information)

AUTHORS: **GEORGE T. DANAKAS, M.D.,** and **RUBEN ALVERO, M.D.**

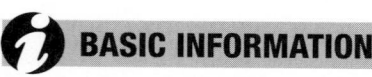

BASIC INFORMATION

DEFINITION

Paget's disease of the bone is a focal disorder of chaotic bone remodeling with increased osteoblastic and osteoclastic activity that results in disorganized woven and lamellar bone in one or more skeletal sites. The end result is bone of poor quality that is enlarged, hypervascular, and susceptible to deformation and fracture.

SYNONYMS

Osteitis deformans

ICD-9CM CODES
731.0 Paget's disease (osteitis deformans)

EPIDEMIOLOGY & DEMOGRAPHICS

Epidemiologic data suggest an origin of Paget's disease in Great Britain spreading to other areas by English colonists beginning in the seventeenth century. Highest prevalence occurs in Eastern and Western Europe and in those who have emigrated to New Zealand, Australia, South Africa, and North America. Rarely seen in Japanese, Chinese, Asian Indians, sub-Saharan Africans, and middle eastern Arabs.

Most commonly diagnosed in those aged >50 yr and rare before 40 yr.

Prevalence estimates of up to 3% of population aged >50 yr and up to 10% in those aged >90 yr.

PREDOMINANT SEX: Variable preponderance of males.
PREDOMINANT AGE: Middle or advanced years.
FAMILIAL INCIDENCE: Common, family history positive in up to 40% of cases.

PHYSICAL FINDINGS & CLINICAL PRESENTATION

- Most common sites of involvement: pelvis, spine, sacrum, femora, skull, tibiae, humeri, scapulae.
- Uncommon: hand, foot, fibula.
- Lesions in one (monostotic) or more bones (polyostotic).
- Gradual progression of disease in affected bone(s) with rare appearance at new site(s).
- Many patients are asymptomatic, but up to 40% of patients who come to medical attention present with bone pain.
- Symptoms and signs include bone and articular pain often related to secondary arthritis, bone deformities and enlargement, increased warmth over pagetic bone, skull enlargement, nerve entrapment or compression syndromes, cranial nerve deficits especially deafness, spinal cord compression and vascular steal syndromes, fissure fractures, fractures, and neoplastic degeneration.

ETIOLOGY

Etiology remains unknown.

Extensive epidemiologic and laboratory data are in keeping with potential role of paramyxo-viral infection of osteoclasts in a genetically susceptible individual with or without documented genetic mutations.

DIAGNOSIS

DIFFERENTIAL DIAGNOSIS

- Osteosclerosis
- Hyperphosphatasia
- Familial expansile osteolysis
- Fibrous dysplasia
- Skeletal neoplasm (primary or metastatic)
- Osteomalacia with secondary hyperparathyroidism

LABORATORY TESTS

- Increase in serum alkaline phosphatase or bone-specific alkaline phosphatase
- Increase in urine NTx/creatinine ratio or plasma CTx
- Bone biopsy may be necessary to rule out sarcomatous degeneration or metastasic disease

IMAGING STUDIES

Bone scintigraphy is the most sensitive test for delineating the extent and site of pagetic lesions but nonspecific in that areas of uptake may be related to arthritis or metastatic lesions. Radiographs (Fig. 1-619) will further delineate characteristic pagetic changes.

TREATMENT

Indications for therapy include extensive or symptomatic disease; neurologic complications; involvement of weight-bearing bones, skull, vertebrae, and other areas of critical involvement, for example, in proximity to joints; and prevention of excess bleeding from an orthopedic procedure on pagetic bone.

NONPHARMACOLOGIC THERAPY

Optimization of calcium and vitamin D intake and appropriate guidance regarding ambulatory needs.

SPECIFIC THERAPY

Bisphosphonates are the mainstay of therapy and include oral alendronate or risedronate and intravenous pamidronate or zoledronic acid.

- SC salmon calcitonin when bisphosphonates are not tolerated or are contraindicated as in those with GFR of <35 ml/min
- Acetaminophen, aspirin, and nonsteroidal drugs for relief of pain

DISPOSITION

- Without treatment, progression of disease is common
- With treatment, remissions of varying duration in most patients. Bisphosphonates can normalize bone turnover in a high proportion of patients, but evidence that long-term suppression of bone turnover prevents complications or improves the clinical outcome is currently inconclusive.
- Careful and regular clinical and biochemical followup at 3- to 6-mo intervals with necessity of retreatment in patients with continued pagetic activity or reactivation
- With first ever intravenous dose of pamidronate or zoledronic acid, patients may experience a flu-like syndrome for several days that may be prevented with acetaminophen

SUGGESTED READINGS

available at www.expertconsult.com

RELATED CONTENT

Paget's Disease of Bone (Patient Information)

AUTHOR: **JOSEPH R. TUCCI, M.D.**

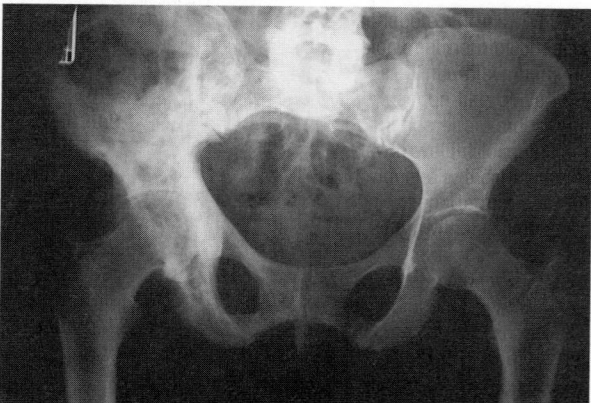

FIGURE 1-619 Paget's disease of the bone. Frontal radiograph of the pelvis shows marked prominence of the trabeculae in the right ilium, ischium, and pubic bones, with small lytic areas identified as compatible with the later stages of Paget's disease. (From Specht N [ed]: *Practical guide to diagnostic imaging*, St Louis, 1998, Mosby.)

BASIC INFORMATION

DEFINITION

Paget's disease of the breast is a malignant disease that presents itself as a scaly, sore, eroding, bleeding ulcer of the nipple. It represents an extension of a ductal adenocarcinoma of the breast. Microscopically, typical large clear cells (Paget's cells) with pale and abundant cytoplasm and hyperchromatic nuclei with prominent nucleoli are found in the epidermal layer. Paget's disease is more often associated with primary invasive or in situ carcinoma of the breast.

ICD-9CM CODES
174.0 Malignant neoplasm of female breast, nipple, and areola

EPIDEMIOLOGY & DEMOGRAPHICS

- Not common
- Found in one in 100 to 200 breast cancer patients

PHYSICAL FINDINGS & CLINICAL PRESENTATION

- Variable; most often reveals an erythematous, irregularly bordered plaque on the nipple.
- Itching or burning nipple and/or reported lump
- Very minimal scaly lesion that may bleed when scales are lifted
- Typical ulcer located on nipple with serous fluid weeping or small amount of bleeding coming from it (Fig. 1-620)
- Palpable carcinoma in the breast of some patients

ETIOLOGY

- Exact origin unknown
- Possibly migration of either in situ or invasive carcinoma cells in breast to nipple skin to produce Paget's disease

DIAGNOSIS

DIFFERENTIAL DIAGNOSIS

- Chronic dermatitis
- Florid papillomatosis of the nipple or nipple adenoma
- Eczema

WORKUP

- Clinically apparent
- Careful breast examination with diagnosis in mind
- Palpable mass or mammographic lesions in 60% to 70% of patients

A clinical algorithm for the evaluation of nipple discharge is described in Section III, "Breast, Nipple Discharge Evaluation."

LABORATORY TESTS

Biopsy of nipple lesion

IMAGING STUDIES

Mammograms to search for possible primary carcinoma

TREATMENT

NONPHARMACOLOGIC THERAPY

- Fewer patients:
  1. Paget's disease of nipple only finding when mammographically negative breast
  2. Consideration of wide excision of nipple with or without radiation
- Other patients: additional invasive or in situ carcinoma recognized
- Either modified mastectomy or breast conservation treatment
- Presence of underlying in situ or invasive carcinoma in mastectomy specimen of majority of patients

ACUTE GENERAL Rx

Systemic adjuvant therapy depending on extent of invasive carcinoma found

DISPOSITION

- Parallel prognosis to that of breast cancer patient without Paget's disease
- Regular follow-up as in other invasive or in situ carcinoma patients

REFERRAL

At outset, all suspicious nipple lesions should be referred for evaluation and treatment.

SUGGESTED READINGS
available at www.expertconsult.com

RELATED CONTENT
Breast Cancer (Related Key Topic)
Fig. 3-33 Breast cancer screening and evaluation (Algorithm)
Paget's Disease of the Breast (Patient Information)

AUTHORS: **TAKUMA NEMOTO, M.D.,** and **RUBEN ALVERO, M.D.**

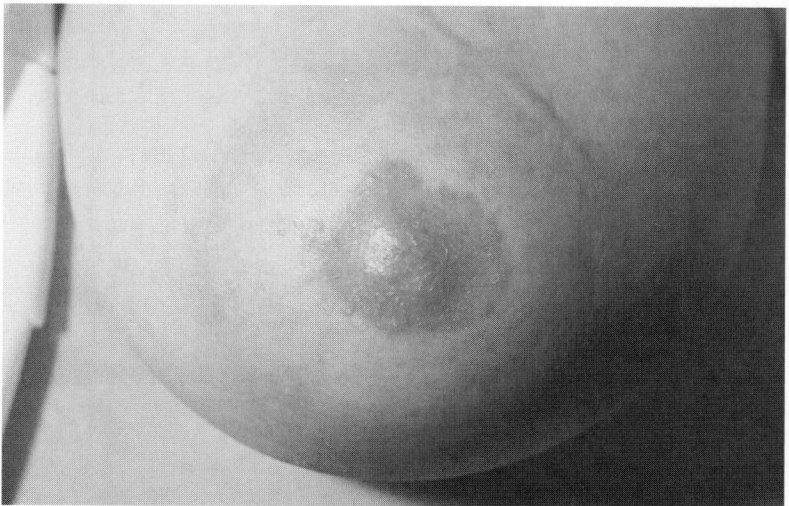

FIGURE 1-620 Paget's disease of the breast. The lesion has insidiously spread for 1 year to infiltrate the areola and surrounding skin. (From Habif TP: *Clinical dermatology: a color guide to diagnosis and therapy,* ed 3, St Louis, 1996, Mosby.)

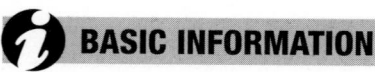

BASIC INFORMATION

DEFINITION

Chronic pain is pain that persists for longer than the expected time frame or that is associated with progressive, nonmalignant disease. Pain is an unpleasant sensory and emotional experience associated with actual or potential tissue damage or described in terms of such damage. The perception of pain is influenced by physiologic, psychological, and social factors.

SYNONYMS

Nonmalignant chronic pain

ICD-9CM CODES	
338.29	Chronic Pain
338.4	Chronic Pain Syndrome
780.96	Generalized Pain
304.7x/304.8x	Opioid Dependence

EPIDEMIOLOGY & DEMOGRAPHICS

Estimates of the prevalence of chronic pain in the United States vary widely. Data from one national survey (1999-2002 National Health and Nutrition Examination Survey [NHANES]) reported a prevalence of chronic regional and widespread pain of 11% and 3.6%, respectively, while the National Center for Health Statistics estimates that 32.8% of the U.S. population suffers from some form of chronic pain. Chronic pain is the third leading cause of physical impairment in the U.S., and related costs are estimated to be tens of billions annually. Patients with chronic pain may also experience changes in mood, depression, sleep disturbances, and fatigue, and decreased overall physical functioning.

CLINICAL PRESENTATION

- History: Comprehensive patient assessment, including history of present illness (cause of pain, location timing, characteristics, exacerbating/relieving factors, triggers), past therapies (pharmacologic and nonpharmacologic and outcomes of these therapies), medical history, family and social history, psychiatric history, substance use history, allergies, and current medications, should be performed on initial evaluation.
- Pain assessment should be performed at each visit; includes pain intensity (1 to 10), response to medication, attributes of pain, and assessment of function (cognitive, emotional, employment, sleep, mobility, and self-care). Standardized templates for both initial and follow-up pain assessment have been developed by various organizations. The website Pain Treatment Topics contains many of these assessment tools (http://pain-topics.org/clinical_concepts/assess.php).
- Physical examination: Directed at systems affected by pain and neurologic examination.

ETIOLOGY

Chronic pain can generally be categorized as originating from one of five etiologies: musculoskeletal, neuropathic, inflammatory, mechanical, or mixed. Chronic pain may include such diagnoses as headache, low back pain, previous trauma, arthritis, neurogenic (e.g., trigeminal neuralgia), psychogenic (related to depression or anxiety), fibromyalgia, reflex sympathetic dystrophy, myofascial pain syndrome, phantom limb pain, idiopathic, or unknown.

DIAGNOSIS

DIFFERENTIAL DIAGNOSIS

- Depends on etiology.
- Depression and anxiety disorders can be both a cause and a result of chronic pain, so temporal association of these disorders is important.

WORKUP

- Laboratory testing, imaging studies, and/or electromyographic studies should be used when etiology of chronic pain is unknown or unclear, when comorbidities are suspected, and as the history and physical examination direct.
- Consider use of random urine drug screens or other tests to screen for presence of illegal drugs, unreported prescribed medications, or alcohol use.

TREATMENT

- Studies increasingly support the application of a multidisciplinary approach that addresses the multiple facets of pain (e.g., physical, psychological, social aspects).
- Therapeutic goal is the reduction of pain (elimination of chronic pain is generally unlikely and providers need to discuss these limitations with patients at outset).

- Fig. E1-621 describes an algorithm for the treatment of pain.

NONPHARMACOLOGIC THERAPY

- Exercise
- Modalities: heat therapy, cold therapy, transcutaneous electrical nerve stimulation (TENS) units, cognitive behavioral therapy, psychological counseling, and physical therapy
- Electrostimulation therapy: TENS units
- Behavioral therapies: cognitive behavioral therapy, hypnosis, biofeedback, relaxation therapy
- Music therapy (in conjunction with other types of therapy)
- Surgery

ACUTE GENERAL Rx

- Short-acting anti-inflammatory and analgesic medications (e.g., acetaminophen/NSAIDs/opioids)
- Trigger point or joint injections (immediate anesthetic plus long-acting corticosteroids)
- Epidural steroid injections
- Nerve blocks

CHRONIC Rx

- Pain management with long-acting pharmacologic agents is considered a key aspect of therapy but is often underused. Fig. 1-622 illustrates a strategy for pharmacologic management of pain using the World Health Organization (WHO) analgesic ladder.
- Long-acting NSAIDs. Table 1-312 describes adjuvant analgesic drugs for chronic pain.
- Sustained-release opioids (used for moderate to severe pain that has failed other therapeutic

WHO ANALGESIC LADDER

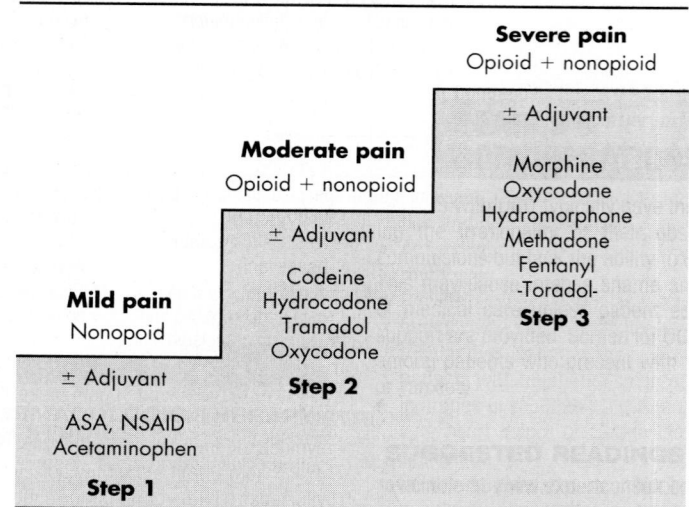

- Advance up the ladder if pain persists

FIGURE 1-622 Strategy for pharmacologic management of pain using the World Health Organization (WHO) analgesic ladder. Multiagent therapy is usually required for optimal pain management. Patients with mild pain should be started on a nonopioid analgesic, and those with moderate pain on a step 2 opioid. Many patients can benefit from the addition of a nonopioid to the opioid (e.g., for bone pain) or an adjuvant agent to the opioid (e.g., for neuropathic pain). If this combination does not produce adequate relief or the patient has severe pain, step 3 opioids should be started initially. Toradol (ketorolac) is a nonsteroidal anti-inflammatory drug *(NSAID)* with the pain-relieving potency of a step 3 opioid. Many patients can benefit from the addition of nonopioid analgesics or adjuvants, if indicated. *ASA,* Aspirin. (From Hoffman R et al: *Hematology, basic principles and practice,* ed 5, Philadelphia, 2009, Churchill Livingstone.)

TABLE 1-312 Adjuvant Analgesic Drugs for Chronic Pain

Drug	Dosage	Indications	Adverse Effects	Comments
Tricyclic Antidepressants				
Amitriptyline, imipramine, desipramine, nortriptyline	10-150 mg/day	Peripheral neuropathy, postherpetic neuralgia, other types of peripheral neuropathic pain, central pain, facial pain, fibromyalgia, headache prophylaxis, irritable bowel syndrome, and chronic low back pain with or without radiculopathy	Sedation, dry mouth, confusion, weight gain, constipation, urinary retention, ataxia, cardiac conduction delay (QTc prolongation)	First-line agents for neuropathic pain and headache prophylaxis Secondary amine drugs (e.g., nortriptyline) have fewer side effects than tertiary amines (e.g., amitriptyline) Contraindicated in glaucoma
Serotonin-Norepinephrine Reuptake Inhibitors				
Venlafaxine	75-225 mg/day	Peripheral neuropathy, headache prophylaxis	Sedation, dry mouth, constipation, ataxia, hypertension, hyperhidrosis	Dose adjustment in patients with renal dysfunction
Duloxetine	60-120 mg/day	Peripheral neuropathy, fibromyalgia, chronic back pain	Sedation, dry mouth, constipation, hyperhidrosis	U.S. Food and Drug Administration (FDA)-approved for fibromyalgia and diabetic neuropathy Contraindicated in glaucoma
Anticonvulsants				
Gabapentin	600-3600 mg/day	Peripheral neuropathy, postherpetic neuralgia, other types of peripheral neuropathic pain, central pain, pelvic pain, headache prophylaxis, radiculopathy, chronic postsurgical pain	Sedation, weight gain, dry mouth, ataxia, edema	First-line agent for neuropathic pain FDA-approved for postherpetic neuralgia Effective preemptively for postoperative pain
Pregabalin	150-600 mg/day	Peripheral neuropathy, postherpetic neuralgia, central pain, fibromyalgia	Sedation, weight gain, dry mouth, ataxia, edema	First-line agent for neuropathic pain FDA-approved for diabetic neuropathy, postherpetic neuralgia, fibromyalgia Effective preemptively for postoperative pain Same mechanism of action as gabapentin
Carbamazepine	200-1600 mg/day	Facial neuralgias, diabetic neuropathy	Sedation, ataxia, diplopia, hyponatremia, agranulocytosis, diarrhea, aplastic anemia, hepatotoxicity, Stevens-Johnson syndrome	First-line agent and FDA-approved for trigeminal and glossopharyngeal neuralgia Contraindicated in patients with porphyria and atrioventricular conduction block
Topiramate	50-400 mg/day	Headache prophylaxis, chronic low back pain with or without radiculopathy	Sedation, ataxia, diplopia, weight loss, diarrhea, metabolic acidosis, kidney stones	First-line agent and FDA-approved for migraine prophylaxis Often used as appetite suppressant
Corticosteroids (Systemic)				
Prednisone	5-60 mg/day	Inflammatory arthritis, other inflammatory pain conditions (e.g., inflammatory bowel disease), traumatic nerve injury, complex regional pain syndrome	Myriad psychiatric, gastrointestinal, neurologic, and cardiac side effects; immunosuppression, weakness, edema, weight gain, elevated glucose, poor wound healing, others	Stronger evidence supports local (i.e., injection) administration More effective for acute pain Strong anti-inflammatory effects
Miscellaneous				
Muscle relaxants	Variable depending on drug	Skeletal muscle spasm, acute spinal pain, temporomandibular disorder Baclofen effective for spasticity, dystonia, and trigeminal neuralgia	Sedation, ataxia, blurred vision, confusion, asthenia, xerostomia and other gastrointestinal effects, palpitations	First-line agents for acute back pain and skeletal muscle spasm
Lidocaine patch	1-3 patches every 12 hr	Postherpetic neuropathy, peripheral neuropathy, other types of neuropathic and possibly myofascial pain associated with allodynia	Minimal systemic side effects when applied appropriately	Second-line agent and FDA-approved for postherpetic neuralgia
Capsaicin cream	0.025% applied three or four times per day	Postherpetic neuralgia, peripheral neuropathy and other types of neuropathic pain, chronic postsurgical pain, arthritis, and other musculoskeletal conditions	Burning on application Minimal systemic side effects when applied appropriately	FDA-approved for arthritis Second-line agent for postherpetic neuralgia and third-line agent for peripheral neuropathy Single application 8% patch providing up to 3 mo of pain relief was recently approved for postherpetic neuralgia
Cannabinoids	Variable depending on drug and delivery route	Strongest evidence is for multiple sclerosis May be effective for peripheral neuropathy and other types of neuropathic pain spasticity	Myriad psychiatric, neurologic, and cardiac effects; xerostomia, abdominal pain, and other gastrointestinal effects	Fourth-line agent with narrow therapeutic index Modest analgesic effect comparable to codeine

From Goldman L, Schafer AI: *Goldman's Cecil medicine*, ed 24, Philadelphia, 2012, Saunders.

interventions): oxycodone, morphine SR, methadone (use with caution), or Duragesic patch; short-acting opioids can be used in conjunction with these agents for management of breakthrough pain. Conversion to a long-acting opioid should be based on an equianalgesic conversion (http://www.acpinternist.org/archives/2008/01/extra/pain_charts.pdf). Table 1-313 provides guidelines for opioid dose selection, conservative initial starting doses for opioid-naïve individuals, and conversion ratios for opioid rotation in patients on chronic opioids.

- Antidepressants (tricyclic and selective serotonin reuptake inhibitor)
- Anticonvulsant medications particularly helpful for neuropathic conditions (e.g., carbamazepine, valproic acid, gabapentin, pregabalin)
- Implantable methods, epidural and intrathecal drug delivery systems, dorsal column stimulators

COMPLEMENTARY & ALTERNATIVE MEDICINE

Acupuncture and massage (evidence based for some indications). Acupuncture is most likely to benefit patients with low back pain, neck pain, chronic idiopathic or tension headache, migraine, and knee osteoarthritis.

REFERRAL

- Pain medicine specialist or multidisciplinary pain clinic: useful when primary therapies

TABLE 1-313 Guidelines for Opioid Dose Selection, Conservative Initial Starting Doses for Opioid-Naïve Individuals, and Conversion Ratios for Opioid Rotation in Patients on Chronic Opioids

Opioid Naïve	Morphine SR	Codeine	Oxycodone	Hydrocodone	Hydromorphone	Methadone	Fentanyl	Oxymorphone
Initial dose and range in opioid-naïve patient (starting dose range for repeated dosing)*	15 mg (15-30 mg q 8-12h)	30 mg (15-60 mg q 4-6h)	5 mg (5-15 mg q 4-6h)	5 mg (5-10 mg q 4-6h)	2 mg (2-4 mg q 4-6h)	2.5 mg q 6-12h	NA	5 mg q 4-6h

Opioid Tolerant Converting from:	Morphine PO	Codeine	Oxycodone	Hydrocodone	Hydromorphone	Methadone	Fentanyl	Oxymorphone
Morphine IM 10 mg (the gold standard for opioid comparisons)	20-30 mg	60-90 mg†	5 mg	5-10 mg q 4-6h	2 mg	2.5 mg	25-µg patch/72 hr	5 mg (the gold standard for opioid comparisons)
Morphine SR 30 mg PO q 8-12h, 60-90 mg/24h		30-90 mg q 4h	3-45 mg/24 hr Oxycodone, approx 50% of morphine dose	30-45 mg/24 hr	12-18 mg/24 hr	24-hr dose morphine 30-90 mg 4:1 conversion 90-300 mg 8:1 conversion >300 mg 12:1	25-mcg patch/72 hr	5 mg q 12h ER
Codeine 30-60 mg q 4h	15-30 mg q 3-4h		5-7.5 mg q 4h	5-10 mg q 4h	12 mg/24 hr	2.5 mg q 8-12h	12.5-µg patch/72 hr	2.5-5 mg q 4-6h IR
Oxycodone 5 mg q 3-4h	10 mg	30-60 mg q 3-4h		5-10 mg q 4h	12 mg/24 hr	2.5 mg q 8-12h	25-µg patch/72 hr	5 mg q 4-6h IR
Hydrocodone 10 mg q 3-4h	15 mg	30-60 mg q 3-4h	5 mg q 3-4h		12 mg/24 hr		12.5-µg patch/72 hr	2.5-5 mg q 4-6h IR
Hydromorphone 2 mg q 4h	10 mg		5 mg	5-10 mg q 4h		2.5 mg q 8-12h	25-µg patch/72 hr	5 mg q 4-6h IR
Methadone 5 mg q 8h	20 mg SR q 8h		10 mg q 3-4h		4 mg q 4-6h		25-µg patch/72 hr	5 mg q 12h ER
Fentanyl 25 µg/hr patch	90 mg morphine per 24-hr (1 µg to 4 mg morphine)					5 mg q 8-12h		5 mg q12h ER
Oxymorphone ER 5 mg q 12h	15 mg SR q 12h		5 mg q 8-12h	10 mg q 4-6h	12 mg/24 hr	5 mg q 8-12h	25-µg patch/72 hr	

Note: Recommended starting doses are low and should be titrated upward slowly to minimize adverse effects. Limitations of equianalgesic tables exist because they are based on single-dose studies in opioid-naïve individuals. Convert opioid 1 to morphine equivalents and calculate dose of opioid 2 according to conversion ratio then reduce the calculated dose for opioid 2 by 1/3 to 1/2 to ensure safety of the 24-hr total daily dose. Rescue dose is 10% to 20% of daily opioid dose given every 3 to 4 hr as needed. Titration upward for unrelieved pain should be by 25% to 30% of the current 24-hr dose, adjusted by daily amount of rescue medications needed over a several-week period.
Equivalent or equianalgesic doses for the different opioid preparations vary in different publications.
ER, Extended release; *IR,* immediate release.
*Conservative low equianalgesic starting doses for opioid-naïve individuals adapted from published recommendations.
†Doses above 1.5 mg/kg not recommended because of increase in side effects.
From Hochberg MC et al: *Rheumatology,* ed 5, St Louis, 2011, Mosby.

fail, in patients with complex pain conditions, or for invasive therapies
- Consider referral to an addiction specialist if patient has a history of substance abuse or addiction
- Psychiatry/psychological services for counseling, if needed

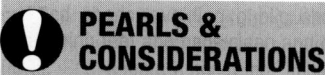

PEARLS & CONSIDERATIONS

- Patient consent should be obtained in the form of a written treatment agreement before initiating treatment. This agreement should outline the goals of therapy, use of a single provider or treatment team and a single pharmacy, limitations on dose and number of prescribed medications, prohibition on use with alcohol or sedating medications, keeping medication safe and secure, prohibition on selling or sharing medication, limitations on refills, compliance with all components of the treatment plan, the role of drug screening, and consequences of nonadherence.

- Follow-up assessment should occur every 1 to 6 mo and include a complete pain assessment (see earlier), review of the type of long-acting analgesic used and dosage, use of breakthrough analgesics, side effects and their management, use of nonpharmacologic therapies, and adjunct medication use.

COMMENTS

- Medication dependence and addiction should not be confused. Most patients receiving chronic opioid therapy can become dependent on these medications for pain relief but opioid addiction does not occur. Patients exhibiting signs of addiction often will seek escalating doses of medication, request refills of prescriptions earlier than planned, and engage in drug-seeking activities (e.g., emergency department visits between prescriptions, seeking multiple prescriptions).
- Side effects need not preclude use of opioid medications and should be anticipated. Antiemetics can aid in controlling nausea. Constipation can be managed with stool softeners and laxatives.

- The emphasis of comprehensive pain management for non–cancer-related chronic pain has led to a fourfold increase in prescribing of opioid medications in the United States. This increase in opiate use has also led to a rise in the misuse and abuse of these medications. Providers should proceed with caution before initiating pain management with opiate medications and should familiarize themselves with processes and tools for pain assessment and medication management. Forty-two states have developed prescription drug monitoring programs (PDMPs) to assist providers in identifying issues of abuse, polypharmacy, and misuse of controlled substances.

PATIENT & FAMILY EDUCATION

National Pain Foundation
(http://www.painconnection.org)
American Pain Foundation
(http://www.painfoundation.org)
National Institutes of Health
(http://www.nih.gov)

SUGGESTED READINGS

available at www.expertconsult.com

AUTHOR: **ANNGENE G. ANTHONY, M.D., M.P.H., F.A.A.F.P.**

BASIC INFORMATION

DEFINITION

Pancreatic cancer is an adenocarcinoma derived from the epithelium of the pancreatic duct.

ICD-9CM CODES
157.9 Pancreatic cancer
157.0 (head)
157.1 (body)
157.2 (tail)
157.3 (duct)
230.9 (in situ)

EPIDEMIOLOGY & DEMOGRAPHICS

INCIDENCE: One case in 10,000 persons annually. In the U.S. there are >35,000 patients diagnosed with pancreatic cancer and >35,000 deaths yearly. It is the fourth leading cause of cancer-related death in the U.S. Less than 20% of patients present with localized, potentially respectable tumors.
PREDOMINANT SEX: Male/female ratio of 2:1
PREDOMINANT AGE: Seventh and eighth decades of life

PHYSICAL FINDINGS & CLINICAL PRESENTATION

Presenting symptoms:
• Jaundice
• Abdominal pain: generally dull upper abdominal pain or vague abdominal discomfort
• Weight loss
• Anorexia/change in taste, asthenia
• Nausea
• Uncommonly: depression, gastrointestinal bleeding, acute pancreatitis (from obstruction of the pancreatic duct), back pain
• Trousseau syndrome (hypercoagulability in the setting of malignancy) may be initial presentation in some patients.
Physical findings:
• Icterus
• Cachexia, temporal wasting
• Ascites, peripheral lymphadenopathy, hepatomegaly
• Excoriations from scratching pruritic skin

ETIOLOGY

Unknown, but several conditions have been associated with pancreatic cancer:
• Smoking
• Alcoholism
• Genetics: 5% to 10% of patients have a family history of the disease
• Gallstones
• Diabetes mellitus
• Chronic pancreatitis
• Diet rich in animal fat
• Occupational exposures: oil refining, paper manufacturing, chemical industry
• Overweight or obesity during early adulthood is associated with a greater risk of pancreatic cancer and a younger age of disease onset. Obesity at an older age is associated with a lower overall survival in patients with pancreatic cancer.

DIAGNOSIS

DIFFERENTIAL DIAGNOSIS

• Common duct cholelithiasis
• Cholangiocarcinoma
• Common duct stricture
• Sclerosing cholangitis
• Primary biliary cirrhosis
• Autoimmune pancreatitis
• Drug-induced cholestasis (e.g., phenothiazines)
• Chronic hepatitis
• Sarcoidosis
• Other pancreatic tumors (islet cell tumor, cystadenocarcinoma, epidermoid carcinoma, sarcomas, lymphomas)

WORKUP

Routine Laboratory Tests	% Abnormal
Alkaline phosphatase	80
Bilirubin	55
Total protein	15
Amylase	15
Hematocrit	60

Ca 19-9: Not useful as a screening tool because it may be elevated in other conditions, such as cholestasis, but is useful for therapeutic monitoring and early detection of recurrent disease after treatment

IMAGING STUDIES

Multidetector helical CT with IV administration of contrast is the imaging procedure of choice for initial evaluation. Endoscopic ultrasonography is useful when there is no identifiable mass on CT and diagnosis is strongly suspected and in obtaining tissue for diagnostic purposes. Fine-needle aspiration biopsy combined with endoscopic ultrasonography is the preferred modality for evaluation of cystic or mass lesions to determine malignancy. Endoscopic retrograde cholangiopancreatography (ERCP) is useful in patients with jaundice needing an endoscopic stent to relieve obstruction.

Noninvasive Imaging	% Abnormal
Abdominal ultrasonography	60
Abdominal CT scan (with contrast) (Fig. 1-623)	90
Abdominal MRI scan	90
Invasive Imaging	
ERCP	90
CT scan or ultrasonography-guided needle aspiration cytology	90-95

STAGING FOR PANCREATIC CANCER

PRIMARY TUMOR (T):
TX	Primary tumor cannot be assessed
T0	No evidence of primary tumor
T1	Tumor <2 cm
T2	Tumor >2 cm, confined to the pancreas
T3	Tumor extends locally beyond the pancreas
T4	Tumor involves celiac or superior mesenteric arteries

LYMPH NODES (N):
NX	Regional lymph nodes cannot be assessed
N0	No regional lymph node metastasis
N1	Regional lymph node metastasis

DISTANT METASTASES (M):
MX	Presence of distant metastasis cannot be assessed
M0	No distant metastasis
M1	Distant metastasis

STAGING GROUP:
IA	T1, N0, M0
IB	T2, N0, M0
IIA	T3, N0, M0
IIB	T1-3, N1, M0
III	T4, N0-1, M0
IV	T1-4, N0-1, M1

A clinical/radiographic staging system for adenocarcinoma of the pancreatic head and uncinate process is described in Table 1-314.

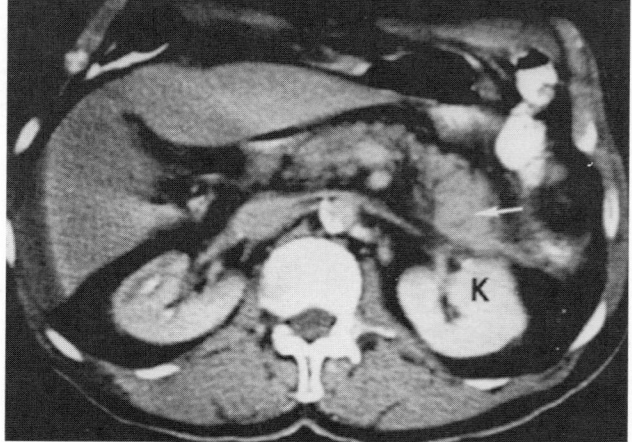

FIGURE 1-623 CT scan of a patient with adenocarcinoma of the body and tail of the pancreas. The tumor *(arrow)* is seen anterior and adjacent to the left kidney *(K)*. At operation, the tumor was invading Gerota's fascia. (From Sabiston D: *Textbook of surgery,* ed 17, Philadelphia, 2005, Saunders.)

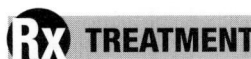

SURGERY

Curative cephalic pancreatoduodenectomy (Whipple's procedure) is appropriate for only 10% to 20% of patients whose lesion is <5 cm, solitary, and without metastases. Surgical mortality rate is 5%. Adjuvant chemotherapy may improve postoperative survival. The addition of gemcitabine to adjuvant fluorouracil and leucovorin chemotherapy has been reported to have a survival benefit for patients with resected pancreatic cancer. An emerging strategy is the use of neoadjuvant preoperative treatment in patients with resectable pancreatic cancer

PALLIATIVE SURGERY (FOR BILIARY DECOMPRESSION/ DIVERSION)

Palliative therapeutic ERCP with stents

CHEMOTHERAPY

In patients with advanced disease an accepted approach is the administration of gemcitabine given alone or combined with a platinum agent, the oral EGFR inhibitor erlotinib, or fluoropyrimidine. Combination therapy consisting of oxaliplatin, irinotecan, fluorouracil, and leucovorin (FOLFIRINOX) offers increased median survival in metastatic pancreatic cancer when compared to gemcitabine (11.1 mo versus 6.8 mo) but increased toxicity.

RADIATION

- External-beam radiation for palliation of pain.
- Combined chemotherapy and radiation provides a median survival of 11 mo.
- Celiac plexus block by an experienced anesthesiologist provides pain relief in 80% to 90% of cases.

DISPOSITION

- Adjunct chemotherapy has a significant survival benefit in patients with resected pancreatic cancer.
- Recent trials have shown that adjuvant postoperative chemotherapy with gemcitabine significantly delays the development of recurrent disease after complete resection of pancreatic cancer.
- Median survival for locally unresectable disease is about 1 yr. Median survival for metastatic cancer is 4-6 mo.

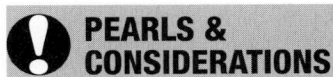

COMMENTS

- The U.S. Preventive Services Task Force (USPSTF) recommends against routine screening for pancreatic cancer in asymptomatic adults by abdominal palpation, ultrasonography, or serologic markers. The USPSTF found no evidence that screening for pancreatic cancer is effective in reducing mortality rates. There is potential for significant harm because of the low prevalence of pancreatic cancer, limited accuracy of available screening tests, invasive nature of diagnostic tests, and poor outcome of treatment. As a result, the USPSTF concluded that the harms of screening for pancreatic cancer exceed any potential benefits.
- Recent trials indicate that pancreatic cancer may have a distinct microRNA (miRNA) expression pattern that may differentiate it from normal pancreas and chronic pancreatitis. Current research is aimed at using miRNA expression patterns to distinguish between long- and short-term survivors.
- Alcohol consumption, specifically liquor consumption of three or more drinks per day, increases pancreatic cancer mortality independent of smoking.

SUGGESTED READINGS

available at www.expertconsult.com

RELATED CONTENT

Fig. 3-131 Diagnostic algorithm for pancreatic cancer (Algorithm)
Pancreatic Cancer (Patient Information)

AUTHOR: **FRED F. FERRI, M.D.**

TABLE 1-314 Clinical/Radiographic Staging System for Adenocarcinoma of the Pancreatic Head and Uncinate Process

Clinical Stage	AJCC Stage	TUMOR-VESSEL RELATIONSHIP ON COMPUTED TOMOGRAPHY			
		SMA	Celiac Axis	CHA*	SMV-PV
Resectable (all four are required to be resectable)[†]	I/II	Normal tissue plane between tumor and vessel	Normal tissue plane between tumor and vessel	Normal tissue plane between tumor and vessel	Patent (may include tumor abutment or encasement)
Borderline resectable (only one of the four required)	III	Abutment	Abutment	Abutment or short segment encasement	May have short segment occlusion if reconstruction possible
Locally advanced (only one of the four required)	III	Encasement	Encasement	Extensive encasement with no technical option for reconstruction	Occluded with no technical option for reconstruction

AJCC, American Joint Commission for Cancer; CHA, common hepatic artery; SMV–PV, superior mesenteric vein–portal vein confluence.
Abutment refers to ≤180 degrees or ≤50% of the vessel circumference; encasement is >180 degrees or >50% of the vessel circumference.
*Assumes normal vascular anatomy; for example, encasement of the CHA is not a limitation in performing PD when there is an uninvolved replaced right hepatic artery arising from the superior mesenteric artery.
[†]Assumes the technical ability to resect and reconstruct the SMV, PV, or SMV-PV confluence when necessary. Others would consider tumor-vein abutment/encasement, which results in deformity of the vein as borderline resectable.
From Cameron JL, Cameron AM: *Current surgical therapy*, ed 10, Philadelphia, 2011, Saunders.

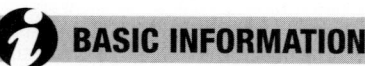

BASIC INFORMATION

DEFINITION

- Acute pancreatitis is an inflammatory process of the pancreas with intrapancreatic activation of enzymes that may also involve peripancreatic tissue and/or remote organ systems.
- Commonly used scoring systems for acute pancreatitis are described in Table 1-315. Severe acute pancreatitis (SAP) is diagnosed by the presence of any of the following four criteria:
  1. Organ failure with one or more of the following: shock (systolic blood pressure <90 mm Hg), pulmonary insufficiency (Pao_2 ≤60 mm Hg), renal failure (serum creatinine >2 mg/dl after rehydration), and gastrointestinal bleeding (>500 ml/24 hr)
  2. Local complications such as necrosis, pseudocyst, or abscess
  3. At least three of Ranson's criteria (see below) *or*
  4. At least eight of the Acute Physiology and Chronic Health Evaluation II (APACHE II) criteria

ICD-9CM CODES
577.0 Acute pancreatitis

EPIDEMIOLOGY & DEMOGRAPHICS

- Acute pancreatitis is most often secondary to biliary tract disease and alcohol. The rate of pancreatitis continues to rise and ranges from 10-45 cases/100,000 in Western countries.
- Incidence in urban areas is twice that of rural areas (20/100,000 persons in urban areas).
- 20% of patients have necrotizing pancreatitis; the remainder have interstitial, or edematous, pancreatitis.
- Acute pancreatitis accounts for >220,000 hospital admissions in the U.S. each year.

PHYSICAL FINDINGS & CLINICAL PRESENTATION

- Epigastric tenderness and guarding, often radiating to the back; pain usually developing suddenly, reaching peak intensity within 10 to 30 min, severe and lasting several hours without relief
- Hypoactive bowel sounds (from ileus)
- Tachycardia, shock (from decreased intravascular volume)
- Confusion (from metabolic disturbances)
- Fever
- Tachycardia, decreased breath sounds (atelectasis, pleural effusions, acute respiratory distress syndrome [ARDS])
- Jaundice (from obstruction or compression of biliary tract)
- Ascites (from tear in pancreatic duct, leaking pseudocyst)
- Palpable abdominal mass (pseudocyst, phlegmon, abscess, carcinoma)
- Evidence of hypocalcemia (Chvostek's sign, Trousseau's sign)
- Evidence of intraabdominal bleeding (hemorrhagic pancreatitis):
  1. Gray-blue discoloration around the umbilicus *(Cullen's sign)*
  2. Bluish discoloration involving the flanks *(Grey Turner's sign)*
- Tender subcutaneous nodules (caused by subcutaneous fat necrosis)

ETIOLOGY

- In >90% of cases: biliary tract disease (calculi or sludge) or alcohol, most common after 5-10 yr of heavy drinking
- Drugs (e.g., thiazides, furosemide, corticosteroids, tetracycline, estrogens, valproic acid, metronidazole, azathioprine, methyldopa, pentamidine, ethacrynic acid, procainamide, sulindac, nitrofurantoin, angiotensin-converting enzyme inhibitors, danazol, cimetidine, piroxicam, gold, ranitidine, sulfasalazine, isoniazid, acetaminophen, cisplatin, opiates, erythromycin, metformin, sitagliptin)
- Abdominal trauma
- Surgery
- Endoscopic retrograde cholangiopancreatography (ERCP)
- Infections (predominantly viral infections)
- Peptic ulcer (penetrating duodenal ulcer)
- Pancreas divisum (congenital failure to fuse of dorsal or ventral pancreas)
- Idiopathic
- Pregnancy
- Vascular (vasculitis, ischemic)
- Hypolipoproteinemia (types I, IV, and V)
- Hypercalcemia
- Pancreatic carcinoma (primary or metastatic)
- Renal failure
- Hereditary pancreatitis
- Occupational exposure to chemicals: methanol, cobalt, zinc, mercuric chloride, creosol, lead, organophosphates, chlorinated naphthalenes
- Others: scorpion bite, obstruction at ampulla region (neoplasm, duodenal diverticula, Crohn's disease), hypotensive shock, autoimmune pancreatitis

DIAGNOSIS

DIFFERENTIAL DIAGNOSIS

- PUD
- Acute cholangitis, biliary colic
- High intestinal obstruction
- Early acute appendicitis
- Mesenteric vascular obstruction
- DKA
- Pneumonia (basilar)
- Myocardial infarction (inferior wall)
- Renal colic
- Ruptured or dissecting aortic aneurysm
- Mesenteric ischemia

LABORATORY TESTS

Pancreatic enzymes:
- Amylase is increased, usually elevated in the initial 3 to 5 days of acute pancreatitis. Isoamylase determinations (separation of pancreatic cell isoenzyme components of amylase) are useful in excluding occasional cases of salivary hyperamylasemia. The use of isoamylase rather than total serum amylase reduces the risk of erroneously diagnosing pancreatitis and is preferred by some as initial biochemical test in patients suspected of having acute pancreatitis.
- Urinary amylase determinations are useful to diagnose acute pancreatitis in patients with lipemic serum, to rule out elevated serum amylase caused by macroamylasemia, and to diagnose acute pancreatitis in patients whose serum amylase is normal.
- Serum lipase levels are elevated in acute pancreatitis; the elevation is less transient than serum amylase; concomitant evaluation of serum amylase and lipase increases diagnostic accuracy of acute pancreatitis. An elevated lipase/amylase ratio is suggestive of alcoholic pancreatitis.
- Elevated serum trypsin levels are diagnostic of pancreatitis (in absence of renal failure).
- Serum C-reactive protein at 48 hr is an excellent laboratory marker of severity.
- Rapid measurement of urinary trypsinogen-2 (if available) is useful in the emergency department as a screening test for acute pancreatitis in patients with abdominal pain; a negative dipstick test for urinary trypsinogen-2 rules out acute pancreatitis with a high degree of probability, whereas a positive test indicates need for further evaluation.

Additional tests:
- Complete blood count: reveals leukocytosis; hematocrit (Hct) may be initially increased as a result of hemoconcentration; decreased Hct may indicate hemorrhage or hemolysis.
- Blood urea nitrogen (BUN) is increased because of dehydration. Serial BUN measurements are the most valuable lab test for predicting mortality during the initial 48 hr.
- Elevation of serum glucose in a previously normal patient correlates with the degree of pancreatic malfunction and may be related to increased release of glycogen, catecholamines, and glucocorticoid release and decreased insulin release.
- Liver profile: aspartate aminotransferase (AST) and lactate dehydrogenase (LDH) are increased as a result of tissue necrosis; bilirubin and alkaline phosphatase may be increased from common bile duct obstruction. A threefold or greater rise in serum alanine aminotransferase concentrations is an excellent indicator (95% probability) of biliary pancreatitis.

- Serum calcium is decreased as a result of saponification, precipitation, and decreased parathyroid hormone response.
- Arterial blood gases: Pao_2 may be decreased as a result of ARDS, pleural effusion(s); pH may be decreased as a result of lactic acidosis, respiratory acidosis, and renal insufficiency.
- Serum electrolytes: potassium may be increased from acidosis or renal insufficiency; sodium may be increased from dehydration.

IMAGING STUDIES

- Abdominal plain films are useful initially to distinguish other conditions that may mimic pancreatitis (perforated viscus). They may reveal localized ileus (sentinel loop), pancreatic calcifications (chronic pancreatitis), blurring of left psoas shadow, dilation of transverse colon, calcified gallstones.
- Chest x-ray may reveal elevation of one or both diaphragms, pleural effusions, basilar infiltrates, or platelike atelectasis.
- Abdominal ultrasonography is useful in detecting gallstones (sensitivity of 60% to 70% for detecting stones associated with pancreatitis). It is also useful for detecting pancreatic pseudocysts. Its availability and noninvasive nature make it the initial imaging study of choice; its major limitation is the presence of distended bowel loops overlying the pancreas.
- CT scan (Fig. 1-624) is superior to ultrasonography in identifying pancreatitis and defining its extent, and it also plays a role in diagnosing pseudocysts (they appear as a well-defined area surrounded by a high-density capsule); gastrointestinal fistulation or infection of a pseudocyst can also be identified by the presence of gas within the pseudocyst. Sequential contrast-enhanced CT is useful for detection of pancreatic necrosis. The severity of pancreatitis can also be graded by CT scan. (A = normal pancreas, B = enlarged pancreas [1 point], C = pancreatic and/or peripancreatic inflammation [2 points], D = single peripancreatic collection [3 points], E = at least

two peripancreatic collections and/or retroperitoneal air [4 points]. Percentage of pancreatic necrosis <30% [2 points], 30% to 50% [4 points], >50% [6 points]. The CT severity index is calculated by adding grade points to points assigned for percentage of necrosis.)
- Magnetic resonance cholangiopancreatography (MRCP) has >90% sensitivity for choledocholithiasis and can identify other anatomic abnormalities.
- Endoscopic ultrasonography (EUS) is a minimally invasive test that provides high-resolution imaging of the pancreas. It is useful to identify anatomic abnormalities of the pancreas and has good sensitivity and specificity for small gallstones (≤5 mm).
- ERCP indications: useful to perform biliary sphincterotomy and stone removal in the presence of a retained bile duct stone seen on imaging.

Rx TREATMENT

NONPHARMACOLOGIC THERAPY

- Bowel rest with avoidance of liquids or solids during the acute illness
- Avoidance of alcohol and any drugs associated with pancreatitis

ACUTE GENERAL Rx

General measures:
- Assess severity of pancreatitis (see Table 1-315). Fig. E1-625 describes an approach to the patient with suspected or proven pancreatitis.
- Maintain adequate intravascular volume with vigorous IV hydration. Aggressive fluid resuscitation is critical in managing acute pancreatitis.
- Patient should remain NPO until clinically improved, stable, and hungry. Enteral feedings are preferred over total parenteral nutrition. Enteral nutrition reduces mortality, multiple organ failure, systemic infections, and

operative interventions more than total parenteral nutrition does in patients with acute pancreatitis. Parenteral nutrition may be necessary in patients who do not tolerate enteral feeding or in whom an adequate infusion rate cannot be reached within 2 to 4 days.
- Nasogastric suction is useful only in severe pancreatitis to decompress the abdomen in patients with ileus.
- Control pain: IV morphine or fentanyl. Meperidine and hydromorphone are also commonly used narcotics for pain control.
- Correct metabolic abnormalities (e.g., replace calcium and magnesium as necessary).

Specific measures:
- Pancreatic or peripancreatic infection develops in 40% to 70% of patients with pancreatic necrosis. However, IV antibiotics should not be used prophylactically for all cases of pancreatitis; their use is justified if the patient has evidence of septicemia, pancreatic abscess, or pancreatitis caused by biliary calculi. Their use should generally be limited to 5 to 7 days to prevent development of fungal superinfection. Appropriate empiric antibiotic therapy should cover:
  ○ *Bacteroides fragilis* and other anaerobes (cefotetan, cefoxitin, metronidazole, or clindamycin plus aminoglycoside)
  ○ *Enterococcus* (ampicillin)
- Surgical therapy has a limited role in acute pancreatitis; it is indicated in the following:
  ○ Gallstone-induced pancreatitis: cholecystectomy when acute pancreatitis subsides. However, randomized trials have shown that patients with mild gallstone pancreatitis can undergo cholecystectomy safely during the first 48 hr of hospitalization.
  ○ Perforated peptic ulcer.
  ○ Necrotizing pancreatitis with infected necrotic tissue is associated with an elevated rate of complications and increased risk of death. Traditional treatment has been open necrosectomy; surgical necrosectomy induces a proinflammatory response and is associated with a high complication rate. Recent trials have shown that a step-up approach consisting of percutaneous drainage followed, if necessary, by minimally invasive retroperitoneal necrosectomy may have a lower rate of complications and death. Endoscopic transgastric necrosectomy, a form of natural orifice transluminal endoscopic surgery, has been shown in recent trials to be effective in reducing the proinflammatory response as well as reducing complications.
- Identification and treatment of complications:
  ○ **Pseudocyst:** round or spheroid collection of fluid, tissue, pancreatic enzymes, and blood.
    ■ Diagnosed by CT scan or sonography
    ■ Treatment: CT scan or ultrasound-guided percutaneous drainage (with a pigtail catheter left in place for continuous drainage) can be used, but the recurrence rate is high; the conservative approach is to reevaluate the pseudocyst (with CT scan or sonography) after 6 to 7 wk and surgically drain it if the pseudocyst has not decreased in size.

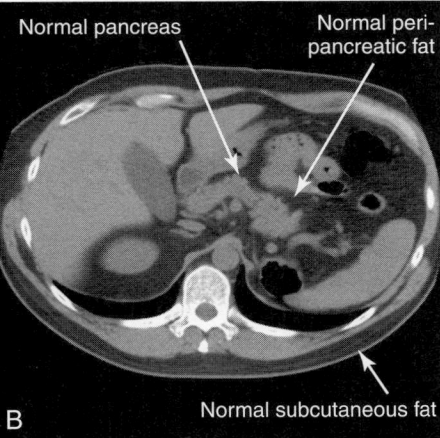

FIGURE 1-624 Gallstone pancreatitis and normal pancreas for comparison, axial CT without contrast. A, Gallstone pancreatitis CT. A dilated gallbladder is visible with a hyperdense dependent lesion consistent with a gal stone. The region of the pancreas shows significant inflammatory stranding. In this patient, the pancreas lies just anterior to the left renal vein, which can be seen crossing anterior to the aorta and entering the inferior vena cava. **B,** A normal pancreas is visible. This pancreas is surrounded by uninflamed fat, which is dark (nearly black). Compare this normal fat with normal subcutaneous fat. (From Broder JS: *Diagnostic imaging for the emergency physician,* Philadelphia, 2011, Saunders.)

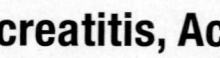
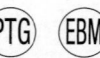

P

Diseases and Disorders

I

Generally, pseudocysts <5 cm in diameter are reabsorbed without intervention, whereas those >5 cm require surgical intervention after the wall has matured.

○ **Phlegmon:** represents pancreatic edema. It can be diagnosed by CT scan or sonography. Treatment is supportive because it usually resolves spontaneously.

○ **Pancreatic abscess:** diagnosed by CT scan (presence of bubbles in the retroperitoneum); Gram staining and cultures of fluid obtained from guided percutaneous aspiration usually identify bacterial organism. Therapy is surgical (or catheter) drainage and IV antibiotics (imipenem-cilastatin is the drug of choice).

○ **Pancreatic ascites:** usually caused by leaking of pseudocyst or tear in pancreatic duct. Paracentesis reveals very high amylase and lipase levels in the pancreatic fluid; ERCP may demonstrate the lesion. Treatment is surgical correction if exuda-

tive ascites from severe pancreatitis does not resolve spontaneously.

○ Gastrointestinal bleeding: caused by alcoholic gastritis, bleeding varices, stress ulceration, or disseminated intravascular coagulation (DIC).

○ Renal failure: caused by hypovolemia, resulting in oliguria or anuria, cortical or tubular necrosis (shock, DIC), or thrombosis of renal artery or vein.

○ Hypoxia: caused by ARDS, pleural effusion, or atelectasis.

THERAPY OF UNCOMMON FORMS OF PANCREATITIS

1. **Autoimmune pancreatitis (AIP):** Fibroinflammatory disease characterized by an IgG4 lymphoplasmacytic infiltrate. It has been associated with other autoimmune disorders (e.g., primary sclerosing cholangitis, Sjögren syndrome). The inflammatory process is generally responsive to corticosteroid therapy. Type II autoimmune hepatitis (idiopathic duct-centric chronic pancreatitis) is

associated with inflammatory bowel disease and not related to IgG4 cell deposition.

2. **Hypertriglyceridemic pancreatitis (HTGP):** Beneficial results have been reported with early (within 48 hr) initiation of apheresis with IV heparin and insulin in addition to conventional treatment modalities for acute pancreatitis when there is concomitant hyperglycemia with severe acute pancreatitis.

DISPOSITION

Prognosis varies with the severity of pancreatitis; overall mortality rate in acute pancreatitis is 5% to 10%. Prognostic criteria for acute pancreatitis are described in Table E1-316.

REFERRAL

● Hospitalization is indicated in moderate to severe cases of pancreatitis.

● Surgical consultation is needed in suspected gallstone pancreatitis, perforated peptic ulcer, or presence of necrotic or infected foci. Acute pancreatitis can generally be attributed to gallstones when patients have both abnormal liver enzymes and gallstones (or sludge) on imaging. Such patients should consider cholecystectomy to prevent recurrent pancreatitis.

● Gastroenterology consultation in severe or recurrent pancreatitis or when the cause of pancreatitis is unclear.

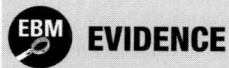

PEARLS & CONSIDERATIONS

● Acute pancreatitis is the most common major complication of ERCP. NSAIDs are potent inhibitors of phospholipase A_2, cyclooxygenase, and neutrophil-endothelial interactions, which play an important role in the pathogenesis of acute pancreatitis. Preliminary trials show that among patients at high risk for post-ERCP pancreatitis, rectal indomethacin (given as two 50 mg indomethacin suppositories administered immediately after ERCP) significantly reduced the incidence of post-ERCP pancreatitis.

● Pancreatic stent placement decreases the risk of post-ERCP pancreatitis.

● Statins reduce risk for pancreatitis in adults. Fibrates do not affect risk for pancreatitis.

TABLE 1-315 Commonly Used Scoring Systems: Advantages and Disadvantages

System	Scoring	Advantages	Disadvantages
Ranson's criteria on admission: 1. Age >55 yr 2. WBC >16 × 10⁹/L 3. LDH >350 U/L 4. AST >250 U/L 5. Glucose >200 mg/dl During initial 48 hr: 1. Hgb falls below 10 mg/dl 2. BUN rises by >5 mg/dl 3. Ca <8 mg/dl 4. Pao₂ <60 mm Hg 5. Base deficit >4 mEq/L 6. Fluid sequestration >6 L	1 point for each factor listed; score >3 indicates SAP	Well known, relatively easy to calculate	Requires 48 hr to complete evaluation
APACHE II*	Score >8 predicts SAP	Can be calculated within 24 hr of admission	Requires large dataset for processing
BISAP 1. BUN >25 mg/dl 2. Altered mental status 3. Presence of SIRS 4. Age >60 yr 5. Pleural effusions	1 point for each factor listed; score >3 indicates SAP	Ease of use, available within 24 hr of admission	Significantly lower sensitivity than either Ranson's or APACHE II; results in greater likelihood of missing severe AP
CTSI	Based on radiographic data	Excellent predictor of local complications; can show infected pancreatic necrosis	Requires 72 to 96 hr, making it a poor test for guiding decisions at admission

*Based on diverse variables, including age, physiology, and long-term health; equation available at www.sfar.org/scores2/apache22.html#calcul. Adding body mass index (BMI) to APACHE II (the APACHE 0 score) increases discrimination (1 point added for BMI 26-30; 2 points for BMI >30).

APACHE, Acute Physiology and Chronic Health Evaluation; AST, Aspartate aminotransferase; BISAP, Bedside Index for Severity in Acute Pancreatitis; BUN, blood urea nitrogen; Ca, serum calcium; CTSI, Computed Tomography Severity Index; Hgb, hemoglobin; LDH, lactate dehydrogenase; SAP, severe acute pancreatitis; SIRS, systemic inflammatory response syndrome; WBC, white blood cell count.

Modified from Cameron JL, Cameron AM: Current surgical therapy, ed 10, Philadelphia, 2011, Saunders.

EBM EVIDENCE

available at www.expertconsult.com

SUGGESTED READINGS

available at www.expertconsult.com

RELATED CONTENT

Acute Pancreatitis (Patient Information)

AUTHOR: **FRED F. FERRI, M.D.**

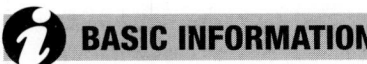

DEFINITION

Chronic pancreatitis is a recurrent or persistent inflammatory process of the pancreas characterized by chronic pain and by pancreatic exocrine and/or endocrine insufficiency.

ICD-9CM CODES
577.1 Chronic pancreatitis

EPIDEMIOLOGY & DEMOGRAPHICS

- Chronic pancreatitis occurs in approximately five to 10 per 100,000 persons in industrialized countries.
- Average age at diagnosis is 35 to 55 yr; male/female ratio is 5:1.

PHYSICAL FINDINGS & CLINICAL PRESENTATION

- Persistent or recurrent epigastric and left upper quadrant pain that may radiate to the back
- Tenderness over the pancreas, muscle guarding
- Significant weight loss
- Bulky, foul-smelling stools, greasy in appearance
- Epigastric mass (10% of patients)
- Jaundice (5% to 10% of patients)

ETIOLOGY

- Chronic alcoholism
- Obstruction (ampullary stenosis, tumor, trauma, pancreas divisum, annular pancreas)
- Hereditary pancreatitis
- Severe malnutrition
- Idiopathic
- Untreated hyperparathyroidism (hypercalcemia)
- Mutations of the cystic fibrosis transmembrane conductance regulator *(CFTR)* gene and the TF genotype
- Autoimmune pancreatitis (AIP) (5% of chronic pancreatitis cases): presents clinically with jaundice (63% of patients) and abdominal pain (35%). CT may reveal diffusely enlarged pancreas, enhanced peripheral rim of hypoattenuation "halo," and low-attenuation mass in head of pancreas. Laboratory values reveal elevated serum immunoglobulin (Ig) G4, elevated serum Ig or gamma-globulin level, presence of antilactoferrin antibody (ALA), anticarbonic anhydrase (ACA) II level, anti-smooth-muscle antibody (ASMA), or antinuclear antibody (ANA).
- Sclerosing pancreatitis: a form of chronic pancreatitis characterized by infrequent attacks of abdominal pain, irregular narrowing of the pancreatic duct, and swelling of the pancreatic parenchyma; patients have high levels of serum immunoglobulins (IgG4). Chronic sclerosing pancreatitis is also known as *autoimmune pancreatitis.*

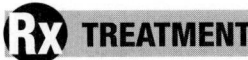

DIFFERENTIAL DIAGNOSIS

- Pancreatic cancer
- Peptic ulcer disease
- Cholelithiasis with biliary obstruction
- Malabsorption from other etiologies
- Recurrent acute pancreatitis
- Renal insufficiency
- Intestinal ischemia or infarction
- Other: Crohn's disease, gastroparesis, inflammatory bowel disease

WORKUP

Medical history with focus on alcohol use, laboratory tests, diagnostic imaging

LABORATORY TESTS

- Serum amylase and lipase may be elevated (normal amylase levels, however, do not exclude the diagnosis).
- Hyperglycemia, glycosuria, hyperbilirubinemia, and elevated serum alkaline phosphatase may also be present.
- 72-hr fecal fat determination (rarely performed) reveals excess fecal fat. Fecal elastase test requires only 20 g of stool.
- Secretin stimulation test is the best test for diagnosing pancreatic exocrine insufficiency.
- Lipid panel: significantly elevated triglycerides can cause pancreatitis.
- Serum calcium: hyperparathyroidism is a rare cause of chronic pancreatitis.
- Elevated levels of serum IgG4 are found in sclerosing pancreatitis and AIP.
- Elevated serum Ig or gamma-globulin level, presence of ALA, ACA II level, ASMA, or ANA in AIP.

IMAGING STUDIES

- Plain abdominal radiographs may reveal pancreatic calcifications (95% specific for chronic pancreatitis).
- Ultrasound of abdomen may reveal duct dilation, pseudocyst, calcification, and presence of ascites.
- Contrast-enhanced CT scan of abdomen is the initial modality of choice. It is useful to detect calcifications, evaluate for ductal dilation, and rule out pancreatic cancer.
- Endoscopic retrograde cholangiopancreatography (ERCP) had been traditionally used to evaluate for the presence of dilated ducts, strictures, pseudocysts, and intraductal stones. However, for the evaluation of pancreatic parenchyma and duct system newer, less invasive modalities such as magnetic resonance cholangiopancreatography and endoscopic ultrasonography (EUS) are preferred. EUS has a sensitivity of 97% and a specificity of 60% for chronic pancreatitis and a very low complication rate. Fine-needle aspiration biopsy combined with EUS is the preferred modality for evaluation of cystic or mass lesions to determine malignancy.

NONPHARMACOLOGIC THERAPY

- Avoidance of alcohol and tobacco
- Frequent, small-volume, low-fat meals

ACUTE GENERAL Rx

- Avoidance of narcotics if possible (simple analgesics or NSAIDs can be used). Fig. E1-626 describes an approach to the patient with painful chronic pancreatitis.
- Treatment of steatorrhea with pancreatic supplements (e.g., Pancrease, Creon, Pancrelipase titrated prn based on the amount of steatorrhea and patient's weight loss). All non–enteric coated enzymes should be used with acid-suppressing medications. Proton pump inhibitors and H_2 blockers reduce inactivation of the enzymes from gastric acid.
- Antioxidants (vitamin A, selenium, vitamin E) may be helpful for pain control in chronic pancreatitis.
- Percutaneous or via EUS celiac plexus blockade with corticosteroids or neurolysis with ethanol may provide temporary pain relief.
- Treatment of complications (e.g., type 1 diabetes mellitus).
- Glucocorticoid therapy in patients with AIP and sclerosing pancreatitis can induce clinical remission and significantly decrease serum concentrations of IgG4, immune complexes, and the IgG4 subclass of immune complexes.

CHRONIC Rx

- Surgical intervention may be necessary to eliminate biliary tract disease and improve flow of bile into the duodenum by eliminating obstruction of pancreatic duct.
- ERCP with endoscopic sphincterectomy and stone extraction is useful in selected patients.
- Transduodenal sphincteroplasty or pancreaticojejunostomy in selected patients. Surgery should also be considered in patients with intractable pain.

DISPOSITION

- Long-term survival is poor (50% of patients die within 10 yr from chronic pancreatitis or malignancy).
- Prognosis is best in patients with recurrent acute pancreatitis resulting from cholelithiasis, hyperparathyroidism, or stenosis of the sphincter of Oddi.

REFERRAL

Gastrointestinal referral for ERCP, surgical referral in selected patients (see "Chronic Rx")

SUGGESTED READINGS
available at www.expertconsult.com

RELATED CONTENT
Chronic Pancreatitis (Patient Information)

AUTHOR: **FRED F. FERRI, M.D.**

BASIC INFORMATION

DEFINITION

- A **panic attack** is a relatively brief, sudden episode of intense fear or apprehension, often associated with a sense of impending doom and various uncomfortable and disquieting physical symptoms. Panic attacks may be uncued ("out of the blue") or cued (i.e., triggered by a particular object or situation). Panic attacks may be present in a variety of different anxiety-related disorders (e.g., phobias, social anxiety, obsessive-compulsive disorder). Table 1-317 describes criteria for diagnosis of panic attack.
- **Panic disorder** is diagnosed at least after two uncued panic attacks have occurred followed by at least 1 mo (or more) of significant concern about future attacks, worry about their implications, or a major change in behavior related to these attacks. The criteria for diagnosis of panic disorder is summarized in Table 1-318. **Agoraphobia** is anxiety about, and avoidance of, places or situations in which the ability to escape is limited or embarrassing or in which help might not be available in the event of having a panic attack.

SYNONYMS

Anxiety attacks
Fear attacks
Ataque de nervios

ICD-9CM CODES
F41.0 Panic disorder without agoraphobia (DSM-IV 300.01)
F40.01 Panic disorder with agoraphobia (DSM-IV 300.21)

EPIDEMIOLOGY & DEMOGRAPHICS

INCIDENCE (IN U.S.): 1% 1-mo incidence of panic attacks

TABLE 1-317 Criteria for Diagnosis of a Panic Attack

A discrete period of intense fear or discomfort, in which ≥4 of the following symptoms developed abruptly and reached a peak within 10 min
- Palpitations, pounding heart, or accelerated heart rate
- Sweating
- Trembling or shaking
- Sensations of shortness of breath or being smothered
- Feeling of choking
- Chest pain or discomfort
- Nausea or abdominal distress
- Feeling dizzy, unsteady, light-headed, or faint
- Derealization (feelings of unreality) or depersonalization (being detached from oneself)
- Fear of losing control or going crazy
- Paresthesias (numbness or tingling sensations)
- Chills or hot flashes

From Kliegman RM et al: *Nelson essentials of pediatrics,* ed 5, Philadelphia, 2006, Saunders.

PREVALENCE (IN U.S.):
- 15% to 20% lifetime prevalence of one or more panic attacks.
- Panic disorder much more uncommon, with a lifetime prevalence of 1.5% to 3.5%; chronicity of condition reflected by a similar 1-yr prevalence rate of 1% to 2%.
- Agoraphobia relatively rare; 0.3% to 1% lifetime prevalence; 30% to 50% of patients diagnosed with panic disorder also have agoraphobia.

PEAK INCIDENCE:
- Chronic condition with a waxing and waning course.
- Bimodal incidence peaks noted, with the first peak between ages 15 and 24 yr and second peak between ages 35 and 44 yr.

PREDOMINANT SEX:
- Women more commonly affected (>85% of clinical population).
- Panic disorder twice as common in women.
- Panic disorder with agoraphobia three times as common in women.

PREDOMINANT AGE:
- Age of onset is typically late adolescence to mid-30s. Onset earlier in males (24 yr) than females (28 yr).
- Onset after age 45 yr is rare and should raise suspicion of different etiology.

GENETICS:
- Risk of developing panic disorder in first-degree relatives of individuals with panic disorder is four to seven times that of general population.
- Findings in twin studies: approximately 60% of contributing factors to panic are genetic.

TABLE 1-318 Criteria for Diagnosis of Panic Disorder

A. Both (1) and (2)
 1. Recurrent unexpected panic attacks
 2. At least 1 of the attacks has been followed by ≥1 mo of ≥1 of the following:
  a. Persistent concern about having additional attacks
  b. Worry about the implications of the attack or its consequences (e.g., losing control, having a heart attack, "going crazy")
  c. A significant change in behavior related to the attacks
B. The presence or absence of agoraphobia
C. The panic attacks are not due to the direct physiologic effects of a drug of abuse or a medication or a general medical condition (e.g., hyperthyroidism)
D. The panic attacks are not better accounted for by another mental disorder, such as social phobia (e.g., occurring on exposure to feared social situations), specific phobia (e.g., on exposure to a specific phobic situation), obsessive-compulsive disorder (e.g., on exposure to dirt in someone with an obsession about contamination), posttraumatic stress disorder (e.g., in response to stimuli associated with a severe stressor), or separation anxiety disorder (e.g., in response to being away from home or close relatives)

From Kliegman RM et al: *Nelson essentials of pediatrics,* ed 5, Philadelphia, 2006, Saunders.

PHYSICAL FINDINGS & CLINICAL PRESENTATION

Panic disorder:
- Present either with a panic attack or with fear and anxiety related to anticipation of a future panic attack or its implications.
- Typical presentation: unexpected, untriggered periods of intense anxiety and fear with associated physiologic changes (e.g., palpitations, sweating, tremulousness, shortness of breath, chest pain, gastrointestinal distress, faintness, derealization, paresthesia). This is accompanied by associated fears of dying, heart attack, stroke, passing out, losing control, or losing one's mind. Panic attacks are often described as "the most terrifying" episode an individual has experienced.
- Emergency or physician visits often occasioned by physical symptoms such as chest pain, dizziness, or difficulty breathing.
Agoraphobia:
- Rare complaints to physician. May manifest in missed office visits or tardiness. Patients may request home visits or telephone care.
- Activities usually self-limited by avoiding public situations where the patient believes he or she might experience a panic attack and would be unable to exit readily, such as the following:
 1. Crowded public areas (stores, public transportation, flying, church)
 2. Individual interactions (hairdresser, dentist, neighborhood meetings)
 3. Driving (especially if alone, far from home over bridges, through tunnels, on highways or on isolated roads)
- On exposure to or anticipation of exposure to feared situations, significant anxiety occurs. Anxiety may generate somatic symptoms that trigger a full-blown panic attack. Patients believe that escape from these situations reduces the alarming symptoms, thus reinforcing future avoidance. In actuality, symptom relief stems from adrenaline breaking down in the body after approximately 20 minutes.

ETIOLOGY

Hypotheses (NOTE: There are sufficient data to support each model. Models are not mutually exclusive.)
1. Central dyscontrol of autonomic arousal (typically localized to the locus ceruleus); similar symptoms may be chemically induced with yohimbine, caffeine, or cholecystokinin.
2. Cognitive overreaction (i.e., "catastrophic misinterpretation") to relatively mild or benign physiologic cues that then triggers a genuine autonomic cascade and further misinterpretations.
3. Dysfunction of a central suffocation alarm mechanism; some signs of compensated respiratory alkalosis. Can be experimentally induced with sodium lactate or carbon dioxide.

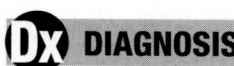 **DIAGNOSIS**

DIFFERENTIAL DIAGNOSIS

Medical conditions:
- Endocrinopathies:
  1. Hyperthyroidism
  2. Hyperparathyroidism
  3. Pheochromocytoma
  4. Carcinoid tumor
- Cardiac and respiratory diseases:
  1. Arrhythmias
  2. Myocardial infarction
  3. Chronic obstructive pulmonary disease
  4. Asthma
  5. Mitral valve prolapse
- Metabolic:
  1. Hypoglycemia
  2. Electrolyte imbalances
  3. Porphyria
- Seizure disorders
- Psychiatric disorders (NOTE: Panic attacks are common in a variety of psychiatric disorders. Panic disorder could be conceptualized as a phobia of the somatic sensations or situations that have become paired with panic attacks.)
  1. Phobias (e.g., specific phobia or social phobia). Note that fear of going on a plane because of crashing would be a specific phobia, whereas fear of going on a plane because one is then trapped and worries about panic is more suggestive of panic disorder with agoraphobia.
  2. Obsessive-compulsive disorder (cued by exposure to the object of the obsession)
  3. Posttraumatic stress disorder (cued by recall of a stressor)
- Therapeutic (theophylline, steroids) and recreational (cocaine, amphetamine, caffeine, diet pills) drugs and drug withdrawal (alcohol, cannabis, barbiturates, benzodiazepines)

WORKUP

- Emergency presentation: cardiac, respiratory, or neurologic symptoms
- History and physical examination to rule out a concomitant medical or substance-related condition

NOTE: Panic disorder and agoraphobia are not diagnoses of exclusion, but exclusion of other conditions is usually required.

LABORATORY TESTS

- Thyroid profile
- Electrolyte measures, including calcium
- Toxicology screen
- ECG
- Acute cases: possible monitoring and cardiac enzymes to rule out arrhythmia or ischemia

IMAGING STUDIES

- For temporal lobe dysfunction (e.g., temporal lesions or as ictal or interictal manifestation of temporal lobe seizures): brain CT scan or MRI or an electroencephalogram in some patients
- Holter monitor to rule out occult or episodic arrhythmias
- Chest x-ray examination, arterial blood gases, or pulmonary function tests if respiratory compromise suspected

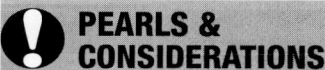 **TREATMENT**

NONPHARMACOLOGIC THERAPY

Cognitive-behavioral therapy (CBT) is generally very effective, with strongest results for cognitive restructuring (i.e., challenging catastrophic misinterpretations of somatic symptoms), in vivo or imaginal exposures (i.e., exposure to panic triggers in a controlled graded hierarchical fashion from least to most difficult with the goal of habituation and extinction of the fear response), and interoceptive exposures (i.e., repeated recreation and management of feared somatic sensations via activities such as chair spinning, straw breathing, and hyperventilation). CBT effect sizes are equal to or larger than for pharmacotherapy, attrition rates are lower, and relapse rates are lower. Treatment may take several sessions spread over weeks and may require referral to a behavioral specialist.

ACUTE GENERAL Rx

- Benzodiazepines, particularly alprazolam: highly effective in the acute setting.
- Low-dose alprazolam for patients with rare panic attacks and asymptomatic periods (0.25 to 0.5 mg PO or sublingually prn).
- Start patient on selective serotonin reuptake inhibitor (SSRI) or similar agent and taper patient off of benzodiazepine by wk 2 to 3.

CHRONIC Rx

- Preferred pharmacologic agents: antidepressants with a significant serotonin reuptake inhibitory action. Generally start at low dose and titrate upward. Minimum treatment duration is 6 to 8 mo, but many patients need to take medications indefinitely.
  1. SSRIs: paroxetine (10 to 60 mg/day), sertraline (50 to 200 mg/day), citalopram (20 to 60 mg/day), escitalopram (5 to 30 mg/day), and fluoxetine (5 to 60 mg/day)

  2. Imipramine (100 to 300 mg/day)
  3. Venlafaxine (75 to 225 mg/day)
- Combination CBT plus SSRI has shown good long-term effects and is somewhat better than antidepressants or CBT alone. Combination CBT plus benzodiazepine does not provide any added benefit and may undermine CBT (interoceptive and in-vivo exposures may be less effective if the benzodiazepine is completely controlling the anxiety).

DISPOSITION

- Typical course is chronic but with significant waxing and waning (common to have long periods of remission).
- Presence of agoraphobia associated with a more chronic course.
- Findings with long-term follow-up studies: 6 to 10 yr after treatment some 30% are in remission, 40% to 50% have improved with residual symptoms, and the remainder are either unchanged or worse.

REFERRAL

- If patients do not respond to an SSRI
- Cognitive-behavioral therapy is the preferred treatment.

 PEARLS & CONSIDERATIONS

- Patient and family education is an important first step in the management of panic disorder. Education provides more adaptive explanations for the benign somatic sensations paired with panic. Presentation of genetic information and explanation of the benign nature of the physiology of each of the symptoms the patient experiences serve as a good start to allay fears and reduce stigma.
- Resumption of avoided activities or situations is a positive prognostic sign and may promote further therapeutic gains.

SUGGESTED READINGS
available at www.expertconsult.com

RELATED CONTENT

Panic Disorder (Patient Information)

AUTHORS: **JEFFREY WINCZE, PH.D,** **JASON M. SATTERFIELD, PH.D.,** and **MITCHELL D. FELDMAN, M.D., M.PHIL.**

BASIC INFORMATION

DEFINITION

Paraneoplastic syndromes are a large group of syndromes caused by hormonal, immunologic, or other soluble factors due to the presence of a malignancy. Findings and symptoms are specific to each syndrome. Paraneoplastic syndromes affect most organ systems, predominantly the central and peripheral nervous systems, endocrine system, kidneys, and skin.

ICD-9CM CODES
275.42 Hypercalcemia of malignancy
253.6   Syndrome of inappropriate antidiuretic hormone (SIADH)
255.0   Cushing's syndrome
323   Limbic encephalitis (LE)
334.9   Paraneoplastic cerebellar degeneration (PCD)
358.1   Lambert-Eaton myasthenia syndrome (LEMS)
358.0   Myasthenia gravis (MG)

EPIDEMIOLOGY & DEMOGRAPHICS

- Paraneoplastic syndromes may affect as many as 8% of cancer patients.
- See Table 1-319 for epidemiology of each syndrome.

PHYSICAL FINDINGS & CLINICAL PRESENTATION

Hypercalcemia of malignancy
- Nausea/vomiting
- Constipation
- Abdominal pain
- Anorexia
- Fatigue
- Altered mental status (from confusion to coma)
- Depression/anxiety
- Renal failure

SIADH
- Headache
- Weakness
- Anorexia
- Nausea
- Vomiting
- Memory impairment, irritability, restlessness
- Mental status changes may progress to obtundation or coma if hyponatremia is <125 mEq/L.

Cushing's syndrome
- Rapid weight gain
- Muscle weakness
- Generalized edema
- Centripetal fat distribution, which often progressed to obesity; limbs are often spared or wasted
- Hypertension
- Characteristic "moon face" due to accumulation of fat deposition in the cheeks
- Skin atrophy, easy bruising, and purple abdominal striae due to skin fragility
- Hyperpigmentation, notably in sun-exposed areas
- Menstrual irregularity, mild hirsutism in women

Limbic encephalitis (LE)
- Slow progression of mood changes
- Hallucinations
- Short-term memory loss
- If hypothalamus is involved, may develop hyperthermia or somnolence.
- Two thirds develop multifocal nervous system involvement.

Paraneoplastic cerebellar degeneration (PCD)
- May develop prodrome of dizziness, nausea, vomiting.
- Ataxia
- Diplopia
- Dysphagia
- Dysarthria

Lambert-Eaton myasthenia syndrome (LEMS)
- Gradual onset of pelvic girdle and lower extremity weakness, progressing in caudocranial direction
- Hyporeflexia
- Fatigue
- Mild bulbar dysfunction
- Dysautonomia, especially erectile dysfunction

Myasthenia gravis (MG)
- Ocular symptoms: ptosis and diplopia
- Weakness of facial muscles, notably with fatigable chewing
- Lower extremity weakness that starts distally and progresses proximally
- May progress to involve muscles of respiration and respiratory crisis

Paraneoplastic dermatologic and rheumatologic syndromes
- Acanthosis nigricans
- Dermatomyositis (DM)
- Erythroderma
- Hypertrophic osteoarthropathy
- Leukocytoclastic vasculitis
- Paraneoplastic pemphigus (PNP)
- Polymyalgia rheumatica (PMR)
- Sweet syndrome (acute febrile neutrophilic dermatosis)

ETIOLOGY

Paraneoplastic endocrine syndromes (PES) are due to tumor production of hormones or peptides that lead to metabolic derangements:

Hypercalcemia of malignancy:
  Humoral hypercalcemia of malignancy (HHM): 80% of hypercalcemia of malignancy cases. Most commonly due to production of parathyroid hormone–related peptide (PTHrP) in lung and breast cancer (also seen in renal, bladder, and ovarian cancer). More rarely, can see 1,25 dihydroxyvitamin D production from increased 1α-hydroxylase activity in Hodgkin and non-Hodgkin lymphomas or ectopic production of parathyroid hormone (PTH) by the tumor.
  Osteolytic activity: 20% of hypercalcemia of malignancy cases. Tumor cells metastasize, infiltrate bone, and produce local factors that stimulate osteoclast activation.

SIADH: production of antidiuretic hormone (arginine vasopressin, atrial natriuretic peptide) by tumor cells

Cushing's syndrome: ectopic ACTH promotes excess production of cortisol and other glucocorticoids from the adrenal glands, which do not respond to normal HPA feedback

Paraneoplastic neurologic syndromes (PNS) are due to immune cross-reactivity between tumor cells and components of the nervous system. Tumor-directed antibodies (onconeural antibodies) are produced by the patient in response to a developing cancer. These onconeural antibodies and associated onconeural antigen-specific T lymphocytes inadvertently attack components of the nervous system because of antigenic similarity:

LE, PCD, LEMS, MG: cross-reactive autoantibodies against various components of the central and peripheral nervous system

---

TABLE 1-319   Epidemiology of Each Paraneoplastic Syndrome

Condition	Prevalence	Risk Factors
Hypercalcemia of malignancy	Up to 10%-20% of all cancer patients	Squamous cell cancers (lung, head, and neck), breast, kidney, bladder, and ovarian cancers, lymphoma
Syndrome of inappropriate antidiuretic hormone (SIADH)	Up to 1-2% of all cancer patients Found in 10-45% of SCLC patients	SCLC
Cushing's syndrome	Approximately 2% in all cancer patients (50% of these are SCLC)	SCLC Pituitary adenoma, benign and malignant adrenal tumors, carcinoid tumors
Limbic encephalitis (LE)	Less than 1%	SCLC Testicular germ cell tumor Breast cancer
Paraneoplastic cerebellar degeneration	Less than 1%	SCLC Hodgkin's lymphoma Breast cancer
Lambert-Eaton myasthenia syndrome (LEMS)	3% of SCLC patients	SCLC, prostate cancer lymphoma
Myasthenia gravis (MG)	15% of thymoma patients	Thymoma

SCLC, Small cell lung cancer.

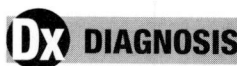 **DIAGNOSIS**

DIFFERENTIAL DIAGNOSIS

Hypercalcemia of malignancy: primary hyperparathyroidism, familial hypocalciuric hypercalcemia, excess calcium intake, vitamin D toxicity, thiazide diuretics. It is important to differentiate between HHM and osteolytic causes of malignancy-associated hypercalcemia because prognosis and response to treatment differ.

SIADH: hypovolemic hyponatremia, reset osmostat, psychogenic polydipsia

Cushing's syndrome: excess glucocorticoid administration, pituitary adenoma, benign or malignant adrenal tumors

LE, PCD, LEMS, MG: multiple sclerosis, stroke, meningitis, encephalitis

WORKUP

- History and physical examination. Box E1-42 summarizes the evaluation and diagnosis of paraneoplastic syndromes.
- Age-appropriate cancer screening
- EEG, EMG

LABORATORY TESTS

Hypercalcemia of malignancy
- Serum calcium and albumin levels to measure corrected calcium (HHM more common when serum Ca^{2+} >13 mg/dl)
- Ionized serum calcium
- PTH (low to normal)
- PTHrP (elevated)
- 1,25 $(OH)_2$ D levels (if the above values are inconclusive)

SIADH
- Serum and urine sodium (serum sodium <135 mEq/L or urine sodium >40 mEq/L)
- Serum and urine osmolality (serum osm <280 mOsm/kg of water and/or urine osm >100 mOsm/kg of water)

Cushing's syndrome
- High-dose dexamethasone suppression: 2 mg dexamethasone by mouth every 6 hr for 72 hr, with measurement of urinary 17-hydroxycorticosteroid at 9 A.M. and midnight days 2 and 3
- Low-dose dexamethasone suppression: 1 mg dexamethasone given with measurement of morning serum cortisol
- Dexamethasone suppression test distinguishes pituitary vs. ectopic source of ACTH
- Potassium and glucose should be monitored closely due to increased risk of hypokalemia and hyperglycemia

LE: Anti-Hu, Anti-Ma2, Anti-CRMP5, anti-amphiphysin, CSF analysis

PCD: Anti-Yo, Anti-Hu, Anti-Ma, Anti-Ri, Anti-VGCC, Anti-mGluR1, CSF analysis

LEMS: Anti-VGCC (P/Q), CSF analysis

MG: Anti-AchR, Anti-MuSk, CSF analysis

IMAGING STUDIES

Hypercalcemia of malignancy: CT imaging to evaluate for breast or lung mass or lymphadenopathy

SIADH: CT imaging to evaluate for brain or lung mass

Cushing's syndrome: CT scan, MRI, or octreotide scan

LE, PCD, LEMS, MG: CT chest, FDG-PET scan, MRI

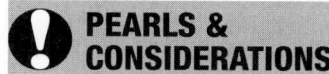 **TREATMENT**

NONPHARMACOLOGIC THERAPY

Hypercalcemia of malignancy
- Treatment of underlying malignancy, either surgical resection or chemotherapy/radiation of identified tumors
- Fluid resuscitation, typically 1 L bolus followed by 200-300 ml/hr to achieve euvolemia; maintenance hydration after euvolemia reached

SIADH
- Surgical resection of identified tumors
- Fluid restriction

Cushing's syndrome
- Surgical resection of identified tumors

LE, PCD, LEMS, MG
- IVIG
- Plasma exchange

ACUTE GENERAL Rx

Hypercalcemia of malignancy
- Furosemide intravenously once euvolemia has been reached, although clinical efficacy is debatable
- Bisphosphonates, either pamidronate acid or zoledronic acid intravenous infusions (treatment side effects are renal dysfunction and osteonecrosis of the jaw)
- Calcitonin weight-based dosing, although tachyphylaxis occurs after 48 hours of administration
- Corticosteroids in cases of myeloma and lymphoma
- Hemodialysis in severe cases

SIADH
- If urine sodium is >308 mOsm/kg and patient develops seizure or obtundation, then sodium replacement with hypertonic saline (3%) is indicated
- Sodium should not be corrected at a rate faster than 1-2 mEq/L/hr to decrease chances of osmotic demyelination syndrome

Cushing's syndrome
- Management of volume status and blood pressure with diuretics and antihypertensive agents

CHRONIC Rx

- Chronic treatment of all is centered on treatment of the underlying malignancy.

Hypercalcemia of malignancy
- Bisphosphonate therapy every 4 weeks in cases of bone metastasis
- Chronic calcitonin use can be considered

SIADH
- Demeclocycline and vasopressin receptor antagonists (conivaptan and tolvaptan, although both are approved for initial administration in hospitalized patients only)

- Cessation of any possible causative medications
- Maintain adequate dietary protein and salt intake

Cushing's syndrome: inhibition of steroid production with ketoconazole, mitotane, metyrapone, aminoglutethimide

LE/PCD: Glucocorticoids, cyclophosphamide, rituximab

LEMS: 3,4-diaminopyridine, pyridostigmine, azathioprine

MG: Pyridostigmine, azathioprine, cyclosporin A, tacrolimus, mycophenolate, rituximab

DISPOSITION

Specific to each condition; however, humoral hypercalcemia of malignancy carries a poor overall prognosis with 30-day mortality of 50%.

REFERRAL

Oncology, endocrinology, neurology, nephrology

⚠ PEARLS & CONSIDERATIONS

COMMENTS

- Signs or symptoms of a paraneoplastic syndrome may manifest prior to the identification of a malignancy.
- If paraneoplastic syndrome is suspected, a thorough workup for a tumor is indicated.
- With treatment of the primary tumor, the clinical effects of hypercalcemia of malignancy, SIADH, and Cushing's syndrome may improve or resolve.
- The effects of the neurologic paraneoplastic syndromes can be long-term, due to permanent CNS or PNS damage. In neurologic paraneoplastic syndromes, tumor detection can be difficult, since the immune system, which is causing the syndrome, is also keeping the tumor in check.

PREVENTION

- Smoking cessation
- Age-appropriate cancer screening

PATIENT & FAMILY EDUCATION

Conditions with autoimmune etiology (LE, PCD, LEMS, MG) symptoms may not improve even if tumor is identified and treated, as damage to the nervous system may be sustained or permanent

SUGGESTED READING

available at www.expertconsult.com

AUTHORS: **JOHN L. REAGAN, M.D.,** and **ANGELA M. TABER (PLETTE), M.D.**

BASIC INFORMATION

DEFINITION

Paranoid personality disorder (PPD) is characterized by a pattern of pervasive distrust and suspiciousness of others that leads the person to assign malevolence to the motives of others. PPD begins by early adulthood and causes significant distress or impairment in multiple domains of functioning. Individuals must meet four or more of the following criteria:

1. Suspect, without justification, that others are exploiting, harming, or deceiving them.
2. Preoccupied with unwarranted doubts about the loyalty or trustworthiness of friends or associates.
3. Reluctant to confide in others because of unjustified fear that the information will be used against them in a malicious fashion.
4. Infer demeaning or threatening statements from benign remarks or events.
5. Bear grudges for extended periods. For example, PPD patients are unforgiving of perceived or real insults and slights.
6. Perceive attacks on their character that are not apparent to others. Quick to react angrily or to counterattack.
7. Recurrent suspicions, without justification, regarding fidelity of spouse or partner.

SYNONYMS

None

ICD-9CM CODES
301.0 Paranoid personality disorder

EPIDEMIOLOGY & DEMOGRAPHICS

PREVALENCE: From 0.5% to 4.4% in the general population, 10% to 30% in inpatient psychiatric settings, and 2% to 10% in outpatient mental health clinics.
PREDOMINANT SEX: More commonly diagnosed in males in clinical samples.
GENETICS: Increased prevalence of PPD in relatives of probands with schizophrenia and delusional disorder, paranoid type.

CLINICAL PRESENTATION

- Signs of PPD in childhood include solitariness, poor peer relationships, social anxiety, underachievement in school, hypersensitivity, peculiar thoughts and language, and idiosyncratic fantasies.
- As children, these patients may have appeared "odd" or "eccentric" and attracted teasing.
- Their excessive suspiciousness often leads to either overt argumentativeness and recurrent complaining or quiet, hostile aloofness.
- These patients maintain interpersonal distance and may refuse to answer personal questions, saying the information is "nobody's business."
- Misinterpret benign actions by others as malicious assaults. PPD patients may, for example, interpret an honest mistake as a deliberate attempt to harm, a casual humorous

remark as a serious character attack, a compliment as a veiled criticism, and an offer of help as a judgment of failure.
- Close relationships are impaired by hypervigilance for threats and associated guardedness. May appear as "cold." Suspiciousness can lead to pathologic jealousy where they gather circumstantial evidence to support contention of betrayal.
- To protect themselves from the perceived malice of others, these patients often maintain a high degree of control of relationships and interactions, constantly questioning the whereabouts, intentions, or actions of the other.
- Often rigid and critical of others but have great difficulty accepting criticism themselves.
- Given their lack of trust of others, PPD patients have an excessive need for self-sufficiency and autonomy.
- Quick to counterattack and may be litigious.
- May join "cults" or groups that share their paranoid belief system.
- In response to stress, may experience very brief psychotic episodes (minutes to hours).

ETIOLOGY

- At this point, limited knowledge about role of genetic loading and neurobiologic vulnerability.
- However, increased prevalence in families of probands with schizophrenia and delusional disorder, paranoid type, suggests possible genetic role.

DIAGNOSIS

DIFFERENTIAL DIAGNOSIS

- Schizophrenia, paranoid type, delusional disorder, paranoid type, and mood disorder with psychotic symptoms: require presence of persistent positive psychotic symptoms such as delusions and hallucinations. To give an additional diagnosis of PPD, the personality disorder must be present before the onset of psychotic symptoms and must persist when the psychotic symptoms are in remission.
- Substance-induced paranoia, especially in the context of cocaine, PCP, or methamphetamine abuse or dependence.
- Personality changes caused by a general medical condition that affects the central nervous system.
- Paranoid traits associated with a sensory disability; for example, hearing impairment.
- Increased risk for major depressive disorder, obsessive-compulsive disorder, agoraphobia, and substance abuse or dependence.
- The most common co-occurring personality disorders are schizotypal, schizoid, narcissistic, avoidant, and borderline:
  1. Schizotypal personality disorder includes magical thinking and unusual perceptual experiences.
  2. Schizoid and borderline personality disorders do not have prominent paranoid ideation.

3. Avoidant personality disorder includes fear of embarrassment.
4. Narcissistic personality disorder includes the fear that hidden "flaws" or "inferiority" may be revealed.

WORKUP

- History: collateral information is essential to establishing the presence of longstanding interpersonal pattern in multiple domains of the patient's life.
- Physical examination
- Mental status examination

LABORATORY TESTS

Those necessary to rule out medical causes of personality changes

IMAGING STUDIES

Those necessary to rule out medical causes of personality changes

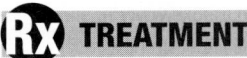 TREATMENT

NONPHARMACOLOGIC THERAPY

- Cognitive-behavioral therapy to help patients control rage, manage perceived criticism, and develop social skills
- Psychodynamic psychotherapy to help patient develop capacity to trust and improve interpersonal functioning.

ACUTE GENERAL Rx

Benzodiazepines or low-dose antipsychotics to control hostility and paranoia

CHRONIC Rx

- Low-dose antipsychotic medication. Increase dose in small increments to minimize risk of side effects.
- Selective serotonin reuptake inhibitors if comorbid depression, obsessive-compulsive disorder, or agoraphobia
- Substance abuse treatment if comorbid dependence

COMPLEMENTARY & ALTERNATIVE MEDICINE

No evidence of efficacy in PPD

DISPOSITION

- Severity is variable and course is chronic. Often lifelong difficulty maintaining intimate relationships.
- At increased risk for major depressive disorder, obsessive-compulsive disorder, agoraphobia, and substance abuse or dependence.
- In some cases, PPD is a prepsychotic antecedent of delusional disorder, paranoid type.

REFERRAL

- If pharmacotherapy or psychotherapy is contemplated
- If patient's social or occupational functioning is impaired

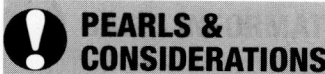

PEARLS & CONSIDERATIONS

COMMENTS

- Illness exacerbates these patients' sense of vulnerability.
- Communicating personal information to the physician challenges the guarded, self-protective approach to others and will often heighten PPD patients' fear that the physician will harm them.
- The encounter with the physician intensifies hypervigilance. As a result, innocuous or even overtly helpful behaviors by the physician may be perceived as manipulating or threatening.
- With the perceived threat, these patients will often confront and challenge the physician on their motives and their rationale for diagnosis and treatment. Conflict and argument are not uncommon.
- Thus establishing an alliance with the patient can be challenging.

- Faced with such a patient, physicians may understandably react defensively to unfounded suspicion or distance and not respond to the patient's concerns. Both responses increase the patient's anxiety and paranoia.
- Management guidelines:
  1. Convey intent "to do no harm."
  2. Address the patient's fears and concerns, no matter how irrational, in a clear, direct, and detailed manner.
  3. Remember that behind the patient's hostility lie fears that are real to him or her.
  4. Maintain a professional and neutral stance.
  5. Responding with too much warmth and friendliness will intensify paranoia.
  6. Give patient detailed and factual information about treatment plan.
  7. Give patient as much control as possible, including maximum participation at each decision node.
  8. Do not personalize patient's hostility and suspicion, but understand his or her distrust as an attempt to manage intense fear.
  9. Validate patient's concerns about the diagnosis or treatment plan.

SUGGESTED READINGS
available at www.expertconsult.com

RELATED CONTENT
Paranoid Personality Disorder (Patient Information)

AUTHOR: **JOHN Q. YOUNG, M.D., M.P.P.**

BASIC INFORMATION

DEFINITION

Idiopathic Parkinson's disease (PD) is a progressive neurodegenerative disorder characterized clinically by rigidity, tremor, postural instability, and bradykinesia.

SYNONYMS

Paralysis agitans

ICD-9CM CODES
332.0 Idiopathic Parkinson's disease, primary
332.1 Parkinson's disease, secondary

EPIDEMIOLOGY & DEMOGRAPHICS

PREVALENCE:
- Affects more than 1 million people in North America.
- In age group <40 yr, <5/100,000 are affected.
- In those aged >70 yr, 700/100,000 are affected.
- Highest incidence in whites, lowest incidence in Asians and African Americans

PHYSICAL FINDINGS & CLINICAL PRESENTATION

- Tremor (Fig. 1-627)—typically a resting tremor with a frequency of 4 to 6 Hz that is often first noted in the hand as a pill-rolling tremor (thumb and forefinger). Can also involve the leg and lip. Tremor improves with purposeful movement. Usually starts asymmetrically.
- Rigidity—increased muscle tone that persists throughout the range of passive movement of a joint. This, too, is usually asymmetric at onset.
- Akinesia/bradykinesia—slowness in initiating movement

- Postural instability—tested by "pull test." Ask patient to stand in place with back to examiner. Examiner pulls patient back by the shoulders, and proper response would be to take no steps back or very few steps back without falling. Retropulsion is a positive test as is falling straight back. This is not usually severe early on. If falls and postural reflexes are greatly impaired early on, then consider other disorders.
- Masked facies—face seems expressionless, giving the appearance of depression. Decreased blink; often there is excess drooling.
- Gait disturbance
- Stooped posture, decreased arm swing
- Difficulty initiating the first step; small shuffling steps that increase in speed (festinating gait). Steps become progressively faster and shorter while the trunk inclines further forward.
- Other complaints and findings early on include micrographia—handwriting becomes smaller, and hypophonia—voice becomes softer and often "gruffer."

ETIOLOGY

- Unknown
- Most cases are sporadic, with age being the most common risk factor, although there is probably a combination of both environmental and genetic factors contributing to disease expression. There are rare familial forms with at least seven different genes identified; these include the parkin gene, which is a significant cause of early-onset autosomal recessive PD and LRRK2, which is the most common cause of familial and sporadic parkinsonism.

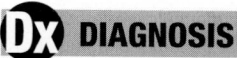 **DIAGNOSIS**

A clinical diagnosis can be made based on a comprehensive history and physical examination. The four cardinal signs used to diagnose PD are (mnemonic = TRAP):
1. **T**remor (resting, typically 4-6 Hz)
2. **R**igidity, of the cogwheel type
3. Bradykinesia/**a**kinesia—slowness of movement
4. **P**ostural instability—failure of postural "righting" reflexes leading to poor balance and falls

One need not demonstrate all four cardinal signs to make a presumptive diagnosis of PD and begin treatment.

DIFFERENTIAL DIAGNOSIS

- Multiple system atrophy—distinguishing features include autonomic dysfunction (including urinary incontinence, orthostatic hypotension, and erectile dysfunction), parkinsonism, cerebellar signs, and normal cognition.
- Diffuse Lewy body disease—parkinsonism with concomitant dementia: patients often have early hallucinations and fluctuations in level of alertness and mental status.
- Corticobasal degeneration—often begins asymmetrically with apraxia, cortical sensory loss in one limb, and sometimes alien limb phenomenon.
- Progressive supranuclear palsy—tends to have axial rigidity greater than appendicular (limb) rigidity. These patients have early and severe postural instability. Hallmark is supranuclear gaze palsy that usually involves vertical gaze (especially downward) before horizontal.
- Essential tremor—bilateral postural and action tremor
- Secondary (acquired) parkinsonism
  1. Iatrogenic—any of the neuroleptics and antipsychotics. The high-potency D_2-blocker neuroleptics are most likely to cause parkinsonism. Quetiapine is an atypical antipsychotic with lower risk of causing parkinsonism. Metoclopramide can also cause parkinsonism. Abuse of methamphetamine has been recently linked to risk of PD.
  2. Postinfectious parkinsonism—von Economo's encephalitis
  3. Parkinson's pugilistica—after repeated head trauma
  4. Toxins (e.g., MPTP, manganese, carbon monoxide)
  5. Cerebrovascular disease "vascular parkinsonism" (basal ganglia infarcts); often lower limbs (especially gait) affected more than upper extremities

WORKUP

- Identification of clinical signs and symptoms associated with PD (see "Physical Findings") and elimination of conditions that may mimic it with a comprehensive history and physical examination
- Routine genetic testing is not recommended.

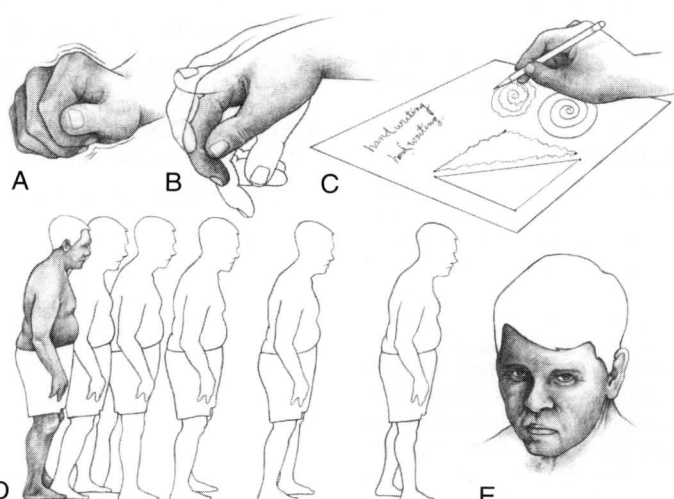

FIGURE 1-627 The parkinsonian syndrome. A, The "pill-rolling" tremor. **B,** Tremor that can worsen with emotional stress. **C,** Handwriting abnormalities, which include micrographia. **D,** Typical posture and gait, which becomes faster (festination). **E,** Lack of facial expression as well as "stare" from decreased blinking. (From Remmel KS et al: *Handbook of symptom oriented neurology,* ed 3, St Louis, 2002, Mosby.)

IMAGING STUDIES

Computed tomographic (CT) scan has almost no role in investigations. Magnetic resonance imaging (MRI) of the head may sometimes distinguish between idiopathic PD and other conditions that present with signs of parkinsonism (see "Differential Diagnosis").

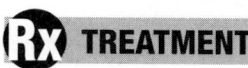 **TREATMENT**

NONPHARMACOLOGIC THERAPY

- Physical therapy, patient education and reassurance, treatment of associated conditions (e.g., depression) are important. Although exercise is routinely encouraged by health care providers, only a few programs have been proven effective. Recent trials reveal that t'ai chi training is effective in reducing balance impairment and falls and improving functional capacity.
- Avoidance of drugs that can induce or worsen parkinsonism: neuroleptics (especially high potency), certain antiemetics (prochlorperazine, trimethobenzamide), metoclopramide, nonselective MAO inhibitors (may induce hypertensive crisis), reserpine, methyldopa

ACUTE GENERAL Rx

- There continues to be controversy whether levodopa or dopamine agonists should be the initial treatment. In younger patients, agonists are usually the drug of choice; in patients >70 yr, levodopa is typically the drug of choice.
- It is appropriate to initiate pharmacotherapy when required by symptoms; prior practice of waiting for limitation of ADLs is now outdated. Fig. E1-628 describes an approach to patients with parkinsonism.
- Motor complications do develop during the course of the disease and likely reflect the combination of disease progression together with the side effects of dopaminergic medications.

CHRONIC Rx

- Levodopa therapy
  1. Cornerstone of symptomatic therapy—should be used with a peripheral dopa decarboxylase inhibitor (carbidopa) to minimize side effects (nausea, light-headedness, postural hypotension). The combination of the two drugs is marketed under the trade name Sinemet. Levodopa therapy has been found to reduce morbidity and mortality in PD patients.
  2. Usual starting dose is 25/100 mg (carbidopa/levodopa) tid 1 hr before meals.
  3. Controlled-release preparations (e.g., Sinemet CR) are available, but their use should be deferred to a neurologist.
  4. Stalevo (combination Sinemet and entacapone, a COMT inhibitor). Useful for patients with motor fluctuations (wearing off); has no role in treating early patients with PD.
- Dopamine receptor agonists (ropinirole and pramipexole) are not as potent as levodopa,

but they are often used as initial treatment in younger patients to attempt to delay the onset of complications (dyskinesias, motor fluctuations) associated with levodopa therapy. These medications are more expensive than levodopa. In general they cause more side effects than levodopa, including nausea, vomiting, light-headedness, peripheral edema, confusion, and somnolence. They can also cause impulse control behaviors such as hypersexuality, binge eating, and compulsive shopping and gambling. Presence of these must be assessed at each visit.
  1. Ropinirole: initial dose is 0.25 mg tid
  2. Pramipexole: initial dose is 0.125 mg tid
- MAO-B inhibitors can be used as monotherapy early in the disease or as adjunctive therapy in later stages; they have been shown to have milder symptomatic benefit than dopamine agonists or levodopa. Well tolerated and easy to titrate. Concurrent use of stimulants and sympathomimetics should be avoided. Certain food restrictions may apply.
  1. Rasagiline: initial dose is 0.5 mg qd, then 1 mg daily. A recent study, ADAGIO, suggests that 1 mg rasagiline may have disease-modifying benefits, but results must be interpreted with caution.
  2. Selegiline: Usual dose, 5 mg bid with breakfast and lunch. Has amphetamine byproduct so has mild stimulant-like effects, which can be beneficial in some patients.
  3. Amantadine can be used alone early in the disease. It is especially useful in the treatment of dyskinesias. Dosage is 100 mg tid (titrate q week from 100 mg qd). Must adjust for elderly and renal impairment. The most notable side effect, especially in the elderly, is confusion.
- Anticholinergic agents are only helpful in treating tremor and drooling in patients with PD. Potential side effects include constipation, urinary retention, memory impairment, and hallucinations. They should be avoided in the elderly.
  1. Trihexyphenidyl: initial dose, 1 mg PO tid
  2. Benztropine: usual dose, 0.5 to 1 mg qd or bid

SURGICAL OPTIONS

- Pallidal (globus pallidus interna) and subthalamic deep-brain stimulation (subthalamic nucleus) are currently the surgical options of choice for patients with advanced PD; similar improvement in motor function and adverse effects has been reported after either procedure. Compared with ablative procedures, DBS has the advantage of being reversible and adjustable. Thalamic DBS may be useful for refractory tremor. It improves the cardinal motor symptoms, extends medication "on" time, and reduces motor fluctuations during the day. In general patients are likely to benefit from this therapy if they show a clear response to levodopa. Therefore, when considering DBS, patients should be evaluated for motor response to levodopa by stopping

levodopa overnight and evaluating motor response before and after a dose of levodopa.
- Surgery is often limited to patients with disabling, medically refractory problems, and patients must still have a good response to L-dopa to undergo surgery. Yet for many patients, earlier stimulation might provide an improved motor benefit before disability from other symptoms has occurred and should be considered at an earlier stage of PD. DBS results in decreased dyskinesias, fluctuations, rigidity, and tremor.

DISPOSITION

PD usually follows a slowly progressive course leading to disability over the course of several years. However, every patient will progress individually, and patients should be reassured that this diagnosis does not, by definition, result in being either wheelchair- or bed-bound.

REFERRAL

- Neurology consultation is recommended at initial diagnosis of PD.
- Exercise is important for all patients with PD.
- Participation in outpatient physical therapy program is recommended for patients with moderate to advanced disease.

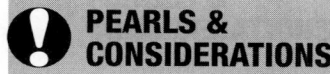 **PEARLS & CONSIDERATIONS**

- Asymmetry of symptoms at onset is very useful in distinguishing PD from other causes of parkinsonism.
- Although resting tremor is a common presenting symptom, up to 25% of patients with idiopathic PD do not have classic resting tremor.

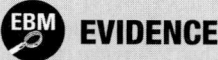 **EVIDENCE**

available at www.expertconsult.com

SUGGESTED READINGS

available at www.expertconsult.com

RELATED CONTENT

Parkinson's Disease (Patient Information)

AUTHOR: **U. SHIVRAJ SOHUR, M.D., PH.D.**

BASIC INFORMATION

DEFINITION

Paronychia is a localized superficial infection or abscess of the lateral and proximal nail fold. Paronychia may be acute or chronic.

SYNONYMS

Nail bed infection
Nail bed abscess

ICD-9CM CODES
681.9 Paronychia

EPIDEMIOLOGY & DEMOGRAPHICS

- Acute paronychia affects males and females equally.
- Chronic paronychia is more common in females than males (9:1).
- Acute paronychia most often occurs in children.
- Chronic paronychia usually presents in the fifth or sixth decade of life.
- Paronychia is the most common infection of the hand.

PHYSICAL FINDINGS & CLINICAL PRESENTATION

- Acute paronychia usually presents with the sudden onset of redness, swelling, and pain with abscess or cellulitis formation in the nail fold. Fluid with purulence is often present.
- Chronic paronychia is insidious, presenting with mild swelling and erythema of the nail folds.
- Acute paronychia usually involves only one finger.
- Chronic paronychia may involve more than one finger.
- Acute paronychia usually involves the thumb.
- Chronic paronychia commonly involves the middle finger.

ETIOLOGY

- Any disruption of the seal between the proximal nail fold and the nail plate can cause paronychial infections.
- Acute paronychia is almost always bacterial in origin (e.g., methicillin-sensitive *Staphylococcus aureus* [most common, but also consider MRSA], *Streptococcus pyogenes*, *Enterococcus faecalis*, *Proteus* and *Pseudomonas* species, and anaerobes).
- Chronic paronychia is commonly caused by *Candida albicans* (70%), with bacterial organisms accounting for the remaining 30%.
- Trauma, nail biting, hangnails, diabetes, and long-term exposure to water are common predisposing features of paronychia.

DIAGNOSIS

The diagnosis of paronychia is self-evident on physical examination.

DIFFERENTIAL DIAGNOSIS

- Herpetic whitlow caused by herpes simplex
- Pyogenic granuloma
- Viral warts
- Ganglions
- Squamous cell carcinoma

WORKUP

A workup is usually not pursued unless there is treatment failure.

LABORATORY TESTS

- Gram stain and culture any purulent drainage.
- Potassium hydroxide mount may show pseudohyphae.

IMAGING STUDIES

Radiographs of the digit if concerned about osteomyelitis.

TREATMENT

NONPHARMACOLOGIC THERAPY

- For acute paronychia without purulent drainage, warm soaks tid or qid are helpful. If pus is present, surgical drainage is required (Fig. 1-629).
- For chronic paronychia, avoid frequent immersion in water or exposure to moisture.

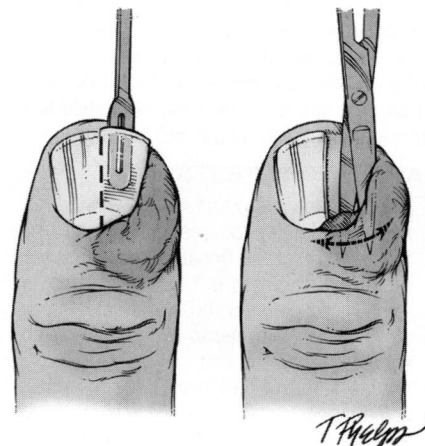
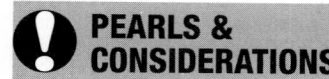

FIGURE 1-629 Surgical drainage of acute paronychia. The lateral nail on the affected side is gently elevated from the nail bed, and a longitudinal strip of nail is removed. If this does not decompress the infection adequately, the margins of the nail fold are opened gently to drain the adjacent soft tissues. (From Cameron JL, Cameron AM: *Current surgical therapy*, ed 10, Philadelphia, 2011, Saunders.)

ACUTE GENERAL Rx

- Trimethoprim-sulfamethoxazole DS † PO bid for 7 days is usually the antibiotic of choice for acute paronychia.
- Alternative antibiotic choices include dicloxacillin 500 mg qid, cephalexin 500 mg qid, clindamycin, and amoxicillin-clavulanate potassium.
- Surgical drainage is indicated if purulent discharge is noted.
- A No. 11 blade scalpel is used to lift the lateral perionychium and proximal eponychium off the nail, facilitating drainage.
- If the pus is located beneath the nail, the lateral edge of the nail can be lifted off the nail bed and excised.

CHRONIC Rx

- If no fungal organism is found, tincture of iodine (2 drops bid) helps keep the nail and skin dry.
- Chronic paronychia caused by *Candida albicans* is treated with topical antifungal agents (e.g., miconazole or ketoconazole applied tid).
- Unresponsive cases may be treated with itraconazole or fluconazole, but this should be done in consultation with dermatology and/or infectious disease.
- Surgery may be needed in refractory cases.

DISPOSITION

- Most acute paronychias with appropriate treatment resolve within 7 to 10 days.
- Osteomyelitis is a potential complication of paronychia.
- Untreated chronic paronychia leads to thickening and discoloration with eventual nail loss.

REFERRAL

Chronic paronychia refractory to topical medical therapy is best referred to dermatology and/or infectious disease. A hand surgeon is consulted if abscess drainage or surgery is being considered.

PEARLS & CONSIDERATIONS

COMMENTS

The gastrointestinal tract, including the mouth and bowel, and the genitourinary tract in women are the usual sources of *C. albicans* in chronic paronychia.

SUGGESTED READINGS

available at www.expertconsult.com

RELATED CONTENT

Paronychia (Patient Information)

AUTHOR: **GLENN G. FORT, M.D., M.P.H.**

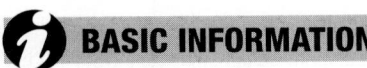

DEFINITION

Paroxysmal cold hemoglobinuria (PCH) is the first, albeit rarest, autoimmune hemolytic anemia to be identified. It is characterized by transient or episodic massive intravascular hemolysis after exposure to cold temperatures. It was first described in patients with secondary or tertiary syphilis, and was classified as acute transient, chronic syphilitic, and chronic nonsyphilitic. In modern times, chronic PCH is very rare, usually occurs in the elderly, and is associated with malignancy. Most cases are of the acute transient type, which is usually idiopathic in adults and secondary to a viral syndrome or immunization in children.

SYNONYMS

PCH
Donath-Landsteiner hemoglobinuria

ICD-9CM CODES
283.2 Hemoglobinuria caused by hemolysis
        from external causes

EPIDEMIOLOGY & DEMOGRAPHICS

INCIDENCE: Estimated at 0.4 cases per 100,000 people
PREVALENCE: Accounts for up to 5% of all adult hemolytic anemias and 30%-40% of childhood cases
PREDOMINANT SEX AND AGE: Mild male sex predilection with reported male-to-female ratio of 2:1 to 5:1
GENETICS: None
RISK FACTORS: Age (most common in young population), infections, and neoplasms have been associated with the development of Donath-Landsteiner antibody.

PHYSICAL FINDINGS & CLINICAL PRESENTATION

- Within minutes to a few hours after cold exposure, there is a sudden onset of fever, rigors, and chills followed by red to brown urination.
- Associated symptoms include back, leg, and abdominal pain.
- Headaches, nausea, vomiting, diarrhea, and esophageal spasm are common. Oliguria and anuria can develop following renal dysfunction.
- May be associated with Raynaud's phenomenon.
- Associated with cold urticaria.
- Transient splenomegaly and hepatomegaly with jaundice may occur.
- Symptoms and gross hemoglobinuria usually resolve within hours.
- Symptoms believed to be mediated by smooth muscle dysfunction as a result of nitric oxide toxicity associated with hemoglobinemia.

ETIOLOGY

- The exact etiology of the D-L antibody is unknown, but the appearance of the antibody is likely related to infection or malignancy.

- The Donath-Landsteiner antibody is a biphasic, usually polyclonal, immunoglobulin (Ig) G. It is known to bind to various antigens such as I-, i-, p-, Pr-, which are normally present on the red blood cell (RBC) surface, yet the glycosphingolipid P antigen is considered its primary target. It sensitizes RBCs in the cold, and as blood warms to 37° C, complement-mediated hemolysis ensues.
- In children, the appearance of the antibody usually follows the onset of a viral respiratory illness by 1 to 3 wk. Symptoms may persist for several weeks.
- PCH has been associated with multiple infectious pathogens, including syphilis, *Haemophilus influenzae*, Epstein-Barr virus (EBV), cytomegalovirus (CMV), influenza A, varicella, measles, mumps, adenovirus, parvovirus B19, coxsackie A9, *Mycoplasma pneumoniae*, and *Klebsiella pneumoniae*.
- Chronic PCH has also been associated with hematologic and solid organ malignancy such as small cell lung cancer and Hodgkin's and non-Hodgkin's lymphoma.

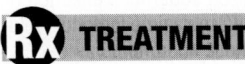

DIFFERENTIAL DIAGNOSIS

- Cold agglutinin disease, paroxysmal nocturnal hemoglobinuria, and malaria
- Other causes of acute massive intravascular hemolysis and myoglobinuria secondary to rhabdomyolysis
- Table 1-320 differentiates various types of autoimmune hemolytic anemias.

WORKUP

U/A, CBC, peripheral blood smear, hemolysis labs (LDH, total bilirubin, haptoglobin), iron studies, reticulocyte count, indirect Coombs and direct Coombs, complement levels, flow cytometry for PNH testing for the presence of CD55 or CD59 on the RBC membrane if clinically indicated, viral studies (if clinically warranted with thick and thin smear to rule out malaria).

LABORATORY TESTS

- The presence of IgG that reacts with the RBC at reduced temperatures but not at body temperature. In the Donath-Landsteiner test, a patient's serum is incubated with papainized pooled donated RBCs and complement at 4° C, then warmed to 37° C. Lysis is observed in a positive test.
- A more sensitive test involves using radiolabeled monoclonal anti-IgG. This is incubated at 4° C with the patient's serum and donor RBCs. The degree of radioactivity on the separated RBCs will be elevated in PCH compared with a control run at 37° C.
- Elevated bilirubin and lactate dehydrogenase, low haptoglobin, free plasma hemoglobin, low complement (C2, C3, C4).
- Abnormal RBC forms on the peripheral blood smear such as poikilocytosis, spherocytosis, anisocytosis, and nucleated RBCs.
- Erythrophagocytosis by neutrophils and monocytes may be seen.

IMAGING STUDIES

If chronic PCH, imaging could be considered to rule out underlying malignancy as the etiology when clinically warranted.

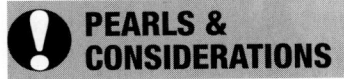

NONPHARMACOLOGIC THERAPY

The mainstay of treatment is the avoidance of exposure to cold and presence of supportive care.

ACUTE GENERAL Rx

- In children in particular, transfusion may be necessary because the anemia may become life threatening and hemolysis may be ongoing for several weeks.
- Testing and treatment for underlying secondary condition.
- Hydration and alkalinization of the urine may be necessary to prevent renal failure.
- Steroids, although commonly used, were not shown to be beneficial.
- Plasma exchange therapy with 5% albumin fluid replacement has been successfully employed.
- Splenectomy is not indicated.
- Treatment with rituximab has resulted in termination of hemolysis in a case report.
- Azathioprine has also been suggested in case reports.

CHRONIC Rx

Several case reports suggest that rituximab and immunosuppressants such as azathioprine may be effective. Treatment of the underlying cause such as infection or malignancy may also help in chronic disease.

COMPLEMENTARY & ALTERNATIVE MEDICINE

None

DISPOSITION

- Postinfectious varieties are self-limited.
- Adult idiopathic form is generally manageable by avoiding environmental exposure.

REFERRAL

To hematologist to aid in diagnosis

PEARLS & CONSIDERATIONS

COMMENTS

- PCH is associated with brown or red discoloration of urine after cold exposure in adults or after a viral infection in children.
- PCH can be associated with viral or bacterial infections, including syphilis, *H. influenzae*, EBV, CMV, influenza A, varicella, measles, mumps, and adenovirus, or malignancy, especially in adults.
- PCH can cause life-threatening hemolysis in children.

PREVENTION

None

TABLE 1-320   Characteristics of Autoimmune Hemolytic Anemia

Characteristic	TYPE OF AUTOIMMUNE HEMOLYTIC ANEMIA		
	Warm Autoimmune Hemolytic Anemia	Cold Agglutinin Disease	Paroxysmal Cold Hemoglobinuria
Antibody isotope	IgG, rare IgA, IgM	IgM	IgG
Direct antiglobulin test (DAT) result	IgG and/or C3	C3	C3
Antigen specificity	Multiple, primarily Rh	i/I, Pr	P
Hemolysis	Primarily extravascular	Primarily extravascular	Intravascular
Common disease associations	B-cell neoplasia/lymphoproliferative, collagen-vascular	Viral, neoplasia	Syphilis, viral

From Hoffman R et al: *Hematology; basic principles and practice,* ed 5, Philadelphia, 2009, Churchill Livingstone.

PATIENT & FAMILY EDUCATION

American Autoimmune Related Diseases Association, Inc.
22100 Gratiot Ave.
East Detroit, MI 48021
Tel: (586) 776-3900
Fax: (586) 776-3903
Tel: (800) 598-4668
Email: aarda@aarda.org
Internet: http://www.aarda.org/
NIH/National Heart, Lung and Blood Institute
P.O. Box 30105
Bethesda, MD 20892-0105
Tel: (301) 592-8573
Fax: (301) 251-1223
Email: nhlbiinfo@rover.nhlbi.nih.gov
Internet: http://www.nhlbi.nih.gov/

Genetic and Rare Diseases (GARD) Information Center
P.O. Box 8126
Gaithersburg, MD 20898-8126
Tel: (301) 251-4925
Fax: (301) 251-4911
Tel: (888) 205-2311
TDD: (888) 205-3223
Internet: http://rarediseases.info.nih.gov/GARD/
Anemia Institute for Research and Education
151 Bloor Street West, Suite 600
Toronto Ontario, M5S 1S4
Canada
Tel: 416-969-7431
Fax: 416-969-7420
Tel: 877-992-6364
Email: info@anemiainstitute.org
Internet: http://www.anemiainstitute.org

AutoImmunity Community
Email: moderator@autoimmunitycommunity.org
Internet: http://www.autoimmunitycommunity.org

SUGGESTED READINGS
available at www.expertconsult.com

AUTHORS: **MATTHEW I. QUESENBERRY, M.D.,** and **MICHAEL MAHER, M.D.**

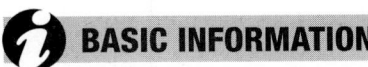

DEFINITION

Paroxysmal nocturnal hemoglobinuria (PNH) is an acquired clonal stem disorder characterized by episodes of intravascular hemolysis and hemoglobinuria usually occurring at night. Thrombocytopenia, leukopenia, and recurrent venous thrombosis are also associated with PNH.

SYNONYMS

PNH

ICD-9CM CODES
283.2 Paroxysmal nocturnal hemoglobinuria

EPIDEMIOLOGY & DEMOGRAPHICS

- Affects patients of any age (reported spectrum 6 to 82 yr) but most common in patients aged 30 to 50 yr
- Affects both sexes (slight female predominance) and all races

PHYSICAL FINDINGS & CLINICAL PRESENTATION

1. Initial manifestations
   - Anemia symptoms (35%)
   - Hemoglobinuria (25%)
   - Bleeding (20%)
   - Aplastic anemia (15%)
   - Gastrointestinal symptoms (10%)
   - Hemolytic anemia (10%)
   - Iron-deficiency anemia (5%)
   - Venous thrombosis (5%)
   - Infections (5%)
   - Neurologic symptoms
2. Hemoglobinuria
   - Typically the first morning void reveals dark urine with progressive clearing during the day. The cause for the circadian rhythm is unknown.
3. Hemolysis
   - In addition to the circadian hemolysis and resulting hemoglobinuria, episodes of hemolytic exacerbations can accompany infections, menstruation, transfusion, surgery, iron therapy, and vaccinations. Symptoms of severe hemolysis include chest, back, or abdominal pain, headache, fever, malaise, and fatigue.
4. Aplastic anemia
   - Aplastic anemia may be the presenting manifestation of PNH (therefore PNH must be in the differential diagnosis of aplastic anemia) or may develop as a later complication of PNH.
5. Thrombosis (leading cause of death in PNH; occurs in 40% of patients)
   - Lower extremity deep vein thrombosis (DVT)
   - Subclavian thrombosis
   - Portal or mesenteric vein thrombosis
   - Hepatic vein thrombosis (Budd-Chiari syndrome)
   - Cerebrovascular thromboses
6. Renal failure
   - Acute renal failure associated with massive hemoglobinuria (acute tubular necrosis)
   - Progressive renal failure associated with thrombosis within renal small veins
7. Dysphagia
8. Infections (associated with leukopenia or steroid treatment)
9. Physical findings include:
   - Pallor (anemia)
   - Jaundice (hemolysis)
   - Splenomegaly
   - Unilateral extremity swelling (DVT)
   - Ascites (Budd-Chiari syndrome)

ETIOLOGY & PATHOGENESIS

- Complement-mediated hemolysis; the erythrocytes are abnormally sensitive to acidified serum.
- Patients have two populations of red blood cells (RBCs): some sensitive to hemolysis (PNH III cells) and others not (PNH I cells), in variable proportions (10% to 75% PNH III cells). Approximately 20% PNH III are required for hemoglobinuria to be detectable.
- The RBC defects in PNH are in the membrane proteins as follows:
   - Decay-accelerating factor deficiency
   - Membrane inhibitor of reactive lysis deficiency
   - C-8 binding protein deficiency
- These protein deficiencies are the result of an acquired mutation located in the X chromosome, which regulates glycosyl phosphatidyl inositol (GPI). GPI anchors the above-mentioned proteins in the RBC membrane; GPI-deficient RBCs proliferate as an abnormal clone. Hemolysis is caused by the absence of decay-accelerating factor (CD55) and the membrane inhibitor of reactive lysis (CD59), which are glycosylphosphatidylinositol-dependent complement regulatory proteins.
- The pathophysiology of the relation of PNH and aplastic anemia is unknown.

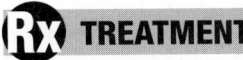 **DIAGNOSIS**

Clinical situations:
- Intravascular hemolysis
- Hemoglobinuria
- Pancytopenia associated with hemolysis
- Iron deficiency associated with hemolysis
- Recurrent venous thrombosis
- Recurrent episodes of abdominal pain, headache, or back pain associated with hemolysis

DIFFERENTIAL DIAGNOSIS

- See "Hemolytic Anemia" in Section I.
- See "Aplastic Anemia" in Section I.
- See "Anemia" algorithm in Section III.

LABORATORY TESTS

- Complete blood count: anemia, leukopenia, thrombocytopenia
- Reticulocytosis
- RBC smear: spherocytes (Fig. E1-630)
- Negative Coombs test
- Low leukocyte alkaline phosphatase
- Elevated lactate dehydrogenase
- Low serum haptoglobin
- Low serum iron saturation, low ferritin
- Elevated urine hemoglobin, urine urobilinogen, urine hemosiderin
- Positive Ham test (acidified serum RBC lysis)
- Normoblastic hyperplasia on bone marrow aspirate or biopsy
- Identification of GPI-anchored protein deficiency on hematopoietic cells by using monoclonal antibodies or flow cytometry; flow cytometric analysis of granulocytes is the best way to diagnose PNH
- Cytogenetic studies are not diagnostic

TREATMENT

- Prednisone (15 to 40 mg qod) helpful to reduce complement activation, but prolonged use should be avoided
- Eculizumab, a humanized antibody that inhibits the activation of terminal complement components, is an effective therapy for PNH; it reduces intravascular hemolysis, hemoglobinuria, and need for transfusion in patients with PNH. It is very expensive and requires lifelong administration. Vaccination against meningococcus is mandatory before eculizumab administration due to increased susceptibility to neisserial infection.
- Iron replacement, folic acid supplementation
- Transfusions
- Treatment and prevention of thrombosis (heparin, Coumadin)
- Avoidance of oral contraceptives
- Bone marrow transplantation

REFERRAL

To hematologist

PROGNOSIS

- Median survival is 10-15 yr.
- 25% survival to 25 yr
- If thrombosis at presentation, only 40% survival to 4 yr
- 1% incidence of leukemia
- 5% incidence of myelodysplastic syndrome
- Death often results from thrombosis or progressive pancytopenia.

SUGGESTED READINGS
available at www.expertconsult.com

AUTHOR: **FRED F. FERRI, M.D.**

BASIC INFORMATION

DEFINITION

Paroxysmal supraventricular tachycardia (SVT) is a group of tachyarrhythmias that originate from within or above the atrioventricular (AV) node and are characterized by sudden onset and abrupt termination. The most common types include AV nodal reentrant tachycardia (AVNRT), AV reentrant tachycardia (AVRT), and paroxysmal atrial tachycardia (PAT).

SYNONYMS

PAT (old terminology for SVT)
PSVT
Supraventricular tachycardia

ICD-9CM CODES

427.0 Paroxysmal atrial tachycardia

PHYSICAL FINDINGS & CLINICAL PRESENTATION

- Patient is usually asymptomatic.
- Patient may be aware of "fast" heartbeat (palpitations) or have presyncope, syncope, or chest pain.
- Hemodynamic status during arrhythmia may vary and can depend on the patient's comorbidities and presence of underlying structural heart disease.

ETIOLOGY

- AVNRT—Dual electrical pathways within or near the AV node
- AVRT—Accessory pathway (concealed [not evident on ECG], only retrograde ventriculoatrial conduction without antegrade atrioventricular conduction)
- Pre-excitation [Wolff-Parkinson-White] syndrome, evident on ECG as described below
- Paroxysmal atrial tachycardia—abnormal automaticity of atrial tissue or triggered activity

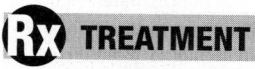 DIAGNOSIS

WORKUP

- Regular rhythm at rate of >100 beats/min is present.

- P waves may or may not be seen (the presence of P waves depends on the relation of atrial to ventricular depolarization).
- Wide QRS complex (>0.12 sec) with initial slurring (delta wave) during sinus rhythm and short PR (<0.12 sec) is characteristic of WPW syndrome.
- QRS complex during SVT is usually narrow; however, may be widened because of intrinsic conduction disease, myocardial disease, or rate-related bundle branch block. It may also be widened if the patient has pre-excitation syndrome.
- Pseudo r and pseudo S waves may be seen in atrioventricular nodal tachycardia (Fig. E1-631).
- Echocardiography is appropriate to assess for the presence of underlying structural heart disease.

 TREATMENT

NONPHARMACOLOGIC THERAPY

- Valsalva maneuver in the supine position is the most effective way to terminate SVT; carotid sinus massage (after excluding occlusive carotid disease) is also commonly used to elicit vagal efferent impulses.
- Synchronized DC shock is used if patient shows signs of hemodynamic instability.
- Table 1-321 describes useful features to differentiate ventricular tachycardia from SVT with aberrancy.

ACUTE GENERAL Rx

- Adenosine is useful for treatment of AVRT and AVNRT, and can uncover the underlying rhythm in paroxysmal atrial tachycardia; it is the first choice of therapy for treatment of almost all episodes of SVT unresponsive to vagal maneuvers. The dose is 6 mg given as a rapid IV bolus; tachycardia is usually terminated within a few seconds. If necessary, may repeat with 12-mg IV bolus. Contraindications are second- or third-degree atrioventricular block, sick sinus syndrome, and atrial fibrillation. Adenosine may cause bronchospasm in asthmatics.

- Verapamil 5 to 10 mg IV is given over 5 min; if no effect, may repeat in 30 min.
  1. Verapamil should be used cautiously in patients with SVT associated with hypotension.
  2. Slow injection of calcium chloride (10 ml of a 10% solution given over 5 to 8 min before verapamil administration) decreases the hypotensive effect without compromising its antiarrhythmic effect.
- Repeat carotid massage after IV verapamil if SVT persists.
- Metoprolol (IV 5 mg/2 min up to 15 mg) or esmolol (500 μg/kg IV bolus, then 50 μg/kg/min) may be effective in the treatment of SVT.
- IV digitalization (0.75 to 1 mg slow IV loading) if other agents are not effective.
  1. Repeat carotid massage 30 min later; if not successful, give additional 0.25 mg IV digoxin and repeat carotid sinus massage 1 hr later.
  2. Digoxin, beta-blockers, and calcium-channel blockers should be avoided in patients with pre-excitation syndrome to avoid increased conduction through the accessory pathway.

DISPOSITION

Most patients respond well with resolution of the paroxysmal atrial tachycardia upon treatment (see "Acute General Rx"). Some patients may need chronic AV blocking agents for recurrence.

REFERRAL

Radiofrequency ablation (RFA) is the procedure of choice in symptomatic patients who are refractory to medical therapy. RFA has high efficacy rates (single procedure success is 93.2%), low all-cause mortality (0.1%), and low adverse events (2.9%). Despite high reported success rates, RFA appears to be underused in clinical practice.

! PEARLS & CONSIDERATIONS

COMMENTS

Accessory pathways occur in 0.1% to 0.3% of the general population.

SUGGESTED READINGS

available at www.expertconsult.com

RELATED CONTENT

Fig. 3-176 Evaluation and management of narrow complex tachycardia (Algorithm)

AUTHORS: **ALEXANDER G. TRUESDELL, M.D., FRED F. FERRI, M.D.,** and **WEN-CHIH WU, M.D., M.P.H.**

TABLE 1-321 Features That May Differentiate Ventricular Tachycardia from Supraventricular Tachycardia with Aberrancy

Helpful Features	Implications
Positive QRS concordance	Diagnostic of VT
Presence of AV dissociation, capture beats, or fusion beats	Diagnostic of VT
Atypical RBBB (monophasic R, QR, RS, or triphasic QRS in V$_1$; R:S ratio < 1, QS or QR, monophasic R in V$_6$)	Suggests VT
Atypical LBBB (R >30 min or R to S [nadir or notch] > 60 min in V$_1$ or V$_2$; R:S ratio < 1, QS or QR in V$_6$)	Suggests VT
Shift of axis from baseline	Suggests VT
History of CAD	Suggests VT
QRS during tachycardia identical to QRS during sinus rhythm	Suggests VT
Termination with adenosine	Suggests SVT
	Suggests SVT

AV, Atrioventricular; *CAD,* coronary artery disease; *LBBB,* left bundle branch block; *RBBB,* right bundle branch block; *SVT,* supraventricular tachycardia; *VT,* ventricular tachycardia.
From Andreoli TG et al (eds): *Andreoli and Carpenter's Cecil essentials of medicine,* ed 8, Philadelphia, 2010, Saunders.

BASIC INFORMATION

DEFINITION

Patellofemoral pain syndrome is overuse or overload of the patellofemoral region leading to anterior knee pain.

SYNONYMS

PFPS
Retropatellar pain syndrome
Runner's knee
Lateral facet compression syndrome
Idiopathic anterior knee pain

ICD-9CM CODES
719.46 Patellofemoral pain syndrome

EPIDEMIOLOGY & DEMOGRAPHICS

PREVALENCE: Estimated >20% of adolescents. PFPS is the most common diagnosis in outpatients presenting with knee pain. PFPS also constitutes 16% to 25% of all injuries to runners.
PREDOMINANT SEX AND AGE: Nearly 2:1 female predominance; disproportionately affects active adolescents and adults in the second and third decades of life
RISK FACTORS: Increase in physical activity intensity or duration, overuse, joint overload, trauma, anatomic abnormalities, malalignment, patellar hypermobility, quadriceps weakness

PHYSICAL FINDINGS & CLINICAL PRESENTATION

- Gradual or acute onset of anterior knee pain
- Sometimes localized under or around the patella
- Also described as a catching sensation under the patella
- Worsened pain with squatting, running, prolonged sitting, or ascending or descending steps
- Effusion implies intraarticular pathology not explained by PFPS
- Pain may be elicited by compression of the patella into the trochlear groove while the leg is extended

ETIOLOGY

No clear consensus; likely multifactorial, including muscle overuse or joint overload with malalignment and/or trauma potentially contributing resulting in imbalances in the forces controlling patellar tracking during knee flexion and extension

DIAGNOSIS

DIFFERENTIAL DIAGNOSIS

- Patellofemoral arthritis
- Patellar instability
- Patellar stress fracture
- Osgood-Schlatter disease
- Articular cartilage injury
- Prepatellar bursitis
- Pes anserine bursitis
- Iliotibial band syndrome
- Plica synovitis
- Chondromalacia
- Bony abnormalities
- Bone tumors
- Patellar tendinopathy
- Other: Referred pain from lumbar spine or hip joint pathology, loose bodies, osteochondritis dissecans, Sinding-Larsen-Johansson syndrome, symptomatic bipartite patella

WORKUP

- PFPS is a clinical diagnosis of exclusion; evaluate and rule out other possibilities on the differential. Dynamic patellar tracking can be assessed by having the patient perform a single leg squat and stand. Physical exam should also include patellar mobility testing (displacement >3 quadrants is considered hypermobile), patellar grind (or inhibition) test (positive test if pain is produced), and patellar tilt test to assess for tightness of the lateral structures.
- Physical exam findings consistent with PFPS include eliciting pain by compression of the patella into the trochlear groove while the leg is extended.

IMAGING STUDIES

- No imaging is necessary in the initial workup.
- Consider plain films if symptoms do not improve after 1 to 2 mo of therapy.

TREATMENT

There is a general lack of consensus. Management should focus on the implementation of a comprehensive rehabilitation program.

NONPHARMACOLOGIC THERAPY

Physical therapy; quadriceps, hamstring, iliotibial band, and calf-stretching exercises; quadriceps and hip abductor strengthening

ACUTE GENERAL Rx

Short-term (2 to 3 wk) nonsteroidal anti-inflammatory drugs or acetaminophen for pain relief; activity modification; ice for 10 to 20 min after activity

CHRONIC Rx

- Physical therapy; strengthening and flexibility exercises; consider arch supports or evaluation for custom orthotics.
- Spontaneous resolution may occur in some cases.

DISPOSITION

Outpatient management

REFERRAL

Consider referral to orthopedics for surgical evaluation as a last resort if conservative therapies fail. Surgical options include release of the lateral retinaculum; articular cartilage procedures; and proximal realignment, usually with anteromedialization of the tibial tubercle.

PEARLS & CONSIDERATIONS

COMMENTS

Treatment is most successful when the patient has a disciplined approach.

PATIENT & FAMILY EDUCATION

The American Academy of Family Practice website www.familydoctor.org contains frequently asked questions, patient information, and example stretching and strengthening exercises. Information is available in English and Spanish.

EVIDENCE

available at www.expertconsult.com

SUGGESTED READING

available at www.expertconsult.com

RELATED CONTENT

Fig. 3-99 Evaluation and management of knee extensor mechanism pain (Algorithm)
Knee Pain (Patient Information)

AUTHOR: **KATE MAVRICH, M.D.**

BASIC INFORMATION

DEFINITION

- Patent foramen ovale (PFO) is a vestige of the fetal circulation, and results from failure of the primum and secundum septa to fuse postnatally. Persistence of the one-way flap valve overlying this foramen ovale allows right to left blood flow when right atrial pressure exceeds that of the left.
- Foramen ovale remains open during intrauterine life, in a valve-like manner, to allow highly oxygenated blood to reach the left atrium from the inferior vena cava. High right atrial pressure in the fetus keeps it open.
- Soon after birth, as the pulmonary circulation fills, the left atrial pressure rises higher than that of the right atrium. This pushes the septum primum against septum secundum, closing the right-to-left pathway through the foramen ovale.

ICD-9CM CODES
745.5 Patent foramen ovale

EPIDEMIOLOGY & DEMOGRAPHICS
- PFO fails to close in as much as a fourth of the population.
- PFO has similar frequency among males and females.

PHYSICAL FINDINGS & CLINICAL PRESENTATION
- Most patients with isolated PFO are asymptomatic.
- It cannot be detected on clinical examination.
COMPLICATIONS
- Cryptogenic stroke (particularly <55 yr).
- The proposed mechanism of stroke with PFO includes paradoxical embolization, in situ thrombosis within the canal of the PFO, associated atrial arrhythmia, and concomitant hypercoagulable state.
- Migraine with aura.
- Decompression sickness and air embolism.
- Increases risk of hypoxemia during sleep in patients with obstructive sleep apnea.
- Platypnea-orthodeoxia syndrome (characterized by both dyspnea and arterial desaturation in the upright position with improvement in supine position).
- Increased risk of postoperative atrial fibrillation and hypoxemia, in off-pump coronary artery bypass surgery.

ETIOLOGY
Unknown

DIAGNOSIS

- Testing for PFO is primarily performed in patients with a cerebral ischemic event of uncertain origin.
- A variety of echocardiography modalities have been used to diagnose PFO. These include:
  1. Transthoracic echocardiography (TTE)
  2. Transesophageal echocardiogram (TEE) (Fig. 1-632)

3. Transmitral Doppler (TMD)
4. Transcranial Doppler (TCD) of middle cerebral artery after injection of agitated saline peripherally
- TEE, especially when performed with contrast injected during a cough or Valsalva, is the most sensitive and preferred test for diagnosing PFO.
- Essentially, a PFO is suggested by the presence of echo dropout in the atrial septum visualized in more than one plane during echocardiography. The appearance of microbubbles in the left atrium within three to five cardiac cycles after injection of agitated saline peripherally is considered diagnostic of PFO with associated right-to-left shunt (RLS).
- The diagnosis of PFO is enhanced with multiple intravenous contrast injections with maneuvers that cause transient elevations of right atrial pressure (cough or Valsalva) to enhance RLS.
- TCD has the advantage of being noninvasive and easy to perform at bedside. But it can only detect a right-to-left shunt, not the location of the shunt or other cardiac structural anomalies.

TREATMENT

- Management guidelines from professional societies are shown in Table 1-322.
- Most patients with a PFO as an isolated finding receive no special treatment. This is because the yearly risk of cryptogenic stroke in healthy persons with PFO may be as low as 0.1%.
- As it is not associated with increased risk for endocarditis, antibiotic prophylaxis is not indicated.

PHARMACOLOGIC TREATMENT

When PFO is associated with an otherwise unexplained neurologic event, traditional treatment has been antiplatelet treatment (e.g., aspirin) therapy alone in low-risk patients and combined with therapeutic anticoagulants (e.g., warfarin) in high-risk patients.

Risk factors associated with a higher risk of complications, particularly stroke, include:
- Coexisting atrial septal aneurysm
- Large PFO
- Spontaneous right-to-left shunting
- Major shunt (>50 bubbles)
- Valsalva-provoking activity preceding the onset of stroke
- Presence of Chiari network (a congenital remnant of the right valve of the sinus venosus)
- Eustachian valves
- Younger age (<55 yr)
- Multiple clinical events or infarcts
- Pulmonary hypertension
- Failure or contraindications to anticoagulants
- High risk for recurrent deep venous thrombosis
- Pulmonary embolism at time of initial event
- Hypercoagulable state

PERCUTANEOUS TRANSCATHETER CLOSURE OF PFO

Percutaneous method of closure is usually preferred over open surgical closure because of invasiveness, procedure time, and patient convenience.
- Indications:
  1. Recurrent cryptogenic stroke due to presumed paradoxical embolism through PFO while on adequate medical treatment with antiplatelets or anticoagulants. The

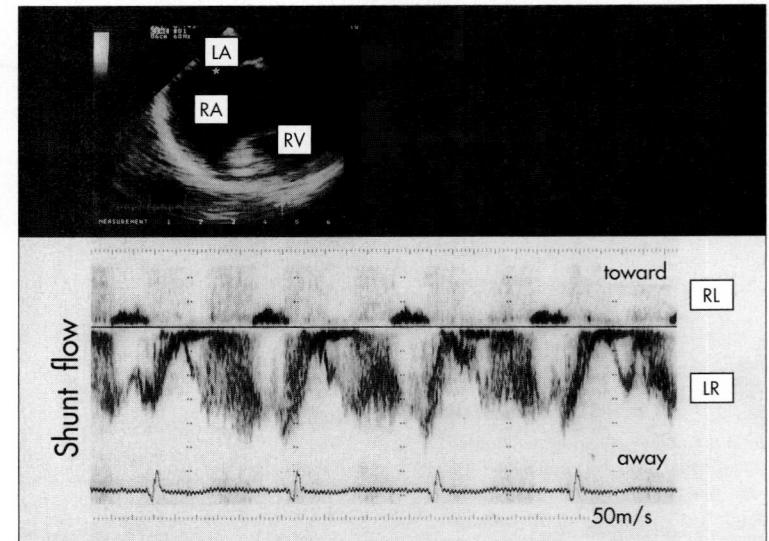

FIGURE 1-632 Transesophageal echocardiography of an internal defect and pulsed Doppler flow signal. Pulsed Doppler echocardiographic signal is consistent with left-to-right level. *LA,* Left atrium; *RA,* right atrium; *RV,* right ventricle; *LR,* left-to-right shunt signal; *RL,* right-to-left shunt signal. (From Crawford MH et al [eds]: *Cardiology,* ed 2, St Louis, 2004, Mosby.)

American Heart Association and American College of Cardiology have discouraged the use of devices to close a PFO as a means of preventing recurrent stroke. A recent trial (CLOSURE I) revealed that in patients with cryptogenic stroke or TIA who had a PFO, closure with a device did not offer a greater benefit than medical therapy alone for the prevention of recurrent stroke or TIA.
2. In presence of contraindications to anticoagulants
- Contraindications:
  1. Presence of thrombus on the implant site or in the venous system used for access
  2. Active endocarditis or bacteremia
  3. Inadequate size of femoral vein for access
  4. Atrial septal anatomy without an adequate rim to hold the device

5. Atrial septal anatomy that may result in the occluder obstructing an intracardiac structure
6. Known hypercoagulable state
7. Presence of an intracardiac mass or vegetation
- The Food and Drug Administration (FDA) has approved CardioSEAL Septal Occlusion System and Amplatzer PFO Occluder devices for percutaneous PFO closure.
- Requires SBE prophylaxis and antiplatelets (aspirin and clopidogrel for first 3 mo, followed by aspirin for another 3 mo) for 6 mo postprocedure. During this period of endothelialization, the risk of recurrent stroke is highest.
- The 1-yr rate of recurrent neurologic events ranged from 0% to 5% with percutaneous closure group vs. 4% to 12% with medical therapy group.
- MRI or metal detectors do not affect these implants, as they are not metallic in nature.

SURGICAL CLOSURE (OPEN THORACOTOMY)

Indications:
1. PFO >25 mm in size
2. Inadequate rim of tissue around the defect
3. Percutaneous device failure
4. In presence of other indication for open heart surgery

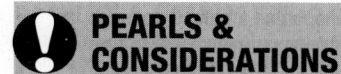

PEARLS & CONSIDERATIONS

COMMENTS

PFO is found on transesophageal echocardiography in about 50% of young survivors of stroke without clear cause for their stroke. In these patients, it is unclear whether the PFO was the cause of the stroke or whether it was an incidental finding. Trials have shown that closure of a PFO for secondary prevention of cryptogenic embolism did not result in a significant reduction in the risk of recurrent embolic events or death as compared with medical therapy.

SUGGESTED READINGS
available at www.expertconsult.com

AUTHOR: **HEMANT K. SATPATHY, M.D.**

TABLE 1-322 Management Guidelines from Professional Societies

	American Academy of Neurology	American College of Chest Physicians
PFO	1. Evidence is insufficient to determine whether warfarin or aspirin is superior in preventing recurrent strokes or death, but minor bleeding is more frequent with warfarin. 2. There is insufficient evidence to evaluate the efficacy of surgical or endovascular closure.	
PFO alone		1. Antiplatelet therapy recommended over no therapy 2. Antiplatelet therapy suggested over warfarin
PFO with other risk factors		Inadequate data available to allow recommendation of optimal medical therapy vs. endovascular or surgical closure
PFO with concomitant deep vein thrombosis or pulmonary embolism	At least 3 mo of anticoagulation	Anticoagulation recommended

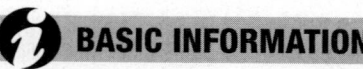

BASIC INFORMATION

DEFINITION

Pediculosis is lice infestation. Human beings can be infested with three kinds of lice: *Pediculus capitis* (head louse), *Pediculus corporis* (body louse), and *Phthirus pubis* (pubic, or crab, louse). Lice feed on human blood and deposit their eggs (nits) on the hair shafts (head lice and pubic lice) and along the seams of clothing (body lice). Nits generally hatch within 7 to 10 days. Lice are obligate human parasites and cannot survive away from their hosts for longer than 7 to 10 days.

SYNONYMS

Lice

ICD-9CM CODES
132.9 Pediculosis

EPIDEMIOLOGY & DEMOGRAPHICS

- There are 6 to 12 million cases of head lice in the U.S. yearly. The estimated annual direct and indirect cost of head louse infestation in the U.S. is $1 billion.
- Lice infestation of the scalp is most common in children (girls affected more often than boys).
- Infestation of the eyelashes is most frequently seen in children and may indicate sexual abuse.
- The chance of acquiring pubic lice from one sexual exposure with an infested partner is >90% (most contagious STD known).
- Body lice is most common in conditions of poor hygiene.

PHYSICAL FINDINGS & CLINICAL PRESENTATION

- Pruritus with excoriation may be caused by hypersensitivity reaction, inflammation from saliva, and fecal material from the lice.
- Nits can be identified by examining hair shafts.
- The presence of nits on clothes is indicative of body lice.
- Lymphadenopathy may be present (cervical adenopathy with head lice, inguinal lymphadenopathy with pubic lice).
- Head lice is most frequently found in the back of the head and neck, behind the ears.
- Scratching can result in pustules and crusting.
- Pubic lice may affect the hair around the anus.

ETIOLOGY

Lice are transmitted by close personal contact or use of contaminated objects (e.g., combs, clothing, bed linen, hats).

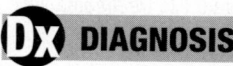

DIAGNOSIS

DIFFERENTIAL DIAGNOSIS

- Seborrheic dermatitis
- Scabies
- Eczema
- Other: pilar casts, trichonodosis (knotted hair), monilethrix

WORKUP

Diagnosis is made by seeing the lice (Fig. 1-633) or their nits. Combing hair with a fine-toothed comb is recommended because visual inspection of the hair and scalp may miss more than 50% of infestations.

LABORATORY TESTS

Wood's light examination is useful to screen a large number of children: live nits fluoresce, empty nits have a gray fluorescence, nits with unborn louse reveal white fluorescence.

Rx TREATMENT

NONPHARMACOLOGIC THERAPY

- Patients with body lice should discard infested clothes and improve their hygiene.
- Combing out nits is a widely recommended but unproven adjunctive therapy.
- Personal items such as combs and brushes should be soaked in hot water for 15 to 30 min.
- Close contacts and household members should also be examined for the presence of lice.

ACUTE GENERAL Rx

The following products are available for treatment of lice:

- Permethrin: available over the counter (1% permethrin [Nix]) or by prescription (5% permethrin [Elimite]); should be applied to the hair and scalp and rinsed out after 10 min. A repeat application 7 days later is generally not necessary in patients with head lice. It can be applied to clean, dry hair and left on overnight (8 to 14 hours) under a shower cap. Resistance to permethrin is now widespread.
- Malathion, an organophosphate, is effective in head lice. It is available by prescription. Use should be avoided in children ≤2 yr. It is not commonly used because of its objection-

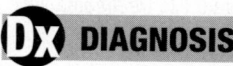

FIGURE 1-633 Body louse, Pediculus humanus var. corporis, as it was obtaining a blood meal from human host. (Courtesy Public Health Image Library, Centers for Disease Control and Prevention. From Vincent JL et al: *Textbook of critical care*, ed 6, Philadelphia, 2011, Saunders.)

able odor, fear of flammability, and prolonged application time (8 to 12 hr).

- Spinosad (Natroba) is a newer FDA-approved product for head lice. It is a topical suspension applied to dry hair for 10 min, then rinsed. It may be repeated 7 days later if necessary. It is more effective than permethrin but also much more expensive. It is safe in pregnancy (category B—no evidence of risk in humans).
- Benzyl alcohol lotion, 5% (Ulesfia) can be used for treatment of head lice in patients >6 mo old. The lotion is applied to dry hair and left on for 10 min. Treatment must be repeated after 7 days because the drug is not ovicidal.
- Eyelash infestation can be treated with the application of petroleum jelly rubbed into the eyelashes three times a day for 5 to 7 days. The application of baby shampoo to the eyelashes and brows three or four times a day for 5 days is also effective. The use of fluorescein drops applied to the lids and eyelashes is also toxic to lice.
- In patients who have previously not responded to treatment or in whom resistance with 1% permethrin cream rinse occurs, a 10-day course of trimethoprim-sulfamethoxazole (TMP-SMX) 8 mg/kg/day in divided doses is an effective treatment for head lice infestation, especially for eyelash infestations with *Phthirus pubis*.
- Ivermectin, an antiparasitic drug, given as an oral dose of 400 mcg/kg of body weight on days 1 and 8, is effective for head lice resistant to other treatments (currently not FDA approved for pediculosis). Ivermectin 0.5% lotion is FDA approved as a single-use topical treatment for head lice in patients 6 mo or older. Cost is more than $200 for 4 oz.

PEARLS & CONSIDERATIONS

COMMENTS

- Patients with pubic lice should notify their sexual contacts. Sex partners within the last month should be treated.
- Parents of patients should also be educated that head lice infestation (unlike body lice) does not indicate poor hygiene.

SUGGESTED READINGS

available at www.expertconsult.com

RELATED CONTENT

Lice (Patient Information)

AUTHOR: **FRED F. FERRI, M.D.**

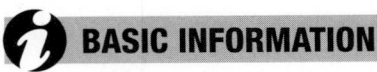

BASIC INFORMATION

DEFINITION

According to the DSM-IV-TR, pedophilia is one of nine possible paraphilias. A paraphilia is an enduring sexual preference that is highly unusual or illegal and results in distress or impairment. The sexual preference of a pedophile is for young children. The pedophile must experience at least 6 mo of intense sexual urges, fantasies, or behaviors involving *prepubescent* children. The pedophile must experience distress or impairment. According to the DSM-IV-TR, if the individual acts upon his/her sexual urge with a child, or if the sexual urge puts the person at odds with society or with the law, the functional impairment criterion has been met. The pedophile must be older than 16 yr and at least 5 yr older than the object of his/her longings. DSM-IV-TR subtypes pedophiles into categories based on his/her victim gender preference (boys, girls, or both), on the exclusivity of his/her sexual urges toward children (children only or affinity for adults and children), and on his/her relationship with the victim (family or extrafamilial).

> **ICD-10CM CODES**
> F65.4 Pedophilia
> **ICD-9CM CODES**
> 302.2 Pedophilia

EPIDEMIOLOGY & DEMOGRAPHICS

PREVALENCE (IN U.S.): Prevalence rates are largely based on self-reports of convicted child molesters, who are not necessarily pedophiles. According to this data, 3% to 9% of men self-report sexual contact or sexual fantasy with prepubescent children. Convenience samples suggest an upper limit of 5% for pedophilia.

ONSET & PREDOMINANT AGE: Pedophilia has an early onset and a chronic course. A study of 4007 self-admitted child molesters (2429 pedophiles) found that 40% of pedophiles molest before age 15 and the majority molest before age 20. Dickey et al reviewed charts of 174 sex offenders, 68 of whom were pedophiles. The pedophiles were distributed across the three age groups as follows: 17.6% were young adults, 38.2% were adults, and 44.1% were older adults, aged 40 to 70 yr old.

PREDOMINANT SEX: The significant majority of pedophiles are men (females comprise 1% to 6% of child molesters).

PHYSICAL FINDINGS & CLINICAL PRESENTATION

According to Abel and Harlow's study of 4007 child molesters:

- Child molesters match the general population with regards to education, marital status, and religion.
- 93% of child molesters reported some sexual interest in adults.
- 51% of men who abuse boys reported being exclusively heterosexual. 8% reported being exclusively homosexual.
- 60% have other paraphilias.

- Sex offenders have higher rates of *general* crime recidivism than *sexual* crime recidivism. When known child molesters are rearrested, ~40% of their rearrests are for sexual offenses.

DIAGNOSIS

DIFFERENTIAL DIAGNOSIS

Pedophilia is often confused with terms such as child molester, sex offender, and hebephile. Not all child molesters are pedophiles. For example, individuals with antisocial personality disorder may have an exclusive sexual preference for adults but may take a child's presence as an opportunity to gratify their sexual impulses. An individual who is hypersexual, indiscriminate, disinhibited, and who has very little opportunity for sexual gratification with their preferred age group may molest a child. A hebephile is one who has a sexual affinity for pubescent adolescents, rather than prepubescent youth. The term "sexual offender" represents a broad group of individuals who sexually offend against either children or adults.

WORKUP

Requires comprehensive data from multiple sources, including self-report, past sexual offense convictions, past and present partner report, psychophysiologic assessments, forensic computer analysis, and/or scales. Deviant sexual preferences and lifestyle instability/criminality are strongly associated with general sexual recidivism. Therefore, clinical interview should explore sexual preferences (sex drive, paraphilic interests, victim characteristics), past sexual behaviors (including inquiry into the use of child pornography), and a history of rule violation, substance abuse, and risk taking. It is also important to explore opportunities that the individual has to be around children as well as exploring an individual's strengths and protective factors (lifestyle stability).

Investigation into comorbid disorders should include substance abuse, antisocial personality disorder, other paraphilias, personality disorders, and also mood, anxiety, and disruptive behavior disorders.

SCALES AND LABORATORY TESTS

- Phallometric/Plethysmographic Testing: The penile volume or circumference is measured in response to a variety of sexual materials. The result is thought to be a predictor of sexual recidivism among sex offenders. However, ~20% to 30% of individuals tested are considered low or nonresponders. Further, in the U.S., possession of the viewing material (child pornography) presents a legal dilemma for researchers. Other limitations include its lack of applicability to females, lack of applicability to males with impotence, and ability of individuals to try to suppress sexual feelings via distraction. This form of testing is not currently admissible in court for the purpose of determining guilt.

- Viewing Time: Viewing time is correlated with self-reported sexual interest and phallometric sexual arousal to children. No studies report that this measure predicts recidivism.
- Scales: For the prediction of general sexual recidivism, the most accurate approach appears to be the use of certain actuarial and mechanical measures. Some of the measures include the Static 99, MnSOST-R, Risk Matrix-2000 sex, and the SVR 20. An individual's likelihood to recidivate is estimated based on the average risk of a group of individuals with similar characteristics.

TREATMENT

NONPHARMACOLOGIC THERAPY

- Many models of sex offender treatment include identification of the offender's "sexual assault cycle." A response prevention intervention is devised. Triggers and relapse cues are identified, high-risk factors are avoided, and skills are taught to interrupt an offending response. An individual's life skills are enhanced via training in anger management, self-regulation, intimacy and relationships, and general coping. Comorbidity such as substance abuse and mania should be treated. Treatment of pedophilia focuses on diminishing the pedophile's likelihood of acting on his/her urges rather than on changing the core sexual orientation. Scales have been developed in order to monitor progress in sex offender treatment.
- Hanson and Morton-Bourgon reported that recidivism rates over 5 to 6 yr for general sexual offenders vary from 13% (sexual recidivism) to 36% (any type of recidivism). Other sources range from 10% to 50% for pedophiles. There is no clear and consistent support for the efficacy of current treatment for sexual offenders. A 2009 Cochrane Collaboration Review on Management for people with disorders of sexual preference and for convicted sexual offenders concluded that the area lacked a strong evidence base.
- Treatment should develop positive life competencies, such as skills and beliefs, that will enhance the likelihood of a prosocial life and that are incompatible with offending behaviors.
- Community interventions might include the education of parents (re: high-risk situations, neighborhood sex offenders) and the education of children (re: assertiveness training, etc).
- Behavioral treatments are controversial interventions that are not the standard of care. They were devised to decrease sexual arousal to children. Examples include the introduction of aversive stimuli, habituation, and increasing sexual arousal to adults. It is unclear how effective these treatments are.

ACUTE GENERAL Rx & CHRONIC Rx

- Cyproterone acetate (CPA), medroxyprogesterone, and leuprolide acetate interfere with

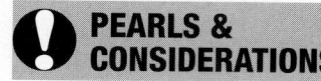

testosterone. These agents may reduce the frequency or intensity of sexual urges and arousal. There are no large well-controlled studies. The agents require close monitoring. Long-term consequences are unknown. Hormone therapy is expensive.

- SSRIs are supported by open label trials and case reports. They may decrease urges and lessen sexual preoccupation.
- Surgical castration involves removal of the testes. A significant minority of surgically castrated individuals continue to be able to have erections and to achieve ejaculation. Testosterone may be purchased by the sex offender in order to circumvent the function of their surgical castration.

REFERRAL
Refer to specialty mental health.

ⓘ PEARLS & CONSIDERATIONS

- Pedophiles with no known risk of prior sexual contacts with children are at unknown risk to offend.
- Physicians should be aware of reporting requirements in their jurisdiction.

SUGGESTED READINGS
available at www.expertconsult.com

RELATED CONTENT
Pedophilia (Patient Information)

AUTHORS: **ELIZABETH A. LOWENHAUPT, M.D.,** and **SARAH L. XAVIER, D.O.**

P

Diseases and Disorders

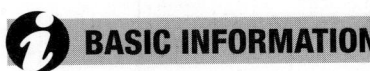

BASIC INFORMATION

DEFINITION

Pelvic inflammatory disease (PID) is a polymicrobial infection of the upper genital tract, including a combination of any of the following:
- Endometritis, salpingitis, tubo-ovarian abscess, or pelvic peritonitis
- Resulting from an ascending lower genital tract infection
- Not related to obstetric or surgical intervention

SYNONYMS

PID
Adnexitis
Pyosalpinx
Salpingitis
Tubo-ovarian abscess

ICD-9CM CODES
614.0 Acute salpingitis and oophoritis
614.2 Salpingitis and oophoritis not specified as acute, subacute, or chronic
614.9 Unspecified inflammatory disease of female pelvic organs and tissue

EPIDEMIOLOGY & DEMOGRAPHICS

INCIDENCE/PREVALENCE:
- Estimated 600,000 to 1 million cases annually (U.S.), affecting primarily young sexually active women
- Diagnosed in 2% to 5% of women seen in sexually transmitted disease clinics
- Most common cause of female infertility and ectopic pregnancy

RISK FACTORS:
- Adolescent sexually active females <20 yr (1:8)
- Previous episode of gonococcal PID
- Multiple sexual partners

PHYSICAL FINDINGS & CLINICAL PRESENTATION

- Lower abdominal pain
- Abnormal vaginal discharge
- Abnormal uterine bleeding
- Dysuria
- Dyspareunia
- Nausea and vomiting (suggestive of peritonitis)
- Fever
- Right upper quadrant tenderness (perihepatitis): 5% of PID cases
- Cervical motion tenderness and adnexal tenderness
- Adnexal mass

ETIOLOGY

- *Chlamydia trachomatis*
- *Neisseria gonorrhoeae*
- Polymicrobial infection: *Bacteroides fragilis, Escherichia coli, Gardnerella vaginalis, Haemophilus influenzae, Mycoplasma hominis, Ureaplasma urealyticum*
- *Mycobacterium tuberculosis* (an important cause in developing countries)
- Cytomegalovirus (CMV)

DIAGNOSIS

DIFFERENTIAL DIAGNOSIS

- Ectopic pregnancy
- Appendicitis
- Ruptured ovarian cyst
- Endometriosis
- Urinary tract infection (cystitis or pyelonephritis)
- Renal calculus
- Adnexal torsion
- Proctocolitis

WORKUP

Diagnostic considerations:
- Clinical diagnosis is difficult and imprecise. The spectrum of disease ranges from asymptomatic to life-threatening tubo-ovarian abscess. PID should be suspected in at-risk patients who present with pelvic or lower abdominal pain.
- Clinical diagnosis of symptomatic PID has a positive predictive value of 65% to 90% compared with laparoscopy as the standard.
- No single historical, physical, or laboratory finding is both sensitive and specific for the diagnosis of PID.
- Empiric treatment for PID should be initiated in sexually active young women and other women at risk for STDs if they are experiencing pelvic or lower abdominal pain, if no cause for the illness other than PID can be identified, and if one or more of the following minimum criteria are present on pelvic examination:
  - Uterine tenderness
  - Adnexal tenderness
  - Cervical motion tenderness
- The requirement that all three minimum criteria be present before the initiation of empiric treatment could result in insufficient sensitivity for the diagnosis of PID. The presence of signs of lower genital tract inflammation (predominance of leukocytes in vaginal secretions), in addition to one of the three minimum criteria, increases the specificity of the diagnosis.
- Additional criteria to increase the specificity of the diagnosis of PID in women with severe clinical signs:
  - Oral temperature >38.3° C (101° F)
  - Abnormal cervical or vaginal discharge
  - Elevated erythrocyte sedimentation rate (ESR)
  - Elevated C-reactive protein
  - Laboratory documentation of cervical infection with *N. gonorrhoeae* or *C. trachomatis*
- Presence of abundant numbers of WBCs on saline microscopy of vaginal fluid.
- Definitive criteria for diagnosing PID warranted in selected cases:
  - Laparoscopic abnormalities consistent with PID
  - Histopathologic evidence of endometritis on biopsy. Endometrial biopsy is warranted in women undergoing laparoscopy who do not have visual evidence of salpingitis because endometritis is the only sign of PID in some women
  - Transvaginal sonography or other imaging techniques showing thickened fluid-filled tubes with or without free pelvic fluid or tubo-ovarian complex

LABORATORY TESTS

- Leukocytosis
- Elevated acute phase reactants: ESR >15 mm/hr, C-reactive protein
- Gram stain of endocervical exudate: >30 polymorphonuclear cells per high-power field correlates with chlamydial or gonococcal infection
- Endocervical cultures for *N. gonorrhoeae* and *C. trachomatis*
- Fallopian tube aspirate or peritoneal exudate culture if laparoscopy performed
- Human chorionic gonadotropin to rule out ectopic pregnancy

IMAGING STUDIES

- Transvaginal ultrasound to look for adnexal mass has sensitivity for PID of 81%, specificity of 78%, and accuracy of 80%.
- MRI has sensitivity for PID of 95%, specificity of 89%, and accuracy of 93%. It is useful for establishing the diagnosis of PID and detecting other processes responsible for the symptoms. Disadvantages are its higher cost and limited availability.
- CT scan (Fig. 1-634).

TREATMENT

NONPHARMACOLOGIC THERAPY

- Most patients are treated as outpatients.
- Criteria for hospitalization (CDC, 2006) as follows:
  - Surgical emergencies such as appendicitis cannot be excluded
  - Tubo-ovarian abscess
  - Pregnant patient
  - Patient is immunodeficient
  - Severe illness, nausea, or vomiting precluding outpatient management
  - Patient unable to follow or tolerate outpatient regimens
  - No clinical response to outpatient therapy

ACUTE GENERAL Rx

Regimens for treatment of PID should also be effective against *N. gonorrhoeae* and *C. trachomatis* because endocervical screening for these organisms does not rule out upper reproductive tract infections.

INPATIENT REGIMENS:
Recommended parenteral regimen A
- Cefotetan 2 g IV q12h
  OR
- Cefoxitin 2 g IV q6h
  PLUS
- Doxycycline 100 mg PO or IV q12h

Recommended parenteral regimen B
- Clindamycin 900 mg IV q8h PLUS
- Gentamicin loading dose IV or IM (2 mg/kg of body weight), followed by a maintenance

dose (1.5 mg/kg) q8h. Single daily dosing (3 to 5 mg/kg) can be substituted.

Alternative parenteral regimens

- Ampicillin/sulbactam 3 g IV q6h PLUS
- Doxycycline 100 mg PO or IV q12h

OUTPATIENT REGIMENS:

Recommended regimen

- Ceftriaxone 250 mg IM in a single dose PLUS
- Doxycycline 100 mg PO bid for 14 days WITH or WITHOUT
- Metronidazole 500 mg PO bid for 14 days OR
- Cefoxitin 2 g IM in a single dose and probenecid, 1 g PO administered concurrently in a single dose PLUS

- Doxycycline 100 mg PO bid for 14 days WITH or WITHOUT
- Metronidazole 500 mg PO bid for 14 days OR
- Other parenteral third-generation cephalosporin (e.g., ceftizoxime or cefotaxime) PLUS
- Doxycycline 100 mg PO bid for 14 days WITH or WITHOUT
- Metronidazole 500 mg PO bid for 14 days

CHRONIC Rx

Hospitalized patients receiving IV therapy:

1. Significant clinical improvement is characterized by defervescence, decreased abdominal tenderness, and decreased uterine, adnexal, and cervical motion tenderness within 3 to 5 days.

2. If no clinical improvement occurs, further diagnostic workup is necessary, including possible surgical intervention.

DISPOSITION

- Long-term sequelae of PID: recurrent PID, chronic pelvic pain, ectopic pregnancy, infertility, Fitz-Hugh-Curtis syndrome (Fig. 1-635)
- Risk of tubal infertility related to episodes of PID: first episode, 8%; second episode, 20%; third episode, 40%
- Essential to evaluate and treat male sex partners

REFERRAL

If there is no clinical improvement with outpatient therapy observed within 72 hr, patient should be hospitalized and gynecology consult requested.

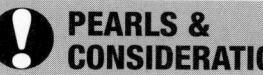

PEARLS & CONSIDERATIONS

COMMENTS

- Maintain a low threshold for the diagnosis of PID.
- Women with documented chlamydial or gonococcal infections have a high rate of re-infection within 6 mo of treatment. Repeat testing of all women who have been diagnosed with chlamydia or gonorrhea is recommended 3 to 6 mo after treatment, regardless of whether their sex partners were treated.
- All women diagnosed with acute PID should be offered HIV testing.
- Male sex partners of women with PID should be examined and treated if they had sexual contact with the patient during 60 days preceding the patient's onset of symptoms. If a patient's last sexual intercourse was >60 days before onset of symptoms or diagnosis, the patient's most recent sex partner should be treated.
- Patients should be instructed to abstain from sexual intercourse until therapy is completed and until they and their sex partners no longer have symptoms.

SUGGESTED READINGS

available at www.expertconsult.com

RELATED CONTENT

Abscess, Pelvic (Related Key Topic)
Chlamydia Genital Infections (Related Key Topic)
Gonorrhea (Related Key Topic)
Pelvic Inflammatory Disease (Patient Information)

AUTHOR: **RUBEN ALVERO, M.D.**

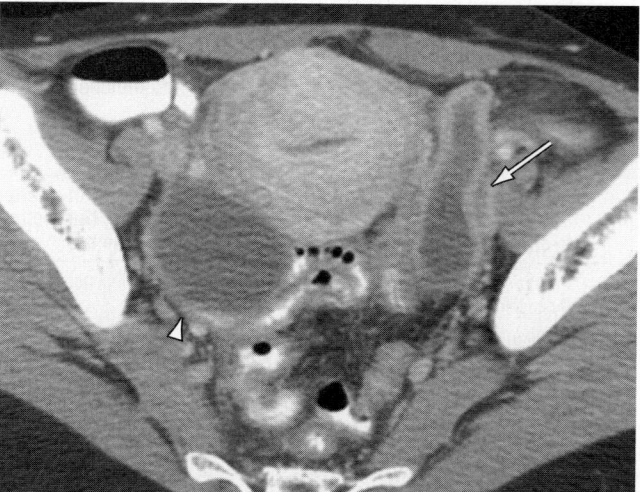

FIGURE 1-634 Pelvic inflammatory disease with pyosalpinx in a 26-yr-old patient. Computed tomographic image through pelvis shows cystic tubular structure with thick enhancing walls *(arrow)* lateral to the uterus, which, in absence of oral contrast, could be mistaken for a loop of small bowel. (From Fielding JR et al: *Gynecologic imaging,* Philadelphia, 2011, Saunders.)

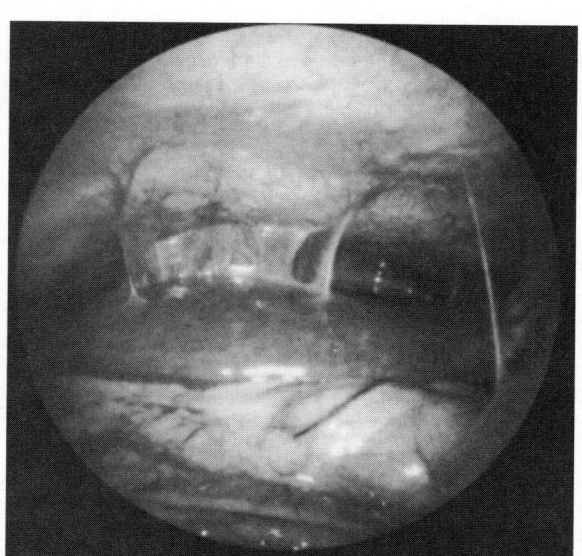

FIGURE 1-635 "Violin string" adhesions are visualized in this patient with Fitz-Hugh-Curtis syndrome. (From Copeland LJ: *Textbook of gynecology,* ed 2, Philadelphia, 2000, Saunders.)

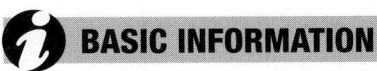

BASIC INFORMATION

DEFINITION

Pelvic organ prolapse (POP) or *uterine prolapse* refers to the protrusion of the uterus into or out of the vaginal canal. In a first-degree uterine prolapse, the cervix is visible when the perineum is depressed. In a second-degree uterine prolapse, the uterine cervix has prolapsed through the vaginal introitus, with the fundus remaining within the pelvis proper. In a third-degree uterine prolapse (i.e., complete uterine prolapse, uterine procidentia), the entire uterus is outside the introitus. Table 1-323 compares the various types of prolapse.

SYNONYMS

Genital prolapse
Uterine descensus
Uterine prolapse
POP

ICD-9CM CODES
618.8 Genital prolapse
618.1 Uterine descensus
618.8 Pelvic organ prolapse

EPIDEMIOLOGY & DEMOGRAPHICS

PREVALENCE: Most prevalent in postmenopausal multiparous women.
RISK FACTORS:
- Pregnancy, especially POP symptoms during pregnancy
- Labor
- Vaginal childbirth
- Obesity
- Chronic coughing
- Constipation
- Pelvic tumors
- Ascites
- Strenuous physical exertion, especially during pregnancy
- Maternal history of prolapse
- Caucasian race

GENETICS: Increased incidence in women with spina bifida occulta.

PHYSICAL FINDINGS & CLINICAL PRESENTATION

- Pelvic pressure
- Bearing-down sensation
- Bilateral groin pain
- Sacral backache
- Coital difficulty
- Protrusion from vagina
- Spotting
- Ulceration
- Bleeding
- Examination of patient in lithotomy, sitting, and standing positions and before, during, and after a maximum Valsalva effort
- Erosion or ulceration of the cervix possible in the most dependent area of the protrusion

ETIOLOGY

- Vaginal childbirth and chronic increases in intraabdominal pressure leading to detachments, lacerations, and denervations of the vaginal support system
- Further weakening of pelvic support system by hypoestrogenic atrophy
- Direct injury to the levator ani, neurologic injury from stretching of the pudendal nerves
- Some cases from congenital or inherited weaknesses within the pelvic support system
- Neonatal uterine prolapse mostly coexistent with congenital spinal defects

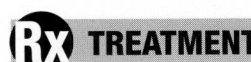

DIAGNOSIS

DIFFERENTIAL DIAGNOSIS

- Occasionally, elongated cervix; body of the uterus remains undescended.
- Diagnosis is based on history and physical examination. Currently there is only one genital tract prolapse classification system that has attained international acceptance and recognition: the patient pelvic organ prolapse quantification (POP-Q) (Boxes 1-43 and 1-44).

WORKUP

- If erosion or ulceration of the cervix is present, a Pap smear followed by a cervical biopsy should be performed if indicated.
- If urinary symptoms are significant, further urodynamic workup is indicated, looking for concurrent cystourethrocele, cystocele, enterocele, or rectocele.

LABORATORY TESTS

Urine culture

IMAGING STUDIES

Ultrasound if concurrent fibroids need further evaluation, CT or MRI (Fig. 1-636) in symptomatic patients with unclear diagnosis

TREATMENT

NONPHARMACOLOGIC THERAPY

- Prophylactic measures
  1. Diagnosis and treatment of chronic respiratory and metabolic disorders

TABLE 1-323   Types of Genital Prolapse

Original Position of Organs	Prolapse	Symptoms (in addition to the general symptoms of discomfort, dragging, the feeling of a "lump" and, rarely, coital problems)
Anterior	Urethrocele Cystocele	Urinary symptoms (stress incontinence, urinary frequency)
Central	Cervix/uterus: 1st, 2nd, and 3rd degree Procidentia	Bleeding and/or discharge from ulceration in association with procidentia
Posterior	Rectocele Enterocele	Bowel symptoms, particularly the feeling of incomplete evacuation and sometimes having to press the posterior wall backwards to pass stool

From Drife J, Magowan B: *Clinical obstetrics and gynaecology*, Philadelphia, 2004, Saunders.

BOX 1-43   Staging of Pelvic Organ Prolapse Based on POP-Q Examination

Stage 0	No prolapse.
Stage I	Most distal prolapse >1 cm above hymenal ring.
Stage II	Most distal point is ≤1 cm above hymenal ring.
Stage III	Most distal point is >1 cm below the hymenal ring but not farther than 2 cm less than the total vaginal length (TVL) (i.e., ≥1 cm but ≤ (TVL − 2) cm.
Stage IV	Complete vaginal eversion.

From Pemberton J (ed): *The pelvic floor*, Philadelphia, 2002, Saunders.

BOX 1-44   Points of Reference for POP-Q

Point A: 3 cm above the hymen on anterior vaginal wall (Aa) or posterior vaginal wall (Ap). Point Aa roughly corresponds with the urethrovesical junction. These points can range from −3 cm (no prolapse) to +3 cm (maximal prolapse).
Point B: The lowest extent of the segment of vagina between point A and the apex of the vagina. Unlike point A, it is not fixed but will be the same as A if point A is the most protruding point. In maximal prolapse it will be the same as point C.
Point C: The most distal part of the cervix or vaginal vault.
Point D: The posterior fornix, which is omitted in women with prior hysterectomy.
Genital hiatus: From midline external urethral meatus to inferior hymenal ring.
Perineal body: From inferior hymenal ring to middle of anal orifice.
Vaginal length: This should be measured without undue stretching of the vagina.

From Pemberton J (ed): *The pelvic floor*, Philadelphia, 2002, Saunders.

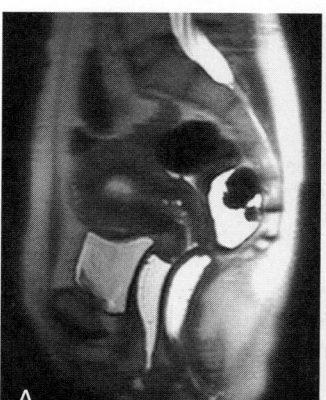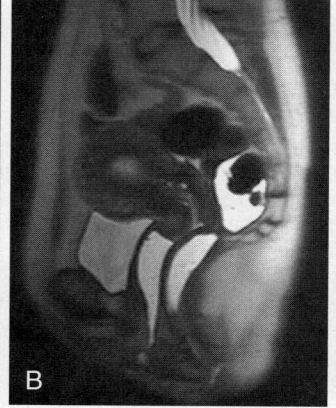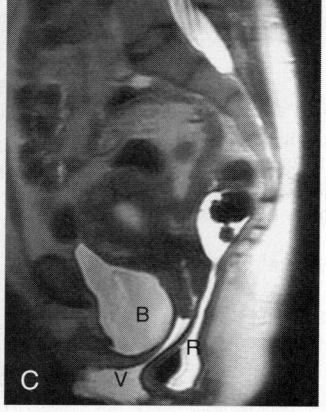

FIGURE 1-636 A, Moderate global pelvic prolapse in a woman with stress urinary incontinence, pelvic heaviness, and constipation after three vaginal deliveries. At rest, all viscera are normally situated in the pelvis. **B,** With Kegel contraction, note that all viscera remain normally situated in the pelvis. **C,** With maximal strain, bladder *(B)*, vagina *(V),* and rectum *(R)* are well below the pelvic floor. (From Fielding JR et al: *Gynecologic imaging,* Philadelphia, 2011, Saunders.)

2. Correction of constipation
3. Weight control, nutrition, and smoking cessation counseling
4. Pelvic muscle exercises
- Supportive pessary therapy
  1. Ring-type pessary useful for first- or second-degree prolapse
  2. Gellhorn pessary preferred for more advanced prolapse
  3. Use of pessaries in conjunction with continuous hormone replacement therapy, unless contraindicated
  4. Perineorrhaphy under local anesthesia possibly needed to support the pessary if the vaginal outlet is very relaxed

ACUTE GENERAL Rx

- Patients who are only infrequently symptomatic: insertion of a tampon or diaphragm for temporary relief when prolonged standing is anticipated
- Neonatal uterine prolapse: simple digital reduction or the use of a small pessary

CHRONIC Rx

- Hormone replacement therapy at the time of menopause helps preserve tissue strength, maintain elasticity of the vagina, and promote the durability of surgical repairs.
- Gold standard for therapy is vaginal hysterectomy.
- Vaginal apex should be well suspended, but a prophylactic sacrospinous ligament fixation is not routinely required.

- If occult enterocele present, McCall culdoplasty is performed.
- If vaginal approach to hysterectomy is contraindicated, abdominal hysterectomy is performed; vaginal apex likewise well supported.
- Colpocleisis is considered for the elderly patient who is sexually inactive and is a high-risk patient from a surgical point of view; can be done rapidly under local anesthesia with mild sedation if necessary.
- For symptomatic women who desire childbearing: management with pessaries or pelvic muscle exercises is recommended; if surgical correction is required, transvaginal sacrospinous fixation is the preferred method.
- Other surgical options are sling operations and sacral cervicopexy.
- Trials have shown that as compared with anterior colporrhaphy, use of a standardized, trocar-guided mesh kit for cystocele repair results in higher short-term rates of successful treatment but also in higher rates of surgical complications and postoperative adverse events.
- Women without stress incontinence undergoing vaginal surgery for POP are at risk for postoperative urinary incontinence. Use of a prophylactic midurethral sling inserted during vaginal prolapse surgery has been shown to result in a lower rate of urinary incontinence at 3 and 12 months but a higher rate of adverse events (UTIs, major bleeding complications, incomplete bladder emptying).

DISPOSITION

If untreated, uterine prolapse progressively worsens.

REFERRAL

To a gynecologist/urologist if pessary fitting or surgical intervention is needed

! PEARLS & CONSIDERATIONS

COMMENTS

Surgery contraindicated in mild or asymptomatic uterine prolapse because the patient will seldom benefit from the operation although exposed to its risks.

SUGGESTED READINGS

available at www.expertconsult.com

RELATED CONTENT

Incontinence, Urinary (Related Key Topic)
Fig. E3-185 Management of vaginal prolapse (Algorithm)
Uterine Prolapse (Patient Information)

AUTHORS: **ARUNDATHI G. PRASAD, M.D.,** and **RUBEN ALVERO, M.D.**

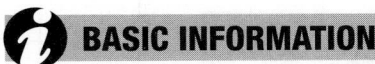

BASIC INFORMATION

DEFINITION

- *Pemphigus* refers to a group of rare, potentially fatal, chronic, autoimmune blistering diseases of the skin and mucous membranes
- Pemphigus has four main subtypes:
  1. Pemphigus vulgaris (PV) (most common) (Fig. 1-637)
     - Pemphigus vegetans, a rare clinical variant of PV
  2. Pemphigus foliaceus (PF)
     - Pemphigus erythematosus, a variant of PF
  3. Paraneoplastic pemphigus
  4. Immunoglobulin (Ig) A pemphigus

SYNONYMS

Pemphigus
Fogo selvagem: endemic pemphigus foliaceus
Senear-Usher syndrome: pemphigus erythematosus

ICD-9CM CODES
694.4 Pemphigus

EPIDEMIOLOGY & DEMOGRAPHICS

- Incidence is approximately one case per 100,000 persons and varies substantially by geographic region.
- More common in Ashkenazi Jews and people of Middle Eastern descent.
- Typically occurs in the fourth and fifth decades of life, although range of ages affected is broad and it may occur in the very young or elderly.
- No gender predilection

PHYSICAL FINDINGS & CLINICAL PRESENTATION

- History:
  1. Multiple oropharyngeal ulcerations and erosions typically occur first, which can then be followed by a more generalized bullous eruption involving the skin within several weeks or months
  2. Blisters are fragile and rupture easily, leaving painful erosions and ulcerations that may be the predominant clinical finding
  3. Pain associated with oral mucosal blistering often results in dysphagia and hoarseness
  4. Not commonly pruritic
- Physical findings:
  1. Anatomic distribution
     a. Oral mucosa
     b. Can also involve the pharynx, larynx, vagina, penis, anus, and conjunctival mucosa
     c. Generalized cutaneous involvement (Figs. 1-638 and 1-639)
  2. Lesion configuration
     a. Any stratified squamous epithelial surfaces can become involved
  3. Lesion morphology
     a. Flaccid bullae and vesicles
     b. Erosion with crusting commonly occurs

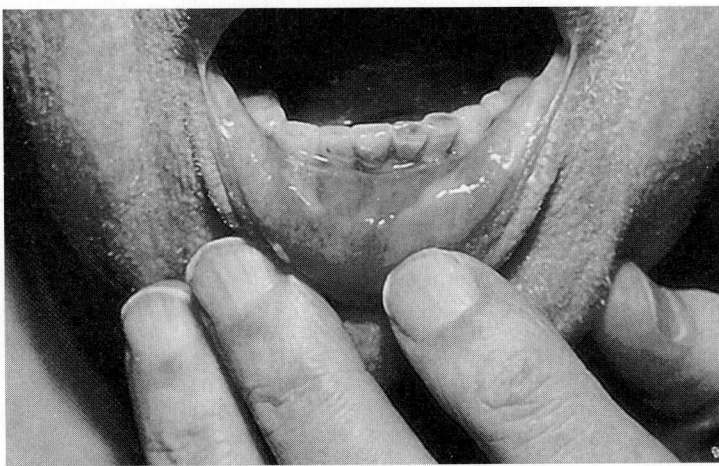

FIGURE 1-637 Pemphigus vulgaris with oral lesions and no intact bullae. (Courtesy Department of Dermatology, University of North Carolina at Chapel Hill. From Goldstein BG, Goldstein AO: *Practical dermatology,* ed 2, St Louis, 1997, Mosby.)

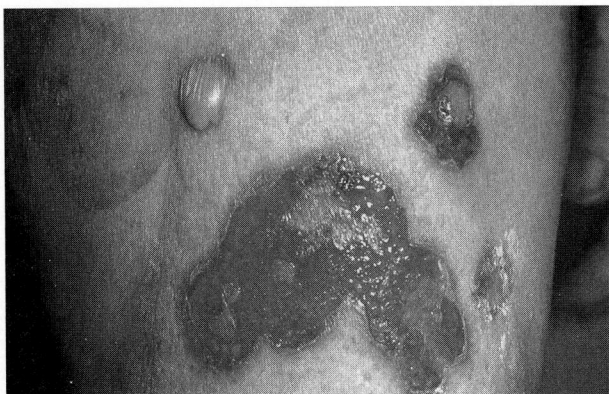

FIGURE 1-638 Pemphigus vulgaris; extensive erosions and blisters are present on the shin. (Courtesy R. A. Marsden, M.D., St. George's Hospital, London. From McKee PH et al [eds]: *Pathology of the skin with clinical correlations,* ed 3, St Louis, 2005, Mosby.)

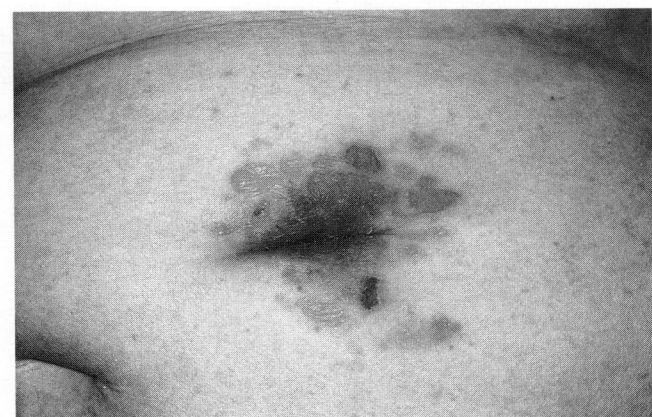

FIGURE 1-639 Pemphigus vulgaris: umbilical lesions showing intact blisters as well as raw erosions. (Courtesy R. A. Marsden, M.D., St. George's Hospital, London. From McKee PH et al [eds]: *Pathology of the skin with clinical correlations,* ed 3, St Louis, 2005, Mosby.)

4. Positive Nikolsky sign: when the clinician applies lateral pressure to normal-appearing skin at the periphery of active lesions, separation of the superficial epidermis occurs

ETIOLOGY

Autoimmune disease caused by autoantibodies against the cell surface of keratinocytes. The predominant antibody in PV is directed against desmoglein 3; in PF it is directed against desmoglein 1.

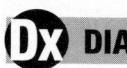 **DIAGNOSIS**

The diagnosis of pemphigus vulgaris should be suspected in patients with painful oral erosions and flaccid bullae or erosions on the skin.

DIFFERENTIAL DIAGNOSIS

- Bullous pemphigoid (Table 1-324)
- Cicatricial pemphigoid
- Behçet's syndrome
- Erythema multiforme
- Hailey-Hailey disease
- Aphthous stomatitis
- Bullous lupus erythematosus
- Drug eruptions
- Dermatitis herpetiformis
- Epidermolysis bullosa acquisita
- IgA pemphigus
- Paraneoplastic pemphigus
- Pemphigus foliaceus

WORKUP

Skin biopsy is diagnostic; specimens should be sent for routine histochemical staining and direct immunofluorescence. Certain laboratory values may also be useful in establishing the diagnosis of pemphigus.

LABORATORY TESTS

- Skin biopsy reveals intraepidermal vesicles, also called *acantholysis* (loss of cell adhesion between the epidermal cells).

- Indirect immunofluorescence may detect circulating autoantibodies.
- Direct immunofluorescence studies of perilesional skin demonstrate IgG directed against keratinocyte surfaces in the epidermis.

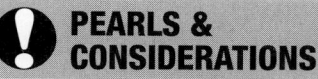 **TREATMENT**

NONPHARMACOLOGIC THERAPY

- Mild soaps and emollients to skin
- Burow's solution may be useful for weeping erosions.
- Soft diet and viscous lidocaine can be used in patients with oral lesions.

ACUTE GENERAL Rx

- For localized disease, topical steroids may be effective.
- For generalized disease, systemic corticosteroids (prednisone) are the mainstay of therapy and often work rapidly to halt blistering.
  - Initial dose of prednisone is usually 1 mg/kg/day, then tapered over weeks as blistering decreases.
  - Steroid-sparing immunosuppressive therapies are often initiated simultaneously with prednisone to minimize the side effects of prolonged corticosteroid therapy.

CHRONIC Rx

- Adjuvant therapy such as immunosuppressants, anti-inflammatories, chemotherapeutic agents, and biologics are useful for disease control and to shorten the length of treatment with oral steroids; treatment duration and dosing are determined by clinical response:
  1. Azathioprine 50 to 100 mg/day
  2. Cyclophosphamide 1 to 3 mg/kg/day
  3. Mycophenolate mofetil 500 mg to 2 g daily
- Refractory disease:
  1. IV Ig
  2. Rituximab (anti-CD20 monoclonal antibody)
  3. Plasmapheresis

DISPOSITION

- Before the use of oral corticosteroids, pemphigus was usually a fatal disease with most patients dying within 5 yr of diagnosis.
- Combined corticosteroids and adjuvant therapy have decreased mortality rates to <10%.
- Death generally occurs from sepsis or complications related to medical therapy.

REFERRAL

Dermatology
Otolaryngology

⚠ PEARLS & CONSIDERATIONS

COMMENTS

- PV, unlike bullous pemphigoid, is a disease of middle-aged persons.
- Early diagnosis of pemphigus is important to initiate prompt treatment.
- Oral corticosteroids have many substantial side effects, and patients should be monitored for osteoporosis, hypertension, and diabetes.

SUGGESTED READINGS

available at www.expertconsult.com

RELATED CONTENT

Pemphigus Vulgaris (Patient Information)

AUTHORS: **JESSICA RISSER, M.D., M.P.H.,** and **KACHIU LEE, B.A.**

P

Diseases and Disorders

I

TABLE 1-324 Differentiation of Pemphigus Vulgaris and Bullous Pemphigoid

Characteristics	Pemphigus Vulgaris	Bullous Pemphigoid
Age	Usually occurs in middle-aged persons	>60 yr
Site	Oral mucosa, face, chest, groin	Flexural areas, groin, axilla; less often involving mucosal surfaces
Findings	Flaccid bullae and erosions, intraepidermal blisters, IgG autoantibodies against keratinocyte surfaces	Intact bullae, subepidermal blisters, IgG autoantibodies against hemidesmosomal antigens
Treatment	Prednisone 1 mg/kg/day with adjuvant immunosuppressant agents; refractory disease may require intravenous immunoglobulin, plasmapheresis, or rituximab	Prednisone 1 mg/kg/day with adjuvant immunosuppressant therapy; localized disease may be controlled with topical steroids
Prognosis	>90% respond; steroid side effects significant	>90% respond; remissions and recurrences common

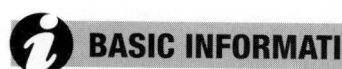

BASIC INFORMATION

DEFINITION

Peptic ulcer disease (PUD) is an ulceration in the stomach or duodenum resulting from an imbalance between mucosal protective factors and various mucosal damaging mechanisms (see "Etiology").

SYNONYMS

PUD
Duodenal ulcer (DU)
Gastric ulcer (GU)

ICD-9CM CODES

536.8 Peptic ulcer disease
531.3 Peptic ulcer, stomach, acute
531.7 Peptic ulcer, stomach, chronic
532.3 Peptic ulcer, duodenum, acute
532.7 Peptic ulcer, duodenum, chronic

EPIDEMIOLOGY & DEMOGRAPHICS

- Incidence: 250,000 to 500,000 (200,000 to 400,000 duodenal; 50,000 to 100,000 gastric) annually; duodenal ulcer/gastric ulcer ratio is 4:1.
- Anatomic location: >90% of duodenal ulcers occur in the first portion of the duodenum; gastric ulcers occur most frequently in the lesser curvature near the incisura angularis.

PHYSICAL FINDINGS & CLINICAL PRESENTATION

- Physical examination is often unremarkable.
- Patient may have epigastric tenderness, tachycardia, pallor, hypotension (from acute or chronic blood loss), nausea and vomiting (if pyloric channel is obstructed), boardlike abdomen and rebound tenderness (if perforated), and hematemesis or melena (with a bleeding ulcer). Box 1-45 describes key symptoms and signs of peptic ulcer.

ETIOLOGY

Often multifactorial. The following are common mucosal damaging factors:

- *Helicobacter pylori* infection. *H. pylori* is the major cause of PUD. It is found in more than 70% of patients with duodenal ulcers and gastric ulcers in the U.S. Rates are much higher (>90%) in other parts of the world. Eradication of *H. pylori* markedly reduces peptic ulcer recurrence.
- Medications (NSAIDs, glucocorticoids). Risk factors for development of NSAID-related ulcers are described in Table 1-325.

TABLE 1-325   Risk Factors for Development of NSAID-Related Ulcers

Definite

Advanced age
History of ulcer
Concomitant corticosteroid therapy
Concomitant anticoagulation therapy
High doses of NSAIDs
Serious systemic disorders

Possible

Concomitant infection with *Helicobacter pylori*
Cigarette smoking
Consumption of alcohol

NSAIDs, Nonsteroidal anti-inflammatory drugs.
From Andreoli TE et al: *Andreoli and Carpenter's Cecil essentials of medicine,* ed 8, Philadelphia, 2010, Saunders.

- Incompetent pylorus or lower esophageal sphincter
- Bile acids
- Impaired proximal duodenal bicarbonate secretion
- Decreased blood flow to gastric mucosa
- Acid secreted by parietal cells and pepsin secreted as pepsinogen by chief cells
- Cigarette smoking
- Alcohol

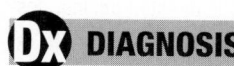

DIAGNOSIS

DIFFERENTIAL DIAGNOSIS

- Gastroesophageal reflux disease
- Cholelithiasis syndrome
- Pancreatitis
- Gastritis
- Nonulcer dyspepsia
- Neoplasm (gastric carcinoma, lymphoma, pancreatic carcinoma)
- Angina pectoris, myocardial infarction, pericarditis
- Dissecting aneurysm
- Other: high small-bowel obstruction, pneumonia, subphrenic abscess, early appendicitis

WORKUP

Comprehensive history and physical exam to exclude other diagnoses. Diagnostic modalities include endoscopy or upper GI series. Endoscopy is preferred.

LABORATORY TESTS

- Routine laboratory evaluation is usually unremarkable.
- Anemia may be present in patients with significant GI bleeding.
- *H. pylori* testing by endoscopic biopsy, urea breath test, stool antigen test (*H. pylori* stool antigen), or specific antibody test is recommended:
  1. Serologic testing for antibodies to *H. pylori* is easy and inexpensive; however, the presence of antibodies demonstrates previous but not necessarily current infection. Antibodies to *H. pylori* can remain elevated for months to years after infection has cleared; therefore antibody levels must be interpreted in light of the patient's symptoms and other test results (e.g., PUD seen on upper GI series).
  2. The urea breath test documents active infection (sensitivity and specificity >90%). The patient ingests a small amount of urea labeled with carbon 13 or carbon 14. If urease is present (produced by the organism), the urea is hydrolyzed and the patient exhales labeled carbon dioxide that is then collected and measured. This test is more expensive and not as readily available. Use of proton pump inhibitors (PPI) within 2 wk of the urea breath test may interfere with test results. Recently a new card test for ¹⁴C urea has been developed, providing a testing option in primary care settings. It uses a flat

---

BOX 1-45   Key Symptoms and Signs of Peptic Ulcer

Uncomplicated Ulcer
No symptoms ("silent ulcer" in up to 40% of cases)
Epigastric pain
Pain may radiate to the back, thorax, other parts of abdomen (cephalad most likely, caudad least likely)
Pain may be nocturnal (most specific), "painful hunger" relieved by food, or continuous (least specific)
Nausea
Vomiting
Heartburn (mimics or associated with gastroesophageal reflex)

Complicated Ulcer
Acute perforation
Severe abdominal pain
Shock
Abdominal boardlike rigidity (and rebound and other signs of peritoneal irritation)
Free intraperitoneal air
Hemorrhage
Hematemesis and/or melena
Hemodynamic changes, anemia
Previous history of ulcer symptoms (80%)
Gastric outlet obstruction
Satiation, inability to ingest food, eructation
Nausea, vomiting (and related disturbances)
Weight loss

From Goldman L, Schafer AI: *Goldman's Cecil medicine,* ed 24, Philadelphia, 2012, Saunders.

breath card that is read by a small analyzer.

3. Histologic evaluation of endoscopic biopsy samples is considered by many the gold standard for accurate diagnosis of *H. pylori* infection. However, detection of *H. pylori* depends on the site and number of biopsy samples, the method of staining, and experience of the pathologist.

4. Stool antigen test is an ELISA that identifies *H. pylori* antigen in a stool specimen through a polyclonal anti–*H. pylori* antibody. It is as accurate as the urea breath test for diagnosis of active infection and follow-up evaluation of patients treated for *H. pylori*. A negative result on the stool antigen test 6 wk after completion of therapy identifies patients in whom eradication of *H. pylori* was successful.

- Additional laboratory evaluation is indicated only in specific cases (e.g., amylase level in suspected pancreatitis, serum gastrin level in suspected Zollinger-Ellison [ZE] syndrome).

IMAGING STUDIES

Conventional upper GI barium studies identify approximately 70% to 80% of PUD; accuracy can be increased to approximately 90% by using double contrast.

Rx TREATMENT

NONPHARMACOLOGIC THERAPY

- Stop smoking; smoking increases the risk of PUD, decreases the healing rate, and increases the frequency of recurrence.
- Avoid NSAIDs and alcohol.
- Special diets have been proved unrelated to ulcer development and healing; however, avoid foods that cause symptoms.

ACUTE GENERAL Rx

Eradication of *H. pylori,* when present, can be accomplished with various regimens:

1. PPI (e.g., omeprazole 20 mg bid or lansoprazole 30 mg bid, esomeprazole 40 mg qd) *plus* clarithromycin 500 mg bid *and* amoxicillin 1000 mg bid for 10 days. This regimen achieves an eradication rate of 80% to 90% and can be used as first-line therapy for patients not allergic to penicillin.

2. PPI bid *plus* amoxicillin 500 mg bid *plus* metronidazole 500 mg bid for 10 days.

3. PPI bid *plus* clarithromycin 500 mg bid *and* metronidazole 500 mg bid for 10 days. This regimen is useful in those with penicillin allergy.

4. A 1-day quadruple therapy may be as effective as a 7-day triple-therapy regimen. The 1-day quadruple-therapy regimen consists of 2 tablets of 262-mg bismuth subsalicylate qid, 1 500-mg metronidazole tablet qid, 2 g of amoxicillin suspension qid, and 2 capsules of 30 mg of lansoprazole.

5. Bismuth compound qid *plus* tetracycline 500 mg qid *and* metronidazole 500 mg qid for 14 days.

6. A combination of levofloxacin 250 mg bid, amoxicillin 1000 mg bid, and a PPI bid for 10 to 14 days can be used as salvage therapy after unsuccessful attempts to eradicate *H. pylori* using other regimens.

A 10-day sequential therapy has been reported to be superior to standard triple therapy for eradication of *H. pylori*. It consists of 5 days of treatment with a PPI and one antibiotic (usually amoxicillin) followed by 5-day treatment with the PPI and two other antibiotics (usually clarithromycin and metronidazole).

PUD patients testing negative for *H. pylori* should be treated with antisecretory agents:

- H_2 receptor antagonists (H_2RAs): cimetidine, ranitidine, famotidine, and nizatidine are all effective; they are usually given in split dose or at nighttime.
- PPIs: can also induce rapid healing; they are usually given 30 min before meals.

Antacids and sucralfate are also effective agents for the treatment and prevention of PUD.

CHRONIC Rx

Maintenance therapy in duodenal ulcer patients is indicated in the following situations:

- Persistent smokers
- Recurrent ulcerations
- Long-term treatment with NSAIDs, glucocorticoids
- Elderly or debilitated patients
- Aggressive or complicated ulcer disease (e.g., perforation, hemorrhage)
- Asymptomatic bleeders

Misoprostol therapy (100 µg qid with food, increased to 200 µg qid if well tolerated) is useful for the prevention of NSAID-induced gastric ulcers in all patients on long-term NSAID therapy; it is contraindicated in women of childbearing age because of its abortifacient properties. PPIs are at least as effective as misoprostol and more effective than H_2 receptor antagonists at healing ulcers and maintaining remission in patients on long-term NSAIDs.

DISPOSITION

- The recurrence rate for untreated PUD is ~60% (>70% in smokers). Treatment decreases the recurrence rate by nearly 30%.
- Patients with recurrent ulcers should be re-treated for an additional 8 wk and then placed on maintenance therapy with H_2RAs, PPIs, sucralfate, or antacids.
- An ulcer is considered refractory to treatment if healing is not evident after 8 wk for duodenal ulcers and 12 wk for gastric ulcers. In these patients maximum acid inhibition (e.g., esomeprazole 40 mg bid) is preferred over continued therapy with standard antiulcer therapy.
- Eradication of *H. pylori* (when present) is indicated in all patients. A negative stool anti-

gen test for *H. pylori* 6 wk after treatment accurately confirms cure of *H. pylori* infection with reasonable sensitivity in initially seropositive healthy subjects.

- Screening for ZE syndrome should also be considered in patients with multiple recurrent ulcers; in patients with ZE, the serum gastrin level is >1000 pg/ml and the basal acid output is usually >15 mEq/hr.
- Surgery for refractory ulcers is now only rarely performed; it consists of highly selective vagotomy for duodenal ulcers or ulcer removal with antrectomy or hemigastrectomy without vagotomy for gastric ulcers.

REFERRAL

- GI referral for patients requiring endoscopy
- Surgical referral for patients with nonhealing ulcers despite appropriate medical therapy

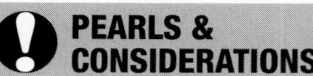

PEARLS & CONSIDERATIONS

COMMENTS

- Patients with gastric ulcers should have repeat endoscopy after 4 to 6 wk of therapy to document healing and test exfoliative cytology for gastric carcinoma.
- After endoscopic treatment of bleeding peptic ulcers, bleeding recurs in up to 20% of patients. PPI administration intravenously by continuous infusion substantially reduces the risk of recurrent bleeding. High-dose IV esomeprazole (80 mg IV bolus followed by 8 mg/hr infusion over 72 hr) given after successful endoscopic therapy to patients with high-risk peptic ulcer bleeding has been reported to reduce recurrent bleeding at 72 hr and to maintain sustained clinical benefits for up to 30 days.
- Among low-dose aspirin recipients who had peptic ulcer bleeding, continuous aspirin therapy may increase the risk for recurrent bleeding; however, mortality was reported higher among those who stopped aspirin therapy and were at risk for cardiovascular events

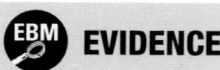

EVIDENCE

available at www.expertconsult.com

SUGGESTED READINGS
available at www.expertconsult.com

RELATED CONTENT
Peptic Ulcer (Patient Information)

AUTHOR: **FRED F. FERRI, M.D.**

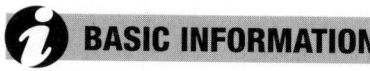

BASIC INFORMATION

DEFINITION

Pericarditis is the inflammation (or infiltration) of the pericardium.

ICD-9CM CODES
420.91 Pericarditis

EPIDEMIOLOGY & DEMOGRAPHICS

- The exact incidence of acute pericarditis is not known. However, it is approximately 0.1% of hospitalized patients, and 5% of patients seen in the emergency room for non-acute myocardial infarction chest pain.
- Increased incidence found in males and in adults compared with children.
- The use of thrombolytic agents and early revascularization has greatly reduced the incidence of both early postinfarction pericarditis and Dressler's syndrome.

PHYSICAL FINDINGS & CLINICAL PRESENTATION

- Severe, constant pain that localizes over the anterior chest and may radiate to the arms and back. As opposed to ischemic pain, the pain is pleuritic and is improved by sitting up and leaning forward.
- A pericardial friction rub is a classic finding, although not present in all patients. When present, it is virtually pathognomonic of acute pericarditis. It is best heard with the patient sitting up and leaning forward and by pressing the diaphragm of the stethoscope firmly against the chest at the lower left sternal border during inspiration. It consists of three short, scratchy sounds, corresponding to a systolic, diastolic, and late diastolic component. In many patients, the rub is not clearly triphasic.
- The physical exam is important in assessing the presence of cardiac tamponade which may occur as a complication of large or rapidly accumulating effusions. Classic tamponade findings include hypotension, jugular venous distention, and muffled heart sounds (Beck's triad). In addition, tachycardia and pulsus paradoxus are usually present.

ETIOLOGY

- Most common causes (most likely 80%-90%) of pericarditis are idiopathic or viral
- Other infectious agents (bacterial [1%-2%], tuberculous [4%], fungal, amebic, toxoplasmosis)
- Collagen-vascular disease (systemic lupus erythematosus, rheumatoid arthritis, scleroderma, vasculitis, dermatomyositis): 3% to 5% of cases
- Neoplasm (primary or metastatic [breast, lung, leukemia, lymphoma]): 7% of cases
- Drug-induced: procainamide, hydralazine, phenytoin, isoniazid, rifampin, doxorubicin, mesalamine
- Acute myocardial infarction and post-MI (Dressler's syndrome, usually 2 weeks post MI)
- Trauma or posttraumatic
- After pericardiotomy
- After mediastinal radiation (e.g., patients with Hodgkin's disease)
- Uremia
- Leakage of aortic aneurysm into pericardial sac

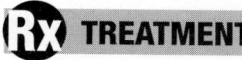

DIAGNOSIS

DIFFERENTIAL DIAGNOSIS

- Angina pectoris
- Pulmonary infarction
- Dissecting aneurysm
- Gastrointestinal abnormalities (e.g., hiatal hernia, esophageal rupture)
- Pneumothorax
- Hepatitis
- Cholecystitis
- Pneumonia with pleurisy

WORKUP

Diagnosis is clinical, based on history and physical examination. ECG may help confirm the diagnosis if typical changes are found. Laboratory tests may help on elucidating the potential cause, and an echocardiogram can assist in ruling out significant pericardial effusion.

LABORATORY TESTS

Laboratory tests will not confirm the diagnosis, but can help determine a specific etiology. Initial blood work should be limited to the following tests:

- Complete blood count with differential
- Erythrocyte sedimentation rate (not specific but may be of value in following the course of the disease and the response to therapy)
- Blood urea nitrogen, creatinine
- Troponin I (plasma troponins are elevated in 35% to 50% of patients with pericarditis, and indicate involvement of the myocardium, i.e., myopericarditis)

The following tests may be useful when specific etiologies of pericarditis are suspected:

- HIV, PPD
- Antinuclear antibody, rheumatoid factor
- Pericardiocentesis is indicated in patients with tamponade physiology, in those with purulent pericarditis, when a neoplastic origin is suspected, and in patients with a significant idiopathic pericardial effusion that has not resolved by 3 mo. The fluid should be analyzed for red and white blood cell counts, cytology, glucose, lactate dehydrogenase, protein, pH, triglyceride level, and cultured. Polymerase chain reaction assays or elevated levels of adenosine deaminase activity (>30 U/L) are useful when suspecting tuberculous pericarditis.
- Pericardial biopsy may be helpful in recurrent pericardial effusion if the diagnosis remains elusive. It should also be considered whenever malignancy or tuberculosis is suspected.

IMAGING STUDIES

- Echocardiogram to detect and determine amount of pericardial effusion; absence of effusion does not rule out the diagnosis of pericarditis. Variation in atrioventricular valve inflow with respiration is present in cardiac tamponade and constrictive pericarditis.
- ECG: the changes vary with the evolutionary stage of pericarditis:
  1. Acute phase: PR-segment depression and diffuse ST-segment elevations (particularly evident in the precordial leads), which can be distinguished from acute MI by the lack of reciprocal changes and the absence of Q waves
  2. Intermediate phase: return of PR and ST segments to baseline, and T-wave inversion in leads previously showing ST-segment elevation (Fig. 1-640)
  3. Late phase: resolution of the T-wave changes
- Chest x-ray: done primarily to rule out abnormalities of the mediastinum or lung fields that may cause chest pain
  1. Cardiac silhouette appears enlarged in patients with pericardial effusion if more than 250 ml of fluid has accumulated.
  2. Calcifications around the heart may be seen with constrictive pericarditis.
- MRI (Fig. E1-641) may be useful in patients with constrictive pericarditis and when malignancy is suspected.

TREATMENT

NONPHARMACOLOGIC THERAPY

- Limitation of activity until the pain abates
- Patient education regarding potential complications (e.g., cardiac tamponade, constrictive pericarditis)

ACUTE GENERAL Rx

- Aspirin 650 mg q4-6h. NSAIDs can be used in place of aspirin. NSAID therapy (e.g., ibuprofen 800 mg tid, naproxen 500 mg bid). NSAIDs are contraindicated in patients with recent MI and CHF.
- Colchicine 0.6 mg bid may be used in combination or as an alternative to NSAIDs. There is evidence of colchicine being effective in both reducing symptoms and the rates of recurrent pericarditis. Its use is recommended for first episodes and recurrent disease.
- Use of corticosteroids is controversial. There is evidence of their use being associated with increased recurrence, side effects, and hospitalizations. The 2004 European Society of Cardiology guidelines recommend that systemic steroid therapy be restricted to patients with acute pericarditis caused by connective tissue disease, autoimmune-mediated pericarditis, and uremic pericarditis. One study found that using a lower dose (0.2 to 0.5 mg/kg per day) maintained for 4 weeks and followed by a slow taper had same efficacy and fewer adverse effects.
- Close observation of patients when there is suspicion for cardiac tamponade.
- Avoidance of anticoagulants (increased risk of hemopericardium).

TREATMENT OF UNDERLYING CAUSE:
- Bacterial pericarditis: systemic antibiotics and surgical drainage of pericardium
- Collagen vascular disease: prednisone
- Uremic: dialysis

POTENTIAL COMPLICATIONS FROM PERICARDITIS:
1. **Chronic constrictive pericarditis:**
   a. Physical examination reveals jugular venous distention, Kussmaul's sign (increase in jugular venous distention during inspiration as a result of increased venous pressure), pericardial knock (early diastolic filling sound heard 0.06 to 0.1 sec after S_2), clear lungs, tender hepatomegaly, pedal edema, ascites, scrotal edema, and possible anasarca.
   b. Chest radiograph: clear lung fields, normal or slightly enlarged heart, pericardial calcification.
   c. ECG: low-voltage QRS complex.
   d. Echocardiography: may show respiratory inflow variation over the mitral and tricuspid valves (due to variations in the diastolic ventricular pressure gradients with respiration), pericardial thickening or may be normal.
   e. Cardiac catheterization to confirm elevation of right-sided filling pressures: shows a prominent y descent in the right atrial tracing, a "dip and plateau" tracing of the right ventricular pressure and discordance of right ventricular and left ventricular systolic pressures during respiration.
   f. Therapy: surgical stripping or removal of both layers of the constricting pericardium.
2. **Cardiac tamponade:** occurs in 15% of patients with idiopathic pericarditis but in nearly 60% of those with neoplastic, tuberculous, or purulent pericarditis.
   a. Signs and symptoms: dyspnea, orthopnea, interscapular pain.
   b. Physical examination: distended neck veins, distant heart sounds, decreased apical impulse, diaphoresis, tachypnea, tachycardia, Ewart's sign (an area of dullness at the angle of the left scapula caused by compression of the lungs by the pericardial effusion), pulsus paradoxus (decrease in systolic blood pressure >10 mm Hg during inspiration), hypotension, narrowed pulse pressure. Of all the clinical signs, a pulsus paradoxus >10 mm Hg in patients with pericardial effusion is the most specific for tamponade.
   c. Chest x-ray: cardiomegaly ("water-bottle" configuration of the cardiac silhouette may be seen) with clear lungs; the chest x-ray film may be normal when acute tamponade occurs rapidly in the absence of prior pericardial effusion.
   d. ECG reveals decreased amplitude of the QRS complex, variation of the R-wave amplitude from beat to beat (electrical alternans). This results from the heart's oscillating motion in the pericardial sac from beat to beat and frequently occurs with neoplastic effusions.
   e. Echocardiography: may show diastolic collapse of the right ventricle and/or the right atrium, respiratory inflow variation over the mitral valve and tricuspid valve (due to transmission of respiratory changes in intrathoracic pressure to the ventricles), and a paradoxical wall motion may also be seen.
   f. Cardiac catheterization: equalization of pressures within chambers of the heart, elevation of right atrial pressure with a prominent x but no significant y descent.
   g. MRI can also be used to diagnose pericardial effusions.
   h. Therapy for pericardial tamponade consists of immediate pericardiocentesis, preferably by needle paracentesis with the use of echocardiography, fluoroscopy, or CT; in patients with recurrent effusions (e.g., neoplasms), placement of a percutaneous drainage catheter or pericardial window draining in the pleural cavity may be necessary.
3. **Effusive-constrictive pericarditis:**
   a. Uncommon pericardial syndrome characterized by concomitant tamponade caused by tense pericardial effusion and constriction caused by the visceral pericardium.
   b. Extensive epicardiectomy is the procedure of choice in symptomatic patients.
4. **Myopericarditis:** myocardial injury unrelated to MI. It occurs in 15% of patients with pericarditis. ECG reveals concave downward ST-segment elevation; cardiac enzymes are positive.

DISPOSITION
- Complete resolution of pain and other signs and symptoms during the initial 3 wk of therapy.
- Recurrence in 10% to 15% of patients within the initial 12 mo. The recurrence rate increases up to 50% after a first recurrence. Colchicine (0.6 mg qd) is safe and effective for secondary prevention of recurrent pancreatitis.
- Recurrent pericarditis in 28% of patients.
- Recurrence of large effusion after pericardiocentesis is common in patients with idiopathic chronic pericardial effusion. Pericardiectomy should be considered in these patients.
- Most cases of pericarditis can be treated in the outpatient setting. Indications for hospitalization are fever >38° C, immunosuppressed state, history of trauma, subacute onset, oral anticoagulant therapy, presence of myocarditis (myopericarditis), large pericardial effusion or tamponade, and failure to respond to 1 week of outpatient treatment.
- In patients with pericardial effusion after cardiac surgery, use of NSAIDs is not recommended because they have not been shown to reduce the size of the effusions or prevent late cardiac tamponade.

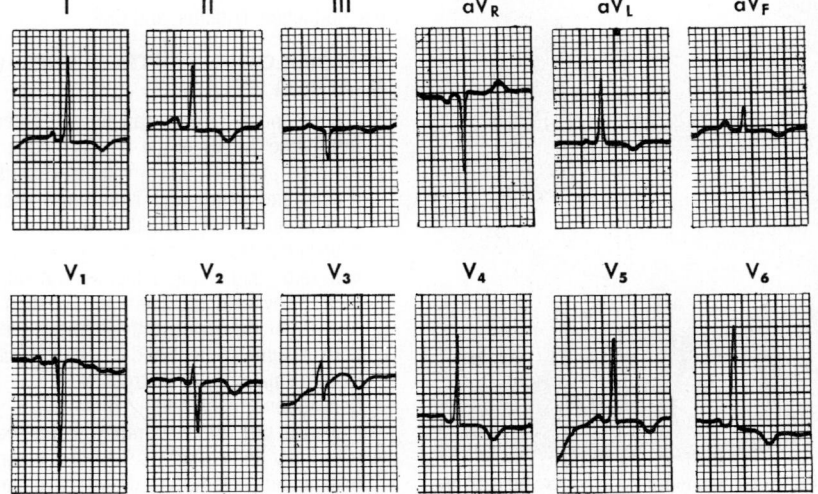

FIGURE 1-640 Pericarditis, evolving pattern. Note the diffuse T-wave inversions in leads I, II, III, aVL, aVF, and V2 to V6. (From Goldberg AL [ed]: *Clinical electrocardiography,* ed 5, St Louis, 1994, Mosby.)

(EBM) **EVIDENCE**

available at www.expertconsult.com

SUGGESTED READINGS

available at www.expertconsult.com

RELATED CONTENT

Pericarditis (Patient Information)

AUTHORS: **ZHE ZHENG, M.D., PH.D., DAVID J. FORTUNATO, M.D., F.A.C.C.,** and **FRED F. FERRI, M.D.**

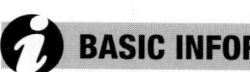 **BASIC INFORMATION**

DEFINITION

Peripheral arterial disease (PAD) refers to atherosclerotic, inflammatory vascular processes, occlusive, and aneurysmal diseases involving the abdominal aorta and its branch arteries. (We will focus on lower extremity PAD.)

SYNONYMS

PAD
Peripheral vascular disease (PVD)
Arteriosclerosis obliterans
Atherosclerotic occlusive disease
Atherosclerosis of the extremities
Peripheral arterial stenosis
Vaso-occlusive disease of the legs
Chronic critical limb ischemia

ICD-9CM CODES
443.9 Peripheral vascular disease

EPIDEMIOLOGY & DEMOGRAPHICS

- ~12% of the adult population has PAD, and the prevalence is equal in men and women. It increases with age, from 0.9% in those aged 40 to 49 yr to 14.5% in those aged 70 to 79 yr, according to the NHANES study.
- Prevalence among smokers age 50-69 is 29% and 16% of patients had PAD and cardiovascular disease.
- Traditional risk factors are similar to coronary artery disease and include tobacco use, diabetes, hyperlipidemia, hypertension, and advanced age.
- African Americans, Hispanics, and those with chronic kidney disease and metabolic syndrome are also at increased risk.
- Patients with newly diagnosed PAD are six times more likely to die within the next 10 yr when compared with patients without PAD.

PHYSICAL FINDINGS & CLINICAL PRESENTATION

- About 20% to 50% of patients are asymptomatic.
- One third of patients present with claudication (aching pain, cramping, or numbness of the calf induced by exercise, relieved by rest).
- However, 40% to 50% of patients present with atypical symptoms of claudication involving the calf, thigh, or buttock, making diagnosis difficult.
- Diminished pedal pulses and/or cool skin temperature of lower extremities.
- Bruits heard over the distal aorta, iliac, or femoral arteries.
- Changes in skin color, especially on feet (rubor with prolonged capillary refill on dependency or delayed pallor).
- Trophic changes of hair loss, brittle nails, and muscle atrophy.
- Nonhealing ulcers (Fig. 1-642), necrotic tissue, and gangrene.

- Weakness, numbness, or a feeling of heaviness in legs.
- Aching or burning in toes and feet during rest and especially while lying flat, which may be a sign of ischemia and more serious PAD.

ETIOLOGY

PAD is primarily the result of atherosclerotic disease and the formation of plaques that consist of a lipid core of cholesterol and inflammatory mediators with a fibrous intravascular covering. Symptoms of claudication are a product of physiologically significant luminal stenoses of the peripheral vessels, limiting blood flow to limb muscles.

Dx **DIAGNOSIS**

DIFFERENTIAL DIAGNOSIS

- Spinal stenosis
- Musculoskeletal disorder
- Lumbar spinal stenosis or nerve root compression (neurogenic or pseudoclaudication)
- Peripheral neuropathy
- Reflex sympathetic dystrophy
- Raynaud's disease
- Compartment syndrome
- Deep venous thrombosis
- Popliteal entrapment syndrome
- Direct vascular injury

WORKUP

- Thorough history, including symptoms regarding walking impairment, claudication, ischemic rest pain, or nonhealing wounds in patients ≥70 yr or those ≥50 yr with a history of smoking and/or diabetes:

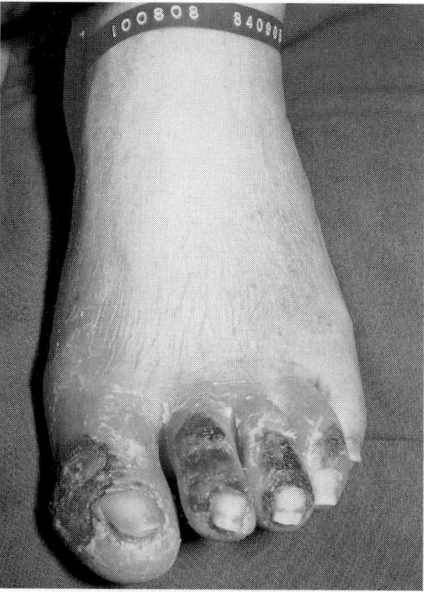

FIGURE 1-642 Ischemic skin ulcer induced by trauma from shoes. This patient with peripheral arterial occlusive disease suffered severe superficial skin necrosis of several toes because of shoes that were too tight. (From Crawford MH et al [eds]: *Cardiology,* ed 2, St Louis, 2004, Mosby.)

- Measurement of blood pressure in both arms and notation of asymmetry.
- Palpation and recording of carotid pulses, upstroke, amplitude, and presence of bruits.
- Auscultation and palpation of abdomen for bruits, aortic pulsation, and diameter.
- Palpation of brachial, radial, ulnar, femoral, popliteal, dorsalis pedis, and posterior tibial pulses. Pulse intensity should be recorded as follows: 0, absent; 1+, diminished; 2+, normal; 3+, bounding.
- Auscultation of femoral arteries for the presence of bruits.
- Feet should be inspected for color, temperature, integrity of the skin.
- Hair loss, trophic skin changes, and hypertrophic nails.
- Measurement of resting ankle-brachial index (ABI) should be performed to establish diagnosis of lower extremity PAD in patients with suspected lower extremity PAD (individuals with one or more of the following exertional leg symptoms: nonhealing wounds, age >65, or age >50 with smoking or diabetes history). ABI should be measured in both legs in all new patients (Fig. 1-643).
- Toe-brachial index should be used in patients suspected of PAD with unreliable ABI due to noncompressible vessels.
- The severity of PAD is based on the ABI at rest and during treadmill exercise (1 to 2 mph, 5 min, or symptom limited).
  - Normal: 1.00 to 1.40 at rest
  - Borderline: 0.91 to 0.99 at rest
  - Mild: ABI at rest 0.71 to 0.90 or ABI during exercise 0.50 to 0.90
  - Moderate: ABI at rest 0.41 to 0.70 or ABI during exercise 0.20 to 0.50
  - Severe: ABI at rest <0.40 or ABI during exercise <0.20

LABORATORY TESTS

Laboratory tests can help identify risk factors and allow for their modification. These include lipid profile, hemoglobin A_{1C}, homocysteine levels, fibrinogen, D-dimer, and CRP.

PHYSIOLOGIC TESTING AND IMAGING STUDIES

- The diagnosis of PAD can be confirmed by measuring the ABI or toe-brachial index.
- Rest or exercise pulse volume recordings (PVRs) and segmental limb pressures are also useful. PVRs measure volume of limb flow per pulse in different segments of the limb (e.g., thigh, calf, ankle, metatarsal, and toes). They help to assess the location and severity of the lesion with alterations in the pulse volume contour and amplitude indicating proximal arterial obstruction.
- Conventional angiography remains the gold standard, but ultrasonography, computed tomography angiography (CTA), and magnetic resonance angiography (MRA) have largely replaced catheter-based angiography in the initial diagnostic evaluation.

- Contrast angiography (Fig. 1-644) is now reserved for patients with PAD who are being considered for endovascular revascularization and can provide physiologic information such as pressure gradients prior to percutaneous intervention.

Rx TREATMENT

The treatment goal in patients with PAD is to focus on cardiovascular risk-factor reduction to decrease morbidity and mortality as well as to improve limb-related symptoms. There are also medical and surgical approaches to management of limb-related symptoms.

CHRONIC MEDICAL Rx
LOWERING CARDIOVASCULAR MORBIDITY AND MORTALITY:
- Medical therapy for PAD is mainly aimed at decreasing cardiovascular risk; however, smoking may decrease progression of PAD.
- Smoking cessation should be emphasized in patients with PAD with assistance of behavioral and pharmacologic treatment (Class I).
- Antiplatelet therapy is indicated to reduce risk of myocardial infarction, stroke, and vascular death in individuals with symptomatic PAD with either aspirin (75 to 325 mg) or clopidogrel (75 mg) (Class I) and in asymptomatic patients (Class IIa).
- Warfarin is not indicated.
- Goal LDL cholesterol is <100 mg/dl and possibly <70 mg/dl in high-risk patients.
- If triglycerides are >200 mg/dl, non-HDL cholesterol should be lowered to <130 mg/dl.

- Management of hypertension with a goal of <140/90 mm Hg or <130/80 mm Hg if the patient has diabetes or chronic renal disease. Ramipril use has been reported to improve walking ability and quality of life in PAD patients with intermittent claudication.
- No clear benefit has been observed with combination aspirin and clopidogrel therapy.

TREATMENT OF CLAUDICATION:
- Exercise therapy: Supervised training should be performed for a minimum of 30 to 45 min, in sessions performed at least three times per week for a minimum of 12 wk. Studies have shown that a rigorous exercise-training program may be as beneficial as lower-extremity bypass surgery in symptomatic improvement. Supervised treadmill training and resistance training improve functional performance measured by treadmill walking and quality of life evaluation.
- Pharmacologic therapy with cilostazol (Pletal) 100 mg bid has been shown to increase pain-free and maximal walking distance by 40% to 60% in symptomatic patients with infrainguinal PAD after 12 to 24 wk of therapy, and has been demonstrated to improve ABI.
- Cilostazol has also been shown to be superior to pentoxifylline but is contraindicated in patients with systolic heart failure.

SURGICAL Rx
- The 2006 ACC/AHA guidelines on PAD have suggested that the following factors be considered prior to revascularization with either percutaneous or surgical methods:
  - The patient has had inadequate response to a supervised exercise training program and pharmacologic therapy.

- Symptoms of claudication have resulted in significant disability resulting in an inability to perform normal work or other activities.
- There is a very favorable risk–benefit ratio, and the characteristics of the lesion allow for intervention at a low risk with a high likelihood of success.
- The patient has more urgent limb-threatening ischemia as manifested by ischemic rest pain, ischemic ulcers, or gangrene.
- Studies have shown no significant difference in outcome between percutaneous transluminal angioplasty (PTA) and bypass surgery for iliac or femoropopliteal disease. Surgery is associated with a higher morbidity, PTA has a higher reintervention rate.
- Features that may favor a surgical strategy include long segments; multifocal segments; long segment occlusions; and eccentric, calcified stenoses.
- The ACC/AHA via the 2006 guidelines have suggested the following guidelines for revascularization therapy:
  - Endovascular intervention is recommended for TransAtlantic Inter-Society Consensus type A iliac and femoropopliteal arterial lesions.
  - Endovascular therapy is preferred in patients aged 50 yr or younger, because they have a higher risk of graft failure after surgical therapy than older patients.
  - Endovascular intervention is not indicated as prophylactic therapy in an asymptomatic patient with lower-extremity PAD, or if there is no significant pressure gradient across a stenosis even after augmentation of flow with vasodilators.
  - Primary stent placement is not recommended in the femoral, popliteal, or tibial arteries.
  - Surgical intervention is not indicated to prevent progression to limb-threatening ischemia in patients with intermittent claudication as generally claudication does not progress to severe ischemia.
  - Surgical interventions are indicated for individuals with claudication symptoms who have a significant functional disability that is vocational or lifestyle limiting. These patients need to also be unresponsive to exercise or pharmacotherapy and should have a reasonable likelihood of symptomatic improvement.
  - Prior to any surgical therapy, patients should have a preoperative cardiovascular risk evaluation.

DISPOSITION

Risk factors for atherosclerosis should be assessed, and appropriate modification instituted. Focus should be placed on smoking cessation, dietary adjustment, and pharmacotherapy for dyslipidemia, hyperglycemia, and hypertension. All patients with PAD should receive aspirin therapy unless contraindicated. Revascularization is performed if the symptoms of PAD do not

How to Perform and Calculate the ABI

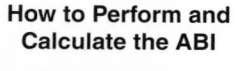

Partners Program ABI Interpretation
Above 0.90— Normal
0.71–0.90— Mild Obstruction
0.41–0.70— Moderate Obstruction
0.00–0.40— Severe Obstruction

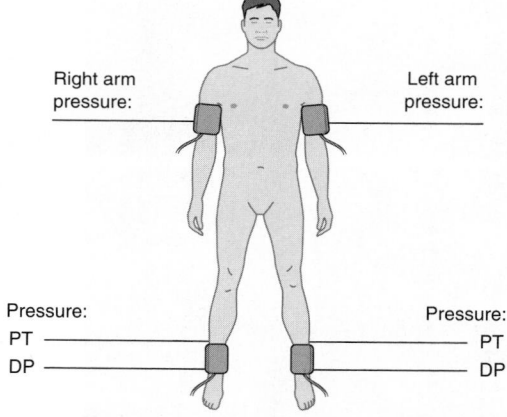

Right arm pressure:

Left arm pressure:

Pressure:
PT ——————————— PT
DP ——————————— DP

RIGHT ABI

LEFT ABI

$$\frac{\text{Higher right ankle pressure}}{\text{Higher arm pressure}} = \frac{\text{mm Hg}}{\text{mm Hg}} \underline{\quad} = \frac{\text{Higher left ankle pressure}}{\text{Higher arm pressure}} = \frac{\text{mm Hg}}{\text{mm Hg}} = \underline{\quad}$$

EXAMPLE

$$\frac{\text{Higher ankle pressure}}{\text{Higher arm pressure}} = \frac{92 \text{ mm Hg}}{164 \text{ mm Hg}} = 0.56 \qquad \text{See ABI Chart}$$

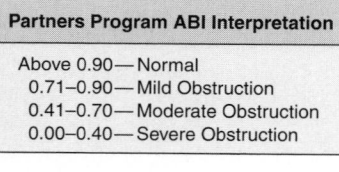

FIGURE 1-643 Performing pressure measurements and calculating the ankle-brachial index (ABI). To calculate the ABI, systolic pressures are determined in both arms and both ankles with the use of a handheld Doppler instrument. The highest readings for the dorsalis pedis (DP) and posterior tibial (PT) arteries are used to calculate the index. (From Goldman L, Schafer AI: *Goldman's Cecil medicine*, ed 24, Philadelphia, 2012, Saunders.)

improve with conservative therapy as discussed previously.

REFERRAL

Consultation with vascular medicine, vascular surgery, or other physicians with expertise in PAD is recommended in patients with rest pain, functional disability from pain, ABI <0.50 at rest, or any physical signs of limb ischemia or gangrene.

PEARLS & CONSIDERATIONS

COMMENTS

- PAD remains underdiagnosed and undertreated.
- Medical treatment is aimed mainly at cardiovascular risk factor modification, except for cilostazol.
- Studies of the natural history of claudication show the relative safety of initial conservative treatment of PAD in the absence of critical limb ischemia.

- When PAD limits a patient's ability to walk and exercise, percutaneous revascularization can be considered.
- Surgical intervention should be considered in patients who meet the criteria for intervention but have lesions that are not amenable to PTA/stenting or in older patients with a low surgical risk. In younger patients, due to the high risk of graft failure and recurrence, surgery should be a last resort.

PREVENTION

Cardiovascular disease is the major cause of death in patients with intermittent claudication. Therefore, the treatment of claudication is directed not only at improving walking distance but also at reducing cardiovascular risk.

PATIENT & FAMILY EDUCATION

The following organizations offer more information about PAD:

- American College of Cardiology (http://www.acc.org)
- Vascular Disease Foundation (http://www.vdf.org)

EBM EVIDENCE

available at www.expertconsult.com

SUGGESTED READINGS

available at www.expertconsult.com

RELATED CONTENT

Peripheral Arterial Disease (Patient Information)

AUTHORS: **HARKAWAL S. HUNDAL, M.D., M.S.,** and **PRANAV M. PATEL, M.D., F.A.C.C., F.S.C.A.I.**

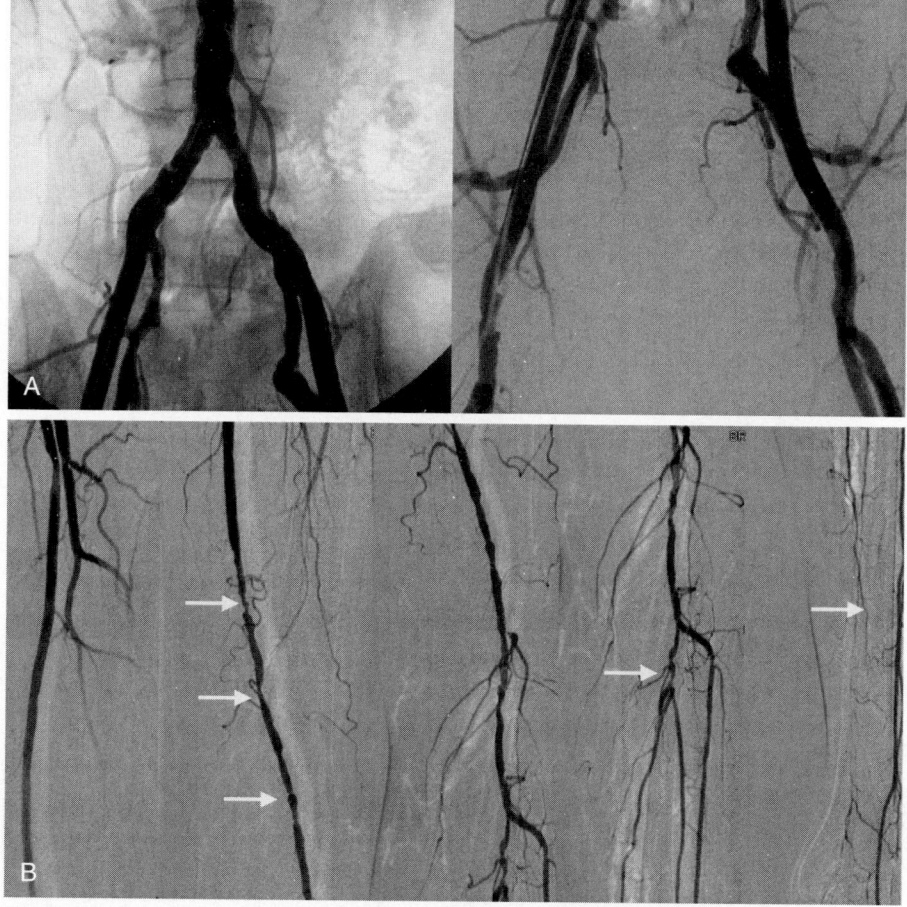

FIGURE 1-644 Angiogram of a patient with disabling left calf claudication. A, The aorta and bilateral common iliac arteries are patent. **B,** The left superficial femoral artery has multiple stenotic lesions *(arrows)*. There is a significant stenosis of the left tibioperoneal trunk and left posterior tibial artery *(arrows)*. (From Zipes DP et al [eds]: *Braunwauld's heart disease,* ed 7, Philadelphia, 2005, Saunders.)

BASIC INFORMATION

DEFINITION

Peritonitis refers to the acute onset of severe abdominal pain caused by peritoneal inflammation.

Secondary peritonitis is a localized (abscess) or diffuse peritonitis originating from a defect in abdominal viscus.

SYNONYMS

Acute abdomen
Surgical abdomen

ICD-9CM CODES
567.2 Peritonitis

EPIDEMIOLOGY & DEMOGRAPHICS

Common presentation as a result of diverse etiologies; for example, 5% to 10% of the population has acute appendicitis at some point in their lives.

PHYSICAL FINDINGS & CLINICAL PRESENTATION

- Acute abdominal pain
- Abdominal distention and ascites
- Abdominal rigidity, rebound, and guarding
- Fever, chills
- Exacerbation with movement
- Anorexia, nausea, and vomiting
- Constipation
- Decreased bowel sounds
- Hypotension and tachycardia
- Tachypnea, dyspnea

ETIOLOGY

- Microbiology: most common is gram-negative bacteria (*Escherichia coli, Enterobacter, Klebsiella, Proteus*), gram-positive bacteria (enterococci, streptococci, staphylococci), anaerobic bacteria (*Bacteroides, Clostridium*), and fungi
- Acute perforation peritonitis: gastrointestinal perforation, intestinal ischemia, pelvic peritonitis, and other forms
- Postoperative peritonitis: anastomotic leak, accidental perforation, and devascularization
- Posttraumatic peritonitis: after blunt or penetrating abdominal trauma

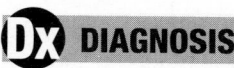 **DIAGNOSIS**

DIFFERENTIAL DIAGNOSIS

- Postoperative: abscess, sepsis, bowel obstruction, injury to internal organs

- Gastrointestinal: perforated viscus, appendicitis, inflammatory bowel disease, infectious colitis, diverticulitis, acute cholecystitis, peptic ulcer perforation, pancreatitis, bowel obstruction
- Gynecologic: ruptured ectopic pregnancy, pelvic inflammatory disease, ruptured hemorrhagic ovarian cyst, ovarian torsion, degenerating leiomyoma
- Urologic: nephrolithiasis, interstitial cystitis
- Miscellaneous: abdominal trauma, penetrating wounds, infections caused by intraperitoneal dialysis

WORKUP

- Acute peritonitis is mainly a clinical diagnosis based on patient history and physical examination.
- Laboratory and imaging studies (see "Laboratory Tests") assist in determining the need for and type of intervention.
- If patient is hemodynamically unstable, immediate diagnostic laparotomy should be performed in lieu of adjuvant diagnostic studies.

LABORATORY TESTS

- Complete blood count: leukocytosis, left shift, anemia
- SMA7: electrolyte imbalances, kidney dysfunction
- Liver function tests: ascites from liver disease, cholelithiasis
- Amylase: pancreatitis
- Blood cultures: bacteremia, sepsis
- Peritoneal cultures: infectious etiology
- Blood gas: respiratory versus metabolic acidosis
- Ascitic fluid analysis: exudate versus transudate
- Urinalysis and culture: urinary tract infection
- Cervical cultures for gonorrhea and *Chlamydia*
- Urine/serum human chorionic gonadotropin

IMAGING STUDIES

- Abdominal series: free air from perforation, small or large bowel dilation from obstruction, identification of fecalith
- Chest x-ray examination: elevated diaphragm, pneumonia
- Pelvic/abdominal ultrasound: abscess formation, abdominal mass, intrauterine versus ectopic pregnancy, identify free fluid suggestive of hemorrhage or ascites
- CT: mass, ascites

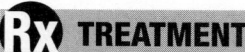 **TREATMENT**

NONPHARMACOLOGIC THERAPY

- IV hydration to correct dehydration, hypovolemia
- Blood transfusion to correct anemia from hemorrhage
- Nasogastric decompression, especially if obstruction is present
- Oxygen: intubation if necessary
- Bed rest

ACUTE GENERAL Rx

- Surgery to correct underlying pathology, such as controlling hemorrhage, correcting perforation, draining abscess
- Broad-spectrum antibiotics to cover both gram-negative aerobic and gram-negative anaerobic bacteria:
  1. Mild-moderate disease: piperacillin-tazobactam 3.375 g IV q6h or 4.5 g IV q8h *or* ticarcillin-clavulanate 3.1 g IV q6h. Alternative agents are ciprofloxacin 400 mg IV q12h or levofloxacin 750 mg IV q24h *plus* metronidazole 1 g IV q12h.
  2. Severe life-threatening disease: imipenem 500 mg IV q6h or meropenem 1 g IV q8h. Alternative agents are ampicillin *plus* metronidazole *plus* ciprofloxacin.
- Pain control: morphine or meperidine as needed (hold until diagnosis confirmed)

DISPOSITION

Depends on etiology of peritonitis, age of patient, coexisting medical disease, and duration of process before presentation

REFERRAL

Surgical consultation is required in all cases of acute peritonitis.

SUGGESTED READINGS
available at www.expertconsult.com

AUTHORS: **ARUNDATHI G. PRASAD, M.D.,** and **RUBEN ALVERO, M.D.**

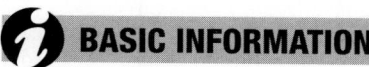

BASIC INFORMATION

DEFINITION

Spontaneous bacterial peritonitis (SBP) is an inflammatory reaction of the peritoneum secondary to the presence of bacteria or other microorganisms. More specifically, SBP is defined as an ascitic fluid infection without an evident intra-abdominal surgically treatable source occurring primarily in patients with advanced cirrhosis of the liver.

SYNONYMS

Primary peritonitis
SBP

ICD-9CM CODES
567.2 Peritonitis

EPIDEMIOLOGY & DEMOGRAPHICS

PREVALENCE: The prevalence of SBP in cirrhotic patients admitted to the hospital has been estimated at 10% to 30%.
PREDOMINANT SEX: Males affected more often than females

PHYSICAL FINDINGS & CLINICAL PRESENTATION

- Acute fever with accompanying abdominal pain/ascites, nausea, vomiting, diarrhea
- In cirrhotic patients, presentation may be subtle with a low-grade temperature (100° F) with or without abdominal abnormalities
- In patients with ascites, a heightened degree of awareness is necessary for detection
- Jaundice and encephalopathy
- Deterioration of mental status and/or renal function

ETIOLOGY

- *Escherichia coli*
- *Klebsiella pneumoniae*
- *Streptococcus pneumoniae*
- *Streptococcus* and *Enterococcus* spp.
- *Staphylococcus aureus*
- Anaerobic pathogens: *Bacteroides, Clostridium* organisms
- Other: fungal, mycobacterial, viral

DIAGNOSIS

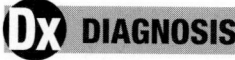

The diagnosis of SBP is established by a positive ascitic fluid bacterial culture and an elevated ascitic fluid absolute polymorphonuclear leukocyte count (≥250 cells/mm³).

DIFFERENTIAL DIAGNOSIS

- Appendicitis (in children)
- Perforated peptic ulcer
- Secondary bacterial peritonitis
- Peritoneal abscess
- Splenic, hepatic, or pancreatic abscess
- Cholecystitis
- Cholangitis

WORKUP

Paracentesis and ascitic fluid analysis will confirm diagnosis (see "Laboratory Tests").

LABORATORY TESTS

Ascitic fluid analysis reveals the following:
- Cell count with an absolute polymorphonuclear cell count >250/mm³
- Presence of bacteria on Gram stain
- pH <7.31
- Lactic acid >32 mg/dl
- Protein <1 g/dl
- Glucose >50 mg/dl
- Lactate dehydrogenase <225 mU/ml
- Positive culture of peritoneal fluid
- Measurement of the serum/ascites/albumin gradient: The serum/ascites/albumin gradient indirectly measures portal pressure. The albumin concentration of ascitic fluid and serum must be obtained on the same day. The ascitic fluid value is subtracted from the serum value to obtain the gradient. If the difference (not a ratio) is >1.1 g/dl, the patient has portal hypertension, with 97% accuracy. If the difference is <1.1 g/dl, portal hypertension is not present. The majority of patients with SBP have portal hypertension as a result of cirrhosis.

IMAGING STUDIES

- Abdominal ultrasound: if there is clinical difficulty in performing paracentesis
- CT scan: to rule out secondary peritonitis (if indicated) and to exclude abscess, mass

TREATMENT

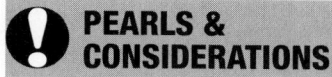

ACUTE GENERAL Rx

- Cefotaxime (2 g IV q12h) or ceftriaxone (2 g IV q24h) or ticarcillin-clavulanate or piperacillin-tazobactam. Continue therapy for 7 days. Repeat diagnostic paracentesis at day 2. Repeat paracentesis at 48 hours will demonstrate a significant decrease in polymorphonuclear count in patients with SBP. If ascites PMN count decreases by at least 25% at day 2, IV therapy can be switched to PO (levofloxacin 250 mg PO bid) to complete 7 days of therapy.

- IV albumin (1 g/kg of body weight) if BUN >30 mg/dL, bilirubin >4 mg/dL; repeat at day 3 if renal dysfunction persists

PROPHYLAXIS

- Oral norfloxacin 400 mg PO qd or ciprofloxacin 500 mg PO qd or levofloxacin 250 mg PO qd
- Alternative therapy: TMP-SMX one double-strength tablet PO qd
- Prophylaxis should be continued until disappearance of ascites or until liver transplantation

DISPOSITION

- The overall mortality rate from an episode of SBP is 20%, and following an episode, the 1-year mortality rate approaches 70%.

REFERRAL

- To a gastroenterologist for management of ascites and prevention of recurrent SBP
- To an infectious disease specialist for management of difficult-to-treat infections, antibiotic-resistant bacterial infections, or antibiotic drug intolerance

PEARLS & CONSIDERATIONS

COMMENTS

- Renal failure is a major cause of morbidity in cirrhotic patients with SBP. The use of IV albumin (1.5 g/kg at the time of diagnosis and 1 g/kg on day 3) may lower the rate of renal failure and mortality in patients with SBP.
- The criteria for the diagnosis of SBP require that abdominal paracentesis be performed and ascitic fluid be analyzed before a diagnosis of SBP can be made.
- Culturing ascitic fluid as if it were blood (with bedside inoculation of at least 10 ml of ascitic fluid directly into blood culture bottles at the bedside) has been shown to significantly increase the culture positivity of the ascitic fluid in the 80% to 100% range.
- Avoid therapeutic paracenteses during active infection
- Positive blood cultures in an individual with ascites require exclusion of a peritoneal source by paracentesis.

SUGGESTED READINGS
available at www.expertconsult.com

AUTHOR: **GLENN G. FORT, M.D., M.P.H.**

BASIC INFORMATION

DEFINITION

Pertussis is a prolonged bacterial infection of the upper respiratory tract characterized by paroxysms of an intense cough.

SYNONYMS

Whooping cough

ICD-9CM CODES
033.9 Pertussis

EPIDEMIOLOGY

INCIDENCE (IN U.S.): Provisional case counts for 2012 have surpassed the last peak year, 2010, with 41,880 pertussis cases and 14 deaths in infants aged <12 months.

PEAK INCIDENCE:
- Childhood
- Usually affects children aged <1 yr

PREDOMINANT AGE:
- 50% in children aged <1 yr
- 20% in children aged >15 yr
- Classically an infection of infants and young children, pertussis is often overlooked as a cause of chronic cough in adults. Recently, a resurgence of pertussis has been observed in adolescents and previously vaccinated adults as immunity wanes

PHYSICAL FINDINGS & CLINICAL PRESENTATION

- Infection is characterized by 3 phases: catarrhal, paroxysmal, and convalescent
- Catarrhal phase: Usually begins with a 1- to 2-wk prodrome that resembles a common cold. This phase may be mild or absent in adolescents and adults given partial immunity from prior immunization
- After this initial phase, increased production of mucus is noted. Excessive lacrimation and conjunctival infection should heighten the suspicion for pertussis
- Paroxysmal phase: Increased mucus production is followed by an intense, paroxysmal cough, ending with gasps and an inspiratory whoop
- In some children, cyanosis and anoxia are noted; posttussive gagging and vomiting are characteristic of pertussis
- When prolonged, frank exhaustion and even apnea occur. The paroxysmal phase lasts from 2 wk to 2 mo
- Convalescent phase: Lasts over 2 months and is characterized by cough of decreasing severity

ETIOLOGY

Gram-negative rod *Bordetella pertussis,* which adheres to human cilia

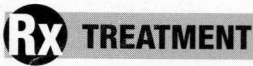

DIAGNOSIS

DIFFERENTIAL DIAGNOSIS

- Croup
- Epiglottitis
- Foreign body aspiration
- Bacterial pneumonia

WORKUP

Pertussis is often overlooked as a cause of chronic cough, especially in adolescents and adults. The presence or absence of posttussive emesis or inspiratory whoop increases the likelihood of pertussis but only modestly. Therefore, clinicians must use their overall impression in pursuing the diagnosis.

- Enzyme-linked immunosorbent assay for detection of antibody to pertussis. Polymerase chain reaction (PCR) is the most sensitive method for rapid detection of pertussis. PCR testing should be used only to confirm a diagnosis in persons with signs and symptoms consistent with pertussis. PCR testing sensitivity declines and is unlikely to be positive after 1 month of infection. PCR testing after 5 days of treatment with antibiotics can cause false-negative results and is generally not recommended
- Blood cultures in hospitalized patients
- Chest x-ray (Fig. 1-645)
- Culture of bacteria, usually from nasopharynx by aspiration or by swabbing the posterior nasopharynx with a polyester-tipped, rayon-tipped, or nylon-flocked swab
- Immunofluorescent staining of nasopharyngeal secretions
- Serologic tests for immunoglobulin G (IgG) or A (IgA) are available. A twofold increase between acute and convalescent sera is considered proof of seroconversion. A single elevated IgG or IgA titer is considered diagnostic when no acute serum is available

LABORATORY TESTS

Complete blood count, which usually demonstrates marked lymphocytosis:
- Up to 18,000 white blood cells
- 70% to 80% lymphocytes

IMAGING STUDIES

Chest x-ray examination is of value if secondary bacterial pneumonia is suspected.

TREATMENT

ACUTE GENERAL Rx

- Intensive supportive care:
  1. Adequate hydration
  2. Control of secretions
  3. Maintenance of airway
- Antibiotics (Table 1-326) are indicated even though their ability to alter the course of the disease is controversial.
  1. Azithromycin 500 mg on day 1, followed by 250 mg for days 2 to 5. Erythromycin

TABLE 1-326 Recommended Antimicrobial Treatment and Postexposure Prophylaxis for Pertussis, by Age Group

Age Group	PRIMARY AGENTS		ALTERNATE AGENT*	
	Azithromycin	Erythromycin	Clarithromycin	TMP-SMZ
<1 mo	Recommended agent. 10 mg/kg/day in a single dose for 5 days (only limited safety data available)	Not preferred Erythromycin is substantially associated with infantile hypertrophic pyloric stenosis Use if azithromycin is unavailable; 40-50 mg/kg/day in 4 divided doses for 14 days	Not recommended (safety data unavailable)	Contraindicated for infants aged <2 mo (risk for kernicterus)
1-5 mo	10 mg/kg/day in a single dose for 5 days	40-50 mg/kg/day in four divided doses for 14 days	15 mg/kg/day in two divided doses for 7 days	Contraindicated at age <2 mo For infants aged ≥2 mo: TMP 8 mg/kg/day plus SMZ 40 mg/kg/day in two divided doses for 14 days
Infants aged ≥6 mo and children	10 mg/kg in a single dose on day 1 (maximum 500 mg), then 5 mg/kg/day (maximum 250 mg) on days 2-5	40-50 mg/kg/day (maximum 2 g/day) in four divided doses for 14 days	15 mg/kg/day in two divided doses (maximum 1 g/day) for 7 days	TMP 8 mg/kg/day plus SMZ 40 mg/kg/day in two divided doses for 14 days
Adults	500 mg in a single dose on day 1 then 250 mg/day on days 2-5	2 g/day in four divided doses for 14 days	1 g/day in two divided doses for 7 days	TMP 320 mg/day, SMZ 1600 mg/day in two divided doses for 14 days

*Trimethoprim-sulfamethoxazole (TMP-SMZ) can be used as an alternative agent to macrolides in patients aged ≥2 mo who are allergic to macrolides, who cannot tolerate macrolides, or who are infected with a rare macrolide-resistant strain of *Bordetella pertussis.*

From Centers for Disease Control and Prevention: Recommended antimicrobial agents for treatment and postexposure prophylaxis of pertussis: 2005 CDC guidelines, *MMWR Morbid Mortal Wkly Rep* 54:1-16, 2005.

50 mg/kg/day for 14 days. Recent literature reports indicate that a 7-day treatment regimen may be as effective as a 14-day course of erythromycin. TMP/SMX 320/1600 mg per day in divided doses can be used in patients with allergy or intolerance to macrolides.

2. Although unproved, dexamethasone 1 mg/kg/day in four doses for severe, life-threatening paroxysms.

3. Ceftriaxone 75 mg/kg/day in two doses for broad coverage of secondary bacterial pneumonias.

- Vaccination is successful in preventing the disease: universal vaccination is advised for all children aged <7 yr. The Advisory Committee on Immunization Practices (ACIP) updated Tdap recommendations to include a single dose of Tdap vaccine in place of routine Td for adults age 19-64 yr and a single-dose Tdap for adults 65 yr and older who have or will have close contact with an infant (<12 mo). The ACIP also recommends that unvaccinated pregnant women receive a dose of Tdap.

- Erythromycin is recommended for all close contacts in the household: TMP/SMX in two oral doses per day for those intolerant to erythromycin.

DISPOSITION

Close attention to accepted vaccination schedules is the best prevention.

REFERRAL

To intensive care setting for life-threatening infections:

- Pulmonologist
- Infectious disease specialist

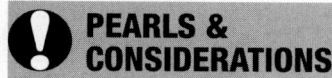

PEARLS & CONSIDERATIONS

- The diagnosis of pertussis in a young child is easily recognized, but in adults pertussis can be a subtle diagnosis and is often missed.

The tip-off is often a persistent, hacking, and productive cough with minor or no fever in a previously healthy person that lasts >2 wk.

- Approximately 11% of pertussis cases in the pediatric population are attributable to vaccine refusal, dispelling the myth that herd immunity protects children whose parents refuse pertussis vaccine.

SUGGESTED READINGS

available at www.expertconsult.com

RELATED CONTENT

Pertussis (Patient Information)

AUTHOR: **GLENN G. FORT, M.D., M.P.H.**

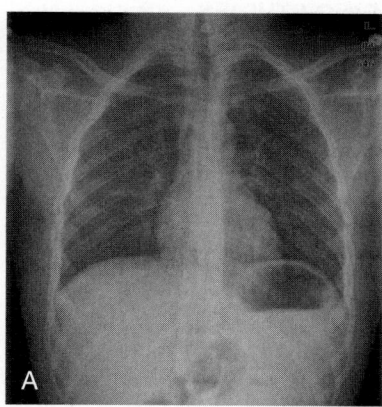
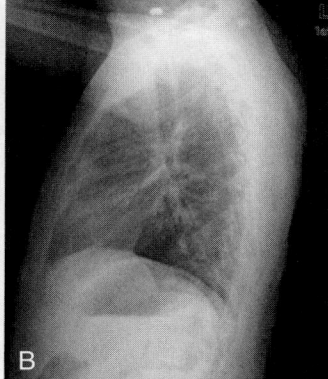
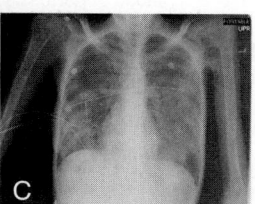

FIGURE 1-645 Pertussis present with a predominantly interstitial pattern of pneumonia with peribronchial cuffing. A and **B,** PA and lateral chest x-rays in a patient with pertussis. This 19-year-old male with sickle cell trait and short gut syndrome presented with cough and emesis. He had been seen multiple times in the emergency department over the past 3 weeks for moderately productive cough, diagnosed with bronchitis, and treated with azithromycin. His current presentation included 5 days of posttussive emesis. His chest x-ray **(C)** showed peribronchial cuffing and prominent interstitial markings but otherwise was near normal. His polymerase chain reaction test and cultures were positive for *Bordetella pertussis,* which does not typically cause a focal infiltrate on chest x-ray. Perhaps the most important point is to consider pertussis even with normal imaging findings when the clinical history is suggestive. (From Broder JS: *Diagnostic imaging for the emergency physician,* Philadelphia, 2011, Saunders.)

BASIC INFORMATION

DEFINITION

- A hamartomatous polyp is a benign intestinal growth that may contain all components of the intestinal mucosa. In gastrointestinal polyposis, multiple such polyps coexist within the intestinal tract, and associated manifestations are usually also present.
- Juvenile polyps are benign polyps composed of cystic dilatations of glandular structures within the fibroblastic stroma of the lamina propria. They may cause bleeding or intussusception.
- Commonly recognized syndromes are Peutz-Jeghers syndrome, juvenile polyposis syndrome, Cowden's disease, Bannagan-Ruvalcaba-Riley syndrome, and Cronkhite-Canada syndrome. Other lesser known inherited hamartomatous polyposis syndromes are hereditary mixed polyposis syndrome, intestinal ganglioneuromatosis and neurofibromatosis (variant of von Recklinghausen's syndrome), Devon family syndrome, basal cell nevus syndrome, and tuberous sclerosis (may involve gastrointestinal tract). Table 1-327 describes general features of some inherited colorectal cancer syndromes.

ICD-9CM CODES
759.6 (Peutz-Jeghers syndrome)
211.3 (Cronkhite-Canada syndrome)

EPIDEMIOLOGY

- Colonic adenomas, the precursors of nearly all colorectal cancers, are found in nearly 40% of patients by age 60 yr.
- 25% of men and 15% of women who undergo colonoscopy are found to have one or more adenomas.
- Detection of any adenoma in patients <60 yr confers an increased risk of colorectal cancer (by a factor of 2.6) in their first-degree relatives.

PHYSICAL FINDINGS & CLINICAL PRESENTATION

PEUTZ-JEGHERS SYNDROME:

- Transmission: autosomal dominant with incomplete penetrance
- Disease expression:
  - Stomach, small and large intestinal hamartomas with bands of smooth muscle in the lamina propria
  - Pigmented lesions around mouth (lips and buccal mucosa), nose, hands, feet, genitals, and perineal areas
  - Ovarian tumors
  - Sertoli cell testicular tumors
  - Airway polyps
  - Pancreatic cancer
  - Breast cancer
  - Urinary tract polyps
- Cumulative lifetime cancer risk
  - Colon cancer: 39%
  - Stomach cancer: 29%
  - Small intestine cancer: 13%
  - Pancreatic cancer: 36%
  - Breast cancer: 54%
  - Ovarian cancer: 10%
  - Sertoli cell tumor: 9%
  - Overall cancer risk: 93%
- Clinical manifestation:
  - Gastrointestinal, small-bowel obstruction, intussusception, gastrointestinal bleeding
  - See chapters on relevant malignancies for their signs and symptoms

JUVENILE POLYPOSIS SYNDROME:

- Transmission: autosomal dominant
- Disease expression
  - Solitary juvenile polyps numbering 10 or more in the rectum or throughout the gastrointestinal tract; the polyps are smooth and covered with normal epithelium
  - Various congenital abnormalities coexist in 20%
- Cumulative cancer risk is increased (may be as high as 50%)

- Clinical manifestation
  - Intestinal obstruction
  - Intussusception
  - Gastrointestinal bleeding

COWDEN'S DISEASE:

- Transmission: autosomal dominant, rare
- Disease expression
  - Juvenile intestinal polyposis
  - Orocutaneous hamartomas
  - Fibrocystic breast disease and breast cancer
  - Goiter and thyroid cancer
  - Facial tricholemmomas (papules) in 83%
- Cumulative cancer risk
  - Gastrointestinal: same as general population
  - Thyroid: 3% to 10%
  - Breast: 25% to 50%

BANNAGAN-RUVALCABA-RILEY SYNDROME:

- Transmission: autosomal dominant, rare
- Disease expression
  - Juvenile intestinal polyposis
  - Macrocephaly
  - Developmental delay
  - Penile pigmented spots
  - Cumulative cancer risk unknown

CRONKHITE-CANADA SYNDROME:

- Transmission: acquired
- Age of onset: midlife
- Disease expression
  - Diffuse gastrointestinal juvenile polyposis (50% to 95% of cases)
  - Chronic diarrhea and protein-losing enteropathy (the entire intestinal mucosa may be inflamed), which leads to abdominal pain, weight loss, and various complications of malnutrition
  - Dystrophic nails
  - Alopecia
  - Hyperpigmentation
- Cumulative cancer risk: same as the average population

TABLE 1-327   General Features of the Inherited Colorectal Cancer Syndromes

Syndrome	Polyp Histology	Polyp Distribution	Age of Onset	Risk of Colon Cancer	Genetic Lesion	Clinical Manifestations	Associated Lesions
Familial adenomatous polyposis	Adenoma	Large intestine, duodenum	16 yr (range, 8-34 yr)	100%	5q (*APC* gene)	Rectal bleeding, abdominal pain, bowel obstruction	Desmoids, CHRPE
Peutz-Jeghers syndrome	Hamartoma	Large and small intestine	First decade	Slightly above average	19p (*STK11*)	Possible rectal bleeding, abdominal pain, intussusception	Orocutaneous melanin pigment spots, other tumors
MUTYH-associated polyposis	Adenoma	Large intestine, duodenum	45-50 yr (range, 13-60 yr)	75% (range, 50%-100%)	1p (*MYH* gene)	Rectal bleeding, abdominal pain, bowel obstruction	CHRPE, osteomas
Juvenile polyposis	Hamartoma (rarely adenoma)	Large and small intestine	First decade	≈9%	*PTEN, SMAD4, BMPR1*	Possible rectal bleeding, abdominal pain, intussusception	Pulmonary AVMs
Hereditary non-polyposis colon cancer	Adenoma	Large intestine	40 yr (range, 18-65 yr)	30%	Mismatch repair genes*	Rectal bleeding, abdominal pain, bowel obstruction	Other tumors (e.g., ovary, uterus, pancreas, stomach)

AVM, Arteriovenous malformation; *CHRPE,* congenital hypertrophy of the retinal pigment epithelium; *MUTYH,* mutY homolog (*Escherichia coli*);.
*Including *hMSH2, hMSH3, hMSH6, hMLH1, hPMS1,* and *hPMS2.*

From Goldman L, Schafer AI: *Goldman's Cecil medicine,* ed 24, Philadelphia, 2012, Saunders.

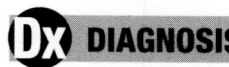

Diagnosis is suggested in many cases by family history and confirmed by colonoscopy and physical findings described previously.

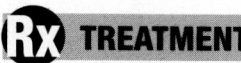

GENERAL Rx

Peutz-Jeghers syndrome:
- Colonoscopies with polypectomies
- Screening for breast cancer, testicular cancer, possibly ovarian cancer

Juvenile polyposis syndrome:
- Colonoscopies with polypectomies if few colon polyps
- Total colectomy if numerous polyps
- Esophagogastroscopies and polypectomies

Cowden's disease:
- Rigorous breast cancer screening or prophylactic simple bilateral mastectomy with reconstruction.

Cronkhite-Canada syndrome:
- Progressive malabsorption syndrome is the hallmark of this syndrome, and no specific treatment exists. Enteral or parenteral feeding is the cornerstone of management and can result in remission.

DISPOSITION

- The screening of first-degree relatives of patients with colonic adenomas detected before 60 yr of age is controversial. Some recommend beginning colonoscopic screening at age 40 yr or 10 yr younger than the age at diagnosis of the youngest person in the family with an adenoma.

- Recommended interval between colonoscopies from the U.S. Consensus Guidelines for Colonoscopic Surveillance after Polypectomy are as follows:
  - 10 yr for small, rectal hyperplastic polyps
  - 5 to 10 yr for one to two low-risk adenomas (tubular adenomas <1 cm)
  - 3 yr for low-risk adenomas or any high-risk adenoma (large [≥1 cm] or histologically advanced adenomas [tubulovillous or villous adenomas or villous adenomas and those with high-grade dysplasia])
  - <3 yr for presence of >10 adenomas
  - 2 to 6 mo for inadequately removed adenomas

SUGGESTED READING
available at www.expertconsult.com

RELATED CONTENT
Peutz-Jeghers Syndrome (Patient Information)

AUTHOR: **FRED F. FERRI, M.D.**

 BASIC INFORMATION

DEFINITION

Peyronie's disease is an abnormal curvature and shortening of the penis during an erection. This is caused by scarring of the tunica albuginea of the corpora cavernosa.

SYNONYMS

Plastic induration of the penis
Penile fibromatosis

ICD-9CM CODES
607.89 Peyronie's disease

EPIDEMIOLOGY & DEMOGRAPHICS

- Peyronie's disease occurs in approximately 1% of men.
- It is commonly seen between the ages of 45 and 60 yr.
- A genetic predisposition has been suggested.
- There are no incidence and prevalence data available in the literature.

PHYSICAL FINDINGS & CLINICAL PRESENTATION

- Painful erections
- Tenderness over the scar tissue area
- Erectile dysfunction
- Curvature of the erected penis interfering with penetration
- Dupuytren's contracture is a commonly associated finding in patients with Peyronie's disease

ETIOLOGY

- Specific cause is unknown. It is believed that scar tissue forms on either the dorsal or ventral midline surface of the penile shaft. The scar restricts expansion at the involved site, causing the penis to bend or curve in one direction.
- The precipitating factor appears to be trauma from repetitive microvascular injury caused by vigorous sexual intercourse, accidents, or prior surgeries (e.g., transurethral or radical prostatectomy, cystoscopy).

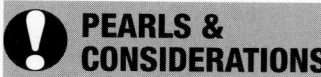 DIAGNOSIS

Diagnosis is based on the clinical findings.

DIFFERENTIAL DIAGNOSIS

- The history differentiates congenital from acquired curvatures of the penis.
- Other causes of erectile dysfunction must be excluded, including metabolic, diabetic, thyroid, and renal causes, in addition to hypogonadism and hyperprolactinemia.

WORKUP

History and physical examination alone will usually establish the diagnosis of Peyronie's disease.

LABORATORY TESTS

There are no specific blood tests to diagnose Peyronie's disease. Electrolytes, blood urea nitrogen, creatinine, glucose, thyroid function tests (thyroid-stimulating hormone, T_3U, T_4), testosterone, and prolactin levels are blood tests to exclude other medical causes of erectile dysfunction.

IMAGING STUDIES

Imaging studies are not specific.

TREATMENT

NONPHARMACOLOGIC THERAPY

A conservative approach of reassurance and observation is taken at first because the disease process may be self-limiting.

ACUTE GENERAL Rx

Although not substantiated by direct randomized, controlled clinical trials, the following treatment modalities have been tried:
- Vitamin E 400 mg bid.
- Paraaminobenzoic acid 12 g/day.
- Colchicine 0.6 mg bid for 2 to 3 wk.
- Fexofenadine 60 mg bid for 3 mo.
- Steroid injection into the scar tissue.
- Collagenase injection into the scar tissue.
- Radiation to the scar tissue area.
- Extracorporeal shockwave therapy (ESWT): Current evidence on the safety, but not the efficacy, of ESWT appears adequate. From comparative studies, the main benefits of ESWT were the alleviation of pain and reduction of angulation of the penis. In one comparative study, 10 of 20 patients receiving ESWT had a decrease in the curvature of at least 30%. Case series evidence also suggested some improvement of sexual performance.
- Other medications that can be helpful include verapamil, tamoxifen, and interferon.

CHRONIC Rx

In patients who have progressed to intractable pain with erection or erectile dysfunction, surgical treatment with excision of the plaque and skin grafting may be indicated.

DISPOSITION

Peyronie's disease evolves slowly and in some cases can resolve on its own. Waiting for 1 yr before proceeding with surgical attempts is recommended.

REFERRAL

A urologic consultation is recommended in patients with progressive symptoms and erectile dysfunction.

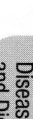 PEARLS & CONSIDERATIONS

COMMENTS

- Peyronie's disease is not commonly seen in younger patients because they are able to sustain intracorporeal pressures high enough to stretch the scar tissue, preventing it from deforming the penis during erection.
- Trauma from buckling of the erected penis is thought to be the precipitant cause of scar formation and Peyronie's disease. It is found more often in men who are sexually very active and vigorous, having sexual intercourse daily or almost daily.
- Sexual positions with the women being on top or thrusting the penis into the anterior vaginal wall are thought to increase the chances of developing Peyronie's disease.

SUGGESTED READINGS
available at www.expertconsult.com

RELATED CONTENT
Peyronie's Disease (Patient Information)

AUTHOR: **TANYA ALI, M.D.**

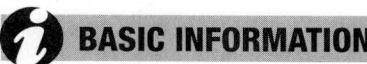

DEFINITION

Inflammation of the pharynx or tonsils

SYNONYMS

Sore throat
Group A streptococci (GAS)

ICD-9CM CODES
462 Pharyngitis

EPIDEMIOLOGY & DEMOGRAPHICS

Acute pharyngitis accounts for 1.3% of outpatient visits to health care providers in the U.S.
PEAK INCIDENCE: Late winter/early spring (GAS infections)
PREDOMINANT SEX: Females = males
PREDOMINANT AGE:
- All ages affected
- Streptococcal pharyngitis most common among school-age children (5-15 yr of age). GAS are responsible for 5%-15% of cases of pharyngitis in adults and 20%-30% of cases in children (5-15 yr of age).

PHYSICAL FINDINGS & CLINICAL PRESENTATION

- Pharynx:
  1. May appear normal to severely erythematous
  2. Tonsillar hypertrophy and exudates commonly seen but do not indicate etiology
- Viral infection:
  1. Rhinorrhea
  2. Conjunctivitis
  3. Cough
- Bacterial infection, especially GAS:
  1. High fever
  2. Systemic signs of infection
- Herpes simplex or enterovirus infection: vesicles
- Streptococcal infection:
  1. Rare complications:
     a. Scarlet fever
     b. Rheumatic fever
     c. Acute glomerulonephritis
  2. Extension of infection: tonsillar, parapharyngeal, or retropharyngeal abscess presenting with severe pain, high fever, trismus
- Streptococcal tonsillitis is manifested as acute onset of fever, headache, neck pain, odynophagia, sore throat, otalgia, red tongue with enlargement of papillae, sore throat, red swollen uvula, and tender anterior cervical adenitis.
- Peritonsillar abscess (accumulation of pus between the tonsil and its capsule) is the most common complication of acute tonsillitis. Clinical signs include deformed posterior pharynx, medial displacement of the uvula, trismus, and muffled voice (hot-potato voice).
- Table 1-328 describes seven danger signs in patients with sore throat.

ETIOLOGY

- Viruses:
  1. Respiratory syncytial virus
  2. Influenza A and B
  3. Epstein-Barr virus
  4. Adenovirus
  5. Herpes simplex
- Bacteria:
  1. GAS: *Streptococcus pyogenes*. β-Hemolytic GAS are the most common cause of acute tonsillitis.
  2. *Neisseria gonorrhoeae*
  3. *Arcanobacterium haemolyticum*
- Other organisms:
  1. *Mycoplasma pneumoniae*
  2. *Chlamydophila pneumoniae*

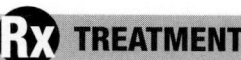 DIAGNOSIS

DIFFERENTIAL DIAGNOSIS

- Sore throat associated with granulocytopenia, thyroiditis
- Tonsillar hypertrophy associated with lymphoma
- Section II describes the differential diagnosis of sore throat.

WORKUP

The Centor criteria to identify patients at risk for GAS consists of (1) fever subjective or measured >38.1° C (100.5° F), (2) absence of cough, (3) tonsilar exudates, (4) tender anterior cervical lymphadenopathy. Patients with ≤1 criteria are at low risk and do not need additional testing. The McIsaac criteria adds 1 point for age 3-14 and subtracts a point for age ≥45 yr.
- Rapid streptococcal antigen test (culture should be performed if rapid test negative)
- Throat swab for culture to exclude *S. pyogenes, N. gonorrhoeae* (requires specific transport medium) in selected cases

LABORATORY TESTS

- Bloodwork is only rarely necessary
- Complete blood count with differential
  1. May help support diagnosis of bacterial infection when diagnosis is unclear
  2. Streptococcal infection suggested by leukocytosis >15,000/mm^3
- Viral cultures, serologic studies rarely needed
- Monospot if diagnosis is unclear

IMAGING STUDIES

Seldom indicated. If necessary to distinguish between tonsillitis and peritonsillar abscess, CT or MRI of the neck can be done.

TABLE 1-328 Seven Danger Signs in Patients with Sore Throat

1. Persistence of symptoms longer than 1 wk without improvement
2. Respiratory difficulty, particularly stridor
3. Difficulty in handling secretions
4. Difficulty in swallowing
5. Severe pain in the absence of erythema
6. A palpable mass
7. Blood, even in small amounts, in the pharynx or ear

From Andreoli TE et al: *Andreoli and Carpenter's Cecil essentials of medicine,* ed 8, Philadelphia, 2010, Saunders.

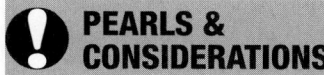 TREATMENT

NONPHARMACOLOGIC THERAPY

- Fluids
- Salt water gargles

ACUTE GENERAL Rx

- Analgesics: aspirin (adults) or acetaminophen or ibuprofen (adults and children)
- If streptococcal infection proven or suspected:
  1. Penicillin V 500 mg PO bid for 10 days or benzathine penicillin 1.2 million U IM once (adults). Children: penicillin V 250 mg bid or tid
  2. Erythromycin 500 mg PO bid or 250 mg qid for 10 days or azithromycin if penicillin allergic
- If gonococcal infection proven or suspected: ceftriaxone 125 mg IM once
- Amoxicillin 500 mg tid for 10 days is the primary antibiotic treatment of streptococcal tonsillitis. Macrolides or clindamycin can be used in penicillin-allergic patients.
- Treatment of peritonsillar abscess is drainage through needle or incision.

CHRONIC Rx

- Recurrent streptococcal infections are common and may represent reinfection from other household members, including pets.
- There is no conclusive evidence from randomized clinical trials that tonsillectomy is superior to antibiotic therapy for recurrent tonsillitis in adults.
- Tonsillopharyngitis is generally managed in an outpatient setting with follow-up arranged in 1 to 2 wk. Admission to the hospital is indicated for local suppurative complications (peritonsillar abscess; lateral pharyngeal or posterior pharyngeal abscess; impending airway closure; or inability to swallow food, medications, or water).

REFERRAL

- To otolaryngologist:
  1. If peritonsillar or other abscess is suspected
  2. If tonsillar hypertrophy persists
- To infectious disease expert if unusual pathogen is suspected

PEARLS & CONSIDERATIONS

COMMENTS

- Antibiotic therapy should be avoided unless bacterial etiology is suspected or proven, especially in adults.

SUGGESTED READINGS

available at www.expertconsult.com

RELATED CONTENT

Tonsillitis (Patient Information)

AUTHOR: **GLENN G. FORT, M.D., M.P.H.**

BASIC INFORMATION

DEFINITION

Pheochromocytomas are catecholamine-producing tumors that originate from chromaffin cells of the adrenergic system. They generally secrete both norepinephrine and epinephrine, but norepinephrine is usually the predominant amine.

SYNONYMS

Paraganglioma

ICD-9CM CODES
194.0 Pheochromocytoma
255.6 Medulloadrenal hyperfunction

EPIDEMIOLOGY & DEMOGRAPHICS

- Incidence: 0.05% of population; peak incidence in 30s and 40s.
- "Rough" rule of 10: 10% are extraadrenal, 10% are malignant, 10% occur in children, 10% involve both adrenals, 10% are multiple (other than bilateral adrenal).
- Approximately 25% of patients with apparently sporadic pheochromocytoma may be carriers of mutations.
- Approximately 25% of pheochromocytomas are familial and associated with genetic disorders. Pheochromocytoma is a feature of two disorders with an autosomal-dominant pattern of inheritance:
  1. Multiple endocrine neoplasia (MEN) type 2
  2. Von Hippel-Lindau disease: angioma of the retina, hemangioblastoma of the central nervous system, renal cell carcinoma, pancreatic cysts, and epididymal cystoadenoma
- Pheochromocytomas occur in 5% of patients with neurofibromatosis type 1.

PHYSICAL FINDINGS & CLINICAL PRESENTATION

- Hypertension: can be sustained (55%) or paroxysmal (45%).
- Headache (80%): usually paroxysmal in nature and described as "pounding" and severe.
- Palpitations (70%): can be present with or without tachycardia.
- Hyperhidrosis (60%): most evident during paroxysmal attacks of hypertension.
- Physical examination may be entirely normal if done in a symptom-free interval; during a paroxysm the patient may demonstrate marked increase in both systolic and diastolic pressure, profuse sweating, visual disturbances (caused by hypertensive retinopathy), dilated pupils (from catecholamine excess), paresthesias in the lower extremities (caused by severe vasoconstriction), tremor, tachycardia.

ETIOLOGY

- Catecholamine-producing tumors that are usually located in the adrenal medulla.
- Specific mutations of the RET protooncogene cause familial predisposition to pheochromocytoma in MEN 2.

- Mutations in the von Hippel-Lindau tumor suppressor gene (*VHL* gene) cause familial disposition to pheochromocytoma in von Hippel-Lindau disease.
- Recently identified genes for succinate dehydrogenase subunit D *(SDHD)* and succinate dehydrogenase subunit B *(SDHB)* predispose carriers to pheochromocytoma and globus tumors.

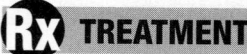
DIAGNOSIS

DIFFERENTIAL DIAGNOSIS

- Anxiety disorder
- Thyrotoxicosis
- Amphetamine or cocaine abuse
- Carcinoid
- Essential hypertension

WORKUP

Laboratory evaluation and imaging studies to locate the neoplasm (Fig. E1-646). Misdiagnosis of pheochromocytoma is not uncommon. Correct interpretation of biochemical tests and imaging is crucial to a correct diagnosis.

LABORATORY TESTS

- Although there is no consensus on the best test, plasma-free metanephrines have been suggested as the test of first choice for excluding or confirming the tumor. Plasma concentrations of normetanephrines >2.5 pmol/ml or metanephrine levels >1.4 pmol/ml indicate a pheochromocytoma with 100% specificity.
- 24-hr urine collection for metanephrines (up to 100% sensitive) will also show increased metanephrines; the accuracy of the 24-hr urinary levels for metanephrines can be improved by indexing urinary metanephrine levels by urine creatinine levels.

IMAGING STUDIES

- Abdominal CT scan with and without contrast (88% sensitivity) is useful in locating pheochromocytomas >0.5 inch in diameter (90% to 95% accurate).
- MRI with contrast: pheochromocytomas demonstrate a distinctive MRI appearance (up to 100% sensitivity); MRI may become the diagnostic imaging modality of choice.
- Scintigraphy with 131 or 1-123 I-MIBG (up to 100% sensitivity): this norepinephrine analog localizes in adrenergic tissue; it is particularly useful in locating extraadrenal pheochromocytomas.
- 6-[^{18}F]Fluorodopamine positron emission tomography is reserved for cases in which clinical symptoms and signs suggest pheochromocytoma and results of biochemical tests are positive but conventional imaging studies cannot locate the tumor. An alternative approach is to use vena caval sampling for plasma catecholamines and metanephrines.

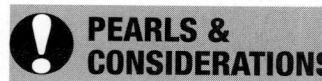
TREATMENT

GENERAL Rx

Laparoscopic adrenalectomy (surgical resection for both benign and malignant disease):
1. Preoperative stabilization with combination of alpha-adrenergic blocking agents (prazosin, doxazosin, terazosin, or phenoxybenzamine), beta-blocker, and liberal fluid and salt intake starting 10 to 14 days before surgery. Beta-blockers should be avoided until patients receive adequate alpha-adrenergic blockade for several days to avoid hypertensive crisis due to unopposed alpha stimulation. Amlodipine or verapamil can be added to beta-blockers if blood pressure control is still inadequate.
2. Hypertensive crisis preoperatively and intraoperatively can be controlled with nitroprusside.

PEARLS & CONSIDERATIONS

COMMENTS

- Obtaining a detailed family history is important because 25% of pheochromocytomas are familial.
- Screening for pheochromocytoma should be considered in patients with any of the following:
  1. Malignant hypertension
  2. Poor response to antihypertensive therapy
  3. Paradoxical hypertensive response
  4. Hypertension during induction of anesthesia, parturition, surgery, or thyrotropin-releasing hormone testing
  5. Hypertension associated with imipramine or desipramine
  6. Neurofibromatosis (increased incidence of pheochromocytoma)
- All patients with pheochromocytoma should be screened for MEN-2 and von Hippel-Lindau disease with pentagastrin test, serum parathyroid hormone, ophthalmoscopy, MRI of the brain, CT scan of the kidneys and pancreas, and ultrasonography of the testes.
- In patients with pheochromocytoma, routine analysis for mutations of *RET, VHL, SDHD,* and *SDHB* is indicated to identify pheochromocytoma-associated syndromes.

SUGGESTED READINGS

available at www.expertconsult.com

RELATED CONTENT

Pheochromocytoma (Patient Information)

AUTHORS: **MARK F. BRADY, M.D., M.P.H.,** and **FRED F. FERRI, M.D.**

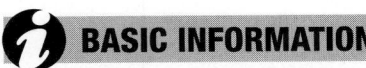

BASIC INFORMATION

DEFINITION

Specific phobias are anxiety disorders characterized by an excessive, persistent fear elicited by a specific object or situation that is then avoided or tolerated with intense distress. The provoking stimulus may be a specific object, such as an animal or insect; natural environments, such as heights or water; or a specific situation, such as the sight of blood, the receipt of an injection, or being in a tunnel or on a bridge. Social phobia is a specific disorder characterized by a fear of being in social or performance situations. Also, those with panic disorder may have agoraphobia, characterized by an intense anxiety about being in a place or situation from which they would not be able to escape in the event of a panic attack.

SYNONYMS

Simple phobia (obsolete name for specific phobia)

Phobias named for the provoking stimulus, such as arachnophobia (fear of spiders) and acrophobia (fear of heights)

Social anxiety disorder (social phobia)

ICD-9CM CODES
F40.2 Specific phobia (DSM-IV: 300.29)
F40.1 Social phobia (DSM-IV: 300.23),
Agoraphobia (DSM-IV: 300.21 [with panic disorder], 300.22 [without panic disorder])

EPIDEMIOLOGY & DEMOGRAPHICS

PEAK INCIDENCE: Specific phobias are often lifelong conditions; some of those with childhood onset (e.g., some animal phobias) tend to remit spontaneously.

PREVALENCE (IN U.S.):
- Specific phobias are prevalent in 5% to 10% of the general population.
- Social phobia is prevalent in approximately 13% of the general population.

PREDOMINANT SEX AND AGE:
- Females with specific phobias outnumber males, though rates vary by phobia.
- More women than men (16% vs. 11%) are affected with social phobia.
- Agoraphobia is more prevalent in women.
- Most specific phobias have childhood onset.
- Situational phobias have two peaks—in childhood and the mid-20s.
- Onset of social phobia usually occurs in the mid-teens, with onset after age 25 being unusual; this disorder is generally lifelong.

GENETICS: Specific and social phobias are more common in first-degree relatives.

PHYSICAL FINDINGS & CLINICAL PRESENTATION

- When approaching the phobic stimulus, the experience of extreme anxiety is often accompanied by autonomic symptoms such as tachycardia, tremor, and diaphoresis; depersonalization may occur. In blood or injection phobias, symptoms are often followed by a parasympathetic response that can cause vasovagal syncope.
- Specific phobias frequently occur with other anxiety disorders.
- Social phobias are distinguished from specific phobias in that what is feared is humiliation or embarrassment rather than a specific object or environment.

ETIOLOGY

There is no clear etiology.

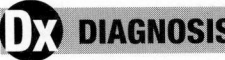

DIAGNOSIS

DIFFERENTIAL DIAGNOSIS

- Panic attacks (with or without agoraphobia): anxiety symptoms seen in specific phobia may resemble symptoms of panic attacks, but the stimulus in the specific or social phobia is clear, whereas panic attacks do not have a clearly associated provoking stimulus.
- Posttraumatic stress disorder (PTSD): anxiety and physiologic arousal associated with specific cues from the traumatic event defining the PTSD may resemble the symptoms induced by a phobia.
- Generalized anxiety disorder (GAD): may be difficult to distinguish from social phobia, but in social phobia the focus is fear of embarrassment or humiliation from other people, whereas GAD has no specific focus for the worry.
- Avoidant personality disorder is often comorbid with social phobia.
- Psychotic disorders can present with a fear of being in public that arises from delusions.

WORKUP

- History: usually diagnostic. This should include information about other medical disorders, medications, any history of past trauma, and substance abuse.
- Physical examination: to confirm absence of cardiovascular abnormalities such as arrhythmias or evidence of endocrinologic reasons for hyperarousal such as an enlarged or tender thyroid gland.

LABORATORY TESTS

No specific laboratory tests are indicated.

IMAGING STUDIES

No specific imaging studies are recommended.

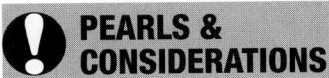

TREATMENT

NONPHARMACOLOGIC THERAPY

- Cognitive-behavioral therapy (CBT) and exposure-based treatments have been effective for treating social phobia in controlled trials.
- Behavioral treatments can involve relaxation training, often paired with visualization and progressive desensitization.
- Success rates in treating specific phobias are higher when the phobia is not complicated by other anxiety disorders.

ACUTE GENERAL Rx

- Benzodiazepines provide rapid relief of anxiety associated with exposure to provoking stimuli, but may be associated with adverse effects including somnolence, accidents, abuse, and dependence.
- Lorazepam or alprazolam can be administered sublingually to increase the rate of absorption.
- Beta-blockers (e.g., propranolol) have been used to decrease autonomic hyperarousal and tremor associated with performance situations (e.g., before public speaking).

CHRONIC Rx

- If the phobic stimulus is rarely encountered, benzodiazepines on an as-needed basis can be an appropriate long-term treatment, although there is a risk of abuse and dependence.
- Selective serotonin reuptake inhibitors are the most effective pharmacologic treatment in reducing symptoms and improving function for people with social phobia.
- Monoamine oxidase inhibitors are also effective for treatment of social phobia.

COMPLEMENTARY & ALTERNATIVE MEDICINE

No definitive evidence supports complementary or alternative medicines in the treatment of phobic disorders.

DISPOSITION

Phobic disorders are generally present for life, although outpatient-based treatment may effectively reduce symptoms.

REFERRAL

Recommended for confirmation of diagnosis and for evaluation for psychotherapy and other treatment modalities.

PEARLS & CONSIDERATIONS

People with social phobia often have low self-esteem and fear being scrutinized by others such that they avoid or are fearful of any situation in which others may assess or evaluate them directly or indirectly. More than half are concurrently affected by another anxiety disorder, and alcohol and other substance dependence is common because these patients often use substances to mask their anxiety.

SUGGESTED READINGS
available at www.expertconsult.com

RELATED CONTENT
Posttraumatic Stress Disorder (Related Key Topic)
Phobias (Patient Information)

AUTHORS: **ILJIE KIM FITZGERALD, M.D., M.S.,** and **SETH A. BERKOWITZ, M.D.**

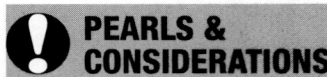

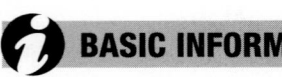 **BASIC INFORMATION**

DEFINITION

From the Latin words *pilus,* meaning "hair," and *nidus,* meaning "nest."

A *pilonidal sinus* is a short tract that extends from the skin surface and most likely represents a distended hair follicle. It is most commonly found in the intergluteal fold sacrococcygeal region, but it can also occur in the interdigital area, umbilicus, chest wall, and scalp. An *acute pilonidal abscess,* which consists of pus and a wall of edematous fat, results from rupture of an infected follicle into fat. A *chronic pilonidal abscess* results when an infected follicle ruptures directly into surrounding tissues; the wall of a chronic pilonidal abscess consists of fibrous tissue. A *pilonidal cyst* develops from a chronic abscess of long duration as a thin and flat lining of epithelium grows into the cavity from the skin surface.

SYNONYMS

Jeep disease

ICD-9CM CODES
685.1 Pilonidal cyst

EPIDEMIOLOGY & DEMOGRAPHICS

INCIDENCE: 26 cases per 100,000 persons
PREDOMINANT SEX: Males are more commonly affected than females (2.2:1).
AVERAGE AGE OF PRESENTATION: 21 yr
RISK FACTORS:
- Male sex
- Caucasian race
- Family predisposition
- Obesity
- Sedentary lifestyle
- Occupation requiring prolonged sitting
- Local hirsutism
- Poor hygiene
- Increased sweat activity

PHYSICAL FINDINGS & CLINICAL PRESENTATION
- May manifest as asymptomatic pits or pores in the natal cleft (Fig. E1-647)
- Tenderness after physical activity or prolonged sitting
- Acute pilonidal abscess in 20% of patients with pilonidal disease
- Presents as a hot, tender, fluctuant swelling just lateral to the midline over the sacrum that may exude pus through the midline pit
- Chronic pilonidal abscess in 80% of patients with pilonidal disease
- Acute suppuration, tenderness, swelling, and heat
- Infrequently, systemic reaction: occasionally fever, leukocytosis, and malaise

ETIOLOGY
- Currently believed to be acquired rather than congenital.
- Drilling of hair shed from the perineum or the head into sebaceous or hair follicles in the natal cleft.

- Drilling is facilitated by the friction of the natal cleft.
- Subsequent infection by skin organisms leads to pilonidal abscess.

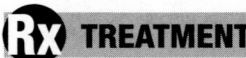 **DIAGNOSIS**

DIFFERENTIAL DIAGNOSIS
- Perianal abscess arising from the posterior midline crypt
- Hidradenitis suppurativa
- Carbuncle
- Furuncle
- Osteomyelitis
- Anal fistula
- Coccygeal sinus

WORKUP
- Diagnosis is based on history and physical examination.
- Midline pits present behind the anus overlying the sacrum and coccyx.
- Broken hairs are often seen extruding from the midline pits.
- Insert probe in pilonidal sinus in path away from the anus.
- Complicated anal fistula may be angulating posteriorly before passing into a retrorectal abscess, but thorough examination of the anal cavity usually discloses point of origin.

LABORATORY TESTS
Complete blood count

IMAGING STUDIES
CT scan in advanced, recurrent cases

Rx **TREATMENT**

NONPHARMACOLOGIC THERAPY
Prevention of exacerbations:
1. Local hygiene
2. Avoidance of prolonged sitting position
3. Weight reduction

ACUTE GENERAL Rx
- Procedure of choice for first-episode acute abscess: simple incision and drainage in an outpatient setting. Box E1-46 describes surgical options for the treatment of pilonidal sinus.
- Cure rate of 76% after 18 mo
- Antibiotics: generally not indicated unless the patient has a medical condition such as rheumatic heart disease or is immunosuppressed

CHRONIC Rx
Elective treatment of pilonidal disease:
1. Minimal surgery:
   a. Remove hair from midline pits and shave buttocks.
   b. May use a fine wire brush with local anesthesia to clear the pits and any lateral openings of granulation tissue and hair.
   c. Keep area clean.

2. Fistulotomy and curettage:
   a. Used when minimal surgery does not control episodes of suppuration
   b. Pass probe to outline the pilonidal sinus and open tract surgically
   c. Curette granulation tissue at the base of the sinus and excise edges of the skin
   d. Keep open granulating wound meticulously clean and allow to heal
   e. If complete healing does not take place, use a skin graft or advancement flap to close the defect
3. Marsupialization:
   a. This is the treatment of choice for chronic pilonidal disease.
   b. Wide excision of the pilonidal area is performed, including all affected skin and subcutaneous tissues down to the presacral fascia.
   c. Wound is left open, allowed to marsupialize, or closed as a primary procedure.
   d. Give antibiotics for 24 hr (particularly those directed against *Staphylococcus* and *Bacteroides* species).
4. Other procedures:
   a. Excision and closure
   b. Excision and skin grafting
   c. Bascom procedure (follicle removal and lateral drainage)
   d. Flaps: *Z*-plasty, V-Y advancement flap, rhomboid flap, gluteus maximus myocutaneous flap

DISPOSITION
- Recurrence rate for excision (most definitive procedure): 1% to 6%
- Incidence of squamous cell carcinoma in a chronic, recurrent pilonidal sinus is rare <1%

REFERRAL
- Emergency department for incision and drainage for an acute abscess
- To a surgeon for elective treatment or management of chronic or recurrent disease

! **PEARLS & CONSIDERATIONS**

COMMENTS
Because of significant associated morbidity, the elective surgical procedures outlined are performed only after the potential risks versus benefits are carefully weighed.

SUGGESTED READINGS
available at www.expertconsult.com

RELATED CONTENT
Pilonidal Cyst (Patient Information)

AUTHORS: **ARUNDATHI G. PRASAD, M.D.,** and **RUBEN ALVERO, M.D.**

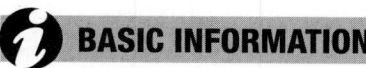

DEFINITION

Pinworms are a noninvasive infestation of the intestinal tract by *Enterobius vermicularis,* a helminth of the nematode family. It is a small (1 cm in length), white, thread-like roundworm that typically inhabits the cecum, appendix, and adjacent areas of the ileum and ascending colon.

SYNONYMS

Enterobiasis

ICD-9CM CODES
127.4 Enterobiasis

EPIDEMIOLOGY & DEMOGRAPHICS

- Most common intestinal nematode; approximately 30,000 cases annually in the U.S.
- Worldwide distribution, but most common in temperate climates.
- The prevalence of pinworm infection is lowest in infants and reaches highest infection rate in school-age children (ages 5 to 14 yr).
- Eggs are infective within 6 hr of oviposition and may remain so for 20 days.
- Clusters are found in families, institutionalized persons, and homosexual men.

PHYSICAL FINDINGS & CLINICAL PRESENTATION

- Most infested persons are asymptomatic.
- Perianal itching is the most common reported symptom, with scratching leading to excoriation and sometimes secondary infection.
- Rarely insomnia, irritability, anorexia, and weight loss are described.
- Granulomas have been described in various organs resulting from worms wandering outside the intestines and dying there.

ETIOLOGY & PATHOGENESIS

- *E. vermicularis* is highly prevalent throughout the world, particularly in countries of the temperate zone. Human beings are the only host for this worm. Infestation is by fecal-oral route; ingested eggs hatch in the stomach and the larvae migrate to the colon, where they mature. Gravid female worms containing an average of 10,000 ova migrate to the perianal skin at night, lay their eggs there, and die. The eggs embryonate within 6 hr and cause itching; scratching causes egg deposition under fingernails, from which they can contaminate food or lead to autoreinfection.
- *E. vermicularis* may be transmitted between sexual partners, especially those engaging in oral-anal sex.

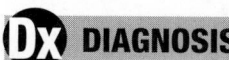 **DIAGNOSIS**

DIFFERENTIAL DIAGNOSIS

- Perianal itching related to poor hygiene
- Hemorrhoidal disease and anal fissures
- Perineal yeast/fungal infections

Section II describes the causes of pruritus ani.

WORKUP

Identification of adult worms or eggs. *E. vermicularis* ova are ovoid but flattened on one side and measure approximately 56×27 micrometers (Fig. 1-648). The eggs can be identified on transparent tape placed on the perianal skin on awakening. (NOTE: Five consecutive negative tests rule out the diagnosis.) A single examination detects 50% of infections, three examinations detect 90%, and five examinations detect 99%.

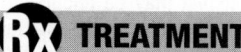 **TREATMENT**

- Single dose of mebendazole (100 mg) with a repeat dose given after 2 wk results in cure rates of 90% to 100%.
- Single dose of albendazole (400 mg) with a second dose given 2 wk later is also highly effective.
- Pyrantel pamoate (11 mg/kg up to 1 g) can prevent against *E. vermicularis.* It is available as a suspension and has minimal toxicity (mild transient gastrointestinal symptoms, headache, drowsiness). A repeat dose after 2 wk is recommended because of the frequency of reinfection and autoinfection.
- Other infected family members, classmates, or residents of long-term care facilities should be treated at the same time as the index case.

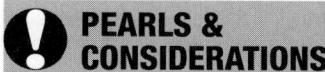 **PEARLS & CONSIDERATIONS**

- Eosinophilia is not observed in most cases because tissue invasion does not occur.
- Good hand hygiene is the most effective method of prevention.
- Frequent changing of underclothes, bed clothes, and bed sheets is helpful to decrease risk of autoinfection.

SUGGESTED READINGS
available at www.expertconsult.com

RELATED CONTENT
Pinworms (Patient Information)

AUTHOR: **FRED F. FERRI, M.D.**

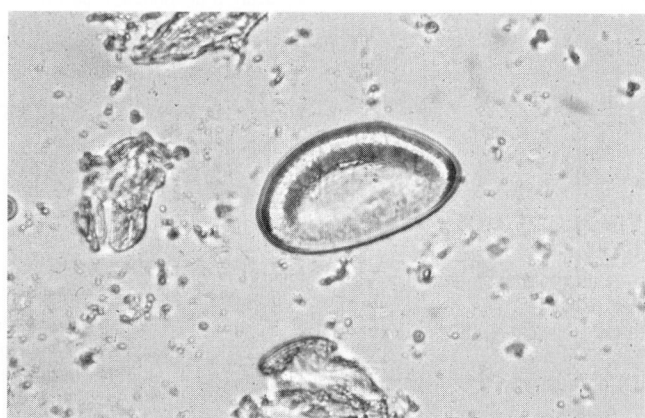

FIGURE 1-648 Enterobius vermicularis embryonated egg. Note larva inside ($40 \times 10 \ \mu m$). (From Gorbach SL et al [eds]: *Infectious diseases,* ed 2, Philadelphia, 1998, Saunders.)

BASIC INFORMATION

DEFINITION

Pituitary adenoma is a benign neoplasm of the anterior lobe of the pituitary that causes symptoms, either by excess secretion of hormones or by a local mass effect as the tumor impinges on other, nearby structures (e.g., optic chiasm, hypothalamus, pituitary stalk). Pituitary adenomas are classified by their size, function, and features that characterize their appearance. Microadenomas are <10 mm in size, and macroadenomas are ≥10 mm in size.

- *Acromegaly* is the disease state characterized by a pituitary adenoma that secretes growth hormone (GH).
- A *prolactinoma* secretes prolactin (PRL).
- *Cushing's disease* is a disease state of hypersecretion of adrenocorticotropic hormone (ACTH).
- *Thyrotropin-secreting pituitary adenomas* secrete primarily thyroid-stimulating hormone (TSH).
- *Nonsecretory pituitary adenomas* are those in which the neoplasm is a space-occupying lesion whose secretory products do not cause a specific disease state.

ICD-9CM CODES
253   Pituitary adenoma
253.0   Acromegaly
253.1   Prolactinoma

EPIDEMIOLOGY & DEMOGRAPHICS

CLASSIFICATION (BY HORMONE SECRETED):
- PRL only: 35%
- No hormone: 30%
- GH only: 20%
- PRL and GH: 7%
- ACTH: 7%
- Luteinizing hormone (LH), follicle-stimulating hormone (FSH), TSH: 1%

PREVALENCE/INCIDENCE:
- Pituitary adenomas: up to 10% to 15% of all intracranial neoplasms; 3% to 27% at autopsy series
- Prolactinomas: up to 20% in women with unexplained primary or secondary amenorrhea
- GH-secreting pituitary adenoma: 50 to 60 cases per 1 million persons
- Thyrotropin-secreting pituitary adenoma: 2.8% of pituitary adenomas with a slight female/male predominance of 1.7:1
- Corticotropin-secreting pituitary adenomas: female/male predominance of 8:1

PHYSICAL FINDINGS & CLINICAL PRESENTATION

PROLACTINOMAS:
- Females:
  1. Galactorrhea
  2. Amenorrhea
  3. Oligomenorrhea with anovulation
  4. Infertility
  5. Estrogen deficiency leading to hirsutism
  6. Decreased vaginal lubrication
  7. Osteopenia
- Males:
  1. Large tumors more common as a result of delayed diagnosis
  2. Possible impotence, decreased libido, or hypogonadism
  3. Galactorrhea rare because males lack the estrogen-dependent breast growth and differentiation

GH-SECRETING PITUITARY ADENOMA: ACROMEGALY
- Coarse facial features
- Oily skin
- Prognathism
- Carpal tunnel syndrome
- Osteoarthritis
- History of increased hat, glove, or shoe size
- Decreased exercise capacity
- Visual field deficits
- Diabetes mellitus

CORTICOTROPIN-SECRETING PITUITARY ADENOMA: CUSHING'S DISEASE
- Usually present when the tumor is small (1 to 2 mm)
- 50% of the tumors <5 mm
- Other symptoms:
  1. Truncal obesity
  2. Round facies (moon face)
  3. Dorsocervical fat accumulation (buffalo hump)
  4. Hirsutism
  5. Acne
  6. Menstrual disorders
  7. Hypertension
  8. Striae
  9. Bruising
  10. Thin skin
  11. Hyperglycemia

THYROTROPIN-SECRETING PITUITARY ADENOMA:
- In males, larger, more invasive, and more rapidly growing tumors that present later in life
- Other symptoms: thyrotoxicosis, goiter, visual impairment

NONSECRETORY PITUITARY ADENOMAS (ENDOCRINE INACTIVE PITUITARY ADENOMA):
- Usually large at the time of diagnosis
- Symptoms:
  1. Bitemporal hemianopsia as a result of compression of the optic chiasm
  2. Hypopituitarism from compression of the pituitary gland
  3. Hypogonadism in men and in premenopausal women
  4. Cranial nerve deficits caused by extension into the cavernous sinus
  5. Hydrocephalus from extension into the third ventricle, compressing the foramen of Monro
  6. Diabetes insipidus resulting from compression of the hypothalamus or pituitary stalk (a rare complication)

ETIOLOGY

Benign neoplasms of epithelial origin

 DIAGNOSIS

DIFFERENTIAL DIAGNOSIS
PROLACTINOMA:
- Pregnancy
- Postpartum puerperium
- Primary hypothyroidism
- Breast disease
- Breast stimulation
- Drug ingestion (especially phenothiazines, antidepressants, haloperidol, methyldopa, reserpine, opiates, amphetamines, and cimetidine)
- Chronic renal failure
- Liver disease
- Polycystic ovarian disease
- Chest wall disorders
- Spinal cord lesions
- Previous cranial irradiation

ACROMEGALY: Ectopic production of GH-releasing hormone from a carcinoid or other neuroendocrine tumor

CUSHING'S DISEASE:
- Diseases that cause ectopic sources of ACTH overproduction (including small-cell carcinoma of the lung, bronchial carcinoid, intestinal carcinoid, pancreatic islet cell tumor, medullary thyroid carcinoma, or pheochromocytoma)
- Adrenal adenomas, adrenal carcinoma
- Nelson's syndrome

THYROTROPIN-SECRETNG PITUITARY ADENOMAS: Primary hypothyroidism

NONSECRETORY PITUITARY ADENOMA: Nonneoplastic mass lesions of various etiologies (e.g., infectious, granulomatous)

WORKUP

See Section III algorithm, "Evaluation of Suspected Pituitary Tumor."
PROLACTINOMA:
First step: measurement of basal PRL levels (practitioners should be aware of discriminatory values in their own institutions)
- Elevated PRL levels are correlated with tumor size.
- Level >200 ng/ml is diagnostic, with levels of 100 to 200 ng/ml being equivocal.
- Basal PRL levels between 20 and 100 suggest a microadenoma as well as other conditions such as psychotropic drug ingestion, recent breast examination, and even a recent meal.
- Basal level <20 ng/ml is usually considered normal. Each laboratory should develop its own normative values, however, and practitioner should refer to these values.
- Threshold level for obtaining imaging such as MRI should be developed by individual providers depending on the level of specificity and sensitivity desired.

ACROMEGALY:
- First screening tests are the measurement of the serum insulin-like growth factor I level, postprandial serum GH, and TRH stimulation test.
- Follow with an oral glucose tolerance test.
- Failure to suppress serum GH to <2 ng/ml with an oral load of 100 g glucose is considered conclusive.

- A GH-releasing hormone level >300 ng/ml is indicative of an ectopic source of GH.

CUSHING'S DISEASE:
- Normal or slightly elevated corticotropin levels ranging from 20 to 200 pg/ml; normal is 10 to 50 pg/ml (normative data should be developed by each institution for its population).
- Level <10 pg/ml usually indicates an autonomously secreting adrenal tumor.
- Level >200 pg/ml suggests an ectopic corticotropin-secreting neoplasm.
- Cushing's disease can be assessed by absence of cortisol suppression with the low-dose dexamethasone test but with the presence of cortisol suppression after the high-dose test. As a method to distinguish Cushing's disease from an ectopic source of ACTH, this test is robust.
- 24-hr urine collection should demonstrate an increased level of cortisol excretion.

THYROTROPIN-SECRETING PITUITARY ADENOMA:
- Highly sensitive thyrotropin assays, which evaluate the presence of thyrotoxicosis, are one way to detect a thyrotropin-secreting tumor.
- Free alpha subunit is secreted by >80% of tumors, with the ratio of the alpha subunit to thyrotropin <1.
- With central resistance to thyroid hormone, ratio is <1 and the sella is normal.
- Laboratory tests show elevated serum levels of both T_3 and T_4.

NONSECRETORY PITUITARY ADENOMA:
- Visual field testing
- Assessment of the pituitary and organ function to determine if there is hypopituitarism or hypersecretion of hormones (even if the effects of hypersecretion are subclinical)
- TRH to provoke secretion of FSH, LH, and LH-beta-subunit; will not elicit response in normal persons
- Exclusion of Klinefelter's syndrome in patient with longstanding primary hypogonadism, elevated gonadotropin levels, and enlargement of the sella

IMAGING STUDIES

Study of choice: MRI of the pituitary (Fig. E1-649) and hypothalamus
- When evaluating Cushing's disease, small size at the onset of symptoms noted
- MRI, in this case, only 60% sensitive at best and may yield false-positive results
- CT scan only when MRI is unavailable or is otherwise contraindicated

Rx TREATMENT

NONPHARMACOLOGIC THERAPY
SURGERY:
- Selective transsphenoidal resection of the adenoma is the treatment of choice for acromegaly, Cushing's disease, and thyrotropin-secreting pituitary adenomas, all of which tend to be microadenomas at the time of onset of symptoms.
- Macroadenomas, such as the nonsecretory pituitary adenoma, may also be surgically removed, but risk of recurrence is greater with these tumors and adjunctive therapy such as irradiation may also be necessary.
- Bilateral adrenalectomy has been performed in patients with Cushing's disease after failure of other therapies; complications requiring lifelong hormone replacement or Nelson's syndrome may occur.

RADIOTHERAPY:
- Radiotherapy is used primarily as adjuvant treatment. It is reserved for patients who have not responded to surgical treatment and who still have symptoms of the adenoma.
- Used with varying degrees of success in all the different pituitary adenomas
- Radiotherapy complications include long-term hypopituitarism (40% of patients) and secondary neoplasms (1.5% of patients).

ACUTE GENERAL Rx
PROLACTINOMA:
- Bromocriptine, a dopamine analog, is generally given orally in divided doses of 1.5 to 10 mg. Cabergoline is given once or twice weekly. It is better tolerated and more effective than bromocriptine for tumor shrinkage but more expensive.
- Side effects include orthostatic hypotension, nausea, and dizziness; avoided by beginning with low-dose therapy.
- Other compounds include pergolide mesylate, a long-acting ergot derivative with dopaminergic properties, as well as other nonergot derivatives.

ACROMEGALY:
- Somatostatin analogues: octreotide, lanreotide administered as monthly injections
- Cabergoline or bromocriptine can also be used. They have modest activity but can be administered orally and are less expensive than somastatin analogues.
- Pegvisomant can also be used to normalize IGF-1 levels.

CUSHING'S DISEASE:
- Ketoconazole, which inhibits the cytochrome P-450 enzymes involved in steroid biosynthesis, is effective in managing mild to moderate disease in daily oral doses of 600 to 1200 mg.
- Metyrapone and aminoglutethimide can be used to control hypersecretion of cortisol but are generally used when preparing a patient for surgery or while waiting for a response to radiotherapy.

THYROTROPIN-SECRETING PITUITARY ADENOMA:
- Ablative therapy with either radioactive iodide or surgery is indicated.
- Treatment directed to the thyroid alone may accelerate growth of the pituitary adenoma.
- Octreotide has been shown to be effective in doses similar to those used for acromegaly.

NONSECRETORY PITUITARY ADENOMA:
- There is no role for medical therapy at this time.
- Surgery and radiotherapy are indicated.

CHRONIC Rx

For all pituitary adenomas:
- Careful follow-up is important. Patients undergoing transsphenoidal microsurgical resection should be seen in 4 to 6 wk to ensure that the adenoma has been completely removed and that the endocrine hypersecretion is resolved.
- If there is good clinical response, patient should be monitored yearly for recurrence and to follow the level of the hypersecreted hormone.
- Patients who have undergone irradiation should have close follow-up with backup medical therapy because response to radiotherapy may be delayed; incidence of hypopituitarism also increases with time.

SUGGESTED READINGS
available at www.expertconsult.com

RELATED CONTENT
Acromegaly (Related Key Topic)
Amenorrhea (Related Key Topic)
Cushing's Disease and Syndrome (Related Key Topic)
Galactorrhea (Related Key Topic)
Prolactinoma (Related Key Topic)
Fig. 3-139 Evaluation of suspected pituitary tumor (Algorithm)
Pituitary Adenoma (Patient Information)

AUTHORS: **BETH J. WUTZ, M.D.,** and **RUBEN ALVERO, M.D.**

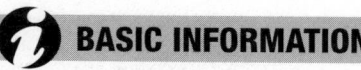

BASIC INFORMATION

DEFINITION

Pityriasis is a common self-limiting skin eruption of unknown etiology.

ICD-9CM CODES
696.3 Pityriasis rosea

EPIDEMIOLOGY & DEMOGRAPHICS

- Most cases of pityriasis rosea occur between ages 10 and 35 yr; mean age is 23 yr.
- The incidence of disease is highest in the fall and spring.
- Female/male ratio is 1.5:1.

PHYSICAL FINDINGS & CLINICAL PRESENTATION

- Initial lesion (herald patch), an annular pink patch with trailing scale, precedes the eruption by approximately 1 to 2 wk; typically measures 3 to 6 cm; it is round to oval in appearance and most frequently located on the trunk (Fig. 1-650).
- Eruptive phase follows within 2 wk and peaks after 7 to 14 days.
- Lesions are most frequently located in the lower abdominal area. They have a salmon-pink appearance in whites and a hyperpigmented appearance in blacks.

- Most lesions are 4 to 5 mm in diameter; center has a "cigarette paper" appearance; border has a characteristic ring of scale (collarette).
- Lesions occur in a symmetric distribution and follow the cleavage lines of the trunk (Christmas tree pattern).
- The number of lesions varies from a few to hundreds.
- Most patients are asymptomatic; pruritus is the most common symptom.
- History of recent fatigue, headache, sore throat, and low-grade fever is present in approximately 25% of cases.

ETIOLOGY

Unknown, possibly viral (picornavirus)

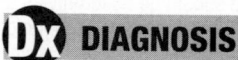

DIAGNOSIS

DIFFERENTIAL DIAGNOSIS

- Tinea corporis (can be ruled out by potassium hydroxide examination)
- Secondary syphilis (absence of herald patch, positive serologic test for syphilis)
- Psoriasis
- Nummular eczema
- Drug eruption: medications that may cause rashes similar to pityriasis rosea include clonidine, captopril, interferon, bismuth, barbiturates, gold, hepatitis B vaccine, and imatinib mesylate

- Viral exanthem
- Eczema
- Lichen planus
- Tinea versicolor (the lesions are more brown and the borders are not as ovoid)
- Erythema migrans

WORKUP

Presence of herald lesion and characteristic rash are diagnostic. Skin biopsy is generally reserved for atypical cases.

LABORATORY TESTS

Generally not necessary; serologic test for syphilis if clinically indicated

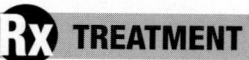

TREATMENT

NONPHARMACOLOGIC THERAPY

The disease is self-limited and generally does not require any therapeutic intervention.

ACUTE GENERAL Rx

- Use calamine lotion or oral antihistamines in patients with significant pruritus.
- Use prednisone tapered over 2 wk in patients with severe pruritus.
- Direct sun exposure or use of ultraviolet light within the first week of eruption is beneficial in decreasing the severity of disease.

DISPOSITION

- Spontaneous complete resolution of the rash within 4 to 8 wk
- Recurrence rare (<2% of cases)

PEARLS & CONSIDERATIONS

COMMENTS

Reassure patient that the disease is not contagious and its course is benign.

SUGGESTED READING
available at www.expertconsult.com

RELATED CONTENT

Pityriasis Rosea (Patient Information)

AUTHOR: **FRED F. FERRI, M.D.**

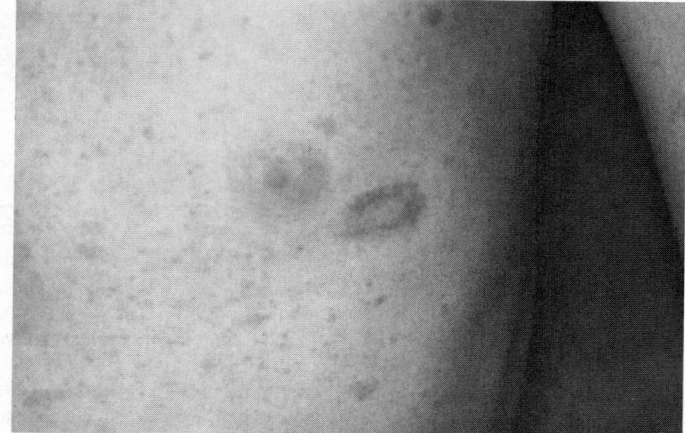

FIGURE 1-650 Herald patch and surrounding pityriasis rosea. (From Kliegman RM et al: *Nelson textbook of pediatrics,* ed 19, Philadelphia, 2011, Saunders.)

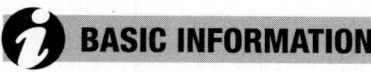

DEFINITION

Placenta previa is the implantation of the placenta over the internal os. Four degrees of this abnormality (Fig. 1-651) have been traditionally defined; however, the accurate localization of the placental edge in relation to the discrete point of the internal os with transvaginal sonography makes the following terms outmoded:

1. Total placenta previa: the internal os is covered completely.
2. Partial placenta previa: the internal os is partially covered.
3. Marginal placenta previa: the edge of the placenta is at the margin of the internal os.
4. Low-lying placenta: the placenta is implanted in the lower uterine segment and, although its edge does not reach the internal os, is in close proximity to it.

ICD-9CM CODES
641.1 Placenta previa

EPIDEMIOLOGY & DEMOGRAPHICS

INCIDENCE: 0.26% to 0.7% of pregnancies
RISK FACTORS:
- Previous cesarean delivery (after one cesarean delivery, the risk is 1% to 4%; after four or more, the risk approaches 10%).
- Multiparity has also been associated with placenta previa.

PHYSICAL FINDINGS & CLINICAL PRESENTATION

The classic presentation of placenta previa is painless vaginal bleeding, usually in the second or third trimester. Uterine contractions may or may not be present. On physical examination, the uterus is soft and pain free. The fetus is often in breech, transverse lie, or high. Fetal distress is usually not present.

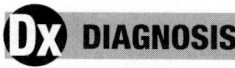 DIAGNOSIS

DIFFERENTIAL DIAGNOSIS
- Placenta accreta
- Placenta percreta
- Placenta increta
- Vasa previa
- Abruptio placentae
- Vaginal or cervical trauma
- Labor
- Local malignancy

WORKUP
- Do *not* perform a digital vaginal examination.
- The diagnosis of placenta previa can seldom be firmly established by physical examination alone. A speculum examination in a hospital setting to exclude any local bleeding may be performed.

- This diagnosis should not be dismissed until thorough evaluation, including sonography, has completely excluded its presence.

LABORATORY TESTS
- A complete blood count can be used to monitor hemoglobin and hematocrit.
- A Kleihauer-Betke preparation of maternal blood in all Rh-negative women and Rh-immune globulin when indicated

IMAGING STUDIES
- The simplest and safest method of placental localization is transabdominal sonography with confirmatory imaging by transvaginal ultrasonography (TVS). Transabdominal ultrasound alone is inaccurate in the diagnosis of placenta previa and should be used only as a screening tool. TVS has become the gold standard for the diagnosis of placenta previa. It is safe even in the presence of active bleeding. A distance of ≤20 mm from placental edge to interior cervical os is becoming a new criterion for performing term cesarean delivery in women with placenta previa.
- MRI has also been effective in detecting placenta previa, although sonography remains the preferred method.

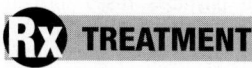 TREATMENT

NONPHARMACOLOGIC THERAPY
- In preterm pregnancies with no active bleeding, close observation and expectant management are indicated. In those with active bleeding, conservative management, including blood transfusions for severe bleeds, is appropriate. The woman should stay in the hospital for at least 48 hr after the bleeding has stopped.
- Bed rest, preferably in a hospital setting, should be prescribed.

ACUTE GENERAL Rx
- Initial assessment for signs of maternal hemodynamic compromise or hemorrhagic

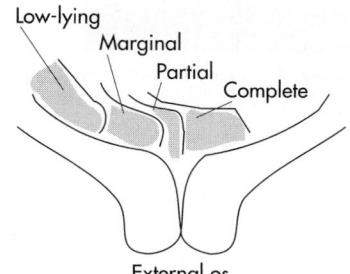

FIGURE 1-651 Depiction of degrees of placenta previa. (From Weissleder R et al: *Primer of diagnostic imaging,* St Louis, 2007, Mosby.)

Labels: Low-lying, Marginal, Partial, Complete, External os

shock; large-bore IV access with crystalloid fluid resuscitation
- Assess fetal status and gestational age by sonogram and continuous fetal heart rate monitoring
- Cross-matched blood should be made available during bleeding episodes; if the hemorrhage is severe, cesarean delivery is indicated despite fetal immaturity
- Tocolytic therapy may be considered in those women in preterm labor, as well as the administration of corticosteroids to enhance fetal lung maturity

CHRONIC Rx
- Cesarean delivery is necessary in nearly all cases of placenta previa.
- Uncontrollable hemorrhage after placental removal should be anticipated as a result of the poorly contractile nature of the lower uterine segment. The need for hysterectomy to control bleeding should be discussed with the patient before delivery, if possible.

DISPOSITION
Because of the unpredictable nature of placenta previa, not all women with placenta previa can be treated expectantly.

REFERRAL
Affected women and their families should be aware of all signs and symptoms that would necessitate immediate transport to the hospital. The possibility of hysterectomy should also be discussed early during pregnancy.

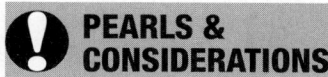 PEARLS & CONSIDERATIONS

COMMENTS
Third-trimester measurement of the distance from the placental edge to the internal cervical os by TVS commonly is used to gauge the likelihood of need for cesarean section. The decision to offer women with a placenta that is situated 11 to 20 mm away a trial of labor remains controversial. Recent reports by Vergani et al indicate that more than two thirds of women with a placental edge to cervical os distance of >10 mm fewer than 28 days before delivery can deliver vaginally without increased risk of hemorrhage

SUGGESTED READINGS
available at www.expertconsult.com

RELATED CONTENT
Vaginal Bleeding During Pregnancy (Related Key Topic)
Placenta Previa (Patient Information)

AUTHORS: **SONYA S. ABDEL-RAZEQ, M.D.,** and **RUBEN ALVERO, M.D.**

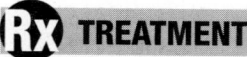
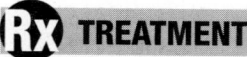 BASIC INFORMATION

DEFINITION

The plantar fascia arises from the calcaneal tuberosity and has various attachments as it travels longitudinally, ending at the digital level (Fig. 1-652). It acts as a tension band supporting the medial longitudinal arch of the foot. Plantar fasciitis describes the local inflammation and subsequent pain occurring at the insertion at the medial calcaneal tuberosity or along the course of the fascial band.

SYNONYMS

Heel pain syndrome

ICD-9CM CODES
728.71 Plantar fasciitis
726.73 Calcaneal spur

EPIDEMIOLOGY & DEMOGRAPHICS

INCIDENCE: Plantar fasciitis affects >1 million persons/yr in the U.S. and two thirds of patients will seek care from their primary care physician for this condition. It is one of the more common causes of heel pain in adults.
PREDOMINANT SEX: Females slightly greater than males, studies vary
PREDOMINANT AGE: Commonly middle aged; any age group possible
RISK FACTORS: Weight gain, obesity (present in 90% of patients), increased activity, change in activity type, prolonged standing, hard surfaces, trauma, certain activities (see "Etiology").

PHYSICAL FINDINGS & CLINICAL PRESENTATION

- Pain is localized to the heel or along the course of the plantar fascia.
- Pain is greatest upon first steps in the morning and upon standing after rest (poststatic dyskinesia).
- Symptoms may improve throughout the day or with ambulation, but may persist or increase with prolonged standing.
- Pain may be elicited with ankle dorsiflexion and simultaneous subtalar eversion.

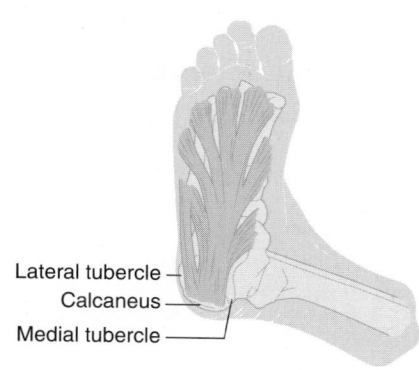

Lateral tubercle —
Calcaneus —
Medial tubercle —

FIGURE 1-652 Plantar view of origin and insertion of plantar fascia. (From Frontera WR: *Essentials of physical medicine and rehabilitation,* ed 2, Philadelphia, 2008, Saunders.)

- Often exquisitely tender upon palpation of the medial calcaneal tuberosity
- May have localized or medial heel edema.

ETIOLOGY

- Any factor that increases the tension at the insertion of the fascia on the medial calcaneal tuberosity, creating local inflammation. Evidence suggests that plantar spurs are secondary rather than an etiology; these are an incidental finding in about 30% of asymptomatic patients.
- Achilles/ankle equinus or pseudoequinus
- Active STJ/rearfoot pronation, such as with calcaneal or forefoot varus
- A strain of the fascia or dorsiflexory force of the forefoot on the midfoot or vice versa. Example: jumping from a height, sprinting from starting blocks, reaching on a ladder.

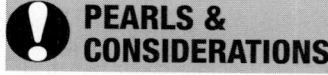 DIAGNOSIS

DIFFERENTIAL DIAGNOSIS

- Calcaneal fracture, including traumatic or stress fracture, or bone bruise
- Tarsal tunnel syndrome
- Calcaneal osteomyelitis
- Bone cyst or bone tumor
- Posterior tibial tendon dysfunction (often misdiagnosed as plantar fasciitis)
- Plantar fascial fibromatosis (thickening/soft tissue mass along the plantar fascial band)
- Systemic cause: gout, Paget's disease of the bone, psoriasis, Reiter's syndrome, etc.
- Plantar fascia rupture

STUDIES

- Weight-bearing x-rays: rule out tumor or trauma (lateral, oblique, calcaneal axial views)
- MRI/bone scan to rule out stress fracture (takes 2 wk to show on x-ray)
- MRI or ultrasound if suspected plantar fascial fibromatosis
- May need to rule out tarsal tunnel syndrome with nerve studies

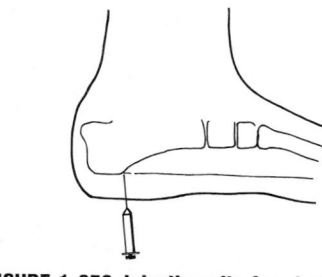

FIGURE 1-653 Injection site for plantar fasciitis. Injection should be through the sole into the area of maximum tenderness. A 25- or 27-gauge needle should be used and the medication injected slowly because some pain may occur. The total volume should be no greater than 1.5 ml. (From Mercier L: *Practical orthopedics,* ed 5, St Louis, 2002, Mosby.)

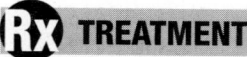 TREATMENT

- Supportive lace-up sneakers with firm, cushioned sole. Weight loss for obese patients
- Ice, stretching exercises, NSAIDs, limit activity
- Low-dye strapping/taping
- Steroid/local anesthetic injections (Fig. 1-653) via several techniques. Although corticosteroid injection is often used to alleviate pain from plantar fasciitis, evidence supporting this treatment is limited. Trials have shown that pain improvement after steroid injection is slightly faster than placebo and benefits are likely to be short lived.
- Custom orthotics will limit subtalar joint overpronation and other faulty biomechanics.
- Add heel cushion to orthotics if acute pain/inflammation.
- Heel lifts if the etiology is Achilles equinus or pseudoequinus
- Night splints maintain ankle dorsiflexion overnight.
- Severe cases may require a cast or cast walker for 4 to 6 wk.
- Recalcitrant cases may require surgical endoscopic or open fasciotomy.

DISPOSITION

Cases that are treated sooner and acute cases with sudden onset have a higher likelihood of resolving completely. Chronic, recalcitrant cases may require surgery.

REFERRAL

- For biomechanical exam or surgical consult (podiatric/orthopedic foot/ankle surgeon)
- Physical therapy is often beneficial when first-line therapy fails.

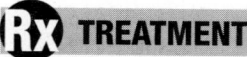 PEARLS & CONSIDERATIONS

COMMENTS

Caution: common, seemingly simple diagnosis. Do not overlook differential diagnosis.

PREVENTION

- Avoid shoes with bendable/flexible soles and shoes without laces/straps.
- Maintain foot/ankle flexibility with stretching exercises.
- Seek treatment at first signs of pain. Faster recovery rate with early diagnosis and treatment.

SUGGESTED READINGS
available at www.expertconsult.com

RELATED CONTENT

Plantar Fasciitis (Patient Information)

AUTHOR: **BROOKE E. KEELEY, D.P.M.**

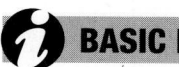 **BASIC INFORMATION**

DEFINITION

Pleurisy refers to the inflammation of the parietal pleura. This inflammation results in pleuritic chest pain that is characteristically worsened with respiration or movement.

SYNONYMS

Pleuritis

ICD-9CM CODES
511.0 Pleurisy

EPIDEMIOLOGY & DEMOGRAPHICS

INCIDENCE: One of the most common causes of pleuritic chest pain is viral pleurisy. However, there are a variety of disorders that may result in pleurisy. Infectious diseases, rheumatologic disorders, thromboembolic events, and trauma may all lead to pleural inflammation. Therefore, the incidence of pleurisy varies in accordance with the underlying etiology.

PHYSICAL FINDINGS & CLINICAL PRESENTATION

- The defining characteristic of pleurisy is chest pain that worsens with respiration, coughing, or sneezing.
- Pleuritic chest pain is typically described as sharp or stabbing. However, pleuritic chest pain may also be described as dull pain, burning pain, or a "catch" while breathing.
- Movements of the trunk or chest wall may exacerbate pain. Patients with pleurisy may locate the position of minimal discomfort and remain still in that position.
- Dyspnea may be associated with pleurisy.
- Physical exam may be remarkable for a pleural friction rub.
- Decreased breath sounds, rales, or egophony may be appreciated if pneumonia is the underlying etiology of the patient's pleurisy.

ETIOLOGY

- Pleurisy is caused by inflammation of the parietal pleura. The visceral pleura is not innervated by nociceptors. However, injury or inflammation at the periphery of the lung parenchyma often results in inflammation of the overlying parietal pleura. The parietal pleura, which lines the rib cage and the lateral portion of each hemidiaphragm, is innervated by intercostal nerves; therefore pain is localized to the cutaneous distribution of those nerves (over the chest wall). The parietal pleura of the central diaphragm is innervated by fibers that travel with the phrenic nerve; therefore pain associated with inflammation in this area is referred to the ipsilateral shoulder or neck.
- Various underlying etiologies may result in pleurisy, including:
  1. Thromboembolism (pulmonary embolism)
  2. Viral infection (coxsackieviruses, respiratory syncytial virus [RSV], cytomegalovirus [CMV], adenovirus, Epstein-Barr virus [EBV], parainfluenza, influenza)
  3. Bacterial infection (pneumonia or tuberculous pleuritis)
  4. Fungal infection (coccidioidomycosis, histoplasmosis)
  5. Rheumatologic disease (rheumatoid arthritis, systemic lupus erythematosus [SLE])
  6. Medications
  7. Malignancy of the lung or pleura
  8. Trauma (rib fracture)
  9. Hereditary (familial Mediterranean fever, sickle cell disease)

DX **DIAGNOSIS**

DIFFERENTIAL DIAGNOSIS

- Cardiac: myocardial infarction, ischemia, pericarditis
- Intraabdominal process: pancreatitis, cholecystitis
- Thromboembolic: pulmonary embolism, infarction of lung parenchyma
- Traumatic/mechanical: rib fracture or pneumothorax
- Viral infection: viral infections may lead to epidemic pleurodynia (also known as Bornholm's disease). Implicated viruses include coxsackieviruses, RSV, CMV, adenovirus, EBV, parainfluenza, influenza. Of note, viral pleurisy is a diagnosis of exclusion.
- Bacterial infection: pneumonia or tuberculous pleurisy
- Fungal infection: coccidioidomycosis, histoplasmosis
- Rheumatologic disease: rheumatoid arthritis, SLE
- Medications: drug-induced lupus
- Hereditary causes: familial Mediterranean fever, sickle cell disease
- Malignancy: malignancy affecting the lung or pleura
- Uremia

WORKUP

- A thorough history and physical exam of all patients presenting with pleuritic chest pain should be taken. The time course of the patient's symptoms can provide valuable diagnostic clues. Acute onset of symptoms is suggestive of traumatic injuries, spontaneous pneumothorax, pulmonary embolism, or myocardial infarction. Subacute onset of symptoms suggests a potential infectious, rheumatologic, or medication-induced cause. Viral pleurisy is often associated with prodromal symptoms of upper respiratory infection. Chronic or recurrent symptoms suggest a potential malignant, tuberculous, or hereditary cause.
- Chest x-ray to evaluate for pneumonia, pneumothorax, or pleural effusion
- ECG to evaluate for infarction, ischemia, or pericarditis
- Evaluation for pulmonary embolism should be undertaken if clinical suspicion exists.

LABORATORY TESTS

- Laboratory testing varies based on suspected underlying etiology.
- If a pleural effusion is present, diagnostic thoracentesis may provide valuable diagnostic clues to the underlying etiology.

IMAGING STUDIES

- Chest x-ray
- ECG

Rx **TREATMENT**

- Treatment of pleurisy consists of pain control as well as treating the underlying condition.
- NSAIDs are the preferred first-line agent to control pain associated with pleurisy. Human studies have been limited to trials using indomethacin for pain control, although an NSAID class effect is presumed.
- Indomethacin 50 mg orally up to three times a day has been found to be effective in relieving pain and is associated with an improvement in mechanical lung function.

SUGGESTED READINGS
available at www.expertconsult.com

AUTHOR: **MARISA E. VAN POZNAK, M.D.**

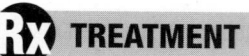

BASIC INFORMATION

DEFINITION

Aspiration pneumonia is a vague term that refers to pulmonary abnormalities following abnormal entry of endogenous or exogenous substances in the lower airways. It is generally classified as:

- Aspiration (chemical pneumonitis)
- Primary bacterial aspiration pneumonia
- Secondary bacterial infection of chemical pneumonitis

ICD-9CM CODES

507.0 Aspiration pneumonia

EPIDEMIOLOGY & DEMOGRAPHICS

INCIDENCE (IN U.S.):
- Few reliable data
- 20% to 35% of all pneumonias
- 5% to 15% of all community-acquired pneumonias

PEAK INCIDENCE: Elderly patients in hospitals or nursing homes

PREVALENCE (IN U.S.): Unknown (unreliable data)

PREDOMINANT SEX: Males and females affected equally

PREDOMINANT AGE: Elderly

PHYSICAL FINDINGS & CLINICAL PRESENTATION

- Shortness of breath, tachypnea, cough, sputum, fever after vomiting, or difficulty swallowing
- Rales, rhonchi, often diffusely throughout lung

ETIOLOGY

Complex interaction of etiologies, ranging from chemical (often acid) pneumonitis after aspiration of sterile gastric contents (generally not requiring antibiotic treatment) to bacterial aspiration

COMMUNITY-ACQUIRED ASPIRATION PNEUMONIA:

- Generally results from predominantly anaerobic mouth bacteria (anaerobic and microaerophilic streptococci, fusobacteria, gram-positive anaerobic non–spore-forming rods), *Bacteroides* species *(melaninogenicus, intermedius, oralis, ureolyticus)*, *Haemophilus influenzae*, and *Streptococcus pneumoniae*
- Rarely caused by *Bacteroides fragilis* (of uncertain validity in published studies) or *Eikenella corrodens*
- High-risk groups: the elderly; alcoholics; IV drug users; patients who are obtunded; stroke victims; and those with esophageal disorders, seizures, poor dentition, or recent dental manipulations.

HOSPITAL-ACQUIRED ASPIRATION PNEUMONIA:

- Often occurs among elderly patients and others with diminished gag reflex; those with nasogastric tubes, intestinal obstruction, or ventilator support; and especially those exposed to contaminated nebulizers or unsterile suctioning.

- High-risk groups: seriously ill hospitalized patients (especially patients with coma, acidosis, alcoholism, uremia, diabetes mellitus, nasogastric intubation, or recent antimicrobial therapy, who are frequently colonized with aerobic gram-negative rods); patients undergoing anesthesia; those with strokes, dementia, or swallowing disorders; the elderly; and those receiving antacids or H_2 blockers (but not sucralfate).
- Hypoxic patients receiving concentrated O_2 have diminished ciliary activity, encouraging aspiration.
- Causative organisms:
  1. Anaerobes listed above, although in many studies gram-negative aerobes (60%) and gram-positive aerobes (20%) predominate.
  2. *E. coli, P. aeruginosa, S. aureus* including MRSA, *Klebsiella, Enterobacter, Serratia, Proteus* spp., *H. influenzae, S. pneumoniae, Legionella,* and *Acinetobacter* spp. (sporadic pneumonias) in two thirds of cases.
  3. Fungi, including *Candida albicans,* in fewer than 1%.

DIAGNOSIS

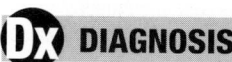

DIFFERENTIAL DIAGNOSIS

- Other necrotizing or cavitary pneumonias (especially tuberculosis, gram-negative pneumonias)
- See "Pulmonary Tuberculosis."

WORKUP

- Chest x-ray examination
- Complete blood count (CBC), blood cultures
- Sputum Gram stain and culture
- Consideration of tracheal aspirate

LABORATORY TESTS

- CBC: leukocytosis often present
- Sputum Gram stain
  1. Often useful when carefully prepared immediately after obtaining suctioned or expectorated specimen, examined by experienced observer.
  2. Only specimens with multiple white blood cells and rare or absent epithelial cells should be examined.
  3. Unlike nonaspiration pneumonias (e.g., pneumococcal), multiple organisms may be present.
  4. Long, slender rods suggest anaerobes.
  5. Sputum from pneumonia caused by acid aspiration may be devoid of organisms.
  6. Cultures should be interpreted in light of morphology of visualized organisms.

IMAGING STUDIES

- Chest x-ray often reveals bilateral, diffuse, patchy infiltrates and posterior segment upper lobes. Chemical pneumonitis typically affects the most dependent regions of the lungs.
- Aspiration pneumonia of several days' or longer duration may reveal necrosis (especially community-acquired anaerobic pneumonias) and even cavitation with air-fluid levels, indicating lung abscess.

TREATMENT

NONPHARMACOLOGIC THERAPY

- Airway management to prevent repeated aspiration
- Ventilatory support if necessary

ACUTE GENERAL Rx

Acute aspiration of acidic gastric contents without bacteria may not require antibiotic therapy; consult infectious disease or pulmonary expert.

- Community-acquired anaerobic aspiration pneumonia: clindamycin (600 mg IV twice daily followed by 300 mg q6h orally). Intravenous penicillin G (1 to 2 million U q4 to 6h) can also still be used. Alternative oral agents include: amoxicillin-clavulanate (875 mg orally twice daily), amoxicillin plus metronidazole or oral moxifloxacin (400 mg orally once daily). Do not use metronidazole alone, as this is associated with high failure rates.
- Nursing home aspirations: levofloxacin 500-750 mg qd or piperacillin-tazobactam 3.375 g q6h or ceftazidime 2 g q8h +/− vancomycin if MRSA suspected or known
- Hospital-acquired aspiration pneumonia:
  ○ Piperacillin-tazobactam 3.375 g IV q6h, or cefoxitin 2 g IV q8h +/− vancomycin IV to cover MRSA. Alternative agents are ceftriaxone 1 g IV q24h *plus* metronidazole 500 mg IV q6h or 1 g IV q12h.
  ○ Knowledge of resident flora in the microenvironment of the aspiration within the hospital is crucial to intelligent antibiotic selection; consult infection control nurses or hospital epidemiologist.
  ○ Confirmed *Pseudomonas* pneumonia should be treated with antipseudomonal beta-lactam agent plus an aminoglycoside until antimicrobial sensitivities confirm that less toxic agents may replace the aminoglycoside.
  ○ Do not use metronidazole alone for anaerobes.

DISPOSITION

Repeat chest x-ray examination in 6 to 8 wk.

REFERRAL

For consultation with infectious disease and/or pulmonary experts for patients with respiratory distress, hypoxia, ventilatory support, pneumonia in more than one lobe, or necrosis or cavitation on x-ray examination or for those not responding to antibiotic therapy within 2 to 3 days.

SUGGESTED READINGS

available at www.expertconsult.com

RELATED CONTENT

Aspiration Pneumonia (Patient Information)

AUTHOR: **GLENN G. FORT, M.D., M.P.H.**

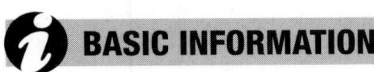 **BASIC INFORMATION**

DEFINITION

Bacterial pneumonia is an infection involving the lung parenchyma.

ICD-9CM CODES
486.0 Pneumonia, acute
507.0 Pneumonia, aspiration
482.9 Pneumonia, bacterial
481   Pneumonia, pneumococcal
482.1 Pneumonia, *Pseudomonas*
482.4 Pneumonia, staphylococcal
482.0 Pneumonia, *Klebsiella*
482.2 Pneumonia, *Haemophilus influenzae*

EPIDEMIOLOGY & DEMOGRAPHICS

- The incidence of community-acquired pneumonia (CAP) is 1 in 100 persons. CAP is the most common infectious cause of death in the U.S.
- The incidence of health care facility–acquired pneumonia (HCAP) is 8 cases per 1000 persons annually.
- Primary care physicians see an average of 10 cases of pneumonia annually.
- Hospitalization rate for pneumonia is 15% to 20%.
- Most cases of pneumonia occur in the winter and in elderly patients.

PHYSICAL FINDINGS & CLINICAL PRESENTATION

- Fever, tachypnea, chills, tachycardia, cough
- Presentation varies with the cause of pneumonia, the patient's age, and the clinical situation:
  - Patients with streptococcal pneumonia usually present with high fever, shaking chills, pleuritic chest pain, cough, and copious production of rusty-appearing purulent sputum. Pleurisy and parapneumonic effusions are also common. Potential complications include bacteremia, empyema, and distant infections (e.g., meningitis).
  - *Mycoplasma pneumoniae:* insidious onset; headache; dry, paroxysmal cough that is worse at night; myalgias; malaise; sore throat; extrapulmonary manifestations (e.g., erythema multiforme, aseptic meningitis, urticaria, erythema nodosum) may be present.
  - *Chlamydia pneumoniae:* persistent, nonproductive cough, low-grade fever, headache, sore throat.
  - *Legionella pneumophila:* high fever, mild cough, mental status change, myalgias, diarrhea, respiratory failure.
  - MRSA pneumonia: often preceded by influenza, may present with shock and respiratory failure.
  - Elderly or immunocompromised hosts with pneumonia may initially present with only minimal symptoms (e.g., low-grade fever, confusion); respiratory and nonrespiratory symptoms are less commonly reported by older patients with pneumonia.
  - In general, auscultation of patients with pneumonia reveals crackles and diminished breath sounds.
  - Percussion dullness is present if the patient has pleural effusion.
  - The clinical impression of pneumonia has an overall sensitivity of 70% to 90%; specificity ranges from 40% to 70%.

ETIOLOGY

- *Streptococcus pneumoniae* (20% to 60% of CAP cases)
- *Haemophilus influenzae* (3% to 10% of CAP cases)
- *L. pneumophila* (1% to 5% of adult pneumonias) (2% to 8% of CAP cases)
- *Klebsiella, Pseudomonas, Escherichia coli*
- *Staphylococcus aureus* (3% to 5% of CAP cases)
- Atypical organisms such as *M. pneumoniae, C. pneumoniae,* and *L. pneumophila* implicated in up to 40% of cases of CAP
- Pneumococcal infection responsible for 50% to 75% of CAPs. Influenza infection is one of the important predisposing factors to *S. pneumoniae* and *S. aureus* pneumonia; gram-negative organisms cause >80% of nosocomial pneumonias
- Predisposing factors:
  1. Chronic obstructive pulmonary disease: *H. influenzae, S. pneumoniae, Legionella*
  2. Seizures: aspiration pneumonia
  3. Compromised hosts: *Legionella,* gram-negative organisms
  4. Alcoholism: *Klebsiella, S. pneumoniae, H. influenzae*
  5. HIV: *S. pneumoniae*
  6. IV drug addicts with right-sided bacterial endocarditis: *S. aureus*
  7. Older patient with comorbid diseases: *C. pneumoniae*

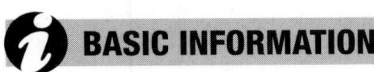 **DIAGNOSIS**

DIFFERENTIAL DIAGNOSIS

- Exacerbation of chronic bronchitis
- Pulmonary embolism or infarction
- Lung neoplasm
- Bronchiolitis
- Sarcoidosis
- Hypersensitivity pneumonitis
- Pulmonary edema
- Drug-induced lung injury
- Viral pneumonias
- Fungal pneumonias
- Parasitic pneumonias
- Atypical pneumonia
- Tuberculosis

WORKUP

Laboratory evaluation and chest x-ray. Table E1-329 summarizes diagnostic testing for CAP. Useful tools for assessing severity of illness are the *CURB-65* (see following) and *Pneumonia Severity Index.* Poor prognostic indicators are hypotension (SBP <90 or DBP <60), respiratory rate >30/min, hyperpyrexia (>40° C), or hypothermia (<35° C). None of these indices is as valuable as clinical judgment of the physician.

LABORATORY TESTS

- Complete blood count with differential; white blood cell count is elevated, usually with left shift
- Blood cultures (hospitalized patients only): positive in approximately 20% of cases of pneumococcal pneumonia
- Pneumococcal urinary antigen test can be used to detect the C-polysaccharide antigen of *S. pneumoniae.* It is a useful tool in the treatment of hospitalized adult patients with CAP.
- Direct immunofluorescent examination of sputum when suspecting *Legionella* (e.g., direct fluorescent antibody stain is a highly specific and rapid test for detecting legionellae in clinical specimen) or urine *Legionella* antigen test
- Serologic testing for HIV in selected patients
- Serum electrolytes (hyponatremia in suspected *Legionella* pneumonia), BUN, creatinine
- Pulse oximetry or arterial blood gases: hypoxemia with partial pressure of oxygen <60 mm Hg while the patient is breathing room air, a standard criterion for hospital admission

IMAGING STUDIES

Chest x-ray: findings vary with the stage and type of pneumonia and the hydration of the patient (Fig. 1-654):

- Classically, pneumococcal pneumonia presents with a segmental lobe infiltrate.
- Diffuse infiltrates on chest x-ray can be seen with *L. pneumophila, M. pneumoniae,* viral pneumonias, *P. jirovecii (carinii),* miliary tuberculosis, aspiration, aspergillosis.
- An initial chest x-ray is also useful to rule out the presence of any complications (pneumothorax, empyema, abscesses).

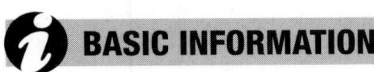 **TREATMENT**

NONPHARMACOLOGIC THERAPY

- Avoidance of tobacco use
- Oxygen to maintain partial oxygen pressure in arterial blood >60 mm Hg
- IV hydration, correction of dehydration
- Assisted ventilation in patients with significant respiratory failure

ACUTE GENERAL Rx

- Initial antibiotic therapy should be based on clinical, radiographic, and laboratory evaluation.
- Macrolides (azithromycin or clarithromycin) or levofloxacin is recommended for empiric outpatient treatment of CAP. Box E1-47 summarizes empirical therapy regimens for severe CAP. Cefotaxime or a beta-lactam/beta-lactamase inhibitor can be added in patients with more severe presentation who insist on outpatient therapy. Duration of treatment ranges from 7 to 14 days. The treatment of choice in suspected *Legionella* pneumonia is either a quinolone (e.g., moxifloxacin) or a macrolide (e.g., azithromycin) antibiotic.
- In the hospital setting, patients admitted to the general ward can be treated empirically

with a second- or third-generation cephalo-sporin (ceftriaxone, ceftizoxime, cefotaxime, or cefuroxime) plus a macrolide (azithromy-cin or clarithromycin) or doxycycline. An an-tipseudomonal quinolone (levofloxacin or moxifloxacin) can be substituted in place of the macrolide or doxycycline.

- Empiric therapy in ICU patients: IV beta-lactam (ceftriaxone, cefotaxime, ampicillin-sulbactam) plus an IV quinolone (levofloxacin, moxifloxacin) or IV azithromycin.
- In hospitalized patients at risk for *P. aeruginosa* infection, empiric treatment should consist of an antipseudomonal beta-lactam (merope-nem, doripenem, imipenem, or piperacillin-tazobactam) plus an aminoglycoside plus an antipseudomonal quinolone.
- In patients with suspected methicillin-resistant *S. aureus,* vancomycin or linezolid is effective.

CHRONIC Rx

Parapneumonic effusion empyema can be man-aged with chest tube placement for drainage. Instillation of fibrinolytic agents (streptokinase, urokinase) by chest tube may be necessary in resistant cases.

DISPOSITION

- Most patients respond well to antibiotic ther-apy. Risk factors for a poor outcome from CAP. are summarized in Box E1-48.
- Indications for hospital admission are:
  1. Hypoxemia (oxygen saturation <90% while patient is breathing room air)

2. Hemodynamic instability
3. Inability to tolerate medications
4. Active coexisting condition requiring hos-pitalization

A criterion often used to determine hospital admission is known as the "CURB-65": **C**on-fusion, **B**UN >19.6 mg/dl, **R**espiratory rate >30 breaths/min, systolic **B**P <90 mg Hg, and diastolic BP ≤60 mm Hg, age ≥**65**. Pa-tients are generally admitted to the hospital if they fulfill 2 or more criteria and to the ICU if they have 3 or more criteria.

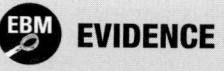 **PEARLS & CONSIDERATIONS**

COMMENTS

- Use of gastric acid suppressive therapy (H₂ receptor antagonists, proton pump inhibi-tors [PPIs]) has been associated with an increased risk of CAP. It appears that PPI therapy started within the previous 30 days is associated with an increased risk for CAP, whereas longer-term current use is not.
- Causes of slowly resolving or nonresolving pneumonia:
  1. Difficult to treat infections: viral pneumo-nia, *Legionella,* pneumococci or staphylo-cocci with impaired host response, tuber-culosis, fungi
  2. Neoplasm: lung, lymphoma, metastasis
  3. Congestive heart failure
  4. Pulmonary embolism

5. Immunologic or idiopathic: Wegener gran-ulomatosis, pulmonary eosinophilic syn-dromes, systemic lupus erythematosus
6. Drug toxicity (e.g., amiodarone)

- If patients with pneumonia are not doing well, repeat films should be taken promptly. In those with complete clinical recovery, it is reasonable to wait 6 to 8 wk before repeating the radiograph to document clearing of the infiltrate. The benefit of routine radiography after pneumonia has been questioned due to the low 1 yr incidence of lung cancer. Oppo-nents propose a selective approach limiting follow-up chest x-ray to middle-aged and older adults.

EBM **EVIDENCE**

available at www.expertconsult.com

SUGGESTED READINGS

available at www.expertconsult.com

RELATED CONTENT

Bacterial Pneumonia (Patient Information)

AUTHOR: **FRED F. FERRI, M.D.**

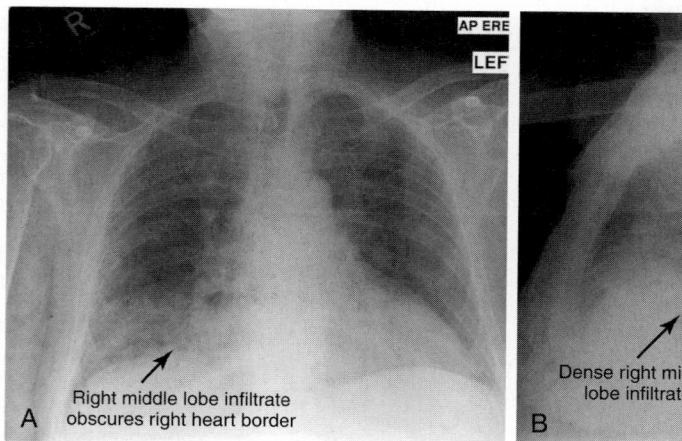
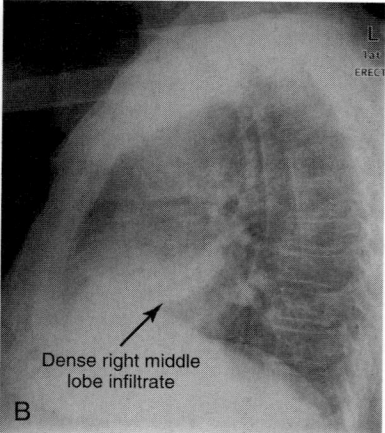

FIGURE 1-654 Pneumonia, right middle lobe. A, Anteroposterior chest x-ray. **B,** Lateral chest x-ray. This 73-year-old man presented with cough and yellow sputum, fever 39.3° C, tachycardia, and oxygen saturation of 93% on room air. His chest x-ray shows classic right middle lobe pneumonia. The opacity in **A** obscures the right heart border, which lies immediately adjacent. On the lateral x-ray **(B),** this appears as a more circumscribed density overlying the heart. (From Broder JS: *Diagnostic imaging for the emergency physician,* Philadelphia, 2011, Saunders.)

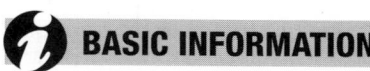

BASIC INFORMATION

DEFINITION

Mycoplasma pneumonia is an infection of the lung parenchyma caused by a small bacterium, *Mycoplasma pneumoniae*.

SYNONYMS

Primary atypical pneumonia
Eaton's pneumonia
Walking pneumonia

ICD-9CM CODES
483 *Mycoplasma* pneumonia

EPIDEMIOLOGY & DEMOGRAPHICS

INCIDENCE (IN U.S.):
- It is a frequent cause of community-acquired pneumonia. CDC estimates 2 million cases a yr with 100,000 pneumonia-related hospitalizations.
- Many cases probably resolve without coming to medical attention.
- Incidence is estimated at one case per 1000 persons annually.
- Incidence is estimated to at least triple every (approximately) 5 yr during epidemics.

PEAK INCIDENCE:
- Some increased incidence in fall to early winter
- Seems more prevalent in temperate climates

PREVALENCE (IN U.S.):
- Estimated to be present in one in every five patients hospitalized for pneumonia (generally a self-limited disease, so its true prevalence is unknown)
- Estimated to cause 7% of all cases of pneumonia and approximately half the cases in those aged 5 to 20 yr

PREDOMINANT SEX: Equal distribution

PREDOMINANT AGE:
- Most commonly affected: school-age children and young adults (ages 5 to 20 yr)
- Occurs in older adults as well, especially with household exposure to a young child
- More severe infections in affected elderly patients

GENETICS: Familial disposition:
- None known
- May be more severe in patients with sickle cell anemia

Neonatal infection: severe respiratory distress, sometimes requiring intubation, attributed to this disease in infants.

PHYSICAL FINDINGS & CLINICAL PRESENTATION

- Nonexudative pharyngitis (common)
- Headache, otalgia common
- Fever may be mild or not present
- Rhonchi or rales without evidence of consolidation (common) in lower lung zones
- Associated with bullous myringitis (nonspecific finding; perhaps no more frequently than in other pneumonias)
- Skin rashes in up to one fourth of patients
  1. Morbilliform
  2. Urticaria
  3. Erythema nodosum (unusual)
  4. Erythema multiforme (unusual)
  5. Stevens-Johnson syndrome (rare)
- Muscle tenderness (<50% of the patients)
- On examination (and confirmed with testing):
  1. Mononeuritis or polyneuritis
  2. Transverse myelitis
  3. Cranial nerve palsies
  4. Meningoencephalitis
- Lymphadenopathy and splenomegaly
- Conjunctivitis
- Table 1-330 summarizes the clinical manifestations of *Mycoplasma pneumoniae*.

ETIOLOGY

Infection is spread person-to-person via respiratory droplets or secretions with an incubation period of 1 to 4 wk.

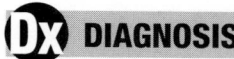 DIAGNOSIS

DIFFERENTIAL DIAGNOSIS

- *Chlamydia* (now known as *Chlamydophila*) *pneumoniae*
- *Chlamydophila psittaci*
- *Legionella* spp.
- *Coxiella burnetii*
- Several viral agents
- Q fever
- *Streptococcus pneumoniae*
- Pulmonary embolism or infarction

WORKUP

- Chest x-ray
- Thorough history and physical examination

- Laboratory tests
- Evaluation guided by symptoms and findings

LABORATORY TESTS

- White blood cells (WBCs):
  1. WBC count $>10,000/mm^3$ in approximately one fourth of patients
  2. Differential count nonspecific
  3. Leukopenia rare
- Cold agglutinins:
  1. Detected in approximately half of the patients
  2. Also may be found in:
     a. Lymphoproliferative diseases
     b. Influenza
     c. Mononucleosis
     d. Adenovirus infections
     e. Occasionally, Legionnaires' disease
  3. Titers typically >1:64
     a. May be detectable with bedside testing
     b. Appear between days 5 and 10 of the illness (so may be demonstrable when patient is first examined) and disappear within 1 mo
- Complement fixation testing assay specific for mycoplasm antigens of paired sera (four-fold rise) or a single titer ≥1:32 in patients with pneumonia and a compatible history:
  1. Considered diagnostic in the appropriate clinical setting
  2. Other assays include ELISA, antigen capture-enzyme immunoassay, and PCR
- Culture of the organism from specimens
  1. Only truly specific test for infection
  2. Technically difficult and done reliably by few laboratories
  3. May require weeks to get results
- Sputum
  1. Often no sputum produced for laboratory testing
  2. When present, Gram-stained specimens show polymorphonuclear cells without organisms
- Infection occasionally complicated by pancreatitis or glomerulitis
- Disseminated intravascular coagulation is a rare complication
- Electrocardiographic evidence of pericarditis or myocarditis may be present

IMAGING STUDIES

- Predilection for lower lobe involvement (upper lobes involved in less than a fourth), with radiographic abnormalities frequently out of proportion to those on physical examination (Fig. 1-655)
- Small pleural effusions in approximately 30% of patients
- Large effusions: rare
- Infiltrates: patchy, unilateral, and with a segmental distribution, although multilobar involvement may be seen
- Evidence of hilar adenopathy on chest radiographs in 20% to 25%
- Rare cases reported:
  1. Associated lung abscess
  2. Residual pneumatoceles
  3. Lobar collapse
  4. Hyperlucent lung syndrome

TABLE 1-330	Clinical Manifestations of *Mycoplasma Pneumoniae* Infection	
Respiratory tract	Pharyngitis, laryngitis, acute bronchitis, bronchopneumonia
Skin and mucosa	Maculopapular and vesicular exanthema, urticaria, purpura, erythema nodosum, erythema multiforme, Stevens-Johnson syndrome
Central nervous system	Meningitis, meningoencephalitis, acute psychosis, cerebellitis, Guillain-Barré syndrome?
Parenchymatous organs	Pancreatitis, diabetes mellitus, nonspecific reactive hepatitis, subacute thyroiditis?
Miscellaneous	Hemorrhagic bullous myringitis, hemolytic anemia, pericarditis, thromboembolism?

Some association remains uncertain.
From Cohen J, Powderly WG: *Infectious diseases,* ed 2, St Louis, 2004, Mosby.

Rx TREATMENT

ACUTE GENERAL Rx

- Therapy: azithromycin 500 mg qd × 3 or 500 mg initially, then 250 mg daily for 4 days for adults. For children: 10 mg/kg in one dose on first day, then 5 mg/kg in one dose for 4 days or clarithromycin: 500 mg bid for 10 days in adults, 15 mg/kg per day in two divided doses for 10 days in children. Alternatives include erythromycin (500 mg qid) for adults or 30 to 40 mg/kg per day in four divided doses in children or doxycycline: 2 to 4 mg/kg per day in one or two divided doses for 10 days, maximum daily dose: 100 to 200 mg, but this agent cannot be used in young children or women of childbearing age. Respiratory fluoroquinolones such as Levaquin or moxifloxacin are alternative agents for treatment in adults but should not be used in young children.
- Therapy shortens the duration and severity of symptoms and may hasten radiographic clearing, but the disease is self-limiting.

CHRONIC Rx

- Effective antimicrobial therapy does not eliminate the organism from the respiratory secretions, which may be positive for weeks.

- Serum antibody response does not necessarily provide lifelong immunity.
- Chronic symptoms do not occur, although clinical relapses may occur 7 to 10 days after the initial response and may be associated with new areas of infiltration.

DISPOSITION

- Clinical improvement is almost universal within 10 days.
- Infiltrates generally clear within 5 to 8 wk.
- Rare deaths are likely attributable to underlying medical diseases.
- Person-to-person spread can be minimized by avoiding open coughing, especially in enclosed areas.

REFERRAL

- Not responding to treatment
- Severe infection
- Severe extrapulmonary manifestations
- Multilobe involvement accompanied by respiratory embarrassment (very rare)

❶ PEARLS & CONSIDERATIONS

COMMENTS

X-ray resolution complete by 8 wk in approximately 90% of patients.

SUGGESTED READINGS

available at www.expertconsult.com

RELATED CONTENT

Mycoplasmal Pneumonia (Patient Information)

AUTHOR: **GLENN G. FORT, M.D., M.P.H.**

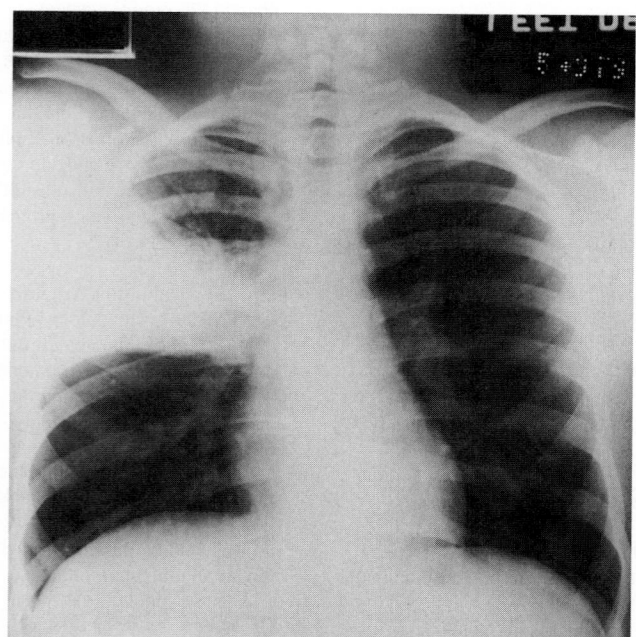

FIGURE 1-655 Localized airspace opacification resulting from ***Mycoplasma pneumoniae.*** (From Specht N [ed]: *Practical guide to diagnostic imaging,* St Louis, 1998, Mosby.)

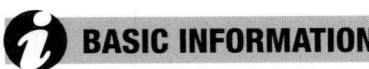
BASIC INFORMATION

DEFINITION

Pneumocystis jirovecii pneumonia (PJP) is a serious respiratory infection caused by the fungal or protozoal organism *P. jirovecii* (formerly known as *P. carinii*).

SYNONYMS

PCP
PJP

ICD-9CM CODES
136.3 *Pneumocystis jirovecii* (*P. carinii*) pneumonia

EPIDEMIOLOGY & DEMOGRAPHICS

INCIDENCE (IN U.S.):
- Seen primarily in the setting of AIDS
- Approximately 11 cases per 100 patient-years among HIV-infected patients with CD4 lymphocyte counts $<100/mm^3$
- Also seen in other immunocompromised patients with severe cell-mediated immune deficiency (congenital T-cell deficiency, acute leukemia, lymphoma, bone marrow or organ transplant deficiency)
- Rituximab use has been associated with *Pneumocystis* pneumonia in HIV-negative patients, most of whom had hematologic cancers.

PEAK INCIDENCE: Age 20 to 40 yr (parallel to AIDS epidemic)
PREDOMINANT SEX: Equal incidence when corrected for HIV status
PREDOMINANT AGE:
- $<$2 yr
- 20 to 40 yr

GENETICS: Neonatal infection:
- Most frequent opportunistic infection among HIV-infected children, occurring in approximately 30%
- Neonatal occurrence unusual

PHYSICAL FINDINGS & CLINICAL PRESENTATION

- Fever, cough, shortness of breath present in almost all cases
- Lungs frequently clear to auscultation, although rales occasionally present
- Cyanosis and pronounced tachypnea in severe cases
- Hemoptysis unusual
- Spontaneous pneumothorax

ETIOLOGY

- *P. jirovecii* (formerly *P. carinii*) recently reclassified as a fungal organism
- Reactivation of dormant infection
- Extrapulmonary involvement rare

DIAGNOSIS

DIFFERENTIAL DIAGNOSIS

- Other opportunistic respiratory infections:
  1. Tuberculosis
  2. Histoplasmosis
  3. Cryptococcosis
- Nonopportunistic infections:
  1. Bacterial pneumonia
  2. Viral pneumonia
  3. Mycoplasmal pneumonia
  4. Legionellosis
- Occurs virtually exclusively in the setting of profound depression of cellular immunity

WORKUP

- Chest x-ray
- Arterial blood gases
- Because *Pneumocystis* cannot be cultured, diagnosis relies on detection of the organism by colorimetric or immunofluorescent stains or PCR.
- Sputum examination for cysts of PJP and to exclude other pathogens
- Bronchoscopy with bronchoalveolar lavage or lung biopsy for diagnosis if sputum examination is negative or equivocal. Stains such as Gomori methenamine silver stain or toluidine blue O are used to identify the organism.

LABORATORY TESTS

- Arterial blood gas monitoring
- Elevated lactate dehydrogenase in majority of cases
- HIV antibody test if cause of underlying immune deficiency state is unclear

IMAGING STUDIES

Diffuse uptake on gallium scanning of the lungs is suggestive but not diagnostic.

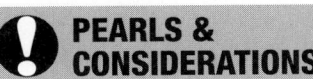
TREATMENT

NONPHARMACOLOGIC THERAPY

- Supplemental oxygen
- Ventilatory support if needed
- Prompt thoracotomy if pneumothorax develops

ACUTE GENERAL Rx

For confirmed or suspected PJP:
- Trimethoprim-sulfamethoxazole (15 to 20 mg/kg trimethoprim and 75 to 100 mg/kg sulfamethoxazole qd) PO or IV per day divided and given q6 to 8h
- Pentamidine (4 mg/kg IV qd)
- Either regimen with prednisone (40 mg PO bid):
  1. If arterial oxygen pressure $<$70 mm Hg
  2. If arterial-alveolar oxygen pressure difference $>$35 mm Hg

  3. Dose tapered to 20 mg bid after 5 days and 20 mg qd after 10 days
- Therapy continued for 3 wk
- Alternative therapies available for patients unable to tolerate conventional therapy:
  1. Dapsone/trimethoprim
  2. Clindamycin/primaquine
  3. Atovaquone

CHRONIC Rx

- After completion of therapy, lifelong prophylaxis should be maintained with trimethoprim-sulfamethoxazole (one single-strength tablet PO qd or double-strength three times weekly).
- Patients intolerant of this therapy should be treated with dapsone (50 mg PO qd) plus pyrimethamine (50 mg PO weekly) plus leucovorin (25 mg PO weekly).
- Inhaled pentamidine (300 mg monthly by standardized nebulizer) is less effective and is reserved for patients intolerant to other forms of prophylaxis.
- Same approach taken to all HIV-infected patients with CD4 lymphocyte counts <200 to $250/mm^3$ or $<20\%$ of the total lymphocyte count because of their high risk of PJP.

DISPOSITION

After completion of therapy, long-term ambulatory follow-up is mandatory to provide secondary prevention of PJP (see "Chronic Rx" above) and management of the underlying immunodeficiency syndrome.

REFERRAL

- To pulmonologist for bronchoscopy if diagnosis cannot be confirmed by sputum examination
- To an infectious disease specialist if case is severe or difficult to manage

PEARLS & CONSIDERATIONS

COMMENTS

All patients, especially those with severe infection or intolerant of conventional therapy, should be followed by a physician experienced in the management of PJP and, if appropriate, in the long-term management of HIV infection or other underlying disease.

Severe and life-threatening hypoglycemia may occur after 1 or 2 wk after start of IV pentamidine. Monitor closely and advise the patient of symptoms of hypoglycemia.

SUGGESTED READINGS
available at www.expertconsult.com

RELATED CONTENT

Pneumocystis Pneumonia (Patient Information)

AUTHOR: **GLENN G. FORT, M.D., M.P.H.**

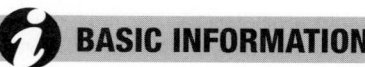

BASIC INFORMATION

DEFINITION

Viral pneumonia is infection of the pulmonary parenchyma caused by any of a large number of viral agents. The most important viruses are discussed.

SYNONYMS

Nonbacterial pneumonia
Atypical pneumonia

ICD-9CM CODES
480.8 Viral pneumonia
487.0 Viral pneumonia due to influenza

EPIDEMIOLOGY & DEMOGRAPHICS

INCIDENCE (IN U.S.):
- Influenza virus:
  1. 10% to 20% of population in temperate zones infected during 1-2 mo epidemics occurring yearly during winter months.
  2. Up to 50% infected during pandemics.
  3. Pneumonia develops in small percentage of infected persons.
- Incidence of other important viral pneumonias is not known precisely.

PEAK INCIDENCE:
- Influenza:
  1. Winter months for influenza A
  2. Year round for influenza B
  3. Peak of pneumonia seen weeks into the outbreak of infection
- Respiratory syncytial virus (RSV) and parainfluenza virus:
  1. Winter and spring
- Adenovirus:
  1. Endemic (military)
- Varicella:
  1. Spring in temperate zones
- Measles:
  1. Year round
- Cytomegalovirus (CMV):
  1. Year round

PREVALENCE (IN U.S.):
- Often related to immune status of the population or presence of an epidemic
- Normal hosts (estimates):
  1. 86% of cases of pneumonia resulting in hospitalization in American adults
  2. 16% of pediatric pneumonias managed as outpatients
  3. 49% of hospitalized infants with pneumonia
- Important problem in hosts with impaired immunity

PREDOMINANT SEX:
- None generally
- Male sex may predispose to more severe respiratory disease in RSV infection

PREDOMINANT AGE:
- Influenza:
  1. Overall incidence greatest at age 5 yr
  2. Lower with increasing age
  3. The most serious sequelae in those with chronic medical illnesses, especially cardiopulmonary disease
  4. Hospitalizations greatest in infants and adults aged >64 yr

- RSV and parainfluenza virus:
  1. Young children (as the major cause of pneumonia)
  2. Occurs throughout life
- Adenoviruses:
  1. Young children
  2. Adults, primarily military recruits
- Varicella:
  1. Approximately 16% of adults (not infected in childhood) who contract chickenpox
  2. Acute varicella during pregnancy more likely to be complicated by severe pneumonia
  3. 90% of reported varicella pneumonia cases are in adults (highest incidence ages 20 to 60 yr)
- Measles:
  1. Young adults and older children who received a single vaccination (5% failure rate)
  2. Measles during pregnancy more likely to be complicated by pneumonia
  3. Underlying cardiopulmonary diseases and immunosuppression predispose to serious pneumonia complicating measles
  4. Before availability of measles vaccine, 90% of pneumonias in those <10 yr
  5. Currently more than one third of U.S. patients >14 yr
  6. 3% to 50% of measles cases are complicated by pneumonia
- CMV:
  1. Neonatal through adult
  2. Immunosuppression is key predisposing factor

GENETICS:
Familial disposition:
- Close contact, not genetics, is important in acquisition
- Congenital anomalies and immunosuppression worsen course of RSV pneumonia
Congenital infection:
- CMV is the most common intrauterine infection in the U.S.
- Pneumonia occurs occasionally in infants with symptomatic congenital infection.
Neonatal infection:
- Severe RSV pneumonia
- Adenovirus pneumonia
  1. 5% to 20% mortality rate
  2. Can lead to residual restrictive or obstructive functional abnormalities
- "Varicella neonatorum"
  1. Disseminated visceral disease including pneumonia
  2. May develop in neonates whose mothers develop peripartum chickenpox
- CMV pneumonia
  1. Generally fatal
  2. Associated with severe cerebral damage in this population

PHYSICAL FINDINGS & CLINICAL PRESENTATION

1. Influenza:
   - Fever, cough, or sore throat (reffered to as influenza-like illness [ILI])
   - Uncomfortable or lethargic appearance
   - Prominent dry cough (rarely hemoptysis)
   - Flushed integument and erythematous mucous membranes

   - Rales or rhonchi
2. RSV and parainfluenza:
   - Fever
   - Tachypnea
   - Prolonged expiration
   - Wheezes and rales
3. Adenoviruses:
   - Hoarseness
   - Pharyngitis
   - Tachypnea
   - Cervical adenitis
4. Measles:
   - Conjunctivitis
   - Rhinorrhea
   - Koplik's spots (white lesions on the buccal mucosa)
   - Exanthem (maculopapular rash that starts on the head, then moves down to rest of body)
   - Pneumonitis
     a. May occur as a complication in 3% to 4% of adolescents and young adults
     b. Coincident with rash
     c. May also develop after apparent recovery from measles
   - Fever
   - Dry cough
5. Varicella:
   - Fever
   - Maculopapular or vesicular rash (all lesions at the same stage)
     a. Becomes encrusted
     b. Pneumonia typical 1 to 6 days after rash appears
     c. Pneumonia accompanied by cough and occasionally hemoptysis
   - Few auscultatory abnormalities noted on examination of the lungs
6. CMV:
   - Fever
   - Paroxysmal cough
   - Occasional hemoptysis
   - Diffuse adenopathy when pneumonia occurs after transfusion

ETIOLOGY

Viral infection can lead to pneumonia in both immunocompetent and immunocompromised hosts.

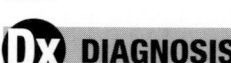

DIAGNOSIS

DIFFERENTIAL DIAGNOSIS

- Bacterial pneumonia, which frequently complicates (i.e., can follow or be simultaneous with) viral pneumonia
- Other causes of atypical pneumonia:
  1. *Mycoplasma* spp.
  2. *Chlamydia* spp.
  3. *Coxiella* spp.
  4. Legionnaires' disease
- Acute respiratory distress syndrome (ARDS)
- Physical findings and associated hypoxemia confused with pulmonary emboli

WORKUP

- Information about the current prevalent strain of influenza virus can be obtained from local

health departments or from the Centers for Disease Control and Prevention.

- Influenza and other viruses may be cultured from respiratory secretions during the initial few days of the illness (special media and techniques necessary).
- Respiratory viral panels that use PCR-based assays to test for a variety of viruses are extremely sensitive and are becoming the test of choice.
- Rapid flu tests have a 50% sensitivity in diagnosing influenza (a negative test does not mean the patient does not have influenza).
- Measles and adenovirus pneumonia are usually diagnosed clinically and can be confirmed with serology.
- CMV may be grown in culture or PCR amplified from bronchoalveolar lavage samples. An algorithm for the workup and management of suspected severe influenza pneumonia in the critical care unit is described in Fig. E1-656. Open lung biopsy is required for a definite diagnosis of CMV pneumonia.

LABORATORY TESTS

- Sputum Gram stain (usually produced in scanty amounts) typically shows few polymorphonuclear leukocytes and few bacteria.
- White blood cell count may vary from leukopenic to modest elevation, usually without a leftward shift.
- Disseminated intravascular coagulation occasionally complicates adenovirus type 7 pneumonia.
- Multinucleated giant cells on Tzanck preparation of an unroofed vesicular lesion are useful in diagnosing varicella in a patient with an infiltrate (also found in herpes simplex).
- Severe immunosuppression is associated with symptomatic CMV pneumonia (usually reactivation of latent infection or in previously seronegative recipients from the donor).
- Hypoxemia may be profound.
- Cultures may be helpful in identifying superinfecting bacterial pathogens.
- When they occur, parapneumonic pleural effusions are exudative.

IMAGING STUDIES

- Chest radiographs may demonstrate a spectrum of findings from ill-defined, patchy, or generalized interstitial infiltrates, which can be associated with ARDS.
- A localized dense alveolar infiltrate suggests a superimposed bacterial pneumonia.
- Small calcified nodules may develop as a radiographic residual of varicella pneumonia.

Rx TREATMENT

NONPHARMACOLOGIC THERAPY

General:
- Measures to diminish person-to-person transmission
- Modified bed rest
- Maintenance of adequate hydration
- Possible ventilatory support for severe pneumonia or ARDS

Influenza:
- Yearly prophylactic strain-specific influenza vaccination (only subvirion vaccine should be used in children <13 yr) can be given to prevent infection.
- Live, attenuated influenza vaccines administered by nose drops as effective as injected inactivated viral vaccines.

RSV:
- Isolation techniques are important in limiting spread of RSV infections.
- Immunoglobulins with a high RSV-neutralizing antibody titer are beneficial in treatment.

Adenoviruses:
- Intestinal inoculation of respiratory adenoviruses has been used to successfully immunize military recruits.
- Although they produce no disease in recipients, the viruses may be shed chronically and may infect others at a later date.
- These vaccines are not available for civilian populations.

Varicella:
- Live, attenuated varicella vaccine has been successfully used in clinical trials.
- Varicella-zoster immune globulin should be administered within 4 days of exposure to prevent or modify the disease in susceptible persons.
- Nonimmunized persons exposed to varicella are potentially infectious between 10 and 21 days after exposure.

Measles:
- Effective measles vaccine is available:
  - The vaccine should be administered at age 15 mo.
  - A second dose should be administered at the time of school entry.
- Live, attenuated vaccine or gamma-globulin can prevent measles in unvaccinated persons if administered early after exposure.
- Vitamin A given PO for 2 days reduces morbidity and mortality rates from measles in exposed children.

Severe acute respiratory syndrome (SARS) = associated coronaviruses:
- No vaccine currently available.
- Supportive care: ribavirin ineffective, use of steroids or interferon-alpha of unclear value.

ACUTE GENERAL Rx

- **General:** Administer appropriate antibiotics for bacterial superinfections.
- **Influenza:**
  - Amantadine and rimantadine for influenza A (not active against influenza B). Early use can speed recovery from small airways dysfunction, but whether it influences the development or course of pneumonia is uncertain.
  - The neuraminidase inhibitors oseltamivir and zanamivir are effective if given in the first 48 hours of symptoms of influenza; their efficacy in established influenza pneumonia is unclear.
  - Aerosolized ribavirin or amantadine may have a role in severe influenza pneumonia but have not been approved for this indication.

- **RSV and parainfluenza:**
  - Ribavirin aerosol is effective for severe RSV pneumonia.
  - There is no approved antiviral therapy for parainfluenza virus pneumonia.
- **Adenoviruses:** no effective agent; some case reports of cidofovir use but unproved.
- **Varicella:**
  - Varicella pneumonia can be treated with IV acyclovir.
  - Adults who develop chickenpox should be considered for acyclovir treatment, which may prevent the development of pneumonia.
- **Measles:** no effective antimeasles agent.
- **CMV:**
  - Acyclovir can prevent CMV infection in renal transplant recipients.
  - Ganciclovir and foscarnet, with or without CMV hyperimmune globulin, show promise in the treatment of serious CMV infection, including pneumonia, in compromised hosts.

DISPOSITION

- Supportive therapy is useful.
- Death is possible during acute illness.
- Residual functional abnormalities may be persistent or develop into or predispose to chronic respiratory diseases in later life.
- Morbidity and mortality rates after most viral pneumonias are increased by bacterial superinfection.

REFERRAL

- Uncertainty about the diagnosis in a compromised host.
- Symptoms or findings are progressive.
- Severe respiratory compromise, diffuse infiltrates, or the development of ARDS.

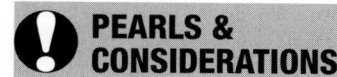
PEARLS & CONSIDERATIONS

COMMENTS

- Influenza spreads by close contact and by small droplets transmitted by cough.
- RSV is effectively transmitted by fomites and by direct contact (little by aerosol).
- Varicella is transmitted by direct contact or by aerosol.
- Of the three major forms of parainfluenza viruses (types 1 to 3), type 3 is the most common cause of viral pneumonia; types 1 and 2 primarily cause laryngotracheitis.
- Recent evidence indicates that a newly discovered virus known as metapneumovirus is a common cause of upper respiratory infections worldwide; this virus can cause pneumonia.

SUGGESTED READINGS

available at www.expertconsult.com

RELATED CONTENT

Viral Pneumonia (Patient Information)

AUTHORS: **PHILIP A. CHAN, M.D.,** and **GLENN G. FORT, M.D., M.P.H.**

BASIC INFORMATION

DEFINITION

A spontaneous pneumothorax (SP) is defined as the accumulation of air into the pleural space, collapsing the lung. This can be primary SP (without any obvious underlying lung disease) or secondary SP (with underlying lung disease).

SYNONYMS

Primary spontaneous pneumothorax
Secondary spontaneous pneumothorax

ICD-9CM CODES

512.0S Spontaneous tension pneumothorax
512.8   Other spontaneous pneumothorax

EPIDEMIOLOGY & DEMOGRAPHICS

- Approximately 20,000 new cases of SP occur each year in the U.S.
- SP is more common in men than women (6:1).
- Incidence of primary SP is 7.4 per 100,000 in men and 1.2 per 100,000 in women.
- Incidence of secondary SP is 6.3 per 100,000 in men and 2.0 per 100,000 in women.
- SP is commonly seen in tall, thin young men aged 20 to 40 yr.
- Risk factors include smoking, family history, Marfan's syndrome, homocystinuria, and thoracic endometriosis.

PHYSICAL FINDINGS & CLINICAL PRESENTATION

- Sudden onset of pleuritic chest pain (90%), usually at rest, which often becomes dull after a few hours
- Pain is usually unilateral and can be sharp and agonizing and associated with considerable apprehension.
- Dyspnea (80%), which often resolves within 24 hr, despite persistence of pneumothorax
- Cough (10%)
- Asymptomatic (5%); may take up to 7 days to come to medical attention
- Tachycardia
- Hypoxemia
- Decreased chest excursion on the affected side
- Diminished breath sounds
- Subcutaneous emphysema may be present.
- Hyperresonance on percussion

ETIOLOGY

- In primary SP, rupture of small blebs, usually located near the apex of the upper lobes, is a common cause. The check-valve mechanism is uncommon in this case; therefore, tension pneumothorax rarely occurs.
- In secondary SP, chronic obstructive pulmonary disease is the most common cause, but it can also be associated with pneumonia, bronchogenic carcinoma, mesothelioma, sarcoidosis, tuberculosis, cystic fibrosis, and many other lung diseases (Fig. 1-657).

DIAGNOSIS

Established by the chest x-ray (Fig. 1-658)

DIFFERENTIAL DIAGNOSIS

- Pleurisy
- Pulmonary embolism
- Myocardial infarction
- Pericarditis
- Asthma
- Pneumonia

WORKUP

Includes CXR and, in some inconclusive cases, CT scan of the chest

LABORATORY TESTS

Arterial blood gases may show hypoxemia and hypocapnia as a result of hyperventilation.

IMAGING STUDIES

- SP is usually confirmed by upright CXR:
  1. A white visceral pleural line. The absence of vessel markings peripheral to this line helps differentiate from mimicking conditions such as an overlying skin fold. A lateral width of 1 cm corresponds to 10% pneumothorax.

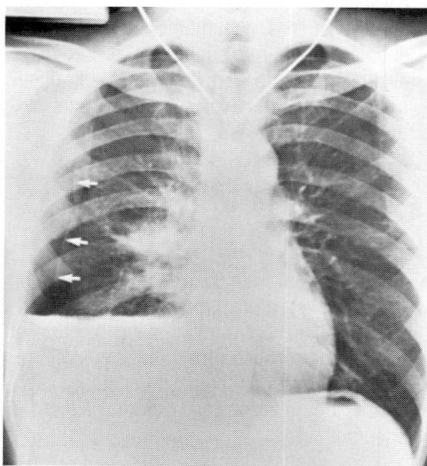

FIGURE 1-658 Chest radiograph shows right hydropneumothorax. Horizontal line in lower right hemithorax is interface between air and liquid in pleural space. *Arrows* point to visceral pleura above level of effusion. There is air in pleural space between visceral pleura and chest wall. (From Weinberg SE et al: *Principles of pulmonary medicine*, ed 5, Philadelphia, 2008, Saunders.)

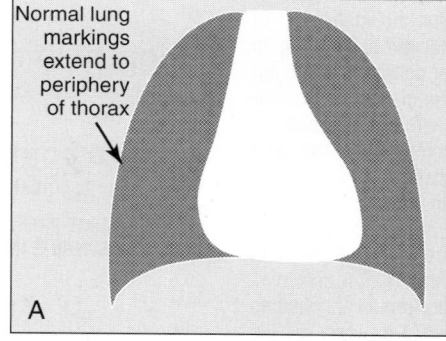
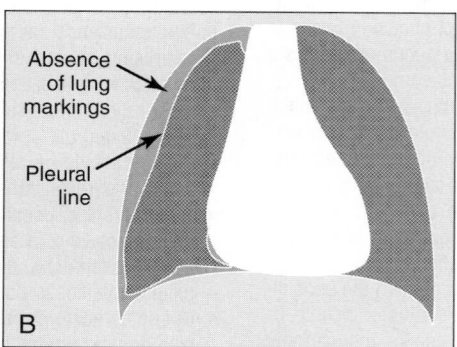

FIGURE 1-657 Pneumothorax. A, Schematic of normal lung. **B,** Schematic of pneumothorax. Pneumothoraces can range in size from tiny to massive. Because of the variability in their size and location, pneumothoraces can be difficult to detect on chest x-ray. For example, a pneumothorax that is anterior or posterior rather than lateral may be hidden on frontal chest x-ray, particularly one taken in the supine position. An upright chest x-ray should be obtained if possible. An expiratory film is thought to be more sensitive, because the lung and thorax decrease in size during expiration, but air trapped in the pleural space remains the same size and thus appears relatively larger. Subtle pneumothoraces may not be visible on chest x-ray. In some cases, subcutaneous air may be the only visible clue to underlying lung injury. CT is extremely sensitive for pneumothorax, although controversy remains over the proper management of pneumothoraces seen only on CT. Ultrasound is also thought to be more sensitive than chest x-ray for detection of pneumothorax, although, again, the management of pneumothorax seen only on ultrasound is uncertain because this is a relatively newly described method of detection. The chest x-ray findings of pneumothorax include a lack of the normal lung markings, which should be visible to the periphery of the chest wall. Sometimes a line marking the boundary of the lung and visceral pleura is visible, although this can be confused with ribs and with the medial margin of the scapula. Depending on the degree of pneumothorax and lung collapse, the lung parenchyma may appear denser than the opposite side. In extreme cases of tension pneumothorax, the pressure exerted by the air in the pleural space may begin to displace other structures, including the diaphragm and mediastinum. In tension pneumothorax, the hyperinflated hemithorax may also have abnormally positioned ribs, with a position more horizontal than usual. (From Broder JS: *Diagnostic imaging for the emergency physician*, Philadelphia, 2011, Saunders.)

Normal lung markings extend to periphery of thorax

Absence of lung markings

Pleural line

A

B

2. The left lateral decubitus position is the most sensitive and the supine position the least sensitive. The increased sensitivity of expiratory films in detecting pneumothorax has never been demonstrated in studies.
3. As little as 50 ml of air can be detected on upright film.

- Tension pneumothorax (Fig. E1-659) is a medical emergency and should be suspected when the patient is hemodynamically unstable or with contralateral tracheal and mediastinal deviation and ipsilateral flattening or inversion of the diaphragm on the CXR (Fig. E1-660).
- CT scan can be done in suspected but difficult-to-visualize pneumothoraces, to differentiate from large subpleural bullae or to evaluate for underlying lung pathology, especially in patients with secondary pneumothorax.

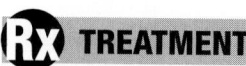

TREATMENT

INITIAL MANAGEMENT

- 100% oxygen administration reduces the partial pressure of nitrogen in pleural capillaries, consequently quadrupling the rate of pneumothorax absorption, and should be administered to all patients with pneumothorax.
- Further treatment is based on the size of the pneumothorax.
  - If the pneumothorax is small (<3 cm between lung and chest wall on CXR), the patient can be treated with observation alone. Repeat imaging should be performed to ensure stability/resorption of the pneumothorax.
  - If the pneumothorax is >3 cm, initial management should focus on removing air from the pleural space. This can be accomplished by either chest tube placement or needle aspiration. Needle aspiration is the treatment of choice in unstable patients with a tension pneumothorax as a bridge to chest tube placement.
  - There is no firm conclusion on the initial optimal treatment (simple aspiration versus chest tube insertion) for a first episode of primary SP. Studies suggest that shorter hospital stay can be achieved with the aspiration technique, but there is a potential risk of lung laceration.
- Needle aspiration can be done at the bedside using a large-bore angiocatheter needle or commercially available needle thoracotomy kit. The needle is introduced in the second

intercostal space midclavicular line. The catheter is left in place and attached to a three-way stopcock and a large syringe. Air is aspirated until resistance is met or the patient experiences significant coughing. Repeat CXR is done immediately after aspiration and again in 4 to 24 hr to document reexpansion of the lung. If the pneumothorax fails to resolve with aspiration, a chest tube should be placed.
- If there is improvement but not complete resolution of pneumothorax after the aspiration, the catheter can be attached to a Heimlich (one-way) valve to allow further lung expansion. Some stable patients can be discharged home with this device in place if close follow-up monitoring can be obtained.
- Chest tube insertion has been recommended for patients with primary SP who do not respond to simple aspiration and for all patients with secondary SP, recurrent pneumothorax, or tension pneumothorax.

PREVENTION

- Multiple techniques have been used to prevent recurrence, including pleurectomy, laser abrasion of parietal pleura, intrapleural instillation of sclerosing agents, and pleural abrasion with dry gauze. The overall recurrence rate is estimated at <5%.
- The current recommended approach is the use of video-assisted thoracoscopy (VATS) with an aim to excise the associated bullae or perform guided pleurodesis or treatment. Most pulmonologists recommend definitive management after the first recurrence. However, high-risk occupations such as divers or pilots should be considered for surgery after their first pneumothorax. Similarly, complex conditions such as patients with persistent bronchopleural fistula suggested by a persistent air leak from the chest tube should also be considered for VATS and early surgical intervention.
- The recurrence rates for the instillation of sclerosing agents (minocycline 5 mg/kg in 50 ml of normal saline or doxycycline 500 mg in 50 ml of normal saline) are higher than for VATS-guided therapy. Therefore this mode of therapy should be reserved for patients who are poor surgical candidates.
- Talc has also been used as a sclerosing agent; however, there are case reports of acute respiratory distress syndrome and pleural calcification occurring after use.
- Open thoracotomy is performed in patients who do not respond to VATS or when VATS is not available.

DISPOSITION

- Approximately 25% to 50% of patients with primary SP will have recurrence within 1 yr.
- Smoking cessation should be advised.
- The rates of recurrence after the second and third episode of SP are 60% and 80%, respectively, with the majority of recurrences occurring on the same side as the first pneumothorax.
- Death from primary SP is uncommon. In patients with secondary SP and chronic obstructive pulmonary disease, mortality rates range from 1% to 16%.

REFERRAL

A pulmonary specialist and surgical consultation are recommended.

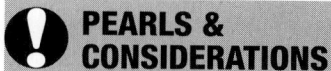

PEARLS & CONSIDERATIONS

- The rate of pleural air absorption is approximately 1.25% of the volume of the hemithorax per day. Therefore the interval for complete resolution of pneumothorax with observation can be estimated.
- Catamenial pneumothorax is a rare condition characterized by recurrent SP coinciding with the onset of menses. It usually affects the right lung and is believed to be caused by endometriosis with involvement of the diaphragm and/or pleura. It is believed to be hormonally related, and treatment is aimed at endometrial suppression.

COMMENTS

- Patients with AIDS and *Pneumocystis carinii* infection have a high incidence of SP. Treatment typically requires chest tube placement and either thoracoscopy or open thoracotomy.

SUGGESTED READINGS

available at www.expertconsult.com

RELATED CONTENT

Pneumothorax (Patient Information)

AUTHORS: **SUNIT-PREET CHAUDHRY, M.D.,** and **RICHARD REGNANTE, M.D.**

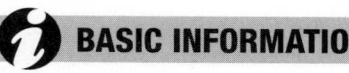

BASIC INFORMATION

DEFINITION

Poison ivy dermatitis is a contact dermatitis caused by exposure to urushiol, the oil of plants of the genus *Toxicodendron,* which includes poison ivy, poison oak, and poison sumac.

SYNONYMS

Rhus dermatitis
Toxicodendron dermatitis

ICD-9CM CODES
692.6 Dermatitis due to plant

EPIDEMIOLOGY & DEMOGRAPHICS

INCIDENCE: Affects 10 million to 40 million Americans annually.
PEAK INCIDENCE: More frequent in months when outdoor activity is more common.
PREVALENCE: From 50% to 75% of the adult population is clinically sensitive to these plants. Sensitivity rates are lower in urban areas. (Tolerance is found in 10% to 15% of the population.)
PREDOMINANT SEX AND AGE: Sensitization occurs most commonly between ages 8 and 14 yr. Sensitivity wanes with age, especially with limited exposure and prior mild reactions.
GENETICS: There is believed to be a genetic susceptibility to sensitivity; however, the rash occurs in all ethnicities and skin types.
RISK FACTORS: Firefighters, forestry workers, farmers, and outdoor workers in general as well as those who participate in outdoor recreation. These plants are indigenous to the United States, Canada, and Mexico, and cases are most common in these areas.

PHYSICAL FINDINGS & CLINICAL PRESENTATION

- Patients typically present with intense pruritus and rash. The patient may not be aware of exposure to the plant.
- Symptoms typically peak from 1 to 14 days after exposure depending on the degree of exposure and thickness of affected skin.
- Dermatitis may initially present as erythema and may develop into papules, vesicles, and bullae.
- Lesions may be found in the classic linear configuration, typically in exposed areas likely to have been in contact with plants (Fig. E1-661). Atypical appearance or location of dermatitis is more common with secondary exposure, such as through pets or infected tools or clothing.
- Face and genital involvement may present with significant edema.
- Inhalation of urushiol aerosolized by fire can cause significant respiratory tract inflamma-

tion. This can be a particular occupational hazard of forest firefighters.
- Postinflammatory hyperpigmentation may occur, more commonly in dark skin types. This usually resolves with treatment.

ETIOLOGY

- Initial contact with oil of plants in this genus, which is released with damage to plant parts, causes a classic T-lymphocyte–mediated delayed-type allergic reaction.
- Subsequent exposures cause a cell-mediated cytotoxic immune response.

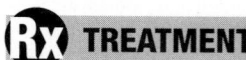

DIAGNOSIS

DIFFERENTIAL DIAGNOSIS

- Allergic contact dermatitis from other plants or nonplant substances
- Irritant contact dermatitis
- Nummular dermatitis
- Arthropod reactions, including scabies and bedbug bites

WORKUP

Typically not needed. Diagnosis is based on characteristic rash and possibly history of exposure.

TREATMENT

Prevention is the most effective treatment.

NONPHARMACOLOGIC THERAPY

- After known exposure, patients should remove contaminated clothing and wash the skin gently with soap and water. Washing after appearance of dermatitis does not prevent further lesions.
- Calamine lotion, cool compresses, baking soda, or colloidal oatmeal baths may provide symptomatic relief.
- Keep nails short and clean to help prevent secondary bacterial infection.
- Exposed clothing, as well as tools, pets, and equipment, should be washed with soap and water to prevent secondary exposure.

ACUTE GENERAL Rx

- Topical steroids generally should be avoided. They may be effective in mild, early cases with erythema and pruritus but no vesiculation.
- Topical antibiotics should be avoided.
- Use of antihistamines for associated pruritus may be effective, but this has not been extensively studied.
- Systemic corticosteroids offer significant relief in moderate to severe *Rhus* dermatitis, including generalized rash or severe facial or genital involvement.

- Effective dosing of oral prednisone is 1 mg/kg/day over 7 to 10 days (maximum 60 mg initial dose), with tapering over an additional 7 to 10 days.
- Inadequate doses or too-rapid tapering of systemic steroids may cause symptom rebound.
- IM treatment with long-acting triamcinolone suspension may be considered for patients intolerant of oral therapy.

CHRONIC Rx

- Recurrence may be caused by repeated exposure to fomites, including contaminated clothing, equipment, or pets.
- Secondary bacterial infection of the skin is the most common complication of *Rhus* dermatitis. Staph and strep are the most common pathogens, but MRSA must be considered.

DISPOSITION

Untreated *Rhus* dermatitis will resolve in 1 to 3 weeks.

REFERRAL

Refer to dermatology if there is diagnostic confusion.

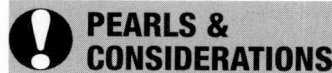

PEARLS & CONSIDERATIONS

PREVENTION

- Patients should be educated regarding identification and avoidance as well as washing to remove the oil after known exposure.
- Total avoidance of the plants may not be practical.
- The use of barrier creams applied before exposure to prevent dermatitis may be of some benefit, particularly in potential occupational (therefore predictable) exposure.
- Products available for postexposure prophylaxis are effective; however, equal efficacy may be obtained from less expensive liquid dishwashing soap.
- Desensitization has not been found to be effective.

PATIENT & FAMILY EDUCATION

- "Leaves of three, let it be," is a helpful reminder for patients.
- Patient education material, including access to photographs of the leaves of these plants in a variety of seasons and conditions, may be useful.

SUGGESTED READINGS
available at www.expertconsult.com

RELATED CONTENT
Poison Ivy (Patient Information)

AUTHOR: **MARGARET TRYFOROS, M.D.**

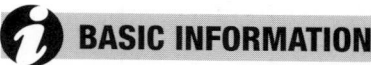

DEFINITION

Polyarteritis nodosa (PAN) is a systemic vasculitic syndrome involving medium-sized to small arteries, characterized histologically by necrotizing inflammation of the arterial media and inflammatory cell infiltration.

SYNONYMS

Periarteritis nodosa
PAN
Necrotizing arteritis

ICD-9CM CODES
446.0 Polyarteritis nodosa

EPIDEMIOLOGY & DEMOGRAPHICS

- Incidence is 1/100,000 persons annually. Increased incidence in patients with hepatitis B surface antigen or hepatitis C virus.
- Male/female ratio of 2:1
- Can occur in any age group, more commonly between 40 yr and 60 yr.
- No racial predilection is observed.
- Prevalence is 2 to 33/1,000,000.
- Is also associated with hairy cell leukemia.

PHYSICAL FINDINGS & CLINICAL PRESENTATION

- Typical presentation is subacute, with the onset of constitutional symptoms over weeks to months in more than 90% of cases
- Nausea, vomiting, headache
- Testicular pain or tenderness
- Myalgias, weakness, or leg tenderness in 24% to 80% of cases
- Neuropathy (mononeuritis multiplex), foot drop
- Skin lesions are observed in one third of patients with tender nodules, livedo reticularis, palpable purpura, ulceration of digits
- Abdominal pain after meals, hematemesis, hematochezia, occasionally with diarrhea and gastrointestinal bleeding in severe cases
- Asymmetric polyarthritis (tending to involve large joints of lower extremities); true synovitis occurs only in a minority of patients
- Presence of lung vasculitis suggests other causes
- Fever (PAN is often a cause of fever of unknown origin) can range from intermittent, low-grade fevers to high fevers with chills
- Chest pain secondary to ischemic infarcts in the coronary arteries, pericarditis, congestive heart failure, and arrhythmias are seen with cardiac involvement
- Tachycardia is common and often striking
- Hypertension can occur due to renal artery involvement

ETIOLOGY

- Unknown
- Hepatitis B virus–associated PAN appears to be an immune complex–mediated disease.
- Hepatitis C and hairy cell leukemia are also associated in some cases.

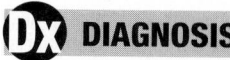 DIAGNOSIS

DIFFERENTIAL DIAGNOSIS

- Cryoglobulinemia
- Systemic lupus erythematosus
- Infections (e.g., subacute bacterial endocarditis, trichinosis, *Rickettsia*)
- Lymphoma
- Henoch-Schönlein purpura
- Wegener granulomatosis
- Microscopic polyangiitis
- Kawasaki disease
- Churg-Strauss syndrome
- Giant cell arteritis
- Human immunodeficiency virus

WORKUP

- Laboratory evaluation, arteriography, and biopsy of small or medium-sized arteries can confirm diagnosis. Clinical manifestations are variable and depend on the arteries involved and the organs affected (e.g., kidney involvement occurs in >80% of cases).
- The presence of any three of the following 10 items allows the diagnosis of PAN with a sensitivity of 82% and a specificity of 86%:
  1. Weight loss >4 kg
  2. Livedo reticularis
  3. Testicular pain or tenderness
  4. Myalgias, weakness, or leg tenderness
  5. Neuropathy
  6. Diastolic blood pressure >90 mm Hg
  7. Elevated blood urea nitrogen (BUN) or creatinine

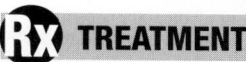

FIGURE 1-662 Superior mesenteric arteriogram in patients with polyarteritis. Several small aneurysms *(arrows)* are present in branches of superior mesenteric artery. (Courtesy Dr. A.W. Stanson. From Harris ED et al: *Kelley's textbook of rheumatology,* ed 7, 2005, Saunders.)

8. Positive test for hepatitis B virus
9. Arteriography revealing small or large aneurysms and focal constrictions between dilated segments
10. Biopsy of small or medium-sized artery containing necrotizing inflammatory infiltrate.

LABORATORY TESTS

- Elevated BUN or creatinine, positive test for hepatitis B virus or hepatitis C.
- Elevated erythrocyte sedimentation rate and C-reactive protein, anemia, elevated platelets, eosinophilia, proteinuria, hematuria.
- Biopsy of small or medium-sized artery of symptomatic sites (muscle, nerve) is >90% specific. Biopsy of the gastrocnemius muscle and sural nerve is commonly performed.
- Circumferential or segmental vessel wall involvement with necrotizing mixed cell inflammation with fibrinoid necrosis is characteristic lesion of active PAN.
- Assays for antinuclear antibody and rheumatoid factor are negative; however, low, nonspecific titers may be detected.
- Serum and urine immunofixation electrophoresis for monoclonal gammopathy and human immunodeficiency virus should also be tested for alternative diagnoses

IMAGING STUDIES

Arteriography can be done in patients with negative biopsies or if there are no symptomatic sites. Mesenteric angiography will reveal aneurysmal dilation of the renal, mesenteric (Fig. 1-662), or hepatic arteries. Less invasive techniques, such as computed tomography (CT) and MRI angiography, also help evaluate the extent and resolution of the disease.

Nerve conduction studies are useful in patients with neuropathy suggesting PAN, helping to evaluate nerves or muscles to biopsy.

Rx TREATMENT

NONPHARMACOLOGIC THERAPY

Low-sodium diet in hypertensive patients

ACUTE GENERAL Rx

- Prednisone 1 to 2 mg/kg/day with higher doses initially, then tapering the doses slowly with overall course of average 9 mo or longer.
- Patients with isolated cutaneous involvement may be treated with steroids alone or in combination with methotrexate.
- Severe PAN with multiorgan involvement treated with a combination of cyclophosphamide 1.5 to 2 mg/kg per day and glucocorticoids has shown good disease outcomes. Once patient achieves stable remission, transition to a less toxic immunomodulatory therapy such as methotrexate or azathioprine, along with tapering doses of oral prednisone, is indicated for chronic therapy.

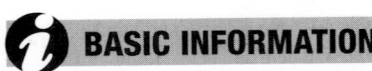

DEFINITION

Polycythemia vera is a chronic myeloproliferative disorder that originates from a pluripotent hematopoietic stem cell and is characterized mainly by erythrocytosis (increase in red blood cell [RBC] mass).

SYNONYMS

Primary polycythemia
Vaquez disease

ICD-9CM CODES
238.4 Polycythemia vera

EPIDEMIOLOGY & DEMOGRAPHICS

INCIDENCE: 1 case per 100,000 persons. Occurs most commonly in patients aged 50 to 75 years. Mean age at onset is 60 yr; men are affected more often than are women.

PHYSICAL FINDINGS & CLINICAL PRESENTATION

Polycythemia vera has a latent, proliferative, and spent phase. The patient generally comes to medical attention because of symptoms associated with increased blood volume and viscosity or impaired platelet function:

- Impaired cerebral circulation resulting in headache, vertigo, blurred vision, dizziness, transient ischemic attack, cerebrovascular accident
- Fatigue, poor exercise tolerance
- Pruritus, particularly after bathing (caused by overproduction of histamine)
- Bleeding: epistaxis, upper gastrointestinal bleeding (increased incidence of peptic ulcer disease)
- Abdominal discomfort from splenomegaly; hepatomegaly may be present
- Hyperuricemia may result in nephrolithiasis and gouty arthritis
- Nearly 20% of patients experience arterial or venous thrombosis as their initial symptom.

The physical examination may reveal:

- Facial plethora, congestion of oral mucosa, ruddy complexion
- Enlargement and tortuosity of retinal veins
- Splenomegaly (found in >75% of patients)

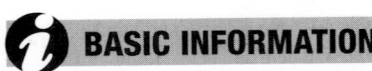 DIAGNOSIS

DIFFERENTIAL DIAGNOSIS

Smoking:

- Polycythemia is caused by increased carboxyhemoglobin, resulting in left shift in the hemoglobin (Hgb) dissociation curve.
- Laboratory evaluation shows increased hematocrit (Hct), RBC mass, erythropoietin level, and carboxyhemoglobin.
- Splenomegaly is not present on physical examination.

Hypoxemia (secondary polycythemia):

- Living for prolonged periods at high altitudes, pulmonary fibrosis, congenital cardiac lesions with right-to-left shunts.

- Laboratory evaluation shows decreased arterial oxygen saturation and elevated erythropoietin level.
- Splenomegaly is not present on physical examination.

Erythropoietin-producing states:

- Renal cell carcinoma, hepatoma, cerebral hemangioma, uterine fibroids, polycystic kidneys.
- The erythropoietin level is elevated in these patients, and the arterial oxygen saturation is normal.
- Splenomegaly may be present with metastatic neoplasms.

Stress polycythemia (Gaisböck's syndrome, relative polycythemia):

- Laboratory evaluation demonstrates normal RBC mass, arterial oxygen saturation, and erythropoietin level; plasma volume is decreased.
- Splenomegaly is not present on physical examination.

Hemoglobinopathies associated with high oxygen affinity:

- An abnormal oxyhemoglobin-dissociation curve (P50) is present.

WORKUP

Recent developments in molecular biology have identified a single, acquired point mutation in the Janus kinase 2 *(JAK2)* gene in the majority of patients with polycythemia vera and other pH-negative myeloproliferative disorders. The *JAK2* mutation is found in >95% of patients with polycythemia vera and can be used for diagnostic purposes. Testing for the *JAK2 V617F* mutation with polymerase chain reaction assay is now available. In patients with high hematocrit (>52% in men or >48% in women) and in the absence of coexisting secondary erythrocytosis, the presence of the *JAK2* mutation is sufficient for the diagnosis of polycythemia vera.

The World Health Organization diagnostic criteria for polycythemia vera are described in Table 1-332.

LABORATORY TESTS

- Elevated RBC count (>6 million/mm³), elevated Hgb (>18 g/dl in men, >16 g/dl in

women), elevated Hct (>54% in men, >49% in women)
- Increased white blood cell count (often with basophilia); thrombocytosis in the majority of patients
- Elevated leukocyte alkaline phosphatase, serum vitamin B_{12}, and uric acid levels
- Low serum erythropoietin level
- Bone marrow aspiration revealing RBC hyperplasia (Fig. E1-667) and absent iron stores

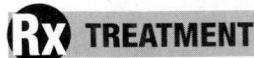 TREATMENT

NONPHARMACOLOGIC THERAPY

Phlebotomy to keep Hct <45% in men and <42% in women is the mainstay of therapy. Phlebotomy, however, has no effect on the development of myelofibrosis.

ACUTE GENERAL Rx

- Hydroxyurea can be used in conjunction with phlebotomy to decrease the incidence of thrombotic events.
- Interferon-alpha-2b is also effective in controlling RBC values without significant side effects.
- Myelosuppressive therapy with chlorambucil is effective but should not be routinely used because of its leukemogenic potential.
- Box 1-49 describes an algorithm for management of patients with polycythemia vera.

CHRONIC Rx

- Patient education regarding need for lifelong monitoring and treatment.
- Adjunctive therapy: treatment of pruritus with antihistamines, control of significant hyperuricemia with allopurinol, reduction of gastric hyperacidity with antacids of H_2 blockers, low-dose aspirin to treat vasomotor symptoms in patients without bleeding diathesis. Low-dose aspirin can safely prevent thrombotic complications in patients with polycythemia vera and should be given to all patients in absence of contraindications.

TABLE 1-332 World Health Organization 2008 Diagnostic Criteria for Polycythemia Vera

Major Criteria

1. Hemoglobin (Hgb) >18.5 g/dl (men), >16.5 (women); *or* Hgb or hematocrit (Hct) >99% reference range for age, sex, or altitude of residence; *or* Hgb >17 g/dl (men), >15 g/dl (women) if associated with a sustained increase of ≥ 2 g/dl from baseline that cannot be attributed to correction of iron deficiency; *or* elevated red cell mass (>25% above mean normal predicted value)
2. Presence of JAK2 V617F or similar mutation

Minor Criteria

1. Bone marrow trilineage myeloproliferation
2. Subnormal serum erythropoietin level
3. Endogenous erythroid colony formation in vitro

Either both major criteria and one minor criterion *or* the first major criterion and two minor criteria must be met for diagnosis of polycythemia vera.

From Andreoli TE et al: *Andreoli and Carpenter's Cecil essentials of medicine*, ed 8, Philadelphia, 2010, Saunders.

BASIC INFORMATION

DEFINITION

Polycystic kidney disease (PKD) refers to a systemic hereditary disorder characterized by the formation of cysts in the cortex and medulla of both kidneys (Figs. 1-663 and 1-664).

SYNONYMS

Autosomal-dominant polycystic kidney disease (ADPKD)

ICD-9CM CODES
753.1   Polycystic kidney, unspecified type
753.13   Polycystic kidney, autosomal
         dominant

EPIDEMIOLOGY & DEMOGRAPHICS

- The most common mendelian disorder of the kidneys
- Affects all racial groups worldwide
- Results in kidney failure in the majority of individuals by the fifth to sixth decade
- PKD occurs in one in 700 to 1000 persons
- Usually presents in the third to fourth decades of life

PHYSICAL FINDINGS & CLINICAL PRESENTATION

- Characterized by focal development of renal and extrarenal cysts in an age-dependent manner, resulting in a slow, gradual, and massive kidney enlargement.

Symptoms:
- Pain (60%): acute pain can be associated with renal hemorrhage, passage of stones (20% of patients; usually uric acid or calcium oxalate), and urinary tract infections
- Palpable flank mass
- Hypertension: >60% of patients; usually develops before the loss of renal function
- Headache
- Nocturia, hematuria

Renal manifestations:
- Kidney and cyst volumes and renal blood flow (or vascular resistance) are the strongest predictors of renal function decline. Kidney function does not decline in individuals with PKD until kidney size is at least five times greater than normal.
- Morphometric analysis of sequential CT was shown to be sufficiently accurate to monitor rates of renal enlargement in PKD, and MRI-based methods have been developed. Two general groups of kidney volume increase: those with rapid rates (>5% increase in total kidney volume per year) and those with rates of progression <5% per year. Intervals between measurements as short as 6 mo may be adequate to determine an effect of treatment that reduces the rates of volume progression >50% in those with rapidly progressive disease.
- All cysts develop from preexisting renal tubule segments, and only a small portion of the nephrons (1%) undergoes cystic formation.
- Renal failure: in most patients renal function is maintained within normal range, despite relentless growth of cysts, until the fourth to sixth decades of life.
- Nephrolithiasis (20%)
- Urinary tract infection

Extrarenal manifestations:
- Associated with liver cysts (50% to 70%), pancreatic cysts (10%), splenic cysts (5%), central nervous system arachnoid cysts (5%), and cerebral aneurysms (20%)
- Polycystic liver disease: most common extrarenal manifestation—associated with both *PKD1* and non-*PKD1* genotypes
- Vascular manifestations: intracranial aneurysms (occur in approximately 6% of patients with a negative family history of aneurysms and 16% of those with a positive history), thoracic aortic and cervicocephalic artery dissection, and coronary artery aneurysms
- Increased incidence of diverticular disease and mitral valve prolapse

ETIOLOGY

- Dominantly inherited heterogenic systemic disease: mutations in *PKD1* (chromosome region 16p13.3; 85% of cases) or *PKD2* (4q21; approximately 15% of cases).
- Polycystin 1 and polycystin 2 are the protein products of PKD1 and PKD2, which interact and coassemble and seem to function together to regulate the morphologic configuration of epithelial cells. Although individuals with PKD1 are clinically indistinguishable from individuals with PKD2, patients with PKD2 have a less severe course of disease with a later mean age of diagnosis, hypertension, and end-stage renal disease (ESRD).
- Disease penetrance is 100%.

DIAGNOSIS

Sonographic imaging or CT scan:
1. In an individual with a family history for the disease, including:
   - Age <30 yr: at least two unilateral or bilateral cysts
   - 30 to 59 yr: two cysts in each kidney
   - ≥60 yr: four cysts in each kidney
2. In the absence of a family history: bilateral renal enlargement or cysts or the presence of multiple bilateral cysts with hepatic cysts together and in the absence of other manifestations suggesting a different renal cyst disease
   - Genetic testing can be used when the imaging results are equivocal and when a definitive diagnosis is required in a younger individual, such as a potential living related kidney donor.

DIFFERENTIAL DIAGNOSIS

- Simple cysts
- Autosomal-recessive PKD in children
- Tuberous sclerosis
- von Hippel-Lindau syndrome
- Acquired cystic kidney disease

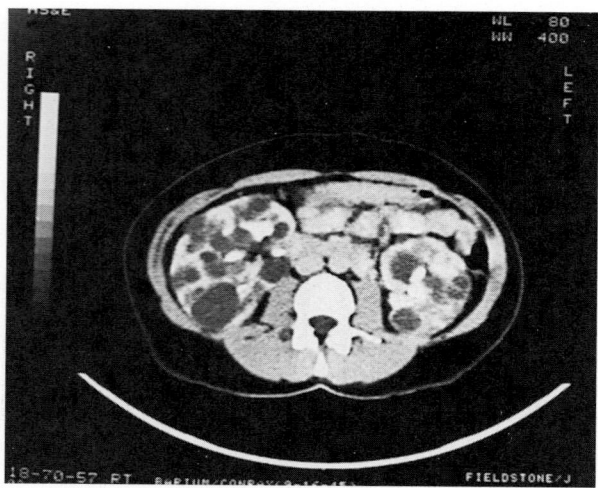

FIGURE 1-663 Tomogram of autosomal-dominant kidney disease. Kidney cysts. (From Stein JH [ed]: *Internal medicine*, ed 5, St Louis, 1998, Mosby.)

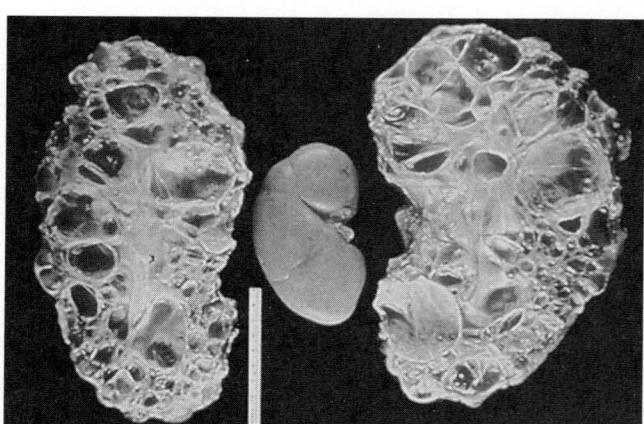

FIGURE 1-664 Markedly enlarged polycystic kidneys from a patient with autosomal-dominant polycystic kidney disease compared with a normal kidney *(middle).* (From Johnson RJ, Feehally J: *Comprehensive clinical nephrology*, ed 2, St Louis, 2000, Mosby.)

LABORATORY TESTS

- Hemoglobin and hematocrit are elevated because of increased secretion of erythropoietin from functioning renal cysts.
- Electrolyte abnormalities commonly seen in any patients with renal insufficiency.
- Blood urea nitrogen and creatinine can be elevated.
- Urinalysis can show microscopic hematuria and proteinuria (seldom >1 g/24 hr). Proteinuria >2 g/day is unusual and suggests the presence of another kidney disease.

IMAGING STUDIES

- A cyst is considered to be present if it measures >2 mm in diameter.
- Abdominal renal ultrasound is the easiest and most cost-efficient test for renal cysts. Renal ultrasound can detect cysts from 1 to 1.5 cm.
- Abdominal CT scan is more sensitive than ultrasound and can detect cysts as small as 0.5 cm.
- Both studies can detect associated hepatic, splenic, and pancreatic cysts.
- MRI is more sensitive than ultrasound and may help distinguish renal cell carcinomas from simple cysts.

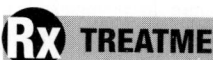 **TREATMENT**

NONPHARMACOLOGIC THERAPY

- Treatment consists of the standard therapies for chronic renal disease, including good blood pressure control and control of hyperlipidemia.
- When conservative measures fail to control the pain, infection, or bleeding, surgical interventions such as cystic decompression by aspiration under ultrasound or CT guidance or laparoscopic or surgical cyst fenestration through lumbotomy or flank incision may be of benefit.
- When above measures fail, nephrectomy should be undertaken in ESRD.
- Combined percutaneous cyst drainage and antibiotic treatment provide the best treatment results for hepatic cyst infection.

ACUTE GENERAL Rx

- Kidney infections should be treated with antibiotics known to penetrate the cyst (e.g., trimethoprim-sulfamethoxazole 1 tablet PO bid or ciprofloxacin 250 mg PO bid).
- Early detection and treatment of hypertension are important because cardiovascular disease is the main cause of death.

CHRONIC Rx

- Dialysis for end-stage renal failure.
- Pretransplant nephrectomy is reserved for patients with a history of infected cyst or frequent bleeding.
- Renal transplantation is the treatment of choice for ESRD.
- Cyst infections are often difficult to treat. Lipophilic agents penetrate the cysts consistently. If fever persists after 1 to 2 wk of appropriate antimicrobial treatment, percutaneous or surgical drainage of the cysts may be needed. Several months of antibiotic treatment may be needed to eradicate the infection.
- Most cases of polycystic liver disease do not need treatment; patients should avoid estrogens and compounds that promote cyclic adenosine monophosphate accumulation (e.g., caffeine).

DISPOSITION

- Most patients with PKD will progress to renal failure.
- Gross hematuria is usually self-limited.

REFERRAL

- Nephrology consultation
- Urology can also be consulted in patients with nephrolithiasis, for recurrent episodes of gross hematuria, or for consideration for nephrectomy before transplantation.
- Counseling should be done before PKD genetic testing. Benefits include certainty of diagnosis that could affect family planning, early detection and treatment of disease complications, and selection of genetically unaffected family members for living related donor transplantation. Potential discrimina-

tion in terms of insurability and employment associated with a positive diagnosis should be discussed.

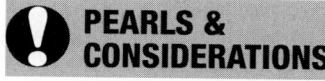 **PEARLS & CONSIDERATIONS**

- ESRD patients with PKD do better on dialysis than do patients with other causes of ESRD.
- There is no difference in patient survival after transplantation between patients with PKD and other ESRD populations.
- Widespread screening is not indicated. Indications for screening include family history of aneurysm, subarachnoid hemorrhage, previous aneurysm rupture, preparation for major elective surgery, high-risk occupations (airplane pilots), and patient anxiety despite adequate information.
- Kidney and cyst volumes are the strongest predictors of renal function decline.

COMMENTS

- Conservative management is recommended for patients with a small (<7 mm) cerebral aneurysm, particularly in the anterior circulation. Rescreening of patients with a family history of intracranial aneurysm after 5 to 10 yr seems reasonable.
- Trials with treatment protocols involving vasopressin antagonists (tolvaptan) are under way to slow the progression of PKD. Results with the rapamycin (mTOR) inhibitors everolimus and sirolimus have been disappointing.

SUGGESTED READINGS

available at www.expertconsult.com

RELATED CONTENT

Polycystic Kidney Disease (Patient Information)

AUTHOR: **SHAHNAZ PUNJANI, M.D.**

P

Diseases and Disorders

I

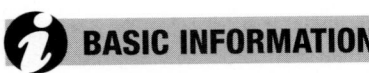

BASIC INFORMATION

DEFINITION

Polycystic ovary syndrome (PCOS) is characterized by an accumulation of incompletely developed follicles in the ovaries due to anovulation and associated with ovarian androgen production. In its complete form, it is associated with polycystic ovaries, amenorrhea, hirsutism, and obesity. Criteria for PCOS according to published definitions are described in Table 1-331.

SYNONYMS

Stein-Leventhal syndrome
PCOS

ICD-9CM CODES
256.4 Polycystic ovary syndrome

EPIDEMIOLOGY & DEMOGRAPHICS

- 5% to 15% of reproductive-age women (most common endocrine disorder in this population).
- Symptoms usually begin around the time of menarche, and the diagnosis is often made during adolescence or young adulthood.
- Increased risk of endometrial and ovarian cancers.
- PCOS is the most common cause of anovulatory infertility

PHYSICAL FINDINGS & CLINICAL PRESENTATION

- Oligomenorrhea or amenorrhea
- Dysfunctional uterine bleeding
- Infertility
- Hirsutism
- Acne, alopecia, acanthosis nigricans
- Obesity (40% only), predominantly abdominal obesity
- Insulin resistance (type 2 diabetes mellitus)
- Hypertension

ETIOLOGY & PATHOGENESIS

Elevated serum luteinizing hormone (LH) concentrations and an increased serum LH/follicle-stimulating hormone (FSH) ratio result either from an increased gonadotropin-releasing hormone hypothalamic secretion or less likely from a primary pituitary abnormality. This results in dysregulation of androgen secretion and increased intraovarian androgen, the effect of which in the ovary is follicular atresia, maturation arrest, polycystic ovaries, and anovulation. Hyperinsulinemia is a contributing factor to ovarian hyperandrogenism, independent of LH excess. A role for insulin growth factor (IGF) receptors has been postulated for the association of PCOS and diabetes.

DIAGNOSIS

The diagnosis of PCOS excludes secondary causes (androgen-producing neoplasm, hyperprolactinemia, adult-onset congenital adrenal hyperplasia).
Clinical:

- The symptoms, signs, and biochemical features of PCOS vary greatly among women and may change over time.
- PCOS is the most common cause of chronic anovulation with estrogen present. A positive progesterone withdrawal test establishes the presence of estrogen. Medroxyprogesterone (Provera) 10 mg qd is administered for 5 days and bleeding occurs if estrogen is present.
- The presence of oligomenorrhea, hirsutism, obesity, and documented polycystic ovaries establishes the diagnosis.

DIFFERENTIAL DIAGNOSIS

Causes of amenorrhea:
- Primary (unusual in PCOS)
  1. Genetic disorder (Turner's syndrome)
  2. Anatomic abnormality (e.g., imperforate hymen)
- Secondary
  1. Pregnancy
  2. Functional (cause unknown, anorexia nervosa, stress, excessive exercise, hyperthyroidism, less commonly hypothyroidism, adrenal dysfunction, pituitary dysfunction, severe systemic illness, drugs such as oral contraceptives, estrogens, or dopamine agonists)

  3. Abnormalities of the genital tract (uterine tumor, endometrial scarring, ovarian tumor)

LABORATORY TESTS

- Glucose tolerance test at the initial presentation and every 2 yr thereafter (rule out diabetes mellitus). Impaired glucose tolerance is very common, occurring in approximately 30% of women with PCOS
- Fasting lipid panel (rule out dyslipidemia), alanine aminotransferase, aspartate aminotransferase (rule out hepatic steatosis)
- Elevated LH/FSH ratio >2.5
- Prolactin level elevation in 25%
- Elevated androgens (testosterone [free and total levels], DHEA-S) (rule out androgen-secreting tumor)
- Other: thyroid-stimulating hormone (rule out hypothyroidism), 17-hydroxyprogesterone (rule out congenital adrenal hyperplasia), 24-hr urine for cortisol and creatinine (rule out Cushing's syndrome)

IMAGING STUDIES

Pelvic ultrasound (Fig. 1-665) (or CT scan) reveals the presence of twofold to fivefold ovarian enlargement with a thickened tunica albuginea, thecal hyperplasia, and 20 or more subcapsular follicles from 1 to 15 mm in diameter (Fig. 1-666). It is important to note that having polycystic ovaries alone does not make the diagnosis of PCOS because 20% of women with polycystic ovaries have no symptoms.

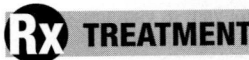 TREATMENT

The goal is to interrupt the self-perpetuating abnormal hormone cycle:

- Reduction of ovarian androgen secretion by laparoscopic ovarian wedge resection. Laparoscopic ovarian surgery (laparoscopic ovarian drilling [LOD]) is a useful alternative that does not trigger ovarian hyperstimulation
- Reduction of ovarian androgen secretion by using oral contraceptives or LH-releasing hormone (LHRH) analogs

---

TABLE 1-331 Criteria for Polycystic Ovary Syndrome according to Published Definitions

	NICHD/NIH/1990	Rotterdam 2003	AE-PCOS/2009
Diagnostic criteria	Requires simultaneous presence of: • Clinical and/or biochemical hyperandrogenism • Menstrual dysfunction	Requires the presence of at least two criteria: • Clinical and/or biochemical hyperandrogenism • Ovulatory dysfunction • PCOM	Requires the presence of: • Hyperandrogenism and/or hyperandrogenemia • Ovarian dysfunction: oligoovulation or anovulation and/or polycystic ovaries
Exclusion criteria	Congenital adrenal hyperplasia, androgen-secreting tumors, Cushing's syndrome, and hyperprolactinemia	Congenital adrenal hyperplasia, androgen-secreting tumors, and Cushing's syndrome	21-hydroxylase-deficient nonclassic adrenal hyperplasia, androgen-secreting neoplasms, androgenic–anabolic drug use or abuse, the hyperandrogenic-insulin resistance-acanthosis nigricans syndrome, thyroid dysfunction, and hyperprolactinemia
Clinical traits	Hirsutism, acne, and alopecia	Hirsutism, acne, and androgenic alopecia	Hirsutism
PCOM	Not included	At least one ovary showing either: • Twelve or more follicles of 2-9 mm in diameter • Ovarian volume, 10 ml	At least one ovary showing either: • Twelve or more follicles of 2-9 mm in diameter • Ovarian volume, 10 ml

AE-PCOS, Androgen Excess and PCOS Society; *NICHD/NIH,* National Institute for Child Health and Human Development/National Institutes of Health; *PCOM,* polycystic morphology.
From Fielding JR et al: *Gynecologic imaging,* Philadelphia, 2011, Saunders.

- Weight reduction for all obese women with PCOS. Loss of abdominal fat seems to be crucial to restore ovulation
- FSH stimulation with clomiphene HMG or pulsatile LHRH
- Urofollitropin (pure FSH) administration
- Metformin improves ovulation, insulin sensitivity, and possibly hyperandrogenemia

Choice of treatment:

- The management of hirsutism without risking pregnancy includes oral contraceptives, glucocorticoids, LHRH analogs, or spironolactone (an antiandrogen). Finasteride and flutamide may be similarly effective in reducing hirsutism as spironolactone.
- Pregnancy can be achieved with clomiphene (alone or with glucocorticoids, human chorionic gonadotropin, or bromocriptine), HMG, urofollitropin, pulsatile LHRH, or ovarian wedge resection. (Metformin may induce ovulation.)
- Psychological screening for depression is recommended. Women with PCOS are fourfold more likely to have abnormal depression scores.

SUGGESTED READINGS
available at www.expertconsult.com

RELATED CONTENT

Polycystic Ovarian Syndrome (Patient Information)

AUTHOR: **FRED F. FERRI, M.D.**

Diseases and Disorders

P

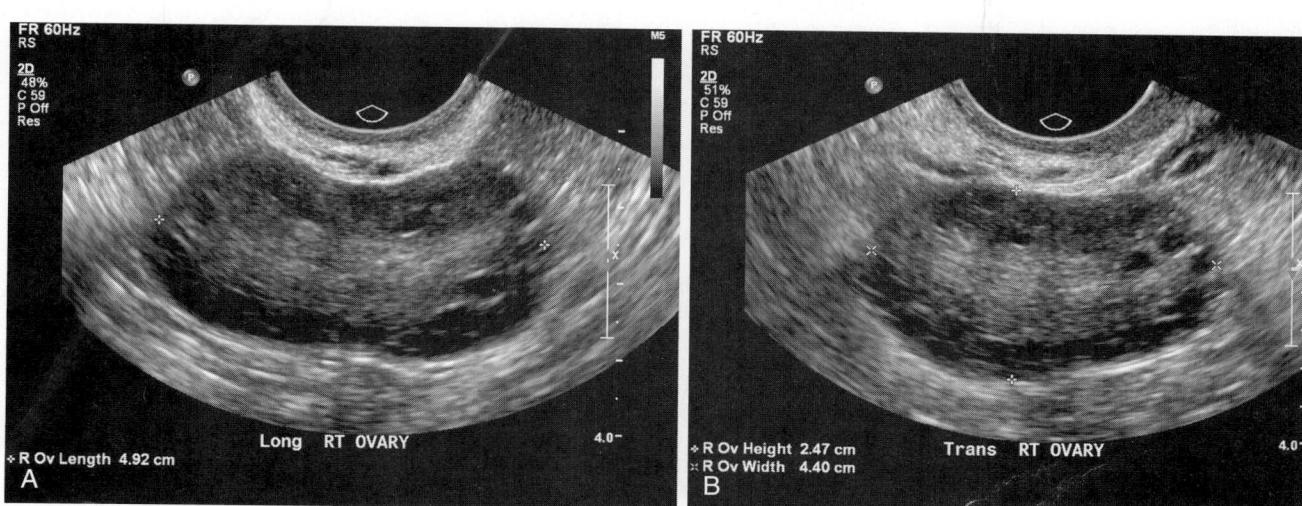

FIGURE 1-665 A, Transvaginal ultrasound in the longitudinal plane showing polycystic ovary morphology. Numerous small follicles surround an echogenic central stroma. **B,** Transvaginal ultrasound in the transverse plane in the same patient. (From Fielding JR et al: *Gynecologic imaging,* Philadelphia, 2011, Saunders.)

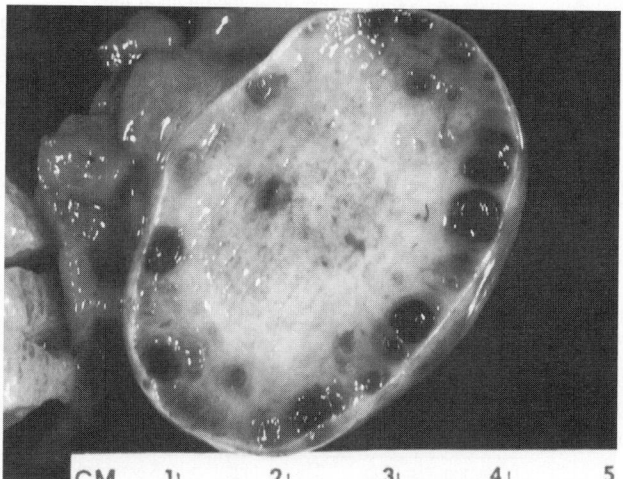

FIGURE 1-666 Sagittal section of a polycystic ovary illustrating large number of follicular cysts and thickened stroma. (From Mishell DR: *Comprehensive gynecology,* ed 3, St Louis, 1997, Mosby.)

- If hepatitis B is identified, then appropriate antiviral treatment (interferon alfa-2b or lamivudine with or without plasma exchange) is initiated.

CHRONIC Rx

Monitoring for infections and potential complications such as thrombosis, infarction, or organ necrosis. Hypertension in patients with renal involvement in PAN is treated with angiotensin-converting enzyme inhibitor.

DISPOSITION

The 5-yr survival is <20% in untreated patients. Treatment with corticosteroids increases survival to approximately 50%. Use of both corticosteroids and immunosuppressive drugs may increase 5-yr survival to >80%. Poor prog-

nostic signs are severe renal or gastrointestinal involvement. Patients on cyclophosphamide should have regular white cell count monitoring for leukopenia. Cyclophosphamide can cause increased risk of infertility, myelodysplsia, lymphoma, bladder malignancy, and when given in combination of high-dose corticosteroids can predispose patients to infection with *Pneumocystis jirovecii (carinii)* pneumonia. Therefore, close follow-up and PCP prophylaxis are recommended.

REFERRAL

Patients with suspected diagnosis of PAN should be immediately referred to a rheumatologist.

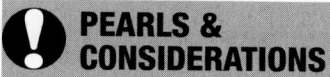

PEARLS & CONSIDERATIONS

- After treatment, patients should be followed up closely for relapse throughout their lifetime.
- Smoking cessation, exercise, and lifestyle modifications should be discussed to decrease vascular complications.

SUGGESTED READINGS

available at www.expertconsult.com

AUTHORS: **SYEDA M. SAYEED, M.D.,** and **HARALD A. HALL, M.D.**

BOX 1-49   Management of Patients with Polycythemia Vera

Low-risk young patients (<60 yr) and no prior history of thrombosis, platelet count <1.5 × 10^6 mm^{-3}

Phlebotomy + low-dose aspirin (81 mg/d) to maintain Hct <45% in males and <42% in females. Aspirin should not be used in patients with histories of hemorrhagic episode or with extreme thrombocytosis (>1.5 × 10^6 mm^{-3}) or acquired von Willebrand syndrome.
↓

Thrombosis or hemorrhage
Systemic symptoms
Severe pruritus refractory to histamine antagonists
Painful splenomegaly
↓

Pegylated interferon 90 to 180 μg/wk or interferon α (3 × 10^6 units three times/wk; alter dose depending on response and toxicity). Consider the use of pegylated interferon, which can be administered once/wk.
↓

If platelet control is inadequate or patient cannot tolerate interferon, one option could be the use of anagrelide. However, the use of this drug is controversial. In this case, supplemental phlebotomy is required to maintain Hct <45% in males and <42% in females, and the use of hydroxyurea should be considered, especially if patient continues to have thrombotic episodes.
↓

If the patient has increasing splenomegaly, systemic symptoms, or repeated thromboses in spite of adequate dose of hydroxyurea (2 to 3 g/d) start busulphan 4 to 6 mg/d PO for 4 to 8 wk. It should be mentioned that the sequential use of hydroxyurea and busulphan may be associated with an increased risk of leukemia. Supplemental phlebotomy may be required.
↓

Painful splenomegaly
Splenectomy + continued systemic therapy
High-risk patients (>60 yr), previous thrombosis, platelet count >1.5 × 10^6 mm^{-3}
Phlebotomy to Hct <42% in females and <45% in males
Aspirin (81 mg/d) to be given only in patients with platelet counts <1.5 × 10^6 mm^{-2}
Myelosuppressive therapy with hydroxyurea 30 mg/kg PO for 1 wk
↓
Then 15 to 20 mg/kg
If patient continues to have thrombotic episodes and has extreme thrombocytosis or cannot tolerate hydroxyurea, consider pegylated interferon 90 to 180 μg/wk or add busulphan 4 to 6 mg/d PO for 4 to 8 wk.
Stop when blood counts are normalized or platelet count is <300,000 mm^{-3}.
Occasional supplemental phlebotomy if Hct is >42% in females and >45% in males; when patient relapses (patient is symptomatic), initiate busulphan therapy again at same dose.
↓

If patient is poorly compliant, consider ^{32}P: 2.3 mCi/m^2 IV every 12 wk as needed (limit 5 mCi per dose).
Increase dose by 25% if no response
Patient age >70 yr
Phlebotomy + low-dose aspirin + hydroxyurea
↓
No response or poor compliance
Busulphan 4 to 6 mg/d PO for 4 to 8 wk. Stop when blood counts are normalized or platelet count is >300,000 mm^{-3}.
↓
No response ^{32}P

From Hoffmann R et al: *Hematology: basic principles and practice*, ed 5, Philadelphia, 2009, Churchill Livingstone.

DISPOSITION

- The median survival time without treatment is 6 to 18 mo after diagnosis; phlebotomy extends the average survival time to 12 yr.
- Patients with polycythemia vera with a hematocrit <45% have a significantly lower rate of cardiovascular death and major thrombosis than those with hematocrit of 45% to 50%.
- Prognosis is worse in patients >60 yr and those with a history of thrombosis.

SUGGESTED READINGS

available at www.expertconsult.com

RELATED CONTENT

Fig. E3-143 Diagnostic algorithm for polycythemia (Algorithm)
Polycythemia Vera (Patient Information)

AUTHOR: **FRED F. FERRI, M.D.**

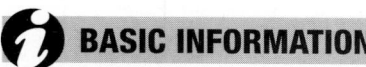

BASIC INFORMATION

DEFINITION

Polymyalgia rheumatica (PMR) is an inflammatory condition characterized by shoulder and pelvic girdle muscle pain and stiffness.

SYNONYMS

Anarthritic rheumatoid syndrome
PMR

ICD-9CM CODES
725.0 Polymyalgia rheumatica

EPIDEMIOLOGY & DEMOGRAPHICS

PREVALENCE: Some geographic variation with rates of 59 per 100,000 in Minnesota; 84 per 100,000 in UK; rare in African Americans
PREDOMINANT SEX: Female/male ratio of 2:1
PREDOMINANT AGE: Age >50 years with greater incidence as age increases

PHYSICAL FINDINGS & CLINICAL PRESENTATION

- In majority of patients, sudden onset of muscle pain and stiffness
- Neck, shoulders, and arms are most often affected. Pelvic girdle and thigh muscles also involved.
- Patients often note severe pain and stiffness.
- Constitutional symptoms of fatigue, malaise, and loss of appetite may accompany pain and stiffness.

BOX 1-50 Disease Entities with Polymyalgias

Rheumatoid arthritis
Rotator cuff syndrome
Osteoarthritis of shoulder and hip joints
Fibromyalgia
Polymyositis/dermatomyositis
Spondyloarthritis
Systemic lupus erythematosus
Vasculitides
Paraneoplastic myalgias
Infection-associated myalgias
RS3PE (remitting seronegative symmetric synovitis and pitting edema)
Parkinson's disease
Hypothyroidism

From Hochberg M: *Rheumatology,* ed 4, Philadelphia, 2007, Mosby.

- Physical exam is fairly benign; passive range of motion is typically preserved; may find minimal joint swelling, and strength testing is normal.
- Presence of fever, chills, night sweats, visual disturbances, headaches, or jaw claudication suggests concomitant giant cell arteritis and warrants further evaluation.

ETIOLOGY

Appears to be related to the presence of HLA-D4 haplotypes, which confer susceptibility to activation of the innate immune system leading to inflammation.

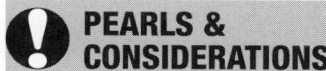

DIAGNOSIS

DIFFERENTIAL DIAGNOSIS

See Box 1-50.

WORKUP

- Elderly patients with PMR symptoms should have initial laboratory evaluation with ESR, CBC, CPK.
- ESR >40 is seen in majority of patients.
- May have a normocytic, normochromic anemia and thrombocytosis.
- Table 1-333 describes diagnostic criteria for PMR.

TREATMENT

ACUTE GENERAL Rx

- Prednisone 10 to 20 mg/day with dramatic improvement in symptoms typically noted in 24 to 48 hr.

- Initial dose of prednisone maintained for 2 to 4 wk with steroid dose reduced by 10% every 4 wk as long as patient remains symptom free.
- It is prudent to start a proton-pump inhibitor at initiation of therapy given the need for gastric protection in an elderly age group at high risk for GI toxicity.
- Attention should be paid to bone health given most patients are on steroids for 1 to 2 yr. Calcium and vitamin D supplementation should be started early on with possible bisphosphonate use if indicated by bone density measurement.

PEARLS & CONSIDERATIONS

Patients with PMR should be monitored carefully for the development of giant cell arteritis. Patients who have incomplete response to treatment with prednisone or have an evolving pattern of pain and swelling should be reevaluated for the possibility of a different diagnosis.

SUGGESTED READINGS

available at www.expertconsult.com

RELATED CONTENT

Giant Cell Arteritis (Related Key Topic)
Vasculitis (Related Key Topic)
Polymyalgia Rheumatica (PMR) (Patient Information)

AUTHOR: **NUHA R. SAID, M.D.**

TABLE 1-333 Polymyalgia Rheumatica: Diagnostic Criteria

Chuang et al 1982	Healey 1984
- Age of onset = 50 yr or older - Erythrocyte sedimentation rate >40 mm/h - Bilateral aching and stiffness for =1 mo and involving two of the following areas: neck or torso, shoulders or proximal regions of the arms, and hips or proximal aspects of the thighs - Exclusion of all other diagnoses causing PMR-like symptoms	- Age of onset = 50 yr or older - Erythrocyte sedimentation rate >40 mm/h - Pain persisting for =1 mo and involving two of the following areas: neck, shoulders and pelvic girdle - Absence of other diseases capable of causing the musculoskeletal symptoms - Morning stiffness lasting more than 1 hr - Rapid response to prednisone (=20 mg/day)

From Hochberg M: *Rheumatology,* ed 4, Philadelphia, 2007, Mosby.

BASIC INFORMATION

DEFINITION

Clinically significant portal hypertension is defined as a portal vein pressure >10 mm Hg, most commonly attributable to liver disease.

SYNONYMS

None

ICD-9CM CODES
572.3 Portal hypertension

EPIDEMIOLOGY & DEMOGRAPHICS

- Incidence of portal hypertension is not known.
- Cirrhosis is the most common cause of portal hypertension in the U.S.
- More than 90% of patients with cirrhosis develop portal hypertension.
- Alcoholic and viral liver diseases are the most common causes of cirrhosis and portal hypertension in the U.S.
- Schistosomiasis is the main cause of portal hypertension outside the U.S.
- Esophageal varices may appear when portal vein pressure rises to >10 mm Hg.
- Variceal hemorrhage is the most serious complication of portal hypertension and may occur when portal pressures rise >12 mm Hg.

PHYSICAL FINDINGS & CLINICAL PRESENTATION

- Jaundice
- Ascites (Fig. 1-668)
- Spider angiomata
- Testicular atrophy
- Gynecomastia
- Palmar erythema

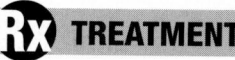

FIGURE 1-668 Ascites secondary to portal hypertension. Note the dilated collateral vein running up the right side of the abdomen. (From Forbes A et al [eds]: *Atlas of clinical gastroenterology,* ed 3, Oxford, 2005, Mosby.)

- Dupuytren's contracture
- Asterixis (with advanced liver failure)
- Irritability, encephalopathy
- Splenomegaly
- Dilated veins in the anterior abdominal wall
- Venous pattern on the flanks
- Caput medusae (tortuous collateral veins around the umbilicus)
- Hemorrhoids
- Hematemesis
- Melena
- Pruritus

ETIOLOGY

Pathophysiologically caused by:
1. Conditions resulting in an increased resistance to flow
   - Prehepatic (e.g., portal vein thrombosis, splenic vein thrombosis, congenital stenosis)
   - Hepatic (e.g., cirrhosis, alcoholic liver disease, primary biliary cirrhosis, schistosomiasis)
   - Posthepatic (e.g., Budd-Chiari syndrome, constrictive pericarditis, inferior vena cava obstruction, cor pulmonale, tricuspid regurgitation)
2. Conditions leading to increase in portal blood flow
   - Splanchnic arterial vasodilation accompanying portal hypertension, mediated by local release of nitric oxide
   - Arterial-portal venous fistulae

Table 1-334 summarizes the etiology of portal hypertension.

DX DIAGNOSIS

- The diagnosis of portal hypertension is made on clinical grounds after a comprehensive history and physical examination.
- Noninvasive and invasive procedures confirm diagnosis and determine the severity of portal hypertension.

DIFFERENTIAL DIAGNOSIS

- Ascites from infection, neoplasm, or other inflammatory processes
- Obesity
- Abdominal organomegaly

WORKUP

The workup of portal hypertension includes blood tests and noninvasive imaging studies to determine if the cause of portal hypertension is prehepatic, hepatic, or posthepatic. Ascitic fluid analysis is a key part of the diagnosis.

LABORATORY TESTS

- Complete blood count with platelets
- Liver function tests with serum albumin
- Prothrombin and partial thromboplastin times
- Hepatitis B surface antigen and antibody
- Hepatitis C antibody
- In selected cases: iron, total iron-binding capacity, and ferritin; antinuclear antibody, anti–smooth muscle antibodies, antimitochondrial antibody, ceruloplasmin, alpha-1 antitrypsin.

- Ascitic fluid analysis: a serum-ascites albumin gradient ≥1.1 mg/dl suggests portal hypertension. Polymorphonuclear cells ≥250 cells/ml or positive Gram stain or culture suggest complicating spontaneous bacterial peritonitis (SBP).

IMAGING STUDIES

- Duplex-Doppler ultrasound is effective in screening for portal hypertension.
- Less commonly, CT/MRI/MRA scanning (Fig. E1-669) or liver-spleen nuclear medicine scanning can be used if the results from ultrasound are equivocal.
- Upper endoscopy is the most reliable test documenting the presence of esophageal varices.

RX TREATMENT

The treatment of portal hypertension is complex and involves measures to reduce the hypertension directly, minimize volume overload, correct underlying disorders, and prevent complications (most notably SBP and variceal bleeding).

NONPHARMACOLOGIC THERAPY

Dietary sodium restriction to generally 2000 mg/day forms the basis of therapy to limit fluid overload.

ACUTE GENERAL Rx

- For tense ascites, serial large-volume paracentesis (LVP) is generally recommended. The use of albumin infusion (8 to 10 g/L of ascites fluid removed) during LVP >5 L has been shown to reduce the incidence of postparacentesis circulatory dysfunction, although its use remains somewhat controversial.
- IV diuretics, typically furosemide and spironolactone, are used to achieve natriuresis and net negative salt and water balance. Renal function and serum electrolytes are monitored frequently, with transition to an oral regimen for long-term therapy.
- SBP is treated with IV antibiotics directed against enteric bacteria.
- Acute variceal hemorrhage is treated with crystalloid and blood product resuscitation, IV octreotide, terlipressin/vasopressin or somatostatin, and urgent upper endoscopy, often with sclerotherapy or band ligation. Patients with acute variceal hemorrhage should receive antibiotic prophylaxis against SBP.
- Traditionally, a transjugular intrahepatic portosystemic shunt (TIPS) or surgical shunt placement may be considered in patients not responding to above measures. However, recent data show early TIPS placement improved outcomes in acute variceal hemorrhage.

CHRONIC Rx

- Dietary sodium restriction in combination with diuretics: the typical ratio of furosemide 40 mg to spironolactone 100 mg retains

normal serum potassium levels in most patients.

- Nonselective beta-blockers (propranolol and nadolol) in dosages sufficient to reduce the resting heart rate by 25% have been shown to be effective in primary prophylaxis for first-time variceal bleeding and for preventing recurrent variceal bleeding. Dosages are usually given bid and decreased if heart rate falls to <55 beats/min or systolic blood pressure drops to <90 mm Hg. The addition of a long-acting nitrate (e.g., isosorbide-5-mononitrate) has been shown to improve portal hemodynamics. Findings of a prospective trial of beta-blockers to prevent the formation of varices were negative. The combination of beta-blockade plus endoscopic esophageal variceal banding is superior to either intervention alone.
- Intermittent LVP may be needed in "diuretic resistant" patients.
- Patients with prior SBP merit lifelong antibiotics for secondary prevention.
- Abstinence from alcohol or treatment for hepatitis B or hepatitis C. Vaccination for hepatitis A and B as appropriate.
- Hepatic transplantation is an option in selected patients.

DISPOSITION

- The most common complication associated with portal hypertension is variceal bleeding. The risk of bleeding from varices is approximately 15% at 1 yr.
- Development of the hepatorenal syndrome (HRS) is associated with high near-term mortality. In particular, HRS may complicate SBP, which emphasizes the importance of making the diagnosis of SBP and instituting appropriate prophylaxis.

REFERRAL

Consultation with a gastroenterologist is recommended in all patients with portal hypertension to screen for esophageal varices.

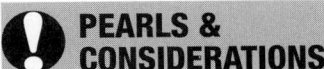

PEARLS & CONSIDERATIONS

Splanchnic arterial vasodilation is increasingly recognized as an important component of the pathophysiology of portal hypertension and ascites. There may be vasodilation in other capillary beds as well; of note, pulmonary arteriolar vasodilation can create a significant shunt fraction and resultant hypoxemia in the absence of chest radiograph or CT chest evidence of parenchymal disease. The diagnosis is suspected when otherwise unexplained hypoxia arises in a patient with cirrhosis, along with platypnea (dyspnea worse when sitting upright) and orthodeoxia (desaturation with upright posture). The diagnosis is confirmed by echocardiography with agitated saline, in which there is delayed appearance of bubbles in the left heart after injection into a peripheral vein.

COMMENTS

Portal hypertension and its complications carry significant morbidity and mortality rates. Emphasize ethanol abstinence, provide vaccinations and prophylactic therapy where indicated, and consider early referral to a specialist for assistance with management and consideration for hepatic transplantation.

SUGGESTED READINGS

available at www.expertconsult.com

AUTHOR: **MEL L. ANDERSON, M.D.**

TABLE 1-334 Etiology of Portal Hypertension

Condition	Site of Increased Resistance	FHVP	WHVP	HVPG	SPP	Liver Disease
Cirrhosis	Intrahepatic sinusoidal	Normal	Increased	Increased	Increased	Yes
Alcoholic hepatitis	Intrahepatic sinusoidal	Normal	Increased	Increased	Increased	Yes
Extrahepatic portal, splenic, or mesenteric vein thrombosis	Extrahepatic presinusoidal	Normal	Normal	Normal	Increased	No
Early primary biliary cirrhosis, PSC, sarcoid, schistosomiasis, congestive heart failure, noncirrhotic portal fibrosis, NRH	Intrahepatic presinusoidal	Normal	Normal/?raised	Normal/?raised	Increased	No
Hemochromatosis, peliosis, infiltrative disease, acute fatty liver of pregnancy	Intrahepatic sinusoidal hypertension	Normal	Increased	Increased	Increased	Yes
Veno-occlusive disease, posttransplant rejection	Intrahepatic postsinusoidal hypertension	Normal	?Increased	?Decreased	Increased	Yes
Budd-Chiari syndrome (noncirrhotic)	Extrahepatic postsinusoidal hypertension	Increased	Increased	Normal	Increased	Depends on severity
Constrictive pericarditis, inferior vena cava obstruction, congenital inferior vena cava web, right heart failure	Extrahepatic postsinusoidal hypertension	Increased	Increased	Normal	Increased	Depends on severity

FHVP, Free hepatic venous pressure; *HVPG,* hepatic venous pressure gradient; *SPP,* systolic pulse pressure; *WHVP,* wedged hepatic venous pressure.

From Vincent JL et al: *Textbook of critical care,* ed 6, Philadelphia, 2011, Saunders.

BASIC INFORMATION

DEFINITION

Portal vein thrombosis (PVT) is thrombotic occlusion of the portal vein. The thrombus can also involve segments of the mesenteric veins and/or the splenic vein.

SYNONYMS

Pylethrombosis
PVT

ICD-9CM CODES
452   Portal vein thrombosis
572.1 Septic portal vein thrombosis

EPIDEMIOLOGY & DEMOGRAPHICS

Occurs with equal frequency in children (peak age: 6 yr) and adults (peak age: 40 yr)

PHYSICAL FINDINGS & CLINICAL PRESENTATION

- Acute PVT may present with sudden onset of fever and abdominal pain (when there is mesenteric extension).
- Upper gastrointestinal hemorrhage (hematemesis and/or melena) caused by esophageal varices

ETIOLOGY & PATHOPHYSIOLOGY

In children: umbilical sepsis (pathophysiology unknown). In adults:
1. Hypercoagulable states
   - Antiphospholipid syndrome
   - Neoplasm (common cause)
   - Paroxysmal nocturnal hemoglobinuria
   - Myeloproliferative diseases
   - Oral contraceptives
   - Polycythemia vera
   - Pregnancy
   - Protein S or C deficiency
   - Sickle cell disease
   - Thrombocytosis
2. Inflammatory diseases
   - Crohn's disease
   - Pancreatitis
   - Ulcerative colitis
3. Complications of medical intervention
   - Ambulatory dialysis
   - Chemoembolization
   - Liver transplantation
   - Partial hepatectomy
   - Sclerotherapy
   - Splenectomy

   - Transjugular intrahepatic portosystemic shunt
4. Infections
   - Appendicitis
   - Diverticulitis
   - Cholecystitis
5. Miscellaneous
   - Cirrhosis (common cause)
   - Bladder cancer

Pathophysiology: PVT results in portal hypertension, leading to esophageal and gastrointestinal varices. The liver sustained by the hepatic artery maintains normal function.

DIAGNOSIS

DIFFERENTIAL DIAGNOSIS

Causes of upper gastrointestinal hemorrhage are covered in Section II.

WORKUP

- Abdominal ultrasound (Fig. 1-670) or MRI may show the PVT. Abdominal ultrasound color Doppler imaging has a 98% negative predictive value and is considered the imaging modality of choice in diagnosing PVT.
- Determination of underlying cirrhosis of the liver should be the foremost step.
- Esophagogastroscopy shows esophageal varices.

TREATMENT

- Anticoagulation data on thrombolytic therapy are inconclusive. In patients with chronic PVT and concomitant cirrhosis, long-term anticoagulation generally not recommended.
- Variceal sclerotherapy or banding
- Surgical mesocaval or splenorenal shunt
- The roles of thrombolysis and transjugular intrahepatic portosystemic shunt continue to evolve

REFERRAL

- To surgeon to rule out intestinal infacrtion
- To gastroenterologist

SUGGESTED READING

available at www.expertconsult.com

AUTHOR: **FRED F. FERRI, M.D.**

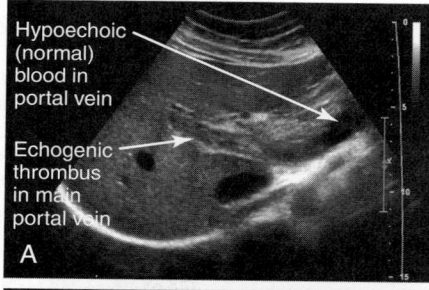

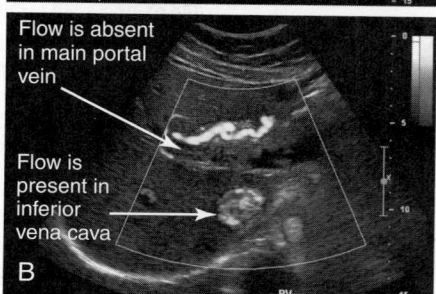

FIGURE 1-670 Portal vein thrombosis: ultrasound. This 22-year-old female, 2 months postpartum, presented with 1 week of right upper quadrant pain. Ultrasound was performed to evaluate for suspected cholecystitis or symptomatic cholelithiasis. Instead, portal vein thrombosis was discovered. The postpartum state is a risk factor for this condition. Hypercoagulable states and inflammatory or neoplastic abdominal conditions, including pancreatitis and abdominal malignancies, also can result in portal vein thrombosis. **A,** Ultrasound gray scale image showing thrombus in the main portal vein. **B,** Doppler ultrasound showing no flow within the portal vein. (From Broder JS: *Diagnostic imaging for the emergency physician,* Philadelphia, 2011, Saunders.)

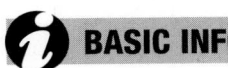

BASIC INFORMATION

DEFINITION

Postconcussive syndrome (PCS) refers to persistent neurologic symptoms that result from traumatic brain injury (TBI). PCS can also follow moderate and severe brain injury, although it is more commonly associated with mild brain injury or concussion. Concussion is an acute trauma-induced alteration of mental function lasting <24 hr, with or without preceding loss of consciousness.

SYNONYMS

PCS
Postconcussion syndrome
Posttraumatic nervous instability or brain injury
Postcontusion syndrome or encephalopathy
Status post commotio cerebri

ICD-9CM CODES
310.2 Postconcussion syndrome

EPIDEMIOLOGY & DEMOGRAPHICS

- Incidence is approximately 27 cases per 100,000 persons/year.
- From 30% to 80% of patients with mild to moderate brain injury will experience some symptoms of PCS.
- Female gender and increasing age are risk factors for PCS.
- Usually seen in the young, ages 20 to 30 yr.

PHYSICAL FINDINGS & CLINICAL PRESENTATION

- Usually present without focal neurologic deficits on examination.
- Symptoms start within a few days after the head injury and usually persist after 3 mo.
- Can be divided into early and late or persistent (>6 mo).
- 15% of patients will have persistent symptoms 1 yr later.
- Symptoms include (at least three of the following after TBI to meet ICD-10 criteria):
  1. Headache (usually of fronto-occipital location and showing characteristics of tension or migraine headache). The International Headache Society suggests that coding and attribution of headaches with characteristics of primary headaches but in the setting of an inciting event should be attributed to the event, unless there was a known history of the headache and the inciting event was seen as aggravating/initiating the preexisting migraine/tension headache.
  2. Fatigue
  3. Dizziness and/or vertigo
  4. Impaired memory
  5. Difficulty in concentrating
  6. Insomnia
  7. Irritability
  8. Lowered tolerance of stress, emotion, or alcohol
- Other associated symptoms: noise sensitivity, neck pain, nondermatomal paresthesias, interference with social role functioning.

ETIOLOGY

- Caused by TBI from events such as falls, motor vehicle accidents, and contact sports.
- Postmortem findings reveal diffuse axonal injury as the primary pathologic finding along with small petechial hemorrhages and local edema.
- Diffuse axon injury is believed to lead to altered neurotransmission and possibly to clinical manifestations.
- A psychogenic origin has been suggested by a number of empiric and clinical observations; however, limitations in methodology and differing definitions preclude firm conclusions.

DIAGNOSIS

A careful history, a nonfocal neurologic examination, and a normal neurologic test will usually establish the diagnosis.

DIFFERENTIAL DIAGNOSIS

- Headache (dissection of the vertebral artery, occipital neuralgia)
- Epidural hematoma
- Subdural hematoma
- Skull fracture
- Cervical spine disk disease
- Whiplash
- Cerebrovascular accident
- Depression
- Anxiety

WORKUP

To exclude other causes of neurologic symptoms after TBI:
- Electroencephalography is normal.
- Evoked potentials are normal.
- Neuropsychological testing is useful because it reveals difficulties in concentration, memory, language, and executive function.

LABORATORY TESTS

Blood tests are not specific.

IMAGING STUDIES

- 10% of CT scans of the head following mild TBI are abnormal, showing mild subarachnoid hemorrhage, subdural hemorrhage, or contusions.
- MRI of the head is abnormal in 30% of patients with normal CT scans and may show irregular brain contours or old cerebral contusions.

TREATMENT

Must be recognized as a physiologic and psychological problem and treated accordingly.

GENERAL Rx

- Must be individualized to the patient's particular symptoms.
- Simple reassurance is often the major treatment.
- Supportive care may include the use of non-narcotic analgesics and antiemetics.
- Pain management.
- Amitriptyline has been widely used for posttraumatic tension-type headaches as well as for nonspecific symptoms such as irritability, dizziness, insomnia, and depression.
- Posttraumatic migraine-type headaches can be treated with a trial of propranolol or amitriptyline alone or in combination.

- Depression can be treated with selective serotonin reuptake inhibitors but may not respond as well when compared with patients without PCS who have depression.
- Some patients may be admitted for severe symptoms; most can be managed as outpatients.
- There may be a role for cognitive behavioral therapy in treating symptoms.

NONPHARMACOLOGIC THERAPY

- Early psychological intervention and cognitive rehabilitation are key for full recovery.
- Physical and occupational therapy.
- Avoidance of alcohol, narcotics, and sleep deprivation.
- Explanation of symptoms and expectations, combined with early follow-up with reassurance, may hasten resolution of symptoms.

DISPOSITION

- Most patients improve after mild TBI without any residual deficits within 3 months.
- Predictors for the development of persistent PCS include:
  - Female sex
  - Ongoing litigation (conflicting studies)
  - Low socioeconomic status
  - Prior headaches
  - Prior TBI
  - Prior psychiatric illnesses

REFERRAL

Early consultations with psychologists, psychiatrists, neurologists, and rehabilitation specialists in an outpatient setting may be beneficial.

PEARLS & CONSIDERATIONS

- PCS starts within a few days after the injury.
- Recognizing depression and treating pain symptoms early in the course may help prevent the development of persistent PCS (>1 yr).
- The severity of the trauma does not clearly predict the risk of PCS.
- The severity of the brain injury is usually documented by the initial Glasgow Coma Scale, the length of unconsciousness, and the duration of amnesia; however, the field may be moving toward more subtle tests of function, such as neuropsychological testing.

COMMENTS

- Attempts to determine how much of a role psychological and/or neurologic factors play in the PCS are important but very difficult.
- No medication at hospital discharge has been proved to change the natural course of the disease.

SUGGESTED READINGS
available at www.expertconsult.com

RELATED CONTENT
Post-concussion Syndrome (Patient Information)

AUTHORS: **WEN Y. WU-CHEN, M.D.,** and **MARK F. BRADY, M.D., M.P.H.**

P

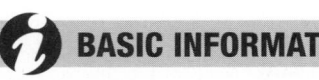 **BASIC INFORMATION**

DEFINITION

Posttraumatic stress disorder (PTSD) is an anxiety disorder that may arise when an individual has witnessed or experienced a potentially fatal or serious injury during which he or she felt helpless or horrified. The individual continues to experience the event in the form of flashbacks (reliving the trauma), intrusive recollections, dreams, or physiologic reactivity. These responses are associated with persistent hyperarousal (e.g., hypervigilance, exaggerated startle response, sleep disturbance, irritability, and difficulty concentrating) and avoidance (both physically and cognitively) of stimuli associated with the traumatic event. In children, the horror may be expressed by disorganized or agitated behavior.

SYNONYMS

Soldier's heart
Effort syndrome
Shell shock
Irritable heart
Traumatic necrosis
Survivor syndrome
Concentration camp syndrome
Gross stress reaction (DSM-I, published in 1952)
Developmental trauma disorder (for children)

ICD-9CM CODES
309.81 Posttraumatic stress syndrome

EPIDEMIOLOGY & DEMOGRAPHICS

INCIDENCE: Fewer than 10% of individuals who have experienced a traumatic event will develop PTSD.
PREVALENCE (IN U.S.):
- One of the most common psychiatric disorders; estimated lifetime prevalence 7.8% to 12.3%
- Prevalence among high-risk populations (e.g., combat veterans or victims of violent crimes) up to 58%
- ~80% have a comorbid psychiatric disorder (depression, anxiety disorder, or substance use)
- Factors most associated with development are subsequent life stress and perceived lack of social support

PREDOMINANT SEX: Twice as many women as men are affected (prevalence 10% to 14% for women and 5% to 6% for men). More than 50% of cases in women are related to sexual assault.
PREDOMINANT AGE: No predisposing age factors
GENETICS: Twin studies have demonstrated genetic vulnerability related to combat.

PHYSICAL FINDINGS & CLINICAL PRESENTATION

- A life-threatening event evoking intense fear or horror (criterion A).
- Reexperiencing of traumatic events in the form of dreams, flashbacks, and intrusive memories (criterion B).

- Depersonalization, detachment, emotional numbing, and dissociation, with avoidance of physical or cognitive reminders of the event (criterion C).
- Hyperarousal, hypervigilance and exaggerated startle response, irritability, anxiety, and difficulty concentrating (criterion D).
- To meet DSM-IV criteria for PTSD, one must meet criterion A plus symptoms from each of the three symptoms clusters A, B, C, and D. A fifth criterion concerns duration of symptoms (>1 mo) and a sixth assesses function (must be impaired).
- Mnenmonic: TRAUMA
  *T*raumatic event (criterion A)
  *R*eexperiencing (criterion B)
  *A*voidance (criterion C)
  *U*nable to function (criterion F)
  *M*onth at least (criterion E)
  *A*rousal (criterion D)

ETIOLOGY

- Interpersonal violence is more likely to give rise to PTSD than events such as motor vehicle accidents or natural disasters.
- Severity of physical injury is a weaker predictor of PTSD than the psychological distress; stress duration is the most important factor.
- Proposed mechanisms include excessive release of norepinephrine in the amygdala, exaggerated negative feedback inhibition of the HPA axis by glucocorticoids, and enhanced postsynaptic alpha-1 response to norepinephrine.
- Hippocampal volumes in adults with PTSD are smaller than normal. Whether this is a result of PTSD or a predisposing factor is unknown.

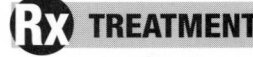 **DIAGNOSIS**

DIFFERENTIAL DIAGNOSIS

- Adjustment disorders: precipitating stress is less catastrophic and psychological reaction is less specific.
- Acute stress disorder: duration of symptoms from 48 hr to 4 wk after trauma.
- Acute PTSD: duration of symptoms is <3 mo
- Chronic PTSD: duration of symptoms is 3 mo or longer
- PTSD with delayed onset: symptoms develop >6 mo after the event.

WORKUP

- Among self-report questionnaires and structured diagnostic instruments, the best validated is the Posttraumatic Diagnostic Scale.
- Laboratory and imaging are not clinically useful.
- Primary care PTSD (PC-PTSD) screen recommended by the Veterans Administration. "Yes" answers to three of four of the questions is a positive screen:
  In your life, have you ever had any experience that was so frightening, horrible, or upsetting that, in the past month, you:
  1. Have had nightmares about it or thought about it when you did not want to? YES NO

  2. Tried hard not to think about it or went out of your way to avoid situations that reminded you of it? YES NO
  3. Were constantly on guard, watchful, or easily startled? YES NO
  4. Felt numb or detached from others, activities, or your surroundings? YES NO

Rx TREATMENT

NONPHARMACOLOGIC THERAPY

- Talk therapy, either psychodynamic or CBT with sensitivity to pacing, readiness, containment, and dissociation, can decrease symptom intensity and frequency. Prolonged exposure (PE), a type of CBT that includes education on stress response, breathing training, and prolonged recounting of the event including sensory details, was found to be more effective than standard CBT in female veterans. There is some controversy regarding appropriateness of exposure therapy for all patients, particularly those with "complex PTSD" from multiple lifetime traumatic events, and the potential for "retraumatization."
- Group therapy is helpful, particularly combat veterans.
- Eye movement desensitization reprocessing (EMDR) has shown efficacy in controlled trials.

ACUTE GENERAL Rx

- Immediate postincident debriefing may worsen outcome.
- A brief course of benzodiazepines may be helpful acutely but has not been shown to decrease development of core symptoms.
- Beta-adrenergic blockers may be helpful if given within hours after the trauma to disrupt the physiologic stress response.
- Sedating antidepressants or sleep aids may be helpful for initial insomnia.

CHRONIC Rx

- SSRIs are agents of choice.
- TCAs are also helpful in reducing symptoms.
- Guanfacine may be helpful in treating arousal symptoms.
- Prazosin may decrease distressing dreams and improve sleep quality.
- Mood stabilizers and antipsychotics may be needed for severe symptoms such as paranoia, extreme anxiety, or angry outbursts.

COMPLEMENTARY & ALTERNATIVE APPROACHES

Acupuncture has been shown to be as effective as CBT in decreasing symptoms of PTSD.

DISPOSITION

- Recovery rates are highest in the first 12 mo after onset.
- Average duration of symptoms is 36 mo for those who undergo treatment and 64 mo for those never treated.
- 50% chance of remission at 2 yr; 50% have chronic symptoms.

Diseases and Disorders

I

- Predictors of chronic course include previous trauma, premorbid psychiatric function, panic reaction at time of event, prolonged terror, or dissociation at time of event.

REFERRAL

Because early intervention improves outcome, refer to psychiatry as soon as diagnosis made.

PEARLS & CONSIDERATIONS

- Screen for comorbid substance abuse.
- Treatment can be effective even if it begins years after the traumatic event occurred.
- PTSD is increasingly being conceived of as a stress-induced fear-circuitry disorder of the limbic system.

SUGGESTED READINGS

available at www.expertconsult.com

RELATED CONTENT

Posttraumatic Stress Disorder (PTSD) (Patient Information)

AUTHORS: **KAILA COMPTON, M.D., Ph.D., RADHIKA A. RAMANAN, M.D., M.P.H.,** and **ALISON C. MAY, M.D.**

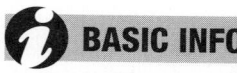

BASIC INFORMATION

DEFINITION

Postural orthostatic tachycardia syndrome (POTS), an underrecognized autonomic disorder, is defined as a form of orthostatic intolerance in which an exaggerated increase in heart rate (HR) occurs during standing, without orthostatic hypotension. Symptoms occur while standing and are relieved by recumbency. It is often misdiagnosed for having panic or anxiety disorders. These symptoms may be profoundly exacerbated by simple activities such as walking or even eating, and thus can be disabling.

SYNONYMS

Orthostatic intolerance
Postural tachycardia syndrome
Orthostatic tachycardia
POTS

ICD-9CM CODES
337.9

EPIDEMIOLOGY & DEMOGRAPHICS

INCIDENCE: Unknown
PREVALENCE: Estimated to be 5-10× as common as orthostatic hypotension; ~500,000 patients in the U.S. (25% are disabled and unable to work)
PREDOMINANT SEX AND AGE: Female/male ratio of 5:1. Mean age is 30 years old (most commonly between 15 and 50 years old).
GENETICS: Possible links with mutations in a norepinephrine transporter have been identified. They result in decreased norepinephrine clearance, causing excessive sympathetic activation.
RISK FACTORS:
- Female sex
- Preceding viral infection or systemic illness (up to 50% of cases)
- Deconditioning and prolonged bed rest
- Medications (e.g., vasodilators, diuretics, antidepressants, anxiolytic agents)
- Predisposition to hypovolemia
- Autoimmune disorders (e.g., multiple sclerosis)
- Excess sympathetic states (e.g., sepsis, trauma, surgery)
- Underlying autonomic neuropathy
- Chronic fatigue syndrome (40% have POTS)

PHYSICAL FINDINGS & CLINICAL PRESENTATION

Symptoms vary, are due to orthstasis (with cerebral hypoperfusion) or sympathetic overaction, and commonly include:
- Palpitations
- Fatigue
- Tremulousness
- Dizziness, lightheadedness, presyncope
- Intolerance to exercise or heat
- Nausea
- Cyclic nature (e.g., worsening with intravascular volume changes during menstrual cycle)

Physical findings are mostly due to the orthostatic hemodynamic changes and may include a reduced pulse pressure with marked beat-to-beat variability of both pulse pressure and HR. Flack sign is the difficulty in palpating a radial pulse with continued standing or Valsalva maneuver. There may be venous prominence with continued standing resulting in blueness and swelling of the feet.

ETIOLOGY

Heterogenous etiologies, which overlap in different types of POTS:
- Hypovolemic POTS: Decreased effective intravascular volume, with peripheral and splanchic venous pooling that worsens with standing. Most patients do not have reduced plasma volume or red cell mass.
- Neuropathic POTS: Patchy sympathetic denervation of lower extremities and kidneys resulting in orthostatic venous pooling and relative hypovolemia with failure of the peripheral vasculature to vasoconstrict upon standing
- Hyperadrenergic POTS: High orthostatic plasma norepinephrine levels (≥600 pg/ml); prominent symptoms are of sympathetic activation
- Deconditioned POTS: Venous pooling in lower extremities due to weak leg "muscle pump"; fibromyalgia-type symptoms with anxiety, exercise intolerance, and prominent fatigue

DIAGNOSIS

DIFFERENTIAL DIAGNOSIS

- Orthostatic hypotension
- Anxiety and panic attacks
- Dehydration
- Medication side effects
- Other forms of autonomic neuropathies
- Other forms of central dysautonomias
- Deconditioning

WORKUP

- Full autonomic system review to evaluate autonomic neuropathies
- Orthostatic vital signs
- Tilt table testing is diagnostic. Continuously monitor HR and blood pressure (BP) for at least 10 min. Findings during head-up tilt include:
  ○ Immediate increase in HR of ≥30 beats/min (HR usually ≥120 beats/min)
  ○ Absence of drop in BP
  ○ Orthostatic intolerance symptoms (see earlier)
- Plasma catecholamines should be measured supine and after standing for 15 minutes. In 50% of patients standing, norepinephrine level was ≥600 pg/ml, signifying a hyperadrenergic response.
- 24-hour urine sodium of <100 mEq signifies a hypovolemic state.

LABORATORY TESTS

Include serum norepinephrine and 24-hour urine sodium to rule out hyperadrenergic and hypovolemic states.

TREATMENT

Education about the pathophysiology of POTS and aggravating and ameliorating factors can help patients better handle the condition. Suspected medications should be discontinued. ~40%-90% of patients respond to a combination of nonpharmacotherapy and pharmacotherapy (mostly β-blockers, then SSRIs, pharmacologic volume expander, or α-1 agonists).

NONPHARMACOLOGIC THERAPY

Cornerstone is increasing vascular tone and effective intravascular volume with prevention of venous pooling.
- Some measures, such as contracting muscles below waist for 30 seconds and wearing abdominal binders or support hose, can reduce venous capacitance and increase total peripheral resistance.
- Drinking two 8-oz glasses of water sequentially can result in sympathetically mediated pressor response lasting for 1-2 hr.
- Hypovolemic patients usually improve with increasing fluid (2 L/day) and sodium intake (10-20 g of salt).
- All patients (especially deconditioned ones) can benefit from an exercise training program (aerobic with lower extremity strengthening).
- Atrioventricular node ablation and pacemaker implantation can be considered for recurrent syncope refractory to therapies.

ACUTE GENERAL Rx

Volume expansion with 1 L of normal saline over 1-3 hours

CHRONIC Rx

- Beta-blockers (propranolol and atenolol) for neuropathic (allow unopposed α-receptor-mediated vasoconstriction) and hyperadrenergic POTS (block β1 receptors in heart)
- SSRIs for neuropathic and hyperadrenergic POTS (decrease central production of serotonin)
- Volume expanders (fludrocortisone and oral vasopressin) for hypovolemic and neuropathic POTS
- Midodrine for neuropathic POTS
- Central sympatholytic agents (clonidine and methyldopa) for hyperadrenergic POTS
- Erythropoietin for refractory neuropathic POTS (increases sensitivity to angiotension II)

SUGGESTED READINGS

available at www.expertconsult.com

AUTHORS: **ALI DAHHAN, M.D.,** and **WEN-CHIH WU, M.D., M.P.H.**

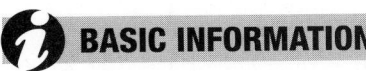

DEFINITION

Precocious puberty is defined as sexual development occurring before age 8 yr in females and 9 yr in males.

SYNONYMS

Pubertas praecox

ICD-9CM CODES
259.1 Precocious puberty

EPIDEMIOLOGY & DEMOGRAPHICS

INCIDENCE: Estimated to be between one in 5000 to 10,000.
PREDOMINANT SEX: Females are affected more often than males for the idiopathic variant; for other causes, dependent on the underlying etiology.
GENETICS: The genetics for some of the etiologies of precocious puberty is known.

PHYSICAL FINDINGS & CLINICAL PRESENTATION

- In females: breast development, pubic hair development, accelerated growth, menarche
- In males: increase in testicular volume and penile length, pubic hair development, accelerated growth, muscular development, acne, change in voice, penile erections

ETIOLOGY

- Idiopathic or true: diagnosis of exclusion
- Central nervous system (CNS) pathology: tumors, hydrocephalus, ventricular cysts, benign lesions
- Severe hypothyroidism
- Posttraumatic head injury
- Genetic disorders: neurofibromatosis, tuberous sclerosis, McCune-Albright syndrome, congenital adrenal hyperplasia
- Gonadal tumors
- Nongonadal tumors: hepatoblastoma
- Exposure to exogenous sex steroids

DIAGNOSIS

DIFFERENTIAL DIAGNOSIS

- Most common diagnoses to consider: premature thelarche and premature adrenarche
- Gonadotropin hormone-releasing hormone (GnRH)-dependent precocious puberty: idiopathic, CNS tumors, hypothalamic hamartomas, neurofibromatosis, tuberous sclerosis, hydrocephalus, status after acute head injury, ventricular cysts, status after CNS infection
- GnRH-independent precocious puberty: congenital adrenal hyperplasia, adrenocortical tumors (males), McCune-Albright syndrome (females), gonadal tumors, ectopic human chorionic gonadotropin (hCG)-secreting tumors (chorioblastoma, hepatoblastoma), exposure to exogenous sex steroids, severe hypothyroidism

WORKUP

Thorough history and physical examination are essential to determine if the patient has true precocious puberty. Particular attention should be paid to growth, development, order of appearance of the secondary sexual characteristics, pubertal development in family members, medications, neurologic symptoms, Tanner staging, abdominal and neurologic examination. Fig. E1-671 describes a clinical approach to precocious puberty.

LABORATORY TESTS

- GnRH testing will help determine if dependent or independent cause
- Sex hormone studies: luteinizing hormone, follicle-stimulating hormone, hCG, testosterone (males), estrogen (females). Levels of sex steroids should be determined in the morning, with use of assays that have detection limits adapted to pediatric values. In girls, serum estradiol levels are highly variable and have a rather low sensitivity for the diagnosis of precocious puberty.
- T_4, thyroid-stimulating hormone

IMAGING STUDIES

- CT scan or MRI of the brain to evaluate for CNS pathology
- Consideration of pelvic ultrasound in female patients to evaluate for cysts or tumors
- Abdominal imaging with CT scan if intraabdominal pathology suspected

TREATMENT

NONPHARMACOLOGIC THERAPY

- Good communication with the parents is essential to care.
- Psychological support for the child may be needed with regard to self-image and problems with peer acceptance.

ACUTE GENERAL Rx

There is no acute therapy for precocious puberty.

CHRONIC Rx

Therapy depends on the etiology of precocious puberty. For the treatment of central or gonadotropin-dependent precocious puberty depot GnRH agonists (leuprorelin, leuprolide, triptorelin, goserelin, histrelin, buserelin) are effective.

- Leuprolide is given 0.25 to 0.3 mg/kg with a 7.5 mg minimum IM every 4 wk. Local side effects include pain, erythema, and inflammatory reactions. Other side effects include headaches and menopausal-like symptoms (asthenia, hot flashes).
- For other CNS lesions and extragonadal tumors, therapy is dependent on the type of lesion, location of the lesion, and the overall prognosis of the underlying problem.
- For severe hypothyroidism, treatment with thyroid hormone will result in regression of the sexual development. The child will subsequently undergo appropriate pubertal development later in life.
- For familial male gonadotropin-independent precocious puberty, the androgen-synthesis inhibitor ketoconazole can be used at doses of 600 mg/day divided tid, or a combination of the aromatase inhibitor testolactone and spironolactone can be used.

DISPOSITION

- For true precocious puberty and some CNS lesions, long-term outcome is usually very good. When drug therapy is instituted, it is continued until a time when further pubertal development is appropriate. It is then discontinued, allowing the child to progress through puberty.
- For other cases, long-term outcomes depend on the prognosis of the underlying cause.

REFERRAL

- Initial workup can be instituted by the primary care provider.
- Referral to an endocrinologist is indicated for most children because they will need long-term management, monitoring, and treatment.
- Attention to the emotional needs of the child is important.

SUGGESTED READING
available at www.expertconsult.com

RELATED CONTENT
Precocious Puberty (Patient Information)

AUTHORS: **BETH J. WUTZ, M.D.,** and **RUBEN ALVERO, M.D.**

BASIC INFORMATION

DEFINITION

Preeclampsia involves the triad of hypertension, proteinuria, and edema that develops after the twentieth week of gestation. Mild preeclampsia is defined as a blood pressure of <140/90 mm Hg. Severe preeclampsia (Table 1-335) is associated with a blood pressure >160/110 mm Hg, proteinuria >5 g in a 24-hr urine collection, oliguria (<400 ml/24 hr), cerebral or visual disturbances, epigastric pain, pulmonary edema, thrombocytopenia, hepatic dysfunction, or severe intrauterine growth restriction. Table 1-336 differentiates preeclampsia from chronic hypertension.

SYNONYMS

Pregnancy-induced hypertension
Toxemia of pregnancy

ICD-9CM CODES
642.6 Preeclampsia

EPIDEMIOLOGY & DEMOGRAPHICS

INCIDENCE: 0% to 14% in primigravidas, 5.7% to 7.3% in multigravidas
RISK FACTORS: Increased incidence and severity with multiple gestations or renal or collagen-vascular diseases. Extremes of reproductive age, <20 or >35 yr, obesity, African American race, thrombophilia, previous preeclampsia.
GENETICS: Positive correlation with maternal and paternal family history

PHYSICAL FINDINGS & CLINICAL PRESENTATION

- Preeclampsia typically presents with hypertension, peripheral edema, and proteinuria, most commonly in the third semester of pregnancy.

TABLE 1-335 Criteria for the Diagnosis of Severe Preeclampsia

In patients with preeclampsia, **severe preeclampsia** can be diagnosed if any one of the following criteria is present:

Blood pressure
  160 mm Hg systolic or 110 mm Hg diastolic or higher on two separate occasions at least 6 hours apart

Proteinuria
  Random urine protein-creatinine ratio ≥5 mg/ml (500 mg/mmol) or proteinuria >5 g/24 h

Oliguria <500 ml in 24 hours

Cerebral or visual disturbances such as cerebrovascular accident, seizures, or visual loss

Pulmonary edema

Epigastric or right upper quadrant pain

Hepatocellular injury (serum transaminases at least twice normal)

Serum lactate dehydrogenase: >600 IU/L

Thrombocytopenia <100 × 10⁹/L

Fetal growth restriction (birth weight less than 10th percentile for the gestational age)

From Floege J et al: *Comprehensive clinical nephrology,* ed 4, Philadelphia, 2010, Saunders.

- Generalized swelling or nondependent edema, possibly manifested by rapid weight gain (>4 lb/wk) even in the absence of edema
- Auscultation of pulmonary rales
- Right upper quadrant pain (HELLP syndrome [hemolysis, elevated liver enzymes, and low platelet count] or subcapsular liver hematoma)
- Hyperreflexia or clonus
- Vaginal bleeding (placental abruption)
- Acute or chronic fetal compromise manifested by intrauterine growth restriction or fetal tachycardia with late decelerations, respectively
- Wide range of symptoms attributable to multiorgan system dysfunction, involving hepatic, hematologic, renal, pulmonary, and central nervous systems
- Possibility of severe disease despite "normal" blood pressure readings, so a high index of suspicion must be maintained in high-risk situations

ETIOLOGY

- Exact etiology or toxic substance is unknown
- Theories:
  - Imbalance between thromboxane A_2 (vasoconstrictor and platelet aggregator) and prostacyclin (vasodilator)
  - Abnormal trophoblastic invasion of spiral arteries
  - Increased sensitivity to angiotensin II by the muscular walls of the arteries
  - Excess circulating soluble fms-like tyrosine kinase 1 (*sFlt1*), which binds placental growth factor (PlGF) and vascular endothelial growth factor (VEGF), may have a pathogenic role
- Potential secondary effects of the metabolic, inflammatory endothelial alternatives in preeclampsia are described in Table 1-337.

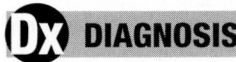 DIAGNOSIS

DIFFERENTIAL DIAGNOSIS

- Acute fatty liver of pregnancy
- Appendicitis
- Diabetic ketoacidosis
- Gallbladder disease
- Gastroenteritis
- Glomerulonephritis
- Hemolytic-uremic syndrome
- Hepatic encephalopathy
- Hyperemesis gravidarum
- Idiopathic thrombocytopenia
- Thrombotic thrombocytopenic purpura
- Nephrolithiasis
- Pyelonephritis
- Peptic ulcer disease
- Systemic lupus erythematosus
- Viral hepatitis

WORKUP

- Two blood pressure measurements with the patient in lateral recumbent position 6 hr apart, with an absolute pressure >140/90 mm Hg or an increase of 30 mm Hg systolic or 15 mm Hg diastolic from baseline, an increase in the mean arterial

TABLE 1-336 Differences between Preeclampsia and Chronic Hypertension

Feature	Preeclampsia	Chronic Hypertension
Age (yr)	Young (<20)	Older (>30)
Parity	Primigravida	Multigravida
Onset	After 20 wk of pregnancy	Before 20 wk of pregnancy
Weight gain and edema	Sudden	Gradual
Systolic blood pressure	<160 mm Hg	>160 mm Hg
Funduscopic findings	Spasm, edema	Arteriovenous nicking, exudates
Left ventricular hypertrophy	Rare	More common
Proteinuria	Present	Absent
Plasma uric acid	Increased	Normal
Blood pressure after delivery	Normal	Elevated

From Zipes DP et al (eds): *Braunwald's heart disease,* ed 7, Philadelphia, 2005, Saunders.

TABLE 1-337 Potential Secondary Effects of the Metabolic, Inflammatory Endothelial Alternatives in Preeclampsia

CVS	Increased peripheral resistance leading to hypertension Increased vascular permeability and reduced maternal plasma volume
Lungs	Laryngeal and pulmonary edema
Renal	Glomerular damage leading to proteinuria, hypoproteinemia, and reduced oncotic pressure, which further exacerbates the hypovolemia. May develop acute renal failure ± cortical necrosis
Clotting	Hypercoagulability, with increased fibrin formation and increased fibrinolysis, i.e., disseminated intravascular coagulation
Liver	HELLP syndrome Hepatic rupture
CNS	Thrombosis and fibrinoid necrosis of the cerebral arterioles Eclampsia (convulsions), cerebral hemorrhage, and cerebral edema
Fetus	Impaired uteroplacental circulation, potentially leading to FGR, hypoxemia, and intrauterine death

CVS, Cardiovascular system; *CNS,* central nervous system; *FGR,* fetal growth restriction; *HELLP,* hemolysis, elevated liver enzymes, low platelets.
From Drife J, Magowan B: *Clinical obstetrics and gynecology,* Philadelphia, 2004, Saunders.

pressure (MAP) of 20 mm Hg, or an absolute MAP >105 mm Hg
- Evaluation for proteinuria as defined by >0.1 g/L on urine dipstick or >300 mg protein on a 24-hr urine collection
- Evaluation of fetal status for evidence of intrauterine growth restriction, oligohydramnios, alteration in umbilical or uterine artery Doppler flow, or acute compromise, such as abruption
- Because of the insidious nature of the disease with potential for multiple organ involvement, complete evaluation for preeclampsia in any pregnant patient presenting with central nervous system derangement or gastrointestinal symptoms after 20 wk of gestation
- Evaluation for associated conditions such as disseminated intravascular coagulation, hepatic dysfunction, or subcapsular hematoma

LABORATORY TESTS
- High-risk patients: baseline assessment of renal function (24-hr urine collection for protein and creatinine clearance), platelets, blood urea nitrogen, creatinine, liver function tests (LFTs), and uric acid should be obtained at the first prenatal visit.
- Complete blood count (hemoglobin, hematocrit, platelets) may show signs of volume contraction or HELLP syndrome.
- LFTs (aspartate aminotransferase, alanine aminotransferase, lactate dehydrogenase) are useful in evaluation for HELLP syndrome or to exclude important differentials.
- Hyperuricemia or increased creatinine may indicate decreasing renal function.
- Prothrombin time, partial thromboplastin time, and fibrinogen should be checked to rule out disseminated intravascular coagulation.
- Peripheral smear may demonstrate microangiopathic hemolytic anemia.
- Complement levels can be used to differentiate from an acute exacerbation of a collagen-vascular disease.
- Increased levels of *sFlt1* and reduced levels of PlGF predict subsequent development of preeclampsia.

IMAGING STUDIES
- CT scan of head if atypical presentation of eclampsia, possibility of intracerebral bleed, or prolonged postictal state
- Sonogram of fetus to evaluate for intrauterine growth restriction (Fig. E1-672), amniotic fluid, placenta
- Sonogram of maternal liver if suspect subcapsular hematoma

 TREATMENT

NONPHARMACOLOGIC THERAPY
Bed rest in left lateral decubitus position

ACUTE GENERAL Rx
Delivery is the treatment of choice and the only cure for the disease. This must be taken in the context of the gestational age of the fetus, severity of the preeclampsia, and the likelihood of a successful induction and reliability of patient.
- Administer magnesium sulfate 6 g IV loading dose, with 2 to 3 g maintenance or phenytoin at 10 to 15 mg/kg loading dose, then 200 mg IV q8h starting 12 hr after loading dose.
- Hydralazine 10 mg IV, labetalol hydrochloride 20 to 40 mg IV, nifedipine 20 mg SL can be used for acute blood pressure control.
- Continuous fetal monitoring is needed.
- Epidural is anesthesia of choice for pain management in labor or cesarean section.
- All patients undergoing induction of labor should receive antiseizure medications regardless of severity of disease.

CHRONIC Rx
- Mild preeclampsia <37 wk: close observation for worsening maternal or fetal condition, with delivery at >37 wk with favorable cervix or at 40 wk regardless of cervical status.
- Severe preeclampsia: delivery in the presence of maternal or fetal compromise, labor, or >34 wk; at 28 to 34 wk consider steroids with close monitoring, and at <24 wk consider termination of pregnancy.
- Methyldopa is drug of choice for long-term blood pressure control during pregnancy.

DISPOSITION
Preeclampsia is a progressive and unpredictable disease process; a course of expectancy should be managed with caution. Up to 20% of patients who have seizures are normotensive.

REFERRAL
Obstetric management is indicated because of the insidious nature of the disease, with transfer of all cases <34 wk to a facility with a level three nursery.

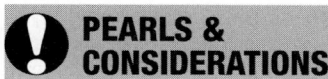 **PEARLS & CONSIDERATIONS**

COMMENTS
- Low-dose aspirin 81 mg qd and calcium supplementation 1500 mg qd can be considered in high-risk patients to decrease the risk of recurrence.
- Begin after first trimester.
- Although the absolute risk of ESRD in women who have had preeclampsia is low, preeclampsia is a marker for an increased risk of subsequent ESRD.
- The development of preeclampsia may be one of the earliest identifiable risk markers for potential future cardiovascular disease in women. It has been shown that women who develop preeclampsia have a higher incidence of cardiovascular risk factors including components of the metabolic syndrome within 1 yr of delivery.

SUGGESTED READINGS
available at www.expertconsult.com

RELATED CONTENT
Eclampsia (Related Key Topic)
Preeclampsia (Patient Information)

AUTHOR: **RUBEN ALVERO, M.D.**

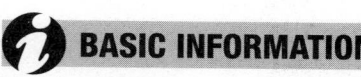

BASIC INFORMATION

DEFINITION

Premature labor is defined as regular contractions that result in cervical dilation or effacement prior to 37 wk gestation.

SYNONYMS

Preterm labor

ICD-9CM CODES
644.0

EPIDEMIOLOGY & DEMOGRAPHICS

INCIDENCE: The incidence of preterm births in the U.S. has increased over the past two decades from 9.5% in 1981 to 12.7% in 2006. Between 40% and 45% of these births follow spontaneous preterm labor; either the remaining preterm births result from premature rupture of membranes (PPROM), or they occur secondary to maternal or fetal indications.
PREDOMINANT SEX AND AGE: Pregnant women at the extremes of reproductive age (<17 yr and >35 yr) are at greatest risk.
GENETICS: A genetic component has been suggested. Women with sisters who have had preterm births and women with grandparents who were born preterm may be at increased risk for having preterm deliveries themselves. Single-nucleotide polymorphisms have also been associated with preterm labor.
RISK FACTORS: Risk factors for premature labor include a prior preterm delivery, intrauterine infection, systemic or genital tract infections, interpregnancy interval (<6 mo), short cervical length (<25 to 30 mm), low pre-pregnancy BMI (<19.8 kg/m^2), age <17 yr or >35 yr, a history of elective pregnancy termination, history of prior stillbirth, African-American ethnicity, vaginal bleeding, polyhydramnios or oligohydramnios, multiple gestation, structural abnormalities of the uterus, history of cervical cone biopsy or loop electrocautery excision, in vitro fertilization or ovulation induction, tobacco use, heavy alcohol consumption, cocaine use, heroin use, and psychological or social stress.

PHYSICAL FINDINGS & CLINICAL PRESENTATION

Presenting symptoms include increased pelvic pressure, abdominal cramping or contractions, increased vaginal discharge, vaginal spotting, or leakage of fluid.

ETIOLOGY

Causes of premature labor are varied and often difficult to determine. Premature labor may be secondary to infection, systemic illness, trauma, anatomic abnormalities (i.e., uterine anomaly), or a combination of factors. It is thought that cervical ripening is the most common first step to premature labor or delivery. Subsequently, decidual-membrane activation occurs, as do contractions.

DIAGNOSIS

DIFFERENTIAL DIAGNOSIS

The differential should include premature labor, preterm rupture of membranes, preterm contractions (contractions prior to 37 wk gestation that do not result in cervical change), and abdominal pain or cramping secondary to other medical conditions. There are many conditions that may cause preterm contractions or premature labor. These include:
- Infection
  - Chorioamnionitis
  - Genital tract infections, including bacterial vaginosis, gonorrhea, chlamydia
  - Urinary tract infections, including pyelonephritis, cystitis, or asymptomatic bacteriuria
  - Gastroenteritis
- Trauma
- Placental abruption
- Illicit drug use
- Preterm premature rupture of membranes
- Appendicitis
- Nephrolithiasis
- Pancreatitis
- Cholelithiasis

WORKUP

- History and physical exam to rule out trauma, abuse, other causes of abdominal pain, and infection
- Fetal heart rate monitoring and tocometry to determine fetal status and contraction frequency
- Speculum exam to visually assess the cervix and assess for rupture of membranes, bleeding, infection, or advanced cervical dilation
  - If the patient is <35 wk gestation, a Fetal Fibronectin (FFN) test should be collected prior to performing a digital exam or transvaginal ultrasound. A FFN test can help predict preterm delivery if the patient has a cervical length on transvaginal ultrasound of <30 mm
- Digital exam to determine cervical dilation and effacement, and fetal station

LABORATORY TESTS

- CBC
- Urine analysis and culture
- Urine toxicology screen
- Collect tests for GBS, gonorrhea, and *Chlamydia*
- Perform a wet prep for yeast, bacterial vaginosis, and *Trichomonas*
- Fetal fibronectin
- Consider PT, PTT, INR, CMP, amylase, and lipase
- Amniocentesis may be performed if an intraamniotic infection is suspected

IMAGING STUDIES

A formal ultrasound is indicated to determine estimated fetal weight, fetal presentation, amniotic fluid volume, placental location and appearance, and cervical length.

TREATMENT

Patients with premature labor should be delivered promptly when an intraamniotic infection is suspected or when they have cervical dilation >5 cm, a persistently nonreassuring fetal heart rate tracing, intrauterine growth restriction, or vaginal bleeding concerning for placental abruption.

NONPHARMACOLOGIC THERAPY

- Smoking cessation
- Bedrest, activity restriction, and pelvic rest are often recommended, but there are insufficient data to support this practice.

ACUTE GENERAL Rx

- Antenatal administration of corticosteroids between 24 wk and 33 6/7 wk gestation is recommended for women at risk of preterm delivery to prevent neonatal respiratory distress syndrome and decrease the incidence of intraventricular hemorrhage and necrotizing enterocolitis.
- Numerous tocolytic agents have been used in an attempt to inhibit contractions. Although efficacy is unclear, they can be utilized during an observation period in an effort to prolong gestation for administration of steroids or to transfer the mother to a facility capable of caring for preterm infants. This, of course, assumes there are no maternal or fetal medical contraindications to use of tocolytic drugs and no indications for rapid delivery. The most commonly used tocolytics are beta-mimetics (terbutaline, ritodrine), magnesium sulfate, calcium channel blockers (nifedipine), or prostaglandin synthetase inhibitors (indomethacin, ketorolac, sulindac).
- Routine antibiotic use has failed to show benefit in the absence of a known infection. But all mothers in preterm labor (without a documented negative group B strep culture) should be given antibiotics to prevent neonatal infection.

CHRONIC Rx

- Patients with a history of prior spontaneous preterm birth may be candidates for prophylactic use of 17 alpha-hydroxyprogesterone caproate between 16 wk and 36 wk gestation.
- Patients with a history of preterm birth and short cervix may also be candidates for prophylactic or rescue cerclage.
- There is no evidence supporting the use of maintenance tocolytic therapy

REFERRAL

- Women who present in preterm labor should be referred to an obstetrician and transferred to a facility with a neonatal intensive care unit.
- For women who present for prenatal care with a history of preterm delivery, early referral to an obstetrician is also recommended

SUGGESTED READINGS

available at www.expertconsult.com

RELATED CONTENT

Abruptio Placentae (Related Key Topic)
Breech Birth (Related Key Topic)
Molar Pregnancy (Related Key Topic)
Uterine Fibroids (Related Key Topic)

AUTHOR: **LAUREN MAY, M.D.**

BASIC INFORMATION

DEFINITION

The *Diagnostic and Statistical Manual of Mental Disorders,* 4th edition, classifies premenstrual dysphoric disorder (PMDD) as a "depressive disorder not otherwise specified" and requires as criteria for definition the presence of five or more of the following symptoms in most menstrual cycles for the past year.

- The symptoms should be present most of the time during the last week of the luteal phase, with remission beginning within a few days after the onset of the follicular phase, and absent during the week after menses, with at least one of the symptoms being either 1, 2, 3, or 4:
  1. Marked depressed mood, feeling of hopelessness, or self-deprecating thoughts
  2. Marked anxiety, tension, feeling of being "keyed up" or "on edge"
  3. Marked affective lability (e.g., feeling suddenly sad or tearful or increased sensitivity to rejection)
  4. Persistent and marked anger or irritability or increased interpersonal conflicts
  5. Decreased interest in usual activities (e.g., work, school, friends, hobbies)
  6. Subjective sense of difficulty in concentrating
  7. Lethargy, easy fatigability, or marked lack of energy
  8. Marked change in appetite, overeating, or specific food cravings
  9. Hypersomnia or insomnia
  10. A subjective sense of being overwhelmed or out of control
  11. Other physical symptoms, such as breast tenderness or swelling, headaches, joint or muscle pain, a sensation of "bloating," or weight gain
- The disturbance markedly interferes with work or school or with usual social activities and relationships with others (e.g., avoidance of social activities, decreased production and efficiency at work or school).
- The disturbance is not merely an exacerbation of the symptoms of another disorder, such as major depressive disorder, panic disorder, dysthymic disorder, or a personality disorder (although it may be superimposed on any of these disorders).
- The first three criteria must be confirmed by prospective daily ratings during at least two consecutive symptomatic cycles (diagnosis may be made provisionally before such confirmation).

NOTE: In menstruating women, the luteal phase corresponds to the period between ovulation and the onset of menses, and the follicular phase begins with menses. In nonmenstruating women (e.g., women who have had a hysterectomy), determination of the timing of the luteal and follicular phases may require measurement of circulating reproductive hormones.

ICD-9CM CODES

625.4 Premenstrual dysphoric syndrome

EPIDEMIOLOGY & DEMOGRAPHICS

- PMDD affects 3% to 5% of women of reproductive age.
- Genetic factors play a significant role (increased incidence in monozygotic twins and in women whose mothers had PMDD).
- 30% to 76% of women with PMDD have a lifetime history of depression.

PHYSICAL FINDINGS & CLINICAL PRESENTATION

- Physical examination may be completely normal.
- Depressed mood, tachycardia, sweating from comorbid disorders (e.g., panic disorder, major depression) may be present.
- Symptoms occur during the last half of the menstrual cycle (the luteal phase) and are absent from the first day of menstruation until ovulation (follicular phase).

ETIOLOGY

- Unknown. Serotonin deficiency and altered sensitivity in serotoninergic system in response to phasic hormone fluctuations in the menstrual cycle are believed to play a role.
- Progesterone appears to be the main precipitating factor in PMDD symptoms, but estrogen may also provoke symptoms.

DIAGNOSIS

DIFFERENTIAL DIAGNOSIS

- Premenstrual syndrome
- Dysthymic syndrome
- Personality disorder
- Panic disorder
- Major depressive disorder
- Hyperthyroidism
- Polycystic ovarian syndrome
- Drug or alcohol abuse
- Irritable bowel syndrome
- Endometriosis

WORKUP

- Diagnosis is based on obtaining a detailed history and ruling out the presence of physical or psychiatric disorders. No objective diagnostic tests exist.
- The diagnosis should be confirmed by using a symptom checklist prospectively for two consecutive menstrual cycles. Commonly used diagnostic instruments include the Calendar of Premenstrual Experiences and the Premenstrual Syndrome Diary.

LABORATORY TESTS

- None are usually necessary.
- A serum thyroid-stimulating hormone test to exclude thyroid problems, complete blood count to rule out anemia, and a chemistry profile to assess electrolytes may be ordered if diagnosis is unclear.

TREATMENT

NONPHARMACOLOGIC THERAPY

- Reduction in intake of caffeine, refined sugars, or sodium may be helpful in some patients.
- Increased aerobic exercise, smoking cessation, alcohol restriction, and regular sleep are often beneficial.
- Stress reduction and management will decrease severity of symptoms.

GENERAL Rx

- Selective serotonin reuptake inhibitors are useful for the treatment of PMDD. Commonly used agents and initial doses are fluoxetine 10 mg qd, sertraline 50 mg qd, paroxetine 10 mg qd, and citalopram 20 mg qd. Many patients will require titration to significantly higher doses to achieve therapeutic benefit. These medications can be administered continuously during the menstrual cycle or only when the patients experience symptoms. Luteal phase or intermittent administration involves initiating medication at the time of ovulation and stopping it at the beginning of menses.
- Other useful agents are benzodiazepines (alprazolam 0.25 mg tid prn) and the tricyclic antidepressant clomipramine (25 mg qd as starting dose).
- Gonadotropin-releasing hormone (GnRH) agonists are effective in treating patients with PMDD. The accelerated bone loss and vasomotor symptoms associated with long-term use of a GnRH agonist will require add-back therapy. Hormonal intervention with monthly intramuscular injections of leuprolide has been reported effective in some patients; however, it should be reserved only for patients unresponsive to first- and second-line agents.
- Nutritional supplementation (vitamin B_6 up to 100 mg/day, vitamin E up to 600 IU/day, calcium carbonate up to 1200 mg/day, and magnesium up to 500 mg/day) are also commonly used for symptom reduction in some patients with limited results.
- Ovariectomy may be considered in severe refractory cases.

SUGGESTED READINGS

available at www.expertconsult.com

AUTHOR: **FRED F. FERRI, M.D.**

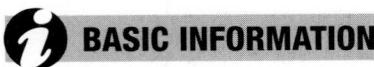

BASIC INFORMATION

DEFINITION

Premenstrual syndrome (PMS) is a cyclic recurrence during the luteal phase of the menstrual cycle of somatic, affective, and behavioral disturbances that are of sufficient severity to affect interpersonal relationships adversely or interfere with normal activities.

SYNONYMS

PMS
PMDD

ICD-9CM CODES
625.4 Premenstrual tension syndromes

EPIDEMIOLOGY & DEMOGRAPHICS

- PMS is believed to be extremely prevalent, intermittently affecting approximately one third of all premenopausal women.
- Severe cases occur in approximately 2% to 10% of women with PMS.
- Those seeking treatment for PMS are usually in their 30s or 40s.
- The natural history of PMS has not been clearly elucidated.

PHYSICAL FINDINGS & CLINICAL PRESENTATION

- Diverse and potentially disabling symptoms. Table 1-338 summarizes common symptoms of cyclic PMS.
- Associated with >150 psychological, physical, and behavioral symptoms
- Most frequent reason for seeking treatment: emotional symptoms
- Most common emotional symptoms: depression, irritability, anxiety, labile moods, anger, crying easily, sadness, extreme sensitivity, nervous tension
- Most common physical symptoms: headache, bloating, cramps, breast tenderness, migraines, fatigue, weight gain, aches and pains, palpitations

- Most common behavior symptom: food cravings
- Other behavioral symptoms: increased appetite, increased alcohol intake, decreased motivation, decreased efficiency, avoidance of activities, staying home, sleep changes, libido changes, forgetfulness, decreased concentration

ETIOLOGY

- Etiology remains obscure.
- Because of the multifactorial, multiorgan nature of PMS, a single etiologic cause is unlikely.

DIAGNOSIS

DIFFERENTIAL DIAGNOSIS

- A diagnosis of exclusion, so other medical or psychological disorders should be ruled out.
- Most common disorders: depression or anxiety, thyroid disease.

WORKUP

- History
- Physical examination
- Laboratory studies to rule out alternative diagnosis
- If no alternative diagnosis confirms diagnosis of PMS, basal body temperature charting is used to determine if the patient is ovulating:
  1. If she is not ovulating, it is not PMS.
  2. If she is ovulating, symptoms should be charted for at least two cycles to determine if the symptoms occur in the luteal phase.
  3. If symptoms are not occurring in the luteal phase, it is not PMS and further investigation is needed.
     a. If symptoms occur in the follicular phase, patient has premenstrual exacerbation of another condition.
     b. If symptoms do not occur in the follicular phase, diagnosis of PMS is confirmed.

LABORATORY TESTS

- None available to specifically confirm the diagnosis of PMS
- Thyroid function tests to rule out thyroid disease

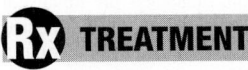

TREATMENT

NONPHARMACOLOGIC THERAPY

- Individualization of the treatment plan to maximize therapeutic response
- Psychosocial intervention:
  ○ Education
  ○ Stress management
  ○ Environmental changes
  ○ Adequate rest and sleep
  ○ Regular exercise
- Nutritional recommendations:
  ○ Regularly eaten, well-balanced meals
  ○ Adequate amounts of protein, fiber, and complex carbohydrates; low fat
  ○ Avoidance of foods that are high in salt and simple sugars; may promote water retention, weight gain, and physical discomfort
  ○ Avoidance of caffeine-containing beverages; stimulant effects of caffeine may worsen tension, irritability, and insomnia
  ○ Avoidance of alcohol and illicit drugs; may worsen emotional lability
  ○ Calcium supplementation (1000 mg/day for women 19 to 50 yr, 1300 mg/day for girls 14 to 18 yr) to reduce the physical and emotional symptoms
  ○ Magnesium (360 mg/day) to reduce water retention and the negative effect associated with PMS
  ○ Pyridoxine (vitamin B_6) 50 mg bid to improve depression, fatigue, irritability, and natural diuretic ability; neurotoxicity observed at higher dosages

ACUTE GENERAL Rx

Suppression of ovulation:
- Oral contraceptives: one pill per day
- Progestin-only oral contraceptive: one pill per day
- Oral micronized progesterone: 100 mg every morning and 200 mg every evening on days 17 through 28 of menstrual cycle
- Progestin suppository: 200 to 400 mg bid on days 17 through 28 of menstrual cycle
- Oral contraceptive containing drosperinone/ethinyl estradiol: very effective in decreasing physical symptoms
- Medroxyprogesterone: 150 mg IM q3mo
- Levonorgestrel implants: surgical insertion every 5 yr
- Transdermal estradiol: one or two 100-μg patches every 3 days
- Danazol: 100 to 200 mg/day (ovulation not suppressed at this dose)
- Gonadotropin-releasing hormone (GnRH) agonists: daily by intranasal spray or monthly by depot injection
Suppression of physical symptoms:
- Spironolactone: 25 to 50 mg bid on days 14 through 28 of menstrual cycle

---

TABLE 1-338 Common Symptoms of Cyclic Premenstrual Syndrome

Somatic Symptoms

Abdominal bloating	Constipation or diarrhea
Acne	Headache
Alcohol intolerance	Peripheral edema
Breast engorgement and tenderness	Weight gain
Clumsiness	

Emotional and Mental Symptoms

Anxiety	Insomnia
Change in libido	Irritability
Depression	Lethargy
Fatigue	Mood swings
Food cravings (especially salt and sugar)	Panic attacks
Hostility	Paranoia
Inability to concentrate	Violence toward self and others
Increased appetite	Withdrawal from others

From Goldman L, Schafer AI: Goldman's Cecil medicine, ed 24, Philadelphia, 2012, Saunders.

- Mefenamic acid
  - For fluid retention: 250 mg tid on days 24 through 28 of cycle
  - For pain: 500 mg tid on days 19 through 28 of cycle
- Bromocriptine: 5 mg/day on days 10 through 26 of cycle
- Danazol: 200 mg/day on days 19 through 28 of cycle
- Naproxen: 550 mg bid on days 17 through 28 of cycle, Naprosyn-500 mg bid on days 17 through 28 of cycle

Suppression of psychological symptoms:
- Nortriptyline: 50 to 125 mg/day
- Fluoxetine: 20 mg/day or 90 mg weekly (this medication has indications for premenstrual dysphoric disorder)
- Buspirone: 10 mg bid or tid on days 16 through 28 of cycle, then taper drug
- Alprazolam: 25 mg tid on days 16 through 28 of cycle, then taper drug

- Clonidine: 0.1 mg bid
- Naltrexone: 0.25 mg/day on days 9 through 18 of cycle
- Atenolol: 50 mg/day
- Paroxetine: 20 mg/day
- Sertraline: 50 to 100 mg/day
- Nefazodone: initial dosage 100 mg bid; after 1 wk increase to 150 mg bid
- Propranolol: 20 to 40 mg bid
- Verapamil: 100 to 320 mg qd

CHRONIC Rx

- Therapy is largely trial and error, with the goal of providing effective treatment with the safest and most simple therapy.
- For severe intractable PMS: bilateral oophorectomy; give trial of GnRH therapy or danazol before surgery (bilateral oophorectomy should be exceedingly rare).
- Estrogen replacement therapy recommended postoperatively to reduce the risk of osteoporosis, heart disease, and genitourinary atrophy.

DISPOSITION

Improved symptoms in 90% of women over time

REFERRAL

- For counseling with a psychologist or psychiatrist if underlying psychiatric disorder is discovered (cognitive-behavioral therapy)
- To a gynecologist if surgical therapy is contemplated

SUGGESTED READINGS
available at www.expertconsult.com

RELATED CONTENT

Dysmenorrhea (Related Key Topic)
Premenstrual Syndrome (Patient Information)
Premenstrual Dysphoric Disorder (Related Key Topic)

AUTHORS: **GEORGE T. DANAKAS, M.D.,** and **RUBEN ALVERO, M.D.**

P

Diseases and Disorders

I

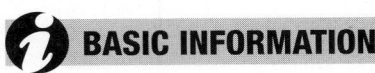

BASIC INFORMATION

DEFINITION

Preoperative evaluation is the clinical risk evaluation for patients undergoing surgery. The goal of the assessment is to identify and treat unrecognized disease and risk factors that may increase the risk of surgery above baseline. Preoperative evaluation should also include functional assessment and determine social support.

SYNONYMS

Preoperative evaluation and risk reduction
Risk reduction in patients undergoing invasive procedures

ICD-9CM CODES
ICD-V72.81–ICD-V72.84

EPIDEMIOLOGY & DEMOGRAPHICS

In the United States, the number of surgical procedures is increasing, although the percentage that occurs in inpatient facilities is decreasing. The scope of the issue is enormous: more than 46 million surgical procedures were performed in 2006 on hospital inpatients (National Health Statistics Report, July 30, 2008).

Some studies have shown the benefits of preoperative testing while others have shown no added benefit. Lack of added benefit has been particularly true for otherwise healthy individuals: the prevalence of significant unrecognized disease and the predictive value of tests are both low for this population–leading to an excess of false positive tests.

Certain risk factors do exist that may be helpful: The nature and extent of surgery appear to play a role, as do increasing age, exercise capacity, and certain medications. Box 1-51 describes stratification of risk of common noncardiac surgical procedures.

There may be other reasons to perform preoperative evaluations: In the United States, individuals undergo an increasing number of surgical procedures of all kinds and seeing patients during the preoperative period may be a good opportunity to reach out to patients about other preventive, screening, and routine health care issues. The primary care physician is uniquely poised to provide an accurate assessment and risk stratification of patients and to develop care plans for follow-up. This information can then be used to help surgeons counsel patients and guide patients' decision making.

PEAK INCIDENCE: When there are adverse consequences from surgery, cardiovascular complications account for the majority of the morbidity and mortality in patients. Perioperative MIs (PMI) is one of the most important predictors of short- and long-term morbidity and mortality associated surgery. The highest incidence of PMI is in the first 3 to 5 days after surgery.

PHYSICAL FINDINGS & CLINICAL PRESENTATION

The history, physical, and other studies need to assess the risks for myocardial infarction, arrhythmias, heart failure, endocarditis, stroke, pulmonary insufficiency, venous thrombosis and pulmonary embolism, hemorrhage, diabetic acidosis, renal or hepatic failure, and infection.

WORKUP

HISTORY

- A thorough medical history is the most valuable tool. Assess the urgency of the surgical procedure. A conversation with the surgical team is helpful for urgent and emergent procedures.
- Age is important to consider because age is often associated with an increasing number of comorbidities, which are in turn associated with an increase in perioperative risk.
- All patients should be asked about their exercise capacity before surgery. Table E1-339 describes the New York Heart Association functional classification. One way to assess functional capacity is in metabolic equivalents (METS) (*Circulation,* 2009). The ability to walk two blocks on level ground or carry two bags of groceries up stairs without symptoms are simple questions that can give an approximate assessment of patient risk. One MET is defined as the energy expenditure for sitting quietly. For the average adult, this is equivalent to an oxygen consumption of 3.5 ml/kg body weight per minute. Studies have shown that those who have a low exercise capacity have twice as much risk for postoperative complications compared to those have high exercise capacity.
  - Can take care of self such as eat, dress, or use toilet = 1 MET
  - Can walk up a flight of steps or hill = 4 METS
  - Can do heavy work around the house = 4 to 10 METS
  - Can participate in strenuous sports such as swimming, tennis, football, and skiing = > 10 METS
- Assess other relevant risk factors by addressing the following questions:
  - What is patient's BMI?
  - Does the patient experience shortness of breath when lying flat?
  - Does the patient have any of the following cardiac conditions: heart disease, heart attack within the past 6 mo, angina, irregular heartbeat, heart failure?
  - Has the patient ever had any rheumatologic conditions, kidney disease, liver disease, diabetes, anemia?
  - Has the patient or any member of the patient's family had any adverse reactions to anesthesia?
  - Any family history of deep venous thrombosis or pulmonary embolism, bleeding problems, diabetes mellitus, elevated cholesterol, hypertension, or heart disease?
  - For female patients, is it possible the patient is pregnant? What was the date of the patient's last menstrual period?
  - Is patient on any medications? Is the patient on any anticoagulants, antiplatelet drugs, or other medications that can increase bleeding risk? Can these medications be safely stopped for surgery?
- Consider further testing based on above risk factors. The decision to order preoperative tests should be guided by the patient's clinical history, comorbidities, and physical examination findings. An algorithm for preoperative evaluation of patients with known or suspected coronary artery disease is described in Fig. E1-673.

PHYSICAL EXAMINATION

- Vital signs: blood pressure, heart rate and rhythm, rate and ease of respirations, and temperature.
- Cardiovascular exam. Auscultate heart to check for heart murmurs, pathologic heart sounds, and ventricular systolic or diastolic dysfunction.
- Respiratory exam. Auscultate lungs for crackles, wheezes, decreased breath sounds.
- Vascular exam. Examine for carotid, abdominal, and femoral bruits.
- Integumentary exam. Check for evidence of venous stasis in lower extremities, petechiae, and unusual bruises.
- Mental status. Conduct a mini-mental exam.

LABORATORY TESTS & IMAGING STUDIES

- Determine the patient's age, height, weight.
- ECG: Although it has often been routine to perform an ECG in patients older than age 55 (except those undergoing low-risk procedures like endoscopy) and in those patients

---

BOX 1-51 Stratification of Risk of Common Noncardiac Surgical Procedures

Higher risk	Emergent and urgent major operations, especially in the elderly
	Aortic and noncarotid major vascular surgery
	Surgery associated with large fluid status change or blood loss
Intermediate risk	Head and neck surgery
	Carotid endarterectomy surgery
	Major thoracic surgery
	Major abdominal surgery
	Orthopedic surgery
	Prostate surgery
Lower risk	Eye and skin surgery
	Endoscopy
	Breast
	Ambulatory procedure

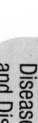

with preexisting cardiac conditions, a more nuanced approach is suggested by the 2007 Guidelines published by the American College of Cardiology (ACC) and the American Health Association, which use Assessment of Risk for CAD and Assessment of Functional Capacity:

Recommendations for Preoperative Resting 12-Lead ECG

Class I

1. Preoperative resting 12-lead ECG is recommended for patients with at least 1 clinical risk factor who are undergoing vascular surgical procedures. (Level of Evidence: B)
2. Preoperative resting 12-lead ECG is recommended for patients with known CHD, peripheral arterial disease, or cerebrovascular disease who are undergoing intermediate-risk surgical procedures. (Level of Evidence: C)

Class IIa

1. Preoperative resting 12-lead ECG is reasonable in persons with no clinical risk factors who are undergoing vascular surgical procedures. (Level of Evidence: B)

Class IIb

1. Preoperative resting 12-lead ECG may be reasonable in patients with at least 1 clinical risk factor who are undergoing intermediate-risk operative procedures. (Level of Evidence: B)

Class III

1. Preoperative and postoperative resting 12-lead ECGs are not indicated in asymptomatic persons undergoing low-risk surgical procedures. (Level of Evidence: B)

- Routine laboratory studies are not necessary unless there is a specific medical indication. (*Anesthesiology*, 2002). Testing need not be repeated if results are recently available, unless there has been a change in clinical status.
  - Low-risk procedures do not require routine basic metabolic panel, blood glucose, liver function, hemostasis evaluation, or a urine analysis.
  - For intermediate- and high-risk procedures as well as in the setting of diabetes,

cardiac, or renal disease, obtain a complete blood count.
  - A CBC is recommended for all patients older than age 65 undergoing major surgery as well as anyone undergoing a surgery with expected large amounts of blood loss.
  - Fasting glucose is recommended for all patients age >45 yr.
  - Coagulation studies are only needed for patients with personal or family history of bleeding or thrombophilia and for those taking anticoagulants.
  - Urine hCG is recommended for all women of childbearing age.
- Chest x-ray is indicated for all patients with new respiratory symptoms, suspected congestive heart failure, valvular heart disease, or previous malignancy, and for patients who are current smokers with a >20-pack year history. Clinicians should not order routine preoperative chest x-rays or pulmonary function tests.

MEDICATIONS

Most medications can be continued through the perioperative period with the exception of aspirin, clopidogrel, ticlopidine, warfarin, and nonsteroidal anti-inflammatory drugs. If the patient is going to be NPO during the procedure, then hypoglycemia-inducing agents should be reduced to half-dose the night before surgery and held the morning of surgery. Many studies have been done on beta-blocker usage during surgical procedures. Based on the results of the POISE Trial (2008), the only class 1 recommendation for perioperative beta-blockade was that it be continued in patients who are receiving long-term beta-blockade therapy.

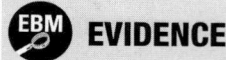

PEARLS & CONSIDERATIONS

COMMENTS

Although most individuals will not require any significant preoperative testing, certain conditions will require further workup.

- Ischemic heart disease
  - If patient has angina, determine frequency, precipitating factors, response to rest and nitroglycerin

  - If patient has had prior cardiac catheterizations or coronary revascularizations, obtain previous records
- Dysrhythmias and pacemakers
  - Examine current and prior ECGs for high-grade atrioventricular block, symptomatic ventricular arrhythmias, supraventricular tachycardias at uncontrolled rates.
  - If patient has a pacemaker, establish the type and mode, date of implantation, and when it was last interrogated.
- Valvular and congenital heart disease
  - Look for signs of severe valvular heart disease on last echocardiographic evaluations.
- Cerebrovascular disease
  - Inquire about prior carotid artery ultrasounds
- Venous thromboembolism
  - Determine results of studies for thrombophilia (factor V Leiden mutation, lupus anticoagulant, antithrombin III, protein C or S).
- Tools for cardiac risk assessment:
  - http://www.statcoder.com
  - http://www.infopoems.com

PATIENT & FAMILY EDUCATION

Advise patients that their preoperative evaluation visit with their PCP is another opportunity for them to bring up concerns or get questions answered about their upcoming procedure.

(EBM) **EVIDENCE**

available at www.expertconsult.com

SUGGESTED READINGS
available at www.expertconsult.com

AUTHOR: **PRIYA SARIN GUPTA, M.D.**

P

Diseases and Disorders

I

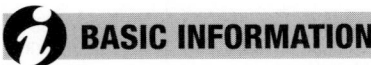

BASIC INFORMATION

DEFINITION

Pressure ulcers are any damage to the skin, the underlying tissue, or both, that results from pressure, friction, or shearing forces that usually occur over bony prominences.

SYNONYMS

Decubitus ulcers
Pressure sores
Bedsores
Decubiti

ICD-9CM CODES
707.0

ICD-10CM CODES
L89 Pressure ulcers
Subcategories of codes determined by stage and location of ulcer
L89.153 Example: Stage 3 ulcer of sacral area

EPIDEMIOLOGY & DEMOGRAPHICS

- Occurs in all health care settings from hospitals to nursing homes and even at home. Incidence approaches as many as 40% of affected individuals. Prevalence has declined among all nursing home residents over the past decade. It is highest in institutions with lower staffing levels of certified nurses and nursing assistants, reflecting emphasis on health care resources more than medical decision-making.
- Associated with decreased quality of life and significant morbidity and mortality. One-year mortality rate approaches 40%.
- Pain occurs in two thirds of patients with stage II or greater pressure ulcers.
- Complicated by cellulitis, osteomyelitis, abscesses, and sepsis.

CLINICAL PRESENTATION

The National Pressure Ulcer Advisory Panel in 2007 has outlined the staging system of pressure ulcers as follows:

Stage I: Nonblanchable erythema of intact skin usually over a bony prominence or boggy, mushy feeling of skin

Stage II: Partial-thickness skin loss involving the epidermis, dermis, or both. May also present as an intact or ruptured serum-filled blister.

Stage III: Full-thickness skin loss involving damage or necrosis of subcutaneous tissue that may extend down to, but not through, underlying fascia or muscle. There may be undermining and tunneling.

Stage IV: Full-thickness skin loss with exposed muscle, bone, or supporting structures (e.g., tendons, joint capsule). Sloughing or eschar may be present. These ulcers often include undermining and tunneling (Fig. 1-674).

Deep tissue injury: Purple or maroon localized area of discolored, intact skin or blood-filled blister due to damage of underlying tissue from pressure and/or shear.

Unstageable: Full-thicknesss tissue loss with the base of the ulcer covered by slough or eschar in the wound bed.

Only pressure ulcers are classified by stage.

ETIOLOGY

Pressure ulcers are ischemic soft tissue injuries caused by constant, unrelieved pressure in tissues over bony prominences. Shearing and friction forces contribute to and cause damage to the tissues, leading to an ulcer. Risk factors include immobility, malnutrition, bowel or bladder incontinence, and dry or damaged skin.

DIAGNOSIS

DIFFERENTIAL DIAGNOSIS

- Venous stasis ulcers
- Arterial ulcers
- Diabetic ulcers
- Skin cancer
- Cellulitis
- Kennedy ulcers (rapidly progressing ulcers that occur at the end of life)

WORKUP

Evaluate ulcer characteristics, including its stage, appearance, location, and size. For stages III and IV, describe the wound bed (epithelialization, granulation tissue, necrotic tissue, eschar); presence of exudates, including type and amount; depth and wound edges (undermining, sinus tracts, tunneling, or fistulas); signs of infection (purulent drainage, odor, surrounding cellulitis); and pain. In addition, pressure ulcer risk factors and causes should be reassessed.

LABORATORY TESTS

- Directed at identifying cause of risk factors or any complications arising from the pressure ulcer (e.g., abscess or osteomyelitis).
- Cultures of wound bed are often not helpful and should not be routinely performed. Deep tissue biopsy is the gold standard if a culture is indicated.
- Markers for malnutrition include prealbumin, albumin, transferrin, lymphocyte count, and total cholesterol level.
- Complete blood count if infection is suspected.

IMAGING STUDIES

- Ultrasound not proven to be effective.
- Plain radiographs, MRI, and bone scan may help identify osteomyelitis when clinically suspected.
- A comparison study of 44 patients scheduled for open biopsy did not show MRI to have superior diagnostic benefit over plain radiography.

PREVENTION & TREATMENT

- Identify high-risk patients using standardized risk assessment scales (e.g., Braden, Norton, and Waterlow scales)
- Routine skin inspection and good skin care for high-risk patients.
- Minimize prolonged skin exposure to moisture, urine, or stool.
- Treat dry, cracking skin.
- Use repositioning and pressure-reducing devices (e.g., foam mattresses, low–air loss beds, pillows, or foam wedges when in bed or in a chair).
  - Patient repositioning:
    Although there is clinical consensus that repositioning is critical, three randomized controlled trials (RCTs) found no evidence that regular manual repositioning prevented pressure ulcers.
  - Bed surface
    Air-fluidized beds
    a. Two RCTs found that use of air-fluidized beds contributed to the healing of a greater number of ulcers after 15 days compared with standard care.
    b. Systematic review revealed no differences in rate of pressure ulcer healing with use of either alternating-pressure mattresses or low–air loss beds compared with standard care.
    Pressure-relieving overlays
    a. One RCT demonstrated that a viscoelastic pad on the operating table significantly reduced incidence of postoperative pressure ulcers compared with a standard operating table.

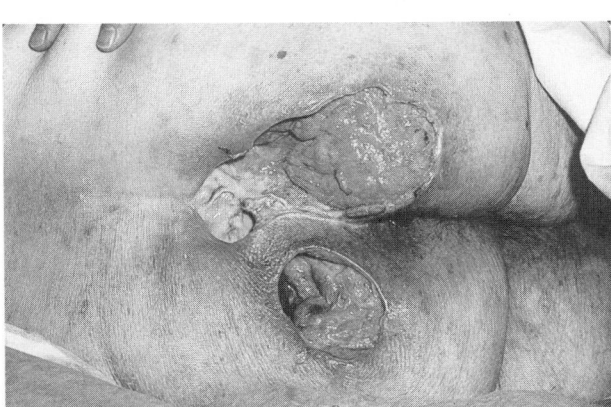

FIGURE 1-674 Natural debridement of pressure injury at 2 weeks. (From Tallis R, Fillit H: *Brockelhurst's textbook of geriatric medicine and gerontology*, ed 6, London, 2003, Churchill Livingstone.)

b. One RCT found that sheepskin overlays plus standard care compared with standard care alone significantly reduced incidence of pressure sores in elderly patients recuperating from hip fracture.

Foam alternatives

a. Four RCTs revealed that foam alternatives versus standard hospital mattresses reduced the incidence of pressure ulcer development in elderly patients in orthopedic hospital wards.

b. Forty-one RCTs demonstrated that patients lying on standard hospital mattresses are more likely to develop pressure ulcers than those patients lying on higher specification foam mattresses.

- Use adequate support surfaces while in bed or in a chair to prevent "bottoming out" (defined as less than 1 inch between patient and support surface; measured by putting hand under support surface and feeling thickness to patient).
- Recent systematic review of pressure ulcer prevention strategies showed poor methodology in most studies. Use of support surfaces, repositioning, optimized nutrition, and sacral skin moisturizing was most appropriate.
  - The 2010 consensus statement from the National Pressure Ulcer Advisory Panel said that not all pressure ulcers are avoidable because there are patient situations where pressure cannot be relieved and perfusion cannot be improved.

NONPHARMACOLOGIC THERAPY

- Should be cleaned at each dressing change; necrotic tissue should be debrided quickly because it delays wound healing (except for heel ulcers).
- Wound irrigation should not exceed 15 psi and is best done with an 18-gauge angiocatheter.
- No single dressing or product is superior; should be used to keep ulcer bed moist and protect it from urine/stool. Silver dressings (which are felt to be antimicrobial), topical phenytoin, and growth factors should be limited to difficult-to-heal wounds, chronic ulcers, and extensive burns given their extra cost and limited scientific validation.
- Avoid agents that are cytotoxic to epithelial cells (e.g., iodine, iodophor, sodium hypochlorite, hydrogen peroxide, acetic acid, alcohol).
- Reduce pressure by using foam mattress, dynamic support surface (e.g., low–air loss bed), and frequent repositioning (e.g., q2h or, in cases of poor perfusion, more frequently).
- Hyperbaric oxygen, ultrasound, ultraviolet, electromagnetic therapy, and low-energy radiation either are ineffective or have not been extensively evaluated for efficacy.
- Negative pressure devices (Vac devices) may help in wounds that have significant drainage. They also may improve healing by promoting angiogenesis, improving tissue perfusion, and decreasing bacterial count. Calcium alginate and foam dressings may also be beneficial for such wounds.
- Although correcting poor nutrition has been shown to be beneficial, a recent large investigation demonstrated that feeding tube insertion did not prevent or heal pressure ulcers, but increased the risk for developing a pressure ulcer.
- Minimize urinary and/or fecal contamination.
- Use a standardized assessment tool to monitor wound healing on weekly basis. Examples of monitoring scales include the Pressure Sore Status Tool (PSST) and Pressure Ulcer Scale for Healing (PUSH).
- No RCTs have compared debridement versus no debridement in the treatment of pressure ulcers.
- Thirty-two RCTs have compared different debridement agents, but there is insufficient evidence to promote the use of one particular agent.
- One RCT demonstrated ulcers treated with collagenase healed significantly more quickly than those treated with hydrocolloid.
- A meta-analysis and one RCT found significant benefit in rates of healing with use of hydrocolloid dressings versus traditional saline gauze dressings but not over other forms such as hydrogels, foam dressings, or collogenase.
- No benefit was found with honey, nutritional and vitamin supplements, artificial nutrition, or ultrasound therapy.

ACUTE GENERAL Rx

- Pain medications are necessary because pressure ulcers could be painful.
- Growth factors appear promising but are second-line treatments if traditional approaches are ineffective.

CHRONIC Rx

- Continue vigilance with pressure reduction because decubitus ulcers can recur with minimal trauma.
- Consider radiologic evaluation for infected ulcer bed, occult osteomyelitis, or abscess.

COMPLEMENTARY & ALTERNATIVE MEDICINE

Vitamin C, zinc, and multivitamin supplements may be of benefit to optimize nutrition.

DISPOSITION

- When systematic risk assessments are done and preventive measures are followed, most pressure ulcers can be prevented. Most ulcers heal when appropriate management strategies are followed.
- Stage IV ulcers in high-risk patients (e.g., paraplegics) can take months or years to heal.

REFERRAL

- Physical and occupational therapists to improve bed and chair mobility.
- Wounds with necrotic tissue need referral to persons trained in sharp debridement.
- To plastic surgeons for operative repair for large stage III or IV ulcers that do not respond to optimal care.
- To a specialty wound center for nonhealing ulcers.

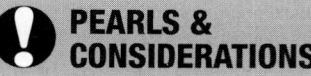 **PEARLS & CONSIDERATIONS**

COMMENTS

- Up to 10% of older persons will have a pressure ulcer.
- Because 70% of pressure ulcers occur in older persons, the approach should be similar to other multifactorial geriatric syndromes with a multidisciplinary team approach. Identify and reduce all modifiable risk factors for pressure ulcers.
- Treat the pain associated with pressure ulcers.
- Proper skin care, use of support surfaces, mobilization, and attention to nutrition are key for prevention and treatment.
- Clinical studies have not revealed if any one dressing product is superior.
- Nonhealing ulcers require assessment for debridement, infection, abscess, and/or referral to a wound center.

PATIENT & FAMILY EDUCATION

- Educate patient and family members on the risk factors for pressure ulcers.
- Encourage mobility and adequate nutritional intake and avoid bed rest.

SUGGESTED READINGS

available at www.expertconsult.com

RELATED CONTENT

Bed Sores (Patient Information)

AUTHORS: **RACHEL ROACH, A.P.R.N.-B.C.,** and **NOEL S. C. JAVIER, M.D.**

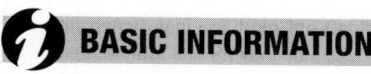

BASIC INFORMATION

DEFINITION

Priapism is the persistent, usually painful erection associated or unassociated with sexual stimulation. There are two major forms: low-flow (veno-occlusive) priapism and high-flow priapism (associated with increased arterial inflow without increased venous outflow resistance).

ICD-9CM CODES
607.3 Priapism

EPIDEMIOLOGY & DEMOGRAPHICS

- Peak incidence is seen from ages 5 to 10 yr and 20 to 50 yr.
- In the younger group, priapism is often associated with sickle cell disease or neoplasm. In the older group it is often caused by pharmacologic agents.
- Low-flow (veno-occlusive priapism [type I]) is much more common than high-flow (type II).

PHYSICAL FINDINGS & CLINICAL PRESENTATION

- In idiopathic priapism the initial erection is associated with prolonged sexual excitement. Previous transient episodes are frequently reported. The erection involves the corpora cavernosa alone. Detumescence does not occur spontaneously.
- In secondary priapism, sexual excitement need not be involved. Otherwise the clinical picture is the same as in idiopathic priapism.
- Table 1-340 compares normal erection and priapism.

ETIOLOGY

Idiopathic: prolonged sexual arousal
Secondary or associated causes:
- Sickle cell disease
- Diabetes
- Leukemia (especially chronic myelogenous leukemia)
- Solid tumor (malignant) penile infiltration
- Spinal cord injury
- Perineal or penile trauma
- Iatrogenic
- Total parenteral nutrition, which includes a fat emulsion
- Hyperosmolar IV contrast
- Spinal or general anesthesia
- Anticoagulant therapy
- Phenothiazines
- Trazodone
- Intracorporeal injection therapy for impotence

- Phosphodiesterase type 5 inhibitors (e.g., sildenafil [Viagra], tadalafil [Cialis], vardenafil [Levitra])

PATHOPHYSIOLOGY

- Low-flow priapism: prolonged erection leads to edema of the cavernosal trabeculae, resulting in a sequence of stasis, thrombosis, venous occlusion, fibrosis, scarring, and possibly impotence.
- High-flow priapism: cavernosal artery rupture leading to an arteriocavernous fistula.

DIAGNOSIS

WORKUP

None if the associated underlying causes are known to be present. Otherwise they should be ruled out. Low-flow priapism can be distinguished from high-flow priapism by obtaining a corporeal blood gas value. A Po_2 <30 mm Hg, Pco_2 >60 mm Hg, and a pH <7.25 are consistent with low-flow priapism. High-flow priapism can be confirmed by a perineal Doppler ultrasound or arteriography (useful to identify arterial-lacunar fistula).

TREATMENT

Goal: achieve detumescence with preservation of potency.
1. Medical therapies:
   - Ice packs
   - Ice water enemas
   - Hot water enemas
   - Pressure dressing
   - Sedatives
   - Analgesics
   - Antispasmodic/anticholinergic drugs
   - Estrogens
   - Anticoagulants

- Procaine
- Amyl nitrite
- Local or general anesthesia
- Ketamine (1 mg/lb)
2. In the patient with sickle cell disease: intravenous hydration, alkalinization, transfusion or exchange transfusion, oxygen.
3. Corporeal irrigation with normal saline may be used for low-flow priapism. The midshaft of the penis can be injected with a small-gauge butterfly needle and irrigated with 10 to 20 ml of normal saline, followed by an intracorporeal injection of an alpha-adrenergic agonist every 5 min until detumescence. Commonly used intracavernous vasoconstrictor agents are epinephrine (10 to 20 mcg), phenylephrine (250 to 500 mcg), and ephedrine (50 to 100 mg). It is mandatory to monitor the patient's blood pressure and pulse when using alpha-adrenergic agonists.
4. Surgery:
   - Cavernospongiosum shunt
   - Glans-cavernosum shunt
   - Cavernosaphenous shunt
   - In the less common situation of high-flow priapism (diagnosed by the finding of bright red arterial blood on aspiration), arterial embolization or surgical ligation is recommended.

PROGNOSIS

Impotence is associated with the duration of priapism, with 36 hr being an important threshold.

REFERRAL

To urologist

RELATED CONTENT

Priapism (Patient Information)

AUTHOR: **FRED F. FERRI, M.D.**

TABLE 1-340   Comparison of Normal Erection and Priapism

Factor	Normal Erection	Priapism
Portion of penis involved	Corpora cavernosa and corpus spongiosum and glans	Corpora cavernosa
Cause	Vasodilatation of penile arteries	Obstruction of venous outflow
		Disturbance of neuroarterial mechanism (imbalance between it and adrenergic activity)
		Increased viscosity
Sexual desire	Present	Absent
Pain	Absent	Present
Duration	Minutes to hours	Hours to days

From Nseyo UO (ed): *Urology for primary care physicians*, Philadelphia, 1999, Saunders.

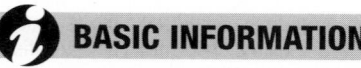 BASIC INFORMATION

DEFINITION

- Woman younger than 40 yr of age with amenorrhea, oligomenorrhea, or dysfunctional uterine bleeding for 4 mo or more along with follicle stimulating hormone (FSH) levels in the menopausal range meet diagnostic criteria for primary ovarian insufficiency.
- Menopause younger than the age of 40 yr.

SYNONYMS

Hypergonadotropic hypogonadism
Premature ovarian failure
Premature menopause
Gonadal dysgenesis

ICD-9CM CODES
256.31 Premature menopause

EPIDEMIOLOGY & DEMOGRAPHICS

INCIDENCE: Affects 1% to 4% of the female population in the U.S.
PREDOMINANT AGE: 1:250 incident cases by age 35 and 1:100 by age 40

PHYSICAL FINDINGS & CLINICAL PRESENTATION

- The most common presentation is disturbance in menstrual pattern due to intermittent ovarian function.
- Between 5% and 30% of affected women have another affected female relative.
- Between 10% and 30% of affected women already have a concurrent autoimmune condition, the most common of which is hypothyroidism.
- Symptoms of estrogen deficiency include hot flashes, night sweat, poor concentration, drying of the vagina, and infertility.
- Physical exam may reveal stigmata of an autoimmune condition such as vitiligo, thyroid enlargement, or Turner's syndrome (webbed neck, short stature, and high-arched palate).

ETIOLOGY (see Table 1-341)
Idiopathic in 95% of cases

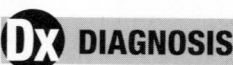 DIAGNOSIS

DIFFERENTIAL DIAGNOSIS

- Pregnancy
- Causes of secondary amenorrhea include polycystic ovarian disease, hypothalamic amenorrhea, hyperprolactinemia.

WORKUP

- After pregnancy is ruled out, the initial evaluation should include the measurement of serum prolactin, FSH, and thyrotropin (TSH) levels.
- If the FSH level is in the menopausal range, the test should be repeated in 1 month along with a serum estradiol measurement to confirm the diagnosis of primary ovarian insufficiency.

LABORATORY TESTS

Once a diagnosis of premature ovarian failure is made, other evaluations include:
- Autoimmune disorders, adrenal insufficiency (seen in 3% of cases): serum anti-adrenal and anti-21 hydroxylase antibodies should be measured.
- Hypothyroidism: serum TSH, T_4, and anti-TPO antibodies
- All cases should be screened for osteoporosis by DXA for bone mineral density.
- A karyotype analysis should be performed for all patients to look for chromosomal defects including Turner's variant or deletions of the X chromosome.
- Permutations for the fragile X syndrome (FMR1 gene) should be checked for as well.

IMAGING STUDIES

Pelvic ultrasound has no proven benefit in the management of these patients.

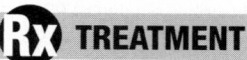 TREATMENT

NONPHARMACOLOGIC THERAPY

Counseling or patient support group should be offered to all women with low self-esteem and depression due to the psychological scar left by the diagnosis.

ACUTE GENERAL Rx

- Physiologic estrogen and progestin replacement is reasonable in the cases of young women until they reach the age of natural menopause.
- A dose of 100 mcg of estradiol per day, administered by transdermal patch, achieves average estradiol level observed in normal menstruating women and effectively treats symptoms.
- Cyclic medroxyprogesterone at a dose of 10 mg per day for 12 days each month is the preferred progestin to provide protection against endometrial cancer.
- Pregnancy may occur while a woman is taking estrogen and progesterone therapy and the therapy should be stopped immediately if the pregnancy test is found to be positive.

CHRONIC Rx

- Intake of 1200 mg of elemental calcium and 800 units of vitamin D_3 per day should be encouraged to prevent bone loss. A serum 25-hydroxyvitamin D level of 30 ng per ml or higher should be maintained.
- Patients with positive tests for adrenal antibodies should be evaluated annually for adrenal insufficiency by corticotropin stimulation test.
- Patients who wish to avoid pregnancy should use a barrier method or an IUD.
- Options for parenthood include adoption, foster parenthood, egg donation, and embryo donation.

DISPOSITION

Women with the known diagnosis should be encouraged to maintain a lifestyle that optimizes bone and cardiovascular health, including regular weight-bearing exercises, adequate intake of calcium (1200 mg daily) and vitamin D (800 IU daily), healthy diet to prevent obesity, and screening for cardiovascular risk factors.

REFERRAL

Referral to gynecologist and reproductive endocrinologist may be helpful in patients who decide to pursue parenthood.

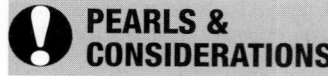 PEARLS & CONSIDERATIONS

COMMENTS

- Common etiologies should be ruled out, including chromosomal abnormalities, fragile X premutations, and autoimmune causes.
- Management directed at symptom resolution and bone protection primarily, but should include psychosocial support for women facing this devastating diagnosis.

PREVENTION

Early diagnosis of primary ovarian insufficiency important for osteoporosis prevention and possibly prevention of coronary artery disease.

PATIENT & FAMILY EDUCATION
www.pofsupport.org

SUGGESTED READINGS
available at www.expertconsult.com

AUTHOR: **PRIYA BANSAL, M.D., M.P.H.**

TABLE 1-341 Mechanisms and Causes of Primary Ovarian Insufficiency

Accelerated Follicular Depletion

Genetic: Turner's syndrome, fragile X premutations, galactosemia
Toxic: Chemotherapy, radiation, infections such as mumps or cytomegalovirus
Autoimmune: Polyglandular failure, hypothyroidism, Addison's disease, vitiligo, myasthenia gravis

Abnormal Follicular Stimulation

Gonadotropin receptor function: follicle stimulating hormone/luteinizing hormone receptor mutation
Enzyme defects: Aromatase deficiency
Luteinized follicles

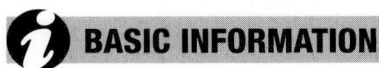

BASIC INFORMATION

DEFINITION

Primary sclerosing cholangitis (PSC) is a chronic progressive cholestatic liver disease characterized by segmental fibrosing and inflammation of intrahepatic and extrahepatic bile ducts complicated by recurrent cholangitis, cholangiocarcinoma, cirrhosis, and portal hypertension.

SYNONYMS

Chronic obliterative cholangitis
Fibrosing cholangitis
Stenosing cholangitis
PSC

ICD-9CM CODES

567.1 Cholangitis
698 Pruritus
780.7 Malaise and fatigue
782.4 Jaundice

EPIDEMIOLOGY & DEMOGRAPHICS

- The incidence and prevalence of PSC are 0.9 to 1.3 cases and 8.5 to 13.6 cases per 100,000 population, respectively.
- About 65% of patients with PSC are men with a M:F ratio of 3:1.
- Mean age of presentation is 40 yr old.
- 70% to 90% of patients with PSC also have inflammatory bowel disease (IBD), particularly with ulcerative colitis (UC). Patients with PSC and UC are at higher risk for developing colon cancer than patients with UC alone.
- PSC can coexist with other autoimmune liver disease. Autoimmune hepatitis and PSC overlap syndrome is mostly seen in young adults and children.
- Cumulative lifetime incidence of cholangiocarcinoma in PSC patients is 10% to 30%.
- The median survival from time of diagnosis is 10 to 15 yr without liver transplantation.

PHYSICAL FINDINGS & CLINICAL PRESENTATION

- Most patients are asymptomatic (15% to 40%) at the time of diagnosis with normal physical findings.
- More than 75% of asymptomatic patients develop symptoms, the most common of which are pruritus (70%) and fatigue (70%). Other complaints include abdominal discomfort, steatorrhea, jaundice, and weight loss, which are concerning for advanced PSC, sepsis or mechanical obstruction (i.e., cholangitis), and malignancy (i.e., cholangiocarcinoma).
- Patients with advanced liver disease can present with decompensated cirrhosis (i.e., ascites, spontaneous bacterial peritonitis, hepatic encephalopathy, and variceal hemorrhage) and hepatic failure.
- Physical findings of symptomatic patients may reveal jaundice, skin excoriation and hyperpigmentation from scratching due to pruritus, hepatosplenomegaly, and xanthelasma. In patients with cirrhosis, physical findings may reveal a shrunken nodular liver and evidence of portal hypertension.

ETIOLOGY

- The cause of PSC is unknown but is thought to be due to a combination of environmental, immunologic, and genetic factors.
- Genetic and immunologic factors are supported by reports of familial occurrence of this disorder and increased frequency of HLA B8 and DR3, which are known to be associated with several autoimmune disorders.
- An environmental factor is implicated in PSC due to the close association of PSC with UC. This has led to the hypothesis that bacterial, viral, or toxic substances in the inflamed colonic mucosa may transmigrate to the biliary tree and cause chronic inflammation and fibrosis.

DIAGNOSIS

Diagnosis is based on characteristic cholangiographic findings in combination with clinical, biochemical, and in some cases histologic features. Table 1-342 describes staging of PSC.

DIFFERENTIAL DIAGNOSIS

- Choledocholithiasis
- Surgical biliary trauma
- Recurrent pyogenic cholangitis
- Ischemic cholangitis
- Cholangiocarcinoma
- IgG4-associated cholangitis
- Intraarterial chemotherapy
- Diffuse intrahepatic metastasis
- Histiocytosis X

WORKUP

History, physical examination, laboratory evaluation, imaging studies +/− liver biopsy

LABORATORY TESTS

- Serum biochemical tests usually indicate cholestasis with predominant elevation in the serum alkaline phosphatase (three to ten times the upper limit of normal). Serum aminotransferase levels are elevated in the majority of patients (two to three times the upper limits of normal). Serum bilirubin is usually normal at the time of diagnosis unless patient has advanced liver disease.
- A wide range of autoantibodies can be detected in patients with PSC; however, they have no role in the routine diagnosis of PSC including the perinuclear antineutrophil cytoplasmic antibody (pANCA), which is nonspecific. However, autoantibodies such as antinuclear antibody (ANA) and/or anti-smooth muscle antibody (ASMA) and/or serum IgG levels are useful in the diagnosis of PSC-autoimmune hepatitis (AIH) overlap syndrome.

IMAGING STUDIES

- Cholangiography is considered to be the "gold standard" for the diagnosis of PSC. Characteristic findings reveal segmental fibrosis of bile ducts with saccular dilatation of normal intervening areas resulting in a "beads-on-a-string" appearance (Fig. 1-675).
- Magnetic resonance cholangiopancreatography (MRCP) has an overall diagnostic accuracy rate of 90%. It is the imaging modality of choice when PSC is suspected due to serious complications associated with endoscopic retrograde cholangiopancreatography (ERCP) (i.e., pancreatitis and cholangitis).
- Liver biopsy is not necessary for the diagnosis of PSC in patients with typical cholangiographic findings. Typical onion skin–type periductal fibrosis is a rare finding. Liver biopsy is recommended for diagnosis in patients with suspected autoimmune hepatitis, PSC overlap syndrome, or small duct PSC (normal cholangiogram) or for prognostication.

TREATMENT

- No medical therapy has been proved to be effective in halting the disease progression of PSC.

TABLE 1-342 Staging of Primary Sclerosing Cholangitis

Stage	Description
I—Portal	Portal edema, inflammation, ductal proliferation; abnormalities do not extend beyond the limiting plate
II—Periportal	Periportal fibrosis with or without inflammation extending beyond the limiting plate
III—Septal	Septal fibrosis, bridging necrosis, or both
IV—Cirrhotic	Biliary cirrhosis

From Cameron JL, Cameron AM: *Current surgical therapy,* ed 10, Philadelphia, 2011, Saunders.

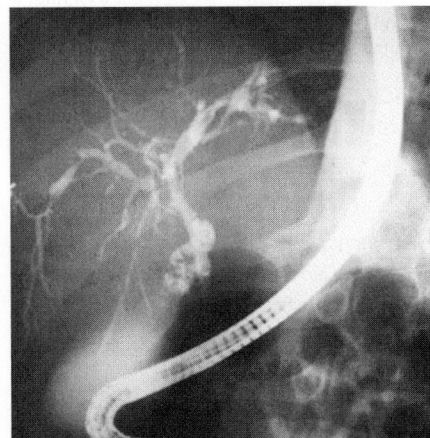

FIGURE 1-675 A 29-year-old male patient who was diagnosed with PSC 5 years previously. Both the intra- and extrahepatic bile ducts are involved at cholangiography. (From Parlak E et al: An endoscopic finding in patients with primary sclerosing cholangitis: retraction of the main duodenal papilla into the duodenum wall, *Gastrointest Endosc* 65(3):535, 2007.)

- Management of PSC patients are aimed at symptom relief and management of complications from PSC (i.e., obstruction/strictures, bacterial cholangitis, metabolic bone disease, portal hypertension, and malignancy).
- There have been mixed data on the use of ursodeoxycholic acid (UDCA) in adults with PSC. It is yet unclear if UDCA slows the progression of PSC-related liver disease and in high doses it has been shown to be harmful. Therefore UDCA is not recommended as medical therapy in patients with PSC.
- The use of corticosteroids and other immunosuppressive agents is not recommended in patients with PSC alone; however, it is recommended in patients with PSC and overlap syndrome.

ACUTE GENERAL Rx

- Bile acid sequestrants (i.e., cholestyramine 16 g/day) are the preferred choice for the initial management of pruritus. Alternative agents for pruritus refractory to bile acid sequestrants include rifampicin 150 to 300 mg twice daily, naltrexone 50 mg daily, and sertraline 75 to 100 mg daily.
- Patients who present with increasing serum bilirubin and/or worsening pruritus, progressive bile duct dilatation on imaging studies, and/or cholangitis need to be evaluated for dominant strictures.
- ERCP with balloon dilatation +/− stenting is recommended in patients with dominant strictures after the exclusion of malignancy. If ERCP is unsuccessful percutaneous cholangiopancreatography +/− stenting should be considered.
- In noncirrhotic patients with dominant strictures refractory to endoscopic and/or percutaneous management, surgery should be

considered, although this may complicate future liver transplantation surgery.
- Antibiotic usage is recommended in patients with dominant strictures/obstructions both acutely and for long-term prophylaxis in patients with recurrent cholangitis.

CHRONIC Rx

- Avoidance of alcohol advised to avoid further insults to the liver.
- All patients need to be vaccinated against hepatitis A and B.
- Patients with PSC are at risk for metabolic bone disease. At time of diagnosis a DEXA scan is recommended to evaluate for osteopenia and osteoporosis. Calcium (1000 to 1500 g) and vitamin D 1000 IU daily are recommended for patients with osteopenia and the addition of bisphosphonate is recommended in patients with osteoporosis.
- Patients with newly diagnosed PSC should have a full colonoscopy with biopsies to exclude concurrent IBD and for surveillance of colorectal cancer. In patients with established PSC and IBD continued surveillance colonoscopy with biopsies at 1 to 2 yr is recommended.
- Annual transabdominal ultrasound is recommended to screen for gallbladder mass due to risk of gallbladder malignancy and if detected cholecystectomy should be performed if underlying liver disease permits.
- Patients with cirrhosis are recommended to have gastroesophageal variceal and hepatocellular carcinoma (HCC) surveillance at regular intervals.
- All patients with deterioration in clinical performance status or liver biochemical parameters should be evaluated for development of cholangiocarcinoma and in patients with cirrhosis the development of hepatocellular car-

cinoma. Depending on underlying liver disease, resection versus liver transplantation would be required.

DISPOSITION

Liver transplantation is the only effective treatment for patients with end-stage liver disease, portal hypertension, liver failure, and recurrent or intractable bacterial cholangitis. The recurrence of PSC after transplant is reportedly 5% to 20%.

REFERRAL

Gastroenterology and/or hepatology for treatment of PSC, management of its complications, surveillance of associated malignancy, and evaluation for liver transplantation.

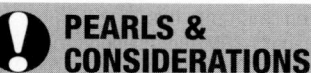

PEARLS & CONSIDERATIONS

- Management of PSC targets symptom relief and complications of PSC and cirrhosis.
- Patients are at increased risk for the development of colorectal cancer, gallbladder cancer, and cholangiocarcinoma.
- In patients with cirrhosis, surveillance for gastroesophageal varices and HCC is recommended.
- Liver transplant remains the only definitive therapy for complications of PSC.

SUGGESTED READINGS

available at www.expertconsult.com

RELATED CONTENT

Ulcerative Colitis (Related Key Topic)

AUTHORS: **CUI LI LIN, M.D., JUDY NEE, M.D.,** and **AMANDA PRESSMAN, M.D.**

P

Diseases and Disorders

I

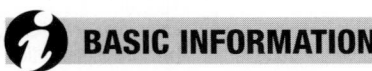

BASIC INFORMATION

DEFINITION

Progressive multifocal leukoencephalopathy (PML) is an uncommon and often fatal subacute demyelinating disease of the white matter, caused by reactivation of the JC virus (JCV) infection in an immunocompromised individual. JCV was isolated in 1971 and is named for the initials of the first patient from whose brain it was isolated.

ICD-9CM CODES

341 Other demyelinating disorders of the central nervous system

EPIDEMIOLOGY & DEMOGRAPHICS

RISK FACTORS: Typically seen in patients with profound immunosuppression and impaired cell mediated immunity. These include patients with AIDS, lymphoproliferative disorders, infections such as tuberculosis, inflammatory diseases such as sarcoidosis, and, more recently, patients using immunosuppressive drugs or immunomodulating agents such as natalizumab and rituximab and efalizumab (Raptiva).

INCIDENCE & PREVALANCE:
- Two population groups—HIV and natalizumab-treated patients—have seen a significant increase in PML.
- HIV: a 50-fold increase in PML cases was reported with HIV epidemic. About 3% to 5% of all HIV patients will develop PML. PML is now classified as an AIDS-defining illness.
- Incidence of PML from treatment with natalizumab is estimated to be 3 to 4/1000 patients and depends on treatment duration.
- Seroepidemiologic studies have shown that asymptomatic primary infection with JCV occurs at an early age, and by adult life 30% to 90% of the population is seropositive.

PREDOMINANT SEX & AGE: Males and females are equally affected. There is no specific age distribution.

GENETICS: Unknown

PHYSICAL FINDINGS & CLINICAL PRESENTATION

- Presentation is usually with subacute neurologic deficits but can present acutely as a stroke mimic.
- Clinical signs and symptoms reflect the affected region of the brain. Lesions usually involve the cerebral hemispheres, but cerebellum and brainstem may be involved, especially in AIDS.
- The clinical course spans weeks to months leading to severe disability and death.
- Non–AIDS-associated PML: early lesions involve occipital subcortical white matter and cause visual-field deficits (homonymous hemianopia) or cortical blindness. Motor weakness and altered mentation may be seen, while headache, seizures, and extrapyramidal syndromes are rare.
- AIDS-related PML: motor weakness is more common. Other common symptoms include abnormalities of speech, cognition, gait, sensation, and visual impairment.
- Natalizumab-associated PML: frontal lobe is commonly involved, leading to cognitive impairment, neurobehavioral changes, motor disorders, language disorders, and visual defects.
- Immune reconstitution inflammatory syndrome (IRIS): a paradoxical clinical deterioration that occurs during immunologic recovery in patients previously immunocompromised, such as antiretroviral therapy–treated HIV-seropositive patients, or cessation of immunomodulating treatment, such as natalizumab. An increase in the number or size of lesions on neuroimaging with contrast enhancement of brain lesions and brain edema may be seen.

ETIOLOGY & PATHOGENESIS

- JCV infection may be acquired through respiratory tissue or oropharyngeal route; seroconversion usually occurs in childhood.
- A cytotoxic-specific response against JCV acts as a containing mechanism for PML. Immunosuppression leads to development of PML either as primary infection of the CNS following immunosuppression or reactivation of a dormant infection. The virus produces lytic infection of the oligodendrocytes and causes demyelination. Neuronal infection does not usually occur except in granule cell neurons of the cerebellum.

DIAGNOSIS

DIFFERENTIAL DIAGNOSIS

- Multiple sclerosis
- Acute disseminated encephalomyelitis
- Vasculitis
- HIV encephalitis
- Mitochondrial encephalopathies (e.g., MELAS)
- Posterior reversible encephalopathy syndrome

WORKUP

- Diagnosis of PML is based on compatible clinical presentation, classic MRI brain features, and detection of JCV in CSF.
- Brain biopsy is the gold standard and demonstrates a triad of histopathologic findings—demyelination, bizarre astrocytes, and enlarged oligodendrocytic nuclei.

LABORATORY TESTS

- CSF examination: usually normal; may show mild lymphocytic pleocytosis (20-25 leukocytes/ml) and elevated protein (<65 mg/dl).
- CSF PCR for JCV has a sensitivity of 95% and specificity of 99% using ultrasensitive PCR techniques, but may be lower depending on the techniques used.

IMAGING STUDIES

- MRI brain is the neuroimaging of choice and shows demyelinating lesions that are hyperintense on T2 and FLAIR sequences, hypointense on T1, and may enhance with gadolinium.
- CT head may show demyelinating lesions as subcortical hypodensities with faint contrast enhancement.
- MR spectroscopy will demonstrate features of demyelination—decreased N-acetyl acetate, increased choline, and increased lactate.

TREATMENT

There is no specific treatment for PML. Treatment is aimed at reversal of the underlying causes of immunosuppression.

NONPHARMACOLOGIC THERAPY

Plasma exchange and immunoadsorption for natalizumab-treated patients to rapidly reduce blood levels of natalizumab and hasten restoration of immune function

ACUTE GENERAL Rx

- HIV-positive patients: antiretroviral therapy should be optimized.
- HIV-negative patients: offending immunosuppressive medication should be discontinued; plasma exchange may be considered for natalizumab-treated patients to restore immune function.
- IRIS: treatment with steroids should be considered.

CHRONIC Rx

No specific pharmacologic therapy exists for chronic treatment.

DISPOSITION

Of all HIV-related cerebral disorders, PML probably has the worst prognosis. Pre-AIDS era survival was 6 months. With advent of antiretroviral therapy treatment, the incidence and prognosis of patients with PML has improved. Individuals with lower CSF JCV load and better CD4 counts have better prognoses. Natalizumab-treated patients have worse prognoses seen with longer time to diagnosis, presence of widespread disease, and brainstem involvement.

REFERRAL

Refer to neurology if patients have neurologic deficits of uncertain etiology, especially in the setting of AIDS or immunosuppression.

PEARLS & CONSIDERATIONS

COMMENTS

PML is a fatal opportunistic cerebral infection that should be considered in all immunosuppressed individuals presenting with neurologic deficits and demyelinating cerebral lesions. Early referral to a center with neurologic expertise, especially neuroimmunology or neuroinfectious diseases, should be considered.

SUGGESTED READINGS

available at www.expertconsult.com

AUTHORS: **PADMAJA SUDHAKAR, M.B.B.S.,** and **SACHIN KEDAR, M.B.B.S., M.D.**

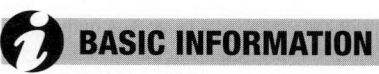

BASIC INFORMATION

DEFINITION

Progressive supranuclear palsy (PSP) is an atypical parkinsonian syndrome characterized by supranuclear gaze impairment, prominent and early postural instability with falls, axial greater than appendicular rigidity, and poor or absent response to levodopa.

SYNONYMS

Steele-Richardson-Olszewski syndrome
Progressive supranuclear ophthalmoplegia

ICD-9CM CODES
333.0 Other degenerative diseases of the basal ganglia

EPIDEMIOLOGY & DEMOGRAPHICS

INCIDENCE: 1.1 per 100,000 (5.3 per 100,000 over age 50)
PREVALENCE: 4.9 per 100,000 (6.4 per 100,000 age-adjusted)
PREDOMINANT SEX AND AGE: Slight male predominance; mean age onset 63 yr, very uncommon for onset <50 yr
GENETICS: Familial cases have been reported only rarely. The vast majority of cases are sporadic.

PHYSICAL FINDINGS & CLINICAL PRESENTATION

Tremorless parkinsonism is the general clinical presentation, and differentiation from idiopathic Parkinson's disease can be challenging early in the disease course. However, there are certain symptoms that can serve as "red flags" to consider PSP:

- Early postural instability and retropulsion leads to frequent falls; falls within the first year of onset of symptoms is typically the rule.
- Supranuclear gaze palsy is often preceded by slowing of vertical saccades; square wave jerks can be present; blepharospasm is common.
- Dystonia of the frontalis and procerus muscles gives the PSP patient a "surprised" or "frightened" expression as opposed to the hypomimia of Parkinson's disease (Fig. 1-676).
- Speech is typically strained, spastic, hypernasal, with a low-pitched dysarthria.
- Pseudobulbar affect and "emotional incontinence" can be seen, with easy crying or laughter.
- Early cognitive impairment, most commonly with apathy, disinhibition, and anxiety.

ETIOLOGY

PSP is caused by neuronal degeneration of nuclei in the midbrain and basal ganglia, as a result of abnormal tau protein accumulation, most commonly in astrocyte inclusions and neurofibrillary tangles.

DIAGNOSIS

DIFFERENTIAL DIAGNOSIS

- Parkinson's disease: responds more robustly to levodopa, progression much slower, and lacks "red flag" symptoms above
- Corticobasal degeneration: also a tauopathy like PSP, but characterized by parkinsonism with prominent asymmetric dystonia, cortical sensory signs such as astereognosis, typically progressing to apraxia and sometimes an "alien hand" syndrome
- Multiple system atrophy: distinguished by autonomic involvement such as orthostatic hypotension, cerebellar ataxia, and inspiratory stridor
- Dementia with Lewy bodies: dementia coincident with parkinsonism, fluctuating mental status, visual hallucinations often preceding onset of dopaminergic treatment

WORKUP

- PSP is a clinical diagnosis, best made by a neurologist familiar with the disorder such as a movement disorders specialist.
- A robust response to a trial of levodopa may help to lead consideration away from PSP.
- MRI scan (see below) can be helpful.

LABORATORY TESTS

There are no diagnostic laboratory tests.

IMAGING STUDIES

- Dorsal midbrain atrophy is commonly seen on MRI.
- MRI regional apparent diffusion coefficients (rADC) in specific nuclei on diffusion-weighted imaging can reliably differentiate

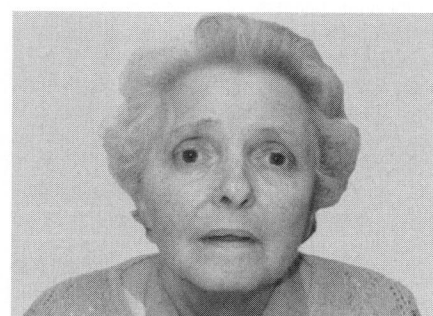

FIGURE 1-676 A patient with progressive supranuclear palsy with staring expression, frontalis overactivity, and retrocolitis. She is wearing a neck sling for a fractured wrist sustained in a fall. (From Burn D, Lees A: Progressive supranuclear palsy: where are we now? *Lancet Neurol* 1:359, 2002.)

PSP from Parkinson's disease, although not from multiple system atrophy.

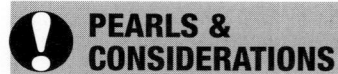

TREATMENT

NONPHARMACOLOGIC THERAPY

- Physical therapy, in particular focusing on fall prevention, is essential for avoiding the morbidity associated with frequent falls. Assistive devices such as a walker or wheelchair should be encouraged.
- Dysphagia is a common finding and should be monitored for closely in conjunction with a speech therapist.
- Prisms can be helpful in some patients for the eye movement abnormalities that can result in misalignment and diplopia.

CHRONIC Rx

- Although classically felt to be unresponsive to levodopa, there is often a transient response to this medication and it can be useful. The poor response to levodopa is most likely due to the loss of postsynaptic dopamine receptors.
- Anticholinergic medications should be avoided.
- Blepharospasm can be effectively treated with botulinum toxin injections.

DISPOSITION

Median latency from symptom onset to wheelchair-bound state is 5 yr and to death is 7 yr.

REFERRAL

Referral to a general neurologist or movement disorders center is appropriate.

PEARLS & CONSIDERATIONS

COMMENTS

Consider PSP in a parkinsonian patient with the onset of falls within 1 yr of diagnosis, vertical eye movement abnormalities, early cognitive impairment, pseudobulbar affect, frontonasal dystonia, or poor response to levodopa.

PATIENT & FAMILY EDUCATION

Patient and caregiver information and resources can be found at www.wemove.org (a comprehensive movement disorders website) as well as the Society for Progressive Supranuclear Palsy at www.curepsp.org.

SUGGESTED READINGS
available at www.expertconsult.com

AUTHOR: **ANDREW DUKER, M.D.**

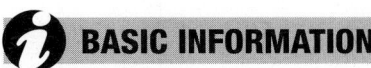

DEFINITION

Prolactinomas are monoclonal tumors that secrete prolactin.

ICD-9CM CODES
253.1 Forbes-Albright syndrome

EPIDEMIOLOGY & DEMOGRAPHICS

INCIDENCE: Most common pituitary tumor; nearly 30% of all pituitary adenomas secrete enough prolactin to cause hyperprolactinemia.
PREDOMINANT SEX: Microadenomas are more common in women; macroadenomas are found more frequently in men.

PHYSICAL FINDINGS & CLINICAL PRESENTATION

- Men: decreased facial and body hair, infertility, small testicles; may also have decreased libido, erectile dysfunction, and delayed puberty (caused by decreased testosterone as a result of inhibition of gonadotropin secretion).
- Women: physical examination may be normal; history may reveal amenorrhea, galactorrhea (Fig. E1-677), oligomenorrhea, and anovulation.
- Both sexes: visual field defects and headache may occur depending on size of tumor and its expansion.

ETIOLOGY

Prolactin-secreting pituitary adenomas: microadenomas (<10 mm diameter) or macroadenomas (>10 mm diameter). No risk factors have been identified for sporadic prolactinomas. Rarely prolactinomas can be part of multiple endocrine neoplasia (MEN) type 1 syndrome.

Dx DIAGNOSIS

DIFFERENTIAL DIAGNOSIS

Secretion of prolactin is under tonic inhibitory control by hypothalamic dopamine. Hyperprolactinemia may be caused by the following:

- Drugs: risperidone, phenothiazines, methyldopa, reserpine, monoamine oxidase inhibitors, androgens, progesterone, cimetidine, tricyclic antidepressants, haloperidol, meprobamate, chlordiazepoxide, estrogens, narcotics, metoclopramide, verapamil, amoxapine, cocaine, oral contraceptives
- Hepatic cirrhosis, renal failure, primary hypothyroidism
- Ectopic prolactin-secreting tumors (hypernephroma, bronchogenic carcinoma)
- Infiltrating diseases of the pituitary (sarcoidosis, histiocytosis)
- Head trauma, chest wall injury, spinal cord injury
- Polycystic ovary disease, pregnancy, nipple stimulation
- Idiopathic hyperprolactinemia, stress, exercise

WORKUP

- The diagnosis of prolactinoma is established by demonstration of an elevated serum prolactin level (after exclusion of other causes of hyperprolactinemia) and radiographic evidence of a pituitary adenoma.
  1. Normal mean prolactin levels are 8 ng/ml in women and 5 ng/ml in men.
  2. Levels >300 ng/ml are virtually diagnostic of prolactinomas.
  3. Prolactin levels can vary with time of day, stress, sleep cycle, and meals. More accurate measurements can be obtained 2 to 3 hr after awakening, preprandially, and when patient is not distressed.
  4. Serial measurements are recommended in patients with mild prolactin elevations.
- TSH, free T_4, BUN, Creat, ALT, AST are useful tests. Pregnancy test in all women of childbearing age.
- All patients with prolactinomas should undergo visual field testing. Serial evaluation is recommended, particularly during pregnancy in patients with macroadenomas.

IMAGING STUDIES

- MRI with gadolinium enhancement is the procedure of choice in the radiographic evaluation of pituitary disease.
- In absence of MRI, a radiographic diagnosis is best accomplished with a high-resolution CT scanner and special coronal cuts through the pituitary region.

Rx TREATMENT

NONPHARMACOLOGIC THERAPY

Pregnancy and breastfeeding should be avoided because they can encourage tumor growth.

ACUTE GENERAL Rx

- Management of prolactinomas depends on their size and encroachment on the optic chiasm and other vital structures, the presence or absence of gonadal dysfunction, and the patient's desires regarding fertility. Fig. E1-678 describes a management algorithm for prolactinomas.
- Medical therapy is preferred when fertility is an important consideration.
  1. Bromocriptine: initial dose is 0.625 mg at bedtime for the first week. After 1 wk, add morning dose of 1.25 mg. Gradually increase dose by 1.25 mg/wk until dose of 5 to 10 mg/day is achieved. Bromocriptine decreases size of the tumor and generally lowers the prolactin level into the normal range when the initial serum prolactin is <500 ng/ml. Side effects of bromocriptine are nausea, constipation, dizziness, and nasal stuffiness. Bromocriptine appears to be safe during pregnancy.
  2. Cabergoline is a longer acting dopamine agonist that is more expensive but may be more effective and better tolerated than bromocriptine; initial dose is 0.25 mg twice weekly.
- Transsphenoidal resection: option in an infertile patient who cannot tolerate bromocriptine or cabergoline or when medical therapy is ineffective. The success rate depends on the location of the tumor (entirely intrasellar),

experience of the neurosurgeon, and size of the tumor (<10 mm in diameter); the recurrence rate may reach 80% within 5 yr. Possible complications of transsphenoidal surgery vary with experience and skill of the neurosurgeon and tumor anatomy and include transient diabetes insipidus, hypopituitarism, cerebrospinal fluid rhinorrhea, and infections (meningitis, wound infection).

- Pituitary irradiation is useful as adjunctive therapy of macroadenomas (>10 mm in diameter) and in patients with persistent hypersecretion after surgery. Potential complications include cranial nerve damage, radionecrosis, and cognitive abnormalities.
- Stereotactic radiosurgery (gamma knife) has become popular as a modality in the treatment of prolactinomas. A high dose of ionizing radiation is delivered to the tumor through multiple ports. Its advantage is minimal irradiation to surrounding tissues. Proximity of the tumor to the optic chiasm limits this therapeutic modality.

CHRONIC Rx

- Patients on medical therapy require periodic measurement of prolactin levels. An attempt to reduce the dose of bromocriptine or cabergoline can be made after the prolactin level has been normal for 2 yr. An MRI scan of the pituitary should be obtained to rule out tumor enlargement within 6 mo of initiation of tapering regimen.
- Evaluation and monitoring of pituitary function are recommended after transsphenoidal surgery.

DISPOSITION

- Transsphenoidal surgery will result in a cure in nearly 50% to 75% of patients with microadenomas and 10% to 20% of patients with macroadenomas.
- Nearly 20% of microprolactinomas resolve during long-term dopamine agonist treatment.

! PEARLS & CONSIDERATIONS

COMMENTS

- Patients must be monitored for several years after surgery because up to 50% of microadenomas and nearly 90% of macroadenomas can recur.
- Pituitary microadenomas are found in 10.9% of autopsies, and 44% of these microadenomas are prolactinomas.

SUGGESTED READINGS
available at www.expertconsult.com

RELATED CONTENT

Prolactinoma (Patient Information)

AUTHOR: **FRED F. FERRI, M.D.**

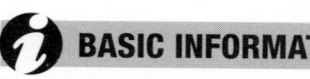

BASIC INFORMATION

DEFINITION

Pronator syndrome is a form of compression neuropathy of the median nerve in the proximal forearm caused primarily by the pronator teres muscle (Fig. 1-679). Occasionally, only the anterior interosseus motor branch is affected, sometimes causing a specific separate clinical presentation.

SYNONYMS

Kiloh-Nevin syndrome (anterior interosseus syndrome)

ICD-9CM CODES
354.1 Median nerve entrapment
354.9 Mononeuritis of upper limb

EPIDEMIOLOGY & DEMOGRAPHICS

PREDOMINANT SEX: Males are affected more often than females.

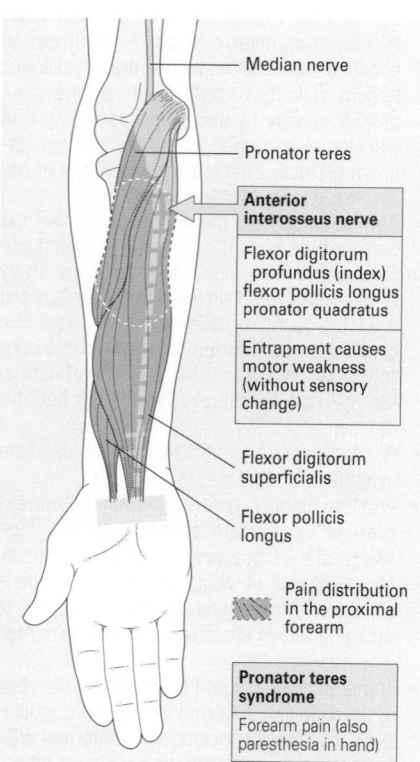

Median nerve

Pronator teres

Anterior interosseus nerve

Flexor digitorum profundus (index) flexor pollicis longus pronator quadratus

Entrapment causes motor weakness (without sensory change)

Flexor digitorum superficialis

Flexor pollicis longus

Pain distribution in the proximal forearm

Pronator teres syndrome

Forearm pain (also paresthesia in hand)

FIGURE 1-679 Forearm entrapment regions. The median nerve may be compressed at several locations in the forearm, most commonly as it traverses the pronator teres muscle. The anterior interosseus branch of the median nerve is solely motor, thus entrapment produces no sensory deficit. (From Hochberg MC et al [eds]: *Rheumatology,* ed 3, St Louis, 2003, Mosby.)

INCIDENCE: Rare (comprises <1% of median nerve entrapment disorders); most common in dominant arm.

PHYSICAL FINDINGS & CLINICAL PRESENTATION

- Forearm discomfort and fatigue, often resulting from repetitive pronation
- Insidious onset
- Nocturnal paresthesias are not typical.
- Vague numbness in hand, primarily in thumb and index finger, may be present.
- Tenderness and enlargement of the pronator teres may be present.
- Tinel's sign may be positive at the site of compression.
- Although there are no reliable provocative tests, painful paresthesias may occasionally be elicited with forced pronation of the forearm against resistance.
- Motor impairment is rare.

Anterior interosseus nerve syndrome:
- Forearm pain and weakness
- Patient may be unable to form a circle when trying to pinch the index finger and thumb because of the inability to flex distal phalanges of thumb and index finger.
- Sensation to the hand is not affected.

ETIOLOGY

- Localized anatomic compression
- Trauma
- Traumatic cutdown or phlebotomy

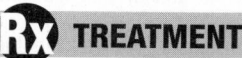

DIAGNOSIS

DIFFERENTIAL DIAGNOSIS

- Carpal tunnel syndrome
- Cervical disc syndrome with radiculopathy
- Tendon rupture
- Tendinitis

WORKUP

- Electrodiagnostic studies may be helpful; they are indicated if symptoms persist >4 to 6 wk or if motor weakness is suspected
- Plain radiography to rule out bony abnormalities causing compression

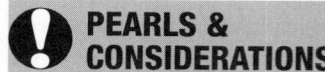

TREATMENT

- Rest, bracing of forearm, sling
- Stretching exercises, physical therapy
- Nonsteroidal anti-inflammatory drugs

DISPOSITION

Patients whose symptoms are mainly subjective often respond to nonsurgical management. Motor deficits may not be reversible despite surgery.

REFERRAL

Surgical referral in cases of failed medical management or when motor weakness is present

PEARLS & CONSIDERATIONS

COMMENTS

Prognosis for recovery is good. When indicated, surgical intervention is most effective if the diagnosis can be firmly established by objective testing.

SUGGESTED READINGS

available at www.expertconsult.com

AUTHOR: **LONNIE R. MERCIER, M.D.**

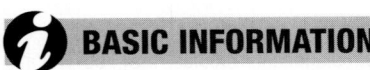

BASIC INFORMATION

DEFINITION & CLASSIFICATION

Prostate cancer is a neoplasm involving the prostate. Various classifications have been developed to evaluate malignancy potential and prognosis.

- The degree of malignancy varies with the stage:
  1. Stage A: Confined to the prostate, no nodule palpable
  2. Stage B: Palpable nodule confined to the gland
  3. Stage C: Local extension
  4. Stage D: Regional lymph nodes or distant metastases
- In the Gleason classification, two histologic patterns are independently assigned numbers 1 to 5 (best to least differentiated). These numbers are added to give a total tumor score between 2 and 10. Prognosis is best for highly differentiated tumors (e.g., Gleason score 2 to 4) compared with most poorly differentiated tumors (Gleason score 7 to 10).
- Another commonly used classification is the Tumor-Node-Metastasis (TNM) classification of prostate cancer.

ICD-9CM CODES
185 Malignant neoplasm of prostate

EPIDEMIOLOGY & DEMOGRAPHICS

- Prostate cancer has surpassed lung cancer as the most common nonskin cancer in men.
- In the U.S. nearly 200,000 cases are diagnosed yearly, and nearly 30,000 males die from prostate cancer each year (second leading cause of death from cancer in U.S. men).
- Incidence of prostate cancer increases with age: uncommon <50 yr; 80% of new cases are diagnosed in patients aged ≥65 yr. Widespread PSA testing has doubled the incidence of prostate cancer and the lifetime risk for prostate cancer to approximately 16%. Prostate cancer is also diagnosed earlier, and the incidence of clinically "silent" T1 tumors has increased from 17% in 1989 to 48% in 2001 since the advent of PSA screening.
- Average age at time of diagnosis is 72 yr.
- Blacks in the U.S. have the highest incidence of prostate cancer in the world (one in every nine males).
- Incidence is low in Asians.
- Approximately 9% of all prostate cancers may be familial. Obesity is a risk factor for prostate cancer. High-fat, low-fiber diet increases risk. High insulin levels may also increase the risk of prostate cancer. Dietary supplementation with vitamin E has been reported to significantly increase the risk of prostate cancer among healthy men. Linkage studies have implicated chromosome 17p21-22 as a possible location of a prostate-cancer susceptibility gene. Germline mutations in *HOXB13* are associated with a significantly increased risk of hereditary prostate cancer.

- Mortality rates of prostate cancer have declined substantially in the past 15 yr from 34% in 1990 to <20% currently.

PHYSICAL FINDINGS & CLINICAL PRESENTATION

- Generally silent disease until it reaches advanced stages.
- Bone pain and pathologic fractures may be initial symptoms of prostate cancer.
- Local growth can cause symptoms of outflow obstruction.
- Digital rectal examination (DRE) may reveal an area of increased firmness; 10% of patients will have a negative DRE.
- Prostate may be hard, fixed, with extension of tumor to the seminal vesicles in advanced stages.

DIAGNOSIS

DIFFERENTIAL DIAGNOSIS

- Benign prostatic hypertrophy
- Prostatitis
- Prostate stones

LABORATORY TESTS

- Fig. E1-680 describes the assessment and treatment of patients with prostate cancer suspected on the grounds of a DRE and PSA. Measurement of prostate-specific antigen (PSA) is controversial in early diagnosis of prostate cancer. PSA screening is associated with psychological harm, and its potential benefits remain uncertain. In asymptomatic men with no history of prostate cancer, screening using PSA does not reduce all-cause mortality or death from prostate cancer. Normal PSA is found in >20% of patients with prostate cancer, whereas only 20% of men with PSA levels between 4 ng/ml and 10 ng/ml have prostate cancer. Most guidelines encourage a shared decision-making approach between patient and physician regarding PSA testing. The American Cancer Society recommends offering the PSA test and DRE yearly to men aged ≥50 yr who have a life expectancy of at least 10 yr. Earlier testing, starting at age 45 yr, is recommended for men at high risk (e.g., blacks, men with family history of prostate cancer). An isolated elevation in PSA level should be confirmed several weeks later before proceeding with further testing, including prostate biopsy. Screening for prostate cancer in men aged ≥75 yr is controversial and generally not recommended. The U.S. Preventive Services Task Force (USPSTF) recommends against PSA-based screening for prostate cancer in all age groups. According to the USPSTF:
  - The magnitude of harms from screening (e.g., falsely high PSA levels, psychological effects, unnecessary biopsies, overdiagnosis of indolent tumors) is "at least small."
  - The magnitude of treatment-associated harms (i.e., adverse effects of surgery,

radiation, and hormonal therapy) is "at least moderate."
  - The 10-yr mortality benefit of PSA-based prostate cancer screening is "small to none."
  - The overall balance of benefits and harms results in "moderate certainty that PSA-based screening has no net benefit."
- Free PSA: the use of serum free PSA for prostate screening has been proposed by some urologists as a means to decrease unwarranted biopsies without missing a significant number of prostate cancers. This approach is based on the higher free PSA in men with benign prostatic hyperplasia and the higher protein-bound PSA levels in men with prostate cancer. For example, in men with total PSA levels of 4 to 10 ng/ml, the cancer probability is 0.25, but if the percentage of free PSA is ≤17%, the probability of cancer increases to 0.45.
- PSA velocity: the rate of increase of serum PSA over time (PSA velocity) can aid in the diagnosis of prostate cancer. A yearly PSA velocity >0.75 ng/ml increases the likelihood of later malignancy when total PSA is still within normal range. Proper interpretation of PSA velocity requires at least three PSA measurements over an 18-month period because most PSA variations are physiologic. Recent trials have cast a doubt on the value of PSA velocity by showing that adding PSA velocity as a trigger for biopsy did not improve predictive accuracy beyond that of using PSA threshold values alone.
- Age-adjusted PSA: there is evidence that the current threshold of 4.0 ng/ml is inadequate for younger men, because in a recent study 22% of men with PSA levels between 2.6 and 4.0 were found to have prostate cancer. The concept of age-related cutoffs remains controversial. Lowering the upper limit of normal for PSA would improve sensitivity but decrease specificity.
- Prostatic acid phosphatase can be used for evaluation of nonlocalized disease.
- Prostate cancer gene 3 *(PCA3)* is overexpressed in prostate cancer cell, and high levels are suggestive of prostate cancer. Measurement of *PCA3* in urine specimens collected after digital exams is helpful to make decisions about prostate biopsy in men with elevated PSA.
- Transrectal biopsy and fine-needle aspiration of prostate can confirm the diagnosis. Indications for biopsy include an abnormal PSA level, an abnormal DRE, or a previous biopsy specimen that showed prostatic intraepithelial neoplasia or prostatic atypia. The number of cores taken is patient specific, typically including a minimum of 10 cores. Prostate volume negatively affects cancer detection rate (23% in glands >50 cm^3, 38% in glands <50 cm^3).

IMAGING STUDIES

- Bone scan is useful to evaluate bone metastasis (present or eventually develops in almost 80% of patients). However, according to

the American Urological Association (AUA), the routine use of bone scanning is not required for staging of prostate cancer in asymptomatic men with clinically localized cancer if the PSA level is ≤20 ng/ml.

- CT scan, MRI, and transrectal ultrasonography may be useful in selected patients to assess extent of prostate cancer. High-resolution MRI with magnetic nanoparticles has been used for the detection of small and otherwise undetectable lymph node metastases in patients with prostate cancer. However, according to the AUA, transrectal ultrasonography adds little to the combination of PSA and DRE. Similarly, CT and MRI imaging are generally not indicated for cancer staging in men with clinically localized cancer and PSA <25 ng/ml. With regard to pelvic lymph node dissection in staging, the AUA states that it may not be required in patients with PSA levels <10 ng/ml and when PSA level is <20 ng/ml and the Gleason score is <6.

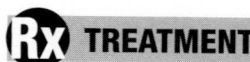 **TREATMENT**

NONPHARMACOLOGIC THERAPY

Watchful waiting is reasonable in selected patients with early-stage (T-IA) and projected life expectancy <10 yr or in patients with focal and moderately differentiated carcinoma.

ACUTE GENERAL Rx

- Therapeutic approach varies with the following:
  1. Stage of the tumor
  2. Patient's life expectancy
  3. General medical condition
  4. Patient's treatment preference (e.g., patient may be opposed to orchiectomy)
- The optimal treatment of clinically localized prostate cancer is unclear. It's important to remember that all forms of treatment have potential adverse effects. Management requires careful consideration of the potential benefits and harms of intervention, the patient's age, health status, and individual preferences.
  1. Radical prostatectomy is generally performed in patients with localized prostate cancer and life expectancy >10 yr. Radical prostatectomy reduces disease-specific mortality, overall mortality, and the risks of metastasis and local progression. The absolute reduction in the risk of death after 10 yr is small, but the reductions in the risks of metastasis and local tumor progression are substantial. Postoperative complications of radical prostatectomy include urinary incontinence (10% to 20% depending on degree of neurovascular bundle and urethral preservation, patient age, and correct mucosal apposition) and erectile dysfunction (percentage exceeds 50% and varies with patient age, preoperative erectile dysfunction, stage of tumor at time of surgery, and preservation of neurovascular bundle). Lower complication rates occur in hospitals that per-

form a large number of prostatectomies. Fewer men will have postsurgical erectile dysfunction after unilateral or bilateral nerve-sparing surgery. In men undergoing prostatectomy, robotic-assisted laparoscopic surgery represents an alternative to open retropubic radical prostatectomy. Despite advertisements that suggest that there are fewer complications after robotic surgery, recent data show that sexual dysfunction occurs postoperatively in about 88% of patients who have undergone robotic-assisted or conventional prostatectomy and that incontinence problems are more prevalent (33%) with robotic surgery than with open retropubic radical prostatectomy (RPP) (27%). Recent trials have shown that prostatectomy is preferred over "watchful waiting" in patients with localized prostate cancer detected by PSA if the PSA level is >10 ng/ml. In this subgroup, the 10-year mortality is 48.4% with prostatectomy versus 61.6% with watchful waiting.

2. Radiation therapy (external-beam irradiation or brachytherapy with implantation of radioactive pellets [iodine-125 or palladium-103 seeds] into the prostate gland) represents an alternative in patients with localized prostate cancer, especially poor surgical candidates or patients with a high-grade malignancy. The efficacy of brachytherapy is comparable to external radiation. In patients receiving external-beam radiation, a total dose of 79.2 Gy (high dose) compared with a total dose of 70.2 Gy (conventional dose) has been reported to lower the risk of recurrence without increased risk of morbidity and mortality. Newer radiation treatments such as intensity-modulated radiation therapy (IMRT) and proton therapy are becoming increasingly popular and replacing the older technique of conformal radiation therapy over the past 10 years. Trials have shown that among patients with nonmetastatic prostate cancer, the use of IMRT compared with conformal therapy is associated with less gastrointestinal morbidity and fewer hip fractures but more erectile dysfunction; IMRT compared with proton therapy is associated with less GI morbidity. Patients with localized prostate cancer and high risk for extraprostatic disease and disease recurrence (e.g., Gleason score ≤7 with multiple positive biopsy cores and clinical stage T1b-T2b) may benefit (increased overall survival) with the addition of 6 mo of androgen suppression therapy to radiation therapy.

3. Watchful waiting is reasonable in patients who are too old or too ill to survive longer than 10 yr. If the cancer progresses to the point where it becomes symptomatic, palliation can be attempted with several methods. Conservative management is also reasonable for patients with Gleason score of 2 to 4 be-

cause these patients do not have a shortened life expectancy and treatment is associated with long-term side effects. Watchful waiting also appears to be safe in older men with less-aggressive disease. Individual preferences play a central role in the decision whether to treat or to pursue active surveillance.

- Patients with advanced disease and projected life expectancy <10 yr are candidates for radiation therapy and hormonal therapy (diethylstilbestrol, luteinizing hormone–releasing hormone analogs, antiandrogens, bilateral orchiectomy).
- Recommended treatment of patients with regional metastatic prostate cancer with projected life expectancy ≥10 yr includes radiation therapy and hormonal therapy.
- Prostate cancer is an androgen-receptor-dependent disease, and the blocking of androgen-receptor signaling is an effective treatment modality. Androgen deprivation therapy (ADT) is the mainstay of treatment for metastatic prostate cancer. Adverse effects of ADT include decreased libido, impotence, hot flashes, osteopenia with increased fracture risk, metabolic alterations, and changes in mood and cognition. Adjuvant treatment with luteinizing hormone-releasing hormone (LHRH) agonists (goserelin, leuprolide, or triptorelin) plus antiandrogens (flutamide, bicalutamide, or nilutamide), when started simultaneously with external-beam radiation, improves local control and survival in patients with locally advanced prostate cancer. Pamidronate inhibits osteoclast-mediated bone resorption and prevents bone loss in the hip and lumbar spine in men receiving treatment for prostate cancer. Gonadotropin-releasing hormone (GnRH) receptor antagonists can be used for rapid medical castration of men with advanced prostate cancer. Degarelix is an injectable GnRH agonist useful to suppress testosterone in patients with prostate cancer who are not good candidates for LHRH agonists and refuse surgical castration. Assessment of bone density and treatment with once-weekly oral alendronate can prevent and improve the bone loss that occurs in men receiving ADT for prostate cancer.
- Docetaxel plus prednisone or docetaxel plus estramustine can be used in metastatic hormone–refractory prostate cancer. Newer treatments for hormone-refractory prostate cancer (castration-resistant cancer) include immunotherapy with sipuleucel and cabazitaxel, a microtubule inhibitor that interferes with cell mitosis and replication. Both agents can prolong survival but adverse effects can be severe and both agents are very expensive. Abiraterone is an oral agent that blocks biosynthesis of androgens by inhibiting CYP17, an enzyme required for androgen biosynthesis. It has been FDA approved for oral treatment, in combination with prednisone, of metastatic castration-resistant prostate cancer in patients previously treated with docetaxel.

- Enzalutamide is a newer nonsteroidal antiandrogen. Trials have shown it to be highly effective in extending survival in patients with metastatic castration-resistant prostate cancer. It can be used sequentially with other agents such as docetaxel, abiraterone, cabazitaxel, and immunotherapy.

CHRONIC Rx

- Patients should be monitored at 3- to 6-mo intervals with clinical examination and PSA for the first year, then every 6 mo for the second year, then yearly if stable. For patients who have undergone radical prostatectomy, a rising PSA level suggests evidence of residual or recurrent prostate cancer. Salvage radiotherapy may potentially cure patients with disease recurrence after radical prostatectomy.
- Chest radiography and bone scan should be performed yearly or sooner if patient develops symptoms.

DISPOSITION

- Prognosis varies with the stage of the disease and the Gleason classification (see "Definition"). For patients between ages 65 and 69 yr at diagnosis and a Gleason score of 2 to 4, the probability of dying from prostate cancer 15 yr after diagnosis is 0.06 and that of dying from other causes is 0.56. If the Gleason score is 7 to 10, the probability of dying from prostate cancer increases to 0.72 and from other causes varies from 0.25 to 0.36.
- The ploidy of the tumor also has prognostic value; prognosis is better with diploid tumor cells and worse with aneuploid tumor cells.

- For grade 1 tumors, the extended 10-yr, disease-specific survival is similar for patients with prostatectomy (94%), radiotherapy (90%), and conservative management (93%); survival rate is better with surgery than with radiotherapy or conservative management in patients with grade 2 or 3 localized prostate cancer.
- Expression of the gene *EZH2* has been identified as an important factor in the determination of the aggressiveness of prostate cancer. A recent study revealed that expression of the *EZH2* gene may be a better predictor of clinical failure than Gleason score, tumor stage, or surgical margin status. Testing for *EZH2* protein in prostate cancer tissue may be useful to determine prognosis and direct treatment.
- Preoperative PSA level and PSA velocity have prognostic significance. Men whose PSA level increases by >2.0 mcg/ml during the year before the diagnosis of cancer may have a relatively high risk of death from prostate cancer despite undergoing radical prostatectomy.
- Extraprostatic disease is detected at radical prostatectomy in 38% to 52% of patients and is associated with a risk of disease recurrence, progression, and death. In these patients, adjuvant radiotherapy results in significantly reduced risk of PSA relapse and disease recurrence; however, the improvements in metastases-free survival and overall survival are not statistically significant.
- The Prostate Cancer Prevention trial revealed that the use of 5-alpha-reductase inhibitors lowers the incidence of prostate cancer but

also increases the incidence of high-grade tumors (Gleason score >7). It is possible that these agents delay diagnosis of prostate cancer by lowering PSA levels and decreasing prostate size. The trade-off inherent in using 5-alpha-reductase inhibitors for prostate cancer prevention is risk of one additional high-grade cancer in order to avert three or four lower grade cancers. Based on these results, the FDA's Oncologic Drugs Advisory Committee concluded that finasteride and dutasteride do not have a favorable risk-benefit profile for chemoprevention of prostate cancer in healthy men.
- Patients undergoing prostatectomy are more likely to have urinary incontinence than those undergoing radiotherapy at 2 years and 5 years. However, at 15 years there are no significant relative differences in disease-specific functional outcomes among men undergoing prostatectomy or radiotherapy.

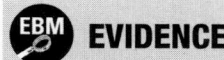 **EVIDENCE**

available at www.expertconsult.com

SUGGESTED READINGS
available at www.expertconsult.com

RELATED CONTENT
Prostate Cancer (Patient Information)

AUTHOR: **FRED F. FERRI, M.D.**

BASIC INFORMATION

DEFINITION

Benign prostatic hyperplasia (BPH) is the benign growth of the prostate, generally originating in the periureteral and transition zones, with subsequent obstructive and irritative voiding symptoms.

SYNONYMS

BPH
Prostatic hypertrophy

ICD-9CM CODES

600 Benign prostatic hyperplasia

EPIDEMIOLOGY & DEMOGRAPHICS

- 80% of men have evidence of BPH by age 80 yr.
- Medical and surgical intervention for problems caused by BPH is required in >20% of males by age 75 yr.
- Transurethral resection of the prostate (TURP) is the tenth most common operative procedure (>400,000/yr in U.S.).
- 10% to 30% of men with BPH have occult prostate cancer.

PHYSICAL FINDINGS & CLINICAL PRESENTATION

- Digital rectal examination (DRE) reveals enlargement of the prostate.
- Focal enlargement may be indicative of malignancy.
- There is poor correlation between size of prostate and symptoms (BPH may be asymptomatic if it does not encroach on the urethral lumen).
- Most patients with BPH report difficulty in initiating urination (hesitancy), decrease in caliber and force of stream, incomplete emptying of bladder often resulting in double voiding (need to urinate again a few minutes after voiding), postvoid "dribbling," and nocturia.

ETIOLOGY

Multifactorial; a functioning testicle is necessary for development of BPH (as evidenced by the absence in males who were castrated before puberty).

DIAGNOSIS

DIFFERENTIAL DIAGNOSIS

- Prostatitis
- Prostate cancer
- Strictures (urethral)
- Medications interfering with the muscle fibers in the prostate and also with bladder function
  - Opiates: impaired autonomic function
  - Decongestants: increased sphincter tone
  - Antihistamines: decreased parasympathetic tone
  - Tricyclic antidepressants: anticholinergic effects
- Neurogenic bladder
- Bladder cancer

WORKUP

Symptom assessment (use of American Urological Association [AUA] Symptom Index for BPH [Table 1-343]), laboratory tests, and imaging studies Fig. E1-681 describes a diagnostic approach to patients with BPH.

LABORATORY TESTS

- Prostate-specific antigen (PSA): protease secreted by epithelial cells of the prostate; elevated in 30% to 50% of patients with BPH. Testing for PSA increases detection rate for prostate cancer and tends to detect cancer at an earlier stage. However, the PSA test does not discriminate well between patients with symptomatic BPH and those with prostate cancer, particularly if the cancer is pathologically localized and curable. The test may also trigger additional evaluation, including ultrasound biopsy of the prostate. Asymptomatic men with PSA levels <2 ng/ml do not need annual testing. According to the AUA, PSA testing and DRE should be offered to any asymptomatic man >50 yr with a life expectancy of 10 yr. PSA testing can also be offered at an earlier age in men at higher risk of prostatic cancer (e.g., first-degree relatives with prostate cancer; African American race).

TABLE 1-343 International Prostate Symptom Score (I-PSS)

Symptom	SCORE						Total Score
	Not at All	Less than 1 Time in 5	Less than Half the Time	About Half the Time	More than Half the Time	Almost Always	
Incomplete emptying: Over the past month, how often have you had a sensation of not emptying your bladder completely after you finished urinating?	0	1	2	3	4	5	
Frequency: Over the past month, how often have you had to urinate again <2 hr after you finished urinating?	0	1	2	3	4	5	
Intermittency: Over the past month, how often have you found you stopped and started again several times when you urinated?	0	1	2	3	4	5	
Urgency: Over the past month, how often have you found it difficult to postpone urination?	0	1	2	3	4	5	
Weak stream: Over the past month, how often have you had a weak urinary stream?	0	1	2	3	4	5	
Straining: Over the past month, how often have you had to push or strain to begin urination?	0	1	2	3	4	5	
	None	1 Time	2 Times	3 Times	4 Times	5 or More Times	
Nocturia: Over the past month, how many times did you most typically get up to urinate from the time you went to bed at night until the time you got up in the morning?	0	1	2	3	4	5	

Total I-PSS score =

- Measurement of "free" PSA is useful to assess the probability of prostate cancer in patients with normal DRE and total PSA between 4 and 10 ng/ml. In these patients the global risk of prostate cancer is 25%. However, if the free PSA is >25%, the risk of prostate cancer decreases to 8%, whereas if the free PSA is <10%, the risk of cancer increases to 56%. Free PSA is also useful to evaluate the aggressiveness of prostate cancer. A low free PSA percentage generally indicates a high-grade cancer, whereas a high free PSA percentage is generally associated with a slower growing tumor.
- Elevated measurement of prostate cancer gene 3 (PCA3) in urine specimens collected after digital exam is helpful in deciding about prostate biopsy in men with elevated PSA (increased PCA3 = increased likelihood of prostate cancer).
- Urinalysis, urine culture, and sensitivity to rule out infection (if suspected).
- Blood urea nitrogen and creatinine to rule out postrenal insufficiency.

IMAGING STUDIES

- Transrectal ultrasound may be indicated in patients with palpable nodules or significant elevation of PSA. It is also useful to estimate prostate size. BPH may also be evident in suprapubic ultrasound and MRI.
- Uroflowmetry may be used to determine relative impact of obstruction on urine flow. Urethral pressure profile is useful to predict prostatic hypertrophy within the urethral lumen.
- Pressure flow studies, although invasive, are particularly helpful in patients whose history and/or examination suggest primary bladder dysfunction as a cause of symptoms of prostatism. They are also useful in patients for whom a distinction between prostatic obstruction and impaired detrusor contractility may affect the choice of therapy. However, pressure flow studies may not be useful in the workup of the usual patient with symptoms of prostatism.
- Postvoid residual urine measurement has not been proved useful in predicting the need for or response to treatment; it may be useful in monitoring the course of the disease in patients who elect nonsurgical treatment.
- Urethral cystoscopy is an option during later evaluation if invasive treatment is being planned.

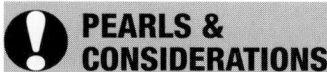 TREATMENT

NONPHARMACOLOGIC THERAPY

- Avoidance of caffeine or any other foods that may exacerbate symptoms
- Avoidance of medications that may exacerbate symptoms (e.g., most cold and allergy remedies)

GENERAL Rx

- Asymptomatic patients with prostate enlargement caused by BPH generally do not require treatment. Patients with mild to moderate symptoms are candidates for pharmacologic treatment (see below). For patients who have specific complications from BPH, prostate surgery is usually the most appropriate form of treatment. However, surgery may result in significant complications (e.g., incontinence, infection).
- Alpha-blockers (e.g., tamsulosin, alfuzosin, doxazosin, prazosin, terazosin) relax smooth muscle of the bladder neck and prostate and can increase peak urinary flow rate. They have no effect on the size of the prostate. Alpha-1 blockers are useful in symptomatic patients to relieve symptoms of obstruction by causing relaxation of smooth muscle tone in the prostatic capsule, urethra, and bladder neck.
- Hormonal manipulation with finasteride, a 5-alpha-reductase inhibitor that blocks conversion of testosterone to dihydrotestosterone, can reduce the size of the prostate. Usual dose is 5 mg qd. Treatment requires ≥6 mo for maximal effect.
- Dutasteride is also a 5-alpha-reductase inhibitor useful to decrease prostate size and improve urinary flow. In addition to inhibiting the isoform of 5-alpha-reductase located in the prostate, the medication inhibits a second isoform and reduces dihydrotestosterone formation in the skin and liver. Usual dose is 0.5 mg qd.
- Tadalafil 5 mg qd has been FDA-approved to treat patients with signs and symptoms of BPH and patients with both ED and signs and symptoms of BPH. Tadalafil can potentiate the hypotensive effect of alpha-blockers and should not be used in combination with alpha-blockers.
- The dietary supplement saw palmetto is commonly used for relief of symptoms of BPH. Recent trials using 160 mg of saw palmetto bid did not improve symptoms of BPH. This contrasts with the positive findings of many previous studies. Trials with higher dose-ranging protocols are currently in progress.
- TURP is the most commonly used surgical procedure for BPH. Transurethral incision of the prostate (TUIP), a procedure almost equivalent in efficacy, is limited to patients whose estimated resection tissue weight would be 30 g or less. TUIP can be performed in an ambulatory setting or during a 1-day hospitalization. Open prostatectomy is typically performed on patients with very large prostates.
- Laser therapy for BPH is a less invasive alternative to TURP; YAG laser enucleation has minimal effect on potency, libido, or patient satisfaction with his sex life and is associated with retrograde ejaculation. However, recent studies indicate that at least in the initial 7 mo after surgery, TURP is moderately more effective than laser therapy in relieving symptoms of BPH.
- Transurethral needle ablation with radiofrequency to remove periurethral prostate tissue is being increasingly used in patients with

prostate volume <60 ml and moderate symptoms. It has a low morbidity rate, but treatment failure is approximately 25% at 5 yr and >80% at 10 yr.
- Balloon dilation of the prostatic urethra is less effective than surgery for relieving symptoms but is associated with fewer complications. It is a reasonable treatment option for patients with smaller prostates and no middle lobe enlargement.
- Surgery need not be the treatment of last resort for most patients; that is, patients need not undergo other treatments for BPH before they can have surgery. However, recommending surgery on the grounds that a patient's surgical risk will "only increase with age" is generally inappropriate.

DISPOSITION

With appropriate therapy, symptoms improve or stabilize in >70% of patients with BPH.

REFERRAL

Urology referral for patients with severe or intolerable symptoms and for any patient suspected of having prostate cancer (10% to 30% of men with BPH)

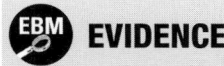 PEARLS & CONSIDERATIONS

COMMENTS

- Emerging technologies for treating BPH, including transurethral holmium laser enucleation, transurethral electrovaporization, and transurethral microwave thermotherapy of the prostate, appear promising; however, long-term effectiveness has not yet been demonstrated.
- The increase in the use of pharmacologic management has resulted in >30% reduction in the total number of TURP procedures.
- Combined drug therapy for BPH with an alpha-blocker and a 5-alpha-reductase inhibitor is superior to monotherapy with either agent.
- Saw palmetto extract is ineffective for BPH symptoms. Trials have shown that even at three times the standard dosing, saw palmetto extract had no greater effect than placebo on improving lower urinary symptoms associated with BPH.

EVIDENCE

available at www.expertconsult.com

SUGGESTED READINGS

available at www.expertconsult.com

RELATED CONTENT

Enlarged Prostate (Patient Information)

AUTHOR: **FRED F. FERRI, M.D.**

BASIC INFORMATION

DEFINITION

Prostatitis refers to inflammation of the prostate gland. There are four major categories:
1. Acute bacterial prostatitis (type I)
2. Chronic bacterial prostatitis (type II)
3. Chronic prostatitis/pelvic pain syndrome (CP/CPPS) (type III): subdivided into type IIIA (inflammatory) and IIIB (noninflammatory)
4. Asymptomatic inflammatory prostatitis (type IV)

ICD-9CM CODES
601.0 Prostatitis (acute)
601.1 Prostatitis (chronic)
099.54 Prostatitis (chlamydial)

EPIDEMIOLOGY & DEMOGRAPHICS

- 50% of men will have symptoms of prostatitis in their lifetime.
- Prostatitis accounts for >8% of visits to urologists and 1% of visits to primary care physicians.
- The prevalence of chronic bacterial prostatitis is 5% to 10%.
- CP/CPPS is the most common of the clinically defined prostatitis syndromes, with prevalence ranging from 9%-12% of men.

PHYSICAL FINDINGS & CLINICAL PRESENTATION

1. Acute bacterial prostatitis:
   - Sudden or rapidly progressive onset of:
     ○ Dysuria
     ○ Frequency
     ○ Urgency
     ○ Nocturia
     ○ Perineal pain that may radiate to the back, rectum, or penis
   - Hematuria or a purulent urethral discharge may occur.
   - Occasionally urinary retention complicates the course.
   - Fever, chills, and signs of sepsis can also be part of the clinical picture.
   - On rectal examination the prostate is typically tender.
2. Chronic bacterial prostatitis:
   - Characterized by positive culture of expressed prostatic secretions. May cause symptoms such as suprapubic, low back, or perineal pain; mild urgency, frequency, and dysuria with urination; and possibly recurrent urinary tract infections.
   - May be asymptomatic when the infection is confined to the prostate.
   - May present as an increase in severity of baseline symptoms of benign prostatic hypertrophy (BPH).
   - When cystitis is also present, urinary frequency, urgency, and burning may be reported.

- Hematuria may be a presenting complaint.
- In elderly men, new onset of urinary incontinence may be noted.
3. CP/CPPS:
   - Presents similarly with pain in the pelvic region lasting >3 mo. Symptoms also can include pain in the suprapubic region, low back, penis, testes, or scrotum.
   - The symptoms can be of variable severity and may include lower urinary tract symptoms, sexual dysfunction, and reduced quality of life.

ETIOLOGY

1. Acute bacterial prostatitis:
   - Acute, usually gram-negative infection of the prostate gland. *E. coli* is the most commonly isolated organism.
     ○ Generally associated with cystitis
     ○ Results from the ascent of bacteria into the urethra
   - Occasionally the route of infection is hematogenous or a lymphatogenous spread of rectal bacteria.
   - Consider *Neisseria gonorrhoeae* or *Chlamydia trachomatis* in young patients (age <35 yr) with risk of sexually transmitted disease (STD).
2. Chronic bacterial prostatitis:
   - Often asymptomatic. *E. coli* is the most commonly isolated organism.
   - Exacerbation of symptoms of BPH caused by the same mechanism as in acute bacterial prostatitis.
3. CP/CPPS:
   - Type IIIA: refers to symptoms of prostatic inflammation associated with the presence of white blood cells in prostatic secretions with no identifiable bacterial organism.
   - *Chlamydia* infection may be etiologically implicated in some cases.
   - Type IIIB: refers to symptoms of prostatic inflammation with no or few white blood cells in the prostatic secretion.
   - Its cause is unknown. Spasm in the bladder neck or urethra may be responsible for the symptoms.

DIAGNOSIS

DIFFERENTIAL DIAGNOSIS
- BPH with lower urinary tract symptoms
- Prostate cancer

WORKUP
- Rectal examination:
  1. Tender prostate most suggestive of acute bacterial prostatitis
  2. Enlarged prostate common in chronic bacterial prostatitis
  3. Normal prostate is consistent with chronic bacterial prostatitis and CP/CPPS.

- Expression of prostatic secretions by prostate massage is contraindicated in acute bacterial prostatitis but is appropriate in the other three situations.

LABORATORY TESTS
- Urinalysis
- Urine culture and sensitivity
- Bacterial localization studies can be performed but are cumbersome and impractical in most clinical settings.
- Cell count and culture of expressed prostatic secretions
- Prostate-specific antigen (PSA) is not used to diagnose prostatitis and is not recommended unless a nodule is present on digital examination. A rapid rise over baseline should raise the possibility of prostatitis even in the absence of symptoms. In such cases, a follow-up PSA after treatment of prostatitis is appropriate.
- Complete blood count and blood cultures if fever, chills, or signs of sepsis exist.

TREATMENT

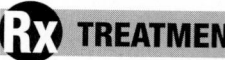

1. Acute bacterial prostatitis:
   - Uncomplicated (with risk of STD, age <35 yr): ceftriaxone 250 mg IM × 1 dose *or* cefixime 400 mg PO × 1 *then* doxycycline 100 mg bid × 10 days
   - Uncomplicated with low risk of STD: levofloxacin 500 mg qd or ciprofloxacin 500 mg bid × 10-14 days
2. Chronic bacterial prostatitis:
   - First-line choice is a quinolone (ciprofloxacin or levofloxacin) for 4 wk.
   - Trimethoprim-sulfamethoxazole (TMP-SMX) is second-line choice for 1-3 mo if the organism is sensitive. Tissue penetration for TMP-SMX is not as good as quinolones, and there is evidence of increasing uropathogenic resistance.
3. CP/CPPS:
   - No specific treatment. A brief course of NSAIDs may be tried until urine localization cultures are completed. Alfuzosin may reduce symptoms in men who have not received prior therapy with an alpha-blocker.
   - Recent trials have shown modest improvement with quinolones (possibly secondary to their anti-inflammatory and analgesic effects), but antibiotics are not generally effective and should be avoided in patients who are afebrile and have normal urinalysis results.

SUGGESTED READINGS
available at www.expertconsult.com

RELATED CONTENT
Prostatitis (Patient Information)

AUTHOR: **FRED F. FERRI, M.D.**

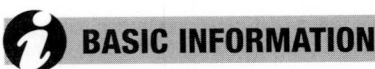

BASIC INFORMATION

DEFINITION

Pruritus ani refers to an intense chronic itching of the anus and perianal skin.

ICD-9CM CODES
698.0 Pruritus ani

EPIDEMIOLOGY & DEMOGRAPHICS

- Any age can be affected.
- Occurs in 1% to 5% of the population.
- Male/female predominance of 4:1

PHYSICAL FINDINGS & CLINICAL PRESENTATION

- Anal itching
- Anal fissures
- Hemorrhoids
- Excoriations
- Pinworms
- Fecal incontinence

ETIOLOGY

Anorectal diseases and fecal contamination:
- Diarrhea
- Anal incontinence
- Hemorrhoids
- Fissures
- Fistulae
- Rectal prolapse
- Malignancy: Bowen's disease, epidermoid cancer, perianal Paget's disease

Infections:
- Fungal: candidiasis, dermatophytes
- Parasitic: pinworms, scabies
- Bacterial: *Staphylococcus aureus,* erythrasma
- Lymphogranuloma venereum
- Granuloma inguinale
- Chancroid
- Molluscum contagiosum
- Trichomoniasis
- Venereal: herpes, gonococcal syphilis, human papillomavirus

Local irritants:
- Moisture, obesity, excessive perspiration
- Soaps, hygiene products
- Toilet paper: perfumed, dyed
- Underwear: irritating fabrics, detergents

- Anal creams, suppositories
- Dietary: coffee, beer, acidic foods
- Drugs: mineral oil, ascorbic acid, hydrocortisone sodium succinate, quinine, colchicine

Dermatologic diseases:
- Psoriasis
- Atopic dermatitis
- Seborrheic dermatitis

Section II also describes the various causes of pruritus ani.

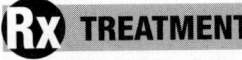

DIAGNOSIS

DIFFERENTIAL DIAGNOSIS

- Allergies
- Anxiety
- Dermatologic conditions
- Infections
- Parasites
- Diabetes mellitus
- Chronic liver disease
- Neoplasia
- Proctalgia fugax

WORKUP

- Detailed history regarding bowel habits, hygiene, use of perfumed products, and medical history
- Inspection of perianal area
- Possible biopsy to exclude neoplasia
- Microscopic inspection of scrapings
- Colposcopy of perineum

LABORATORY TESTS

- Chemistry profile
- Urinalysis
- Cultures
- Stool for ova and parasites
- Tape test
- Glucose tolerance test, if necessary

TREATMENT

NONPHARMACOLOGIC THERAPY

- Avoidance of tight, nonbreathable clothing and underclothing
- Discontinuation or curtailment of coffee, beer, citrus fruits, tomatoes, chocolate, and tea. Dietary modification is frequently recommended, although its effectiveness has not been established.

- Cleansing of anal area after bowel movements with a premoistened pad or tissue and avoidance of perfumes and dyes present in toilet paper and soaps
- Avoidance of excessive perspiration
- Aggressive management of fecal leakage or incontinence to avoid soiling of perianal skin

ACUTE GENERAL Rx

- Minimization of frequent loose stools with antidiarrheals and fiber agents if appropriate
- Use of a 1% hydrocortisone cream sparingly bid during the acute phase of pruritus ani but not for >2 wk to avoid atrophy
- Protective ointments such as zinc oxide may be helpful.
- Treatment of predisposing factors, such as parasites, diabetes, liver disease, hemorrhoids, and other infections

CHRONIC Rx

- Possible complications: excoriation and secondary bacterial infection; must be treated aggressively
- Longstanding, intractable pruritus ani: good response to intracutaneous injections of methylene blue and other agents, steroid injection

DISPOSITION

- Usually good results with total resolution of symptoms
- In some, persistent and recurrent symptoms

REFERRAL

To colorectal specialist if conservative measures fail or if patient experiences rectal bleeding or change in bowel movements

SUGGESTED READING
available at www.expertconsult.com

RELATED CONTENT
Hemorrhoids (Related Key Topic)
Anal Itching (Patient Information)

AUTHORS: **MARIA A. CORIGLIANO, M.D.,** and **RUBEN ALVERO, M.D.**

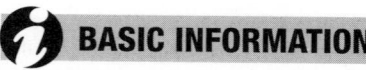 BASIC INFORMATION

DEFINITION

Pruritus vulvae refers to intense itching of the female external genitalia.

SYNONYMS

Vulvodynia

ICD-9CM CODES

698.1 Pruritus of genital organs

EPIDEMIOLOGY & DEMOGRAPHICS

- A female disorder that can affect women at any age
- Young girls: infection is usually causative
- Postmenopausal women: frequently affected because of hypoestrogenic state

PHYSICAL FINDINGS & CLINICAL PRESENTATION

Constant, intense itching or burning of the vulva

ETIOLOGY

- Approximately 50% are caused by monilial infection or trichomoniasis.
- Other infectious causes are herpes simplex, condylomata acuminata, and molluscum contagiosum.
- Other causes:
  1. Infestations with scabies, pediculosis pubis, and pinworms
  2. Dermatoses such as hypertrophic dystrophy, lichen sclerosus, lichen planus, and psoriasis
  3. Neoplasms such as Bowen's disease, Paget's disease, and squamous cell carcinoma
  4. Allergic or chemical dermatitis caused by dyes in clothing or toilet paper, detergents, contraceptive gels, vaginal medications, douches, or soaps
  5. Vulvar or vaginal atrophy
- Severe pruritus is probably caused by degeneration and inflammation of terminal nerve fibers.
- Most intense itching occurs with hyperplastic lesions.
- Children typically (75%) have nonspecific pruritus, lichen sclerosus, bacterial infections, yeast infection, or pinworm infestation.

Dx DIAGNOSIS

DIFFERENTIAL DIAGNOSIS

- Vulvitis
- Vaginitis
- Lichen sclerosus
- Squamous cell hyperplasia
- Pinworms
- Vulvar cancer
- Syringoma of the vulva

WORKUP

- Inspection of vulva, vagina, and perianal area for infection, fissures, ulcerations, induration, or thick plaques
- Must rule out trichomoniasis, candidiasis, bacterial vaginosis, allergy, vitamin deficiencies, diabetes. Fig. E1-682 describes a diagnostic approach to the diagnosis of vulvar pruritus.

LABORATORY TESTS

- Wet prep of saline and potassium hydroxide of vaginal discharge
- Tape test to look for pinworms
- Vaginal cultures
- Biopsy when needed (punch biopsy commonly used)

Rx TREATMENT

NONPHARMACOLOGIC THERAPY

- Keep vulva clean and dry.
- Wear white cotton panties.
- Avoid perfumes and body creams over vulvar area because they can cause irritation.
- Reduce stress.
- Apply wet dressings with aluminum acetate (Burow's) solution frequently.
- Avoid coffee and caffeine-containing beverages, chocolate, and tomatoes.
- Sitz baths may be helpful.

ACUTE GENERAL Rx

Need to treat underlying problem:
- Yeast infection: any of the vaginal creams or difluconazole 150-mg one-time dose
- Trichomoniasis or *Gardnerella vaginalis:* metronidazole 500 mg or 375 mg PO bid for 7 days
- Urinary tract infection: treatment of specific organism

- Estrogen replacement therapy if atrophy is the cause of pruritus
- Pinworms: mebendazole 100 mg 1 tablet at diagnosis and repeated in 1 to 2 wk; also treat other members in family aged >2 yr
- Squamous cell hyperplasia: local application of corticosteroids
  1. One of the high- or medium-potency corticosteroids (0.025% or 0.01% fluocinolone acetonide or 0.01% triamcinolone acetonide) can be used to relieve itching.
  2. Rub into vulva bid or tid for 4 to 6 wk.
  3. Once itching is controlled, fluorinated steroid can be discontinued and patient can be switched to hydrocortisone preparation.
- Lichen sclerosus: topical 2% testosterone in petrolatum massaged into the vulvar tissue bid or tid; clobetasol propionate gel 0.05% tid for 5 days is effective
- Treatment with immune response modifiers

CHRONIC Rx

- If not relieved by topical measures: intradermal injection of triamcinolone (10 mg/ml diluted 2:1 saline); 0.1 ml of the suspension injected at 1-cm intervals and tissue gently massaged
- If symptoms still uncontrollable: SC injection of absolute alcohol 0.1 ml at 1-cm intervals

DISPOSITION

Usually controlled with conservative measures and topical steroids

REFERRAL

To a gynecologist for further workup if conservative measures do not give relief

SUGGESTED READINGS

available at www.expertconsult.com

RELATED CONTENT

Vaginitis, Bacterial (Related Key Topic)
Vaginitis, Estrogen-Deficient (Related Key Topic)
Vaginitis, Fungal (Related Key Topic)
Vaginitis, Prepubescent (Related Key Topic)
Vaginitis, Trichomonas (Related Key Topic)

AUTHORS: **MARIA A. CORIGLIANO, M.D.,** and **RUBEN ALVERO, M.D.**

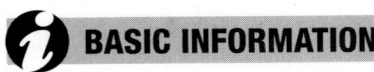

DEFINITION

Pseudogout refers to an acute synovitis caused by calcium pyrophosphate dihydrate (CPPD) crystals. CPPD deposition diseases comprise a spectrum of clinical syndromes including pseudogout, chondrocalcinosis, and pyrophosphate arthropathy. *Chondrocalcinosis* (CC) refers to the presence of calcification in cartilage by radiograph and does not confirm the diagnosis of pseudogout as it can be present in other types of crystal deposition diseases or asymptomatic. Pyrophosphate arthropathy is the term used for a chronic structural arthropathy related to CPPD deposition.

SYNONYMS

Calcium pyrophosphate dihydrate crystal deposition disease (CPPD crystal deposition disease)
Chondrocalcinosis
Pyrophosphate arthropathy

ICD-9CM CODES
275.4 Chondrocalcinosis

EPIDEMIOLOGY & DEMOGRAPHICS

PREVALENCE:
- The epidemiology of CPPD crystal deposition is described in Table 1-344.
- Most linked with advancing age (average age of 70)

GENETICS: Associated with *ANKH* (ankylosis human) gene, which functions to transport inorganic pyrophosphate (PPi) out of cells. Familial mutations can increase extracellular PPi and lead to onset of CPPD disease in third or fourth decade of life.

PHYSICAL FINDINGS & CLINICAL PRESENTATION

- Acute pseudogout: monoarticular attacks most commonly involve the knee but can be polyarticular. Patients, especially the elderly, can have systemic manifestations such as fever and altered mental status. Situations that may trigger acute CPPD crystal arthritis are described in Box 1-52.

TABLE 1-344 Epidemiology of Calcium Pyrophosphate Dihydrate Crystal Deposition

Age association	Rises with age
Sex distribution	(F : M) 1 : 1
Chondrocalcinosis prevalence	8.1% (age range 63-93)
Pyrophosphate arthropathy prevalence	3.4% (age range 40-89)
Geography	Appears ubiquitous
Genetic associations	Mutations of *ANKH* gene on chromosome 5p (CCAL2) and unknown genes on chromosome 8q (CCAL1)

From Hochberg MC et al: *Rheumatology*, ed 5, St Louis, 2011, Mosby.

- Asymptomatic CC
- Pyrophosphate arthropathy: chronic arthritis with osteoarthritic features
- "Pseudo–polymyalgia rheumatica (pseudo-PMR)": pain and stiffness in the neck and shoulder girdle mimicking PMR
- "Pseudo–rheumatoid arthritis (pseudo-RA)": symmetric polyarthritis
- Crowned-dens syndrome caused by crystal deposition in the ligamentum flavum of the cervical spine either asymptomatic or causing acute neck pain

ETIOLOGY

- Idiopathic
- Metabolic: hyperparathyroidism, hypophosphatasia, hypomagnesemia, hemochromatosis, ochronosis, familial hypocalciuric hypercalcemia, X-linked hypophosphatemic rickets

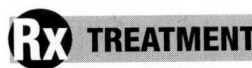

DIFFERENTIAL DIAGNOSIS

- Gouty arthritis
- Septic arthritis
- RA
- PMR

BOX 1-52 Situations That May Trigger Acute Calcium Pyrophosphate Dihydrate Crystal Arthritis

Definite
Direct trauma to joint
Intercurrent medical illness (e.g., chest infection, myocardial infarction)
Surgery (especially parathyroidectomy)
Blood transfusion, parenteral fluid administration
Joint lavage

Possible
Institution of thyroxine replacement therapy
Intra-articular injection of hyaluronan
Bisphosphonate treatment

Note: Most cases of pseudogout develop spontaneously.
From Hochberg MC et al: *Rheumatology*, ed 5, St Louis, 2011, Mosby.

Table 1-345 describes metabolic diseases predisposing to CPPD disposition. Section II describes the differential diagnosis of acute monoarticular and oligoarticular arthritis and crystal-induced arthritides. An algorithm for evaluation and treatment of CPPD is shown in Fig. 1-683.

LABORATORY TESTS

- Arthrocentesis with presence of weakly positive birefringent rhomboid-shaped crystals (yellow perpendicular and blue parallel to polarizer axis) (Fig. 1-684)
- Synovial fluid should always be analyzed for cell count with differential, crystals, Gram stain, and culture because gout and septic arthritis can coexist with pseudogout.
- Evaluate for possible metabolic cause, especially in younger patients aged <55 yr or patients with florid polyarticular disease. Box 1-53 describes screening blood tests for metabolic diseases associated with CPPD crystal deposition.

IMAGING STUDIES

Plain radiographs often reveal CC located parallel to subchondral bone.
- Classic locations for CC include knee menisci, wrist triangular fibrocartilage, and symphysis pubis (Fig. 1-685).

NONPHARMACOLOGIC THERAPY

General measures such as immobilization of inflamed joint

ACUTE GENERAL Rx

- Monoarticular pseudogout:
  - Aspiration with corticosteroid injection (often superior to systemic treatment in the elderly)
- Polyarticular pseudogout:
  - Oral corticosteroids or NSAIDs if not contraindicated

CHRONIC GENERAL Rx

Prophylaxis: daily low-dose colchicine 0.6 mg twice daily or once daily as tolerated

TABLE 1-345 Metabolic Diseases Predisposing to Calcium Pyrophosphate Dihydrate Deposition

	CC	Pseudogout	Chronic PA
Hemochromatosis	Yes	Yes	Yes
Hyperparathyroidism	Yes	Yes	No
Hypophosphatasia	Yes	Yes	No
Hypomagnesemia	Yes	Yes	No
Hypothyroidism	No	No	No
Gout	Possibly	Possibly	No
Acromegaly	Possibly	No	No
Ochronosis	Yes	Yes	No
Familial hypocalciuric hypercalcemia	Possibly	No	No
X-linked hypophosphatemic rickets	Possibly	Possibly	Possibly

CC, Chondrocalcinosis; *PA*, pyrophosphate arthropathy.

- Pseudo-RA or refractory disease: hydroxy-chloroquine or methotrexate
- Treat underlying metabolic disease

DISPOSITION
Structural joint damage may occasionally occur, requiring arthroplasty in rare cases.

REFERRAL
Rheumatology

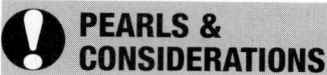

PEARLS & CONSIDERATIONS

COMMENTS
Acute pseudogout attacks have been reported to occur in the setting of surgical procedures, diuresis, bisphosphonate administration, and hyaluronate joint injections.

SUGGESTED READINGS
available at www.expertconsult.com

RELATED CONTENT
Gout (Related Key Topic)
Pseudogout (Patient Information)

AUTHOR: **ELISABETH B. MATSON, D.O.**

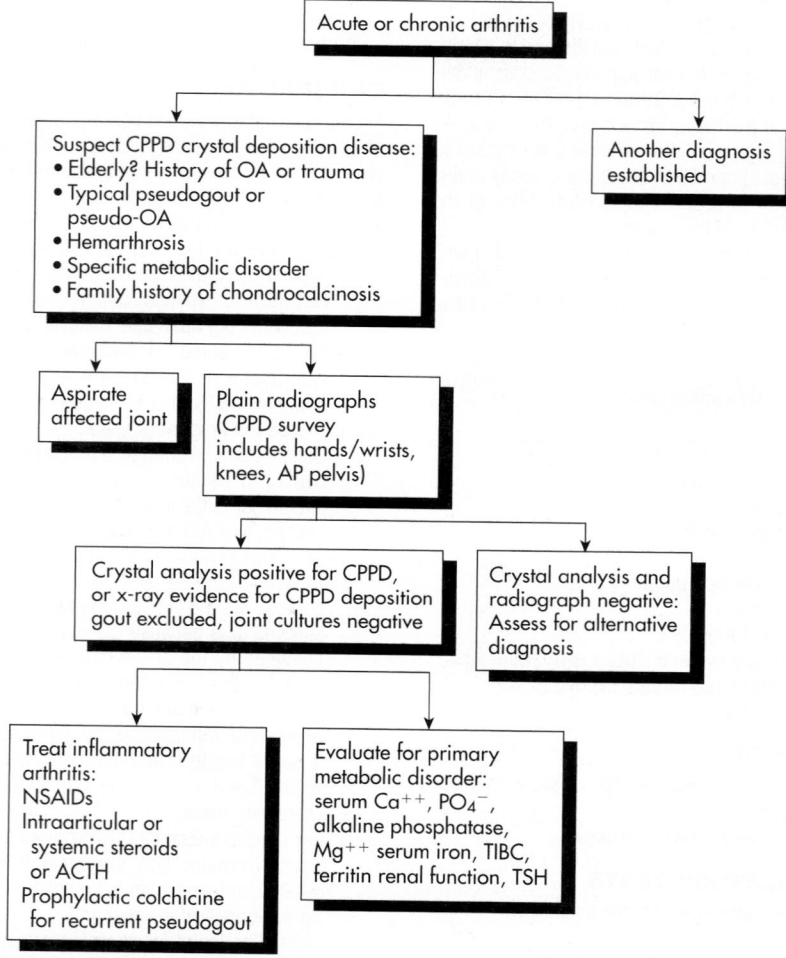

FIGURE 1-683 Algorithm for evaluation and treatment of calcium pyrophosphate dihydrate disease. *ACTH,* Adrenocorticotropic hormone; *AP,* anteroposterior; *CPPD,* calcium pyrophosphate deposition; *NSAIDs,* nonsteroidal anti-inflammatory drugs; *OA,* osteoarthritis; *TIBC,* total iron-binding capacity; *TSH,* thyroid-stimulating hormone. (From Harris ED et al: *Kelley's textbook of rheumatology,* ed 7, Philadelphia, 2005, Saunders.)

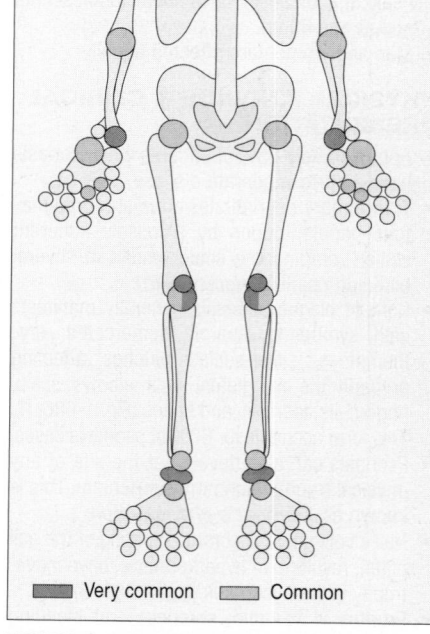

FIGURE 1-685 **Chronic arthropathy.** Common sites of involvement of chronic pyrophosphate. (From Hochberg MC et al: *Rheumatology,* ed 5, St Louis, 2011, Mosby.)

FIGURE 1-684 **Synovial fluid calcium pyrophosphate crystals.** (From Hochberg M et al: *Rheumatology,* Philadelphia, 2011, Mosby.)

BOX 1-53 Screening Blood Tests for Metabolic Diseases Associated with Calcium Pyrophosphate Dihydrate Crystal Deposition

Calcium
Alkaline phosphatase
Magnesium
Ferritin
Liver function
Thyroid-stimulating hormone

From Hochberg MC et al: *Rheumatology,* ed 5, St. Louis, 2011, Mosby.

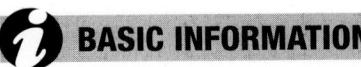

DEFINITION

Psoriasis is a chronic skin disorder characterized by excessive proliferation of keratinocytes, resulting in the formation of thickened scaly plaques, itching, and inflammatory changes of the epidermis and dermis. The various forms of psoriasis include guttate, pustular, and arthritis variants.

ICD-9CM CODES
696.0 Psoriasis, arthritis, arthropathic
696.1 Psoriasis, any type except arthropathic

EPIDEMIOLOGY & DEMOGRAPHICS

- Psoriasis affects 1% to 3% of the world's population. Most patients have limited psoriasis involving <5% of their body surface.
- There is a strong association between psoriasis and human leukocyte antigens (HLAs) B13, B17, and B27 (pustular psoriasis).
- Peak age of onset is bimodal (adolescents and at age 60 yr).
- Men and women are affected equally.

PHYSICAL FINDINGS & CLINICAL PRESENTATION

- Approximately 85% of patients with psoriasis have mild-to-moderate disease.
- The primary psoriatic lesion is an erythematous papule topped by a loosely adherent scale. Scraping the scale results in several bleeding points **(Auspitz sign)**.
- Chronic plaque psoriasis generally manifests with symmetric, sharply demarcated, erythematous, silver-scaled patches affecting primarily the intergluteal folds, elbows, scalp, fingernails, toenails, and knees (Fig. 1-686, *A*). This form accounts for 80% of psoriasis cases.
- Psoriasis can also develop at the site of any physical trauma (sunburn, scratching). This is known as **Koebner's phenomenon**.
- Nail involvement is common (pitting of the nail plate), resulting in hyperkeratosis, onychodystrophy with onycholysis (Fig. 1-686, *B*).
- Pruritus is variable; soreness and bleeding may occur.

- Joint involvement can result in sacroiliitis and spondylitis.
- Guttate psoriasis is generally preceded by streptococcal pharyngitis and manifests with multiple droplike lesions on the extremities and the trunk (Fig. 1-686, *C*).
- Adverse effect on psychological and social functioning, with affected persons often feeling stigmatized.

ETIOLOGY

- Unknown, but there is a strong genetic component and high heritability. There are at least nine chromosomal loci with linkage to psoriasis. These loci are called psoriasis susceptibility 1 through 9 (PSORS1-PSORS9). PSORS1 locus in the major histocompatibility complex (MHC) region on chromosome 6 is considered the most important susceptibility locus and is believed to account for 35% to 50% of the heritability of the disease.
- Familial clustering (genetic transmission with a dominant mode with variable penetrants).
- One third of persons affected have a positive family history.

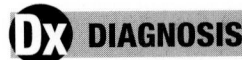

DIFFERENTIAL DIAGNOSIS

- Contact dermatitis
- Atopic dermatitis
- Stasis dermatitis
- Tinea
- Nummular dermatitis
- Candidiasis
- Mycosis fungoides
- Cutaneous systemic lupus erythematosus
- Secondary and tertiary syphilis
- Drug eruption

WORKUP

- Diagnosis is clinical. Blood work is rarely needed.
- Skin biopsy is rarely necessary.

LABORATORY TESTS

Generally not necessary for diagnosis

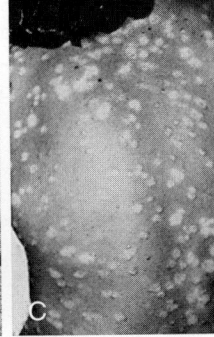

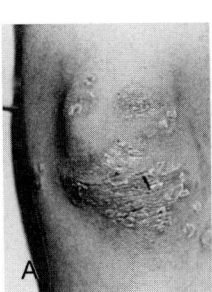
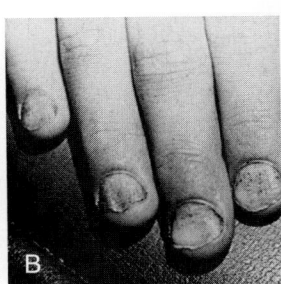

FIGURE 1-686 A, Chronic psoriatic plaques on the knee. **B,** Psoriatic nail changes of pitting and dystrophy. **C,** Guttate psoriasis in widespread distribution over the trunk. (From Behrman RE: *Nelson textbook of pediatrics*, ed 17, Philadelphia, 2004, Saunders.)

TREATMENT

NONPHARMACOLOGIC THERAPY

- Sunbathing generally leads to improvement.
- Eliminate triggering factors (e.g., stress, certain medications [e.g., lithium, beta-blockers, antimalarials]).
- Patients with psoriasis benefit from a daily bath in warm water followed by application of a cream or ointment moisturizer. Regular use of an emollient moisturizer limits evaporation of water from the skin and allows the stratum corneum to rehydrate itself.

GENERAL Rx

Therapeutic options vary according to the extent of disease. Approximately 70% to 80% of all patients can be treated adequately with topical therapy.

- Patients with limited disease (<20% of the body) can be treated with the following:
  1. Topical steroids: disadvantages are brief remissions, expense, and decreased effect with continued use. Salicylic acid can be compounded by pharmacist in concentrations of 2% to 10% and used in combination with a corticosteroid to decrease the amount of scale.
  2. Calcipotriene: a vitamin D analogue effective for moderate plaque psoriasis. Adults should comb the hair, apply solution to the lesions, and rub it in, avoiding uninvolved skin. Disadvantages include its cost and potential burning and skin irritation. It should not be used concurrently with salicylic acid because calcipotriene is inactivated by the acidic nature of salicylic acid. Taclonex ointment is a combination of calcipotriene and the high-potency corticosteroid betamethasone dipropionate. It is well tolerated and more effective than either agent used alone but also much more expensive.
  3. Tar products (Estar, LCD, Psorigel) can be used overnight and are most effective when combined with ultraviolet B (UVB) light (Goeckerman regimen).
  4. Anthralin: useful for chronic plaques; can result in purple-brown staining; best used with UVB light.
  5. Retinoids such as tazarotene 0.05%, 0.1% cream or gel, are effective in thinning plaques but are expensive and can cause irritation.
  6. Other useful measures include tape or occlusive dressing, UVB and lubricating agents, and interlesional steroids.
- Therapeutic options for persons with generalized disease (affecting >20% of the body) and for those with inadequate response to topical agents:
  1. UVB light exposure three times a week: this therapy does not require administration of a systemic drug (unlike psoralen plus ultraviolet A [PUVA]), but to be effective, it requires removal of scale with keratolytic agents and emollients.

2. Oral PUVA administered two to three times weekly is effective for generalized disease. It is often considered in patients for whom narrow-band UVB therapy is ineffective. However, many PUVA treatments are required, necessitating frequent office visits, and it may be associated with phototoxicity, such as erythema and blistering, and increased risk of skin cancer.

- Systemic treatments include methotrexate 25 mg/wk for severe psoriasis. Etretinate (a synthetic retinoid) is most effective for palmar-plantar pustular psoriasis. Dose is 0.5 to 1 mg/kg/day. It can cause liver enzyme and lipid abnormalities and is teratogenic.
- Cyclosporine is also effective in severe psoriasis; however, relapses are common.
- Chronic plaque psoriasis may be treated with alefacept, a recombinant protein that selectively targets T lymphocytes. Treatment with alefacept for 12 wk (0.025, 0.075, or 0.150 mg/kg of body weight IV weekly) may result in significant improvement. Some patients also demonstrate a sustained clinical response after the cessation of treatment. This medication is very expensive (a 12-wk course costs >$8000).
- TNF inhibitors: Treatment with etanercept, a tumor necrosis factor (TNF) antagonist, for 24 wk can also lead to a reduction in severity of plaque psoriasis. Efalizumab, a humanized monoclonal antibody that inhibits the activation of T cells, has also been reported to produce significant improvement in plaque psoriasis over a 24-wk treatment period. Adalimumab—a fully human, anti-TNF-alpha monoclonal antibody—has been reported to be effective for joint and skin manifestations of psoriasis.
- Newer biologic agents in patients with moderate to severe plaque psoriasis are ustekinumab (an interleukin-12 and interleukin-23 blocker), brodalumab, an anti–interleukin-17 receptor antibody, and briakinumab, a monoclonal antibody against the p40 molecule shared by interleukin-12 and interleukin-23, which is overexpressed in psoriatic skin lesions. Trials have shown efficacy in the treatment of moderate-to-severe psoriasis.

DISPOSITION
The course of psoriasis is chronic, and the disease may be refractory to treatment.

REFERRAL
- Dermatology referral is recommended in all patients with generalized disease.

- Hospital admission may be necessary for severe diffuse or poorly responsive psoriasis. The Goeckerman regimen combines daily application of tar with UVB exposure and can result in prolonged remissions.

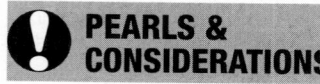 PEARLS & CONSIDERATIONS

COMMENTS
Psoriasis is more emotionally than physically disabling for most patients. Counseling may be indicated, particularly when it affects younger patients.

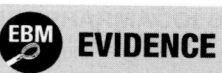 EVIDENCE

available at www.expertconsult.com

SUGGESTED READINGS
available at www.expertconsult.com

RELATED CONTENT
Psoriasis (Patient Information)

AUTHOR: **FRED F. FERRI, M.D.**

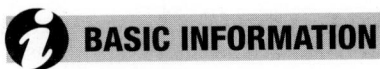

BASIC INFORMATION

DEFINITION

Psoriatic arthritis is an inflammatory arthropathy occurring in association with skin psoriasis and generally in the absence of rheumatoid factor (RF). It is often included in a class of disorders called the *seronegative spondyloarthropathies,* a family of diseases characterized by inflammation of the spine, peripheral joints, and enthesial sites (sites of insertion of tendon into bone). Classifications of psoriatic arthritis are described in Table 1-346.

ICD-9CM CODES
696.0 Psoriatic arthritis

EPIDEMIOLOGY & DEMOGRAPHICS

PREVALENCE: 0.1% to 0.2% overall, variable estimates of 7% to 30% of patients with psoriasis (psoriasis incidence varies by population but overall estimated prevalence of 1% to 2% of general population)
PREDOMINANT SEX: Equal male/female distribution of 1:1
PREDOMINANT AGE: Symptom onset generally age 30 to 55 yr

PHYSICAL FINDINGS & CLINICAL PRESENTATION

- Variably arthritis, dactylitis, spondylitis, and enthesitis occur in the setting of known psoriasis although joint symptoms may predate skin psoriasis in ~15% of patients.
  - Arthritis is inflammatory in nature, commonly characterized by prolonged morning stiffness, joint erythema, warmth, or swelling including joint effusions.
- Distribution of joint involvement follows five classically described patterns (Box 1-54).
- Often more than one classical pattern will occur simultaneously and patterns can evolve over time in an individual patient. Subtypes of psoriatic arthritis are described in Box 1-24.
- Dactylitis refers to diffuse swelling of a digit, either finger or toe, which is typically the result of inflammation in both small joints of the digit as well as associated tenosynovitis of digital tendons. Dactylitis is common in psoriatic arthritis and occurs in approximately 30% to 40% of patients during the course of disease.
- Enthesitis commonly occurs at the Achilles tendon insertion into the calcaneus as well as the insertion of the plantar fascia. Findings on physical exam may include swelling and tenderness.

- Dystrophic changes of the nails (pitting, onycholysis) may occur in association with joint inflammation in involved digits.
- Spondyloarthritis may include sacroiliitis as well as inflammation of the axial spine, but is generally less likely to cause contiguous fusion to the extent seen in ankylosing spondylitis.

ETIOLOGY
Unknown

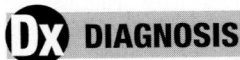

DIAGNOSIS

DIFFERENTIAL DIAGNOSIS
- Rheumatoid arthritis
- Erosive osteoarthritis
- Crystal arthritis including gout and pseudo-gout
- Other seronegative spondyloarthropathies, including reactive arthritis, enteropathic arthritis, and ankylosing spondylitis
- The differential diagnosis of spondyloarthropathies is described in Section III

WORKUP
- Diagnosis generally made on clinical grounds based on history, exam, and radiographic findings given lack of specific lab findings.

TABLE 1-346 Classifications of Psoriatic Arthritis

| Moll and Wright | CLASSIFICATION CRITERIA FOR PSORIATIC ARTHRITIS (CASPAR)* | | |
	Points	Category	Description
Presence of psoriasis and: 1) An inflammatory arthritis (peripheral arthritis and/or sacroiliitis or spondylitis) 2) The (usual) absence of serologic tests for rheumatoid factor	2	Current psoriasis or personal or family history of psoriasis	Psoriatic skin or scalp disease confirmed by dermatologist or rheumatologist; history of psoriasis from patient, family physician, dermatologist, rheumatologist, or other qualified practitioner; patient-reported history of psoriasis in first- or second-degree relative
	1	Psoriatic nail dystrophy on current physical examination	Includes onycholysis, pitting, and hyperkeratosis
	1	Negative for rheumatoid factor	Enzyme-linked immunosorbent assay or nephelometry preferred (no latex) using local laboratory reference range
	1	Current dactylitis or history of dactylitis documented by a rheumatologist	Swelling of entire digit
	1	Radiographic evidence of juxta-articular new bone formation	Ill-defined ossification near joint margins excluding osteophyte formation on plain radiographs of hand or foot

*Psoriatic arthritis is diagnosed when ≥3 points are assigned in the presence of inflammatory articular disease (joint, spine, or entheseal).
From Hochberg MC et al: *Rheumatology,* ed 5, St Louis, 2011, Mosby.

BOX 1-54 Subtypes of Psoriatic Arthritis

Distal interphalangeal joint–predominant arthritis (10%) (Fig. 1-687)
Symmetric polyarthritis–predominant arthritis (5%-20%)
Asymmetric oligoarthritis or monoarthritis (70%-80%)
Axial disease–predominant (spondylitis and/or sacroiliitis) (5%-20%)
Arthritis mutilans (rare)

From Hochberg MC et al: *Rheumatology,* ed 5, St Louis, 2011, Mosby.

- Early diagnosis may be difficult to establish when the arthritis develops before skin lesions appear.

LABORATORY TESTS

- No specific/diagnostic lab tests
- Acute phase reactants such as ESR and CRP may be elevated although less commonly than in patients with rheumatoid arthritis.
- Anemia of chronic disease may be seen.
- RF, while generally negative, can be present in ~10% of patients.
- *HLA B27* is significantly more common in patients with axial inflammation (note that *HLA B27* positivity is present in up to 8% of general population).
- Arthrocentesis of active joint generally demonstrates inflammatory synovial fluid and absence of crystals.

IMAGING STUDIES

- Radiographic findings of involved joints may include soft tissue swelling, joint space narrowing, subluxation, erosive changes, and new bone formation such as periostitis and fusion.
- Severe digital erosive change with adjacent heterotopic bone formation may give rise to "pencil in cup" deformity seen in arthritis mutilans.
- Findings in patients with spondylitis may include sacroiliitis and development of vertebral syndesmophytes that often bridge adjacent vertebral bodies.
- Musculoskeletal ultrasound may be helpful in the evaluation of an inflamed enthesis or joint.
- MRI may be helpful in the evaluation of sacroiliitis or spinal involvement.

Rx TREATMENT

ACUTE GENERAL Rx

- NSAIDs may be used for mild symptoms or limited involvement.
- Intraarticular corticosteroid injections can be used as adjunctive therapy in involved joints.

CHRONIC Rx

- NSAIDs for mild or limited disease
- In patients with several sites of active peripheral disease, elevated acute phase reactants, or with evidence of erosive changes on imaging, traditional DMARDs such as methotrexate, sulfasalazine, and leflunamide should be considered early in disease.
- In patients with peripheral arthritis who fail to respond to traditional DMARD therapy, additional therapy with a tumor necrosis factor (TNF) inhibitor should be considered.
- In patients with predominant axial disease not responsive to NSAIDs, anti-TNF therapy should be considered for initial disease-modifying therapy.
- Enthesitis and dactylitis are poorly responsive to oral DMARD therapy but like spondylitis will often respond to anti-TNF therapy.

REFERRAL

Rheumatology for confirmation of diagnosis and management

! PEARLS & CONSIDERATIONS

- Patients frequently have a positive family history of psoriasis or psoriatic arthritis.
- Severity of skin psoriasis and activity of inflammatory arthritis are frequently discordant.

SUGGESTED READING

available at www.expertconsult.com

RELATED CONTENT

Fig. 3-170 Algorithm for diagnosis of the spondyloarthropathies (Algorithm)
Fig. 3-171 Treatment algorithm for patients with spondyloarthropathy (Algorithm)
Psoriatic Arthritis (Patient Information)

AUTHOR: **HARALD A. HALL, M.D.**

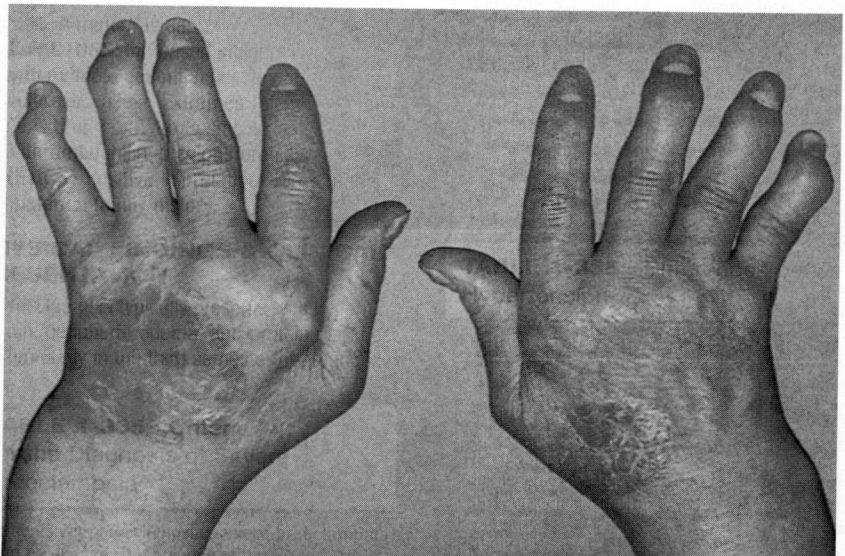

FIGURE 1-687 The hands of a woman with symmetric polyarthritis. Initially, this was indistinguishable from rheumatoid disease, but note the distal interphalangeal joint involvement, which is uncommon in rheumatoid arthritis, as well as the skin psoriasis. (From Klippel J et al [eds]: *Primary care rheumatology,* London, 1999, Mosby.)

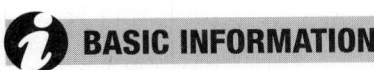

DEFINITION

Psychosis is a state in which external reality is distorted by delusions and/or hallucinations (a delusion is a fixed false idiosyncratic belief; a hallucination is a false auditory, visual, olfactory, tactile, or taste perception).

SYNONYMS

Psychosis is a key finding in many mental illnesses, such as brief psychotic disorder, delusional disorder, schizoaffective disorder, schizophrenia, schizophreniform disorder, or shared psychotic disorder. Psychosis can also present as part of the evolution of a mood disorder (depression and bipolar disorder) or a sign of an underlying medical condition.

EPIDEMIOLOGY & DEMOGRAPHICS

One-year prevalence: 4.5 per 1000. The demographics of psychosis depends on the underlying disorder.

PHYSICAL FINDINGS & CLINICAL PRESENTATION

History:
- Past and current medical history important to identify potential medical etiologies
- Medication use
- Use of illicit substances or alcohol
- Identification of functional and social impairment
- Behavior that is odd or unpredictable; patient may clearly be responding to internal stimuli

Examination:
- Examine for symptoms of:
  - Mood disorder: delusions or hallucinations are usually congruent with the mood (e.g., auditory hallucinations in a depressed patient may tell the patient what a terrible person he is)
  - Altered or disorganized thought pattern: usually reflected in disorganized speech (including word salad, thought blocking, rhyming, clang associations)
  - Lack of insight into problems
  - Signs of Parkinson's disease, dementia

ETIOLOGY

- Involves an interaction among:
  1. Dopaminergic overactivity (particularly in the mesolimbic, nigrostriatal, and mesocortical systems)
  2. Environmental, social, or childhood factors
  3. Genetic predisposition

DIAGNOSIS

WORKUP

- Evaluate for potential confounding factors. Fig. E1-688 describes an algorithmic approach to evaluation of the psychotic patient.

- Underlying mental disorder: schizophrenia, major depression, brief psychotic disorder, delusional disorder, schizoaffective disorder, schizophreniform disorder, shared psychotic disorder
- Underlying personality disorder: borderline, paranoid, schizoid, schizotypal
- Underlying medical conditions: Infections ranging from UTIs to HIV/AIDS, Parkinson's disease, Huntington's disease, leprosy, malaria, sarcoidosis, systemic lupus erythematosus, prion disease, hypoglycemia, postpartum state, cerebrovascular event, temporal lobe epilepsy, brain neoplasm
- Medications: systemic steroids, anticonvulsants, antiparkinsonian medications, some chemotherapy, scopolamine
- Underlying dementia: Alzheimer's disease, Lewy body dementia, vascular dementia
- Illicit drugs (usually with chronic use; can be caused by intoxication or withdrawal): LSD, PCP, cocaine, gamma-hydroxybutyrate (GHB; withdrawal), alcohol, amphetamines, marijuana. New substances of abuse (e.g., "bath salts", synthetic cannabinoids) may not be detected by current toxicology panels.
- Traumatic brain injury
- Intensive care unit stay: hypoxia, decreased cardiac output, infection, medications, sleep deprivation, alteration of diurnal cycle, sensory deprivation or overload, pain
- Emotional stress

LABORATORY TESTS

Consider checking chemistry panel (calcium), complete blood count, UA, liver function tests, cortisol, HIV, rapid plasma reagin, thyroid-stimulating hormone, toxicology screen, lumbar puncture (LP).

IMAGING STUDIES

Consider chest x-ray (rule out sarcoid), electroencephalography, head CT or MRI.

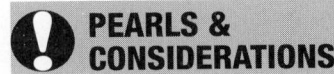

TREATMENT

NONPHARMACOLOGIC THERAPY

- Cognitive-behavioral therapy
- Social and behavioral skills training
- Training for self-management of disease
- Aforementioned strategies favored over psychoanalytic techniques given the relative inability for abstract thought and lack of insight in psychotic patients
- Family intervention, including education and strategies to reduce emotional expression
- Counseling for substance abuse

ACUTE GENERAL Rx

- Antipsychotics, such as haloperidol combined with anticholinergics like benztropine to reduce side effects; low doses should control first episode. Use with caution in elderly patients because adverse effects limit effectiveness. Second-generation antipsychotics are also useful starting with low doses. Newer formulations are available in rapid injectable form or oral disintegrating tablets.
- Benzodiazepines if agitation is severe
- Discontinue offending medication if present.

CHRONIC Rx

Second-generation antipsychotics may reduce the incidence of tardive dyskinesia but may increase incidence of metabolic disorders compared with first-generation antipsychotics. Recent multicenter trial showed similar efficacy between first and second generation. Consider economic, including insurance formulary, factors when selecting a maintenance regimen.

DISPOSITION

Prognosis varies according to etiology of psychosis. In general, the more severe and longer the psychotic episode, the worse the prognosis.

REFERRAL

Patient should be admitted for acute stabilization if actively psychotic to prevent harm to self and others as well as ensure administration of medications.

PEARLS & CONSIDERATIONS

- Delusions and/or hallucinations are hallmarks of psychosis.
- Rule out medical or drug causes of psychosis.
- Antipsychotics are the mainstay of acute and chronic treatment.
- Consider alternatives to antipsychotics in elderly or intellectually disabled patients (see "Nonpharmacologic Therapy").

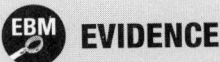 **EVIDENCE**

available at www.expertconsult.com

SUGGESTED READINGS
available at www.expertconsult.com

RELATED CONTENT

Psychosis (Patient Information)

AUTHORS: **ARNOLD A. BERGES, M.D., RICHARD J. GOLDBERG, M.D.,** and **MICHAEL K. ONG, M.D., PH.D.**

BASIC INFORMATION
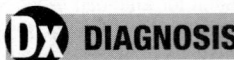

DEFINITION
Acute cardiogenic pulmonary edema (ACPE) is a life-threatening condition that may occur when there is elevated left ventricular (LV) filling pressure related to systolic or diastolic LV dysfunction.

SYNONYMS
Cardiogenic pulmonary edema
Acute cardiogenic pulmonary edema
ACPE

ICD-9CM CODES
428.1 Acute pulmonary edema with heart disease

EPIDEMIOLOGY & DEMOGRAPHICS
- Leading cause of hospitalization (6.5 million hospital days in the U.S. each year)
- In-hospital mortality rate is 10% to 20%, particularly when associated with acute MI.

PHYSICAL FINDINGS & CLINICAL PRESENTATION
- Dyspnea with rapid, shallow breathing
- Diaphoresis, perioral and peripheral cyanosis
- Pink, frothy sputum
- Moist, bilateral pulmonary rales
- Increased pulmonary second sound, S_3 gallop
- Hypertension (unless in cardiogenic shock and hypotensive)
- Tachycardia
- Bulging neck veins

ETIOLOGY
Increased pulmonary capillary pressure attributable to:
- Acute myocardial infarction
- Exacerbation of chronic congestive heart failure
- Valvular regurgitation (e.g., mitral regurgitation)
- Ventricular septal defect
- Severe myocardial ischemia
- Mitral stenosis
- Other: cardiac tamponade, endocarditis, myocarditis, arrhythmias, cardiomyopathy, hypertensive crisis

DIAGNOSIS
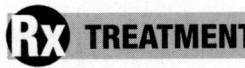

DIFFERENTIAL DIAGNOSIS
- Noncardiogenic pulmonary edema (see Fig. 1-689)
- Pulmonary embolism
- Exacerbation of asthma
- Exacerbation of chronic obstructive pulmonary disease
- Sarcoidosis
- Pulmonary fibrosis
- Lymphangitic carcinomatosis
- Pulmonary fibrosis
- Viral pneumonitis and other pulmonary infections

LABORATORY TESTS
- Arterial blood gases (ABGs): respiratory and metabolic acidosis, decreased Pao_2, increased $Paco_2$, low pH. (NOTE: The patient may initially show respiratory alkalosis as a result of hyperventilation in attempts to maintain Pao_2.)
- Measurement of plasma brain natriuretic peptide (elevated).
- Cardiac biomarkers: evaluate for possible acute myocardial infarction.
- Basic chemistries: hyponatremia is common in chronic heart failure; evaluate renal function.

IMAGING STUDIES
- ECG:
  1. May have evidence of ischemia, arrhythmias, or LV hypertrophy (often seen in diastolic dysfunction)
- Chest x-ray (Fig. 1-690):
  1. Pulmonary congestion with Kerley B lines; fluffy perihilar infiltrates in the early stages; bilateral interstitial alveolar infiltrates
  2. Pleural effusions
  3. Enlarged cardiac silhouette
- Echocardiogram:
  1. Useful to evaluate valvular abnormalities, diastolic versus systolic dysfunction
  2. Can help differentiate cardiogenic versus noncardiogenic pulmonary edema
  3. Can also estimate pulmonary capillary wedge pressure and rule out presence of myxoma or atrial thrombus
- Right heart catheterization (selected patients): increased pulmonary artery diastolic pressure and pulmonary capillary wedge pressure (PCWP) generally ≥ 25 mm Hg; low mixed venous oxyhemoglobin saturation

TREATMENT

ACUTE GENERAL Rx
All the following steps can be performed concomitantly:
- 100% oxygen by face mask. Noninvasive ventilation (continuous positive airway pressure [CPAP]) or bilevel noninvasive positive-pressure ventilation [NPPV]) reduces dyspnea and corrects metabolic abnormalities more rapidly than does standard oxygen therapy, and may reduce the need for endotracheal intubation. Both CPAP and bilevel NPPV systems can improve oxygenation and lower carbon dioxide tensions. Monitor ABGs; if marked hypoxemia or severe respiratory acidosis, intubate the patient and place on a mechanical ventilator. Positive pressure ventilation (invasive or noninvasive) decreases preload and afterload and reduces the work of breathing, while positive end expiratory pressure improves oxygenation.
- Pharmacologic preload reducers:
  1. Furosemide: 1 mg/kg IV bolus (typically 40 to 100 mg) to rapidly establish diuresis and decrease venous return through its venodilator action; may double the dose in 30 min if no effect.
  2. Nitrates: particularly useful if the patient has concomitant chest pain or is hypertensive.

Signs	Cardiac	Renal	Lung Injury
Heart size	Enlarged	Normal	Normal
Blood flow	Inverted	Balanced	Normal
Kerley lines	Common	Common	Absent
Edema	Basilar	Central: butterfly	Diffuse
Air bronchograms	Not common	Not common	Very common
Pleural effusions	Very common	Common	Not common

FIGURE 1-689 Types of pulmonary edema. (From Weissleder R et al: *Primer of diagnostic imaging*, St Louis, 2007, Mosby.)

a. Nitroglycerin: 150 to 600 mcg SL or nitroglycerin spray may be given immediately on arrival and repeated multiple times if the patient remains symptomatic and blood pressure remains stable.

b. 2% nitroglycerin ointment: 1 to 3 inches out of the tube applied continuously; absorption may be erratic.

c. IV nitroglycerin: 100 mg in 500 ml of D_5W solution; start at 6 mcg/min (2 ml/hr).

3. Morphine: 2 to 4 mg IV, SC, or IM; may repeat q15min prn. It decreases venous return, anxiety, and systemic vascular resistance (naloxone should be available at bedside to reverse the effects of morphine if respiratory depression occurs). However, potential adverse effects of morphine administration may outweigh these physiologic benefits, and the role of morphine in treatment of ACPE has recently been questioned.

- Vasodilator therapy:
1. Angiotensin-converting enzyme (ACE) inhibitors: captopril 25 mg PO tablet can be used for SL administration (placing a drop or two of water on the tablet and placing it under the tongue helps dissolve it); on-

set of action is <10 min, peak effect can be reached in 30 min. ACE inhibitors can also be given IV (e.g., enalaprilat 1 mg IV given q2h prn).

2. Nitroprusside: useful for afterload reduction in hypertensive patients with decreased cardiac index (CI).

a. Increases the CI and decreases LV filling pressure.

b. Nitroprusside use in patients with acute myocardial infarction is controversial because it may increase ischemia by decreasing blood flow to the myocardium.

- Inotropes:
1. Dobutamine: parenteral inotropic agent of choice in severe cases of cardiogenic pulmonary edema. It can be administered at a dosage of 2.5 to 10 mcg/kg/min IV.

2. IV phosphodiesterase inhibitors (amrinone, milrinone) may be useful in refractory cases.

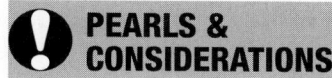

PEARLS & CONSIDERATIONS

COMMENTS

Accumulated evidence still favors the use of noninvasive ventilation, especially CPAP, in patients with ACPE, especially as this therapy reduces dyspnea and helps correct metabolic abnormalities more rapidly than standard oxygen therapy. The role of morphine in the treatment of ACPE has come into question.

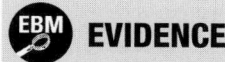

EVIDENCE

available at www.expertconsult.com

SUGGESTED READINGS

available at www.expertconsult.com

AUTHORS: **MATTHEW D. JANKOWICH, M.D.,** and **FRED F. FERRI, M.D.**

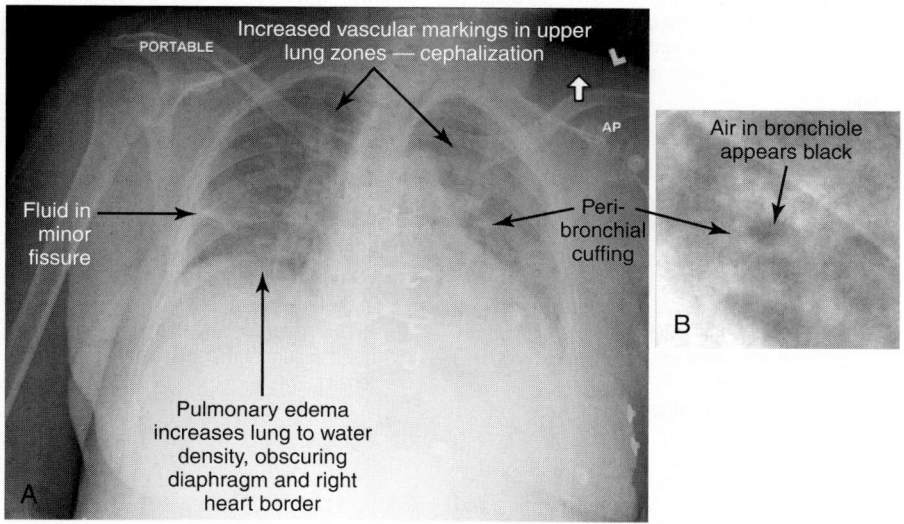

FIGURE 1-690 Pulmonary edema. A, Anterior-posterior chest x-ray. **B,** Close-up from **A.** This 53-year-old female with end-stage renal disease missed dialysis and presented to the emergency department. Her examination demonstrated bilateral rales. Her x-ray shows mild cardiomegaly, bilateral interstitial opacities, and cephalization of the pulmonary vascular markings. The minor fissure appears thickened. These findings are consistent with pulmonary edema. In addition, peribronchial cuffing is present. As discussed elsewhere, this is a nonspecific thickening of the bronchial wall that can occur from edema in the setting of heart failure, asthma, viral illness, or even infections such as pertussis. The thickened wall appears white, whereas the air-filled bronchiole appears black and has a circular short-axis cross section. (From Broder JS: *Diagnostic imaging for the emergency physician,* Philadelphia, 2011, Saunders.)

BASIC INFORMATION

DEFINITION

Pulmonary embolism (PE) refers to the lodging of a thrombus or other embolic material from a distant site in the pulmonary circulation.

SYNONYMS

Pulmonary thromboembolism
PE

ICD-9CM CODES

415.1 Pulmonary embolism and infarction

EPIDEMIOLOGY & DEMOGRAPHICS

- 650,000 cases of PE occur in the U.S. each year (increased incidence in women and with advanced age); annually, as many as 300,000 people in the U.S. die from acute PE, and the diagnosis is often not made until after autopsy. The incidence of PE is increasing with the increasing use of spiral CT scans, with a lower severity of illness and lower mortality, suggesting the increase is caused by earlier diagnosis.
- More than 90% of pulmonary emboli originate in the deep venous system of the lower extremities.
- Pulmonary thromboembolism is associated with >200,000 hospitalizations each yr in the U.S.
- 8% to 10% of victims of PE die within the first hr.

PHYSICAL FINDINGS & CLINICAL PRESENTATION

- Most common symptom: dyspnea (82% to 85%)
- Tachypnea (30% to 60%)
- Chest pain: may be nonpleuritic or pleuritic (infarction) (40% to 49%)
- Syncope (massive PE) (10% to 14%)
- Fever, diaphoresis, apprehension
- Hemoptysis (2%)
- Evidence of DVT may be present (e.g., swelling and tenderness of extremities)

- Cardiac examination may reveal: tachycardia (23%), increased pulmonic component of S2, murmur of tricuspid insufficiency, right ventricular heave, right-sided S3
- Pulmonary examination: may demonstrate rales, localized wheezing, friction rub

ETIOLOGY

- Thrombus, fat, or other foreign material
- Risk factors for PE:
  1. Prolonged immobilization, reduced mobility
  2. Postoperative state, major surgery
  3. Trauma to lower extremities, immobilizer, or cast
  4. Estrogen-containing birth control pills, hormone replacement therapy
  5. Prior history of DVT or PE
  6. CHF
  7. Pregnancy and early puerperium
  8. Visceral cancer (lung, pancreas, alimentary and genitourinary tracts)
  9. Spinal cord injury
  10. Advanced age
  11. Obesity
  12. Hematologic disease (e.g., factor V Leiden mutation, antithrombin III deficiency, protein C deficiency, protein S deficiency, lupus anticoagulant, polycythemia vera, dysfibrinogenemia, paroxysmal nocturnal hemoglobinuria, acquired protein C resistance without factor V Leiden, G20210A prothrombin mutation)
  13. COPD, diabetes mellitus, acute medical illness
  14. Prolonged air travel
  15. Central venous catheterization
  16. Autoimmune diseases (SLE, IBD, RA)

Dx DIAGNOSIS

DIFFERENTIAL DIAGNOSIS

- Myocardial infarction
- Pericarditis
- Pneumonia
- Pneumothorax
- Chest wall pain

- GI abnormalities (e.g., peptic ulcer, esophageal rupture, gastritis)
- CHF
- Pleuritis
- Anxiety disorder with hyperventilation
- Pericardial tamponade
- Dissection of aorta
- Asthma

WORKUP

- Clinical assessment alone is insufficient to diagnose or rule out PE. It is also important to remember that no single noninvasive test has both high sensitivity and high specificity for PE. Consequently, in addition to clinical assessment, most patients require an imaging test to diagnose PE. Figs. E1-691 and E1-692 are diagnostic algorithms for suspected PE. The Wells prediction rules can be used to estimate the probability of PE. Each of the following findings is assigned a score:
  1. Clinical signs/symptoms of deep vein thrombosis (score = 3.0)
  2. No alternate diagnosis as likely or more likely than PE (score = 3.0)
  3. Heart rate >100/min (score = 1.5)
  4. Immobilization or surgery in last 4 weeks (score = 1.5)
  5. Previous history of DVT or PE (score = 1.5)
  6. Hemoptysis (score = 1.0)
  7. Cancer actively treated within last 6 months (score = 1.0)
- The probability of PE is high if total score is >6, moderate if 2-6; and low if <2.
- A low clinical probability of PE in association with a normal plasma D-dimer measurement essentially rules out PE, and further imaging is not needed. If clinical probability is intermediate or high, and/or the D-dimer measurement is abnormal, further workup with imaging is needed.
- Spiral chest CT with contrast (see Fig. 1-693) is an excellent diagnostic modality.
- V/Q scan is reserved for patients with clinically significant contrast allergies or renal insufficiency.

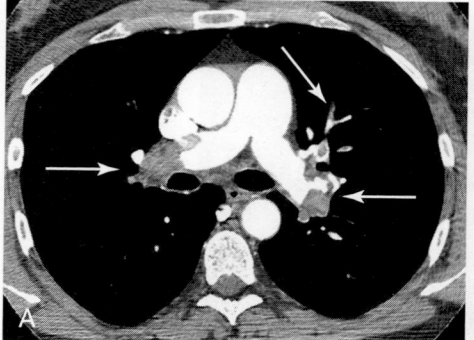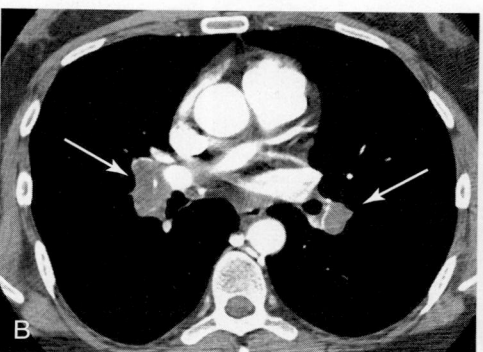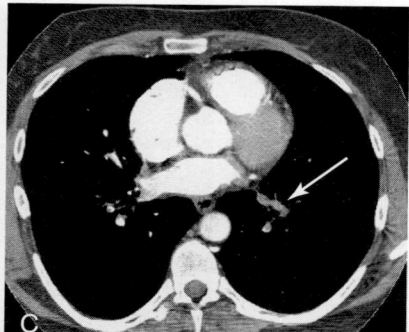

FIGURE 1-693 A 46-year-old woman presented with acute shortness of breath and hypoxia. Chest radiograph was normal. **A,** Chest computed tomography shows a low-attenuation filling defect in left and right main pulmonary arteries *(arrows)* and left upper lobe segmental artery *(arrow),* representing massive pulmonary embolism. Emboli extend to left and right interlobar arteries *(arrows),* as well as a left lower lobe segmental artery *(arrow),* seen in **B** and **C,** respectively. (From Vincent JL et al: *Textbook of critical care,* ed 6, Philadelphia, 2011, Saunders.)

- Pulmonary angiogram (when indicated) will confirm the diagnosis.
- Serial compressive duplex ultrasonography of lower extremities can be used in patients with "low-probability" lung scan and high clinical suspicion (see "Imaging Studies"). It is useful if positive; negative results do not exclude PE.

LABORATORY TESTS

- ABGs may reveal hypoxemia and respiratory alkalosis (decreased Pao_2 and $Paco_2$ and increased pH); normal results do not rule out PE.
- Alveolar-arteriolar (A-a) oxygen gradient, a measure of the difference in oxygen concentration between alveoli and arterial blood, may be elevated. However, a normal A-a gradient does not rule out PE.
- Plasma D-dimer measurement: D-dimer assays by ELISA detect the presence of plasmin-mediated degradation products of fibrin that contain cross-linked D fragments in the whole blood or plasma. A normal plasma D-dimer level is useful to exclude PE in patients with a low pretest probability of PE. However, it cannot be used to "rule in" the diagnosis because it increases with many other disorders (e.g., metastatic cancer, trauma, sepsis, postoperative state). Plasma D-dimer can also be used in conjunction with lower-extremity compression ultrasonography in patients with indeterminate V/Q and spiral CT scans. Absence of DVT and presence of a normal D-dimer level in these settings generally rules out clinically significant PE.
- Elevated cardiac troponin levels also occur in patients with PE because of right ventricular dilation and myocardial injury; therefore, PE should be considered in the differential diagnosis of all patients presenting with chest pain or dyspnea and elevated cardiac troponin levels.
- Elevated serum BNP levels in patients with acute PE may reflect RV overload.
- ECG is abnormal in 85% of patients with acute PE. Frequent abnormalities are sinus tachycardia; nonspecific ST-segment or T-wave changes; S-1, Q-3, T-3 pattern (10% of patients); S-1, S-2, S-3 pattern; T-wave inversion in V_1 to V_6; acute RBBB; new-onset atrial fibrillation; ST segment depression in lead II; right ventricular strain. A right ventricular strain pattern on ECG in patients with PE and normal blood pressure is associated with adverse short-term outcome and adds incremental prognostic value to echocardiographic evidence of right ventricular function.

IMAGING STUDIES

- Chest x-ray may be normal; suggestive findings include elevated diaphragm, pleural effusion, dilation of pulmonary artery, infiltrate or consolidation, abrupt vessel cut-off, oligemia distal to the PE (**Westermark sign**), or atelectasis. A wedge-shaped consolidation in the middle and lower lobes is suggestive of a pulmonary infarction and is known as "**Hampton's hump.**"
- CT angiography is an accurate, noninvasive tool in the diagnosis of PE at the main, lobar, and segmental pulmonary artery levels. A major advantage of CT angiography over standard pulmonary angiography is its ability to diagnose intrathoracic disease other than PE that may account for the patient's clinical picture. It is also less invasive, less costly, and more widely available. Its major shortcoming is its poor sensitivity for subsegmental emboli.
- Lung scan (in patient with normal chest x-ray examination):
  1. A normal lung scan rules out PE.
  2. A ventilation-perfusion mismatch is suggestive of PE, and a lung scan interpretation of high probability is confirmatory (Fig. 1-694).
  3. If the clinical suspicion of PE is high and the lung scan is interpreted as low probability, moderate probability, or indeterminate, a pulmonary arteriogram is diagnostic; a positive arteriogram confirms diagnosis; a positive compressive duplex ultrasonography for DVT obviates the need for an arteriogram, because treatment with IV anticoagulants is indicated in these patients; the overall sensitivity of compressive ultrasonography for DVT in patients with PE is 29%, specificity 97%; adding ultrasonography in patients with a nondiagnostic lung scan prevents 9% of angiographies; however, this improvement in efficacy is achieved at the cost of unnecessary anticoagulant therapy in 26% of patients who have false-positive ultrasonography results.
- Angiography: pulmonary angiography is the historic gold standard; however, it is invasive, expensive, and not readily available in some clinical settings. False-positive pulmonary angiograms may result from mediastinal disorders such as radiation fibrosis and tumors.
- Gadolinium-enhanced magnetic resonance angiography (MRA) of the pulmonary arteries has a moderate sensitivity and high specificity for the diagnosis of PE at experienced centers, but obtaining acceptable images is technically challenging and should only be performed if other imaging tests are contraindicated.
- Echocardiography: useful for identifying patients with PE who may have poor prognosis. Moderate or severe hypokinesis, persistent pulmonary hypertension, patent foramen ovale, and free-floating right heart thrombus are markers for increased risk of death or

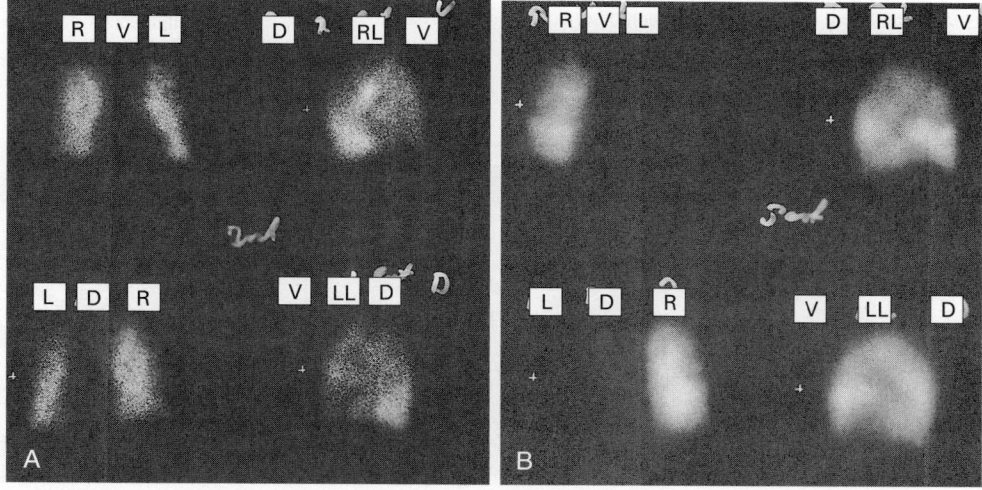

FIGURE 1-694 Ventilation-perfusion lung scan in massive pulmonary embolism. A, A normal pattern on the ventilation scan. **B,** The complete disappearance of the entire left lung from the perfusion scan indicates proximal occlusion of the left pulmonary artery. *D,* Dorsal; *L,* left; *LL,* left lobe; *R,* right; *RL,* right lobe; *V,* ventral. (From Crawford MH et al [eds]: *Cardiology,* ed 2, St Louis, 2004, Mosby.)

recurrent thrombosis. Such patients should be considered for thrombolysis or embolectomy.

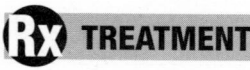

TREATMENT

NONPHARMACOLOGIC THERAPY

Correction of risk factors (see "Etiology") to prevent future PE

ACUTE GENERAL Rx

- Anticoagulant drugs for initial treatment of PE are described in Table E1-347. Unfractionated heparin (UFH) (IV or subcutaneous), subcutaneous low-molecular-weight heparin (LMWH), or subcutaneous fondaparinux is recommended for the initial treatment for at least 5 days. If IV unfractionated heparin is used, a bolus dose (80 U/kg) followed by a weight-based (18 U/kg/hr) continuous infusion to achieve therapeutic anti-factor Xa (or aPTT) levels should be used. LMWH and fondaparinux should be avoided in patients with severe renal failure.
- Oral rivaroxaban, a factor Xa inhibitor (15 mg bid for 3 wk, then 20 mg/d), has been studied as a treatment for DVT and for PE, without prior parenteral therapy. For both DVT and PE, treatment with rivaroxaban alone was noninferior to treatment with LMWH followed by a vitamin K antagonist with regard to the endpoint of recurrent venous thromboembolism. Use of rivaroxaban should be avoided in patients with severe renal failure.
- Thrombolytic agents (urokinase, tPA, streptokinase): provide rapid resolution of clots; thrombolytic agent are the treatment of choice in patients with massive PE who are hemodynamically unstable and with no contraindication to their use. The use of thrombolytic agent in the treatment of hemodynamically stable patients with acute submassive PE remains controversial. Use of the thrombolytic agents alteplase (100 mg IV over 2-hr period) in normotensive patients with moderate or severe right ventricular dysfunction identified by ECG has been advocated by some physicians. Use of alteplase in conjunction with heparin has been shown to improve the clinical course of stable patients who have acute submassive PE without internal bleeding, mainly by reducing need for subsequent thrombolytic use. Additional studies are needed to confirm these findings before recommending routine use of this therapeutic approach.

- Long-term treatment for PE not associated with malignancy can be carried out with warfarin therapy or rivaroxaban.
- For PE associated with malignancy, LMWH is recommended for long-term therapy.
- For PE occurring in the setting of a reversible risk factor, anticoagulation should be continued for 3 mo. For patients with an unprovoked PE, longer term anticoagulation should be considered, and indefinite long-term anticoagulation should be used in patients with recurrent unprovoked PE. Important factors to consider in the decision to extend anticoagulation include the patient's risk of bleeding and patient preferences after an informed discussion of risks and benefits.
- If thrombolytics and anticoagulants are contraindicated (e.g., GI bleeding, recent CNS surgery, recent trauma) or if the patient continues to have recurrent PE despite anticoagulation therapy, vena caval interruption is indicated by transvenous placement of an inferior vena caval filter.
- IVC filters are also strongly associated with reduced in-hospital fatality rate in stable patients who received thrombolytic therapy. It seems prudent to consider a vena cava filter in patients with PE who are receiving thrombolytic therapy.
- Acute pulmonary artery surgical embolectomy or catheter-based thrombectomy may be indicated in a patient with massive PE who cannot receive thrombolytic therapy. Pulmonary embolectomy is also recommended for those whose critical status does not allow sufficient time for thrombolytic therapy to be effective and for those who remain unstable after receiving fibrinolysis.

CHRONIC Rx

- Elimination of risk factors (see "Etiology")
- Patients with unprovoked DVT/PE have a high rate of recurrent VTE. Longer durations of chronic anticoagulation after unprovoked DVT/PE result in lower rates of recurrent DVT/PE while anticoagulation is in use, but benefits are lost once anticoagulation is halted. The use of indefinite anticoagulation in selected individuals with apparently unprovoked DVT/PE must be weighed against ongoing bleeding risk and other factors.
- A recent study demonstrated that aspirin (100 mg daily) is superior to placebo in preventing recurrence of venous thromboembolism in patients with a first-ever unprovoked

venous thromboembolism (VTE) who had already completed 6 to 18 months of oral anticoagulation. This suggests that aspirin could be offered as an alternative to oral anticoagulants for prevention of recurrent VTE in patients who refuse to or cannot continue oral anticoagulant therapy but who have a high risk of recurrent VTE.

DISPOSITION

- Mortality can be reduced to <10% by rapid and effective treatment. Stratification of risk of death associated with PE and severity-adjusted treatment is described in Table E1-348.
- Mortality from recurrent pulmonary emboli is 8% with effective treatment and >30% in patients with untreated pulmonary emboli.

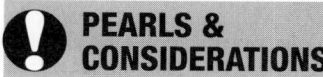

PEARLS & CONSIDERATIONS

COMMENTS

- Use of clinical prediction rules in association with D-dimer testing may reduce the use of unnecessary imaging in patients in whom PE is unlikely.
- Massive PE (PE associated with hypotension, shock, or circulatory arrest) remains the clearest situation in which thrombolytics should be employed. Submassive PE (PE associated with right ventricular dysfunction or injury but without hypotension) remains an area of controversy with regards to thrombolytic use.

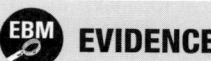

EVIDENCE

available at www.expertconsult.com

SUGGESTED READINGS

available at www.expertconsult.com

RELATED CONTENT

Pulmonary Embolism (PE) (Patient Information)
Deep Vein Thrombosis (Related Key Topic)
Hypercoagulable State (Related Key Topic)

AUTHORS: **MATTHEW D. JANKOWICH, M.D.,** and **FRED F. FERRI, M.D**

P

Diseases and Disorders

I

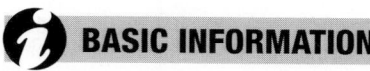

BASIC INFORMATION

DEFINITION

Pulmonary hypertension (PH) is defined as the presence of an abnormally elevated pulmonary arterial pressure. A mean pulmonary artery pressure (PAP) >25 mm Hg at rest is considered abnormal. Pulmonary arterial hypertension (PAH) is a syndrome with various causes and is defined as a mean PAP >25 mm Hg, with a pulmonary capillary wedge pressure, left atrial pressure, or left ventricular end diastolic pressure ≤5 mm Hg, and a pulmonary vascular resistance greater than 3 Wood units. Idiopathic pulmonary arterial hypertension (IPAH) is diagnosed when PAH is present without any apparent cause. Sustained elevation in PAP from increased pulmonary venous pressure, hypoxic pulmonary vasoconstriction, or increased flow is often referred to as *secondary pulmonary hypertension,* although the current classification system discourages use of this term in favor of grouping of PH by etiology.

SYNONYMS

Idiopathic pulmonary arterial hypertension (IPAH)
Secondary pulmonary hypertension

ICD-9CM CODES
416.0 Primary pulmonary hypertension
416.8 Secondary pulmonary hypertension

EPIDEMIOLOGY & DEMOGRAPHICS

- IPAH is rare, occurring in one to two cases per 1 million people per year, with an overall prevalence estimated at 1300 per 1 million.
- IPAH is more common in women than men (1.7:1), usually presenting in the third to fourth decades of life.
- Secondary PH is more common than IPAH.
- Secondary PH is the common pathophysiologic mechanism leading to cor pulmonale in patients with underlying pulmonary disease (e.g., chronic obstructive pulmonary disease [COPD], pulmonary embolism).

PHYSICAL FINDINGS & CLINICAL PRESENTATION

IPAH:
- Insidious, may go undetected for years
- Exertional dyspnea most common presenting symptom (60%)
- Fatigue and weakness
- Syncope, classically exertion-related or after a warm shower with peripheral vasodilation
- Chest pain
- Hoarse voice from compression of recurrent laryngeal nerve by an enlarged pulmonary artery (Ortner's syndrome)
- Loud P2 component of the second heart sound and paradoxical splitting of second heart sound
- Right-sided S4
- Jugular venous distention
- Abdominal distention and ascites
- Prominent parasternal (right ventricular [RV] impulse

- Holosystolic tricuspid regurgitation murmur heard best along the left fourth parasternal line that increases in intensity with inspiration
- Peripheral edema

SECONDARY PH: Similar to IPAH but from an underlying cause (e.g., left-sided congestive heart failure, mitral stenosis, COPD)

ETIOLOGY

- The etiology of IPAH is unknown. Most cases are sporadic, but there is a 6% to 12% familial incidence.
- PH is associated with several known risk factors: connective tissue disorders, portal hypertension and liver cirrhosis, appetite-suppressant drugs (fenfluramine), hemoglobinopathies, and infections including schistosomiasis and HIV disease. It is estimated that 10% of patients with hemoglobinopathies and 0.5% of patients with HIV infection develop moderate to severe PH. Schistosomiasis, sickle cell disease, and HIV disease may be the most common causes of PH worldwide, although pulmonary venous hypertension from left ventricular failure and PH related to COPD are more common causes of PH in developed nations.
- Several genetic abnormalities have been associated with the familial form of IPAH, many of which are mutations in the genes that code for members of the tumor growth factor-beta family of receptors (BMPR-II, ALK-1, endoglin) on chromosome 2q33.
- Familial PAH is an autosomal-dominant disease with variable penetrance, affecting only about 10% to 20% of carriers.
- Several factors play a role in the pathogenesis of PAH, including a genetic predisposition, endothelial cell dysfunction, abnormalities in vasomotor control, thrombotic obliteration of the vascular lumen, and vascular remodeling through cell proliferation and matrix production.
- SSRI use in late pregnancy is associated with increased persistent PH in newborns.
- The updated clinical classification of PAH is described in Table 1-349.

DIAGNOSIS

- PAH is a hemodynamic diagnosis involving the detection of elevated pressure in the pulmonary arteries and elevated pulmonary vascular resistance in the pulmonary vascular bed, occurring in the absence of significant pulmonary venous hypertension; characterization of this abnormality determines its etiology.
- Right-sided heart catheterization must be performed in all patients suspected of having PAH to establish the diagnosis and to assess pulmonary hemodynamics and acute vasoreactivity response testing.
- IPAH is a diagnosis of exclusion.

DIFFERENTIAL DIAGNOSIS

The differential diagnosis is as listed under "Etiology."

TABLE 1-349 Updated Clinical Classification of Pulmonary Hypertension

Group 1

Pulmonary arterial hypertension
Idiopathic pulmonary arterial hypertension
Heritable
  BMPR2
  ALK1, endoglin (with or without hereditary hemorrhagic telangiectasia)
  Unknown
Drug- and toxin-induced
Associated with:
  Connective tissue diseases
  HIV infection
  Portal hypertension
  Congenital heart diseases
  Schistosomiasis
  Chronic hemolytic anemia
Persistent pulmonary hypertension of the newborn
Pulmonary veno-occlusive disease with left to right shunts and/or pulmonary capillary hemangiomatosis

Group 2

Pulmonary hypertension owing to left heart disease
Systolic dysfunction
Diastolic dysfunction
Valvular disease

Group 3

Pulmonary hypertension owing to lung diseases and/or hypoxia
Chronic obstructive pulmonary disease
Interstitial lung disease
Other pulmonary diseases with mixed restrictive and obstructive pattern
Sleep-disordered breathing
Alveolar hypoventilation disorders
Chronic exposure to high altitude
Developmental abnormalities

Group 4

Chronic thromboembolic pulmonary hypertension

Group 5

Pulmonary hypertension with unclear multifactorial mechanisms
Hematologic disorders: myeloproliferative disorders, splenectomy
Systemic disorders: sarcoidosis, pulmonary Langerhans cell histiocytosis: lymphangioleiomyomatosis, neurofibromatosis, vasculitis
Metabolic disorders: glycogen storage disease, Gaucher's disease, thyroid disorders
Others: tumoral obstruction, fibrosing mediastinitis, chronic renal failure on dialysis

ALK1, Activin receptor-like kinase type 1; *BMPR2,* bone morphogenetic protein receptor type 2; *HIV,* human immunodeficiency virus.
From Simonneau G et al: Updated clinical classification of pulmonary hypertension, *J Am Coll Cardiol* 54:S43-S54, 2009.

EVALUATION

- Consists of establishing the diagnosis and etiology.
- Echocardiography with Doppler technique can provide a noninvasive but limited estimation of systolic PAP. Common findings include tricuspid regurgitation, right heart enlargement, abnormal movement of septum and, rarely, pericardial effusion. However, the diagnosis of PH cannot be established by echocardiography alone, as echocardiography can overestimate or underestimate PAP.
- ECG shows RV enlargement, strain pattern, and right axis deviation.
- Chest radiograph (Fig. 1-695) shows enlarged central pulmonary arteries and right heart enlargement. Chest radiography is abnormal in 90% of patients at diagnosis.
- A normal chest radiograph does not rule out the diagnosis. High-resolution computed tomography (CT) (Fig. 1-696) can assist in the evaluation for emphysema or interstitial lung disease. Ventilation-perfusion lung scan has high sensitivity for chronic thromboembolic disease. The diagnosis should be confirmed by pulmonary angiography, which has high specificity.
- Pulmonary function tests may show obstructive (airway disease) and/or restrictive disease (parenchymal disease) depending on etiology. Diffusion capacity of carbon monoxide in the lung is reduced due to pulmonary vascular destruction in PAH.
- Right heart catheterization is required to assess pulmonary hemodynamics, exclude shunts and left heart disease, and perform acute vasoreactivity response testing.
- Screening for the presence of PAH with Doppler echocardiography is warranted in individuals with a known predisposing genetic mutation or first-degree relative with IPAH, connective tissue diseases (especially scleroderma), congenital heart disease with left-to-right shunt, or portal hypertension undergoing evaluation for orthotopic liver transplantation.

- Determining the degree of functional impairment, as assessed by the WHO functional classification system (Classes I-IV) and the 6-min walk test (6MWT), is a useful way to monitor disease progression and assess response to treatment.

LABORATORY TESTS

- Complete blood count is usually normal in PAH but may show secondary polycythemia.
- Arterial blood gases show low PO_2 and oxygen saturation.
- Overnight oximetry and/or sleep study to rule out sleep apnea or hypopnea.
- Other blood tests: antinuclear antibody (ANA), antineutrophil cytoplasmic antibodies (ANCA), anti-Scl-70, anticentromere, ribonucleoprotein antibody levels, and rheumatoid factor (RF) to screen for underlying connective tissue disease, HIV serology, liver function tests, and antiphospholipid antibodies.
- Brain natriuretic peptide (BNP) level can provide prognostic information, with elevation in BNP level being associated with increased mortality.
- Ventilation-perfusion lung scan has high sensitivity for chronic thromboembolic PAH. The diagnosis should be confirmed by pulmonary angiography, which has high specificity.

(Rx) TREATMENT

- Most of the evidence in management of PAH is limited to IPAH. There is some evidence in treatment of PAH associated with connective tissue disease, especially scleroderma, and congenital heart disease. The recommendations for treating PAH associated with other causes are limited to case studies and expert opinions.
- There is some evidence for the use of advanced therapies for sarcoidosis-associated PH. The heterogeneity of sarcoid-associated PH complicates the interpretation.

NONPHARMACOLOGIC THERAPY

- Oxygen therapy to improve alveolar oxygen flow in both idiopathic and secondary PH. Goal oxygen saturation >90%
- Avoidance of vigorous exercise and pregnancy

GENERAL TREATMENT:

1. Diuretics (e.g., furosemide 40 to 80 mg qd) improve dyspnea by reducing preload and peripheral edema.
2. Digoxin 0.25 mg qd has been used in patients with IPAH with inconclusive benefits.
3. Oral anticoagulation with warfarin B for IPAH, C for other PAH. Recommended INR is 1.5 to 2.5.

CHRONIC Rx

- Acute vasoreactivity response testing should be done in all patients at the time of right heart catheterization. Epoprostenol, adenosine, or nitric oxide is generally used to assess the response. A positive response is a fall in mean PAP of >10 mm Hg to a value of <40 mm Hg, with increased or unchanged

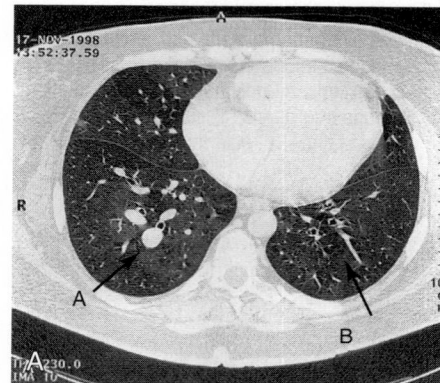

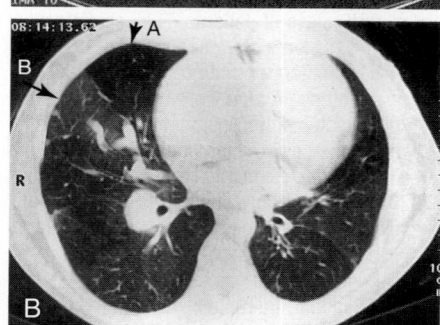

FIGURE 1-696 Chest computed tomographic scans in a patient with chronic thromboembolic pulmonary hypertension. A, Helical scan with contrast medium enhancement of the pulmonary vasculature shows a marked disparity in vessel size between the involved vessels *(A),* which are enlarged from thrombus, and the uninvolved vessels *(B).* **B,** Non-contrast-enhanced high-resolution scan illustrates a marked mosaic pattern manifest by differences in density of regions of the lung parenchyma reflecting the perfused areas *(B)* and the nonperfused areas *(A),* also consistent with underlying thromboembolic disease. (From Zipes DP et al [eds]: *Braunwald's heart disease,* ed 7, Philadelphia, 2005, Saunders.)

FIGURE 1-695 Progressive pulmonary arterial hypertension. This patient initially presented with a relatively normal chest radiograph **(A).** However, several years later **(B)** there is increasing heart size and marked dilation of the main pulmonary artery *(MPA)* and right pulmonary artery *(RPA).* Rapid tapering of the arteries as they proceed peripherally is suggestive of pulmonary hypertension and is sometimes referred to as pruning. (From Mettler FA [ed]: *Primary care radiology,* Philadelphia, 2000, Saunders.)

cardiac output. Fewer than 10% of patients are responders.

- The positive responders may benefit from treatment with calcium channel blockers (diltiazem, amlodipine, or nifedipine). Verapamil is not recommended because of its negative inotropic effects. All patients should be reassessed in 6 to 8 wk to demonstrate sustained benefit from the calcium channel blocker.
- Nonresponders or nonsustained responders are eligible for selective pulmonary vasodilators.
- Prostanoids (epoprostenol, treprostinil, iloprost, and beraprost) act as potent vasodilators of pulmonary arteries and inhibitors of platelet aggregation. Ideal for class IV patients.
  1. Epoprostenol: IV formulation with very short half-life. Requires long-term IV access with associated risks of infection and thrombosis. Rapid tachyphylaxis, and therefore dose escalation, is seen. Common side effects include jaw pain, abdominal cramping, and diarrhea. Limited evidence exists for use in secondary PAH patients.
  2. Treprostinil: IV and SQ formulation with longer half-life. Main disadvantage is pain at SQ pump site (no long-term evidence for IV formulation). Treprostinil is also available as a nebulized inhaled solution.
  3. Iloprost: aerosolized formulation with short half-life requiring 6 to 8 treatments/day.
  4. Beraprost: PO formulation. Not approved in U.S.
- Endothelin receptor antagonists:
  1. Bosentan (nonselective endothelin A and B receptor blocker): oral pulmonary vasodilator, requires monthly liver function tests, often response delay by weeks. Thus, it is not an ideal starting therapy for WHO class IV patients. They are effective in class II and III patients.
  2. Sitaxsentan and ambrisentan (selective endothelin A receptor blockers).
- Phosphodiesterase inhibitors (sildenafil and tadalafil): act by increasing concentration of nitric oxide. Sildenafil is administered as 20 mg PO tid up to 80 mg PO tid. Tadalafil dose is 40 mg once daily. Highly effective in WHO class II patients, both in IPAH and scleroderma-associated PAH.
- Combination therapies: considered when there is no improvement or deterioration on monotherapy.
- Bosentan + inhaled iloprost (STEP trial) showed some benefit over monotherapy.
- IV epoprostenol + oral bosentan (BREATH-2 trial) did not show much difference.
- IV epoprostenol + oral sildenafil (PACES trial) showed benefit over monotherapy.
- Lung transplantation and heart-lung transplantation are other options in patients with end-stage class IV disease. Atrial septostomy may be performed as a bridge to transplant.

The defect can be closed at the time of transplantation.

- Atrial septostomy is recommended for individuals with a room air SaO_2 >90% who have severe right-sided heart failure (with refractory ascites) despite maximal diuretic therapy, or who have signs of impaired systemic blood flow (such as syncope) from reduced left heart filling.
- Lung transplant recipients with IPAH had survival rates of 73% at 1 yr, 55% at 3 yr, and 45% at 5 yr.

TREATMENT OF SECONDARY PAH:
- Directed toward cause. Some situations merit mention.
- PAH with uncorrected congenital heart disease: Eisenmenger's syndrome. Medical treatment generally ineffective. Heart-lung transplantation required in most patients. PH may persist after surgical correction of congenital heart disease, and pulmonary vasodilators can be effective therapies in this patient population.
- PAH with scleroderma: selective pulmonary vasodilators are effective.
- PAH with lung disease or hypoxia: oxygen therapy, for hypoxemia, CPAP (for OSA), control of primary disease process.
- PAH with chronic thromboembolic disease: may consider pulmonary vasodilators after anticoagulation and pulmonary thromboendarterectomy (or if thromboendarterectomy is not an option) if continued symptoms and elevation in PVR and transpulmonary gradient.
- PAH with HIV: control of viral load by antiretroviral therapy.

FOLLOW-UP
Regular follow-up at 3-mo intervals with clinical assessment: WHO class and 6MWT, 6- to 12-mo objective assessment of RV function by ECG and cardiac catheterization studies.

DISPOSITION
- The 6MWT is predictive of survival in patients with idiopathic PAH. A baseline 6MWT less than 250 m is associated with a 50% risk of death at 2 yr. Drop in O_2 saturation >10% during the test increases mortality risk 2.9 times over a median follow-up of 26 mo.
- A BNP level ≥350 pg/ml at baseline evaluation is associated with a 25% risk of death at 2 yr.
- WHO class II and III patients with PAH have a mean survival of 3.5 yr.
- WHO class IV patients have a mean survival of 6 mo.

REFERRAL
If the diagnosis of IPAH is suspected, a consultation with a pulmonary specialist is recommended. Secondary causes of PH may require disease-specific consultations.

PEARLS & CONSIDERATIONS
- The exertional dyspnea of PAH is typically described by patients as being relentlessly progressive over several months to a year, often out of proportion to, or in the absence of, underlying heart or lung disease.
- Over 20% of patients in the Registry to Evaluate Early and Long-term PAH Disease Management had symptoms for more than 2 years before PAH was recognized. Consideration of the diagnosis of PAH in the differential diagnosis of unexplained dyspnea, especially in younger individuals, is essential.
- Chest x-ray may reveal evidence of interstitial fluid or fibrosis within the lungs in cases of secondary PH. IPAH is not associated with infiltrates on chest radiograph.

COMMENTS
- RV systolic pressure (RVSP) as estimated by echocardiography is not a good indicator of the presence of PAH because RVSP increases with age and body mass index. Athletically conditioned men also have a higher resting RVSP. Thus, these measurements can be misleading.
- Abrupt development of pulmonary edema during acute vasodilator testing suggests pulmonary veno-occlusive disease or pulmonary capillary hemangiomatosis and is a contraindication to long-term vasodilator treatment.
- In advanced PAH, heart rate increase is the main compensatory mechanism and reflects increased sympathetic tone. A higher heart rate at rest is an important marker of prognosis and should be assessed at frequent intervals after initiation of treatment for PAH.

FUTURE TREATMENTS
- Serotonin receptor modulators, platelet-derived growth factor and Rho kinase inhibitors
- Potential of cardiac MRI in assessment of RV function

SUGGESTED READINGS
available at www.expertconsult.com

RELATED CONTENT
Pulmonary Hypertension (Patient Information)

AUTHORS: **MATTHEW D. JANKOWICH, M.D.,**
DOUGLAS W. MARTIN, M.D., and
GAURAV CHOUDHARY, M.D.

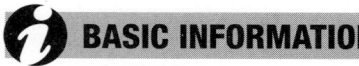

BASIC INFORMATION

DEFINITION

Pulseless electrical activity (PEA) is defined as the presence of organized electrical activity without sufficient mechanical contraction of the heart to produce a palpable pulse or measurable blood pressure.

SYNONYMS

Electromechanical dissociation (EMD)

ICD-9CM CODES
427.5 Cardiac arrest

EPIDEMIOLOGY & DEMOGRAPHICS

- Accounts for about 35% of cardiac arrest cases
- Increasingly recognized as the cause of sudden cardiac death in patients with implantable cardioverter-defibrillators

PHYSICAL FINDINGS & CLINICAL PRESENTATION

PRIMARY PEA:
- Organized electrical activity (not VT/VF)
- No detectable pulse

SECONDARY PEA: As in primary PEA and may also have:
- Bradycardia: drug overdose
- Tachycardia: hypovolemia, massive PE
- Decreased jugular venous pressure (JVP): hypovolemia
- Elevated JVP and no pulse with CPR: cardiac tamponade, massive PE, tension pneumothorax
- Absent unilateral breath sounds and tracheal deviation: tension pneumothorax
- Cyanosis: hypoxia

ETIOLOGY

PRIMARY PEA: Myocardial electromechanical uncoupling secondary to advanced heart muscle disease
SECONDARY PEA: Because of changes in the loading conditions of the heart, ischemia, myocardial depressants
- Massive MI
- Massive PE
- Hypovolemia
- Cardiac tamponade
- Tension pneumothorax
- Hypoxia
- Hypothermia
- Acidosis
- Hyperkalemia/hypokalemia
- Drug overdose: β-blockers, calcium channel blockers, digoxin, tricyclic antidepressants, benzodiazepines, opioids

DIAGNOSIS

WORKUP

- Stabilizing patient and workup to establish etiology should proceed simultaneously
- History, physical examination, laboratory tests, imaging studies

LABORATORY TESTS

- CBC, potassium, CK-MB, troponin
- Arterial blood gas
- ECG (Fig. 1-697):
  Low voltage: tamponade
  Right heart strain: PE, pneumothorax
  Arrhythmias: MI, metabolic abnormalities, drug effects
  ST changes, Q waves: MI

IMAGING STUDIES

- Chest radiograph: rule out pneumothorax
- Chest CT/pulmonary arteriogram: rule out PE
- Echocardiogram: rule out tamponade, ischemia (LV contractility, wall motion), valve dysfunction, tumors, and clots. May help diagnose aortic dissection and PE and assess intravascular volume status
- Abdominal radiograph: rule out ruptured abdominal aortic aneurysm

TREATMENT

Identifying and treating a reversible cause is critical.

Physiologic parameters can help monitor quality of CPR and detect the return of spontaneous circulation (ROSC). Suggested methods include quantitative waveform capnography (if intubated), arterial relaxation "diastolic" pressure (if arterial catheter in place), or central venous oxygen saturation (if central venous catheter in superior vena cava).

NONPHARMACOLOGIC THERAPY

- Activate emergency response service
- Begin CPR; minimize interruptions. Perform CPR for 2 min between pulse checks
- Attach cardiac monitor/defibrillator
- Obtain IV/intraosseous (IO) access
- Consider advanced airway placement
- Confirm absence of blood flow with Doppler ultrasound, arterial line, or bedside echocardiogram

ACUTE GENERAL Rx

- Treat specific cause if known
- Give 100% oxygen
- Epinephrine 1 mg IV push/IO, q3 to 5min; vasopressin 40 U IV/IO may be used to replace the first or second dose of epinephrine
- Give normal saline (20 ml) bolus after peripheral IV administration of medication to improve its distribution
- Medication can be given via endotracheal tube if IV/IO access cannot be obtained; IV/IO routes preferred because they provide more predictable drug delivery and pharmacologic effects. Give 2 to 2.5× the IV dose in 10 ml of sterile water.
- If rhythm changes to VF or pulseless VT
  - Defibrillate
  - For refractory VF or pulseless VT consider amiodarone
- If achieve ROSC, initiate post–cardiac arrest care

DISPOSITION

Of hospitalized patients who develop PEA, <15% survive to discharge. Survival rates much lower in patients with prehospital PEA. Survivors often have poor neurologic outcomes.

REFERRAL

As needed for underlying condition

PEARLS & CONSIDERATIONS

- 2010 American Heart Association guidelines for cardiopulmonary resuscitation and emergency cardiovascular care recommend the use of epinephrine in PEA resuscitation. New data suggest that epinephrine use may be associated with increased mortality.
- Termination of resuscitation guidelines exist for out-of-hospital cardiac arrest. Similar guidelines for in-hospital cardiac arrest are not available; termination of resuscitation is based on multiple patient factors.
- Therapeutic hypothermia (32° to 34° C for 12 to 24 hr) may improve neurologic outcomes and reduce mortality in comatose cardiac arrest survivors.
- Prognosis may be guided by median nerve somatosensory-evoked potentials (24 hr), EEG (24 hr), or corneal and pupillary reflexes (72 hr) after cardiac arrest. Prognostication is more difficult in patients treated with hypothermia; wait >72 hr before attempting to predict outcome.

SUGGESTED READINGS

available at www.expertconsult.com

AUTHOR: **SUDEEP KAUR AULAKH, M.D.**

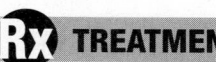

FIGURE 1-697 Sinus rhythm with pulseless electrical activity (PEA). Although the ECG showed sinus rhythm, the patient had no pulse or blood pressure. In this case the PEA was a result of depressed myocardial function after a cardiac arrest. (From Goldberg AL: *Clinical electrocardiography,* ed 5, St Louis, 1994, Mosby.)

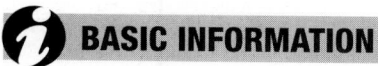

BASIC INFORMATION

DEFINITION

Pyelonephritis is an infection, usually bacterial in origin, of the upper urinary tract.

SYNONYMS

Acute pyelonephritis
Pyonephrosis
Renal carbuncle
Lobar nephronia
Acute bacterial nephritis

ICD-9CM CODES
590.81 Pyelonephritis
599.0 Urinary tract infection
595.9 Cystitis

EPIDEMIOLOGY & DEMOGRAPHICS

INCIDENCE (IN U.S.): Extremely common
PREDOMINANT SEX: Female
PREDOMINANT AGE:
- Sexually active years in women
- Usually age >50 yr in men

GENETICS: Congenital urologic structural disorders may predispose to infections at an early age.

PHYSICAL FINDINGS & CLINICAL PRESENTATION

- Fever, rigors, chills
- Flank pain
- Dysuria
- Polyuria
- Hematuria
- Toxic feeling and appearance
- Nausea and vomiting
- Headache
- Diarrhea
- Physical examination notable
  1. Costovertebral angle tenderness
  2. Exquisite flank pain

ETIOLOGY

- Gram-negative bacilli such as *Escherichia coli* and *Klebsiella* spp. in more than 95% of cases
- Other, more unusual gram-negative organisms, especially if instrumentation of the urinary system has occurred
- Resistant gram-negative organisms or even fungi in hospitalized patients with indwelling catheters
- Gram-positive organisms such as enterococci
- *Staphylococcus aureus:* presence in urine indicates hematogenous origin
- Viruses: rarely, but these are usually limited to the lower tract

DIAGNOSIS

DIFFERENTIAL DIAGNOSIS

- Nephrolithiasis
- Appendicitis
- Ovarian cyst torsion or rupture
- Acute glomerulonephritis
- Pelvic inflammatory disease

- Endometritis
- Other causes of acute abdomen
- Perinephric abscess
- Hydronephrosis

WORKUP

- No workup usually indicated in sexually active women
- Poorly responding infections, especially with azotemia and frank bacteremia
- Renal sonogram or CT scan (Fig. 1-699) to assess for underlying urologic pathology such as hydronephrosis

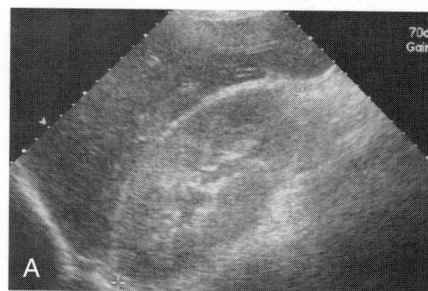
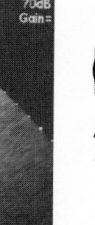
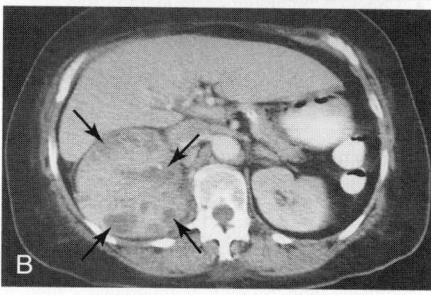

FIGURE 1-699 Acute pyelonephritis. A, Ultrasound image demonstrates an enlarged echogenic kidney. Bipolar length of kidney is 12.9 cm. **B,** CT scan with contrast enhancement obtained 24 hours later demonstrates multiple nonenhancing abscesses *(arrows)*. (From Floege J et al: *Comprehensive clinical nephrology,* ed 4, Philadelphia, 2010, Saunders.)

- Urologic imaging studies in all young men and boys
- Prostate assessment in older men

LABORATORY TESTS

- Complete blood count with differential
- Renal panel
- Blood cultures
- Gram stain of urine, urinalysis, and urine cultures
- Urgent renal sonography if obstruction or closed space infection suspected
- CT scans may better define the extent of collections of pus and can identify emphysematous pyelonephritis (Fig. 1-700)
- Helical CT scans excellent to detect calculi

TREATMENT

ACUTE GENERAL Rx

- Hospitalization for:
  1. Toxic patients
  2. Complicated infections
  3. Diabetes
  4. Suspected bacteremia
- Keep patients well hydrated.
- IV fluids are indicated for those unable to take adequate amounts of liquids.
- Give antipyretics such as acetaminophen when necessary.
- Antibiotic therapy should be initiated after cultures are obtained and guided by the results of culture and sensitivity testing.
  1. Oral quinolones such as ciprofloxacin (500 mg PO bid usually for 10 to 14 days) or Levaquin (500 or 750 mg for 10 to 14 days) are typically used for stable patients who can tolerate oral medications with sensitive pathogens. The optimum duration of therapy for acute pyelonephritis is unclear. Recent trials have shown that a short course (7 days) is not inferior to a 14-day course in women with uncomplicated pyelonephritis.

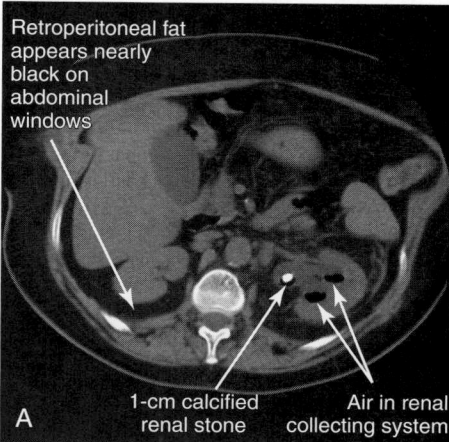
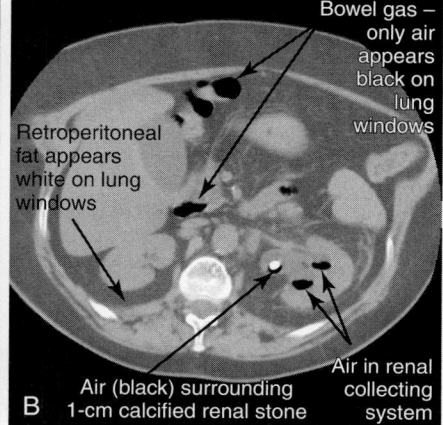

FIGURE 1-700 Emphysematous pyelonephritis noncontrast CT. A and B, Emphysematous pyelonephritis is a urologic emergency in which infection with gas-forming organisms affects the kidney. This patient has a large stone in the left renal pelvis. Notably, air is filling the renal collecting system. On typical soft-tissue windows, the black appearance of air may be difficult to distinguish from dark retroperitoneal and peritoneal fat. Lung windows make every tissue type except air white, leaving black air in stark relief. (From Broder JS: *Diagnostic imaging for the emergency physician,* Philadelphia, 2011, Saunders.)

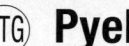

2. IV antibiotic options for more toxic patients pending cultures include ceftriaxone (1 to 2 g q day), IV cipro (400 mg q12h) or IV Levaquin (500 to 750 mg IV q day), piperacillin/tazobactam (3.375 g IV q6h) or carbapenems such as meropenem or imipenem (500 mg IV q6-8h)

3. Ceftazidime 1 to 2 g IV 8h, piperacillin/tazobactam, and carbapenems are best choices for *Pseudomonas*. There is increasing resistance of *Pseudomonas* to ciprofloxacin

4. Aminoglycosides such as gentamicin (2 mg/kg IV load followed by 1 mg/kg IV q8h adjusted for renal function) added, but nephrotoxicity possible, especially in diabetics with azotemia

5. Vancomycin 1 g IV q12h or linezolid to cover gram-positive cocci such as enterococci or staphylococci

6. Ampicillin 1 to 2 g IV q4 to 6h to cover enterococci with an aminoglycoside for synergy

- Prompt drainage with nephrostomy tube placement for obstruction.
- Surgical drainage of large collections of pus to control infection.
- Diabetic patients, as well as those with indwelling catheters, are especially prone to complicated infections and abscess formation.

CHRONIC Rx

- Repair underlying structural problems, especially when renal function is compromised.
  1. Reflux
  2. Obstruction
  3. Nephrolithiasis should be considered
- Patients with diabetes mellitus and indwelling urinary catheters are at particular risk of severe and complicated infections.
- When possible, remove catheters.

DISPOSITION

Most patients with uncomplicated pyelonephritis are now treated as outpatients or in short hospitalizations. Indications to admit a patient with pyelonephritis include pregnancy, suspected urinary obstruction, suspected renal abscess or perinephric abscess, bacterial sepsis, diabetes or other immunocompromised states, recurrent or refractory pyelonephritis, or infection with an unusual or antibiotic-resistant microorganism.

REFERRAL

- To a surgeon for correction of underlying urologic problems (e.g., reflux and hydronephrosis)
- To a pediatrician for detection of reflux to avoid recurrent urinary tract infection and loss of renal function
- To an internist for aggressive metabolic and urologic evaluation for patients with nephrolithiasis

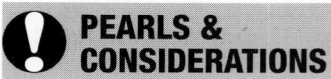

PEARLS & CONSIDERATIONS

Pyelonephritis is a systemic illness and may be a source of bacteremia and sepsis, especially if accompanied by urinary obstruction. Workup for abscess, obstruction, papillary necrosis, and other local complications of pyelonephritis should be initiated if the patient is septic, if patient does not respond to antibiotic therapy after 72 hr of treatment, or if infection is accompanied by worsening renal function.

SUGGESTED READINGS

available at www.expertconsult.com

RELATED CONTENT

Pyelonephritis (Patient Information)

AUTHOR: **GLENN G. FORT, M.D., M.P.H.**

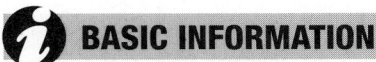

BASIC INFORMATION

DEFINITION

Pyogenic granuloma is a benign vascular lesion of the skin and mucous membranes. The lesions are caused by capillary proliferation, generally the result of trauma.

SYNONYMS

Granuloma pyogenicum
Tumor of pregnancy
Eruptive hemangioma
Lobular capillary hemangioma
Granulation tissue–type hemangioma

ICD-9CM CODES

686.1 Pyogenic granuloma

EPIDEMIOLOGY & DEMOGRAPHICS

- Common in children and young adults. Also found more frequently in pregnant women.
- Equally prevalent in males and females, with no racial or familial predisposition.
- Caused by trauma or surgery.
- Gingival lesions occur more frequently during pregnancy.

PHYSICAL FINDINGS & CLINICAL PRESENTATION

- Small (<1 cm), yellow to red, dome-shaped lesions
- May have surrounding scale at base (Fig. 1-702)
- Most commonly found on the head, neck, and extremities
- Often found on the gingiva during pregnancy (called *epulis*)
- Extremely friable, can easily ulcerate, and may bleed profusely with minor trauma

ETIOLOGY

Trauma causing focal capillary growth. These lesions are neither infectious in etiology nor granulomatous in histology.

DIAGNOSIS

DIFFERENTIAL DIAGNOSIS

- Amelanotic melanoma
- Bacillary angiomatosis
- Glomus tumor
- Hemangioma
- Irritated nevus
- Wart
- Kaposi's sarcoma

WORKUP

Diagnosis is based on clinical history and appearance. Generally begins with trauma followed by the development of an erythematous papule. The lesion tends to bleed easily and develops over several days to weeks.

LABORATORY TESTS

Pathologic examination should be performed after excision to rule out melanoma.

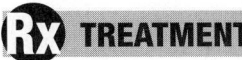

TREATMENT

ACUTE GENERAL Rx

- Excision: using 1% lidocaine for anesthesia, shave or curette at base and border. Follow with electrocauterization or cryotherapy.
- Pulsed-dye laser is also a safe and effective treatment modality.
- Pregnancy epulis generally resolves spontaneously after childbirth.

REFERRAL

Dermatology referral recommended if lesion recurs or multiple satellite lesions occur after excision

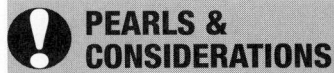

PEARLS & CONSIDERATIONS

COMMENTS

- Removal of entire lesion is essential because lesions may recur at the site of residual tissue.
- Patients and parents should be alerted to the possibility of recurrence after removal.
- Multiple satellite lesions occasionally develop near a primary pyogenic granuloma, usually after destruction of that lesion.

AUTHOR: **FRED F. FERRI, M.D.**

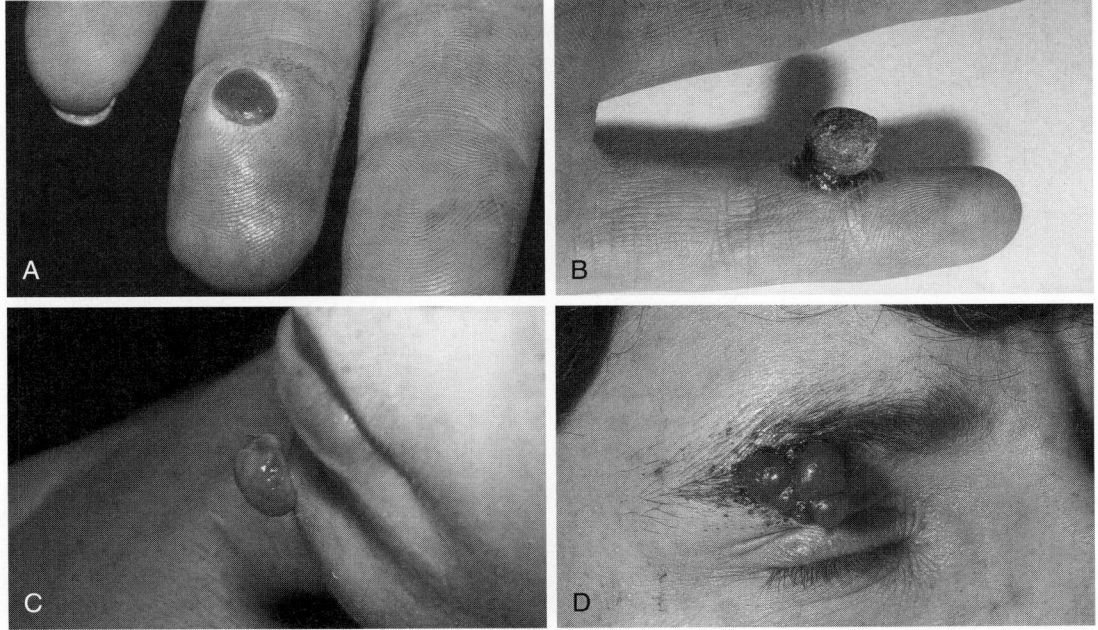

FIGURE 1-702 Pyogenic granuloma. A, This is the classic appearance of a red, friable nodule growing rapidly on the finger. There is often a portion that extends under the skin laterally. **B,** Pyogenic granuloma on the finger. This lesion is more dry and crusted. **C,** Pyogenic granuloma on the chin of an adult. The fingers, lip, palms, soles, and face are typical sites. **D,** Pyogenic granuloma of the eyebrow. (From White GM, Cox NH [eds]: *Diseases of the skin, a color atlas and text,* ed 2, St Louis, 2006, Mosby.)

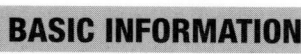

BASIC INFORMATION

DEFINITION

Radiation is the emission of energy as electromagnetic waves or moving subatomic particles. It can be natural or man-made. Natural radiation can come from a cosmic source, such as the sun, or a terrestrial source, such as naturally occurring radionuclides. Man-made radiation can come from nuclear reactors and x-ray machines. Radiation with the potential for human tissue injury is called ionizing radiation. Examples of ionizing radiation include x-rays, gamma rays, and photons.

UNITS OF RADIATION

- Roentgen (R): unit of exposure in air
- Radiation absorbed dose (rad): amount of radiation absorbed in a material; 100 rad =1 gray (Gy)
- Roentgen equivalent man (rem): amount of radiation biologic damage; 100 rem = 1 Sievert (Sv). It takes into account differential sensitivity among tissues (quality factor) (Table 1-354).

SYNONYMS

For large exposures (deterministic, or non-stochastic, effects of radiation):
  Acute radiation syndrome
  Radiation sickness
Chronic low-dose exposures produce stochastic effects. This has no common synonyms.

ICD-9CM CODES
990 Radiation exposure

EPIDEMIOLOGY & DEMOGRAPHICS

- High-dose radiation doses are limited to nuclear disasters.
- Epidemiology of cumulative low-level radiation is not well understood and is based on the following two theories:
  - Stochastic effects of radiation exposure: there is a probability of damage-increased effect with dose, but there is no dose threshold and severity is not dose related.
  - Deterministic effects: severity of damage is dose related but with a threshold below which there is no negative outcome.

PHYSICAL FINDINGS & CLINICAL PRESENTATION

- Low-level radiation: Low-level radiation over time may present clinically with various malignancies that may be at increased incidence compared with background rates of malignancies, but there remains much controversy.
- Acute radiation syndrome: Effects of acute radiation exposure are better studied based on previous nuclear disasters and are summarized in Table 1-355. Rapidly dividing cells such as hematopoietic cells are most prone to radiation. Radiation sickness symptoms are most apparent with doses >1 Gy.
  1. Stage 1 (prodromal phase): flulike syndrome with anorexia, apathy, nausea, vomiting, diarrhea, fever, tachycardia, and/or headache, usually occurring in the first 48 hours.
  2. Stage 2 (latent phase): a short period characterized by improvement in symptoms, lasting for several days to a month.
  3. Stage 3 (manifest illness phase): if the person survives this stage, recovery is likely.
     - Hematopoietic syndrome: effects can occur with exposure >1 Gy and include pancytopenia, increased infection risk, and bleeding disorders.
     - GI syndrome: radiation induces loss of intestinal crypts, resulting in abdominal pain, nausea, vomiting, anorexia, and diarrhea.
     - Central nervous system: symptoms occur with a very high level of acute radiation (>5 Gy) and include ataxia, confusion, and coma.
  4. Stage 4: recovery, lasting weeks to months. If patients survive, they will need lifelong follow-up because of the potential for unusual infections, organ dysfunction, and carcinogenesis.
     - Radiation "burn": Prolonged exposure from fluoroscopy can lead to acute radiodermatitis presenting as red patches but over a few weeks can lead to tissue necrosis.

TABLE 1-355 Dose Estimates for Common Life and Medical Activities

Activity	Dose Estimate
Natural background and man-made radiation (annual average dose equivalent, including radon)	360 mrem
Diagnostic chest x-ray	6-10 mrem
Flight from Los Angeles to Paris	800 mrem
Barium enema	5 mrem
Smoking 1.5 packs per day for 1 year	16,000 mrem = 16 rem
Heart catheterization	45,000 mrad = 45 rad = 0.45 Gy
Mild acute radiation syndrome	200 rad = 2 Gy
LD_{50} for acute whole body irradiation	450 rad = 4.5 Gy
Occupational limit for a radiation worker	5 rem = 0.05 Sv
Limit of a member of the public	0.1 rem = 0.001 Sv = 1 mSv

Gy, Gray; LD_{50}, median lethal dose; mrad, millirad; mrem, millirem; mSv, millisievert; rad, radiation absorbed dose; rem, roentgen equivalent man; Sv, sievert.
Modified from Goans RE: Medical management of radiation incidents. In Shannon MW et al (eds): *Haddad and Winchester's clinical management of poisoning and drug overdose*, ed 4, Philadelphia, 2007, Saunders.

TABLE 1-354 Symptoms, Therapy, and Prognosis of Whole Body Ionizing Radiation Injury

	0-1 SV	1-2 SV	2-6 SV	6-10 SV	10-20 SV	>50 SV
Therapeutic needs	None	Observation	Specific treatment	Possible treatment	Palliative	Palliative
Vomiting	None	5%-50%	>3 Gy, 100%	100%	100%	100%
Time to nausea, vomiting	—	3 hr	2 hr	1 hr	30 min	<30 min
Main locus of injury	None	Lymphocytes	Bone marrow	Bone marrow	Small bowel	Brain
Symptoms and signs	—	Moderate leukopenia, epilation	Leukopenia, hemorrhage, epilation	Leukopenia, hemorrhage, epilation	Diarrhea, fever, electrolyte imbalance	Ataxia, coma, convulsions
Critical period	—	—	4-6 wk	4-6 wk	5-14 days	1-4 hr
Therapy	Reassurance	Observation	Transfusion of granulocytes, platelets	Transfusion, antibiotics, bone marrow transplantation	Fluids and salts, possible bone marrow transplantation	Palliative
Prognosis	Excellent	Excellent	Guarded	Guarded	Poor	Hopeless
Lethality	0	0	0-80%	80%-100%	100%	100%
Time of death	—	—	2 mo	1-2 mo	2 wk	1-2 days
Cause of death	—	—	Infection, hemorrhage	Hemorrhage, infection, pneumonitis	Enteritis, infection	Cerebral edema

Modified from Phillips TL: Radiation injury. In Wyngaarden JB et al (eds): *Cecil textbook of medicine*, ed 24, Philadelphia, 2012, Saunders.

PROGNOSIS

ACUTE RADIATION SYNDROME

- Exposure <1 Gy: almost certain survival
- Exposure 1 to 2 Gy: 90% survival with medical care
- Exposure 2 to 3.5 Gy: probable survival with medical care
- Exposure 3.5 to 5.5 Gy: 50% survival with medical care
- Exposure 5.5 to 10 Gy: probable death
- Exposure >10 Gy: certain death

CHRONIC LOW-DOSE EXPOSURE: excess cancer not detected below 100 mSv

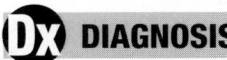
DIAGNOSIS

ACUTE RADIATION SYNDROME

- Diagnosis usually accompanies a nuclear disaster and therefore suspicion is already very high.
- Workup can include measuring radiation levels at site.
- Laboratory studies: in the acute setting, CBC, brain imaging

CHRONIC LOW-DOSE EXPOSURE: Currently impossible to determine whether a subsequently diagnosed malignancy is radiation induced. Workup is for underlying malignancy evaluation.

ETIOLOGY

ACUTE RADIATION SYNDROME: usually nuclear disaster

CHRONIC LOW-DOSE EXPOSURE: The average annual dose to residents of the U.S. is approximately 3.6 mSv.

- Cosmic: positive-charged ions that interact with atmosphere to create secondary radiation
- Terrestrial: radon, potassium-40, thorium, and uranium
- Man-made: medical radiation including x-rays, CT scans, PET scans, nuclear stress tests, nuclear weapon fallout, fluoroscopy, and smoking

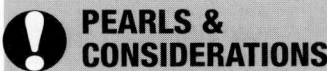
TREATMENT

- For all accidental radiation contamination, such as nuclear medicine materials, the following decontamination steps are considered mandatory:
  1. Perform at site of exposure unless there is continued radiation exposure.
  2. Remove all clothing (and treat as radioactive waste). Providers should use strict isolation precautions, including donning of gown, mask, cap, double gloves, and shoe covers, when evaluating and treating contaminated patients.
  3. Wash patient with mild soap (neutral pH) and tepid water. Dispose of contaminated water as radioactive waste.
  4. Scrub any open wound.
  5. Depending on the situation, the regional emergency response system should be called for additional measures such as evacuation.
- Management of acute radiation syndrome:
  1. Establish IV access.
  2. Monitor physiologic signs.
  3. Manage the airway.
  4. Manage burns.
  5. Identify and treat other injuries.
  6. Provide analgesia.
  7. Give antiemetics (e.g., ondansetron).
  8. Manage bleeding and transfuse if necessary.
  9. Diagnose and treat sepsis. Administration of antibiotics reduces the mortality rate. In nonneutropenic patients, use of antibiotics should be reserved for obvious foci of infection secondary to extensive burns, penetrating wounds, and/or abdominal/visceral trauma.
  10. Confirm initial dose estimate using chromosome aberration cytogenetic bioassay when possible.
  11. Consider colony-stimulating factors (CSFs). In any adult with whole-body or significant partial body exposure >3 Gy, treatment with CSFs should be rapidly initiated (e.g., G-CSF or filgrastim, 5 mcg/kg of body weight per day). CSFs may be withdrawn when the absolute neutrophil count reaches a level greater than 1.0×10^9 after recovery from the nadir.
  12. Consider stem cell transplantation in people with exposure dose of 7 to 10 Gy who do not have significant burns or other major organ toxicity and who have an appropriate donor.
  13. Provide counseling; 75% of individuals exposed to nuclear weapon denotations exhibit some form of psychological symptoms, ranging from insomnia to difficulty concentrating and social withdrawal.
- Chronic low-dose exposures: Treatment of radiation-induced organ damages would not differ significantly from non–radiation-induced cancers, cataracts, or skin lesions.

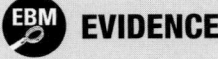
PEARLS & CONSIDERATIONS

COMMENTS

- It is difficult to make a link between exposure to chronic low-level radiation and a specific malignancy in an individual.
- Positioning patients for fluoroscopy procedures and monitoring amount of x-ray radiation are very important to prevent radiation burns.
- Humans are consistently exposed to background/naturally occurring radiation.
- Ionizing radiation from medical imaging procedures is not negligible. Since the early 1980s, the per capita dose of radiation from medical imaging has increased by a factor of nearly 6. Radiation exposure from imaging at current rates is predicted to be responsible for 2% of future cancers.

EVIDENCE

available at www.expertconsult.com

SUGGESTED READINGS

available at www.expertconsult.com

AUTHORS: **HARKAWAL S. HUNDAL, M.D., M.S., FRED F. FERRI, M.D.,** and **PRANAV M. PATEL, M.D., F.A.C.C., F.S.C.A.I.**

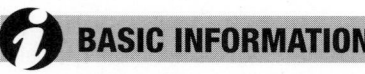

BASIC INFORMATION

DEFINITION

Ramsay Hunt syndrome is a localized herpes zoster infection involving the seventh nerve and geniculate ganglia, resulting in hearing loss, vertigo, and facial nerve palsy.

SYNONYMS

Herpes zoster oticus
Geniculate herpes
Herpetic geniculate ganglionitis

ICD-9CM CODES
053.11 Ramsay Hunt syndrome

EPIDEMIOLOGY & DEMOGRAPHICS

PREDOMINANT SEX: Equal sex distribution
PREDOMINANT AGE:
- Increasingly common with advancing age
- Rare in childhood

PHYSICAL FINDINGS & CLINICAL PRESENTATION

- Characteristic vesicles:
  1. On pinna
  2. In external auditory canal (Fig. 1-704)
  3. In distribution of the facial nerve and, occasionally, adjacent cranial nerves
- Facial paralysis on the involved side

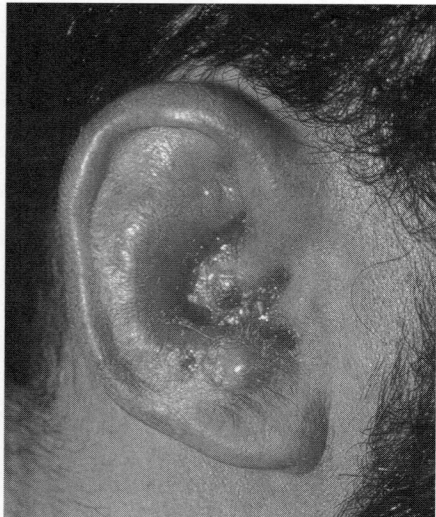

FIGURE 1-704. Herpes zoster of the geniculate ganglion resulting in vesicles on the ear (as shown here) and tympanic membrane occurs in Ramsay Hunt syndrome. Both seventh and eighth cranial nerve functions may be affected. (From White GM, Cox NH [eds]: *Diseases of the skin: color atlas and text,* ed 2, St Louis, 2006, Mosby.)

ETIOLOGY

Reactivation of dormant infection with varicella-zoster virus after primary varicella

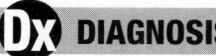

DIAGNOSIS

- Usually made by recognition of the clinical features detailed previously
- Viral culture and/or microscopic examination of specimens taken from active vesicles

DIFFERENTIAL DIAGNOSIS

- Herpes simplex
- External otitis
- Impetigo
- Enteroviral infection
- Bell's palsy of other etiologies
- Acoustic neuroma (before appearance of skin lesions)

The differential diagnosis of headache and facial pain is described in Section II.

WORKUP

If the diagnosis is in doubt, confirm varicella-zoster virus infection.

LABORATORY TESTS

- Generally not necessary
- Viral culture of specimens of vesicular fluid and scrapings of the vesicle base
- Tzanck preparation, which may reveal multi-nucleated giant cells
- Direct immunofluorescent staining of scrapings

IMAGING STUDIES

MRI may demonstrate enhancement of the facial and vestibulocochlear nerves before appearance of vesicles.

TREATMENT

ACUTE GENERAL Rx

- Prednisone (40 mg PO for 2 days, 30 mg for 7 days, followed by tapering course) is recommended by some authors.
- Acyclovir (800 mg PO five times qd for 10 days), famciclovir (500 mg tid for 7 days), or valacyclovir (1 g q8h for 7 days) may hasten healing.
- Analgesics should be used as indicated.

CHRONIC Rx

- Duloxetine and amitriptyline are effective in postherpetic pain.
- Other agents for postherpetic pain include gabapentin and pregabalin.
- Narcotic analgesics may occasionally be necessary.

DISPOSITION

Recurrences are unusual.

REFERRAL

To otolaryngologist: patients with persistent facial paralysis for potential surgical decompression of the facial nerve

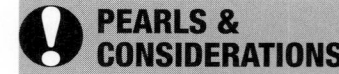

PEARLS & CONSIDERATIONS

COMMENTS

Immunodeficiency states, particularly HIV infection, should be considered in:
- Younger patients
- Severe cases
- Patients with a history of specific risk behavior

SUGGESTED READINGS
available at www.expertconsult.com

RELATED CONTENT

Ramsay Hunt Syndrome (Patient Information)

AUTHOR: **GLENN G. FORT, M.D., M.P.H.**

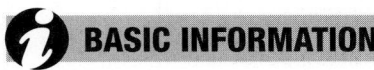

DEFINITION

Raynaud's phenomenon (RP) is a vasospastic disorder that causes an exaggerated response to cold temperatures and/or emotional stress, resulting in episodic digital ischemia. It presents as a cold-induced, symmetric, sharply demarcated white or blue discoloration of the distal fingers or toes, followed by erythema at a variable time after rewarming.

SYNONYMS

Primary Raynaud's phenomenon or Raynaud's disease
Secondary Raynaud's phenomenon

ICD-9CM CODES
443.0 Raynaud's syndrome, Raynaud's disease, Raynaud's phenomenon (secondary)
785.4 If gangrene present

EPIDEMIOLOGY & DEMOGRAPHICS

- RP is classified clinically into primary or secondary forms and affects approximately 3% to 5% of the general population, 15% of children younger than 12 yr, and less than 1% of adults older than 60 yr.
- Primary RP usually occurs between the ages of 12 and 25 yr. It is more likely to affect women than men (4:1) and appears to be more common in colder climates.
- 5% to 15% of patients with primary Raynaud's phenomenon develop a secondary cause later in the course of the disease (mostly a connective tissue disorder).
- Secondary RP tends to begin after age 35 to 40 yr.
- Secondary RP occurs in more than 90% of patients with scleroderma and in approximately 30% of patients with systemic lupus erythematosus or Sjögren's syndrome.
- There is also some suggestion that secondary RP may be associated with drugs (nicotine, caffeine, ergotamine, vinyl chloride) or trauma to the hands from vibrating tools such as jackhammers.

PHYSICAL FINDINGS & CLINICAL PRESENTATION

- The typical manifestation of RP is the biphasic color response of the digits to cold exposure and rewarming, which may or may not be accompanied by pain. RP most often affects the hand (Fig. 1-705).
  1. White (pallor) or blue (cyanotic) discoloration of the digit(s) resulting from vasospasm on cold or vibration exposure.
  2. Red (rubor) with or without pain and paresthesia when vasospasm resolves and blood returns to the digit.
- Color changes can sometimes be induced by placing the hand in an ice bath, although this is not recommended as a diagnostic maneuver because responses may be inconsistent even in patients with definite RP.

- Color changes are well delineated, symmetric, and usually bilateral, involving the fingers and toes. The index, middle, and ring fingers are commonly involved and the thumb infrequently; however, if the thumb is involved, that suggests secondary causes of RP.
- Fingertips are most often involved, but feet, ears, nose, tongue, and nipples can also be affected.
- Patients with RP may exhibit livedo reticularis during cold response, which is a violaceous or reticular pattern of skin of arms and legs, sometimes with regular, unbroken circles.
- Duration of attacks can range from seconds to hours and averages 15 to 20 min.
- Chronic skin changes resulting from repeated attacks may include skin thickening and brittle nails. Ulcerations and, rarely, gangrene may occur.
- Physical examination should also include examination for symptoms associated with autoimmune disease, such as fever, rash, arthritis, dry eyes, dry mouth, myalgias, or cardiopulmonary abnormalities.

ETIOLOGY

- Primary RP can also be called idiopathic Raynaud's phenomenon, primary Raynaud's syndrome, or Raynaud's disease. It occurs in the absence of any associated disease.
- With primary RP, the possibility that another first-degree family member is affected is reported as approximately 25%.
- Secondary RP is associated with an underlying pathologic condition or disorder, use of certain drugs, or related occupation. Secondary RP is associated with:
  1. CREST syndrome (calcinosis, RP, esophageal involvement, sclerodactyly, and telangiectasia)
  2. Scleroderma, Sjögren's syndrome
  3. Mixed connective tissue disease, polymyositis, and dermatomyositis
  4. Systemic lupus erythematosus, arteritis
  5. Rheumatoid arthritis
  6. Thromboangiitis obliterans (Buerger's disease)
  7. Drugs (beta-blockers, ergotamine, methysergide, vinblastine, bleomycin, oral contraceptives, nicotine, clonidine, cocaine, caffeine, vinyl chloride, tegafur, interferon alfa, interferon beta)
  8. Hematologic disorders (polycythemia, cryoglobulinemia, cold agglutinins, paraproteinemia, cryofibrinogenemia)
  9. Carpal tunnel syndrome
  10. Use of tools that vibrate
  11. Endocrine disorders (hypothyroidism, carcinoid syndrome, pheochromocytoma, metabolic syndrome)
  12. Estrogen replacement therapy without progesterone
  13. Hypercoagulable states, protein C, protein S, antithrombin III deficiency, factor V Leiden deficiency, and antiphospholipid syndrome
  14. Poliomyelitis is a rare cause
  15. Primary biliary cirrhosis
  16. Vasospastic disorders (migraines, Prinzmetal angina)
  17. Malignancies (angiocentric lymphoma, ovarian cancer)
  18. Primary pulmonary hypertension
  19. Peripheral emboli

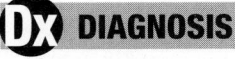 DIAGNOSIS

Clinical criteria:
- Definite RP: repeated episodes of biphasic color change on cold exposure
- Possible RP: Uniphasic color changes plus numbness or paresthesia on cold exposure
- No RP: No color change on cold exposure

The suggested criteria for primary RP are:
- Symmetric attacks
- Absence of tissue necrosis, ulceration, gangrene, or peripheral vascular disease
- Absence of a secondary cause on the basis of a patient's history and general physical examination
- Negative nail-fold capillary examination
- Negative test for antinuclear antibody (ANA)
- Normal erythrocyte sedimentation rate (ESR)

Secondary RP is suggested by the following findings:
- Onset of symptoms after age 30 yr
- Male gender
- Episodes that are painful, asymmetric, or associated with ischemic skin lesions
- Clinical features suggestive of a connective-tissue disease
- Elevated specific autoantibody tests and ESR
- Evidence of microvascular disease on microscopy of nail-fold capillaries

DIFFERENTIAL DIAGNOSIS

- Neurogenic thoracic outlet syndrome or carpal tunnel syndrome
- Frostbite or cold weather injury
- Medication reaction (ergotamine, chemotherapeutic agents)
- Atherosclerosis, thromboembolic disease
- Buerger's disease, embolic disease
- Acrocyanosis
- Livedo reticularis
- Injury from repetitive motion

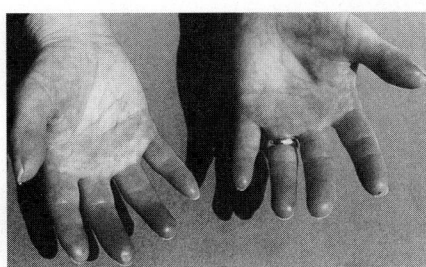

FIGURE 1-705 Raynaud's phenomenon. Sharply demarcated cyanosis of the fingers with proximal venular congestion (livedo reticularis) is seen. (From Klippel J et al [eds]: *Primary care rheumatology,* London, 1999, Mosby.)

WORKUP

- Once the diagnosis of RP is established, differentiating primary from secondary is helpful in treatment and prognosis.
- Patients who are younger when their symptoms occur, have a normal history and physical examination and normal nail-fold capillaries, and have no history of digital ischemic lesions can be considered as having primary RP. These patients can be monitored clinically without any further testing.
- If a secondary cause of RP is suspected, appropriate laboratory testing is recommended (see "Laboratory Tests"). Secondary RP has associated abnormal nail-fold microscopy.

LABORATORY TESTS

- CBC, serum electrolytes, blood urea nitrogen, creatinine, ESR, ANAs, VDRL antibody test, rheumatoid factor, and urinalysis should be included in the initial evaluation.
- If the history, physical examination, and initial laboratory tests suggest a possible secondary cause, specific serologic testing (e.g., anti-centromere antibodies, anti-Scl 70, cryoglobulins, complement testing, and serum protein electrophoresis) may be indicated.
- Noninvasive vascular testing includes finger systolic blood pressures, segmental blood pressure measurements, cold recovery time (measure vasoconstrictor and vasodilator responses of finger to cold), fingertip thermography, and laser Doppler with thermal challenge (measures relative change in skin blood flow with ambient warming).

IMAGING STUDIES

- The diagnosis of RP should not be made on the basis of laboratory tests, and imaging studies should not replace a good history and physical examination.
- Duplex ultrasound can image the palmar arch and digital arteries for patency.
- Magnetic resonance angiography is useful for imaging larger arteries.
- Contrast angiography is the gold standard for arterial imaging.
- Nail-fold capillary microscopy can differentiate primary from secondary RP.
- Videomicroscopy and thermography are also useful for diagnosis of RP.

Rx TREATMENT

NONPHARMACOLOGIC THERAPY

- Avoid drugs that may precipitate RP (see "Etiology").
- Avoid cold exposure and sudden temperature shifts. Use warm gloves, hats, and garments during the winter months or before going into cold environments (e.g., air-conditioned rooms).
- Avoid stressful situations, and use relaxation techniques in preventing RP attacks.

ACUTE GENERAL Rx

- Acute measures to terminate an attack include rotating the arms in a windmill pattern, placing the hands under warm water or in a warm body fold such as the axilla, and the swing-arm maneuver.
- Medications are indicated in the treatment of RP if there are signs of critical ischemia or if the quality of life of the patient is affected to the degree that activities of normal living are no longer possible and preventive techniques do not work.

CHRONIC Rx

- Dihydropyridine calcium channel blockers (e.g., nifedipine, amlodipine, felodipine, nisoldipine, isradipine) are the most effective pharmacologic treatment for RP and are the drugs of choice. Verapamil is ineffective for patients with severe RP.
- Nifedipine is most often prescribed at a dose of 10 to 20 mg 30 min before cold exposure. If symptoms occur with long duration, nifedipine XL 30 to 180 mg PO qd is often effective. Nifedipine also decreases skin temperature recovery time after cold-induced vasospasm.
- Patients who do not tolerate or do not respond to calcium channel blocker therapy can sometimes benefit from other drugs that directly or indirectly cause vasodilation, either alone or in combination, although data for these therapies are less robust. Some potential therapeutic options include direct vasodilators such as nitroprusside, hydralazine, papaverine, minoxidil, niacin, and griseofulvin. Topical 1% nitroglycerin or topical L-arginine, ethyl nicotinate, hexyl nicotinate, thurfyl salicylate may also be useful, particularly if low blood pressure is a concern.
- Phosphodiesterase inhibitors (cilostazol, pentoxifylline, and sildenafil), angiotensin 2 receptor antagonists (losartan), and selective serotonin reuptake inhibitors (fluoxetine) have been used with some limited success.
- Alpha receptor antagonists such as prazosin and phenoxybenzamine have shown some effectiveness in treating RP.
- The prostaglandins, including inhaled iloprost, IV epoprostenol, alprostadil, and tadalafil, may be promising in severe RP. However, additional experience and controlled studies are needed.
- Antioxidants like zinc gluconate have been used to decrease tissue damage.
- N-Acetylcysteine and probucol have been shown to lead to improvement in RP.
- Anticoagulation with IV unfractionated heparin or subcutaneous low-molecular-weight heparin and addition of aspirin can be considered during the acute phase of a severe ischemic event. Aspirin (81 mg/day) therapy can be considered in all patients with secondary RP with a history of ischemic ulcers or thrombotic events; however, caution should be exercised because aspirin can theoretically worsen vasospasm by the inhibition of prostacyclin. Long-term anticoagulation with heparin or warfarin is not recommended unless there is evidence of a hypercoagulable state.
- Bypass surgery can be performed for severe RP associated with reconstructible arterial occlusive disease.

- Sympathectomy is available for unreconstructible occlusive disease or pure vasospastic disease refractory to medical treatment.
- Microsurgical revascularization of the hand and digital reconstruction may improve digital vascular perfusion and heal digital ulcers when proximal arterial occlusion is associated with digital vasospasm.
- Ischemic digital lesions should be treated with topical antibiotics and daily cleansing with soap and water. Digits that progress to dry gangrene should be permitted to undergo autoamputation. Surgical amputation is limited for intractable pain or deep tissue infection.

DISPOSITION

The prognosis of patients with RP depends on the etiology.

- Primary RP is fairly benign, usually remaining stable and controlled with nonpharmacologic medical treatment.
- Remission of primary RP can occur spontaneously.
- Patients with secondary RP, specifically those with scleroderma, CREST syndrome, or thromboangiitis obliterans, may develop severe ischemic digits with ulceration, gangrene, and autoamputation.

REFERRAL

- Rheumatology consult is indicated if secondary collagen vascular disease is diagnosed.
- Vascular surgery consult is indicated if ulcers, gangrene, or threatened digit loss is noted.

⚠ PEARLS & CONSIDERATIONS

- Most patients with RP can be managed by a primary care provider.
- It is important to differentiate primary from secondary forms. Secondary forms may become manifest as far out as 10 yr from the diagnosis of RP. It is important to take immediate action during an attack, and patients are encouraged to:
  1. Keep warm
  2. Not use tobacco products
  3. Avoid aggravating medications
  4. Control stress
  5. Exercise
  6. Follow up with a physician

SUGGESTED READINGS

available at www.expertconsult.com

RELATED CONTENT

Raynaud's Phenomenon (Patient Information)

AUTHORS: **SYEDA M. SAYEED, M.D.**, and **FRED F. FERRI, M.D.**

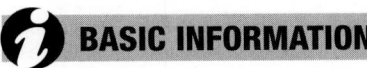

DEFINITION

Reiter's syndrome is one of the seronegative spondyloarthropathies, so called because serum rheumatoid factor is not present in these forms of inflammatory arthritis. There is an international consensus that the term *reactive arthritis* (ReA) should replace the name "Reiter's syndrome" to describe this constellation of signs and symptoms. Unfortunately, the original name is still associated with the syndrome. Reiter's syndrome is an asymmetric polyarthritis that affects mainly the lower extremities and is associated with one or more of the following:
- Urethritis
- Cervicitis
- Dysentery
- Inflammatory eye disease
- Mucocutaneous lesions

SYNONYMS

Reiter's disease
Reactive arthritis
Seronegative spondyloarthropathy

ICD-9CM CODES
099.3 Reiter's syndrome

EPIDEMIOLOGY & DEMOGRAPHICS

INCIDENCE (IN U.S.): 0.0035% annually of men ≤50 yr
PEAK INCIDENCE: Most common in the third decade
PREDOMINANT SEX: Male
PREDOMINANT AGE: 20 to 40 yr
GENETICS: Familial disposition: strongly associated with HLA-B27 (63% to 96%)

PHYSICAL FINDINGS & CLINICAL PRESENTATION

- Polyarthritis
  1. Affecting the knee and ankle
  2. Commonly asymmetric
- Heel pain and Achilles tendinitis, especially at the insertion of the Achilles tendon
- Plantar fasciitis
- Large effusions
- Dactylitis, or "sausage toe"
- Urethritis
- Uveitis or conjunctivitis; uveitis can progress to blindness without treatment
- Keratoderma blennorrhagicum, circinate balanitis
  1. Hyperkeratotic lesions on soles of the feet (Fig. E1-706), toes, penis (Fig. E1-707), hands
  2. Closely resembles psoriasis
- Aortic regurgitation similar to that seen in ankylosing spondylitis

ETIOLOGY

- Epidemic Reiter's syndrome after outbreaks of dysentery has been well described.
- Genetically susceptible HLA-B27 individuals are at risk for developing Reiter's syndrome after infection with certain pathogens:
  - *Salmonella*
  - *Shigella*
  - *Yersinia enterocolitica*
  - *Chlamydia trachomatis*
- Symptom complex indistinguishable from Reiter's syndrome has been described in association with HIV infection.

DIAGNOSIS

DIFFERENTIAL DIAGNOSIS

- Ankylosing spondylitis
- Psoriatic arthritis
- Rheumatoid arthritis
- Gonococcal arthritis-tenosynovitis
- Rheumatic fever

WORKUP

- X-ray examination of affected joints
- Synovial fluid examination and culture
- Careful examination of eyes and skin
- Cultures for gonococcus (urethral, cervical, stool)

LABORATORY TESTS

- Elevated but nonspecific erythrocyte sedimentation rate
- No specific laboratory tests to diagnose Reiter's syndrome
- Do not use HLA-B27 testing as a diagnostic tool

IMAGING STUDIES

Plain radiographs:
- Juxtaarticular osteopenia of affected joints
- Erosions and joint space narrowing in more advanced disease
- Periostitis and reactive new bone formation at the insertions of the Achilles tendon and the plantar fascia
- Sacroiliitis:
  1. Unilateral or bilateral
  2. Indistinguishable from ankylosing spondylitis
- Vertebral bridging osteophytes

TREATMENT

NONPHARMACOLOGIC THERAPY

Physical therapy to maintain range of motion of the spine and other joints

ACUTE GENERAL Rx

- Flares treated with nonsteroidal anti-inflammatory drugs such as indomethacin (25 to 50 mg PO tid).

- Enteric or urethral infection should be treated with appropriate antibiotic coverage.
- Uveitis should be treated with steroid eye drops in consultation with an ophthalmologist.
- Achilles tendinitis and plantar fasciitis should be treated with injections of methylprednisolone (40 to 80 mg).
- Sulfasalazine (2 to 3 g PO tid) may be effective.
- Careful monitoring for the following is essential:
  - Gastrointestinal toxicity
  - Hypersensitivity
  - Bone marrow suppression
- Persistent and uncontrolled disease should be managed with cytotoxic drugs (methotrexate, azathioprine) in consultation with a rheumatologist.

CHRONIC Rx

Chronic disease is best managed by a team approach with the collaboration of a rheumatologist or other experienced physician and physical therapist.

DISPOSITION

- Recurrences are frequent, even with treatment.
- Long-term sequelae:
  - Persistent polyarthritis
  - Chronic back pain
  - Heel pain
  - Progressive iridocyclitis
  - Aortic regurgitation

REFERRAL

- To ophthalmologist if uveitis is suspected
- To rheumatologist if arthritis and tendinitis fail to improve rapidly after a course of nonsteroidal anti-inflammatory drugs

PEARLS & CONSIDERATIONS

COMMENTS

- Infection with HIV is associated with particularly severe cases of Reiter's syndrome.
- HIV testing is recommended, especially if risk factors such as unprotected sexual activity or IV drug use are identified.

SUGGESTED READINGS
available at www.expertconsult.com

RELATED CONTENT
Reiter's Syndrome (Patient Information)

AUTHOR: **GLENN G. FORT, M.D., M.P.H.**

BASIC INFORMATION

DEFINITION

Renal artery stenosis (RAS) is the progressive narrowing of the renal artery, which is generally due to either atherosclerosis or fibromuscular dysplasia. RAS is an important, potentially reversible cause of hypertension and ischemic nephropathy. Acute renal artery occlusion usually results from cardioemboli, vascular emboli, or in situ thrombosis.

SYNONYMS

Acute:
    Renal artery thrombosis
    Renal artery embolism
Chronic:
    Renovascular hypertension

ICD-9CM CODES
593.81 Renal artery occlusion
440.1   Renal artery stenosis
405.01 Renovascular hypertension,
        secondary
447.9   Renal artery hyperplasia

EPIDEMIOLOGY & DEMOGRAPHICS

- Chronic RAS:
    1. Atherosclerotic renovascular disease accounts for about 90% of chronic RAS. True prevalence is unknown.
        a. General population autopsy studies show prevalence of 4% and 2% to 5% in hypertensive patients.
        b. In the general population >65 yr of age, the prevalence is 6.8% (5.5% of women, 9.1% of men, 6.7% of African Americans, and 6.9% of Caucasians). Of those with RAS, 12% had bilateral disease.
        c. In patients with malignant hypertension, the prevalence is 43% in Caucasians and 7% in African Americans. In patients with mild hypertension, the prevalence is <1%.
        d. In patients with peripheral artery disease, the prevalence is 22% to 59%.
    2. Fibromuscular dysplasia accounts for approximately 10% of chronic RAS. It is typically seen in women aged <50 yr and typically involves the distal main renal artery and intrarenal branches.
        - Acute renal artery occlusion: epidemiology depends on the underlying cause. The incidence on autopsy study was 1.4%.

PHYSICAL FINDINGS & CLINICAL PRESENTATION

Progressive RAS:
- Majority of patients with RAS are asymptomatic.
- Fibromuscular dysplasia: new-onset hypertension at age <50 yr or hypertension in any patient without family history or risk factors
- Atherosclerotic renal artery disease: new-onset hypertension at age >55 yr, with risk factors for or evidence of atherosclerotic disease
- Uncontrolled hypertension refractory to three or more medications including a diuretic
- Abdominal bruit (40% of cases)
- Chronic kidney disease
- Hypertensive retinopathy
- Pulmonary edema in a hypertensive patient
- Hypokalemia
- Acute kidney injury (AKI) after the administration of an ACE inhibitor (ACEI) has previously been considered a marker for bilateral RAS but is neither sensitive nor specific.

Acute renal artery occlusion:
- Flank or abdominal pain
- Fever
- Nausea and/or vomiting
- Leukocytosis
- Hematuria (microscopic or gross)
- Elevated aspartate aminotransferase, lactate dehydrogenase, and alkaline phosphatase
- Oliguric renal failure if occlusion is bilateral; normal or near-normal renal function in unilateral occlusion
- Cholesterol or septic emboli: depending on distribution of emboli, patients may have multisystem manifestations such as visual disturbance, painful distal extremities, abdominal pain, signs of organ or limb ischemia; laboratory findings include eosinophiluria, proteinuria, AKI, elevated erythrocyte sedimentation rate

ETIOLOGY

RAS and thrombosis:

- Atherosclerosis: risk factors for atherosclerosis include family history, smoking, diabetes, hypertension, and hyperlipidemia
- Fibromuscular dysplasia (Fig. 1-708): etiology unknown. Classified into three categories based on the layer of arterial wall affected: medial (>90%), intimal (<10%), adventitial (<1%). Typically involves the distal main renal artery and intrarenal branches.
- Extrinsic compression (e.g., neoplasm)
- Neurofibromatosis and fibrous bands
- Vasculitides, including autoimmune (Takayasu's, antiphospholipid syndrome), infectious (syphilis)
- Renal artery aneurysm
- Hypercoagulable state
- Complication of renal transplantation (role of cyclosporine)

Renal artery embolism (cardiac conditions contribute 90%):
- Left ventricular thrombus (may be the result of myocardial infarction or other cardiomyopathy)
- Atrial fibrillation
- Endocarditis
- Paradoxical emboli from deep vein thrombosis in patient with atrioventricular or ventricular septal defect
- Atheromatous plaques (cholesterol emboli)

PATHOGENESIS

- Pathogenesis of fibromuscular dysplasia is unknown.
- The pathogenesis of hypertension is related to the neurohormonal cascade resulting from renal ischemia. The macula densa of the

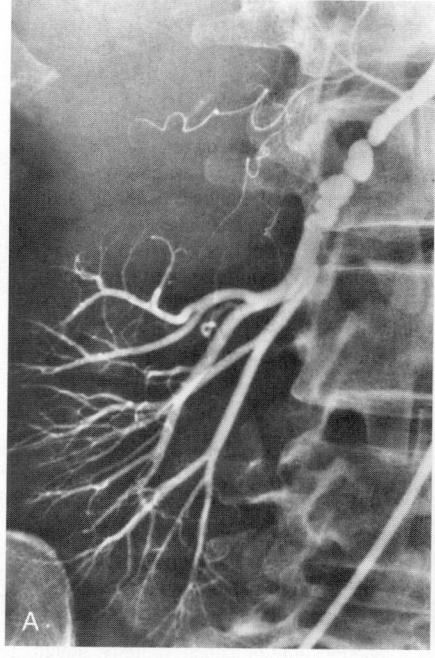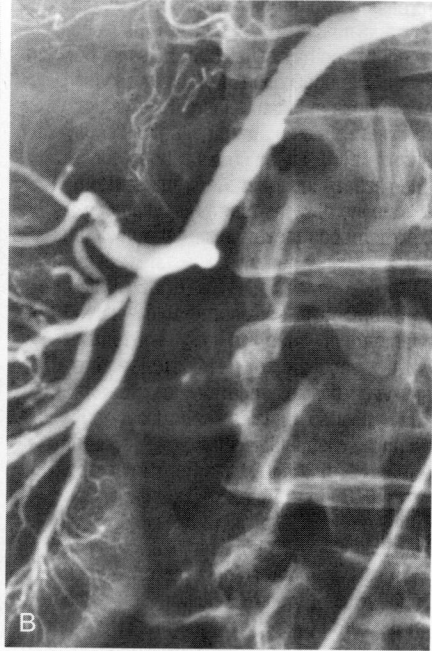

FIGURE 1-708 Fibromuscular dysplasia. A, Selective renal arteriogram illustrating the beaded appearance of fibromuscular dysplasia with multiple webs characteristic of medial fibroplasia in a 39-yr-old woman. **B,** Selective injection of the same renal artery after technically successful percutaneous transluminal renal angioplasty. (Courtesy Michael McKusick, M.D., Mayo Clinic, Rochester, Minnesota. From Floege J et al: *Comprehensive clinical nephrology,* ed 4, Philadelphia, 2010, Saunders.)

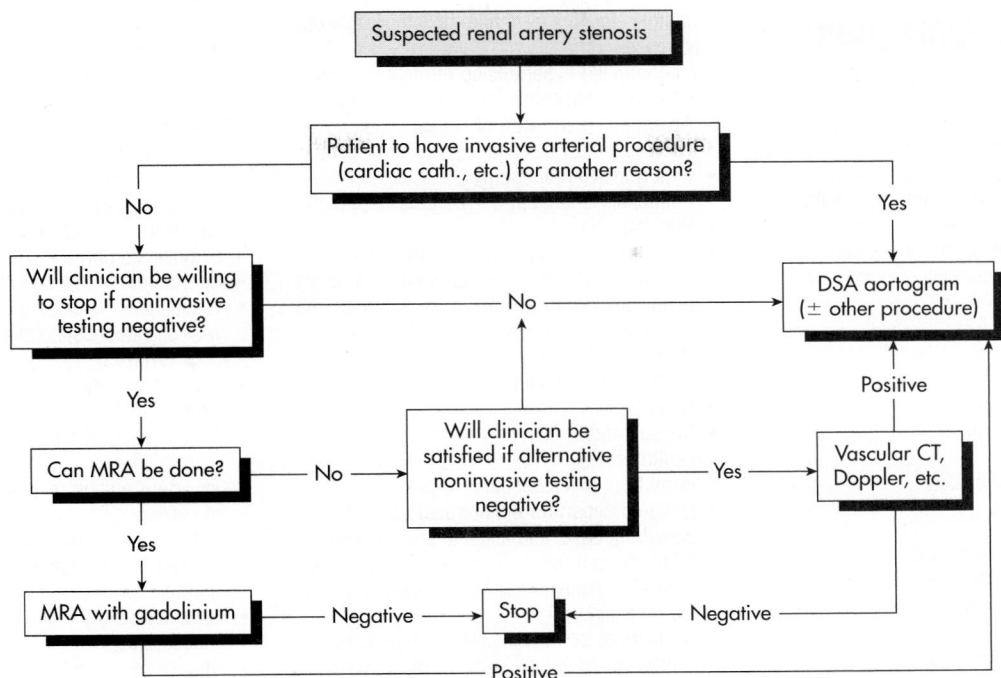

FIGURE 1-709 Approach to the anatomic evaluation of renal artery stenosis. Once stenosis is suspected, if the patient is to have another invasive arterial procedure, noninvasive imaging is deferred and a low-volume digital subtraction aortogram *(DSA)* is done at the time of that procedure. In other cases, the clinician should assess whether a negative noninvasive test would be sufficient evidence to acquit the renal arteries. If so, noninvasive testing should be performed. If not, consideration should be given to DSA and selective angiography. *Cath,* Catherization; *CT,* computed tomography; *MRA,* magnetic resonance angiography. (From Zipes DP et al [eds]: *Braunwald's heart disease,* ed 7, Philadelphia, 2005, Saunders.)

kidney senses a decreased systemic blood pressure caused by the reduced blood flow through the stenotic artery leading to a decrease in the glomerular filtration rate. Renal hypoperfusion or ischemia produces an increase in plasma renin that stimulates the conversion of angiotensin I to angiotensin II, causing vasoconstriction and aldosterone secretion, sodium retention, and potassium wasting. Hypertension results and can be self-sustaining, even in the case of unilateral RAS, because of hypertensive damage to the contralateral kidney.

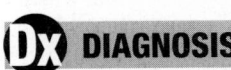 **DIAGNOSIS**

SCREENING

American College of Cardiology and American Heart Association (ACC/AHA) guidelines for identifying patients who should be screened for RAS:
- Onset of hypertension at age <30 yr or severe hypertension at age >55 yr
- Clinical findings that suggest secondary hypertension as opposed to essential hypertension in the absence of another more likely cause of secondary hypertension such as pheochromocytoma
- Malignant hypertension: hypertension with coexistent evidence of acute end-organ damage (acute renal failure, acute decompensated heart failure, new visual or neurologic disturbance, and/or retinopathy)

- Accelerated hypertension: sudden and persistent worsening
- Resistant hypertension: full doses of a three-drug regimen that includes a diuretic
- Sudden unexpected pulmonary edema
- New azotemia or acute renal failure after ACEI or angiotensin receptor blockers (ARBs)

LABORATORY TESTS
- Basic chemistry, including sodium, potassium, blood urea nitrogen, and creatinine
- Glomerular filtration rate
- Urinalysis and urine cultures
- Electrocardiogram to evaluate for atrial fibrillation and signs of coronary artery disease/myocardial infarction
- Hypercoaguable workup in setting of thrombosis or embolic disease

IMAGING STUDIES
- Duplex Doppler ultrasonography, CT angiography, and magnetic resonance angiography (MRA) are effective diagnostic screening methods. The choice of imaging modality will depend on the availability of the diagnostic tool, the experience and local accuracy of each modality, and patient characteristics, including body size, renal function, contrast allergy, and presence of prior stents. Fig. 1-709 describes an approach to the anatomic evaluation of RAS. An approach to the angiographic evaluation and treatment of RAS is described in Fig. E1-710.

- Duplex Doppler ultrasonography is safe and inexpensive. When compared with angiography, duplex ultrasound has a sensitivity of 84% to 98% and a specificity of 62% to 99% for detecting RAS. An end-diastolic velocity of >150 cm/sec predicts severe RAS. Duplex Doppler ultrasonography may be used to measure the renal dimensions and the renal resistive index. When renal ultrasound examination shows size discrepancy >1.5 cm, this suggests significant RAS involving the smaller kidney. Limitations include operator-dependent imaging, patient body habitus, and poor visualization of accessory renal arteries.
- MRA (Fig. 1-711) provides good visualization of both main and accessory renal arteries. Limitations include the associated risk of nephrogenic systemic fibrosis with gadolinium infusion, high cost, inability to image within a previously placed metallic stent, and lack of widespread availability.
- CT angiography is fast and effective but requires radiation exposure and infusion of potentially nephrotoxic iodinated contrast.
- IV digital subtraction catheter angiography (88% sensitivity, 90% specificity) is the gold standard for anatomic diagnosis of RAS. It is not a first-line screening tool but is recommended, if noninvasive tests are inconclusive but clinical suspicion is high. Renal fractional flow reserve (FFR) at the time of catheter angiography can be used to assess severity

of RAS using maximal vasodilatation. A hyperemeic systolic gradient of at least 21 mm Hg or renal fractional flow reserve of <0.90 can be considered hemodynamically significant. This modality should be reserved for patients with a high likelihood of intervention.

(Rx) TREATMENT

ACUTE GENERAL Rx

Acute renal artery thrombosis:
- Thrombolytic therapy
- Anticoagulation
- Revascularization (endovascular therapy or surgery). Endovascular renal artery stenting is favored over surgery, and has shown better clinical results when compared with balloon angioplasty (without stenting). Primary open revascularization can be considered selectively for nonatherosclerotic renal artery disease (NARAD) in some young patients or patients who need complex renal reconstructions.
- Acute blood pressure control with IV antihypertensives

CHRONIC Rx

Renal artery thrombosis/emboli: anticoagulation based upon underlying condition. If the patient has atrial fibrillation with therapeutic INR, consider INR 2.5 to 3.5.
Cholesterol emboli:
- Supportive care
RAS:
- Because of the activation of the renin-angiotensin-aldosterone system in RAS, ACEI/ARBs are recommended for the treatment of renovascular hypertension. Renal function should be monitored carefully when initiating or titrating these medications, particularly in patients with bilateral RAS or unilateral stenosis with solitary kidney, so as to avoid precipitating AKI.
- Beta-blockers are recommended for the treatment of hypertension in patients with RAS of all types.
- Antiplatelet therapy and statin therapy in patients with atherosclerotic RAS.
- Percutaneous intervention or surgical revascularization should be reserved for patients whose blood pressure control with medication is difficult and for patients with progressive disease. The ACC/AHA guidelines for clinical indications of renal artery revascularization in the presence of significant stenosis include:
  1. Accelerated, resistant, or malignant hypertension
  2. Hypertension with unilateral small kidney
  3. Hypertension with intolerance to medication

  4. Treatment of cardiac destabilization syndromes such as unexplained heart failure exacerbations, episodes of flash pulmonary edema, and refractory or unstable angina
  5. Progressive chronic kidney disease with bilateral RAS or RAS associated with a solitary functioning kidney
- Randomized control trials (e.g., ASTRAL and DRASTIC) have shown no benefit to percutaneous therapy when compared with medical therapy, with endpoints of blood pressure control, renal function, and cardiovascular events. The DRASTIC trial found no difference in blood pressure but did show decrease in daily doses of antihypertensive drugs and number of drugs in the intervention group. The ASTRAL trial found no difference in blood pressure control or the number of antihypertensives but had increased risks associated with intervention. However, these trials did have several inherent limitations and further trials are ongoing.

NATURAL HISTORY
- RAS caused by fibromuscular dysplasia generally does not progress. Fibromuscular dysplasia RAS responds well to angioplasty with long-term patency of the lesion typically observed.
- RAS associated with atherosclerosis is progressive. Of patients with >60% stenosis, 5% progress to total occlusion in 1 yr and 11% progress in 2 yr.
- An increased pulse pressure (PP), defined as systolic minus diastolic blood pressure, has been implicated in the development and progression of small-vessel disease and has been shown to reflect more advanced renal disease. It can help identify patients who are less likely to benefit from percutaneous interventions.

DISPOSITION & REFERRAL
- Patients with uncontrolled hypertension on multiple agents should be referred for management by a specialist.
- Decision for percutaneous intervention for atherosclerotic RAS requires weighing the risks and benefits in detail and should be reserved for selected patients until further data are available.

(!) PEARLS & CONSIDERATIONS

- Symptoms for acute renal artery occlusion are nonspecific and can be confused with nephrolithiasis and pyelonephritis among other causes. Evaluation with LDH and liver enzymes can be very helpful. LDH four times the normal range without significant transaminitis is consistent with renal infarction.
- Renal artery stenting currently requires more data to address its utility in both unilateral and bilateral RAS.
- The modality for the type of imaging should depend on the expertise of the institution.

SUGGESTED READINGS

available at www.expertconsult.com

RELATED CONTENT

Renal Artery Stenosis (Patient Information)
Hypertension (Related Key Topic)

AUTHORS: **ELLIOTT GROVES, M.D., M.ENG., FRED F. FERRI, M.D.,** and **PRANAV M. PATEL, M.D., F.A.C.C., F.S.C.A.I.**

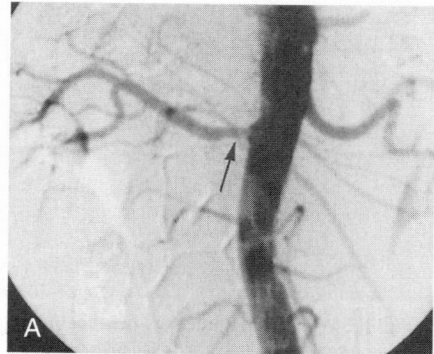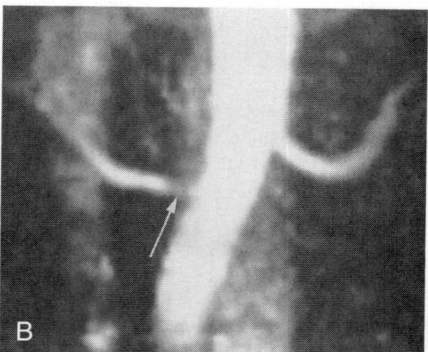

FIGURE 1-711 Renal arteriograms. A, Conventional renal digital subtraction (DSA) showing mild renal stenosis *(arrows)* on the right. **B,** Magnetic resonance angiogram (MRA) of the same patient. The stenosed segment *(arrows)* is clearly seen in this coronal projection. (Courtesy Dr. W. Gedroyc. From Souhami RL, Moxham J: *Textbook of medicine,* ed 4, London, 2002, Churchill Livingstone.)

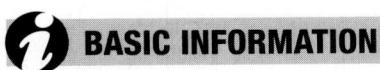

BASIC INFORMATION

DEFINITION

Renal cell adenocarcinoma (RCA) is a primary adenocarcinoma originating in the renal parenchyma from the malignant transformation of proximal renal tubular epithelial cells. Most renal cell cancers are of clear cell type. Papillary tumors comprise 15% of renal cancers, and chromophobe tumors make up 10%.

SYNONYMS

Hypernephroma
Clear cell carcinoma of the kidney
Grawitz tumor

ICD-9CM CODES
189.0 Adenocarcinoma of kidney
189.1 (Renal pelvis)

EPIDEMIOLOGY & DEMOGRAPHICS

INCIDENCE: Approximately one in 10,000 persons annually (3% of all adult malignancies). In the U.S., renal cancer is the seventh leading malignant condition among men and twelfth among women. Two percent of cases of renal cancer are associated with inherited syndromes.
PREDOMINANT SEX: Male/female ratio of 2:1
PREDOMINANT AGE: Peaks at age 50 to 70 yr

PHYSICAL FINDINGS & CLINICAL PRESENTATION

The classic presentation of RCA includes the triad of flank pain, hematuria, and a palpable abdominal mass. This now represents an unusual presentation. Current presenting findings in RCA patients now include:

Hematuria	50% to 60%
Elevated erythrocyte sedimentation rate	50% to 60%
Abdominal mass	25% to 45%
Anemia	20% to 40%
Flank pain	35% to 40%
Hypertension	20% to 40%
Weight loss	30% to 35%
Fever	5% to 15%
Hepatic dysfunction	10% to 15%
Classic triad (hematuria, abdominal mass, flank pain)	5% to 10%
Hypercalcemia	3% to 6%
Erythrocytosis	3% to 4%
Varicocele	2% to 3%

ETIOLOGY

Hereditary forms:
- Familial renal carcinoma
- Renal carcinoma associated with von Hippel-Lindau disease
- Hereditary papillary renal cell carcinoma

Risk factors:
- Cigarette smoking
- Obesity
- Use of diuretics
- Phenacetin-containing analgesics
- Asbestos exposure
- Gasoline and other petroleum products
- Lead
- Cadmium
- Thorotrast
- Role of the *VHL* gene on chromosome 3

DIAGNOSIS

DIFFERENTIAL DIAGNOSIS

- Transitional cell carcinomas of the renal pelvis (8% of all renal cancers)
- Wilms' tumor
- Other rare primary renal carcinomas and sarcomas
- Renal cysts
- All causes of hematuria (see Section II)
- Retroperitoneal tumors

WORKUP

Laboratory tests and imaging studies

LABORATORY TESTS

- Urinalysis: hematuria
- Complete blood count: anemia or erythrocytosis
- Nonmetastatic hepatic dysfunction with elevated alkaline phosphatase, prolonged prothrombin time, and hypoalbuminemia
- Hypercalcemia (caused by parathyroid-related protein)
- Other: elevated ferritin, elevated insulin and glucagon levels, elevated alpha-fetoprotein, and elevated beta–human chorionic gonadotropin
- Recent reports indicate that urine AQP1 and ADFP concentrations quantified by Western blot appear to be sensitive and specific biomarkers of kidney cancers of proximal tubule origin and may be useful to diagnose an imaged renal mass and screen for kidney cancer at an early stage. Additional investigations are under way to determine if these tests should become standard tumor markers in the investigation of renal masses.

IMAGING STUDIES

Nearly 50% of renal cancers are now detected because a renal mass is incidentally detected on radiographic evaluation.
- Renal ultrasound
- Abdominal CT scan with contrast (Figs. 1-712 and 1-713); CT-guided biopsy is generally not necessary for diagnosis of solid masses >4 cm (high likelihood of cancer)
- MRI
- Renal arteriogram
- Intravenous pyelography

STAGING

See Table 1-356.

COMMON SITES OF METASTASES

Lung	50% to 60%
Bone	30% to 40%
Regional nodes	15% to 30%
Main renal vein	15% to 20%
Perirenal fat	10% to 20%
Adrenal (ipsilateral)	10% to 15%
Vena cava	10% to 15%
Brain	10% to 15%
Adjacent organs (colon, pancreas)	10%
Kidney (contralateral)	2%

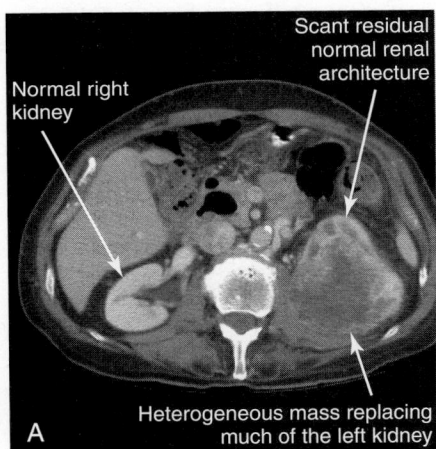
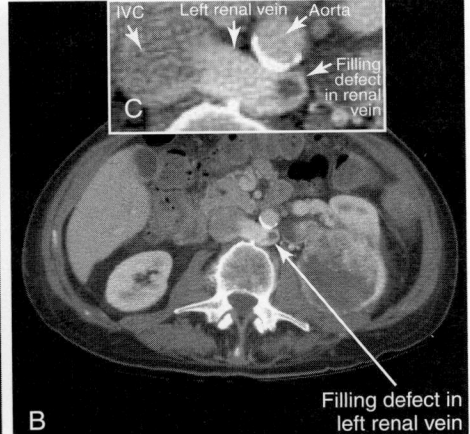

FIGURE 1-712 Renal masses: renal cell carcinoma. Noncontrast CT performed for assessment of urinary stone disease sometimes reveals underlying renal malignancies. When a malignancy is suspected, intravenous contrast should be administered to further characterize the lesion. Flank pain and painless hematuria are both sometimes presenting symptoms of renal cell carcinomas (hypernephromas). **A through C,** In this patient, an aggressive renal cell carcinoma has nearly replaced the left kidney. A small amount of relatively normal renal architecture can be seen anteriorly, whereas the bulk of the tumor is heterogeneously enhancing, likely because of a degree of necrosis. Incidentally, the patient has a retroaortic left renal vein (the normal course being anterior to the aorta). This vein deserves attention because renal cell carcinomas are known to invade the renal vein, enter the inferior vena cava *(IVC)*, and embolize to the lungs. In this patient, a filling defect is seen in the left renal vein, likely representing tumor invasion. The IVC is just beginning to fill with contrast and has a heterogeneous appearance due to mixing of contrast and normal blood, so it cannot be assessed for tumor invasion. Delayed images could be obtained to identify filling defects in the IVC once the contrast appearance of the IVC has become more uniform. (From Broder JS: *Diagnostic imaging for the emergency physician,* Philadelphia, 2011, Saunders.)

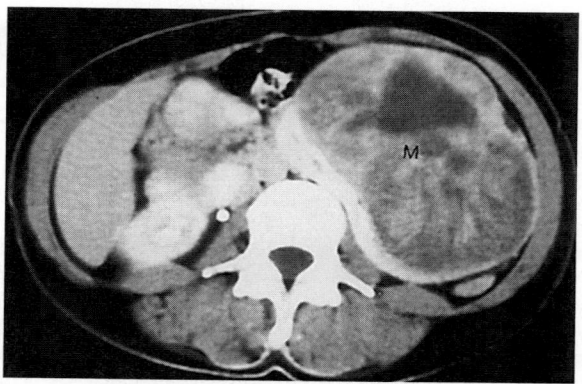

FIGURE 1-713 Large renal cell carcinoma. Large mass *(M)* containing areas of high enhancement, low enhancement, and necrosis. (From Stein JH [ed]: *Internal medicine*, ed 5, St Louis, 1998, Mosby.)

TABLE 1-356 Comparison of Conventional and TNM Staging Classification of Renal Cell Carcinomas

Robson Stage	T	N	M
I: Tumor confined by capsule	T_1 (tumor ≤2.5 cm) T_2 (tumor >2.5 cm, limited to kidney)		
II: Tumor extension to perirenal fat or ipsilateral adrenal but confined by Gerota's fascia	T_3a (tumor invades adrenal gland or perinephric fat but not beyond Gerota's fascia)		
IIIa: Renal vein or inferior vena caval involvement	T_3b (renal vein or caval involvement below diaphragm)	N_0 (nodes negative)	M_0 (no distant metastases)
IIIb: Lymphatic involvement	T_{1-4}	N_1 (single lymph node ≤2 cm) N_2 (single node 2 to 5 cm, or multiple) N_3 (single or multiple nodes >5 cm)	T_3c (caval involvement above nodes <5 cm)
IIIc: Combination of IIIa and IIIb	$T_{3,\,4}$		
IVa: Spread to contiguous	T_4 (tumor extends beyond organs except ipsilateral adrenal Gerota's fascia)		
IVb: Distant metastases	T_{1-4}		M_1 (distant metastases)

(Rx) TREATMENT

- Surgery
  - Surgical nephrectomy (open procedure or laparoscopic approach) is the only effective management for stages I, II, and some stage III tumors. Although radical nephrectomy had long been the standard treatment, retrospective studies have shown that partial rather than radical nephrectomy is associated with improved survival and is appropriate for patients with renal cell neoplasms <4 cm that are not adjacent to renal pelvis.
  - Various forms of partial nephrectomy may be available for patients with bilateral cancers or with a solitary kidney.
  - The role of nephrectomy in patients with metastatic renal cell carcinoma is controversial and should probably be reserved for patients who have a solitary metastasis amenable to surgical resection. However, there are data showing that nephrectomy before immunotherapy improves survival in patients with metastatic renal cell cancer compared with immunotherapy alone.

- Angioinfarction (for palliation)
- Radiotherapy (for palliation)
- Chemotherapy: In patients with unresectable disease, inhibitors of vascular endothelial growth factor (VEGF) such as the antivascular endothelial growth factor antibody bevacizumab, mTOR kinase inhibitors such as everolimus and temsirolimus, and the tyrosine kinase inhibitors axitinib, sunitinib, pazopanib, and sorafenib can be used as first-line therapy.
- Hormonal therapy (high-dose progesterone may achieve a 15% to 20% response rate)
- Immunotherapy: interleukin-2 may achieve a 15% to 30% response rate; alpha-, beta-, and gamma-interferons are somewhat less effective and now used less frequently

PROGNOSIS

Prognosis of surgically treated patients:

TNM Stage	5-yr Survival (%)
I	95
II	88
III (renal vein or vena cava)	50 to 60
III (nodal involvement)	15 to 25
IV	5 to 20

REFERRAL

To urologist

SUGGESTED READINGS

available at www.expertconsult.com

RELATED CONTENT

Kidney Cancer (Patient Information)

AUTHOR: **FRED F. FERRI, M.D.**

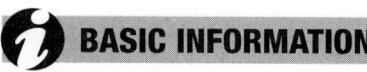

BASIC INFORMATION

DEFINITION

Renal tubular acidosis (RTA) is a disorder characterized by inability to excrete H^+ or inadequate generation of new HCO_3^-. RTA syndromes are summarized in Table E1-357. Factors differentiating types of RTA are described in Table E1-358. Four main types of RTA are described in the medical literature:

- Type I (classic, distal RTA): abnormality in distal hydrogen secretion, resulting in hypokalemic hyperchloremic metabolic acidosis.
- Type II (proximal RTA): decreased proximal bicarbonate reabsorption, resulting in hypokalemic hyperchloremic metabolic acidosis.
- Type III (RTA of glomerular insufficiency): normokalemic hyperchloremic metabolic acidosis as a result of impaired ability to generate sufficient NH_3 in the setting of decreased glomerular filtration rate (<30 ml/min). This type of RTA is described in older textbooks and is considered by many not to be a distinct entity.
- Type IV (hyporeninemic hypoaldosteronemic RTA): aldosterone deficiency or antagonism, resulting in decreased distal acidification and decreased distal sodium reabsorption with subsequent hyperkalemic hyperchloremic acidosis.

SYNONYMS

RTA

ICD-9CM CODES
588.8 Renal tubular acidosis

EPIDEMIOLOGY & DEMOGRAPHICS

RTA type IV affects mostly adults, whereas RTA types I and II are more frequent in children.

PHYSICAL FINDINGS & CLINICAL PRESENTATION

- Examination may be normal.
- Poor skin turgor may be present from dehydration.
- Muscle weakness and muscle aches from hypokalemia may occur.
- Low back pain and bone pain may be present in patients with abnormalities of calcium metabolism (RTA II).
- There is failure to thrive in children (RTA II).

ETIOLOGY

- Type I RTA: autoimmune disorders, primary biliary cirrhosis and other liver diseases, medications (amphotericin, nonsteroidals), systemic lupus erythematosus, Sjögren's syndrome, genetic disorders (Ehlers-Danlos syndrome, Marfan syndrome, hereditary elliptocytosis), toxins (toluene), disorders with nephrocalcinosis (hyperparathyroidism, vitamin D intoxication, idiopathic hypercalciuria),

tubulointerstitial disease (obstructive uropathy, renal transplantation)
- Type II RTA: Fanconi's syndrome, primary hyperparathyroidism, multiple myeloma, medications (acetazolamide)
- Type IV RTA: diabetes mellitus, sickle cell disease, Addison's disease, urinary obstruction

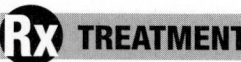

DIAGNOSIS

DIFFERENTIAL DIAGNOSIS

- Diarrhea with significant bicarbonate loss
- Other causes of metabolic acidosis
- Respiratory acidosis

WORKUP

Detection of hyperchloremic metabolic acidosis with arterial blood gases (ABGs) and serum electrolytes and evaluation of potential causes (see "Etiology"). Fig. E1-714 describes an approach to the patient with RTA.

LABORATORY TESTS

- ABGs reveal metabolic acidosis; serum potassium is low in RTA types I and II, normal in type III, and high in type IV.
- Minimal urine pH is >5.5 in RTA type I and <5.5 in types II, III, and IV.
- Urinary anion gap is 0 or positive in all types of RTA.
- Additional useful studies include serum calcium level and urine calcium.
- Anion gap is normal.
- Parathyroid hormone measurement is useful in patients suspected of primary hyperparathyroidism (may be associated with type II RTA).

IMAGING STUDIES

- Plain abdominal radiography is useful to evaluate for nephrocalcinosis.
- Renal sonogram can be used to evaluate renal size or presence of stones.
- Intravenous pyelogram in patients with nephrocalcinosis or nephrolithiasis.

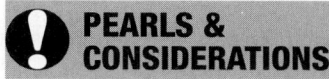

TREATMENT

ACUTE GENERAL Rx

- Types I and II are treated with oral sodium bicarbonate (1 to 2 mEq/kg/day in RTA I, 2 to 4 mEq/kg/day in RTA type II) titrated to correct acidosis.
- Potassium supplementation is needed in hypokalemic patients.
- Type IV RTA can be treated with furosemide to lower elevated potassium levels and sodium bicarbonate to correct significant acidosis. Fludrocortisone 100 to 300 μg/day can be used to correct mineralocorticoid deficiency.

CHRONIC Rx

- Frequent monitoring of potassium levels in RTA type IV
- Monitoring for bone disease in RTA type II
- Monitoring for nephrocalcinosis and nephrolithiasis in RTA type I

DISPOSITION

- Prognosis varies with the presence of associated conditions (see "Etiology").
- Untreated distal RTA may result in hypercalcemia, hyperphosphaturia, nephrolithiasis, and nephrocalcinosis.

PEARLS & CONSIDERATIONS

COMMENTS

Patient education material can be obtained from the National Kidney and Urologic Diseases Information Clearinghouse, Box NKUDIC, Bethesda, MD 20893.

AUTHOR: **FRED F. FERRI, M.D.**

TABLE 1-358 Factors Differentiating Type 1, Type 2, and Type 4 Renal Tubular Acidosis (RTA)

	Type 1 RTA	Type 2 RTA	Type 4 RTA
Serum K^+	Low	Low	High
Renal function	Normal or near normal	Normal or near normal	Stage 3, 4, or 5 chronic kidney disease
Urine pH during acidosis	High	Low	Low or high
Serum HCO_3^- (mmol/L)	10-20	16-18	16-22
Urine pCO_2 (mm Hg)	<40	<40	>70
Urine citrate	Low	High	Low
Fanconi syndrome	No	May be present	No

From Floege J et al: *Comprehensive clinical nephrology*, ed 4, Philadelphia, 2010, Saunders.

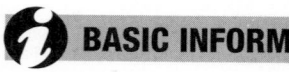

BASIC INFORMATION

DEFINITION

Renal vein thrombosis is the thrombotic occlusion of one or both renal veins.

ICD-9CM CODES
453.3 Renal vein thrombosis

EPIDEMIOLOGY & DEMOGRAPHICS

- Incidence unknown; probably an underdiagnosed condition
- May occur at any age with no gender preference
- Epidemiology tied to the underlying cause

PHYSICAL FINDINGS & CLINICAL PRESENTATION

Acute bilateral renal vein thrombosis:
- Back and bilateral flank pain
- Acute renal failure

Acute unilateral renal vein thrombosis:
- Flank pain
- Decline in renal function
- Hematuria
- Increase in the amount of proteinuria if associated with nephrotic syndrome

Chronic unilateral renal vein thrombosis:
- May be silent
- Pulmonary emboli and hemolysis
- Back pain
- Deep vein thrombosis in lower extremities
- Edema
- Glycosuria
- Hyperchloremic acidosis
- Left varicocele (if the left renal vein is thrombosed)
- Dilated abdominal veins

ETIOLOGY & PATHOGENESIS

- Extrinsic compression by a tumor or retroperitoneal mass
- Invasion of the renal vein or inferior vena cava by tumor (almost always renal cell cancer)
- Trauma
- Hypercoagulable states
- Dehydration
- Glomerulopathies (membranous glomerulonephritis, crescentic glomerulonephritis, systemic lupus erythematosus, amyloidosis) especially in the presence of nephrotic syndrome when the serum albumin is <2 g/dl
- NOTE: For unknown reasons, diabetic nephropathy is not commonly associated with renal vein thrombosis even if the nephrotic syndrome is present

A controversy has existed regarding whether the renal vein thrombosis association with nephrotic syndrome is a complication of nephrotic syndrome or whether renal vein thrombosis occurring in the setting of increased renal vein pressure (e.g., with congestive heart failure, constrictive pericarditis, or extrinsic compression) can independently cause proteinuria. Current evidence is that renal vein thrombosis does not cause nephrotic syndrome.

DIAGNOSIS

DIFFERENTIAL DIAGNOSIS

The diagnosis of renal vein thrombosis does not include any differential consideration. The differential diagnosis is that of proteinuria. Renal vein thrombosis should be considered if proteinuria worsens or if renal function worsens in a patient with glomerulonephritis. Renal vein thrombosis should also be considered in patients with pulmonary emboli and no lower-extremity deep vein thrombosis.

WORKUP

Clinical suspicion (see "Differential Diagnosis") and imaging studies

IMAGING STUDIES

- Abdominal ultrasound
- Abdominal MRI or CT with contrast (Fig. 1-715)
- Renal arteriography (delayed films during venous phase)
- Selective renal vein venography (inferior venacavogram images should be obtained before advancing the catheter in the vena cava because clots, if present, could be dislodged)
- Renal biopsy may be indicated if evidence of nephritis is present (e.g., active urinary sediment)

TREATMENT

- Anticoagulation in acute renal vein thrombosis to prevent pulmonary emboli and in attempt to improve renal function and decrease proteinuria
- Thrombolytic therapy or surgical thrombectomy has also been reported to be effective
- The value of anticoagulation in chronic renal vein thrombosis is dubious except in nephrotic patients with membranous glomerulonephritis with profound hypoalbuminemia where prolonged prophylactic anticoagulation may be of benefit even if renal vein thrombosis has not been documented

PROGNOSIS

Probable worsening of the underlying glomerulonephritis by acute renal vein thrombosis; the effect of chronic renal vein thrombosis is unclear.

AUTHOR: **FRED F. FERRI, M.D.**

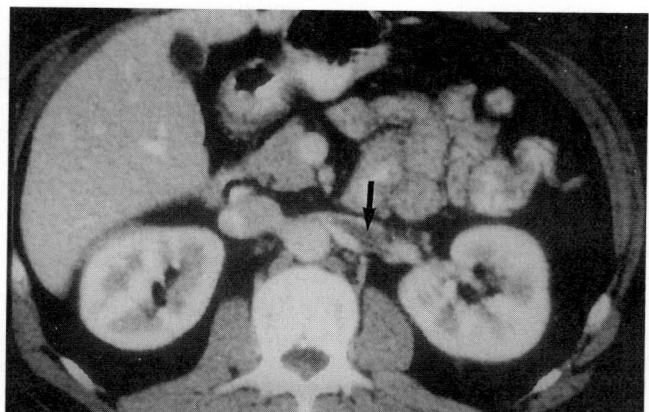

FIGURE 1-715 Renal vein thrombus in a patient with nephritic syndrome. Contrast medium–enhanced CT at the level of the renal vein shows thrombus in the left renal vein *(arrow)*. (From Grainger RG et al [eds]: *Grainger & Allison's diagnostic radiology*, ed 4, Philadelphia, 2001, Churchill Livingstone.)

BASIC INFORMATION

DEFINITION Restless legs syndrome (RLS) is an awake phenomenon consisting of an urge to move legs, usually associated with feeling of discomfort in legs.

SYNONYMS

RLS
Wittmaack-Ekbom syndrome

ICD-9CM CODES
333.94 Restless leg syndrome

EPIDEMIOLOGY & DEMOGRAPHICS

PREVALENCE: Average prevalence rate is 1% to 29%. Prevalence estimates in Europe are around 10%, and 0.1% to 12% in East Asian population.
PEAK PREVALENCE: 10% in persons aged 30 to 79 and 19% in persons aged 80 or above.
PREDOMINANT SEX: Early onset RLS is more common in females, with 2:1 female/male ratio.
PREDOMINANT AGE: Prevalence of RLS increases with age, and it is more commonly seen in elderly population.
GENETICS: Genetic basis of RLS has been reported, particularly in early onset RLS.
- Autosomal dominant disorder
- Common among first-degree relatives
- RLS associated with certain sequences in chromosome 6p,12q, 14q, 9p, 20p, 2p, 16p
RISK FACTORS: Diabetes mellitus (most consistent risk factor for RLS), iron deficiency anemia (IDA), end-stage renal disease (ESRD) requiring hemodialysis, pregnancy, rheumatoid arthritis, Parkinson's disease, neuropathy, and myelopathy

CLASSIFICATION

- Primary RLS is without any obvious cause, with no associated disorder.
- Secondary RLS results from other medical conditions; the most frequently found associations are pregnancy, IDA, ESRD, and Parkinson disease.

PHYSICAL FINDINGS & CLINICAL PRESENTATION

- Wide spectrum of severity of clinical manifestations has been reported in RLS.
- Most common symptom is unpleasant sensations in legs ("dysesthesias"), reported as discomfort or "creepy-crawling" sensations, mostly bilateral. Arms are occasionally involved.
- There is an extreme urge to move legs and relief is sustained as long as the movement continues.
- Symptoms are worse at night or evening. Best sleep is usually early in the morning.

ETIOLOGY The exact etiology remains unknown. Pharmacologic, pathologic, physiologic, and imaging studies have implicated dopaminergic pathways, brain iron metabolism, and endogenous opioid pathways.

DIAGNOSIS

DIFFERENTIAL DIAGNOSIS

- Periodic limb movement disorder (PLMD)
- Nocturnal leg cramps
- Painful peripheral neuropathy
- Akathisias
- Positional discomfort
- Volitional movements, foot tapping, leg rocking

WORKUP

- Diagnosis of RLS is based on established clinical criteria (Table 1-359) and normal neurologic examination.
- Testing is done to determine possible cause of secondary RLS.
- Polysomnography to document periodic limb movements during sleep
- Leg activity monitors to determine limb movements during sleep but they are unable to distinguish periodic limb movements from periodic movements associated with sleep apnea.
- Nerve conduction studies and electromyography for associated peripheral neuropathy

LABORATORY TESTS

- Iron status: serum ferritin, total iron binding capacity, percent saturation
- CBC for anemia in case of iron deficiency
- Metabolic panel: blood urea nitrogen and serum creatinine for renal insufficiency

IMAGING STUDIES No imaging studies are required for diagnosis for RLS.

TREATMENT

Treatment options for RLS include:
- Dopaminergic agents, levodopa, and dopamine agonists help to ameliorate RLS symptoms, decrease periodic limb movements, and improve sleep. Dopamine agonists, pramipexole and ropinirole, are first-line agents in the treatment of RLS.
- Anticonvulsants, such as gabapentin, have been shown to be effective in multiple studies. Limited case reports reveal use of lamotrigine, Gabatril, and topiramate in patients who are intolerant to other agents.
- Opiates, mostly methadone, are generally reserved as last line of treatment.
- Iron replacement should be started in case of iron deficiency.

NONPHARMACOLOGIC THERAPY

- Avoidance of caffeine, alcohol, nicotine, and medications that exacerbate RLS
- Physical and mental activity
- Good sleep hygiene

ACUTE GENERAL Rx Once the diagnosis of RLS is considered based on clinical criteria as mentioned in Table 1-359 and causes impairment of quality of life, a dopamine agonist (bromocriptine, pramipexole, or ropinirole) should be started at low dose and then gradually tapered up depending on tolerance. Recently a new extended-release preparation of gabapentin (gabapentin anapranil ER [Horizant]) has been FDA approved for treatment of moderate-to-severe RLS.

CHRONIC Rx Dopamine agonists or gabapentin are given daily on chronic basis. Oral iron replacement is added to the regimen in case of iron deficiency.

DISPOSITION It is usually a life-long disorder, presenting with relapses and remissions. Usually, medications are able to control symptoms and improve sleep quality.

REFERRAL Refer to neurologist if diagnosis is uncertain or an underlying disorder is suspected.

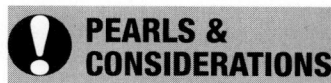

PEARLS & CONSIDERATIONS

COMMENTS RLS is diagnosed based on patient's history and physical exam. Laboratory tests are done only to exclude secondary RLS. Neurologic exam in idiopathic RLS is normal unless another neurologic diagnosis is suspected with it. Pharmacologic therapy should be limited to individuals who meet the specific diagnostic criteria. Severity of the disease, subjective complaints, age, and desire of the patient for treatment should be considered.

SUGGESTED READINGS

available at www.expertconsult.com

RELATED CONTENT

Restless Legs Syndrome (Patient Information)

AUTHOR: **FARIHA ZAHEER, M.D.**

TABLE 1-359 Diagnostic Criteria for Restless Legs Syndrome

Minimal Criteria

1. Desire to move the legs usually associated with paresthesias.
2. Motor restlessness, as characterized by floor pacing, leg rubbing, stretching, and flexing.
3. Worse at rest, with relief by activity.
4. Worse at night.

Additional Criteria

1. Sleep disturbances, as difficulty in sleep onset and maintaining sleep, daytime fatigue, or somnolence.
2. Involuntary movements, as periodic limb or leg movements in sleep and periodic or aperiodic limb movements while awake.
3. Neurologic examination is normal in idiopathic restless legs syndrome.
4. Clinical course may begin at any age but most severe in middle and older age.
5. Family history suggests autosomal dominant mode of inheritance in 1/3 of the cases.

From Stiansy K et al: Clinical symptomatology and treatment of restless leg syndrome and periodic limb movement disorder, *Sleep Med Rev* 6(4):253-265, 2002.

BASIC INFORMATION

DEFINITION

Retinal detachment is the separation of the neurosensory retina (NSR) from the retinal pigment epithelium (RPE). This results in the accumulation of subretinal fluid (SRF) in the potential space between the NSR and the RPE. The main types of retinal detachment are rhegmatogenous, tractional, exudating, and combined tractional-rhegmatogenous.

SYNONYMS

Inflammatory lesions of choroid
Uveitis
Tumor
Vascular lesions
Congenital disorders

ICD-9CM CODES
361 Retinal detachment and defects

EPIDEMIOLOGY & DEMOGRAPHICS

INCIDENCE (IN U.S.):
- 0.02% of the population
- Particularly common in patients with high myopia of 5 diopters or more

PEAK INCIDENCE: Incidence increases with increasing age or increasing myopia.

PREVALENCE (IN U.S.): Busy ophthalmologists may see one or two acute retinal detachments per month.

PREDOMINANT AGE:
- Congenital in younger patients
- Usually trauma in patients aged 30 to 40 yr and older

- High myopia a predisposition

PHYSICAL FINDINGS & CLINICAL PRESENTATION

- Elevation of retina and vessels associated with tears in the retina (Fig. 1-716 and Fig. 1-717), fluid, and/or hemorrhage beneath the retina and changes in the vitreous.
- Reports of flashing lights and floaters.
- After a variable period of time, the patient notices a relative peripheral visual field defect that may progress to involve central vision.

ETIOLOGY

- Trauma
- Tears in the retina
- Uveitis
- Fluid accumulation beneath the retina
- Tumors
- Scleritis
- Inflammatory disease
- Diabetes
- Collagen-vascular disease
- Vascular abnormalities
- Oral fluoroquinolones (higher risk of retinal detachment compared with nonusers, although the absolute risk is small)

DIAGNOSIS

DIFFERENTIAL DIAGNOSIS

- Degenerative retinoschisis
- Uveal effusion syndrome
- Choroidal detachment
- Hemorrhage
- Tumors

WORKUP

- Full eye examination
- Fluorescein angiography
- Visual fields
- Ultrasonography to show the retinal detachment or tumors beneath it
- Medical workup only when inflammation or systemic disease considered

LABORATORY TESTS

Usually not necessary

IMAGING STUDIES

B scan ultrasonography (US) of the eye

TREATMENT

NONPHARMACOLOGIC THERAPY

Immediate surgery. The three principal methods for reattachment of the retina in patients with primary retinal detachment are scleral buckling, vitrectomy, and pneumatic retinopexy. There is a paucity of randomized trials comparing these procedures and the choice remains subjective. Some data suggest that vitrectomy may be preferable for detachment in pseudophakic eyes, whereas primary detachment in phakic eyes with complexity exceeding the original indications for rheumatic retinopexy may be treated with scleral buckling or vitrectomy.

ACUTE GENERAL Rx

- Early surgery to repair the detachment
- Treatment of the underlying disorder

CHRONIC Rx

Occasionally, steroids or other treatment of underlying disease is indicated.

DISPOSITION

- Immediately refer to an ophthalmologist.
- Early intervention improves outcomes.

REFERRAL

Immediately

PEARLS & CONSIDERATIONS

COMMENTS

If treated early, most patients will recover a substantial portion of their vision.

SUGGESTED READINGS
available at www.expertconsult.com

AUTHOR: **MELVYN KOBY, M.D.**

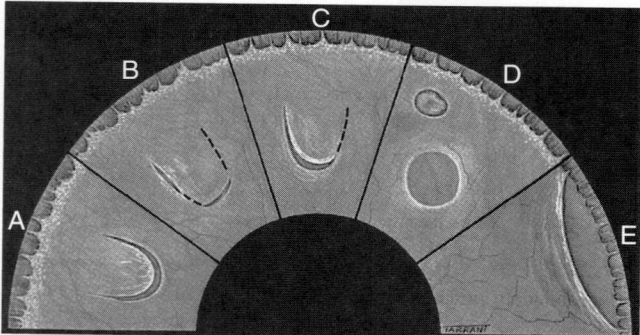

FIGURE 1-716 Retinal tears. A, Complete U-shaped; **B,** linear; **C,** L-shaped; **D,** operculated; **E,** dialysis. (From Kanski JJ, Bowling B: *Clinical ophthalmology: a systematic approach,* ed 7, Philadelphia, 2010, Saunders.)

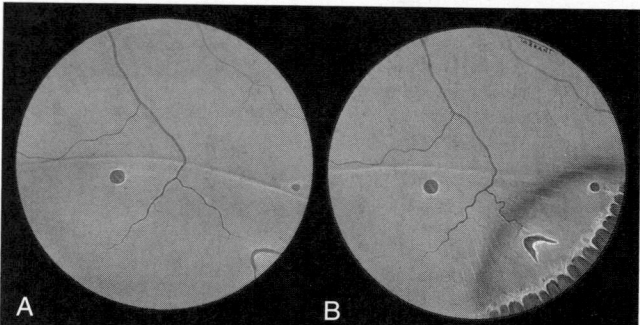

FIGURE 1-717 Appearance of retinal breaks in detached retina. A, Without scleral indentation; **B,** with indentation. (From Kanski JJ, Bowling B: *Clinical ophthalmology, a systematic approach,* ed 7, Philadelphia, 2010, Saunders.)

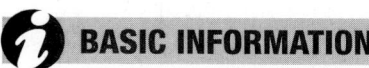

BASIC INFORMATION

DEFINITION

In a retinal hemorrhage, blood accumulates in the retinal and subretinal areas as a result of multiple causes (see "Etiology").

SYNONYMS

Pseudoxanthoma elasticum
Coats' disease
Retinal trauma
High-altitude retinopathy

ICD-9CM CODES
362.81 Retinal hemorrhage

EPIDEMIOLOGY & DEMOGRAPHICS

INCIDENCE (IN U.S.): Busy ophthalmologists see one or two cases a month.
PEAK INCIDENCE:
- In children: associated primarily with trauma and hematologic disorders (must consider shaken baby syndrome)
- Associated with trauma, diabetes, vascular disease, macular degeneration, altitude changes (mountain climbing)

PREDOMINANT AGE: Degenerative disease in older patients

PHYSICAL FINDINGS & CLINICAL PRESENTATION

- Hemorrhage within the retina or subretinal area (Fig. 1-718)
- Evidence of retinal tears, tumors, and inflammation; macular degeneration, drugs, diabetes

ETIOLOGY

- Diabetes
- Hypertension
- Trauma
- Inflammation
- Tumors
- Subretinal neovascularization
- Associated with diabetes and aging
- Rapid changes in altitude (mountain climbing or scuba diving)

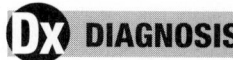

DIAGNOSIS

DIFFERENTIAL DIAGNOSIS

- Evaluate patients for local and systemic diseases.
- Trauma in children or adults
- Venous or arterial occlusion associated with atherosclerotic or heart disease may cause retinal hemorrhage.
- Rule out malignant melanoma, trauma, hypertensive cardiovascular disease.

Section II describes the differential diagnosis of acute painless loss of vision.

WORKUP

Complete general physical examination, evaluate for trauma; look for systemic diseases and medication etiologies.

LABORATORY TESTS

- Minimum: complete blood count, erythrocyte sedimentation rate, complete blood chemistries
- Fluorescein
- Angiography
- Visual field testing

IMAGING STUDIES

- Usually not necessary
- Trauma: skull radiographs or head CT
- Ultrasound
- Fluorescein angiography

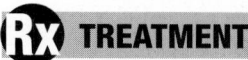

TREATMENT

NONPHARMACOLOGIC THERAPY

- Laser or treatment of underlying disorder
- Treat medical problems (age-related macular degeneration, etc.)

ACUTE GENERAL Rx

- Laser treatment is often indicated.
- Steroids may be indicated with macular degeneration (intravitreal injection).
- Treat underlying disease.
- Repair any damage from trauma.

CHRONIC Rx

- Laser treatment if hemorrhage is recurrent
- Vitamin therapy: high in zinc and antioxidants

DISPOSITION

Consider this condition an emergency.

REFERRAL

Immediate referral to an ophthalmologist; early treatment significantly affects outcome

PEARLS & CONSIDERATIONS

COMMENTS

- Vision may return substantially.
- Complete recovery depends on amount of scar tissue formed.
- Chronic situations have poor prognosis.

SUGGESTED READINGS
available at www.expertconsult.com

RELATED CONTENT

Diabetic Retinopathy (Patient Information)

AUTHOR: **MELVYN KOBY, M.D.**

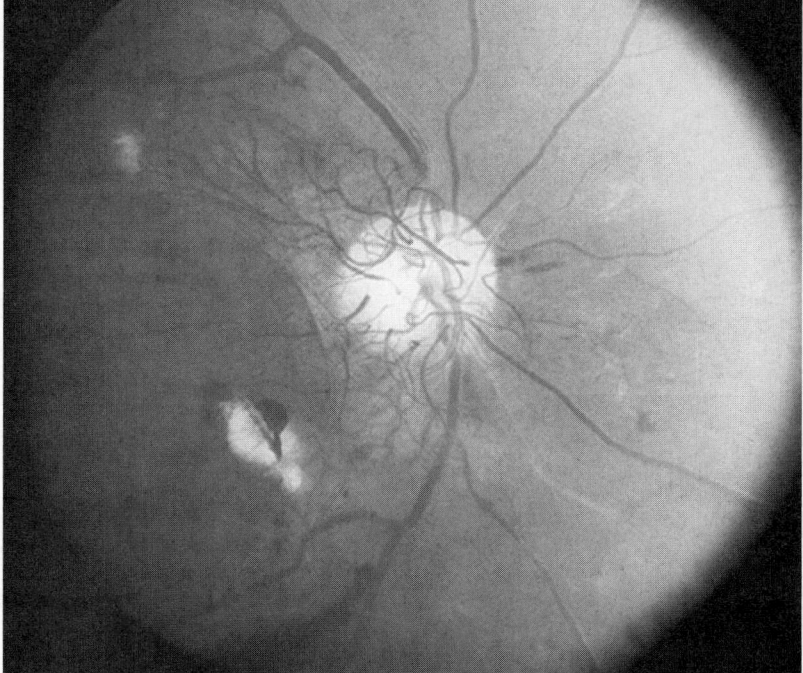

FIGURE 1-718 Fronds of neovascularization on the disc are present in this right eye. Temporally, two cotton-wool spots have adjacent intraretinal hemorrhage and preretinal hemorrhage. Native retinal arteries are narrowed and show evidence of sclerosis. (From Palay D [ed]: *Ophthalmology for the primary care physician,* St Louis, 1997, Mosby.)

BASIC INFORMATION

DEFINITION

Retinitis pigmentosa (RP) refers to a clinically and genetically diverse group of diffuse retinal dystrophies initially predominantly affecting the rod photoreceptor cells with subsequent degeneration of cones (rod-cone dystrophy).

ICD-9CM CODES
362.74 Retinitis pigmentosa, pigmentary retinal dystrophy

EPIDEMIOLOGY & DEMOGRAPHICS

PEAK INCIDENCE:
- Recessive incidence: in the 20s
- Dominant form: in the 40s

PREVALENCE (IN U.S.): One in 5000 persons. It is the most commonly encountered hereditary fundus dystrophy.

PREDOMINANT SEX: Depends on inheritance

PREDOMINANT AGE: The age of onset, rate of progression, eventual vision loss, and associated ocular features are frequently related to the mode of inheritance.

GENETICS:
- 19% dominant
- 19% recessive
- 8% X-linked
- 46% not known to be genetically related (mutations)
- 8% undetermined cause

PHYSICAL FINDINGS & CLINICAL PRESENTATION

- Deposition of retinal pigment in midperiphery and centrally in the retina (Fig. E1-719) with a pale optic nerve and narrowing of blood vessels (Fig. 1-720)
- Possible cataracts and macular edema
- Decrease in night vision and peripheral vision. Patients typically lose night vision to a greater extent than they lose day vision, and they lose peripheral vision before losing central vision.

ETIOLOGY

RP may occur as an isolated sporadic disorder, or may be inherited as AD, AR, or XL. Many cases are due to mutation of the rhodopsin gene. XL is the least common but most severe form, and may result in complete blindness by the third or fourth decade.

DIAGNOSIS

DIFFERENTIAL DIAGNOSIS

- Syphilis
- Old inflammatory scars
- Old hemorrhage
- Diabetes
- Toxic retinopathies (phenothiazines, chloroquine)

WORKUP

- Electrophysiologic studies
- Dark adaptation studies
- Visual fields

LABORATORY TESTS

- Usually not necessary
- VDRL (syphilis), glucose (selected patients)

IMAGING STUDIES

- Usually not necessary
- Rate of decline of vision for different groups cannot be accurately determined; decline rates are fastest with patients with mutations

TREATMENT

CHRONIC Rx

- No proven effective therapy
- Correction of biochemical abnormalities. Some success has been reported with subretinal gene therapy in which patients with mutations in the gene encoding RPE65 were treated with delivery under the retina of a normal RPE65 gene by intraocular injection
- Nutritional supplements: sometimes vitamin E or vitamin A may be helpful
- In patients with advanced disease, treatment options may include attempts to regenerate photoreceptors by transplantation or genetic manipulation of nonphotoreceptor retinal cell types

DISPOSITION

Disease may be either mild or severe, but if the patient is expected to progress to total blindness, counseling and early education are important.

REFERRAL

To ophthalmologist to confirm diagnosis

PEARLS & CONSIDERATIONS

COMMENTS

- The spider web–like appearance of macular degeneration should not be confused with the extra pigments sometimes seen in dark-skinned individuals.
- Patient education material can be obtained from the Retinitis Pigmentosa Foundation Fighting Blindness, 1401 Mt. Royal Avenue, 4th Floor, Baltimore, MD 21217.
- Research in fetal retinal pigment transplantation and computer chip implantation is ongoing.

SUGGESTED READINGS
available at www.expertconsult.com

RELATED CONTENT
Retinitis Pigmentosa (Patient Information)

AUTHOR: **MELVYN KOBY, M.D.**

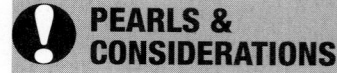

FIGURE 1-720 Retinitis pigmentosa. (From Behrman RE [ed]: *Nelson textbook of pediatrics*, Philadelphia, 2005, Saunders.)

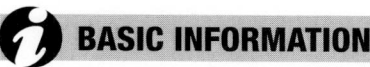

BASIC INFORMATION

DEFINITION

Retinoblastoma is an inherited, highly malignant congenital neoplasm arising from the neural layers of the retina.

ICD-9CM CODES
190.5 Retinoblastoma, malignant neoplasm of eyes, retina

EPIDEMIOLOGY & DEMOGRAPHICS

INCIDENCE (IN U.S.): Retinoblastoma affects 1 in 15,000 children, with ~300 children newly diagnosed each year in the United States. It is the most common primary intraocular malignancy of childhood.

PEAK INCIDENCE:
- 6 to 13 mo. Mean age at diagnosis is 12 mo for bilateral tumors and 24 mo for unilateral tumors.
- 72% diagnosed by age 3 yr
- 90% diagnosed by age 4 yr

PREDOMINANT AGE: 8 mo

GENETICS:
- Gene mutation or an autosomal-dominant gene with 80% to 95% penetration
- 5% mutations

PHYSICAL FINDINGS & CLINICAL PRESENTATION

- Leukocoria (white reflex or white pupil) (Fig. 1-721)
- White elevated retinal masses
- Strabismus
- Glaucoma
- Uveitis
- Vitreous masses and opacity

ETIOLOGY

The retinoblastoma gene is a tumor suppressor gene located on the long arm of chromosome 13 at region 14 that codes for the RB protein. ~60% of retinoblastomas are attributable to somatic, nonhereditary mutations.

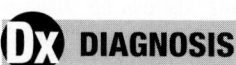

DIAGNOSIS

DIFFERENTIAL DIAGNOSIS

Examination of eye
- Strabismus
- Retinal detachment
- Uveitis
- Other tumors
- Glaucoma
- Coats' disease (pathologic telangiectatic retinal vessels that leak and lead to accumulation of subretinal fluid and lipid)
- Endophthalmitis
- Cataract
- Infectious

WORKUP

Diagnosis is by ophthalmologic examination. An awake examination to determine if the patient can fixate and extent of eye mobility should be done. Examination should also include visual acuity, papillary examination, extraocular movements, slit-lamp examination for evidence of iris neovascularization, hyphema or hypopyon, indirect ophthalmoscopy with 360 degrees of scleral depression, and fundus photographs documenting all lesions. Ophthalmologic examination is followed by ultrasonography of the eye and MRI of the orbits and brain to exclude extraocular extension and trilateral retinoblastoma.

CLASSIFICATION

Retinoblastoma is separated into intraocular and extraocular disease. The Reese-Ellsworth classification system became outdated as chemoreduction strategies became widely used for salvage therapy and a new international classification system for intraocular retinoblastoma was formulated in 2003, which more accurately reflects response to standardized chemotherapy regimen used in conjunction with focal consolidative therapy. The international classification system is subdivided into group A (small), group B (medium), group C (confined, medium), group D (diffuse, large), and group E (enucleation, advanced)

IMAGING STUDIES

- MRI: may show calcifications in retina
- Ultrasonography: good delineation of mass

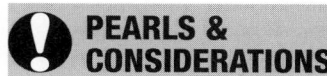

TREATMENT

Usually treated by a multidisciplinary team consisting of a pediatrician, an ophthalmologist, a pediatric oncologist, and pediatric radiation oncologist. Treatment depends on location and stage of tumor when diagnosed:
- Chemotherapy for larger tumors usually with carboplatin, etoposide, and vincristine. The goal of chemotherapy is to reduce the tumor volume for focal therapy with cryotherapy, laser, thermotherapy, or plaque bracytherapy.
- Radioactive plaque brachytherapy with iodine 125 or ruthenium 106 plaques and cryotherapy
- Surgical enucleation of the eye
- Radiation and chemotherapy

DISPOSITION

Overall there is a high cure rate (93% 5-yr survival in the United States) for retinoblastoma. Group A tumors generally have good visual and survival prognosis with focal consolidative therapy alone, groups B and C are treated with chemotherapy and focal therapy with good results (vision salvage rates up to 93%), group D patients often eventually require enucleation despite treatment.

REFERRAL

- To ophthalmologist, pediatric oncologist, and pediatric radiation oncologist
- Prospective parents with a family history of retinoblastoma should be referred for genetic counseling. Genetic testing should be carried out for most retinoblastoma patients unless it is declined.

PEARLS & CONSIDERATIONS

COMMENTS

- High incidence of second tumor in survivors compared with general population
- High incidence of lung cancer, bladder cancer, and other epithelial cancers

SUGGESTED READINGS
available at www.expertconsult.com

RELATED CONTENT
Retinoblastoma (Patient Information)

AUTHORS: **MELVYN KOBY, M.D.,** and **FRED F. FERRI, M.D.**

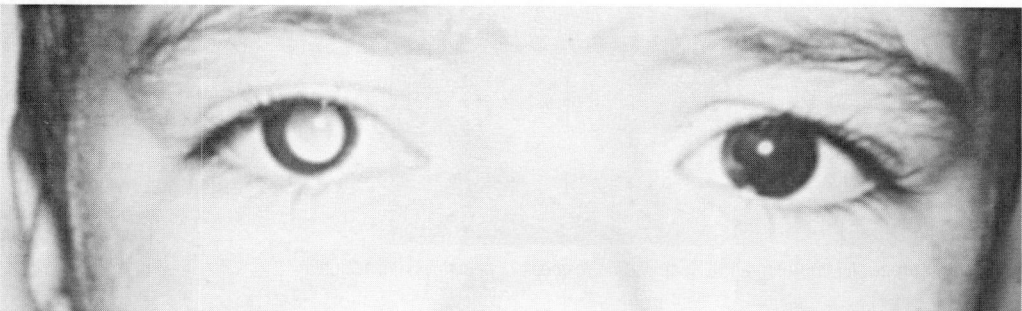

FIGURE 1-721 Leukocoria. White papillary reflex in a child with retinoblastoma. (From Behrman RE [ed]: *Nelson textbook of pediatrics,* Philadelphia, 2005, Saunders.)

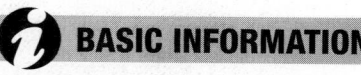

BASIC INFORMATION

DEFINITION

Rh incompatibility occurs when an absence of the D antigen on maternal red blood cells (RBCs) and its presence on fetal RBCs cause risk of isoimmunization.

ICD-9CM CODES
656.1 Rh incompatibility

EPIDEMIOLOGY & DEMOGRAPHICS

INCIDENCE:
- The absence of the D antigen (Rh− blood type) occurs in 15% of whites, 8% of blacks, and virtually no Asians or Native Americans. If the father's blood type is not known, the chance that an Rh− pregnant woman is bearing an Rh+ fetus is approximately 60%.
- Of those pregnancies complicated by Rh incompatibility, the risk of maternal isoimmunization to the D antigen is approximately 8% for each ABO-compatible pregnancy if no prophylaxis is given.
- Maternal-fetal ABO incompatibility is somewhat protective against Rh isoimmunization.

GENETICS: Five major loci determine Rh status: C, D, E, c, e. The presence of the D antigen results in an Rh+ individual. Its absence results in an Rh− individual. Of Rh+ fathers, 45% are homozygotes, and 55% are heterozygotes. For homozygous Rh+ fathers, the probability of an Rh+ offspring is 100%. The probability for heterozygotes is approximately 50%.

RISK FACTORS:
- Antepartum: fetal-to-maternal transfusion
- Intrapartum: fetal-to-maternal transfusion, spontaneous abortion, ectopic pregnancy, abruptio placentae, abdominal trauma, chorionic villus sampling, amniocentesis, percutaneous umbilical blood sampling (PUBS), external cephalic version, manual removal of the placenta, therapeutic abortion, autologous blood product administration

ETIOLOGY

The initial response to D antigen exposure is production of immunoglobulin (Ig) M (molecular weight 900,000) that does not cross the placenta. With a repeated exposure, IgG (MW 160,000) is produced. IgG can cross the placenta and enter the fetal circulation, producing hemolysis in the fetus. This may produce erythroblastosis fetalis or hemolytic disease in the newborn, resulting in antepartum or neonatal death or neurologic damage to the fetus because of hyperbilirubinemia and kernicterus.

DIAGNOSIS

LABORATORY TESTS

ABO and Rh blood type and an antibody screen as part of the initial prenatal profile
- If antibody screen negative:
  1. Repeat antibody screen at 28 wk gestation.
  2. Obtain neonatal blood type after delivery.
  3. If Rh incompatibility is confirmed by the neonatal blood type, a Kleihauer-Betke or rosette test should be performed to determine the amount of fetomaternal transfusion in the following high-risk circumstances: abruptio placentae, placenta previa, cesarean delivery, intrauterine manipulation, manual removal of the placenta.
- If anti-D antibody screen is positive:
  1. Maternal indirect Coombs test is needed to determine antibody titer.
  2. Determine paternal Rh status and zygosity.
  3. If father is heterozygous, PUBS or amniotic fluid is needed to determine fetal Rh status.

IMAGING STUDIES

Ultrasound evaluation can diagnose hydrops fetalis, but it cannot predict it.

TREATMENT

PREVENTION OF D ISOIMMUNIZATION

- 50 mcg of D immunoglobulin: after spontaneous or induced abortion or ectopic pregnancy <13 wk gestation.
- 300 mcg of D immunoglobulin (protects against 30 ml of fetal blood):
  1. After spontaneous or induced abortion >13 wk gestation, amniocentesis, chorionic villous sampling, PUBS, external cephalic version, or other intrauterine manipulation.
  2. As antepartum prophylaxis at 28 wk gestation. Maternal anti-D prophylaxis does not cause hemolysis in the fetus or newborn.
  3. At delivery if the neonate is D- or Du-positive.
  4. If Kleihauer-Betke or rosette test confirms >30 ml of fetal red blood in maternal circulation, additional D immunoglobulin is indicated. Confirm adequacy of therapy by a maternal indirect Coombs test 48 to 72 hr after Rh immune globulin is given.

MANAGEMENT OF D ISOIMMUNIZED PREGNANCIES

- Serial amniocentesis for assessment of OD_{450} after 25 wk gestation with interpretation of the Delta OD_{450} according to criteria established by Liley
- PUBS if ultrasonographic evidence of hydrops, rising zone II Delta OD_{450} values on amniocentesis, or maternal history of a severely affected child
- Intrauterine exchange transfusion if severe anemia is documented remote from term
- Initiation of steroids for lung maturation at 28 wk in severely affected pregnancies with delivery at lung maturity
- Delivery as soon as lung maturation is achieved in mild to moderately affected pregnancies

DISPOSITION

Survival of nonhydropic infants is 90%. Of infants with hydrops, 82% survive.

REFERRAL

Refer all Rh isoimmunized pregnancies to a tertiary care center before 18 to 20 wk gestation.

SUGGESTED READING
available at www.expertconsult.com

AUTHOR: **LAUREL M. WHITE, M.D.**

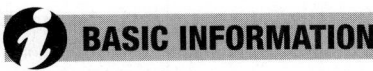

BASIC INFORMATION

DEFINITION

Rhabdomyolysis is the dissolution or disintegration of muscle, which causes membrane lysis and leakage of muscle constituents, resulting in the excretion of myoglobin in the urine. In general CK levels in excess of 5× normal and the presence of myoglobinuria with the appropriate clinical presentation (see below) are sufficient criteria for the diagnosis of rhabdomyolysis. Renal damage can occur as a result of tubular obstruction by myoglobin as well as hypovolemia.

ICD-9CM CODES
728.89 Rhabdomyolysis

EPIDEMIOLOGY & DEMOGRAPHICS

PREDOMINANT AGE: Rare in children. Increased risk in advanced age (>80 yr).
MORTALITY RATE: 8%
ONSET: The average length of time on statin therapy before rhabdomyolysis is 1 yr. Average time for onset of rhabdomyolysis after addition of fibrate to statin therapy is 32 days.

PHYSICAL FINDINGS & CLINICAL PRESENTATION

- Variable muscle tenderness. Rhabdomyolysis apart from statin use presents with muscle symptoms only 50% of the time.
- Weakness
- Muscular rigidity
- Fever
- Altered consciousness
- Muscle swelling
- Malaise, fatigue. In statin-induced rhabdomyolysis, fatigue (74%) is nearly as common as muscle pain (88%).

TABLE 1-362 Genetic Mutations Associated with Exertional Rhabdomyolysis

Gene	
Ryanodine receptor 1	*RyR1*
Myoadenylate deaminase	*AMPDA1*
Carnitine palmitoyltransferase II	*CPT2*
Myophosphorylase	*PYGM*
Phosphofructokinase	*PFKM*
Phosphorylase *b* kinase	*PHKA1*
Very long chain acyl coenzyme-A dehydrogenase	*ACAD9*
Phosphoglycerate mutase	*PGAMM*
Phosphoglycerate kinase	*PGK1*
Lactate dehydrogenase	*LDHA*
Cytochrome *c* oxidase	*COX I, II,* and *III*
Cytochrome *b* (complex III)	*CYTB*
Mitochondrial tRNA	*Mt-tRNA*
β-Sarcoglycan	*SGCB*

From Goldman L, Schafer AI: *Goldman's Cecil medicine,* ed 24, Philadelphia, 2012, Saunders.

- Dark urine: myoglobinuria may cause the urine to be reddish-brown

ETIOLOGY

- Exertion (exercise-induced). Genetic mutations associated with exertional rhabdomyolysis are described in Table 1-362.
- Electrical injury
- Drug-induced (statins, combination of statins with fibrates, or erythromycin, simvastatin and amiodarone, amphetamines, haloperidol)
- Compartment syndrome
- Multiple trauma
- Malignant hyperthermia
- Limb ischemia
- Reperfusion after revascularization procedures for ischemia
- Extensive surgical (spinal) dissection, bariatric surgery
- Tourniquet ischemia
- Prolonged static positioning during surgery
- Infectious and inflammatory myositis
- Metabolic myopathies
- Hypovolemia and urinary acidification are important precipitating causes in the development of acute renal failure
- Sickle cell trait is a predisposing condition
- Hypothyroidism
- Alcoholism
- Seizures
- Table 1-363 summarizes the various causes of rhabdomyolysis.

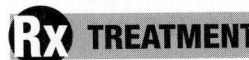

DIAGNOSIS

DIFFERENTIAL DIAGNOSIS

"Creatine Kinase Elevation" in Section IV describes a clinical algorithm for the evaluation of creatine phosphokinase (CPK) elevation.

LABORATORY TESTS

- Screening for myoglobinuria with a simple urine dipstick test using orthotoluidine or benzidine. Myoglobinuria does not occur in the absence of rhabdomyolysis; therefore, when present, it is the best marker and diagnostic cornerstone of rhabdomyolysis
- Blood urea nitrogen, creatinine
- Increased CK: CK levels typically peak 2 to 5 days after the initial insult (Fig. 1-723).

- Levels above 15,000 U/L are more likely to be associated with renal injury
- Hyperkalemia
- Hypocalcemia: due to influx and deposition of of Ca^{2+} in damaged muscle tissue. Hypercalcemia may follow resolution of rhabdomyolysis with subsequent release of calcium back into the circulation
- Hyperphosphatemia
- Elevations in serum myoglobin precede the rise in CK, but it is rapidly eliminated, making this test a less reliable marker of muscle injury
- Pigmented granular casts
- Hyperuricemia
- Anion gap metabolic acidosis may be present due to the release of organic acids from damaged muscle

TREATMENT

ACUTE GENERAL Rx

- Early, aggressive, high-volume IV fluid replacement. Fluid repletion reduces the accumulation of toxic intracellular contents caused by the rapid breakdown of muscle and subsequent renal damage.

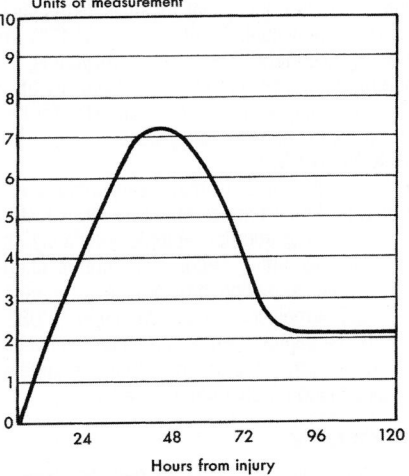

FIGURE 1-723 Typical creatine kinase elimination curve. (From Rosen P [ed]: *Emergency medicine,* ed 4, St Louis, 1998, Mosby.)

TABLE 1-363 Causes of Rhabdomyolysis

Muscle injury/ischemia	Trauma, pressure necrosis, electric shock, burns, acute vascular disease
Myofiber exhaustion	Seizures, excessive exercise, heat exhaustion
Toxins	Alcohol, cocaine, heroin, amphetamines, Ecstasy, phencyclidine, snakebite
Drugs	Statins, fibrates, zidovudine, neuroleptic malignant syndrome, azathioprine, theophylline, lithium, diuretics
Electrolyte disorders	Hypophosphatemia, hypokalemia, excess water shifts (hyperosmolality)
Infections	Viral (influenza, HIV, Coxsackievirus, Epstein-Barr virus), bacterial (*Legionella, Francisella, Streptococcus pneumoniae, Salmonella, Staphylococcus aureus*)
Familial	McArdle's disease, carnitine palmitoyl transferase deficiency, malignant hyperthermia
Other	Hypothyroidism, polymyositis, dermatomyositis

From Floege J et al: *Comprehensive clinical nephrology,* ed 4, Philadelphia, 2010, Saunders.

- Initiate volume repletion with normal saline at a rate of 200 to 1000 ml/hour depending on the setting and severity. Consider treatment with mannitol (up to 200 g/day and cumulative dose up to 800 g) to induce diuresis to prevent acute renal failure. Typically a 20% mannitol infusion at a dose of 0.5 g/kg is given over a 15-min period followed by an infusion at 0.1 g/kg/hr. Fluids should be administered at a rate that results in a urine output of 200 ml/hr until CK levels begin to decrease. Check for plasma osmolality and plasma osmolal gap. Discontinue mannitol if diuresis (>20 ml/hr) is not established. Maintain volume repletion until myoglobinuria is cleared (negative urine dipstick for blood).
- Monitor serum potassium frequently. Correct electrolyte imbalances. Correct hypocalcemia only if symptomatic or if severe hyperkalemia occurs.
- Treatment of electrolyte imbalances
- Alkalinization of urine (to maintain urine pH between 6 and 7 and keep serum pH at 7.50) is controversial but appears helpful in research models when administered early in the course of rhabdomyolysis. Urine alkalinization may trap myoglobin, thereby preventing toxic myoglobin precipitation, and lowers lipid peroxidation, reactive oxygen species formation, and myoglobin-induced vasoconstriction.
- Fasciotomy is indicated in compartment syndrome for preservation of muscle and nerve function. Fasciotomy can lead to rapid decompression of compartment syndrome.

DISPOSITION

Early diagnosis and management are necessary to avoid renal failure, which occurs in 30% of cases. Rhabdomyolysis accounts for 7% to 10% of all cases of acute kidney injury.

REFERRAL

Renal consultation

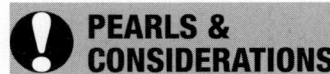

PEARLS & CONSIDERATIONS

COMMENTS

- A clinical algorithm for the evaluation of muscle cramps and aches is described in Section III.
- Statin-induced rhabdomyolysis is 12× more frequent when statins are combined with fibrates compared with statin monotherapy.

- Short-term high-dose corticosteroids (500 to 1000 mg of methylprednisolone) have been successfully used in the treatment of alcohol-induced rhabdomyolysis unresponsive to fluid repletion and may be reasonable in cases of severe rhabdomyolysis refractory to conventional treatment. Corticosteroids block the response of neutrophils to damage tissues and inhibit the chemotaxis of monocytes and neutrophils to sites of inflammation. It has been hypothesized that corticosteroid administration may help diminish the inflammatory exacerbation of muscle damage.

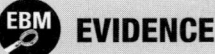

EVIDENCE

available at www.expertconsult.com

SUGGESTED READINGS

available at www.expertconsult.com

RELATED CONTENT

Statin-Induced Muscle Syndromes (Related Key Topic)
Rhabdomyolysis (Patient Information)

AUTHOR: **FRED F. FERRI, M.D.**

R

Diseases and Disorders

I

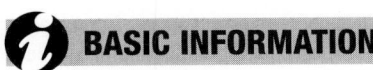

BASIC INFORMATION

DEFINITION

Rheumatoid arthritis (RA) is a systemic autoimmune disease characterized by inflammatory polyarthritis, which affects peripheral joints, especially the small joints of the hands and feet. Chronic untreated inflammation may lead to joint erosions and joint destruction.

ICD-9CM CODES
714.0 Rheumatoid arthritis

EPIDEMIOLOGY & DEMOGRAPHICS

INCIDENCE: Annual incidence in northern Europe and U.S. 0.15 to 0.60 per 1000
PEAK INCIDENCE: Steadily increases with age until the mid-70s
PREVALENCE: 0.5% to 1.0% of the worldwide population
PREDOMINANT SEX AND AGE: Male/female ratio of 1:2; prevalence increases with age
GENETICS: Genetic factors account for more than 50% of risk of disease. RA is polygenic; identified genetic associations include *HLA-DRB1, PTPN22,* and *PADI4.*
RISK FACTORS: Female sex, age, tobacco use, silica exposure, obesity

PHYSICAL FINDINGS & CLINICAL PRESENTATION

Initial presentation:
>6 wk of pain, swelling, warmth in one or more peripheral joints, frequently with symmetric joint involvement involving wrists, hands, and/or feet, and often associated with >1 hr of morning stiffness.
Most common joints involved include metacarpophalangeal (MCP), proximal interphalangeal (PIP), wrists, metatarsophalangeal (MTP), and ankles.
Also elbows, shoulders, hips, and knees.
Distal interphalangeal (DIP) joints are spared.
Sacroiliac and vertebral joints are spared except for C1 to C2.

Chronic longstanding disease:
"Swan-neck" (DIP flexion and PIP hyperextension) and "boutonniere" PIP flexion and DIP hyperextension) deformities (Fig. 1-724), as well as MCP subluxation resulting in ulnar drift (Fig. 1-725).
C1 to C2 inflammation can lead to odontoid erosion and transverse ligament laxity, resulting in atlantoaxial subluxation and cord compression.
Joint damage of wrists, elbows, shoulders, hips, and knees can lead to severe osteoarthritis, necessitating joint surgery and/or replacement.
Extraarticular manifestations:
Secondary Sjögren's syndrome (~35%): immune-mediated inflammation of lacrimal and salivary glands resulting in dry mouth and eyes (sicca syndrome).
Rheumatoid nodules (25%): on extensor surfaces and pressure points, in rheumatoid factor positive (RF+) disease. Histopathology demonstrates palisading histiocytes surrounding fibrinoid necrosis.
Normocytic normochromic anemia
Felty's syndrome: RA with splenomegaly and leukopenia
Pulmonary disease
Pleural disease (effusions, pleuritis)
Interstitial lung disease (up to 10% clinically significant)
Vasculitis
Cardiac disease
Pericarditis
↑ Risk cardiovascular disease
Ocular disease
Keratoconjunctivitis sicca (dry eye, without dry mouth/secondary Sjögren's) (10%)
Episcleritis, scleritis
Amyloidosis: longstanding RA. Can affect heart, kidney, liver, spleen, intestines, and skin.

ETIOLOGY

Unknown. It is likely that a combination of genetic and environmental factors leads to aberrant immune activation and inflammatory response in the joint. Stages of disease development presumably include:
- Initiation of immune response (trigger unknown, but environmental exposures such as tobacco and silica have been implicated.)
- Perpetuation of inflammatory response, with migration of inflammatory cells into joint space, activation of macrophage-like and fibroblast-like synoviocytes, and development of "synovial pannus," a thickened synovial membrane
- The pannus releases proinflammatory cytokines (TNF-α, IL-1, IL-6, IL-8), as well as proteases, which erode cartilage and bone
- Many of the new "biologic" disease-modifying antirheumatic drugs (DMARDs) are engineered to target these cytokines

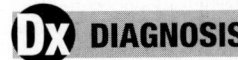

DIAGNOSIS

The American College of Rheumatology and the European League Against Rheumatism have developed new classification criteria for RA. Four variables constitute the new criteria:
1. The number and size of involved joints (score 0 to 5, with higher scores for a larger number of small joints affected)
2. Results of rheumatoid factor (RF) and anticitrullinated protein antibody testing (score 0 to 3, with more points for a high positive RF or anti-CCP)
3. Abnormal sedimentation rate or elevated C-reactive protein (1 point)
4. Symptom duration >6 wk (1 point)
Scores ≥6 points are considered to have "definite RA." Maximum score is 10 points.

DIFFERENTIAL DIAGNOSIS

- Infections: parvovirus B19, hepatitis B, hepatitis C, poststreptococcal reactive arthritis, acute rheumatic fever
- Systemic lupus erythematosus
- Seronegative spondyloarthropathies
- Calcium pyrophosphate deposition (CPPD or "pseudo-RA")
- Polymyalgia rheumatica
- Hemochromatosis
- Scleroderma

LABORATORY TESTS

- RF. An immunoglobulin directed against the Fc region of the IgG

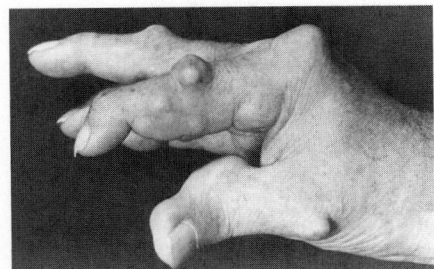

FIGURE 1-725 Rheumatoid arthritis. Hand of a 60-year-old man with seropositive rheumatoid arthritis. There are fixed deformities and gross rheumatoid nodules. (From Canoso JJ: *Rheumatology in primary care,* Philadelphia, 1997, Saunders.)

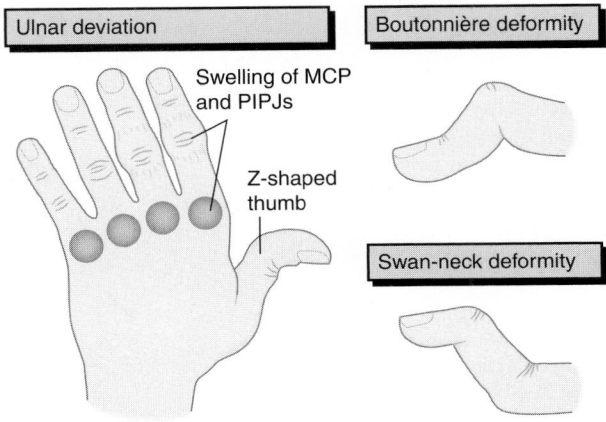

FIGURE 1-724 Characteristic hand deformities in rheumatoid arthritis. *MCP,* Metacarpophalanges; *PIPJs,* proximal interphalangeal joints. (From Ballinger A: *Kumar & Clark's essentials of clinical medicine,* ed 6, Edinburgh, 2012, Saunders.)

○ Sensitivity ~60%
○ Specificity ~80%. False positives are seen with hepatitis C, subacute bacterial endocarditis, sarcoidosis, malignancy, Sjögren's, SLE, increasing age
• Anti-cyclic citrullinated peptide (anti-CCP) antibodies. More specific than RF for RA (up to 95% to 98%). Sensitivity similar to RF. The presence of either RF or anti-CCP ("seropositive RA") is associated with more severe RA.
• ↑ Erythrocyte sedimentation rate (ESR), ↑ C-reactive protein (CRP)
• CBC with differential: possible mild anemia and leukocytosis
• Synovial fluid: inflammatory, with >2000 PMNs.

IMAGING STUDIES

Plain radiography:
• Earlier changes include soft tissue swelling, joint space narrowing, and periarticular osteopenia.
• Later changes include periarticular erosions, especially in MCPs, PIPs, MTPs, and wrist. This reflects cartilage and bone destruction secondary to pannus (Fig. 1-726).
• MRI and musculoskeletal ultrasound are more sensitive for detecting erosive disease and joint effusion/synovitis.

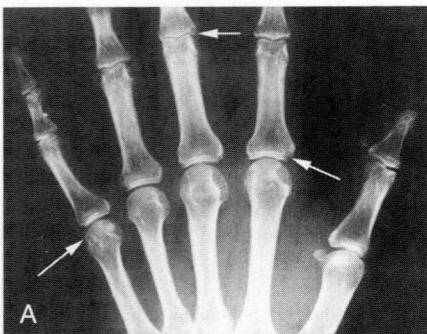
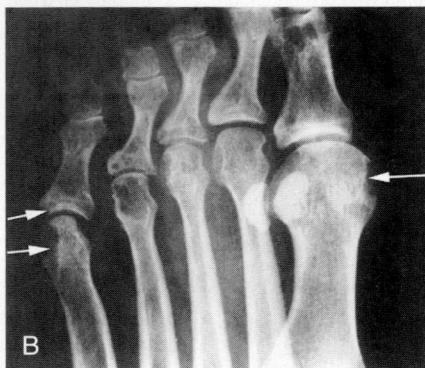

FIGURE 1-726 Rheumatoid arthritis. A, Periarticular osteopenia and marginal erosions in metacarpophalangeal joints and a proximal interphalangeal *(arrows)*. **B,** In the same patient, marginal erosions at metatarsal heads. (From Canoso JJ [ed]: *Rheumatology in primary care,* Philadelphia, 1997, Saunders.)

Rx TREATMENT

Early identification and treatment of RA with DMARDs are crucial. More than half of patients have radiographic joint damage within 2 yr of disease onset, but early aggressive treatment (with DMARDs) is associated with less damage.

ACUTE GENERAL Rx

• NSAIDs: Sometimes used initially to relieve pain and mild inflammation, or used later in the disease course for additional control of mild pain. NSAIDs are NOT disease modifying.
• Corticosteroids: oral or intraarticular, frequently used initially to reduce inflammation rapidly until oral DMARD treatments take effect. They may also be used during acute flares or in low doses for additional control of inflammation. They have many side effects, including but not limited to weight gain, increased risk of diabetes, osteoporosis, and avascular necrosis.

CHRONIC Rx

DMARDs: Can be classified into "nonbiologic" and "biologic" treatments.
  Nonbiologic DMARDs: commonly used agents are methotrexate (MTX), hydroxychloroquine (HCQ), sulfasalazine (SSZ), and leflunomide. Most of these are associated with potential toxicity and require close monitoring. They are also slow-acting drugs that require >8 wk to become fully effective.
    MTX is the most commonly used DMARD worldwide for the treatment of RA.
    "Triple therapy"—MTX, HCQ, and SSZ are superior to MTX alone.
  Biologic DMARDs: newer biologically engineered therapies, which target cytokines and cells involved in the RA inflammatory response. Major side effects include an increased risk of severe infection, most notably reactivation of tuberculosis with anti-TNF agents. A negative PPD is prerequisite to initiate therapy. Biologic DMARDs are most effective when used in combination with a nonbiologic DMARD, usually MTX.
    Tumor necrosis factor α inhibitors (TNFI). Includes infliximab, etanercept, adalimumab, certolizumab pegol, and golimumab.
    Abatacept (CTLA-4Ig). A recombinant protein that prevents costimulatory binding of antigen presenting cell to T cell, preventing T cell activation.
    Tocilizumab (anti–IL-6). A monoclonal antibody against the IL-6 receptor.
    Rituximab (anti-CD20). A monoclonal antibody against CD20 antigen on B lymphocytes.

DISPOSITION

• Remissions and exacerbations are common, but condition is chronically progressive in the majority of cases.
• Joint degeneration and deformity often lead to disability. Joint replacement is indicated for patients with severe joint damage whose symptoms are poorly controlled by medical management.
• Early and aggressive diagnosis and treatment are crucial in preventing or slowing joint destruction.

REFERRAL

• Early referral to rheumatologist
• Orthopedic consultation for corrective surgery

❗ PEARLS & CONSIDERATIONS

RA sometimes develops acutely in the postpartum patient; conversely, many patients with RA will experience remission during pregnancy.

EBM EVIDENCE

available at www.expertconsult.com

SUGGESTED READINGS

available at www.expertconsult.com

RELATED CONTENT

Rheumatoid Arthritis (Patient Information)

AUTHOR: **KERRI BATRA, M.D.**

R

Diseases and Disorders

I

BASIC INFORMATION

DEFINITION

Allergic rhinitis is an IgE-mediated hypersensitivity response to nasally inhaled allergens that causes sneezing, rhinorrhea, nasal pruritus, and congestion. It may be seasonal or perennial.

SYNONYMS

Hay fever
IgE-mediated rhinitis
Seasonal allergic rhinitis
SAR

ICD-9CM CODES
477.9 Allergic rhinitis

EPIDEMIOLOGY & DEMOGRAPHICS

- Allergic rhinitis affects approximately 10% to 20% of the U.S. population and 40% of children.
- Mean age of onset is 8 to 12 yr.
- The prevalence of allergic rhinitis in patients presenting to their primary care provider with nasal symptoms is estimated to be 30% to 60%.

PHYSICAL FINDINGS & CLINICAL PRESENTATION

- Pale or violaceous mucosa of the turbinates caused by venous engorgement (this can distinguish it from erythema present in viral rhinitis)
- Nasal polyps
- Lymphoid hyperplasia in the posterior oropharynx with cobblestone appearance
- Erythema of the throat, conjunctival and scleral injection
- Clear nasal discharge
- Clinical presentation: usually consists of sneezing, nasal congestion, cough, postnasal drip, loss of or alteration of smell, and sensation of plugged ears

ETIOLOGY

- Pollens in the springtime, ragweed in fall, grasses in the summer
- Dust, mites, animal allergens
- Smoke or any irritants
- Perfumes, detergents, soaps
- Emotion, changes in atmospheric pressure or temperature

DIAGNOSIS

DIFFERENTIAL DIAGNOSIS

- Infections (sinusitis; viral, bacterial, or fungal rhinitis)
- Rhinitis medicamentosa (cocaine, sympathomimetic nasal drops)
- Vasomotor rhinitis (e.g., secondary to air pollutants)
- Septal obstruction (e.g., deviated septum), nasal polyps, nasal neoplasms
- Systemic diseases (e.g., Wegener's granulomatosis, hypothyroidism [rare])

WORKUP

- The initial strategy should be to determine whether patients should undergo diagnostic testing or receive empirical treatment.
- Workup is often unnecessary if the diagnosis is apparent. A detailed medical history is useful in identifying the culprit allergen.
- Selected patients with allergic rhinitis that is not controlled with standard therapy may benefit from allergy testing to target allergen avoidance measures or guide immunotherapy. Allergy testing can be performed using skin testing or radioallergosorbent (RAST) testing. Immunoglobulin E (IgE) testing using newest generation assays is also an excellent tool for diagnosing the cause of symptoms related to rhinitis. Allergy testing with skin or blood testing is most useful as confirmatory tests when the patient's history is compatible with an IgE-mediated reaction and should generally be reserved for ambiguous or complicated cases.
- Examination of nasal smears for the presence of neutrophils to rule out infectious causes and the presence of eosinophils (suggestive of allergy) may be useful in selected patients.
- Peripheral blood eosinophil counts are not useful in allergy diagnosis.

TREATMENT

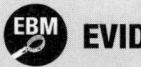

NONPHARMACOLOGIC THERAPY

- Maintain allergen-free environment by covering mattresses and pillows with allergen-proof casings, eliminating carpeting, eliminating animal products, and removing dust-collecting fixtures.
- Use of air purifiers and dust filters is helpful.
- Maintain humidity in the environment below 50% to prevent dust mites and mold.
- Use air conditioners, especially in the bedroom.
- Remove pets from homes of patients with suspected sensitivity to animal allergens.
- Use of acupuncture to treat seasonal allergic rhinitis is controversial. A recent trial showed that acupuncture led to statistically significant improvement in disease-specific quality of life and antihistamine use measures after 8 weeks of treatment compared with sham acupuncture and with rescue medication alone.

ACUTE GENERAL Rx

- Determine if the patient is troubled by swollen turbinates (best treated with decongestants) or blockages secondary to mucus (effectively treated by antihistamines).
- Topical nasal steroids are very effective and are preferred by many as first-line treatment for allergic rhinitis in adults. Patients should be instructed on proper use and informed that improvement might not occur for at least 1 wk after initiation of therapy. Commonly available inhalers follow.
  - Beclomethasone dipropionate: one to two sprays in each nostril bid
  - Fluticasone: initially two sprays in each nostril qd or one spray in each nostril bid, decreasing to one spray in each nostril qd based on response
  - Flunisolide: initially two sprays in each nostril bid
  - Budesonide: two sprays in each nostril bid or four sprays in each nostril qam
- Most first-generation antihistamines can cause considerable sedation and anticholinergic symptoms. The second-generation antihistamines (loratadine, fexofenadine, cetirizine, levocetirizine, desloratadine) are preferred because they do not have any significant anticholinergic or sedative effects.
- Montelukast, a leukotriene receptor antagonist commonly used for asthma, is also effective for allergic rhinitis. Usual adult dose is 10 mg qd.
- Azelastine is an antihistamine nasal spray effective for seasonal allergic rhinitis. Olopatadine is an intranasal H_1-antihistamine alternative to azestaline in mild to moderate seasonal allergic rhinitis.

CHRONIC Rx

- Cromolyn sodium: one spray to each nostril three to four times daily can be used for prophylaxis (mast cell stabilizer).
- Immunotherapy is generally reserved for patients responding poorly to the above treatments.

DISPOSITION

Most patients experience significant relief with avoidance of allergens and proper use of medications.

REFERRAL

Allergy testing in patients with severe symptoms who are unresponsive to therapy or when the diagnosis is uncertain

EVIDENCE

available at www.expertconsult.com

SUGGESTED READINGS
available at www.expertconsult.com

RELATED CONTENT
Allergic Rhinitis (Patient Information)

AUTHOR: **FRED F. FERRI, M.D.**

BASIC INFORMATION

DEFINITION

Rickets is a result of deficient mineralization causing softening and weakening of bones in infants and children. The mineralization impairment may be secondary to abnormal calcium, phosphorus, or vitamin D metabolism leading to accumulation of osteoid before epiphyseal closure, compromising bone stability. When this occurs in adulthood after epiphyseal closure, it is referred to as osteomalacia. Renal osteodystrophy is a term used to describe a similar condition in patients with chronic kidney disease. Certain forms of the disorder may respond only to high doses of vitamin D and are referred to as vitamin D–resistant rickets (VDRR).

ICD-9CM CODES
268.0 Active rickets
268.1 Late effect rickets
275.3 Vitamin D–resistant rickets, familial hypophosphatemia
588.0 Renal rickets (renal osteodystrophy)
268.2 Osteomalacia

RISK FACTORS:
- Children ages 6 to 24 months
- Premature infants
- Residents of northern latitudes with inadequate sunlight exposure
- Solely breastfed infants
- Darker skin pigmentation
- Use of anticonvulsants

PHYSICAL FINDINGS & CLINICAL PRESENTATION

The classic clinical presentation of children with rickets includes the following:
- Apathy, muscle weakness, delayed growth
- Skeletal pain and swollen joints
- Protuberant abdomen due to muscle hypotonia
- Widened sutures, delayed closure of fontanelles, and frontal bossing of head
- Craniotabes (softening of skull bones)
- Delayed eruption and poorly mineralized teeth
- Bowing deformity of lower extremities, specifically femur and tibia (Fig. 1-727)
- Rachitic rosary (enlargement and cupping of the costochondral junctions)
- Harrison's groove (indentation of the lower ribs)
- Pathologic fractures

The less pronounced clinical presentation of adults with osteomalacia includes the following:
- Skeletal pain and bone tenderness
- Muscle hypotonia and proximal muscle weakness
- Pathologic fractures
- Gait disturbances

ETIOLOGY

The most common cause of rickets and osteomalacia is vitamin D deficiency. This may arise from various conditions, including inadequate dietary intake, malabsoption, and the additional risk factors listed previously. Malabsorption that causes inefficient mineralization is observed in such diseases as cystic fibrosis and celiac disease. Vitamin D is required for adequate calcium absorption in the GI tract. If a deficiency of vitamin D is present, dietary calcium is not absorbed properly, and this leads to hypocalcemia.

Other causes specifically include vitamin D–dependent rickets, VDRR, and hereditary hypophosphatemic rickets.
- VDRR type I results from abnormalities in the gene coding for 25 (OH)D3-1-alpha-hydroxylase, and type II results from defective vitamin D receptors.
- Chronic renal failure can produce renal osteodystrophy (renal rickets). This results in decreased excretion of phosphate, therefore elevating serum phosphorus, along with elevated parathyroid hormone (PTH) and low levels of 1,25-OH vitamin D.

DIAGNOSIS

DIFFERENTIAL DIAGNOSIS
- Osteoporosis
- Hyperparathyroidism
- Hyperthyroidism
- Hypophosphatasia
- Metaphyseal dysostoses

WORKUP

Diagnosis is clinically based, and it is often challenging to determine the exact cause. A dietary and medication history for children is important. Bone biopsy is generally not performed; however, it is the diagnostic gold standard.

LABORATORY TESTS
- Requires a high degree of interest because many of the conditions are so similar that only a complicated laboratory evaluation may establish the diagnosis.
- Blood testing would include serum calcium, inorganic phosphorus (Pi), alkaline phosphate, PTH, 25-OH vitamin D, creatinine, and liver enzymes.

IMAGING STUDIES
- In rickets, characteristic radiologic findings include irregular epiphyseal-metaphyseal junctions with widening and flaring of the epiphyses of long bones, causing bowing.

- Pseudofractures (Looser zones) and narrow radiolucent lines may be seen as a result of microfractures at high stress points or at the location of entry of blood vessels into the bone and are observed in severe rickets and osteomalacia.

TREATMENT

- Treatment is dependent on the underlying cause.
- VDRR type I is treated with vitamin D. The earliest biochemical change after initiation of treatment is an increase in the level of phosphorus followed by a rise in calcium level. Serum calcium, phosphorus, alkaline phosphatase, and calcidiol levels and urine calcium and phosphorus levels should be obtained within 2 wk of initiation of therapy and periodically. The treatment of type II is more complex and requires the expertise of an endocrinologist and/or nephrologists.
- Familial hypophosphatemic rickets is treated with calcitriol and oral phosphorus.
- Oral phosphorus alone is the treatment of choice for hereditary hypophosphatemic rickets with hypercalciuria.

REFERRAL
- Because of the complex nature of many of these disorders, a qualified endocrinologist and nephrologist should be consulted for treatment.
- Orthopedic consultation may be required for some cases of bowlegs or spinal deformities, which may require specific bracing for long-term growth of the bones. If the deformity is very severe, it may require surgery.
- Surgical care is indicated for slipped capital femoral epiphysis, which is fairly common in renal rickets.

SUGGESTED READINGS
available at www.expertconsult.com

RELATED CONTENT
Vitamin D Deficiency (Patient Information)

AUTHOR: **STEPHANIE A. CURRY, M.D.**

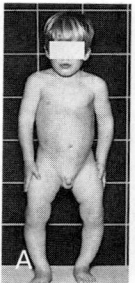 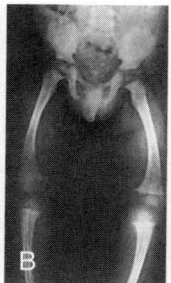 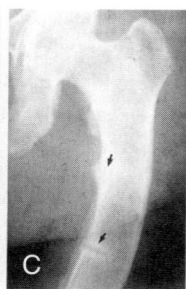

FIGURE 1-727 A, A typical example of rickets. Note the bowing of the femurs and tibiae, which may result from vitamin D deficiency, phosphate deficiency, or other causes. **B,** A skeletal radiograph of a child with rickets. Note that the weight-bearing bones of the lower extremities are bowed and that the epiphyses are open, mottled, and overgrown. **C,** Looser zones or pseudofractures that are characteristic of osteomalacia or rickets. Because the epiphyses are closed, the patient is an adult. This radiograph is diagnostic of osteomalacia. (From Stewart A: Metabolic bone diseases. In Andreoli TE et al [eds]: *Cecil essentials of medicine*, ed 8, Philadelphia, 2010, Saunders.)

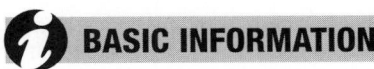

BASIC INFORMATION

DEFINITION

Rocky Mountain spotted fever (RMSF) is a life-threatening, tick-borne febrile illness caused by infection with *Rickettsia rickettsii*. The infection occurs when *R. rickettsii* in the salivary glands of a vector tick is transmitted into the dermis, spreading and replicating in the cytoplasm of endothelial cells and eliciting widespread vasculitis and end-organ damage.

ICD-9CM CODES
082.0 Rocky Mountain spotted fever

EPIDEMIOLOGY & DEMOGRAPHICS

INCIDENCE: 0.18 to 0.32 cases per 100,000 person-years
PREVALENCE: Most prevalent in the Southeast, followed by the South Central states, but seen anywhere (Fig. E1-728). It has recently been reported in eastern Arizona, with common brown dog ticks (*Rhipicephalus sanguineus*) implicated as a vector of *R. rickettsii*.
PREDOMINANT SEX: Affects both genders equally
PREDOMINANT AGE: Occurs at any age, but more likely in children ages 5 to 14 yr

PHYSICAL FINDINGS & CLINICAL PRESENTATION

- Incubation: 2 to 14 days
- First symptoms: fever, headache, malaise, myalgias

Common History, Signs, or Symptoms	%
Tick bite	65
Fever	100
Rash	90
Rash on palms and soles (Fig. E1-729)	80
Headache	90
Myalgia	75
Nausea or vomiting	60
Abdominal pain	40
Conjunctivitis	30
Edema	20
Pneumonitis	15
Any severe neurologic complication (including stupor, delirium, seizures, ataxia, papilledema, focal neurologic deficits, and coma)	30

- Rash:
  - Appears during first 3 days in 50%; by day 5, 80% have it. No rash in 10%.
  - Initial appearance: blanching erythematous macules on wrists and ankles that then spread to trunk, palms, and soles.
  - Lesions may evolve into papules and eventually become nonblanching (petechiae or palpable purpura).
- Gastrointestinal symptoms:
  - Nausea, vomiting, and abdominal pain are common
  - Occasionally may mimic an "acute abdomen" (e.g., appendicitis, cholecystitis)
  - Mild hepatitis
- Cardiopulmonary involvement:
  - Interstitial pneumonitis
  - Myocarditis
- Renal problems:
  - Prerenal azotemia
  - Interstitial nephritis
  - Glomerulonephritis
- Neurologic involvement:
  - Encephalitis (confusion, lethargy, delirium)
  - Ataxia
  - Convulsion
  - Cranial nerve palsy
  - Speech impediment
  - Hemiparesis or paraparesis
  - Spasticity
- Fulminant RMSF:
  - Early, widespread vascular necrosis leading to multisystem illness and death

ETIOLOGY & PATHOGENESIS

- Infectious agent: *R. rickettsii* (an intracellular bacterium)
- Vector: dog tick and wood tick (vertical transmission exists in ticks, but horizontal transmission involving rodents represents an important reservoir for the agent). In the United States *R. rickettsii* is transmitted mainly by the American dog tick (*Dermacentor variabilis*) and the Rocky Mountain wood tick (*D. andersoni*).
- Pathogenesis: the spread of *R. rickettsii* is hematogenous with attachment to the vascular endothelium, causing a vasculitis. The manifestations of this illness are caused by increased vascular permeability.

DIAGNOSIS

DIFFERENTIAL DIAGNOSIS

Influenza A, enteroviral infection, typhoid fever, leptospirosis, infectious mononucleosis, viral hepatitis, sepsis, ehrlichiosis, gastroenteritis, acute abdomen, bronchitis, pneumonia, meningococcemia, disseminated gonococcal infection, secondary syphilis, bacterial endocarditis, toxic shock syndrome, scarlet fever, rheumatic fever, measles, rubella, typhus, rickettsialpox, Lyme disease, drug hypersensitivity reactions, idiopathic thrombocytopenic purpura, thrombotic thrombocytopenic purpura, Kawasaki disease, immune complex vasculitis, connective tissue disorders.

WORKUP

Consider RMSF in any patient with an acute febrile illness with headache and myalgia, especially with an associated history of tick exposure. Absence of rash does not rule out the diagnosis.

LABORATORY TESTS

Routine Tests	%
White cell count	
$<10,000/mm^3$	72
>10% bands	69
Platelet count	
$<150,000/mm^3$	52
$<99,000/mm^3$	32
Serum sodium value <132 mEq/L	56
Aspartate aminotransferase $\geq 2\times$ normal	62
Alanine aminotransferase $\geq 2\times$ normal	39
Bilirubin value >1.4 mg/dl	30
Cerebrospinal fluid	
Opening pressure ≥ 250 mm H_2O	14
Glucose value ≤ 50 mg/dl	8
Protein value ≥ 50 mg/dl	35
White cell count $\geq 5/mm^3$	38
Mononuclear cell predominance	46
Polymorphonuclear cell predominance	50

- Etiologic tests:
  - Antibody titers to *R. rickettsii* (by indirect fluorescent antibody test). The diagnosis of RMSF requires a fourfold increase 2 wk apart and thus is not helpful in the care of the patients despite a sensitivity and specificity of near 100%.
  - The only test that can provide a timely diagnosis is the immunohistologic demonstration of *R. rickettsii* in skin biopsy specimens.

TREATMENT

- Oral or IV doxycycline, 200 mg/day in 2 divided doses for 7 days or for 2 days after defervescence
- Chloramphenicol, 50 mg/kg/day in 4 divided doses; chloramphenicol may be preferred during pregnancy because of the effects of doxycycline on fetal bones and teeth; therapy continued for at least 2 days after defervescence

PROGNOSIS

Fatality rate: 1% to 4% (five times greater if treatment is initiated after day 5 of illness, which is more likely in the absence of rash and during seasonal nonpeak tick activity). Long-term sequelae seen in patients who recover from severe RMSF: paraparesis, hearing loss; peripheral neuropathy; bladder and bowel incontinence; cerebellar, vestibular, and motor dysfunction; language disorders; limb amputation; and scrotal pain after cutaneous necrosis.

SUGGESTED READINGS
available at www.expertconsult.com

RELATED CONTENT
Rocky Mountain Spotted Fever (Patient Information)

AUTHOR: **FRED F. FERRI, M.D.**

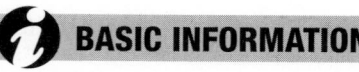 **BASIC INFORMATION**

DEFINITION

Rosacea is a chronic skin disorder characterized by papules and pustules affecting the face and often associated with flushing and erythema.

SYNONYMS

Acne rosacea

ICD-9CM CODES

695.3 Rosacea

EPIDEMIOLOGY & DEMOGRAPHICS

- Rosacea occurs in one in 20 Americans
- Onset often between ages 30 and 50 yr
- More common in people of Celtic origin; however, this disease may be overlooked in nonwhites because skin pigmentation results in atypical presentation
- Female/male ratio of 3:1

PHYSICAL FINDINGS & CLINICAL PRESENTATION

- Facial erythema, presence of papules, pustules, and telangiectasia.
- Excessive facial warmth and redness are the predominant presenting symptoms.
- Itching is generally absent.
- Comedones are absent (unlike acne).
- Women are more likely to show symptoms on the chin and cheeks, whereas in men the nose is commonly involved.
- Ocular findings (mild dryness and irritation with blepharitis, conjunctival injection, burning, stinging, tearing, eyelid inflammation, swelling, and redness) are present in 50% of patients.

Rosacea can be classified into four major subtypes:
1. Erythematotelangiectatic (vascular): erythema in central part of face, telangiectasia, flushing
2. Papulopustular (inflammatory): presence of dome-shaped erythematous papules and small pustules, in addition to facial erythema, flushing, and telangiectasia
3. Phymatosis (Fig. E1-730): presence of thickened skin with prominent pores that may affect the nose (rhinophyma), chin (gnathophyma), forehead (metophyma), eyelids (blepharophyma), and ears (otophyma)
4. Ocular: conjunctival injection, sensation of foreign body in the eye, telangiectasia and erythema of lid margins, scaling.

ETIOLOGY

- Unknown but believed to involve the vasculature
- Hot drinks, alcohol, and sun exposure may accentuate the erythema by causing vasodilation of the skin.
- Flare-ups may also result from reactions to medications (e.g., simvastatin, angiotensin-converting enzyme inhibitors, vasodilators, fluorinated corticosteroids), stress, extreme heat or cold, wind, humidity, strenuous exercise, spicy drinks, menstruation.

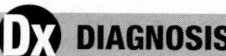 **DIAGNOSIS**

DIFFERENTIAL DIAGNOSIS

- Drug eruption
- Acne vulgaris
- Contact dermatitis
- Systemic lupus erythematosus
- Carcinoid flush
- Idiopathic facial flushing
- Seborrheic dermatitis
- Facial sarcoidosis
- Photodermatitis
- Mastocytosis
- Perioral dermatitis
- Granulomas of the skin

WORKUP

Diagnosis is based on clinical findings. Distinguishing features between acne and rosacea are the presence of telangiectasia and deep diffuse erythema and absence of comedones in rosacea.

 TREATMENT

NONPHARMACOLOGIC THERAPY

- Avoid alcohol, excessive sun exposure, and hot drinks of any type.
- Use of mild, nondrying soap is recommended; local skin irritants should be avoided.
- Reassure patient that rosacea is completely unrelated to poor hygiene.
- Vascular laser surgery is effective for telangiectasia.
- Surgical options are available for rhinophyma.

GENERAL Rx

- Several classes of drugs are used in treatment of rosacea, including the metronidazole family, the tetracycline family, and azelaic acid.
- Vascular rosacea: topical therapy with metronidazole aqueous gel (MetroGel) applied bid is effective as initial therapy for mild cases. A new 1% formulation of metronidazole (Noritate) applied daily may improve patient compliance. Clindamycin lotion (Cleocin), sulfacetamide, or erythromycin 2% solution may also be effective.
- Pustular and ocular rosacea: systemic antibiotics (doxycycline 100 mg qd or tetracycline 250 mg qid until symptoms diminish, then taper off). Minocycline 50 to 100 mg qd should be used only in resistant cases because this medication is expensive. Oral metronidazole (200 mg qd to bid) for 4 to 6 wk is also effective.
- Isotretinoin (Accutane) 0.5 to 1 mg/kg/day in two divided doses for 15 to 20 wk can be used for refractory papular and pustular rosacea; use of retinoids may, however, worsen erythema and telangiectasis.
- Laser treatment is an option for progressive telangiectasias or rhinophyma.
- Erythema and flushing may respond to low-dose clonidine (0.05 mg bid).
- Treatment of phymatous rosacea: oral tetracyclines, oral isotretinoin, ablative/pulsed dye laser therapy, electrosurgery.
- Treatment of ocular rosacea: topical or oral tetracyclines, artificial tears, and/or lid cleansing for eyelid hygiene.

DISPOSITION

- Rosacea is often resistant to initial treatment and recurrent. Periods of remission and relapse are common.
- The progression of rosacea is variable. Typical stages include:
  1. Facial flushing
  2. Erythema and/or edema and ocular symptoms
  3. Papules and pustules
  4. Rhinophyma

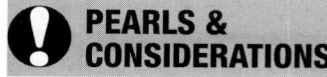 **PEARLS & CONSIDERATIONS**

COMMENTS

- The course of the disease is typically chronic, with remissions and relapses.
- Patients with resistant cases may have *Demodex folliculorum* mite infestation or tinea infection (diagnosis can be confirmed with potassium hydroxide examination); the role of *D. folliculorum* in rosacea is unclear. These mites can sometimes be found in large numbers in the lesions; however, their numbers do not generally decline with treatment.
- Rosacea can result in emotional and social stigmas, especially because many people associate rosacea and rhinophyma with alcohol abuse.
- Early consultation with an ophthalmologist is recommended in patients with suspected ocular involvement.

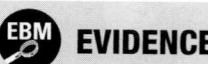 **EVIDENCE**

available at www.expertconsult.com

SUGGESTED READINGS

available at www.expertconsult.com

RELATED CONTENT

Rosacea (Patient Information)

AUTHOR: **FRED F. FERRI, M.D.**

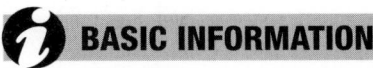

DEFINITION

Roseola is a benign viral illness found in infants and characterized by high fevers that last 3 or 4 days, followed by defervescence and development of a macular or maculopapular rash.

SYNONYMS

Exanthem subitum
Sixth disease
Roseola infantum
Pseudorubella
Human herpesvirus 6 (HHV-6), human herpesvirus 7 (HHV-7)

ICD-9CM CODES
057.8 Roseola

EPIDEMIOLOGY & DEMOGRAPHICS

- Nearly one third of all infants develop roseola before the age of 2 yr.
- Peak prevalence is between 7 and 13 mo.
- More than 90% of children older than 2 yr of age are seropositive for the virus causing roseola.
- Roseola is spread from person to person. It is not known how it is spread, but it must be very efficiently spread and presumably via the respiratory tract.
- There is no predilection for gender or time of year.

PHYSICAL FINDINGS & CLINICAL PRESENTATION

- Typically the child develops a high fever, usually up to 104° F (40° C), that lasts for 3 to 5 days
- Fever may be associated with a runny nose, irritability, and fatigue
- A rash appears within 48 hr of defervescence, begins on the neck or trunk and then spreads to extremities, and persists for a few hours to 2 days.
- Faint pink maculopapular rash that blanches when palpated (Fig. E1-731) and generally nonpruritic
- Other common findings: cervical and/or occipital adenopathy, erythematous tympanic membranes, anorexia
- Nagayama spots: red papules on the soft palate or base of the uvula
- Seizures
- Less common: febrile seizures (≤6% of cases), cough, diarrhea, aseptic meningitis

ETIOLOGY

- Roseola is usually caused by human herpesvirus-6 (HHV-6) in the great majority of cases but other causes include human herpesvirus-7, enteroviruses, adenoviruses, and parainfluenza virus type 1. A small percentage of children may have primary infection with HHV-7.
- The incubation period is between 5 and 15 days.

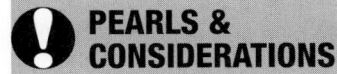 **DIAGNOSIS**

The diagnosis of roseola is usually made by the clinical presentation as stated previously. It can be confirmed serologically by indirect immunofluorescence assays, ELISA, neutralization assays, and immunoblot. Viral culture is the gold standard to document active viral replication but is expensive, time consuming, and available only in research laboratories.

DIFFERENTIAL DIAGNOSIS

- Rubeola (measles)
- Rubella
- Fifth disease (erythema infectiosum) caused by parvovirus B19
- Enteroviral infections
- Drug eruption
- Mononucleosis
- All causes of fever (e.g., otitis media, pneumonia, and urinary tract infection)
- Meningitis

WORKUP

- If unsure of the diagnosis of roseola in a febrile infant, a fever workup is done to rule out other infectious causes.
- The decision to proceed with a fever workup is a clinical judgment call.

LABORATORY TESTS

- CBC with differential usually shows relative neutropenia and mild atypical lymphocytosis.
- Erythrocyte sedimentation rate (ESR), blood cultures as indicated
- Urinalysis and urine cultures
- Stool cultures if diarrhea is present
- Lumbar puncture if needed to rule out meningitis in patients with mental status changes
- Commercial assays can be used to detect HHV-6-specific IgG antibody responses but IgM assays are not always reliable for acute infection

IMAGING STUDIES

Chest x-ray to rule out pneumonia

Rx **TREATMENT**

NONPHARMACOLOGIC THERAPY

- Supportive care
- Maintain hydration by drinking clear fluids: water, fruit juice, lemonade, and so forth
- Sponge bathe with lukewarm water if febrile

ACUTE GENERAL Rx

- Acetaminophen 10 to 15 mg/kg per dose at 4-hr intervals for fever

- Ibuprofen 5 to 10 mg/kg per dose at 6-hr intervals (maximal dose 600 mg)

CHRONIC Rx

Roseola is a viral disease that is short lasting; chronic treatment is usually not an issue.

DISPOSITION

- Roseola is generally a benign, self-limited disease that usually lasts approximately 1 wk.
- Complications, although rare, can occur and include:
  1. Febrile seizures
  2. Meningitis
  3. Encephalitis
  4. Pneumonitis
  5. Hepatitis

REFERRAL

Subspecialty consultation is made with the appropriate discipline if any of the previously mentioned complications occur (e.g., neurology for seizures).

! **PEARLS & CONSIDERATIONS**

COMMENTS

- A child with fever and rash should be excluded from day care.
- HHV-6 is named accordingly because it is the sixth herpesvirus discovered after herpes simplex 1 (HSV-1), HSV-2, cytomegalovirus (CMV), Epstein-Barr virus (EBV), and varicella-zoster virus (VZV).
- Roseola is called sixth disease because it represents the sixth childhood "exanthem"; the other five are measles, scarlet fever, rubella, Dukes disease, and erythema infectiosum.

SUGGESTED READINGS
available at www.expertconsult.com

AUTHOR: **GLENN G. FORT, M.D., M.P.H.**

BASIC INFORMATION

DEFINITION

- The rotator cuff syndrome is a spectrum of afflictions involving the four rotator cuff muscles of the shoulder: supraspinatus, infraspinatus, teres minor, and subscapularis.
- It consists of subacromial bursitis, rotator cuff tendinopathy, and partial- or full-thickness muscle or tendon tear.

SYNONYMS

Shoulder impingement syndrome
Painful arc syndrome
Supraspinatus syndrome

ICD-9CM CODES
726.10 Rotator cuff syndrome
727.61 Rotator cuff rupture

EPIDEMIOLOGY & DEMOGRAPHICS

PREVALENCE: 5% to 10% of the population
PREDOMINANT SEX: Males more than females
PREDOMINANT AGE: >40 yr
RISK FACTORS: Repetitive overhead activity, advanced age, obesity, smoking, trauma

PHYSICAL FINDINGS & CLINICAL PRESENTATION

- Lateral shoulder pain with overhead activity
- Pain at night when lying on the shoulder
- Muscle weakness would indicate a tear
- Atrophy and sunken appearance of the scapular muscles with longstanding disease
- Tenderness over the affected mucle or localized under the acromion (Fig. E1-732)
- Useful clinical tests:
  - *Hawkins-Kennedy sign:* shoulder and elbow are flexed at 90 degrees; shoulder pain is elicited with passive internal rotation (Fig. 1-733, *A*)
  - *Painful arc sign:* pain with active abduction of the shoulder between 70% to 120%
  - *Drop arc sign:* failure to smoothly control shoulder adduction
  - Painful resisted external rotation and forced passive full-forward flexion (Fig. 1-733, *B, C*)

- The combination of Hawkins-Kennedy sign, the painful arc sign, and weakness in external rotation yields the best probability (95%) for any degree of impingement
- The combination of drop arc sign, painful arc sign, and weakness in external rotation accurately predicts full-thickness tears (91%)
- A subacromial lidocaine injection can be used to distinguish weakness from rotator cuff tendinopathy and true tears—normal strength after injection indicates tendinopathy

ETIOLOGY

A combination of tendon overload, microvascular compromise, and compression by surrounding structures

DIAGNOSIS

DIFFERENTIAL DIAGNOSIS

- Bicipital tendinitis, labrum tears, adhesive capsulitis, glenohumeral osteoarthritis, acromioclavicular injury, subscapular bursitis, avascular necrosis. Table E1-364 describes the differential diagnosis of shoulder pain.
- Neurologic and visceral etiologies need to be ruled out.

IMAGING STUDIES

- Plain radiography: not routinely needed; can reveal tendon calcifications and migration of humeral head, indicating a large tear
- Ultrasonography: acurate tool for initial evaluation but has limitations; partial tears are difficult to identify; highly operator-dependent
- MRI is the test of choice for shoulder soft tissue lessions

TREATMENT

ACUTE GENERAL Rx

- Ice and rest without overhead activity
- Physical therapy
- NSAIDs for 7 to 10 days, then as needed
- Subacromial glucocorticoid injections can be used in patients with severe pain that is refractory to oral medications

- Surgery is reserved for healthy patients with acute full-thickness tears or with chronic partial tears who fail conservative management

DISPOSITION

Return to work or sport should be gradual and is based upon the ability to exhibit full ROM and appropriate strength without discomfort.

REFERRAL

Orthopedic consultation should be obtained in patients with a clinically significant rotator cuff tear and in patients who fail to improve with medical management.

PEARLS & CONSIDERATIONS

COMMENTS

- Supraspinatus is the most commonly injured muscle.
- Rotator cuff tears can be asymptomatic.
- Identification of partial tears remains a clinical challenge and imaging is often needed.
- It is important to differentiate tears from tendinopathy because they require different management.
- Most patients respond to conservative management.
- Untreated, longstanding rotator cuff tendinopathy can cause significant loss in range of motion and adhesive capsulitis.

EVIDENCE

available at www.expertconsult.com

SUGGESTED READINGS

available at www.expertconsult.com

RELATED CONTENT

Bursitis (Related Key Topic)
Rotator Cuff Tendinitis (Patient Information)

AUTHOR: **DAN A. CRISTESCU, M.D.**

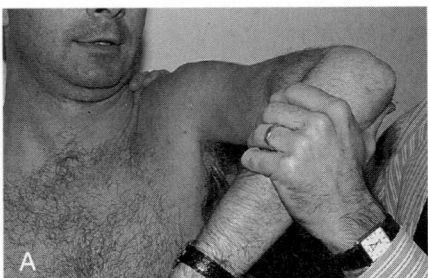
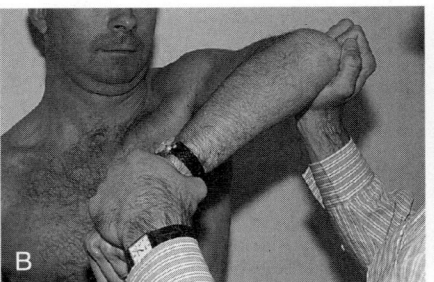
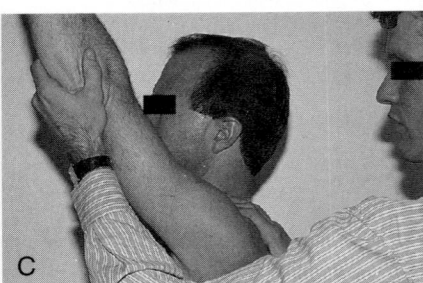

FIGURE 1-733 Impingement tests. A, Forced passive internal rotation. **B,** Resisted external rotation. **C,** Forced passive full forward flexion. (From Hochberg MC et al: *Rheumatology*, ed 5, St Louis, 2011, Mosby.)

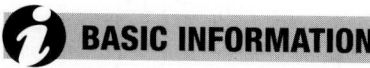

BASIC INFORMATION

DEFINITION

Salivary gland neoplasms are benign or malignant tumors of a salivary gland (parotid, submandibular, or sublingual).

SYNONYMS

These tumors are often named according to their histologic type (see "Diagnosis").

ICD-9CM CODES
142.9 Salivary gland neoplasm
142.0 (Parotid)
142.1 (Submandibular)
142.2 (Sublingual)

EPIDEMIOLOGY & DEMOGRAPHICS

INCIDENCE: One to two cases per 100,000 person-years (1% of all head and neck tumors)
DISTRIBUTION:
- Parotid gland, 85% (80% are benign)
- Submandibular gland, 10% (55% are benign)
- Sublingual and minor glands, 5% (35% are benign)

PHYSICAL FINDINGS & CLINICAL PRESENTATION

- Parotid gland:
  1. Painless swelling overlying the masseter muscle (under the temporomandibular joint)
  2. Pain
  3. Facial nerve palsy
  4. Cervical lymph nodes
  5. Mass in oral cavity
- Submandibular gland: swelling under anterior portion of the mandible
- Sublingual gland: intraoral swelling under the tongue, medial to the mandible

DIAGNOSIS

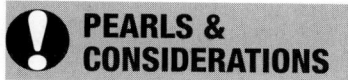

PATHOLOGY

HISTORY:
Benign Tumors:
- Mixed tumor (usually parotid)
- Adenolymphoma (Warthin's tumor)

- Pleomorphic adenoma
- Capillary hemangioma, lymphangioma (in children)
- Intraductal papilloma
- Other (e.g., myoepithelioma, canalicular adenoma, basal cell adenoma)

Malignant Tumors:
- Mucoepidermoid carcinoma (most common malignant tumor of the parotid gland)
- Adenoid cystic carcinoma
- Adenocarcinoma
- Malignant mixed tumor
- Squamous cell carcinoma
- Other

STAGE (TNM):
T_0 No evidence of primary tumor
T_1 Tumor <2 cm
T_2 Tumor 2 to 4 cm
T_3 Tumor 4 to 6 cm
T_4 Tumor >6 cm
All subdivided into
- Without local extension
- With local extension
N_0 No lymph node metastasis
N_1 Single ipsilateral node <3 cm
N_2 Ipsilateral, contralateral, or bilateral node <6 cm
N_3 Any node >6 cm
M_0 No distant metastasis
M_1 Distant metastasis
Stage I T_{1a} or $_{2a}N_0M_0$
Stage II $T_{1b,2b,3a} N_0M_0$
Stage III $T_{3b,4a} N_0M_0$ or any T except $_{4b}N_1M_0$
Stage IV T_{4b} any N any M or any T $N_{2,3}M_0$ or any T, any N_1M_1

WORKUP

- Fine-needle aspiration. The sensitivity, specificity, and accuracy of parotid gland aspirates are approximately 92%, 100%, and 98%, respectively
- Imaging by CT scan or MRI
- Open biopsy (rarely indicated)

TREATMENT

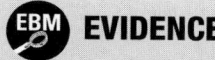

Malignant tumors:
- Surgery is the mainstay of treatment; gland resection and neck dissection if lymph nodes are involved.

- A lateral lobectomy with preservation of facial nerve should be considered for tumors confined to the superficial lobe of the parotid gland. Gross tumor should not be left in situ, but if the facial nerve is able to be preserved by "peeling" tumor off the nerve, it should be attempted, followed by radiation therapy for microscopic disease.
- Postoperative radiation is indicated for high-grade malignancies demonstrating extra-glandular disease, perineural invasion, direct invasion of surrounding tissues, or regional metastases.
- Chemotherapy.

Benign tumors: surgery for tumor resection

PROGNOSIS OF MALIGNANT TUMORS

Five-year survival rates:
- Mucoepidermoid carcinoma: 75% to 95%
- Adenoid cystic carcinoma: 40% to 80%
- Adenocarcinoma: 20% to 75%
- Malignant mixed tumor: 35% to 75%
- Squamous cell carcinoma: 25% to 60%

PEARLS & CONSIDERATIONS

COMMENTS

Salivary gland neoplasms most often present as slow-growing, well-circumscribed masses. Pain, rapid growth, nerve weakness, fixation to skin or underlying muscle, and paresthesias usually are indicative of malignancy.

EVIDENCE

available at www.expertconsult.com

SUGGESTED READING
available at www.expertconsult.com

RELATED CONTENT
Salivary Gland Tumors (Patient Information)

AUTHOR: **FRED F. FERRI, M.D.**

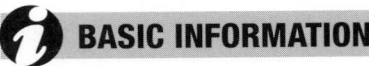

BASIC INFORMATION

DEFINITION

Salmonellosis is an infection caused by one of several serotypes of a gram-negative bacillus of the genus *Salmonella*. Current *Salmonella* nomenclature is described in Table 1-366.

SYNONYMS

Typhoid fever
Paratyphoid fever
Enteric fever

ICD-9CM CODES
003.0 Salmonellosis

EPIDEMIOLOGY & DEMOGRAPHICS

INCIDENCE (IN U.S.):
- Epidemiologically, the clinical syndromes are divided into those that cause a typhoidal type of infection (systemic illness with fever and abdominal pain) such as *Salmonella typhi* and those that do not: nontyphoidal *Salmonella* infections (gastroenteritis) such as *S. enteritidis*, *S. newport*, and *S. typhimurium*.
- Estimated 1 million cases/yr of nontyphoidal salmonellosis in the U.S.
- Approximately 500 cases of *Salmonella typhi* infection reported each yr. In 2009 contaminated peanut butter and peanut products caused a nationwide *Salmonella typhimurium* outbreak in 46 states, affecting more than 700 individuals.
- Largest outbreak: 200,000 people who ingested contaminated milk

PEAK INCIDENCE: Summer and fall
PREDOMINANT AGE:
- <20 yr old
- >70 yr old
- Highest rates of infection in infants, especially neonates

GENETICS:
Neonatal infection:
- Highly susceptible to infection with nontyphoidal *Salmonella*

PHYSICAL FINDINGS & CLINICAL PRESENTATION
- Infections
  1. Localized to GI tract (gastroenteritis)
  2. Systemic (typhoid fever)
  3. Localized outside of GI tract

- Gastroenteritis
  1. Incubation period: 12 to 48 hr
  2. Nausea, vomiting
  3. Diarrhea, abdominal cramps
  4. Fever
  5. Bacteremia: occurs mostly in the immunocompromised host or those with underlying conditions, including HIV infection
  6. Self-limited illness lasting 3 or 4 days
  7. Colonization of GI tract persistent for months, especially in those treated with antibiotics
- Typhoid fever
  1. Incubation period of few days to several wk
  2. Prolonged fever, often with a stepwise-increasing temperature pattern
  3. Myalgias
  4. Headache, cough, sore throat
  5. Malaise, anorexia
  6. Abdominal pain
  7. Hepatosplenomegaly
  8. Diarrhea or constipation early in the course of illness
  9. Rose spots (faint, maculopapular, blanching lesions) sometimes seen on chest or abdomen
- Untreated disease
  1. Fever lasting 1 to 2 mo
  2. Main complication: GI bleeding caused by perforation from ulceration of Peyer's patches in the ileum
  3. Rare complications:
     a. Mental status changes
     b. Shock
  4. Relapse rate of approximately 10%
- Infections outside GI tract
  1. Can occur in virtually any location
  2. Usually occur in patients with underlying diseases
  3. Endocarditis, endovascular infections are caused by seeding of atherosclerotic plaques or aneurysms
  4. Hepatic or splenic abscesses in patients with underlying disease in these organs
  5. Urinary tract infections in patients with renal TB or schistosomiasis
  6. Salmonellae are a frequent cause of gram-negative meningitis in neonates
  7. Osteomyelitis in children with hemoglobinopathies (particularly sickle cell disease)

ETIOLOGY
- More than 2000 serotypes of *Salmonella* exist, but only a few cause disease in humans. Host factors and conditions predisposing to

the development of systemic disease with nontyphoidal *Salmonella* strains are described in Table 1-367.
- Raw produce is an increasingly recognized vehicle for salmonellosis. In 2008 there was a large outbreak of *Salmonella* Saintpaul involving 1500 persons, of whom 21% were hospitalized and 2 died. It was due to contaminated jalapeno and serrano peppers. More recently outbreaks of human *Salmonella* infections have been increasingly associated with contact with live poultry.
- Some found only in humans are the cause of enteric fever.
  1. *S. typhi*
  2. *S. paratyphi*
- Some responsible for gastroenteritis and frequently isolated from raw meat and poultry and uncooked or undercooked eggs.
  1. *S. typhimurium*
  2. *S. enteritidis*
- *S. choleraesuis* is a prototype organism that causes extraintestinal nontyphoidal disease.
- Transmission generally via ingestion of contaminated food or drink.
- Outbreaks of gastroenteritis related to contaminated poultry, meat, and dairy products are common.
- Typhoid fever is a systemic illness caused by serotypes exclusive to humans.
  1. Acquisition by ingestion of food or water contaminated by other humans
  2. Most cases in the U.S. are:
     a. Acquired during foreign travel
     b. Acquired by ingestion of food prepared by chronic carriers, many of whom have acquired the organism outside of the U.S.

DIAGNOSIS

DIFFERENTIAL DIAGNOSIS
- Other causes of prolonged fever:
  1. Malaria
  2. TB

TABLE 1-367 Host Factors and Conditions Predisposing to the Development of Systemic Disease with Nontyphoidal *Salmonella* Strains

Neonates and young infants (≤3 mo of age)
HIV/AIDS
Other immunodeficiencies and chronic granulomatous disease
Immunosuppressive and corticosteroid therapies
Malignancies, especially leukemia and lymphoma
Hemolytic anemia, including sickle cell disease, malaria, and bartonellosis
Collagen vascular disease
Inflammatory bowel disease
Achlorhydria or use of antacid medications
Impaired intestinal motility
Schistosomiasis, malaria
Malnutrition

From Kliegman RM et al: *Nelson textbook of pediatrics*, ed 19, Philadelphia, 2011, Saunders.

TABLE 1-366 Salmonella Nomenclature

Traditional Usage	Formal Name	CDC Designation
S. typhi	*S. enterica** subsp. enterica ser. Typhi	*S.* ser. Typhi
S. dublin	*S. enterica* subsp. enterica ser. Dublin	*S.* ser. Dublin
S. typhimurium	*S. enterica* subsp. enterica ser. Typhimurium	*S.* ser. Typhimurium
S. choleraesuis	*S. enterica* subsp. enterica ser. Choleraesuis	*S.* ser. Choleraesuis
S. marina	*S. enterica* subsp. houtenae ser. Marina	*S.* ser. Marina

CDC, Centers for Disease Control and Prevention; *ser.*, serovar; *subsp.*, subspecies.
*Some authorities prefer *S. choleraesuis* or *S. enteritidis* rather than *S. enterica* to describe the species.
From Kliegman RM et al: *Nelson textbook of pediatrics*, ed 19, Philadelphia, 2011, Saunders.

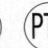

3. Brucellosis
4. Amebic liver abscess
- Other causes of gastroenteritis:
  1. Bacterial: *Shigella, Yersinia, Campylobacter* spp.
  2. Viral: Norwalk virus, rotavirus
  3. Parasitic: *Entamoeba histolytica, Giardia lamblia*
  4. Toxic: enterotoxigenic *E. coli, Clostridium difficile*

WORKUP

- Typhoid fever
  1. Cultures of blood, stool, urine; repeat if initially negative.
  2. Blood cultures are more likely to be positive early in the course of illness.
  3. Stool and urine cultures are more commonly positive in the second and third wk of illness.
  4. Highest yield with bone marrow biopsy cultures: 90% positive.
  5. Serology using Widal's test is helpful in retrospect, showing a fourfold increase in convalescent titers.
- Gastroenteritis: stool cultures
- Extraintestinal localized infection:
  1. Blood cultures
  2. Cultures from the site of infection

LABORATORY TESTS

- Neutropenia is common
- Transaminitis is possible
- Culture to grow organism: blood, body fluids, biopsy specimens

IMAGING STUDIES

- Not routinely indicated
- Radiographs of bone may be suggestive of osteomyelitis (particularly in patients with sickle cell disease and bone infarctions).
- CT scan or sonogram of abdomen:
  1. May reveal hepatic or splenic abscesses or pleural involvement
  2. May reveal aortic aneurysm

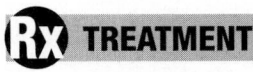 **TREATMENT**

NONPHARMACOLOGIC THERAPY

Adequate hydration and electrolyte replacement in people with diarrhea

ACUTE GENERAL Rx

- Typhoid fever:
  1. Ciprofloxacin 500 mg PO bid or 400 mg IV bid *or* levofloxacin 750 mg PO/IV q24h for 7-10 days. Should not be used as first line in patients from South Asia due to resistance unless known to be susceptible.
  2. Ceftriaxone 2 g IV qd for 7-14 days or cefixime (20-30 mg/kg/day orally divided into q12h dosing for 7-14 days)
  3. Another alternative agent: azithromycin (1 g orally then 500 mg daily for 5-7 days)
  4. Children: see Table 1-368. In general, quinolones are avoided in children unless a multidrug-resistant strain is involved due to concerns of possible cartilage damage. Another alternative for children: azithromycin (10-20 mg/kg to 1 g maximum once daily for 5-7 days)
  5. If tests show susceptibility, can also use amoxicillin or Bactrim in adults and children
  6. Dexamethasone 3 mg IV initially, followed by 1 mg IV q6h for eight doses for patients with shock or mental status changes
- Gastroenteritis:
  1. Usually not indicated for gastroenteritis alone because this illness usually self-limited
  2. Treatment may prolong the carrier state and is discouraged for healthy patients <50 yr of age who have relatively mild disease.
  3. Prophylactic treatment for patients who are at high risk of developing complications from bacteremia (see Table 1-368)
     a. Neonates
     b. Patients with hemoglobinopathies
     c. Patients with atherosclerosis
     d. Patients with aneurysms
     e. Patients with prosthetic devices
     f. Immunocompromised patients

CHRONIC Rx

- Carrier states are possible in those with typhoid fever.
- More common in people >60 yr of age and in people with gallstones.
- Usual site of colonization is the gallbladder.
- Treatment should be considered for those with persistently positive stool cultures and for food handlers.

- Suggested regimens for eradication of carrier state:
  1. Ciprofloxacin 500 mg PO bid for 4 wk
  2. SMX/TMP 1 to 2 DS tabs PO bid for 6 wk (if susceptible)
  3. Amoxicillin 2 g PO q8h for 6 wk (if susceptible)
- Cholecystectomy may be required in carriers with gallstones who fail medical therapy, but this is rarely indicated for nontyphoidal salmonellosis currently.
- Prolonged course of oral therapy or lifetime suppression for patients with AIDS who have chronic infection.

DISPOSITION

- Typhoid fever
  1. Treated patients usually respond to therapy; small percentage of chronic carriers.
  2. Untreated patients may have serious complications.
- Gastroenteritis
  1. Usually self-limited
  2. May be recurrent or persistent in AIDS patients

REFERRAL

- If gastroenteritis is persistent or recurrent
- If there is evidence of extraintestinal infection, typhoid fever, or chronic carriers

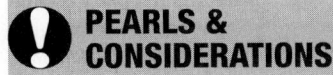 **PEARLS & CONSIDERATIONS**

COMMENTS

- Quinolones should not be used in children or pregnant women.
- Infections should be reported to local health departments.
- Recent outbreaks in the U.S. have been traced back to raw tomatoes, peanut butter, pet turtles, and frozen pot pies.

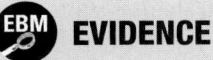 **EVIDENCE**

available at www.expertconsult.com

SUGGESTED READINGS

available at www.expertconsult.com

RELATED CONTENT

Salmonellosis (Patient Information)

AUTHOR: **GLENN G. FORT, M.D., M.P.H.**

TABLE 1-368 Treatment of *Salmonella* Gastroenteritis	
Organism and Indication	**Dose and Duration of Treatment**
Salmonella infections in infants <3 mo of age or immunocompromised persons (in addition to appropriate treatment for underlying disorder)	Cefotaxime 100-200 mg/kg/day every 6 hr for 5-14 days *or* Ceftriaxone 75 mg/kg/day once daily for 7 days *or* Ampicillin 100 mg/kg/day every 6 hr for 7 days *or* Cefixime 15 mg/kg/day for 7-10 days

From Kliegman RM et al: *Nelson textbook of pediatrics*, ed 19, Philadelphia, 2011, Saunders.

BASIC INFORMATION

DEFINITION Sarcoidosis is a chronic multisystem granulomatous disease characterized histologically by the presence of nonspecific, noncaseating granulomas.

SYNONYMS Boeck's sarcoid

ICD-9CM CODES
135.0 Sarcoidosis

EPIDEMIOLOGY & DEMOGRAPHICS

INCIDENCE (IN U.S.): 11 in 100,000 whites and 35 in 100,000 blacks; presents most commonly in the winter and early spring
PREDOMINANT SEX: Increased incidence in females
PREDOMINANT AGE: 20 to 40 yr
GENETICS: Familial clustering has been described. Having a first-degree relative with sarcoidosis increases the risk for disease fivefold.

PHYSICAL FINDINGS & CLINICAL PRESENTATION

- Clinical manifestations often vary with the stage of the disease and degree of organ involvement. Patients may be asymptomatic, but a chest radiograph may demonstrate findings consistent with sarcoidosis (see "Imaging Studies"). Nearly 50% of patients with sarcoidosis are diagnosed by incidental findings on chest radiograph. Thoracic involvement occurs in >90% of patients with sarcoidosis.
- Frequent manifestations:
  1. Pulmonary manifestations: dry, nonproductive cough; dyspnea; chest discomfort
  2. Constitutional symptoms: fatigue, weight loss, anorexia, malaise
  3. Visual disturbances: blurred vision, ocular discomfort, conjunctivitis, iritis, uveitis (65% of patients)
  4. Dermatologic manifestations (30% of patients): erythema nodosum (10% of patients), macules, papules, subcutaneous nodules, hyperpigmentation, lupus pernio (indurated violaceous lesions on the nose, lips, ears, and cheeks that can erode into underlying cartilage and bone) (Fig. E1-736)
  5. Myocardial disturbances, arrhythmias, cardiomyopathy. Cardiac sarcoidosis is much more common than clinically appreciated and is found in up to 25% of patients in the United States
  6. Splenomegaly, hepatomegaly
  7. Rheumatologic manifestations: arthralgias have been reported in up to 40% of patients
  8. Neurologic and other manifestations: cranial nerve palsies, diabetes insipidus, meningeal involvement, parotid enlargement, hypothalamic and pituitary lesions, peripheral adenopathy. Neurosarcoidosis is detected in up to 25% of patients and can occur in the absence of apparent disease elsewhere

ETIOLOGY Unknown. A cardinal feature of sarcoidosis is the presence of CD4+ T cells that interact with antigen-presenting cells to initiate the formation and maintenance of granulomas. Multiple lines of evidence suggest that sarcoidosis may result from the interaction of multiple genes with environmental exposures or infection.

DIAGNOSIS

DIFFERENTIAL DIAGNOSIS

- Tuberculosis
- Lymphoma
- Hodgkin's disease
- Metastases
- Pneumoconioses
- Enlarged pulmonary arteries
- Infectious mononucleosis
- Lymphangitic carcinomatosis
- Idiopathic hemosiderosis
- Alveolar cell carcinoma
- Pulmonary eosinophilia
- Hypersensitivity pneumonitis
- Fibrosing alveolitis
- Collagen disorders
- Parasitic infection

Section II describes the differential diagnosis of granulomatous lung disease and a classification of granulomatous disorders.

WORKUP

- No pathognomonic diagnostic test exists for sarcoidosis, so the diagnosis remains one of exclusion. Workup is aimed at excluding critical organ involvement, determining extent and severity of disease, and excluding other disease. The presence of noncaseating granulomas does not establish the diagnosis, because conditions such as tuberculosis and malignancies, among others, can cause granulomas. A complete neurologic and ophthalmologic examination is mandatory. A complete occupational and environmental exposure history is recommended.
- Initial laboratory evaluation should include complete blood count, serum chemistries (alanine aminotransferase, aspartate aminotransferase, alkaline phosphatase, electrolytes, blood urea nitrogen, creatinine, serum calcium), urinalysis, 24-hour urinary excretion of calcium, CRP, ESR, and tuberculin skin test.
- Chest radiograph and ECG should also be obtained in all patients with sarcoidosis.
- Pulmonary function testing: spirometry, diffusion capacity of carbon monoxide–single breath.
- Biopsy should be done on accessible tissues suspected of sarcoid involvement (conjunctiva, skin, lymph nodes); bronchoscopy with transbronchial biopsy (85% diagnostic yield) is the procedure of choice in patients without any readily accessible site. Endobronchial ultrasound-guided fine-needle aspiration of intrathoracic lymph nodes also has high diagnostic yield and makes use of mediastinoscopy mostly unnecessary.

LABORATORY TESTS

Laboratory abnormalities:
- Hypergammaglobulinemia, anemia, leukopenia may be present
- Liver function test abnormalities are common

- Hypercalcemia (11% of patients), hypercalciuria (40% of patients; attributable to increased gastrointestinal absorption, abnormal vitamin D metabolism, and increased calcitriol production by sarcoid granuloma)
- Angiotensin-converting enzyme: elevated in approximately 60% of patients with sarcoidosis; nonspecific and generally not useful as a diagnostic tool and in following the course of the disease

IMAGING STUDIES

- Chest radiograph (Fig. 1-737): adenopathy of the hilar and paratracheal nodes is a frequent finding. Parenchymal changes may also be present, depending on the stage of the disease (stage 0, normal radiograph; stage I, bilateral hilar adenopathy; stage II, stage I plus pulmonary infiltrate; stage III, pulmonary infiltrate without adenopathy; stage IV, advanced fibrosis with evidence of "honeycombing," hilar retraction, bullae, cysts, and emphysema).
- Pulmonary function tests (spirometry and diffusing capacity of the lung for carbon dioxide): may be normal or may reveal a restrictive ventilatory defect with reduced forced vital capacity, reduced DLCO, or both.
- For patients without apparent lung involvement, ^{18}F-fluorodeoxyglucose positron emission tomography (FDG-PET) is useful in identifying sites for diagnostic biopsy.
- CT imaging is generally unnecessary for most patients with sarcoidosis. It is indicated when the chest radiograph is atypical for sarcoidosis or if the patient has hemoptysis.
- FDG-PET and MRI with gadolinium are useful in patients with suspected cardiac and neurologic involvement.
- Gallium-67 scan: represents an older testing modality. It will localize in areas of granulomatous infiltrates; however, it is not specific and not necessary. The "panda" sign (localization in the lacrimal and salivary glands, giving a "panda" appearance to the face) is suggestive of sarcoidosis.

TREATMENT

GENERAL Rx

- Many patients with sarcoidosis will not require any treatment. In general, treatment should be instituted when organ function is threatened. Corticosteroids (Table 1-369) are the mainstay of therapy when treatment is required (e.g., prednisone 40 mg qd for 8 to 12 wk with gradual tapering of the dose to 10 mg qod over 8 to 12 mo); corticosteroids should be considered in patients with severe symptoms (e.g., dyspnea, chest pain); hypercalcemia; ocular, central nervous system, or cardiac involvement; or progressive pulmonary disease. Patients with interstitial lung disease benefit from oral steroid therapy for 6 to 24 mo.
- A lack of benefit from steroid therapy may be due to the presence of irreversible fibrotic disease. Patients with progressive disease refractory to corticosteroids may be treated with methotrexate 7.5 to 15 mg once per week or another immunosuppressant such as azathioprine or mycophenolate mofetil.

- Hydroxychloroquine is effective for chronic disfiguring skin lesions, hypercalcemia, and neurologic involvement.
- Nonsteroidal anti-inflammatory drugs are useful for musculoskeletal symptoms and erythema nodosum.
- Pulmonary rehabilitation in patients with significant respiratory insufficiency. Consider liver and lung transplantation in patients unresponsive to conventional treatment.

DISPOSITION

- The majority of patients with sarcoidosis have spontaneous remission within 2 yr and do not require treatment. Their course can be followed by periodic clinical evaluation, chest radiographs, and pulmonary function tests.
- Blacks have increased rates of pulmonary involvement, a worse long-term prognosis, and more frequent relapses.
- Up to one third of patients have unrelenting disease, leading to clinically significant organ impairment. Adverse prognostic factors in sarcoidosis include age of onset >40 yr, cardiac involvement, neurosarcoidosis, progressive pulmonary fibrosis, chronic hypercalcemia, chronic uveitis, involvement of nasal mucosa, nephrocalcinosis, and presence of cystic bone lesions and lupus pernio.

REFERRAL Ophthalmologic examination is indicated in all patients with suspected sarcoidosis because ocular findings (iridocyclitis, uveitis, conjunctivitis, and keratopathy) are found in ≥25% of documented cases.

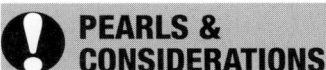

COMMENTS

- Serial spirometry and measurement of DLCO can be useful in following response to therapy and disease progression.
- Approximately 15% to 20% of patients with lung involvement advance to irreversible lung impairment (bronchiectasis, cavitation, progressive fibrosis, pneumothorax, and respiratory failure). Death from pulmonary failure occurs in 5% to 7% of patients with sarcoidosis.
- Newer treatment approaches are aimed at targeting mechanisms involving CD4 type 1 helper T cells.
- The diagnosis of sarcoidosis should be reconsidered in the presence of atypical manifestations or persistent/progressive disease despite appropriate therapy.

SUGGESTED READINGS
available at www.expertconsult.com

RELATED CONTENT
Sarcoidosis (Patient Information)

AUTHOR: **FRED F. FERRI, M.D.**

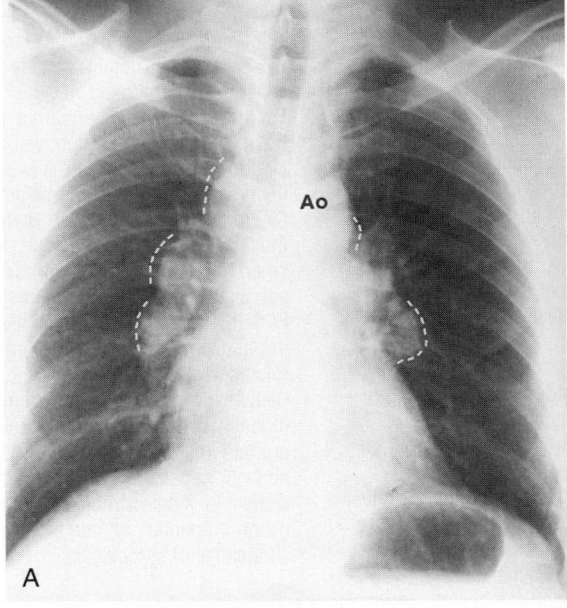
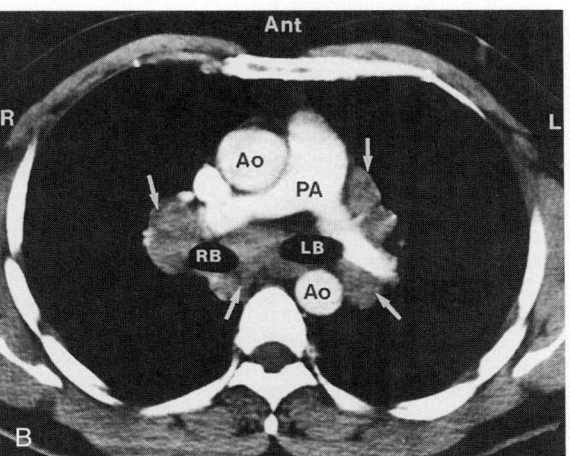

FIGURE 1-737 Sarcoid. Marked lymphadenopathy *(dotted lines)* is seen in the region of both hila in the right paratracheal region **(A)**. The transverse contrast-enhanced CT scan of the upper chest **(B)** clearly shows the ascending and descending aorta *(Ao)* as well as the pulmonary artery *(PA)* and superior vena cava. The right and left mainstem bronchus area is also seen. The arrows indicate the extensive lymphadenopathy. *LB,* Left bronchus; *RB,* right bronchus. (From Mettler FA [ed]: *Primary care radiology,* Philadelphia, 2000, Saunders.)

TABLE 1-369 Indications for Use of Corticosteroids in Sarcoidosis

Disorder	Treatment
Iridocyclitis	Corticosteroid eye drops; local subconjunctival deposit of cortisone
Posterior uveitis	Oral prednisone
Pulmonary involvement	Steroids rarely recommended for stage I; typically used if infiltrate remains static or worsens over 3-mo period or the patient is symptomatic
Upper airway obstruction	Rare indication for intravenous steroids
Lupus pernio	Oral prednisone shrinks the disfiguring lesions
Hypercalcemia	Responds well to corticosteroids
Cardiac involvement	Corticosteroids usually recommended if patient has arrhythmias or conduction disturbances
Central nervous system involvement	Response is best in patients with acute symptoms
Lacrimal/salivary gland involvement	Corticosteroids recommended for disordered function, not gland swelling
Bone cysts	Corticosteroids recommended if symptomatic

From Andreoli TE (ed): *Cecil essentials of medicine,* ed 8, Philadelphia, 2010, Saunders.

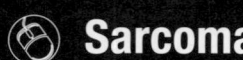
BASIC INFORMATION

DEFINITION

Sarcomas are heterogenous groups of malignant tumors of connective tissue. They show a wide range of differentiation—blood vessels (angiosarcoma), fat tissue (liposarcoma), bone (osteosarcoma). Sarcomas occur in soft tissues and bones, but are more common in soft tissues. They affect virtually all tissues, but 75% occur in the limbs. Sarcomas of bone are extremely rare. There are three histiogenic types: osteosarcoma, Ewing's sarcoma, and chondrosarcoma.

ICD-9CM CODES
171.0 Malignant neoplasm of connective and other soft tissue of head, face, and neck (depends on type)

EPIDEMIOLOGY & DEMOGRAPHICS
INCIDENCE:
Soft tissue sarcoma: 30 cases per million per annum.
Sarcoma of bone: 8 cases per million per annum.
Soft tissue sarcoma can occur at any age.
- In the United States there are 7800 new cases per year.
- Incidence increases with age.
- Average age of diagnosis is 57 yr.
- Men and women are affected equally.
- Soft tissue sarcomas represent <1% of all newly diagnosed malignancies.
Sarcomas of bone represent 0.2% of all new cancers.
- About 2600 new cases in the United States each year.
- Osteosarcoma and Ewing's sarcoma (the two most common bone tumors) occur predominantly during childhood and adolescence.
GENETICS: See "Etiology."

PHYSICAL FINDINGS & CLINICAL PRESENTATION
- Bone sarcomas. Clinical presentation usually includes:
  - Pain—at rest or at night
  - Swelling or mass at the site
  - Pathologic fractures
- Soft tissue sarcomas:
Present with painless mass (usually >5 cm). Mass grows slowly for months or years.

ETIOLOGY
- Most sarcomas arise sporadically.
- Genetic predispositions:
  1. Familial retinoblastoma (mutation of the *RB1* gene at 13q14) predisposes to osteosarcoma.
  2. Neurofibromatosis type 1 (mutation of *NF1* gene at 17q11) predisposes to malignant peripheral nerve sheath tumor.
  3. Diaphyseal aclasis (an autosomal inherited condition) is associated with increased risk of peripheral chondrosarcoma.

- Environmental causes:
  1. Previous radiotherapy (e.g., for cervical or breast cancer): predisposes to sarcoma 4 yr or so later.
  2. Chronic lymphedema: associated with the development of angiosarcoma.
  3. Exposure to chemicals (e.g., dioxins, phenoxyacetic herbicides, vinyl choride).
  4. Viruses (e.g., human herpesvirus 8 causes Kaposi's sarcoma).
  5. Foreign body (shrapnel, medical implants)

DIAGNOSIS

WORKUP
- Soft tissue sarcoma: any unexplained superficial soft tissue mass >5 cm or deep-seated, soft tissue mass should be regarded as malignant until proven otherwise.
- Bone sarcoma: patients with unexplained bone pain, persistent bone tenderness, or nonmechanical bone pain (especially when it disturbs sleep or rest) have bone cancer until proven otherwise.
- Patients with suspected spontaneous fracture or recurrence of the fracture with minor trauma should be considered as having bone cancer.
- Referral to a sarcoma treatment center of all patients with a suspected sarcoma is recommended.

IMAGING STUDIES
- A chest spiral CT scan is compulsory for staging purposes. Chest spiral CT helps de-

tect lung metastasis, since metastasis through blood to the lungs is the principal form of spread.
- Staging aids in estimating prognosis, survival, and plan management.
- The American Joint Committee on Cancer (AJCC) and International Union Against Cancer (IUCC) are widely used for staging classification.

Soft tissue sarcoma
- Magnetic resonance imaging (MRI) is the initial imaging modality of choice, especially for soft tissue sarcoma of the extremities, trunk, and head and neck. CT with IV contrast (Fig. 1-738) is also useful for diagnosis.
- Ultrasound is used to help differentiate between benign and suspicious lesions.
Bone sarcoma
- Radiograph (Fig. 1-739) is the initial imaging of choice. It helps to rule out bone tumor, shows calcification, and reveals bone erosions.
- A multidisciplinary approach is essential. The team should include radiologist, surgeons, pathologist, medical oncologist, and radiation therapists.

BIOPSY
- In nearly all cases a biopsy is needed to establish a tissue diagnosis.
- Multiple core needle biopsies are usually done.
- An excisional biopsy may be used for superficial lesions <5 cm.

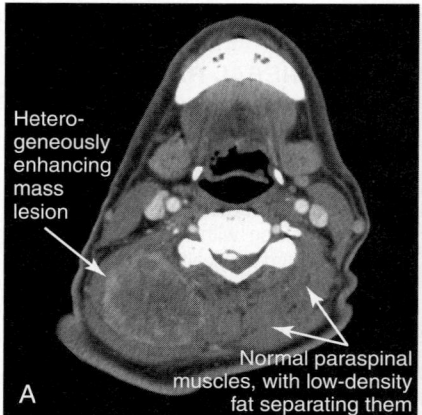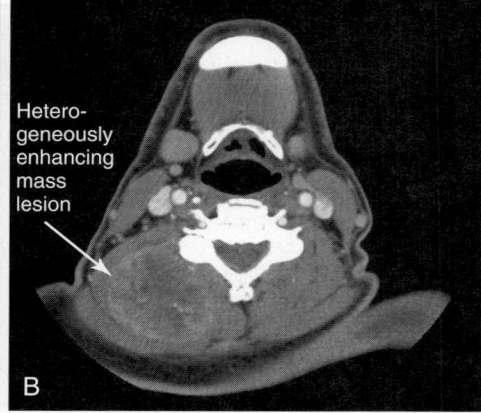

FIGURE 1-738 Neck mass. A and **B,** This 70-year-old patient presented with progressive right posterior neck swelling over a period of 1 mo following a dental procedure. Asymmetry and a palpable mass were present on exam. Computed tomography (CT) with intravenous contrast was performed to assess for abscess or mass. A heterogeneously enhancing mass is visible in the right posterior paraspinous muscles, measuring approximately 5.2 by 4.2 cm in axial dimension. The mass does not have the appearance of an abscess, which most often would have a lower density (fluid density, darker gray) center. Note how the mass has obliterated the normal planes separating paraspinal muscles; compare this with the patient's left side, which is normal. Without contrast, these asymmetric features and the overall size of the mass would be appreciated, but the discrete margins of the mass would not be seen without enhancement because the mass shares the same density with normal muscle. CT does not identify the exact etiology of the mass, although the differential diagnosis for a muscle density mass lesion includes sarcoma. Biopsy or excision would be needed to prove the diagnosis. Interestingly, the patient underwent fine-needle aspiration that showed gram-negative rods and spindle-shaped cells initially thought to represent reactive myositis or fasciitis, possibly an infection caused by the reported dental procedure. Unfortunately, surgical pathology showed an undifferentiated sarcoma. (From Broder JS: *Diagnostic imaging for the emergency physician,* Philadelphia, 2011, Saunders.)

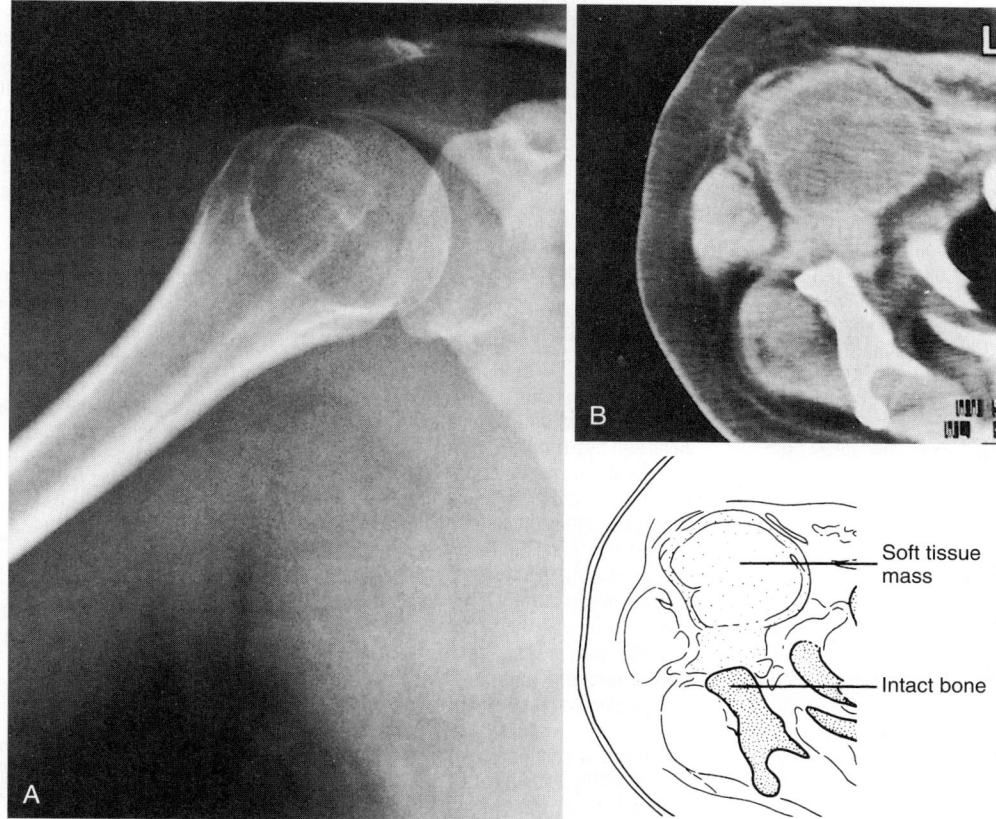

FIGURE 1-739 Fibrosarcoma. A, Anteroposterior plain film of the shoulder of a 40-year-old woman with a history of an enlarging mass in the right axilla shows an ill-defined mass adjacent to the lateral border of the scapula. **B,** CT section with contrast enhancement shows the extent of the mass and the lack of bone involvement. The tumor proved to be a fibrosarcoma. (From Skarin AT: *Atlas of diagnostic oncology,* ed 3, St Louis, 2003, Mosby.)

- In carefully selected cases an open biopsy may be done (rarely used because of its high complication rate).
- For difficult to palpate or necrotic soft sarcomas, ultrasound or computed tomography (CT)–guided biopsies are performed.
- Biopsy results are interpreted collaboratively by the specialist sarcoma pathologist, surgeon, and radiologist together.

HISTOLOGIC DIAGNOSIS

- Treatment planning is guided by a histologic diagnosis.
- Histologic diagnosis is made according to the World Health Organization (WHO) classification.
- WHO has defined more than 50 histologic subtypes of soft tissue sarcoma.
- Newer methods such as immunocytochemistry and cytogenetics can aid diagnosis. They identify tumor lineage.

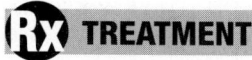 **TREATMENT**

Treatment depends on the extent of the disease and falls into several groups.

ACUTE GENERAL Rx

- Tumors treated by surgery: for example, in most adults soft tissue sarcoma and sarcoma of bone are not sensitive to chemotherapy.
  1. Surgery must be done by surgeon trained to treat this disease.
  2. Wide excision with negative margins is the standard surgical procedure.
  3. For bone sarcomas amputation has been the standard procedure. Recent advances permit the avoidance of amputation with limb-sparing surgery followed by reconstruction by endoprosthetic replacement.
- Chemotherapy followed by local therapy: for example, osteosarcoma.
  1. Early chemotherapy to reduce disseminated micrometastasis and tumor size.
- Follow-up of bone sarcoma after treatment includes:
  ○ Periodic monitoring with radiographs and other imaging modalities
  ○ CT scan of the chest
  ○ Bone scan
- Follow-up of soft tissue sarcoma (extremities):
  ○ Physical exam detects 97% of recurrence.

○ Physical exam is done every 3-6 mo for 3 yr, then every 6 mo for the next 2 yr for stage II and III cancers, then annually.
○ Imaging
  ■ Stage I: CXR every 6-12 mo
  ■ Stages II and III: image the primary site with MRI or CT
  ■ Chest x-ray or chest CT every 3-6 mo for 5 yr, then annually

REFERRAL

- Because sarcomas are relatively uncommon yet comprise a wide variety of different entities, evaluation by oncology teams who have expertise in the field is recommended.
- Treatment and follow-up guidelines have been published by the National Comprehensive Cancer Network (www.nccn.org).

SUGGESTED READINGS

available at www.expertconsult.com

AUTHOR: **DANIEL K. ASIEDU, M.D., PH.D., F.A.C.P.**

BASIC INFORMATION

DEFINITION

Scabies is a contagious disease caused by the mite *Sarcoptes scabiei*.

ICD-9CM CODES
133.0 Scabies

EPIDEMIOLOGY & DEMOGRAPHICS

- Scabies is generally acquired by sleeping with or in the bedding of infested individuals.
- It is generally associated with poor living conditions and is also common in hospitals and nursing homes.

PHYSICAL FINDINGS & CLINICAL PRESENTATION

- Primary lesions are caused when the female mite burrows within the stratum corneum, laying eggs within the tract she leaves behind; burrows (linear or serpiginous tracts, see Fig. 1-740) end with a minute papule or vesicle.
- Primary lesions are most commonly found in the web spaces of the hands, wrists, buttocks, scrotum, penis, breasts, axillae, and knees. They are often confused with eczema (Fig. 1-741).
- Secondary lesions result from scratching or infection.
- Intense pruritus, especially nocturnal, is common; it is caused by an acquired sensitivity to the mite or fecal pellets and is usually noted 1 to 4 wk after the primary infestation.
- Examination of the skin may reveal burrows, tiny vesicles, excoriations, inflammatory papules.
- Widespread and crusted lesions (Norwegian or crusted scabies) may be seen in elderly and immunocompromised patients.

ETIOLOGY

Human scabies is caused by the mite *S. scabiei*, var. *hominis* (Fig. 1-742). After impregnation on the skin surface, the gravid female burrows in the stratum corneum within 30 min and gradually extends the tract along the boundary with the stratum granulosum depositing 10 to 25 oval eggs in a 4- to 5-wk period. The eggs hatch in 3 to 5 days, and larvae move to the skin surface and mature in 2 to 3 wk, resuming the cycle.

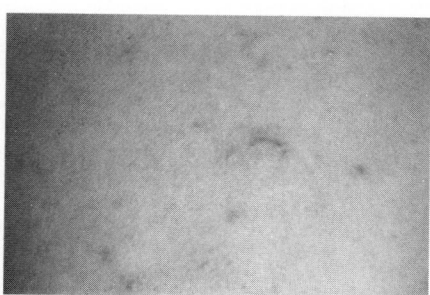

FIGURE 1-740 Classic scabies burrow. (From Kliegman RM et al: *Nelson textbook of pediatrics*, ed 19, Philadelphia, 2011, Saunders.)

DIAGNOSIS

DIFFERENTIAL DIAGNOSIS

- Pediculosis
- Atopic dermatitis
- Flea bites
- Seborrheic dermatitis
- Dermatitis herpetiformis
- Contact dermatitis
- Nummular eczema
- Syphilis
- Other insect infestation

WORKUP

Diagnosis is made on the clinical presentation and on the demonstration of mites, eggs, or mite feces.

LABORATORY TESTS

- Microscopic demonstration of the organism, feces, or eggs: a drop of mineral oil may be placed over the suspected lesion before re-

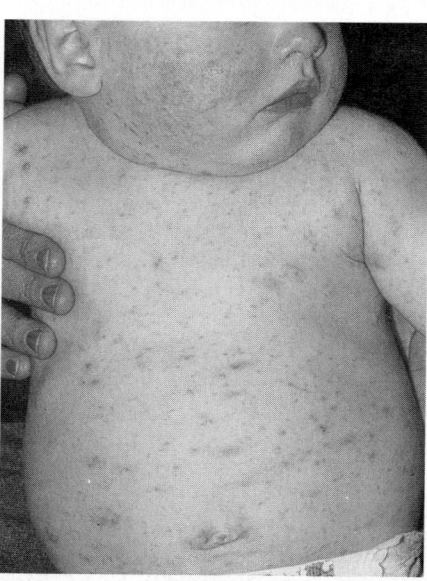

FIGURE 1-741 Scabies in an infant. Diffuse pruritic, eczematous lesions on an infant are often confused with eczema. (From White GM, Cox NH [eds]: *Diseases of the skin: a color atlas and text,* ed 2, St Louis, 2006, Mosby.)

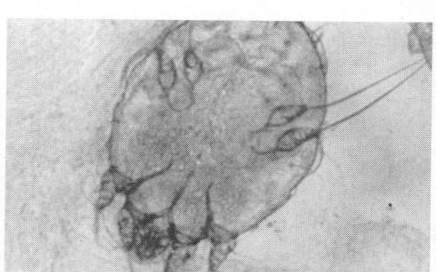

FIGURE 1-742 Scabies organism in a wet mount preparation. (From Mandell GL: *Mandell, Douglas, and Bennett's principles and practice of infectious diseases*, ed 5, New York, 2000, Churchill Livingstone.)

moval; the scrapings are transferred directly to a glass slide; a drop of potassium hydroxide is added and a cover slip is applied.
- Skin biopsy is rarely necessary to make the diagnosis.

TREATMENT

NONPHARMACOLOGIC THERAPY

Clothing, underwear, and towels used in the 48 hr before treatment must be laundered.

ACUTE GENERAL Rx

- Permethrin 5% cream (Elimite) is usually effective with one treatment; it should be massaged into the skin from head to soles of feet and applied under fingernails and toenails; remove 8 to 14 hr later by washing. Repeat in 1 to 2 wk. Permethrin is safe for children >2 mo old.
- A single dose (150 to 200 micrograms/kg in 6-mg tablets) of ivermectin, an antihelmintic agent, is also effective for the treatment of scabies. It is the best treatment for generalized crusted scabies.
- Pruritus generally abates 24 to 48 hr after treatment but can last up to 2 wk; oral antihistamines are effective in decreasing post-scabietic pruritus.
- Topical corticosteroid creams may hasten the resolution of secondary eczematous dermatitis.
- If the patient is a resident of an extended care facility, it is important to educate the patients, staff, family, and frequent visitors about scabies and the need to have full cooperation in treatment. Scabicide should be applied to all patients, staff, and frequent visitors, whether symptomatic or not; symptomatic family members of staff and visitors should also receive treatment.

DISPOSITION

Refractory cases usually are seen with immunocompromised hosts or patients with underlying skin diseases. ***Norwegian scabies*** refers to a highly contagious variant often found in institutions caring for physically and mentally disabled individuals.

PEARLS & CONSIDERATIONS

COMMENTS

- Lindane is potentially neurotoxic and should not be used on infants or pregnant women (permethrin is safe and effective in these situations).
- Sexual partners should be notified and treated.

SUGGESTED READING

available at www.expertconsult.com

RELATED CONTENT

Scabies (Patient Information)

AUTHOR: **FRED F. FERRI, M.D.**

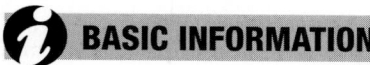

BASIC INFORMATION

DEFINITION

Scarlet fever is a rash involving the skin and tongue and complicating streptococcal group A pharyngitis.

SYNONYMS

Scarlatina
SF

ICD-9CM CODES
034.1 Scarlet fever

EPIDEMIOLOGY & DEMOGRAPHICS

- Same as streptococcal pharyngitis; namely, children ages 5 to 15 yr. May also complicate impetigo.
- Most common in cooler climates during the late fall, winter, and early spring.
- Most cases follow tonsillitis or pharyngitis; however, it has also been reported after wounds ("surgical scarlet fever"), burns, and pelvic or puerperal infections.

PHYSICAL FINDINGS & CLINICAL PRESENTATION

- Diffuse erythema, beginning on face and spreading to neck, back, chest, rest of trunk, and extremities (Fig. 1-743, A). Most intense on inner aspects of arms and thighs.
- Erythema blanches, but nonblanching petechiae may be present or produced by a tourniquet.
- Strawberry or raspberry tongue (Fig. 1-743 B, C).
- Rash lasts approximately 1 wk and then desquamates.
- Febrile illness with headache, malaise, anorexia, and pharyngitis begins after a 2- to 4-day incubation period.
- Scarlatinal rash begins 1 or 2 days after the onset of pharyngitis.

ETIOLOGY

Caused by group A beta-hemolytic *Streptococcus* infection, which produces one of three erythrogenic toxins (NOTE: *Some streptococcal species have the ability to cause both scarlet fever and rheumatic fever*).

DIAGNOSIS

DIFFERENTIAL DIAGNOSIS

- Viral exanthems (covered in Section II)
- Kawasaki disease
- Toxic shock syndrome
- Drug rashes

See differential diagnosis of "Pharyngitis" in Section I.

WORKUP

- Identification of group A *Streptococcus* by throat culture
- Streptolysin O antibody titers

TREATMENT

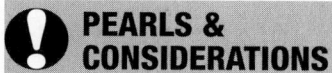

- Penicillin 250 mg PO qid for 10 days or erythromycin 250 mg PO qid for 10 days in penicillin-allergic patients. A clinical response can be expected in 24 to 48 hr.
- Benzathine penicillin 1 to 2 million U IM once; may be used for a patient who cannot swallow pills.

COMPLICATIONS (RARE)

- Peritonsillar abscess
- Mastoiditis
- Otitis media
- Pneumonia
- Sepsis and distant foci of infection
- Acute rheumatic fever
- Inability to swallow liquids or upper airway obstruction requiring hospitalization

NOTE: Failure to respond to penicillin should raise doubt about the diagnosis because *Streptococcus* may be carried in the pharynx without causing infection.

PEARLS & CONSIDERATIONS

COMMENTS

Patients with antibodies against the toxin are spared the rash but still develop other symptoms of the infection (e.g., sore throat).

RELATED CONTENT

Scarlet Fever (Patient Information)

AUTHOR: **FRED F. FERRI, M.D.**

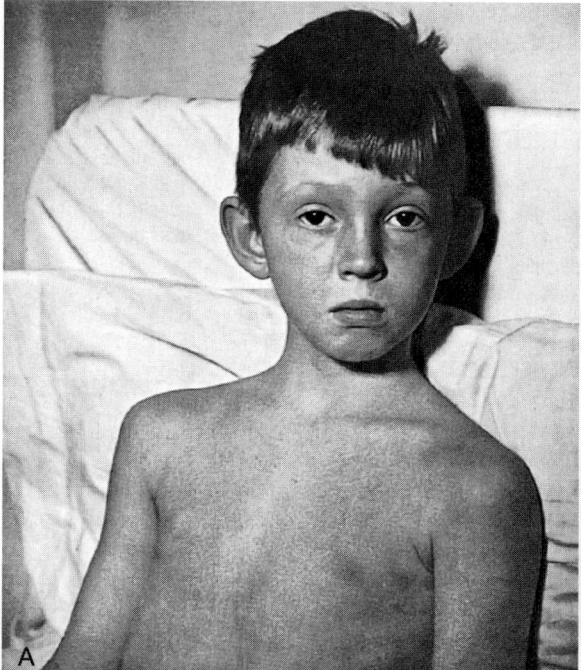
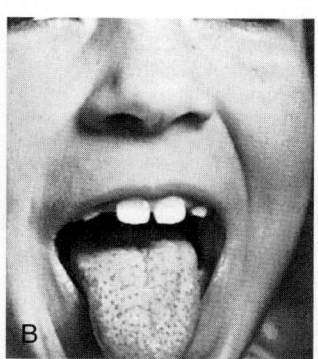
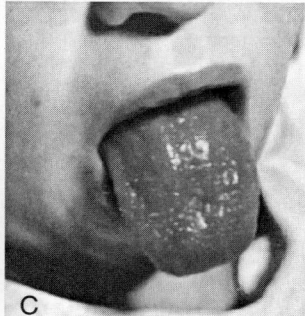

FIGURE 1-743 Scarlet fever.   A, Punctate, erythematous rash (2nd day). **B,** White strawberry tongue (1st day). **C,** Red, strawberry tongue (3rd day). (Courtesy Dr. Franklin H. Top, Professor and Head of the Department of Hygiene and Preventive Medicine, State University of Iowa, College of Medicine, Iowa City, IA; and Parke, Davis & Company's Therapeutic Notes. From Gershon AA et al: *Krugman's infectious diseases of children*, ed 11, Philadelphia, 2004, Mosby.)

BASIC INFORMATION

DEFINITION

Schizophrenia is a disorder that causes significant distortions in thinking, perception, speech, and behavior. Characteristics include psychosis, apathy, social withdrawal, and cognitive impairment, which result in significant social impairment.

SYNONYMS

Dementia praecox

ICD-9CM CODES
295.9 Schizophrenia

EPIDEMIOLOGY & DEMOGRAPHICS

INCIDENCE: 0.2 per 1000
PREVALENCE: 0.5%; lifetime prevalence risk, 0.4%
PREDOMINANT SEX: Males have a more severe illness with earlier onset. Prevalence in males approximately 1.4 times higher.
PREDOMINANT AGE:
- Age of onset of psychotic symptoms is the early 20s for males and the late 20s for females.
- Age of onset of negative symptoms is usually earlier (i.e., the mid-teenage years).
PEAK INCIDENCE: Between ages of 16 and 30 yr
GENETICS:
- Genetics accounts for 70% of risk; the remaining 30% associated with other factors such as urban environments, migration, or cannabis use.
- First-degree relatives have a 10 times greater chance of becoming schizophrenic.
- Discordant rates among identical twins are higher than expected with the simple inheritance pattern.
- Associations with several chromosomes have been described, but none has been replicated.
- Evidence exists that triplet nucleotide repeat expansion (e.g., such as that seen with Huntington's disease) may play a role in the inheritance of the disease.

PHYSICAL FINDINGS & CLINICAL PRESENTATION

- Schizophrenia is best defined as a dementing illness that begins early in life and that progresses slowly throughout the lifetime.
- Frequent structural brain imaging findings include the enlargement of the ventricular system, a loss of brain volume and cortical gray matter, and an alteration of the white matter tracts.
- The initial "negative" symptoms of adolescence (prodromal phase)—cognitive decline, social withdrawal and awkwardness, loss of motivation and pleasure, and loss of emotional expressiveness—begin after a period of normal development.
- During early adulthood, positive symptoms of psychosis and thought disturbance occur;

psychotic symptoms then wax and wane throughout life. Treatment ameliorates positive symptoms but generally does little for negative ones.
- The condition is also accompanied by cognitive impairment, including problems with attention and concentration, psychomotor speed, learning, memory, and executive functions (e.g., abstract thinking, problem solving).
- Social and occupational dysfunction can be profound.

ETIOLOGY

- The basic determination of whether this is a degenerative or developmental condition has not been made.
- The major hypothesis is that abnormality of the mesocortical pathways produces the hypofrontality and the negative symptoms. This occurs along with a compensatory hyperactivation of the mesolimbic pathways, which produces the positive symptoms of psychosis.

DIAGNOSIS

DIFFERENTIAL DIAGNOSIS

- Schizophrenia is diagnosed when an individual has experienced at least 6 mo (1 mo if using ICD-10 criteria) of hallucinations, delusions, thought disorders, catatonia, or negative symptoms (e.g., avolition, anhedonia, social isolation, affective flattening).
- Any medical condition, medicine, or substance that can affect brain homeostasis can cause psychosis; this is distinguished from schizophrenia by a relatively brief course and an alteration in mental status that suggests an underlying delirium.
- Other neurologic conditions that have psychosis as the initial presentation (e.g., Huntington's disease) need to be ruled out.
- Mood disorders with psychosis: these are indistinguishable from schizophrenia cross-sectionally but have a longitudinal course that includes full recovery.
- Delusional disorder involves nonbizarre delusions and lacks the thought disturbance, hallucinations, and negative symptoms of schizophrenia.
- Autism in the adult has an early age of onset and lacks significant hallucinations or delusions.

WORKUP

- History and physical examination to help determine whether the psychosis is primary or secondary
- Neurologic examination to uncover the soft neurologic signs (e.g., clumsiness, cortical thumb, loss of fine motor movements) that are common with schizophrenia

LABORATORY TESTS

- No laboratory tests are specific.
- Laboratory examinations (e.g., chemistry profile, blood count, sedimentation rate, toxi-

cology screen, urinalysis) are geared toward excluding a primary medical condition.

IMAGING STUDIES

- CT or MRI of the brain during the initial workup; repeated if the course of the illness varies from what is expected
- EEG may reveal slowing when psychosis is the result of an encephalopathy. Findings can be similar as a result of common medication use for treatment of psychosis

TREATMENT

NONPHARMACOLOGIC THERAPY

- Significant social support is required by most schizophrenic patients, but available support services are grossly inadequate. Schizophrenic patients constitute nearly one third of all homeless individuals. They usually require help with basic social, occupational, and interactive skills.
- Family stress can precipitate relapse and rehospitalization. Family interventions can reduce morbidity.
- Cognitive behavioral therapy can reduce the severity of both psychotic and negative symptoms.
- Illness management training for patients can increase medication adherence and reduce symptom distress.
- Integrated treatment that includes assertive community treatment, family involvement programs, and social skills training reduces the severity of both psychotic and negative symptoms, reduces comorbid substance misuse, reduces hospital days, increases adherence to treatment, and increases satisfaction with treatment.

ACUTE GENERAL Rx

- Acute psychosis is usually adequately controlled with antipsychotic agents.
- Few differences in effectiveness exist between first-generation antipsychotics (e.g., haloperidol, perphenazine, fluphenazine, chlorpromazine) and second-generation antipsychotics (e.g., risperidone, olanzapine, quetiapine, ziprasidone, aripiprazole, clozapine, lurasidone) for nonrefractory patients. First-generation antipsychotics are slightly more likely than second-generation antipsychotics to cause a parkinsonian state and eventual tardive dyskinesia (rate of tardive dyskinesia, 15% to 30%). Antiparkinsonian drugs (e.g., benztropine, amantadine) are used to ameliorate the parkinsonism. Risperidone has been shown to be superior to haloperidol for the prevention of acute psychotic relapse.
- Sedatives (i.e., benzodiazepines and, to a lesser degree, barbiturates) can be used transiently if a patient is in an agitated state.

CHRONIC RX

- Relapse prevention is a major goal of treatment. Noncompliance is common and leads to high relapse rates. Antipsychotic agents usually must be continued at the same doses

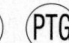
that controlled psychosis. For noncompliant patients, long-acting injectable preparations given biweekly or monthly can be used.

- Most patients frequently switch among antipsychotics; there is considerable individual variability with regard to antipsychotic response and vulnerability to specific adverse effects.
- Clozapine is more effective than other agents for treatment-refractory patients. However, it requires monitoring to prevent life-threatening adverse effects. Olanzapine may also be more effective than less expensive first-generation drugs but has substantial adverse metabolic effects. Lurasidone is a newer second-generation antipsychotic that appears to be better tolerated, but longer-term studies are needed.
- Neurocognitive improvement associated with antipsychotic treatment among patients with schizophrenia is small and does not differ between first-generation and second-generation antipsychotics.
- Antiparkinsonian agents may also need to be continued for the long term.
- Tardive dyskinesia (i.e., choreoathetoid movements of the muscles of tongue and face and occasionally of other muscle groups) can occur in as many as 30% of patients with the long-term use of neuroleptics.
- The negative symptoms of schizophrenia can resemble depression. In addition, depressive disorders may occur in schizophrenic patients. Antidepressant treatment of the negative symptoms is usually not effective. However, antidepressants can improve the symptoms of a comorbid depressive episode.
- Mood stabilizers (e.g., lithium, valproate, carbamazepine) are of little use unless the patient has a comorbid impulse control disorder.

- Substance abuse is a major problem for more than a third of schizophrenic patients. More than half of these patients smoke cigarettes. Unfortunately, these individuals do poorly in traditional substance abuse treatment programs. Specialized "dual-diagnosis" programs with highly structured aftercare are required.
- Specific antipsychotic medications have been associated with weight gain (i.e., olanzapine and clozapine) and QT prolongation. Hyperlipidemia and diabetes mellitus are associated with second-generation antipsychotics, and hyperprolactinemia is associated with first-generation antipsychotics. (Risperidone, a second-generation antipsychotic, can also produce hyperprolactinemia). Clozapine is associated with agranulocytosis.

DISPOSITION

- The positive symptoms of as many as 20% to 30% of schizophrenic patients do not respond to available treatments. A much higher fraction of patients experience relapse as a result of poor compliance.
- Negative symptoms are responsible for the 50% to 70% of patients in whom deterioration in occupational and social function continues.
- Approximately 10% of schizophrenic patients will complete suicide.
- The course of the illness is most strongly predicted by level of social development attained at the onset of psychosis.
- Schizophrenic patients die 12 to 15 yr sooner than the average population, mostly as a result of physical causes related to a lack of access to health care or as a result of health risk factors (e.g., smoking, obesity).

REFERRAL

- If hospitalization is required
- If patient is noncompliant
- If patient is resistant to treatment

PEARLS & CONSIDERATIONS

- Rule out delirium caused by medical conditions, medications, or substance abuse before diagnosing an individual's psychotic behavior as schizophrenia.
- All antipsychotic medications have high discontinuation rates in chronic schizophrenia treatment. Olanzapine and clozapine may be more effective than other antipsychotics for chronic treatment, but they have significant side effects.
- Significant social support is required for most patients with schizophrenia. Nonpharmacologic therapy should be used in conjunction with pharmacotherapy.

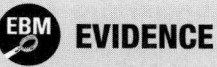

available at www.expertconsult.com

SUGGESTED READINGS
available at www.expertconsult.com

RELATED CONTENT

Schizophrenia (Patient Information)

AUTHORS: **ARNALDO A. BERGES, M.D., RICHARD J. GOLDBERG, M.D.,** and **MICHAEL K. ONG, M.D., PH.D.**

BASIC INFORMATION

DEFINITION

Scleritis is inflammation of the sclera (the fibrous layer of the eye underlying the conjunctiva and episclera). It is characterized by edema and cellular infiltration of the entire thickness of the sclera.

Classification of immune:

1. Anterior nonnecrotizing scleritis: can be subdivided into diffuse or nodular
2. Anterior necrotizing scleritis with inflammation: subdivided into vasoocclusive, granulomatous, surgically induced. Aggressive form of scleritis. Average age of onset is 60 yr. Bilateral in 60% of patients
3. Scleromalacia perforans: typically affects elderly women with longstanding rheumatoid arthritis
4. Posterior scleritis: involves the deeper tissues of the eye and is potentially blinding. Age of onset is often under 40 yr. Bilateral in 35% of cases

SYNONYMS

Anterior scleritis
Diffuse nodular, necrotizing scleritis
Scleromalacia perforans
Scleral melt syndrome

ICD-9CM CODES
379.0 Scleritis and episcleritis

EPIDEMIOLOGY & DEMOGRAPHICS

PEAK INCIDENCE: Increases with increasing age
INCIDENCE (IN U.S.): Busy ophthalmologists may see one or two cases a year
PREVALENCE (IN U.S.): Relatively rare
PREDOMINANT SEX: 61% women
PREDOMINANT AGE: 52 yr

PHYSICAL FINDINGS & CLINICAL PRESENTATION

- Deep, boring (dull) eye pain that may awaken patient from sleep
- Photophobia
- Tearing
- Conjunctival injection (Fig. 1-746)
- Thinning of the sclera
- More than 50% of patients have an underlying systemic autoimmune disease. Most common rheumatic problem is rheumatoid arthritis. Most patients with systemic disease are diagnosed before development of scleritis.

ETIOLOGY

- Inflammatory (seen with rheumatoid arthritis, granulomatosis with polyangiitis [Wegener granulomatosis], relapsing polychondritis, polyarteritis nodosa)
- Allergic
- Bisphosponates: risk of scleritis is 50% higher among new bisphosphonate users than among nonusers.
- Infectious scleritis (herpes zoster, tuberculosis, Lyme disease, syphilis, *Pseudomonas aeruginosa, Nocardia*, leprosy) is uncommon, accounting for 4% to 18% of cases
- Approximately 50% of patients with scleritis have an underlying systemic disease (vasculitis, infectious disease).

DIAGNOSIS

DIFFERENTIAL DIAGNOSIS

- Most common causes are rheumatoid arthritis and other collagen-vascular diseases.
- Occasionally there are allergic, infectious, or traumatic causes.
- Conjunctivitis, iritis, and episcleritis should be considered in the differential diagnosis. Patients with episcleritis generally have less pain and vision is unaffected.

WORKUP

- Fluorescein angiography
- Eye examination
- Visual field examination
- Workup for autoimmune disease
- Workup for vasculitis
- Collagen vascular workup

LABORATORY TESTS

Rheumatoid factor, antinuclear antibody, erythrocyte sedimentation rate, ANCA (c-ANCA, p-ANCA), antiphospholipid antibodies, may be useful for underlying etiology

IMAGING STUDIES

Usually not necessary; CT scan of orbit may be useful in selected patients for collagen vascular disease or vasculitis

TREATMENT

NONPHARMACOLOGIC THERAPY

- Bandage lenses
- Surgery if thinning of the sclera is severe to prevent eye rupture

ACUTE GENERAL Rx

Immunotherapy:

- Steroids (topical, periocular, and systemic)
- Cycloplegic drops
- Nonsteroidal anti-inflammatory drugs (topical and systemic); systemic more effective than topical
- Cytotoxic agents (cyclophosphamide, azathioprine, mycophenolate mofetil, methotrexate)
- Immune modulators (cyclosporin, tacrolimus)
- Specific antibodies (infliximab, rituximab)

CHRONIC Rx

- Systemic steroids can be given for the underlying disease.
- Local steroids may be helpful.
- Control underlying disease.

DISPOSITION

Urgent referral to ophthalmologist because this disorder can be a sight-threatening condition

REFERRAL

If not referred to an ophthalmologist early, patients may develop uveitis and other complications.

PEARLS & CONSIDERATIONS

COMMENTS

An ominous diagnosis because these patients often have other severe underlying debilitating disease processes.

SUGGESTED READINGS

available at www.expertconsult.com

AUTHORS: **MELVYN KOBY, M.D.**, and **FRED F. FERRI, M.D.**

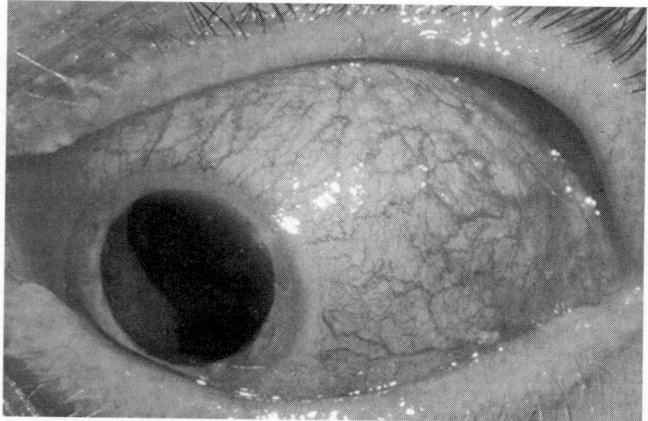

FIGURE 1-746 In diffuse anterior scleritis, widespread injection of the conjunctival and deep episcleral vessels occurs. (From Palay D [ed]: *Ophthalmology for the primary care physician*, St Louis, 1997, Mosby.)

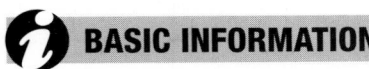

DEFINITION

Scleroderma (systemic sclerosis [SSc]) is a connective tissue disorder that is characterized by thickening and fibrosis of the skin and variably severe involvement of diverse internal organs. It can be subdivided into two major subgroups: (1) limited cutaneous SSc (lcSSc), which involves mainly the face, neck, arms, and hands; and (2) diffuse cutaneous SSc (dcSSc), which affects the skin in a more generalized distribution including the entire extremities, face, neck, and trunk. Both subgroups typically have characteristic internal organ involvement. Table 1-370 compares localized scleroderma and SSc. A classification of scleroderma is described in Box 1-56.

SYNONYMS

Systemic sclerosis
Morphea applies to localized scleroderma that affects only the skin
Scleredema is a disease of the skin that is distinct from scleroderma.

ICD-9CM CODES
710.1 Scleroderma
701.0 Morphea

EPIDEMIOLOGY & DEMOGRAPHICS

INCIDENCE: There are 2.3 to 22.8 cases per 1 million persons per yr, but many mild cases go unrecognized.
PREVALENCE: 50 to 300 cases per 1 million persons
PREDOMINANT SEX: Female/male ratio of 4:1
PREDOMINANT AGE: 30 to 50 yr
DISTRIBUTION: Worldwide

BOX 1-56 Classification of Scleroderma

I. Localized scleroderma
  A. Morphea
  B. Linear scleroderma
  C. Scleroderma en coup de sabre
II. Systemic sclerosis
  A. Limited cutaneous systemic sclerosis
  B. Diffuse cutaneous systemic sclerosis

From Hochberg MC et al: *Rheumatology,* ed 5, St Louis, 2011, Mosby.

TABLE 1-370 Comparison of Localized Scleroderma and Systemic Sclerosis

Feature	Localized Scleroderma/Morphea	Systemic Sclerosis
Skin findings	Patches or linear distribution of thickened skin	Sclerodactyly ± proximal skin thickening
Raynaud's phenomenon	Absent	Present
Digital ischemic changes	Absent	Usually present (digital pitting scars or ulcers, loss of fingerpad substance)
Internal organ disease	Absent	Present
Antinuclear antibody	Positive in ≥50% of cases	Positive in ≥85% of cases
Scleroderma-specific autoantibodies*	Negative	Positive in 60% of cases
Biopsy—histologic findings	Dermal fibrosis	Dermal fibrosis

*Scleroderma-specific antibodies include antibodies to centromere, topoisomerase-1 (Scl 70), and RNA polymerase III.
From Hochberg MC et al: *Rheumatology,* ed 5, St Louis, 2011, Mosby.

PHYSICAL FINDINGS & CLINICAL PRESENTATION

PHYSICAL FINDINGS:
1. Skin
   - Tightening of the skin begins on the hands and then progresses to the forearms, face, and neck; the skin is shiny, taut, and sometimes red, with a loss of creases and hair.
   - Later, skin tightening may limit movement by causing flexion contractures of the fingers, wrists, and elbows.
   - Pigmentary changes may occur.
   - Skin atrophy and digital gangrene of fingertips (Fig. 1-747) occurs during later stages.
2. Musculoskeletal
   - Joint pain and swelling
   - Symmetric inflammatory arthritis
   - Myopathy
3. Gastrointestinal involvement
   - Esophageal dysmotility with heartburn, dysphagia, and odynophagia
   - Delayed gastric emptying
   - Small-bowel dysmotility with abdominal cramps and diarrhea
   - Colon dysmotility with constipation
   - Primary biliary cirrhosis (see "Cirrhosis, Primary Biliary" in Section I)
4. Pulmonary manifestations
   - Pulmonary fibrosis with symptoms of dyspnea and nonproductive cough as well as fine inspiratory crackles on examination
   - Pulmonary hypertension
5. Cardiac involvement
   - Myocardial fibrosis that leads to congestive heart failure
6. Renal involvement
   - Malignant hypertension
   - Rapidly progressive renal failure
7. Other organ involvement
   - Hypothyroidism
   - Erectile dysfunction
   - Sjögren's syndrome
   - Entrapment neuropathies
8. CREST syndrome (term now replaced by lcSSc)
   - **C**alcinosis, **R**aynaud's syndrome, **E**sophageal dysmotility, **S**clerodactyly (Fig. 1-748), **T**elangiectasias—with CREST syndrome, scleroderma is limited to the distal extremities. This acronym is now considered obsolete by many because it does not accurately reflect the burden of internal organ involvement.

CLINICAL PRESENTATION:
- Raynaud's phenomenon: initial complaint in 70% of patients (NOTE: The prevalence of Raynaud's phenomenon is 5% to 10% in the general population; most cases do not progress to scleroderma.)
- Finger or hand swelling that is sometimes associated with carpal tunnel syndrome
- Arthralgias/arthritis
- Internal organ involvement

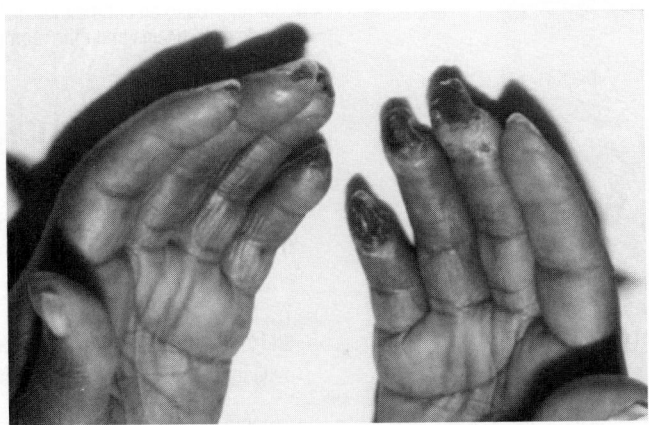

FIGURE 1-747 Digital gangrene on the fingertips of a patient with scleroderma. (From Hochberg MC et al: *Rheumatology*, ed 5, St Louis, 2011, Mosby.)

ETIOLOGY

The etiology of this condition is unknown. Genetic profiles show clustering of different alleles acoording to the subtype of SSc. There is abnormal selection of fibroblasts and aberrant control of connective tissue synthesis by fibroblasts and other cells. Although there are characteristic autoantibodies detected, it is not clear that they directly participate in the pathogenesis of the disease.

- Extracellular connective tissue activation
- Frequent immunologic abnormalities including autoantibodies
- Inflammation in the early stages of disease
- Vasoconstriction

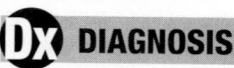 **DIAGNOSIS**

DIFFERENTIAL DIAGNOSIS

DERMATOLOGIC:
- Scleredema
- Amyloidosis
- Porphyria cutanea tarda
- Eosinophilic fasciitis
- Reflex sympathetic dystrophy
- Nephrogenic systemic fibrosis

SYSTEMIC:
- Idiopathic pulmonary fibrosis
- Primary pulmonary hypertension
- Primary biliary cirrhosis
- Cardiomyopathies
- Gastrointestinal dysmotility problems
- Systemic lupus erythematosus and overlap syndromes

WORKUP

Laboratory tests and imaging studies

LABORATORY TESTS

- Antinuclear antibodies (homogeneous, speckled, or nucleolar patterns)
- Negative antibody to native DNA
- Negative anti–smooth muscle antibody
- Autoantibodies against ribonucleoprotein positive in 20% of patients

- Rheumatoid factor positive in 20% of patients
- Anticentromere antibodies in one third of patients with lcSSc
- Positive extractable nuclear antibody to Scl-70 in 40% of patients with dcSSc
- Routine biochemistry tests may indicate specific organ involvement (e.g., liver, kidney, muscle)

IMAGING AND OTHER STUDIES

1. Arthritis: joint radiographs
2. Gastrointestinal
   - Endoscopy (diagnostic procedure of choice; may be therapeutic)
   - Cine-esophagography (in rare circumstances)
   - Barium swallow (occasionally indicated)
   - Esophageal manometry (almost never necessary)
3. Pulmonary
   - Chest x-ray
   - Pulmonary function tests (especially single-breath diffusion capacity for CO)
   - Chest computed tomography (CT) scan
   - Bronchoscopy with biopsy
   - Gallium lung scan
   - Bronchoalveolar lavage
4. Heart
   - ECG
   - Ambulatory (Holter) ECG monitoring
   - Echocardiography
   - Cardiac catheterization
5. Kidney: renal biopsy
6. Skin: skin biopsy

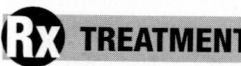 **TREATMENT**

1. Fig. E1-749 illustrates management strategies in SSc. No disease-modifying therapy available. Immunosuppressive agents used in individual patients. Prednisone should be used with extreme caution, especially in doses >20 mg/day
2. Raynaud's syndrome:

- Calcium channel blockers (i.e., long-acting dihydropyridines)
- Peripheral α_1-adrenergic blockers
- Angiotensin II receptor blockers
- Pentoxifylline
- Phosphodiesterase inhibitors
- Stellate ganglionic blockades
- Digital sympathectomy

3. Arthralgias: nonsteroidal anti-inflammatory drugs
4. Skin: for extensive skin fibrosis, immunomodulatory drugs have been used such as methotrexate, mycophenalate mofetil, and cyclophosphamide but have not been proved to be beneficial
5. Esophageal reflux
   - H_2-receptor blockers
   - Proton pump inhibitors
6. Pulmonary hypertension and fibrosis
   - Oxygen
   - Diuretics (with caution)
   - Endothelin-1 receptor inhibitors (bosentan, ambrisentan)
   - Sildenafil, tadalafil
   - Prostacyclin analogues (epoprostenol, iloprost, treprostinil)
   - Lung transplantation
   - Cyclophosphamide chemotherapy for symptomatic scleroderma-related interstitial lung disease
7. Renal involvement
   - Angiotensin-converting enzyme inhibitors
   - Dialysis
   - Renal transplantation

REFERRAL

Rheumatology consultation

RELATED CONTENT

Scleroderma (Patient Information)

AUTHORS: **EDWARD V. LALLY, M.D.,** and **FRED F. FERRI, M.D.**

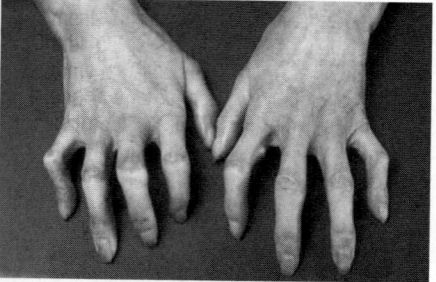

FIGURE 1-748 Sclerodactyly in a patient with systemic sclerosis. (From Hochberg MC et al: *Rheumatology,* ed 5, St Louis, 2011, Mosby.)

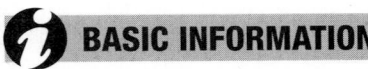

DEFINITION

Scoliosis is a lateral curvature of the spine in the upright position, usually 10 degrees or greater. Scoliosis may be classified as either structural (fixed, nonflexible) or nonstructural (flexible, correctable).

ICD-9CM CODES
737.30 Idiopathic scoliosis
737.39 Paralytic scoliosis
754.2 Congenital scoliosis
724.3 Sciatic scoliosis
737.43 Associated with neurofibromatosis

EPIDEMIOLOGY & DEMOGRAPHICS (IDIOPATHIC FORM)

PREDOMINANT SEX: Females are affected more often than males (7:1)
PREVALENCE: Four cases per 1000 persons. Idiopathic scoliosis is present in 2% of adolescents.
PREDOMINANT AGE:
- Onset variable
- Most curves found in adolescents (age ≥11 yr)

PHYSICAL FINDINGS & CLINICAL PRESENTATION

- Record patient age (in years plus months) and height.
- Perform neurologic examination to rule out neuromuscular disease.
- Inspect the shoulders and iliac crests to determine if they are level.
- Palpate the spinous processes to determine their alignment.

- Have the patient bend forward symmetrically at the waist with the arms hanging free (Adams' position); observe from the back or front to detect abnormal spine rotation (Fig. 1-750).

ETIOLOGY

- 90% unknown, usually referred to as *idiopathic* (genetic)
- Congenital spine deformity
- Neuromuscular disease
- Leg-length inequality
- Local inflammation or infection
- Acute pain (disk disease)
- Chronic degenerative disk disease with asymmetric disk narrowing
  Curves of an idiopathic nature or those accompanying congenital deformity or neuromuscular disease are associated with structural changes. The nonstructural types (leg-length discrepancy, inflammation, or acute pain) disappear when the offending disorder is corrected.

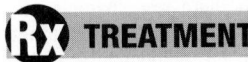

DIAGNOSIS

WORKUP

- Curvatures associated with congenital spine abnormalities, neuromuscular disease, and other less common forms of scoliosis can usually be identified by history or associated radiographic or physical findings.
- The diagnosis of scoliosis is suspected on the basis of physical examination and confirmed by radiography performed while the patient is in a standing position. Scoliosis screening is described in Fig. E1-751.

IMAGING STUDIES

- Diagnosis of idiopathic scoliosis is confirmed by a standing roentgenogram of the spine.

- Severity of the curve is measured in degrees, usually by the Cobb method (Fig. E1-752).
- MRI is usually not indicated unless there is pain, a neurologic deficit, or a left thoracic curve (which is often associated with an underlying spinal disorder).

TREATMENT

ACUTE GENERAL Rx

- Treatment or correction of cause if curve is nonstructural
- Early detection is key in treating genetic curve
- Regular observation for curves <20 degrees
- Bracing for idiopathic curves of 25 to 45 degrees in patients with an immature skeleton to prevent progression
- Surgery for idiopathic curves >45 degrees in patients with an immature skeleton

DISPOSITION

- The larger the curve at detection, the greater the chance of progression.
- Progression is more common in young children who are beginning their growth spurt.
- Curves in females are more likely to progress.
- Curves <20 degrees will improve spontaneously >50% of the time.
- Failure to diagnose and treat these curves may allow progressive deformity, pain, and cardiopulmonary compromise to develop.
- Spinal deformities >50 degrees in adults may progress and eventually become painful.
- There is no difference in the rate of back pain in the general population and patients with adolescent idiopathic scoliosis.

REFERRAL

For orthopedic consultation if structural curve is present

PEARLS & CONSIDERATIONS

COMMENTS

- Congenital scoliosis has a high incidence of cardiac and urinary tract abnormalities.
- Bracing is not intended to completely straighten the idiopathic curve. It may improve the curvature but is mainly used to stabilize and prevent progression.

SUGGESTED READINGS
available at www.expertconsult.com

RELATED CONTENT
Scoliosis (Patient Information)

AUTHORS: LONNIE R. MERCIER, M.D., and **HARALD A. HALL, M.D.**

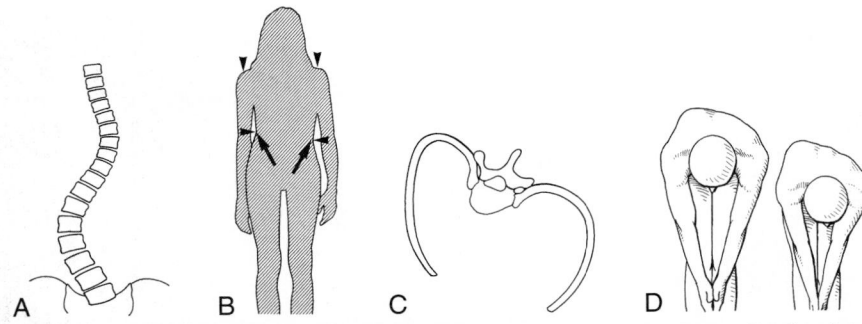

FIGURE 1-750 Structural changes in idiopathic scoliosis. A, As curvature increases, alterations in body configuration develop in both the primary and compensatory curve regions. **B,** Asymmetries of shoulder height, waistline, and the elbow-to-flank distance are common findings. **C,** Vertebral rotation and associated posterior displacement of the ribs on the convex side of the curve are responsible for the characteristic deformity of the chest wall in scoliosis patients. **D,** In the school screening examination for scoliosis, the patient bends forward at the waist. Rib asymmetry of even a small degree is obvious. (From Scoles PV: Spinal deformity in childhood and adolescence. In Behrman RE, Vaughn VC III [eds]: *Nelson textbook of pediatrics*, ed 5, Philadelphia, 1989, Saunders.)

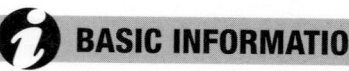

BASIC INFORMATION

DEFINITION

Recurrent depressive episodes during autumn and winter alternating with nondepressive episodes during spring and summer. Patients with seasonal affective disorder (SAD) have experienced two episodes of major depression in the past 2 yr that demonstrate the temporal seasonal relations and have had no nonseasonal episodes over this period.

SYNONYMS

SAD
Seasonal depression
Winter depression
Wintertime blues

ICD-9CM CODES
296.30 Seasonal affective disorder

EPIDEMIOLOGY & DEMOGRAPHICS

- Climate, genetic vulnerability, and sociocultural factors all play a role. The risk of seasonal mood swings is clearly associated with northern latitudes. The prevalence of SAD is estimated to be 0.5% to 1.5% in northern European populations, but up to 10% to 20% of these populations report milder, recurrent episodes consistent with subsyndromal SAD. In the U.S. it is estimated that about 5% of the population experiences SAD.
- As with other depressive disorders, women are affected disproportionately.

PHYSICAL FINDINGS & CLINICAL PRESENTATION

- The symptoms of SAD can be identical to those of other depressive episodes but tend to include features associated with atypical major depression, including low energy, irritability, weight gain, and overeating.
- Average duration is 5 mo, generally beginning in November.

ETIOLOGY

- Explanations focus on biologic models. Retinal sensitivity anomalies and emotional reactivity to light stimuli, circadian rhythm disturbance, and irregularities in melatonin and melatonin-serotonin interaction have been identified as potential risk factors. Shorter photoperiod and decrease in sunlight are hypothesized to be the triggers.
- Several neurotransmitters implicated, including dopamine, serotonin, and norepinephrine.
- Elevated rumination and low activity and exercise levels, which are also implicated in nonseasonal depression, have been shown in some studies to characterize SAD.

DIAGNOSIS

Diagnostic workup similar to that for major depression

DIFFERENTIAL DIAGNOSIS

- Major depressive disorder
- Minor depression or adjustment disorder
- Bipolar affective disorder
- Evaluate for substance use (especially alcohol)
- Medical illness or medications that may contribute to depression (e.g., endocrine disorders, neurologic disease)

WORKUP

- As with major depression, consider medical etiologies and rule out as indicated by the presenting signs and symptoms. Consider endocrine evaluation, especially thyroid function; sleep studies and a toxicology screen might be considered.
- Structured Interview Guide for the Hamilton Depression Rating Scale–Seasonal Affective Disorders Version (SIGH-SAD) used in research settings.
- In patients with major depressive disorder treated longitudinally, the routine use of depression scales to monitor outcome can help identify seasonal fluctuations of symptoms.

LABORATORY TESTS

As directed by presenting symptoms

IMAGING STUDIES

Generally not indicated

TREATMENT

NONPHARMACOLOGIC THERAPY

- Phototherapy presupposes that artificial light at a similar strength to natural sunlight will prevent the biologic changes that mediate SAD.
- Many studies have demonstrated efficacy of light therapy; however, not all studies have been able to demonstrate a benefit over placebo.
- Light therapy may be used as a first-line treatment; choice of light therapy vs. medication or psychotherapy depends on various factors, however, including severity of symptoms and suicidality, prior response to medication or light therapy, feasibility, and patient preference.
- Some studies showing retinal sensitivity anomalies in SAD normalize following phototherapy.

- Phototherapy tends to use 2500 to 10,000 lux delivered by a commercial light box or a portable head-mounted unit. Phototherapy is recommended to begin within 2 wk of the start of symptoms and continue through the winter months. Patients are instructed to sit ~18 in from the light box for 30 min up to several hours once or twice per day for a minimum of 1 wk.
- Some studies have found efficacy for high-density negative ions, although negative studies and studies demonstrating superior efficacy of light therapy also exist and more research is needed.
- Small trials have demonstrated the efficacy of cognitive-behavioral therapy, either alone or with possible additive effects to light therapy.

PHARMACOLOGIC THERAPY

Bupropion effective in preventing recurrence

ACUTE GENERAL Rx

Necessary if patient is suicidal

CHRONIC Rx

- Growing support for use of SSRIs for SAD (e.g., fluoxetine, sertraline), although more research is needed.
- Preliminary studies demonstrated efficacy of novel antidepressants that act on melatonin (i.e., agomelatine), but further research is needed.

DISPOSITION

Psychiatric referral may be helpful to confirm diagnosis. Recommended for high-risk and suicidal patients.

REFERRAL

For active suicidal ideation, psychosis, symptoms suggestive of bipolar disorder

PEARLS & CONSIDERATIONS

Patients with SAD may present with a complaint of overeating, particularly food high in carbohydrates.

SUGGESTED READINGS

available at www.expertconsult.com

RELATED CONTENT

Seasonal Affective Disorder (SAD) (Patient Information)

AUTHORS: **MARK ZIMMERMAN, M.D., CATHERINE D'AVANZATO, M.S.,** and **MITCHELL D. FELDMAN, M.D., M.PHIL.**

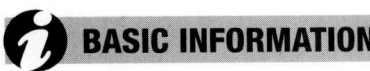

BASIC INFORMATION

DEFINITION

Seborrheic dermatitis (SD) is a common, inflammatory skin condition characterized by a mild to severe rash with scaling and erythema that occurs in areas of the skin rich in sebaceous glands.

SYNONYMS

SD
Dandruff
Cradle cap (Fig. 1-753)
Sebopsoriasis
Seborrheic eczema
Pityriasis capitis
Seborrhea

ICD-9CM CODES
690.10 Seborrheic dermatitis

EPIDEMIOLOGY & DEMOGRAPHICS

PREVALENCE: Affects between 3% and 5% of otherwise healthy adults.
PREDOMINANT SEX AND AGE: Can occur from infancy through old age, with peak incidence in adolescents and young adults and increasing again after age 50 yr. More common in men than women.
RISK FACTORS: More common in patients with HIV/AIDS, Parkinson's disease, other neurologic disorders, mood disorders, chronic alcoholic pancreatitis, hepatitis, cancer, and genetic disorders (e.g., Down syndrome). Occurs more often during winter season.

PHYSICAL FINDINGS & CLINICAL PRESENTATION

Mild, greasy scaling of the scalp and nasolabial folds, postauricular skin, beard area, eyebrows, trunk, and sometimes the central face. Blepharitis, otitis externa, and coexisting acne vulgaris or pityriasis may also be present. Itching and sting-ing of lesions can occur. Increased occurrence during times of stress or sleep deprivation.

ETIOLOGY

Actual etiology is unknown but has been linked to hormone levels, fungal infections, altered immune function, nutritional deficits, and neurogenic factors. Fungal infections of the *Malassezia* species have been associated with SD.

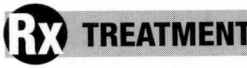 DIAGNOSIS

DIFFERENTIAL DIAGNOSIS

- Atopic dermatitis
- Candidiasis
- Dermatophytosis
- Langerhans cell histiocytosis
- Psoriasis
- Rosacea
- Systemic lupus erythematosus
- Tinea infection

WORKUP

- Diagnosis usually based on clinical identification of lesions
- Skin biopsies can be performed, if warranted, to distinguish SD from similar disorders

LABORATORY TESTS

Microscopic examination with special stains can be used to determine if yeast cells are present in keratinocytes

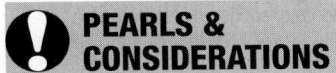 TREATMENT

NONPHARMACOLOGIC THERAPY

- Patient education that SD is a chronic condition and treatment is aimed at resolving lesions but does not prevent recurrence.

- General recommendations: wash skin regularly, soften and remove scales, and apply moisturizing emollients after washing.
- Scale removal can be accomplished through the application of mineral or olive oil and removed with a comb or brush after 1 hr.

ACUTE GENERAL Rx

- Topical steroids: can be in the form of shampoos, creams, or ointments. Can be used alone or in more severe SD with antifungals.
- Antifungals (e.g., Nizoral, selenium sulfide, ketoconazole [the most evidence for effectiveness among antifungals], ciclopirox, fluconazole). Reserve oral antifungal therapy for patients with widespread SD or SD that is refractory to topical therapy. Itraconazole 200 mg/day for 7 days is a sample oral regimen
- Calcineurin inhibitors (e.g., tacrolimus ointment, pimecrolimus cream): good when face and ears are affected
- Keratolytics (e.g., tar, salicylic acid, zinc pyrithione)
- Treatment of any secondary bacterial infection with oral antibiotics

CHRONIC Rx

Recalcitrant SD: topical azole combined with desonide regimen (limit use to 2 wk)

COMPLEMENTARY & ALTERNATIVE MEDICINE

Tea tree oil (Melaleuca oil)

REFERRAL

Consider referral to dermatology for recalcitrant cases or uncertain diagnosis

PEARLS & CONSIDERATIONS

- Use a combination of topical steroids and antifungal cream for severe SD
- Limit use of steroids to 2-wk course of treatment due to risk of cutaneous atrophy and telangiectasias
- SD of the scalp can be treated with an antifungal (e.g., 2% ketoconazole) or keratolytic shampoo. Limit use of antifungal shampoos to twice a week to prevent drying of the scalp. Alternate the use of antifungal shampoos with a moisturizing shampoo.
- In patients with widespread SD, consider testing for HIV infection

SUGGESTED READINGS
available at www.expertconsult.com

AUTHOR: ANNGENE ANTHONY, M.D., M.P.H., F.A.A.F.P.

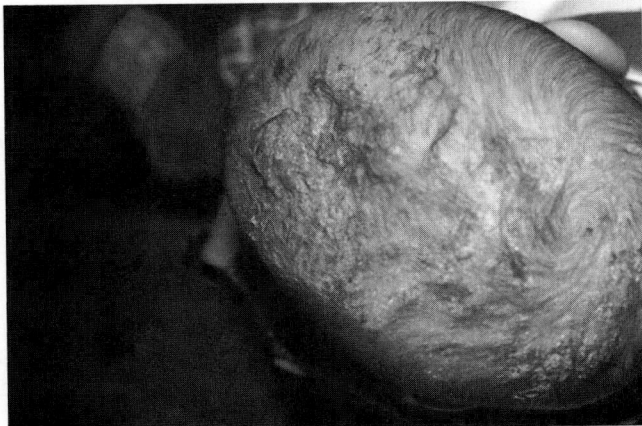

FIGURE 1-753 Cradle cap in an infant. (From Kliegman RM et al: *Nelson textbook of pediatrics,* ed 19, Philadelphia, 2011, Saunders.)

Diseases
and Disorders

I

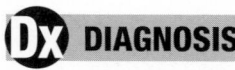
BASIC INFORMATION

DEFINITION
Absence seizures are a type of generalized seizures, characterized by brief episodes of staring with impairment of consciousness (absence). They usually last a few seconds, up to 20 to 30 sec. The onset and the end of the seizures are sudden. Usually the patients are not aware of them and resume the activity they were doing prior to the seizure. The electroencephalogram signature of absence seizures consists of generalized 3-Hz spike and slow wave discharges.

SYNONYMS
Childhood absence epilepsy
Petit mal epilepsy

ICD-9CM CODES
345.0 Generalized nonconvulsive epilepsy

EPIDEMIOLOGY & DEMOGRAPHICS
INCIDENCE: 1 to 10 cases per 100,000 population
PEAK INCIDENCE: 6 to 7 yr
PREVALENCE: Represent up to 18% of all pediatric epilepsy syndromes
PREDOMINANT SEX AND AGE: More common in girls than in boys, absences typically begin between 4 and 8 yr

PHYSICAL FINDINGS & CLINICAL PRESENTATION
- Patients with absence seizures usually have normal physical and neurologic examinations.
- During the seizures, the patients are unresponsive and can have motor phenomena (automatisms, eye blinks, mouth and hand movements).
- Tonic clonic seizures are not usually a feature of this syndrome. If this is the case, other etiologies should be investigated such as juvenile absence epilepsy, juvenile myoclonic epilepsy, etc.

ETIOLOGY
Genetic

DIAGNOSIS

DIFFERENTIAL DIAGNOSIS
- Juvenile absence epilepsy
- Juvenile myoclonic epilepsy
- Complex partial seizures

WORKUP
- EEG with hyperventilation and photic stimulation is crucial in the diagnosis.
- Ambulatory EEG and video EEG are recommended for patients with diagnostic uncertainty.

LABORATORY TESTS
No specific studies needed

IMAGING STUDIES
- MRI of the brain should be performed in all epilepsy patients, especially if the EEG does not show the typical characteristic of absence seizures (3-Hz spike and slow wave discharges).
- CT scans of the head should be avoided in children due to unnecessary exposure to radiation and the low yield of the test except when MRI cannot be obtained.

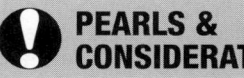
TREATMENT

The medication of choice based on the best current data available is ethosuximide, followed by valproic acid and lamotrigine.

NONPHARMACOLOGIC THERAPY
Not applicable

GENERAL Rx
- Ethosuximide: initial dose: 10 mg/kg/day; then after 7 days, 20 mg/kg
- Valproic acid (Depakote): initial dose: 5-10 mg/kg/day (divided bid), maximum dose 60 mg/kg/day
- Lamotrigine: dose for patients on no other antiepileptic drugs. Wk 1 and 2: 0.3 mg/kg/day. Wk 3 and 4: 0.6 mg/kg/day. Wk 5 onward: increase every 1 to 2 wk by 0.6 mg/kg/day. Maintenance: 4.5 to 7.5 mg/kg/day. Warning: should be used with caution due to the potential for toxicity and Stevens-Johnson syndrome. Patients on other antiepileptic drugs can also have severe adverse reactions.

CHRONIC Rx
- Children with recurrent seizures require chronic treatment.
- If children are seizure free for a period of 1 to 2 yr, a trial on no medications should be considered; children, unlike adults, can "outgrow" seizures.

COMPLEMENTARY & ALTERNATIVE MEDICINE
Not applicable

DISPOSITION
- Response to treatment is excellent.
- Absence seizures tend to remit in teenage years.

REFERRAL
Patients with epilepsy and seizures should be referred for a consultation by a neurologist, preferably one specializing in epilepsy.

PEARLS & CONSIDERATIONS

COMMENTS
- Absence seizures can be present in other epilepsy syndromes.
- Valproic acid should be avoided in girls and women with childbearing potential due to the risk of teratogenicity.
- Carbamazepine and phenytoin should be avoided in the treatment of absence seizures, since these medications may worsen seizures and could provoke absence status epilepticus.
- All women of childbearing age taking antiepileptic drugs should take folic acid supplementation (1 to 4 mg/day) for the prevention of neural tube defects.

PREVENTION
Sleep deprivation and alcohol consumption should be avoided.

PATIENT & FAMILY EDUCATION
- Patients with epilepsy have normal lives.
- The goal of treatment is no seizures and no side effects to medications.
- Patient education and information can be obtained from the Epilepsy Foundation: www.epilepsyfoundation.org
- Pregnant women with epilepsy should visit the Antiepileptic Drug Pregnancy Registry website for information and assistance: www2.massgeneral.org/aed
- Patients with ongoing seizures are forbidden from driving; check state regulations and laws regarding driving and epilepsy.

SUGGESTED READINGS
available at www.expertconsult.com

RELATED CONTENT
Absence Seizures (Patient Information)

AUTHOR: **PATRICIO SEBASTIAN ESPINOSA, M.D., M.P.H.**

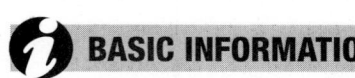 BASIC INFORMATION

DEFINITION

Febrile seizures are seizures that occur in febrile children (fever of at least 100.4° F [38° C]) between the ages of 6 and 60 mo in the absence of intracranial infection, metabolic disturbance, or history of a febrile seizure. Febrile seizures are subdivided into 2 categories: simple and complex. Simple febrile seizures last <15 min, are generalized (without a focal component), and occur once in a 24-hr period, whereas complex febrile seizures are prolonged (>15 min), show focal neurologic signs, or occur more than once in 24 hr.

SYNONYMS

Febrile convulsions

ICD-9CM CODES
780.6 Febrile seizures

EPIDEMIOLOGY & DEMOGRAPHICS

INCIDENCE: Febrile seizures are the most common seizures of childhood. 2% to 5% of children will have a febrile seizure by age 60 mo. Simple febrile seizures represent 65% to 90% of febrile seizures.
PREDOMINANT SEX AND AGE: Slightly more common in boys than girls.
PEAK INCIDENCE: 6 to 60 mo
PREVALENCE: Represent up to 18% of all pediatric epilepsy syndromes

PHYSICAL FINDINGS & CLINICAL PRESENTATION

- Children with febrile seizures have normal physical and neurologic examinations.
- Viral illnesses are the predominant cause of febrile seizures.

ETIOLOGY

- Most causes of febrile seizures are multifactorial, with two or more genetic and contributing environmental factors.
- Viral infections are a common cause of fever that triggers febrile seizures.
- There are case-control studies suggesting that iron and zinc deficiencies may be risk factors for febrile seizures.

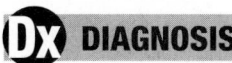 DIAGNOSIS

DIFFERENTIAL DIAGNOSIS
- CNS infection (i.e., meningitis)
- Epilepsy

WORKUP
- It is important to first investigate whether an underlying infection exists. Fig. E1-754 describes guidelines for febrile seizure evaluation.
- In patients with simple self-limited febrile seizures with rapid return to consciousness and a normal neurologic examination, further workup is not routinely recommended.
- In patients with complex febrile seizures, laboratory workup and brain imaging are recommended.
- EEG is not routinely recommended in the evaluation of a neurologically healthy child with simple partial seizures.

LABORATORY TESTS
- Routine blood workup (CBC with differential, CMP, electrolytes), blood and urine cultures are often performed but there is no evidence that these tests are necessary for identifying the cause of a simple febrile seizure.
- CSF analysis: lumbar puncture guidelines (American Academy of Pediatrics)
  ○ Lumbar puncture should be performed in children with febrile seizures and signs and symptoms of meningitis (e.g., neck stiffness, Kernig sign, Brudzinski sign), or if the patient history or examination suggests the presence of meningitis or intracranial infection.
  ○ In infants 6 to 12 months of age with febrile seizures, lumbar puncture is an option if they have not received the recommended *Haemophilus influenza* type b (Hib) or pneumococcal vaccinations, or if their immunization status is unknown.
  ○ Lumbar puncture is also considered an option in children with febrile seizures pretreated with antibiotics.

IMAGING STUDIES
- MRI of the brain is not required in the routine evaluation of patients with simple febrile seizures.
- Imaging of the brain should be considered in children with complex febrile seizures and in children with focal neurologic deficits.
- CT scans of the head should be avoided in children, if possible, due to exposure to radiation and the relative low yield of the test compared to MRI. CT scans of the head are reserved for neurologic emergencies and are adjusted for weight in children.

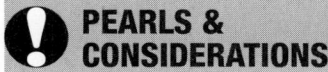 TREATMENT

Febrile seizures do not usually require antiepileptic drug treatment.

NONPHARMACOLOGIC THERAPY
Not applicable

GENERAL Rx
Treat the cause of the fever.

CHRONIC Rx
No chronic treatment for febrile seizures is recommended.

COMPLEMENTARY & ALTERNATIVE MEDICINE
Not applicable

DISPOSITION
- Treatment is not recommended.
- Febrile seizures should stop by age 60 mo.
- Risk of recurrence in the first 2 years after an initial febrile seizure is 15% to 70%.

REFERRAL
Patients with recurrent febrile seizures need to be referred for a consultation by a pediatric neurologist.

PEARLS & CONSIDERATIONS

COMMENTS
- It is crucial to find out the etiology of the fever and to treat it appropriately.
- Patient with seizures and fever after age 60 mo are not classified as febrile seizures.

PREVENTION
Antipyretics do not reduce the recurrence risk of febrile seizures. However, fever should be treated and worked up independently of the diagnosis of febrile seizures.

PATIENT & FAMILY EDUCATION
- Children with febrile seizures do not need antiepileptic drug treatment.
- Patient education and information can be obtained at the Epilepsy Foundation: www.epilepsyfoundation.org. Parents should be reassured that children without underlying developmental problems will usually not have lasting neurologic effects from febrile seizures.

SUGGESTED READINGS
available at www.expertconsult.com

AUTHOR: **PATRICIO SEBASTIAN ESPINOSA, M.D., M.P.H.**

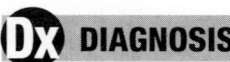

BASIC INFORMATION

DEFINITION

Tonic clonic seizures are characterized by sudden loss of consciousness, muscle contraction (tonic phase) followed by rhythmic jerking activity (clonic phase).

SYNONYMS

Convulsive seizures
Grand mal seizures

ICD-9CM CODES

345.1 Generalized convulsive epilepsy

EPIDEMIOLOGY & DEMOGRAPHICS

INCIDENCE: 30 to 50 cases per 100,000 person-yr (epilepsy incidence)
PEAK INCIDENCE: Not applicable
PREVALENCE: 5 to 8 cases per 1000 persons (epilepsy incidence)
PREDOMINANT SEX AND AGE: No gender preference

PHYSICAL FINDINGS & CLINICAL PRESENTATION

- Patients with tonic clonic seizures usually have normal physical and neurologic examinations (interictally).
- During the seizures, the patients are unresponsive and can have violent postures with severe repetitive muscle contractions.
- After the seizure, the patients are usually lethargic and confused.
- Tonic clonic seizures are associated with injuries, bladder incontinence, and tongue biting.
- Focal postictal weakness may point toward a focal neurologic lesion (Todd's paralysis).

ETIOLOGY

- Seizures are a cardinal sign of cortical neurologic injury.
- The etiology of seizures can be idiopathic (likely genetic), cryptogenic (possibly genetic), and symptomatic (due to a neurologic injury).

 DIAGNOSIS

DIFFERENTIAL DIAGNOSIS

- Convulsive syncope
- Nonepileptic spells

WORKUP

- EEG
- Ambulatory EEG and/or video EEG recommended for patients with diagnostic uncertainty
- MRI of the brain

LABORATORY TESTS

- Routine blood workup (CBC, CMP, glucose, electrolytes)
- Urine drug screen
- Lumbar puncture is recommended in patients with the suspicion of meningitis

IMAGING STUDIES

- Neurodiagnostic imaging studies such as CT of the head or, preferably, MRI of the brain should be performed in all patients with first unprovoked seizure.
- CT scans of the head should be avoided in children due to unnecessary exposure to radiation and the low yield of the test. CT scans of the head are reserved for neurologic emergencies and are adjusted for weight in children.

TREATMENT

- Treatment is based on the type and etiology of seizures (i.e., metabolic disturbance, infectious, etc.).
- Levetiracetam is an effective and well-tolerated antiepileptic drug for treating generalized tonic clonic seizures.
- Valproic acid is better tolerated than topiramate and more efficacious than lamotrigine in patients with generalized and unclassified epilepsy types.
- Valproic acid should be avoided in girls and women with childbearing potential due to the risk of teratogenicity.

NONPHARMACOLOGIC THERAPY

Not applicable

GENERAL Rx

- First unprovoked seizure with normal imaging, EEG, and laboratory workup requires no treatment.
- Recurrent seizures and seizures with abnormal studies require treatment depending on the etiology.
- Valproic acid (Depakote): Initial dose: 10 to 15 mg/kg/day (divided bid), maximum dose 60 mg/kg/day.
- Levetiracetam (Keppra): Initial dose 250 to 500 bid, maximum dose 1500 mg bid.

CHRONIC Rx

Chronic treatment with antiepileptic drugs is indicated for ≥2 nonprovoked seizures or in patients with one seizure with abnormal workup.

COMPLEMENTARY & ALTERNATIVE MEDICINE

Not applicable

DISPOSITION

- Response to treatment is excellent.
- No driving until seizure freedom in accordance with local laws and regulations.

REFERRAL

Patients with epilepsy and seizures should be referred for a consultation by a neurologist, preferably one with epilepsy training.

PEARLS & CONSIDERATIONS

COMMENTS

- It is crucial to understand that tonic clonic seizures can occur in variety of acute neurologic diseases.
- Successful treatment depends on the correct choice of antiepileptic drugs based on the type (partial vs. generalized in onset) and etiology of the seizures.
- Valproic acid should be avoided in girls and women with childbearing potential due to the risk of teratogenicity.
- All women of childbearing age taking antiepileptic drugs should take folic acid supplementation (1-4 mg/day) for the prevention of neural tube defects.

PREVENTION

Sleep deprivation and alcohol consumption should be avoided.

PATIENT & FAMILY EDUCATION

- Patients with epilepsy have normal lives.
- The goal of treatment is no seizures and no side effects to medications.
- Patient education and information can be obtained at the Epilepsy Foundation: www.epilepsyfoundation.org
- Pregnant women with epilepsy should visit the Antiepileptic Drug Pregnancy Registry website for information and assistance: www2.massgeneral.org/aed
- Patients with ongoing seizures are forbidden from driving; check your state regulations and laws regarding driving and epilepsy.

SUGGESTED READINGS

available at www.expertconsult.com

RELATED CONTENT

Generalized Tonic-Clonic Seizures (Patient Information)

AUTHOR: **PATRICIO SEBASTIAN ESPINOSA, M.D., M.P.H.**

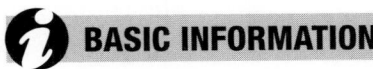

BASIC INFORMATION

DEFINITION

Partial seizures are characterized by focal cortical discharges that provoke seizure symptoms related to the area of the brain involved. Simple partial seizures do not cause impairment of consciousness.

SYNONYMS

Simple partial seizures
Focal seizures

ICD-9CM CODES

345.5 Localization-related (focal) (partial) epilepsy and epileptic syndromes with simple partial seizures

EPIDEMIOLOGY & DEMOGRAPHICS

INCIDENCE: 30 to 50 cases per 100,000 person-yr
PREVALENCE: 5 to 8 cases per 1000 persons
PREDOMINANT SEX AND AGE: No gender preference

PHYSICAL FINDINGS & CLINICAL PRESENTATION

- Patients with partial seizures usually have normal physical and neurologic examinations unless the focal seizures are due to a structural abnormality such as a stroke, wherein the patient will have a neurologic exam consistent with the area of CNS structural damage.
- During partial seizures the patients are conscious, unless there is spread of the epileptic focus causing secondary generalization and unresponsiveness. A focal seizure can evolve to a generalized tonic clonic seizure.
- Patients with partial seizures can experience postictal weakness/paralysis that usually resolves within 24 hr (Todd's paralysis). However, focal neurologic deficits may also be indicative of a structural brain lesion.

ETIOLOGY

- Seizures in general are a cardinal sign of cortical neurologic injury.
- The etiology of partial seizures can be idiopathic (likely genetic), cryptogenic (unknown, possibly genetic), and symptomatic (due to a neurologic injury).
- Frequent causes of partial seizures are tumor, stroke, CNS infections (cysticercosis, abscesses), arteriovenous malformations (AVMs), traumatic brain injury, cortical malformations, and others.

DIAGNOSIS

DIFFERENTIAL DIAGNOSIS

- Transient ischemic attack
- Movement disorders
- Nonepileptic spells

WORKUP

- EEG
- Ambulatory EEG and/or video EEG recommended for patients with diagnostic uncertainty

LABORATORY TESTS

Routine blood workup (CBC, CMP, glucose, electrolytes) may be considered in appropriate clinical situations.

IMAGING STUDIES

- In the acute setting, a CT scan of the head is high yield to rule out space-occupying lesions.
- MRI of the brain with a defined epilepsy protocol should be performed in all patients with recurrent seizures.
- CT scans of the head should be avoided in children if possible, unless in an emergency setting.

TREATMENT

- Carbamazepine traditionally has been the standard initial drug treatment for partial seizures.
- Lamotrigine and levetiracetam are effective and well-tolerated antiepileptic drugs for treating partial seizures.
- Other antiepileptic drugs (e.g., lacosamide, oxcarbazepine, ezogabine) may be used by an epilepsy specialist in specific cases.
- Surgical treatments (e.g., temporal lobectomy in mesial temporal sclerosis) may be indicated in refractory cases of partial seizures.

GENERAL Rx

- After a first unprovoked seizure with normal examination, imaging, and EEG, no treatment is required.
- Recurrent seizures and seizures with abnormal studies require treatment.

DISPOSITION

- Response to treatment often depends on the etiology of the partial seizures.
- 47% of patients become seizure free with monotherapy and 67% with polytherapy.

- No driving until seizure freedom in accordance with local laws and regulations.

REFERRAL

Patients with epilepsy and seizures should be referred for a consultation by a neurologist, preferably one with a special interest in epilepsy.

PEARLS & CONSIDERATIONS

COMMENTS

- It is crucial to understand that partial seizures can be due to a variety of neurologic diseases.
- Successful treatment depends on the correct choice of antiepileptic drugs based on patient's gender and comorbidities.
- Valproic acid should be avoided in girls and women with childbearing potential due to the risk of teratogenicity.
- All women in childbearing age taking antiepileptic drugs should take folic acid supplementation (1 to 4 mg/day) for the prevention of neural tube defects.

PREVENTION

- Sleep deprivation and alcohol consumption should be avoided.
- Drug compliance is compulsory to prevent seizure recurrence.

PATIENT & FAMILY EDUCATION

- People with epilepsy can lead normal lives.
- The goal of treatment is no seizures and no side effects to medications.
- Patient education and information can be obtained at the Epilepsy Foundation: www.epilepsyfoundation.org
- Pregnant women with epilepsy should visit the Antiepileptic Drug Pregnancy Registry website for information and assistance: www2.massgeneral.org/aed
- Patients with ongoing seizures are forbidden from driving; check your state regulations and laws regarding driving and epilepsy.
- Patients should be counseled on general seizure precautions such as swimming, bathing, and heights.

SUGGESTED READINGS
available at www.expertconsult.com

RELATED CONTENT
Partial Motor Seizures (Patient Information)

AUTHOR: **PATRICIO SEBASTIAN ESPINOSA, M.D., M.P.H.**

BASIC INFORMATION

DEFINITION

Sepsis is an exaggerated inflammatory response to an infectious stimulus. It is generally caused by generalized bacterial or fungal infection and characterized by evidence of infection, fever or hypothermia, hypotension, and evidence of end-organ compromise.

SYNONYMS

Septicemia
Sepsis syndrome
Severe sepsis
Systemic inflammatory response syndrome
Septic shock

ICD-9CM CODES
038.9 Sepsis
038.40 Sepsis, gram-negative bacteremia
038.1 Sepsis, *Staphylococcus*

EPIDEMIOLOGY & DEMOGRAPHICS

INCIDENCE (IN U.S.):
- Exact incidence is unknown
- Approximately 750,000 cases of severe sepsis occur among hospitalized patients each year in the U.S.
- Complicates a minority of bacteremia cases and may occur in the absence of documented bacteremia

PREDOMINANT SEX: Males slightly more commonly affected than females

PREDOMINANT AGE:
- Neonatal period
- Patients >65 yr of age account for 60% of all cases of severe sepsis

GENETICS:
- Familial disposition: a great variety of congenital immunodeficiency states and other inherited disorders may predispose to septicemia.
- Neonatal infection: incidence is high in neonatal period.

PHYSICAL FINDINGS & CLINICAL PRESENTATION

- Fever or hypothermia
- Hypotension
- Tachycardia
- Tachypnea
- Altered mental status
- Bleeding diathesis
- Skin rashes
- Symptoms that reflect primary site of infection: urinary tract, GI tract, CNS, respiratory tract
- Table 1-371 describes some clinical signs and symptoms of sepsis.

ETIOLOGY

- Disseminated infection with a great variety of bacteria:
  A. Gram-negative bacteria
    1. *Escherichia coli*
    2. *Klebsiella* spp.
    3. *Pseudomonas aeruginosa*
    4. *Proteus* spp.
    5. *Neisseria meningitidis*
  B. Gram-positive bacteria
    1. *Staphylococcus aureus* (including MRSA)
    2. *Streptococcus* spp.
    3. *Enterococcus* spp.
- Less common infections:
  1. Fungal
  2. Viral
  3. Rickettsial
  4. Parasitic
- Sepsis is a complex dysregulation of both inflammation and coagulation. There is activation of coagulation, inflammatory cytokines, complement, and kinin cascades with release of a variety of vasoactive endogenous mediators
- Predisposing host factors:
  1. General medical condition
  2. Extremes of age
  3. Immunosuppressive therapy
  4. Recent surgery
  5. Granulocytopenia
  6. Hyposplenism
  7. Diabetes
  8. Instrumentation

DIAGNOSIS
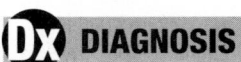

DIFFERENTIAL DIAGNOSIS

- Cardiogenic shock
- Acute pancreatitis
- Pulmonary embolism
- Systemic vasculitis
- Toxic ingestion
- Exposure-induced hypothermia
- Fulminant hepatic failure
- Collagen-vascular diseases

WORKUP

- Evaluation should focus on identifying a specific pathogen and localizing the site of primary infection. Fig. E1-755 illustrates workup following results of blood cultures.
- Hemodynamic, metabolic, coagulation disorders should be carefully characterized.
- Intensive monitoring, including the use of central venous catheters.

LABORATORY TESTS

- Cultures of blood and examination and culture of sputum, urine, wound drainage, stool, and CSF
- CBC with differential, coagulation profile
- Routine chemistries, LFTs
- ABGs, lactic acid level; procalcitonin might be useful as a general marker of infection/sepsis
- Urinalysis

IMAGING STUDIES

- Chest x-ray examination
- Other radiographic and radioisotope procedures according to suspected site of primary infection

TREATMENT

NONPHARMACOLOGIC THERAPY

- Tissue oxygenation: mixed venous oxygen saturation maintained >70% if possible; early mechanical ventilation
- Focal infection should be drained if possible, and potentially infected catheters should be removed

ACUTE GENERAL Rx

- Blood pressure support, rapid IV fluid resuscitation and vasopressors, if needed, with the goal of reestablishing a mean arterial blood pressure >65 mm Hg; reduction in blood lactate and mixed venous oxygen saturation >70% within 6 hr of recognition of septic shock is associated with improved survival. Measure vena cava oxygen saturation (ScvO$_2$) to assess adequacy of resuscitation. If the ScvO$_2$ is <70%, consider packed red blood cell transfusion to achieve Hct >30%. Start inotropic agents if ScvO$_2$ is <70% despite transfusion.
  1. IV hydration; crystalloids are as effective as colloids as resuscitation fluids. Most patients need 4 to 6 L of fluid in the first 6 hours.
  2. Therapy with vasopressors (e.g., dopamine, norepinephrine, vasopressin) if mean blood pressure of 70 to 75 mm Hg cannot be maintained by hydration alone. A recent trial comparing low-dose vasopressin with norepinephrine revealed that low-dose vasopressin did not reduce mortality rates as compared with norepinephrine among patients with septic shock who were treated with catecholamine vasopressors.
- Correction of acidosis by improving the tissue perfusion, not by giving bicarbonate
  1. Mechanical ventilation
- Antibiotics
  1. Directed at the most likely sources of infection. Table 1-372 describes initial antibiotic recommendations for septic patients.
  2. Should generally provide broad coverage of gram-positive and gram-negative bacteria (or fungi if clinically indicated).
  3. Antibiotics should be administered within 1 hr of the diagnosis of septic shock—this is a medical emergency.

4. The role of corticosteroids in the acute management of septicemia has long been debated. Previous trials had shown that corticosteroid therapy improved hemodynamic outcomes in patients with severe septic shock. Patients with relative adrenal insufficiency may benefit from low-dose therapy with hydrocortisone (50 mg IV q6h) and fludrocortisone (50 micrograms daily PO) given together for 7 days. Recent trials, however, revealed that hydrocortisone did not improve survival or reversal of shock, either overall or in patients who did not have a response to corticotropin, although hydrocortisone hastened reversal of shock in patients in whom shock was reversed. Until definitive data are available, the decision to administer corticosteroids for septic shock should be based on the individual patient's severity of illness versus risk of corticosteroid administration. The corticotropin (ACTH) stimulation test is not helpful and should not be used to determine the need for corticosteroid in these patients.

CHRONIC Rx
- Adjust antibiotic therapy on the basis of culture results.
- In general, continue therapy for a minimum of 2 wk.

DISPOSITION
All patients with suspected septicemia should be hospitalized and given access to intensive monitoring and nursing care.

REFERRAL
- To infectious diseases expert
- To physician experienced in critical care

⚠ PEARLS & CONSIDERATIONS

COMMENTS
- Mortality rises quickly if antibiotic therapy is not instituted promptly (preferably within 1 hr of onset of shock) and metabolic derangements are not treated aggressively.

- Human recombinant activated protein C (drotrecogin alfa activated) was taken off the market as a treatment for sepsis after follow-up studies showed no added benefit to standard sepsis care.

SUGGESTED READINGS
available at www.expertconsult.com

AUTHOR: **STEVEN M. OPAL, M.D.**

TABLE 1-371   Clinical Signs and Symptoms of Sepsis

Infection	General	Inflammatory	Hemodynamic	Tissue Perfusion
Documented or suspected	Temperature >38°C or < 36°C Heart rate >90 beats/min Respiratory rate ≥20 breaths/min Altered mental status Hyperglycemia Third spacing of fluid	WBC count <4000 or >12,000 cells/mcL or ≥10% bands	Hypotension: systolic blood pressure <90 mm Hg MAP <70 mm Hg SVo_2 >70 CI >3.5 L/min/m^2	Hypoxemia: (Pao_2/Fio_2 <300) Acute oliguria (urine output <0.5 ml/kg/hr) Coagulopathy Abnormal liver function tests Platelet count <100,000 cells/μL Lactic acidosis Skin mottling

CI, Cardiac index; *MAP*, mean arterial pressure; *SVo₂*, mixed venous oxygen saturation; *WBC*, white blood cell.
From Cameron, JL, Cameron AM: *Current surgical therapy*, ed 10, Philadelphia, 2011, Saunders.

TABLE 1-372   Initial Antibiotic Recommendations for Septic Patients*

Empiric coverage	Vancomycin 15 mg/kg q12h plus either piperacillin-tazobactam† 3.375 g IV q6h or imipenem 0.5 g IV q6h or meropenem 1.0 g IV q8h with or without an aminoglycoside (e.g., tobramycin 5 mg/kg IV q24).‡
Community-acquired pneumonia	Ceftriaxone 1 g IV q24h plus azithromycin 500 mg IV q24h or a fluoroquinolone (e.g., moxifloxacin 400 mg IV q24h or levofloxacin 750 mg IV q24h).§
Community-acquired urosepsis	Ciprofloxacin 400 mg IV q24h or ampicillin 2 g IV q6h plus gentamicin 5 mg/kg IV q24h.
Meningitis	Vancomycin 500-750 mg IV q6h plus ceftriaxone 2 g IV q12h plus dexamethasone 0.15 mg/kg IV q6h × 2-4 days preferably before antibiotics; add ampicillin 2 g IV q4h if *Listeria* is suspected.
Nosocomial pneumonia	Vancomycin 15 mg/kg q12h plus either piperacillin-tazobactam 4.5 g IV q6h or imipenem 0.5 g IV q6h or meropenem 1 g IV q8h or cefepime 2 g IV q12h plus either an aminoglycoside (e.g., amikacin 15 mg/kg IV q24h or tobramycin 7 mg/kg IV q24h) or levofloxacin 750 mg IV q24h. Some authorities would substitute linezolid 600 mg IV q12h for vancomycin if methicillin-resistant *Staphylococcus aureus* is of significant concern or known to be the cause.
Neutropenia	Cefepime 2 g IV q8h; add vancomycin 15 mg/kg IV q12h if a central line is present and infection is a concern. Add antifungal coverage with liposomal amphotericin B 3-5 mg/kg q24h or caspofungin 70 mg IV × 1 then 50 mg IV q24h if fever persists ≥5 days. If invasive aspergillosis is highly suspected or proven, voriconazole 6 mg/kg IV q12h × 2 then 4 mg/kg IV q12h should be used.
Cellulitis and skin infections	Vancomycin 15 mg/kg IV q12h. Add piperacillin-tazobactam 4.5 g IV q6h in diabetics or immunocompromised patients. If necrotizing fasciitis is suspected, add clindamycin 900 mg IV; surgical debridement is crucial.

*Assumes normal renal function; dose adjustments required with impaired creatinine clearance.
†Substitute aztreonam 2 g IV q8h if penicillin allergic.
‡Monitor drug levels of aminoglycosides (i.e., peak and trough).
§Use ceftriaxone and azithromycin if the patient is admitted to the intensive care unit.
From Andreoli TE et al: *Andreoli and Carpenter's Cecil essentials of medicine*, ed 8, Philadelphia, 2010, Saunders.

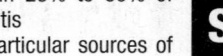

 BASIC INFORMATION

DEFINITION

Septic arthritis is a highly destructive form of joint disease most often caused by hematogenous spread of organisms from a distant site of infection. Direct penetration of the joint as a result of trauma or surgery and spread from adjacent osteomyelitis may also cause bacterial arthritis. Any joint in the body may be affected.

SYNONYMS

Infectious arthritis
Bacterial arthritis
Pyogenic arthritis

ICD-9CM CODES
711 Pyogenic arthritis, site unspecified

EPIDEMIOLOGY & DEMOGRAPHICS

INCIDENCE (IN U.S.): Unknown
PREVALENCE (IN U.S.): Unknown
PREDOMINANT SEX: Gonococcal arthritis in females
PREDOMINANT AGE: Gonococcal arthritis in sexually active adults
PEAK INCIDENCE:
- Gonococcal arthritis: young adults
- Other bacterial causes: all ages

PHYSICAL FINDINGS & CLINICAL PRESENTATION

- Hallmark: acute onset of monoarticular joint pain, erythema, heat, and immobility
- Limited range of motion of the joint
- Effusion, with varying degrees of erythema and increased warmth around the joint
- Single joint affected in 80% to 90% of cases of nongonococcal arthritis
- Gonococcal dermatitis-arthritis syndrome
  - Typical pattern is a migratory polyarthritis or tenosynovitis
  - Small pustules on the trunk or extremities
- Febrile patient at presentation
- Most commonly affected joints in adult: knee and hip, but any joint may be involved; in children: hip

ETIOLOGY

- Bacteria spread from another locus of infection
  - Highly vascular synovium is invaded by hematogenously spread bacteria.
  - WBC enzymes cause necrosis of synovium, cartilage, and bone.
  - Extensive joint destruction is rapid if infection is not treated with appropriate IV antibiotics and drainage of necrotic material.
- Predisposing factors: rheumatoid arthritis, prosthetic joints, advanced age, immunodeficiency (HIV, DM, immunosuppressive drugs), sexual activity (gonococcal arthritis), skin infections, cutaneous ulcers (contiguous spread), recent joint surgery, recent intraarticular infection. Fig. E1-756 illustrates routes by which bacteria can reach the joint.

- The most common nongonococcal organisms are staphylococci (40%), streptococci (28%), and gram-negative bacilli (19%). Less common are mycobacteria (8%), gram-negative cocci (3%), anaerobes (1%), and gram-positive bacilli (1%).
- Staphylococci (S. aureus and coagulase-negative staphylococcal species) account for >50% of prosthetic-hip and prosthetic-knee infections. S. aureus is very common in patients with rheumatoid arthritis.

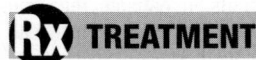 **DIAGNOSIS**

DIFFERENTIAL DIAGNOSIS

- Gout
- Pseudogout
- Trauma
- Hemarthrosis
- Rheumatic fever
- Adult or juvenile rheumatoid arthritis
- Spondyloarthropathies such as reactive arthritis (Reiter's syndrome)
- Osteomyelitis
- Viral arthritides
- Septic bursitis
- Lyme disease caused by *Borrelia burgdorferi*

WORKUP

- Joint aspiration, Gram stain, and culture of the synovial fluid. Fig. E1-757 describes an algorithm for synovial fluid analysis in septic arthritis.
- Immediate arthrocentesis before other studies are undertaken or antibiotics instituted. Synovial fluid should be evaluated at bedside and then sent for lab evaluation

LABORATORY TESTS

- Joint fluid analysis
  - Synovial fluid leukocyte count is usually elevated >50,000 cells/mm^3 with >80% polymorphonuclear cells.
  - Counts are highly variable, with similar findings in gout, pseudogout, or rheumatoid arthritis. Lower WBC counts can occur in joint replacement, disseminated gonococal disease, and peripheral leukopenia.
  - Synovial fluid glucose or protein is not helpful because results are not specific for septic arthritis. The differential diagnosis of synovial fluid abnormalities is described in Section III.
  - PCR testing: useful for detection of uncommon organisms (e.g., Lyme disease)
  - Crystal analysis: septic arthritis can coexist with crystal arthropathy; therefore, the presence of crystals does not preclude a diagnosis of septic arthritis.

- Blood cultures: positive in 25% to 50% of patients with septic arthritis
- Culture of possible extraarticular sources of infection
- Elevated peripheral WBC count, ESR (nonspecific), C-reactive protein (CRP) (nonspecific). When elevated, ESR and CRP may be useful to monitor therapeutic response.
- If gonococcus is suspected, perform nucleic acid amplification tests (NAATs) on synovial fluid.

IMAGING STUDIES

- Radiograph of the affected joint: useful to rule out osteomyelitis, fractures, chondrocalcinosis, or inflammatory arthritis
- MRI: findings that suggest an acute intraarticular infection include the combination of bony erosions with marrow edema
- CT scan: useful for early diagnosis of infections of the spine, hips, and sternoclavicular and sacroiliac joints
- Ultrasound: can be useful for detecting effusions in joints that are more difficult to examine (e.g., hip)

TREATMENT

NONPHARMACOLOGIC THERAPY

- Affected joints aspirated daily to remove necrotic material and to follow serial WBC counts and cultures
- If no resolution with IV antibiotics and closed drainage: open debridement and lavage, particularly in nongonococcal infections
- Prevention of contractures:
  - After acute stage of inflammation, range-of-motion exercises of the affected joint
  - Physical therapy helpful

ACUTE GENERAL Rx

- IV antibiotics immediately after joint aspiration and Gram stain of the synovial fluid. Empiric antibiotic therapy is based on organism found on Gram stain of synovial fluid:
  - Gram-positive cocci: vancomycin
  - Gram-negative cocci: ceftriaxone
  - Gram-negative rods: ceftazidime, cefepime, piperacillin-tazobactam. Aztreonam or fluoroquinolones can be used in patients with allergy to penicillin or cephalosporins
  - Negative Gram stain: vancomycin plus either ceftazidime or a carbapenem such as meropenem or ertapenem.

SUGGESTED READINGS
available at www.expertconsult.com

RELATED CONTENT
Septic Arthritis (Patient Information)

AUTHOR: **GLENN G. FORT, M.D., M.P.H.**

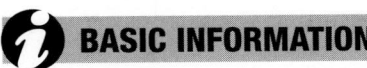

BASIC INFORMATION

DEFINITION

Serotonin syndrome (SS) refers to a group of symptoms resulting from increased activity of serotonin (5-hydroxytryptamine) in the CNS. SS is a drug-induced disorder that is classically characterized by a change in mental status and alteration in neuromuscular activity and autonomic function.

SYNONYMS

SS
Hyperserotonemia
Serotonergic syndrome
Serotonin toxicity

ICD-9CM CODES
333.99 Syndrome serotonin

EPIDEMIOLOGY & DEMOGRAPHICS

- The incidence of SS is not known.
- SS is seen in all age groups, from neonates to elderly.
- SS classically occurs in patients receiving two or more serotonergic drugs, but it can also occur with monotherapy—selective serotonin reuptake inhibitor (SSRI) monotherapy has an incidence of 0.5 to 0.9 cases of SS per 1000 patient-mo. Although there is an FDA alert, it has been argued that there is a lack of sufficient evidence showing that SSRIs and triptans cause serious SS.
- Concomitant use of an SSRI with a monoamine oxidase inhibitor (MAOI) poses the greatest risk of developing SS.
- Combination of SSRIs with other serotonergic drugs (e.g., tryptophan, illicit drugs like cocaine and MDMA, "Ecstasy") or drugs with serotonergic properties (e.g., lithium, meperidine, triptans, linezolid) may also lead to SS.

PHYSICAL FINDINGS & CLINICAL PRESENTATION

- Findings of clonus with hyperreflexia in the setting of recent (<5 wk) use of serotonergic agents strongly suggests the diagnosis of SS.
- Symptoms can manifest within minutes to hours after starting a new psychopharmacologic treatment, increasing the dose of a serotonergic drug, or administering a second serotonergic drug.
- Clonus (inducible, spontaneous, and ocular) is the key finding in establishing a diagnosis of SS.
- Other pertinent findings include:
  - Confusion, agitation, hypomania
  - Fever >38° C (100° F), tachycardia, and tachypnea
  - Nausea, vomiting, abdominal pain, and diaphoresis
  - Diarrhea, tremors, shivering, and seizures
  - Hyperreflexia and muscle rigidity

ETIOLOGY

- Hyperstimulation of the brainstem and spinal cord serotonin receptors leading to the neuromuscular and autonomic symptoms.

- Psychopharmacologic drugs—in particular, fluoxetine and sertraline co-administered with MAOI (e.g., tranylcypromine and phenelzine)—have been cited in the literature as a common cause of SS. Triptans (serotonin-receptor agonists used in the treatment of migraines) may also precipitate the SS when used in combination with SSRIs and serotonin-norepinephrine reuptake inhibitors (SNRIs). Box 1-57 describes classes of medications that produce SS in psychiatric patients.

DIAGNOSIS

- The diagnosis of SS is made on clinical grounds. There are no specific laboratory tests for SS. A high index of suspicion along with a detailed medication history is the mainstay of diagnosis.
- Diagnostic criteria: most accurate is Hunter Serotonin Toxicity Criteria (sensitivity 84%, specificity 97%, confirmation by toxicologist).
- To fulfill Hunter criteria a patient must have consumed a serotonergic drug and have one of the following:
  1. Spontaneous clonus
  2. Inducible clonus plus agitation or diaphoresis
  3. Ocular clonus plus agitation or diaphoresis
  4. Tremor and hyperreflexia
  5. Temperature greater than 38° C (100° F) plus hypertonia plus ocular clonus or inducible clonus

DIFFERENTIAL DIAGNOSIS

- Neuroleptic malignant syndrome (NMS), substance abuse (e.g., cocaine, amphetamines), anticholinergic toxicity, thyroid storm, infection (e.g., meningitis, encephalitis), alcohol and opioid withdrawal.
- Classic features in differentiation of NMS from SS are that SS develops over 24 hr, involves neuromuscular hyperactivity, and begins to resolve within 24 hr with appropriate therapy, whereas NMS develops gradually

---

BOX 1-57 Classes of Medications That Produce Serotonin Syndrome in Psychiatric Patients

Selective serotonin reuptake inhibitors
Monoamine oxidase inhibitors
Atypical antipsychotics
Heterocyclic antidepressants
Trazodone
Dual-uptake inhibitors
Psychostimulants
Buspirone
Mood stabilizers
Analgesics
Antiemetics
Cough suppressants
Dietary supplements

From Goldman L, Schafer AI: *Goldman's Cecil medicine*, ed 24, Philadelphia, 2012, Saunders.

---

over days to weeks, involves sluggish neuromuscular response, and resolves over an average period of 1 wk to 10 days.

WORKUP

- Because SS is a clinical diagnosis, there is no laboratory test that confirms the diagnosis, and serum serotonin concentration does not correlate with clinical picture. Other causes are described in "Differential Diagnosis." Thus, all patients should have blood tests and diagnostic imaging studies to rule out infectious, toxic, and metabolic causes.
- Additional laboratory tests are performed to exclude complicating features of SS (e.g., renal failure secondary to rhabdomyolysis).

LABORATORY TESTS

- CBC with differential to rule out sepsis
- Electrolytes, BUN, and creatinine to rule out acidosis and renal failure
- Blood and urine toxicology screen
- Thyroid function tests
- Creatine-phosphokinase (CPK) with isoenzymes
- Urine and blood cultures
- ECG because ventricular rhythm disturbance is a potentially fatal complication

IMAGING STUDIES

Imaging studies are not specific in the diagnosis of SS and are only ordered to exclude other causes with similar clinical presentations as SS.

TREATMENT

- Once a diagnosis of SS is established, appropriate consultation with a medical toxicologist, clinical pharmacologist, and/or poison control center should be sought.
- Management includes:
  - Discontinue use of all potential precipitating drugs
  - Provide supportive management
  - Control agitation
  - Administer serotonin antagonists
  - Control autonomic instability
  - Control hyperthermia
  - Reassess the need to resume the use of the serotonergic agent once the symptoms have resolved

NONPHARMACOLOGIC THERAPY

- Discontinuation of the drug is the mainstay of therapy.
- Treatment is supportive: maintaining oxygenation and blood pressure and monitoring respiratory status. Hypotensive patients may require both IV fluids and vasopressor therapy.
- Patients who are severely hyperthermic with temperatures greater than 41° C (106° F) should be given IV sedation, paralyzed, and intubated. Cooling blankets can be used for patients with mild to moderate hyperthermia. There is no role for acetaminophen here.
- Intubation is recommended for patients unable to protect their airways as a result of mental status changes or seizures.

ACUTE GENERAL Rx

- Benzodiazepines for control of agitation are preferred to physical restraints.
  1. Lorazepam 1 to 2 mg IV every 30 min has been used effectively in treating agitation, muscle rigidity, myoclonus, and seizure complications.
  2. Diazepam is an alternative choice.
- Blood pressure management with short-acting agents such as esmolol and nitroprusside.
- Serotonin antagonists should be titrated to clinical effectiveness in patients for whom nonpharmacologic therapy and benzodiazepines are not achieving adequate response, although substantial and rigorous data are lacking.
  1. Cyproheptadine 4-mg tablet or 2 mg/5 ml syrup is given 12 mg initially followed by 2 mg every 2 hr until therapeutic response is achieved in adults (up to 32 mg/day); children ages 7 to 14 should receive 4 mg every 6 hr (up to 16 mg/day), children ages 2 to 6 should receive 2 mg every 6 hr (up to 12 mg/day), and children younger than 2 yr should receive a maximum of 0.25 mg/kg/day as 0.06 mg/kg every 6 hr.

2. Atypical antipsychotic agents with serotonin antagonist properties (e.g., olanzapine 10 mg SL) have been tried with some success.
3. Chlorpromazine 50 to 100 mg IM may be considered in severe cases.

CHRONIC Rx

For patients not requiring hospital admission, cyproheptadine and lorazepam can be given in an oral dose on a prn basis with close follow-up.

DISPOSITION

- SS is a potentially life-threatening condition if not recognized early, although it does exist on a spectrum.
- Prompt diagnosis and withdrawal of the medication result in improvement of symptoms within 24 hr.
- Seizures, rhabdomyolysis, hyperthermia, ventricular arrhythmia, respiratory arrest, and coma are all complicating features of SS.

REFERRAL

All cases of SS secondary to psychotropic medications should be referred to a psychiatrist.

PREVENTION

Modify prescription practices by avoiding multidrug regimens.

ⓘ PEARLS & CONSIDERATIONS

The combined use of SSRIs and MAOIs is contraindicated.

COMMENTS

- The use of SSRIs and other serotonergic agents is not an absolute contraindication; however, prompt withdrawal of the medication is recommended if any symptoms suggesting SS occur.
- SS is usually found in patients being treated for depression, bipolar disorders, obsessive-compulsive disorder, attention-deficit disorder, and Parkinson's disease.

SUGGESTED READINGS

available at www.expertconsult.com

AUTHOR: **MARK F. BRADY, M.D., M.P.H., M.M.S.**

Diseases and Disorders

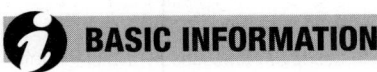

DEFINITION

Sexual assault is any sexual act performed by one person on another without consent, resulting from the use of force, the threat of force or from the victim's inability to give consent.

SYNONYMS

Rape

ICD-9CM CODES
E960.1 Rape

EPIDEMIOLOGY & DEMOGRAPHICS

INCIDENCE: 17.6% of women, 3% of men
PEAK INCIDENCE: As high as 25%
PREVALENCE (IN U.S.): 17.7 million women, 2.8 million men
PREDOMINANT SEX AND AGE: Female, age 16-24
RISK FACTORS: Alcohol/drug consumption, prior history of being sexually/physically abused, multiple sexual partners, involvement in sex work, poverty, incarceration/institutionalization, mental retardation

PHYSICAL FINDINGS & CLINICAL PRESENTATION

- Extragenital trauma: 70%: bruises, abrasions, erythema on thigh, arms, face, neck
- Anogenital trauma: 27%: injury to breasts, external genitalia, vagina, anus, rectum
- Physical findings more likely if examined within 72 hr of event, if event occurred outdoors, and if perpetrator was unknown

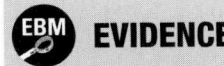 **DIAGNOSIS**

WORKUP

- History
  - Circumstances of assault: date, time, location
  - Physical description of perpetrator
  - Areas of trauma, specifically details of oral, vaginal, anorectal contact, or penetration
  - Condom use
  - Ejaculation: presence or absence
  - Presence of bleeding in victim or perpetrator
  - Recent consensual sexual activity
  - Showering, bathing, changing of clothes since event
- Physical examination
  - Ideally performed by individual trained to perform sexual assault examinations, i.e., SANE (Sexual Assault Nurse Evaluation) providers: www.sane-sart.com
  - Physical exam can take 3-6 hr to complete
  - Components
    - Physical examination of entire body
    - Forensic evidence collection
    - STD evaluation and treatment
    - Pregnancy risk evaluation
    - Care of injuries

- General physical exam components
  - Documentation of any physical trauma, including photographs
  - Colposcopy: may reveal areas of minor genital trauma
  - Wood's light: to reveal foreign debris or semen
- Forensic evaluation: not required, but should be offered; written informed consent needed
  - Commercially made specimen collection kits available: once completed, kits need to be sealed and handled according to kit instructions
  - U.S.: States required to provide free specimen collection
  - Samples of blood, saliva, mucosal swabs: buccal/vaginal/rectal, fingernail scrapings/clippings, hair specimens
  - Clothing: if unchanged since event

LABORATORY TESTS

- Pregnancy test (if applicable)
- STD testing
  - GC/CT: recommended for all, may be excluded if individual elects for prophylactic treatment
  - Wet mount or vaginal swab for *Trichomonas*
  - Baseline HIV/hepatitis/syphilis testing: individual basis
    - Retest for HIV/syphilis at 6 wk, 3 mo, and 6 mo from incident

IMAGING STUDIES

Use of imaging studies as dictated by other injuries sustained for diagnosis/treatment of fractures, soft tissue, and other traumatic injuries

TREATMENT

NONPHARMACOLOGIC THERAPY

Acute crisis counseling: to support mental health needs of victim in immediate post-assault period

ACUTE GENERAL Rx

- Sexually transmitted infections
  - Empiric treatment recommended secondary to poor follow-up rates
  - Gonorrhea: ceftriaxone 250 mg IM *or* cefixime 400 mg PO
  - *Chlamydia:* azithromycin 1 g (single dose) *or* doxycycline 100 mg bid × 7 days
  - Trichomoniasis: metronidazole 2 g PO (single dose)
- Hepatitis B
  - If perpetrator known to be infected: HBIG + Hep B vaccination
  - If perpetrator disease status unknown: Hep B vaccination alone
  - If victim has already been vaccinated with documented immunity: no treatment necessary

- HIV
  - Use of antiretrovirals after sexual assault is controversial.
  - Overall risk of acquiring HIV is unknown but higher in certain situations.
    - Male-on-male rapists
    - Assault occurring in area with high local prevalence
    - Multiple assailants
    - Anal sexual assault
    - Presence of trauma, bleeding, or genital lesions in either victim/assailant
  - Antiretroviral drugs should be offered in all situations.
  - Ideally, antiretrovirals are initiated within 4 hr; should not start if >72 hr.
- Pregnancy
  - Pregnancy risk is estimated to be 5% per rape in women age 12-45.
  - Emergency contraception should be offered in all cases.
    - Levonorgestrel: 0.75 mg q12h for two doses or 1.5 mg single dose
    - Yuzpe regimen: 100 mcg ethinyl estradiol + 0.5 mg levonorgestrel, repeated in 12 hr
    - Ulipristal: preferred method when >72 hr from assault
  - Antiemetics: EC + antibiotics for STD prophylaxis commonly causes nausea.

CHRONIC Rx

- No chronic prescriptions
- Long-term psychiatric counseling may be needed.

REFERRAL

Mental health professional

RELATED CONTENT

Chlamydia Genital Infections (Related Key Topic)
Contraception (Related Key Topic)
Gonorrhea (Related Key Topic)
Syphilis (Related Key Topic)

AUTHOR: **SARAH L. CHISHOLM, M.D.**

BASIC INFORMATION

DEFINITION

A sexual dysfunction in a woman is any disorder that interferes with female sexuality and that causes marked distress to that person. These disorders are generally categorized into four types:

1. Disorders of desire (most common)
2. Disorders of arousal
3. Orgasmic disorders
4. Sexual pain disorders (including dyspareunia, vaginismus, and vulvodynia)

Female sexual dysfunction is also further categorized as lifelong (primary) or acquired (secondary), situational (e.g., current partner) or generalized (all partners and settings).

SYNONYMS

Female sexual dysfunction

ICD-9CM CODES
302.70 Decreased libido
302.72 Disorders of arousal
302.73 Orgasmic disorders
625.x   Sexual pain disorders

EPIDEMIOLOGY & DEMOGRAPHICS

INCIDENCE: According to the National Health and Social Life Survey, in 1999, ~20% to 50% of women reported some form of sexual dysfunction during their lifetimes. One third of women reported a decrease in sexual interest, and one fourth reported an inability to achieve orgasm.

PREVALENCE: A more recent survey of women 18 yr of age and older found an age-adjusted prevalence of any sexual problem to be ~43%.

PREDOMINANT AGE: Sexually related personal distress was more common in middle-aged women (aged 45 to 64) than in younger or older women.

RISK FACTORS:
- Correlates of distressing sexual problems include poor self-assessed health, low education level, depression, anxiety, thyroid conditions, and urinary incontinence.
- Obesity and overweight body status have been associated with lower sexual satisfaction and desire.

PHYSICAL FINDINGS & CLINICAL PRESENTATION

- History:
  - Important to obtain the patient's definition of the dysfunction, including its onset and duration; to determine whether the dysfunction is situational or global; and to determine whether more than one dysfunction exists and the interrelationship among the dysfunctions
  - Related medical and gynecologic conditions (including prior gynecologic surgery)
  - Psychosocial factors, including sexual abuse, sexual orientation, depression and anxiety, status of current relationships and

sexual activity, personal and family beliefs about sexuality
  - Current medications including OTC and herbal preparations, alcohol, tobacco and drug use, and birth control method
- Physical examination:
  - The gynecologic examination can aid in identifying signs of decreased estrogen and androgen levels, infection, endometriosis, pelvic floor dysfunction, and systemic disease
  - Other body systems as indicated (e.g., cardiovascular, thyroid)

ETIOLOGY

- Chronic medical conditions (e.g., diabetes, coronary vascular disease, arthritis, urinary incontinence)
- Medication induced (e.g., antihypertensives, selective serotonin reuptake inhibitors [SSRIs])
- Gynecologic conditions (e.g., cystitis, posthysterectomy, gynecologic cancers, breast cancer [femininity/self-image issues; chemotherapy effects], postpregnancy, postmenopausal)
- Psychosocial (e.g., religion, taboos, identity conflicts, guilt, relationship problems, abuse, rape, life stressors)

 DIAGNOSIS

DIFFERENTIAL DIAGNOSIS

- Depression
- Psychosocial stressors
- Medical disease (e.g., thyroid dysfunction)

LABORATORY TESTS

- Cervical cultures and vaginal swabs for infectious disease
- Pap smear
- Appropriate laboratory tests if comorbid or chronic disease is suspected

IMAGING STUDIES

Appropriate imaging studies if comorbid or chronic disease is suspected

 TREATMENT

NONPHARMACOLOGIC THERAPY

- Education including a discussion of normal sexual behavior
- Stress management
- Activities to enhance stimulation and eliminate routine
- Distraction techniques
- Noncoital behavior
- Position changes (e.g., female astride)
- Lubricants (e.g., nonpetroleum based). There are several over-the-counter lubricants and massage oils, some of which are hypoallergenic, that can be safely applied to female genitalia

ACUTE GENERAL Rx

NSAIDs before intercourse for sexual pain disorders

CHRONIC Rx

- Treat underlying medical, gynecologic, or psychological conditions.
- Reduce comorbidities, including weight loss.
- Increase physical activity (associated with increased satisfaction and sexual engagement).
- For medication-induced conditions, decrease dose or change medication.
- For postmenopausal women or those with hypoestrogenism, try estrogen replacement therapy with or without progesterone.
- Testosterone therapy (still in Phase III clinical trials): results show increase in satisfying sexual activity and sexual desire.
- Sildenafil (evidence from RCTs for use in patients with neurodegenerative disease and antidepressant-induced FSD after traditional therapy has failed). Data are conflicting. Phosphodiesterase inhibitors may increase blood flow to the genitalia but generally appear to have little benefit in treating arousal disorders.
- Bupropion 300 to 400 mg/day was shown to increase sexual arousal and orgasm completion in a recent trial. In addition, adjunctive treatment with bupropion significantly improved key aspects of sexual function in women with SSRI-induced sexual dysfunction.
- Behavioral therapy (e.g., cognitive-behavioral therapy to reduce anxiety).

REFERRAL

- Gynecologic referral for conditions that may be amenable to surgical therapy
- Psychological referral for conditions (e.g., depression, abuse) that may benefit from counseling or psychotherapy
- Social services referrals for active abuse issues

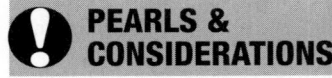 **PEARLS & CONSIDERATIONS**

COMMENTS

Identify the earliest cause in the chain and treat that first.

PATIENT & FAMILY EDUCATION

When appropriate, involve the patient's partner or significant other in treatment.

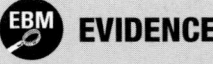 **EVIDENCE**

available at www.expertconsult.com

SUGGESTED READINGS
available at www.expertconsult.com

RELATED CONTENT

Fig. E3-158 Evaluation of sexual dysfunction (Algorithm)
Female Sexual Dysfunction (Patient Information)

AUTHOR: **ANNGENE ANTHONY, M.D., M.P.H., F.A.A.F.P.**

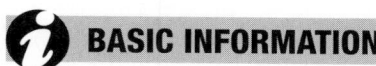

BASIC INFORMATION

DEFINITION

Shaken baby syndrome is violent shaking that causes severe injury in infants. It is a potentially life-threatening head injury in children <2 yr of age. Intracranial injury is caused by rapid acceleration and rotation of the cranium (sometimes associated with impact on a solid object, which leads to rapid angular deceleration). The diagnosis of shaken baby syndrome is often tough to make because of the lack of obvious external signs. Head injury, especially subdural hemorrhage, and retinal hemorrhages are the hallmarks of the syndrome (Fig. 1-758).

SYNONYMS

Shaken infant syndrome
Abusive head trauma
Nonaccidental head injury

ICD-9CM CODES
995.55 Shaken infant syndrome

EPIDEMIOLOGY & DEMOGRAPHICS

INCIDENCE: Shaken baby syndrome is the most common cause of death or serious neurologic injury resulting from child abuse. It is specific to infancy, when children have unique anatomic features. Subdural and retinal hemorrhages are markers of shaking injury. A 15-yr retrospective study in Scotland suggested an estimated incidence of nonaccidental head injury of 11.2 per 100,000 children under 1 yr. This may even be an underestimate.
PEAK INCIDENCE: Shaken babies are typically younger than 1 yr old; most are under 6 mo of age.
PREVALENCE: About 25% of clinically diagnosed babies with shaken baby syndrome die, and about 80% of the remaining suffer lifelong neurologic damage.
PREDOMINANT SEX: About 60% of identified victims of shaking injury are male. Children of families who live at or below the poverty level are at an increased risk for these injuries as well as any type of child abuse.
RISK FACTORS: History of abuse, history of domestic violence, and low socioeconomic status are all risk factors. Experts believe that the perpetrators in 65%-90% of cases are males.

PHYSICAL FINDINGS & CLINICAL PRESENTATION

Increased drowsiness, lethargy, or decreased feeding. One study of 364 children with shaken baby syndrome found that 40% had no signs of external injury on initial evaluation. Shaken baby syndrome should be considered in infants presenting with seizures, failure to thrive, vomiting associated with lethargy or drowsiness, hypothermia, bradycardia, hypertension or hypotension, respiratory irregularities, coma, or death.

ETIOLOGY

Improved neuropathology and imaging techniques have established the cause of brain injury as hypoxic ischemic encephalopathy.

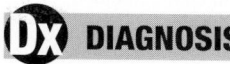

DIAGNOSIS

DIFFERENTIAL DIAGNOSIS

Head trauma from other etiology vs. infection vs. other etiology

WORKUP

Imaging of the brain

LABORATORY TESTS

CBC, chemistry

IMAGING STUDIES

Diffusion-weighted magnetic resonance imaging is the most sensitive, and specific method of confirming a shaking injury.

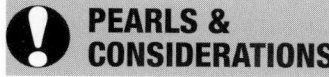

TREATMENT

Treatment is focused on targeting the specific injuries and also focusing on prevention of future injuries.

NONPHARMACOLOGIC THERAPY

Treatment involves admission to a hospital for observation.

ACUTE GENERAL Rx

Supportive care and interventions as dictated by the clinical, laboratory, and imaging findings

CHRONIC Rx

Counseling, working with the child's school to optimize academic development

REFERRAL

Neurologist and neurosurgery (if needed)

PEARLS & CONSIDERATIONS

PREVENTION

The National Center on Shaken Baby Syndrome offers a prevention program. Additionally, researchers like Harvey Karp have suggested ideas.

PATIENT & FAMILY EDUCATION

Shaken baby syndrome can result in lifelong, irreversible injuries. Prevention is a key component. Infants crying most commonly leads to shaking. Therefore the National Center on Shaken Baby Syndrome offers a prevention program, the **Period of Purple Crying,** which seeks to help parents and other caregivers understand crying in normal infants. By defining and describing the sometimes inconsolable infant crying that can sometimes cause stress, anger, and frustration in parents and caregivers, the program hopes to educate and empower people to prevent abusive head trauma.

Another method that may help is one suggested by author Dr. Harvey Karp's "five S's":
1. Shushing: use "white noise" or rhythmic sounds that mimic the constant whir of noise in the womb.
2. Side/stomach positioning: place the baby on the left side to help digestion.
3. Sucking: let the baby breast-feed or bottle-feed, or give the baby a pacifier or finger to suck on.
4. Swaddling: wrap the baby up snugly in a blanket to help him or her feel more secure.
5. Swinging gently: rock in a chair, use an infant swing, or take a car ride to help duplicate the constant motion the baby felt in the womb.

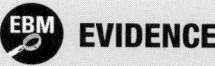

EVIDENCE

available at www.expertconsult.com

SUGGESTED READINGS

available at www.expertconsult.com

AUTHOR: **PRIYA SARIN GUPTA, M.D, M.P.H.**

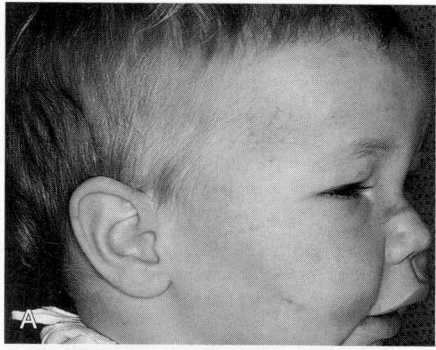

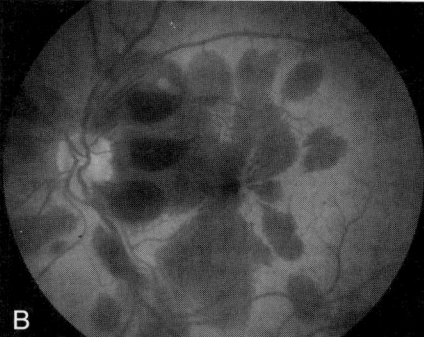

FIGURE 1-758 Shaken baby syndrome. A, Facial bruising. **B,** Fundus hemorrhages involving different levels. (Courtesy R. Bates. From Kanski JJ, Bowling B: *Clinical ophthalmology, a systematic approach,* ed 7, Philadelphia, 2010, Saunders.)

BASIC INFORMATION

DEFINITION

Sheehan's syndrome is a state of hypopituitarism resulting from an infarct of the pituitary secondary to postpartum hemorrhage or shock, causing partial or complete loss of the anterior pituitary hormones (adrenocorticotropic hormone [ACTH], follicle-stimulating hormone [FSH], luteinizing hormone [LH], growth hormone [GH], prolactin [PRL], thyroid-stimulating hormone [TSH]) and their target organ functions.

ICD-9CM CODES
253.2 Sheehan's syndrome

EPIDEMIOLOGY & DEMOGRAPHICS

INCIDENCE: One case in 10,000 deliveries (perhaps more rare in the U.S.)
PREDOMINANT SEX: Affects only females
RISK FACTORS:
- Hypovolemic shock
- Type 1 (insulin-dependent) diabetes mellitus (secondary to microvascular disease)
- Sickle cell anemia (secondary to occlusion of the small vessels in the pituitary)

ONSET OF SYMPTOMS: Presentation is subacute with progressive hypopituitarism, inability to lactate (due to prolactin deficiency), and amenorrhea. Average delay of 5 to 7 yr between onset of symptoms and diagnosis of disease.

PHYSICAL FINDINGS & CLINICAL PRESENTATION

- Failure of lactation
- Infertility
- Failure to resume menses after delivery
- Failure to regrow shaved pubic or axillary hair
- Skin depigmentation (including areola)
- Rapid breast involution
- Superinvolution of the uterus
- Hypothyroidism
- Adrenal cortical insufficiency
- Diabetes insipidus (rare)

ETIOLOGY

- Compromise of the blood supply to the low-pressure pituitary sinusoidal system may occur with postpartum hemorrhage or shock, resulting in pituitary infarct and/or necrosis.
- It is hypothesized that locally released factors may mediate vascular spasm of the pituitary blood supply.
- Severity of postpartum hemorrhage does not always correlate with the presence of Sheehan's syndrome.

DIAGNOSIS

DIFFERENTIAL DIAGNOSIS

- Chronic infections
- HIV
- Sarcoidosis
- Amyloidosis
- Rheumatoid disease
- Hemochromatosis
- Metastatic carcinoma
- Lymphocytic hypophysitis

WORKUP

- Target gland deficiency should be investigated by measuring levels of ACTH, FSH, LH, TSH (which may be normal or low), and T_4. Cortisol and estradiol (which may be low) should also be measured.
- Provocative testing of pituitary hormone reserves (e.g., metyrapone test, insulin tolerance test, and cosyntropin test): normal, subnormal, or delayed responses may suggest the presence of islands of pituitary cells that no longer have the support of the hypothalamic-portal circulation.
- Measurement of insulin-like growth factor-I to screen for GH deficiency: subnormal levels suggest decreased GH.
- Impaired prolactin response to TRH or dopamine antagonist stimulation is frequently found.
- During pregnancy, adjustments must be made in interpreting both hormone levels and responses to various stimuli because of normal physiologic changes.

IMAGING STUDIES

- Study of choice: MRI of the pituitary
  1. Sella turcica partially or totally empty
  2. Rules out mass lesion
- CT scan of the pituitary when MRI is unavailable or contraindicated

TREATMENT

ACUTE GENERAL Rx

- Acute form can be lethal, presenting with hypotension, tachycardia, failure to lactate, and hypoglycemia.
- A high degree of suspicion is required with any woman who has undergone postpartum hemorrhage and shock.

- IV corticosteroids and fluid replacement should be given initially.
- Diagnosis is confirmed with a full endocrinologic workup.
- Thyroid hormone is replaced as levothyroxine in doses of 0.1 to 0.2 mg qd.

CHRONIC Rx

- With late-onset disease (symptoms of general hypopituitarism, such as oligomenorrhea or amenorrhea, vaginal atrophic changes, and loss of libido): a full endocrinologic workup and replacement of the appropriate hormones are needed.
- With symptoms of adrenal insufficiency: corticosteroids should be given.
  1. A maintenance dose of cortisone acetate or prednisone may be given.
  2. Because adrenal production of cortisol is not entirely dependent on ACTH, replacement of mineralocorticoids is rarely necessary.
  3. Stress doses of glucocorticoids should be administered during surgery or during labor and delivery.

DISPOSITION

- Patients who receive early diagnosis and adequate hormonal replacement may expect favorable outcomes, including subsequent pregnancy.
- Central adrenal insufficiency is the primary cause of mortality in Sheehan's syndrome.

REFERRAL

Patients should have yearly examinations by an endocrinologist.

SUGGESTED READING
available at www.expertconsult.com

RELATED CONTENT
Hypopituitarism (Related Key Topic)

AUTHORS: **BETH J. WUTZ, M.D.,** and **RUBEN ALVERO, M.D.**

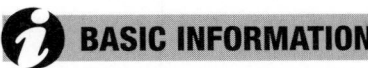

BASIC INFORMATION

DEFINITION

Shigellosis is an inflammatory disease of the bowel caused by one of several species of *Shigella*. It is the third most common cause of diarrhea in the U.S. after *Salmonella* and *Campylobacter* and the most common cause of bacillary dysentery in the U.S.

SYNONYMS

Bacillary dysentery

ICD-9CM CODES
004.9 Shigellosis

EPIDEMIOLOGY & DEMOGRAPHICS

INCIDENCE (IN U.S.): 6.59 cases per 100,000 population with approximately 450,000 cases/yr
PREDOMINANT SEX: Male homosexuals at increased risk
PREDOMINANT AGE: Shigellosis predominantly affects children with 28 cases per 100,000 population in children less than 4 yr old and 25.67 cases per 100,000 population in children aged 4 to 11.
PEAK INCIDENCE: Summer
GENETICS: Neonatal infection: rare but severe

PHYSICAL FINDINGS & CLINICAL PRESENTATION

- Possibly asymptomatic, but incubation period can range from 1 to 7 days with an average of 3 days
- Mild illness that is usually self-limited, resolving in a few days
- High fever
- Watery diarrhea
- Bloody diarrhea
- Dysentery (abdominal cramps, tenesmus, and numerous, small-volume stools with blood, mucus, and pus)
- Descending intestinal tract illness, reflecting infection of small bowel first and then the colon
- Severe disease is more common in children and elderly and outside of U.S.
- Complications of severe illness:
  1. Seizures
  2. Megacolon
  3. Intestinal perforation
  4. Death
- Extraintestinal manifestations are rare
- Bacteremia is more common in children; in adults it has been described in patients with AIDS, the elderly, and diabetics

- Hemolytic-uremic syndrome (HUS): can be caused by *S. dysenteriae* 1.
- Reactive arthritis, sometimes as part of Reiter's syndrome following *S. flexneri* infection

ETIOLOGY

- *Shigella:* gram-negative rod bacteria that are less susceptible to stomach acid and thus as few as 10 to 100 bacteria can cause disease. The bacteria invade colonic tissue and cause inflammation.
  1. *S. flexneri*
  2. *S. dysenteriae*
  3. *S. sonnei*
  4. *S. boydii*
- *S. sonnei* is the most commonly isolated species in the U.S. (over 75% of cases), and it usually causes a mild watery diarrhea.
- Direct person-to-person transmission is thought to be the most common route. Outbreaks among men who have sex with men have occurred because of direct or indirect oral-anal contact.
- Contaminated food or water may transmit disease.
- Outbreaks have occurred in day care centers, a community wading pool frequented by toddlers, and residential institutions.

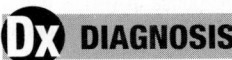

DIAGNOSIS

DIFFERENTIAL DIAGNOSIS

- May mimic other bacterial gastroenteritis, such as *Clostridium difficile, Salmonella, Campylobacter,* and *Yersinia*.
- Dysentery can also be caused by *Entamoeba histolytica*.
- Bloody diarrhea may resemble disease caused by invasive *E. coli* (IEC).
- Hemolytic-uremic syndrome caused by enterohemorrhagic *E. coli* (0157:H7).

LABORATORY TESTS

- The diagnosis is established by bacterial stool culture.
- Stool should be cultured from fresh samples, because the yield is increased by processing the specimen soon after passage. The best yield is from the mucoid part of the stool.
- Serology is available but rarely useful.
- Polymerase chain reaction (PCR) is available but due to cost used mainly for outbreak investigations.
- Fecal leukocyte preparation may show WBCs.
- Total WBCs may be low, normal, or high. Leukemoid reactions can occur in children.

IMAGING STUDIES

Abdominal radiographs may suggest megacolon or perforation in rare, severe cases.

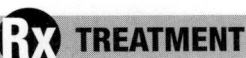

TREATMENT

NONPHARMACOLOGIC THERAPY

- Adequate hydration
- Electrolyte replacement

ACUTE GENERAL Rx

Antibiotics:
- To shorten course of illness
- To limit transmission of illness
- For adults: Pending susceptibilities, ciprofloxacin 750 mg PO bid for 3 days or levofloxacin 500-750 mg q day for 3 days should be used. An alternative is azithromycin 500 mg q day for 3 days.
- For children: IV ceftriaxone (50 mg/kg/day) for 5 days in cases of severe disease. For oral therapy, can use cefixime: 8 mg/kg/day as single daily dose or divided q12h for 5 days *or* azithromycin: 10 mg/kg/day in a single daily dose for 3 days. A short course of an oral quinolone can also be used safely although they are not approved for children.

DISPOSITION

- Most disease is self-limited.
- Severe illness may be fatal.

REFERRAL

For severe illness or complications

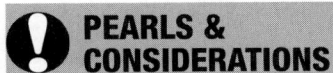

PEARLS & CONSIDERATIONS

COMMENTS

- *Shigella* is one cause of "gay bowel syndrome."
- Illness is worsened by agents that decrease intestinal motility.
- Food handlers, child care providers, and health care workers should have a negative stool culture documented following treatment.

SUGGESTED READINGS
available at www.expertconsult.com

AUTHOR: **GLENN G. FORT, M.D., M.P.H.**

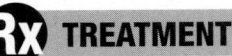

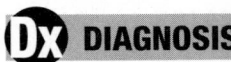 **BASIC INFORMATION**

DEFINITION

Short bowel syndrome (SBS) is a malabsorption syndrome that results from extensive small intestinal resection or congenital causes (Table 1-373).

SYNONYMS

Short bowel
SBS

ICD-9CM CODES

579.3 (Postsurgical malabsorption)

EPIDEMIOLOGY & DEMOGRAPHICS

- Parallels Crohn's disease (see "Crohn's Disease" in Section I), which is the most common cause of the syndrome in adults.
- In children, two thirds of short bowels are related to congenital abnormalities (intestinal atresia, gastroschisis, volvulus, aganglionosis) and one third are related to necrotizing enterocolitis.
- Prevalence: 10,000 to 20,000 cases are estimated to exist in the U.S.

PHYSICAL FINDINGS & CLINICAL PRESENTATION

- Diarrhea and steatorrhea
- Weight loss
- Anemia related to iron or vitamin B_{12} absorption
- Bleeding diathesis related to vitamin K malabsorption
- Osteoporosis/osteomalacia related to vitamin D and calcium malabsorption
- Hyponatremia, hypokalemia
- Hypovolemia
- Other macronutrient or micronutrient deficiency states

ETIOLOGY

- Extensive bowel resection for treatment of the conditions mentioned previously (see "Epidemiology").
- Congenital (Table 1-373).

TABLE 1-373 Causes of Short Bowel Syndrome

Congenital

Congenital short bowel syndrome

Multiple atresias

Gastroschisis

Bowel Resection

Necrotizing enterocolitis

Volvulus with or without malrotation

Long-segment Hirschsprung disease

Meconium peritonitis

Crohn's disease

Trauma

From Kliegman RM et al: *Nelson textbook of pediatrics,* ed 19, Philadelphia, 2011, Saunders.

The human intestine is 3 to 8 m in length. Removal of up to half of the small intestine produces no disruption in nutrient absorption, and most patients can maintain nutritional balance on oral feeding if they have more than 100 cm (3 ft) of jejunum. Similarly, 100 cm of intact jejunum can maintain a normal water, sodium, and potassium balance under normal circumstances. The presence of an intact colon can compensate for some small intestine loss.

Site-specific functions:

- Calcium, magnesium, phosphorus, iron, and vitamins are absorbed in the duodenum and proximal jejunum.
- Vitamin B_{12} and bile acids are absorbed in the ileum. The resection of more than 60 cm of ileum results in vitamin B_{12} malabsorption. The loss of more than 100 cm results in fat malabsorption (from the loss of bile acids).
- The loss of gastrointestinal endocrine hormones can affect intestinal motility.
- Intestinal bacterial overgrowth may also occur, especially if the ileocecal valve is lost.

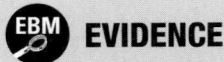 **DIAGNOSIS**

Presence of macronutrient and/or micronutrient loss in a patient with a known history of bowel resection

DIFFERENTIAL DIAGNOSIS

Because the history of significant bowel resection is typically known, there is no differential diagnosis. If that history is not known, all causes of weight loss, malabsorption, and diarrhea must be considered.

TABLE 1-374 Management Strategies for Short Bowel Syndrome

1. Acute phase
   a. Treat postoperative complications
   b. Maintain full support via the parenteral route
   c. Initiate low-rate trophic enteral feeds
   d. Document amount and site of remaining bowel and underlying disease
2. Early adaptation (up to 1 yr postsurgery)
   a. Increase enteral nutrition to tolerance; supplement with glutamine
   b. Achieve permanent parenteral access, if indicated
   c. Maximize antiperistaltic agents
   d. Octreotide for high-output ostomy or fistula
   e. Dietary counseling
   f. Clinical trials of trophic growth factors
3. Long-term adaptation (>1 yr postsurgery)
   a. Recruit bypassed bowel
   b. Bowel-lengthening procedure (Bianchi or STEP)
   c. Monitor for development of TPN-associated complications, and refer for transplant prior to recurrent sepsis, thrombosis, or end-stage liver disease

From Cameron JL, Cameron AM: *Current surgical therapy,* ed 10, Philadelphia, 2011, Saunders.

RX TREATMENT

Extensive small bowel resection with colectomy (<100 cm of jejunum)

- Rx: long-term total parenteral nutrition (TPN). Some patients can switch to oral intake after 1 to 2 yr of TPN. In jejunostomy patients, excessive fluid loss can be reduced with H_2 blockers, proton pump inhibitors, or octreotide. Micronutrients are supplemented.

Extensive small bowel resection with partial colectomy (usually patients with Crohn's disease)

- Rx: oral intake alone is possible in all patients with >100 cm of jejunum. In addition to vitamin B_{12} deficiency, these patients often have diarrhea. Consider lactose malabsorption and bacterial overgrowth treated, respectively, with lactose restriction and antibiotics (tetracycline 250 mg tid or metronidazole 500 mg tid for 2 wk). Nonspecific antidiarrheal agents may also be indicated (e.g., Imodium or codeine). The patient must be monitored for micronutrient losses.
- Table 1-374 summarizes management strategies for SBS. Intestinal transplantation is performed mostly in children at selective centers.
- FDA-approved medications for SBS in patients receiving nutritional support are:
  - Recombinant growth hormone somatropin (Zorbtive): effective in increasing weight and reducing parenteral nutrition volume. These effects do not persist when the drug is stopped.
  - Teduglutide (Gattex), a recombinant DNA analog of glucagon-like peptide-2. It promotes mucosal growth in the small bowel through stimulation of crypt cell proliferation and inhibition of enterocyte apoptosis. This drug may have to be continued indefinitely for effects to persist.

COMPLICATIONS

- Oxalate kidney stones
- Cholesterol gallstones
- D-Lactic acidosis

PROGNOSIS

- Directly dependent on the extent of the bowel resection and in the case of Crohn's disease by the underlying illness
- Whether the colon remains in continuity with the small bowel is an important factor in the patient's ability to adapt after significant small bowel resection.

EBM EVIDENCE

available at www.expertconsult.com

RELATED CONTENT

Short-Bowel Syndrome (Patient Information)

AUTHOR: **FRED F. FERRI, M.D.**

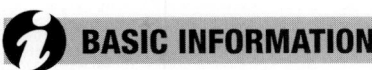

BASIC INFORMATION

DEFINITION

Sialadenitis is an inflammation of the salivary glands.

ICD-9CM CODES
527.2 Sialadenitis

EPIDEMIOLOGY & DEMOGRAPHICS

Parotid or submandibular glands are most frequently affected (Fig. 1-759).

PHYSICAL FINDINGS & CLINICAL PRESENTATION

- Pain and swelling of the affected salivary gland
- Increased pain with meals
- Erythema, tenderness at the duct opening
- Purulent discharge from duct orifice
- Induration and pitting of the skin, with involvement of the masseteric and submandibular spatial planes in severe cases

ETIOLOGY

- Ductal obstruction is generally from a mucus plug caused by stasis of saliva with increased viscosity with subsequent stasis and infection.

- Most frequent infecting organisms are *Staphylococcus aureus, Pseudomonas, Enterobacter, Klebsiella, Enterococcus, Proteus,* and *Candida* spp.
- Sjögren's syndrome, trauma, radiation therapy, chemotherapy, dehydration, and chronic illness are predisposing factors.

DIAGNOSIS

DIFFERENTIAL DIAGNOSIS

- Salivary gland neoplasm
- Ductal stricture
- Sialolithiasis
- Decreased salivary secretion as a result of medications (e.g., amitriptyline, diphenhydramine, anticholinergics)

WORKUP

- Generally not necessary
- Ultrasound or CT scan in patients not responding to medical treatment

LABORATORY TESTS

- Generally not indicated
- Complete blood count with differential to possibly reveal leukocytosis with left shift

IMAGING STUDIES

- Ultrasound or CT scan may be needed in patients not responding to medical therapy.
- Sialography should not be performed during the acute phase.

TREATMENT

NONPHARMACOLOGIC THERAPY

- Massage of the gland: may express pus and relieve some of the pressure
- Rehydration
- Warm compresses
- Oral cavity irrigations

ACUTE GENERAL Rx

- Amoxicillin-clavulanate 500 to 875 mg or cefuroxime 250 to 500 mg bid should be given for 10 days. Clindamycin is an alternative choice in patients allergic to penicillin.
- IV antibiotics (e.g., cefoxitin, nafcillin) can be given in severe cases.

DISPOSITION

Complete recovery unless the patient has underlying obstruction (e.g., ductal stricture, tumor, or stone)

REFERRAL

- To ear-nose-throat specialist for nonresolving cases despite appropriate antibiotic therapy
- For salivary gland incision and drainage, which may be necessary in resistant cases

PEARLS & CONSIDERATIONS

COMMENTS

Prevention of dehydration will decrease the risk of sialadenitis.

RELATED CONTENT

Salivary Gland Inflammation (Patient Information)

AUTHOR: **FRED F. FERRI, M.D.**

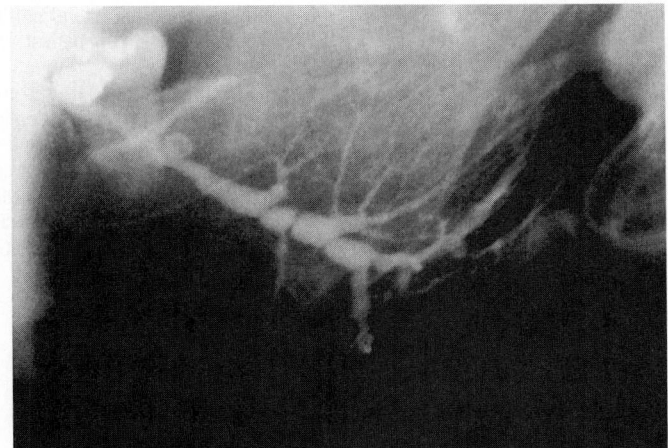

FIGURE 1-759 Sialogram of patient with chronic sialadenitis showing sausage link–like patterns and massive duct dilation. (From Blitzer CE et al: Sialadenitis. In Johnson JT, Yu VL [eds]: *Infectious diseases and antimicrobial therapy of the ears, nose, and throat,* Philadelphia, 1997, Saunders.)

BASIC INFORMATION

DEFINITION

Sialolithiasis is the existence of hardened intraluminal deposits in the ductal system of a salivary gland.

SYNONYMS

Salivary gland stone
Salivary calculus

ICD-9CM CODES
527.5 Sialolithiasis

EPIDEMIOLOGY & DEMOGRAPHICS

Affects patients mostly in the fifth to eighth decades and occurs most commonly in the submandibular gland (80%); only 14% are located in a parotid gland.

PHYSICAL FINDINGS & CLINICAL PRESENTATION

- Symptoms: colicky postprandial pain and swelling of a salivary gland. Tends to have a remitting/relapsing course.
- Signs: swelling and tenderness of a salivary gland. The stone may be felt by palpation of the floor of the mouth (Fig. 1-760).

ETIOLOGY

- The cause is unknown. Contributing factors include saliva stagnation, sialadenitis (inflammation of a salivary gland), ductal inflammation, or injury.
- Salivary calculus composition is mainly calcium phosphate and carbonate, often combined with small proportions of magnesium, zinc, ammonium salts, and organic materials or debris.

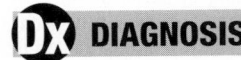 DIAGNOSIS

DIFFERENTIAL DIAGNOSIS

- Lymphadenitis
- Salivary gland tumor
- Salivary gland bacterial (*Staphylococcus* or *Streptococcus*), viral (mumps), or fungal infection (sialadenitis)
- Noninfectious salivary gland inflammation (e.g., Sjögren's syndrome, sarcoidosis, lymphoma)
- Salivary duct stricture
- Dental abscess

IMAGING STUDIES

- Plain radiograph
- Sialography

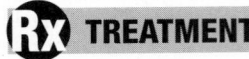 TREATMENT

- Warm soaks to area
- Antibiotics if associated bacterial sialadenitis is present
- Bland diet; avoid citrus fruit and spices
- Manual stone extraction sometimes associated with incisional enlargement of the ductal orifice
- Surgical salivary gland removal for retained hilar calculi

REFERRAL

To otorhinolaryngologist

RELATED CONTENT

Salivary Gland Stones (Patient Information)

AUTHOR: **FRED F. FERRI, M.D.**

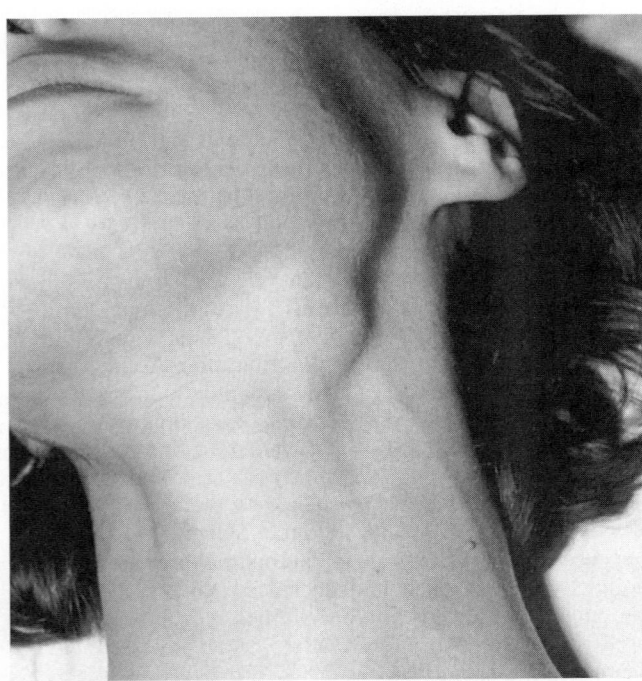

FIGURE 1-760 Patient with large calculus and obstruction of the left submandibular gland. (From Blitzer CE et al: Sialadenitis. In Johnson JT, Yu VL [eds]: *Infectious diseases and antimicrobial therapy of the ears, nose, and throat,* Philadelphia, 1997, Saunders.)

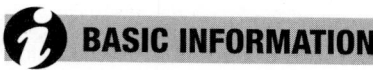

BASIC INFORMATION

DEFINITION

Sickle cell disease is a hemoglobinopathy characterized by the production of hemoglobin S caused by substitution of the amino acid valine for glutamic acid in the sixth position of the gamma-globin chain. When exposed to lower oxygen tension, red blood cells (RBCs) assume a sickle shape, resulting in stasis of RBCs in capillaries. Painful crises are caused by ischemic tissue injury resulting from obstruction of blood flow produced by sickled erythrocytes. Vasoocclusive crises are the main reason for hospital admission of children with sickle cell disease.

SYNONYMS

Sickle cell anemia
SCA
SCD
Hemoglobin S disease

ICD-9CM CODES
286.60 Sickle cell anemia

EPIDEMIOLOGY & DEMOGRAPHICS

- Sickle cell hemoglobin S is transmitted by an autosomal-recessive gene. In African Americans, the incidence of sickle cell anemia at birth is 1 in 600 and the incidence of all genotypes of sickle cell disease is 1 in 300.
- Sickle cell trait occurs in approximately 300 million people worldwide, with the highest prevalence of approximately 30% to 40% in sub-Saharan Africa. In the United States, it is found in nearly 10% of black Americans.
- It is estimated that 2000 babies are born with sickle cell disease in the U.S. each year.
- There is no predominant sex.

PHYSICAL FINDINGS & CLINICAL PRESENTATION

- Physical examination is variable depending on the degree of anemia and presence of acute vasoocclusive syndromes or neurologic, cardiovascular, genitourinary, and musculoskeletal complications. Pain in adults with sickle cell disease is the rule rather than the exception and is far more prevalent and severe than reported in older large-scale surveys.
- There is no clinical laboratory finding that is pathognomonic of painful crisis of sickle cell disease. The diagnosis of a painful episode is made solely on the basis of the medical therapy and physical examination.
- Bones are the most common site of pain. Dactylitis, or hand-foot syndrome (acute, painful swelling of the hands and feet), is the first manifestation of sickle cell disease in many infants. Irritability and refusal to walk are other common symptoms. After infancy, musculoskeletal pain can be symmetric, asymmetric, or migratory, and it may or may

not be associated with swelling, low-grade fever, redness, or warmth.
- In both children and adults, sickle vaso-occlusive episodes are difficult to distinguish from osteomyelitis, septic arthritis, synovitis, rheumatic fever, or gout.
- When abdominal or visceral pain is present, care should be taken to exclude sequestration syndromes (spleen, liver) or the possibility of an acute condition such as appendicitis, pancreatitis, cholecystitis, urinary tract infection, pelvic inflammatory disease, or malignancy.
- Pneumonia develops during the course of 20% of painful events and can present as chest and abdominal pain. In adults chest pain may be a result of vasoocclusion in the ribs and often precedes a pulmonary event. The lower back is also a frequent site of painful crisis in adults.
- The acute chest syndrome manifests with chest pain, fever, wheezing, tachypnea, and cough. Chest radiograph may reveal pulmonary infiltrates (Fig. 1-761). Common causes include infection (*Mycoplasma, Chlamydia,* viruses), infarction, and fat embolism.
- Musculoskeletal and skin abnormalities seen in sickle cell anemia include leg ulcers (particularly on the malleoli) and limb-girdle deformities caused by avascular necrosis of the femoral and humeral heads. Osteonecrosis of the heads of the femur and humerus is found in nearly 50% of adults with sickle cell disease.
- Endocrine abnormalities include delayed sexual maturation and late physical maturation, especially evident in boys.

- Neurologic abnormalities on examination may include seizures and altered mental status. Strokes occur in about 10% of children and adults with sickle cell anemia.
- Infections, particularly involving *Salmonella, Mycoplasma,* and *Streptococcus,* are relatively common.
- Severe splenomegaly as a result of sequestration often occurs in children before splenic atrophy.

DIAGNOSIS

DIFFERENTIAL DIAGNOSIS

- Thalassemia
- Iron-deficiency anemia, leukemia
- The differential diagnosis of patients presenting with a painful crisis is discussed in "Physical Findings"

WORKUP

- Screening of all newborns regardless of racial background is performed in the United States. Screening can be performed with sodium metabisulfite reduction test (Sickledex test).
- Hemoglobin electrophoresis will also confirm the diagnosis and is useful to identify hemoglobin variants such as fetal hemoglobin and hemoglobin A_2.
- Sickle cell disease encompasses genotypes associated with hemolysis and vasoocclusive crisis. Hemoglobin electrophoresis results, mean corpuscular volume, erythrocyte morphology, and degree of anemia can be used

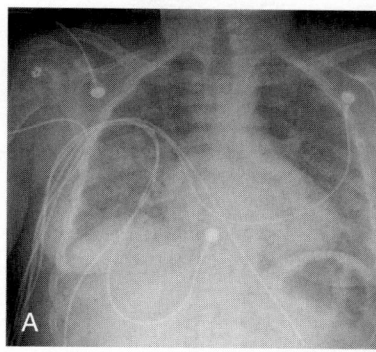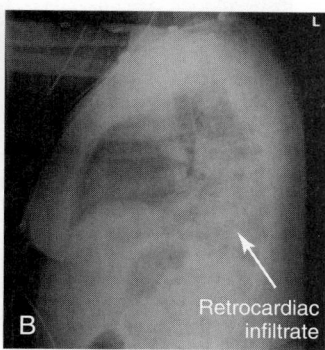

Retrocardiac infiltrate

FIGURE 1-761 Acute chest syndrome of sickle cell anemia does not have a single pathognomonic appearance on chest x-ray. The condition is caused by microvascular sludging of sickled red blood cells, resulting in infarction of the lung from small vessel occlusion. In the face of parenchymal necrosis, fluid accumulates within alveoli, increasing the density of lung tissue from air density to soft tissue density (fluid density).
The radiographic appearance is indistinguishable from that of other pneumonias. Because the infarction occurs in small vessels, the distribution of infarction is not in the territory of a large vessel as might be seen with pulmonary embolism, where infarction of an entire lung segment distal to the point of thrombotic occlusion may be seen. Thus the distribution of lung infiltrates in acute chest syndrome may be patchy or may follow a lobar distribution. Because alveoli fill with fluid, air bronchograms may be seen, as in bacterial pneumonia. Making the diagnosis even more indistinct, patients with sickle cell anemia may have bacterial pneumonia with negative blood and sputum cultures, so a pulmonary infection may be wrongly labeled as acute chest syndrome. With these caveats, this x-ray is from a 24-year-old male with sickle cell anemia disease, presenting with fever and an oxygen saturation of 60% on room air. He improved with oxygen, fluids, and antibiotic administration, although antigen testing for *Streptococcus pneumoniae, Legionella,* and influenza were negative, as were cultures. **A,** The posterior-anterior chest x-ray demonstrates patchy bilateral infiltrates. The right lower lobe shows particular density, and increased density is seen in the retrocardiac space on the lateral x-ray. **B,** Note the absence of the usual decrease in density toward the diaphragm. (From Broder JS: *Diagnostic imaging for the emergency physician,* Philadelphia, 2011, Saunders.)

to differentiate among the sickle cell syndromes.
- For prenatal diagnosis, initial step is identification of parenteral globin gene mutation by DNA-based testing. If positive, then DNA-based testing of chorionic villus sampling or amniotic fluid cells is performed.

LABORATORY TESTS
- Anemia (resulting from chronic hemolysis), reticulocytosis, leukocytosis, and thrombocytosis are common.
- Elevations of bilirubin and lactate dehydrogenase are also common.
- Peripheral blood smear may reveal sickle cells, target cells, poikilocytosis, and hypochromia (Fig. 1-762).
- Elevated blood urea nitrogen and creatinine may be present in patients with progressive renal insufficiency.
- Urinalysis may reveal hematuria and proteinuria.

IMAGING STUDIES
- Chest x-ray is useful in patients presenting with chest syndrome. Cardiomegaly may be present on chest x-ray.
- MRI or bone scan is useful to rule out osteomyelitis (usually the result of *Salmonella*).
- CT scan or MRI of brain is often needed in patients with neurologic complications such as transient ischemic attack, cerebrovascular accident, seizures, or altered mental status.
- Transcranial Doppler ultrasonograhy (TCD) is a useful commodity to identify children with sickle cell anemia who are at risk for stroke. There should be an initial screening starting at age 2. Patients determined to be at risk should be enrolled in long-term transfusion programs. These are effective in reducing risk of stroke by >90%. In adults magnetic resonance angiography (MRA) can be used instead of TCD to identify those at risk for stroke.
- Doppler echocardiography may be helpful in diagnosing pulmonary hypertension but has a low positive predictive value. Screening for vasculopathy is done by estimating the tricuspid regurgitant jet velocity (TRV). Elevated

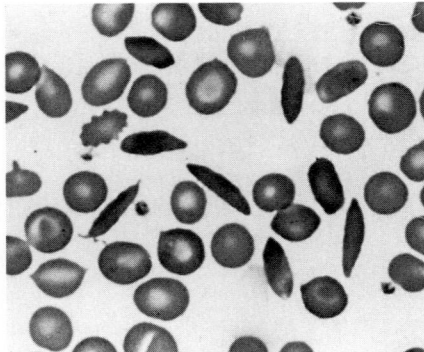

FIGURE 1-762 Photomicrograph of peripheral blood smear with sickle cells, typical of sickle cell anemia. (From Andreoli TE [ed]: *Cecil essentials of medicine,* ed 4, Philadelphia, 1997, Saunders.)

values are predictive of early mortality. The prevalence of pulmonary hypertension when right heart catheterization is performed is approximately 6% in adults with sickle cell disease.

Rx TREATMENT

NONPHARMACOLOGIC THERAPY
- Patients should be instructed to avoid conditions that may precipitate sickling crisis, such as hypoxia, infections, acidosis, and dehydration.
- Maintain adequate hydration (PO or IV).
- Correct hypoxia.

ACUTE GENERAL Rx
- Aggressively diagnose and treat suspected infections (*Salmonella* osteomyelitis and pneumococcal infections occur more often in patients with sickle cell anemia because of splenic infarcts and atrophy). Combination therapy with a cephalosporin and erythromycin plus incentive spirometry and bronchodilators is useful in patients with acute chest syndrome.
- Provide pain relief during the vasoocclusive crisis. The fear of creating or perpetuating addiction or being deceived by patients often causes physicians to prescribe subtherapeutic dosages of opioids. However, available evidence suggests that the prevalence of drug addiction among patients with sickle cell anemia is no higher than in the overall U.S. population. Medications should be administered on a fixed time schedule with a dosing interval that does not extend beyond the duration of the desired pharmacologic effect.
  1. Meperidine is contraindicated in patients with renal dysfunction or central nervous system disease because its metabolite, normeperidine (which is excreted by the kidneys), can cause seizures.
  2. Narcotics (e.g., morphine 0.1 mg/kg IV q3-4h or 0.3 mg/kg PO q4h) should be given on a fixed schedule (not prn for pain), with rescue dosing for breakthrough pain as needed.
  3. Except when contraindications exist, concomitant use of nonsteroidal anti-inflammatory drugs should be standard treatment.
  4. Nurses should be instructed not to give narcotics if the patient is heavily sedated or respirations are depressed.
  5. When the patient shows signs of improvement, narcotic drugs should be tapered gradually to prevent withdrawal syndrome. It is advisable to observe the patient on oral pain relief medications for 12 to 24 hr before discharge from the hospital.
  6. Analgesic medications should be used in combination with psychological, behavioral, and physical modalities in the management of sickle cell disease.

- Aggressively diagnose and treat any potential complications (e.g., septic necrosis of the femoral head, priapism, bony infarcts, and acute chest syndrome).
- Overall strategies for the management of acute chest syndrome are described in Table 1-375.
- Hydroxyurea (15 mg/kg body weight per day in patients with normal creatinine clearance) increases hemoglobin F levels and reduces the incidence of vasoocclusive complications. It is generally well tolerated. Side effects consist primarily of mild, reversible neutropenia. It should be avoided in patients with existing leukopenia, thrombocytopenia, or severe hypoplastic anemia. It is indicated for adults with sickle cell anemia who have moderate to severe disease, typically those with three or more acute painful crises or episodes of the acute chest syndrome in the previous year.
- Replace folic acid (1 mg PO qd) due to loss from increased utilization of folic acid stores due to chronic hemolysis. Sickle cell patients also often have mineral and vitamin deficiencies (calcium, zinc, and vitamins A, C, D, and E) and may need vitamin and nutritional supplementation.

TABLE 1-375 Overall Strategies for the Management of Acute Chest Syndrome

Prevention

Incentive spirometry and periodic ambulation in patients admitted for vasoocclusive crises, surgery, or febrile episodes

Watchful waiting in any hospitalized child or adult with sickle cell disease (pulse oximetry monitoring and frequent respiratory assessments)

Avoidance of overhydration

Intense education and optimum care of patients who have sickle cell anemia and asthma

Diagnostic Testing and Laboratory Monitoring

Blood cultures

Nasopharyngeal samples for viral culture (respiratory syncytial virus, influenza)

Blood counts every day and appropriate chemistries

Continuous pulse oximetry

Chest radiographs

Treatment

Blood transfusion (simple or exchange)

Supplemental O_2 for drop in pulse oximetry by 4% over baseline, or values <90%

Empirical antibiotics (cephalosporin and macrolide)

Continued respiratory therapy (incentive spirometry and chest physiotherapy as necessary)

Bronchodilators and steroids for patients with asthma

Optimum pain control and fluid management

From Kliegman RM et al: *Nelson textbook of pediatrics,* ed 19, Philadelphia, 2011, Saunders.

CHRONIC Rx

- Guidelines for prompt management of fever, infections, pain, and specific complications should be reviewed.
- Genetic counseling is recommended in all cases.
- Avoid unnecessary transfusions. Exchange transfusions may be necessary for patients with acute neurologic signs, in aplastic crisis, or undergoing surgery. The target hemoglobin level is 10 to 11 g/dl (hematocrit 30%). Transfusing to a higher Hb/Hct should be avoided due to associated hyperviscosity if there is a substantial portion of HbS in the blood. Indications for transfusion in sickle cell disease are described in Table 1-376. Iron overload due to blood transfusions (transfusional hemosiderosis) can be treated with chelating agents (deferoxamine [SC infusion], deferasirox [PO], and deferiprone [PO]).
- Allogeneic stem cell transplantation can be curative in young patients with symptomatic sickle cell disease; however, the death rate from the procedure is nearly 10%, the marrow recipients are likely to be infertile, and there is an undefined risk of chemotherapy-induced malignancy. Myeloablative stem cell transplantation is generally limited to children under age 16 with severe disease.
- Penicillin V 125 mg PO bid should be administered by age 2 mo and increased to 250 mg bid by age 3 yr. Penicillin prophylaxis can be discontinued after age 5 yr except in children who have had splenectomy.

REFERRAL

- Hospitalization is generally recommended for most crises and complications.
- Psychosocial counseling and support structures should be developed.
- At least yearly evaluation by a hematologist competent in sickle cell anemia is recommended in all patients with sickle cell anemia.
- Patients with pulmonary hypertension should follow up with a cardiologist and a pulmonologist.

❗ PEARLS & CONSIDERATIONS

COMMENTS

- Pain in adults with sickle cell disease is the rule rather than the exception and needs to be treated appropriately.
- Patients and their families should receive genetic counseling and should be made aware of the difference between sickle cell trait and sickle cell disease.
- Regular immunizations and pneumococcal vaccination are recommended. The prophylactic administration of penicillin soon after birth and the timely administration of pneumococcal and *Haemophilus influenzae* type b vaccines have resulted in a significant decline in the incidence of these infections. The heptavalent conjugated pneumococcal vaccine (Prevan) should be administered from 2 mo of age. The 23-valent unconjugated pneumococcal vaccine is given from age 2 yr

and can be boosted once 3 yr later. Influenza vaccination can be given after 6 mo of age.
- Patients should be instructed on a well-balanced diet and appropriate folic acid supplementation.
- The presence of dactylitis, Hb 7, or leukocytosis in the absence of infection during the first 2 yr of life indicates a higher risk of severe sickle cell disease later in life.
- Among patients with sickle cell disease, acute chest syndrome is commonly precipitated by fat embolism and infection, especially community-acquired pneumonia. Among older patients and those with neurologic symptoms, the syndrome often progresses to respiratory failure.
- Poloxamer 188, a nonionic surfactant with hemorrheologic and antithrombotic properties, has been reported to produce a significant but relatively small decrease in the duration of painful episodes and an increase in the proportion of patients who achieved resolution of the symptoms. A more significant effect was observed in patients who received concomitant hydroxyurea.
- Pulmonary hypertension is a complication of chronic hemolysis and is associated with a high risk of death. It can be detected by Doppler echocardiography in more than 30% of adult patients with sickle cell disease. Cardiac catheterization will confirm the diagnosis. It is resistant to hydroxyurea therapy.
- Neurocognitive brain dysfunction is common in sickle cell disease. Trials have shown that compared with healthy controls, adults with sickle cell disease have a poorer cognitive performance, which is associated with anemia and age.
- Among patients with sickle cell disease hospitalized with vasoocclusive pain crisis, the use of inhaled nitric oxide compared with placebo did not improve time to crisis resolution.
- The average life span of individuals with sickle cell trait is similar to that of the general population. However, it is associated with a higher incidence of renal medullary cancer.

SUGGESTED READINGS

available at www.expertconsult.com

RELATED CONTENT

Sickle Cell Anemia (Patient Information)

AUTHOR: **FRED F. FERRI, M.D.**

TABLE 1-376   Indications for Transfusion in Sickle Cell Disease

	Duration	Consensus	Method	Goal*
Stroke, acute	Single	+	Ex	HbS <30%
Stroke, ongoing care	Chronic	+	Either	HbS <30%
High-velocity transcranial Doppler	Chronic	+	Either	HbS <30%
ACS, initial episode	Single	+	Dir > Ex	Hgb 10
ACS, recurrent	6-12 mo	+	Either	
Pulmonary hypertension	Chronic	+	Either	
Multiorgan failure	Single	+	Ex	
Major surgery	Single	+	Dir	Hgb 10
Acute anemia	Single	+	Dir	
Recurrent spleen sequestration	Chronic	+		
Sepsis/meningitis	Single	+	Dir	
Severe chronic pain	6-12 mo	+		
Congestive heart failure	Chronic	+		
Silent infarct with abnormal neuropsychology	Chronic	−		
Pregnancy		−		
Anemia/renal failure	Chronic	−		
Leg ulcers	6-12 mo	−		
Severe growth delay		−		
Severe eye disease		−		
Priapism		−		

ACS, Acute chest syndrome; *Dir,* direct; *Ex,* exchange; *Hb,* hemoglobin type; *Hgb,* hemoglobin concentration; +, consensus reached; −, consensus not reached.
*Goal of transfusion if a consensus has been reached.
From Fuhrman BP et al: *Pediatric critical care,* ed 4, Philadelphia, 2011, Saunders.

BASIC INFORMATION

DEFINITION

Silicosis is a lung disease attributable to the inhalation of silica (silicon dioxide) in crystalline form (quartz) or in cristobalite or tridymite forms.

SYNONYMS

Pneumoconiosis caused by silica

ICD-9CM CODES
502 Silicosis, occupational
503 Pneumoconiosis caused by other inorganic dust

EPIDEMIOLOGY & DEMOGRAPHICS

- Occupational disease affecting men and women involved in gathering, milling, processing, or using silica-containing rock or sand. Jobs that can lead to silicosis are described in Box 1-58.
- An estimated 1 million Americans are exposed.

PHYSICAL FINDINGS & CLINICAL PRESENTATION

- Dyspnea
- Cough
- Wheezing
- Abnormal chest radiograph in an asymptomatic person

ETIOLOGY

- Silica particles are ingested by alveolar macrophages, which in turn release oxidants causing cell injury and cell death, attract fibroblasts, and activate lymphocytes, increasing immunoglobulins in the alveolar space.
- Hyperplasia of alveolar epithelial cells occurs.
- Collagen accumulates in the interstitium.

- Neutrophils also accumulate and secrete proteolytic enzymes, which leads to tissue destruction and emphysema.
- Silica dust may be carcinogenic (not proven).
- Exposure to silicosis predisposes to tuberculosis.
- Some patients develop rheumatoid silicotic pulmonary nodules and may have arthritic symptoms of rheumatoid arthritis (Caplan's syndrome). Scleroderma has also been associated with silicosis.

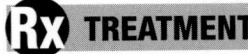

DIAGNOSIS

DIFFERENTIAL DIAGNOSIS

- Other pneumoconiosis, berylliosis, hard metal disease, asbestosis
- Sarcoidosis
- Tuberculosis
- Interstitial lung disease
- Hypersensitivity pneumonitis
- Lung cancer
- Langerhans' cell granulomatosis (histiocytosis X)
- Granulomatous pulmonary vasculitis

WORKUP

- History of occupational exposure
- Chest radiograph (Fig. 1-763)

Chronic silicosis:
- Most common clinical presentation. Onset is after decades of repeated exposure.
- Characteristic finding: small, rounded lung parenchymal opacities
- Hilar lymphadenopathy with "eggshell" calcifications
- Pleural plaques (uncommon)

Accelerated silicosis (progressive massive fibrosis):
- Develops <10 years after initial exposure.
- Large parenchymal lesions resulting from coalesced small nodules
- Higher risk for progressive massive fibrosis

Acute silicosis:
- Develops several weeks to <5 years after silica exposure.
- Ground-glass appearance of the lung fields
- Chest CT scan
- Pulmonary function tests
- Combination of obstructive and restrictive changes with or without reduction in diffusing capacity
- Bronchoscopy with lung biopsy in uncertain cases

COURSE

Chronic silicosis:
- May not progress with absence of further exposure
- Accelerated silicosis: progressive respiratory failure and cor pulmonale

Acute silicosis:
- Fatal course from respiratory failure over several months to a few years

TREATMENT

- Treatment is symptomatic (supplemental O_2 for hypoxemia, bronchodilators, antibiotics for infections).
- Prevention (industrial hygiene)
- Treatment of associated tuberculosis if present
- Supportive measures (oxygen, bronchodilators)
- Consider lung transplant for patients who develop chronic respiratory failure.

RELATED CONTENT

Silicosis (Patient Information)

AUTHOR: **FRED F. FERRI, M.D.**

BOX 1-58   Jobs That Can Lead to Silicosis

Mining: surface or underground mining (tunneling)
Milling: ground silica for abrasives and filler
Quarrying
Sandblasting (e.g., of buildings, preparing steel for painting)
Pottery; ceramic or clay work
Grinding, polishing using silica wheels
Stone work
Foundry work: grinding, molding, chipping
Refractory brick work
Glass making: to polish and as an abrasive
Boiler work: cleaning boilers
Manufacture of abrasives

From Goldman L, Schafer AI: *Goldman's Cecil medicine,* ed 24, Philadelphia, 2012, Saunders.

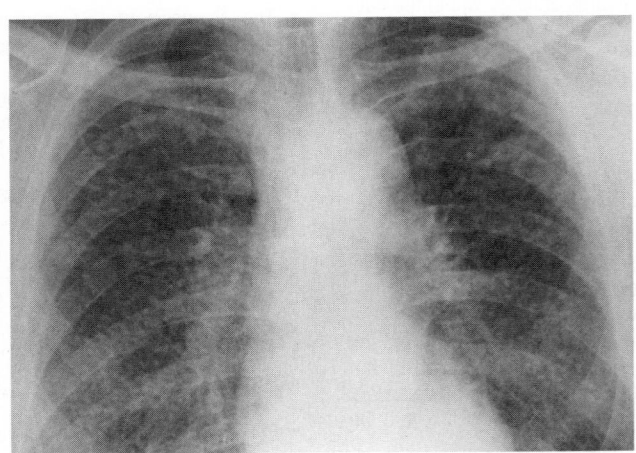

FIGURE 1-763 Simple silicosis. There are multiple small (2- to 4-mm) nodules distributed throughout the lungs, with an upper lobe predominance. (From McLoud TC: *Thoracic radiology: the requisites,* St Louis, 1998, Mosby.)

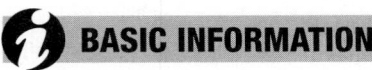

DEFINITION

Cavernous sinus thrombosis (CST) is a late complication of facial or paranasal sinus infection, resulting in thrombosis of the cavernous sinus and inflammation of its surrounding anatomic structures, including cranial nerves III, IV, V (ophthalmic and maxillary branch), and VI, and the internal carotid artery.

SYNONYMS

CST
Intracranial venous sinus thrombosis or thrombophlebitis
Dural sinus thrombosis

ICD-9CM CODES

325 Phlebitis and thrombophlebitis of intracranial venous sinuses

EPIDEMIOLOGY & DEMOGRAPHICS

- CST is rare in the postantibiotic era.
- Before antibiotics the mortality rate was 80% to 100%.
- With antibiotics and early diagnosis, mortality rates have fallen to ~20%.
- Reported morbidity rates have also declined from between 50% and 70% to only 22% with advances in imaging modalities and aggressive medical care.

PHYSICAL FINDINGS & CLINICAL PRESENTATION

- Can be either an acute and fulminant disease or an indolent and subacute presentation.
- Headache, although not specific, is the most common presenting symptom and may precede fever and periorbital edema by several days. Elderly patients, however, may only demonstrate alteration in mental status without antecedent headache. A classic presentation is abrupt onset of unilateral periorbital edema progressing to bilateral eye involvement, headache, photophobia, and proptosis. These signs and symptoms are related to the anatomic structures affected within the cavernous sinus, notably cranial nerves III to VI, as well as impaired venous drainage from the orbit and the eye.

Other common signs and symptoms include:
- Ptosis
- Chemosis
- Cranial nerve palsies (III, IV, V, VI)
  1. Sixth nerve palsy is the most common (abducens nerve is located medially in the cavernous sinus and is surrounded by blood, making it more susceptible to inflammatory changes).
  2. Hypoesthesia or hyperesthesia of the ophthalmic and maxillary branch of the fifth nerve is common. Periorbital sensory loss and impaired corneal reflex may be noted.

- Papilledema, retinal hemorrhages, and decreased visual acuity progressing to blindness may occur from venous congestion within the retina.
- Pupil may be dilated and sluggishly reactive.
- Fever, tachycardia, and sepsis may be present.
- Headache with nuchal rigidity and changes in mental status may occur.
- Infection can spread to the contralateral cavernous sinus through the intercavernous sinuses within 24 to 48 hr of initial presentation.

ETIOLOGY

- CST most commonly results from contiguous spread of an infection from the sinuses (sphenoid, ethmoid, or frontal) or the medial third of the face (areas around the eyes and nose that drain to the ophthalmic vein). Nasal furuncles are the most common facial infection to produce this complication. Less-common primary sites of infection include dental abscess, tonsils, soft palate, middle ear, or orbit (orbital cellulitis).
- CST also can result from hematogenous spread of infection to the cavernous sinus by the superior and inferior ophthalmic veins or through the lateral and sigmoid sinuses. It can spread in a retrograde direction depending on the pressure gradients, because the dural sinuses are valveless.
- *Staphylococcus aureus* is the most commonly identified pathogen, found in 60% to 70% of the cases.
- *Streptococcus* is the second leading cause.
- Gram-negative rods and anaerobes may also lead to CST.
- Rarely, *Aspergillus fumigatus* and mucormycosis cause CST.
- Risk factors for dural sinus thrombosis include venous hypercoagulable disorders, infections (see above), trauma, malignancies, systemic inflammatory disorders, pregnancy, and dehydration.

DIAGNOSIS

- The diagnosis of CST is made by clinical suspicion and confirmed by appropriate imaging studies.
- Proptosis, ptosis, chemosis, and cranial nerve palsy beginning in one eye and progressing to the other eye establish the diagnosis.

DIFFERENTIAL DIAGNOSIS

- Orbital or periorbital cellulitis
- Internal carotid artery aneurysm or fistula
- Cerebrovascular disease
- Migraine headache
- Allergic blepharitis
- Thyroid ophthalmopathy
- Orbital neoplasm
- Meningitis
- Epidural and subdural infections

- Epidural and subdural hematoma
- Subarachnoid hemorrhage
- Acute angle-closure glaucoma
- Trauma

WORKUP

CST is a clinical diagnosis, with laboratory tests and imaging studies confirming the clinical impression.

LABORATORY TESTS

- Complete blood count, erythrocyte sedimentation rate, blood cultures, and sinus cultures help establish and identify an infectious primary source.
- Lumbar puncture (LP) helps to distinguish CST from more localized processes (e.g., sinusitis, orbital cellulitis). LP reveals inflammatory cells in 75% of cases. In half of these cases, the cerebrospinal fluid profile is typical for a parameningeal focus (high white blood cells with polymorphonuclear and/or mononuclear cells, normal glucose, normal protein, culture negative), and in one third may be similar to that of a bacterial meningitis.

IMAGING STUDIES

- MRI with gadolinium, including magnetic resonance angiography (Fig. 1-764), is more sensitive than CT scan and is the imaging study of choice to diagnose CST. Findings may include deformity of the internal carotid artery within the cavernous sinus and an obvious signal hyperintensity within thrombosed vascular sinuses on all pulse sequences.
- Noncontrast CT scan of the head and orbits may demonstrate increased density in the region of the cavernous sinus but has relatively low sensitivity. Contrast-enhanced CT scan may reveal underlying sinusitis, thickening of the superior ophthalmic vein, and irregular filling defects within the cavernous sinus ("empty delta sign"); however, findings may be normal early in the disease course.

TREATMENT

NONPHARMACOLOGIC THERAPY

Recognizing the primary source of infection (i.e., facial cellulitis, middle ear, and sinus infections) and treating the primary source expeditiously is the best way to prevent CST.

ACUTE GENERAL Rx

- Appropriate therapy should take into account the primary source of infection as well as possible associated complications such as brain abscess, meningitis, or subdural empyema.
- Broad-spectrum intravenous antibiotics are used as empiric therapy until a definite pathogen is found. Treatment should include vancomycin to cover hospital or community

acquired methicillin-resistant *Staphylococcus aureus* or resistant *Streptococcus pneumoniae* plus a third- or fourth-generation cephalosporin:

1. Vancomycin (1 g q12h with normal renal function) plus either ceftriaxone (2 g q12h) or cefepime (2 g q8 to 12h).
2. Metronidazole 500 mg IV q6h should be added if anaerobic bacterial infection is suspected (dental or sinus infection).

- Most experts recommend anticoagulation with heparin after the diagnosis is confirmed, unless surgical intervention is planned or there is evidence of an expanding hematoma. Cerebral infarction or intracranial hemorrhage should first be ruled out before initiating heparin therapy. Early heparinization has been suggested in patients with unilateral CST to prevent clot propagation. Coumadin therapy should be avoided in the acute phase of the illness but should ultimately be instituted to achieve an INR of 2 to 3 and continued until the infection, symptoms, and signs of CST have resolved or significantly improved. A nonrandomized prospective cohort study found treatment with low-molecular-weight heparin led to more functional independence at 6 mo without significant differences in complete recovery and mortality compared to unfractionated heparin.
- Steroid therapy is also controversial but may prove helpful in reducing cranial nerve dysfunction or when progression to pituitary insufficiency occurs. Corticosteroids should only be instituted after appropriate antibiotic coverage. Dexamethasone 10 mg q6h is the treatment of choice.
- Emergent surgical drainage with sphenoidotomy is indicated if the primary site of infection is believed to be the sphenoid sinus.

CHRONIC Rx

- Patients with CST are usually treated with prolonged courses (3 to 4 wk) of IV antibiotics. If there is evidence of complications such as intracranial suppuration, 6 to 8 wk of total therapy may be warranted.
- All patients should be monitored for signs of complicated infection, continued sepsis, or septic emboli while antibiotic therapy is being administered.

DISPOSITION

- CST can be a life-threatening, rapidly progressive infectious disease with high morbidity and mortality rates (30%) despite antibiotic use. Morbidity and mortality rates are increased in cases of sphenoid sinus infection.
- Complications of untreated CST include extension of thrombus to other dural sinuses, carotid thrombosis with concomitant strokes, subdural empyema, brain abscess, or meningitis. Septic embolization may also occur to the lungs, resulting in acute respiratory distress syndrome, pulmonary abscess, empyema, and pneumothorax.
- Thirty percent of treated patients develop long-term sequelae, including cranial nerve palsies, blindness, pituitary insufficiency, and hemiparesis.

REFERRAL

If CST is suspected, it should be considered a medical emergency. Depending on the primary site of infection, appropriate consultation should be made (i.e., ear-nose-throat, ophthalmology, and infectious disease).

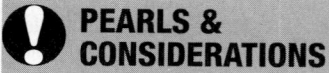
PEARLS & CONSIDERATIONS

COMMENTS

The clinical findings and diagnosis are easier to understand when the anatomy is realized: the cavernous sinus lies just above and lateral to the sphenoid sinus and drains the middle portion of the face by the superior and inferior ophthalmic veins; cranial nerves III, IV, V, and VI pass alongside or through the cavernous sinus.

SUGGESTED READINGS
available at www.expertconsult.com

RELATED CONTENT
Cavernous Sinus Thrombosis (Patient Information)

AUTHORS: **MARK F. BRADY, M.D., M.P.H.**, and **WEN Y. WU-CHEN, M.D.**

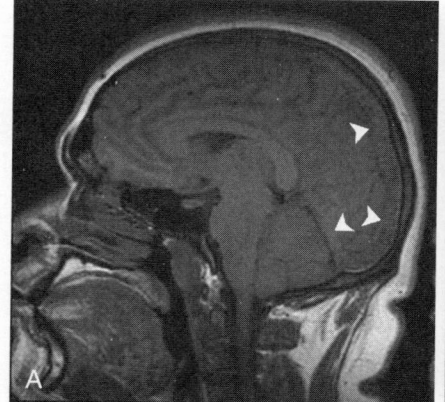
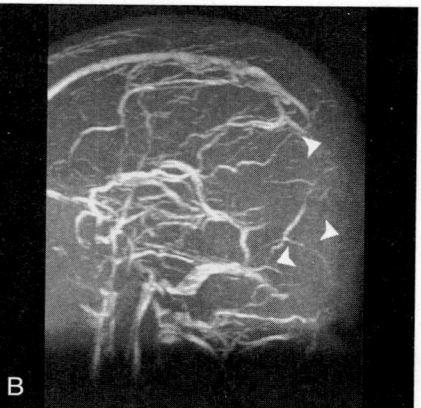
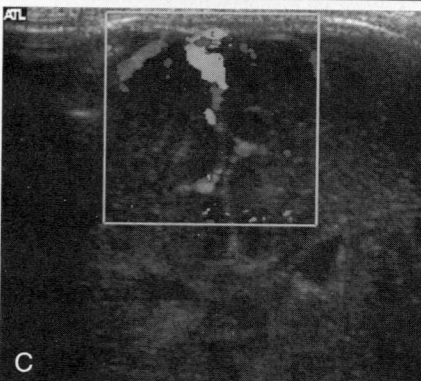

FIGURE 1-764 Superior sagittal sinus (SSS) thrombosis on magnetic resonance venogram (MRV). Sagittal T1 magnetic resonance imaging **(A)** shows intermediate signal intensity in sagittal and straight sinuses *(arrowheads)*. No flow is seen on MRV **(B)** in these vessels *(arrowheads)*, which is consistent with thrombosis. Color Doppler evacuation **(C)** of the SSS in another 6-mo-old patient with suspected thrombosis demonstrated a patent SSS with normal draining cortical veins. (From Fuhrman BP et al: *Pediatric critical care*, ed 4, Philadelphia, 2011, Saunders.)

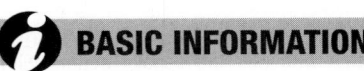

BASIC INFORMATION

DEFINITION

Sinusitis is inflammation of the mucous membranes lining one or more of the paranasal sinuses. The various presentations are:
- Acute sinusitis: infection lasting <4 wk, with complete resolution of symptoms.
- Subacute infection: lasts from 4 to 12 wk, with complete resolution of symptoms.
- Recurrent acute infection: episodes of acute infection lasting <30 days, with resolution of symptoms, which recur at intervals at least 10 days apart.
- Chronic sinusitis: inflammation lasting >12 wk, with persistent upper respiratory symptoms.
- Acute bacterial sinusitis superimposed on chronic sinusitis: new symptoms that occur in patients with residual symptoms from prior infection(s). With treatment, the new symptoms resolve but the residual ones do not.

SYNONYMS

Rhinosinusitis: sinusitis is almost always accompanied by inflammation of the nasal mucosa; thus it is now the preferred term.

ICD-9CM CODES
473.9 Sinusitis (accessory) (nasal) (hyperplastic) (nonpurulent) (purulent) (chronic)
461.9 Acute sinusitis

EPIDEMIOLOGY & DEMOGRAPHICS

INCIDENCE (IN U.S.): Seems to correlate with the incidence of upper respiratory tract infections and higher in women than men; 30 million cases a year in the U.S.
PEAK INCIDENCE:
- Fall, winter, spring: September through March
- In adults: greatest incidence between 45 and 74 years of age

PHYSICAL FINDINGS & CLINICAL PRESENTATION

- Patients often give a history of a recent upper respiratory illness with some improvement, then a relapse.
- Mucopurulent secretions in the nasal passage:
  1. Purulent nasal and postnasal discharge lasting 7 to 10 days
  2. Facial tightness, pressure, or pain
  3. Nasal obstruction
  4. Headache
  5. Decreased sense of smell
  6. Purulent pharyngeal secretions, brought up with cough, often worse at night
- Erythema, swelling, and tenderness over the infected sinus in a small proportion of patients:
  1. Diagnosis cannot be excluded by the absence of such findings.
  2. These findings are not common, and do not correlate with number of positive sinus aspirates.

- Intermittent low-grade fever in about half of adults with acute bacterial sinusitis.
- Toothache is a common complaint when the maxillary sinus is involved.
- Periorbital cellulitis and excessive tearing with ethmoid sinusitis:
  1. Orbital extension of infection: chemosis, proptosis, impaired extraocular movements
- Characteristics of acute sinusitis in children with upper respiratory tract infections:
  1. Persistence of symptoms
  2. Cough
  3. Bad breath
- Symptoms of chronic sinusitis (may or may not be present):
  1. Nasal or postnasal discharge
  2. Fever
  3. Facial pain or pressure
  4. Headache
- Nosocomial sinusitis is typically seen in patients with nasogastric tubes or nasotracheal intubation.

ETIOLOGY

- Each of the four paranasal sinuses is connected to the nasal cavity by narrow tubes (ostia), 1 to 3 mm in diameter; these drain directly into the nose through the turbinates. The sinuses are lined with a ciliated mucous membrane (mucoperiosteum).
- Acute viral infection:
  1. Infection with the common cold or influenza
  2. Mucosal edema and sinus inflammation
  3. Decreased drainage of thick secretions/obstruction of the sinus ostia
  4. Subsequent entrapment of bacteria
     a. Multiplication of bacteria
     b. Secondary bacterial infection
- Other predisposing factors:
  1. Tumors
  2. Polyps
  3. Foreign bodies
  4. Congenital choanal atresia
  5. Other entities that cause obstruction of sinus drainage
  6. Allergies
  7. Asthma
- Dental infections lead to maxillary sinusitis.
- Viruses recovered alone or in combination with bacteria (in 16% of cases):
  1. Rhinovirus
  2. Coronavirus
  3. Adenovirus
  4. Parainfluenza virus
  5. Respiratory syncytial virus
- The principal bacterial pathogens in sinusitis are *Streptococcus pneumoniae*, nontypeable *Haemophilus influenzae*, and *Moraxella catarrhalis*.
- In the remainder of cases *Streptococcus pyogenes*, *Staphylococcus aureus*, beta-hemolytic streptococci, and mixed anaerobic infections (*Peptostreptococcus, Fusobacterium, Bacteroides, Prevotella* spp.) are found.
- Infection is polymicrobial in about one third of cases.

- Anaerobic infections are seen more often in cases of chronic sinusitis and in cases associated with dental infection; anaerobes are unlikely pathogens in sinusitis in children.
- Fungal pathogens are isolated with increasing frequency in immunocompromised patients but remain uncommon pathogens in the paranasal sinuses. Fungal pathogens include: *Phaeohyphomycosis, Aspergillus, Pseudallescheria, Sporothrix,* and *Zygomycetes* spp.
- Nosocomial infections: occur in patients with nasogastric tubes, nasotracheal intubation, cystic fibrosis, and immunocompromised state.
  1. *S. aureus* (including MRSA)
  2. *Pseudomonas aeruginosa*
  3. *Klebsiella pneumoniae*
  4. *Enterobacter* spp.
  5. *Proteus mirabilis*
- Organisms typically isolated in chronic sinusitis:
  1. *S. aureus*
  2. *S. pneumoniae*
  3. *H. influenzae*
  4. *P. aeruginosa*
  5. Anaerobes

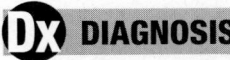

DIAGNOSIS

DIFFERENTIAL DIAGNOSIS

- Temporomandibular joint disease
- Migraine headache
- Cluster headache
- Dental infection
- Trigeminal neuralgia
- Allergic rhinitis
- Drugs (cocaine, decongestant overuse)
- Gastroesophageal reflux disease
- Wegener granulomatosis
- Cystic fibrosis

WORKUP

- The diagnosis is generally based on clinical signs and symptoms (purulent rhinorrhea and facial pain). Radiologic tests and cultures are not recommended initially and should be considered only when treatment is ineffective and sinusitis persists.
- In the normal healthy host, the paranasal sinuses should be sterile. Although the contiguous structures are colonized with bacteria and likely contaminate the sinuses, the mucociliary lining functions to remove these bacteria.
- Gold standard for diagnosis: recovery of bacteria in high-density ≥10^4 colony-forming units/ml from a paranasal sinus, in the setting of a patient with history of upper respiratory infection and symptoms persisting for 7 to 10 days. Sinus aspiration is the best method for obtaining cultures; however, it must be performed by an otorhinolaryngologist and is not practical for the primary care practitioner. Therefore, most diagnoses are based on the clinical history and presentation, possibly supported by radiologic evaluations.

1. Standard four-view sinus radiographs
   a. Complete opacification and air-fluid levels are most specific findings (average 85% and 80%, respectively)
   b. Mucosal thickening has low specificity (40% to 50%)
   c. Absence of all three of the previous findings has estimated sensitivity of 90%
   d. Overall, standard radiographs are of limited use in diagnosis, although negative films are strong evidence against the diagnosis
2. CT scans:
   a. Much more sensitive than plain radiographs in detecting acute changes and disease in the sinuses
   b. Recommended for patients requiring surgical intervention, including sinus aspiration; it is a useful adjunct to guide therapy
3. Transillumination:
   a. Used for diagnosis of frontal and maxillary sinusitis
   b. Place transilluminator in the mouth or against cheek to assess maxillary sinuses, under medial aspect of the supraorbital ridge to assess frontal sinuses
   c. Absence of light transmission indicates that sinus is filled with fluid
   d. Dullness (decreased light transmission) is less helpful in diagnosing infection
4. Endoscopy:
   a. Used to visualize secretions coming from the ostia of infected sinuses
   b. Culture collection via endoscopy often contaminated by nasal flora; not nearly as good as sinus puncture
5. Sinus puncture:
   a. Gold standard for collecting sinus cultures
   b. Generally reserved for treatment failures, suspected intracranial extension, and nosocomial sinusitis

Rx TREATMENT

NONPHARMACOLOGIC THERAPY
To help promote sinus drainage:
- Air humidification with vaporizers (for steam) or humidifiers (for a cool mist)
- Application of hot, wet towel over the face
- Sipping hot beverages
- Hydration

ACUTE GENERAL Rx
- Sinus drainage:
  1. Nasal vasoconstrictors, such as phenylephrine nose drops, 0.25% or 0.5%
  2. Topical decongestants should not be used for more than a few days because of the risk of rebound congestion
  3. Systemic decongestants
  4. Nasal or systemic corticosteroids, such as nasal beclomethasone, short-course oral prednisone

5. Nasal irrigation, with hypertonic or normal saline (saline may act as a mild vasoconstrictor of nasal blood flow)
6. Use of antihistamines has no proven benefit, and the drying effect on the mucous membranes may cause crusting, which blocks the ostia, thus interfering with sinus drainage
- Analgesics, antipyretics
Antimicrobial therapy:
- Most cases of acute sinusitis have a viral cause and will resolve within 2 wk without antibiotics.
- Current treatment recommendations favor symptomatic treatment for those with mild symptoms. Physicians grossly overprescribe antibiotics for presumed bacterial sinusitis despite a much higher prevalence of viral infections.
- Antibiotics should not be prescribed for mild to moderate sinusitis within the first week of illness. They should be reserved for those with severe symptoms who meet the criteria for diagnosis of sinusitis.
- Antibiotic therapy is usually empiric, targeting the common pathogens:
  1. First-line antibiotics in children include amoxicillin or amoxicillin/clavulanate. For adults amoxicillin/clavulanate or doxycycline is first-line agent, with quinolones (levofloxacin or moxifloxacin) reserved as second-line agents unless patient is penicillin allergic.
  2. Second-line antibiotics include the newer macrolides: clarithromycin, azithromycin, and oral cephalosporins: cefuroxime axetil, cefprozil, cefaclor, loracarbef, but high rate of resistance of *S. pneumoniae* is a concern with these agents as is *H. influenzae* resistance with TMP-SMX such that it is no longer used as a first-line agent.
  3. For patients with uncomplicated acute sinusitis, the less expensive first-line agents appear to be as effective as the costlier second-line agents.
- Hospitalization and IV antibiotics may be required for more severe infection and those with suspected intracranial complications. Broader-spectrum antibiotic coverage may be indicated in severe cases, to cover for MRSA, *Pseudomonas,* and fungal pathogens.
- Duration of therapy generally 5 to 7 days rather than 10 to 14 days as recommended in the past.
Surgery:
- Surgical drainage indicated
  1. If intracranial or orbital complications suspected
  2. Many cases of frontal and sphenoid sinusitis
  3. Chronic sinusitis recalcitrant to medical therapy
- Surgical debridement imperative in the treatment of fungal sinusitis
Complications:
- Untreated, sinusitis may lead to a number of serious, life-threatening complications.

- Intracranial complications include meningitis, brain abscess, and epidural and subdural empyema.
- Intracranial sequelae are more common with frontal and ethmoid infections.
- Extracranial complications include orbital cellulitis, blindness, orbital abscess, osteomyelitis.
- Extracranial sequelae are more commonly seen with ethmoid sinusitis.

CHRONIC Rx
- Broad-spectrum antibiotics that cover both aerobes and anaerobes
- Duration of therapy not clearly established: range 3 to 6 wk
- Adjunctive therapy: one or more of the various options listed previously
- Surgical intervention may be necessary in nonresponders

DISPOSITION
Appropriate diagnosis and treatment are necessary to avoid the various sequelae that can occur without proper therapy.

REFERRAL
- To infectious disease specialist if failure to respond to initial therapy
- To otorhinolaryngologist for:
  1. Failure to respond to therapy
  2. Suspected fungal infection
  3. Suspected intracranial or orbital complications

① PEARLS & CONSIDERATIONS

- Recurrent sinusitis is usually related to anatomic defects, poor drainage, or immunocompromised states; such patients deserve a thorough workup by an ENT specialist and/or an infectious disease specialist.
- Nosocomial sinusitis from obstruction by nasotracheal or nasogastric tubes is not uncommon and can be difficult to recognize in patients in the critical care units.

SUGGESTED READINGS
available at www.expertconsult.com

RELATED CONTENT
Sinusitis (Patient Information)

AUTHOR: **GLENN G. FORT, M.D., M.P.H.**

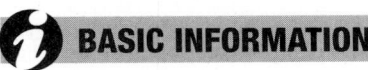

DEFINITION

Sjögren's syndrome (SS) is an autoimmune disorder that targets exocrine glands. It is characterized by lymphocytic and plasma cell infiltration and destruction of salivary and lacrimal glands with subsequent diminished lacrimal and salivary gland secretions. It can occur in both primary and secondary forms.

- Primary: dry mouth (xerostomia) and dry eyes (xerophthalmia) develop as isolated entities.
- Secondary: associated with other autoimmune connective tissue diseases.

SYNONYMS

Sicca syndrome
Sicca complex

ICD-9CM CODES
710.2 Sjögren's syndrome

EPIDEMIOLOGY & DEMOGRAPHICS

INCIDENCE: 3.9 per 100,000
PREVALENCE: Prevalence is 0.3% to 0.6% of population; secondary SS is also common and can affect up to 15% of patients with systemic lupus erythematosus (SLE) and nearly 25% of rheumatoid arthritis (RA) and scleroderma patients.
PREDOMINANT SEX: Female predominance with a female/male ratio of approximately 9:1
PREDOMINANT AGE: Peak incidence is in the fourth and fifth decade, but SS can occur in all ages.
RISK FACTOR: Seen in all races/ethnicities, but more common in Caucasians.

PHYSICAL FINDINGS & CLINICAL PRESENTATION

- Diagnosis of SS is based on the presence of at least two of three objective diagnostic tests below:
  1. Positive serum levels of anti-SS-A/Ro and/or anti-SS-B/La or a positive rheumatoid factor and antinuclear antibody (ANA) titer of at least 1:320

2. Salivary gland biopsy exhibiting focal sites of inflammation. One or more sites of inflammation per 4 mm^2 is considered to be positive.
3. Keratoconjunctivitis sicca with ocular staining score of three or more (the dissipation rate of a specialized dye that is applied to the tear film that bathes the surface of the eye; a score of three or more is considered to be positive).
- Dry mouth with dry lips (cheilosis), erythema of tongue (Fig. 1-765) and other mucosal surfaces, carious teeth
- Dry eyes (conjunctival injection, corneal ulceration, blurred vision, decreased luster, enlargement of lacrimal glands, and irregularity of the corneal light reflex)
- Possible salivary gland enlargement and dysfunction, with subsequent difficulty in chewing and swallowing food and in speaking without frequent water intake, thickened saliva, and burning sensation in mouth
- Leukocytoclastic vasculitis may be present.
- Skin ulceration, photosensitivity, and allergic drug eruptions
- Extraglandular involvement occurs in 50% of patients. There are multiple systemic manifestations associated with SS, which include the following:
  - Dyspareunia can occur secondary to vaginal dryness
  - Pulmonary involvement includes chronic obstructive pulmonary disease, lymphocytic interstitial pneumonitis, fibrosis, and xerotrachea
  - Gastrointestinal conditions such as esophageal dysmotility, hepatitis, and pancreatitis can occur
  - Renal manifestations include renal tubular acidosis, Fanconi syndrome, and interstitial nephritis
  - Neurologic involvement including peripheral neuropathy and trigeminal neuropathy
  - Musculoskeletal symptoms including arthralgias and polymyopathy
  - Hematologic conditions such as lymphoma and leukopenia. Nearly 5% of patients develop B-cell lymphoma.

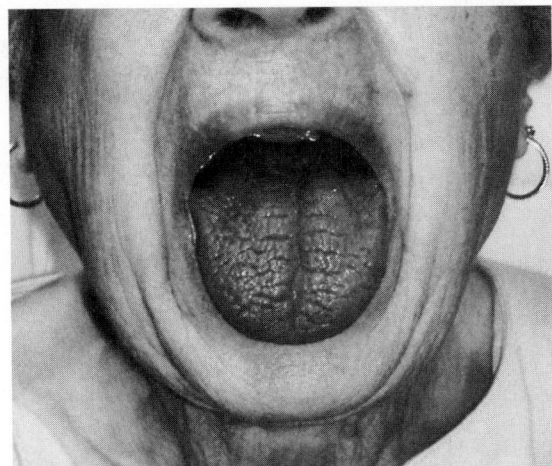

FIGURE 1-765 "Crocodile tongue" in a patient with Sjögren's syndrome. (From Noble J: *Primary care medicine*, ed 3, St Louis, 2001, Mosby.)

- RA and other connective tissue diseases are present in secondary SS.
- Hypothyroidism may be observed in patients with SS.

ETIOLOGY

Autoimmune disorder of unclear etiology. It is associated with certain HLA-DQ alleles. It has been postulated that viral agents (e.g., hepatitis C) may trigger the clinical presentation.

DX DIAGNOSIS

DIFFERENTIAL DIAGNOSIS

- Medication-related dryness (e.g., anticholinergics)
- Age-related exocrine gland dysfunction
- Mouth breathing
- Anxiety
- HIV infection
- Hepatitis C infection
- Diabetes mellitus
- Chronic sialadenitis
- Acromegaly
- Hyperlipidemia
- Graft-versus-host disease
- Other: sarcoidosis, primary salivary hypofunction, radiation injury, amyloidosis
- IgG4-related disease
- Ocular herpetic lesions
- An algorithm for the diagnosis of SS is provided in Fig. 1-766.

WORKUP

Workup involves ocular and oral examination and laboratory and radiographic testing to demonstrate the following criteria for diagnosis of primary and secondary SS.
PRIMARY:
- Symptoms and objective signs of ocular dryness:
  1. Schirmer's test (Fig. E1-767): <8 mm wetting per 5 min
  2. Positive rose bengal or fluorescein staining of cornea and conjunctiva to demonstrate keratoconjunctivitis sicca
  3. Tear breakup time and tear osmolality measured after instillation of fluorescein
- Symptoms and objective signs of dry mouth:
  1. Decreased parotid flow using Lashley cups or other methods
  2. Abnormal biopsy result of minor salivary gland (focus score >2 based on average of four assessable lobules)
  3. Assessment of rate of saliva production in which collection of ≤1.5 ml after two expectorations 15 min apart is considered positive
- Evidence of systemic autoimmune disorder:
  1. Elevated rheumatoid factor (70%-90% of patients)
  2. Elevated titer of ANA >1:320 (80% of patients)
  3. Presence of anti-SS-A (Ro) (>60% of patients) or anti-SS-B (La) antibodies (40% of patients)
SECONDARY:
- Characteristic signs and symptoms of SS
- Clinical features sufficient to allow a diagnosis of RA, SLE, polymyositis, or scleroderma

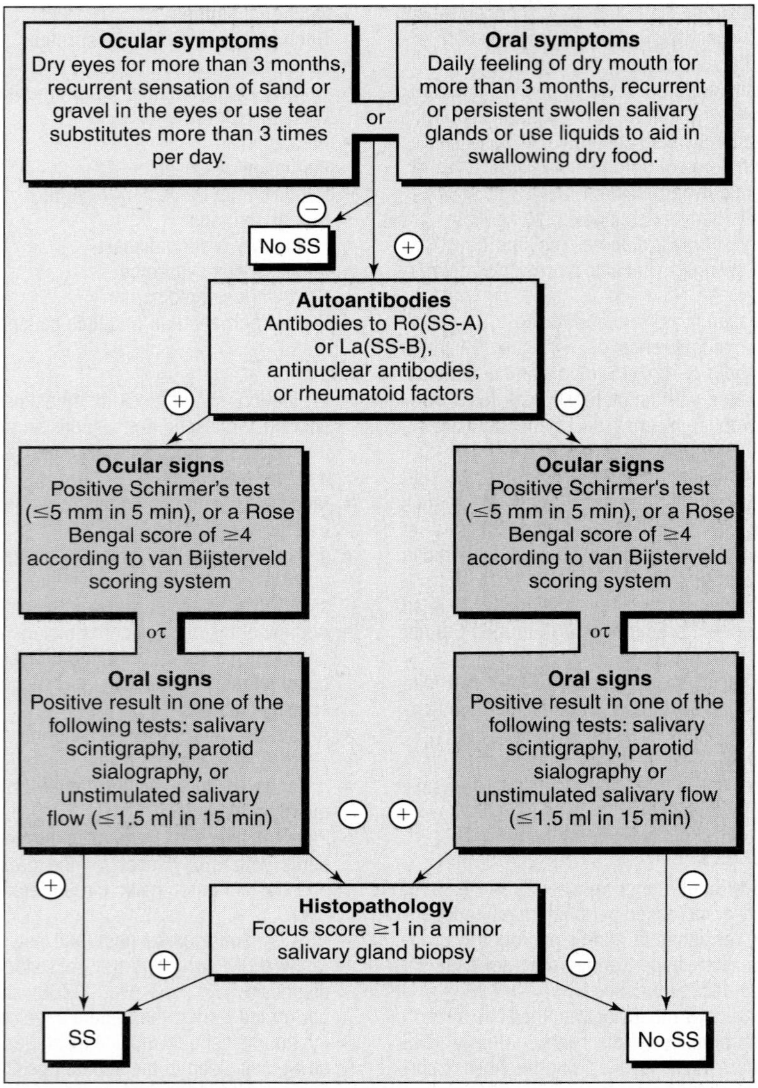

Ocular symptoms
Dry eyes for more than 3 months, recurrent sensation of sand or gravel in the eyes or use tear substitutes more than 3 times per day.

or

Oral symptoms
Daily feeling of dry mouth for more than 3 months, recurrent or persistent swollen salivary glands or use liquids to aid in swallowing dry food.

(−) → No SS

(+)

Autoantibodies
Antibodies to Ro(SS-A) or La(SS-B), antinuclear antibodies, or rheumatoid factors

(+) | (−)

Ocular signs
Positive Schirmer's test (≤5 mm in 5 min), or a Rose Bengal score of ≥4 according to van Bijsterveld scoring system

Ocular signs
Positive Schirmer's test (≤5 mm in 5 min), or a Rose Bengal score of ≥4 according to van Bijsterveld scoring system

oτ | oτ

Oral signs
Positive result in one of the following tests: salivary scintigraphy, parotid sialography, or unstimulated salivary flow (≤1.5 ml in 15 min)

Oral signs
Positive result in one of the following tests: salivary scintigraphy, parotid sialography or unstimulated salivary flow (≤1.5 ml in 15 min)

(−) (+)

(+) | (−)

Histopathology
Focus score ≥1 in a minor salivary gland biopsy

(+) | (−)

SS | No SS

FIGURE 1-766 Suggested algorithm for the diagnosis of Sjögren's syndrome. Exclusion criteria include hepatitis C or human immunodeficiency virus infection, sarcoidosis, graft-versus-host disease, preexisting lymphoma, previous head or neck irradiation, and use of anticholinergic drugs. (From Hochberg MC et al: *Rheumatology*, ed 5, St Louis, 2011, Mosby.)

- Periodic dental and ophthalmologic evaluations to screen for complications

GENERAL Rx
- Use artificial tears frequently.
- The muscarinic agonist pilocarpine (5 mg PO qid) is useful to improve dryness. A cyclosporine 0.05% ophthalmic emulsion (Restasis) may also be useful for dry eyes.
- Cevimeline (Evoxac), a cholinergic agent with muscarinic agonist activity, 30 mg PO tid is effective for the treatment of dry mouth in patients with SS.
- Methotrexate and oral cyclosporine only improve the symptoms of subjective dryness.
- Hydroxychloroquine may be useful for arthralgias. Antitumor necrosis factor agents have not shown significant clinical efficacy and larger controlled trials are needed to establish the efficacy of rituximab for severe inflammatory manifestations.
- Propionic acid gel can be used for vaginal dryness.
- Systemic manifestations are treated according to symptoms and complications.
- Cyclophosphamide, azathioprine, chlorambucil are generally reserved for life-threatening extraglandular manifestations.

REFERRAL
- Rheumatology referral is generally indicated.
- Referral should be made to an oncologist when lymphoma is suspected.

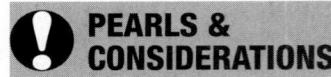

! PEARLS & CONSIDERATIONS

COMMENTS
- Unusual presentations of SS may occur in association with polymyalgia rheumatica, chronic fatigue syndrome, fever of unknown origin, and inflammatory myositis.
- The most serious complication of primary SS is the development of non-Hodgkin's lymphoma and other lymphoproliferative disorders, which occur at a 44-fold increased rate as compared to age-matched controls.

SUGGESTED READINGS
available at www.expertconsult.com

RELATED CONTENT
Sjögren's Syndrome (Patient Information)

AUTHORS: **SYEDA M. SAYEED, M.D.**, and **HARALD A. HALL, M.D.**

LABORATORY TESTS
- Positive ANA (>80% of patients) with autoantibodies anti-SS-A and anti-SS-B may be present.
- Additional laboratory abnormalities may include elevated erythrocyte sedimentation rate, anemia (normochromic, normocytic), abnormal liver function studies, elevated serum $beta_2$ microglobulin levels, rheumatoid factor, hypergammaglobulinemia, and cryoglobulins (30% of patients).
- A definite diagnosis of SS can be made with a salivary gland biopsy.

Rx TREATMENT

NONPHARMACOLOGIC THERAPY
- Adequate fluid replacement. Ameliorate skin dryness by gently blotting dry after bathing, leaving a small amount of moisture, and then applying a moisturizer.
- Increased environmental moisture by using humidifiers
- Proper oral hygiene (daily topical fluoride use and antimicrobial mouth rinses) to reduce the incidence of caries. Sugar-free chewing gum and sour lemon lozenges to stimulate salivary secretion.

BASIC INFORMATION

DEFINITION

The *International Classification of Sleep Disorders, Second Edition*, classifies sleep-disordered breathing disorders into three categories: central sleep apnea syndrome, obstructive sleep apnea (OSA), and sleep-related hypoventilation/hypoxic syndromes. The American Academy of Sleep Disorders defines OSA as repetitive episodes of upper airway obstruction that occur during sleep and that are typically associated with oxyhemoglobin desaturations.

SYNONYMS

Sleep apnea syndrome
Sleep-disordered breathing
Obstructive sleep apnea syndrome
Obstructive sleep apnea–hypopnea syndrome
OSA

ICD-9CM CODES
327.2   Organic sleep apnea
327.21 Organic sleep apnea, unspecified
327.23 Obstructive sleep apnea (adult)
       (pediatric)

EPIDEMIOLOGY & DEMOGRAPHICS

OSA is a common disease in the U.S. Data from the Wisconsin Cohort Study indicated that the prevalence of OSA in people between the ages of 30 and 60 yr is 9% to 24% for men and 4% to 9% for women. The estimated prevalence of OSA is 4% for men and 2% for women. The prevalence of OSA increases from 18 to 45 years of age, with a plateau occurring at 55 to 65 years of age. The prevalence is higher in obese and hypertensive patients. ~2% of children have OSA, which develops more commonly between the ages of 2 and 8 yr when adenotonsillar size is largest relative to size of the airway. Definite risk factors include obesity and craniofacial and upper airway soft tissue abnormalities, while potential risk factors include heredity, current tobacco smoking, nasal congestion, and diabetes.

PHYSICAL FINDINGS & CLINICAL PRESENTATION

- Nocturnal symptoms, including nocturia and angina pectoris
- Snoring that can be loud, habitual, and bothersome to others
- Witnessed apneas that often interrupt snoring and end with a snort
- Gasping, choking, or smothering sensations that arouse the patient from sleep
- Restless sleep associated with frequent arousals
- Daytime symptoms:
  - Nonrestorative sleep
  - Not feeling refreshed upon awakening
  - Morning headache
  - Dry mouth or throat upon awakening
  - Excessive daytime sleepiness, typically during quiet activities
  - Daytime fatigue or tiredness
  - Problems with memory, concentration, and cognitive function, especially with executive functioning
  - Easily angered, short tempered, and inattentive
  - Hyperactivity in children
  - Symptoms of fibromyalgia
- Systemic hypertension (HTN)
- Obesity (body mass index >30 kg/m^2)
- History of type 2 diabetes mellitus
- Mood swings, irritability, anxiety, and depression
- Decreased libido and impotence
- Neck circumference of >43 cm (17 in) in men and >37 cm (15 in) in women has been associated with an increased risk for OSA.
- The oropharynx may be erythematous as a result of snoring.
- Adenotonsillar hypertrophy, excessive soft tissue, high-arched hard palate, pendulous uvula, prominent tongue, large degree of overjet, and retrognathia or micrognathia can be present.
- A narrowing of the lateral airway walls is an independent predictor of OSA in men but not in women.
- Craniofacial skeletal abnormalities can lead to OSA, particularly among children and non-obese adults.
- A positive family history increases an individual's risk with each additional close family member with OSA.

ETIOLOGY

- Narrowing of upper airway as a result of obesity or increased peripharyngeal fat deposition, retrognathia and/or micrognathia, adenotonsillar hypertrophy, macroglossia, or neuromuscular weakness
- Upper airway muscular weakness as a result of neuromuscular disorders, primary CNS disorders (e.g., stroke), or metabolic disorders
- Other diseases associated with the development of OSA (e.g., hypothyroidism, acromegaly)

DIAGNOSIS

DIFFERENTIAL DIAGNOSIS

- Anemia
- Anxiety or panic disorder
- Behaviorally induced insufficient sleep syndrome
- Cardiac or heart disease
- Central sleep apnea
- Circadian rhythm disorder
- Depression
- Drug or alcohol abuse
- Gastroesophageal reflux
- Hypothyroidism
- Idiopathic hypersomnia with long or short sleep time
- Inadequate sleep hygiene
- Insomnia
- Medication effect
- Narcolepsy
- Nocturnal asthma
- Nocturnal gastroesophageal reflux
- Nocturnal seizures
- Obesity-hypoventilation syndrome (i.e., Pickwickian syndrome)
- Parasomnias
- Parkinson's disease
- Periodic limb movement disorder
- Primary snoring
- Pulmonary or lung disease
- Restless legs syndrome
- Shift work sleep disorder
- Sleep fragmentation (multiple causes)

WORKUP

- Evaluation should include questions about snoring, witnessed apneas, gasping or choking episodes, restless sleep, and excessive daytime sleepiness.
- Mood swings and personality changes should be addressed.
- Job performance and difficulty driving or previous motor vehicle accidents related to excessive daytime sleepiness should be discussed.
- Additional historic concerns include morning dry mouth or throat, morning headaches, alcohol intake, weight gain, and mood or personality changes.
- A thorough drug history should include muscle relaxants and sedatives.
- A family history should target any family members with OSA.
- Physical exam is frequently normal in patients with OSA except for the presence of obesity, enlarged neck circumference, and HTN.
- OSA is confirmed by nocturnal polysomnography (PSG), which is the gold standard for diagnosis. The PSG (Fig. 1-768) should be performed during the patient's typical sleeping hours; it should include all stages of sleep as well as sleep in the supine position.
- The severity of the OSA is determined by the apnea-hypopnea index (AHI), which is derived from the total number of apneas and hypopneas divided by the total sleep time.
- Recommended severity cutoff levels for the AHI in adult patients are as follows:
  - Mild: 5-15 episodes/hr (with symptoms)
  - Moderate: 15 to 30 episodes per hr
  - Severe: >30 episodes per hr
- Criteria for the treatment of mild OSA often require symptoms, including excessive daytime sleepiness, cardiovascular disease, HTN, and mood swings.
- In-home respiratory monitoring is an effective alternative to PSG for the evaluation of OSA.

LABORATORY TESTS

- Arterial blood gas testing should be performed if a patient has suspected pulmonary HTN or cor pulmonale to rule out daytime hypoxemia or hypercapnia.
- Thyroid-stimulating hormone level should be obtained if hypothyroidism is suspected.
- Fasting glucose level is recommended because OSA increases the risk of developing diabetes independent of other risk factors.

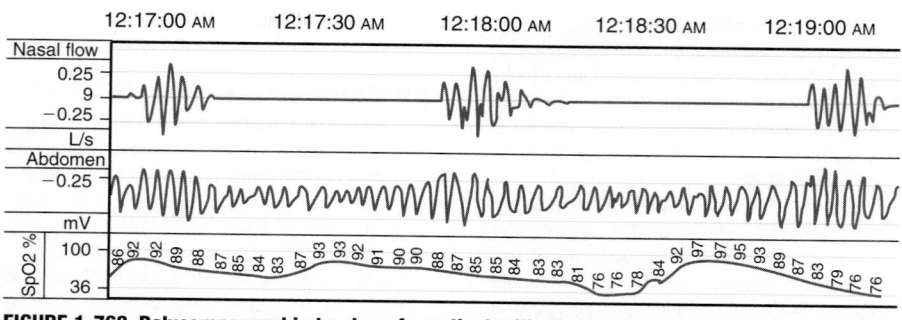

FIGURE 1-768 **Polysomnographic tracing of a patient with obstructive sleep apnea during 2 minutes of non–rapid eye movement sleep.** Displayed are airflow in the upper airway ("nasal flow"), recorded with a nasal pressure transducer, respiratory effort ("abdomen"), recorded by inductance plethysmography; and oxygen saturation of hemoglobin (SpO₂) recorded with pulse oximetry. (From Goldman L, Schafer AI: *Goldman's Cecil medicine,* ed 24, Philadelphia, 2012, Saunders.)

- CBC is helpful to look for anemia, and iron studies are indicated if anemia is detected.
- Pulmonary function testing is indicated if a pulmonary disorder is suspected or to assess the severity of neuromuscular disease, if present.
- ECG or echocardiogram is indicated if a cardiac disorder (e.g., arrhythmia, pulmonary HTN) is suspected.

IMAGING STUDIES
- Plain radiography of the neck can be helpful to assess the soft tissues of patients with suspected anatomic abnormalities.
- Chest x-ray is indicated if pulmonary disease is suspected.

Rx TREATMENT

NONPHARMACOLOGIC THERAPY
- Behavioral modifications:
  - Weight loss in overweight and obese patients. Weight loss is effective for reducing the severity of OSA, and if significant, it may potentially allow some patients to discontinue continuous positive airway pressure (CPAP) therapy.
  - Weight loss with bariatric surgery may improve OSA in some patients, but its definitive role remains unclear. In a recent trial in obese patients with OSA, the use of bariatric surgery compared with conventional weight loss therapy did not result in a statistically greater reduction in AHI despite major differences in weight loss.
  - Exercise without weight loss may improve OSA.
  - Avoid alcohol for 4-6 hr before bedtime.
  - Avoid muscle relaxants and sedating medications.
  - Sleep hygiene training
  - Avoid or eliminate supine sleeping positions.
  - Avoid medications that may worsen OSA.
- Medical treatment:
  - CPAP is the primary therapy for OSA. This method of treatment delivers a constant airway pressure that acts as a pneumatic splint that relieves the upper airway obstruction.
  - Other methods of delivering positive pressure include:
    - Bilevel positive airway pressure (BiPAP), which delivers a preset inspiratory and expiratory airway pressure.
    - Autotitrating positive airway pressure (APAP), which increases or decreases the level of pressure in response to change in airflow, a vibratory snore, or change in circuit pressure.
    - Adaptive servoventilation provides a varying amount of inspiratory pressure superimposed on a low level of CPAP.
  - Oral appliance constructed by a reputable and qualified dentist may be effective for the treatment of mild OSA in certain patients, especially those with retrognathia.
  - Optimal treatment of allergic rhinitis is needed; nasal irrigation with saline followed by nasal corticosteroids is often helpful.
  - Symptoms of excessive daytime sleepiness may linger and require further investigation or medical therapy.
  - Patients should be considered for surgery if multiple attempts at CPAP therapy have failed and if an oral appliance is not an option. If the patient opts for surgery, ensure that the surgery is performed by a reputable and qualified otolaryngologist and that the surgery is based on the location of airway collapse.
- Surgical treatment:
  - Adenotonsillectomy is often curative for children with OSA.
  - Nasal septoplasty should be considered for patients with nasoseptal deformities.
  - Uvulopalatopharyngoplasty, which involves the resection of the uvula and the soft palate, is effective for a small number of patients. However, predicting which patients will benefit from the procedure is difficult.
  - Tracheostomy is typically reserved for patients with very severe OSA who failed medical therapy or who have cor pulmonale.

DISPOSITION
- The short-term prognosis for excessive daytime sleepiness and snoring is good to excellent with the regular use of nasal CPAP, but no studies have been performed to address the long-term effects in a large population of patients.

- Residual symptoms of excessive daytime sleepiness can occur in some patients with OSA despite regular CPAP use. This has led the FDA to approve modafinil for the management of residual sleepiness.

REFERRAL
- Highly trained sleep specialists with expertise in caring for patients with OSA are recommended, especially for complex cases.
- Surgical referral to otolaryngology should be considered for children and for adults who are unresponsive to weight loss and CPAP therapy.
- Referral to a qualified dentist for treatment with an oral appliance may be useful for certain patients with mild OSA.

ⓘ PEARLS & CONSIDERATIONS
- OSA is a common disorder that is underrecognized and underdiagnosed, so the identification of risk factors is crucial for making the correct diagnosis.
- The prevalence of OSA increases among women after menopause. OSA affects about 2% to 3% of middle-aged women in the general population and is associated with increased cardiovascular death.
- The degree of tonsillar hypertrophy does not correlate with the presence of OSA in children.
- A 10% weight loss can decrease the AHI of a patient with OSA by as much as 50%.
- The single most effective therapy for OSA is nasal CPAP.
- Patients with OSA are more vulnerable than healthy persons to the effects of alcohol consumption and sleep restriction with regard to various driving performance variables.
- OSA is a risk factor for HTN. In patients with untreated HTN and OSA, the use of CPAP results in small but statistically significant reductions in blood pressure.
- OSA may also be an independent risk factor for peptic ulcer bleeding.

EBM EVIDENCE

available at www.expertconsult.com

SUGGESTED READINGS
available at www.expertconsult.com

RELATED CONTENT
Fig. 3-167, *A,* Patient with sleep disturbance (Algorithm)
Fig. 3-167, *B,* Hypersomnia (Algorithm)
Fig. 3-167, *C,* Sleep-associated affective and behavioral disturbance (Algorithm)
Sleep Apnea (Patient Information)

AUTHOR: **DON HAYES, JR., M.D.**

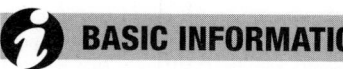

DEFINITION

Slipped capital femoral epiphysis (SCFE) is defined as displacement of the capital femoral epiphysis (femoral head) posteriorly on the metaphysis (femoral neck) at the level of the physis (growth plate)

- Commonly unilateral but can present with bilateral hip involvement
- Classified as stable or unstable
- Stable SCFE: slipped capital femoral epiphysis in a child who is able to walk with minimal or no symptoms
- Unstable SCFE: slipped capital femoral epiphysis resulting in a child who cannot walk or who cannot walk without crutches and is associated with severe pain of acute onset

SYNONYMS

Slipped capital femoral epiphysis, nontraumatic
Slipped upper femoral epiphysis
Slipped upper femoral epiphysis, nontraumatic

ICD-10CM CODES
732.2 Nontraumatic slipped upper femoral
epiphysis

EPIDEMIOLOGY & DEMOGRAPHICS

INCIDENCE: Reported incidence in male children is 13.35 cases per 100,000 children, and reported incidence in female children is 8.07 cases per 100,000 children.
PEAK INCIDENCE: Average age at diagnosis is 13.5 yr for boys and 12.0 yr for girls.
PREVALENCE: 10.8 cases per 100,000 children
PREDOMINANT SEX: More common in boys than girls
GENETICS: More commonly seen in blacks and Hispanic populations; no strong evidence of genetic predisposition
RISK FACTORS: Obesity by far the greatest risk factor

PHYSICAL FINDINGS & CLINICAL PRESENTATION

- The slip occurs at the weakest part of the physeal plate and results in the head being displaced from the metaphysis.
- Typical presentation of pain in the knee, hip, groin, thigh, or all; external rotation of the extremity and limp are commonly seen. Few patients present with painless limp; <10% report inciting trauma; even fewer complain of severe hip pain and inability to bear weight.
- Important physical exam findings include limited range of motion of the affected hip on internal rotation; involved hip typically will go into obligatory external rotation if passively flexed up to 90 degrees.
- Patients with unstable SCFE are unable to bear weight, their leg is in external rotation, and any hip motion is painful.

ETIOLOGY

- Multifactorial
- The slip itself usually occurs during the preadolescent growth spurt.

- 25%-40% are bilateral slips.
- Obesity: of children diagnosed with SCFE, 63% are at the 90th percentile for weight or higher.
- Growth surges: varying levels of hormonal activity associated with the adolescent growth spurt may also contribute to the causes of SCFE.
- Endocrine disorders: related endocrine disorders include hypothyroidism, growth hormone supplementation, hypogonadism, and panhypopituitarism; consider an endocrinopathy in SCFE with unusual presentations, including patients who are younger than 8 yr, older than 15 yr, or underweight.

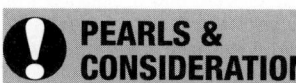

DIAGNOSIS

DIFFERENTIAL DIAGNOSIS

- Apophyseal avulsion fracture
- Avascular necrosis
- Hip apophysitis
- Transient synovitis
- Stress fracture
- Septic arthritis
- Osteomyelitis
- Legg-Calvé-Perthes disease
- Adductor muscle strain (groin pull)

WORKUP

- Diagnosis is based on physical exam and radiologic findings.
- Laboratory testing can be done to look for secondary causes.

LABORATORY TESTS

Check renal, endocrine, growth hormone, thyroid function tests in patients <10 yr of age and body weight <50th percentile or less.

IMAGING STUDIES

- Plain radiographs are sensitive and specific to make the diagnosis of SCFE.
- B/L hip x-rays: both AP and frog-leg lateral views should be done; 60% of patients have bilateral hip involvement at presentation.
- The frog-leg lateral view is more sensitive.
- Physical blurring of the epiphysis or widening can be seen.
- Bone scans may be helpful in predicting prognosis; "cold spots" on technetium bone scan in acute SCFE may represent ischemia and/or avascular necrosis.

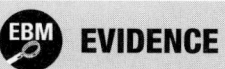

TREATMENT

- Once diagnosis is confirmed, the patient should be placed on non–weight-bearing crutches or in a wheelchair and quickly referred to an orthopedic surgeon for surgical management.
- The initial goals of treatment are to prevent slip progression and avoid complications.
- A recent open-label observational trial suggested a potential role for intravenous bisphosphonates as adjunctive therapy for acute SCFE that has been operatively fixed but had "cold spots" on bone scan indicating ischemia or necrosis; rationale for bisphos-

phonate use was to decrease necrotic bone resorption and allow for revascularization.

NONPHARMACOLOGIC THERAPY

- The standard treatment of SCFE is surgery.
- The standard surgical procedure of stable SCFE is in situ fixation with a single screw.
- For unstable SCFE, treatment goals are similar to those of stable SCFE with in situ fixation, but there is controversy as to the specifics of treatment, including timing of surgery, value of reduction, and whether traction should be used.
- Prophylactic treatment of the contralateral hip in SCFE is controversial and not recommended in most patients.
- Prophylactic pinning may be indicated in high-risk patients such as those with obesity or an endocrine disorder.

DISPOSITION

- SCFE is a common preadolescent disorder with little short-term morbidity and rare long-term sequelae if diagnosed and treated before the development of a severe deformity.
- The two most feared complications of SCFE are osteonecrosis/avascular necrosis and chondrolysis.
- Osteonecrosis/avascular necrosis: occurs in up to 60% of unstable SCFE; factors associated include overreduction of unstable SCFE, reduction of stable SCFE, pin penetration of posterior quadrant, and multiplicity of pin; often leads to advanced and early degenerative osteoarthritis.
- Chondrolysis: acute dissolution of articular cartilage in association with rapid progressive joint stiffness and pain; usually as a complication of surgery but can occur in untreated SCFE as well; incidence has decreased to 1%-2% with improvement in surgical techniques.

PEARLS & CONSIDERATIONS

- Physicians should consider SCFE when a child between the ages of 10-15 yr presents with limping and groin, hip, thigh, or knee pain.
- Physical exam usually shows decreased internal rotation of the hip and obligatory external rotation.
- Radiography to rule out SCFE should include anteroposterior lateral views of the hips (frog-lateral views for stable SCFE; cross-table views for unstable SCFE).
- The standard treatment of stable SCFE is in situ fixation with a single screw.

EBM EVIDENCE

available at www.expertconsult.com

SUGGESTED READINGS
available at www.expertconsult.com

AUTHOR: **WAFFIYAH AFRIDI, M.D.**

BASIC INFORMATION

DEFINITION

Social anxiety disorder (SAD) is a persistent and intense fear of being embarrassed, humiliated, or negatively evaluated in social situations. SAD commonly presents as excessive anxiety or fear in situations involving social interactions (e.g., conversing with one or a group of other individuals, with sexually attractive others, with authority figures), performance situations (e.g., public speaking, acting/performing in front of an audience), or situations in which one is being observed (e.g., while eating). The anxiety must persist in these situations for at least 6 mo in individuals younger than age 18. The anxiety often results in avoidance of these situations, thus leading to significant occupational, academic, and/or social impairment as well as marked distress. Currently two subtypes are described: specific (fear of one or only a few situations) and generalized (fear of many social situations). However, revisions to these specifiers are being considered for the DSM-5.

SYNONYMS

Social phobia
SAD

ICD-9CM CODES
F40.1 (DSM-IV Code 300.23)

EPIDEMIOLOGY & DEMOGRAPHICS

INCIDENCE (IN U.S.): Ranges from 4 to 5 to 9/1000 person-yrs; cumulative incidence of 11.0% in first three decades of life
PEAK INCIDENCE: Highest standardized incidence rates per person-yr between 10 and 19 yr of age
PREVALENCE (IN U.S.): Lifetime prevalence of 12% in epidemiologic samples; point prevalence of up to 30% in outpatient clinical settings
PREDOMINANT SEX: More common in women than in men (ratio of 3:2) in epidemiologic samples; the two genders are equally represented in clinical settings
PREDOMINANT AGE: Mean age of onset ~16 yr of age; onset rarely occurs after age 25
GENETICS:
- Heritability ranges from 20% to 50%.
- 15% to 26% risk of SAD among first-degree relatives of those with SAD.

PHYSICAL FINDINGS & CLINICAL PRESENTATION

- Physical symptoms during social interactions such as heart palpitations, sweating, shaking, and/or blushing, which may take the form of a panic attack.
- Fear that others will observe these physical symptoms in social situations and negatively judge them; fears that they will "say something stupid," make a mistake, or offend others also are common.
- Report being "shy" most of their lives.
- Comorbid psychiatric disorders (e.g., major depression, other anxiety disorders) and substance abuse (e.g., alcohol/cannabis) are common.
- Few seek treatment specifically for SAD, and instead initially seek treatment for other psychiatric disorders (e.g., major depression, other anxiety disorders).
- The onset of SAD often precedes that of the other comorbid psychiatric conditions.

ETIOLOGY

- There is no clear etiology and likely is a combination of multiple factors.
- Research has examined developmental psychology factors (e.g., lack of modeling of socialization by parents), temperamental factors (e.g., behavioral inhibition), and occurrence of prior traumatic social experiences (e.g., significant teasing by peers, being embarrassed or humiliated in a social or performance situation).
- The risk of SAD also may be increased with family history.

DIAGNOSIS

DIFFERENTIAL DIAGNOSIS

- Other anxiety disorders (e.g., panic disorder with agoraphobia).
- As a consequence of mood disorders (e.g., avoidance of social situations associated with major depression).
- Pervasive developmental disorder (e.g., Asperger's disorder).
- Personality disorders (e.g., schizoid personality disorder); however, in the case of avoidant personality disorder, both may be diagnosed.
- Anxiety associated with medical conditions such as stuttering or Parkinson's disease.

WORKUP

- Psychiatric history is required for a diagnosis.
- Screening measures may improve detection of SAD as it is a chronic, disabling condition for which many individuals do not seek treatment.
- Physical examination may be useful in ruling out other explanations for physical symptoms that are present, and to rule out presence of social anxiety due to a medical condition.

TREATMENT

NONPHARMACOLOGIC THERAPY

- Cognitive-behavior therapy (CBT)
- Exposure therapy
- Social skills training

PHARMACOLOGIC THERAPY

- SSRIs/SNRIs
- Benzodiazepines (less favored)
- MAOIs (less favored)
- Beta-blockers (e.g., propanolol, atenolol: for performance-related anxiety)

ACUTE GENERAL Rx

- SAD is a chronic condition; therefore acute treatment is rarely indicated.
- However, benzodiazepines or beta-blockers may be prescribed on an as-needed basis for acute performance anxiety; caution should be taken when prescribing benzodiazepines due to the possibility of dependence or misuse and high incidence of relapse following discontinuation.
- Beta-blockers may also be prescribed on an as-needed basis, particularly for physical symptoms experienced during performance situations. However, evidence does not support its use for more generalized forms of SAD.

CHRONIC Rx

- CBT is effective and an appropriate first-line treatment.
- SSRIs/SNRIs (e.g., paroxetine, sertraline, venlafaxine) are also effective in the treatment of SAD and are a first-line pharmacologic treatment.
- MAOIs previously were considered gold standard treatment for SAD, but currently are less favorable due to side effects and dietary restrictions.
- Combination treatment of SSRI/SNRI and CBT is effective for SAD; however, some research has suggested that CBT alone may result in greater long-term benefit compared to combination treatment.

DISPOSITION

- SAD is a chronic condition, typically unremitting without treatment.
- Treatment may significantly improve SAD, although symptoms and impairment may continue to be present for some individuals following treatment.

REFERRAL

- If comorbid psychiatric conditions are present
- If the symptoms do not improve upon treatment or response to treatment is not optimal

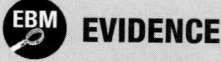 EVIDENCE

available at www.expertconsult.com

SUGGESTED READINGS
available at www.expertconsult.com

RELATED CONTENT
Generalized Anxiety Disorder (Related Key Topic)

AUTHOR: **KRISTY L. DALRYMPLE, PH.D.**

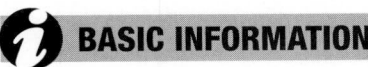

BASIC INFORMATION

DEFINITION

Somatization disorder refers to a pattern of recurring multiple somatic complaints that begin before the age of 30 yr and persist over several years. Patients complain of multiple sites of pain (a minimum of four), gastrointestinal symptoms (a minimum of two), a sexual or reproductive symptom, and a pseudoneurologic symptom. These cannot be explained by a medical condition or are in excess of an expected disability from a coexisting medical condition.

SYNONYMS

Briquet's syndrome
Nonorganic physical symptoms
Medically unexplained symptoms
Functional somatic symptoms

ICD-9CM CODES
300.81 Somatization disorder

EPIDEMIOLOGY & DEMOGRAPHICS

PREVALENCE (IN U.S.): Lifetime rates of 0.25% to 2% in women, ≤0.2% in men
PEAK INCIDENCE: Typically before age 25 yr
PREDOMINANT SEX: Women are more commonly affected in the U.S. (10:1 ratio)
PREDOMINANT AGE: Onset occurs before age 30 yr and usually in adolescence.
GENETICS: In males, there is a high risk of associated substance abuse or antisocial personality disorder.

PHYSICAL FINDINGS & CLINICAL PRESENTATION

- Onset is characteristically in the teens; course is marked by frequent, unexplained, and frequently disabling pain symptoms and physical complaints.
- Patient frequently undergoes multiple procedures and seeks treatment from multiple physicians. Symptom focus rotates periodically with new physicians sought for new complaints.
- Patient often has a comorbid psychiatric disorder, most commonly generalized anxiety, panic disorder, or depression.

ETIOLOGY

- Believed to be the physical expression of psychological distress; there appears to be a biologic predisposition.
- May be more common in individuals without sufficient verbal or intellectual capacity to communicate psychological distress, individuals with alexithymia (inability to describe emotional states), or individuals from cultural backgrounds that consider emotional distress as an undesirable quality.
- Some aspects of somatization behavior possibly learned from somatizing parents.

DIAGNOSIS

DIFFERENTIAL DIAGNOSIS

- Undifferentiated somatoform disorder (ICD-10 F45.1, DMS-IV 300.81): one or more physical complaints that cannot be explained by a medical condition are present for at least 6 mo (NOTE: Somatization disorder is more severe and less common).
- Conversion disorder: an alteration or loss of voluntary motor or sensory function without demonstrable physical cause and related to a psychological stress or a conflict (NOTE: With multiple complaints, the diagnosis of conversion is not made).
- Pain disorder associated with psychological factors: distinguished from somatization disorder by the latter featuring multiple nonpain symptoms.
- Factitious disorder (e.g., Munchausen's syndrome) and malingering: the psychological basis of the complaints in somatization disorder is not conscious as in factitious disorder, in which the goal is to be in the patient role, and malingering, in which symptoms are also produced consciously but for some secondary gain like a monetary award in litigation or opioids.

WORKUP

- Rule out a general medical condition.
- If somatization is suspected on the basis of a history of repeated, multiple, unexplained complaints, restraint in ordering tests is recommended.

LABORATORY TESTS

No specific laboratory tests are required.

IMAGING STUDIES

No specific imaging studies are required.

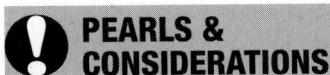

TREATMENT

NONPHARMACOLOGIC THERAPY

- Legitimize patient's complaints.
- Minimize diagnostic investigation and symptomatic treatment. Only do invasive testing or procedures when there are clear-cut signs, not just symptom reports.
- Set attainable treatment goals. Patients may benefit from realizing that even though they cannot be cured, that they will be cared for. This may help reassure them that they will continue to have a relationship with the caregiver.
- Treat coexisting psychiatric conditions such as depression and anxiety.

ACUTE GENERAL Rx

- At each visit do a brief physical examination focusing on the area of complaint.

- Gently praise increased functioning rather than focusing on symptoms.
- Explore recent life events and ask how the patient is handling these.
- Convey empathy with the patient's suffering and psychosocial difficulties.
- No specific pharmacologic therapy has been clearly proven effective, although a number of agents, including gabapentin and St. John's wort, have been useful in some studies.

CHRONIC Rx

- Provide one primary care practitioner to manage care.
- Avoid confronting the patient regarding the psychological origin of symptoms.
- Ensure follow-up visits at regular intervals (e.g., 2- to 4-wk intervals that are not symptom contingent; maintain the regularity even if the symptoms improve so that the patient does not need new symptoms to continue the relationship).
- Avoid invasive or expensive diagnostic procedures unless there are clear signs of new illness, not just symptoms.
- Diagnose and treat mood or anxiety disorders.
- Cognitive behavior therapy groups have been helpful for patients with unexplained somatic symptoms and can dramatically improve functioning.

DISPOSITION

A chronic condition with frequent exacerbations

REFERRAL

If the patient is open to discussing psychological issues, a referral for psychotherapy can be made.

PEARLS & CONSIDERATIONS

Patients with somatization disorder respond best to establishing a regular, working relationship with a primary care provider. Avoiding confrontations about the origins of symptoms, investigating symptoms when related to actual signs of disease, and gently investigating concurrent stressors will help avoid most of the common problems with this population.

Patients with subsyndromal symptoms (i.e., failing to meet the full criteria but having three or more medically unexplained symptoms) may be just as challenging and chronic. They warrant similar approaches as utilized for the full syndrome.

SUGGESTED READINGS
available at www.expertconsult.com

RELATED CONTENT
Somatization Disorder (Patient Information)

AUTHOR: **STUART J. EISENDRATH, M.D.**

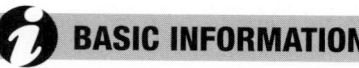

BASIC INFORMATION

DEFINITION

Spasticity is an exaggerated tone that displays a velocity-dependent increase in resistance of muscles to a passive stretch stimulus.

SYNONYMS

Hypertonicity

ICD-9CM CODES

782.85 Spasm of muscle
342.1, 343.0-344.9 Spastic paralysis
781.0 Abnormal involuntary movements/ Spasms NOS
781.2 Abnormality of gait/spastic
342.1 Spastic hemiplegia
344.0-344.9 Spastic paralysis specified as noncongenital or noninfantile
343 Infantile cerebral palsy/spastic infantile paralysis

EPIDEMIOLOGY & DEMOGRAPHICS

INCIDENCE: Spasticity affects between 47% and 70% of people with multiple sclerosis, 32% to 36% of those with spinal cord injury, approximately 20% of those with stroke, more than 90% with cerebral palsy, and approximately 50% of patients with traumatic brain injury.
PREDOMINANT SEX AND AGE: Spasticity is not affected by sex, race, or age group, nor is it more prevalent in any of those groups.
RISK FACTORS: Multiple sclerosis, stroke, spinal cord injury, cerebral palsy, traumatic brain injury

TABLE 1-377 Modified Ashworth Scale

0	No increase in muscle tone
1	Slight increase in muscle tone, manifested by a catch and release or by minimal resistance at the end range of motion when the part is moved in flexion or extension/ abduction or adduction
1+	Slight increase in muscle tone, manifested by a catch, followed by minimal resistance throughout the remainder (less than half) of the range of motion
2	More marked increase in muscle tone through most of the range of motion, but the affected part is easily moved
3	Considerable increase in muscle tone, passive movement is difficult
4	Affected part is rigid in flexion or extension (abduction or adduction)

From Stein J: Spasticity. In Frontera WR et al (eds): *Essentials of physical medicine and rehabilitation,* ed 2, Philadelphia, 2008, Saunders.

PHYSICAL FINDINGS & CLINICAL PRESENTATION

- Patient may present with impaired gait, impaired limb function, decreased mobility, or discomfort due to increased muscle tone.
- While increased muscle tone may preserve strength in the affected muscles, function may be impaired, especially fine motor. Examine active and passive motion, reflexes, and functions:
  ○ Strength may be normal or decreased. Isometric strength is typically greater than concentric strength.
  ○ Tone may be variably increased to passive range of motion (modified Ashworth scale; see Table 1-377).
  ○ Reflexes are typically brisk.
  ○ Patient may have accompanying extensor plantar signs, clonus, or spontaneous flexor spasms.
  ○ Function may be impaired or enhanced due to increased tone.

ETIOLOGY

Upper motor neuron injury, most commonly due to multiple sclerosis, stroke, spinal cord injury, cerebral palsy, traumatic brain injury

 DIAGNOSIS

DIFFERENTIAL DIAGNOSIS

Rigidity, clonus, dystonia, dyskinesia, myotonia, tetanus, muscle contracture, cramps

WORKUP

- A diagnosis is established clinically.
- Investigate reversible exacerbating causes of spasticity: underlying infection, bladder distention, bowel impaction, fracture, pain.

LABORATORY TESTS

Urinalysis, complete blood count, metabolic panel

IMAGING STUDIES

Chest x-ray, abdominal x-ray series, bladder ultrasound

Rx TREATMENT

First treat reversible causes of worsened spasticity (see "Workup"), then proceed to physical and pharmacologic therapeutics. Lastly, consider surgical intervention in severe, refractory cases.

NONPHARMACOLOGIC THERAPY

- Physical therapeutics include range of motion and muscle stretching, serial casting or orthotics, muscle cooling, electrical stimulation.
- Surgical procedures include tenotomy, tendon lengthening, and tendon transfers. More invasive surgical interventions include peripheral neurectomy, myelotomy, and rhizotomy.

ACUTE GENERAL Rx

- Oral medications: baclofen, tizanidine, diazepam, dantrolene (Table E1-378)
- Other interventions: intrathecal baclofen, botulism toxin intramuscular injections, chemical nerve blocks (with bupivacaine, phenol, or ethyl alcohol)

COMPLEMENTARY & ALTERNATIVE MEDICINE

EMG biofeedback

DISPOSITION

Typically nonprogressive, but medications may lose efficacy after long duration of use. Drug holidays (with use of alternate spasmolytic) may be beneficial.

REFERRAL

- Physicians: neurologist or physiatrist with expertise in botulism toxin injection and/or intrathecal spasmolytic therapy is recommended when oral medications are ineffective or not tolerated.
- Physical and occupational therapy

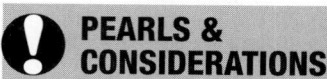 PEARLS & CONSIDERATIONS

- Assess whether the spasms recently increased in severity or intensity (as would occur with reversible exacerbating causes).
- Consider whether patient's tone is beneficial or detrimental to patient's functionality or overall health status.
- Spasticity may assist posture and mobility, as well as maintain muscle mass and bone mineralization, reduce dependent edema, and prevent deep venous thromboses.
- Spasticity may impair patient's functionality, interfere with activities of daily living, interfere with sleep, and cause discomfort.
- Monitor liver function with dantrolene and tizanidine, as these drugs may cause hepatotoxicity.

SUGGESTED READINGS

available at www.expertconsult.com

AUTHOR: **KARA A. KENNEDY FISTER, D.O.**

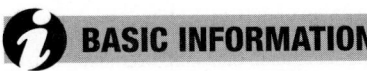

BASIC INFORMATION

DEFINITION Spinal cord compression is the neurologic loss of spine function. Fig. 1-773 illustrates a schematic demarcation of levels of principal dermatomes shown as distinct segments. Lesions may be complete or incomplete and develop gradually or acutely. Incomplete lesions often present as distinct syndromes, as follows:

- Central cord syndrome
- Anterior cord syndrome
- Brown-Séquard syndrome
- Conus medullaris syndrome
- Cauda equina syndrome

ICD-9CM CODES
344.89 Brown-Séquard syndrome
344.60 Cauda equina syndrome
336.8 Conus medullaris syndrome
Other lesions listed by site

EPIDEMIOLOGY Spinal cord injury (SCI) typically occurs in males at the peak of their productive lives.
INCIDENCE: 11,000 new cases/yr
PREVALENCE: 171,000 persons
COST (IN U.S.): >$5 billion/yr

PHYSICAL FINDINGS & CLINICAL PRESENTATION Clinical features reflect the amount of spinal cord involvement:

- Motor loss and sensory abnormalities
- Babinski testing usually positive
- Clonus

- Gradual compression, often manifested by progressive difficulty walking, clonus with weight bearing, and involuntary spasm; development of sensory symptoms; bladder dysfunction (late)
- *Central cord syndrome:* results in a variable quadriparesis with the upper extremities more severely involved than the lower extremities; some sensory sparing
- *Anterior cord syndrome:* results in motor, pain, and temperature loss below the lesion
- *Brown-Séquard syndrome:*
  1. Spinal cord syndrome caused by injury to either half of the spinal cord and resulting in the loss of motor function, position, vibration, and light touch on the affected side
  2. Pain and temperature sense loss on the opposite side
- *Conus medullaris syndrome:* results in variable motor loss in the lower extremities with loss of bowel and bladder function
- *Cauda equina syndrome:* typical low back pain, weakness in both lower extremities, saddle anesthesia, and loss of voluntary bladder and bowel control

ETIOLOGY

- Trauma. Most SCIs result from high-speed motor vehicle accidents, falls, and work-related injuries.
- Tumor
- Infection
- Inflammatory processes
- Degenerative disk conditions with spinal stenosis

- Acute disk herniation
- Cystic abnormalities

DIAGNOSIS

DIFFERENTIAL DIAGNOSIS

- See "Etiology."
- Section II describes the differential diagnosis of paraplegia.

WORKUP

- Spinal cord compression: requires an immediate referral for radiographic and neurologic assessment
- With respect to airway management, suspected SCI dictates in-line immobilization of the spine at all times, so hyperextension of the neck is contraindicated. A jaw thrust must be used to open the airway, and required intubation must be done with the head/neck in a neutral position.
- Lab results usually unremarkable unless infectious or inflammatory causes suspected

IMAGING STUDIES

- Depend on the suspected etiology
- After initial resuscitative efforts, fine-cut helical CT scan with coronal and sagittal reconstructions have supplanted plain radiographs in most trauma centers as an initial evaluation in detecting spine fractures.
- MRI usually required to rule out ligamentous injury

TREATMENT

- Urgent surgical decompression is usually indicated as soon as the etiology is established.
- Corticosteroids: The administration of methylprednisolone reduces the amount of secondary injury that occurs after SCI and has become an important tool in the treatment of SCI.

DISPOSITION Important indicators regarding prognosis:
- The greater the distal motor and sensory sparing, the greater the expected recovery.
- When a plateau of recovery is reached, no further improvement is expected.
- The quicker the recovery, the greater the recovery.

REFERRAL Immediate referral for radiographic and neurologic evaluation and treatment in all suspected cases of spinal cord compression

SUGGESTED READINGS
available at www.expertconsult.com

RELATED CONTENT
Spinal Stenosis (Patient Information)

AUTHOR: **LONNIE R. MERCIER, M.D.**

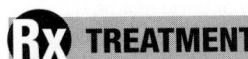

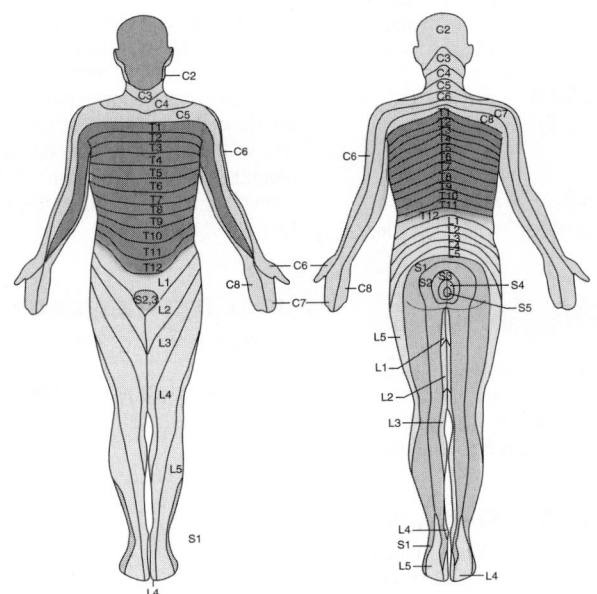

Levels of principal dermatomes

C5	Clavicles
C5,6,7	Lateral parts of upper limbs
C8, T1	Medial sides of upper limbs
C6	Thumb
C6,7,8	Hand
C8	Ring and little fingers
T4	Level of nipples
T10	Level of umbilicus
T12	Inguinal or groin regions
L1,2,3,4	Anterior and inner surfaces of lower limbs
L4,5 S1	Foot
L4	Medial side of great toe
S1,2, L5	Posterior and outer surfaces of lower limbs
S1	Lateral margin of foot and little toe
S2,3,4	Perineum

FIGURE 1-773 Schematic demarcation of levels of principal dermatomes shown as distinct segments. There is actually considerable overlap between any two adjacent dermatomes. (From Goldman L, Schafer AI: *Goldman's Cecil medicine,* ed 24, Philadelphia, 2011, Saunders.)

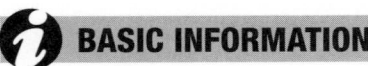 BASIC INFORMATION

DEFINITION

A spinal epidural abscess (SEA) is a focal suppurative infection occurring in the spinal epidural space.

ICD-9CM CODES
324.1 Spinal epidural abscess

EPIDEMIOLOGY & DEMOGRAPHICS
INCIDENCE (IN U.S.):
- 2 to 25 cases/100,000 hospitalized patients/yr
- May be increasing over the past 3 decades

PREDOMINANT AGE:
- Median age of onset approximately 50 yr (35 yr in intravenous drug users)
- Peak incidence in seventh and eighth decades of life

PHYSICAL FINDINGS & CLINICAL PRESENTATION
- The presentation of SEA can be nonspecific.
- Fever, malaise, and back pain are the most consistent early symptoms.
- Pain is often focal. It may initially be mild but can progress to become severe.
- As the disease progresses, root pain can occur, followed by motor weakness, sensory changes, bladder and bowel dysfunction, and paralysis.
- Physical findings may be limited to fever or spinal tenderness.
- The evolution to neurologic deficits can occur as quickly as a few hours, or over weeks to months.
- Once paralysis occurs, it may quickly become irreversible without the appropriate intervention.

ETIOLOGY
- Pyogenic bacteria account for the majority of cases in the U.S. Immigrants from TB-endemic areas may present with tuberculous SEAs. Fungi and parasites can also cause this condition. The most common causative organism is *Staphylococcus aureus*. Gram-negative bacilli and anaerobes may be seen if the infection has a urinary or GI source.

- Most posterior SEAs are thought to originate from distant focus (e.g., skin and soft tissue infections), while anterior SEAs are commonly associated with diskitis or vertebral osteomyelitis. No source was found in approximately one third of cases.
- Associated predisposing conditions include diabetes mellitus, alcoholism, cancer, AIDS, and chronic renal failure, or following epidural anesthesia, spinal surgery or trauma, or IV drug use. No predisposing condition is found in approximately 20% of patients.
- Damage to the spinal cord can be caused by direct compression of the spinal cord, vascular compromise, bacterial toxins, and inflammation.

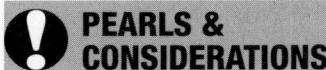 DIAGNOSIS

DIFFERENTIAL DIAGNOSIS
- Herniated disk
- Vertebral osteomyelitis and diskitis
- Metastatic tumors
- Meningitis

LABORATORY TESTS
- WBC may be normal or elevated.
- ESR is usually elevated over 30 mm/hr.
- Blood cultures are positive in approximately 60% of patients with SEA.
- CSF cultures are positive in 19%, but lumbar puncture is unnecessary, and may be contraindicated.
- Once imaging is done, CT-guided aspiration or open biopsy should be done to determine causative organism. Abscess content culture is positive in 90% of patients.

IMAGING STUDIES
- MRI with gadolinium is the imaging modality of choice (Fig. 1-774); CT scan with contrast may show the abscess (Fig. 1-775) but is less sensitive than MRI.
- CT with myelography is more sensitive for cord compression.

TREATMENT

NONPHARMACOLOGIC THERAPY
- Surgical decompression is the mainstay of treatment. Decompression within the first

24 hr has been related to an improved prognosis.
- Nonsurgical treatment is effective in some patients, but failure rate may be excessive. This approach should not be considered and should only be attempted in the absence of signs of compressive myelopathy and with very careful follow-up.

ACUTE GENERAL Rx
- In addition to surgery, antibiotics directed at the most likely organism should be initiated. Fig. E1-776 describes an algorithm for the management of patients with SEA.
- If the organism is unknown, broad coverage against staphylococci, streptococci, and gram-negative bacilli should be initiated. Empiric antimicrobial therapy typically includes vancomycin plus an antipseudomonal cephalosporin or carbapenem. The regimen can be adjusted according to culture results. Therapy should continue for at least 4 to 6 wk.

CHRONIC Rx
Neurologic deficits may remain despite aggressive treatment.

DISPOSITION
Irreversible paralysis and death can occur in up to 25% of patients.

REFERRAL
All cases should be referred to a neurosurgeon and an infectious disease specialist.

PEARLS & CONSIDERATIONS

- It is critically important to recognize this process early; the prognosis is generally excellent if treatment is initiated while symptoms are localized and before evidence of myelopathy develops.
- The likelihood of success postsurgery is low in patients who have developed complete paralysis for longer than 36 hours.

SUGGESTED READINGS
available at www.expertconsult.com

AUTHOR: **GLENN G. FORT, M.D., M.P.H.**

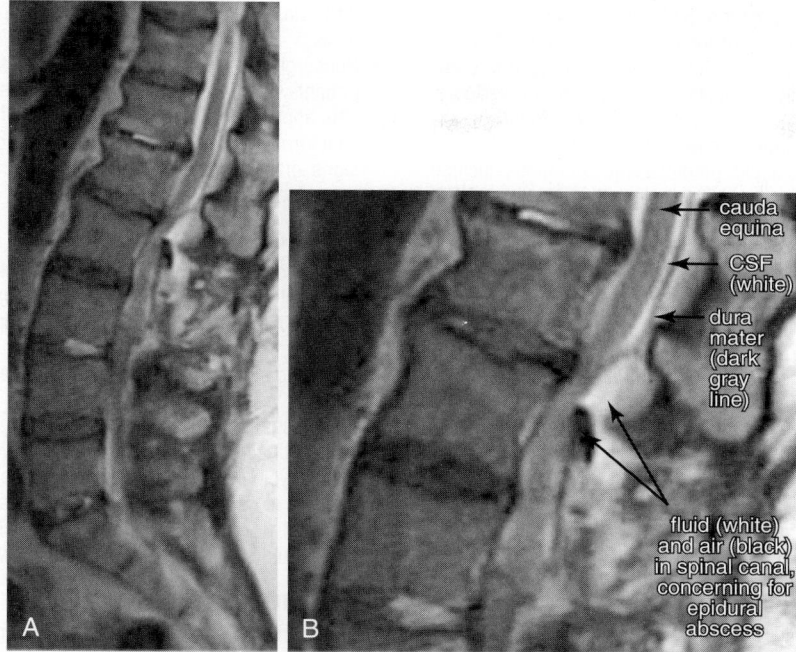

FIGURE 1-774 Same patient as in Fig. 1-775, in whom noncontrast computed tomography showed air in the spinal canal, concerning for epidural abscess. Magnetic resonance imaging (MRI) of the lumbar spine without contrast was performed, as the patient was in acute renal failure. **A,** This T_2-weighted sagittal MR image provides useful information even without gadolinium contrast. **B,** Close-up. On T_2-weighted MRI sequences, fluid including cerebrospinal fluid *(CSF)* appears white. Fat-containing tissues such as bone marrow and the spinal cord or cauda equina appear dark gray. Calcified bone appears nearly black due to an absence of resonating protons. Air appears completely black for the same reason. The midline sagittal image shows the cauda equina to be impinged upon by an epidural fluid collection containing air—an epidural abscess. The dura mater is visible as a thin, dark gray line parallel to the spinal cord. It is indented in the region of the epidural abscess. (From Broder JS: *Diagnostic imaging for the emergency physician*, Philadelphia, 2011, Saunders.)

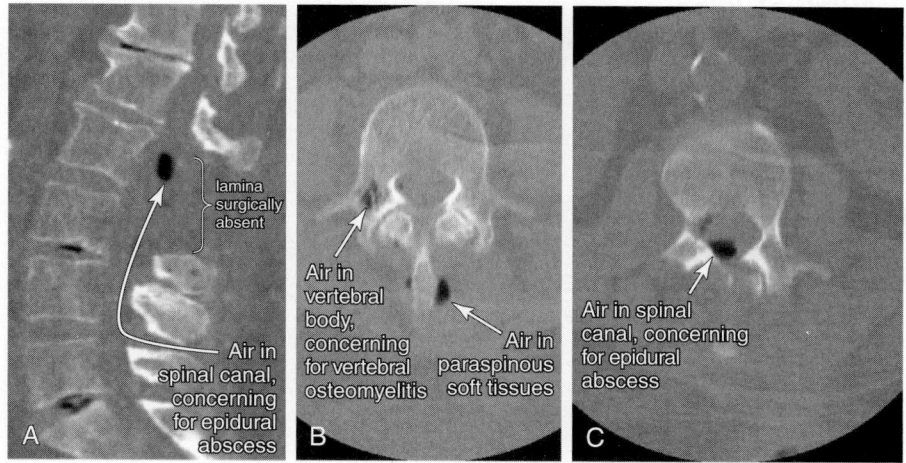

FIGURE 1-775 This 67-year-old female presented with delirium and fever. Three months prior, she had undergone lumbar laminectomy, and her wound had been treated with a wound VAC dressing. Magnetic resonance imaging was not initially available, so noncontrast computed tomography (CT) was performed. Noncontrast CT is excellent at delineating air, which appears black on bone windows. **A,** The midsagittal view demonstrates air *(black)* in the spinal canal at the L2 and L3 levels. On the axial views **(B, C),** air is visible in the spinal canal, in paraspinal soft tissues, and within the vertebral body. These findings are concerning for a paraspinal infection that has developed into an epidural abscess with vertebral osteomyelitis. (From Broder JS: *Diagnostic imaging for the emergency physician*, Philadelphia, 2011, Saunders.)

BASIC INFORMATION

DEFINITION

Spinal stenosis is the pathologic condition caused by the compressing or narrowing of the spinal canal, nerve root canal, or intervertebral foramina at the lumbar region.

SYNONYMS

Central spinal stenosis
Lateral spinal stenosis
Spondylosis

ICD-9CM CODES

724.02 Spinal stenosis lumbar, lumbosacral

EPIDEMIOLOGY & DEMOGRAPHICS

More common between 50 and 60 yr of age

PHYSICAL FINDINGS & CLINICAL PRESENTATION

- Symptoms caused by direct mechanical compression or indirect vascular compression of the nerve roots or the cauda equina.
- Neurogenic claudication: leg, buttock, or back pain precipitated by walking and relieved by sitting.
- Pain may radiate down to ankles and is associated with numbness, tingling, and weakness.
- Taking a flexed posture reduces symptoms because it increases the available space in the lumbar spinal canal.
- Decreased lumbar extension.
- Normal peripheral pulses.
- Positive Romberg's sign (decreased proprioception).
- Wide-based gait.
- Reduced knee and ankle reflex.
- Urine incontinence.

ETIOLOGY

Spinal stenosis may be primary or secondary
- Primary stenosis (congenital or developmental narrowing)
  1. Idiopathic
  2. Achondroplasia
  3. Morquio-Ullrich syndrome
- Secondary stenosis (acquired)
  1. Degenerative (hypertrophy of the articular processes, disk degeneration, ligamentum flavum hypertrophy, spondylolisthesis)
  2. Fracture/trauma
  3. Postoperative (postlaminectomy)
  4. Paget's disease
  5. Ankylosing spondylitis
  6. Tumors
  7. Acromegaly

DIAGNOSIS

DIFFERENTIAL DIAGNOSIS

- Osteoarthritis of the knee or hip
- Acute cauda equina syndrome, resulting from compression by epidural abscess or tumors
- Pain and weakness caused by multiple myeloma or osteomyelitis
- Intermittent claudication—peripheral vascular disease

- Peripheral neuropathy such as that caused by a herniated nucleus pulposus
- Scoliosis or spondylolisthesis
- Rheumatoid diseases: ankylosing spondylitis, Reiter's syndrome, fibromyalgia
- Table 1-379 compares clinical features of spinal stenosis, peripheral vascular disease, and disk disease.

WORKUP

History, physical examination, and specific imaging studies

IMAGING STUDIES

- Lumbar spine film sensitivity 66%, specificity 93%.
- Ultrasound of the spinal canal has also been used.
- CT scan of the lumbosacral spine: sensitivity (75% to 85%), specificity (80%).
- MRI of the lumbosacral spine: sensitivity (80% to 90%), specificity (95%).
- Myelogram: sensitivity (77%), specificity (72%). Absolute stenosis is defined as the anterior-posterior (AP) diameter of the spinal canal <10 mm. Relative stenosis: 10 to 12 mm AP diameter.
- Electromyography (EMG) and nerve conduction velocity (NCV) are additional studies particularly useful in differentiating peripheral neuropathy from lumbar spinal stenosis.

TREATMENT

NONPHARMACOLOGIC THERAPY

- Physiotherapy
- Lumbar corsets
- Back exercises
- Abdominal muscle strengthening
- Aquatic exercises

ACUTE GENERAL Rx

- Surgery is indicated in patients with significant compression of nerve roots as determined by MRI or CT and incapacitating symptoms limiting activities of daily living or bladder and bowel incontinence.
- Surgical procedures include decompressive laminectomy, arthrodesis, hemilaminectomy, and medial facetectomy.
- Lumbar interspinous process decompression using X-STOP device: a titanium oval spacer placed between the two adjacent spinous

processes of the affected level; provides an unloading distractive force to the stenotic middle column part of the motion segment.

CHRONIC Rx

- Conservative therapy with NSAIDs (ibuprofen 800 mg PO tid, naproxen 500 mg PO bid) may be tried for symptomatic relief in addition to acetaminophen 1 g PO qid.
- Epidural steroid injections may provide temporary relief.

DISPOSITION

- Approximately 20% of patients having surgery require repeat surgery within 10 yr. Nearly one third of these patients continue to experience pain.
- The natural history of spinal stenosis is one of slow progression. Although not very common, cord compression with resultant bowel and bladder incontinence and paresis can occur.
- Operative treatment is more effective in reducing pain and disability than nonoperative treatment.

REFERRAL

- Patients who have spinal stenosis should be referred to an orthopedic surgeon specializing in back surgery or to a neurosurgeon.
- Pain clinic referrals should be made if surgery is contraindicated or if the patient does not want surgery.

PEARLS & CONSIDERATIONS

COMMENTS

- Approximately one third of patients have coexisting peripheral vascular disease.
- The severity of cauda equina constriction is directly related to the walking ability and the pain intensity in the legs and back.
- Spinal stenosis is also a cause of chronic low back pain in the young.

SUGGESTED READINGS

available at www.expertconsult.com

RELATED CONTENT

Spinal Stenosis (Patient Information)

AUTHOR: **JORGE A. VILLAFUERTE, M.D.**

TABLE 1-379 Comparative Clinical Features of Spinal Stenosis, Peripheral Vascular Disease, and Disc Disease

Feature	Spinal Stenosis	Disc Prolapse	Peripheral Vascular Disease
Reduced straight leg raise	Rarely	Usually	No
Neurologic deficit	Sometimes	Often	No
Leg pain on walking	Yes	Usually	Yes
Leg pain on sitting	No	Yes	No
Pain relief on standing still	No	No	Yes
Pain relief on sitting	Yes	No	Yes
Numbness/paresthesia	Yes	Yes	Sometimes

From Carr A, Hamilton W: *Orthopedics in primary care*, ed 2, Philadelphia, 2005, Butterworth-Heinemann.

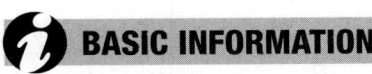

BASIC INFORMATION

DEFINITION

The spinocerebellar ataxias (SCAs) are a heterogeneous group of autosomal dominantly inherited genetic conditions that cause progressive ataxia and other neurologic symptoms.

SYNONYMS

Autosomal-dominant cerebellar ataxia (ADCA)
Machado-Joseph disease (eponym for SCA3; this may be the most common SCA)

ICD-9CM CODES
334.2 Primary cerebellar degeneration

EPIDEMIOLOGY & DEMOGRAPHICS

PREVALENCE: The prevalence of the condition is approximately 3 persons per 100,000. The most common SCAs are 1, 2, 3, 6, and 7.
PREDOMINANT SEX: SCA demonstrates no gender preference.
PREDOMINANT AGE: The age of onset is often during the 30s or 40s. However, this can be highly variable, even within family groups; SCAs can occur anytime from childhood to late adulthood.
GENETICS: All SCAs are inherited in an autosomal dominant fashion; however, reduced penetrance can be present.

PHYSICAL FINDINGS & CLINICAL PRESENTATION

- Chronically progressive ataxia is the predominant symptom of all of the SCAs. It typically presents as a combination of balance and gait difficulty, limb incoordination, and dysarthria.
- More than 36 different genetic subtypes of SCA have been described to date. Although certain clinical characteristics are common to specific SCA subtypes, there is significant overlap among and variability within these conditions, so making a diagnosis on the basis of the clinical presentation alone can be challenging and sometimes impossible without genetic testing. Some of the more common SCAs and their possible distinguishing features in addition to ataxia include the following:
  - SCA1 can be characterized by nystagmus, spasticity, and neuropathy.
  - SCA2 can be characterized by slow saccades, gaze palsy, neuropathy, and sometimes parkinsonism or dementia.
  - SCA3, which is also known as *Machado-Joseph disease,* can be characterized by neuropathy, amyotrophy, parkinsonism, and dystonia.
  - SCA6 is generally felt to be a pure cerebellar syndrome with ataxia and nystagmus (gaze evoked and downbeat) as well as a frequently later age of onset.
  - SCA7 is characterized by dementia, vision loss caused by a pigmentary maculopathy, and spasticity.
  - Knowledge in this area is constantly expanding and being updated. Online sources of information (e.g., Online Mendelian Inheritance in Man [http://www.ncbi.nlm.nih.gov/omim]) can be invaluable for tracking new developments.

ETIOLOGY

Several of the SCAs are the result of polyglutamine CAG repeat expansions; this causes the accumulation of mutant proteins inside neurons, which is thought to cause dysfunction and cell death. Higher numbers of repeats are correlated with an earlier onset of symptoms, and anticipation may be present. Other types of repeat expansions and point mutations have been found with several SCAs; for others, the affected gene has not been identified.

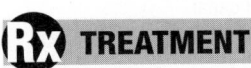

DIAGNOSIS

DIFFERENTIAL DIAGNOSIS

- Structural cerebellar abnormality: includes cerebellar tumor, inflammation (e.g., multiple sclerosis), stroke, or hemorrhage; the time course for these causes is typically more acute or subacute than chronic
- Endocrine dysfunction: hypothyroidism or hypoparathyroidism can uncommonly cause ataxia
- Alcoholic cerebellar degeneration: caused by heavy alcohol use; gait ataxia predominates
- Other toxin-induced ataxias: antiepileptic medications, lithium, and chemotherapeutic agents
- Creutzfeldt-Jakob disease: rapidly progressive ataxia, dementia, and myoclonus
- Paraneoplastic cerebellar degeneration: found in association with primary malignancies (e.g., small cell lung cancer, breast cancer); subacute-onset ataxia that progresses rapidly
- Celiac disease: gluten-sensitive enteropathy with malabsorption may be associated with ataxia; autoantibodies such as antigliadin or antiendomysial antibodies are typically present
- Multiple system atrophy: cerebellar variant of this disorder causes ataxia; there is typically associated parkinsonism with some degree of autonomic dysfunction (e.g., orthostatic hypotension, urinary incontinence)
- Friedreich's ataxia: autosomal recessive inheritance, generally younger age of onset (i.e., mean 15 yr of age), lower limb areflexia, and posterior column dysfunction
- Ataxia associated with vitamin E deficiency: can be an autosomal recessive disorder or acquired; clinically resembles Friedreich's ataxia, with areflexia and loss of position sense
- Ataxia telangiectasia: autosomal recessive inheritance, childhood onset, oculocutaneous telangiectases, and immunodeficiency
- Wilson's disease: can cause hepatic dysfunction and a variety of movement disorders, including ataxia; particularly important to screen for this in patients who are young at onset because it is treatable
- Dentatorubral-pallidoluysian atrophy: autosomal dominant like SCA but typically has ataxia with associated choreoathetosis, myoclonus, epilepsy, and dementia
- Fragile X–associated tremor/ataxia syndrome: premutation of the fragile X mutation gene; more common among males than females; late onset of ataxia (i.e., >50 yr), tremor, and sometimes parkinsonism; MRI often shows T_2 hyperintensity in the middle cerebellar peduncle
- Box 1-61 shows the classification of the various causes of ataxia.

LABORATORY TESTS

- Rule out acquired causes of ataxia, depending on the clinical scenario, with thyroid studies, toxicology screening, and the determination of the vitamin E level or presence of paraneoplastic antibodies.
- Screen for Wilson's disease with ceruloplasmin and, if indicated, a 24-hour urinary copper determination.
- Genetic testing is commercially available for many but not all of the SCAs.

IMAGING STUDIES

- MRI of the brain should be performed to exclude structural abnormalities.
- Cerebellar or brain stem atrophy can be seen with several of the SCA subtypes.

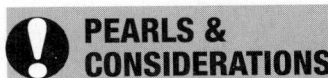

TREATMENT

NONPHARMACOLOGIC THERAPY

- Speech therapy for dysarthria and dysphagia
- Physical therapy
- Occupational therapy

CHRONIC Rx

Treatment is symptomatic and supportive. In some cases, parkinsonism can respond to levodopa. Clonazepam can be helpful if tremor is prominent. Spasticity can be treated with baclofen or tizanidine. Dystonia may benefit from botulinum toxin injections.

DISPOSITION

All SCA disorders are progressive, although the speed is variable from subtype to subtype and from patient to patient. On average, patients become wheelchair bound 15 yr after the onset of ataxia, and death can occur after 20 to 25 yr.

REFERRAL

Referral to a general neurologist or to a movement disorders center is appropriate.

PEARLS & CONSIDERATIONS

COMMENTS

- Genetic testing can have consequences for both the patient and the family. These issues

BOX 1-61   Classification of Ataxia

Congenital Ataxias

Hereditary Ataxias

Autosomal Recessive Ataxias

- Friedreich's ataxia
- Ataxia–telangiectasia
- Ataxia with oculomotor apraxia type 1
- Ataxia with oculomotor apraxia type 2
- Autosomal recessive spastic ataxia of Charlevoix-Saguenay
- Abetalipoproteinemia
- Ataxia with isolated vitamin E deficiency
- Refsum's disease
- Cerebrotendinous xanthomatosis
- Marinesco-Sjögren syndrome
- Autosomal recessive ataxia with known gene locus
- Early-onset cerebellar ataxia

X-Linked Ataxias

- Fragile X tremor ataxia syndrome

Autosomal Dominant Ataxias

- Spinocerebellar ataxias
- Dentatorubral-pallidoluysian atrophy
- Episodic ataxias

Nonhereditary Degenerative Ataxias

- Multiple system atrophy, cerebellar type
- Sporadic adult-onset ataxia of unknown etiology

Acquired Ataxias

- Alcoholic cerebellar degeneration
- Ataxia as a result of other toxic causes (e.g., antiepileptic medications, lithium, solvents)
- Paraneoplastic cerebellar degeneration
- Other immune-mediated ataxias (e.g., gluten ataxia, ataxia associated with anti-glutamic acid decarboxylase antibodies)
- Acquired vitamin E deficiency
- Hypothyroidism
- Ataxia as a result of physical causes (e.g., heat stroke, hyperthermia)

From Goetz CG: *Textbook of clinical neurology,* ed 3, Philadelphia, 2007, Saunders.

should be discussed during the informed consent process. Patients who desire asymptomatic testing as a result of a relevant family history should undergo genetic counseling before testing.

- In symptomatic patients with a family history of dominantly inherited ataxia, the diagnostic process is relatively straightforward. Genetic testing that is directed toward likely mutations by phenotype and ethnic origin should be the first step rather than an extensive workup for other causes.

PATIENT & FAMILY EDUCATION

Patient educational materials as well as contact information for support and advocacy groups are available on the website of the National Ataxia Foundation: http://www.ataxia.org.

SUGGESTED READINGS
available at www.expertconsult.com

AUTHOR: **ANDREW DUKER, M.D.**

S

Diseases
and Disorders

I

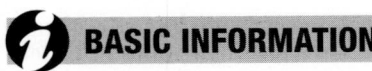

BASIC INFORMATION

DEFINITION

Spontaneous miscarriage is fetal loss before week 20 of pregnancy, calculated from the patient's last menstrual period or the delivery of a fetus weighing <500 g. Early loss is before menstrual week 12, whereas late loss refers to losses from weeks 12 to 20.

Miscarriage can also be classified as incomplete (partial passage of fetal tissue through partially dilated cervix), complete (spontaneous passage of all fetal tissue), threatened (uterine bleeding without cervical dilation or passage of tissue), inevitable (bleeding with cervical dilation without passage of fetal tissue), or missed abortion (intrauterine fetal demise without passage of tissue).

Recurrent miscarriage involves three or more spontaneous pregnancy losses before week 20.

SYNONYMS

Abortion

ICD-9CM CODES
634.0 Spontaneous abortion

EPIDEMIOLOGY & DEMOGRAPHICS

INCIDENCE: 5% to 20% of clinically recognized pregnancies, with 80% of miscarriages occurring in the first trimester. Recurrent miscarriage occurs in less than 1% of couples attempting to have children.

GENETICS:
- Distribution of abnormal karyotypes: autosomal trisomy (50%), monosomy 45,X (20%), triploidy (15%), tetraploidy (10%), structural chromosomal abnormalities (5%).
- With two or more spontaneous miscarriages, a karyotype should be performed to evaluate for balanced translocation, which has 80% risk for abortion, and, if the pregnancy is carried to term, has 3% to 5% risk for unbalanced karyotype.

RISK FACTORS: Prior pregnancy history (risk after live birth, 5%; prior pregnancy aborted, 20% subsequent risk) is the most significant risk factor. Vaginal bleeding, especially >3 days, carries with it a 15% to 20% chance of miscarriage.

PHYSICAL FINDINGS & CLINICAL PRESENTATION

- Profuse bleeding and cramping have a higher association with miscarriage than bleeding without cramping, which is more consistent with a threatened miscarriage.
- Cervical dilation with history or finding of fetal tissue at cervical os may be present.
- In cases of missed abortion, uterine size may be smaller than menstrual dating, in contrast to molar gestation, where size may be greater than dates.

ETIOLOGY

- In a general overview the etiology can be classified in terms of maternal (environmental) and fetal (genetic) factors, with the majority of miscarriages being related to genetic or chromosomal causes.
- Causes: uterine anomalies (unicornuate uterus risk, 50%; bicornuate or septate uterus risk, 25% to 30%); incompetent cervix (iatrogenic or congenital, associated with 20% of mid-trimester losses); diethylstilbestrol exposure in utero (T-shaped uterus); submucous leiomyomas; intrauterine adhesions or synechiae; luteal phase or progesterone deficiency; autoimmune disease such as anticardiolipin antibodies; uncontrolled diabetes mellitus. Rare or controversial causes include human leukocyte antigen associations between mother and father; infections such as tuberculosis, *Chlamydia,* and *Ureaplasma;* smoking and alcohol use; irradiation; and environmental toxins.

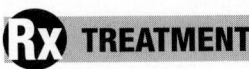

DIAGNOSIS

DIFFERENTIAL DIAGNOSIS

- Normal pregnancy
- Hydatidiform molar gestation
- Ectopic pregnancy
- Dysfunctional uterine bleeding
- Pathologic endometrial or cervical lesions

WORKUP

- All patients with bleeding in the first trimester should have an evaluation for possible ectopic pregnancy.
- If there are three early, prior pregnancy losses, a workup and treatment for recurrent miscarriage should begin before next conception. If there is a strong history for second-trimester loss, consideration for cerclage should be given if the history is consistent with incompetent cervix (e.g., painless cervical dilation).
- Most providers will initiate an evaluation for couples who have had only two previous losses.

LABORATORY TESTS

- Type and antibody screen are used to evaluate the need for Rh immune globulin.
- During the preconception period, hemoglobin A_{1c}, anticardiolipin antibody, lupus anticoagulant, MTHFR, antithrombin III, prothrombin gene 2210A, karyotyping, endometrial biopsy (rarely performed currently because of poor predictive value), progesterone level, and cervical cultures or serum antibodies can be checked for suspected disease processes.
- Progesterone level <5 mg/dl suggests nonviable gestation vs. >25 mg/dl, which suggests a good prognosis.

IMAGING STUDIES

Transabdominal or transvaginal sonogram (preferably) (Fig. E1-777) can be used in combination with menstrual dating and serum quantitative human chorionic gonadotropin to document pregnancy location, fetal heart presence, gestational sac size, and adnexal pathology.

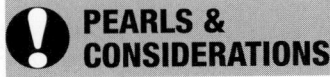

TREATMENT

NONPHARMACOLOGIC THERAPY

Depending on the patient's clinical status, desire to continue the pregnancy, and certainty of the diagnosis, expectant management can be considered. In pregnancies <6 wk or >14 wk, complete expulsion of fetal tissue usually occurs and surgical intervention such as dilation and curettage (D&C) can be avoided.

ACUTE GENERAL Rx

- Incomplete miscarriage between 6 and 14 wk can be associated with large amounts of blood loss; thus these patients should undergo D&C.
- In cases of missed abortion, if fetal demise has occurred >6 wk before or gestational age is >14 wk, there is an increased risk of hypofibrinogenemia with disseminated intravascular coagulation. Thus D&C or manual vacuum aspiration should be performed early in the disease course. Consider use of misoprostol (Cytotec) 200 mg PO q6h as an alternative approach if patient desires a less invasive approach.
- Rh-negative patients should be given Rhogam 300 mcg IM to prevent Rh isoimmunization.

REFERRAL

Refer to obstetrician/gynecologist.

PEARLS & CONSIDERATIONS

Spontaneous pregnancy loss is recommended as a replacement for the term *abortion* and to acknowledge the emotional aspects of losing a pregnancy.

SUGGESTED READINGS
available at www.expertconsult.com

RELATED CONTENT
Ectopic Pregnancy (Related Key Topic)
Molar Pregnancy (Related Key Topic)
Vaginal Bleeding during Pregnancy (Related Key Topic)

AUTHORS: **SCOTT J. ZUCCALA, D.O.,** and **RUBEN ALVERO, M.D.**

BASIC INFORMATION

DEFINITION

Squamous cell carcinoma (SCC) is a malignant tumor of the skin arising in the epithelium.

SYNONYMS

SCC
Skin cancer

ICD-9CM CODES
173.9 Skin neoplasm, site unspecified

EPIDEMIOLOGY & DEMOGRAPHICS

- SCC is the second most common cutaneous malignancy, comprising 20% of all cases of nonmelanoma skin cancer.
- Incidence is highest in lower latitudes (e.g., southern U.S., Australia).
- Male/female ratio is 2:1.
- Incidence increases with age and sun exposure.
- Average age at diagnosis is 66 yr.

PHYSICAL FINDINGS & CLINICAL PRESENTATION

- SCC commonly affects the scalp, neck region, back of hands, superior surface of the pinna, and the lip (Fig. E1-779).
- The lesion may have a scaly, erythematous macule or plaque.
- Telangiectasia, central ulceration may also be present (Fig. 1-780).

- Most SCCs present as exophytic lesions that grow over a period of months.
- Although most SCCs are relatively slow growing and nonaggressive, some (2%-5%) can exhibit rapid growth and metastases. Aggressive tumors are more common in immunocompromised patients and when arising from scars, burns, or prior injury (Marjolin's ulcer). Presence of SCC on ears, lips, or size >2 cm are high risk features of SCC.

ETIOLOGY

Risk factors include ultraviolet B radiation, immunosuppression (kidney transplant recipients have a threefold increased risk), arsenic exposure, HPV infection, and tobacco abuse.

DIAGNOSIS

DIFFERENTIAL DIAGNOSIS

- Keratoacanthomas
- Actinic keratosis
- Amelanotic melanoma
- Basal cell carcinoma
- Benign tumors
- Healing traumatic wounds
- Spindle cell tumors
- Warts

WORKUP

Diagnosis is made by full-thickness skin biopsy (incisional or excisional).

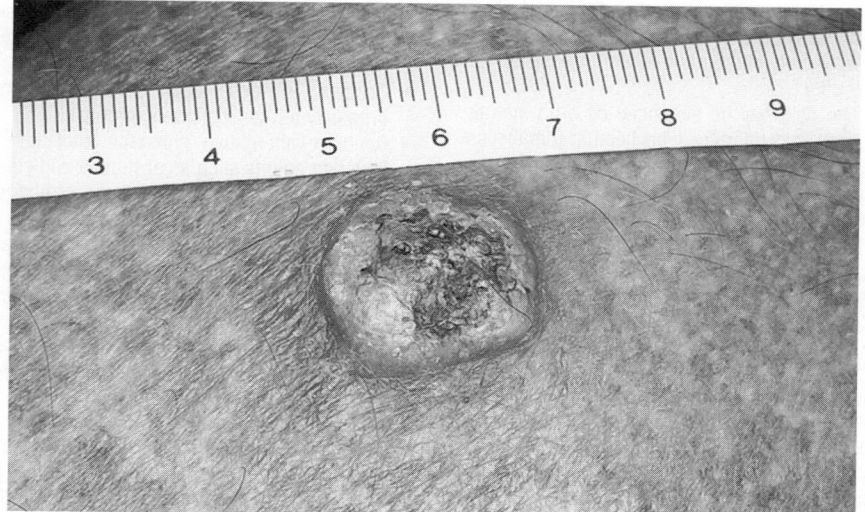

FIGURE 1-780 Squamous cell carcinoma. Nodular hyperkeratotic lesion with central erosion. (From Noble J et al: *Textbook of primary care medicine,* ed 3, St Louis, 2001, Mosby.)

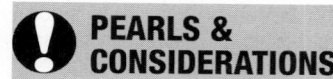

TREATMENT

ACUTE GENERAL Rx

- Electrodesiccation and curettage for small SCCs (<2 cm in diameter), superficial tumors, and lesions located in extremity and trunk.
- Tumors thinner than 4 mm can be managed by simple local removal.
- Lesions between 4 and 8 mm thick or those with deep dermal invasion should be excised.
- Tumors penetrating the dermis can be treated with several modalities, including excision and Mohs' surgery, radiation therapy, and chemotherapy. Mohs' surgery is commonly used for lesions on the face.
- Metastatic SCC can be treated with cryotherapy and combination of chemotherapy using 13-*cis*-retinoic acid and interferon-alpha 2A.

DISPOSITION

- Survival is related to size, location, degree of differentiation, immunologic status of the patient, depth of invasion, and presence of metastases. Risk factors for metastasis include lesions on the lip or ear, increasing lesion depth, and poor cell differentiation.
- Patients whose tumors penetrate through the dermis or exceed 8 mm in thickness are at risk of tumor recurrence.
- The most common metastatic locations are regional lymph nodes, liver, and lung.
- Tumors on the scalp, forehead, ears, nose, and lips also carry a higher risk.
- SCCs originating in the lip and pinna metastasize in 10% to 20% of cases.
- Five-year survival for metastatic SCC is 34%.

REFERRAL

Oncology referral for metastatic SCC

PEARLS & CONSIDERATIONS

COMMENTS

SCC arising in areas of prior radiation, thermal injury, and areas of chronic ulcers or chronic draining sinuses are more aggressive and have a higher frequency of metastasis than those originating in actinic damaged skin.

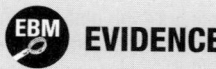

EVIDENCE

available at www.expertconsult.com

SUGGESTED READING

available at www.expertconsult.com

RELATED CONTENT

Squamous Cell Carcinoma (Patient Information)

AUTHOR: **FRED F. FERRI, M.D.**

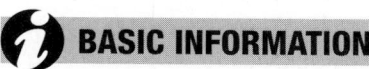

DEFINITION

Statin-induced muscle syndromes (SIMS) include myopathy, myalgia, myositis, and rhabdomyolysis. Definitions for these syndromes are inconsistent in the medical literature.

- Myopathy: a general term defined as any disease of muscles.
- Myalgia: muscle weakness or pain without serum creatinine kinase elevation.
- Myositis: muscle weakness or pain with an increased serum creatinine kinase level.
- Rhabdomyolysis: muscle weakness or pain and a marked serum creatinine kinase level usually greater than 10 times the upper limit of normal and serum creatinine elevation as well as signs of brown urine and elevated urine myoglobin.

SYNONYMS

Statin-induced myopathies
Statin-induced myositis
Statin-induced myalgias
Statin-induced rhabdomyolysis

ICD-9CM CODES
729.1   Myalgia and myositis
728.8   Rhabdomyolysis
359.4   Toxic myopathy
359.9   Myopathy, unspecified
359.81 Critical illness myopathy
359.89 Other myopathies

EPIDEMIOLOGY & DEMOGRAPHICS

INCIDENCE & PREVALENCE: Risk of statin-induced rhabdomyolysis is 1.2 per 10,000 persons/yr increasing to 0.9% in patients taking high-dose statins. Rhabdomyolysis risk of death is 0.15 deaths per 1 million prescriptions. SIMS most commonly occur in people aged 51 to 75, which may reflect the pattern of statin use. The prevalence of statin-induced myalgias is about 1% to 5%, similar to placebo in clinical trials, although observational studies have suggested a prevalence of 10% or higher. Statins may cause elevated transaminases (ALT, AST) at a prevalence of 0.5% to 2.0% and rhabdomyolysis ~0.08%.

PREDOMINANT SEX AND AGE: The mean age of hospitalized patients with statin-induced myopathy or rhabdomyolysis was 64 yr. Slightly more common in women (56%).

GENETICS: There is interpatient variability in the activity of the *CYP3A4* gene for the metabolism of simvastatin, atorvastatin, and lovastatin. Homozygous carriers of CYP2D6 (poor metabolizers) had a higher rate of discontinuation of simvastatin due to muscle syndromes compared with the CYP2D6 wild-type genotype; patients taking atorvastatin and having a muscle event were more likely to have the CYP2D6*4 allele. SLCO1B1 polymorphisms encode for the organic anion transport of statins into the liver cells. Some data exist on deficiencies in ubiquinone (coenzyme Q10) in patients with a mutation in the *COQ2* gene.

RISK FACTORS: Small body frame; age over 80 yr; frail elderly women; patients taking multiple drugs, especially gemfibrozil, cyclosporine, itraconazole, ketoconazole, erythromycin, clarithromycin, verapamil, amiodarone; renal or liver impairment; pharmacogenetic variability; hypothyroidism; excessive alcohol intake; vigorous exercise; severe infections; excessive grapefruit juice ingestion; inherited defects of muscle metabolism such as carnitine palmityl transferase II deficiency, McArdle's disease, and myoadenylate deaminase deficiency; acquired myopathies such as postpoliomyelitis syndrome; lipophilic statins (simvastatin, atorvastatin, lovastatin); multiple conditions such as diabetes; and drugs of abuse (amphetamines, heroin, cocaine, phencyclidine).

PHYSICAL FINDINGS & CLINICAL PRESENTATION

- Myopathy can occur at any time, although it is more common within the first 4 weeks of therapy.
- Proximal generalized muscle aches, body aches, and pains, and may be mild or severe.
- Dark-colored urine
- Muscle cramps, spasms, tenderness, or stiffness
- Unusually tired or weak
- Nocturnal cramping
- Tendon pain

ETIOLOGY

- History of current statin use
- May be explained by one of three deficiencies of end products of the 3-hydroxy-3-methyl-glutaryl-coA reductase pathway: cell signaling and apoptosis, mitochondrial respirations and ubiquinone concentrations, and cholesterol concentrations and cell membrane integrity.
- The risk may be enhanced by drug interactions that interfere with hepatic metabolism and gut wall transport of interacting medications and by pharmacodynamic effects.
- Underlying metabolic muscle disorder may predispose a patient to develop myopathy.

DIAGNOSIS

DIFFERENTIAL DIAGNOSIS

Bursitis, tendinitis, radiculopathy, osteoarthritis, muscle strain, myofascial pain, hypothyroidism, proton-pump inhibitor-induced polymyositis, viral illness, polymyositis, and polymyalgia rheumatica

WORKUP

Workup consists of a thorough history, including exercise history, urine color, medication history, and physical exam to palpate tenderness and obtain blood tests to evaluate muscle and kidney damage.

LABORATORY TESTS

If severe myopathy or rhabdomyolysis is suspected:

- Elevated CPK, positive serum myoglobin, elevated BUN, serum creatinine, AST, ALT, LDH, and potassium
- Urine creatinine, positive casts, and hemoglobin in urine with absence of red blood cells
- Consider electrocardiogram and assessment of calcium, phosphate, and uric acid.

If mild to moderate myopathy is suspected:

- Monitor TSH and CPK levels; CPK may only be elevated when sudden severe myopathy occurs.
- If the patient has brown or dark urine or elevated CPK, monitor BUN and serum creatinine.

IMAGING STUDIES

- Not recommended

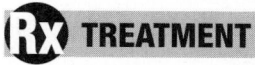

- Discontinue statin therapy immediately if muscle symptoms occur. An algorithm for monitoring and management of suspected statin-associated myopathy is described in Fig. E1-781.
- Depending on severity of the syndrome, consider switching to another statin once muscle condition resolves, which may take up to 4 months.
- Consider alternate-day therapy or once or twice weekly therapy for long-acting statins such as atorvastatin and rosuvastatin.
- Patient willingness to rechallenge with lower dose, or if not, or if symptoms recur, consider alternative statin such as pravastatin or atorvastatin.
- Consider fluvastatin 80 mg extended release, which may be effective in reducing myalgia symptoms.
- Consider low-dose statin once weekly and gradually titrate at monthly intervals.
- Consider alternative nonstatin cholesterol-lowering agents such as ezetimibe and colesevelam. Box 1-62 describes recommendations regarding statin and muscle safety.
- Consider alternative nonpharmacologic treatment such as plant stanols and sterols, although no data exist specifically for statin-tolerant patients.
- Although controversial, consider red yeast rice as an alternative to statin therapy for statin-intolerant patients.

NONPHARMACOLOGIC THERAPY

- Treatment of rhabdomyolysis is generally supportive in nature (see "Rhabdomyolysis" topic).
- Use of coenzyme Q10, although data are conflicting, may be of some benefit for mild symptoms of myalgias due to the potential decrease in coenzyme Q10 concentrations secondary to the use of statins.

ACUTE GENERAL Rx

- Stop statin therapy; check history, potential drug-drug interactions, CPK, TSH, renal function, hepatic function, and urinalysis.

- If patients have suspected rhabdomyolysis, they should be hospitalized and treated with supportive therapy and monitoring of complications.
- If CPK < 10× the upper limit of normal without symptoms, continue statin therapy at the same or lower dosage
- If CPK < 10× the upper limit of normal with intolerable symptoms, discontinue statin.
- If CPK > 10× the upper limit of normal, discontinue statin.

CHRONIC Rx

- After stopping the statin and symptom or CPK resolution, consider the same statin at a lower dosage or a different statin at the same or lower dosage.
- When restarting therapy, consider statins with a lower risk of myopathy such as low-dose rosuvastatin; long-acting fluvastatin; and alternate-day dosing of rosuvastatin, atorvastatin, or long-acting fluvastatin.
- If patient had rhabdomyolysis secondary to statin therapy, consider nonstatin treatments.
- If the patient develops myopathy after a second trial of therapy, statin treatment should be permanently discontinued and nonstatin cholesterol-lowering therapy initiated, such as bile acid sequestrants or ezetimibe.

COMPLEMENTARY & ALTERNATIVE MEDICINE

- The effects of coenzyme Q10 on reducing or preventing SIMS remain controversial with evidence both supporting and refuting its potential benefits. Given its general safety, coenzyme Q10 can be recommended if the actions listed under "Chronic Rx" are insufficient to continue the use of the statin and if the muscle symptoms have been limited generally to myalgias and not rhabdomyolysis. Use coenzyme Q10 with caution in patients taking warfarin, as its anticoagulant effect may be decreased.
- Several observational studies have suggested an association between vitamin D deficiency and statin-induced myopathy. Data are conflicting. The effects of supplementing vitamin D in patients with statin myopathy are limited and such supplement cannot be recommended unless a documented vitamin D deficiency is present.

DISPOSITION

- Usually resolves within 1 wk up to 4 mo after discontinuing statin therapy.
- Once the patient has a full recovery, an alternative statin can be tried.

REFERRAL

- If rhabdomyolysis is suspected, immediate referral for hospitalization is suggested.

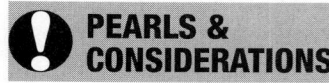

PEARLS & CONSIDERATIONS

COMMENTS

SIMS are usually mild and will resolve within a few wk after discontinuing statin therapy. However, such syndromes may progress to rhabdomyolysis.

PREVENTION

- Use the lowest statin dosage to achieve target lipid levels, and titrate dosage slowly to minimize myopathy risk.
- Avoid risk of potentiating myopathy with drugs known to increase the risk of myopathy such as macrolide antibiotics, cyclosporine, protease inhibitors, fibrates, amiodarone, P-glycoprotein inhibitors (i.e., colchicine).
- Discontinue statin therapy prior to and during surgical procedures.
- If patient requires a short-term therapy with an interacting medication such as an azole antifungal, temporarily discontinue statin therapy until interacting therapy is completed.
- If statin–fibric acid therapy is warranted, fenofibrate is preferred over gemfibrozil to decrease risk of myopathy; consider fluvastatin for a combination with gemfibrozil, if desired.
- Baseline liver function testing before initiation of statin therapy and only if clinically indicated thereafter

PATIENT & FAMILY EDUCATION

- Inform patients to promptly report muscle weakness, unexpected muscle pain, or brownish urine.
- Ensure that the pharmacist and/or primary care physician checks for drug-drug interactions with every new prescription, including those from dentists and physicians from other specialties.
- Coenzyme Q10 may lessen some of the milder muscle symptoms from statins, but patients should inform their physician and pharmacist if they decide to use this supplement.

SUGGESTED READINGS

available at www.expertconsult.com

AUTHORS: **LISA COHEN, PHARM.D.**, and **ANNE L. HUME, PHARM.D.**

BOX 1-62 Recommendations to Health Care Professionals Regarding Statin and Muscle Safety

- Whenever muscle symptoms or an increased CK level is encountered in patients receiving statin therapy, health professionals should attempt to rule out other causes, because these are most likely to explain the findings. Other common causes include increased physical activity, trauma, falls, accidents, seizure, shaking chills, hypothyroidism, infections, carbon monoxide poisoning, polymyositis, dermatomyositis, alcohol abuse, and drug abuse (cocaine, amphetamines, heroin, or PCP).
- Obtaining a pretreatment, baseline CK level can be considered in patients who are at high risk of experiencing muscle toxicity (e.g., older patients or those combining a statin with an agent known to increase myotoxicity), but this is not routinely necessary in other patients.
- It is unnecessary to measure CK levels in asymptomatic patients during the course of statin therapy, because marked, clinically important CK elevations are rare and are usually related to physical exertion or other causes.
- Patients receiving statin therapy should be counseled about the increased risk of muscle symptoms, particularly if initiation of vigorous, sustained endurance exercise or a surgical operation is being contemplated; they should be advised to report such muscle symptoms to a health professional.
- Creatine kinase measurements should be obtained in symptomatic patients to help gauge the severity of muscle damage and facilitate decision of whether to continue therapy or alter doses.
- In patients who develop intolerable muscle symptoms with or without CK elevation and for whom other etiologies have been ruled out, the statin should be discontinued. Once symptoms disappear, the same or different statin at the same or a lower dose can be restarted to test the reproducibility of symptoms. Recurrence of symptoms with multiple statins and doses requires initiation of other lipid-altering therapy.
- In patients who develop tolerable muscle symptoms or have no symptoms but have a CK level <10 × ULN, statin therapy may be continued at the same or reduced doses and symptoms may be used as the clinical guide to stop or continue therapy.
- In patients who develop rhabdomyolysis (CK >10,000 IU/L or >10 × ULN with an elevation in serum creatinine or need for intravenous hydration therapy), statin therapy should be stopped. Intravenous hydration therapy in a hospital should be instituted if indicated for patients experiencing rhabdomyolysis. Once patients recover, risk vs. benefit of statin therapy should be carefully reconsidered.

CK, Creatine kinase; PCP, phencyclidine; ULN, upper limit of normal.
From McKenney JM et al: Final conclusions and recommendations of the National Lipid Association Statin Safety Assessment Task Force, Am J Cardiol 97(suppl 8A):89C-94C, 2006.

S

Diseases and Disorders

I

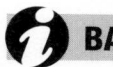
BASIC INFORMATION

DEFINITION

Status epilepticus is a medical neurologic emergency. It is historically defined as 30 min of continuous seizure activity or two or more seizures without full recovery of consciousness between seizures. However, in practice a continuous seizure that lasts >5 min should be treated as status epilepticus.

SYNONYMS

Convulsive status epilepticus
Nonconvulsive status epilepticus

ICD-9CM CODES
345.3 Grand mal status
345.2 Petit mal status

EPIDEMIOLOGY & DEMOGRAPHICS

INCIDENCE: 40 to 100 cases per 100,000 persons
PEAK INCIDENCE: It is most common among children younger than 1 yr and adults older than 60 yr.
PREDOMINANT SEX AND AGE: No gender preference

PHYSICAL FINDINGS & CLINICAL PRESENTATION

- Patients can present with repetitive tonic clonic movements of the body (convulsive status epilepticus); other patients are comatose and nonresponsive (nonconvulsive status epilepticus).
- Patients may also present with lethargy, intermittent confusion, and involuntary movements.

ETIOLOGY

- Status epilepticus can be the result of an acute neurologic injury, such as stroke, meningitis, etc.
- In patients with epilepsy, abrupt discontinuation of antiepileptic drugs can result in status epilepticus.
- See Table 1-380 for causes of status epilepticus.

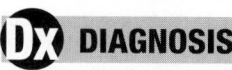
DIAGNOSIS

DIFFERENTIAL DIAGNOSIS

- Convulsive syncope
- Nonepileptic spells

TABLE 1-380 Causes of Status Epilepticus

- Stroke (ischemic/hemorrhagic)
- CNS infections
- Traumatic head injury
- CNS toxicity: certain medications, drugs, ethanol
- Brain tumors or other mass lesions
- Metabolic disturbances: hypoglycemia, hyponatremia
- Abrupt discontinuation of antiepileptic drugs in patient with epilepsy
- Cryptogenic

CNS, Central nervous system.

- Encephalopathies: metabolic, infectious, toxic, etc.

WORKUP

- ABCs
- ICU admission
- Emergent electroencephalogram (EEG)
- Continuous video EEG in refractory cases
- Investigation of the patient with status epilepticus is summarized in Box E1-63.

LABORATORY TESTS

- Routine blood workup (CBC, CMP, glucose, electrolytes)
- Urine drug screen
- Lumbar puncture and CSF analysis in patients with suspected meningitis

IMAGING STUDIES

- Immediate CT scan of the head
- MRI of the brain should be performed once the patient is in a stable condition.

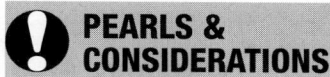
TREATMENT

- Patients with continuous seizure activity over 3 min need intravenous lorazepam 0.1 mg/kg at 2 mg/min (or diazepam 0.2 mg/kg at 5 mg/min only when lorazepam is not available).
- Lorazepam is followed by intravenous fosphenytoin 20 mg/kg (PE) at a rate not greater than 150 mg/min.
- An alternate to fosphenytoin is phenytoin 20 mg/kg IV at up to 50 mg/min as tolerated. Vital signs should be monitored during the infusion.
- If seizures continue, intravenous phenobarbital, midazolam, or propofol is an alternative. Other agents used include intravenous valproic acid and intravenous levetiracetam.
- Results of recent trials comparing intramuscular midazolam vs. intravenous lorazepam for prehospital status epilepticus show that IM midazolam may be as good as lorazepam, with successful termination of seizures in 73% of patients in the IM midazolam group vs. 63% in the IV lorazepam group. This difference was attributed to the more rapid administration of the IM medication (1.2 min vs. 4.8 min with the IV route). Fig. E1-782 describes guidelines for the treatment of prolonged seizures and status epilepticus in infants (>1 mo), children, and adolescents and refractory status epilepticus.

NONPHARMACOLOGIC THERAPY
None

GENERAL Rx

It is important to find out the etiology of the status epilepticus (e.g., metabolic disturbance, infection). The appropriate treatment/understanding of the underlying cause of the status epilepticus will impact the successful treatment.

CHRONIC Rx

- The chronic treatment of patient with status epilepticus depends on the etiology.

- Patient with status epilepticus due to epilepsy will need chronic treatment.

COMPLEMENTARY & ALTERNATIVE MEDICINE
Not applicable

DISPOSITION

- Response to treatment depends on the etiology of the status epilepticus.
- When there is no CNS injury as a cause or result of the status epilepticus, the prognosis is good.
- No driving until seizure freedom in accordance with local laws and regulations.

REFERRAL

Status epilepticus is a neurologic emergency; therefore immediate neurologic consultation is warranted.

PEARLS & CONSIDERATIONS

COMMENTS

- Status epilepticus is a medical emergency that carries a high risk of mortality. Mortality among patients who present in status epilepticus is 15% to 22%. Among those who survive, functional ability will decline in 25% of cases.
- Continuous video EEG is crucial in the treatment of these patients because some of them may not be clinically seizing (convulsing) but electrographically they may still have subclinical repetitive seizures or subclinical status epilepticus.

PREVENTION

Medication compliance is crucial in patients with epilepsy.

PATIENT & FAMILY EDUCATION

- Patients with epilepsy have normal lives.
- The goal of treatment is no seizures and no side effects to medications.
- Patient education and information can be obtained at the Epilepsy Foundation: www.epilepsyfoundation.org
- Pregnant women with epilepsy should visit the Antiepileptic Drug Pregnancy Registry website for information and assistance: www2.massgeneral.org/aed
- Patients with ongoing seizures are forbidden from driving; check state regulations and laws regarding driving and epilepsy.

SUGGESTED READINGS
available at www.expertconsult.com

AUTHOR: **PATRICIO SEBASTIAN ESPINOSA, M.D., M.P.H.**

BASIC INFORMATION

DEFINITION Stevens-Johnson syndrome (SJS) is a rare, severe vesiculobullous form of erythema multiforme (EM) affecting the skin, mouth, eyes, and genitalia. SJS is defined as affecting <10% of body surface area (BSA). When it affects 10%-30% of BSA, it is known as SJS–toxic epidermal necrolysis (TEN) overlap syndrome. TEN affects >30% of BSA.

SYNONYMS

SJS
Herpes iris
Febrile mucocutaneous syndrome

ICD-9CM CODES
695.1 Stevens-Johnson syndrome

EPIDEMIOLOGY & DEMOGRAPHICS

- SJS affects predominantly children and young adults.
- Male/female ratio is 2:1.
- Prevalence: 1:100,000 for SJS and 1:1,000,000 for TEN

PHYSICAL FINDINGS & CLINICAL PRESENTATION

- The cutaneous eruption generally occurs within 8 wk of drug initiation and is generally preceded by vague, nonspecific symptoms of low-grade fever and fatigue occurring 1 to 14 days before the skin lesions. Cough is often present. Fever may be high during the active stages.
- Enlarging red-purple macules or papules and bullae generally occur on the conjunctiva, mucous membranes of the mouth (Fig. 1-783), nares, and genital regions.
- Corneal ulcerations may result in blindness.
- Ulcerative stomatitis results in hemorrhagic crusting.
- Nikolsky sign (shearing off of epidermis with pressure on skin) can be present.
- Flat, atypical target lesions or purpuric maculae may be distributed on the trunk or be widespread (Fig. 1-784).

- The pain from oral lesions may compromise fluid intake and result in dehydration.
- Thick, mucopurulent sputum and oral lesions may interfere with breathing.

ETIOLOGY

- Drugs (e.g., phenytoin, sulfonamides, lamotrigine, sertraline, NSAIDs, tramadol, allopurinol, β-lactam antibiotics, phenobarbital) are the most common cause.
- Upper respiratory tract infections (e.g., *Mycoplasma pneumoniae*) and HSV infections have also been implicated.

DIAGNOSIS

DIFFERENTIAL DIAGNOSIS

- Toxic erythema (drugs or infection)
- Pemphigus
- Pemphigoid
- Urticaria
- Hemorrhagic fevers
- Serum sickness
- *Staphylococcus* scalded-skin syndrome
- Behçet's syndrome

WORKUP

- Diagnosis is generally based on clinical presentation and characteristic appearance of the lesions.
- Skin biopsy is generally reserved for when classic lesions are absent and diagnosis is uncertain. Biopsy reveals epidermal necrolysis but cannot distinguish between SJS, TEN, and EM.

LABORATORY TESTS
CBC with differential, cultures in cases of suspected infection

IMAGING STUDIES
Chest x-rays may show patchy changes in patients with pulmonary involvement.

TREATMENT

NONPHARMACOLOGIC THERAPY

- Withdrawal of any potential drug precipitants
- Careful skin nursing to prevent secondary infection

ACUTE GENERAL Rx

- Treatment of associated conditions (e.g., acyclovir for HSV infection, azithromycin for *Mycoplasma* infection)
- Antihistamines for pruritus
- Treatment of the cutaneous blisters with cool, wet Burow's compresses
- Relief of oral symptoms by frequent rinsing with lidocaine (Xylocaine Viscous)
- Liquid or soft diet with plenty of fluids to ensure proper hydration
- Treatment of secondary infections with antibiotics
- Corticosteroids: use remains controversial; should be used only in severe cases early in the disease; when used, prednisone 20 to 30 mg bid until new lesions no longer appear, then rapidly tapered
- Topical steroids: may use to treat papules and plaques; however, should not be applied to eroded areas
- Vitamin A: may be used for lacrimal hyposecretion
- Consider IVIG in severe cases.

DISPOSITION

- Prognosis varies with severity of disease. It is generally good in patients with limited disease; however, mortality rate may approach 10% in patients with extensive involvement. A severity of illness score known as SCORE-TEN that incorporates increased glucose level (>252 mg/dl), increased BUN (>28 mg/dl), electrolytes (serum bicarbonate <20 mEq/L), age (>40 yr), immunosuppression (presence of cancer), involvement >10% of BSA, and increased heart rate (>120 beats/min) can be used to calculate mortality risk.
- Oral lesions may continue for several months.
- Scarring and corneal abnormalities may occur in 20% of patients.

REFERRAL

- Hospital admission in a unit used for burn care is recommended in severe cases.
- Urethral involvement may necessitate catheterization.
- Ocular involvement should be monitored by an ophthalmologist.

SUGGESTED READING
available at www.expertconsult.com

RELATED CONTENT
Stevens-Johnson Syndrome (Patient Information)

AUTHOR: **FRED F. FERRI, M.D.**

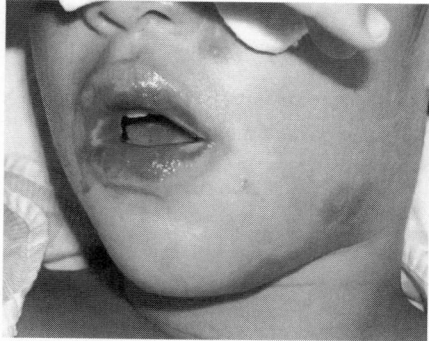

FIGURE 1-783 Lip changes found in Stevens-Johnson syndrome associated with *Mycoplasma pneumoniae* infection. (From Kliegman RM et al: *Nelson textbook of pediatrics*, ed 19, Philadelphia, 2011, Saunders.)

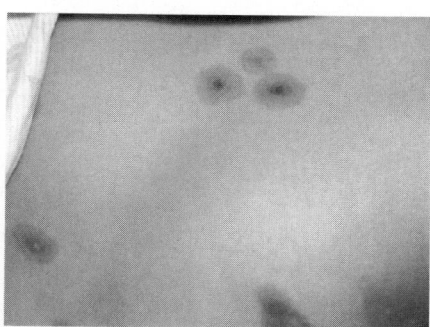

FIGURE 1-784 Classic erythema multiforme skin lesions found in Stevens-Johnson syndrome associated with *Mycoplasma pneumoniae* infection. (From Kliegman RM et al: *Nelson textbook of pediatrics*, ed 19, Philadelphia, 2011, Saunders.)

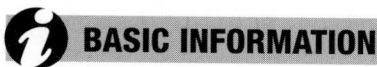

DEFINITION

Stomatitis is inflammation involving the oral mucous membranes.

SYNONYMS

Heterogeneous grouping of unrelated illnesses, each with its own designation(s)

ICD-9CM CODES
528.0 Stomatitis
054.2 (herpetic)
528.2 (aphthous)
112.0 (monilial)

PHYSICAL FINDINGS & CLINICAL PRESENTATION

WHITE LESIONS:
- Candidiasis (thrush)
- Caused by yeast infection *(Candida albicans)*
- Examination: white, curdlike material that when wiped off leaves a raw bleeding surface
- Epidemiology: seen in the very young and the very old, those with immunodeficiency (AIDS, cancer), persons with diabetes, and patients treated with antibacterial agents
- Other
  1. Leukoedema: filmy opalescent-appearing mucosa, which can be reverted to normal appearance by stretching. This condition is benign.
  2. White sponge nevus: thick, white corrugated folds involving the buccal mucosa. Appears in childhood as an autosomal dominant trait. Benign condition.
  3. Darier's disease (keratosis follicularis): white papules on the gingivae, alveolar mucosa, and dorsal tongue. Skin lesions also present (erythematous papules). Inherited as an autosomal dominant trait.
  4. Chemical injury: white sloughing mucosa.
  5. Nicotine stomatitis: whitened palate with red papules.
  6. Lichen planus: linear, reticular, slightly raised striae on buccal mucosa. Skin is involved by pruritic violaceous papules on forearms and inner thighs.
  7. Discoid lupus erythematosus: lesion resembles lichen planus.
  8. Leukoplakia: white lesions that cannot be scraped off; 20% are premalignant epithelial dysplasia or squamous cell carcinoma.
  9. Hairy leukoplakia: shaggy white surface that cannot be wiped off; seen in HIV infection, caused by Epstein-Barr virus.

RED LESIONS:
- Candidiasis may present with red lesions instead of the more frequent white. Median rhomboid glossitis is a chronic variant.

- Benign migratory glossitis (geographic tongue): area of atrophic depapillated mucosa surrounded by a keratotic border. Benign lesion, no treatment required.
- Hemangiomas.
- Histoplasmosis: ill-defined, irregular patch with a granulomatous surface, sometimes ulcerated.
- Allergy.
- Anemia: atrophic reddened glossal mucosa seen with pernicious anemia.
- Erythroplakia: red patch usually caused by epithelial dysplasia or squamous cell carcinoma.
- Burning tongue (glossopyrosis): normal examination; sometimes associated with denture trauma, anemia, diabetes, vitamin B_{12} deficiency, psychogenic problems.

DARK LESIONS (BROWN, BLUE, BLACK):
- Coated tongue: accumulation of keratin; harmless condition that can be treated by scraping
- Melanotic lesions: freckles, lentigines, lentigo, melanoma, Peutz-Jeghers syndrome, Addison's disease
- Varices
- Kaposi's sarcoma: red or purple macules that enlarge to form tumors; seen in patients with AIDS

RAISED LESIONS:
- Papilloma
- Verruca vulgaris
- Condyloma acuminatum
- Fibroma
- Epulis
- Pyogenic granuloma
- Mucocele
- Retention cyst

BLISTERS:
- Primary herpetic gingivostomatitis (Fig. 1-785)
- Caused by herpes simplex virus type 1 or, less frequently, type 2
- Course: day 1: malaise, fever, headache, sore throat, cervical lymphadenopathy; days 2 and 3: appearance of vesicles that develop into painful ulcers of 2 to 4 mm in diameter; duration of up to 2 wk

- Recurrent intraoral herpes: rare; recurrences typically involve only the keratinized epithelium (lips)
- Pemphigus and pemphigoid
- Hand-foot-mouth disease: caused by coxsackievirus group A
- Erythema multiforme
- Herpangina: caused by echovirus
- Traumatic ulcer
- Primary syphilis
- Perlèche (or angular cheilitis)
- Recurrent aphthous stomatitis (canker sores): most common oral mucosa lesion; may be associated with many systemic diseases
- Behçet's syndrome (aphthous ulcers, uveitis, genital ulcerations, arthritis, and aseptic meningitis)
- Reiter's syndrome (conjunctivitis, urethritis, and arthritis with occasional oral ulcerations)
- Unknown cause

Course: solitary or multiple painful ulcers may develop simultaneously and heal over 10 to 14 days. The size of the lesions and the frequency of recurrences are variable.

DX DIAGNOSIS

WORKUP
- White lesions: candidiasis (thrush) diagnosis: ovoid yeast and hyphae seen in scrapings treated with KOH culture
- Blisters:
  - Exfoliative cytology
  - Viral culture
  - Immunofluorescence for herpes antigen

RX TREATMENT

White lesions: candidiasis (thrush) treatment:
- Topical with nystatin or clotrimazole
- Systemic with ketoconazole or fluconazole

Blisters:
- Supportive
- Consider acyclovir

Recurrent intraoral herpes/aphthous ulcerations: topical corticosteroids (dexamethasone ointment applied to the identified ulcer tid) or systemic steroids for severe cases

SUGGESTED READINGS
available at www.expertconsult.com

RELATED CONTENT
Stomatitis (Patient Information)

AUTHOR: **FRED F. FERRI, M.D.**

FIGURE 1-785 Herpetiform mouth ulcers. This patient had lost 10 kg because of inability to eat. He gained 4 kg within a month of starting tetracycline. (From White GM, Cox NH [eds]: *Diseases of the skin, a color atlas and text,* ed 2, St Louis, 2006, Mosby.)

BASIC INFORMATION

DEFINITION
Strabismus is a condition of the eyes in which the visual axes of the eyes are not straight in the primary position or in which the eyes do not follow each other in the different positions of gaze.

SYNONYMS
Esotropia
Exotropia
Restrictive eye movement

ICD-9CM CODES
378.9 Strabismus

EPIDEMIOLOGY & DEMOGRAPHICS
INCIDENCE (IN U.S.): 2% of all children
PEAK INCIDENCE: Childhood
PREDOMINANT SEX: None
PREDOMINANT AGE: Birth to age 5 yr
GENETICS: None known

PHYSICAL FINDINGS & CLINICAL PRESENTATION
- Conjugate gaze loss in both eyes with the eyes focusing independently
- Amblyopia (a decrease in best-corrected visual acuity in an otherwise structurally healthy eye) may occur with untreated strabismus.

ETIOLOGY
- Many cases are congenital.
- Accommodative cases occur later with focusing.
- Rarely, there is neurologic disease or severe refractive errors.
- Hereditary form is common, with hyperopia (far-sightedness) the most common.

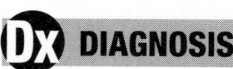
DIAGNOSIS

DIFFERENTIAL DIAGNOSIS
- Measuring eye position and movement
- Vision testing
- Refractive errors
- Central nervous system (CNS) tumors
- Orbital tumors
- Brain and CNS dysfunction

WORKUP
- Eye examination. Fig. E1-786 illustrates diagnostic tests that help differentiate between common causes of strabismus. Strabismus is classified according to the type and magnitude of misalignment. Esotropia refers to an inward deviation of the nonfixing eye and exotropia to the outward deviation of the nonfixing eye. Hypertropia is a vertical deviation in which the nonfixing eye is higher, and hypotropia is a

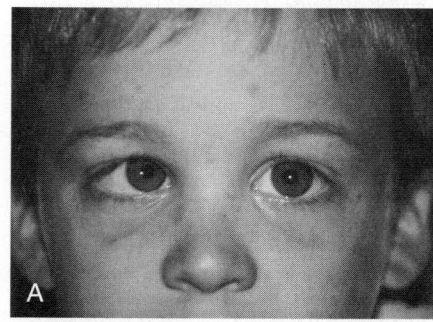
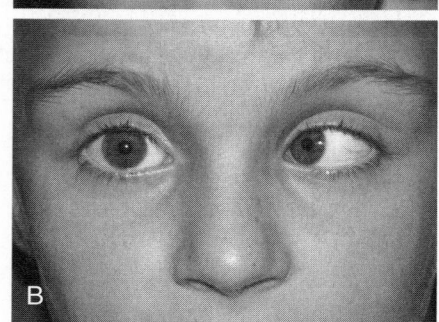
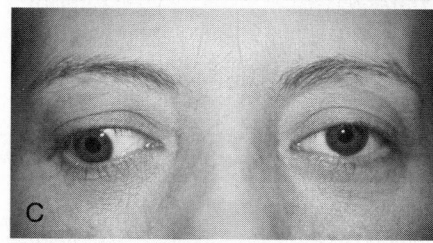

FIGURE 1-787 Hirschberg test. A, The right corneal reflex is near the temporal border of the pupil, indicating an angle of about 15°. **B,** The left corneal reflex is at the limbus, indicating an angle of about 45°. **C,** The right corneal reflex is at the limbus in a divergent squint. (**A** courtesy J. Yanguela. From Kanski JJ, Bowling B: *Clinical ophthalmology, a systematic approach,* ed 7, Philadelphia, 2010, Saunders.)

vertical deviation in which the nonfixing eye is lower.
- Measurement of deviation: the *Hirschberg test* (Fig. 1-787) gives a rough estimate of the angle of a manifest strabismus and is especially useful in young or uncooperative patients or when fixation in the deviating eye is poor.
- Visual field
- MRI to rule out tumors that develop later with no apparent cause

LABORATORY TESTS
Generally not needed

IMAGING STUDIES
Necessary only if other neurologic findings are found

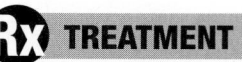
TREATMENT

NONPHARMACOLOGIC THERAPY
- Glasses
- Patching: best between age 3 and 7 yr; vision most improved by 3 to 6 mo
- Prisms
- Atropine: same as patching most of the time, although patching may give better results in resistant cases

CHRONIC Rx
- Glasses
- Alternate eye patching
- Surgery
- Prisms

DISPOSITION
- The earlier the condition is treated, the more likely the child will have normal vision in both eyes.
- After age 7 yr, visual loss is usually permanent from amblyopia.

REFERRAL
- Early for full rehabilitation of eye cosmetically and functionally
- To an ophthalmologist for management (usually)

SUGGESTED READING
available at www.expertconsult.com

RELATED CONTENT
Strabismus (Patient Information)

AUTHOR: **MELVYN KOBY, M.D.**

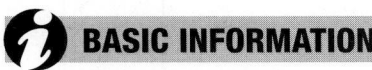

BASIC INFORMATION

DEFINITION

Ischemic stroke is the sudden onset of a focal neurologic deficit as a result of ischemia. Acute ischemic stroke may be defined as relating to the first few days after onset. However, the purpose of this chapter is to help the provider to make decisions regarding the acute stroke patient within the first several hours of symptoms; this is the crucial time for definitive treatment interventions.

SYNONYMS

Stroke
Brain attack
Cerebrovascular accident (this is a nonspecific term and should not be used.)

ICD-9CM CODES
494.31 Ischemic stroke
436   Acute stroke

EPIDEMIOLOGY & DEMOGRAPHICS

INCIDENCE:
- ~800,000 new or recurrent strokes occur each year in the U.S.
- Stroke is the number three cause of death and the leading cause of long-term disability in the U.S.

PREVALENCE: There are ~4.5 million stroke survivors in the U.S.

RISK FACTORS: Hypertension, dyslipidemia, diabetes mellitus, and smoking are the four major risk factors. Other risk factors include atrial fibrillation, mechanical heart valve, patent foramen ovale, recent myocardial infarction, carotid stenosis, hypercoagulable states, subclinical atrial tachyarrhythmias without clinical atrial fibrillation, and sickle cell disease.

GENETICS: Multifactorial

PHYSICAL FINDINGS & CLINICAL PRESENTATION

The presentation of ischemic stroke varies with the artery involved and the region of the central nervous system affected. Following are some common syndromic presentations. Please note that this list is not comprehensive and that all findings for a particular syndrome may not be listed here.

- Large- to medium-sized arteries:
  - Left middle cerebral artery: right face, arm, and leg weakness and sensory loss with aphasia (expressive, receptive, or both); possible hemianopia
  - Right middle cerebral artery: right face, arm, and leg weakness and sensory loss with hemineglect; possible hemianopia
  - Basilar artery: typically an acute loss of consciousness preceded by vertigo, nausea, vomiting, and diplopia; quadriparesis or quadriplegia may be seen, including the "locked-in" syndrome
  - Posterior cerebral artery: unilateral hemianopia
  - Anterior cerebral artery: unilateral leg weakness and sensory loss
  - Cerebellum: ataxia (typically of the limbs), often with vertigo, nausea, and vomiting

- Small arteries (common lacunar syndromes)
  - Lateral medullary (Wallenberg's) syndrome
  - Posterior limb internal capsule

ETIOLOGY

Etiologies include atherosclerosis, cardioembolism, artery-to-artery embolism, small-vessel lipohyalinosis, arteritis, arterial dissection, and vasospasm.

DIAGNOSIS
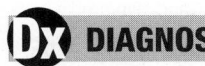

DIFFERENTIAL DIAGNOSIS

The differential diagnosis of acute ischemic stroke includes hemorrhagic stroke (primarily intracerebral hemorrhage), seizure with postictal paralysis, migraine with hemiparesis, syncope, hypoglycemia, hypertensive encephalopathy, and conversion disorder.

LABORATORY TESTS

- Immediate (Box 1-64): CBC, metabolic panel that includes blood glucose and renal function, PT/INR, aPTT, troponin I, and urinalysis
- National Institutes of Health Stroke Scale: a brief, focused neurologic examination aimed at providing a numeric estimate of the severity of stroke; can be performed by any health care provider trained in its use; may increase the likelihood of the correct assessment of stroke
- ECG and telemetry monitoring

IMAGING STUDIES

- Immediate (Fig. 1-788): computed tomography (CT) of the head without contrast or MRI of the brain with stroke protocol to rule out hemorrhage and, if possible, to assess the extent of stroke. (Because CT typically will not show an ischemic stroke for several

---

BOX 1-64 Immediate Diagnostic Studies: Evaluation of a Patient with Suspected Acute Ischemic Stroke

All Patients	Selected Patients
Noncontrast brain computed tomographic scan or magnetic resonance image	Hepatic function tests
Blood glucose level	Toxicology screen
Serum electrolyte and renal function tests	Blood alcohol level
Electrocardiography	Pregnancy test
Markers of cardiac ischemia	Arterial blood gas tests (if hypoxia is suspected)
Complete blood count, including platelet count*	Chest radiography (if lung disease is suspected)
Prothrombin time/international normalized ratio*	Lumbar puncture (if subarachnoid hemorrhage is suspected and computed tomography scan is negative for blood)
Activated partial thromboplastin time*	Electroencephalogram (if seizures are suspected)
Oxygen saturation	

*Although it is desirable to know the results of these tests before giving a patient tissue plasminogen activator, thrombolytic therapy should not be delayed while awaiting the results unless (1) there is clinical suspicion of a bleeding abnormality or thrombocytopenia; (2) the patient has received heparin or warfarin; or (3) the patient's use of anticoagulants is not known.

From Christensen H et al: Abnormalities on ECG and telemetry predict stroke outcome at 3 months, *J Neurol Sci* 234:99-103, 2005.

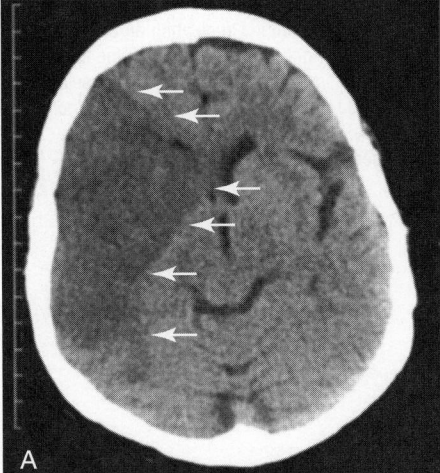
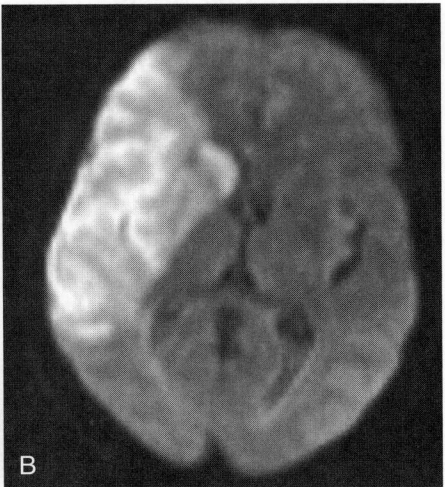

FIGURE 1-788 Large right middle cerebral artery infarct on an unenhanced computed tomographic scan **(A)** and a diffusion-weighted magnetic resonance image **(B)**. There is a mass effect, and this patient is at risk for cerebral herniation syndromes.

hours, it may also be useful to estimate how long ischemia has been present for cases in which the time of onset is unclear.)

- Several other neuroimaging studies are useful during the early stages of acute stroke to assess whether there is a thrombus that is amenable to intervention (Table 1-381).

Cross reference: see "Transient Ischemic Attack" for general workup, which is identical to that for ischemic stroke.

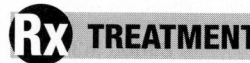 TREATMENT

NONPHARMACOLOGIC THERAPY

GENERAL CONSIDERATIONS:
- Airway and breathing should be maintained.
- Supplemental oxygen should be provided to keep the oxygen saturation at ≥92%.
- Fever is harmful during acute stroke. Ascertaining and addressing the cause while lowering an elevated temperature is strongly advised.
- Pneumatic compression devices or pharmacologic means should be applied to help prevent deep venous thromboses.
- Avoid any and all oral intake until swallowing is clearly unimpaired; this helps to avoid aspiration pneumonia.
- Early mobilization for rehabilitation is desirable.
- Consider neurosurgical intervention for craniectomy in select cases. Typical cases in which craniectomy may be performed include cerebellar ischemia with compression of the brain stem and/or the fourth ventricle as well as large right middle cerebral artery ischemia.

IMMEDIATE CATHETER CEREBRAL ANGIOGRAPHY FOR ENDOVASCULAR INTERVENTION

(Figs. 1-789 and 1-790): Methods available:
1. The Merci clot retrieval system is approved by the U.S. FDA for use up to 8 hr after the onset of symptoms.
2. The Penumbra System is also available at some centers.
3. Intraarterial tissue plasminogen activator (TPA) is used routinely for up to 6 hr after the onset of symptoms, although it is not approved by the U.S. FDA for this purpose.

Pearls and caveats:
- Multimodal therapy (i.e., thrombectomy and intraarterial TPA) is sometimes performed.
- Endovascular treatment may be performed for select cases in which intravenous (IV) TPA has failed to recanalize an occluded artery.
- Endovascular intervention may be an option for cases in which there are systemic contraindications to IV TPA.
- Endovascular intervention is useful only for large, accessible thrombi. Therefore, if a stroke patient is a candidate for IV TPA, then he or she should probably receive IV TPA.
- One can reasonably expect an endovascular recanalization rate of 60% in appropriate patients.
- Complications can ensue from the endovascular procedure itself, including an intracerebral hemorrhage rate that is similar to that associated with IV TPA.
- Endovascular intervention is typically available only at select large stroke centers.

- Some practitioners are making use of perfusion imaging (i.e., CT perfusion and magnetic resonance perfusion) to assess whether there is salvageable brain tissue before performing the procedure. In some cases, this may lead to a dramatic expansion of traditional time windows; this practice is currently being studied in clinical trials.

ACUTE GENERAL Rx
INTRAVENOUS THROMBOLYSIS:
- IV TPA is the only medical therapy approved by the U.S. FDA for the treatment of acute ischemic stroke. Recent trials involving tenecteplase, a genetically engineered mutant TPA, have shown significantly better reperfusion and clinical outcomes than alteplase in patients with stroke who were selected on the basis of CT perfusion imaging.
- The time window for administration is within 3 hr of symptom onset.
- There are strict criteria for the administration of IV TPA (see Box 1-65).
- The protocol is weight based, with 90 mg being the maximum allowable dose.

TABLE 1-381 Imaging Modalities for Stroke

Imaging Modality	Advantage	Disadvantage
Cerebral catheter angiography	• Allows for the definitive assessment of cerebral circulation (gold standard) • Allows for the deployment of intra-arterial thrombolysis and thrombectomy devices if a thrombus is found • Allows for the assessment of collateral circulation	• Invasive (significant risks) • High cost • Not available at all facilities
Doppler studies	• Noninvasive • May be performed at the patient's bedside	• Can be limited by the patient's body habitus • Operator dependent
Magnetic resonance angiography	• Excellent view of the large arteries of the neck and brain • No contrast material needed	• Cannot be performed in patients who are critically ill, who are unable to tolerate supine positioning, who have a pacemaker or other ferromagnetic hardware, or who are claustrophobic
Magnetic resonance perfusion	• Assesses cerebral hemodynamics • May show ischemic penumbra (i.e., the area of the brain that may be saved by timely intervention)	• Not commonly available • Not well standardized
CT angiography	• Excellent view of the large arteries of the neck and brain • Similar to magnetic resonance angiography with regard to resolution	• Requires intravenous contrast
CT perfusion	• Assesses cerebral hemodynamics • May show ischemic penumbra (i.e., the area of the brain that may be saved by timely intervention)	• Challenging to interpret in some cases • Not routinely available at many facilities • Requires intravenous contrast

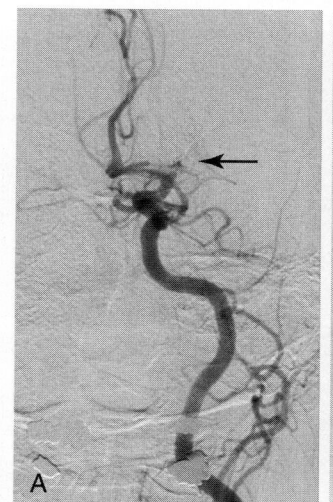
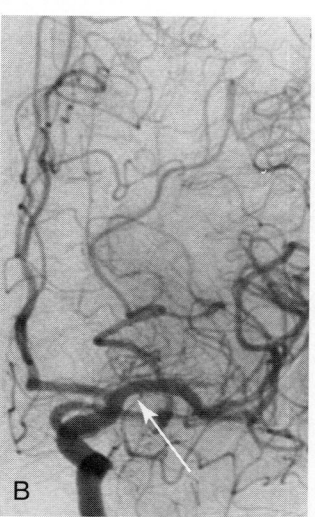

FIGURE 1-789 A, A catheter angiogram showing left middle cerebral artery occlusion, which caused severe stroke symptoms for several hours. **B,** The artery was opened with the Merci clot retrieval system, and this resulted in normal flow.

- The risk of brain hemorrhage with IV TPA is about 5% in stroke patients.
- Recent data suggest that IV TPA can be administered safely and with benefit in select patients up to 4.5 hours after symptom onset. There are additional exclusion criteria if IV TPA is given beyond the 3-hr window.

HYPERTENSION: Elevated blood pressure is common during acute stroke, and it often subsides without specific therapy. In general, hypertension is not treated acutely unless it is extremely high (e.g., >220 mm Hg systolic blood pressure); there is evidence of organ damage caused by the hypertension; or thrombolysis is being considered, in which case the blood pressure needs to come down (if it can be safely accomplished) to <185/110 mm Hg. It is risky to severely decrease blood pressure in the presence of acute ischemic stroke as it can cause an extension of the stroke into the ischemic penumbra. A 15% to 25% decrease over the first 24 hours is recommended.

HYPOGLYCEMIA: Hypoglycemia can mimic stroke. Prompt assessment of serum glucose level and replacement as necessary are important.

HYPERGLYCEMIA: The presence of hyperglycemia worsens ischemic stroke outcome. Hyperglycemia should be managed aggressively.

HYPOTENSION: The presence of systemic hypotension in acute ischemic stroke portends a poor outcome. The cause should be sought, and volume depletion should be corrected with normal saline. Cardiac arrhythmias should be treated. Induced hypertension with vasopressor agents may be useful for select cases with an ischemic penumbra that is at risk, but caution is strongly advised.

ANTIPLATELET THERAPY: Oral or feeding tube administration of aspirin (325 mg/day) within 48 hours of stroke onset is advised to decrease the likelihood of a repeat ischemic stroke. Other oral antiplatelet regimens approved for secondary stroke prophylaxis (e.g., clopidogrel, aspirin plus extended-release dipyridamole) will also suffice and may be superior in the long term.

DISPOSITION

Patients with acute ischemic stroke should be cared for in a stroke unit or an intensive care unit. Nurses with skills in stroke care and telemetry monitoring should be routine. Once the patient is stable and the workup is complete, rehabilitation should be arranged.

REFERRAL

Patients with acute ischemic stroke should be transported to a hospital in which providers are skilled in stroke care. Depending on the severity and duration of symptoms, the patient may qualify for immediate endovascular intervention at a comprehensive stroke center, even if he or she is not a candidate for IV TPA. If complications from brain edema develop, further evaluation by a neurosurgeon may be helpful during the acute phase.

BOX 1-65 Three-Hour Criteria for Tissue Plasminogen Activator (Alteplase [Activase]) Use in Patients with Thromboembolic Stroke

Criteria for considering TPA as a treatment option:
- Noncontrast CT scan without evidence of hemorrhage
- Time since onset of symptoms clearly <3 hr before TPA administration would begin

Criteria for excluding TPA as a treatment option:
- Historic and clinical findings:
  - Clinical presentation suggestive of subarachnoid hemorrhage, even if CT scan is normal
  - Sudden, severe headache, often with a loss of consciousness at onset
  - Vomiting
- Active internal bleeding, increased risk of bleeding, or known bleeding diathesis, including as a result of the following:
  - Recent use of warfarin with an INR of ≥1.7
  - Use of heparin within 48 hr with a prolonged aPTT
  - Platelet count of <100,000/mm³
  - History of intracranial hemorrhage
  - Known arteriovenous malformation or aneurysm

  - GI or GU bleeding within the past 21 days
  - Arterial puncture within the past 7 days
- Recent lumbar puncture
- Stroke, intracranial surgery, or head trauma within the previous 3 mo
- Major surgery or serious trauma within the preceding 14 days
- Systolic blood pressure >185 mm Hg or diastolic blood pressure >110 mm Hg that does not decrease below that range with treatment
- Seizure at stroke onset
- Rapidly improving neurologic signs
- Isolated mild neurologic deficits
- Acute myocardial infarction
- Post–myocardial infarction pericarditis
- Blood glucose <50 mg/dl or >400 mg/dl
- Patient who is pregnant or lactating
- CT findings:
  - Evidence of intracranial hemorrhage
  - Hypodensity or effacement of the sulci in one third of the territory of the middle cerebral artery

aPTT, Activated partial thromboplastin time; *CT,* computed tomography; *GI,* gastrointestinal; *GU,* genitourinary; *INR,* international normalized ratio; *TPA,* tissue plasminogen activator.
From Rakel RE [ed]: *Principles of family practice,* ed 6, Philadelphia, 2002, Saunders.

(!) PEARLS & CONSIDERATIONS

PREVENTION

The prevention of acute ischemic stroke depends on the aggressive management of risk factors in individual patients.

Cross reference: stroke, secondary prevention

PATIENT & FAMILY EDUCATION

Patients and families need to be taught about ways to reduce the risk for recurrent stroke, including lifestyle modifications. Education about rehabilitation goals, when appropriate, should also be accomplished.

(EBM) EVIDENCE

available at www.expertconsult.com

SUGGESTED READINGS

available at www.expertconsult.com

RELATED CONTENT

Fig. E3-173 Algorithm for the emergency evaluation of a patient with suspected stroke (Algorithm)
Stroke (Patient Information)

AUTHOR: **MICHAEL R. DOBBS, M.D.**

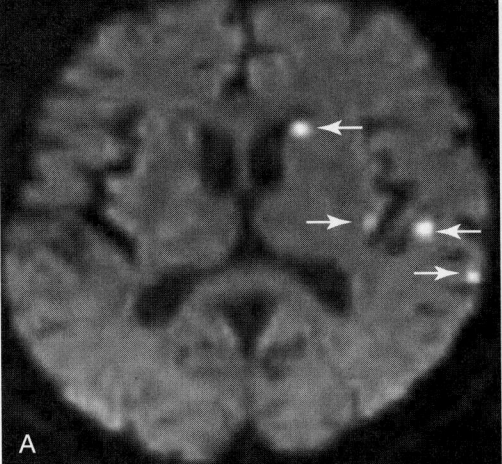
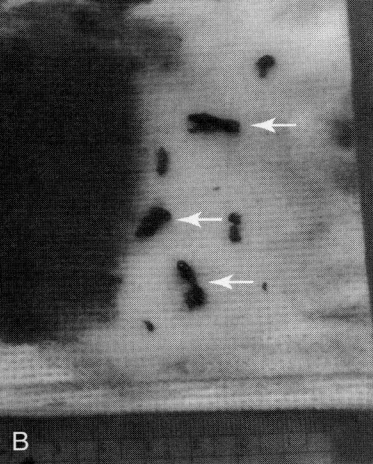

FIGURE 1-790 A, A diffusion-weighted magnetic resonance image of the same patient as shown in previous figure, this time showing only mild left cerebral ischemia after intervention. The patient was clinically normal. **B,** Thrombi removed from the middle cerebral artery with the use of the Merci clot retrieval system.

BASIC INFORMATION

DEFINITION

Hemorrhagic stroke is the sudden onset of a focal neurologic deficit caused by hemorrhage into or around the brain.

SYNONYMS

Intracerebral hemorrhage
Intracranial hemorrhage
Cerebrovascular attack (This is a nonspecific term and should not be used.)
The term *subarachnoid hemorrhage* refers to a specific location for hemorrhage, which commonly occurs as a result of a ruptured aneurysm. Please see "Subarachnoid Hemorrhage" for additional information.

ICD-9CM CODES
431 Intracerebral hemorrhage
432.9 Unspecified intracranial hemorrhage

EPIDEMIOLOGY & DEMOGRAPHICS

INCIDENCE: There are approximately 800,000 new or recurrent strokes per year in the United States, of which ~10% to 15% are hemorrhagic.
RISK FACTORS:
- Hypertension
- Anticoagulant use
- Thrombolysis
- Alcoholism
- Illicit drug use (e.g., cocaine)
- Cerebral amyloid angiopathy
GENETICS: Multifactorial

PHYSICAL FINDINGS & CLINICAL PRESENTATION

The presentation varies with the region of the brain that is affected. The following are common locations for hemorrhage:
- Basal ganglia
- Cerebellum
- Pons
- Lobar (i.e., amyloid angiopathy)

ETIOLOGY
- Rupture of vessels
- Aneurysm
- Arteriovenous malformation
- Brain tumor
- Amyloid angiopathy

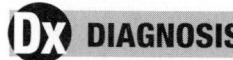

DIAGNOSIS

DIFFERENTIAL DIAGNOSIS
- Ischemic stroke
- Seizure with postictal paralysis
- Migraine with hemiparesis
- Syncope
- Conversion disorder

LABORATORY TESTS
- CBC, metabolic panel including blood glucose and renal function, PT/INR, aPTT, urinalysis, and toxicology screens
- ECG and telemetry monitoring

IMAGING STUDIES
- Immediate: CT scanning of the head without contrast is highly sensitive for hemorrhage (Fig. 1-791).
- MRI of the brain with a gradient echo sequence is also highly sensitive for hemorrhage, including intracerebral microhemorrhages that may not be visible with computed tomography scanning.

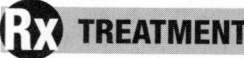

TREATMENT

NONPHARMACOLOGIC THERAPY
- Surgery should be performed promptly for cases of cerebellar hemorrhage of >3 cm when the patient is deteriorating clinically, showing brain stem edema or hydrocephalus.
- Surgery for lobar or deep brain clots may be considered for select cases, although the level of evidence for efficacy is not high.
- Pneumatic compression devices should be applied to help prevent deep venous thromboses.
- Early mobilization for rehabilitation is desirable.

ACUTE GENERAL Rx
- Hypertension (Box 1-66): blood pressure should be quickly lowered by 15% and then gradually and safely brought to the individual patient's target range. In theory, this may diminish the expansion of the hematoma.
- Hyperglycemia: a high blood glucose level predicts a worse outcome. Markedly elevated glucose levels should be lowered to <300 mg/dl.
- Seizures: if seizures occur, they should be treated aggressively, including with intravenous medications, if needed.
- Elevated intracranial pressure: this condition should be treated with a graded approach, which may include the elevation of the head of the bed, analgesia/sedation, hyperventilation, and osmotic therapy.
- Antipyretics should be administered for fever in addition to searching for a cause of the fever.
- Protamine sulfate is used to treat cases of heparin-induced intracerebral hemorrhage.
- Vitamin K is given for warfarin-associated intracerebral hemorrhage. In addition, recombinant factor VIIa and fresh frozen plasma are sometimes used.
- Recommendations for thrombolytic-associated intracerebral hemorrhage treatment include the consideration of the infusion of platelets and cryoprecipitate.

DISPOSITION

For large hemorrhages or unstable patients, immediate referral to a stroke center

REFERRAL

Patients with hemorrhagic stroke should be transported to a hospital where providers are skilled in the treatment of stroke and cerebrovascular diseases including the availability of neurosurgery services and neurocritical care. Depending on the severity and duration of symptoms, the patient may require neurosurgical intervention.

PEARLS & CONSIDERATIONS

- Outcomes are inversely correlated with hemorrhage size.
- Specific reversal agents may be useful for warfarin-, heparin-, or thrombolysis-associated hemorrhage.
- No procoagulant medications have yet been shown to be safe and effective for the mitigation of spontaneous intracerebral hemorrhage in placebo-controlled trials.

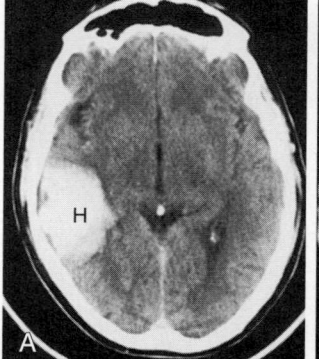
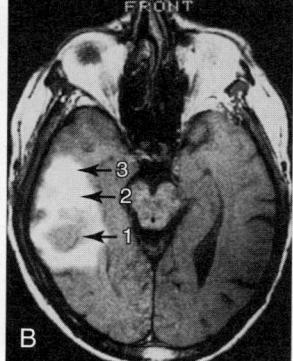
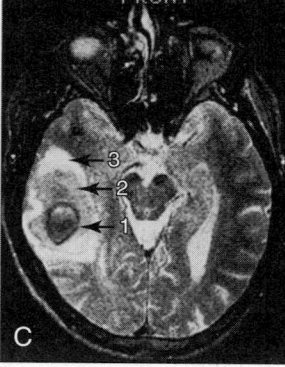
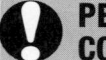

FIGURE 1-791 Hemorrhage. Axial CT image **(A)** demonstrates a large area of acute hemorrhage *(H)* in right temporal lobe. T_1-weighted **(B)** and T_2-weighted **(C)** MRI scans demonstrate the hemorrhage in various stages of breakdown. Center of lesion is dark on T_1- and T_2-weighted images, indicating oxyhemoglobin *(1)*. Intermediate zone is bright on T_1-weighted image and gray on T_2-weighted image, indicating intracellular methemoglobin *(2)*. Outer rim is bright on both T_1- and T_2-weighted images, indicating extracellular methemoglobin *(3)*. (From Vincent JL et al: *Textbook of critical care*, ed 6, Philadelphia, 2011, Saunders.)

PREVENTION

Prevention depends on the aggressive management of risk factors in individual patients, including hypertension, smoking, alcohol use, and cocaine use.

PATIENT & FAMILY EDUCATION

Patients and families need to understand that most patients will not soon achieve functional independence and that rehabilitation will be a long process. Education about avoiding antithrombotic agents should be stressed as appropriate for individual circumstances.

SUGGESTED READING

available at www.expertconsult.com

RELATED CONTENT

Fig. E3-173 Algorithm for the emergency evaluation of a patient with suspected stroke (Algorithm)
Stroke (Patient Information)

AUTHOR: **MICHAEL R. DOBBS, M.D.**

BOX 1-66 Suggested Recommended Guidelines for the Treatment of Elevated Blood Pressure in Patients with Spontaneous Intracerebral Hemorrhage

1. SBP of >200 mm Hg or MAP of >150 mm Hg: Consider the aggressive reduction of BP with continuous intravenous infusion, with BP monitoring every 5 min.
2. SBP of >180 mm Hg or MAP of >130 mm Hg with evidence or suspicion of elevated ICP: Consider ICP monitor and reducing BP with intermittent or continuous intravenous medications to keep cerebral perfusion pressure >60 to 80 mm Hg.
3. SBP of >180 mm Hg or MAP of >130 mm Hg without evidence or suspicion of elevated ICP: Consider a modest reduction of BP (e.g., MAP of 110 mm Hg or target blood pressure of 160/90 mm Hg) with intermittent or continuous intravenous medications, and clinically reexamine the patient every 15 min.

BP, Blood pressure; *ICP,* intracranial pressure; *MAP,* mean arterial pressure; *SBP,* systolic blood pressure.
Modified from Broderick J et al: Guidelines for the management of spontaneous intracerebral hemorrhage in adults: 2007 update, *Stroke* 38:2001-2023, 2007.

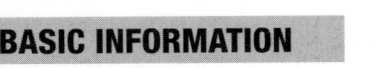

BASIC INFORMATION

DEFINITION

Secondary prevention of stroke involves preventing the recurrence of a cerebral vascular ischemic or hemorrhagic stroke after a primary event.

SYNONYMS

Brain attack
Stroke
Cerebral thrombosis
Cerebral hemorrhage
Brain infarct

ICD-9CM CODES

433 Precerebral vessel occlusion
434 Cerebral vessel thrombosis or occlusion

EPIDEMIOLOGY

Stroke is the third leading cause of death in the U.S. and the leading cause of morbidity. Each year, there are a total of 750,000 strokes, of which approximately 200,000 are recurrent strokes. Thus, secondary prevention of ischemic stroke remains good treatment strategy. Secondary prevention is specifically targeted toward modifiable risk factors.

RISK FACTORS: Age is the most important non-modifiable risk factor for stroke. Modifiable risk factors include hypertension, hyperlipidemia, cigarette smoking, excessive alcohol consumption, physical inactivity, obesity (i.e., a body mass index of >25 kg/m^2), and diabetes mellitus.

GENETICS: Multifactorial

PHYSICAL FINDINGS & CLINICAL PRESENTATION

- Stroke can have a varied presentation. Typically, the individual has a sudden definable loss of motor, sensory, visual, or cognitive functions that have a clear time of onset and that are noticed by others or by the individuals themselves.
- Physical findings such as weakness and/or numbness in one limb or on one side of the body, facial droop, visual field loss, or the inability to understand or communicate with others raises one's suspicion of a stroke event.

ETIOLOGY

- Strokes are broadly divided into ischemic or hemorrhagic (i.e., intraparenchymal or subarachnoid hemorrhage)
- Ischemic strokes can be caused by large-vessel atherosclerosis, cardioembolism such as in atrial fibrillation or cardiomyopathy, or small vessel disease such as lacunar stroke. Rare causes such as recreational drug use (e.g., cocaine abuse); arterial dissection; and hypercoagulable states need to be considered when ischemic stroke occurs in younger individuals.

- The most common cause of intracerebral hemorrhage is uncontrolled hypertension. Spontaneous rupture of a brain aneurysm causes subarachnoid hemorrhage.

DIAGNOSIS

DIFFERENTIAL DIAGNOSIS

- Seizure and postictal states
- Complicated migraine
- Hypoglycemia
- Brain tumor
- Somatization disorder

WORKUP

- Blood glucose level at the bedside or in the office
- aPTT, PT/INR, CBC, and CMP
- Fasting lipid panel
- Hypercoagulability tests for young stroke patients with no obvious risk factors

IMAGING STUDIES

- Computed tomography scanning of the head without contrast can differentiate between ischemic and hemorrhagic stroke. MRI of the brain is a more specific test.
- Carotid ultrasound and transcranial Doppler are used to detect large-vessel atherosclerosis. Magnetic resonance and computed tomography angiography are good alternatives.
- Echocardiogram and ECG can be used to detect a cardioembolic source.

TREATMENT

The secondary prevention of stroke is targeted toward modifiable risk factors. These include lifestyle modifications such as appropriate diet, exercise, weight loss, and smoking cessation, and risk factor modification as listed below. All patients with noncardioembolic ischemic stroke or transient ischemic attack (TIA), should be on aspirin (50 to 325 mg/day), a combination of aspirin and extended-release dipyridamole, or clopidogrel. Both a combination of aspirin and extended-release dipyridamole or clopidogrel. were found to be superior to aspirin in comparison trials. A consultation with a neurologist should be considered for young stroke patients and for patients with no obvious cause or with stroke from unusual causes (e.g., hypercoagulable states, dissections).

PREVENTING STROKE IN SPECIFIC CONDITIONS

1. Cardioembolic strokes as a result of atrial fibrillation have two first-line drug therapies: warfarin and dabigatran. Warfarin remains a first-line therapy with an international normalized ratio (INR) between 2.0 and 3.0. Dabigatran has equal efficacy as warfarin without the need for routine monitoring of INR. Dabigatran is approved by the U.S. Food and Drug Administration at a dosing regimen of 150 mg twice a day. For patients

with contraindications to anticoagulants, aspirin (325 mg/day) is recommended. The Active-A trial suggested that a combination of aspirin and clopidogrel is slightly better than aspirin alone for those unable to tolerate warfarin.

2. Cardioembolic strokes as a result of a prosthetic metallic valve: anticoagulant therapy with warfarin is recommended with a goal INR between 2.5 and 3.5.

3. Strokes as a result of large-vessel atherosclerois (i.e., symptomatic carotid stenosis): for patients with recent TIA or ischemic stroke within the last 6 months and ipsilateral severe (70% to 99%) carotid artery stenosis, carotid endarterectomy (CEA) performed by a surgeon is recommended and results in a perioperative morbidity and mortality rate of $<6\%$. For patients with recent TIA or ischemic stroke and ipsilateral moderate (50% to 69%) carotid stenosis, CEA is recommended. When the degree of stenosis is $<50\%$, there is no indication for CEA. Carotid stenting is not indicated except for cases in which surgery is high risk. Current trials are comparing carotid endarterectomy versus carotid stenting.

4. Symptomatic intracranial atherosclerosis: treatment with aspirin has proven effective and just as efficacious as warfarin in both the WASID and WARSS studies. The utility of angioplasty and stenting in patients with symptomatic intracranial atherosclerosis is available at several stroke centers but remains investigational (Fig. 1-792). In April 2011 the NINDS stopped enrollment into the symptomatic intracranial artery stenosis stenting trial, SAMMPRIS.

5. Patent foramen ovale (PFO): the American Academy of Neurology recommends medical therapy for stroke patients with PFO. Trials are under way to evaluate if endovascular PFO closure reduces the risk of recurrent transient ischemic attacks or strokes.

6. Intracerebral hemorrhage: for immediate management, please refer to the chapter on intracerebral hemorrhage. Antiplatelet agents should be held for 3 to 4 weeks and can be restarted if there is a compelling indication such as nonvalvular atrial fibrillation. The American Stroke Association/American Heart Association 2010 guideline recommends avoiding long-term anticoagulation (e.g., warfarin, heparin) after spontaneous lobar intracerebral hemorrhage, but antiplatelet therapy (e.g., aspirin, clopidogrel, Aggrenox) may be considered in all cases of intracerebral hemorrhage where there is a definite indication. Consider a neurology consultation in these cases.

PREVENTING LONG-TERM COMPLICATIONS AFTER A STROKE

Rehabilitation is integral to the reduction of morbidity and mortality of persons suffering

from a stroke with residual motor or speech deficits. Evaluation by a physical, occupational, and speech therapist will reduce the long-term disability that can follow a stroke event. The American Stroke Association 2010 guideline recommends a multidisciplinary approach to rehabilitation. Studies have shown an improved survival and recovery. Home-based rehabilitation can be considered after discussion with the rehabilitation specialist.

RISK FACTOR MODIFICATION

1. Hypertension: antihypertensive treatment is recommended for both the prevention of recurrent stroke and the prevention of other vascular events in persons who have had an ischemic stroke or a TIA. An absolute target blood pressure level and reduction are uncertain and should be individualized. Blood pressure should be lowered gradually over a period of months to prevent cerebral hypoperfusion and extension of stroke. Lifestyle modifications as listed above should be included as part of a comprehensive antihypertension treatment plan.
2. Diabetes: the goal for the hemoglobin A_{1c} level should be <7%. For type 2 diabetics, diet and exercise can prove very beneficial. Type 1 diabetics can also benefit from diet and compliance with their insulin regimen. Uncontrolled hyperglycemia can lead to acceleration of both intracranial and extracranial arteriosclerosis. Always consider consulting a diabetic educator.
3. Hyperlipidemia: for patients with ischemic stroke or TIA with elevated cholesterol levels, statin agents are recommended. The target goals for cholesterol lowering are an LDL-C level of <100 mg/dl and an LDL-C

level of <70 mg/dl for very high-risk persons with multiple risk factors (e.g., both coronary artery disease and diabetes).
4. Cigarette smoking: absolute cessation is required. Try to offer pharmacologic therapy or counseling services to the patient. Secondhand tobacco exposure is just as dangerous, so inquire about secondhand exposure.
5. Obesity: weight reduction may be considered for all overweight ischemic stroke and TIA patients to maintain the goal of a body mass index of between 18.5 and 24.9 kg/m^2 and a waist circumference of <35 in for women and <40 in for men.
6. Excessive alcohol consumption: patients with ischemic stroke or TIA who are heavy drinkers should eliminate or reduce their consumption of alcohol. Light to moderate levels of no more than two drinks per day for men and one drink per day for nonpregnant women may be considered.

DISPOSITION

Secondary stroke prevention is a multifaceted approach of lifestyle modification and pharmacologic intervention that is aimed at preventing or limiting disability.

REFERRAL

For complicated recurrent strokes, a referral to a neurologist who specializes in stroke is recommended.

PEARLS & CONSIDERATIONS

The modification of risk factors is the best preventive measure for stroke. Lifestyle modification is a very important aspect of secondary stroke prevention. Always consider the patient's

ability to afford the therapy and prescribed follow-up tests. Experience teaches us that patients sometimes will not let us know about their ability to afford therapies unless we inquire.

PREVENTION

Prevention is the goal of treatment, and compliance is the most important factor. Review risk factor reduction and pharmacologic therapy as previously discussed.

PATIENT/FAMILY EDUCATION

More information can be obtained from the following sources:
- American Heart Association, National Center, 7272 Greenville Avenue, Dallas, TX 75231
- American Stroke Association, 1-888-4-STROKE or 1-888-478-7653
- H.O.P.E. for Stroke, 250 Duck Pond Drive, Wantagh, NY 11793, 516-804-8495

EBM EVIDENCE

available at www.expertconsult.com

SUGGESTED READINGS

available at www.expertconsult.com

RELATED CONTENT

Stroke (Patient Information)

AUTHOR: **NAWAZ HACK, M.D.**

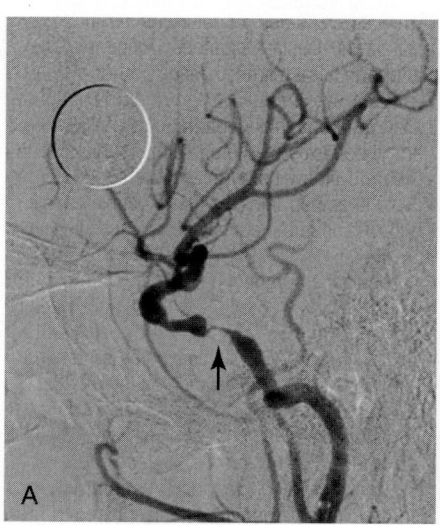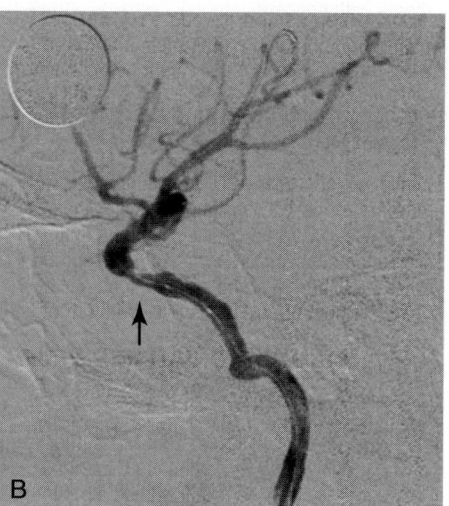

FIGURE 1-792 A, Intracranial high-grade symptomatic stenosis. **B,** This patient failed aggressive medical therapy and responded only to angioplasty and stenting.

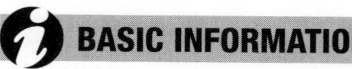

BASIC INFORMATION

DEFINITION

Stuttering is a problem of speech fluency, usually starting in early childhood. Stuttered speech is broken by repetitions, prolongations or abnormal stoppages of sounds, syllables, or words.

SYNONYMS

Speech dysfluency

ICD-9CM CODES
307.00 Stuttering

EPIDEMIOLOGY & DEMOGRAPHICS

INCIDENCE: Approximately 5% of children have stuttered 6 months or more. About 1% of the population is affected by stuttering at any given time.
PREDOMINANT SEX AND AGE: During childhood, twice as many boys stutter as girls. More girls than boys outgrow stuttering, which results in four times as many men stuttering as women.
GENETICS: Studies show higher rates of stuttering within families of those who stutter and a higher concordance for stuttering in identical twins compared to fraternal twins.
RISK FACTORS: Presence of other speech or language disorder, family history of stuttering, onset after 3.5 years of age, male sex, and stuttering over 6 months in duration.

PHYSICAL FINDINGS & CLINICAL PRESENTATION

- Stuttering usually presents between the ages of 2 and 5, when normal language development begins and children are transitioning from using simple phrases to more complex sentences. Stuttered speech is characterized by at least one of the following: repetitions (for for for example), prolongations (fffffffor example), interjections, broken words, audible or silent blocking, and circumlocutions.
- If stuttering is left untreated, it can lead to significant impairment in academic, social, and occupational spheres. Affected individuals show fear and embarrassment around speech and may avoid speaking in some situations. Compensatory maladaptive behaviors may also develop such as eyelid closing, involuntary movements, and some physical tension around the mouth during speech.
- Differentiating stuttering from normal developmental dysfluency is important. Normal dysfluency occurs in many children, is self-limited, and does not need treatment. It is characterized by occasional stuttering events (once every 10 sentences) and brief stuttering events (<0.5 second). The child does not seem concerned about the dysfluency and the disrupted speech tends to come and go based on whether the child is tired, excited, or talking about new or complex topics. Stuttering, in comparison, is defined by more frequent ($>3\%$ to 10% of speech) and longer stuttering events (>0.5 second). Also, the repetitions are greater in number ("for for for for example" as opposed to "for for for

example") and the prolongations are longer ("Forrrrrrrrrrrrrrrr example" as opposed to "Forrrrr example").

ETIOLOGY

- Stuttering arises from a combination of genetic and environmental influences.
- Although several specific chromosomal abnormalities have been found to explain a few cases of stuttering, the genetic causes of most cases are still being investigated. Susceptibility to nonsyndromic stuttering is associated with variations in genes governing lysosomal metabolism.
- Stuttering might be related to abnormal elevations of cerebral dopamine activity.
- Brain imaging studies show distinct differences in sensorimotor integration centers in the brains of those who stutter compared to controls.
- Although parents do not cause their child's stuttering, a critical, impatient, or interrupting speech environment can lead to worsening stuttered speech.

DIAGNOSIS

DIFFERENTIAL DIAGNOSIS

Stuttering is classified as neurogenic, psychogenic, or developmental. Neurogenic stuttering can result from traumatic brain injuries (TBIs) or cerebrovascular accidents. Psychogenic stuttering is usually preceded by an emotional stressor. Those affected by psychogenic stuttering are usually not overly concerned about the dysfluency and their stuttering does not improve when singing or when reciting something in a chorus, as is the case in developmental stuttering. Developmental stuttering, known simply as stuttering, is the most common form and usually presents in the preschool years.

WORKUP

- The clinical interview should include assessment of symptoms (onset, context, quality, frequency, duration, etc.) and impact on academic, social, or occupational spheres. A developmental history and family history of stuttering should be obtained, as well as assessing for family discord or recent emotional stressors. One should also try to assess parental response to the child's stuttering (intrusive/critical/anxious vs. accepting/patient/calm).
- A full physical exam should be conducted with special attention to the mental status exam and neurologic exam.
- No laboratory tests or imaging studies are indicated unless neurogenic stuttering is suspected.
- Evaluation by an audiologist for a formal hearing assessment to rule out hearing loss or discrimination disorder may be beneficial in some cases.

TREATMENT

NONPHARMACOLOGIC THERAPY

- Typically, the treatment of choice for stuttering is Speech and Language Therapy (SALT). Medications are not a first-line treatment.

- SALT consists of the following treatment modalities: fluency-shaping mechanisms, stuttering modification, delayed auditory feedback devices, and the Lidcombe approach (parental involvement).
- The above therapies help the child reduce fear about stuttering and produce speech more easily. The child is helped to speak slower and without increased physical tension and struggle. Families are encouraged to create an atmosphere of acceptance and calm for their child to speak and to model slower speech.
- After about a year of speech therapy, children's stuttering will gradually decrease in frequency and duration.

ACUTE GENERAL Rx

- There have been no large-scale pharmacologic treatment trials for stuttering. Smaller-scale trials and case studies have been conducted with a variety of agents, including clonidine, antipsychotics, and GABA-A partial agonists. Clonidine was found to be ineffective in reducing speech dysfluency. Weaker studies involving antipsychotic medications have found some positive effects, but almost all of these studies have serious methodologic problems and the associated side-effect profile makes using these agents for the long-term treatment of stuttering prohibitive. In some instances (e.g., a TBI patient with resulting neurogenic stuttering and psychosis), an antipsychotic might work well. A recent double-blind, randomized, placebo-controlled study of the GABA-A partial agonist, pagoclone, showed a modest reduction in speech dysfluency in adults.
- Case reports of deep brain stimulation of the ventral intermediate nucleus of the thalamus have shown some reduction in speech dysfluency in adults with severe stuttering.

DISPOSITION

Although adults who stutter improve in treatment, the best results occur when children are referred early.

REFERRAL

Those with severe stuttering should be referred immediately to a speech-language pathologist for further evaluation and treatment. Those with mild stuttering should be referred if the stuttering continues for longer than 6 weeks or if there is significant concern by the parent or child.

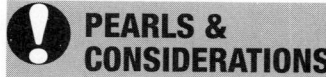

PEARLS & CONSIDERATIONS

Further information for patients and families can be found through the Stuttering Foundation of America (www.stutteringhelp.org).

SUGGESTED READINGS
available at www.expertconsult.com

AUTHOR: JAMISON ROGERS, M.D.

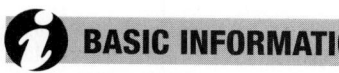

DEFINITION

Subarachnoid hemorrhage (SAH) is defined as hemorrhage into the subarachnoid space. Box 1-67 describes the Hunt and Hess clinical classification of SAH.

SYNONYMS

Subarachnoid bleed

ICD-9CM CODES

430 Subarachnoid hemorrhage

EPIDEMIOLOGY & DEMOGRAPHICS

INCIDENCE: ~6 to 8 cases/100,000 persons per yr

PREDOMINANT SEX: Women aged >55 yr were found to have a 25% greater risk of developing SAH compared with men of the same age.

PREDOMINANT AGE: The mean age at onset is 55 yr.

PEAK INCIDENCE: Most aneurysmal SAH occurs in people who are between the ages of 55 and 60 yr.

GENETICS:
- First-degree relatives have a 5 to 12 times greater risk of developing SAH compared with the general population.
- Autosomal dominant polycystic kidney disease is known to be associated with cerebral aneurysms in 8% of cases; screening is recommended in families with this condition in which one family member has experienced a ruptured aneurysm.

RISK FACTORS: Although genetics seem to play a factor in SAH, lifestyle factors are more important for determining overall risk. These risk factors include smoking, hypertension, oral contraception, pregnancy, and cocaine use.

PHYSICAL FINDINGS & CLINICAL PRESENTATION

- The primary symptom is a sudden, severe headache in 97% of cases. This is classically described as the "worst headache of my life" and also called a thunderclap headache.
- 30% to 60% of patients report a history of sentinel bleeds with short-lasting headaches during the weeks before the hemorrhage.
- The onset of the headache may be associated with a brief loss of consciousness, seizure, nausea or vomiting, and meningismus.
- Altered mental status and coma may result from the direct effect of the SAH causing a mass effect and increased intracranial pressure.
- A posterior communication aneurysm may cause third cranial nerve palsy.
- Table E1-382 describes the World Federation of Neurologic Surgeons clinical classification of SAH.

ETIOLOGY

- Trauma is the most common cause of SAH; a ruptured aneurysm is the most common cause of spontaneous SAH (75%-80% of spontaneous SAH).
- Idiopathic SAH, also known as angiogram-negative SAH, accounts for 15% to 20% of spontaneous SAH. In these cases, no angiographic cause of the hemorrhage is found.
- Other causes of spontaneous SAH include arteriovenous malformations, bleeding into preexisting tumors, vasculitis, and cerebral artery dissection.
- Cocaine abuse, sickle cell anemia, coagulopathies, and pituitary apoplexy can also result in SAH.

DIAGNOSIS

DIFFERENTIAL DIAGNOSIS

- Intracerebral hemorrhage as a result of trauma, tumors, and stroke with hemorrhagic conversion
- Other causes: thunderclap headaches such as idiopathic thunderclap headache, sexual headache, cough headache, exertional headache, secondary causes including pituitary apoplexy, acute hydrocephalus, etc.

WORKUP

- Computed tomography (CT) of the head: shows hemorrhage in more than 95% of cases, especially during the acute phase (i.e., 24 to 48 hr) after the onset of bleeding. Box 1-68 describes the Fisher grade of SAH on initial CT. About 3%-5% of SAH may be missed on initial CT of the head.
- Lumbar puncture should be performed in all cases of suspected SAH with "normal CT of the head." The following suggest SAH:
  - An RBC count of more than 100,000/m^3 in tubes 1 and 4.
  - Presence of xanthochromia or bilirubin in the cerebrospinal fluid.
- CT angiogram or a cerebral angiogram is imperative for determining the origin of the SAH. Angiography may also be extremely useful, because it may offer a therapeutic benefit via the coiling of the aneurysm.

LABORATORY TESTS

- Basic laboratory values, including CBC, chemistry panel, prothrombin time, partial thromboplastin time, and platelet count
- Serum troponin and sodium levels are important to guide management; elevated troponins indicate cardiac ischemia and a poor outcome.
- Sodium levels should be monitored frequently and patients should be kept normonatremic to slightly hypernatremic, especially when they enter the vasospasm window.

IMAGING STUDIES

- High-resolution CT scanning (Fig. 1-795) correctly identifies more than 95% of SAH cases, with blood appearing hyperdense in the subarachnoid spaces.
- Cerebral angiography is the gold standard for diagnosis and may offer a therapeutic option via coiling.

BOX 1-67 Hunt and Hess Clinical Classification of Subarachnoid Hemorrhage

I	Asymptomatic or mild headache and neck stiffness
II	Moderate to severe headache and neck stiffness ± cranial nerve palsy
III	Mild focal deficit, lethargy, or confusion
IV	Stupor, moderate to severe hemiparesis
V	Deep coma, extensor posturing

From Vincent JL et al: *Textbook of critical care,* ed 6, Philadelphia, 2011, Saunders.

BOX 1-68 Fisher Grade of Subarachnoid Hemorrhage on Initial Computed Tomography

1	No blood detected
2	Diffuse or vertical layers <1 mm thick
3	Localized subarachnoid clot and/or vertical layers ≥1 mm thick
4	Intraparenchymal or intraventricular clot with diffuse or no SAH

Modified Fisher CT Rating Scale

1	Minimal or diffuse thin SAH without IVH
2	Minimal or thin SAH with IVH
3	Thick cisternal clot without IVH
4	Thick cisternal clot with IVH

CT, Computed tomography; *IVH,* intraventricular hemorrhage; *SAH,* subarachnoid hemorrhage.
From Vincent JL et al: *Textbook of critical care,* ed 6, Philadelphia, 2011, Saunders.

- MRI is not a good imaging modality during the acute phase; however, its sensitivity increases after 4 to 7 days.

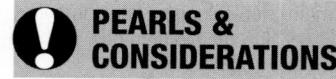 TREATMENT

NONPHARMACOLOGIC THERAPY
- Patients with a depressed level of consciousness may need to be intubated and mechanically ventilated in an intensive care unit setting.
- A lumbar drain or a ventriculostomy is required should the patient develop hydrocephalus and increased intracranial pressure.

ACUTE GENERAL Rx
- Critical care management: initial management strategies are geared toward stabilizing the patient and preventing rehemorrhage and hydrocephalus.
- Blood pressure control: tight blood pressure control is paramount, before securing the aneurysm to protect against rerupture. This can be done with the use of antihypertensive infusions or as-needed medications. A systolic blood pressure of 120 to 150 mm Hg is recommended. Placement of arterial line is recommended.
- Pain control: using short-acting and less-sedating medications (e.g., codeine, low-dose morphine).
- Seizures occur in about 3% of patients during the acute phase; however, the use of prophylactic antiepileptics is controversial.
- Vasospasm: cerebral vasospasm is a dreaded complication leading to cerebral ischemia, disability, and death after SAH. It typically develops around day 3 after the hemorrhage

and reaches a peak on day 6 to 8. Treatment strategies include:
  - "Triple H" therapy—*H*ypertension, *H*ypervolemia, and *H*emodilution—is used in an attempt to provide adequate cerebral perfusion. Recent studies have, however, recommended the use of euvolemia instead of hypervolemia as the latter was found to lead to significant cardiopulmonary and hemodynamic complications.
  - Nimodipine: has been shown to improve outcomes if it is administered between days 4 and 21 after the hemorrhage, even if it does not significantly reduce the amount of vasospasm detected on angiography.
- The underlying aneurysm should be treated by:
  - Clipping: performed through a craniotomy by placing a clip around the neck of the aneurysm.
  - Coiling: performed via intraarterial angiography; it consists of deploying platinum coils or liquid embolics (Onyx) inside the aneurysm to cause thrombosis of the aneurysmal sac.

CHRONIC Rx
- Management of reversible risk factors mentioned above (smoking, hypertension)
- Management of neurologic disability through physical therapy and rehabilitation.

DISPOSITION
- SAH is often associated with a poor outcome with a death rate between 40% and 50%; 10% to 15% of patients die before they reach the hospital.

- More than 46% of those who survive hospitalization have cognitive impairments that affect their lifestyles.

REFERRAL
Patients should be managed in a critical care setting with neurosurgical care.

PEARLS & CONSIDERATIONS

COMMENTS
- All thunderclap headaches should be considered SAH till proven otherwise and evaluated by CT of the head and/or LP.
- All SAH should be managed in a critical care setting (preferably neurocritical care unit) with neurosurgical care available.
- All anticoagulation and antiplatelet therapy should be withheld, and coagulopathy should be corrected.
- Measures to prevent rebleeding include adequate control of blood pressure and aneurysm treatment with the use of coiling or clipping.

PREVENTION
Controlling some of the modifiable risk factors, including smoking and blood pressure, may help to decrease the risk of aneurysmal rupture.

PATIENT & FAMILY EDUCATION
- SAH is a devastating condition, with most survivors developing significant cognitive deficits. A good support system and an adequate physical and cognitive rehabilitation program may prove useful to survivors.
- Screening may be useful for patients with two or three relatives with SAH.

EBM EVIDENCE
available at www.expertconsult.com

SUGGESTED READINGS
available at www.expertconsult.com

AUTHOR: **WISSAM S. Z. ASFAHANI, M.D.**

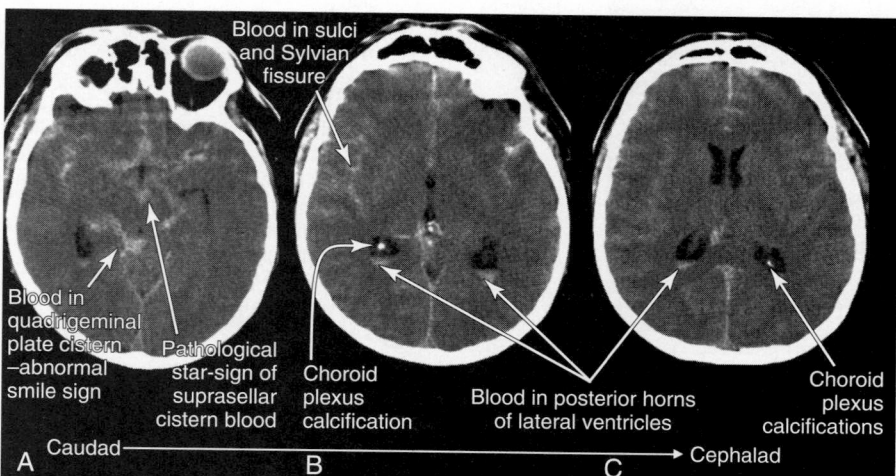

FIGURE 1-795 Subarachnoid hemorrhage (SAH), noncontrast CT, brain windows. Acute SAH appears white on noncontrast computed tomography (CT) brain windows. **A** through **C,** nonconsecutive axial slices, progressing from caudad to cephalad. In this case of diffuse SAH, note the presence of subarachnoid blood filling the sulci, as well as extending into the cisterns, Sylvian fissures, and even lateral ventricles. In **A,** blood *(white)* fills the suprasellar cistern. This star-shaped structure is normally filled with CSF *(black)*. The quadrigeminal plate cistern is normally a smile-shaped black crescent, filled with CSF, but in this case is filled with blood. Extremely bright calcifications in the choroid plexus of the posterior horns of the lateral ventricles are common, normal findings—do not mistake these for hemorrhage. Note their similarity in density to bone of the calvarium. (From Broder JS: *Diagnostic imaging for the emergency physician,* Philadelphia, 2011, Saunders.)

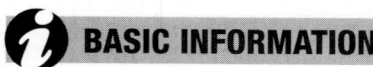 **BASIC INFORMATION**

DEFINITION

Subclavian steal syndrome is an occlusion or severe stenosis of the proximal subclavian artery leading to decreased antegrade flow or retrograde flow in the ipsilateral vertebral artery and neurologic symptoms referable to the posterior circulation.

SYNONYMS

Proximal subclavian (or innominate) artery stenosis or occlusion

ICD-9CM CODES
435.2 Subclavian steal syndrome

EPIDEMIOLOGY & DEMOGRAPHICS

- Similar to that of other manifestations of atherosclerosis (coronary artery disease, cerebrovascular disease, or peripheral vascular disease)
- Affects middle-aged persons (men somewhat younger than women on average) with arteriosclerotic risk factors, including family history, smoking, diabetes mellitus, hyperlipidemia, hypertension, and sedentary lifestyle

PHYSICAL FINDINGS & CLINICAL PRESENTATION

Symptoms:
- Many patients are asymptomatic.
- Upper extremity ischemic symptoms: fatigue, exercise-related aching, coolness, numbness of the involved upper extremity.
- Neurologic symptoms are reported by 25% of patients with known unilateral subclavian steal. These include brief spells of:
  1. Vertigo
  2. Diplopia
  3. Decreased vision
  4. Oscillopsia
  5. Gait unsteadiness

These spells are only occasionally provoked by exercising the ischemic upper extremity (classic subclavian steal). Left subclavian steal is more common than right, but the latter is more serious.
- Posterior circulation stroke related to subclavian steal is rare.
- Innominate artery stenosis can cause decreased right carotid artery flow and cerebrovascular symptoms of the anterior cerebral circulation, but this is uncommon.

Physical findings:
- Delayed and smaller volume pulse (wrist or antecubital) in the affected upper extremity

- Lower blood pressure in the affected upper extremity
- Supraclavicular bruit

NOTE: Inflating a blood pressure cuff will increase the bruit if it originates from a vertebral artery stenosis and decrease the bruit if it originates from a subclavian artery stenosis.

ETIOLOGY & PATHOGENESIS

Etiology:
- Atherosclerosis
- Arteritis (Takayasu's disease and temporal arteritis)
- Embolism to the subclavian or innominate artery
- Cervical rib
- Long-term use of a crutch
- Occupational (baseball pitchers and cricket bowlers)

Pathogenesis: the vertebral artery originates from the subclavian artery. For subclavian steal to occur, the occlusion must be proximal to the takeoff of the vertebral artery. On the right side, only a small distance separates the bifurcation of the innominate artery and the takeoff of the vertebral artery, explaining why the condition occurs less commonly on the right side. Occlusion of the innominate artery must affect right carotid artery flow.

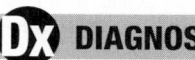 **DIAGNOSIS**

The carotid arteries should be evaluated at least noninvasively in all cases.

DIFFERENTIAL DIAGNOSIS

- Posterior circulation transient ischemic attack or stroke
- Upper extremity ischemia
  1. Distal subclavian artery stenosis or occlusion
  2. Raynaud's syndrome
  3. Thoracic outlet syndrome

WORKUP

- Noninvasive upper extremity arterial flow studies
- Doppler sonography of the vertebral, subclavian, and innominate arteries
- Arteriography, magnetic resonance arteriogram (Fig. 1-796)

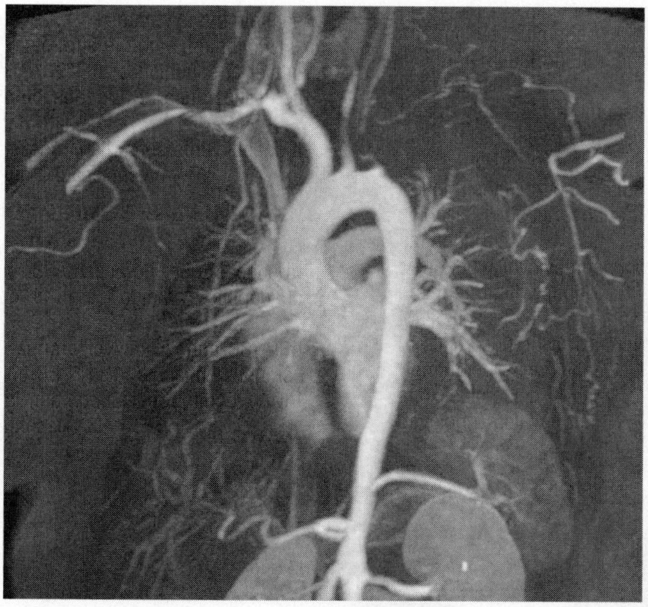

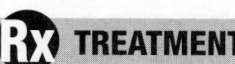 **TREATMENT**

- In most patients the disease is benign and requires no treatment other than atherosclerosis risk factor modification and aspirin. Symptoms tend to improve over time as collateral circulation develops.
- Vascular surgical reconstruction requires a thoracotomy; it may be indicated in innominate artery stenosis or when upper extremity ischemia is incapacitating.

AUTHOR: **FRED F. FERRI, M.D.**

FIGURE 1-796 Magnetic resonance arteriogram demonstrating diffuse moderate stenosis of the proximal left common carotid and proximal occlusion of the left subclavian artery coming off the aortic arch with development of an extensive collateral network. (From Hochberg MC et al: *Rheumatology,* ed 5, St Louis, 2011, Mosby.)

BASIC INFORMATION

DEFINITION

A subdural hematoma (SDH) is a collection of blood or blood products between the arachnoidal (superficial) layer of the brain and the dura or meningeal layer of the brain. Subdural hematomas can be acute (ASDH) or chronic (CSDH).

SYNONYMS

Subdural hemorrhage

ICD-9CM CODES
852.10 Subdural hematoma

EPIDEMIOLOGY & DEMOGRAPHICS

INCIDENCE:
- The exact incidence of ASDH is unknown, but it is very common in trauma patients.
- CSDH is most common in the elderly with an incidence of 1.72 to 13.1 per 100,000.
- Patients on warfarin have a reported incidence between 21% and 36%.

PREVALENCE: Unknown

PREDOMINANT AGE AND SEX:
- Patients with cerebral atrophy such as the elderly (>70 yr) and alcoholic populations
- Infant population (e.g., shaken baby)

RISK FACTORS:
- Trauma and antithrombotic therapy are the most common risk factors for ASDH and CSDH.
- Brain atrophy secondary to advanced age and alcoholism are common risk factors, especially with the coagulopathy seen in chronic alcoholics.
- Intracranial hypotension associated with CSF shunts or leaks is uncommon but important.

PHYSICAL FINDINGS & CLINICAL PRESENTATION

Symptoms vary on the basis of acuity, size, and location. Acute traumatic SDHs are often seen in comatose patients. When associated with a midline shift (i.e., >5 mm), they can cause signs of cerebral herniation (e.g., ipsilateral pupil dilation, contralateral weakness) requiring prompt surgical evacuation.
- Patients with CSDH may present with diverse nonspecific symptoms such as headaches, confusion, aphasia, hemiparesis, TIA-like symptoms, and seizures.

ETIOLOGY

SDH is usually the result of shearing and tearing of a bridging vein between the brain parenchyma and the dura mater. Other causes of bleeding into the subdural space include contusion, extension of parenchymal hemorrhage, rarely other vascular abnormalities (e.g., AV malformation, aneurysm, dural AV fistula).

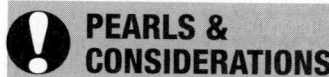 **DIAGNOSIS**

DIFFERENTIAL DIAGNOSIS

Other causes of subdural collections, such as hygromas, abscesses, and tumor infiltrations

WORKUP

- Clinical assessment: patient history, including medications with anticoagulant properties, alcohol abuse, trauma, cancer, and recent bacterial infections
- Physical examination, including alertness, pupil and facial symmetry, and motor weakness (i.e., pronator drift)
- Noncontrast CT scan of the head

LABORATORY TESTS

Assessment of the patient's coagulation status including CBC with platelet count, prothrombin time, partial thromboplastin time and liver function test (especially with a history of alcoholism or liver failure)

IMAGING STUDIES

CT scan of the head (Fig. 1-797): demonstrates the classic crescentic collection between the brain and the inner table. For comatose and trauma patients, include a cervical spine CT scan. ASDH is usually hyperdense, whereas a CSDH is usually hypodense on noncontrast CT. Contrast is only needed if there are concerns about tumor or infection.

TREATMENT

- Correction of underlying coagulopathy, if present (e.g., Coumadin reversal)
- The majority of SDH can be managed without surgery in awake patients with normal neurologic examinations.

NONPHARMACOLOGIC THERAPY

Surgical treatment is indicated in:
- All ASDHs measuring >10 mm in thickness with a midline shift >5 mm on CT scan should be evacuated.
- CSDH with a mass effect, a clear change in the neurologic examination from baseline, or enlargement of the hematoma size, evacuation via craniotomy or burr hole should be considered.

DISPOSITION

Depending on the size and location of the SDH and the examination of the patient, observation can range from the ICU to outpatient management. When observation of the patient is considered, clinical examinations should be serially performed. Patient baseline and follow-up clinical examinations are more important than CT scan findings.

REFERRAL

Neurosurgical and operative consultation should be made available.

PEARLS & CONSIDERATIONS

COMMENTS

- Many elderly patients have small CSDHs or hygromas. Unless these are associated with seizures or clinical or radiographic progression, they are usually not emergent. The important thing is to recognize the cause (e.g., medication, fall risk).
- Recurrence after surgical management for CSDH is common.
- SDHs in elderly patients can have a mixed hyperdense and hypodense appearance on noncontrast CT scan; this is suggestive of acute and chronic components.

PATIENT & FAMILY EDUCATION

Individuals with SDHs are at higher risk for seizure, so surveillance is important.

RELATED CONTENT

Subdural Hematoma (Patient Information)

AUTHOR: **WISSAM S. Z. ASFAHANI, M.D.**

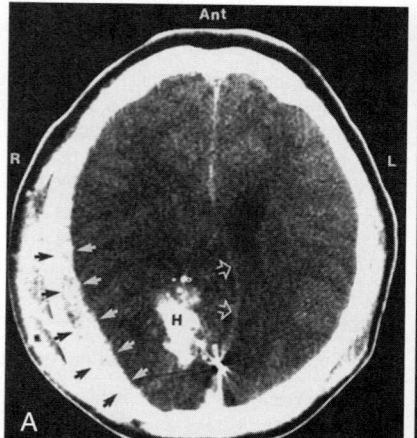
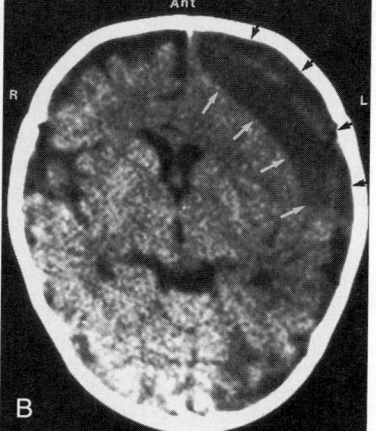

FIGURE 1-797 A, Noncontrast CT scan of an acute subdural hematoma shows a crescentic area of increased density in the right posterior parietal region between the brain and the skull *(black and white arrows)*. An area of intraparenchymal hemorrhage (H) is also seen. **B,** A chronic subdural hematoma for a different patient is shown. There is an area of decreased density in the left frontoparietal region *(arrows)* that effaces the sulci, compresses the anterior horn of the left lateral ventricle, and shifts the midline somewhat to the right. (From Mettler FA [ed]: *Primary care radiology*, Philadelphia, 2000, Saunders.)

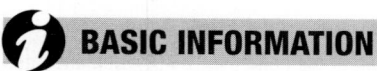

BASIC INFORMATION

DEFINITION
Suicide is the intentional ending of one's own life.

SYNONYMS
Self-murder

ICD-9CM CODES
Categorized by method

EPIDEMIOLOGY & DEMOGRAPHICS
INCIDENCE (IN U.S.): Mortality (CDC, 2007 data)

All suicides
- Number of deaths: 34,598
- Deaths per 100,000 population: 11.5
- Cause of death rank: 11th leading cause of death

Firearm suicides
- Number of deaths: 17,352
- Deaths per 100,000 population: 5.8

Suffocation suicides
- Number of deaths: 8161
- Deaths per 100,000 population: 2.7

Poisoning suicides
- Number of deaths: 6358
- Deaths per 100,000 population: 2.1

Suicidal deaths are only part of the problem. More people survive suicide attempts than actually die. They are often seriously injured and need medical care.

AGE-RELATED DATA:
- Incidence of suicide increases with age (13.1 cases/100,000 persons ages 15 to 24 yr, 16.9 cases/100,000 persons ages 65 to 74 yr, and 23.5 cases/100,000 persons ages 75 to 84 yr)
- During 2002 to 2006, the greatest percentage of suicides occurred by firearm among all race/ethnicity groups for persons ages 65 yr and older. Except for Asian/Pacific Islanders, suffocation accounted for the highest percentage of suicides among those 65 yr and older (52.6%).

GENDER DIFFERENCES:
- Women attempt suicide about two to three times as often as men.
- Males succeed at taking their own lives at nearly four times the rate of females and represent 79% of all U.S. suicides.
- Suicide is the seventh leading cause of death for males and sixteenth leading cause for females.

- Firearms are the most common method of suicide among males (56%).
- Poisoning is the most common method in women (40.3%).

ENVIRONMENTAL FACTORS:
- Suicide rates traditionally decrease in times of war and increase in times of economic crises.
- After adjusting for age, suicide rates are highest in the western and northwestern regions of the United States.

MARITAL STATUS: Suicide rates are highest among the divorced, separated, and widowed and lowest among the married.

SUBSTANCE USE: CDC data: 33.3% of suicides tested positive for alcohol and 16.4% for opiates.

RISK FACTORS (Table 1-383):
- Previous suicide attempt(s).
- History of depression or other mental illness (bipolar, psychosis, PTSD, and others).
- Anxiety.
- Alcohol or drug abuse.
- Family history of suicide or violence.
- Physical illness. Patients who have recently received a cancer diagnosis have increased risk of suicide.
- Feeling alone.
- Individuals with a mental or substance use disorder account for >90% of suicides.
- The concurrence of more than one condition (e.g., depression and alcohol abuse) greatly increases the risk.
- Hopelessness is a strong predictor of suicide potential.
- Rates are higher in developing countries.
- Rates vary by occupation, ethnicity, and employment status.

SUICIDAL BEHAVIOR:
- All suicidal behavior should be taken seriously, as a failed attempt may lead to a completed suicide in the future.
- Nearly half of suicides are preceded by an attempt that does not end in death.
- Those with a history of attempts are 23 times more likely to eventually end their own lives than those without.
- A suicidal gesture does not have death as a goal, but can serve as a dramatic way of alerting others to some type of ongoing distress.
- Risky behaviors such as speeding or disregarding traffic laws, or abusing drugs, are considered parasuicide when the person

shows total disregard for whether the actions might result in his or her death.
- Unsuccessful suicide attempts may also result from miscalculations in the plan. These people are at high risk for attempting suicide again.

EVALUATION:
- The provider must directly inquire into the presence of suicidal ideation. Approximately one half to two thirds of individuals who commit suicide visit physicians within 1 mo of taking their lives.
- Explicit suicidal intent, hopelessness, and a well-formulated plan indicate high risk. Clinicians can use the mnemonic SAL: Is the method specific? Is it available? Is it lethal?
- The concurrence of multiple psychiatric problems, substance abuse, and multiple physical problems increases the risk.
- Covert suicidal ideation occurs in patients primarily with multiple vague physical complaints, depression, anxiety, or substance abuse.

ACUTE INTERVENTIONS
- Place patient in a safe environment (usually hospitalization in a psychiatric unit or a medical unit with continuous observation).
- Emergency medical stabilization and clearance as required, related to severity and lethality of attempt, age, comorbid medical issues, and overall clinical presentation.

ACUTE PSYCHOPHARMACOLOGIC INTERVENTIONS
- Benzodiazepines may be useful in reducing extreme anxiety and dysphoria in an acutely suicidal patient; however, these agents should not be prescribed until the means of the suicidal attempt are known (not a benzodiazepine overdose) and patient is medically stable (i.e., respiratory system, vital signs, cognitive functioning are stable).
- Antipsychotics (typicals or atypicals) can be used if psychosis is present (e.g., voices telling patient to hurt self) and to manage acute agitation.
- If indicated, mood stabilizers and antidepressants can be started in the acute setting but may have up to a 2-wk latency period. However, awareness of increased risk of suicidal thoughts/behavior with these medications in some populations is required.

TABLE 1-383 Suicide and Risk Factors: A Summary

Primary Diagnosis	Demographics	Personality Factors	Comorbidities	Social Factors	Other Factors
Bipolar	Male	Borderline	Substance abuse	Divorced	Means available
Schizophrenia	Older age	Narcissistic	Panic disorder	Widower	History of child abuse
Major depressive disorder	White race	Antisocial	Anxiety	Lives alone	Few reasons to live
Dysthymia	Homosexuality	Conduct disorder	Axis III dx	Isolated	Lots of adverse events
Adjustment disorder	History of attempt	Impulsive		Money worries	Change in grades
Conduct disorder	Family history			Other losses	Change in friends
Psychosis	Suicidal ideas			No religion	Giving things away
	Hopeless				Guns in the home
	Helpless				

From Sadock BJ et al: *Kaplan & Sadock's comprehensive textbook of psychiatry*, ed 9, Philadelphia, 2009, Wolters Kluwer Health/Lippincott Williams & Wilkins.

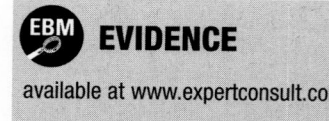

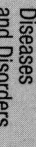

THERAPY

- Long-term: psychotherapy aimed at factors that underlie the decision to pursue suicide or at the risk factors contributing to suicidal behavior
- Substance abuse treatment (e.g., Alcoholics Anonymous, Narcotics Anonymous) when substance use disorder is present
- Therapy should be aimed at the underlying condition (e.g., antidepressants for depression, anxiolytics or antidepressants for anxiety, substance abuse treatment, or psychotherapy for chronic low self-esteem, hopelessness).
- In elderly, loneliness and medical disability are major reasons for suicide and therefore major targets for intervention.
- Involvement of family members, spouse, loved one, caregivers if possible for therapy and management.

EBM EVIDENCE

available at www.expertconsult.com

SUGGESTED READINGS

available at www.expertconsult.com

AUTHOR: **ALI KAZIM, M.D.**

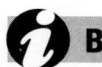

DEFINITION

Superior vena cava (SVC) syndrome is a set of symptoms that results when a mediastinal mass compresses the SVC or the veins that drain into it, resulting in obstruction of blood flow from the head, neck, upper torso, or extremities to the right atrium.

ICD-9CM CODES
453.2 Vena cava thrombosis

EPIDEMIOLOGY & DEMOGRAPHICS

- SVC syndrome occurs in 15,000 persons in the U.S. every year.
- More than 50% of patients present with SVC at the initial manifestation of a previously undiagnosed malignancy.
- Mirrors lung cancer (especially small cell carcinoma) and lymphoma (see "Lung Neoplasm" and "Lymphoma" in Section I).

PHYSICAL FINDINGS & CLINICAL PRESENTATION

The pathophysiology of the syndrome involves the increased pressure in the venous system draining into the SVC, producing edema of the head, neck, and upper extremities. Symptoms develop over a period of 2 wk in one third of patients and include:

- Shortness of breath
- Chest pain
- Cough
- Dysphagia, hoarseness, stridor
- Headache
- Syncope
- Visual trouble

Signs:
- Chest wall vein distention (Fig. 1-798)
- Neck vein distention
- Facial edema, facial plethora
- Upper extremity swelling
- Cyanosis

ETIOLOGY

- Lung cancer (65% of all cases, of which half are small cell lung cancer)
- Lymphoma (15%)
- Thymoma
- Tuberculosis
- Goiter
- Aortic aneurysm (arteriosclerotic or syphilitic)
- SVC thrombosis
  1. Primary: associated with a central venous catheter
  2. Secondary: as a complication of SVC syndrome associated with one of the above-mentioned causes
- Inflammatory process, fibrosing mediastinitis
- Table 1-384 summarizes common malignancies associated with SVC syndrome in adults.

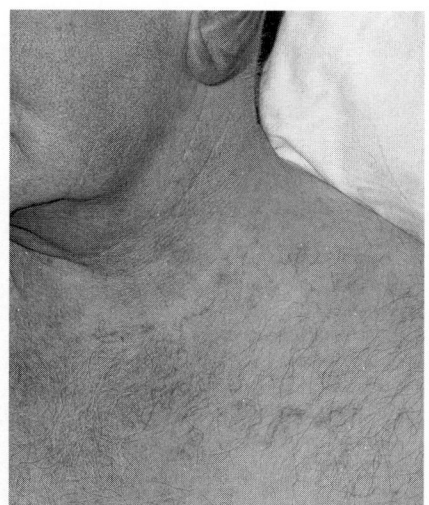

FIGURE 1-798 Superior vena cava obstruction causing dilated veins and plethora of the upper trunk and neck in a patient with bronchial carcinoma. Patients with superior vena cava obstruction are occasionally referred to dermatologists with suspected contact allergy (eyelid swelling) or angioedema (facial or hand swelling). (From White GM, Cox NH [eds]: *Diseases of the skin, a color atlas and text*, ed 2, St Louis, 2006, Mosby.)

DIAGNOSIS

CT scan of the chest with contrast is the most useful diagnostic study. MRI is usually adequate to establish the diagnosis of SVC obstruction and to assist in the differential diagnosis of probable cause.

DIFFERENTIAL DIAGNOSIS

The syndrome is characteristic enough to exclude other diagnoses. The differential diagnosis concerns the underlying etiologies listed above.

WORKUP

- Chest radiograph (mediastinal widening, pleural effusion)
- Chest CT with contrast or MRI (in patient who cannot tolerate contrast medium)
- Venography: warranted only when an intervention (e.g., stent or surgery) is planned
- Percutaneous needle biopsy or mediastinoscopy are usually the initial diagnostic modalities used to establish a histologic diagnosis

TREATMENT

- Although invasive procedures such as mediastinoscopy are associated with higher than usual risk of bleeding, a tissue diagnosis is usually needed before commencing therapy.
- Management is guided by the severity of the symptoms and the underlying etiology.
- Emergency empiric radiation is indicated in critical situations such as respiratory failure or central nervous system signs associated with increased intracranial pressure.
- Treatment of the underlying malignancy:
  1. Radiotherapy: the majority of tumors causing SVC syndrome are sensitive to radiotherapy
  2. Systemic chemotherapy
- Anticoagulant or fibrinolytic therapy in patients who do not respond to cancer treatment within a week or if an obstructing thrombus has been documented.
- Loop diuretics are often used, but their effect is limited.
- Upright positioning and fluid restriction until collateral channels develop and allow for clinical regression are useful modalities for SVC syndrome secondary to benign disease.
- Steroids (dexamethasone 4 mg q6h) may be useful in reducing the tumor burden in lymphoma and thymoma.
- Percutaneous self-expandable stents that can be placed under local anesthesia with radiologic manipulation are useful in the treatment of SVC syndrome to bypass the obstruction, especially in cases associated with malignant tumors.
- Surgical bypass grafting is infrequently used to treat SVC syndrome.

REFERRAL

To a thoracic surgeon, pulmonary specialist, or oncologist

AUTHOR: **FRED F. FERRI, M.D.**

TABLE 1-384 Malignancies Associated with Superior Vena Cava (SVC) Syndrome in Adults*

Neoplastic Diagnosis	Percentage of SVC	Percentage of Disease-Associated SVC
Lung cancer, stage 3B or 4:	48-81	
Small cell lung cancer		15-45
Squamous cell cancer		20-25
Adenocarcinoma		5-25
Large cell carcinoma		4-30
Lymphoma:	2-21	
Diffuse large cell lymphoma		64
Lymphoblastic lymphoma		33
Breast cancer	11	

*Include lung cancer, lymphomas, and metastases from other solid tumors. 75% to 85% of patients with SVC have neoplastic disease.
From Zipes DP et al (eds): *Braunwald's heart disease*, ed 7, Philadelphia, 2005, Saunders.

BASIC INFORMATION

DEFINITION

Syncope is the transient loss of consciousness with spontaneous recovery that results from an acute global reduction in cerebral blood flow. Syncope is a symptom, and the goal is to distinguish lethal causes from benign causes of transient loss of consciousness.

ICD-9CM CODES
780.2 Syncope

EPIDEMIOLOGY & DEMOGRAPHICS

- Syncope accounts for 3% to 5% of emergency department visits.
- 30% of the adult population will experience at least one syncopal episode during their lifetimes.
- Incidence of syncope is highest in elderly men and young women.

PHYSICAL FINDINGS & CLINICAL PRESENTATION

- Blood pressure: if low, consider orthostatic hypotension; if unequal in both arms (difference >20 mm Hg), consider subclavian steal or dissecting aneurysm. (NOTE: Blood pressure [BP] and heart rate should be recorded in the supine and standing positions, waiting at least 5 minutes between each position.) If there is a drop in BP but no change in heart rate (HR), the patient may be taking a beta-blocker or may have an autonomic neuropathy.
- Pulse: if patient has tachycardia, bradycardia, or irregular rhythm, consider arrhythmia.
- Heart: if there are murmurs present, consider syncope attributable to left ventricular outflow obstruction (aortic stenosis or idiopathic hypertrophic subaortic stenosis); if there are jugular venous distention and distal heart sounds, consider cardiac tamponade.
- Carotid sinus pressure: can be diagnostic if it reproduces symptoms and other causes are excluded; a pause >3 sec or a systolic BP drop >50 mm Hg without symptoms or <30 mm Hg with symptoms when sinus pressure is applied separately on each side for <5 sec is considered abnormal. This test should be avoided in patients with carotid bruits or cerebrovascular disease. ECG monitoring, IV access, and bedside atropine should be available when carotid sinus pressure is applied.

ETIOLOGY

- Neurally mediated syncope
  1. Psychophysiologic (emotional upset, panic disorders, hysteria, hyperventilation)
  2. Visceral reflex (micturition, defecation, food ingestion, coughing, ventricular contraction, glossopharyngeal neuralgia)
  3. Carotid sinus pressure
  4. Reduction of venous return caused by Valsalva maneuver
- Orthostatic hypotension
  1. Hypovolemia
  2. Vasodilator medications
  3. Autonomic neuropathy (diabetes, amyloid, Parkinson's disease, multisystem atrophy)

4. Pheochromocytoma
5. Carcinoid syndrome
- Cardiac
  1. Reduced cardiac output
     a. Left ventricular outflow obstruction (aortic stenosis, hypertrophic cardiomyopathy)
     b. Obstruction to pulmonary flow (pulmonary embolism, pulmonic stenosis, primary pulmonary hypertension)
     c. Myocardial infarct with pump failure
     d. Cardiac tamponade
     e. Mitral stenosis
     f. Reduction of venous return (atrial myxoma, valve thrombus)
     g. Beta-blocker therapy
  2. Arrhythmias or asystole
     a. Extreme tachycardia (>160 to 180 beats/min)
     b. Severe bradycardia (<30 to 40 beats/min)
     c. Sick sinus syndrome
     d. Atrioventricular block (second or third degree)
     e. Ventricular tachycardia or fibrillation
     f. Long QT syndrome
     g. Pacemaker malfunction
     h. Psychotropic medications and beta-blockers

DIAGNOSIS

DIFFERENTIAL DIAGNOSIS

1. Seizure (see "Workup")
2. Vertebrobasilar transient ischemic attack (TIA) usually manifests as diplopia, vertigo, or ataxia but not loss of consciousness. Isolated episodes of transient loss of consciousness (TLOC) without accompanying neurologic symptoms are unlikely to be TIAs.
3. Recreational drugs or alcohol.
4. Functional causes, such as stress and somatoform disorders.
5. Sleep disorders, such as sleep attacks and narcolepsy, are also in the differential for TLOC.
6. Head trauma.

WORKUP

The history is crucial to diagnosing the cause of syncope and may suggest a diagnosis that can be evaluated with directed testing. History is also important to determine other etiologies for TLOC, such as seizure. Fig. E1-799 describes an algorithm for syncope evaluation.
- Sudden LOC: consider cardiac arrhythmias.
- Gradual LOC: consider orthostatic hypotension, vasodepressor syncope, hypoglycemia.
- History of aura before LOC or prolonged confusion (>1 min), amnesia, or lethargy after LOC suggests seizure rather than syncope.
- Patient's activity at the time of syncope:
  1. Micturition, coughing, defecation: consider syncope caused by decreased venous return.
  2. Turning head or while shaving: consider carotid sinus syndrome.
  3. Physical exertion in a patient with murmur: consider aortic stenosis.

4. Arm exercise: consider subclavian steal syndrome.
5. Assuming an upright position: consider orthostatic hypotension.
- Associated events:
  1. Chest pain: consider myocardial infarction, pulmonary embolism.
  2. Palpitations: consider arrhythmias.
  3. Incontinence (urine or fecal) and tongue biting are associated with seizure or syncope.
  4. Brief, transient shaking after LOC may represent myoclonus from global cerebral hypoperfusion and not seizures. However, sustained tonic/clonic muscle action is more suggestive of seizure.
  5. Focal neurologic symptoms or signs point to a neurologic event such as a seizure with residual deficits (e.g., Todd's paralysis) or cerebral ischemic injury.
  6. Psychological stress: syncope may be vasovagal.
- Review current medications, particularly antihypertensive and psychotropic drugs.
- All patients presenting with syncope require electrocardiography, orthostatic vital signs, and QT interval monitoring.

LABORATORY TESTS

Routine blood tests rarely yield diagnostically useful information and should be done only if they are specifically suggested by the results of the history and physical examination. Box E1-69 describes possibly useful tests. The following are commonly ordered tests:
- Pregnancy test in women of childbearing age
- Complete blood count to look for anemia and signs of infection
- Electrolytes, blood urea nitrogen, creatinine, magnesium, and calcium to look for electrolyte abnormalities and evaluate fluid status
- Serum glucose level
- Cardiac troponins, especially if the patient gives a history of chest pain before the syncopal episode
- Drug and alcohol levels with suspected toxicity

IMAGING STUDIES

- ECG to rule out arrhythmias; may be diagnostic in 5% to 10% of patients.
- Echocardiography.
- If seizure is suspected, CT scan and/or MRI of the head and electroencephalogram may be useful.
- If head trauma or neurologic signs on examination, CT or MRI may be helpful.
- If arrhythmias are suspected, a 24-hr Holter monitor or admission to a telemetry unit is appropriate. In general, Holter monitoring is rarely useful, revealing a cause for syncope in <3% of cases. Loop recorders that can be activated after syncopal episode to retrieve information about the cardiac rhythm during the preceding 4 min add considerable diagnostic yield in patients with unexplained syncope.
- Implantable cardiac monitors that function as permanent loop recorders or implantable cardioverter-defibrillators, which are placed

subcutaneously in the pectoral region with the patient under local anesthesia, are useful in patients with cardiac syncope.

- Electrophysiologic studies may be indicated in patients with structural heart disease and/or recurrent syncope.

TILT-TABLE TESTING

- Useful to support a diagnosis of neurally mediated syncope. Patients age >50 yr should have stress testing before tilt-table testing. Positive results would preclude tilt-table testing.
- Indicated in patients with recurrent episodes of unexplained syncope as well as patients in high-risk occupations (e.g., pilots, bus drivers) (Fig. 1-800). The test is also useful for identifying patients with prominent bradycardic response who may benefit from implantation of a permanent pacemaker.
- It is performed by keeping the patient in an upright posture on a tilt table with footboard support. The angle of the tilt table varies from 60 to 80 degrees. The duration of upright posture during tilt-table testing varies from 25 to 45 min.

- The hallmark of neurally mediated syncope is severe hypotension associated with a paradoxic bradycardia triggered by a specific stimulus. The diagnosis of neurally mediated syncope is likely if upright tilt testing reproduces these hemodynamic changes in <15 min and causes presyncope or syncope.

PSYCHIATRIC EVALUATION

- May be indicated in young patients without heart disease who have frequently recurring transient loss of consciousness and other somatic symptoms.
- Generalized anxiety disorder, pain disorder, and major depression predispose patients to neurally mediated reactions and may result in syncope.

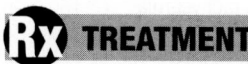 **TREATMENT**

NONPHARMACOLOGIC THERAPY

- Ensure proper hydration; consider compression stockings and salt tablets in appropriate patients.
- Eliminate medications that may induce hypotension.

ACUTE GENERAL Rx

- Varies with the underlying etiology of syncope (e.g., pacemaker in patients with syncope resulting from complete heart block).
- Syncope caused by orthostatic hypotension is treated with volume replacement in patients with intravascular volume depletion. Also consider midodrine to promote venous return by adrenergic-mediated vasoconstriction and Florinef for its mineralocorticoid effects to increase intravascular volume.

DISPOSITION

Prognosis varies with the age of the patient and the etiology of the syncope. In general:
- Benign prognosis (very low 1-yr morbidity rate) in patients:
  1. Age <30 yr and having noncardiac syncope
  2. Age <70 yr and having vasovagal or psychogenic syncope or syncope of unknown cause
- Poor prognosis (high mortality and morbidity rates) in patients with cardiac syncope, with presenting systolic BP <90 mm Hg.
- Patients with the following risk factors have a higher 1-yr mortality rate: abnormal ECG, history of ventricular arrhythmia, history of congestive heart failure.

REFERRAL

Hospital admission in elderly patients without prior history of syncope or unknown etiology of their syncope and in any patients suspected of having cardiac syncope, with presenting systolic BP <90 mm Hg..

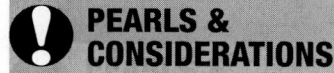 **PEARLS & CONSIDERATIONS**

COMMENTS

- Section III, "Palpitations, Dizziness, and/or Syncope," describes an algorithmic approach to the patient.
- The etiology of syncope is identified in <50% of cases during the initial evaluation.
- A thorough history and physical examination are the most productive means of establishing a diagnosis in patients with syncope.

SUGGESTED READINGS

available at www.expertconsult.com

RELATED CONTENT

Fig. 3-129 Algorithm for evaluating patients with symptoms of palpitation, dizziness, or syncope (Algorithm)
Syncope (Patient Information)

AUTHOR: **TZU-CHING (TEDDY) WU, M.D.**

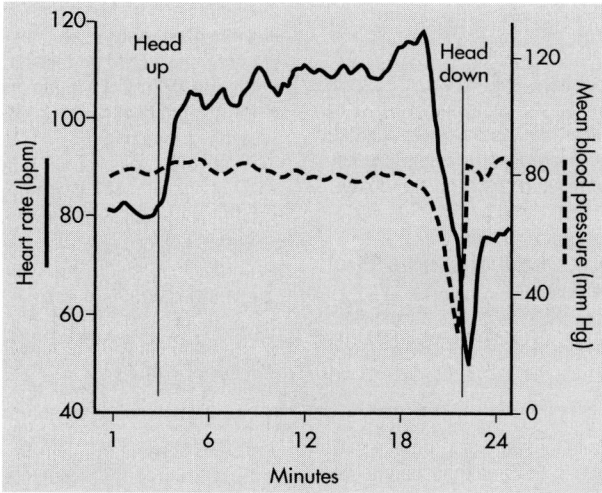

FIGURE 1-800 Head-up tilt test performed on an 18-year-old woman with a history of syncope associated with pain, preceded by a prodrome of dizziness, graying vision, and diaphoresis. A similar prodrome preceded syncope during the test. Note the precipitous and nearly simultaneous decline of heart rate and blood pressure after an initial rise in heart rate. Vital signs returned to normal rapidly after the head was lowered. (Courtesy Robert F. Sprung, University of Utah. In Goldman L, Ausiello D [eds]: *Cecil textbook of medicine,* ed 22, Philadelphia, 2004, Saunders.)

BASIC INFORMATION

DEFINITION

Syndrome of inappropriate antidiuresis (SIAD) is a syndrome characterized by excessive secretion of antidiuretic hormone (ADH) in absence of normal osmotic or physiologic stimuli (increased serum osmolarity, decreased plasma volume, hypotension).

SYNONYMS

SIAD
SIADH
Syndrome of inappropriate antidiuretic hormone secretion
Syndrome of inappropriate ADH release
Inappropriate secretion of antidiuretic hormone

ICD-9CM CODES
276.9 Inappropriate secretion of antidiuretic hormone

EPIDEMIOLOGY & DEMOGRAPHICS

SIAD is the most frequent cause of hyponatremia. Nearly 50% of hyponatremia detected in the hospital setting is caused by SIAD.

PHYSICAL FINDINGS & CLINICAL PRESENTATION

- The patient is generally normovolemic or slightly hypervolemic; edema is absent.
- Delirium, lethargy, and seizures may be present if the hyponatremia is severe or of rapid onset.
- Manifestations of the underlying disease may be evident (e.g., fever from an infectious process or headaches and visual field defects from an intracranial mass).
- Diminished reflexes and extensor plantar responses may occur with severe hyponatremia.

ETIOLOGY

- Neoplasm: lung, oropharynx, stomach, duodenum, pancreas, brain, thymus, bladder, prostate, endometrium, mesothelioma, lymphoma, Ewing's sarcoma
- Pulmonary disorders: pneumonia, aspergillosis, pulmonary abscess, TB, bronchiectasis, emphysema, cystic fibrosis, status asthmaticus, respiratory failure associated with positive-pressure breathing.
- Intracranial pathology: trauma, neoplasms, infections (meningitis, encephalitis, brain abscess), hemorrhage, hydrocephalus, MS, Guillain-Barré syndrome
- Postoperative period: surgical stress, ventilators with positive pressure, anesthetic agents
- Drugs: nicotine, chlorpropamide, thiazide diuretics, vasopressin, desmopressin, oxytocin, chemotherapeutic agents (vincristine, vinblastine, cyclophosphamide), carbamazepine, phenothiazines, MAO inhibitors, tricyclic antidepressants, narcotics, nicotine, clofibrate, haloperidol, SSRIs, NSAIDs

- Other: acute intermittent porphyria, myxedema, psychosis, delirium tremens, ACTH deficiency (hypopituitarism), general anesthesia, endurance exercise

DIAGNOSIS

DIFFERENTIAL DIAGNOSIS

- Hyponatremia associated with hypervolemia (congestive heart failure, cirrhosis, nephrotic syndrome)
- Factitious hyponatremia (hyperglycemia, abnormal proteins, hyperlipidemia)
- Hyponatremia associated with hypovolemia (e.g., burns, GI fluid loss)

WORKUP

- Demonstration through laboratory evaluation (see "Laboratory Tests") of excessive secretion of ADH in absence of appropriate osmotic or physiologic stimuli (abnormal result on test of water load, elevated plasma arginine vasopressin levels despite the presence of hypotonicity and clinical euvolemia)
- Demonstration of normal thyroid, adrenal, and cardiac function
- No recent or concurrent use of diuretics
- Failure to correct hyponatremia after 0.9% saline infusion
- Correction of hyponatremia through fluid restriction
- Diagnostic criteria for SIADH are decribed in Table 1-385

LABORATORY TESTS

- Hyponatremia
- Decreased effective osmolality (<275 mOsm/kg of water)

TABLE 1-385 Diagnostic Criteria for the Syndrome of Inappropriate Antidiuretic Hormone Release

Essential Diagnostic Criteria

Decreased extracellular fluid effective osmolality (<270 mOsm/kg H_2O)
Inappropriate urinary concentration (>100 mOsm/kg H_2O)
Clinical euvolemia
Elevated urinary Na^+ concentration under conditions of normal salt and water intake
Absence of adrenal, thyroid, pituitary, or renal insufficiency or diuretic use

Supplemental Criteria

Abnormal water-load test (inability to excrete at least 90% of a 20-ml/kg water load in 4 hours and/or failure to dilute urine osmolality to <100 mOsm/kg)
Plasma vasopressin level inappropriately elevated relative to the plasma osmolality
No significant correction of plasma Na^+ level with volume expansion, but improvement after fluid restriction

From Floege J et al: *Comprehensive clinical nephrology*, ed 4, Philadelphia, 2010, Saunders.

- Urine osmolality >100 mOsm/kg of water during hypotonicity
- Urinary osmolarity > serum osmolarity
- Urinary sodium usually >40 mEq/L with normal dietary salt intake
- Normal BUN, creatinine (indicative of normal renal function and absence of dehydration), normal TSH
- Decreased uric acid

IMAGING STUDIES

Chest radiograph to rule out neoplasm or infectious process

TREATMENT
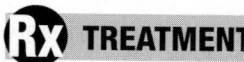

NONPHARMACOLOGIC THERAPY

Fluid restriction to 500 to 800 ml/day with close monitoring of levels of urinary and plasma electrolytes. Adequate intake of dietary protein and salt should be encouraged.

ACUTE GENERAL Rx

- In emergency situations (seizures, coma) SIAD can be treated with combination of:
  1. Hypertonic saline solution (slow infusion of 250 ml of 3% NaCl). Infuse 3% saline (513 mmol/L) at a rate of 1 to 2 ml/kg of body weight per hour to increase the serum sodium level by 1 to 2 mmol/L/hr.
  2. Furosemide, 20 to 40 mg IV. This combination increases the serum sodium by causing diuresis of urine that is more dilute than plasma and prevents extracellular fluid volume expansion.
- The rapidity of correction varies depending on the degree of hyponatremia and if the hyponatremia is acute or chronic; generally the serum sodium should be corrected only halfway to normal in the initial 24 hr. A prudent approach is to increase serum sodium by <0.5 mEq/L/hr and limit the total increase to 8 to 12 mmol/L during the first 24 hr.
- Close monitoring of the rate of correction (every 2 to 3 hr) is recommended to avoid overcorrection. In patients with hyponatremia of chronic duration, correction of serum sodium level by >12 mmol/L over a period of 24 hr increases the risk of osmotic demyelination.
- Conivaptan (20 to 40 mg/day IV) or tolvaptan (15 mg/day PO initially) are selective arginine-vasopressin (AVP) antagonists useful in selected hospitalized patients with moderate-to-severe hypervolemic and euvolemic hyponatremia. Their direct antagonism of the renal V_2 receptors increases urine water excretion, resulting in an increase in free water clearance (aquaresis). With these agents there is a significant increase in serum sodium concentration in as early as 8 hours and the change is maintained for several days. Potential problems associated with these agents are risk of osmotic demyelination if serum sodium levels are corrected too rapidly and are infusion-site reactions (50% of patients) with conivaptan.

CHRONIC Rx

- Depending on the underlying etiology, fluid restriction may be needed indefinitely. Monthly monitoring of electrolytes is recommended in patients with chronic SIAD.
- Demeclocycline 300 to 600 mg PO bid reduces urinary osmolality and increases serum sodium levels. It may be useful in patients with chronic SIAD (e.g., secondary to neoplasm) but use with caution in patients with hepatic disease; its side effects include nephrogenic diabetes insipidus (DI) and photosensitivity. This medication is also very expensive.
- Successful treatment of chronic nephrogenic SIAD with urea to induce osmotic diuresis has been reported in children and adults. However, oral intake of urea (30 g/day) is generally poorly tolerated.

DISPOSITION

- Prognosis varies depending on the cause. Generally, prognosis is benign when SIAD is caused by an infectious process.
- Morbidity and mortality are high (>40%) when serum sodium concentration is <110 mEq/L.

REFERRAL

Hospital admission depending on severity of symptoms and degree of hyponatremia

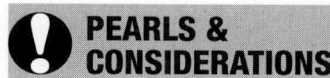

COMMENTS

- Use of hypertonic (3%) saline is contraindicated in patients with CHF, nephrotic syndrome, or cirrhosis.

- Too rapid correction of hyponatremia can cause demyelination and permanent central nervous system damage. When considering the use of vasopressor receptor antagonists, their perceived short-term benefits of improving serum sodium need to be weighed against the risks involved with overcorrection of hyponatremia.

SUGGESTED READING

available at www.expertconsult.com

RELATED CONTENT

Syndrome of Inappropriate Secretion of Antidiuretic Hormone (Patient Information)

AUTHOR: **FRED F. FERRI, M.D.**

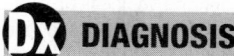 BASIC INFORMATION

DEFINITION

Syphilis is a systemic sexually transmitted treponemal disease, with acute and chronic manifestations, characterized by primary skin lesions; secondary eruption involving skin and mucous membranes; long periods of latency; and late lesions of the skin, bone, viscera, central nervous system, and cardiovascular system.

SYNONYMS

Lues

ICD-9CM CODES
097.9 Syphilis, acquired unspecified

EPIDEMIOLOGY & DEMOGRAPHICS

- Widespread, primarily involving ages 20 to 35 yr. Racial differences in incidence are related to social factors. Usually more prevalent in urban areas. Estimated annual incidence of 90,000 cases in the U.S. Rates reached historic lows in the U.S. in 2000 but began increasing among males in 2001 and increase has continued. Rates are disproportionately higher among black and Hispanic men who have sex with men (MSM) compared with white MSM and among young MSM.
- Communicability is indefinite and variable. Communicable during primary, secondary, and latent mucocutaneous lesions in up to first 4 yr of latency. Most probable congenital transmission occurs in early maternal syphilis. Adequate penicillin treatment ends infectivity within 24 to 48 hr.

PHYSICAL FINDINGS & CLINICAL PRESENTATION

PRIMARY SYPHILIS: Characteristic lesion is a painless chancre on genitalia, mouth, or anus (Fig. 1-801); atypical primary lesions may occur. Usually appears 3 wk after exposure and may spontaneously involute.

SECONDARY SYPHILIS:
- Localized or diffuse mucocutaneous lesions and generalized lymphadenopathy. Common to have constitutional symptoms, flulike symptoms. May begin approximately 4 to 6 wk after appearance of primary lesion. Manifestations may resolve in 1 wk to 12 mo.
- 60% to 80% of patients have maculopapular lesions on their palms and soles.
- Condylomata lata intertriginous papules form at areas of friction and moisture, such as the vulva.
- 21% to 58% have mucocutaneous or mucosal lesions (pharyngitis, tonsillitis, "mucous patch" lesion on oral and genital mucosa).

EARLY LATENT (≤1 YR): Generally asymptomatic

LATE LATENT (>1 YR):
- Characterized by gummas (nodular, ulcerative lesions) that can involve the skin, mucous membranes, skeletal system, and viscera.
- Manifestations of cardiovascular syphilis include aortitis, aneurysm, or aortic regurgitation.

- Neurosyphilis may be asymptomatic or symptomatic. Tabes dorsalis, meningovascular syphilis, general paralysis, or insanity may occur. Iritis, choroidoretinitis, and leukoplakia may also occur.

ETIOLOGY

- *Treponema pallidum,* a spirochete
- Spread by sexual intercourse or by intrauterine transfer

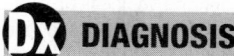 DIAGNOSIS

DIFFERENTIAL DIAGNOSIS

- Other genitoulcerative diseases such as herpes, chancroid (see Section II)
- See Section III for a clinical algorithm for the evaluation of genital ulcer disease

WORKUP

Confirmation is primarily through laboratory diagnosis. An algorithm for interpretation of reactive serologic tests for syphilis is described in Fig. E1-802.

LABORATORY TESTS

- Dark-field microscopy of fluid from lesion to look for treponeme is the definitive method for diagnosis of early syphilis.
- Serologic testing, both nontreponemal (VDRL, RPR) and treponemal (FTA, MHA). Many labs now screen patients for syphilis with automated treponemal antibody immunoassays and then confirm positive results with nontreponemal tests. The use of only one type of serologic test is insufficient for diagnosis because each type of test has limitations, including the possibility of false-positive test results in persons without syphilis. False-positive nontreponemal test results can be associated with various medical conditions unrelated to syphilis, including autoimmune conditions, older age, and injection-drug use; therefore, persons with a reactive nontreponemal test should receive a treponemal test to confirm the diagnosis of syphilis. Positive results on both treponemal and nontreponemal testing indicate new untreated syphilis. When the nontreponemal test is negative despite a positive screen, an additional treponemal screen may be helpful. Trials have shown that two positive treponemal screens help identify a population with likely prior or current syphilis, and treatment of these patients may be justifiable.
- In patients with neurosyphilis, serologic criteria for response to therapy is a fourfold or greater decrease in VDRL titer over 6 to 12 months.
- Lumbar puncture (LP) for cerebrospinal fluid VDRL (CSF-VDRL) in patients with evidence of latent syphilis. When reactive in the absence of substantial contamination of CSF with blood, it is considered diagnostic of neurosyphilis. The Centers for Disease Control and Prevention indications for LP are neurologic symptoms, treatment failure, any eye or ear involvement, or evidence of active syphilis (aortitis, gumma, iritis).

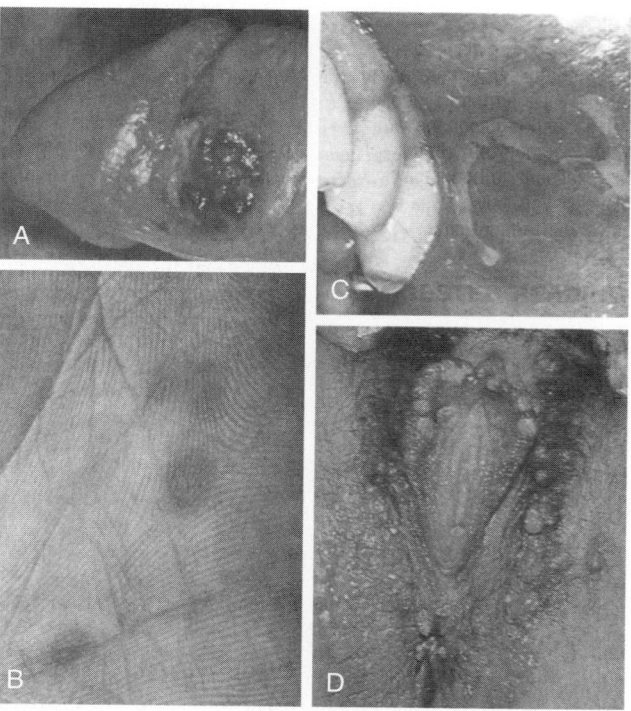

FIGURE 1-801 Syphilis lesions. A, Chancre in primary syphilis. **B,** Palmar lesions of a coppery color in secondary syphilis. **C,** Mucous patch in secondary syphilis. **D,** Condylomata lata in secondary syphilis. (**A, C,** and **D** from Forbes CD, Jackson WF: *Color atlas and text of clinical medicine,* ed 3, London, 2003, Mosby. **B** from Habif TP et al: *Skin disease: diagnosis and treatment,* St Louis, 2001, Mosby.)

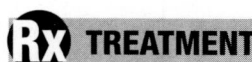

ACUTE GENERAL Rx

- Early (primary, secondary, early latent): penicillin G benzathine 2.4 million U IM × 1 *or* azithromycin 2 g PO × 1 dose
- Late (late latent, cardiovascular, gumma): penicillin G benzathine 2.4 million U IM q wk × 3 wk or doxycycline 100 mg PO bid × 4 wk
- Neurosyphilis: aqueous crystalline penicillin G 18 to 24 million U/day, administered as 3 to 4 million U IV q4h × 10 to 14 days or procaine penicillin 2.4 million U IM/day plus probenecid 500 mg PO qid, both for 10 to 14 days
- Congenital syphilis: aqueous crystalline penicillin G 50,000 U/kg/dose IV q12h × first 7 days of life and q8h after that for total of 10 days or procaine penicillin G 50,000 U/kg/dose IM/day × 10 days
- Penicillin-allergic patients with primary or secondary syphilis: doxycycline 100 mg PO bid × 14 days, or tetracycline 500 mg PO qid × 14 days, or ceftriaxone 1 g IM or IV qd × 10 to 14 days. A recent large study has shown that a single oral dose of azithromycin (2 g administered as 4 500-mg tablets) can be curative in patients with early syphilis
- Latent syphilis in penicillin-allergic patient: doxycycline 100 mg PO bid or tetracycline 500 mg qid for 28 days
- Tetracyclines are contraindicated in pregnancy. If pregnant and penicillin allergic, must be desensitized prior to treatment

DISPOSITION

- Repeat quantitative nontreponemal tests at 3, 6, and 12 mo. Pregnancy requires monthly tests until delivery.
- If a fourfold increase in titer occurs, if initial high titer fails to drop by fourfold within a year, or signs persist, retreatment may be indicated. Use treatment regimen for late syphilis.
- Pregnant women without a fourfold drop in titer in a 3-mo period need to be retreated.
- Cases should be reported to local or state health department for referral, follow-up, and partner notification.

REFERRAL

- Pregnant and possible congenital syphilis
- Pregnant and allergic to penicillin, with need to be desensitized
- Late latent syphilis with serious central nervous system, cardiovascular, or other organ system compromise

PEARLS & CONSIDERATIONS

- Jarisch-Herxheimer reaction (fever, myalgia, tachycardia, hypotension) may occur within 24 hr of treatment.
- One third of untreated patients develop central nervous system and/or cardiovascular sequelae.
- Up to 80% of those treated during late stages remain seropositive indefinitely.
- Treponemal tests remain positive even after adequate therapy.

- Male circumcision does not decrease the incidence of syphilis (unlike HIV, HSV-2, and HPV infection).
- Partner notification and treatment:
  ○ Persons who are exposed within 90 days preceding the diagnosis of primary, secondary, or early latent syphilis in a sex partner might be infected even if seronegative; therefore, such persons should be treated presumptively.
  ○ Persons who were exposed ≥90 days before the diagnosis of syphilis in a sex partner should be treated presumptively if serologic test results are not available immediately and the opportunity for follow-up is uncertain.

SUGGESTED READINGS

available at www.expertconsult.com

RELATED CONTENT

Chancroid (Related Key Topic)
Condyloma Acuminatum (Related Key Topic)
Granuloma Inguinale (Related Key Topic)
Lymphogranuloma Venereum (Related Key Topic)
Fig. 3-73 Evaluation of patients with genital lesions or ulcers (Algorithm)
Syphilis (Patient Information)

AUTHOR: **RUBEN ALVERO, M.D.**

BASIC INFORMATION

DEFINITION

Syringomyelia is a disease of the spine characterized by the formation of fluid-filled cavities within the spinal cord, sometimes extending into the brain stem.

ICD-9CM CODES
336.0 Syringomyelia

PHYSICAL FINDINGS & CLINICAL PRESENTATION

- Onset is usually insidious, with symptoms often not beginning until the third or fourth decade.
- Cervical spine is the most commonly affected area.
  1. Neuropathic joints (Fig. 1-803), intrinsic hand atrophy, weakness, and anesthetic sensory loss may develop.
  2. The latter may lead to unnoticed burns or other injuries in the hand.
  3. Loss of pain and temperature sensation may occur, but tactile sense in the upper extremity is preserved.
  4. Sharp testing elicits no pain, but patient often perceives the sharpness of the object.
  5. A Charcot joint in the shoulder or elbow may develop.
- Reflexes are absent in the upper extremity.
- Spasticity and hyperreflexia are present in the lower extremity.
- Scoliosis is common.
- Nystagmus and Horner's syndrome may also occur.

- Trophic skin changes eventually develop in many cases.

ETIOLOGY

- Cause is unknown, but condition is believed to result from obstruction of the outlet of the fourth ventricle, often associated with a Chiari I malformation, which causes fluid to be diverted down the central cord.
- A history of birth injury often exists.
- Syringes later in life may be the result of trauma or an intramedullary tumor.

DIAGNOSIS

DIFFERENTIAL DIAGNOSIS

- Amyotrophic lateral sclerosis
- Multiple sclerosis
- Spinal cord tumor
- Tabes dorsalis
- Progressive spinal muscular atrophy

WORKUP

- Plain radiographs usually reveal widening of the bony canal in the region of involvement.
- Bony anomalies are often present at the base of the skull and at the C1-C2 spinal segments.
- MRI (Fig. 1-804).

TREATMENT

Drainage and operative repair of any bony anomalies are undertaken, often with decompression laminectomy of C1 and C2.

DISPOSITION

- Condition is slowly progressive in most cases but course may be quite variable, ranging from death in a few months to slow incapacitation over several years; progression may halt at any time.
- Surgical intervention often stops progression but frequently does not lead to improvement in neurologic findings.

REFERRAL

For neurosurgical consultation when diagnosis is suspected

SUGGESTED READINGS

available at www.expertconsult.com

RELATED CONTENT

Syringomyelia (Patient Information)

AUTHOR: **LONNIE R. MERCIER, M.D.**

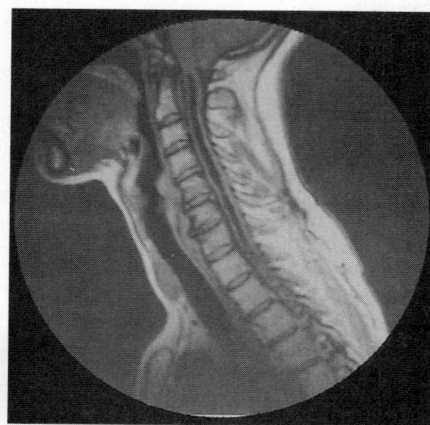

FIGURE 1-804 **Magnetic resonance imaging of cervical spine in syringomyelia, showing the fluid-filled syrinx in the center of the spinal cord.** (From Hochberg MC et al: *Rheumatology*, ed 5, St Louis, 2011, Mosby.)

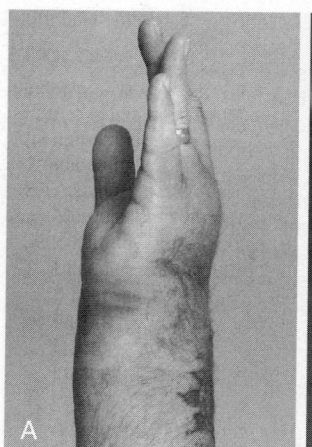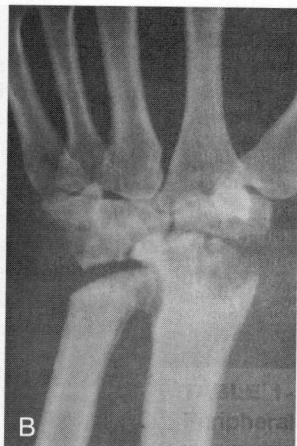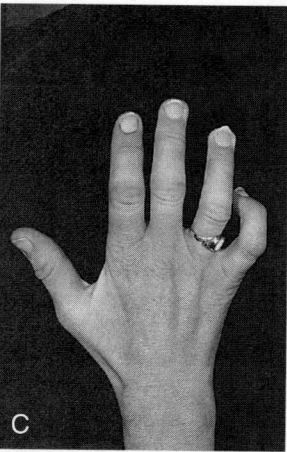

FIGURE 1-803 **Syringomyelia. A,** A neuropathic wrist joint in a patient with mild syringomyelia. Note the swelling and deformity of the joint. **B,** Radiograph showing the gross destruction of the proximal carpal row with attrition and simplification of the bony margins. Residual fragments of bone and considerable soft tissue swelling can also be seen. **C,** Wasting of the intrinsic muscle of the hand and "claw" deformity. (From Hochberg MC et al: *Rheumatology*, ed 5, St Louis, 2001, Mosby.)

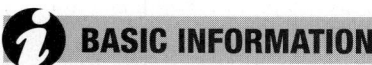

BASIC INFORMATION

DEFINITION

Systemic lupus erythematosus (SLE) is a chronic, multisystemic disease characterized by production of autoantibodies and protean clinical manifestations.

SYNONYMS

SLE

ICD-9CM CODES

710.0 Systemic lupus erythematosus

EPIDEMIOLOGY & DEMOGRAPHICS

INCIDENCE: 20 to 70 cases per 100,000 persons. Certain ethnic groups, including those of African, Hispanic, or Asian ancestry, are at an increased risk of developing the disorder.
PREDOMINANT SEX: Female/male ratio is 9:1.
PREDOMINANT AGE: Predominant age ranges from 20 to 45 yr (childbearing age).

PHYSICAL FINDINGS & CLINICAL PRESENTATION

- Constitutional: unexplained fever, fatigue, malaise (see Table 1-386)

TABLE 1-386 Potential Clinical Manifestations of Systemic Lupus Erythematosus

Target Organ	Potential Clinical Manifestations
Constitutional	Fatigue, anorexia, weight loss, fever, lymphadenopathy
Musculoskeletal	Arthritis, myositis, arthralgias, myalgias, avascular necrosis, osteoporosis
Skin	Malar rash, discoid rash, photosensitive rash, cutaneous vasculitis, livedo reticularis, periungual capillary abnormalities, Raynaud's phenomenon, alopecia, oral and nasal ulcers
Renal	Hypertension, proteinuria, hematuria, edema, nephrotic syndrome, renal failure
Cardiovascular	Pericarditis, myocarditis, conduction system abnormalities, Libman-Sacks endocarditis
Neurologic	Seizures, psychosis, cerebritis, stroke, transverse myelitis, depression, cognitive impairment, headaches, pseudotumor, peripheral neuropathy, chorea, optic neuritis, cranial nerve palsies
Pulmonary	Pleuritis, interstitial lung disease, pulmonary hemorrhage, pulmonary hypertension, pulmonary embolism
Hematologic	Immune-mediated cytopenias (hemolytic anemia, thrombocytopenia or leukopenia), anemia of chronic inflammation, hypercoagulability, thrombocytopenic thrombotic microangiopathy
Gastroenterology	Hepatosplenomegaly, pancreatitis, vasculitis affecting bowel, protein-losing enteropathy
Ocular	Retinal vasculitis, scleritis, episcleritis, papilledema

Modified from Kliegman RM et al: *Nelson textbook of pediatrics*, ed 19, Philadelphia, 2011, Saunders.

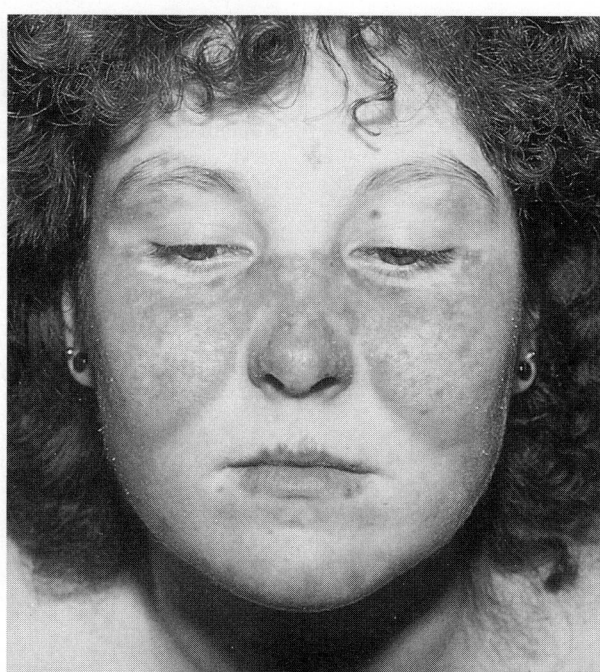

FIGURE 1-805 Acute cutaneous lupus erythematosus (LE) (systemic LE). The classic butterfly rash occurs in 10% to 50% of patients with acute LE. (From Habif TP: *Clinical dermatology: a color guide to diagnosis and therapy,* ed 3, St Louis, 1996, Mosby.)

- Skin: malar rash sparing nasolabial folds (acute cutaneous lupus) (Fig. 1-805); annular or papulosquamous rash (subacute cutaneous lupus) (Fig. 1-806); raised erythematous patches with subsequent edematous plaques and adherent scales (discoid cutaneous lupus) (Fig. 1-807); alopecia, nasal, or oropharyngeal ulcerations; Raynaud's phenomenon; petechiae, palpable purpura, skin ulceration, or digital ischemia (vasculitis); livedo reticularis or livedo racemosa (secondary antiphospholipid antibody syndrome)
- Musculoskeletal: arthritis (tenderness, swelling, effusion) typically affecting peripheral joints; myositis
- Cardiac: pericardial rub (pericarditis), heart murmur (Libman-Sacks endocarditis and other valvular heart disease), congestive heart failure (myocarditis), premature atherosclerotic heart disease
- Pulmonary: pleuritis, pneumonitis, diffuse alveolar hemorrhage
- Gastrointestinal: abdominal pain, intestinal vasculitis, ascites
- Neurologic: headache, psychosis, seizure, acute confusional states, peripheral or cranial neuropathy, transverse myelitis, cerebral vascular accident, chronic cognitive impairment
- Hematologic: anemia (hemolytic, anemia chronic disease, aplastic anemia), thrombocytopenia, leukopenia, lymphadenopathy, secondary antiphospholipid antibody syndrome
- Renal: acute renal failure, proteinuria, nephritic syndrome, nephrotic syndrome

ETIOLOGY

Exact etiology and pathogenesis are uncertain. Genetic susceptibility to lupus is likely inherited as a polygenic trait. Multiple genetic linkages including 1q23, 2q35-37, 6p21-11, and 12q24 show strong associations with SLE. Environmental factors such as ultraviolet light exposure and Epstein-Barr virus infection may have a triggering role. Autoantibodies can be present years before the diagnosis of SLE. Evidence supports the improper processing of nuclear proteins and nucleic acid from programmed cell death. This leads to the presentation of self-DNA to plasmacytoid dendritic cells. Plasmacytoid dendritic cells propagate antibody and immune complex production and other arms of specific autoimmunity.

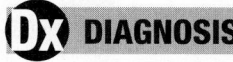 DIAGNOSIS

DIFFERENTIAL DIAGNOSIS

- Rheumatologic disorder
- Rheumatoid arthritis, mixed connective tissue disease, systemic vasculitis
- Neoplastic disorder
- Hematologic malignancy, paraneoplastic syndrome
- Systemic infection
- Other: thrombotic thrombocytopenic purpura/hemolytic uremic syndrome, primary antiphospholipid antibody syndrome

WORKUP

The diagnosis of SLE is suspected when any *four or more* of the following 1997 American College of Rheumatology criteria are present:
- Malar rash
- Discoid rash
- Photosensitivity (recurrence of unusual skin rash in sun-exposed areas)
- Oral or nasopharyngeal painless ulceration, observed by physician
- Arthritis, nonerosive
- Serositis (pleuritis, pericarditis)
- Renal disorder (persistent proteinuria >0.5 g/day, or 3+ on dipstick if quantitation not performed; cellular casts)
- Neurologic disorder (seizures, psychosis [in absence of offending drugs or metabolic derangement])
- Hematologic disorder:
  - Hemolytic anemia with reticulocytosis
  - Leukopenia (<4000/mm^3 total on two or more occasions)
  - Lymphopenia (<1500/mm^3 on two or more occasions)
  - Thrombocytopenia (<100,000/mm^3 in the absence of offending drugs)
- Immunologic disorder:
  - Anti–double-stranded DNA antibody (anti-dsDNA)
  - Anti-Smith antibody (anti-Sm)
  - Antiphospholipid antibodies (anticardiolipin IgM or IgG, lupus anticoagulant, or false-positive fluorescent treponemal antibody absorption test or *Treponema pallidum* immobilization for 6 months)
- Antinuclear antibody (ANA): an abnormal titer of ANA by immunofluorescence or equivalent assay at any time in the absence of drugs known to be associated with drug-induced lupus syndrome

LABORATORY TESTS

Suggested initial laboratory evaluation of suspected SLE:
- Complete blood count with differential, blood urea nitrogen and serum creatinine, urinalysis, ESR, PT, PTT, complements (C3, C4, CH50)
- ANA

Consider additional laboratory testing:
- Anti-dsDNA, anti-Sm, anti-SSA, anti-SSB, anti-RNP antibodies
- Lupus anticoagulant, anticardiolipin antibodies especially in patients with thrombotic events
- Random spot urine protein to urine creatinine ratio, 24-hour urine protein collection if proteinuria

IMAGING STUDIES

- Chest x-ray for evaluation of pulmonary involvement (pleural effusion, pulmonary infiltrates)
- Electrocardiogram for complaint of unexplained chest pain
- Echocardiogram if unexplained murmur, evidence of new or unexplained congestive heart failure, or suspected pericarditis

(Rx) TREATMENT

NONPHARMACOLOGIC THERAPY

- Patients with SLE should avoid sunlight and use high-SPF sunscreen.
- Screening and counseling for modifiable cardiovascular risk factors like cigarette cessation are necessary for the prevention of atherosclerotic disease.
- Counseling for pregnancy planning should be performed for patients of childbearing age.
- Calcium carbonate and vitamin D$_3$ supplementation for prevention of early osteoporosis.

GENERAL Rx

- Defined courses of corticosteroids are useful for a variety of SLE symptoms.
- Immunosuppressive drugs such as methotrexate or azathioprine are used as steroid-sparing drugs.
- Joint pain and mild serositis are generally well controlled with nonsteroidal anti-inflammatory drugs or low-dose corticosteroids. Hydroxychloroquine and methotrexate are also effective for arthritis. Leflunomide or anti-TNF agents may be considered for difficult arthritis.
- Cutaneous manifestations
  - Topical or intradermal corticosteroids are helpful for individual discoid lesions, especially in the scalp.
  - Hydroxychloroquine is efficacious. Some studies support a combination of quinacrine and hydroxychloroquine for refractory skin disease.
- Hematologic manifestations
  - Corticosteroids are first-line therapy.
  - Azathioprine can be used for thrombocytopenia or hemolytic anemia.
  - Intravenous immunoglobulin or rituximab may be considered for severe leukopenia, autoimmune hemolytic anemia, or autoimmune thrombocytopenia
- Central nervous system manifestations.
  - Headaches are treated symptomatically.
  - Anticonvulsants and antipsychotics may be indicated.
  - Standard therapy for other neuropsychiatric SLE symptoms is not established.

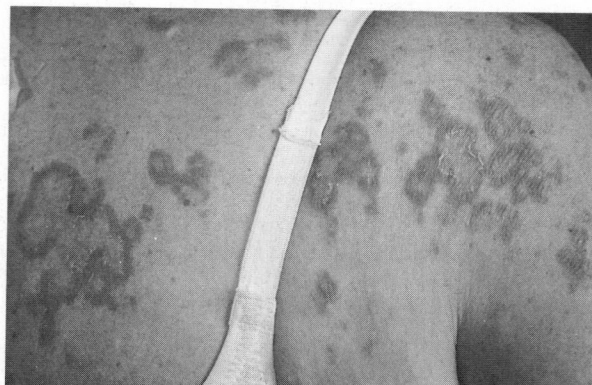

FIGURE 1-806 Subacute cutaneous lupus. (From Hochberg MC et al: *Rheumatology*, ed 4, St Louis, 2008, Mosby.)

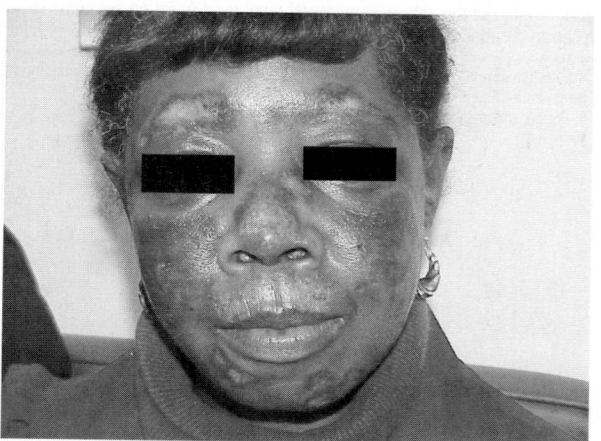

FIGURE 1-807 Discoid lupus erythematosus. (From Firestein GS et al: *Kelley's textbook of rheumatology*, ed 8, Philadelphia, 2008, Saunders.)

- Renal disease (Class III, IV, V lupus nephritis; see Table 1-387)
  - The use of high doses of intravenous cyclophosphamide with corticosteroids given at monthly intervals is more effective in preserving renal function than is treatment with glucocorticoids alone.
  - Increasingly, mycophenolate mofetil (target dose 3000 mg daily) has become the induction treatment of choice due to its improved tolerability and better fertility profile. Studies show that patients treated with mycophenolate mofetil as induction therapy had similar renal and nonrenal outcomes as compared to high-dose intravenous cyclophosphamide.
- Mycophenolate mofetil or azathioprine is used for maintenance therapy.
- Severe nonrenal organ disease
  - Evidence from systematic randomized controlled trials for nonrenal lupus treatment is comparatively limited.
  - High-dose intravenous cyclophosphamide is used as induction treatment. Azathioprine or mycophenolate mofetil may be used as maintenance drugs.
- Intravenous immunoglobulin may be considered in severe disease when concomitant infection is present.
- Plasmapheresis may be considered in critical situations, but efficacy is not proved in controlled trials and infectious complication is a substantial consideration.
- New therapy
  - Rituximab: randomized controlled trials for rituximab as an adjunct induction agent were negative in terms of both renal and nonrenal outcomes. Other clinical trials have shown an improvement in certain SLE parameters with rituximab.
  - Belimumab: in March 2011, the U.S. Food and Drug Administration approved belimumab for treatment of active SLE in adults. When used in addition to standard therapy, patients on belimumab showed increased efficacy compared to placebo based on a newly defined clinical benchmark. A majority of study patients had primary dermatologic or joint disease. Patients with CNS or serious kidney disease were excluded. Belimumab-treated patients had a reduced time to disease flare and lower glucocorticoid exposure.

DISPOSITION

- Most patients with SLE experience remissions and exacerbations.
- Five-year survival rate has improved to over 90% in patients with newly diagnosed SLE since the advent of potent immunosuppressive therapy.
- African Americans, Asian Americans, and Hispanic Americans in general have a worse prognosis.
- The leading cause of death in SLE patients in developed countries is premature atherosclerosis.
- The quality of life for SLE patients is poor due to fatigue, chronic pain, and cognitive impairment.

REFERRAL

- Rheumatology consultation for all patients with SLE
- Hematology consultation for patients with significant hematologic abnormalities (e.g., severe hemolytic anemia or thrombocytopenia)
- Nephrology consultation in patients with significant renal involvement
- Dermatology consultation for patients with unexplained or unusual skin rash
- Cardiology consultation for patients with lupus carditis, arrhythmias

 EVIDENCE

available at www.expertconsult.com

SUGGESTED READINGS

available at www.expertconsult.com

RELATED CONTENT

Systemic Lupus Erythematosus (Patient Information)

AUTHOR: **SAMUEL H. POON, M.D.**

TABLE 1-387   Severity of Lupus Nephritis*

Proliferative Disease

Mild	Type III without severe histologic features (e.g., crescents, fibrinoid necrosis); low chronicity index (i.e., ≤3); normal renal function; nonnephrotic-range proteinuria
Moderately severe	Mild disease as defined above with partial or no response after the initial induction therapy or delayed remission (>12 months), or Focal proliferative nephritis with adverse histologic features or reproducible increase of at least 30% in serum creatinine levels, or Diffuse proliferative nephritis (class IV) without adverse histologic features
Severe	Moderately severe as defined above but not remitting after 6 to 12 months of therapy, or Proliferative disease with impaired renal function and fibrinoid necrosis or crescents in >25% of glomeruli, or Mixed membranous and proliferative nephritis, or Proliferative nephritis with high chronicity alone or in combination with high activity (chronicity index >4 or chronicity index >3 and activity index >10), or Rapidly progressive glomerulonephritis (doubling of serum creatinine within 2 to 3 months)

Membranous Nephropathy

Mild	Nonnephrotic-range proteinuria with normal renal function
Moderate	Nephrotic-range proteinuria with normal renal function at presentation
Severe	Nephrotic-range proteinuria with impaired renal function at presentation (at least 30% increase in serum creatinine)

*Concomitant therapy with corticosteroids or other immunosuppressive drugs may modify urinary sediment and/or histologic findings and should be taken into consideration.
From Hochberg MC et al: *Rheumatology*, ed 5, St Louis, 2011, Mosby.

BASIC INFORMATION

DEFINITION

Tachycardia-bradycardia syndrome is a group of cardiac rhythm disturbances characterized by abnormalities of the sinus node, including (1) chronic, inappropriate bradycardia, (2) sinus pauses, arrest, or exit block, (3) combinations of sinoatrial or atrioventricular conduction defects, and (4) alternating with paroxysmal supraventricular tachyarrhythmias. Sick sinus syndrome is present when sinus node dysfunction is associated with symptoms.

SYNONYMS

Sick sinus syndrome

ICD-9CM CODES
427.81 Sick sinus syndrome

EPIDEMIOLOGY & DEMOGRAPHICS

- In children: associated with congenital and acquired heart disease, particularly after cardiac surgery.
- In adults: it is primarily a disease of the elderly secondary to idiopathic degenerative disease.

PHYSICAL FINDINGS & CLINICAL PRESENTATION

- Light-headedness, syncope, presyncope, palpitations. Other manifestations include dyspnea on exertion and worsening angina.
- Physical examination may be normal or reveal abnormalities (e.g., heart murmurs or gallop sounds) associated with the underlying heart disease.

ETIOLOGY

- Sinus node fibrosis is the primary etiology, which may also affect the atrioventricular node, the His bundle, or its branches.
- In addition, acute coronary syndromes, diseases of the SA nodal artery, inflammatory and infiltrative diseases such as hemochromatosis, amyloidosis, collagen vascular diseases (SLE and scleroderma), epicardial and pericardial diseases, medications (beta-blockers, calcium channel blockers, methyldopa, cimetidine, clonidine, lithium and antiarrhythmics), trauma following cardiac surgery, hypothyroidism, hypothermia, hypoxia, sepsis, muscular dystrophies (myotonic dystrophy, Friedreich ataxia), infectious etiologies such as Lyme disease, increased intracranial pressure.

DIAGNOSIS

DIFFERENTIAL DIAGNOSIS

- Bradycardia: atrioventricular block
- Tachycardia: atrial fibrillation
- Atrial flutter
- Paroxysmal atrial tachycardia
- Sinus tachycardia

WORKUP

- ECG (Fig. 1-809)
- Ambulatory cardiac rhythm monitoring
- 24-hour ambulatory ECG (Holter) with diary to correlate symptoms to findings
- Event recorder or a loop recorder
- Exercise stress testing to evaluate the severity of chronotropic incompetence
- Electrophysiologic testing, including sinus nodal recovery time and sinoatrial conduction time

TREATMENT

- Permanent pacemaker placement is primarily indicated if bradycardia is symptomatic. Indications for sinus node dysfunction are described in Table 1-388.
- In bradycardia-tachycardia syndrome, drug treatment is indicated for tachycardia, primarily with AV node blocking agents.
- Bradycardia is treated with permanent pacemaker placement.

REFERRAL

To cardiologist

SUGGESTED READINGS

available at www.expertconsult.com

RELATED CONTENT

Fig. 3-31 General approach to the patient with bradycardia (Algorithm)

AUTHORS: **ABDULRAHMAN ABDULBAKI, M.D., FRED F. FERRI, M.D.,** and **WEN-CHIH WU, M.D., M.P.H.**

TABLE 1-388 Indications for Permanent Pacing in Sinus Node Dysfunction

Class	Indications
I	Sinus node dysfunction with documented symptomatic bradycardia. In some patients the bradycardia is iatrogenic and will occur as a consequence of essential long-term therapy of a type and dose for which there are no acceptable alternatives.
IIa	Sinus node dysfunction, occurring spontaneously or as a result of necessary drug therapy, with a heart rate of less than 40 beats/min when a clear association between significant symptoms consistent with bradycardia has not been documented.
IIb	A chronic heart rate of less than 30 beats/min, while awake, in the minimally symptomatic patient.
III	Sinus node dysfunction in asymptomatic patients, including those in whom substantial sinus bradycardia (heart rate of less than 40 beats/min) is a consequence of long-term drug treatment. Sinus node dysfunction in which symptoms suggestive of bradycardia are clearly documented as not associated with a slow heart rate.

From Crawford MH et al (eds): *Cardiology,* ed 2, St Louis, 2004, Mosby.

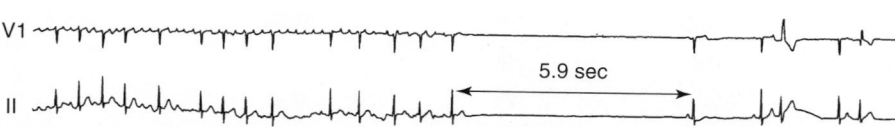

V1

5.9 sec

II

FIGURE 1-809 Tachycardia-bradycardia syndrome. Two surface ECG leads show atrial fibrillation that spontaneously terminates followed by a 5.9-second pause before sinus rhythm resumes. The patient became light-headed during this period. (From Issa Z et al: *Clinical arrhythmology and electrophysiology,* ed 2, Philadelphia, 2012, Saunders.)

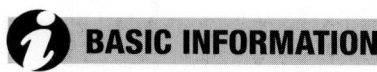

BASIC INFORMATION

DEFINITION

Takayasu's arteritis is a chronic systemic granulomatous large-vessel vasculitis. It often presents as a pulseless disease caused by widespread arterial stenosis.

SYNONYMS

Pulseless disease
Aortitis syndrome
Aortic arch arteritis
Nonspecific aortoarteritis

ICD-9CM CODES
446.7 Takayasu disease or syndrome

EPIDEMIOLOGY & DEMOGRAPHICS

Takayasu's arteritis is the third most common vasculitis in childhood worldwide, although relatively uncommon in Europe and North America. Most cases have been reported in Japan, China, India, and Mexico. There has been considerable delay to diagnosis in Western populations as opposed to Asian countries, owing in large part to the increased incidence in those areas.
INCIDENCE: Incidence in the U.S. is 2.6/1 million persons.
PREDOMINANT SEX AND AGE: The female/male ratio is 8:1. The age of onset is usually between 10 and 40 yr. The disease commonly presents between the age of 10 and 20 yr, with three quarters of the patients presenting during this time.

PHYSICAL FINDINGS & CLINICAL PRESENTATION

- Takayasu's arteritis is typically divided into systemic and occlusive stages, with the occlusive stage characterized by ischemia and symptoms from arterial occlusion. Table 1-389 summarizes common symptoms and signs in Takayasu's arteritis.
- The systemic stage of Takayasu's arteritis often manifests as nonspecific symptoms, including the following:
  1. Low-grade fever
  2. Malaise
  3. Weight loss
  4. Fatigue
  5. Arthralgia and myalgia
  6. Carotidynia
- In the occlusive stage, Takayasu's arteritis may progress to stenosis or aneurysm of the aorta and its primary branches, and may therefore manifest as follows:
  1. Arm or leg claudication, weakness, and numbness
  2. Amaurosis fugax, diplopia, headache, orthostasis, vertigo, or syncope
  3. Angina or myocardial infarction
  4. Vascular bruits of the carotid artery, subclavian artery, and aorta
  5. Discrepancy of blood pressures between the upper extremities, typically of >10 mm Hg
  6. Diminished or absent pulses, ischemic ulcerations, or gangrene in advanced disease
  7. Hypertension
  8. Retinopathy
  9. Aortic insufficiency as a result of aortic root dilatation and aneurysm formation
  10. Weakness of the arterial walls may give rise to localized aneurysms/dissection.

ETIOLOGY

- The cause of Takayasu's arteritis is poorly understood. Cell-mediated mechanisms are thought to be important to the pathogenesis.
- The infiltration of inflammatory cells (lymphocytes, macrophages, and multinucleated giant cells) into the vasa vasorum and media of the large elastic arteries leads to fibrosis, thickening, and narrowing or obliteration. Patients with Takayasu's arteritis have stenoses in >90% of cases, and aneurysms in ~25% of cases. Release of metalloproteinases and reactive oxygen species may result in local aneurysms.
- Infection, and in particular, tuberculosis, has been implicated in the pathogenesis with several studies reporting an increased incidence of caseating granulomas in those with Takayasu's disease. Additional immunologic studies are also lending support to a pathogenic role of CD4 and CD8 T-cells in this patient population.

DIAGNOSIS

Diagnostic criteria for Takayasu's arteritis were established by the American College of Rheumatology in 1990 and include the following:
- Age of disease onset <40 yr
- Claudication of extremities
- Decreased brachial artery pulse
- Systolic blood pressure difference >10 mm Hg between left and right arms
- Bruit over subclavian arteries or abdominal aorta

TABLE 1-389 Common Symptoms and Signs (%) in Takayasu's Arteritis

Symptom/Sign	Japan (n = 52)	India (n = 106)	China (n = 530)	Korea (n = 129)	USA (n = 60)	Mexico (n = 107)
			STUDY			
Fatigue/constitutional	27%	—	—	34%	43%	78%
Weight loss	—	9%	—	11%	20%	22%
Musculoskeletal	6%	5%	—	—	53%	53%
Claudication	13%	—	25%	21%	90%	29%
Headache	31%	44%	—	60%	42%	57%
Visual changes	6%	12%	10%	20%	30%	8%
Syncope/dizziness	40%	26%	14%	36%	35%	13%
Palpitations	23%	19%	—	23%	10%	43%
Dyspnea	21%	26%	11%	42%	—	72%
Carotidynia	21%	—	—	2%	32%	—
Hypertension	33%	77%	60%	40%	35%	72%
Bruit	—	35%	58%	37%	80%	94%
Decreased pulses	62%	—	37%	55%	60%	96%
Asymmetric blood pressure	—	—	—	—	47%	—

From Hochberg MC et al: *Rheumatology*, ed 5, St Louis, 2011, Mosby.

TABLE 1-390 Pathologic Characteristics of Selected Forms of Vasculitis

	Takayasu's Arteritis	Polyarteritis Nodosa	Wegener's Granulomatosis	Churg-Strauss Syndrome	Henoch-Schönlein Purpura	Cutaneous Leukocytoclastic Angiitis
Vessels involved	Elastic (large) or muscle (medium-sized) arteries	Medium-sized and small muscle arteries	Small arteries and veins; sometimes medium-sized vessels	Small arteries and veins; sometimes medium-sized vessels	Capillaries, venules, arterioles	Capillaries, venules, arterioles
Organ involvement	Aorta, aortic arch and major branches, pulmonary arteries	Skin, peripheral nerve, gastrointestinal tract, other viscera	Upper respiratory tract, lungs, kidneys, skin, eyes	Upper respiratory tract, lungs, heart, peripheral nerves	Skin, joints, gastrointestinal tract, kidneys	Skin, joints
Type of vasculitis and inflammatory cells	Granulomatous with some giant cells; fibrosis in chronic stages	Necrotizing, with mixed cellular infiltrate	Necrotizing or granulomatous (or both); mixed cellular infiltrate plus occasional eosinophils	Necrotizing or granulomatous (or both); prominent eosinophils and other mixed infiltrate	Leukocytoclastic, with some lymphocytes and variable eosinophils; IgA deposits in affected tissues	Leukocytoclastic, with occasional eosinophils

From Goldman L, Schafer AI: *Goldman's Cecil medicine*, ed 24, Philadelphia, 2012, Saunders.

- Abnormal arteriogram, not related to arteriosclerosis or fibromuscular dysplasia
- Takayasu's arteritis is diagnosed if at least three of the six criteria are present; this results in a sensitivity of 91% and specificity of 98%

DIFFERENTIAL DIAGNOSIS

Table 1-390 describes pathologic characteristics of selected forms of vasculitis. Other causes of inflammatory aortitis must be excluded:
- Temporal arteritis (giant cell arteritis)
- Syphilis
- Tuberculosis
- Systemic lupus erythematosus
- Rheumatoid arthritis
- Buerger's disease
- Behçet's disease
- Cogan's syndrome
- Kawasaki disease
- Spondyloarthropathies

WORKUP

Any young patient with findings of absent pulses and loud bruits merits a workup for Takayasu's arteritis. The workup generally includes blood testing to look for signs of inflammation as well as imaging studies, with the angiogram being the diagnostic gold standard.

LABORATORY TESTS

- Erythrocyte sedimentation rate (ESR) and serum C-reactive protein levels are usually elevated, but can be normal even in the setting of active vasculitis.
- A CBC may reveal a normal or elevated white blood cell count as well as anemia.
- Immunologic studies may include elevated immunoglobulins (IgG and IgA) and complement components (C3 and C4).
- Hypercoagulation and increase in platelet activity
- A positive association with HLA-B52 and HLA-B39 has been identified.
- Recent studies have attempted to establish a link between elevated levels of various interleukins and active disease.

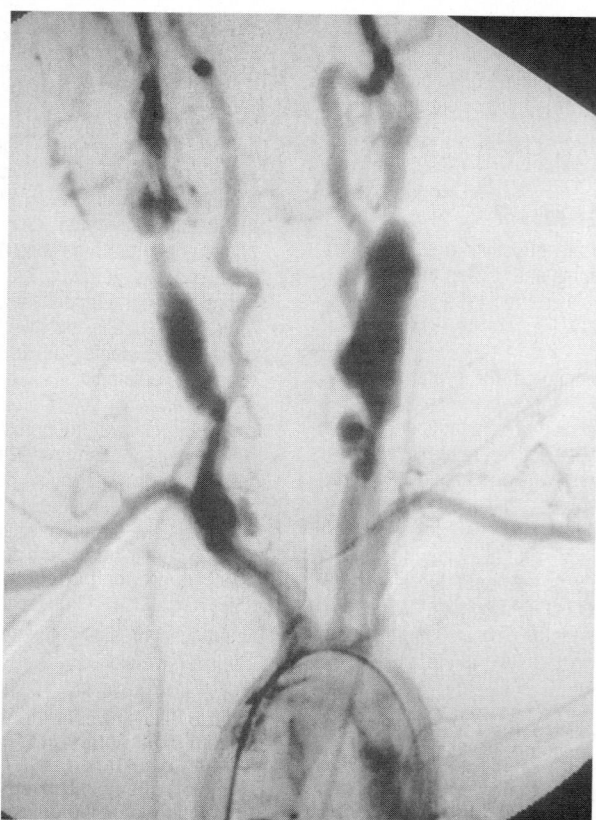

FIGURE 1-810 Angiogram of a child with Takayasu's arteritis that shows massive bilateral carotid dilation, stenosis, and poststenotic dilation. (From Behrman RE: *Nelson textbook of pediatrics*, ed 16, Philadelphia, 2000, Saunders.)

IMAGING STUDIES

- Imaging of the entire aorta and major branch vessels using angiography, CT angiography, or MR angiography
- Computed tomographic (CT) angiography can detect vessel wall changes and assist with vessel luminography.
- Cardiovascular magnetic resonance (CMR) provides information on vessel lumen and wall thickening, cardiac morphology and function, and myocardial tissue characterization.

- Angiography (Fig. 1-810) can show the narrowing of the aorta and its branches, aneurysm formation, and poststenotic dilation. Collateral circulation may also be visualized. Angiographic findings are classified into five types:
  1. Type I: lesions that involve only branches of the aortic arch
  2. Type IIa: lesions that involve the ascending aorta, the aortic arch, and its branches
  3. Type IIb: lesions from IIa plus the thoracic descending aorta

4. Type III: lesions that involve the thoracic descending aorta, abdominal aorta, and/or renal arteries
5. Type IV: lesions that involve the abdominal aorta and/or renal arteries
6. Type V: lesions that involve the entire aorta and its branches
- Chest radiograph: pathologic changes of the aorta are often visible, with areas of alternating stenosis and dilation seen. Segmental calcification outlining areas of aortic narrowing is characteristic of Takayasu's disease.
- Ultrasound: carotid, thoracic, and abdominal ultrasound are useful adjunctive imaging studies to diagnose the occlusive disease that results from Takayasu's arteritis.
- Doppler and noninvasive upper and lower extremity studies are helpful to assess blood flow and absent pulses.
- Positron emission tomography using radioisotope fluorodeoxyglucose (FDG-PET) as a marker for tissue with high glucose uptake has shown promising results in terms of specificity and sensitivity.

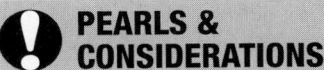 **TREATMENT**

ACUTE GENERAL Rx

- Glucocorticoids are effective in suppressing systemic symptoms and to stop the progression of Takayasu's arteritis. Prednisone (40 to 60 mg PO daily or 1 mg/kg/day) can be used for 3 months.
- Patients are monitored for symptoms and ESR. Attempts to taper prednisone can be made with resolution of constitutional symptoms, ESR and C-reactive protein levels, and in accordance with imaging studies. Patients often relapse when prednisone is tapered.
- Second-line agents such as cyclophosphamide, methotrexate, and azathioprine can be added if there is no response to glucocorticoids or as corticosteroid-sparing agents.
- Tumor necrosis factor (TNF)-alpha inhibitors have also shown promise as corticosteroid-sparing agents.

CHRONIC Rx

- Long-term low-dose prednisone may be necessary to stop the progression of arterial stenoses.

- Although there have been no randomized controlled trials, use of steroid-sparing immunosuppressants is increasing. Methotrexate is the most commonly used agent, although there are also data supporting the use of azathioprine or antitumor necrosis factor as adjunctive or alternative therapy with glucocorticoids to patients who are in relapse or resistant to other treatments. There is limited experience with cyclophosphamide.
- Treatment of hypertension in these patients can be difficult, especially since typically there is concurrent glucocorticoid therapy. Special monitoring should be employed when using ACE inhibitors as there is a high frequency of renal artery stenosis in this population.
- Percutaneous angioplasty or bypass grafts should be considered for irreversible arterial stenoses with severe ischemia (cardiac or cerebral), severe hypertension in renal artery stenosis, or aneurysmal enlargement with risk of rupture. Five-year arterial complication rate after surgical or endovascular revascularization is 44%; the likelihood of complications increases sevenfold when inflammation is present at the time of revascularization.
- Studies of coronary artery angioplasty in this population are limited, due to the high frequency of coronary lesions that are near the ostia, making them surgical interventions as opposed to percutaneous interventions.
- There have been positive data regarding drug-eluting stents, and in particular sirolimus-covered stents, likely related to the synergistic effect of its antiproliferative and immunosuppressive properties.
- Aortic regurgitation may require valve replacement or repair by surgery, although the need to manipulate friable tissue can lead to complications such as valvular detachment after replacement.

DISPOSITION

- Immunosuppressant therapy may achieve clinical remission.
- No studies have proved that treatment results in regression of stenosis, although there are limited case reports describing the return of pulses with treatment.

- With the addition of a second agent for patients with treatment resistance or relapse, 50% remission has been seen.
- Quality of life is comparable to that of patients with rheumatoid arthritis or ankylosing spondylitis.
- Mortality results are mixed, with high rates in reports from Asia and lower rates in studies performed in the United States (2%). In the absence of major complications (MI, stroke, severe HTN, heart failure, aneurysm), 5-year survival rates reach 95%. In the presence of major complications, 5-year survival is 50% to 70%.
- Death can occur suddenly from a ruptured aneurysm, a myocardial infarction, or a stroke.

REFERRAL

Whenever the diagnosis of vasculitis is suspected, a rheumatology consultation is appropriate. Vascular surgery and cardiology consultations are recommended for any evidence of carotid, peripheral, or coronary artery disease or if a large abdominal aneurysm is found.

❶ PEARLS & CONSIDERATIONS

With long-term glucocorticoid use, consider measures to protect against bone loss. Bisphosphonates have been studied prospectively with corticosteroid use in this fashion; remember to ensure adequate dietary calcium and vitamin D intake as well.

COMMENTS

The long-term prognosis of patients with treated Takayasu's disease varies by geography, and 10-yr survival ranges from 80% to 96%.

RELATED CONTENT

Vasculitis (Related Key Topic)

SUGGESTED READINGS
available at www.expertconsult.com

AUTHORS: **AILIN BARSEGHIAN EL-FARRA, M.D.,** and **PRANAV M. PATEL, M.D., F.A.C.C., F.S.C.A.I.**

BASIC INFORMATION

DEFINITION

Four species of adult tapeworm (cestodes) may infect humans as the definitive host: *Taenia saginata* (beef tapeworm), *Taenia solium* (pork tapeworm), *Diphyllobothrium latum* (fish tapeworm), and *Hymenolepis nana*. In addition, *T. solium* may infect humans in its larval form (cysticercosis), and several animal tapeworms (see "Echinococcosis" in Section I) may cause infection in an analogous manner.

SYNONYMS

Cysticercosis (larval infection by *T. solium*)

ICD-9CM CODES
123.9 Tapeworm infestation

EPIDEMIOLOGY & DEMOGRAPHICS

INCIDENCE (IN U.S.):
- Diagnosed primarily in immigrants
- Varies widely by country of origin and dietary practices

PREVALENCE (IN U.S.):
- *T. saginata:* <0.1%
- *D. latum:* <0.05%
- *T. solium:* <0.1%
- *H. nana:* sporadic, often in setting of outbreak

PREDOMINANT SEX: Equal sex distribution

PREDOMINANT AGE:
- *T. saginata, T. solium, D. latum:* 20 to 39 yr of age
- *H. nana* in setting of institution outbreaks: children

PHYSICAL FINDINGS & CLINICAL PRESENTATION

Adult worms
1. Attach to bowel mucosa via suckers, hooks, or grooves depending on species
2. Feed and grow
3. Cause minimal or no symptoms or sequelae but occasionally can cause nausea, anorexia, or epigastric pain.

Cysticercosis: larval infection by *T. solium*
1. Mass lesions of brain (neurocysticercosis), soft tissue, viscera
2. Neurocysticercosis may cause seizures, hydrocephalus

Prolonged infection with *D. latum*
1. Vitamin B$_{12}$ deficiency
2. Megaloblastic anemia

ETIOLOGY

TAPEWORM:
- Adult worms consist of a head, neck, and hundreds or thousands of body segments known as proglottids. Each proglottid contains a complete set of reproductive organs and thus eggs.
- Adult worm resides in small or large bowel; proglottids and eggs are passed in stool.
- *T. saginata* may produce up to 100,000 eggs per proglottid and *T. solium* may produce up to 50,000 eggs per proglottid.

- Eggs are ingested by the animal intermediate host.
- Eggs hatch into larvae.
- Larvae disseminate largely in skeletal muscle, brain, viscera.
- Humans eat infected beef *(T. saginata),* infected pork *(T. solium),* or infected fish *(D. latum).*
- Larvae mature into adults within the GI lumen.
- *H. nana* infection is acquired by ingesting eggs in human or rodent feces.

CYSTICERCOSIS:
- Humans ingest eggs of *T. solium* in food contaminated with human feces that contain the eggs.
- Eggs hatch into larvae in gut.
- Larvae disseminate widely through tissues (particularly soft tissue and CNS) forming cystic lesions containing either viable or nonviable larvae.

DIAGNOSIS

WORKUP

- Stool examination for eggs or proglottids (tapeworm)
  1. Eggs of *Taenia* spp. cannot be differentiated by microscopy, but the species can be identified through examination of the proglottids in stool.
  2. Eggs of *Taenia* spp. are round and measure 30 to 40 micrometers.
- Cerebral CT scan (neurocysticercosis)
- Serum antibody (neurocysticercosis) with high sensitivity with multiple cysts (94%) but low with a single cyst or calcified cysts (as low as 28%)

IMAGING STUDIES

- Tapeworm: incidental finding on upper GI series
- Neurocysticercosis:
  1. Cerebral cysts are readily demonstrated by CT scan or MRI.
  2. Calcified lesions are an incidental finding.

TREATMENT

ACUTE GENERAL Rx

- All adults and children with intestinal tapeworm infections should be treated with a single oral dose of praziquantel.
  1. *T. solium:* 5-10 mg/kg
  2. *T. saginata:* 5-10 mg/kg
  3. *D. latum:* 5-10 mg/kg
  4. *H. nana:* 25 mg/kg and a repeat dose 7-10 days later if heavy infection
- Praziquantel acts by causing changes in the teguments of the worms, allowing increased permeability to calcium ions, which then accumulate inside worm and cause paralysis.
- Follow-up stool screening is recommended at 1 and 3 mo to confirm cure.

- An alternative therapy to praziquantel for tapeworm infections is niclosamide, 2 g PO once for adults and 1 g for children 11-34 kg and 1.5 g for children over 34 kg.
- Therapy that may be considered for symptomatic cysticercosis:
  1. May regress spontaneously
  2. Surgery
  3. Albendazole 10-15 mg/kg/day PO divided in two doses for 8 days
  4. Praziquantel 50-100 mg/kg/day PO for 15-30 days divided in three doses
  5. Use of steroids in neurocysticercosis may reduce CNS inflammation and increase levels of albendazole in CNS.
- Therapy contraindicated with:
  1. Ocular infections
  2. Cerebral infections in which local inflammation caused by destruction of the parasite may cause significant damage

CHRONIC Rx

- Retreatment if required
- Avoidance of undercooked pork, meat, or fish
- Cysticercosis: proper hand washing, proper disposal of human waste

DISPOSITION

- Neurologic follow-up for patients with neurocysticercosis
- Ophthalmologic follow-up for patients with ocular involvement

REFERRAL

Patients treated for neurocysticercosis should be evaluated by a physician experienced in managing this infection, if possible.

PEARLS & CONSIDERATIONS

COMMENTS

T. solium is the most dangerous of the tapeworms because of the potential for cysticercosis by means of autoinfection.

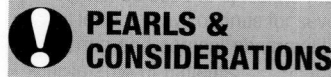

SUGGESTED READINGS
available at www.expertconsult.com

RELATED CONTENT
Cysticercosis (Related Key Topic)
Tapeworm Infection (Patient Information)

AUTHOR: **GLENN G. FORT, M.D., M.P.H.**

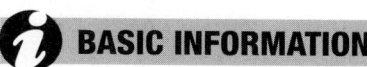

BASIC INFORMATION

DEFINITION

Tardive dyskinesia (TD) is a syndrome of involuntary movements associated with the long-term use of antipsychotic medication, particularly first-generation antipsychotics. Patients exhibit rapid, repetitive, stereotypic movements that mostly involve the oral, lingual, trunk, and limb areas.

SYNONYMS

Orofacial dyskinesia
Tardive syndrome
TD

ICD-9CM CODES
333.85 Tardive dyskinesia

EPIDEMIOLOGY & DEMOGRAPHICS

- The disorder is caused by dopamine-blocking antipsychotics (e.g., haloperidol) and antiemetics (e.g., metoclopramide, prochlorperazine, and promethazine).
- With first-generation antipsychotics, at least 20% of patients are affected with TD, and ~5% are expected to develop TD with each year of antipsychotic treatment.
- The incidence of TD is declining with the increased use of second-generation antipsychotics. ~0.5% to 1% of all adults develop TD yearly while taking these medications.
- Risk increases with the duration of antipsychotic treatment, in female and in elderly patients, in patients with brain damage or dementia, with concurrent anticholinergic use, and in patients with nonschizophrenia diagnoses.

PHYSICAL FINDINGS & CLINICAL PRESENTATION

- TD is classically described as a chronic condition of insidious onset, but symptoms are variable over time and may even improve despite continued antipsychotic therapy.
- The condition typically appears with the reduction or withdrawal of the antipsychotic medications.
- TD primarily involves stereotypic movements of the mouth and tongue, including lip smacking and puckering, tongue twisting and protrusion, and facial grimacing.
- TD may also involve slow, writhing movements of the trunk or choreoathetotic movements of the fingers and toes.
- The involuntary mouth movements associated with TD may be suppressed by voluntary actions (e.g., putting food in the mouth, talking).
- Variants of TD with similar treatment include tardive dystonia (e.g., torticollis, blepharospasm), tardive myoclonus, tardive akathisia, and tardive tics.

ETIOLOGY

TD is generally thought to result from chronic exposure to dopamine receptor–blocking agents, which are primarily used to treat psychosis. TD has not been reported with dopamine depleters (e.g., reserpine), and it is less common with second-generation antipsychotic drugs. Some drugs used to treat nausea (e.g., metoclopramide, prochlorperazine) can also cause TD. TD is believed to be caused by the upregulation and increased sensitivity of dopamine receptors in the basal ganglia and by antipsychotic-induced damage to striatal cholinergic neurons. Destruction of striatal GABAergic neurons has also been implicated.

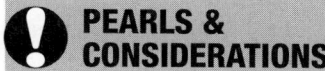

DIAGNOSIS

DIFFERENTIAL DIAGNOSIS

- Acute extrapyramidal symptoms (e.g., short-term withdrawal dyskinesias, parkinsonism, akathisia)
- Basal ganglia movement disorders (e.g., Huntington's chorea, Tourette's syndrome, levodopa-induced dyskinesia in Parkinson's disease, Wilson's disease)
- Autoimmune diseases (Sydenham's chorea, multiple sclerosis)
- Other causes of neurologic damage (e.g., lead or mercury toxicity, HIV, neurosyphilis, head injury, neurodegeneration from illicit substances)
- Mannerisms associated with disorganized type or catatonic type schizoprenia
- Hyperthyroidism-induced choreoathetosis
- Edentulous dyskinesias and improperly fitted dentures
- Rabbit syndrome (a rare variant of extrapyramidal symptoms) with vertical orofacial movements without tongue involvement; may respond to anticholinergic agents

WORKUP

TD is a diagnosis of exclusion, with emphasis on a complete neuropsychiatric and medication history and a thorough physical examination.

IMAGING STUDIES

Standard brain imaging is normal in patients with TD.

TREATMENT

ACUTE GENERAL Rx

- Treatment is predicated on prevention: limit the indications for antipsychotics; use the lowest effective dose; discontinue the drugs, when feasible; and monitor patients frequently. Anticholinergic medications may worsen symptoms.
- Switch to second-generation antipsychotics, if possible.

CHRONIC Rx

- Clozapine has the best evidence for improving the symptoms of TD, although olanzapine and amisulpride may also be of benefit.
- Tetrabenazine, benzodiazepines, vitamin B_6, donepezil, piracetam, amantadine, and melatonin may be helpful, although controlled trial evidence is weak.
- For disabling TD, deep brain stimulation of the subthalamic nucleus or internal globus pallidus has been reported to provide significant symptom reduction without exacerbation of psychiatric symptoms.
- TD is potentially irreversible in nearly two thirds of patients; thus, patients undergoing long-term treatment with dopamine receptor–blocking medications require frequent monitoring and aggressive management at the onset of TD symptoms.

REFERRAL

Movement disorder specialist consultation if symptoms are severe

PEARLS & CONSIDERATIONS

- First-generation antipsychotics should be resumed to treat TD in the absence of active psychosis only as a last resort for persistent, disabling, and treatment-resistant TD.
- Avoid the use of anticholinergic medications (e.g., benztropine), which may exacerbate TD symptoms.
- A worsening of the overall psychopathology in patients with schizophrenia is longitudinally associated with the emergence of TD and suggestive of a worse prognosis.
- Recent evidence suggests increased overall mortality among patients with TD, which highlights the need for referral for more aggressive specialized interventions.

SUGGESTED READINGS

available at www.expertconsult.com

RELATED CONTENT

Tardive Dyskinesia (Patient Information)

AUTHOR: **JOHN A. GRAY, M.D., PH.D.**

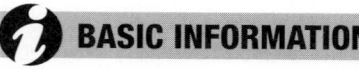

BASIC INFORMATION

DEFINITION

Tarsal tunnel syndrome is the most common compressive neuropathy in the foot and ankle. The syndrome is secondary to a pathologic, structural, or biomechanical factor that causes compression of the posterior tibial nerve or its branches (medial calcaneal, medial plantar, lateral plantar branches), within or distal to the tarsal canal (Fig. 1-811).

ICD-9CM CODES
355.5 Tarsal tunnel syndrome

EPIDEMIOLOGY & DEMOGRAPHICS

PREVALENCE: Most common entrapment neuropathy in the foot/ankle
PREDOMINANT SEX: Relatively equal

PHYSICAL FINDINGS & CLINICAL PRESENTATION

- Symptoms can vary widely in location and nature. One or many symptoms can occur.
- Common presentations: medial ankle pain, localized heel pain, distal numbness/shooting pain, and generalized foot/ankle pain that keeps the patient awake at night
- Percussion over the porta pedis resulting in Tinel's sign (distal radiation of symptoms)
- Valleix phenomenon (producing proximal symptomatology) is consistent with tarsal tunnel syndrome.

- In cases of mechanical etiology, holding the foot in a dorsiflexed and everted subtalar joint position may reproduce symptoms.
- Look for: localized edema, varicosities, palpable soft tissue masses, biomechanical abnormalities, and signs of trauma.
- Loss of motor function and permanent loss of sensation are extremely rare.

ETIOLOGY

- Inflammatory (adjacent tendonitis, recent ankle trauma)
- Compressive pathology (ganglion cyst, lipoma, varicosities)
- Structural (osseous): exostosis, severe arthritis, fracture of rearfoot/ankle
- Biomechanical: abnormal calcaneal eversion or inversion, subtalar joint pronation
- Systemic causes of neuropathy: diabetes, hypothyroidism, Reiter's syndrome, and more

DIAGNOSIS

DIFFERENTIAL DIAGNOSIS

- Plantar fasciitis
- Calcaneal fracture/other osseous trauma.
- Ankle sprain/strain or chronic ST injury. Posterior tibial tendonitis often overlooked
- Systemic causes of peripheral neuropathy: diabetes, hypothyroidism, Reiter's syndrome
- Radiculopathy
- Peripheral vascular disease

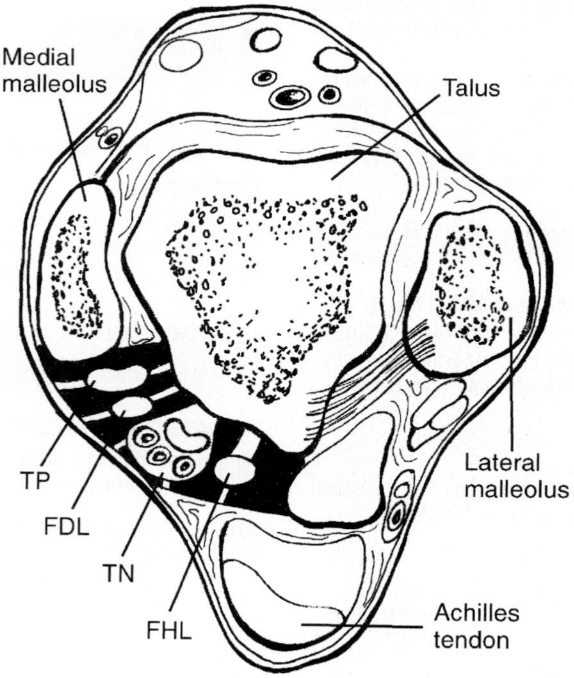

DIAGNOSTIC STUDIES

- X-rays: rule out trauma, bone tumor, structural deformity.
- Biomechanical exam
- MRI: look for soft tissue mass, edema, trauma.
- EMG/nerve conduction studies support clinical diagnosis, but false negatives are common.
- Local diagnostic injections: evaluate local versus proximal source of neuropathy.

TREATMENT

- First line: rest, ice, limit aggravating activity
- Address shoegear problems: in structural cases, tight shoegear will exacerbate symptoms, while in functional cases symptoms may be aggravated by loose/unstable rearfoot fit.
- Nonsteroidal anti-inflammatory drugs
- Biomechanical: custom orthotics for optimal biomechanical function/stabilization. Heel lifts assist by promoting ankle plantar flexion, supinating the foot, and reducing pressure within the tarsal tunnel.
- Ankle bracing if ankle instability present and contributing factor
- Physical therapy (iontophoresis, other therapeutic modalities, strength/flexibility work)
- Local steroid injection
- If persistent, offloading with cast or cast walker may yield resolution in 3 to 6 wk
- Surgical: release of retinaculum, mass excision, etc.

DISPOSITION

Can yield lifelong, chronic pain with unknown specific etiology or can follow a limited course once causative factor resolved (mechanical, healed ankle sprain, soft tissue mass resection, etc.).

REFERRAL

- Physical therapy for various treatment modalities
- Podiatric or foot/ankle orthopedic surgeon for biomechanical evaluation, orthotic treatment, diagnostic/therapeutic injection, and surgery if necessary.

PEARLS & CONSIDERATIONS

- Be sure to rule out etiologies such as calcaneal fracture and bone or soft tissue tumor.
- Differentiation from plantar fasciitis is often difficult, yet the initial therapy can be identical (refer to "Plantar Fasciitis").

SUGGESTED READINGS
available at www.expertconsult.com

RELATED CONTENT
Tarsal Tunnel Syndrome (Patient Information)

AUTHOR: **BROOKE E. KEELEY, D.P.M.**

Diseases and Disorders

FIGURE 1-811 Anatomy of tarsal tunnel syndrome. Transverse view of ankle. Tendons and neurovascular elements are included in individual fibrous septa that connect periosteum with the deep fascia. *FDL,* Flexor digitorum longus; *FHL,* flexor hallucis longus tendon; *TN,* tibial nerve (single contour), posterior tibial artery, veins; *TP,* tibialis posterior tendon. (From Canoso J: *Rheumatology in primary care,* Philadelphia, 1997, Saunders.)

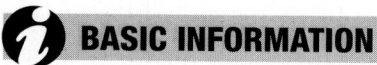 **BASIC INFORMATION**

DEFINITION

Temporomandibular joint (TMJ) syndrome refers to a group of disorders leading to symptoms of the TMJ.

SYNONYMS

Temporomandibular dysfunction
Painful temporomandibular joint
TMJ

ICD-9CM CODES

524.60 Temporomandibular joint pain-dysfunction syndrome

EPIDEMIOLOGY & DEMOGRAPHICS

- 15% of the population have TMJ disorders.
- Females are affected more often than males (4:1 ratio).
- Occurs between the second and fourth decades of life.
- Usually unilateral, affecting either side with equal frequency

PHYSICAL FINDINGS & CLINICAL PRESENTATION

- Often unilateral pain in the muscles of mastication, usually described as a "dull" ache
- Otalgia
- Odontalgia
- Headaches (frontal, temporal, retro-orbital)
- Tinnitus
- Dizziness
- Clicking or popping sounds with movement of the TMJ
- Joint locking
- Application of mild anterior pressure with a finger placed posteriorly to each tragus may result in tenderness, clicking, or crepitus.
- Limited range of motion of the TMJ
- Symptoms usually appear in association with a stressful life event

ETIOLOGY

- Multifactorial, encompassing local anatomic anomalies to systemic disease processes.
- Myofascial pain-dysfunction syndrome: the most common cause of TMJ syndrome and results from teeth grinding and clenching the jaw (bruxism)
- Internal TMJ derangement: abnormal connection of the articular disk to the mandibular condyle
- Degenerative joint disease
- Rheumatoid arthritis
- Gouty arthritis
- Pseudogout
- Ankylosing spondylitis
- Trauma
- Prior surgery (orthodontic, intraarticular steroid injection)
- Tumors

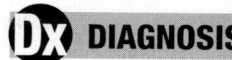 **DIAGNOSIS**

Can be made based on history and physical examination in most cases.

DIFFERENTIAL DIAGNOSIS

Includes the list provided above. Myofascial pain-dysfunction syndrome, internal TMJ derangement, and degenerative joint disease represent >90% of all causes of TMJ syndrome. Others not mentioned include dental problems such as loss of posterior teeth support and Eagle's syndrome (stylohyoid syndrome, carotidynia, and trigeminal neuralgia). Alternative diagnoses such as otitis, mastoiditis, salivary gland disorders, and temporal arteritis should always be excluded.

WORKUP

Radiographic imaging evaluation is used to exclude anatomic or systemic causes of disease when conservative management has failed.

LABORATORY TESTS

Laboratory examination is not very helpful.

IMAGING STUDIES

- Plain radiographs: the most common views are the panoramic, transorbital, and transpharyngeal in both opened and closed positions.
- Arthrography is helpful in looking for meniscus involvement but is seldom performed anymore.
- CT scan is highly accurate in diagnosing meniscal and osseous derangements of the TMJ.
- MRI is the procedure of choice and has replaced arthrography in cases of disabling pain or if locking occurs. It is used to determine disc position and morphology along with degenerative bony changes.

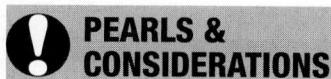 **TREATMENT**

NONPHARMACOLOGIC THERAPY

- Soft diet to rest the muscles of mastication
- Heat 15 to 20 min four to six times per day
- Massage of the masseter and temporalis muscles
- Formed splints or bite appliances
- Range-of-motion exercises
- Cognitive-behavioral therapy and biofeedback have been shown to reduce pain.

ACUTE GENERAL Rx

- Nonsteroidal anti-inflammatory drugs: ibuprofen 800 PO mg tid prn, naproxen 500 mg PO bid prn, titrated to relieve symptoms
- Muscle relaxants at bedtime: diazepam 2.5 to 5 mg PO tid prn or amitriptyline 5 to 100 mg PO qd prn
- In degenerative joint disease of the TMJ, intraarticular steroid injection can be tried
- Botulism toxin injections into the masticatory muscles

CHRONIC Rx

- Most of the above treatments are used for myofascial pain-dysfunction syndrome; however, they can be applied to other causes of TMJ syndrome. Surgery is usually a measure of last resort in patients who do not respond to nonpharmacologic and acute general treatment.
- Surgical procedures include:
  1. Meniscoplasty
  2. Meniscectomy
  3. Subcondylar osteotomy
  4. TMJ reconstruction

DISPOSITION

The course depends on the underlying etiology; however, less than 5% of adults with temporomandibular symptoms develop chronic symptoms.

REFERRAL

All patients with TMJ syndrome refractory to conservative nonpharmacologic and acute therapy should be referred to a periodontist, oral maxillofacial surgeon, or ear-nose-throat surgeon.

PEARLS & CONSIDERATIONS

Patients with rheumatoid arthritis involving the TMJ usually have bilateral involvement.

COMMENTS

Frequently, emotional stress initiates the myofascial pain-dysfunction, which accounts for 85% of all cases of TMJ syndrome.

SUGGESTED READINGS

available at www.expertconsult.com

RELATED CONTENT

Temporomandibular Joint (TMJ) Syndrome (Patient Information)

AUTHORS: **RYAN W. ZUZEK, M.D.,** and **DOUGLAS BURTT, M.D.**

BASIC INFORMATION
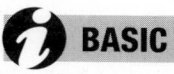

DEFINITION

Testicular neoplasms are primary cancers originating in a testis.

SYNONYMS

Testis tumor
Testicular neoplasms

ICD-9CM CODES	
186.9	Testicular neoplasm
M906/3	(seminoma)
M9101/3	(embryonal carcinoma or teratoma)
M9100/3	(choriocarcinoma)

EPIDEMIOLOGY & DEMOGRAPHICS

INCIDENCE: 5.4 cases per 100,000 men annually. White men have the highest incidence at 6.3 cases/100,000 men. Testicular cancer is the most common cancer diagnosis in men between the ages of 15 and 35 yr. The incidence has been gradually increasing since 1975.
PREVALENCE: 1% to 2% of all cancers in males
PREDOMINANT AGE: Can occur in any age but most common in young adults; average age for embryonal cell carcinoma: 30 yr; average age for seminoma: 36 yr

PHYSICAL FINDINGS & CLINICAL PRESENTATION

- Testicular cancer typically presents as a painless mass in the testis. Any mass within the testicle should be considered cancer until proven otherwise. It may be found by the patient, who brings it to the attention of a physician, or it may be found by a physician on a routine examination.
- Symptoms other than scrotal or testicular swelling are typically absent unless the cancer has metastasized (10% of patients at diagnosis). Occasionally a patient may report scrotal fullness or heaviness. About 10% of patients present with acute pain. Gynecomastia from tumors that secrete beta-human chorionic gonadotropin (hCG) is found in 5% of men with testicular cancer.
- Testicular palpation should be performed with two hands. Transillumination may distinguish a solid mass (e.g., cancer) and a fluid-filled lesion (e.g., hydrocele or spermatocele). The mass is nontender; indeed, it is less sensitive than a normal testicle.

ETIOLOGY, CLASSIFICATION, & PATHOLOGY

- Cryptorchidism (undescended testes) is a major risk factor even if corrected by orchiopexy; however, treatment of undescended testis before puberty decreases the risk of testicular cancer from fivefold to twofold. Other risk factors are family history, Klinefelter's syndrome, infertility, tobacco use, and white race.
- Classification: testicular cancers can be classified as pure seminomas or nonseminomatous germ cell tumors (embryonic carcinoma, choriocarcinoma, yolk sac carcinoma, teratoma)
- Pathology: germ cell tumors account for >95% of testicular cancers

Cell Type	Frequency (%)
Seminoma	42
Embryonal cell carcinoma	26
Teratocarcinoma	26
Teratoma	5
Choriocarcinoma	1

- Other rare types:
  - Yolk sac carcinoma
  - Mixed germ cell tumors
  - Carcinoid tumor
  - Sertoli cell tumors
  - Leydig cell tumors
  - Lymphoma
  - Metastatic cancer to the testes
- TNM staging system for testicular cancer
  - T_0: No apparent primary
  - T_1: Testis only (excludes rete testis)
  - T_2: Beyond the tunica albuginea
  - T_3: Rete testis or epididymal involvement
  - T_4: Spermatic cord
    1. Spermatic cord
    2. Scrotum
  - N_0: No nodal involvement
  - N_1: Ipsilateral regional nodal involvement
  - N_2: Contralateral or bilateral abdominal or groin nodes
  - N_3: Palpable abdominal nodes or fixed groin nodes
  - N_4: Juxtaregional nodes
  - M_0: No distant metastases
  - M_1: Distant metastases present

The clinical stages consist of stage I, with tumor confined to the testis; stage II, with positive regional lymph nodes; and stage III, with metastases.

DIAGNOSIS

DIFFERENTIAL DIAGNOSIS

- Spermatocele
- Varicocele
- Hydrocele
- Epididymitis
- Epidermoid cyst of the testicle
- Epididymis tumors

WORKUP

Physical examination, laboratory tests, and imaging studies (see Section III, "Testicular Mass")

LABORATORY TESTS

- Serum hCG
- Serum alpha-fetoprotein (AFP): elevated in nonseminoma tumors
One or both of these tumor markers will be elevated in 70% of cases of testicular cancer.
- Serum lactate dehydrogenase (LDH) level: elevated with rapid turnover of malignant cells
- Testicular biopsy contraindicated

IMAGING STUDIES

- Testicular ultrasound
- CT scan or MRI of pelvis and abdomen
- Chest radiograph
- CT of the chest in patients with abnormal chest x-ray or in those with suspected mediastinal, hilar, or lung parenchymal disease; MRI of the brain in patients with neurologic symptoms
- PET scan is not recommended (frequent false positives).

TREATMENT
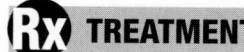

- Seminoma
  1. Stage I: Radical orchiectomy plus one cycle of single agent carboplatin chemotherapy or radiation therapy (RT) to the paraaortic lymph nodes
  2. Stage IIA or IIB: RT or cisplatin-based chemotherapy (e.g., cisplatin, bleomycin, etoposide)
- Nonseminoma
  1. Stage IA: radical orchiectomy plus retroperitoneal lymph node dissection (RPLND)
  2. Stage IB: Same as stage IA plus two cycles of chemothapy (cisplatin, bleomycin, etoposide)
  3. Advanced stages: cisplatin-based chemotherapy or RPLND
- Posttreatment surveillance for testicular cancer survivors (annually)
  1. Fertility assessment
  2. Skin examination (increased risk of dysplastic nevi)
  3. Testicular examination (3% to 4% risk of second testicular cancer)
  4. Serum tumor markers (hCG, AFP)
  5. Chest CT 4 months postoperatively

DISPOSITION

The overall cure for testicular cancer is >95% (80% for metastatic disease). Patients with pure seminomas have a better prognosis. Because treatment produces favorable outcomes even in advanced stages, the U.S. Preventive Services Task Force recommends against screening asymptomatic men for testicular cancer.

SUGGESTED READINGS

available at www.expertconsult.com

RELATED CONTENT

Fig. 3-179 Diagnosis, staging, and risk assessment of patients with testicular germ cell tumor (Algorithm)
Testicular Cancer (Patient Information)

AUTHOR: **FRED F. FERRI, M.D.**

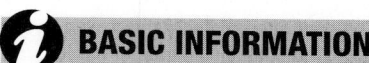

BASIC INFORMATION

DEFINITION

Testicular torsion is a twisting of the spermatic cord leading to cessation of testicular blood flow, ischemia, and infarction if left untreated.

SYNONYMS

Spermatic cord torsion

ICD-9CM CODES
608.2 Testicular torsion

EPIDEMIOLOGY & DEMOGRAPHICS

INCIDENCE: Affects one in 4000 males aged <25 yr
PREDOMINANT AGE: Two thirds of all cases occur between the ages of 12 and 18 yr, but may occur at any age, including antenatally.

PHYSICAL FINDINGS & CLINICAL PRESENTATION

- Typical sequence is sudden onset of hemiscrotal pain, then swelling, nausea, and vomiting without fever or urinary symptoms.
- Physical examination may reveal a tender firm testis, high-riding testis, horizontal lie of testis, absent cremasteric reflex, and no pain with elevation of testis. Absence of the cremasteric reflex (stroking or pinching the medial thigh normally causes contraction of the cremaster muscle and elevation of the testis) is the most sensitive physical finding.
- Painless testicular swelling occurs in 10%.
- One out of three patients reports previous episodes of spontaneously remitting scrotal pain.
- In the neonate, testicular torsion should be presumed in patients with a painless, discolored hemiscrotal swelling.
- In rare cases, torsion may involve an undescended testicle. In such situations an empty hemiscrotum is palpated together with a tender lump in the inguinal area.

ETIOLOGY

- There are two types of testicular torsion: extravaginal, caused by nonadherence of the tunica vaginalis to the dartos layer, and intravaginal, caused by malrotation of the spermatic cord with the tunica vaginalis. Intravaginal torsion accounts for 90% of cases.
- Torsion usually occurs in the absence of any precipitating events. Trauma accounts for <10% of cases.

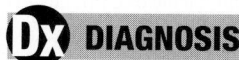

DIAGNOSIS

Diagnosis is made mainly by clinical suspicion. Color Doppler ultrasound evaluation (Fig. 1-812) or a nuclear testicular scan (Fig. E1-813) may help with the diagnosis. Ultrasonography will show absent or decreased blood flow; scintigraphy reveals decreased perfusion on symptomatic side.

DIFFERENTIAL DIAGNOSIS

See also Section II.
- Torsion of the testicular appendages (appendix testis)
- Testicular tumor
- Epididymitis
- Incarcerated inguinoscrotal hernia
- Orchitis
- Spermatocele
- Hydrocele, varicocele

WORKUP

The diagnosis is usually based on history and physical examination.

IMAGING STUDIES

- Radionuclide scrotal scanning (technetium-99m): cold testicle
- Doppler ultrasonic stethoscope (Doppler flowmetry)

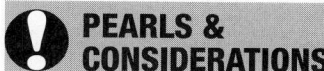

TREATMENT

Surgical derotation of the spermatic cord followed by bilateral testicular fixation with nonabsorbable sutures. If the affected testis is nonviable, orchiectomy of the affected testis and orchiopexy of the contralateral side are performed. Attempts at manual detorsion should not delay surgical consultation.

PROGNOSIS

- The degree of ischemia depends on the duration of torsion and the degree of rotation of the spermatic cord.

- There is an 80% testicular salvage rate if detorsion occurs within 12 hr of onset.
- After 24 hr, irreversible testicular infarction is expected.
- Because the contralateral testes can be affected (immunologic process), when treatment is delayed and return of blood flow does not occur after detorsion, some recommend orchiectomy of the infarcted testicle.

REFERRAL

To urologist

PEARLS & CONSIDERATIONS

- Manual detorsion by external rotation of the testis toward the thigh can be attempted for adolescent intravaginal torsion if an operating facility is not readily available.
- Extravaginal torsion is diagnosed in the newborn. Intravaginal torsion can occur at any age but is usually diagnosed in males ages 12 to 18 yr.

SUGGESTED READING

available at www.expertconsult.com

RELATED CONTENT

Testicular Torsion (Patient Information)

AUTHOR: **FRED F. FERRI, M.D.**

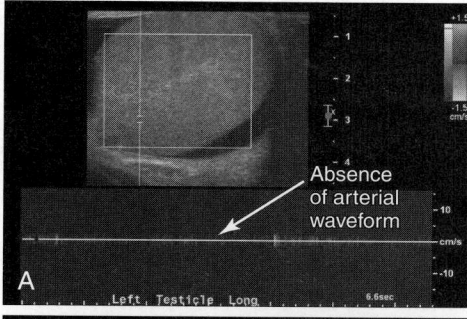

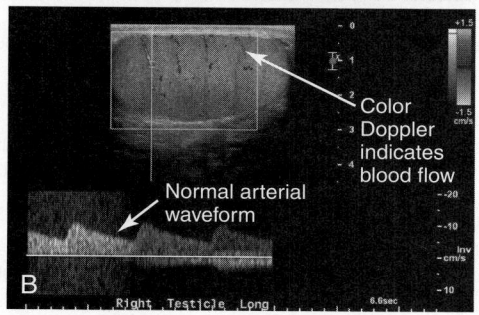

FIGURE 1-812 Testicular torsion ultrasound. A and **B,** Ultrasound has become the standard modality to assess for testicular torsion. In this 20-yr-old male with left testicular pain, the left testicle has no blood flow, whereas the right testicle has normal arterial and venous blood flow by color Doppler assessment and a normal arterial waveform. The patient was taken to the operating suite, where left testicular torsion was confirmed. After rapid detorsion and orchiopexy, the left testicle reperfused and was viable. (From Broder JS: *Diagnostic imaging for the emergency physician,* Philadelphia, 2011, Saunders.)

BASIC INFORMATION

DEFINITION

Tetralogy of Fallot (TOF) is a congenital heart deformity that consists of the following four features (Fig. 1-818):
1. Ventricular septal defect (VSD)
2. Infundibular stenosis that leads to the obstruction of the right ventricular (RV) outflow tract or pulmonary valve stenosis
3. An aorta that overrides the VSD by <50% of its diameter with deviation to the right
4. Concentric RV hypertrophy

SYNONYMS

None

ICD-9CM CODES
745.2 Tetralogy of Fallot

EPIDEMIOLOGY & DEMOGRAPHICS

INCIDENCE:
- TOF is the most common cyanotic congenital heart malformation that is diagnosed in patients after the age of 1 yr.
- TOF accounts for nearly 7% to 10% of all cases of congenital heart disease.
- Occurs in approximately 3.9/10,000 live births in the U.S.
- It is the most common cyanotic malformation to reach adulthood without reparative surgery.

PREDOMINANT SEX: Slightly higher incidence in males than females

GENETICS: Genetic influence is suspected.

PHYSICAL FINDINGS & CLINICAL PRESENTATION

- Of the four major features of TOF, infundibular stenosis that leads to RV outflow tract obstruction and VSD are the primary defects that result in clinical manifestations. The degree of RV outflow obstruction determines the age and symptoms at presentation. RV outflow tract obstruction and the VSD result in the following:
  - Right-to-left shunting and hypoxemia
  - Altered RV hemodynamics
  - Decreased pulmonary blood flow
- The aforementioned pathophysiologic concepts result in common manifestations of TOF, including the following:
  - Cyanosis of the nail beds and lips
  - Dyspnea on exertion
  - Digital clubbing
  - The child assuming a squatting position after exercise to increase systemic vascular resistance, thereby decreasing right-to-left shunting
  - Low birth weight and growth rate
  - Palpable RV impulse
  - Systolic thrill along the left sternal border
  - Single second heart sound comprised of aortic component only
  - A grade 3 to 5 crescendo/decrescendo murmur is heard along the left mid to upper sternal border with posterior radiation
- Murmur is softened in deeply cyanotic neonates with TOF with pulmonary atresia.
- Paroxymal episodes of rapid and deep breathing (tet spells) with increased cyanosis would occur with almost complete right ventricular outflow tract obstruction. Tet spells, and sometimes syncope are noticed especially after feeding and defecation.
- Presentation depends on the degree of RV outflow obstruction. May present at birth with cyanosis in severe cases with insufficient pulmonary blood flow. Cases with mild to moderate obstruction and compensated pulmonary flow are usually diagnosed while patient is being evaluated for murmur or heart failure.
- After repair, patients may have a low-pitched diastolic murmur at the pulmonic area that is consistent with pulmonary regurgitation or a pansystolic murmur that is consistent with a VSD patch leak. If the patient only has a palliative shunt, a continuous murmur may be heard from the site of the shunt.

ETIOLOGY

TOF likely results from the maldevelopment of the embryologic conotruncus and is associated with some genetic disorders but the exact mechanism is unknown.

DIAGNOSIS

- The diagnosis of TOF is suspected in any neonate, infant, or child who presents with cyanosis and a heart murmur (see "Physical Findings & Clinical Presentation").
- VSD is associated with other cardiac defects:
  - Persistent foramen ovale/atrial septal defect
  - Pulmonary artery anomalies
  - Right aortic arch
  - Left superior vena cava to coronary sinus
  - Additional VSDs
  - Coronary artery anomalies
  - Aortic valve regurgitation
- Associated anomalies and syndromes include the following:
  - DiGeorge
  - de Lange

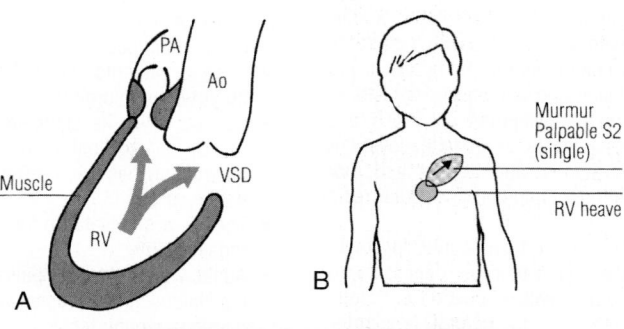
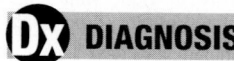
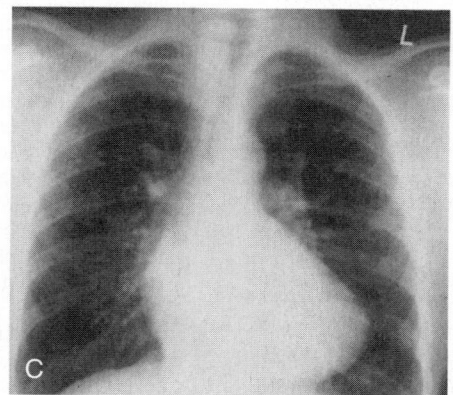
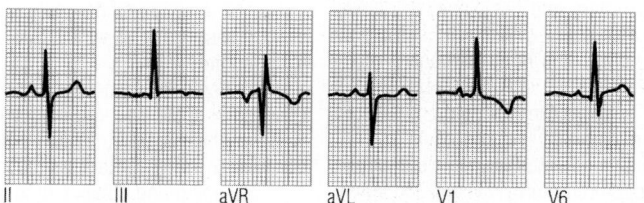

FIGURE 1-818 Features of Fallot tetralogy. A, Diagram of abnormality. *Ao,* Aorta; *PA,* pulmonary artery; *VSD,* ventricular septal defect. **B,** Physical signs. **C,** Chest x-ray showing right ventricular hypertrophy, typical "coeur en sabot." **D,** ECG showing right atrial and ventricular hypertrophy and right axis deviation. (From Souhami RL, Moxham J: *Textbook of medicine,* ed 4, London, 2002, Churchill Livingstone.)

- ○ Goldenhar
- ○ Klippel-Feil
- ○ VACTERL
- ○ CHARGE
- ○ Pierre Robin
- ○ Trisomies 21, 13, and 18
- ○ Fetal alcohol
- ○ Alagille
- ○ MTHFR polymorphism

DIFFERENTIAL DIAGNOSIS

- Asthma
- Isolated VSD
- Pulmonary atresia
- Patent ductus arteriosus
- Aortic stenosis
- Pneumothorax

WORKUP

- Detailed history and physical examination, including pulse oximetry
- Echocardiogram, chest radiograph, 12-lead ECG, and routine laboratory tests

LABORATORY TESTS

- Pulse oximetry to determine oxygenation.
- The CBC shows polycythemia from long-standing hypoxemia.
- Arterial blood gas levels show hypoxemia, normal pH, and pCO_2 (carbon dioxide levels).
- ECG commonly demonstrates right axis deviation, RV hypertrophy, and right atrial enlargement.
- Exercise testing may help to evaluate functional capacity and exertional arrhythmias.

IMAGING STUDIES

- Chest radiography reveals a boot-shaped heart that is commonly described as *coeur en sabot;* a prominent RV with decreased pulmonary vascularity; and a heart size that is usually normal. However, in patients with increased aortopulmonary collateral blood flow or with associated large patent ductus arteriosus, the heart size is increased with increased pulmonary vascularity.
- Echocardiography demonstrates VSD(s), anatomy and severity of right ventricular outflow tract obstruction, aortic arch anatomy, and other associated anomalies.
- Cardiac catheterization and angiography help to determine hemodynamics, the severity of right-to-left shunting, the localization of the VSD, coronary artery anatomy, right ventricular outflow obstruction, pulmonary artery stenosis, aortopulmonary collaterals. Interventions are also possible, such as the elimination of collateral vessels or systemic-pulmonic artery shunts, dilation or stent implantation for obstructed pulmonary arteries, and possible percutaneous pulmonic valve replacement.
- Cardiac MRI is used for the localization of the VSD, the anatomic assessment of the RV outflow tract, the assessment of RV function, the quantification of pulmonary regurgitation, and the detection of RV myocardial fibrosis.

Magnetic resonance angiography can be a noninvasive alternative to cardiac catheterization for the evaluation of pulmonary vascular anatomy and the ascending aorta.
- Multislice spiral computed tomography can be used for diagnosis, and it is extremely important during the planning of the repair procedure. Its use may be limited by the risks associated with radiation exposure in children. It can also be used to make assessments that are similar to those usually made by MRI for patients who are unable to undergo MRI.

Rx TREATMENT

NONPHARMACOLOGIC THERAPY

- Oxygen
- Prostaglandins at time of birth to keep a patent ductus and to maintain ductal flow to the lungs
- Knee-chest position during hypoxemic spells to help reduce venous return and to increase systemic vascular resistance, thereby decreasing right-to-left shunting

ACUTE GENERAL Rx

- The acute treatment of any infant or child with TOF who is cyanotic with respiratory distress is aimed at increasing systemic vascular resistance and decreasing right-to-left shunting (e.g., phenylephrine 0.1 to 0.5 mcg/kg/min intravenously to increase systemic vascular resistance, and oxygen and morphine to decrease pulmonary vascular resistance).
- Intravenous sodium bicarbonate for metabolic acidosis and, if more is necessary, respiratory support with intubation and sedation are required to control respiratory distress in cyanotic spells.
- Intravenous β-blockers (e.g., propranolol 0.15 to 0.25 mg/kg via slow intravenous push) are used to decrease RV outflow tract contractility.
- Emergent complete surgical repair or aortopulmonary shunt (Blalock-Taussig shunt) is required if all of the above treatments fail.

CHRONIC Rx

- Palliative repair includes procedures to increase pulmonary blood flow, thus reducing right-to-left shunting and allowing for pulmonary development. Examples of palliative procedures include the Blalock-Taussig shunt, in which a shunt is made between the subclavian artery and the pulmonary artery; the Waterston shunt, which attaches the ascending aorta to the right pulmonary artery; and the Potts shunt, which attaches the descending aorta to the left pulmonary artery. These are generally performed in patients who are not candidates for complete surgical repair due to prematurity, hypoplastic pulmonary arteries, and/or other anomalies in the coronary anatomy.

- Complete surgical repair has good success and involves closing the VSD with a Dacron patch and relieving the RV outflow tract obstruction by simple resection of the infundibular stenosis, patch augmentation of the RV outflow, or the placement of a transannular patch. Patients who have the repair before the age of 2 yr are usually symptom free and can generally lead a normal life. If the repair is performed during adulthood, pulmonary valve replacement may be required.
- Postoperative issues include the following:
  - ○ Residual pulmonic regurgitation
  - ○ RV dilation and dysfunction from pulmonary regurgitation
  - ○ Residual RV outflow tract obstruction
  - ○ Branch pulmonary artery stenosis or hypoplasia
  - ○ Sustained ventricular tachycardia
  - ○ Sudden cardiac death
  - ○ Atrioventricular block, atrial flutter, and atrial fibrillation
  - ○ Progressive aortic regurgitation
  - ○ Syndromal associations

DISPOSITION

- Almost all patients with TOF have either palliative or complete surgical repair before they reach adulthood.
- <3% of patients with TOF reach the age of 40 yr without surgery.
- Survival after the complete operative repair of TOF is excellent if the RV outflow tract obstruction has been relieved and the VSD has been closed.
- The 35-yr survival rate for patients after TOF repair is 85%.
- Adults who underwent palliative surgery during childhood can present with polycythemia, pulmonary hypertension, cyanosis, aortic regurgitation, and clubbing.
- Conduction disturbances; tricuspid, aortic, and pulmonary regurgitation; pulmonary stenosis; and cardiomegaly may present in patients who underwent complete surgical repair during childhood.
- Ventricular arrhythmia can lead to sudden cardiac death in 8.3% of surgically repaired patients by the age of 35 yr. Monomorphic ventricular tachycardia is likely the result of a reentry circuit from a scar caused by the surgery.
- A prolonged QRS duration on the preoperative ECG predicts an increased risk of postoperative supraventricular or ventricular arrhythmia. Prolongation of the QRS beyond 180 msec identifies patients who are at increased risk of ventricular tachycardia after surgery.
- Patients with signs or symptoms of arrhythmia should undergo hemodynamic and electrophysiologic testing, including pulmonic valve replacement, residual VSD closure, mapping and ablation of an arrhythmia, antiarrhythmic medication, or the placement of an implantable cardiac defibrillator.

- Reduced exercise capacity is usually the result of chronic pulmonary regurgitation or residual RV outflow tract obstruction.
- Patients with left ventricular dysfunction may benefit with angiotensin-converting enzyme inhibitors, diuretics, and digoxin.
- Women with repaired TOF should be assessed by a cardiologist before considering pregnancy to determine if pulmonic valve replacement is needed first.
- The offspring of patients with TOF are more likely than the general population to have congenital anomalies.
- Selected patients with normal RV pressures and function without evidence of residual shunt and without atrial or ventricular tachyarrhythmia are eligible to participate in competitive sports.

REFERRAL

- Infants and children with cyanotic heart disease should be referred to a pediatric cardiologist for further diagnostic evaluation. After being diagnosed with TOF, patients should be referred to centers with experience in palliative and complete surgical repair.
- Adult patients with repaired TOF should be comanaged with a cardiologist who specializes in adults with congenital heart disease.

! PEARLS & CONSIDERATIONS

- TOF was first described by the French physician Etienne Fallot in 1888.
- The first palliative surgical treatment for TOF was performed by Dr. Alfred Blalock at Johns Hopkins University in 1945 (i.e., the Blalock-Taussig shunt).
- The first surgical repair for TOF was performed by Dr. C. Walton Lillehei at the University of Minnesota in 1954.

COMMENTS

- The severity of RV outflow tract obstruction is the primary determinant of clinical symptoms and outcomes.

- There is a 3% increased risk of congenital heart disease in the children of parents with TOF.
- TOF requires subacute bacterial endocarditis prophylaxis before any dental work or nonsterile surgical procedures (e.g., surgery of the bowel or bladder).
- Children with TOF are at risk for neurodevelopmental delay when they reach school age.

SUGGESTED READINGS
available at www.expertconsult.com

RELATED CONTENT
Tetralogy of Fallot (Patient Information)

AUTHORS: **SYEDA M. SAYEED, M.D.,** and **WEN-CHIH WU, M.D., M.P.H.**

T

Diseases and Disorders

I

BASIC INFORMATION

DEFINITION

Thalassemias are a heterogeneous group of disorders of hemoglobin synthesis that have in common a deficient synthesis of one or more of the polypeptide chains of the normal human hemoglobin, resulting in a quantitative abnormality of the hemoglobin thus produced. Table 1-392 describes the various thalassemias. There are no qualitative changes such as those encountered in the hemoglobinopathies (e.g., sickle cell disease).

SYNONYMS

Mediterranean anemia
Cooley's anemia

ICD-9CM CODES
282.4 Thalassemia

EPIDEMIOLOGY & DEMOGRAPHICS

- Thalassemia is among the most common genetic disorders worldwide. Approximately 4.83% of the world's population carry globin variants, including 1.67% of the population that are heterozygous for alpha-thalassemia and beta-thalassemia.
- The highest concentration of alpha-thalassemia is found in Southeast Asia and the African west coast. For example, the prevalence is 5% to 10% in Thailand. It is also common among blacks, with a prevalence of approximately 5%.
- The worldwide prevalence of beta-thalassemia is approximately 3%; in certain regions of Italy and Greece the prevalence reaches 15% to 30%. This high prevalence can be found in Americans of Italian or Greek descent.
- The distribution of thalassemia in Europe and Africa parallels that of malaria, suggesting that thalassemic persons are more resistant to the parasite, thus permitting evolutionary survival advantage.

CLASSIFICATION

Beta-thalassemia:
- Beta (+) thalassemia (suboptimal beta-globin synthesis)
- Beta (o) thalassemia (total absence of beta-globin synthesis)
- Delta-beta-thalassemia (total absence of both delta-globin and beta-globin synthesis)

- Lepore hemoglobin (synthesis of small amounts of fused delta-beta-globin and total absence of delta- and beta-globin)
- Hereditary persistence of fetal hemoglobin (HPHF) (increased hemoglobin F synthesis and reduced or absence of delta- and beta-globin)

Alpha-thalassemia:
- Silent carrier (three alpha-globin genes present)
- Alpha-thalassemia trait (two alpha-globin genes present)
- Hemoglobin H disease (one alpha-globin gene present)
- Hydrops fetalis (no alpha-globin gene)
- Hemoglobin constant sprint (elongated alpha-globin chain)

Thalassemic hemoglobinopathies:
- Hb Terre Haute, Hb Quong Sze, HbE, Hb Knossos

PHYSICAL FINDINGS & CLINICAL PRESENTATION

Beta-thalassemia:
- Heterozygous beta-thalassemia (thalassemia minor): no or mild anemia, microcytosis and hypochromia, mild hemolysis manifested by slight reticulocytosis and splenomegaly

TABLE 1-392 The Thalassemias

Thalassemia	Globin Genotype	Features	Expression	Hemoglobin Analysis
α-Thalassemia				
1 gene deletion	-,α/α,α	Normal	Normal	Newborn: Bart's 1%-2%
2 gene deletion trait	-,α/-,α -, -/α,α	Microcytosis, mild hypochromasia	Normal, mild anemia	Newborn: Bart's: 5%-10%
3 gene deletion hemoglobin H	-,-/-,α	Microcytosis, hypochromic	Mild anemia, transfusions not required	Newborn: Bart's: 20%-30%
2 gene deletion + Constant Spring	-,-/α,α$^{Constant Spring}$	Microcytosis, hypochromic	Moderate to severe anemia, transfusion, splenectomy.	2%-3% Constant Spring, 10%-15% hemoglobin H
4 gene deletion	-,-/-,-	Anisocytosis, poikilocytosis	Hydrops fetalis	Newborn: 89%-90% Bart's with Gower 1 and 2 and Portland
Nondeletional	α,α/α,α^{variant}	Microcytosis, mild anemia	Normal	1%-2% variant hemoglobin
β-Thalassemia				
β^0 or β$^+$ heterozygote: trait	β^0/A, β$^+$/A	Variable microcytosis	Normal	Elevated A$_2$, variable elevation of F
β^0-Thalassemia	β^0/β^0, β$^+$/β^0, E/β^0	Microcytosis, nucleated RBC	Transfusion dependent	F 98% and A$_2$ 2% E 30%-40%
β$^+$-Thalassemia severe	β$^+$/β$^+$	Microcytosis nucleated RBC	Transfusion dependent/thalassemia intermedia	F 70%-95%, A$_2$ 2%, trace A
Silent	β$^+$/A	Microcytosis	Normal with only microcytosis	A$_2$ 3.3%-3.5%
β$^+$/β$^+$		Hypochromic, microcytic	Mild to moderate anemia	A$_2$ 2%-5%, F 10%-30%
Dominant (rare)	B^0/A	Microcytosis, abnormal RBCs	Moderately severe anemia, splenomegaly	Elevated F and A$_2$
δ-Thalassemia	A/A	Normal	Normal	A$_2$ absent
(δβ)^0-Thalassemia	(δβ)^0/A	Hypochromic	Mild anemia	F 5%-20%
(δβ)$^+$-Thalassemia Lepore	β^{Lepore}/A	Microcytosis	Mild anemia	Lepore 8%-20%
Lepore	β^{Lepore}/β^{Lepore}	Microcytic, hypochromic	Thalassemia intermedia	F 80%, Lepore 20%
γδβ-Thalassemia	(Υ^{A}δβ)^0/A	Microcytosis, microcytic, hypochromic	Moderate anemia, splenomegaly, homozygote: thalassemia intermedia	Decreased F and A$_2$ compared with δβ-thalassemia
Υ-Thalassemia	(Υ^{A}Υ^G)^0/A	Microcytosis	Insignificant unless homozygote	Decreased F
Hereditary Persistence of Fetal Hemoglobin				
Deletional	A/A	Microcytic	Mild anemia	F 100% homozygotes
Nondeletional	A/A	Normal	Normal	F 20%-40%

From Kliegman RM et al: *Nelson textbook of pediatrics*, ed 19, Philadelphia, 2011, Saunders.

- Homozygous beta-thalassemia (thalassemia major): intense hemolytic anemia; transfusion dependency; bone deformities (skull and long bones); hepatomegaly; splenomegaly; iron overload leading to cardiomyopathy, diabetes mellitus, and hypogonadism; growth retardation; pigment gallstones; susceptibility to infection
- Thalassemia intermedia caused by combination of beta- and alpha-thalassemia or beta-thalassemia and Hb Lepore: resembles thalassemia major but is milder

Alpha-thalassemia:
- Silent carrier: no symptoms.
- Alpha-thalassemia trait: microcytosis only.
- Hemoglobin H disease: moderately severe hemolysis with microcytosis and splenomegaly.
- The loss of all four alpha-globin genes is incompatible with life (stillbirth of hydropic fetus). NOTE: Pregnancies with hydrops fetalis are associated with a high incidence of toxemia.

ETIOLOGY

- Beta-thalassemia: it is caused by more than 200 point mutations and, rarely, by deletions. The reduction of beta-globin synthesis results in redundant alpha-globin chains (Heinz bodies), which are cytotoxic and cause intramedullary hemolysis and ineffective erythropoiesis. The pathophysiology of beta-thalassemia is illustrated in Fig. E1-819. Fetal hemoglobin may be increased.
- Alpha-thalassemia: several mutations can result in insufficient amounts of alpha-globin available for combination with non–alpha-globins.

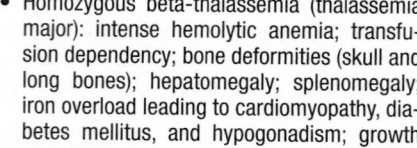 DIAGNOSIS

LABORATORY TESTS

Beta-thalassemia:
- Microcytosis (mean cell volume: 55 to 80 fL)
- Normal red blood cell (RBC) distribution width index (RDW)
- Smear: nucleated RBCs, anisocytosis, poikilocytosis, polychromatophilia, Pappenheimer and Howell-Jolly bodies
- Hemoglobin electrophoresis: absent or reduced hemoglobin A, increased fetal hemoglobin, variable increase in the amount of hemoglobin A_2
- Markers of hemolysis: elevated indirect bilirubin and lactate dehydrogenase, decreased haptoglobin

Alpha-thalassemia:
- Microcytosis in the absence of iron deficiency
- Hemoglobin electrophoresis normal except for the presence of hemoglobin H in hemoglobin H disease

TREATMENT

- Thalassemia minor: no treatment, but avoid iron administration for incorrect diagnosis of iron deficiency.
- Beta-thalassemia major (and hemoglobin H disease):
  1. Transfusion as required together with chelation of iron with desferrioxamine (by IV or subcutaneous administration, 8 to 12 hr nightly, 5 to 6 days a week at a dose of 2 to 6 g/day with a portable infusion pump). Deferiprone, an oral chelating agent, can be used as a second-line treatment of iron overload caused by blood transfusions (transfusional hemosiderosis).
  2. Splenectomy for hypersplenism if present.
  3. Bone marrow transplantation. Although hematopoietic stem cell transplantation is the only curative approach for thalassemia, it has been limited by the high cost and scarcity of human leukocyte antigen–matched donors. Before transplantation, it is necessary to administer myeloablative regimens to eradicate the endogenous thalassemic bone marrow. Commonly used agents are hydroxyurea, azathioprine, fludarabine, busulfan, and cyclophosphamide.
  4. Hydroxyurea may increase the level of hemoglobin F.

PEARLS & CONSIDERATIONS

- Polymerase chain reaction can be used to detect point mutations or deletions in chorionic villous samples, enabling first-trimester, DNA-based testing for thalassemia.
- Preimplantation genetic diagnosis can be extended to human leukocyte antigen typing on embryonic biopsies, allowing the selection of an embryo that is not affected by thalassemia and that may also serve as a stem cell donor for a previously affected child within the same family.

SUGGESTED READING
available at www.expertconsult.com

AUTHOR: **FRED F. FERRI, M.D.**

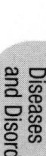
Diseases and Disorders

T

BASIC INFORMATION

DEFINITION

Thoracic outlet syndrome describes a condition producing upper extremity symptoms believed to result from neurovascular compression at the thoracic outlet. Three types are described on the basis of point of compression: (1) cervical rib and scalenus syndrome, in which abnormal scalene muscles or the presence of a cervical rib may cause compression; (2) costoclavicular syndrome, in which compression may occur under the clavicle; and (3) hyperabduction syndrome, in which compression may occur in the subcoracoid area.

ICD-9CM CODES
353.0 Thoracic outlet syndrome

EPIDEMIOLOGY & DEMOGRAPHICS

PREVALENCE: Varies from source to source; presence of cervical ribs in 0.5% to 1% of population (50% bilateral), but most are asymptomatic
PREDOMINANT SEX: Females affected more often than males (ratio of 3.5:1)
PREDOMINANT AGE: Rare in those aged <20 yr

PHYSICAL FINDINGS & CLINICAL PRESENTATION

- Symptoms and signs are related to the degree of involvement of each of the various structures at the level of the first rib.
- True venous or arterial involvement is not common.
- Diagnosis is most often used in the consideration of neural pain affecting the arm, which suggests involvement of the brachial plexus.
  1. Arterial compression: pallor, paresthesias, diminished pulses, coolness, digital gangrene, and a supraclavicular bruit or mass
  2. Venous compression: edema and pain; thrombosis causing superficial venous dilation in the shoulder area
  3. "True" neural compression: lower trunk (C8, T1) findings with intrinsic weakness and diminished sensation to the ring finger and small fingers and ulnar aspect of the forearm
  4. Possible supraclavicular tenderness
  5. Provocative tests (Adson's, Wright's): may reproduce pain but are of disputed usefulness

ETIOLOGY

- Congenital cervical rib or fibrous extension of cervical rib (Fig. 1-820)
- Abnormal scalene muscle insertion
- Drooping of shoulder girdle from generalized hypotonia or trauma
- Narrowed costoclavicular interval as a result of downward and backward pressure on shoulder (sometimes seen in individuals who carry heavy backpacks)
- Acute venous thrombosis with exercise (effort thrombosis)
- Bony abnormalities of first rib
- Abnormal fibromuscular bands
- Malunion of clavicle fracture

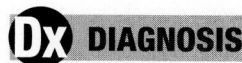

DIAGNOSIS

DIFFERENTIAL DIAGNOSIS

- Carpal tunnel syndrome
- Cervical radiculopathy
- Brachial neuritis
- Ulnar nerve compression
- Reflex sympathetic dystrophy
- Superior sulcus tumor

WORKUP

Fig. E1-821 describes a diagnostic algorithm for thoracic outlet syndrome. Except for venous or arterial pathology, no ancillary diagnostic tests are reliable for diagnostic confirmation.

IMAGING STUDIES

- Arteriography or venography when vascular pathology is strongly suspected clinically
- Cervical spine radiographs to rule out cervical disk disease
- Chest radiograph to rule out lung tumor
- Electromyography, nerve conduction velocity studies to rule out carpal tunnel syndrome, cervical radiculopathy

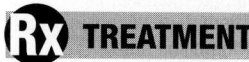

TREATMENT

ACUTE GENERAL Rx

- Sling for pain relief
- Physical therapy modalities plus shoulder girdle–strengthening exercises
- Postural reeducation
- Nonsteroidal anti-inflammatory drugs

DISPOSITION

- Surgery: generally successful for vascular disorders
- Nonsurgical treatment: often successful for patients with pain as the primary symptom

REFERRAL

For vascular surgery consultation when venous or arterial impairment is present

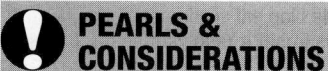

PEARLS & CONSIDERATIONS

COMMENTS

- True thoracic outlet syndrome is probably an uncommon condition.
- Diagnosis is often used to describe a wide variety of clinical symptoms.
- Considerable disagreement exists regarding the frequency of this disorder.

SUGGESTED READINGS
available at www.expertconsult.com

RELATED CONTENT
Thoracic Outlet Syndrome (Patient Information)

AUTHOR: **LONNIE R. MERCIER, M.D.**

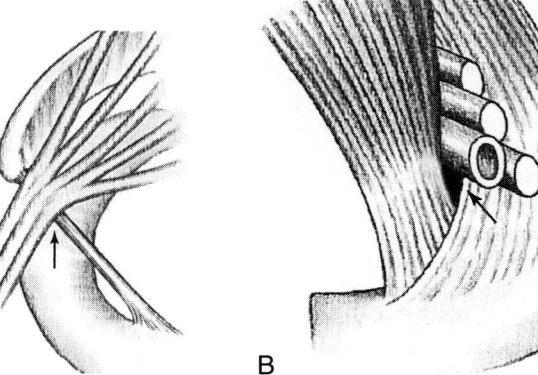

FIGURE 1-820 A, Compression caused by a cervical rib *(arrow).* **B,** Abnormal scalene muscle insertions that may cause compression at the cervicobrachial region *(arrow).* (From Mercier LR: *Practical orthopedics,* ed 5, St Louis, 2000, Mosby.)

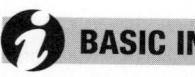

BASIC INFORMATION

DEFINITION

Thrombocytosis is defined by an elevated platelet count (>450,000/μL) in peripheral blood. It is caused by overproduction of platelets (reactive thrombocytosis), or it may be caused by clonal expansion of megakaryocytes (autonomous thrombocytosis). Reactive thrombocytosis is driven by excessive cytokines induced by various stimuli, such as trauma or inflammation. The latter is defined as chronic myeloproliferative disorders (CMPD), of which four subgroups are well characterized: chronic myelogenous leukemia (CML), polycythemia vera (PV), primary myelofibrosis (PMF), and essential thrombocythemia (ET). In addition, platelet count can be spuriously elevated in some conditions (see differential diagnosis). Extreme thrombocytosis is defined as platelet count >1 million/μL.

SYNONYMS

Thrombocythemia

ICD-9CM CODES
289.9   Unspecified diseases of blood and blood-forming organs
238.71   Essential thrombocytosis

EPIDEMIOLOGY & DEMOGRAPHICS

Reactive thrombocytosis is much more frequent than autonomous thrombocytosis (70% vs. 22% in one series).
INCIDENCE: 2.5 new cases/100,000 population/yr
PREVALENCE: Estimated as 24 cases/100,000 population
PREDOMINANT SEX AND AGE: The median age at diagnosis is 60 yr. Female/male ratio is 2:1.

PHYSICAL FINDINGS & CLINICAL PRESENTATION

- Regardless of the cause, a high platelet count may be associated with vasomotor symptoms such as headache, visual disturbances, dizziness, atypical chest pain, acral dysesthesia, and erythromelalgia.
- Thrombotic and bleeding complications can occur.
- Symptoms and complications are much more likely to occur in association with autonomous thrombocytosis than reactive thrombocytosis.
- The degree of thrombocytosis does not predict the likelihood of autonomous thrombocytosis, and does not generally correlate to the risk of thrombosis.
- Splenomegaly is common with CMPD.
- Coexistent leukocytosis and erythrocytosis are common with CML and PV.
- Disease transformation from ET to PV, PMF, and acute myeloid leukemia (AML) is uncommon.

ETIOLOGY

- *JAK2* mutation is frequent in CMPD (95%-97% in PV, 50% in ET, and 40% to 60% in PMF).
- *MPL* mutation in 1% to 4% of ET patients

These mutations may play a role in pathogenesis of CMPD.

DIAGNOSIS

DIFFERENTIAL DIAGNOSIS

- Spurious thrombocytosis
  - Mixed cryoglobulinemia
  - Circulating cytoplasmic fragments in patients with leukemia, lymphoma, or severe hemolysis or burns can be counted as platelets
- Reactive thrombocytosis
  - Benign hematologic disorders
  - Acute hemorrhage, iron deficiency anemia, hemolytic anemia
  - Chronic infection, such as tuberculosis
  - Acute and chronic inflammatory disorders
  - Rheumatologic disorders
  - Inflammatory bowel disease
  - Celiac disease
  - Functional and surgical asplenia
  - Tissue damage
  - Trauma, thermal burn
  - Myocardial infarction
  - Acute pancreatitis
  - Recent surgery
  - Renal failure, nephrotic syndrome
  - Exercise
  - Medications, such as vincristine, epinephrine
- Autonomous thrombocytosis
  - CML
  - PV
  - PMF
  - Myelodysplastic syndrome (5q-syndrome)
  - AML with inv(3), t(3;3)
  - Essential thrombocytosis (Box 1-72)

WORKUP

- Comprehensive history and physical examination to exclude many of the common causes of reactive thrombocytosis: history and physical examination suggestive of acute blood loss, iron deficiency, acute or chronic infection/inflammation, medication use, asplenia, malignancy, and trauma should be looked for. Fig. E1-825 describes a diagnostic algorithm for thrombocytosis. Laboratory tests are summarized in Box E1-73. The diagnosis of ET requires platelet counts >600 x 10⁹/L on two separate occasions >4 weeks apart, absence of Philadelphia chromosome, and exclusion of secondary causes of thrombocytosis.
- Repeat CBC with peripheral blood smear and bone marrow biopsy (Figs. E1-823 and E1-824) to exclude spurious thrombocytosis.

LABORATORY TESTS

- CBC with peripheral blood smear: Howell-Jolly bodies and target cells are present in patients with asplenia; nucleated RBC, teardrop RBC and WBC precursors in patients with PMF
- Serum ferritin level: low ferritin level suggests iron deficiency
- Serum C-reactive protein (CRP), ESR, and plasma fibrinogen: nonspecific markers of infection or inflammation
- Philadelphia chromosome or BCR-ABL rearrangement: positive in CML
- Serum erythropoietin assay: low to normal in PV and ET
- *JAK2* mutation analysis: PV and ET; JAK2 V617F mutation is found in about 50% of patients with ET and indicates a more aggressive course

---

BOX 1-72   World Health Organization Diagnostic Criteria for Essential Thrombocythemia

Diagnosis requires that all of the following criteria be met:
- Sustained platelet count ≥450 × 10⁹/Lᵃ
- Bone marrow biopsy specimen showing proliferation mainly of the megakaryocytic lineage, with increased numbers of enlarged, mature megakaryocytes; no significant increase or left shift of neutrophil granulopoiesis or erythropoiesis
- Failure to meet the WHO criteria for polycythemia vera,ᵇ primary myelofibrosis,ᶜ BCR-ABL1–positive chronic myelogenous leukemia,ᵈ myelodysplastic syndrome,ᵉ or other myeloid neoplasms
- Demonstration of JAK2 V617F or other clonal marker; or, in the absence of JAK2 V617F, no evidence of reactive thrombocytosisᶠ

ᵃSustained during the workup process.
ᵇRequires the failure of iron replacement therapy to increase the hemoglobin level to the polycythemia vera range in the presence of decreased serum ferritin. Exclusion of polycythemia vera is based on hemoglobin and hematocrit levels; red cell mass measurement is not required.
ᶜRequires the absence of relevant reticulin fibrosis, collagen fibrosis, peripheral blood leukoerythroblastosis, or markedly hypercellular marrow accompanied by megakaryocyte morphology typical for primary myelofibrosis—small to large megakaryocytes with an aberrant nuclear-to-cytoplasmic ratio and hyperchromatic, bulbous, or irregularly folded nuclei and dense clustering.
ᵈRequires the absence of BCR-ABL1.
ᵉRequires the absence of dyserythropoiesis and dysgranulopoiesis.
ᶠCauses of reactive thrombocytosis include iron deficiency, splenectomy, surgery, infection, inflammation, connective tissue disease, metastatic cancer, and lymphoproliferative disorders. However, the presence of a condition associated with reactive thrombocytosis does not exclude the possibility of essential thrombocythemia if other criteria are met.
From Swerdlow SH et al (eds): *WHO classification of tumours of haematopoietic and lymphoid tissues*, Lyon, France, 2008, IARC Press.

- Bone marrow chromosome analysis: 5q-syndrome and other myelodysplastic syndrome, CML
- Bone marrow exam in ET may show clusters of abnormal megakaryocytes and increased reticulin fibrosis (see Fig. E1-824).

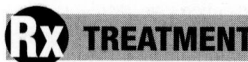

TREATMENT

Treatment for ET will be addressed in this chapter. Reactive thrombocytosis has been rarely associated with thrombosis or bleeding and generally does not require specific therapy.

ACUTE GENERAL Rx

- Vasomotor symptoms easily manageable with low-dose aspirin (<100 mg/day)
- Bleeding
  - Discontinue any platelet antiaggregating agent, such as aspirin or nonsteroidal anti-inflammatory agents.
  - Evaluate for disseminated intravascular coagulopathy and coagulation factor deficiency. Acquired factor V deficiency is occasionally present in association with autonomous thrombocytosis. In that case, treat with fresh frozen plasma infusion.
  - In case of extreme thrombocytosis, acquired von Willebrand disease may occur. Immediate platelet apheresis with definitive therapy with a platelet-lowering agent is essential in this instance.
- Thrombosis
  - Arterial or venous thrombosis occurs in 20% to 30% of patients.
  - If the platelet count is >800,000/μL, platelet apheresis coupled with a platelet-lowering agent should be considered with the goal of platelet count <400,000/μL.

- Initial workup should include additional thrombophilic diseases, such as proteins C and S abnormality, antithrombin, anticardiolipin antibody, mutations of factor V and II, and plasma homocysteine.
- Anticoagulant therapy for 3 to 9 mo based on the presence or absence of additional thrombophilic defects.

CHRONIC Rx

Treatment strategies for ET are based on the presence or absence of risk factors for thrombosis. Smoking cessation and obesity management should be discussed with all patients with ET. In low-risk patients (age <60 yr, no history of thrombosis or hemorrhage, a platelet count <1 million/μL), observation may be adequate. The cytoreductive therapy is indicated in high-risk patients (aged ≥65 yr and/or with previous history of thrombosis).

- Low-dose aspirin (81 mg/day) may be safe and possibly effective in preventing vascular events. It is also effective in preventing recurrent vascular events in high-risk patients and in treating the vasomotor symptoms.
- Cytoreductive therapy
  - Hydroxyurea (HU) versus anagrelide: HU plus aspirin is suggested to be safer and more effective than anagrelide plus aspirin in regard to thrombosis, bleeding, and transformation to PMF at 5 yr in a randomized trial. Monitor liver function tests and the degree of neutropenia or anemia with HU therapy.
  - The incidence of leukemic conversion in patients with ET treated with HU alone is reported as <1%. Interferon alpha may be effective for controlling platelet count in patients failing treatment with HU.

DISPOSITION

Most patients with ET have a normal life expectancy without disease-related complications.

REFERRAL

Refer to hematologist/oncologist when platelet count is consistently elevated >450,000/μL without causes for reactive thrombocytosis.

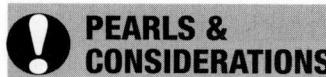

PEARLS & CONSIDERATIONS

COMMENTS

- Some patients with clinically apparent ET have Philadelphia chromosome or *BCR-ABL* rearrangement, even in the absence of other features of CML. It is suggested that it should be tested in all ET patients due to its potential therapeutic implications.
- The risk of bleeding with aspirin use in patients with ET is increased when the platelet count is >1 million/μL.
- Leukocytosis may be a better predictor of thrombosis risk than the platelet count.

PATIENT & FAMILY EDUCATION

Smoking cessation is encouraged in both patients with ET and reactive thrombocytosis.

SUGGESTED READINGS

available at www.expertconsult.com

AUTHOR: **ETSUKO AOKI, M.D., PH.D.**

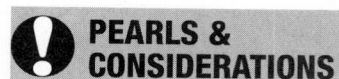

BASIC INFORMATION

DEFINITION

Superficial venous thrombophlebitis (SVT) is an inflammation of a vein with subsequent secondary thrombus formation. SVT most frequently involves superficial veins of the leg, but any superficial vein can be affected. SVT has been reported to occur in 125,000 people in the U.S. per year; however, the actual incidence is likely far greater. SVT is not always a benign condition. SVT should be regarded as the superficial venous manifestation of a systemic process known as venous thromboembolism (DVT, PE).

SYNONYMS

SVT
Superficial phlebitis
Superficial suppurative thrombophlebitis
Suppurative thrombophlebitis

ICD-9CM CODES
451.0 Thrombophlebitis, superficial

EPIDEMIOLOGY & DEMOGRAPHICS

- Approximately 30% to 45% of patients diagnosed with SVT are men with an average age of 54 yr.
- Approximately 55% to 70% of patients diagnosed with SVT are women with an average age of 58 yr.
- The overall recurrence of SVT is 18% over an average observation period of 15 mo, equally involving varicose and nonvaricose veins.
- The lifetime incidence of SVT in those with untreated varicose veins has been estimated at 25% to 50%.

PHYSICAL FINDINGS & CLINICAL PRESENTATION

- Subcutaneous vein is palpable as a tender cord or "wormlike" mass with increased warmth and erythema.
- Induration, redness, and tenderness are localized along the course of the vein. This linear appearance rather than circular appearance is useful to distinguish thrombophlebitis from other conditions (cellulitis, erythema nodosum).
- There is some swelling of the overlying skin and subcutaneous tissue but without generalized edema of the limb.
- Low-grade fever may be present.

ETIOLOGY

- In the lower extremity, 70% of SVT occurs in patients with varicose veins, with the great saphenous vein being most commonly involved (60% to 80%).
- Intravenous catheters and infusion of caustic drugs are the most common cause of upper extremity SVT.
- Malignancy
- Pregnancy/puerperium
- Hypercoagulable states
- Previous
- DVT/SVT

- OCP (oral contraceptive pill)/HRT (hormone replacement therapy)

DIAGNOSIS

DIFFERENTIAL DIAGNOSIS

- Lymphangitis
- Cellulitis
- Erythema nodosum
- Panniculitis
- Acute lipodermatosclerosis

WORKUP

The clinical investigation includes not only the local findings but also the presence of varicose veins with or without the stigmata of chronic venous insufficiency. Today, duplex ultrasound is the most important additional diagnostic tool.

IMAGING STUDIES

- Duplex ultrasound offers the advantage of being inexpensive, noninvasive, and repeatable for follow-up examination.
- Ultrasonography confirms the diagnosis, shows the location of the thrombus and its location regarding the saphenofemoral and/or saphenopopliteal junctions.
- Ultrasound examination of patients with SVT has revealed that a concomitant DVT can exist in 15% to 20%.
- In up to 25% of these patients, the DVT may not be contiguous with the SVT and may be found in the contralateral leg.
- Therefore bilateral duplex exam is recommended in all cases of SVT that involve the main trunk of the great saphenous vein (GSV) or small saphenous vein (SSV).

TREATMENT

NONPHARMACOLOGIC THERAPY

- Warm, moist compresses
- Do not restrict activity. Immediate mobilization with walking exercises.

ACUTE GENERAL Rx

- Treatment guidelines for SVT are not well established because of the lack of controlled clinical trials. In general, the primary goal of management should be to prevent thrombus extension and the risk of venous thromboembolism. All other therapy is directed at patient comfort.
- In patients with migratory SVT, recurrent SVT, or SVT without varicose veins, the underlying condition should be investigated and treatment directed accordingly.
- The most common cause of upper extremity SVT is an intravenous catheter. Treatment starts with removal of the cannula and application of warm compresses. The resultant lump may persist for months. No anticoagulant therapy is required.
- In patients with lower extremity SVT in a varicose vein branch, control of pain with analgesics and the use of gradient compression stockings are usually sufficient. Patients

are encouraged to continue their usual daily activities.
- Many investigators favor systemic anticoagulation when there is superficial thrombosis of 5 cm or more in length, the thrombus is within 1 cm of the saphenous junctions, or more than 5 cm of the saphenous trunk is involved, as shown by duplex ultrasonography.
- The 2012 American College of Chest Physicians guidelines recommend the use of fondaparinux (1 mg/kg/day) for 45 days over no anticoagulation in patients with lower extremity SVT within 1 cm of the saphenofemoral or saphenopopliteal junction.
- In the case of patients with varicose veins secondary to saphenous vein reflux, a catheter vein ablation procedure should be performed only after the acute SVT episode is over in order to avoid the thromboembolic complications induced by such procedures.

DISPOSITION

Clinical improvement within 10 to 14 days

REFERRAL

Referral to vascular surgeon or phlebologist with vascular lab

PEARLS & CONSIDERATIONS

SUPERFICIAL SUPPURATIVE THROMBOPHLEBITIS

- Superficial suppurative thrombophlebitis is associated with an intravenous catheter or multiple puncture sites secondary to IV drug abuse and is located primarily in the upper extremity.
- Clinical presentation is similar to that of nonsuppurative SVT but with associated fever, leukocytosis, and/or septicemia.
- Most cases of intravenous catheter sepsis are not complicated by suppurative thrombophlebitis; local IV catheter site infections occur in about 7% of cases and septicemia is found in only 1 of every 400 IV catheterizations.
- The incidence of peripheral vein suppurative thrombophlebitis is highest in patients with specific risk factors such as burns, steroids, and IV drug abuse.
- Treatment consists of antibiotics with adequate coverage of gram-negative rods and *Staphylococcus aureus*, including MRSA. Initial empirical treatment is with IV vancomycin 1 g q12h *plus* ceftriaxone 1 g IV q24h. Alternative regimen consists of daptomycin 6 mg/kg IV q 12h *plus* ceftriaxone 1 g IV q24h.

SUGGESTED READINGS

available at www.expertconsult.com

RELATED CONTENT

Thrombophlebitis (Patient Information)

AUTHOR: **GLENN G. FORT, M.D., M.P.H.**

BASIC INFORMATION

DEFINITION

Thrombotic thrombocytopenic purpura (TTP) is a rare disorder characterized by thrombocytopenia (often accompanied by purpura) and microangiopathic hemolytic anemia; neurologic impairment, renal dysfunction, and fever may also be present.

SYNONYMS

TTP

ICD-9CM CODES
446.6 Thrombotic thrombocytopenic purpura

EPIDEMIOLOGY & DEMOGRAPHICS

- TTP primarily affects females between ages 10 and 50 yr.
- Frequency is 11 cases annually per 1 million persons. There is increased incidence in HIV/AIDS and during pregnancy.

PHYSICAL FINDINGS & CLINICAL PRESENTATION

- Most patients present with nonspecific constitutional symptoms (weakness, nausea, abdominal pain, vomiting)
- Purpura (secondary to thrombocytopenia)
- Jaundice, pallor (from hemolysis)
- Mucosal bleeding
- Fever
- Fluctuating levels of consciousness (caused by thrombotic occlusion of the cerebral vessels)
- Renal failure and neurologic events are usually end-stage features

ETIOLOGY

- TTP is caused in some patients by autoantibodies or, in rare cases, by a hereditary deficiency of the protease ADAMTS13, which cleaves the high-molecular-weight multimers of von Willebrand factor. This results in abnormal platelet adhesion and activation.
- Many drugs, including clopidogrel, penicillin, antineoplastic agents (gemcitabine, mitomycin C, cyclosporine) oral contraceptives, quinine, and ticlopidine, have been associated with TTP. Other precipitating causes include infectious agents, pregnancy, malignancies, allogeneic bone marrow transplantation, and neurologic disorders.

DIAGNOSIS

DIFFERENTIAL DIAGNOSIS

- Disseminated intravascular coagulation (DIC)
- Malignant hypertension
- Vasculitis
- Eclampsia or preeclampsia
- Hemolytic-uremic syndrome (typically encountered in children, often after a viral infection)
- Gastroenteritis as a result of a serotoxin-producing serotype of *Escherichia coli*
- Medications: clopidogrel, ticlopidine, penicillin, antineoplastic chemotherapeutic agents, oral contraceptives

WORKUP

- A comprehensive history, physical examination, and laboratory evaluation usually confirm the diagnosis. Fig. E1-826 is an algorithm for diagnosis of TTP.
- The disease often begins as a flulike illness ultimately followed by clinical and laboratory abnormalities.

LABORATORY TESTS

- Severe anemia and thrombocytopenia (platelet count <50,000 or >50% reduction from previous counts). Peripheral blood smear (Fig. E1-827) reveals numerous red cell fragments (schistocytes).
- Elevated blood urea nitrogen and creatinine
- Evidence of hemolysis: elevated reticulocyte count, indirect bilirubin, lactate dehydrogenase, decreased haptoglobin
- Urinalysis: hematuria (red blood cells [RBCs] and RBC casts in urine sediment) and proteinuria
- Peripheral smear: severely fragmented RBCs (schistocytes). More than 4% RBC fragments in the peripheral blood.
- No laboratory evidence of DIC (normal fibrin degradation product, fibrinogen)
- The ADAMTS13 level is not necessary and metalloproteinase deficiency need not be proved for diagnosis of TTP

TREATMENT

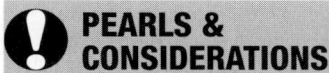

ACUTE GENERAL Rx

- Discontinue potential offending agents.
- The American Association of Blood Banks, the American Society for Apheresis, and the British Committee for Standards in Haematology recommend daily plasma exchange with replacement of 1.0 to 1.5 times the predicted plasma volume of the patient as standard therapy for TTP. The British guidelines recommend that plasma exchange therapy be continued for a minimum of 2 days after the platelet count returns to normal (>150,000 cells/m³).
- Corticosteroids (prednisone 1 to 2 mg/kg/day) use is controversial. They may be effective alone in patients with mild disease or may be administered concomitantly with plasmapheresis plus plasma exchange with fresh frozen plasma.
- High-dose plasma infusion (25 ml/kg/day) may be useful only if plasma exchange cannot be promptly started and for patients with very severe or refractory disease between plasma exchange sessions. High-dose plasma infusions can cause volume overload in patients with renal insufficiency.
- The monoclonal antibody rituximab has also been used for treatment of TTP.
- Platelet transfusions are contraindicated except in severely thrombocytopenic patients with documented bleeding.
- Use of antiplatelet agents (acetylsalicylic acid, dipyridamole) is controversial.
- Splenectomy is performed in refractory cases.

CHRONIC Rx

- Relapsing TTP may be treated with plasma exchange.
- Remission of chronic TTP that is unresponsive to conventional therapy has been reported after treatment with cyclophosphamide and the monoclonal antibody rituximab.
- Splenectomy done while the patients are in remission has been used in some centers to decrease the frequency of relapse in TTP.

DISPOSITION

- Survival of patients with TTP currently exceeds 80% with plasma exchange therapy.
- Relapse occurs in 20% to 40% of patients who have TTP in remission.

REFERRAL

Surgical referral for splenectomy in selected patients (see "Acute General Rx" and "Chronic Rx").

PEARLS & CONSIDERATIONS

COMMENTS

The diagnosis of TTP/hemolytic-uremic syndrome should be considered in pregnant women with vague neurologic, gastrointestinal, or renal symptoms in either the obstetric triage or emergency department areas.

SUGGESTED READINGS
available at www.expertconsult.com

RELATED CONTENT

Hemolytic Uremic Syndrome (Related Key Topic)

AUTHOR: **FRED F. FERRI, M.D.**

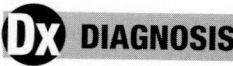
BASIC INFORMATION

DEFINITION

Thyroid carcinoma is a primary neoplasm of the thyroid. There are four major types of thyroid carcinoma: papillary, follicular, anaplastic, and medullary.

SYNONYMS

Papillary carcinoma of thyroid
Follicular carcinoma of thyroid
Anaplastic carcinoma of thyroid
Medullary carcinoma of thyroid

ICD-9CM CODES
193 Malignant neoplasm of thyroid

EPIDEMIOLOGY & DEMOGRAPHICS

- Thyroid cancer is the most common endocrine cancer, with over 48,000 new cases in the U.S. and approximately 1100 deaths.
- Female/male ratio is 3:1.
- Median age at diagnosis: 45 to 50 yr

PHYSICAL FINDINGS & CLINICAL PRESENTATION

- Presence of thyroid nodule
- Hoarseness and cervical lymphadenopathy
- Painless swelling in the region of the thyroid

ETIOLOGY

- Risk factors: prior neck irradiation
- Multiple endocrine neoplasia II (medullary carcinoma)
- Inherited syndromes associated with thyroid cancer are described in Table 1-393.
- Exenatide, a once-weekly GLP-1 receptor agonist for the treatment of type 2 DM, can increase the risk of medullary thyroid carcinoma (MTC).

DIAGNOSIS

DIFFERENTIAL DIAGNOSIS

- Multinodular goiter
- Lymphocytic thyroiditis
- Ectopic thyroid

WORKUP

The workup of thyroid carcinoma includes laboratory evaluation and diagnostic imaging. However, diagnosis is confirmed with fine-needle aspiration or surgical biopsy. The characteristics of thyroid carcinoma vary with the type:
- Papillary carcinoma (85%):
  1. Most frequently occurs in women during second or third decades
  2. Histologically, psammoma bodies (calcific bodies present in papillary projections) are pathognomonic; found in 35% to 45% of papillary thyroid carcinomas
  3. Majority are not papillary lesions but mixed papillary follicular carcinomas
  4. Spread is by lymphatics and by local invasion
- Follicular carcinoma (10%):
  1. More aggressive than papillary carcinoma
  2. Incidence increases with age
  3. Tends to metastasize hematogenously to bone, producing pathologic fractures
  4. Tends to concentrate iodine (useful for radiation therapy)
- Anaplastic carcinoma (1%):
  1. Very aggressive neoplasm
  2. Two major histologic types: small cell (less aggressive, 5-yr survival approximately 20%) and giant cell (death usually within 6 mo of diagnosis)
- MTC (4%):
  1. Unifocal lesion: found sporadically in elderly patients
  2. Bilateral lesions: associated with pheochromocytoma and hyperparathyroidism; this combination is known as MEN-II and is inherited as an autosomal-dominant disorder

LABORATORY TESTS

- Thyroid function studies are generally normal. Thyroid-stimulating hormone (TSH), T_4, and serum thyroglobulin levels should be obtained before thyroidectomy in patients with confirmed thyroid carcinoma.
- Increased plasma calcitonin assay in patients with medullary carcinoma (tumors produce thyrocalcitonin). RET proto-oncogene sequencing and measurement of plasma free metanephrine and normetanephrine levels to rule out coexistent pheochromocytoma are recommended in all patients with medullary thyroid cancer.
- Fine-needle aspiration biopsy is the best method to assess a thyroid nodule (see "Thyroid Nodule" in Section I).

IMAGING STUDIES (Fig. 1-828)

- Thyroid ultrasound can detect solitary solid nodules that have a high risk of malignancy. However, a negative ultrasound does not exclude diagnosis of thyroid carcinoma.
- Thyroid scanning with iodine-123 or technetium-99m can identify hypofunctioning (cold) nodules, which are more likely to be malignant. However, warm nodules can also be malignant.

STAGING

- Stage I: thyroid cancer of any size without distal spread in patient under age 45. In patients 45 years or older, tumor size ≤2 cm without local invasion or positive cervical lymph nodes
- Stage II: distal spread in patient younger than 45 years. In patients 45 years or older, tumors >2 cm but <4 cm without local invasion or positive cervical lymph nodes
- Stage III: tumors >4 cm in patient over 45 years of age
- Stage IV: distal spread in patient over 45 years of age

TREATMENT

ACUTE GENERAL Rx

- Papillary carcinoma:
  1. Total thyroidectomy is indicated if the patient has:
     a. Extrapyramidal extension of carcinoma
     b. Papillary carcinoma limited to thyroid but a positive history of irradiation to the neck
     c. Lesion >2 cm

TABLE 1-393 Inherited Syndromes Associated with Thyroid Cancer

Multiple endocrine neoplasia (MEN) 2A and 2B
Isolated familial medullary thyroid cancer
Gardner syndrome
Familial adenomatous polyposis
Carney complex
Cowden syndrome
Familial nonmedullary thyroid cancer

From Cameron JL, Cameron AM: *Current surgical therapy*, ed 10, Philadelphia, 2011, Saunders.

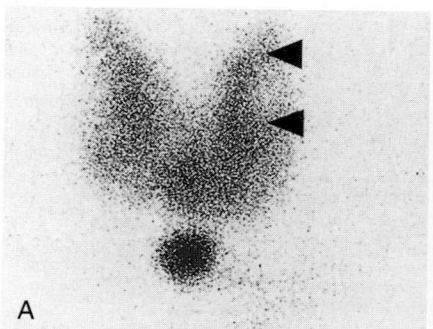
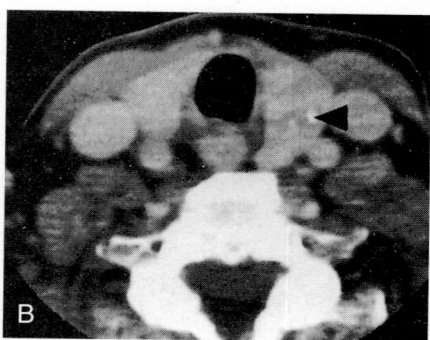

FIGURE 1-828 Papillary adenocarcinoma. A 74-year-old woman presented with a thyroid nodule. **A,** An ^{123}I thyroid scan (anterior view) demonstrates a "cold" nodule *(arrows)* in the upper portion of the left thyroid lobe. The "hot" spot below the thyroid is a suprasternal marker. **B,** An axial CT scan demonstrates an irregular density within the left thyroid lobe at the level of the lesion seen on the radionuclide scan. The lesion contains a single area of calcification *(arrow)* and is not sharply demarcated from normal thyroid tissue. At operation, there proved to be extracapsular extension. (From Skarin AT: *Atlas of diagnostic oncology,* ed 3, St Louis, 2003, Mosby.)

2. Lobectomy with isthmectomy may be considered in patients with intrathyroid papillary carcinoma <2 cm and no history of neck or head irradiation; surgery should be followed with suppressive therapy with thyroid hormone because these tumors are TSH responsive. The accepted practice is to suppress serum TSH concentrations to <0.1 microunit/ml in patients with persistent disease, suppression to 0.1-0.5 microunit/ml in patients who are disease free but are at high risk of recurrence, and a goal TSH level of 0.3-2.0 microunits/ml in patients who are disease free and have a low risk of recurrence.
3. Radioiodine ablation reduces rates of death and recurrence. Radioiodine is administered for stages III and IV disease.
- Follicular carcinoma:
  1. Total thyroidectomy followed by TSH suppression, as previously noted
  2. Radiotherapy with iodine-131 followed by thyroid suppression therapy with triiodothyronine is useful in patients with metastasis
- Anaplastic carcinoma:
  1. At diagnosis, this neoplasm is rarely operable; palliative surgery is indicated for extremely large tumor compressing the trachea.
  2. Management is usually restricted to radiation therapy or chemotherapy (combination of doxorubicin, cisplatin, and other antineoplastic agents); these measures rarely provide significant palliation.

- Medullary carcinoma:
  1. Thyroidectomy should be performed, followed by TSH suppression.
  2. Vandetanib, an oral tyrosine kinase inhibitor, was recently FDA-approved for treatment of symptomatic or progressive, unresectable, locally advanced or metastatic medullary thyroid cancer. It is not recommended for treatment of asymptomatic or less aggressive disease due to its many serious side effects. It is also very expensive ($10,000 for one month of therapy).
  3. Patients and their families should be screened for pheochromocytoma and hyperparathyroidism.

DISPOSITION

Prognosis varies with the type of thyroid carcinoma: 5-yr survival approaches 80% for follicular carcinoma and is approximately 5% with anaplastic carcinoma (see Table 1-394).

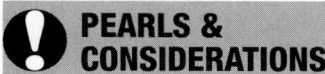 **PEARLS & CONSIDERATIONS**

COMMENTS

- Family members of patients with medullary carcinoma should be screened; DNA analysis for the detection of mutations in the *RET* gene structure permits the identification of *MEN IIA* gene carriers.
- Motesanib, an oral inhibitor of vascular endothelial growth factor (VEGF) receptors, has been reported effective in inducing partial responses in patients with advanced or metastatic differentiated thyroid cancer that is progressive.
- While there is little controversy regarding the benefit of radioactive iodine in iodine-avid advanced-stage well-differentiated thyroid cancer, the indications for radioactive iodine following total thyroidectomy in patients with very low risk disease is controversial. Proponents argue that its use may destroy microscopic metastases while opponents counter that the risk of secondary cancer due to radioactive iodine is not warranted in patients whose prognosis is typically excellent.
- Metastatic thyroid cancers that are refractory to radioiodine (iodine-131) are associated with a poor prognosis. Recent trials have shown that the selective mitogen-activated protein kinase (MAPK) pathway antagonist selumetinib produces clinically meaningful increases in iodine uptake and retention in some patients with thyroid cancer that is refractory to radioiodine.

SUGGESTED READINGS

available at www.expertconsult.com

RELATED CONTENT

Thyroid Cancer (Patient Information)

AUTHOR: **FRED F. FERRI, M.D.**

Type of Cancer	Percentage of Thyroid Cancers	Age of Onset (Yr)	Treatment	Prognosis
Papillary	88	40-80	Thyroidectomy, followed by radioactive iodine ablation and TSH suppression	Good
Follicular	10	45-80	Thyroidectomy, followed by radioactive iodine ablation and TSH suppression	Fair to good
Medullary	3-4	20-50	Thyroidectomy and central compartment lymph node dissection and TSH suppression	Fair
Anaplastic	1	50-80	Isthmusectomy followed by palliative x-ray treatment	Poor
Lymphoma	<1	25-70	X-ray therapy and/or chemotherapy	Fair

TABLE 1-394 Characteristics of Thyroid Cancers

From Andreoli TE et al: *Andreoli and Carpenter's Cecil essentials of medicine,* ed 8, Philadelphia, 2010, Saunders.

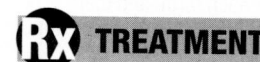 BASIC INFORMATION

DEFINITION

A thyroid nodule is an abnormality found on physical examination of the thyroid gland; nodules can be benign (70%) or malignant.

ICD-9CM CODES
241.0 Nodule, thyroid

EPIDEMIOLOGY & DEMOGRAPHICS

- Palpable thyroid nodules occur in 4% to 7% of the population.
- Thyroid nodules can be found in 50% of autopsies; however, only one in 10 is palpable.
- Malignancy is present in 5% to 15% of all thyroid nodules and in 5% to 30% of palpable nodules.
- Incidence of thyroid nodules increases after age 45 yr. They are found more frequently in women.
- History of prior head and neck irradiation increases the risk of thyroid cancer.
- Increased likelihood that nodule is malignant: nodule increasing in size or >3 cm, regional lymphadenopathy, fixation to adjacent tissues, age <40 yr, symptoms of local invasion (dysphagia, hoarseness, neck pain, male sex, family history of thyroid cancer or polyposis [Gardner syndrome]), rapid growth during levothyroxine therapy microcalcification within the nodule, and high intranodular vascular flow.

PHYSICAL FINDINGS & CLINICAL PRESENTATION

- Palpable, firm, and nontender nodule in the thyroid area should prompt suspicion of carcinoma. Signs of metastasis are regional lymphadenopathy and inspiratory stridor.
- Signs and symptoms of thyrotoxicosis can be found in functioning nodules.

ETIOLOGY

- History of prior head and neck irradiation
- Family history of pheochromocytoma, carcinoma of the thyroid, and hyperparathyroidism (medullary carcinoma of the thyroid is a component of MEN-II)

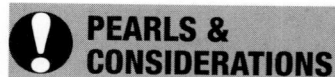 DIAGNOSIS

DIFFERENTIAL DIAGNOSIS

- Thyroid carcinoma
- Multinodular goiter
- Thyroglossal duct cyst
- Epidermoid cyst
- Laryngocele
- Nonthyroid neck neoplasm
- Branchial cleft cyst

WORKUP

- Fine-needle aspiration (FNA) biopsy is the best diagnostic study; the accuracy can be >90%, but it is directly related to the level of experience of the physician and the cytopathologist interpreting the aspirate. FNA is not routinely recommended for thyroid nodules <1 cm in diameter unless there are significant risk factors (see above).
- FNA biopsy is less reliable with thyroid cystic lesions; surgical excision should be considered for most thyroid cysts not abolished by aspiration.
- A diagnostic approach to thyroid nodule is described in Fig. E1-829. Preoperative, ultrasonically guided FNA accurately classifies 62% to 85% of thyroid nodules as benign; however, 15% to 30% of aspirations yield indeterminate cytologic findings.

LABORATORY TESTS

- Serum TSH should be obtained in all patients with thyroid nodules. If suppressed, obtain free T4 and free T3 and thyroid scan to rule out "hot nodule," indicative of hyperthyroid adenoma. Less than 1% of hyperfunctioning nodules are malignant.
- Thyroid-stimulating hormone (TSH), T_4, and serum thyroglobulin levels should be obtained before thyroidectomy in patients with confirmed thyroid carcinoma on FNA biopsy.
- Serum calcitonin at random or after pentagastrin stimulation is useful when suspecting medullary carcinoma of the thyroid and in anyone with a family history of medullary thyroid carcinoma.
- Serum thyroid autoantibodies (see "Thyroiditis" in Section I) are useful in patients with multinodular goiter and when suspecting thyroiditis.
- Molecular analysis of thyroid tissue for the presence of BRAF and RAS mutations and for RET/PTC and PAX8-PPAR gamma 1 gene rearrangements can be used as a diagnostic tool, since 60% to 70% of thyroid cancers harbor at least one genetic mutation. The gene expression classifier profile can be used to identify a subpopulation of patients with a low likelihood of cancer, thereby avoiding unnecessary surgery in patients with indeterminate FNA. The gene expression classifier test has a high negative predictive value for cytologically indeterminate nodules (95% for an atypical or follicular lesion of undetermined significance, 94% for a follicular neoplasm, and 85% for a lesion suggestive of cancer).

IMAGING STUDIES

- Thyroid ultrasound is useful to evaluate the size of the thyroid and the number, composition (solid vs. cystic), and dimensions of the thyroid nodule; solid thyroid nodules have a higher incidence of malignancy, but cystic nodules can also be malignant.
- Thyroid scan can be performed with technetium-99m pertechnetate, iodine-123, or iodine-131. Iodine isotopes are preferred because up to 35% of nodules that appear functioning on pertechnetate scanning may appear nonfunctioning on radioiodine scanning. A thyroid scan:
  1. Classifies nodules as hyperfunctioning (hot), normally functioning (warm), or nonfunctioning (cold); cold nodules have a higher incidence of malignancy.
  2. Scan has difficulty evaluating nodules near the thyroid isthmus or at the periphery of the gland.
  3. Normal tissue over a nonfunctioning nodule might mask the nodule as "warm" or normally functioning.
- Both thyroid scan and ultrasound provide information about the risk of malignant neoplasia based on the characteristics of the thyroid nodule, but their value in the initial evaluation of a thyroid nodule is limited because neither provides a definite tissue diagnosis.

Rx TREATMENT

GENERAL Rx

- Evaluation of results of FNA:
  1. Normal cells: may repeat biopsy during present evaluation or reevaluate patient after 3 to 6 mo of suppressive therapy (L-thyroxine, prescribed in doses to suppress the TSH level to 0.1 to 0.5)
     a. Failure to regress indicates increased likelihood of malignancy.
     b. Reliance on repeat FNA biopsy is preferable to routine surgery for nodules not responding to thyroxine.
  2. Indeterminate: use of gene expression classifier profile. If suspicious, perform surgery; if benign, monitor with subsequent repeat FNA and gene expression classifier profile.
  3. Malignant cells: surgery

DISPOSITION

Variable with results of FNA biopsy

REFERRAL

Surgical referral for FNA biopsy

! PEARLS & CONSIDERATIONS

COMMENTS

- Most solid, benign nodules grow; therefore an increase in nodule volume alone is not a reliable predictor of malignancy.
- Surgery is indicated in hard or fixed nodule, presence of dysphagia or hoarseness, and rapidly growing solid masses regardless of "benign" results on FNA.
- Suppressive therapy of malignant thyroid nodules postoperatively with thyroxine is indicated. The use of suppressive therapy for benign solitary nodules is controversial.

SUGGESTED READINGS
available at www.expertconsult.com

RELATED CONTENT
Thyroid Nodule (Patient Information)

AUTHOR: **FRED F. FERRI, M.D.**

BASIC INFORMATION

DEFINITION

Thyroiditis is an inflammatory disease of the thyroid. It is a multifaceted disease with various etiologies, different clinical characteristics (depending on the stage), and distinct histopathology. Thyroiditis can be subdivided into three common types (Hashimoto's, painful, and painless) and two rare forms (suppurative and Riedel's). To add to the confusion, there are various synonyms for each form, and there is no internationally accepted classification of autoimmune thyroid disease.

SYNONYMS

Hashimoto's thyroiditis: chronic lymphocytic thyroiditis, chronic autoimmune thyroiditis, lymphadenoid goiter

Painful subacute thyroiditis: subacute thyroiditis, giant cell thyroiditis, de Quervain's thyroiditis, subacute granulomatous thyroiditis, pseudogranulomatous thyroiditis

Painless postpartum thyroiditis: subacute lymphocytic thyroiditis, postpartum thyroiditis

Painless sporadic thyroiditis: silent sporadic thyroiditis, subacute lymphocytic thyroiditis

Suppurative thyroiditis: acute suppurative thyroiditis, bacterial thyroiditis, microbial inflammatory thyroiditis, pyogenic thyroiditis

Riedel's thyroiditis: fibrous thyroiditis

ICD-9CM CODES
245.2 Hashimoto's thyroiditis
245.1 Subacute thyroiditis
245.9 Silent thyroiditis
245.0 Suppurative thyroiditis
245.3 Riedel's thyroiditis

PHYSICAL FINDINGS & CLINICAL PRESENTATION

- Hashimoto's: patients may have signs of hyperthyroidism (tachycardia, diaphoresis, palpitations, weight loss) or hypothyroidism (fatigue, weight gain, delayed reflexes) depending on the stage of the disease. Usually there is diffuse, firm enlargement of the thyroid gland; the gland may also be of normal size (atrophic form with clinically manifested hypothyroidism).
- Painful subacute: exquisitely tender, enlarged thyroid, fever; signs of hyperthyroidism are initially present; signs of hypothyroidism can subsequently develop.
- Painless thyroiditis: clinical features are similar to subacute thyroiditis except for the absence of tenderness of the thyroid gland.
- Suppurative: patient is febrile with severe neck pain, focal tenderness of the involved portion of the thyroid, erythema of the overlying skin.
- Riedel's: slowly enlarging hard mass in the anterior neck; often mistaken for thyroid cancer; signs of hypothyroidism occur in advanced stages.

ETIOLOGY

- Hashimoto's: autoimmune disorder that begins with the activation of CD4 (helper) T-lymphocytes specific for thyroid antigens. The etiologic factor for the activation of these cells is unknown.
- Painful subacute: possibly postviral; usually follows a respiratory illness not considered to be a form of autoimmune thyroiditis
- Painless thyroiditis: frequently occurs postpartum
- Suppurative: infectious etiology, generally bacterial, although fungi and parasites have also been implicated; often occurs in immunocompromised hosts or after a penetrating neck injury
- Riedel's: fibrous infiltration of the thyroid; etiology unknown
- Drug induced: lithium, interferon-alfa, amiodarone, interleukin-2

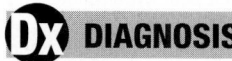

DIAGNOSIS

DIFFERENTIAL DIAGNOSIS

- The hyperthyroid phase of Hashimoto's, subacute, and silent thyroiditis can be mistaken for Graves' disease.
- Riedel's thyroiditis can be mistaken for carcinoma of the thyroid.
- Painful subacute thyroiditis can be mistaken for infections of the oropharynx and trachea or for suppurative thyroiditis.
- Factitious hyperthyroidism can mimic silent thyroiditis.

WORKUP

- The diagnostic workup includes laboratory and radiologic evaluation to rule out other conditions that may mimic thyroiditis (see above) and differentiate the various forms of thyroiditis.
- The patient's medical history may be helpful in differentiating the various types of thyroiditis (e.g., presentation after childbirth is suggestive of silent [postpartum, painless] thyroiditis; occurrence after a viral respiratory infection suggests subacute thyroiditis; history of penetrating injury to the neck indicates suppurative thyroiditis).

LABORATORY TESTS

- Thyroid-stimulating hormone, free T_4: may be normal or indicative of hypothyroidism or hyperthyroidism depending on the stage of the thyroiditis.
- White blood cell (WBC) with differential: increased WBC with left shift occurs with subacute and suppurative thyroiditis.
- Antimicrosomal antibodies: detected in >90% of patients with Hashimoto's thyroiditis and 50% to 80% of patients with silent thyroiditis.
- Serum thyroglobulin levels are elevated in patients with subacute and silent thyroiditis; this test is nonspecific but may be useful in monitoring the course of subacute thyroiditis and distinguishing silent thyroiditis from factitious hyperthyroidism (low or absent serum thyroglobulin level).

IMAGING STUDIES

Twenty-four-hour radioactive iodine uptake (RAIU) is useful to distinguish Graves' disease (increased RAIU) from thyroiditis (normal or low RAIU).

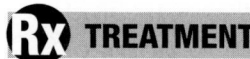

TREATMENT

ACUTE GENERAL Rx

- Treat hypothyroid phase with levothyroxine 25 to 50 mcg/day initially and monitor serum thyroid-stimulating hormone initially every 6 to 8 wk.
- Control symptoms of hyperthyroidism with beta-blockers (e.g., propranolol 20 to 40 mg PO q6h).
- Control pain in patients with subacute thyroiditis with nonsteroidal anti-inflammatory drugs. Prednisone 20 to 40 mg qd may be used if nonsteroidals are insufficient, but it should be gradually tapered off over several weeks.
- Use IV antibiotics and drain abscess (if present) in patients with suppurative thyroiditis.

DISPOSITION

- Hashimoto's thyroiditis: long-term prognosis is favorable; most patients recover their thyroid function.
- Painful subacute thyroiditis: permanent hypothyroidism occurs in 10% of patients.
- Painless thyroiditis: 6% of patients have permanent hypothyroidism.
- Suppurative thyroiditis: there is usually full recovery after treatment.
- Riedel's thyroiditis: hypothyroidism occurs when fibrous infiltration involves the entire thyroid.

REFERRAL

Surgical referral in patients with compression of adjacent neck structures and in some patients with suppurative thyroiditis

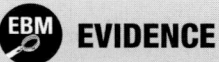

available at www.expertconsult.com

SUGGESTED READINGS
available at www.expertconsult.com

RELATED CONTENT
Fig. 3-181 Painful thyroid (Algorithm)
Thyroiditis (Patient Information)

AUTHOR: **FRED F. FERRI, M.D.**

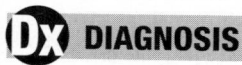 BASIC INFORMATION

DEFINITION

Thyrotoxic storm is the abrupt and severe exacerbation of thyrotoxicosis. It is an acute, life-threatening complication of hyperthyroidism.

ICD-9CM CODES
242.9 Thyrotoxic storm
242.0 With goiter
242.2 Multinodular
242.3 Adenomatous
242.8 Thyrotoxicosis factitia

PHYSICAL FINDINGS & CLINICAL PRESENTATION

- Tremor, tachycardia/tachyarrhythmias, fever (as high as 105.8° F)
- Sweating, diarrhea, vasodilation
- Lid lag, lid retraction, proptosis
- Altered mental status (psychosis, coma, seizures)
- Goiter
- Other: evidence of precipitating factors (infection, trauma), CHF, hepatosplenomegaly, jaundice

ETIOLOGY

- Precipitating factors: surgery, infection, myocardial infarction or cardiac disease, diabetic ketoacidosis, labor, iodinated IV contrast agents, radioactive iodine therapy
- Inadequate therapy in a hyperthyroid patient

DIAGNOSIS

The clinical presentation is variable. The patient may present with the following signs and symptoms:
- Fever
- Marked anxiety and agitation, psychosis
- Hyperhidrosis, heat intolerance
- Marked weakness and muscle wasting
- Tachyarrhythmias, palpitations
- Diarrhea, nausea, vomiting
- Elderly patients may have a combination of tachycardia, congestive heart failure (CHF), and mental status changes

DIFFERENTIAL DIAGNOSIS

- Psychiatric disorders
- Alcohol or other drug withdrawal
- Pheochromocytoma
- Metastatic neoplasm

WORKUP

- Laboratory evaluation to confirm hyperthyroidism (elevated free T_4, decreased thyroid-stimulating hormone [TSH])
- Evaluation for precipitating factors (e.g., ECG and cardiac enzymes in suspected MI, blood and urine cultures to rule out sepsis)
- Elimination of disorders noted in the differential diagnosis (e.g., psychiatric history, evidence of drug and alcohol abuse)

LABORATORY TESTS

- Free T_4, TSH
- Complete blood count with differential
- Blood and urine cultures
- Glucose
- Liver enzymes
- Blood urea nitrogen, creatinine
- Serum calcium
- Creatine phosphokinase

IMAGING STUDIES

Chest x-ray to exclude infectious process, neoplasm, CHF in suspected cases

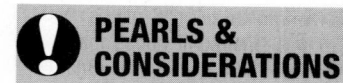 TREATMENT

NONPHARMACOLOGIC THERAPY

- Nutritional care: replace fluid deficit aggressively (daily fluid requirement may reach 6 L); use solutions containing glucose and add multivitamins to the hydrating solution.
- Monitor for fluid overload and CHF in the elderly and in those with underlying cardiovascular or renal disease.
- Treat significant hyperthermia with cooling blankets.

ACUTE GENERAL Rx

- Inhibition of thyroid hormone synthesis:
  1. Administer propylthiouracil (PTU) 800 mg initially (PO or by nasogastric tube)/PR, then 200 to 300 mg PO/PR q6h.
  2. If the patient is allergic to PTU, use methimazole 80 to 100 mg PO/PR followed by 40 mg PO/PR q8h.
- Inhibition of stored thyroid hormone from the gland:
  1. Iodide can be administered as Telepaque (iopanoic acid) 1 g PO once daily or sodium iodine 250 mg IV q6h or saturated solution of potassium iodide (SSKI), 5 gtt PO q8h, or Lugol's solution, 10 gtt PO q8h. It is important to administer PTU or methimazole 1 hr

before the iodide to prevent the oxidation of iodide to iodine and its incorporation in the synthesis of additional thyroid hormone.
  2. Corticosteroids: dexamethasone 1-2 mg IV q6h or hydrocortisone 100 mg IV q6h for approximately 48 hr is useful to inhibit thyroid hormone release, impair peripheral conversion of T_3 from T_4, and provide additional adrenocortical hormone to correct deficiency (if present).
- Suppression of peripheral effects of thyroid hormone:
  1. Beta-adrenergic blockers: administer propranolol 80 to 120 mg PO q4-6h. Propranolol may also be given IV 1 mg/min for 2 to 10 min under continuous ECG and blood pressure monitoring. Beta-adrenergic blockers must be used with caution in patients with severe CHF or bronchospasm. Cardioselective beta-blockers (e.g., esmolol or metoprolol) may be more appropriate for patients with bronchospasm, but these patients must be closely monitored for exacerbation of bronchospasm because these agents lose their cardioselectivity at high doses.
- Control of fever with acetaminophen 325 to 650 mg q4h; avoidance of aspirin because it displaces thyroid hormone from its binding protein
- Consider digitalization of patients with CHF and atrial fibrillation (these patients may require higher than usual digoxin doses)
- Treatment of any precipitating factors (e.g., antibiotics if infection is strongly suspected)

DISPOSITION

Patients with thyrotoxic crisis should be treated and appropriately monitored in the ICU.

REFERRAL

Endocrinology referral is appropriate in patients with thyrotoxic crisis.

PEARLS & CONSIDERATIONS

COMMENTS

If the diagnosis is strongly suspected, therapy should be started immediately without waiting for laboratory confirmation.

AUTHOR: **FRED F. FERRI, M.D.**

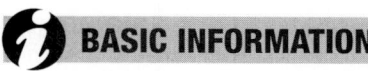
DEFINITION

Tinea capitis is a dermatophyte infection of the scalp most commonly caused by fungal species such as *Microsporum audouinii* and *Trichophyton tonsurans*.

SYNONYMS

Ringworm of the scalp, ringworm of the head, gray patch tinea capitis, black dot tinea capitis, tinea tonsurans, superficial mycosis, dermatophytosis, kerion

ICD-9CM CODES
110.0 Tinea capitis

EPIDEMIOLOGY & DEMOGRAPHICS

Tinea capitis is the most common dermatophytosis of childhood, primarily affecting children between 3 and 7 yr of age. About 3% to 8% of American children are affected, although it is more common among black children, and 34% of household contacts are asymptomatic carriers. Adult and geriatric populations are less frequently affected, possibly because of the fungistatic effect of the sebum found in older persons. In urban populations, large family size, low socioeconomic status, and crowded living conditions may contribute to an increased incidence of tinea capitis. Infection of the scalp with *Trichophyton tonsurans* results from person-to-person transmission. Transmission occurs via infected persons or asymptomatic carriers, fallen infected hairs, animal vectors, and fomites. *Microsporum audouinii* is commonly spread by dogs and cats. Infectious fungal particles may remain viable for many months.

PHYSICAL FINDINGS & CLINICAL PRESENTATION

- Triad of scalp scaling, alopecia, and cervical adenopathy
- Most forms of tinea capitis begin with one or few round patches of scale or alopecia
- Primary lesions including plaques, papules, pustules, or nodules on the scalp (usually occipital region)
- Secondary lesions include scales, alopecia (usually reversible), erythema, exudates, and edema

- Two distinctly different forms:
  - Gray patch: Lesions are scaly and well demarcated. The hairs within the patch break off a few millimeters above the scalp. One or several lesions may be present; sometimes the lesions join to form larger ones.
  - Black dot: Early lesions with erythema and scaling patch are easily overlooked until areas of alopecia develop. Hairs within the patches break at the surface of the scalp, leaving behind a pattern of swollen black dots.
- Scalp pruritus may be present.
- Fever, pain, and lymphadenopathy (commonly postcervical) with inflammatory lesions
- Kerion (Fig. 1-830): inflamed, exudative, pustular, boggy, tender nodules exhibiting marked edema, and hair loss seen in severe tinea capitis. Caused by immune response to the fungus. May lead to some scarring.
- Favus: production of scutula (hair matted together with dermatophyte hyphae and keratin debris), characterized by yellow cup-shaped crusts around hair shafts. A fetid odor may be present.

ETIOLOGY

Although the organism remains viable on combs, hairbrushes, and other fomites for long periods of time, the role of fomites in causative organisms may vary in different geographic areas. *T. tonsurans* is the predominant cause of tinea capitis, present in more than 90% of cases in North and Central America. *Microsporum canis, M. audouinii,* and *Trichophyton mentagrophytes* are less common. Most common causative species for black dot tinea capitis is *T. tonsurans* and for gray patch tinea capitis are *M. andouinii* and *M. canis.* The infection of the hair shaft is preceded by invasion of the stratum corneum of the scalp.

DIAGNOSIS

DIFFERENTIAL DIAGNOSIS

Seborrhea dermatitis and psoriasis may be confused with tinea of the scalp. Alopecia areata, impetigo, pediculosis, trichotillomania, traction alopecia, folliculitis, pseudopelade, seborrhea/atopic dermatitis, psoriasis, carbuncles, pyo-

derma, lichen ruber planus, lupus erythematosus. Table 1-395 summarizes the differential diagnosis of tinea capitis.

WORKUP

- KOH testing of hair shaft extracted from the lesion, not the scale, because the *T. tonsurans* spores attach to or reside inside hair shafts and will rarely be found in the scales.
- Wood's ultraviolet light fluoresces blue-green on hair shafts for *Microsporum* infections but will fail to identify *T. tonsurans*.
- Fungal culture of hairs and scales on fungal medium such as Sabouraud's agar may be used to confirm the diagnosis, especially if uncertain.
- Histology of biopsies with fungal staining in cases where mycology tests are negative because of treatment initiation.

Rx TREATMENT

- Griseofulvin is the gold standard FDA-approved treatment, which costs less than other treatments and has an excellent long-term safety profile. Micronized and ultramicronized preparations are absorbed better, and side effects are infrequent, especially when administered with fatty meals. Periodic monitoring of hematologic, liver, and renal function may be indicated, especially in prolonged treatment over 8 wk. However, a metaanalysis published in 2012 reported that a species-specific approach to treating tinea capitis may be more efficacious. The metaanalysis looked at randomized controlled trials comparing 8 wk of griseofulvin (6.25-12.5 mg/kg/day) to 4 wk of terbinafine (3.125-6.25 mg/kg/day) in the treatment of tinea capitis. The results of the analysis did not show a significant difference in the overall efficacy of the two drugs at the doses specified, but specific efficacy differences were observed based on the infectious species. For tinea capitis caused by *Microsporum* spp., griseofulvin is superior ($p = .04$), whereas terbinafine is superior for *Trichophyton* spp. infection ($p = .04$).
  Children: Griseofulvin is approved for children age >2: microsize griseofulvin 10 to 25 mg/kg per day (maximum, 1 g) or ultramicrosize griseofulvin, 5 to 15 mg/kg per day (maximum, 750 mg), is given orally once daily. Optimally, griseofulvin is given after a meal containing fat (e.g., peanut butter or ice cream). Treatment for 6 to 8 wk typically is necessary and should be continued 2 wk beyond clinical resolution (until hair regrowth occurs). Some children may require higher doses to achieve clinical cure.
  Adults: 250 mg orally bid or 500 mg qd (or 250 mg tid for a few cases of black dot type) for 4 to 12 weeks.
- New alternative treatments: oral terbinafine, itraconazole, or fluconazole are comparable in efficacy and safety to griseofulvin, with possibly shorter treatment and better patient compliance. Preferred when resistant or

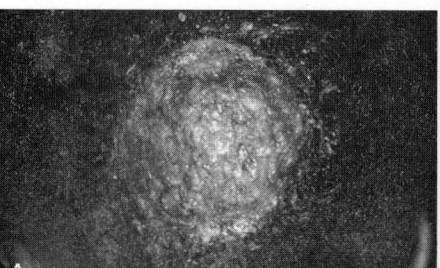
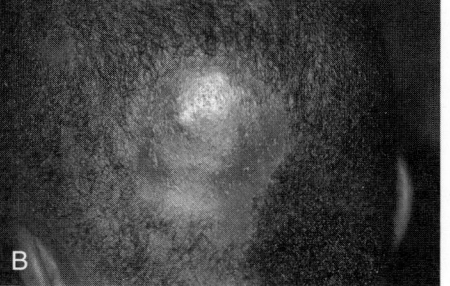

FIGURE 1-830 A, Kerion. Boggy granulomatous mass of the scalp. **B,** Scarring after kerion. (From Kliegman RM et al: *Nelson textbook of pediatrics,* ed 19, Philadelphia, 2011, Saunders.)

when an allergy to griseofulvin is of concern. Monitoring of CBC, liver function tests, and renal function may be indicated.

- Terbinafine—4-wk course of therapy as effective as with griseofulvin. Dosages are 67.5 mg/day for patients weighing <20 kg; 125 mg/day for patients weighing 20 to 40 kg; and 250 mg for patients weighing >40 kg.
- Itraconazole—3.5 mg/kg daily for 4 to 6 wk or pulse therapy of 5 mg/kg daily for 1 wk each month for 2 to 3 mo (not approved for children)
- Fluconazole—the only oral antifungal agent approved for children <2 yr, 6 mg/kg/day for 6 wk in children (3 to 6 wk in adults) or 8 mg/kg weekly for 8 to 12 wk (cap at 150 mg weekly for adults)

- The adjuvant use of antifungal shampoos may be recommended for all patients and household contacts. Shampoo like selenium sulfide 2.5% used for 5 min or ketoconazole shampoo used 2 to 3 times/wk can help prevent infection or eradicate asymptomatic carrier state by inhibiting fungal growth.
- Severe inflammatory kerion can be managed with additional prednisone 40 mg daily (1 mg/kg/day in children) and tapering over 2 wk.

PEARLS & CONSIDERATIONS

- Systemic antifungal therapy is required for tinea capitis because topical antifungal medications are not effective.
- Prompt treatment is indicated, as is examination of siblings and other household contacts for evidence of tinea capitis.
- Shaving of the head, haircuts, or wearing a cap or scarf during treatment is unnecessary.
- Sharing of combs, hair ribbons, and hairbrushes should be discouraged. Children receiving treatment for tinea capitis may attend school once they start therapy with griseofulvin or other effective systemic agent.

COMMENTS

- Confirming the diagnosis of tinea capitis with a laboratory specimen is important because misdiagnosis will result in delay or improper treatment.
- Patients and their families should look for sources of infections and disinfect contaminated objects such as combs, brushes, towels, and headgear. Avoid sharing personal hygiene utensils.

- Culture of hairs and scalp dander facilitates carrier identification and prevention.
- Pets that are infected or asymptomatic carriers should be treated.
- Recommend follow-up visit every 2 to 4 wk with Wood's light, microscopic study, and fungal culture. A mycologic documented cure is the goal of treatment.

SUGGESTED READINGS
available at www.expertconsult.com

AUTHORS: **MARIE ELIZABETH WONG, M.D., JEFFREY BORKAN, M.D., PH.D.,** and **PRIYA SARIN GUPTA, M.D., M.P.H.**

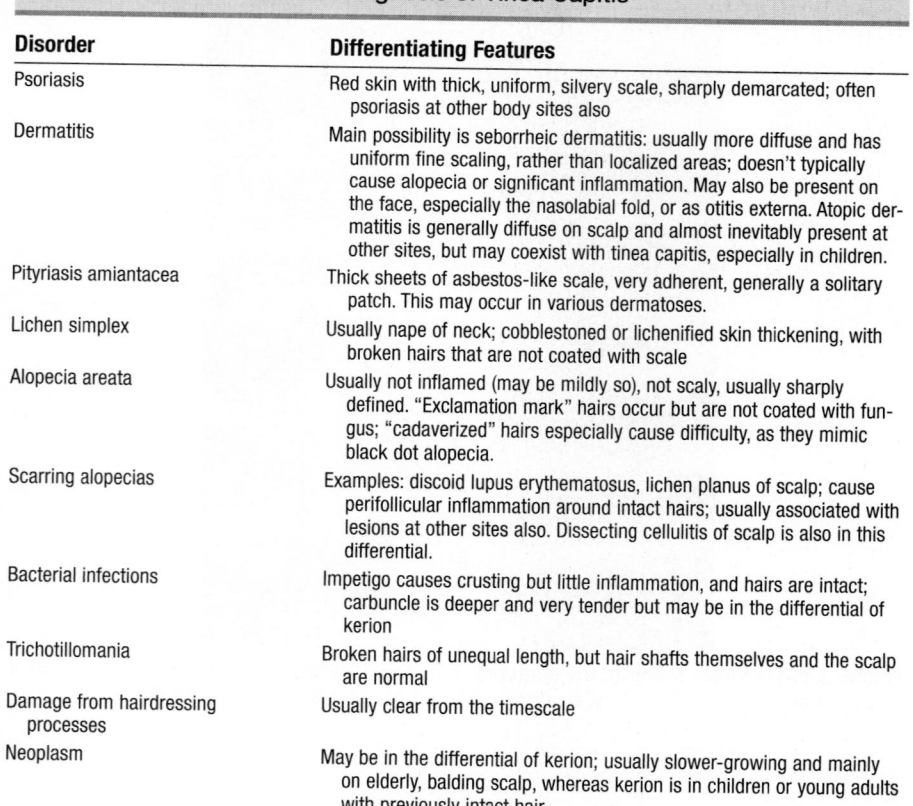

TABLE 1-395 Differential Diagnosis of Tinea Capitis

Disorder	Differentiating Features
Psoriasis	Red skin with thick, uniform, silvery scale, sharply demarcated; often psoriasis at other body sites also
Dermatitis	Main possibility is seborrheic dermatitis: usually more diffuse and has uniform fine scaling, rather than localized areas; doesn't typically cause alopecia or significant inflammation. May also be present on the face, especially the nasolabial fold, or as otitis externa. Atopic dermatitis is generally diffuse on scalp and almost inevitably present at other sites, but may coexist with tinea capitis, especially in children.
Pityriasis amiantacea	Thick sheets of asbestos-like scale, very adherent, generally a solitary patch. This may occur in various dermatoses.
Lichen simplex	Usually nape of neck; cobblestoned or lichenified skin thickening, with broken hairs that are not coated with scale
Alopecia areata	Usually not inflamed (may be mildly so), not scaly, usually sharply defined. "Exclamation mark" hairs occur but are not coated with fungus; "cadaverized" hairs especially cause difficulty, as they mimic black dot alopecia.
Scarring alopecias	Examples: discoid lupus erythematosus, lichen planus of scalp; cause perifollicular inflammation around intact hairs; usually associated with lesions at other sites also. Dissecting cellulitis of scalp is also in this differential.
Bacterial infections	Impetigo causes crusting but little inflammation, and hairs are intact; carbuncle is deeper and very tender but may be in the differential of kerion
Trichotillomania	Broken hairs of unequal length, but hair shafts themselves and the scalp are normal
Damage from hairdressing processes	Usually clear from the timescale
Neoplasm	May be in the differential of kerion; usually slower-growing and mainly on elderly, balding scalp, whereas kerion is in children or young adults with previously intact hair

From White GM, Cox NH (eds): *Diseases of the skin, a color atlas and text,* ed 2, St Louis, 2006, Mosby.

BASIC INFORMATION

DEFINITION

Tinea corporis is a dermatophyte fungal infection caused by the genera *Trichophyton* or *Microsporum*.

SYNONYMS

Ringworm
Body ringworm
Tinea circinata

ICD-9CM CODES
110.5 Tinea corporis

EPIDEMIOLOGY & DEMOGRAPHICS

- The disease is more common in warm climates.
- There is no predominant age or sex.

PHYSICAL FINDINGS & CLINICAL PRESENTATION

- Typically appears as single or multiple annular lesions with an advancing scaly border; the margin is slightly raised, reddened, and may be pustular.
- The central area becomes hypopigmented and less scaly as the active border progresses outward (Fig. 1-831).
- The trunk and legs are primarily involved.
- Pruritus is variable.
- It is important to remember that recent topical corticosteroid use can significantly alter the appearance of the lesions.

ETIOLOGY

Trichophyton rubrum is the most common pathogen.

DIAGNOSIS

DIFFERENTIAL DIAGNOSIS

- Pityriasis rosea
- Erythema multiforme
- Psoriasis
- Cutaneous systemic lupus erythematosus
- Secondary syphilis
- Nummular eczema
- Eczema
- Granuloma annulare
- Lyme disease
- Tinea versicolor
- Contact dermatitis

WORKUP

Diagnosis is usually made on clinical grounds. It can be confirmed by direct visualization under the microscope of a small fragment of the scale using wet mount preparation and potassium hydroxide solution; dermatophytes appear as translucent branching filaments (hyphae) with lines of separation appearing at irregular intervals.

LABORATORY TESTS

- Microscopic examination of hyphae
- Mycotic culture is usually not necessary.
- Biopsy is indicated only when the diagnosis is uncertain and the patient has not responded to treatment.

TREATMENT

NONPHARMACOLOGIC THERAPY

Affected areas should be kept clean and dry.

ACUTE GENERAL Rx

- Various creams are effective; the application area should include normal skin approximately 2 cm beyond the affected area:
  1. Butenafine cream applied qd for 14 days
  2. Terbinafine cream applied bid for 14 days
- Systemic therapy is reserved for severe cases and is usually given up to 4 wk; commonly used agents:
  1. Fluconazole, 200 mg qd
  2. Terbinafine, 250 mg qd

DISPOSITION

Majority of cases resolve without sequelae within 3 to 4 wk of therapy.

REFERRAL

Dermatology referral in patients with persistent or recurrent infections

SUGGESTED READINGS
available at www.expertconsult.com

RELATED CONTENT

Ringworm (Patient Information)

AUTHOR: **FRED F. FERRI, M.D.**

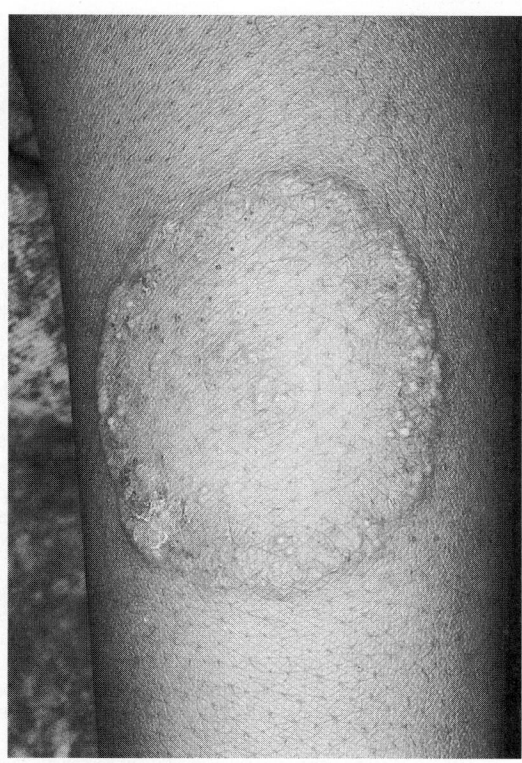

FIGURE 1-831 Annular lesion (tinea corporis). Note raised erythematous, scaling border and central clearing. (From Noble J et al: *Textbook of primary care medicine,* ed 3, St Louis, 2001, Mosby.)

BASIC INFORMATION

DEFINITION
Tinea cruris is a dermatophyte infection of the groin.

SYNONYMS
Jock itch
Ringworm

ICD-9CM CODES
110.3 Tinea cruris

EPIDEMIOLOGY & DEMOGRAPHICS
- Most common during the summer in adolescent and young adult males.
- Males are affected more frequently than females; however, it has become more common in postpubertal females who are overweight or who often wear tight jeans or pantyhose.
- The infection often coexists with tinea pedis.

PHYSICAL FINDINGS & CLINICAL PRESENTATION
- Erythematous plaques have a half-moon shape and a scaling border.
- The acute inflammation tends to move down the inner thigh and usually spares the scrotum; in severe cases the fungus may spread onto the buttocks.
- Itching may be severe.
- Red papules and pustules may be present.
- An important diagnostic sign is the advancing well-defined border with a tendency toward central clearing (Fig. 1-832).

ETIOLOGY
- Dermatophytes of the genera *Trichophyton, Epidermophyton,* and *Microsporum. T. rubrum* and *E. floccosum* are the most common infecting agents.
- Transmission from direct contact (e.g., infected persons, animals). The patient's feet should be evaluated as a source of infection because tinea cruris is often associated with tinea pedis.

DIAGNOSIS

DIFFERENTIAL DIAGNOSIS
- Candidal intertrigo
- Psoriasis
- Seborrheic dermatitis
- Erythrasma
- Contact dermatitis
- Tinea versicolor

WORKUP
Diagnosis is based on clinical presentation and demonstration of hyphae microscopically using potassium hydroxide.

LABORATORY TESTS
- Microscopic examination
- Cultures are generally not necessary.

TREATMENT

NONPHARMACOLOGIC THERAPY
- Keep infected area clean and dry.
- Boxer shorts are preferred to briefs.

ACUTE GENERAL Rx
- Various topical antifungal agents are available:
  1. Butenafine cream, applied qd × 14 days
  2. Terbinafine cream, applied bid × 14 days
- Drying powders (e.g., miconazole nitrate) may be useful in patients with excessive perspiration.
- Oral antifungal therapy is generally reserved for cases unresponsive to topical agents or can be used along with topical agents in severe cases. Effective medications are fluconazole 200 mg qd × 10 days and terbinafine 250 mg qd × 30 days.

DISPOSITION
Most cases respond promptly to therapy with complete resolution within 2 to 3 wk.

SUGGESTED READINGS
available at www.expertconsult.com

RELATED CONTENT
Tinea Cruris (Patient Information)

AUTHOR: **FRED F. FERRI, M.D.**

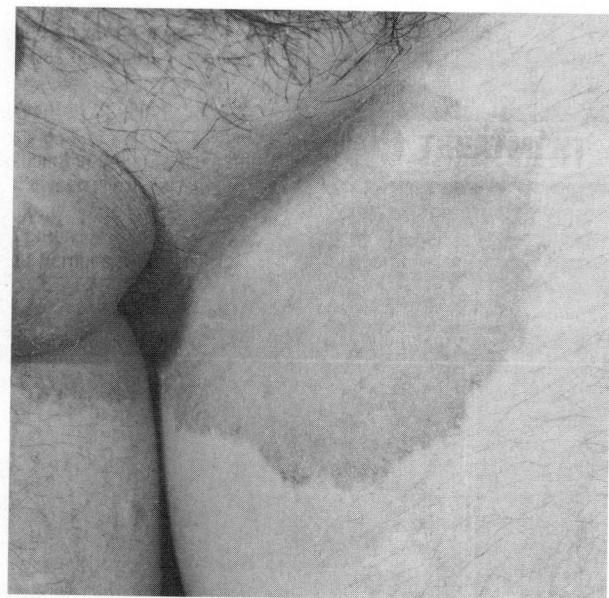

FIGURE 1-832 Tinea cruris. A half-moon–shaped plaque has a well-defined, scaling border. (From Habif TB: *Clinical dermatology: a color guide to diagnosis and therapy,* ed 3, St Louis, 1996, Mosby.)

BASIC INFORMATION

DEFINITION

Tinea pedis is a dermatophyte infection of the feet.

SYNONYMS

Athlete's foot

ICD-9CM CODES
110.4 Tinea pedis

EPIDEMIOLOGY & DEMOGRAPHICS

- Most common dermatophyte infection
- Increased incidence in hot humid weather; occlusive footwear is a contributing factor
- Occurrence is rare before adolescence
- More common in adult males

PHYSICAL FINDINGS & CLINICAL PRESENTATION

- Typical presentation is variable and ranges from erythematous scaling plaques (Fig. 1-833) and isolated blisters to interdigital maceration.

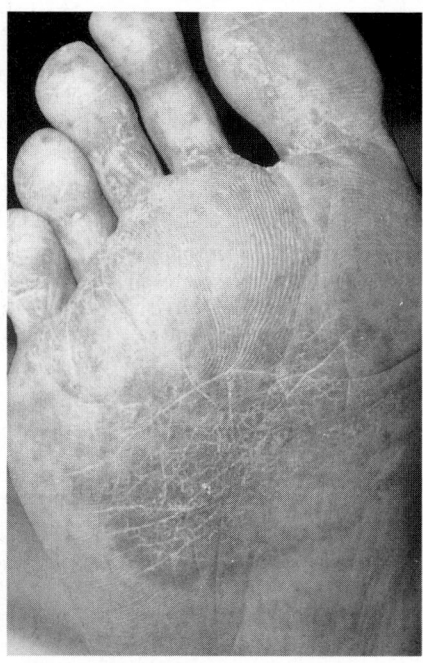

FIGURE 1-833 **Tinea pedis.** (From Goldstein BG, Goldstein AO: *Practical dermatology,* ed 2, St Louis, 1997, Mosby.)

- The infection usually starts in the interdigital spaces of the foot. Most infections are found in the toe webs or on the soles.
- Fourth or fifth toes are most commonly involved.
- Pruritus is common and is most intense after removal of shoes and socks.
- Infection with *Trichophyton rubrum* often manifests with a "moccasin" distribution affecting the soles and lateral feet.

ETIOLOGY

Dermatophyte infection caused by *T. rubrum, Trichophyton mentagrophytes,* or less commonly *Epidermophyton floccosum*

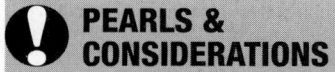

DIAGNOSIS

DIFFERENTIAL DIAGNOSIS

- Contact dermatitis
- Toe web infection (bacterial or candidal infection)
- Eczema
- Psoriasis
- Keratolysis exfoliativa
- Juvenile plantar dermatosis

WORKUP

- Diagnosis is usually made by clinical observation.
- Laboratory testing, when performed, generally consists of a simple potassium hydroxide preparation with mycologic examination under a light microscope to confirm the presence of dermatophytes.

LABORATORY TESTS

- Microscopic examination of a scale or the roof of a blister with 10% KOH under low or medium power will reveal hyphae.
- Mycologic culture is rarely indicated in the diagnosis of tinea pedis.
- Biopsy is reserved for when the diagnosis remains in question after testing or failure to respond to treatment.

TREATMENT

NONPHARMACOLOGIC THERAPY

- Keep infected area clean and dry. Aerate feet by using sandals when possible.

- Use 100% cotton socks rather than nylon socks to reduce moisture.
- Areas likely to become infected should be dried completely before being covered with clothes.

ACUTE GENERAL Rx

- Benzylamines: butenafine HCl 1% cream applied bid for 1 wk or qd for 4 wk is effective in interdigital tinea pedis.
- Allylamines: terbinafine cream applied bid × 14 days, or naftifine 1% cream applied qd or naftifine gel applied bid for 4 wk produces a significantly high cure rate.
- Imidazoles: econazole, ketoconazole, miconazole, and clotrimazole cream are also effective agents. Clotrimazole 1% cream is an over-the-counter treatment. It should be applied to affected and surrounding area bid for up to 4 wk.
- Ciclopirox and tolnaftate are other antifungal agents available in cream, suspension, or gel. Tolnaftate is also available as a lotion, spray, or powder.
- When using topical preparations, the application area should include normal skin approximately 2 cm beyond the affected area.
- Areas of maceration can be treated with Burow's solution soaks for 10 to 20 min bid followed by foot elevation.
- Oral agents (fluconazole 150 mg once per week for 4 wk) can be used in combination with topical agents in resistant cases.

PEARLS & CONSIDERATIONS

Combination therapy of antifungal and corticosteroid (clotrimazole/betamethasone [Lotrisone]) should only be used when the diagnosis of fungal infection is confirmed and inflammation is a significant issue.

SUGGESTED READING

available at www.expertconsult.com

RELATED CONTENT

Athlete's Foot (Patient Information)

AUTHOR: **FRED F. FERRI, M.D.**

BASIC INFORMATION

DEFINITION

Tinea versicolor is a fungal infection of the skin caused by the yeast *Pityrosporum orbiculare (Malassezia furfur)*.

SYNONYMS

Pityriasis versicolor

ICD-9CM CODES
111.0 Tinea versicolor

EPIDEMIOLOGY & DEMOGRAPHICS

- Increased incidence in adolescence and young adulthood
- More common during the summer (hypopigmented lesions are more evident when the skin is tanned)

PHYSICAL FINDINGS & CLINICAL PRESENTATION

- Most lesions begin as multiple small, circular macules of various colors.
- The macules may be darker or lighter than the surrounding normal skin and will scale with scraping.
- Most frequent site of distribution is trunk.
- Facial lesions are more common in children (forehead is most common facial site).
- Eruption is generally of insidious onset and asymptomatic.
- Lesions may be hyperpigmented in blacks.
- Lesions may be inconspicuous in fair-complexioned individuals, especially during the winter.
- Most patients become aware of the eruption when the involved areas do not tan (Fig. 1-834).

ETIOLOGY

The infection is caused by the lipophilic yeast *P. orbiculare* (round form) and *P. ovale* (oval form), which are normal inhabitants of the skin flora. Factors that favor proliferation are pregnancy, malnutrition, immunosuppression, oral contraceptives, and excess heat and humidity.

DIAGNOSIS

DIFFERENTIAL DIAGNOSIS

- Vitiligo
- Pityriasis alba
- Secondary syphilis
- Pityriasis rosea
- Seborrheic dermatitis
- Postinflammatory hyperpigmentation or hypopigmentation

WORKUP

Diagnosis is based on clinical appearance; identification of hyphae and budding spores ("spaghetti and meatballs" appearance) with microscopy confirms diagnosis.

LABORATORY TESTS

Microscopic examination with potassium hydroxide confirms diagnosis.

TREATMENT

NONPHARMACOLOGIC THERAPY

Sunlight accelerates repigmentation of hypopigmented areas.

ACUTE GENERAL Rx

- Topical treatment: selenium sulfide 2.5% suspension (Selsun or Exsel) applied daily for 30 min for 7 consecutive days results in a cure rate of 80% to 90%.
- Antifungal topical agents (e.g., miconazole, ciclopirox, clotrimazole) are also effective.
- Oral treatment can be given along with topical agents but is generally reserved for resistant cases. Effective agents are ketoconazole 200 mg qd for 5 days, or single 400-mg dose (cure rate >80%), fluconazole 400 mg given as a single dose (cure rate >70% at 3 wk after treatment), or itraconazole 200 mg/day for 5 days.

DISPOSITION

The prognosis is good, with death of the fungus usually occurring within 3 to 4 wk of treatment; however, recurrence is common.

PEARLS & CONSIDERATIONS

COMMENTS

Patients should be informed that the hypopigmented areas will not disappear immediately after treatment and that several months may be necessary for the hypopigmented areas to regain their pigmentation.

RELATED CONTENT

Tinea Versicolor (Patient Information)

AUTHOR: **FRED F. FERRI, M.D.**

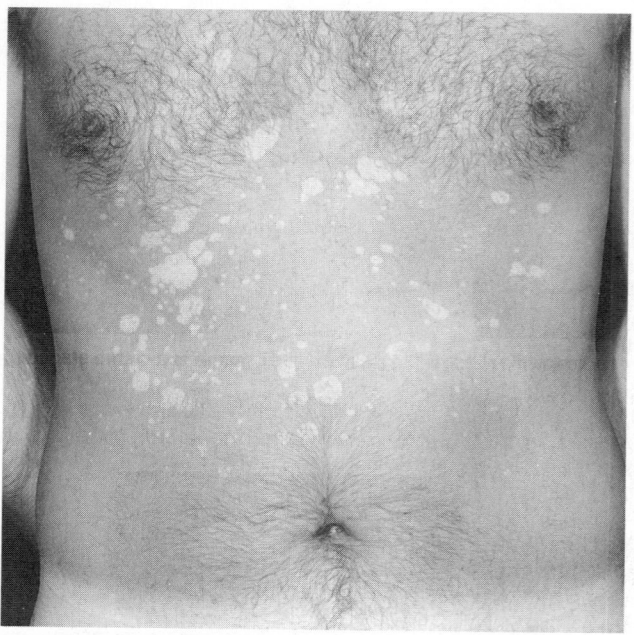

FIGURE 1-834 The classic presentation of tinea versicolor with white, oval, or circular patches on tan skin. (From Habif TB: *Clinical dermatology: a color guide to diagnosis and therapy,* ed 3, St Louis, 1996, Mosby.)

BASIC INFORMATION

DEFINITION

Tinnitus is perceived sound in absence of acoustic stimulus external to the head. It may be unilateral, bilateral, or lateral dominant. It is commonly described as ringing, buzzing, roaring, hissing, whistling, humming, cricket-like, and pulsing. It is frequently a symptom associated with hearing loss, Meniere's disease, acoustic neuroma, drug toxicity, depression, or autoimmune inner ear disease. The sound may be internal and perceived only by the patient, called subjective or tonal tinnitus, or it may be heard by both patient and examiner, called objective or nontonal tinnitus.

SYNONYMS

Ringing in the ear(s)

ICD-9CM CODES
388.3   Tinnitus
388.30 Tinnitus, unspecified
388.31 Subjective tinnitus
388.32 Objective tinnitus

ICD-10CM CODES
H93.1 Tinnitus
H93.2 Other abnormal auditory perceptions

EPIDEMIOLOGY & DEMOGRAPHICS

PREVALENCE:
- The American Tinnitus Association reports that 50 million Americans have tinnitus.
- Prevalence increases with age, peaking for persons aged 65-74 years.
- Prevalence in U.S. based on National Health Interview Survey (NHIS) in 1996:
  - 2.98% all ages
  - 0.26% for persons <18 yr old
  - 1.6% for persons aged 18-44 yr
  - 5.96% for persons aged 45-64 yr: 7.7% males, 4.3% females
  - 9.6% for persons aged 65-74 yr: 12% males, 7.7% females
  - 7.6% for persons >75 yr old: 11.4% males, 5.3% females
  - 2:1 South/Northeast regions
- Up to 18% of people in industrialized societies are mildly affected by chronic tinnitus, and 0.5% report tinnitus having a severe effect on their daily life.

PREDOMINANT SEX AND AGE: Persons most affected are male, Caucasian, elderly, persons with hearing impairment, persons living in southern U.S. For military veterans, tinnitus is the third most common service-related disability

RISK FACTORS: Any condition causing hearing loss or damage to the auditory system can produce tinnitus. Cochlear damage from exposure to noise is most common cause. Exposure to ototoxic drugs.

PHYSICAL FINDINGS & CLINICAL PRESENTATION

- History should focus on exposure to loud noises, evidence of hearing loss, ototoxic drugs.
- Patient should be screened for depression.
- Patient complains of sounds in ear, may complain of ear pain or fullness.
- Objective tinnitus is pulsatile and coincides with patient's pulse.
- PE should focus on HEENT, neck, neurologic exams.
- May have no significant physical findings.

ETIOLOGY

- Mechanism is poorly understood; central in origin; may originate at any point along the auditory pathway. Includes injured cochlear hair cells, spontaneous activity in auditory nerve fibers, hyperactivity in the auditory nuclei in the brain stem, or a reduction in the suppressive activity of the central auditory cortex.
- Medications implicated in tinnitus: salicylates, NSAIDs, aminoglycosides, loop diuretics, valproate, quinine, chemotherapeutic agents, cisplatin, vincristine, heavy metals such as lead.

DIAGNOSIS

DIFFERENTIAL DIAGNOSIS

- Subjective/tonal tinnitus:
  - Otologic: tympanic membrane disorder, inner ear disorder (hair cells, organ of Corti), Meniere's disease
  - Ototoxic medications (inflammatory?)
  - Neurologic: multiple sclerosis, head trauma, cochlear nerve lesion, acoustic schwannoma, neurofibroma, meningioma
  - Metabolic: thyroid disorder, hyperlipidemia (leading to plaque formation), vitamin B_{12} deficiency
  - Psychogenic: depression, anxiety, fibromyalgia
  - Infectious: otitis media, Lyme disease, meningitis, syphilis
- Objective/nontonal tinnitus:
  - Vascular: arterial bruit, venous hum, arteriovenous malformation, vascular tumors
  - Neurologic: contraction of muscles of eustachian tube, contraction of stapedius muscle, contraction of tensor tympani muscles, palatal myoclonus, glomus jugulare tumor
  - Conductive: patulous (wide-open) eustachian tube

WORKUP

- Audiometry, tympanometry
- Electronystagmography, to evaluate for Meniere's disease
- Box E1-74 describes useful diagnostic tests. An algorithm for tinnitus evaluation is described in Fig. E1-835.

LABORATORY TESTS

Evaluate for metabolic abnormalities: TSH, CBC, B_{12}, lipid panel.

IMAGING STUDIES

- CT/MRI: consider to evaluate for subjective tinnitus
- MRI/MRA: for evaluation of objective tinnitus

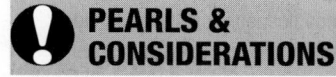

TREATMENT

NONPHARMACOLOGIC THERAPY

Avoid exposure to excessive noise, ototoxic agents. Ear protective equipment in noisy environments. Mask the tinnitus through amplification of normal sounds with a hearing aid. Habituation techniques—tinnitus retraining therapy. Cognitive behavioral therapy to improve coping, biofeedback to improve tinnitus distress.

ACUTE GENERAL Rx

- If the tinnitus is severe enough to cause suicidal symptoms, immediate referral to a psychiatrist and an otolaryngologist is recommended to minimize time to diagnosis and optimize treatment.
- Patients with persistent symptoms, or those with tinnitus accompanied by visual changes or headache, should be evaluated for the presence of tumors such as acoustic neuroma.

CHRONIC Rx

There is insufficient evidence to support use of any medication, vitamin, or nutritional supplement to treat tinnitus.

COMPLEMENTARY & ALTERNATIVE MEDICINE

Possibly effective: acupuncture, relaxation therapy, hypnosis (based on systematic review)

DISPOSITION

The clinical course is variable. 20% to 25% of patients with chronic tinnitus consider it a significant problem. Individualized tinnitus management programs can be beneficial in most patients.

REFERRAL

ENT, neurology, neurosurgery

PEARLS & CONSIDERATIONS

COMMENTS

- Be aware of high prevalence of tinnitus in population.
- Be aware of concurrent depression and screen for it.

PREVENTION

Avoid loud, chronic noise and ototoxic drugs.

PATIENT & FAMILY EDUCATION

- American Tinnitus Association: 800-634-8978, http://www.ata.org
- American Academy of Audiology: 800-AAA-2336, http://www.audiology.org

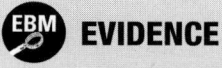 **EVIDENCE**

available at www.expertconsult.com

SUGGESTED READINGS
available at www.expertconsult.com

RELATED CONTENT

Tinnitus (Patient Information)

AUTHOR: **DAWN HOGAN, M.D.**

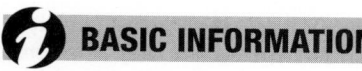 BASIC INFORMATION

DEFINITION

Torticollis is a contraction or contracture of the muscles of the neck that causes the head to be tilted to one side. It is usually accompanied by rotation of the chin to the opposite side with flexion (Fig. 1-836). Usually it is a symptom of some underlying disorder. This term is often used incorrectly in cases when the torticollis may simply be positional.

SYNONYMS

Twisted neck
"Wry neck"
Spasmodic torticollis

ICD-9CM CODES	
723.5	Spastic (intermittent) torticollis
754.1	Congenital muscular (sternocleidomastoid)
300.11	Hysterical
714.0	Rheumatoid
333.83	Spasmodic

PHYSICAL FINDINGS & CLINICAL PRESENTATION

- Congenital muscular torticollis:

1. Palpable soft tissue "mass" in the sterno-cleidomastoid shortly after birth
2. Mass gradually subsides, leaving a shortened, contracted sternocleidomastoid muscle
3. Head characteristically tilted toward the side of the mass and rotated in the opposite direction
4. Facial asymmetry and other secondary changes persisting into adulthood
- Spasmodic torticollis:
   1. "Spasms" in the cervical musculature; may be bilateral and uncontrollable
   2. Head often tilted toward the affected side
- Findings in other cases depend on etiology

ETIOLOGY

Torticollis has been found to have more than 50 different causes:
- Localized fibrous shortening of unknown cause involving the sternocleidomastoid, leading to the condition termed *congenital muscular torticollis*
- Spasmodic torticollis: of uncertain etiology, possibly a variant of dystonia musculorum deformans
- Infection, specifically pharyngitis, tonsillitis, retropharyngeal abscess

- Miscellaneous rare causes: congenital musculoskeletal deformities, trauma, inflammation from rheumatoid arthritis, vestibular disturbances, posterior fossa tumor, syringomyelia, neuritis of spinal accessory nerve, and drug reactions

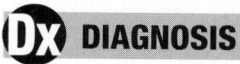 DIAGNOSIS

DIFFERENTIAL DIAGNOSIS

- Usually involves separating each disorder from the others
- Acquired positional disorders (e.g., ocular disturbances, acute disk herniation)

WORKUP

- Workup depends on the clinical situation.
- Laboratory studies are usually not helpful unless infection or rheumatoid disease is suspected.
- Section II describes a differential diagnosis for the evaluation and therapy of neck pain.
- Any child with a gradually increasing torticollis should have a complete eye examination.

IMAGING STUDIES

- Plain radiographs in cases of trauma or to rule out congenital abnormalities
- MRI in appropriate cases
- Electrodiagnostic studies: only rarely indicated to rule out neurologic causes

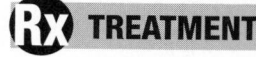 TREATMENT

- Congenital muscular torticollis: gentle stretching exercises carried out by the parent
- Spasmodic torticollis: physical therapy, psychotherapy, cervical braces, biofeedback, and pain control
- Focal dystonia responds well to injections of botulinum toxin A or B.
- Other forms: treated according to etiology

DISPOSITION

- Most patients with congenital muscular torticollis respond well to conservative treatment.
- Spasmodic torticollis is often resistant to normal conservative treatment.
- Prognosis of other forms of torticollis depends on etiology.

REFERRAL

- Torticollis often requires a multidisciplinary approach unless the etiology is obvious.
- Children usually do not require any specific studies; however, an orthopedic consultation is recommended.
- Fixed deformity in the child; may need orthopedic referral for surgical release.

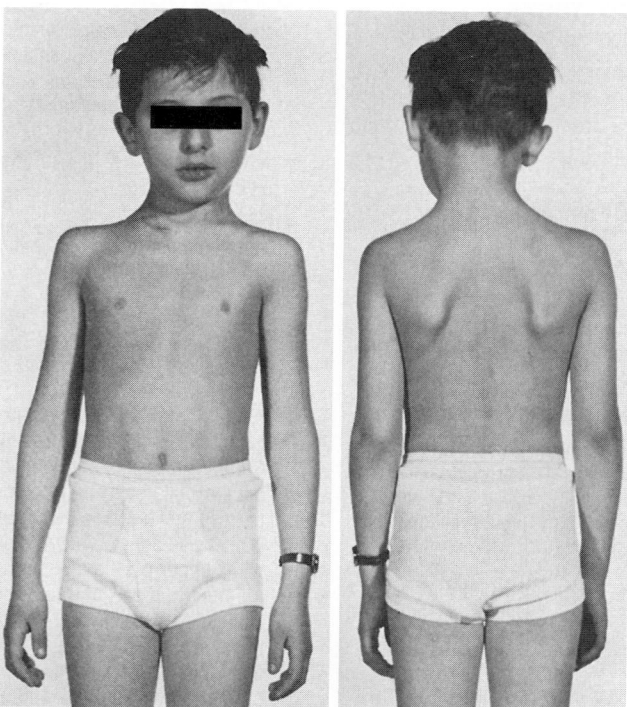

FIGURE 1-836 Torticollis. In this child, the right sternocleidomastoid muscle is contracted. (From Brinker MR, Miller MD: *Fundamentals of orthopaedics*, Philadelphia, 1999, Saunders.)

SUGGESTED READINGS

available at www.expertconsult.com

RELATED CONTENT

Torticollis (Patient Information)

AUTHOR: **LONNIE R. MERCIER, M.D.**

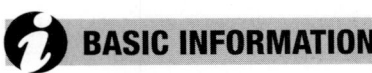

BASIC INFORMATION

DEFINITION

Tics are sudden, brief, intermittent involuntary or semivoluntary movements (motor tics) or sounds (phonic or vocal tics) that mimic fragments of normal behavior.

Tourette's syndrome (TS) is an inherited neuropsychiatric disorder characterized by motor, vocal, and phonic tics that change during the course of illness. Onset is typically before age 18 (new-onset tics can occasionally occur after age 18 yr, but for DSM-IV criteria of TS, they must begin before this age).

SYNONYMS

Gilles de la Tourette syndrome
TS
Tourette's disorder

ICD-9CM CODES
307.23 Gilles de la Tourette disorder

EPIDEMIOLOGY & DEMOGRAPHICS

PREVALENCE (IN U.S.): Unknown; estimates range from 0.7% to 5%
PREDOMINANT SEX: Approximate male/female ratio of 3:1
PREDOMINANT AGE: Typical age of onset is between 2 and 15 yr (mean 5 to 7 yr)

PHYSICAL FINDINGS & CLINICAL PRESENTATION

- Neurologic examination is normal.
- Vocal and/or phonic tics could be simple (clearing of throat, sniffing, grunting or sucking sounds) or complex (repetitive short phrases, e.g., "you bet," swearing [coprolalia]).
- Motor tics can be simple (e.g., blinking, grimacing, head jerking) or complex (e.g., gesturing). Tics wax, wane, and change over time. Often they can be suppressed for short periods. Commonly they are preceded by an urge to perform the tic.
- TS is often associated with a variety of behavioral symptoms, most commonly attention deficit hyperactivity disorder (ADHD) and obsessive-compulsive disorder (OCD).

TS can be diagnosed using the DSM-IV-TR criteria as follows:

1. Both multiple motor and one or more vocal tics must be present at some time during the illness.
2. Tics occur many times a day (usually in bouts over >1 yr, during which time there must be no tic-free period of >3 consecutive mo.
3. Age at onset is <18 yr.
4. Disturbance is not attributable to the direct physiologic effects of a substance (e.g., stimulants) or a general medical condition (e.g., Huntington's disease or postviral encephalitis).

ETIOLOGY

Exact pathogenesis is unknown. Genetic predisposition is likely as there is a strong family history of OCD or TS in patients with tics, and twin studies provide evidence for the importance of genetic factors. Recent analysis of linkage in a two-generation pedigree has led to the identification of a mutation in the HDC gene encoding L-histidine decarboxylase, the rate-limiting enzyme in histamine biosynthesis, pointing to a role for histaminergic neurotransmission in the mechanism and modulation of Tourette's syndrome and tics. Immunologic dysfunction is being explored in the pathogenesis of this complex disorder.

DIAGNOSIS

DIFFERENTIAL DIAGNOSIS

- Sydenham's chorea: occurs after infection with group A *Streptococcus*
- PANDAS: pediatric autoimmune neuropsychiatric disorder associated with streptococcal infection
- Sporadic tic disorders: tend to be motor or vocal but not both
- Head trauma
- Drug intoxication: many drugs are known to induce or exacerbate tic disorder, including methylphenidate, amphetamines, pemoline, anticholinergics, and antihistamines
- Postinfectious encephalitis
- Inherited disorders: Huntington's disease, Hallervorden-Spatz disease, and neuroacanthocytosis. All these conditions should have other observed abnormalities on neurologic examination.

WORKUP

Clinical observation and history to confirm diagnosis

LABORATORY TESTS

No definitive laboratory tests

IMAGING STUDIES

CT scan and MRI of brain are normal and unnecessary in the absence of abnormal neurologic examination.

TREATMENT

NONPHARMACOLOGIC THERAPY

Multidisciplinary: education of parents, teachers, psychologists, and school nurses is essential. Cognitive behavioral therapy termed habit-reversal treatment is efficacious in suppressing tics

ACUTE GENERAL Rx

Dopamine-blocking agents may be used to reduce severity of tics acutely (e.g., haloperidol 0.25 mg PO qhs initially). There are risks of side effects, such as acute dystonic reactions.

CHRONIC Rx

Tics only require treatment when they interfere with psychosocial, educational, and occupational functioning of a person.

TICS:

- Alpha-2 agonists like clonidine and guanfacine are used for treatment of motor tics and are considered by some experts as first-line medications because of their favorable adverse effect profile. However, they are more beneficial for treatment of behavioral symptoms and should be preferred for patients with predominant psychiatric problems.
- Haloperidol and pimozide are the only neuroleptics that are approved by U.S. FDA for the treatment of tics in TS. Pimozide is started as 0.5-1.0 mg at night and increased every 5 to 7 days to therapeutic dose of 2-8 mg. Halo-

peridol is started as 0.25-0.5 mg and can be increased to 1-4 mg depending on response and side effects. Use of neuroleptics carries a small but significant risk of tardive dyskinesia.
- Tetrabenazine: dopamine-depleting agent can be used effectively in TS patients for control of tics. It does not cause many of the typical side effects of the neuroleptics but is not readily available. Severe depression may occur with use of this medication.
- Dopamine agonists: a few small, open-label studies have found that ropinirole and pramipexole in low doses may be effective in reducing tic severity.
- Botulinum toxin local injection is effective for focal tics like eye blinking and neck and shoulder tics. The benefits are temporary, lasting 3 to 6 mo.
- Surgical treatment with deep brain stimulation has also been reported effective in some patients with disabling tics that are refractory to medications.

ADHD:
Stimulants (dextroamphetamine, methylphenidate) are useful for symptoms of ADHD but may exacerbate tics in 25% of patients, but should be used if troublesome behavioral symptoms persist.

OCD:
Selective serotonin reuptake inhibitors, such as fluoxetine, are the most effective.

DISPOSITION

- In the later teen years, intensity and frequency of tics typically diminish.
- One third of patients will achieve significant remission, although complete, lifelong remission is rare.
- One third will have mild, persistent, but "non-impairing" tics.

REFERRAL

To a neurologist to confirm initial diagnosis and for treatment in difficult cases

PEARLS & CONSIDERATIONS

- Tics do not need treatment unless they interfere with an individual's ability to function.
- Greater improvement in symptom severity among children with Tourette's and chronic tic disorder has been reported with a comprehensive behavioral intervention compared with supportive therapy and education.
- An important part of treatment is appropriate evaluation and therapy of coexisting conditions (e.g., ADHD, OCD).
- Deep brain stimulation (DBS) has shown some promising results as an alternative therapy in patients with medically refractory disease.

COMMENTS

Patient education may be obtained from the Tourette's Syndrome Association, 4240 Bell Blvd., Bayside, NY 11361-2864; 800-237-0717 or 718-224-2999; http://www.tsa-usa.org.

SUGGESTED READINGS

available at www.expertconsult.com

RELATED CONTENT

Tourette's Syndrome (Patient Information)

BASIC INFORMATION

DEFINITION

Toxic shock syndrome (TSS) is an acute febrile illness resulting in multiple organ system dysfunction caused most commonly by a bacterial exotoxin. Disease characteristics also include hypotension, vomiting, myalgia, watery diarrhea, vascular collapse, and an erythematous sunburnlike cutaneous rash that desquamates during recovery.

SYNONYMS

TSS

ICD-9CM CODES
040.89 Toxic shock syndrome

EPIDEMIOLOGY & DEMOGRAPHICS

- Case reported incidence peak: 14 cases per 100,000 menstruating women annually in 1980; has since fallen to one case per 100,000 persons
- Occurs most commonly between ages 10 and 30 yr in healthy, young, menstruating white females
- Case fatality ratio of 3%

PHYSICAL FINDINGS & CLINICAL PRESENTATION

- Fever (>38.0° C)
- Diffuse macular erythrodermatous rash that involves both skin and mucous membranes, resembles sunburn, and also involves the palms and soles. The rash then desquamates 1 to 2 wk after disease onset in survivors
- Orthostatic hypotension
- Gastrointestinal symptoms: vomiting, diarrhea, abdominal tenderness
- Constitutional symptoms: myalgia, headache, photophobia, rigors, altered sensorium, conjunctivitis, arthralgia
- Respiratory symptoms: dysphagia, pharyngeal hyperemia, strawberry tongue
- Genitourinary symptoms: vaginal discharge, vaginal hyperemia, adnexal tenderness
- End-organ failure
- Severe hypotension and acute renal failure
- Hepatic failure
- Cardiovascular symptoms: disseminated intravascular coagulation, pulmonary edema, acute respiratory distress syndrome (ARDS), endomyocarditis, heart block

ETIOLOGY

- Menstruation-associated TSS: 45% of cases associated with tampons, diaphragm, or vaginal sponge use.
- Non–menstruation-associated TSS: 55% of cases associated with puerperal sepsis, post–cesarean section endometritis, mastitis, sinusitis, wound or skin infection, septorhinoplasty, pelvic inflammatory disease, respiratory infections following influenza, enterocolitis, and burns.
- Causative agent: *Staphylococcus aureus* infection of a susceptible individual (10% of population lacking sufficient levels of anti-toxin antibodies), which liberates the disease mediator TSST-1 (exotoxin). While most cases are caused by methicillin-susceptible *S. aureus* (MSSA), cases of TSS from methicillin-resistant *S. aureus* (MRSA) have occurred, particularly those due to the more virulent community-associated MRSA strains.
- *S. aureus* exotoxins are superantigens that can activate large numbers of T cells (up to 20% at one time) resulting in a massive cytokine production: interleukin (II-1), II-2, TNF, and interferon gamma that then mediate the signs and symptoms of the disease.
- Other causative agents: coagulase-negative streptococci producing enterotoxins B or C, and exotoxin A–producing group A beta-hemolytic streptococci.

DIAGNOSIS

DIFFERENTIAL DIAGNOSIS

- Staphylococcal food poisoning
- Septic shock
- Mucocutaneous lymph node syndrome
- Scarlet fever
- Rocky Mountain spotted fever
- Meningococcemia
- Toxic epidermal necrolysis
- Kawasaki syndrome
- Leptospirosis
- Legionnaires' disease
- Hemolytic-uremic syndrome
- Stevens-Johnson syndrome
- Scalded skin syndrome
- Erythema multiforme
- Acute rheumatic fever

WORKUP

Broad-spectrum syndrome with multiorgan system involvement and variable but acute clinical presentation, including the following:
- Fever (>38° C)
- Classic desquamating rash (1 to 2 wk)
- Hypotension/orthostatic systolic blood pressure ≤90 mm Hg
- Syncope
- Negative throat and cerebrospinal fluid cultures
- Negative serologic test for Rocky Mountain spotted fever, rubeola, and leptospirosis
- Clinical involvement of three or more of the following:
  ○ Cardiopulmonary: ARDS, pulmonary edema, endomyocarditis, second- or third-degree atrioventricular block
  ○ Central nervous system: altered sensorium without focal neurologic findings
  ○ Hematologic: thrombocytopenia (platelets <100,000)
  ○ Liver: elevated liver function test results
  ○ Renal: >5 cells/high-power field, negative urine cultures, azotemia, and increased creatinine (double normal)
  ○ Mucous membrane involvement: vagina, oropharynx, conjunctiva
  ○ Musculoskeletal: myalgia, creatine phosphokinase twice normal
  ○ Gastrointestinal: vomiting, diarrhea

LABORATORY TESTS

- Pan culture (cervix and vagina, throat, nasal passages, urine, blood, cerebrospinal fluid, wound) for *Staphylococcus, Streptococcus* (Table 1-396), and other pathogenic organisms
- Electrolytes to detect hypokalemia, hyponatremia
- Complete blood count with differential and clotting profile for anemia (normocytic or normochromic), thrombocytopenia, leukocytosis, coagulopathy, and bacteremia
- Chemistry profile to detect decreased protein, increased aspartate aminotransferase, increased alanine aminotransferase, hypocalcemia, elevated blood urea nitrogen and creatinine, hypophosphatemia, increased lactate dehydrogenase, increased creatine phosphokinase
- Urinalysis to detect white blood cells (>5 cells/high-power field), proteinemia, microhematuria
- Arterial blood gases to assess respiratory function and acid-base status
- Serologic tests considered for Rocky Mountain spotted fever, rubeola, and leptospirosis

TABLE 1-396 Staphylococcal versus Streptococcal Toxic Shock Syndrome

Feature	Staphylococcal	Streptococcal
Age	Primarily 15-35 yr	Primarily 20-50 yr
Gender	Higher frequency in women	Men and women equally affected
Severe pain	Rare	Common
Hypotension	100%	100%
Erythroderma rash	Very common	Less common
Renal failure	Common	Common
Bacteremia	Low frequency	60%
Tissue necrosis	Rare	Common
Predisposing factors	Tampons, surgery	Cuts, burns, varicella
Thrombocytopenia	Common	Common
Mortality rate	<3%	30%-70%

From Mandell GL et al: *Principles and practice in infectious diseases*, ed 7, Philadelphia, 2008, Churchill Livingstone.

IMAGING STUDIES

- Chest x-ray examination to evaluate pulmonary edema
- ECG to evaluate arrhythmia
- Sonography, CT scan, or MRI considered if pelvic abscess or tubo-ovarian abscess suspected

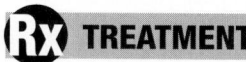 **TREATMENT**

NONPHARMACOLOGIC THERAPY

- For optimal outcome: high index of suspicion and early and aggressive supportive management in an ICU setting
- Aggressive fluid resuscitation (maintenance of circulating volume, cardiac output, systolic blood pressure)
- Thorough search for a localized infection or nidus: incision and drainage, debridement, removal of tampon or vaginal sponge
- Central hemodynamic monitoring, Swan-Ganz catheter, and arterial line for surveillance of hemodynamic status and response to therapy
- Foley catheter to monitor hourly urine output
- Possible military antishock trousers as temporary measure
- Acute ventilator management if severe respiratory compromise
- Renal dialysis for severe renal impairment
- Surgical intervention for indicated conditions (i.e., ruptured tubo-ovarian abscess, wound abscess, mastitis)

ACUTE GENERAL Rx

- Isotonic crystalloid (normal saline solution) for volume replacement following "7-3" rule (refers to the response in millimeters of mercury [mm Hg] of the pulmonary artery wedge pressure to volume replacement).
- Electrolyte replacement (K^+, C^+)
- Packed red blood cells, coagulation factor replacement, fresh frozen plasma to treat anemia or dilation and curettage.
- Vasopressor therapy for hypotension refractory to fluid volume replacement (e.g., dopamine beginning at 2 to 5 μg/kg/min)
- Steroids have been used but are not generally recommended due to lack of evidence of benefit.

- It is not clear whether antibiotics alter the course of acute TSS. Most authors recommend that patients receive 10 to 14 days of combination antibiotic therapy. In staphylococcal TSS, effective agents are clindamycin (900 mg IV every 8 hr in adults or 25 to 40 mg/kg per day in children) plus vancomycin (adults: 30 mg/kg per day IV in two divided doses; children: 40 mg/kg per day IV in four divided doses). Oxacillin or nafcillin sodium (2 g IV every 4 hr in adults; children: 100 to 150 mg/kg per 24 hr divided in four doses) can be used instead of vancomycin if TSS due to MSSA. An alternative to vancomycin is linezolid.
- In streptococcal TSS, effective agents are penicillin G 24 million units/day in divided doses *plus* clindamycin 900 mg IV q8h. Alternative agents are ceftriaxone 2 g IV q24h *plus* clindamycin 900 mg IV q8h.
- Broad-spectrum antibiotic including gram-negative coverage added if concurrent sepsis suspected with TSS.
- Intravenous immune globulin (IVIG): while no controlled trials exist, most authors recommend IVIG (400 mg/kg in a single dose administered over several hours) in severe cases of TSS that are not responding to fluids or vasopressors. It may neutralize superantigen and decrease tissue damage.
- Tetracycline added if considering Rocky Mountain spotted fever.

CHRONIC Rx

- Severely ill patient: may require prolonged hospitalization and supportive management with gradual recovery and/or sequelae from severe end-organ involvement (ARDS or renal failure requiring dialysis)
- Majority of patients: complete recovery
- Early-onset complications (within 2 wk):
  - Skin desquamation
  - Impaired digit sensation
  - Denuded tongue
  - Vocal cord paralysis
  - Acute tubular necrosis
  - ARDS
- Late-onset complications (after 8 wk):
  - Nail splitting and loss
  - Alopecia

- Central nervous system sequelae
- Renal impairment
- Cardiac dysfunction
- Recurrent TSS:
  - More common in menstruation-related cases.
  - Less common in patients treated with beta-lactamase–resistant antistaphylococcal antibiotics.
  - Patients with history of TSS: if suspect signs and symptoms occur, have high index of suspicion and low threshold for evaluation and treatment.
  - Screen for nasal carriage of *S. aureus* in patients with *S. aureus* TSS and treat with mupirocin in those with positive cultures.

PREVENTION

- Avoidance of tampons or use of low-absorbency tampons only (<4 hr in situ) and alternate with napkins
- Education for patients concerning signs and symptoms of TSS
- Avoidance of tampons for patients with history of TSS

DISPOSITION

- Complete recovery for most patients
- Long-term management of early- and late-onset complications for minority of patients

REFERRAL

- For multidisciplinary management, involving primary physician, gynecologist, internist, infectious disease specialist, and other supportive care specialists
- To tertiary-level hospital

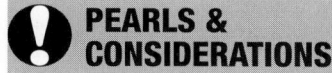 **PEARLS & CONSIDERATIONS**

COMMENTS

Patient information is available from American College of Gynecologists and Obstetricians.

SUGGESTED READINGS

available at www.expertconsult.com

RELATED CONTENT

Toxic Shock Syndrome (Patient Information)

AUTHOR: **GLENN G. FORT, M.D., M.P.H.**

BASIC INFORMATION

DEFINITION

Toxoplasmosis is an infection caused by the protozoal parasite *Toxoplasma gondii.*

ICD-9CM CODES
130.9 Toxoplasmosis

EPIDEMIOLOGY & DEMOGRAPHICS

INCIDENCE (IN U.S.):
- 3% to 70% of healthy adults
- Increases with age
- Increases with certain activities
  1. Slaughterhouse workers
  2. Cat owners
- Increases with certain geographic locations: high prevalence of cats

PREDOMINANT SEX: Equal gender distribution

PREDOMINANT AGE:
- Infancy (congenital infection)
- Prevalence increases with age

PEAK INCIDENCE: Temperate climates

GENETICS: Congenital infection: 400 to 4000 cases/yr in the U.S.
- Incidence and severity vary with the trimester of gestation during which the mother acquired infection.
  1. 10% to 25% (first trimester)
  2. 30% to 54% (second trimester)
  3. 60% to 65% (third trimester)
- Congenital infection occurring in the first trimester is the most severe.
- 89% to 100% of infections in the third trimester are asymptomatic.
- Risk to the fetus is not correlated with symptoms in the mother.

PHYSICAL FINDINGS & CLINICAL PRESENTATION

- Acquired (immunocompetent host)
  1. 80% to 90% asymptomatic
  2. Adenopathy (usually cervical)
  3. Fever
  4. Myalgias
  5. Malaise
  6. Sore throat
  7. Maculopapular rash
  8. Hepatosplenomegaly
  9. Chorioretinitis rare
- Acquired (in patients with AIDS)
  1. 89% of symptomatic cases
     a. Encephalitis
     b. Intracerebral mass lesions
  2. Pneumonitis
  3. Chorioretinitis
  4. Other end organ
- Acquired (immunocompromised patients)
  1. Encephalitis
  2. Myocarditis (especially in heart transplant patients)
  3. Pneumonitis
- Ocular infection in the immunocompetent host
  1. Congenital infection
  2. Blurred vision
  3. Photophobia
  4. Pain
  5. Loss of central vision if macula involved
  6. Focal necrotizing retinitis
  7. Typically presents in second or third decade
- Congenital
  1. Results from acute infection acquired by the mother within 6 to 8 wk before conception or during gestation
  2. Usually, asymptomatic mother
  3. No sign of disease
  4. Chorioretinitis
  5. Blindness
  6. Epilepsy
  7. Psychomotor or mental retardation
  8. Intracranial calcifications
  9. Hydrocephalus
  10. Microcephaly
  11. Encephalitis
  12. Anemia
  13. Thrombocytopenia
  14. Hepatosplenomegaly
  15. Lymphadenopathy
  16. Jaundice
  17. Rash
  18. Pneumonitis
  19. Most infected infants are asymptomatic at birth

ETIOLOGY

- *Toxoplasma gondii*
  1. Ubiquitous intracellular protozoan
  2. Present worldwide
  3. Cat is definitive host (Fig. E1-837)
- Human infection
  1. Ingestion of oocysts shed by cats in soil, litter boxes, vegetables
  2. Ingestion of inadequately cooked meat containing tissue cysts
  3. Vertical transmission

DIAGNOSIS

DIFFERENTIAL DIAGNOSIS

- Lymphadenopathy
  1. Infectious mononucleosis
  2. Cytomegalovirus (CMV) mononucleosis
  3. Cat-scratch disease
  4. Sarcoidosis
  5. Tuberculosis
  6. Lymphoma
  7. Metastatic cancer
- Cerebral mass lesions in immunocompromised host
  1. Lymphoma
  2. Tuberculosis
  3. Bacterial abscess
- Pneumonitis in immunocompromised host
  1. *Pneumocystis jirovecii (carinii)* pneumonia
  2. Tuberculosis
  3. Fungal infection
- Chorioretinitis
  1. Syphilis
  2. Tuberculosis
  3. Histoplasmosis (competent host)
  4. CMV
  5. Syphilis
  6. Herpes simplex
  7. Fungal infection
  8. Tuberculosis (AIDS patient)
- Myocarditis
  1. Organ rejection in heart transplant recipients
- Congenital infection
  1. Rubella
  2. CMV
  3. Herpes simplex
  4. Syphilis
  5. Listeriosis
  6. Erythroblastosis fetalis
  7. Sepsis

WORKUP

- Acute infection, immunocompetent host
  1. CBC
  2. *Toxoplasma* serology (IgG, IgM) in serial blood specimens 3 wk apart
  3. Lymph node biopsy if diagnosis uncertain
- Immunocompromised host
  1. CNS symptoms
     a. Cerebral CT scan or MRI if CNS symptoms present
     b. Spinal tap, if safe
     c. Brain biopsy if no response to empiric therapy
  2. Ocular symptoms
     a. Funduscopic examination
     b. Serologic studies
     c. Rarely, vitreous tap
  3. Pulmonary symptoms
     a. Chest x-ray examination
     b. Bronchoalveolar lavage
     c. Transbronchial or open-lung biopsy
  4. Myocarditis
     a. Cardiac enzymes
     b. Electrocardiogram
     c. Endomyocardial biopsy for definitive diagnosis
- Toxoplasmosis in pregnancy
  1. Initial maternal screening with IgM and IgG
     a. If negative, mother at risk of acute infection and should be retested monthly
     b. If both IgG and IgM positive, obtain IgA and IgE ELISA, AC/HS test
     c. IgA and IgE ELISA, AC/HS test elevated in acute infection
     d. Ig high for 1 yr or more
     e. IgG repeated 3 to 4 wk later to determine if titer is stable
  2. Acute maternal infection not excluded or documented
     a. Fetal blood sampling (for culture, Ig, IgA, IgE)
     b. Amniotic fluid polymerase chain reaction (PCR)
  3. Fetal ultrasound every other wk if maternal infection documented
- Congenital toxoplasmosis
  1. Placental histology
  2. Specific IgM or IgA in infant's blood

LABORATORY TESTS

- Antibody studies
  1. More than one test necessary to establish diagnosis of acute toxoplasmosis

2. IgM antibody
   a. Appears 5 days into infection
   b. Peaks at 2 wk
   c. Falls to low level or disappears within 2 mo
   d. May persist at low levels for 1 yr or more
3. Antibody not measurable
   a. Ocular toxoplasmosis
   b. Reactivation
   c. Immunocompromised hosts
4. IgA ELISA, IgE ELISA, and IgE ASAGA
   a. More sensitive tests
   b. Disappear more rapidly than Ig, establishing diagnosis of acute infection
5. IgG antibody
   a. Appears 1 to 2 wk after infection
   b. Peaks at 6 to 8 wk
   c. Gradually declines over months to years

IMAGING STUDIES

- Chest x-ray if pulmonary involvement suspected
- Cerebral CT scan (Fig. 1-838) or MRI if encephalitis suspected

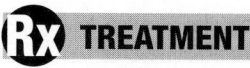

TREATMENT

NONPHARMACOLOGIC THERAPY

- Selected cases of ocular infection
  1. Photocoagulation
  2. Vitrectomy
  3. Lentectomy
- Selected cases of congenital cerebral infection
  1. Ventricular shunting

ACUTE GENERAL Rx

- Acute infection, immunocompetent host
  1. No treatment, unless severe and persistent symptoms or vital organ damage

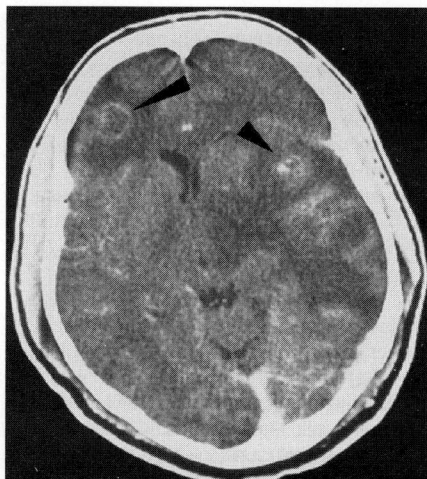

FIGURE 1-838 Toxoplasmic encephalitis in person who has AIDS. A cranial CT scan shows bilateral contrast-enhanced ring lesions with peripheral edema and mass effect. (From Cohen J, Powderly WG: *Infectious diseases,* ed 2, St Louis, 2004, Mosby.)

- Acute infection, immunocompromised host, non-AIDS
  1. Treat even if asymptomatic
  2. Duration
     a. Until 4 to 6 wk after resolution of all signs and symptoms
     b. Usually 6 mo or longer
- Reactivated infection, immunocompromised host, non-AIDS
  1. Treat if symptomatic
- Acute or reactivated infection, AIDS
  1. Treat in all cases
  2. Induction course
     a. 3 to 6 wk.
     b. Maintenance therapy continued for life; consider discontinuation of suppressive therapy if the patient has a good response to antiretroviral therapy and if the CD4 count remains >200 cell/mm³ for more than 3 mo.
  3. Empiric therapy
     a. AIDS with positive IgG
     b. Multiple ring-enhancing lesions on cerebral CT scan or MRI
     c. Response seen by day 7 in 71% and day 14 in 91%
- Ocular infection
  1. Treat in all cases
  2. Therapy continued for 1 mo or longer if needed
  3. Response seen in 70% within 10 days
  4. Retreat as needed
  5. Steroids may be indicated in patients with signs or symptoms of increased intracranial pressure
  6. Surgical treatment in selected cases
- Treatment regimens
  1. Pyrimethamine 200 mg loading dose once PO, then 50 mg (<60 kg) to 75 mg (>60 kg) q day; plus
  2. Leucovorin 10 to 20 mg PO qid, plus
  3. Sulfadiazine 1 (<60 kg) to 1.5 g (>60 kg) PO q6h
  Other treatment options (if sulfahypersensitivity or allergy is present): pyrimethamine 50 to 75 mg/day PO with leucovorin 10 to 20 mg/day PO and either (1) clindamycin 600 mg q6h PO or IV (up to 1200 mg IV) q6h, or (2) clarithromycin 1 g PO bid, or (3) dapsone 100 mg/day PO, or (4) atovaquone 750 mg PO q6h.
- Acute infection in pregnancy
  1. Treat immediately
  2. Risk of fetal infection reduced by 60% with treatment
     a. First trimester
        i. Spiramycin 3 g PO qid in two to four divided doses
        ii. Sulfadiazine 4 g PO qid in four divided doses
     b. Second and third trimester
        i. Sulfadiazine as previously described, *plus*
        ii. Pyrimethamine 25 mg PO qid, *plus*
        iii. Leucovorin 5 to 15 mg PO qid
        iv. Spiramycin as previously described
- Congenital infection
  1. Sulfadiazine 50 mg/kg PO bid, *plus*
  2. Pyrimethamine 2 mg/kg PO for 2 days, then 1 mg/kg PO, three times weekly, *plus*

3. Leucovorin 5 to 20 mg PO three times weekly
4. Minimum duration of treatment: 12 mo

CHRONIC Rx

Maintenance therapy in AIDS patients because of the high risk (80%) of relapse
1. Pyrimethamine 25 mg PO qid
2. Sulfadiazine 500 mg PO qid
3. Leucovorin 10 to 20 mg PO qid

DISPOSITION

- Prognosis
  1. Excellent in the immunocompetent host
  2. Good in ocular infection (although relapses are common)
- Treatment of acute infection in pregnancy
  1. Reduces incidence and severity of congenital toxoplasmosis
- Treatment of congenital infection
  1. Improvement in intellectual function
  2. Regression of retinal lesions
- AIDS
  1. 70% to 95% response to therapy

REFERRAL

- To infectious disease expert:
  1. Immunocompromised hosts
  2. Pregnant women
  3. Difficulty in making a diagnosis or deciding on treatment
- To pediatric infectious disease expert:
  1. Congenital infection
- To obstetrician:
  1. Pregnant seronegative mother
  2. Acute seroconversion
- To ophthalmologist:
  1. Congenital infection
  2. Any case of ocular infection

PEARLS & CONSIDERATIONS

COMMENTS

- Prevention of toxoplasmosis is most important in seronegative pregnant women and immunocompromised hosts.
- Patient instructions:
  1. Cook meat to 66° C.
  2. Cook eggs.
  3. Do not drink unpasteurized milk.
  4. Wash hands thoroughly after handling raw meat.
  5. Wash kitchen surfaces that come in contact with raw meat.
  6. Wash fruits and vegetables.
  7. Avoid contact with materials potentially contaminated with cat feces.

SUGGESTED READINGS
available at www.expertconsult.com

RELATED CONTENT
Toxoplasmosis (Patient Information)

AUTHOR: **GLENN G. FORT, M.D., M.P.H.**

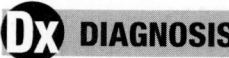

BASIC INFORMATION

DEFINITION

Acute hemolytic transfusion reaction (AHTR) is acute intravascular hemolysis caused by mismatches in the ABO system. It is caused by complement-fixing immunoglobulin (Ig) and IgG antibodies to group A and B red blood cells. Hemolytic transfusion reactions can also be caused by minor antigen systems; however, they are usually less severe. In delayed serologic transfusion reactions, hemolysis with hemoglobinemia is unusual; in delayed reactions the only manifestations may be the development of a newly positive Coombs test and fever. The clinical severity of an ABO-incompatible blood transfusion is significantly influenced by the degree of complement activation and cytokine stimulation.

SYNONYMS

AHTR
Acute hemolytic transfusion reaction

ICD-9CM CODES
999.8 Other transfusion reaction

EPIDEMIOLOGY & DEMOGRAPHICS

- Acute intravascular hemolysis occurs in one to five per 50,000 transfusions.

PHYSICAL FINDINGS & CLINICAL PRESENTATION

- Hypotension
- Pain at the infusion site
- Fever, tachycardia, chest pain, dyspnea, dizziness, bronchospasm
- Lower back pain due to ischemic muscle pain or vasospasm rather than kidney pain from developing renal failure
- Severe reactions often occur in surgical patients under anesthesia who are unable to give any warning signs.
See Table 1-397.

ETIOLOGY

Most fatal hemolytic reactions are caused by clerical errors and mislabeled specimens.

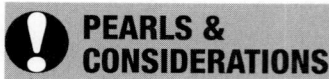

DIFFERENTIAL DIAGNOSIS

- Bacterial contamination of blood
- Hemoglobinopathies

WORKUP

The transfusion must be stopped immediately. The blood bank must be notified, and the donor transfusion bag must be returned to the blood bank along with a freshly drawn posttransfusion specimen.

LABORATORY TESTS

- Positive Coombs test, elevated BUN, creatinine, LDH, bilirubin (especially indirect bilirubin).
- Analyze urine for hemoglobinuria (wine-colored urine), observe plasma for hemoglobinemia (pink plasma).
- Decreased hematocrit and serum haptoglobin (haptoglobin low to 0 mg/dl).
- The direct antiglobulin test (DAT) usually becomes positive in an immune hemolytic reaction (if tested before all the incompatible RBCs are destroyed). Preparation of an antibody eluate is necessary to identify the offending antibody.
- Monitor coagulation status (PT, aPTT, fibrinogen).

TREATMENT

NONPHARMACOLOGIC THERAPY

- Stop transfusion immediately. Test anticoagulated blood from the recipient for the presence of free hemoglobin in the plasma.
- Monitor vital signs closely, and maintain IV access and adequate airway.

ACUTE GENERAL Rx

- Treatment is supportive and consists of fluid resuscitation, vasopressor support, and mannitol.
- Vigorous IV hydration (0.9% NaCl or some other suitable crystalloid solution) to maintain urine flow at >100 ml/hr until hypotension is corrected and hemoglobinuria clears. IV furosemide may be necessary to maintain adequate renal flow.
- The addition of mannitol may prevent renal damage (controversial). Mannitol, if chosen, must be used with caution; if acute tubular necrosis occurs before mannitol infusion, pulmonary edema may occur as a result of the acute increase in intravascular volume secondary to fluid expansion.
- Monitor for the presence of disseminated intravascular coagulation. PT, aPTT, and fibrinogen levels should be closely monitored.
- If sepsis is suspected, culture as appropriate.

DISPOSITION

Mortality rate exceeds 50% in severe transfusion reactions.

PEARLS & CONSIDERATIONS

COMMENTS

Hemolysis caused by minor antigen systems is generally less severe and may be delayed 5 to 10 days after transfusion.

SUGGESTED READING
available at www.expertconsult.com

AUTHOR: **FRED F. FERRI, M.D.**

TABLE 1-397   Signs and Symptoms of Acute Adverse Reactions to Blood Transfusion

Reaction	Fever	Chills/ Rigors	Nausea/ Vomiting	Chest Discomfort/ Pain	Facial Flushing	Wheezing/ Dyspnea	Back/ Lumbar Pain	Discomfort at Infusion Site	Hypotension
Acute hemolytic	X	X	X	X	X	X	X	X	X
Febrile nonhemolytic	X	X		X	X				
Nonimmune hemolysis									
Acute lung injury	X			X		X			X
Allergic									
Massive transfusion complications									
Anaphylaxis	X	X	X	X	X	X	X	X	X
Passive cytokine infusion	X	X	X			X			
Hypervolemia						X			
Bacterial sepsis	X	X	X				X	X	X
Air embolus				X		X			

From Goldman L, Bennett JC (eds): *Cecil textbook of medicine*, ed 22, Philadelphia, 2004, Saunders.

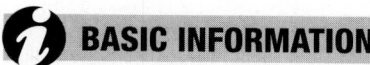

BASIC INFORMATION

DEFINITION

Transient ischemic attack (TIA) is a transient episode of neurologic dysfunction caused by focal brain, spinal cord, or retinal ischemia without acute infarction noted on MRI. TIA symptoms typically resolve within 60 min and almost always within 24 hr.

SYNONYMS

TIA
Amaurosis fugax
"Mini-stroke"
Pre-stroke

ICD-9CM CODES
435.9 Unspecified transient cerebral ischemia

EPIDEMIOLOGY & DEMOGRAPHICS

INCIDENCE: 49 to 83 cases per 100,000 persons annually
PEAK INCIDENCE: After age 60 yr
PREVALENCE: 200,000 to 500,000 persons in the United States
PREDOMINANT SEX AND RACE: Males > females; African American > Caucasian
RISK FACTORS: Same as for ischemic stroke

PHYSICAL FINDINGS & CLINICAL PRESENTATION

TIAs often present with ipsilateral transient monocular blindness (amaurosis fugax), contralateral numbness or weakness, contralateral homonymous hemianopsia, and/or aphasia.

ETIOLOGY

Embolic (cardioembolism in 10% to 15%), large vessel atherothrombotic disease (20% to 25%), lacunar disease, hypoperfusion, hypercoagulable state, arteritis

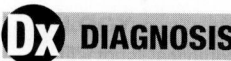 DIAGNOSIS

DIFFERENTIAL DIAGNOSIS

Seizures, hypoglycemia, complicated migraine, intracranial hemorrhage, mass lesion, vestibular disease, Bell's palsy, meningitis, multiple sclerosis, subdural hematoma, brain abscess, cervical or lumbar spine disease, conversion disorder

WORKUP

Given the high risk of stroke within the first 48 hr following TIA (up to 10%), hospital admission for workup is advised. Fig E1-839 describes a TIA algorithm. The American Heart Association recommends that the ABCD2 score be used in the evaluation of TIA. It consists of 1 point for age ≥60 years, 1 point for BP ≥140 mm Hg systolic or ≥90 mm Hg diastolic, clinical features (2 points for unilateral weakness, 1 point for speech impairment), duration of TIA (2 points for duration ≥60 min, 1 point for duration 10-59 min), presence of diabetes mellitus (1 point). According to the guidelines, it is reason-able to hospitalize patients with TIA if they present within 72 hours and have an ABCD^2 score ≥3.

LABORATORY TESTS

Complete blood count, basic metabolic panel, prothrombin time, activated partial thromboplastin time, sedimentation rate, fasting lipid panel, serum glucose and hemoglobin A_{1c} (to detect latent diabetes mellitus)

IMAGING STUDIES

- CT scan should be obtained to exclude hemorrhage; MRI with diffusion weighting if immediately available.
- Imaging of the vessels should be obtained via magnetic resonance angiography (MRA), computed tomography angiography (CTA), or carotid Dopplers/transcranial Dopplers (CD/TCD).
  - If symptoms are referable to the posterior circulation, MRA or CTA should be obtained in lieu of CD/TCD.
  - Transthoracic echocardiogram should be obtained.
    An echocardiogram with bubble should be obtained in all patients younger than 50 yr with TIA symptoms.
- Electrocardiogram should be obtained to exclude the presence of arrhythmias, namely atrial fibrillation.
- At least 24 hr of heart rhythm monitoring should be accomplished to screen for arrhythmia.

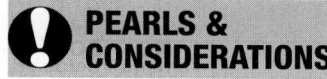 TREATMENT

NONPHARMACOLOGIC THERAPY

- Carotid endarterectomy or carotid stenting should be considered for patients found to have carotid stenosis as the cause for TIA. Please refer to "Carotid Stenosis" chapter for more information.
- Intracranial angioplasty and stenting may be considered in cases of symptomatic intracranial atherosclerosis. Clinical trials are ongoing.

ACUTE GENERAL Rx

- In the absence of contraindications, patients who are identified to have atrial fibrillation should be considered for anticoagulation with intravenous heparin (or therapeutic lovenox) along with warfarin until target INR between 2.0 and 3.0 is achieved.
- Although no compelling evidence exists for the use of heparin in the acute treatment of TIAs without cardioembolic source, patients who develop recurrent symptoms within the same vascular territory that increase in duration, severity, and/or frequency (crescendo TIA/stuttering TIA) may benefit from its use.

CHRONIC Rx

- Chronic therapy should be aimed at modifying the four major risk factors: blood pressure control, control of dyslipidemia, control of blood sugars, and smoking cessation.

- Antiplatelet therapy should be used to reduce the risk of recurrent TIAs or subsequent stroke. Three antiplatelet agents are commonly used in stroke prevention: aspirin, aspirin/dipyridamole, and clopidogrel. All are reasonable choices but practitioners should consider their individual patient's comorbidities when selecting an antiplatelet agent.
- Dose-adjusted warfarin (INR 2.0 to 3.0) is indicated for prevention of future strokes in atrial fibrillation patients. The direct thrombin inhibitor dabigatran and the direct factor Xa inhibitors apixaban and rivaroxaban have been approved as an alternative treatment to warfarin for stroke prevention in atrial fibrillation.

DISPOSITION

Disposition and prognosis depend on the duration of symptoms and underlying etiology.

REFERRAL

Neurology consultation

PEARLS & CONSIDERATIONS

Despite complete symptom resolution, 20% to 50% of patients with TIA have evidence of acute tissue infarction on MRI.

PREVENTION

Prevention of carotid stenosis should be guided at pursuing a healthy lifestyle and management of risk factors.

PATIENT/FAMILY EDUCATION

Patients should be counseled on the early signs of stroke symptoms and instructed to promptly seek medical attention if they develop symptoms concerning for stroke. Patients should be encouraged to pursue a healthy lifestyle to include exercise and smoking cessation. In addition, patients should take an active role in controlling blood pressure and blood glucose. Further educational materials can be found online at http//www.strokecenter.org/education.

SUGGESTED READINGS
available at www.expertconsult.com

RELATED CONTENT

Transient Ischemic Attack (TIA) (Patient Information)

AUTHOR: **JOSEPH R. OWENS, M.D.**

BASIC INFORMATION

DEFINITION

Demyelination in a transverse region of the spinal cord due to an inflammatory process that leads to sensory and motor changes below the lesion. The pathologic hallmark of transverse myelitis is the presence of focal collections of lymphocytes and monocytes with varying degrees of demyelination, axonal injury, and astroglial and microglial activation within the spinal cord.

SYNONYMS

None

ICD-9CM CODES
323.82 Other causes of myelitis, Transverse myelitis NOS
341.2 Acute (transverse) myelitis

EPIDEMIOLOGY & DEMOGRAPHICS

INCIDENCE: Annual incidence of idiopathic or postinfectious transverse myelitis ranges from 1.3 to 8 cases per million. The incidence increases to 24.6 cases per million annually if acquired demyelination causes such as multiple sclerosis (MS) are included.
PREVALENCE: Unknown
PREDOMINANT SEX: None
GENETICS: No genetic predisposition has been shown.
PEAK INCIDENCE: Bimodal peak in the incidence between 10 to 19 yr and 30 to 39 yr
RISK FACTORS: Infection, vaccination

PHYSICAL FINDINGS & CLINICAL PRESENTATION

- The clinical signs are caused by an interruption in ascending and descending neuroanatomic pathways in the transverse plane of the spinal cord, and a resulting sensory level is characteristic of transverse myelitis.
- Rapid onset of symmetric or asymmetric paraparesis or paraplegia of the lower extremities over a few days, ascending paresthesia, trunk sensory level, back pain, sphincter dysfunction, and positive Babinski with upgoing toes bilaterally. The arms may also be involved but less than the legs in most cases.
- One third to one half of patients present with localizing back pain.
- There is progression to nadir of clinical deficits between 4 hr and 21 days after symptom onset.
- Urinary incontinence or retention, GI disturbances (incontinence or constipation), and sexual dysfunction are common.

ETIOLOGY

- Demyelination due to the body's immune response to infection, post-vaccination, may be onset of MS, or may be idiopathic (15% to 30% of cases).
- About 50% of patients have had a recent upper respiratory infection.
- Epstein-Barr virus and cytomegalovirus are most common viral infections.
- Hepatitis B, varicella, enterovirus, rhinovirus, mycoplasma, syphilis, measles, Lyme disease are less common.

DIAGNOSIS

DIFFERENTIAL DIAGNOSIS

- MS
- Neuromyelitis optica (NMO)
- Tumor of spinal cord
- Herniated or slipped discs
- Spinal stenosis
- Abscess
- Vascular malformation

WORKUP

- Transverse myelitis should be suspected in patients with a history of rapid (hours to days) onset of motor weakness, sensory abnormalities referable to the spinal cord, and bladder or bowel dysfunction. The dysfunction is bilateral (not necessarily symmetric) and there is a clearly defined sensory level.
- Lumbar puncture looking for oligoclonal bands for MS or infection.
- Magnetic resonance imaging (MRI) of brain and MRI of spine at level of suspected involvement (Fig. E1-840).
- Computed tomography (CT) if MRI is unavailable; may use myelography with CT.

LABORATORY TESTS

- ANA, hepatitis B serology, Lyme disease titer, VDRL
- Cerebrospinal fluid (CSF) may show increased protein/normal protein, lymphocytes, and normal glucose.
- Serum NMO-IgG to evaluate for neuromyelitis optica.

IMAGING STUDIES

- MRI shows demyelinating lesion on T_2 with contrast enhancement.
- Chest and joint radiology
- CT or PET scan as indicated by history and examination

TREATMENT

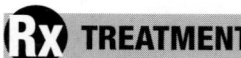

Corticosteroids are the first-line treatment for transverse myelitis; IVIG and plasma exchange can be considered in intractable cases, although there is no evidence-based medicine for use of corticosteroids, plasma exchange, or IVIG. A referral to a neurologist is recommended for treatment.

NONPHARMACOLOGIC THERAPY

- Physical therapy
- Respiratory and oropharyngeal support

ACUTE GENERAL Rx

- High-dose IV corticosteroid (e.g., methylprednisolone 1000 mg/day for 3 to 5 days)
- Rescue therapy with plasma exchange may be helpful in patients who do not respond to corticosteroids
- Combination therapy with plasmapheresis and immunosuppressive agents (e.g., cyclophosphamide) may also be effective
- Naproxen, ibuprofen for pain

CHRONIC Rx

- Baclofen, tizanidine, or some other muscle relaxant for muscle spasms
- Gabapentin for pain
- Low-molecular-weight heparin for DVT prophylaxis in patients with immobility

DISPOSITION

- One third of patients with transverse myelitis will have complete recovery, one third will have fair recovery, and one third have permanent disability and do not recover. Some people will have recurrence or relapse.
- Patients who need further care including Foley catheters may need home nursing assistance. Some patients may benefit from a rehab center placement or outpatient physical therapy services.

REFERRAL

- Consider physical therapy.
- Consider occupational therapy.
- Consider rehab services.
- Consider psychiatric consultation (high incidence of long-term mood and anxiety disorders).

SUGGESTED READINGS
available at www.expertconsult.com

AUTHOR: **SHARLISA HUTSON, M.D.**

BASIC INFORMATION

DEFINITION

Tricuspid regurgitation (TR) refers to an abnormal flow of blood from the right ventricle to the right atrium (Fig. 1-842.)

SYNONYMS

Tricuspid insufficiency
Tricuspid incompetence

ICD-9CM CODES
397.0 Diseases of the tricuspid valve
424.2 Tricuspid valve disorders, specified as non-rheumatic

EPIDEMIOLOGY & DEMOGRAPHICS

- In the adult population, TR is usually functional rather than structural.
- In adolescents and young adults, most cases of TR are the result of congenital cardiac abnormalities.
- In patients with rheumatic heart disease, TR rarely occurs alone; it is usually associated with mitral or aortic valve disease.
- A small degree (i.e., trace to mild) of TR is present in approximately 70% of normal adults. On echocardiography, this "normal" degree of regurgitation is localized to a small region adjacent to valve closure, it often does not extend throughout systole, and it has a low signal strength.

PHYSICAL FINDINGS & CLINICAL PRESENTATION

- Isolated TR can cause nonspecific symptoms (e.g., exercise intolerance).
- Signs and symptoms in the presence of TR are usually the result of an underlying cause.
- Signs and symptoms may be caused by accompanying right-sided heart failure (e.g., jugular venous distention, peripheral edema, ascites, hepatomegaly, right-sided S_3).
- A lower-left parasternal holosystolic murmur may be found; the murmur becomes louder during inspiration (Carvallo's sign) and during maneuvers that increase venous return.
- Prominent V waves in the jugular venous waveform can occur.
- Severe TR may produce systolic propulsion of the eyeballs, pulsatile varicose veins, a venous systolic thrill and murmur in the neck, a mid-diastolic murmur in severe regurgitation, and systolic hepatic pulsation.
- Atrial fibrillation or flutter is common as a result of right atrial enlargement.

ETIOLOGY

- Tricuspid valve dysfunction can occur with structurally normal (functional TR) or abnormal valves (structural TR).
- Functional TR involves conditions that lead to the dilation of the tricuspid annulus or right ventricular enlargement, including the following:
  - Any cause of pulmonary hypertension (e.g., chronic obstructive pulmonary disease, pulmonary embolism, restrictive lung disease, collagen vascular disease, primary pulmonary hypertension, left to right shunts [i.e., ASD, VSD, anomalous pulmonary venous return])
  - Left-sided heart failure that leads to right-sided heart failure
  - Dilated cardiomyopathy
  - Right ventricular infarction
- Structural TR involves conditions directly affecting the tricuspid valve apparatus, including the following:
  - Rheumatic valvulitis
  - Congenital conditions (e.g., Ebstein's anomaly, tricuspid atresia)
  - Endocarditis, either bacterial (particularly related to intravenous drug use) or marantic (e.g., systemic lupus erythematosus, rheumatoid arthritis)
  - Tricuspid valve prolapse or chordae rupture
  - Carcinoid syndrome
  - Marfan's syndrome
  - Iatrogenic damage to the valve (e.g., pacemaker, implantable cardioverter-defibrillator, myocardial biopsy, anorectic drugs)
  - External trauma (e.g., deceleration injury)
  - Right atrial myxoma
  - Collagen vascular diseases
  - Radiation injury

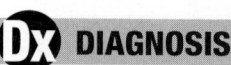 DIAGNOSIS

The diagnosis of TR is made noninvasively by physical examination and imaging techniques (e.g., echocardiography) and invasively by right-sided heart catheterization in selected cases.

DIFFERENTIAL DIAGNOSIS

On the basis of heart auscultation, the diagnosis of TR may be confused with other causes of systolic murmurs, such as mitral regurgitation, aortic stenosis, pulmonary stenosis, ventricular septal defect, and hypertrophic cardiomyopathy.

WORKUP

Any patient suspected of having significant TR should undergo the following:
- Chest x-ray
- ECG
- Echocardiogram (confirmatory)
- Right-sided cardiac heart catheterization (in selected cases)
- CMR (in selected cases)

LABORATORY TESTS

ECG may show evidence of the following:
- Right atrial enlargement (e.g., P-wave amplitude in leads II or III or aVF of >2.5 mV)
- Right ventricular enlargement or hypertrophy (e.g., R:S ratio >1 in V_1, or R >7 mm in V_1, deep S in V_5 and V_6)
- Right axis deviation of >90 degrees
- Atrial fibrillation

IMAGING STUDIES

- A chest x-ray may show the following:
  - Evidence of chronic obstructive pulmonary disease (e.g., flattened diaphragms, barrel chest, dilated pulmonary arteries, increased retrosternal air space) or restrictive lung disease
  - Enlarged right atrium
  - Enlarged right ventricle
- An echocardiogram (either transthoracic or transesophageal) will do the following:
  - Assess tricuspid valve structure and motion, measure annular size, and identify other cardiac abnormalities

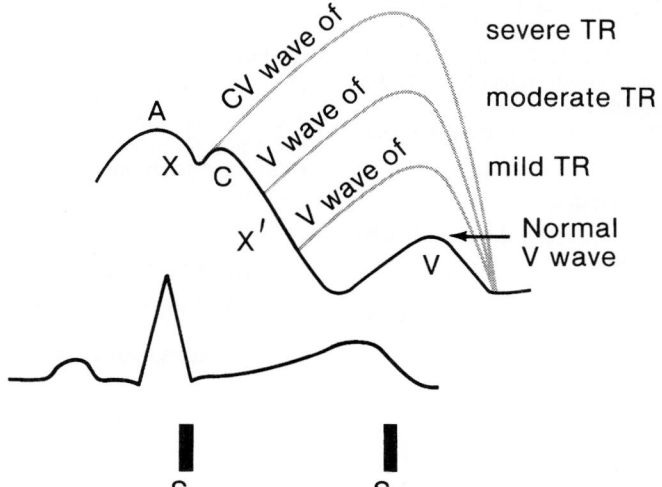

FIGURE 1-842 The jugular venous pulse in tricuspid regurgitation. The jugular venous pulse wave normally drops during ventricular systole. As tricuspid regurgitation becomes more severe, the CV wave becomes more obvious during ventricular systole. (From Conn R: *Current diagnosis,* ed 9, Philadelphia, 1997, Saunders.)

- Estimate the severity of TR (vena contracta width >0.7 cm and systolic flow reversal in hepatic veins)
- Estimate the pulmonary artery pressure
- Exclude vegetation, mass, or prolapse
- Assess left and right ventricular function
- CMR (cardiovascular magnetic resonance)
  - If echocardiographic evaluation is poor
  - Quantitative measurements of TR volume
  - RV volumes
  - Ejection fraction
- Right-sided cardiac heart catheterization shows the following:
  - Elevated right atrial and right ventricular systolic and end-diastolic pressures
  - Large V waves

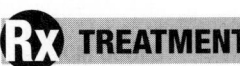 **TREATMENT**

The treatment of TR is usually directed at the underlying cause.

NONPHARMACOLOGIC THERAPY
Oxygen therapy is beneficial for patients with functional TR caused by underlying pulmonary hypertension provoked by alveolar hypoxia.

ACUTE GENERAL Rx
- Functional TR caused by left-sided heart failure is treated in the standard way with preload reduction, afterload reduction, or inotropic therapy (see "Congestive Heart Failure").
- The reversal of pulmonary hypertension with vasodilators or pulmonary thromboendarterectomy has been shown to reverse functional TR.
- Structural TR treatment depends on the underlying cause of heart disease.

CHRONIC Rx
- The 2006 American College of Cardiology/American Heart Association Guidelines Pertaining to the Surgical Management of Tricuspid Valve Disease/Regurgitation include the following:
  - Class I: Tricuspid valve repair is beneficial for severe TR in patients with mitral valve (MV) disease that requires MV surgery. ❸

- Class IIa: Tricuspid valve replacement or annuloplasty is reasonable for a symptomatic patient with severe primary TR and for severe TR as a result of diseased or abnormal tricuspid valve leaflets that are not amenable to annuloplasty or repair. ❻
- Class IIb: Tricuspid annuloplasty may be considered for less-than-severe TR in patients who are undergoing MV surgery when there is pulmonary hypertension or tricuspid annular dilatation (usually >21 mm/m² body surface area [BSA]). ❻
- Class III: Tricuspid valve replacement or annuloplasty is not indicated for asymptomatic patients with TR whose pulmonary artery pressure is <60 mm Hg in the presence of a normal MV or for those with mild TR. ❻
- Patients with severe TR of any cause have poor long-term outcomes as a result of right ventricular dysfunction or systemic venous congestion.
- During recent years, annuloplasty has become an established surgical approach to significant TR. A recent study showed that tricuspid valve (TV) repair with an annuloplasty ring results in improved long-term outcomes.
- When the valve leaflets themselves are diseased, abnormal, or destroyed, valve replacement with a low-profile mechanical valve or bioprosthesis is often necessary.
- A biologic prosthesis is preferred because of the high rate of thromboembolic complications that occur with mechanical prostheses in the tricuspid position.

DISPOSITION
- Regardless of the cause, a greater-than-mild degree of TR is associated with decreased survival.
- Clinically insignificant TR can be detected by color Doppler imaging in many normal people. This is not an indication for either routine follow-up or prophylaxis against bacterial endocarditis.
- Isolated TR should not pose a significant problem during pregnancy, although greater care may be necessary for protection from diuretic-induced hypoperfusion.

- Isolated TR with normal right ventricular function does not preclude an individual's involvement in competitive sports.

REFERRAL
For patients with significant symptomatic TR, a cardiology consultation is recommended.

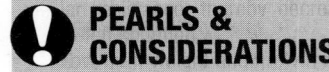 **PEARLS & CONSIDERATIONS**

- TR that results from tricuspid valve prolapse is often associated with concurrent MV prolapse.
- Secondary TR commonly occurs in combination with left-sided valvular heart disease. It often does not improve, despite correction of the left-sided valve dysfunction.
- Functional tricuspid insufficiency, if left uncorrected, carries serious long-term consequences.

COMMENTS
- Antibiotic prophylaxis for dental, gastrointestinal, or genitourinary procedures is no longer recommended for patients with only structural tricuspid valve abnormalities.
- Tricuspid annuloplasty at the time of MV surgery results in improved functional capacity without any increase in perioperative morbidity or mortality.
- During TR of the donor heart after cardiac transplantation, tricuspid valve replacement with a biologic prosthesis is a safe, durable, and effective method of treating TR after transplantation. This allows for future endomyocardial biopsies to be performed. Mechanical valves should be avoided.

SUGGESTED READINGS
available at www.expertconsult.com

RELATED CONTENT
Tricuspid Regurgitation (Patient Information)

AUTHORS: **ARAVIND RAO KOKKIRALA, M.D., VIKRAM BEHERA, M.D.,** and **GAURAV CHOUDHARY, M.D.**

Diseases and Disorders

T

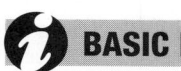 **BASIC INFORMATION**

DEFINITION

Tricuspid stenosis (TS) is an uncommon valvular pathology that is caused by the narrowing of the tricuspid valve orifice, which results in the restriction of right atrial emptying. TS is most often rheumatic in origin, and it often presents with a combination of regurgitation and stenosis.

SYNONYMS

Tricuspid valve stenosis
TS

ICD-9CM CODES
397.0 Disease of the tricuspid valve

EPIDEMIOLOGY & DEMOGRAPHICS

- TS is most commonly caused by rheumatic heart disease, and it almost always occurs with associated mitral or aortic valve disease.
- Antibiotic therapy has made rheumatic heart disease and TS in the U.S. very rare.
- TS is present at autopsy in 15% of patients with rheumatic heart disease, but it is clinically significant in only 5%.

PHYSICAL FINDINGS & CLINICAL PRESENTATION

- Obstruction to tricuspid flow limits cardiac output.
- Symptoms and physical examination findings usually depend on the presence and severity of concomitant mitral or aortic valve disease.
- Symptoms of right heart failure include fatigue, right upper quadrant abdominal pain (from hepatic congestion), ascites, hepatomegaly, peripheral edema, and clear lungs.
- Jugular venous distention, a prominent a wave, slow rate of y descent, and a palpable hepatic pulsation are noted during the sinus rhythm.
- A right atrial pulsation may be palpated to the right of the sternum, and a diastolic thrill that increases with inspiration may be felt over the left sternal edge.
- An opening snap and a low-frequency diastolic murmur are best heard along the left sternal border of the fourth intercostal space. The murmur is softer, high-pitched, and shorter in duration as compared to mitral stenosis. These are augmented by inspiration (i.e., Carvallo's sign), leg raises, isotonic exercise, and squatting.

ETIOLOGY

- Rheumatic heart disease results in the scarring of the valve leaflets, the shortening of the chordae tendineae, and the fusion of the commissures, thereby leading to the immobility of the valve leaflets and the narrowing of the tricuspid valve orifice.
- Other causes are congenital, infectious (e.g., endocarditis), metabolic, and enzymatic abnormalities (e.g., carcinoid syndrome, Whipple's disease, Fabry's disease); right atrial or metastatic tumors; and, rarely, scarring and adhesions as a result of complications of pacemaker placement.

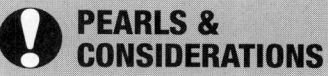 **DIAGNOSIS**

DIFFERENTIAL DIAGNOSIS

- Congenital tricuspid atresia
- Right heart diastolic dysfunction: endomyocardial fibrosis or constrictive pericarditis
- Extrinsic compression of the right ventricle: severe pectum excavatum, massive ascites, pleural effusion, pericardial effusion, or tumor
- Obstruction of right atrial emptying: right atrial myxoma, metastatic tumor, right atrial thrombi, or tricuspid valve vegetation (particularly in association with a permanent pacemaker lead)

WORKUP

- Echocardiography is the diagnostic test of choice to evaluate the tricuspid valve.
- ECG is recommended to look for atrial arrhythmias, atrial fibrillation, or atrial flutter as a result of an enlarged right atrium.
- Chest x-ray.
- Right heart catheterization is an option when echocardiography cannot be used to make a definitive diagnosis.

IMAGING STUDIES

- Echocardiography reveals the thickening and shortening of the tricuspid valve leaflets, the restriction of the movement of the leaflets and the leaflet tips, a reduction in the diameter of the annulus, and diastolic doming of the valve. Evidence of right atrial enlargement and dilated IVC is present in most cases. For severe TS the mean gradient is >5 mm Hg.
- Doppler echocardiography or cardiac catheterization demonstrates a reduced tricuspid valve area (severe when <1 cm²) and a diastolic pressure gradient across the tricuspid valve (normal gradient, <1 mm Hg).
- Chest radiography may reveal an enlarged right atrium and a reduced pulmonary blood volume.

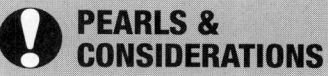 **TREATMENT**

NONPHARMACOLOGIC THERAPY

Salt and fluid restriction is essential to decrease peripheral edema.

ACUTE GENERAL Rx

- Assess and treat the underlying cause of the valvular pathology.
- Treat bacterial endocarditis with antibiotics.
- Manage right atrium volume overload with diuretics.
- Prescribe rate-controlling atrioventricular nodal blockers and anticoagulants, especially for patients with atrial arrhythmia.

CHRONIC Rx

- Symptoms of systemic venous hypertension and congestion can be controlled with diuretics and angiotensin-converting enzyme inhibitors or angiotensin receptor antagonists.
- Balloon valvuloplasty or dilation of the stenosed tricuspid valve has been shown to be effective. Patients with clinical evidence of systemic venous hypertension and congestion should be considered for valvotomy. Tricuspid regurgitation that is more than mild is generally considered a contraindication to valvotomy. Tumor masses, vegetations, and thrombi are also contraindications to valvotomy.
- Surgery for TS is usually recommended when the valve is not treatable by balloon valvuloplasty and the valve area is <2 cm² with a mean diastolic gradient across the tricuspid valve of >5 mm Hg.
- Isolated tricuspid valve replacement surgery almost never occurs. It is typically performed in the setting of concomitant mitral or aortic valve surgery.
- Surgical procedures for TS include commissurotomy and tricuspid valve replacement.

DISPOSITION

The natural course of severe TS is not well known.

REFERRAL

TS may be difficult to diagnose, so consultation with a cardiologist is recommended.

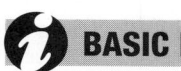 **PEARLS & CONSIDERATIONS**

- Rheumatic heart disease accounts for >90% of stenotic tricuspid valves.
- Rheumatic TS almost always occurs in association with mitral valve disease and sometimes with aortic valve disease.
- The majority of cases present with tricuspid regurgitation or a combination of regurgitation and stenosis.

COMMENTS

Tricuspid valve replacement carries a 30-day operative morbidity and mortality rate of 5% to 7% in addition to a high risk of right heart thrombus formation. Therefore, surgical procedures are reserved for patients who are not candidates for balloon dilation techniques. Unlike patients with mitral stenosis, patients with TS typically do not report dyspnea, orthopnea, or paroxysmal nocturnal dyspnea.

SUGGESTED READINGS
available at www.expertconsult.com

RELATED CONTENT
Tricuspid Stenosis (Patient Information)

AUTHORS: **ARAVIND RAO KOKKIRALA, M.D., VIKRAM BEHERA, M.D.,** and **GAURAV CHOUDHARY, M.D.**

BASIC INFORMATION

DEFINITION
Trigeminal neuralgia is an intense, usually unilateral, paroxysmal, stabbing pain in the distribution of the fifth cranial nerve.

SYNONYMS
Tic douloureux ("painful tics/spasms")

ICD-9CM CODES
350.1 Trigeminal neuralgia

EPIDEMIOLOGY & DEMOGRAPHICS
INCIDENCE: 4 per 100,000
PEAK INCIDENCE: Incidence increases with age, peaks at 67 yr; onset is after age 40 in 90% of patients.
PREVALENCE: 155 in 1 million
PREDOMINANT SEX AND AGE: Male/female ratio is 1:1.5.
RISK FACTORS: Most cases are idiopathic; age and multiple sclerosis are risk factors.

PHYSICAL FINDINGS & CLINICAL PRESENTATION
- Patients present with paroxysmal, unilateral facial pain that is usually described as shock-like, stabbing, or electric (Fig. 1-844).
- Pain can be spontaneous or triggered by touching, air current, or activities such as shaving, eating, or brushing teeth.
- In severe cases, facial spasms can accompany the pain.
- Pain is usually described in distribution of the second (V2-maxillary) and third (V3-mandibular) divisions of the trigeminal nerve.
- The pain seldom lasts more than a few seconds to a minute.
- There is usually no sensory or motor loss.

ETIOLOGY
- Idiopathic or "classic": cause usually unknown, likely an aberrant artery or vein compressing cranial nerve V at or near the pons
- Secondary: caused by nonvascular lesions such as a demyelinating plaque from multiple sclerosis, compression from meningioma, arachnoid cyst, etc.

DIAGNOSIS

DIFFERENTIAL DIAGNOSIS
- Glossopharyngeal neuralgia
- Temporomandibular joint pain
- Unilateral, neuralgiform headache
- Postherpetic neuralgia
- Dental pain

WORKUP
Trigeminal neuralgia is a clinical diagnosis (see above)

IMAGING STUDIES
Neuroimaging (MRI/magnetic resonance angiogram [MRA]) should be considered in young patient with atypical symptoms (sensory loss, bilateral symptoms)

TREATMENT

NONPHARMACOLOGIC THERAPY
Patients with refractory pain eventually need secondary intervention, such as nerve root de-

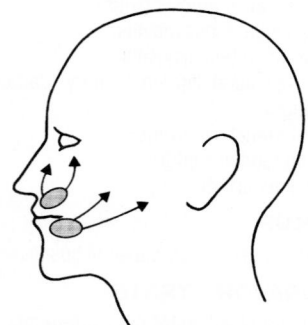

FIGURE 1-844 Trigeminal neuralgia. The two most common sites of origin and radiation of pain are shown: mouth-ear and nose-orbit. Pain usually starts in the region of the encircled area and radiates in the directions shown. (From Souhami RL, Moxham J: *Textbook of medicine,* ed 4, London, 2002, Churchill Livingstone.)

compression, selective nerve fiber destruction (rhizotomy), glycerol injection, thermal lesioning, chemical ablation, or gamma knife radiosurgery.

CHRONIC Rx
- Carbamazepine 100 to 200 mg bid is the recommended initial treatment. This can be titrated to pain relief by 200 mg daily to a maximum of 1200 mg divided bid.
- Oxcarbazepine can be used if carbamazepine is not tolerated due to side effects. Other medications include baclofen, gabapentin, clonazepam, levetiracetam, lamotrigine, and phenytoin.
- Drug combinations can be tried when one medication is partially effective prior to proceeding with secondary intervention.
- In the elderly population, caution should be used when initiating and titrating the above medications.

DISPOSITION
- Most patients are very responsive to pharmacologic treatment. Spontaneous remission is possible.
- Medical management is ineffective in 30% of patients.

REFERRAL
Referral to a neurologist is appropriate if uncertain about diagnosis or refractory to conservative management.

PEARLS & CONSIDERATIONS

In secondary disease, no medications have been established for treatment. Initial therapy should address underlying secondary causes.

SUGGESTED READINGS
available at www.expertconsult.com

RELATED CONTENT
Trigeminal Neuralgia (Patient Information)

AUTHOR: **WILLIAM F. DOTSON II, M.D.**

BASIC INFORMATION

DEFINITION

Trigger finger, or digital stenosing tenosynovitis, refers to an inflammatory process of the digital flexor tendon sheath that can lead to nodule formation of the flexor tendon. These changes lead to pain and difficulty or inability to extend the digit due to inability of the flexor tendon to glide through the A1 pulley.

SYNONYMS

Digital stenosing tenosynovitis

ICD-9CM CODES
727.03 Trigger finger (acquired)

EPIDEMIOLOGY & DEMOGRAPHICS

In adults, the middle finger is most often affected (Fig. 1-845). In children, the thumb is most often affected.
PREDOMINANT SEX AND AGE: Female/male ratio of 4:1. Trigger finger can be found in all age groups but is commonly found in patients aged >45 yr.
RISK FACTOR: Repetitive use occupations, such as meat cutters, seamstresses, tailors, and dentists.

PHYSICAL FINDINGS & CLINICAL PRESENTATION

- Tenosynovitis of the flexor tendon always precedes the mechanical symptoms of triggering pain over the flexor tendon with palpation, passive stretching, or resisting flexion isometrically.
- A palpable tender nodule is noted at the metacarpophalangeal (MCP) joint of the affected digit.

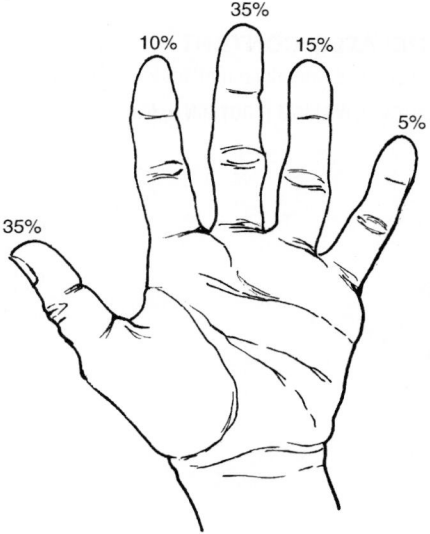

FIGURE 1-845 Trigger finger. Frequency of trigger finger according to digit in adults. In children, virtually all cases occur in the thumb. (From Canoso J: *Rheumatology in primary care,* Philadelphia, 1997, Saunders.)

- Painful triggering or snapping with flexion of the affected digit.
- Locking or loss of active digital extension.
- The digit can be fixed in flexion (trapped or incarcerated).
- Usually affects one digit. If more digits are involved, a systemic cause is most likely present (e.g., diabetes, rheumatoid arthritis).

ETIOLOGY

Trigger finger is described as being primary or secondary:
- Primary (idiopathic)
- Secondary
  - Diabetes
  - Rheumatoid arthritis
  - Hypothyroidism
  - Histiocytosis
  - Amyloidosis
  - Gout

DIAGNOSIS

Clinical history and physical examination

DIFFERENTIAL DIAGNOSIS

- Dupuytren's contracture
- De Quervain's tenosynovitis
- Acute digital tenosynovitis
- Proliferative tenosynovitis
- Ulnar collateral ligament injury (gamekeeper's thumb)
- Carpal tunnel syndrome
- Flexion tendon rupture
- MCP osteoarthritis

WORKUP

Pursued if a secondary cause is suspected

LABORATORY TESTS

- Complete blood count with differential
- Electrolytes, blood urea nitrogen, creatinine
- Blood glucose, Hb_{A1c}
- Thyroid function tests
- Rheumatoid factor/anti-CCP antibody
- Uric acid

IMAGING STUDIES

- Radiograph studies are not helpful unless a secondary cause has affected other organs (e.g., rheumatoid lung).

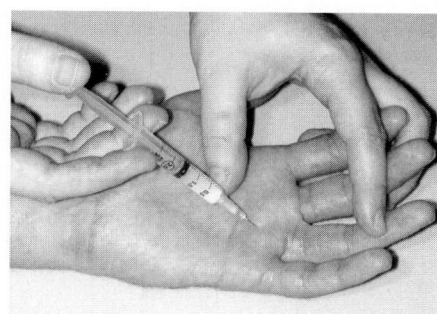

FIGURE 1-846 Injection into the palm for trigger finger. (From Carr A, Hamilton W: *Orthopedics in primary care,* ed 2, Philadelphia, 2005, Saunders.)

- Musculoskeletal ultrasonography (MSKUS) can be useful in characterizing the lesion and guiding treatment.

TREATMENT

The goals of treatment are to reduce swelling and inflammation in the flexor tendon sheath and allow smooth movement of the tendon under the A1 pulley of the MCP joint.

NONPHARMACOLOGIC THERAPY

- Splinting or buddy taping to the adjacent finger for 4 to 6 wk.
- Preventive measures include the use of gloves and damping tape to widen grips.
- Physiotherapy with stretching and heat.

ACUTE GENERAL Rx

- In idiopathic trigger finger, different steroid preparations with local anesthetics are used if patients have not responded to conservative treatment (Fig. 1-846).
- If symptoms do not resolve in 6 wk, a repeat injection can be tried.
- Pain control.

CHRONIC Rx

- Surgical release is indicated in patients with refractory symptoms (e.g., locked digits) despite nonpharmacologic and acute treatment.
- Surgery is also indicated in patients with recurrent symptoms despite two steroid injections.

DISPOSITION

- After steroid injection, symptoms usually resolve in 3 to 5 days, and locking resolves in 60% of the cases in 2 to 3 wk.
- If symptoms recur, a repeat steroid injection improves the symptoms in ≥80% of patients.
- Diabetic patients do not have the same success rate with steroid injections as the idiopathic group.

REFERRAL

If steroid injection therapy is considered, a rheumatology or hand surgery consult is requested.

PEARLS & CONSIDERATIONS

COMMENTS

If more than one digit is involved, a workup for a secondary systemic cause is in order.

SUGGESTED READINGS
available at www.expertconsult.com

RELATED CONTENT

Trigger Finger (Patient Information)

AUTHORS: **RYAN W. ZUZEK, M.D.,**
PAUL GORDON, M.D., and
DANIEL MENDEZ, M.D.

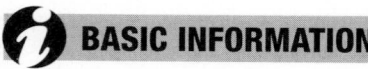 BASIC INFORMATION

DEFINITION

Trochanteric bursitis reflects inflammation or irritation of the bursa or bursae located at the insertion of the gluteal muscles at the greater trochanter of the femur (Fig. 1-847).

SYNONYMS

Greater trochanteric pain syndrome
Greater trochanteric bursitis

ICD-9CM CODES

726.5 Bursitis trochanteric area
726.5 Enthesopathy of hip region (Bursitis of hip, Trochanteric tendinitis)

EPIDEMIOLOGY & DEMOGRAPHICS

- Trochanteric bursitis can be associated with other conditions, including osteoarthritis of the hip, lumbar spinal degenerative joint disease, and rheumatoid arthritis.
- Incidence peaks between the fourth and sixth decades of life but can occur at any age group.
- Occurs in females more often than males (ratio of 4:1).
- Prevalence is 3200/100,000.

PHYSICAL FINDINGS & CLINICAL PRESENTATION

- Lateral hip pain is the most common symptom. The pain is chronic, intermittent, and located over the outer lateral hip and thigh.
- Pain is precipitated with prolonged lying or standing on the affected side.
- Walking, climbing, and running exacerbate the pain.
- Point tenderness over the greater trochanter is noted.
- Pain is reproduced with resisted hip abduction.

ETIOLOGY

- The specific cause of trochanteric bursitis is not known, although repetitive high-intensity use of the tensor fasciae and gluteus medius over the outer femur, trauma, infection (tuberculosis and bacterial), and crystal deposition can precipitate the disease.

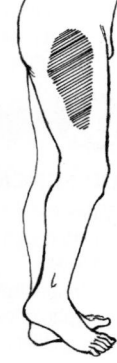

FIGURE 1-847 Typical location of pain in trochanteric bursitis syndrome. This is also a frequent pain radiation site for lumbar spine lesion, various nerve compression syndromes, and hip disease, particularly in osteonecrosis of the femoral head. (From Canoso JJ: *Rheumatology in primary care,* Philadelphia, 1997, Saunders.)

- Trochanteric bursitis can occur when other conditions such as osteoarthritis of the knee and hip, sacroiliac joint disorders, leg length discrepancy, ankle sprain, and bunions of the feet cause changes in the patient's gait, placing varus stress on the hip joint.

DX DIAGNOSIS

A detailed physical examination and clinical presentation usually make the diagnosis of trochanteric bursitis. X-ray images are helpful adjunctive studies used to exclude other conditions either associated with or mimicking trochanteric bursitis.

DIFFERENTIAL DIAGNOSIS

- Osteoarthritis of the hip
- Osteonecrosis of the hip
- Stress fracture of the hip
- Osteoarthritis of the lumbar spine
- Meralgia paresthetica
- Iliotibial band syndrome
- Fibromyalgia
- Iliopsoas bursitis
- Trochanteric tendonitis
- Trauma
- Osteomyelitis
- Tuberculosis of the greater trochanter
- Metastatic bone disease
- Septic arthritis

WORKUP

A workup is indicated if suspected associated conditions exist; otherwise treatment can be started on clinical grounds alone.

LABORATORY TESTS

Lab evaluation is generally not indicated in clear cases.

IMAGING STUDIES

- Standing anteroposterior pelvic x-rays and specific views of hip and back are used to evaluate associated symptoms such as leg length discrepancy, lumbar spondylosis, and sacroiliac joint diseases causing the bursitis. Sometimes calcifications may be seen around the greater trochanter in the areas of bursal development.
- Bone scan can be done but is usually not necessary.
- CT and MRI may show bursitis but are usually not warranted unless associated conditions are suspected, which would affect treatment decisions. MRI results would show increased signal in bursitis.

RX TREATMENT

NONPHARMACOLOGIC THERAPY

- Physical therapy and iliotibial band stretching exercises can reduce irritation of the trochanteric bursa area.
- Ultrasound therapy
- Rest

- Treat gait disturbance by knee brace, shoe lift, ankle supports, foot orthotics for the specific underlying conditions

ACUTE GENERAL Rx

- Nonsteroidal anti-inflammatory drugs (NSAIDs) for pain relief: ibuprofen 800 mg PO tid or naproxen 500 mg PO bid for the initial 4 wk
- Using ultrasound to enhance absorption of topical corticosteroids percutaneously (phonophoresis)
- Corticosteroid injection

CHRONIC Rx

Although rarely done, surgical removal of the bursa or with also lengthening of iliotibial band with bursectomy is possible for patients with refractory symptoms or infection.

DISPOSITION

- Most patients respond to NSAIDs and/or non-pharmacologic therapy.
- If steroid injection is used, approximately 70% of patients respond after the first injection and more than 90% respond to two injections.
- 25% of patients receiving steroid injection may develop a relapse.

REFERRAL

A rheumatology or orthopedics referral is made if steroid injection therapy is needed or if the etiology is believed to be infectious.

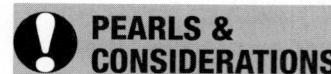 PEARLS & CONSIDERATIONS

Patients with trochanteric bursitis will commonly report "hip" pain. The physical examination readily distinguishes true hip pain from trochanteric bursitis. Relief of pain with local corticosteroid injection is helpful in differentiating pain of trochanteric bursitis from that of referred pain.

COMMENTS

- The absence of pain with flexion and extension differentiates trochanteric bursitis from degenerative joint disease of the hip.
- Localization of pain over the lateral hip and thigh differentiates trochanteric bursitis from pain caused by meralgia paresthetica located over the anterolateral thigh and pain from osteoarthritis located over the inner thigh groin area.

SUGGESTED READINGS

available at www.expertconsult.com

RELATED CONTENT

Trochanteric Bursitis (Patient Information)

AUTHORS: **SYEDA M. SAYEED, M.D.**

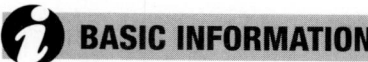

DEFINITION

Miliary tuberculosis (TB) is an infection of disseminated hematogenous disease, caused by the bacterium *Mycobacterium tuberculosis* (Mtb), and is often characterized as resembling millet seeds on pathologic or radiologic examination. Extrapulmonary disease may occur in virtually every organ site.

SYNONYMS

Disseminated TB

ICD-9CM CODES

018.94 Miliary tuberculosis

EPIDEMIOLOGY & DEMOGRAPHICS

INCIDENCE (IN U.S.): >38% of AIDS patients with TB have disseminated disease, often with concurrent pulmonary and extrapulmonary active sites. (See "Tuberculosis, Pulmonary" in Section I.)

PREVALENCE (IN U.S.):
- Undetermined
- Highest prevalence
  1. AIDS patients
  2. Minorities
  3. Children
  4. Foreign-born persons
  5. Elderly

PREDOMINANT SEX:
- No specific predilection
- Male predominance in AIDS, shelters, and prisons reflected in disproportionate male TB incidence

PREDOMINANT AGE: Predominantly among 24- to 45-yr-olds

PEAK INCIDENCE: HIV-positive patients, regardless of age

PHYSICAL FINDINGS & CLINICAL PRESENTATION

- See also "Etiology"
- Common symptoms
  1. High intermittent fever (93%)
  2. Night sweats (79%)
  3. Weight loss (85%)
  4. Dyspnea (64%)
  5. Cough (82%)
- Symptoms referable to individual organ systems may predominate
  1. Meninges
  2. Pericardium
  3. Liver
  4. Kidney
  5. Bone
  6. GI tract
  7. Lymph nodes
  8. Serous spaces
     a. Pleural
     b. Pericardial
     c. Peritoneal
     d. Joint
  9. Skin
  10. Lung: cough, shortness of breath
- Adrenal insufficiency possible, caused by infection of adrenal gland

- Pancytopenia
  1. With fever and weight loss *or*
  2. Without other localizing symptoms or signs *or*
  3. With only splenomegaly
- TB hepatitis
  1. Tender liver
  2. Obstructive enzymes (alkaline phosphatase) elevated out of proportion to minimal hepatocellular enzymes (SGOT, SGPT) and bilirubin
- TB meningitis
  1. Gradual-onset headache
  2. Minimal meningeal signs
  3. Malaise
  4. Low-grade fever (may be absent)
  5. Sudden stupor or coma
  6. Cranial nerve VI palsy
- TB pericarditis
  1. Effusions resembling TB pleurisy
  2. Cardiac tamponade
- Skeletal TB
  1. Large joint arthritis (with effusions resembling TB pericarditis)
  2. Bone lesions (especially ribs)
  3. Pott's disease
     a. TB spondylitis, especially of lower thoracic spine
     b. Paraspinous TB abscess
     c. Possible psoas abscess
     d. Frequent cord compression (often relieved by steroids)
- Genitourinary TB
  1. Renal TB
     a. Papillary necrosis
     b. Destruction of renal pelvis
     c. Strictures of upper third of ureters
     d. Hematuria
     e. Pyuria with misleading bacterial cultures
     f. Preserved renal function
  2. TB orchitis or epididymitis
     a. Scrotal mass
     b. Draining abscess
  3. Chronic prostatic TB
- GI TB
  1. Diarrhea
  2. Pain
  3. Obstruction
  4. Bleeding
  5. Especially common with AIDS
  6. Bowel lesions
     a. Circumferential ulcers
     b. Short strictures
     c. Calcified granulomas
     d. TB mesenteric caseous adenitis
     e. Abscess, but rare fistula formation
     f. Often difficult to distinguish from granulomatous bowel disease (Crohn's disease)
- TB peritonitis
  1. Fluid resembles TB pleurisy
  2. PPD often negative
  3. Tender abdomen
  4. Doughy peritoneal consistency, often with ascites
  5. Peritoneal biopsy indicated for diagnosis
- TB lymphadenitis (scrofula)
  1. May involve all node groups

  2. Common adenopathies
     a. Cervical
     b. Supraclavicular
     c. Axillary
     d. Retroperitoneal
  3. Biopsy generally needed for diagnosis
  4. Surgical resection of nodes may be necessary
  5. Especially common with AIDS
- Cutaneous TB
  1. Skin infection from autoinoculation or dissemination
  2. Nodules or abscesses
  3. Tuberculids (possibly allergic reactions)
  4. Erythema nodosum
- Miscellaneous presentations
  1. TB laryngitis
  2. TB otitis
  3. Ocular TB
     a. Choroidal tubercles
     b. Iritis
     c. Uveitis
     d. Episcleritis
  4. Adrenal TB
  5. Breast TB

ETIOLOGY

- See also "Pulmonary Tuberculosis" in Section I.
- Mtb, a slow-growing, aerobic, non–spore forming, nonmotile acid-fast bacillus
- Humans are the only reservoir for Mtb.
- Pathogenesis:
  1. Acid-fast bacilli (AFB) (Mtb) are ingested by macrophages in alveoli, then transported to regional lymph nodes where spread is contained.
  2. Some AFB reach the bloodstream and disseminate widely.
  3. Immediate active disseminated disease may ensue or a latent period may develop.
  4. During latent period, T-cell immune mechanisms contain infection in granulomas until later reactivation occurs as a result of immunosuppression or other undefined factors in conjunction with reactivated pulmonary TB or alone.
- Miliary TB may occur as a consequence of the following:
  1. Primary infection: inability to contain primary infection leads to a hematogenous spread and progressive disseminated disease.
  2. In late chronic TB and in those with advanced age or poor immunity, a continuous seeding of the blood may develop and lead to disseminated disease.

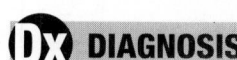 **DIAGNOSIS**

DIFFERENTIAL DIAGNOSIS

Widespread sites of possible dissemination associated with myriad differential diagnostic possibilities:
- Lymphoma
- Typhoid fever
- Brucellosis

- Other tumors
- Collagen-vascular disease

WORKUP

- Prompt evaluation is essential
- Sputum for AFB stain and culture and chest x-ray
- High-resolution CT is more sensitive for miliary TB than CXR
- PPD, which may be negative in immunocompromised patients
- Fluid analysis and mycobacterial culture wherever available
  1. Sputum
  2. Blood: particularly helpful in patients with AIDS
  3. Urine
  4. CSF
  5. Pleural
  6. Pericardial
  7. Peritoneal
  8. Gastric aspirates
- Biopsy of any involved tissue is advisable to make immediate diagnosis
  1. Transbronchial biopsy preferred and easily accessible
  2. Bone marrow
  3. Lymph node
  4. Scrotal mass if present
  5. Any other involved site
  6. Positive granuloma or AFB on biopsy specimen is diagnostic
- Imaging studies as needed

LABORATORY TESTS

- Culture and fluid analysis as described previously

- Smear-negative sputum often is positive weeks later on culture
- CBC is usually normal
- ESR is usually elevated

IMAGING STUDIES

- Chest x-ray examination (may or may not be positive) (see "Tuberculosis, Pulmonary" in Section I)
- CT scan or MRI of brain and spinal cord (Fig. 1-848)
  1. Tuberculoma
  2. Basilar arachnoiditis
- Barium studies of bowel

 TREATMENT

NONPHARMACOLOGIC THERAPY

- Bed rest during acute phase of treatment
- High-calorie, high-protein diet to reverse malnutrition and enhance immune response to TB
- Isolation in negative-pressure rooms with high-volume air replacement and circulation (with health care provider wearing proper protective 0.5- to 1-micron filter respirators)
  1. Until three consecutive sputum AFB smears are negative, if pulmonary disease coexists
  2. Isolation not required for closed-space TB infections

ACUTE GENERAL Rx

- See "Tuberculosis, Pulmonary" in Section I.
- Therapy should be initiated immediately. Do not wait for definitive diagnosis.
- More rapid response to chemotherapy by disseminated TB foci than cavitary pulmonary TB.
- Treatment for 6 mo with INH plus rifampin plus PZA.
  1. Treatment for 12 mo often required for bone and renal TB.

2. Prolonged treatment often required for CNS and pericardial.
3. Prolonged treatment often required for all disseminated TB in infants.
- Compliance (rigid adherence to treatment regimen) is the chief determinant of success.
  1. Supervised directly observed therapy (DOT) is recommended for all patients.
  2. Supervised DOT is mandatory for unreliable patients.
- Steroids are often helpful additions in fulminant miliary disease with the hypoxemia and DIC.

CHRONIC Rx

- Generally not indicated beyond treatment described previously
- Prolonged treatment supervised by infectious disease expert required in a few complicated infections caused by resistant organisms

DISPOSITION

- Monthly follow-up by physician experienced in TB treatment
- Confirm sensitivity testing, and alter treatment appropriately (see "Tuberculosis, Pulmonary" in Section I)

REFERRAL

- To infectious disease expert for:
  1. HIV-positive patient
  2. Patient with suspected drug-resistant TB
  3. Patient previously treated for TB
  4. Patient whose fever has not decreased and sputum (if positive) has not converted to negative in 2 to 4 wk
  5. Patients with overwhelming pulmonary or extrapulmonary TB
- To pulmonary, orthopedic, or GI physicians for examinations or biopsy

❗ PEARLS & CONSIDERATIONS

COMMENTS

- Consider acute TB in critically ill patients with enigmatic acute respiratory distress syndrome, shock, or DIC.
- All contacts (especially close household contacts and infants) should be properly tested for PPD conversions >3 mo following exposure.
- Those with positive PPD should be evaluated for active TB and properly treated or given prophylaxis.

SUGGESTED READINGS

available at www.expertconsult.com

AUTHORS: **GLENN G. FORT, M.D., M.P.H.**

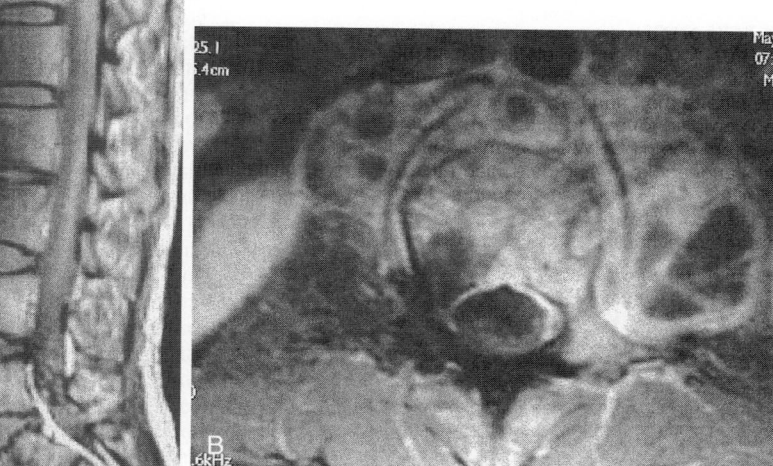

FIGURE 1-848 A and B, Magnetic resonance MR images of tuberculous spinal osteomyelitis with scalloping of the vertebrae (tuberculous caries) and paraspinal "cold" abscesses. (From Grainger RG, Allison D: *Grainger & Allison's diagnostic radiology, a textbook of medical imaging,* ed 4, London, 2001, Churchill Livingstone.)

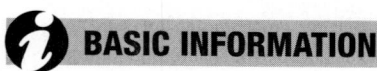

BASIC INFORMATION

DEFINITION

Pulmonary tuberculosis (TB) is an infection of the lung and, occasionally, surrounding structures, caused by the bacterium *Mycobacterium tuberculosis* (Mtb). Multidrug-resistant (MDR) TB is defined as disease caused by strains of Mtb that are at least resistant to treatment with isoniazid and rifampin; extensively drug-resistant (XDR) TB refers to disease caused by MDR strains that are also resistant to treatment with any fluoroquinolone and any of the injectable drugs used in the treatment of second-line anti-TB drugs.

SYNONYMS

TB

ICD-9CM CODES

011.9 Pulmonary tuberculosis

EPIDEMIOLOGY & DEMOGRAPHICS

INCIDENCE (WORLDWIDE):

In 2011 there were:

- 8.7 million new cases of active tuberculosis; 13% involved coinfection with HIV
- 1.4 million deaths from TB, including 430,000 among HIV-infected patients 310,000 incident cases of multidrug-resistant TB
- Sub-Saharan Africa has the highest rates of active TB per capita.
- Absolute number of cases is highest in Asia, with India and China having the greatest burden of disease globally.

INCIDENCE (IN U.S.):

- In 2010, there were 11,181 cases of TB in the U.S. for a rate of 3.6 cases/100,000 persons—the lowest reported rate since recording began in 1953.
- >90% of new cases each yr from reactivated prior infections
- 9% newly infected
- Only 10% of patients with purified protein derivative (PPD) conversions (higher [8%/yr] in HIV-positive patients) will develop TB, most within 1 to 2 yr
- Two thirds of all new cases in racial and ethnic minorities
- 80% of new cases in children in racial and ethnic minorities
- Occurs most frequently in geographic areas and among populations with highest AIDS prevalence
  1. Urban blacks and Hispanics between 25 and 45 yr old
  2. Poor, crowded urban communities
- Nearly 36% of new cases from new immigrants
- In 2008 in the U.S., 8.2% of cases were MDR TB.

PREVALENCE (IN U.S.):

- Estimated 10 million people infected
- Varies widely among population groups

PREDOMINANT SEX:

- No specific predilection
- Male predominance in AIDS, shelters, and prisons reflected in disproportionate male incidence

PREDOMINANT AGE:

- 24 to 45 yr old
- Childhood cases common among minorities
- Nursing home outbreaks among elderly

PEAK INCIDENCE:

- Infancy
- Teenage years
- Pregnancy
- Elderly
- HIV-positive patients, regardless of age, at highest risk

GENETICS:

- Populations with widespread low native resistance have been intensely infected when initially exposed to TB.
- Following elimination of those with least native resistance, incidence and prevalence of TB tend to decline.

PHYSICAL FINDINGS & CLINICAL PRESENTATION

- See "Etiology"
- Primary pulmonary TB infection generally asymptomatic
- Reactivation pulmonary TB
  1. Fever
  2. Night sweats
  3. Cough
  4. Hemoptysis
  5. Scanty nonpurulent sputum
  6. Weight loss
- Progressive primary pulmonary TB disease: same as reactivation pulmonary TB
- TB pleurisy
  1. Pleuritic chest pain
  2. Fever
  3. Shortness of breath
- Rare massive, suffocating, fatal hemoptysis secondary to erosion of pulmonary artery within a cavity (Rasmussen's aneurysm)
- Chest examination
  1. Not specific
  2. Usually underestimates extent of disease
  3. Rales accentuated following a cough (posttussive rales)

ETIOLOGY

- Mtb, a slow-growing, aerobic, non-sporeforming, nonmotile bacillus, with a lipid-rich cell wall:
  1. Lacks pigment
  2. Produces niacin
  3. Reduces nitrate
  4. Produces heat-labile catalase
  5. Mtb staining, acid-fast and acid-alcohol fast by Ziehl-Neelsen method, appearing as red, slightly bent, beaded rods 2 to 4 microns long (acid-fast bacilli [AFB]), against a blue background
  6. Polymerase chain reaction (PCR) to detect <10 organisms/ml in sputum (compared with the requisite 10,000 organisms/ml for AFB smear detection)
  7. Culture
     a. Growth on solid media (Löwenstein-Jensen; Middlebrook 7H11) in 2 to 6 wk
     b. Growth in liquid media (BACTEC, using a radioactive carbon source for early growth detection) often in 9 to 16 days

  c. Enhanced in a 5% to 10% carbon dioxide atmosphere
  8. DNA fingerprinting (based on restriction fragment length polymorphism [RFLP])
     a. Facilitates immediate identification of Mtb strains in early growing cultures
     b. False negatives possible if growth suboptimal
  9. Humans are the only reservoir for Mtb
  10. Transmission
      a. Facilitated by close exposure to high-velocity cough (unprotected by proper mask or respirators) from patient with AFB-positive sputum and cavitary lesions, producing aerosolized droplets containing AFB, which are inhaled directly into alveoli
      b. Occurs within prisons, nursing homes, and hospitals
- Pathogenesis
  1. AFB (Mtb) ingested by macrophages in alveoli, then transported to regional lymph nodes, where spread is contained
  2. Some AFB may reach bloodstream and disseminate widely
  3. Primary TB (asymptomatic, minimal pneumonitis in lower or midlung fields, with hilar lymphadenopathy) essentially an intracellular infection, with multiplication of organisms continuing for 2 to 12 wk after primary exposure, until cell-mediated hypersensitivity (detected by positive skin test reaction to tuberculin PPD) matures, with subsequent containment of infection
  4. Local and disseminated AFB thus contained by T-cell-mediated immune responses
     a. Recruitment of monocytes
     b. Transformation of lymphocytes with secretion of lymphokines
     c. Activation of macrophages and histiocytes
     d. Organization into granulomas, where organisms may survive within macrophages (Langhans' giant cells), but within which multiplication essentially ceases (95%) and from which spread is prohibited
  5. Progressive primary pulmonary disease
     a. May immediately follow the asymptomatic phase
     b. Necrotizing pulmonary infiltrates
     c. Tuberculous bronchopneumonia
     d. Endobronchial TB
     e. Interstitial TB
     f. Widespread miliary lung lesions
  6. Postprimary TB pleurisy with pleural effusion
     a. Develops after early primary infection, although often before conversion to positive PPD
     b. Results from pleural seeding from a peripheral lung lesion or rupture of lymph node into pleural space
     c. May produce a large (sometimes hemorrhagic) exudative effusion (with polymorphonuclear cells early, rapidly

replaced by lymphocytes), frequently without pulmonary infiltrates
   d. Generally resolves without treatment
   e. Portends a high risk of subsequent clinical disease, and therefore must be diagnosed and treated early (pleural biopsy and culture) to prevent future catastrophic TB illness
   f. May result in disseminated extrapulmonary infection
7. Reactivation pulmonary TB
   a. Occurs months to years following primary TB
   b. Preferentially involves the apical posterior segments of the upper lobes and superior segments of the lower lobes
   c. Associated with necrosis and cavitation of involved lung, hemoptysis, chronic fever, night sweats, weight loss
   d. Spread within lung occurs via cough and inhalation
8. Reinfection TB
   a. May mimic reactivation TB
   b. Ruptured caseous foci and cavities, which may produce endobronchial spread
9. Mtb in both progressive primary and reactivation pulmonary TB
   a. Intracellular (macrophage) lesions (undergoing slow multiplication)
   b. Closed caseous lesions (undergoing slow multiplication)
   c. Extracellular, open cavities (undergoing rapid multiplication)
   d. INH and rifampin are cidal in all three sites
   e. Pyrazinamide (PZA) especially active within acidic macrophage environment
   f. Extrapulmonary reactivation disease also possible
10. Rapid local progression and dissemination in infants with devastating illness before PPD conversion occurs
11. Most symptoms (fever, weight loss, anorexia) and tissue destruction (caseous necrosis) from cytokines and cell-mediated immune responses
12. Mtb has no important endotoxins or exotoxins
13. Granuloma formation related to tumor necrosis factor (TNF) secreted by activated macrophages

Dx DIAGNOSIS

DIFFERENTIAL DIAGNOSIS

- Necrotizing pneumonia (anaerobic, gram-negative)
- Histoplasmosis
- Coccidioidomycosis
- Melioidosis
- Interstitial lung diseases (rarely)
- Cancer
- Sarcoidosis
- Silicosis
- Rare pneumonias

1. *Rhodococcus equi* (cavitation)
2. *Bacillus cereus* (50% hemoptysis)
3. *Eikenella corrodens* (cavitation)

WORKUP

- Sputum for AFB stains
- Chest x-ray (Fig. 1-849)
- PPD (tuberculin skin test [TST])
   1. Recent conversion from negative to positive within 3 mo of exposure is highly suggestive of recent infection.
   2. Single positive PPD is not helpful diagnostically.
   3. Negative PPD never rules out acute TB.
   4. Be certain that positive PPD does not reflect "booster phenomenon" (prior positive PPD may become negative after several yr and return to positive only after second repeated PPD; repeat second PPD within 1 wk), which thus may mimic skin test conversion.
   5. Positive PPD reaction is determined as follows:
      a. Induration after 72 hr of intradermal injection of 0.1 ml of 5 TU-PPD
      b. 5-mm induration if HIV-positive (or other severe immunosuppressed state affecting cellular immune function), close contact of active TB, fibrotic chest lesions
      c. 10-mm induration if in high–medical risk groups (immunosuppressive disease or therapy, renal failure, gastrectomy, silicosis, diabetes), foreign-born high-risk group (Southeast Asia, Latin America, Africa, India), low socioeconomic groups, IV drug addict, prisoner, healthcare worker
      d. 15-mm induration if low risk

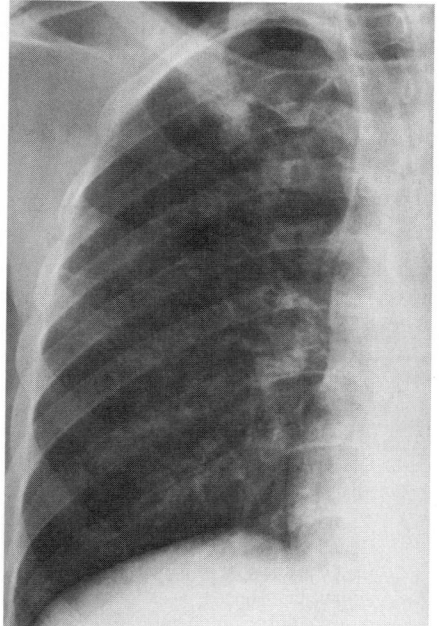

FIGURE 1-849 Miliary pattern in tuberculosis consists of numerous nodules of uniform size. (From Grainger RG et al [eds]: *Grainger & Allison's diagnostic radiology*, ed 4, Philadelphia, 2001, Churchill Livingstone.)

6. Anergy antigen testing (using mumps, *Candida*, tetanus toxoid) may identify patients who are truly anergic to PPD and these antigens, but results are often confusing. Not recommended.
7. Patients with TB may be selectively anergic only to PPD.
8. Positive PPD indicates prior infection but does not itself confirm active disease.
- Interferon gamma release assays (IGRAs): diagnostic test for latent TB infection, known as the quantaferon test (QFT-G). This is a blood test that measures interferon response to specific Mtb antigens. The test is FDA approved and is available in some large TB centers and state health departments. It may assist in distinguishing true positive reactions, from individuals with latent TB, from PPD reactions related to nontuberculous mycobacteria; prior BCG vaccination; or difficult-to-interpret skin test results from people with dermatologic conditions or immediate allergic reactions to PPD. The diagnostic utility of the test as a replacement or supplement to the standard PPD is not yet fully determined. When IGRA is used for routine screening, positive results should be repeated routinely due to a high rate of false-positive results. The enzyme-linked immunospot assay (Elispot plus) incorporating a novel antigen, RV3879c, when used in combination with tuberculin testing, has been reported to enable rapid exclusion of active infection in patients with moderate to high pretest probability of TB. Other IGRAs now available for detection of TB using blood include QFT-GIT and T-spot.
- The Xpert MTB/RIF is an automated molecular test for *Mycobacterium tuberculosis* (MTB) and resistance to rifampin (RIF) that provides sensitive detection of TB and rifampin resistance directly from untreated sputum in less than 2 hr with minimal hands-on time.

LABORATORY TESTS

- Sputum for AFB stains and culture
   1. Induced sputum if patient not coughing productively
- Sputum from bronchoscopy if high suspicion of TB with negative expectorated induced sputum for AFB
   1. Positive AFB smear is essential before or shortly after treatment to ensure subsequent growth for definitive diagnosis and sensitivity testing
   2. Consider lung biopsy if sputum negative, especially if infiltrates are predominantly interstitial
- AFB stain-negative sputum may grow Mtb subsequently
- Gastric aspirates reliable, especially in HIV-negative patients
- CBC
   1. Variable values
      a. WBCs: low, normal, or elevated (including leukemoid reaction: >50,000)
      b. Normocytic, normochromic anemia often
   2. Rarely helpful diagnostically
- ESR usually elevated
- Thoracentesis

1. Exudative effusion
   a. Elevated protein
   b. Decreased glucose
   c. Elevated WBCs (polymorphonuclear leukocytes early, replaced later by lymphocytes)
   d. May be hemorrhagic
2. Pleural fluid usually AFB-negative
3. Pleural biopsy often diagnostic—may need to be repeated for diagnosis
4. Culture pleural biopsy tissue for AFB
- Bone marrow biopsy is often diagnostic in difficult-to-diagnose cases, especially miliary TB

IMAGING STUDIES

- Chest radiograph
  1. Primary infection reflected by calcified peripheral lung nodule with calcified hilar lymph node
  2. Reactivation pulmonary TB
     a. Necrosis
     b. Cavitation (especially on apical lordotic views)
     c. Fibrosis and hilar retraction
     d. Bronchopneumonia
     e. Interstitial infiltrates
     f. Miliary pattern
     g. Many of previous findings may also accompany progressive primary TB
  3. TB pleurisy
     a. Pleural effusion, often rapidly accumulating and massive
  4. TB activity not established by single chest x-ray examination
  5. Serial chest x-ray examinations are excellent indicators of progression or regression

Rx TREATMENT

NONPHARMACOLOGIC THERAPY

- Increased rest during acute phase of treatment
- High-calorie, high-protein diet to reverse malnutrition and enhance immune response to TB
- Isolation in negative-pressure rooms with high-volume air replacement and circulation, with health care provider wearing proper protective 0.5- to 1-micron filter respirators, until three consecutive sputum AFB smears are negative

ACUTE GENERAL Rx

- Compliance (rigid adherence to treatment regimen) chief determinant of success.
  1. Supervised directly observed therapy (DOT) recommended for all patients and mandatory for unreliable patients
- Preferred adult regimen: DOT.
  1. Isoniazid (INH) 15 mg/kg (max 900 mg), rifampin 600 mg, ethambutol (EMB) 30 mg/kg (max 2500 mg), and pyrazinamide (PZA) (2 g [<50 kg]; 2.5 g [51 to 74 kg]; 3 g [>75 kg]) thrice weekly for 6 mo
  2. Alternative, more complicated DOT regimens
- Rifapentine, a rifampin derivative with a much longer serum half-life, was shown to be as effective when administered weekly

(with weekly isoniazid) as conventional regimens for drug-sensitive pulmonary TB in non–HIV-infected patients.
- Short-course daily therapy: adult.
  1. HIV-negative patient: 6 mo total therapy (2 mo INH 300 mg, rifampin 600 mg, and EMB 15 mg/kg [max 2500 mg]) and PZA (1.5 g [<50 kg]; 2 g [51 to 74 kg]; 2.5 g [>75 kg]) daily and until smear negative and sensitivity confirmed; then INH and rifampin daily for 4 mo
  2. HIV-positive patient: 9 mo total therapy (2 mo INH, rifampin, EMB, and PZA daily until smear negative and sensitivity confirmed; then INH and rifampin qid for 7 mo)
  3. Continue treatment at least 3 mo following conversion to negative cultures
- Drug resistance (often multiple drug resistance TB [MDRTB]) increased by:
  1. Prior treatment
  2. Acquisition of TB in developing countries
  3. Homelessness, incarceration
  4. AIDS, IVDA
  5. Known contact with MDRTB
- Never add single drug to failing regimen.
- Never treat TB with fewer than two to three drugs or two to three new additional drugs.
- Other medications used in MDR or XDRTB include: moxifloxacin, cycloserine, aminoglycosides such as amikacin or kanamycin, clarithromycin, PAS, and ethionamide.
- Monitor for clinical toxicity (especially hepatitis).
  1. Patient and physician awareness that anorexia, nausea, right upper quadrant pain, and unexplained malaise require immediate cessation of treatment
  2. Evaluation of liver function testing
     a. Minimal SGOT/SGPT elevations without symptoms generally transient and not clinically significant
- Preventive treatment for PPD conversion only (infection without disease).
  1. Must be certain that chest x-ray examination is negative and patient has no symptoms of TB
  2. Most important groups:
     a. HIV-positive and other severely immunocompromised patients
     b. Close contact with active TB
     c. Recent converter
     d. Old TB on chest x-ray examination
     e. IV drug addict
     f. Medical risk factor
     g. High-risk foreign country
     h. Homeless
  3. The traditional preventive therapy for persons with latent M. tuberculosis consists of INH 300 mg daily for 9 to 12 mo; at least 12 mo if HIV-positive patient. The CDC has issued recommendations for a new regimen consisting of isoniazid and rifapentine administered once a week for 12 weeks as directly observed therapy. Studies have demonstrated that this regimen is as effective as 9 months of isoniazid therapy for preventing tuberculosis. Patients who should not receive this regimen include children younger than 2 years, persons

with HIV infection taking antiretroviral therapy, pregnant women or those who may become pregnant during the course of treatment, and patients who have latent M. tuberculosis infection that is presumed to be resistant to isoniazid or rifampin.
- Infants generally given prophylaxis immediately if recent contact with active TB (even if infant PPD negative), then retested with PPD in 3 mo (continuing INH if PPD becomes positive and stopping INH if PPD remains negative).
- Chronic, stable PPD (several yr) given INH prophylaxis generally only if patient is <35 yr old.
  1. INH toxicity may outweigh benefit
  2. Individualize decision
- Preventive therapy for suspected INH-resistant organisms is unclear.

CHRONIC Rx

- Generally not indicated beyond treatment described previously
- Prolonged treatment, supervised by infectious disease expert, in a few very complicated infections caused by resistant organisms

DISPOSITION

- Monthly follow-up by physician experienced in TB treatment
- Confirm sensitivity testing and alter treatment appropriately
- Frequent sputum samples until culture is negative
- Confirm chest x-ray regression at 2 to 3 mo

REFERRAL

- To infectious disease expert for:
  1. HIV-positive patient
  2. Patient with suspected drug-resistant TB
  3. Patients previously treated for TB
  4. Patients whose fever has not decreased and sputum has not converted to negative in 2 to 4 wk
  5. Patients with overwhelming pulmonary or extrapulmonary TB
- To pulmonologist for bronchoscopy or pleural biopsy

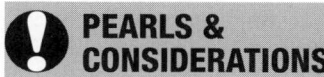

PEARLS & CONSIDERATIONS

COMMENTS

- All contacts (especially close household contacts and infants) should be properly tested for PPD conversions during 3 mo following exposure.
- Those with positive PPD should be evaluated for active TB and properly treated or given prophylaxis.
- Previous treatment is a common risk factor for XDR and MDR TB.

SUGGESTED READINGS

available at www.expertconsult.com

RELATED CONTENT

Tuberculosis (TB) (Patient Information)

AUTHOR: **GLENN G. FORT, M.D., M.P.H.**

BASIC INFORMATION

DEFINITION

Acute tubular necrosis (ATN) refers to damage caused by hypoperfusion or direct toxic injury to renal parenchymal cells, particularly tubular epithelial cells, that results in an acute decrease in renal function.

SYNONYMS

ATN
Acute tubular injury
Ischemic or nephrotoxic acute renal failure (ARF)

ICD-9CM CODES	
586	Renal failure, unspecified
584.5	Acute renal failure with lesion of tubular necrosis
997.5	Urinary complications

EPIDEMIOLOGY & DEMOGRAPHICS

- Most common cause of intrinsic renal failure among hospitalized patients, especially on surgical services in patients undergoing major cardiovascular surgery or in intensive care units in patients suffering severe trauma, hemorrhage, sepsis, or volume depletion.
- Hospital-acquired ARF is often caused by more than one insult.
- Early identification is important because causes are often reversible.

PHYSICAL FINDINGS & CLINICAL PRESENTATION

No apparent physical findings. Clinical features include recent hemorrhage, hypotension, or surgery, thereby suggesting ischemic ARF. Recent radiocontrast study, nephrotoxic drugs, history suggestive of rhabdomyolysis, hemolysis, or myeloma may suggest toxin-mediated ARF.

- The classic progression of ATN includes three phases, but can be highly variable:
  1. Initiation phase (hours to days)—renal hypoperfusion, evolving ischemia. Acute decrease in GFR (glomerular filtration rate), sudden can rise in BUN and serum creatinine, and decrease in urine output.
  2. Maintenance phase (1 to 2 wk)—renal cell injury established, GFR stabilizes at its nadir (5 to 10 ml/min), urine output at its lowest (usually 40 to 400 cc/day), and complications can arise such as hyperkalemia, metabolic acidosis, uremia, and salt and water overload. Some patients have nonoliguric ATN, where urine output does not decrease, which usually signifies a more benign course.
  3. Recovery phase (>2 wk)—renal parenchymal cell repair and regeneration, gradual return of GFR to premorbid levels; may be complicated by a marked diuretic phase due to excretion of retained salt and water and other solutes, or delayed recovery of epithelial cell function (solute and water reabsorption) relative to glomerular filtration.

PATHOLOGIC FINDINGS

- Ischemic ARF—patchy and focal necrosis of tubule epithelium with detachment from its basement membrane and occlusion of tubule lumens with casts composed of epithelial cells, cellular debris, Tamm-Horsfall mucoprotein (represents the matrix of all urinary casts), and pigments. Also present is leukocyte accumulation in vasa recta (capillaries that return the NaCl and water reabsorbed in the loop of Henle and medullary collecting tubule to the systemic circulation). Morphology of glomeruli and renal vasculature remain normal. Necrosis most severe in pars recta (straight portion of proximal tubule and thick ascending limb of loop of Henle).
- Nephrotoxic ARF-morphologic changes in convoluted and straight portion of proximal tubule. Tubule cell necrosis less pronounced than in ischemic ARF.

ETIOLOGY

- Ischemia from any cause, including hypotension or shock, prolonged prerenal azotemia, and postoperative sepsis syndrome. Hypoperfusion may occur without clinically apparent hypotension, so ischemic ARF should be considered even in patients who have had normal blood pressures.
- Medications: NSAIDs, antimicrobial drugs (acyclovir, foscarnet, aminoglycosides, amphotericin B, pentamidine, cephalosporins), calcineurin inhibitors, cisplatin, ifosfamide, thiazides, anesthetics
- Radiocontrast (contrast nephropathy)
- Hemoglobin and myoglobin (rhabdomyolysis, transfusion reactions)
- Heavy metals
- Crystals (urate, oxalate, acute phosphate nephropathy)
- Hypercalcemia
- Immunoglobulin light chain disease (amyloidosis, multiple myeloma, MGUS)

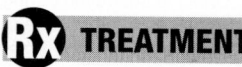

DIAGNOSIS

DIFFERENTIAL DIAGNOSIS

Allergic interstitial nephritis, acute bilateral pyelonephritis

LABORATORY TESTS

- Urinalysis for specific gravity (SG), U_{Na}, P_{Cr}, P_{Na}, U_{Cr}.
- Urine microscopic analysis.
- Calculate fractional excretion of sodium $(FE_{Na}) = [(U_{Na} \times P_{Cr}) / (P_{Na} \times U_{Cr})] \times 100$.
- Trial of fluid repletion can distinguish prerenal azotemia from ATN. Improvement in urine output and renal function with intravenous fluids suggests prerenal disease.
- Potential biomarkers for early diagnosis of ATN are currently under investigation.

LABORATORY FINDINGS

- $FE_{Na} > 1\%$
- $U_{Na} > 20$ mmol/L
- Urinalysis: "muddy brown" granular and epithelial cell casts
- SG < 1.015

IMAGING STUDIES

Not necessary

TREATMENT

ACUTE GENERAL Rx

Should focus on providing etiology-specific supportive care or correction of primary hemodynamic abnormality. Peritoneal or hemodialysis for replacement of renal function may be necessary until regeneration and repair restore renal function. Diuretic use is not recommended.

DISPOSITION

Recovery typically takes 1 to 2 wk after normalization of renal perfusion as it requires repair and regeneration of renal cells. Prognosis depends heavily on clinical context, but patients who do not have complications or underlying illness can have a 95% chance of recovery. However, with sepsis or multiorgan failure mortality can be more than 50%.

REFERRAL

Renal consultation for severe cases of ATN requiring dialysis

PEARLS & CONSIDERATIONS

COMMENTS

Prevention is paramount.

PREVENTION

- Aggressive restoration of intravascular volume in surgical/trauma patients to prevent ischemic ARF.
- Tailoring dosage of potential nephrotoxins to body size and GFR to limit renal injury.
- Low-volume contrast, pre-study intravenous fluids, and acetylcysteine (600 mg PO bid × 2 days or 600 to 1200 mg IV bid) may help prevent contrast-induced nephropathy.

SUGGESTED READINGS
available at www.expertconsult.com

RELATED CONTENT

Acute Kidney Injury (Related Key Topic)

AUTHOR: **ELIZABETH BROWN, M.D.**

BASIC INFORMATION

DEFINITION

- Tumor lysis syndrome is a constellation of metabolic derangements that can occur after starting cancer treatment.
- It usually occurs in patients with bulky, rapidly proliferating, and treatment-responsive tumors.
- It is associated with acute leukemias, high-grade non-Hodgkin's lymphoma, solid tumors, and hematologic cancers.
- Tumor lysis syndrome occurs when large numbers of cancer cells are destroyed during cancer treatment. The result is the release of large amounts of intracellular ions and other metabolic products into the blood. This leads to:
  - Hyperkalemia
  - Hypocalcemia
  - Hyperphosphatemia
  - Hyperuricemia
  - Acute renal failure

ICD-9CM CODES
277.88   Other specified disorders of metabolism

EPIDEMIOLOGY & DEMOGRAPHICS
INCIDENCE: Unknown
PREVALENCE:
- Varies
- Increased frequency is associated with bulky, aggressive, and treatment-sensitive tumors.

PREDOMINANT SEX AND AGE:
- No sex predilection exists.
- Occurs in all age groups. The elderly are more susceptible because of impaired renal function with age.

GENETICS: No known racial predilection
RISK FACTORS: Risk factors for developing tumor lysis syndrome include:
- Large tumor burden, as in:
  - Acute leukemias with elevated WBC count
  - Large, bulky, rapidly proliferating solid tumors
  - High-grade lymphomas
- Tumors sensitive to treatment
- Elevated pretreatment lactate dehydrogenase (LDH)
- Baseline renal insufficiency
- Older patients (due to these patients having a lower glomerular filtration rate)

PHYSICAL FINDINGS & CLINICAL PRESENTATION

CLINICAL PRESENTATION
Patients may present with a number of symptoms either before starting chemotherapy or commonly within 3 days after initiating cytotoxic treatment. Common symptoms include:
- Nausea
- Vomiting
- Edema
- Shortness of breath (from fluid overload or CHF)
- Lethargy/weakness
- Seizure
- Syncope
- Muscle cramps
- Tetany

PHYSICAL FINDINGS
Physical findings usually reflect the effects of specific metabolic derangement. Patients with tumor lysis syndrome present with hyperkalemia, hyperuremia, hypocalcemia, and hyperphosphatemia.
- Hyperkalemia causes:
  - Weakness
  - Paresthesia
  - Paralysis
  - ECG changes
  - Cardiac arrhythmias
  - Cardiac arrest
- Hyperuremia:
  - Weakness
  - Malaise
  - Vomiting
  - Pruritus
  - Restless legs
  - Ecchymoses
  - Hiccups
  - Paresthesia
  - Pericarditis
  - Dyspnea
  - Hypertension
- Hypocalcemia:
  - Paresthesia
  - Tetany
  - Bronchospasm
  - Heart block
  - Muscle twitching
- Hyperphosphatemia:
  - Oliguria
  - Anuria
  - Renal failure

ETIOLOGY
- Can occur spontaneously or after initiation of therapy in patients with:
  - Acute leukemias
  - Bulky solid tumors
  - High-grade lymphomas
- Administration of certain agents:
  - Paclitaxel
  - Hydroxyurea
  - Etoposide
  - Fludarabine
- It has been reported in some cancer patients who received:
  - Corticosteroids
  - Monoclonal antibodies
  - Radiation therapy
  - Hormonal compounds
- Intrathecal administration of chemotherapy
- Rare causes: pregnancy, fever, some patients under general anesthesia

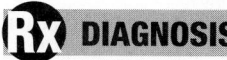
DIAGNOSIS

DIFFERENTIAL DIAGNOSIS
See "Acute Kidney Injury" topic in Section I.

LABORATORY TESTS
- Monitor BUN, creatinine phosphate, potassium, calcium, uric acid, LDH in high-risk patients before and up to 72 hr after initiating therapy. If evidence of tumor lysis syndrome develops, check these at least twice a day.
- Closely monitor urine output (for signs of oliguria).
- Perform frequent ECG or continuous cardiac monitoring to look for lethal arrhythmia (that can be caused by K or Ca abnormalities).

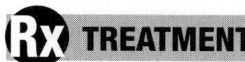
TREATMENT

GENERAL PRINCIPLES
- It is very important to identify high-risk patients (by assessing the extent of tumor burden, renal function, and pathologic findings) in order to initiate prophylactic measures before starting treatment. Delay in doing this may lead to life-threatening conditions.
- In patients with pretreatment tumor lysis syndrome:
  - Correct all metabolic derangement before starting cancer treatment, if possible.
- Careful and frequent laboratory and clinical monitoring. Check:
  - Baseline ECG/continuous cardiac monitoring
  - Renal/fluid status by checking vital signs, daily weights, fluid intake/output
  - For high-risk patients and those with overt tumor lysis syndrome, check the following at least twice daily:
    - Basic metabolic panel
    - Calcium
    - Uric acid
    - Phosphate
    - LDH

TREATMENT OPTIONS (PREVENTIVE MEASURES) FOR HIGH-RISK PATIENTS WITHOUT TUMOR LYSIS SYNDROME
- **Hydration:** prevent volume depletion and help correct electrolyte derangement
  - Start 24-48 hr before initiating cancer treatment and continue for up to 72 hr after treatment.
  - May use D_5W plus 2 amps of $NaCO_3$.
- **Control of hyperuricemia:** use allopurinol or rasburicase.
  - Allopurinol (xanthine oxidase inhibitor prevents the conversion of xanthine and hypoxanthine to uric acid)
    - Give 600 mg/day PO or IV for prophylaxis and 600-900 mg/day PO or IV to treat tumor lysis syndrome.
  - Rasburicase (recombinant urate oxidase) is used when uric acid levels cannot be lowered by standard procedures.
  - Given IV or IM at dosages from 50-100 U/kg/day for 1-5 days.
    - Do not give together with allopurinol.
    - Alkalization is not necessary.
    - Contraindicated in glucose-6-phosphate dehydrogenase deficiency and pregnancy.
- Diuretics: indicated for well-hydrated patients with poor/inadequate diuresis.

○ Furosemide may be used in well-hydrated patients with elevated potassium or in patients with fluid overload.

TREATMENT OF PATIENTS WITH TUMOR LYSIS SYNDROME

- **Principles:**
  - General and preventive measures as mentioned in General Principles and Treatment Options
  - Aggressively treating electrolyte disturbances
  - Treat renal failure if above fail
- Treating electrolyte disturbances:
  - Hyperuricemia: as outlined above
  - Hyperkalemia:
    - Restrict dietary potassium
    - Stop potassium in IV fluid
    - IV infusion of glucose and insulin (to move K to intracellular space)
    - IV gluconate (cardioprotective effect)
    - PO potassium-exchange resins
    - If above measures fail, then immediate dialysis is needed.

- Hyperphosphatemia
  - Decrease dietary intake
  - IV glucose plus insulin
  - Oral phosphate binders
- Hypocalcemia
  - Treat only if symptomatic (e.g., neuromuscular irritability as in positive Chvostek or Trousseau sign).
  - Calcium gluconate only when symptomatic
  - Calcitrol can be used only if serum phosphate level is normal.

TREAT RENAL FAILURE

- Consider early dialysis if above methods fail.
- Dialysis prevents life-threatening complications and irreversible renal failure.
- Hemodialysis is the preferred procedure.

REFERRAL

- Nephrology
- Critical care

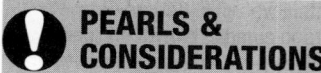 **PEARLS & CONSIDERATIONS**

COMMENTS

- High-risk patients should have prophylactic measures 24-48 hr before starting cytotoxic drugs.
- Prophylactic measures include:
  - IV hydration
  - Administration of allopurinol
  - Urinary alkalization
- Monitor blood chemistry and fluid status.
- Complications of tumor lysis syndrome include:
  - Uremia
  - Renal failure
  - Electrolyte disturbances
  - Cardiac arrhythmia
  - Pulmonary edema secondary to aggressive hydration
  - Metabolic alkalosis from IV bicarbonate administration

SUGGESTED READING

available at www.expertconsult.com

AUTHOR: **DANIEL K. ASIEDU, M.D., PH.D., F.A.C.P.**

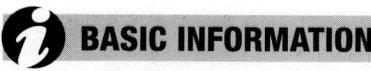

BASIC INFORMATION

DEFINITION

Ulcerative colitis (UC) is a chronic inflammatory bowel disease of undetermined etiology. Accumulating evidence suggests that it may result from an inappropriate inflammatory response to environmental triggers and immune dysregulation involving $CD4^+$ T-cell Th2 response in a genetically susceptible host.

SYNONYMS

UC
Inflammatory bowel disease (IBD)
Idiopathic proctocolitis
Pancolitis

ICD-9CM CODES
556.9 Ulcerative colitis

EPIDEMIOLOGY & DEMOGRAPHICS

INCIDENCE: The incidence of UC is 1.2 to 20.3 cases per 100,000 persons per year; most common between ages 15 and 40 yr, with a second peak between 50 and 80 yr. The disease affects men and women at similar rates.
PREVALENCE: The prevalence of UC is 7.6 to 246.0 cases per 100,000 per year. Higher prevalence in Ashkenazi Jewish descendants.
GEOGRAPHIC DISTRIBUTION: The highest incidence and prevalence of IBD are seen in northern Europe and North America, and the lowest in continental Asia.

GENETICS:
- Both specific and nonspecific gene variants are associated with UC.
- There are 47 loci associated with UC, of which 19 are specific for UC and 28 are shared with Crohn's disease.
- Abnormalities in humoral and cellular adaptive immunity are also found in UC.

PHYSICAL FINDINGS & CLINICAL PRESENTATION

- Patients with UC often present with acute onset of bloody diarrhea accompanied by tenesmus, fever, and dehydration. At presentation 40% of adults have proctitis, 40% have left-sided colitis, and 20% have pancolitis.
- Abdominal distention and tenderness may indicate the presence of complications such as toxic megacolon.
- The onset of symptoms is typically acute and is generally followed by periods of spontaneous remission and frequent relapses.
- Fever, evidence of dehydration may be present during the acute flare-up.
- Evidence of extraintestinal manifestations may be present in nearly 25% of patients: liver disease, sclerosing cholangitis, iritis, uveitis, episcleritis, arthritis, erythema nodosum, pyoderma gangrenosum, aphthous stomatitis.

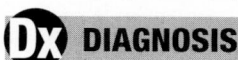

DIAGNOSIS

DIFFERENTIAL DIAGNOSIS
- Crohn's disease (Table 1-402)
- Bacterial infections (Table 1-403)

1. Acute: *Campylobacter, Yersinia, Salmonella, Shigella, Chlamydia, Escherichia coli, Clostridium difficile,* gonococcal proctitis
2. Chronic: Whipple's disease, tuberculosis, enterocolitis
- Irritable bowel syndrome
- Protozoal and parasitic infections (amebiasis, giardiasis, cryptosporidiosis)
- Neoplasm (intestinal lymphoma, carcinoma of colon)
- Ischemic bowel disease
- Diverticulitis
- Celiac sprue, lymphocytic or collagenous colitis, radiation enteritis, endometriosis
- Solitary rectal ulcer
- Acute self-limited colitis
- Medication (NSAIDs, chemotherapy)

WORKUP

An accurate diagnosis of UC should define the extent and severity of inflammation. Diagnostic workup includes:
- Comprehensive history, physical examination
- Laboratory tests (see "Laboratory Tests")
- Colonoscopy to establish the presence of mucosal inflammation; typical endoscopic findings in UC are areas of continuous friable mucosa; diffuse, uniform erythema replacing the usual mucosal vascular pattern; and pseudopolyps. The transition from abnormal to normal tissue tends to be abrupt. Rectal involvement is invariably present if the disease is active. Pathologic findings suggestive of UC include crypt abscesses and atrophy, mucin depletion, basal plasmacytosis, basal lymphoid aggregates, increased lamina propria cellularity, and Paneth cell metaplasia.

LABORATORY TESTS

- Anemia and high erythrocyte sedimentation rate (in severe colitis) are common.
- Potassium, magnesium, calcium, and albumin may be decreased.
- Antineutrophil cytoplasmic antibodies (ANCA) with a perinuclear staining pattern (pANCA) can be found in >45% of patients; there is an increased frequency in treatment-resistant left-sided colitis, suggesting a possible association between these antibodies and a relative resistance to medical therapy in patients with UC.
- Calprotectin is a protein that is measured in feces as a marker of intestinal mucosa leukocyte activity that may be useful for screening of patients with suspected IBD. Trials have shown that based on a pretest probability of IBD of 32% in adults, an abnormal fecal calprotectin test would increase the posttest probability to 91% and a normal result would reduce the probability to 3%.
- Stool examinations for ova and parasites, stool culture, and testing for *Clostridium difficile* toxin and *E. coli* 0157:H7 may be useful to eliminate other causes of diarrhea in selected patients with risk factors.

IMAGING STUDIES

Image studies (plain radiography, CT scan) are generally reserved for suspected complications such as perforation of bowel or toxic megacolon.

TABLE 1-402 Comparison of Crohn's Disease and Ulcerative Colitis

Feature	Crohn's Disease	Ulcerative Colitis
Rectal bleeding	Sometimes	Common
Diarrhea, mucus, pus	Variable	Common
Abdominal pain	Common	Variable
Abdominal mass	Common	Not present
Growth failure	Common	Variable
Perianal disease	Common	Rare
Rectal involvement	Occasional	Universal
Pyoderma gangrenosum	Rare	Present
Erythema nodosum	Common	Less common
Mouth ulceration	Common	Rare
Thrombosis	Less common	Present
Colonic disease	50%-75%	100%
Ileal disease	Common	None except backwash ileitis
Stomach-esophageal disease	More common	Chronic gastritis can be seen
Strictures	Common	Rare
Fissures	Common	Rare
Fistulas	Common	Rare
Toxic megacolon	None	Present
Sclerosing cholangitis	Less common	Present
Risk for cancer	Increased	Greatly increased
Discontinuous (skip) lesions	Common	Not present
Transmural involvement	Common	Unusual
Crypt abscesses	Less common	Common
Granulomas	Common	None
Linear ulcerations	Uncommon	Common

From Kliegman RM et al: *Nelson textbook of pediatrics,* ed 19, Philadelphia, 2011, Saunders.

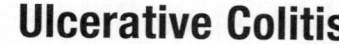

℞ TREATMENT

NONPHARMACOLOGIC THERAPY

- Correct nutritional deficiencies; total parenteral nutrition with bowel rest may be necessary in severe cases. Folate supplementation may reduce the incidence of dysplasia and cancer in chronic UC.
- Avoid oral feedings during acute exacerbation to decrease colonic activity; a low-roughage diet may be helpful in early relapse.
- Psychotherapy is useful in most patients. Referral to self-help groups is also important because of the chronicity of the disease and the young age of the patients.

ACUTE GENERAL Rx

The therapeutic options vary with the degree of disease (mild, severe, fulminant) and areas of involvement (distal, extensive).

- Mild disease can be treated with 5-amino-salicylate agents (mesalamine, olsalazine, balsalazide, sulfasalazine). It can be administered as an enema (40 mg once daily at bedtime for 3 to 6 wk) or suppository (500 mg bid) for patients with distal colonic disease. Oral forms in which the 5-acetyl salicylic acid is in a slow-release or pH-dependent matrix (Pentasa 1 g qid, Asacol 800 mg PO tid) can deliver therapeutic concentrations to the more proximal small bowel or distal ileum. Olsalazine can be useful for maintenance of remission of UC in patients intolerant to sulfasalazine. Usual dose is 500 mg bid taken with food. Balsalazide is indicated for mild to moderately active UC. Usual dose is three 750-mg capsules tid. Probiotics may also be helpful in inducing remission in mild-to-moderate UC.
- Mild-to-moderate UC is often treated with a combination of rectal and oral 5-aminosalicylate. Refractory patients are candidates for oral glucocorticoids or immunosuppressive agents (e.g., cyclosporine).
- Severe disease usually responds to oral corticosteroids (e.g., prednisone 40 to 60 mg/day); corticosteroid suppositories or enemas are also useful for distal colitis. The immunosuppressant azathioprine also provides effective long-term treatment for Crohn's disease.
- Infliximab, a chimeric monoclonal antibody, has been shown to be effective in patients who have not responded to corticosteroid therapy. Newer therapeutic modalities include the use of adalimumab (ADA), a recombinant human monoclonal antibody against tumor necrosis factor-α (TNF-α), for the induction of clinical remission in anti–TNF-α naïve patients with moderately to severely active UC and use of tofacitinib, an oral Janus kinase inhibitor, for patients with moderately to severely active UC.
- Fulminant disease generally requires hospital admission and parenteral corticosteroids (e.g., IV hydrocortisone 100 mg q6h). When bowel movements have returned to normal and the patient is able to eat normally, oral prednisone is resumed. IV cyclosporine can also be used in severe refractory cases; renal toxicity is a potential complication.
- Surgery is indicated in patients who do not respond to intensive medical therapy. Proctocolectomy is usually curative in these patients and also eliminates the high risk of developing adenocarcinoma of the colon (10% to 20% of patients develop it after 10 yr with the disease). Total proctocolectomy with ileal pouch-anal anastomatosis (IPAA) is the procedure of choice for most patients who require elective surgery, since it preserves anal sphincter function. Continent ileostomy is an alternative procedure.

CHRONIC Rx

- Colonoscopic surveillance and multiple biopsies should be instituted approximately 10 yr

TABLE 1-403 Infectious Agents Mimicking Inflammatory Bowel Disease

Agent	Manifestations	Diagnosis	Comments
Bacterial			
Campylobacter jejuni	Acute diarrhea, fever, fecal blood, and leukocytes	Culture	Common in adolescents, may relapse
Yersinia enterocolitica	Acute → chronic diarrhea, right lower quadrant pain, mesenteric adenitis-pseudoappendicitis, fecal blood, and leukocytes Extraintestinal manifestations, mimics Crohn's disease	Culture	Common in adolescents as fever of unknown origin, weight loss, abdominal pain
Clostridium difficile	Postantibiotic onset, watery → bloody diarrhea, pseudomembrane on sigmoidoscopy	Cytotoxin assay	May be nosocomial Toxic megacolon possible
Escherichia coli O157:H7	Colitis, fecal blood, abdominal pain	Culture and typing	Hemolytic-uremic syndrome
Salmonella	Watery → bloody diarrhea, food borne, fecal leukocytes, fever, pain, cramps	Culture	Usually acute
Shigella	Watery → bloody diarrhea, fecal leukocytes, fever, pain, cramps	Culture	Dysentery symptoms
Edwardsiella tarda	Bloody diarrhea, cramps	Culture	Ulceration on endoscopy
Aeromonas hydrophila	Cramps, diarrhea, fecal blood	Culture	May be chronic Contaminated drinking water
Plesiomonas	Diarrhea, cramps	Culture	Shellfish source
Tuberculosis	Rarely bovine, now *Mycobacterium tuberculosis* Ileocecal area, fistula formation	Culture, purified protein derivative, biopsy	Can mimic Crohn's disease
Parasites			
Entamoeba histolytica	Acute bloody diarrhea and liver abscess, colic	Trophozoite in stool, colonic mucosal flask ulceration, serologic tests	Travel to endemic area
Giardia lamblia	Foul-smelling, watery diarrhea, cramps, flatulence, weight loss; no colonic involvement	"Owl"-like trophozoite and cysts in stool; rarely duodenal intubation	May be chronic
AIDS-Associated Enteropathy			
Cryptosporidium	Chronic diarrhea, weight loss	Stool microscopy	Mucosal findings not like inflammatory bowel disease
Isospora belli	As in *Cryptosporidium*		Tropical location
Cytomegalovirus	Colonic ulceration, pain, bloody diarrhea	Culture, biopsy	More common when on immunosuppressive medications

From Kliegman RM et al: *Nelson textbook of pediatrics,* ed 19, Philadelphia, 2011, Saunders.

U

Diseases and Disorders

I

after diagnosis because of the increased risk of colon carcinoma.

- Erythropoietin is useful in patients with anemia refractory to treatment with iron and vitamins.
- In patients on long-term steroid therapy, periodic bone density scans are recommended to screen for glucocorticoid-induced osteoporosis.

DISPOSITION

The clinical course is variable. ~66% of patients will achieve clinical remission with medical therapy, and nearly 80% of treatment compliant patients maintain remission. 15% to 20% of patients eventually require colectomy. Pouchitis is the most common long-term complication of IPAA (up to 40% of patients). >75% of patients treated medically will experience relapse.

REFERRAL

- Gastrointestinal consultation for initial diagnostic sigmoidoscopy/colonoscopy in suspected cases
- Surgical referral for patients with severe disease unresponsive to medical therapy

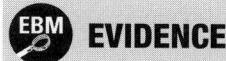

EVIDENCE

available at www.expertconsult.com

SUGGESTED READINGS

available at www.expertconsult.com

RELATED CONTENT

Ulcerative Colitis (Patient Information)

AUTHOR: **FRED F. FERRI, M.D.**

BASIC INFORMATION

DEFINITION

Urethritis is a well-defined clinical syndrome manifested by dysuria, a urethral discharge, or both.

ICD-9CM CODES
597.80 Urethritis, unspecified
098.20 Gonococcal

EPIDEMIOLOGY & DEMOGRAPHICS

- The major single specific etiology of acute urethritis is *Neisseria gonorrhoeae*, producing gonococcal urethritis (GCU). Urethritis of all other etiologies is called *nongonococcal urethritis* (NGU).
- NGU is twice as common as GCU in the U.S. NGU is the most common sexually transmitted disease (STD) syndrome occurring in men, accounting for 6 million office visits annually. NGU is more frequently encountered in higher socioeconomic groups. GCU is more common in homosexual males than heterosexual males with acute urethritis.
- *N. gonorrhoeae* is a gram-negative, kidney-shaped diplococcus with flattened opposed margins. The urethra is the most common site of infection in all men. In the United States, the rates of gonorrhea are 40 times higher in black adolescent males than in white adolescent males. In heterosexual men, the pharynx is infected in 7%, and in homosexual men the pharynx is infected in 40% and the rectum in 25%. A single episode of intercourse with an infected partner carries a transmission risk of 20% for males; female partners of an infected male will contract the disease 80% of the time.

PHYSICAL FINDINGS & CLINICAL PRESENTATION

- Symptoms of GCU: urethral discharge and dysuria are the most common symptoms. There is complaint of urethral itching. Prostatic involvement can cause frequency, urgency, and nocturia. It can involve the epididymis through spreading down the vas deferens, causing acute epididymitis.
- Incubation period: 3 to 10 days. Without treatment urethritis persists for 3 to 7 wk, with 95% of men becoming asymptomatic after 3 mo. GCU is asymptomatic in up to 60% of contacts.
- Signs of GCU: yellow-brown discharge, meatal edema, urethral tenderness to palpation. Rectal bleeding with pus is seen with gonococcal proctitis. Periurethritis leading to urethral stenosis can occur. Disseminated infection can occur. Tenosynovitis and arthritis can occur. Rarely, hepatitis, myocarditis, endocarditis, and meningitis can occur.

DIAGNOSIS

DIFFERENTIAL DIAGNOSIS

- NGU
- Herpes simplex virus

LABORATORY TESTS

- Nucleic acid amplification tests (NAATs): these tests have largely replaced culture in many settings where persons are screened for asymptomatic genital infection. They are not more sensitive than culture for detecting *N. gonorrhoeae* in cervical or urethral specimen; however, they have specificities of >99% and retain sensitivity when used to test voided urine or self-collected vaginal swabs.
- Calcium alginate or rayon swab on a metal shaft (not cotton-tipped swabs, which are bactericidal) of the urethra should be performed anywhere from 2 to 4 hr after voiding to prevent bacterial washout with voiding. Gram staining with modified Thayer-Martin media is indicated. Cultures of the pharynx and rectum when indicated.
- Concomitant serologic testing for syphilis on all patients.
- Concomitant *Chlamydia* testing on all patients.
- Offer of HIV counseling and testing to all patients.

TREATMENT

NONPHARMACOLOGIC THERAPY

Behavioral management: avoid intercourse until cure has been attained and sexual partners have been evaluated and treated.

ACUTE GENERAL Rx

- Ceftriaxone 250 mg IM x 1 dose *plus* azithromycin 1 g orally single dose *or* doxycycline 100 mg orally twice/day for 7 days

Alternative regimens:
- Cefixime 400 mg PO x 1 dose *plus* azithromycin 1 g orally single dose *or* doxycycline 100 mg orally twice/day for 7 days *plus* test of cure in 1 wk
- If the patient has severe cephalosporin allergy: azithromycin 2 g in a single oral dose *plus* test of cure in 1 wk
- Resistance to penicillins, fluoroquinolones, sulfonamides, and tetracyclines is now widespread.
- The use of azithromycin as the second antimicrobial is preferred over doxycycline due to the high prevalence of tetracycline resistance.
- The proportion of gonorrhea cases in heterosexual men that are fluoroquinolone resistant (QRNG) has reached 6.7%, an elevenfold increase from 0.6% in 2001. Fluoroquinolone

antibiotics are no longer recommended to treat gonorrhea in the U.S.
- Dual treatment for gonococcal and chlamydial infections is based on theory and expert opinion rather than evidence from clinical trials.

CHRONIC Rx

Postgonococcal urethritis (PGU): reinfection is the most common cause of recurrence. Repeat swab and culture of the urethra, pharynx, and rectum (where applicable) are mandatory. Persistence of polymorphonuclear cells (PMNs) with the absence of gram-negative intracellular diplococci suggests a diagnosis of PGU. This occurs when GCU is treated with a regimen that is ineffective against coincident chlamydial infection; it represents NGU after GCU. The syndrome should be treated as NGU. Persistence of *N. gonorrhoeae* by smear or culture requires treatment for *N. gonorrhoeae*.

PEARLS & CONSIDERATIONS

COMMENTS

- Partner notification: the names and contact information of sexual partners should be gathered at the time of the visit and referred to the health department or the patient notifies the contact directly. Expedited partner treatment is recommended by the Centers for Disease Control and Prevention (CDC) and approved in several states. This consists of giving prescriptions to the infected patient for their partner(s) who has not been evaluated by a physician and is unlikely to seek medical care.
- On examination of the urethral smear, the presence of small numbers of PMNs provides objective evidence of urethritis. The complete absence of PMNs on a urethral smear argues against urethritis. If in addition to the PMNs there are gram-negative, intracellular diplococci, the diagnosis of gonorrhea is established.

SUGGESTED READINGS

available at www.expertconsult.com

RELATED CONTENT

Fig. E1-862 Urethral discharge (Algorithm)
Fig. 3-60 Evaluation of patients with dysuria and/or urethral discharge (Algorithm)
Gonococcal Urethritis (Patient Information)

AUTHORS: **PHILIP J. ALIOTTA, M.D., M.S.H.A.,** and **RUBEN ALVERO, M.D.**

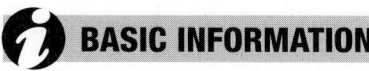

BASIC INFORMATION

DEFINITION

Nongonococcal urethritis (NGU) is urethral inflammation caused by any of several organisms.

SYNONYMS

NGU

ICD-9CM CODES
099.40 Nongonococcal
099.41 Chlamydial

EPIDEMIOLOGY & DEMOGRAPHICS

- Occurrence is 50% in sexually transmitted disease clinics.
- NGU most commonly affects men in a higher socioeconomic class, affecting heterosexual men more frequently than homosexual men.
- NGU carries a greater morbidity rate than gonococcal urethritis (GCU).

PHYSICAL FINDINGS & CLINICAL PRESENTATION

- Incubation period: 2 to 35 days
- Symptoms: dysuria, whitish-clear urethral discharge (Fig. 1-857), and urethral itching. The onset of symptoms in NGU is less acute than GCU.
- Signs: whitish-clear urethral discharge, meatal edema, and erythema. Infected women

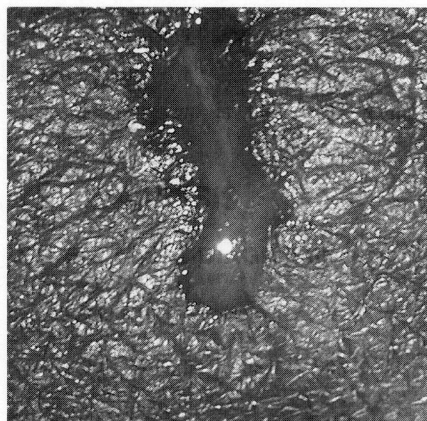

FIGURE 1-857 Urethral discharge from a man with nongonococcal urethritis. (From Mandell GL et al: *Principles and practice of infectious diseases,* ed 7, Philadelphia, 2009, Churchill Livingstone.)

manifest pyuria, and the disease can present as acute urethral syndrome.

COMPLICATIONS

Epididymitis in heterosexual men may be linked to nonbacterial prostatitis, proctitis in homosexual men, or Reiter's syndrome.

ETIOLOGY

- Most common agent is *Chlamydia* spp., an obligate intracellular parasite possessing both DNA and RNA, which replicates by binary fission. It causes 20% to 50% of NGU cases. Two species exist:
  - *Chlamydia psittaci*
  - *Chlamydia trachomatis* with its 15 serotypes
    Serotypes A through C cause hyperendemic-blinding trachoma.
    Serotypes D through K cause genital tract infection.
    Serotypes L1 through L3 cause lymphogranuloma venereum.
- Other causes of NGU: *Mycoplasma genitalium* (found in 44% of treatment failures); *Ureaplasma urealyticum,* causing 15% to 30% of the cases of NGU; *Trichomonas vaginalis;* and herpes simplex virus. The cause of 20% of the cases of NGU has not been identified.
- Asymptomatic infection occurs in 28% of the contacts of women with chlamydial cervical infection.

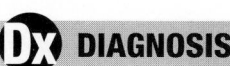 DIAGNOSIS

DIFFERENTIAL DIAGNOSIS

- GCU
- Herpes simplex virus
- Trichomoniasis

LABORATORY TESTS

- Requires demonstration of urethritis and exclusion of infection with *N. gonorrhoeae*.
- Nucleic acid amplification tests (NAATs): these tests have largely replaced culture in many settings where persons are screened for asymptomatic genital infection.
- The appearance of PMNs on urethral smear confirms the diagnosis of urethritis. Because *Chlamydia* is an intracellular parasite of the columnar epithelium, the best specimen for culture is an endourethral swab taken from an area 2 to 4 cm inside the urethra. For culture, a Dacron-tipped swab is used; avoid

calcium alginate or cotton swabs. The organism can only be grown in tissue culture, which is expensive.

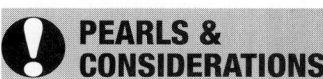 TREATMENT

Because it is impossible to differentiate among the common etiologies of NGU, the condition is treated syndromically, including in the initial treatment regimen those drugs effective against the common causative agents. In patients with isolated uncomplicated NGU, recommended regimens are azithromycin 1 g orally single dose or doxycycline 100 mg bid × 7 days. In patients with confirmed urethritis and unclear etiology, concurrent treatment for gonorrhea and *Chlamydia* is recommended. In these patients, uncomplicated infections of the urethra can be treated with combination of a single 1-g dose of oral azithromycin or 100 mg doxycycline bid × 7 days *plus*
- Cefixime 400 mg PO × 1 dose or
- Ceftriaxone 125 mg IM × 1 dose
Recommended regimen in pregnancy is azithromycin, 1 g orally as a single dose. Repeat test 3 weeks after completion of treatment to confirm cure.

PEARLS & CONSIDERATIONS

COMMENTS

Partner notification: The names and contact information of sexual partners should be gathered at the time of the visit and referred to the health department or the patient notifies the contact directly. Expedited partner treatment is recommended by the CDC and approved in several states. This consists of giving prescriptions to the infected patient for their partner(s) who has not been evaluated by a physician and is unlikely to seek medical care.

SUGGESTED READINGS

available at www.expertconsult.com

RELATED CONTENT

Cervicitis (Related Key Topic)
Chlamydia Genital Infections (Related Key Topic)
Nongonococcal Urethritis (Patient Information)

AUTHORS: **PHILIP J. ALIOTTA, M.D., M.S.H.A.,** and **RUBEN ALVERO, M.D.**

BASIC INFORMATION

DEFINITION

Urinary tract infection (UTI) is a term that encompasses a broad range of clinical entities that have in common a positive urine culture. A conventional threshold is growth of >100,000 colony-forming units per milliliter from a midstream-catch urine sample. In symptomatic patients, a smaller number of bacteria (between 100 and 10,000 colony-forming units per milliliter of midstream urine) is recognized as an infection.

SYNONYMS

UTI

ICD-9CM CODES
595.0 Acute cystitis
595.3 Trigonitis
595.2 Chronic cystitis
590.1 Acute pyelonephritis
590.0 Chronic pyelonephritis
590.8 Nonspecific pyelonephritis

CLASSIFICATION

- Uncomplicated UTI: occurs in a normal urinary tract and resolves rapidly with conventional antimicrobials.
- Complicated UTI: occurs in patients with coexisting pathology (strictures, stones, comorbidities [diabetes mellitus, multiple sclerosis, spinal cord injuries]).
- First infection: the first documented UTI; tends to be uncomplicated and is easily treated.
- Unresolved bacteriuria: UTI in which the urinary tract is not sterilized during therapy. Main causes are bacterial resistance, patient noncompliance with medication, mixed bacterial infection, rapid reinfection, azotemia, infected stones, Münchausen syndrome, and papillary necrosis.
- Bacterial persistence: UTI in which the urine cultures become sterile during therapy, but a persistent source of infection from a site within the urinary tract that was excluded from the high urinary concentrations gives rise to reinfection by the same organism. Causes include infected stone, chronic bacterial prostatitis, atrophic infected kidney, vesicovaginal or enterovesical fistulas, obstructive uropathy, infected pyelocaliceal diverticula, infected ureteral stump after nephrectomy, infected necrotic papillae from papillary necrosis, infected urachal cysts, infected medullary sponge kidney, urethral diverticula, and foreign bodies.
- Reinfection: UTI in which a new infection occurs with new pathogens at variable intervals after a previous infection has been eradicated.
- Relapse: the less common form of recurrent infection; occurs within 2 wk of treatment when the same organism reappears in the same site as the previous infection. Relapsing infections of the urinary tract most commonly occur in pyelonephritis, kidney obstruction from a stone, and prostatitis.

EPIDEMIOLOGY & DEMOGRAPHICS

INCIDENCE:

- UTI is the most common bacterial infection encountered in the ambulatory care setting in the U.S. The self-reported annual incidence of UTI in women is 12%, and by age 32 half of all women report having had at least one UTI.
- In neonates: more common in boys as a result of anatomic abnormalities.
- In preschool children: more common in girls (4.5% vs. 0.5% for boys).
- In adulthood: more common in women, with a 1% to 3% prevalence in nonpregnant women. Table 1-404 describes factors modulating risk for acute uncomplicated UTIs in women. In pregnancy at 12 wk, the incidence of asymptomatic bacteriuria is similar to nonpregnant women, at 2% to 10%. However, 25%-30% of pregnant women with untreated asymptomatic bacteriuria develop acute pyelonephritis, especially in the second and third trimesters, and have a pyelonephritic recurrence rate of 10%. In adults aged ≥65 yr, at least 10% of men and 20% of women have bacteriuria.

PHYSICAL FINDINGS & CLINICAL PRESENTATION

- UTI presentation is inconsistent and cannot be relied on to diagnose UTI accurately or to localize the site of infection. Patients report:
  - Urinary frequency, urgency
  - Dysuria
  - Urge incontinence
  - Suprapubic pain
  - Gross or microscopic hematuria
- When negative cultures are associated with significant pyuria, vaginal discharge, or hematuria, infections with Chlamydia trachomatis, Neisseria gonorrhoeae, and Trichomonas vaginalis should be considered.
- Acute pyelonephritis presents with fever, flank or abdominal pain, chills, malaise, vomiting, and diarrhea. It is these systemic symptoms that distinguish pyelonephritis from cystitis. Complications of acute pyelonephritis are renal abscess, perinephric abscess, emphysematous pyelonephritis, and pyonephrosis.

ETIOLOGY & PATHOGENESIS

- Four major pathways:
  - Ascending from the urethra
  - Lymphatic
  - Hematogenous
  - Direct extension from another organ system
- Other risk factors: neurologic diseases, renal failure, diabetes, anatomic abnormalities, bladder outlet obstruction, urethral stricture, vesicoureteral reflux, fistula, urinary diversion, megacystis, infected stones, age, pregnancy, instrumentation, poor patient compliance, poor hygiene, infrequent voiding, diaphragm contraceptives, tampon use, douches, and catheters.
- Catheters: all patients who require a long-term Foley catheter eventually develop significant levels of bacteriuria. Treatment is reserved for individuals who become symptomatic (leukocytosis, fever, chills, malaise, loss of appetite, etc.) Using prophylactic antibiotics to treat patients who have chronic catheters is to be discouraged because of the risk of acquiring bacteria resistant to antibiotic therapy.
- Once bacteria reach the urinary tract, three factors determine whether the infection occurs (Box E1-75). These factors also determine the anatomic level of the UTI:
  - Virulence of the microorganism
  - Inoculum size
  - Adequacy of the host defense mechanisms
- Urinary pathogens: in 95% of UTIs the infecting organism is a member of the Enterobacteriaceae, enterococci, or, in young women, Staphylococcus saprophyticus. Escherichia coli is the most common pathogen (85% of UTI cases). In contrast, the organisms that commonly colonize the distal urethra and skin of both men and women and the vagina of women are Staphylococcus epidermidis, diphtheroids, lactobacilli, Gardnerella vaginalis, and a variety of anaerobes that rarely cause UTIs. In general, the isolation of two or more bacterial species from a urine culture signifies a contaminated specimen unless the patient is being managed with an indwelling catheter or urinary diversion or has a chronic complicated infection.
- Defense mechanisms against cystitis: low pH and high osmolarity, mucopolysaccharide glycosaminoglycan protective layer, normal bladder that empties completely and has no incontinence, and the presence of estrogen.

TABLE 1-404 Factors Modulating Risk for Acute Uncomplicated Urinary Tract Infections in Women

Host Determinants	Uropathogen Determinants
Behavioral: sexual intercourse, use of spermicidal products, recent antimicrobial use, suboptimal voiding habits	Escherichia coli virulence determinants: P, S, Dr, and type I fimbriae; hemolysin; aerobactin; serum resistance
Genetic: innate and adaptive immune response, enhanced epithelial cell adherence, antibacterial factors in urine and bladder mucosa, nonsecretor of ABO blood group antigens, P₁ blood group phenotype, reduced CXCR1 expression, previous history of recurrent cystitis	
Biologic: estrogen deficiency in postmenopausal women, micturition	

From Floege J et al: Comprehensive clinical nephrology, ed 4, Philadelphia, 2010, Saunders.

Dx DIAGNOSIS

DIFFERENTIAL DIAGNOSIS

- Interstitial cystitis
- Vaginitis
- Urethritis (gonococcal, nongonococcal, *Trichomonas*)
- Frequency-urgency syndrome, prostatitis (acute and chronic)
- Obstructive uropathy
- Infected stones
- Fistulas
- Papillary necrosis
- Vesicoureteral reflux
- Irritation

LABORATORY TESTS

- Urinalysis with microscopic evaluation of clean-catch urine for bacteria and pyuria. The presence of ≥10 leukocytes/μl of unspun urine from a midstream catch indicates UTI. If urine dipsticks are used, the presence of positive nitrite and positive leukocyte esterase is indicative of UTI in a symptomatic patient.
- Urine culture and sensitivity are useful in complicated UTIs but generally not needed in uncomplicated UTIs.
- Complete blood count with differential (shows leukocytosis)
- Antibody-coated bacteria are seen with pyelonephritis
- An approach to the management of UTI is described in Fig. E1-858.

IMAGING STUDIES

- Warranted only if renal infection or genitourinary abnormality is suspected
- KUB (kidneys, ureter, and bladder); voiding cystourethrogram; renal sonogram; intravenous pyelogram; CT scan; nuclear scan
- Specialty examination: cystoscopy with occasional retrograde pyelography to rule out obstructive uropathy; stenting the obstruction possibly required

Rx TREATMENT

NONPHARMACOLOGIC THERAPY

- Hot sitz baths, anticholinergics, urinary analgesics
- For pyelonephritis: bed rest, analgesics, antipyretics, and IV hydration

ACUTE GENERAL Rx

- Conventional therapy of 7 days; short-term therapy of 3 or 5 days (Fig. E1-859).
- Agents of choice: nitrofurantoin, fluoroquinolones, trimethoprim plus sulfonamide (TMP-SMX), amoxicillin/clavulanate, and cephalosporins. Drug resistance needs to be considered when choosing antibiotic therapy. Currently, in the U.S., fluoroquinolone resistance exceeds 20% and TMP-SMX resistance 40% in some regions, but resistance is much lower for nitrofurantoin.
- For pyelonephritis: hospitalization until afebrile and stable, then at home by home care agency with IV antibiotic composed of aminoglycoside plus cephalosporin for 1 wk followed by oral agents (based on sensitivity) for 2 wk. Moderate forms of pyelonephritis may be successfully treated with fluoroquinolone therapy for 21 days without requiring hospitalization. Most important, complicating factors such as obstructive uropathy or infected stones must be identified and treated.
- A urinary analgesic (e.g., phenazopyridine) can also be used along with antibiotics in patients with significant dysuria.

! PEARLS & CONSIDERATIONS

COMMENTS

- Asymptomatic bacteriuria: occurs in both anatomically normal and abnormal urinary tracts. This can clear spontaneously, persist, or lead to symptomatic kidney infection. Treatment is recommended in patients with vesicoureteral reflux, stones, obstructive uropathy, parenchymal renal disease, or diabetes mellitus and in pregnant or immunocompromised patients.
- Pregnancy: 25% to 30% of pregnant women with asymptomatic untreated bacteriuria develop pyelonephritis. This is associated with prematurity and low-birth-weight infants. Confirmed significant bacteriuria should be treated with an aminopenicillin and cephalosporin.
- Recurrent UTI: caused by an unresolved infection, vaginal colonization of the originally infecting organism, or reinfection with a new strain. Management of recurrent UTI includes continuous antibiotic prophylaxis, intermittent self-treatment, and postcoital prophylaxis. Prophylaxis is recommended for women who have two or more symptomatic UTIs over a 6-mo period or three or more episodes over a 12-mo period.

- Changes after menopause: lower levels of lactobacilli, decreased estrogen, senile atrophy of the genitalia, and loss of bladder elasticity (compliance).
- Biologic factors altering defense systems: the presence of sialosyl galactosyl globoside on the surface of the kidney acts as a powerful receptor for *Escherichia coli* and increases the risk for UTI; the presence of the blood group P_1 causes increased binding of *E. coli* that is resistant to normal infection-fighting mechanisms in the body. It is believed that some individuals are deficient in a compound called human beta-defensin-1, a naturally occurring antibiotic that fights *E. coli* within the urinary tract.
- Cranberry juice is often used as a remedy for the prevention of UTIs, however, randomized placebo-controlled trials have shown that it is no better than placebo for preventing UTIs.

RESISTANCE:

- Because of the overuse of antibiotics, organisms once sensitive to a number of antimicrobial agents are now increasingly more resistant, making effective management of UTI and pyelonephritis more difficult and potentially more dangerous. Most important has been the increasing resistance to trimethoprim plus sulfamethoxazole (TMP-SMX), the current primary care provider drug of choice for acute uncomplicated UTI in women.
- When choosing a treatment regimen, physicians should consider such factors as:
  - In vitro susceptibility
  - Adverse effects
  - Cost effectiveness
  - Resistance rates in their respective communities

EBM EVIDENCE
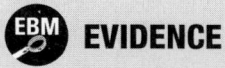

available at www.expertconsult.com

SUGGESTED READINGS
available at www.expertconsult.com

RELATED CONTENT

Pyelonephritis (Related Key Topic)
Urinary Tract Infection (Patient Information)
Urinary Tract Infection Child (Patient Information)

AUTHORS: **PHILIP J. ALIOTTA, M.D., M.S.H.A.,** and **RUBEN ALVERO, M.D.**

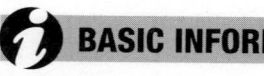 BASIC INFORMATION

DEFINITION

Urolithiasis is the presence of calculi within the urinary tract. The five major types of urinary stones are calcium oxalate (>50%), calcium phosphate (10% to 20%), uric acid (7%), struvite (7%), and cystine (3%) (Table 1-405).

SYNONYMS

Kidney stones
Renal colic
Nephrolithiasis

ICD-9CM CODES
592.9 Urinary calculus

EPIDEMIOLOGY & DEMOGRAPHICS

- In the U.S., the lifetime prevalence of nephrolithiasis is 13% in men and 7% in women, annually.
- Between 1% and 1.7% of emergency department visits (1 to 2 million visits annually) are accounted for by a primary diagnosis of renal colic or renal calculus.
- The incidence of symptomatic nephrolithiasis is greatest during the summer as a result of increased humidity and temperatures with a concomitant increased risk of dehydration and concentrated urine.
- Calcium oxalate or mixed calcium oxalate/calcium phosphate stones account for nearly 70% of uroliths. Supersaturation, often expressed as the ratio of urinary calcium oxalate or calcium phosphate concentration to its solubility, is the driving force in stone formation. At levels above 1, crystals can nucleate and grow, promoting stone formation.

PHYSICAL FINDINGS & CLINICAL PRESENTATION

Stones may be asymptomatic, or they may cause the following signs and symptoms as a result of obstruction:
- Sudden onset of flank tenderness

- Nausea and vomiting
- The patient being in constant movement in an attempt to lessen the pain. (Patients with an acute abdomen are usually still because movement exacerbates the pain.)
- Pain that is referred to the testes or labium by the progression of stone down the urinary ureter
- Fever and chills that accompany the acute colic if there is superimposed infection
- Pain that may radiate anteriorly over to the abdomen and result in intestinal ileus

ETIOLOGY

- Supersaturation, often expressed as the ratio of urinary calcium oxalate or calcium phosphate concentration to its solubility, is the driving force in calcium kidney stone formation
- Increased absorption of calcium in the small bowel: type I absorptive hypercalciuria (i.e., independent of calcium intake)
- Idiopathic hypercalciuria nephrolithiasis. (This is the most common diagnosis for patients with calcium stones; the diagnosis is made only if there is no hypercalcemia and no known cause of the hypercalciuria.)
- Increased vitamin D synthesis (e.g., as a result of renal phosphate loss: type III absorptive hypercalciuria)
- Renal tubular malfunction with inadequate reabsorption of calcium and resulting hypercalciuria
- Heterozygous mutations in the NPT2a gene that result in hypophosphatemia and urinary phosphate loss
- Hyperparathyroidism with resulting hypercalcemia
- Elevated uric acid level (e.g., metabolic defects, dietary excess) (Box E1-76)
- Chronic diarrhea (e.g., inflammatory bowel disease) with increased oxalate absorption
- Type I (distal tubule) renal tubular acidosis (<1% of calcium stones)
- Long-term hydrochlorothiazide treatment

- Chronic infections with urease-producing organisms (e.g., *Proteus, Providencia, Pseudomonas, Klebsiella*). (Struvite, or magnesium ammonium phosphate crystals, is produced when the urinary tract is colonized by bacteria, thus producing elevated concentrations of ammonia [Box E1-77])
- Abnormal excretion of cystine
- Chemotherapy for malignancies
- Estrogen supplements

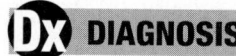 DIAGNOSIS

DIFFERENTIAL DIAGNOSIS

- Urinary tract infection
- Pyelonephritis
- Diverticulitis
- Pelvic inflammatory disease
- Ovarian pathology
- Factitious (i.e., in drug addicts)
- Appendicitis
- Small-bowel obstruction
- Ectopic pregnancy

The differential diagnosis of obstructive uropathy is described in Section II.

WORKUP

- Fig. E1-860 describes an algorithm for evaluation of suspected renal colic.
- Stone analysis should be performed on recovered stones.
- A clinical algorithm for the evaluation of nephrolithiasis is described in Fig. E1-861.
- Box 1-78 describes events in the medical history that may be significant with regard to urolithiasis.

LABORATORY TESTS

- Urinalysis: Hematuria may be present; however, its absence does not exclude urinary stones. The evaluation of the urinary pH is of value for the identification of the type of stone: a pH of >7.5 is associated with struvite stones, whereas a pH of <5 generally is

---

TABLE 1-405 Stone Composition and Relative Occurrence

Stone Composition	Occurrence (%)
Calcium-containing stones	
Ca oxalate	60
Mixed Ca oxalate/ hydroxyapatite	20
Brushite	2
Non–calcium containing stones	
Uric acid	7
Magnesium ammonium phosphate (struvite)	7
Cystine	1-3 (10% of stones in children)
Xanthine	<1
Medication-related stones	<1

From Lipshultz LI et al: *Urology and the primary care practitioner*, ed 3, Philadelphia, 2008, Elsevier.

BOX 1-78 Components of the Medical History That Are Significant for Urolithiasis

- Diseases associated with disturbances of calcium metabolism: primary hyperparathyroidism, Wilson's disease, medullary sponge kidney, osteoporosis, immobilization, sarcoidosis, osteolytic metastases, plasmacytoma, neuroendocrine tumors, Paget's disease
- Dietary history: purine gluttony, calcium excess, milk alkali, oxalate excess, sodium excess, low citrus fruit intake
- Medications: uricosurics, diuretics, analgesics, vitamins C and D, antacids (especially phosphorus-binding agents), acetazolamide, calcium channel blockers, triamterene, estrogens, theophylline, protease inhibitors (indinavir), sulfonamides
- Diseases associated with disturbances of oxalate metabolism: primary hyperoxaluria types I and II, Crohn's disease, ulcerative colitis, intestinal bypass surgery (especially jejunoileal bypass), ileal resection
- Diseases associated with disturbances of purine metabolism
- Intrinsic metabolic disorders: anemia, neoplastic disorders (especially leukemias), intoxication, myocardial infarction, irradiation, cytotoxic chemotherapy
- Enzyme deficiency: primary gout, Lesch-Nyhan syndrome
- Altered excretion: renal insufficiency, metabolic acidosis
- Infectious history: organisms (particularly *Proteus* and *Klebsiella*), febrile, upper tract involvement, and dates (if hospitalized)

Modified from Nseyo UO (ed): *Urology for primary care physicians*, Philadelphia, 1999, Saunders.

seen with uric acid or cystine stones. A low serum bicarbonate concentration with a urine pH of ≥6 is suggestive of renal tubular acidosis.

- Urine culture and sensitivity results should be obtained for all patients.
- Serum chemistries should include calcium, electrolytes, phosphate, and uric acid.
- Additional tests: 24-hr urine collection for calcium, uric acid, phosphate, oxalate, and citrate excretion is generally reserved for patients with recurrent stones.

IMAGING STUDIES

- Common diagnostic modalities for renal colic are summarized in Table 1-406.
- Plain films of the abdomen can identify radiopaque stones (e.g., calcium, uric acid) of ≥5 mm in diameter.
- Renal sonogram (Fig. 1-862) is generally not sensitive for very small calculi, but it may be

helpful for identifying associated hydronephrosis. Accuracy in detecting distal ureteral stones can be high but is variable with size of the calculus and expertise of the technician and radiologist.

- Unenhanced (noncontrast) helical computed tomography scanning can be used to visualize the calculus (Fig. E1-863), which is identified by the "rim sign" or "halo" that represents the edematous ureteral wall around the stone. The test is fast and accurate (sensitivity nearly 100%; specificity, 94% to 96%), and it can be used to readily identify all stone types in all locations. This modality is being used increasingly during the initial assessment of renal colic.
- Intravenous pyelography demonstrates the size and location of the stone as well as the degree of obstruction. However, this modality is now rarely used and has largely been replaced by computed tomography.

Rx TREATMENT

NONPHARMACOLOGIC THERAPY

- An increase in water or other fluid intake is recommended; in fact, a doubling of previous fluid intake should occur unless the patient has a history of congestive heart failure or fluid overload. Generally, patients at increased risk for the development of stones should increase their fluid intake to >2 L/day (68 oz/day) to maintain a urine volume of >2 L/day.
- Normal dietary calcium intake is recommended. If one does not consume enough calcium, less is available to bind to dietary oxalate; as a result, more oxalate reaches the colon, is absorbed into the bloodstream, and excreted as calcium oxalate, thus setting the stage for calcium urolithiasis.

TABLE 1-406 Common Diagnostic Imaging Modalities for Renal Colic

Modality	Information Provided	Radiation Dose	Contrast	Approximate Cost	Time
CT	Renal stones, including size and position of stones and evidence of obstruction Alternative diagnoses, such as AAA, appendicitis, and free air	4-10 mSv	No	$750-$1000	Less than 5 min to perform, 30 min for interpretation
CT with IV contrast	Same as noncontrast CT Delineation of renal mass lesions Additional information about vascular dissections and mesenteric ischemia	4-10 mSv	Yes	$750-$1000	Less than 5 min, after delay to measure creatinine
CT with IV and oral contrast	Same as CT with IV contrast Potentially improved diagnosis of bowel abnormalities	4-10 mSv	Yes	$750-$1000	Less than 5 min, after delay of approximately 2 hr to ingest oral contrast
Intravenous urogram	Structural and functional information about obstruction Rarely, identification of other pathology, such as AAA	1.5 mSv	Yes	$350	Approximately 75 min
X-ray	Possible identification of stone, but not useful for hydronephrosis or most other pathology	0.5-1 mSv	No	$250	Less than 5 min
Ultrasound	Identification of hydronephrosis or hydroureter Possible identification of stone Used to assess for AAA or biliary disease	No	No	$150	Approximately 15-30 min—bedside ultrasound is quicker

CT, Computed tomography; *IV,* intravenous.

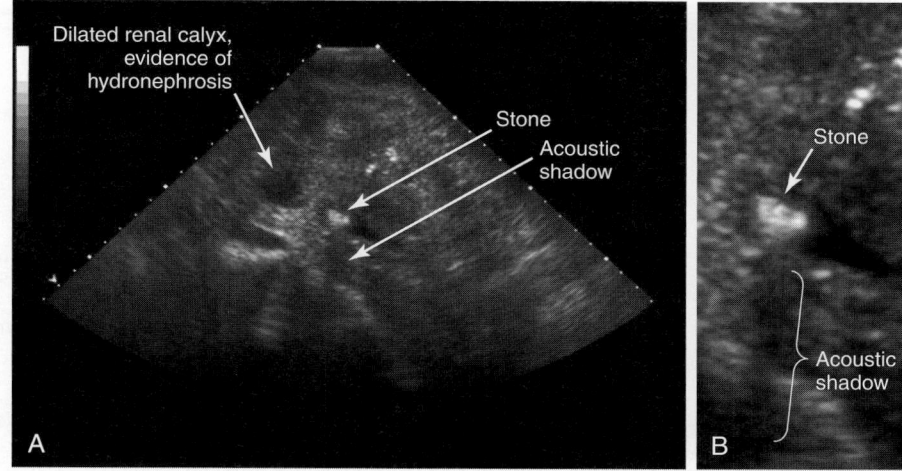

FIGURE 1-862 Ultrasound of renal stone. Ultrasound can be used to assess for renal stones and complications such as hydronephrosis. Stones can be difficult to detect, whereas hydronephrosis is usually readily observed. Because stones are dense, they reflect sound and prevent its through transmission. As a result, stones are echogenic (bright) on ultrasound, and cast an acoustic shadow (black). **A,** Short-axis view of kidney. **B,** Close-up. (From Broder JS: *Diagnostic imaging for the emergency physician,* Philadelphia, 2011, Saunders.)

- Sodium restriction to decrease calcium excretion and decreased protein intake to 1 g/kg/day to decrease uric acid, calcium, and oxalate excretion should be considered.
- Increasing the amount of bran in the diet may decrease bowel transit time with an increased binding of calcium and a subsequent decrease in urinary calcium.

ACUTE GENERAL Rx

- Pain control: ketorolac (60 mg intramuscularly) can be used for moderate pain. However, the use of narcotics is generally indicated because of the severity of pain.
- Specific therapy is tailored to the stone type:
  - ○ Uric acid calculi: control of hyperuricosuria with allopurinol 100 to 300 mg/day; increase urinary pH with potassium citrate 10-mEq tablets tid. Alkalinization of the urine may help prevent uric acid stones and cystine stones.
  - ○ Calcium stones:
    1. Hydrochlorothiazide 25 to 50 mg qd in patients with type I absorptive hypercalciuria
    2. Decrease bowel absorption of calcium with cellulose phosphate 10 g/day in patients with type I absorptive hypercalciuria
    3. Orthophosphates to inhibit vitamin B synthesis in patients with type III absorptive hypercalciuria
    4. Potassium citrate supplementation for patients with hypocitraturic calcium nephrolithiasis
    5. Purine dietary restrictions or allopurinol for patients with hyperuricosuric calcium nephrolithiasis
    6. Paradoxically, calcium restriction is not warranted for patients who have had calcium stones and may even be harmful
  - ○ Struvite stones:
    1. Most of these stones are large and cause obstruction and bleeding.
    2. Extracorporeal shock wave lithotripsy (ESWL) and percutaneous nephrolithotomy are generally necessary. Percutaneous nephrolithotomy is very effective for large stones in the kidney and is especially indicated for struvite stones.
    3. The prolonged use of antibiotics directed against the predominant urinary tract organism may be beneficial to prevent recurrence.
  - ○ Cystine stones: hydration and alkalinization of the urine to pH >6.5; penicillamine

and tiopronin can be used to reduce the formation of cystine; captopril is also beneficial and causes fewer side effects.
- Possibly useful medications to help with the passage of distal ureteral stones of <10 mm in diameter are tamsulosin (alpha-adrenergic antagonist) and nifedipine (calcium channel blocker used for ureteral dilatation and relaxation). Side effects may include dizziness with tamsulosin and hypotension with nifedipine.
- Administer antibiotics if fever or pyuria (>5 to 20 leukocytes/high-power field) is present.
- Surgical treatment for patients with severe pain that is unresponsive to medication and patients with persistent fever or nausea or significant impediment of urine flow:
  - ○ Ureteroscopic stone extraction. Indications for percutaneous nephrolithotomy are described in Table E1-407.
  - ○ ESWL for most renal stones. In 2011 the European Association of Urology recommended shock wave lithotripsy as first-line therapy for non-lower pole renal calculi <2 cm in diameter and for lower pole renal calculi <1 cm in diameter. Several types of lithotripters are in clinical use and differ from one another primarily in the way they generate shock waves. Contraindications to shock wave lithotripsy include pregnancy, active UTI, coagulopathies, and distal obstruction. Spinal or orthopedic deformities and morbid obesity may also preclude lithotripsy due to inability to properly position patient or inadequate visualization of the stone.
- Fig. E1-864 describes the management of ureteral stones.
- In 1997, the American Urological Association issued the following guidelines for the treatment of ureteral stones:
  - ○ Proximal ureteral stones <1 cm in diameter: the options are ESWL, percutaneous nephroureterolithotomy, and ureteroscopy.
  - ○ Proximal ureteral stones >1 cm in diameter: the options are ESWL, percutaneous nephroureterolithotomy, and ureteroscopy. The placement of a ureteral stent should be considered if the stone is causing high-grade obstruction.
  - ○ Distal ureteral stones <1 cm in diameter: most of these stones pass spontaneously. ESWL and ureteroscopy are two accepted modes of therapy.
  - ○ Distal ureteral stones >1 cm in diameter: the options are watchful waiting, ESWL, and ureteroscopy (after stone fragmentation).

Fig. E1-864 describes an approach to the management of ureteral calculi.

CHRONIC Rx

The maintenance of proper hydration and dietary restrictions (see "Acute General Rx")

DISPOSITION

- >50% of patients will pass the stone within 48 hr.
- Stones will recur in approximately 50% of patients within 5 yr if no medical treatment is provided.

REFERRAL

A urology referral should be undertaken for patients with complicated or recurrent urolithiasis. Most patients with small uncomplicated ureteral or renal calculi can be followed up as outpatients, whereas patients with persistent vomiting, suspected urinary tract infection, pain that is unresponsive to oral analgesics, or obstructing calculus associated with a solitary kidney should be admitted.

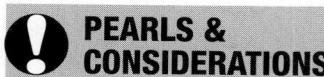
PEARLS & CONSIDERATIONS

COMMENTS

- The early identification and aggressive treatment of urinary tract infections is indicated for all patients with struvite stones.
- The alkalinization of urine (i.e., getting to a pH of >7.5 with the use of penicillamine) is useful for patients with recurrent cystine stones.
- Stones <5 mm in diameter often pass spontaneously whereas stones >10 mm generally do not.
- An algorithmic approach to the management of ureteral calculi is described in Fig. E1-864.

SUGGESTED READINGS
available at www.expertconsult.com

RELATED CONTENT
Urinary Tract Infection (Patient Information)
Kidney Stones (Patient Information)

AUTHORS: **PHILIP J. ALIOTTA, M.D., M.S.H.A.,** and **RUBEN ALVERO, M.D.**

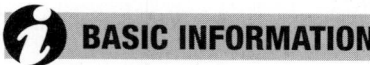

DEFINITION

Urticaria is a pruritic rash involving the epidermis and the upper portions of the dermis caused by localized capillary vasodilation and followed by transudation of protein-rich fluid in the surrounding tissue and manifesting clinically with the presence of hives. Urticaria is classified according to its chronicity into acute (<6-wk duration) and chronic (>6-wk duration).

SYNONYMS

Hives
Wheals

ICD-9CM CODES
708.8 Other unspecified urticaria

EPIDEMIOLOGY & DEMOGRAPHICS

- 15% to 20% of the population will have one episode of hives during their lifetime.
- Incidence is increased in atopic patients.
- The etiology of chronic urticaria (hives lasting >6 wk) is determined in only 5% to 20% of cases.

PHYSICAL FINDINGS & CLINICAL PRESENTATION

- Presence of elevated, erythematous, or white nonpitting plaques that change in size and shape over time; they generally last a few hours and disappear without a trace.
- Annular configuration with central pallor (Fig. 1-865).
- Angioedema occurs in approximately 40% of cases of urticaria and is caused by mast cell mediator release in the subcutaneous tissue and deep dermis.

ETIOLOGY

- Foods (e.g., shellfish, eggs, strawberries, nuts)
- Drugs (e.g., penicillin, aspirin, sulfonamides)
- Systemic diseases (e.g., systemic lupus erythematosus, serum sickness, autoimmune thyroid disease, polycythemia vera)
- Food additives (e.g., salicylates, benzoates, sulfites)
- Infections (viral infections, fungal infections, chronic bacterial infections); viral upper

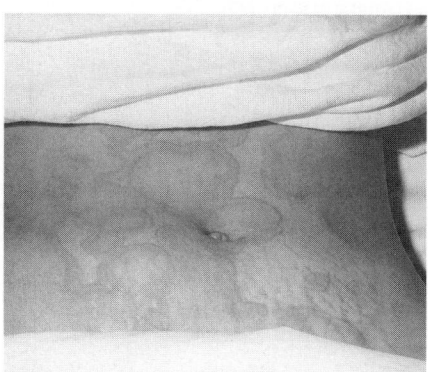

FIGURE 1-865 Wheal (urticaria). Note central clearing, giving annular configuration. (From Noble J et al: *Textbook of primary care medicine,* ed 3, St Louis, 2001, Mosby.)

respiratory infections are the predominant cause

- Physical stimuli (e.g., pressure urticaria, exercise-induced, solar urticaria, cold urticaria)
- Inhalants (e.g., mold spores, animal dander, pollens)
- Contact (nonimmunologic) urticaria (e.g., caterpillars, plants)
- Other: hereditary angioedema, urticaria pigmentosa, pregnancy, cryoglobulinemia, hair bleaches, chemicals, saliva, cosmetics, perfumes, pemphigoid, emotional stress, malignancy (lymphomas, endocrine tumors)
- Idiopathic urticaria is diagnosed in 50% of patients with chronic urticaria.

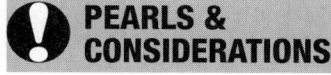 **DIAGNOSIS**

DIFFERENTIAL DIAGNOSIS

- Erythema multiforme
- Erythema marginatum
- Erythema infectiosum
- Urticarial vasculitis
- Herpes gestationis
- Drug eruption
- Multiple insect bites
- Bullous pemphigoid

WORKUP

- It is useful to determine whether hives are acute or chronic; a medical history focused on various etiologic factors is necessary before embarking on extensive laboratory testing.
- Most cases of acute urticaria resolve spontaneously and diagnostic testing is not required. However, in patients with acute urticaria it is crucial to rule out anaphylaxis.
- A diagnostic approach to chronic urticaria is described in Fig. E1-866.

LABORATORY TESTS

- Complete blood count with differential.
- Stool for ova and parasites in patients with chronic urticaria and suspected parasitic infestations.
- Skin testing with allergic extracts and screening for dermatographism by attempting to elicit a wheal after application of linear skin pressure should be performed only after withholding antihistamines for 36 to 72 hr to prevent false-negative results.
- Antinuclear antibody, erythrocyte sedimentation rate, thyroid-stimulating hormone, antithyroid antibodies, *Helicobacter pylori* serology, liver function tests, and eosinophil count are indicated only in patients with chronic urticaria. However, even with extensive testing, the cause of chronic urticaria is rarely established.
- Measurement of C_4 may be helpful in patients who present with angioedema alone. In these patients, C1 inhibitor deficiency should be considered.
- Skin biopsy is helpful in patients with fever, arthralgias, and elevated erythrocyte sedimentation rate. Histologic evidence of leukocytoclasia (neutrophilic infiltration with fragmentation of nuclei) is indicative of urticarial vasculitis.
- When food allergy is suspected in acute urticaria, testing can be performed using skin prick, immunoCAP, and radioallergosorbent testing.

 TREATMENT

NONPHARMACOLOGIC THERAPY

- Remove suspected etiologic agents (e.g., stop aspirin and all nonessential drugs), and restrict diet (e.g., elimination of tomatoes, nuts, eggs, shellfish).
- Elimination of yeast should be attempted in patients with chronic urticaria (*Candida albicans* sensitivity may be a factor in patients with chronic urticaria).

ACUTE GENERAL Rx

- Oral antihistamines: use of nonsedating antihistamines (e.g., loratadine 10 mg qd, cetirizine 10 mg qd, fexofenadine 180 mg qd, levocetirizine 5 mg qd) is preferred over first-generation antihistamines (e.g., hydroxyzine, diphenhydramine).
- Doxepin (a tricyclic antidepressant that blocks both H_1 and H_2 receptors) 25 to 75 mg qhs may be effective in patients with chronic urticaria.
- Oral corticosteroids should be reserved for refractory cases (e.g., prednisone 20 mg qd or 20 mg bid).
- H_2 receptor antagonists (cimetidine, ranitidine, famotidine) can be added to H_1 antagonists in refractory cases.

CHRONIC Rx

- Use of nonsedating antihistamines, doxepin, and/or oral corticosteroids (see "Acute General Rx").
- Low dose of the immunosuppressant cyclosporine (2.5 to 3 mg/kg body weight/day) has been shown to be effective and corticosteroid sparing in chronic urticaria. Algorithms for the evaluation and management of chronic urticaria are described in Figs. E1-867 and E1-868, respectively.
- Omalizumab, a monoclonal antibody that inactivates free IgE and down-regulates surface IgE receptors, has been shown effective in trials for refractory chronic urticaria. It is, however, expensive and not currently FDA approved for this indication.
- There are insufficient data to support use of leukotriene antagonists (zafirlukast, montelukast) in patients with chronic urticaria.

DISPOSITION

- Most cases of urticaria resolve within 6 wk.
- Only 25% of patients with a history of chronic urticaria are completely cured after 5 yr.

PEARLS & CONSIDERATIONS

COMMENTS

Local treatment (e.g., starch baths or oatmeal baths) may be helpful in selected patients; however, local treatment is generally not rewarding.

SUGGESTED READINGS
available at www.expertconsult.com

RELATED CONTENT
Hives (Patient Information)
AUTHOR: **FRED F. FERRI, M.D.**

BASIC INFORMATION

DEFINITION

Uterine fibroids are benign tumors of muscle cell origin. They are discrete nodular tumors that vary in size and number and that may be found as subserosal, intramural, or submucosal masses. They can also be located in the cervix, broad ligament, or on a stalk (pedunculated) (Fig. 1-869). They can also be parasitic, acquiring a blood supply from a nonuterine source.

SYNONYMS

Uterine leiomyomas
Uterine myomas

ICD-9CM CODES
218.9 Leiomyomas, fibroids

EPIDEMIOLOGY & DEMOGRAPHICS

- Estimated prevalence of 20% to 40% of reproductive age women
- The most common benign uterine tumor
- More common in black women than white women
- Asymptomatic fibroids may be present in 40% to 50% of women aged >40 yr
- May occur singly but are often multiple
- Less than half of all fibroids are estimated to produce symptoms
- Frequently diagnosed incidentally on pelvic examination
- There is increased familial incidence
- Potential to enlarge during pregnancy as well as regress after menopause
- Infrequent primary cause of infertility in <3% of infertile patients
- Symptomatic fibroids are the primary indication for approximately 30% of all hysterectomies

PHYSICAL FINDINGS & CLINICAL PRESENTATION

- Enlarged, irregular uterus on pelvic examination

- Presenting symptoms:
  1. Menorrhagia (most common)
  2. Chronic pelvic pain (dysmenorrhea, dyspareunia, pelvic pressure)
  3. Acute pain (torsion of pedunculated fibroid, infarction, and degeneration)
  4. Urinary symptoms (frequency from bladder pressure, partial ureteral obstruction, complete ureteral obstruction)
  5. Rectosigmoid compression with constipation or intestinal obstruction
  6. Prolapse through cervix of pedunculated submucosal tumor
  7. Venous stasis of lower extremities
  8. Polycythemia
  9. Ascites

ETIOLOGY

Incompletely understood. It is suggested that fibroids arise from an original single smooth muscle cell in the myometrium. Each individual fibroid is monoclonal (all the cells are derived from one progenitor myocyte). Malignant degeneration of preexisting leiomyoma is extremely uncommon (<0.5%).

DIAGNOSIS

DIFFERENTIAL DIAGNOSIS

Leiomyosarcoma, ovarian mass (neoplastic, non-neoplastic, endometrioma), inflammatory mass, pregnancy

WORKUP

- Complete pelvic examination, rectovaginal examination, Pap test
- Estimation of size of mass in centimeters and location of fibroids
- Endometrial sampling may be indicated (biopsy or dilation and curettage) when abnormal bleeding and pelvic mass are present
- If urinary symptoms are prominent, cystometry, cystoscopy to rule out bladder lesions, intravenous pyelogram to rule out impingement on urinary system

LABORATORY TESTS

- Pregnancy test
- Pap smear
- Complete blood count, erythrocyte sedimentation rate
- Fecal occult blood

IMAGING STUDIES

- Pelvic ultrasound (Fig. 1-870) is useful as a primary diagnostic modality. Transvaginal ultrasound commonly has higher diagnostic accuracy.
- MRI scan is helpful in planning treatment if malignancy is strongly suspected. Also important to localize fibroids, especially if myomectomy is contemplated. Size, number, and location of fibroids are also important if a minimally invasive myomectomy is considered.
- Saline infusion sonography is helpful in determining location and degree of intrusion into uterine cavity. Important if hysteroscopic resection is contemplated. Typically at least 50% of the fibroid must be intracavitary for a hysteroscopic approach to be successful.
- Hysteroscopy may provide direct evidence of intrauterine pathology or submucosal leiomyoma that distorts uterine cavity, and surgical resection may be performed during the same procedure.

TREATMENT

Management should be based on primary symptoms and may include observation with close follow-up, temporizing surgical therapies, embolization, medical management, or definitive surgical procedures. Treatment is generally indicated only when symptoms are present and are severe enough to be unacceptable to the patient.

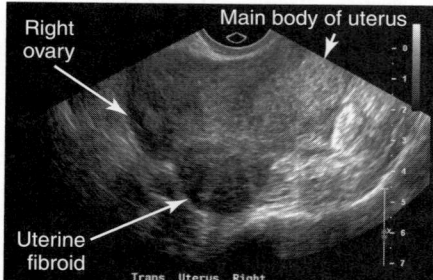

FIGURE 1-870 Fibroid uterus: endovaginal ultrasound. Ultrasound is the primary modality used for evaluation of uterine fibroids (leiomyomas). Typical features include a well-circumscribed appearance. Fibroids may be hypoechoic or hyperechoic relative to the uterus. They may be exophytic or intramural, or they may project into the uterine cavity. Malignant uterine tumors may invade adjacent structures, whereas a fibroid is contained within the uterine serosa. Uterine tumors, both benign and malignant, can show central necrosis, which usually appears hypoechoic with ultrasound. In this 38-year-old woman, the fibroid is exophytic. The right ovary lies adjacent and is difficult to distinguish in this case. (From Broder JS: *Diagnostic imaging for the emergency physician,* Philadelphia, 2011, Saunders.)

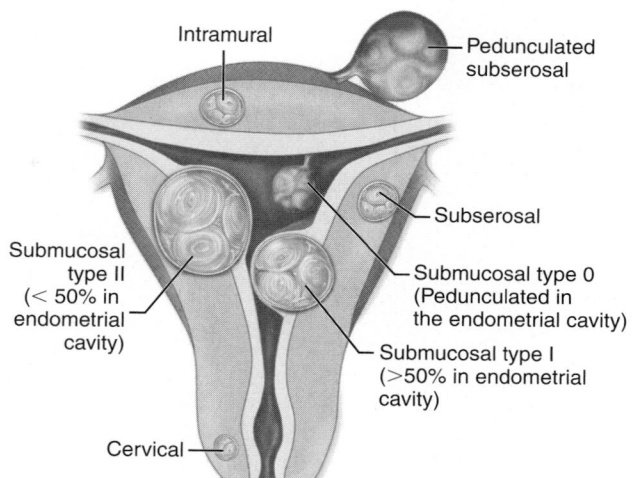

FIGURE 1-869 Drawing of uterus in the coronal plane, illustrating possible location of uterine leiomyomas. (From Fielding JR et al: *Gynecologic imaging,* Philadelphia, 2011, Saunders.)

NONSURGICAL Rx

- Patient observation and follow-up with periodic repeat pelvic examinations to ensure that tumors are not growing rapidly.
- Gonadotropin-releasing hormone (GnRH) agonist use results in 40% to 60% reduction in uterine volume. Hypoestrogenism, reversible bone loss, and hot flushes are associated with use. Limit to short-term use and consider low-dose hormonal replacement to minimize hypoestrogenic effects.
- Regrowth occurs in approximately 50% of women treated within a few months after cessation.
- Indications for GnRH:
  1. Fertility preservation in women with large myomas before attempting conception or preoperative myectomy treatment
  2. Anemia treatment to normalize hemoglobin before surgery
  3. Women approaching menopause to avoid surgery
  4. Preoperative for large myomas to make vaginal hysterectomy, hysteroscopic resection/ablation, or laparoscopic destruction more feasible
  5. Women with medical contraindications for surgery
  6. Personal or medical indications for delaying surgery
- Use of GnRH agonists may alter the consistency of the fibroid, making myomectomy more challenging.
- Progestational agents may also result in decrease in uterine size and amenorrhea, allowing iron therapy to treat anemia with limited success. Ulipristal acetate is a selective progesterone-receptor modulator that acts on progesterone receptors in myometrial and endometrial tissue and inhibits ovulation without causing large effects on estradiol levels or antiglucocorticoid activity. Recent trials have shown that treatment with ulipristal acetate for 13 wk effectively controlled excessive bleeding due to uterine fibroids and reduced the size of the fibroids.
- Other drugs used and under investigation:
  1. Danazol: androgen and multienzyme inhibitor of steroidogenesis
  2. Mifepristone: antiprogestogen shown to reduce the fibroid volume by 40% to 50% with amenorrhea
  3. Raloxifene: selective estrogen receptor modulator, either alone or with a GnRHa, shown to reduce the fibroid volume 70% up to 1 yr but only in postmenopausal women
  4. Fadrozole: aromatase inhibitor reported to have produced a 71% reduction in volume

SURGICAL Rx

- Indications
  1. Abnormal uterine bleeding with anemia refractory to hormonal therapy
  2. Chronic pain with severe dysmenorrhea, dyspareunia, or lower abdominal pressure/pain
  3. Acute pain, torsion, or prolapsing submucosal fibroid
  4. Urinary symptoms or signs such as hydronephrosis
  5. Rapid uterine enlargement premenopausal or any growth after menopause
  6. Infertility or recurrent pregnancy loss with submucous leiomyoma as only finding
  7. Enlarged uterus with compression symptoms or discomfort
- Procedures
  1. Hysterectomy (definitive procedure): Nearly 15% of women with uterine fibroids and a mean age of 45 yr require hysterectomy
  2. Abdominal myomectomy (to preserve fertility)
  3. Vaginal myomectomy for prolapsed pedunculated submucous fibroid
  4. Hysteroscopic resection
  5. Laparoscopic/robotic myomectomy
  6. Uterine artery embolization (UAE): safe and effective short-term alternative to surgery, but its less invasive nature should be balanced against a higher rate for treatment failure or complications at 5 yr (32%) versus the surgery group (4%). Age 40 years and under at embolization and history of previous myomectomy are significant predictors of embolization failure.

COMPLICATIONS

- Red degeneration
- Leiomyosarcoma ($<0.1\%$)

REFERRAL

Consultation with gynecologic oncologist if suspicion of malignancy

SUGGESTED READINGS

available at www.expertconsult.com

RELATED CONTENT

Dysfunctional Uterine Bleeding (Related Key Topic)
Premature Labor (Related Key Topic)
Uterine Fibroids (Patient Information)

AUTHORS: **ARUNDATHI G. PRASAD, M.D.,** and **RUBEN ALVERO, M.D.**

BASIC INFORMATION

DEFINITION

Uterine malignancy includes tumors from the endometrium and sarcomas. Uterine sarcoma is an abnormal proliferation of cells originating from the mesenchymal, or connective tissue, elements of the uterine wall.

SYNONYMS

Leiomyosarcomas
Endometrial stromal sarcoma
Malignant mixed Müllerian tumors
Adenosarcomas

ICD-9CM CODES

182.0 Malignant neoplasm of body of uterus (corpus uteri), except isthmus
182.1 Malignant neoplasm of body of uterus, isthmus
182.8 Malignant neoplasm of body of uterus, other specified sites of body of uterus

---

BOX 1-79   Risk Factors for Uterine Sarcoma

Nulliparity
Obesity
History of pelvic radiation
Exposure to tamoxifen

From Fielding JR et al: *Gynecologic imaging*, Philadelphia, 2011, Saunders.

BOX 1-80   Uterine Sarcoma Prognostic Factors

Tumor stage
Tumor grade
Tumor size
Patient age
Vascular space involvement
Mitotic count
Residual disease at surgery
Adjuvant chemotherapy

From Fielding JR et al: *Gynecologic imaging*, Philadelphia, 2011, Saunders.

EPIDEMIOLOGY & DEMOGRAPHICS

INCIDENCE: 17.1 cases per 1 million females. Endometrial cancer remains the most common gynecologic malignancy in the U.S.
PREVALENCE: Uterine sarcoma accounts for 4.3% of all cancers of the uterine corpus and is the most lethal gynecologic malignancy.
MEAN AGE AT DIAGNOSIS: 52 yr
RISK FACTORS: Box 1-79 describes risk factors for uterine sarcoma

PHYSICAL FINDINGS & CLINICAL PRESENTATION

- Abnormal vaginal bleeding is the most common symptom
- May also present as pelvic pain or pressure and pelvic mass on examination
- May appear as tumor protruding through the cervix
- Vaginal discharge may also be a presenting symptom
- Rapidly enlarging uterus

ETIOLOGY

- The exact etiology is unknown.
- Prior pelvic radiation is a risk factor for sarcoma.
- Black women may be at higher risk.

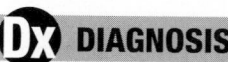

DIAGNOSIS

DIFFERENTIAL DIAGNOSIS

Leiomyoma

WORKUP

Diagnosis is made histologically by biopsy for abnormal bleeding.

BOX 1-81   Uterine Sarcoma: Key Points

The disease mainly affects postmenopausal women.
Most patients present early with postmenopausal bleeding.
The primary treatment is hysterectomy.
Adjuvant radiotherapy to the pelvis is used if poor prognosis features in stage 1 or if spread has occurred beyond the corpus.

From Greer IA et al: *Mosby's color atlas and text of obstetrics and gynecology*, London, 2001, Harcourt.

LABORATORY TESTS

Chest radiography, CT scans, and MRI are used to evaluate metastatic lesions.

IMAGING STUDIES

- Chest x-ray is usually done as routine preoperative testing.
- CT scans (Fig. E1-871) and MRI are useful for assessing tumor spread once diagnosis is made.

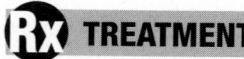

TREATMENT

NONPHARMACOLOGIC THERAPY

- Surgical excision is the mainstay of treatment.
- Grade and stage of tumor affect prognosis.
- The benefit of adjuvant radiotherapy in stage I endometrial adenocarcinoma to improve pelvic disease control and improve survival remains controversial despite several phase 3 trials.
- Chemotherapeutic agents have produced only partial and short-term responses.

DISPOSITION

- Survival varies with each type of sarcoma but is generally very poor. Box 1-80 describes uterine prognostic factors.
- Five-year survival for leiomyosarcoma ranges from 48% for stage I to 0% for stage IV.
- Five-year survival for malignant mixed mesodermal tumor ranges from 36% for stage I to 6% for stage IV.

REFERRAL

Uterine sarcoma should be managed by a gynecologic oncologist and radiation oncologist. Key points in the management of uterine sarcoma are described in Box 1-81.

SUGGESTED READINGS
available at www.expertconsult.com

RELATED CONTENT

Endometrial Cancer (Related Key Topic)
Uterine Cancer (Patient Information)

AUTHORS: **GIL M. FARKASH, M.D.,** and **RUBEN ALVERO, M.D.**

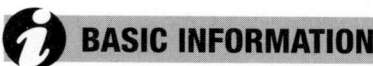

DEFINITION

Uveitis is inflammation of the uveal tract, including the iris, ciliary body, and choroid. It may also involve other closed structures such as the sclera, retina, and vitreous humor (Fig. E1-872).

SYNONYMS

Anterior uveitis
Posterior uveitis
Acute or chronic uveitis
Granulomatous or nongranulomatous uveitis
Iritis
Choroiditis
Pars planitis
Iridocyclitis

ICD-9CM CODES
364.3 Unspecified iridocyclitis, uveitis

EPIDEMIOLOGY & DEMOGRAPHICS

INCIDENCE (IN U.S.): Common; busy ophthalmologist will see two or more cases per week.
PEAK INCIDENCE: Middle age or older.
PREVALENCE (IN U.S.): 17 cases per 100,000 persons
PREDOMINANT SEX: None
PREDOMINANT AGE: 38 yr. Although uveitis is less common in children than adults, it is believed to be more severe with an increased risk for vision-threatening complications.

PHYSICAL FINDINGS & CLINICAL PRESENTATION

- Symptoms of uveitis depend on the site of involvement and whether process is acute or insidious:
  - Acute anterior uveitis: pain and photophobia. Vision may not be affected initially.
  - Posterior uveitis: floaters, hazy vision. Involvement of the retina may produce blind spots or flashing lights.
  - Insidious anterior uveitis: symptoms may not be present until scarring cataracts and loss of vision occur.
- Photophobia
- Blurred visual acuity
- Irregular pupil
- Hazy cornea
- Abnormal cells and flare in anterior chamber or vitreous humor ("flare cells") note with slit lamp examination
- Retinal hemorrhage, vascular sheathing
- Conjunctival injection
- Ciliary flush
- Keratitic precipitates (precipitates on the cornea)
- Hazy vitreous
- Retinal inflammation
- Iris nodules

ETIOLOGY

- Infections: herpes simplex virus, cytomegalovirus, toxoplasmosis, tuberculosis, syphilis, HIV
- Systemic disorders: sarcoidosis, Behçet's syndrome, HLA-B27–associated diseases (e.g., ankylosing spondylitis, reactive arthritis), inflammatory bowel disease, juvenile idiopathic arthritis
- There is also an association between oral bisphosphonates and uveitis, with risk of uveitis being 50% higher among new bisphosphonate users than among nonusers.
- Idiopathic (>50% of patients)

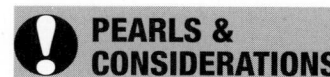 **DIAGNOSIS**

DIFFERENTIAL DIAGNOSIS

- Glaucoma
- Conjunctivitis
- Retinal detachment
- Retinopathy
- Keratitis
- Scleritis
- Episcleritis
- Masquerading syndromes: lymphoma, uveal melanoma, metastases (breast, lung, renal), leukemia, retinitis pigmentosa, retinoblastoma

WORKUP

- Slit lamp examination, indirect ophthalmoscopy
- Visual field testing

LABORATORY TESTS

- Complete blood count
- Laboratory tests for specific inflammatory causes cited previously in "Workup" (e.g., antinuclear antibody, erythrocyte sedimentation rate, syphilis (VDRL), HLA-B27, purified protein derivative, Lyme titer)

IMAGING STUDIES

- Chest radiograph in suspected sarcoidosis, tuberculosis, histoplasmosis
- Sacroiliac radiograph in suspected ankylosing spondylitis

TREATMENT

ACUTE GENERAL Rx

- Corticosteroids are the mainstay of therapy for noninfectious causes. The route of administration depends on the location of inflammation, the severity, and the presence of systemic disease. Cycloplegic drops (cyclopentolate) or cycloplegic agents (homatropine hydrobromide 1 gtt q3 to 4h while awake) and topical steroids (prednisone acetate 1% 1 gtt qh during day, prn at night until favorable response,

then q4 to 6h); avoid topical corticosteroids in infectious uveitis. Periocular corticosteroid injections can be used for posterior disease; they have the advantage of achieving high intraocular levels of steroids without the systemic side effects of oral corticosteroids.
- Antibiotics for bacterial infections and antiviral agents, when infection is suspected, should be started to prevent retinal damage.
- Systemic steroids if appropriate for the underlying disease. Systemic corticosteroid therapy is generally reserved for patients with systemic disorders and those with bilateral disease that is refractory to local medication or those with major ocular disability or retinitis.
- Antimetabolites when indicated. Immunosuppressive medications used in steroid-dependent or refractory uveitis include methotrexate, sulfasalazine, azathioprine, cyclosporine, and tacrolimus. These medications can have significant toxicity and should be prescribed only by physicians experienced with their use.
- High-dose IV daclizumab has been reported as effective in reducing active inflammation in active juvenile idiopathic arthritis (JIA)-associated anterior uveitis. Additional trials are needed to better assess efficacy and safety.

REFERRAL

Urgent referral to ophthalmologist for diagnosis and treatment

PEARLS & CONSIDERATIONS

COMMENTS

Chronic anterior uveitis is the most common form of intraocular inflammation in children. JIA is the most common cause.

SUGGESTED READINGS
available at www.expertconsult.com

AUTHORS: **MELVYN KOBY, M.D.,** and **FRED F. FERRI, M.D.**

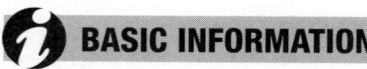

BASIC INFORMATION

DEFINITION

Bleeding per vagina at any time during pregnancy must be regarded as abnormal and is associated with an increased likelihood of pregnancy complications.

SYNONYMS

Hemorrhage

ICD-9CM CODES

634.9	Spontaneous abortion
633.9	Ectopic pregnancy
630/631	Molar pregnancy
640.0	Threatened abortion
622.7	Cervical polyps
180.9/180.0/180.8	Cervical dysplasia/cancer
616.0	Cervicitis
616.10	Vulvovaginitis
184.0	Vaginal cancer
644.2	Early onset of delivery
641.1	Placenta previa
641.2	Placental abruption

EPIDEMIOLOGY & DEMOGRAPHICS

- Common in U.S.; 20% to 25% of patients have vaginal spotting/bleeding in first trimester; of those, miscarriage occurs in 50%.
- Occurs in women of childbearing age.
- Between 1% and 2% of all pregnancies in the U.S. are ectopic.
- After one ectopic pregnancy, the chance of another is 7% to 15%.
- Ectopic pregnancy is the leading cause of maternal mortality in the first trimester.
- Average reported frequency for placental abruption is about 1 in 150 deliveries (0.3%).
- Incidence of placenta previa is <1 in 200 deliveries (0.5%).

PHYSICAL FINDINGS & CLINICAL PRESENTATION

- Bleeding: ranges from scant to life-threatening with hemodynamic instability
- Color: brown to bright red
- Can be painless or painful (cramps, back pain, severe abdominal pain)
- Fetal compromise: ranges from none to fetal demise

ETIOLOGY

- Influenced by gestational age
- Vaginal
- Cervical
- Uterine

DIAGNOSIS

DIFFERENTIAL DIAGNOSIS

- Any gestational age:
  1. Cervical lesions: polyps, decidual reaction, neoplasia
  2. Vaginal trauma
  3. Cervicitis/vulvovaginitis
  4. Postcoital trauma
  5. Bleeding dyscrasias
- Gestation <20 wk:
  1. Spontaneous abortion
  2. Presence of intrauterine device
  3. Ectopic pregnancy
  4. Molar pregnancy
  5. Implantation bleeding
  6. Low-lying placenta
- Gestation >20 wk:
  1. Molar pregnancy
  2. Placenta previa
  3. Placental abruption
  4. Vasa previa
  5. Marginal separation of the placenta
  6. Bloody show at term
  7. Preterm labor
- Section II describes the differential diagnosis of vaginal bleeding in pregnancy.

WORKUP

- Gestation <20 wk (Section III, "Bleeding, Early Pregnancy")
  1. Pelvic examination
  2. Culdocentesis
  3. Laparoscopy
  4. Laparotomy
  5. Ultrasound to verify viable intrauterine pregnancy
- Gestation >20 wk:
  1. Ultrasound to locate placenta before pelvic examination
  2. If placenta previa, no speculum or bimanual examination
  3. If preterm labor, appropriate evaluation done

LABORATORY TESTS

- Urine pregnancy test: if positive, get quantitative β human chorionic gonadotropin (hCG). The following are typical although not entirely exclusive patterns:
  1. Early pregnancy: follow serially every 48 hr
  2. Normal pregnancy: hCG doubles approximately every 48 hr
  3. Spontaneous abortion: hCG level will fall
  4. Ectopic pregnancy: hCG level will rise inappropriately
  5. Molar pregnancy: hCG level is extremely high

- CBC
- Blood type and screen (Rh-negative patients need RhoGAM)
- Coagulation profile (useful in missed abortion and abruption)
- Cervical cultures/wet mount
- Pap smear for cervical malignancy; caution with biopsy, because cervix can bleed extensively

IMAGING STUDIES

Ultrasound:
- 5 to 6 wk: gestational sac (transvaginally); hCG >1500 mIU/ml is discriminatory level for seeing a singleton gestation
- 6 to 7 wk: fetal cardiac activity
- Molar pregnancy: characteristic cluster of cysts
- Location of placenta
- Degree of placental separation: difficult to assess
- Evidence of subchorionic hemorrhage

TREATMENT

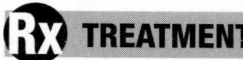

NONPHARMACOLOGIC THERAPY

- Pelvic rest: no coitus, douching, or tampons
- Bed rest, if >20 wk
- Counseling: genetic, bereavement

ACUTE GENERAL Rx

- Hemodynamic stabilization
- Emergency D&C, laparotomy, or cesarean section as necessary

CHRONIC Rx

Depends on diagnosis

DISPOSITION

Depends on diagnosis

REFERRAL

- If patient is unstable and needs emergency ob/gyn management and/or surgery
- If patient has diagnosis of ectopic or molar pregnancy, because immediate surgical treatment is indicated
- Perinatal consultation for high-risk pregnancy

SUGGESTED READING

available at www.expertconsult.com

RELATED CONTENT

Abruptio Placentae (Related Key Topic)
Ectopic Pregnancy (Related Key Topic)
Molar Pregnancy (Related Key Topic)
Placenta Previa (Related Key Topic)
Sheehan's Syndrome (Related Key Topic)
Spontaneous Miscarriage (Related Key Topic)

AUTHORS: **GEORGE T. DANAKAS, M.D.,** and **RUBEN ALVERO, M.D.**

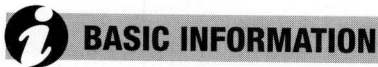

BASIC INFORMATION

DEFINITION
Vaginal malignancy is an abnormal proliferation of vaginal epithelium demonstrating malignant cells below the basement membrane.

SYNONYMS
Squamous cell carcinoma of the vagina
Adenocarcinoma of the vagina
Melanoma of the vagina
Sarcoma of the vagina
Endodermal sinus tumor

ICD-9CM CODES
184.0 Vagina, vaginal neoplasm

EPIDEMIOLOGY & DEMOGRAPHICS
INCIDENCE: 0.42 cases per 100,000 persons
PREVALENCE: Vaginal cancer is the second rarest gynecologic cancer. It comprises 2% of malignancies of the female genital tract.
MEAN AGE AT DIAGNOSIS: Predominantly a disease of menopause. Mean age at diagnosis is 60 yr.

PHYSICAL FINDINGS & CLINICAL PRESENTATION
- Majority of cases are asymptomatic
- Postmenopausal vaginal bleeding and/or vaginal discharge are the most common symptoms
- May also present as pelvic pain or pressure, dyspareunia, dysuria, malodor, or postcoital bleeding
- May present as a vaginal lesion or abnormal Pap smear

ETIOLOGY
- The exact etiology is unknown.
- Vaginal intraepithelial neoplasia is believed to be a precursor for squamous cell carcinoma of the vagina.
- Long-term pessary use has been associated with vaginal malignancy.
- Prior pelvic radiation may be a risk factor.
- Clear-cell adenocarcinoma is related to in utero diethylstilbestrol exposure.

DIAGNOSIS

DIFFERENTIAL DIAGNOSIS
- Extension from other primary carcinoma more common than primary vaginal cancer
- Vaginitis

WORKUP
- Diagnosis is made histologically by biopsy.
- Colposcopy and biopsy should follow suspicious Pap smear.
- Cystoscopy, proctosigmoidoscopy, chest radiography, IV urography, and barium enema may be used for clinical staging.
- CT scan (Fig. 1-873), FDG, PET scan, and MRI are used to evaluate spread.
- Staging I to IV (Fig. 1-874).

IMAGING STUDIES
- Chest radiography, IV urography, and barium enema are used for staging.
- CT scan and MRI are good for assessing tumor spread.

TREATMENT

NONPHARMACOLOGIC THERAPY
- Radiation therapy is the mainstay of treatment.
- Stage I tumors that are small and confined to the posterior, upper third of the vagina may be treated with radical surgery.
- Other stages require a whole-pelvis, interstitial, and/or intracavitary radiation therapy.
- Chemotherapy is used in conjunction with radiotherapy in rare select cases.

DISPOSITION
Five-year survival ranges from 80% for stage I to 17% for stage IV.

REFERRAL
Vaginal cancer should be managed by a gynecologic oncologist and radiation oncologist.

SUGGESTED READING
available at www.expertconsult.com

RELATED CONTENT
Vaginal Cancer (Patient Information)

AUTHORS: **GIL M. FARKASH, M.D.,** and **RUBEN ALVERO, M.D.**

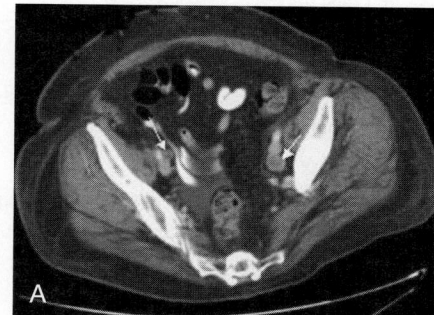
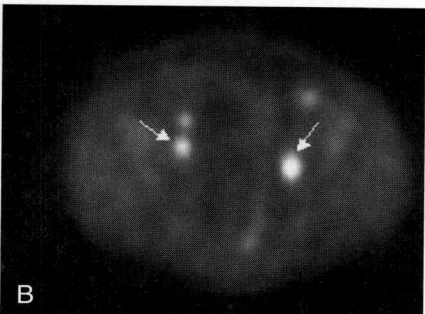

FIGURE 1-873 Vaginal cancer with lymphadenopathy. A, CT of pelvis showing mildly enlarged external iliac nodes suggestive of metastases *(arrows).* **B,** Axial FDG PET scan showing hypermetabolic nodes as hyperintense spots confirming metastases. (From Abeloff MD: *Clinical oncology,* ed 3, Philadelphia, 2004, Churchill Livingstone.)

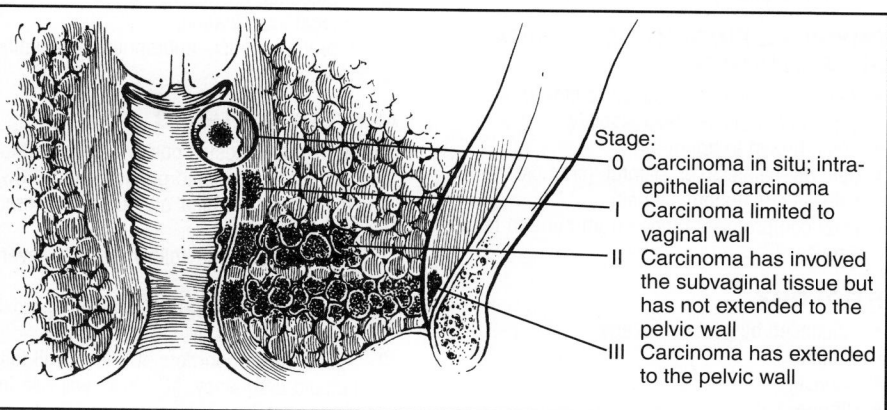

Stage:
0 Carcinoma in situ; intraepithelial carcinoma
I Carcinoma limited to vaginal wall
II Carcinoma has involved the subvaginal tissue but has not extended to the pelvic wall
III Carcinoma has extended to the pelvic wall

FIGURE 1-874 Staging system for vaginal cancer. Metastatic disease that involves the bladder or rectum is stage IV-a. Metastatic disease beyond the pelvis is stage IV-b. (From Copeland LJ: *Textbook of gynecology,* ed 2, Philadelphia, 2000, Saunders.)

BASIC INFORMATION

DEFINITION

Vaginismus refers to the involuntary spasm of the vaginal, introital, and/or levator ani muscles, preventing penetration or causing painful intercourse.

ICD-9CM CODES

300.11 Hysterical vaginismus
306.51 Psychogenic or functional vaginismus
625.1 Reflex vaginismus

EPIDEMIOLOGY & DEMOGRAPHICS

INCIDENCE: Estimated at 11.7% to 42% of women presenting to sexual dysfunction clinics
PREVALENCE: Affects approximately 1 in 200 women
PREDOMINANT SEX: Affects only females
RISK FACTORS: Any previous sexual trauma, including incest or rape

PHYSICAL FINDINGS & CLINICAL PRESENTATION

- Fear of pain with coitus
- Dyspareunia
- Orgasmic dysfunction

ETIOLOGY

- Learned conditioned response to real or imagined painful vaginal experience (e.g., traumatic speculum examination, incest, rape)
- Vaginitis
- Pelvic inflammatory disease
- Endometriosis
- Anatomic anomalies
- Atrophic vaginitis
- Mucosal tears
- Inadequate lubrication
- Focal vulvitis
- Painful hymenal tags
- Scarring secondary to episiotomy
- Skin disorders
- Topical allergies
- Postherpetic neuralgia

DIAGNOSIS

WORKUP

- Thorough history (including sexual history)
- Careful pelvic examination
- Behavioral therapy

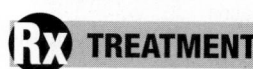

TREATMENT

NONPHARMACOLOGIC THERAPY

- Deconditioning the response by systematic self-administered progressive dilation techniques using fingers or dilators
- Behavioral and/or psychosexual therapy

ACUTE GENERAL Rx

- Botulinum toxin therapy given locally has been shown to relieve the perineal muscle spasms associated with vaginismus, allowing resumption of intercourse.
  1. Acts by preventing neuromuscular transmission, causing muscle weakness
  2. Considered experimental treatment for vaginismus at this time
- Cause should be determined by history and explained to the patient so that she understands the mechanics of the muscle spasms.
- Patient must be motivated to desire painless vaginal insertion for such reasons as pleasurable coitus, tampon insertion, or gynecologic examination.
- Patient (and her partner) must be willing to patiently undergo the process of systematic desensitization and counseling.

DISPOSITION

A high percentage of successfully treated patients

REFERRAL

To a gynecologist or sex therapist

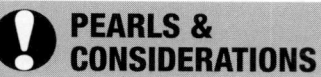

PEARLS & CONSIDERATIONS

COMMENTS

- May uncover early sexual abuse or an aversion to sexuality in general
- American Association of Sex Educators, Counselors and Therapists, 11 Dupont Circle, NW, Washington, DC, 20036.
- Sex Information and Education Council of the U.S. (SIECUS), 90 John St., New York, NY 10038.

SUGGESTED READINGS

available at www.expertconsult.com

AUTHORS: **BETH J. WUTZ, M.D.,** and **RUBEN ALVERO, M.D.**

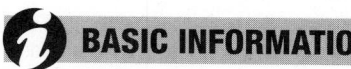

BASIC INFORMATION

DEFINITION

Bacterial vaginitis, also known as bacterial vaginosis (BV), is a polymicrobial infection affecting the vagina caused by anaerobic bacteria.

SYNONYMS

Bacterial vaginosis
BV
Gardnerella vaginalis
Haemophilus vaginalis
Corynebacterium vaginalis

ICD-9CM CODES

616.10 Vulvovaginitis

EPIDEMIOLOGY & DEMOGRAPHICS

- Most prevalent form of vaginal infection of reproductive age women in the U.S.
- 32% to 64% in patients visiting STD clinics
- 12% to 25% in other clinic populations
- 10% to 26% in patients visiting obstetric clinics
- More common in women with multiple sexual partners. Douching also increases risk.
- May be associated with adverse pregnancy outcomes: premature rupture of membranes, preterm labor, preterm birth
- Organisms frequently found in postpartum or postcesarean endometritis

PHYSICAL FINDINGS & CLINICAL PRESENTATION

- >50% of all women may be without symptoms.
- Unpleasant, fishy, or musty vaginal odor in about 50% to 70% of all patients. Odor exacerbated immediately after intercourse or during menstruation.
- Vaginal discharge is increased and may have a white or gray homogeneous appearance.
- Vaginal itching and irritation occur.

ETIOLOGY

- Synergistic polymicrobial infection characterized by an overgrowth of anaerobic bacteria normally found in the vagina with significant reduction of the normal vaginal hydrogen peroxide producing lactobacilli

- Anaerobes: *Bacteroides* spp., *Peptostreptococcus* spp., *Mobiluncus* spp.
- Facultative anaerobes: *G. vaginalis*, *Mycoplasma hominis*
- Concentration of anaerobic bacteria increased to 100 to 1000 times normal
- Lactobacilli are absent or greatly reduced

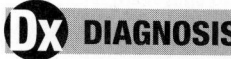

DIAGNOSIS

DIFFERENTIAL DIAGNOSIS

- Fungal vaginitis
- *Trichomonas* vaginitis
- Atrophic vaginitis
- Cervicitis

WORKUP

- Pelvic examination
- Speculum examination
- Normal saline and 10% KOH slide of discharge
- Amsel criteria for diagnosis (three of four should be present):
  1. pH >4.5
  2. Clue cells (epithelial cells covered with bacteria) on saline solution slide
  3. Positive whiff test on 10% KOH (fishy odor when KOH added to vaginal sample)
  4. Homogeneous, white, adherent discharge
- Sensitivity of Amsel criteria is >90%, specificity >75%.
- Section III, "Vaginal Discharge," describes the evaluation of discharge. Culture for *G. vaginalis* is not recommended in suspected BV (low specificity).

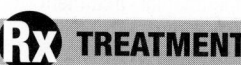

TREATMENT

ACUTE GENERAL Rx

- Metronidazole 500 mg PO bid × 7 days, >90% cure rate
- Metronidazole 2 g PO × 1 day, 67% to 92% cure rate
- Metronidazole gel 5 g, intravaginal bid × 5 days
- Clindamycin 2% cream 5 g, intravaginal qd × 7 days
- Clindamycin 300 mg PO bid × 7 days; cure rate similar to those achieved with metronidazole

- Good hygiene: avoidance of douching, harsh shower gels, bubble baths; cotton underwear

DISPOSITION

- Reevaluate if not cured with treatment
- Recurrence fairly common

REFERRAL

Refer to obstetrician/gynecologist for recurrence or pregnant patient with BV.

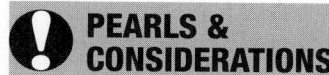

PEARLS & CONSIDERATIONS

COMMENTS

- Treating sexual partners has failed to demonstrate a benefit.
- Recurrence rate of BV is 30% within 3 months.

SUGGESTED READINGS

available at www.expertconsult.com

RELATED CONTENT

Candidiasis, Vulvovaginal (Related Key Topic)
Pruritus Vulvae (Related Key Topic)
Vaginitis, Fungal (Related Key Topic)
Vaginitis, Prepubescent (Related Key Topic)
Vaginitis, *Trichomonas* (Related Key Topic)
Vaginosis, Bacterial (Related Key Topic)
Bacterial Vaginal Infection (Patient Information)

AUTHORS: **JULIE ANNE SZUMIGALA, M.D.**, and **RUBEN ALVERO, M.D.**

BASIC INFORMATION

DEFINITION

Estrogen-deficient vulvovaginitis is the irritation and/or inflammation of the vulva and vagina because of progressive thinning and atrophic changes secondary to estrogen deficiency (Fig. 1-875).

SYNONYMS

Atrophic vaginitis
Vulvovaginal atrophy

ICD-9CM CODES
616.10 Vulvovaginitis

EPIDEMIOLOGY & DEMOGRAPHICS

- Seen most often in postmenopausal women
- Average age of menopause is 52 yr
- Up to half of postmenopausal women are symptomatic, but a quarter of these will not seek treatment

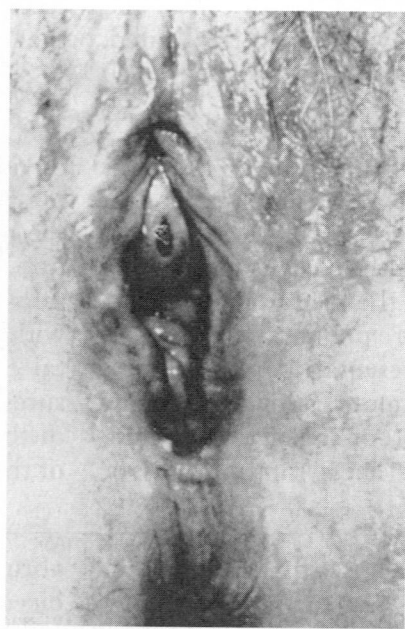

FIGURE 1-875 Advanced postmenopausal atrophy of the vulva in a 72-year-old woman. (From Symonds EM, Macpherson MBA: *Color atlas of obstetrics and gynecology,* St Louis, 1994, Mosby.)

PHYSICAL FINDINGS & CLINICAL PRESENTATION

- Thinning of pubic hair, labia minora and majora
- Decreased secretions from the vestibular glands, with vaginal dryness
- Regression of subcutaneous fat
- Vulvar and vaginal itching
- Dyspareunia
- Dysuria and urinary frequency
- Vaginal spotting

ETIOLOGY

- Estrogen deficiency. Estrogen is essential to maintaining the urogenital environment. Postmenopausal thinning of the vaginal epithelium and increase in subepithelial connective tissue results in loss of rugal folds and elasticity. Reduced blood flow also contributes to a decline in vaginal secretions.
- Smoking and use of antiestrogen medications (e.g., aromatase inhibitors) increase the risk of vulvovaginal atrophy.

DIAGNOSIS

DIFFERENTIAL DIAGNOSIS

- Infectious vulvovaginitis
- Squamous cell hyperplasia
- Lichen sclerosus
- Vulvar malignancy
- Vaginal malignancy
- Cervical and endometrial malignancy
- Irritant contact dermatitis

WORKUP

- Pelvic examination
- Speculum examination
- Pap smear
- Possible endometrial biopsy if bleeding

LABORATORY TESTS

FSH and estradiol: generally after menopause, estradiol <15 pg and FSH >40 mIU/ml (diagnosis of menopause usually made on a clinical basis and does not usually require FSH and/or estradiol testing)

TREATMENT

NONPHARMACOLOGIC THERAPY

- Avoidance of contact irritants such as scented soaps and feminine hygiene products
- Avoidance of synthetic undergarments, tight-fitting clothing

GENERAL Rx

- Regular use of vaginal moisturizers (e.g., Replens) can decrease vaginal itching and irritation.
- Use of water or silicone-based personal lubricants (e.g., Astroglide) during intercourse is useful to reduce dyspareunia.
- Conjugated estrogen vaginal cream intravaginally. Estradiol vaginal cream (0.625 mg estrogen/gram).
  2 to 4 g/day × 2 wk then
  1 to 2 g/day × 2 wk then
  1 to 2 g × 3 days/wk
- Vagifem (estradiol vaginal tablets) 25 mg inserted intravaginally daily for 2 wk then twice weekly. May take up to 12 wk to feel the full benefits of the medication.
- Conjugated estrogen vaginal cream: 2 to 4 g qd (3 wk on, 1 wk off) for 3 to 5 mo.
- Hormone replacement therapy (HRT): use ultra-low doses. Estrogen use should be reviewed every 3 to 6 mo, with an attempt to taper or discontinue its use.
- Estraderm patch 0.05 mg × 2 per week.
- If uterus present:
  1. Estrogen + 2.5 mg PO Provera qd *or*
  2. Estrogen + 5 to 10 mg PO Provera × 14 days each mo

DISPOSITION

The symptoms should be improved with the therapy. Caution for vaginal bleeding if uterus present.

REFERRAL

To obstetrician/gynecologist if vaginal bleeding

SUGGESTED READINGS
available at www.expertconsult.com

RELATED CONTENT

Candidiasis, Vulvovaginal (Related Key Topic)
Pruritus Vulvae (Related Key Topic)
Vaginitis, Bacterial (Related Key Topic)
Vaginitis, Fungal (Related Key Topic)
Vaginitis, Prepubescent (Related Key Topic)
Vaginitis, *Trichomonas* (Related Key Topic)

AUTHORS: **JULIE ANNE SZUMIGALA, M.D.,** and **RUBEN ALVERO, M.D.**

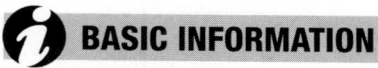
BASIC INFORMATION

DEFINITION

Fungal vulvovaginitis is the inflammation of vulva and vagina caused by *Candida* spp.

SYNONYMS

Monilial vulvovaginitis
Vulvovaginal candidiasis
VVC

ICD-9CM CODES

112.1 Vulvovaginitis, monilial

EPIDEMIOLOGY & DEMOGRAPHICS

- Second most common cause of vaginal infection
- 75% of women will have at least one episode during their childbearing years, and ~40% to 50% of these will have a second attack.
- No symptoms in 20% to 40% of women who have positive cultures

PHYSICAL FINDINGS & CLINICAL PRESENTATION

- Intense vulvar and vaginal pruritus
- Edema and erythema of vulva
- Thick, curd-like vaginal discharge ("cottage cheese" discharge)
- Adherent, dry, white, curdy patches attached to vaginal mucosa

ETIOLOGY

- *Candida albicans* is responsible for 80% to 95% of vaginal fungal infections.
- *Candida tropicalis* and *Torulopsis glabrata* (*Candida glabrata*) are the most common nonalbicans *Candida* species that can induce vaginitis.

PREDISPOSING HOST FACTORS

- Pregnancy
- Oral contraceptives (high-estrogen)
- Diabetes mellitus
- Antibiotics
- Immunosuppression (e.g., HIV)
- Tight, poorly ventilated, nylon underclothing, with increased local perineal moisture and temperature

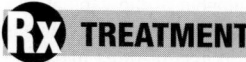
DIAGNOSIS

DIFFERENTIAL DIAGNOSIS

- Bacterial vaginosis
- *Trichomonas* vaginitis
- Atrophic vaginitis

Section II describes the differential diagnosis of vaginal discharges and infections.

WORKUP

- Pelvic examination
- Speculum examination
- Hyphae or budding spores on 10% KOH preparation (positive in 50% to 70% of individuals with yeast infection)
- Normal vaginal pH

Section III, "Vaginal Discharge," describes the evaluation of discharge.

LABORATORY TESTS

Culture, especially recurrence for identification

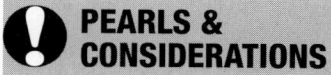
TREATMENT

ACUTE GENERAL Rx

- Cure rate of the various azole derivatives 85% to 90%; little evidence of superiority of one azole agent over another
- No significant differences in persistent symptoms with oral or vaginal treatment
- Fluconazole 150 mg PO × 1 is preferred treatment
- Cure rate of polyene cream, and suppositories: 75% to 80%
- Miconazole 200-mg suppository, one suppository × 3 days or 2% vaginal cream, one applicator full intravaginally qhs × 7
- Clotrimazole 200-mg vaginal tablet, one tablet intravaginally qhs × 3 or 100-mg vaginal tablet one tablet intravaginally qhs × 7, or 1% vaginal cream intravaginally qhs × 7
- Butoconazole 2% cream one applicator intravaginally qhs × 3
- Terconazole 80-mg suppository or 0.8% vaginal cream, one suppository or one applicator intravaginally qhs × 3 or 0.4% vaginal cream, one applicator intravaginally qhs × 7
- Gynecazole-1 vaginal cream, one applicator intravaginally × 1
- Tioconazole 6.5% ointment (Vagi-stat), one applicator intravaginally × 1
- In pregnant patient, treat with 7-day course of topical imidazole.

CHRONIC Rx (FOUR OR MORE SYMPTOMATIC EPISODES ANNUALLY)

- Resistance or recurrence
  ○ 14- to 21-day course of 7-day regimens mentioned in "Acute General Rx" above
  ○ Fluconazole 150 mg PO × 2, 3 days apart
  ○ Ketoconazole 200 mg PO bid × 5 to 14 days
  ○ Itraconazole 200 mg PO qd × 3 days
  ○ Boric acid 600-mg capsule intravaginally bid × 14 days

- Prophylactic regimens
  ○ Clotrimazole one 500-mg vaginal tablet each month
  ○ Ketoconazole 200 mg PO bid × 5 days each month
  ○ Fluconazole 150 mg PO × 1 each month
  ○ Miconazole 100-mg vaginal tablet × 2 weekly

DISPOSITION

- If symptoms do not resolve completely with treatment, or if they recur within a 2- to 3-mo period, further evaluation is indicated.
- Reexamination and possibly culture are necessary.
- Positive culture in absence of symptoms should not lead to treatment. Approximately 30% of women harbor *Candida* spp. and other species in the vagina.

REFERRAL

To obstetrician/gynecologist for recurrence

PEARLS & CONSIDERATIONS

COMMENTS

- No evidence that treating a woman's male sexual partner significantly improves woman's infection or reduces her rate of relapse.
- Many *Candida albicans* strains produce hyaluronidase, which is an enzyme that degrades hyaluronan. Elevated hyaluronan levels in vaginal secretions are associated with increased itching, burning, and discharge in women with recurrent vulvovaginal candidiasis.
- Twenty percent of cases of recurrent vulvovaginal candidiasis are due to *Candida* species other than *C. albicans*.

SUGGESTED READING

available at www.expertconsult.com

RELATED CONTENT

Candidiasis, Vulvovaginal (Related Key Topic)
Pruritus Vulvae (Related Key Topic)
Vaginitis, Bacterial (Related Key Topic)
Vaginitis, Estrogen-Deficient (Related Key Topic)
Vaginitis, Prepubescent (Related Key Topic)
Vaginitis, *Trichomonas* (Related Key Topic)
Candidiasis (Patient Information)

AUTHORS: **JULIE ANNE SZUMIGALA, M.D.,** and **RUBEN ALVERO, M.D.**

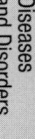

BASIC INFORMATION

DEFINITION

Prepubescent vulvovaginitis is an inflammatory condition of the vulva and vagina.

ICD-9CM CODES
616.10 Vulvovaginitis

EPIDEMIOLOGY & DEMOGRAPHICS

- Most common gynecologic problem of the premenarcheal female.
- Prepubertal girl is susceptible to irritation and trauma because of the absence of protective hair and labial fat pads and the lack of estrogenization with atrophic vaginal mucosa.
- Symptoms of vulvovaginitis and introital irritation and discharge account for 80% to 90% of gynecologic visits.
- Nonspecific etiology in approximately 75% of children with vulvovaginitis.
- Majority of vulvovaginitis in children involves a primary irritation of the vulva with secondary involvement of the lower third of the vagina.

PHYSICAL FINDINGS & CLINICAL PRESENTATION

Vulvar pain, dysuria, pruritus
1. Discharge is not a primary symptom.
2. If present, vaginal discharge may be foul smelling or bloody.

ETIOLOGY

- Infections
  1. Bacterial
  2. Protozoal
  3. Mycotic
  4. Viral
- Endocrine disorders
- Labial adhesions
- Poor hygiene
- Sexual abuse
- Allergic substance
- Trauma
- Foreign body
- Masturbation
- Constipation

Section II describes the differential diagnosis of vaginal discharge in prepubertal girls.

DIAGNOSIS

DIFFERENTIAL DIAGNOSIS

- Physiologic leukorrhea
- Foreign body
- Bacterial vaginosis
- Gonorrhea
- Fungal vulvovaginitis
- *Trichomonas* vulvovaginitis
- Sexual abuse
- Pinworms

WORKUP

- Pelvic, genital examination
- Speculum examination
- Rectal examination
- Vaginoscopy if considering a foreign body
- KOH and normal saline preparation of discharge
- Knee-chest position for examination may be less difficult for the child to tolerate during an examination

Section III, "Vaginal Discharge," describes the evaluation of discharge.

LABORATORY TESTS

- Urinalysis to rule out urinary tract infection and diabetes
- Cultures including sexually transmitted diseases

TREATMENT

NONPHARMACOLOGIC THERAPY

- Avoid tight clothing
- Perineal hygiene
- Avoid irritant chemicals
- Reassurance

ACUTE GENERAL Rx

- Group A beta *Streptococcus* and *Streptococcus pneumoniae*: penicillin V potassium 125 to 250 mg PO qid × 10 days
- *Chlamydia trachomatis*: azithromycin 1 g PO single dose
- *Neisseria gonorrhoeae*: ceftriaxone 250 mg IM × 1 day
  - Children >8 yr should also be given doxycycline 100 mg bid PO × 7 days
- *Staphylococcus aureus*: amoxicillin-clavulanate 20 to 40 mg/kg/day PO × 7 to 10 days
- *Haemophilus influenzae*: amoxicillin 20 to 40 mg/kg/day PO × 7 days
- *Trichomonas*: metronidazole 125 mg (15 mg/kg/day) tid PO × 7 to 10 days
- Pinworms: mebendazole 100-mg tablet chewable, repeat in 2 wk
- Labial agglutination: spontaneous resolution or topical estrogen cream for 7 to 10 days

CHRONIC Rx

See "Referral."

DISPOSITION

Further education:
- Young child: hygiene
- Adolescent: pregnancy prevention and safe sexual practices

REFERRAL

- To obstetrician/gynecologist
- To pediatrician

SUGGESTED READING

available at www.expertconsult.com

RELATED CONTENT

Pruritus Vulvae (Related Key Topic)
Vaginitis, Bacterial (Related Key Topic)
Vaginitis, Fungal (Related Key Topic)
Vaginitis, *Trichomonas* (Related Key Topic)
Vaginosis, Bacterial (Related Key Topic)

AUTHORS: **JULIE ANNE SZUMIGALA, M.D.,** and **RUBEN ALVERO, M.D.**

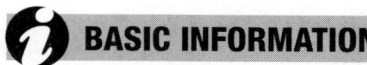 BASIC INFORMATION

DEFINITION

Trichomonas vulvovaginitis is the inflammation of vulva and vagina caused by *Trichomonas* spp.

SYNONYMS

Trichomonas vaginalis
Trichomoniasis
TV

ICD-9CM CODES
131.01 Vulvovaginitis, trichomonal

EPIDEMIOLOGY & DEMOGRAPHICS

- Acquired through sexual contact
- Diagnosed in
  - 50% to 75% of prostitutes
  - 5% to 15% of women visiting gynecology clinics
  - 7% to 32% of women in sexually transmitted disease (STD) clinics
  - 5% of women in family planning clinics

PHYSICAL FINDINGS & CLINICAL PRESENTATION

- Profuse, yellow, malodorous vaginal discharge and severe vaginal itching
- Vulvar itching
- Dysuria
- Dyspareunia
- Intense erythema of the vaginal mucosa
- Cervical petechiae ("strawberry cervix")
- Asymptomatic in ~50% of women and 90% of men

ETIOLOGY

Single-cell protozoan *Trichomonas vaginalis*

RISK FACTORS

- Multiple sexual partners
- History of previous STDs

Dx DIAGNOSIS

DIFFERENTIAL DIAGNOSIS
(Table 1-408)

- Bacterial vaginosis
- Fungal vulvovaginitis
- Cervicitis
- Atrophic vulvovaginitis

WORKUP

- Pelvic examination
- Speculum examination
- Mobile trichomonads seen on normal saline preparation (Fig. 1-876): 70% sensitivity
- Elevated pH (>5) of vaginal discharge
- Culture is considered the traditional gold standard laboratory test for diagnosis of TV.
- Nucleic acid amplification tests (NAATs) have been developed that combine excellent performance characteristics with a more rapid turnaround time compared with culture.

- APTIMA assays utilize target capture and transcription-mediated amplification (TMA) to selectively purify, amplify, and detect species-specific 16 S ribosomal RNA. APTIMA *Trichomonas vaginalis* transcription-mediated amplification may be a better laboratory test than culture based on sensitivity and time frame for results.

LABORATORY TESTS

- Culture (modified Diamond media): 90% sensitivity
- Direct enzyme immunoassay
- Fluorescein-conjugated monoclonal antibody test
- Pap test 40% detected

Rx TREATMENT

NONPHARMACOLOGIC THERAPY
Condom use

ACUTE GENERAL Rx

Metronidazole 2 g PO × 1 *or* Tindamax (tinidazole) single 2-g oral dose in both sexes. Treatment of the sexual partner is essential to prevent reinfection.

CHRONIC Rx

- Metronidazole gel: less likely to achieve therapeutic levels; therefore not recommended.
- Metronidazole (retreat): 500 mg PO bid × 7 days.
- Treatment of future recurrences: metronidazole 2 g PO qd × 3 to 5 days.

- Allergy, intolerance, or adverse reactions: alternatives to metronidazole are not available. Patients who are allergic to metronidazole can be managed by desensitization.
- Pregnancy:
  - Associated with adverse outcomes (i.e., premature rupture of membranes)
  - Metronidazole 2 g PO × 1 day

DISPOSITION

Trichomonas infection is considered an STD; therefore treatment of the sexual partner is necessary.

REFERRAL

To obstetrician/gynecologist for recurrence and pregnancy

SUGGESTED READINGS
available at www.expertconsult.com

RELATED CONTENT

Pruritus Vulvae (Related Key Topic)
Vaginitis, Bacterial (Related Key Topic)
Vaginitis, Fungal (Related Key Topic)
Vaginitis, Prepubescent (Related Key Topic)
Vaginosis, Bacterial (Related Key Topic)
Trichomoniasis (Patient Information)

AUTHORS: **JULIE ANNE SZUMIGALA, M.D.**, and **RUBEN ALVERO, M.D.**

TABLE 1-408 Differential Diagnosis of Vaginitis

Characteristics of Vaginal Discharge	*C. Aalbicans* Vaginitis	*T. vaginalis* Vaginitis	Bacterial Vaginosis
pH	4.5	>5.0	>5.0
White curd	Usually	No	No
Odor with KOH	No	Yes	Yes
Clue cells	No	No	Usually
Motile trichomonads	No	Usually	No
Yeast cells	Yes	No	No

From Goldman L, Ausiello D (eds): *Cecil textbook of medicine,* ed 22, Philadelphia, 2004, Saunders.

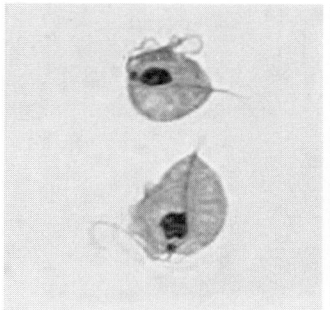 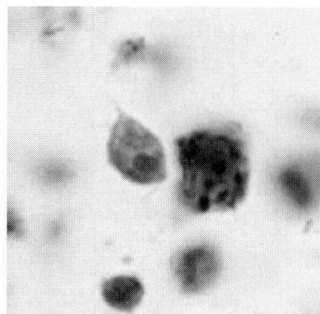

FIGURE 1-876 *Trichomonas vaginalis* trophozoites stained with Giemsa *(left)* and iron hematoxylin *(right).* (From the Centers for Disease Control and Prevention: *Laboratory identification of parasites of public health concern, Trichomoniasis.* www.dpd.cdc.gov/dpdx/HTML/ImageLibrary/Trichomoniasis_il.htm. Accessed August 30, 2010.)

BASIC INFORMATION

DEFINITION

Bacterial vaginosis (BV) is a thin, gray, homogeneous, malodorous vaginal discharge that results from a shift in the vaginal flora from a predominance of lactobacilli to high concentrations of anaerobic bacteria.

SYNONYMS

Before 1955: nonspecific vaginitis
1955: *Haemophilus vaginalis* vaginitis
1963: *Corynebacterium vaginalis* vaginitis
1980: *Gardnerella vaginalis* vaginitis
1990: Bacterial vaginosis

ICD-9CM CODES

616.10 Vaginitis, bacterial

EPIDEMIOLOGY & DEMOGRAPHICS

- Most common vaginal infection
- *Gardnerella, Mycoplasma,* and *Mobiluncus* are harbored in the urethra of male partners; however:
  1. Male partners are asymptomatic.
  2. There is no improved cure rate or lower reinfection rate if the infected patient's male partner is treated.
  3. Abstinence from intercourse or condom use while the patient completes her treatment regimen may improve cure rates and lessen recurrences.

PHYSICAL FINDINGS & CLINICAL PRESENTATION

- 50% of patients are asymptomatic
- A thin, dark, or dull gray homogeneous discharge that adheres to the vaginal walls
- An offensive, "fishy" odor that is accentuated after intercourse or menses
- Pruritus (only in 13%)

ETIOLOGY

- *Gardnerella vaginalis* is detected in 40% to 50% of vaginal secretions.
  1. Increase in vaginal pH caused by decrease in hydrogen peroxide–producing lactobacilli

2. Anaerobes predominate and produce amines
- Amines, when alkalinized by semen, menstrual blood, the use of alkaline douches, or the addition of 10% potassium hydroxide, volatilize and cause the unpleasant "fishy" odor. This amine-whiff test is one of the diagnostic approaches used for BV.
- In BV:
  1. *Bacteroides* (anaerobes) species are increased 1000× the usual concentration.
  2. *G. vaginalis* are 100× normal.
  3. *Peptostreptococcus* are 10× normal.
  4. *Mycoplasma hominis* and Enterobacteriaceae members are present in increased concentrations.

DIAGNOSIS

WORKUP

Seattle Group criteria:
- The presence of three of the four following signs will diagnose 90% correctly, with <10% false-positive results:
  1. Thin, gray, homogeneous, malodorous discharge that adheres to the vaginal walls
  2. Elevated pH >4.5
  3. Positive potassium hydroxide whiff test
  4. Clue cells present on wet mount
- Cultures are unnecessary.
- Pap smear will not identify *G. vaginalis.*
- Gram stain of vaginal secretions will reveal clue cells and abnormal mixed bacteria (Fig. 1-877).

TREATMENT

ACUTE GENERAL Rx

- Recommended regimens (equal efficacy):
  1. Metronidazole 500 mg PO bid for 7 days
  2. 0.75% metronidazole gel in vagina bid for 5 days
  3. 2% clindamycin cream qd for 7 days
- Alternate regimens (lower efficacy for BV):
  1. Clindamycin ovules 100 g intravaginally qhs for 3 days
  2. Clindamycin 300 mg PO bid for 7 days (increased incidence of diarrhea)

3. Metronidazole ER 750 mg PO qd for 7 days
  4. Metronidazole 2 g PO single dose (higher relapse rate)
- Patients should be advised to avoid alcohol while taking metronidazole and for 24 hr thereafter due to disulfiram-type reaction when taken concurrently with alcohol.
- Treatment in pregnancy:
  ○ All pregnant patients proved to have BV should be treated because of its association with preterm labor, chorioamnionitis, and premature rupture of membranes (PROM).
- Recommended regimens:
  1. Metronidazole 250 mg PO tid for 7 days
  2. Clindamycin 300 mg PO bid for 7 days
- Existing data do not support the use of topical agents during pregnancy.
- Multiple studies and meta-analyses have not demonstrated associations between metronidazole use during pregnancy and teratogenic effects in newborns.
  3. Tinidazole, an oral antiprotozoal drug, is now FDA approved for treatment of BV. Dosage is 2 g once/day for 2 days or 1 g qd × 5 days
- Recurrent BV:
  1. Condom use may help reduce the risk of recurrence.
  2. Concurrent treatment of male partner is controversial. Consider treating the male partner if there is recurrent vaginitis or any suspicion of associated upper genital tract infection.

PEARLS & CONSIDERATIONS

- BV has been associated with pelvic inflammatory disease, cystitis, posthysterectomy vaginal cuff cellulitis, postabortal infection, preterm delivery, PROM, amnionitis, chorioamnionitis, and postpartum endometritis. New evidence also shows BV increases women's risk of acquiring HIV.
- Higher cumulative cure rates have been found at 3 to 4 wk for a 7-day regimen of metronidazole (500 mg twice daily) than with a single dose (2 g).
- Persistent BV is associated with several bacteria in the Clostridiales order, *Megasphaera* phylotype 2, and *P. lacrimalis.*

SUGGESTED READINGS

available at www.expertconsult.com

RELATED CONTENT

Vaginitis, Estrogen-Deficient (Related Key Topic)
Vaginitis, Fungal (Related Key Topic)
Vaginitis, Prepubescent (Related Key Topic)
Vaginitis, *Trichomonas* (Related Key Topic)
Vaginal Bacterial Infection (Patient Information)

AUTHORS: **ARUNDATHI G. PRASAD, M.D.,**
and **RUBEN ALVERO, M.D.**

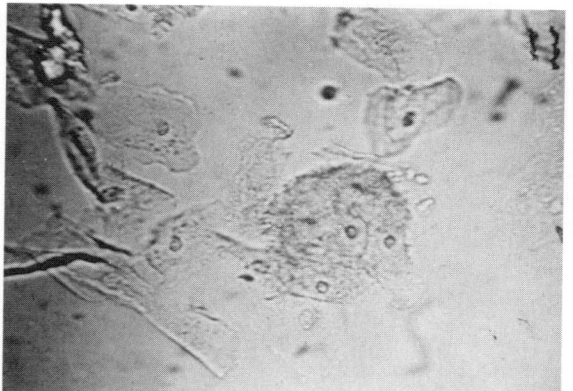

FIGURE 1-877 Clue cells characteristic of bacterial vaginosis, squamous epithelial cells whose borders are obscured by bacteria. (From Carlson K [ed]: *Primary care of women,* St Louis, 1995, Mosby.)

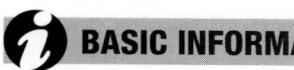

BASIC INFORMATION

DEFINITION

Enterococci are gram-positive, facultative, anaerobic organisms usually oval in shape and can be seen as single cells, pairs, or chains. Vancomycin-resistant *Enterococcus* (VRE) are enterococci that have become resistant to vancomycin and several antibiotics normally used to treat enterococcal infections.

SYNONYMS

VRE

ICD-9CM CODES

V09.8 Infection with microorganisms resistant to other specified drugs

EPIDEMIOLOGY & DEMOGRAPHICS

INCIDENCE: VRE may be associated with the use of specific classes of antibiotics.
PEAK INCIDENCE: VRE was first reported in Europe in 1986, and there has been a steady rise in the incidence of enterococcal strains resistant to vancomycin. In 2007, 80% of *E. faecium* isolates and 7% of *E. faecalis* isolates were resistant to vancomycin.
PREVALENCE: 80% of *E. faecium* are VRE; 69% of *E. faecalis* are VRE.
RISK FACTORS:
- Prior antimicrobial therapy, especially vancomycin
- Prolonged hospitalization
- Chronic medical conditions, renal failure
- Invasive devices
- ICU stay
- Colonization: VRE colonize the gastrointestinal tract; can be found on skin or perirectal swab culture or stool culture

PHYSICAL FINDINGS & CLINICAL PRESENTATION

Patients may be asymptomatic and have gastrointestinal colonization; it can be associated with diarrhea. In hospitalized patients, infection is associated with colonization and can cause wound infections, bacteremia, abscesses (intraabdominal), and, rarely, pneumonia and urinary tract infections.

ETIOLOGY

- Enterococci are primarily found in the human digestive tract and female genital tract, where they make up a significant portion of the normal bacterial population in healthy people. Enterococci can cause urinary tract, wound, bloodstream, heart valve, and brain infections. In the great majority of cases, VRE infections occur in hospitalized patients who have compromised immune systems. Most cases of VRE are caused by the *E. faecium* strains that have acquired resistance when they came in contact with other bacteria and shared genetic information.
- VRE is most commonly transmitted from one patient to another by healthcare workers whose hands have become contaminated inadvertently with feces or fluids of a person carrying the organism. VRE are not airborne but can survive on surfaces for several weeks.

DIAGNOSIS

DIFFERENTIAL DIAGNOSIS

- Other bacterial pathogens in blood, wounds, or urine
- Once colonized, increased incidence to become infected

LABORATORY TESTS

- VRE rectal culture
- VRE stool culture
- Blood, urine, and wound cultures

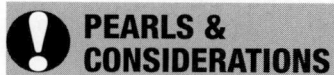

TREATMENT

- For rectal or stool colonization, therapy is not recommended
- Therapy is complicated by the fact that strains exhibit inherent resistance to many commonly used antibiotics.
- More than 80% of vancomycin-resistant *E. faecium* strains are also resistant to ampicillin.
- In symptomatic patients, if VRE strains are known to be susceptible, potential therapeutic agents include
  1. Linezolid: 600 mg IV or PO q12h
  2. Daptomycin: 4 mg/kg/day IV
  3. Quinupristin-dalfopristin (Synercid) only effective for *E. faecium* strains with no activity for *E. faecalis* strains: 7.5 mg/kg q8-12h. Can cause severe myalgias and arthralgias and venous irritation that often requires use of a central line, which has limited the use of this antibiotic.

REFERRAL

To infectious disease specialist

PEARLS & CONSIDERATIONS

COMMENTS

- Incidence increases with comorbidity and hospitalization.
- The number of patients already colonized with VRE in a defined geographic area (colonization pressure) is the most significant factor for predicting new acquisition of VRE.
- An association between VRE colonization and *Clostridium difficile* infection has been reported in patients with hematologic malignancies.

PREVENTION

Hand hygiene–isolation techniques, cleaning contaminated objects or surfaces, gowns and gloves, antibiotic management (prudent vancomycin use), surveillance

SUGGESTED READINGS

available at www.expertconsult.com

AUTHOR: **GLENN G. FORT, M.D., M.P.H.**

BASIC INFORMATION

DEFINITION

Varicella is a common viral illness that is characterized by the acute onset of a generalized vesicular rash and fever.

SYNONYMS

Chickenpox

ICD-9CM CODES
052.9 Varicella

EPIDEMIOLOGY & DEMOGRAPHICS

- Varicella is extremely contagious. More than 90% of unvaccinated contacts become infected.
- The incubation period of chickenpox ranges from 9 to 21 days.
- The peak incidence is during the springtime.
- The predominant age is 5 to 10 yr.
- The infectious period begins 2 days before the onset of clinical symptoms and lasts until all of the lesions have crusted.
- Most patients will have lifelong immunity after an attack of chickenpox; protection from the virus after a varicella vaccine is approximately 6 yr.

PHYSICAL FINDINGS & CLINICAL PRESENTATION

- Findings vary with the clinical course. Initial symptoms consist of fever, chills, backache, generalized malaise, and headache.
- Symptoms are generally more severe in adults.
- Initial lesions generally occur on the trunk (centripetal distribution) and occasionally on the face; these lesions consist primarily of 3- to 4-mm red papules with an irregular outline and a clear vesicle on the surface (i.e., the appearance of dewdrops on a rose petal).
- Intense pruritus generally accompanies the initial stage.
- New lesion development generally ceases by the fourth day, with subsequent crusting by the sixth day.
- Lesions generally spread to the face and the extremities (i.e., centrifugal spread).
- Patients generally present with lesions that are in different stages at the same time.
- Crusts generally fall off within 5 to 14 days.
- The fever is usually highest during the eruption of the vesicles; the patient's temperature generally returns to normal after the disappearance of vesicles.
- Signs of potential complications (e.g., bacterial skin infections, neurologic complications, pneumonia, hepatitis) may be present on physical examination.

- Mild constitutional symptoms (e.g., anorexia, myalgias, headaches, restlessness) may be present; these are most common among adults.
- Excoriations may be present if scratching is prominent.

ETIOLOGY

Varicella-zoster virus is a human herpes virus III that can manifest with either varicella or herpes zoster (i.e., shingles, which is a reactivation of varicella).

DIAGNOSIS

DIFFERENTIAL DIAGNOSIS

- Other viral infection
- Impetigo
- Scabies
- Drug rash
- Urticaria
- Dermatitis herpetiformis
- Smallpox

WORKUP

The diagnosis is usually made on the basis of the patient's history and clinical presentation.

LABORATORY TESTS

- Laboratory evaluation is generally not necessary.
- The CBC may reveal leukopenia and thrombocytopenia.
- Serum varicella titers (i.e., a significant rise in the serum varicella immunoglobulin G antibody level), skin biopsies, or Tzanck smears are used only when diagnosis is in question.

TREATMENT

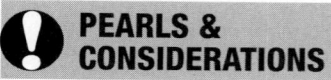

NONPHARMACOLOGIC THERAPY

- Use antipruritic lotions for symptomatic relief.
- Avoid scratching to prevent excoriations and superficial skin infections.
- Use a mild soap for bathing.
- Hands should be washed often.

ACUTE GENERAL Rx

- Use acetaminophen for fever and myalgias; aspirin should be avoided because of the associated increased risk for Reye's syndrome.
- Oral acyclovir (20 mg/kg qid for 5 days) initiated at the earliest sign (i.e., within 24 hr of illness) is useful for healthy, nonpregnant individuals 13 yr old or older to decrease the duration and severity of signs and symptoms. Immunocompromised hosts should be treated with intravenous acyclovir 500 mg/m^2 or 10 mg/kg q8h for 7 to 10 days.

- Varicella is most contagious from 2 days before to a few days after the onset of the rash. Varicella vaccine is available for children and adults; protection lasts at least 6 yr. Healthy, nonimmune adults and children exposed to varicella-zoster virus should receive prophylaxis with live attenuated varicella vaccine (Varivax). Patients with HIV or other immunocompromised patients should not receive the live attenuated vaccine.
- Exposed patients with contraindications to varicella vaccine can be treated with varicella-zoster immunoglobulin (VariZIG), which effectively prevents varicella in susceptible individuals. The dose is 12.5 U/kg IM up to a maximum of 625 U. VariZIG must be administered as early as possible after presumed exposure (i.e., within 10 days) for postexposure prophylaxis of varicella.
- Pruritus from chickenpox can be controlled with antihistamines (e.g., hydroxyzine 25 mg q6h) and oral antipruritic lotions (e.g., calamine).
- Oral antibiotics are not routinely indicated and should be used only in patients with secondary infection and infected lesions; the most common infective organisms are *Streptococcus* sp. and *Staphylococcus* sp.

DISPOSITION

- The course is generally benign in immunocompetent adults and children.
- Infants who develop chickenpox are incapable of controlling the infection and should be given varicella-zoster immunoglobulin or gamma globulin if VariZIG is not available.

PEARLS & CONSIDERATIONS

COMMENTS

- VariZIG can be obtained from the nearest regional Red Cross Blood Center or the Centers for Disease Control and Prevention in Atlanta.
- Varicella immunization is recommended for all who have not had chickenpox; the dosage for adults and adolescents (>13 yr old) is two 0.5-ml doses 4 to 8 wk apart.

EVIDENCE

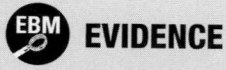

available at www.expertconsult.com

RELATED CONTENT

Chickenpox (Patient Information)

AUTHOR: **FRED F. FERRI, M.D.**

BASIC INFORMATION

DEFINITION

A varicocele is a collection of dilated and tortuous veins in the pampiniform plexus surrounding the spermatic cord in the scrotum.

SYNONYMS

Sometimes referred to as "bag of worms" (Fig. 1-878)

ICD-9CM CODES
456.4

EPIDEMIOLOGY & DEMOGRAPHICS

PREVALENCE: A varicocele is present in up to 20% of all males. It occurs in approximately 40% of infertile men. However, only 10% to 15% of males with varicoceles have fertility problems.
RISK FACTORS: There are no reliable data on epidemiologic risk factors for varicocele, such as a family history or environmental exposures.

PHYSICAL FINDINGS & CLINICAL PRESENTATION

- Patients may report a mass lying posterior to and above the testis. When the patient is supine, dilation of the veins is generally decreased. Dilation and tortuosity of the veins are increased when the patient is upright and when the patient performs a Valsalva maneuver.
- The majority of cases (90%) occur more commonly on the left side because the left spermatic vein enters the left renal vein at a 90-degree angle, whereas the right testicular vein drains directly into the vena cava.

- Physical examination reveals a soft scrotal mass that increases in size when standing and is typically described as a "bag of worms."
- Most varicoceles are painless.

ETIOLOGY

Varicoceles are caused by dysfunction of the valves in the spermatic vein, which allows pooling of blood in the pampiniform plexus.

DIAGNOSIS

DIFFERENTIAL DIAGNOSIS

- Hydrocele
- Spermatocele
- Epididymal orchitis
- Testicular tumor

WORKUP

Patient should undergo a testicular exam in the upright and supine position.

LABORATORY TESTS

Semen analysis may be performed if a varicocele is detected and the patient is infertile.

IMAGING

High-resolution color-flow Doppler ultrasound and Doppler ultrasound (Fig. E1-879) are the most common and least invasive techniques to confirm a varicocele and differentiate from other scrotal abnormalities. Follow-up studies may be considered to assess progression and testicular size.

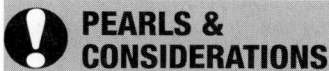

TREATMENT

Once a varicocele is identified, providers must document bilateral testicular size at regular intervals. If the testicle on the affected side is small, spermatogenesis may have been adversely affected.

SURGERY

- Surgical treatment is indicated when there is significant disparity in testicular size or pain. Also, surgery should be performed if the contralateral testis is diseased or absent. Surgery may be considered if the varicocele is large, even without a disparity in testicular size.
- Should surgery be advisable, varicocelectomy is performed by ligation of the veins of the pampiniform plexus through an inguinal incision or by ligating the internal spermatic vein in the retroperitoneum. This is generally performed as an ambulatory surgery.
- The goal of varicocelectomy is to maximize chances for fertility.
- Postoperatively the involved testis typically enlarges and catches up to the uninvolved side in 1 to 2 yr. Semen parameters also improve significantly in 65%.
- The success rate of surgical repair is close to 98%; that of percutaneous repair is significantly lower.
- Sclerotherapy represents a less invasive option but is less effective in symptom reduction.

PEARLS & CONSIDERATIONS

- Varicocele repair has been shown to reverse a spectrum of effects contributing to impaired fertility, but studies have demonstrated variable effects on postoperative sperm parameters and pregnancy rates. Some of this variability may be due to methodologic issues, but additional studies are warranted with improved microsurgical techniques.
- A varicocele in a boy <10 yr or on the right side may be indicative of an abdominal or retroperitoneal mass. Ultrasound should be performed.
- The sudden occurrence of a left-sided varicocele in an older man indicates occlusion of the spermatic vein and should prompt evaluation for a renal tumor.

EVIDENCE

available at www.expertconsult.com

SUGGESTED READINGS

available at www.expertconsult.com

RELATED CONTENT

Varicocele (Patient Information)

AUTHORS: **BETH NOWAK, M.D.,** and **JANICE PATACSIL-TRULL, M.D.**

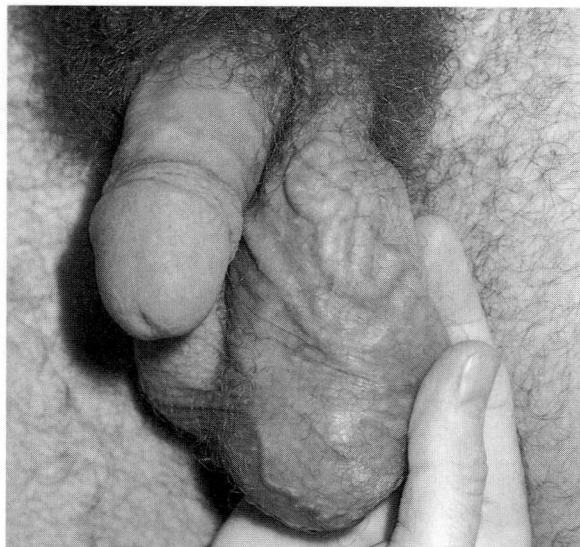

FIGURE 1-878 Varicocele. (From Swartz MH: *Textbook of physical diagnosis,* ed 5, Philadelphia, 2006, Saunders.)

BASIC INFORMATION

DEFINITION

Veins in the leg are soft, thin-walled tubes that return blood back to the heart. This is accomplished by the presence of one-way valves and the action of the calf pump. Superficial venous insufficiency develops when venous return is impaired by valvular incompetence, obstruction, or calf muscle pump failure.

Varicose veins, the most common clinical manifestation of chronic venous disease, are bulging (>3 mm in diameter), tortuous conduits (Fig. 1-880). Reticular veins, often called "feeder veins," are bluish subdermal veins about 1 to 3 mm in diameter that give rise to telangiectasia. Spider veins or telangiectasias are very small (≤1 mm in diameter) thread veins found commonly in cluster on the surface of the skin.

SYNONYMS

Chronic venous disorder

ICD-9CM CODES
448.1 Spider veins/telangiectasias
454.9 Varicose veins
454.8 Varicose veins with symptoms

EPIDEMIOLOGY

PREVALENCE: One large U.S. cohort study found the biannual incidence of varicose veins was 3% in women and 2% in men.

The prevalence of varicose veins in Western populations was estimated in one study to be about 25% to 30% in women and 10% to 20% in men.
RISK FACTORS:
Gender: female
Genetics: family history of varicose veins
Increasing age
Multiple pregnancies

SYMPTOMS AND PHYSICAL FINDINGS

Leg complaints consistent with chronic venous disease include aching, heaviness, subjective swelling, cramps, itching, tingling, and pain. These symptoms can be exacerbated by menses, heat, and prolonged standing.

CLINICAL PRESENTATION

- Chronic vein disease is the result of the introduction of high pressures into a normal low-pressure superficial venous system.
- This increased pressure or venous hypertension causes superficial veins to distend to such a degree that vein valves fail to close, causing reflux and pooling of blood in surface veins.
- Manifested clinically by two syndromes:
  - Junctional: failure of the terminal valve at the intersection between the saphenous vein trunks and the deep system. If the great saphenous vein is involved, large varicose veins are found mainly above medial knee or calf. When the small saphenous vein is involved, large varicose veins are found in posterior knee or calf

area. If the anterior accessory of great saphenous vein is involved, large varicose veins are found mainly in anterior or lateral thigh.
  - Perforator: failure of valves located in perforating vein. Large varicose veins are found most commonly in medial calf and proximal thigh region.

CLASSIFICATION

Chronic venous disease can now be classified using the Clinical-Etiology-Anatomy-Pathophysiology (CEAP) criteria to allow a precise description of the type of venous disease being discussed and provide an orderly framework for decision making (Table 1-409).

ETIOLOGY

- The underlying etiology of varicose veins remains uncertain.
- Important structural changes that occur: failure of vein valve function and vein wall dilation from fragmentation of the muscle layer.

COMPLICATIONS

- Superficial venous thrombophlebitis (SVT): a very common disorder with an incidence of 125,000 new cases per year in the U.S. The most frequent predisposing risk factors are varicose veins. The clinical findings include the presence of erythema, tenderness, and a palpable cord. Pain, increased warmth, and swelling are also present. Diagnosis is made by ultrasonography, which is useful to identify associated deep vein thrombosis that can occur in approximately 15% of patients. The location of the SVT determines the course of

---

TABLE 1-409 CEAP Classification of Chronic Venous Disease

C: Clinical

C_0: no visible or palpable signs of venous disease
C_1: telangiectasias or reticular veins
C_2: varicose veins
C_3: edema
C_4: pigmentation or eczema
C_5: healed venous ulcer
C_6: active venous ulcer

E: Etiology

c: congenital
p: primary
s: secondary or post thrombotic
n: no venous cause identified

A: Anatomy

s: superficial veins
p: perforator veins
d: deep veins
n: no venous location identified

P: Pathophysiology

r: reflux
o: obstruction
r,o: reflux and obstruction
n: no venous pathophysiology identified

---

treatment; if the proximal great saphenous vein (GSV) is involved, a 1-mo course of low-molecular-weight heparin plus compression stockings has been found to be more effective than vein ligation. If SVT involves branch varicosities, treatment is usually symptomatic (control of pain).
- Bleeding is a more common complication than traditionally suspected. It is associated with thin-walled ectatic veins known as "blue blebs" that are found predominantly in the medial lower calf and ankle region. The best emergency treatment consists of pressure wrapping and not suture ligation, which results in delayed healing of the bleeding site. Sclerotherapy of these veins is the definitive treatment to prevent further bleeding.
- Dermal pathology of prolonged chronic venous disease (CEAP classes 4, 5, and 6).
  - Varicose eczema: see "Venous Ulcers" section.
  - Atrophie blanche: see "Venous Ulcers" section.
  - Lipodermosclerosis: see "Venous Ulcers" section.
  - Venous stasis ulcer: see "Venous Ulcers" section.

DIAGNOSIS

DIFFERENTIAL DIAGNOSIS

Other conditions that cause leg pain:
- Stress fracture
- Arthritis hip/knee joint
- Gout
- Degenerative disk disease of lower back
- Intermittent claudication secondary to peripheral arterial disease (PAD)
- Medications such as allopurinol and statins
Other conditions that cause leg swelling:
- Cellulitis
- Soft tissue injury to leg/ankle/foot
- Obesity
- Diabetes
- Advancing age
- Medications such as calcium channel blockers, steroids, MAO inhibitors, and tricyclics

WORKUP

The diagnosis of chronic venous disorders is predominantly clinical. Initial evaluation consists of a thorough history and physical exam with classification of disease according to the CEAP criteria.

LABORATORY TESTS

Laboratory tests are not useful in patients with varicose veins.

IMAGING STUDIES

Duplex ultrasonography:
- Gold-standard imaging modality for the diagnosis, prognostic evaluation, pretreatment mapping, and posttreatment assessment of therapeutic intervention.
- Duplex ultrasound is used to identify and quantify points of valvular reflux within the superficial venous system.

- Assessment of valvular reflux is done with patient in the upright position, which physiologically approximates the condition in which valvular reflux occurs.
- Reverse flow of greater than 0.5 sec after distal compression is considered abnormal.

Other tests:

- Air plethysmography: may be useful in patients who have reflux in both superficial and deep venous systems or in patients with an unusual presentation of leg pain.
- Venography: has been largely replaced by duplex ultrasonography but still retains a critical role in the evaluation of chronic venous insufficiency prior to venous reconstruction.

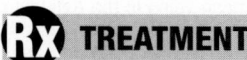 TREATMENT

CONSERVATIVE THERAPY:
- Aerobic exercise regularly for 30 min a day.
- Elevate legs above heart level to reduce swelling.
- Flex ankles frequently at work and during air travel or long car travel.
- Maintain proper weight.
- Graduated compression stockings (below knee) to alleviate symptoms in patients who are not candidates or do not desire to undergo treatment of their varicose veins.

SCLEROTHERAPY:
- Small- to medium-sized varicose veins such as spider veins and reticular varices in the absence of reflux in saphenous trunks are best treated with liquid sclerotherapy.

- The three principal sclerosants used in the U.S. are hypertonic saline, sodium tetradecyl-sulfate, and the newly FDA-approved solution, polidocanol.
- These agents are injected into vessels using 27-gauge or 30-gauge needles at concentrations of 23.4%, 0.1%, or 0.5%, respectively, causing injury to the endothelium with the resultant disappearance of the vein over period of time (usually 8 to 12 wk).

AMBULATORY PHLEBECTOMY:
- A procedure in which large varicose vein branches are removed with special hook instruments through a small puncture—incisions are made with an 18-gauge needle or No. 11 blade
- Performed safely under local anesthesia in an office setting and offers excellent cosmetic results and relief of symptoms
- Most commonly performed in conjunction with endovenous ablation procedures

ENDOVENOUS ABLATION:
- Ablation of diseased saphenous vein trunks, large incompetent tributaries, or perforating veins can be achieved by using:
  ○ Radiofrequency energy
  ○ Laser energy
  ○ Ultrasound-guided foam sclerotherapy.
- The first two accomplish thermal injury to the vein in situ via an intraluminal catheter or bare-tipped laser wire. Chemical ablation uses a solution (polidocanol or sodium tetradecylsulfate) that is injected directly into the vein in the form of foam.

- Endovenous ablation can be performed in an office setting using local anesthesia. Patients can return to their normal daily activities immediately.
- The efficacy of these endovenous ablation procedures have been borne out by numerous published reports with occlusion rates over 95% and reflux free rates over 5-yr follow-up of 86%.

DISPOSITION

- It is important that the physician educate the patient to understand that varicose veins are a chronic and progressive disease.
- Any treatment is at best palliative, as patients in time will develop varicose veins in other areas.

REFERRAL

To either a phlebologist, preferably board certified by the newly created American Board of Phlebology, or a residency-trained vascular surgeon

SUGGESTED READINGS
available at www.expertconsult.com

RELATED CONTENT

Varicose Veins (Patient Information)

AUTHOR: **FRANK G. FORT, M.D., F.A.C.S.**

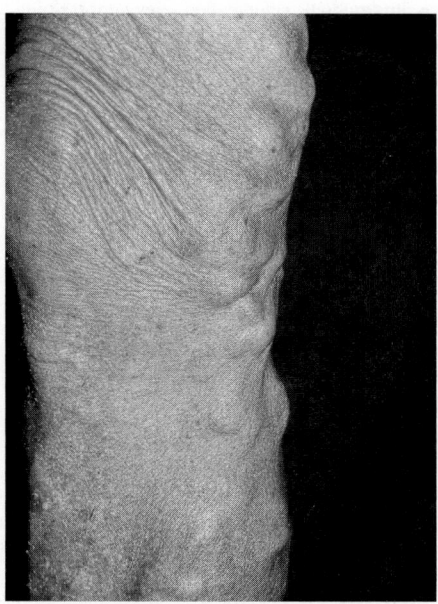

FIGURE 1-880 Varicose veins. (From White GM, Cox NH [eds]: *Diseases of the skin, a color atlas and text,* ed 2, St Louis, 2006, Mosby.)

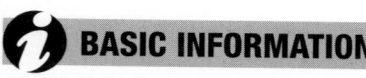

BASIC INFORMATION

DEFINITION

Vasculitis refers generically to inflammation occurring within the walls of blood vessels. Blood vessel inflammation can result in either perforation of affected vessels with hemorrhage into adjacent structures or thrombosis with subsequent ischemia and infarction of supplied tissues. Vasculitis can occur as a primary process or secondary to another connective tissue disease, infection, or drug exposure. The systemic vasculitides are a heterogeneous group of disorders characterized by blood vessel inflammation affecting vessels of varying size and location resulting in a wide range of clinical manifestations dictated largely by which vessels are affected (Fig. E1-881). They are traditionally classified according to the size of the blood vessels predominantly affected (Table 1-410). Several of

---

TABLE 1-410 Classification Scheme of Vasculitides According to Size of Predominant Blood Vessels Involved

Primary vasculitides
Predominantly large vessel vasculitides
Takayasu's arteritis
Giant cell arteritis (temporal arteritis)
Cogan's syndrome
Behçet's disease*
Predominantly medium-sized vessel vasculitides
Polyarteritis nodosa
Cutaneous polyarteritis nodosa
Buerger's disease
Kawasaki's disease
Primary angiitis of the central nervous system
Predominantly small vessel vasculitides
Immune complex mediated
Goodpasture's disease (anti–glomerular basement membrane disease)[†]
  Cutaneous leukocytoclastic angiitis ("hypersensitivity vasculitis")
  Henoch-Schönlein purpura
  Hypocomplementemic urticarial vasculitis
  Essential cryoglobulinemia[‡]
  Erythema elevatum diutinum
ANCA-associated disorders[§]
  Wegener's granulomatosis[‡]
  Microscopic polyangiitis[‡]
  Churg-Strauss syndrome[‡]
  Renal-limited vasculitis
Secondary forms of vasculitis
Miscellaneous small vessel vasculitides
Connective tissue disorders[‡] (rheumatoid vasculitis, lupus erythematosus, Sjögren's syndrome, inflammatory myopathies)
Inflammatory bowel disease
Paraneoplastic
Infection
Drug-induced vasculitis: ANCA-associated, other

*May involve small, medium-sized, and large blood vessels.
[†]Immune complexes formed in situ, in contrast to other forms of immune complex–mediated vasculitis.
[‡]Frequent overlap of small and medium-sized blood vessel involvement.
[§]Not all forms of these disorders are always associated with ANCA.
ANCA, Antineutrophil cytoplasmic antibody.
From Firestein G et al: *Kelley's textbook of rheumatology,* ed 8, Philadelphia, 2008, Saunders.

---

these are covered in individual chapters including chapters on granulomatosis with polyangiitis (GPA), polyarteritis nodosa (PAN), giant cell arteritis (GCA), Takayasu's arteritis, and Henoch-Schönlein purpura (HSP). Severity varies between and within specific vasculitides from a relatively benign, self-limited process to severe, life-threatening multisystem organ involvement with significant morbidity and mortality.

SYNONYMS

None

ICD-9CM CODES
446.0 Polyarteritis nodosa
446.1 Kawasaki disease
446.4 Wegener's granulomatosis, Churg-Strauss syndrome
446.5 Giant cell arteritis
446.7 Takayasu's arteritis

EPIDEMIOLOGY & DEMOGRAPHICS

- The epidemiology and demographics of the various vasculitides vary by the individual disease and where applicable are covered under the relevant disease chapters.
- The most common form of systemic vasculitis in the United States is giant cell arteritis, with an approximate incidence of 170 cases per 1 million per year in individuals older than 50 years.
- Antineutrophil cytoplasmic antibodies (ANCA)-associated vasculitis is significantly less common with aggregate incidence estimated at approximately 20 per million in the U.S.
- Age distribution can demonstrate significant variability between the vasculitides as demonstrated by the fact that GCA generally does not occur before age 50, while 90% of cases of HSP occur in the pediatric population and 80% of patients with Kawasaki disease are under age 5.
- While genetics clearly plays a role in disease susceptibility, familial cases of vasculitis are rare.

PHYSICAL FINDINGS & CLINICAL PRESENTATION

- Clinical presentation often includes nonspecific constitutional symptoms including fever, malaise, headache, and weight loss.
- Signs and symptoms are generally dictated by the tropism of involved vessels.
- Skin manifestations of vasculitis include petechiae, palpable purpura (Fig. 1-882), subcutaneous nodules, livedo reticularis, ulcerations, and digital ischemia.
- Kidney involvement of medium-sized and large vessel vasculitis is often in the form of renovascular hypertension, as opposed to glomerulonephritis in small vessel vasculitis.
- Pulmonary small vessel involvement can cause alveolar hemorrhage, which can present with cough, dyspnea, and alveolar hemorrhage.
- Mononeuritis multiplex is the characteristic finding of vasculitis affecting the vasa nervorum of the peripheral nervous system.

- Gastrointestinal involvement of the mesenteric vasculature can cause postprandial pain, bleeding, and perforation.
- Arthritis, while nonspecific, can be present.
- Significant clinical variability exists between the various vasculitides, although overlapping symptoms may be seen.

ETIOLOGY

Most forms of systemic vasculitis are of unknown etiology. Cryoglobulinemic vasculitis is often secondary to hepatitis C infection, and cutaneous leukocytoclastic vasculitis can often be related to a drug exposure.

DIAGNOSIS

DIFFERENTIAL DIAGNOSIS

- Infective endocarditis
- Atrial myxoma
- Cholesterol emboli
- Malignancy

WORKUP

- The diagnosis of most forms of systemic vasculitis relies on the history and physical examination as well as supportive laboratory testing. Table E1-411 describes differential diagnostic features of selected forms of small-vessel vasculitis.

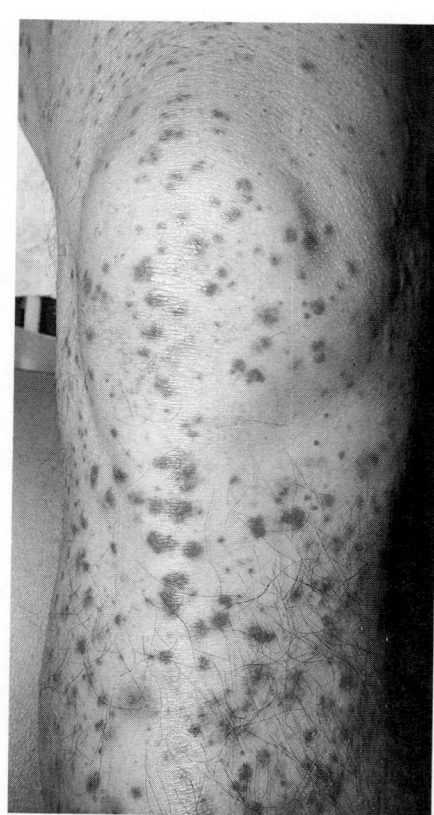

FIGURE 1-882 Leukocytoclastic vasculitis, palpable purpura. (From James W et al: *Andrews' diseases of the skin, clinical dermatology,* ed 10, Philadelphia, 2005, Saunders.)

- Tissue biopsy is important in establishing an accurate diagnosis; biopsy sites should target affected tissues.
- Imaging such as mesenteric angiography in the setting of PAN affecting the mesenteric vasculature can be supportive and can at times obviate the need for tissue biopsy.

LABORATORY TESTS

- Generic laboratory markers of systemic inflammation include an elevated erythrocyte sedimentation rate (ESR), C-reactive protein (CRP), and an anemia of chronic disease.
- ANCA targeting myeloperoxidase (MPO) and proteinase 3 (PR3) are frequently found in several small vessel vasculitides, including GPA (Wegener's), microscopic polyangiitis (MPA), and Churg-Strauss syndrome (CSS). Table 1-412 describes antibody profiles for vasculitis associated with various autoimmune diseases.
- Hepatitis C antibodies and rheumatoid factor are often present in cryoglobulinemic vasculitis.
- Urinalysis in patients with glomerulonephritis due to small vessel ANCA-associated vasculitis will generally demonstrate hematuria with an active urinary sediment with red blood cell casts and proteinuria without significant immune deposits (pauci-immune) on biopsy.

IMAGING STUDIES

- Angiography can demonstrate vascular narrowing and aneurysm formation in suspected medium-size and large vessel vasculitis.
- Pulmonary and sinus CT scans can demonstrate active pulmonary and upper airway disease in ANCA-associated vasculitis.

Rx TREATMENT

Treatment of vasculitis depends on the specific type of vasculitis and is tailored to the severity of disease activity.

ACUTE GENERAL Rx

- Systemic corticosteroids are generally required to gain initial control of active disease although mild cases of drug-induced cutaneous leukocytoclastic vasculitis can often be treated with NSAIDs and cessation of the offending medication.
- GCA, HSP, and vasculitis limited to the skin including cutaneous PAN can often be managed without further immunosuppression.
- Major organ-threatening disease in systemic vasculitis has traditionally been treated with oral or intravenous cyclophosphamide.
- Recent studies have demonstrated noninferiority of rituximab compared to cyclophosphamide in ANCA-associated vasculitis with major organ involvement.
- Less severe disease such as granulomatosis with polyangiitis (Wegener's) limited to the upper airways can be managed with methotrexate rather than cyclophosphamide.
- The goal of acute therapy is to induce remission of disease activity and is generally continued for 1 to 2 months once this is achieved, at which point chronic therapy is used to prevent disease relapse.

CHRONIC Rx

- The goal of chronic therapy is to prevent disease relapse and minimize medication side effects.

- Steroids are gradually tapered as allowed by disease activity.
- Immunomodulatory agents such as methotrexate or azathioprine are used for maintenance therapy in place of cyclophosphamide to reduce side effects.
- Cryoglobulinemic vasculitis due to chronic hepatitis C will often improve with treatment of the underlying viral infection.
- The role and dosing of rituximab for maintenance therapy are not yet established.

DISPOSITION

Varies widely among the various vasculitides

REFERRAL

Systemic vasculitis care is generally coordinated by a rheumatologist. Renal, pulmonary, neurologic, and gastrointestinal consultation is often needed when vasculitis involves these organ systems. Isolated cutaneous leukocytoclastic vasculitis is often managed by dermatology.

SUGGESTED READINGS
available at www.expertconsult.com

RELATED CONTENT

Churg-Strauss Syndrome (Related Key Topic)
Cogan's Syndrome (Related Key Topic)
Giant Cell Arteritis (Related Key Topic)
Henoch-Schönlein Purpura (Related Key Topic)
Kawasaki Disease (Related Key Topic)
Takayasu's Arteritis (Related Key Topic)
Granulomatosis with Polyangiitis (Related Key Topic)
Polyarteritis Nodosa (Related Key Topic)

AUTHOR: **HARALD A. HALL, M.D.**

TABLE 1-412	Autoantibody Profiles for Vasculitis Associated with Various Autoimmune Diseases				
	ANA	**ds-DNA**	**Smith**	**ANCA**	**Complements**
SLE	+++	+ in 40%-80%	+ 50%-60%	Usually −	Low
WG	− or weakly +	−	−	0% + (PR3)	Normal
MPA	− or weakly +	−	−	90% + (MPO)	Normal
Polyarteritis	−	−	−	Usually −	Normal
Takayasu's arteritis	−	−	−	−	Normal
SJIA	−	−	−	−	Normal-high

+, Positive; −, negative; *ANA*, antinuclear antibody; *ANCA*, antineutrophil cytoplasmic antibody; *ds-DNA*, double-stranded deoxyribonucleic acid; *MPA*, microscopic polyangiitis; *MPO*, myeloperoxidase; *SJIA*, systemic juvenile idiopathic arthritis; *SLE*, systemic lupus erythematosus; *WG*, Wegener's granulomatosis.
From Fuhrman BP et al: *Pediatric critical care*, ed 4, Philadelphia, 2011, Saunders.

BASIC INFORMATION

DEFINITION

The spectrum of chronic venous disease (CVD) ranges from varicose veins to leg edema and skin manifestations consissiting of hyperpigmentation, eczema, lipodermatosclerosis, and venous ulcer. These latter venous specific skin changes constitute an advanced form of CVD known as chronic venous insufficiency (CVI).

SYNONYMS

Stasis dermatitis
Post-thrombotic syndrome (PTS)

ICD-9CM CODES
454.1 Varicose veins of lower extremities with inflammation

EPIDEMIOLOGY & DEMOGRAPHICS

- From 10% to 35% of adults in the U.S. have some form of CVI.
- Venous ulcers are the complication of CVI that results in the greatest morbidity and affects 4% of people over the age of 65
- The population-based costs to the U.S. government for CVI treatment and venous ulcer care have been estimated at >$1 billion a year.
- In addition, 4.6 million workdays per year are lost to chronic venous-related diseases.

PHYSICAL FINDINGS & CLINICAL PRESENTATION

The spectrum of cutaneous changes of CVI in the affected leg include:
- Varicose eczema: the most common and earliest sign, this involves the skin above the medial ankle and consists of pruritic, red, and scaly eczematous patches and plaques (Fig. 1-883).
- Hyperpigmentation: caused by the breakdown of red blood cells and leads to hemosiderin deposition and dark staining of the skin (Fig. 1-884).
- Atrophie blanche: usually presents as hypopigmented white patches with focal red punctate dots or telangiectasia surrounded by hyperpigmentation. Skin in this condition is avascular and prone to ulceration (Fig. 1-885).
- Lipodermatosclerosis: a chronic, brawny induration of the skin and underlying fat that usually involves the skin from medial malleolus up to the lower border of the calf. Progression of the disease leads to an "inverted champagne bottle" appearance. The induration and lack of perfusion of the skin in this area make it susceptible to ulcer formation (Fig. 1-886).

ETIOLOGY

- CVI occurs as a result of sustained venous hypertension in the leg, which can be caused by the following:
  1. Primary: vein valve failure with reflux in the superficial venous system or perforating veins (most common cause of CVI)
  2. Secondary: post-thrombotic syndrome in which a deep vein thrombosis causes outflow obstruction or
  3. Combination of the two above processes
- This sustained elevation in venous pressure or venous hypertension results in pathologic effects in the skin and subcutaneous tissues such as edema, eczema, hyperpigmentation, fibrosis, and ultimately venous ulceration.

DIAGNOSIS

The diagnosis and evaluation of CVI are directed primarily by a detailed history and physical examination.

DIFFERENTIAL DIAGNOSIS

- Contact dermatitis
- Atopic dermatitis
- Cellulitis
- Dermatophyte infection
- Pretibial myxedema
- Nummular eczema
- Xerosis
- Asteatotic eczema

WORKUP

The primary goal is to identify the cause of sustained venous hypertension.

LABORATORY TESTS

Generally not indicated

IMAGING STUDIES

- Evaluation of the patient is performed in the standing position with duplex ultrasonography to identify reflux in the superficial, deep, and perforating veins as well as obstruction of the deep veins.
- No exam of a leg with CVI is complete without palpation of pulses and/or determination of ankle-brachial index (ABI).

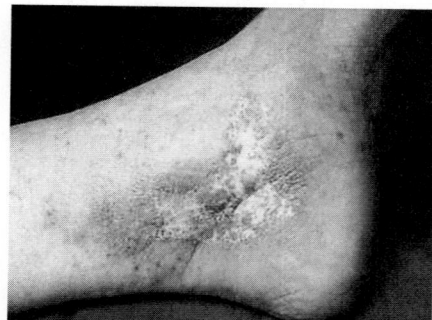

FIGURE 1-885 Atrophie blanche.

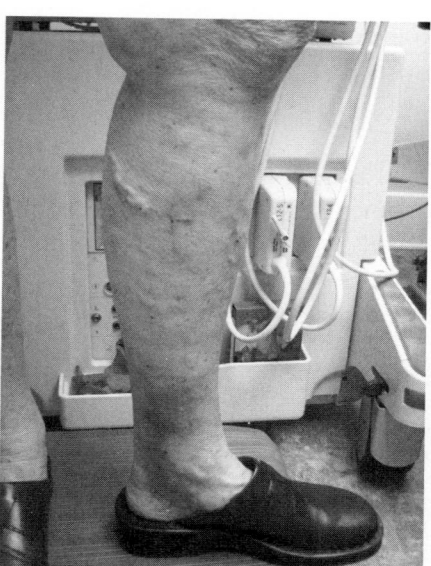

FIGURE 1-883 Varicose eczema.

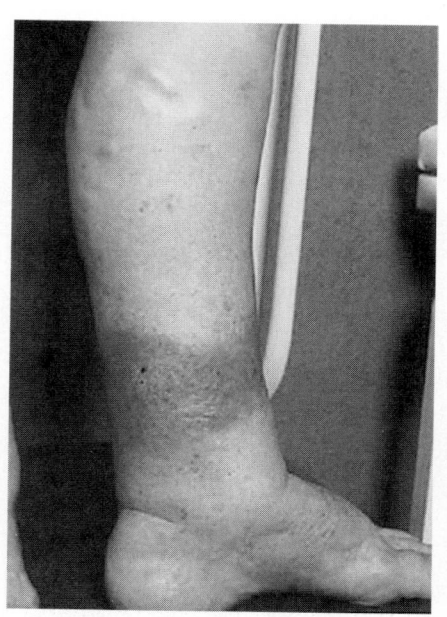

FIGURE 1-884 Hyperpigmentation.

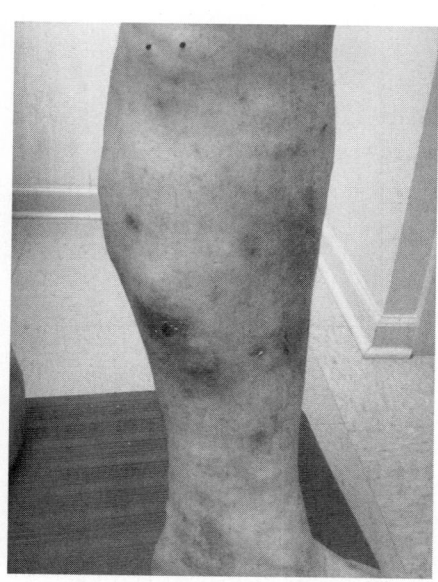

FIGURE 1-886 Lipodermosclerosis.

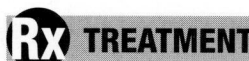 **TREATMENT**

NONPHARMACOLOGIC THERAPY

- Leg elevation above heart level for 30 min 3 to 4 times a day
- Weight reduction because obesity is a risk factor for DVT and CVI
- Walking exercises to improve calf function
- Physical therapy to improve ankle joint mobility
- For weeping skin lesions, wet-to-dry dressing changes

ACUTE GENERAL Rx

- The fundamental role of compression in the treatment of CVI is well recognized and has been validated by randomized controlled trials (RCTs).
- The beneficial effects of gradient compression stockings (decrease in edema and control of discomfort) are due to their effect on microvascular hemodynamics and Starling forces.
- Below-knee compression stocking with a gradient of at least 20 to 30 mm Hg will control edema, alleviate pain, and improve the quality of life in CVI patients.
- Compression stockings are contraindicated in patients with an ABI of <0.6.
- Some patients (acute lipodermatosclerosis) may benefit from nonelastic compression with the Unna gel paste gauze boot to alleviate their symptoms and acute increase in their swelling. The Unna boot is changed once a week.
- Topical corticosteroid creams or ointments (e.g., triamcinolone 0.12% bid) may be used to help reduce inflammation and itching. Steroids should never be applied to ulcer.
- Antibiotics should only be used when treating a clinically apparent, culture-proved infection. Most secondary infections are the result of *Staphylococcus* or *Streptococcus* organisms.
- Diuretics have no role in the treatment of CVI-related edema.

CHRONIC Rx

- While conservative care is fundamental, patients with CVI should be considered for correction of their underlying venous hypertension.
- The majority of patients with CVI have superficial vein or perforator vein reflux as their underlying pathology and would benefit from the newer vein ablation procedures listed below.
  - ○ Endovenous ablation of superficial (saphenous) or perforator vein reflux
  - ○ RF ablation with VNUS closure
  - ○ Endovenous laser therapy (EVLT)
  - ○ Ultrasound-guided foam sclerotherapy

COMPLEMENTARY & ALTERNATIVE MEDICINE

Several groups of drugs have been evaluated in the treatment of CVI, including coumarins, flavinoids, and saponosides (horse chestnut extracts). These drugs have venoactive properties and are widely used in Europe but are not approved for use in the U.S. The precise mechanism of action is not known. Horse chestnut seed extract has been found, in the short term, to be as effective as compression stockings in reducing pain and edema, but long-term efficacy has not been established.

REFERRAL

- Phlebology
- Vascular surgery
- Indications for referral
  - ○ Skin and subcutaneous changes consistent with CVI
  - ○ Associated peripheral arterial insufficiency (PAD)
  - ○ Longstanding varicose vein disease
  - ○ Consideration for vein ablation procedure

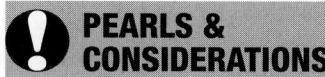 **PEARLS & CONSIDERATIONS**

COMMENTS

- Inflammatory skin changes from CVI are irreversible. The goal of therapy is to eliminate venous hypertension and prevent progression.
- Venous ulcers are often an end-stage manifestation of CVI. Refer to section on "Venous Ulcers" for more information.

SUGGESTED READINGS
available at www.expertconsult.com

RELATED CONTENT

Stasis Dermatitis (Patient Information)

AUTHOR: **FRANK G. FORT, M.D., F.A.C.S.**

BASIC INFORMATION

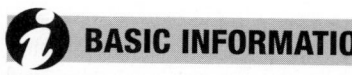

DEFINITION

Venous ulcers are defined as chronic defects of the skin that fail to heal spontaneously and persist for longer than 4 weeks. Venous ulcers account for about 70% of all lower extremity ulcerations. They are usually located in the "gaiter" region and can be accompanied by varicose veins, edema, hyperpigmentation, and lipodermatosclerosis. Venous ulceration develops in patients as a result of sustained venous hypertension.

SYNONYMS

Stasis ulcers

ICD-9CM CODES
459.3   Chronic venous hypertension, including stasis edema
459.81 Peripheral venous insufficiency
707.1   Ulcer of the lower limb (calf: 2, ankle: 3)

EPIDEMIOLOGY & DEMOGRAPHICS

In industrialized nations, up to 1.5% of the population will suffer from venous ulcers. In patients ≥65 yr old, the incidence increases to 4%. In the U.S., more than 500,000 people suffer from stasis ulcers.

RISK FACTORS

- Obesity
- Increasing age
- Family history of chronic venous insufficiency
- History of deep venous thromboembolism

PHYSICAL FINDINGS & CLINICAL PRESENTATION

Venous ulcers are most commonly located in the lower leg just above the ankle (gaiter region). They are a partial-thickness, irregularly shaped wound with well-defined borders with granulation tissue and fibrin present in the ulcer base (Fig. E1-887). Venous ulcers are relatively painless and are surrounded by brown-stained skin and/or dry, itchy, and reddened skin. In about 50% of patients, there are visible varicose veins in an aching, swollen leg.

ETIOLOGY

The exact mechanism of the role of venous hypertension in the etiology of venous ulcers is not certain. Hemodynamic forces such as venous hypertension, circulatory stasis, and modified conditions of shear stress appear to play an important role in an inflammatory reaction accompanied by leukocyte activation that clinically leads to fibrosclerotic remodeling of the skin and then to ulceration.

DIAGNOSIS

DIFFERENTIAL DIAGNOSIS

- Arterial ulcer
- Neurotrophic ulcers (located predominantly in the foot)
- Vasculitis
- Pyoderma gangrenosum
- Ulcerated skin tumors like basal cell or squamous cell carcinoma (Marjolin's ulcer)
- Rheumatoid arthritis

WORKUP

- The history and clinical signs and symptoms of leg ulcers are often misleading and may not differentiate venous ulcers from other leg ulcers; about 30% of leg ulcers are not of venous origin.
- Measurement of the ankle-brachial index (ABI) is essential in excluding peripheral arterial disease (PAD), which can be present in 20% of patients and is required before starting compression therapy. Arterial insufficiency is suggested by an ABI <0.9.
- Patients with lower-extremity ulcers should also be evaluated for diabetes.
- Coagulation defects have been found in 40% of patients with leg ulcers. This finding suggests that many patients with leg ulcers have a known or suspected history of deep venous thrombosis and a thrombophilia workup is indicated.
- If vasculitis is suspected, a biopsy of the edge of the ulcer can confirm the diagnosis.
- Any wound that has failed to improve after therapy of 4 wk should have a biopsy to rule out malignancy.

IMAGING STUDIES

- Evaluation of patients with venous leg ulcer should include duplex sonography to identify reflux in the superficial, deep, and perforating veins as well as possible obstruction of the deep veins.
- If the ulcer appears to be infected, consider tissue for culture, plain x-ray films, and bone scan to evaluate for osteomyelitis.

TREATMENT

NONPHARMACOLOGIC THERAPY

- Surgical debridement to remove all nonviable material can be accomplished in the office setting with the use of a topical Xylocaine gel. Debridement produces the release of growth factors that allow the development of healthy granulation tissue and the initiation of the healing process.
- The first-line treatment of ulcers includes below-knee compression stockings to improve venous return to the heart, thereby decreasing edema, inflammation, and tissue ischemia (used only if the ABI is between 0.6 and 0.85 because compression can cause limb ischemia).
- There is Level A evidence that graduated compression stockings alone can lead to healing of a venous ulcer. The stockings should be worn during the day and removed at night.
- Regular, brisk walking 30 min a day, five times a week is recommended.
- Elevate leg above heart level and raise the foot of bed with 3-in blocks to reduce edema.
- Role of surgery: in a randomized controlled trial, endovenous catheter ablation of superficial reflux showed no improvement in the healing rate of ulcers but did demonstrate a reduction of ulcer recurrence from 28% to 12% at 12 mo.

ACUTE GENERAL Rx

- Dressings are used under compression stockings to provide a clean, moist environment to promote healing.
- Modern, more complex dressings have been developed and include occlusive and semi-occlusive dressings, classified according to their physical composition and ability to control wound drainage.
- Semiocclusive dressings have varying ability to absorb wound drainage. Some examples of this type are hydrocolloids (DuoDerm), hydrogels (Duoderm hydrogel), foam dressings (Allevyn), and alginates.
- Biologic wound dressings (Apligraf) and tissue-engineered products (Oasis) have been developed, and these products can either directly provide growth factors or indirectly stimulate growth factors in the ulcer bed.
- Pentoxifylline (800 mg tid) has been shown to be an effective adjuvant to compression therapy as reported in a meta-analysis of nine clinical trials.
- Skin grafting should be considered for large or refractory ulcers as long as the wound is clean and there is healthy granulation tissue.
- Published randomized clinical trials on the value of the different types of dressings in the management of leg ulcers have not shown effects on ulcer healing. Despite the lack of evidence to support their use, modern dressings remain a part of the standard of care. Decisions regarding their use should be based on local cost of the dressings and the physician's clinical experience.
- Trials involving the use of weekly, low-dose, high-frequency ultrasound for hard-to-heal venous leg ulcers do not support adding therapeutic ultrasound to standard care for venous leg ulcers.

DISPOSITION

The overall prognosis for this condition is poor; the healing rate depends on the initial size of the ulcer. Although 65% to 70% of venous ulcers are healed within 6 mo, the 5-yr recurrence rate of healed venous ulcers can be as high as 40%. Maintenance of lifelong compression therapy is recommended.

REFERRAL

All patients should be evaluated weekly during the first month of therapy. Nonhealing ulcers with little to no improvement should also be referred to a wound care clinic.

EVIDENCE

available at www.expertconsult.com

SUGGESTED READINGS

available at www.expertconsult.com

AUTHOR: FRANK G. FORT, M.D., F.A.C.S.

BASIC INFORMATION

DEFINITION

- *Ventricular septal defect* (VSD) refers to an abnormal communication through the septum that separates the right and left ventricles of the heart.
- VSDs may be large or small, single or multiple.
- VSDs are located at various anatomic regions of the septum and classified as follows:
  - Membranous (75% to 80%): This is the most common type of defect, and it extends into the membranous portion of the interventricular septum. The septal leaflet of the tricuspid valve may become adherent and form a "pouch" of the septum that can limit the left-to-right shunting and lead to self-closure.
  - Muscular or trabecular (5% to 20%): This defect is entirely surrounded by muscular tissue. Spontaneous closure is common.
  - Canal or inlet (8%): This defect commonly lies beneath the septal leaflet of the tricuspid valve; associated with Down syndrome.
  - Subarterial, outlet, infundibular, or supracristal (5% to 7%): This is the least common type of defect. It is usually found beneath the aortic valve, and it may lead to aortic regurgitation. High prevalence in Asian population.

SYNONYMS

VSD

ICD-9CM CODES
745.4 Ventricular septal defect

EPIDEMIOLOGY & DEMOGRAPHICS

- VSDs are one of the most common congenital heart abnormalities, accounting for 30% of all congenital cardiac defects.
- VSD accounts for ~25% of all congenital heart defects in children and for approximately 10% of defects in adults (the decrease is a result of spontaneous closure that occurs by adulthood).
- The prevalence of VSD is 3 to 3.5 infants per 1000 live births and 0.5/1000 adults.
- VSD is found with equal frequency among both males and females.
- VSD may be associated with the following conditions:
  - Atrial septal defect (35%)
  - Patent ductus arteriosus (22%)
  - Coarctation of the aorta (17%)
  - Subvalvular aortic stenosis (4%)
  - Subpulmonic stenosis, usually associated with progressive aortic regurgitation caused by prolapse of the aortic cusp through the defect
- Multiple VSDs are more prevalent among patients with tetralogy of Fallot and double-outlet right ventricular defects.

PHYSICAL FINDINGS & CLINICAL PRESENTATION

- Clinical presentation depends on the direction and volume of the VSD shunt, which is dictated by the size of the defect and the ratio of the pulmonary vascular resistance. Fig. 1-888 illustrates the physiology of VSD.
  - Defects of ≤25% of the aortic annulus diameter are small defects. These typically involve small left-to-right shunts, no left ventricular volume overload, and no pulmonary artery hypertension (PAH).
  - Defects that are 25% to 75% of aortic annulus diameter are considered to be moderate in size. Small to moderate left-to-right shunting, mild to moderate left ventricular volume overload, and mild or no pulmonary artery hypertension are seen. Patients may have symptoms of congestive heart failure that may improve with medical therapy or with age as the defect decreases in size relative to increasing body size.
  - Defects of ≥75% of the aortic annulus diameter usually have moderate to large left-to-right shunting, left ventricular volume overload, and pulmonary artery hypertension. These patients usually have a history of congestive heart failure, or they may possibly develop right-to-left shunting in the setting of Eisenmenger's syndrome during late childhood, adolescence, or young adulthood.
- Infants may be asymptomatic at birth because of elevated pulmonary artery resistance. During the first few weeks of life, pulmonary arterial resistance decreases, thereby allowing for more left-to-right shunting through the VSD. This results in a subsequent increase in flow into the lungs, the left atrium, and the left ventricle, which can potentially cause left ventricular volume overload. Tachypnea, failure to thrive, and congestive heart failure may then ensue.
- In adults with VSD, the shunt is left to right in the absence of pulmonary stenosis and pulmonary hypertension. Patients typically manifest symptoms of left-sided heart failure from left ventricular volume overload (e.g., shortness of breath, orthopnea, dyspnea on exertion).
- A spectrum of physical findings may be seen, including the following:
  - Machinelike holosystolic murmur that is heard best along the left sternal border
  - Murmur becomes shorter as right heart pressures increase
  - Systolic thrill
  - Mid-diastolic rumble heard at the apex
  - S_3 heart sound
  - Rales
- With the development of pulmonary hypertension, the following occur:
  - An augmented pulmonic component of the S_2 heart sound
  - Cyanosis, clubbing, right ventricular heave, and signs of right heart failure (i.e., as seen with Eisenmenger's complex, with a reversal of the shunt in a right-to-left direction)

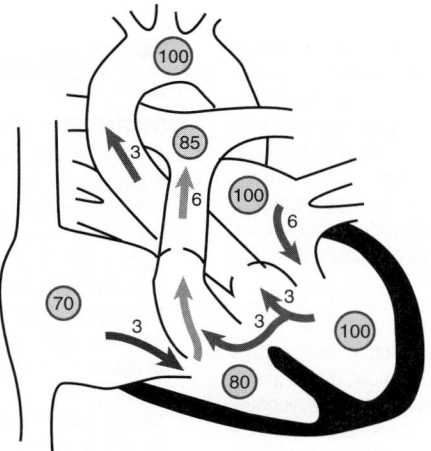

FIGURE 1-888 Physiology of a large ventricular septal defect (VSD). Circled numbers represent oxygen saturation values. The numbers next to the arrows represent volumes of blood flow (in L/min/m²). This illustration shows a hypothetical patient with a pulmonary-to-systemic blood flow ratio (Qp:Qs) of 2:1. Desaturated blood enters the right atrium from the vena cava at a volume of 3 L/min/m² and flows across the tricuspid valve. An additional 3 L of blood shunts left to right across the VSD, the result being an increase in oxygen saturation in the right ventricle. Six liters of blood is ejected into the lungs. Pulmonary arterial saturation may be further increased because of incomplete mixing at right ventricular level. Six liters returns to the left atrium, crosses the mitral valve, and causes a mid-diastolic flow rumble. Three liters of this volume shunts left to right across the VSD, and 3 L is ejected into the ascending aorta (normal cardiac output). (From Kliegman RM et al: *Nelson textbook of pediatrics,* ed 19, Philadelphia, 2011, Saunders.)

ETIOLOGY

- VSD is usually congenital but can be acquired.
- Acquired VSD may result from postsurgical residual leak, trauma, or myocardial infarction.
- Postinfarct ventricular septal defect (PIVSD) typically occurs 1 to 5 days after the event in 0.2% of patients in the current fibrinolytic, primary angioplasty era.

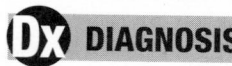 **DIAGNOSIS**

The diagnosis of VSD can be suspected during a physical examination. Imaging studies—particularly transthoracic echocardiography with color Doppler—establish the diagnosis.

DIFFERENTIAL DIAGNOSIS

On the basis of the physical examination alone, the diagnosis of VSD may be confused with other causes of systolic murmurs, such as mitral regurgitation, tricuspid regurgitation, aortic stenosis, pulmonary stenosis, and hypertrophic cardiomyopathy.

WORKUP

Any person who is suspected of having a VSD should undergo an ECG, a chest radiograph, and an echocardiogram.

LABORATORY TESTS

- Laboratory tests are not specific but may offer insight into the severity of the disease.
- The CBC may show polycythemia, especially in patients with Eisenmenger's complex.
- Arterial blood gas results may demonstrate hypoxemia.

IMAGING STUDIES

- ECG findings vary in accordance with the size of the VSD and depending on whether pulmonary hypertension is present. With large VSDs with pulmonary hypertension, right-axis deviation is seen, along with evidence of right ventricular hypertrophy.
- Chest x-ray findings in patients with VSD include the following:
  - Cardiomegaly that results from left ventricular volume overload that directly relates to the magnitude of the shunt
  - The enlargement of the proximal pulmonary arteries along with the redistribution and pruning of the distal pulmonary vessels as a result of sustained pulmonary hypertension (Fig. 1-889, *A*)
- Echocardiography is the imaging modality of choice for the diagnosis of VSD:
  - Two-dimensional echocardiography and color Doppler display the size and location of the VSD (Fig. 1-889, *B*), the chamber sizes, ventricular function, the presence of aortic valve prolapse or regurgitation, outflow tract obstruction, and the presence of tricuspid regurgitation.
  - Continuous-wave Doppler approximates the gradient between the left and right ventricles and estimates the pulmonary artery pressure.
  - The magnitude of the shunt can be determined by the calculation of the pulmonary-to-systemic flow ratio with the use of echocardiography.
- Heart catheterization is primarily indicated to assess operability of VSD patients with PAH, and in patients in whom the noninvasive testing was inconclusive, and further information, such as quantification of shunting and assessment of pulmonary pressures, is required.
- Ventriculography may help to locate the VSD:
  - MRI and computed tomography scanning can be useful to assess the pulmonary artery, the pulmonary vein, and the aortic anatomy and to confirm the anatomy of unusual VSDs (e.g., inlet or apical defects) that are not seen well with echocardiography.

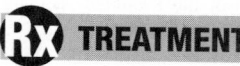 **TREATMENT**

The decision to close a VSD depends on the type, size, and shunt severity as well as the patient's pulmonary vascular resistance, functional capacity, and associated valvular abnormalities.

NONPHARMACOLOGIC THERAPY

- Young children and adults with a small, asymptomatic VSD with a large left-to-right ventricular pressure gradient, a pulmonary-to-systemic blood flow ratio of less than 1.5:1, and no evidence of pulmonary hypertension can be observed (i.e., restrictive defect).

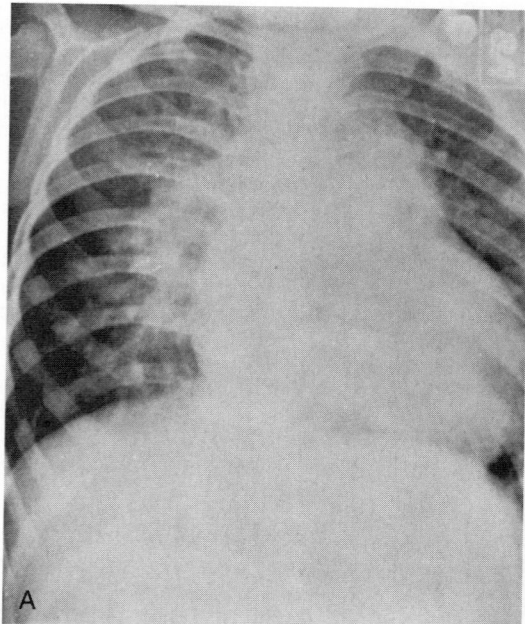
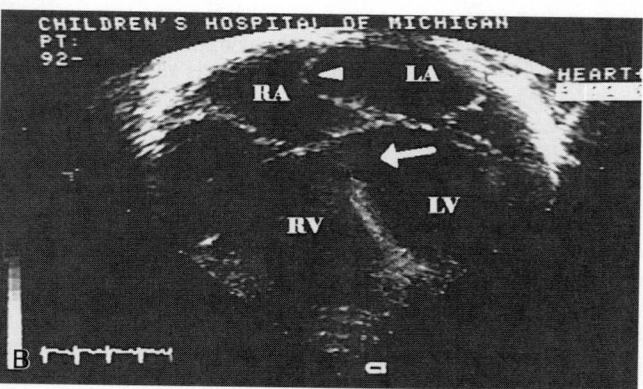

FIGURE 1-889 A, Chest roentgenogram of a child with a large ventricular septal defect, large pulmonary blood flow, and pulmonary hypertension but only mild elevation of peripheral vascular resistance. This is reflected in the evidence of left and right ventricular enlargement, the enlargement of the main pulmonary artery, and a marked increase in pulmonary blood flow. **B,** Apical four-chamber echocardiographic view of ventricular septal defect *(large arrow)*. The small arrow points to the interatrial septum. *LA,* Left atrium; *LV,* left ventricle; *RA,* right atrium; *RV,* right ventricle. (**A** from Pacifico AD et al: Surgical treatment of ventricular septal defect. In Sabiston DC Jr, Spencer FC [eds]: *Surgery of the chest,* ed 5, Philadelphia, 1990, Saunders. **B** courtesy of Richard Humes, M.D., Children's Hospital of Michigan, Detroit.)

- Oxygen for hypoxemia and a low-salt diet are recommended for patients with congestive heart failure.

ACUTE GENERAL & CHRONIC RX

Closure is indicated for the following patients:
- Infants with congestive heart failure
- Children between the ages of 1 and 6 yr with persistent VSD and a pulmonary-to-systemic blood flow ratio (Qp/Qs) of >2:1
- Adults with a Qp/Qs of ≥2 and clinical evidence of left ventricular volume overload (class I):
  - Positive history of infective endocarditis (IE) (class I)
  - Adults with a Qp/Qs of >1.5 with pulmonary artery pressure that is less than two thirds of the systemic pressure and pulmonary vascular resistance that is less than two thirds of the systemic vascular resistance (class IIa)
  - Adults with a Qp/Qs of >1.5 in the presence of left ventricular systolic or diastolic failure (class IIa)
  - Surgical closure is not indicated for VSD with severe irreversible PAH.

Surgical closure with Dacron or Gore-Tex patches or primary surgical closure has long been the gold standard of therapy. However, with improvements in cardiac imaging and catheter devices, percutaneous transcatheter closure has risen in popularity. Some studies have shown similar success rates for both surgical and percutaneous closures, and there are significantly fewer complications, days in the hospital, and blood transfusions after percutaneous closures.

Catheter-based closure in muscular VSD may be considered, especially if the VSD is remote from the tricuspid valve and the aorta, if the VSD is associated with severe left-sided heart chamber enlargement, or if there is PAH (class IIb). Device closure is indicated in residual defects after prior attempts at surgical closure, restrictive VSDs with either a significant left-to-right shunt (Qp/Qs >1.5:1) or hx of IE, trauma, or iatrogenic artifacts after surgical replacement of the aortic valve.

PIVSDs usually carry a high mortality rate, and surgical closure remains the gold standard in the acute setting or for large (>15 mm) septal ruptures. In the subacute or chronic setting, small or medium PIVSD (<15 mm) can be treated with percutaneous closure with comparable mortality to surgery.

DISPOSITION

- The natural history of an isolated VSD depends on the type of defect, its size, and any associated abnormalities.
- ~75% to 80% of small VSDs close spontaneously by the time the patient reaches the age of 10 yr.

- Only 10% to 15% of large VSDs will close spontaneously.
- Large VSDs that are left untreated may lead to arrhythmias, congestive heart failure, pulmonary hypertension, and Eisenmenger's complex.
- Eisenmenger's complex carries a poor prognosis, with most patients dying before the age of 40 yr.
- Issues to monitor in adults with unrepaired or repaired and catheter-closed VSDs include the following:
  - Development of aortic regurgitation
  - Assessment of associated coronary artery disease
  - Development of tricuspid regurgitation
  - Assessment of the degree of left-to-right shunting (in unrepaired or residual VSD after repair)
  - Ventricular dysfunction
  - Assessment of pulmonary pressure
  - Development of subpulmonary stenosis (usually as a result of a double-chambered right ventricle)
  - Development of discrete subaortic stenosis
  - Development of arrhythmia or heart block
  - Thromboembolic complications
  - Infective endocarditis
- After closure, late survival is excellent when ventricular function is normal. Pulmonary artery hypertension may improve, progress, or remain the same. Late operations may be required for tricuspid or aortic regurgitation.

REFERRAL

All infants and children diagnosed with VSD should be referred to a pediatric cardiologist. Adults with VSD should be referred to an adult cardiologist. Cardiothoracic surgeons who have experience with congenital heart disease surgery should be consulted if surgery is indicated.

FOLLOW-UP

- Adults with no residual VSD, no associated lesions, and normal pulmonary artery pressure do not require continued follow-up at a regional adult congenital heart disease (ACHD) center except on referral from the patient's cardiologist or physician.
- Adults with VSD with residual heart failure, shunts, PAH, AR, or RV outflow tract (RVOT) or LV outflow tract (LVOT) obstruction should be seen at least annually at an ACHD regional center (level of evidence: C).
- Adults with a small residual VSD and no other lesions should be seen every 3 to 5 yr at an ACHD regional center (level of evidence: C).
- Adults with device closure of a VSD should be followed up every 1 to 2 yr at an ACHD center depending on the location of the VSD and other factors.

- Patients who develop bifascicular block or transient trifascicular block after VSD closure are at risk in later years for the development of complete heart block and should be followed up yearly by history and ECG and have periodic ambulatory monitoring and/or exercise testing.

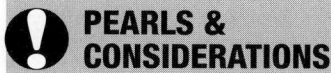

PEARLS & CONSIDERATIONS

COMMENTS

- A loud murmur does not imply a large VSD. Small, hemodynamically insignificant VSDs can cause loud murmurs.
- In patients with Eisenmenger's complex, the right-to-left shunting across the VSD is usually not associated with an audible murmur.
- The risk of patients with unrepaired VSD developing infective endocarditis is 4%. The risk is higher if aortic insufficiency is present.
- For patients with endocarditis, routine antibiotic prophylaxis for dental or surgical procedures is no longer indicated for isolated VSDs, except in the following circumstances:
  - In the presence of complex congenital heart disease with cyanosis
  - In the presence of a residual VSD after surgical closure
  - During the first 6 mo after surgical patch or percutaneous transcatheter closure
- Any patient with a newly diagnosed murmur or hemodynamic compromise after a myocardial infarction should undergo evaluation for possible VSD.
- Pregnancy with a VSD is generally well tolerated in women with small VSDs, no pulmonary artery hypertension, and no associated lesions. Women with large shunts may experience arrhythmias, ventricular dysfunction, and the progression of pulmonary hypertension.
- Women with VSDs and severe pulmonary artery hypertension or Eisenmenger's physiology should be counseled against pregnancy because of associated excessive maternal and fetal mortality.
- Minimally invasive periventricular device closure of VSD without cardiopulmonary bypass under guidance of transesophageal echocardiography is a promising technique, but it needs long-term follow-up.

SUGGESTED READINGS

available at www.expertconsult.com

RELATED CONTENT

Ventricular Septal Defect (VSD) (Patient Information)

AUTHORS: **AKINNIRAN A. ABISOGUN, M.D.,** and **WEN-CHIH WU, M.D.**

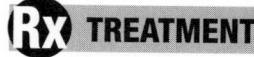 BASIC INFORMATION

DEFINITION

Vertebral compression fractures (VCFs) are defined as fractures of spinal vertebrae in which a bony surface is driven toward another bony surface. These fractures are classified as radiographic reductions in vertebral body height of more than 15% to 20%.

SYNONYMS

Thoracolumbar vertebral compression fractures
Osteoporotic fractures

ICD-9CM CODES
805.8   Compression fracture, spine
805.4   Compression fracture, lumbar vertebra
805.2   Compression fracture, thoracic vertebra
733.13 Compression fracture, L2 vertebra

EPIDEMIOLOGY & DEMOGRAPHICS

~750,000 VCFs occur in the United States each year, and they affect up to 25% of postmenopausal women. The prevalence increases with age, reaching a peak of 40% to 50% among women aged >80 yr. Compression fractures are also a major concern among men, although their rates of VCF are lower.

RISK FACTORS:
- Modifiable: tobacco or alcohol use, osteoporosis, estrogen deficiency (i.e., early menopause, bilateral ovariectomy, premenopausal amenorrhea for >1 yr), frailty, impaired vision, abusive situations, inadequate physical activity, low body mass index, and dietary deficiency of vitamin D or calcium
- Nonmodifiable: advanced age, female gender, dementia, Caucasian, history of fractures in adulthood and among first-degree relatives, and falls

PHYSICAL FINDINGS & CLINICAL PRESENTATION

- Asymptomatic: Most VCFs are asymptomatic, except for height loss or kyphosis (i.e., dowager's hump [Fig. 1-890]), which is often a sign of multiple VCFs.
- Symptomatic: Many VCFs often present as acute back pain after activity (e.g., bending, lifting) or coughing; neck strain and rib pain may also be present.

ETIOLOGY

- VCFs take place when the combination of bending and the axial load on the spine exceed the strength of the vertebral body.
- The primary etiology of VCF is osteoporosis.

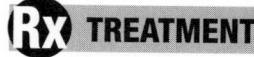 DIAGNOSIS

DIFFERENTIAL DIAGNOSIS

- Hyperparathyroidism
- Osteomalacia
- Granulomatous diseases (e.g., tuberculosis)

- Hematologic/oncologic diseases (e.g., multiple myeloma, malignancy)

WORKUP

- Only one third of VCFs are diagnosed. Guidelines for patient selection for vertebral fractural assessment are described in Box 1-82.
- VCF can be clinically suspected from the history and physical alone.
- There may or may not be a specific injury or a remembered event that led to the VCF.

LABORATORY TESTS

Tests to rule out infection or cancer may be helpful, such as a CBC, an erythrocyte sedimentation rate, an alkaline phosphatase level, and a C-reactive protein level; these tests can be reserved for individuals for whom there is clinical suspicion.

IMAGING STUDIES

- Plain frontal and lateral radiographs (x-rays) are the initial imaging method (Fig. 1-890) and may be sufficient, particularly when no neurologic abnormalities are present. MRI and computed tomography (CT) scans may be uncomfortable or painful for the patient, especially during the acute phase.
- Although CT scans are not routinely necessary, they can be helpful for visualizing fractures that are not seen on plain films, for evaluating the integrity of the posterior vertebral wall, for ruling out other causes of back pain, for detecting spinal canal narrowing, and for assessing instability.

- MRI may be useful when spinal cord compression is suspected, if neurologic symptoms are present, or to distinguish malignancy from osteoporosis (e.g., in patients <55 yr with VCF after minimal or no trauma).
- Bone density studies may be helpful to determine the severity of osteoporosis, which is a key risk factor for future fractures.

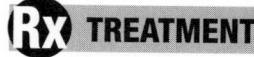 TREATMENT

NONPHARMACOLOGIC THERAPY

- Physical therapy
- External back braces
- Exercise programs: Getting the person active as soon as possible is extremely important for both the short and long term.

ACUTE GENERAL Rx

- Analgesics for pain control, including acetaminophen and opioids (oral or parenteral). The prevention of constipation is important with opioids.
- Nonsteroidal anti-inflammatory drugs are helpful but must be used with caution among elderly patients or when contraindicated.
- Muscle relaxants should be used judiciously.
- The efficacy of vertebroplasty versus kyphoplasty versus conservative treatment is controversial: percutaneous vertebroplasty involves the injection of acrylic bone cement into the affected vertebral body in an effort to stabilize the fracture and reduce pain, while in kyphoplasty a high-pressure inflatable

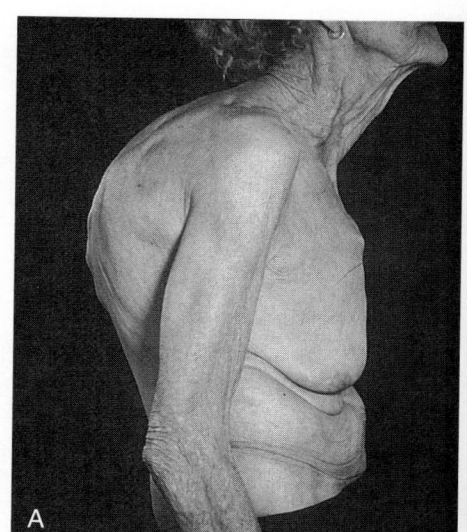
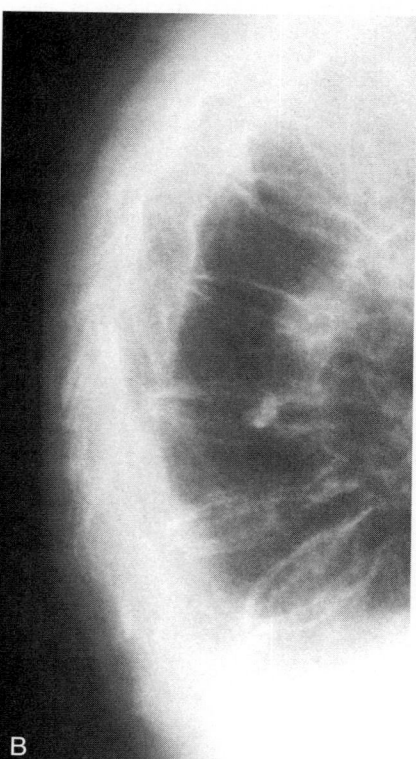

FIGURE 1-890 Dowager's hump. A, Marked thoracic kyphosis due to multiple osteoporotic fractures in an elderly woman with corresponding radiograph (**B**). (From Hochberg MC et al [eds]: *Rheumatology,* ed 3, St Louis, 2003, Mosby.)

bone tamp or balloon is expanded before the injection of bone cement into the cavity in the fractured vertebral body. These two procedures were thought to be helpful in patients who did not respond to conservative therapy; however, further studies showed them to be no more effective than sham procedures (Buchbinder et al., 2009; Kallmes et al., 2009). Nonetheless, Klazen et al. (2010) demonstrated in an open-label prospective randomized trial that for the subgroup of patients with acute osteoporotic VCFs fractures and persistent pain, percutaneous vertebroplasty may provide immediate pain relief, sustained for at least a year, which may be significantly greater than that achieved with conservative treatment. Zampiri (2011) showed in a nonrandomized cohort study that elderly patients who underwent kyphoplasty were more likely to be discharged home. These procedures are still in their infancy, and more answers should be forthcoming as to their efficacy, as well as questions regarding the amount of time that conservative therapy alone should be pursued and which procedure, if any, should be advised.

CHRONIC Rx

Osteoporosis should be treated with the reduction of risk factors (e.g., smoking, alcohol), diet, exercise, calcium and vitamin D supplements, and potentially the use of medications that are more commonly used to treat osteoporosis (e.g., bisphosphonates).

REFERRAL

Referral is indicated for neurologic abnormalities, unremitting pain, instability, continued disability, or when the investigation of the cause of the fracture reveals serious underlying pathology.

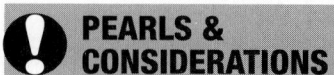

PEARLS & CONSIDERATIONS

Prevention of osteoporosis and conservative therapy remain the mainstays.

COMMENTS

- VCFs should be suspected in anyone aged >50 yr with the acute onset of low back pain. There are many opportunities for diagnosis and treatment that are easy to miss, especially for males.
- Solitary vertebral fractures higher than T7 are unusual and may raise suspicion for other pathologic causes.
- Diagnosing and treating osteoporosis reduce the incidence of VCFs.
- Getting people with VCF physically active as soon as possible will be efficacious both acutely and in the long term.
- In general, VCF can perhaps be best managed through a partnership of the patient, the primary care physician, an orthopedist, a physical therapist, a dietitian, and a social worker.

PREVENTION

Reducing the effects of modifiable risk factors is key.

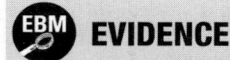

EVIDENCE

available at www.expertconsult.com

SUGGESTED READINGS

available at www.expertconsult.com

BOX 1-82 2007 ISCD Guidelines for Patient Selection for Vertebral Fractural Assessment

- Postmenopausal women with low bone mass (osteopenia) by BMD criteria, *plus* any one of the following: age ≥70 yr, historical height loss >4 cm (1.6 in), or prospective height loss >2 cm (0.8 in), self-reported vertebral fracture (not previously documented)
- Two or more of the following: age 60 to 69 yr, self-reported prior non-vertebral fracture, historical height loss of 2 to 4 cm, or chronic systemic diseases associated with increased risk of vertebral fractures (e.g., moderate to severe COPD or COAD, seropositive rheumatoid arthritis, Crohn's disease)
- Men with low bone mass (osteopenia) by BMD criteria, *plus* any one of the following: age ≥80 yr, historical height loss >6 cm (2.4 in), prospective height loss >3 cm (1.2 in), self-reported vertebral fracture (not previously documented)
- Two or more of the following: age 70 to 79 yr, self-reported prior non-vertebral fracture, historical height loss of 3 to 6 cm, on pharmacologic androgen deprivation therapy or following orchiectomy, chronic systemic diseases associated with increased risk of vertebral fractures (e.g., moderate to severe COPD or COAD, seropositive rheumatoid arthritis, Crohn's disease)
- Women or men on chronic glucocorticoid therapy (equivalent to 5 mg or more of prednisone daily for 3 mo or longer)
- Postmenopausal women or men with osteoporosis by BMD criteria, if documentation of one or more vertebral fractures will alter clinical management

BMD, Bone mineral density; *COAD,* chronic obstructive airways disease; *COPD,* chronic obstructive pulmonary disease; *ISCD,* International Society for Clinical Densitometry.
Reproduced with permission from the International Society for Clinical Densitometry.
From Hochberg MC et al: *Rheumatology,* ed 5, St Louis, 2011, Mosby.

AUTHOR: **JEFFREY BORKAN, M.D., PH.D.**

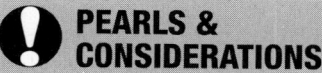

BASIC INFORMATION

DEFINITION

Vestibular neuronitis is a syndrome of sudden-onset dysfunction of the peripheral vestibular system, often severe, with prolonged vertigo, nausea, and vomiting.

SYNONYMS

Vestibular neuritis
Acute neuritis
Neurolabyrinthitis
Vestibular neuropathy

ICD-9CM CODES

078.81 Vestibular neuronitis
386.12 Neuronitis, vestibular

EPIDEMIOLOGY & DEMOGRAPHICS

Vestibular neuritis is the second most common cause of peripheral vestibular vertigo with an incidence of about 3.5:100,000 population. Although etiology remains uncertain, thought to result from selective inflammation of the vestibular nerve, the etiology is presumed to be viral. Viral origin is supported by the fact that it occurs in epidemics, may affect several family members, and occurs more commonly in spring and early summer. The male-to-female ratio is nearly 1:1. There is selective damage to the superior part of the vestibular labyrinth, supplied by the superior division of the vestibular nerve.

PHYSICAL FINDINGS & CLINICAL PRESENTATION

Course: develops over period of hours and resolves over periods of days or weeks, although long-term sequelae may occur. Symptoms include vertigo, spontaneous peripheral nystagmus, positive head-thrust test, and imbalance. Patient reports intense sensation of rotation and difficulty standing and walking and tends to veer toward affected side; autonomic symptoms occur with pallor, sweating, nausea, and vomiting.

ETIOLOGY

Etiology remains uncertain. It is thought to be viral in origin, possibly due to herpes zoster, reactivation of herpes simplex, or other viruses, but evidence is circumstantial.

DIAGNOSIS

DIFFERENTIAL DIAGNOSIS

- Labyrinthitis: similar symptoms of vertigo, with the addition of unilateral hearing loss
- Labyrinthine infarction
- Acoustic neuroma
- Perilymph fistula
- Brain stem and cerebellar infarction
- Migraine-associated vertigo
- Meniere disease
- Multiple sclerosis

WORKUP

- Patient may fall toward affected side when attempting ambulation or during Romberg tests.
- Hallpike maneuver: checking for nystagmus and asking about recreation of vertigo symptoms
- Head-thrust test: grasp patient's head, apply brief small-amplitude rapid head turn, first to one side and then the other; patient fixates on examiner's nose: positive test is lack of corrective eye movements ("saccades") on affected side
- Laboratory testing and imaging are generally not indicated but may help rule out other etiologies

LABORATORY TESTS

- Electronystagmography (ENG): a battery of eye movement tests that may provide an objective assessment of the vestibular and oculomotor systems and may help localize the lesion's site
- Audiogram: normal

IMAGING STUDIES

Brain imaging: CT or MRI—normal

TREATMENT

NONPHARMACOLOGIC THERAPY

Vestibular exercises, when tolerated, will accelerate recovery.

ACUTE GENERAL Rx

Most treatments are empirical and related to symptoms. Further studies are needed.

- Corticosteroids: corticosteroids are often prescribed, although a recent Cochrane Review finds that there is insufficient evidence for administration. Some studies have shown that glucocorticoids administered within 3 days after onset of vestibular neuronitis may improve long-time recovery of vestibular function and reduce the length of hospital stay and may improve the caloric extent and recovery of canal paresis.

- Antihistamines: e.g., meclizine, dimenhydrinate, promethazine
- Anticholinergics: scopolamine
- Antiemetics: droperidol, prochlorperazine
- Benzodiazepines: e.g., diazepam, valium, lorazepam
- Valacyclovir, either alone or in combination, is likely ineffective in treating vestibular neuronitis.

CHRONIC Rx

- Vestibular rehabilitation exercises
- Anti-GABA agents
- Antihistamines

DISPOSITION

Most patients can be treated as outpatients, but inpatient care may be required in cases where vomiting is uncontrollable. If dehydrated because of severe vomiting, sufferers may require brief parenteral therapy.

REFERRAL

- ENT: if diagnosis uncertain, and if these patients are at risk for benign paroxysmal positional vertigo (BPPV) subsequently; also if symptoms linger
- Neurology: if question of central origin or migraine

PEARLS & CONSIDERATIONS

COMMENTS

- Diagnosis unlikely to be vestibular neuronitis if hearing is impaired or other neurologic signs and symptoms are present.
- Although patients may recover from dramatic acute symptoms, subtle vestibular deficits may linger for prolonged period, if not indefinitely.
- Program of vestibular habituation head movement exercises can reduce imbalance symptoms.

PATIENT & FAMILY EDUCATION

Vestibular Disorders Association: http://www.vestibular.org

SUGGESTED READINGS

available at www.expertconsult.com

AUTHOR: **JEFFREY M. BORKAN, M.D., PH.D.**

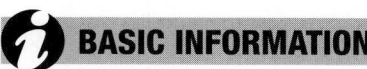

BASIC INFORMATION

DEFINITION

Vitamins are organic compounds that cannot be synthesized by humans but are required as nutrients in minute amounts. Vitamins have several different functions: They may regulate cell growth and differentiation, as catalysts, as antioxidants, and as co-enzymes. Vitamins are classified as either fat soluble (vitamins A, D, E, K) or water soluble (B group of vitamins and C). Deficiency of most vitamins is rare in Western countries. Certain groups may be prone to vitamin deficiency, and these are discussed here. Vitamin D deficiency is discussed in a separate topic.

SYNONYMS

Vitamin A: retinol
Vitamin E: alpha tocopherol
Vitamin K: phytonadione or menadiol
Vitamin B_1: thiamine
Vitamin B_2: riboflavin
Niacin: vitamin B_3; nicotinic acid
Vitamin B_5: pantothenic acid
Vitamin B_6: pyridoxine; pyridoxal phosphate
Folic acid: vitamin B_9; folate
Vitamin B_{12}: cyanocobalamin
Vitamin C: ascorbic acid

ICD-9CM CODES
264.8   Vitamin A deficiency
269.1   Vitamin E deficiency
260.0   Vitamin K deficiency
265.1   Vitamin B_1 deficiency
266.0   Vitamin B_2 deficiency
265.2   Niacin deficiency
266.1   Pyridoxine deficiency
266.2   Folic acid deficiency
266.2   Cyanocobalamin deficiency
267   Ascorbic acid deficiency

EPIDEMIOLOGY & DEMOGRAPHICS

Deficiency can occur in all age groups but is most common in the elderly.

Vitamin A deficiency: Affects 250 million preschool children worldwide.

Vitamin K deficiency: Varies by geographic regions; no race predilection; affects both sexes equally.

Vitamin B_1 (thiamine) deficiency: Incidence is unknown; no sex, race, or age predilection.

Vitamin B_5 (pantothenic acid) deficiency: Rare, as it is present in all foods.

Vitamin B_{12} (cobalamin) deficiency: Relatively common. Occurs in all age groups but more common in the elderly.

Vitamin B_9 (folic acid) deficiency: Mandatory fortification started in 1998. Prevalence before fortification 16% and after 0.5%. Neural tube defect associated with low maternal folate status during pregnancy. Pregnant women and the elderly are at greatest risk of folic acid deficiency.

Vitamin C (ascorbic acid) deficiency: Smokers and low-income persons are at increased risk.

PHYSICAL FINDINGS & CLINICAL PRESENTATION

- **Vitamin A:** xerophthalmia; xerosis of the cornea; keratomalacia; Bitot's spots (abnormal squamous cell proliferation and keratinization of the conjunctiva); nyctalopia (poor adaptation to darkness)/night blindness; poor bone growth; dry skin and hair
- **Vitamin E:** nerve dysfunction (ataxia; hyporeflexia, peripheral neuropathy); bone weakness.
- **Vitamin B_1 (thiamine):**
  - Nervous system (dry beriberi): peripheral neuropathy, Wernicke encephalopathy, Korsakoff syndrome.
  - Cardiovascular (wet beriberi): edema, chest pain, increased heart rate (HR), lowered blood pressure (BP).
  - Gastrointestinal (GI): anorexia; constipation.
- **Vitamin B_2 (riboflavin):**
  - Cheilosis (chapping and fissure of the lip)
  - Glossitis (sore red tongue)
  - Oily, scaly rashes on nasolabial folds, eyelids, scrotum, labia majoris
  - Red itchy eyes
  - Anemia
  - Peripheral neuropathy
- **Vitamin B_3 (niacin):**
  - Pellagra (4 *Ds*—diarrhea, dermatitis, dementia, and ultimately death).
  - Hyperpigmentation of sun-exposed skin.
  - "Raw beef" swollen and painful tongue.
- **Vitamin B_6:** seborrheic dermatitis; glossitis, cheilosis, impaired proprioception; sensory ataxia, seizure.
- **Vitamin B_{12}:** Neurologic symptoms including peripheral neuropathy, ataxia, paresthesia; subacute degeneration of the spinal cord (demyelination of the dorsal column). Patients may also have dementia, depression, and weakness. Glossitis and GI symptoms such as nausea, vomiting, and anorexia are also common.
- **Vitamin B_9 (folic acid):**
  - Patchy hyperpigmentation of skin (especially between fingers and toes) and mucous membranes
  - Moderate fever (temp <102° F) despite the absence of infection
  - Neural tube defect
  - Angular stomatitis
  - Red, beefy, smooth and shiny tongue.
- **Vitamin C:** scurvy (poor wound healing, petechiae, follicular hyperkeratosis, fatigue, bleeding gums, weight loss).

ETIOLOGY

- Fat-soluble vitamins (vitamins A, D, E, K):
  1. Decreased ingestion, malnutrition, eating disorders.
  2. Diseases that affect fat absorption decrease the absorption of fat-soluble vitamins—for example, cystic fibrosis, celiac sprue, inflammatory bowel disease, cholestasis, hepatobiliary disease, small bowel surgery.

  3. Change in vitamin metabolism:
     - Alcoholism
     - Drugs such as cholestyramine, Coumadin
  4. Increased risk in:
     - Vegans
     - Recent immigrants
     - Refugees
     - Toddlers/preschoolers living below the poverty line
- Water-soluble vitamins (the B group of vitamins and viitamin C)—there are several etiologic factors, including:
  - Inadequate intake
  - Decreased absorption
  - Alcoholism
  - Pregnancy/lactation
  - Peritoneal dialysis
  - Medications (e.g., isoniazide, phenothiazides, tricyclic antidepressants)
  - Malabsorption
  - Low income
  - Advanced age
- Vitamin B_{12} deficiency—caused by:
  - Insufficient dietary intake, as in strict vegans
  - Decreased absorption secondary to intrinsic factor deficiency, decreased intrinsic factor secretion, gastric atrophy, gastrectomy
  - Terminal ileum disease such as celiac disease, enteritis, tropical sprue
- Folic acid deficiency—increased needs can lead to deficiency (e.g., pregnancy, lactation, malignancy).
- Derangement of folate metabolism by:
  - Medication (e.g., methotrexate)
  - Disease (e.g., hypothyroidism)
  - Increased excretion: as seen in alcoholics

DIAGNOSIS

WORKUP/LABORATORY TESTS

- General initial laboratory tests include:
  1. Complete blood cell count (CBC).
     Liver function tests (LFTs).
     Basic metabolic panel (BMP).
     Albumin.
  2. Measurement of serum levels of the specific vitamin in question.
- Specific tests may be considered in the following cases:
  - Vitamin A:
    Retinol binding protein.
    Dark-adaptation threshold test.
  - Vitamin K:
    Prothrombin time/partial thromboplastin time (PT/PTT).
    Prothrombin.
    Des-gamma-carboxy prothrombin (most sensitive test).
  - Niacin: urine-*N*-methylnicotinamide (level <0.8 mg/day indicates niacin deficiency).
  - Vitamin B_{12}:
    Serum vitamin B_{12} <100 pg/ml is diagnostic of vitamin B_{12} deficiency.

Serum methylmalonic acid, which is elevated in B_{12} deficiency.

Antiparietal antibody.

Intrinsic factor antibody is decreased.

Blood smear shows macrocytosis and hypersegmentation of megaloblasts.

CBC shows increased mean corpuscle volume (MCV).

Megaloblastic anemia.

○ Folic acid:

Check serum folate level

Additional testing includes checking for serum homocysteine level, which will be elevated.

Red cell folate level shows chronic folate status.

Rx TREATMENT

Most of the vitamins are available over the counter individually or in different multivitamin formulations.

Specific vitamins:
- Vitamin A deficiency: treat with oral supplementation 10,000 IU daily.
  - ○ Consume vitamin A–rich foods such as liver, beef, carrots, oranges, mangoes.
  - ○ 5 servings of fruit and vegetables give enough carotenoids for a day.
- Vitamin K deficiency: treatment depends on the severity of bleeding, administered subcutaneously (SQ) or intramuscularly (IM).
- Vitamin B_1 (thiamine) deficiency: give intramuscular thiamine 50 mg for several days.
  - ○ If B_1 deficiency is suspected and patient needs intravenous glucose, give thiamine first before intravenous glucose. This prevents the development of Korsakoff psychosis.
- Vitamin B_{12} deficiency: give 1000 mcg IM daily for 7 days, then once a week for 1 month, then once a month indefinitely.
  - ○ A potential option is oral supplementation.

- Folic acid deficiency: daily requirement is 400 to 1000 mcg (1 mg) daily.
  - ○ Centers for Disease Control and Prevention (CDC) recommend that women of childbearing age take 400 mcg of folic acid daily.

SUGGESTED READINGS

available at www.expertconsult.com

RELATED CONTENT

Anemia, Pernicious (Related Key Topic)
Rickets (Related Key Topic)
Vitamin D Deficiency (Related Key Topic)
Wernicke Syndrome (Related Key Topic)

AUTHOR: **DANIEL K. ASIEDU, M.D., PH.D., F.A.C.P.**

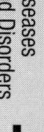

Diseases and Disorders

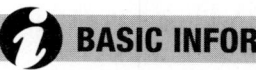

- Vitamin D is a hormone and a steroid and, by definition, not a vitamin. There are two forms of vitamin D: vitamin D_2 and vitamin D_3.
- Vitamin D_2 is mainly found in some plant foods.
- Vitamin D_3 is produced in skin exposed to ultraviolet (UV) B radiation from sunlight (Fig. E1-891). Gloson, Whistler, and DeBoot independently described rickets in the mid-seventeenth century. Sniadecki first reported the association of rickets with inadequate exposure to sunlight in 1822.
- The major functions of vitamin D include:
  - Increasing calcium and phosphorus absorption from the small intestines
  - Promoting the maturation of osteoclast to resorb calcium from bones

DEFINITION

Vitamin D deficiency is characterized by impaired bone mineralization. It is classified as a serum 25-hydroxyvitamin D (25[OH]D) level of <20 ng/ml (50 nmol/L).

SYNONYMS

The sunshine vitamin
The antirachitic factor
Cholecalciferol

ICD-9CM CODES
268.9 Vitamin D deficiency unspecified

EPIDEMIOLOGY & DEMOGRAPHICS

INCIDENCE:
- Worldwide deficiency and insufficiency affect about 1 billion people.
- Children and young adults: 40% to 50% of preadolescent Caucasian girls, and Hispanic and African American adolescents, are vitamin D deficient.

PEAK INCIDENCE: In the United States, 40% to 100% of the elderly are vitamin D deficient.

PREVALENCE: 42% of African American girls and women 15 to 49 yr old have 25(OH)D levels <20 ng/dl.

PREDOMINANT SEX AND AGE:
- Decreased skin production of vitamin D with age
- Increased prevalence among darker skinned individuals

RISK FACTORS:
1. Age (due to decreased ability to produce D_3)
2. Sunshine-deficient areas (geographic location, living in higher latitudes)
3. Dark-skinned individuals (melanin competes with vitamin D_3 precursors for UV photons and thus decreases pre-D_3 formation)
4. Institutionalized individuals
5. Use of sunscreen (sun radiation that causes skin cancer also produces pre-vitamin D_3 in skin)
6. Patients on certain medications that antagonize vitamin D action (phenobarbital, phenytoin)

7. Intestinal resection
8. Severe chronic liver diseases (such as cirrhosis)
9. Kidney disease (e.g., nephritic syndrome).
10. Sarcoidosis and lymphomas (increased catabolism of 25[OH]D to 1,25[OH]$_2$D)
11. Intestinal malabsorption disease (caused by celiac sprue, cystic fibrosis, Whipple's disease)

PHYSICAL FINDINGS & CLINICAL PRESENTATION

- Rickets—seen in children; caused by defective mineralization in the skeleton (Fig. 1-892)
  - Bowing of the legs
  - Leg bone pain
  - Delayed growth
  - Seizure due to hypocalcemia
- Osteomalacia—seen in adults
  - Periosteal bone pain (best detected by putting a firm pressure on tibia or sternal bones)
  - Proximal muscle weakness
  - Chronic muscle aches/pain
- Fracture with very minimal trauma (brittle and easily broken bones)
- Severe hypocalcemia—especially in late vitamin D deficiency leading to seizure tetany
- Hypophosphatemia
- Neuromuscular
  - Paresthesia
  - Tetany
  - Muscle cramps

ETIOLOGY

- Inadequate exposure to sunlight, such as:
  - During winter
  - In nursing home and health care institution residents
  - With excessive use of sunscreen
- Medications:
  - Individuals on certain medications, such as phenobarbital, phenytoin, and rifampin (antagonize vitamin D action/increase vitamin D catabolism)
- Diseases and disease states:
  - Diseases causing vitamin D malabsorption:
    Cystic fibrosis
    Whipple's disease
    Celiac sprue
  - Diseases increasing vitamin D catabolism:
    Lymphoma
    Sarcoidosis
  - Intestinal resection
  - Decreased 25(OH)D production:
    Kidney disease
    Liver cirrhosis

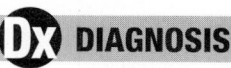 **DIAGNOSIS**

DIFFERENTIAL DIAGNOSIS
- Arthritis
- Fibromyalgia

WORKUP
- Population-wide screening for vitamin D deficiency is not recommended because evidence to support this practice is lacking.

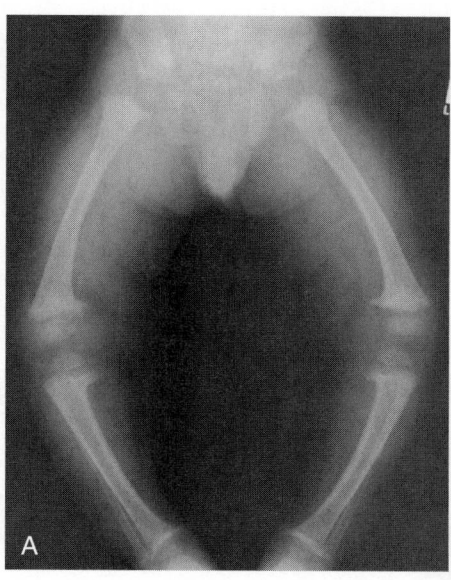
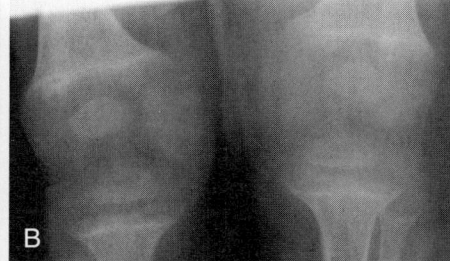
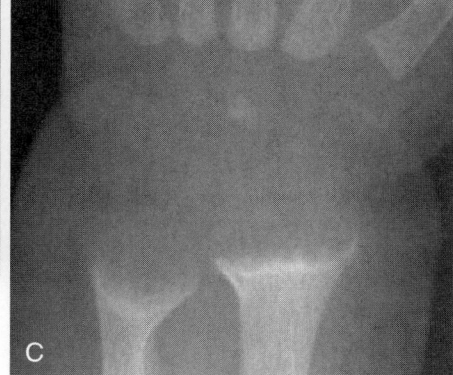

FIGURE 1-892 Radiographs of a child with vitamin D–deficiency rickets demonstrating bowing of the femurs and tibias **(A)** and widened, frayed, demineralized epiphyseal plates **(B and C)**. (From Hochberg MC et al: *Rheumatology,* ed 5, St Louis, 2011, Mosby.)

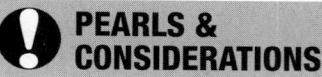
- Screening is needed for individuals at risk (osteoporosis, history of falls, obese persons, pregnant and lactating women, diseases causing vitamin D malabsorption, African Americans). Workup involves blood and urine tests as well as radiography, as outlined in the next section.

LABORATORY TESTS

- Serum 25(OH)D: this is the best test to determine vitamin D status.
- Parathyroid hormone (PTH): increased levels in vitamin D insufficiency. It is a marker of vitamin D insufficiency.
- Increased (serum or bone) alkaline phosphatase
- Decreased 24-hour urine calcium (patient should not be on a thiazide)

IMAGING STUDIES

- Radiographs may show:
  - Pseudofractures of the pelvis, femur, metatarsals.
  - Nontraumatic fractures.
- Bone density:
  - Decreased bone mineral density (osteopenia or osteoporosis)

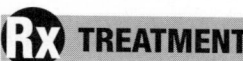 **TREATMENT**

NONPHARMACOLOGIC THERAPY

- Natural sources of vitamin D. These include:
  - Exposure to sunlight
  - Dietary sources are not enough to meet daily requirements. Oily fish such as salmon, cod, and mackerel are rich sources of vitamin D_3.
- Foods fortified with vitamin D
  - Mainly fortified dairy products
  - Fortified orange juice

ACUTE GENERAL Rx

- Treating deficiency (general population):
  - 50,000 IU of vitamin D every week for 8 weeks, or
  - 6000 IU daily to achieve a serum level of 25(OH)D of at least 30 ng/ml
- Maintenance measures after treatment (general population): 1500 to 2000 IU daily
- Treating deficiency (obese patients, patients with malabsorption syndromes, or those taking certain medications, as indicated earlier)
  - 6000 to 10,000 IU daily
- Maintenance measures after treatment (obese patients, patients with malabsorption syndromes, or those taking certain medications, as indicated earlier):
  - 3000 to 6000 IU daily
- After treating deficiency, recheck 25(OH)D in 12 to 14 weeks.

REFERRAL

Referral to an endocrinologist is recommended if there is no response to treatment.

PREVENTION

- Food fortification with vitamin D_2 or vitamin D_3
- Adequate sun exposure
- Vitamin D supplementation (per the Endocrine Society):
  - Infants (age range 1-12 mo) require at least 400 IU/day of vitamin D.
  - Children (age range 1-18 yr) require 600 IU/day of vitamin D.
  - Adult supplementation (adults age 19 to 70 yr): 600 IU of vitamin D daily
  - Adult supplementation (persons 70 yr and older): 800 IU of vitamin D daily
  - Exceptions: pregnant or lactating women, obese persons, and patients on antiseizure medications, steroids, antifungals, and AIDS medications should be given 2× to 3× more vitamin D.
- Screening: recommended only for individuals at high risk for vitamin D deficiency such as blacks and Hispanics, obese individuals (BMI >30 kg/m²), patients with osteoporosis, the elderly, and patients with certain chronic diseases (see "Risk Factors").

PEARLS & CONSIDERATIONS

- In the U.S., vitamin D supplements are available by prescription as vitamin D_2 (ergocalciferol) or over the counter as vitamin D_3 (cholecalciferol, usually in 400-1000 IU doses). Both vitamin D_2 and vitamin D_3 are acceptable as supplements. On average, oral vitamin D_3 raises blood levels more than does vitamin D_2.
- Upper limit of maintenance tolerability in healthy adults is 4000 IU a day. More than 4000 IU of vitamin D daily in nondeficient individuals increases the risk of harm. High-level supplements (more than 10,000 IU daily) are associated with kidney and tissue damage.
- Vitamin D supplementation is recommended for fall prevention. High-dose vitamin D supplementation (≥800 IU daily) has been shown to be favorable in the prevention of hip fracture and any nonvertebral fracture in persons 65 years of age and older.
- Prescribing more than the recommended daily amount to improve quality of life or prevent cardiovascular disease or death is not advised.
- Trials have shown that low vitamin D levels are associated with depressive symptoms, especially in persons with a history of depression. These findings suggest that vitamin D levels may be useful in patients with a history of depression.
- Vitamin D supplementation, administered with calcium, has been shown to lower the risk for falling and improve muscle strength in the elderly, especially in older vitamin D–deficient women who are at high baseline risk for falling.
- The treatment of vitamin D insufficiency decreases the risk of nonvertebral and hip fractures.
- Recent data suggest that vitamin D deficiency is associated with the risk of developing certain cancers (including breast, colon, and prostate).
- Vitamin D deficiency is associated with some autoimmune diseases (types 1 and 2 diabetes, metabolic syndrome, multiple sclerosis).

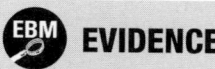 **EVIDENCE**

available at www.expertconsult.com

SUGGESTED READINGS
available at www.expertconsult.com

RELATED CONTENT
Vitamin D Deficiency (Patient Information)

AUTHOR: **DANIEL K. ASIEDU, M.D., PH.D., F.A.C.P.**

DEFINITION Vitiligo is the acquired loss of epidermal pigmentation that is characterized histologically by the absence of epidermal melanocytes. There are two major forms: nonsegmental (generalized) vitiligo, which accounts for >80% of cases, and segmental vitiligo, which accounts for 30% of childhood cases.

ICD-9CM CODES
709.1 Vitiligo

EPIDEMIOLOGY & DEMOGRAPHICS
PREVALENCE: Vitiligo affects 0.5% to 1% of the population; it is the most common depigmenting disorder.
PREDOMINANT AGE: Vitiligo can begin at any age, but the age at onset is <20 yr for half of patients.
GENETICS: A positive family history is present in 25% to 30% of patients, and both sexes are equally affected. There are no differences in the rates of occurrence with regard to skin type or race.

PHYSICAL FINDINGS & CLINICAL PRESENTATION
- Hypopigmented and depigmented lesions (Fig. 1-893) favor sun-exposed regions, intertriginous areas, genitalia, and sites over bony prominences (i.e., nonsegmental or type A vitiligo).
- Areas around the body orifices are also frequently involved.
- The lesions tend to be symmetric.
- Occasionally the lesions are linear or pseudodermatomal (i.e., segmental or type B vitiligo).
- Vitiligo lesions may occur at trauma sites (i.e., Koebner's phenomenon).
- The hair in affected areas may be white.
- The margins of the lesions are usually well demarcated; when a ring of hyperpigmentation is seen, the term *trichrome vitiligo* is used.
- The term *marginal inflammatory vitiligo* is used to describe lesions with raised borders.
- Initially the disease is limited, but the lesions tend to become more extensive over time.

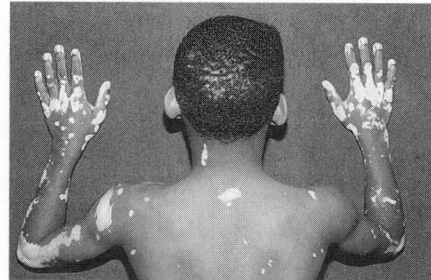

FIGURE 1-893 Multiple, sharply demarcated, symmetric, depigmented areas of vitiligo. (From Behrman RE: *Nelson textbook of pediatrics,* Philadelphia, 2006, Saunders.)

- Type B vitiligo is more common among children.
- Vitiligo may begin around pigmented nevi and produce a halo (i.e., Sutton's nevus); in such cases, the central nevus often regresses and disappears over time.

ETIOLOGY & PATHOGENESIS
- Three pathophysiologic theories:
  1. Autoimmune theory (i.e., autoantibodies against melanocytes)
  2. Neural theory (i.e., neurochemical mediators selectively destroy melanocytes)
  3. Self-destructive process in which melanocytes fail to protect themselves against cytotoxic melanin precursors
- Although vitiligo is considered to be an acquired disease, 25% to 30% of cases are familial. The mode of transmission is unknown; the condition seems to be polygenic or autosomal dominant with incomplete penetrance and variable expression.
- Associated disorders:
  - Alopecia areata
  - Type 1 diabetes mellitus
  - Adrenal insufficiency
  - Hyperthyroidism and hypothyroidism
  - Mucocutaneous candidiasis
  - Pernicious anemia
  - Polyglandular autoimmune syndromes
  - Melanoma

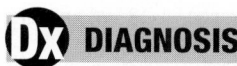 **DIAGNOSIS**

DIFFERENTIAL DIAGNOSIS
- Acquired hypopigmentation disorders:
  - Chemical-induced (e.g., chloroquine, imatinib, phenolic-catecholic derivatives [e.g., adhesives, deodorants, latex gloves, lacquer resins, varnish, soap antioxidants, insecticides, printing ink, paints, motor oil additives, disinfectants])
  - Halo nevus
  - Idiopathic guttate hypomelanosis
  - Leprosy
  - Leukoderma associated with melanoma
  - Pityriasis alba
  - Postinflammatory hypopigmentation
  - Tinea versicolor
  - Vogt-Koyanagi syndrome (i.e., vitiligo, uveitis, and deafness)
  - Melasma
  - Mycosis fungoides
- Congenital hypopigmentation disorders:
  - Albinism, partial (piebaldism)
  - Albinism, total
  - Nevus anemicus
  - Nevus depigmentosus
  - Tuberous sclerosis
  - Ito's hypomelanosis

WORKUP
- Inquire about a personal and family history of autoimmune disease.
- Perform a physical examination.

- A Wood's light examination may enhance the lesions of light-skinned individuals.

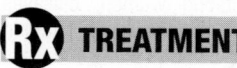 **TREATMENT**

Treatment is indicated primarily for cosmetic purposes when depigmentation causes emotional or social distress. Depigmentation is more noticeable among patients with darker complexions.
- Cosmetic masking agents (e.g., Dermablend, Covermark) or stains (e.g., DY-O-Derm, Vitadye)
- Sunless tanning lotions (e.g., dihydroxyacetone)
- Repigmentation (This is achieved by the activation and migration of melanocytes from hair follicles; therefore, skin with little or no hair responds poorly to treatment.)
- Narrow-band ultraviolet B radiation (This is the preferred treatment for nonsegmental vitiligo. It is given twice weekly [not on successive days] during sessions that last from 5 to 10 min. The best results are achieved on the face, trunk, and limbs.)
- Psoralens and sunlight (e.g., PUVAsol)
- Topical mid-potency steroids (e.g., triamcinolone 0.1% or desonide 0.05% cream qd for 3 to 4 mo)
- Topical calcineurin inhibitors for face and neck lesions
- Intralesional steroid injection
- Systemic steroids (e.g., betamethasone 5 mg qd on two consecutive days per wk for 2 to 4 mo)
- Total depigmentation in cases of extensive vitiligo with 20% monobenzyl ether or hydroquinone (This is a permanent procedure, and patients will require lifelong protection from sun exposure.)
- Topical immunomodulators (e.g., tacrolimus, pimecrolimus) (These substances can also induce the repigmentation of vitiliginous skin lesions. However, their potential for systemic immunosuppression or for increasing the risk of skin or other malignancies remains to be defined.)
- Calcipotriol, which is a synthetic analog of vitamin D_3 (This has also been used in combination with ultraviolet light or clobetasol, with limited results.)
- Surgical techniques

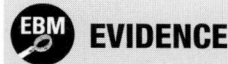 **EVIDENCE**

available at www.expertconsult.com

SUGGESTED READING
available at www.expertconsult.com

RELATED CONTENT
Vitiligo (Patient Information)

AUTHOR: **FRED F. FERRI, M.D.**

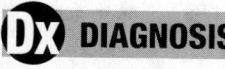

BASIC INFORMATION

DEFINITION

Von Willebrand's disease is a congenital disorder of hemostasis characterized by defective or deficient von Willebrand factor (vWF). There are several subtypes of von Willebrand's disease. The most common type (80% of cases) is type I, which is caused by a quantitative decrease in vWF; type IIA and type IIB are results of qualitative protein abnormalities; and type III is a rare, autosomal recessive disorder characterized by a near-complete quantitative deficiency of vWF. Acquired von Willebrand's disease is a rare disorder that usually occurs in elderly patients and usually presents with mucocutaneous bleeding abnormalities and no clinically meaningful family history. It is often accompanied by a hematoproliferative or autoimmune disorder. Successful treatment of the associated illness can reverse the clinical and laboratory manifestations.

SYNONYMS

Pseudohemophilia
vWD

ICD-9CM CODES
286.4 von Willebrand's disease

EPIDEMIOLOGY & DEMOGRAPHICS

- Autosomal-dominant disorder
- Most common inherited bleeding disorder
- Prevalence is 1% to 2% in general population, according to screening studies; estimates based on referral for symptoms of bleeding suggest a prevalence of 30 to 100 cases per million

PHYSICAL FINDINGS & CLINICAL PRESENTATION

- Generally normal physical examination
- Mucosal bleeding (gingival bleeding, epistaxis) and gastrointestinal bleeding may occur
- Easy bruising
- Postpartum bleeding, bleeding after surgery or dental extraction, menorrhagia

ETIOLOGY

Quantitative or qualitative deficiency of vWF (see "Definition")

DIAGNOSIS

The diagnosis of von Willebrand's disease generally requires two criteria: (1) a personal history, family history, or physical evidence of mucocutaneous bleeding and (2) a qualitative or quantitative decrease in functional activity of von Willebrand's disease. The American Society of Hematology states that a definitive diagnosis of vWD may be made if vWF antigen levels are less than 30 IU/dl. It also describes a gray zone of 30 to 50 IU/dl, designated as "low vWF."

DIFFERENTIAL DIAGNOSIS

Platelet function disorders, clotting factor deficiencies

WORKUP

- Laboratory evaluation (see "Laboratory Tests")
- Initial testing includes partial thromboplastin time (increased), platelet count (normal), and bleeding time (prolonged)
- Subsequent tests include vWF level (decreased), factor VIII:C (decreased), and ristocetin agglutination (increased in type IIB) (Table 1-415)

LABORATORY TESTS

- Decreased factor VIII coagulant activity
- Decreased vWF antigen or ristocetin cofactor
- Normal platelet number and morphology
- Prolonged bleeding time
- Normal platelet aggregation studies
- Type IIA von Willebrand's disease can be distinguished from type I by absence of ristocetin cofactor activity and abnormal multimer
- Type IIB von Willebrand's disease is distinguished from type I by abnormal multimer

TREATMENT

NONPHARMACOLOGIC THERAPY

- Avoidance of aspirin and other nonsteroidal anti-inflammatory drugs
- Evaluation for likelihood of bleeding (with measurement of bleeding time) before surgical procedures. When a patient undergoes surgery or receives repeated therapeutic doses of concentrates, factor VIII activity should be assayed every 12 hr on the day a dose is administered and every 24 hr thereafter.

GENERAL Rx

- The mainstay of treatment in von Willebrand's disease is the replacement of the deficient protein at the time of spontaneous bleeding or before invasive procedures are performed.

- Desmopressin acetate (DDAVP) is useful to release stored vWF from endothelial cells. It is used to cover minor procedures and traumatic bleeding in mild type I von Willebrand's disease. Dose is 0.3 mcg/kg in 100 ml of normal saline solution IV infused >20 min. DDAVP is also available as a nasal spray (dose of 150 mcg spray administered to each nostril) as a preparation for minor surgery and management of minor bleeding episodes. DDAVP is not effective in type IIA von Willebrand's disease and is potentially dangerous in type IIB (increased risk of bleeding and thrombocytopenia).
- In patients with severe disease, replacement therapy in the form of cryoprecipitate is the method of choice. The standard dose is 1 bag of cryoprecipitate per 10 kg of body weight.
- Factor VIII concentrate rich in vWF (Humate-P) is useful to correct bleeding abnormalities in type IIA, IIB, and type III von Willebrand's disease without alloantibodies. Alloantibodies that inactivate vWF and form circulating immune complexes develop in 15% of patients with type III von Willebrand's disease who have received multiple transfusions. In these patients, recombinant factor VIII is preferred because autoantibodies can elicit life-threatening anaphylactic reactions because of complement activation by immune complexes.
- Life-threatening hemorrhage unresponsive to therapy with cryoprecipitate or factor VIII concentrate may require transfusion of normal platelets.

SUGGESTED READINGS
available at www.expertconsult.com

RELATED CONTENT
von Willebrand's Disease (Patient Information)

AUTHOR: **FRED F. FERRI, M.D.**

TABLE 1-415 Genetic and Laboratory Findings in von Willebrand's Disease

Parameter Type	BT	VIII-C	vW-Ag	R-Cof	RIPA	Multimer Structure	Mode of Inheritance
I (classic)	P	R	R	R	R	Normal	AD
II							
A	P	N/R	N/R	R	R	Abnormal	AD
B	P	N/R	N/R	N/R	I	Abnormal	AD
III	P	R	R	R	R	Variable	AR

AD, Autosomal dominant; *AR*, autosomal recessive; *BT*, bleeding time; *I*, increased; *N/R*, normal or reduced; *P*, prolonged; *R*, reduced; *R-Cof*, ristocetin cofactor; *RIPA*, ristocetin-induced platelet aggregation (agglutination); *vW-Ag*, von Willebrand antigen (protein); *VIII-C*, factor VIII coagulant activity.
From Behrman RE: *Nelson textbook of pediatrics*, ed 17, Philadelphia, 2004, Saunders.

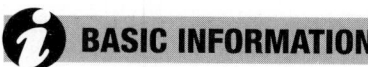

BASIC INFORMATION

DEFINITION

Vulvar cancer is an abnormal cell proliferation arising on the vulva and exhibiting malignant potential. The majority are of squamous cell origin; however, other types include adenocarcinoma, basal cell carcinoma, sarcoma, and melanoma.

SYNONYMS

Squamous cell carcinoma of the vulva (90%)
Basal cell carcinoma of the vulva
Adenocarcinoma of the vulva
Melanoma of the vulva
Bartholin gland carcinoma
Verrucous carcinoma of the vulva
Vulvar sarcoma

ICD-9CM CODES
184.4 Vulvar neoplasm

EPIDEMIOLOGY & DEMOGRAPHICS

INCIDENCE: 2.2 cases per 100,000 persons
PREVALENCE: Vulvar cancer is uncommon. It comprises 4% of malignancies of the female genital tract. It is the fourth most common gynecologic malignancy.
MEAN AGE AT DIAGNOSIS: Predominantly a disease of menopause. Mean age at diagnosis is 65 yr.

PHYSICAL FINDINGS & CLINICAL PRESENTATION

- Vulvar pruritus or pain is present.
- May produce a malodorous discharge or present as bleeding.

- Raised lesion that may have fleshy (Fig. E1-895), ulcerated, leukoplakic, or warty appearance; may have multifocal lesions.
- Lesions are usually located on labia majora but may be seen on labia minora, clitoris, and perineum.
- The lymph nodes of groin may be palpable.

ETIOLOGY

- The exact etiology is unknown.
- Vulvar intraepithelial neoplasia has been reported in 20% to 30% of invasive squamous cell carcinoma of the vulva, but the malignant potential is unknown.
- Human papillomavirus is found in 30% to 50% of vulvar carcinoma, but its exact role is unclear.
- Chronic pruritus, wetness, industrial wastes, arsenicals, hygienic agents, and vulvar dystrophies have been implicated as causative agents.
- Vulvar cancer in younger women is more directly dependent on HPV infection, vulvar dysplasia, and tobacco use.

DIAGNOSIS

DIFFERENTIAL DIAGNOSIS

- Lymphogranuloma inguinale
- Tuberculosis
- Vulvar dystrophies
- Vulvar atrophy
- Paget's disease

WORKUP

- Diagnosis is made histologically by biopsy
- Thorough examination of the lesion and assessment of spread. Table 1-416 describes FIGO staging of vulvar cancer

- Possible colposcopy of adjacent areas
- Cytologic smear of vagina and cervix
- Cystoscopy and proctosigmoidoscopy may be necessary

IMAGING STUDIES

- Chest radiography
- CT scan and MRI for assessing local tumor spread

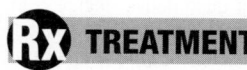 TREATMENT

NONPHARMACOLOGIC THERAPY

- Treatment is individualized depending on the stage of the tumor. Fig. E1-896 describes a treatment algorithm for management of patients with vulvar cancer.
- Stage I tumors with <1 mm stromal invasion are treated with complete local excision without groin node dissection. Imiquimod 5% cream, a topical immune response modulator, is also effective in the treatment of vulvar intraepithelial neoplasia.
- Stage I tumors with >1 mm stromal invasion are treated with complete local excision with groin node dissection.
- Stage II tumors require radical vulvectomy with bilateral groin node dissection.
- Advanced-stage disease may require the addition of radiation and chemotherapy to the surgical regimen.
- Fig. E1-896 describes a treatment algorithm for management of vulvar cancer.

DISPOSITION

Five-year survival ranges from 90% for stage I to 15% for stage IV.

REFERRAL

Vulvar cancer should be managed by a gynecologic oncologist and radiation oncologist.

SUGGESTED READINGS
available at www.expertconsult.com

RELATED CONTENT

Vulvar Cancer (Patient Information)

AUTHORS: **GIL M. FARKASH, M.D.,** and **RUBEN ALVERO, M.D.**

TABLE 1-416 FIGO Staging of Vulval Cancer

Stage I	Tumor confined to the vulva—2 cm or less in diameter. Nodes are not involved. A. Lesions less than 1 mm depth invasion B. Other lesions less than 2 cm in diameter
Stage II	Tumor confined to the vulva—more than 2 cm in diameter. Nodes are not involved.
Stage III	Tumor of any size with: Adjacent spread to the lower urethra and/or the vagina, the perineum and the anus, and/or unilateral lymph node involvement.
Stage IV	Tumor of any size with bilateral groin lymph node involvement: A. Infiltrating the bladder mucosa or the rectal mucosa, or both, including the upper part of the urethral mucosa B. Fixed to the bone or other distant metastases. Fixed or ulcerated nodes in either one or both groins.

From Symonds EM, Symonds IM: *Essential obstetrics and gynecology,* ed 4, London, 2004, Churchill Livingstone.

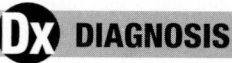

BASIC INFORMATION

DEFINITION

Waldenström's macroglobulinemia (WM) is a plasma cell dyscrasia (B-cell malignancy) characterized by lymphoplasmacytic infiltration in the bone marrow or lymphatic tissue and a monoclonal immunoglobulin M protein (IgM) in the serum.

SYNONYMS

WM
Monoclonal macroglobulinemia
Lymphoplasmacytic lymphoma

ICD-9CM CODES
273.3 Waldenström's macroglobulinemia

EPIDEMIOLOGY & DEMOGRAPHICS

- Accounts for 2% of all hematologic cancers
- 1500 people diagnosed every year in the United States
- Overall incidence: 3.4 per million person-yr in men, 1.7 per million person-yr in women
- Median age approximately 63 yr
- More common among men than women and among whites than blacks

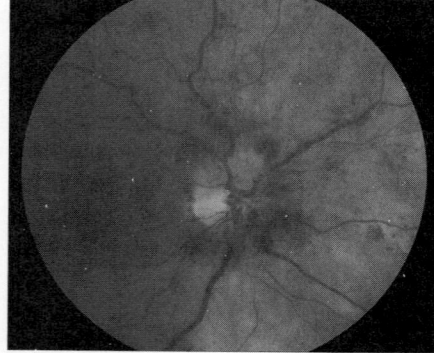

FIGURE 1-897 Hyperviscosity syndrome. Right eye retinal image in a patient with Waldenström's macroglobulinemia and hyperviscosity syndrome showing sausaging (focal venular dilations), intraretinal hemorrhages, microaneurysms, and peripapillary cotton wool spots and disc swelling (papilledema). (From Goldman L, Schafer AI: *Goldman's Cecil medicine,* ed 24, Philadelphia, 2011, Saunders.)

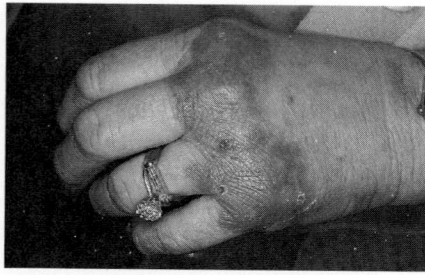

FIGURE 1-898 Nonpalpable purpura of hyperglobulinemic purpura of Waldenström's hypergammaglobulinemia. (From Hochberg MC et al: *Rheumatology,* ed 5, St Louis, 2011, Mosby.)

PHYSICAL FINDINGS & CLINICAL PRESENTATION

- Weakness
- Fatigue
- Weight loss
- Pallor
- Headache, dizziness, vertigo, deafness, and seizures (hyperviscosity syndrome)
- Easy bleeding (e.g., epistaxis)
- Retinal vein link-sausage shaped (Fig. 1-897)
- Lymphadenopathy (15%)
- Hepatomegaly (20%)
- Most commonly encountered neurologic presentation is symmetric polyneuropathy (5%)
- Splenomegaly (15%)
- Purpura (Fig. 1-898)
- Fever and night sweats

ETIOLOGY

- WM is an IgM-secreting lymphoplasmacytic lymphoma (LPL). The underlying mutation in this disorder has not been delineated.
- Multiple reports suggest familial clustering, which indicates a genetic predisposition. In one study, chromosomal deletions in 6q21–22.1 were confirmed in 42% of WM patients, regardless of family history. In another study, the strongest evidence of linkage was found on chromosomes 1q and 4q.
- The main risk factor for development of WM is having IgM monoclonal gammopathy of unknown significance (MGUS).
- Radiation exposure, occupational chemicals, viral infection, and chronic inflammatory stimulation have been suggested, but there is insufficient evidence to substantiate these hypotheses.
- There is a twofold to threefold increased risk of WM in people with a personal history of autoimmune diseases with autoantibodies. There is also increased risk with HIV, hepatitis, and rickettsiosis.

DIAGNOSIS

The diagnosis of WM is usually established by laboratory blood tests and by bone marrow biopsy. Diagnosis requires demonstration of lymphoplasmacytic lymphoma comprising ≥10% of the bone marrow cellularity and the presence of an IgM M protein. MYD88 L265P is a commonly recurring mutation in WM that can be useful in differentiating it and non-IgM lymphoplasmacytic lymphoma (LPL) from B-cell disorders that have some of the same features.

DIFFERENTIAL DIAGNOSIS

- MGUS
- Multiple myeloma
- Chronic lymphocytic leukemia
- Hairy-cell leukemia
- Lymphoma
- Smoldering macroglobulinemia

WORKUP

In any patient suspected of having WM, specific blood tests (CBC, erythrocyte sedimentation rate [ESR], serum or urine protein electrophoresis [SPEP or UPEP, respectively], IgM level, beta 2-microglobulin, serum viscosity) should be ordered. Bone marrow biopsy confirms the diagnosis.

LABORATORY TESTS

- CBC with differential:
  - Anemia is a common finding, with a median hemoglobin value of approximately

TABLE 1-417 Physicochemical and Immunologic Properties of Monoclonal Immunoglobulin Protein in Waldenström's Macroglobulinemia

Properties of Monoclonal Immunoglobulin Protein	Diagnostic Condition	Clinical Manifestations
Pentameric structure	Hyperviscosity	Headaches, blurred vision, epistaxis, retinal hemorrhages, leg cramps, impaired mentation, and intracranial hemorrhage
Prescription on cooling	Cryoglobulinemia (type I)	Raynaud's phenomenon, acrocyanosis, ulcers, purpura, and cold urticaria
Autoantibody activity to myelin-associated glycoprotein, ganglioside M1, and sulfatide moieties on peripheral nerve sheaths	Peripheral neuropathies	Sensorimotor neuropathies, painful neuropathies, ataxic gait, and bilateral foot drop
Autoantibody activity to immunoglobulin G	Cryoglobulinemia (type II)	Purpura, arthralgias, renal failure, and sensorimotor neuropathies
Autoantibody activity to red blood cell antigens	Cold agglutinins	Hemolytic anemia, Raynaud's phenomenon, acrocyanosis, and livedo reticularis
Tissue deposition as amorphous aggregates	Organ dysfunction	Skin: bullous skin disease, papules, and Schnitzler syndrome; Gastrointestinal: diarrhea, malabsorption, and bleeding; Kidney: proteinuria and renal failure (light-chain component)
Tissue deposition as amyloid fibrils (light-chain fibrils commonly the largest component)	Organ dysfunction	Fatigue, weight loss, edema, periorbital purpura, hepatomegaly, macroglossia, and organ dysfunction of the involved organs: heart, kidney, liver, and peripheral sensory and autonomic nerves

From Hoffman R et al: *Hematology, basic principles and practice,* ed 5, Philadelphia, 2009, Churchill Livingstone.

10 g/dl. WBC count is usually normal; thrombocytopenia can occur.

- Peripheral smear may reveal "stacked coin" rouleaux formations and malignant lymphoid cells in terminal patients.
- Elevated ESR.
- SPEP: homogeneous M spike (monoclonal gammopathy).
- Immunoelectrophoresis: confirms IgM responsible for the M spike. Table 1-417 describes physicochemical and immunologic properties of the monoclonal IgM protein in WM.
- Urine immunoelectrophoresis: monoclonal light chains are usually kappa chains. Bence Jones protein can be seen, but is not the typical finding in WM.
- IgM levels are high, generally >3 g/dl.
- Beta 2-microglobulin: elevated in 55%; high levels are associated with poor prognosis.
- Serum viscosity: symptoms usually occur when the serum viscosity is four times the viscosity of normal serum; classic feature although present in only 15% of cases.
- Cryoglobulins, rheumatoid factor, or cold agglutinins may be present.
- Bone marrow biopsy: lymphoplasmacytoid cells are characteristic.

IMAGING STUDIES

Chest x-ray can be obtained to rule out pulmonary involvement.

Rx TREATMENT

- Because of the incurable nature of WM, the aim of treatment is to relieve symptoms and reduce the risk of organ damage. Patients with smoldering or asymptomatic WM and preserved hematologic function should be observed without therapy. Considerations for the initiation of treatment include the following: hemoglobin concentration less than 100 × 10⁹/L, significant adenopathy or organomegaly, symptomatic hyperviscosity, severe neuropathy, amyloidosis, cryoglobulinemia, cold-agglutinin disease, or evidence of disease transformation.
- Treatment is directed at both hyperviscocity and the lymphoproliferative disorder itself.

NONPHARMACOLOGIC THERAPY

Asymptomatic patients do not require treatment, and these patients should be monitored periodically for the onset of symptoms or changes in blood tests (e.g., worsening anemia, thrombocytopenia, rising IgM, and serum viscosity).

ACUTE GENERAL Rx

- Treatment of the lymphoproliferative disorder includes single or combination therapy; although guidance has been suggested in the Mayo Stratification of Macroglobulinemia and Risk-Adapted Therapy (mSMART) Guidelines, there is no universally agreed upon standard of care:
  - Rituximab, a monoclonal anti-CD20 antibody, can be used in symptomatic patients with modest hematologic compromise, IgM-related neuropathy, or hemolytic anemia unresponsive to corticosteroids.
  - Plasmapheresis should be initial treatment in patients with symptoms of hyperviscosity.
  - DRC regimen (dexamethasone, rituximab, cyclophosphamide) in patients with severe constitutional symptoms, symptomatic bulky disease, hyperviscosity, or profound hematologic compromise.

CHRONIC Rx

- Refractory patients can be retried on original therapy if length of response from initial therapy is >2 yr. If the response from the initial therapy was <2 yr, alternative first-line agents such as fludarabine or cladribine can be used.
- Other treatment options: interferon alpha, thalidomide, and autologous stem cell transplantation.

DISPOSITION

- The onset of WM is slow and insidious. Most patients die from progression of the disease with hyperviscosity, hemorrhage, and infection, or from congestive heart failure.
- Some patients develop acute myelogenous leukemia, immunoblastic sarcoma, or chronic myelogenous leukemia as a preterminal event.

- Median survival in patients with WM is about 4 to 5 yr.
- ~10% of patients will achieve complete remission, with prognosis being more favorable (median survival 11 yr).
- A staging system using serum beta 2-microglobulin concentration, hemoglobin concentration, and serum IgM concentration before treatment provides insight into prognosis and survival.
- Other factors can negatively affect the survival: age >65, male gender, the presence of organomegaly, and the presence of cytopenias.

REFERRAL

If WM is suspected, a hematology consultation is helpful in guiding future workup, treatment, and monitoring. Autologous stem cell transplantation should be considered in all eligible patients with relapsed disease.

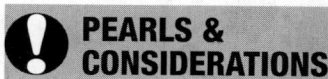

PEARLS & CONSIDERATIONS

COMMENTS

- WM was first described in 1944 by the Swedish physician Jan Gosta Waldenström.
- Amyloidosis is rare, occurring in 5% of patients with WM.

SUGGESTED READINGS

available at www.expertconsult.com

AUTHOR: **MARK F. BRADY, M.D., M.P.H., M.M.S.**

BASIC INFORMATION

DEFINITION

Warts are benign epidermal lesions caused by human papillomavirus (HPV).

SYNONYMS

Verruca vulgaris (common warts)
Verruca plana (flat warts)
Condyloma acuminatum (venereal warts)
Verruca plantaris (plantar warts)
Mosaic warts (cluster of many warts)

ICD-9CM CODES
078.10 Viral warts
078.19 Venereal wart (external genital organs)

EPIDEMIOLOGY & DEMOGRAPHICS

- Risk factors include use of communal showers, occupational handling of meat, and immunosuppression. Common warts occur most frequently in children and young adults.
- Anogenital warts are most common in young, sexually active patients. Genital warts are the most common viral sexually transmitted disease in the United States, with up to 24 million Americans carrying the causative virus.
- Common warts are longer lasting and more frequent in immunocompromised patients (e.g., lymphoma, AIDS, immunosuppressive drugs).
- Plantar warts occur most frequently at points of maximal pressure (over the heads of the metatarsal bones or on the heels).

PHYSICAL FINDINGS & CLINICAL PRESENTATION

- Common warts (Fig. 1-899) have an initial appearance of a flesh-colored papule with a rough surface; they subsequently develop a hyperkeratotic appearance with black dots on the surface (thrombosed capillaries). They may be single or multiple and are most common on the hands.
- Warts obscure normal skin lines (important diagnostic feature). Cylindrical projections from the wart may become fused, forming a mosaic pattern.
- Flat warts generally are pink or light yellow, slightly elevated, and often found on the forehead, back of hands, mouth, and beard area. They often occur in lines corresponding to trauma (e.g., a scratch), are often misdiagnosed (particularly when present on the face), and are inappropriately treated with topical corticosteroids.
- Filiform warts have a fingerlike appearance with various projections; they are generally found near the mouth, beard, or periorbital and paranasal regions.
- Plantar warts are slightly raised and have a roughened surface; they may cause pain when walking; as they involute, small hemorrhages (caused by thrombosed capillaries) may be noted.
- Genital warts are generally pale pink with several projections and a broad base. They may coalesce in the perineal area to form masses with a cauliflower-like appearance. Intraanal warts occur predominantly in patients who have had receptive anal intercourse, in contrast with perianal warts (Fig. 1-900), which may occur in men and women without a history of anal sex.
- Genital warts on the cervical epithelium can produce subclinical changes that may be noted on Pap smear or colposcopy.

ETIOLOGY

- HPV infection; >60 types of viral DNA have been identified. Transmission of warts is by direct contact.
- Genital warts: 90% are caused by HPV types 6 or 11. HPV types 16, 18, 31, 33, and 35 are found occasionally in visible genital warts (usually as coinfections with HPV 6 or 11) and can be associated with foci of high-grade, intraepithelial neoplasia, particularly in persons who are infected with HIV infection. In addition to warts on genital areas, HPV types 6 and 11 have been associated with conjunctival, nasal, oral, and laryngeal warts.

DIAGNOSIS

DIFFERENTIAL DIAGNOSIS

- Molluscum contagiosum
- Condyloma latum
- Acrochordon (skin tags) or seborrheic keratosis

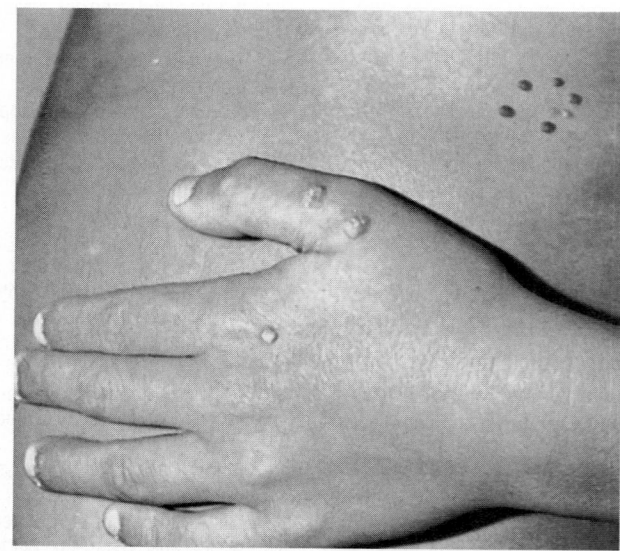

FIGURE 1-899 Common warts of the left hand and the chest wall. (From Meneghini CL, Bonifaz E: *An atlas of pediatric dermatology,* Chicago, 1986, Year Book Medical Publishers.)

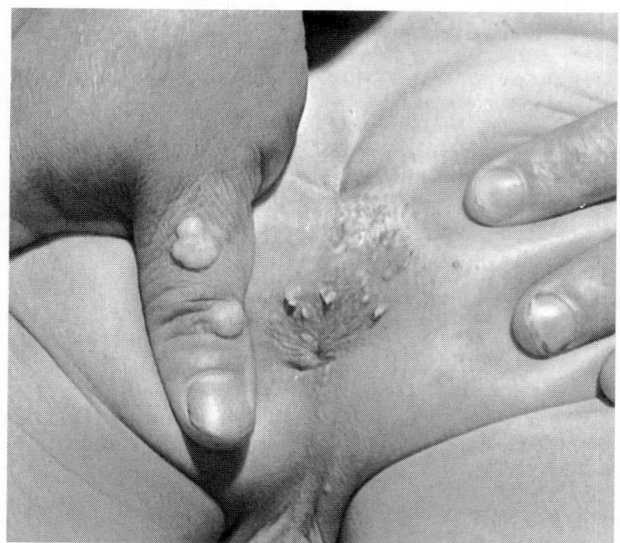

FIGURE 1-900 Common warts of the hand in a mother and perianal condylomata acuminata in her son. (From Meneghini CL, Bonifaz E: *An atlas of pediatric dermatology,* Chicago, 1986, Year Book Medical Publishers.)

- Epidermal nevi
- Hypertrophic actinic keratosis
- Squamous cell carcinomas
- Acquired digital fibrokeratoma
- Varicella-zoster virus in patients with AIDS
- Recurrent infantile digital fibroma
- Plantar corns (may be mistaken for plantar warts)

WORKUP

- Diagnosis is generally based on clinical findings.
- Suspect lesions should be biopsied.
- The application of 3% to 5% acetic acid, which causes skin color to turn white, has been used by some providers to detect HPV-infected genital mucosa. However, acetic acid application is not a specific test for HPV infection. Therefore, the routine use of this procedure for screening to detect mucosal changes attributed to HPV infection is not recommended.

LABORATORY TESTS

- Screening for cervical cancer with cytology, which is performed by either Pap smear or liquid-based cytology. Screening guidelines recommend starting screening at age 21. Annual cytology is recommended until at least three normal cytology results are obtained.
- Colposcopy with biopsy is recommended in patients with cervical squamous cell changes.

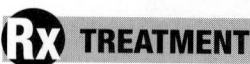 **TREATMENT**

NONPHARMACOLOGIC THERAPY

- Importance of use of condoms to reduce transmission of genital warts should be emphasized.
- Watchful waiting is an acceptable option in the treatment of nongenital cutaneous warts because many warts will disappear without intervention over time. However, many patients often request treatment because of social stigma or discomfort.
- Plantar warts that are not painful do not need treatment.
- Factors that influence selection of treatment include wart size, wart number, anatomic site of the wart, wart morphology, patient preference, cost of treatment, convenience, adverse effects, and provider experience. Factors that might affect response to therapy include the presence of immunosuppression and compliance with therapy.

GENERAL Rx

- Common warts:
  - Application of topical salicylic acid 17%. Soak area for 5 min in warm water and dry. Apply thin layer once or twice daily for up to 12 wk, avoiding normal skin. Bandage.
  - Liquid nitrogen and electrocautery are also common methods of removal. Cure rates for cryotherapy are 50% to 70% after three to four treatments.

- Blunt dissection can be used in large lesions or resistant lesions.
  - Duct tape occlusion is also effective for treating common warts. It is cut to cover warts and left in place for 6 days. It is removed after 6 days and the warts are soaked in water and then filed with pumice stones. New tape is applied 12 hr later. This treatment can be repeated until warts resolve.
  - Recalcitrant warts can be treated with injection of *Candida* or mumps skin antigen into the wart every 3 to 4 wk for up to three treatments, photodynamic therapy with aminolevulinic acid, pulsed dye laser, and intralesional bleomycin.
- Filiform warts: surgical removal is necessary.
- Flat warts: generally more difficult to treat.
  - Tretinoin cream applied at bedtime over the involved area for several weeks may be effective.
  - Application of liquid nitrogen.
  - Electrocautery.
  - 5-Fluorouracil cream applied once or twice a day for 3 to 5 wk is also effective. Persistent hyperpigmentation may occur after Efudex use.
- Plantar warts:
  - Salicylic acid therapy (e.g., Occlusal-HP). Soak wart in warm water for 5 min, remove loose tissue, dry. Apply to area, allow to dry, reapply. Use once or twice daily; maximum 12 wk. Use of 40% salicylic acid plasters (Mediplast) is also a safe, nonscarring treatment; it is particularly useful in treating mosaic warts covering a large area.
  - Blunt dissection is also a fast and effective treatment modality.
  - Laser therapy can be used for plantar warts and recurrent warts; however, it leaves open wounds that require 4 to 6 wk to fill with granulation tissue.
  - Interlesional bleomycin is also effective but generally used when all other treatments fail.
- Genital warts:
  - Can be effectively treated with 20% podophyllin resin in compound tincture of benzoin applied with a cotton tip applicator by the treating physician and allowed to air dry. The treatment can be repeated weekly if necessary.
  - Podofilox (Condylox 0.5% gel) is available for application by the patient. Local adverse effects include pain, burning, and inflammation at the site.
  - Cryosurgery with liquid nitrogen delivered with a probe or as a spray is effective for treating smaller genital warts.
  - Carbon dioxide laser can also be used for treating primary or recurrent genital warts (cure rate >90%).
  - Imiquimod cream, 5%, is a patient-applied immune response modifier effective in the treatment of external genital and perianal warts (complete clearing of genital warts

in >70% of females and >30% of males in 4 to 16 wk). Sexual contact should be avoided while the cream is on the skin. It is applied 3 times per wk before normal sleeping hours and is left on the skin for 6 to 10 hr.
  - Sinecatechins (Veregen), a botanical drug product, is also effective for treatment of external genital and perianal warts. Formulation is a 15% ointment applied to affected area tid for up to 16 wk.
- Application of trichloroacetic acid or bichloracetic acid 80% to 90% is also effective for external genital warts. A small amount should be applied only to warts and allowed to dry, at which time a white "frosting" develops. This treatment can be repeated weekly if necessary.

DISPOSITION

- Warts can be effectively treated with the previous modalities with complete resolution in the majority of patients; however, the recurrence rate is high.
- Cervical carcinomas and precancerous lesions in women are associated with genital papillomavirus infection.
- Squamous cell anal cancer is also associated with a history of genital warts.

REFERRAL

- Dermatology referral for warts resistant to conservative therapy
- Surgical referral in selected cases
- Sexually transmitted disease counseling for patients with anogenital warts

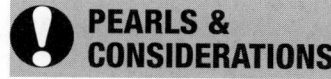 **PEARLS & CONSIDERATIONS**

COMMENTS

- Subungual and periungual warts are generally more resistant to treatment. Dermatology referral for cryosurgery is recommended in resistant cases.
- Examination of sex partners is not necessary for the management of genital warts because no data indicate that reinfection plays a role.
- Sexually transmitted HPV infections contribute to nearly 20,000 cases of invasive cancer in the U.S. affecting cervix, anus, vagina, penis, and oral cavity. HPV vaccination is available for females aged 11 to 26 and males aged 9 to 26.

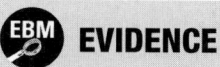 **EVIDENCE**

available at www.expertconsult.com

SUGGESTED READINGS
available at www.expertconsult.com

RELATED CONTENT

Warts (Patient Information)

AUTHOR: **FRED F. FERRI, M.D.**

BASIC INFORMATION

DEFINITION

Wernicke syndrome is an acute neuropsychiatric disorder characterized by the classic triad of ophthalmoplegia, ataxia, and disturbances of mental activity or consciousness due to a deficiency of thiamine often associated with chronic alcoholism.

SYNONYMS

Wernicke encephalopathy (WE)
Gayet-Wernicke encephalopathy
Cerebral beriberi
Wernicke's superior hemorrhagic polioencephalitis

ICD-9CM CODES

265.1 Wernicke's encephalopathy, disease, or syndrome (superior hemorrhagic polioencephalitis)
294.0 Wernicke-Korsakoff's syndrome or psychosis, non-alcoholic
291.1 Wernicke-Korsakoff's syndrome or psychosis, alcoholic

EPIDEMIOLOGY & DEMOGRAPHICS

- A higher prevalence of WE noted on autopsy studies (0.8% to 2.8%) compared to clinical studies (0.04% to 0.13%)
  - WE lesions on autopsy of alcoholic abusers: 12.5%
  - WE lesions on autopsy patients with alcohol-related deaths: 29% to 59%

PREDOMINANT SEX AND AGE:
- Male-to-female ratio of 1.7 to 1
- Estimated mortality: 17%

GENETICS:
- Biochemical studies in fibroblasts from patients with WE show thiamine-dependent enzyme, transketolase, to have a decreased affinity for thiamine pyrophosphate.
- Thiamine deficiency causes wet (cardiovascular) beriberi more commonly in the Asian population and dry beriberi (polyneuropathy and WE) in the European population.

RISK FACTORS:
- Alcohol abuse/misuse
- Diet
  - Malnutrition/unbalanced nutrition/infant formulas
  - Intravenous hyperalimentation without thiamine supplementation
  - Magnesium depletion–cofactor required by enzymes: transketolase and thiamine pyrophosphokinase
- Gastrointestinal disorders including recurrent vomiting or chronic diarrhea such as hyperemesis gravidarum
- Gastrointestinal surgical procedures (gastrointestinal resection) that cause malabsorption secondary to reduced surface area of gastric and duodenal mucosa such as bariatric surgery

- Systemic cancers
  - Most common underlying disorder onset for WE in children
  - Consumption of thiamine by fast-growing neoplastic cells
- Chemical compounds/drugs or chemotherapeutic treatments
- Systemic diseases
  - Peritoneal or hemodialysis
  - HIV/AIDS
  - Prolonged infectious febrile disease
  - Hypermetabolic states
  - Thyrotoxicosis

PHYSICAL FINDINGS & CLINICAL PRESENTATION

- WE is a clinical diagnosis with a classic triad of ophthalmoplegia, ataxia, and disturbances of mental activity or consciousness—although this triad is only seen in 16% of all patients.
- Eye movement abnormalities include nystagmus, external rectus palsies, and reduced conjugate gaze.
- Ophthalmoscopic findings include swelling of the optic discs and retinal hemorrhages.
- Clinical suspicion must remain high in patients with risk factors listed above, especially in the setting of poor nutrition.
- Diagnosis is confirmed by improvement of neurologic signs after administration of parenteral thiamine.
- Labs and radiologic studies may aid diagnosis, but these should not delay a trial of parenteral administration of thiamine.

ETIOLOGY

- The biologically active form of vitamin B_1, thiamine pyrophosphate (TP), a coenzyme for several important biochemical pathways involved in energy production, lipid metabolism, and production of amino acids and glucose-derived neurotransmitters.
- Body's reserve for thiamine is sufficient for 18 days.
- Malnutrition for 2 to 3 wk or a diet disproportionately high in carbohydrates and low in thiamine intake can lead to an impaired function of enzymes requiring TP.

DIAGNOSIS

DIFFERENTIAL DIAGNOSIS

- Other acute encephalopathies (Table 1-418)
- Paramedian thalamic infarction
- Ventriculoencephalitis, paraneoplastic encephalitis, herpes simplex encephalitis
- Miller-Fisher syndrome
- Primary cerebral lymphoma
- Multiple sclerosis, Behcet's disease, Leigh's disease
- Variant Creutzfeldt-Jakob disease

WORKUP

- WE is a clinical diagnosis based on the triad of features listed above.
- Laboratory tests and radiologic studies as listed below may be obtained to confirm diagnosis.

LABORATORY TESTS

- Blood thiamine concentration.
- Functional measurement of erythrocyte thiamine transketolase (ETKA) before and after administration of parenteral thiamine. A diagnosis may be confirmed if ETKA is low followed by a 25% increase after thiamine supplementation.
- High-performance liquid chromatography for assessment of thiamine, thiamine mono- and di-phosphate in human erythrocytes.
- Serum magnesium concentration (depletion of magnesium may mimic features of WE).

IMAGING STUDIES

MRI of brain may show bilaterally symmetric increase in T2 signal at the paraventricular regions of the thalamus and mammillary bodies. Other areas include hypothalamus, periaqueductal region, floor of the fourth ventricle, and midline cerebellum.

TABLE 1-418 Acute and Subacute Presentation of Nutritional Deficiency Syndromes

Syndrome	Clinical Setting
Wernicke-Korsakoff syndrome	Administration of intravenous glucose to a thiamine-deficient alcoholic patient
Wernicke-Korsakoff syndrome	Intractable vomiting due to hyperemesis gravidarum or gastroplasty
Postgastroplasty neuropathy	Intractable vomiting and severe weight loss in patients following weight reduction surgical procedures
Vitamin B_{12} myeloneuropathy	Nitrous oxide administration in cobalamin-deficient patients
Central pontine myelinolysis	Sudden change in tissue osmolarity in critically ill patients or alcoholics

From Goetz CG: *Textbook of clinical neurology*, ed 3, Philadelphia, 2007, Saunders.

Rx TREATMENT

ACUTE GENERAL Rx

- Treatment should be initiated in all patients with clinical suspicion of WE. Thiamine supplementation should precede glucose administration in all patients at risk for WE.
- Alcoholics with WE: treat with 500 mg of thiamine hydrochloride (dissolved in 100 ml of normal saline) infused intravenously over 30 min, 3 times daily for 2 to 3 days.
- If a response is observed, continue with 250 mg of thiamine hydrochloride intravenously or intramuscularly daily until clinical improvement ceases.
- Nonalcoholics with WE: treat with 200 mg of thiamine hydrochloride (dissolved in 100 ml of normal saline) infused intravenously over 30 min, 3 times daily for 2 to 3 days.
- Parenteral side effects may include generalized pruritus, transient local irritation, or rarely, anaphylactic or anaphylactoid reactions.
- Parenteral magnesium must be infused concurrently with thiamine.

CHRONIC Rx

Recommended oral dose after treatment for WE: thiamine 30 to 100 mg twice daily

DISPOSITION

- If prompt treatment with thiamine is not administered during the potential reversible stages of WE, Korsakoff's syndrome may develop consisting of a typical pattern of memory loss emerging after the acute global confusional state of WE resolves.
- Approximately 80% who survive WE develop Korsakoff's syndrome.

REFERRAL

In cases of altered mental status, ophthalmoplegia or ataxia of gait, consider neurology consultation. Treatment should be initiated as soon as WE is suspected.

! PEARLS & CONSIDERATIONS

COMMENTS

- WE should be suspected in all patients with poor nutrition.
- WE is a clinical diagnosis composed of a triad of confusion, ataxia, and ophthalmoplegia.
- Thiamine infusion should be initiated upon clinical suspicion of WE.
- Thiamine infusion should precede infusion of fluids with glucose in all patients with poor nutrition or clinical suspicion of WE.

PREVENTION

- Prophylactic treatment for patient with severe alcohol withdrawal, poor nourishment, or signs of malnutrition: thiamine 250 mg intramuscular daily for 3 to 5 days.

- In individuals susceptible to WE, 100 mg of intravenous thiamine should precede any glucose infusion.
- Recommended daily dose of thiamine for an average, healthy adult: 1.4 mg or 0.5 mg per 1000 kcal of carbohydrates consumed.
- Higher dose recommended for children, in critically ill conditions, and during pregnancy and lactation.

PATIENT & FAMILY EDUCATION

In cases of known alcohol abuse or severe illness, the patient and family should be counseled on the importance of proper nutrition, including vitamin supplementation.

SUGGESTED READINGS

available at www.expertconsult.com

RELATED CONTENT

Alcoholism (Related Key Topic)
Korsakoff's Psychosis (Related Key Topic)
Vitamin Deficiency (Related Key Topic)

AUTHOR: **D. BRANDON BURTIS, D.O.**

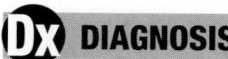

BASIC INFORMATION

DEFINITION

West Nile virus (WNV) infection is an illness affecting the central nervous system (CNS) caused by the mosquito-borne WNV.

SYNONYMS

West Nile virus fever
West Nile virus encephalitis
Neuroinvasive West Nile virus infection
Nonneuroinvasive West Nile virus infection

ICD-9CM CODES
066.4 West Nile virus infection

EPIDEMIOLOGY & DEMOGRAPHICS

- Before 1999, WNV infection was confined to areas in the Middle East, with occasional outbreaks in Europe. The infection began being diagnosed in the Western Hemisphere in 1999. First seen in the northeast and mid-Atlantic states, WNV virus infection has spread steadily each year to new regions of the U.S., with a general westward migration pattern. In 2003, a record number of cases were reported from the U.S., with over 7000 cases reported, resulting in several hundred deaths. Most deaths occur in elderly patients with WNV encephalitis. In 2003, Illinois, Ohio, Michigan, and Louisiana were hardest hit. Since 2004 the incidence of WNV infection diminished gradually as it spread to the western states. Human cases of WNV infection have now been reported across all the contiguous continental U.S. (sparing only Hawaii and Alaska). A total of 720 neuroinvasive and nonneuroinvasive cases, with 33 deaths from WNV, were reported in the U.S. in 2009.
- The virus is carried by a number of species of birds, as well as horses and several other animals. It is transmitted to humans through the bite of an infected mosquito. For this reason, WNV infection is seen primarily from mid-summer to mid-autumn, the period of maximum mosquito intensity.
- The majority of severe cases have been reported among individuals >50 yr of age. There is no gender predilection. Certain HLA haplotypes appear to predispose to severe disease (e.g., HLA-A68 and HLA-C08).
- Person-to-person transmission is fortunately rare but has been reported to occur by blood transfusion, organ transplantation, breast-feeding, and perhaps perinatal transmission; the blood supply is now routinely tested by nucleic acid testing methods to reduce the risk of transmission-acquired WNV in the U.S.

PHYSICAL FINDINGS & CLINICAL PRESENTATION

- Less than 20% of infected individuals develop symptomatic disease. The initial phase of illness is nonspecific, with abrupt onset of fever (West Nile fever) accompanied by malaise, eye pain, anorexia, headache, and, occasionally, rash and lymphadenopathy. Less commonly, myocarditis, hepatitis, or pancreatitis may occur.
- Encephalitis is the most common neurologic manifestation of West Nile virus infection. Aseptic meningitis may also occur.
- In approximately 1 in 150 cases, especially among elderly patients, severe neurologic sequelae will occur (West Nile neuroinvasive disease [WNND]). Most common among these are ataxia, cranial nerve palsies, optic neuritis, seizures, myelitis, and polyradiculitis.

ETIOLOGY

The WNV is a member of the flavivirus group, along with the yellow fever, dengue, St. Louis, and Japanese encephalitis viruses. It has a large reservoir in nature, infecting many species of birds, as well as certain mammals, and is spread to humans primarily by the bite of an infected *Culex* mosquito or other various species of mosquito with a peak incidence in the late summer and early fall. Neurologic disease is caused by direct invasion of the CNS.

DIAGNOSIS

DIFFERENTIAL DIAGNOSIS

- Meningitis or encephalitis caused by more common viruses (e.g., enteroviruses, herpes simplex)
- Bacterial meningitis
- Vasculitis
- Fungal meningitis (e.g., cryptococcal infection)
- Tuberculous meningitis

LABORATORY TESTS

- CBC, electrolytes (hyponatremia common)
- Spinal tap and CSF examination: typically demonstrates lymphocytic pleocytosis with normal level of glucose and elevated level of protein
- CSF WNV IgM antibody level: detection in symptomatic patients is diagnostic of West Nile neuronivasive disease. The antibody can be detected within 9 days of fever onset and can persist for several months. There can be rare false-positive results in people recently vaccinated against Japanese encephalitis or yellow fever viruses.

IMAGING STUDIES

MRI of the brain to exclude mass lesions and cerebral edema

TREATMENT

W

NONPHARMACOLOGIC THERAPY

Hospitalization, IV hydration, ventilator support may be necessary.

ACUTE GENERAL Rx

No specific therapy has been established in clinical trials. Ribavirin and interferon alfa-2b have been shown to have in vitro activity against the virus. IV immunoglobulin (IVIG) from convalescent patient plasma is under study but no controlled trials have been reported as yet.

CHRONIC Rx

Chronic rehabilitation therapy usually necessary for patients with severe neurologic impairment. Mental status defects following WNV neuroinvasive disease appear to be more common and severe than initially recognized.

DISPOSITION

Chronic rehabilitation as needed following recovery from acute infection. Physical and mental outcome measures seem to normalize within approximately 1 yr in patients with WNV. The presence of preexisting comorbid conditions is associated with longer recovery.

REFERRAL

- Infectious disease consultant
- Public health authorities

PEARLS & CONSIDERATIONS

COMMENTS

- Diagnosis requires a high index of suspicion, because disease course may be nonspecific and may mimic other, more common disorders.
- Specific laboratory diagnostic studies are available only through public-health laboratories.

EVIDENCE

available at www.expertconsult.com

SUGGESTED READINGS
available at www.expertconsult.com

RELATED CONTENT
West Nile Virus Infection (Patient Information)

AUTHOR: **STEVEN M. OPAL, M.D.**

Diseases and Disorders

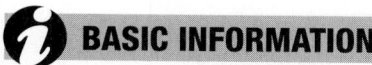

BASIC INFORMATION

DEFINITION

Whiplash refers to a hyperextension injury to the neck, often the result of being struck from behind by a fast-moving vehicle.

SYNONYMS

Acceleration flexion-extension neck injury

ICD-9CM CODES

847.0 Whiplash injury or syndrome

EPIDEMIOLOGY & DEMOGRAPHICS

- Whiplash occurs in more than 1 million people each year.
- Most injuries (40%) are the result of rear-end motor vehicle accidents.
- Whiplash occurs at all ages, in both sexes, and at all socioeconomic levels.
- Incidence is 4 per 1000 persons and is higher in women than men.
- Nearly 50% of patients with whiplash seek legal advice.
- Whiplash is also seen in shaken baby syndrome.

PHYSICAL FINDINGS & CLINICAL PRESENTATION

- Most present with a history of being involved in a motor vehicle accident and being rear-ended by another vehicle
- Pain not present initially but usually develops hr to a few days later
- Neck tightness and stiffness
- Occipital headache
- Shoulder, arm, and back pain
- Numbness in the arms
- Tinnitus
- Temporomandibular joint (TMJ) pain
- Dysphagia (retropharyngeal hematoma)
- Decreased range of motion of the neck
- Depressive symptoms

ETIOLOGY

- The mechanism of injury is the result of the sudden acceleration of the body forward, forcing the neck to hyperextend backward, causing injury to ligaments, muscles, bone, and/or intervertebral disk. At the end of the accident the head is thrust forward in a flexion position, sometimes causing injury to the cervical spine: C5-C6-C7.
- Motor vehicle accidents, trauma from falls, contact sports, physical abuse, and altercations are all possible causes of whiplash.
- The incidence of whiplash injury following polytrauma is low.
- Low-velocity crashes constitute a major cause of whiplash injury.

DIAGNOSIS

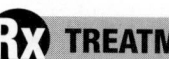

DIFFERENTIAL DIAGNOSIS

- Osteoarthritis
- Cervical disk disease
- Fibrositis
- Neuritis
- Torticollis
- Spinal cord tumor
- TMJ syndrome
- Tension headache
- Migraine headache

WORKUP

Any patient who presents with symptoms of whiplash and musculoskeletal or neurologic signs merits a workup to exclude cervical spine fractures or herniated disk disease.

LABORATORY TESTS

Laboratory studies are not helpful.

IMAGING STUDIES

- Plain C-spine films (anteroposterior, lateral, and odontoid views)
- Flexion/extension x-rays
- CT scan to exclude fracture
- MRI as alternative or in addition to CT in selected cases

TREATMENT

NONPHARMACOLOGIC THERAPY

- Soft cervical collar for no longer than 72 hr
- Moist heat 15 to 20 min four to six times per day.
- Continue with usual activities.

TABLE 1-419 Factors Associated with Persistent and Severe Whiplash Injuries

Severe Whiplash Injury

High-speed injury
Intense and rapid onset of pain
Severe restriction of movement at presentation
Abnormal neurology
Bony injuries

Persistent Whiplash Injury

High-speed injury
Intense and rapid onset of pain
Severe restriction of movement at presentation
Abnormal neurology
Bony injuries
Increasing age
Upper limb paresthesias
Cervical spondylosis

From Carr A, Hamilton W: *Orthopedics in primary care*, ed 2, Philadelphia, 2005, Saunders.

ACUTE GENERAL Rx

- Analgesics
  1. Ibuprofen 800 mg PO tid
  2. Naproxen 500 mg PO bid
  3. Acetaminophen 1 g PO qid
- Muscle relaxants (short-term use)
  1. Cyclobenzaprine 10 mg PO tid
  2. Methocarbamol 1 g PO qid
  3. Carisoprodol 350 mg PO qid

CHRONIC Rx

NSAIDs can be used long term.

DISPOSITION

- Most patients recover from the acute whiplash injury within weeks.
- Factors associated with persistent and severe whiplash injuries are described in Table 1-419.
- 20% to 40% may develop chronic whiplash syndrome (symptoms of headache, neck pain, and psychiatric complaints that persist for 6 mo).
- Older age, female gender, lawyer involvement, and work status (employed at time of entry to the clinic) were found to be prognostic factors associated with a negative outcome.

REFERRAL

Orthopedic, physical therapy

PEARLS & CONSIDERATIONS

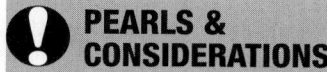

- Nearly one third of all personal injury cases involve cervical injuries.
- There is no dose-response relationship between trauma severity and incidence of whiplash injury.

COMMENTS

The entity of chronic whiplash syndrome remains elusive. Some authorities argue that financial motivation is a factor leading to persistent neck symptoms. Other studies do not substantiate this, showing a true chronic injury to the soft tissues of the neck.

SUGGESTED READINGS

available at www.expertconsult.com

RELATED CONTENT

Whiplash (Patient Information)

AUTHOR: **JORGE A. VILLAFUERTE, M.D.**

BASIC INFORMATION

DEFINITION

Wilson's disease is an autosomal recessive disorder of copper transport with inadequate biliary copper excretion, leading to an accumulation of the metal in liver, brain, kidneys, and corneas.

SYNONYMS

Progressive hepatolenticular degeneration

ICD-9CM CODES
275.1 Wilson's disease

EPIDEMIOLOGY & DEMOGRAPHICS

PREVALENCE: One case in 30,000
PREDOMINANT SEX: Affects men and women equally (autosomal recessive gene)
ONSET OF SYMPTOMS: Ages 3 to 40 yr

PHYSICAL FINDINGS & CLINICAL PRESENTATION

Hepatic presentation:
- Acute hepatitis with malaise, anorexia, nausea, jaundice, elevated transaminase, prolonged prothrombin time; rarely fulminant hepatic failure
- Chronic active (or autoimmune) hepatitis with fatigue, malaise, rashes, arthralgia, elevated transaminase, elevated serum immunoglobulin G, positive antinuclear antibody and anti-smooth muscle antibody
- Chronic liver disease/cirrhosis with hepatosplenomegaly, ascites, low serum albumin, prolonged prothrombin time, portal hypertension

Neurologic presentation:
- Movement disorder: tremors, ataxia
- Spastic dystonia: masklike facies, rigidity, gait disturbance, dysarthria, drooling, dysphagia

Ophthalmic:
- Kayser-Fleischer ring; indicates copper deposition in the Descemet's membrane of the iris
- Sunflower cataracts

Psychiatric presentation:
- Depression, obsessive-compulsive disorder, psychopathic behaviors, neuroses

Other organs:
- Hemolytic anemia
- Renal disease (i.e., Fanconi's syndrome with hematuria, phosphaturia, renal tubular acidosis, vitamin D–resistant rickets)
- Cardiomyopathy
- Arthritis
- Hypoparathyroidism
- Hypogonadism

PHYSICAL FINDINGS:
- Ocular: the Kayser-Fleischer ring is a gold-yellow ring seen at the periphery of the iris (Fig. 1-901); these should be sought with slit-lamp examination by a skilled examiner.
- Stigmata of acute or chronic liver disease.
- Neurologic abnormalities: see previous.

ETIOLOGY & PATHOGENESIS

- Dietary copper is transported from the intestine to the liver, where normally it is metabolized into ceruloplasmin. In Wilson's disease, defective incorporation of copper into ceruloplasmin and a decrease of biliary copper excretion lead to accumulation of this mineral.
- The gene for Wilson's disease is located in chromosome 13.

DIAGNOSIS

DIFFERENTIAL DIAGNOSIS

- Hereditary hypoceruloplasminemia
- Menkes' disease
- Consider the diagnosis of Wilson's disease in all cases of acute or chronic liver disease for which another cause has not been established.
- Consider Wilson's disease in patients with movement disorders or dystonia even without symptomatic liver disease.

LABORATORY TESTS

- Low serum copper (<65 mcg/L)
- 24-hr urinary copper excretion greater than 100 mcg (normal <30 mcg); increases to greater than 1200 mcg/24 hr after 500 mg of D-penicillamine (normal <500 mcg/24 hr)
- Abnormal liver function tests (note that aspartate aminotransferase may be higher than alanine aminotransferase)
- Low serum ceruloplasmin level (<200 mg/L)
- Low serum uric acid and phosphorus
- Abnormal urinalysis (hematuria)

BIOPSY

- Early:
  - Steatosis, focal necrosis, glycogenated hepatocyte nuclei
  - May reveal inflammation and piecemeal necrosis
- Late: cirrhosis
- Hepatic copper content (>250 mcg/g of dry weight) (normal is 20 to 50 mcg)
- Histochemical confirmation of excess copper can be helpful in diagnosis, but if absent, does not exclude Wilson's disease. The lack of immunoreactivity to copper-binding protein can occur because of the diffuse presence of copper in the cytoplasm and because of the assay's low sensitivity. Rhodamine and rubeanic acid stains can show dense granular lysosomal copper deposition in hepatocytes at the stage of cirrhotic nodular regeneration.

TREATMENT

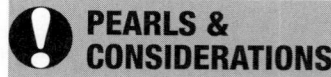

- Penicillamine: (chelator therapy)
  - 0.75 to 1.5 g/day divided bid (with pyridoxine 25 mg/day)
  - Monitor complete blood count (CBC) and urinalysis weekly
- Trientine (triethylene tetramine): (chelator therapy)
  - 1 to 2 g/day divided tid
  - Monitor CBC
- Zinc: (inhibits intestinal copper absorption)
  - 50 mg tid
  - Monitor zinc level
- Ammonium tetrathiomolybdate for neurologic symptoms
- Antioxidants
- Liver transplantation (for severe hepatic failure unresponsive to chelation); liver transplantation corrects the underlying pathophysiology and can be lifesaving

PROGNOSIS

Good with early chelation treatment

REFERRAL

To gastroenterologist, neurologist

PEARLS & CONSIDERATIONS

COMMENTS

Family screening of first-degree relatives must be undertaken. Genetic diagnosis is also useful in patients with indeterminate clinical and biochemical features.

SUGGESTED READING
available at www.expertconsult.com

RELATED CONTENT

Wilson's Disease (Patient Information)

AUTHOR: **FRED F. FERRI, M.D.**

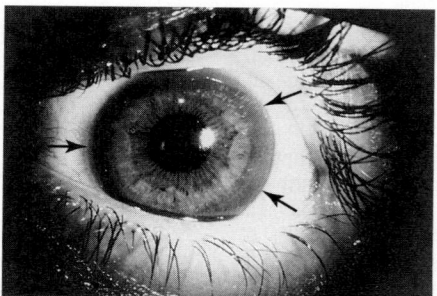

FIGURE 1-901 Deposition of copper (Kayser-Fleischer ring, *arrows*) in the periphery of the cornea as seen in hepatolenticular degeneration (Wilson's disease). (From Haines DE: *Fundamental neuroscience for basic and clinical applications,* ed 3, Philadelphia, 2005, Churchill Livingstone.)

DEFINITION

Wolff-Parkinson-White (WPW) syndrome is defined as the presence of preexcitation of the ventricles of the heart due to an abnormal electrical communication from the atria to the ventricles through an accessory pathway. Patients with WPW syndrome have both ventricular preexcitation and arrhythmias, which may be atrial fibrillation (AF), atrioventricular (AV) reentrant tachycardia, or both. Patients with WPW pattern have characteristic ECG findings of preexcitation: short PR interval <120 ms and the presence of a delta wave but no subjective or objective evidence of arrhythmia.

SYNONYMS

Preexcitation syndrome
WPW

ICD-9CM CODES
426.7   Wolff-Parkinson-White syndrome
426.81 Lown-Ganong-Levine syndrome

EPIDEMIOLOGY & DEMOGRAPHICS

- The prevalence of a WPW pattern on the surface ECG is 0.15% to 0.25% in the general population. The prevalence is increased to 0.55% in first-degree relatives of affected patients.
- In a study of a presumed healthy population of more than 20,000 patients, the WPW pattern was recognized in 0.25%. Of these patients, only 1.8% had documented arrhythmias that were consistent with the WPW syndrome.
- The prevalence of WPW is higher among males and decreases with age.
- Most patients with WPW syndrome have structurally normal hearts, but associations with mitral valve prolapse, cardiomyopathies, and Ebstein's anomaly have been reported.

PHYSICAL FINDINGS & CLINICAL PRESENTATION

- The physical examination may be entirely normal.
- Symptoms are typically related to tachyarrhythmias, including the following:
  - Palpitations, anxiety dyspnea, chest pain or tightness
  - Syncope or near syncope
  - Sudden cardiac death (rarely)
- Over time, 25% of cases become asymptomatic and remain symptom free if past age 40.
- The type of tachycardia can be any of the following:
  - Supraventricular tachycardia: AV reentrant tachycardia (AVRT) most common arrhythmia, further classified as orthodromic (narrow complex and occurs in 70% of symptomatic patients), or antidromic (wide complex, in 4%-5% of patients)
  - AF (~10% to 38%), the second most common tachycardia, can be complicated by a very rapid ventricular response via conduction over the accessory pathway (AP), which can lead to ventricular fibrillation and sudden death. This risk is dependent on the antegrade refractory period of AP during AF.
    - Atrial flutter (~5%)
- Presence of WPW can be associated with other congenital cardiac defects.
- Incidence of sudden cardiac death in WPW syndrome is estimated at 0.15% per patient per yr. The risk of death is lower in asymptomatic patients.
- Left free wall accessory pathways are most common, followed by posteroseptal, right free wall, and anteroseptal locations.

ETIOLOGY & PATHOGENESIS

- The existence of an accessory pathway allows for conduction from the atria to the ventricles while bypassing the AV node.
- If the accessory pathway is capable of anterograde conduction, two parallel routes of AV conduction are possible: one is subject to delay through the AV node, and the other occurs without delay through the accessory pathway and results in preexcitation of the ventricle. The resulting QRS complex is a fusion beat, as a portion of the ventricle is activated via the accessory pathway giving rise to the delta wave, and the remainder of the ventricle is activated by the normal activation pathway (Fig. 1-902).
- Tachycardias occur when conduction is anterograde in one pathway (usually the normal AV pathway) and retrograde in the other (usually the accessory pathway) as a result of different refractory periods. Some patients (~5% to 10%) with WPW syndrome have multiple accessory pathways.

WPW: Sinus Rhythm

FIGURE 1-902 With Wolff-Parkinson-White *(WPW)* syndrome, an abnormal accessory conduction pathway called a *bypass tract (BT)* connects the atria and the ventricles. (From Goldberger AL [ed]: *Clinical electrocardiography: a simplified approach,* ed 6, St Louis, 1999, Mosby.)

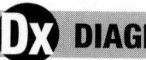

- Three basic features characterize the ECG abnormalities associated with WPW pattern (Fig. 1-903):
  1. PR interval <120 msec
  2. QRS complex >120 msec with a slurred, slowly rising onset of QRS in some leads (delta wave) and a normal terminal QRS portion
  3. Secondary ST-T wave changes directed in an opposite direction to the major delta and QRS vectors.
- ECG patterns with abnormal QRS complexes and ST and T changes can mask or mimic myocardial infarction, bundle branch block, or ventricular hypertrophy.
- Most commonly seen tachycardia is characterized by a normal QRS with a regular rate of 150-250 bpm. Onset and termination are abrupt.
- Variants of preexcitation:
  - Lown-Ganong-Levine syndrome: fibers from the atrium to the His bundle bypass the physiologic delay of the AV node (atriohisian pathways) with a short PR interval and a normal QRS complex on ECG (no delta wave)
  - Atriofascicular accessory pathways: duplication of the AV node and distal conducting system with normal baseline ECG
  - The only way to be certain of the accessory pathways' properties and propensity for rapid conduction is via an electrophysiology (EP) study.

RISK STRATIFICATION

- Intermittent loss or appearance of preexcitation on a beat-to-beat basis is indicative of lower risk, assessed with Holter monitoring or with exercise testing.

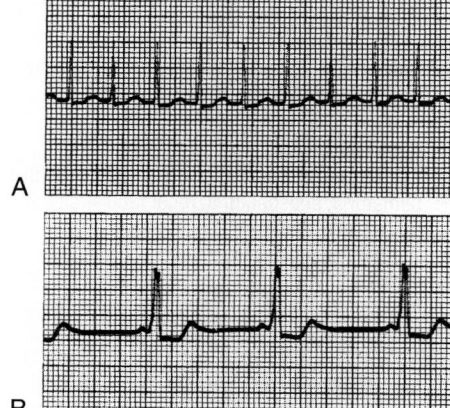

FIGURE 1-903 A, Supraventricular tachycardia in a child with Wolff-Parkinson-White syndrome. Note the normal QRS complexes during the tachycardia. **B,** Later, the typical features of Wolff-Parkinson-White syndrome are apparent: a short P-R interval, a delta wave, and a wide QRS. (From Behrman RE: *Nelson textbook of pediatrics,* ed 18, Philadelphia, 2007, Saunders.)

- In patients with a persistent preexcitation pattern, EP study is the procedure of choice for risk stratification by inducing AF, indicating high risk.

Rx TREATMENT

- Goals of electrophysiologic evaluation in patients with WPW syndrome are described in Box 1-83.
- Urgent cardioversion, for an acute tachycardia episode with hemodynamic instability
- Stable patients treated medically
  - Narrow QRS width tachycardias:
  1. Carotid sinus massage or vagal maneuvers
  2. Atrial pacing (transvenous or transesophageal)
  3. Adenosine, use with caution (may induce AF in 15% of cases)
  4. AF is potentially life threatening
  - Wide QRS complex tachycardias (WCTs):
  1. Because atrial arrhythmias (Aflutter/AF) with antegrade conduction down an AP are *not* AV node dependent, AV nodal blocking therapies are ineffective and potentially dangerous.
  2. Beta-blockers, calcium channel blockers, digoxin, and adenosine should be avoided. Can try procainamide. If tachycardia persists, synchronized DCCV is the treatment of choice.
- Long-term management:
  - Priority of therapy:
  1. Asymptomatic: no therapy unless high risk or family history of sudden death, competitive athletes, high-risk occupation (pilots)
  2. Symptomatic, prior AF, aborted sudden death: further study/therapy

  - Medical therapy (asymptomatic high risk):
  1. Single drug: amiodarone, sotalol, flecainide, propafenone
  2. Combination AV nodal blocker (beta-blocker/calcium channel blocker) and drugs that exclusively work on AP (class IA arrhythmics [quinidine, procainamide, and disopyramide])
  - Recommendations for radiofrequency catheter ablation of accessory pathways:
  1. Class 1: patients with symptomatic AVRT and AF (or other atrial tachyarrhythmia) with a rapid ventricular rates (RVR) via the AP when the tachycardia is drug resistant or the patient is intolerant or does not desire long-term drug therapy.
- For the acute termination of narrow complex regular tachyarrhythmias, carotid sinus massage or the Valsalva maneuver may be successful. First-line pharmacologic therapy includes adenosine or verapamil for patients *without* AF or flutter.
- For patients with a rapid ventricular response with hemodynamic compromise, urgent electrical cardioversion is warranted.
- Digitalis should not be used as a single drug in patients who have atrial flutter or AF, because it can reduce refractoriness in the accessory pathway and accelerate the tachycardia.
- Drug therapy for the chronic prevention of narrow complex regular tachyarrhythmias includes class IC antiarrhythmics, β-blockers, calcium channel blockers, amiodarone, or sotalol. The choice of drug therapy is dictated by the underlying mechanism of the tachyarrhythmia.

- For the treatment of AF in patients with WPW, the administration of AV nodal–blocking agents may not slow the ventricular rate, because the accessory pathways capable of rapid conduction do not respond to AV-blocking agents. Procainamide is the drug of choice for controlling the ventricular rate and restoring the sinus rhythm in patients with WPW who have AF.
- For long-term therapy to prevent recurrence, radiofrequency catheter ablation has become the first-line therapy for most patients. When medical therapy fails or patients are drug intolerant, or for those patients who do not wish to take drugs, or cannot tolerate the tachyarrhythmias, radiofrequency ablation should be performed (class 1 indication).

SUGGESTED READINGS
available at www.expertconsult.com

RELATED CONTENT
Wolff-Parkinson-White Syndrome (Patient Information)

AUTHORS: **SHAHNAZ PUNJANI, M.D.,**
FRED F. FERRI, M.D., and
WEN-CHIH WU, M.D., M.P.H.

BOX 1-83 Goals of Electrophysiologic Evaluation in Patients with Wolff-Parkinson-White Syndrome

- Confirmation of the presence of an atrioventricular bypass tract (BT)
- Evaluation for the presence of multiple BTs
- Localization of the BT(s)
- Evaluation of the refractoriness of the BT and its implications for life-threatening arrhythmias
- Induction and evaluation of tachycardias
- Demonstration of the BT role in the tachycardia
- Evaluation of other tachycardias not dependent on the presence of the BT
- Termination of the tachycardias

From Issa Z et al: *Clinical arrhythmology and electrophysiology,* ed 2, Philadelphia, 2012, Saunders.

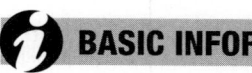

DEFINITION

Zenker's diverticulum (ZD) refers to the acquired physiologic obstruction of the esophageal introitus that results from mucosal herniation posteriorly between the cricopharyngeus muscle and the inferior pharyngeal constrictor muscle (Fig. 1-904).

SYNONYMS

Pharyngoesophageal diverticulum
Pulsion diverticulum

ICD-9CM CODES
530.6 Zenker's diverticulum (esophagus)

EPIDEMIOLOGY & DEMOGRAPHICS

- The most common type of diverticulum of the upper gastrointestinal tract
- Rare disease with annual incidence estimated 1/50,000 per year
- Most commonly presents after the age of 60 yr, more commonly seen in males
- Peak incidence is seventh to ninth decades
- Associated with gastroesophageal reflux disease (GERD) and hiatal hernia

PHYSICAL FINDINGS & CLINICAL PRESENTATION

A small ZD may be asymptomatic. As it becomes larger, symptoms may include:
- Dysphagia to solids and liquids (most common)
- Regurgitation of undigested food
- Sensation of globus or fullness in the neck
- Cough
- Halitosis
- Aspiration pneumonia
- Weight loss
- Voice changes
- Sialorrhea (excessive drooling)

ETIOLOGY

- The specific cause is not known. The leading hypothesis suggests a discoordination of the swallowing muscles (specifically, incomplete relaxation of the cricopharyngeus muscle) that leads to an increased pressure on the mucosa of the hypopharynx, resulting in a progressive distention of that mucosa in its weakest area (posterior wall in "Killian's triangle," the point between the oblique fibers of the inferior pharyngeal muscle and the horizontal fibers of the cricopharyngeus muscle). The end result is the formation of a false diverticulum where food elements and secretions may be lodged, causing the symptoms listed previously.
- ZD may also occur after anterior spinal surgery or cervical spine injury.

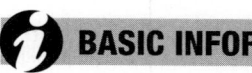

- Clinical presentation and barium swallow typically make the diagnosis of ZD.
- Neck ultrasound can also be used.
- Esophageal manometry can help elucidate the pathogenesis but not required for diagnosis

DIFFERENTIAL DIAGNOSIS

The differential diagnosis is similar to anyone presenting with dysphagia:
- Achalasia
- Esophageal spasm
- Esophageal carcinoma
- Esophageal webs
- Peptic stricture
- Lower esophageal (Schatzki) ring
- Foreign bodies
- Central nervous system disorders (stroke, Parkinson's disease, amyotrophic lateral sclerosis, multiple sclerosis, myasthenia gravis, muscular dystrophies)

- Dermatomyositis
- Infection

WORKUP

Barium swallow is the test of choice. Upper endoscopy runs the risk of perforation.

LABORATORY TESTS

Not specific

IMAGING STUDIES

- Barium swallow: demonstrates a herniated sac with a narrow diverticular neck that typically originates proximal to the cricopharyngeus at the level of C5-C6 (Fig. 1-905).
- Endoscopy is only indicated if barium studies show mucosal irregularities to rule out neoplasia.
- Oropharyngeal-esophageal scintigraphy has recently been shown to be an effective, sensitive, and simple diagnostic study for both qualitative and quantitative analyses.
- A chest x-ray is performed in cases of suspected aspiration pneumonia.

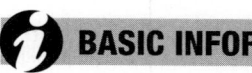

NONPHARMACOLOGIC THERAPY

- Soft mechanical diet can be tried in patients with symptoms of dysphagia.
- Avoid seeds, skins, and nuts.

ACUTE GENERAL Rx

- Surgical repair is the conventional treatment for symptomatic patients (dysphagia, cough, aspiration) with excellent relief of symptoms in nearly all patients and low procedural mortality (<1.5%). Procedures include:
  1. Cervical diverticulectomy with cricopharyngeal myotomy (most common approach)
  2. Diverticulopexy or diverticular inversion with cricopharyngeal myotomy
  3. Diverticulectomy alone
  4. Cricopharyngeal myotomy alone
- Endoscopic techniques (esophagodiverticulostomy) have largely replaced conventional surgery and include:
  1. Endoscopic stapler diverticulotomy (may be the initial treatment of choice)
  2. Microendoscopic carbon dioxide laser surgical diverticulotomy
  3. Diverticulum <3 cm is a contraindication to endosurgical approach.
  4. Head-to-head comparison with surgical repairs showed endoscopic techniques to be similar in results, relief of symptoms, and patient satisfaction.

CHRONIC Rx

In patients not having surgery, treatment is directed toward any complications that may occur:
- Antibiotics for aspiration pneumonia
- H₂ antagonists for ulcerations that can develop within the diverticulum
- Botulinum toxin for temporary relief of dysphagia

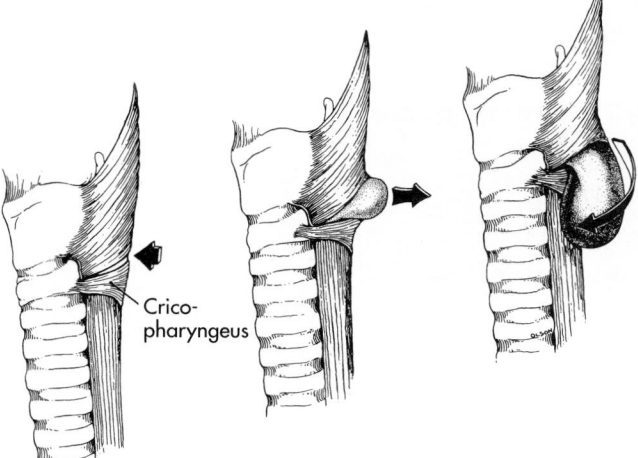

FIGURE 1-904 Formation of pharyngoesophageal (Zenker's) diverticulum. *Left,* Herniation of the pharyngeal mucosa and submucosa occurs at the point of transition *(arrow)* between the oblique fibers of the thyropharyngeus muscle and the more horizontal fibers of the cricopharyngeus muscle. *Center and right,* As the diverticulum enlarges, it dissects toward the left side and downward into the superior mediastinum in the prevertebral space. (From Sabiston D: *Textbook of surgery,* ed 15, Philadelphia, 1997, Saunders.)

Crico-pharyngeus

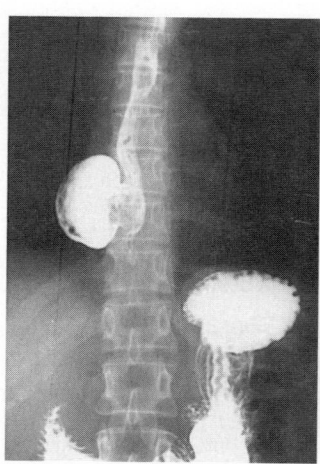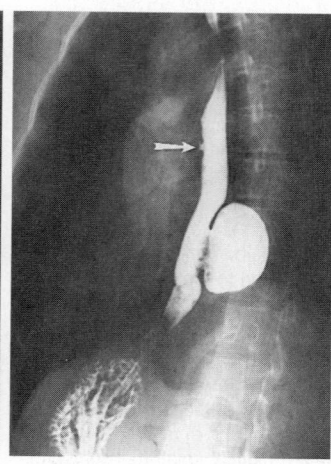

FIGURE 1-905 Posteroanterior *(left)* and oblique *(right)* views from barium esophagogram showing both a typical diverticulum of the junction of the mid-esophagus and distal esophagus and a small traction diverticulum *(arrow)* of the mid-esophagus. (From Sabiston D: *Textbook of surgery,* ed 15, Philadelphia, 1997, Saunders.)

DISPOSITION
- If left untreated, progressive enlargement of the diverticulum occurs.
- The risk of complications (e.g., aspiration pneumonia) increases with the size of the diverticulum.
- Postsurgical recurrence can occur (4%); however, these are usually asymptomatic.

REFERRAL
Any patient with dysphagia requires a gastroenterology consultation. A thoracic surgical, ENT, or head and neck surgeon may be consulted if surgery is considered.

COMMENTS
The association with cancer is rare (0.4%).

SUGGESTED READINGS
available at www.expertconsult.com

RELATED CONTENT
Zenker's Diverticulum (Patient Information)

AUTHORS: **ROBERT M. KIRCHNER, M.D.,** and **PAUL GORDON, M.D.**

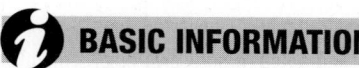

BASIC INFORMATION

DEFINITION

Zollinger-Ellison (ZE) syndrome is a hypergastrinemic state caused by a pancreatic or extrapancreatic non–beta islet cell tumor (gastrinoma) resulting in peptic acid disease.

SYNONYMS

Gastrinoma

ICD-9CM CODES
251.5 Zollinger-Ellison syndrome

EPIDEMIOLOGY & DEMOGRAPHICS

- Incidence is unknown, but 0.1% of all duodenal ulcers are believed to be caused by ZE.
- Occurs in both genders and at any age (most common in ages 30 to 50 yr).
- Two thirds of gastrinomas are sporadic, and one third are associated with multiple endocrine neoplasia type 1 (MEN-1), an autosomal-dominant genetic disorder that also includes hyperparathyroidism and pituitary tumors.
- Approximately 60% of gastrinomas are malignant.
- The incidence and prevalence of pancreatic neuroendocrine tumors are increasing. They represent 1.3% of all cases of pancreatic cancer.

PHYSICAL FINDINGS & CLINICAL PRESENTATION

- The majority of patients (95%) present with symptoms of peptic ulcer (see Section I, "Peptic Ulcer Disease").
- 60% of patients have symptoms related to gastroesophageal reflux disease (see Section I, "Gastroesophageal Reflux Disease").
- One third of patients with ZE have diarrhea and, less commonly, steatorrhea.

The following circumstances warrant suspicion of ZE syndrome:
- Ulcers distal to the first portion of the duodenum
- Multiple peptic ulcers
- Ineffective treatment for peptic ulcer disease with the usual drug doses and schedules
- Peptic ulcer and diarrhea
- Familial history of peptic ulcer

- Patients with a personal or family history suggesting parathyroid or pituitary tumors or dysfunction
- Peptic ulcer and urinary tract calculi
- Patients with peptic ulcer who are negative for *Helicobacter pylori* and do not have a history of nonsteroidal anti-inflammatory drug use

ETIOLOGY

- The pathophysiologic manifestations of ZE syndrome are related to the effects of hypergastrinemia. Gastrin stimulates gastric acid secretion, which in turn is responsible for the development of duodenal ulcers and diarrhea. Gastrin also promotes gastric mucosal epithelial cell growth and resulting parietal cell hyperplasia.
- Gastrinomas are usually small (0.1 to 2 cm) but sometimes large (>20 cm) tumors.
- 60% of gastrinomas are malignant, with liver and regional lymph nodes the most common site of metastases. Histology is not a good predictor of the biology of gastrinomas.
- 60% of patients with MEN-1 have gastrinomas.
- 10% of patients with ZE syndrome have islet cell hyperplasia rather than gastrinomas; in 10% to 20% of patients with gastrinoma the tumors cannot be located because of small size.

DIAGNOSIS

DIFFERENTIAL DIAGNOSIS

- Peptic ulcer disease (see Section I, "Peptic Ulcer Disease")
- Gastroesophageal reflux disease (see Section I, "Gastroesophageal Reflux Disease")
- Diarrhea (see Section III, "Diarrhea, Acute" and "Diarrhea, Chronic")

WORKUP

- Diagnosis of peptic ulcer:
  - Upper gastrointestinal series (may also show prominent gastric rugal folds)
  - Endoscopy
- Gastric acid secretion:
  - Serum gastrin level (fasting) >150 pg/ml (criterion for diagnosis is serum gastrin >1000 pg/ml) (causes of false-positive results: pernicious anemia, renal failure, retained gastric antrum syndrome, diabetes mellitus, rheumatoid arthritis)

- Provocative gastrin level tests:
  - Secretin stimulation
  - Calcium stimulation
  - Standard test meal stimulation
- Gastrinoma localization:
  - Arteriography
  - Abdominal sonography
  - Abdominal CT scan
  - Abdominal MRI
  - Selective portal vein branch gastrin level
  - Octreotide scan

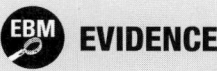

TREATMENT

- Surgical resection of the gastrinoma (NOTE: 90% of gastrinomas can be located, resulting in a 40% overall cure rate)
- Total gastrectomy or vagotomy (palliative in some patients)
- Medical treatment
  - Proton pump inhibitors (e.g., omeprazole, lansoprazole)
  - Somatostatin or octreotide
  - Chemotherapy for metastatic gastrinoma with streptozotocin, 5-fluorouracil, and doxorubicin
  - Early trials with everolimus, an oral inhibitor of mammalian target of rapamycin (mTOR) have shown antitumor activity in patients with advanced pancreatic neuroendocrine tumors with significant prolongation of progression-free survival and low rates of severe adverse events
  - Preliminary trials with the tyrosine kinase inhibitor sunitinib have shown encouraging results on prolongation of survival

PROGNOSIS

Five-year survival:
- Two thirds of all patients
- 20% with liver metastases
- 90% without liver metastases

REFERRAL

To gastroenterologist and surgeon

EVIDENCE

available at www.expertconsult.com

SUGGESTED READINGS
available at www.expertconsult.com

RELATED CONTENT
Zollinger-Ellison Syndrome (Patient Information)

AUTHOR: **FRED F. FERRI, M.D.**

Differential Diagnosis

ABDOMINAL DISTENTION
ICD-9CM # 787.3

NONMECHANICAL OBSTRUCTION
Excessive intraluminal gas.
Intraabdominal infection.
Trauma.
Retroperitoneal irritation (renal colic, neoplasms, infections, hemorrhage).
Vascular insufficiency (thrombosis, embolism).
Mechanical ventilation.
Extraabdominal infection (sepsis, pneumonia, empyema, osteomyelitis of spine).
Metabolic/toxic abnormalities (hypokalemia, uremia, lead poisoning).
Chemical irritation (perforated ulcer, bile, pancreatitis).
Peritoneal inflammation.
Severe pain, pain medications.

MECHANICAL OBSTRUCTION
Neoplasm (intraluminal, extraluminal).
Adhesions, endometriosis.
Infection (intraabdominal abscess, diverticulitis).
Gallstones.
Foreign body, bezoars.
Pregnancy.
Hernias.
Volvulus.
Stenosis at surgical anastomosis, radiation stenosis.
Fecaliths.
Inflammatory bowel disease.
Gastric outlet obstruction.
Hematoma.
Other: parasites, superior mesenteric artery (SMA) syndrome, pneumatosis intestinalis, annular pancreas, Hirschsprung's disease, intussusception, meconium.

ABDOMINAL PAIN, ADOLESCENCE[26]
ICD-9CM # 789.67

Acute gastroenteritis.
Irritable bowel syndrome (IBS).
Anxiety.
Mittelschmerz.
Appendicitis.
Inflammatory bowel disease.
Peptic ulcer disease (PUD).
Cholecystitis.
Neoplasm.
Diabetic ketoacidosis.
Functional abdominal pain.
Pelvic inflammatory disease (PID).
Pregnancy.
Pyelonephritis.
Renal stone.
Trauma.

ABDOMINAL PAIN, CHILDHOOD[26]
ICD-9CM # 789.67

Acute gastroenteritis.
Appendicitis.
Constipation.

Cholecystitis, acute.
Intestinal obstruction.
Pancreatitis.
Neoplasm.
Inflammatory bowel disease.
Other:
  Functional abdominal pain.
  Pyelonephritis.
  Pneumonia.
  Diabetic ketoacidosis.
  Heavy metal poisoning.
  Sickle cell crisis.
  Trauma.
  Anxiety.
  Sexual abuse.

ABDOMINAL PAIN, CHRONIC LOWER[38]
ICD-9CM # 789.64 Abdominal Pain, Left Lower Quadrant
789.63 Abdominal Pain, Right Lower Quadrant
789.85 Abdominal Pain, Suprapubic

ORGANIC DISORDERS
Common
Gynecologic disease.
Lactase deficiency.
Diverticulitis/diverticulosis.
Crohn's disease.
Intestinal obstruction.
Uncommon
Chronic intestinal pseudoobstruction.
Mesenteric ischemia.
Malignancy (e.g., ovarian carcinoma).
Abdominal wall pain.
Spinal disease.
Testicular disease.
Metabolic diseases (e.g., diabetes mellitus, familial Mediterranean fever, C1 esterase deficiency [angioneurotic edema], porphyria, lead poisoning, tabes dorsalis, renal failure).

FUNCTIONAL DISORDERS
Common
Irritable bowel syndrome.
Functional abdominal bloating.
Uncommon
Functional abdominal pain.

ABDOMINAL PAIN, DIFFUSE
ICD-9CM # 789.67

Early appendicitis.
Aortic aneurysm.
Gastroenteritis.
Intestinal obstruction.
Diverticulitis.
Peritonitis.
Mesenteric insufficiency or infarction.
Pancreatitis.
Inflammatory bowel disease.
Irritable bowel.
Mesenteric adenitis.
Metabolic: toxins, lead poisoning, uremia, drug overdose, diabetic ketoacidosis (DKA), heavy metal poisoning.

Sickle cell crisis.
Pneumonia (rare).
Trauma.
Urinary tract infection, PID.
Other: anxiety, acute intermittent porphyria, tabes dorsalis, periarteritis nodosa, Henoch-Schönlein purpura, adrenal insufficiency.

ABDOMINAL PAIN, EPIGASTRIC
ICD-9CM # 789.66

Gastric: PUD, gastric outlet obstruction, gastric ulcer.
Duodenal: PUD, duodenitis.
Biliary: cholecystitis, cholangitis, biliary dyskinesia.
Hepatic: hepatitis.
Pancreatic: pancreatitis.
Intestinal: high small bowel obstruction, early appendicitis.
Cardiac: angina, MI, pericarditis.
Pulmonary: pneumonia, pleurisy, pneumothorax.
Subphrenic abscess.
Vascular: dissecting aneurysm, mesenteric ischemia.
Psychiatric: anxiety.

ABDOMINAL PAIN, INFANCY[26]
ICD-9CM # 789.67

Acute gastroenteritis.
Appendicitis.
Intussusception.
Volvulus.
Meckel diverticulum.
Other: colic, trauma.

ABDOMINAL PAIN, LEFT LOWER QUADRANT
ICD-9CM # 789.64

Intestinal: diverticulitis, diverticulosis, intestinal obstruction, perforated ulcer, inflammatory bowel disease, perforated descending colon, inguinal hernia, neoplasm, appendicitis.
Reproductive: ectopic pregnancy, ovarian cyst, torsion of ovarian cyst, tuboovarian abscess, mittelschmerz, endometriosis, seminal vesiculitis.
Renal: renal or ureteral calculi, pyelonephritis, neoplasm.
Vascular: leaking aortic aneurysm.
Psoas abscess.
Trauma.

ABDOMINAL PAIN, LEFT UPPER QUADRANT
ICD-9CM # 789.32

Gastric: PUD, gastritis, pyloric stenosis, hiatal hernia.
Pancreatic: pancreatitis, neoplasm, stone in pancreatic duct or ampulla.
Cardiac: MI, angina pectoris.
Splenic: splenomegaly, ruptured spleen, splenic abscess, splenic infarction.

Differential Diagnosis
II

Renal: calculi, pyelonephritis, neoplasm.
Pulmonary: pneumonia, empyema, pulmonary infarction.
Vascular: ruptured aortic aneurysm.
Cutaneous: herpes zoster.
Trauma.
Intestinal: high fecal impaction, perforated colon, diverticulitis.

ABDOMINAL PAIN, NONSURGICAL CAUSES

ICD-9CM # 789.9

Irritable bowel syndrome.
Urinary tract infection, pyelonephritis, salpingitis, PID.
Gastroenteritis, gastritis, peptic ulcer.
Diverticular spasm.
Hepatitis, mononucleosis.
Pancreatitis.
Inferior wall myocardial infarction.
Basilar pneumonia, pulmonary embolism.
Diabetic ketoacidosis.
Strain or hematoma of rectus muscle.
Ruptured Graafian follicle.
Herpes zoster.
Nerve root compression.
Sickle cell crisis.
Acute adrenal insufficiency.
Other: acute porphyria, familial Mediterranean fever, tabes dorsalis, anxiety, sexual abuse.

ABDOMINAL PAIN, PERIUMBILICAL

ICD-9CM # 789.65

Intestinal: small bowel obstruction or gangrene, early appendicitis.
Vascular: mesenteric thrombosis, dissecting aortic aneurysm.
Pancreatic: pancreatitis.
Metabolic: uremia, DKA.
Trauma.

ABDOMINAL PAIN, POORLY LOCALIZED[26]

ICD-9CM # 789.60

EXTRAABDOMINAL

Metabolic
DKA, acute intermittent porphyria, hyperthyroidism, hypothyroidism, hypercalcemia, hypokalemia, uremia, hyperlipidemia, hyperparathyroidism.
Hematologic
Sickle cell crisis, leukemia or lymphoma, Henoch-Schönlein purpura.
Infectious
Infectious mononucleosis, Rocky Mountain spotted fever, acquired immunodeficiency syndrome (AIDS), streptococcal pharyngitis (in children), herpes zoster.
Drugs and Toxins
Heavy metal poisoning, black widow spider bites, withdrawal syndromes, mushroom ingestion.
Referred Pain
Pulmonary: pneumonia, pulmonary embolism, pneumothorax.

Cardiac: angina, MI, pericarditis, myocarditis.
Genitourinary: prostatitis, epididymitis, orchitis, testicular torsion.
Musculoskeletal: rectus sheath hematoma.
Functional
Somatization disorder, malingering, hypochondriasis, Munchausen syndrome.

INTRAABDOMINAL

Early appendicitis, gastroenteritis, peritonitis, pancreatitis, abdominal aortic aneurysm, mesenteric insufficiency or infarction, intestinal obstruction, volvulus, ulcerative colitis.

ABDOMINAL PAIN, PREGNANCY

ICD-9CM # 789.67

GYNECOLOGIC (GESTATIONAL AGE IN PARENTHESES)

Miscarriage	(<20 wk; 80% <12 wk)
Septic abortion	(<20 wk)
Ectopic pregnancy	(<14 wk)
Corpus luteum cyst rupture	(<12 wk)
Ovarian torsion	(especially <24 wk)
Pelvic inflammatory disease	(<12 wk)
Chorioamnionitis	(>16 wk)
Abruptio placentae	(>16 wk)

NONGYNECOLOGIC

Appendicitis	(Throughout)
Cholecystitis	(Throughout)
Hepatitis	(Throughout)
Pyelonephritis	(Throughout)
Preeclampsia	(>20 wk)

ABDOMINAL PAIN, RIGHT LOWER QUADRANT

ICD-9CM # 789.63

Intestinal: acute appendicitis, regional enteritis, incarcerated hernia, cecal diverticulitis, intestinal obstruction, perforated ulcer, perforated cecum, Meckel diverticulitis.
Reproductive: ectopic pregnancy, ovarian cyst, torsion of ovarian cyst, salpingitis, tuboovarian abscess, mittelschmerz, endometriosis, seminal vesiculitis.
Renal: renal and ureteral calculi, neoplasms, pyelonephritis.
Vascular: leaking aortic aneurysm.
Cutaneous: herpes zoster.
Psoas abscess.
Trauma.
Cholecystitis.

ABDOMINAL PAIN, RIGHT UPPER QUADRANT

ICD-9CM # 789.61

Biliary: calculi, infection, inflammation, neoplasm.
Hepatic: hepatitis, abscess, hepatic congestion, neoplasm, trauma.

Gastric: PUD, pyloric stenosis, neoplasm, alcoholic gastritis, hiatal hernia.
Pancreatic: pancreatitis, neoplasm, stone in pancreatic duct or ampulla.
Renal: calculi, infection, inflammation, neoplasm, rupture of kidney.
Pulmonary: pneumonia, pulmonary infarction, right-sided pleurisy.
Intestinal: retrocecal appendicitis, intestinal obstruction, high fecal impaction, diverticulitis.
Cardiac: myocardial ischemia (particularly involving the inferior wall), pericarditis.
Cutaneous: herpes zoster.
Trauma.
Fitz-Hugh-Curtis syndrome (perihepatitis).

ABDOMINAL PAIN, SUPRAPUBIC

ICD-9CM # 789.85

Intestinal: colon obstruction or gangrene, diverticulitis, appendicitis.
Reproductive system: ectopic pregnancy, mittelschmerz, torsion of ovarian cyst, PID, salpingitis, endometriosis, rupture of endometrioma.
Cystitis, rupture of urinary bladder.

ABDOMINAL WALL MASSES[38]

ICD-9CM # varies with specific diagnosis

LUMPS ARISING IN THE SKIN AND SUBCUTANEOUS FAT (THAT COULD OCCUR ANYWHERE ON THE BODY)

Lipoma.
Sebaceous cyst.

LUMPS ARISING IN THE SKIN AND SUBCUTANEOUS FAT (SPECIFIC TO THE ANTERIOR ABDOMINAL WALL)

Tumor nodule of the umbilicus (secondary to the intraperitoneal malignancy, also called *Sister Mary Joseph nodule*).

LUMPS ARISING IN THE FASCIA AND MUSCLE

Rectus sheath hematoma (usually painful).
Desmoid tumor (associated with Gardner's syndrome).

HERNIA

Incisional	It has an overlying scar. The sac may be very much larger than the neck of the hernia.
Umbilical	The hernia is through the umbilical scar. Those presenting at birth commonly resolve in the first years of life.
Paraumbilical	The neck is just lateral to the umbilical scar. Patients usually present later in life.

Epigastric	It occurs in the midline between the xiphoid process and the umbilicus. They are usually small (<2 cm). They result when a knuckle of extraperitoneal fat extrudes through a small defect in the linea alba. Commonly irreducible and without an expansile cough impulse.
Spigelian	A rare hernia found along the linea semilunaris at the lateral edge of the rectus sheath, most commonly a third of the way between the umbilicus and the pubis.

DIVARICATION OF THE RECTI

Supraumbilical elliptical swelling of the attenuated linea alba (no cough impulse).

ABORTION, RECURRENT

ICD-9CM # 761.8

Congenital anatomic abnormalities.
Adhesions (uterine synechiae).
Uterine fibroids.
Endometriosis.
Endocrine abnormalities (luteal phase insufficiency, hypothyroidism, uncontrolled diabetes mellitus [DM]).
Parenteral chromosome abnormalities.
Maternal infections (cervical mycoplasma, ureaplasma, chlamydia).
DES exposure, heavy metal exposure.
Thrombocytosis.
Allogenic immunity, autoimmunity, lupus anticoagulant.

ACHES AND PAINS, DIFFUSE

ICD-9CM # 719.49

Postviral arthralgias/myalgias.
Bilateral soft tissue rheumatism.
Overuse syndromes.
Fibrositis.
Hypothyroidism.
Metabolic bone disease.
Paraneoplastic syndrome.
Myopathy (polymyositis, dermatomyositis).
Rheumatoid arthritis (RA).
Sjögren's syndrome.
Polymyalgia rheumatica.
Hypermobility.
Benign arthralgias/myalgias.
Chronic fatigue syndrome.
Hypophosphatemia.

ACIDOSIS, HYPERCHLORIC METABOLIC[38b]

ICD-9CM # 276.2

GASTROINTESTINAL BICARBONATE LOSS

Diarrhea.
External pancreatic or small bowel drainage.

Ureterosigmoidostomy, jejunal loop.
Drugs:
Calcium chloride (acidifying agent).
Magnesium sulfate (diarrhea).
Cholestyramine (bile acid diarrhea).

RENAL ACIDOSIS

Hypokalemic:
Proximal RTA (type 2).
Distal (classic) RTA (type 1).
Drug-induced hypokalemia:
- Acetazolamide (proximal RTA).
- Amphotericin B (distal RTA).

Hyperkalemic:
Generalized distal nephron dysfunction (type 4 RTA).
Mineralocorticoid deficiency or resistance (pseudohypoaldosteronism type 1) PHA-I, PHA-II.
↓ Na^+ delivery to distal nephron.
Tubulointerstitial disease.
Ammonium excretion defect.
Drug-induced hyperkalemia:
- Potassium-sparing diuretics (amiloride, triamterene, spironolactone).
- Trimethoprim.
- Pentamidine.
- Angiotensin-converting enzyme inhibitors and angiotensin II receptor blockers.
- Nonsteroidal anti-inflammatory drugs.
- Cyclosporine, tacrolimus.

Normokalemic:
Early renal insufficiency.

OTHER

Acid loads (ammonium chloride, hyperalimentation).
Loss of potential bicarbonate: ketosis with ketone excretion.
Dilution acidosis (rapid saline administration).
Hippurate.
Cation-exchange resins.

ACIDOSIS, LACTIC[38b]

ICD-9CM # 276.2

CAUSES OF LACTIC ACIDOSIS

L-Lactic Acidosis
Conditions associated with type A lactic acidosis:
Poor tissue perfusion.
Shock:
- Cardiogenic.
- Hemorrhagic.
- Septic.
Profound hypoxemia:
- Severe asthma.
- Severe anemia.
Carbon monoxide poisoning.
Conditions associated with type B lactic acidosis:
Liver disease.
Diabetes mellitus.
Catecholamine excess:
- Endogenous
- Exogenous
Thiamine deficiency.

Ketoacidosis.
Seizure.
Malignancy.
Intracellular inorganic phosphate depletion.
Intravenous (IV) fructose.
IV xylose.
IV sorbitol.
Alcohols metabolized by alcohol dehydrogenase:
- Ethanol.
- Methanol.
- Ethylene.
- Propylene glycol.
Mitochondrial toxins:
- Salicylate intoxication.
- Cyanide poisoning.
- 2,4-Dinitrophenol ingestion.
- Nonnucleoside antireverse transcriptase drugs.
Metformin.
Inborn errors of metabolism.
Pyroglutamic acidosis.
Kombucha tea.

D-Lactic Acidosis
Short bowel syndrome.
Ischemic bowel.
Small bowel obstruction.

ACIDOSIS, METABOLIC

ICD-9CM # 276.2

METABOLIC ACIDOSIS WITH INCREASED Anion Gap (AG ACIDOSIS)

Lactic acidosis.
Ketoacidosis (DM, alcoholic ketoacidosis).
Uremia (chronic renal failure).
Ingestion of toxins (paraldehyde, methanol, salicylate, ethylene glycol).
High-fat diet (mild acidosis).

METABOLIC ACIDOSIS WITH NORMAL AG (HYPERCHLOREMIC ACIDOSIS)

Renal tubular acidosis (including acidosis of aldosterone deficiency).
Intestinal loss of HCO_3^- (diarrhea, pancreatic fistula).
Carbonic anhydrase inhibitors (e.g., acetazolamide).
Dilutional acidosis (as a result of rapid infusion of bicarbonate-free isotonic saline).
Ingestion of exogenous acids (ammonium chloride, methionine, cystine, calcium chloride).
Ileostomy.
Ureterosigmoidostomy.
Drugs: amiloride, triamterene, spironolactone, β-blockers.

ACIDOSIS, RESPIRATORY

ICD-9CM # 276.2

Pulmonary disease (COPD, severe pneumonia, pulmonary edema, interstitial fibrosis).
Airway obstruction (foreign body, severe bronchospasm, laryngospasm).
Thoracic cage disorders (pneumothorax, flail chest, kyphoscoliosis).

Defects in muscles of respiration (myasthenia gravis, hypokalemia, muscular dystrophy).

Defects in peripheral nervous system (amyotrophic lateral sclerosis, poliomyelitis, Guillain-Barré syndrome, botulism, tetanus, organophosphate poisoning, spinal cord injury).

Depression of respiratory center (anesthesia, narcotics, sedatives, vertebral artery embolism or thrombosis, increased intracranial pressure).

Failure of mechanical ventilator.

ACUTE KIDNEY INJURY AND LIVER DISEASE, CAUSES[12a]

ICD-9CM # varies with specific diagnosis

Prerenal uremia	Diuretic use, gastrointestinal loss, peritoneal aspiration, hypoalbuminemia
Hepatorenal syndrome	
Acute tubular necrosis	Hyperbilirubinemia, sepsis, toxic shock syndrome
Drugs	Acetaminophen (paracetamol), NSAIDs, tetracycline, rifampicin, isoniazid, anesthetic agents, sulfonamides, allopurinol, methotrexate
Infections	Hepatitis C and cryoglobulinemia, hepatitis B and polyarteritis nodosa, leptospirosis, hantavirus, Epstein-Barr virus, gram-negative sepsis, spontaneous bacterial peritonitis
Other	Papillary necrosis and obstruction, inhalation of chlorinated hydrocarbons, mushroom poisoning (Amanita phalloides)

ACUTE KIDNEY INJURY, HIV PATIENT, CAUSES[12a]

ICD-9CM # varies with specific diagnosis

Prerenal	Diarrhea, nausea and vomiting, cirrhosis and hepatorenal syndrome, sepsis
Vascular	Thrombotic microangiopathy
Glomerular	Immune complex glomerulonephritis (MPGN secondary to hepatitis C virus, postinfectious glomerulonephritis), HIVAN
Acute tubular necrosis	Sepsis, hypotension, nephrotoxins (aminoglycosides, amphotericin, acyclovir, cidofovir, tenofovir, pentamidine)
Acute interstitial nephritis	Drug-induced (co-trimoxazole), rifampicin, foscarnet, nevirapine), CMV infection, DILS

Drug-induced intratubular obstruction	Sulfadiazine, indinavir, foscarnet, acyclovir
Postrenal obstruction	Stones, tuberculosis, fungal ball, tumor
Associated with IV drug use	Sepsis, endocarditis, heroin-associated nephropathy (FSGS), rhabdomyolysis

CMV, Cytomegalovirus; *DILS*, diffusive infiltrative lymphocytosis syndrome; *FSGS*, focal segmental glomerulosclerosis; *HIVAN*, HIV-associated nephropathy; *MPGN*, membranoproliferative glomerulonephritis

ACUTE SCROTUM

ICD-9CM # 608.9

Testicular torsion.
Epididymitis.
Testicular neoplasm.
Orchitis.
Trauma.

ADNEXAL MASS[26]

ICD-9CM # varies with specific disorder

Ovary (neoplasm, endometriosis, functional cyst).
Fallopian tube (ectopic pregnancy, neoplasm, tuboovarian abscess, hydrosalpinx, paratubal cyst).
Uterus (fibroid, neoplasm).
Retroperitoneum (neoplasm, abdominal wall hematoma or abscess).
Urinary tract (pelvic kidney, distended bladder, urachal cyst).
Inflammatory bowel disease.
GI tract neoplasm.
Diverticular disease.
Appendicitis.
Bowel loop with feces.

ADRENAL MASSES[36]

ICD-9CM # 194.0 Adrenocortical Carcinoma
255.8 Adrenal Hyperplasia

UNILATERAL ADRENAL MASSES

Functional Lesions
Adrenal adenoma.
Adrenal carcinoma.
Pheochromocytoma.
Primary aldosteronism, adenomatous type.

Nonfunctional Lesions
Incidentaloma of adrenal.
Ganglioneuroma.
Myelolipoma.
Hematoma.
Adenolipoma.
Metastasis.

BILATERAL ADRENAL MASSES

Functional Lesions
ACTH-dependent Cushing's syndrome.
Congenital adrenal hyperplasia.
Pheochromocytoma.
Conn's syndrome, hyperplastic variety.
Micronodular adrenal disease.

Idiopathic bilateral adrenal hypertrophy.

Nonfunctional Lesions
Infection (tuberculosis, fungi).
Infiltration (leukemia, lymphoma).
Replacement (amyloidosis).
Hemorrhage.
Bilateral metastases.

ADRENOCORTICAL HYPERFUNCTION[1]

ICD-9CM # 255.1

SYNDROMES OF ADRENOCORTICAL HYPERFUNCTION

States of Glucocorticoid Excess
Physiologic states
Stress.
Strenuous exercise.
Last trimester of pregnancy.
Pathologic states
Psychiatric conditions (pseudo-Cushing's disorders).
  Depression.
  Alcoholism.
  Anorexia nervosa.
  Panic disorders.
  Alcohol and drug withdrawal.
ACTH-dependent states.
  Pituitary adenoma (Cushing's disease).
  Ectopic ACTH syndrome.
  • Bronchial carcinoid.
  • Thymic carcinoid.
  • Islet cell tumor.
  • Small cell lung carcinoma.
  Ectopic CRH secretion.
ACTH-independent states.
  Adrenal adenoma.
  Adrenal carcinoma.
  Micronodular adrenal disease.
Exogenous sources
Glucocorticoid intake.
ACTH intake.
States of Mineralocorticoid Excess
Primary aldosteronism
Aldosterone-secreting adenoma.
Bilateral adrenal hyperplasia.
Aldosterone-secreting carcinoma.
Glucocorticoid-suppressible hyperaldosteronism.
Adrenal Enzyme Deficiencies
11β-Hydroxylase deficiency.
17α-Hydroxylase deficiency.
11β-Hydroxysteroid dehydrogenase, type II.
Exogenous Mineralocorticoids
Licorice.
Carbenoxolone.
Fludrocortisone.
Secondary hyperaldosteronism
Associated with hypertension.
  Accelerated hypertension.
  Renovascular hypertension.
  Estrogen administration.
  Renin-secreting tumors.
Without hypertension.
  Bartter syndrome.
  Sodium-wasting nephropathy.
  Renal tubular acidosis.

Diuretic and laxative abuse.
Edematous states (cirrhosis, nephrosis, congestive heart failure).

ACTH, Adrenocorticotropin hormone; *CRH,* corticotropin-releasing hormone.

ADRENOCORTICAL HYPOFUNCTION
ICD-9CM # 255.4

SYNDROMES OF ADRENOCORTICAL HYPOFUNCTION

Primary Adrenal Disorders
Combined glucocorticoid and mineralocorticoid deficiency
Autoimmune:
  Isolated autoimmune disease (Addison disease).
  Polyglandular autoimmune syndrome, type I.
  Polyglandular autoimmune syndrome, type II.
Infectious:
  Tuberculosis.
  Fungal.
  Cytomegalovirus.
  Human immunodeficiency virus.
Vascular:
  Bilateral adrenal hemorrhage.
  Sepsis.
  Coagulopathy.
  Thrombosis; embolism.
  Adrenal infarction.
Infiltration:
  Metastatic carcinoma and lymphoma.
  Sarcoidosis.
  Amyloidosis.
  Hemochromatosis.
Congenital:
  Congenital adrenal hyperplasia.
  • 21-Hydroxylase deficiency.
  • 3β-ol Dehydrogenase deficiency.
  • 20,22-Desmolase deficiency.
  Adrenal unresponsiveness to ACTH.
  Congenital adrenal hypoplasia.
  Adrenoleukodystrophy.
  Adrenomyeloneuropathy.
Iatrogenic
Bilateral adrenalectomy.
Drugs: metyrapone, aminoglutethimide, trilostane, ketoconazole, o,p'-DDD, mifepristone.
Mineralocorticoid deficiency without glucocorticoid deficiency:
Cortiscosterone methyl oxidase deficiency.
Isolated zona glomerulosa defect.
Heparin therapy.
Critical illness.
Converting-enzyme inhibitors.
Secondary Adrenal Disorders
Secondary adrenal insufficiency
Hypothalamic-pituitary dysfunction.
Exogenous glucocorticoids.
After removal of an ACTH-secreting tumor.
Hyporeninemic Hypoaldosteronism
Diabetic nephropathy.
Tubulointerstitial diseases.
Obstructive uropathy.

Autonomic neuropathy.
Nonsteroidal anti-inflammatory drugs.
β-Adrenergic drugs.

ACTH, Adrenocorticotropic hormone.

ADVERSE FOOD REACTIONS, DIFFERENTIAL DIAGNOSIS[22a]
ICD-9CM # varies with specific diagnosis

GASTROINTESTINAL DISORDERS (WITH VOMITING AND/OR DIARRHEA)
Structural abnormalities (pyloric stenosis, Hirschsprung's disease).
Enzyme deficiencies (primary or secondary):
  Disaccharidase deficiency—lactase, fructase, sucrase-isomaltase.
  Galactosemia.
Other: pancreatic insufficiency (cystic fibrosis), peptic disease.

CONTAMINANTS AND ADDITIVES
Flavorings and preservatives—rarely cause symptoms: Sodium metabisulfite, monosodium glutamate, nitrites.
Dyes and colorings—very rarely cause symptoms (urticaria, eczema): Tartrazine.
Toxins: Bacterial, fungal (aflatoxin), fish-related (scombroid, ciguatera).
Infectious organisms:
  Bacteria *(Salmonella, Escherichia coli, Shigella).*
  Virus (rotavirus, enterovirus).
  Parasites *(Giardia, Akis simplex* [in fish]).
Accidental contaminants: Heavy metals, pesticides.
Pharmacologic agents: Caffeine, glycosidal alkaloid solanine (potato spuds), histamine (fish), serotonin (banana, tomato), tryptamine (tomato), tyramine (cheese).

PSYCHOLOGIC REACTIONS
Food phobias.

ADYNAMIC ILEUS[26]
ICD-9CM # 560.1

Abdominal trauma.
Infection (retroperitoneal, pelvic, intrathoracic).
Laparotomy.
Metabolic disease (hypokalemia).
Renal colic.
Skeletal injury (rib fracture, vertebral fracture).
Medications (e.g., narcotics).

AEROPHAGIA (BELCHING, ERUCTATION)
ICD-9CM # 787.3

Anxiety disorders.
Rapid food ingestion.
Carbonated beverages.
Nursing infants (especially when nursing in horizontal position).
Eating or drinking in supine position.
Gum chewing.

Poorly fitting dentures, orthodontic appliances.
Hiatal hernia, gastritis, nonulcer dyspepsia.
Cholelithiasis, cholecystitis.
Ingestion of legumes, onions, peppers.

AIR-SPACE OPACIFICATION ON X-RAY[16a]
ICD-9CM # varies with specific diagnosis

CAUSES OF AIR-SPACE OPACIFICATION
Edema
Cardiogenic.
Non-cardiogenic.
Inflammation/Infection
Wegener's granulomatosis.
Cryptogenic organizing pneumonia.
Blood
Idiopathic pulmonary hemosiderosis.
Antibasement membrane antibody disease.
Systemic lupus erythematosus.
Miscellaneous Causes
Eosinophilic pneumonia.
Alveolar proteinosis.
Alveolar cell carcinoma.
Alveolar microlithiasis.
Lymphoma (MALToma).
Sarcoidosis.

AIRWAY OBSTRUCTION, PEDIATRIC AGE[19]

ICD-9CM #	
496	Obstruction Due to Bronchospasm
934.9	Obstruction Due to Foreign Body
478.75	Obstruction Due to Laryngospasm
506.9	Obstruction Due to Inhalation of Fumes or Vapors

CONGENITAL CAUSES
Craniofacial dysmorphism.
Hemangioma.
Laryngeal cleft/web.
Laryngoceles, cysts.
Laryngomalacia.
Macroglossia.
Tracheal stenosis.
Vascular ring.
Vocal cord paralysis.

ACQUIRED INFECTIOUS CAUSES
Acute laryngotracheobronchitis.
Epiglottitis.
Laryngeal papillomatosis.
Membranous croup (bacterial tracheitis).
Mononucleosis.
Retropharyngeal abscess.
Spasmodic croup.
Diphtheria.

ACQUIRED NONINFECTIOUS CAUSES
Anaphylaxis.
Foreign body aspiration.

Differential Diagnosis

II

Supraglottic hypotonia.
Thermal/chemical burn.
Trauma.
Vocal cord paralysis.
Angioneurotic edema.

AKINETIC/RIGID SYNDROME[1]

ICD-9CM # code not available

Parkinsonism (idiopathic, drug-induced).
Catatonia (psychosis).
Progressive supranuclear palsy.
Multisystem atrophy (Shy-Drager syndrome, olivopontocerebellar atrophy).
Diffuse Lewy-body disease.
Toxins (MPTP, manganese, carbon monoxide).
Huntington's disease and other hereditary neurodegenerative disorders.

ALKALOSIS, METABOLIC

ICD-9CM # 276.3

CAUSES OF METABOLIC ALKALOSIS

Exogenous HCO_3^- Loads
Acute alkali administration.
Milk-alkali syndrome.
Effective Extracellular Volume Contraction, Normotension, Hypokalemia, and Secondary Hyperreninemic Hyperaldosteronism
Gastrointestinal origin:
    Vomiting.
    Gastric aspiration.
    Congenital chloridorrhea.
    Villous adenoma.
    Combined administration of sodium polystyrene sulfonate (Kayexalate and aluminum hydroxide).
Renal origin:
    Diuretics (especially thiazides and loop diuretics).
    • Acute.
    • Chronic.
    • Edematous states.
    • Posthypercapnic state.
    • Hypercalcemia-hypoparathyroidism.
    • Recovery from lactic acidosis or ketoacidosis.
    • Nonreabsorbable anions such as penicillin, carbenicillin.
    • Mg^{++} deficiency.
    • K^+ depletion.
    • Bartter syndrome (loss-of-function mutation of Cl^- transport in thick ascending limb of Henle loop).
    • Gitelman syndrome (loss-of-function mutation in Na^+/Cl^- cotransporter).
    • Carbohydrate refeeding after starvation.
Extracellular Volume Expansion, Hypertension, K^+ Deficiency, and Hypermineralocorticoidism
Associated with high renin:
    Renal artery stenosis.
    Accelerated hypertension.
    Renin-secreting tumor.
    Estrogen therapy.
Associated with low renin:
    Primary aldosteronism.

Adenoma.
Hyperplasia.
Carcinoma.
Glucocorticoid suppressible.
Adrenal enzymatic defects:
    11_β-Hydroxylase deficiency.
    17_α-Hydroxylase deficiency.
Cushing syndrome or disease:
    Ectopic corticotropin.
    Adrenal carcinoma.
    Adrenal adenoma.
    Primary pituitary.
Other:
    Licorice.
    Carbenoxolone.
    Chewer's tobacco.
    Lydia Pinkham tablets.
Gain-of-function Mutation of ENaC with Extracellular Fluid Volume Expansion, Hypertension, K^+ Deficiency, and Hyporeninemic Hypoaldosteronism
Liddle syndrome.

ALKALOSIS, RESPIRATORY

ICD-9CM # 276.3

Hypoxemia (pneumonia, pulmonary embolism, atelectasis, high-altitude living).
Drugs (salicylates, xanthenes, progesterone, epinephrine, thyroxine, nicotine).
Central nervous system (CNS) disorders (tumor, cerebrovascular accident [CVA], trauma, infections).
Psychogenic hyperventilation (anxiety, hysteria).
Hepatic encephalopathy.
Gram-negative sepsis.
Hyponatremia.
Sudden recovery from metabolic acidosis.
Assisted ventilation.

ALOPECIA[14][28]

ICD-9CM #		
704.00	Alopecia NOS	
704.01	Alopecia, Androgenic	
704.01	Alopecia Areata	
757.4	Alopecia, Congenital	
316	Alopecia, Psychogenic	

SCARRING ALOPECIA

Congenital (aplasia cutis).
Tinea capitis with inflammation (kerion).
Bacterial folliculitis.
Discoid lupus erythematosus.
Lichen planopilaris.
Folliculitis decalvans.
Neoplasm.
Trauma.

NONSCARRING ALOPECIA

Cosmetic treatment.
Tinea capitis.
Structural hair shaft disease.
Trichotillomania (hair pulling).
Anagen arrest.
Telogen arrest.
Alopecia areata.
Androgenetic alopecia.

ALOPECIA AND HYPOTRICHOSIS, IN CHILDREN AND ADOLESCENTS

ICD-9CM # 704.00

Congenital total alopecia: atrichia with papules, Moynahan alopecia syndrome.
Congenital localized alopecia: aplasia cutis, triangular alopecia, sebaceous nevus.
Hereditary hypotrichosis: Marie-Unna syndrome, hypotrichosis with juvenile macular dystrophy, hypotrichosis–Mari type, ichthyosis with hypotrichosis, cartilage-hair hypoplasia, Hallermann-Streiff syndrome, trichorhinophalangeal syndrome, ectodermal dysplasia ("pure" hair and nail and other ectodermal dysplasias).
Diffuse alopecia of endocrine origin: hypopituitarism, hypothyroidism, hypoparathyroidism, hyperthyroidism.
Alopecia of nutritional origin: marasmus, kwashiorkor, iron deficiency, zinc deficiency (acrodermatitis enteropathica), gluten-sensitive enteropathy, essential fatty acid deficiency, biotinidase deficiency.
Disturbances of the hair cycle: telogen effluvium.
Toxic alopecia: anagen effluvium.
Autoimmune alopecia: alopecia areata.
Traumatic alopecia: traction alopecia, trichotillomania.
Cicatricial alopecia: lupus erythematosus, lichen planopilaris, pseudopelade, morphea (en coup de saber), dermatomyositis, infection (kerion, favus, tuberculosis, syphilis, folliculitis, leishmaniasis, herpes zoster, varicella), acne keloidalis, follicular mucinosis, sarcoidosis.
Hair shaft abnormalities: monilethrix, pili annulati, pili torti, trichorrhexis invaginata, trichorrhexis nodosa, woolly hair syndrome, Menkes disease, trichothiodystrophy, trichodento-osseous syndrome, uncombable hair syndrome (spun-glass hair, pili trianguli et canaliculi).

ALOPECIA, DRUG-INDUCED

ICD-9CM # 704.00

DRUGS REPORTED TO INDUCE HAIR LOSS

ACE inhibitors (captopril, enalapril, moexipril, ramipril).
Allopurinol.
Amiodarone.
Amphetamines.*†
Analgesics, anti-inflammatories (ibuprofen, indomethacin, naproxen).
Androgens.*¶
Anticoagulants (coumarin, dextran, heparin/heparinoids).*†
Antiepileptics (carbamazepine, hydantoins, lamotrigine, troxidone, valproic acid, vigabatrin).*†
Antipsychotics (flupenthixol decanoate, fluphenazine decanoate).
Antithyroid drugs (carbimazole, iodine, thiouracil).*
Appetite suppressants.

Aromatase inhibitors (fadrozole, 4-OHA, vorozole).*¶

Benzimidazoles (albendazole, mebendazole)

β-Blockers (levobunolol, metoprolol, nadolol, propranolol, timolol).*

Bromocriptine.

Buspirone.

Butyrophenones.

Cantharidin.

Chloramphenicol.

Cholestyramine.

Cidofovir.

Cimetidine.

Clonazepam.

Clotrimazole.

Colchicine.

Contraceptives (oral).ǁ

Danazol.

Diazoxide.

Diclofenac.

Dixyrazine.

Ethambutol.

Ethionamide.

Fibrates (clofibrate, fenofibrate).

G-CSF (granulocyte-colony stimulating factor)

Gefitinib.‡

Gentamicin.

Glatiramer acetate.

Glibenclamide.

Gold salts.

Haloperidol.

Immunoglobulins.

Indanediones.

Indinavir.*

Interferons.*†

Isonicotinic acid hydrazide.§

Leflunomide.*

Levodopa.

Lithium.*

Maprotiline.

Mesalazine.

Methyldopa.

Methysergide.

Metyrapone.

Minoxidil.ǁ

Nicotinic acid.

Nitrofurantoin.

Octreotide.

Olanzapine.

Pentosan polysulfate.

Phenindione.

Potassium thiocyanate.

Pyridostigmine.

Radiation (<700 Gy).*§

Retinoids (acitretin, etretinate, isotretinoin).*†

Retinol (vitamin A).*

Risperidone.

Salicylates.

Serotonin reuptake inhibitors (fluoxetine, fluvoxamine, paroxetine, sertraline).*

Sorafenib.

Spironolactone.

Strontium ranelate.*†

Sulfasalazine.

Tamoxifen.

Terbinafine.

Terfenadine.

Thiamphenicol.

Thyroxine.

Tocopherol (vitamin E).

Trazodone.

Triazoles (fluconazole, itraconazole).

Tricyclic antidepressants (amitriptyline, desipramine, doxepin, imipramine, maprotiline).

Trimethadione.

Triparanol.

Vasopressin.

---

*Established by multiple reports or proved by rechallenge.

†Hair loss usually severe.

‡May produce permanent alopecia.

§May produce anagen effluvium.

ǁMay produce telogen effluvium 3 months after discontinuation.

¶May produce androgenetic alopecia.

ALVEOLAR CONSOLIDATION
ICD-9CM # 514

Infection.

Neoplasm (bronchoalveolar carcinoma, lymphoma).

Aspiration.

Trauma.

Hemorrhage (Wegener's, Goodpasture's, bleeding diathesis).

ARDS.

CHF.

Renal failure.

Eosinophilic pneumonia.

Bronchiolitis obliterans.

Pulmonary alveolar proteinosis.

ALVEOLAR HEMORRHAGE[28]
ICD-9CM # 770.3

Hematologic disorders (coagulopathies, thrombocytopenia).

Goodpasture's syndrome (anti–basement-membrane antibody disease).

Wegener's vasculitis.

Immune complex–mediated vasculitis.

Idiopathic pulmonary hemosiderosis.

Drugs (penicillamine).

Lymphangiogram contrast.

Mitral stenosis.

AMENORRHEA
ICD-9CM # 626.0

PREGNANCY

EARLY MENOPAUSE

HYPOTHALAMIC DYSFUNCTION: defective synthesis or release of LHRH, anorexia nervosa, stress, exercise.

PITUITARY DYSFUNCTION: neoplasm, postpartum hemorrhage, surgery, radiotherapy.

OVARIAN DYSFUNCTION: gonadal dysgenesis, 17α-hydroxylase deficiency, premature ovarian failure, polycystic ovarian disease, gonadal stromal tumors.

UTEROVAGINAL ABNORMALITIES

Congenital: imperforate hymen, imperforate cervix, imperforate or absent vagina, Müllerian agenesis.

Acquired: destruction of endometrium with curettage (Asherman's syndrome), closure of cervix or vagina caused by traumatic injury, hysterectomy.

OTHER

Metabolic diseases (liver, kidney), malnutrition, rapid weight loss, exogenous obesity, endocrine abnormalities (Cushing's syndrome, Graves' disease, hypothyroidism).

AMNESIA
ICD-9CM # 292.83 Drug Induced
      300.12 Hysterical
      780.9 Retrograde
      437.7 Transient Global

Degenerative diseases (e.g., Alzheimer's, Huntington's disease).

CVA (especially when involving thalamus, basal forebrain, and hippocampus).

Head trauma.

Postsurgical (e.g., mammillary body surgery, bilateral temporal lobectomy).

Infections (herpes simplex encephalitis, meningitis).

Wernicke-Korsakoff syndrome.

Cerebral hypoxia.

Hypoglycemia.

CNS neoplasms.

Creutzfeldt-Jakob disease.

Medications (e.g., midazolam and other benzodiazepines).

Psychosis.

Malingering.

AMNIOTIC FLUID ALPHA-FETOPROTEIN ELEVATION[16a]
ICD-9CM # V28.1

CAUSES OF ELEVATED AMNIOTIC FLUID α-FETOPROTEIN

Craniospinal defect (open neural tube defect).

Omphalocele.

Gastroschisis.

Duodenal atresia.

Congenital nephrosis.

Cystic hygroma.

Unbalanced D/G dislocation.

Down, Tay–Sachs, Klinefelter's, Turner's syndromes.

Fetal tumors.

Epidermolysis bullosa.

Pilonidal sinus.

Rhesus disease.

Fetal demise.

Incorrect dates.

Multiple pregnancy.

ANAL ABSCESS AND FISTULA[38]
ICD-9CM # 566

Primary anal gland infection.

Secondary abscess:

  Inflammatory bowel disease:

    • Crohn's disease.

    • Ulcerative colitis.

Infection:
- Tuberculosis.
- Actinomycosis.
- Threadworm.

Trauma.
Leukopenia.
Immunosuppression:
- HIV.
- Drugs.

Rectal cancer.
Diabetes mellitus.

ANAL INCONTINENCE[26]
ICD-9CM # 787.6

TRAUMATIC
Nerve injured in surgery.
Spinal cord injury.
Obstetric trauma.
Sphincter injury.

NEUROLOGIC
Spinal cord lesions.
Dementia.
Autonomic neuropathy (e.g., DM).
Obstetrics: pudendal nerve stretched during surgery.
Hirschsprung's disease.

MASS EFFECT
Carcinoma of anal canal.
Carcinoma of rectum.
Foreign body.
Fecal impaction.
Hemorrhoids.

MEDICAL
Procidentia.
Inflammatory disease.
Diarrhea.
Laxative abuse.

PEDIATRIC
Congenital.
Meningocele.
Myelomeningocele.
Spina bifida.
After corrective surgery for imperforate anus.
Sexual abuse.
Encopresis.

ANAPHYLAXIS[21]
ICD-9CM # 995.0

PULMONARY
Laryngeal edema.
Epiglottitis.
Foreign body aspiration.
Pulmonary embolus.
Asphyxiation.
Hyperventilation.

CARDIOVASCULAR
Myocardial infarction.
Arrhythmia.
Hypovolemic shock.
Cardiac arrest.

CNS
Vasovagal reaction.
CVA.
Seizure disorder.
Drug overdose.

ENDOCRINE
Hypoglycemia.
Pheochromocytoma.
Carcinoid syndrome.
Catamenial (progesterone-induced anaphylaxis).

PSYCHIATRIC
Vocal cord dysfunction syndrome.
Munchausen syndrome.
Panic attack/globus hystericus.

OTHER
Hereditary angioedema.
Cord urticaria.
Idiopathic urticaria.
Mastocytosis.
Serum sickness.
Idiopathic capillary leak syndrome.
Sulfite exposure.
Scombroid poisoning (tuna, blue fish, mackerel).

ANDROGEN EXCESS, REPRODUCTIVE-AGE WOMAN
ICD-9CM # varies with specific disorder

Polycystic ovary syndrome.
Idiopathic.
Medications (e.g., anabolizing agents, testosterone, danazol).
Pregnancy (luteoma, hyperreactio luteinalis).
Sertoli-Leydig ovarian neoplasm.
Adrenal adenoma or hyperplasia.
Cushing's syndrome.
Glucocorticoid resistance.
Hypothyroidism.
Hyperprolactinemia.

ANEMIA, APLASTIC[20]
ICD-9CM # 284

ACQUIRED APLASTIC ANEMIA
Secondary aplastic anemia.
Irradiation.
Drugs and chemicals.
Regular effects.
Cytotoxic agents.
Benzene.
Idiosyncratic reactions.
Chloramphenicol.
Nonsteroidal anti-inflammatory drugs.
Antiepileptics.
Gold.
Other drugs and chemicals.
Viruses.
Epstein-Barr virus (infectious mononucleosis).
Hepatitis virus (non-A, non-B, non-C, non-G hepatitis).
Parvovirus (transient aplastic crisis, some pure red cell aplasia).
Human immunodeficiency virus (acquired immunodeficiency syndrome).

Immune diseases.
Eosinophilic fasciitis.
Hyperimmunoglobulinemia.
Thymoma and thymic carcinoma.
Graft-versus-host disease in immunodeficiency.
Paroxysmal nocturnal hemoglobinuria.
Pregnancy.
Idiopathic aplastic anemia.

INHERITED APLASTIC ANEMIA
Fanconi anemia.
Dyskeratosis congenita.
Shwachman-Diamond syndrome.
Reticular dysgenesis.
Amegakaryocytic thrombocytopenia.
Familial aplastic anemias.
Preleukemia (e.g., monosomy 7).
Nonhematologic syndromes (e.g., Down, Dubowitz, Seckel).

ANEMIA, APLASTIC, DUE TO DRUGS AND CHEMICALS[1]
ICD-9CM # 284.89

Agents that regularly produce marrow depression as a major toxic effect when used in commonly employed doses or normal exposures:
Cytotoxic drugs used in cancer chemotherapy.
Alkylating agents (busulfan, melphalan, cyclophosphamide).
Antimetabolites (antifolic compounds, nucleotide analogs), antimitotics (vincristine, vinblastine, colchicine).
Some antibiotics (daunorubicin, doxorubicin [Adriamycin]).
Benzene (and less often benzene-containing chemicals; kerosene, carbon tetrachloride, Stoddard's solvent, chlorophenols).

Agents probably associated with aplastic anemia but with a relatively low probability relative to their use:
Chloramphenicol.
Insecticides.
Antiprotozoals (quinacrine and chloroquine).
Nonsteroidal anti-inflammatory drugs (including phenylbutazone, indomethacin, ibuprofen, sulindac, diclofenac, naproxen, piroxicam, fenoprofen, fenbufen, aspirin).
Anticonvulsants (hydantoins, carbamazepine, phenacemide, ethosuximide).
Gold, arsenic, and other heavy metals such as bismuth and mercury.
Sulfonamides as a class.
Antithyroid medications (methimazole, methylthiouracil, propylthiouracil).
Antidiabetes drugs (tolbutamide, carbutamide, chlorpropamide).
Carbonic anhydrase inhibitors (acetazolamide, methazolamide, mesalazine).
D-Penicillamine.
2-Chlorodeoxyadenosine.

Agents more rarely associated with aplastic anemia:
Antibiotics (streptomycin, tetracycline, methicillin, ampicillin, mebendazole and albendazole, sulfonamides, flucytosine, mefloquine, dapsone).
Antihistamines (cimetidine, ranitidine, chlorpheniramine).

Sedatives and tranquilizers (chlorpromazine, prochlorperazine, piperacetazine, chlordiazepoxide, meprobamate, methyprylon, remoxipride).

Antiarrhythmics (tocainide, amiodarone).

Allopurinol (can potentiate marrow suppression by cytotoxic drugs).

Ticlopidine.

Methyldopa.

Quinidine.

Lithium.

Guanidine.

Canthaxanthin.

Thiocyanate.

Carbimazole.

Cyanamide.

Deferoxamine.

Amphetamines.

ANEMIA, DRUG-INDUCED[17]

ICD-9CM # 283.0

DRUGS THAT MAY INTERFERE WITH RED CELL PRODUCTION BY INDUCING MARROW SUPPRESSION OR APLASIA

Alcohol.

Antineoplastic drugs.

Antithyroid drugs.

Antibiotics.

Oral hypoglycemic agents.

Phenylbutazone.

Azidothymidine (AZT).

DRUGS THAT INTERFERE WITH VITAMIN B$_{12}$, FOLATE, OR IRON ABSORPTION OR UTILIZATION

Nitrous oxide.

Anticonvulsant drugs.

Antineoplastic drugs.

Isoniazid, cycloserine A.

DRUGS CAPABLE OF PROMOTING HEMOLYSIS

Immune Mediated

Penicillins.

Quinine.

Alpha-methyldopa.

Procainamide.

Mitomycin C.

Oxidative Stress

Antimalarials.

Sulfonamide drugs.

Nalidixic acid.

DRUGS THAT MAY PRODUCE OR PROMOTE BLOOD LOSS

Aspirin.

Alcohol.

Nonsteroidal anti-inflammatory agents.

Corticosteroids.

Anticoagulants.

ANEMIA, HYPOCHROMIC[20]

ICD-9CM # varies with specific diagnosis
280.9 Iron Deficiency
285.0 Sideroblastic

DECREASED BODY IRON STORES

Iron-deficiency anemia.

NORMAL OR INCREASED BODY IRON STORES

Impaired iron metabolism.

Anemia of chronic disease.

Defective absorption, transport, or use of iron.

Disorders of globin synthesis:

- Thalassemia.
- Other microcytic hemoglobinopathies.

Disorders of heme synthesis: sideroblastic anemias:

- Hereditary.
- Acquired.

ANEMIA, LOW RETICULOCYTE COUNT[1]

ICD-9CM # 285.9

MICROCYTIC ANEMIA (MCV <80)

Iron deficiency.

Thalassemia minor.

Sideroblastic anemia.

Lead poisoning.

MACROCYTIC ANEMIA (MCV >100)

Megaloblastic anemias.

Folate deficiency.

Vitamin B$_{12}$ deficiency.

Drug-induced megaloblastic anemia.

Nonmegaloblastic macrocytosis.

Liver disease.

Hypothyroidism.

NORMOCYTIC ANEMIA (MCV 80-100)

Early iron deficiency.

Aplastic anemia.

Myelophthisic disorders.

Endocrinopathies.

Anemia of chronic disease.

Uremia.

Mixed nutritional deficiency.

ANEMIA, MEGALOBLASTIC[36]

ICD-9CM # 281.0 Pernicious Anemia
281.1 B$_{12}$ Deficiency
281.2 Folate Deficiency
281.3 B$_{12}$ with Folate Deficiency
281.4 Protein or Amino Acid Deficiency
281.8 Nutritional
281.9 NOS

COBALAMIN (CBL) DEFICIENCY

NUTRITIONAL CBL DEFICIENCY (INSUFFICIENT CBL INTAKE): vegetarians, vegans, breastfed infants of mothers with pernicious anemia.

ABNORMAL INTRAGASTRIC EVENTS (INADEQUATE PROTEOLYSIS OF FOOD CBL): atrophic gastritis, partial gastrectomy with hypochlorhydria.

LOSS/ATROPHY OF GASTRIC OXYNTIC MUCOSA (DEFICIENT INTRINSIC FACTOR [IF] MOLECULES): total or partial gastrectomy, pernicious anemia (PA), caustic destruction (lye).

ABNORMAL EVENTS IN SMALL BOWEL LUMEN:

Inadequate pancreatic protease (R-CBL not degraded, CBL not transferred to IF).

- Insufficiency of pancreatic protease—pancreatic insufficiency.
- Inactivation of pancreatic protease—Zollinger-Ellison syndrome.

Usurping of luminal CBL (inadequate CBL binding to IF).

- By bacteria—stasis syndromes (blind loops, pouches of diverticulosis, strictures, fistulas, anastomoses); impaired bowel motility (scleroderma, pseudoobstruction), hypogammaglobulinemia.
- By *Diphyllobothrium latum.*

DISORDERS OF ILEAL MUCOSA/IF RECEPTORS (IF-CBL NOT BOUND TO IF RECEPTORS):

Diminished or absent IF receptors—ileal bypass/resection/fistula.

Abnormal mucosal architecture/function—tropical/nontropical sprue, Crohn's disease, TB ileitis, infiltration by lymphomas, amyloidosis.

IF-/post IF-receptor defects—Imerslund-Graesbeck syndrome, TC II deficiency.

Drug-induced effects (slow K, biguanides, cholestyramine, colchicine, neomycin, PAS).

DISORDERS OF PLASMA CBL TRANSPORT (TC II-CBL NOT DELIVERED TO TC II RECEPTORS)

Congenital TC II deficiency, defective binding of TC II-CBL to TC II receptors (rare).

METABOLIC DISORDERS (CBL NOT UTILIZED BY CELL)

Inborn enzyme errors (rare).

Acquired disorders: (CBL oxidized to cob[III]alamin)—N$_2$O inhalation.

FOLATE DEFICIENCY

Nutritional Causes

Decreased dietary intake—poverty and famine (associated with kwashiorkor, marasmus), institutionalized individuals (psychiatric/nursing homes), chronic debilitating disease/goats' milk (low in folate), special diets (slimming), cultural/ethnic cooking techniques (food folate destroyed) or habits (folate-rich foods not consumed).

Decreased diet and increased requirements:

- Physiologic: pregnancy and lactation, prematurity, infancy.
- Pathologic: intrinsic hematologic disease (autoimmune hemolytic disease), drugs, malaria; hemoglobinopathies (SS, thalassemia), RBC membrane defects (hereditary spherocytosis, paroxysmal nocturnal hemoglobinopathy); abnormal hematopoiesis (leukemia/lymphoma, myelodysplastic syndrome, agnogenic myeloid metaplasia with myelofibrosis); infiltration with malignant disease; dermatologic (psoriasis).

Folate Malabsorption

With normal intestinal mucosa:

- Some drugs (controversial).
- Congenital folate malabsorption (rare).

With mucosal abnormalities—tropical and non-tropical sprue, regional enteritis.

Defective Cellular Folate Uptake—Familial Aplastic Anemia (Rare), Inadequate Cellular Utilization

Folate antagonists (methotrexate).

Hereditary enzyme deficiencies involving folate.

Drugs (Multiple Effects on Folate Metabolism)

Alcohol, sulfasalazine, triamterene, pyrimethamine, trimethoprim-sulfamethoxazole, diphenylhydantoin, barbiturates.

MISCELLANEOUS MEGALOBLASTIC ANEMIAS (NOT CAUSED BY CBL OR FOLATE DEFICIENCY)

Congenital Disorders of DNA Synthesis (Rare)

Orotic aciduria, Lesch-Nyhan syndrome, congenital dyserythropoietic anemia.

Acquired Disorders of DNA Synthesis

Thiamine-responsive megaloblastosis (rare).

Malignancy—erythroleukemia—refractory sideroblastic anemias—all antineoplastic drugs that inhibit DNA synthesis.

Toxic—alcohol.

ANERGY, CUTANEOUS[36]
ICD-9CM # 279.9

IMMUNOLOGIC
Acquired (AIDS, acute leukemia, carcinoma, CLL, Hodgkin's lymphoma, NHL).

Congenital (ataxia-telangiectasia, Di George's syndrome, severe combined immunodeficiency, Wiskott-Aldrich syndrome).

INFECTIONS
Bacterial (bacterial pneumonia, brucellosis).

Disseminated mycotic infections.

Mycobacterial (lepromatous leprosy, TB).

Viral (varicella, hepatitis, influenza, mononucleosis, measles, mumps).

IMMUNOSUPPRESSIVE MEDICATIONS
Systemic corticosteroids.

Methotrexate, cyclophosphamide.

Rifampin.

OTHER
Alcoholic cirrhosis, biliary cirrhosis, sarcoidosis, rheumatic disease.

Diabetes, Crohn's disease, uremia.

Anemia, pyridoxine deficiency, sickle cell anemia.

Burns, malnutrition, pregnancy, old age, surgery.

ANEURYSMS, THORACIC AORTA
ICD-9CM # 441.2

Trauma.

Infection.

Inflammatory (syphilis, Takayasu's disease).

Collagen vascular disease (RA, ankylosing spondylitis).

Annuloaortic ectasia (Marfan's syndrome, Ehlers-Danlos syndrome).

Congenital.

Coarctation.

Cystic medial necrosis.

ANHIDROSIS
ICD-9CM # 705.1

Drugs (anticholinergics).

Dehydration.

Hysteria.

Obstruction of sweat ducts (e.g., inflammation, miliaria).

Local radiant heat or pressure.

CNS lesions (medulla, hypothalamus, pons).

Spinal cord lesions.

Lesions of sympathetic nerves.

Congenital sweat gland disturbances.

ANION GAP ACIDOSIS[38b]
ICD-9CM # 276.9

CLINICAL CAUSES OF HIGH ANION GAP AND NORMAL ANION GAP ACIDOSIS

High Anion Gap

Ketoacidosis:

Diabetic ketoacidosis (acetoacetate).

Alcoholic (β-hydroxybutyrate).

Starvation.

Lactic acid acidosis:

L-Lactic acid acidosis (types A and B).

D-Lactic acid acidosis.

Renal failure: sulfate, phosphate, urate, hippurate.

Ingestions (toxins and their metabolites):

Ethylene glycol → glycolate, oxalate.

Methyl alcohol → formate.

Salicylate → ketones, lactate, salicylate.

Paraldehyde → organic anions.

Toluene → hippurate (commonly presents with normal anion gap).

Propylene glycol → lactate.

Pyroglutamic acidosis (acetaminophen use) → 5-oxoproline.

Normal Anion Gap

Gastrointestinal loss of HCO_3^- (negative urine anion gap):

Diarrhea.

Fistula, external.

Renal loss of HCO_3^- or failure to excrete NH_4^+ (positive urine anion gap):

Proximal renal tubular acidosis (RTA type 2).

Acetazolamide.

Classic distal renal tubular acidosis (low serum K^+) RTA type 1.

Generalized distal renal tubular defect (high serum K^+) RTA type 4.

Miscellaneous:

NH_4Cl ingestion.

Sulfur ingestion.

Dilutional acidosis.

Late stages in treatment of diabetic ketoacidosis.

ANION GAP INCREASE
ICD-9CM # 276.9

Uremia.

Ketoacidosis (diabetic, starvation, alcoholic).

Lactic acidosis.

Ethylene glycol poisoning.

Salicylate overdose.

Methanol poisoning.

ANISOCORIA
ICD-9CM # 379.41

Mydriatic or miotic drugs.

Prosthetic eye.

Inflammation (keratitis, iridocyclitis).

Infections (herpes zoster, syphilis, meningitis, encephalitis, TB, diphtheria, botulism).

Subdural hemorrhage.

Cavernous sinus thrombosis.

Intracranial neoplasm.

Cerebral aneurysm.

Glaucoma.

CNS degenerative diseases.

Internal carotid ischemia.

Toxic polyneuritis (alcohol, lead).

Adie's syndrome.

Horner's syndrome.

DM.

Trauma.

Congenital.

ANOREXIA[38]
ICD-9CM # 783.0

SELECTED CAUSES OF ANOREXIA

Gastrointestinal Tract/Liver

Gastric outlet obstruction or small bowel obstruction.

Gastric cancer.

Hepatic metastases.

Acute viral hepatitis.

Metabolic

Addison's disease.

Hypopituitarism.

Hyperparathyroidism.

Functional

Extremely unpleasant sight/smell.

Systemic

Chronic pain.

Renal failure.

Severe congestive heart failure.

Respiratory failure.

Psychiatric

Depression.

Anorexia nervosa.

Medications

Digoxin.

Narcotic analgesics.

Diuretics.

Antihypertensives.

Chemotherapeutic agents.

Amphetamines.

Miscellaneous

Excessive smoking.

Excessive alcohol intake.

Oral cavity disease.

Thiamine deficiency.

Early pregnancy.

Hypogeusia or dysgeusia.

ANOVULATION

ICD-9CM # 628.0

Anorexia and bulimia.
Strenuous exercise.
Weight loss/malnutrition.
Empty sella syndrome.
Pituitary disorders (infarction, infection, trauma, irradiation, surgery, microadenomas, macroadenomas).
Idiopathic hypopituitarism.
Drug induced.
Thyroid dysfunction (hypothyroidism, hyperthyroidism).
Systemic diseases (e.g., liver disease).
Adrenal hyperfunction (Cushing's syndrome, congenital adrenal hyperplasia).
Polycystic ovarian syndrome.
Isolated gonadotropin deficiency.

APPETITE LOSS IN INFANTS AND CHILDREN[19]

ICD-9CM # 783.0   Appetite Loss
          307.59 Appetite Loss, Psychogenic Origin

ORGANIC DISEASE

Infection (Acute or Chronic)
Neurologic
Congenital degenerative disease.
Hypothalamic lesion.
Increased intracranial pressure (including a brain tumor).
Swallowing disorders (neuromuscular).
Gastrointestinal
Oral lesions (e.g., thrush or herpes simplex).
Gastroesophageal reflux.
Obstruction (especially with gastric or intestinal distention).
Inflammatory bowel disease.
Celiac disease.
Constipation.
Cardiac
Congestive heart failure (especially associated with cyanotic lesions).
Metabolic
Renal failure and/or renal tubule acidosis.
Liver failure.
Congenital metabolic disease.
Lead poisoning.
Nutritional
Marasmus.
Iron deficiency.
Zinc deficiency.
Fever
RA.
Rheumatic fever.
Drugs
Morphine.
Digitalis.
Antimetabolites.
Methylphenidate.
Amphetamines.
Miscellaneous
Prolonged restriction of oral feedings, beginning in the neonatal period.
Systemic lupus erythematosus (SLE).
Tumor.

PSYCHOLOGIC FACTORS

Anxiety, fear, depression, mania (limbic influence on the hypothalamus).
Avoidance of symptoms associated with meals (abdominal pain, diarrhea, bloating, urgency, dumping syndrome).
Anorexia nervosa.
Excessive weight loss and food aversion in athletes, simulating anorexia nervosa.

ARTERIAL OCCLUSION[15]

ICD-9CM # 444.22 Arterial Occlusion, Lower Extremities
          444.21 Arterial Occlusion, Upper Extremities

Thromboembolism (post-MI, mitral stenosis, rheumatic valve disease, atrial fibrillation, atrial myxoma, marantic endocarditis, bacterial endocarditis, Libman-Sacks endocarditis).
Atheroembolism (microemboli composed of cholesterol, calcium, and platelets from proximal atherosclerotic plaques).
Arterial thrombosis (endothelial injury, altered arterial blood flow, trauma, severe atherosclerosis, acute vasculitis).
Vasospasm.
Trauma.
Hypercoagulable states.
Miscellaneous (irradiation, drugs, infections, necrotizing).

ARTHRITIS AND ABDOMINAL PAIN

ICD-9CM # varies with specific disorder

Viral syndrome.
Inflammatory bowel disease.
Celiac disease.
Vasculitis.
SLE.
RA.
Scleroderma.
Amyloidosis.
Chronic hepatitis C.
Whipple's disease.
Polyarteritis nodosa.
Behçet's disease.
Familial Mediterranean fever.
Blind loop syndrome.
Babesiosis.
Lyme disease.
Ehrlichiosis.

ARTHRITIS AND DIARRHEA

ICD-9CM # varies with specific disorder

Viral syndrome.
Inflammatory bowel disease.
Celiac disease.
Whipple's disease.
Enterogenic (bacterial) reactive arthritis.
Collagenous colitis.
Behçet's disease.
Hyperthyroidism.
Spondyloarthropathy.
Blind loop syndrome.

ARTHRITIS AND EYE LESIONS[6]

ICD-9CM # varies with specific diagnosis

SLE.
Sjögren's syndrome.
Behçet's syndrome.
Sarcoidosis.
Subacute bacterial endocarditis (SBE).
Lyme disease.
Wegener's granulomatosis.
Giant cell arteritis.
Takayasu's arteritis.
RA, JRA.
Scleroderma.
Inflammatory bowel disease.
Whipple's disease.
Ankylosing spondylitis.
Reactive arthritis.
Psoriatic arthritis.

ARTHRITIS AND HEART MURMUR[6]

ICD-9CM # varies with specific diagnosis

SBE.
Cardiac myxoma.
Ankylosing spondylitis.
Reactive arthritis.
Acute rheumatic fever.
RA.
SLE with Libman-Sacks endocarditis.
Relapsing polychondritis.

ARTHRITIS AND MUSCLE WEAKNESS[8]

ICD-9CM # varies with specific diagnosis

RA.
Ankylosing spondylitis.
Polymyositis.
Dermatomyositis.
SLE, scleroderma, mixed connective tissue disease.
Sarcoidosis.
HIV-associated arthritis.
Whipple's disease.

ARTHRITIS AND RASH[6]

ICD-9CM # varies with specific diagnosis

Chronic urticaria.
Vasculitic urticaria.
SLE.
Dermatomyositis.
Polymyositis.
Psoriatic arthritis.
Reactive arthritis.
Chronic sarcoidosis.
Serum sickness.
Sweet's syndrome.
Leprosy.

Differential Diagnosis

II

ARTHRITIS AND SUBCUTANEOUS NODULES[6]

ICD-9CM # varies with specific diagnosis

RA.
Gout.
Pseudogout (rare).
Sarcoidosis.
Light chain (LA) amyloidosis (primary, multiple myeloma).
Acute rheumatic fever (ARF).
Hemochromatosis.
Whipple's disease.
Multicentric reticulohistiocytosis.

ARTHRITIS AND WEIGHT LOSS[6]

ICD-9CM # varies with specific diagnosis

Severe RA.
RA with vasculitis.
Reactive arthritis.
RA or psoriatic arthritis or ankylosing spondylitis with amyloidosis.
Cancer.
Enteropathic arthritis (Crohn's, ulcerative colitis).
HIV infection.
Whipple's disease.
Blind loop syndrome.
Scleroderma with intestinal bacterial overgrowth.

ARTHRITIS OR EXTREMITY PAIN, IN CHILDREN AND ADOLESCENTS[22a]

ICD-9CM # varies with specific diagnosis

CAUSES OF ARTHRITIS OR EXTREMITY PAIN IN CHILDREN AND ADOLESCENTS

Rheumatic and Inflammatory Diseases
Juvenile idiopathic arthritis.
Systemic lupus erythematosus.
Juvenile dermatomyositis.
Polyarteritis.
Vasculitis.
Scleroderma.
Sjögren syndrome.
Behçet disease.
Overlap syndromes.
Wegener granulomatosis.
Sarcoidosis.
Kawasaki syndrome.
Henoch-Schönlein purpura.
Chronic recurrent multifocal osteomyelitis.
Seronegative Spondyloarthropathies
Juvenile ankylosing spondylitis.
Inflammatory bowel disease.
Psoriatic arthritis.
Reactive arthritis associated with urethritis, iridocyclitis, and mucocutaneous lesions.
Infectious Illnesses
Bacterial arthritis (septic arthritis, *Staphylococcus aureus,* pneumococcus, gonococcus, *Haemophilus influenzae*).

Lyme disease.
Viral illness (parvovirus, rubella, mumps, Epstein-Barr virus, hepatitis B).
Fungal arthritis.
Mycobacterial infection.
Spirochetal infection.
Endocarditis.
Reactive Arthritis
Acute rheumatic fever.
Reactive arthritis (postinfectious due to *Shigella, Salmonella, Yersinia, Chlamydia,* or meningococcus).
Serum sickness.
Toxic synovitis of the hip.
Postimmunization.
Immunodeficiencies
Hypogammaglobulinemia.
Immunoglobulin A deficiency.
Human immunodeficiency virus.
Congenital and Metabolic Disorders
Gout.
Pseudogout.
Mucopolysaccharidoses.
Thyroid disease (hypothyroidism, hyperthyroidism).
Hyperparathyroidism.
Vitamin C deficiency (scurvy).
Hereditary connective tissue disease (Marfan syndrome, Ehlers-Danlos syndrome).
Fabry disease.
Farber disease.
Amyloidosis (familial Mediterranean fever).
Bone and Cartilage Disorders
Trauma.
Patellofemoral syndrome.
Hypermobility syndrome.
Osteochondritis dissecans.
Avascular necrosis (including Legg-Calvé-Perthes disease).
Hypertrophic osteoarthropathy.
Slipped capital femoral epiphysis.
Osteolysis.
Benign bone tumors (including osteoid osteoma).
Histiocytosis.
Rickets.
Neuropathic Disorders
Peripheral neuropathies.
Carpal tunnel syndrome.
Charcot joints.
Neoplastic Disorders
Leukemia.
Neuroblastoma.
Lymphoma.
Bone tumors (osteosarcoma, Ewing sarcoma).
Histiocytic syndromes.
Synovial tumors.
Hematologic Disorders
Hemophilia.
Hemoglobinopathies (including sickle cell disease).
Miscellaneous Disorders
Pigmented villonodular synovitis.
Plant-thorn synovitis (foreign body arthritis).
Myositis ossificans.
Eosinophilic fasciitis.
Tendinitis (overuse injury).
Raynaud phenomenon.

Pain Syndromes
Fibromyalgia.
Growing pains.
Depression (with somatization).
Reflex sympathetic dystrophy.
Regional myofascial pain syndromes.

ARTHRITIS, AXIAL SKELETON

ICD-9CM # 720.0 Arthritis, Rheumatoid, Spine
696.0 Arthritis, Psoriatic
715.9 Arthritis, Degenerative, NOS
720.0 Ankylosing Spondylitis

RA.
Psoriatic arthritis.
Reiter's syndrome.
Ankylosing spondylitis.
Juvenile RA.
Degenerative disease of the nucleus pulposus.
Spondylosis deformans.
Diffuse idiopathic skeletal hyperostosis (DISH).
Alkaptonuria.
Infection.

ARTHRITIS, FEVER, AND RASH[6]

ICD-9CM # varies with specific diagnosis

Rubella, parvovirus B19.
Gonococcemia, meningococcemia.
Secondary syphilis, Lyme borreliosis.
Adult acute rheumatic fever, adult Still's disease, adult Kawasaki disease.
Vasculitic urticaria.
Acute sarcoidosis.
Familial Mediterranean fever.
Hyperimmunoglobulinemia D and periodic fever syndrome.

ARTHRITIS, MONOARTICULAR AND OLIGOARTICULAR[2]

ICD-9CM # 715.3 Osteoarthritis, Localized
711.9 Infectious Arthritis
716.6 Monoarticular Arthritis; 5th digit to be added to the above depending on site of arthritis
0. Site Unspecified
1. Shoulder Region
2. Upper Arm
3. Forearm
4. Hand
5. Pelvic Region and Thigh
6. Lower Leg
7. Ankle and/or Foot
8. Other Specified Except Spine

Septic arthritis (*S. aureus, Neisseria gonorrhoeae,* meningococci, streptococci, *Streptococcus pneumoniae,* enteric gram-negative bacilli).
Crystalline-induced arthritis (gout, pseudogout, calcium oxalate, hydroxyapatite and other basic calcium/phosphate crystals).

Traumatic joint injury.
Hemarthrosis.
Monoarticular or oligoarticular flare of an inflammatory polyarticular rheumatic disease (RA, psoriatic arthritis, Reiter's syndrome, SLE).

ARTHRITIS, PEDIATRIC AGE[19]

ICD-9CM # 711.9 Infectious Arthritis
714.30 Juvenile Chronic or Unspecified
714.31 Juvenile Rheumatoid Polyarticular Acute
714.32 Juvenile Rheumatoid Pauciarticular
714.33 Juvenile Rheumatoid Monoarticular

RHEUMATIC DISEASES OF CHILDHOOD

Acute rheumatic fever.
SLE.
Juvenile ankylosing spondylitis.
Polymyositis and dermatomyositis.
Vasculitis.
Scleroderma.
Psoriatic arthritis.
Mixed connective tissue disease and overlap syndromes.
Kawasaki disease.
Behçet's syndrome.
Familial Mediterranean fever.
Reiter's syndrome.
Reflex sympathetic dystrophy.
Fibromyalgia (fibrositis).

INFECTIOUS DISEASES

Bacterial arthritis.
Viral or postviral arthritis.
Fungal arthritis.
Osteomyelitis.
Reactive arthritis.

NEOPLASTIC DISEASES

Leukemia.
Lymphoma.
Neuroblastoma.
Primary bone tumors.

NONINFLAMMATORY DISORDERS

Trauma.
Avascular necrosis syndromes.
Osteochondroses.
Slipped capital femoral epiphysis.
Diskitis.
Patellofemoral dysfunction (chondromalacia patellae).
Toxic synovitis of the hip.
Overuse syndromes.

GENETIC OR CONGENITAL SYNDROMES

Hematologic Disorders
Sickle cell disease.
Hemophilia.

INFLAMMATORY BOWEL DISEASE

Miscellaneous
Growing pains.
Psychogenic arthralgias (conversion reactions).
Hypermobility syndrome.
Villonodular synovitis.
Foreign body arthritis.

ARTHRITIS, POLYARTICULAR

ICD-9CM # 715.09 Generalized Osteoarthritis, Multiple Sites
716.89 Arthritis, Multiple Sites
714.31 Juvenile Rheumatoid, Polyarticular, Acute

RA, juvenile (rheumatoid) polyarthritis.
SLE, other connective tissue diseases, erythema nodosum, palindromic rheumatism, relapsing polychondritis.
Psoriatic arthritis, ankylosing spondylitis.
Sarcoidosis.
Lyme arthritis, bacterial endocarditis, *Neisseria gonorrhoeae* infection, rheumatic fever, Reiter's disease.
Crystal deposition disease.
Hypersensitivity to serum or drugs.
Hepatitis B, HIV, rubella, mumps.
Other: serum sickness, leukemias, lymphomas, enteropathic arthropathy, Whipple's disease, Behçet's syndrome, Henoch-Schönlein purpura, familial Mediterranean fever, hypertrophic pulmonary osteoarthropathy.

ASCITES

ICD-9CM # 789.5 Ascites NOS
197.6 Ascites, Cancerous (Malignant)
457.8 Ascites, Chylous

Hypoalbuminemia: nephrotic syndrome, protein-losing gastroenteropathy, starvation.
Cirrhosis.
Hepatic congestion: CHF, constrictive pericarditis, tricuspid insufficiency, hepatic vein obstruction (Budd-Chiari syndrome), inferior vena cava or portal vein obstruction.
Peritoneal infections: TB and other bacterial infections, fungal diseases, parasites.
Neoplasms: primary hepatic neoplasms, metastases to liver or peritoneum, lymphomas, leukemias, myeloid metaplasia.
Lymphatic obstruction: mediastinal tumors, trauma to the thoracic duct, filariasis.
Ovarian disease: Meigs' syndrome, struma ovarii.
Chronic pancreatitis or pseudocyst: pancreatic ascites.
Leakage of bile: bile ascites.
Urinary obstruction or trauma: urine ascites.
Myxedema.
Chylous ascites.

ASPIRATION LUNG INJURY, CHILDREN[22a]

ICD-9CM # 507.0

CONDITIONS PREDISPOSING TO ASPIRATION LUNG INJURY IN CHILDREN

Anatomic and Mechanical
Tracheoesophageal fistula.
Laryngeal cleft.
Vascular ring.
Cleft palate.
Micrognathia.
Macroglossia.
Achalasia.
Esophageal foreign body.
Tracheostomy.
Endotracheal tube.
Nasoenteric tube.
Collagen vascular disease (scleroderma, dermatomyositises).
Gastroesophageal reflux disease.
Obesity.
Neuromuscular
Altered consciousness.
Immaturity of swallowing/prematurity.
Dysautonomia.
Increased intracranial pressure.
Hydrocephalus.
Vocal cord paralysis.
Cerebral palsy.
Muscular dystrophy.
Myasthenia gravis.
Guillain-Barré syndrome.
Werdnig-Hoffmann disease.
Ataxia-telangiectasia.
Cerebral vascular accident.
Miscellaneous
Poor oral hygiene.
Gingivitis.
Prolonged hospitalization.
Gastric outlet or intestinal obstruction.
Poor feeding techniques (bottle propping, overfeeding, inappropriate foods for toddlers).
Bronchopulmonary dysplasia.
Viral infection.

ASTHENIA

ICD-9CM # 780.79

Depression.
Chronic fatigue syndrome.
Sleep disorders.
Anemia.
Hypothyroidism.
Sedentary lifestyle.
Medications (e.g., narcotics, sedatives).
Infections.
Dehydration/electrolyte disorders.
COPD and other pulmonary disorders.
Renal failure.
CHF.
Diabetes.
Addison's disease.
Paraneoplastic syndrome.

Differential Diagnosis

II

ASTHMA, CHILDHOOD[4]

ICD-9CM # 493.0 use 5th digit
0 Without Mention of Status Asthmaticus
1 With Status Asthmaticus

INFECTIONS

Bronchiolitis (RSV).
Pneumonia.
Croup.
Tuberculosis, histoplasmosis.
Bronchiectasis.
Bronchiolitis obliterans.
Bronchitis.
Sinusitis.

ANATOMIC, CONGENITAL

Cystic fibrosis.
Vascular rings.
Ciliary dyskinesia.
B-lymphocyte immune defect.
Congestive heart failure.
Laryngotracheomalacia.
Tumor, lymphoma.
H-type tracheoesophageal fistula.
Repaired tracheoesophageal fistula.
Gastroesophageal reflux.

VASCULITIS, HYPERSENSITIVITY

Allergic bronchopulmonary aspergillosis.
Allergic alveolitis, hypersensitivity pneumonitis.
Churg-Strauss syndrome.
Periarteritis nodosa.

OTHER

Foreign body aspiration.
Pulmonary thromboembolism.
Psychogenic cough.
Sarcoidosis.
Bronchopulmonary dysplasia.
Vocal cord dysfunction.

ATAXIA

ICD-9CM # 781.3   Ataxia NOS
303.0   Alcoholic, Acute
303.9   Alcoholic, Chronic
334.3   Cerebellar
331.89   Cerebral
334.0   Friedreich's
300.11   Hysterical

Vertebral-basilar artery ischemia.
Diabetic neuropathy.
Tabes dorsalis.
Vitamin B_{12} deficiency.
Multiple sclerosis and other demyelinating diseases.
Meningomyelopathy.
Cerebellar neoplasms, hemorrhage, abscess, infarct.
Nutritional (Wernicke's encephalopathy).
Paraneoplastic syndromes.
Parainfectious: Guillain-Barré syndrome, acute ataxia of childhood and young adults.
Toxins: phenytoin, alcohol, sedatives, organophosphates.
Wilson's disease (hepatolenticular degeneration).
Hypothyroidism.
Myopathy.

Cerebellar and spinocerebellar degeneration: ataxia/telangiectasia, Friedreich's ataxia.
Frontal lobe lesions: tumors, thrombosis of anterior cerebral artery, hydrocephalus.
Labyrinthine destruction: neoplasm, injury, inflammation, compression.
Hysteria.
AIDS.

ATAXIA, ACUTE OR RECURRENT[11]

ICD-9CM # varies with specific diagnosis
781.3   Ataxia NOS
0.94   Locomotor Ataxia
334.0   Friedreich's Ataxia
334.2   Cerebellar Ataxia, Primary
334.3   Other Cerebellar Ataxia
334.8   Ataxia-telangiectasia

Drug ingestion (e.g., phenytoin, carbamazepine, sedatives, hypnotics, and phencyclidine) or intoxication (e.g., alcohol, ethylene glycol, hydrocarbon fumes, lead, mercury, or thallium).
Postinfectious (cerebellitis [e.g., varicella], acute disseminated encephalomyelitis).
Head trauma.
Basilar migraine.
Benign paroxysmal vertigo (migraine equivalent).
Brain tumor or neuroblastoma (if accompanied by opsoclonus or myoclonus [i.e., "dancing eyes, dancing feet"]).
Hydrocephalus.
Infection (e.g., labyrinthitis, abscess).
Seizure (ictal or postictal).
Vascular events (e.g., cerebellar hemorrhage or stroke).
Miller-Fisher variant of Guillain-Barré syndrome (ataxia, ophthalmoplegia, and areflexia). Warning: If bulbar signs present, disease is likely progressive; patient may lose ability to protect airway and/or ability to breathe.
Inherited ataxias.
Inborn errors of metabolism (e.g., mitochondrial disorders, amino-acidopathies, urea cycle defects).
Conversion reaction.
Multiple sclerosis.

ATAXIA, CEREBELLAR, ADULT ONSET[34a]

ICD-9CM # 334.2

CAUSES OF ADULT ONSET CEREBELLAR ATAXIA

Inherited
Later onset SCA syndromes.
Rarely Friedreich's ataxia.
Congenital
Arnold–Chiari malformation (cerebellar ectopia).
Inflammatory
Multiple sclerosis.
Sarcoidosis.
Infections (TB, viral).
Neoplastic
Often metastatic in adults.
Meningioma, neurofibroma.

Hemangioblastoma.
Paraneoplastic
Usually with small cell bronchial carcinoma.
Vascular
Infarction, hemorrhage.
Arteriovenous malformations.
Trauma
Head injury.
Postsurgical.
Toxic
Alcohol, phenytoin, solvent abuse.
Endocrine
Hypothyroidism (very rare).
Degenerative
Multiple system atrophy (MSA).

ATAXIA, CEREBELLAR, CHILDREN[34a]

ICD-9CM # 334.2

CAUSES OF CEREBELLAR ATAXIA IN CHILDREN

Congenital Malformations
Cerebellar agenesis/hypoplasia.
Dandy–Walker syndrome.*
Arnold–Chiari malformation.**
Hereditary Ataxias
Friedreich's ataxia.
Trauma
Birth trauma.*
Head injury in childhood.*
Infectious
Secondary to bacterial meningitis.
Secondary to encephalitis.
*Hydrocephalus**
Tumors
Medulloblastoma.
Astrocytoma.
Hemangioblastoma.

*May persist into adult life.
**May present in adult life.

ATAXIA, CHRONIC OR PROGRESSIVE[11]

ICD-9CM # varies with specific diagnosis
781.3   Ataxia NOS
0.94   Locomotor Ataxia
334.0   Friedreich's Ataxia
334.2   Cerebellar Ataxia, Primary
334.3   Other Cerebellar Ataxia
334.8   Ataxia-telangiectasia

Hydrocephalus.
Hypothyroidism.
Tumor or paraneoplastic syndrome.
Low vitamin E levels (e.g., cystic fibrosis).
Wilson disease.
Inborn errors of metabolism.
Inherited ataxias (e.g., ataxia-telangiectasia, Friedreich's ataxia).

ATELECTASIS

ICD-9CM # 518.0

Lung neoplasm (primary or metastatic).
Infection (pneumonia, TB, fungal, histoplasmosis).

Postoperative (lower lobes).
Sarcoidosis.
Mucoid impaction.
Foreign body.
Postinflammatory (middle lobe syndrome).
Pneumothorax.
Pleural effusion.
Pneumoconiosis.
Interstitial fibrosis.
Bulla.
Mediastinal or adjacent mass.

ATRIAL ENLARGEMENT, LEFT ATRIUM[16a]

ICD-9CM # varies with specific diagnosis

CAUSES OF LARGE LEFT ATRIUM

Causes Due to Volume Overload
Mitral regurgitation (often with left ventricular failure).
Ventricular septal defect.
Patent ductus arteriosus.
Atrial septal defect with shunt reversal (i.e., pulmonary hypertension).
ASD with tricuspid atresia (obligatory shunt reversal).
Aortopulmonary window.
Causes Due to Pressure Overload
Mitral stenosis.
Noncompliant left ventricle: hypertension, hypertrophic cardiomyopathy, aortic stenosis.
Left ventricular failure (often with secondary mitral regurgitation).
Left atrial myxoma.
Other Causes (Both Rare)
Atrial fibrillation.
Isolated/idiopathic.

ATRIAL ENLARGEMENT, RIGHT ATRIUM

ICD-9CM # varies with specific disorder

Right ventricular failure.
Atrial septal defect.
Tricuspid regurgitation.
Tricuspid stenosis.
Pulmonary hypertension.
Restrictive cardiomyopathy.
Right atrial myxoma.
Ebstein's anomaly.
Anomalous pulmonary venous drainage to the right atrium.
Endomyocardial fibrosis.
Sinus of Valsalva fistula.
Arrhythmogenic right ventricular dysplasia.

ATYPICAL LYMPHOCYTOSIS, HETEROPHIL NEGATIVE, INFECTIOUS CAUSES[1]

ICD-9CM # 288.61

MOST COMMON INFECTIOUS CAUSES OF HETEROPHIL-NEGATIVE ATYPICAL LYMPHOCYTOSIS

Babesiosis.
Cytomegalovirus.

Epstein-Barr virus (particularly in children).
Human herpesvirus 6.
Human immunodeficiency virus (especially during acute seroconversion).
Infectious mononucleosis.
Malaria.
Measles.
Toxoplasmosis.
Varicella.
Infectious hepatitis.

AV NODAL BLOCK[15]

ICD-9CM # 426.10 AV Block (Incomplete, Partial)
426.0 AV Block, Complete

Idiopathic fibrosis (Lenègre's disease).
Sclerodegenerative processes (e.g., Lev's disease with calcification of the mitral and aortic annuli).
AV node radiofrequency ablation procedure.
Medications (e.g., digoxin, beta-blockers, calcium channel blockers, class III antiarrhythmics).
Acute inferior wall MI.
Myocarditis.
Infections (endocarditis, Lyme disease).
Infiltrative diseases (e.g., hemochromatosis, sarcoidosis, amyloidosis).
Trauma (including cardiac surgical procedures).
Collagen vascular diseases.
Aortic root diseases (e.g., spondylitis).
Electrolyte abnormalities (e.g., hyperkalemia).

BACK PAIN

ICD-9CM # 724.5 Back Pain (Postural)
724.2 Low Back Pain
307.89 Back Pain Psychogenic
724.8 Stiff Back
847.9 Back Strain
724.6 Backache, Sacroiliac

Trauma: injury to bone, joint, or ligament.
Mechanical: pregnancy, obesity, fatigue, scoliosis.
Degenerative: osteoarthritis.
Infections: osteomyelitis, subarachnoid or spinal abscess, TB, meningitis, basilar pneumonia.
Metabolic: osteoporosis, osteomalacia.
Vascular: leaking aortic aneurysm, subarachnoid or spinal hemorrhage/infarction.
Neoplastic: myeloma, Hodgkin's disease, carcinoma of pancreas, metastatic neoplasm from breast, prostate, lung.
GI: penetrating ulcer, pancreatitis, cholelithiasis, inflammatory bowel disease.
Renal: hydronephrosis, calculus, neoplasm, renal infarction, pyelonephritis.
Hematologic: sickle cell crisis, acute hemolysis.
Gynecologic: neoplasm of uterus or ovary, dysmenorrhea, salpingitis, uterine prolapse.
Inflammatory: ankylosing spondylitis, psoriatic arthritis, Reiter's syndrome.
Lumbosacral strain.
Psychogenic: malingering, hysteria, anxiety.
Endocrine: adrenal hemorrhage or infarction.

BACK PAIN, CHILDREN AND ADOLESCENTS[22a]

ICD-9CM # 724.2

INFLAMMATORY OR INFECTIOUS

Diskitis.
Vertebral osteomyelitis (pyogenic, tuberculous).
Spinal epidural abscess.
Pyelonephritis.
Pancreatitis.

RHEUMATOLOGIC

Pauciarticular juvenile rheumatoid arthritis.
Reiter syndrome.
Ankylosing spondylitis.
Psoriatic arthritis.

DEVELOPMENTAL

Spondylolysis.
Spondylolisthesis.
Scheuermann disease.
Scoliosis.

TRAUMATIC (ACUTE VERSUS REPETITIVE)

Hip-pelvis anomalies.
Herniated disk.
Overuse syndromes.
Vertebral stress fractures.
Upper cervical spine instability.

NEOPLASTIC

Vertebral Tumors
Benign
Eosinophilic granuloma.
Aneurysmal bone cyst.
Osteoid osteoma.
Osteoblastoma.
Malignant
Osteogenic sarcoma.
Leukemia.
Lymphoma.
Metastatic tumors.
Spinal Cord, Ganglia, and Nerve Roots
Intramedullary spinal cord tumor.
Sympathetic chain.
Ganglioneuroma.
Ganglioneuroblastoma.
Neuroblastoma.

OTHER

Intraabdominal or pelvic pathology.
Following lumbar puncture.
Conversion reaction.
Juvenile osteoporosis.

BACK PAIN, LOW, ACUTE[2]

ICD-9CM # 724.2

DIFFERENTIAL CONSIDERATIONS IN ACUTE LOW BACK PAIN

Emergent
Aortic dissection.
Cauda equina syndrome.
Epidural abscess or hematoma.
Meningitis.
Ruptured/expanding aortic aneurysm.

Differential Diagnosis

II

Spinal fracture or subluxation with cord or root impingement.

Urgent
Back pain with neurologic deficits.
Disk herniation causing neurologic compromise.
Malignancy.
Sciatica with motor nerve root compression.
Spinal fractures without cord impingement.
Spinal stenosis.
Transverse myelitis.
Vertebral osteomyelitis.

Common or Stable
Acute ligamentous injury.
Acute muscle strain.
Ankylosing spondylitis.
Degenerative joint disease.
Intervertebral disk disease without impingement.
Pathologic fracture without impingement.
Seropositive arthritis.
Spondylolisthesis.

Referred or Visceral
Cholecystitis.
Esophageal disease.
Nephrolithiasis.
Ovarian torsion, mass, or tumor.
Pancreatitis.
Peptic ulcer disease.
Pleural effusion.
Pneumonia.
Pulmonary embolism.
Pyelonephritis.
Retroperitoneal hemorrhage or mass.

BACK PAIN, VISCEROGENIC ORIGIN

ICD-9CM # varies with specific disorder

Urolithiasis.
Aortic aneurysm.
Colorectal carcinoma.
Endometriosis.
Tubal pregnancy.
Prostatitis.
Peptic ulcer.
Pancreatitis.
Diverticular spasm.
Metastatic neoplasm (e.g., bladder, uterus, ovary, kidney).

BACTERIAL OVERGROWTH, SMALL INTESTINE[38]

ICD-9CM # varies with specific diagnosis

Gastric surgery—Billroth II.
Small bowel diverticula.
Small bowel stricture:
- Crohn's disease.
- Radiation enteritis.

Impaired small intestinal motility:
- Scleroderma.
- Diabetes mellitus.
- Chronic intestinal pseudoobstruction.

Miscellaneous/multifactorial
- Elderly.
- Immune deficiency syndrome.
- Chronic pancreatitis.
- Cirrhosis.

BALLISM

ICD-9CM # 333.5

Cerebral infarction or hemorrhage.
Medications (e.g., dopamine agonists, phenytoin).
CNS neoplasm (primary or metastatic).
Nonketotic hyperosmolar state.

*Violent, flinging, nonpatterned rapid movements

BILE DUCT, DILATED[38]

ICD-9CM # varies with specific diagnosis

Normal variant.
Post-cholecystectomy.
Unsuspected bile duct stone.
Sphincter of Oddi stenosis.
Occult bile duct stricture.
Previous bile duct injury.
Early carcinoma of the pancreas, carcinoma of the bile duct, or carcinoma of the ampulla.
Extrinsic compression of the bile duct by a primary or secondary neoplasm.

BLEEDING, LOWER GI

ICD-9CM # 578.9

(ORIGINATING BELOW THE LIGAMENT OF TREITZ)
Small Intestine
Ischemic bowel disease (mesenteric thrombosis, embolism, vasculitis, trauma).
Small bowel neoplasm: leiomyomas, carcinoids.
Hereditary hemorrhagic telangiectasia (Rendu-Osler-Weber syndrome).
Meckel diverticulum and other small intestine diverticula.
Aortoenteric fistula.
Intestinal hemangiomas: blue rubber-bleb nevi, intestinal hemangiomas, cutaneous vascular nevi.
Hamartomatous polyps: Peutz-Jeghers syndrome (intestinal polyps, mucocutaneous pigmentation).
Infections of small bowel: tuberculous enteritis, enteritis necroticans.
Volvulus.
Intussusception.
Lymphoma of small bowel, sarcoma, Kaposi's sarcoma.
Irradiation ileitis.
AV malformation of small intestine.
Inflammatory bowel disease.
Polyarteritis nodosa.
Other: pancreatoenteric fistulas, Henoch-Schönlein purpura, Ehlers-Danlos syndrome, SLE, amyloidosis, metastatic melanoma.
Colon
Carcinoma (particularly left colon).
Diverticular disease.
Inflammatory bowel disease.
Ischemic colitis.
Colonic polyps.
Vascular abnormalities: angiodysplasia, vascular ectasia.
Radiation colitis.
Infectious colitis.

Uremic colitis.
Aortoenteric fistula.
Lymphoma of large bowel.
Hemorrhoids.
Anal fissure.
Trauma, foreign body.
Solitary rectal/cecal ulcers.
Long-distance running.

BLEEDING, LOWER GI, PEDIATRIC[2]

ICD-9CM # 578.9

<3 MO
Swallowed maternal blood.
Infectious colitis.
Milk allergy.
Bleeding diathesis.
Intussusception.
Midgut volvulus.
Meckel diverticulum.
Necrotizing enterocolitis.

<2 YR
Anal fissure.
Infectious colitis.
Milk allergy.
Colitis.
Intussusception.
Meckel diverticulum.
Polyp.
Duplication.
Hemolytic-uremic syndrome.
Inflammatory bowel disease.
Pseudomembranous enterocolitis.

<5 YR
Infectious colitis.
Anal fissure.
Polyp.
Intussusception.
Meckel diverticulum.
Henoch-Schönlein purpura.
Hemolytic-uremic syndrome.
Inflammatory bowel disease.
Pseudomembranous enterocolitis.

5 TO 18 YR
Infectious colitis.
Inflammatory bowel disease.
Pseudomembranous enterocolitis.
Polyp.
Hemolytic-uremic syndrome.
Hemorrhoid.

BLEEDING, RECTAL[38]

ICD-9CM # 578.9

IN PATIENTS <40 YR
Very Common:
Hemorrhoids.
Anal fissure.
Inflammatory bowel disease (mainly proctitis).
Less Common:
Polyps (hamartomatous or adenomatous).
Infective colitis.
Meckel's diverticulum.

Intussusception.
Rare:
Colorectal cancer.

IN PATIENTS >40 YR

Hemorrhoids.
Anal fissure.
Colorectal cancer.
Colorectal polyps (mostly adenomas).
Angiodysplasia.
Diverticular disease.
Inflammatory bowel disease.
Ischemic colitis.
Infective colitis.

BLEEDING, UPPER GI

ICD-9CM # 578.9

(ORIGINATING ABOVE THE LIGAMENT OF TREITZ)

Oral or pharyngeal lesions: swallowed blood from nose or oropharynx.
Swallowed Hemoptysis
Esophageal: varices, ulceration, esophagitis, Mallory-Weiss tear, carcinoma, trauma.
Gastric: peptic ulcer (including Cushing and Curling's ulcers), gastritis, angiodysplasia, gastric neoplasms, hiatal hernia, gastric diverticulum, pseudoxanthoma elasticum, Rendu-Osler-Weber syndrome.
Duodenal: peptic ulcer, duodenitis, angiodysplasia, aortoduodenal fistula, duodenal diverticulum, duodenal tumors, carcinoma of ampulla of Vater, parasites (e.g., hookworm), Crohn's disease.
Biliary: hematobilia (e.g., penetrating injury to liver, hepatobiliary malignancy, endoscopic papillotomy).

BLEEDING, UPPER GI, PEDIATRIC[2]

ICD-9CM # 578.9

<3 MO

Swallowed maternal blood.
Gastritis.
Ulcer, stress.
Bleeding diathesis.
Foreign body (NG tube).
Vascular malformation.
Duplication.

<2 YR

Esophagitis.
Gastritis.
Ulcer.
Pyloric stenosis.
Mallory-Weiss syndrome.
Vascular malformation.
Duplication.

<5 YR

Esophagitis.
Gastritis.
Ulcer.
Esophageal varices.
Foreign body.

Mallory-Weiss syndrome.
Hemophilia.
Vascular malformations.

5 TO 18 YR

Esophagitis.
Gastritis.
Ulcer.
Esophageal varices.
Mallory-Weiss syndrome.
Inflammatory bowel disease.
Hemophilia.
Vascular malformation.

BLINDNESS, GERIATRIC AGE

ICD-9CM # 369.4

Cataracts.
Glaucoma.
Diabetic retinopathy.
Macular degeneration.
Trauma.
CVA.
Corneal scarring.
Giant cell arteritis.
Ocular herpes zoster.

BLINDNESS, MONOCULAR, TRANSIENT

ICD-9CM # 369.67

Migraine (vasospasm).
Embolic cerebrovascular disease.
Intermittent angle-closure glaucoma.
Partial retinal vein occlusion.
Hyphema.
Optic disc edema.
Giant cell arteritis.
Psychogenic.
Hypotension.
Hypercoagulopathy disorders.
Multiple sclerosis.

BLINDNESS, PEDIATRIC AGE[23]

ICD-9CM # varies with specific disorder

CONGENITAL

Optic nerve hypoplasia or aplasia.
Optic coloboma.
Congenital hydrocephalus.
Hydranencephaly.
Porencephaly.
Microencephaly.
Encephalocele, particularly occipital type.
Morning glory disc.
Aniridia.
Anterior microphthalmia.
Peter's anomaly.
Persistent pupillary membrane.
Glaucoma.
Cataracts.
Persistent hyperplastic primary vitreous.

PHAKOMATOSES

Tuberous sclerosis.
Neurofibromatosis (special association with optic glioma).

Sturge-Weber syndrome.
von Hippel–Lindau disease.

TUMORS

Retinoblastoma.
Optic glioma.
Perioptic meningioma.
Craniopharyngioma.
Cerebral glioma.
Posterior and intraventricular tumors when complicated by hydrocephalus.
Pseudotumor cerebri.

NEURODEGENERATIVE DISEASES

Cerebral storage disease.
Gangliosidoses, particularly Tay-Sachs disease (infantile amaurotic familial idiocy), Sandhoff's variant, generalized gangliosidosis.
Other lipidoses and ceroid lipofuscinoses, particularly the late-onset amaurotic familial idiocies such as those of Jansky-Bielschowsky and of Batten-Mayou-Spielmeyer-Vogt.
Mucopolysaccharidoses, particularly Hurler's syndrome and Hunter's syndrome.
Leukodystrophies (dysmyelination disorders), particularly metachromatic leukodystrophy and Canavan's disease.
Demyelinating sclerosis (myelinoclastic diseases), especially Schilder's disease and Devic's neuromyelitis optica.
Special types: Dawson's disease, Leigh's disease, Bassen-Kornzweig syndrome, Refsum's disease.
Retinal degenerations: retinitis pigmentosa and its variants, Leber's congenital type.
Optic atrophies: congenital autosomal recessive type, infantile and congenital autosomal dominant types, Leber's disease, and atrophies associated with hereditary ataxias—the types of Behr, of Marie, and of Sanger-Brown.

INFECTIOUS PROCESSES

Encephalitis, especially in the prenatal infection syndromes caused by *Toxoplasma gondii,* cytomegalovirus, rubella virus, *Treponema pallidum,* herpes simplex.
Meningitis, arachnoiditis.
Chorioretinitis.
Endophthalmitis.
Keratitis.

HEMATOLOGIC DISORDERS

Leukemia with central nervous system involvement.

VASCULAR AND CIRCULATORY DISORDERS

Collagen vascular diseases.
Arteriovenous malformations—intracerebral hemorrhage, subarachnoid hemorrhage.
Central retinal occlusion.

TRAUMA

Contusion or avulsion of optic nerves, chiasm, globe, cornea.
Cerebral contusion or laceration.
Intracerebral, subarachnoid, or subdural hemorrhage.

DRUGS AND TOXINS
Other
Retinopathy of prematurity.
Sclerocornea.
Conversion reaction.
Optic neuritis.
Osteopetrosis.

BLISTERS, SUBEPIDERMAL
ICD-9CM # 919.2

Burns.
Porphyria cutanea tarda.
Bullous pemphigoid.
Bullous drug reaction.
Arthropod bite reaction.
Toxic epidermal necrosis.
Dermatitis herpetiformis.
Polymorphous light eruption.
Variegate porphyria.
SLE.
Epidermolysis bullosa.
Pseudoporphyria.
Acute graft-versus-host reaction.
Linear IgA disease.
Leukocytoclastic vasculitis.
Pressure necrosis.
Urticaria pigmentosa.
Amyloidosis.

BONE DENSITY, DECREASED, GENERALIZED[16a]
ICD-9CM # 733.00

DISORDERS ASSOCIATED WITH GENERALIZED LOSS OF BONE DENSITY
Disorders of Multiple or Uncertain Cause
Senile osteoporosis.*
Juvenile osteoporosis.
Osteogenesis imperfecta.†
Secondary Bone Disorders
Endocrine
Adrenal cortex.†
　Cushing's disease.
　Addison's disease.
Gonadal disorders.
　Postmenopausal osteoporosis.*
　Hypogonadism.†
Pituitary.
　Acromegaly.
　Hypopituitarism.
Pancreas.
　Diabetes mellitus.*
Thyroid.
　Hyperthyroidism.
　Hypothyroidism.
Parathyroid.
　Hyperparathyroidism.*
Marrow replacement and expansion
Myeloma.
Leukemia.
Lymphoma.
Metastatic disease.*
Gaucher's disease.
Anemias (sickle cell, thalassaemia, hemophilia).†

Drugs and other substances
Steroids.*†
Heparin (osteoporosis).
Anticonvulsants (osteomalacia).
Immunosuppressants.
Alcohol.*
Chronic disease
Chronic renal disease.†
Hepatic insufficiency.†
GI malabsorption syndromes.
Chronic inflammatory polyarthropathies.
Chronic debility or immobilization.

---

*Common cause of decrease in bone density in adults.
†Common cause of decrease in bone density in children.

BONE DENSITY, DECREASED, LOCALIZED[16a]
ICD-9CM # V17.81

DISORDERS ASSOCIATED WITH LOCALIZED LOSS OF BONE DENSITY
Disuse osteoporosis.*
Reflex sympathetic dystrophy (Sudeck's).*
Osteolytic syndromes.
　Acro-osteolysis, primary and secondary.
　Massive osteolysis of Gorham.
　Carpotarsal osteolysis.
Transient regional osteoporosis.
Neuromuscular disorders.
Infection.*
Arthropathies.*
Tumors, primary and secondary, myelomatosis.

*Common causes.

BONE LESIONS, PREFERENTIAL SITE OF ORIGIN[35]
ICD-9CM # 170.0 Skull and Face
　　　　　170.1 Mandible
　　　　　170.2 Vertebral Column
　　　　　170.3 Ribs, Sternum, Clavicle
　　　　　170.4 Scapula, Long Bones, Upper Limb
　　　　　170.5 Short Bones and Upper Limb
　　　　　170.6 Pelvic Bones, Sacrum, Coccyx
　　　　　170.7 Long Bones, Lower Limb
　　　　　170.8 Short Bones, Lower Limb
　　　　　170.9 Bone Cancer NOS
　　　　　198.5 Bone Cancer, Metastatic

EPIPHYSIS
Chondroblastoma.
Giant cell tumor—after fusion of growth plate.
Langerhans' cell histiocytosis.
Clear cell chondrosarcoma.
Osteosarcoma.

METAPHYSIS
Parosteal sarcoma.
Chondrosarcoma.

Fibrosarcoma.
Nonossifying fibroma.
Giant cell tumor—before fusion of growth plate.
Unicameral bone cyst.
Aneurysmal bone cyst.

DIAPHYSIS
Myeloma.
Ewing's tumor.
Reticulum cell sarcoma.

METADIAPHYSEAL
Fibrosarcoma.
Fibrous dysplasia.
Enchondroma.
Osteoid osteoma.
Chondromyofibroma.

BONE MARROW FAILURE SYNDROMES, INHERITED[20]
ICD-9CM # 284

BI-LINEAGE AND TRI-LINEAGE CYTOPENIAS
Fanconi anemia.
Shwachman-Diamond syndrome.
Dyskeratosis congenita.
Amegakaryocytic thrombocytopenia:
- Other inherited thrombocytopenia disorders.

Other genetic syndromes:
- Down syndrome.
- Dubowitz syndrome.
- Seckel syndrome.
- Reticular dysgenesis.
- Schimke immunoosseous dysplasia.
- Noonan syndrome.
- Cartilage-hair hypoplasia.
- Familial marrow failure (non-Fanconi).

UNI-LINEAGE CYTOPENIA
Diamond-Blackfan anemia.
Kostmann syndrome/Congenital neutropenia:
- *ELA2* mutations.
- *HAX1* mutations.
- *GFI1* mutations.
- *WASP* mutations.
- Constitutive cell surface G-CSF-R mutations.

Other inherited neutropenia syndromes:
- Barth syndrome.
- Glycogen storage disease 1b.
- Miscellaneous.

Thrombocytopenia with absent radii.
Congenital dyserythropoietic anemias (CDAs):
- Types I, II, III, IV.
- Variants.
- Nonclassifiable CDAs.
- Groups IV, V, VI, VII.

BONE MARROW FIBROSIS[14]
ICD-9CM # 289.9

MYELOID DISORDERS
Myelofibrosis with myeloid metaplasia.
Metastatic cancer.
Chronic myeloid leukemia.
Myelodysplastic syndrome.
Atypical myeloid disorder.

Acute megakaryocytic leukemia.
Other acute myeloid leukemias.
Gray platelet syndrome.

LYMPHOID DISORDERS

Hairy cell leukemia.
Multiple myeloma.
Lymphoma.

NONHEMATOLOGIC DISORDERS

Connective tissue disorder.
Infections (tuberculosis, kala-azar).
Vitamin D–deficiency rickets.
Renal osteodystrophy.

BONE MASS, LOW[1]

ICD-9CM # varies with specific diagnosis

SECONDARY CAUSES OF LOW BONE MASS

Endocrine Diseases
Female hypogonadism.
Hyperprolactinemia.
Hypothalamic amenorrhea.
Anorexia nervosa.
Premature and primary ovarian failure.
Female athlete triad.
Male hypogonadism.
Primary gonadal failure (e.g., Klinefelter's syndrome).
Secondary gonadal failure (e.g., idiopathic hypogonadotropic hypogonadism, androgen deprivation therapy for prostate cancer).
Hyperthyroidism.
Hyperparathyroidism.
Hypercortisolism.
Vitamin D insufficiency or deficiency.
Gastrointestinal Diseases
Subtotal gastrectomy.
Gastric bypass surgery.
Malabsorption syndromes.
Chronic obstructive jaundice.
Primary biliary cirrhosis and other cirrhoses.
Bone Marrow Disorders
Multiple myeloma.
Monoclonal gammopathy of unknown significance (MGUS).
Lymphoma.
Leukemia.
Hemolytic anemias.
Systemic mastocytosis.
Disseminated carcinoma.
Connective Tissue Diseases
Osteogenesis imperfecta.
Ehlers-Danlos syndrome.
Marfan's syndrome.
Homocystinuria.
Drugs
Alcohol.
Antiseizure medications.
Aromatase inhibitors.
Chemotherapy.
Cyclosporine.
Depo-medroxyprogesterone.
Excess thyroid hormone.
Glucocorticoids.
Gonadotropin-releasing hormone agonists.
Heparin.

Miscellaneous Causes
Immobilization.
Rheumatoid arthritis.
Chronic obstructive pulmonary disease.
Weight loss.

BONE MINERAL DENSITY, INCREASED

ICD-9CM # 733.99

Paget's disease of bone.
Skeletal metastases.
DISH.
Osteonecrosis.
Sarcoidosis.
Hypoparathyroidism, pseudohypoparathyroidism.
Milk-alkali syndrome.
Osteopetrosis.
Hypervitaminosis A or D.
Dysplasias (craniodiaphyseal, craniometaphyseal, frontometaphyseal).
Endosteal hyperostosis.
Fluorosis.
Heavy metal poisoning.
Ionizing radiation.
Other: lymphoma, leukemia, mastocytosis, multiple myeloma, polycythemia vera.

BONE PAIN

ICD-9CM # varies with specific diagnosis

Trauma.
Neoplasm (primary or metastatic).
Osteoporosis with compression fracture.
Paget's disease of bone.
Infection (osteomyelitis, septic arthritis).
Osteomalacia.
Viral syndrome.
Sickle cell disease.
Anxiety.

BONE RESORPTION[35]

ICD-9CM # 733.90 Bone Disorder

DISTAL CLAVICLE

Hyperparathyroidism.
RA.
Scleroderma.
Posttraumatic osteolysis.
Progeria.
Pycnodysostosis.
Cleidocranial dysplasia.

INFERIOR ASPECT OF RIBS

Vascular impression, associated with but not limited to coarctation of the aorta.
Hyperparathyroidism.
Neurofibromatosis.

TERMINAL PHALANGEAL TUFTS

Scleroderma.
Raynaud's phenomenon.
Vascular disease.
Frostbite, electrical burns.
Psoriasis.
Tabes dorsalis.
Hyperparathyroidism.

GENERALIZED RESORPTION

Paraplegia.
Myositis ossificans.
Osteoporosis.

BOW LEGS (GENU VARUM), CLASSIFICATION[22a]

ICD-9CM # 736.42 Bow Legs (Genu Varum)

PHYSIOLOGIC

ASYMMETRIC GROWTH

Tibia vara (Blount disease).
- Infantile.
- Juvenile.
- Adolescent.
Focal fibrocartilaginous dysplasia.
Physeal injury.
Trauma.
Infection.
Tumor.

METABOLIC DISORDERS

Vitamin D deficiency (nutritional rickets).
Vitamin D–resistant rickets.
Hypophosphatasia.

SKELETAL DYSPLASIA

Metaphyseal dysplasia.
Achondroplasia.
Enchondromatosis.

BRADYCARDIA, SINUS[15]

ICD-9CM # 427.89

Idiopathic.
Degenerative processes (e.g., Lev's disease, Lenègre's disease).
Medications
Beta-blockers.
Some calcium channel blockers (diltiazem, verapamil).
Digoxin (when vagal tone is high).
Class I antiarrhythmic agents (e.g., procainamide).
Class III antiarrhythmic agents (amiodarone, sotalol).
Clonidine.
Lithium carbonate.
Acute Myocardial Ischemia and Infarction
Right or left circumflex coronary artery occlusion or spasm.
High vagal tone (e.g., athletes).

BREAST INFLAMMATORY LESION[12]

ICD-9CM # 611.0 Acute Mastitis
610.1 Chronic Cystic Mastitis
771.5 Neonatal Infective Mastitis
778.7 Neonatal Noninfective Mastitis

Mastitis (*S. aureus,* beta-hemolytic *Streptococcus*).
Trauma.
Foreign body (sutures, breast implants).
Granuloma (TB, fungal).

Differential Diagnosis

II

Fat necrosis post biopsy.
Necrosis or infarction (anticoagulant therapy, pregnancy).
Breast malignancy.

BREAST MASS

ICD-9CM # 611.72

Fibrocystic breasts.
Benign tumors (fibroadenoma, papilloma).
Mastitis (acute bacterial mastitis, chronic mastitis).
Malignant neoplasm.
Fat necrosis.
Hematoma.
Duct ectasia.
Mammary adenosis.

BREATH ODOR[34]

ICD-9CM # 784.9 Halitosis

Sweet, fruity: DKA, starvation ketosis.
Fishy, stale: uremia (trimethylamines).
Ammonia-like: uremia (ammonia).
Musty fish, clover: fetor hepaticus (hepatic failure).
Foul, feculent: intestinal obstruction/diverticulum.
Foul, putrid: nasal/sinus pathology (infection, foreign body, cancer), respiratory infections (empyema, lung abscess, bronchiectasis).
Halitosis: tonsillitis, gingivitis, respiratory infections, Vincent's angina, gastroesophageal reflux, achalasia, certain foods (garlic, onions, protein drinks, etc.)
Cinnamon: pulmonary TB.

BREATHING, NOISY[34]

ICD-9CM # 786.09 Breathing, Labored
789.09 Snoring, Wheezing
786.1 Stridor

Infection: upper respiratory infection, peritonsillar abscess, retropharyngeal abscess, epiglottitis, laryngitis, tracheitis, bronchitis, bronchiolitis.
Irritants and allergens: hyperactive airway, asthma (reactive airway disease), rhinitis, angioneurotic edema.
Compression from outside of the airway: esophageal cysts or foreign body, neoplasms, lymphadenopathy.
Congenital malformation and abnormality: vascular rings, laryngeal webs, laryngomalacia, tracheomalacia, hemangiomas within the upper airway, stenoses within the upper airway, cystic fibrosis.
Acquired abnormality (at every level of the airway): nasal polyps, hypertrophied adenoids and/or tonsils, foreign body, intraluminal tumors, bronchiectasis.
Neurogenic disorder: vocal cord paralysis.

BRONCHIAL OBSTRUCTION[16a]

ICD-9CM # varies with specific diagnosis

CAUSES OF BRONCHIAL OBSTRUCTION

Outside the Bronchus
Lymph nodes and other masses.

In the Wall of the Bronchus
Tumors
Lung carcinoma (commonly squamous cell).
Bronchial carcinoid.
Metastasis.
Hamartoma.
Inflammation
Tuberculosis.
Sarcoidosis.
Wegener's granulomatosis.
Inflammatory bowel disease.
Bronchomalacia
Broncholith.
Inside the Bronchus
Mucus plug.
Inhaled foreign body.

BRONCHOPLEURAL FISTULA[16a]

ICD-9CM # 510.0

CAUSES OF BRONCHOPLEURAL FISTULA

Trauma
Penetrating.
Iatrogenic (especially post-pneumonectomy, post-lobectomy, post-biopsy).
Infection
Necrotizing pneumonia.
Empyema.
Tuberculosis.
Septic embolus.
Infected pulmonary infarct.

BROWN URINE

ICD-9CM # 788.69

Bile pigments.
Myoglobin.
Concentrated urine.
Use of multivitamin supplements.
Medications (antimalarials, metronidazole, nitrofurantoin, levodopa, methyldopa, phenazopyridine).
Diet rich in fava beans.
Urinary tract infection.

BRUISING

ICD-9CM # 459.89

Medication-induced (warfarin, aspirin, NSAIDs, prednisone).
Alcohol abuse.
Senile purpura.
Purpura simplex.
Physical abuse.
Vasculitis.
Platelet disorders.
Coagulation factor deficiencies.
Cushing's disease.
Vitamin C deficiency.
Marfan's syndrome.
Ehlers-Danlos syndrome.
Disseminated intravascular coagulation.
Leukemia.
Hereditary hemorrhagic telangiectasia.

BULLOUS DISEASES

ICD-9CM # 694.9 Bullous Dermatoses
694.5 Bullous Pemphigoid
694.4 Pemphigus Vulgaris
694.4 Pemphigus Foliaceus

Bullous pemphigoid.
Pemphigus vulgaris.
Pemphigus foliaceus.
Paraneoplastic pemphigus.
Cicatricial pemphigoid.
Erythema multiforme.
Dermatitis herpetiformis.
Herpes gestationis.
Impetigo.
Erosive lichen planus.
Linear IgA bullous dermatosis.
Epidermolysis bullosa acquisita.

CAFÉ-AU-LAIT SPOTS[22a]

ICD-9CM # 709

Neurofibromatosis types 1 and 2.
McCune-Albright syndrome.
Russell-Silver syndrome.
Ataxia-telangiectasia.
Fanconi anemia.
Tuberous sclerosis.
Bloom syndrome.
Basal cell nevus syndrome.
Gaucher disease.
Chédiak-Higashi syndrome.
Hunter syndrome.
Maffucci syndrome.
Multiple mucosal neuroma syndrome.
Watson syndrome.
Proteus syndrome.
Turner syndrome.
Ring chromosome syndrome.
Jaffe-Campanacci syndrome.

CALCIFICATION ON CHEST X-RAY

ICD-9CM # 722.92

Lung neoplasm (primary or metastatic).
Silicosis.
Idiopathic pulmonary fibrosis.
Tuberculosis.
Histoplasmosis.
Disseminated varicella infection.
Mitral stenosis (end-stage).
Secondary hyperparathyroidism.

CALCIFICATIONS, ABDOMINAL, NONVISCERAL ON X-RAY[16a]

ICD-9CM # 728.10

NONVISCERAL ABDOMINAL CALCIFICATION

Common
Atherosclerosis.
Mesenteric lymph nodes.
Phleboliths.
Aneurysm.
Dermoid cyst.

Differentiate
Rib cartilage.
Injections in the buttocks.

Uncommon
Infestations.
Armillifer armillatus.
Cysticercosis.
Guinea worm.
Hydatid.
Tumors.
Lipoma.
Hemangioma.
Neuroblastoma.
Osteo/chondrosarcoma of soft tissues.
Retroperitoneal sarcoma of soft tissues.
Peritoneal metastases.
Pheochromocytoma.
Tuberculosis.
Peritonitis.
Psoas abscess.
Meconium peritonitis.

Pseudomyxoma Peritonei
Mesenteric cyst.
Pancreatitis with saponification.
Lithopedion.

Appendices Epiploicae
Ligaments.
Foreign bodies.
Posttraumatic buttock cysts.

CALCIFICATIONS, ADRENAL GLAND ON X-RAY[16a]
ICD-9CM # 275.49

ADRENAL GLAND CALCIFICATION

Common
Idiopathic.
Hemorrhage.
Tuberculosis.
Neuroblastoma/ganglioneuroma.
Pheochromocytoma.

Uncommon
Other tumors:
Adenoma.
Carcinoma.
Dermoid.
Addison's disease.
Cyst.
Histoplasmosis.

CALCIFICATIONS, CARDIAC ON X-RAY[16a]
ICD-9CM # 275.49

CAUSES OF VISIBLE CALCIFICATION WITHIN THE HEART

Coronary Artery
Atherosclerosis.

Aortic Root
Atherosclerotic aorta.
Thrombus.
Syphilis.
Ankylosing spondylitis.
Homograft calcification.

Pericardium
Chronic pericarditis, tuberculosis, hemopericardium, pyogenic or viral pericarditis.
Posttraumatic.
Postoperative.
Uremic pericarditis.
Asbestosis (may be pleural calcification applied to pericardium).

Myocardium
Ventricular aneurysm (may mimic pericardial calcification).
Calcified myocardial infarction.
Postmyocarditis.

Endocardium
Endomyocardial fibrosis.
Thrombus.

Valve Cusps
Calcified valves (particularly mitral and aortic valves).
Mitral annulus calcification.
Homograft calcification.
Old vegetation.

Valve Annulus
Submitral.
Mitral.
Aortic.

Left Atrium
Wall.
Thrombus.
Atrial myxoma.

Pulmonary Artery
Pulmonary hypertension.
Postoperative.

Postoperative Serumoma

Calcified Hydatid Cyst

CALCIFICATIONS, CUTANEOUS
ICD-9CM # 709.3

Calcification, Raynaud's phenomenon, esophageal dysmotility, sclerodactyly, and telangiectasia (CREST) syndrome.
Trauma.
Pancreatitis or pancreatic cancer.
Chronic renal failure.
Sarcoidosis.
Hyperparathyroidism.
Milk-alkali syndrome.
Hypervitaminosis D.
Panniculitis.
Idiopathic.
Iatrogenic (e.g., application of calcium alginate dressing to skin).
Multiple myeloma.
Dermatomyositis.
Parasitic infections.
Leukemia.
Lymphoma.

CALCIFICATIONS, GENITAL TRACT, FEMALE ON X-RAY[16a]
ICD-9CM # 275.49

FEMALE GENITAL TRACT CALCIFICATION

Uterus
Leiomyomas.
Squamous cell carcinoma.
Adenocarcinoma of endometrium.
Leiomyosarcoma.
Lithopedion.

Fallopian Tubes
Ovary.
Dermoid cyst.
Serous cystadenoma/carcinoma.
Tuberculosis.
Cysts.
Autoamputation.

CALCIFICATIONS, LIVER ON X-RAY[16a]
ICD-9CM # 573

LIVER CALCIFICATION

Common
Granuloma (tuberculosis, histoplasmosis, brucellosis).
• Multiple scattered round densities.
Hydatid cyst.
• Fine curvilinear in wall, or dense and irregular if contracted.
Primary liver tumor (hemangioma, hepatoblastoma, hepatoma, cholangiocarcinoma).
• Irregular patterns or multiple nodules.
Metastases (mucinous primary of colon or breast, cystadenocarcinoma of ovary).
• Finely stippled, may be extensive.

Uncommon
Hepatic artery aneurysm.
Armillifer armillatus infestation.
Chronic granulomatous disease of childhood.
Cyst (congenital or acquired).
Hematoma.
Intrahepatic gallstones.
Old liver abscess.
Portal vein thrombosis.

Differentiate
Hemochromatosis.
Thorotrast, thallium, iron.

CALCIFICATIONS, PANCREAS ON X-RAY[16a]
ICD-9CM # 275.49

PANCREATIC CALCIFICATION

Common
Chronic pancreatitis.

Uncommon
Acute pancreatitis (saponification).
Tumors.
Cystadenoma.
Cystadenocarcinoma.
Islet cell tumor.
Metastases.

Differential Diagnosis

II

Hereditary pancreatitis (large clumps).
Hemorrhage.
Hyperparathyroidism.
Pseudocyst.
Cavernous lymphangioma.
Mucoviscidosis.
Kwashiorkor.

CALCIFICATIONS, SPLEEN ON X-RAY[16a]

ICD-9CM # 275.49

SPLENIC CALCIFICATION

Larger than 10 mm
Splenic artery aneurysm.
Splenic artery atheroma.
Cyst.
  Posttraumatic.
  Dermoid.
  Epidermoid.
  Hydatid.
Hematoma.
Infarct.
Abscess.
Tuberculosis.
Smaller than 10 mm
Histoplasmosis.
Tuberculosis.
Phleboliths.
Armillifer armillatus infestation.
Brucellosis.
Infarcts.

CALCIFICATIONS, VALVULAR ON X-RAY[16a]

ICD-9CM # 275.49

CAUSES OF RADIOGRAPHICALLY VISIBLE VALVE CALCIFICATION

Aortic Valve
Rheumatic aortic valve disease.
Bicuspid aortic valve.
Age/degenerate aortic valve.
Syphilis.
Ankylosing spondylitis.
Homograft calcification.
Mitral Valve
Rheumatic mitral valve disease.
Mitral annulus calcification.
Old vegetation (may only be visible on CT).
Homograft calcification.
Pulmonary Valve
Congenital pulmonary valve stenosis.
Rheumatic pulmonary valve disease (rare).
Fallot's tetralogy (usually after repair).
Pulmonary hypertension.
Homograft calcification.
Tricuspid Valve
Rheumatic tricuspid valve disease.
Old vegetation (may only be visible on ultrafast CT).

CALCIUM STONES

ICD-9CM # 592.9

Medications (e.g., antacids, loop diuretics, vitamin D, acetazolamide, glucocorticoids).

Primary hyperparathyroidism.
Hypercalcemia from malignancy.
Sarcoidosis.
Prolonged immobilization.
Hyperoxaluria (e.g., Crohn's disease, celiac disease, chronic pancreatitis).
Hyperuricosuria (e.g., hyperuricemia, excessive dietary purine, allopurinol, probenecid).
Renal tubular acidosis.
Milk-alkali syndrome.
Thyrotoxicosis.
Hypocitraturia (e.g., metabolic acidosis, hypomagnesemia, hypokalemia).

CARDIAC ARREST, NONTRAUMATIC[26]

ICD-9CM # 427.5 Cardiac Arrest NOS

Cardiac (coronary artery disease, cardiomyopathies, structural abnormalities, valve dysfunction, arrhythmias).
Respiratory (upper airway obstruction, hypoventilation, pulmonary embolism, asthma, COPD exacerbation, pulmonary edema).
Circulatory (tension pneumothorax, pericardial tamponade, PE, hemorrhage, sepsis).
Electrolyte abnormalities (hypokalemia or hyperkalemia, hypomagnesemia or hypermagnesemia, hypocalcemia).
Medications (tricyclic antidepressants, digoxin, theophylline, calcium channel blockers).
Drug abuse (cocaine, heroin, amphetamines).
Toxins (carbon monoxide, cyanide).
Environmental (drowning/near-drowning, electrocution, lightning, hypothermia or hyperthermia, venomous snakes).

CARDIAC DEATH, SUDDEN[1]

ICD-9CM # varies with specific disorder

Ventricular tachycardia.
Bradyarrhythmia, sick sinus syndrome.
Aortic stenosis.
Tetralogy of Fallot.
Pericardial tamponade.
Cardiac tumors.
Complications of infective endocarditis.
Hypertrophic cardiomyopathy (arrhythmia or obstruction).
Myocardial ischemia.
Atherosclerosis.
Prinzmetal's angina.
Kawasaki's arteritis.

CARDIAC ENLARGEMENT[15]

ICD-9CM # 429.3 Cardiomegaly, Idiopathic
746.89 Cardiomegaly, Congenital
402.0 Cardiomegaly, Malignant
402.1 Cardiomegaly, Benign

CARDIAC CHAMBER ENLARGEMENT

Chronic Volume Overload
Mitral or aortic regurgitation.
Left-to-right shunt (PDA, VSD, AV fistula).
Cardiomyopathy
Ischemic.
Nonischemic.

Decompensated Pressure Overload
Aortic stenosis.
Hypertension.
High-Output States
Severe anemia.
Thyrotoxicosis.
Bradycardia
Severe sinus bradycardia.
Complete heart block.

LEFT ATRIUM

LV failure of any cause.
Mitral valve disease.
Myxoma.

RIGHT VENTRICLE

Chronic volume overload.
Tricuspid or pulmonic regurgitation.
Left-to-right shunt (ASD).
Decompensated pressure overload:
  Pulmonic stenosis.
  Pulmonary artery hypertension:
  • Primary.
  • Secondary (PE, COPD).
  Pulmonary venoocclusive disease.

RIGHT ATRIUM

RV failure of any cause.
Tricuspid valve disease.
Myxoma.
Ebstein's anomaly.

MULTICHAMBER ENLARGEMENT

Hypertrophic cardiomyopathy.
Acromegaly.
Severe obesity.

PERICARDIAL DISEASE

Pericardial effusion with or without tamponade.
Effusive constrictive disease.
Pericardial cyst, loculated effusion.

PSEUDOCARDIOMEGALY

Epicardial fat.
Chest wall deformity (pectus excavatum, straight back syndrome).
Low lung volumes.
AP chest x-ray.
Mediastinal tumor, cyst.

CARDIAC MURMURS

ICD-9CM # varies with specific disorder

SYSTOLIC

Mitral regurgitation (MR).
Tricuspid regurgitation (TR).
Ventricular septal defect (VSD).
Aortic stenosis (AS).
Idiopathic hypertrophic subaortic stenosis (IHSS).
Pulmonic stenosis (PS).
Innocent murmur of childhood.
Coarctation of aorta.
Mitral valve prolapse (MVP).

DIASTOLIC

Aortic regurgitation (AR).
Atrial myxoma.
Mitral stenosis (MS).

Pulmonary artery branch stenosis.
Tricuspid stenosis (TS).
Graham Steell murmur (diastolic decrescendo murmur heard in severe pulmonary hypertension).
Pulmonic regurgitation (PR).
Severe mitral regurgitation (MR).
Austin Flint murmur (diastolic rumble heard in severe AR).
Severe VSD and patent ductus arteriosus.

CONTINUOUS

Patent ductus arteriosus.
Pulmonary AV fistula.

CARDIAC TUMORS[14a]

ICD-9CM # 164 Cardiac Tumors

PRIMARY

Benign.
  Myxoma.
  Lipoma.
  Fibroma.
  Rhabdomyoma.
  Fibroelastoma.
Malignant.
  Sarcoma.
  Mesothelioma.
  Lymphoma.

SECONDARY

Direct Extension
Lung cancer.
Breast cancer.
Mediastinal tumors.
Metastatic Tumors
Malignant melanoma.
Leukemia.
Lymphoma.
Venous Extension
Renal cell cancer.
Adrenal cancer.
Liver cancer.

CARDIOEMBOLISM

ICD-9CM # 410.9

Acute MI.
Atrial fibrillation.
Left ventricular aneurysm.
Valvular heart disease (e.g., rheumatic mitral valve disease, mitral valve prolapse).
Dilated cardiomyopathy.
Atrial septal defect.
Patent foramen ovale.
Cardioversion for atrial fibrillation.
Infective endocarditis.
Atrial septal aneurysm.
Sick sinus syndrome and cardiac arrhythmias.
Nonbacterial thrombotic endocarditis.
Prosthetic heart valves.
Atrial myxoma and other intracardiac tumors.
Cyanotic heart disease.
Balloon angioplasty.
Coronary artery bypass grafting.
Aneurysms of sinus of Valsalva.
Other: VVI pacing, ventricular support devices, heart transplantation, intracardiac defects with paradoxical embolism.

CARDIOGENIC SHOCK

ICD-9CM # 785.51

Myocardial infarction.
Arrhythmias.
Pericardial effusion/tamponade.
Chest trauma.
Valvular heart disease.
Myocarditis.
Cardiomyopathy.
CHF, end-stage.

CATARACTS, PEDIATRIC AGE

ICD-9CM # 366

DEVELOPMENTAL VARIANTS

Prematurity (Y-suture vacuoles) with or without retinopathy of prematurity.

GENETIC DISORDERS

Simple Mendelian Inheritance
Autosomal dominant (most common).
Autosomal recessive.
X-linked.
Major Chromosomal Defects
Trisomy disorders (13, 18, 21).
Turner syndrome (45X).
Deletion syndromes (11p13, 18p, 18q).
Duplication syndromes (3q, 20p, 10q).
Multisystem Genetic Disorders
Alport syndrome (hearing loss, renal disease).
Alström syndrome (nerve deafness, diabetes mellitus).
Apert disease (craniosynostosis, syndactyly).
Cockayne syndrome (premature senility, skin photosensitivity).
Conradi disease (chondrodysplasia punctata).
Crouzon disease (dysostosis craniofacialis).
Hallermann-Streiff syndrome (microphthalmia, small pinched nose, skin atrophy, hypotrichosis).
Hypohidrotic ectodermal dysplasia (anomalous dentition, hypohidrosis, hypotrichosis).
Ichthyosis (keratinizing disorder with thick, scaly skin).
Incontinentia pigmenti (dental anomalies, mental retardation, cutaneous lesions).
Lowe syndrome (oculocerebrorenal syndrome: hypotonia, renal disease).
Marfan syndrome.
Marinesco-Sjögren syndrome (cerebellar ataxia, hypotonia).
Meckel-Gruber syndrome (renal dysplasia, encephalocele).
Myotonic dystrophy.
Nail-patella syndrome (renal dysfunction, dysplastic nails, hypoplastic patella).
Nevoid basal cell carcinoma syndrome (autosomal dominant, basal cell carcinoma erupts in childhood).
Peters anomaly (corneal opacifications with iris-corneal dysgenesis).
Reiger syndrome (iris dysplasia, myotonic dystrophy).
Rothmund-Thomson syndrome (poikiloderma: skin atrophy).

Rubinstein-Taybi syndrome (broad great toe, mental retardation).
Smith-Lemli-Opitz syndrome (toe syndactyly, hypospadias, mental retardation).
Sotos syndrome (cerebral gigantism).
Spondyloepiphyseal dysplasia (dwarfism, short trunk).
Werner syndrome (premature aging in 2nd decade of life).
Inborn Errors of Metabolism
Abetalipoproteinemia (absent chylomicrons, retinal degeneration).
Fabry disease (α-galactosidase A deficiency).
Galactokinase deficiency.
Galactosemia (galactose-1-phosphate uridyl transferase deficiency).
Homocystinemia (subluxation of lens, mental retardation).
Mannosidosis (acid α-mannosidase deficiency).
Niemann-Pick disease (sphingomyelinase deficiency).
Refsum disease (phytanic acid α-hydrolase deficiency).
Wilson disease (accumulation of copper leads to cirrhosis and neurologic symptoms).

ENDOCRINOPATHIES

Hypocalcemia (hypoparathyroidism).
Hypoglycemia.
Diabetes mellitus.

CONGENITAL INFECTIONS

Toxoplasmosis.
Cytomegalovirus infection.
Syphilis.
Rubella.
Perinatal herpes simplex infection.
Measles (rubeola).
Poliomyelitis.
Influenza.
Varicella-zoster.

OCULAR ANOMALIES

Microphthalmia.
Coloboma.
Aniridia.
Mesodermal dysgenesis.
Persistent papillary membrane.
Posterior lenticonus.
Persistent hyperplastic primary vitreous.
Primitive hyaloid vascular system.

MISCELLANEOUS DISORDERS

Atopic dermatitis.
Drugs (corticosteroids).
Radiation.
Trauma.

IDIOPATHIC

CAVITARY LESION ON CHEST X-RAY[16]

ICD-9CM # 793.1 Chest X-Ray Lung Shadow

NECROTIZING INFECTIONS

Bacteria: anaerobes, *Staphylococcus aureus*, enteric gram-negative bacteria, *Pseudomonas aeruginosa*, *Legionella* species, *Haemophilus in-*

Differential Diagnosis

fluenzae, Streptococcus pyogenes, Streptococcus pneumoniae (?), Rhodococcus, Actinomyces.
Mycobacteria: Mycobacterium tuberculosis, Mycobacterium kansasii, MAI.
Bacteria-like: Nocardia species.
Fungi: Coccidioides immitis, Histoplasma capsulatum, Blastomyces hominis, Aspergillus species, Mucor species.
Parasitic: Entamoeba histolytica, Echinococcus, Paragonimus westermani.

CAVITARY INFARCTION

Bland infarction (with or without superimposed infection).
Lung contusion.

SEPTIC EMBOLISM

S. aureus, anaerobes, others.

VASCULITIS

Wegener's granulomatosis, periarteritis.

NEOPLASMS

Bronchogenic carcinoma, metastatic carcinoma, lymphoma.

MISCELLANEOUS LESIONS

Cysts, blebs, bullae, or pneumatocele with or without fluid collections.
Sequestration.
Empyema with air-fluid level.
Bronchiectasis.

CEREBRAL INFARCTION SECONDARY TO INHERITED DISORDERS
ICD-9CM # 434.91

Homocystinuria.
Marfan's syndrome.
Ehlers-Danlos syndrome.
Rendu-Osler-Weber syndrome.
Pseudoxanthoma elasticum.
Fabry's disease.

CEREBRAL VASCULITIS, CAUSES[12b]
ICD-9CM # varies with specific diagnosis

PRIMARY CEREBRAL VASCULITIDES

Takayasu arteritis.
Primary cerebral vasculitis.
Polyarteritis nodosa.

SECONDARY VASCULITIDES

Immune Disorders
Systemic lupus erythematosus.
Wegner granulomatosis.
Kawasaki syndrome.
Sarcoidosis.
Henoch-Schönlein purpura.
Primary Intracranial Infections
Bacterial meningitis (especially *Diplococcus pneumoniae*).
Tuberculous meningitis.
Mycotic infections.

Cat-scratch disease.
Human immunodeficiency virus/acquired immunodeficiency syndrome.
Malaria.
Lyme disease.
Rickettsial infections.
Brucellosis.

CEREBROVASCULAR DISEASE, ISCHEMIC[40]
ICD-9CM # 437.9

VASCULAR DISORDERS

Large-vessel atherothrombotic disease.
Lacunar disease.
Arterial-to-arterial embolization.
Carotid or vertebral artery dissection.
Fibromuscular dysplasia.
Migraine.
Venous thrombosis.
Radiation.
Complications of arteriography.
Multiple, progressive intracranial arterial occlusions.

INFLAMMATORY DISORDERS

Giant cell arteritis.
Polyarteritis nodosa.
SLE.
Granulomatous angiitis.
Takayasu's disease.
Arteritis associated with amphetamine, cocaine, or phenylpropanolamine.
Syphilis, mucormycosis.
Sjögren's syndrome.
Behçet's syndrome.

CARDIAC DISORDERS

Rheumatic heart disease.
Mural thrombus.
Arrhythmias.
Mitral valve prolapse.
Prosthetic heart valve.
Endocarditis.
Myxoma.
Paradoxical embolus.

HEMATOLOGIC DISORDERS

Thrombotic thrombocytopenic purpura.
Sickle cell disease.
Hypercoagulable states.
Polycythemia.
Thrombocytosis.
Leukocytosis.
Lupus anticoagulant.

CERVICAL INSTABILITY, PEDIATRIC
ICD-9CM # 722.2

CONGENITAL

Vertebral (Bony Anomalies)
Cranio-occipital defects (occipital vertebrae, basilar impression, occipital dysplasias, condylar hypoplasia, occipitalized atlas).
Atlantoaxial defects (aplasia of atlas arch, aplasia of odontoid process).

Subaxial anomalies (failure of segmentation and/or fusion, spina bifida, spondylolisthesis).
Ligamentous or Combined Anomalies
Found at birth as an element of somatogenic aberration.
Syndromic Disorders
Down syndrome.
Klippel-Feil syndrome.
22q11.2 deletion syndrome.
Larsen syndrome.
Marfan syndrome.
Ehlers-Danlos syndrome.

ACQUIRED

Trauma.
Infection (pyogenic, granulomatous).
Tumor (including neurofibromatosis).
Inflammatory conditions (e.g., juvenile rheumatoid arthritis).
Osteochondrodysplasias (e.g., achondroplasia, diastrophic dysplasia, metatropic dysplasia, spondyloepiphyseal dysplasia).
Storage disorders (e.g., mucopolysaccharidoses).
Metabolic disorders (rickets).
Miscellaneous (including osteogenesis imperfecta, sequela of surgery).

CHEST PAIN, CHILDREN[4]
ICD-9CM # 786.50 Chest Pain NOS
786.59 Chest Pressure
786.52 Chest Pain, Pleuritic

MUSCULOSKELETAL (COMMON)

Trauma (accidental, abuse).
Exercise, overuse injury (strain, bursitis).
Costochondritis (Tietze's syndrome).
Herpes zoster (cutaneous).
Pleurodynia.
Fibrositis.
Slipping rib.
Sickle cell anemia vasoocclusive crisis.
Osteomyelitis (rare).
Primary or metastatic tumor (rare).

PULMONARY (COMMON)

Pneumonia.
Pleurisy.
Asthma.
Chronic cough.
Pneumothorax.
Infarction (sickle cell anemia).
Foreign body.
Embolism (rare).
Pulmonary hypertension (rare).
Tumor (rare).

GASTROINTESTINAL (LESS COMMON)

Esophagitis (gastroesophageal reflux).
Esophageal foreign body.
Esophageal spasm.
Cholecystitis.
Subdiaphragmatic abscess.
Perihepatitis (Fitz-Hugh-Curtis syndrome).
Peptic ulcer disease.

CARDIAC (LESS COMMON)

Pericarditis.
Postpericardiotomy syndrome.
Endocarditis.
Mitral valve prolapse.
Aortic or subaortic stenosis.
Arrhythmias.
Marfan's syndrome (dissecting aortic aneurysm).
Anomalous coronary artery.
Kawasaki disease.
Cocaine, sympathomimetic ingestion.
Angina (familial hypercholesterolemia).

IDIOPATHIC (COMMON)

Anxiety, hyperventilation.
Panic disorder.

OTHER (LESS COMMON)

Spinal cord or nerve root compression.
Breast-related pathologic condition.
Castleman's disease (lymph node neoplasm).

CHEST PAIN (NONPLEURITIC)[9]

ICD-9CM # 786.50 Chest Pain NOS
786.59 Chest Discomfort

Cardiac: myocardial ischemia/infarction, myocarditis.
Esophageal: spasm, esophagitis, ulceration, neoplasm, achalasia, diverticula, foreign body.
Referred pain from subdiaphragmatic GI structures.
Gastric and duodenal: hiatal hernia, neoplasm, PUD.
Gallbladder and biliary: cholecystitis, cholelithiasis, impacted stone, neoplasm.
Pancreatic: pancreatitis, neoplasm.
Dissecting aortic aneurysm.
Pain originating from skin, breasts, and musculoskeletal structures: herpes zoster, mastitis, cervical spondylosis.
Mediastinal tumors: lymphoma, thymoma.
Pulmonary: neoplasm, pneumonia, pulmonary embolism/infarction.
Psychoneurosis.
Chest pain associated with mitral valve prolapse.

CHEST PAIN (PLEURITIC)

ICD-9CM # 786.52 Chest Pain, Pleuritic

Cardiac: pericarditis, postpericardiotomy/ Dressler's syndrome.
Pulmonary: pneumothorax, hemothorax, embolism/infarction, pneumonia, empyema, neoplasm, bronchiectasis, pneumomediastinum, TB, carcinomatous effusion.
GI: liver abscess, pancreatitis, esophageal rupture, Whipple's disease with associated pericarditis or pleuritis.
Subdiaphragmatic abscess.
Pain originating from skin and musculoskeletal tissues: costochondritis, chest wall trauma, fractured rib, interstitial fibrositis, myositis, strain of pectoralis muscle, herpes zoster, soft tissue and bone tumors.
Collagen vascular diseases with pleuritis.

Psychoneurosis.
Familial Mediterranean fever.

CHEST WALL TUMORS, PRIMARY[5a]

ICD-9CM # varies with specific diagnosis

SOFT TISSUE

Benign
Lipoma
Hemangioma
Lymphangioma
Fibroma
Rhabdomyoma
Neurofibroma
Desmoid tumor
Malignant
Malignant fibrous histiocytoma
Rhabdosarcoma
Liposarcoma
Neurofibrosarcoma
Leiomyosarcoma

BONY AND CARTILAGINOUS

Benign
Fibrous dysplasia
Osteochondroma
Chondroma
Askin tumor
Plasmacytoma
Malignant
Chondrosarcoma
Osteogenic sarcoma
Ewing sarcoma

CHILDHOOD EOSINOPHILIA

ICD-9CM # 288.3

PHYSIOLOGIC

Prematurity.
Infants receiving hyperalimentation.
Familial.

INFECTIOUS

Parasitic (with tissue-invasive helminths, e.g., trichinosis, strongyloidiasis, pneumocystosis, filariasis, cysticercosis, cutaneous and visceral larva migrans, echinococcosis).
Bacterial (brucellosis, tularemia, cat-scratch disease, *Chlamydia*).
Fungal (histoplasmosis, blastomycosis, coccidioidomycosis, allergic bronchopulmonary aspergillosis).
Mycobacterial (tuberculosis, leprosy).
Viral (hepatitis A, hepatitis B, hepatitis C, Epstein-Barr virus).

PULMONARY

Allergic (rhinitis, asthma).
Loeffler syndrome.
Hypersensitivity pneumonitis.
Eosinophilic pneumonia.
Pulmonary interstitial eosinophilia.

DERMATOLOGIC

Atopic dermatitis.
Pemphigus.

Dermatitis herpetiformis.
Infantile eosinophilic pustular folliculitis.
Episodic angioedema and urticaria.
Eosinophilic fasciitis (Schulman syndrome).
Eosinophilic cellulitis (Wells syndrome).
Kimura disease.

ONCOLOGIC

Neoplasm (lung, gastrointestinal, uterine).
Hodgkin disease.
Leukemia.
Myelofibrosis.

IMMUNOLOGIC

T-cell immunodeficiencies.
Hyperimmunoglobulin E (Job) syndrome.
Wiskott-Aldrich syndrome.
Graft-versus-host disease.
Drug hypersensitivity.
Post-irradiation.
Post-splenectomy.

ENDOCRINE

Post-adrenalectomy.
Addison disease.
Panhypopituitarism.

CARDIOVASCULAR

Loeffler disease (fibroplastic endocarditis).
Congenital heart disease.
Hypersensitivity vasculitis.

GASTROINTESTINAL

Milk protein allergy.
Inflammatory bowel disease.
Eosinophilic esophagitis.
Eosinophilic gastroenteritis.

CHOLANGITIS, ACUTE[5a]

ICD-9CM # 576.1 Cholangitis

NONIATROGENIC

Benign Conditions
Choledocholithiasis.
  Primary.
  Secondary.
Pancreatitis (chronic/acute), including pancreatic pseudocyst.
Papillary stenosis.
Mirizzi syndrome.
Choledochal cysts (type V, Caroli disease).
Primary sclerosing cholangitis.
Malignancies
Pancreatic cancer.
Cholangiocarcinoma.
Porta hepatis tumor/metastasis.

IATROGENIC

Obstructed biliary endoprosthesis.
Iatrogenic biliary stricture.
Direct surgical trauma.
Ischemia-induced stricture.
Anastomotic stricture (biliobiliary/bilioenteric anastomosis).

CHOLESTASIS[14]
ICD-9CM # 574.71

EXTRAHEPATIC
Choledocholithiasis.
Bile duct stricture.
Cholangiocarcinoma.
Pancreatic carcinoma.
Chronic pancreatitis.
Papillary stenosis.
Ampullary cancer.
Primary sclerosing cholangitis.
Choledochal cysts.
Parasites (e.g., ascaris, clonorchis).
AIDS.
Cholangiography.
Biliary atresia.
Portal lymphadenopathy.
Mirizzi's syndrome.

INTRAHEPATIC
Viral hepatitis.
Alcoholic hepatitis.
Drug induced.
Ductopenia syndromes.
Primary biliary cirrhosis.
Benign recurrent intrahepatic cholestasis.
Byler's disease.
Primary sclerosing cholangitis.
Alagille's syndrome.
Sarcoid.
Lymphoma.
Postoperative.
Total parenteral nutrition.
Alpha-1-antitrypsin deficiency.

CHOLESTASIS, NEONATAL AND INFANTILE, DIFFERENTIAL DIAGNOSIS[22a]
ICD-9CM # varies with specific diagnosis

INFECTIOUS
Generalized bacterial sepsis.
Viral hepatitis.
- Hepatitis A, B, C, D.
- Cytomegalovirus.
- Rubella virus.
- Herpesvirus: herpes simplex, human herpesvirus 6 and 7.
- Varicella virus.
- Coxsackievirus.
- Echovirus.
- Reovirus type 3.
- Parvovirus B19.
- HIV.
- Adenovirus.

Others.
- Toxoplasmosis.
- Syphilis.
- Tuberculosis.
- Listeriosis.
- Urinary tract infection.

TOXIC
Sepsis.
Parenteral nutrition related.
Drug related.

METABOLIC
Disorders of amino acid metabolism.
- Tyrosinemia.

Disorders of lipid metabolism.
- Wolman disease.
- Niemann-Pick disease (type C).
- Gaucher disease.

Cholesterol ester storage disease.
Disorders of carbohydrate metabolism.
- Galactosemia.
- Fructosemia.
- Glycogenosis IV.

Disorders of bile acid biosynthesis.
Other metabolic defects.
- α1-Antitrypsin deficiency.
- Cystic fibrosis.
- Hypopituitarism.
- Hypothyroidism.
- Zellweger (cerebrohepatorenal) syndrome.
- Neonatal iron storage disease.
- Indian childhood cirrhosis/infantile copper overload.
- Congenital disorders of glycosylation.
- Mitochondrial hepatopathies.
- Citrin deficiency.

GENETIC OR CHROMOSOMAL
Trisomy 17, 18, 21.
Donahue syndrome.

INTRAHEPATIC CHOLESTASIS SYNDROMES
"Idiopathic" neonatal hepatitis.
Alagille syndrome (arteriohepatic dysplasia).
Nonsyndromic bile duct paucity syndrome.
Intrahepatic cholestasis (PFIC):
- FIC-1 deficiency.
- BSEP deficiency.
- MDR3 deficiency.

Familial benign recurrent cholestasis associated with lymphedema (Aagenaes).
Congenital hepatic fibrosis.
Caroli disease (cystic dilatation of intrahepatic ducts).

EXTRAHEPATIC DISEASES
Biliary atresia.
Sclerosing cholangitis.
Bile duct stricture/stenosis.
Choledochal-pancreaticoductal junction anomaly.
Spontaneous perforation of the bile duct.
Choledochal cyst.
Mass (neoplasia, stone).
Bile/mucous plug ("inspissated bile").

MISCELLANEOUS
Shock and hypoperfusion.
Associated with enteritis.
Associated with intestinal obstruction.
Neonatal lupus erythematosus.
Myeloproliferative disease (trisomy 21).
Hemophagocytic lymphohistiocytosis (HLH).
Arthrogryposis cholestatic pigmentary (ARC) syndrome.

CHOREA
ICD-9CM # 333.5

Medications (e.g., neuroleptics, tricyclics, antiparkinsonian drugs).
Cerebral palsy.
Huntington's disease.
Benign hereditary chorea.
Thyroid disorder (hyperthyroidism, hypothyroidism).
Friedreich's ataxia.
Ataxia-telangiectasia.
Hypoglycemia, hyperglycemia.
Electrolyte abnormalities (hyponatremia, hypocalcemia, hypomagnesemia, hypernatremia).
Vitamin B_{12} deficiency.
SLE.
Wilson's disease.
Alcohol.
Cocaine.
Carbon monoxide poisoning.
Mercury poisoning.

CHOREOATHETOSIS[28]
ICD-9CM # 275.1 Choreoathetosis-Agitans Syndrome
33.5 Choreoathetosis, Paroxysmal

SYSTEMIC DISEASES
SLE.
Polycythemia.
Thyrotoxicosis.
Rheumatic fever.
Cirrhosis of the liver (acquired hepatocerebral degeneration).
DM.
Wilson's disease.

PRIMARY DEGENERATIVE BRAIN DISEASES
Huntington's chorea.
Olivopontocerebellar atrophies.
Neuroacanthocytosis.

FOCAL BRAIN DISEASES
Hemichorea.
Stroke.
Tumor.
Arteriovenous malformation.

DRUG-INDUCED CHOREOATHETOSIS
Parkinson's Disease Drugs
Levodopa.
Epilepsy Drugs
Phenytoin.
Carbamazepine.
Phenobarbital.
Gabapentin.
Valproate.
Psychostimulant Drugs
Cocaine.
Amphetamine.
Methamphetamine.
Dextroamphetamine.
Methylphenidate.
Pemoline.

Psychotropic Drugs
Lithium.
Tricyclic antidepressant drugs.
Oral Contraceptive Drugs
Cimetidine

CHYLOTHORAX

ICD-9CM # 457.8

Post lymph node dissection of neck or chest.
Subclavian venous catheterization.
Thoracic aneurysm repair.
Trauma to chest and neck.
Mediastinal tumor resection.
Esophagectomy, pneumonectomy.
Lymphangitis, mediastinitis.
Neoplasms (lymphoma, carcinoma of esophagus, lung, mediastinal malignancies).
Sympathectomy.
Venous thrombosis.
Congenital.

CLOUDY URINE

ICD-9CM # 788.69

Concentrated urine.
Use of multivitamin supplements.
Diet high in purine-rich foods.
Pyuria.
Phosphaturia.
Urinary tract infection.
Lipiduria.
Chyluria.
Hyperoxaluria.

CLUBBING

ICD-9CM # 781.5 Clubbing Finger

Pulmonary neoplasm (lung, pleura).
Other neoplasm (GI, liver, Hodgkin's, thymus, osteogenic sarcoma).
Pulmonary infectious process (empyema, abscess, bronchiectasis, TB, chronic pneumonitis).
Extrapulmonary infectious process (subacute bacterial endocarditis, intestinal TB, bacterial or amebic dysentery, arterial graft sepsis).
Pneumoconiosis.
Cystic fibrosis.
Sarcoidosis.
Cyanotic congenital heart disease.
Endocrine (Graves' disease, hyperparathyroidism).
Inflammatory bowel disease.
Celiac disease.
Chronic liver disease, cirrhosis (particularly biliary and juvenile).
Pulmonary AV malformations.
Idiopathic.
Thyroid acropachy.
Hereditary (pachydermoperiostosis).
Chronic trauma (jackhammer operators, machine workers).

COBALAMIN DEFICIENCY[20]

ICD-9CM # 266.2

ETIOPATHOPHYSIOLOGIC CLASSIFICATION OF COBALAMIN DEFICIENCY

Nutritional cobalamin deficiency (i.e., insufficient cobalamin intake):
Vegetarians, poverty-imposed near-vegetarians, breastfed infants of mothers with pernicious anemia.
Abnormal intragastric events (i.e., inadequate proteolysis of food cobalamin):
Atrophic gastritis, partial gastritis with hypochlorhydria, proton-pump inhibitors, H_2 blockers.
Loss or atrophy of gastric oxyntic mucosa (i.e., deficient intrinsic factor [IF] molecules):
Total or partial gastrectomy, pernicious anemia, caustic destruction (lye).
Abnormal events in small bowel lumen:
Inadequate pancreatic protease (e.g., R-cobalamin not degraded, cobalamin not transferred to IF):
• Insufficient pancreatic protease (i.e., pancreatic insufficiency).
• Inactivation of pancreatic protease (i.e., Zollinger–Ellison syndrome).
Usurping of luminal cobalamin (i.e., inadequate cobalamin binding to IF):
• By bacteria, during stasis syndromes (e.g., blind loops, pouches of diverticulosis, strictures, fistulas, anastomosis), impaired bowel motility (e.g., scleroderma), hypogammaglobulinemia.
• By *Diphyllobothrium latum* (fish tapeworm).
Disorders of ileal mucosa/IF–cobalamin receptors (i.e., IF–cobalamin not bound to IF–cobalamin receptors):
Diminished or absent IF–cobalamin receptors (e.g., ileal bypass, resection, fistula).
Abnormal mucosal architecture/function (e.g., tropical or nontropical sprue, Crohn's disease, tuberculosis ileitis, infiltration by lymphomas, amyloidosis).
IF-/post-IF–cobalamin receptor defects (e.g., Imerslund–Gräsbeck syndrome, transcobalamin II [TC II] deficiency).
Drug effects (e.g., slow K, metformin, cholestyramine, colchicine, neomycin).
Disorders of plasma cobalamin transport (i.e., TC II–cobalamin not delivered to TC II receptors):
Congenital TC II deficiency, defective binding of TC II–cobalamin to TC II receptors (rare).
Metabolic disorders (i.e., cobalamin not used by cells):
Inborn enzyme errors (rare).
Acquired disorders (e.g., cobalamin functionally inactivated by irreversible oxidation, N_2O inhalation).

COLIC, ACUTE ABDOMINAL[38]

ICD-9CM # 789.0

Acute gastroenteritis.
Food poisoning.
Nonspecific causes.
Constipation.

Gastric outlet obstruction:
• Chronic peptic ulceration.
• Gastric cancer.
Small bowel obstruction:
Adhesions:
• Postsurgical.
• Inflammatory (e.g., diverticular).
• Radiation.
• Meckel's diverticulum.
• Metastatic.
Stricture:
• Ischemic.
• Radiation.
• Inflammatory (e.g., Crohn's disease).
Volvulus intussusception:
• Tumor (e.g., Peutz-Jegher's syndrome).
• Superior mesenteric artery syndrome.
Intraluminal bolus:
• Gallstone.
• Bezoar.
Hernia:
• Abdominal wall.
• Internal.
Neoplasm:
• Benign (e.g., leiomyoma).
• Malignant (e.g., carcinoid tumor, adenocarcinoma).
Large bowel obstruction:
• Colon cancer.
• Diverticular disease.
• Volvulus.
Uterine:
• Missed abortion.
• Parturition.
• Period pain.

COLOR CHANGES, CUTANEOUS[34]

ICD-9CM # 709.00 Pigmentation Anomaly

BROWN

Generalized: pituitary, adrenal, liver disease, ACTH-producing tumor (e.g., oat cell lung carcinoma).
Localized: nevi, neurofibromatosis.

WHITE

Generalized: albinism.
Localized: vitiligo, Raynaud's syndrome.

RED (ERYTHEMA)

Generalized: fever, polycythemia, urticaria, viral exanthems.
Localized: inflammation, infection, Raynaud's syndrome.

YELLOW

Generalized: liver disease, chronic renal disease, anemia.
Generalized (except sclera): hypothyroidism, increased intake of vegetables containing carotene.
Localized: resolving hematoma, infection, peripheral vascular insufficiency.

BLUE

Lips, mouth, nail beds: cardiovascular and pulmonary diseases, Raynaud's.

Differential Diagnosis

II

COMA
ICD-9CM # 780.01

Vascular: hemorrhage, thrombosis, embolism.
CNS infections: meningitis, encephalitis, cerebral abscess.
Cerebral neoplasms with herniation.
Head injury: subdural hematoma, cerebral concussion, cerebral contusion.
Drugs: narcotics, sedatives, hypnotics.
Ingestion or inhalation of toxins: CO, alcohol, lead.
Metabolic disturbances.
Hypoxia.
Acid-base disorders.
Hypoglycemia, hyperglycemia.
Hepatic failure.
Electrolyte disorders.
Uremia.
Hypothyroidism.
Hypothermia, hyperthermia.
Hypotension, malignant hypertension.
Postictal.

COMA, NORMAL COMPUTED TOMOGRAPHY[1]
ICD-9CM # 780.01

MENINGEAL DISORDERS
Subarachnoid hemorrhage (uncommon).
Bacterial meningitis.
Encephalitis.
Subdural empyema.

EXOGENOUS TOXINS
Sedative drugs and barbiturates.
Anesthetics and γ-hydroxybutyrate.*
Alcohols.
Stimulants:
  Phencyclidines.[†]
  Cocaine and amphetamines.[‡]
Psychotropic drugs:
  Cyclic antidepressants.
  Phenothiazines.
  Lithium.
Anticonvulsants.
Opioids.
Clonidine.[§]
Penicillins.
Salicylates.
Anticholinergics.
Carbon monoxide, cyanide, and methemoglobinemia.

ENDOGENOUS TOXINS/ DEFICIENCIES/DERANGEMENTS
Hypoxia and ischemia.
Hypoglycemia.
Hypercalcemia.
Osmolar:
  Hyperglycemia.
  Hyponatremia.
  Hypernatremia.
Organ system failure:
  Hepatic encephalopathy.
  Uremic encephalopathy.
  Pulmonary insufficiency (carbon dioxide narcosis).

SEIZURES
Prolonged postictal state.
Spike-wave stupor.

HYPOTHERMIA OR HYPERTHERMIA
Brain stem ischemia.
Basilar artery stroke.
Brain stem or cerebellar hemorrhage.
Conversion or malingering.

---

*General anesthetic, similar to γ-aminobutyric acid; recreational drug and body building aid. Rapid onset, rapid recovery often with myoclonic jerking and confusion. Deep coma (2-3 hr; Glasgow Coma Scale = 3) with maintenance of vital signs.
†Coma associated with cholinergic signs: lacrimation, salivation, bronchorrhea, and hyperthermia.
‡Coma after seizures or status (i.e., a prolonged postictal state).
§An antihypertensive agent active through the opiate receptor system; frequent overdose when used to treat narcotic withdrawal.

COMA, PEDIATRIC POPULATION[31]
ICD-9CM # 780.01

ANOXIA
Birth asphyxia.
Carbon monoxide poisoning.
Croup/epiglottitis.
Meconium aspiration.

INFECTION
Hemolysis.
Blood loss.
Hydrops fetalis.
Infection.
Meningoencephalitis.
Sepsis.
Postimmunization encephalitis.

INCREASED INTRACRANIAL PRESSURE
Anoxia.
Inborn metabolic errors.
Toxic encephalopathy.
Reye's syndrome.
Head trauma/intracranial bleed.
Hydrocephalus.
Posterior fossa tumors.

HYPERTENSIVE ENCEPHALOPATHY
Coarctation of aorta.
Nephritis.
Vasculitis.
Pheochromocytoma.

ISCHEMIA
Hypoplastic left heart.
Shunting lesions.
Aortic stenosis.
Cardiovascular collapse (any cause).

PURPURIC CAUSES
Disseminated intravascular coagulation.
Hemolytic-uremic syndrome.
Leukemia.
Thrombotic purpura.

HYPERCAPNIA
Cystic fibrosis.
Bronchopulmonary dysplasia.
Congenital lung anomalies.

NEOPLASM
Medulloblastoma.
Glioma of brain stem.
Posterior fossa tumors.

DRUGS/TOXINS
Maternal sedation.
Alcohol.
Any drug.
Lead.
Salicylism.
Arsenic.
Pesticides.

ELECTROLYTE ABNORMALITIES
Hypernatremia (diarrhea, dehydration, salt poisoning).
Hyponatremia (SIADH, androgenital syndrome, gastroenteritis).
Hyperkalemia (renal failure, salicylism, androgenitalism).
Hypokalemia (diarrhea, hyperaldosteronism, salicylism, DKA).
Hypocalcemia (vitamin D deficiency, hyperparathyroidism).
Severe acidosis (sepsis, cold injury, salicylism, DKA).

HYPOGLYCEMIA
Birth injury or stress.
Diabetes.
Alcohol.
Salicylism.
Hyperinsulinemia.
Iatrogenic.

POSTSEIZURE
Renal Causes
Nephritis.
Hypoplastic kidneys.
Hepatic Causes
Acute hepatitis.
Fulminant hepatic failure.
Inborn metabolic errors.
Bile duct atresia.

CONGESTIVE HEART FAILURE AND CARDIOMYOPATHY[1]
ICD-9CM # 428.0 Congestive Heart Failure
425.9 Cardiomyopathy, Secondary, Unspecified

CAUSES OF CONGESTIVE HEART FAILURE AND CARDIOMYOPATHY
Coronary Artery Disease
Acute ischemia.
Myocardial infarction.
Ischemic cardiomyopathy with hibernating myocardium.

Idiopathic
Idiopathic dilated cardiomyopathy.*
Idiopathic restrictive cardiomyopathy.
Peripartum.
Pressure Overload
Hypertension.
Aortic stenosis.
Volume Overload
Mitral regurgitation.
Aortic insufficiency.
Anemia.
Atrioventricular fistula.
Toxins
Ethanol.
Cocaine.
Doxorubicin (Adriamycin).
Methamphetamine.
Metabolic-Endocrine
Thiamine deficiency.
Diabetes.
Hemochromatosis.
Thyrotoxicosis.
Obesity.
Infiltrative
Amyloidosis.
Inflammatory
Viral myocarditis.
Hereditary
Hypertrophic.
Dilated.

*Genetic bases for these cardiomyopathies have been identified in a large number of individual patients and families. Most of the mutations have been found in cardiac contractile or structural proteins.

CONJUNCTIVAL NEOPLASM

ICD-9CM # varies with specific disorder

MALIGNANT
Squamous cell carcinoma.
Melanoma.
Sebaceous carcinoma.
Kaposi's sarcoma.
Metastatic neoplasms.

BENIGN
Melanocytic nevus.
Squamous papilloma.
Hemangioma.
Lymphangioma.
Myxoma.

CONSCIOUSNESS IMPAIRMENT, ACUTE, IN CRITICALLY ILL PATIENT

ICD-9CM # 293.1

GENERAL CAUSES OF ACUTELY IMPAIRED CONSCIOUSNESS IN THE CRITICALLY ILL
Infection
Sepsis encephalopathy.
Central nervous system infection.
Drugs
Narcotics.
Benzodiazepines.

Anticholinergics.
Anticonvulsants.
Tricyclic antidepressants.
Selective serotonin uptake inhibitors.
Phenothiazines.
Steroids.
Immunosuppressants (cyclosporine, FK-506, OKT3).
Anesthetics.
Electrolyte and Acid-Base Disturbances
Hyponatremia.
Hypernatremia.
Hypercalcemia.
Hypermagnesemia.
Severe acidemia and alkalemia.
Organ System Failure
Shock.
Renal failure.
Hepatic failure.
Pancreatitis.
Respiratory failure (hypoxia, hypercapnia).
Endocrine Disorders
Hypoglycemia.
Hyperglycemia.
Hypothyroidism.
Hyperthyroidism.
Pituitary apoplexy.
Drug Withdrawal
Alcohol.
Opiates.
Barbiturates.
Benzodiazepines.
Vascular Causes
Shock.
Hypotension.
Hypertensive encephalopathy.
Central nervous system vasculitis.
Cerebral venous sinus thrombosis.
Central Nervous System Disorders
Hemorrhage.
Stroke.
Brain edema.
Hydrocephalus.
Increased intracranial pressure.
Meningitis.
Ventriculitis.
Brain abscess.
Subdural empyema.
Seizures.
Vasculitis.
Seizures
Convulsive and nonconvulsive status epilepticus.
Miscellaneous
Fat embolism syndrome.
Neuroleptic malignant syndrome.
Thiamine deficiency (Wernicke encephalopathy).
Psychogenic unresponsiveness.

CONSTIPATION

ICD-9CM # 564.0

Intestinal obstruction.
Fecal impaction.
Diverticular disease.
GI neoplasm.
Strangulated femoral hernia.
Gallstone ileus.
Tuberculous stricture.

Adhesions.
Ameboma.
Volvulus.
Intussusception.
Inflammatory bowel disease.
Hematoma of bowel wall, secondary to trauma or anticoagulants.
Poor dietary habits: insufficient bulk in diet, inadequate fluid intake.
Change from daily routine: travel, hospital admission, physical inactivity.
Acute abdominal conditions: renal colic, salpingitis, biliary colic, appendicitis, ischemia.
Hypercalcemia or hypokalemia, uremia.
Irritable bowel syndrome, pregnancy, anorexia nervosa, depression.
Painful anal conditions: hemorrhoids, fissure, stricture.
Decreased intestinal peristalsis: old age, spinal cord injuries, myxedema, diabetes, multiple sclerosis, Parkinsonism and other neurologic diseases.
Drugs: codeine, morphine, antacids with aluminum, verapamil, anticonvulsants, anticholinergics, disopyramide, cholestyramine, alosetron, iron supplements.
Hirschsprung's disease, meconium ileus, congenital atresia in infants.

CONSTIPATION, ADULT PATIENT[38]

ICD-9CM # 564

NO GROSS STRUCTURAL ABNORMALITY
Inadequate fiber intake.
Irritable bowel syndrome (associated with abdominal pain) or functional constipation.
Idiopathic slow-transit constipation.
"Obstructed defecation"—pelvic floor dysfunction (or dyssynergia).

STRUCTURAL DISORDERS
Anal fissure, infection, or stenosis.
Colon cancer or stricture.
Aganglionosis and/or abnormal myenteric plexus:
- Hirschsprung's disease.
- Chagas' disease.
- Neuropathic pseudoobstruction.
Abnormal colonic muscle:
- Myopathy.
- Dystrophia myotonica.
- Systemic sclerosis.
Idiopathic megarectum and/or megacolon.
Proximal megacolon.

NEUROLOGIC CAUSES
Diabetic autonomic neuropathy.
Damage to the sacral parasympathetic outflow.
Spinal cord damage or disease (e.g., multiple sclerosis).
Parkinson's disease.
Blunting of consciousness, mental retardation, psychosis.
Pain induced by straining (e.g., sciatic nerve compression).

Differential Diagnosis

II

ENDOCRINE OR METABOLIC CAUSES

Hypothyroidism.
Hypercalcemia.
Porphyria.
Pregnancy.

PSYCHOLOGIC DISORDERS

Depression.
Anorexia nervosa.
Denied bowel habit.

DRUG SIDE EFFECTS

CORNEAL SENSATION, DECREASED

ICD-9CM # 371.89

Herpes (simplex, zoster).
Contact lens wear.
Topical agents (NSAIDs, anesthetics, beta-blockers).
Diabetes.
Eye trauma.
Postsurgery.

COUGH

ICD-9CM # 786.2

Infectious process (viral, bacterial).
Postinfectious.
"Smoker's cough."
Rhinitis (allergic, vasomotor, postinfectious).
Asthma.
Exposure to irritants (noxious fumes, smoke, cold air).
Drug-induced (especially ACE inhibitors, beta-blockers).
GERD.
Interstitial lung disease.
Lung neoplasms.
Lymphomas, mediastinal neoplasms.
Bronchiectasis.
Cardiac (CHF, pulmonary edema, mitral stenosis, pericardial inflammation).
Recurrent aspiration.
Inflammation of larynx, pleura, diaphragm, mediastinum.
Cystic fibrosis.
Anxiety.
Other: pulmonary embolism, foreign body inhalation, aortic aneurysm, Zenker's diverticulum, osteophytes, substernal thyroid, thyroiditis, PMR.

CUTANEOUS INFECTIONS, ATHLETES

ICD-9CM # 686.9

Tinea pedis.
Tinea cruris.
Molluscum contagiosum.
Herpes simplex.
Verruca vulgaris.
Folliculitis.
Impetigo.
Furuncles.
Otitis externa.
Erythrasma.

CYANOSIS[2]

ICD-9CM # 782.5

DIFFERENTIAL DIAGNOSIS OF CYANOSIS

Peripheral Cyanosis
Low cardiac output states
Shock.
Left ventricular failure.
Hypovolemia.
Environmental exposure (cold)
Air or water.
Arterial occlusion
Thrombosis.
Embolism.
Vasospasm (Raynaud's phenomenon).
Peripheral vascular disease.
Venous obstruction
Redistribution of blood flow from extremities
Central Cyanosis
Decreased arterial oxygen saturation
High altitude (>8000 ft).
Impaired pulmonary function.
  Hypoventilation.
  Impaired oxygen diffusion.
  Ventilation-perfusion mismatching.
  • Pulmonary embolism.
  • Acture respiratory distress syndrome.
  • Pulmonary hypertension.
  Respiratory compromise.
  • Upper airway obstruction.
  • Pneumonia.
  • Diaphragmatic hernia.
  • Tension pneumothorax.
  • Polycythemia.
Anatomic Shunts
Pulmonary arteriovenous fistulae and intrapulmonary shunts.
Cerebral, hepatic, peripheral arteriovenous fistulae.
Cyanotic congenital heart disease.
  Endocardial cushion defects.
  Ventricular septal defects.
  Coarctation of aorta.
  Tetralogy of Fallot.
  Total anomalous pulmonary venous drainage.
  Hypoplastic left ventricle.
  Pulmonary vein stenosis.
  Tricuspid atresia and anomalies.
  Premature closure of foramen ovale.
  Dextrocardia.
  Pulmonary stenosis of atrial septal defect.
  Patent ductus arteriosus with reversed shunt.
Abnormal Hemoglobin
Methemoglobinemia.
  Hereditary.
  Acquired.
Sulfhemoglobinemia.
Mutant hemoglobin with low oxygen affinity (e.g., hemoglobin Kansas).

DAYTIME SLEEPINESS

ICD-9CM # varies with specific disorder

Sleep deprivation.
Medication induced (e.g., benzodiazepines, beta-blockers, narcotics, sedative antidepressants, gabapentin).

Depression.
Obstructive sleep apnea.
Medical illness (e.g., severe anemia, hypothyroidism, COPD, hepatic failure, renal insufficiency, CHF, electrolyte disturbances).
Circadian rhythm abnormalities (e.g., jet lag, shift work sleep disorder).
Restless legs syndrome.
Posttrauma.
Narcolepsy.
Neurologic disorders (e.g., neurodegenerative disorders; parkinsonism; multiple sclerosis; lesions affecting thalamus, hypothalamus, or brain stem).

DELAYED PASSAGE OF MECONIUM[16a]

ICD-9CM # 777.1

Ileal atresia.
Meconium ileus.
Functional immaturity of the colon.
Colon atresia.
Anorectal malformations.
Hirschsprung's disease.
Megacystis-microcolon-intestinal hypoperistalsis syndrome.
Extrinsic compression of the distal bowel by a mass lesion.
  Mesenteric cyst.
  Enteric duplication cyst.
Paralytic ileus, sepsis, drugs, and metabolic upset.

DELIRIUM[26]

ICD-9CM # 780.09 Delirium NOS
293.0 Acute Delirium

PHARMACOLOGIC AGENTS

Anxiolytics (benzodiazepines).
Antidepressants (e.g., amitriptyline, doxepin, imipramine).
Cardiovascular agents (e.g., methyldopa, digitalis, reserpine, propranolol, procainamide, captopril, disopyramide).
Antihistamine.
Cimetidine.
Corticosteroids.
Antineoplastics.
Drugs of abuse (alcohol, cannabis, amphetamines, cocaine, hallucinogens, opioids, sedative-hypnotics, phencyclidine).

METABOLIC DISORDERS

Hypercalcemia.
Hypercarbia.
Hypoglycemia.
Hyponatremia.
Hypoxia.

INFLAMMATORY DISORDERS

Sarcoidosis.
SLE.
Giant cell arteritis.

ORGAN FAILURE

Hepatic encephalopathy.
Uremia.

NEUROLOGIC DISORDERS

Alzheimer's disease.
CVA.
Encephalitis (including HIV).
Encephalopathies.
Epilepsy.
Huntington's disease.
Multiple sclerosis.
Neoplasms.
Normal-pressure hydrocephalus.
Parkinson's disease.
Pick's disease.
Wilson's disease.

ENDOCRINE DISORDERS

Addison's disease.
Cushing's disease.
Panhypopituitarism.
Parathyroid disease.
Postpartum psychosis.
Recurrent menstrual psychosis.
Sydenham's chorea.
Thyroid disease.

DEFICIENCY STATES

Niacin.
Thiamine, vitamin B_{12}, and folate.

DELIRIUM AND AGITATION, DRUG-INDUCED

ICD-9CM # 293.1

COMMONLY USED DRUGS ASSOCIATED WITH DELIRIUM AND AGITATION

Benzodiazepines.
Opiates (especially meperidine).
Anticholinergics.
Antihistamines.
H_2 blockers.
Antibiotics.
Corticosteroids.
Metoclopramide.

DELIRUM, AGITATED[2]

ICD-9CM # 293.1

Metabolic causes:
   Electrolyte abnormalities.
   Hypoglycemia.
   Hypoxia.
   Uremia/hyperammonemia.
Structural lesions of the CNS:
   Trauma.
   Stroke.
   Hemorrhage.
   Mass.
Endocrine disease:
   Thyrotoxicosis.
Infections:
   Bacterial/viral meningitis/encephalitis.
Toxicologic causes:
   Sympathomimetic/stimulants.
   • Cocaine.
   • Amphetamines and derivatives.
   • Caffeine.
   • Phencyclidine/ketamine.

   Anticholinergics.
   Serotonin syndrome.
   Sedative-hypnotic withdrawal.
Heatstroke.
Postictal state.

CNS, Central nervous system.

DELIRIUM, DIALYSIS PATIENT[26]

ICD-9CM # 293.0 Acute Delirium
             293.9 Encephalopathy from Dialysis

STRUCTURAL

Cerebrovascular accident (particularly hemorrhage).
Subdural hematoma.
Intracerebral abscess.
Brain tumor.

METABOLIC

Disequilibrium syndrome.
Uremia.
Drug effects.
Meningitis.
Hypertensive encephalopathy.
Hypotension.
Postictal state.
Hypernatremia or hyponatremia.
Hypercalcemia.
Hypermagnesemia.
Hypoglycemia.
Severe hyperglycemia.
Hypoxemia.
Dialysis dementia.

DEMYELINATING DISEASES[40]

ICD-9CM # 341.9

MULTIPLE SCLEROSIS

Relapsing and chronic progressive forms.
Acute multiple sclerosis.
Neuromyelitis optica (Devic's disease).

DIFFUSE CEREBRAL SCLEROSIS

Schilder's encephalitis periaxialis diffusa.
Baló's concentric sclerosis.

ACUTE DISSEMINATED ENCEPHALOMYELITIS

After measles, chickenpox, rubella, influenza, mumps.
After rabies or smallpox vaccination.

NECROTIZING HEMORRHAGIC ENCEPHALITIS

Hemorrhagic leukoencephalitis.

LEUKODYSTROPHIES

Krabbe's globoid leukodystrophy.
Metachromatic leukodystrophy.
Adrenoleukodystrophy.
Adrenomyeloneuropathy.
Pelizaeus-Merzbacher leukodystrophy.
Canavan's disease.
Alexander's disease.

DIAPHRAGM ELEVATION, BILATERAL, SYMMETRICAL[16a]

ICD-9CM # 519.4

CAUSES OF BILATERAL SYMMETRICAL ELEVATION OF THE DIAPHRAGM

Supine position.
Poor inspiration.
Obesity.
Pregnancy.
Abdominal distention (ascites, intestinal obstruction, abdominal mass).
Diffuse pulmonary fibrosis.
Lymphangitis carcinomatosa.
Disseminated lupus erythematosus.
Bilateral basal pulmonary emboli.
Painful conditions (after abdominal surgery).
Bilateral diaphragmatic paralysis.

DIAPHRAGM ELEVATION, UNILATERAL[16a]

ICD-9CM # 519.4

CAUSES OF UNILATERAL ELEVATION OF THE DIAPHRAGM

Posture—lateral decubitus position (dependent side).
Gaseous distention of stomach or colon.
Dorsal scoliosis.
Pulmonary hypoplasia.
Pulmonary collapse.
Phrenic nerve palsy.
Eventration.
Pneumonia or pleurisy.
Pulmonary thromboembolism.
Rib fracture and other painful conditions.
Subphrenic infection.
Subphrenic mass.

DIARRHEA, ACUTE WATERY AND BLOODY[38]

ICD-9CM # varies with specific diagnosis
       009.3   Infectious Diarrhea
       558.9   Non-infectious Diarrhea
       564.5   Functional Diarrhea
       787.91 Diarrhea

ACUTE WATERY DIARRHEA

Gastrointestinal infections:
• Protozoal (e.g., *Giardia*).
• Bacterial (e.g., enterotoxigenic *Escherichia coli,* cholera).
• Viral (e.g., rotavirus, Norwalk virus).
Drugs.
Toxins.
Dietary constituents (e.g., lactose intolerance).
Onset of chronic diarrheal illness.

ACUTE BLOODY DIARRHEA

Infectious colitis:
• Confluent proctocolitis (e.g., *Shigella, Campylobacter, Salmonella, Entamoeba histolytica*).

Differential Diagnosis

II

- Segmental colitis (e.g., *Campylobacter*, *Salmonella*, enteroinvasive *E. coli*, *Aeromonas*, *E. histolytica*).

Drug-induced colitis (e.g., nonsteroidal anti-inflammatory drugs [NSAIDs]).

Inflammatory bowel disease.

Ischemic colitis (usually elderly patient with underlying heart disease or arrhythmias).

Antibiotic-associated colitis.

DIARRHEA, INFECTIOUS[2]
ICD-9CM # 009.2

ETIOLOGIC AGENTS OF INFECTIOUS DIARRHEA

Viral (60% of Cases)

Astrovirus.
Calicivirus.
Coronavirus.
Cytomegalovirus.*
Enteric adenovirus.
Hepatitis A through G.
Herpes simplex virus.
HIV enteropathy.
Norwalk-like agents.
Pararotavirus.
Norwalk virus.
Picomavirus.
Rotavirus.
Small round viruses.

Bacterial (20% of Cases)

Invasive*

Aeromonas spp.
Campylobacter spp.
Clostridium difficile.
Enteroinvasive *E. coli.*
Mycobacterium spp.
Plesiomonas shigelloides.
Salmonella spp.
Shigella spp.
Vibrio fluvialis.
Vibrio parahaemolyticus.
Vibrio vulnificus.
Yersinia enterocolitica.
Yersinia pseudotuberculosis.

Toxigenic

Food poisoning with preformed toxins.
   Bacillus cereus.
   Clostridium botulinum.
   Staphylococcus aureus.
Toxin formation after colonization.
   Aeromonas hydrophila.
   Clostridium perfringens.
   Enterohemorrhagic *E. coli* O157:H7.*
   Enterotoxigenic *E. coli.*
   Klebsiella pneumoniae.
   Shigella spp.
   Vibrio cholerae.

Other bacteria

Parasitic (5% of Cases)

Protozoa

*Balantidium coli.**
Blastocystis hominis.
Cryptosporidium.
Cyclospora.
Dientamoeba fragilis.
*Entamoeba histolytica.**
Entamoeba polecki.

Enteromonas hominis.
Giardia lamblia.
Isospora belli.
Microsporidia.
Sarcocystis hominis.

Helminths

Angiostrongylus costaricense.
Anisakiasis.
Ascaris lumbricoides.
Diphyllobothrium latum.
Enterobius vermicularis.
Hookworms.
Schistosoma spp.
Strongyloides stercoralis.
Taenia spp.
Trichinella spiralis.
Trichuris trichiura.

---

*Associated with fever, abdominal pain, and fecal red blood cells or white blood cells. % indicates the estimated contribution to total cases.

DIARRHEA, NONINFECTIOUS[2]
ICD-9CM # 564.5

CAUSES OF NONINFECTIOUS DIARRHEA

Toxins

Drugs

ACE inhibitors.
Alprazolam.
Antacids (Mg).
Antibiotics.
Antidepressants.
Antiepileptic drugs.
Antihypertensives.
Antiparkinson drugs.
Beta-blockers.
Caffeine.
Cardiac antiarrhythmics.
Chemotherapy agents.
Cholesterol-lowering drugs.
Cholinergic agents.
Cholinesterase inhibitors.
Colchicine.
Digitalis.
Diuretics.
Flurouracil.
Fluoxetine.
Histamine H_2-receptor antagonists.
Hydralazine.
Lactulose.
Laxatives/cathartics.
Levodopa.
Lithium.
NSAIDs.
Neomycin.
Podophyllin.
Procainamide.
Prostaglandins.
Quinidine.
Ricinoleic acid.
Theophylline.
Thyroid hormone.
Valproic acid.

Dietetic foods

Mannitol.
Sorbitol.
Xylitol.

Fish-associated toxins

Amnestic shellfish poisoning.
Ciguatera.
Echinoderms.
Neurotoxic shellfish poisoning.
Paralytic shellfish poisoning.
Scombroid.
Tetroton.

Plant-associated toxins

Herbal preparations.
Horse chestnut.
Mushrooms—*Amanita* spp.
Nicotine.
Other plant toxins:
   Pesticides—organophosphates.
   Pokeweed.
   Rhubarb.
Miscellaneous:
   Allergic reactions.
   Carbon monoxide poisoning.
   Ethanol.
   Heavy metals.
   Monosodium glutamate (MSG).
   Opiate withdrawal.

Gastrointestinal Pathology

Appendicitis.
Autonomic dysfunction.
Bile acid malabsorption.
Blind loop.
Bowel obstruction.
Celiac disease.
Cirrhosis.
Defects in amino acid transport.
Diverticular disease.
Familial dysautonomia.
Fecal impaction.
Fecal incontinence.
GI bleed.
GI cancer.
Hirschsprung's disease.
Inflammatory bowel disease (ulcerative colitis, Crohn's disease).
Intussusception.
Irritable bowel syndrome.
Ischemic bowel.
Lactose/fructose intolerance.
Malabsorption syndromes.
Malrotation.
Postsurgical.
Postvagotomy.
Radiation therapy.
Short gut syndrome.
Small bowel resection.
Strictures.
Toxic megacolon.
Tropical sprue.
Volvulus.
Whipple's disease.

Endocrine-related

Carcinoid syndrome (serotonin).
Hormonal hypersecretion.
Hyperthyroidism (thyroid hormone).
Medullary carcinoma of the thyroid (calcitonin).
Pancreatic cholera (VIP).
Somatostatinoma (somatostatin).
Systemic mastocytosis (histamine).
Zollinger-Ellison syndrome (gastrin).

Endocrine pathology

Adrenal insufficiency.

Diabetes enteropathy.
Hypoparathyroidism.
Pancreatic insufficiency.
Systemic Illness/Other
Alcoholism.
Amyloidosis.
Connective tissue disease.
Cystic fibrosis.
Ectopic pregnancy.
Hemolytic-uremic syndrome.
Henoch-Schönlein purpura.
Lymphoma.
Otitis media—infants.
Pelvic inflammatory disease.
Pneumonia/sepsis.
Pyelonephritis.
Scleroderma/SLE.
Severe malnutrition.
Stevens-Johnson syndrome.
Toxic shock syndrome.
Wilson's disease.
Miscellaneous:
    Factitious diarrhea.
    Runner's diarrhea.

ACE, Angiotensin-converting enzyme; *GI,* gastrointestinal; *NSAIDs,* nonsteroidal anti-inflammatory drugs; *SLE,* systemic lupus erythematosus; *VIP,* vasoactive intestinal polypeptide.

DIARRHEA, TUBE-FED PATIENT[14]
ICD-9CM # 564.4

COMMON CAUSES UNRELATED TO TUBE FEEDING
Elixir medications containing sorbitol.
Magnesium-containing antacids.
Antibiotic-induced sterile gut.
Pseudomembranous colitis.

POSSIBLE CAUSES RELATED TO TUBE FEEDING
Inadequate fiber to form stool bulk.
High fat content of formula (in the presence of fat malabsorption syndrome).
Bacterial contamination of enteral products and delivery systems (causal association with diarrhea not documented).
Rapid advancement in rate (after the GI tract is unused for prolonged periods).

UNLIKELY CAUSES RELATED TO TUBE FEEDING
Formula hyperosmolality (proven not to be the cause of diarrhea).
Lactose (absent from nearly all enteral feeding formulas).

DIPLOPIA, BINOCULAR
ICD-9CM # 368.2

Cranial nerve palsy (3rd, 4th, 6th).
Thyroid eye disease.
Myasthenia gravis.
Decompensated strabismus.
Orbital trauma with blowout fracture.
Orbital pseudotumor.
Cavernous sinus thrombosis.

DIPLOPIA, MONOCULAR
ICD-9CM # 368.2

Postoperative corrected longstanding tropia.
Defective contact lenses.
Poorly fitting bifocals.
Trauma to iris.
Corneal disorder (e.g., dry eye, astigmatism).
Cataracts.
Lens subluxation.
Nystagmus.
Eyelid twitching.
Foreign body in aqueous or vitreous media.
Migraine.
Lesions of occipital cortex.
Psychogenic.

DIPLOPIA, VERTICAL
ICD-9CM # 368.2

Myasthenia.
Superior oblique palsy.
Myositis or pseudotumor with orbital involvement.
Lymphoma or metastases affecting the orbits.
Brain stem or cerebellar lesions.
Hydrocephalus.
Third nerve palsy.
Botulism.
Wernicke's encephalopathy.
Dysthyroid orbitopathy (muscle infiltration).

DIZZINESS
ICD-9CM # 780.4

Viral syndrome.
Anxiety, hyperventilation.
Benign positional paroxysmal vertigo.
Medications (e.g., sedatives, antihypertensives, analgesics).
Withdrawal from medications (e.g., benzodiazepines, SSRIs).
Alcohol or drug abuse.
Postural hypotension.
Hypoglycemia, hyperglycemia.
Hematologic disorders (e.g., anemia, polycythemia, leukemia).
Head trauma.
Menière's disease.
Vertebrobasilar ischemia.
Cervical osteoarthritis.
Cardiac abnormalities (arrhythmias, cardiomyopathy, CHF, pericarditis).
Multiple sclerosis.
Peripheral vestibulopathy.
Air or sea travel.
Electrolyte abnormalities.
Eye problems (cornea, lens, retina).
Migraine.
Brain stem infarct.
Autonomic neuropathy.
Chronic otomastoiditis.
Complex partial seizures.
Ramsey Hunt syndrome.
Arteritis.
Syncope and presyncope.
Perilymph fistula.
Cerebellopontine tumor.
Hepatic or renal disease.

DRY EYE
ICD-9CM # 375.15

Contacts.
Medications (antihistamines, clonidine, beta-blockers, ibuprofen, scopolamine).
Keratoconjunctivitis sicca.
Trauma.
Environmental causes (air conditioning in patient with contacts).

DYSPAREUNIA[12]
ICD-9CM # 625.0   Dyspareunia
           608.89 Dyspareunia, Male
           302.76 Dyspareunia, Psychogenic

INTROITAL
Vaginismus.
Intact or rigid hymen.
Clitoral problems.
Vulvovaginitis.
Vaginal atrophy: hypoestrogen.
Vulvar dystrophy.
Bartholin or Skene gland infection.
Inadequate lubrication.
Operative scarring.

MIDVAGINAL
Urethritis.
Trigonitis.
Cystitis.
Short vagina.
Operative scarring.
Inadequate lubrication.

DEEP
Endometriosis.
Pelvic infection.
Uterine retroversion.
Ovarian pathology.
GI.
Orthopedic.
Abnormal penile size or shape.

DYSPHAGIA
ICD-9CM # 787.2

Esophageal obstruction: neoplasm, foreign body, achalasia, stricture, spasm, esophageal web, diverticulum, Schatzki's ring.
Peptic esophagitis with stricture, Barrett's stricture.
External esophageal compression: neoplasms (thyroid neoplasm, lymphoma, mediastinal tumors), thyroid enlargement, aortic aneurysm, vertebral spurs, aberrant right subclavian artery (dysphagia lusoria).
Hiatal hernia, GERD.
Oropharyngeal lesions: pharyngitis, glossitis, stomatitis, neoplasms.
Hysteria: globus hystericus.
Neurologic and/or neuromuscular disturbances: bulbar paralysis, myasthenia gravis, ALS, multiple sclerosis, Parkinsonism, CVA, diabetic neuropathy.
Toxins: poisoning, botulism, tetanus, postdiphtheritic dysphagia.

Differential Diagnosis

II

Systemic diseases: scleroderma, amyloidosis, dermatomyositis.
Candida and herpes esophagitis.
Presbyesophagus.

DYSPHAGIA, OROPHARYNGEAL[38]
ICD-9CM # 787.22

FUNCTIONAL DISORDERS
Central Nervous System
Stroke.
Head injury.
Parkinson's disease.
Motor neuron disease.
Multiple sclerosis.
Tumor.
Drugs (e.g., phenothiazines).
Malformations (e.g., syrinx, Arnold–Chiari).
Neural
Motor neuron disease.
Myasthenia gravis.
Radiotherapy.
Poliomyelitis.
Familial dysautonomia.
Muscle
Autoimmune myopathy (polymyositis, dermatomyositis, systemic lupus erythematosus).
Thyrotoxic myopathy.
Guillain-Barré motor neuropathy.
Muscular dystrophies.

STRUCTURAL DISORDERS
Head/neck surgery.
Stricture.
Radiotherapy.
Tumor.
Pharyngeal pouch.
Web.
Extrinsic (e.g., osteophytes).

MISCELLANEOUS
Xerostomia.

DYSPNEA
ICD-9CM # 786.00

Upper airway obstruction: trauma, neoplasm, epiglottitis, laryngeal edema, tongue retraction, laryngospasm, abductor paralysis of vocal cords, aspiration of foreign body.
Lower airway obstruction: neoplasm, COPD, asthma, aspiration of foreign body.
Pulmonary infection: pneumonia, abscess, empyema, TB, bronchiectasis.
Pulmonary hypertension.
Pulmonary embolism/infarction.
Parenchymal lung disease.
Pulmonary vascular congestion.
Cardiac disease: ASHD, valvular lesions, cardiac dysrhythmias, cardiomyopathy, pericardial effusion, cardiac shunts.
Space-occupying lesions: neoplasm, large hiatal hernia, pleural effusions.
Disease of chest wall: severe kyphoscoliosis, fractured ribs, sternal compression, morbid obesity.
Neurologic dysfunction: Guillain-Barré syndrome, botulism, polio, spinal cord injury.

Interstitial pulmonary disease: sarcoidosis, collagen vascular diseases, DIP, Hamman-Rich pneumonitis, etc.
Pneumoconioses: silicosis, berylliosis, etc.
Mesothelioma.
Pneumothorax, hemothorax, pleural effusion.
Inhalation of toxins.
Cholinergic drug intoxication.
Carcinoid syndrome.
Hematologic: anemia, polycythemia, hemoglobinopathies.
Thyrotoxicosis, myxedema.
Diaphragmatic compression caused by abdominal distention, subphrenic abscess, ascites.
Lung resection.
Metabolic abnormalities: uremia, hepatic coma, DKA.
Sepsis.
Atelectasis.
Psychoneurosis.
Diaphragmatic paralysis.
Pregnancy.

DYSURIA
ICD-9CM # 788.1 Dysuria
306.53 Dysuria, Psychogenic

Urinary tract infection.
Estrogen deficiency (in postmenopausal female).
Vaginitis.
Genital infection (e.g., herpes, condyloma).
Interstitial cystitis.
Chemical irritation (e.g., deodorant aerosols, douches).
Meatal stenosis or stricture.
Reiter's syndrome.
Bladder neoplasm.
GI etiology (diverticulitis, Crohn's disease).
Impaired bladder or sphincter action.
Urethral carbuncle.
Chronic fibrosis posttrauma.
Radiation therapy.
Prostatitis.
Urethritis (gonococcal, *Chlamydia*).
Behçet's syndrome.
Stevens-Johnson syndrome.

EARACHE[33]
ICD-9CM # 388.70 Earache
388.72 Ear Pain, Referred

Otitis media.
Serous otitis media.
Eustachitis.
Otitis externa.
Otitic barotrauma.
Mastoiditis.
Foreign body.
Impacted cerumen.
Referred otalgia, as with TMJ dysfunction, dental problems, and tumors.

ECTOPIC ACTH SECRETION[14]
ICD-9CM # 255.0

Small cell carcinoma of lung.
Endocrine tumors of foregut origin.
  Thymic carcinoid.
  Islet cell tumor.

Medullary carcinoid, thyroid.
Bronchial carcinoid.
Pheochromocytoma.
Ovarian tumors.

EDEMA, CHILDREN[19]
ICD-9CM # 782.3 Edema NOS

CARDIOVASCULAR
Congestive heart failure.
Acute thrombi or emboli.
Vasculitis of many types.

RENAL
Nephrotic syndrome.
Glomerulonephritis of many types.
End-stage renal failure.

ENDOCRINE OR METABOLIC
Thyroid disease.
Starvation.
Hereditary angioedema.

IATROGENIC
Drugs (diuretics and steroids).
Water or salt overload.

HEMATOLOGIC
Hemolytic disease of the newborn.

GASTROINTESTINAL
Hepatic cirrhosis.
Protein-losing enteritis.
Lymphangiectasis.
Cystic fibrosis.
Celiac disease.
Enteritis of many types.

LYMPHATIC ABNORMALITIES
Congenital (gonadal dysgenesis).
Acquired.

EDEMA, GENERALIZED
ICD-9CM # 782.3 Edema NOS

Congestive heart failure (CHF).
Cirrhosis.
Nephrotic syndrome.
Pregnancy.
Idiopathic.
Acute nephritic syndrome.
Myxedema.
Medications (NSAIDs, estrogens, vasodilators).

EDEMA, LEG, UNILATERAL[26]
ICD-9CM # 782.3

WITH PAIN
DVT.
Postphlebitic syndrome.
Popliteal cyst rupture.
Gastrocnemius rupture.
Cellulitis.
Psoas or other abscess.

WITHOUT PAIN
DVT.
Postphlebitic syndrome.

Other venous insufficiency (after saphenous vein harvest, varicosities).

Lymphatic obstruction/lymphedema (carcinoma, lymphoma, sarcoidosis, filariasis, retroperitoneal fibrosis).

EDEMA OF LOWER EXTREMITIES

ICD-9CM # 782.3

CHF (right-sided).
Hepatic cirrhosis.
Nephrosis.
Myxedema.
Lymphedema.
Pregnancy.
Abdominal mass: neoplasm, cyst.
Venous compression from abdominal aneurysm.
Varicose veins.
Bilateral cellulitis.
Bilateral thrombophlebitis.
Vena cava thrombosis, venous thrombosis.
Retroperitoneal fibrosis.

EJECTION SOUND OR CLICK

ICD-9CM # 785.3

Aortic regurgitation.
Aortic root dilatation.
Systemic hypertension.
Chronic pulmonary hypertension.
Tetralogy of Fallot.
Atrial septal defect.
Pulmonary valve stenosis.
Aortic aneurysm.

ELBOW PAIN

ICD-9CM # 719.42

Trauma.
Infection.
Inflammatory arthritis.
Lateral or medial epicondylitis.
Entrapment neuropathy.
Olecranon bursitis.
Osteoarthritis.
Gout.
Cervical disease (referred pain).
Shoulder disease (referred pain).
Partial subluxation.
Synovial osteochondromatosis.
Loose body.

ELEVATED HEMIDIAPHRAGM

ICD-9CM # 519.4 Diaphragm Disorder
519.4 Diaphragm Paralysis
756.6 Diaphragm Eventration, Congenital

Neoplasm (bronchogenic carcinoma, mediastinal neoplasm, intrahepatic lesion).
Substernal thyroid.
Infectious process (pneumonia, empyema, TB, subphrenic abscess, hepatic abscess).
Atelectasis.
Idiopathic.
Eventration.

Phrenic nerve dysfunction (myelitis, myotonia, herpes zoster).
Trauma to phrenic nerve or diaphragm (e.g., surgery).
Aortic aneurysm.
Intraabdominal mass.
Pulmonary infarction.
Pleurisy.
Radiation therapy.
Rib fracture.

EMBOLI, ARTERIAL[26]

ICD-9CM # 444.22 Embolism, Artery, Lower Extremity
444.21 Embolism, Artery, Upper Extremity

Myocardial infarction with mural thrombi.
Atrial fibrillation.
Cardiomyopathies.
Prosthetic heart valves.
CHF.
Endocarditis.
Left ventricular aneurysm.
Left atrial myxoma.
Sick sinus syndrome.
Paradoxical embolus from venous thrombosis.
Aneurysms of large blood vessels.
Atheromatous ulcers of large blood vessels.

EMESIS, PEDIATRIC AGE[19]

ICD-9CM # 787.03

INFANCY

Gastrointestinal Tract
Congenital:
Regurgitation—chalasia, gastroesophageal reflux.
Atresia—stenosis (tracheoesophageal fistula, prepyloric diaphragm, intestinal atresia).
Duplication.
Volvulus (errors in rotation and fixation, Meckel diverticulum).
Congenital bands.
Hirschsprung's disease.
Meconium ileus (cystic fibrosis), meconium plug.
Acquired:
Acute infectious gastroenteritis, food poisoning (staphylococcal, clostridial).
Pyloric stenosis.
Gastritis, duodenitis.
Intussusception.
Incarcerated hernia—inguinal, internal secondary to old adhesions.
Cow's milk protein intolerance, food allergy, eosinophilic gastroenteritis.
Disaccharidase deficiency.
Celiac disease—presents after introduction of gluten in diet; inherited risk.
Adynamic ileus—the mediator for many nongastrointestinal causes.
Neonatal necrotizing enterocolitis.
Chronic granulomatous disease with gastric outlet obstruction.
Nongastrointestinal Tract
Infectious—otitis, urinary tract infection, pneumonia, upper respiratory tract infection, sepsis, meningitis.

Metabolic—aminoaciduria and organic aciduria, galactosemia, fructosemia, adrenogenital syndrome, renal tubular acidosis, diabetic ketoacidosis, Reye's syndrome.
Central nervous system—trauma, tumor, infection, diencephalic syndrome, rumination, autonomic responses (pain, shock).
Medications—anticholinergics, aspirin, alcohol, idiosyncratic reaction (e.g., codeine).

CHILDHOOD

Gastrointestinal Tract
Peptic ulcer—vomiting is a common presentation in children younger than 6 yr old.
Trauma—duodenal hematoma, traumatic pancreatitis, perforated bowel.
Pancreatitis—mumps, trauma, cystic fibrosis, hyperparathyroidism, hyperlipidemia, organic acidemias.
Crohn's disease.
Idiopathic intestinal pseudoobstruction.
Superior mesenteric artery syndrome.
Nongastrointestinal Tract
Central nervous system—cyclic vomiting, migraine, anorexia nervosa, bulimia.

ENCEPHALOMYELITIS, NONVIRAL CAUSES[25]

ICD-9CM # varies with specific disorder

Subacute bacterial endocarditis.
Rocky Mountain spotted fever.
Typhus.
Ehrlichia.
Q fever.
Chlamydia.
Mycoplasma.
Legionella.
Brucellosis.
Listeria.
Whipple's disease.
Cat-scratch disease.
Syphilis (meningovascular).
Relapsing fever.
Lyme disease.
Leptospirosis.
Nocardia.
Actinomycosis.
Tuberculosis.
Cryptococcus.
Histoplasma.
Toxoplasma.
Plasmodium falciparum.
Trypanosomiasis.
Behçet's disease.
Vasculitis.
Carcinoma.
Drug reactions.

ENCEPHALOPATHY, HYPERTENSIVE

ICD-9CM # 293.9

Cerebral infarction.
Subarachnoid hemorrhage.
Intracerebral hemorrhage.
Subdural or epidural hematoma.
Brain tumor or other mass lesion.
Seizure disorder.

Differential Diagnosis

II

Central nervous system vasculitis.
Encephalitis/meningitis.
Drug ingestion.
Drug withdrawal.

ENCEPHALOPATHY, METABOLIC[36]

ICD-9CM # 291.2   Alcoholic Encephalopathy
          572.2   Hepatic Encephalopathy
          251.2   Hypoglycemic
                  Encephalopathy
       349.82   Toxic Encephalopathy
         984.9   Lead Encephalopathy
         293.9   Encephalopathy

Substrate deficiency: hypoxia/ischemia, carbon monoxide poisoning, hypoglycemia.
Cofactor deficiency: thiamine, vitamin B_{12}, pyridoxine (INH administration).
Electrolyte disorders: hyponatremia, hypercalcemia, carbon dioxide narcosis, dialysis, hypermagnesemia, disequilibrium syndrome.
Endocrinopathies: DKA, hyperosmolar coma, hypothyroidism, hyperadrenocorticism, hyperparathyroidism.
Endogenous toxins: liver disease, uremia, porphyria.
Exogenous toxins: drug overdose (sedative/hypnotics, ethanol, narcotics, salicylates, tricyclic antidepressants), drug withdrawal, toxicity of therapeutic medications, industrial toxins (e.g., organophosphates, heavy metals), sepsis.
Heat stroke.
Epilepsy (postictal).

ENTHESOPATHY

ICD-9CM # code not available

Viremia or bacteremia.
Ankylosing spondylitis.
Psoriatic arthritis.
Drug-induced (quinolones, etretinate).
Reactive arthritis.
DISH.
Reiter's syndrome.

EOSINOPHILIC LUNG DISEASE[16a]

ICD-9CM # 495.8

IDIOPATHIC

Simple pulmonary eosinophilia (Löffler's syndrome).
Acute eosinophilic pneumonia.
Chronic eosinophilic pneumonia.
Hypereosinophilic syndrome.

DRUG-INDUCED

Aminosalicylic acid.
Para-arminosalicylic acid.
NSAIDs.
Captopril.
Cocaine.
Minocycline.
Nitrofurantoin.
Phenytoin.

INFECTION

Parasitic (ascariasis, paragonimiasis. tropical eosinophilia).

Fungal (aspergillus).
Bacterial (TB, atypical mycobacterial infection, brucella).
Viral (respiratory syncytial virus).

IMMUNOLOGIC DISEASES

Wegener's granulomatosis.
Churg–Strauss syndrome.
Rheumatoid disease.
Sarcoidosis.

NEOPLASMS

Bronchogenic carcinoma.
Bronchial carcinoid.
Lymphoma (Hodgkin's, non-Hodgkin's).

EPIGASTRIC PAIN[38]

ICD-9CM # 789.66

Peptic ulceration (uncomplicated).*
Peptic ulceration (perforated).*
Biliary colic.*
Acute pancreatitis.*
Abdominal aortic aneurysm.
Anxiety.
Inferior wall MI.

---

*Conditions that also cause right upper quadrant pain.

EPILEPSY

ICD-9CM # 345.9 Epilepsy NOS

Psychogenic spells.
Transient ischemic attack.
Hypoglycemia.
Syncope.
Narcolepsy.
Migraine.
Paroxysmal vertigo.
Arrhythmias.
Drug reaction.

EPISTAXIS

ICD-9CM # 784.7

Trauma.
Medications (nasal sprays, NSAIDs, anticoagulants, antiplatelets).
Nasal polyps.
Cocaine use.
Coagulopathy (hemophilia, liver disease, DIC, thrombocytopenia).
Systemic disorders (hypertension, uremia).
Infections.
Anatomic malformations.
Rhinitis.
Nasal polyps.
Local neoplasms (benign and malignant).
Desiccation.
Foreign body.

ERECTILE DYSFUNCTION, ORGANIC[31]

ICD-9CM # 607.84

Neurogenic abnormalities: Somatic nerve neuropathy, central nervous system abnormalities.

Psychogenic causes: Depression, performance anxiety, marital conflict.
Endocrine causes: Hyperprolactinemia, hypogonadotropic hypogonadism, testicular failure, estrogen excess.
Trauma: Pelvic fracture, prostate surgery, penile fracture.
Systemic disease: DM, renal failure, hepatic cirrhosis.
Medications: Diuretics, antidepressants, H_2 blockers, exogenous hormones, alcohol, antihypertensives, nicotine abuse, finasteride, etc.
Structural abnormalities: Peyronie's disease.

EROSIONS, GENITALIA

ICD-9CM # 599.84

Candidiasis.
Intraepithelial neoplasia.
Squamous cell carcinoma.
Lichen planus.
Pemphigus vulgaris.
Erythema multiforme.
Lichen sclerosus.
Bullous pemphigoid.
Extramammary Paget's disease.
Impetigo.

ERYTHEMATOUS ANNULAR SKIN LESIONS

ICD-9CM # varies with diagnosis

Tinea corporis.
Warfarin plaques.
Erythema multiforme.
Erythema annulare.
Cutaneous lupus.
Cutaneous sarcoidosis.
Trauma.
Acute febrile neutrophilic dermatosis (Sweet's syndrome).

ERYTHROCYTOSIS[20]

ICD-9CM # 289.6

CAUSES OF ERYTHROCYTOSIS

Relative or Spurious Erythrocytosis (Normal Red Cell Mass)
Hemoconcentration secondary to dehydration (diarrhea, diaphoresis, diuretics, water deprivation, emesis, ethanol, hypertension, preeclampsia, pheochromocytoma, carbon monoxide intoxication).
True or Absolute Erythrocytosis
Polycythemia vera.
Primary congenital polycythemia.
Secondary erythrocytosis caused by:
     Congenital causes (e.g., activating mutation of erythropoietin receptor).
     Hypoxia caused by carbon monoxide poisoning, high oxygen affinity hemoglobin, high-altitude residence, chronic pulmonary disease, hypoventilation syndromes such as sleep apnea, right to left cardiac shunt, neurologic defects involving the respiratory center.

Nonhypoxic causes with pathologic erythropoietin production.
- Renal disease (cysts, hydronephrosis, renal artery stenosis, focal glomerulonephritis, renal transplantation).
- Tumors (renal cell cancer, hepatocellular carcinoma, cerebellar hemangioblastoma, uterine fibromyoma, adrenal tumors, meningioma, pheochromocytoma).

Drug-associated causes:
- Androgen therapy.
- Exogenous erythropoietin growth factor therapy.

ERYTHRODERMA

ICD-9CM # 695.9   Secondary
696.2   Maculopapular
696.1   Psoriaticum
695.89 Exfoliative
778.8   Neonatorum

Drug reaction (e.g., allopurinol, ampicillin, phenytoin, vancomycin, dapsone, omeprazole, carbamazepine).
Atopic dermatitis.
Psoriasis.
Contact dermatitis.
Idiopathic.
Pityriasis rubra.
Chronic actinic dermatitis.
Bullous pemphigoid.
Paraneoplastic.
Cutaneous T-cell lymphoma.
Connective tissue disease.
Hypereosinophilia syndrome.

ESOPHAGEAL PERFORATION[26]

ICD-9CM # 530.4   Perforation, Nontraumatic
862.22 Injury, Traumatic

Trauma.
Caustic burns.
Iatrogenic.
Foreign bodies.
Spontaneous rupture (Boerhaave's syndrome).
Postoperative breakdown of anastomosis.

ESOPHAGITIS[25]

ICD-9CM # 530.12

INFECTIOUS
Candidiasis.
Cytomegalovirus.
Herpes simplex virus.
HIV infection, acute.

NONINFECTIOUS
Gastroesophageal reflux.
Mucositis from cancer chemotherapy.
Mucositis from radiation therapy.
Aphthous ulcers.

ESOTROPIA

ICD-9CM # 378.00 Nonaccommodative
378.35 Accommodative
378.05 Alternating

Congenital.
Accommodative esotropia.
Myasthenia gravis.
Abducens palsy.
Pseudo-sixth nerve palsy.
Medial rectus entrapment (e.g., blowout fracture).
Posterior internuclear ophthalmoplegia.
Wernicke's encephalopathy.
Thyroid myopathy.
Chiari malformation.

EXANTHEMS[28]

ICD-9CM # 782.1

Measles.
Rubella.
Erythema infectiosum (fifth disease).
Roseola exanthema.
Varicella.
Enterovirus.
Adenovirus.
Epstein-Barr virus.
Kawasaki disease.
Staphylococcal scalded skin.
Scarlet fever.
Meningococcemia.
Rocky Mountain spotted fever.

EYELID NEOPLASM

ICD-9CM # varies with specific disorder

MALIGNANT
Melanoma.
Basal cell carcinoma.
Squamous cell carcinoma.
Bowen's disease.
Sebaceous cell carcinoma.
Metastatic lymphoma/leukemia.

BENIGN
Melanocytic nevus.
Pilar, eccrine, or apocrine tumor.
Neurofibroma.
Keratosis.
Squamous papilloma.
Keratoacanthoma.

EYELID RETRACTION

ICD-9CM # 374.89

Congenital.
Graves' ophthalmopathy.
Myasthenia gravis.
Postsurgical.
Guillain-Barré syndrome.
Cerebellar disease.
Horizontal gaze palsy.
Partial palsy of superior rectus muscle.
Encephalitis.
Closed head injury.
Disseminated sclerosis.
Eye trauma.
Contact lens wear.

Proptosis.
Eyelid neoplasm.
Atopic dermatitis.
Herpes zoster ophthalmicus.
Botulinum toxin injection.
Cyclic oculomotor paralysis.
Spheroid wing meningioma.
Hepatic cirrhosis.
Down syndrome.
Essential hypertension.
Meningitis.
Paget's disease of bone.

EYE PAIN

ICD-9CM # 379.91

Foreign body.
Herpes zoster.
Trauma.
Conjunctivitis.
Iritis.
Iridocyclitis.
Uveitis.
Blepharitis.
Ingrown lashes.
Orbital or periorbital cellulitis/abscess.
Sinusitis.
Headache.
Glaucoma.
Inflammation of lacrimal gland.
Tic douloureux.
Cerebral aneurysm.
Cerebral neoplasm.
Entropion.
Retrobulbar neuritis.
UV light.
Dry eyes.
Irritation or inflammation from eye drops, dust, cosmetics, etc.

FACIAL PAIN

ICD-9CM # 784.0

Infection, abscess.
Postherpetic neuralgia.
Trauma, posttraumatic neuralgia.
Tic douloureux.
Cluster headache, "lower-half headache."
Geniculate neuralgia.
Anxiety, somatization syndrome.
Glossopharyngeal neuralgia.
Carotidynia.

FACIAL PARALYSIS[28]

ICD-9CM # 351.0 Facial (7th Nerve) Palsy

INFECTION
Bacterial: otitis media, mastoiditis, meningitis, Lyme disease.
Viral: herpes zoster, mononucleosis, varicella, rubella, mumps, Bell's palsy.
Mycobacterial: TB, meningitis, leprosy.
Miscellaneous: syphilis, malaria.

TRAUMA
Temporal bone fracture, facial laceration.
Surgery.

Differential Diagnosis

II

NEOPLASM

Malignant: squamous cell carcinoma, basal cell and adenocystic tumors, leukemia, parotid neoplasms, metastatic tumors.

Benign: facial nerve neuroma, vestibular schwannoma, congenital cholesteatoma.

IMMUNOLOGIC

Guillain-Barré syndrome, periarteritis nodosa.
Reaction to tetanus antiserum.

METABOLIC

Pregnancy.
Hypothyroidism.
DM.

FAILURE TO THRIVE

ICD-9CM # 783.4

PSYCHOSOCIAL/BEHAVIORAL

Inadequate diet because of poverty/food insufficiency, errors in food preparation.
Poor parenting skills (lack of knowledge of sufficient diet).
Child/parent interaction problems (autonomy struggles, coercive feeding, maternal depression).
Food refusal.
Rumination.
Parental cognitive or mental health problems.
Child abuse or neglect; emotional deprivation.

NEUROLOGIC

Cerebral palsy.
Hypothalamic and other CNS tumors (diencephalic syndrome).
Neuromuscular disorders.
Neurodegenerative disorders.

RENAL

Recurrent urinary tract infection.
Renal tubular acidosis.
Renal failure.

ENDOCRINE

Diabetes mellitus.
Diabetes insipidus.
Hypothyroidism/hyperthyroidism.
Growth hormone deficiency.
Adrenal insufficiency.

GENETIC/METABOLIC/ CONGENITAL

Sickle cell disease.
Inborn errors of metabolism (organic acidosis, hyperammonemia, storage disease).
Fetal alcohol syndrome.
Skeletal dysplasias.
Chromosomal disorders.
Multiple congenital anomaly syndromes (VATER [vertebral defects, imperforate anus, tracheoesophageal fistula, radial and renal dysplasia], CHARGE [coloboma, heart disease, atresia choanae, retarded growth and retarded development and/or central nervous system anomalies, genital hypoplasia, ear anomalies and/or deafness]).

GASTROINTESTINAL

Pyloric stenosis.
Gastroesophageal reflux.
Repair of tracheoesophageal fistula.
Malrotation.
Malabsorption syndromes.
Celiac disease.
Milk intolerance: lactose, protein.
Pancreatic insufficiency syndromes (cystic fibrosis).
Chronic cholestasis.
Inflammatory bowel disease.
Chronic congenital diarrhea states.
Short bowel syndrome.
Pseudoobstruction.
Hirschsprung disease.
Food allergy.

CARDIAC

Cyanotic heart lesions.
Congestive heart failure.
Vascular rings.

PULMONARY/RESPIRATORY

Severe asthma.
Cystic fibrosis; bronchiectasis.
Chronic respiratory failure.
Bronchopulmonary dysplasia.
Adenoid/tonsillar hypertrophy.
Obstructive sleep apnea.

MISCELLANEOUS

Collagen vascular disease.
Malignancy.
Primary immunodeficiency.
Transplantation.

INFECTIONS

Perinatal infection (TORCHES [toxoplasma, other, rubella, cytomegalovirus, herpes simplex]).
Occult/chronic infections.
Parasitic infestation.
Tuberculosis.
HIV.

FATIGUE

ICD-9CM # 780.7 Fatigue NOS
　　　　　300.5 Fatigue Psychogenic
　　　　　780.7 Chronic Fatigue Syndrome

Depression.
Anxiety, emotional stress.
Inadequate sleep.
Chronic fatigue syndrome.
Prolonged physical activity.
Pregnancy and postpartum period.
Anemia.
Hypothyroidism.
Medications (beta-blockers, anxiolytics, antidepressants, sedating antihistamines, clonidine, methyldopa).
Viral or bacterial infections.
Sleep apnea syndrome.
Dieting.
Renal failure, CHF, COPD, liver disease.

FATIGUE, CHRONIC

ICD-9CM # 780.7

CHRONIC INFECTIONS

Hepatitis C.
Lyme disease.
Parasitic and fungal infections.
Tuberculosis.
Human immunodeficiency virus.
Xenotropic murine leukemia retrovirus.

SLEEP DISORDERS

Obstructive sleep apnea.
Restless leg syndrome.
Circadian rhythm disorder.
Upper airway resistance syndrome.
Narcolepsy/parasomnias.
Alpha-delta sleep disorder.

ENDOCRINE/METABOLIC DISORDERS

Addison's disease.
Cushing's syndrome.
Poorly controlled diabetes.
Thyroid disorders.
Hemochromatosis.
Hypopituitarism.
Diabetes insipidus.

GENERAL MEDICAL DISORDERS

Anemia (any cause).
Chronic renal/hepatic failure.
Malnutrition.
Medication side effects.
Chronic pain disorders.

PSYCHOLOGICAL

Mood disorders (depression, anxiety, bipolar).
Schizophrenia.
Posttraumatic stress disorder.
Anorexia nervosa/bulimia.
Childhood abuse and/or neglect.

CHRONIC INFLAMMATION

Rheumatoid arthritis.
Systemic lupus erythematosus.
Sjögren's syndrome.
Polymyositis/dermatomyositis.
Vasculitis.
Sarcoidosis.

CARDIOPULMONARY

Congestive heart failure.
Neurally mediated hypotension.
Postural orthostatic tachycardia syndrome.
Pulmonary hypertension.
Chronic obstructive pulmonary disease.
Mitral valve prolapse.

GASTROINTESTINAL

Celiac disease.
Inflammatory bowel disease.
Autoimmune hepatitis.
Hepatic cirrhosis.

MALIGNANCY

Lymphoma and occult malignancies.
Postchemotherapy syndrome.

NEUROLOGIC DISORDERS

Multiple sclerosis.
Myasthenia gravis.
Muscular dystrophies.
Parkinson's disease.
Early dementia.

LIFESTYLE FACTORS

Chronic overwork.
Persistent unresolved stress.
Inadequate exercise.
Morbid obesity (body mass index >40).
Alcoholism/drug abuse.

FATTY LIVER

ICD-9CM # 571.8

Obesity.
Alcohol abuse.
DM.
Acute fatty liver of pregnancy.
Medications (tetracycline, valproic acid, glucocorticoids, amiodarone, estrogen, methotrexate).
Reye's syndrome.
Wilson's disease.
Nonalcoholic steatosis.

FEVER AND JAUNDICE

ICD-9CM # 789.6

Bacterial sepsis.
Cholangitis.
Hepatic abscess.
Leptospirosis.
Malaria.
Viral hepatitis.
Yellow fever.

FEVER AND LYMPHADENOPATHY

ICD-9CM # 780.60

Regional
Cervical
Streptococci.
Tuberculosis.
Viral upper respiratory infection.
Peripheral
Bartonella henselae.
Herpesviruses.
Lymphoma.
Metastatic cancer.
Sporotrichosis.
Streptococci.
Inguinal
Chancroid.
Herpes.
Lymphogranuloma venereum.
Syphilis (primary).
GENERALIZED
Cytomegalovirus.
Epstein-Barr virus.
HIV.
Lymphoma.
Sarcoidosis.
Syphilis (secondary).
Toxoplasmosis.
Viral hepatitis.

FEVER AND RASH

ICD-9CM # 782.1 Exanthem
57.9 Exanthem, Viral
789.6 Fever

Drug hypersensitivity: penicillin, sulfonamides, thiazides, anticonvulsants, allopurinol.
Viral infection: measles, rubella, varicella, erythema infectiosum, roseola, enterovirus infection, viral hepatitis, infectious mononucleosis, acute HIV.
Other infections: meningococcemia, staphylococcemia, scarlet fever, typhoid fever, *Pseudomonas* bacteremia, Rocky Mountain spotted fever, Lyme disease, secondary syphilis, bacterial endocarditis, babesiosis, brucellosis, listeriosis.
Serum sickness.
Erythema multiforme.
Erythema marginatum.
Erythema nodosum.
SLE.
Dermatomyositis.
Allergic vasculitis.
Pityriasis rosea.
Herpes zoster.

FEVER AND RASH IN ICU

ICD-9CM # 782.1 Exanthem
789.6 Fever

DIFFERENTIAL DIAGNOSTIC CLINICAL FEATURES OF FEVER AND RASH IN THE ICU

Rash with Shock
Infectious causes: toxic shock syndrome, meningococcemia, postsplenectomy sepsis, overwhelming *Staphylococcus aureus* bacteremia/acute bacterial endocarditis, arboviral hemorrhagic fevers, hemorrhagic smallpox, *Vibrio vulnificus,* gas gangrene, dengue fever.
Noninfectious cause: systemic lupus erythematosus (on steroids).
Rash with Mental Changes
Infectious causes: Rocky Mountain spotted fever, meningococcemia (with meningitis), *S. aureus* acute bacterial endocarditis, Chikungunya fever, typhus.
Noninfectious cause: systemic lupus erythematosus.
Rash with Conjunctival Suffusion
Infectious causes: Rocky Mountain spotted fever, dengue fever, arboviral hemorrhagic fevers, toxic shock syndrome.
Noninfectious cause: adult Kawasaki's disease.
Rash with Relative Bradycardia
Infectious causes: Rocky Mountain spotted fever, typhus, dengue fever, typhoid, arboviral hemorrhagic fevers.
Noninfectious cause: drug rash.
Rash with Abdominal Pain
Infectious causes: *V. vulnificus,* gas gangrene, *Clostridium sordelli,* scarlet fever.
Noninfectious causes: cholesterol emboli syndrome, systemic lupus erythematosus.

Rash on Palms and Soles
Infectious causes: Rocky Mountain spotted fever, toxic shock syndrome, chickenpox, smallpox, monkeypox, scarlet fever.
Noninfectious cause: drug rash.
Rash with Diarrhea
Infectious causes: *V. vulnificus,* gas gangrene, toxic shock syndrome, dengue fever, arboviral hemorrhagic fevers.
Noninfectious cause: none.
Rash with Edema of Dorsum of Hands/Feet
Infectious causes: Rocky Mountain spotted fever, toxic shock syndrome.
Noninfectious cause: adult Kawasaki's disease.
Rash with Bullae
Infectious causes: *V. vulnificus, S. aureus* complicated skin/skin structure infection, gas gangrene.
Noninfectious cause: none.
Rash with Heart Murmur
Infectious cause: acute bacterial endocarditis.
Noninfectious cause: systemic lupus erythematosus.
Rash with Gangrene of Nose Tip
Infectious cause: *S. aureus* acute bacterial endocarditis.
Noninfectious causes: systemic lupus erythematosus, vasculitis.
Rash with Cerebrovascular Accident
Infectious causes: cholesterol emboli syndrome, *S. aureus* acute bacterial endocarditis.
Noninfectious cause: none.
Rash with Splenomegaly
Infectious causes: Rocky Mountain spotted fever, typhus.
Noninfectious causes: systemic lupus erythematosus, adult Kawasaki's disease.
Rash with Deafness
Infectious causes: Rocky Mountain spotted fever, typhus, meningococcal meningitis.
Noninfectious cause: none.
Rash with Hepatosplenomegaly
Infectious causes: Rocky Mountain spotted fever, typhus.
Noninfectious cause: atypical measles.
Rash with Hepatomegaly
Infectious cause: typhus.
Noninfectious cause: none.

FEVER, AFTER TRAVEL TO THE TROPICS[1a]

ICD-9CM # 789.6

CAUSES OF FEVER AFTER TRAVEL TO THE TROPICS
80% of Specific Infections Causing Fever (Includes Respiratory and Urinary Tract Infection)
Malaria.
Viral hepatitis.
Febrile illness unrelated to foreign travel.
Dengue fever.
Enteric fever (typhoid and paratyphoid fevers).

Other Causes
Gastroenteritis.
Rickettsia.
Leptospirosis.
Schistosomiasis.
Amebic liver abscess.
Tuberculosis.
Acute HIV infection.
Others.

FEVER, DRUG-INDUCED[14a]

ICD-9CM # 789.6

SELECTED AGENTS ASSOCIATED WITH DRUG-INDUCED FEVER

Common
Antimicrobial:
    Amphotericin B.
    β-Lactams.
    Sulfonamides.
Cardiovascular:
    Procainamide.
    Quinidine.
Central nervous system:
    Carbamazepine.
    Phenytoin.
Miscellaneous:
    Bleomycin.
    Interferon-α.
    Interleukin-2.
Less Common
Antimicrobial:
    Clindamycin.
    Fluoroquinolones.
    Rifampin.
Cardiovascular:
    Diltiazem.
    Hydralazine.
Central nervous system:
    Haloperidol.
    Serotonin reuptake inhibitors.
Miscellaneous:
    Allopurinol.
    Cimetidine.
    Tacrolimus.

FEVER, HOSPITAL ASSOCIATED[14a]

ICD-9CM # 780.60 Fever

SELECTED CAUSES OF HOSPITAL-ASSOCIATED FEVER

Common
Infectious:
    Clostridium difficile enterocolitis.
    Pneumonia.
    Surgical wound.
    Urinary tract.
    Vascular catheter.
Noninfectious:
    Drug-induced fever.
    Hematoma.
    Immediate postoperative state.
    Transfusion reaction.
    Venous thromboembolism.

Less Common
Infectious:
    Biliary tract disease.
    Endometritis.
    Intraabdominal abscess.
    Mediastinitis.
    Sinusitis.
Noninfectious:
    Adrenal insufficiency.
    Gout.
    Myocardial infarction.
    Organ infarction.
    Pancreatitis.

FEVER IN RETURNING TRAVELERS AND IMMIGRANTS[28]

ICD-9CM # varies with specific disorder

Differential diagnosis of some selected systemic febrile illnesses to consider in returned travelers and immigrants.*

COMMON

Acute respiratory tract infection (worldwide).
Gastroenteritis (worldwide) [foodborne, waterborne, fecal-oral].
Enteric fever, including typhoid (worldwide) [food, water].
Urinary tract infection (worldwide) [sexual contact].
Drug reactions [antibiotics, prophylactic agents, other] {rash frequent}.
Malaria (tropics, limited areas of temperate zones) [mosquitoes].
Arboviruses (Africa; tropics) [mosquitoes, ticks, mites].
Dengue (Asia, Caribbean, Africa) [mosquitoes].
Viral hepatitis (worldwide).
Hepatitis A (worldwide) [food, fecal-oral].
Hepatitis B (worldwide, especially Asia, sub-Saharan Africa) [sexual contact] {long incubation period}.
Hepatitis C (worldwide) [blood or sexual contact].
Hepatitis E (Asia, North Africa, Mexico, others) [food, water].
Tuberculosis (worldwide) [airborne, milk] {long period to symptomatic infection}.
Sexually transmitted diseases (worldwide) [sexual contact].

LESS COMMON

Filariasis (Asia, Africa, South America) [biting insects] {long incubation period, eosinophilia}.
Measles (developing world) [airborne] {in susceptible individual}.
Amebic abscess (worldwide) [food].
Brucellosis (worldwide) [milk, cheese, food, animal contact].
Listeriosis (worldwide) [foodborne] {meningitis}.
Leptospirosis (worldwide) [animal contact, open fresh water] {jaundice, meningitis}.
Strongyloidiasis (warm and tropical areas) [soil contact] {eosinophilia}.
Toxoplasmosis (worldwide) [undercooked meat].

RARE

Relapsing fever (western Americas, Asia, northern Africa) [ticks, lice].
Hemorrhagic fevers (worldwide) [arthropod and nonarthropod transmitted].
Yellow fever (tropics) [mosquitoes] {hepatitis}.
Hemorrhagic fever with renal syndrome (Europe, Asia, North America) [rodent urine] {renal impairment}.
Hantavirus pulmonary syndrome (western North America, other) [rodent urine] {respiratory distress syndrome}.
Lassa fever (Africa) [rodent excreta, person to person] {high mortality rate}.
Other—chikungunya, Rift Valley, Ebola-Marburg, etc. (various) [insect bites, rodent excreta, aerosols, person to person] {often severe}.
Rickettsial infections {rashes and eschars}.
Leishmaniasis, visceral (Middle East, Mediterranean, Africa, Asia, South America) [biting flies] {long incubation period}.
Acute schistosomiasis (Africa, Asia, South America, Caribbean) [fresh water].
Chagas' disease (South and Central America) [reduviid bug bites] {often asymptomatic}.
African trypanosomiasis (Africa) [tsetse fly bite] {neurologic syndromes, sleeping sickness}.
Bartonellosis (South America) [sandfly bite] {skin nodules}.
HIV infection/AIDS (worldwide) [sexual and blood contact].
Trichinosis (worldwide) [undercooked meat] {eosinophilia}.
Plague (temperate and tropical plains) [animal exposures and fleas].
Tularemia (worldwide) [animal contact, fleas, aerosols] {ulcers, lymph nodes}.
Anthrax (worldwide) [animal, animal product contact] {ulcers}.
Lyme disease (North America, Europe) [tick bites] {arthritis, meningitis, cardiac abnormalities}.

---

*Diagnoses for which particular symptoms are indicative are in *italics*. Exposure to regions of the world that are most likely to be significant to the diagnosis are presented in (parentheses). Vectors, risk behaviors, and sources associated with acquisition are presented in [brackets]. Special clinical characteristics are listed within {braces}.

FEVER, NONINFECTIOUS CAUSES[2]

ICD-9CM # 780.60

DIFFERENTIAL DIAGNOSIS— NONINFECTIOUS CAUSES OF FEVER

Critical Diagnoses
Acute myocardial infarction.
Pulmonary embolism/infarction.
Intracranial hemorrhage.
Cerebrovascular accident.
Neuroleptic-malignant syndrome.
Thyroid storm.
Acute adrenal insufficiency.
Transfusion reaction.
Pulmonary edema.

Emergent Diagnoses
Congestive heart failure.
Dehydration.
Recent seizure.
Sickle cell disease.
Transplant rejection.
Pancreatitis.
Deep vein thrombosis.
Nonemergent Diagnoses
Drug fever.
Malignancy.
Gout.
Sarcoidosis.
Crohn's disease.
Postmyocardiotomy syndrome.

FEVER, RECURRENT OR PERIODIC, IN CHILDREN[22a]
ICD-9CM # 780.60 Fever

INFECTIOUS DISEASES
Brucellosis.
Rat-bite fever.
Relapsing fever.

RHEUMATIC DISEASES
Juvenile idiopathic arthritis (systemic onset).
Behçet disease.
Systemic lupus erythematosus.
Relapsing polychondritis.
Crohn's disease.

HEREDITARY AUTOINFLAMMATORY SYNDROMES
Familial Mediterranean fever (FMF).
Cryopyrinopathies:
   Familial cold autoinflammatory syndrome (FCAS).
   Muckle-Wells syndrome (MWS).
   Chronic infantile neurologic cutaneous and articular (CINCA) syndrome, also called neonatal-onset multisystem inflammatory disease (NOMID).
Tumor necrosis factor receptor–associated periodic syndrome (TRAPS).
Hyperimmunoglobulinemia D with periodic fever syndrome (HIDS).

CYCLIC HEMATOPOIESIS
Hereditary form.
Acquired form.

IDIOPATHIC CONDITIONS
Periodic fever with aphthous stomatitis, pharyngitis, and adenitis (PFAPA).

FINGER LESIONS, INFLAMMATORY
ICD-9CM # varies with specific disorder

Paronychia.
Herpes simplex type 1 (herpetic whitlow).
Dyshidrotic eczema (pompholyx).
Herpes zoster.
Bacterial endocarditis (Osler's nodes).
Psoriatic arthritis.

FLACCID PARALYSIS, ACUTE, DIFFERENTIAL DIAGNOSIS[22a]
ICD-9CM # 344.9   Flaccid Paralysis

Brain stem stroke.
Brain stem encephalitis.
Acute anterior poliomyelitis.
- Caused by poliovirus.
- Caused by other neurotropic viruses.
Acute myelopathy.
- Space-occupying lesions.
- Acute transverse myelitis.
Peripheral neuropathy.
- Guillain-Barré syndrome.
- Post-rabies vaccine neuropathy.
- Diphtheritic neuropathy.
- Heavy metals, biologic toxins, or drug intoxication.
- Acute intermittent porphyria.
- Vasculitic neuropathy.
- Critical illness neuropathy.
- Lymphomatous neuropathy.
Disorders of neuromuscular transmission.
- Myasthenia gravis.
- Biologic or industrial toxins.
- Tic paralysis.
Disorders of muscle.
- Hypokalemia.
- Hypophosphatemia.
- Inflammatory myopathy.
- Acute rhabdomyolysis.
- Trichinosis.
- Periodic paralyses.

FLATULENCE AND BLOATING[33]
ICD-9CM # 787.3

Ingestion of nonabsorbable carbohydrates.
Ingestion of carbonated beverages.
Malabsorption: pancreatic insufficiency, biliary disease, celiac disease, bacterial overgrowth in small intestine.
Lactase deficiency.
Irritable bowel syndrome.
Anxiety disorders.
Food poisoning, giardiasis.

FLUSHING[27]
ICD-9CM # 782.62

Physiologic flushing: menopause, ingestion of monosodium glutamate (Chinese restaurant syndrome), ingestion of hot drinks.
Drugs: alcohol (with or without disulfiram, metronidazole, or chlorpropamide), nicotinic acid, diltiazem, nifedipine, levodopa, bromocriptine, vancomycin, amyl nitrate.
Neoplastic disorders: carcinoid syndrome, VIPoma syndrome, medullary carcinoma of thyroid, systemic mastocytosis, basophilic chronic myelocytic leukemia, renal cell carcinoma.
Anxiety.
Agnogenic flushing.

FOLATE DEFICIENCY[20]
ICD-9CM # 281.2

ETIOPATHOPHYSIOLOGIC CLASSIFICATION OF FOLATE DEFICIENCY
Nutritional causes:
  Decreased dietary intake:
- Poverty and famine.
- Institutionalized individuals (e.g., psychiatric, nursing homes), chronic debilitating disease.
- Prolonged feeding of infants with goat's milk, special slimming diets or food fads (i.e., folate-rich foods not consumed), cultural or ethnic cooking techniques (i.e., food folate destroyed).
  Decreased diet and increased requirements:
- Physiologic (e.g., pregnancy and lactation, prematurity, hyperemesis gravidarum, infancy).
- Pathologic (e.g., intrinsic hematologic diseases involving hemolysis with compensatory erythropoiesis, abnormal hematopoiesis, or bone marrow infiltration with malignant disease and dermatologic disease such as psoriasis).
Folate malabsorption:
  With normal intestinal mucosa:
- Some drugs (controversial).
- Congenital folate malabsorption (rare).
  With mucosal abnormalities (e.g., tropical and nontropical sprue, regional enteritis).
Defective cellular folate uptake:
  Familial aplastic anemia (rare).
  Acute cerebral folate deficiency.
Inadequate cellular use:
  Folate antagonists (e.g., methotrexate).
  Hereditary enzyme deficiencies involving folate.
Drugs:
  Multiple effects on folate metabolism (e.g., alcohol, sulfasalazine, triamterene, pyrimethamine, trimethoprim-sulfamethoxazole, diphenylhydantoin, barbiturates).
Acute folate deficiency:
  Intensive care unit setting.
  Uncertain origin.

FOOT AND ANKLE PAIN, IN DIFFERENT AGE GROUPS[8]
ICD-9CM # varies with specific diagnosis

COMMON CAUSES OF FOOT AND ANKLE PAIN IN DIFFERENT AGE GROUPS
Childhood (2-10 yr)
Intraarticular:
Club foot.
Congenital midfoot and forefoot deformities.
Septic arthritis.
Periarticular:
Osteomyelitis.
Adolescence (10-18 yr)
Intraarticular:
Arch disorders (pes cavus, pes planus).

Periarticular:
Osteomyelitis.
Tumors.
Early Adulthood (18-30 yr)
Intraarticular:
Metatarsalgia.
Hallux valgus.
Hallux rigidus.
Osteochondritis.
Accessory ossicles.
Periarticular:
Achilles tendonitis.
Achilles tendon rupture.
Fasciitis.
Referred:
Lumbar spine.
Knee.
Adulthood (30-50 yr)
Intraarticular:
Osteoarthritis.
Inflammatory arthritis.
Gout.
Metatarsalgia.
Hallux valgus.
Hallux rigidus.
Osteochondritis.
Accessory ossicles.
Periarticular:
Ischemic foot pain.
Diabetes.
Bursitis.
Tendonitis.
Plantar fasciitis.
Corns.
Referred:
Lumbar spine.
Knee.
Old Age (> 50 yr)
Intraarticular:
Osteoarthritis.
Inflammatory arthritis.
Gout.
Metatarsalgia.
Hallux valgus.
Hallux rigidus.
Periarticular:
Ischemic foot pain.
Diabetes.
Bursitis.
Tendonitis.
Plantar fasciitis.
Corns.
Referred:
Lumbar spine.
Knee.

FOOT DERMATITIS
ICD-9CM # varies with specific disorder

Tinea pedis.
Dyshidrotic eczema.
Tylosis (mechanically induced hyperkeratosis, fissuring, and dryness).
Allergic contact dermatitis.
Psoriasis.
Peripheral vascular insufficiency.
Neuropathic foot ulcers (DM, poorly fitting shoes).
Acquired plantar keratoderma.
Sézary's syndrome.

FOOTDROP
ICD-9CM # varies with specific disorder

Peripheral neuropathy.
L5 radiculopathy.
Peroneal nerve compression.
Sciatic nerve palsy.
Scapuloperoneal syndromes.
Spasticity.
Peroneal nerve compression.
Myopathy.
Dystonia.

FOOT LESION, ULCERATING
ICD-9CM # 917.9

Cellulitis.
Plantar wart.
Squamous cell carcinoma.
Actinomycosis (Madura foot).
Plantar fibromatosis.
Pseudoepitheliomatous hyperplasia.

FOOT PAIN
ICD-9CM # varies with specific diagnosis

Trauma (fractures, musculoskeletal and ligamentous strain).
Inflammation (plantar fasciitis, Achilles tendonitis or bursitis, calcaneal apophysitis).
Arterial insufficiency, Raynaud's phenomenon, thromboangiitis obliterans.
Gout, pseudogout.
Calcaneal spur.
Infection (cellulitis, abscess, lymphangitis, gangrene).
Decubitus ulcer.
Paronychia, ingrown toenail.
Thrombophlebitis, postphlebitic syndrome.

FOOT PAIN BY AGE[22a]
ICD-9CM # varies with specific diagnosis

0-6 YEARS
Poorly fitting shoes.
Foreign body.
Fracture.
Osteomyelitis.
Leukemia.
Puncture wound.
Drawing of blood.
Dactylitis.
Juvenile rheumatoid arthritis (JRA).

6-12 YEARS
Poorly fitting shoes.
Sever disease.
Enthesopathy (JRA).
Foreign body.
Accessory navicular.
Tarsal coalition.
Ewing sarcoma.
Hypermobile flatfoot.
Trauma (sprains, fractures).
Puncture wound.

12-20 YEARS
Poorly fitting shoes.

Stress fracture.
Foreign body.
Ingrown toenail.
Metatarsalgia.
Plantar fasciitis.
Osteochondroses (avascular necrosis).
Freiberg.
Köhler.
Achilles tendinitis.
Trauma (sprains).
Plantar warts.
Tarsal coalition.

FOREARM AND HAND PAIN
ICD-9CM # 959.3 Forearm Injury
959.4 Hand Injury

Epicondylitis.
Tenosynovitis.
Osteoarthritis.
Cubital tunnel syndrome.
Carpal tunnel syndrome.
Trauma.
Herpes zoster.
Peripheral vascular insufficiency.
Infection (cellulitis, abscess).

GAIT ABNORMALITY
ICD-9CM # 781.2 Gait Abnormality

Parkinsonism.
Degenerative joint disease (hips, back, knees).
Multiple sclerosis.
Trauma, foot pain.
CVA.
Cerebellar lesions.
Infections (tabes, encephalitis, meningitis).
Sensory ataxia.
Dystonia, cerebral palsy, neuromuscular disorders.
Metabolic abnormalities.

GALACTORRHEA[28]
ICD-9CM # 611.6

Prolonged suckling.
Drugs (INH, phenothiazines, reserpine derivatives, amphetamines, spironolactone and tricyclic antidepressants).
Major stressors (surgery, trauma).
Hypothyroidism.
Pituitary tumors.

GASTRIC DILATATION[16a]
ICD-9CM # 536.1

CAUSES OF A MASSIVELY DILATED STOMACH
Mechanical Gastric Outlet Obstruction
Duodenal or pyloric canal ulceration.
Carcinoma of pyloric antrum.
Extrinsic compression.
Paralytic Ileus
Surgery.
Trauma.
Peritonitis.
Pancreatitis.
Cholecystitis.
Diabetes.

Hepatic coma.
Drugs.
Gastric Volvulus
Intubation.
Air swallowing.

GASTRIC EMPTYING, DELAYED[1]

ICD-9CM # 578.89

CAUSES OF DELAYED GASTRIC EMPTYING

Mechanical Causes
Peptic ulcer disease, scarred pylorus.
Malignancy: gastric cancer, gastric lymphoma, pancreatic cancer.
Gastric surgery: vagotomy, gastric resection, Roux-en-Y anastomosis.
Crohn's disease.

Endocrine and Metabolic Causes
Diabetes mellitus.
Hypothyroidism.
Hypoadrenal states.
Electrolyte abnormalities.
Chronic renal failure.
Medications.
Anticholinergics.
Opiates.
Dopamine agonists.
Tricyclic antidepressants.

Abnormalities of Gastric Smooth Muscle
Scleroderma.
Polymyositis, dermatomyositis.
Amyloidosis.
Pseudo-obstruction.
Myotonic dystrophy.
Neuropathy.
Scleroderma.
Amyloidosis.
Autonomic neuropathy.

Central Nervous System or Psychiatric Disorders
Brain stem tumors.
Spinal cord injury.
Anorexia nervosa.
Stress.

Miscellaneous
Idiopathic gastroparesis.
Gastroesophageal reflux disease.
Nonulcer (functional) dyspepsia.
Cancer cachexia or anorexia.

GASTRIC EMPTYING, RAPID

ICD-9CM # 536.8 Gastric Motility Disorder

Pancreatic insufficiency.
Dumping syndrome.
Peptic ulcer.
Celiac disease.
Promotility agents.
Zollinger-Ellison disease.

GENITAL DISCHARGE, FEMALE[12]

ICD-9CM # 629.9

Physiologic discharge: cervical mucus, vaginal transudation, bacteria, squamous epithelial cells.

Individual variation.
Pregnancy.
Sexual response.
Menstrual cycle variation.
Infection.
Foreign body: tampon, cervical cap, other.
Neoplasm.
Fistula.
IUD.
Cervical ectropion.
Spermicide.
Nongenital causes: urinary incontinence, urinary tract fistula, Crohn's disease, rectovaginal fistula.

GENITAL SORES[1]

ICD-9CM # 054.10 Genital Herpes
        91.0 Genital Syphilis
        078.11 Condyloma Acuminatum
        099.0 Chancroid
        099.2 Granuloma Inguinale
        099.1 Lymphogranuloma Venereum
        629.8 Ulcer, Genital Site, Female
        608.89 Ulcer, Genital Site, Male

Herpes genitalis.
Syphilis.
Chancroid.
Lymphogranuloma venereum.
Granuloma inguinale.
Condyloma acuminatum.
Neoplastic lesion.
Trauma.

GLOMERULONEPHRITIS, RAPIDLY PROGRESSIVE[1]

ICD-9CM # 583.4

DIFFERENTIAL DIAGNOSIS OF RAPIDLY PROGRESSIVE GLOMERULONEPHRITIS

Linear Immune Staining
Anti-GBM disease.
Goodpasture's syndrome.
Rarely membranous glomerulonephritis.

Granular Immune Staining
Subacute bacterial endocarditis (past infectious).
Lupus nephritis.
Cryoglobulinemia.
Membranoproliferative glomerulonephritis (type II more than type I).
Immunoglobulin A nephropathy, Henoch-Schönlein purpura.
Idiopathic.

No Immune Staining (Pauci-immune)
Antineutrophil cytoplasmic antibody-associated vasculitis (Wegener granulomatosis, microscopic polyangiitis, Churg-Strauss syndrome).
Idiopathic.

GLOMERULOPATHIES, THROMBOTIC, MICROANGIOPATHIC[1]

ICD-9CM # 446.6

THROMBOTIC MICROANGIOPATHIC GLOMERULOPATHIES

Thrombotic thrombocytopenic purpura.
Hemolytic-uremic syndrome.
Malignant hypertension.
Scleroderma renal crisis.
Preeclampsia, eclampsia.
HELLP syndrome (hemolysis, elevated liver enzymes, low platelets).
Antiphospholipid antibody syndrome.
Drugs: oral contraceptives, quinine, cyclosporine, tacrolimus, ticlopidine, clopidogrel.

GLOMERULOSCLEROSIS, FOCAL SEGMENTAL[1]

ICD-9CM # 582.1

ETIOLOGY OF FOCAL SEGMENTAL GLOMERULOSCLEROSIS (FSGS)

Primary idiopathic FSGS.
Secondary FSGS.
HIV (usually collapsing variant).
Reflux nephropathy.
Heroin abuse.
Sickle cell disease.
Oligomeganephronia.
Renal dysgenesis or agenesis (low nephron mass).
Radiation nephritis.
Familial podocytopathies.
NPHS1 (nephrin) mutation.
NPHS2 (podocin) mutation.
TRPC6 (cation channel) mutation.
ACTN4 (α-actinin 4 mutation).

GLOSSODYNIA[38]

ICD-9CM # 529.6

DENTURE-RELATED

Dentures (ill-fitting, monomer from denture base).
Dental plaque.
Oral parafunction.

INFECTIVE/DERMATOLOGIC

Candidiasis.
Lichen planus.

DEFICIENCY STATES

Iron, B_{12}, folate, B_2 (riboflavin), B_6 (pyridoxine), zinc.

ENDOCRINE

Diabetes.
Myxedema.*
Hormonal changes occurring during menopause.*

NEUROLOGICALLY MEDIATED
Referred from tonsils, teeth.
Lingual nerve neuropathy.
Glossopharyngeal neuralgia.
Esophageal reflux.*

IATROGENIC
Mouthwash.

XEROSTOMIA

PSYCHOGENIC

IDIOPATHIC

*Unproven associations

GLUCOCORTICOID DEFICIENCY[14]
ICD-9CM # 255.4

ACTH-independent causes.
TB.
Autoimmune (idiopathic).
Other rare causes:
  Fungal infection.
  Adrenal hemorrhage.
  Metastases.
  Sarcoidosis.
  Amyloidosis.
  Adrenoleukodystrophy.
  Adrenomyeloneuropathy.
  HIV infection.
  Congenital adrenal hyperplasia.
  Medications (e.g., ketoconazole).
ACTH-dependent causes:
Hypothalamic-pituitary-adrenal suppression.
  Exogenous.
  Glucocorticoid.
  ACTH.
  Endogenous—cure of Cushing's syndrome.
Hypothalamic-pituitary lesions.
  Neoplasm:
  • Primary pituitary tumor.
  • Metastatic tumor.
  • Craniopharyngioma.
  Infection:
  • Tuberculosis.
  • Actinomycosis.
  • Nocardiosis.
  Sarcoid.
  Head trauma.
  Isolated ACTH deficiency.

GOITER
ICD-9CM # 240.9 Goiter, Unspecified
241.9 Goiter, Adenomatous
246.1 Goiter, Congenital
240.9 Goiter, Nontoxic Diffuse
241.1 Goiter, Nontoxic Multinodular
240.0 Simple Goiter
242.1 Thyrotoxic Goiter

Thyroiditis.
Toxic multinodular goiter.
Graves' disease.

Medications (PTU, methimazole, sulfonamides, sulfonylureas, ethionamide, amiodarone, lithium, etc.).
Iodine deficiency.
Sarcoidosis, amyloidosis.
Defective thyroid hormone synthesis.
Resistance to thyroid hormone.

GRANULOMATOUS DERMATITIDES
ICD-9CM # varies with specific disorder

Granuloma annulare.
Sarcoidosis.
Necrobiosis lipoidica diabeticorum.
Cutaneous Crohn's disease.
Rheumatoid nodules.
Annular elastolytic giant cell granuloma (actinic granuloma).
Foreign body granuloma.

GRANULOMATOUS DISORDERS[32]
ICD-9CM # 446.4 Granulomatosis
288.1 Granulomatous Disease

INFECTIONS
Fungi
Histoplasma.
Coccidioides.
Blastomyces.
Sporothrix.
Aspergillus.
Cryptococcus.
Protozoa
Toxoplasma.
Leishmania.
Metazoa
Toxocara.
Schistosoma.
Spirochetes
Treponema pallidum.
T. pertenue.
T. carateum.
Mycobacteria
M. tuberculosis.
M. leprae.
M. kansasii.
M. marinum.
M. avian.
Bacille Calmette-Guérin (BCG) vaccine.
Bacteria
Brucella.
Yersinia.
Other Infections
Cat scratch.
Lymphogranuloma.

NEOPLASIA
Carcinoma.
Reticulosis.
Pinealoma.
Dysgerminoma.
Seminoma.
Reticulum cell sarcoma.
Malignant nasal granuloma.

CHEMICALS
Beryllium.
Zirconium.
Silica.
Starch.

IMMUNOLOGIC ABERRATIONS
Sarcoidosis.
Crohn's disease.
Primary biliary cirrhosis.
Wegener's granulomatosis.
Giant cell arteritis.
Peyronie's disease.
Hypogammaglobulinemia.
SLE.
Lymphomatoid granulomatosis.
Histiocytosis X.
Hepatic granulomatous disease.
Immune complex disease.
Rosenthal-Melkersson syndrome.
Churg-Strauss allergic granulomatosis.

LEUKOCYTE OXIDASE DEFECT
Chronic granulomatous disease of childhood.

EXTRINSIC ALLERGIC ALVEOLITIS
Farmer's lung.
Bird fancier's.
Mushroom worker's.
Suberosis (cork dust).
Bagassosis.
Maple bark stripper's.
Paprika splitter's.
Coffee bean.
Spatlese lung.

OTHER DISORDERS
Whipple's disease.
Pyrexia of unknown origin.
Radiotherapy.
Cancer chemotherapy.
Panniculitis.
Chalazion.
Sebaceous cyst.
Dermoid.
Sea urchin spine injury.

GRANULOMATOUS LIVER DISEASE
ICD-9CM # 572.8

Sarcoidosis.
Wegener's granulomatosis.
Vasculitis.
Inflammatory bowel disease.
Allergic granulomatosis.
Erythema nodosum.
Infections (fungal, viral, parasitic).
Primary biliary cirrhosis.
Lymphoma.
Hodgkin's disease.
Drugs (e.g., allopurinol, hydralazine, sulfonamides, penicillins).
Toxins (copper sulfate, beryllium).

GREEN OR BLUE URINE
ICD-9CM # 788.69

Pseudomonal urinary tract infection
Medications: triamterene, amitriptyline, IV cimetidine, IV promethazine.
Biliverdin.
Dyes (methylene blue, indigo carmine).

GROIN LUMP[38]
ICD-9CM # varies with specific diagnosis

COMMON CAUSES

Inguinal hernia.
Femoral hernia.
Lymph node.

OTHER CAUSES

Saphena varix.
Femoral artery aneurysm/pseudoaneurysm.
Psoas abscess.
Lipoma of the cord.
Encysted hydrocele of the cord (male).
Testicular maldescent (male).
Hydrocele of canal of Nuck (female).

GROIN MASSES
ICD-9CM # 959.1

Hernia (inguinal, femoral).
Hydrocele.
Varicocele.
Sebaceous cyst.
Hidradenitis of inguinal apocrine glands.
Neoplasm: lymphoma, metastases.
Lipoma.
Hematoma.
Reactive inguinal adenopathy, femoral adenitis.
Folliculitis, psoas abscess.
Epididymitis, testicular torsion, ectopic testes.
Aneurysm or pseudoaneurysm of femoral artery.

GROIN PAIN[5a]
ICD-9CM # 338   Groin Pain

DIFFERENTIAL DIAGNOSIS OF GROIN PAIN

Surgery
Workers' Compensation.
Hernia.
Recurrent hernia.
Posthernia.
Orthopedic
Hip disorders.
  Acetabular labral tears.
  Avascular necrosis.
  Chondritis dissecans.
  Legg-Calvé-Perthes disease.
  Osteoarthritis.
  Pelvic stress fractures.
  Slipped femoral capital epiphysis.
  Synovitis.
Urology
Cystitis.
Epididymitis.
Nephrolithiasis.
Prostate cancer.

Prostatitis.
Torsion of testes.
Urethral extravasation.
Urinary tract infection.
Vas granuloma/fibrosis.
Dermatology
Lymphadenitis.
Psoriasis/burn.
Sebaceous cyst/hidradenitis.
Thrombophlebitis/cellulitis.
Neurosurgery
Disk disease.
Spinal injuries, inflammation, tumors.
Spondylolisthesis.
Spondylolysis.
Rheumatology
Connective tissue disorders.
Iliopsoas bursitis.
Osteitis pubis.
Systemic lupus erythematosus.
Neurology
Lumbosacral disorders.
Neurofibromatosis.
Infectious Disease
Herpes zoster.
HIV/tuberculosis.
Lyme disease.
Psoas abscess.
Sports Medicine
"Sports hernia" (adductor strains).
Gilmore's groin.
Vascular
Abscess hematoma.
Post-vein stripping.
Pseudoaneurysm.
Vascular graft.
Gastroenterology
Appendicitis/adhesions.
Diverticulitis.
Inflammatory retroperitoneal phlegmon (pancreatitis).
Meckel diverticulum.
Granulomatous colitis.
Gynecology
Cesarean section.
Cervical cancer.
Endometriosis.
Tubal/ovarian disorders.

GROIN PAIN, ACTIVE PATIENT[37]
ICD-9CM # 959.1 Groin Injury
           848.8 Groin Pain

MUSCULOSKELETAL

Avascular necrosis of the femoral head.
Avulsion fracture (lesser trochanter, anterior superior iliac spine, anterior inferior iliac spine).
Bursitis (iliopectineal, trochanteric).
Entrapment of the ilioinguinal or iliofemoral nerve.
Gracilis syndrome.
Muscle tear (adductors, iliopsoas, rectus abdominis, gracilis, sartorius, rectus femoris).
Myositis ossificans of the hip muscles.
Osteitis pubis.
Osteoarthritis of the femoral head.
Slipped capital femoral epiphysis.

Stress fracture of the femoral head or neck and pubis.
Synovitis.

HERNIA-RELATED

Avulsion of the internal oblique muscle in the conjoined tendon.
Defect at the insertion of the rectus abdominis muscle.
Direct inguinal hernia.
Femoral ring hernia.
Indirect inguinal hernia.
Inguinal canal weakness.

UROLOGIC

Epididymitis.
Fracture of the testis.
Hydrocele.
Kidney stone.
Posterior urethritis.
Prostatitis.
Testicular cancer.
Torsion of the testis.
Urinary tract infection.
Varicocele.

GYNECOLOGIC

Ectopic pregnancy.
Ovarian cyst.
Pelvic inflammatory disease.
Torsion of the ovary.
Vaginitis.

LYMPHATIC ENLARGEMENT IN GROIN

GYNECOMASTIA
ICD-9CM # 611.1 Gynecomastia,
                Nonpuerperal

Physiologic (puberty, newborns, aging).
Drugs (estrogen and estrogen precursors, 5-alpha reductase inhibitors, digitalis, testosterone and exogenous androgens, clomiphene, cimetidine, spironolactone, ketoconazole, amiodarone, ACE inhibitors, isoniazid, phenytoin, methyldopa, metoclopramide, phenothiazine).
Increased prolactin level (prolactinoma).
Liver disease.
Adrenal disease.
Thyrotoxicosis.
Increased estrogen production (hCG-producing tumor, testicular tumor, bronchogenic carcinoma).
Secondary hypogonadism.
Primary gonadal failure (trauma, castration, viral orchitis, granulomatous disease).
Defects in androgen synthesis.
Testosterone deficiency.
Klinefelter's syndrome.

HALITOSIS
ICD-9CM # 784.9

Tobacco use.
Alcohol use.
Dry mouth (mouth breathing, inadequate fluid intake).
Foods (onion, garlic, meats, nuts, protein drinks).

Disease of mouth or nose (infections, cancer, inflammation).
Medications (antihistamines, antidepressants).
Systemic disorders (diabetes, uremia).
GI disorders (esophageal diverticula, hiatal hernia, GERD, achalasia).
Sinusitis.
Pulmonary disorders (bronchiectasis, pneumonia, neoplasms, TB).

HAND PAIN AND SWELLING[6]

ICD-9CM # varies with specific diagnosis

Trauma.
Gout.
Pseudogout.
Cellulitis.
Lymphangitis.
DVT of upper extremity.
Thrombophlebitis.
RA.
Remitting seronegative symmetrical synovitis with pitting edema (RS3PE).
Polymyalgia rheumatica.
Mixed connective tissue disease.
Scleroderma.
Rupture of the olecranon bursa.
Metzger's syndrome (neoplasia).
The puffy hand of drug addiction.
Reflex sympathetic dystrophy.
Eosinophilic fasciitis.
Sickle cell (hand-foot syndrome).
Leprosy.
Factitial (the rubber band syndrome).

HEADACHE[13]

ICD-9CM # 784.0	Headache NOS
307.81	Headache, Tension
346.2	Headache, Cluster
346.9	Headache, Migraine
784.0	Headache, Vascular

Vascular: migraine, cluster headaches, temporal arteritis, hypertension, cavernous sinus thrombosis.
Musculoskeletal: neck and shoulder muscle contraction, strain of extraocular and/or intraocular muscles, cervical spondylosis, temporomandibular arthritis.
Infections: meningitis, encephalitis, brain abscess, sepsis, sinusitis, osteomyelitis, parotitis, mastoiditis.
Cerebral neoplasm.
Subdural hematoma.
Cerebral hemorrhage/infarct.
Pseudotumor cerebri.
Normal-pressure hydrocephalus (NPH).
Postlumbar puncture.
Cerebral aneurysm, arteriovenous malformations.
Posttrauma.
Dental problems: abscess, periodontitis, poorly fitting dentures.
Trigeminal neuralgia, glossopharyngeal neuralgia.
Otitis and other ear diseases.
Glaucoma and other eye diseases.
Metabolic: uremia, carbon monoxide inhalation, hypoxia.

Pheochromocytoma, hypoglycemia, hypothyroidism.
Effort induced: benign exertional headache, cough, headache, coital cephalalgia.
Drugs: alcohol, nitrates, histamine antagonists.
Paget's disease of the skull.
Emotional, psychiatric.

HEADACHE, ACUTE[11]

ICD-9CM # 784.0

DIFFERENTIAL DIAGNOSIS OF ACUTE HEADACHE

Evaluation of the first acute headache should exclude pathologic causes listed here before consideration of more common etiologies.
Increased intracranial pressure (ICP): Trauma, hemorrhage, tumor, hydrocephalus, pseudotumor cerebri, abscess, arachnoid cyst, cerebral edema.
Decreased ICP: After ventriculoperitoneal shunt, lumbar puncture, cerebrospinal fluid leak from basilar skull fracture.
Meningeal inflammation: Meningitis, leukemia, subarachnoid or subdural hemorrhage.
Vascular: Vasculitis, arteriovenous malformation, hypertension, cerebrovascular accident.
Bone, soft tissue: Referred pain from scalp, eyes, ears, sinuses, nose, teeth, pharynx, cervical spine, temporomandibular joint.
Infection: Systemic infection, encephalitis, sinusitis, etc.
First migraine.

HEADACHE AND FACIAL PAIN[36]

ICD-9CM # 784.0	Headache NOS
784.0	Facial Pain

VASCULAR HEADACHES

Migraine
Migraine with headaches and inconspicuous neurologic features:
- Migraine without aura ("common migraine").
Migraine with headaches and conspicuous neurologic features:
- With transient neurologic symptoms:
  Migraine with typical aura ("classic migraine").
  Sensory, basilar, and hemiplegic migraine.
- With prolonged or permanent neurologic features ("complicated migraine"):
  Ophthalmoplegic migraine.
  Migrainous infarction.
Migraine without headaches but with conspicuous neurologic features ("migraine equivalents"):
- Abdominal migraine.
- Benign paroxysmal vertigo of childhood.
- Migraine aura without headache ("isolated auras," transient migrainous accompaniments).

Cluster Headaches
Episodic cluster headache ("cyclic cluster headaches").
Chronic cluster headaches.
Chronic paroxysmal hemicrania.

Other Vascular Headaches
Headaches of reactive vasodilation (fever, drug-induced, postictal, hypoglycemia, hypoxia, hypercarbia, hyperthyroidism).
Headaches associated with arterial hypertension:
- Chronic severe hypertension (diastolic 120 mm Hg).
- Paroxysmal severe hypertension (pheochromocytoma, some coital headaches).
Headaches caused by cranial arteritis:
- Giant cell arteritis ("temporal arteritis").
- Other vasculitides.

HEADACHES ASSOCIATED WITH DEMONSTRABLE MUSCLE SPASM

Headache caused by posturally induced or perilesional muscle spasm:
- Headaches of sustained or impaired posture (e.g., prolonged close work, driving).
- Headaches associated with cervical spondylosis and other diseases of cervical spine.
- Myofascial pain dysfunction syndrome (headache or facial pain associated with disorders of teeth, jaws, and related structures, or "TMJ syndrome").
Headaches caused by psychophysiologic muscular contraction ("muscle contraction headaches," or tension-type headache associated with disorder of pericranial muscles).

HEADACHES AND FACIAL PAIN WITHOUT DEMONSTRABLE PHYSICAL SUBSTRATE

Headaches of uncertain etiology:
- "Tension headaches" (tension-type headache unassociated with disorder of pericranial muscles).
- Some forms of posttraumatic headache.
Psychogenic headaches (e.g., hypochondriacal, conversional, delusional, malingered).
Facial pain of uncertain etiology ("atypical facial pain").

COMBINED TENSION-MIGRAINE HEADACHES

Episodic migraine superimposed on chronic tension headaches.
Chronic daily headaches:
- Associated with analgesic and/or ergotamine overuse ("rebound headaches").
- Not associated with drug overuse.

HEADACHES AND HEAD PAINS CAUSED BY DISEASES OF EYES, EARS, NOSE, SINUSES, TEETH, OR SKULL

HEADACHES CAUSED BY MENINGEAL INFLAMMATION

Subarachnoid hemorrhage.
Meningitis and meningoencephalitis.
Others (e.g., meningeal carcinomatosis).

HEADACHES ASSOCIATED WITH ALTERED INTRACRANIAL PRESSURE ("TRACTION HEADACHES")

Increased Intracranial Pressure
Intracranial mass lesions (neoplasm, hematoma, abscess, etc.).
Hydrocephalus.
Benign intracranial hypertension.
Venous sinus thrombosis.

Decreased Intracranial Pressure
Post–lumbar puncture headaches.
Spontaneous hypoliquorrheic headaches.

HEADACHES AND HEAD PAINS CAUSED BY CRANIAL NEURALGIAS

Presumed Irritation of Superficial Nerves
Occipital neuralgia.
Supraorbital neuralgia.

Presumed Irritation of Intracranial Nerves
Trigeminal neuralgia ("tic douloureux").
Glossopharyngeal neuralgia.

HEADACHE, CHRONIC[11]
ICD-9CM # 784.0

DIFFERENTIAL DIAGNOSIS OF RECURRENT OR CHRONIC HEADACHES
Migraine (with or without aura).
Tension.
Analgesic rebound.
Caffeine withdrawal.
Sleep deprivation (e.g., in children with sleep apnea) or chronic hypoxia.
Tumor.
Psychogenic: Conversion disorder, malingering.
Cluster headache.

HEAD AND NECK, SOFT TISSUE MASSES
ICD-9CM # varies with specific diagnosis

Lipoma.
Pilar cyst.
Epidermal inclusion cyst.
Dermoid cyst.
Bone cyst.
Hemangioma.
Eosinophilic granuloma.
Other: facial nerve neuroma, teratoma, rhabdomyoma, rhabdomyosarcoma, branchial cleft cyst.

HEARING LOSS, ACUTE[26]
ICD-9CM # 388.2

Infectious: mumps, measles, influenza, herpes simplex, herpes zoster, CMV, mononucleosis, syphilis.
Vascular: macroglobulinemia, sickle cell disease, Berger's disease, leukemia, polycythemia, fat emboli, hypercoagulable states.
Metabolic: diabetes, pregnancy, hyperlipoproteinemia.
Conductive: cerumen impaction, foreign bodies, otitis media, otitis externa, barotrauma, trauma.

Medications: aminoglycosides, loop diuretics, antineoplastics, salicylates, vancomycin.
Neoplasm: acoustic neuroma, metastatic neoplasm.

HEARTBURN AND INDIGESTION[33]
ICD-9CM # 787.1 Heartburn
         536.8 Indigestion

Reflux esophagitis.
Gastritis.
Nonulcer dyspepsia.
Functional GI disorder (anxiety disorder, social/environmental stresses).
Excessive intestinal gas (ingestion of flatulogenic foods, GI stasis, constipation).
Gas entrapment (hepatitis or splenic flexure syndrome).
Neoplasm (adenocarcinoma of stomach or esophagus, lymphoma).
Gallbladder disease.

HEART FAILURE WITH PRESERVED LEFT VENTRICULAR EJECTION FRACTION[14a]
ICD-9CM # 428.9

CAUSES OF (AND ALTERNATIVE EXPLANATIONS FOR) HEART FAILURE WITH PRESERVED LEFT VENTRICULAR EJECTION FRACTION (>45%-50%)
Inaccurate diagnosis of heart failure (e.g., pulmonary disease, obesity).
Inaccurate measurements of ejection fraction.
Systolic function overestimated by ejection fraction (e.g., mitral regurgitation).
Episodic, unrecognized systolic dysfunction.
Intermittent ischemia.
Arrhythmia.
Severe hypertension.
Alcohol abuse.
Diastolic dysfunction.
Abnormalities of myocardial relaxation:
  Ischemia.
  Hypertrophy.
Abnormalities of myocardial compliance:
  Hypertrophy.
  Aging.
  Fibrosis.
  Diabetes.
  Infiltrative disease (amyloidosis, sarcoidosis).
  Storage disease (hemochromatosis).
  Endomyocardial disease (endomyocardial fibrosis, radiation, anthracyclines).
Pericardial disease (constriction, tamponade).

HEART FAILURE, ACUTE[2]
ICD-9CM # 428.9

COMMON PRECIPITATING CAUSES OF ACUTE HF
Systemic hypertension.
Myocardial infarction or ischemia.

Dysrhythmia.
Systemic infection.
Anemia.
Dietary, physical, environmental, and emotional excesses.
Pregnancy.
Thyrotoxicosis or hypothyroidism.
Acute myocarditis.
Acute valvular dysfunction.
Pulmonary embolus.
Pharmacologic complications.

HEART FAILURE, PATHOGENIC CAUSES[14a]
ICD-9CM # 428.9

IMPAIRED SYSTOLIC (CONTRACTILE) FUNCTION
Ischemic damage or dysfunction:
  Myocardial infarction.
  Persistent or intermittent myocardial ischemia.
  Hypoperfusion (shock).
Chronic pressure overloading:
  Hypertension.
  Obstructive valvular disease.
Chronic volume overload:
  Regurgitant valvular disease.
  Intracardiac left-to-right shunting.
  Extracardiac shunting.
Nonischemic dilated cardiomyopathy:
  Familial/genetic disorders.
  Toxic/drug-induced damage
  Immunologically mediated necrosis.
  Infectious agents.
  Metabolic disorders.
  Infiltrative processes.
  Idiopathic conditions.

IMPAIRED DIASTOLIC FUNCTION (RESTRICTED FILLING, INCREASED STIFFNESS)
Pathologic myocardial hypertrophy:
  Primary (hypertrophic cardiomyopathies).
  Secondary (hypertension).
Aging.
Ischemic fibrosis.
Restrictive cardiomyopathy:
  Infiltrative disorders (amyloidosis, sarcoidosis).
  Storage diseases (hemochromatosis, genetic abnormalities).
Endomyocardial disorders.

MECHANICAL ABNORMALITIES
Intracardiac:
  Obstructive valvular disease.
  Regurgitant valvular disease.
  Intracardiac shunts.
  Other congenital abnormalities.
Extracardiac:
  Obstructive (coarctation, supravalvular aortic stenosis).
  Left-to-right shunting (patent ductus arteriosus).

Differential Diagnosis

II

DISORDERS OF RATE AND RHYTHM

Bradyarrhythmias (sinus node dysfunction, conduction abnormalities).
Tachyarrhythmias (ineffective rhythms, chronic tachycardia).

PULMONARY HEART DISEASE

Cor pulmonale.
Pulmonary vascular disorders.

HIGH-OUTPUT STATES

Metabolic disorders:
Thyrotoxicosis.
Nutritional disorders (beriberi).
Excessive blood flow requirements:
Chronic anemia.
Systemic arteriovenous shunting.

HEART FAILURE, PREGNANCY

ICD-9CM # 428.90

Congenital valvular heart disease exacerbated by pregnancy.
Peripartum cardiomyopathy.
Untreated thyrotoxicosis.
Hypothyroidism.
Pulmonary hypertension.
Myocardial infarction.

HEEL PAIN

ICD-9CM # varies with specific diagnosis

Achilles tendonitis/tendinopathy (insertional, noninsertional).
Retrocalcaneal bursitis (superficial, deep).
Plantar fasciopathy.
Neuropathy (tarsal tunnel, posterior tibial nerve [medial calcaneal branch], abductor digiti quinti).
Calcaneal stress fracture.
Puncture wound, foreign body.
Cellulitis.
Spondyloarthropathy.
Fat pad atrophy.
Soft tissue tumor.
S1 radiculopathy.
Paget's disease of bone.
Haglund deformity.
Primary or metastatic bone tumor.

HEEL PAIN, PLANTAR[24]

ICD-9CM # 729.5

SKIN

Keratoses.
Verruca.
Ulcer.
Fissure.

CONNECTIVE TISSUE

Fat
Atrophy.
Panniculitis.
Dense Connective Tissue
Inflammatory fasciitis.
Fibromatosis.
Enthesopathy.
Bursitis.

Bone (Calcaneus)
Stress fracture.
Paget's disease.
Benign bone cyst/tumor.
Malignant bone tumor.
Metabolic bone disease (osteopenia).
Nerve
Tarsal tunnel.
Plantar nerve entrapment.
S1 nerve root radiculopathy.
Painful peripheral neuropathy.

INFECTION

Dermatomycoses.
Acute osteomyelitis.
Plantar abscess.

MISCELLANEOUS

Foreign body.
Nonunion calcaneus fracture.
Psychogenic.
Idiopathic.

HEMARTHROSIS

ICD-9CM # 848.9 Hemarthrosis (Sprain) NOS

Trauma.
Anticoagulant therapy.
Thrombocytopenia, thrombocytosis.
Bleeding disorders (e.g., von Willebrand's disease).
Charcot's joint.
Idiopathic.
Other: pigmented villonodular synovitis, hemangioma, synovioma, AV fistula, ruptured aneurysm.

HEMATEMESIS[38]

ICD-9CM # 578.0

CAUSES OF HEMATEMESIS

Very Common
Gastric or duodenal ulcer or erosions.
Common
Mallory-Weiss tear (a laceration at the gastro-esophageal junction).
Ulcerative esophagitis.
Esophageal varices.
Uncommon
Vascular malformations.
Ulcerated gastrointestinal stromal tumor.
Carcinoma of esophagus or stomach.
Aortoenteric fistula.

HEMATURIA

ICD-9CM # 599.7 Hematuria, Benign (Essential)

Use the mnemonic TICS:
T (trauma): blow to kidney, insertion of Foley catheter or foreign body in urethra, prolonged and severe exercise, very rapid emptying of overdistended bladder.
(tumor): hypernephroma, Wilms' tumor, papillary carcinoma of the bladder, prostatic and urethral neoplasms.
(toxins): turpentine, phenols, sulfonamides and other antibiotics, cyclophosphamide, NSAIDs.

I (infections): glomerulonephritis, TB, cystitis, prostatitis, urethritis, *Schistosoma haematobium,* yellow fever, blackwater fever.
(inflammatory processes): Goodpasture's syndrome, periarteritis, postirradiation.
C (calculi): renal, ureteral, bladder, urethra.
(cysts): simple cysts, polycystic disease.
(congenital anomalies): hemangiomas, aneurysms, AVM.
S (surgery): invasive procedures, prostatic resection, cystoscopy.
(sickle cell disease and other hematologic disturbances): hemophilia, thrombocytopenia, anticoagulants.
(somewhere else): bleeding genitals, factitious (drug addicts).

HEMATURIA, DIFFERENTIAL BASED ON AGE AND SEX

ICD-9CM # 599.7 Hematuria Benign (Essential)
other codes vary with cause

0 TO 20 YR

Acute urinary tract infections.
Acute glomerulonephritis.
Congenital urinary tract anomalies with obstruction.
Trauma to genitals.

20 TO 40 YR

Acute urinary tract infection.
Trauma to genitals.
Urolithiasis.
Bladder cancer.

40 TO 60 YR (WOMEN)

Acute urinary tract infection.
Bladder cancer.
Urolithiasis.

40 TO 60 YR (MEN)

Acute urinary tract infection.
Bladder cancer.
Urolithiasis.

60 YR AND OLDER (WOMEN)

Acute urinary tract infection.
Bladder cancer.
Vaginal trauma or irritation.
Urolithiasis.

60 YR AND OLDER (MEN)

Acute urinary tract infection.
Benign prostatic hyperplasia.
Bladder cancer.
Urolithiasis.
Trauma.

HEMATURIA, IN CHILDREN[2]

ICD-9CM # 599.7

EXTRARENAL

Trauma.
Meatal stenosis or posterior urethral valves.
Exercise.
Menstruation or rectal bleeding.

Foreign bodies.
Cystitis, urethritis, or epididymitis.

INTRARENAL

Pyelonephritis.
Renal or bladder stones or tumors.
Poststrepotococcal or idiopathic glomerulone-
phritis.
Acute interstitial nephritis.
Acute tubular necrosis.
Basement membrane glomerular disease.
Renal vein or arterial thrombosis.
Recurrent familial hematuria.
Polycystic kidney disease.

SYSTEMIC

Henoch-Schönlein purpura.
Systemic lupus erythematosus.
Hemolytic-uremic syndrome.
Infectious mononucleosis.
Sickle cell disease or other hemoglobinopathies.
Bacterial endocarditis or artificial cardiac valves.
Bleeding disorders, warfarin, or aspirin.
Medications such as amitriptyline or chlorprom-
azine, radiocontrast dyes.
Munchausen syndrome or factitious.

HEMIPARESIS/HEMIPLEGIA

ICD-9CM # 436.0 Acquired Due to Acute
CVA, Flaccid
436.1 Acquired Due to CVA,
Acute, Spastic

CVA.
Transient ischemic attack.
Cerebral neoplasm.
Multiple sclerosis or other demyelinating dis-
order.
CNS infection.
Migraine.
Hypoglycemia
Subdural hematoma.
Vasculitis.
Todd's paralysis.
Epidural hematoma.
Metabolic (hyperosmolar state, electrolyte im-
balance).
Psychiatric disorders.
Congenital disorders.
Leukodystrophies.

HEMOLYSIS AND HEMOGLOBINURIA

ICD-9CM # 773.2 Hemolysis
791.2 Hemoglobinuria

Erythrocyte trauma (prosthetic cardiac valves,
marching and severe trauma, extensive
burns).
Infections (malaria, *Bartonella*, *Clostridium
welchii*).
Brown recluse spider bite.
Incompatible blood transfusions.
Hemolytic-uremic syndrome.
Thrombotic thrombocytopenic purpura (TTP).
Paroxysmal nocturnal hemoglobinuria (PNH).
Drugs (penicillins, quinidine, methyldopa, sul-
fonamides, nitrofurantoin).

Erythrocyte enzyme deficiencies (e.g., exposure
to fava beans in patients with glucose-
6-phosphate dehydrogenase deficiency).

HEMOLYSIS, INTRAVASCULAR

ICD-9CM # 283.2

Infections.
Exertional hemolysis (e.g., prolonged march).
Valve hemolysis.
Microangiopathic hemolytic anemia.
Osmotic and chemical agents.
Thermal injury.
Cold agglutinins.
Venoms (snakes, spiders).
Paroxysmal nocturnal hemoglobinuria (PNH).

HEMOLYSIS, MECHANICAL

ICD-9CM # 283.19

Prosthetic heart valves.
Aortic stenosis.
Malignant hypertension.
Metastatic adenocarcinoma.
Traumatic exercise.
Renal transplants.
Renal cortical necrosis.
Glomerulonephritis.
Thrombotic thrombocytopenic purpura (TTP),
hemolytic-uremic syndrome (HUS).
Renal vasculitis.
Scleroderma.
Diabetes.

HEMOPERITONEUM

ICD-9CM # 568.81

Ruptured Graafian follicle.
Ruptured spleen.
Ectopic pregnancy.
Traumatic laceration of liver.
Ruptured aneurysm.
Ruptured bladder.
Traumatic laceration of bowel, pancreas, uterus.

HEMOPTYSIS

ICD-9CM # 786.3

CARDIOVASCULAR

Pulmonary embolism/infarction.
Left ventricular failure.
Mitral stenosis.
AV fistula.
Severe hypertension.
Erosion of aortic aneurysm.

PULMONARY

Neoplasm (primary or metastatic).
Infection.
Pneumonia: *Streptococcus pneumoniae*, *Kleb-
siella pneumoniae*, *Staphylococcus aureus*,
Legionella pneumophila.
Bronchiectasis.
Abscess.
TB.
Bronchitis.

Fungal infections (aspergillosis, coccidioidomy-
cosis).
Parasitic infections (amebiasis, ascariasis, para-
gonimiasis).
Vasculitis: Wegener's granulomatosis, Churg-
Strauss syndrome, Henoch-Schönlein pur-
pura.
Goodpasture's syndrome.
Trauma (needle biopsy, foreign body, right-sided
heart catheterization, prolonged and severe
cough).
Cystic fibrosis, bullous emphysema.
Pulmonary sequestration.
Pulmonary AV fistula.
SLE.
Idiopathic pulmonary hemosiderosis.
Drugs: aspirin, anticoagulants, penicillamine.
Pulmonary hypertension.
Mediastinal fibrosis.

OTHER

Epistaxis, trauma.
Laryngeal bleeding (laryngitis, laryngeal neo-
plasm).
Hematologic disorders (clotting abnormalities,
DIC, thrombocytopenia).

HEPATIC CYSTS[36]

ICD-9CM # 751.62 Hepatic Cyst, Congenital
122.8 *Echinococcus* Infection,
Liver

CONGENITAL HEPATIC CYSTS

Parenchymal: solitary cyst, polycystic disease.
Ductal: localized dilatation, multiple cystic dilatations of intrahepatic ducts (Caroli's disease).

ACQUIRED HEPATIC CYSTS

Inflammatory cysts: retention cysts, echinococ-
cal cyst, amebic cyst.
Neoplastic cyst.
Peliosis hepatis.

HEPATIC GRANULOMAS[1]

ICD-9CM # 572.8

INFECTIONS

Bacterial, spirochetal: TB and atypical mycobacterial infections, tularemia, brucellosis, leprosy, syphilis, Whipple's disease, listeriosis.
Viral: mononucleosis, CMV.
Rickettsial: Q fever.
Fungal: coccidioidomycosis, histoplasmosis, cryptococcal infections, actinomycosis, aspergillosis, nocardiosis.
Parasitic: schistosomiasis, clonorchiasis, toxocariasis, ascariasis, toxoplasmosis, amebiasis.

HEPATOBILIARY DISORDERS

Primary biliary cirrhosis, granulomatous hepatitis, jejunoileal bypass.

SYSTEMIC DISORDERS

Sarcoidosis, Wegener's granulomatosis, inflammatory bowel disease, Hodgkin's disease,
lymphoma.

Differential
Diagnosis

II

DRUGS/TOXINS

Beryllium, parenteral foreign material (starch, talc, silicone, etc.), phenylbutazone, α-methyldopa, procainamide, allopurinol, phenytoin, nitrofurantoin, hydralazine.

HEPATITIS, ACUTE[25]

ICD-9CM # varies with specific disorder

Infectious:
  Hepatitis A, B, C, D, G.
  Epstein-Barr virus.
  Cytomegalovirus.
  Herpes simplex virus.
  Yellow fever.
  Leptospirosis.
  Q fever.
  HIV.
  Brucellosis.
  Lyme disease.
  Syphilis.
Noninfectious:
  Drug induced.
  Autoimmune.
  Ischemic.
  Acute fatty liver of pregnancy.
  Acute Budd-Chiari syndrome.
  Wilson's disease.

HEPATITIS, CHRONIC[25]

ICD-9CM # 571.40 Hepatitis, Noninfectious, Chronic
          072.22 Hepatitis B, Chronic
          070.44 Hepatitis C, Chronic

Chronic viral hepatitis:
  Hepatitis B.
  Hepatitis C.
  Hepatitis D.
Autoimmune hepatitis and variant syndromes.
Hereditary hemochromatosis.
Wilson's disease.
α₁-Antitrypsin deficiency.
Fatty liver and nonalcoholic steatohepatitis.
Alcoholic liver disease.
Drug-induced liver disease.
Hepatic granulomas:
  Infectious.
  Drug induced.
  Neoplastic.
  Idiopathic.

HEPATITIS, IN CHILDREN[22a]

ICD-9CM # varies with specific diagnosis

CAUSES AND DIFFERENTIAL DIAGNOSIS OF HEPATITIS IN CHILDREN

Infectious
Hepatotropic viruses:
- HAV.
- HBV.
- HCV.
- HDV.
- HEV.
- Hepatitis non–A-E viruses.

Systemic infection that can include hepatitis:
- Adenovirus.
- Arbovirus.
- Coxsackievirus.
- Cytomegalovirus.
- Enterovirus.
- Epstein-Barr virus.
- "Exotic" viruses (e.g., yellow fever).
- Herpes simplex virus.
- Human immunodeficiency virus.
- Paramyxovirus.
- Rubella.
- Varicella zoster.
Other.

Nonviral liver infections
Abscess.
Amebiasis.
Bacterial sepsis.
Brucellosis.
Fitz-Hugh-Curtis syndrome.
Histoplasmosis.
Leptospirosis.
Tuberculosis.
Other.

Autoimmune
Autoimmune hepatitis.
Sclerosing cholangitis.
Other (e.g., systemic lupus erythematosus, juvenile rheumatoid arthritis).

Metabolic
α1-Antitrypsin deficiency.
Tyrosinemia.
Wilson disease.
Other.

Toxic
Iatrogenic or drug induced (e.g., acetaminophen).
Environmental (e.g., pesticides).

Anatomic
Choledochal cyst.
Biliary atresia.
Other.

Hemodynamic
Shock.
Congestive heart failure.
Budd-Chiari syndrome.
Other.

Nonalcoholic fatty liver disease
Idiopathic.
Reye syndrome.
Other.

HEPATOMEGALY

ICD-9CM # 789.1

FREQUENT JAUNDICE
Infectious hepatitis.
Toxic hepatitis.
Carcinoma: liver, pancreas, bile ducts, metastatic neoplasm to liver.
Cirrhosis.
Obstruction of common bile duct.
Alcoholic hepatitis.
Biliary cirrhosis.
Cholangitis.
Hemochromatosis with cirrhosis.

INFREQUENT JAUNDICE
CHF.
Amyloidosis.
Liver abscess.
Sarcoidosis.
Infectious mononucleosis.
Alcoholic fatty infiltration.
Nonalcoholic steatohepatitis.
Lymphoma.
Leukemia.
Budd-Chiari syndrome.
Myelofibrosis with myeloid metaplasia.
Familial hyperlipoproteinemia type 1.
Other: amebiasis, hydatid disease of liver, schistosomiasis, kala-azar (*Leishmania donovani*), Hurler's syndrome, Gaucher's disease, kwashiorkor.

HEPATOMEGALY, BY SHAPE OF LIVER[38]

ICD-9CM # 789.1

DIFFUSELY ENLARGED AND SMOOTH
Massive
Metastatic disease.
Alcoholic liver disease with fatty infiltration.
Myeloproliferative diseases (e.g., polycythemia rubra vera, myelofibrosis).
Moderate
The above causes.
Hemochromatosis.
Hematologic disease (e.g., chronic myeloid leukemia, lymphoma).
Fatty liver (e.g., diabetes mellitus, obesity).
Infiltrative disorders (e.g., amyloid).
Mild
The above causes.
Hepatitis (viral, drugs).
Cirrhosis.
Biliary obstruction.
Granulomatous disorders (e.g., sarcoid).
HIV infection.

DIFFUSELY ENLARGED AND IRREGULAR
Metastatic disease.
Cirrhosis.
Hydatid disease.
Polycystic liver disease.

LOCALIZED SWELLINGS
Riedel's lobe (a normal variant—the lobe may be palpable in the right lumbar region).
Metastasis.
Large simple hepatic cyst.
Hydatid cyst.
Hepatoma.
Liver abscess (e.g., amebic abscess).

HERMAPHRODITISM[4]

ICD-9CM # 752.7 Hermaphroditism, Congenital

FEMALE PSEUDOHERMAPHRODITISM
Androgen exposure:

Fetal source:
- 21-Hydroxylase (P450 c21) deficiency.
- 11β-Hydroxylase (P450 c11) deficiency.
- 3β-Hydroxysteroid dehydrogenase II (3β-HSD II) deficiency.
- Aromatase (P450arom) deficiency.

Maternal source.
Virilizing ovarian tumor.
Virilizing adrenal tumor.
Androgenic drugs.
Undetermined origin:
    Associated with genitourinary and GI tract defects.

MALE PSEUDOHERMAPHRODITISM

Defects in testicular differentiation:
    Denys-Drash syndrome (mutation in WT1 gene).
    WAGR syndrome (Wilms tumor, aniridia, genitourinary malformation, retardation).
    Deletion of 11p13.
    Camptomelic syndrome (autosomal gene at 17q24.3-q25.1) and SOX 9 mutation.
    XY pure gonadal dysgenesis (Swyer syndrome).
- Mutation in SRY gene.
- Unknown cause.

    XY gonadal agenesis.
Deficiency of testicular hormones:
    Leydig cell aplasia.
    Mutation in LH receptor.
    Lipoid adrenal hyperplasia (P450 scc) deficiency; mutation in StAR (steroidogenic acute regulatory protein).
    3α-HSD II deficiency.
    17-Hydroxylase/17, 20-lyase (P450 c17) deficiency.
    Persistent Müllerian duct syndrome.
- Gene mutations, Müllerian-inhibiting substance (MIS).
- Receptor defects for MIS.

Defect in androgen action:
    5α-Reductase II mutations.
    Androgen receptor defects:
- Complete androgen insensitivity syndrome.
- Partial androgen insensitivity syndrome.
- Reifenstein and other syndromes.
- Smith-Lemli-Opitz syndrome.

Defect in conversion of 7-dehydrocholesterol to cholesterol.

TRUE HERMAPHRODITISM

XX.
XY.
XX/XY chimeras.

HICCUPS[21]

ICD-9CM # 786.8

TRANSIENT HICCUPS

Sudden excitement, emotion.
Gastric distention.
Esophageal obstruction.
Alcohol ingestion.
Sudden change in temperature.

PERSISTENT OR CHRONIC HICCUPS

Toxic/metabolic: uremia, DM, hyperventilation, hypocalcemia, hypokalemia, hyponatremia, gout, fever.
Drugs: benzodiazepines, steroids, α-methyldopa, barbiturates.
Surgery/general anesthesia.
Thoracic/diaphragmatic disorders: pneumonia, lung cancer, asthma, pleuritis, pericarditis, myocardial infarction, aortic aneurysm, esophagitis, esophageal obstruction, diaphragmatic hernia or irritation.
Abdominal disorders: gastric ulcer or cancer, hepatobiliary or pancreatic disease, IBD, bowel obstruction, intraabdominal or subphrenic abscess, prostatic infection or cancer.
Central nervous system disorders: traumatic, infectious, vascular, structural.
Ear, nose, and throat disorders: pharyngitis, laryngitis, tumor, irritation of auditory canal.
Psychogenic disorders.
Idiopathic disorders.

HILAR AND MEDIASTINAL LYMPH NODE ENLARGEMENT[14a]

ICD-9CM # 785.6

DISORDERS ASSOCIATED WITH HILAR AND MEDIASTINAL LYMPH NODE ENLARGEMENT

Sarcoidosis.
Lymphoma.
Fungal disease.
Tuberculosis.
Metastatic cancer.
Silicosis, coal worker's pneumoconiosis, beryllium lung.

HIP PAIN, CHILDREN[26]

ICD-9CM # 959.6   Hip Injury
             719.95 Hip Joint Disorder
             843.9 Hip Strain

TRAUMA

Hip or pelvis fractures.
Overuse injuries.

INFECTION

Septic arthritis.
Osteomyelitis.

INFLAMMATION

Transient synovitis.
Juvenile RA.
Rheumatic fever.

NEOPLASM

Leukemia.
Osteogenic or Ewing's sarcoma.
Metastatic disease.

HEMATOLOGIC DISORDERS

Hemophilia.
Sickle cell anemia.

MISCELLANEOUS

Legg-Calvé-Perthes disease.
Slipped capital femoral epiphysis.

HIP PAIN, DIFFERENTIAL DIAGNOSIS[18b]

ICD-9CM # varies with specific diagnosis

ARTICULAR

Inflammatory joint diseases.
    Rheumatoid arthritis.
    Spondyloarthropathies.
    Polymyalgia rheumatica.
Degenerative joint disease.
    Primary osteoarthritis.
    Secondary osteoarthritis.
Metabolic joint diseases.
    Gout.
    Pseudogout.
    Ochronosis.
    Hemochromatosis.
    Wilson's disease.
    Acromegaly.
Femoroacetabular impingement.
Acetabular labral tear.
Infections.
Tumors.
    Benign.
- Pigmented villonodular sclerosis.
- Osteochondromatosis.

    Malignant.
- Synovial sarcoma.
- Synovial metastasis.

Hemarthrosis.
In children:
    Toxic synovitis.
    Juvenile chronic arthritis.

REFERRED PAIN

Thoracolumbar spine.
Intraabdominal structures.
Retroperitoneal structures.

PERIARTICULAR

Bursitis.
    Trochanteric.
    Iliopsoas.
    Ischiogluteal.
Tendinitis.
    Trochanteric.
    Adductor.
Acute calcific periarthritis.
Heterotropic ossification.

OSSEOUS

Bone lesions.
Fractures.
Neoplasms.
Infection.
Osteonecrosis of the femoral head.
Paget's disease.
Metabolic bone disease.
Stress fracture.
Transient osteoporosis.
In children:
    Congenital dislocation of the hip.
    Acetabular dysplasia.

Coxa vara.
Slipped capital femoral epiphysis.
Legg-Calvé-Perthes disease.
Rickets.

NEUROLOGIC

Entrapment neuropathies.
Lateral femoral cutaneous nerve (meralgia paresthetica).
Lumbar nerve root compression.
L2, L3, and L4.

VASCULAR

Atherosclerosis of aorta, iliac vessels.

HIP PAIN, IN DIFFERENT AGE GROUPS[8]

ICD-9CM # 719.45

COMMON CAUSES OF HIP PAIN IN DIFFERENT AGE GROUPS

Childhood (2-10 yr)
Intraarticular:
Developmental dislocation of the hip.
Perthes' disease.
Irritable hip.
Rickets.
Periarticular:
Osteomyelitis.
Referred:
Abdominal.
Adolescence (10-18 yr)
Intraarticular:
Slipped upper femoral epiphysis.
Torn labrum.
Periarticular:
Trochanteric bursitis.
Snapping hip.
Osteomyelitis.
Tumors.
Referred:
Abdominal.
Lumbar spine.
Early Adulthood (18-30 yr)
Intraarticular:
Inflammatory arthritis.
Torn labrum.
Periarticular:
Bursitis.
Referred:
Abdominal.
Lumbar spine.
Adulthood (30-50 yr)
Intraarticular:
Osteoarthritis.
Inflammatory arthritis.
Osteonecrosis.
Transient osteoporosis.
Periarticular:
Bursitis.
Referred:
Abdominal.
Lumbar spine.
Old Age (>50 yr)
Intraarticular:
Osteoarthritis.
Inflammatory arthritis.

Referred:
Abdominal.
Lumbar spine.

HIP PAIN WITHOUT OBVIOUS FRACTURE[2]

ICD-9CM # 338

DIFFERENTIAL DIAGNOSIS OF A PAINFUL HIP WITHOUT OBVIOUS FRACTURE

Referred pain (lumbar spine, hip, or knee).
Avascular necrosis of the femoral head.
Degenerative joint disease or osteoarthritis.
Herniation of a lumbar disk.
Diskitis.
Toxic synovitis of the hip.
Septic arthritis.
Bursitis.
Tendonitis.
Ligamentous injuries of the knee or hip.
Occult fracture.
Slipped capital femoral epiphysis.
Perthes' disease.
Tumor (lymphoma).
Deep venous thrombosis.
Arterial insufficiency.
Osteomyelitis.
Iliopsoas abscess.
Retroperitoneal hematoma.
Inguinal hernia.
Inguinal lymphadenopathy.
Genitourinary complaints.
Sports-related hernia.

HIRSUTISM

ICD-9CM # 704.1

Idiopathic: familial, possibly increased sensitivity to androgens.
Menopause.
Polycystic ovarian syndrome.
Drugs: androgens, anabolic steroids, methyltestosterone, minoxidil, diazoxide, phenytoin, glucocorticoids, cyclosporine.
Congenital adrenal hyperplasia.
Adrenal virilizing tumor.
Ovarian virilizing tumor: arrhenoblastoma, hilus cell tumor.
Pituitary adenoma.
Cushing's syndrome.
Hypothyroidism (congenital and juvenile).
Acromegaly.
Testicular feminization.

HIV INFECTION, ANORECTAL LESIONS[26]

ICD-9CM # 042 HIV Infection, Symptomatic
V08 HIV Infection, Asymptomatic

COMMON CONDITIONS

Anal fissure.
Abscess and fistula.
Hemorrhoids.
Pruritus ani.
Pilonidal disease.

COMMON STDs

Gonorrhea.
Chlamydia.
Herpes.
Chancroid.
Syphilis.
Condylomata acuminata.

ATYPICAL CONDITIONS

Infectious: TB, CMV, actinomycosis, cryptococcus.
Neoplastic: lymphoma, Kaposi's sarcoma, squamous cell carcinoma.
Other: idiopathic and ulcer.

HIV INFECTION, CHEST RADIOGRAPHIC ABNORMALITIES[26]

ICD-9CM # 042 HIV Infection, Symptomatic
V08 HIV Infection, Asymptomatic

DIFFUSE INTERSTITIAL INFILTRATION

Pneumocystis jiroveci.
Cytomegalovirus.
Mycobacterium tuberculosis.
Mycobacterium avium complex.
Histoplasmosis.
Coccidioidomycosis.
Lymphoid interstitial pneumonitis.

FOCAL CONSOLIDATION

Bacterial pneumonia.
Mycoplasma pneumoniae.
Pneumocystis jiroveci.
Mycobacterium tuberculosis.
Mycobacterium avium complex.

NODULAR LESIONS

Kaposi's sarcoma.
Mycobacterium tuberculosis.
Mycobacterium avium complex.
Fungal lesions.
Toxoplasmosis.

CAVITARY LESIONS

Pneumocystis jiroveci.
Mycobacterium tuberculosis.
Bacterial infection.

PLEURAL EFFUSION

Kaposi's sarcoma.
(Small effusion may be associated with any infection).

ADENOPATHY

Kaposi's sarcoma.
Lymphoma.
Mycobacterium tuberculosis.
Cryptococcus.

PNEUMOTHORAX

Kaposi's sarcoma.

HIV INFECTION, COGNITIVE IMPAIRMENT[25]

ICD-9CM # 042 HIV Infection, Symptomatic

EARLY TO MID-STAGE HIV DISEASE

Depression.
Alcohol and substance abuse.
Medication-induced cognitive impairment.
Metabolic encephalopathies.
HIV-related cognitive impairment.

ADVANCED HIV DISEASE (CD4+ <100/mm³)

Opportunistic infection of CNS.
Neurosyphilis.
CNS lymphoma.
Progressive multifocal leukoencephalopathy.
Depression.
Metabolic encephalopathies.
Medication-induced cognitive impairment.
Stroke.
HIV dementia.

HIV INFECTION, CUTANEOUS MANIFESTATIONS[21]

ICD-9CM # 042 HIV Infection, Symptomatic
V08 HIV Infection, Asymptomatic

BACTERIAL INFECTION

Bacillary angiomatosis: Numerous angiomatous nodules associated with fever, chills, weight loss.
Staphylococcus aureus: Folliculitis, ecthyma, impetigo, bullous impetigo, furuncles, carbuncles.
Syphilis: May occur in different forms (primary, secondary, tertiary); chancre may become painful because of secondary infection.

FUNGAL INFECTION

Candidiasis: Mucous membranes (oral, vulvovaginal), less commonly candida intertrigo or paronychia.
Cryptococcoses: Papules or nodules that strongly resemble molluscum contagiosum; other forms include pustules, purpuric papules, and vegetating plaques.
Seborrheic dermatitis: Scaling and erythema in the hair-bearing areas (eyebrows, scalp, chest, and pubic area).

ARTHROPOD INFESTATIONS

Scabies: Pruritus with or without rash, usually generalized but can be limited to a single digit.

VIRAL INFECTION

Herpes simplex: Vesicular lesion in clusters; perianal, genital, orofacial, or digital; can be disseminated.
Herpes zoster: Painful dermatomal vesicles that may ulcerate or disseminate.
HIV: Discrete erythematous macules and papules on the upper trunk, palms, and soles are the most characteristic cutaneous finding of acute HIV infection.

Human papillomavirus: Genital warts (may become unusually extensive).
Kaposi's sarcoma (herpesvirus): Erythematous macules or papules; enlarge at varying rates; violaceous nodules or plaques; occasionally painful.
Molluscum contagiosum: Discrete umbilicated papules commonly on the face, neck, and intertriginous sites (axilla, groin, or buttocks).

NONINFECTIOUS

Drug reactions: More frequent and severe in HIV patients.
Nutritional deficiencies: Mainly seen in children and patients with chronic diarrhea; diffuse skin manifestations, depending upon the deficiency.
Psoriasis: Scaly lesions; diffuse or localized; can be associated with arthritis.
Vasculitis: Palpable purpuric eruption (can resemble septic emboli).

HIV INFECTION, ESOPHAGEAL DISEASE

ICD-9CM # varies with specific diagnosis

Candida infection.
Cytomegalovirus infection.
Aphthous ulcer.
Herpes simplex.

HIV INFECTION, HEPATIC DISEASE[25]

ICD-9CM # 042 HIV Infection, Symptomatic

VIRUSES

Hepatitis A.
Hepatitis B.
Hepatitis C.
Hepatitis D (with HBV).
Epstein-Barr virus.
Cytomegalovirus.
Herpes simplex virus.
Adenovirus.
Varicella-zoster virus.

MYCOBACTERIA

Mycobacterium avium complex.
Mycobacterium tuberculosis.

FUNGI

Histoplasma capsulatum.
Cryptococcus neoformans.
Coccidioides immitis.
Candida albicans.
Pneumocystis jiroveci.
Penicillium marneffei.

PROTOZOA

Toxoplasma gondii.
Cryptosporidium parvum.
Microsporida.
Schistosoma.

BACTERIA

Bartonella henselae (peliosis hepatis).

MALIGNANCY

Kaposi's sarcoma (HHV-8).
Non-Hodgkin's lymphoma.
Hepatocellular carcinoma.

MEDICATIONS

Zidovudine.
Didanosine.
Ritonavir.
Other HIV-1 protease inhibitors.
Fluconazole.
Macrolide antibiotics.
Isoniazid.
Rifampin.
Trimethoprim-sulfamethoxazole.

HIV INFECTION, LOWER GI TRACT DISEASE[25]

ICD-9CM # 042 HIV Infection, Symptomatic

CAUSES OF ENTEROCOLITIS

Bacteria
Campylobacter jejuni and other spp.
Salmonella spp.
Shigella flexneri.
Aeromonas hydrophila.
Plesiomonas shigelloides.
Yersinia enterocolitica.
Vibrio spp.
Mycobacterium avium complex.
Mycobacterium tuberculosis.
Escherichia coli (enterotoxigenic, enteroadherent).
Bacterial overgrowth.
Clostridium difficile (toxin).
Parasites
Cryptosporidium parvum.
Microsporida (*Enterocytozoon bieneusi, Septata intestinalis*).
Isospora belli.
Entamoeba histolytica.
Giardia lamblia.
Cyclospora cayetanensis.
Viruses
Cytomegalovirus.
Adenovirus.
Calicivirus.
Astrovirus.
Picobirnavirus.
Human immunodeficiency virus.
Fungi
Histoplasma capsulatum.

CAUSES OF PROCTITIS

Bacteria
Chlamydia trachomatis.
Neisseria gonorrhoeae.
Treponema pallidum.
Viruses
Herpes simplex.
Cytomegalovirus.

HIV INFECTION, OCULAR MANIFESTATIONS[36]

ICD-9CM # 042 HIV Infection, Symptomatic
              V08 HIV Infection, Asymptomatic

EYELIDS

Molluscum contagiosum.
Kaposi's sarcoma.

CORNEA/CONJUNCTIVA

Keratoconjunctivitis sicca.
Bacterial/fungal ulcerative keratitis.
Herpes simplex.
Herpes zoster ophthalmicus.
Conjunctival microvasculopathy.
Kaposi's sarcoma.

RETINA, CHOROID, AND VITREOUS

Microvasculopathy.
Endophthalmitis.
Cytomegalovirus retinitis.
Acute retinal necrosis.
Syphilis.
Toxoplasmosis.
Pneumocystis choroidopathy.
Cryptococcosis.
Mycobacterial infection.
Intraocular lymphoma.
Candidiasis.
Histoplasmosis.

DRUGS ASSOCIATED WITH OCULAR TOXICITY

Rifabutin.
Didanosine.

NEUROOPHTHALMIC

Disc edema.
Primary or secondary optic neuropathy.
Cranial nerve palsies.

ORBITAL

Lymphoma.
Infection.
Pseudotumor.

HIV INFECTION, PULMONARY DISEASE[25]

ICD-9CM # 042 HIV Infection, Symptomatic

MYCOBACTERIAL

M. tuberculosis.
M. kansasii.
M. avium complex.
Other nontuberculous mycobacteria.

OTHER BACTERIAL

Streptococcus pneumoniae.
Staphylococcus aureus.
Haemophilus influenzae.
Enterobacteriaceae.
Pseudomonas aeruginosa.
Moraxella catarrhalis.
Group A Streptococcus.
Nocardia spp.
Rhodococcus equi.
Chlamydia pneumoniae.

FUNGAL

Pneumocystis carinii.
Cryptococcus neoformans.
Histoplasma capsulatum.
Coccidioides immitis.
Aspergillus spp.
Blastomyces dermatitidis.
Penicillium marneffei.

VIRAL

Cytomegalovirus.
Herpes simplex virus.
Adenovirus.
Respiratory syncytial virus.
Influenza viruses.
Parainfluenza virus.

OTHER

Toxoplasma gondii.
Strongyloides stercoralis.
Kaposi's sarcoma.
Lymphoma.
Lung cancer.
Lymphocytic interstitial pneumonitis.
Nonspecific interstitial pneumonitis.
Bronchiolitis obliterans with organizing pneumonia.
Pulmonary hypertension.
Emphysema-like or bullous disease.
Pneumothorax.
Congestive heart failure.
Diffuse alveolar damage.
Pulmonary embolus.

HOARSENESS

ICD-9CM # 784.49

Allergic rhinitis.
Infections (laryngitis, epiglottitis, tracheitis, croup).
Vocal cord polyps.
Voice strain.
Irritants (tobacco smoke).
Vocal cord trauma (intubation, surgery).
Neoplastic involvement of vocal cord (primary or metastatic).
Neurologic abnormalities (multiple sclerosis, ALS, parkinsonism).
Endocrine abnormalities (puberty, menopause, hypothyroidism).
Other (laryngeal webs or cysts, psychogenic, muscle tension abnormalities).

HYDROCEPHALUS

ICD-9CM # 331.4

Head trauma.
Brain neoplasm (primary or metastatic).
Spinal cord tumor.
Cerebellar infarction.
Exudative or granulomatous meningitis.
Cerebellar hemorrhage.
Subarachnoid hemorrhage.
Aqueductal stenosis.
Third ventricle colloid cyst.
Hindbrain malformation.
Viral encephalitis.
Metastases to leptomeninges.

HYPERCALCEMIA

ICD-9CM # 275.42 Hypercalcemia Disorder

Malignancy: increased bone resorption via osteoclast-activating factors, secretion of PTH-like substances, prostaglandin E_2, direct erosion by tumor cells, transforming growth factors, colony-stimulating activity. Hypercalcemia is common in the following neoplasms:
    Solid tumors: breast, lung, pancreas, kidneys, ovary.
    Hematologic cancers: myeloma, lymphosarcoma, adult T-cell lymphoma, Burkitt's lymphoma.
Hyperparathyroidism: increased bone resorption, GI absorption, and renal absorption; etiology:
    Parathyroid hyperplasia, adenoma.
    Hyperparathyroidism or renal failure with secondary hyperparathyroidism.
Granulomatous disorders: increased GI absorption (e.g., sarcoidosis).
Paget's disease: increased bone resorption, seen only during periods of immobilization.
Vitamin D intoxication, milk-alkali syndrome; increased GI absorption.
Thiazides: increased renal absorption.
Other causes: familial hypocalciuric hypercalcemia, thyrotoxicosis, adrenal insufficiency, prolonged immobilization, vitamin A intoxication, recovery from acute renal failure, lithium administration, pheochromocytoma, disseminated SLE.

HYPERCALCEMIA, MALIGNANCY-INDUCED

ICD-9CM # 275.42

Lung carcinoma	(6% frequency, 35% of hypercalcemic cases)
Breast carcinoma	(10% frequency, 25% of hypercalcemic cases)
Multiple myeloma	(33% frequency, 10% of hypercalcemic cases)
Lymphoma	(4% of hypercalcemic cases)
Genitourinary cancer	(6% of hypercalcemic cases)

HYPERCAPNIA, PERSISTENT[36]

ICD-9CM # 786.09

Hypercapnia with normal lungs: CNS disturbances (CVA, parkinsonism, encephalitis), metabolic alkalosis, myxedema, primary alveolar hypoventilation, spinal cord lesions.
Diseases of the chest wall (e.g., kyphoscoliosis, ankylosing spondylitis).
Neuromuscular disorders (e.g., myasthenia gravis, Guillain-Barré syndrome, amyotrophic lateral sclerosis, muscular dystrophy, poliomyelitis).
COPD.

HYPERCOAGULABLE STATE, ASSOCIATED DISORDERS[20]
ICD-9CM # 289.82

Systemic lupus erythematosus in association with the presence of a lupus anticoagulant or antiphospholipid antibodies.
Malignancy:
  Disease-related: includes migratory superficial thrombophlebitis (Trousseau syndrome), nonbacterial thrombotic endocarditis, thrombosis associated with chronic DIC, thrombotic microangiopathy.
  Treatment-related: associated with the administration of various chemotherapeutic agents (L-asparaginase, mitomycin, some adjuvant chemotherapeutic agents for treatment of breast cancer, thalidomide or lenalidomide in conjunction with high doses of dexamethasone).
Infusion of prothrombin complex concentrates.
Nephrotic syndrome.
Heparin-induced thrombocytopenia.
Myeloproliferative disorders.
Paroxysmal nocturnal hemoglobinuria.

DIC, Disseminated intravascular coagulopathy.

HYPERGASTRINEMIA
ICD-9CM # varies with specific disorder

Decreased gastrin release inhibition from medications (proton pump inhibitors [PPIs], H_2 receptor antagonists), vagotomy.
Chronic renal failure.
Hypochlorhydria due to atrophic gastritis, gastric carcinoma, pernicious anemia.
Gastrinoma (Zollinger-Ellison syndrome).
Pyloric obstruction.
Hyperplasia of antral G cells.
RA.

HYPERHIDROSIS[4]
ICD-9CM # 780.8 Hyperhidrosis

CORTICAL
Emotional.
Familial dysautonomia.
Congenital ichthyosiform erythroderma.
Epidermolysis bullosa.
Nail-patella syndrome.
Jadassohn-Lewandowsky syndrome.
Pachyonychia congenita.
Palmoplantar keratoderma.

HYPOTHALAMIC
Drugs
Antipyretics.
Emetics.
Insulin.
Meperidine.
Exercise Infection
Defervescence.
Chronic illness.
Metabolic
Debility.
DM.

Hyperpituitarism.
Hyperthyroidism.
Hypoglycemia.
Obesity.
Porphyria.
Pregnancy.
Rickets.
Infantile scurvy.
Cardiovascular
Heart failure.
Shock.
Vasomotor
Cold injury.
Raynaud phenomenon.
RA.
Neurologic
Abscess.
Familial dysautonomia.
Postencephalitic.
Tumor.
Miscellaneous
Chédiak-Higashi syndrome.
Compensatory.
Phenylketonuria.
Pheochromocytoma.
Vitiligo.
Medullary
Physiologic gustatory sweating.
Encephalitis.
Granulosis rubra nasi.
Syringomyelia.
Thoracic sympathetic trunk injury.
Spinal
Cord transection.
Syringomyelia.
Changes in Blood Flow
Mallucci syndrome.
Arteriovenous fistula.
Klippel-Trenaunay syndrome.
Glomus tumor.
Blue rubber bleb nevus syndrome.

HYPERKALEMIA
ICD-9CM # 276.7

Pseudohyperkalemia.
  Hemolyzed specimen.
  Severe thrombocytosis (platelet count 0.106 ml).
  Severe leukocytosis (white blood cell count 0.105 ml).
  Fist clenching during phlebotomy.
Excessive potassium intake (often in setting of impaired excretion).
  Potassium replacement therapy.
  High-potassium diet.
  Salt substitutes with potassium.
  Potassium salts of antibiotics.
Decreased renal excretion.
  Potassium-sparing diuretics (e.g., spironolactone, triamterene, amiloride).
  Renal insufficiency.
  Mineralocorticoid deficiency.
  Hyporeninemic hypoaldosteronism (DM).
  Tubular unresponsiveness to aldosterone (e.g., SLE, multiple myeloma, sickle cell disease).
  Type 4 RTA.

ACE inhibitors.
Heparin administration.
NSAIDs.
Trimethoprim-sulfamethoxazole.
Beta-blockers.
Pentamidine.
Redistribution (excessive cellular release).

  Acidemia (each 0.1 decrease in pH increases the serum potassium by 0.4 to 0.6 mEq/L). Lactic acidosis and ketoacidosis cause minimal redistribution.
  Insulin deficiency.
  Drugs (e.g., succinylcholine, markedly increased digitalis level, arginine, beta-adrenergic blockers).
  Hypertonicity.
  Hemolysis.
  Tissue necrosis, rhabdomyolysis, burns.
  Hyperkalemic periodic paralysis.

HYPERKALEMIA, DRUG-INDUCED[38b]
ICD-9CM # 276.7

IMPAIRED RENIN-ALDOSTERONE ELABORATION/FUNCTION
Cyclooxygenase inhibitors (NSAIDs).
β-Adrenergic antagonists.
Spironolactone.
Angiotensin-converting enzyme inhibitors and angiotensin II receptor blockers.
Heparin.

INHIBITORS OF RENAL POTASSIUM SECRETION
Potassium-sparing diuretics (amiloride, triamterene).
Trimethoprim.
Pentamidine.
Cyclosporine.
Digitalis overdose.
Lithium.

ALTERED POTASSIUM DISTRIBUTION
Insulin antagonists (somatostatin, diazoxide).
β-Adrenergic antagonists.
α-Adrenergic agonists.
Hypertonic solutions.
Digitalis.
Succinylcholine.
Arginine hydrochloride, lysine hydrochloride.

HYPERKINETIC MOVEMENT DISORDERS[30]
ICD-9CM # 314.8 Hyperkinetic Syndrome
275.1 Choreoathetosis
335.5 Hemiballism
333.7 Dystonia Due to Drugs
333.6 Dystonia, Idiopathic

Chorea, choreoathetosis: drug-induced, Huntington's chorea, Sydenham's chorea.
Tardive dyskinesia (e.g., phenothiazines).
Hemiballismus (lacunar CVA near subthalamic nuclei in basal ganglia, metastatic lesions, toxoplasmosis [in AIDS]).

Differential Diagnosis

II

Dystonia (idiopathic, familial, drug-induced [prochlorperazine, metoclopramide]), Wilson's disease.
Liver failure.
Thyrotoxicosis.
SLE, polycythemia.

HYPERMAGNESEMIA
ICD-9CM # 275.2

Renal failure (decreased GFR).
Decreased renal excretion secondary to salt depletion.
Abuse of antacids and laxatives containing magnesium in patients with renal insufficiency.
Endocrinopathies (deficiency of mineralocorticoid or thyroid hormone).
Increased tissue breakdown (rhabdomyolysis).
Redistribution: acute DKA, pheochromocytoma.
Other: lithium, volume depletion, familial hypocalciuric hypercalcemia.

HYPEROSTOSIS, CORTICAL BONE[16a]
ICD-9CM # varies with specific diagnosis

DISORDERS ASSOCIATED WITH HYPEROSTOSIS OF CORTICAL BONE
Progressive diaphyseal dysplasia.
Endosteal hyperostosis.
Pachydermoperiostosis.
Hypertrophic oseoarthropathy.
Thyroid acropachy.
Hypervitaminosis A.
Paget's disease.
Infantile cortical hyperostosis.

HYPERPHOSPHATEMIA
ICD-9CM # 275.3

Excessive phosphate administration.
Excessive oral intake or IV administration.
Laxatives containing phosphate (phosphate tablets, phosphate enemas).
Decreased renal phosphate excretion.
Acute or chronic renal failure.
Hypoparathyroidism or pseudohypoparathyroidism.
Acromegaly, thyrotoxicosis.
Bisphosphonate therapy.
Tumor calcinosis.
Sickle cell anemia.
Transcellular shift out of cells.
Chemotherapy of lymphoma or leukemia, tumor lysis syndrome, hemolysis.
Acidosis.
Rhabdomyolysis, malignant hyperthermia.
Artifact: in vitro hemolysis.
Pseudohyperphosphatemia: hyperlipidemia, paraproteinemia, hyperbilirubinemia.

HYPERPIGMENTATION[5]
ICD-9CM # 709.00

Addison's disease.*
Arsenic ingestion.

ACTH- or MSH-producing tumors (e.g., oat cell carcinoma of the lung).*
Drug induced (i.e., antimalarials, some cytotoxic agents).
Hemochromatosis ("bronze" diabetes).
Malabsorption syndrome (Whipple's disease and celiac sprue).
Melanoma.
Melanotropic hormone injection.*
Pheochromocytoma.
Porphyrias (porphyria cutanea tarda and variegate porphyria).
Pregnancy.
Progressive systemic sclerosis and related conditions.
PUVA therapy (psoralen administration) for psoriasis and vitiligo.*

ACTH, Adrenocorticotropic hormone; *MSH*, melanocyte-stimulating hormone; *PUVA*, psoralen plus ultraviolet A.
*Accentuation on sun-exposed surfaces.

HYPERSPLENISM, ASSOCIATED CONDITIONS
ICD-9CM # 289.4

Cirrhosis.
Portal vein thrombosis.
Myeloproliferative diseases.
Lymphomas.
Leukemias.
Splenic vein thrombosis.
Autoimmune disease.
Sickle cell disease.
Thalassemias.
Gaucher's disease.
Niemann-Pick disease.

HYPERTENSION, IN CHILDREN[2]
ICD-9CM # 401

PRIMARY
Essential hypertension.

SECONDARY
Renal
Glomerulonephritis.
Henoch-Schönlein purpura.
Pyelonephritis.
Obstruction of reflux.
Polycystic kidney disease.
Diabetic nephropathy.
Trauma.
Renal transplant or hemodialysis.
Tuberous sclerosis.
Systemic lupus nephritis.
Endocrine
Pheochromocytoma.
Cushing's syndrome.
Congenital adrenal hyperplasia.
Corticosteroid treatment.
Hyperthyroidism.
Neuroblastoma.
Ovarian tumor.
Cardiac
Congestive heart failure.
Coarctation of the aorta.

Vascular
Hemolytic-uremic syndrome.
Kawasaki syndrome.
Renal artery thrombosis or stenosis.
Neurologic
Central nervous system tumor or infection.
Central nervous system trauma or abuse.
Increased intracranial pressure.
Guillain-Barré syndrome.
Neoplastic
Neuroblastoma.
Wilms' tumor.
Pheochromocytoma.
Adrenal carcinoma.
Drugs
Corticosteroids.
Cocaine.
Sympathomimetics.
Oral contraceptives.
Phencyclidine.
Beta-blocker or clonidine withdrawal.
Lead, mercury.
Others
Iatrogenic fluid overload.
Volume overload from end-stage renal disease.

HYPERTENSIVE CRISIS SYNDROMES[38b]
ICD-9CM # 997.91

Malignant hypertension.
Nonmalignant hypertension with target organ disorders:
  Patient requiring emergency surgery with poorly controlled hypertension.
  Hyperviscosity syndrome.
  Postoperative patient.
  Renal transplant patient: acute rejection, transplant renal artery stenosis.
  Quadriplegic patient with autonomic hyperreflexia.
  Severe burns.
  Acute aortic dissection.
  Intracranial hemorrhage, ischemic stroke, or subarachnoid hemorrhage.
  Hypertensive encephalopathy.
  Myocardial ischemia/acute left ventricular failure.
  Preeclampsia/eclampsia.
  Antiphospholipid antibody syndrome.
  Acute renal failure:
  • Scleroderma renal crisis.
  • Chronic glomerulonephritis.
  • Reflux nephropathy.
  • Analgesic nephropathy.
  • Acute glomerulonephritis.
  • Radiation nephritis.
  • Ask-Upmark kidney.
  • Chronic lead intoxication.
  Renovascular hypertension:
  • Fibromuscular dysplasia.
  • Atherosclerosis.
  Endocrine hypertension:
  • Congenital adrenal hyperplasia.
  • Pheochromocytoma.
  • Oral contraceptives.
  • Aldosteronism.
  • Cushing disease/syndrome.

Systemic vasculitis.
Atheroembolic renal crisis.
Drugs:
- Oral contraceptives.
- Nonsteroidal antiinflammatory agents.
- Atropine.
- Corticosteroids.
- Sympathomimetics.
- Erythropoietin.
- Lead intoxication.
- Cyclosporine.

Catecholamine excess states:
- Pheochromocytoma.
- MAO/tyramine interaction.
- Antihypertensive withdrawal.
- Cocaine intoxication, sympathomimetic overdose.

HYPERTRICHOSIS[7]

ICD-9CM # 704.1 Hypertrichosis NOS
       757.4 Hypertrichosis, Congenital

DRUGS

Dilantin.
Streptomycin.
Hexachlorobenzene.
Penicillamine.
Diazoxide.
Minoxidil.
Cyclosporine.

SYSTEMIC ILLNESS

Hypothyroidism.
Anorexia nervosa.
Malnutrition.
Porphyria.
Dermatomyositis.

IDIOPATHIC

HYPERTROPHIC OSTEOARTHROPATHY

ICD-9CM # 731.2

Idiopathic.
Pulmonary disease (e.g., pulmonary fibrosis, cystic fibrosis, sarcoidosis).
Bronchogenic carcinoma.
AIDS.
GI neoplasm (e.g., esophagus, colon).
Hepatic neoplasm, cirrhosis.
Cardiovascular diseases, aortic aneurysm, aortic prosthesis.
Congenital cyanotic heart disease, patent ductus arteriosus.
Pulmonary infections, bacterial endocarditis, amebic dysentery.
Inflammatory bowel disease.
Connective tissue diseases.
Lymphomas.
Thyroid acropachy.

HYPERVENTILATION, PERSISTENT[36]

ICD-9CM # 786.01

Fibrotic lung disease.
Metabolic acidosis (e.g., diabetes, uremia).

CNS disorders (midbrain and pontine lesions).
Hepatic coma.
Salicylate intoxication.
Fever.
Sepsis.
Psychogenic (e.g., anxiety).

HYPOCALCEMIA

ICD-9CM # 275.41

Renal insufficiency: hypocalcemia caused by:
    Increased calcium deposits in bone and soft tissue secondary to increased serum phosphate level.
    Decreased production of 1,25-dihydroxyvitamin D.
    Excessive loss of 25-OHD (nephrotic syndrome).
Hypoalbuminemia: each decrease in serum albumin (g/L) will decrease serum calcium by 0.8 mg/dl but will not change free (ionized) calcium.
Vitamin D deficiency:
    Malabsorption (most common cause).
    Inadequate intake.
    Decreased production of 1,25-dihydroxyvitamin D (vitamin D–dependent rickets, renal failure).
    Decreased production of 25-OHD (parenchymal liver disease).
    Accelerated 25-OHD catabolism (phenytoin, phenobarbital).
    End-organ resistance to 1,25-dihydroxyvitamin D.
Hypomagnesemia: hypocalcemia caused by:
    Decreased PTH secretion.
    Inhibition of PTH effect on bone.
Pancreatitis, hyperphosphatemia, osteoblastic metastases: hypocalcemia is secondary to increased calcium deposits (bone, abdomen).
Pseudohypoparathyroidism (PHP): autosomal recessive disorder characterized by short stature, shortening of metacarpal bones, obesity, and mental retardation; the hypocalcemia is secondary to congenital end-organ resistance to PTH.
Idiopathic hypoparathyroidism, surgical removal of parathyroids (e.g., neck surgery).
"Hungry bones syndrome": rapid transfer of calcium from plasma into bones after removal of a parathyroid tumor.
Sepsis.
Massive blood transfusion (as a result of EDTA in blood).

HYPOCAPNIA

ICD-9CM # 786.01

Hyperventilation.
Pneumonia, pneumonitis.
Fever, sepsis.
Medications (salicylates, beta-adrenergic agonists, progesterone, methylxanthines).
Pulmonary disease (asthma, interstitial fibrosis).
Pulmonary embolism.
Hepatic failure.
Metabolic acidosis.
High altitude.
CHF.

Pregnancy.
Pain.
CNS lesions.

HYPOGLYCEMIA

ICD-9CM # 251.2 Spontaneous
      250.3 Diabetic
      251.0 Due to Insulin
      579.3 Postoperative
      251.2 Reactive

Oral hypoglycemics (therapeutic, factitious).
Exogenous insulin (therapeutic, factitious).
Postoperative gastric emptying (alimentary hyperinsulinism).
Severe malnutrition.
Liver disease.
Hypermetabolic state (sepsis).
Ketotic hypoglycemia.
Insulinoma.
Antibodies to endogenous insulin.
Hormone deficiencies (glucagon, growth hormone, hypoadrenalism).
Enzyme disorders in metabolism of glycogen, hexose, glycolysis, and Krebs cycle.
Idiopathic.

HYPOGLYCEMIA, IN INFANTS AND CHILDREN[22a]

ICD-9CM # 251.2   Hypoglycemia

CLASSIFICATION OF HYPOGLYCEMIA IN INFANTS AND CHILDREN

NEONATAL TRANSIENT HYPOGLYCEMIA
Associated with Inadequate Substrate or Immature Enzyme Function in Otherwise Normal Neonates
Prematurity.
Small for gestational age.
Normal newborn.
Transient Neonatal Hyperinsulinism Also Present in:
Infant of diabetic mother.
Discordant twin.
Birth asphyxia.
Infant of toxemic mother.
NEONATAL, INFANTILE, OR CHILDHOOD PERSISTENT HYPOGLYCEMIAS
Hormonal Disorders
Hyperinsulinism.
Recessive K_{ATP} channel HI.
Recessive HADH (hydroxyl acyl CoA dehydrogenase) mutation HI.
Recessive UCP2 (mitochondrial uncoupling protein 2) mutation HI.
Focal K_{ATP} channel HI.
Dominant K_{ATP} channel HI.
Dominant glucokinase HI.
Dominant glutamate dehydrogenase HI (hyperinsulinism/hyperammonemia syndrome).
Dominant mutation in HNF4A (hepatic nuclear factor 4 alpha) HI with MODY later in life.
Dominant mutation in SLC16A1 (the pyruvate transporter)-exercise-induced hypoglycemia.
Acquired islet adenoma.
Beckwith-Wiedemann syndrome.

Insulin administration (Munchausen syndrome by proxy).

Oral sulfonylurea drugs.

Congenital disorders of glycosylation.

Counter-Regulatory Hormone Deficiency

Panhypopituitarism.

Isolated growth hormone deficiency.

Addison disease.

Epinephrine deficiency.

Glycogenolysis and Gluconeogenesis Disorders

Glucose-6-phosphatase deficiency (GSD 1a).

Glucose-6-phosphate translocase deficiency (GSD 1b).

Amylo-1,6-glucosidase (debranching enzyme) deficiency (GSD 3).

Liver phosphorylase deficiency (GSD 6).

Phosphorylase kinase deficiency (GSD 9).

Glycogen synthetase deficiency (GSD 0).

Fructose-1,6-diphosphatase deficiency.

Pyruvate carboxylase deficiency.

Galactosemia.

Hereditary fructose intolerance.

Lipolysis Disorders

Fatty Acid Oxidation Disorders

Carnitine transporter deficiency (primary carnitine deficiency).

Carnitine palmitoyltransferase-1 deficiency.

Carnitine translocase deficiency.

Carnitine palmitoyltransferase-2 deficiency.

Secondary carnitine deficiencies.

Very long, long-, medium-, short-chain acyl-CoA dehydrogenase deficiency.

OTHER ETIOLOGIES

Substrate-Limited

Ketotic hypoglycemia.

Poisoning—drugs.

Salicylates.

Alcohol.

Oral hypoglycemic agents.

Insulin.

Propranolol.

Pentamidine.

Quinine.

Disopyramide.

Ackee fruit (unripe)—hypoglycin.

Vacor (rat poison).

Trimethoprim-sulfamethoxazole (with renal failure).

Liver Disease

Reye syndrome.

Hepatitis.

Cirrhosis.

Hepatoma.

Amino Acid and Organic Acid Disorders

Maple syrup urine disease.

Propionic acidemia.

Methylmalonic acidemia.

Tyrosinosis.

Glutaric aciduria.

3-Hydroxy-3-methylglutaric aciduria.

Systemic Disorders

Sepsis.

Carcinoma/sarcoma (secreting—insulin-like growth factor II).

Heart failure.

Malnutrition.

Malabsorption.

Anti-insulin receptor antibodies.

Anti-insulin antibodies.

Neonatal hyperviscosity.

Renal failure.

Diarrhea.

Burns.

Shock.

Postsurgical.

Pseudohypoglycemia (leukocytosis, polycythemia).

Excessive insulin therapy of insulin-dependent diabetes mellitus.

Factitious.

Nissen fundoplication (dumping syndrome).

Falciparum malaria.

GSD, Glycogen storage disease; *HI,* hyperinsulinemia; K_{ATP}, regulated potassium channel.

HYPOGONADISM

ICD-9CM # 256.3 Female
257.2 Male
256.3 Ovarian
253.4 Pituitary
257.2 Testicular

HYPERGONADOTROPIC HYPOGONADISM

Hormone resistance (androgen, LH insensitivity).

Gonadal defects (e.g., Klinefelter's syndrome, myotonic dystrophy).

Drug-induced (e.g., spironolactone, cytotoxins).

Alcoholism, radiation-induced.

Mumps orchitis.

Anatomic defects, castration.

HYPOGONADOTROPIC HYPOGONADISM

Pituitary lesions (neoplasms, granulomas, infarction, hemochromatosis, vasculitis).

Drug-induced (e.g., glucocorticoids).

Hyperprolactinemia.

Genetic disorders (Laurence-Moon-Biedl syndrome, Prader-Willi).

Delayed puberty.

Other: chronic disease, nutritional deficiency, Kallmann's syndrome, idiopathic isolated LH or FSH deficiency.

HYPOKALEMIA

ICD-9CM # 276.8

Cellular shift (redistribution) and undetermined mechanisms.

Alkalosis (each 0.1 increase in pH decreases serum potassium by 0.4 to 0.6 mEq/L).

Insulin administration.

Vitamin B_{12} therapy for megaloblastic anemias, acute leukemias.

Hypokalemic periodic paralysis: rare familial disorder manifested by recurrent attacks of flaccid paralysis and hypokalemia.

Beta-adrenergic agonists (e.g., terbutaline), decongestants, bronchodilators, theophylline, caffeine.

Barium poisoning, toluene intoxication, verapamil intoxication, chloroquine intoxication.

Correction of digoxin intoxication with digoxin antibody fragments (Digibind).

Increased renal excretion.

Drugs:

Diuretics, including carbonic anhydrase inhibitors (e.g., acetazolamide).

Amphotericin B.

High-dose sodium penicillin, nafcillin, ampicillin, or carbenicillin.

Cisplatin.

Aminoglycosides.

Corticosteroids, mineralocorticoids.

Foscarnet sodium.

RTA: distal (type 1) or proximal (type 2).

Diabetic ketoacidosis (DKA), ureteroenterostomy.

Magnesium deficiency.

Postobstruction diuresis, diuretic phase of ATN.

Osmotic diuresis (e.g., mannitol).

Bartter's syndrome: hyperplasia of juxtaglomerular cells leading to increased renin and aldosterone, metabolic alkalosis, hypokalemia, muscle weakness, and tetany (seen in young adults).

Increased mineralocorticoid activity (primary or secondary aldosteronism), Cushing's syndrome.

Chronic metabolic alkalosis from loss of gastric fluid (increased renal potassium secretion).

GI loss:

Vomiting, nasogastric suction.

Diarrhea.

Laxative abuse.

Villous adenoma.

Fistulas.

Inadequate dietary intake (e.g., anorexia nervosa).

Cutaneous loss (excessive sweating).

High dietary sodium intake, excessive use of licorice.

HYPOMAGNESEMIA

ICD-9CM # 275.2

GASTROINTESTINAL AND NUTRITIONAL

Defective GI absorption (malabsorption).

Inadequate dietary intake (e.g., alcoholics).

Parenteral therapy without magnesium.

Chronic diarrhea, villous adenoma, prolonged nasogastric suction, fistulas (small bowel, biliary).

EXCESSIVE RENAL LOSSES

Diuretics.

RTA.

Diuretic phase of ATN.

Endocrine disturbances (DKA, hyperaldosteronism, hyperthyroidism, hyperparathyroidism), SIADH, Bartter's syndrome, hypercalciuria, hypokalemia.

Cisplatin, alcohol, cyclosporine, digoxin, pentamidine, mannitol, amphotericin B, foscarnet, methotrexate.

Antibiotics (gentamicin, ticarcillin, carbenicillin).

Redistribution: hypoalbuminemia, cirrhosis, administration of insulin and glucose, theophylline, epinephrine, acute pancreatitis, cardiopulmonary bypass.

Miscellaneous: sweating, burns, prolonged exercise, lactation, "hungry-bones" syndrome.

HYPONATREMIA
ICD-9CM # 276.1

Renal loss from renal disease, diuretics.
GI loss (diarrhea, vomiting, suction).
Hypertonic hyponatremia (e.g., increased serum osmolality from hyperglycemia).
Transcutaneous loss (extensive burns, excessive sweating).
Fluid sequestration (e.g., ascites).
Osmotic diuresis (e.g., mannitol, glucose).
Dilutional (psychogenic polydipsia, iatrogenic).
Syndrome of inappropriate antidiuretic hormone secretion.
Edema with water and sodium retention.
Artifact (e.g., severe hyperlipidemia).
Laboratory error.
Adrenal insufficiency.

HYPOPHOSPHATEMIA
ICD-9CM # 275.3

Decreased intake (prolonged starvation [alcoholics], hyperalimentation, or IV infusion without phosphate).
Malabsorption.
Phosphate-binding antacids.
Renal loss:
    RTA.
    Fanconi syndrome, vitamin D–resistant rickets.
    ATN (diuretic phase).
    Hyperparathyroidism (primary or secondary).
    Familial hypophosphatemia.
    Hypokalemia, hypomagnesemia.
    Acute volume expansion.
    Glycosuria, idiopathic hypercalciuria.
    Acetazolamide.
Transcellular shift into cells:
    Alcohol withdrawal.
    DKA (recovery phase).
    Glucose-insulin or catecholamine infusion.
    Anabolic steroids.
    Total parenteral nutrition.
    Theophylline overdose.
    Severe hyperthermia; recovery from hypothermia.
    "Hungry bones" syndrome.

HYPOPIGMENTATION
ICD-9CM # 709.00

Vitiligo.
Tinea versicolor.
Atopic dermatitis.
Chemical leukoderma.
Idiopathic hypomelanosis.
Sarcoidosis.
SLE.
Scleroderma.
Oculocutaneous albinism.
Phenylketonuria.
Nevoid hypopigmentation.

HYPOTENSION, POSTURAL
ICD-9CM # 458.0

Antihypertensive medications (especially α-blockers, diuretics, ACE inhibitors).
Volume depletion (hemorrhage, dehydration).
Impaired cardiac output (constrictive pericarditis, aortic stenosis).
Peripheral autonomic dysfunction (DM, Guillain-Barré).
Idiopathic orthostatic hypotension.
Central autonomic dysfunction (Shy-Drager syndrome).
Peripheral venous disease.
Adrenal insufficiency.

HYPOTHYROIDISM, CONGENITAL[22a]
ICD-9CM # 243

ETIOLOGIC CLASSIFICATION OF CONGENITAL HYPOTHYROIDISM
PRIMARY HYPOTHYROIDISM
Defect of fetal thyroid development (dysgenesis):
    Aplasia.
    Hypoplasia.
    Ectopia.
Defect in thyroid hormone synthesis (dyshormonogenesis):
    Iodide transport defect: mutation in thyroglobulin gene.
    Thyroid organification, or coupling defect: mutation in thyroid peroxidase gene.
    Defects in H_2O_2 generation: mutations in DUOXA2 maturation factor or *DUOX2* gene.
    Thyroglobulin synthesis defect: mutation in thyroglobulin gene.
    Deiodination defect: mutation in *DEHAL1* gene.
TSH unresponsiveness:
    $G_s\alpha$ mutation (e.g., type 1A pseudohypothyroidism).
    Mutation in TSH receptor.
Defect in thyroid hormone transport: mutation in monocarboxylate transporter 8 *(MCT8)* gene.
Iodine deficiency (endemic goiter).
Maternal antibodies: thyrotropin receptor–blocking antibody (TRBAb, also termed *thyrotropin-binding inhibitor immunoglobulin*).
Maternal medications:
    Iodides, amiodarone.
    Propylthiouracil, methimazole.
    Radioiodine.
CENTRAL (HYPOPITUITARY) HYPOTHYROIDISM
PIT-1 mutations:
    Deficiency of thyroid-stimulating hormone (TSH).
    Deficiency of growth hormone.
    Deficiency of prolactin.
PROP-1 mutations:
    Deficiency of TSH.
    Deficiency of growth hormone.
    Deficiency of prolactin.
    Deficiency of luteinizing hormone.
    Deficiency of follicle-stimulating hormone.
    ±Deficiency of adrenocorticotropic hormone.

TSH deficiency: mutation in TSH β subunit gene (manifests as primary hypothyroidism with elevated TSH level).
Multiple pituitary deficiencies (e.g., craniopharyngioma).
Thyroid-releasing hormone (TRH) deficiency:
    Isolated.
    Multiple hypothalamic deficiencies (e.g., septooptic dysplasia).
TRH unresponsiveness.
Mutations in TRH receptor.

HYPOTONIA, INFANTILE, DIFFERENTIAL DIAGNOSIS[22a]
ICD-9CM # 360.30 Hypotonia

Cerebral hypotonia.
    Benign congenital hypotonia.
    Chromosome disorders.
    • Prader-Willi syndrome.
    • Trisomy.
    Chronic nonprogressive encephalopathy.
    • Cerebral malformation.
    • Perinatal distress.
    • Postnatal disorders.
    Peroxisomal disorders.
    • Cerebrohepatorenal syndrome (Zellweger syndrome).
    • Neonatal adrenoleukodystrophy.
    Other genetic defects.
    • Familial dysautonomia.
    • Oculocerebrorenal syndrome (Lowe syndrome).
    Other metabolic defects.
    • Acid maltase deficiency (see "Metabolic Myopathies").
    • Infantile G_M, gangliosidosis.
Spinal cord disorders.
Spinal muscular atrophies.
    Acute infantile.
    • Autosomal dominant.
    • Autosomal recessive.
    • Cytochrome-*c* oxidase deficiency.
    • X-linked.
    Chronic infantile.
    • Autosomal dominant.
    • Autosomal recessive.
    • Congenital cervical spinal muscular atrophy.
    • Infantile neuronal degeneration.
    • Neurogenic arthrogryposis.
Polyneuropathies.
    Congenital hypomyelinating neuropathy.
    Giant axonal neuropathy.
    Hereditary motor-sensory neuropathies.
Disorders of neuromuscular transmission.
    Familial infantile myasthenia.
    Infantile botulism.
    Transitory myasthenia gravis.
Fiber-type disproportion myopathies.
    Central core disease.
    Congenital fiber-type disproportion myopathy.
    Myotubular (centronuclear) myopathy.
    • Acute.
    • Chronic.
    Nemaline (rod) myopathy.
    • Autosomal dominant.
    • Autosomal recessive.

Metabolic myopathies.
  Acid maltase deficiency.
  Cytochrome-*c* oxidase deficiency.
Muscular dystrophies.
  • Bethlem myopathy.
  • Congenital dystrophinopathy.
  Congenital muscular dystrophy.
  • Merosin deficiency, primary.
  • Merosin deficiency, secondary.
  • Merosin positive.
  Congenital myotonic dystrophy.

HYPOVOLEMIC SHOCK, PEDIATRIC POPULATION[12b]

ICD-9CM # 785.59 Hypovolemic Shock

ETIOLOGIES OF HYPOVOLEMIC SHOCK

Whole blood loss.
• Absolute loss: hemorrhage.
  External bleeding.
  Internal bleeding.
  • Gastrointestinal.
  • Intraabdominal (spleen, liver).
  • Major vessel injury.
  • Intracranial (in infants).
  • Fractures.
• Relative loss.
  Pharmacologic (barbiturates, vasodilators).
  Positive pressure ventilation.
  Spinal cord injury.
  Sepsis.
  Anaphylaxis.
Plasma loss.
• Burns.
• Capillary leak syndromes.
  Inflammation, sepsis.
  Anaphylaxis.
• Protein-losing syndromes.
Fluid and electrolyte loss.
• Vomiting and diarrhea.
• Excessive diuretic use.
• Endocrine:
  Adrenal insufficiency.
  Diabetes insipidus.
  Diabetes mellitus.

ILIAC FOSSA PAIN, LEFT SIDED[38]

ICD-9CM # varies with specific diagnosis

GASTROINTESTINAL CAUSES OF ACUTE LEFT ILIAC FOSSA PAIN

Nonspecific left iliac fossa pain including constipation.
Acute gastroenteritis.
Acute diverticulitis.
Colonic carcinoma.
Colonic ischemia.
Localized small bowel perforation.

ILIAC FOSSA PAIN, RIGHT SIDED[38]

ICD-9CM # varies with specific diagnosis

DIFFERENTIAL DIAGNOSIS OF RIGHT ILIAC FOSSA PAIN

Gastrointestinal Causes
Nonspecific right iliac fossa pain.
Acute appendicitis.
Mesenteric adenitis.
Terminal ileitis.
Acute inflammation of Meckel's diverticulum.
Crohn's disease of the terminal ileum.
Cecal carcinoma.
Inflammatory cecal lesion (e.g., diverticulitis in a solitary cecal diverticulum).
Inflammatory lesion of the terminal ileum (e.g., foreign body perforation).

Non-Gastrointestinal Causes
Ruptured ovarian follicle (mittelschmerz).
Acute salpingitis (pelvic inflammatory disease).
Rupture/torsion or hemorrhage of an ovarian cyst.
Endometriosis.
Ectopic pregnancy.
Urinary tract infection.

IMMUNODEFICIENCY, CONGENITAL (PRIMARY)

ICD-9CM # 279.2

CONGENITAL (PRIMARY) CAUSES OF IMMUNODEFIENCY

T-lymphocyte Deficiencies
DiGeorge syndrome (thymic aplasia with reduced CD4 and CD3 cells).
Purine nucleoside phosphorylase deficiency (marked T-cell depletion).

B-lymphocyte Deficiencies
Bruton X-linked agammaglobulinemia (absence of B cells, plasma cells, and antibody).
Selective immunoglobulin G (IgG) subclass deficiencies.
Selective IgA deficiency.
Hyper-IgM immunodeficiency (elevated IgM but reduced IgG and IgA).

Mixed T- and B-lymphocyte Deficiencies
Common variable immunodeficiency (leads to various B-cell activation or differentiation defects and gradual deterioration of T-cell number and function).
Severe combined immunodeficiency (severe reduction in IgG and absence of T cells).
Wiskott-Aldrich syndrome (decreased T-cell number and function, low IgM, occasionally low IgG).
Ataxia-telangiectasia (decreased T-cell number and function; IgA, IgE, IgG$_2$, and IgG$_4$ deficiency).

Disorders of Complement
C3 deficiency (congenital absence of C3 or consumption of C3 due to deficiency of C3b inactivator).

Phagocyte Defects
Chronic granulomatous disease (defect in nicotinamide adenine dinucleotide phosphate oxidase in phagocytic cells).

Chédiak-Higashi syndrome (impaired microbicidal activity of phagocytes).
Kostmann syndrome, Shwachman-Diamond syndrome, cyclic neutropenia (low neutrophil count).

IMPOTENCE[27]

ICD-9CM # 302.72 Psychosexual
           607.84 Organic
           997.99 Organic
                  Postprostatectomy

Psychogenic.
Endocrine: hyperprolactinemia, DM, Cushing's syndrome, hypothyroidism or hyperthyroidism, abnormality of hypothalamic-pituitary-testicular axis.
Vascular: arterial insufficiency, venous leakage, AV malformation, local trauma.
Medications.
Neurogenic: autonomic or sensory neuropathy, spinal cord trauma or tumor, CVA, multiple sclerosis, temporal lobe epilepsy.
Systemic illness: renal failure, COPD, cirrhosis of liver, myotonic dystrophy.
Peyronie's disease.
Prostatectomy.

INCONTINENCE, FECAL[38]

ICD-9CM # 787.6

NORMAL SPHINCTER
Diarrhea.
Anorectal conditions:
  • Rectal carcinoma.
  • Inflammatory bowel disease.
  • Hemorrhoids.
  • Mucosal prolapse.
  • Fissure-in-ano.
  • Abnormal rectal sensation.

ABNORMAL SPHINCTER
Congenital abnormalities.
Anal sepsis.
Neurologic conditions.
Rectal prolapse.
Sphincter trauma.
Neurogenic (idiopathic) incontinence.

INFERTILITY, FEMALE[14]

ICD-9CM # 628.9

FALLOPIAN TUBE PATHOLOGY
PID or puerperal infection.
Congenital anomalies.
Endometriosis.
Secondary to past peritonitis of nongenital origin.
Amenorrhea and anovulation.
Minor anovulatory disturbances.

CERVICAL AND UTERINE FACTORS
Leiomyomas and polyps.
Uterine anomalies.
Intrauterine synechiae (Asherman's syndrome).
Destroyed endocervical glands (postsurgery or postinfection).

VAGINAL FACTORS

Congenital absence of vagina.
Imperforate hymen.
Vaginismus.
Vaginitis.

IMMUNOLOGIC FACTORS

Sperm-immobilizing antibodies.
Sperm-agglutinating antibodies.

NUTRITIONAL AND METABOLIC FACTORS

Thyroid disorders.
DM.
Severe nutritional disturbances.

INFERTILITY, MALE[14]

ICD-9CM # 606.9

DECREASED PRODUCTION OF SPERMATOZOA

Varicocele.
Testicular failure.
Endocrine disorders.
Cryptorchidism.
Stress, smoking, caffeine, nicotine, recreational drugs.

DUCTAL OBSTRUCTION

Epididymal (postinfection).
Congenital absence of vas deferens.
Ejaculatory duct (postinfection).
Postvasectomy.

INABILITY TO DELIVER SPERM INTO VAGINA

Ejaculatory disturbances.
Hypospadias.
Sexual problems (i.e., impotence), medical or psychological.

ABNORMAL SEMEN

Infection.
Abnormal volume.
Abnormal viscosity.
Abnormal sperm motion.

IMMUNOLOGIC FACTORS

Sperm-immobilizing antibodies.
Sperm-agglutinating antibodies.

INSOMNIA[33]

ICD-9CM # 780.52 Insomnia NOS
307.42 Insomnia, Chronic Associated with Anxiety or Depression
780.51 Insomnia with Sleep Apnea

Anxiety disorder, psychophysiologic insomnia.
Depression.
Drugs (e.g., caffeine, amphetamines, cocaine), hypnotic-dependent sleep disorder.
Pain, fibromyalgia.
Inadequate sleep hygiene.
Restless leg syndrome.
Obstructive sleep apnea.
Sleep bruxism.

Medical illness (e.g., GERD, sleep-related asthma, parkinsonism and movement disorders).
Narcolepsy.
Other: periodic leg movement of sleep, central sleep apnea, REM behavioral disorder.

INTESTINAL PSEUDOOBSTRUCTION[36]

ICD-9CM # 560.1 Adynamic Intestinal Obstruction
564.9 Intestinal Disorder, Functional

"PRIMARY" (IDIOPATHIC INTESTINAL PSEUDOOBSTRUCTION)

Hollow visceral myopathy:
Familial.
Sporadic.
Neuropathic:
Abnormal myenteric plexus.
Normal myenteric plexus.

SECONDARY

Scleroderma.
Myxedema.
Amyloidosis.
Muscular dystrophy.
Hypokalemia.
Chronic renal failure.
DM.
Drug toxicity caused by:
Anticholinergics.
Opiate narcotics.
Ogilvie's syndrome.

INTRAABDOMINAL MASS LESION, NEONATAL[16a]

ICD-9CM # 789.3

CAUSES OF A NEONATAL INTRA-ABDOMINAL MASS LESION

Complicated meconium ileus.
Dilated bowel proximal to an obstruction.
Mesenteric or duplication cyst.
Abscess.
GU causes:
Hydronephrosis.
Renal cystic disease.
Mesoblastic nephroma.
Wilms' tumor.
Adrenal hemorrhage.
Neuroblastoma.
Retroperitoneal teratoma.
Ovarian cyst.
Hydrometrocolpos.
Hemangioendothelioma.
Hepatoblastoma.
Choledochal, hepatic, or splenic cysts.

INTRACEREBRAL HEMORRHAGE, NONHYPERTENSIVE CAUSES

ICD-9CM # 431

Trauma.
Anticoagulation.

Intracranial tumors.
Vascular malformations.
Bleeding disorders.
Vasculitides (e.g., polyarteritis nodosa, granulomatous angiitis).
Cocaine and other sympathomimetic agents.
Cerebral amyloid angiopathy.

INTRACRANIAL LESION

ICD-9CM # 348.8

Tumor (primary or metastatic).
Abscess.
Stroke.
Intracranial hemorrhage.
Angioma.
Multiple sclerosis (initial single lesion).
Granuloma.
Herpes encephalitis.
Artifact.

INTRAOCULAR NEOPLASM

ICD-9CM # varies with specific disorder

MALIGNANT

Retinoblastoma.
Melanoma.
Reticulum cell sarcoma.
Metastatic tumor.

BENIGN

Melanocytic nevus.
Hemangioma.
Reactive lymphoid hyperplasia.

IRON OVERLOAD[20]

ICD-9CM # 275.0

HEREDITARY IRON OVERLOAD

Hereditary hemochromatosis:
HFE-associated (type 1).
Non–HFE-associated:
• Transferrin receptor 2–associated (type 3).
Juvenile hemochromatosis (type 2):
Hemojuvelin-associated (type 2A).
Hepcidin-associated (type 2B).
Autosomal dominant hemochromatosis:
Ferroportin-associated (type 4).
DMT1-associated hemochromatosis.
Atransferrinemia.
Aceruloplasminemia.

ACQUIRED IRON OVERLOAD

Iron-loading anemias (refractory anemias with hypercellular erythroid marrow).
Chronic liver disease.
Porphyria cutanea tarda.
Insulin resistance–associated hepatic iron overload.
African dietary iron overload.[a]
Medical iron ingestion.[a]
Parenteral iron overload:
Transfusional iron overload.
Inadvertent iron overload from therapeutic injections.

PERINATAL IRON OVERLOAD

Neonatal hemochromatosis.
Trichohepatoenteric syndrome.
Cerebrohepatorenal syndrome.
GRACILE[b] (Fellman) syndrome.

FOCAL SEQUESTRATION OF IRON

Idiopathic pulmonary hemosiderosis.
Renal hemosiderosis.
Associated with neurologic abnormalities:
  Pantothenate kinase–associated neurodegeneration (formerly called Hallervorden-Spatz syndrome).
  Neuroferritinopathy.
  Friedreich's ataxia.

---

[a]May have a genetic component.
[b]GRACILE, Growth retardation, aminoaciduria, cholestasis, iron overload, lactic acidosis, and early death.

ISCHEMIA, UPPER EXTREMITY, CAUSES[5a]

ICD-9CM # 903.8 Ischemia, Upper Extremity

VASOSPASM

Raynaud disease.
Medication induced: vasopressors, β-blockers.
Ergot poisoning.

INTRINSIC ARTERIAL DISEASE

Atherosclerosis.
Radiation arteritis.
Azotemic arteriopathy.
Spontaneous dissection.
Fibromuscular dysplasia.

INFLAMMATORY DISEASES

Connective tissue disorders.
Buerger disease.
Takayasu arteritis.
Temporal (giant cell) arteritis.
Hypersensitivity angiitis.

NONINFLAMMATORY MEDICAL DISEASE

Thrombophilic states.
Myeloproliferative disorders.
Cold injury.
Hepatitis-associated vasculitis.
Cryoglobulinemia.
Vinyl chloride exposure.

EMBOLISM

Cardiac (most common).
Proximal aneurysm.
Arterial thoracic outlet syndrome.
Atheroembolism.
Paradoxic embolus (with accompanying septal defect).

TRAUMA

Iatrogenic.
Blunt arterial injury.
Penetrating arterial injury.
Hypothenar hammer syndrome.
Vibration.

ISCHEMIC COLITIS, NONOCCLUSIVE[21]

ICD-9CM # 557.1

ACUTE DIMINUTION OF COLONIC INTRAMURAL BLOOD FLOW

Small Vessel Obstruction

Collagen-vascular disease.
Vasculitis, diabetes.
Oral contraceptives.

Nonocclusive Hypoperfusion

Hemorrhage.
CHF, MI, arrhythmias.
Sepsis.
Vasoconstricting agents: vasopressin, ergot.
Increased viscosity: polycythemia, sickle cell disease, thrombocytosis.

INCREASED DEMAND ON MARGINAL BLOOD FLOW

Increased Motility

Mass lesion, stricture.
Constipation.

Increased Intraluminal Pressure

Bowel obstruction.
Colonoscopy.
Barium enema.

ISCHEMIC NECROSIS OF CARTILAGE AND BONE[14]

ICD-9CM # 733.90

ENDOCRINE/METABOLIC

Ethanol abuse.
Glucocorticoid therapy.
Cushing's disease.
DM.
Hyperuricemia.
Osteomalacia.
Hyperlipidemia.

STORAGE DISEASES (E.G., GAUCHER'S DISEASE)

Hemoglobinopathies (e.g., sickle cell disease).
Trauma (e.g., dislocation, fracture).
HIV infection.
Dysbaric conditions (e.g., caisson disease).
Collagen-vascular disorders.
Irradiation.
Pancreatitis.
Organ transplantation.
Hemodialysis.
Burns.
Intravascular coagulation.
Idiopathic, familial.

JAUNDICE

ICD-9CM # 782.4 Jaundice NOS
576.8 Jaundice, Obstructive
277.4 Bilirubin Excretion Disorders

PREDOMINANCE OF DIRECT (CONJUGATED) BILIRUBIN

Extrahepatic obstruction.
Common duct abnormalities: calculi, neoplasm, stricture, cyst, sclerosing cholangitis.
Metastatic carcinoma.
Pancreatic carcinoma, pseudocyst.
Ampullary carcinoma.
Hepatocellular disease: hepatitis, cirrhosis.
Drugs: estrogens, phenothiazines, captopril, methyltestosterone, labetalol.
Cholestatic jaundice of pregnancy.
Hereditary disorders: Dubin-Johnson syndrome, Rotor's syndrome.
Recurrent benign intrahepatic cholestasis.

PREDOMINANCE OF INDIRECT (UNCONJUGATED) BILIRUBIN

Hemolysis: hereditary and acquired hemolytic anemias.
Inefficient marrow production.
Impaired hepatic conjugation: chloramphenicol.
Neonatal jaundice.
Hereditary disorders: Gilbert's syndrome, Crigler-Najjar syndrome.

JAUNDICE, CLASSIFICATION[1]

ICD-9CM # 782.4

PREHEPATIC (PREDOMINANTLY UNCONJUGATED HYPERBILIRUBINEMIA)

Overproduction

Hemolysis (e.g., spherocytosis, sickle cell disease, hemolysis of the newborn, autoimmune disorders).
Ineffective erythropoiesis (e.g., megaloblastic anemias).
Hematomas.
Pulmonary emboli.

HEPATIC (UNCONJUGATED HYPERBILIRUBINEMIA)

Decreased Hepatic Uptake

Gilbert syndrome.
Drugs (e.g., rifampin, radiographic contrast agents).
Neonatal jaundice.
Posthepatitis.
Decreased cystolic binding proteins (e.g., newborn or premature infants).
Portacaval shunt.
Prolonged fasting.

Decreased Conjugation Due to Limited Glucuronyl Transferase Activity

Gilbert's disease.
Crigler-Najjar syndrome, types I and II.
Neonatal jaundice.
Breast-milk jaundice.
Chronic persistent hepatitis.
Wilson's disease.
Noncirrhotic portal fibrosis.
Drug inhibition (e.g., chloramphenicol).

PREDOMINANTLY CONJUGATED HYPERBILIRUBINEMIA

Impaired Hepatic Excretion

Familial disorders (Dubin-Johnson syndrome, Rotor syndrome, benign recurrent cholestasis, cholestasis of pregnancy).
Hepatocellular infiltrative disorders.
Liver metastasis.
Liver cirrhosis.

Hepatitis (viral, bacterial, parasitic, autoimmune, ethanol, and drug-induced).

Drug-induced cholestasis (especially chlorpromazine, erythromycin estolate, isoniazid, halothane).

Primary biliary cirrhosis.

Primary sclerosing cholangitis.

Pericholangitis.

Congestive heart failure.

Shock.

Toxemia of pregnancy.

Sarcoidosis.

Hepatic trauma.

Amyloidosis.

Autoimmune cholangiopathy.

Vanishing bile duct syndrome.

Sepsis.

Postoperative complications.

EXTRAHEPATIC

Extrahepatic Biliary Obstruction

Gallstones, choledocholithiasis.

Cholecystitis.

Tumors of the head of the pancreas (adenocarcinoma, mucinous duct ectasia, neuroendocrine tumors, metastasis).

Tumors of bile ducts (cholangiocarcinoma, Klatskin tumor: cholangiocarcinoma at the bifurcation).

Gallbladder cancer.

Tumors of the ampulla of Vater (adenoma, adenocarcinoma).

Tumors of the duodenum (adenocarcinoma, lymphoma).

Hemobilia (blood in the biliary tree).

Biliary strictures (postcholecystectomy, post-liver transplantation, primary sclerosing cholangitis).

Congential disorders (biliary atresia, idiopathic dilation of common bile duct, cystic fibrosis).

Metastasis to the hepatic hilum.

Primary bile duct lymphoma.

Cholangiopathy of acquired immunodeficiency syndrome.

Choledochal cysts.

Infectious cholangiopathy (Clonorchis sinensis, Ascaris lumbricoides, Fasciola hepatica).

Chronic pancreatitis (fibrosis of the head of the pancreas).

JAUNDICE, NEONATAL[1]

ICD-9CM # 774.6

PREHEPATIC

Hereditary spherocytosis.

Nonspherocytic hemolytic anemia (glucose-6-phosphate dehydrogenase deficiency, α-thalassemia, vitamin K_3–induced hemolysis, pyruvate kinase deficiency).

HEPATIC

Crigler-Najjar syndrome, types I and II.

α_1-Antitrypsin deficiency.

Sepsis.

Drug-induced.

Hypothyroidism.

Breast-milk jaundice.

Fetomaternal blood group incompatibility (Rhesus, Landsteiner groups ABO).

POSTHEPATIC

Extrahepatic biliary obstruction.

Biliary atresia.

Bile duct paucity.

Alagille syndrome.

JOINT PAIN, ANTERIOR HIP, MEDIAL THIGH, KNEE[28]

ICD-9CM # 719.4 add 5th digit
    0 Site NOS
    1 Shoulder Region
    2 Upper Arm (Elbow, Humerus)
    3 Forearm (Radius, Wrist, Ulna)
    4 Hand
    5 Pelvic Region and Thigh
    6 Lower Leg (Fibula, Patella, Tibia)
    7 Ankle and/or Foot

ACUTE

Acute rheumatic fever.

Adductor muscle strain.

Avascular necrosis.

Crystal arthritis.

Femoral artery (pseudo) aneurysm.

Fracture (femoral neck or intertrochanteric).

Hemarthrosis.

Hernia.

Herpes zoster.

Iliopectineal bursitis.

Iliopsoas tendinitis.

Inguinal lymphadenitis.

Osteomalacia.

Painful transient osteoporosis of hip.

Septic arthritis.

SUBACUTE AND CHRONIC

Adductory muscle strain.

Amyloidosis.

Acute rheumatic fever.

Femoral artery aneurysm.

Hernia (inguinal or femoral).

Iliopectineal bursitis.

Iliopsoas tendinitis.

Inguinal lymphadenopathy.

Osteochondromatosis.

Osteomyelitis.

Osteitis deformans (Paget's disease).

Osteomalacia (pseudofracture).

Postherpetic neuralgia.

Sterile synovitis (e.g., RA, psoriatic, SLE).

JOINT PAIN, HIP, LATERAL THIGH[28]

ICD-9CM # 959.6   Hip Injury
          719.95 Hip Joint Disorder
          843.9 Hip Strain

ACUTE

Herpes zoster.

Iliotibial tendinitis.

Impacted fracture of femoral neck.

Lateral femoral cutaneous neuropathy (meralgia paresthetica).

Radiculopathy: L4-5.

Trochanteric avulsion fracture (greater trochanter).

Trochanteric bursitis.

Trochanteric fracture.

SUBACUTE AND CHRONIC

Lateral femoral cutaneous neuropathy (meralgia paresthetica).

Osteomyelitis.

Postherpetic neuralgia.

Radiculopathy: L4-5.

Tumors.

JOINT PAIN, POLYARTICULAR

ICD-9CM # 719.40

Osteoarthritis.

RA.

Fibromyalgia.

Viral syndrome (e.g., human parvovirus B19 infection).

SLE.

Psoriatic arthritis.

Ankylosing spondylitis.

JOINT PAIN, POSTERIOR HIPS, THIGH, BUTTOCKS[28]

ICD-9CM # 719.4 add 5th digit
    0 Site NOS
    1 Shoulder Region
    2 Upper Arm (Elbow, Humerus)
    3 Forearm (Radius, Wrist, Ulna)
    4 Hand
    5 Pelvic Region and Thigh
    6 Lower Leg (Fibula, Patella, Tibia)
    7 Ankle and/or Foot

ACUTE

Gluteal muscle strain.

Herpes zoster.

Ischial bursitis.

Ischial or sacral fracture.

Osteomalacia (pseudofracture).

Sciatic neuropathy.

Radiculopathy: L5-S1.

SUBACUTE AND CHRONIC

Gluteal muscle strain.

Ischial bursitis.

Lumbar spinal stenosis.

Osteoarthritis of hip.

Osteitis deformans (Paget's disease).

Osteomyelitis.

Osteochondromatosis.

Osteomalacia (pseudofracture).

Postherpetic neuralgia.

Radiculopathy: L5-S1.

Tumors.

Differential Diagnosis

II

JOINT SWELLING

ICD-9CM # 719.0 add 5th digit
0 Site NOS
1 Shoulder Region
2 Upper Arm (Elbow, Humerus)
3 Forearm (Radius, Wrist, Ulna)
4 Hand
5 Pelvic Region and Thigh
6 Lower Leg (Fibula, Patella, Tibia)
7 Ankle and/or Foot

Trauma.
Osteoarthritis.
Gout.
Pyogenic arthritis.
Pseudogout.
RA.
Viral syndrome.

JUGULAR VENOUS DISTENTION

ICD-9CM # 459.89 Increased Venous Pressure

Right-sided heart failure.
Cardiac tamponade.
Constrictive pericarditis.
Goiter.
Tension pneumothorax.
Pulmonary hypertension.
Cardiomyopathy (restrictive).
Superior vena cava syndrome.
Valsalva maneuver.
Right atrial myxoma.
COPD.

KERATITIS, NONINFECTIOUS

ICD-9CM # 370.9

Collagen vascular disease.
Atopic keratoconjunctivitis.
Chemical injury.
Thermal injury.
Ectropion/entropion.
Lid defects.
Exophthalmos.
Keratoconjunctivitis sicca.
Erythema multiforme.
Mucous membrane pemphigoid.
DM (delayed epithelial healing).
Neuroparalytic (cranial nerve VII).
Neurotrophic (diabetes, cranial nerve V).

KIDNEY ENLARGEMENT, UNILATERAL[38]

ICD-9CM # 591

Hydronephrosis (may be bilateral).
Polycystic kidney (may be bilateral).
Simple cyst of kidney.
Renal cell carcinoma.
Pyonephrosis (may be bilateral).
Acute renal vein thrombosis.

KNEE PAIN[28]

ICD-9CM # 844.1 Collateral Ligament Sprain, Medial
844.2 Cruciate Ligament Sprain
716.96 Knee Inflammation
959.7 Knee Injury
718.86 Knee Instability
836.1 Lateral Meniscus Tear
836.0 Medial Meniscus Tear
844.8 Patellar Sprain
719.56 Knee Stiffness
719.06 Knee Swelling

DIFFUSE

Articular.
Anterior.
Prepatellar bursitis.
Patellar tendon enthesopathy.
Chondromalacia patellae.
Patellofemoral osteoarthritis.
Cruciate ligament injury.
Medial plica syndrome.

MEDIAL

Anserine bursitis.
Spontaneous osteonecrosis.
Osteoarthritis.
Medial meniscal tear.
Medial collateral ligament bursitis.
Referred pain from hip and L3.
Fibromyalgia.

LATERAL

Iliotibial band syndrome.
Meniscal cyst.
Lateral meniscal tear.
Collateral ligament.
Peroneal tenosynovitis.

POSTERIOR

Popliteal cyst (Baker's cyst).
Tendinitis.
Aneurysms, ganglions, sarcoma.

KNEE PAIN, IN DIFFERENT AGE GROUPS[8]

ICD-9CM # 719.46

COMMON CAUSES OF KNEE PAIN IN DIFFERENT AGE GROUPS

Childhood (2-10 yr)
Intraarticular:
Juvenile arthritis.
Osteochondritis dissecans.
Infection.
Torn discoid meniscus.
Periarticular:
Osteomyelitis.
Referred:
Perthes' disease.
Irritable hip.
Adolescence (10-18 yr)
Intraarticular:
Osteochondritis dissecans.
Torn meniscus.
Anterior knee pain syndrome.
Patellar instability.

Periarticular:
Osgood–Schlatter disease.
Sinding–Larsen–Johansson syndrome.
Osteomyelitis.
Bone tumors.
Referred:
Slipped upper femoral epiphysis.
Early Adulthood (18-30 yr)
Intraarticular:
Torn meniscus.
Patellar instability.
Anterior knee pain syndrome.
Inflammatory arthritis.
Periarticular:
Ligament injuries.
Bursitis.
Adulthood (30-50 yr)
Intraarticular:
Degenerate meniscal tears.
Osteoarthritis.
Inflammatory arthritis.
Periarticular:
Bursitis.
Referred:
Osteoarthritis of hip.
Spinal disorders.
Old Age (>50 yr)
Intraarticular:
Osteoarthritis.
Inflammatory arthritis.
Periarticular:
Bursitis.
Referred:
Osteoarthritis of hip.
Spinal disorders.

LARGE BOWEL STRICTURE[16a]

ICD-9CM # 751.2

CAUSES OF LARGE BOWEL STRICTURES

Physiologic:
  Spasm.
  Distended bladder.
Maligant:
  Annular carcinoma.
  Scirrhous carcinoma.
  Lymphoma.
Diverticular disease:
  Muscle thickening.
  Pericolic abscess.
  Superimposed malignancy.
Ischemia.
Radiation colitis.
Inflammatory bowel disease:
  Ulcerative colitis.
  Crohn's disease.
  Tuberculosis.
  Lymphogranuloma venereum.
  Amebiasis.
Extrinsic disease:
  Intraabdominal masses.
  Melastatic carcinoma.
  Endometriosis.
  Pelvic lipomatosis.
  Cholecystitis.
  Pancreatitis.
Miscellaneous:

Postoperative anastomosis.
Trauma.
Hirschsprung's disease.

LEFT AXIS DEVIATION[22]

ICD-9CM # 426.3 Left Bundle Branch Block
426.2 Left Bundle Branch
Hemiblock
429.3 Left Ventricular
Hypertrophy

Normal variation.
Left anterior fascicular block (hemiblock).
Left bundle branch block.
Left ventricular hypertrophy.
Mechanical shifts causing a horizontal heart, high diaphragm, pregnancy, ascites.
Some forms of ventricular tachycardia.
Endocardial cushion defects and other congenital heart disease.

LEFT BUNDLE BRANCH BLOCK

ICD-9CM # 426.3

Ischemic heart disease.
Electrolyte abnormalities (e.g., hyperkalemia).
Cardiomyopathy.
Idiopathic.
LVH.
Pulmonary embolism.
Cardiac trauma.
Bacterial endocarditis.

LEG CRAMPS, NOCTURNAL

ICD-9CM # 729.82 Muscle Cramps

Diabetic neuropathy.
Medications.
Electrolyte abnormalities (hypokalemia, hyponatremia, hypocalcemia, hyperkalemia, hypophosphatemia).
Respiratory alkalosis.
Uremia.
Hemodialysis.
Peripheral nerve injury.
ALS.
Alcohol use.
Heat cramps.
Vitamin B_{12} deficiency.
Hyperthyroidism.
Contractures.
DVT.
Hypoglycemia.
Peripheral vascular insufficiency.
Baker's cyst.

LEG LENGTH DISCREPANCIES[23]

ICD-9CM # 736.81 Leg Length Discrepancy, Acquired
755.30 Leg Length Discrepancy, Congenital

CONGENITAL

Proximal femoral local deficiency.
Coxa vara.

Hemiatrophy-hemihypertrophy (anisomelia).
Developmental dysplasia of the hip.

DEVELOPMENTAL

Legg-Calvé-Perthes disease.

NEUROMUSCULAR

Polio.
Cerebral palsy (hemiplegia).

INFECTIOUS

Pyogenic osteomyelitis with physeal damage.

TRAUMA

Physeal injury with premature closure.
Overgrowth.
Malunion (shortening).

TUMOR

Physeal destruction.
Radiation-induced physeal injury.
Overgrowth.

LEG MOVEMENT WHEN STANDING, INVOLUNTARY

ICD-9CM # varies with specific disorder

Benign essential tremor.
Orthostatic tremor.
Spastic ataxia.
Cerebellar truncal tremor.
Postanoxic myoclonus.

LEG PAIN WITH EXERCISE

ICD-9CM # 729.82 Muscle Cramps

Shin splints.
Arteriosclerosis obliterans.
Neurogenic (spinal cord compression or ischemia).
Venous claudication.
Popliteal cyst.
DVT.
Thromboangiitis obliterans.
Adventitial cysts.
Popliteal artery entrapment syndrome.
McArdle syndrome.

LEG ULCERS[28]

ICD-9CM # 440.23 Lower Limb, Arteriosclerotic
707.1 Lower Limb, Chronic
707.1 Lower Limb, Neurogenic
250.70 Lower Limb, Chronic DM Type 2
250.71 Lower Limb, Chronic DM Type 1

VASCULAR

Arterial: arteriosclerosis, thromboangiitis obliterans, AV malformation, cholesterol emboli.
Venous: superficial varicosities, incompetent perforators, DVT, lymphatic abnormalities.

VASCULITIS HEMATOLOGIC

Sickle cell anemia, thalassemia, polycythemia vera, leukemia, cold agglutinin disease.

Macroglobulinemia, protein C and protein S deficiency, cryoglobulinemia, lupus anticoagulant, antiphospholipid syndrome.

INFECTIOUS

Fungal: Blastomycosis, coccidioidomycosis, histoplasmosis, sporotrichosis.
Bacterial: Furuncle, ecthyma, septic emboli.
Protozoal: leishmaniasis.

METABOLIC

Necrobiosis lipoidica diabeticorum.
Localized bullous pemphigoid.
Gout, calcinosis cutis, Gaucher's disease.

TUMORS

Basal cell carcinoma, squamous cell carcinoma, melanoma.
Mycosis fungoides, Kaposi's sarcoma, metastatic neoplasms.

TRAUMA

Burns, cold injury, radiation dermatitis.
Insect bites.
Factitial, excessive pressure.

NEUROPATHIC

Diabetic trophic ulcers.
Tabes dorsalis, syringomyelia.

DRUGS

Warfarin, IV colchicine extravasation, methotrexate, halogens, ergotism, hydroxyurea.

PANNICULITIS

Weber-Christian disease.
Pancreatic fat necrosis, alpha-antitrypsinase deficiency.

LEPTOMENINGEAL LESIONS

ICD-9CM # varies with specific disorder

Metastases.
Multiple sclerosis.
Bacterial or viral meningitis.
Vasculitis.
Lyme disease.
Tuberculosis.
Fungal infections (e.g., *Cryptococcus*).
Sarcoidosis.
Wegener's granulomatosis.
Neurocysticercosis.
Rheumatoid nodules.
Histiocytosis.

LEUKOCORIA

ICD-9CM # 379.90

Cataract.
Retinal detachment.
Retinoblastoma.
Retinal telangiectasia.
Retrolenticular vascularized membrane.
Familial exudative vitreoretinopathy.

Differential Diagnosis

II

LID RETRACTION, CAUSES[20a]

ICD-9CM # 374.41 Lid Retraction

Thyroid eye disease.
Neurogenic.
  Contralateral unilateral ptosis.
  Unopposed levator action due to facial palsy.
  3rd nerve misdirection.
  Marcus Gunn jaw-winking syndrome.
  Collier sign of the dorsal midbrain (Parinaud syndrome).
  Infantile hydrocephalus (setting sun sign).
  Parkinsonism.
  Sympathomimetic drops.
Mechanical.
  Surgical over-correction of ptosis.
  Scarring of upper lid skin.
Congenital.
  Isolated.
  Duane retraction syndrome.
  Down syndrome.
  Transient "eye popping" reflex in normal infants.
Miscellaneous.
  Prominent globe (pseudo-lid retraction).
  Uremia (Summerskill sign).
  Idiopathic.

LIMB ISCHEMIA, ACUTE, NONTRAUMATIC[5a]

ICD-9CM # 903.8

CAUSES OF NONTRAUMATIC ACUTE LIMB ISCHEMIA

Atherosclerotic
In situ thrombosis.
Atheroembolism from thoracic aortic aneurysm/ abdominal aortic aneurysm.
Femoral/popliteal aneurysm with or without compression.
Dissection.
Nonatherosclerotic
Embolism from cardiac thrombosis (atrial fibrillation, post–myocardial infarction akinesis).
Graft thrombosis, graft aneurysm.
Mycotic emboli.
Raynaud syndrome.
Arteritis with thrombosis.
Inherited and acquired hypercoagulable states.
Drug-induced vasospasm.
External compression (Baker cyst, popliteal entrapment).
Mimics
Phlegmasia cerulea dolens.
Acute neuropathy.
Hypovolemia.
Systemic shock.

LIMP

ICD-9CM # 781.2   Gait Abnormality
          719.75 Gait Disorder Due to Joint Abnormality in Hip, Buttock, or Femur
          719.76 Gait Disorder Due to Joint Abnormality in Lower Leg
          719.77 Gait Disorder Due to Joint Abnormality in Ankle and/ or Foot
          300.11 Hysterical Gait Disorder

Degenerative joint disease, osteochondritis dissecans, chondromalacia patellae.
Trauma to extremities, vertebral disk, hips.
Poorly fitting shoes, foreign body in shoe, unequal leg length.
Splinter in foot.
Joint infection (septic arthritis, osteomyelitis), viral arthritis.
Abdominal pain (e.g., appendicitis, incarcerated hernia), testicular torsion.
Polio, neuromuscular disorders, Guillain-Barré syndrome, multiple sclerosis.
Osgood-Schlatter disease.
Legg-Calvé-Perthes disease.
Factitious, somatization syndrome.
Neoplasm (local or metastatic).
Other: diskitis, periostitis, sickle cell disease, hemophilia.

LIMPING, PEDIATRIC AGE[23]

ICD-9CM # 781.2 Gait Abnormality

TODDLER (1-3 YR)

Infection:
  Septic arthritis:
    • Hip.
    • Knee.
  Osteomyelitis.
  Diskitis.
Occult trauma:
  Toddler's fracture.
Neoplasia.

CHILDHOOD (4-10 YR)

Infection:
  Septic arthritis:
    • Hip.
    • Knee.
  Osteomyelitis.
  Diskitis.
  Transient synovitis, hip.
LCPD.
Tarsal coalition.
Rheumatologic disorder:
  JRA.
Trauma.
Neoplasia.

ADOLESCENCE (11 + YR)

SCFE.
Rheumatologic disorder:
  JRA.
Trauma.
Tarsal coalition.
Hip dislocation (DDH).
Neoplasia.

DDH, Developmental dysplasia of the hip; *JRA,* juvenile RA; *LCPD,* Legg-Calvé-Perthes disease; *SCFE,* slipped capital femoral epiphysis.

LIVEDO RETICULARIS

ICD-9CM # code not available

Emboli (SBE, left atrial myxoma, cholesterol emboli).
Thrombocythemia or polycythemia.
Antiphospholipid antibody syndrome.
Cryoglobulinemia, cryofibrinogenemia.
Leukocytoclastic vasculitis.

SLE, RA, dermatomyositis.
Pancreatitis.
Drugs (quinine, quinidine, amantadine, catecholamines).
Physiologic (cutis marmorata).
Congenital.

LIVER DISEASE, PREGNANCY[38]

ICD-9CM # varies with specific diagnosis

INCIDENTAL TO PREGNANCY

Viral hepatitis.
Alcohol related.
Autoimmune chronic active hepatitis.

RELATED TO PREGNANCY (possibly influenced by hormones present in pregnancy)

Complicated gallstone disease.
Hepatic adenoma.
Focal nodular hyperplasia.
Budd-Chiari syndrome.

SPECIFIC TO PREGNANCY

Severe hyperemesis gravidarum.
Benign intrahepatic cholestasis.
Acute fatty liver of pregnancy.
Preeclampsia (HELLP).

LIVER LESIONS, BENIGN, OFTEN CONFUSED WITH MALIGNANCY

ICD-9CM # 573.8

Fatty infiltration.
Adenoma.
Hemangioma.
Cysts.
Flow artifacts.
Focal nodular hyperplasia.
Nonenhanced vessels.

LOW-VOLTAGE ECG

ICD-9CM # 794.31

Hypothyroidism.
Obesity.
Pericardial effusion.
Anasarca.
Pleural effusion.
Pneumothorax.
Amyloidosis.
Aortic stenosis.

LUNG CANCER, OCCUPATIONAL CAUSES[16a]

ICD-9CM # 162.9

CAUSES OF OCCUPATIONAL LUNG CANCER

Asbestos	Lagging, insulation
Arsenic	Metal smelting, pesticide manufacture
Beryllium	Electronics, dental prosthetic manufacture
Chromium	Coloring pigment production, electroplating

Nickel	Electroplating
Silica	Grinding, quarrying, sandblasting
Radon	Mining
Uranium	Mining

LUNG VOLUMES IN DIFFUSE LUNG DISEASE[14a]

Large Lung Volumes
Emphysema.
Chonic asthma.
Diffuse bronchiolitis obliterans.
Highly trained athletes.
Lymphangioleiomyomatosis.

Small Lung Volumes
End-stage lung fibrosis.
Bilateral diaphragmatic paralysis.
Massive ascites.

Normal Lung Volumes
Sarcoidosis.
Langerhans cell histiocytosis.
Neurofibromatosis.
Emphysema with pulmonary fibrosis.

LYMPHADENOPATHY[14]
ICD-9CM # 785.6

GENERALIZED
AIDS.
Lymphoma: Hodgkin's disease, non-Hodgkin's lymphoma.
Leukemias, reticuloendotheliosis.
Infectious mononucleosis, CMV, and other viral infections.
Diffuse skin infection: generalized furunculosis, multiple tick bites.
Parasitic infections: toxoplasmosis, filariasis, leishmaniasis, Chagas' disease.
Serum sickness.
Collagen vascular diseases (RA, SLE).
Dengue (arbovirus infection).
Sarcoidosis and other granulomatous diseases.
Drugs: INH, hydantoin derivatives, antithyroid and antileprosy drugs.
Secondary syphilis.
Hyperthyroidism, lipid-storage diseases.

LOCALIZED

Cervical Nodes
Infections of the head, neck, ears, sinuses, scalp, pharynx.
Mononucleosis.
Lymphoma.
TB.
Malignancy of head and neck.
Rubella.

Scalene/Supraclavicular Nodes
Lymphoma.
Lung neoplasm.
Bacterial or fungal infection of thorax or retroperitoneum.
GI malignancy.

Axillary Nodes
Infections of hands and arms.
Cat-scratch disease.
Neoplasm (lymphoma, melanoma, breast carcinoma).
Brucellosis.

Epitrochlear Nodes
Infections of the hand.
Lymphoma.
Tularemia.
Sarcoidosis, secondary syphilis (usually bilateral).

Inguinal Nodes
Infections of leg or foot, folliculitis (pubic hair).
LGV, syphilis.
Lymphoma.
Pelvic malignancy.
Pasteurella pestis.

Hilar Nodes
Sarcoidosis.
TB.
Lung carcinoma.
Fungal infections, systemic.

Mediastinal Nodes
Sarcoidosis.
Lymphoma.
Lung neoplasm.
TB.
Mononucleosis.
Histoplasmosis.

Abdominal/Retroperitoneal Nodes
Lymphoma.
TB.
Neoplasm (ovary, testes, prostate, and other malignancies).

LYMPHANGITIS[25]
ICD-9CM # 457.2

Acute:
 Group A streptococci.
 Staphylococcus aureus.
 Pasteurella multocida.
Chronic:
 Sporothrix schenckii (sporotrichosis).
 Mycobacterium marinum (swimming pool granuloma).
 Mycobacterium kansasii.
 Nocardia brasiliensis.
 W. bancrofti.

LYMPHOCYTOSIS, ATYPICAL[25]
ICD-9CM # 288.8

Epstein-Barr virus primary infection (infectious mononucleosis).
Cytomegalovirus primary infection (heterophile-negative mono).
Human herpesvirus 6 primary infection (roseola).
Primary HIV infection.
Toxoplasmosis.
Acute viral hepatitis.
Rubella, mumps.
Drug reactions (e.g., phenytoin, sulfa).

MACROTHROMBOCYTOPENIA, INHERITED[20]
ICD-9CM # varies with specific diagnosis

Bernard-Soulier syndrome.
MHY9-related disorders:
• May-Hegglin anomaly.
• Sebastian syndrome.
• Fechtner syndrome.
• Epstein syndrome.
Gray platelet syndrome.

Montreal platelet syndrome.
Mediterranean macrothrombocytopenia.
Mediterranean stomatocytosis/macrothrombocytemia.
GATA1 mutations.
Sialyl-Lewis-S antigen deficiency.
Paris-Trousseau syndrome.
Platelet-type von Willebrand's disease.

MALABSORPTION[38]
ICD-9CM # 579

CAUSES OF MALABSORPTION

More Common
Celiac disease.
Chronic pancreatitis.
Post gastrectomy.
Crohn's disease.
Small bowel resection.
Small intestinal bacterial overgrowth.
Lactase deficiency.

Less Common
AIDS (Myobacterium avium intracellulare, AIDS enteropathy).
Whipple's disease.
Intestinal lymphoma.
Immunoproliferative small intestinal disease (alpha heavy chain disease).
Radiation enteritis.
Collagenous sprue.
Tropical sprue.
Non-granulomatous ulcerative jejunoileitis.
Eosinophilic gastroenteritis.
Amyloidosis.
Zollinger-Ellison syndrome.
Intestinal lymphangiectasia.
Systemic mastocytosis.
Chronic mesenteric ischemia.
Abetalipoproteinemia (autosomal recessive).

MALNUTRITION, CAUSES IN EARLY LIFE[22a]
ICD-9CM # V 77.2

0-6 MO
Breastfeeding difficulties.
Improper formula preparation.
Impaired parent/child interaction.
Congenital syndromes.
Prenatal infections or teratogenic exposures.
Poor feeding (sucking, swallowing) or feeding refusal (aversion).
Maternal psychological disorder (depression or attachment disorder).
Congenital heart disease.
Cystic fibrosis.
Neurologic abnormalities.
Child neglect.
Recurrent infections.

6-12 MO
Celiac disease.
Food intolerance.
Child neglect.
Delayed introduction of age-appropriate foods or poor transition to food.
Recurrent infections.
Food allergy.

Differential Diagnosis

II

AFTER INFANCY

Acquired chronic diseases.
Highly distractible child.
Inappropriate mealtime environment.
Inappropriate diet (e.g., excessive juice consumption, avoidance of high-calorie foods).
Recurrent infections.

MEDIASTINAL COMPARTMENTS, ANATOMY AND PATHOLOGY[39]

ICD-9CM # varies with specific diagnosis

ANTERIOR

Normal Structures
Lymph nodes.
Connective tissue.
Thymus (remnant in adults).
Masses
Thymoma.
Germ cell neoplasm.
Lymphoma.
Thyroid enlargement (intrathoracic goiter).
Other tumors.

MIDDLE

Normal Structures
Pericardium.
Heart.
Vessels: Ascending aorta, venae cavae, main pulmonary arteries.
Trachea.
Lymph nodes.
Nerves: Phrenic, upper vagus.
Masses
Carcinoma.
Lymphoma.
Pericardial cyst.
Bronchogenic cyst.
Benign lymph node enlargement (granulomatous disease).

POSTERIOR

Normal Structures
Vessels: Descending aorta.
Esophagus.
Vertebral column.
Nerves: Sympathetic chain, lower vagus.
Lymph nodes.
Connective tissue.
Masses
Neurogenic tumor.
Diaphragmatic hernia.

MEDIASTINAL MASSES OR WIDENING ON CHEST X-RAY

ICD-9CM # 785.6 Adenopathy
519.3 Disease NEC
793.2 Shift (CXR)

Lymphoma: Hodgkin's disease and non-Hodgkin's lymphoma.
Sarcoidosis.
Vascular: aortic aneurysm, ectasia, or tortuosity of aorta or bronchocephalic vessels.
Carcinoma: lungs, esophagus.
Esophageal diverticula.
Hiatal hernia.

Achalasia.
Prominent pulmonary outflow tract: pulmonary hypertension, pulmonary embolism, right-to-left shunts.
Trauma: mediastinal hemorrhage.
Pneumomediastinum.
Lymphadenopathy caused by silicosis and other pneumoconioses.
Leukemias.
Infections: TB, viral (rare), *Mycoplasma* (rare), fungal, tularemia.
Substernal thyroid.
Thymoma.
Teratoma.
Bronchogenic cyst.
Pericardial cyst.
Neurofibroma, neurosarcoma, ganglioneuroma.

MEDIASTINITIS, ACUTE[25]

ICD-9CM # 519.2

Esophageal perforation.
Iatrogenic.
EGD, esophageal dilation, esophageal variceal sclerotherapy, nasogastric tube, Sengstaken-Blackmore tube, endotracheal intubation, esophageal surgery, paraesophageal surgery, transesophageal echocardiography, anterior stabilization of cervical vertebral bodies.
Swallowed foreign bodies.
Trauma.
Spontaneous perforation (e.g., emesis, carcinoma).
Head and neck infections (e.g., tonsillitis, pharyngitis, parotitis, epiglottitis, odontogenic).
Infections originating at another site (e.g., TB, pneumonia, pancreatitis, osteomyelitis of sternum, clavicle, ribs).
Cardiothoracic surgery (median sternotomy) (e.g., CABG, valve replacement, other types of cardiothoracic surgery).

MELANONYCHIA

ICD-9CM # varies with specific disorder

Pregnancy.
Trauma.
Medications (e.g., AZT, 5-fluorouracil, doxorubicin, psoralens).
Nail matrix nevus.
HIV infection.
Onychomycosis.
Melanocyte hyperplasia.
Verrucae.
Pustular psoriasis.
Lichen planus.
Basal cell carcinoma.
Nail matrix melanoma.
Subungual keratosis.
Addison's disease.
Bowen's disease.

MEMORY LOSS SYMPTOMS, ELDERLY PATIENTS

ICD-9CM # varies with specific disorder

Age-related mild cognitive impairment.
Depression (pseudodementia).

Medications (e.g., anticholinergics, sedatives).
Hypothyroidism.
Chronic hypoxia.
Cerebrovascular infarcts.
Alzheimer's disease.
Hepatic disease.
Chronic renal failure.
Hyperthyroidism.
Frontotemporal dementia.
Lewy body dementia.

MENINGITIS, CHRONIC[26]

ICD-9CM # 322.2

TB.
Fungal CNS infection.
Tertiary syphilis.
CNS neoplasm.
Metabolic encephalopathies.
Multiple sclerosis.
Chronic subdural hematoma.
SLE cerebritis.
Encephalitides.
Sarcoidosis.
NSAIDs.
Behçet's syndrome.
Anatomic defects (traumatic, congenital, postoperative).
Granulomatous angiitis.

MENINGITIS, RECURRENT[25]

ICD-9CM # varies with specific disorder

Drug induced (with rechallenge).
Parameningeal focus.
Infection (sinusitis, mastoiditis, osteomyelitis, brain abscess).
Tumor (epidermoid cyst, craniopharyngioma).
Posttraumatic (bacterial).
Mollaret's meningitis.
SLE.
Herpes simplex virus.

MENTAL STATUS CHANGES AND COMA[2]

ICD-9CM # 780.97

METABOLIC/SYSTEMIC ETIOLOGY OF ALTERED MENTAL STATUS AND COMA

Hypoxia
Severe pulmonary disease (hypoventilation).
Severe anemia.
Environmental/toxin:
Methemoglobinemia.
Cyanide.
Carbon monoxide.
Decreased atmospheric oxygen (high altitude).
Near-drowning.
Disorders of Glucose
Hypoglycemia:
Chronic alcohol abuse and liver disease.
Excessive use of insulin or other hypoglycemic agents.
Insulinoma.
Hyperglycemia:
Diabetic ketoacidosis.
Nonketotic hyperosmolar coma.

Decreased Cerebral Blood Flow
Hypovolemic shock.
Cardiac:
- Vasovagal syncope.
- Arrhythmias.
- Myocardial infarction.
- Valvular disorders.
- Congestive heart failure.
- Pericardial effusion/tamponade.
- Myocarditis.

Infectious:
- Septic shock.
- Bacterial meningitis.

Vascular/hematologic:
- Hypertensive encephalopathy.
- Pseudotumor cerebri.
- Hyperviscosity (sickle cell, polycythemia).
- Hyperventilation.
- Cerebral lupus vasculitis.
- Thrombotic thrombocytopenic purpura.
- Disseminated intravascular coagulation.

Metabolic Cofactor Deficiency
Thiamine (Wernicke-Korsakoff syndrome).
Pyridoxine (isoniazid overdose).
Folic acid (chronic alcohol abuse).
Cyanocobalamin.
Niacin.

Electrolye/pH Disturbances
Acidosis/alkalosis.
Hypernatremia/hyponatremia.*
Hypercalcemia/hypocalcemia.
Hypophosphatemia.
Hypermagnesemia/hypomagnesemia.

Endocrine Disorders
Myxedema coma, thyrotoxicosis.
Hypopituitarism.
Addison's disease (primary or secondary).
Cushing's disease.
Pheochromocytoma.
Hyperparathyroidism/hypoparathyroidism.

Endogenous Toxins
Hyperammonemia (liver failure).
Uremia (renal disease).
Carbon dioxide narcosis (pulmonary disease).
Porphyria.

Exogenous Toxins
Alcohols:
- Ethanol, isopropyl alcohol, methanol, ethylene glycol.

Acid poisons:
- Salicylates.
- Paraldehyde.
- Ammonium chloride.

Antidepressant medications:
- Lithium.
- Tricyclic antidepressants (TCAs).
- Selective serotonin reuptake inhibitors (SSRIs).
- Monamine oxidase inhibitors (MAOIs).

Stimulants:
- Amphetamines/methamphetamines.
- Cocaine.
- Over-the-counter sympathomimetics.

Narcotics/opiates:
- Morphine.
- Heroin.
- Codeine, oxycodone, meperidine, hydrocodone.
- Methadone.
- Fentanyl.
- Propoxyphene.

Sedative-hypnotics:
- Benzodiazepines.
- Barbiturates.
- Rohypnol.
- Bromide.

Hallucinogens:
- Lysergic acid diethylamide (LSD).
- Marijuana.
- Mescaline, peyote.
- Mushrooms.
- Phencyclidine (PCP).

Herbs/plants:
- Aconite.
- Jimson weed.
- Morning glory.

Volatile substances:
- Hydrocarbons (gasoline, butane, toluene, benzene, chloroform).
- Nitrites.
- Anesthetic agents (nitrous oxide, ether).

Other:
- γ-Hydroxybutyrate (GHB).
- Ketamine.
- Penicillin.
- Cardiac glycosides.
- Anticonvulsants.
- Steroids.
- Heavy metals.
- Cimetidine.
- Organophosphates.

Disorders of Temperature Regulation/Environmental
Hypothermia.
Heat stroke.
Malignant hyperthermia.
Neuroleptic malignant syndrome.
High-altitude cerebral edema (HACE).
Dysbarism.

Primary Glial or Neuronal Disorders
Adrenoleukodystrophy.
Creutzfeldt-Jakob disease.
Progressive multifocal leukoencephalopathy.
Marchiava-Bignami disease.
Gliomatosis cerebri.
Central pontine myelinolysis.

Other Disorders of Unknown Etiology
Seizures.
Postictal states.
Reye's syndrome.[†]
Intussuception.[†]

*Can be associated with dilution of formula in infant feeding.
[†]Prominent in the pediatric population.

MESENTERIC ARTERIAL EMBOLISM, ASSOCIATED FACTORS[2]
ICD-9CM # 557.0

FACTORS ASSOCIATED WITH MESENTERIC ARTERIAL EMBOLISM
Coronary artery disease.
- Post-myocardial infarction mural thrombi.
- Congestive heart failure.
- Valvular heart disease.
  - Rheumatic mitral valve disease.
  - Nonbacterial endocarditis.
- Arrhythmias.
  - Chronic atrial fibrillation.
- Aortic aneurysms or dissections.
- Coronary angiography.

MESENTERIC ISCHEMIA, NONOCCLUSIVE[26]

ICD-9CM #	557.0	Mesenteric Artery Embolism or Infarction
	557.1	Mesenteric Artery Insufficiency, Chronic
	902.39	Mesenteric Vein Injury

Cardiovascular disease resulting in low-flow states (CHF, cardiogenic shock, post cardiopulmonary bypass, dysrhythmias).
Septic shock.
Drug induced (cocaine, vasopressors, ergot alkaloid poisoning).

MESENTERIC VENOUS THROMBOSIS[26]
ICD-9CM # 557.0

Hypercoagulable states (protein C or S deficiency, antithrombin III deficiency, Factor V Leyden, malignancy, polycythemia vera, sickle cell disease, homocystinemia, lupus anticoagulant, cardiolipin antibody).
Trauma (operative venous injury, abdominal trauma, postsplenectomy).
Inflammatory conditions (pancreatitis, diverticulitis, appendicitis, cholangitis).
Other: CHF, renal failure, portal hypertension, decompression sickness.

METASTATIC NEOPLASMS

ICD-9CM #	198.5 Bone and Bone Marrow
	198.3 Brain and Spinal Cord
	197.7 Liver
	197.0 Lung

To: Bone	To: Brain
Breast	Lung
Lung	Breast
Prostate	Melanoma
Thyroid	GU tract
Kidney	Colon
Bladder	Sinuses
Endometrium	Sarcoma
Cervix	Skin
Melanoma	Thyroid
To: Liver	**To: Lung**
Colon	Breast
Stomach	Colon
Pancreas	Kidney
Breast	Testis
Lymphomas	Stomach
Bronchus	Thyroid
Lung	Melanoma
Sarcoma	
Choriocarcinoma	
Kidney	

Differential Diagnosis

II

MICROCEPHALY[4]

ICD-9CM # 742.1 Microcephalus

PRIMARY (GENETIC)

Familial (autosomal recessive).
Autosomal dominant.
Syndromes:
    Down (21-trisomy).
    Edward (18-trisomy).
    Cri-du-chat (5 p-).
    Cornelia de Lange.
    Rubinstein-Taybi.
    Smith-Lemli-Opitz.

SECONDARY (NONGENETIC)

Radiation.
Congenital infections:
    Cytomegalovirus.
    Rubella.
    Toxoplasmosis.
Drugs:
    Fetal alcohol.
    Fetal hydantoin.
Meningitis/encephalitis.
Malnutrition.
Metabolic.
Hyperthermia.
Hypoxic-ischemic encephalopathy.

MICROPENIS[27]

ICD-9CM # 752.69 Penile Agenesis or Atresia
           607.89 Penile Atrophy
           752.64 Micropenis (Congenital)

HYPOGONADOTROPIC HYPOGONADISM (HYPOTHALAMIC OR PITUITARY DEFICIENCIES)

Kallmann's syndrome: autosomal dominant; associated with hyposmia.
Prader-Willi syndrome: hypotonia, mental retardation, obesity, small hands and feet.
Rud syndrome: hyposomia, ichthyosis, mental retardation.
De Morsier's syndrome (septooptic dysplasia): hypopituitarism, hypoplastic optic discs, absent septum pellucidum.

HYPERGONADOTROPIC HYPOGONADISM

Primary testicular defect: disorders of testicular differentiation or inborn errors of testosterone synthesis.
Klinefelter's syndrome.
Other X polysomies (i.e., XXXXY, XXXY).
Robinow's syndrome: brachymesomelic dwarfism, dysmorphic facies.

PARTIAL ANDROGEN INSENSITIVITY

Idiopathic
Defective morphogenesis of the penis.

MIOSIS

ICD-9CM # 379.42 Miosis, Persistent Not
           Due to Miotics

Medications (e.g., morphine, pilocarpine).
Neurosyphilis.

Congenital.
Iritis.
CNS pontine lesion.
CNS infections.
Cavernous sinus thrombosis.
Inflammation/irritation of cornea or conjunctiva.

MONOARTHRITIS, ACUTE

ICD-9CM # 716.60

Overuse.
Trauma.
Gout.
Pseudogout.
Osteoarthritis.
Infectious arthritis (e.g., gonococcal, Lyme disease, viral, mycobacteria, fungi).
Osteomyelitis.
Avascular necrosis of bone.
Hemarthrosis.
Bowel disease–associated arthritis.
Bone malignancy.
Psoriatic arthritis.
Juvenile RA.
Sarcoidosis.
Hemoglobinopathies.
Vasculitic syndromes.
Behçet's syndrome.
Foreign body synovitis.
Hypertrophic pulmonary osteoarthropathy.
Amyloidosis, familial Mediterranean fever.

MONOCYTOSIS[20]

ICD-9CM # 288.63

Inflammatory diseases:
  Infectious diseases:
    • Tuberculosis.
    • Syphilis.
    • Subacute bacterial endocarditis.
    • Fever of unknown origin.
  Autoimmune/granulomatous.
  Systemic lupus erythematosus.
  Rheumatoid arthritis.
  Temporal arteritis.
  Myositis.
  Polyarteritis.
  Ulcerative colitis.
  Regional enteritis.
  Sarcoidosis.
Malignant disorders:
  Preleukemia.
  Nonlymphocytic leukemia.
  Histiocytoses.
  Hodgkin's disease.
  Non-Hodgkin's lymphoma.
  Carcinomas.
Miscellaneous:
  Chronic neutropenia.
  Post splenectomy.

MONONEUROPATHY

ICD-9CM # 355.9

Herpes zoster.
Herpes simplex.
Vasculitis.
Trauma, compression.

Diabetes.
Postinfectious or inflammatory.

MONONEUROPATHY, ISOLATED[2]

ICD-9CM # varies with specific diagnosis

UPPER EXTREMITY

Radial nerve.
  Axilla.
  Humerus.
  Elbow (posterior interosseous neuropathy).
  Wrist (superficial cutaneous radial neuropathy).
Ulnar nerve.
  Axilla.
  Humerus.
  Elbow.
  Condylar groove.
  Cubital tunnel.
Wrist (Guyon's canal).
Hand.
  Superficial terminal ulnar neuropathy.
  Deep terminal ulnar neuropathy.
  • Proximal hypothenar.
  • Distal hypothenar.
Median nerve.
Axilla.
Humerus (musculocutaneous mononeuropathy).
Forearm.
  Anterior interosseus.
  Pronator syndrome (?).
Wrist (carpal tunnel).
Hand (recurrent motor branch).
Suprascapular mononeuropathy.
  Axillary mononeuropathy.

LOWER EXTREMITY

Sciatic nerve.
Femoral nerve.
  Iliacus compartment (proximal).
  Saphenous mononeuropathy (distal).
Lateral femoral cutaneous (meralgia paresthetica).
Peroneal nerve.
  Common peroneal mononeuropathy (fibular head, popliteal fossa).
  Deep peroneal mononeuropathy (anterior compartment).
Tibial nerve.
  Popliteal fossa (proximal).
  Tarsal tunnel (distal).
Sural nerve.
  Popliteal fossa, calf (proximal).
  Fifth metatarsal base (distal).
Plantar nerve.
  Distal to tarsal tunnel.
  Interdigital neuropathies (Morton's neuroma).
Obturator mononeuropathy.

MONONUCLEOSIS, MONOSPOT NEGATIVE[1]

ICD-9CM # 075

DIFFERENTIAL DIAGNOSIS OF MONOSPOT-NEGATIVE MONONUCLEOSIS

Acute HIV infection.
EBV mononucleosis (particularly in children).

Cytomegalovirus.
Acute toxoplasmosis.
Streptococcal pharyngitis.
Acute hepatitis B infection.

EBV, Epstein-Barr virus; *HIV*, human immunodeficiency virus.

MUSCLE DISEASE[34a]

ICD-9CM # 728

CLASSIFICATION OF MUSCLE DISEASE

Muscular Dystrophies
Duchenne.
Becker.
Limb girdle.
Childhood.
Facioscapulohumeral.
Myotonic Disorders
Dystrophia myotonica.
Myotonica congenita.
Inflammatory
Infective: bacterial, viral, parasitic.
Unknown cause: polymyositis, dermatomyositis, sarcoidosis.
Endocrine
Thyroid disease—hyper- and hypothyroidism.
Cushing's disease.
Addison's disease.
Hyperparathyroidism.
Metabolic
Glycogen storage diseases.
Periodic paralyses.
Mitochondrial diseases.
Drug-induced
Corticosteroids.
Chloroquine.
Amiodarone.
Penicillamine.
Alcohol.
Zidovudine.
Clofibrate.
Other
Inclusion body myositis.

MUSCLE WEAKNESS

ICD-9CM # 728.9

Physical deconditioning.
Impaired cardiac output (e.g., mitral stenosis, mitral regurgitation).
Uremia, liver failure.
Electrolyte abnormalities (hypokalemia, hyperkalemia, hypophosphatemia, hypercalcemia), hypoglycemia.
Drug induced (e.g., statin myopathy).
Muscular dystrophies.
Steroid myopathy.
Alcoholic myopathy.
Myasthenia gravis, Lambert-Eaton syndrome.
Infections (polio, botulism, HIV, hepatitis, diphtheria, tick paralysis, neurosyphilis, brucellosis, TB, trichinosis).
Pernicious anemia, other anemias, beriberi.
Psychiatric illness (depression, somatization syndrome).
Organophosphate or arsenic poisoning.

Inflammatory myopathies (e.g., collagen vascular disease, RA, sarcoidosis).
Endocrinopathies (e.g., adrenal insufficiency, hypothyroidism), diabetic neuropathy.
Other: motor neuron disease, mitochondrial myopathy, L-tryptophan (eosinophilia-myalgia), rhabdomyolysis, glycogen storage disease, lipid storage disease.

MUSCLE WEAKNESS, LOWER MOTOR NEURON VERSUS UPPER MOTOR NEURON[40]

ICD-9CM # 728.9

LOWER MOTOR NEURON

Weakness, usually severe.
Marked muscle atrophy.
Fasciculations.
Decreased muscle stretch reflexes.
Clonus not present.
Flaccidity.
No Babinski sign.
Asymmetric and may involve one limb only in the beginning to become generalized as the disease progresses.

UPPER MOTOR NEURON

Weakness, usually less severe.
Minimal disuse muscle atrophy.
No fasciculations.
Increased muscle stretch reflexes.
Clonus may be present.
Spasticity.
Babinski sign.
Often initial impairment of only skilled movements.
In the limbs the following muscles may be the only ones weak or weaker than the others: triceps; wrist and finger extensors; interossei; iliopsoas; hamstrings; and foot dorsiflexors, inverters, and extroverters.

MYDRIASIS

ICD-9CM # 379.43 Mydriasis, Persistent Not Due to Mydriatics

Coma.
Medications (cocaine, atropine, epinephrine, etc.).
Glaucoma.
Cerebral aneurysm.
Ocular trauma.
Head trauma.
Optic atrophy.
Cerebral neoplasm.
Iridocyclitis.

MYELIN DISORDERS

ICD-9CM # varies with specific disorder

Multiple sclerosis.
Vitamin B_{12} deficiency.
Radiation.
Hypoxia.
Toxicity from carbon monoxide, alcohol, mercury.
Progressive multifocal encephalopathy.

Acute disseminated encephalomyelitis.
Acute hemorrhagic leukoencephalopathy.
Phenylketonuria.
Adrenoleukodystrophy.
Krabbe's disease.

MYELOPATHY AND MYELITIS[36]

ICD-9CM # 722.70 Myelopathy, Discogenic Intervertebral NOS
       336.9 Myelopathy, Nondiscogenic Unspecified

INFLAMMATORY

Infectious: spirochetal TB, zoster, rabies, HIV, polio, rickettsial, fungal, parasitic.
Noninfectious: idiopathic transverse myelitis, multiple sclerosis.

TOXIC/METABOLIC

DM, pernicious anemia, chronic liver disease, pellagra, arsenic.

TRAUMA COMPRESSION

Spinal neoplasm, cervical spondylosis, epidural abscess, epidural hematoma.

VASCULAR

AV malformation, SLE, periarteritis nodosa, dissecting aortic aneurysm.

PHYSICAL AGENTS

Electrical injury, irradiation.

NEOPLASTIC

Spinal cord tumors, paraneoplastic myelopathy.

MYOCARDIAL ISCHEMIA[36]

ICD-9CM # 414.8 Ischemia (Chronic)
       411.89 Ischemia, Acute without MI

Atherosclerotic obstructive coronary artery disease.
Nonatherosclerotic coronary artery disease:
Coronary artery spasm.
Congenital coronary artery anomalies:
   Anomalous origin of coronary artery from pulmonary artery.
   Aberrant origin of coronary artery from aorta or another coronary artery.
   Coronary arteriovenous fistula.
   Coronary artery aneurysm.
Acquired disorders of coronary arteries:
   Coronary artery embolism.
   Dissection:
- Surgical.
- During percutaneous coronary angioplasty.
- Aortic dissection.
- Spontaneous (e.g., during pregnancy).
   Extrinsic compression:
- Tumors.
- Granulomas.
- Amyloidosis.
   Collagen-vascular disease:
- Polyarteritis nodosa.
- Temporal arteritis.

- RA.
- SLE.
- Scleroderma.

Miscellaneous disorders:
- Irradiation.
- Trauma.
- Kawasaki disease.

Syphilis.

Hereditary disorders:
Pseudoxanthoma elasticum.
Gargoylism.
Progeria.
Homocystinuria.
Primary oxaluria.

"Functional" causes of myocardial ischemia in absence of anatomic coronary artery disease:
Syndrome X.
Hypertrophic cardiomyopathy.
Dilated cardiomyopathy.
Muscle bridge.
Hypertensive heart disease.
Pulmonary hypertension.
Valvular heart disease; aortic stenosis, aortic regurgitation.

MYOCLONUS

ICD-9CM # 333.2

Physiologic (e.g., exercise or anxiety induced).
Renal failure.
Hepatic failure.
Hyponatremia.
Hypoglycemia or severe hyperglycemia.
Postdialysis.
Epileptic myoclonus.
Postencephalitis.
CNS lesion (stroke, neoplasm).
CNS trauma.
Parkinson's disease.
Medications (e.g., tricyclics, L-dopa).
Friedreich's ataxia.
Ataxia-telangiectasia.
Wilson's disease.
Huntington's disease.
Progressive supranuclear palsy.
Heavy metal poisoning.
Benign familial.

MYOPATHIC SYNDROMES, DRUG-INDUCED[18b]

ICD-9CM # 359.9　Myopathic Syndromes

TYPE OF MYOPATHY

Necrotizing myopathy
Inflammatory myopathy
Mitochondrial myopathy
Hypokalemic myopathy
Antimicrotubular myopathy
Lysosomal storage myopathy
Corticosteroid myopathy
Others

DRUGS

HMG-CoA reductase inhibitors (statins), fibrates, alcohol
Penicillamine, interferon-α, procainamide
Zidovudine
Diuretics, laxatives, licorice, amphotericin B, alcohol

Colchicine, vincristine
Chloroquine, hydroxychloroquine, quinacrine, amiodarone, perhexiline
Corticosteroids, especially fluorinated
Ipecac syrup, emetine

MYOPATHIES ASSOCIATED WITH REST PAIN[18b]

ICD-9CM # 359.9　Myopathies

Childhood dermatomyositis.
Hypothyroid myopathy.
Acute alcoholic myopathy.
Drug-induced myopathies.
Infectious myopathies.
Myopathies associated with metabolic bone disease.
Carnitine palmitoyl transferase deficiency.
Rhabdomyolysis from any cause.

MYOPATHIES, INFECTIOUS

ICD-9CM # 359.8

HIV.
Viral myositis.
Trichinosis.
Toxoplasmosis.
Cysticercosis.

MYOPATHIES, INFLAMMATORY

ICD-9CM # 359.9

SLE, RA.
Sarcoidosis.
Paraneoplastic syndrome.
Polymyositis, dermatomyositis.
Polyarteritis nodosa.
Mixed connective tissue disease.
Scleroderma.
Inclusion body myositis.
Sjögren's syndrome.
Cimetidine, D-penicillamine.

MYOPATHIES, METABOLIC[18b]

ICD-9CM # 359.9　Myopathies

DISORDERED GLYCOGEN METABOLISM

- Myophosphorylase deficiency (McArdle disease).
- Phosphorylase b kinase deficiency.
- Phosphofructokinase deficiency.
- Debrancher enzyme deficiency.
- Brancher enzyme deficiency.
- Phosphoglycerate kinase deficiency.
- Phosphoglycerate mutase deficiency.
- Lactate dehydrogenase deficiency.
- Acid maltase deficiency.
- Aldolase deficiency.
- β-Enolase deficiency.

DISORDERED LIPID METABOLISM

- Carnitine deficiencies.
- Carnitine palmitoyltransferase deficiency.
- Fatty acid acyl-CoA dehydrogenase deficiencies.

MITOCHONDRIAL MYOPATHIES

- Coenzyme Q10 deficiency.
- Respiratory chain complex deficiencies.

ENDOCRINE

- Acromegaly.
- Hypothyroidism.
- Hyperthyroidism.
- Hyperparathyroidism.
- Cushing disease.
- Addison disease.
- Hyperaldosteronism.

METABOLIC-NUTRITIONAL

- Uremia.
- Hepatic failure.
- Malabsorption.
- Periodic paralysis.
- Vitamin D deficiency.
- Vitamin E deficiency.

ELECTROLYTE DISORDERS

- Sodium: hypernatremia and hyponatremia.
- Potassium: hyperkalemia and hypokalemia.
- Calcium: hypercalcemia and hypocalcemia.
- Phosphate: hypophosphatemia.
- Magnesium: hypomagnesemia.

MYOPATHIES, TOXIC[1]

ICD-9CM # 359.4

Inflammatory: cimetidine, D-penicillamine.
Noninflammatory necrotizing or vacuolar: cholesterol-lowering agents, chloroquine, colchicine.
Acute muscle necrosis and myoglobinuria: cholesterol-lowering drugs, alcohol, cocaine.
Malignant hyperthermia: halothane, ethylene, others; succinylcholine.
Mitochondrial: zidovudine.
Myosin loss: nondepolarizing neuromuscular blocking agents; glucocorticoids.

MYOSITIS, INFECTIOUS CAUSES[18b]

ICD-9CM # 728.0　Myositis

VIRAL

Influenza A and B viruses.
Enteroviruses (coxsackieviruses, echoviruses).
Human immunodeficiency virus.
Human T-cell lymphotrophic virus type 1.
Hepatitis B and C viruses.
Cytomegalovirus.
Epstein-Barr virus.
Adenovirus.
Varicella-zoster virus.
Parainfluenza.

PARASITIC

Trichinella species.
Echinococcus species.
Schistosoma species.
Toxoplasma gondii.
Trypanosoma cruzi.
Sarcocystis species.

BACTERIAL

Staphylococcus aureus.
Streptococcus, groups A and B.
Aeromonas hydrophila.
Borrelia burgdorferi.
Clostridium perfringens.
Anaerobic streptococci.
Mycobacterium species.
Rickettsia species.

FUNGAL

Candida species.
Cryptococcus neoformans.
Microsporida.

MYOSITIS, INFLAMMATORY[1]
ICD-9CM # 729.1

INFECTIOUS

Viral myositis:
    Retroviruses (HIV, HTLV-I).
    Enteroviruses (echovirus, Coxsackievirus).
    Other viruses (influenza, hepatitis A and B,
       Epstein-Barr virus).
Bacterial: pyomyositis.
Parasites: trichinosis, cysticercosis.
Fungi: candidiasis.

IDIOPATHIC

Granulomatous myositis (sarcoid, giant cell).
Eosinophilic myositis.
Eosinophilia-myalgia syndrome.

ENDOCRINE/METABOLIC DISORDERS

Hypothyroidism.
Hyperthyroidism.
Hypercortisolism.
Hyperparathyroidism.
Hypoparathyroidism.
Hypocalcemia.
Hypokalemia.

METABOLIC MYOPATHIES

Myophosphorylase deficiency (McArdle's disease).
Phosphofructokinase deficiency.
Myoadenylate deaminase deficiency.
Acid maltase deficiency.
Lipid storage diseases.
Acute rhabdomyolysis.

DRUG-INDUCED MYOPATHIES

Alcohol.
D-Penicillamine.
Zidovudine.
Colchicine.
Chloroquine, hydroxychloroquine.
Lipid-lowering agents.
Cyclosporine.
Cocaine, heroin, barbiturates.
Corticosteroids.

NEUROLOGIC DISORDERS

Muscular dystrophies.
Congenital myopathies.
Motor neuron disease.
Guillain-Barré syndrome.
Myasthenia gravis.

NAIL CLUBBING
ICD-9CM # 703.9

COPD.
Pulmonary malignancy.
Cirrhosis.
Inflammatory bowel disease.
Chronic bronchitis.
Congenital heart disease.
Endocarditis.
AV malformations.
Asbestosis.
Trauma.
Idiopathic.

NAIL, HORIZONTAL WHITE LINES (BEAU'S LINES)
ICD-9CM # 703.8

Malnutrition.
Idiopathic.
Trauma.
Prolonged systemic illnesses.
Pemphigus.
Raynaud's disease.

NAIL KOILONYCHIA
ICD-9CM # 703.8

Trauma.
Iron deficiency.
SLE.
Hemochromatosis.
Raynaud's disease.
Nail-patella syndrome.
Idiopathic.

NAIL ONYCHOLYSIS
ICD-9CM # 703.8

Infection.
Trauma.
Psoriasis.
Connective tissue disorders.
Sarcoidosis.
Hyperthyroidism.
Amyloidosis.
Nutritional deficiencies.

NAIL PITTING
ICD-9CM # 703.8

Psoriasis.
Alopecia areata.
Reiter's syndrome.
Trauma.
Idiopathic.

NAIL SPLINTER HEMORRHAGE
ICD-9CM # 703.8

SBE.
Trauma.
Malignancies.
Oral contraceptives.
Pregnancy.

SLE.
Antiphospholipid syndrome.
Psoriasis.
RA.
Peptic ulcer disease.

NAIL STRIATIONS
ICD-9CM # 703.8

Psoriasis.
Alopecia areata.
Trauma.
Atopic dermatitis.
Vitiligo.

NAIL TELANGIECTASIA
ICD-9CM # 703.8

RA.
Scleroderma.
Trauma.
SLE.
Dermatomyositis.

NAIL WHITENING (TERRY'S NAILS)
ICD-9CM # 703.8

Malnutrition.
Trauma.
Liver disease (cirrhosis, hepatic failure).
DM.
Hyperthyroidism.
Idiopathic.

NAIL YELLOWING
ICD-9CM # 703.8

Tobacco abuse.
Nephrotic syndrome.
Chronic infections (TB, sinusitis).
Bronchiectasis.
Lymphedema.
Raynaud's disease.
RA.
Pleural effusions.
Thyroiditis.
Immunodeficiency.

NASAL AND PARANASAL SINUS TUMORS[16a]
ICD-9CM # 873.23

BENIGN AND MALIGNANT NASAL AND PARANASAL SINUS TUMORS

Epithelial Tumors
Benign
Papilloma.
Adenoma.
Inverting papilloma.
Malignant
Squamous carcinoma.
Adenocarcinoma.
Melanoma.
Adenoid cystic carcinoma.
Malignant salivary tumors.

Mesenchymal Tumors
Benign
Osteoma.
Ossifying fibroma complex.
Angiofibroma.
Chondroma.
Malignant
Osteogenic sarcoma.
Fibrosarcoma.
Angiosarcoma.
Chondrosarcoma.
Lymphoma.
Rhabdomyosarcoma.

NASAL MASSES, CONGENITAL[16a]

ICD-9CM # 478.19

Dermoid.
Nasal cerebral heterotopia (glioma).
Frontal meningoencephalocele.
Nasolacrimal duct mucocele.
Nasal hamartoma.
Nasal hemangioma.

NAUSEA AND VOMITING

ICD-9CM # 787.01

Infections (viral, bacterial).
Intestinal obstruction.
Metabolic (uremia, electrolyte abnormalities, DKA, acidosis, etc.).
Severe pain.
Anxiety, fear.
Psychiatric disorders (bulimia, anorexia nervosa).
Pregnancy.
Medications (NSAIDs, erythromycin, morphine, codeine, aminophylline, chemotherapeutic agents, etc.).
Withdrawal from substance abuse (drugs, alcohol).
Head trauma.
Vestibular or middle ear disease.
Migraine headache.
CNS neoplasms.
Radiation sickness.
PUD.
Carcinoma of GI tract.
Reye's syndrome.
Eye disorders.
Abdominal trauma.

NECK AND ARM PAIN

ICD-9CM # 723.1   Neck Pain
         847.0   Neck Strain
         959.09 Neck Injury
         959.2   Arm Injury
         840.9   Arm Strain

Cervical disk syndrome.
Trauma, musculoskeletal strain.
Rotator cuff syndrome.
Bicipital tendonitis.
Glenohumeral arthritis.
Acromioclavicular arthritis.
Thoracic outlet syndrome.
Pancoast tumor.
Infection (cellulitis, abscess).
Angina pectoris.

NECK MASS[28]

ICD-9CM # 784.2

CONGENITAL ANOMALIES

Thyroglossal duct cyst.
Bronchial apparatus anomalies.
Teratomas.
Ranula.
Dermoid cysts.
Hemangioma.
Laryngoceles.
Cystic hygroma.

NONNEOPLASTIC INFLAMMATORY ETIOLOGIES

Folliculitis.
Adenopathy secondary to peritonsillar abscess.
Retropharyngeal or parapharyngeal abscess.
Salivary gland infections.
Viral infections (mononucleosis, HIV, CMV).
TB.
Cat-scratch disease.
Toxoplasmosis.
Actinomyces.
Atypical mycobacterium.
Jugular vein thrombus.

NEOPLASM (PRIMARY OR METASTATIC)

Lipoma.

NECK PAIN[28]

ICD-9CM # 723.1   Neck Pain
                  (Nondiscogenic)
         959.09 Neck Injury

INFLAMMATORY DISEASES

RA.
Spondyloarthropathies.
Juvenile RA.

NONINFLAMMATORY DISEASE

Cervical osteoarthritis.
Diskogenic neck pain.
Diffuse idiopathic skeletal hyperostosis.
Fibromyalgia or myofascial pain.

INFECTIOUS CAUSES

Meningitis.
Osteomyelitis.
Infectious diskitis.

NEOPLASMS

Primary.
Metastatic.

REFERRED PAIN

Temporomandibular joint pain.
Cardiac pain.
Diaphragmatic irritation.
GI sources (gastric ulcer, gallbladder, pancreas).

NECROTIZING PNEUMONIAS[1]

ICD-9CM # 482.8

COMMON

Tuberculosis.
Staphylococcus.
Gram-negative bacilli.
Anaerobes.
Fungi.
Pneumocystis jirovecii.

RARE

Streptococcus pneumoniae.
Legionella.
Viruses.
Mycoplasma pneumoniae.

NEPHRITIC SYNDROME, ACUTE[1]

ICD-9CM # 580.89

LOW SERUM COMPLEMENT LEVEL

Acute postinfectious glomerulonephritis.
Membranoproliferative glomerulonephritis.
SLE.
Subacute bacterial endocarditis.
Visceral abscess "shunt" nephritis.
Cryoglobulinemia.

NORMAL SERUM COMPLEMENT LEVEL

IgA nephropathy.
Idiopathic rapidly progressive glomerulonephritis.
Antiglomerular basement membrane disease.
Polyarteritis nodosa.
Wegener's glomerulonephritis.
Henoch-Schönlein purpura.
Goodpasture's syndrome.

NEPHROCALCINOSIS

ICD-9CM # 275.49

Sarcoidosis.
Hyperparathyroidism.
Chronic glomerulonephritis.
Milk-alkali syndrome.
Distal renal tubular acidosis.
Medullary sponge kidney.
Bartter's syndrome.
Hypervitaminosis D.
Idiopathic hypercalciuria.
Hyperoxaluria.
Cortical necrosis.
Tuberculosis.
Idiopathic hypercalciuria.
Rapidly progressive osteoporosis.

NEUROGENIC BLADDER[29]

ICD-9CM # 396.54

SUPRATENTORIAL

CVA.
Parkinson's disease.
Alzheimer's disease.
Cerebral palsy.

SPINAL CORD

Spinal cord injury.
Spinal stenosis.
Central cord syndrome.
ALS.

Multiple sclerosis.
Myelodysplasia.

PERIPHERAL NEUROPATHY

Diabetes.
Alcohol.
Shingles.
Syphilis.

NEUROLOGIC DEFICIT, FOCAL[26]

ICD-9CM # 436   CVA
          435.9 TIA

TRAUMATIC: INTRACRANIAL, INTRASPINAL

Subdural hematoma.
Intraparenchymal hemorrhage.
Epidural hematoma.
Traumatic hemorrhagic necrosis.

INFECTIOUS

Brain abscess.
Epidural and subdural abscesses.
Meningitis.

NEOPLASTIC

Primary central nervous system tumors.
Metastatic tumors.
Syringomyelia.
Vascular.
Thrombosis.
Embolism.
Spontaneous hemorrhage: arteriovenous malformation, aneurysm, hypertensive.

METABOLIC

Hypoglycemia.
B_{12} deficiency.
Postseizure.
Hyperosmolar nonketotic.

OTHER

Migraine.
Bell's palsy.
Psychogenic.

NEUROLOGIC DEFICIT, MULTIFOCAL[26]

ICD-9CM # 436   CVA
          435.9 TIA

Acute disseminated encephalomyelitis: postviral or postimmunization.
Infectious encephalomyelitis: poliovirus, enteroviruses, arbovirus, herpes zoster, Epstein-Barr virus.
Granulomatous encephalomyelitis: sarcoid.
Autoimmune: SLE.
Other: familial spinocerebellar degenerations.

NEUROMUSCULAR JUNCTION DYSFUNCTION[1]

ICD-9CM # varies with specific diagnosis

DISORDERS OF THE NEUROMUSCULAR JUNCTION

Autoimmune
Myasthenia gravis.
Lambert-Eaton myasthenic syndrome.
Congenital
Presynaptic defects in ACh resynthesis, packaging, or release.
Synaptic defect: congenital end plate AChE deficiency.
Postsynaptic defects: slow-channel syndromes.
Postsynaptic defects: decreased response to ACh.
   Fast-channel syndromes.
   AChR deficiency without kinetic abnormality.
Familial limb-girdle myasthenia.
Toxic
Botulism.
Drug-induced disorders.
Organophosphate intoxication.

Ach, Acetylcholine; *AChE,* acetylcholinesterase; *AChR,* acetylcholine receptor.

NEURONOPATHIES, SENSORY (GANGLIONOPATHIES)[2]

ICD-9CM # varies with specific diagnosis

Herpes:
   Herpes simplex I and II.
   Varicella zoster (shingles).
Inflammatory sensory polyganglionopathy (ISP).
Paraneoplastic.
Primary biliary cirrhosis.
Sjögren's syndrome (keratoconjunctivitis sicca).
Toxin-induced:
   Pyridoxine (vitamin B_6) overdose.
   Metals:
     • Platinum (cisplatin).
     • Methyl mercury.
Vitamin E deficiency.

NEUROPATHIC BLADDER

ICD-9CM # 596.59

Diabetes.
Stroke.
Multiple sclerosis.
Parkinson's disease.
Dementia.
Encephalopathy.
Brain trauma.
Spinal cord trauma.
Pelvic surgery.
Spina bifida.

NEUROPATHIES WITH FACIAL NERVE INVOLVEMENT

ICD-9CM # varies with specific disorder

Sarcoidosis.
HIV.
Lyme disease.
Guillain-Barré.

Others: chronic inflammatory polyneuropathy, Tangier disease, amyloidosis.

NEUROPATHIES, AUTONOMIC[22a]

ICD-9CM # 357 Neuropathies

GUILLAIN-BARRÉ SYNDROME

Non–Guillain-Barré syndrome autoimmunity.
• Paraneoplastic (type I antineuronal nuclear antibody).
• Lambert-Eaton syndrome.
• Antibodies to neuronal nicotinc acetylcholine receptors.
• Antibodies to P/Q type calcium channels.
• Other autoantibodies.
• Systemic lupus erythematosus.

HEREDITARY

• Type I autosomal dominant.
• Type II autosomal recessive (Morvan disease).
• Type III autosomal recessive (Riley-Day).
• Type IV autosomal recessive (congenital insensitivity to pain with anhidrosis).
• Type V absence of pain.

METABOLIC

• Fabry disease.
• Diabetes mellitus.
• Tangier disease.
• Porphyria.

INFECTIOUS

• HIV.
• Chagas' disease.
• Botulism.
• Leprosy.
• Diphtheria.

OTHER

• Triple A (Allgrove) syndrome.
• Navajo Indian neuropathy.
• Multiple endocrine neoplasia type 2b.

TOXINS

NEUROPATHIES, AUTONOMIC, PERIPHERAL, CAUSES[14a]

ICD-9CM # 337.00 Neuropathies

METABOLIC

Diabetes mellitus.
Alcohol.
Acute intermittent porphyria.
Uremia.

AUTOIMMUNE

Autoimmune autonomic ganglionopathy.
Guillain-Barré syndrome.
Morvan's syndrome.
Lambert-Eaton myasthenic syndrome.
Chronic inflammatory demyelinating polyradiculoneuropathy.
Sjögren syndrome.
Systemic lupus erythematosus.
Mixed connective tissue diseases.

PARAPROTEINEMIC
Amyloidosis.

NUTRITIONAL
Cyanocobalamin deficiency.
Thiamine deficiency.
Gluten-sensitive neuropathy.

TOXIC
Heavy metals.
Organic solvents.
Organophosphates.
Vacor.
Acrylamide.

DRUG INDUCED
Cisplatin.
Vincristine.
Amiodarone.
Metronidazole.
Perhexiline.
Paclitaxel.

INFECTIOUS
Human immunodeficiency virus.
Leprosy.
Chagas' disease.
Botulism.
Diphtheria.
Lyme disease.

GENETIC
Hereditary sensory and autonomic neuropathies.
- Types I and II.
- Type III (familial dysautonomia).
- Type IV (congenital insensitivity to pain).
- Type V.
Fabry disease.

IDIOPATHIC
Adie's syndrome.
Ross' syndrome.
Acute cholinergic neuropathy.
Chronic idiopathic anhidrosis.
Amyotrophic lateral sclerosis.

NEUROPATHIES, PAINFUL[40]

ICD-9CM #		
	355.9	Neuropathy NOS
	357.5	Alcoholic
	357.8	Chronic Progressive or Relapsing
	356.2	Congenital Sensory
	356.0	Dejerine-Sottas
	356.60	Diabetic Polyneuropathy, Type II
	356.61	Diabetic Polyneuropathy Type I

MONONEUROPATHIES
Compressive neuropathy (carpal tunnel, meralgia paresthetica).
Trigeminal neuralgia.
Ischemic neuropathy.
Polyarteritis nodosa.
Diabetic mononeuropathy.
Herpes zoster.
Idiopathic and familial brachial plexopathy.

POLYNEUROPATHIES
DM.
Paraneoplastic sensory neuropathy.
Nutritional neuropathy.
Multiple myeloma.
Amyloid.
Dominantly inherited sensory neuropathy.
Toxic (arsenic, thallium, metronidazole).
AIDS-associated neuropathy.
Tangier disease.
Fabry's disease.

NEUROPATHIES, PERIPHERAL, ASYMMETRICAL PROXIMAL/DISTAL[2]

ICD-9CM # varies with specific diagnosis

BRACHIAL PLEXOPATHY
Open
Direct plexus injury (knife or gunshot wound).
Neurovascular (plexus ischemia).
Iatrogenic (central line insertion).
Closed
Traction injuries:
   "Stingers."
   Traction neurapraxia.
   Partial or complete nerve root avulsion.
Radiation.
Neoplastic.
Idiopathic brachial plexitis.
Throracic outlet.

LUMBOSACRAL PLEXOPATHIES
Open
Closed
Traction injuries:
   Pelvic double vertical shearing fracture.
   Posterior hip dislocation.
   Retroperitoneal hemorrhage.
Vasospastic (deep buttock injection).
Neoplastic.
Radiation.
Idiopathic lumbosacral plexitis.
Infectious:
   Herpesvirus (sacrococcygeal).
   Herpes simplex II.
   Herpes zoster.
Cytomegalovirus (CMV) polyradiculopathy (HIV).

NEUROPATHIES, TOXIC AND METABOLIC[22a]

ICD-9CM # 337.00 Neuropathies

METALS
Arsenic (insecticide, herbicide).
Lead (paint, batteries, pottery).
Mercury (metallic, vapor).
Thallium (rodenticides).
Gold.

OCCUPATIONAL OR INDUSTRIAL CHEMICALS
Acrylamide (grouting, flocculation).
Carbon disulfide (solvent).
Cyanide.

Dichlorophenoxyacetate.
Dimethylaminopropionitrite.
Ethylene oxide (gas sterilization).
Hexacarbons (glue, solvents).
Organophosphates (insecticides, petroleum additive).
Polychlorinated biphenyls.
Tetrachlorbiphenyl.
Trichloroethylene.

DRUGS
Amiodarone.
Chloramphenicol.
Chloroquine.
Cisplatin.
Colchicine.
Dapsone.
Ethambutol.
Ethanol.
Gold.
Hydralazine.
Isoniazid.
Metronidazole.
Nitrofurantoin.
Nitrous oxide.
Nucleosides (antiretroviral agents ddC, ddI, d4T, others).
Penicillamine.
Pentamidine.
Phenytoin.
Pyridoxine (excessive).
Statins.
Stilbamidine.
Suramin.
Taxanes (paclitaxel, docetaxel).
Thalidomide.
Tryptophan (eosinophilia-myalgia syndrome).
Vincristine.

METABOLIC DISORDERS
Fabry disease.
Krabbe disease.
Leukodystrophies.
Porphyria.
Tangier disease.
Tyrosinemia.
Uremia.

NEUTROPENIA WITH DECREASED MARROW RESERVE[20]

ICD-9CM # 288.09

PRIMARY
Severe congenital neutropenia.
Shwachman–Diamond syndrome.
Cyclic neutropenia.

SECONDARY
Lymphoproliferative disorder of granular lymphocytes.
Chemotherapy.
Drug induced (nonimmune).
Nutritional.
Viral infection (varicella, EBV, measles, CMV, hepatitis, HIV).

NEUTROPENIA WITH NORMAL MARROW RESERVE[20]

ICD-9CM # 288.0

Chronic benign neutropenia of infancy and childhood.
Ethnic or benign familial neutropenia.
Autoimmune neutropenia.
Alloimmune neutropenia.
Drug-induced neutropenia.
Infection-related neutropenia.
Hypersplenism.

NEUTROPENIA, IN CHILDHOOD

ICD-9CM # 288.09

ACQUIRED

Infection.
Immune mediated.
Hypersplenism.
Vitamin B_{12}, folate, copper deficiency.
Drugs or toxic substances.
Aplastic anemia.
Malignancies or preleukemic disorders.
Ionizing radiation.

CONGENITAL

Cyclic neutropenia.
Severe congenital neutropenia (Kostmann syndrome).
Chronic benign neutropenia of childhood.
Shwachman-Diamond syndrome.
Fanconi anemia.
Metabolic disorders (amino acidopathies, Barth syndrome, glycogen storage disorders).
Osteopetrosis.
Neutropenia with pigmentation abnormalities, e.g., Chédiak-Higashi.

NEUTROPHILIA[20]

ICD-9CM # 288.60

CLASSIFICATION OF NEUTROPHILIA

Primary (No Other Evident Associated Disease)

Hereditary neutrophilia.
Chronic idiopathic neutrophilia.
Chronic myelogenous leukemia (CML) and other myeloproliferative diseases.
Familial myeloproliferative disease.
Congenital anomalies and leukemoid reaction.
Leukocyte adhesion factor deficiency (LAD).
Familial cold urticaria and leukocytosis.

Secondary

Infection.
Stress neutrophilia.
Chronic inflammation.
Drug induced.
Nonhematologic malignancy.

Generalized marrow stimulation as in hemolysis.
Asplenia and hyposplenism.

NIPPLE LESIONS

ICD-9CM # varies with specific disorder

Contact dermatitis.
Trauma.
Paget's disease.
Sebaceous hyperplasia.
Neurofibroma.
Accessory nipple.
Papillary adenoma.
Nevoid hyperkeratosis.
Cellulitis.

NODULAR LESIONS, SKIN

ICD-9CM # 782.2

Lipoma.
Cherry angioma.
Angiokeratoma.
Hemangioma.
Classic Kaposi's sarcoma.
Nodular melanoma.
Pyogenic granuloma.
Angiosarcoma.
Eccrine poroma.

NODULES, PAINFUL

ICD-9CM # varies with specific disorder

Arthropod bite or sting.
Erythema nodosum.
Glomus tumor.
Neuroma.
Leiomyoma.
Angiolipoma.
Dermatofibroma.
Osler's node.
Blue rubber bleb nevus.
Vasculitis.
Sweet's syndrome.

NYSTAGMUS

ICD-9CM # 379.50 Nystagmus NOS
     386.11 Benign Positional
     386.2   Central Positional
     379.59 Congenital

Medications (meperidine, barbiturates, phenytoin, phenothiazines, etc.).
Multiple sclerosis.
Congenital.
Neoplasm (cerebellar, brain stem, cerebral).
Labyrinthine or vestibular lesions.
CNS infections.
Optic atrophy.
Other: Arnold–Chiari malformation, syringobulbia, chorioretinitis, meningeal cysts.

NYSTAGMUS, MONOCULAR

ICD-9CM # 379.50

Amblyopia.
Strabismus.
Multiple sclerosis.

Monocular blindness.
Internuclear ophthalmoplegia.
Lid fasciculations.
Brain stem infarct.

ODYNOPHAGIA[38]

ICD-9CM # varies with specific diagnosis

CAUSES OF ODYNOPHAGIA

Infections

Herpes simplex virus.
Cytomegalovirus.
Candidiasis.

Chemical, Inflammatory

Gastroesophageal reflux.
Drug induced (Slow-K, tetracyclines, quinidine).
Radiation.
Graft-versus-host disease.
Crohn's disease.
Dermatologic diseases (pemphigus and pemphigoid).

OPACIFICATION OF HEMIDIAPHRAGM ON X-RAY[16a]

ICD-9CM # 419.4

CAUSES OF OPACIFICATION OF A HEMITHORAX

Pleural effusion.
Consolidation.
Collapse.
Massive tumor.
Fibrothorax.
Combination of above lesions.
Pneumonectomy.
Lung agenesis.

OPHTHALMOPLEGIA[1]

ICD-9CM # 378.9   Ophthalmoplegia NOS
     378.52 Cerebellar Ataxia
         Syndrome
     376.22 Exophthalmic

BILATERAL

Botulism.
Myasthenia gravis.
Wernicke's encephalopathy.
Acute cranial polyneuropathy.
Brain stem stroke.

UNILATERAL

Carotid-posterior (3rd cranial nerve, pupil involved communicating aneurysm).
Diabetic-idiopathic (3rd or 6th cranial nerve, pupil spared).
Myasthenia gravis.
Brain stem stroke.

OPSOCLONUS*

ICD-9CM # 379.59

Multiple sclerosis.
Encephalitis.
CNS lymphoma.
Hydrocephalus.

Pontine hemorrhage.
Thalamic disorder (glioma, hemorrhage).
Hyperosmolar coma.
Carcinoma, paraneoplastic.
Cocaine.
Medications (e.g., phenytoin, haloperidol, amitriptyline, diazepam, vidarabine).

---

*Spontaneous, multivector, chaotic eye movement

OPTIC ATROPHY[34a]

ICD-9CM # 377.1

CAUSES OF OPTIC ATROPHY

Optic Nerve Compression
Pituitary tumor.
Carotid aneurysm.
Glaucoma.
Optic nerve tumor.
Sphenoid meningioma.
Olfactory groove meningioma.
Optic Neuritis
Following Longstanding Papilledema
Central Retinal Artery Occlusion
Toxic/Metabolic
Diabetes.
Methyl alcohol.
Tobacco.
Quinine.
Ethambutol.
Lead and arsenic.
Anemia.
Secondary to Retinal Disease
Senile macular degeneration.
Retinitis pigmentosa.
Severe chorioretinitis.
Secondary to Trauma
Orbital fracture.
Hereditary
Leber's optic atrophy.
Hereditary ataxias.
Spinocerebellar degeneration.

ORAL MUCOSA, ERYTHEMATOUS LESIONS[9]

ICD-9CM # 528.3 Oral Abscess
528.9 Oral Disease (Soft Tissue)
528.8 Hyperplasia (Tongue)

Allergy.
Erythroplakia.
Candidiasis.
Geographic tongue.
Stomatitis areata migrans.
Plasma cell gingivitis.
Pemphigus vulgaris.

ORAL MUCOSA, PIGMENTED LESIONS[9]

ICD-9CM # 528.3 Oral Abscess
528.9 Oral Disease (Soft Tissue)
528.8 Hyperplasia (Tongue)

Racial pigmentation.
Oral melanotic macule.
Peutz-Jeghers syndrome.
Neurofibromatosis.

Albright's syndrome.
Addison's disease.
Chloasma.
Drug reaction: quinacrine, Minocin, chlorpromazine, Myleran.
Amalgam tattoo.
Lead line.
Smoker's melanosis.
Nevi.
Melanoma.

ORAL MUCOSA, PUNCTATE EROSIVE LESIONS[9]

ICD-9CM # 528.3 Oral Abscess
528.9 Oral Disease (Soft Tissue)
528.8 Hyperplasia (Tongue)

Viral lesion: Herpes simplex, coxsackievirus (A, B, A16), herpes zoster.
Aphthous stomatitis.
Sutton's disease (giant aphthae).
Behçet's syndrome.
Reiter's syndrome.
Neutropenia.
Acute necrotizing ulcerative gingivostomatitis (ANUG).
Drug reaction.
Inflammatory bowel disease.
Contact allergy.

ORAL MUCOSA, WHITE LESIONS[9]

ICD-9CM # 528.3 Oral Abscess
528.9 Oral Disease (Soft Tissue)
528.8 Hyperplasia (Tongue)

Leukoplakia.
White, hairy leukoplakia.
Squamous cell carcinoma.
Lichen planus.
Stomatitis nicotinica.
Benign intraepithelial dyskeratosis.
White spongy nevus.
Leukoedema.
Darier-White disease.
Pachyonychia congenital.
Candidiasis.
Allergy.
SLE.

ORAL ULCERS, ACUTE

ICD-9CM # varies with diagnosis
528.9 Traumatic Ulcer of Oral Mucosa

Trauma (including thermal trauma).
Aphthous stomatitis.
Syphilis.
Herpes simplex infection.
Herpes zoster.

ORAL VESICLES AND ULCERS[1]

ICD-9CM # 528.9

Aphthous stomatitis.
Primary herpes simplex infection.

Vincent's stomatitis.
Syphilis.
Coxsackievirus A (herpangina).
Fungi (histoplasmosis).
Behçet's syndrome.
SLE.
Reiter's syndrome.
Crohn's disease.
Erythema multiforme.
Pemphigus.
Pemphigoid.

ORBITAL LESIONS, CALCIFIED

ICD-9CM # 376.89

Chronic inflammation.
Phlebolith.
Dermoid cyst.
Mucocele walls.
Tumors (lacrimal gland, fibro-osseous).
Meningioma (optic sheath).
Lymphangioma.
Orbital varix.

ORBITAL LESIONS, CYSTIC

ICD-9CM # 376.9

Sweat gland cyst.
Dermoid cyst.
Lacrimal gland cyst.
Abscess.
Conjunctival cyst.
Lymphangioma.
Schwannoma.

ORGASM DYSFUNCTION[12]

ICD-9CM # 302.73 Orgasm Inhibited, Female Psychosexual
302.74 Orgasm Inhibited, Male Psychosexual

Anorgasmia: inadequate stimulation or learning.
Spinal cord lesion or injury.
Multiple sclerosis.
Alcoholic neuropathy.
Amyotrophic lateral sclerosis.
Spinal cord accident.
Spinal cord trauma.
Peripheral nerve damage.
Radical pelvic surgery.
Herniated lumbar disk.
Hypothyroidism.
Addison's disease.
Cushing's disease.
Acromegaly.
Hypopituitarism.
Pharmacologic agents (e.g., SSRIs, beta-blockers).
Psychogenic.

OROFACIAL PAIN

ICD-9CM # 784.0

Dental abscess.
Sinusitis.
Otitis media.
Otitis externa.

Wisdom tooth eruption.
Sialoadenitis.
Herpes zoster.
Trigeminal neuralgia.
Parotitis.
Anxiety disorder.
Malingering.

OSTEOPOROSIS, SECONDARY CAUSES

ICD-9CM # 733.00

Medication induced (e.g., glucocorticoids, anti-convulsants, heparin, LHRH agonists or antagonists).
Hyperparathyroidism.
Hyperthyroidism.
Prolonged immobilization.
Chronic renal failure.
Sickle cell disease.
Multiple myeloma.
Myeloproliferative diseases.
Leukemias and lymphomas.
Acromegaly.
Prolactinoma.
DM.
Total parenteral nutrition.
Malabsorption.
Chronic hypophosphatemia.
Connective tissue disorders (e.g., osteogenesis imperfecta, Marfan's syndrome, Ehlers-Danlos).
Hepatobiliary disease.
Postgastrectomy.
Aluminum-containing antacids.
Systemic mastocytosis.
Homocystinuria.

OSTEOSCLEROSIS, DIFFUSE[16a]

ICD-9CM # varies with specific diagnosis

DISORDERS ASSOCIATED WITH DIFFUSE OSTEOSCLEROSIS

*Neoplastic Causes**
Prostate carcinoma, breast carcinoma, gastrointestinal adenocarcinoma, carcinoid tumors, transitional cell carcinoma of the bladder, myeloma, lymphoma, leukemia.
*Hematologic Causes**
Sickle cell disorders, mastocytosis, myelofibrosis, polycythemia vera.
*Metabolic Causes**
Renal osteodystrophy, primary hyperparathyoidism, familial hypophosphatemic osteomalacia, hypervitaminosis D, fluorosis, hypoparathyroidism, pseudohypoparathyroidism.
Primary Osseous Disorders[†]
Osteoporosis.
Pyknodysostosis.
Paget's disease.

*Involvement principally of cancellous bone
[†]Involvement of cancellous and cortical bone

OVULATORY DYSFUNCTION[21]

ICD-9CM # 628.0 Anovulatory Cycle
626.5 Ovulation Pain

HYPERANDROGENIC ANOVULATION

Polycystic ovarian syndrome.
Late-onset congenital adrenal hyperplasias.
Ovarian hyperthecosis.
Androgen-producing ovarian tumors.
Androgen-producing adrenal tumors.
Cushing's syndrome.

HYPOESTROGENIC ANOVULATION (HYPOTHALAMIC OR PITUITARY ETIOLOGY)

Hypogonadotropic Hypoestrogenic States
Reversible:
  Functional hypothalamic amenorrheas:
    • Eating disorders (anorexia nervosa, excessive weight loss).
    • Excessive athletic training.
  Neoplastic:
    Craniopharyngioma.
    Pituitary stalk compression.
  Infiltrative diseases:
    Histiocytosis-X.
    Sarcoidosis.
  Hypophysitis.
  Pituitary adenomas:
    Hyperprolactinemia.
    Euprolactinemic galactorrhea.
  Endocrinopathies:
    Hypothyroidism/hyperthyroidism.
    Cushing's disease.
Irreversible:
  Kallmann's syndrome.
  Isolated gonadotropin deficiency (hypothalamic or pituitary origin).
  Panhypopituitarism/pituitary insufficiency:
    • Sheehan's syndrome, pituitary apoplexy.
    • Pituitary irradiation or ablation.
Hypergonadotropic Hypoestrogenic States
Physiologic states:
  Menopause.
  Perimenopause.
Premature ovarian failure.
Immune-related:
  Radiation/chemotherapy-induced.
Ovarian dysgenesis.
Turner's syndrome.
46XX with mutations of X.
Androgen insensitivity syndrome.

MISCELLANEOUS

Endometriosis.
Luteal phase defect.

PAIN, MIDFOOT

ICD-9CM # 719.47

MEDIAL ASPECT

Tendonitis of posterior tibialis.
Tendonitis of flexor digitorum longus.
Tendonitis of flexor hallucis longus.
Infection (osteomyelitis, septic arthritis, cellulitis) of foot.
Peripheral vascular insufficiency.

Fracture.
Osteoarthritis.
Gout, pseudogout.
Neuropathy.
Tumor.

LATERAL ASPECT

Peroneus longus tendonitis.
Peroneus brevis tendonitis.
Infection (osteomyelitis, septic arthritis, cellulitis) of foot.
Peripheral vascular insufficiency.
Fracture.
Osteoarthritis.
Gout, pseudogout.
Neuropathy.
Tumor.

PAIN, PLANTAR ASPECT, HEEL

ICD-9CM # 719.47

Plantar fasciitis.
Tarsal tunnel syndrome.
Neuroma.
Infection (osteomyelitis, septic arthritis, cellulitis) of foot.
Peripheral vascular insufficiency.
Fracture.
Bone cyst.
Osteoarthritis.
Gout, pseudogout.
Neuropathy.
Tumor.
Heel pad atrophy.
Plantar fascia rupture.

PAIN, POSTERIOR HEEL

ICD-9CM # 729.5

Achilles tendonitis.
Retrocalcaneal bursitis.
Retroachilles bursitis.
Infection (osteomyelitis, septic arthritis, cellulitis) of foot.
Peripheral vascular insufficiency.
Fracture.
Osteoarthritis.
Gout, pseudogout.
Neuropathy.
Tumor.

PALINDROMIC RHEUMATISM[6]

ICD-9CM # 719.3 use 5th digit
  0 Site Unspecified
  1 Shoulder Region
  2 Upper Arm (Elbow, Humerus)
  3 Forearm (Radius, Wrist, Ulna)
  4 Hand (Carpal, Metacarpal, Fingers)
  5 Pelvic Region and Thigh
  6 Lower Leg
  7 Ankle and Foot
  8 Other
  9 Multiple

Palindromic RA.
Essential palindromic rheumatism.

Differential Diagnosis

II

Crystal synovitis (gout, CPPD, pseudogout, calcific periarthritis).
Lyme borreliosis, stages 2 and 3.
Sarcoidosis.
Whipple's disease.
Acute rheumatic fever.
Reactive arthritis (rare).

PALMOPLANTAR HYPERKERATOSIS

ICD-9CM # 701.1

Superficial skin infection.
Chronic eczema.
Repeated trauma.
Psoriasis.
Reiter's syndrome.
Paraneoplastic acrokeratosis.

PALPITATIONS[33]

ICD-9CM # 785.1 Palpitations

Anxiety.
Electrolyte abnormalities (hypokalemia, hypomagnesemia).
Exercise.
Hyperthyroidism.
Ischemic heart disease.
Ingestion of stimulant drugs (cocaine, amphetamines, caffeine).
Medications (digoxin, beta-blockers, calcium channel antagonists, hydralazines, diuretics, minoxidil).
Hypoglycemia in type 1 DM.
Mitral valve prolapse.
Wolff-Parkinson-White (WPW) syndrome.
Sick sinus syndrome.

PANCREATIC CALCIFICATIONS

ICD-9CM # 577.8

Chronic pancreatitis.
Hyperparathyroidism.
Metastatic neoplasm.
Pseudocyst.
Hereditary pancreatitis.
Cystoadenoma.
Cystoadenocarcinoma.
Cavernous lymphangioma.
Hemorrhage.
Acute pancreatitis (saponification).

PANCREATITIS, ACUTE, IN CHILDREN

ICD-9CM # 577.0

CAUSES OF ACUTE PANCREATITIS IN CHILDREN

Drugs and Toxins
Acetaminophen overdose.
Alcohol.
L-Asparaginase.
Azathioprine.
Carbamazepine.
Cimetidine.
Corticosteroids.
Enalapril.

Erythromycin.
Estrogen.
Furosemide.
Isoniazid.
Lisinopril.
6-Mercaptopurine.
Methyldopa.
Metronidazole.
Organophosphate poisoning.
Pentamidine.
Retrovirals: DDC, DDI, tenofovir.
Sulfonamides: mesalamine, 5-aminosalicylates, sulfasalazine, trimethoprim/sulfamethoxazole.
Sulindac.
Tetracycline.
Thiazides.
Valproic acid.
Venom (spider, scorpion, Gila monster lizard).
Vincristine.

Genetic
Cationic trypsinogen gene (PRSS1).
Chymotrypsin C gene (CTRC).
Cystic fibrosis gene (CFTR).
Trypsin inhibitor gene (SPINK1).

Infectious
Ascariasis.
Coxsackie B virus.
Epstein-Barr virus.
Hepatitis A, B.
Influenza A, B.
Leptospirosis.
Malaria.
Measles.
Mumps.
Mycoplasma.
Reye syndrome: varicella, influenza B.
Rubella.
Rubeola.
Septic shock.

Obstructive
Ampullary disease.
Ascariasis.
Biliary tract malformations.
Choledochal cyst.
Choledochocele.
Cholelithiasis, microlithiasis, and choledocholithiasis (stones or sludge).
Duplication cyst.
Endoscopic retrograde cholangiopancreatography (ERCP) complication.
Pancreas divisum.
Pancreatic ductal abnormalities.
Postoperative.
Sphincter of Oddi dysfunction.
Tumor.

Systemic Disease
Autoimmune pancreatitis.
Brain tumor.
Collagen vascular diseases.
Crohn disease.
Diabetes mellitus.
Head trauma.
Hemochromatosis.
Hemolytic-uremic syndrome.
Hyperlipidemia: type I, IV, V.
Hyperparathyroidism/Hypercalcemia.
Kawasaki disease.
Malnutrition.

Organic acidemia.
Peptic ulcer.
Periarteritis nodosa.
Renal failure.
Systemic lupus erythematosus.
Transplantation: bone marrow, heart, liver, kidney, pancreas.
Vasculitis.

Traumatic
Blunt injury.
Burns.
Child abuse.
Hypothermia.
Surgical trauma.
Total body cast.

PANCREATITIS, DRUG-INDUCED[2]

ICD-9CM # 577.0

DEFINITE
Acetaminophen.
Azathioprine.
Cimetidine.
Cisplatin.
Corticosteroids.
Didanosine.
Erythromycin.
Estrogens.
Ethyl alcohol.
Furosemide.
L-Asparaginase.
Mercaptopurine.
Metronidazole.
Methyldopa.
Nitrofurantoin.
Octreotide.
Organophosphates.
Pentamidine.
Ranitidine.
Tetracycline.
Salicylates.
Sulfonamides, trimethoprim-sulfamethoxazole, sulfasalazine.
Sulindac.
Valproic acid.

POSSIBLE
Bumetanide.
Carbamazepine.
Chlorthalidone.
Clonidine.
Colchicine.
Cyclosporine.
Cytarabine.
Diazoxide.
Enalapril.
Ergotamine.
Ethacrynic acid.
Indomethacin.
Isoniazid.
Isotretinoin.
Mefenamic acid.
Opiates.
Phenformin.
Piroxicam.
Procainamide.
Rifampin.
Thiazides.

PANCYTOPENIA[20]
ICD-9CM # 284.1

PANCYTOPENIA WITH HYPOCELLULAR BONE MARROW

Acquired aplastic anemia.
Inherited aplastic anemia (Fanconi anemia and others).
Some myelodysplasia syndromes.
Rare aleukemic leukemia (acute myelogenous leukemia).
Some acute lymphoblastic leukemias.
Some lymphomas of bone marrow.

PANCYTOPENIA WITH CELLULAR BONE MARROW

Primary bone marrow diseases.
Myelodysplasia syndromes.
Paroxysmal nocturnal hemoglobinuria.
Myelofibrosis.
Some aleukemic leukemias.
Myelophthisis.
Bone marrow lymphoma.
Hairy cell leukemia.
Secondary to systemic diseases.
Systemic lupus erythematosus, Sjögren syndrome.
Hypersplenism.
Vitamin B_{12}, folate deficiency (familial defect).
Overwhelming infection.
Alcohol.
Brucellosis.
Ehrlichiosis.
Sarcoidosis.
Tuberculosis and atypical mycobacteria.

HYPOCELLULAR BONE MARROW ± CYTOPENIA

Q fever.
Legionnaires disease.
Mycobacteria.
Tuberculosis.*
Anorexia nervosa, starvation.
Hypothyroidism.

*Pancytopenia in tuberculosis only rarely is associated with a hypocellular bone marrow at biopsy or autopsy. Marrow failure in the setting of tuberculosis is almost always fatal; exceptional patients probably had underlying myelodysplasia or acute leukemia.

PANCYTOPENIA SYNDROME, INHERITED
ICD-9CM # 284.1

Fanconi anemia.
Shwachman-Diamond syndrome.
Dyskeratosis congenita.
Congenital amegakaryocytic thrombocytopenia.
Unclassified inherited bone marrow failure syndromes.
Other genetic syndromes:
 Down syndrome.
 Dubowitz syndrome.
 Seckel syndrome.
 Reticular dysgenesis.
 Schimke immunoosseous dysplasia.

Familial aplastic anemia (non-Fanconi).
Cartilage-hair hypoplasia.
Noonan syndrome.

PAPILLEDEMA
ICD-9CM # 377.00 Papilledema NOS
377.02 With Decreased Ocular Pressure
377.01 With Increased Intracranial Pressure
377.03 With Retinal Disorder

CNS infections (viral, bacterial, fungal).
Medications (lithium, cisplatin, corticosteroids, tetracycline, etc.).
Head trauma.
CNS neoplasm (primary or metastatic).
Pseudotumor cerebri.
Cavernous sinus thrombosis.
SLE.
Sarcoidosis.
Subarachnoid hemorrhage.
Carbon dioxide retention.
Arnold–Chiari malformation and other developmental or congenital malformations.
Orbital lesions.
Central retinal vein occlusion.
Hypertensive encephalopathy.
Metabolic abnormalities.

PAPULOSQUAMOUS DISEASES[14]
ICD-9CM # 709.8

Psoriasis.
Pityriasis rubra pilaris.
Pityriasis rosea.
Lichen planus.
Lichen nitidus.
Secondary syphilis.
Pityriasis lichenoides.
Parapsoriasis.
Mycosis fungoides.
Dermatophytosis.
Tinea versicolor.

PARANEOPLASTIC NEUROLOGIC SYNDROMES
ICD-9CM # varies with specific disorder

Lambert-Eaton myasthenic syndrome.
Myasthenia gravis.
Guillain-Barré syndrome.
Amyotrophic lateral sclerosis.
Dermatomyositis.
Carcinoid myopathy.
Cerebellar degeneration.
Encephalomyelitis.
Optic neuritis, uveitis, retinopathy.
Stiff-man syndrome.
Autonomic neuropathy.
Brachial neuritis.
Sensory neuropathy.
Progressive multifocal leukoencephalopathy.

PARANEOPLASTIC SYNDROMES, ENDOCRINE[36]
ICD-9CM # varies with specific disorder

Hypercalcemia.
Syndrome of inappropriate secretion of antidiuretic hormone.
Hypoglycemia.
Zollinger-Ellison syndrome.
Ectopic secretion of human chorionic gonadotropin.
Cushing's syndrome.

PARANEOPLASTIC SYNDROMES, NONENDOCRINE[36]
ICD-9CM # varies with specific disorder

CUTANEOUS
Dermatomyositis.
Acanthosis nigricans.
Sweet's syndrome.
Erythema gyratum repens.
Systemic nodular panniculitis (Weber-Christian disease).

RENAL
Nephrotic syndrome.
Nephrogenic diabetes insipidus.

NEUROLOGIC
Subacute cerebellar degeneration.
Progressive multifocal leukoencephalopathy.
Subacute motor neuropathy.
Sensory neuropathy.
Ascending acute polyneuropathy (Guillain-Barré syndrome).
Myasthenic syndrome (Eaton-Lambert syndrome).

HEMATOLOGIC
Microangiopathic hemolytic anemia.
Migratory thrombophlebitis (Trousseau's syndrome).
Anemia of chronic disease.

RHEUMATOLOGIC
Polymyalgia rheumatica.
Hypertrophic pulmonary osteoarthropathy.

PARAPARESIS, ACUTE OR SUBACUTE[34a]
ICD-9CM # varies with specific diagnosis

CAUSES OF ACUTE OR SUBACUTE PARAPARESIS
Trauma to a Previously Normal Spine
Vertebral disease
Metastatic carcinoma.
Cervical spondylosis.
Dorsal disk prolapse.
Paget's disease.
Rheumatoid arthritis.
Pott's disease of spine.

Differential Diagnosis

II

Tumors
Extradural or intradural carcinoma, lymphoma, myeloma, leukemia.
Dorsal meningioma.
Neurofibroma.
Hematologic disease
Any cause of thrombocytopenia.
Other clotting disorders.
Leukemia.
Anticoagulant treatment.
Epidural or intramedullary hemorrhage.
Infection
Epidural abscess.
TB abscess.
Syphilitic myelitis.
HIV infection.
Vascular myelopathy.
Vascular
Anterior spinal artery occlusion.
Infarction secondary to hypotension.
Embolic infarction.
Infarction secondary to aortic dissection.
Arteriovenous malformation: infarction or hemorrhage.
Primary intramedullary hemorrhage.
Vasculitis—polyarteritis nodosa (PAN).
Inflammatory
Myelitis of unknown cause.
Multiple sclerosis.
Systemic lupus erythematosus.
Sarcoidosis.
Metabolic
Subacute degeneration of the cord.

PARAPARESIS, CHRONIC PROGRESSIVE[34a]

ICD-9CM # varies with specific diagnosis

CAUSES OF CHRONIC PROGRESSIVE PARAPARESIS

Vertebral Disease
Cervical spondylosis.
Dorsal disk prolapse.
Rheumatoid arthritis.
Pott's disease of spine.
Ankylosing spondylitis.
Tumors
Meningioma.
Neurofibroma.
Glioma.
Ependymoma.
Chordoma.
Lipoma.
Syringomyelia
With Arnold–Chiari malformation.
With tumor.
Posttraumatic.
Infection
Tropical spastic paraparesis (HTLV 1 infection).
Syphilitic myelitis.
Vascular
Arteriovenous malformation.
Inflammatory
Multiple sclerosis.
Sarcoidosis.
Radiation myelopathy.
Arachnoiditis.

Metabolic
Subacute combined degeneration of the cord.
Paget's disease.
Degenerative
Motor neuron disease.
Hereditary
Hereditary spastic paraplegia.

PARAPLEGIA

ICD-9CM # 344.1 Paraplegia, Acquired
343.0 Paraplegia, Congenital
438.50 Paraplegia, Late Effect of CVA

Trauma: penetrating wounds to motor cortex, fracture-dislocation of vertebral column with compression of spinal cord or cauda equina, prolapsed disk, electrical injuries.
Neoplasm: parasagittal region, vertebrae, meninges, spinal cord, cauda equina, Hodgkin's disease, NHL, leukemic deposits, pelvic neoplasms.
Multiple sclerosis and other demyelinating disorders.
Mechanical compression of spinal cord, cauda equina, or lumbosacral plexus: Paget's disease, kyphoscoliosis, herniation of intervertebral disk, spondylosis, ankylosing spondylitis, RA, aortic aneurysm.
Infections: spinal abscess, syphilis, TB, poliomyelitis, leprosy.
Thrombosis of superior sagittal sinus.
Polyneuritis: Guillain-Barré syndrome, diabetes, alcohol, beriberi, heavy metals.
Heredofamilial muscular dystrophies.
ALS.
Congenital and familial conditions: syringomyelia, myelomeningocele, myelodysplasia.
Hysteria.

PARESTHESIAS

ICD-9CM # 782.0

Multiple sclerosis.
Nutritional deficiencies (thiamin, vitamin B_{12}, folic acid).
Compression of spinal cord or peripheral nerves.
Medications (e.g., INH, lithium, nitrofurantoin, gold, cisplatin, hydralazine, amitriptyline, sulfonamides, amiodarone, metronidazole, dapsone, disulfiram, chloramphenicol).
Toxic chemicals (e.g., lead, arsenic, cyanide, mercury, organophosphates).
DM.
Myxedema.
Alcohol.
Sarcoidosis.
Neoplasms.
Infections (HIV, Lyme disease, herpes zoster, leprosy, diphtheria).
Charcot-Marie-Tooth syndrome and other hereditary neuropathies.
Guillain-Barré neuropathy.

PARKINSONISM-PLUS SYNDROMES

ICD-9CM # varies with specific disorder

Parkinson's disease.
Shy-Drager syndrome.
Corticobasal degeneration.
Olivo-ponto-cerebellar atrophy.
Dementia with Lewy bodies.
Progressive supranuclear palsy.
Striatonigral degeneration.

PAROTID SWELLING[3]

ICD-9CM # 527.2 Allergic Parotitis
72.9 Infectious Parotitis
527.8 Salivary Gland Obstruction
527.5 Salivary Gland Obstruction with Calculus
527.8 Salivary Gland Stricture
527.3 Salivary Gland Abscess
235.1 Salivary Gland Neoplasm

INFECTIOUS

Mumps.
Parainfluenza.
Influenza.
Cytomegalovirus infection.
Coxsackievirus infection.
Lymphocytic choriomeningitis.
Echovirus infection.
Suppuration (bacterial).
Actinomyces infection.
Mycobacterial infection.
Cat-scratch disease.

NONINFECTIOUS

Drug hypersensitivity (thiouracil, phenothiazines, thiocyanate, iodides, copper, isoprenaline, lead, mercury, phenylbutazone).
Sarcoidosis.
Tumors, mixed.
Hemangioma, lymphangioma.
Sialectasis.
Sjögren's syndrome.
Mikulicz's syndrome (scleroderma, mixed connective tissue disease, SLE).
Recurrent idiopathic parotitis.
Pneumoparotitis.
Trauma.
Sialolithiasis.
Foreign body.
Cystic fibrosis.
Malnutrition (marasmus, alcohol cirrhosis).
Dehydration.
DM.
Waldenström's macroglobulinemia.
Reiter's syndrome.
Amyloidosis.

NONPAROTID SWELLING

Hypertrophy of masseter muscle.
Lymphadenopathy.
Rheumatoid mandibular joint swelling.
Tumors of jaw.
Infantile cortical hyperostosis.

PELVIC MASS

ICD-9CM # 789.39

Hemorrhagic ovarian cyst.
Simple ovarian cyst (follicle or corpus luteum).
Ovarian carcinoma, carcinoma of fallopian tube, colorectal carcinoma, metastatic carcinoma, prostate carcinoma, bladder carcinoma, lymphoma, Hodgkin's disease.
Cystadenoma, teratoma, endometrioma.
Leiomyoma.
Leiomyosarcoma.
Diverticulitis, diverticular abscess.
Appendiceal abscess, tuboovarian abscess.
Ectopic pregnancy, intrauterine pregnancy.
Paraovarian cyst.
Hydrosalpinx.

PELVIC PAIN, CAUSES IN WOMEN[2]

ICD-9CM # 338.4

POTENTIAL CAUSES OF PELVIC PAIN IN WOMEN

Reproductive Tract
Ovarian torsion.
Ovarian cyst.
Salpingitis/tubo-ovarian abscess.
Septic pelvic thrombophlebitis.
Endometritis.
Endometriosis.
Uterine perforation.
Uterine fibroids.
Dysmenorrhea.
Pregnancy-related
First trimester
Ectopic pregnancy.
Threatened abortion.
Nonviable pregnancy.
Ovarian hyperstimulation syndrome.
Second and third trimesters
Placenta previa.
Placental abruption.
Round ligament pain.
Intestinal Tract
Appendicitis.
Diverticulitis.
Ischemic bowel.
Perforated viscus.
Bowel obstruction.
Incarcerated/strangulated hernia.
Inflammatory bowel disease.
Gastroenteritis.
Urinary Tract
Pyelonephritis.
Cystitis.
Ureteral stone.

PELVIC PAIN, CHRONIC[7]

ICD-9CM # 625.9 Pelvic Pain, Female
            789.09 Pelvic Pain, Male

GYNECOLOGIC DISORDERS

Primary dysmenorrhea.
Endometriosis.
Adenomyosis.
Adhesions.
Fibroids.
Retained ovary syndrome after hysterectomy.
Previous tubal ligation.
Chronic pelvic infection.

MUSCULOSKELETAL DISORDERS

Myofascial pain syndrome.

GASTROINTESTINAL DISORDERS

Irritable bowel syndrome.
Inflammatory bowel disease.

URINARY TRACT DISORDERS

Interstitial cystitis.
Nonbacterial urethritis.

PELVIC PAIN, GENITAL ORIGIN[26]

ICD-9CM # 625.9 Pelvic Pain, Female
            789.09 Pelvic Pain, Male

PERITONEAL IRRITATION

Ruptured ectopic pregnancy.
Ovarian cyst rupture.
Ruptured tuboovarian abscess.
Uterine perforation.

TORSION

Ovarian cyst or tumor.
Pedunculated fibroid.

INTRATUMOR HEMORRHAGE OR INFARCTION

Ovarian cyst.
Solid ovarian tumor.
Uterine leiomyoma.

INFECTION

Endometritis.
Pelvic inflammatory disease.
Trichomonas cervicitis or vaginitis.
Tuboovarian abscess.

PREGNANCY-RELATED

First Trimester
Ectopic pregnancy.
Abortion.
Corpus luteum hematoma.
Late Pregnancy
Placental problems.
Preeclampsia.
Premature labor.

MISCELLANEOUS

Endometriosis.
Foreign objects.
Pelvic adhesions.
Pelvic neoplasm.
Primary dysmenorrhea.

PENILE RASH

ICD-9CM # 782.1

Herpes simplex 2.
Balanitis (candida).
Condyloma acuminatum.
Molluscum contagiosum.
Scabies.
Pediculosis pubis.
Pearly penile papules.
Lichen nitidus.
Fox-Fordyce disease (follicular papules).
Trauma.

PERIANAL PAIN[38]

ICD-9CM # 569.42

Fissure-in-ano
Anal sepsis
- Anal abscess
- Anal fistula
Hemorrhoids
- Internal hemorrhoids
- External hemorrhoids
Pruritus ani
Proctalgia fugax
Chronic perianal pain syndromes
- Coccygodynia
- Descending perineum syndrome
- Levator ani syndrome
- Idiopathic perineal pain

PERICARDIAL EFFUSION

ICD-9CM # 420.90

Pericarditis.
Uremia.
Myxedema.
Neoplasm (leukemia, lymphoma, metastatic).
Hemorrhage (trauma, leakage of thoracic aneurysm).
SLE, rheumatoid disease.
Myocardial infarction.

PERIODIC PARALYSIS, HYPERKALEMIC

ICD-9CM # 344.9

Chronic renal failure.
Renal insufficiency with excessive potassium supplementation.
Potassium-sparing diuretics.
Endocrinopathies (hypoaldosteronism, adrenal insufficiency).

PERIODIC PARALYSIS, HYPOKALEMIC

ICD-9CM # 344.9

Chronic diarrhea (laxative abuse, sprue, villous adenoma).
Potassium-depleting diuretics.
Medications (amphotericin B, corticosteroids).
Chronic licorice ingestion.
Thyrotoxicosis.
Renal tubular acidosis.
Conn's syndrome.
Barter's syndrome.
Barium intoxication.

PERITONEAL CARCINOMATOSIS[14]
ICD-9CM # 197.6

PRIMARY DISORDERS OF THE PERITONEUM: MESOTHELIOMA

Metastatic spread from:
Stomach.
Colon.
Pancreas.
Carcinoid.
Other Intraabdominal Organs
Ovary.
Pseudomyxoma peritonei.
Extraabdominal Primary Tumors
Breast.
Lung.
Hematologic Malignancy
Lymphoma.

PERITONEAL EFFUSION[18]
ICD-9CM # 792.9

TRANSUDATES

Increased hydrostatic pressure or decreased plasma oncotic pressure.
Congestive heart failure.
Hepatic cirrhosis.
Hypoproteinemia.

EXUDATES

Increased capillary permeability or decreased lymphatic resorption.
Infections (TB, spontaneous bacterial peritonitis, secondary bacterial peritonitis).
Neoplasms (hepatoma, metastatic carcinoma, lymphoma, mesothelioma).
Trauma.
Pancreatitis.
Bile peritonitis (e.g., ruptured gallbladder).

CHYLOUS EFFUSION

Damage or obstruction to thoracic duct.
Trauma.
Lymphoma.
Carcinoma.
Tuberculosis.
Parasitic infection.

PERIUMBILICAL SWELLING
ICD-9CM # 789.3

Umbilical hernia.
Lipoma.
Epigastric hernia.
Umbilical granuloma.
Omphalocele.
Gastroschisis.
Caput medusae.

PHOTODERMATOSES[14]
ICD-9CM # 692.72

Polymorphous light eruption.
Chronic actinic dermatitis.
Solar urticaria.
Phototoxicity and photoallergy.
Porphyrias.

PHOTOSENSITIVITY
ICD-9CM # 692.72

Solar urticaria.
Photoallergic reaction.
Phototoxic reaction.
Polymorphous light eruption.
Porphyria cutanea tarda.
SLE.
Drug induced (e.g., tetracyclines).

PIGMENTURIA[2]
ICD-9CM # varies with specific diagnosis

HEMOGLOBINURIA

Hemolysis.

HEMATURIA

Renal causes.
Trauma.

ACUTE INTERMITTENT PORPHYRIA

Bilirubinuria
Food
Beets.
Drugs
Vitamin B_{12}.
Rifampin.
Phenytoin.
Laxatives.

PITUITARY REGION TUMORS[16a]
ICD-9CM # varies with specific diagnosis

PRIMARY TUMORS IN THE SELLAR AND PARASELLAR REGION

Tumor
Pituitary macroadenoma.
Meningioma.
Schwannoma (e.g., of fifth nerve).
Chordoma.
Chondrosarcoma.
Crangiopharyngioma.
Rathke's cleft cyst.
Dermoid.
Epidermoid.
Tuber cinerum hamartoma.
Optic glioma.
Germ cell tumors.

PLEURAL EFFUSIONS
ICD-9CM # 511.9 Pleural Effusion, Unspecified

EXUDATIVE

Neoplasm: bronchogenic carcinoma, breast carcinoma, mesothelioma, lymphoma, ovarian carcinoma, multiple myeloma, leukemia, Meigs' syndrome.
Infections: viral pneumonia, bacterial pneumonia, *Mycoplasma,* TB, fungal and parasitic diseases, extension from subphrenic abscess.
Trauma.

Collagen vascular diseases: SLE, RA, scleroderma, polyarteritis, Wegener's granulomatosis.
Pulmonary infarction.
Pancreatitis.
Postcardiotomy/Dressler's syndrome.
Drug-induced SLE (hydralazine, procainamide).
Postabdominal surgery.
Ruptured esophagus.
Chronic effusion secondary to congestive failure.

TRANSUDATIVE

CHF.
Hepatic cirrhosis.
Nephrotic syndrome.
Hypoproteinemia from any cause.
Meigs' syndrome.

PLEURAL EFFUSIONS, MALIGNANCY-ASSOCIATED
ICD-9CM # 197.2

Lung cancer	(30% to 40%)
Breast cancer	(20% to 25%)
Lymphoma	(10% to 15%)
Leukemia	(5% to 10%)
GI tract	(5%)
GU tract	(5%)
Reproductive	(3%)

PNEUMATOSIS INTESTINALIS IN NEONATE AND OLDER CHILD[16a]
ICD-9CM # varies with specific diagnosis

CAUSES OF PNEUMATOSIS INTESTINALIS IN THE NEONATE AND THE OLDER CHILD

Necrotizing enterocolitis.
Bowel ischemia, inflammation, and obstruction.
Cyanotic congenital heart disease.
Hirschsprung's disease.
Gastroschisis.
Anorectal atresia.
Inflammatory bowel disease.
Lymphoma.
Leukemia.
CMV and rotavirus gastroenteritis.
Colonoscopy.
Caustic ingestion.
Short bowel syndrome.
Congenital immune deficiency states.
Clostridium infection.
Chronic steroid use.
Posthepatic, renal, or bone marrow transplant.
Collagen vascular disease.
Graft-versus-host disease.
AIDS.

PNEUMONIA, RECURRENT
ICD-9CM # 482.9 Bacterial Pneumonia
480.9 Viral Pneumonia
484.1 Fungal Pneumonia
485 Segmental Pneumonia

Mechanical obstruction from neoplasm.

Chronic aspiration (tube feeding, alcoholism, CVA, neuromuscular disorders, seizure disorder, inability to cough).
Bronchiectasis.
Kyphoscoliosis.
COPD, CHF, asthma, silicosis, pulmonary fibrosis, cystic fibrosis.
Pulmonary TB, chronic sinusitis.
Immunosuppression (HIV, corticosteroids, leukemia, chemotherapy, splenectomy).

PNEUMOPERITONEUM, NEONATAL[16a]

ICD-9CM # varies with specific diagnosis

CAUSES OF NEONATAL PNEUMOPERITONEUM

Necrotizing enterocolitis.
Spontaneous perforation of a hollow viscus.
  Stomach.
  Duodenum.
  Ileum.
  Colon.
Malrotation and volvulus.
Distal obstruction.
Perforation of Meckel's diverticulum.
Anterior abdominal wall defects.
  Pentalogy of Cantrell.
  Omphalocele.
  Gastroschisis.
  Cloacal exstrophy.
Stress and peptic ulcers.
Mechanical ventilation (air leak) or resuscitation ("bagging").
Post-laparotomy.
Iatrogenic gastric perforation with an orogastric tube.
Iatrogenic colon perforation.
  Thermometer.
  During an enema.
Indomethacin.
Dexamethasone treatment.

PNEUMOTHORAX, IN CHILDREN[22a]

ICD-9CM # 512   Pneumothorax

SPONTANEOUS

Primary idiopathic—usually resulting from ruptured subpleural blebs.
Secondary blebs.
Congenital lung disease:
- Congenital cystic adenomatoid malformation.
- Bronchogenic cysts.
- Pulmonary hypoplasia.

Conditions associated with increased intrathoracic pressure:
- Asthma.
- Bronchiolitis.
- Air-block syndrome in neonates.
- Cystic fibrosis.
- Airway foreign body.

Infection:
- Pneumatocele.
- Lung abscess.
- Bronchopleural fistula.

Diffuse lung disease:
- Langerhans cell histiocytosis.
- Tuberous sclerosis.
- Marfan syndrome.
- Ehlers-Danlos syndrome.

Metastatic neoplasm—usually osteosarcoma (rare).

TRAUMATIC

Noniatrogenic.
- Penetrating trauma.
- Blunt trauma.
- Loud music (air pressure).

Iatrogenic.
- Thoracotomy.
- Thoracoscopy, thoracentesis.
- Tracheostomy.
- Tube or needle puncture.

Mechanical ventilation.

POLYCYTHEMIA

ICD-9CM # 790.0

Tobacco abuse.
Chronic lung disease.
High altitude.
Sleep apnea.
Right-to-left cardiac shunts.
Erythropoietin administration.
Androgens/anabolic steroids.
Polycystic kidney disease.
Renal cell carcinoma.
Hepatocellular carcinoma.
Polycythemia vera.
Carbon monoxide exposure.
Primary familial and congenital polycythemia.
High-oxygen–affinity hemoglobins.
Uterine leiomyoma, meningioma, pheochromocytoma, parathyroid carcinoma.
Cobalt exposure.

POLYCYTHEMIA, RELATIVE VERSUS ABSOLUTE[20]

ICD-9CM # 790.0

RELATIVE OR SPURIOUS POLYCYTHEMIA

Decreased plasma volume—reduced fluid intake, marked loss of body fluids (diaphoresis, vomiting, diarrhea, "third-spacing").
Gaisböck syndrome.
Overfilling of blood in collection vacuum tubes.

ABSOLUTE POLYCYTHEMIA

Primary Congenital and Familial Polycythemia
Secondary Polycythemia:
Acquired:
  Hypoxia:
- Pulmonary disease.
- Cyanotic congenital heart disease.
- Hypoventilation syndromes—sleep apnea, Pickwickian syndrome.

  High altitude.
  Smokers' polycythemia, carbon monoxide intoxication due to industrial exposure.
Postrenal transplantation erythrocytosis.
Aberrant erythropoietin production:

- Tumors—renal cell carcinoma, Wilms' tumor, hepatic carcinoma, uterine leiomyomata, virilizing ovarian tumors, vascular cerebellar tumors.
- Miscellaneous renal and hepatic disorders—solitary renal cysts, polycystic kidney disease, renal artery stenosis, hydronephrosis, viral hepatitis.

Endocrine disorders—Cushing's syndrome, primary aldosteronism.
Androgen use.
Erythropoietin use.
Congenital:
  Abnormal high-affinity hemoglobin variants.
  Bisphosphoglycerate deficiency.
  Congenital methemoglobinemia.
  Chuvash polycythemia (von Hippel–Lindau mutations).
  Prolyl hydroxylase mutations.
Polycythemia Vera

POLYMYALGIAS[18b]

ICD-9CM # varies with specific diagnosis

DISEASE ENTITIES WITH POLYMYALGIAS

Rheumatoid arthritis.
Rotator cuff syndrome.
Osteoarthritis of shoulder and hip joints.
Fibromyalgia.
Polymyositis/dermatomyositis.
Spondyloarthritis.
Systemic lupus erythematosus.
Vasculitides.
Paraneoplastic myalgias.
Infection-associated myalgias.
Statin therapy.
RS3PE (remitting seronegative symmetric synovitis and pitting edema).
Parkinson's disease.
Hypothyroidism.

POLYNEUROPATHY[40]

ICD-9CM # 357.9

PREDOMINANTLY MOTOR

Guillain-Barré syndrome.
Porphyria.
Diphtheria.
Lead.
Hereditary sensorimotor neuropathy, types I and II.
Paraneoplastic neuropathy.

PREDOMINANTLY SENSORY

Diabetes.
Amyloidosis.
Leprosy.
Lyme disease.
Paraneoplastic neuropathy.
Vitamin B_{12} deficiency.
Hereditary sensory neuropathy, types I-IV.

PREDOMINANTLY AUTONOMIC

Diabetes.
Amyloidosis.
Alcoholic neuropathy.
Familial dysautonomias.

MIXED SENSORIMOTOR

Systemic diseases: renal failure, hypothyroidism, acromegaly, RA, periarteritis nodosa, SLE, multiple myeloma, macroglobulinemia, remote effect of malignancy.

Medications: isoniazid, nitrofurantoin, ethambutol, chloramphenicol, chloroquine, vincristine, vinblastine, dapsone, disulfiram, diphenylhydantoin, cisplatin, 1-tryptophan.

Environmental toxins: N-hexane, methyl N-butyl ketone, acrylamide, carbon disulfide, carbon monoxide, hexachlorophene, organophosphates.

Deficiency disorders: malabsorption, alcoholism, vitamin B_1 deficiency, Refsum's disease, metachromatic leukodystrophy.

POLYNEUROPATHY, DEMYELINATING[2]

ICD-9CM # varies with specific diagnosis

Guillain-Barré syndrome.
 Acute inflammatory demyelinating polyradiculoneuropathy (AIDP).
 Acute motor axonal neuropathy (AMAN).
 Acute motor and sensory axonal neuropathy (AMSAN).
 Miller Fisher syndrome.
Chronic inflammatory demyelinating polyradiculoplexo-neuropathy.
Malignancy.
HIV.
Hepatitis B.
Buckthorn.
Diphtheria.

POLYNEUROPATHY, DISTAL SENSORIMOTOR[2]

ICD-9CM # varies with specific diagnosis

Diabetes mellitus.
Alcoholism.
Neoplastic or paraneoplastic.
Hereditary motor and sensory neuropathies (Charcot-Marie-Tooth).
Cryptogenic sensorimotor polyneuropathies (CSPN).
HIV.
Toxins:
 Organic or industrial agents:
 • Acrylamide.
 • Allyl chloride.
 • Carbon disulfide.
 • Ethylene oxide.
 • Hexacarbons.
 • Methyl bromide.
 • Organophosphate-induced delayed polyneuropathy (OPIDP).
 • Polychlorinated biphenyls (PCBs).
 • Trichloroethylene.
 • Vacor.
 Metals:
 • Arsenic.
 • Gold.
 • Mercury (inorganic).
 • Thallium.
 Therapeutic agents:
 • Amiodarone.

• Antiretrovirals.
• Dapsone.
• Disulfiram.
• Isoniazid.
• Metronidazole.
• Nitrofurantoin.
• Paclitaxel (Taxol).
• Phenytoin.
• Statins (HMG-CoA reductase inhibitors).
• Thalidomide.
• Vinca alkaloids (vincristine, vinblastine).
Nutritional:
• Beriberi (thiamine or vitamin B_1).
• Pellagra (niacin, B vitamins).
• Pernicious anemia (vitamin B_{12}).
• Pyridoxine deficiency (vitamin B_6).
End-organ dysfunction:
• Acromegaly.
• Chronic pulmonary disease.
• Hypothyroidism.
• Renal failure (uremic neuropathy).
Paraproteinemias:
• Amyloidosis.
• Monoclonal gammopathy of unknown significance (MGUS).
• Multiple myeloma.
• Waldenström's macroglobulinemia.
Porphyria.

HMG-CoA, Hydroxymethylglutaryl coenzyme A.

POLYNEUROPATHY, DRUG-INDUCED[40]

ICD-9CM # 357.6

DRUGS IN ONCOLOGY

Vincristine.
Procarbazine.
Cisplatin.
Misonidazole.
Metronidazole (Flagyl).
Taxol.

DRUGS IN INFECTIOUS DISEASES

Isoniazid.
Nitrofurantoin.
Dapsone.
ddC (dideoxycytidine).
ddI (dideoxyinosine).

DRUGS IN CARDIOLOGY

Hydralazine.
Perhexiline maleate.
Procainamide.
Disopyramide.

DRUGS IN RHEUMATOLOGY

Gold salts.
Chloroquine.

DRUGS IN NEUROLOGY AND PSYCHIATRY

Diphenylhydantoin.
Glutethimide.
Methaqualone.

MISCELLANEOUS

Disulfiram (Antabuse).
Vitamin: pyridoxine (megadoses).

POLYNEUROPATHY, SYMMETRIC[40]

ICD-9CM # 357.9

ACQUIRED NEUROPATHIES

Toxic:
 Drugs.
 Industrial toxins.
 Heavy metals.
 Abused substances.
Metabolic/endocrine:
 Diabetes.
 Chronic renal failure.
 Hypothyroidism.
 Polyneuropathy of critical illness.
Nutritional deficiency:
 Vitamin B_{12} deficiency.
 Alcoholism.
 Vitamin E deficiency.
Paraneoplastic:
 Carcinoma.
 Lymphoma.
Plasma cell dyscrasia:
 Myeloma, typical, atypical, and solitary forms.
 Primary systemic amyloidosis.
Idiopathic chronic inflammatory demyelinating polyneuropathies.
Polyneuropathies associated with peripheral nerve autoantibodies.
Acquired immunodeficiency syndrome.

INHERITED NEUROPATHIES

Neuropathies with Biochemical Markers
Refsum's disease.
Bassen-Kornzweig disease.
Tangier disease.
Metachromatic leukodystrophy.
Krabbe's disease.
Adrenomyeloneuropathy.
Fabry's disease.
Neuropathies without Biochemical Markers or Systemic Involvement
Hereditary motor neuropathy.
Hereditary sensory neuropathy.
Hereditary sensorimotor neuropathy.

POLYURIA

ICD-9CM # 788.42

DM.
Diabetes insipidus.
Primary polydipsia (compulsive water drinking).
Hypercalcemia.
Hypokalemia.
Postobstructive uropathy.
Diuretic phase of renal failure.
Drugs: diuretics, caffeine, alcohol, lithium.
Sickle cell trait or disease, chronic pyelonephritis (failure to concentrate urine).
Anxiety, cold weather.

POPLITEAL SWELLING

ICD-9CM # 459.2   Venous Obstruction
747.4   Vein Anomaly, Lower Limb Vessel
442.3   Artery Aneurysm
904.41   Artery Injury
447.8   Entrapment Syndrome
727.51   Baker's Cyst
451.2   Phlebitis, Lower Extremity
727.67   Rupture of Achilles Tendon

Phlebitis (superficial).
Lymphadenitis.
Trauma: fractured tibia or fibula, contusion, traumatic neuroma.
DVT.
Ruptured varicose vein.
Baker's cyst.
Popliteal abscess.
Osteomyelitis.
Ruptured tendon.
Aneurysm of popliteal artery.
Neoplasm: lipoma, osteogenic sarcoma, neurofibroma, fibrosarcoma.

PORTAL HYPERTENSION[1]

ICD-9CM # 572.3

INCREASED RESISTANCE TO FLOW

Presinusoidal
Portal or splenic vein occlusion (thrombosis, tumor).
Schistosomiasis.
Congenital hepatic fibrosis.
Sarcoidosis.
Sinusoidal
Cirrhosis (all causes).
Alcoholic hepatitis.
Postsinusoidal
Venoocclusive disease.
Budd-Chiari syndrome.
Constrictive pericarditis.

INCREASED PORTAL BLOOD FLOW

Splenomegaly not caused by liver disease.
Arterioportal fistula.

POSTMENOPAUSAL BLEEDING

ICD-9CM # 627.1

Hormone replacement therapy.
Neoplasm (uterine, ovarian, cervical, vaginal, vulvar).
Atrophic vaginitis.
Vaginal infection.
Polyp.
Extragenital (GI, urinary).
Tamoxifen.
Trauma.

POSTURAL HYPOTENSION, NONNEUROLOGIC CAUSES

ICD-9CM # 458.0

Diuretics and hypertensive agents.

GI hemorrhage.
Alcohol.
Excessive heat.
Rapid volume loss from diarrhea, vomiting.
Hemodialysis.
Extensive burns.
Pyrexia.
Aortic stenosis (impaired output).
Constrictive pericarditis, atrial myxoma (impaired cardiac filling).
Adrenal insufficiency.
Diabetes insipidus.
Vasodilatory agents (e.g., nitrates).

PREMATURE GRAYING, SCALP HAIR

ICD-9CM # varies with specific disorder

Chemical exposure (e.g., phenol/catechol derivatives, sulfhydryls, arsenic).
Physical agents (e.g., ionizing radiation, lasers).
Hyperthyroidism.
Vitamin B_{12} deficiency.
Down's syndrome.
Chronic and severe protein deficiency.
Vitiligo.
Idiopathic.
Myotonic dystrophy.
Ataxia-telangiectasia.
Progeria.
Werner's syndrome.

PREMATURE VENTRICULAR CONTRACTIONS AND VENTRICULAR TACHYCARDIA[2]

ICD-9CM # 427.6

CAUSES OF PREMATURE VENTRICULAR CONTRACTIONS AND VENTRICULAR TACHYCARDIA

Acute or previous myocardial infarction/ischemia.
Hypokalemia.
Hypoxemia.
Ischemic heart disease.
Valvular disease.
Catecholamine excess.*
Other drug intoxications (especially cyclic antidepressants).
Idiopathic causes.†
Digitalis toxicity.
Hypomagnesemia.
Hypercapnia.
Class I antidysrhythmic agents.
Ethanol.
Myocardial contusion.
Cardiomyopathy.
Acidosis.
Alkalosis.
Methylxanthine toxicity.

*Relative increase in sympathetic tone from drugs (direct or indirect) or conditions that augment catecholamine release or decrease parasympathetic tone.

†Isolated premature ventricular contractions (PVCs) can occur in up to 50% of young subjects without obvious cardiac or noncardiac disease; however, multiform and repetitive PVCs and ventricular tachycardia are rarely seen in this population.

PROPTOSIS[30]

ICD-9CM # 376.30

Thyrotoxicosis.
Orbital pseudotumor.
Optic nerve tumor.
Cavernous sinus AV fistula, cavernous sinus thrombosis.
Cellulitis.
Metastatic tumor to orbit.

PROPTOSIS AND PALATAL NECROTIC ULCERS

ICD-9CM # 528.9   Ulcer of Palate
376.30   Proptosis

Cavernous sinus thrombosis.
Bacterial orbital cellulitis.
Metastatic neoplasm.
Rhinocerebral mucormycosis.
Ecthyma gangrenosum.
CNS aspergillosis.

PROTEIN-LOSING ENTEROPATHY, PEDIATRIC AGE

ICD-9CM # 579.8

CAUSES OF PROTEIN-LOSING ENTEROPATHY

Mucosal inflammation:
Infection:
- Cytomegalovirus.
- Bacterial overgrowth.
- Invasive bacterial infection.
Gastric inflammation:
- Ménétrier disease.
- Eosinophilic gastroenteropathy.
Intestinal inflammation:
- Celiac disease.
- Crohn disease.
Eosinophilic gastroenteropathy:
- Tropical sprue.
- Radiation enteritis.
Primary intestinal lymphangiectasia.
Secondary intestinal lymphangiectasia:
Constrictive pericarditis.
Congestive heart failure.
Post–Fontan procedure.
Malrotation.
Lymphoma.
Sarcoidosis.
Radiation therapy.
Colonic inflammation:
- Inflammatory bowel diseases.
- Necrotizing enterocolitis.
Congenital disorders of glycosylation.

PROTEINURIA

ICD-9CM # 791.0

Nephrotic syndrome as a result of primary renal diseases.
Malignant hypertension.
Malignancies: multiple myeloma, leukemias, Hodgkin's disease.
CHF.

Differential Diagnosis

II

DM.
SLE, RA.
Sickle cell disease.
Goodpasture's syndrome.
Malaria.
Amyloidosis, sarcoidosis.
Tubular lesions: cystinosis.
Functional (after heavy exercise).
Pyelonephritis.
Pregnancy.
Constrictive pericarditis.
Renal vein thrombosis.
Toxic nephropathies: heavy metals, drugs.
Radiation nephritis.
Orthostatic (postural) proteinuria.
Benign proteinuria: fever, heat, or cold exposure.

PRURITUS

ICD-9CM # 698.9 Pruritus NOS
698.1 Pruritus, Genital Organs

Dry skin.
Drug-induced eruption, fiberglass exposure.
Scabies.
Skin diseases.
Myeloproliferative disorders: mycosis fungoides, Hodgkin's lymphoma, multiple myeloma, polycythemia vera.
Cholestatic liver disease.
Endocrine disorders: DM, thyroid disease, carcinoid, pregnancy.
Carcinoma: breast, lung, gastric.
Chronic renal failure.
Iron deficiency.
AIDS.
Neurosis.
Sjögren's syndrome.

PRURITUS ANI[26]

ICD-9CM # 697.0

FECAL IRRITATION

Poor hygiene.
Anorectal conditions (fissure, fistula, hemorrhoids, skin tags, perianal clefts).
Spicy foods, citrus foods, caffeine, colchicine, quinidine.

CONTACT DERMATITIS

Anesthetic agents, topical corticosteroids, perfumed soap.

DERMATOLOGIC DISORDERS

Psoriasis, seborrhea, lichen simplex or sclerosus.

SYSTEMIC DISORDERS

Chronic renal failure, myxedema, DM, thyrotoxicosis, polycythemia vera, Hodgkin's disease.

SEXUALLY TRANSMITTED DISEASES

Syphilis, herpes simplex virus, human papillomavirus.

OTHER INFECTIOUS AGENTS

Pinworms.
Scabies.
Bacterial infection, viral infection.

PRURITUS VULVAE[34a]

ICD-9CM # 698.1

CAUSES OF PRURITUS VULVAE

Diseases Special to Vulval Skin
Lichen sclerosus et atrophicus.
Leukoplakia.
Carcinoma.
Skin Disease
Psoriasis.
Atopic dermatitis.
Irritant and allergic contact dermatitis (especially medicaments).
Infection
Candidiasis.
Trichomonas.
Infestation
Pediculosis.
Psychogenic
Anxiety.
Depression.
Unknown

PSEUDOCYANOSIS, ETIOLOGY

ICD-9CM # varies with etiology

Medications: amiodarone, minocycline, chlorpromazine.
Heavy metals:
  Gold (systemic absorption).
  Silver (systemic absorption).
Local contact with color dyes, gold, silver.

PSEUDOHERMAPHRODITISM, FEMALE

ICD-9CM # 255.2 Adrenal
752.7 Without Adrenocortical Disorder

Congenital adrenal hyperplasia.
Maternal use of testosterone or related steroids.
Virilizing ovarian or adrenal tumor.
Virilizing luteoma of pregnancy.
Disturbances in differentiation of urogenital structures, non-androgen related.
Maternal virilizing adrenal hyperplasia.
Fetal P450 aromatase deficiency.

PSEUDOHERMAPHRODITISM, MALE

ICD-9CM # 255.2 Adrenal
752.7 Without Adrenocortical Disorder

Maternal ingestion of progestogens.
End-organ resistance to androgenic hormones.
5-Alpha-reductase-2 deficiency.
XY gonadal dysgenesis.
Testicular regression syndrome.
Defects in testosterone metabolism by peripheral tissues.
Testosterone biosynthesis defects.

PSEUDOINFARCTION[22]

ICD-9CM # code varies with specific diagnosis

Cardiac tumors, primary and secondary.

Cardiomyopathy (particularly hypertrophic and dilated).
Chagas' disease.
Chest deformity.
COPD (particularly emphysema).
HIV infection.
Hyperkalemia.
Left anterior fascicular block.
Left bundle branch block.
Left ventricular hypertrophy.
Myocarditis and pericarditis.
Normal variant.
Pneumothorax.
Poor R wave progression, rotational changes, and lead placement.
Pulmonary embolism.
Trauma to chest (nonpenetrating).
Wolff-Parkinson-White syndrome.
Rare causes: pancreatitis, amyloidosis, sarcoidosis, scleroderma.

PSYCHOSIS[28]

ICD-9CM # 298.9 Psychosis NOS
298.90 Psychosis, Affective
291.0 Psychosis, Alcoholic
290.41 Psychosis, Acute Arteriosclerotic

PRIMARY

Schizophrenia related.*
Major depression.
Dementia.
Bipolar disorder.

SECONDARY

Drug use.[†]
Drug withdrawal.[‡]
Drug toxicity.[§]
Charles Bonnet syndrome.
Infections (pneumonia).
Electrolyte imbalance.
Syphilis.
Congestive heart failure.
Parkinson's disease.
Trauma to temporal lobe.
Postpartum psychosis.
Hypothyroidism/hyperthyroidism.
Hypomagnesemia.
Epilepsy.
Meningitis.
Encephalitis.
Brain abscess.
Herpes encephalopathy.
Hypoxia.
Hypercarbia.
Hypoglycemia.
Thiamine deficiency.
Postoperative states.

---

*Includes schizophrenia, schizophreniform disorder, brief reactive psychosis.

†Includes hypnotics, glucocorticoids, marijuana, phencyclidine, atropine, dopaminergic agents (e.g., amantadine, bromocriptine, L-dopa), immunosuppressants.

‡Includes alcohol, barbiturates, benzodiazepines.

§Includes digitalis, theophylline, cimetidine, anticholinergics, glucocorticoids, catecholaminergic agents.

PTOSIS

ICD-9CM # 374.30 Ptosis NOS
743.61 Congenital
374.33 Mechanical
374.32 Myogenic
374.31 Paralytic

Third nerve palsy.
Myasthenia gravis.
Horner's syndrome.
Senile ptosis.

PUBERTY, DELAYED[27]

ICD-9CM # 259.0

NORMAL OR LOW SERUM GONADOTROPIN LEVELS

Constitutional delay in growth and development.
Hypothalamic and/or pituitary disorders:
Isolated deficiency of growth hormone.
Isolated deficiency of Gn-RH.
Isolated deficiency of LH and/or FSH.
Multiple anterior pituitary hormone deficiencies.
Associated with congenital anomalies: Kallmann's syndrome; Prader-Willi syndrome; Laurence-Moon-Biedl syndrome; Friedreich's ataxia.
Trauma.
Postinfection.
Hyperprolactinemia.
Postirradiation.
Infiltrative disease (histiocytosis).
Tumor.
Autoimmune hypophysitis.
Idiopathic.
Functional:
Chronic endocrinologic or systemic disorders.
Emotional disorders.
Drugs: cannabis.

INCREASED SERUM GONADOTROPIN LEVELS

Gonadal abnormalities:
Congenital:
• Gonadal dysgenesis.
• Klinefelter's syndrome.
• Bilateral anorchism.
• Resistant ovary syndrome.
• Myotonic dystrophy in males.
• 17-Hydroxylase deficiency in females.
• Galactosemia.
Acquired:
• Bilateral gonadal failure resulting from trauma or infection or after surgery, irradiation, or chemotherapy.
• Oophoritis: isolated or with other autoimmune disorders.
Uterine or vaginal disorders:
Absence of uterus and/or vagina.
Testicular feminization: complete or incomplete androgen insensitivity.

PUBERTY, PRECOCIOUS

ICD-9CM # 255.2

Idiopathic.
Congenital virilizing adrenal hyperplasia.

Hypothalamic tumors.
Head trauma.
Hydrocephalus.
Degenerative CNS disease.
Arachnoid cyst.
Sex chromosome abnormalities (e.g., 47, XXY, 48, XXXY).
Perinatal asphyxia.
CNS infection (e.g., meningitis, encephalitis).

PULMONARY CRACKLES

ICD-9CM # code not available

Pneumonia.
Left ventricular failure.
Asbestosis, silicosis, interstitial lung disease.
Chronic bronchitis.
Alveolitis (allergic, fibrosing).
Neoplasm.

PULMONARY CYSTS ON X-RAY[16a]

ICD-9CM # 793.1

CAUSES OF CYSTS IN THE LUNG ON CHEST RADIOGRAPH

Cystic fibrosis.
Cystic bronchiectasis.
Bronchopulmonary dysplasia (neonate and older).
Tuberculosis (apical thick walled).
Pulmonary abscess (thick wall, fluid level).
Empyema.
Streptococcal pneumatocele (thin wall, postinfective).
Cavitating pneumonia.
Mycetoma (apical cyst with contents).
Cystic congenital adenomatoid malformation (basal cysts of varying size).
Diaphragmatic hernia (cysts of similar size).
Hiatal hernia (posterior).
Morgagni hernia (midline anterior).
Bronchopulmonary sequestration (basal).
Congenital lobar emphysema.
Hydatid disease (in endemic areas).
Kerosene inhalation (pneumatocele).
Histiocytosis and other causes of interstitial disease.

PULMONARY EDEMA, NONCARDIOGENIC[16a]

ICD-9CM # 518.4

CAUSES OF NONCARDIOGENIC PULMONARY EDEMA

Adult respiratory distress syndrome.
Drowning.
Asphyxia.
Upper airway obstruction (usually with cardiomegaly).
High altitude.
Increased intracranial pressure.
Postictal.
Noxious gases:
Smoke.
Nitrous dioxide (silo filler's disease).
Sulfur dioxide.

Nitrogen mustard.
Drugs:
Asprin.
Diazepam, chlordiazepoxide, barbiturates.
Narcotics (heroin, methadone, morphine).
Beta-adrenergic drugs (terbutaline).
Contrast media.
Colchicine.
Fluorescein.
Hydrochlorothiazide.
Nitrofurantoin.
Propoxyphene.
Poisons:
Parathion.
Transfusion reactions.
Renal failure: transplantation.
Bone marrow transplantation.
Fat embolism.
Pancreatitis.

PULMONARY HEMORRHAGE, PEDIATRIC AGE

ICD-9CM # 770.3

CAUSES OF PULMONARY HEMORRHAGE (HEMOPTYSIS)

Focal Hemorrhage
Bronchitis and bronchiectasis (especially cystic fibrosis related).
Infection (acute or chronic), pneumonia, abscess.
Tuberculosis.
Trauma.
Pulmonary arteriovenous malformation.
Foreign body (chronic).
Neoplasm including hemangioma.
Pulmonary embolus with or without infarction.
Bronchogenic cysts.
Diffuse Hemorrhage
Idiopathic of infancy.
Congenital heart disease (including pulmonary hypertension, venoocclusive disease, congestive heart failure).
Prematurity.
Cow's milk hyperreactivity (Heiner syndrome).
Goodpasture syndrome.
Collagen vascular diseases (systemic lupus erythematosus, rheumatoid arthritis).
Henoch-Schönlein purpura and vasculitic disorders.
Granulomatous disease (Wegener granulomatosis).
Celiac disease.
Coagulopathy (congenital or acquired).
Malignancy.
Immunodeficiency.
Exogenous toxins.
Hyperammonemia.
Pulmonary hypertension.
Pulmonary alveolar hemosiderosis.
Tuberous sclerosis.
Lymphangiomyomatosis or lymphangioleiomyomatosis.
Physical injury or abuse.

Differential Diagnosis

II

PULMONARY HEMORRHAGIC SYNDROMES, DIFFUSE[16a]

ICD-9CM # 770.3

CLASSIFICATION OF DIFFUSE PULMONARY HEMORRHAGE SYNDROMES

Non-immunocompromised patients

Antibasement membrane antibody disease/ Goodpasture's syndrome.

Diseases of presumed immune etiology, with or without nephropathy:
Systemic lupus erythematosus.
Rheumatoid arthritis.
Systemic sclerosis.
Systemic necrotizing vasculitis.
Wegener's granulomatosis.
Microscopic polyarteritis.

Diseases with no known immune etiology:
Idiopathic pulmonary hemosiderosis.
Rapidly progressive glomerulonephritis without immune complexes.
Fibrillary glomerulonephritis.
Drug-induced (anticoagulants, trimellitic anhydride, cocaine, lymphangiography).
Valvular heart disease.
Disseminated intravascular coagulation.
Acute lung injury.
Tumors.

Immunocompromised Patients

Blood dyscrasias.
Infection.
Tumors.

PULMONARY INFILTRATES, IMMUNOCOMPROMISED HOST[39]

ICD-9CM # 518.3

CAUSES OF PULMONARY INFILTRATES IN THE IMMUNOCOMPROMISED HOST

Infections:
Bacteria:
- Gram-positive cocci, especially *Staphylococcus.*
- Gram-negative bacilli.
- *Mycobacterium tuberculosis.*
- Nontuberculous mycobacteria.
- *Nocardia.*

Viruses:
- Cytomegalovirus.
- Herpesvirus.

Fungi:
- *Aspergillus.*
- *Cryptococcus.*
- *Candida.*
- *Mucor.*
- *Pneumocystis jiroveci.*

Protozoa:
- *Toxoplasma gondii* (rare).

Pulmonary effects of therapy:
Chemotherapeutic agents.
Radiation therapy.
Pulmonary hemorrhage.
Congestive heart failure.

Disseminated malignancy.
Nonspecified interstitial pneumonitis (no defined etiology).

PULMONARY LESIONS

ICD-9CM # 518.3   Pulmonary Infiltrate
518.89 Pulmonary Nodule
508.9   Pulmonary Disorder Due to Unspecified External Agent
861.20 Pulmonary Injury NOS

TB.
Legionella pneumonia.
Mycoplasma pneumonia.
Viral pneumonia.
Pneumocystis carinii.
Hypersensitivity pneumonitis.
Aspiration pneumonia.
Fungal disease (aspergillosis, histoplasmosis).
ARDS associated with pneumonia.
Psittacosis.
Sarcoidosis.
Septic emboli.
Metastatic cancer.
Multiple pulmonary emboli.
Rheumatoid nodules.

PULMONARY MASS, SOLITARY, CAUSES[16a]

ICD-9CM # 793.1

CAUSES OF A SOLITARY PULMONARY MASS

Bronchial carcinoma.
Bronchial carcinoid.
Granuloma.
Hamartoma.
Metastasis.
Chronic pneumonia or abscess.
Hydatid cyst.
Pulmonary hematoma.
Bronchocele.
Fungus ball.
Massive fibrosis in coal workers.
Bronchogenic cyst.
Sequestration.
Arteriovenous malformation.
Pulmonary infarct.
Round atelectasis.

PULMONARY MASS, SOLITARY, MIMICS[16a]

ICD-9CM # varies with specific diagnosis

SIMULANTS OF A SOLITARY PULMONARY MASS

Extrathoracic artifacts.
Cutaneous masses.
Bony lesions.
Pleural tumors or plaques.
Encysted pleural fluid.
Pulmonary vessels.

PULMONARY NODULE, SOLITARY

ICD-9CM # 518.89

Bronchogenic carcinoma.
Granuloma from histoplasmosis.
TB granuloma.
Granuloma from coccidioidomycosis.
Metastatic carcinoma.
Bronchial adenoma.
Bronchogenic cyst.
Hamartoma.
AV malformation.
Other: fibroma, intrapulmonary lymph node, sclerosing hemangioma, bronchopulmonary sequestration.

PULMONARY–RENAL SYNDROMES, CAUSES[12a]

ICD-9CM # varies with specific diagnosis

Systemic vasculitis	Anti-GBM disease (Goodpasture's) ANCA associated
	• Wegener's granulomatosis
	• Microscopic polyarteritis
	• Churg-Strauss syndrome
	• Drugs (penicillamine, hydralazine, propylthiouracil)
	Immune complex disease
	• Lupus erythematosus
	• Henoch-Schönlein purpura
	• Mixed cryoglobulinemia
	• Rheumatoid vasculitis
Infection	Severe bacterial pneumonia; postinfectious glomerulonephritis; *Legionella;* hantavirus; opportunistic infection in immunocompromised patients; infective endocarditis
Pulmonary edema and AKI	Volume overload; severe left ventricular failure
Multiorgan failure	Acute respiratory distress syndrome and AKI
Other	Paraquat poisoning; renal vein or IVC thrombosis with pulmonary emboli

AKI, Acute kidney injury; *ANCA,* anti-neutrophil cytoplasmic antibody; *GBM,* glomerular basement membrane; *IVC,* inferior vena cava.

PULSELESS ELECTRICAL ACTIVITY

ICD-9CM # 427.5

Hypovolemia.
Hypoxia.
Hyperkalemia.
Acidosis.
Cardiac tamponade.
Tension pneumothorax.
Pulmonary embolus.
Drug overdose.
Hypothermia.

PUPILLARY DILATATION, POOR RESPONSE TO DARKNESS

ICD-9CM # varies with specific disorder

Drugs (narcotics, general anesthetics, cholinergics).
Acute trauma (spasm from prostaglandin release).
Inflammation, infection (interruption of inhibitory fibers to the Edinger-Westphal nucleus).
Old age (loss of inhibition at midbrain from reticular activating formation).
Horner's syndrome (sympathetic neuron interruption).
Adie's syndrome tonic pupil.
Lymphoma.
Congenital miosis.

PURPURA

ICD-9CM # 287.2 Purpura NOS
287.0 Autoimmune
287.0 Henoch-Schönlein
287.3 Idiopathic
Thrombocytopenic
446.6 Thrombocytopenic

THROMBOTIC

Trauma.
Septic emboli, atheromatous emboli.
DIC.
Thrombocytopenia.
Meningococcemia.
Rocky Mountain spotted fever.
Hemolytic-uremic syndrome.
Viral infection: echo, coxsackie.
Scurvy.
Other: left atrial myxoma, cryoglobulinemia, vasculitis, hyperglobulinemic purpura.

PURPURA, NONPALPABLE[20]

ICD-9CM # 287.2

INCREASED TRANSMURAL PRESSURE GRADIENT

Acute (Valsalva, coughing, vomiting, high altitude, weight lifting).
Chronic—Venous stasis.

DECREASED MECHANICAL INTEGRITY OF MICROCIRCULATION AND SUPPORTING TISSUES

Age related (infancy and actinic purpura).
Glucocorticoid excess—Cushing syndrome and glucocorticoid therapy.
Vitamin C deficiency (scurvy).
Abnormal connective tissue—Ehlers-Danlos syndrome.
Amyloid infiltration of blood vessels.
Colloid milium.
Hormonal—Female easy bruising syndrome (purpura simplex).
Lorenzo's oil.
MELAS syndrome.

TRAUMA TO BLOOD VESSELS

Physical:
- Injuries.
- Child abuse.
- Factitial purpura.

Ultraviolet purpura:
- Purpuric sunburn.
- Solar purpura.

Infectious:
- Bacterial.
- Rickettsial.
- Fungal.
- Viral.
- Parasitic.

Embolic:
- Infectious organisms.
- Atheroemboli (cholesterol crystal emboli).
- Fat emboli.

Allergic and/or inflammatory:
- Serum sickness.
- Pigmented purpuric eruptions.
- Pyoderma gangrenosum.
- Contact dermatitis.
- Familial Mediterranean fever.

Neoplastic.
Metabolic:
- Erythropoietic porphyria.
- Calciphylaxis.

Immunoglobulin related (hyperglobulinemic purpura of Waldenström and light-chain vasculitis).
Drug related.
Thrombotic:
- Disseminated intravascular coagulation.
- Warfarin (Coumadin)-induced skin necrosis.
- Protein C or protein S deficiency, factor V Leiden, prothrombin G20201A.
- Purpura fulminans.
- Paroxysmal nocturnal hemoglobinuria.
- Antiphospholipid antibody syndrome.
- Hemangioma with thrombocytopenia and consumptive coagulopathy (Kasabach-Merritt syndrome).

UNKNOWN CAUSE— PSYCHOGENIC PURPURA

PURPURA, NONPURPURIC DISORDERS SIMULATING PURPURA[1]

ICD-9CM # varies with specific diagnosis

Disorders with telangiectasias:
Cherry angiomas.
Hereditary hemorrhagic telangiectasia.
Chronic actinic telangiectasia.
Scleroderma.
CREST syndrome.
Ataxia-telangiectasia.
Chronic liver disease.
Pregnancy-related telangiectasia.
Kaposi sarcoma and other vascular sarcomas.
Fabry disease.
Neonatal extramedullary hematopoiesis.
Angioma serpiginosum.

PURPURA, PALPABLE[20]

ICD-9CM # 287.2

Cutaneous vasculitis:
Systemic vasculitides.
Paraneoplastic vasculitis.
Henoch-Schönlein purpura.
Acute hemorrhagic edema of infancy.
Livedoid vasculitis.
Idiopathic.
Urticarial.
Cryoglobulinemia.
Cryofibrinogenemia.
Primary cutaneous diseases.

QT INTERVAL PROLONGATION[22]

ICD-9CM # 794.31

Drugs:
Class I antiarrhythmics (e.g., disopyramide, procainamide, quinidine).
Class III antiarrhythmics.
Tricyclic antidepressants.
Phenothiazines.
Astemizole.
Terfenadine.
Adenosine.
Antibiotics (e.g., erythromycin and other macrolides).
Antifungal agents.
Pentamidine, chloroquine.
Ischemic heart disease.
Cerebrovascular disease.
Rheumatic fever.
Myocarditis.
Mitral valve prolapse.
Electrolyte abnormalities.
Hypocalcemia.
Hypothyroidism.
Liquid protein diets.
Organophosphate insecticides.
Congenital prolonged QT syndrome.

RECTAL MASS, PALPABLE[38]

ICD-9CM # varies with specific diagnosis

Rectal carcinoma.
Rectal polyp.
Hypertrophied anal papilla.
Diverticular phlegmon (prolapsing into the pouch of Douglas).
Sigmoid colon carcinoma (prolapsing into the pouch of Douglas).
Metastatic deposits at the pelvic reflection (Blumer's shelf).
Primary pelvic malignancy (uterine, ovarian, prostatic, or cervical).
Mesorectal lymph nodes.
Endometriosis.
Solitary rectal ulcer syndrome.
Foreign body.
Feces.
Presacral cyst.
Amebic granuloma.
Vaginal tampon and even the pubic bone may be mistaken for a rectal mass.

Differential Diagnosis

II

RECTAL PAIN
ICD-9CM # 569.42

Anal fissure.
Thrombosed hemorrhoid.
Anorectal abscess.
Foreign bodies.
Fecal impaction.
Endometriosis.
Neoplasms (primary or metastatic).
Pelvic inflammatory disease.
Inflammation of sacral nerves.
Compression of sacral nerves.
Prostatitis.
Other: proctalgia fugax, uterine abnormalities, myopathies, coccygodynia.

RED BLOOD CELL APLASIA, ACQUIRED, ETIOLOGY
ICD-9CM # 284.0

Idiopathic (>50% of cases).
Medications (most frequent with phenytoin).
Non-Hodgkin's lymphoma.
Viral infections (parvovirus B19, EB virus, mumps, hepatitis).
Myelodysplastic syndromes.
Thymoma.
Autoimmune diseases.
Allogenic bone marrow transplant from ABO incompatible donor.
Pregnancy.

RED EYE
ICD-9CM # 379.93

Infectious conjunctivitis (bacterial, viral).
Allergic conjunctivitis.
Acute glaucoma.
Keratitis (bacterial, viral).
Iritis.
Trauma.

RED HOT JOINT
ICD-9CM # varies with specific disorder

Trauma.
Gout.
Infection (septic joint).
Pseudogout (calcium pyrophosphate dehydrate crystal deposition).
Psoriatic arthropathy.
Reactive arthritis.
Palindromic rheumatism.

RED URINE
ICD-9CM # 788.69

Hematuria.
Porphyrins.
Hemoglobinuria.
Myoglobinuria.
Medications (phenazopyridine, aminosalicylic acid, deferoxamine, phenazopyridine, phenolphthalein, NSAIDs, rifampin, phenytoin, methyldopa, doxorubicin, phenacetin).
Foods (beets, berries, maize).
Urate crystalluria.

RENAL ALLOGRAFT DYSFUNCTION[14a]
ICD-9CM # 593.9

IMMEDIATE/DELAYED GRAFT FUNCTION (1-3 DAYS)
Acute tubular necrosis.
Hyperacute humoral rejection.
Urinary leak or obstruction.
Renal artery or vein thrombosis.
Recurrence of disease (e.g., focal segmental glomerulosclerosis).

EARLY POSTTRANSPLANTATION PERIOD (FIRST MONTH)
Acute cellular rejection.
Acute humoral rejection.
Calcineurin inhibitor toxicity.
Urinary tract obstruction.
Volume depletion.
Recurrence of disease.

LATE ACUTE DYSFUNCTION
Acute rejection.
Cyclosporine or tacrolimus toxicity.
Recurrence of primary disease.
Tubulointerstitial nephritis, drug-induced.
Renal artery stenosis.
Infection (bacterial urinary tract infection [UTI], cytomegalovirus, BK virus).
Hemodynamic (volume; use of angiotensin-converting enzyme inhibitor, angiotensin II receptor blocker).

CHRONIC DYSFUNCTION
Chronic rejection.
Cyclosporine or tacrolimus toxicity.
Recurrent renal disease.
De novo renal disease.
Urinary tract obstruction.
Bacterial UTI.
Hypertensive nephrosclerosis.

RENAL ARTERY OCCLUSION, CAUSES
ICD-9CM # 593.81

Atrial fibrillation.
Angiography or stent placement.
Abdominal aortic surgery.
Trauma.
Renal artery aneurysm/dissection.
Vasculitis.
Thrombosis in patient with fibromuscular dysplasia.
Atherosclerosis.
Septic embolism.
Mural thrombus thromboembolism.
Atrial myxoma thromboembolism.
Mitral stenosis thromboembolism.
Prosthetic valve thromboembolism.
Renal cell carcinoma.

RENAL CYSTIC DISORDERS
ICD-9CM # varies with specific disorder

Simple cysts.
Acquired cystic kidney disease.

Autosomal dominant polycystic kidney disease.
Autosomal recessive polycystic kidney disease.
Medullary cystic disease.
Medullary sponge kidney.

RENAL FAILURE, ACUTE, PIGMENT-INDUCED[2]
ICD-9CM # 586

CAUSES OF PIGMENT-INDUCED ACUTE RENAL FAILURE
Rhabdomyolysis and myoglobinuria.
Vigorous exercise.
Arterial embolization.
Status epilepticus.
Status asthmaticus.
Coma-induced and pressure-induced myonecrosis.
Heat stress.
Diabetic ketoacidosis.
Myopathy.
Alcoholism.
Hypokalemia.
Hypophosphatemia.
Hemoglobinuria.
Transfusion reactions.
Snake envenomation.
Malaria.
Mechanical destruction of RBCs by prosthetic valves.
G6PD deficiency.

G6PD, Glucose-6-phosphate dehydrogenase; *RBCs*, red blood cells.

RENAL FAILURE, CHRONIC[14a]
ICD-9CM # 585.9

CAUSES OF CHRONIC RENAL FAILURE
Diabetic glomerulosclerosis (systemic disease involving the kidney).
Hypertensive nephrosclerosis.
Glomerular disease:
  Glomerulonephritis.
  Amyloidosis, light chain disease (systemic disease involving the kidney).
  Systemic lupus erythematosus, Wegener granulomatosis (systemic disease involving the kidney).
Tubulointerstitial disease:
  Reflux nephropathy (chronic pyelonephritis).
  Analgesic nephropathy.
  Obstructive nephropathy (stones, benign prostatic hypertrophy).
  Myeloma kidney (systemic disease involving the kidney).
Vascular disease:
  Scleroderma (systemic disease involving the kidney).
  Vasculitis (systemic disease involving the kidney).
  Renovascular renal failure (ischemic nephropathy).
  Atheroembolic renal disease (systemic disease involving the kidney).
Cystic disease:

Autosomal dominant polycystic kidney disease.
Medullary cystic kidney disease.

RENAL FAILURE, INTRINSIC OR PARENCHYMAL CAUSES[36]

ICD-9CM # 584 Acute, use 4th digit
- 5   With Acute Tubular Necrosis
- 6   With Cortical Necrosis
- 7   With Medullary Necrosis
- 8   With Other Unspecified Pathologic Condition in Kidney
- 9   Renal Failure Unspecified
- 585 Renal Failure, Chronic

ABNORMALITIES OF THE VASCULATURE

Renal arteries: atherosclerosis, thromboembolism, arteritis.
Renal veins: thrombosis.
Microvasculature: vasculitis, thrombotic microangiopathy.

ABNORMALITIES OF GLOMERULI (ACUTE GLOMERULONEPHRITIS)

Antiglomerular membrane disease (Goodpasture's syndrome).
Immune complex glomerulonephritis: SLE, postinfectious, idiopathic, membranoproliferative.

ABNORMALITIES OF INTERSTITIUM (ACUTE INTERSTITIAL NEPHRITIS)

Drugs (e.g., antibiotics, NSAIDs, diuretics, anticonvulsants, allopurinol).
Infectious pyelonephritis.
Infiltrative: lymphoma, leukemia, sarcoidosis.

ABNORMALITIES OF TUBULES

Physical obstruction (uric acid, oxalate, light chains).
Acute tubular necrosis:
- Ischemic.
- Toxic (antibiotics, chemotherapy, immunosuppressives, radiocontrast dyes, heavy metals, myoglobin, hemolysed RBCs).

RENAL FAILURE, POSTRENAL CAUSES[36]

ICD-9CM # 584 Acute, use 4th digit
- 5   With Acute Tubular Necrosis
- 6   With Cortical Necrosis
- 7   With Medullary Necrosis
- 8   With Other Unspecified Pathologic Condition in Kidney
- 9   Renal Failure Unspecified
- 585 Renal Failure, Chronic

URETER AND RENAL PELVIS

Intrinsic obstruction:
- Blood clots.
- Stones.
- Sloughed papillae: diabetes, sickle cell disease, analgesic nephropathy.
- Inflammatory: fungus ball.

Extrinsic obstruction:
- Malignancy.
- Retroperitoneal fibrosis.
- Iatrogenic: inadvertent ligation of ureters.

BLADDER

Prostatic hypertrophy or malignancy.
Neuropathic bladder.
Blood clots.
Bladder cancer.
Stones.

URETHRAL

Strictures.
Congenital valves.

RENAL FAILURE, PRERENAL CAUSES[36]

ICD-9CM # 584 Acute, use 4th digit
- 5   With Acute Tubular Necrosis
- 6   With Cortical Necrosis
- 7   With Medullary Necrosis
- 8   With Other Unspecified Pathologic Condition in Kidney
- 9   Renal Failure Unspecified
- 585 Renal Failure, Chronic

DECREASED CARDIAC OUTPUT

CHF.
Arrhythmias.
Pericardial constriction or tamponade.
Pulmonary embolism.

HYPOVOLEMIA

GI tract loss (vomiting, diarrhea, nasogastric suction).
Blood losses (trauma, GI tract surgery).
Renal losses (diuretics, mineralocorticoid deficiency, postobstructive diuresis).
Skin losses (burns).

VOLUME REDISTRIBUTION (DECREASE IN EFFECTIVE BLOOD VOLUME)

Hypoalbuminemic states (cirrhosis, nephrosis).
Sequestration of fluid in "third" space (ischemic bowel, peritonitis, pancreatitis).
Peripheral vasodilation (sepsis, vasodilators, anaphylaxis).

ALTERED RENAL VASCULAR RESISTANCE

Increase in afferent vascular resistance (NSAIDs, liver disease, sepsis, hypercalcemia, cyclosporine).
Decrease in efferent arteriolar tone (ACE inhibitors).

RENAL INFARCTION[12a]

ICD-9CM # 593.81 Renal Infarction

CAUSES OF RENAL INFARCTION

Thrombosis: Spontaneous
Atherosclerotic disease of aorta and renal artery.
Fibromuscular dysplasia of renal artery.
Aneurysms of aorta or renal artery.
Dissection of aorta or renal artery.

Marfan's syndrome.
Ehlers-Danlos syndrome.
Vasculitis involving renal artery.
- Polyarteritis nodosa.
- Takayasu's arteritis.
- Kawasaki disease.
- Thromboangiitis obliterans.
- Other necrotizing vasculitides.
Inflammatory disease of the aorta or renal artery.
- Syphilis.
- Tuberculosis.
- Mycoses.
Hypercoagulable states.
- Nephrotic syndrome.
- Antiphospholipid syndrome.
- Antithrombin III deficiency.
- Homocystinuria.
Thrombotic microangiopathies.
- Hemolytic-uremic syndrome.
- Thrombotic thrombocytopenic purpura.
- Antiphospholipid syndrome.
- Malignant hypertension.
- Scleroderma.
- Sickle cell nephropathy.
- Polycythemia vera.
- Postpartum hemolytic-uremic syndrome.
- Hyperacute vascular allograft rejection.

Thrombosis: Induced
Traumatic.
Following endovascular intervention.
Post renal transplantation.

Embolism
Cardiac source.
- Atrial fibrillation or other arrhythmias.
- Native and prosthetic valvular heart disease.
- Infective endocarditis.
- Marantic endocarditis.
Myocardial infarction with mural thrombi.
- Left atrial myxoma or other tumor.
Noncardiac sources.
- Atheromatous embolic disease.
- Paradoxical emboli.
- Fat emboli.
- Tumor emboli.
Therapeutic renal embolization.
Segmental renal infarction of childhood.
Cisplatinum and gemcitabine.
Sickle cell disease or sickle cell trait.

RENAL PARENCHYMAL DISEASE, CHRONIC[16a]

ICD-9CM # 593.9

DIFFERENTIAL DIAGNOSIS OF CHRONIC RENAL PARENCHYMAL DISEASE

No Papillary/Caliceal Abnormality
Diffuse parenchymal loss
Bilateral:
- Chronic glomerulonephritis.
- Diffuse small-vessel disease.
- Hereditary nephropathies.
Unilateral:
- Renal artery stenosis.
- Postirradiation.
- Rare:
  - Hypoplastic kidney.
  - Postobstructive atrophy.

Focal parenchymal loss
Infarct.
Previous trauma.
Papillary/Caliceal Abnormality
Diffuse parenchymal loss
Obstructive nephropathy.
Generalized reflux nephropathy.
No Parenchymal Loss
Papillary necrosis.
TB.
Medullary sponge kidney.
Megacalices.
Pelvicaliceal cyst.
Focal Parenchymal Loss
Focal reflux nephropathy (chronic atrophic py-elonephritis).
TB.
Calculus disease.

RENAL VEIN THROMBOSIS, CAUSES
ICD-9CM # 453.3

Nephrotic syndrome.
Renal cell carcinoma.
Aortic aneurysm causing compression.
Lymphadenopathy.
Retroperitoneal fibrosis.
Estrogen therapy.
Pregnancy.
Renal cell carcinoma with vein invasion.
Severe dehydration.

RESPIRATORY FAILURE, HYPOVENTILATORY[28]
ICD-9CM # 518.81 Respiratory Failure

ABNORMAL RESPIRATORY CAPACITY (NORMAL RESPIRATORY WORKLOADS)
Acute depression of central nervous system:
  Various causes.
Chronic central hypoventilation syndromes:
  Obesity-hypoventilation syndrome.
  Sleep apnea syndrome.
  Hypothyroidism.
  Shy-Drager syndrome (multisystem atrophy syndrome).
Acute toxic paralysis syndromes:
  Botulism.
  Tetanus.
  Toxic ingestion or bites.
  Organophosphate poisoning.
Neuromuscular disorders (acute and chronic):
  Myasthenia gravis.
  Guillain-Barré syndrome.
  Drugs.
  Amyotrophic lateral sclerosis.
  Muscular dystrophies.
  Polymyositis.
  Spinal cord injury.
  Traumatic phrenic nerve paralysis.

ABNORMAL PULMONARY WORKLOADS
Chronic obstructive pulmonary disease:
  Chronic bronchitis.
  Asthmatic bronchitis.
  Emphysema.

Asthma and acute bronchial hyperreactivity syn-dromes.
Upper airway obstruction.
Interstitial lung diseases.

ABNORMAL EXTRAPULMONARY WORKLOADS
Chronic thoracic cage disorders:
  Severe kyphoscoliosis.
  After thoracoplasty.
  After thoracic cage injury.
Acute thoracic cage trauma and burns.
Pneumothorax.
Pleural fibrosis and effusions.
Abdominal processes.

RETINOPATHY, HYPERTENSIVE
ICD-9CM # 362.11

Retinal venous obstruction.
Diabetic retinopathy.
Ocular ischemic syndrome.
Hyperviscosity.
Tortuosity of retinal artery.

RHINITIS
ICD-9CM # 472.0

Allergic rhinitis.
Infectious rhinitis.
Vasomotor rhinitis.
Exercise-induced rhinitis.
Emotional rhinitis.
Rhinitis medicamentosa.
Hormone-mediated rhinitis (menses, pregnancy, oral contraceptives, hypothyroidism).
GERD.
Chemical- or irritant-induced rhinitis.
Rhinitis mimics:
  Deviated septum.
  Enlarged adenoids.
  Nasal polyps/tumors.
  Foreign bodies.
  CSF rhinorrhea.
  Sarcoidosis.
  Midline granuloma.
  Wegener's granulomatosis.
  SLE.
  Sjögren's syndrome.

RIB DEFECTS ON X-RAY[16a]
ICD-9CM # varies with specific diagnosis

CAUSES OF SUPERIOR MARGINAL RIB DEFECTS
Normal
Isolated defects.
Projectional artifacts (due to lordosis).
Neurologic
Paralytic poliomyelitis.
Quadriparesis.
Collagen Vascular Disease
Rheumatoid arthritis.
SLE.
Systemic sclerosis.
Local Pressure
Chest drainage tube.
Osteochondroma.

Neural tumor.
Coarctation of aorta.
Hyperparathyroidism
Miscellaneous
Osteogenesis imperfecta.
Marfan's syndrome.

RIB NOTCHING ON X-RAY[16a]
ICD-9CM # varies with specific diagnosis

CAUSES OF INFERIOR RIB NOTCHING
Arterial
Aortic obstruction
Aortic coarctation.
Aortic thrombosis.
Aortitis.
Subclavian artery obstruction
Blalock-Taussig operation.
Arteritis.
Atherosclerotic occlusion.
Pulmonary oligemia
Pulmonary atresia.
Tetralogy of Fallot.
Multiple pulmonary arterial stenoses.
Venous
Chronic superior vena caval obstruction
Arteriovenous
Arteriovenous malformation
Pulmonary.
Chest wall.
Neural
Neurofibromas

RIGHT AXIS DEVIATION[22]
ICD-9CM # varies with specific diagnosis

Normal variation.
Right ventricular hypertrophy.
Left posterior fascicular block.
Lateral myocardial infarction.
Pulmonary embolism.
Dextrocardia.
Mechanical shifts or emphysema causing a vertical heart.

SALIVARY GLAND ENLARGEMENT
ICD-9CM # 527.1

Neoplasm.
Sialolithiasis.
Infection (mumps, bacterial infection, HIV, TB).
Sarcoidosis.
Idiopathic.
Acromegaly.
Anorexia/bulimia.
Chronic pancreatitis.
Medications (e.g., phenylbutazone).
Cirrhosis.
DM.

SALIVARY GLAND SECRETION, DECREASED
ICD-9CM # 527.7

Medications (antihistamines, antidepressants, neuroleptics, antihypertensives).

Dehydration.
Anxiety.
Sjögren's syndrome.
Sarcoidosis.
Mumps.
Amyloidosis.
CNS disorders.
Head and neck radiation.

SCLERODERMA-LIKE SYNDROMES[1]

ICD-9CM # varies with specific diagnosis

OTHER DISEASES

Morphea.
Eosinophilic fasciitis.
Scleredema (of Buschke).
Scleromyxedema.
Graft-versus-host disease.
Nephrogenic-fibrosing dermopathy.

ENVIRONMENTAL AGENTS AND DRUGS

Bleomycin.
L-Tryptophan.
Organic solvents.
Pentazocine.
Toxic oil syndrome.
Vinyl chloride disease.
Gadolinium.

SCROTAL MASSES, BOYS AND ADOLESCENTS[22a]

ICD-9CM # varies with specific diagnosis

PAINFUL

Testicular torsion.
Torsion of appendix testis.
Epididymitis.
Trauma: ruptured testis, hematocele.
Inguinal hernia (incarcerated).
Mumps orchitis.

PAINLESS

Hydrocele.
Inguinal hernia.*
Varicocele.*
Spermatocele.*
Testicular tumor.*
Henoch-Schönlein purpura.*
Idiopathic scrotal edema.

*May be associated with discomfort.

SCROTAL PAIN[28]

ICD-9CM #		
878.2	Scrotal Injury, Traumatic	
608.9	Scrotal Disorder NOS	
608.4	Scrotal Cellulitis	
608.83	Scrotal Hemorrhage, Nontraumatic	
608.4	Scrotal Nodule, Inflammatory	

Torsion:
  Appendages.
  Spermatic cord.
Infection:

Orchitis.
Abscess.
Epididymitis.
Neoplasia:
  Benign.
  Malignant.
Incarcerated hernia.
Trauma.
Hydrocele.
Spermatocele.
Varicocele.

SCROTAL SWELLING

ICD-9CM # 608.86

Hydrocele.
Varicocele.
Neoplasm.
Acute epididymitis.
Orchitis.
Trauma.
Hernia.
Torsion of spermatic cord.
Torsion of epididymis.
Torsion of testis.
Insect bite.
Folliculitis.
Sebaceous cyst.
Thrombosis of spermatic vein.
Other: lymphedema, dermatitis, fat necrosis, Henoch-Schönlein purpura, idiopathic scrotal edema.

SEIZURE

ICD-9CM # 780.39

Syncope.
Alcohol abuse/withdrawal.
TIA.
Hemiparetic migraine.
Psychiatric disorders.
Carotid sinus hypersensitivity.
Hyperventilation, prolonged breath holding.
Hypoglycemia.
Narcolepsy.
Movement disorders (tics, hemiballismus).
Hyponatremia.
Brain tumor (primary or metastatic).
Tetanus.
Strychnine, phencyclidine poisoning.

SEIZURE, PEDIATRIC[2]

ICD-9CM # 780.39 Infantile Seizures
779.0 Seizures, Newborn

FIRST MONTH OF LIFE

First Day
Hypoxia.
Drugs.
Trauma.
Infection.
Hyperglycemia.
Hypoglycemia.
Pyridoxine deficiency.
Day 2-3
Infection.
Drug withdrawal.
Hypoglycemia.

Hypocalcemia.
Developmental malformation.
Intracranial hemorrhage.
Inborn error of metabolism.
Hyponatremia or hypernatremia.
Day >4
Infection.
Hypocalcemia.
Hyperphosphatemia.
Hyponatremia.
Developmental malformation.
Drug withdrawal.
Inborn error of metabolism.

1 TO 6 MO

As above.

6 MO TO 3 YR

Febrile seizures.
Birth injury.
Infection.
Toxin.
Trauma.
Metabolic disorder.
Cerebral degenerative disease.

>3 YR

Idiopathic.
Infection.
Trauma.
Cerebral degenerative disease.

SEIZURE MIMICS[1]

ICD-9CM # varies with specific diagnosis

NON-EPILEPTIC EPISODIC DISORDERS THAT MAY RESEMBLE SEIZURES

Movement disorders: myoclonus, paroxysmal choreoathetosis, episodic ataxias, hyperexplexia (startle disease).
Migraine: confusional, vertebrobasilar, visual auras.
Syncope.
Behavioral and psychiatric: psychogenic non-epileptic attacks (pseudoseizures), hyperventilation syndrome, panic or anxiety disorder, dissociative states.
Cataplexy (usually associated with narcolepsy).
Transient ischemic attack.
Alcoholic blackouts.
Hypoglycemia.

SEXUAL DYSFUNCTION, FEMALE[1]

ICD-9CM # 302.7

FACTORS THAT MAY INFLUENCE SEXUAL FUNCTIONING IN WOMEN

Biological
Medications (e.g., antidepressants, antihypertensives).
Vaginal atrophy, pain with intercourse.
Low testosterone levels (e.g., bilateral oophorectomy).
Illness (e.g., diabetes, hypothyroidism, cerebrovascular accident).

Sleep disturbances, fatigue.
Disability or pain from illness (e.g., arthritis).
Incontinence.
Psychological
Depression.
Body image.
Interpersonal
Marital issues.
Poor communication.
Partner's sexual problems (e.g., erectile dysfunction).
Partner's health problems (e.g., myocardial infarction).
Sociocultural
Ageism ("too old" to want sex).
Multiple other obligations and commitments.
Lack of partner.

SEXUALLY TRANSMITTED DISEASES, ANORECTAL REGION[26]

ICD-9CM # 569.49 Infection and Region

ULCERATIVE

Lymphogranuloma venereum.
Herpes simplex virus.
Early (primary) syphilis.
Chancroid *(Haemophilus ducreyi).*
Cytomegalovirus.
Idiopathic (usually HIV positive).

NONULCERATIVE

Condyloma acuminatum.
Gonorrhea.
Chlamydia *(Chlamydia trachomatis).*
Syphilis.

SEXUAL PRECOCITY[41]

ICD-9CM # 259.1

TRUE PRECOCIOUS PUBERTY

Premature reactivation of LHRH pulse generator.

INCOMPLETE SEXUAL PRECOCITY

(Pituitary gonadotropin independent).
Males
Chorionic gonadotropin-secreting tumor.
Leydig cell tumor.
Familial testotoxicosis.
Virilizing congenital adrenal hyperplasia.
Virilizing adrenal tumor.
Premature adrenarche.
Females
Granulosa cell tumor (follicular cysts may be manifested similarly).
Follicular cyst.
Feminizing adrenal tumor.
Premature thelarche.
Premature adrenarche.
Late-onset virilizing congenital adrenal hyperplasia.
In Both Sexes
McCune-Albright syndrome.
Primary hypothyroidism.

SHOULDER PAIN

ICD-9CM # 952.2 Shoulder Injury
718.81 Shoulder Instability
726.19 Shoulder Ligament or Muscle Instability
840.9 Shoulder Strain, Site Unspecified

WITH LOCAL FINDINGS IN SHOULDER

Trauma: contusion, fracture, muscle strain, trauma to spinal cord.
Arthrosis, arthritis, RA, ankylosing spondylitis.
Bursitis, synovitis, tendinitis, tenosynovitis.
Aseptic (avascular) necrosis.
Local infection: septic arthritis, osteomyelitis, abscess, herpes zoster, TB.

WITHOUT LOCAL FINDINGS IN SHOULDER

Cardiovascular disorders: ischemic heart disease, pericarditis, aortic aneurysm.
Subdiaphragmatic abscess, liver abscess.
Cholelithiasis, cholecystitis.
Pulmonary lesions: apical bronchial carcinoma, pleurisy, pneumothorax, pneumonia.
GI lesions: PUD, gastric neoplasm, peptic esophagitis.
Pancreatic lesions: carcinoma, calculi, pancreatitis.
CNS abnormalities: neoplasm, vascular abnormalities.
Multiple sclerosis.
Syringomyelia.
Polymyositis/dermatomyositis.
Psychogenic.
Polymyalgia rheumatica.
Ectopic pregnancy.

SHOULDER PAIN BY LOCATION

ICD-9CM # 952.2 Shoulder Injury
726.19 Shoulder Ligament or Muscle Instability
840.8 Shoulder Separation

TOP OF SHOULDER (C4)

Cervical source.
Acromioclavicular.
Sternoclavicular.
Diaphragmatic.

SUPEROLATERAL (C5)

Rotator cuff tendinitis.
Impingement.
Adhesive capsulitis.
Glenohumeral arthritis.

ANTERIOR

Bicipital tendinitis and rupture.
Glenoid labral tear.
Adhesive capsulitis.
Glenohumeral arthritis.
Osteonecrosis.

AXILLARY

Neoplasm (Pancoast's, mediastinal).
Herpes zoster.

SHOULDER PAIN, IN DIFFERENT AGE GROUPS[8]

ICD-9CM # 719.41

COMMON CAUSES OF SHOULDER PAIN IN DIFFERENT AGE GROUPS

Childhood (2-10 yr)
Intraarticular:
Instability.
Periarticular:
Osteochondromas.
Adolescence (10-18 yr)
Intraarticular:
Instability.
Early Adulthood (18-30 yr)
Intraarticular:
Instability.
Acromioclavicular joint sprain.
Periarticular:
Calcific tendonitis.
Impingement.
Referred:
Cervical.
Adulthood (30-60 yr)
Intraarticular:
Osteochondritis.
Osteoarthritis.
Frozen shoulder.
Inflammatory arthritis.
Periarticular:
Calcific tendonitis.
Impingement.
Rotator cuff tear.
Bicipital tendonitis.
Referred:
Cervical.
Old Age (>60 yr)
Intraarticular:
Osteochondritis.
Osteoarthritis.
Frozen shoulder.
Inflammatory arthritis.
Periarticular:
Impingement.
Rotator cuff tear.
Referred:
Cervical.

SINUS NODE DYSFUNCTION[14a]

ICD-9CM # 427.81

CAUSES OF SINUS NODE DYSFUNCTION

Intrinsic
Hypothyroidism.
Fibrocalcific degeneration.
Increased vagal tone, especially in sleep apnea.
Congenital mutations.
Scleroderma.
Amyloidosis.
Chagas disease.
Extrinsic
Trauma, including cardiac surgery.
Drugs:
   Calcium-channel blockers.

β-Blockers.
Digoxin.
Antiarrhythmic medications (amiodarone, dronedarone, sotalol, flecainide, propafenone).
Lithium.

SKIN INDURATION, CHRONIC[18b]

ICD-9CM # varies with specific diagnosis

CONDITIONS ASSOCIATED WITH CHRONIC SKIN INDURATION

Systemic sclerosis.
Localized scleroderma.
Scleroderma variants.
Scleredema.
  Scleredema adultorum of Buschke.
  Scleredema diabeticorum.
  Scleredema neonatorum.
Scleromyxedema.
Nephrogenic fibrosing dermopathy.
Eosinophilic syndromes.
  Eosinophilic fasciitis (diffuse fasciitis with eosinophilia, Schulman disease).
  Eosinophilia-myalgia syndrome.
  Toxic oil syndrome.
Chronic graft-versus-host disease.
Pseudoscleroderma (local injection of vitamin K, bleomycin, pentazocine).
Metabolic diseases.
  Porphyria cutanea tarda.
  Phenylketonuria.
  Werner syndrome.
  Acromegaly.
Pachydermoperiostitis.
Polyneuropathy, organomegaly, endocrinopathy, monoclonal gammopathy (POEMS).
Stiff skin syndrome.
Reflex sympathetic dystrophy.
Hemiplegia.

SMALL BOWEL MASSES[38]

ICD-9CM # varies with specific diagnosis

Cyst:
  Mesenteric cyst.
Tumor:
  Benign.
  Malignant.
Intussusception.
Inflammation:
  Crohn's disease.

SMALL BOWEL OBSTRUCTION[26]

ICD-9CM # 751.1 Small Intestine Obstruction, Congenital
         560.81 Small Intestine Obstruction Due to Adhesion

INTRINSIC

Congenital (atresia, stenosis).
Inflammatory (Crohn's, radiation enteritis).
Neoplasms (metastatic or primary).
Intussusception.
Traumatic (hematoma).

EXTRINSIC

Hernias (internal and external).
Adhesions.
Volvulus.
Compressing masses (tumors, abscesses, hematomas).

INTRALUMINAL

Foreign body.
Gallstones.
Bezoars.
Barium.
Ascaris infestation.

SMALL INTESTINE ULCERATION

ICD-9CM # 569.82

Inflammatory bowel disease.
Celiac disease.
Vasculitis, SLE, Behçet's syndrome.
Uremia.
Infections (Campylobacter, TB, Yersinia, parasites, typhoid, cytomegalovirus [CMV], Clostridium).
Mesenteric insufficiency.
Neoplasms.
Radiation.
Drugs (salicylates, potassium, indomethacin, antimetabolites).
Meckel diverticulum.
Zollinger-Ellison syndrome.
Lymphocytic enterocolitis.
Stomal ulceration.

SMELL DISTURBANCE

ICD-9CM # varies with specific disorder

Upper respiratory tract infection.
Nasal or paranasal sinus disease.
Exposure to noxious vapors.
Head trauma.
Idiopathic.
Dental caries, periodontal disease.
Medications.

SORE THROAT[2]

ICD-9CM # 484.1

DIFFERENTIAL DIAGNOSIS FOR SORE THROAT

Infectious Causes
Aerobes
Common:
  Streptococcus pyogenes (GABHS).
  GABHS.
  Peptostreptococcus spp.
  Non–group A streptococcus.
  Neisseria gonorrhoeae.
  Neisseria meningitides.
  Mycoplasma pneumoniae.
  Arcanobacterium hemolyticum.
  Chlamydia trachomatis.
  Staphylococcus aureus.
Uncommon:
  Haemophilus influenzae.
  Haemophilus parainfluenzae.
  Coccidioides spp.

Corynebacterium diphtheriae.
Streptococcus pneumoniae.
Yersinia enterocolitica.
Treponema pallidum.
Francisella tularensis.
Legionella pneumophila.
Mycobacterium spp.
Anaerobes
Bacteroides spp.
Peptococcus spp.
Clostridium spp.
Fusobacterium spp.
Prevotella spp.
Other
Candida spp.
Viral
Rhinovirus.
Adenovirus.
Coronavirus.
Herpes simplex 1,2.
Influenza A, B.
Parainfluenza.
Cytomegalovirus.
Epstein-Barr.
Varicella-zoster.
Hepatitis virus.
Noninfectious Causes
Systemic
Kawasaki disease.
Stevens-Johnson syndrome.
Cyclic neutropenia.
Thyroiditis.
Connective tissue disease
Trauma, miscellaneous
Penetrating injury.
Angioneurotic edema.
Retained foreign body.
Anomalous aortic arch.
Laryngeal fracture.
Calcific retropharyngeal tendinitis.
Retropharyngeal hematoma.
Caustic exposure.
Tumor
Tongue.
Larynx.
Thyroid.
Leukemia.

SPASTIC PARAPLEGIAS

ICD-9CM # 344.1

Cervical spondylosis.
Friedreich's ataxia.
Multiple sclerosis.
Spinal cord tumor.
HIV.
Tertiary syphilis.
Vitamin B_{12} deficiency.
Spinocerebellar ataxias.
Syringomyelia.
Spinal cord AV malformations.
Adrenoleukodystrophy.

SPINAL CORD COMPRESSION, EPIDURAL

ICD-9CM # varies with specific disorder

Osteoarthritis.

Differential Diagnosis

II

Meningioma.
Spinal epidural abscess.
Spinal epidural hematoma.
Spinal epidural vascular malformations.
RA.
Metastatic cancer (vertebral, intramedullary, leptomeninges).
Radiation myelopathy.
Neurofibroma.
Sarcoidosis.
Paraneoplastic myelopathy.
Histiocytosis.

SPINAL CORD DYSFUNCTION

ICD-9CM # 336.9   Spinal Cord Compression
336.9   Spinal Cord Disease NOS
742.9   Spinal Cord Disease, Congenital
281.1   Spinal Cord Degeneration, B_{12} Deficiency Anemia
336.8   Spinal Cord Atrophy, Acute
336.10 Spinal Cord Atrophy, Adult

Trauma.
Multiple sclerosis.
Transverse myelitis.
Neoplasm (primary, metastatic).
Syringomyelia.
Spinal epidural abscess.
HIV myelopathy.
Diskitis.
Spinal epidural hematoma.
Spinal cord infarction.
Spinal AV malformation.
Subarachnoid hemorrhage.

SPINAL CORD DYSFUNCTION, NONTRAUMATIC[2]

ICD-9CM # 742.9

NONTRAUMATIC ETIOLOGIES OF SPINAL CORD DYSFUNCTION

Processes Affecting the Spinal Cord or Blood Supply Directly
Multiple sclerosis.
Transverse myelitis.
Spinal arteriovenous malformation/subarachnoid hemorrhage.
Syringomyelia.
HIV myelopathy.
Other myelopathies.
Spinal cord infarction.
Compressive Lesions Affecting the Spinal Cord
Spinal epidural abscess.
Spinal epidural hematoma.
Diskitis.
Neoplasm.
Metastatic.
Primary CNS.

HIV, Human immunodeficiency virus; *CNS,* central nervous system.

SPINAL CORD ISCHEMIC SYNDROMES

ICD-9CM # varies with specific disorder

Systemic hypotension.
Venous or arterial occlusion.
Arterial dissection.
Thromboembolism.
Endovascular procedures.
Vasculitis.
Fibrocartilaginous embolism.
Regional hemodynamic compromise.

SPINAL TUMORS[14]

ICD-9CM # 299.7

EXTRADURAL

Metastases.
Primary bone tumors arising in spine.

INTRADURAL EXTRAMEDULLARY

Meningiomas.
Neurofibromas.
Schwannomas.
Lipomas.
Arachnoid cysts.
Epidermoid cysts.
Metastasis.

INTRAMEDULLARY

Ependymoma.
Glioma.
Hemangioblastoma.
Lipoma.
Metastases.

SPLENIC CYSTS, CLASSIFICATION[5a]

ICD-9CM # 289.59 Splenic Cysts

Primary (true).
Parasitic.
Nonparasitic.
Congenital.
Epidermoid.
Dermoid.
Mesothelial (serous).
Transitional.
Neoplastic.
Secondary (false): pseudocysts.
Traumatic.
Degenerative.
Inflammatory.
Hemorrhagic.

SPLENIC TUMORS, CLASSIFICATION[5a]

ICD-9CM # 159.1   Splenic Tumors

Malignant.
Lymphoproliferative disease.
Non-Hodgkin lymphoma.
Hodgkin disease.
Hairy cell leukemia.
Chronic lymphocytic leukemia.
Myeloproliferative disease.
Chronic myelogenous leukemia.

Myelofibrosis.
Primary tumors.
Angiosarcoma.
Metastatic tumors.
Benign.
Hemangiomas.
Hamartomas.
Lymphangiomas.
Sclerosing angiomatoid nodular transformation (SANT).

SPLENOMEGALY

ICD-9CM # 789.2   Splenomegaly Unspecified
289.51 Chronic Congestive
759.0   Congenital
789.2   Unknown Origin

Hepatic cirrhosis.
Neoplastic involvement: CML, CLL, lymphoma, multiple myeloma.
Bacterial infections: TB, infectious endocarditis, typhoid fever, splenic abscess.
Viral infections: infectious mononucleosis, viral hepatitis, HIV.
Gaucher's disease and other lipid storage diseases.
Sarcoidosis.
Parasitic infections (malaria, kala-azar, histoplasmosis).
Hereditary and acquired hemolytic anemias.
Idiopathic thrombocytopenic purpura (ITP).
Collagen vascular disorders: SLE, RA (Felty's syndrome), polyarteritis nodosa.
Serum sickness, drug hypersensitivity reaction.
Splenic cysts and benign tumors: hemangioma, lymphangioma.
Thrombosis of splenic or portal vein.
Polycythemia vera, myeloid metaplasia.

SPLENOMEGALY AND HEPATOMEGALY[38]

ICD-9CM # 789.2   Splenomegaly
789.1   Hepatomegaly

CAUSES OF SPLENOMEGALY AND HEPATOSPLENOMEGALY

Massive Splenomegaly
Hematologic disease (e.g., chronic myeloid leukemia, myelofibrosis).
Moderate Splenomegaly
The above causes.
Portal hypertension.
Hematologic disease (e.g., lymphoma, leukemia, thalassemia).
Storage disease (e.g., Gaucher's disease).
Small Splenomegaly
The above causes.
Infective (hepatitis, leptospirosis, malaria, bacterial endocarditis).
Hematologic disease (e.g., hemolytic anemias, essential thrombocythemia, polycythemia rubra vera).
Connective tissue diseases or vasculitis (e.g., rheumatoid arthritis, systemic lupus erythematosus, polyarteritis nodosa).
Solitary cyst, polycystic syndrome, hydatid cyst.
Infiltration (amyloid, sarcoid).

Hepatosplenomegaly

Chronic liver disease with portal hypertension.
Hematologic disease (e.g., myeloproliferative disease, lymphoma).
Infection (e.g., amyloid, sarcoid).
Connective tissue disease (e.g., systemic lupus erythematosus).

SPLENOMEGALY, CHILDREN[20]

ICD-9CM # 782.2

DISORDERS OF THE BLOOD

Hemolytic anemia: congenital/acquired.
Thalassemia.
Sickle cell disease.
Leukemia.
Osteopetrosis.
Myelofibrosis/myeloid metaplasia/thrombocythemia.

INFECTIONS: ACUTE AND CHRONIC

Viral:
    Congenital (e.g., TORCH association).
    Mononucleosis (e.g., EBV, CMV infection).
    Virus-associated hemophagocytic syndrome.
    Human immunodeficiency virus.
Bacterial:
    Sepsis/abscess.
    Brucellosis.
    Salmonellosis.
    Tularemia.
    Tuberculosis.
    Subacute bacterial endocarditis.
    Syphilis.
    Lyme disease.
Fungal:
    Histoplasmosis (disseminated).
Rickettsial:
    Rocky Mountain spotted fever.
    Cat scratch disease.
Parasitic:
    Toxoplasmosis.
    Malaria.
    Leishmaniasis (kala-azar).
    Schistosomiasis.
    Echinococcosis.

HEPATIC/PORTAL SYSTEM DISORDERS

Acute/chronic active hepatitis.
Cirrhosis/hepatic fibrosis/biliary atresia.
Portal or splenic venous obstruction (Banti syndrome).

AUTOIMMUNE DISEASE

Juvenile rheumatoid arthritis.
Systemic lupus erythematosus.
Autoimmune lymphoproliferative syndrome (Canale–Smith syndrome).

NEOPLASMS/CYSTS

Lymphomas (Hodgkin and non-Hodgkin).
Hemangiomas/lymphangiomas.
Hamartomas.
Congenital or acquired (posttraumatic) cysts.

STORAGE DISEASES/INBORN ERRORS OF METABOLISM

Lipidoses: Gaucher disease, Niemann–Pick disease, others.
Mucopolysaccharidoses.
Defects in carbohydrate metabolism: galactosemia, fructose intolerance.
Sea-blue histiocyte syndrome.

MISCELLANEOUS DISORDERS

Histiocytoses:
    Reactive.
    Langerhans cell.
    Malignant.
Sarcoidosis.
Congestive heart failure.
Familial Mediterranean fever.

CMV, Cytomegalovirus; *EBV,* Epstein-Barr virus; *TORCH,* toxoplasmosis, other infections, rubella, cytomegalovirus infection, herpes simplex.

STEATOHEPATITIS

ICD-9CM # 571.8

Alcohol abuse.
Obesity.
DM.
Parenteral nutrition.
Medications (high-dose estrogen, amiodarone, corticosteroids, methotrexate, nifedipine).
Jejunoileal bypass.
Abetalipoproteinemia.
Wilson's disease, Weber-Christian disease.

STOMATITIS, BULLOUS

ICD-9CM # 528.0

Erythema multiforme.
Erosive lichen planus.
Bullous pemphigoid.
SLE.
Pemphigus vulgaris.
Mucous membrane pemphigoid.

STRIDOR, PEDIATRIC AGE[4]

ICD-9CM # 786.1 Stridor
            748.3 Stridor, Laryngeal, Congenital

RECURRENT

Allergic (spasmodic) croup.
Respiratory infections in a child with otherwise asymptomatic anatomic narrowing of the large airways.
Laryngomalacia.

PERSISTENT

Laryngeal obstruction:
    Laryngomalacia.
    Papillomas, other tumors.
    Cysts and laryngoceles.
    Laryngeal webs.
    Bilateral abductor paralysis of the cords.
    Foreign body.
Tracheobronchial disease:
    Tracheomalacia.
    Subglottic tracheal webs.
    Endotracheal, endobronchial tumors.
    Subglottic tracheal stenosis.
    Congenital.
    Acquired.
    Extrinsic masses.
    Mediastinal masses.
    Vascular ring.
    Lobar emphysema.
    Bronchogenic cysts.
    Thyroid enlargement.
    Esophageal foreign body.
    Tracheoesophageal fistulas.
    Other.
    Gastroesophageal reflux.
    Macroglossia, Pierre Robin syndrome.
    Cri-du-chat syndrome.
    Hysterical stridor.
    Hypocalcemia.

STROKE[36]

ICD-9CM # 436 Acute Stroke

Hypoglycemia.
Drug overdose or intoxication.
Hysterical conversion reaction.
Hyperventilation.
Metabolic encephalopathy.
Migraine.
Syncope.
Transient global amnesia.
Seizures.
Vestibular vertigo.

STROKE, PEDIATRIC AGE[23]

ICD-9CM # 436 Stroke, Acute

CARDIAC DISEASE

Congenital:
    Aortic stenosis.
    Mitral stenosis; mitral prolapse.
    Ventricular septal defects.
    Patent ductus arteriosus.
    Cyanotic congenital heart disease involving right-to-left shunt.
Acquired:
    Endocarditis (bacterial, SLE).
    Kawasaki disease.
    Cardiomyopathy.
    Atrial myxoma.
    Arrhythmia.
    Paradoxical emboli through patent foramen ovale.
    Rheumatic fever.
    Prosthetic heart valve.

HEMATOLOGIC ABNORMALITIES

Hemoglobinopathies:
    Sickle cell (SS) disease.
    Sickle (SC) disease.
Polycythemia.
Leukemia/lymphoma.
Thrombocytopenia.
Thrombocytosis.
Disorders of coagulation:
    Protein C deficiency.
    Protein S deficiency.

Differential Diagnosis

II

Factor V Leiden.
Antithrombin III deficiency.
Lupus anticoagulant.
Oral contraceptive pill use.
Pregnancy and the postpartum state.
Disseminated intravascular coagulation.
Paroxysmal nocturnal hemoglobinuria.
Inflammatory bowel disease (thrombosis).

INFLAMMATORY DISORDERS

Meningitis:
Viral.
Bacterial.
Tuberculosis.
Systemic infection:
Viremia.
Bacteremia.
Local head and neck infections.
Drug-induced inflammation:
Amphetamine.
Cocaine.
Autoimmune disease:
SLE.
Juvenile RA.
Takayasu's arteritis.
Mixed connective tissue disease.
Polyarteritis nodosum.
Primary CNS vasculitis.
Sarcoidosis.
Behçet's syndrome.
Wegener's granulomatosis.

METABOLIC DISEASE ASSOCIATED WITH STROKE

Homocystinuria.
Pseudoxanthoma elasticum.
Fabry's disease.
Sulfite oxidase deficiency.
Mitochondrial disorders:
MELAS.
Leigh syndrome.
Ornithine transcarbamylase deficiency.

INTRACEREBRAL VASCULAR PROCESSES

Ruptured aneurysm.
Arteriovenous malformation.
Fibromuscular dysplasia.
Moyamoya disease.
Migraine headache.
Postsubarachnoid hemorrhage vasospasm.
Hereditary hemorrhagic telangiectasia.
Sturge-Weber syndrome.
Carotid artery dissection.
Postvaricella.

TRAUMA AND OTHER EXTERNAL CAUSES

Child abuse.
Head trauma/neck trauma.
Oral trauma.
Placental embolism.
ECMO therapy.

CNS, Central nervous system; *ECMO*, extracorporeal membrane oxygenation; *MELAS*, mitochondrial encephalomyopathy, lactic acidosis, and stroke.

STROKE, YOUNG ADULT, CAUSES[1]

ICD-9CM # 436

Cardiac factors (ASD, MVP, patent foramen ovale).
Inflammatory factors (SLE, polyarteritis nodosa).
Infections (endocarditis, neurosyphilis).
Drugs (cocaine, heroin, oral contraceptives, decongestants).
Arterial dissection.
Hematolic factors (DIC, TTP, deficiency of protein S, protein C, antithrombin III).
Migraine.
Postpartum angiopathy.
Other: premature atherosclerosis, fibromuscular dysplasia.

ST SEGMENT ELEVATIONS, NONISCHEMIC

ICD-9CM # 794.31

Early repolarization.
Acute pericarditis.
LVH.
Normal pattern variant.
LBBB.
Pulmonary embolism.
Hyperkalemia.
Postcardioversion.

SUDDEN DEATH, PEDIATRIC AGE[4]

ICD-9CM # varies with specific disorder

SIDS AND SIDS "MIMICS"

SIDS.
Long QT syndromes.
Inborn errors of metabolism.
Child abuse.
Myocarditis.
Duct-dependent congenital heart disease.

CORRECTED OR UNOPERATED CONGENITAL HEART DISEASE

Aortic stenosis.
Tetralogy of Fallot.
Transposition of great vessels (postoperative atrial switch).
Mitral valve prolapse.
Hematologic left heart syndrome.
Eisenmenger's syndrome.

CORONARY ARTERIAL DISEASE

Anomalous origin.
Anomalous tract.
Kawasaki disease.
Periarteritis.
Arterial dissection.
Marfan's syndrome.
Myocardial infarction.

MYOCARDIAL DISEASE

Myocarditis.
Hypertrophic cardiomyopathy.
Dilated cardiomyopathy.
Arrhythmogenic right ventricular dysplasia.

CONDUCTION SYSTEM ABNORMALITY/ARRHYTHMIA

Long Q-T syndromes.
Proarrhythmic drugs.
Preexcitation syndromes.
Heart block.
Commotio cordis.
Idiopathic ventricular fibrillation.
Heart tumor.

MISCELLANEOUS

Pulmonary hypertension.
Pulmonary embolism.
Heat stroke.
Cocaine.
Anorexia nervosa.
Electrolyte disturbances.

SIDS, Sudden infant death syndrome.

SUDDEN DEATH, YOUNG ATHLETE

ICD-9CM # varies with specific diagnosis

Hypertrophic cardiomyopathy.
Coronary artery anomalies.
Myocarditis.
Ruptured aortic aneurysm (Marfan's syndrome).
Arrhythmias.
Aortic valve stenosis.
Asthma.
Trauma (cerebral, cardiac).
Drug and alcohol abuse.
Heat stroke.
Cardiac sarcoidosis.
Atherosclerotic coronary artery disease.
Dilated cardiomyopathy.

SWOLLEN LIMB

ICD-9CM # 729.81 Swollen Arm or Hand
729.81 Swollen Leg or Foot

Trauma.
Insect bite.
Abscess.
Lymphedema.
Thrombophlebitis.
Lipoma.
Neurofibroma.
Postphlebitic syndrome.
Myositis ossificans.
Nephrosis, cirrhosis, CHF.
Hypoalbuminemia.
Varicose veins.

TALL STATURE[27]

ICD-9CM # 253.0 Growth Hormone
Overproduction, Gigantism

Constitutional (familial or genetic)—most common cause

ENDOCRINE CAUSES

Growth hormone excess—gigantism.
Sexual precocity (tall as children, short as adults):
True sexual precocity.
Pseudosexual precocity.

Androgen deficiency:
  Klinefelter's syndrome.
  Bilateral anorchism.

GENETIC CAUSES

Klinefelter's syndrome.
Syndromes of XYY, XXYY.

MISCELLANEOUS SYNDROMES AND DISORDERS

Cerebral gigantism or Sotos' syndrome: prominent forehead, hypertelorism, high arched palate, dolichocephaly, mental retardation, large hands and feet, and premature eruption of teeth. Large at birth, with most rapid growth in first 4 yr of life.

Marfan's syndrome: disorder of mesodermal tissues, subluxation of the lenses, arachnodactyly, and aortic aneurysm.

Homocystinuria: same phenotype as Marfan's syndrome.

Obesity: tall as infants, children, and adolescents.

Total lipodystrophy: large hands and feet, generalized loss of subcutaneous fat, insulin-resistant DM, and hepatomegaly.

Beckwith-Wiedemann syndrome: neonatal tallness, omphalocele, macroglossia, and neonatal hypoglycemia.

Weaver-Smith syndrome: excessive intrauterine growth, mental retardation, megalocephaly, widened bifrontal diameter, hypertelorism, large ears, micrognathia, camptodactyly, broad thumbs, and limited extension of elbows and knees.

Marshall-Smith syndrome: excessive intrauterine growth, mental retardation, blue sclerae, failure to thrive, and early death.

TARDIVE DYSKINESIA[13]

ICD-9CM # 781.3 Dyskinesia
          300.11 Hysterical Dyskinesia
          333.82 Orofacial Dyskinesia
          307.9 Psychogenic Dyskinesia

DIFFERENTIAL DIAGNOSIS:

Medications (antidepressants, anticholinergics, amphetamines, lithium, L-dopa, phenytoin).
Brain neoplasms.
Ill-fitting dentures.
Huntington's disease.
Idiopathic dystonias (tics, blepharospasm, aging).
Wilson's disease.
Extrapyramidal syndrome (postanoxic or postencephalitic).
Torsion dystonia.

TASTE AND SMELL LOSS[1]

ICD-9CM # 781.1 Smell and Taste
          Disturbance of Sensation

TASTE

Local: radiation therapy.
Systemic: cancer, renal failure, hepatic failure, nutritional deficiency (vitamin B_{12}, zinc), Cushing's syndrome, hypothyroidism, DM, infection (influenza), drugs (antirheumatic and antiproliferative).

Neurologic: Bell's palsy, familial dysautonomia, multiple sclerosis.

SMELL

Local: allergic rhinitis, sinusitis, nasal polyposis, bronchial asthma.
Systemic: renal failure, hepatic failure, nutritional deficiency (vitamin B_{12}), Cushing's syndrome, hypothyroidism, DM, infection (viral hepatitis, influenza), drugs (nasal sprays, antibiotics).
Neurologic: head trauma, multiple sclerosis, Parkinson's disease, frontal brain tumor.

TELANGIECTASIA

ICD-9CM # 448.9

Oral contraceptive agents.
Pregnancy.
Rosacea.
Varicose veins.
Trauma.
Drug induced (corticosteroids, systemic or topical).
Spider telangiectases.
Hepatic cirrhosis.
Mastocytosis.
SLE, dermatomyositis, systemic sclerosis.

TENDINOPATHY[26]

ICD-9CM # 727.9

INTRINSIC FACTORS

Anatomic Factors
Malalignment.
Muscle weakness or imbalance.
Muscle inflexibility.
Decreased vascularity.
Systemic Factors
Inflammatory conditions (e.g., SLE).
Pregnancy.
Quinolone-induced tendinopathy.
Age-Related Factors
Tendon degeneration.
Increased tendon stiffness.
Tendon calcification.
Decreased vascularity.

EXTRINSIC FACTORS

Repetitive Mechanical Load
Excessive duration.
Excessive frequency.
Excessive intensity.
Poor technique.
Workplace factors.
Equipment Problems
Footwear.
Athletic field surface.
Equipment factors (e.g., racquet size).
Protective gear.

TESTICULAR FAILURE[10]

ICD-9CM # 257.1 Testicular Failure

PRIMARY

Klinefelter's syndrome (XXY).
XYY.
Vanishing testes syndrome (in utero or early postnatal torsion).

Noonan's syndrome.
Varicocele.
Myotonic dystrophy.
Orchitis (mumps, gonorrhea).
Cryptorchidism.
Chemical exposure.
Irradiation to testes.
Spinal cord injury.
Polyglandular failure.
Idiopathic oligospermia or azoospermia.
Germinal cell aplasia (Sertoli cell–only syndrome).
Idiopathic testicular failure.
Testicular torsion.
Testicular trauma.
Diethylstilbestrol (maternal use during pregnancy leading to in utero estrogen exposure).
Testicular tumor with subsequent irradiation therapy, chemotherapy, or surgery (retroperitoneal lymph node dissection or orchiectomy).

SECONDARY

Delayed puberty.
Kallmann's syndrome.
Isolated gonadotropin deficiency.
Prader-Labhart-Willi syndrome.
Lawrence-Moon-Biedl syndrome.
Central nervous system irradiation.
Prepubertal panhypopituitarism.
Postpubertal panhypopituitarism.
Hypogonadism secondary to hyperprolactinemia.
Adrenogenital syndrome.
Chronic liver disease.
Chronic renal failure/uremia.
Hemochromatosis.
Cushing's syndrome.
Malnutrition.
Massive obesity.
Sickle cell anemia.
Hyper/hypothyroidism.
Anabolic steroid use.

TESTICULAR PAIN

ICD-9CM # 608.9

Testicular torsion.
Trauma.
Epididymitis.
Orchitis.
Neoplasm.
Urolithiasis.
Inguinal hernia.
Infection (cellulitis, abscess, folliculitis).
Anxiety.

TESTICULAR SIZE VARIATIONS[10]

ICD-9CM # 608.3 Testicular Atrophy
          608.89 Testicular Mass
          257.2 Hypogonadism

SMALL TESTES

Hypothalamic-pituitary dysfunction.
Gonadotropin deficiency.
Growth hormone deficiency.
Normal variant.
Primary hypogonadism.

Autoimmune destruction, chemotherapy, cryptorchidism, irradiation, Klinefelter's syndrome, orchiditis, testicular regression syndrome, torsion, trauma.

LARGE TESTES

Adrenal rest tissue.
Compensatory.
Fragile X syndrome.
Idiopathic.
Tumor.

TETANUS[26]

ICD-9CM # 037

Acute abdomen.
Black widow spider bite.
Dental abscess.
Dislocated mandible.
Dystonic reaction.
Encephalitis.
Head trauma.
Hyperventilation syndrome.
Hypocalcemia.
Meningitis.
Peritonsillar abscess.
Progressive fluctuating muscular rigidity (stiff-man syndrome).
Psychogenic.
Rabies.
Sepsis.
Subarachnoid hemorrhage.
Status epilepticus.
Strychnine poisoning.
Temporomandibular joint syndrome.

THROMBOCYTOPENIA

ICD-9CM # 287.3 Congenital or Primary
287.4 Secondary
287.5 Thrombocytopenia NOS

INCREASED DESTRUCTION
Immunologic
Drugs: quinine, quinidine, digitalis, procainamide, thiazide diuretics, sulfonamides, phenytoin, aspirin, penicillin, heparin, gold, meprobamate, sulfa drugs, phenylbutazone, nonsteroidal anti-inflammatory drugs (NSAIDs), methyldopa, cimetidine, furosemide, INH, cephalosporins, chlorpropamide, organic arsenicals, chloroquine, platelet glycoprotein IIb/IIIa receptor inhibitors, ranitidine, indomethacin, carboplatin, ticlopidine, clopidogrel.
Idiopathic thrombocytopenic purpura (ITP).
Transfusion reaction: transfusion of platelets with plasminogen activator (PLA) in recipients without PLA-1.
Fetal/maternal incompatibility.
Collagen vascular diseases (e.g., SLE).
Autoimmune hemolytic anemia.
Lymphoreticular disorders (e.g., CLL).
Nonimmunologic
Prosthetic heart valves.
Thrombotic thrombocytopenic purpura (TTP).
Sepsis.
DIC.
Hemolytic-uremic syndrome (HUS).
Giant cavernous hemangioma.

DECREASED PRODUCTION

Abnormal marrow.
Marrow infiltration (e.g., leukemia, lymphoma, fibrosis).
Marrow suppression (e.g., chemotherapy, alcohol, radiation).
Hereditary disorders.
Wiskott-Aldrich syndrome: X-linked disorder characterized by thrombocytopenia, eczema, and repeated infections.
May-Hegglin anomaly: increased megakaryocytes but ineffective thrombopoiesis.
Vitamin deficiencies (e.g., vitamin B_{12}, folic acid).

SPLENIC SEQUESTRATION, HYPERSPLENISM

DILUTIONAL, AS A RESULT OF MASSIVE TRANSFUSION

THROMBOCYTOPENIA, IN PREGNANCY[20]

ICD-9CM # 287.4

Incidental thrombocytopenia of pregnancy (gestational thrombocytopenia).
Preeclampsia/eclampsia.*
Disseminated intravascular coagulation (DIC) secondary to:
Abruptio placentae.
Endometritis.
Amniotic fluid embolism.
Retained fetus.
Preeclampsia/eclampsia:*
Peripartum/postpartum thrombotic microangiopathy.
Thrombotic thrombocytopenic purpura.
Hemolytic-uremic syndrome.

---

*Preeclampsia/eclampsia usually is not associated with overt DIC.

THROMBOCYTOPENIA, INHERITED DISORDERS[1]

ICD-9CM # 287.3

Amegakaryocytic thrombocytopenia.
Thrombocytopenia–absent radii.
MYH9-related thrombocytopenia:
May-Hegglin anomaly.
Fechtner syndrome.
Epstein syndrome.
Sebastian syndrome.
X-linked macrothrombocytopenia.
Wiskott-Aldrich syndrome.
X-linked thrombocytopenia.
Thrombocytopenia and radioulnar synostosis.
Familial platelet disorder—AML.
Familial dominant thrombocytopenia.
Paris-Trousseau thrombocytopenia.
Bernard-Soulier syndrome.
Bernard-Soulier carrier/Mediterranean macrothrombocytopenia.

THROMBOCYTOSIS

ICD-9CM # 289.9 Thrombocytosis, Essential

Iron deficiency.

Posthemorrhage.
Neoplasms (GI tract).
CML.
Polycythemia vera.
Myelofibrosis with myeloid metaplasia.
Infections.
After splenectomy.
Postpartum.
Hemophilia.
Pancreatitis.
Cirrhosis.
Idiopathic.

THROMBOSIS OR THROMBOTIC DIATHESIS[1]

ICD-9CM # 444

DIFFERENTIAL DIAGNOSIS OF THE PATIENT PRESENTING WITH THROMBOSIS OR THROMBOTIC DIATHESIS
Inherited (Primary) Hypercoagulable States
Activated protein C resistance caused by factor V Leiden mutation.
Prothrombin gene mutation (G to A transition at position 20210 in the 3-untranslated region).
Antithrombin III deficiency.
Protein C deficiency.
Protein S deficiency.
Dysfibrinogenemias (rare).
Acquired (Secondary) Hypercoagulable States
In association with physiologic or thrombogenic stimuli:
Pregnancy (especially the postpartum period).
Estrogen use (oral contraceptives, hormone replacement therapy).
Immobilization.
Trauma.
Postoperative state.
Advancing age.
Obesity.
Prolonged air travel.
Lupus anticoagulant or antiphospholipid antibody syndrome.
In association with other clinical disorders.
Mixed/Unknown
Activated protein C resistance in the absence of factor V Leiden.
Elevated factor VIII level.
Elevated factor XI level.
Elevated factor IX level.
Elevated thrombin activatable fibrinolysis inhibitor (TAFI) level.
Decreased free tissue factor pathway inhibitor (TFPI) level.
Decreased plasma fibrinolytic activity.

THYROMEGALY

ICD-9CM # varies with specific diagnosis

Goiter.
Graves' disease.
Thyroiditis (lymphocytic, granulomatous, suppurative).
Toxic adenoma.
Neoplasm (primary, metastatic).

TICK-RELATED INFECTIONS

ICD-9CM # 082.0   Rocky Mountain Spotted Fever
066.1   Colorado Tick Fever
088.82   Babesiosis
082.8   Ehrlichiosis
088.81   Lyme Disease

Lyme disease.
Rocky Mountain spotted fever.
Babesiosis.
Tularemia.
Q fever.
Colorado tick fever.
Ehrlichiosis.
Relapsing fever.

TICS

ICD-9CM # 307.20

Tourette's syndrome.
Physiologic tic.
Anxiety disorder.
Huntington's disease.
Medications (e.g., antipsychotics, carbamazepine, phenytoin, phenobarbital).
Encephalitis.
Head trauma.
Schizophrenia.
Carbon monoxide poisoning.
Stroke.
Sydenham's chorea.
Creutzfeldt-Jakob disease.

TORSADES DE POINTES[22]

ICD-9CM # code not available

Antiarrhythmics known to increase the QT interval (e.g., quinidine, procainamide, amiodarone, disopyramide, sotalol).
Tricyclic antidepressants and phenothiazines.
Histamine (H_1) antagonists (e.g., astemizole, terfenadine).
Antiviral and antifungal agents and antibiotics.
Hypokinemia.
Hypomagnesemia.
Insecticide poisoning.
Bradyarrhythmias.
Congenital long QT syndrome.
Subarachnoid hemorrhage.
Chloroquinine, pentamidine.
Cocaine abuse.

TOXIC MEGACOLON, CAUSES[5a]

ICD-9CM # 564.7   Toxic Megacolon

INFLAMMATORY
Ulcerative colitis.
Crohn's disease.

INFECTIOUS
Bacterial.
- *Clostridium difficile* pseudomembranous colitis.
- *Salmonella* (typhoid and nontyphoid).
- *Shigella*.

- *Campylobacter*.
- *Yersinia*.
Parasitic.
- *Entamoeba histolytica*.
- *Cryptosporidium*.
Viral.
- Cytomegalovirus colitis.

OTHER
- Ischemia.
- Kaposi sarcoma.

TRACHEOBRONCHIAL NARROWING ON X-RAY[16a]

ICD-9CM # varies with specific diagnosis

CAUSES OF TRACHEOBRONCHIAL NARROWING

Long-segment/Diffuse Narrowing
Sarcoidosis.
Amyloidosis.
Wegener's granulomatosis.
Relapsing polychondritis.
Tracheobronchopathia osteochondroplastica.
Pemphigoid.
Short-segment Narrowing
Previous intubation or tracheostomy.
Congenital stenosis or web.
Extrinsic compression (from thyroid).
Adenoid cystic carcinoma.
Squamous carcinoma.

TREMOR

ICD-9CM # 781.0 Tremor NOS
333.1 Benign Essential Tremor
333.1 Familial Tremor

REST TREMORS
Parkinson's disease.
Other parkinsonian syndromes (less commonly).
Midbrain (rubral) tremor: rest < postural < kinetic.
Wilson's disease (also acquired hepatocerebral degeneration).
Essential tremor—only if severe: rest < postural and action.

POSTURAL AND ACTION (TERMINAL) TREMORS
Physiologic tremor.
Exaggerated physiologic tremor (these factors can also aggravate other forms of tremor).
  Stress, fatigue, anxiety, emotion.
  Endocrine: hypoglycemia, thyrotoxicosis, pheochromocytoma, adrenocorticosteroids.
  Drugs and toxins: β-agonists, dopamine agonists, amphetamines, lithium, tricyclic antidepressants, neuroleptics, theophylline, caffeine, valproic acid, alcohol withdrawal, mercury (Hatter's shakes), lead, arsenic, others.
Essential tremor (familial or sporadic)
Primary writing tremor.
With other CNS disorders.
  Parkinson's disease.
  Other akinetic-rigid syndromes.
  Idiopathic dystonia, including focal dystonias.

With peripheral neuropathy.
  Charcot-Marie-Tooth syndrome (controversial whether to call this the Roussy-Levy syndrome).
  Variety of other peripheral neuropathies (especially dysgammaglobulinemia).
Cerebellar tremor.

KINETIC (INTENTION) TREMOR
Disease of cerebellar outflow (dentate nucleus and superior cerebellar peduncle): multiple sclerosis, trauma, tumor, vascular disease, Wilson's acquired hepatocerebral degeneration, drugs, toxins (e.g., mercury), others.

MISCELLANEOUS RHYTHMICAL MOVEMENT DISORDERS
Psychogenic tremor.
Orthostatic tremor.
Rhythmical movements in dystonia (dystonic tremor).
Rhythmical myoclonus (segmental myoclonus—e.g., palatal or branchial myoclonus, spinal myoclonus, limb myorhythmia).
Oscillatory myoclonus.
Asterixis.
Clonus.
Epilepsia partialis continua.
Hereditary chin quivering.
Spasmus nutans.
Head bobbing with third ventricular cysts.
Nystagmus.

TREMOR, IN CHILDREN, CAUSES[22a]

ICD-9CM # 781.0   Tremor

BENIGN
Enhanced physiologic tremor.
Shuddering attacks.
Jitteriness.
Spasmus nutans.

STATIC INJURY/STRUCTURAL
Cerebellar malformation.
Stroke (particularly in the midbrain or cerebellum).
Multiple sclerosis.

HEREDITARY/DEGENERATIVE
Familial essential tremor.
Fragile X premutation.
Wilson disease.
Huntington disease.
Juvenile parkinsonism (tremor is rare).
Pallidonigral degeneration.

METABOLIC
Hyperthyroidism.
Hyperadrenergic state (including pheochromocytoma and neuroblastoma).
Hypomagnesemia.
Hypocalcemia.
Hypoglycemia.
Hepatic encephalopathy.
Vitamin B_{12} deficiency.
Inborn errors of metabolism.
Mitochondrial disorders.

DRUGS/TOXINS

Valproate, phenytoin, carbamazepine, lamotrigine, gabapentin, lithium, tricyclic antidepressants, stimulants (cocaine, amphetamine, caffeine, thyroxine, bronchodilators), neuroleptics, cyclosporin, toluene, mercury, thallium, amiodarone, nicotine, lead, manganese, arsenic, cyanide, naphthalene, ethanol, lindane, serotonin reuptake inhibitors.

PERIPHERAL NEUROPATHIES

PSYCHOGENIC

TUBULOINTERSTITIAL DISEASE, ACUTE[14]

ICD-9CM # 584.5

DRUGS

Antibiotics, penicillins, cephalosporins, rifampin.
Sulfonamides: cotrimoxazole, sulfamethoxazole.
NSAIDs: propionic acid derivatives.
Miscellaneous: phenytoin, thiazides, allopurinol, cimetidine, ifosfamide.

INFECTIONS

Invasion of renal parenchyma.
Reaction to systemic infections: streptococcal, diphtheria, hantavirus.

SYSTEMIC DISEASES

Immune mediated: SLE, transplanted kidney, cryoglobulinemias.
Metabolic: Urate, oxalate.
Neoplastic: Lymphoproliferative diseases.

IDIOPATHIC

TUBULOINTERSTITIAL KIDNEY DISEASE[14]

ICD-9CM # 584.5

Ischemic and toxic acute tubular necrosis.
Allergic interstitial nephritis.
Interstitial nephritis secondary to immune complex-related collagen vascular disease (e.g., SLE, Sjögren's).
Granulomatous diseases (sarcoidosis, uveitis).
Pigment-related tubular injury (myoglobinuria, hemoglobinuria).
Hypercalcemia with nephrocalcinosis.
Tubular obstruction (drugs such as indinavir, uric acid in tumor lysis syndrome).
Myeloma kidney or cast nephropathy.
Infection-related interstitial nephritis: *Legionella, Leptospira*.
Infiltrative diseases (e.g., lymphoma).

TUMOR MARKERS ELEVATION[38]

ICD-9CM # 795.8

CAUSES OF ELEVATED LEVELS OF TUMOR MARKERS

Carcinoembryonic Antigen (CEA)

Colonic cancer (higher levels if the tumor is more differentiated or is extensive or has spread to the liver).

Lung or breast cancer; seminoma.
Cigarette smokers.
Cirrhosis, inflammatory bowel disease, rectal polyps, pancreatitis.
Advanced age.

Alpha-Fetoprotein

Hepatocellular cancer: very high titers or a rising titer is strongly suggestive, but >10% of patients do not have an elevated level.
Hepatic regeneration (e.g., cirrhosis, alcoholic or viral hepatitis).
Cancer of the stomach, colon, pancreas, or lung.
Teratocarcinoma or embryonal cell carcinoma (testis, ovary, extragonadal).
Pregnancy.
Ataxia-telangiectasia.
Normal variant.

Prostate-Specific Antigen

Prostate carcinoma (localized disease).
Prostatic hyperplasia.
Prostatitis.
Prostatic infarction.

Cancer-Associated Antigen (CA-19-9)*

Pancreatic carcinoma (80% with advanced, well-differentiated cancer have an elevated level).
Other gastrointestinal cancers: colon, stomach, bile duct.
Acute or chronic pancreatitis.
Chronic liver disease.
Biliary tract disease.

---

*Patients who cannot synthesize Lewis blood group antigens (~5% of the population) do not produce CA-19-9 antigen.

UREMIC ENCEPHALOPATHY, DIFFERENTIAL DIAGNOSIS[12a]

ICD-9CM # 348.30 Uremic Encephalopathy

Differential Diagnosis	Comment
Hypertensive encephalopathy	
Systemic inflammatory response syndrome (SIRS)	Observed in septic patients
Systemic vasculitis	Vasculitis or lupus with cerebral involvement
Drug-induced neurotoxicity	
Analgesics	Meperidine, codeine, morphine, gabapentin
Antibiotics	High-dose penicillins (may cause seizures), acyclovir, ethambutol (optic nerve damage), erythromycin and aminoglycosides (may cause ototoxicity), nitrofurantoin and isoniazid (peripheral neuropathy)
Psychotropics	Lithium, haloperidol, clonazepam, diazepam, chlorpromazine
Immunosuppressants	Cyclosporine, tacrolimus
Chemotherapeutics	Cisplatinum, ifosfamide
Others	High doses of loop diuretics (ototoxic), ephedrine, methyldopa, aluminum
Cerebral atheroembolic disease	Follows recent aortic or cardiac angiography; associated with peripheral manifestations, including lower extremity cyanosis, livedo reticularis, and eosinophilia
Subdural hematoma Posterior leukoencephalopathy	Observed particularly following renal transplantation due to reversible, abnormal permeability of the blood-brain barrier
	Often manifests as headache followed by mental depression, visual loss, and seizures in the context of volume expansion, acute hypertension, and often treatment with corticosteroids or calcineurin inhibitors
	Lesions in the parietal, temporal, and occipital lobes may be seen on imaging studies

URETERAL COLIC[24a]

ICD-9CM # 788.0

DIAGNOSTIC DIFFERENTIALS OF RENAL OR URETERAL COLIC

Acute cholecystitis, acute cholelithiasis.
Acute appendicitis.
Pelvic inflammatory disease.
Diverticulosis and/or diverticulitis.
Intestinal obstruction.
Leaking abdominal aortic aneurysm.
Musculoskeletal sprains.
Herniated disk.
Hepes zoster (shingles).
Gastrointestinal dysfunction with ileus and/or toxic colonic dilatation.

URETERIC OBSTRUCTION, CONGENITAL[16a]

ICD-9CM # 593.4

CONGENITAL CAUSES OF URETERIC OBSTRUCTION

Primary megaureter.
Ureterocele (ectopic and orthotopic).
Ureteric valve.
Distal ureteric stenosis.
Ureteric atresia.
Circumcaval ureter and variants.
Bladder diverticulum.

URETHRAL DISCHARGE AND DYSURIA

ICD-9CM # 788.7 Urethral Discharge
599.9 Urethral Discharge, Bloody
788.1 Dysuria

Urethritis (gonococcal, chlamydial, trichomonal).
Cystitis.
Prostatitis.
Vaginitis (candidiasis, chemical).
Meatal stenosis.
Interstitial cystitis.
Trauma (foreign body, masturbation, horseback or bike riding).

URETHRAL OBSTRUCTION, CHILDREN[16a]

ICD-9CM # 593.4

CAUSES OF URETHRAL OBSTRUCTION IN CHILDREN

Intrinsic Lesions
Valve (posterior, anterior, saccular diverticulum).
Stenosis, atresia.
Inflammatory stricture.
Traumatic stricture:
  External trauma (saddle injury, and so on).
  Iatrogenic trauma (catheter, cystoscopy, surgery).
Urethral "tumors":
  Girls: leiomyoma.
  Boys: polyp, rhabdomyosarcoma.
Miscellaneous (epidemolysis bullosa).
Extrinsic Lesions
Presacral mass dissecting inferiorly (tumor, cyst).
Fecal impaction (Hirschsprung's, postrepair anal atresia, habitual constipation, neuropathy).
Mass originating in genital organs:
  Boys: utricle cyst, prostate rhabdomyosarcoma, seminal vesicle cyst, Cowper's duct cyst.
  Girls: hydrometrocolpos, hydrocolpos, fused labia.

URIC ACID STONES

ICD-9CM # 792.9

Hyperuricemia.
Excessive dietary purine.
Medications (salicylates, allopurinol, probenecid).
Urine pH <5.5 (e.g., diarrhea, high animal protein diet).

Decreased urine output (dehydration, malabsorption, diarrhea, inadequate fluid intake).
Tumor lysis.
Hemolytic anemia.
Myeloproliferative disorders.

URINARY INCONTINENCE, CHILDREN[22a]

ICD-9CM # 788.3 Urinary Incontinence

CAUSES OF URINARY INCONTINENCE IN CHILDHOOD

Overactive bladder.
Infrequent voiding.
Detrusor-sphincter dyssynergia.
Non-neurogenic neurogenic bladder (Hinman syndrome).
Vaginal voiding.
Giggle incontinence.
Cystitis.
Bladder outlet obstruction (posterior urethral valves).
Ectopic ureter and fistula.
Sphincter abnormality (epispadias, exstrophy; urogenital sinus abnormality).
Neuropathic.
Overflow incontinence.
Traumatic.
Iatrogenic.
Behavioral.
Combination.

URINARY RETENTION[24a]

ICD-9CM # 788.20

COMMON CAUSES OF URINARY RETENTION

Obstructive Cause
Urethral stricture.
Enlarged prostate.
Lower genitourinary tract malignancy.
Pelvic malignancy.
Bladder stones.
Foreign body.
Blood clot.
Posterior urethral valves.
Ureterocele.
Primary Detrusor Insufficiency
Detrusor areflexia.
Multiple sclerosis.
Iatrogenic injury during abdominal or back surgery.
Spinal cord injury.
Myelomeningocele.

URINARY RETENTION, ACUTE

ICD-9CM # 788.20

Mechanical obstruction: urethral stone, foreign body, urethral stricture, BPH, prostate carcinoma, prostatitis, trauma with hematoma formation.
Neurogenic bladder.
Neurologic disease (MS, parkinsonism, tabes dorsalis, CVA).
Spinal cord injury.
CNS neoplasm (primary or metastatic).

Spinal anesthesia.
Lower urinary tract instrumentation.
Medications (antihistamines, antidepressants, narcotics, anticholinergics).
Abdominal or pelvic surgery.
Alcohol toxicity.
Pregnancy.
Anxiety.
Encephalitis.
Postoperative pain.
Spina bifida occulta.

URINARY TRACT OBSTRUCTION[14a]

ICD-9CM # varies with specific diagnosis

INTRARENAL

Uric acid nephropathy.
Sulfonamide precipitates.
Acyclovir, indinavir precipitates.
Multiple myeloma.

URETERAL

Intrinsic
Intraluminal.
  Nephrolithiasis.
  Papillary necrosis.
  Blood clots.
  Fungus balls.
Intramural.
  Ureteropelvic junction dysfunction.
  Ureterovesical junction dysfunction.
  Ureteral valve, polyp, or tumor.
  Ureteral stricture.
  • Schistosomiasis.
  • Tuberculosis.
  • Scarring from instrumentation.
  • Drugs (e.g., nonsteroidal anti-inflammatory agents).
Extrinsic
Vascular system.
  Aneurysm: abdominal aorta or iliac vessels.
  Aberrant vessels: ureteropelvic junction.
  Venous: retrocaval ureter.
Gastrointestinal tract.
  Crohn's disease.
  Diverticulitis.
  Appendiceal abscess.
  Colon cancer.
  Pancreatic tumor, abscess, or cyst.
Reproductive system.
  Uterus: pregnancy, prolapse, tumor, endometriosis.
  Ovary: abscess, tumor, ovarian remnants.
  Gartner's duct cyst, tubo-ovarian abscess.
Retroperitoneal disease.
  Retroperitoneal fibrosis: radiation, drugs, idiopathic.
  Inflammatory: tuberculosis, sarcoidosis.
  Hematoma.
  Primary tumor (e.g., lymphoma, sarcoma).
  Metastatic tumor (e.g., cervix, ovarian, bladder, colon).
  Lymphocele.
  Pelvic lipomatosis.

BLADDER
Neurogenic bladder.

Diabetes mellitus.
Spinal cord defect.
Trauma.
Multiple sclerosis.
Stroke.
Parkinson's disease.
Spinal anesthesia.
Anticholinergics.
Bladder neck dysfunction.
Bladder calculus.
Bladder cancer.

URETHRA

Urethral stricture.
Prostate hypertrophy or cancer.
Obstruction from instrumentation.

URINE CASTS
ICD-9CM # 791.7

Normal finding.
Pyelonephritis.
Chronic renal disease.
Nephrotic syndrome.
Acute tubular necrosis.
Interstitial nephritis.
Nephritic syndrome.
Glomerulonephritis.
Eclampsia.
Heavy metal ingestion.
Allograft rejection.
Hypothyroidism.

URINE COLOR ABNORMALITIES[24a]
ICD-9CM # 791.9

COMMON CAUSES OF ABNORMAL URINE COLOR
Colorless
Disease
- Diabetes mellitus.
- Diabetes insipidus.

Drug
- Ethyl alcohol.
- Diuretics.

Miscellaneous
- Overhydration.

Yellow-orange
Drug
- Tetracycline.
- Flutamide.
- Pyridium.
- Azo Gantrisin (Roche Labs, Nutley, NJ).
- Sulfasalazine.
- Vitamin B.

Miscellaneous
- Dehydration.

Milky White
Disease
- Urinary tract infection/pyuria.

Blue-green
Disease
- *Pseudomonas* urinary tract infection.

Drug
- Methylene blue.
- Urised (Polymedica Pharmaceuticals, Woburn, MA).

- Indigo carmine.
- Doan's pills (Novartis Consumer Health, Parsippany, NJ).
- Clorets (Cadbury Adams, Parsippany, NJ).
- Amitriptyline.

Red-brown
Disease
- Hematuria.
- Hemolytic anemia.
- Hemoglobinuria.
- Lead poisoning.
- Mercury poisoning.
- Porphyria.

Drug
- Rifampin.
- Ex-Lax (Novartis Consumer Health, Parsippany, NJ).
- Phenolphthalein.
- Phenothiazines.
- Nitrofurantoin.
- Doxorubicin.

Miscellaneous
- Beets.
- Blackberries.
- Rhubarb.

Brown-black
Disease
- Fecaluria.
- Methemoglobinuria.
- Melaninuria.

Drug
- Metronidazole.
- Methyldopa.
- Methocarbamol.

Miscellaneous
- Fava beans.
- Aloe.

URINE, RED[29]
ICD-9CM # varies with specific diagnosis

WITH A POSITIVE DIPSTICK
Hematuria.
Hemoglobinuria: negative urinalysis.
Myoglobinuria: negative urinalysis.

WITH A NEGATIVE DIPSTICK
Drugs
Aminosalicylic acid.
Deferoxamine mesylate.
Ibuprofen.
Phenacetin.
Phenolphthalein.
Phensuximide.
Rifampin.
Anthraquinone laxatives.
Doxorubicin.
Methyldopa.
Phenazopyridine.
Phenothiazine.
Phenytoin.

Dyes
Azo dyes.
Eosin.

Foods
Beets, berries, maize.
Rhodamine B.

Metabolic
Porphyrins.
Serratia marcescens (red diaper syndrome).
Urate crystalluria.

UROPATHY, OBSTRUCTIVE[36]
ICD-9CM # 599.6

INTRINSIC CAUSES
Intraluminal
Intratubular deposition of crystals (uric acid, sulfas).
Stones.
Papillary tissue.
Blood clots.
Intramural
Functional.
Ureter (ureteropelvic or ureterovesical dysfunction).
Bladder (neurogenic): spinal cord defect or trauma, diabetes, multiple sclerosis, Parkinson's disease, cerebrovascular accidents.
Bladder neck dysfunction.
Anatomic
Tumors.
Infection, granuloma.
Strictures.

EXTRINSIC CAUSES
Originating in the Reproductive System
Prostate: benign hypertrophy or cancer.
Uterus: pregnancy, tumors, prolapse, endometriosis.
Ovary: abscess, tumor, cysts.
Originating in the Vascular System
Aneurysms (aorta, iliac vessels).
Aberrant arteries (ureteropelvic junction).
Venous (ovarian veins, retrocaval ureter).
Originating in the Gastrointestinal Tract
Crohn's disease.
Pancreatitis.
Appendicitis.
Tumors.
Originating in the Retroperitoneal Space
Inflammations.
Fibrosis.
Tumor, hematomas.

UROSEPSIS[24a]
ICD-9CM # 995.91

COMMON CAUSES OF UROSEPSIS
Obstructing ureteral stone with pyonephrosis.
Staghorn calculus with urinary tract infection.
Ureteral obstruction with proximal urinary tract infection.
Urinary retention with urinary tract infection.
Acute prostatitis with prostatic abscess.
Perinephric abscess or renal carbuncle.
Urethral stricture with periurethral abscess.
Fournier gangrene.
Foreign body within urinary tract (e.g., Foley catheter).

UTERINE BLEEDING, ABNORMAL[12]
ICD-9CM # 626.9

PREGNANCY
Threatened abortion.
Incomplete abortion.

Complete abortion.
Molar pregnancy.
Ectopic pregnancy.
Retained products of conception.

OVULATORY

Vulva: infection, laceration, tumor.
Vagina: infection, laceration, tumor, foreign body.
Cervix: polyps, cervical erosion, cervicitis, carcinoma.
Uterus: fibroids (submucous fibroids most likely to cause abnormal bleeding), polyps, adenomyosis, endometritis, intrauterine device, atrophic endometrium.
Pregnancy complications: ectopic pregnancy; threatened, incomplete, complete abortion; retained products of conception.
Abnormality of clotting system.
Midcycle bleeding.
Halban's disease (persistent corpus luteum).
Menorrhagia.
Pelvic inflammatory disease.

ANOVULATORY

Physiologic causes:
    Puberty.
    Perimenopausal.
Pathologic causes:
    Ovarian failure (FSH over 40 IU/ml).
    Hyperandrogenism.
    Hyperprolactinemia.
    Obesity.
    Hypothalamic dysfunction (polycystic ovaries); LH/FSH ratio greater than 2:1.
    Hyperplasia.
    Endometrial carcinoma.
    Estrogen-producing tumors.
    Hypothyroidism.

UVEITIS, PEDIATRIC AGE

ICD-9CM # 364.3

ANTERIOR UVEITIS

Juvenile rheumatoid arthritis (pauciarticular).
Sarcoidosis.
Trauma.
Tuberculosis.
Kawasaki disease.
Ulcerative colitis.
Postinfectious (enteric or genital) with arthritis and rash.
Spirochetal (syphilis, leptospiral).
Heterochromic iridocyclitis (Fuchs).
Viral (herpes simplex, herpes zoster).
Ankylosing spondylitis.
Stevens-Johnson syndrome.
Idiopathic.
Drugs.

POSTERIOR UVEITIS (CHOROIDITIS—MAY INVOLVE RETINA)

Toxoplasmosis.
Parasites (toxocariasis).
Sarcoidosis.
Tuberculosis.
Viral (rubella, herpes simplex, HIV, cytomegalovirus).

Subacute sclerosing panencephalitis.
Idiopathic.

ANTERIOR AND/OR POSTERIOR UVEITIS

Sympathetic ophthalmia (trauma to other eye).
Vogt-Koyanagi-Harada syndrome (uveo-otocutaneous syndrome: poliosis, vitiligo, deafness, tinnitus, uveitis, aseptic meningitis, retinitis).
Behçet syndrome.
Lyme disease.

VAGINAL BLEEDING, PREGNANCY[7]

ICD-9CM # 626.6 Irregular Vaginal Bleeding

FIRST TRIMESTER

Implantation bleeding.
Abortion.
    Threatened.
    Complete.
    Incomplete.
    Missed.
Ectopic pregnancy.
Neoplasia.
Hydatidiform mole.
Cervix.

THIRD TRIMESTER

Placenta previa.
Placental abruption.
Premature labor.
Choriocarcinoma.

VAGINAL DISCHARGE, PREPUBERTAL GIRLS[19]

ICD-9CM # 623.5 Vaginal Discharge

Irritative (bubble baths, sand).
Poor perineal hygiene.
Foreign body.
Associated systemic illness (group A streptococci, chickenpox).
Infections.
Escherichia coli with foreign body.
Shigella organisms.
Yersinia organisms.
Infections (consider sexual abuse).
    Chlamydia trachomatis.
    Neisseria gonorrhoeae.
    Trichomonas vaginalis.
Tumor (rare).

VALVULAR HEART DISEASE[1]

ICD-9CM # varies with specific diagnosis

MAJOR CAUSES OF VALVULAR HEART DISEASE IN ADULTS

Aortic Stenosis
Bicuspid aortic valve.
Rheumatic fever.
Degenerative stenosis.
Aortic Regurgitation
Bicuspid aortic valve.
Aortic dissection.
Endocarditis.

Rheumatic fever.
Aortic root dilation.
Mitral Stenosis
Rheumatic fever.
Mitral Regurgitation
Chronic
Mitral valve prolapse.
Left ventricular dilation.
Posterior wall myocardial infarction.
Rheumatic fever.
Endocarditis.
Acute
Posterior wall or papillary muscle ischemia.
Papillary muscle or chordal rupture.
Endocarditis.
Prosthetic valve dysfunction.
Systolic anterior motion of mitral valve.
Tricuspid Regurgitation
Functional (annular) dilation.
Tricuspid valve prolapse.
Endocarditis.
Carcinoid heart disease.

VASCULITIS, CLASSIFICATION[26]

ICD-9CM # 447.6

LARGE VESSEL DISEASE

Arteritis
Giant cell arteritis.
Takayasu's arteritis.
Arteritis associated with Reiter's syndrome, ankylosing spondylitis.

MEDIUM AND SMALL VESSEL DISEASE

Polyarteritis Nodosa
Primary (idiopathic).
Associated with viruses (hepatitis B or C, CMV, HIV, herpes zoster).
Associated with malignancy (hairy cell leukemia).
Familial Mediterranean fever.
Granulomatous Vasculitis
Wegener's granulomatosis.
Lymphomatoid granulomatosis.
Behçet's Disease
Kawasaki Disease (Mucocutaneous Lymph Node Syndrome)

PREDOMINANTLY SMALL VESSEL DISEASE

Hypersensitivity Vasculitis (Leukocytoclastic Vasculitis)
Henoch-Schönlein purpura.
Mixed cryoglobulinemia.
Serum sickness.
Vasculitis associated with connective tissue diseases (SLE, Sjögren's syndrome).
Vasculitis associated with specific syndromes:
    Primary biliary cirrhosis.
    Lyme disease.
    Chronic active hepatitis.
    Drug-induced vasculitis.

Differential Diagnosis

II

Churg-Strauss Syndrome
Goodpasture's Syndrome
Erythema Nodosum
Panniculitis
Buerger's Disease (Thrombophlebitis Obliterans)

VASCULITIS (DISEASES THAT MIMIC VASCULITIS)[28]

ICD-9CM # varies with specific disease

EMBOLIC DISEASE

Infectious or marantic endocarditis.
Cardiac mural thrombus.
Atrial myxoma.
Cholesterol embolization syndrome.

NONINFLAMMATORY VESSEL WALL DISRUPTION

Atherosclerosis.
Arterial fibromuscular dysplasia.
Drug effects (vasoconstrictors, anticoagulants).
Radiation.
Genetic disease (neurofibromatosis, Ehlers-Danlos syndrome).
Amyloidosis.
Intravascular malignant lymphoma.

DIFFUSE COAGULATION

Disseminated intravascular coagulation.
Thrombotic thrombocytopenic purpura.
Hemolytic-uremic syndrome.
Protein C and S deficiencies, factor V/Leiden mutation.
Antiphospholipid syndrome.

VEGETATIVE STATE, PERSISTENT[1]

ICD-9CM # 780.03

PERSISTENT VEGETATIVE STATE: COMMON CAUSES*

Trauma (diffuse axonal injury).
Cardiac arrest and hypoperfusion (laminar necrosis of cortical mantle and/or thalamic necrosis).
Bihemispheric infarctions.
Purulent meningitis or encephalitis (cortical injury).
Carbon monoxide.
Prolonged hypoglycemic coma.

---

*A vegetative state may not necessarily begin with coma but can also develop as the end stage of neurodegenerative diseases (e.g., Alzheimer's disease) of adults or children and can accompany severe congenital developmental abnormalities of the brain such as anencephaly.

VENTILATION–PERFUSION MISMATCH ON LUNG SCAN

ICD-9CM # varies with specific disorder

Pulmonary embolism.
Emphysema.
Irradiation.
Pulmonary hypertension.

AV malformations.
Pulmonary thrombosis.
External compression of pulmonary artery (neoplasm, cysts, fibrosing mediastinitis).
Vasculitis.
Tuberculosis.
Pulmonary thrombosis.
Congenital (pulmonary artery hypoplasia, congenital heart disease with upper lobe diversion).
Sequestered segment.
Parasitic lung disease.
Intraluminal obstruction from catheter fragments.

VENTRICULAR FAILURE

ICD-9CM # 429.9 Ventricular Dysfunction

LEFT VENTRICULAR FAILURE

Systemic hypertension.
Valvular heart disease (AS, AR, MR).
Cardiomyopathy, myocarditis.
Bacterial endocarditis.
Myocardial infarction.
Idiopathic hypertrophic subaortic stenosis.

RIGHT VENTRICULAR FAILURE

Valvular heart disease (mitral stenosis).
Pulmonary hypertension.
Bacterial endocarditis (right-sided).
Right ventricular infarction.

BIVENTRICULAR FAILURE

Left ventricular failure.
Cardiomyopathy.
Myocarditis
Arrhythmias.
Anemia.
Thyrotoxicosis.
Arteriovenous fistula.
Paget's disease.
Beriberi.

VERRUCOUS LESIONS

ICD-9CM # varies with specific disorder

Warts.
Seborrheic keratosis.
Lichen simplex.
Acanthosis nigricans.
Scabies (Norwegian, crusted).
Verrucous carcinoma.
Nevus sebaceous.
Deep fungal infection.

VERTIGO

ICD-9CM # 780.4   Vertigo NOS
        386.11 Benign Paroxysmal Positional
        386.2   Central Origin
        386.10 Peripheral
        386.12 Vestibular (Neuronitis)

PERIPHERAL

Otitis media.
Acute labyrinthitis.
Vestibular neuronitis.
Benign positional vertigo.
Meniere's disease.

Ototoxic drugs: streptomycin, gentamicin.
Lesions of the eighth nerve: acoustic neuroma, meningioma, mononeuropathy, metastatic carcinoma.
Mastoiditis.

CNS OR SYSTEMIC

Vertebrobasilar artery insufficiency.
Posterior fossa tumor or other brain tumors.
Infarction/hemorrhage of cerebral cortex, cerebellum, or brain stem.
Basilar migraine.
Metabolic: drugs, hypoxia, anemia, fever.
Hypotension/severe hypertension.
Multiple sclerosis.
CNS infections: viral, bacterial.
Temporal lobe epilepsy.
Arnold–Chiari malformation, syringobulbia.
Psychogenic: ventilation, hysteria.

VESICULOBULLOUS DISEASES[14]

ICD-9CM # 709.8

IMMUNOLOGICALLY MEDIATED DISEASES

Bullous pemphigoid.
Herpes gestationis.
Mucous membrane pemphigoid.
Epidermolysis bullosa acquisita.
Dermatitis herpetiformis.
Pemphigus (vulgaris, foliaceus, paraneoplastic).

HYPERSENSITIVITY DISEASES

Erythema multiforme minor.
Erythema multiforme major (Stevens-Johnson syndrome).
Toxic epidermal necrolysis.

METABOLIC DISEASES

Porphyria cutanea tarda.
Pseudoporphyria.
Diabetic blisters.

INHERITED GENETIC DISORDERS

Epidermolysis bullosa.
  Simplex.
  Junctional.
  Dystrophic.

INFECTIOUS DISEASES

Impetigo.
Staphylococcal scalded skin syndrome.
Herpes simplex.
Varicella.
Herpes zoster.

VISION LOSS, ACUTE, PAINFUL

ICD-9CM # 368.11 Vision Loss, Sudden

Acute angle-closure glaucoma.
Corneal ulcer.
Uveitis.
Endophthalmitis.
Factitious.
Somatization syndrome.
Trauma.

VISION LOSS, ACUTE, PAINLESS

ICD-9CM # 368.11 Vision Loss, Sudden

Retinal artery occlusion.
Optic neuritis.
Retinal vein occlusion.
Vitreous hemorrhage.
Retinal detachment.
Exudative macular degeneration.
CVA.
Ischemic optic neuropathy.
Factitious.
Somatization syndrome, anxiety reaction.

VISION LOSS, CHILDREN

ICD-9CM # 368.9

Craniopharyngioma.
Hereditary optic atrophy.
Optic nerve glioma.
Glioma of chiasm.
Albinism.
Optic nerve hypoplasia.

VISION LOSS, CHRONIC, PROGRESSIVE

ICD-9CM # 369.9 Vision Loss NOS

Cataract.
Macular degeneration.
Cerebral neoplasm.
Refractive error.
Open-angle glaucoma.

VISION LOSS, MONOCULAR, TRANSIENT

ICD-9CM # 369.9

Thromboembolism.
Vasculitis.
Migraine (vasospasm).
Anxiety reaction.
CNS tumor.
Temporal arteritis.
Multiple sclerosis.

VITREOUS HEMORRHAGE[20a]

ICD-9CM # 379.23 Vitreous Hemorrhage

CAUSES OF VITREOUS HEMORRHAGE

Acute posterior vitreous detachment associated either with a retinal tear or avulsion of a peripheral vessel.
Proliferative retinopathies.
- Diabetic.
- Following retinal vein occlusion.
- Sickle cell disease.
- Eales disease.
- Vasculitis.
Miscellaneous retinal disorders.
- Macroaneurysm.
- Telangiectasis.
- Capillary hemangioma.

Trauma.
- Blunt.
- Penetrating.
- Iatrogenic.
Systemic.
- Bleeding disorders.
- Terson syndrome.

VOCAL CORD PARALYSIS

ICD-9CM # 478.30 Unspecified
478.31 Unilateral Partial
478.32 Unilateral Complete
478.33 Bilateral Partial
478.34 Bilateral Complete

Neoplasm: primary or metastatic (e.g., lung, thyroid, parathyroid, mediastinum).
Neck surgery (parathyroid, thyroid, carotid endarterectomy, cervical spine).
Idiopathic.
Viral, bacterial, or fungal infection.
Trauma (intubation, penetrating neck injury).
Cardiac surgery.
RA.
Multiple sclerosis.
Parkinsonism.
Toxic neuropathy.
CVA.
CNS abnormalities: hydrocephalus, Arnold–Chiari malformation, meningomyelocele.

VOLUME DEPLETION[1]

ICD-9CM # 276.5

GI losses:
Upper: bleeding, nasogastric suction, vomiting.
Lower: bleeding, diarrhea, enteric or pancreatic fistula, tube drainage.
Renal losses:
Salt and water: diuretics, osmotic diuresis, postobstructive diuresis, acute tubular necrosis (recovery phase), salt-losing nephropathy, adrenal insufficiency, renal tubular acidosis.
Water loss: diabetes insipidus.
Skin and respiratory losses:
Sweat, burns, insensible losses.
Sequestration without external fluid loss:
Intestinal obstruction, peritonitis, pancreatitis, rhabdomyolysis, internal bleeding.

VOLUME EXCESS[1]

ICD-9CM # varies with specific diagnosis

PRIMARY RENAL SODIUM RETENTION (INCREASED EFFECTIVE CIRCULATING VOLUME)

Renal failure, nephritic syndrome, acute glomerulonephritis.
Primary hyperaldosteronism.
Cushing's syndrome.
Liver disease.

SECONDARY RENAL SODIUM RETENTION (DECREASED EFFECTIVE CIRCULATING VOLUME)

Heart failure.
Liver disease.
Nephrotic syndrome (minimal change disease).
Pregnancy.

VOMITING

ICD-9CM # 787.03

GI disturbances:
Obstruction: esophageal, pyloric, intestinal.
Infections: viral or bacterial enteritis, viral hepatitis, food poisoning, gastroenteritis.
Pancreatitis.
Appendicitis.
Biliary colic.
Peritonitis.
Perforated bowel.
Diabetic gastroparesis.
Other: gastritis, PUD, IBD, GI tract neoplasms.
Drugs: morphine, digitalis, cytotoxic agents, bromocriptine.
Severe pain: MI, renal colic.
Metabolic disorders: uremia, acidosis/alkalosis, hyperglycemia, DKA, thyrotoxicosis.
Trauma: blows to the testicles, epigastrium.
Vertigo.
Reye's syndrome.
Increased intracranial pressure.
CNS disturbances: trauma, hemorrhage, infarction, neoplasm, infection, hypertensive encephalopathy, migraine.
Radiation sickness.
Nausea and vomiting of pregnancy, hyperemesis gravidarum.
Motion sickness.
Bulimia, anorexia nervosa.
Psychogenic: emotional disturbances, offensive sights or smells.
Severe coughing.
Pyelonephritis.
Boerhaave's syndrome.
Carbon monoxide poisoning.

VULVAR LESIONS[12]

ICD-9CM # 625.8 Vulvar Mass
098.0 Vulvar Ulcer, Gonococcal
091.0 Vulvar Ulcer, Syphilitic
616.51 Behçet's
624.0 Leukoplakia
624.8 Dysplasia
233.3 Carcinoma
616.9 Inflammatory Lesion
624.4 Vulvar Scar (Old)
624.1 Vulvar Atrophy

RED LESION

Infection/Infestation
Fungal infection:
Candida.
Tinea cruris.
Intertrigo.
Pityriasis versicolor.
Sarcoptes scabiei.
Erythrasma: *Corynebacterium minutissimum.*

Differential Diagnosis

Granuloma inguinale: Calymmatobacterium granulomatis.
Folliculitis: *Staphylococcus aureus.*
Hidradenitis suppurativa.
Behçet's syndrome.

Inflammation

Reactive vulvitis.
Chemical irritation:
  Detergent.
  Dyes.
  Perfume.
  Spermicide.
  Lubricants.
  Hygiene sprays.
  Podophyllum.
  Topical 5-FU.
  Saliva.
  Gentian violet.
  Semen.
Mechanical trauma: scratching.
Vestibular adenitis.
Essential vulvodynia.
Psoriasis.
Seborrheic dermatitis.

Neoplasm

Vulvar intraepithelial neoplasia (VIN):
  Mild dysplasia.
  Moderate dysplasia.
  Severe dysplasia.
  Carcinoma-in-situ.
Vulvar dystrophy.
Bowen's disease.
Invasive cancer:
  Squamous cell carcinoma.
  Malignant melanoma.
  Sarcoma.
  Basal cell carcinoma.
  Adenocarcinoma.
  Paget's disease.
  Undifferentiated.

WHITE LESION

Vulvar dystrophy:
  Lichen sclerosus.
  Vulvar dystrophy.
  Vulvar hyperplasia.
  Mixed dystrophy.
VIN.
Vitiligo.
Partial albinism.
Intertrigo.
Radiation treatment.

DARK LESION

Lentigo.
Nevi (mole).
Neoplasm (see "Neoplasm, Vulvar," below).
Reactive hyperpigmentation.
Seborrheic keratosis.
Pubic lice.

ULCERATIVE LESION

Infection

Herpes simplex.
Vaccinia.
Treponema pallidum.
Granuloma inguinale.
Pyoderma.
Tuberculosis.

Noninfectious

Behçet's disease.
Crohn's disease.
Pemphigus.
Pemphigoid.
Hidradenitis suppurativa (see "Neoplasm, Vulvar," below).

Neoplasm

Basal cell carcinoma.
Squamous cell carcinoma.
Vulvar tumor <1 cm:
  Condyloma acuminatum.
  Molluscum contagiosum.
  Epidermal inclusion.
  Vestibular cyst.
  Mesonephric duct.
  VIN.
  Hemangioma.
  Hidradenoma.
  Neurofibroma.
  Syringoma.
  Accessory breast tissue.
  Acrochordon.
  Endometriosis.
  Fox-Fordyce disease.
  Pilonidal sinus.
Vulvar tumor >1 cm:
  Bartholin cyst or abscess.
  Lymphogranuloma venereum.
  Fibroma.
  Lipoma.
  Verrucous carcinoma.
  Squamous cell carcinoma.
  Hernia.
  Edema.
  Hematoma.
  Acrochordon.
  Epidermal cysts.
  Neurofibromatosis.
  Accessory breast tissue.

WEAKNESS, ACUTE, EMERGENT[26]

ICD-9CM # 780.7

Demyelinating disorders (Guillain-Barré, chronic inflammatory demyelinating polyneuropathy [CIDP]).
Myasthenia gravis.
Infectious (poliomyelitis, diphtheria).
Toxic (botulism, tick paralysis, paralytic shellfish toxin, puffer fish, newts).
Metabolic (acquired or familial hypokalemia, hypophosphatemia, hypermagnesemia).
Metal poisoning (arsenic, thallium).
Porphyria.

WEAKNESS, GRADUAL ONSET

ICD-9CM # 780.7

Depression.
Malingering.
Anemia.
Hypothyroidism.
Medications (e.g., sedatives, antidepressants, narcotics).
CHF.

Renal failure.
Liver failure.
Respiratory insufficiency.
Alcoholism.
Nutritional deficiencies.
Disorders of motor unit.
Basal ganglia disorders.
Upper motor neuron lesions.

WEAKNESS, NONNEUROMUSCULAR CAUSES

ICD-9CM # 780.79

Anxiety disorder.
Infectious process.
Anemia.
Renal insufficiency.
Hyperventilation.
Malignancy.
Hypothyroidism.
Hypotension.
Hypercapnia.
Hypoglycemia.
Cardiac arrhythmias.
Hepatic insufficiency.
Electrolyte imbalance.
Malnutrition.
Cerebrovascular insufficiency.

WEIGHT GAIN

ICD-9CM # 783.1 Abnormal Weight Gain
278.00 Obesity

Sedentary lifestyle.
Fluid overload.
Discontinuation of tobacco abuse.
Endocrine disorders (hypothyroidism, hyperinsulinism associated with maturity-onset DM, Cushing's syndrome, hypogonadism, insulinoma, hyperprolactinemia, acromegaly).
Medications (nutritional supplements, oral contraceptives, glucocorticoids, etc.).
Anxiety disorders with compulsive eating.
Laurence-Moon-Biedl syndrome, Prader-Willi syndrome, other congenital diseases.
Hypothalamic injury (rare; <100 cases reported in medical literature).

WEIGHT LOSS

ICD-9CM # 783.2 Abnormal Weight Loss

Malignancy.
Psychiatric disorders (depression, anorexia nervosa).
New-onset DM.
Malabsorption.
COPD.
AIDS.
Uremia, liver disease.
Thyrotoxicosis, pheochromocytoma, carcinoid syndrome.
Addison's disease.
Intestinal parasites.
Peptic ulcer disease.
Inflammatory bowel disease.
Food faddism.
Postgastrectomy syndrome.

WHEEZING
ICD-9CM # 786.09

Asthma.
COPD.
Interstitial lung disease.
Infections (pneumonia, bronchitis, bronchiolitis, epiglottitis).
Cardiac asthma.
GERD with aspiration.
Foreign body aspiration.
Pulmonary embolism.
Anaphylaxis.
Obstruction of airway (neoplasm, goiter, edema or hemorrhage from trauma, aneurysm, congenital abnormalities, strictures, spasm).
Carcinoid syndrome.

WHEEZING, PEDIATRIC AGE[4]
ICD-9CM # 786.09 Wheezing

Reactive airways disease.
Atopic asthma.
Infection-associated airway reactivity.
Exercise-induced asthma.
Salicylate-induced asthma and nasal polyposis.
Asthmatic bronchitis.
Other hypersensitivity reactions:
  Hypersensitivity pneumonitis.
  Tropical eosinophilia.
  Visceral larva migrans.
  Allergic bronchopulmonary aspergillosis.
Aspiration:
  Foreign body.
  Food, saliva, gastric contents.
  Laryngotracheoesophageal cleft.
  Tracheoesophageal fistula, H-type.
  Pharyngeal incoordination or neuromuscular weakness.
Cystic fibrosis.
Primary ciliary dyskinesia.
Cardiac failure.
Bronchiolitis obliterans.
Extrinsic compression of airways:
  Vascular ring.
  Enlarged lymph node.
  Mediastinal tumor.
  Lung cysts.
Tracheobronchomalacia.
Endobronchial masses.
Gastroesophageal reflux.
Pulmonary hemosiderosis.
Sequelae of bronchopulmonary dysplasia.
"Hysterical" glottic closure.
Cigarette smoke, other environmental insults.

WRIST AND HAND PAIN, IN DIFFERENT AGE GROUPS[8]
ICD-9CM # 959.3

COMMON CAUSES OF WRIST AND HAND PAIN IN DIFFERENT AGE GROUPS

Childhood (2-10 yr)
Intraarticular:
Infection.

Periarticular:
Fracture.
Osteomyelitis.
Adolescence (10-18 yr)
Intraarticular:
Infection.
Periarticular:
Trauma.
Osteomyelitis.
Tumors.
Ganglion.
Idiopathic wrist pain.
Early Adulthood (18-30 yr)
Intraarticular:
Inflammatory arthritis.
Infection.
Osteoarthritis.
Periarticular:
Peripheral nerve entrapment.
Tendonitis.
Referred:
Cervical.
Adulthood (30-50 yr)
Intraarticular:
Inflammatory arthritis.
Infection.
Osteoarthritis.
Periarticular:
Peripheral nerve entrapment.
Tendonitis.
Referred:
Cervical.
Chest.
Cardiac.
Old age (>50 yr)
Intraarticular:
Inflammatory arthritis.
Osteoarthritis.
Periarticular:
Peripheral nerve entrapment.
Tendonitis.
Referred:
Cervical.
Chest.
Cardiac.

WRIST PAIN
ICD-9CM # 959.3

MECHANICAL
Osteoarthritis.
Ligament tear.
Fracture.
Ganglion.
De Quervain's tenosynovitis.
Avascular necrosis (scaphoid, lunate).
Nonunion of scaphoid or lunate.
Neoplasm.

METABOLIC
Pregnancy.
Diabetes.
Gout.
Pseudogout.
Paget's disease.
Acromegaly.
Hypothyroidism.
Hyperparathyroidism.

INFECTIOUS
Osteomyelitis.
Septic arthritis.
Cat-scratch disease.
Tick bite (Lyme disease, babesiosis).
Tuberculosis.

NEUROLOGIC
Peripheral neuropathy.
Nerve injury (median, ulnar, radial nerve).
Thoracic outlet compression syndrome.
Distal posterior interosseous nerve syndrome.

RHEUMATOLOGIC
Psoriasis.
RA.
SLE, mixed connective tissue disorder (MCTD).
Scleroderma.

MISCELLANEOUS
Granulomatous (sarcoidosis).
Amyloidosis.
Multiple myeloma.
Leukemia.

XEROPHTHALMIA[28]
ICD-9CM # 372.53 Xerophthalmia

MEDICATIONS
Tricyclic antidepressants: amitriptyline (Elavil), doxepin (Sinequan).
Antihistamines: diphenhydramine (Benadryl), chlorpheniramine (Chlor-Trimeton), promethazine (Phenergan), and many cold and decongestant preparations.
Anticholinergic agents: antiemetics such as scopolamine, antispasmodic agents such as oxybutynin chloride (Ditropan).

ABNORMALITIES OF EYELID FUNCTION
Neuromuscular disorders.
Aging.
Thyrotoxicosis.

ABNORMALITIES OF TEAR PRODUCTION
Hypovitaminosis A.
Stevens-Johnson syndrome.
Familial diseases affecting sebaceous secretions.

ABNORMALITIES OF CORNEAL SURFACES
Scarring from past injuries and herpes simplex infection.

XEROSTOMIA[28]
ICD-9CM # 527.7

MEDICATIONS
Tricyclic antidepressants: amitriptyline (Elavil), doxepin (Sinequan).
Antihistamines: diphenhydramine (Benadryl), chlorpheniramine (Chlor-Trimeton), promethazine (Phenergan), and many cold and decongestant preparations.

Differential Diagnosis

II

Anticholinergic agents: antiemetics such as scopolamine, antispasmodic agents such as oxybutynin chloride (Ditropan).

DEHYDRATION

Debility.
Fever.

POLYURIA

Alcohol intake.
Arrhythmia.
Diabetes.

PREVIOUS HEAD AND NECK IRRADIATION SYSTEMIC DISEASES

Sjögren's syndrome.
Sarcoidosis.
Amyloidosis.
Human immunodeficiency virus (HIV) infection.
Graft-versus-host disease.

YELLOW URINE

ICD-9CM # 788.69

Normal coloration.
Concentrated urine.
Use of multivitamin supplements.
Diet rich in carrots.
Use of Cascara.
Urinary tract infection

REFERENCES

1. Andreoli TE (ed): *Cecil essentials of medicine,* ed 5, Philadelphia, 2001, Saunders.
1a. Ballinger A: *Kumar & Clark's essentials of clinical medicine,* ed 6, Edinburgh, 2012, Saunders.
2. Barkin RM, Rosen P: *Emergency pediatrics: a guide to ambulatory care,* ed 5, St Louis, 1998, Mosby.
3. Baude AI: *Infectious diseases and medical microbiology,* ed 2, Philadelphia, 1986, Saunders.
4. Behrman RE: *Nelson textbook of pediatrics,* ed 16, Philadelphia, 2000, Saunders.
5. Callen JP: *Color atlas of dermatology,* ed 2, Philadelphia, 2000, WB Saunders.
5a. Cameron JL, Cameron AM: *Current surgical therapy,* ed 10, Philadelphia, 2011, Saunders.
6. Canoso J: *Rheumatology in primary care,* Philadelphia, 1997, Saunders.

7. Carlson KJ: *Primary care of women,* ed 2, St Louis, 2000, Mosby.
8. Carr A, Hamilton W: *Orthopedics in primary care,* ed 2, Philadelphia, 2005, Saunders.
9. Conn R: *Current diagnosis,* ed 9, Philadelphia, 1997, Saunders.
10. Copeland LJ: *Textbook of gynecology,* ed 2, Philadelphia, 2000, Saunders.
11. Custer JW, Rau RE: *The Harriet Lane handbook,* ed 18, St Louis, Mosby, 2009.
12. Danakas G (ed): *Practical guide to the care of the gynecologic/obstetric patient,* St Louis, 1997, Mosby.
12a. Floege J et al: *Comprehensive clinical nephrology,* ed 4, Philadelphia, 2010, Saunders.
12b. Fuhrman BP et al: *Pediatric critical care,* ed 4, Philadelphia, 2011, Saunders.
13. Goldberg RJ: *The care of the psychiatric patient,* ed 3, St Louis, 2006, Mosby.
14. Goldman L, Ausiello D: *Cecil textbook of medicine,* ed 21, Philadelphia, 2004, Saunders.
14a. Goldman L, Schafer AI: *Goldman's Cecil medicine,* ed 24, Philadelphia, 2012, Saunders.
15. Goldman L, Braunwauld E (eds): *Primary cardiology,* Philadelphia, 1998, Saunders.
16. Gorbach SL: *Infectious diseases,* ed 2, Philadelphia, 1998, Saunders.
16a. Grainger RG, Allison D: *Grainger & Allison's diagnostic radiology, a textbook of medical imaging,* ed 4, London, 2001, Churchill Livingstone.
17. Harrington J: *Consultation in internal medicine,* ed 2, St Louis, 1997, Mosby.
18. Henry JB: *Clinical diagnosis and management by laboratory methods,* ed 20, Philadelphia, 2001, Saunders.
18b. Hochberg MC et al: *Rheumatology,* ed 5, St. Louis, 2011, Mosby.
19. Hoekelman R: *Primary pediatric care,* ed 3, St Louis, 1997, Mosby.
20. Hoffmann R et al: *Hematology: basic principles and practice,* ed 5, Philadelphia, 2009, Churchill Livingstone.
20a. Kanski JJ, Bowling B: *Clinical ophthalmology, a systematic approach,* ed 7, Philadelphia, 2011, Saunders.
21. Kassirer J (ed): *Current therapy in adult medicine,* ed 4, St Louis, 1998, Mosby.
22. Khan MG: *Rapid ECG interpretation,* Philadelphia, 2003, Saunders.
22a. Kliegman RM et al: *Nelson textbook of pediatrics,* ed 19, Philadelphia, 2011, Saunders.

23. Kliegman R: *Practical strategies in pediatric diagnosis and therapy,* Philadelphia, 1996, Saunders.
24. Klippel J (ed): *Practical rheumatology,* London, 1995, Mosby.
24a. Lipshultz LI, Khera M, Atwal DT: *Urology and the primary care practitioner,* ed 3, Philadelphia, 2008, Elsevier.
25. Mandell GL: *Mandell, Douglas, and Bennett's principles and practice of infectious diseases,* ed 6, New York, 2005, Churchill Livingstone.
26. Marx J (ed): *Rosen's emergency medicine: concepts and clinical practice,* ed 5, St Louis, 2002, Mosby.
27. Moore WT, Eastman RC: *Diagnostic endocrinology,* ed 2, St Louis, 1996, Mosby.
28. Noble J (ed): *Primary care medicine,* ed 3, St Louis, 2001, Mosby.
29. Nseyo UO: *Urology for primary care physicians,* Philadelphia, 1999, Saunders.
30. Palay D (ed): *Ophthalmology for the primary care physician,* St Louis, 1997, Mosby.
31. Rakel RE: *Principles of family practice,* ed 6, Philadelphia, 2002, Saunders.
32. Schwarz MI: *Interstitial lung disease,* ed 2, St Louis, 1993, Mosby.
33. Seller RH: *Differential diagnosis of common complaints,* ed 4, Philadelphia, 2000, Saunders.
34. Siedel HM (ed): *Mosby's guide to physical examination,* ed 4, St Louis, 1999, Mosby.
34a. Souhami RL, Moxham J: *Textbook of medicine,* ed 4, London, 2002, Churchill Livingstone.
35. Specht N: *Practical guide to diagnostic imaging,* St Louis, 1998, Mosby.
36. Stein JH (ed): *Internal medicine,* ed 5, St Louis, 1998, Mosby.
37. Swain R, Snodgrass JG: Managing groin pain, *Phys Sportmed* 23:56, 1995.
38. Talley NJ, Martin CJ: *Clinical gastroenterology,* ed 2, Sydney, 2006, Churchill Livingstone.
38a. Tschudy MM, Arcara KM: *The Harriet Lane handbook,* ed 19, Philadelphia, 2012, Mosby.
38b. Vincent JL et al: *Textbook of critical care,* ed 6, Philadelphia, 2011, Saunders.
39. Weinberg SE et al: *Principles of pulmonary medicine,* ed 5, Philadelphia, 2008, Saunders.
40. Wiederholt WC: *Neurology for non-neurologists,* ed 4, Philadelphia, 2000, Saunders.
41. Wilson JD: *Williams textbook of endocrinology,* ed 9, Philadelphia, 1998, Saunders.

Clinical Algorithms

SECTION III

Clinical Algorithms

PLEASE NOTE: These algorithms are designed to assist clinicians in the evaluation and treatment of patients. They may not apply to all patients with a particular disorder and are not intended to replace the clinician's individual judgment.

Additional algorithms available at www.expertconsult.com:

Clinical Algorithms

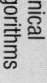

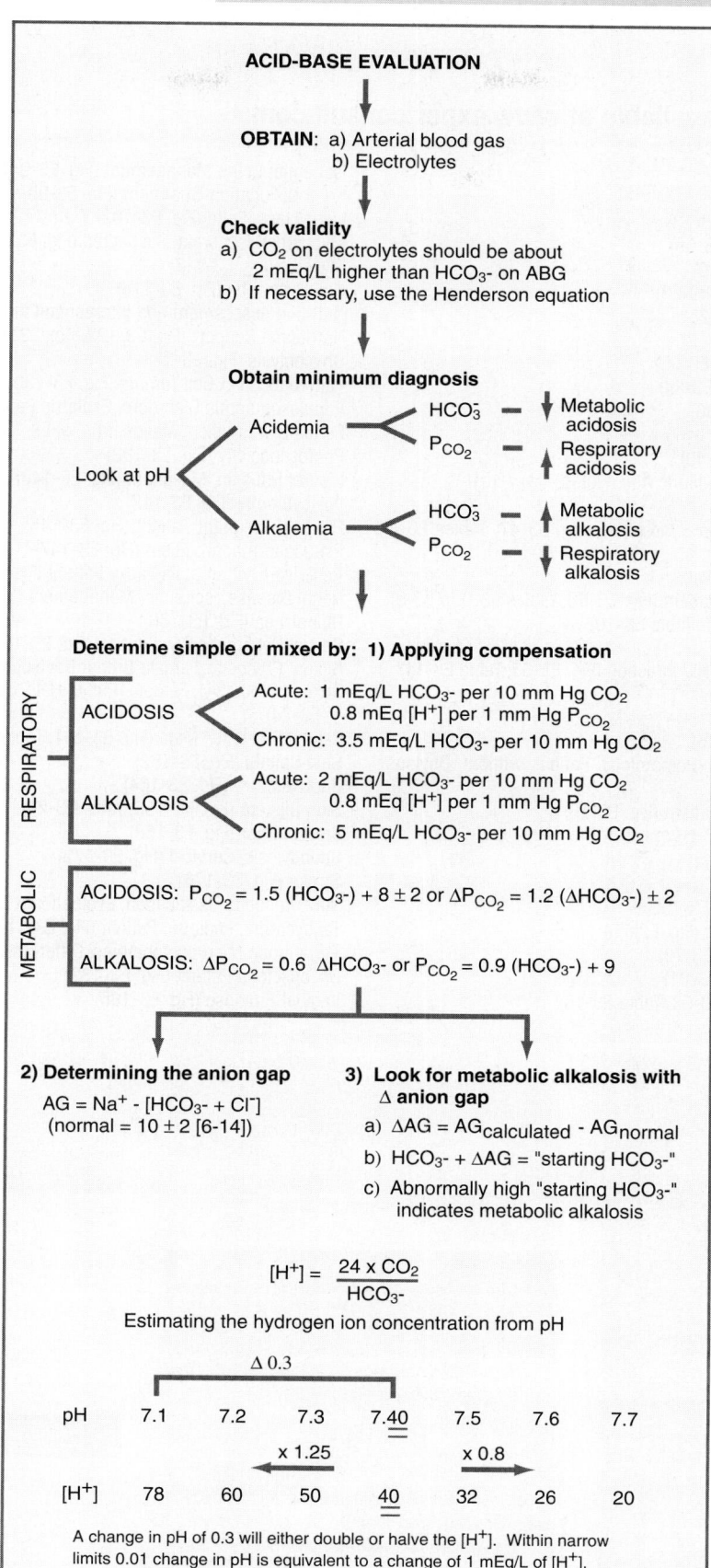

FIGURE 3-1 Scheme for assessing acid-base homeostasis. (From Andreoli TE [ed]: *Cecil essentials of medicine*, ed 7,

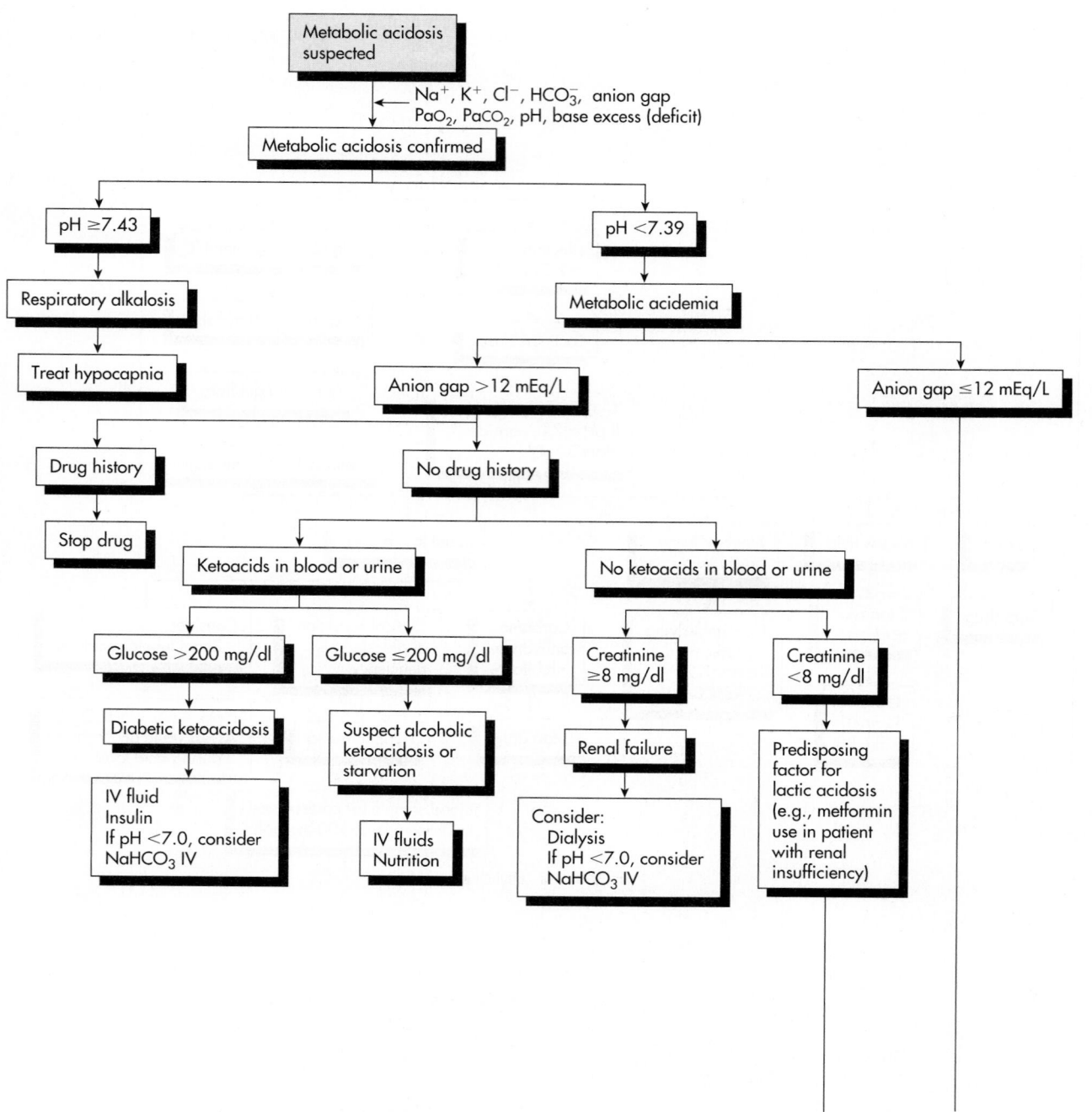

FIGURE 3-2 Suspected metabolic acidosis. (Modified from Greene HL, Johnson WP, Lemcke D [eds]: *Decision making in medicine*, ed 2, St Louis, 1998, Mosby.)

(Continued on next page)

FIGURE 3-2 (Continued)

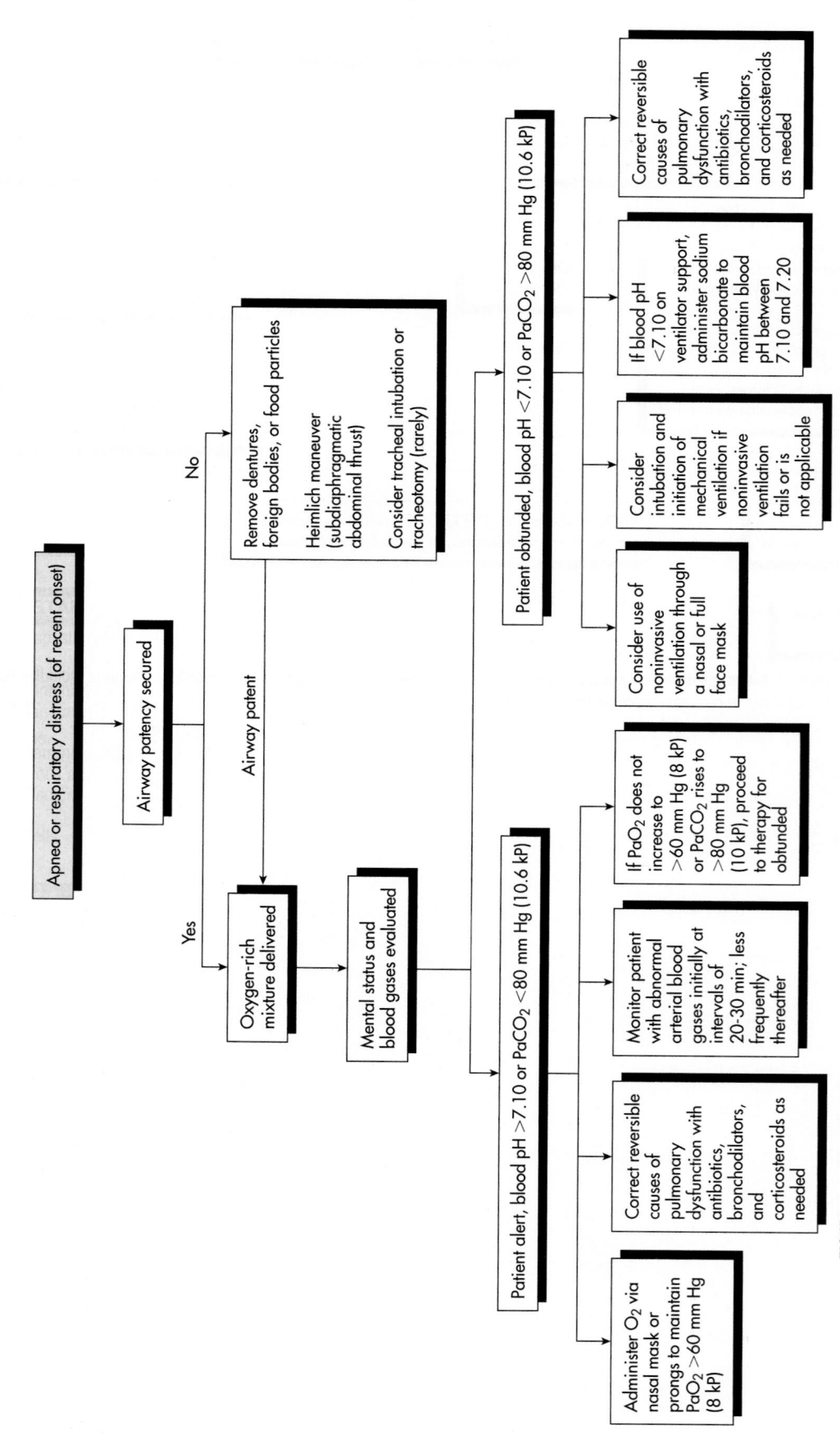

FIGURE 3-3 Algorithm for management of acute respiratory acidosis. (From Feehally J, Floege J, Johnson RJ: *Comprehensive clinical nephrology*, ed 3, St Louis, 2007, Mosby.)

Apnea or respiratory distress (of recent onset)

Airway patency secured

No

Remove dentures, foreign bodies, or food particles

Heimlich maneuver (subdiaphragmatic abdominal thrust)

Consider tracheal intubation or tracheotomy (rarely)

Airway patent

Yes

Oxygen-rich mixture delivered

Mental status and blood gases evaluated

Patient obtunded, blood pH <7.10 or $PaCO_2$ >80 mm Hg (10.6 kP)

Correct reversible causes of pulmonary dysfunction with antibiotics, bronchodilators, and corticosteroids as needed

If blood pH <7.10 on ventilator support, administer sodium bicarbonate to maintain blood pH between 7.10 and 7.20

Consider intubation and initiation of mechanical ventilation if noninvasive ventilation fails or is not applicable

Consider use of noninvasive ventilation through a nasal or full face mask

Patient alert, blood pH >7.10 or $PaCO_2$ <80 mm Hg (10.6 kP)

If PaO_2 does not increase to >60 mm Hg (8 kP) or $PaCO_2$ rises to >80 mm Hg (10 kP), proceed to therapy for obtunded

Monitor patient with abnormal arterial blood gases initially at intervals of 20-30 min; less frequently thereafter

Correct reversible causes of pulmonary dysfunction with antibiotics, bronchodilators, and corticosteroids as needed

Administer O_2 via nasal mask or prongs to maintain PaO_2 >60 mm Hg (8 kP)

Clinical Algorithms

III

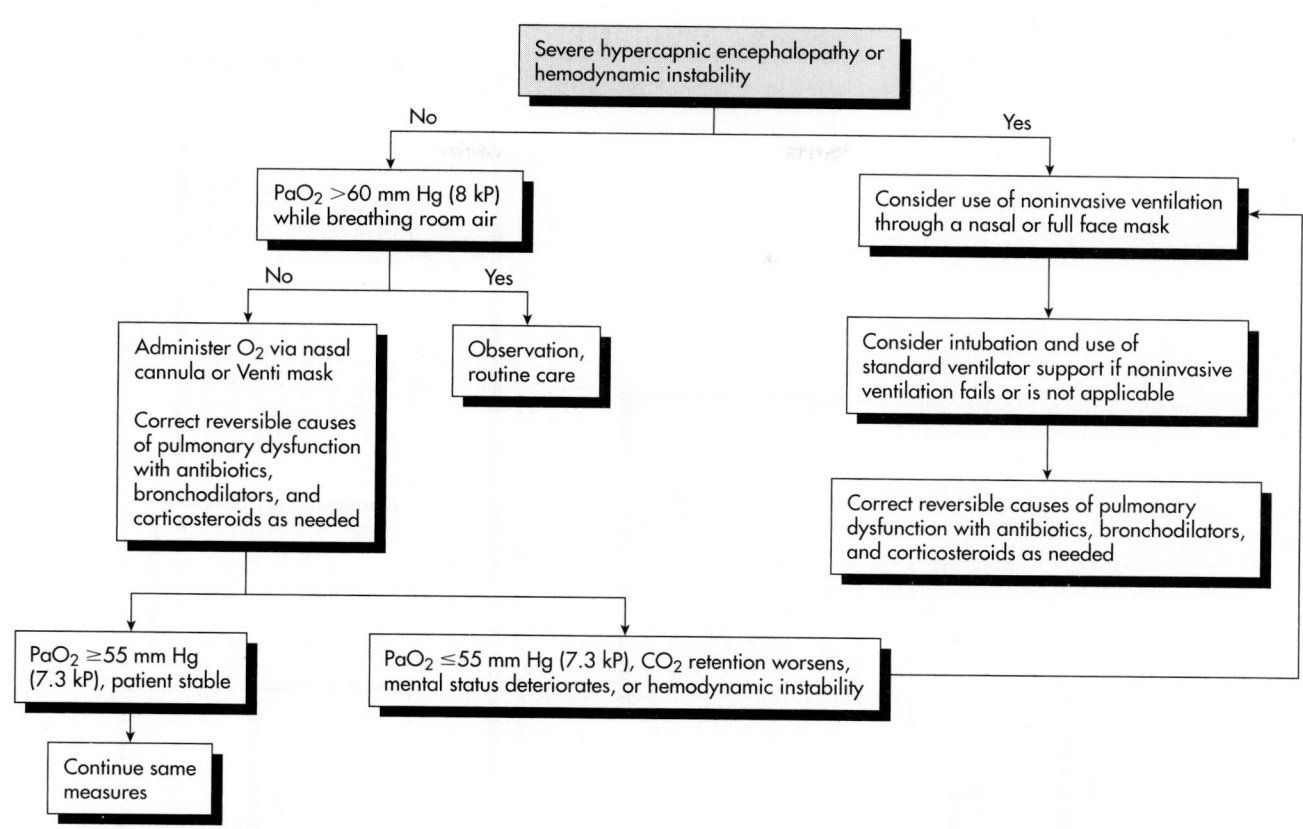

FIGURE 3-4 Algorithm for management of chronic respiratory acidosis. (From Feehally J, Floege J, Johnson RJ: *Comprehensive clinical nephrology,* ed 3, St Louis, 2007, Mosby.)

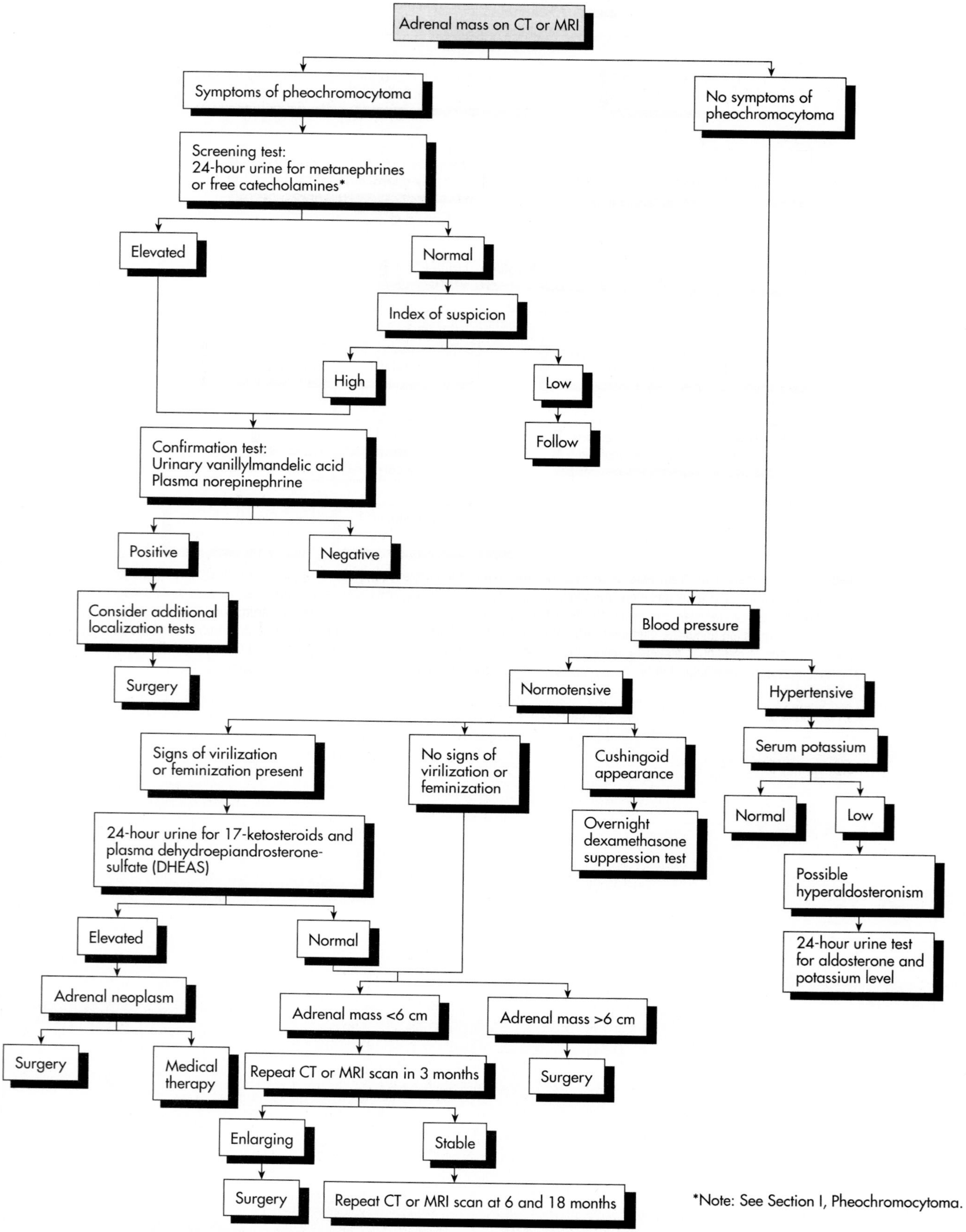

Adrenal mass on CT or MRI

Symptoms of pheochromocytoma

No symptoms of pheochromocytoma

Screening test:
24-hour urine for metanephrines
or free catecholamines*

Elevated

Normal

Index of suspicion

High

Low

Follow

Confirmation test:
Urinary vanillylmandelic acid
Plasma norepinephrine

Positive

Negative

Consider additional
localization tests

Surgery

Blood pressure

Normotensive

Hypertensive

Signs of virilization
or feminization present

No signs of
virilization or
feminization

Cushingoid
appearance

Serum potassium

24-hour urine for 17-ketosteroids and
plasma dehydroepiandrosterone-
sulfate (DHEAS)

Overnight
dexamethasone
suppression test

Normal

Low

Elevated

Normal

Possible
hyperaldosteronism

Adrenal neoplasm

Adrenal mass <6 cm

Adrenal mass >6 cm

24-hour urine test
for aldosterone and
potassium level

Surgery

Medical
therapy

Repeat CT or MRI scan in 3 months

Surgery

Enlarging

Stable

Surgery

Repeat CT or MRI scan at 6 and 18 months

*Note: See Section I, Pheochromocytoma.

FIGURE 3-6 Evaluation of adrenal mass. *CT,* Computed tomography; *MRI,* magnetic resonance imaging. (Modified from
Greene HL, Johnson WP, Lemcke D [eds]: *Decision making in medicine,* ed 2, St Louis, 1998, Mosby.)

Clinical
Algorithms

III

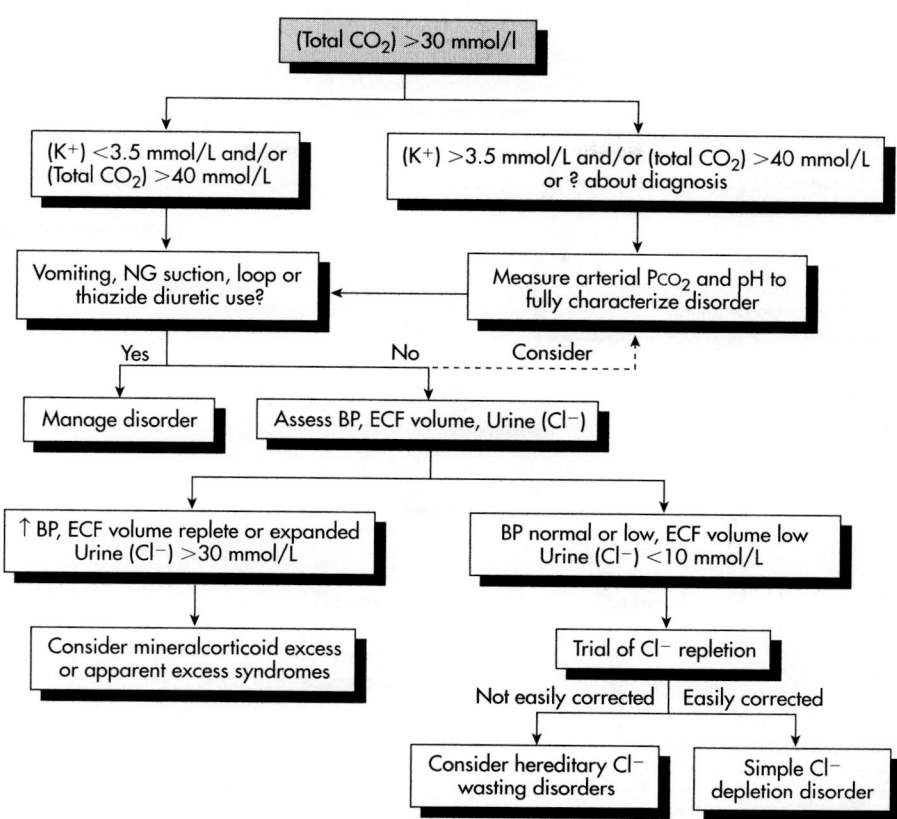

FIGURE 3-7 Approach to diagnosis of metabolic alkalosis. If the increase in [total CO_2] (or serum [HCO_3^-]) is mild and hypokalemia is present, arterial gas measurements are usually not necessary, and a simple algorithm can be used to diagnose Cl^--responsive and Cl^--resistant metabolic alkalosis. If hypokalemia is not present, if the increase in serum [total CO_2] is severe, or if there is a question about the diagnosis, arterial measurement of pH and Pco_2 is recommended to determine whether the condition is due to metabolic alkalosis, respiratory acidosis, or a mixed disorder. *BP,* blood pressure; *ECF,* extracellular fluid; *NG,* nasogastric. (From Floege J et al: *Comprehensive clinical nephrology,* ed 4, Philadelphia, 2010, Saunders.)

ALKALOSIS, RESPIRATORY TREATMENT—cont'd

ICD-9CM # 276.3

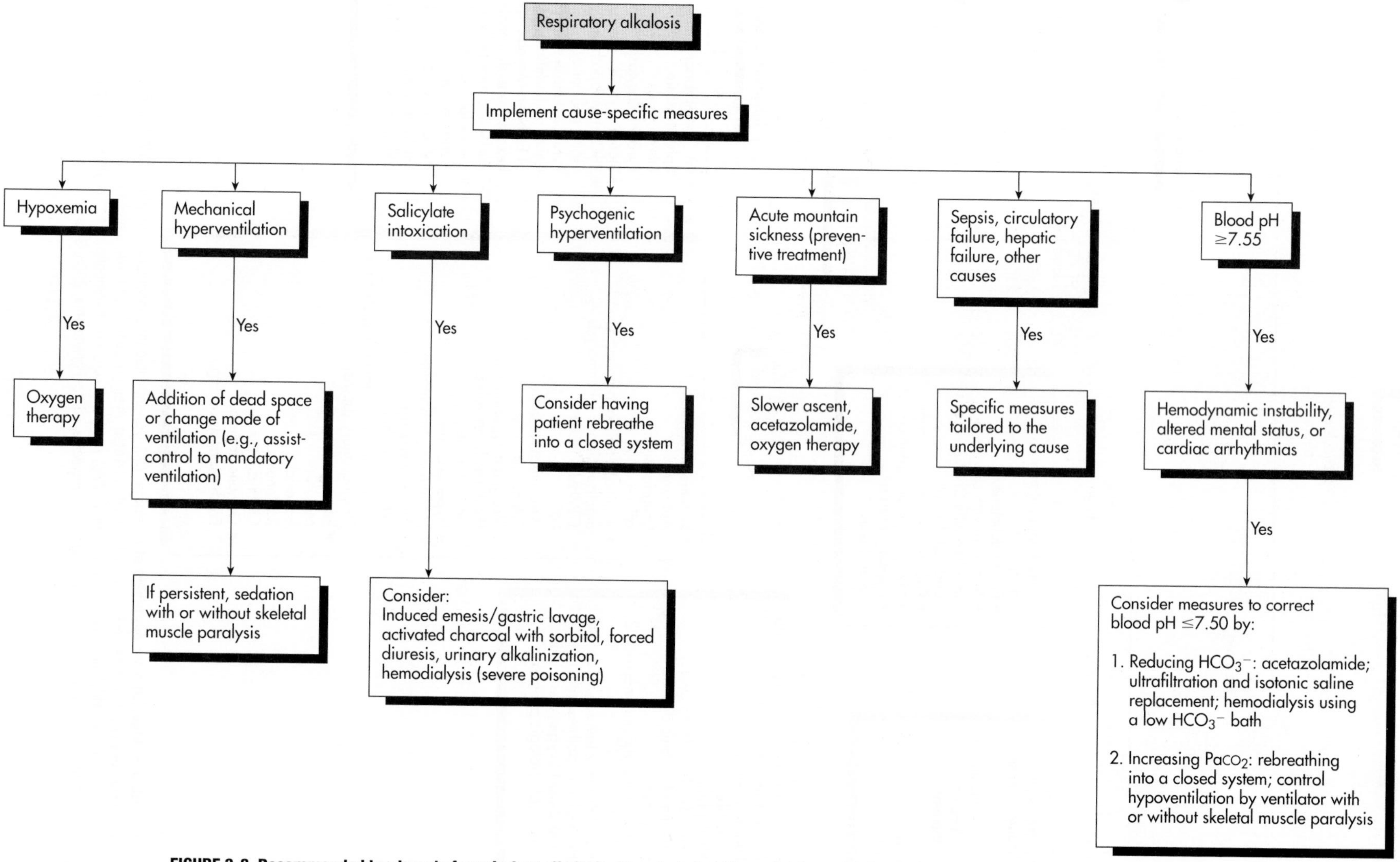

Respiratory alkalosis

Implement cause-specific measures

Hypoxemia
Yes → Oxygen therapy

Mechanical hyperventilation
Yes → Addition of dead space or change mode of ventilation (e.g., assist-control to mandatory ventilation) → If persistent, sedation with or without skeletal muscle paralysis

Salicylate intoxication
Yes → Consider: Induced emesis/gastric lavage, activated charcoal with sorbitol, forced diuresis, urinary alkalinization, hemodialysis (severe poisoning)

Psychogenic hyperventilation
Yes → Consider having patient rebreathe into a closed system

Acute mountain sickness (preventive treatment)
Yes → Slower ascent, acetazolamide, oxygen therapy

Sepsis, circulatory failure, hepatic failure, other causes
Yes → Specific measures tailored to the underlying cause

Blood pH ≥7.55
Yes → Hemodynamic instability, altered mental status, or cardiac arrhythmias
Yes → Consider measures to correct blood pH ≤7.50 by:
1. Reducing HCO_3^-: acetazolamide; ultrafiltration and isotonic saline replacement; hemodialysis using a low HCO_3^- bath
2. Increasing $PaCO_2$: rebreathing into a closed system; control hypoventilation by ventilator with or without skeletal muscle paralysis

FIGURE 3-8 Recommended treatment of respiratory alkalosis. (From Feehally J, Floege J, Johnson RJ: *Comprehensive clinical nephrology*, ed 3, St Louis, 2007, Mosby.)

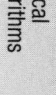

Clinical Algorithms

III

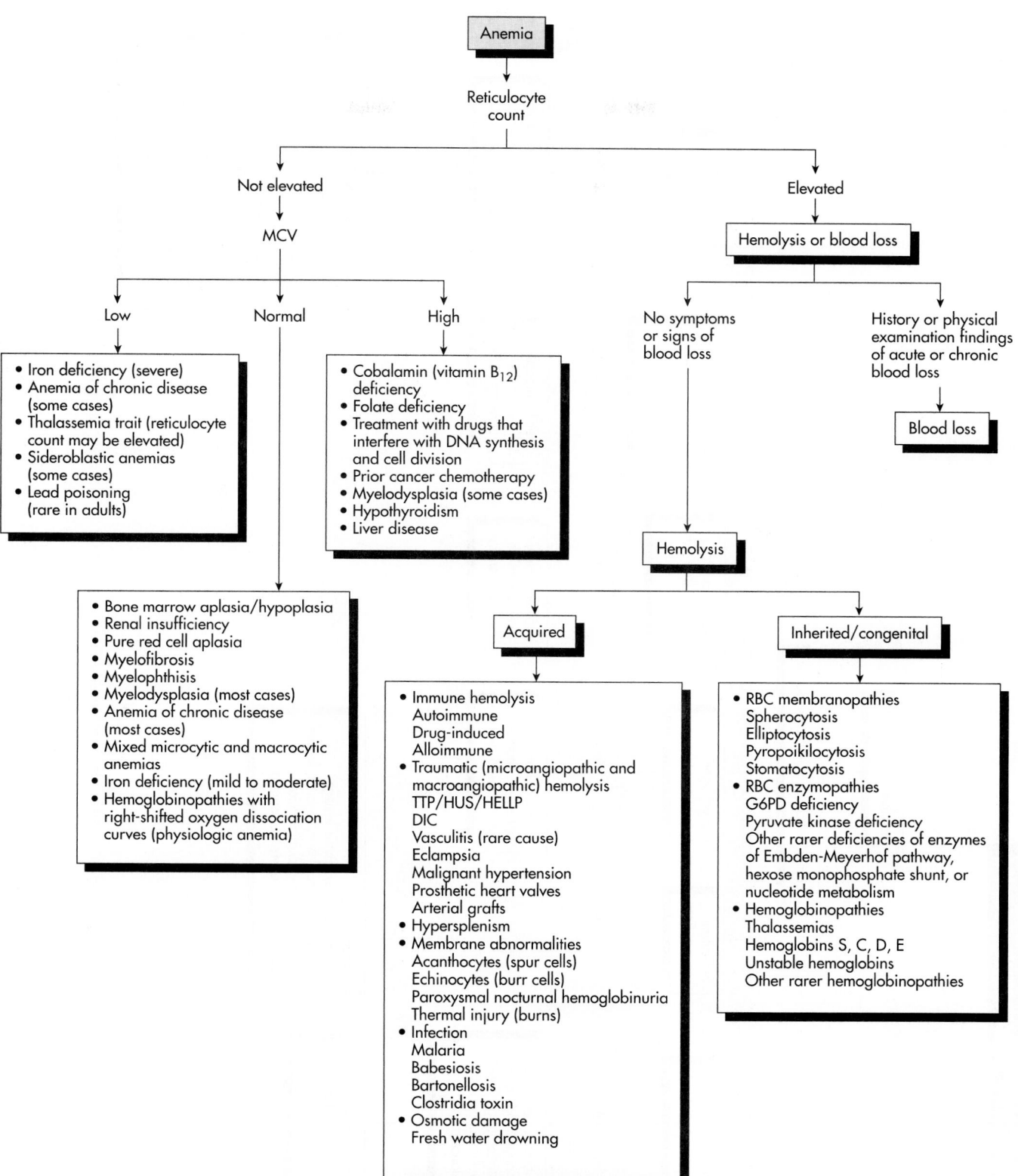

FIGURE 3-9 Algorithm for diagnosis of anemias. *DIC,* Disseminated intravascular coagulation; *G6PD,* glucose-6-phosphate-dehydrogenase; *HELLP, h*epatomegaly-*e*levated *l*iver (function tests)-*l*ow *p*latelets; *HUS,* hemolytic-uremic syndrome; *MCV,* mean corpuscular volume; *RBC,* red blood cell; *TTP,* thrombotic thrombocytopenic purpura. (From Goldman L, Ausiello D [eds]: *Cecil textbook of medicine,* ed 23, Philadelphia, 2008, Saunders.)

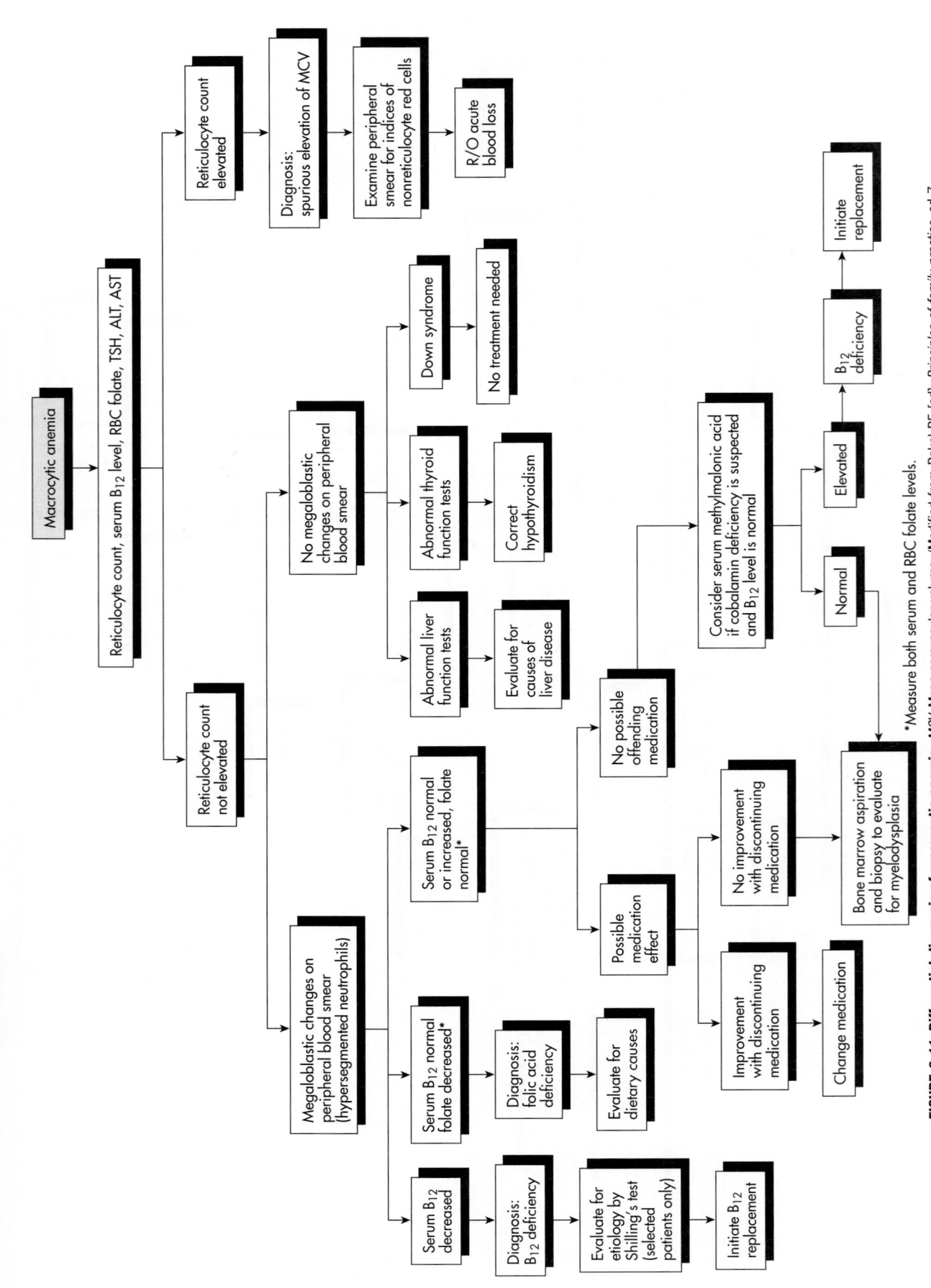

FIGURE 3-11 Differential diagnosis of macrocytic anemia. *MCV,* Mean corpuscular volume. (Modified from Rakel RE [ed]: *Principles of family practice,* ed 7, Philadelphia, 2007, Saunders.)

*Measure both serum and RBC folate levels.

Clinical Algorithms

III

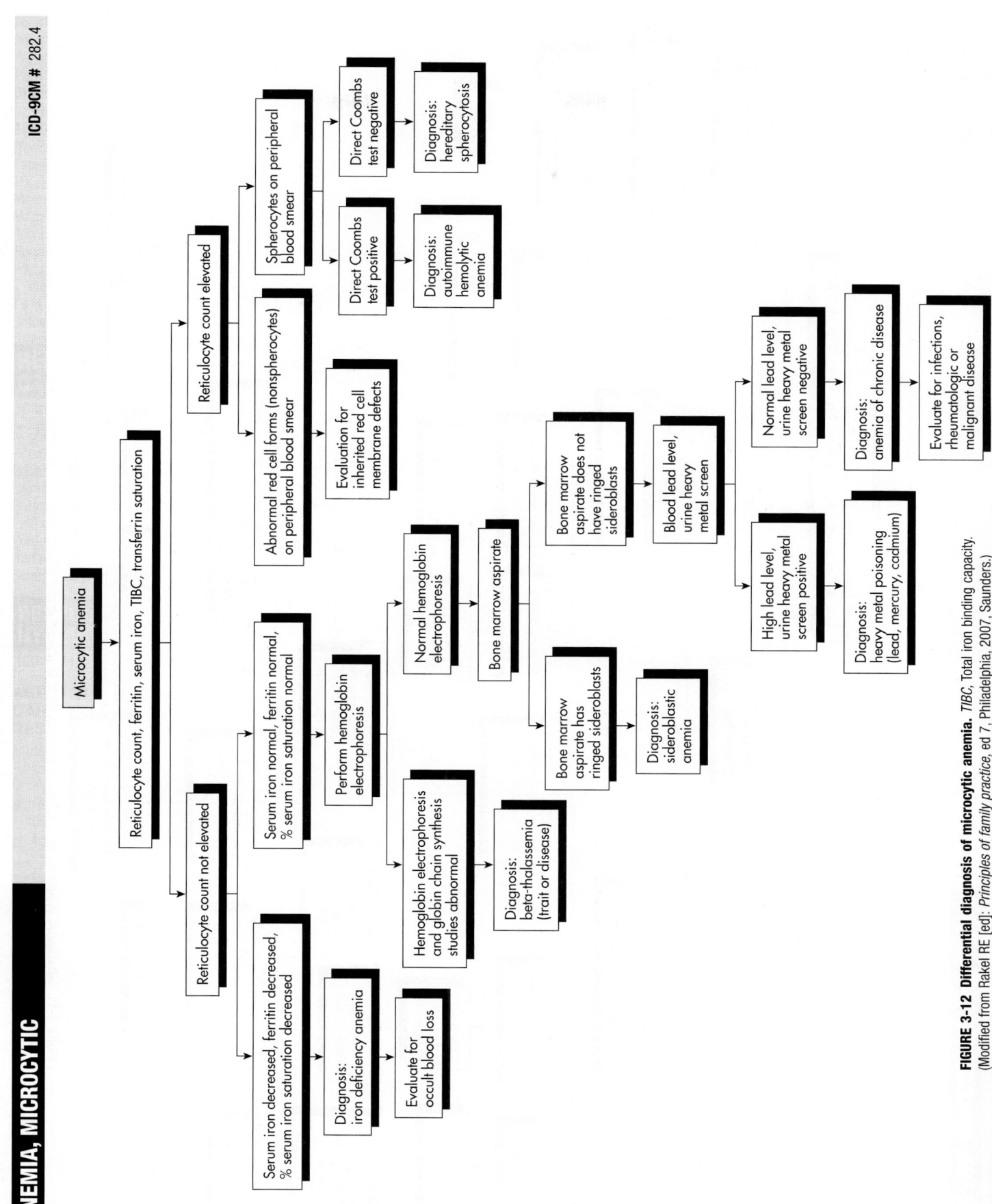

FIGURE 3-12 Differential diagnosis of microcytic anemia. *TIBC*, Total iron binding capacity. (Modified from Rakel RE [ed]: *Principles of family practice*, ed 7, Philadelphia, 2007, Saunders.)

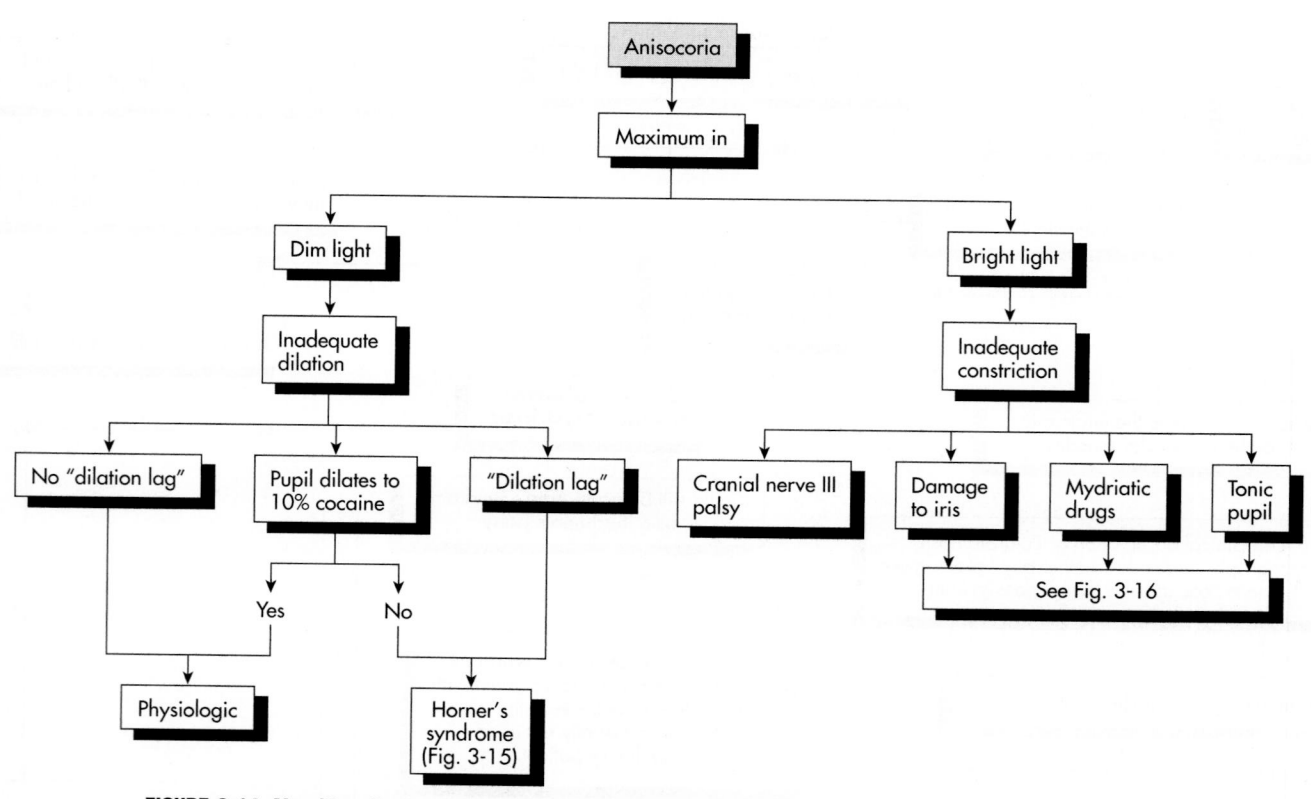

FIGURE 3-14 Algorithm for the approach to unequal pupils (anisocoria). (From Andreoli TE [ed]: *Cecil essentials of medicine,* ed 7, Philadelphia, 2008, Saunders.)

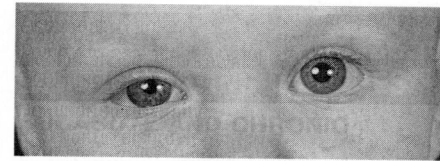

FIGURE 3-15 Horner's syndrome clearly acquired in infancy must be evaluated for neuroblastoma, a treatable tumor. This baby, with a right ptosis and miosis, developed a flush during cycloplegia that made the vasomotor abnormality very clear—the Horner's side remained pale. The baby had no sign of Horner's syndrome during her first 8 months, but at 16 months Horner's syndrome is obvious (ptosis, miosis, and upside-down ptosis). Because the syndrome was acquired, a chest radiograph was ordered; it showed a mass in the pulmonary apex. Magnetic resonance imaging confirmed the lesion. Surgery showed it to be a neuroblastoma. (From Yanoff M, Duker JS: *Ophthalmology,* ed 2, St Louis, 2004, Mosby.)

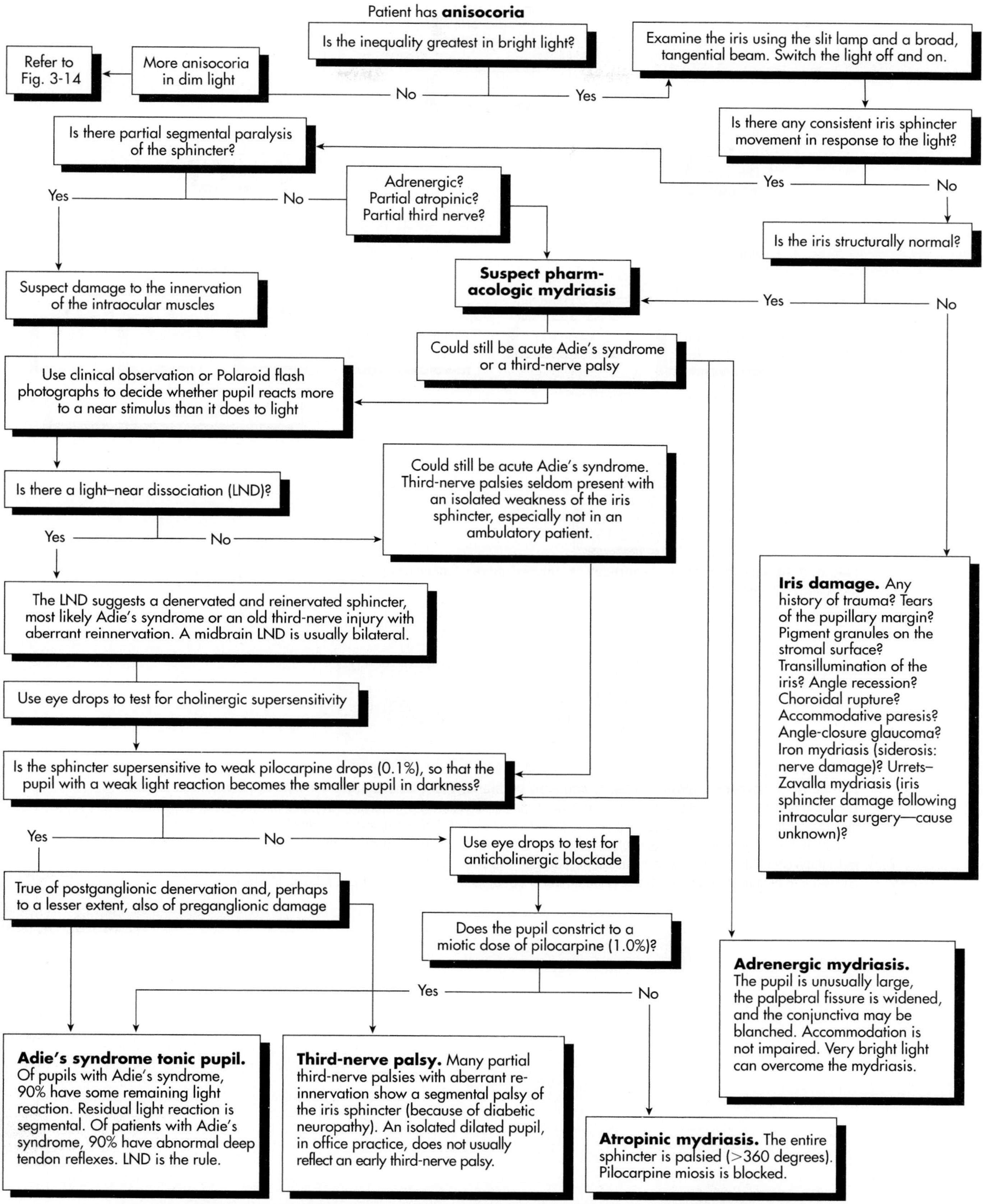

Patient has **anisocoria**

Is the inequality greatest in bright light?

Examine the iris using the slit lamp and a broad, tangential beam. Switch the light off and on.

Refer to Fig. 3-14 ← More anisocoria in dim light

No ——— Yes

Is there any consistent iris sphincter movement in response to the light?

Yes ——— No

Is there partial segmental paralysis of the sphincter?

Adrenergic? Partial atropinic? Partial third nerve?

Is the iris structurally normal?

Yes ——————— No

Suspect damage to the innervation of the intraocular muscles

Suspect pharmacologic mydriasis

Yes ——— No

Could still be acute Adie's syndrome or a third-nerve palsy

Use clinical observation or Polaroid flash photographs to decide whether pupil reacts more to a near stimulus than it does to light

Could still be acute Adie's syndrome. Third-nerve palsies seldom present with an isolated weakness of the iris sphincter, especially not in an ambulatory patient.

Is there a light–near dissociation (LND)?

Yes ——————— No

The LND suggests a denervated and reinnervated sphincter, most likely Adie's syndrome or an old third-nerve injury with aberrant reinnervation. A midbrain LND is usually bilateral.

Iris damage. Any history of trauma? Tears of the pupillary margin? Pigment granules on the stromal surface? Transillumination of the iris? Angle recession? Choroidal rupture? Accommodative paresis? Angle-closure glaucoma? Iron mydriasis (siderosis: nerve damage)? Urrets–Zavalla mydriasis (iris sphincter damage following intraocular surgery—cause unknown)?

Use eye drops to test for cholinergic supersensitivity

Is the sphincter supersensitive to weak pilocarpine drops (0.1%), so that the pupil with a weak light reaction becomes the smaller pupil in darkness?

Yes ——————— No

True of postganglionic denervation and, perhaps to a lesser extent, also of preganglionic damage

Use eye drops to test for anticholinergic blockade

Does the pupil constrict to a miotic dose of pilocarpine (1.0%)?

Yes ——— No

Adrenergic mydriasis. The pupil is unusually large, the palpebral fissure is widened, and the conjunctiva may be blanched. Accommodation is not impaired. Very bright light can overcome the mydriasis.

Adie's syndrome tonic pupil. Of pupils with Adie's syndrome, 90% have some remaining light reaction. Residual light reaction is segmental. Of patients with Adie's syndrome, 90% have abnormal deep tendon reflexes. LND is the rule.

Third-nerve palsy. Many partial third-nerve palsies with aberrant re-innervation show a segmental palsy of the iris sphincter (because of diabetic neuropathy). An isolated dilated pupil, in office practice, does not usually reflect an early third-nerve palsy.

Atropinic mydriasis. The entire sphincter is palsied (>360 degrees). Pilocarpine miosis is blocked.

FIGURE 3-16 Diagnosis of pupillary abnormalities in which anisocoria increases in bright light. Initial pupillary inequality is greater in bright light than in darkness, which indicates that the sphincter of the large pupil is weak or that a parasympathetic lesion is present on that side. (From Yanoff M, Duker JS: *Ophthalmology,* ed 2, St Louis, 2004, Mosby.)

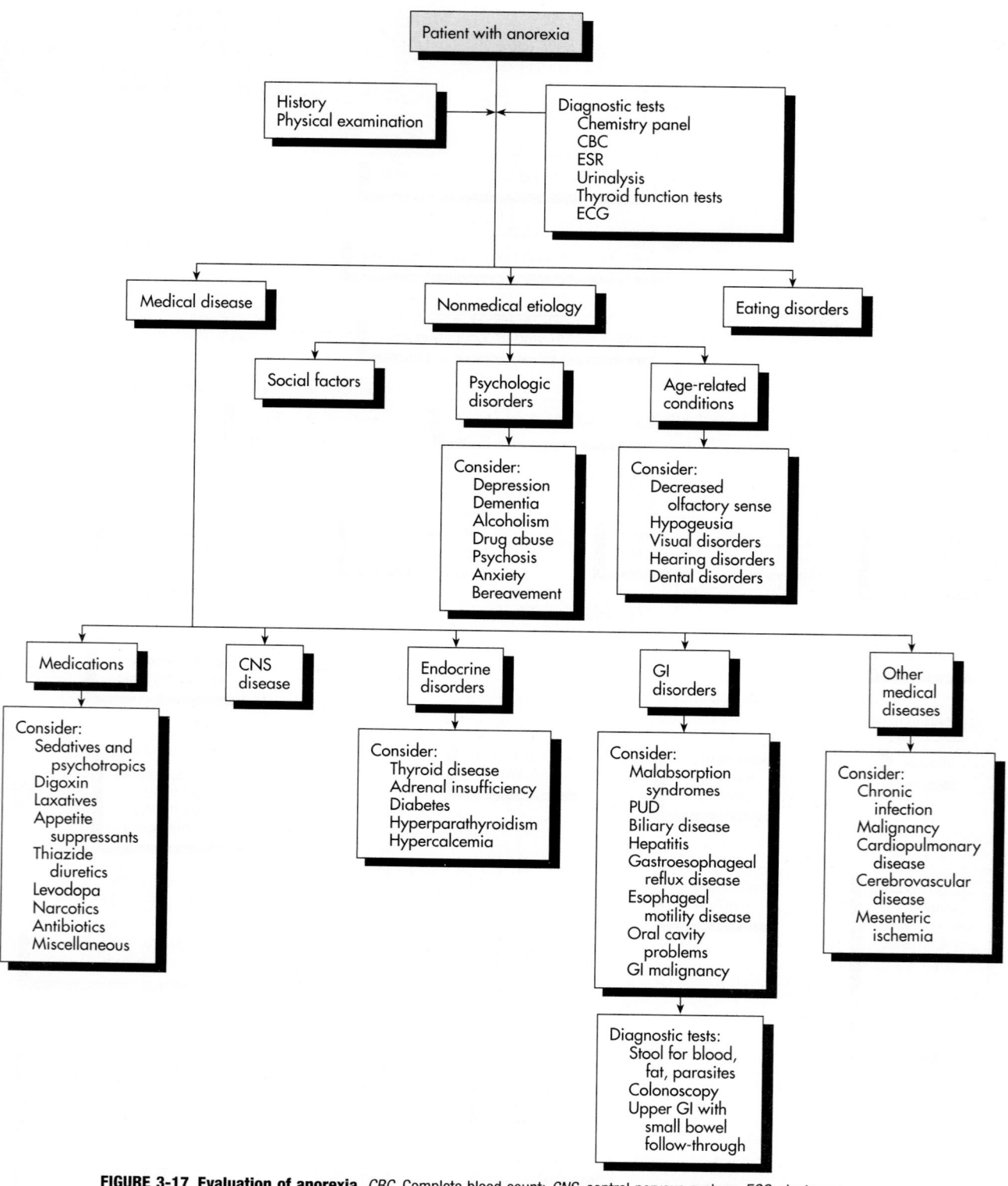

FIGURE 3-17 Evaluation of anorexia. *CBC,* Complete blood count; *CNS,* central nervous system; *ECG,* electrocardiogram; *ESR,* erythrocyte sedimentation rate; *GI,* gastrointestinal; *PUD,* peptic ulcer disease. (Modified from Greene HL, Johnson WP, Lemcke D [eds]: *Decision making in medicine,* ed 2, St Louis, 1998, Mosby.)

Clinical
Algorithms

III

ICD-9CM # 719.40 Arthralgia site NOS
719.41 Arthralgia, shoulder region
719.42 Arthralgia, upper arm
719.43 Arthralgia, forearm
719.44 Arthralgia, hand
719.45 Arthralgia, pelvic region and thigh
719.46 Arthralgia, lower leg
719.47 Arthralgia, ankle and/or foot

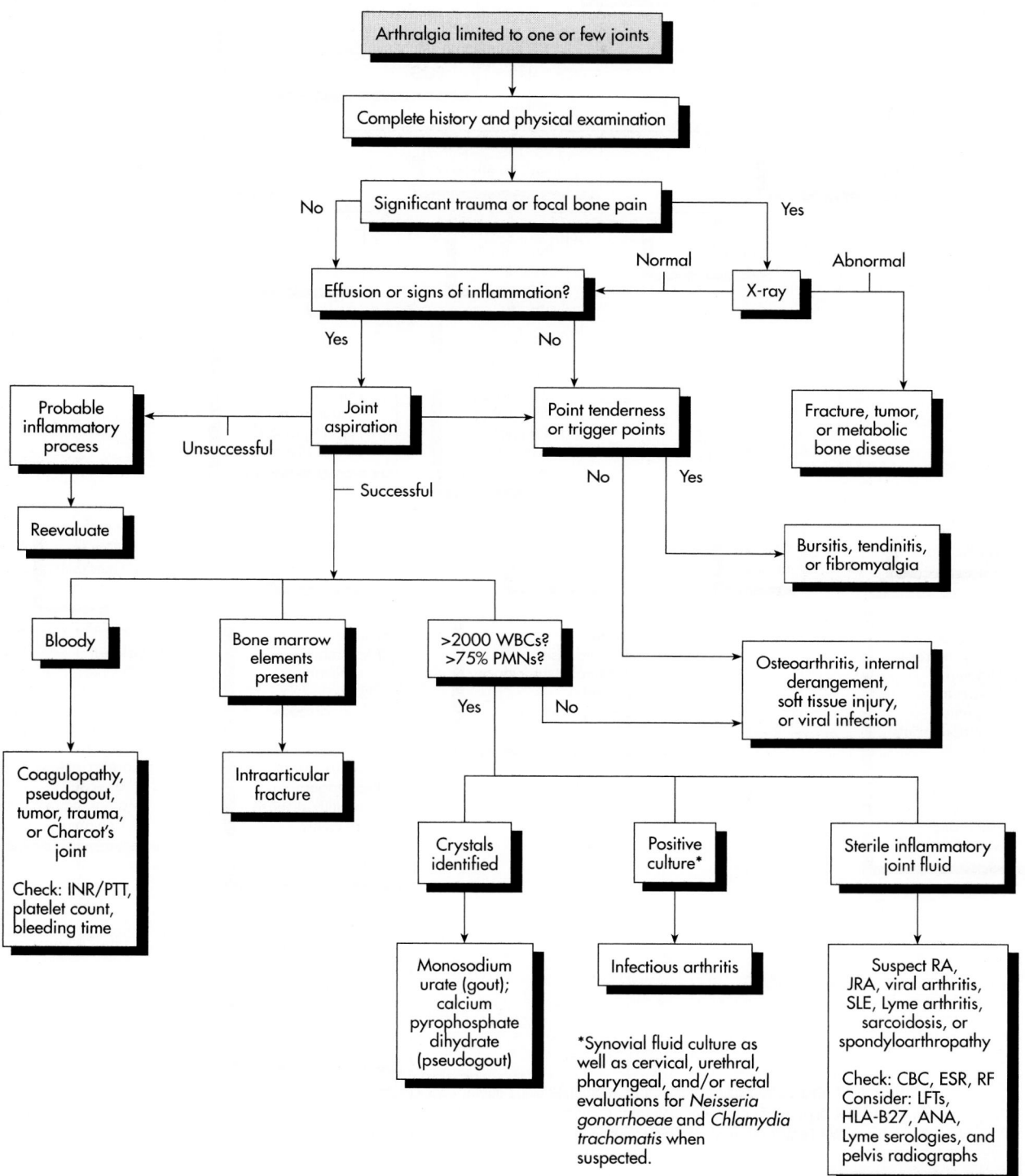

FIGURE 3-18 A diagnostic approach to arthralgia in a few joints. *ANA,* Antinuclear antibodies; *CBC,* complete blood count; *ESR,* erythrocyte sedimentation rate; *JRA,* juvenile rheumatoid arthritis; *LFTs,* liver function tests; *PMNs,* polymorphonuclear neutrophils; *PT,* prothrombin time; *PTT,* partial thromboplastin time; *RA,* rheumatoid arthritis; *RF,* rheumatoid factor; *SLE,* systemic lupus erythematosus; *WBCs,* white blood cells. (Modified from American College of Rheumatology Ad Hoc Committee on Clinical Guidelines: *Arthritis Rheum* 39:1, 1996.)

ATAXIA, PROGRESSIVE

ICD-9CM # 781.3 Ataxia NOS
303.9 Alcoholic, chronic
334.3 Cerebellar
331.89 Cerebral
334.0 Friedreich's

1321

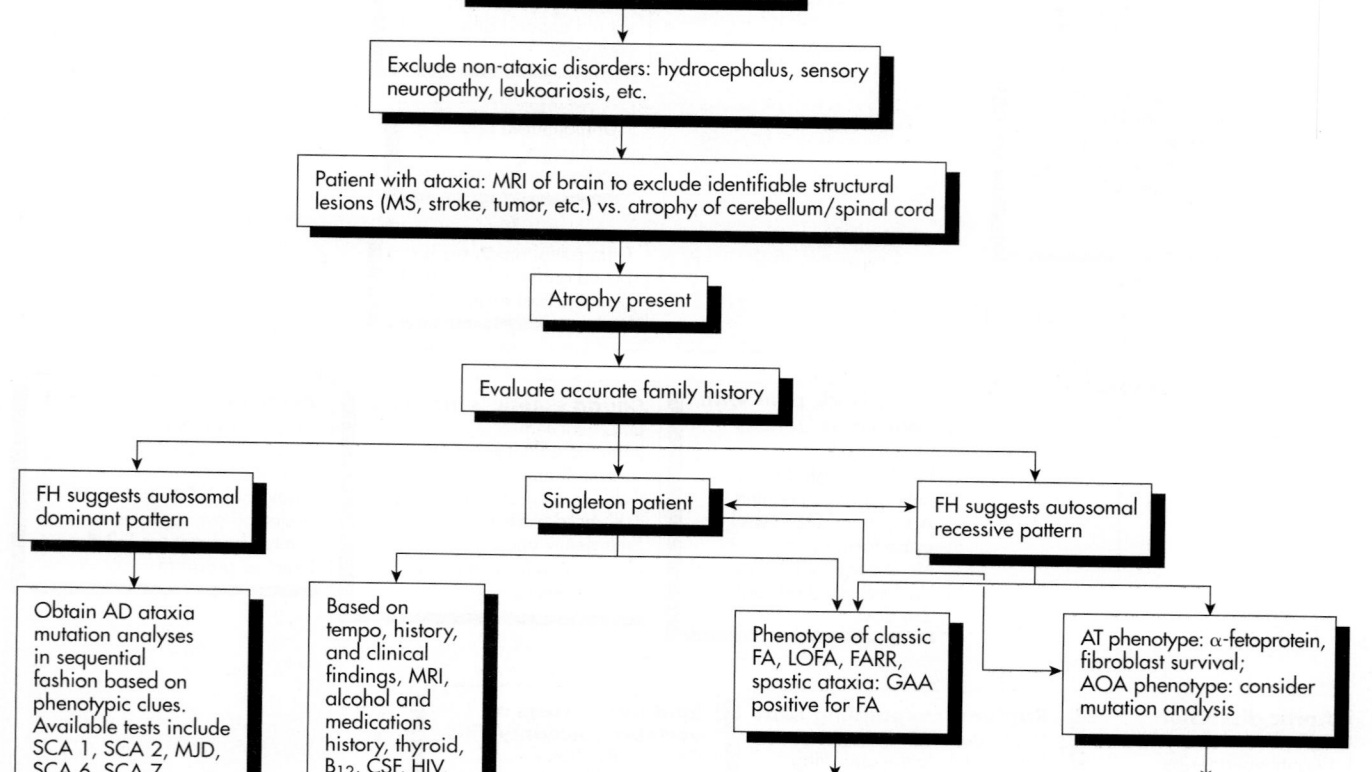

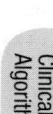

Clinical
Algorithms

III

FIGURE 3-21 An algorithm for a diagnostic approach to patients with progressive ataxia. *AD,* Autosomal dominant; *AOA,* ataxia with oculomotor apraxia; *AR,* autosomal recessive; *AT,* ataxia-telengiectasia; *CSF,* cerebrospinal fluid; *DRPLA,* dentatorubral-pallidoluysian atrophy; *EMG,* electromyelography; *FA,* Friedreich's ataxia; *FH,* family history; *GAD,* glutamate decarboxylase; *HIV,* human immunodeficiency virus; *MRI,* magnetic resonance imaging; *MS,* multiple sclerosis; *SCA,* spinocerebellar ataxia. (From Bradley WG et al [eds]: *Neurology in clinical practice,* ed 4, Philadelphia, 2004, Butterworth Heinemann.)

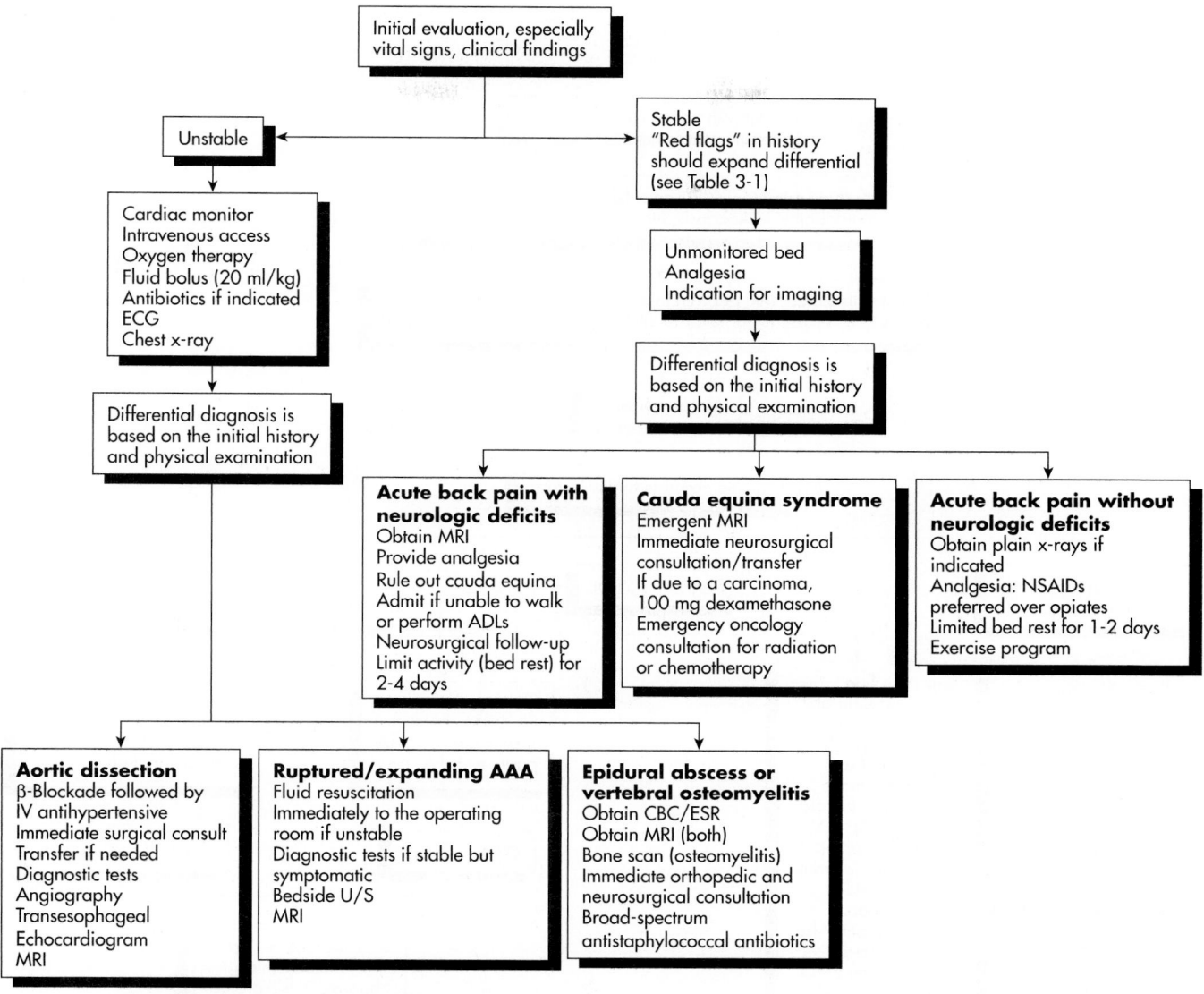

FIGURE 3-22 Management of acute low back pain. *AAA,* Abdominal aortic aneurysm; *ADL,* activities of daily living; *CBC,* complete blood count; *ECG,* electrocardiogram; *ESR,* erythrocyte sedimentation rate; *IV,* intravenous; *MRI,* magnetic resonance imaging; *NSAIDs,* nonsteroidal anti-inflammatory drugs; *U/S,* ultrasound. (From Marx JA [ed]: *Rosen's emergency medicine,* ed 6, St Louis, 2006, Mosby.)

TABLE 3-1 Red Flags for Potentially Serious Conditions

Possible Fracture	Possible Tumor or Infection	Possible Cauda Equina Syndrome
From Medical History		
Major trauma, such as vehicle accident or fall from height	Age over 50 or under 20 yr	Saddle anesthesia
Minor trauma or even strenuous lifting (in older or potentially osteoporotic patient)	History of cancer	Recent onset of bladder dysfunction, such as urinary retention, increased frequency, or overflow incontinence
	Constitutional symptoms, such as recent fever or chills or unexplained weight loss	Severe or progressive neurologic deficit in the lower extremity
	Risk factors for spinal infection: recent bacterial infection (e.g., urinary tract infection), intravenous drug abuse, or immune suppression (from steroids, transplant, or human immunodeficiency virus)	
	Pain that worsens when supine; severe nighttime pain	

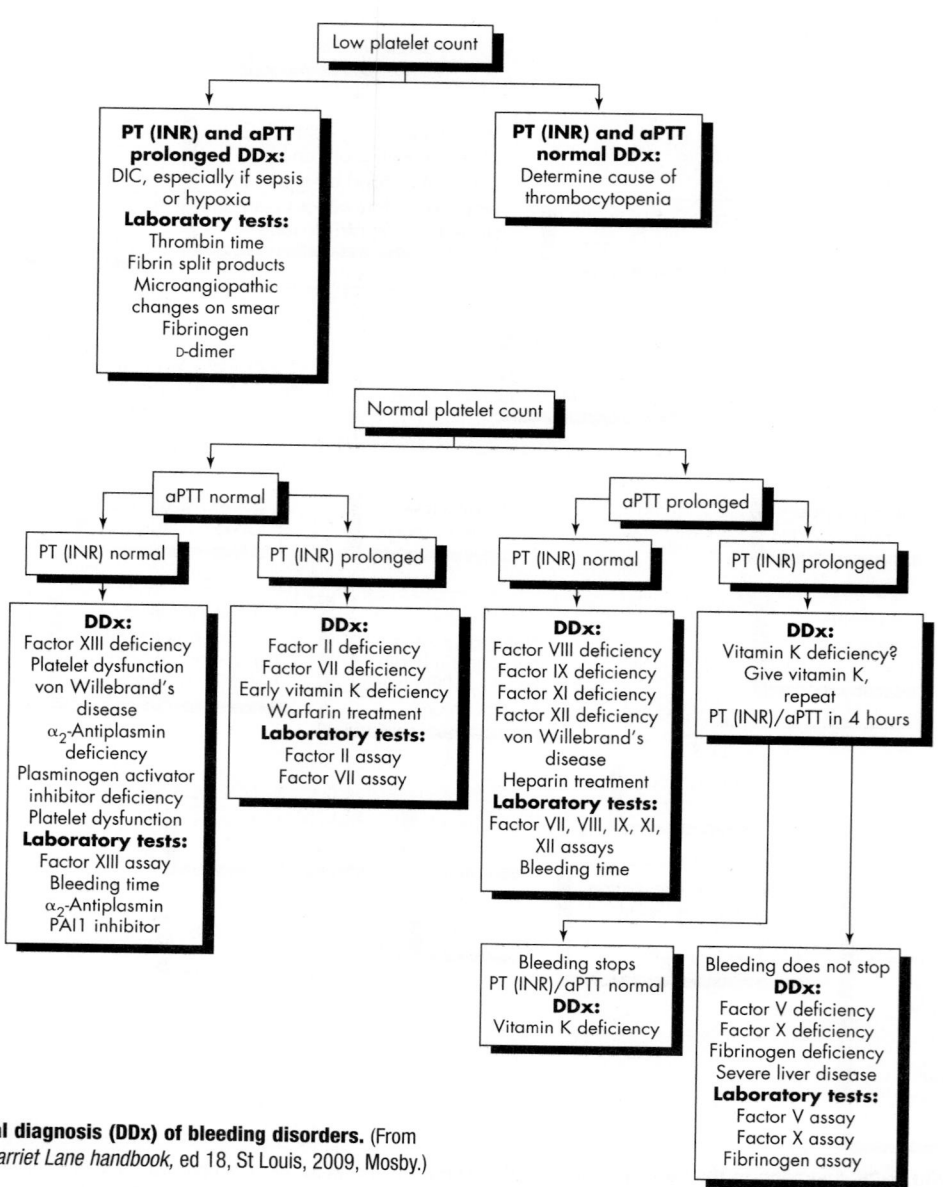

FIGURE 3-24 Differential diagnosis (DDx) of bleeding disorders. (From Cluster JW, Rau RE: *The Harriet Lane handbook,* ed 18, St Louis, 2009, Mosby.)

BOX 3-1   Bleeding Disorders

Congenital
Disorder of platelet number or function
Thrombocytopenia: Secondary to bone marrow disease or defective megakaryocyte maturation
Disorders of platelet function: Bernard-Soulier syndrome, Glanzmann thrombasthenia, storage pool diseases
Factor VIII deficiency: See text (Section I)
Factor IX deficiency: See text (Section I)
von Willebrand's disease: See text (Section I)

Acquired
Disseminated intravascular coagulation: Characterized by prolonged PT and aPTT, decreased fibrinogen and platelets, increased fibrin degradation products, and elevated D-dimers. Treatment includes identifying and treating underlying disorder. Replacement of depleted coagulation factors with FFP may be necessary in severe cases, especially when bleeding is present; 10-15 ml/kg will raise clotting factors 20%. Fibrinogen, if depleted, can be given as cryoprecipitate. Platelet transfusions may also be necessary.

Liver disease: The liver is the major site of synthesis of factors V, VII, IX, X, XI, XII, XIII, prothrombin, plasminogen, fibrinogen, protein C and S, and ATIII. Treatment with FFP and platelets may be needed, but this will increase hepatic protein load. Vitamin K should be given to patients with liver disease and clotting abnormalities.

Vitamin K deficiency: Factors II, VII, IX, X, protein C, and protein S are vitamin K dependent. Early vitamin K deficiency may present with isolated prolonged PT because factor VII has the shortest half-life. Fibrinogen should be normal.

Hemolytic-uremic syndrome/thrombotic thrombocytopenic purpura (HUS/TTP): Characterized by the triad of microangiopathic hemolytic anemia, uremia, and thrombocytopenia. HUS/TTP is often triggered by bacterial enteritis, especially caused by *Escherichia coli* O157:H7, although there are a variety of causes. HUS does not typically include coagulation abnormalities, such as those seen in DIC. Avoid blood products in patients with HUS thought to be secondary to pneumococcal infection. TTP includes the triad of HUS in addition to fever and CNS changes and is more common in older adolescents and adults.

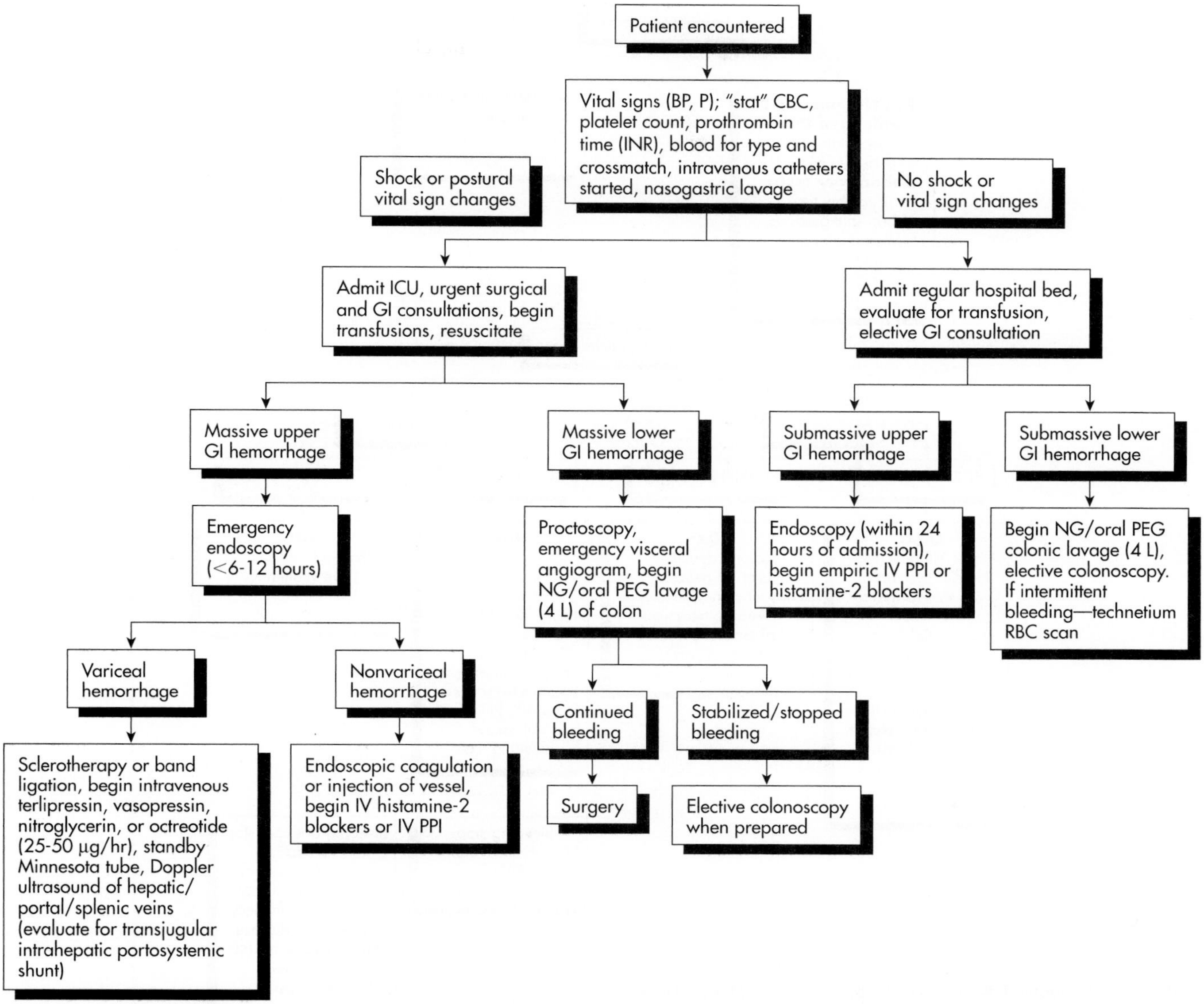

FIGURE 3-26 Approach to the patient with gastrointestinal hemorrhage. *BP*, Blood pressure; *CBC*, complete blood count; *GI*, gastrointestinal; *ICU*, intensive care unit; *IV*, intravenous; *INR*, International Normalized Ratio; *NG*, nasogastric; *P*, weight; *PEG*, percutaneous endoscopic gastrostomy; *PPI*, proton pump inhibitor; *RBC*, red blood cell. (Modified from Goldman L, Ausiello D [eds]: *Cecil textbook of medicine*, ed 23, Philadelphia, 2008, Saunders.)

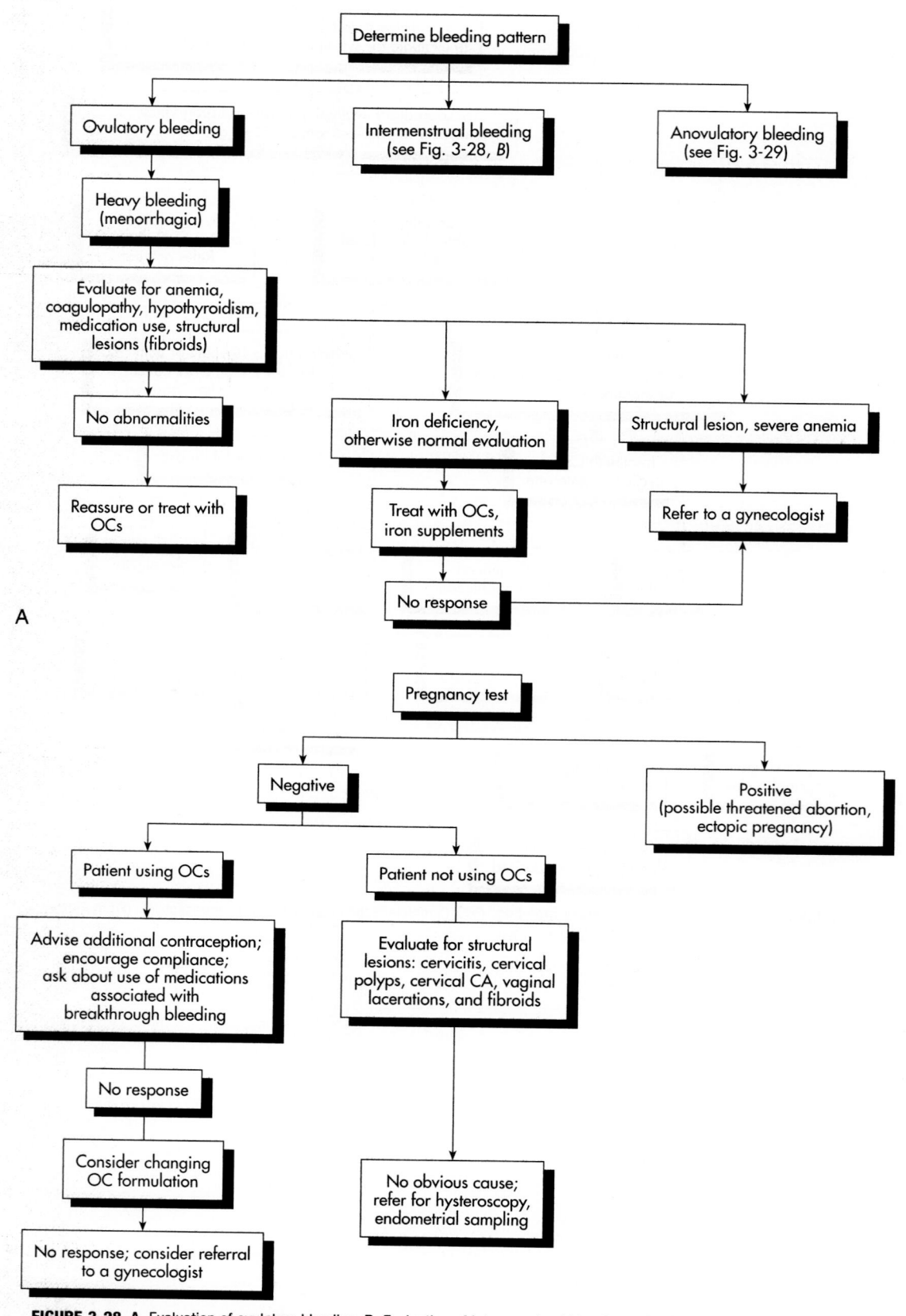

FIGURE 3-28 A, Evaluation of ovulatory bleeding. **B,** Evaluation of intermenstrual bleeding. *OCs,* Oral contraceptives. (Modified from Appleby J, Henderson M, Wathen PI: *Intern Med* Sept:17, 1996.)

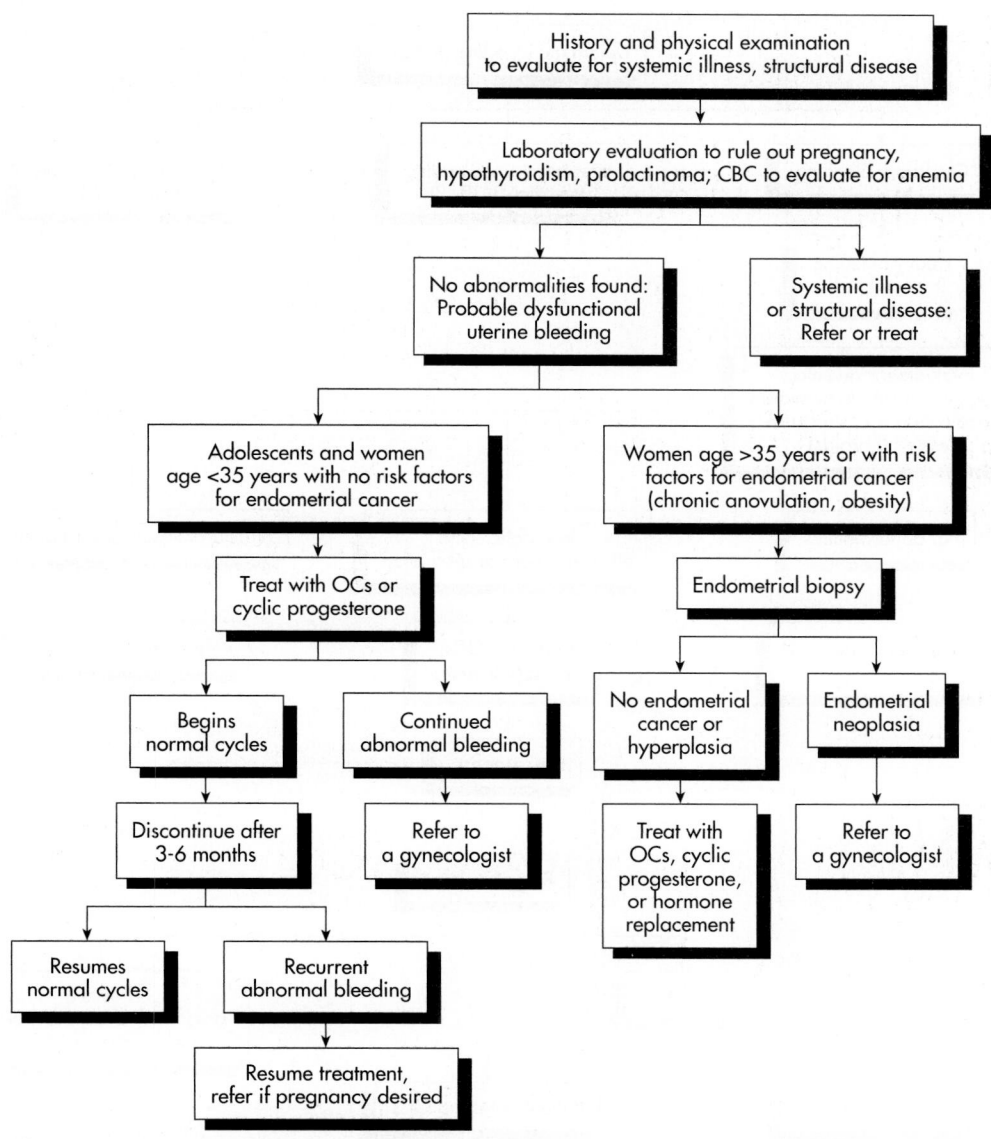

FIGURE 3-29 Evaluation of anovulatory bleeding. *CBC,* Complete blood count; *OCs,* oral contraceptives. (From Appleby J, Henderson M, Wathen PI: *Intern Med,* Sept:17, 1996.)

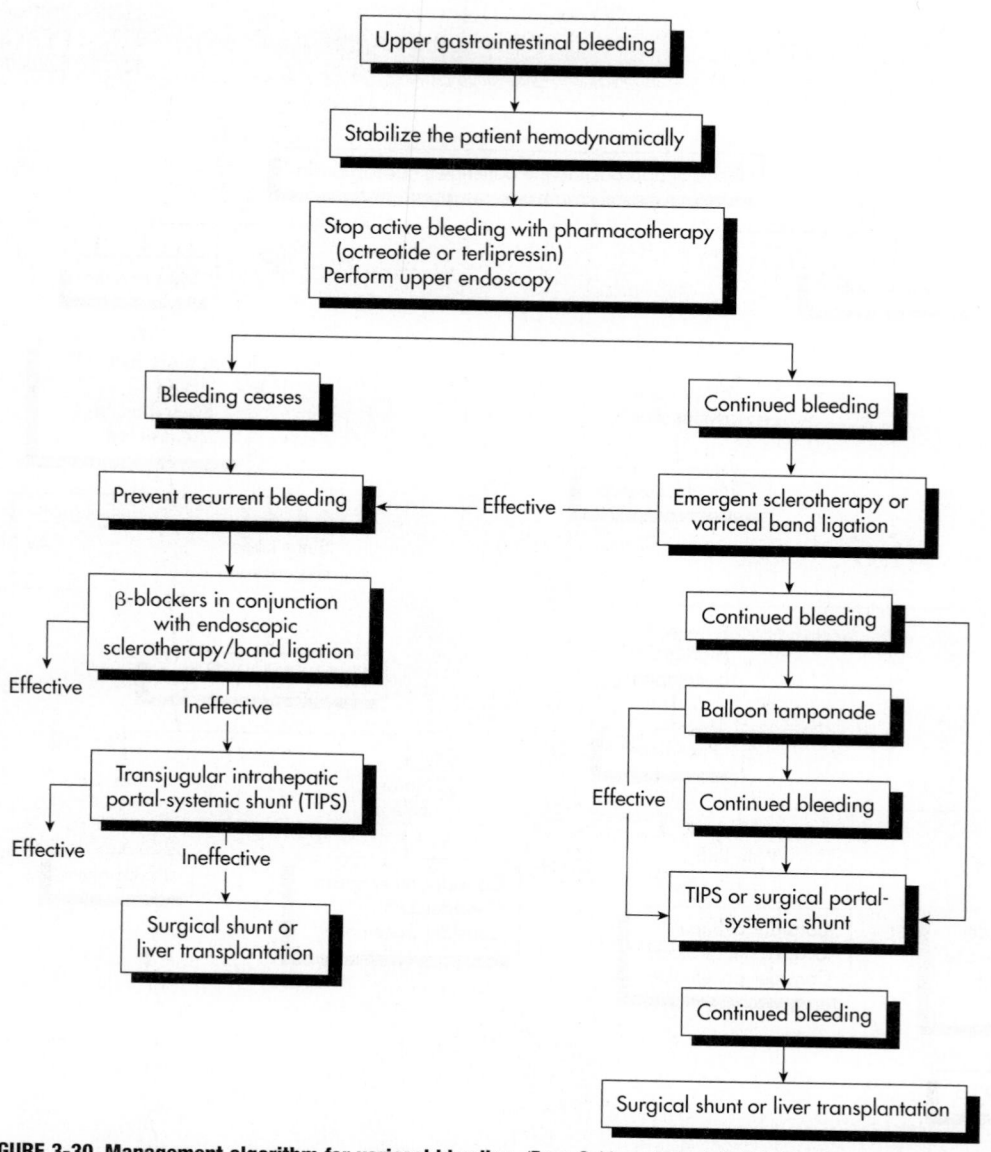

FIGURE 3-30 Management algorithm for variceal bleeding. (From Goldman L, Ausiello D [eds]: *Cecil textbook of medicine,* ed 23, Philadelphia, 2008, Saunders.)

ICD-9CM # 427.89 Unspecified bradycardia
427.81 Chronic bradycardia
770.8 Newborn bradycardia
427.89 Postoperative bradycardia
337 Reflex bradycardia
427.89 Sinus bradycardia

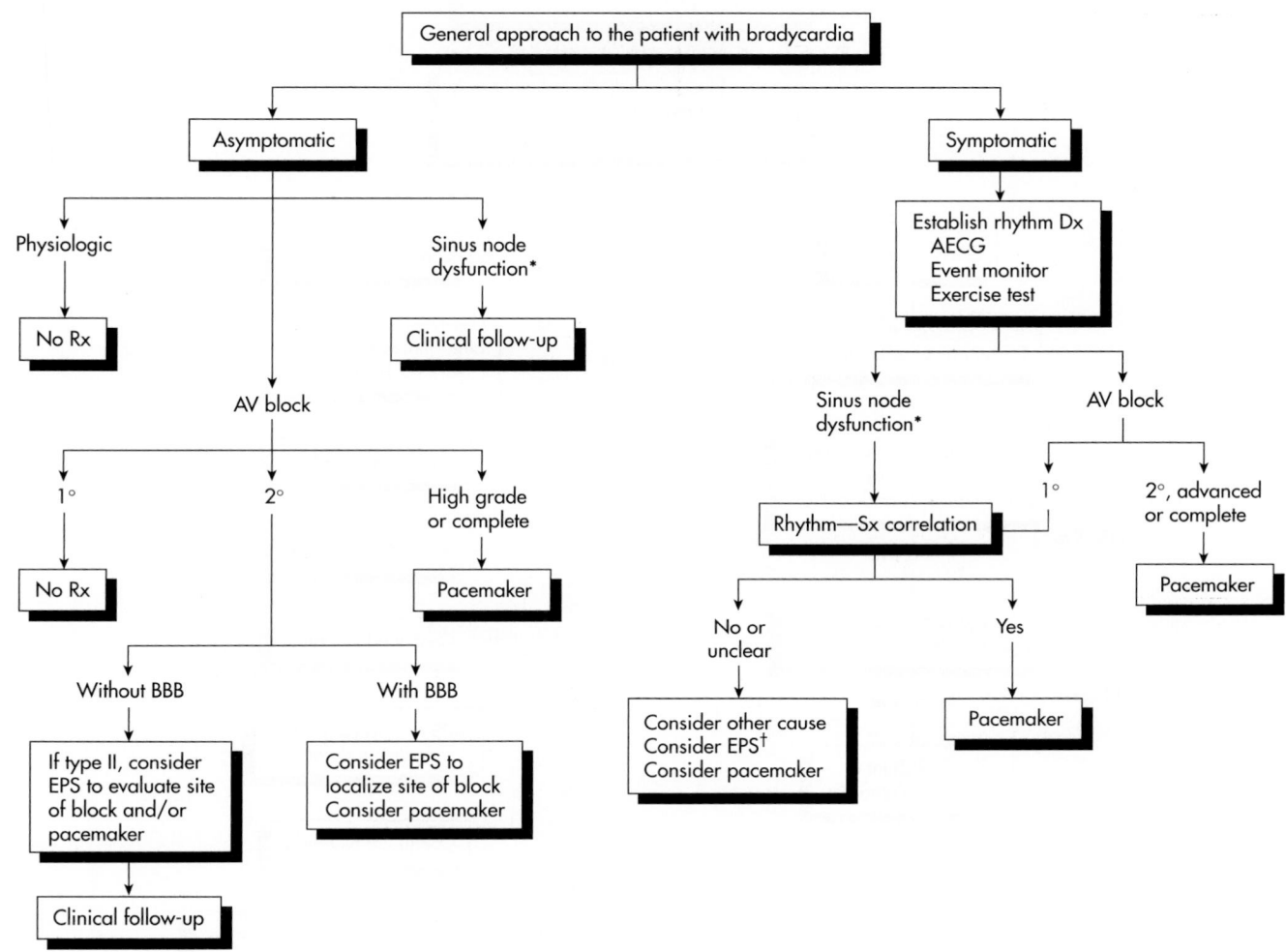

*Includes bradycardia-tachycardia syndrome.
†EPS includes sinus node function and ventricular arrhythmia induction studies.

FIGURE 3-31 General approach to the patient with bradycardia. *AECG,* Ambulatory electrocardiography; *AV,* atrioventricular; *BBB,* bundle branch block; *Dx,* diagnostic; *EPS,* electrophysiologic study; *Rx,* treatment; *Sx,* symptoms; *1°,* first-degree; *2°,* second-degree. (From Goldman L, Braunwald E [eds]: *Primary cardiology,* ed 2, Philadelphia, 2003, Saunders.)

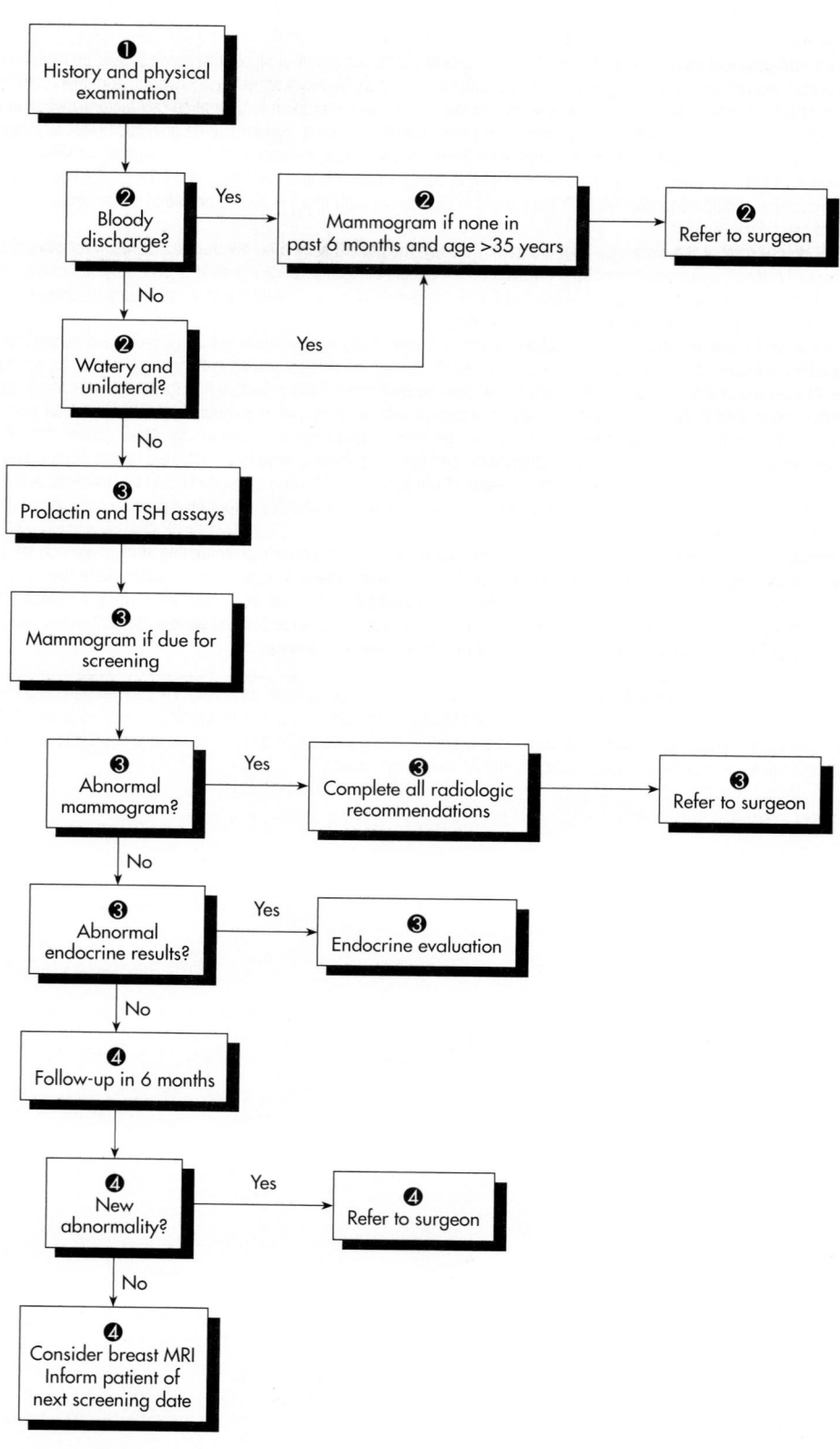

*Without palpable mass.

FIGURE 3-33 Breast cancer screening and evaluation. (Modified from Institute for Clinical Systems Integration, Minneapolis: *Postgrad Med* 100:182, 1996.)

FIGURE 3-33 (Continued)

1. **History and physical examination.*** Patients who present with a complaint of nipple discharge should be evaluated with breast-related history taking and a physical examination. History taking is aimed at uncovering and characterizing any other breast-related symptom. A risk assessment should also be undertaken for identified risk factors, including patient age over 50 years, any past personal history of breast cancer, history of hyperplasia on previous breast biopsies, and family history of breast cancer in first-degree relatives (mother, sister, daughter). Physical examination should include inspection of the breast for any evidence of ulceration or contour changes and inspection of the nipple for Paget's disease. Palpation should be performed with the patient in both the upright and the supine positions to determine the presence of any palpable mass.

2. **Bloody discharge?** If the discharge appears frankly bloody, the patient should be referred to a surgeon for evaluation. At the time of referral, a mammogram of the involved breast should be obtained if the patient is over 35 years of age and has not had a mammogram within the preceding 6 months. Similarly, patients with a watery, unilateral discharge should be referred to a surgeon for evaluation and possible biopsy.

3. **Endocrine tests. Mammogram.** If the discharge appears frankly milky or is bilateral, serum prolactin and serum thyroid-stimulating hormone *(TSH)* assays should be performed to rule out the presence of an endocrinologic basis for the symptoms. At the time of that visit, a mammogram should also be performed if the patient is due for routine mammographic screening according to the recommended intervals. A patient with an abnormal mammogram should be further evaluated radiologically to better characterize the lesion and then be referred to a surgeon if appropriate. Make certain that all recommended additional views, ultrasound examinations, and follow-up studies have been obtained before referral to a surgeon. Should the mammogram appear normal, results of the assays for TSH and prolactin should be reviewed. If the results are abnormal, the patient should undergo appropriate evaluation for etiology, either by a primary care physician or by an endocrinologist.

4. **Six-month follow-up results.** If results of the mammogram and the endocrinologic screening studies are normal, the patient should return for a follow-up visit in 6 months to ensure that there has been no specific change in the character of the discharge, such as development of frank bleeding or Paget's disease, that would warrant surgical evaluation. If the evaluation at that follow-up visit fails to reveal any palpable or visible abnormalities, the patient should be returned to the routine screening process with studies performed at the recommended intervals.

*ICSI health care guidelines are designed to assist clinicians by providing an analytic framework for the evaluation and treatment of patients. They are not intended either to replace a clinician's judgment or to establish a protocol for all patients with a particular condition. A guideline will rarely establish the only approach to a problem. In addition, guidelines are "living documents" that are expected to be imperfect and are subject to annual review and revision.

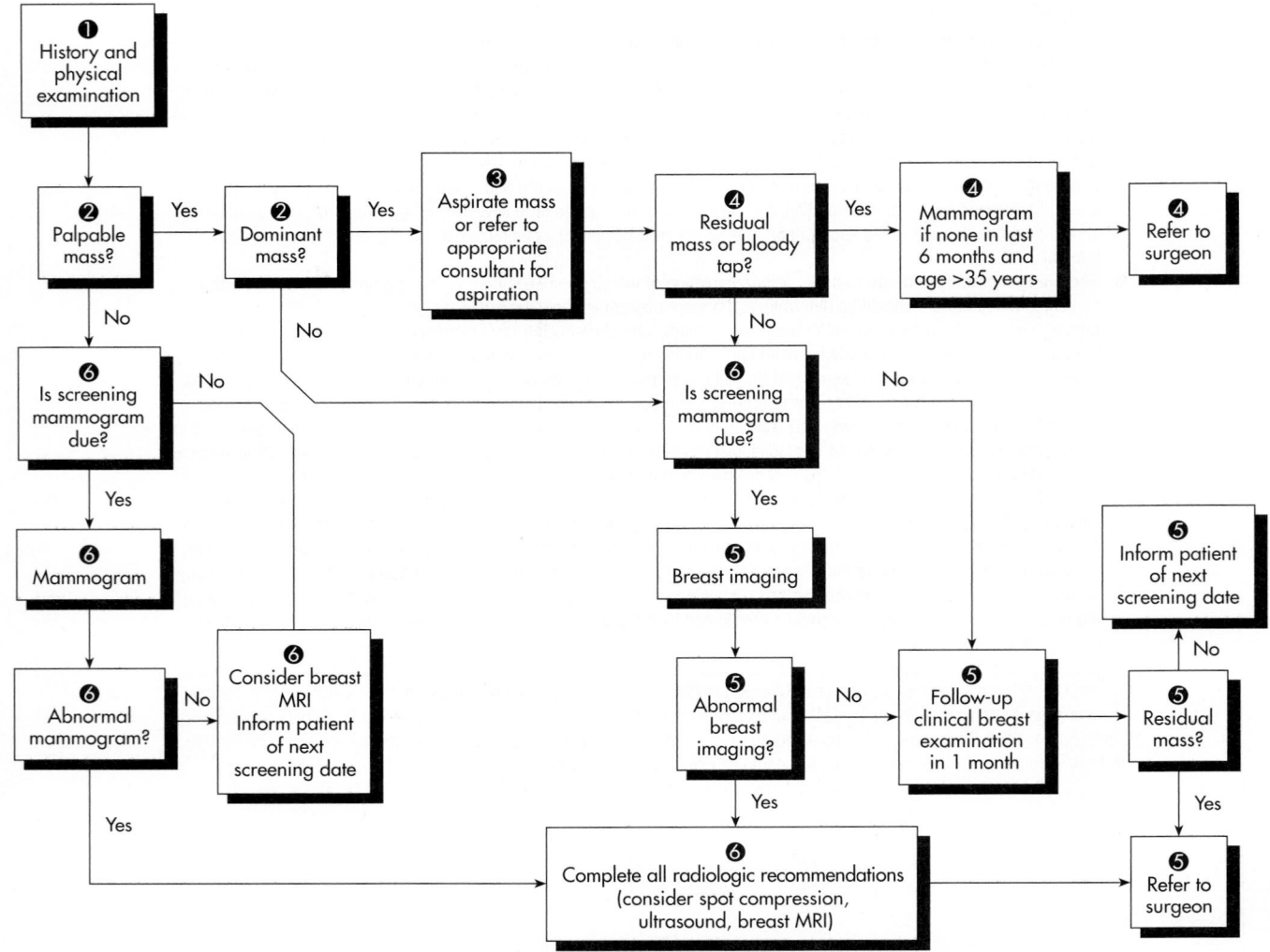

FIGURE 3-35 Breast cancer screening and evaluation. (Modified from Institute for Clinical Systems Integration, Minneapolis: *Postgrad Med* 100:182, 1996.)

1. **History and physical examination.*** Primary care evaluation is initiated with history taking aimed at uncovering and characterizing any breast-related symptom. A risk assessment should also be undertaken for identified risk factors, including patient age over 50 years, any past personal history of breast cancer, history of hyperplasia on previous breast biopsies, and family history of breast cancer in first-degree relatives (mother, sister, daughter). Physical examination should include inspection of the breast for any evidence of ulceration or contour changes and inspection of the nipple for Paget's disease. Palpation should be performed with the patient in both the upright and supine positions to determine the presence of any palpable mass.

2. **Palpable mass? Dominant mass?** A dominant mass is a palpable finding that is discrete and clearly different from the surrounding parenchyma. If a palpable mass is identified, it should be determined whether it represents a dominant (i.e., discrete) mass, which requires immediate evaluation. The primary care physician or appropriate consultant should attempt to aspirate any dominant mass because a simple cyst may be uncovered, in which case aspiration completes the evaluation process.

3. **Aspirate mass or refer for aspiration.** Aspiration of a dominant palpable mass should be performed by the primary care physician or by the appropriate consultant. The breast skin is prepped with alcohol. Then, with the lesion immobilized by the nonoperating hand, an 18- to 25-gauge needle mounted on a 10-ml syringe is directed to the central portion of the mass for a single attempt at aspiration. Successful aspiration of a simple cyst would yield a nonbloody fluid with complete resolution of the dominant mass. Typical watery fluid may be discarded. However, cyst fluid that is bloody or unusually tenacious should be examined cytologically.

4. **Residual mass or bloody tap? Mammogram if none in past 6 months. Refer to surgeon.** Should the mass remain after the attempt at aspiration or should frank blood be aspirated during the process, the presence of a malignant process cannot be ruled out. Patients with a residual mass or bloody tap should be referred to a surgeon for possible biopsy. Before the referral, a mammogram should be obtained for any patient over age 35 years who has not had a mammogram within the preceding 6 months. In patients 35 years and under, obtaining any other breast-imaging studies should be left to the discretion of the surgeon or radiologist.

Continued on following page

FIGURE 3-35 (Continued)

5. **Is screening mammogram due? Breast imaging. Follow-up clinical breast examination. Refer to surgeon.** Should physical examination demonstrate a palpable mass that is not clearly a discrete and dominant mass, its size, location, and character should be documented in anticipation of a follow-up examination. A screening mammogram should be obtained if one has not been done within the recommended interval. If no mammogram is required or if a required mammogram demonstrates no abnormality, a follow-up examination in 1 month is indicated. Breast MRI should be considered. Should any residual mass be identified, the patient should be referred to a surgeon for possible biopsy. Patients with a persisting nondominant palpable mass that does not resolve within 1 month and those with any recurring cystic mass should be referred for surgical evaluation. If no mass is apparent at the time of the follow-up examination, the patient should then be informed of the appropriate date for her next screening examination, according to the recommended intervals.

6. **Screening mammogram and results.** After completion of the physical examination, the appropriateness of a routine screening mammogram should be determined. If a mammogram is done, the radiologist should provide the results to the primary care physician for reporting to the patient. Should any abnormalities be uncovered, it will be the responsibility of the radiologist to complete any additional imaging studies required for the complete radiographic characterization of the lesion. The radiologist should make certain that all recommended additional views, follow-up studies, and ultrasound examinations have been completed before referral to a surgeon. However, it is important that the primary care physician who ordered the mammogram review the results of these studies to understand fully the opinion of the radiologist and to ensure that all recommendations of the radiologist have been completed. Should the radiologist recommend that surgical consultation is warranted, it will be the responsibility of the primary care physician to establish this referral.

NOTE: The importance of communication between the surgical consultant and the primary care physician cannot be overstated. Biopsy results should be reported both to the surgeon and to the primary care physician. More important, patients who do not require biopsy after surgical consultation should be returned to the routine screening process. This process is under the supervision of the primary care physician. Therefore it is absolutely necessary for the primary care physician to know when the patient reenters the routine screening population. In the event that new symptoms arise during the screening interval, the patient should be evaluated by the primary care physician using the primary care evaluation process of this guideline.

*ICSI health care guidelines are designed to assist clinicians by providing an analytic framework for the evaluation and treatment of patients. They are not intended either to replace a clinician's judgment or to establish a protocol for all patients with a particular condition. A guideline will rarely establish the only approach to a problem. In addition, guidelines are "living documents" that are expected to be imperfect and are subject to annual review and revision.

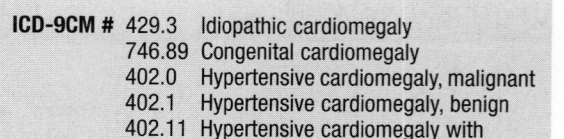

ICD-9CM # 429.3   Idiopathic cardiomegaly
746.89 Congenital cardiomegaly
402.0   Hypertensive cardiomegaly, malignant
402.1   Hypertensive cardiomegaly, benign
402.11 Hypertensive cardiomegaly with
        congestive heart failure

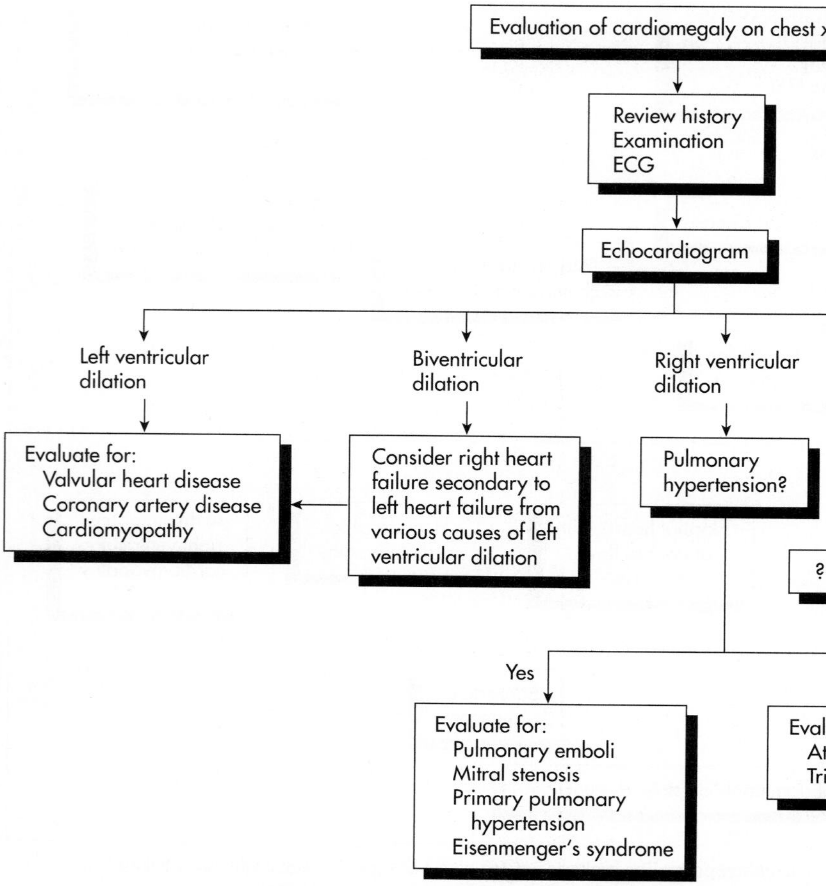

Evaluation of cardiomegaly on chest x-ray

↓

Review history
Examination
ECG

↓

Echocardiogram

Left ventricular dilation → Evaluate for:
    Valvular heart disease
    Coronary artery disease
    Cardiomyopathy

Biventricular dilation → Consider right heart failure secondary to left heart failure from various causes of left ventricular dilation

Right ventricular dilation → Pulmonary hypertension?

    Yes → Evaluate for:
        Pulmonary emboli
        Mitral stenosis
        Primary pulmonary hypertension
        Eisenmenger's syndrome

    No → Evaluate for:
        Atrial septal defect
        Tricuspid regurgitation

Pericardial effusion/thickening/mass
    R/O tamponade → ? Pericardiocentesis
    ? Cause → Consider:
        CT
        MRI
        Surgery/biopsy

No abnormalities → No further workup

FIGURE 3-38 Approach to the patient with cardiomegaly. When cardiomegaly is found on the chest radiograph, the history and physical examination should be reviewed and an electrocardiogram *(ECG)* performed before obtaining a two-dimensional Doppler echocardiographic study. Cardiomegaly may be explained by left ventricular dilation, biventricular dilation, right ventricular dilation, or pericardial abnormalities, or it may be found to be spurious on the echocardiogram. Rarely, isolated abnormalities of the atrium, particularly the left atrium, may cause abnormalities on the chest radiograph but will not cause true cardiomegaly. Depending on the echocardiographic findings, further tests can help elucidate the cause of echocardiographically confirmed cardiomegaly. *CT,* Computed tomography; *MRI,* magnetic resonance imaging; *R/O,* rule out. (From Goldman L, Braunwald E [eds]: *Primary cardiology,* ed 2, Philadelphia, 2003, Saunders.)

Clinical Algorithms

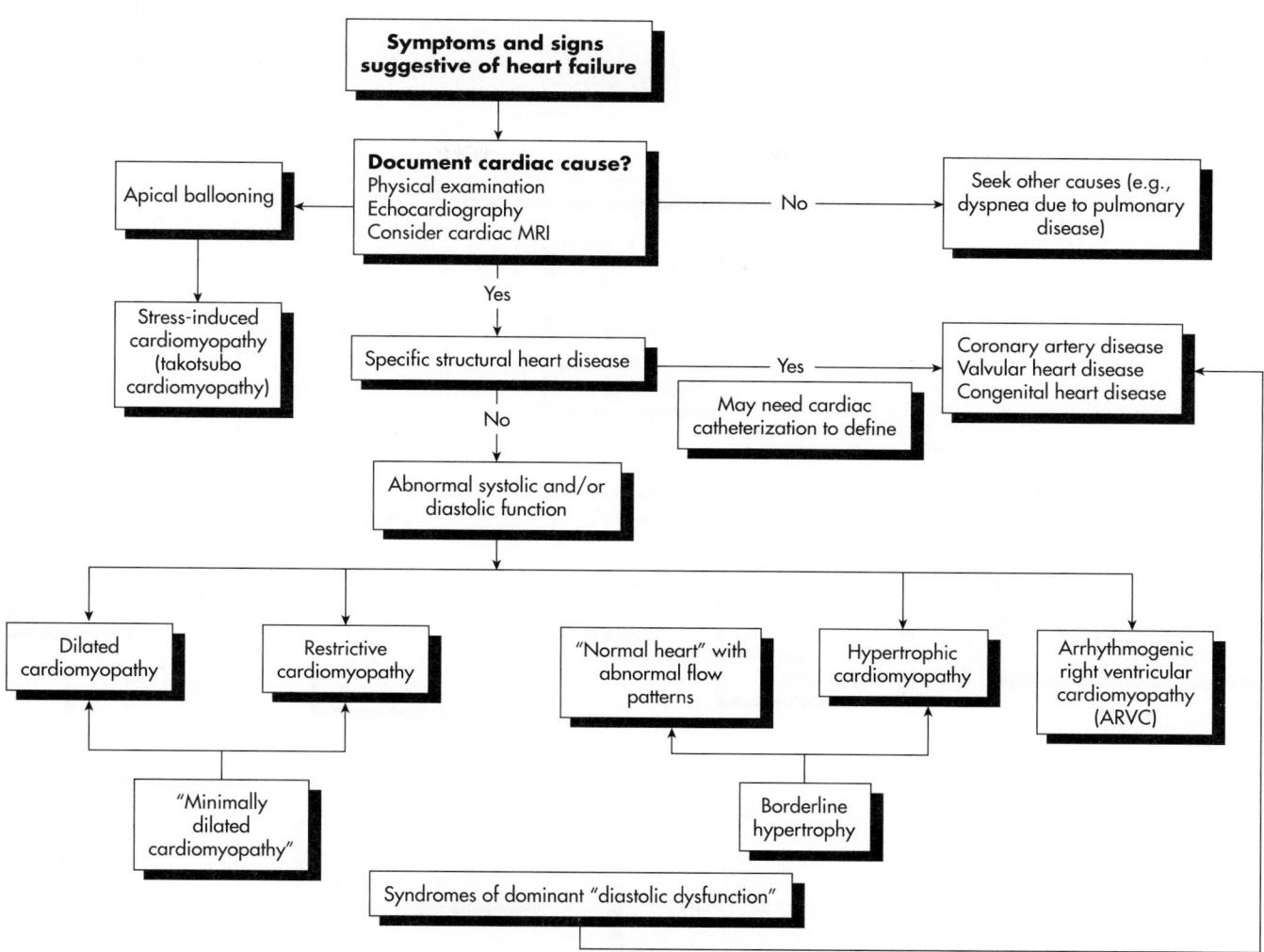

FIGURE 3-39 Initial approach to classification of cardiomyopathy. The evaluation of symptoms or signs consistent with heart failure first includes confirmation that they can be attributed to a cardiac cause. Although this conclusion is often apparent from routine physical examination, echocardiography serves to confirm cardiac disease and provides clues to the presence of other cardiac disease, such as focal abnormalities, suggesting primary valve disease or congenital heart disease. Having excluded these conditions, cardiomyopathy is generally considered to be dilated, restrictive, or hypertrophic. Patients with apparently normal cardiac structure and contraction are occasionally found to demonstrate abnormal intracardiac flow patterns consistent with diastolic dysfunction but should also be evaluated carefully for other causes of their symptoms. Most patients with so-called diastolic dysfunction also demonstrate at least borderline criteria for left ventricular hypertrophy, frequently in the setting of chronic hypertension and diabetes. A moderately decreased ejection fraction without marked dilation or a pattern of restrictive cardiomyopathy is sometimes referred to as "minimally dilated cardiomyopathy," which may represent either a distinct entity or a transition between acute and chronic disease. (From Goldman L, Ausiello D [eds]: *Cecil textbook of medicine,* ed 23, Philadelphia, 2008, Saunders.)

TABLE 3-2   Profiles of Myocardial Disease

	Hypertrophic	Dilated	Restrictive	ARVC
Causes	Genetic	Myocarditis Metabolic/endocrine Genetic	Infiltrative or storage diseases Endomyocardial (e.g., Löffler's, carcinoid) Genetic	Genetic
Ejection fraction	Increased	Reduced	25%-50%	Normal until end stage 30% regional LV disease
Left ventricular End-diastolic dimension	Usually decreased	Increased	Normal	Normal until end stage Right ventricle dilated
Left ventricular wall thickness	Increased	Normal	Normal or mildly increased	Normal
Atrial size	Increased	Increased	Increased; may be massive	Left atrium normal; right dilated in severe disease
Valvular disease	Mitral regurgitation (SAM)	Mitral (functional); tricuspid regur- gitation in late stages	Mitral and tricuspid regurgitation, rarely severe	Tricuspid regurgitation in severe disease
Common symptoms	Dyspnea; chest pain, syncope Late: orthopnea, PND	Dyspnea, fatigue Late: orthopnea, PND	Dyspnea Late: orthopnea, PND, right heart failure	Palpitations, syncope Late: right heart failure
Arrhythmia	Atrial fibrillation, ventricular tachycardia; conduction block in PRKAG2, mitochondrial; Fabry's disease	Ventricular tachyarrhythmias; heart block in Chagas' disease, giant cell myocarditis, laminopathies	Atrial fibrillation; conduction block in sarcoid, amyloidosis, desminopathy	Ventricular ectopy and tachycardia

ARVC, Arrhythmogenic right ventricular cardiomyopathy; *LV,* left ventricular; *SAM,* systolic anterior motion of mitral valve; *PND,* paroxysmal nocturnal dyspnea.
From Goldman L, Schafer AI: *Goldman's Cecil medicine,* ed 24, Philadelphia, 2012, Saunders.

Clinical
Algorithms

III

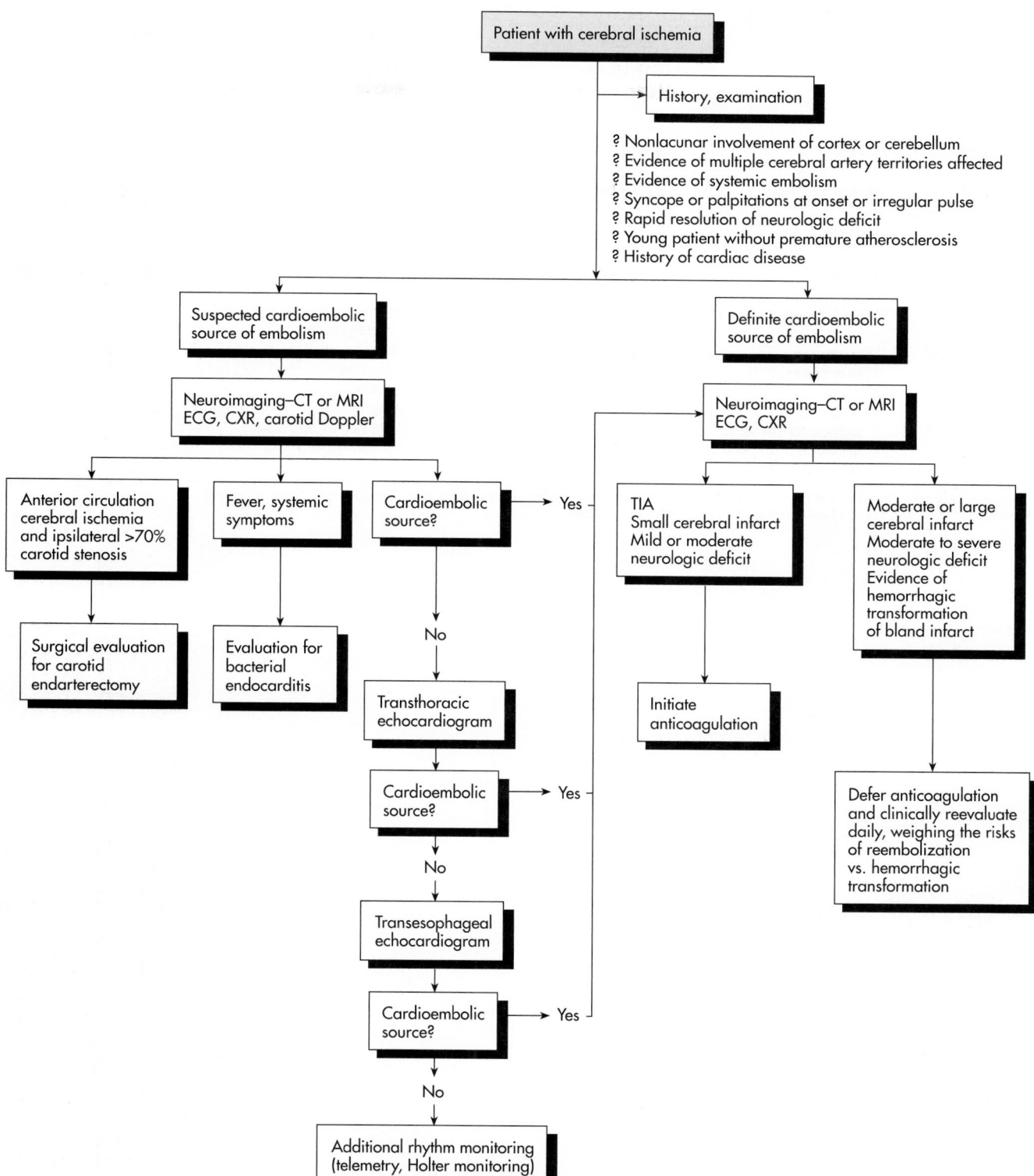

FIGURE 3-41 Evaluation of patients with cerebral ischemia for a cardioembolic source. *CT,* Computed tomography; *CXR,* chest radiograph; *ECG,* electrocardiogram; *MRI,* magnetic resonance imaging; *TIA,* transient ischemic attack. (Modified from Johnson R [ed]: *Current therapy in neurologic disease,* ed 5, St Louis, 1997, Mosby.)

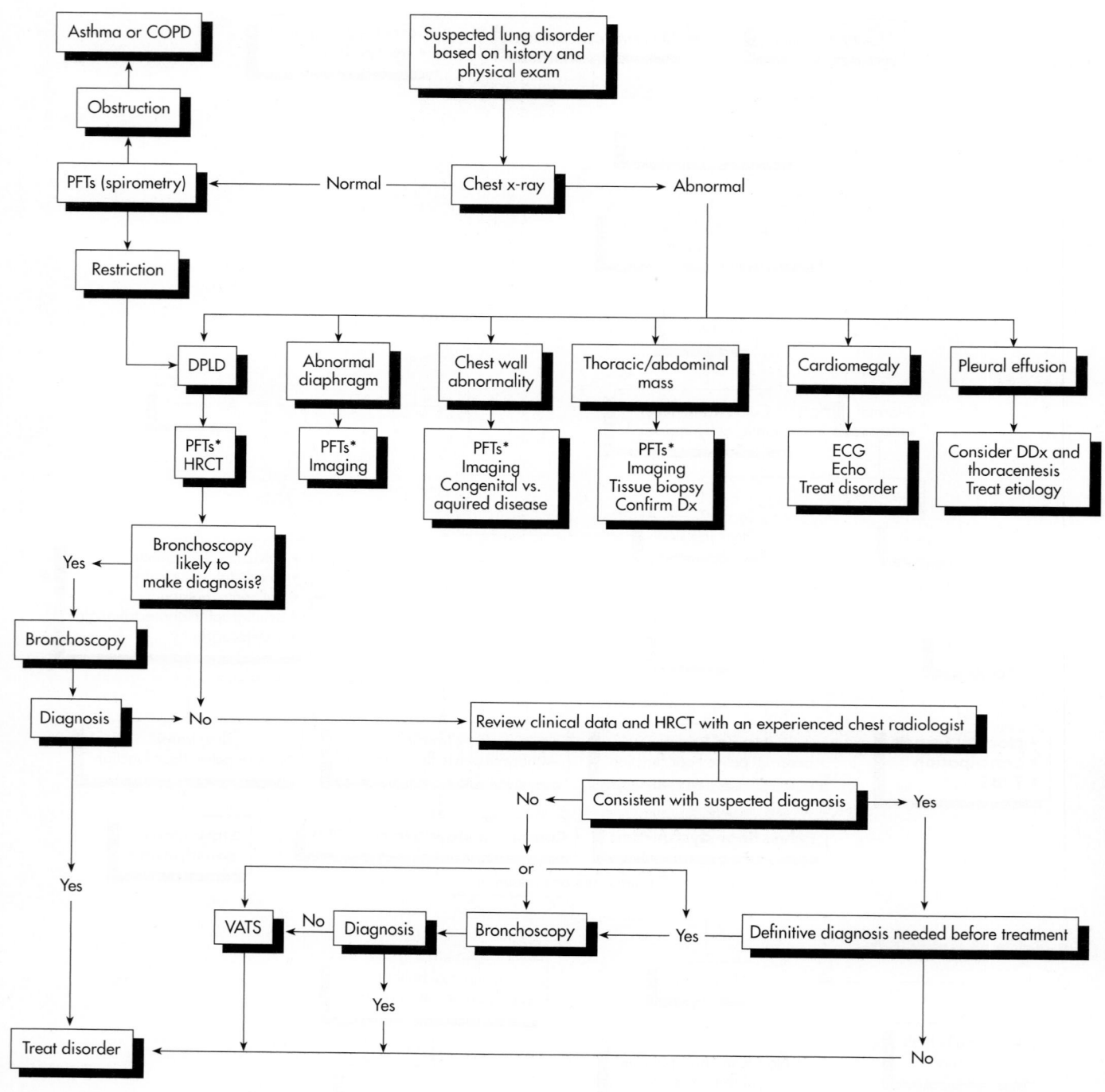

PFTs* = Full set including lung volumes and D<small>LCO</small>

FIGURE 3-42 Diagnostic algorithm. *COPD,* Chronic obstructive pulmonary disease; *DDx,* differential diagnosis; *D<small>LCO</small>,* diffusion capacity; *DPLD,* diffuse parenchymal lung disease; *ECG,* electrocardiogram; *HRCT,* high-resolution computed tomography; *PFTs,* pulmonary function tests; *VATS,* video-assisted thoracoscopic surgery. (Modified from Runge MS, Greganti MA: *Netter's internal medicine,* Philadelphia, 2008, Saunders.)

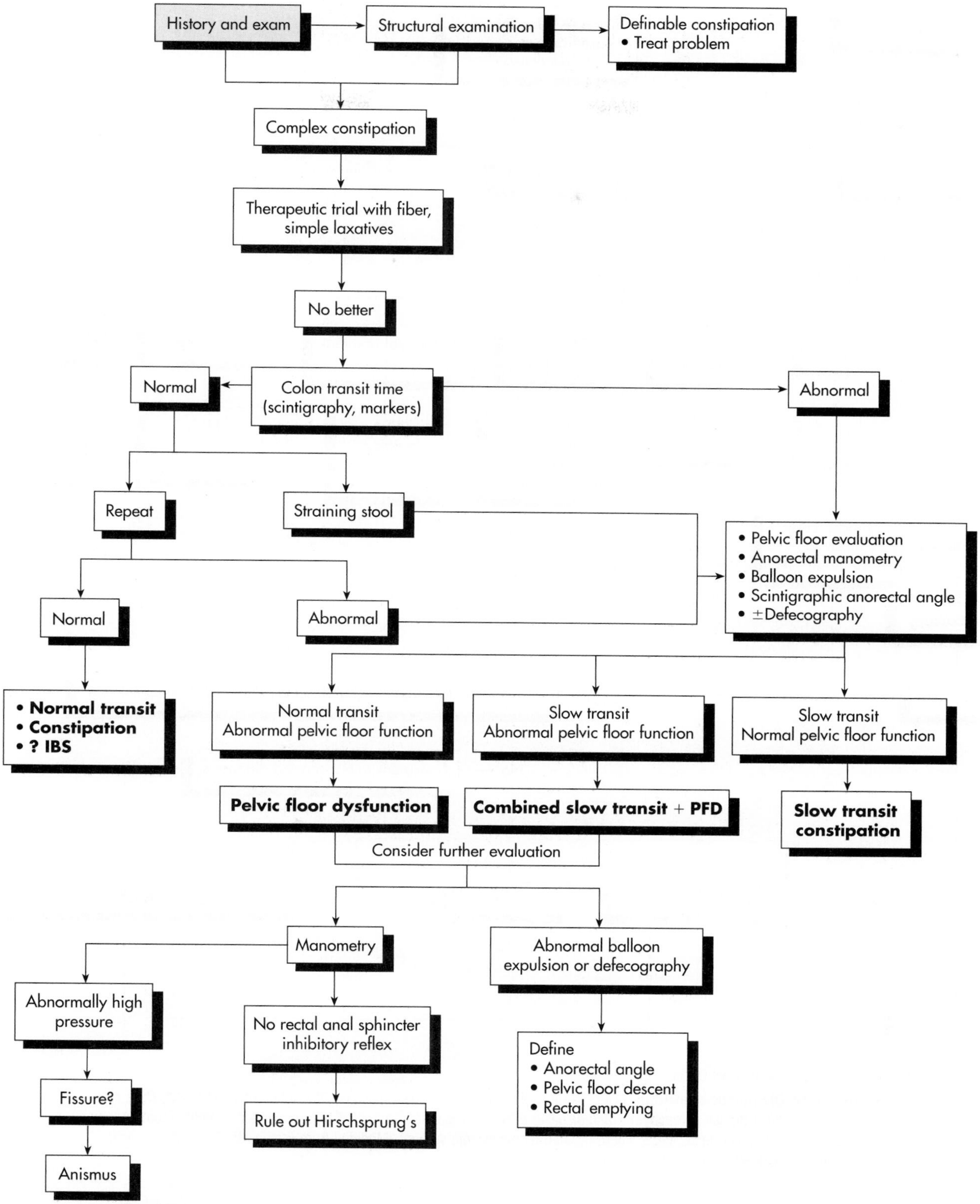

FIGURE 3-43 Evaluation of constipation. *IBS,* Irritable bowel syndrome; *PFD,* pelvic floor dysfunction. (From Pemberton JH et al: *The pelvic floor: its functions and disorders,* Philadelphia, 2001, Saunders.)

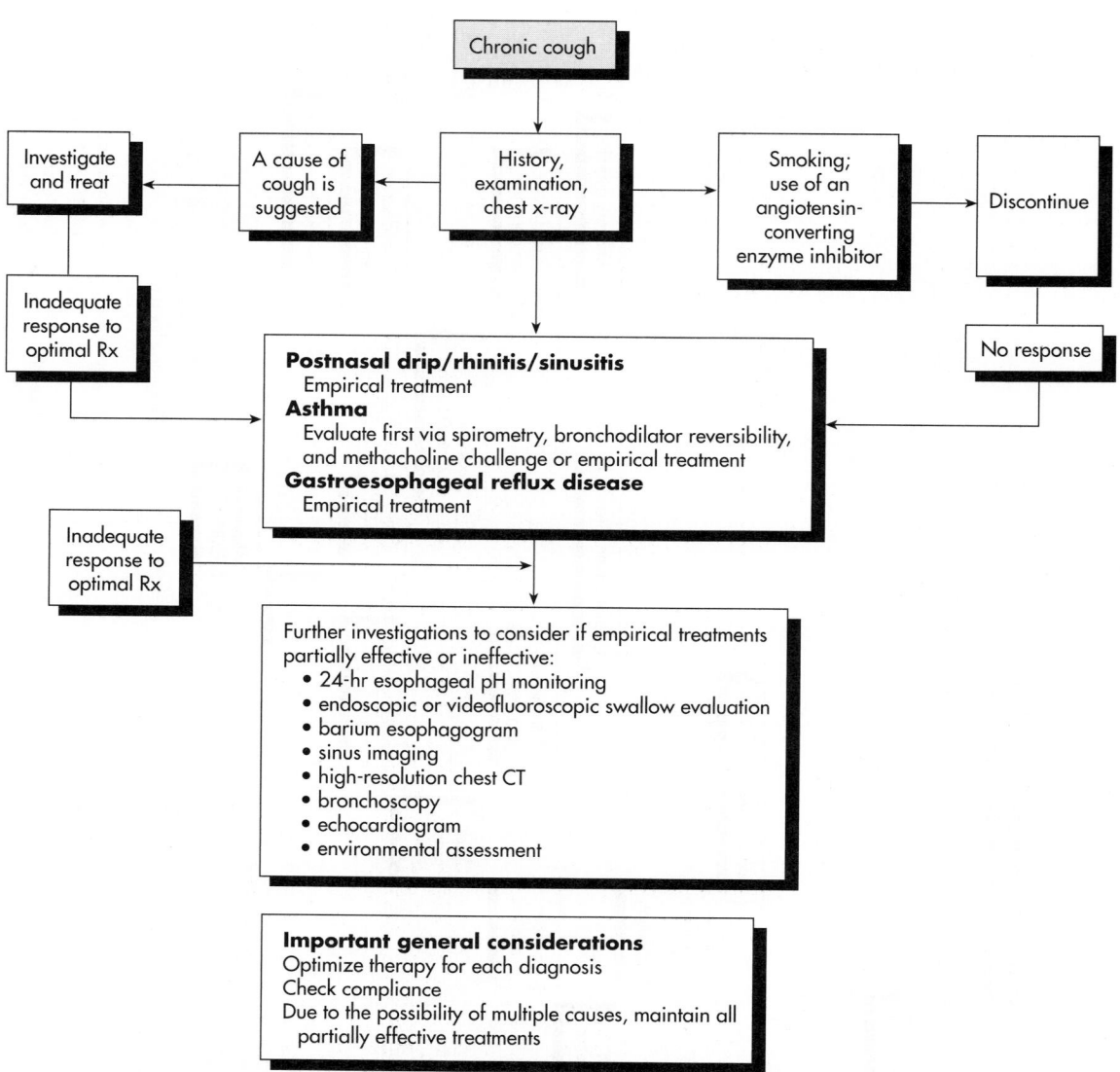

FIGURE 3-46 Algorithm for the management of chronic cough lasting >8 weeks. *CT,* Computed tomography; *Rx,* prescription. (From Goldman L, Schafer AI: *Goldman's Cecil medicine,* ed 24, Philadelphia, 2012, Saunders.)

TABLE 3-3   Testing Characteristics of Diagnostic Protocol for Evaluation of Chronic Cough

Tests	Diagnosis	Positive Predictive Value (%)	Negative Predictive Value (%)
Sinus radiograph	Sinusitis	57-81	95-100
Methacholine inhalation challenge	Asthma	60-82	100
Modified barium esophagography	GERD, esophageal stricture	38-63	63-93
Esophageal pH*	GERD	89-100	>100
Bronchoscopy	Endobronchial mass/lesion	50-89	100

*24-Hour esophageal pH monitoring. *GERD,* Gastroesophageal reflux disease.
From Goldman L, Schafer AI: *Goldman's Cecil medicine,* ed 24, Philadelphia, 2012, Saunders.

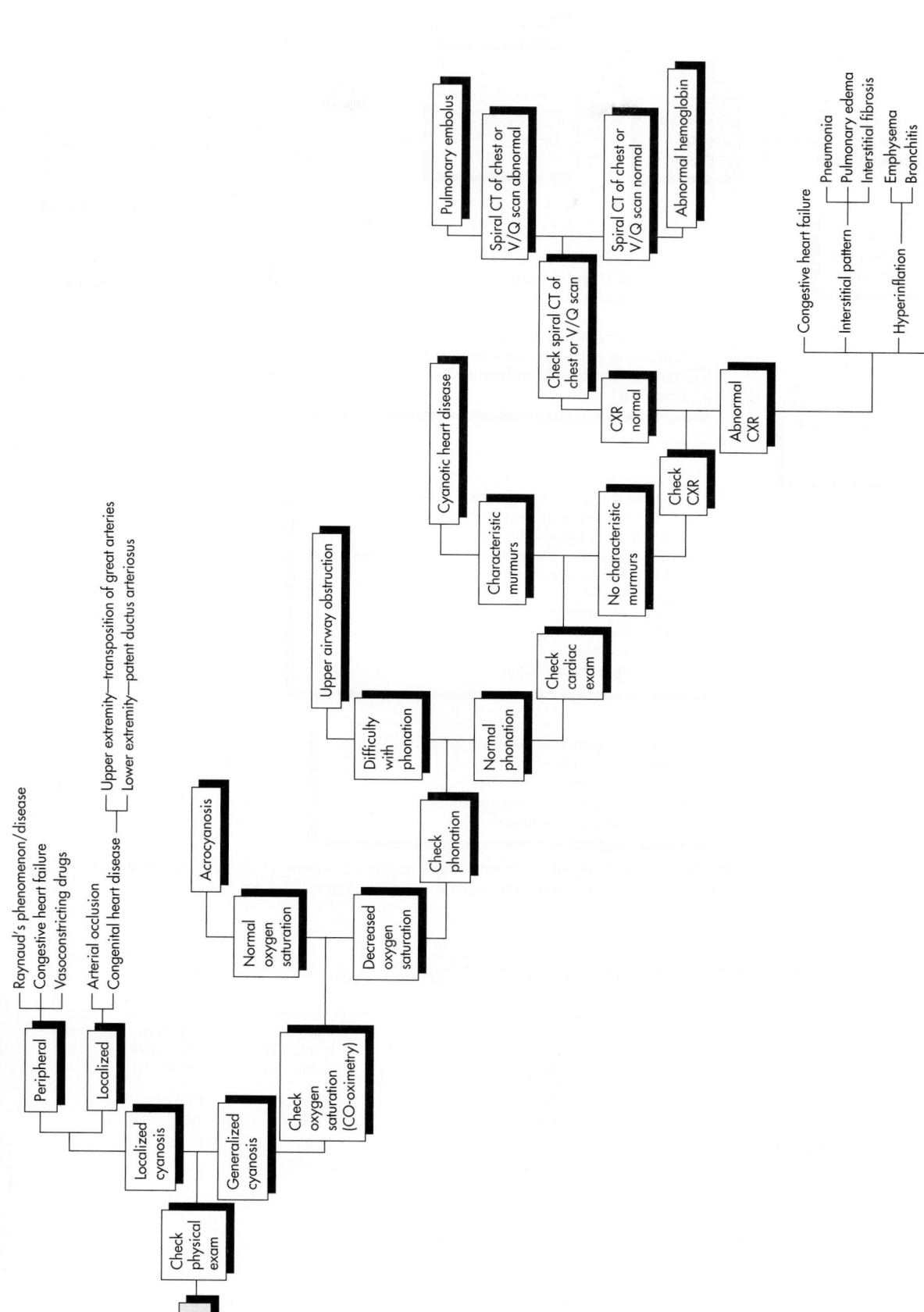

FIGURE 3-48 Cyanosis. *A-V,* Arteriovenous; *CXR,* chest x-ray; *V/Q,* ventilation-perfusion. (From Healey PM: *Common medical diagnosis: an algorithmic approach,* ed 3, Philadelphia, 2000, Saunders.)

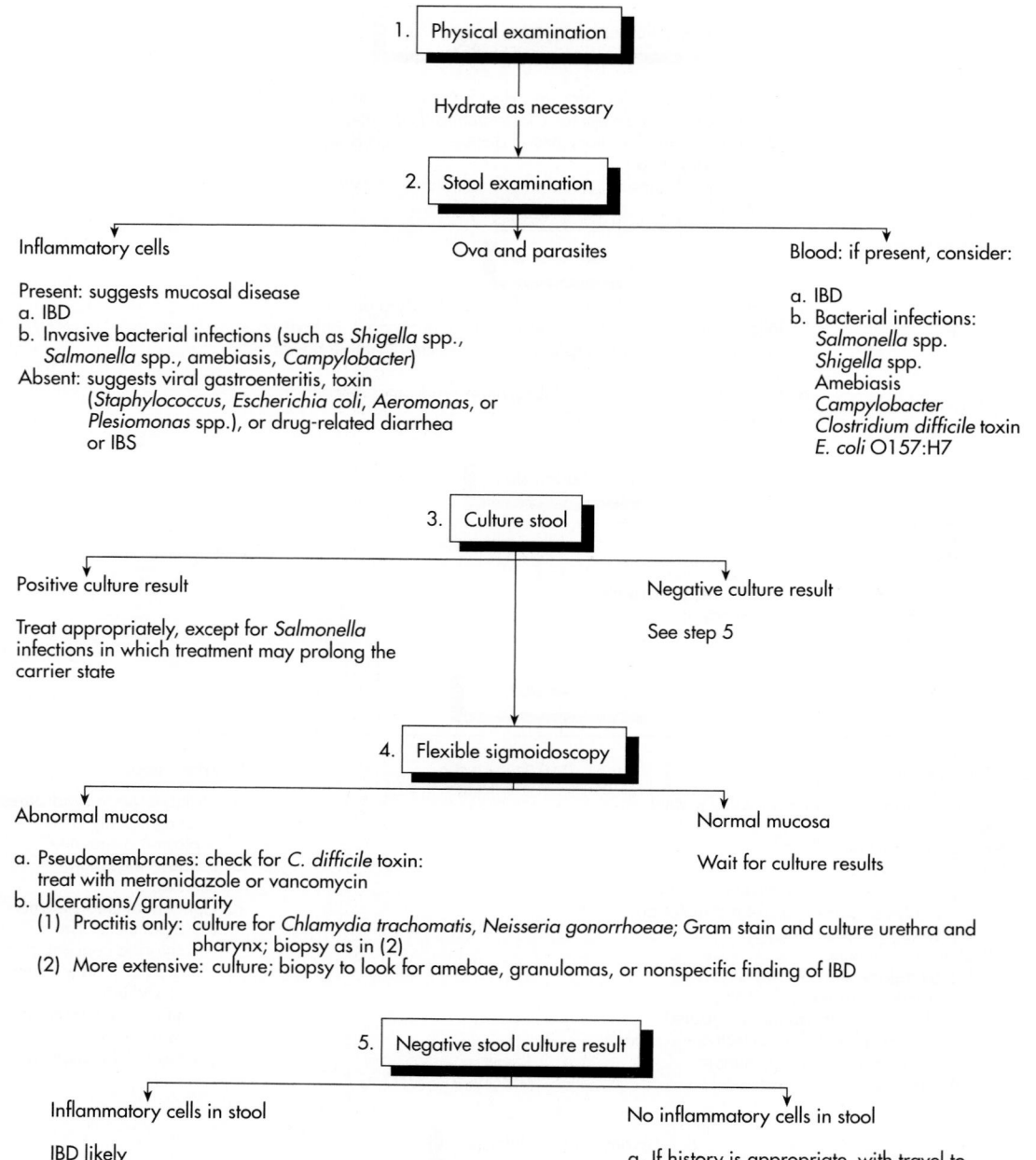

FIGURE 3-53 Diagnostic steps in the assessment of acute diarrhea. *IBD,* Inflammatory bowel disease; *IBS,* irritable bowel syndrome. (Modified from Stein JH [ed]: *Internal medicine,* ed 5, St Louis, 1998, Mosby.)

1. Diagnostic steps 1 to 4 as in Fig. 3-53

   a. Results diagnostic for infectious diarrhea (uncommon in chronic diarrhea except for *Clostridium difficile* after antibiotics), inflammatory bowel disease, or overt drug-induced diarrhea
   b. Results nondiagnostic; usually without inflammatory cells in stool

2. Stool volume

   a. Small volume: usually seen in infectious diarrhea or inflammatory bowel disease (consider colonoscopy), but can also be seen in malabsorption syndromes and irritable bowel syndrome
   b. Large volume: suggests malabsorption syndromes, secretory diarrhea, or laxative abuse

3. Stool Sudan stain

   Positive

   Suggests malabsorption syndrome, pancreatic insufficiency, bile salt insufficiency, or mucosal disease

   Negative

   See step 4

4. Oral intake stopped

   Diarrhea continues

   a. Secretory diarrhea: stool osmolality = stool $(Na^+ + K^+) \times 2$
   b. Nasogastric suction
      (1) Diarrhea stops
         (a) Zollinger-Ellison syndrome: gastric analysis, gastrin, secretin stimulation
         (b) Laxative abuse: see step 5
      (2) Diarrhea continues
         (a) Secretory diarrhea: plasma VIP, calcitonin, urinary 5-HIAA; abdominal ultrasound, computed tomography and/or selective mesenteric angiogram to identify tumor
         (b) Laxative abuse: see step 5

   Diarrhea stops

   a. Malabsorption syndromes: stool osmolality > plasma osmolality
   b. Laxative ingestion: see step 5
   c. Congenital chloridorrhea
      (1) Stool electrolytes: chloride concentration greater than the sum of sodium and potassium concentrations in stool water
      (2) No fecal osmotic gap

5. Laxative abuse detection

   a. Screening tests
      (1) Detailed history
      (2) Colonoscopy and biopsy for melanosis coli
   b. Specific tests (if available)
      (1) Urine screening test for senna
      (2) Chromatographic test for bisacodyl
      (3) Stool test for fecal sulfate and phosphate
      (4) Magnesium concentration in fecal water (atomic absorption spectrophotometry)

6. Radiologic studies

   Perform barium studies only after stool examination, culture, and studies requiring quantitative measurements of the stool have been completed.

FIGURE 3-54 Diagnostic approach to the patient with chronic diarrhea (patients who are HIV negative). *5-HIAA,* 5-Hydroxyindoleacetic acid; *VIP,* vasoactive intestinal polypeptide. (Modified from Stein JH [ed]: *Internal medicine,* ed 5, St Louis, 1998, Mosby.)

DILATED PUPIL

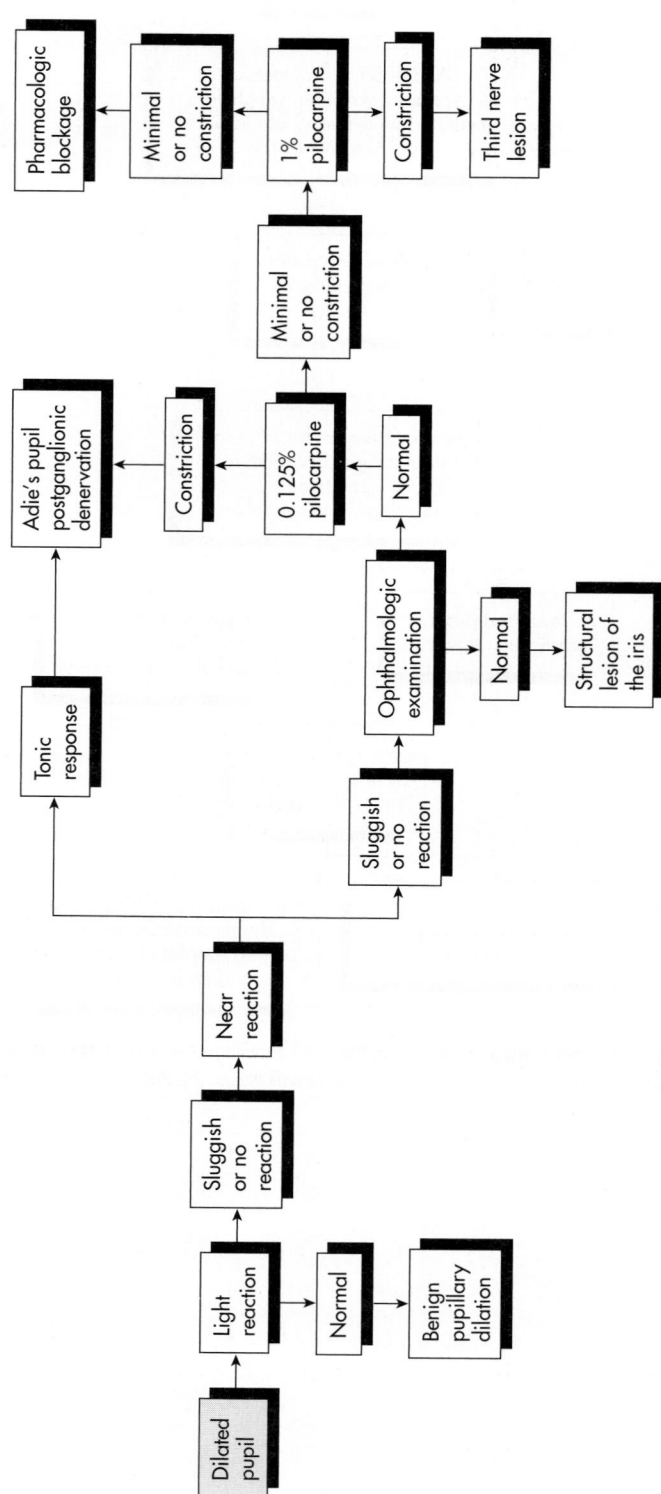

FIGURE 3-57 Use of pilocarpine to help differentiate between different causes of a dilated pupil. (From Goldman L, Ausiello D [eds]: *Cecil textbook of medicine,* ed 23, Philadelphia, 2008, Saunders.)

Clinical Algorithms

III

ICD-9CM # 563.3 Dyspepsia atonic
536.8 Dyspepsia disorders other unspecified function of stomach
306.4 Dyspepsia, psychogenic

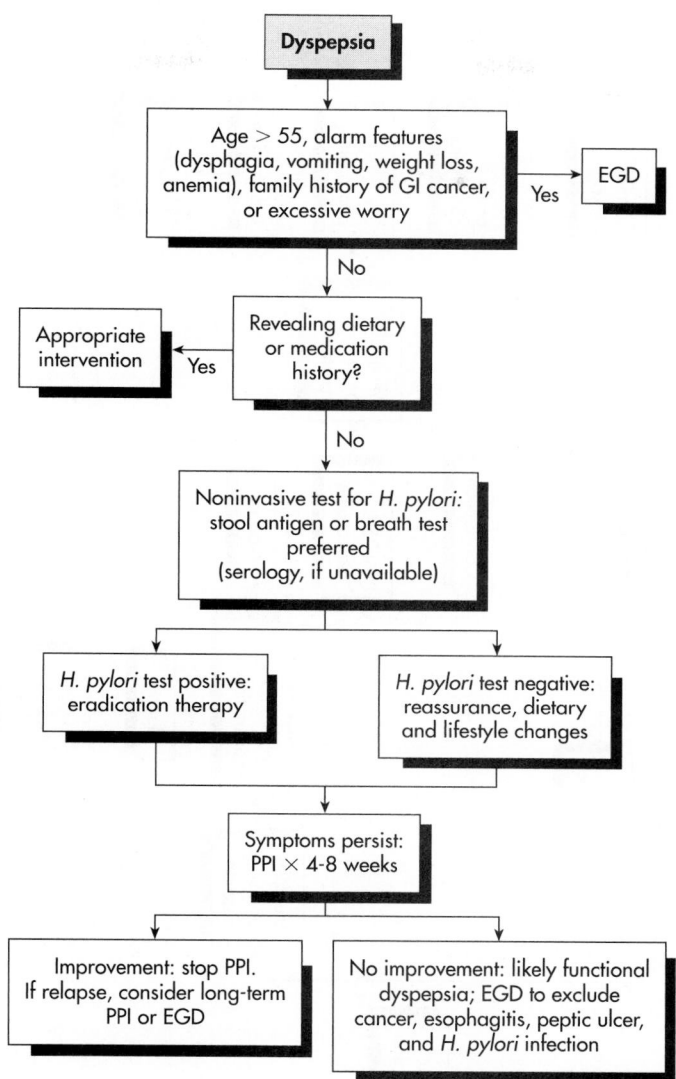

FIGURE 3-58 Approach to the patient with dyspepsia. *EGD,* Esophagastroduodenoscopy; *GI,* gastrointestinal; *PPI,* proton pump inhibitor. (From Goldman L, Schafer AI: *Goldman's Cecil medicine,* ed 24, Philadelphia, 2012, Saunders.)

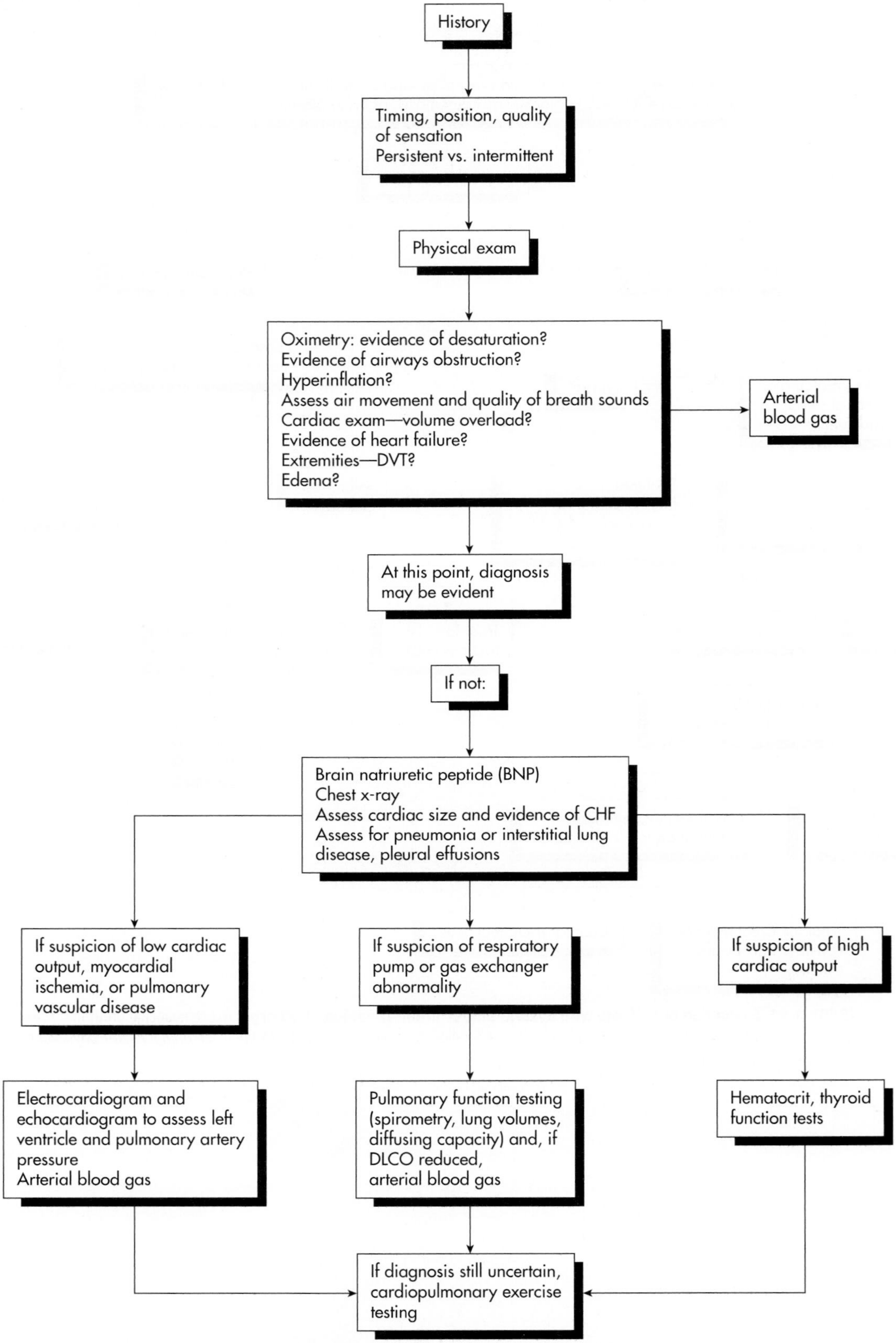

History

↓

Timing, position, quality
of sensation
Persistent vs. intermittent

↓

Physical exam

↓

Oximetry: evidence of desaturation?
Evidence of airways obstruction?
Hyperinflation?
Assess air movement and quality of breath sounds
Cardiac exam—volume overload?
Evidence of heart failure?
Extremities—DVT?
Edema?   →   Arterial
                                                    blood gas

↓

At this point, diagnosis
may be evident

↓

If not:

↓

Brain natriuretic peptide (BNP)
Chest x-ray
Assess cardiac size and evidence of CHF
Assess for pneumonia or interstitial lung
disease, pleural effusions

If suspicion of low cardiac output, myocardial ischemia, or pulmonary vascular disease	If suspicion of respiratory pump or gas exchanger abnormality	If suspicion of high cardiac output
↓	↓	↓
Electrocardiogram and echocardiogram to assess left ventricle and pulmonary artery pressure Arterial blood gas	Pulmonary function testing (spirometry, lung volumes, diffusing capacity) and, if DLCO reduced, arterial blood gas	Hematocrit, thyroid function tests

↓

If diagnosis still uncertain,
cardiopulmonary exercise
testing

FIGURE 3-59 Algorithm for the evaluation of the patient with dyspnea. The pace and completeness with which one approaches this framework depends on the intensity and acuity of the patient's symptoms. In a patient with severe, acute dyspnea, for example, an arterial blood gas measurement may be one of the first laboratory evaluations, whereas this measurement might not be obtained until much later in the workup in a patient with chronic breathlessness of unclear cause. A therapeutic trial of a medication, for example, a bronchodilator, may be instituted at any point if one is fairly confident of the diagnosis based on the data available at that time. *CHF,* Congestive heart failure; *DLCO,* diffusing capacity of the lung for carbon monoxide; *DVT,* deep venous thrombosis. (Modified from Schwartzstein RM, Feller-Kopman D: Approach to the patient with dyspnea. In Braunwald E, Goldman L [eds]: *Primary cardiology,* ed 2, Philadelphia, 2003, Saunders.)

Clinical
Algorithms

III

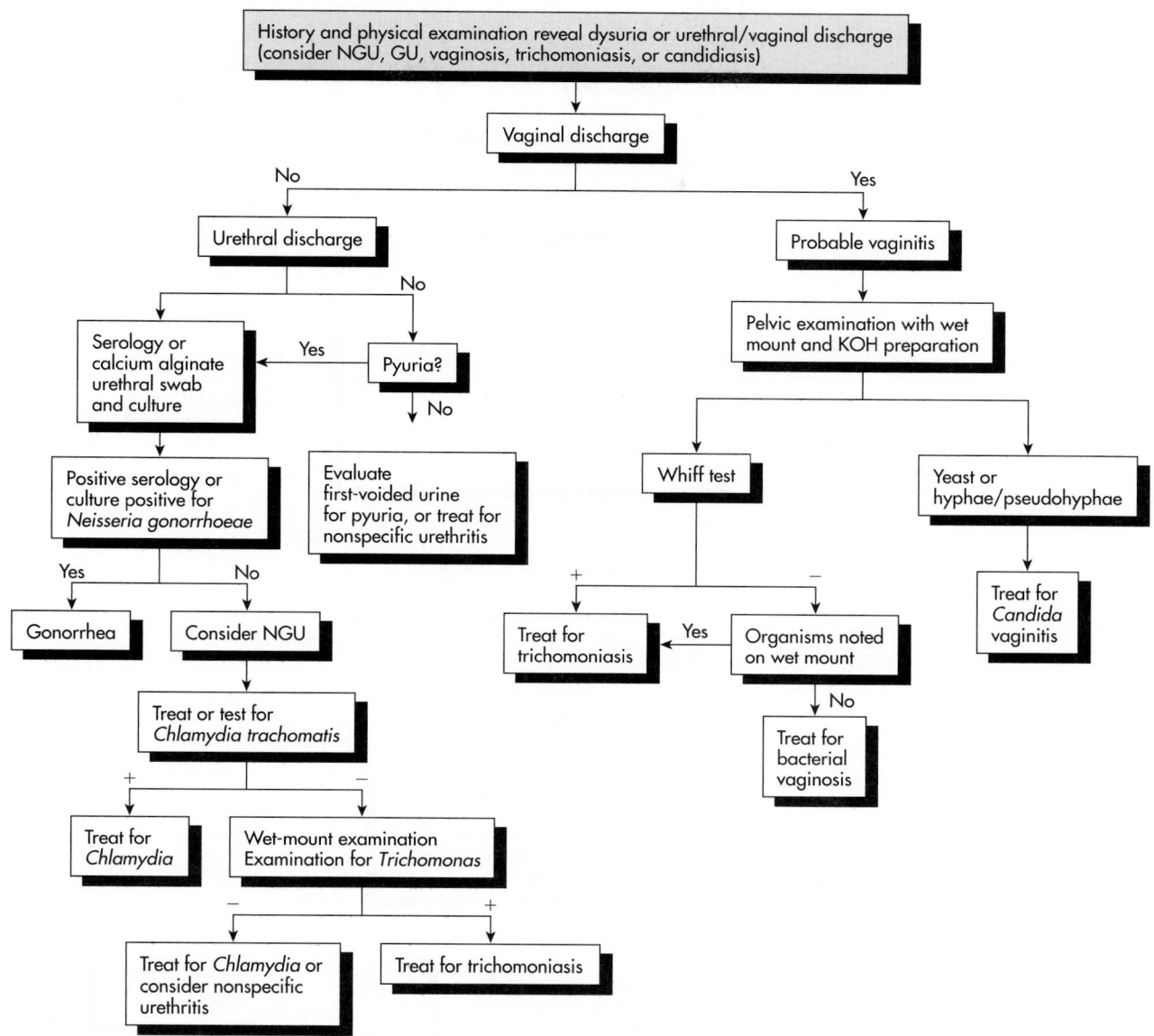

FIGURE 3-60 Evaluation of patients with dysuria and/or urethral/vaginal discharge. *GU*, Gonococcal urethritis; *KOH*, potassium hydroxide; *NGU*, nongonococcal urethritis. (Modified from Nseyo UO [ed]: *Urology for primary care physicians*, Philadelphia, 1999, Saunders.)

Management of Ear Pain

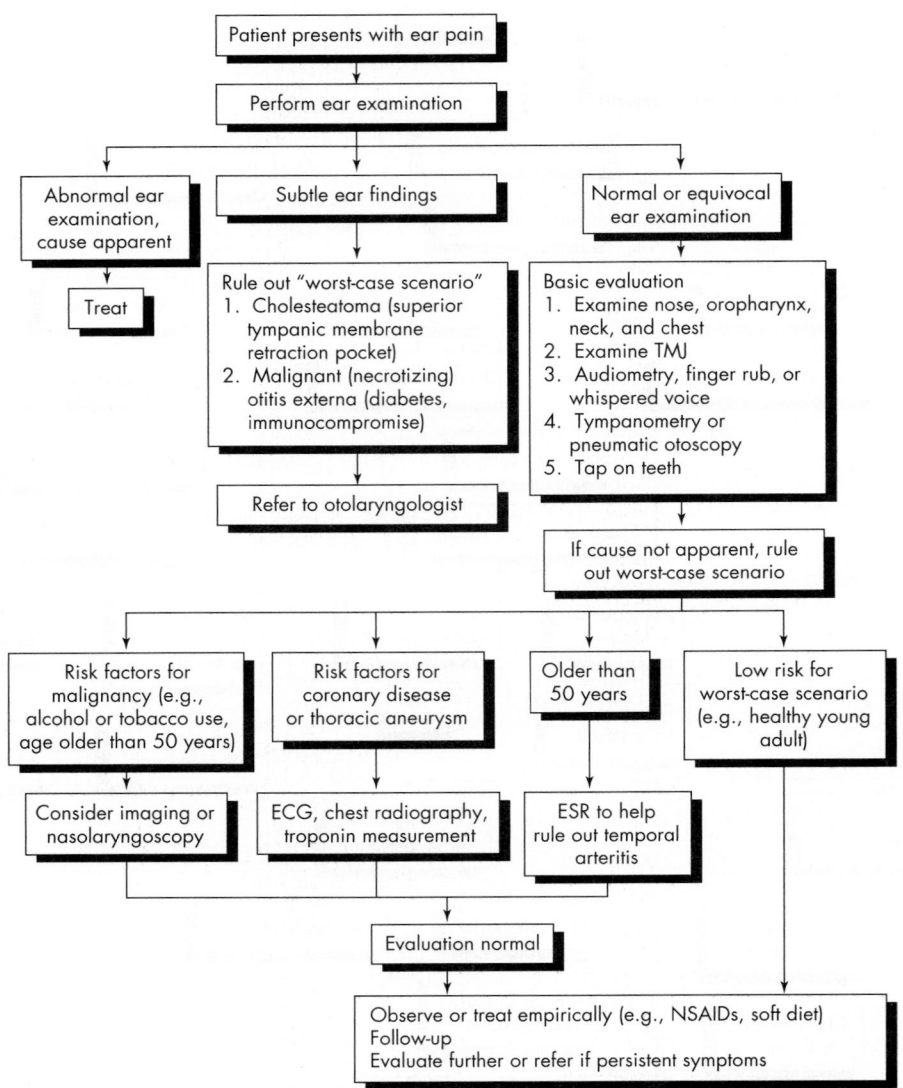

FIGURE 3-61 Management of ear pain. *ECG,* Electrocardiography; *ESR,* erythrocyte sedimentation rate; *NSAIDs,* nonsteroidal anti-inflammatory drugs; *TMJ,* temporomandibular joint. (From Ely JW et al: Diagnosis of ear pain, *Am Fam Physician* 77[5]:622, 2008.)

Clinical
Algorithms

III

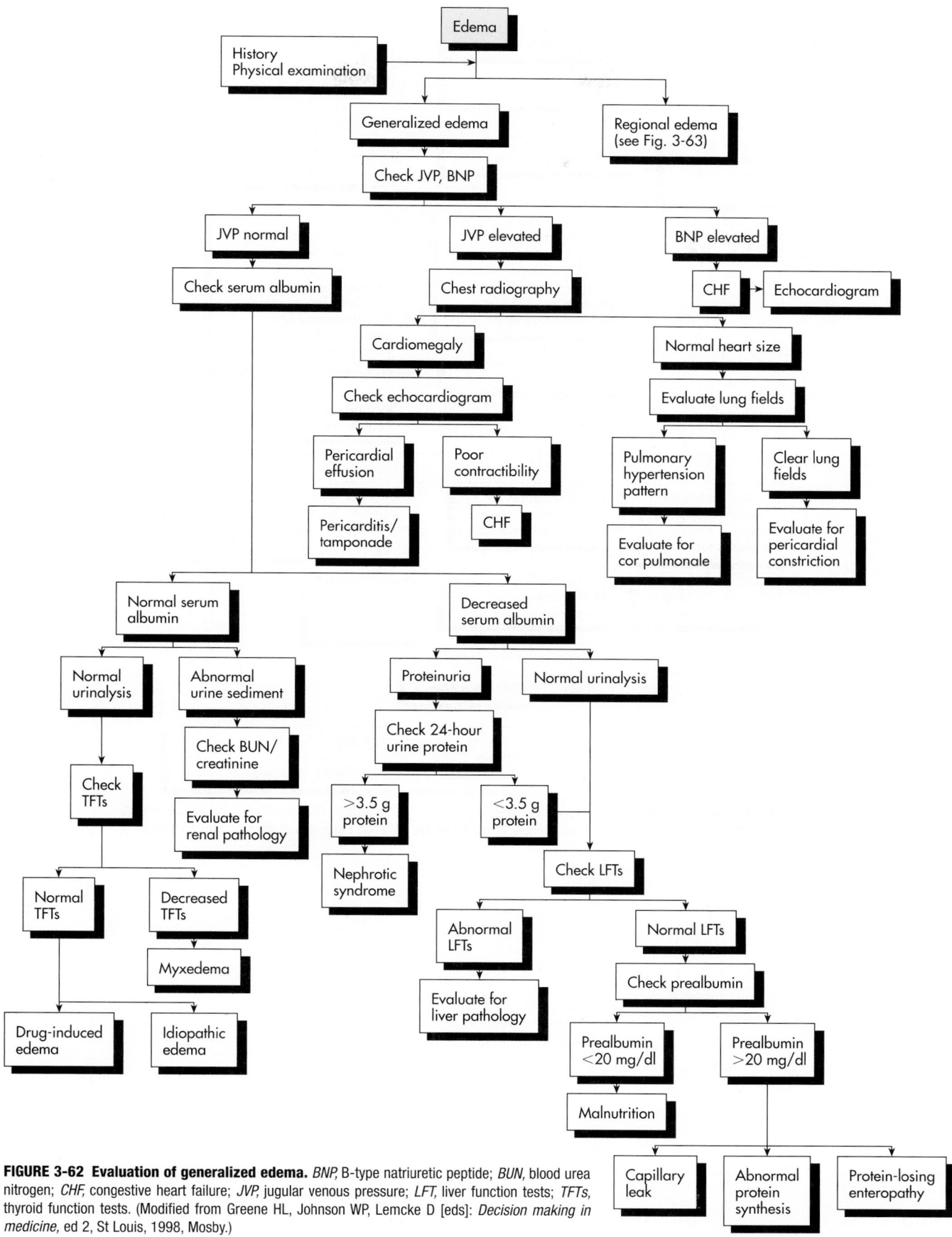

FIGURE 3-62 Evaluation of generalized edema. *BNP,* B-type natriuretic peptide; *BUN,* blood urea nitrogen; *CHF,* congestive heart failure; *JVP,* jugular venous pressure; *LFT,* liver function tests; *TFTs,* thyroid function tests. (Modified from Greene HL, Johnson WP, Lemcke D [eds]: *Decision making in medicine,* ed 2, St Louis, 1998, Mosby.)

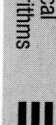

Clinical
Algorithms

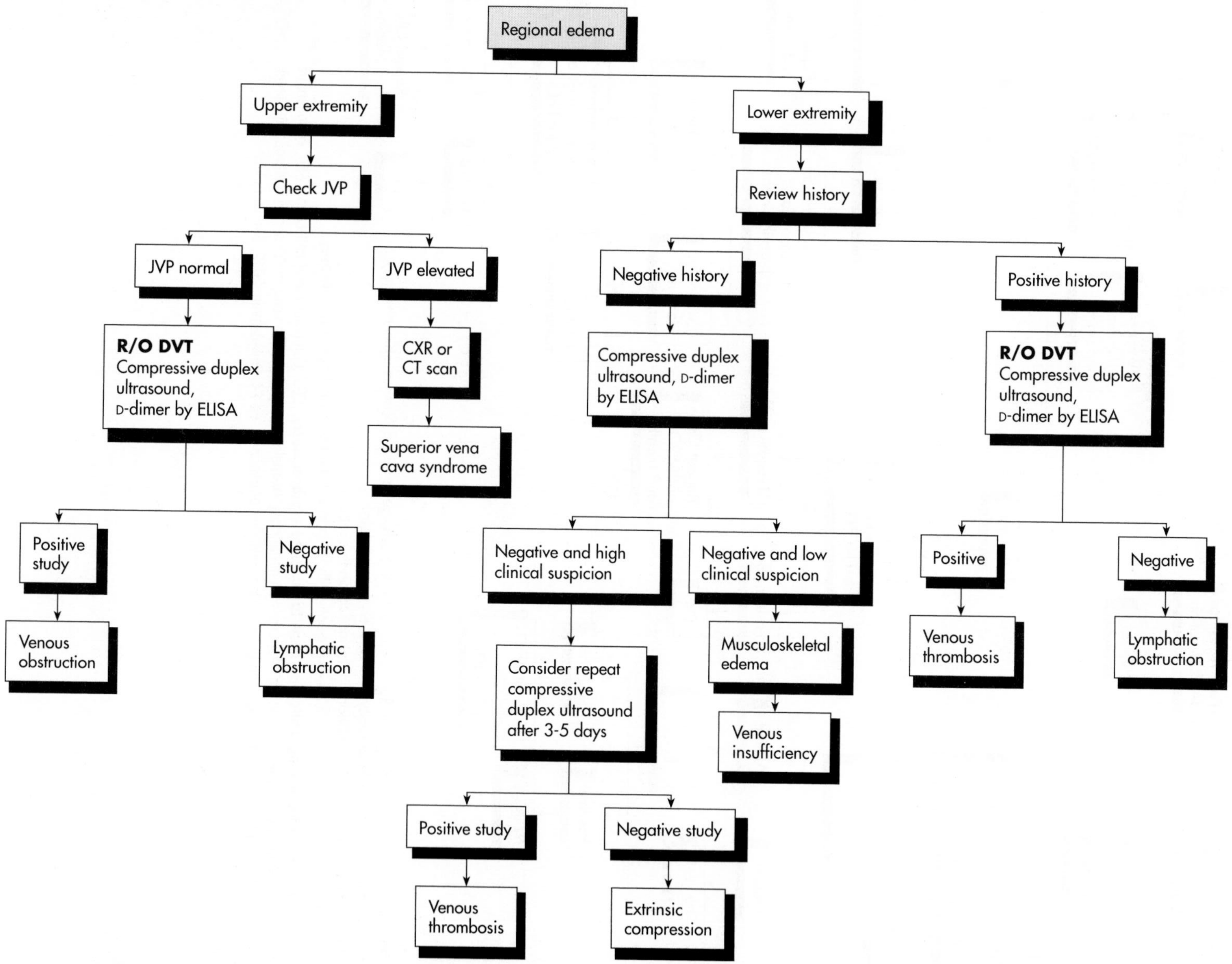

FIGURE 3-63 Evaluation of regional edema. *CT,* Computed tomography; *CXR,* chest x-ray examination; *DVT,* deep venous thrombosis; *ELISA,* enzyme-linked immunosorbent assay; *JVP,* jugular venous pressure. (Modified from Greene HL, Johnson WP, Lemcke D [eds]: *Decision making in medicine,* ed 2, St Louis, 1998, Mosby.)

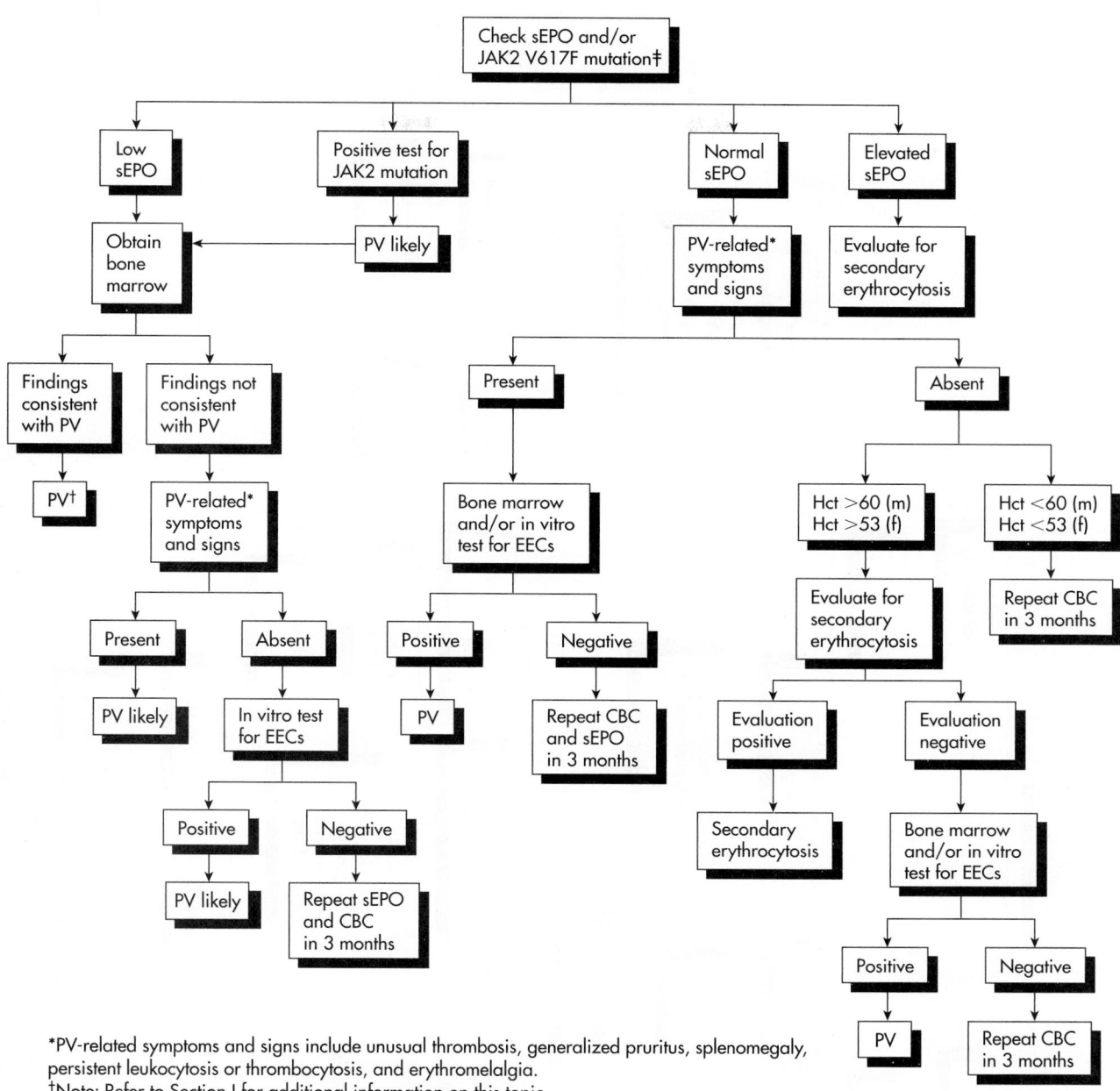

*PV-related symptoms and signs include unusual thrombosis, generalized pruritus, splenomegaly, persistent leukocytosis or thrombocytosis, and erythromelalgia.
†Note: Refer to Section I for additional information on this topic.
‡The JAK2 mutation is found in >95% of patients with PV and can be used for diagnostic purposes.

FIGURE 3-66 A diagnostic approach to acquired erythrocytosis. *CBC,* Complete blood cell count; *EEC,* endogenous (spontaneous) erythroid colonies; *f,* female; *Hct,* hematocrit; *m,* male; *PV,* polycythemia vera; *sEPO,* serum erythropoietin level. (Modified from Goldman L, Ausiello D [eds]: *Cecil textbook of medicine,* ed 24, Philadelphia, 2012, Saunders.)

ERYTHRODERMA

ICD-9CM #	695.9	Secondary
	695.89	Exfoliative
	696.2	Maculopapular
	696.1	Psoriaticum
	695.89	Infantum

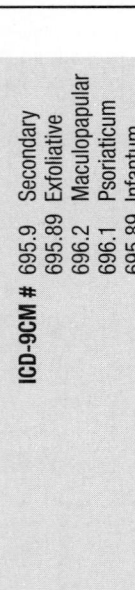

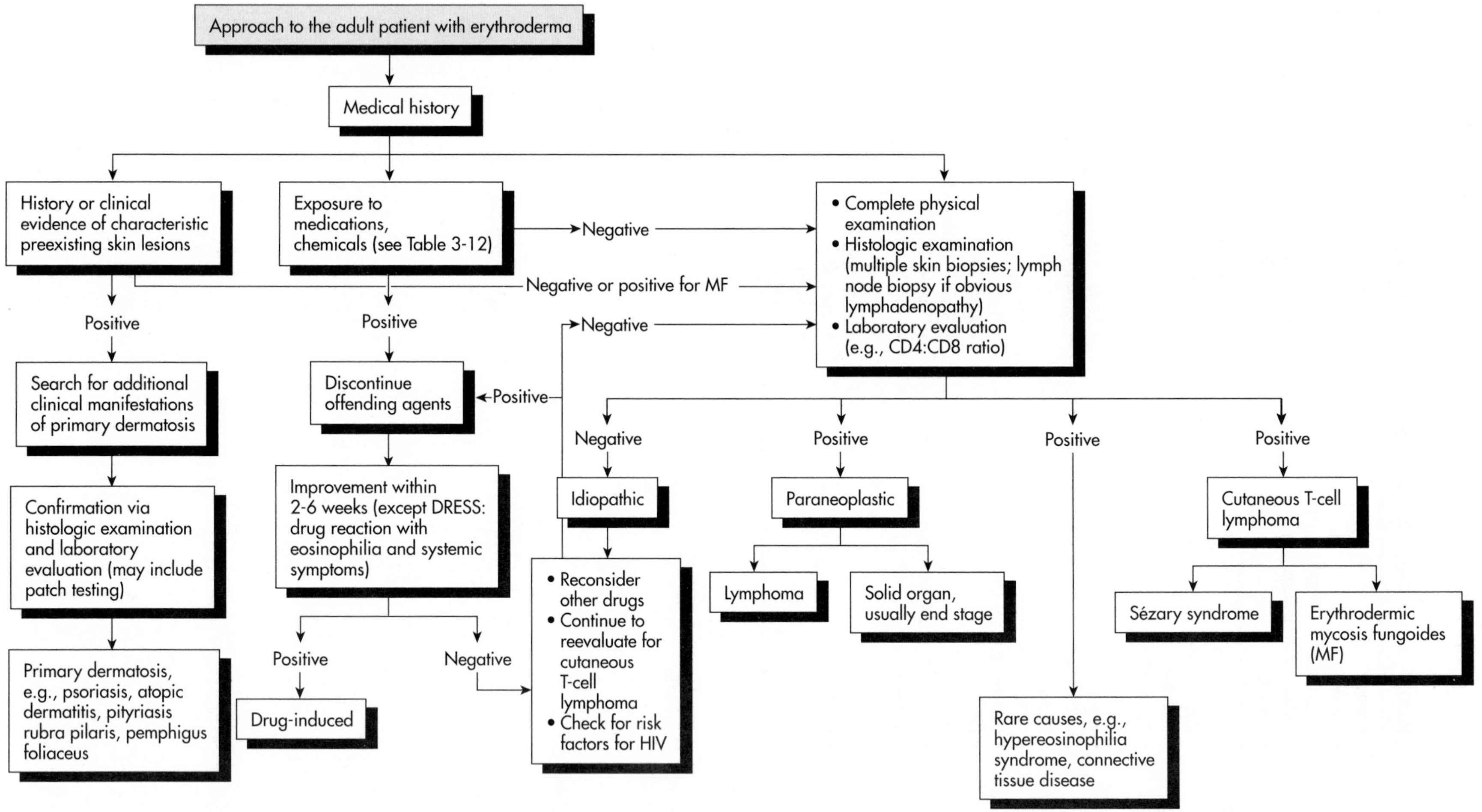

FIGURE 3-67 Approach to the differential diagnosis of adult erythroderma. (From Bolognia JL et al [eds]: *Dermatology*, ed 2, St Louis, 2008, Mosby.)

Clinical
Algorithms

III

ICD-9CM # 695.9 Secondary
695.89 Exfoliative
696.2 Maculopapular
696.1 Psoriaticum
695.89 Infantum

TABLE 3-12 Drugs Associated with Erythroderma

Common

- Allopurinol
- Ampicillin/amoxicillin/penicillin G
- Carbamazepine/oxcarbazepine
- Dapsone
- Omeprazole/lansoprazole
- Phenobarbital
- Phenothiazines
- Phenytoin
- Sulfasalazine
- Sulfonamides
- Vancomycin

Less Common

- Captopril
- Carboplatin/cisplatin
- Cytokines (IL-2/GM-CSF)
- Diflunisal
- Gold
- Hydroxychloroquine/mefloquine
- Isoniazid
- Mercury
- Minocycline
- Nifedipine
- Thalidomide

Rare

- Amiodarone
- Aztreonam
- Cimetidine
- Chlorpromazine
- Clofazimine
- Codeine
- Diltiazem
- Erythropoietin
- Fluorouracil
- Indinavir sulfate
- Lithium
- Mitomycin C
- Pentostatin
- Piroxicam
- Practolol
- Ranitidine
- Rifampin (rifampicin)
- Tear gas (CS gas)
- Teicoplanin
- Terbinafine
- Tobramycin
- Tramadol
- Vinca alkaloids
- Zidovudine

FATIGUE

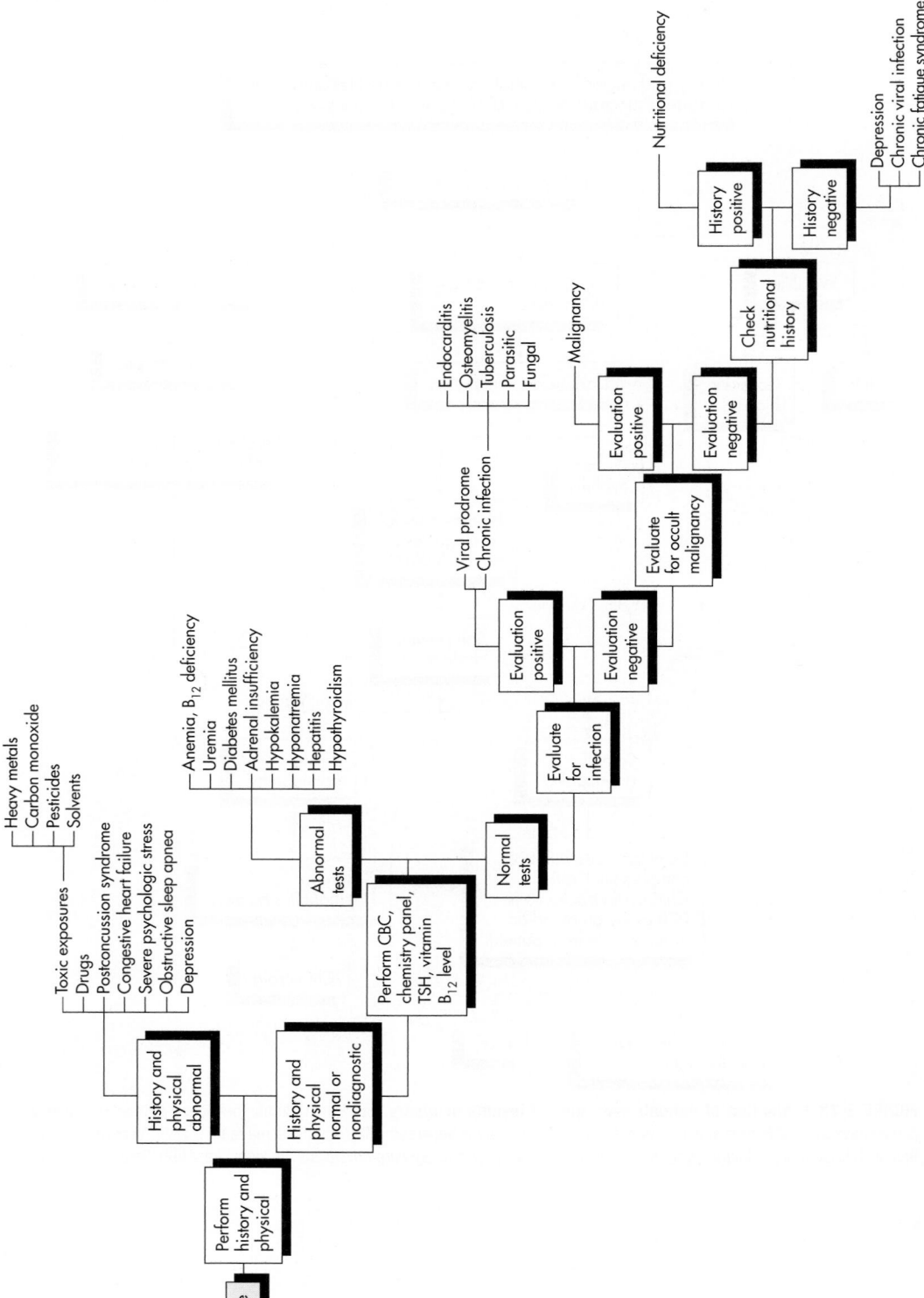

FIGURE 3-68 Evaluation of fatigue. *CBC,* Complete blood count. (Modified from Healey PM: *Common medical diagnosis: an algorithmic approach,* ed 3, Philadelphia, 2000, Saunders.)

Clinical
Algorithms

III

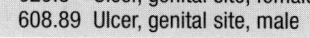

ICD-9CM # 054.10 Genital herpes
91.0 Genital syphilis
078.11 Condyloma acuminatum
099.0 Chancroid
099.2 Granuloma inguinale
099.1 Lymphogranuloma venereum
629.8 Ulcer, genital site, female
608.89 Ulcer, genital site, male

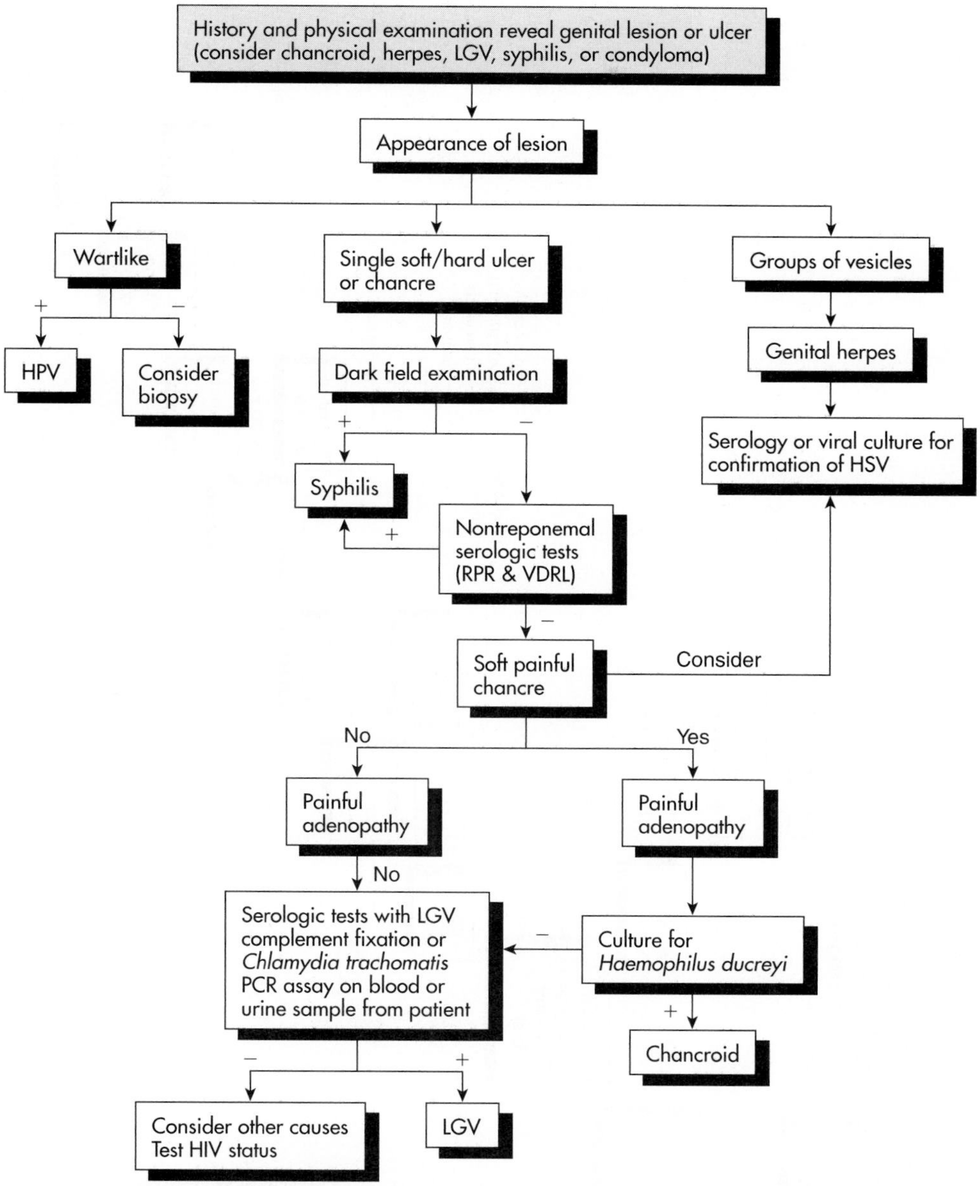

History and physical examination reveal genital lesion or ulcer
(consider chancroid, herpes, LGV, syphilis, or condyloma)

Appearance of lesion

Wartlike

+ HPV

− Consider biopsy

Single soft/hard ulcer or chancre

Dark field examination

+ Syphilis

− Nontreponemal serologic tests (RPR & VDRL)

+ → Syphilis

− Soft painful chancre

Consider

Groups of vesicles

Genital herpes

Serology or viral culture for confirmation of HSV

No — Painful adenopathy

Yes — Painful adenopathy

No → Serologic tests with LGV complement fixation or *Chlamydia trachomatis* PCR assay on blood or urine sample from patient

− Culture for *Haemophilus ducreyi*

+ Chancroid

− Consider other causes Test HIV status

+ LGV

FIGURE 3-73 Evaluation of patients with genital lesions or ulcers. *HIV*, Human immunodeficiency virus; *HPV*, human papillomavirus; *HSV*, herpes simplex virus; *LGV*, lymphogranuloma venereum; *RPR*, rapid plasma reagin; *VDRL*, Venereal Disease Research Laboratory. (Modified from Nseyo UO [ed]: *Urology for primary care physicians*, Philadelphia, 1999, Saunders.)

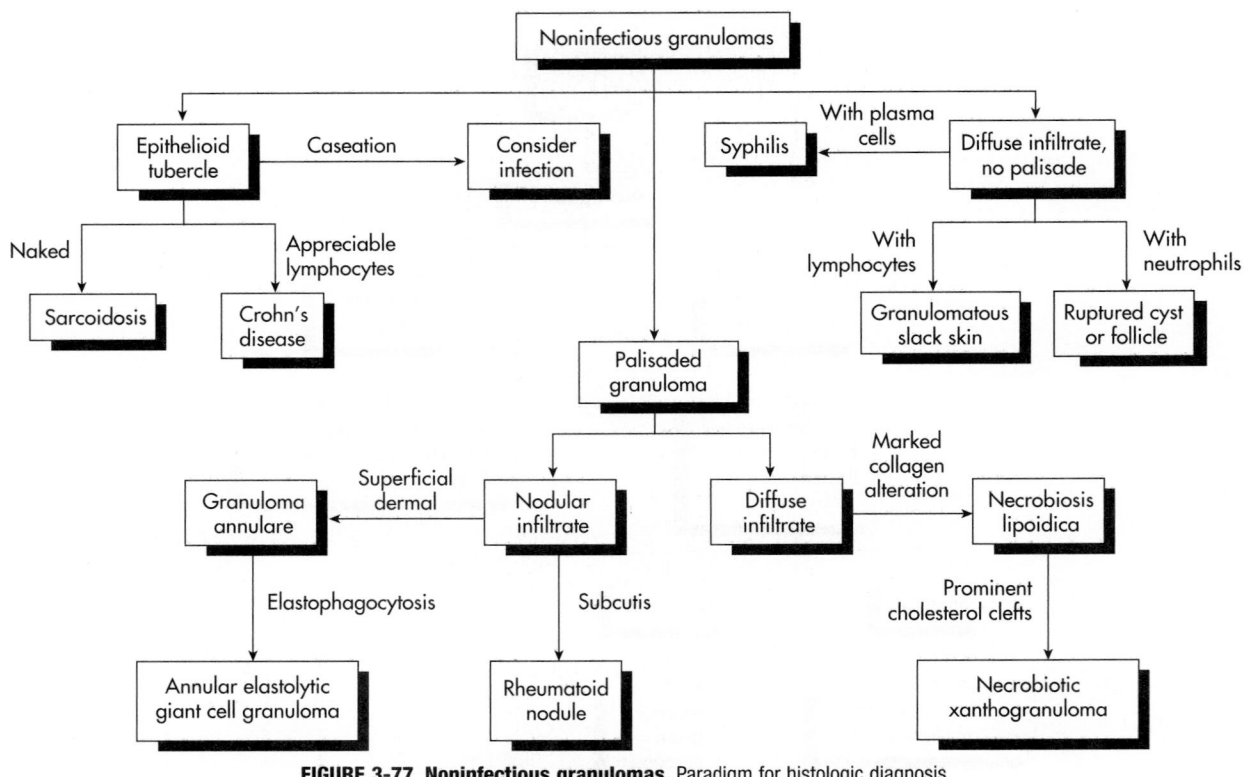

FIGURE 3-77 Noninfectious granulomas. Paradigm for histologic diagnosis.

TABLE 3-13 Clinical Features of the Major Granulomatous Dermatitides

	Sarcoidosis	Classic GA*	NLD	AEGCG	Crohn's Disease	Rheumatoid Nodule
Average age (years)	25-35, 45-65	<30		40	35	30-40
Sex	Female	Female	Female	Female	Female	Female
Racial predilection in United States	African American	None	None	Caucasian	None	None
Site	Symmetric on face, neck, upper trunk, extremities	Hands, feet, extremities	Anterior and lateral distal lower extremities	Face, neck, forearms	Genital areas, lower > upper extremities	Juxtaarticular areas, elbows, hands, ankles, feet
Appearance	Red to red-brown papules and plaques	Papules coalescing into annular plaques	Plaques with elevated borders, telangiectasias centrally	Annular plaques	Dusky erythema and swelling, ulceration	Skin-colored, firm, mobile subcutaneous nodules
Size of lesions	1-5 cm	1-2 mm papules, <5 cm annular plaques	>10 cm	1-6 cm	Variable	1-3 cm
Number of lesions	Variable	1-10	1-10	1-10	1-5	1-10
Associations	Systemic manifestations of sarcoidosis	Rare diabetes mellitus, malignancy	Diabetes mellitus	Actinic damage	Intestinal Crohn's disease	Rheumatoid arthritis
Special clinical characteristics	Occasional central atrophy and hypopigmentation	Central hyperpigmentation	Yellow-brown atrophic centers, ulceration	Central atrophy and hypopigmentation	Draining sinuses and fistulae	Occasional ulceration, especially at site of trauma

From Bolognia JL et al: *Dermatology,* ed 2, St Louis, 2008, Mosby.
AEGCG, Annular elastolytic giant cell granuloma; *GA,* granuloma annulare; *NLD,* necrobiosis lipoidica diabeticorum.
*Clinical variants include generalized, micropapular, nodular, perforating, subcutaneous, and patch GA.

Clinical Algorithms

III

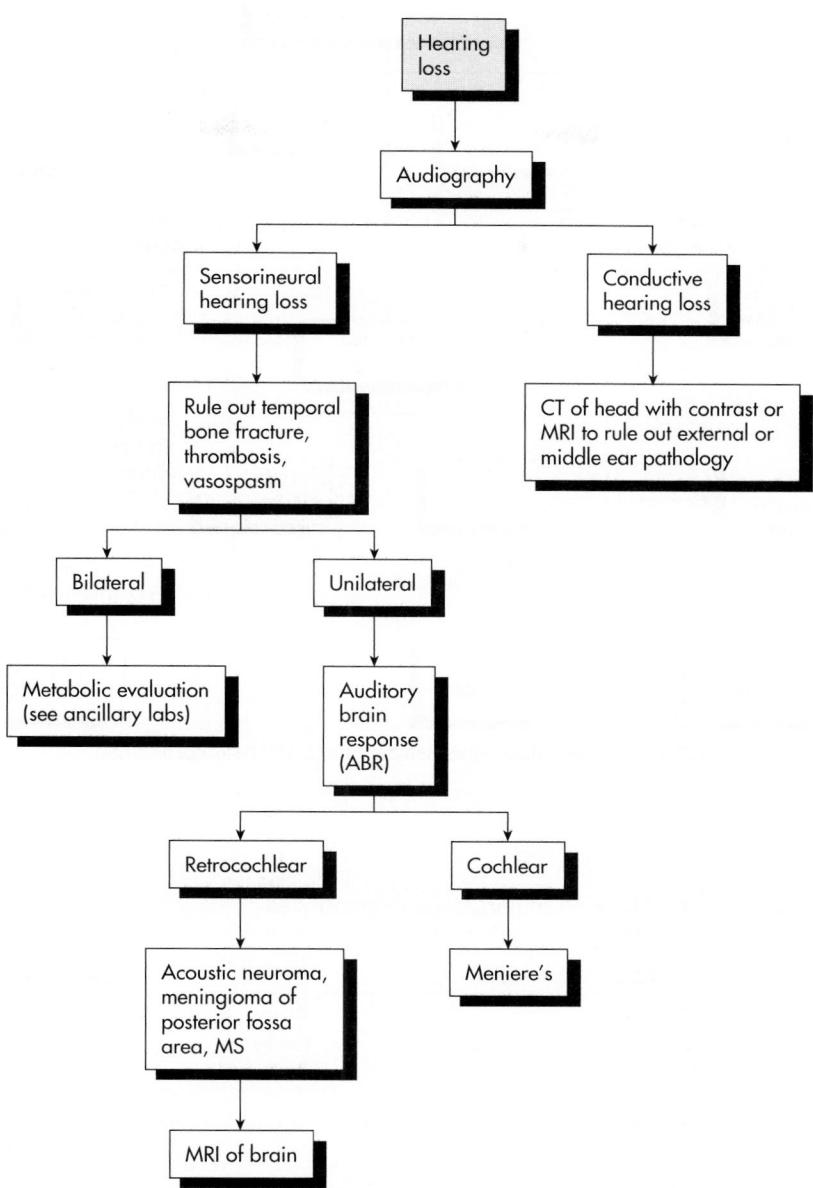

FIGURE 3-78 Evaluation of hearing loss. *CT,* Computed tomography; *MRI,* magnetic resonance imaging; *MS,* multiple sclerosis. (From Ferri FF: *Ferri's best test: a practical guide to clinical laboratory medicine and diagnostic imaging,* ed 2, Philadelphia, 2009, Mosby.)

BOX 3-2   Hearing Loss

Diagnostic imaging	**Lab evaluation**
Best test	***Best test***
None	None
Ancillary tests	***Ancillary tests***
CT of head with contrast or MRI with contrast	CBC
CT of temporal bone without contrast	ALT, AST
	ANA, VDRL
	TSH

From Ferri FF: *Ferri's best test: a practical guide to clinical laboratory medicine and diagnostic imaging,* ed 2, Philadelphia, 2009, Mosby.
ALT, Alanine aminotransferase; *ANA,* antibody to nuclear antigens; *AST,* angiotensin sensitivity test; *CBC,* complete blood count; *CT,* computed tomography; *TSH,* thyroid-stimulating hormone; *VDRL,* Venereal Disease Research Laboratory.

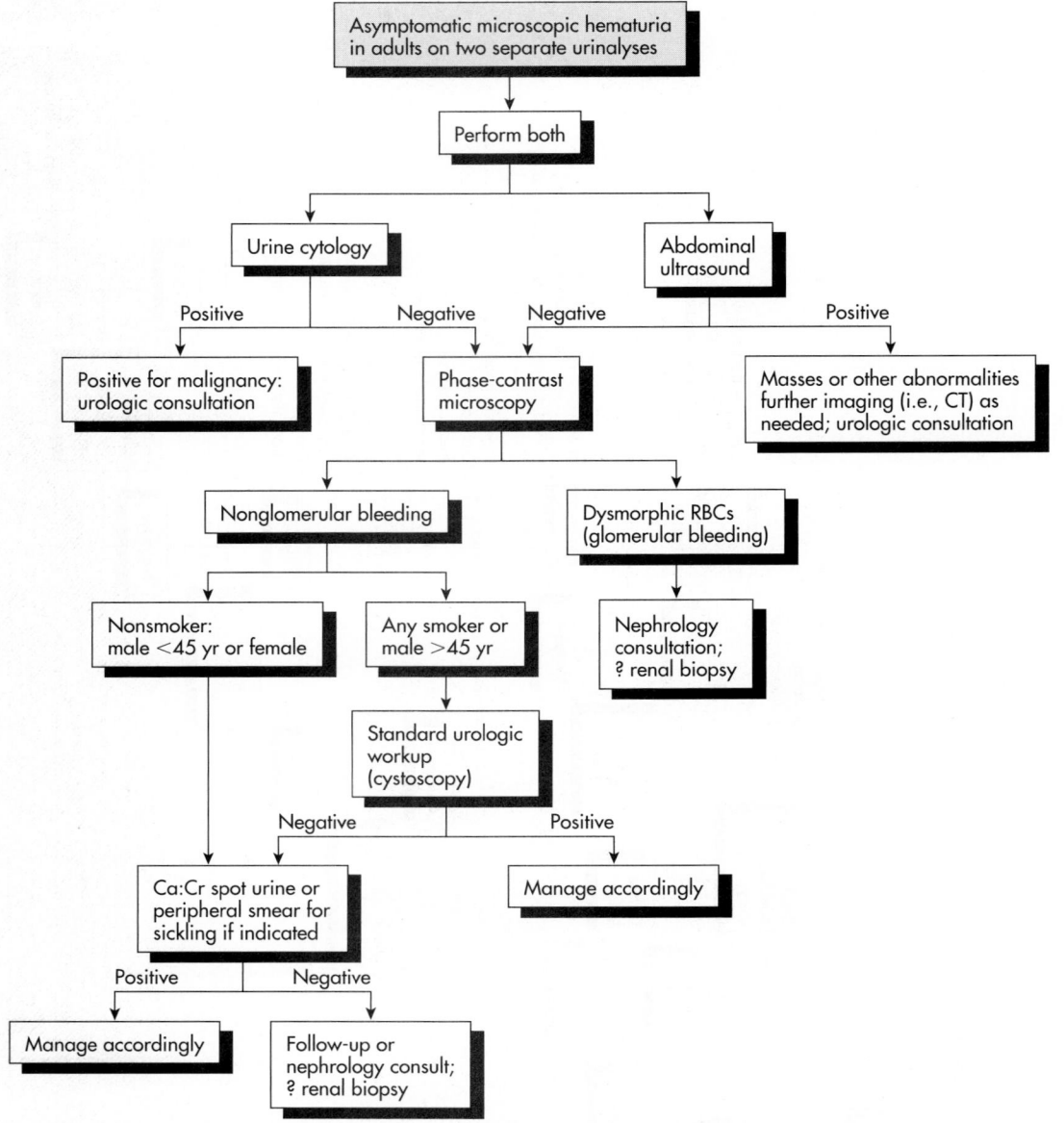

FIGURE 3-80 Suggested algorithm for the evaluation of adult asymptomatic microscopic hematuria. These patients must have no symptoms referable to the hematuria and a negative urinalysis except for red blood cells *(RBCs)*. Adults with gross hematuria require a full urologic evaluation. *Ca:Cr,* Calcium:creatinine ratio. (Modified from Nseyo UO [ed]: *Urology for primary care physicians,* Philadelphia, 1999, Saunders.)

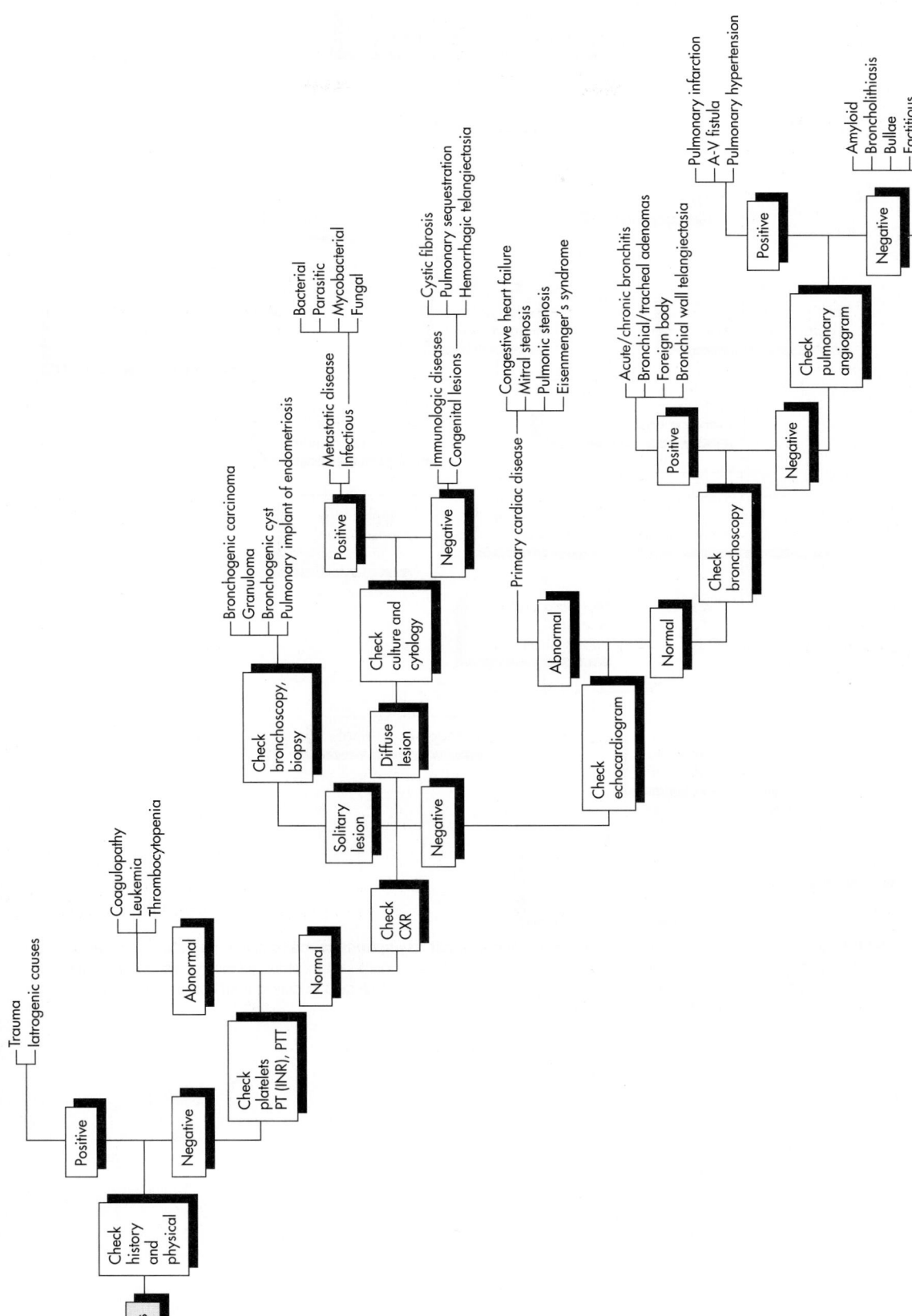

FIGURE 3-82 Evaluation of hemoptysis. *A-V,* Arteriovenous; *CXR,* chest x-ray; *INR,* International Normalized Ratio; *PT,* prothrombin time; *PTT,* partial thromboplastin time. (From Healey PM: *Common medical diagnosis: an algorithmic approach,* ed 3, Philadelphia, 2000, Saunders.)

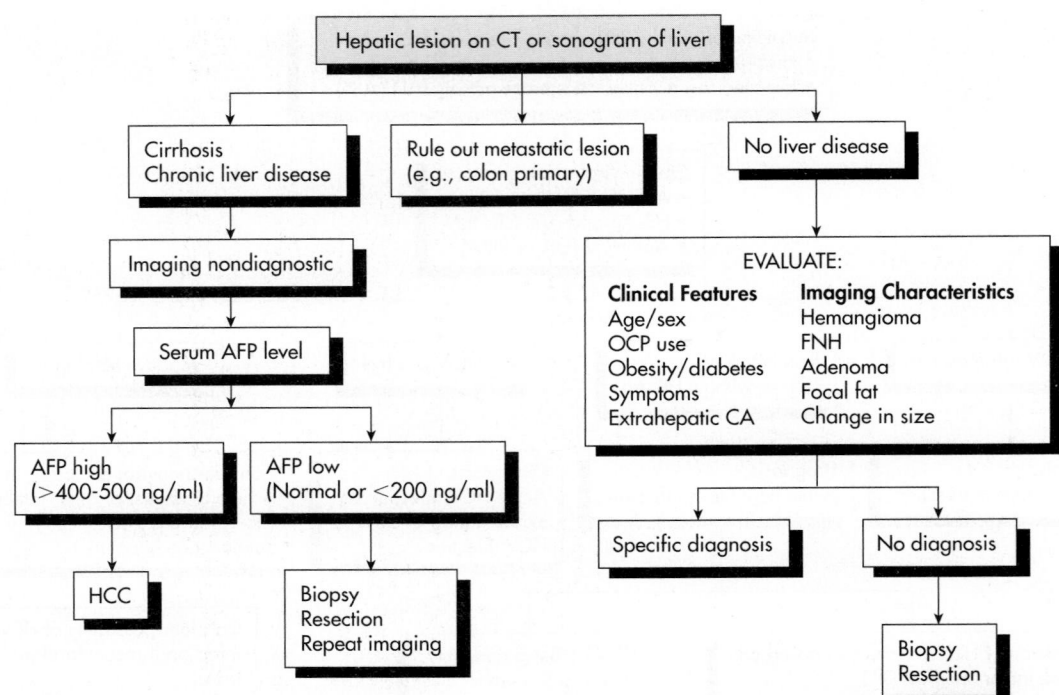

FIGURE 3-83 Diagnostic approach to space-occupying lesions of the liver. *AFP,* α-Fetoprotein; *CA,* cancer antigen; *FNH,* focal nodular hyperplasia; *HCC,* hepatocellular carcinoma; *OCP,* oral contraceptives. (Modified from Goldman L, Ausiello D [eds]: *Cecil textbook of medicine,* ed 23, Philadelphia, 2008, Saunders.)

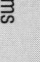

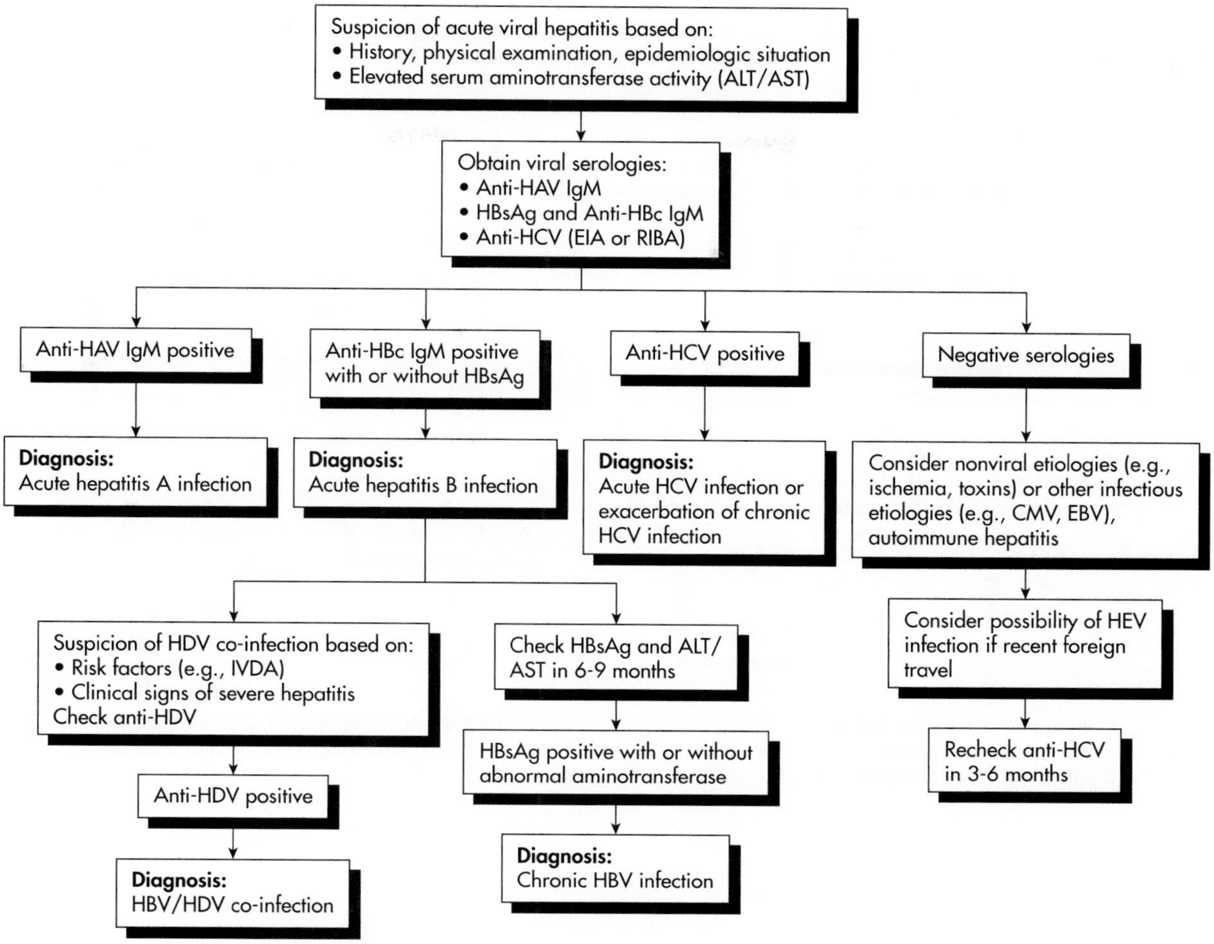

Suspicion of acute viral hepatitis based on:
- History, physical examination, epidemiologic situation
- Elevated serum aminotransferase activity (ALT/AST)

Obtain viral serologies:
- Anti-HAV IgM
- HBsAg and Anti-HBc IgM
- Anti-HCV (EIA or RIBA)

Anti-HAV IgM positive

Anti-HBc IgM positive with or without HBsAg

Anti-HCV positive

Negative serologies

Diagnosis:
Acute hepatitis A infection

Diagnosis:
Acute hepatitis B infection

Diagnosis:
Acute HCV infection or exacerbation of chronic HCV infection

Consider nonviral etiologies (e.g., ischemia, toxins) or other infectious etiologies (e.g., CMV, EBV), autoimmune hepatitis

Suspicion of HDV co-infection based on:
- Risk factors (e.g., IVDA)
- Clinical signs of severe hepatitis
Check anti-HDV

Check HBsAg and ALT/AST in 6-9 months

Consider possibility of HEV infection if recent foreign travel

Anti-HDV positive

HBsAg positive with or without abnormal aminotransferase

Recheck anti-HCV in 3-6 months

Diagnosis:
HBV/HDV co-infection

Diagnosis:
Chronic HBV infection

FIGURE 3-84 A flow diagram showing the use of specific serologic tests for the diagnosis of acute viral hepatitis in relation to the clinical and epidemiologic setting. Co-infections and superinfections of chronic hepatitis B or C patients should always be considered in cases that do not fit well with the clinical or serologic picture. *CMV,* Cytomegalovirus; *EBV,* Epstein-Barr virus; *EIA,* enzyme immunoassay; *HBV,* hepatitis B virus; *HCV,* hepatitis C virus; *HDV,* hepatitis D virus; *HEV,* hepato-encephalomyelitis virus; *IVDA,* intravenous drug abuse; *RIBA,* recombinant immunoblot assay. (Modified from Mandell GL: *Mandell, Douglas, and Bennett's principles and practice of infectious diseases,* ed 7, New York, 2008, Churchill Livingstone.)

HEPATOMEGALY

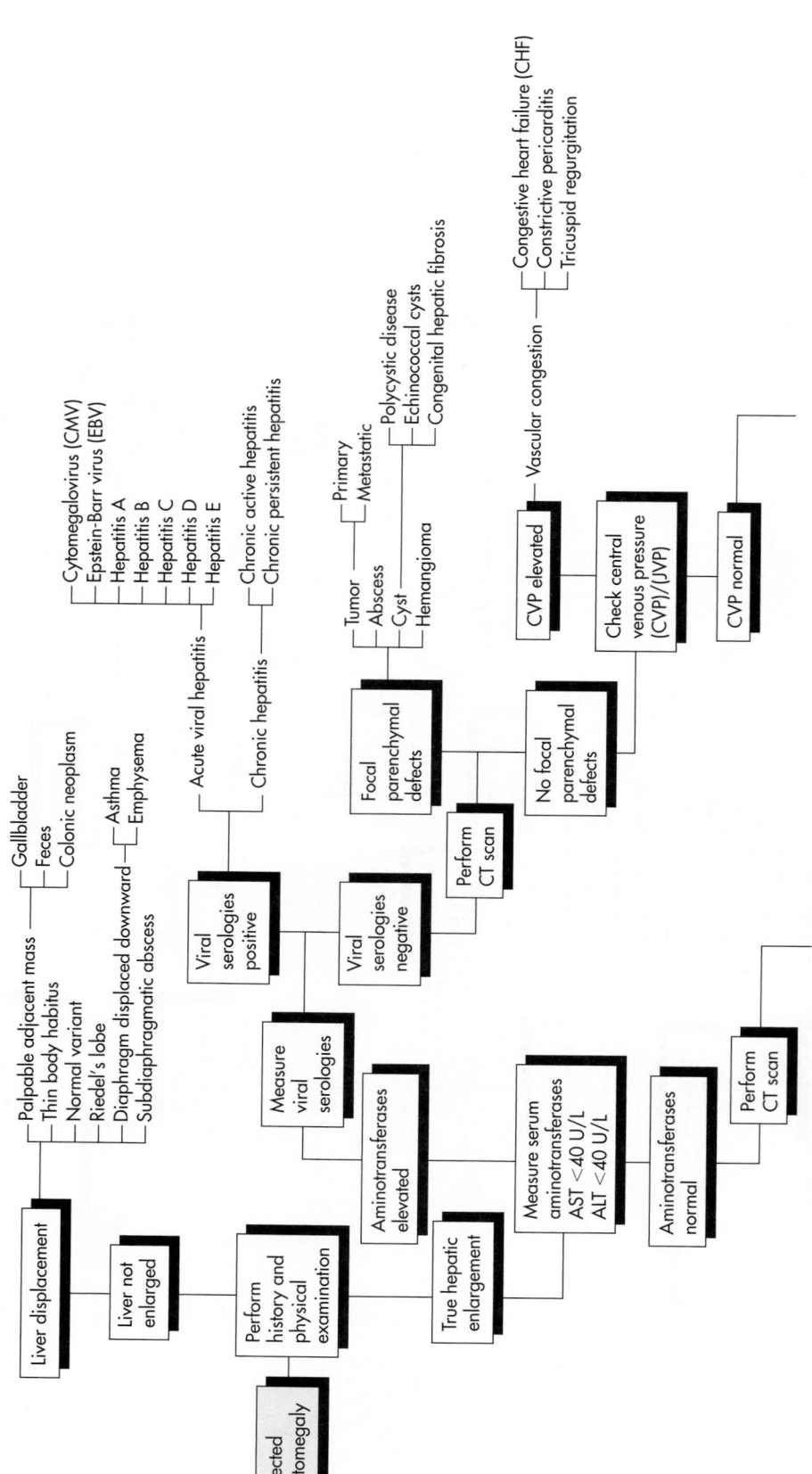

FIGURE 3-85 Hepatomegaly. *ALT,* Alanine aminotransferase; *AST,* aspartate aminotransferase; *CT,* computed tomography; *JVP,* jugular venous pressure. (Modified from Healey PM: *Common medical diagnosis: an algorithmic approach,* ed 3, Philadelphia, 2000, Saunders.)

(Continued on next page)

HEPATOMEGALY—cont'd

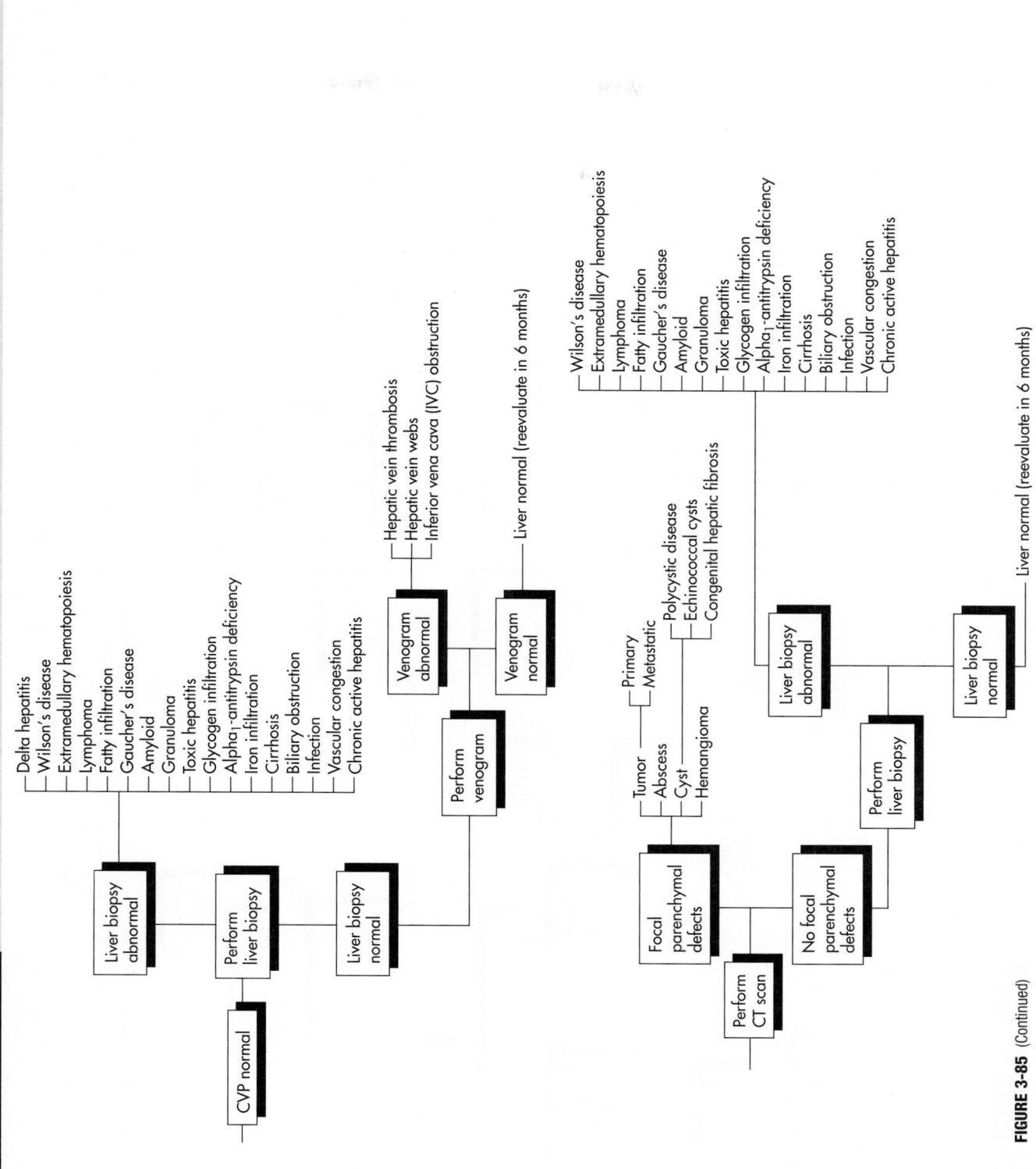

FIGURE 3-85 (Continued)

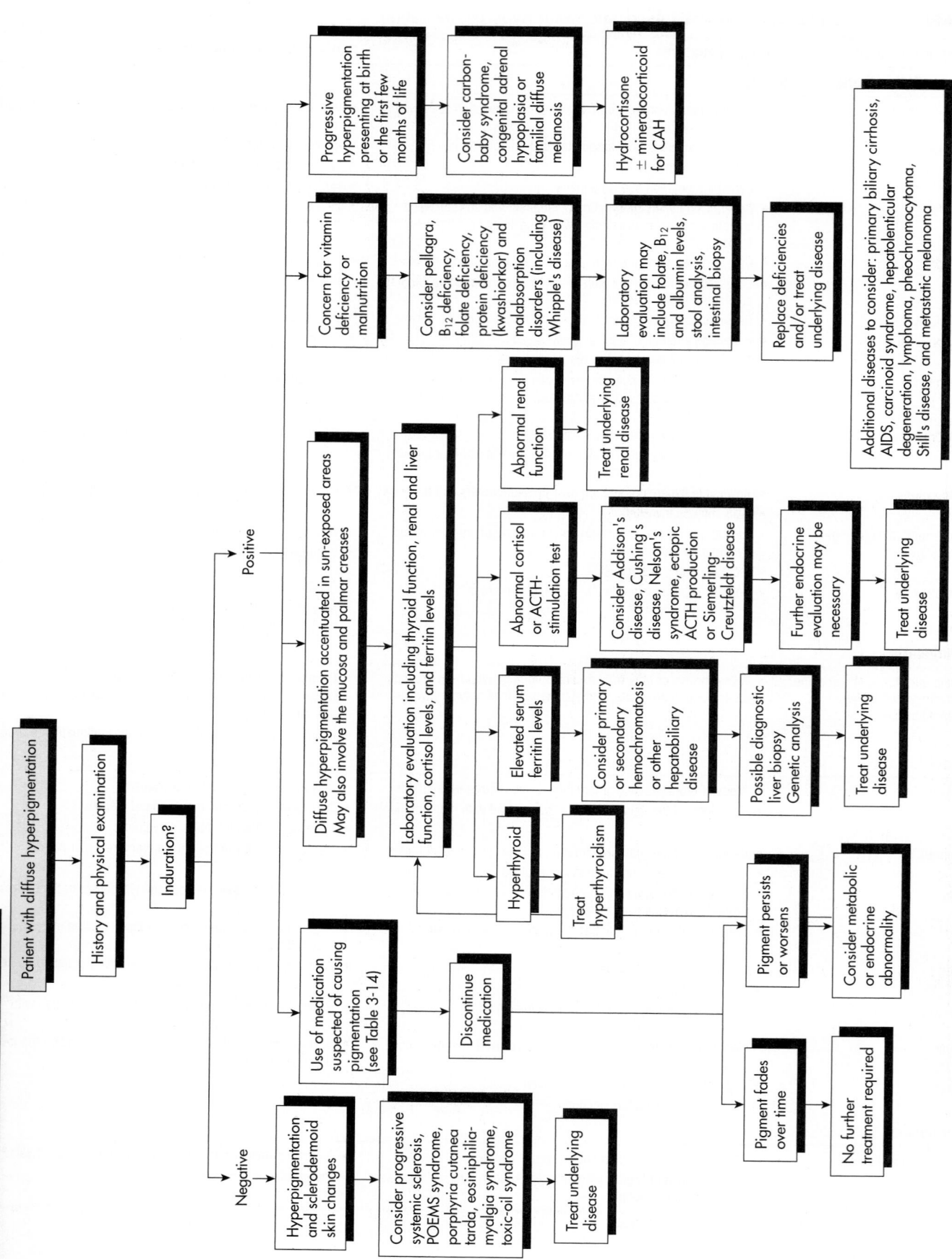

FIGURE 3-86 Approach to the adult patient with diffuse hyperpigmentation. *ACTH,* Adrenocorticotropic hormone; *AIDS,* acquired immunodeficiency syndrome; *CAH,* congenital adrenal hyperplasia; *POEMS,* polyneuropathy, organomegaly, endocrinopathies, monoclonal gammopathy, skin changes. (From Bolognia JL et al [eds]: *Dermatology,* ed 2, St Louis, 2008, Mosby.)

TABLE 3-14 Drugs and Chemicals Associated with Hyperpigmentation

Drug or Chemical	Clinical Features	Histopathology/Comment
Cancer Chemotherapeutic Agents		
BCNU (Topical)	• Hyperpigmentation at site of application (no reaction seen with parenteral administration)	• Hyperplasia of basal melanocytes consistent with postinflammatory hyperpigmentation
Bleomycin	• Linear, flagellate bands, associated with minor trauma	• Increased epidermal melanin
	• Nails may be involved	• Little dermal pigment incontinence
	• Hyperpigmentation overlying joints	• No increase in epidermal melanocytes
Busulfan	• Generalized hyperpigmentation resembling Addison's disease; sometimes seen in association with drug-induced pulmonary fibrosis	• Increased melanin in basal keratinocytes and in dermal macrophages
Cyclophosphamide	• Diffuse hyperpigmentation of the skin and mucous membranes	• Pigmentation usually regresses within 6 to 12 months after therapy is discontinued
	• Localized pigment of the nails (transverse or longitudinal bands), palms and soles, or teeth	
Dactinomycin	• Generalized hyperpigmentation, most prominent on the face	• Pigmentation fades after treatment discontinued
Daunorubicin	• Hyperpigmentation of light-exposed areas	• Structurally similar to doxorubicin
	• Transverse brown-black nail bands	
Doxorubicin	• Pigmentation of the nails; hyperpigmentation of the palmar creases, palms, soles, buccal mucosa, dorsae of the knuckles and tongue	• Increased epidermal melanin
		• Increased number of melanocytes
5-Fluorouracil	• Hyperpigmentation in sun-exposed areas	• Synergistic hyperpigmentation of irradiation portal sites
	• Increased pigmentation of skin overlying veins used for infusion, dorsae of the hands and trunk	
Hydroxyurea	• Reversible hyperpigmentation over pressure points and the back	• Lichenoid eruption with secondary hyperpigmentation
	• Nails may be involved	
Mechlorethamine (nitrogen mustard)	• Topical use for cutaneous lymphoma may result in generalized hyperpigmentation	• Disaggregation of melanosomes within keratinocytes
	• More intense in lesional skin	• Increased number of melanocytes
Methotrexate	• Uniform hyperpigmentation in sun-exposed areas	• Uncommon
		• May be postinflammatory hyperpigmentation secondary to photosensitivity reaction
Antimalarials		
Amino quinolones (chloroquine, hydroxychloroquine, amodiaquine)	• Yellow-brown or gray to blue-black pigment, usually in pretibial areas; face, hard palate, and subungual areas may be involved	• Dyspigmentation in up to 25% of patients
		• Dermal deposition of melanin-drug complexes; hemosiderin around capillaries
		• May fade, but rarely resolves, upon discontinuation of drug
Heavy Metals		
Arsenic	• Areas of bronze hyperpigmentation ± superimposed raindrops	• May appear 1-20 years after exposure
	• Keratoses on the palms and soles associated with pigmentation	• Dermal and epidermal deposition of arsenic
		• Increased epidermal melanin synthesis
Bismuth	• Generalized blue-gray discoloration of face, neck, dorsal hands	• Bismuth granules in the papillary and reticular dermis
	• Oral mucosa and gingivae may be involved	
Gold	• Permanent blue-gray discoloration in sun-exposed areas, mostly around the eyes (chrysiasis)	• Gold particles within macrophage lysosomes in the dermis
Iron	• Permanent brown pigment at injection or application sites	• Pigment coats collagen fibers and is deposited in dermal macrophages
Lead	• "Lead line" in gingival margin	• Lead line is due to subepithelial deposition of lead granules
	• Nail pigmentation	
Mercury	• Slate-gray pigmentation, particularly in skin folds	• Brown-black granules free in dermis, in association with elastic fibers, and within macrophages
Silver	• Generalized slate-gray pigmentation, increased in sun-exposed areas	• Silver granules in the basement membrane and on the membrana propria of eccrine glands
	• Nails and sclerae may also be involved	
	• Localized at sites of application	
Hormones		
Oral contraceptives	• Melasma; increased pigment of nipples and nevi	• Increased melanocytes and increased melanin synthesis
ACTH/MSH	• Diffuse brown or bronze pigmentation; seen in Addison's disease and Cushing's syndrome	• Increased melanin synthesis

From Bolognia JL et al [eds]: *Dermatology*, ed 2, St Louis, 2008, Mosby.

TABLE 3-14   Drugs and Chemicals Associated with Hyperpigmentation—cont'd

Drug or Chemical	Clinical Features	Histopathology/Comment
Miscellaneous Compounds		
Amiodarone	• Slate-gray to violaceous discoloration of sun-exposed skin	• Yellow-brown granules in dermis, mostly perivascular • Lysosomal inclusions with a lipid-like substance
Azidothymidine (zidovudine, AZT)	• Nail and mucocutaneous hyperpigmentation	• Skin biopsy shows increased epidermal and dermal melanin
Clofazimine	• Diffuse red to red-brown discoloration of skin • Violet-brown to bluish discoloration, especially lesional skin	• Redness secondary to drug in fat • Phagolysosomes with lipofuscin material
Dioxins	• Chloracne most common skin finding • Hyperpigmentation may occur in sun-exposed areas	• Rare, except in accidental exposure
Hydroquinone	• Hyperpigmentation in areas of application due to exogenous ochronosis	• Yellow-brown banana-shaped fibers in papillary dermis
Minocycline	• Blue-black discoloration in old acne scars or sites of inflammation as well as lower extremities • May also involve nails, sclerae, oral mucosa, bones, and teeth • Generalized "muddy brown" pigmentation pattern in some patients	• Iron-containing granules and/or increased melanin, depending on clinical type
Psoralens	• Increased pigmentation after exposure to UVA light (PUVA)	• Proliferation of follicular melanocytes • Increased synthesis and transfer of melanin
Psychotropic drugs (phenothiazine, chlorpromazine, imipramine, desipramine)	• Slate-gray discoloration in sun-exposed areas	• Golden-brown granules in the upper dermis • Electron-dense inclusion bodies

Clinical
Algorithms

III

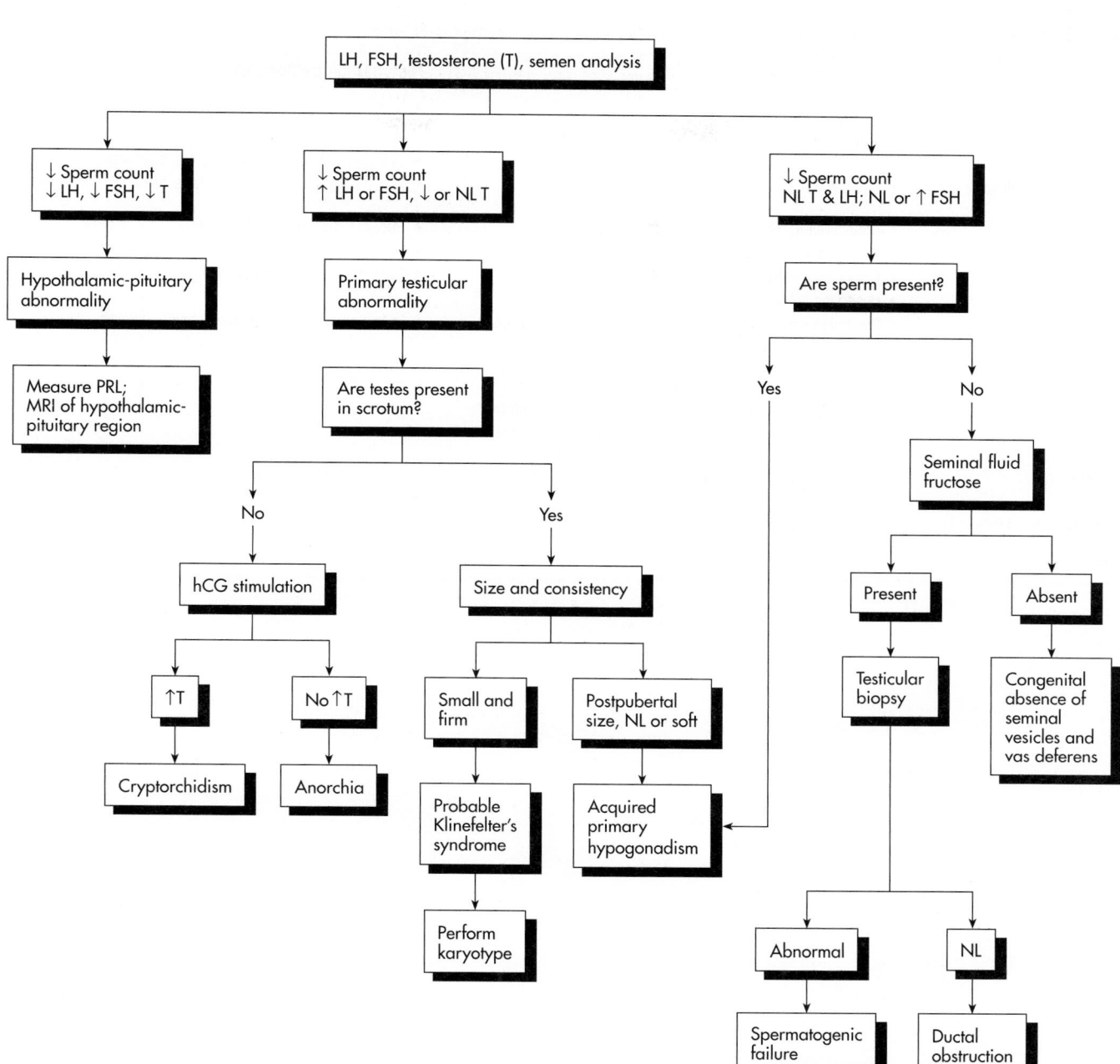

FIGURE 3-87 Laboratory evaluation of hypogonadism. *FSH,* Follicle-stimulating hormone; *hCG,* human chorionic gonadotropin; *LH,* luteinizing hormone; *MRI,* magnetic resonance imaging; *NL,* normal; *PRL,* prolactin; ↑, elevated; ↓, decreased or low. (From Andreoli TE [ed]: *Cecil essentials of medicine,* ed 7, Philadelphia, 2008, Saunders.)

HYPOTENSION

ICD-9CM # 458.9 Hypotension, NOS
458.1 Hypotension, chronic
458.2 Hypotension, iatrogenic
458.0 Hypotension, orthostatic or postural

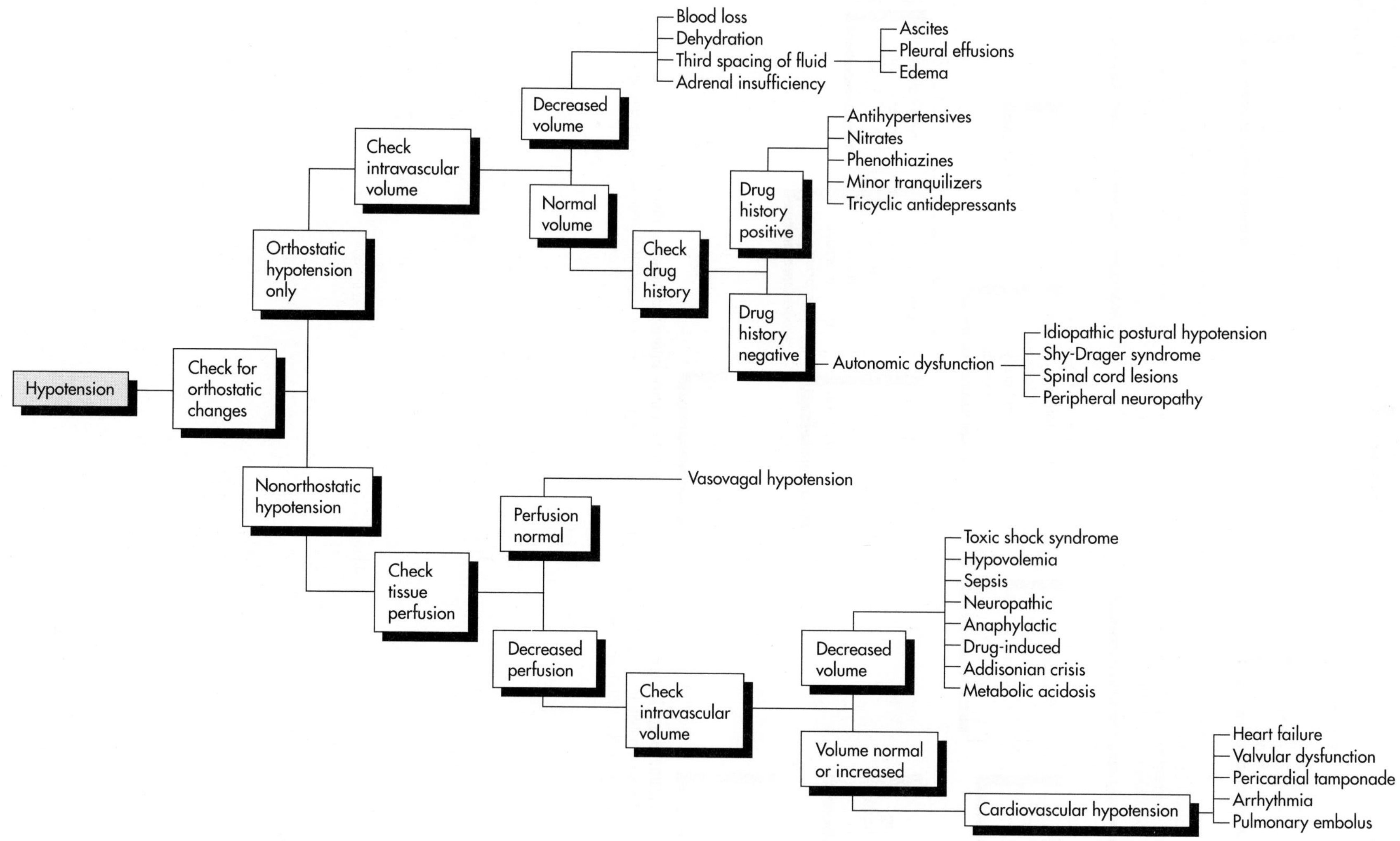

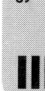

FIGURE 3-88 Hypotension. (From Healey PM: *Common medical diagnosis: an algorithmic approach,* ed 3, Philadelphia, 2000, Saunders.)

Clinical
Algorithms

III

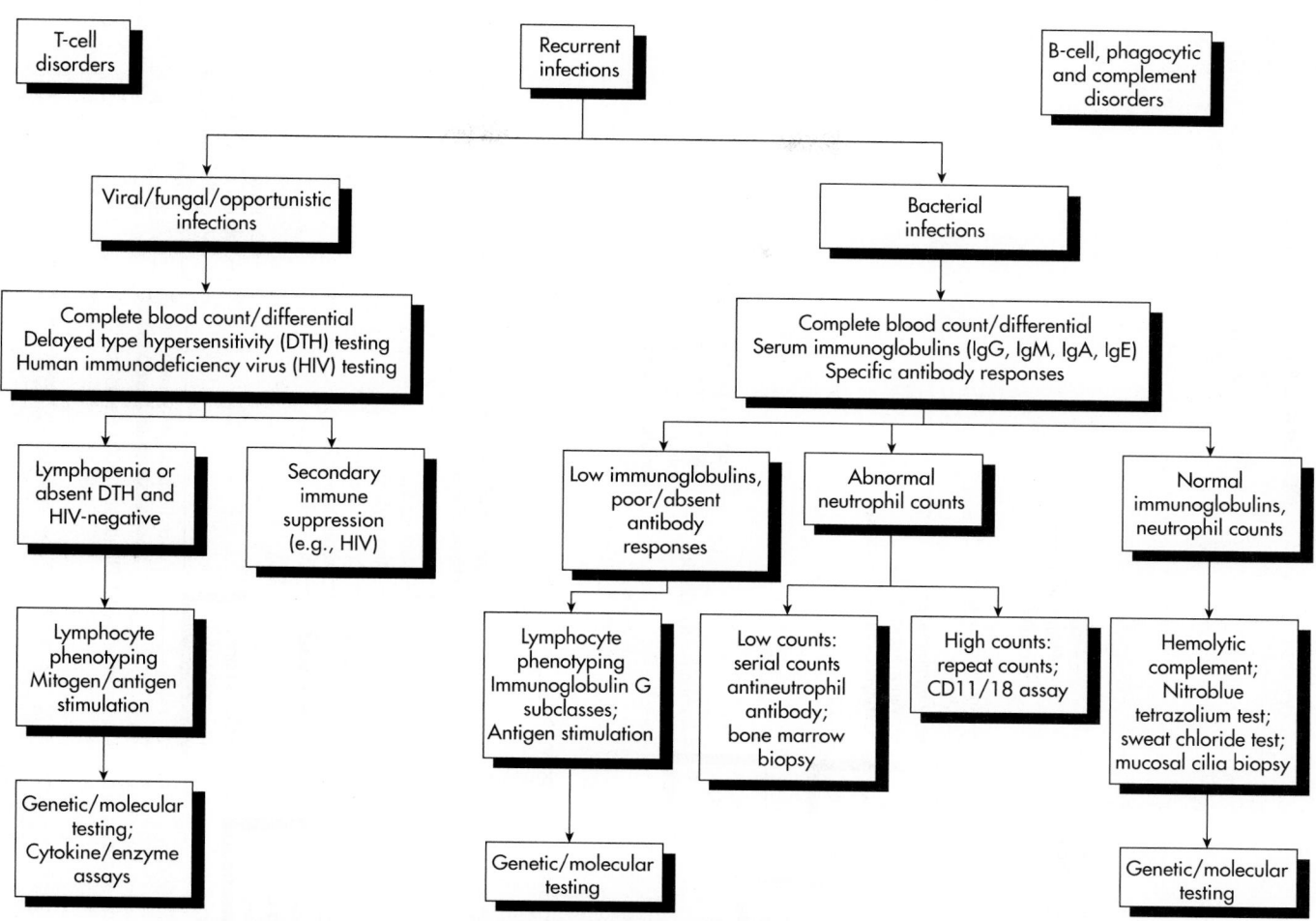

FIGURE 3-89 A diagnostic testing algorithm for primary immunodeficiency diseases. (From Lindegren ML et al: Applying public health strategies to primary immunodeficiency diseases: a potential approach to genetic disorders, *MMWR Recomm Rep* 53[RR-1]:1-29,2004.)

Soft tissue

↓

Erythema
Swelling
Warmth
Tenderness

↓

ESR
CBC with differential
Gram stain
Tissue and blood cultures
with sensitivity

↓

Imaging studies to
determine extent and/or
joint/bone involvement

↓

Positive Gram stain
and/or culture

Joint

Monoarthritis

Pain
Limitation of
active/passive motion
Fever
Effusion

↓

Suspect
nongonococcal septic
arthritis (NGSA),
gonococcal arthritis
(GA), crystal, and
reactive arthritis

Evaluation of risk
factors

↓

Old age
Trauma
Diabetes
RA, OA
HIV
Complement
deficiency
IV drug use
Indwelling catheters
Sickle cell anemia
Immunosuppression

Polyarthritis

Fever
Skin lesions
Tenosynovitis

↓

Consider NGSA, GA,
bacterial, crystal, viral,
and reactive arthritis

Bone

↓

Pain
Swelling
Erythema
Drainage
Fever
Risk factors

↓

CBC with differential
ESR
Blood cultures
Imaging: ultrasound,
PET, CT,
and MRI scans

↓

If bony involvement
present, referral for
needle biopsy and
aspiration

↓

Culture and
sensitivity if positive

Arthrocentesis
Synovial fluid appearance: cloudy-purulent-bloody
Crystal analysis
Leukocyte count: >50,000-100,000/mm³
>75% PMN
Other → Gram stain + aerobic, anaerobic culture
and sensitivity studies
Blood culture: NGSA: up to 90% +
GA: up to 50% +
If GA suspected: culture and PCR for *N. gonorrhoeae*
from cervix, urethra, rectum, throat (80% +)

Start antibiotic therapy

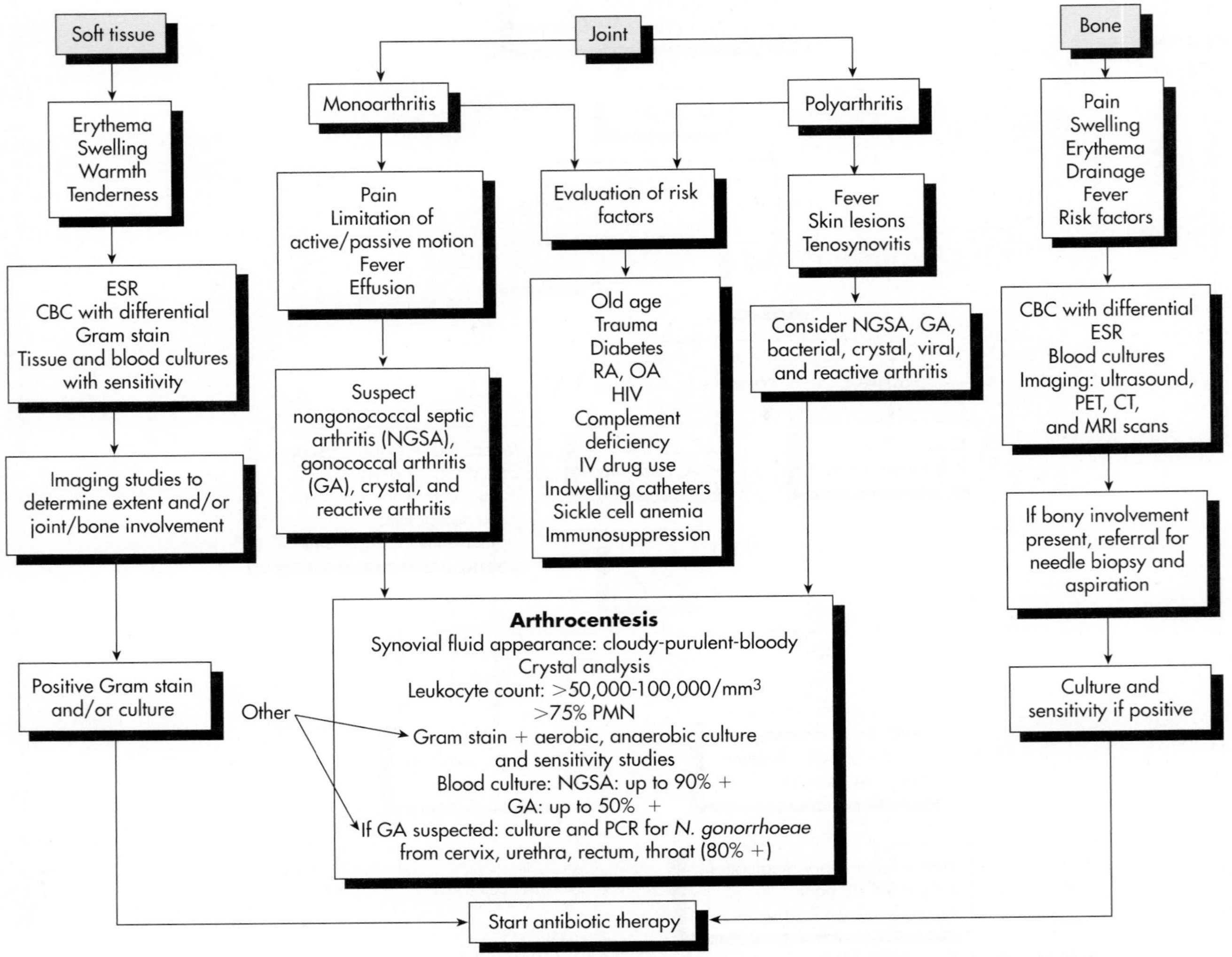

FIGURE 3-90 Clinical evaluation of infections of soft tissues, joints, and bone. *CBC*, Complete blood count; *CT*, computed tomography; *ESR*, erythrocyte sedimentation rate; *GA*, gonococcal arthritis; *HIV*, human immunodeficiency virus; *IV*, intravenous; *MRI*, magnetic resonance imaging; *NGSA*, nongonococcal septic arthritis; *OA*, osteoarthritis; *PCR*, polymerase chain reaction; *PET*, positron emission tomography; *PMN*, polymorphonuclear leukocyte; *RA*, rheumatoid arthritis. (From Goldman L, Schafer AI: *Goldman's Cecil medicine*, ed 24, Philadelphia, 2012, Saunders.)

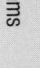

Clinical
Algorithms

III

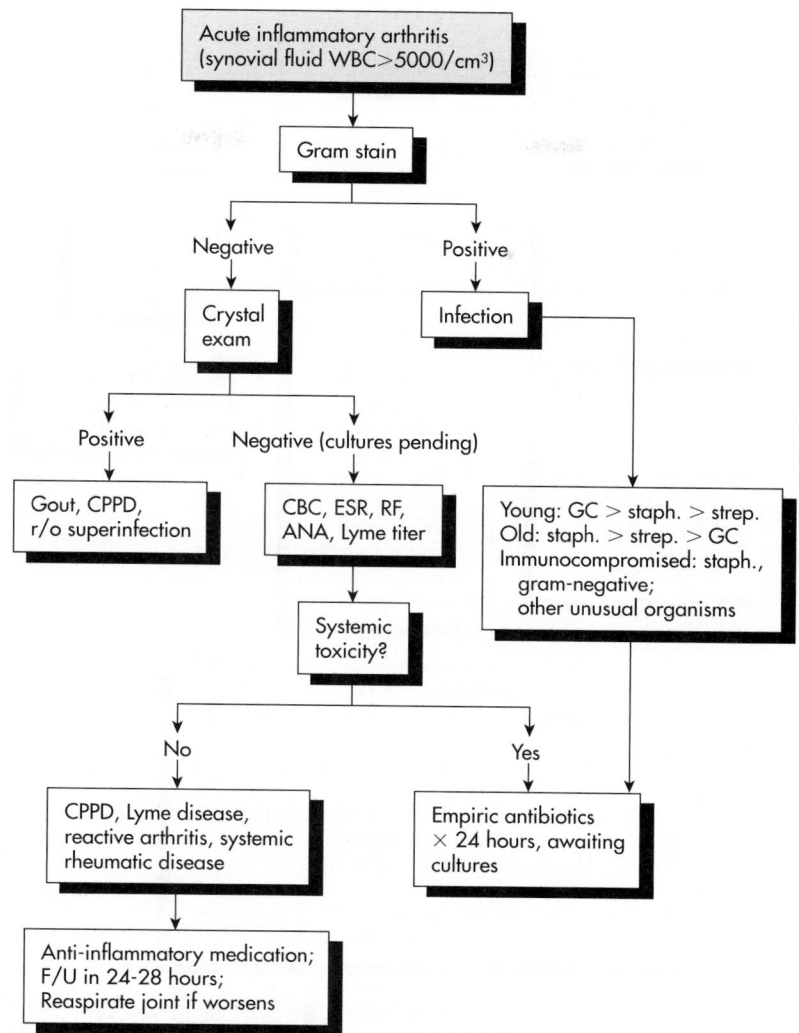

FIGURE 3-91 Approach to acute inflammatory arthritis. *ANA,* Antinuclear antibody test; *CBC,* complete blood count; *CPPD;* calcium pyrophosphate deposition disease; *ESR,* erythrocyte sedimentation rate; *F/U,* follow-up; *GC,* gonococcal infection; *RF,* rheumatoid factor; *r/o,* rule out; *staph.,* staphylococcal infection; *strep.,* streptococcal infection; *WBC,* white blood cell count. (From Harris ED et al [eds]: *Kelley's textbook of rheumatology,* ed 7, Philadelphia, 2005, Saunders.)

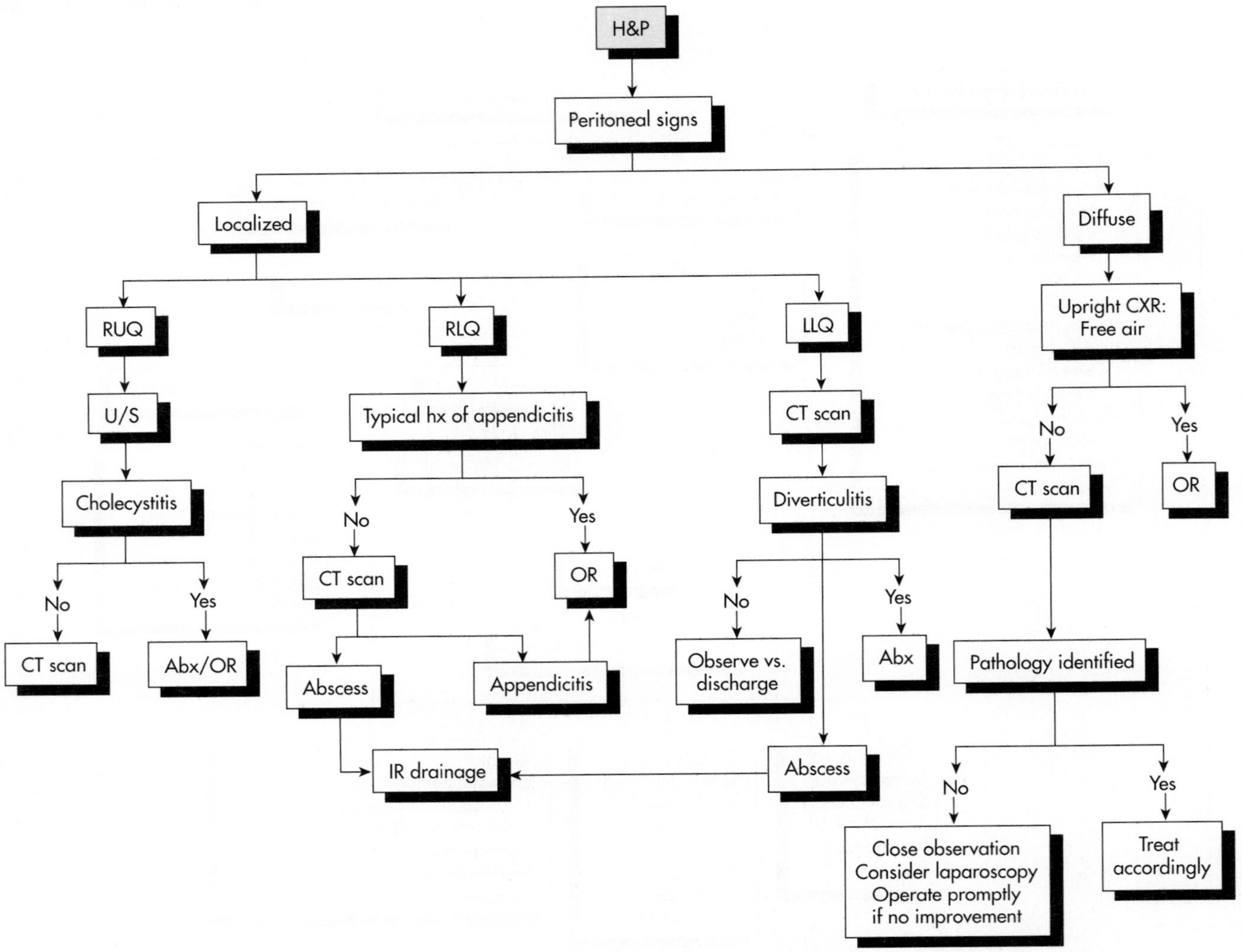

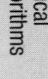

FIGURE 3-92 Algorithm for the diagnosis and management of patients with suspected IAI. *H&P,* History and physical exam; *RUQ,* right upper quadrant; *RLQ,* right lower quadrant; *LLQ,* left lower quadrant; *U/S,* ultrasound; *Abx,* antibiotics; *hx,* history; *IR,* interventional radiology; *CXR,* chest radiograph. (From Cameron JL, Cameron AM: *Current surgical therapy,* ed 10, Philadelphia, 2011, Saunders.)

Clinical Algorithms

ICD-9CM # 774.6   Jaundice neonatal, NOS
           773.1   ABO reaction perinatal
           774.1   Hemolytic perinatal
           773.0   RH reaction perinatal
          751.61 Bile duct obstruction, congenital

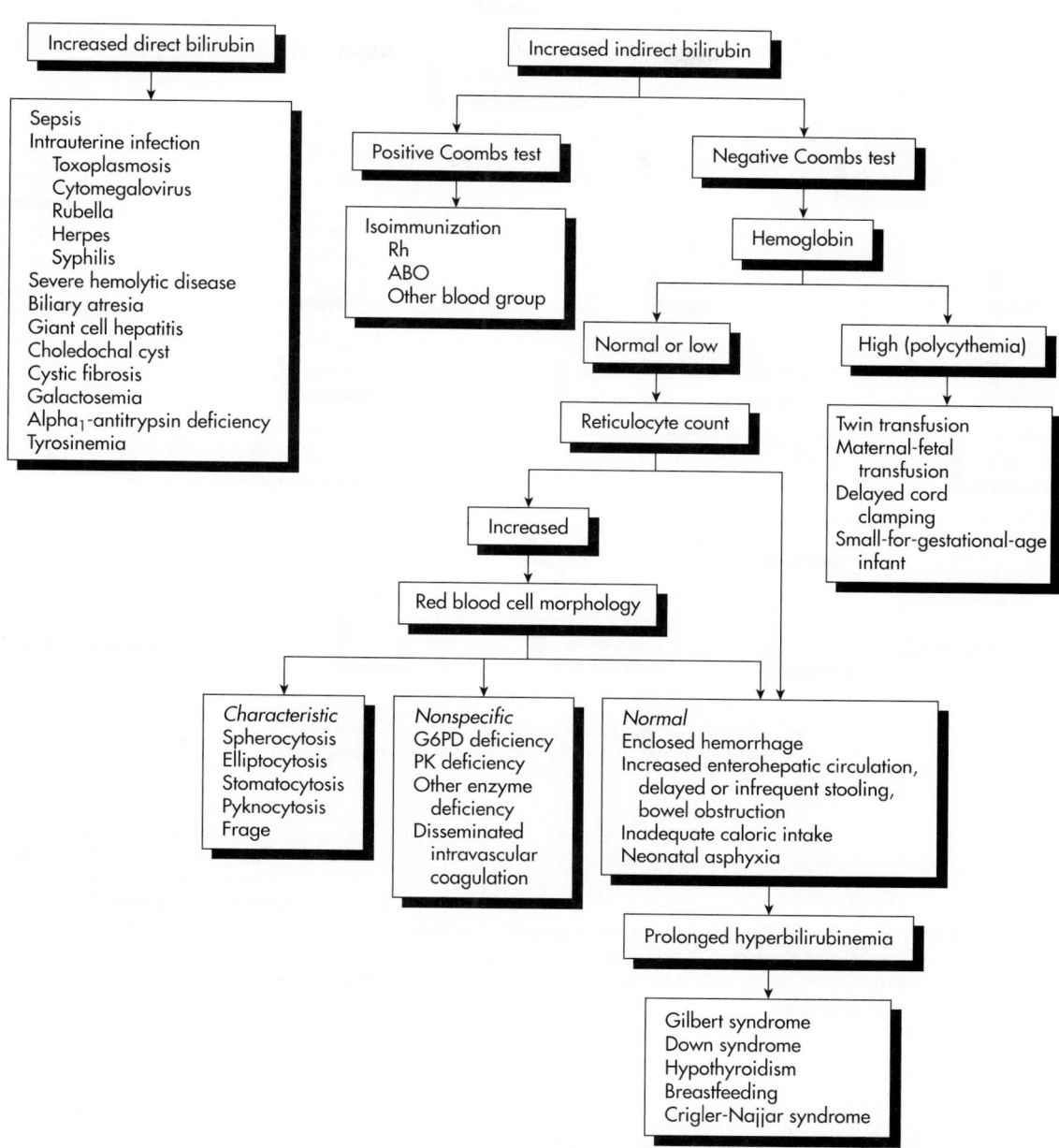

FIGURE 3-95 Schematic approach to the diagnosis of neonatal jaundice. *G6PD,* Glucose-6-phosphate dehydrogenase; *PK,* pyruvate kinase. (From Oski FA: Differential diagnosis of jaundice. In Taeusch HW, Ballard RA, Avery MA [eds]: *Schaffer and Avery's diseases of the newborn,* ed 6, Philadelphia, 1991, Saunders.)

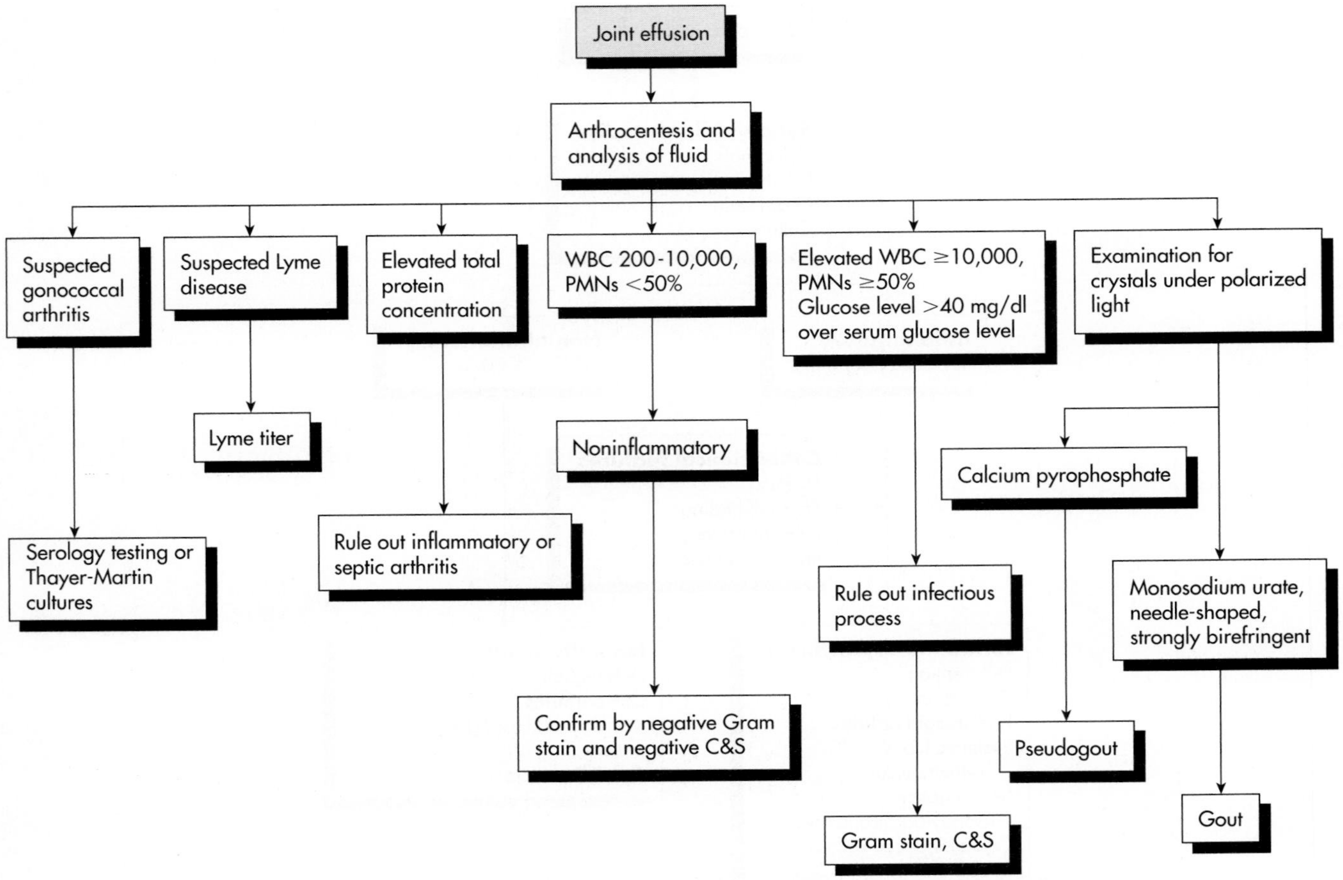

Joint effusion
↓
Arthrocentesis and analysis of fluid
↓

- Suspected gonococcal arthritis → Serology testing or Thayer-Martin cultures
- Suspected Lyme disease → Lyme titer
- Elevated total protein concentration → Rule out inflammatory or septic arthritis
- WBC 200-10,000, PMNs <50% → Noninflammatory → Confirm by negative Gram stain and negative C&S
- Elevated WBC ≥10,000, PMNs ≥50% Glucose level >40 mg/dl over serum glucose level → Rule out infectious process → Gram stain, C&S
- Examination for crystals under polarized light
  - Calcium pyrophosphate → Pseudogout
  - Monosodium urate, needle-shaped, strongly birefringent → Gout

FIGURE 3-96 Joint effusion. *C&S*, Culture and sensitivity; *PMNs*, polymorphonuclear leukocytes; *WBC*, white blood cell count.

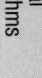

Clinical Algorithms

III

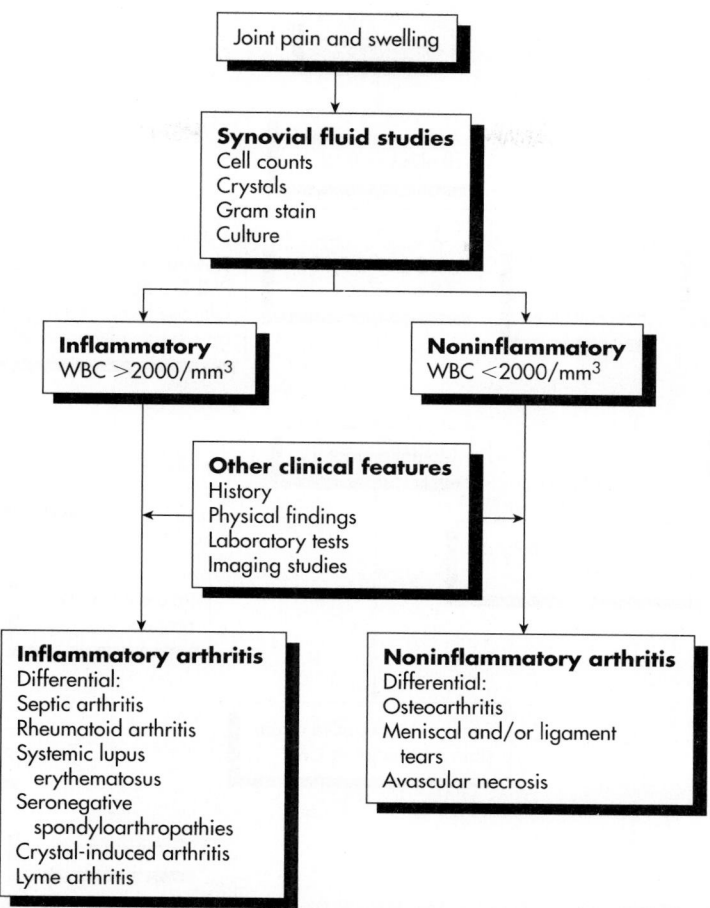

FIGURE 3-97 Diagnostic approach for swollen joints. *WBC,* White blood cell count. (From Goldman L, Ausiello D [eds]: *Cecil textbook of medicine,* ed 24, Philadelphia, 2012, Saunders.)

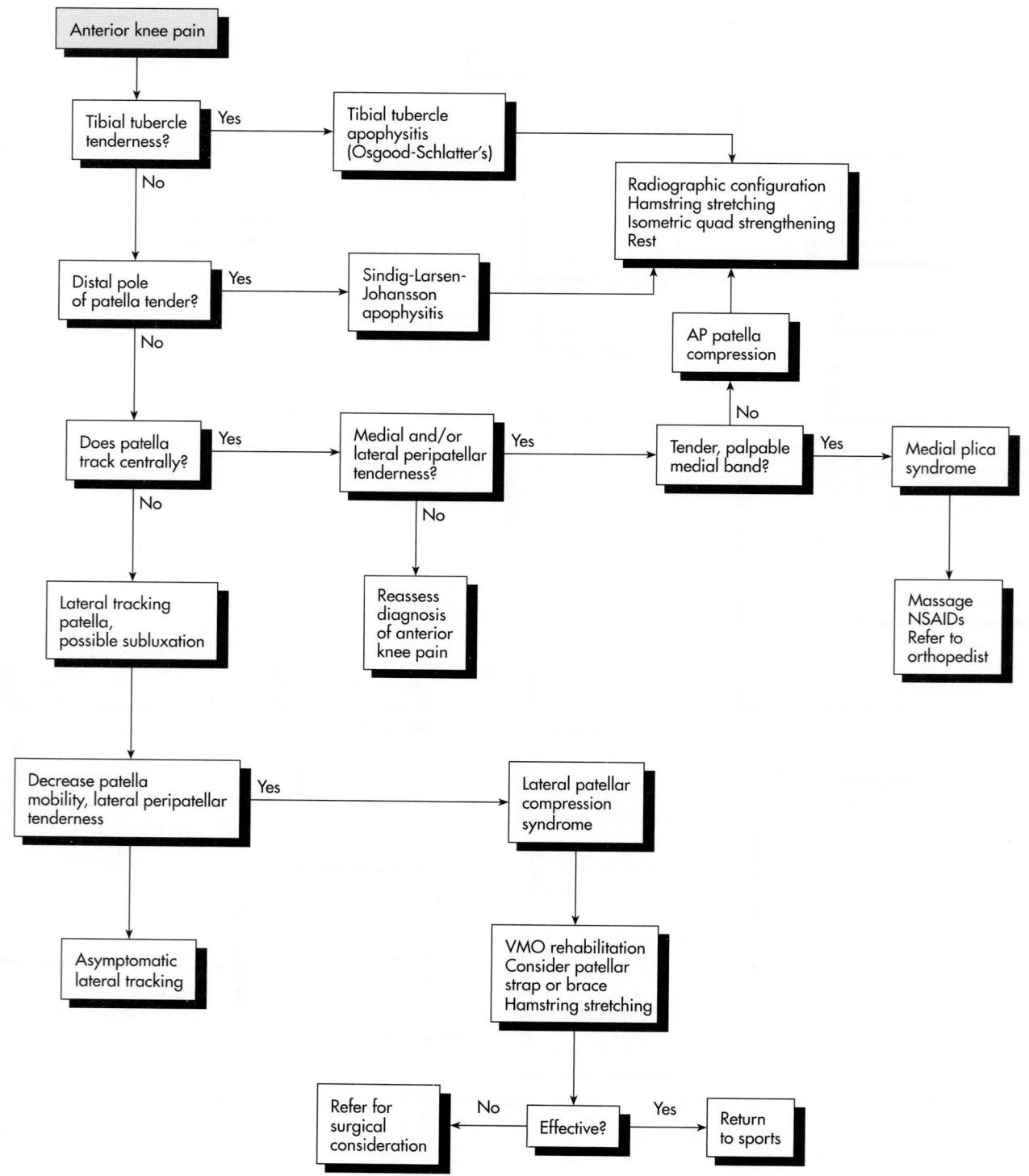

FIGURE 3-99 Evaluation and management of knee extensor mechanism pain. Focused treatment based on specific etiology will prevent recurrence. *AP,* Anteroposterior; *NSAIDs,* nonsteroidal anti-inflammatory drugs; *VMO,* vastus medialis obliquus muscle. (From Scudieri G [ed]: *Sports medicine, principles of primary care,* St Louis, 1997, Mosby.)

ICD-9CM # 440.23 Ulcer, lower limb, arteriosclerotic
707.1 Ulcer, lower limb, chronic
707.1 Ulcer, lower limb, neurogenic
707.9 Ulcer, non-healing
707.0 Pressure ulcer

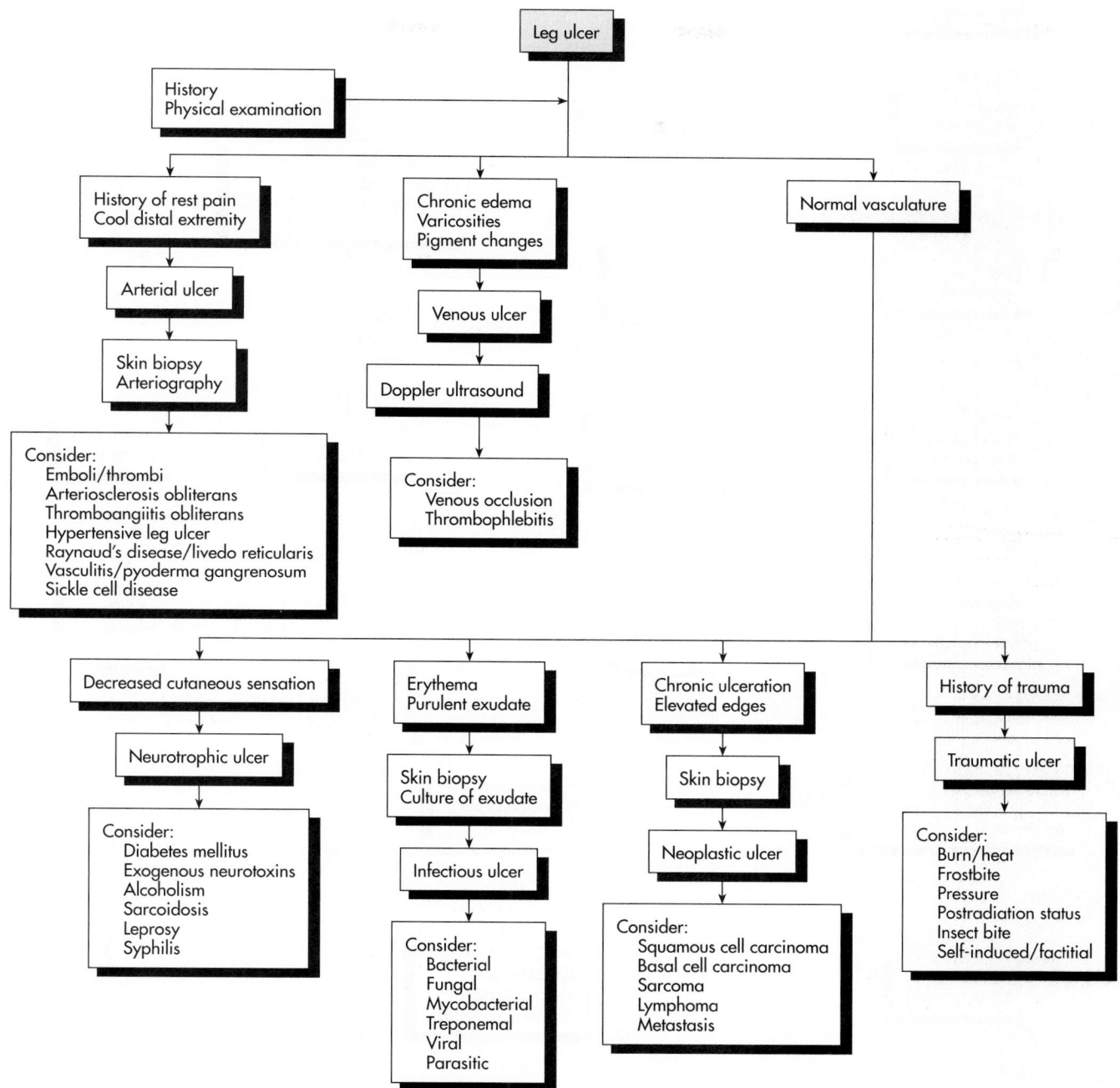

FIGURE 3-100 Leg ulcer. (From Greene HL, Johnson WP, Lemcke D [eds]: *Decision making in medicine,* ed 2, St Louis, 1998, Mosby.)

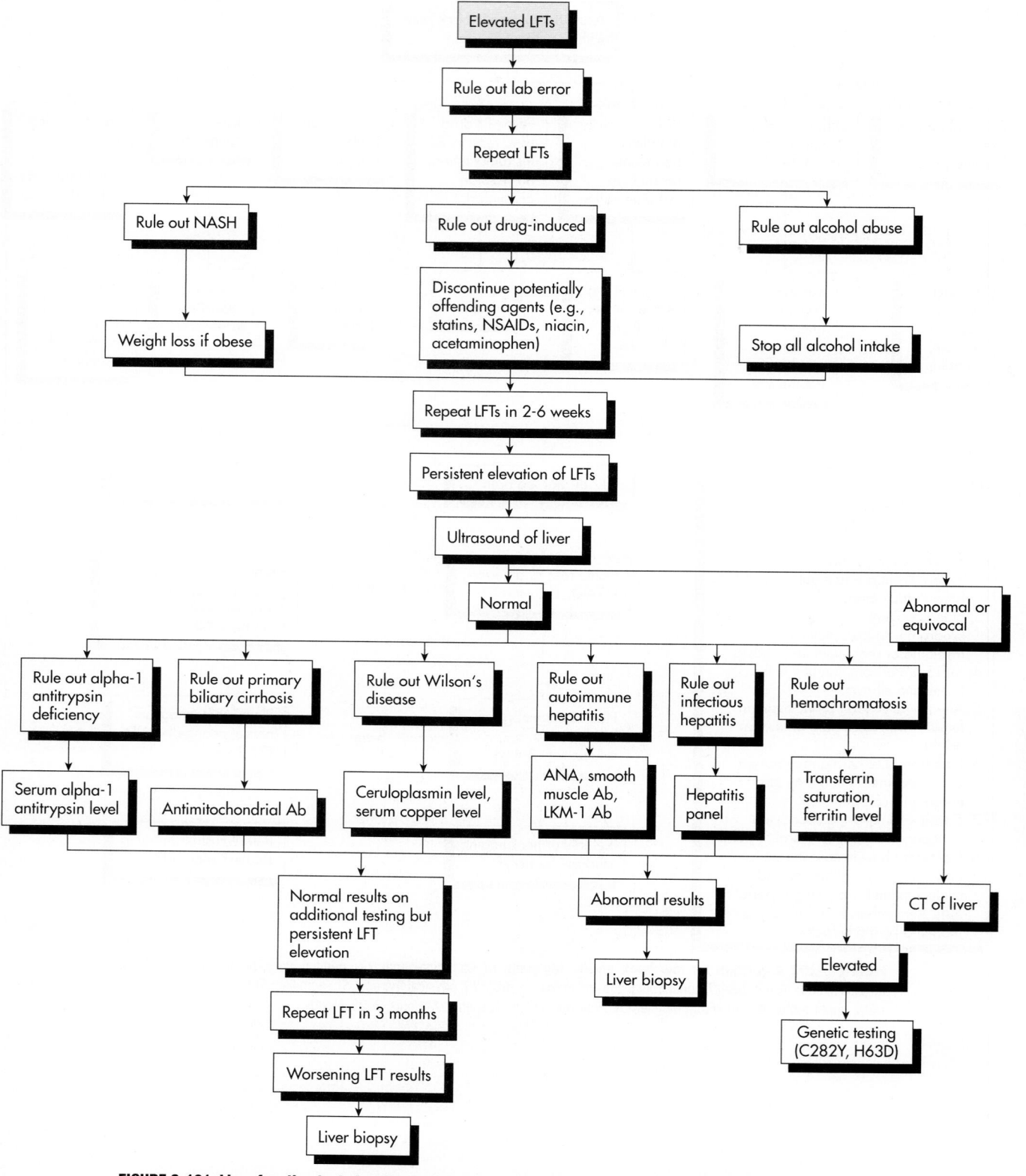

FIGURE 3-101 Liver function test elevations. *Ab,* Antibody; *ANA,* antibody to nuclear antigens; *CT,* computed tomography; *IEP,* immuno-electrophoresis; *LFTs,* liver function tests; *LKM,* liver-kidney microsome; *NASH,* nonalcoholic steatohepatitis; *NSAIDs,* nonsteroidal anti-inflammatory drugs.

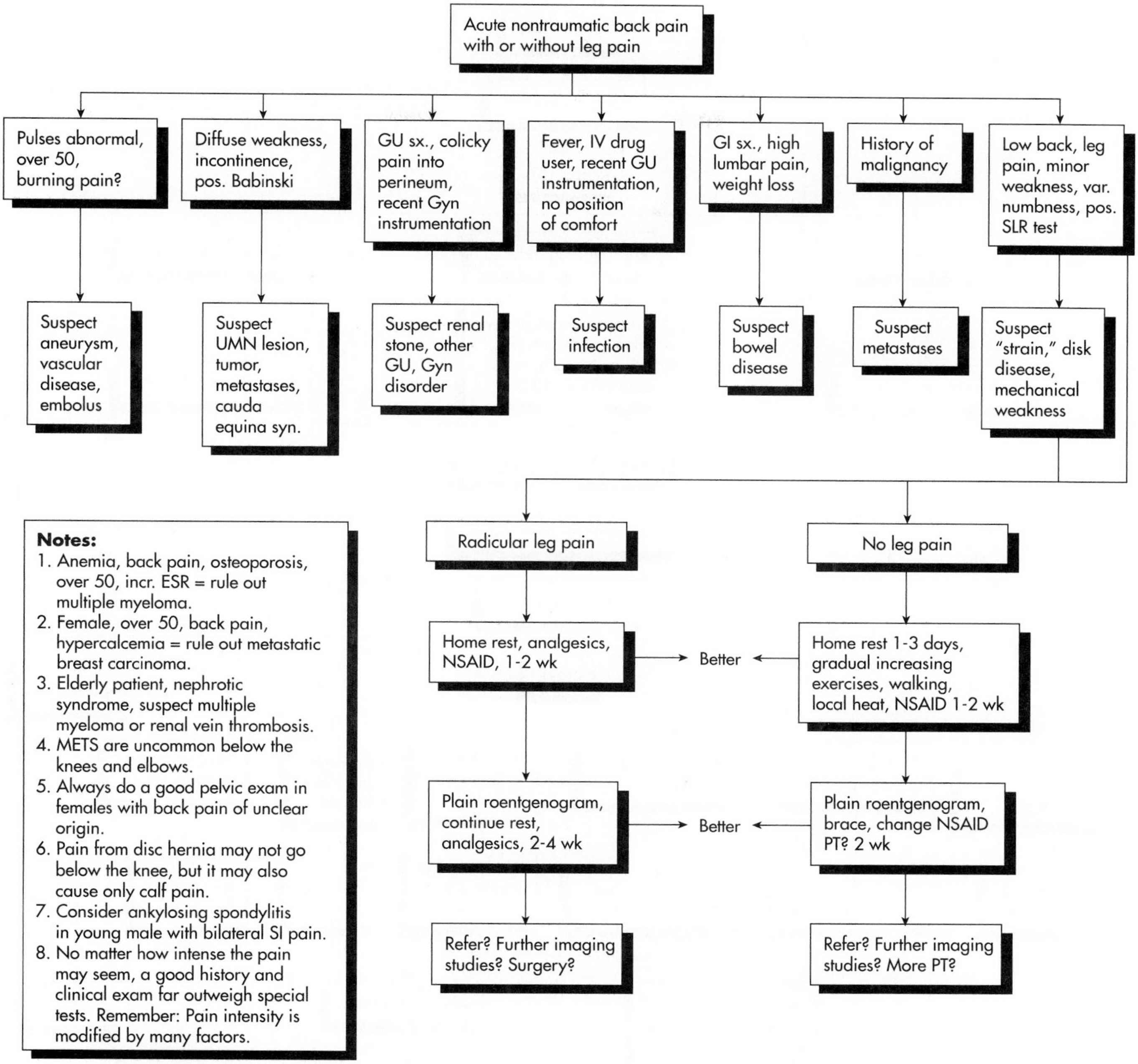

Acute nontraumatic back pain with or without leg pain

Pulses abnormal, over 50, burning pain?

Diffuse weakness, incontinence, pos. Babinski

GU sx., colicky pain into perineum, recent Gyn instrumentation

Fever, IV drug user, recent GU instrumentation, no position of comfort

GI sx., high lumbar pain, weight loss

History of malignancy

Low back, leg pain, minor weakness, var. numbness, pos. SLR test

Suspect aneurysm, vascular disease, embolus

Suspect UMN lesion, tumor, metastases, cauda equina syn.

Suspect renal stone, other GU, Gyn disorder

Suspect infection

Suspect bowel disease

Suspect metastases

Suspect "strain," disk disease, mechanical weakness

Radicular leg pain

No leg pain

Home rest, analgesics, NSAID, 1-2 wk

→ Better ←

Home rest 1-3 days, gradual increasing exercises, walking, local heat, NSAID 1-2 wk

Plain roentgenogram, continue rest, analgesics, 2-4 wk

→ Better ←

Plain roentgenogram, brace, change NSAID PT? 2 wk

Refer? Further imaging studies? Surgery?

Refer? Further imaging studies? More PT?

Notes:
1. Anemia, back pain, osteoporosis, over 50, incr. ESR = rule out multiple myeloma.
2. Female, over 50, back pain, hypercalcemia = rule out metastatic breast carcinoma.
3. Elderly patient, nephrotic syndrome, suspect multiple myeloma or renal vein thrombosis.
4. METS are uncommon below the knees and elbows.
5. Always do a good pelvic exam in females with back pain of unclear origin.
6. Pain from disc hernia may not go below the knee, but it may also cause only calf pain.
7. Consider ankylosing spondylitis in young male with bilateral SI pain.
8. No matter how intense the pain may seem, a good history and clinical exam far outweigh special tests. Remember: Pain intensity is modified by many factors.

FIGURE 3-103 Algorithm for low back and/or leg pain. *GI*, Gastrointestinal; *GU*, genitourinary; *IV*, intravenous; *METS*, metabolic equivalents; *NSAID*, nonsteroidal anti-inflammatory drug; *PT*, physical therapy; *SI*, sacroiliac; *SLR*, straight-leg raising; *UMN*, upper motor neuron. (From Mercier LR: *Practical orthopedics*, ed 2, St Louis, 2000, Mosby.)

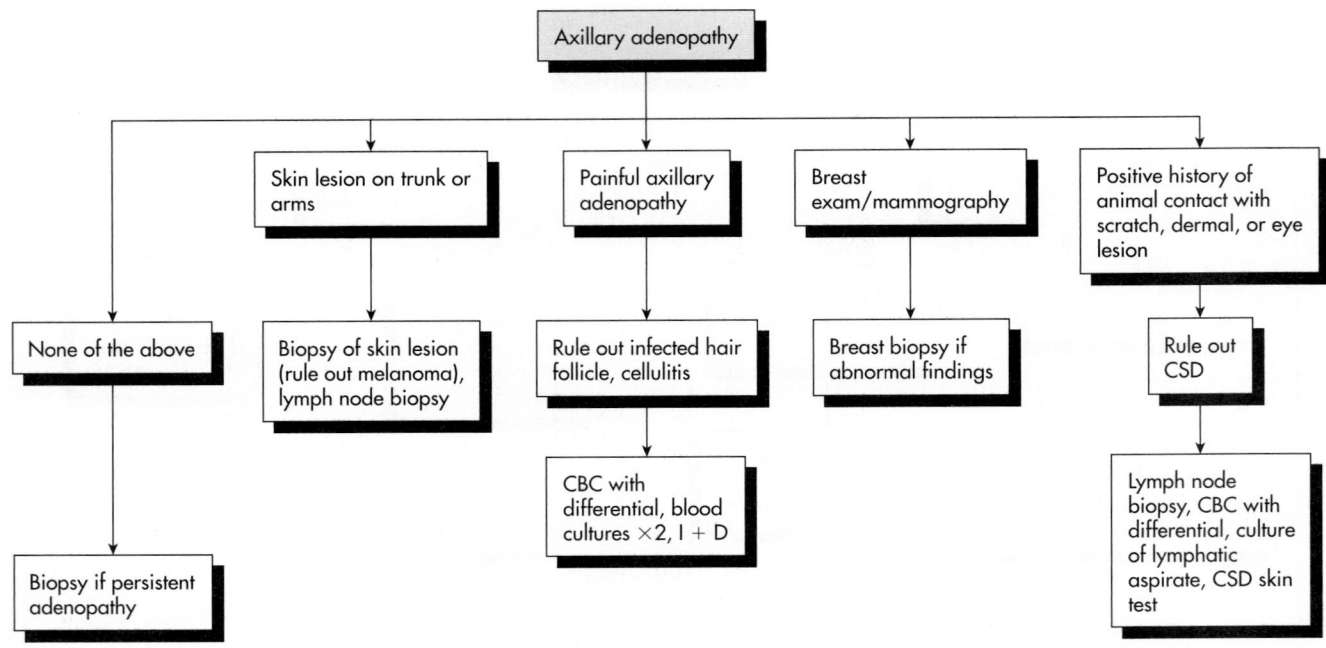

FIGURE 3-104 Lymphadenopathy, axillary. *CBC*, Complete blood count; *CSD*, cat-scratch disease.

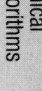

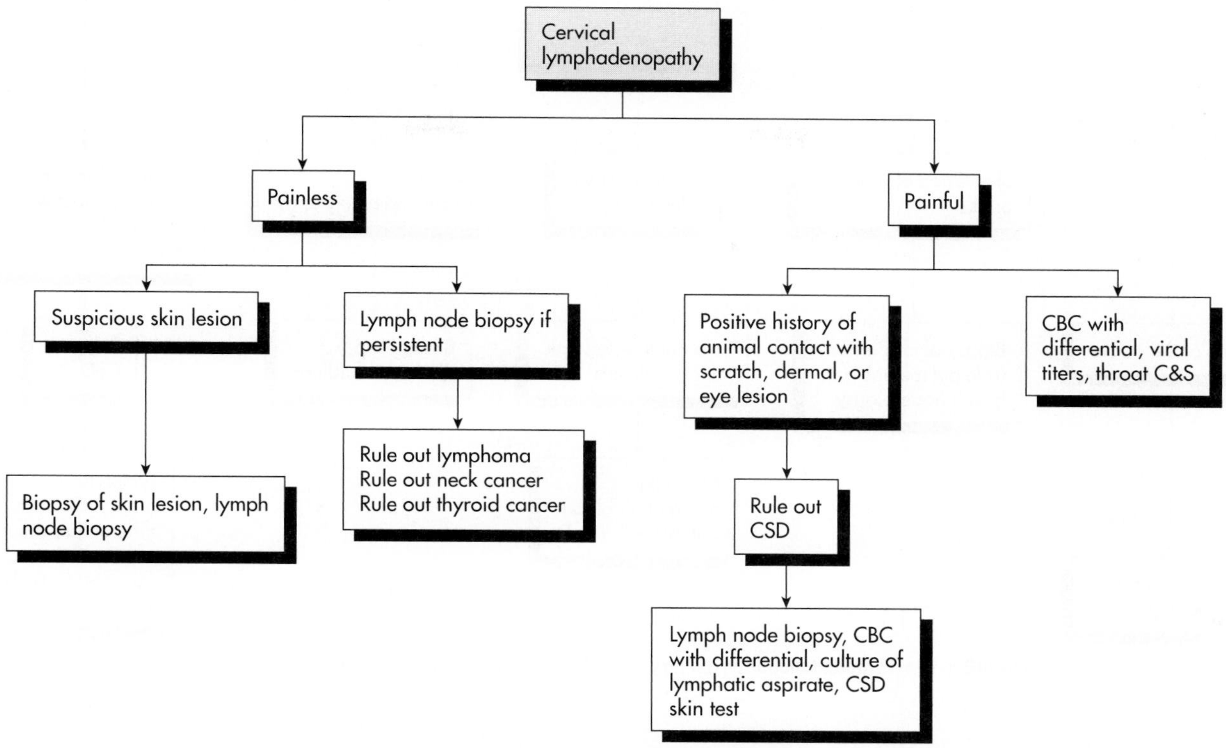

FIGURE 3-105 Lymphadenopathy, cervical. *CBC,* Complete blood count; *C&S,* culture and sensitivity; *CSD,* cat-scratch disease.

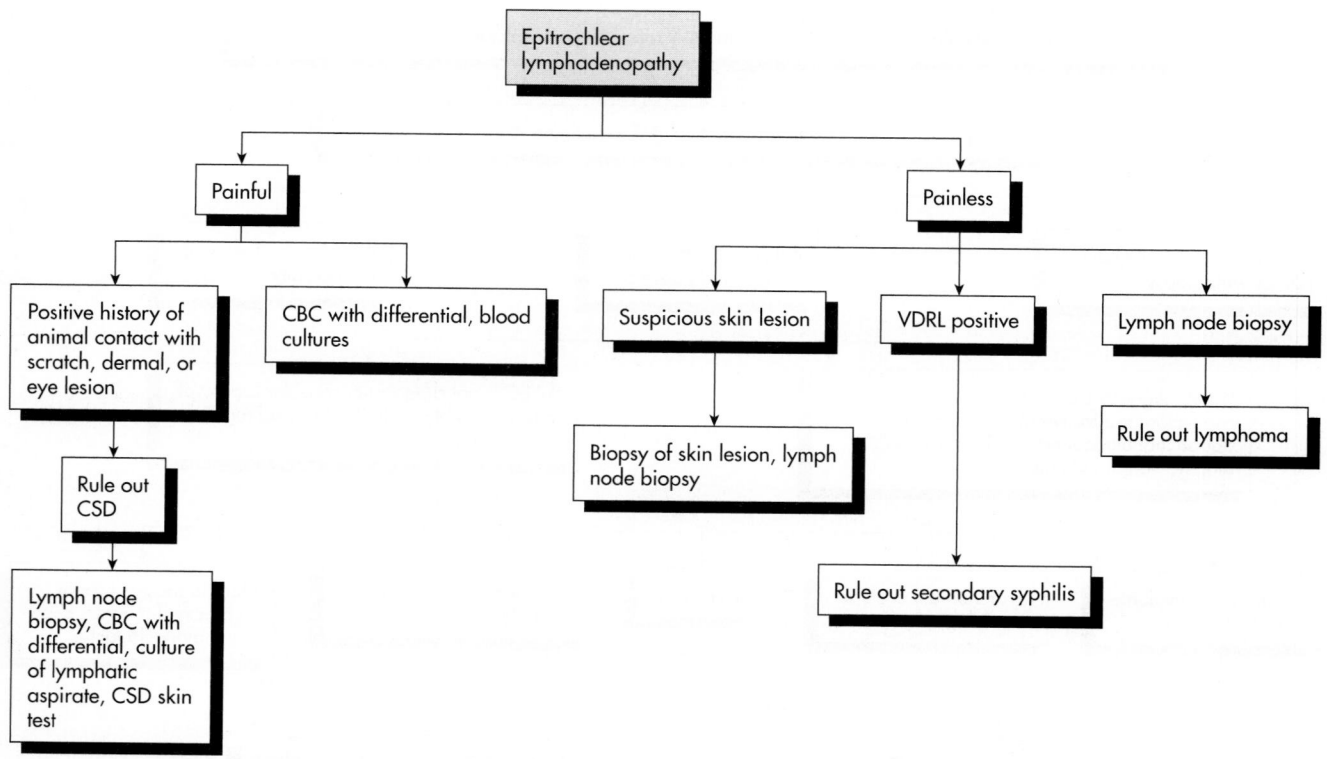

FIGURE 3-106 Lymphadenopathy, epitrochlear. *CBC*, Complete blood count; *CSD*, cat-scratch disease; *VDRL*, Venereal Disease Research Laboratory.

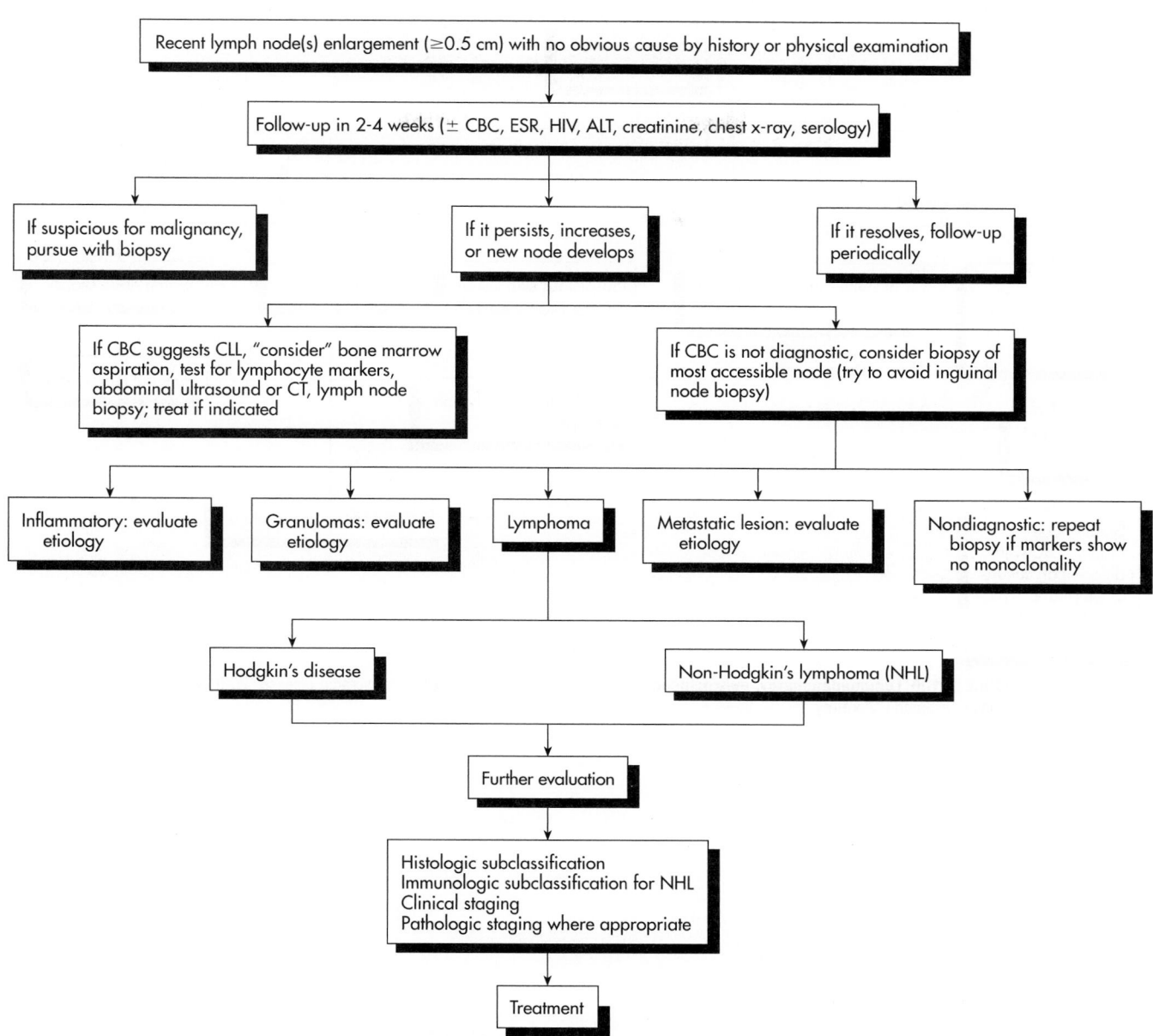

FIGURE 3-107 Workup of lymphadenopathy. *ALT,* Alanine aminotransferase; *CBC,* complete blood count; *CLL,* chronic lymphocytic leukemia; *CT,* computed tomography; *ESR,* erythrocyte sedimentation rate. (Modified from Noble J [ed]: *Primary care medicine,* ed 3, St Louis, 2001, Mosby.)

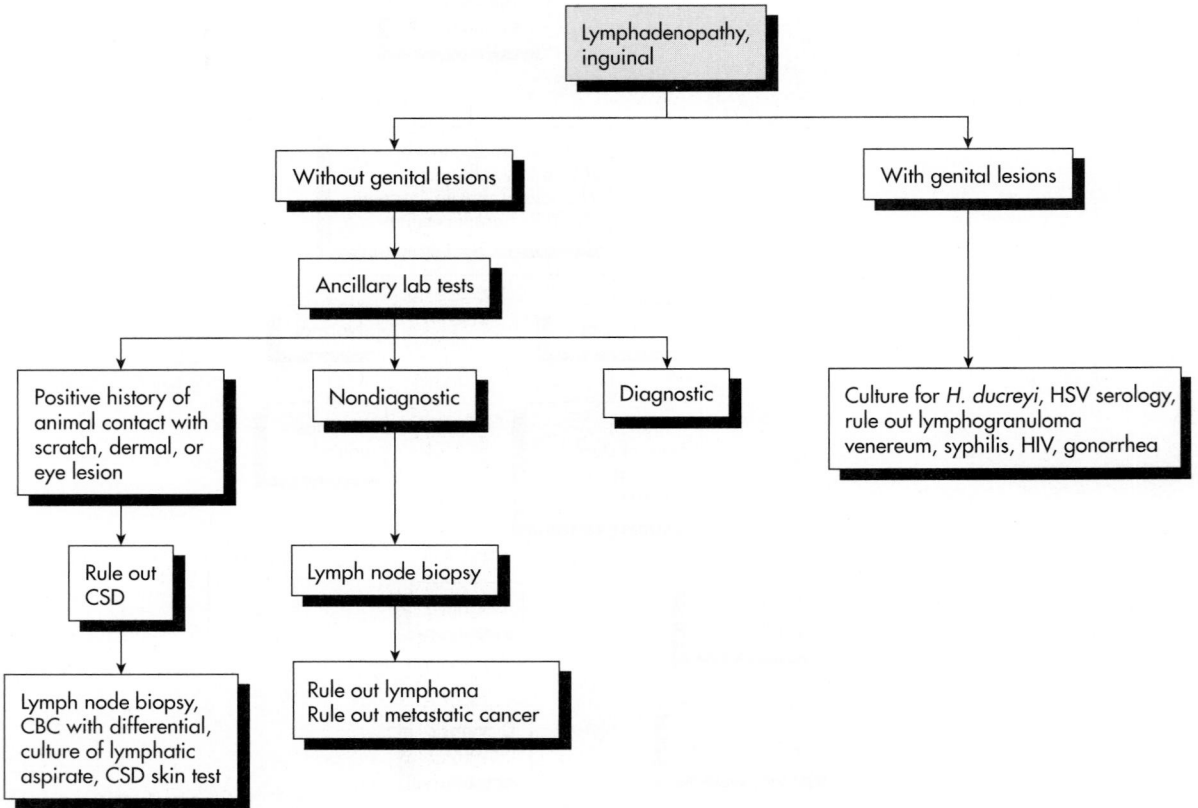

FIGURE 3-108 **Lymphadenopathy, inguinal.** *CBC*, Complete blood count; *CSD*, cat-scratch disease; *HSV*, herpes simplex virus.

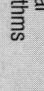

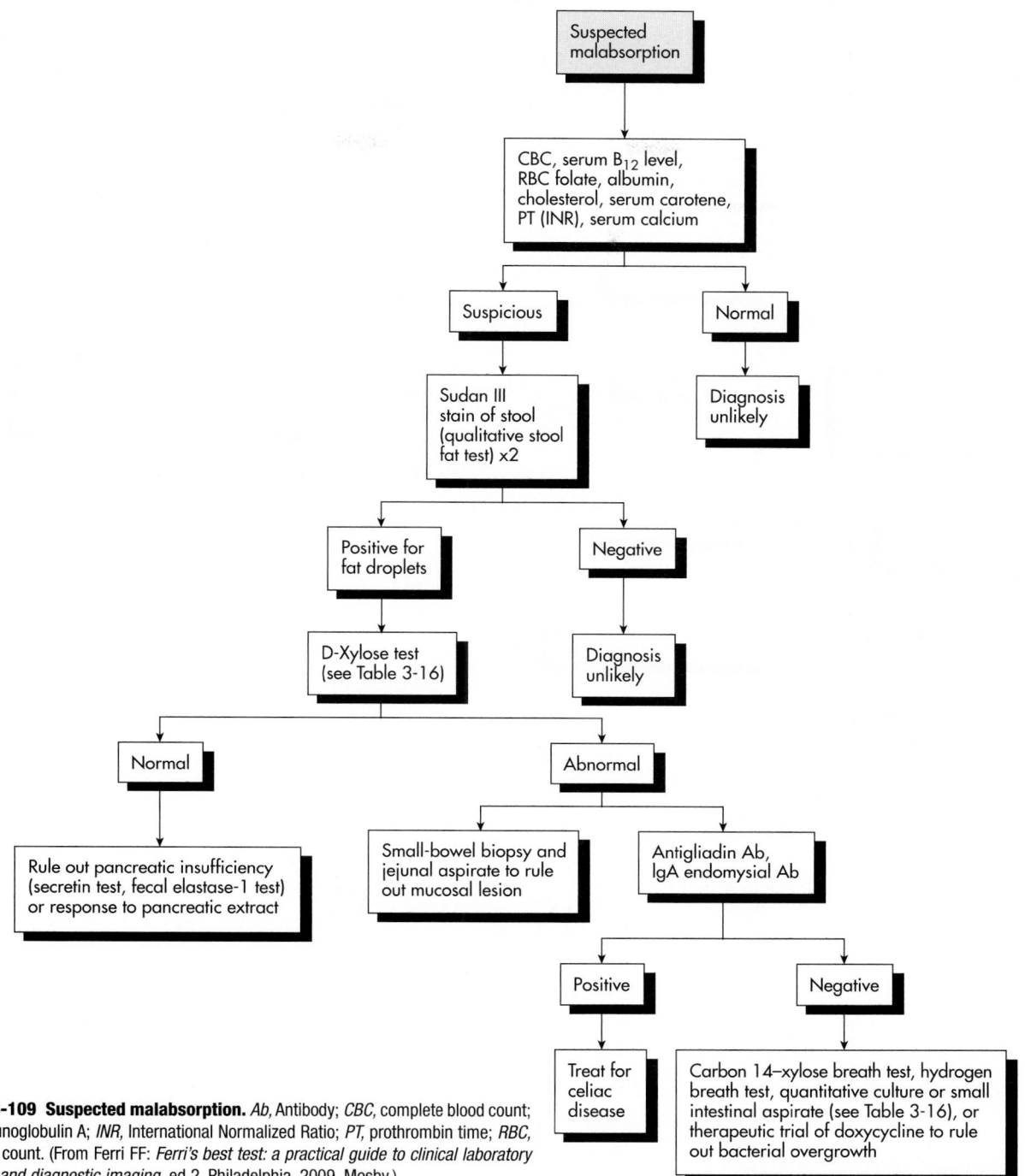

FIGURE 3-109 Suspected malabsorption. *Ab,* Antibody; *CBC,* complete blood count; *IgA,* immunoglobulin A; *INR,* International Normalized Ratio; *PT,* prothrombin time; *RBC,* red blood count. (From Ferri FF: *Ferri's best test: a practical guide to clinical laboratory medicine and diagnostic imaging,* ed 2, Philadelphia, 2009, Mosby.)

BOX 3-3   Malabsorption, Suspected

Diagnostic imaging	**Ancillary tests**
Best test	Albumin, total protein
Small-bowel series	ALT, AST, PT
	Serum lytes, BUN, creatinine
Ancillary test	Sudan III stain of stool for fecal leukocytes
CT of pancreas with IV contrast	CBC, RBC folate, serum iron, serum carotene, cholesterol, serum calcium
Lab evaluation	Hydrogen 14-C xylose breath test
Best test	D-Xylose test, secretin test
Biopsy of small bowel	Quantitative fecal test
	Antigliadin antibody, IgA endomysial antibody

From Ferri FF: *Ferri's best test: a practical guide to clinical laboratory medicine and diagnostic imaging,* ed 2, Philadelphia, 2009, Elsevier Mosby.
   ALT, Alanine aminotransferase; *AST,* aspartate aminotransferase; *BUN,* blood urea nitrogen; *CBC,* complete blood count; *CT,* computed tomography; *IgA,* immunoglobulin A; *IV,* intravenous; *PT,* prothrombin time; *RBC,* red blood count.

TABLE 3-16   Tests for the Evaluation of Malabsorption*

Test	Comments
General Tests of Absorption	
Quantitative stool fat test	Gold standard test of fat malabsorption, with which all other tests are compared. Requires ingestion of a high-fat diet (100 g) for 2 days before and during the collection. Stool is collected for 3 days. Normally, <7 g/24 hr is excreted on a high-fat diet. Borderline abnormalities of 8-14 g/24 hr may be seen in secretory or osmotic diarrheas that are not caused by malabsorption. There are false-negative findings if fat intake is inadequate. False-positive results can occur if mineral oil laxatives or rectal suppositories (e.g., cocoa butter) are given to the patient before stool collection.
Qualitative stool fat test	Sudan stain of a stool sample for fat. Many fat droplets per medium-power field (×40) constitute a positive test result. The nuclear magnetic resonance method determines the percentage of fat in the stool (normal, <20%). The test depends on an adequate fat intake (100 g/day). There is high sensitivity (90%) and specificity (90%) with fat malabsorption of >10 g/24 hr. Sensitivity drops with stool fat in the range of 6-10 g/24 hr.
D-Xylose test	A test of small intestinal mucosal absorption, used to distinguish mucosal malabsorption from malabsorption due to pancreatic insufficiency. An oral dose of D-xylose (24 g/500 ml water) is administered, and D-xylose excretion is measured in a 5-hr urine collection. Normally, >4 g of D-xylose is excreted in the urine over 5 hr. The test also may be positive in bacterial overgrowth owing to metabolism of D-xylose by bacteria in the intestinal lumen. False-positive test results occur with renal failure, ascites, and an incomplete urine collection. Blood levels at 1 and 3 hr improve sensitivity. May be normal with mild or limited mucosal disease.
Hydrogen breath test	Most useful in the diagnosis of lactase deficiency. An oral dose of lactose (1 g/kg body weight) is administered after measurement of basal breath H_2 levels. The sole source of H_2 in the mammal is bacterial fermentation; unabsorbed lactose makes its way to colonic bacteria, resulting in excess breath H_2. A *late peak* (within 3-6 hr) of >20 ppm of exhaled H_2 after lactose ingestion suggests lactose malabsorption. Absorption of other carbohydrates (e.g., sucrose, glucose, fructose) also can be tested.
Specific Tests for Malabsorption	
Tests for Pancreatic Function	
Secretin stimulation test	The gold standard test of pancreatic function. Requires duodenal test intubation with a double-lumen tube and collection of pancreatic juice in response to IV secretin. Allows measurement of bicarbonate (HCO_3-) and pancreatic enzymes. A sensitive test of pancreatic function, but labor intensive and invasive.
Fecal elastase-1 test	Stool test for pancreatic function. Equal sensitivity to the secretin stimulation test for the diagnosis of moderate-to-severe pancreatic insufficiency. More specific than the fecal chymotrypsin test. Unreliable with mild insufficiency. False-positive results occur with increased stool volume and intestinal mucosal diseases.
Tests for Bacterial Overgrowth	
Quantitative culture of small intestinal aspirate	Gold standard test for bacterial overgrowth. Greater than 10^5 colony-forming units (CFU)/ml in the jejunum suggests bacterial overgrowth. Requires special anaerobic sample collection, rapid anaerobic and aerobic plating, and care to avoid oropharyngeal contamination. False-negative results occur with focal jejunal diverticula and when overgrowth is distal to the site aspirated.
Hydrogen breath test	The 50-g glucose breath test has a sensitivity of 90% for growth of 10^5 colonic-type bacteria in the small intestine. If bacterial overgrowth is present, increased H_2 is excreted in the breath. A hydrogen level (within 2 hr) of >20 ppm suggests bacterial overgrowth. False-negative results occur with non-hydrogen-producing organisms.
^{14}C-D-xylose breath test	This test uses 1 g of carbon 14–labeled D-xylose. It has a sensitivity and specificity >90% for growth of 10^5 test colonic-type bacteria in the small intestine. Bacteria metabolize D-xylose with release of $^{14}CO_2$, which is absorbed and exhaled. Non-degraded D-xylose is absorbed in the small bowel and does not reach the colon, yielding a greater specificity than the lactulose H_2 breath test. A nonradioactive ^{13}C-D-xylose breath test is suitable for children and pregnant women.
Tests for Mucosal Disease	
Small bowel biopsy	Obtained for a specific diagnosis when there is a high index of suspicion for small intestinal disease. Several biopsy specimens (4-5) must be obtained to maximize the diagnostic yield. Distal duodenal biopsy specimens are usually adequate for diagnosis, but occasionally enteroscopy with jejunal biopsy specimens is necessary. Small intestinal biopsy provides a specific diagnosis in some diseases (e.g., intestinal infection, Whipple's disease, abetalipoproteinemia, agammaglobulinemia, lymphangiectasia, lymphoma, amyloidosis). In other conditions, such as celiac disease and tropical sprue, the biopsy specimens show characteristic findings, but the diagnosis is made on improvement after treatment.
Tests of Ileal Function	
Schilling test	A test of vitamin B_{12} absorption
^{75}SeHCAT test	This is a test of bile acid absorption. Seven days after ingestion of radiolabeled synthetic selenium-homocholic acid conjugated with taurine (^{75}SeHCAT), whole body retention is measured by a gamma-counting device. The result is expressed as a fraction of baseline ingestion. Retention values of less than 10% are abnormal and indicate bile acid malabsorption with a sensitivity of 80-90% and specificity of 70%-100%. The radiation dose is equivalent to a plain chest x-ray. Liver disease and bacterial overgrowth may give false results. Not approved for use in the United States.

From Goldman L, Schafer AI: *Goldman's Cecil Medicine,* ed 24, Philadelphia, 2012, Saunders.

*Not all these tests are readily available. A strong suspicion for any disease may warrant foregoing an extensive work-up and obtaining the test with highest diagnostic yield. In some cases, empirical treatment, such as removing lactose from the diet of an otherwise healthy individual with lactose intolerance, is warranted without any testing.

Clinical Algorithms

III

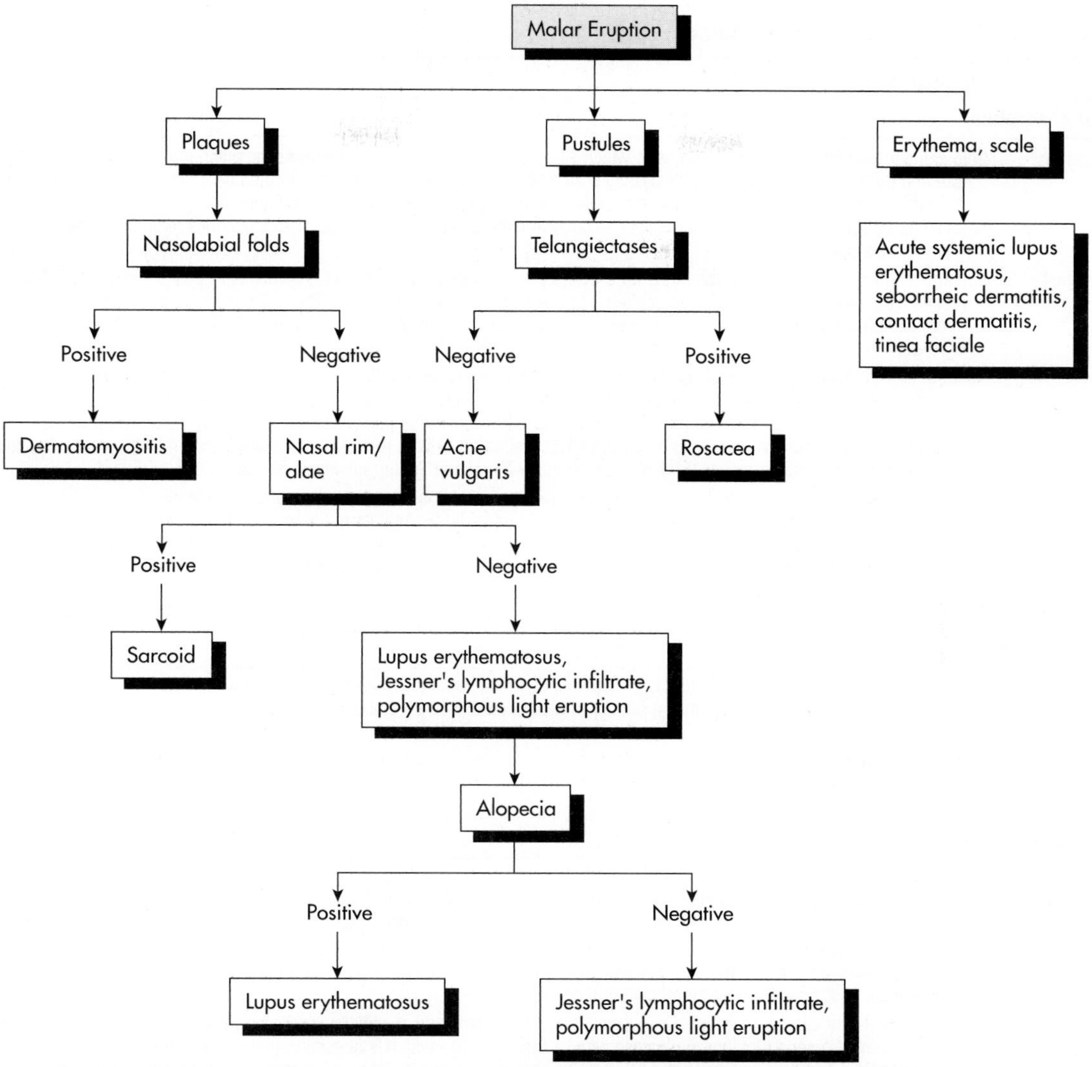

FIGURE 3-110 Clinical algorithm for diagnosis of a malar eruption, which must be confirmed by appropriate cultures, serology, and biopsy. (From Harris ED et al [eds]: *Kelley's textbook of rheumatology,* ed 7, Philadelphia, 2005, Saunders.)

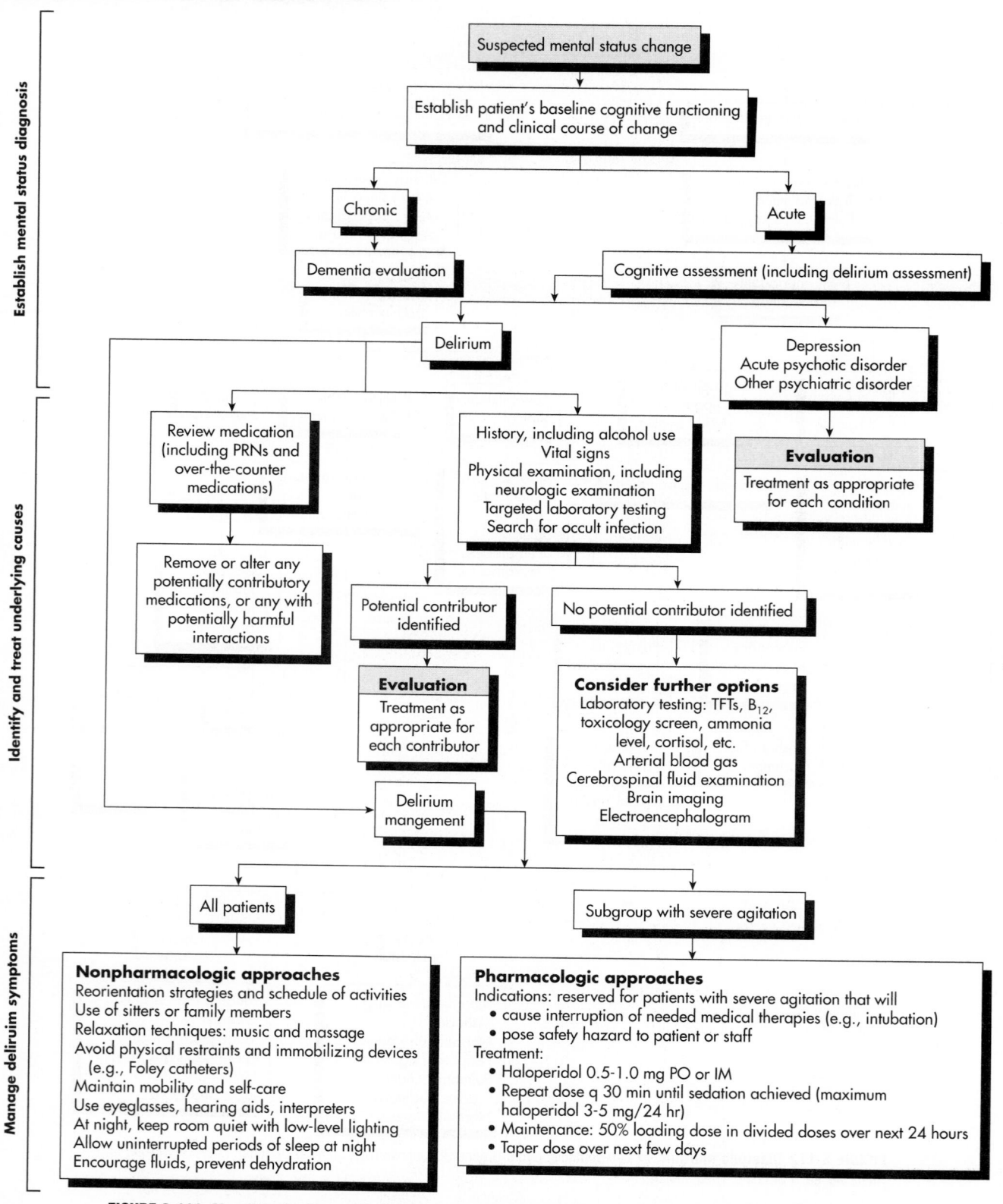

FIGURE 3-111 Algorithm for the evaluation of suspected mental status change in older patients. *PRN,* As needed; *TFTs,* thyroid function tests. (From Goldman L, Schafer AI: *Goldman's Cecil medicine,* ed 24, Philadelphia, 2012, Saunders.)

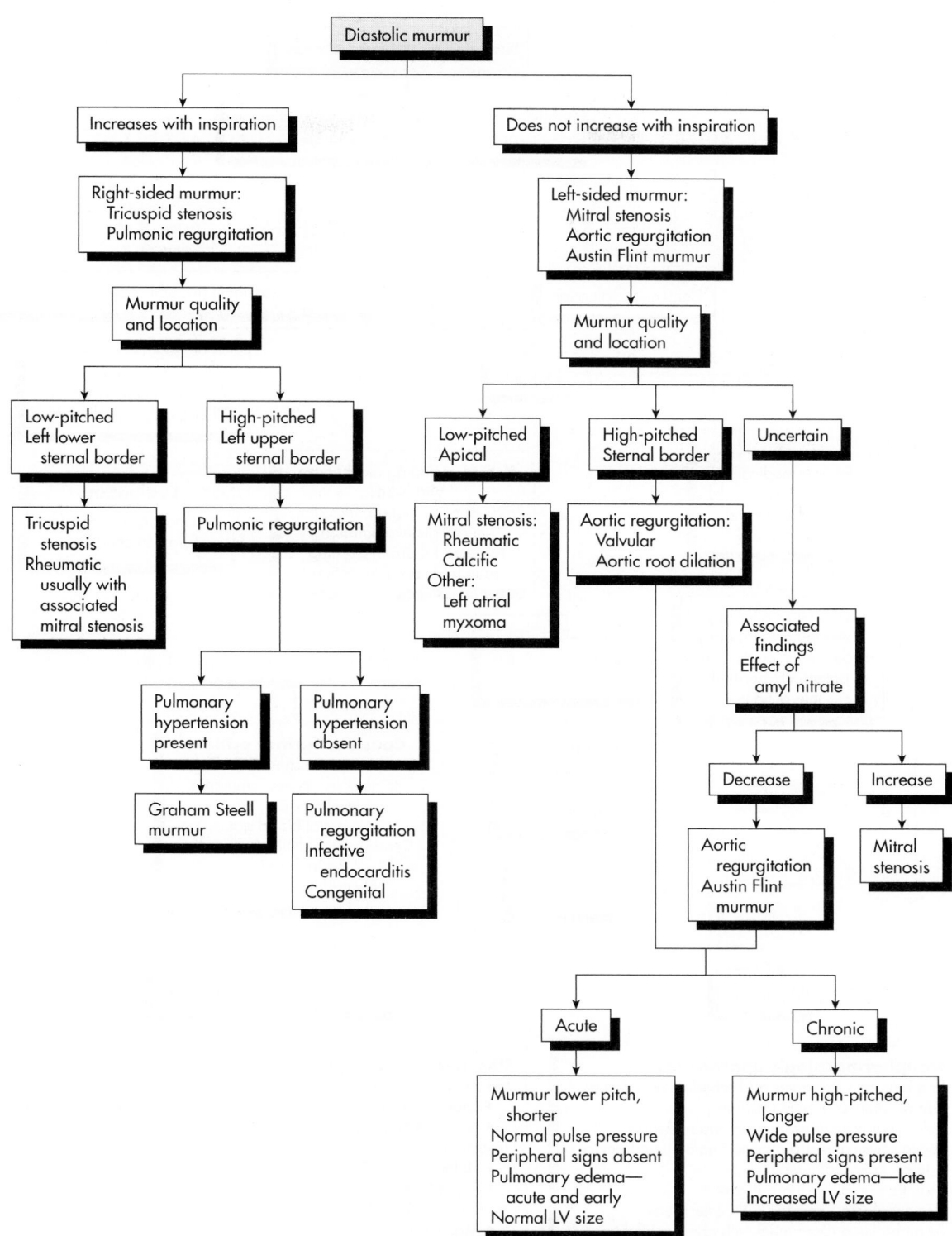

FIGURE 3-112 Diastolic murmur. *LV,* Left ventricle. (From Greene HL, Johnson WP, Lemcke DL [eds]: *Decision making in medicine,* ed 2, St Louis, 1998, Mosby.)

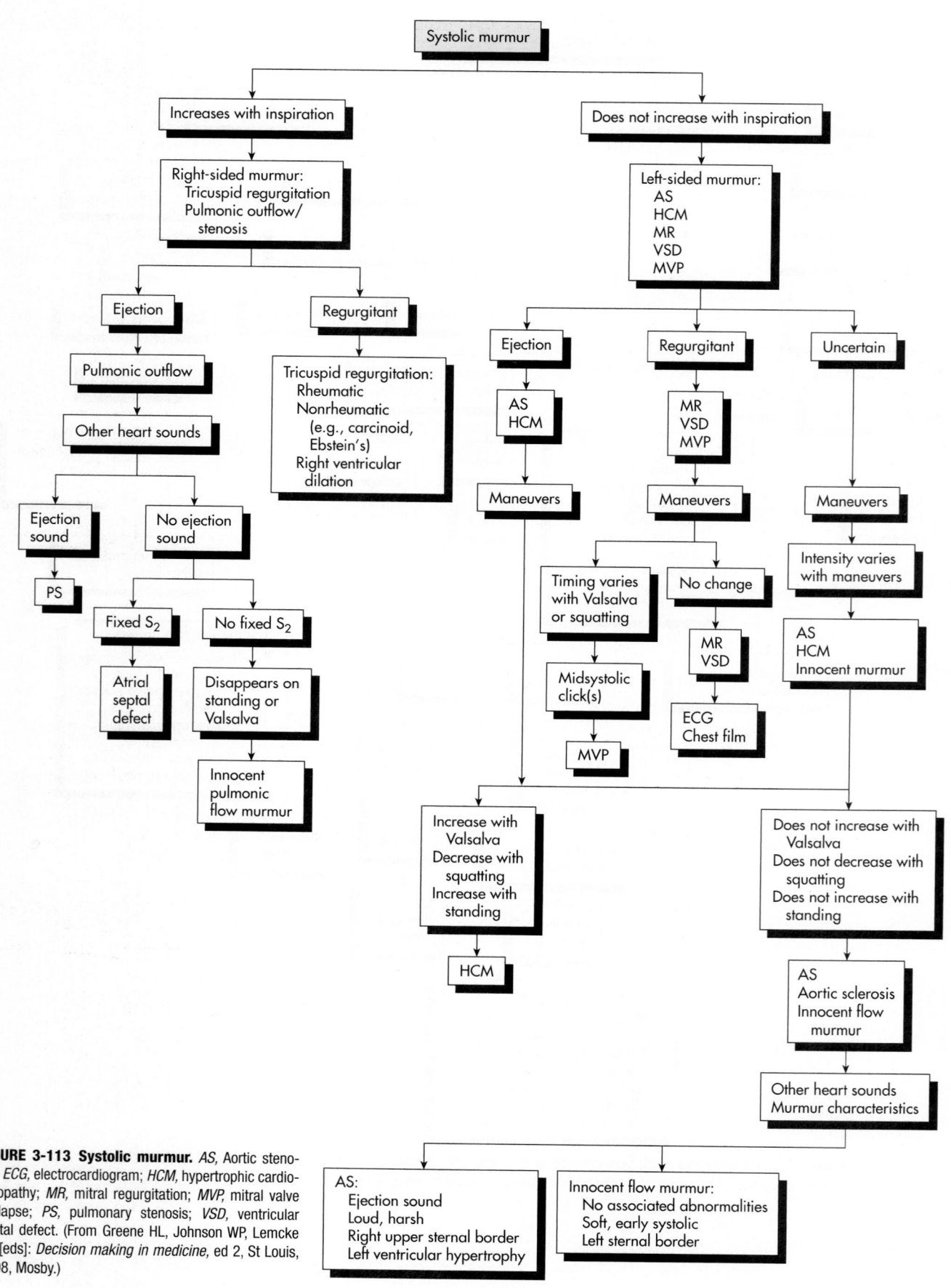

Clinical Algorithms

III

FIGURE 3-113 Systolic murmur. *AS,* Aortic stenosis; *ECG,* electrocardiogram; *HCM,* hypertrophic cardiomyopathy; *MR,* mitral regurgitation; *MVP,* mitral valve prolapse; *PS,* pulmonary stenosis; *VSD,* ventricular septal defect. (From Greene HL, Johnson WP, Lemcke DL [eds]: *Decision making in medicine,* ed 2, St Louis, 1998, Mosby.)

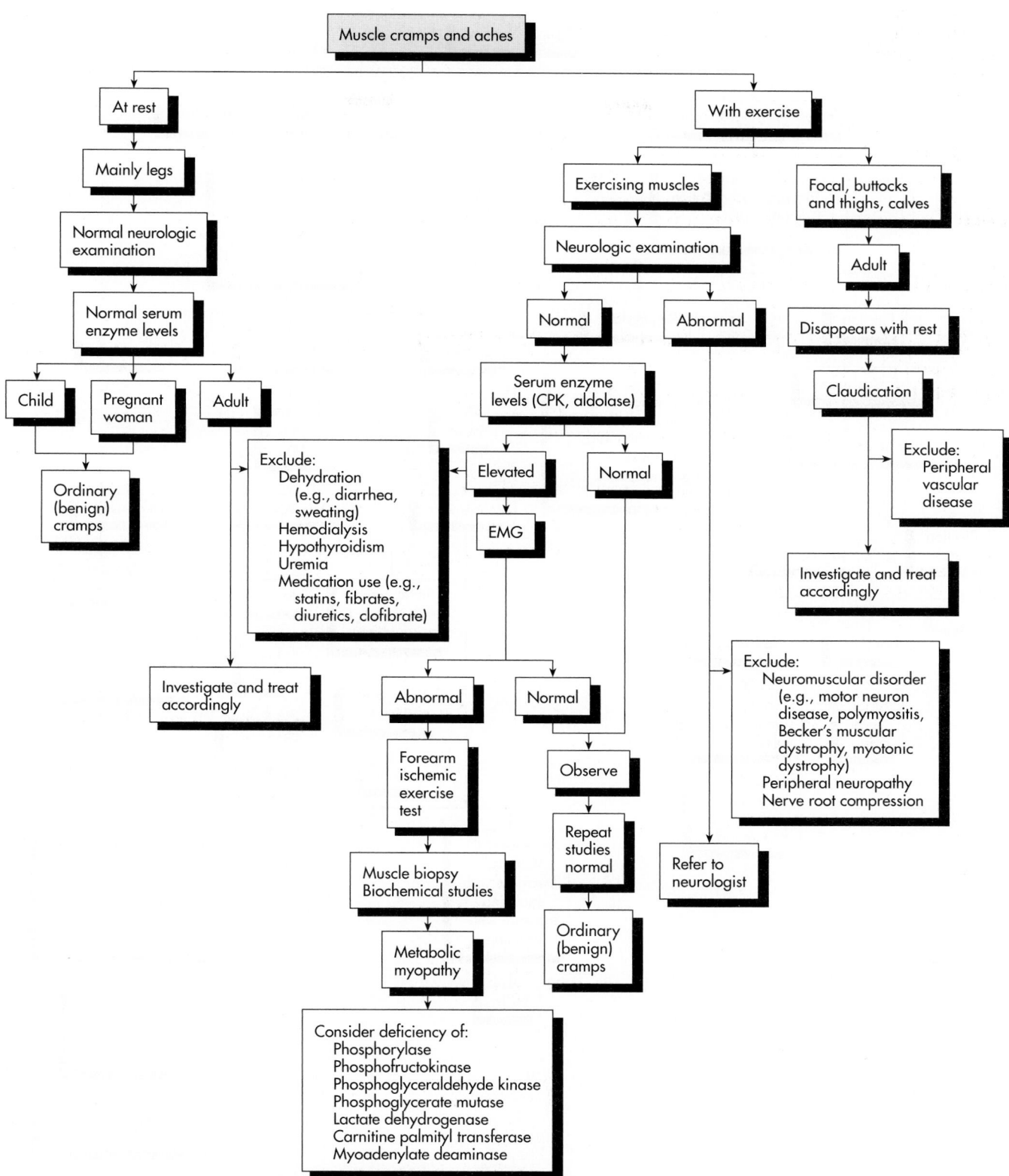

FIGURE 3-114 Evaluation of muscle cramps and aches. *CPK,* Creatine phosphokinase; *EMG,* electromyography. (From Greene HL, Johnson WP, Lemcke D [eds]: *Decision making in medicine,* ed 2, St Louis, 1998, Mosby.)

MUSCLE WEAKNESS

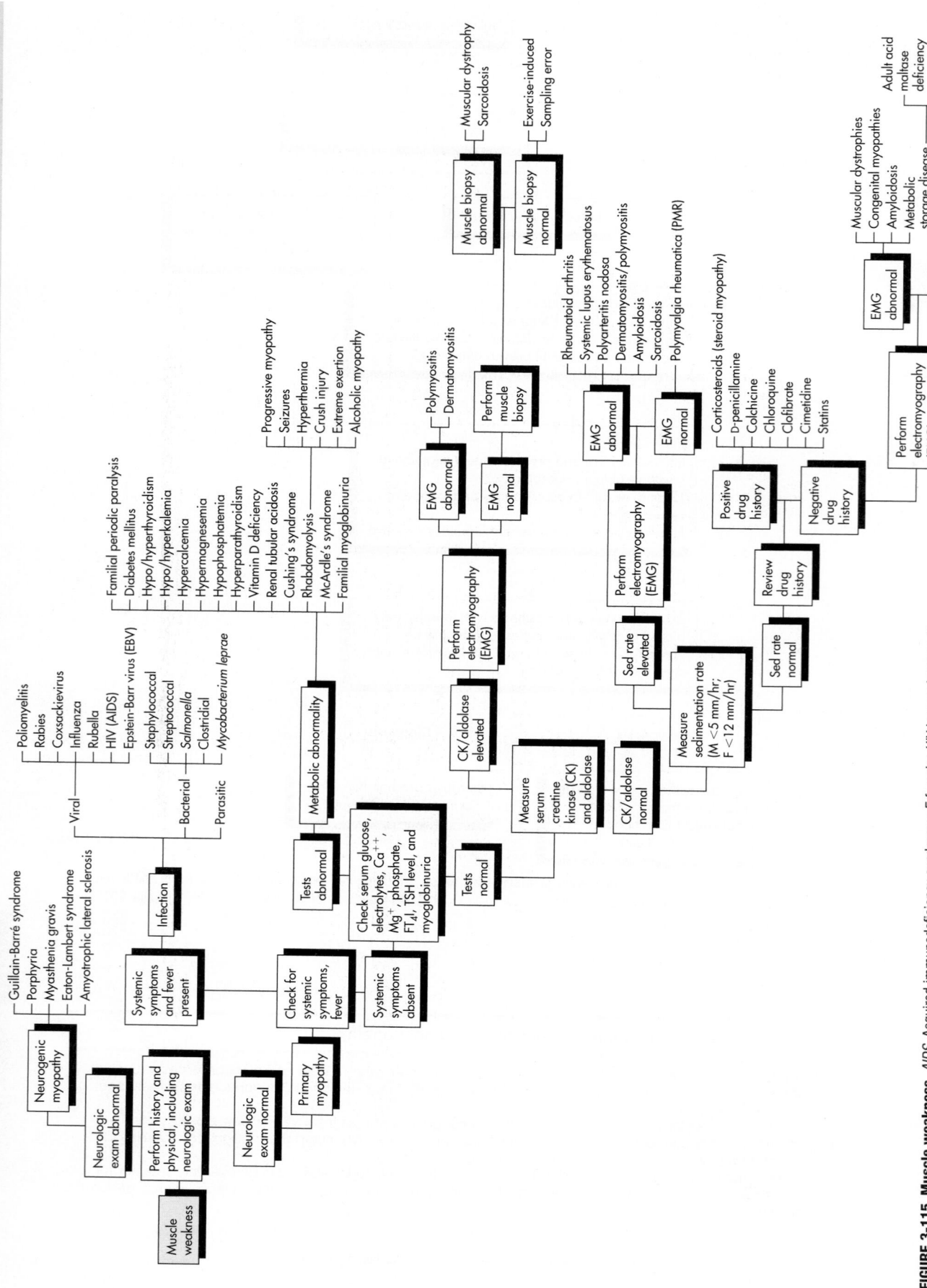

FIGURE 3-115 Muscle weakness. *AIDS,* Acquired immunodeficiency syndrome; *F,* female; *HIV,* human immunodeficiency virus; *M,* male. (From Healey PM: *Common medical diagnosis: an algorithmic approach,* ed 3, Philadelphia, 2000, Saunders.)

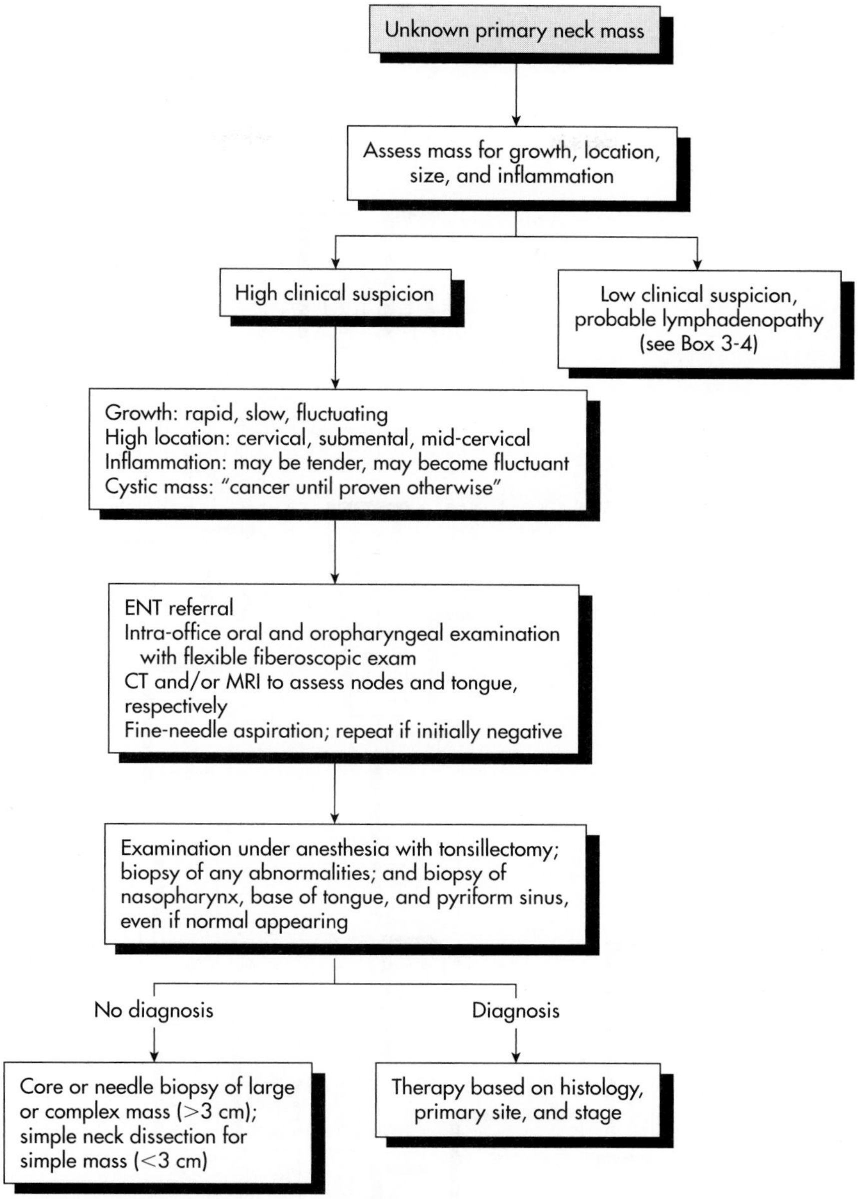

FIGURE 3-119 Evaluation of an unknown primary neck mass. *CT,* Computed tomography; *ENT,* ear, nose, and throat; *MRI,* magnetic resonance imaging. (From Goldman L, Ausiello D [eds]: *Cecil textbook of medicine,* ed 24, Philadelphia, 2012, Saunders.)

BOX 3-4   An Approach to the Patient with Lymphadenopathy

1. Does the patient have a known illness that causes lymphadenopathy? Treat and monitor for resolution.
2. Is there an obvious infection to explain the lymphadenopathy (e.g., infectious mononucleosis)? Treat and monitor for resolution.
3. Are the nodes very large and/or very firm and thus suggestive of malignancy? Perform a biopsy.
4. Is the patient very concerned about malignancy and unable to be reassured that malignancy is unlikely? Perform a biopsy.
5. If none of the preceding are true, perform a complete blood cell count and if it is unrevealing, monitor for a predetermined period (usually 2 to 6 weeks). If the nodes do not regress or if they increase in size, perform a biopsy.

From Goldman L, Ausiello D (eds): *Cecil textbook of medicine,* ed 23, Philadelphia, 2008, Saunders.

What Is the Origin of the Neck Pain?

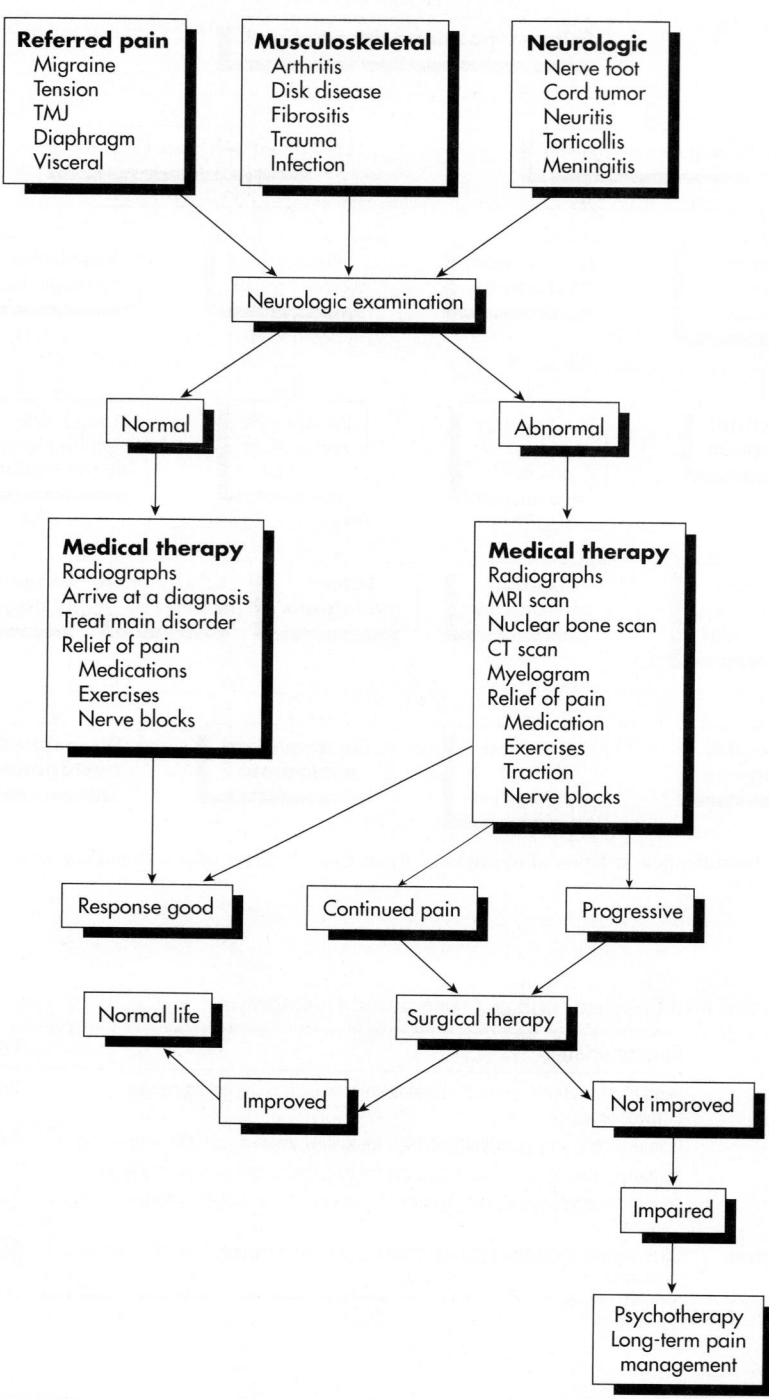

FIGURE 3-120 Neck pain algorithm for diagnosis and treatment. *CT,* Computed tomography; *MRI,* magnetic resonance imaging; *TMJ,* temporomandibular joint. (Modified from Nakano KK: Neck and back pain. In Stein JH [ed]: *Internal medicine,* ed 5, St Louis, 1998, Mosby, pp 963-971.)

Identification of Types of Nystagmus

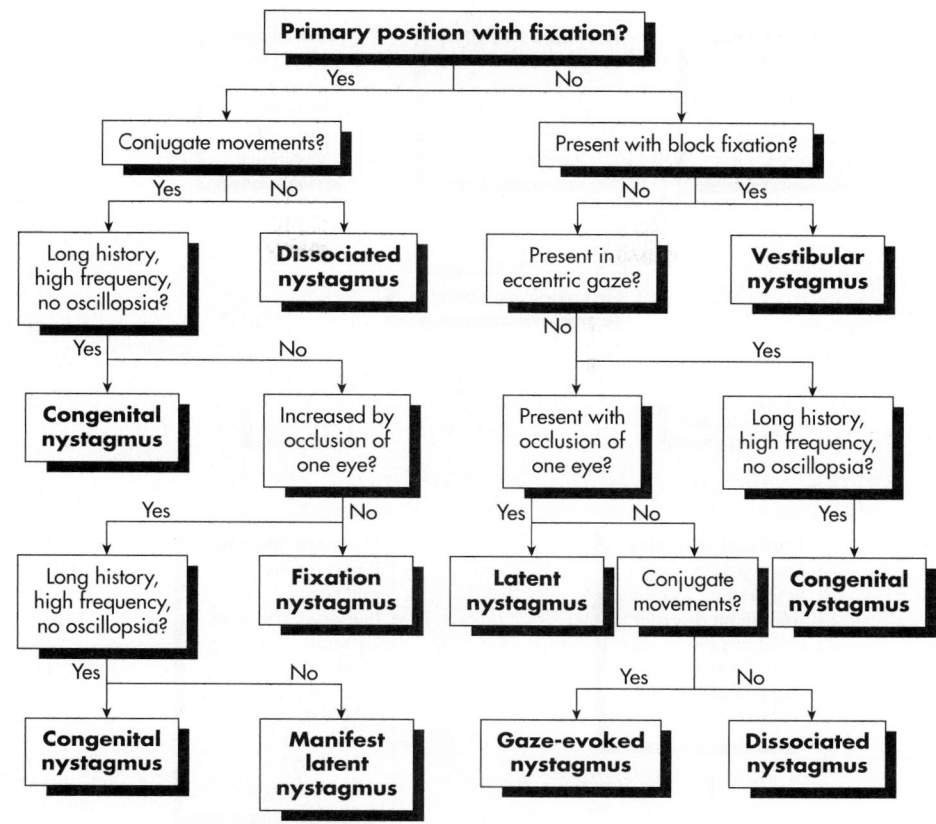

FIGURE 3-123 Identification of types of nystagmus. (From Yanoff M, Duker JS: *Ophthalmology,* ed 2, St Louis, 2004, Mosby.)

TABLE 3-17 Characteristics and Localizations of Dissociated Nystagmus

Nystagmus	Characteristics	Localization
Acquired pendular in adults	Pendular, horizontal, vertical, torsional, disconjugate (coexisting palatal myoclonus)	Brain stem, cerebellum
Superior oblique myokymia	Pendular, jerk, torsional, vertical, high frequency, small amplitude, monocular	Trochlear nucleus
See-saw	Pendular, vertical, torsional, rising eye intorts, falling eye extorts; rarely jerk	Midbrain (interstitial nucleus of Cajal)
Abducting "nystagmus" of internuclear ophthalmoplegia	Jerk, horizontal, decreasing velocity slow components, larger in abducting eye	Medial longitudinal fasciculus in pons, midbrain horizontal gaze
Abducting nystagmus of myasthenia gravis	Gaze-paretic nystagmus in horizontal gaze, greater paresis of medial rectus muscle	Myoneural junction—myasthenia gravis

From Yanoff M, Duker JS: *Ophthalmology,* ed 2, St Louis, 2004, Mosby.

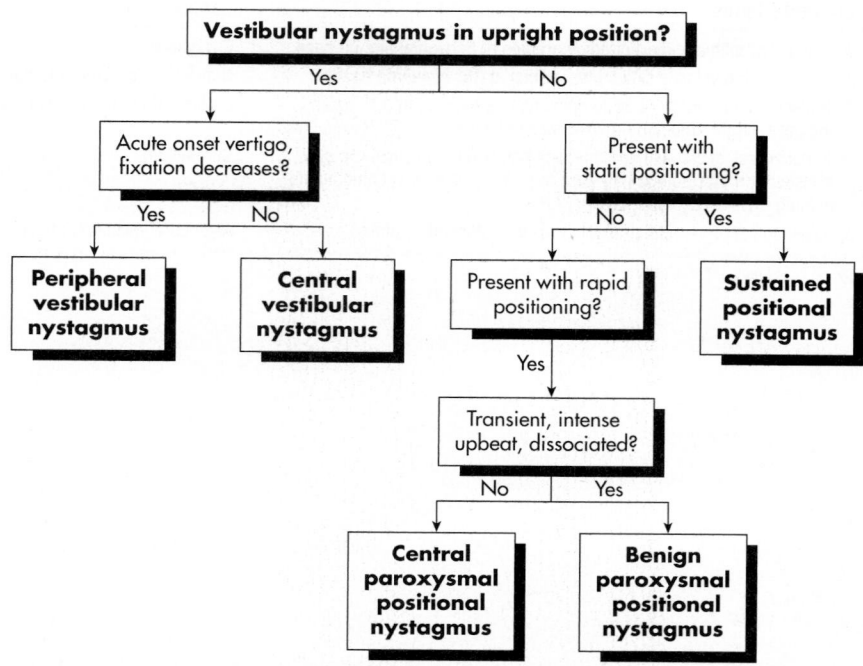

FIGURE 3-124 Identification of types of vestibular nystagmus. (From Yanoff M, Duker JS: *Ophthalmology,* ed 2, St Louis, 2004, Mosby.)

TABLE 3-18 Characteristics and Localizations of Vestibular Nystagmus

Nystagmus	Characteristics	Localization
Spontaneous peripheral vestibular	Jerk, horizontal, small torsional, inhibited by fixation	Labyrinth, eighth nerve (acute)
Central vestibular (fixation) nystagmus	Jerk, pendular, horizontal, vertical, torsional, not inhibited by fixation	Brain stem, cerebellum
Sustained positional vestibular	Jerk, horizontal, small torsional, direction fixed, direction changing (static positioning)	Labyrinth, eighth nerve or brain stem, cerebellum
Benign paroxysmal positional	Jerk, dissociated upbeat, latency, not inhibited by fixation, fatigue (Nylen–Barany maneuver)	Posterior vertical canal
Central paroxysmal positional	Jerk, symmetric, upbeat, downbeat	Brain stem, cerebellum

From Yanoff M, Duker JS: *Ophthalmology,* ed 2, St Louis, 2004, Mosby.

Clinical
Algorithms

III

TABLE 3-19 Characteristics and Localizations of Gaze-Evoked Nystagmus

Nystagmus	Characteristics	Localization
Physiologic, endpoint	Jerk, small amplitude, intermittent, extremes of horizontal and up gaze	Physiologic
Gaze-paretic (symmetric)	Jerk (decreasing velocity slow components) at 30° eccentric gaze	Nonlocalizing (drugs, mental fatigue)
Gaze-paretic (asymmetric)	Jerk (decreasing velocity slow components), horizontal, at 30° eccentric gaze, larger amplitude toward side of lesion	Lesions of brain stem, cerebellum, cerebral hemisphere
Rebound	Jerk, horizontal, decreases and direction can reverse in eccentric gaze, transient jerk nystagmus on return to primary gaze, fast components beating toward eccentric gaze	Cerebellum
Myasthenia gravis	Jerk, horizontal or vertical, gradual onset in prolonged eccentric gaze	Myoneural junction (fatigue—increasing transmission block)

From Yanoff M, Duker JS: *Ophthalmology,* ed 2, St Louis, 2004, Mosby.

**Identification
of Types of Gaze-Evoked Nystagmus**

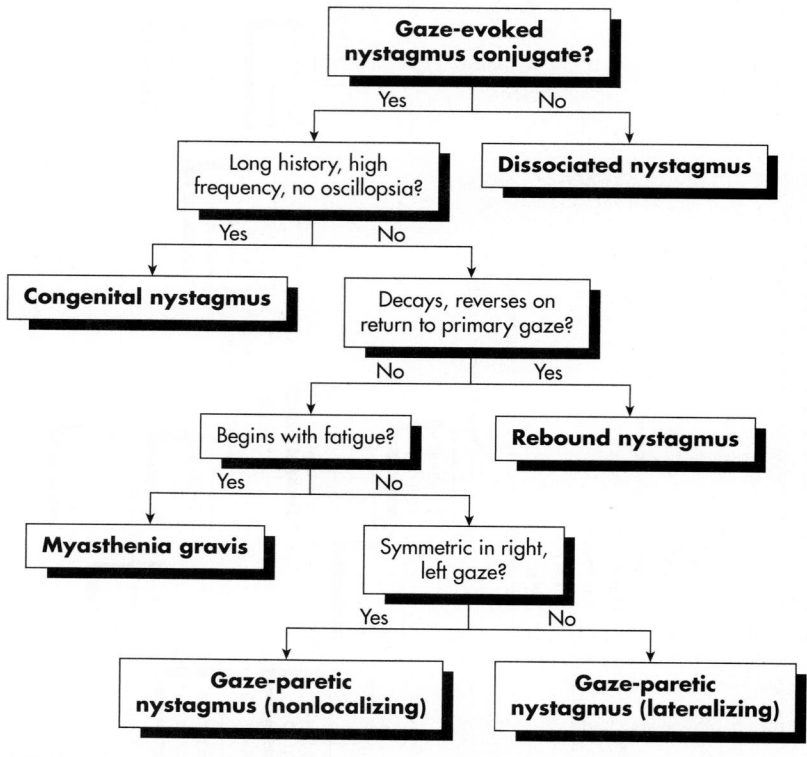

FIGURE 3-125 Identification of types of gaze-evoked nystagmus. (From Yanoff M, Duker JS: *Ophthalmology,* ed 2, St Louis, 2004, Mosby.)

**Identification
of Types of Dissociated Nystagmus**

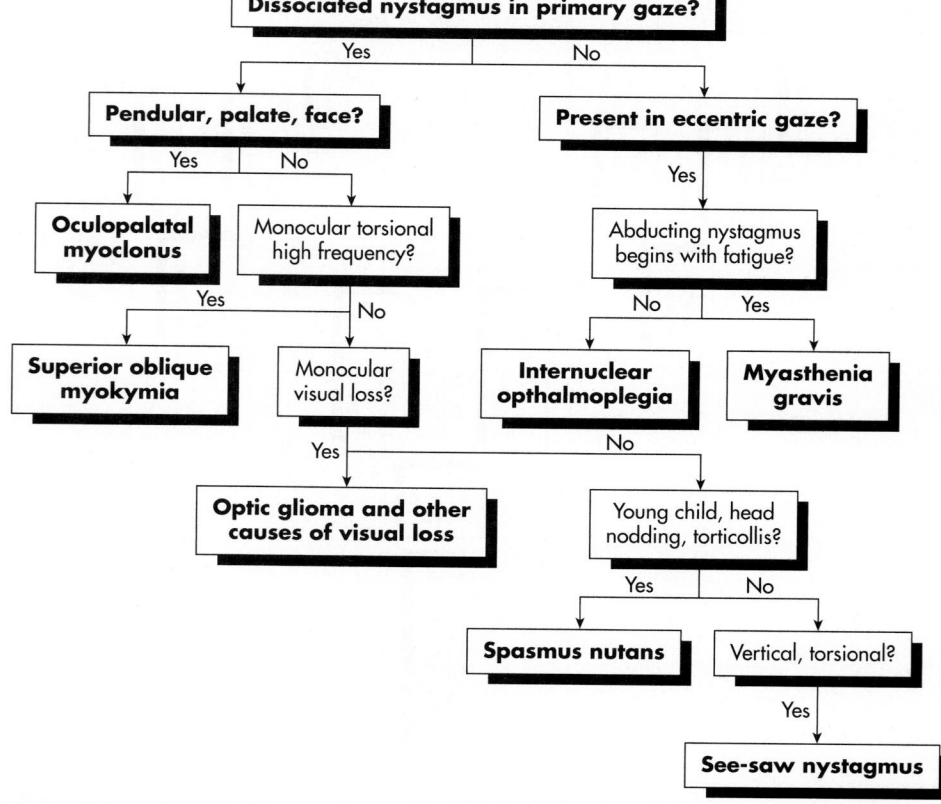

FIGURE 3-126 Identification of types of dissociated nystagmus. (From Yanoff M, Duker JS: *Ophthalmology,* ed 2, St Louis, 2004, Mosby.)

Clinical
Algorithms

III

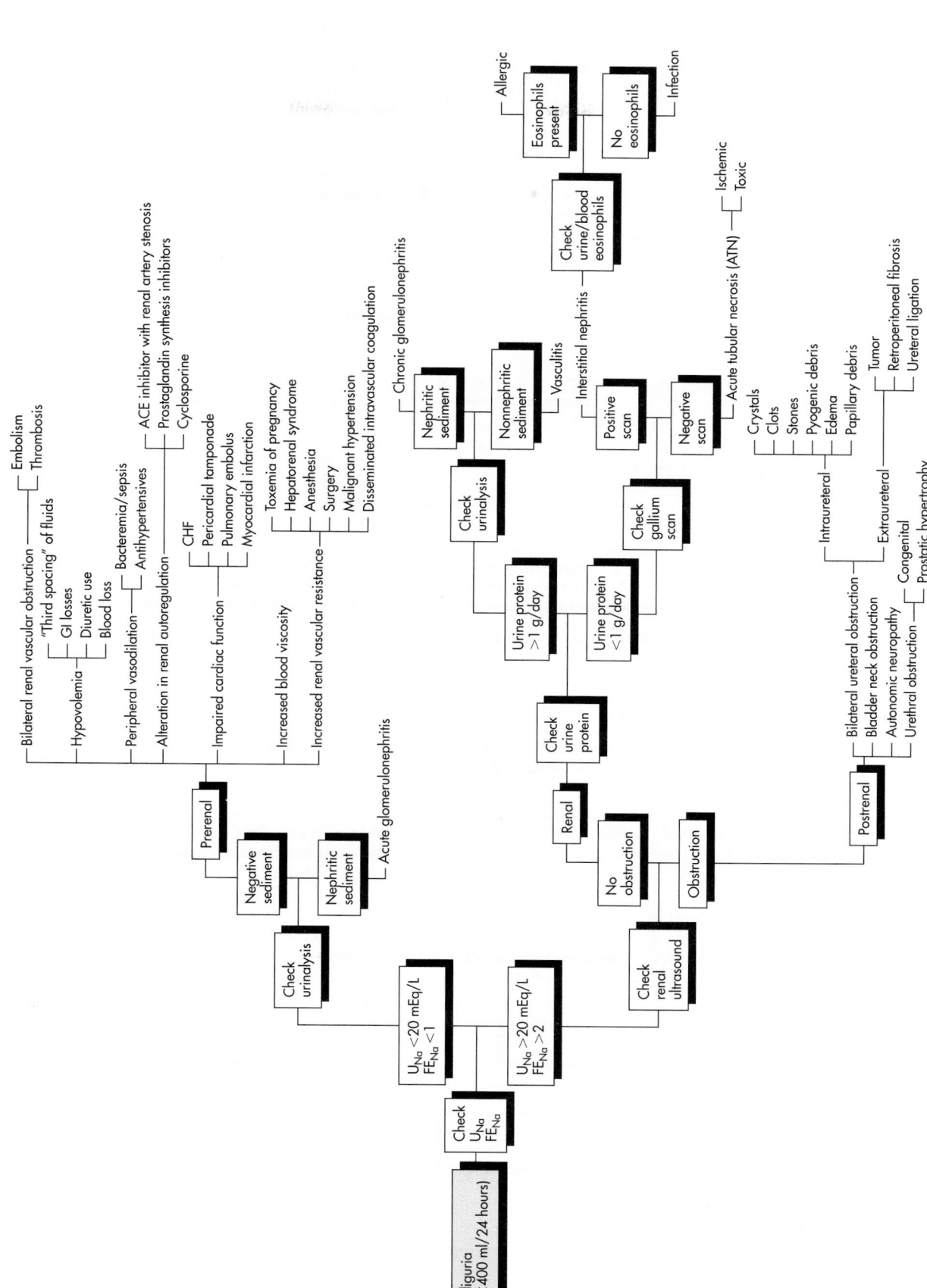

FIGURE 3-127 Evaluation of oliguria. *ACE,* Angiotensin-converting enzyme; *CHF,* congestive heart failure; *GI,* gastrointestinal. (From Healey PM: *Common medical diagnosis: an algorithmic approach,* ed 3, Philadelphia, 2000, Saunders.)

Evaluation of Patients with Palpitations, Dizziness, and/or Syncope

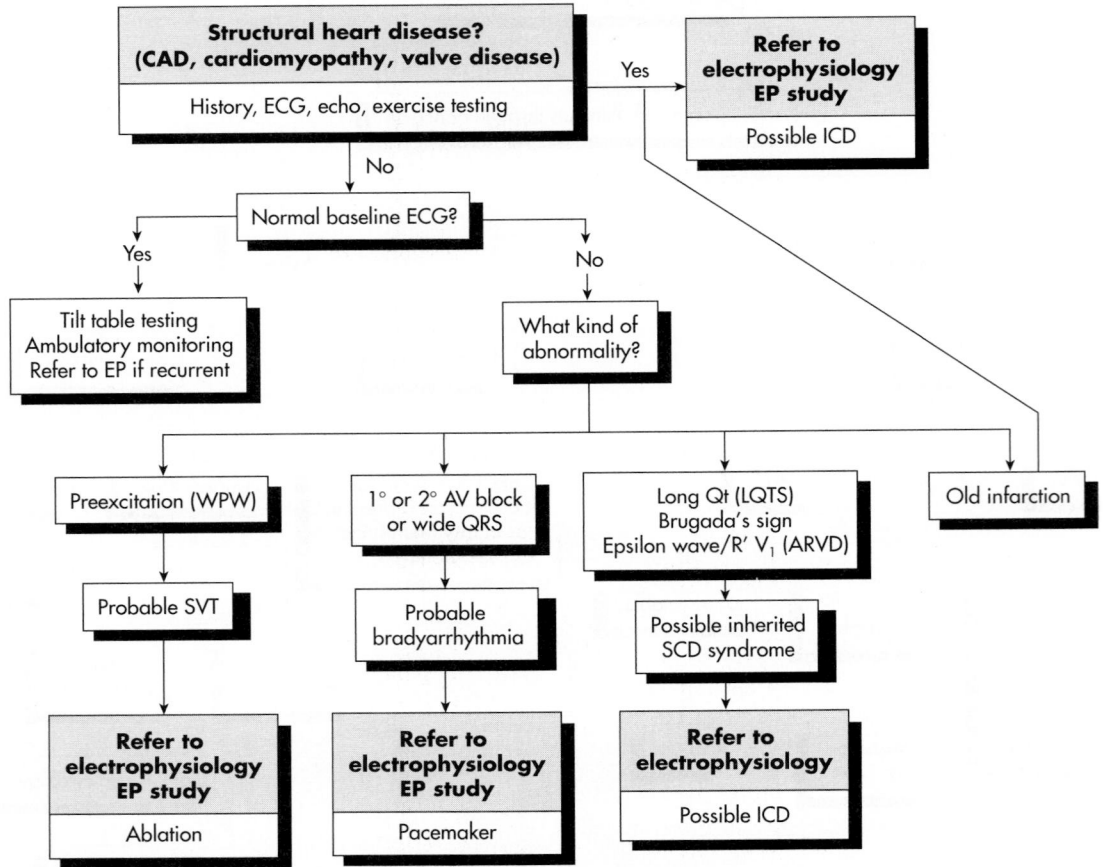

FIGURE 3-129 Algorithm for evaluating patients with symptoms of palpitation, dizziness, or syncope. *ARVD,* Arrhythmogenic right ventricular dysplasia; *AV,* atrioventricular; *CAD,* coronary artery disease; *ECG,* electrocardiogram; *echo,* echocardiogram; *EP,* electrophysiology; *ICD,* implantable cardioverter-defibrillator; *LQTS,* long QT syndrome; *SCD,* sudden cardiac death; *SVT,* supraventricular tachycardia; *WPW,* Wolff-Parkinson-White syndrome. (From Goldman L, Schafer AI: *Goldman's Cecil medicine,* ed 24, Philadelphia, 2012, Saunders.)

TABLE 3-20   Items to be Covered in History of Patient with Palpitation

Does the Palpitation Occur:	If So, Suspect:
As isolated "jumps" or "skips"?	Extrasystoles
In attacks known to be of abrupt beginning, with a heart rate of 120 beats/min or over, with regular or irregular rhythm?	Paroxysmal rapid heart action
Independent of exercise or excitement adequate to account for the symptom?	Atrial fibrillation, atrial flutter, thyrotoxicosis, anemia, febrile states, hypoglycemia, anxiety state
In attacks developing rapidly though not absolutely abruptly, unrelated to exertion or excitement?	Hemorrhage, hypoglycemia, tumor of the adrenal medulla
In conjunction with the taking of drugs?	Tobacco, coffee, tea, alcohol, epinephrine, ephedrine, aminophylline, atropine, thyroid extract, monoamine oxidase inhibitors
On standing?	Postural hypotension
In middle-aged women, in conjunction with flushes and sweats?	Menopausal syndrome
When the rate is known to be normal and the rhythm regular?	Anxiety state

From Goldman L, Braunwald E: Chest discomfort and palpitation. In Isselbacher KJ, Braunwald E et al [eds]: *Harrison's principles of internal medicine,* ed 13, New York, 1994, McGraw-Hill.

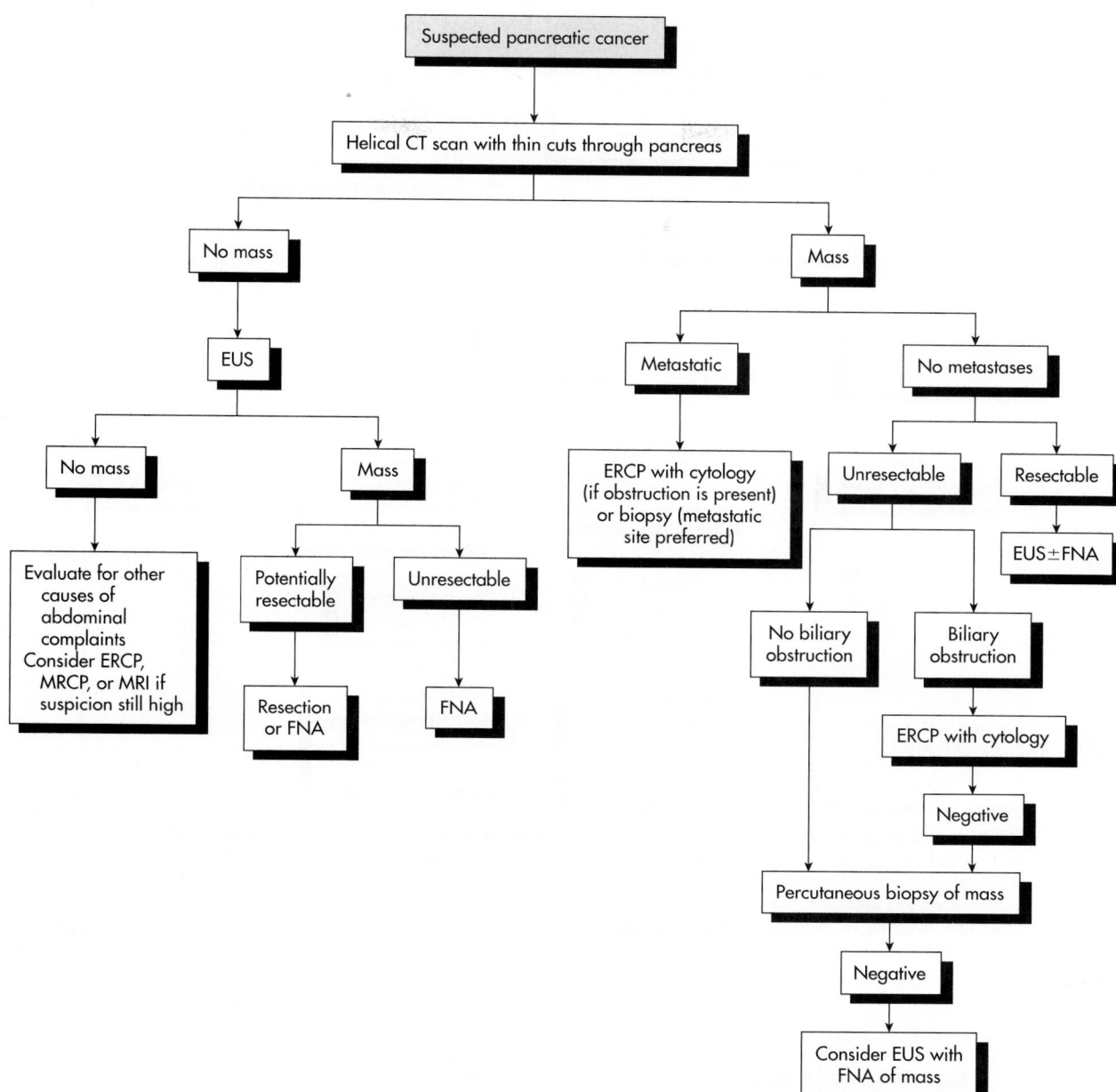

FIGURE 3-131 Diagnostic algorithm for pancreatic cancer. Intraoperative fine-needle aspiration (FNA) if found inoperable during surgery. *CT*, Computed tomography; *ERCP*, endoscopic retrograde cholangiopancreatography; *EUS*, endoscopic ultrasonography; *MRI*, magnetic resonance imaging. (From Goldman L, Ausiello D [eds]: *Cecil textbook of medicine*, ed 24, Philadelphia, 2012, Saunders.)

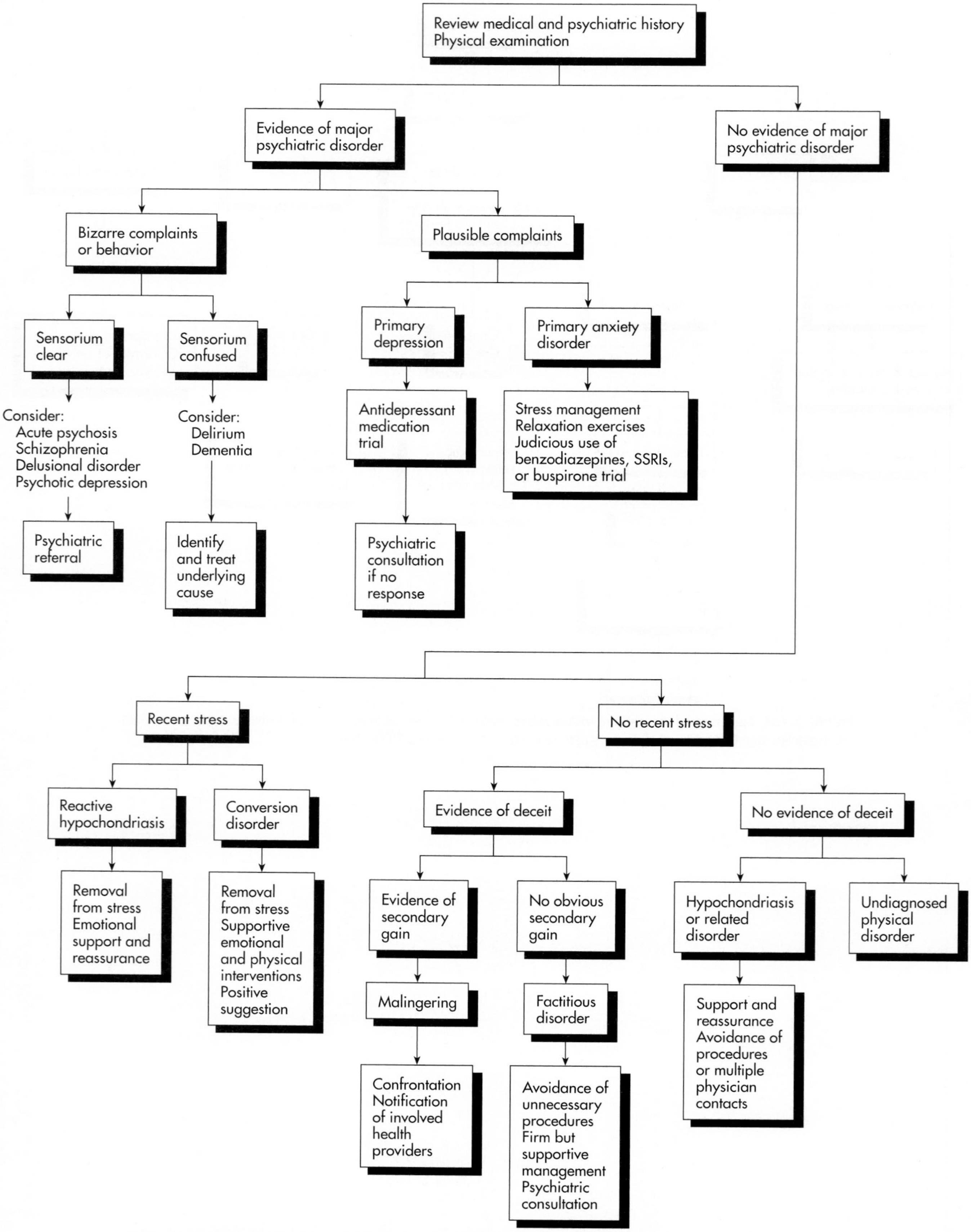

Review medical and psychiatric history
Physical examination

Evidence of major psychiatric disorder

No evidence of major psychiatric disorder

Bizarre complaints or behavior

Plausible complaints

Sensorium clear

Sensorium confused

Primary depression

Primary anxiety disorder

Consider:
Acute psychosis
Schizophrenia
Delusional disorder
Psychotic depression

Consider:
Delirium
Dementia

Antidepressant medication trial

Stress management
Relaxation exercises
Judicious use of benzodiazepines, SSRIs, or buspirone trial

Psychiatric referral

Identify and treat underlying cause

Psychiatric consultation if no response

Recent stress

No recent stress

Reactive hypochondriasis

Conversion disorder

Evidence of deceit

No evidence of deceit

Removal from stress
Emotional support and reassurance

Removal from stress
Supportive emotional and physical interventions
Positive suggestion

Evidence of secondary gain

No obvious secondary gain

Hypochondriasis or related disorder

Undiagnosed physical disorder

Malingering

Factitious disorder

Support and reassurance
Avoidance of procedures or multiple physician contacts

Confrontation
Notification of involved health providers

Avoidance of unnecessary procedures
Firm but supportive management
Psychiatric consultation

Clinical Algorithms

FIGURE 3-133 Patient with ill-defined physical complaints. Previous or recent evaluations are noncontributory. *SSRIs,* Selective serotonin reuptake inhibitors. (From Greene H, Johnson WP, Lemcke D [eds]: *Decision making in medicine,* ed 2, St Louis, 1998, Mosby.)

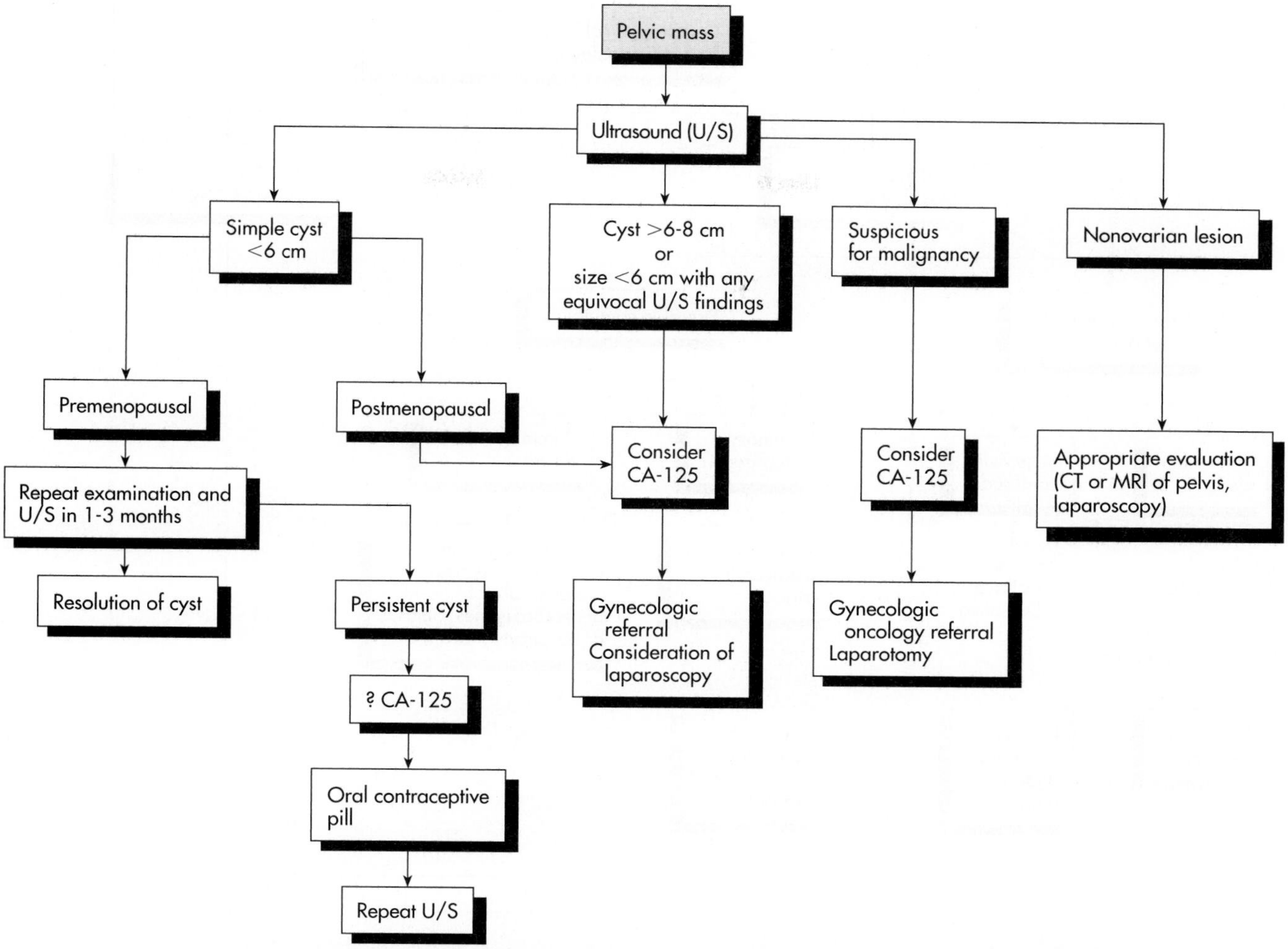

FIGURE 3-134 Approach to the patient with a pelvic mass. *CT,* Computed tomography; *MRI,* magnetic resonance imaging. (Modified from Carlson KJ et al: *Primary care of women,* ed 2, St Louis, 2002, Mosby.)

1. Rapid history and external abdominal examination

- **If surgical abdomen:** Consider early ob/gyn/surgery consultation
  - Rupture (ectopic, cyst, abscess)
  - Torsion (adnexal, fibroid)
  - Perforation (uterine)
  - Appendicitis

2. Vital signs

- **If unstable:** Establish venous access and administer fluid bolus
  Spin Hct, type and crossmatch blood as needed
  Consider early ob/gyn/surgery consult without ultrasound
  - Rupture (ectopic, cyst)
  - Septic (abortion, abscess)
  - Placental (previa, abruptio)

3. Complete history and physical examination, and perform pelvic examination

- **If obvious abortion:** Consult obstetrician and consider ultrasound
  - Abortion (incomplete, septic)

- **If late pregnancy:** Forego pelvic exam
  Check for fetal heart tones
  Consider ultrasound followed by ob/gyn consultation
  - Placenta previa or abruptio
  - Premature labor contractions

4. Laboratory diagnostic workup (pregnancy test, CBC, UA/micro)

- **If pregnant:** Consider ultrasound followed by ob/gyn consultation
  - R/I viable intrauterine gestation
  - R/O ectopic pregnancy, abortion, placental problems
  - R/O free intraperitoneal fluid, abscess formation

- **If not pregnant:** Consider ultrasound and ob/gyn/surgery consultation
  - R/O gynecologic surgical problems
  - Ovarian cyst rupture, hemorrhage
  - Tubo-ovarian abscess rupture
  - Adnexal or fibroid torsion
  - Uterine perforation

  - Consider nonsurgical gynecologic problems
  - PID, pelvic adhesions, endometriosis, neoplasm, menstrual

  - R/O general surgery problems
  - Appendicitis and complications
  - Other, GI, GU, vascular, orthopedic surgery problems

  - Consider nonsurgical nongynecologic problems
  - Systemic illnesses

Clinical Algorithms

FIGURE 3-135 Evaluation and management of reproductive-age women with acute pelvic pain. *CBC,* Complete blood count; *GI,* gastrointestinal; *GU,* genitourinary; *Hct,* hematocrit; *PID,* pelvic inflammatory disease; *UA/micro,* urinalysis with microscopy. (From Marx JA [ed]: *Rosen's emergency medicine,* ed 6, St Louis, 2006, Mosby.)

ICD-9CM # 356.9 Peripheral nerve neuropathy
355.10 Lower extremity neuropathy
354.11 Upper extremity neuropathy

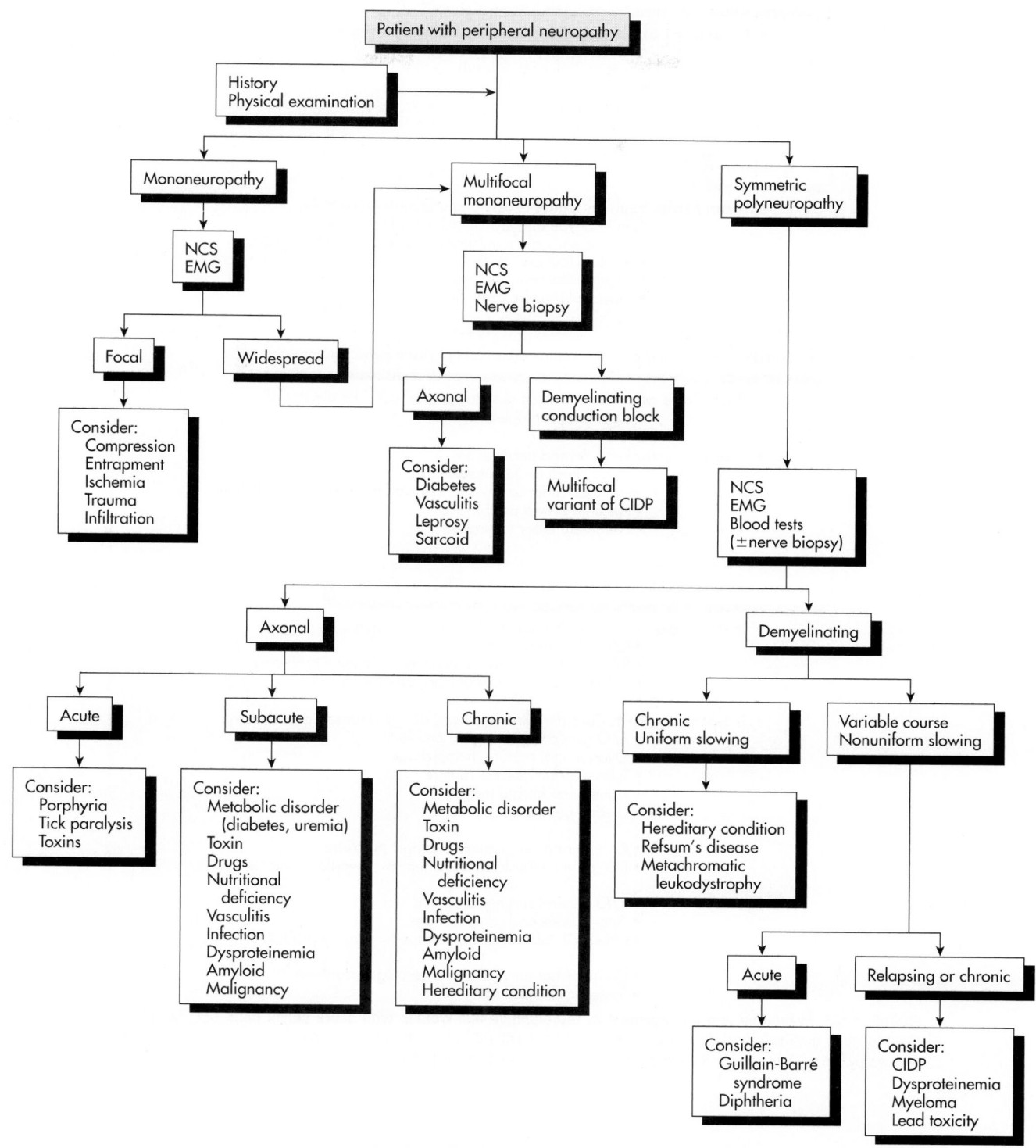

FIGURE 3-137 Approach to the patient with peripheral neuropathy. *CIDP,* Chronic inflammatory demyelinating polyradiculopathy; *EMG,* electromyogram; *NCS,* nerve conduction studies. (From Greene HL, Johnson WP, Lemcke DL: *Decision making in medicine,* ed 2, St Louis, 1988, Mosby.)

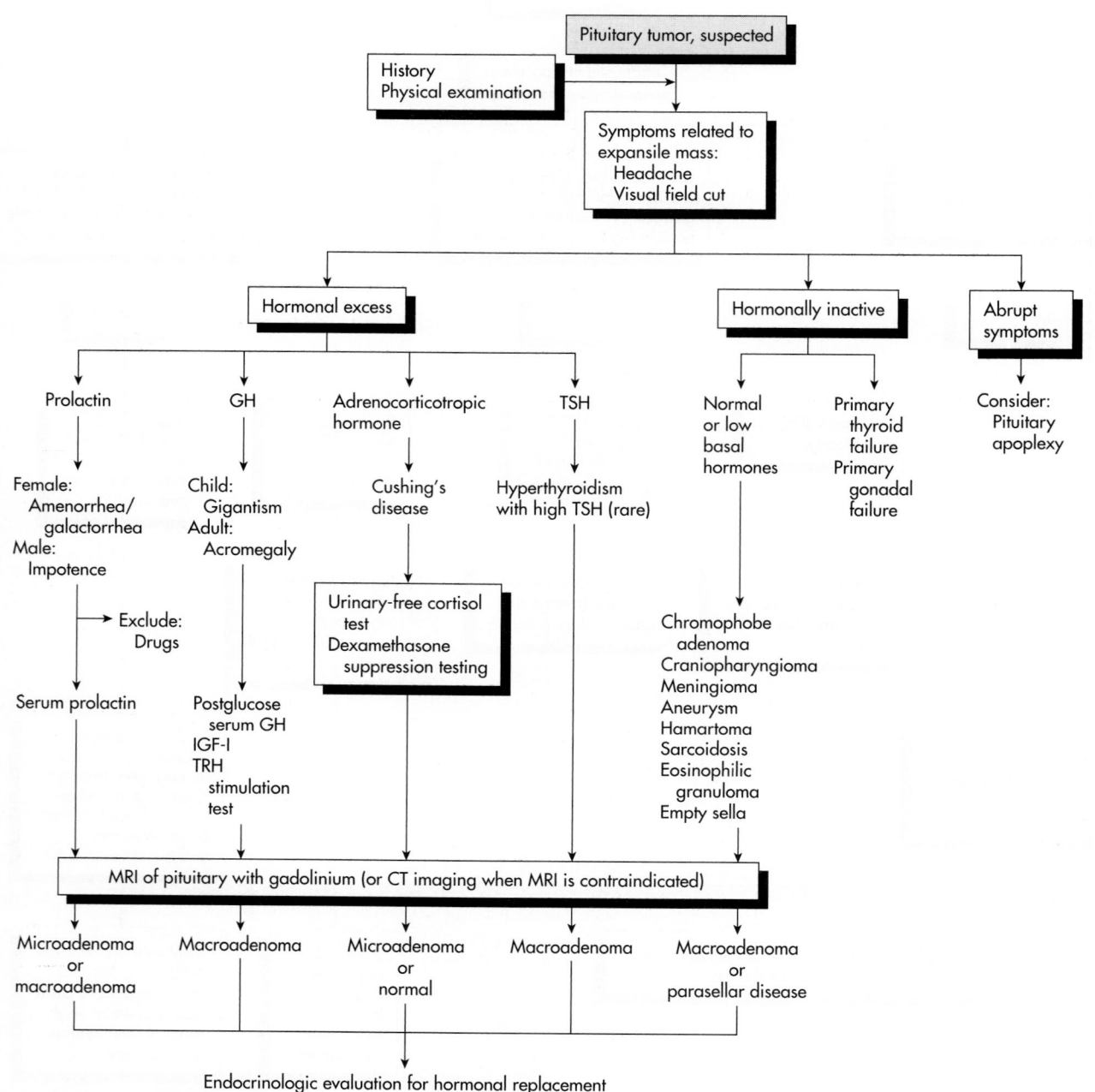

FIGURE 3-139 Evaluation of suspected pituitary tumor. *CT,* Computed tomography; *GH,* growth hormone; *IGF-I,* one of the insulin-like growth factors; *MRI,* magnetic resonance imaging; *TRH,* thyrotropin-releasing hormone; *TSH,* thyroid-stimulating hormone. (From Greene HL, Johnson WP, Lemcke DL: *Decision making in medicine,* ed 2, St Louis, 1998, Mosby.)

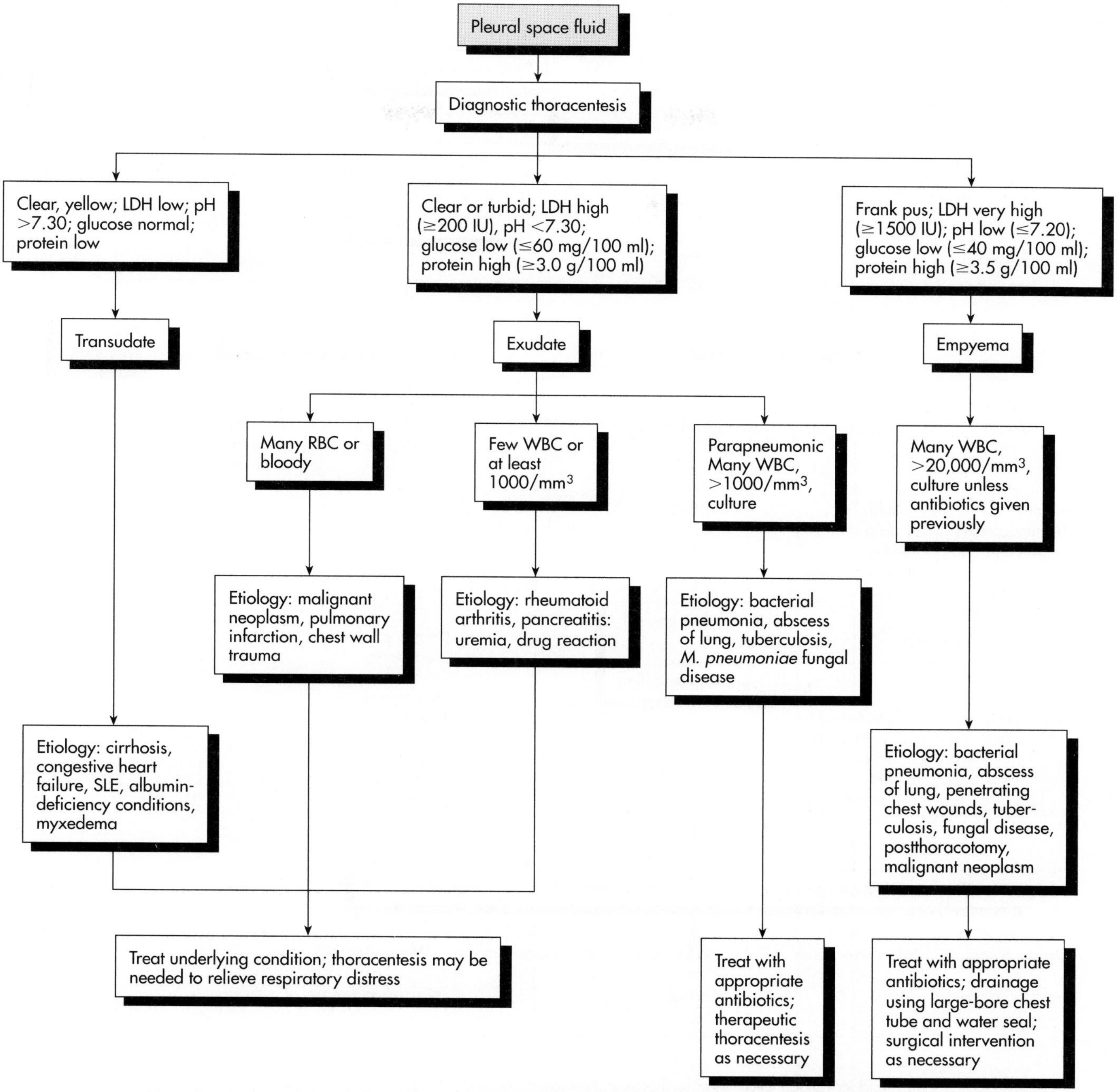

FIGURE 3-141 Evaluation, common etiologies, and management of pleural effusion and empyema. *LDH,* Lactate dehydrogenase; *RBC,* red blood cells; *SLE,* systemic lupus erythematosus; *WBC,* white blood cells. (From Kassirer J [ed]: *Current therapy in adult medicine,* ed 4, St Louis, 1998, Mosby.)

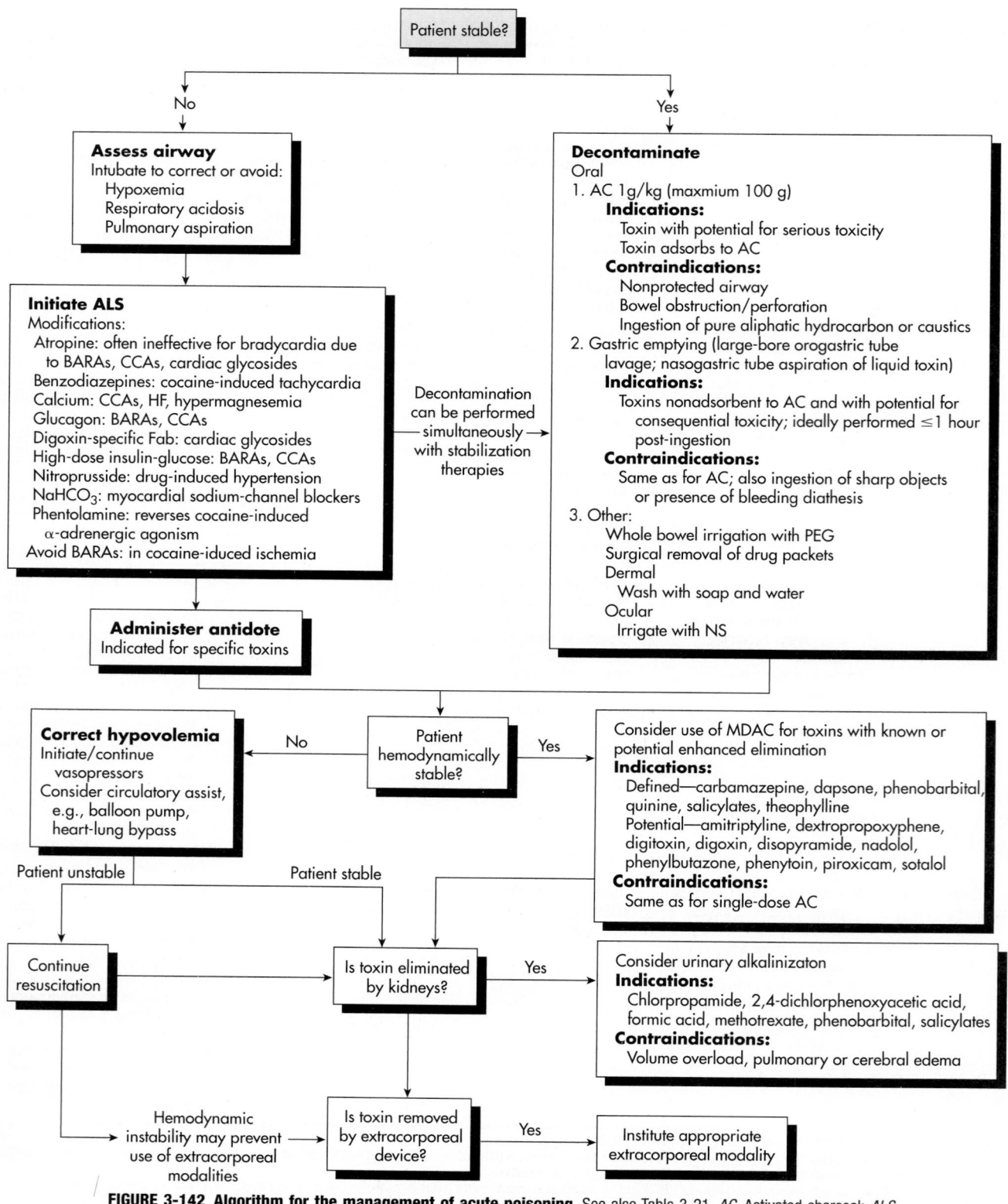

FIGURE 3-142 Algorithm for the management of acute poisoning. See also Table 3-21. *AC,* Activated charcoal; *ALS,* advanced life support; *BARAs,* β-adrenergic receptor antagonists; *CCAs,* L-type calcium-channel antagonists; *HF,* hydrofluoric acid; *MDAC,* multidose activated charcoal; *NS,* 0.9% saline solution; *PEG,* nonabsorbable polyethylene glycol solution. (From Goldman L, Schafer AI: *Goldman's Cecil medicine,* ed 24, Philadelphia, 2012, Saunders.)

Clinical
Algorithms

III

TABLE 3-21 Pathophysiology, Clinical Effects, and Management of Specific Drugs and Toxicants

Drug or Toxicant	Pathophysiology	Clinical Effects	Laboratory	Specific Therapy
Acetaminophen	NAPQI (toxic metabolite) binds hepatic and renal tubular cells; acetaminophen itself induces transient decrease in functional factor VII	Initial: nausea, vomiting, coma, lactic acidosis in severe cases Days 1-3: elevated INR, aminotransferase, and bilirubin levels; RUQ tenderness; increased creatinine level in severe cases Days 4-14: gradual recovery or continued increase in INR and creatinine, lactic acidosis, coma, cerebral edema, death	Potentially toxic level ≥150 μg/ml 4 hr after ingestion* INR may be transiently elevated in first 24 hr because of decrease in functional factor VII; further increases indicate hepatic necrosis; elevated aminotransferase and bilirubin levels not predictive of hepatic failure Creatinine elevated in severe cases	NAC can increase INR but not aPTT†
Amphetamines	Increased release of presynaptic norepinephrine and dopamine Increased seratonin release (especially MDMA, PMA, DOB, other synthetic amphetamines)	Mild: euphoria, decreased appetite, repetitive behavior Moderate: vomiting, agitation, hypertension, tachycardia, mydriasis, bruxism, diaphoresis Severe: hypertension or hypotension, arrhythmias, hyperthermia, seizures, coma, hepatotoxicity, rhabdomyolysis, DIC, hyponatremia (SIADH), renal failure, cerebral infarction or hemorrhage	Not helpful; many false-positives and false-negatives on screening tests	IV crystalloids External cooling Benzodiazepines or barbiturates to control agitation or seizures Benzodiazepines or nitroprusside for hypertension See SSRIs/SRIs for features and treatment of serotonin syndrome
β-Adrenergic receptor antagonists	Blocks catecholamines from β-adrenergic receptors α- and β-adrenergic receptor antagonism: carvedilol, labetalol Delayed rectifier potassium-channel blockade: sotalol	Bradyarrhythmias, decreased myocardial contractility, hypotension, respiratory depression, decreased consciousness with seizures or coma (lipophilic agents, e.g., propranolol), prolonged QT interval (sotalol)	ECG No specific tests	IV glucagon, 3.5-5 mg over 2-min period; if no increase in BP or HR, can repeat up to 10 mg; if effective, immediately start continuous infusion at 2-10 mg/hr; if still unstable, options include (1) regular insulin, 1 U/kg by IV bolus, followed by 1 U/kg/hr, plus dextrose to maintain euglycemia; (2) norepinephrine or dobutamine infusion titrated to desirable BP and HR; (3) IV milrinone, 50 μg/kg over 10-min period, then 0.375-0.75 μg/kg/min based on hemodynamic status‡ Electrical pacing and IABP in refractory cases
L-type calcium-channel antagonists	Blocks L-type voltage-sensitive calcium channels, thereby decreasing calcium entry into myocardial and vascular smooth muscle cells Decreases pancreatic insulin release and increases insulin resistance	Bradyarrhythmias (verapamil, diltiazem), hypotension, hyperglycemia	ECG No specific tests	IV 10% calcium chloride, 10-20 mg/kg (0.1-0.2 ml/kg); can repeat once; if BP improves, continuous infusion at 0.2-0.5 ml/kg/hr (20-50 mg/kg/hr) Ionized Ca²⁺ levels should not exceed 2× normal (severe cases will be refractory to calcium therapy) Glucagon, high-dose insulin and dextrose, catecholamines, and milrinone (as for β-adrenergic antagonists)

From Goldman L, Schafer AI: *Goldman's Cecil medicine,* ed 24, Philadelphia, 2012, Saunders.

*A nomogram to evaluate the potential toxicity of levels drawn more than 4 hours after ingestion is provided in Fig. 3-3, from Rumack BH, Matthew H: Acetaminophen poisoning and toxicity, *Pediatrics* 1975(55):871-876. The nomogram is valid only for levels drawn after a single acute ingestion.

†NAC can be discontinued in patients with uncomplicated disease after a loading dose plus six maintenance doses if hepatic aminotransferase levels are normal and acetaminophen is not detected; otherwise, the full regimen should be administered.

‡Adjust infusion for reduced renal function.

TABLE 3-21   Pathophysiology, Clinical Effects, and Management of Specific Drugs and Toxicants—cont'd

Drug or Toxicant	Pathophysiology	Clinical Effects	Laboratory	Specific Therapy

Cardiac glycosides, including digoxin, bufadienolides (toxic toad venom), or cardenolides (e.g., oleander, lily of the valley, dogbane)	Inhibits Na^+,K^+-ATPase
	Decreased CNS sympathetic output
	Decreased baroreceptor sensitivity
	Increased vagal acetylcholine discharge
		Bradyarrhythmias, including second- and third-degree AV block and asystole
		Ventricular ectopy, tachycardia, fibrillation
		Junctional tachycardia, paroxysmal atrial tachycardia with block
		Weakness, visual disturbances, nausea, vomiting
			Serum digoxin level
			Serum potassium (hyperkalemia occurs in acute poisoning; hypokalemia may be present in chronic poisoning), magnesium, and creatinine levels
				Correct hypokalemia and hypomagnesemia; do not give calcium
				Digoxin-specific antibody fragments (Fab) indicated if patient has hemodynamically significant arrhythmias, serum potassium $\geq$5 mg/L, Mobitz II or third-degree AV block, ingestion of bufadienolide- or cardenolide-containing agents, or renal insufficiency
				Empirical dose
				  Chronic: 2-5 vials
				  Acute: 10-20 vials
				Calculated dose
				  Chronic: number of vials = 2 × serum digoxin level (ng/ml) × 5.6 × weight (kg)/1000
				  Acute: number of vials = 2 × oral digoxin dose (mg) × 0.8

Cyclic antidepressants	Myocardial sodium- and potassium-channel blockade Blockade of α-adrenergic and cholinergic muscarinic receptors Inhibition of norepinephrine re-uptake	Decreased level of consciousness (can develop rapidly), myoclonus, seizures, coma Anticholinergic toxidrome Sinus tachycardia, ventricular conduction delays, ventricular arrhythmias, asystole Hypotension	Serum levels not helpful in management	Intermittent IV boluses of $NaHCO_3$ (1 mEq/kg) to maintain arterial pH at 7.5 because acidemia can worsen cardiovascular complications Intubation and neuroparalytic drugs may be useful to ameliorate acidemia from muscular hyperactivity while seizures are being treated Contraindicated drugs: types IA and IC antiarrhythmic agents; physostigmine, flumazenil
Ethylene glycol, methanol (e.g., antifreeze, window cleaners, camping stove fuels)	Ethylene glycol: toxic metabolites produce cytotoxicity in CNS, kidneys, lungs, heart, liver, muscles; metabolic acidosis is due to glycolate accumulation; oxalate complexes with calcium, so hypocalcemia can develop Methanol: metabolized to formic acid, which is responsible for metabolic acidosis and inhibition of cytochrome aa_3; target organs include retina, optic nerve, CNS	Ethylene glycol: CNS depression, cerebral edema, seizures, anion gap metabolic acidosis, renal failure with acute tubular necrosis, pulmonary edema, myositis Methanol: nausea, vomiting; cerebral edema, hemorrhage, infarcts; necrosis of thalamus and putamen; anion gap metabolic acidosis; visual disturbances, papilledema, hyperemic optic disc, nonreactive pupils	Serum ethylene glycol and methanol levels; levels may be low or undetectable if significant metabolism has occurred Ethylene glycol: serum calcium, creatinine, BUN levels; examine urine for calcium oxalate crystals; false hyperlactatemia occurs with certain analyzers using L-lactate oxidase, which cross-reacts with glycolic and glyoxylic acids	For both: fomepizole (which inhibits alcohol dehydrogenase and blocks formation of toxic metabolites), 15 mg/kg IV loading dose, then 10 mg/kg IV for 4 doses during the next 48 hr, then 15 mg/kg for subsequent doses; interval dosing is q12h (q4h during hemodialysis, with dosing interval adjustments at start and finish); continue until ethylene glycol or methanol is no longer detectable Use of ethanol is no longer recommended Hemodialysis: initiate if level is $\geq$50 mg/dl or metabolic acidosis with end-organ toxicity; continue until acidosis resolves and serum level of ethylene glycol or methanol is undetectable Monitor for cerebral edema with possible herniation Ethylene glycol: IV calcium for symptomatic hypocalcemia Methanol: folinic acid, 50 mg IV q4h until methanol not detectable and acidosis cleared
γ-Hydroxybutyrate (GHB) and its precursors (γ-butyrolactone and 1,4-butanediol [1,4-BD])	Agonist effect on CNS GHB receptors; indirect action with opioid receptors (may increase proenkephalins); metabolized to GABA, interacts with $GABA_B$ receptors; decreases dopamine release	CNS: rapid loss of consciousness, with recovery typical within 2-4 hr; myoclonus (possible seizures) Respiratory depression; bradycardia; nausea, vomiting	No specific tests	Supportive care, including respiratory support as needed Withdrawal resembles sedative-hypnotic withdrawal and can be treated with benzodiazepines or pentobarbital

TABLE 3-21 Pathophysiology, Clinical Effects, and Management of Specific Drugs and Toxicants—cont'd

Drug or Toxicant	Pathophysiology	Clinical Effects	Laboratory	Specific Therapy
Lithium	Decreases brain inositol; alters CNS serotonin, dopamine, and norepinephrine; inhibits adenylate cyclases, including those that mediate vasopressin-induced renal concentration and thyroid function	Chronic toxicity usually more severe than acute toxicity: tremor, hyperreflexia, drowsiness, incoordination, clonus, confusion, ataxia; in severe cases, seizures, coma, death; recovery may take weeks, and CNS deficits may persist Sinus node dysfunction, QT prolongation, T wave abnormalities, U waves Nephrogenic diabetes insipidus, hypothyroidism, hyperthyroidism, hypercalcemia, pseudotumor cerebri Acute toxicity: nausea, vomiting, diarrhea, and milder neurologic findings	Peak serum levels: Normal dose 2-3 hr; up to 5 hr for sustained-release lithium Acute overdose: peak may be delayed ≥4-12 hr	Replenish intravascular volume, maintain urinary output at 1-2 ml/kg/hr Consider GI decontamination with oral polyethylene glycol electrolyte solution within 1-2 hr after acute overdose of sustained-release drug Hemodialysis§ in patients with altered mental status, ataxia, seizures, or coma or in patients with mild symptoms in the setting of acute overdose or renal insufficiency Ineffective or contraindicated therapies include oral activated charcoal, diuretics, and aminophylline
Opioids (e.g., heroin, morphine, oxycodone, fentanyl)	Agonist effect at CNS μ, κ, and δ opioid receptors; result is cell hyperpolarization and decreased neurotransmitter release	CNS depression, respiratory depression, miosis Dextromethorphan increases CNS serotonin and inhibits NMDA receptors, which causes hallucinations Propoxyphene and its metabolite norpropoxyphene block sodium channels and can cause seizures and wide-complex arrhythmias similar to cyclic antidepressants; $NaHCO_3$ treats arrhythmias Seizure risk with tramadol, meperidine, propoxyphene Rapid, powerful heroin-like effect when sustained-release oxycodone is crushed before ingestion, snorting, or smoking QTc prolongation and torsades de pointes with methadone	Rapid urine drug screens detect morphine and codeine but may not detect semisynthetic and synthetic opioids; some interferents/irrelevants	IV naloxone, 0.4-2 mg; can repeat up to 10 mg if no response Continuous infusion for recurrent symptoms or sustained-release opioid ingestion; give 50% of dose that produces desired effect 15 min after initial effect is obtained, then infuse two thirds of this dose every hr; infusion rate can be increased or decreased to maintain normal respiration and avoid withdrawal symptoms Contraindicated therapies: nalmefene and naltrexone should not be used for acute opioid reversal
Organophosphorus compounds and carbamates (e.g., diazinon, mevinphos, fenthion, aldicarb)	Inhibits acetylcholinesterase, resulting in excessive acetylcholine stimulation of nicotinic and muscarinic receptors in autonomic and somatic motor nervous systems and CNS	Nicotinic-mediated effects: tachycardia, mydriasis, hypertension, delirium, coma, seizures, muscle weakness, fasciculations Muscarinic-mediated effects: salivation, lacrimation, urination, vomiting, defecation, miosis, bronchorrhea, bronchospasm, bradycardia	Serum (butyrylcholinesterase) or RBC (acetylcholinesterase) activity <50% of normal Clinical recovery occurs before serum cholinesterase levels normalize	Atropine, 1-2 mg by initial IV bolus; double the dose every 5 min (2 mg, 4 mg, 8 mg, 16 mg, etc.) until drying of bronchial secretions, adequate oxygenation, pulse >80 bpm, systolic blood pressure >80 mm Hg achieved; continuous infusion at 10%-20% of total stabilizing dose per hr; stop infusion if patient develops any signs or symptoms of anticholinergic toxidrome; restart infusion at lower rate when signs or symptoms abate Pralidoxime‖ chloride 30 mg/kg (maximum 2 g) IV bolus over 30 min, then 8-10 mg/kg/hr (maximum 650 mg/hr) continuous infusion; administer as soon as possible after poisoning; continue 12-24 hr after atropine no longer required and symptoms resolve

§Continue hemodialysis until the serum lithium level is less than 1 mEq/L. Recheck the level 8 hr after dialysis, and restart hemodialysis if the level is higher than 1 mEq/L. Repeat this cycle until the serum lithium level remains lower than 1 mEq/L.

‖A double-blind, randomized, placebo-controlled trial of pralidoxime in acute organophosphorus poisoning found no significant difference in mortality rates or need for intubation.

TABLE 3-21 Pathophysiology, Clinical Effects, and Management of Specific Drugs and Toxicants—cont'd

Drug or Toxicant	Pathophysiology	Clinical Effects	Laboratory	Specific Therapy
Salicylates	Inhibits cyclooxygenase; decreases formation of prostaglandins and thromboxane A_2; stimulates CNS medullary respiratory receptor and chemoreceptor trigger zone; impairs platelet function; disrupts carbohydrate metabolism; uncouples oxidative phosphorylation; increases vascular permeability	Acute toxicity Mild: nausea, vomiting, diaphoresis, tinnitus, decreased hearing, hyperpnea, tachypnea Moderate–severe: confusion, delirium, coma, seizures, hyperthermia, ALI; death can occur within hours of overdose Chronic toxicity: same as acute, but may not have diaphoresis or vomiting Consider diagnosis in patients with new-onset confusion, anion gap metabolic acidosis, or ALI	Serum salicylate level: toxic ≥30 mg/dl; level ≥100 mg/dL indicates life-threatening toxicity with possible sudden, rapid clinical deterioration; in chronic toxicity, levels may be minimally elevated (>30 mg/dl), and clinical evaluation is more reliable for gauging degree of toxicity Arterial blood gases: respiratory alkalosis with metabolic acidosis Anion gap metabolic acidosis Prolonged PT and PTT, ketonuria, ketonemia	Multidose activated charcoal q2-3h in acute overdose with progressive symptoms or rising salicylate level
SSRIs/SRIs	Inhibits re-uptake of serotonin SRIs have additional effects (e.g., duloxetine inhibits norepinephrine re-uptake, nefazodone inhibits serotonergic 5-HT2 receptors, trazodone inhibits peripheral α-adrenergic receptors, venlafaxine inhibits norepinephrine and dopamine re-uptake)	Vomiting, blurred vision, CNS depression, tachycardia Seizures and coma rare Torsades de pointes reported with citalopram Serotonin syndrome: clonus, agitation, tremor, diaphoresis, hyperreflexia; hyperthermia and hypertonicity in severe cases	No specific tests If serotonin syndrome suspected: electrolytes, BUN, glucose, liver enzymes, coagulation panel, blood gases, chest radiograph	Respiratory support as needed Benzodiazepines for agitation or seizures Serotonin syndrome: consider cyproheptadine, 12 mg PO initial dose then 2 mg PO q2h (to a maximum of 32 mg/day) until symptoms resolve Critical care therapies for hyperthermia, rhabdomyolysis, DIC, ARDS, renal and hepatic dysfunction, torsades de pointes

ALI, Acute lung injury; *aPTT,* activated partial thromboplastin time; *ARDS,* acute respiratory distress syndrome; *AV,* atrioventricular; *BP,* blood pressure; *bpm,* beats per minute; *BUN,* blood urea nitrogen; *CNS,* central nervous system; *DIC,* disseminated intravascular coagulation; *DOB,* 4-bromo-2,5-dimethoxyamphetamine; *ECG,* electrocardiogram; *GABA,* γ-aminobutyric acid; *GI,* gastrointestinal; *HR,* heart rate; *IABP,* intra-aortic balloon counterpulsation; *INR,* international normalized ratio; *IV,* intravenous; *MDMA,* 3,4-methylenedioxymethamphetamine; *Na^1,K^1-ATPase,* sodium, potassium adenosine triphosphatase; *NAC,* N-acetylcysteine; *NAPQI,* N-acetyl-p-benzoquinone imine; *NMDA,* N-methyl-D-aspartate; *PMA,* paramethoxyamphetamine; *PT,* prothrombin time; *PTT,* partial thromboplastin time; *RBC,* red blood cell; *RUQ,* upper right quadrant (abdomen); *SIADH,* syndrome of inappropriate antidiuretic secretion; *SRI,* serotonin re-uptake inhibitor; *SSRI,* selective serotonin re-uptake inhibitor.

Clinical
Algorithms

III

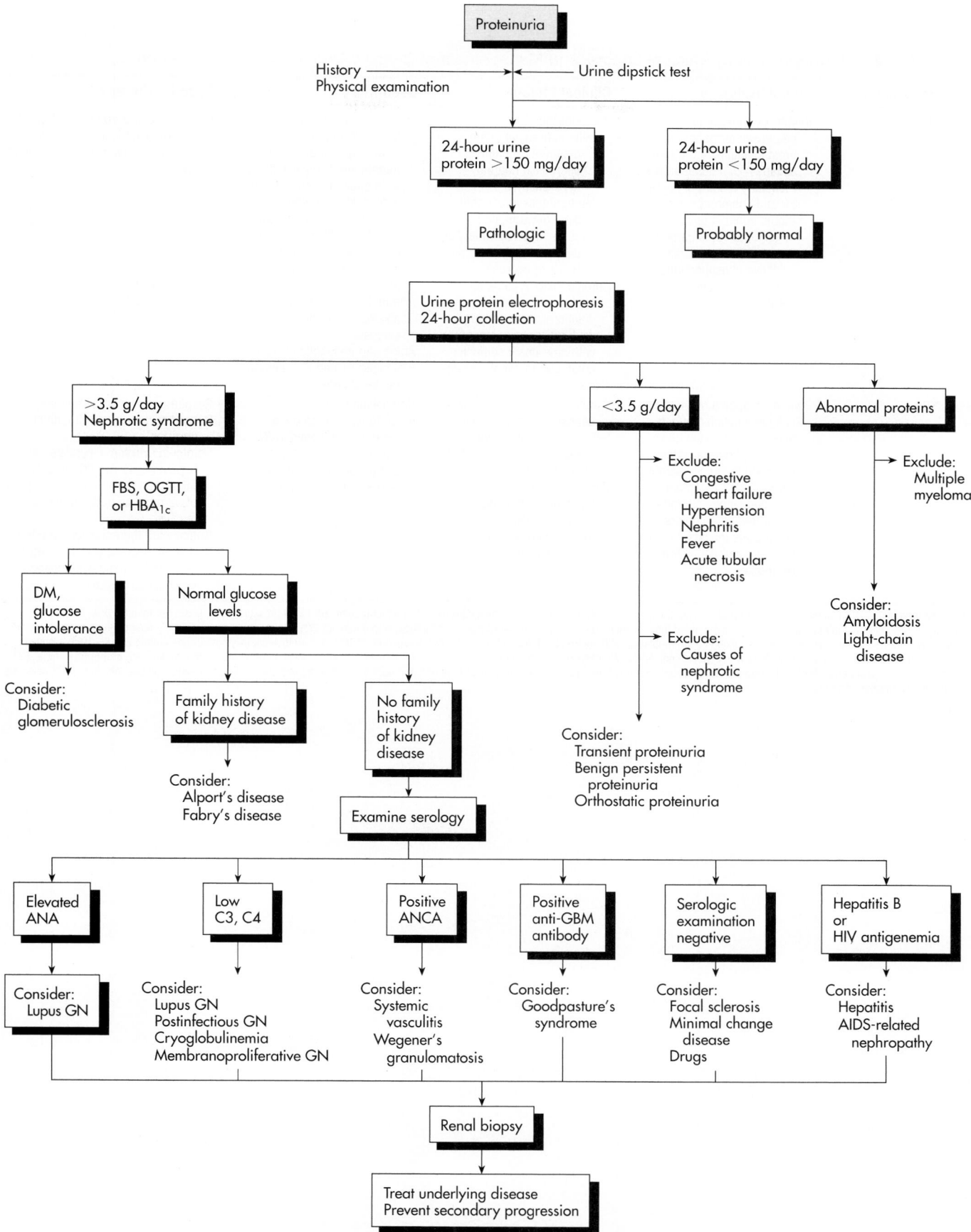

FIGURE 3-144 Proteinuria. *AIDS,* Acquired immunodeficiency syndrome; *ANA,* antinuclear antibody; *ANCA,* antineutrophil cytoplasmic autoantibody; *anti-GBM,* anti-glomerular basement membrane; *FBS,* fasting blood sugar; *GN,* glomerulonephritis; *OGTT,* oral glucose tolerance test. (Modified from Greene HL, Johnson WP, Lemcke DL [eds]: *Decision making in medicine,* ed 2, St Louis, 1998, Mosby.)

PRURITUS, GENERALIZED

ICD-9CM # 698.9 Pruritus NOS

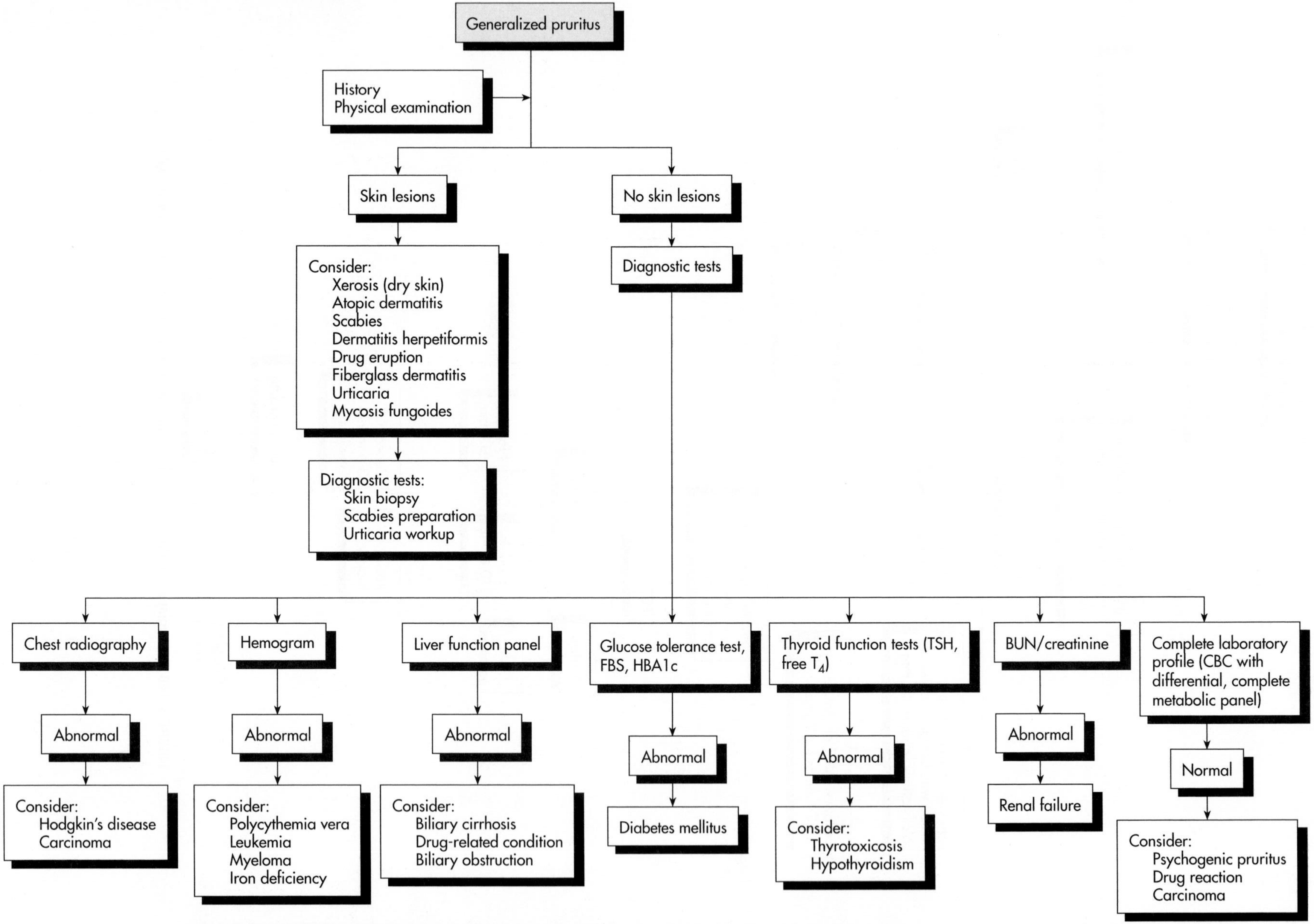

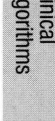

FIGURE 3-145 Evaluation of generalized pruritus. *BUN,* Blood urea nitrogen; *CBC,* complete blood count; *FBS,* fasting blood sugar; *HBA1c,* hemoglobin A1c; *T₄,* thyroxine; *TSH,* thyroid-stimulating hormone. (From Greene HL, Johnson WP, Lemcke DL [eds]: *Decision making in medicine,* ed 2, St Louis, 1998, Mosby.)

Generalized pruritus

History
Physical examination

Skin lesions → Consider:
Xerosis (dry skin)
Atopic dermatitis
Scabies
Dermatitis herpetiformis
Drug eruption
Fiberglass dermatitis
Urticaria
Mycosis fungoides
→ Diagnostic tests:
Skin biopsy
Scabies preparation
Urticaria workup

No skin lesions → Diagnostic tests

Chest radiography → Abnormal → Consider:
Hodgkin's disease
Carcinoma

Hemogram → Abnormal → Consider:
Polycythemia vera
Leukemia
Myeloma
Iron deficiency

Liver function panel → Abnormal → Consider:
Biliary cirrhosis
Drug-related condition
Biliary obstruction

Glucose tolerance test, FBS, HBA1c → Abnormal → Diabetes mellitus

Thyroid function tests (TSH, free T₄) → Abnormal → Consider:
Thyrotoxicosis
Hypothyroidism

BUN/creatinine → Abnormal → Renal failure

Complete laboratory profile (CBC with differential, complete metabolic panel) → Normal → Consider:
Psychogenic pruritus
Drug reaction
Carcinoma

Clinical Algorithms

III

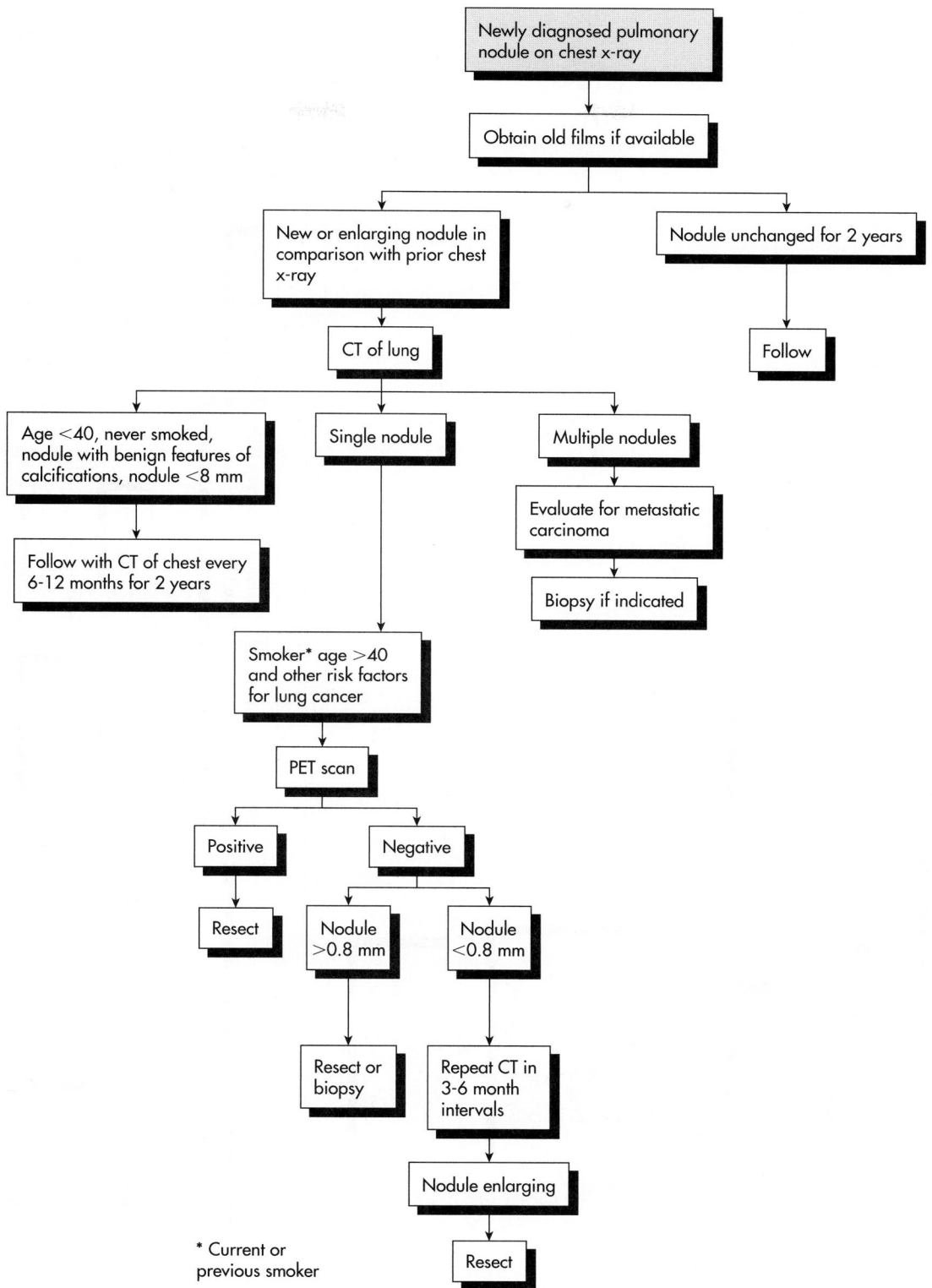

FIGURE 3-148 Pulmonary nodule. *CT,* Computed tomography; *PET,* positron emission tomography.

FIGURE 3-149 Differential diagnosis of purpura. (From Bologna JL, Jorizzo JL, Rapini RP: *Dermatology,* St Louis, 2003, Mosby.)

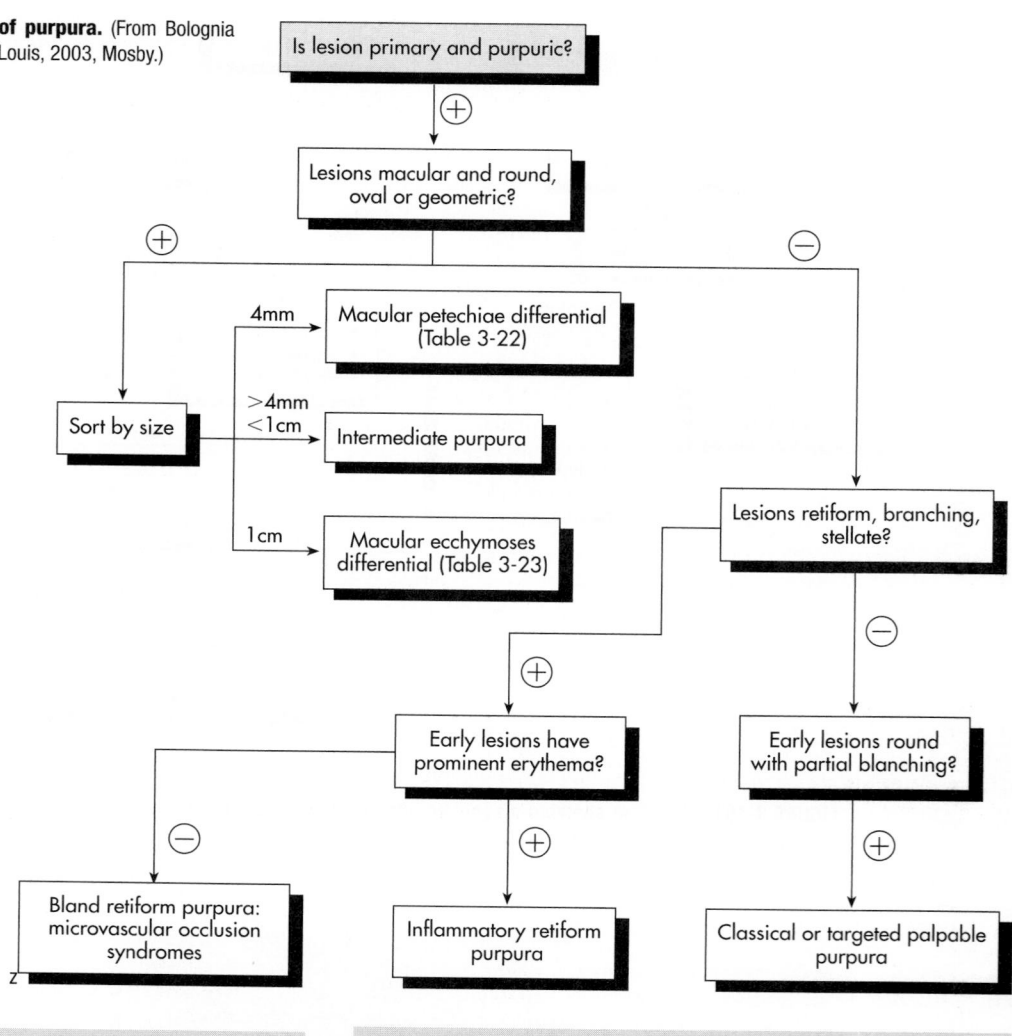

TABLE 3-22 Differential Diagnosis of Petechial Hemorrhage—Non-Palpable, Non-Retiform and ≤4 mm in Diameter

Pathophysiology: Hemostatically Relevant Thrombocytopenia (<550,000/mm³) **

Major etiologies*
1. Idiopathic thrombocytopenic purpura
2. Thrombotic thrombocytopenic purpura
3. Disseminated intravascular coagulation
4. Other acquired thrombocytopenias, including drug-related
   a. Peripheral destruction (e.g., quinine, quinidine)
   b. Decreased production, idiosyncratic or dose-related (e.g., chemotherapy)
   c. Bone marrow infiltration, fibrosis or failure

Pathophysiology: Abnormal Platelet Function

Major etiologies*
1. Congenital or hereditary platelet function defects
2. Acquired platelet function defects
   a. Aspirin, NSAIDs
   b. Renal insufficiency
   c. Monoclonal gammopathy
3. Thrombocytosis in myeloproliferative disease (often >1,000,000/mm³)

Pathophysiology: Non-Platelet Etiologies

Major etiologies*
1. Spiking elevations of intravascular venous pressure (Valsalva maneuver-like, e.g., repetitive vomiting, childbirth, paroxysmal coughing, seizure)
2. Fixed increased pressure (e.g., stasis, ligatures)
3. Trauma (often linear)
4. Perifollicular (vitamin C deficiency)
5. Mildly inflammatory conditions
   a. Chronic pigmented purpura
   b. Hypergammaglobulinemic purpura of Waldenström

TABLE 3-23 Differential Diagnosis for Macular Purpura and Ecchymoses—Non-Palpable and Non-Retiform

Intermediate Macular Purpura (>4 mm, <1 cm in diameter)

Major etiologies*
1. Hypergammaglobulinemic purpura of Waldenström
2. Infection/inflammation in patients with thrombocytopenia
3. Rarely, minimally inflamed immune complex vasculitis (usually dependent distribution)

Ecchymoses (≥1 cm in diameter)

A. Pathophysiology: procoagulant defect plus minor trauma*
   1. Anticoagulant use
   2. Hepatic insufficiency with poor procoagulant synthesis
   3. Vitamin K deficiency
   4. Disseminated intravascular coagulation (some)
B. Pathophysiology: poor dermal support of vessels plus minor trauma*
   1. Actinic (solar, senile) purpura
   2. Corticosteroid therapy, topical or systemic
   3. Vitamin C deficiency (scurvy)
   4. Systemic amyloidosis (light chain-related, some familial types)
   5. Ehlers-Danlos syndrome (primarily type IV)
C. Pathophysiology: other causes plus minor trauma*
   1. Hypergammaglobulinemic purpura of Waldenström
   2. Platelet function defects, including von Willebrand disease, medications, metabolic diseases
   3. Acquired or congenital thrombocytopenia

*Partial list.
**Most patients do not have petechiae until platelets ≤20,000/mm³.

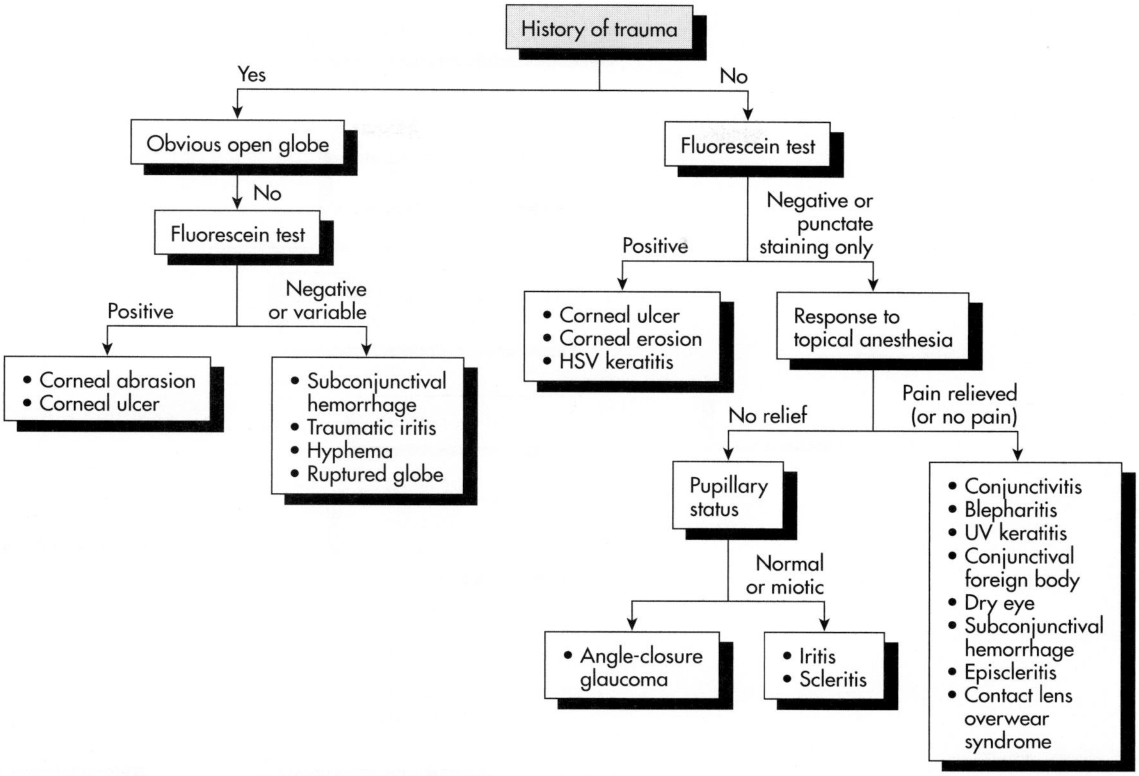

History of trauma

Yes → Obvious open globe

No → Fluorescein test

Obvious open globe — No → **Fluorescein test**

Positive:
- Corneal abrasion
- Corneal ulcer

Negative or variable:
- Subconjunctival hemorrhage
- Traumatic iritis
- Hyphema
- Ruptured globe

Fluorescein test

Positive:
- Corneal ulcer
- Corneal erosion
- HSV keratitis

Negative or punctate staining only → **Response to topical anesthesia**

No relief → **Pupillary status**

Normal or miotic:
- Angle-closure glaucoma
- Iritis
- Scleritis

Pain relieved (or no pain):
- Conjunctivitis
- Blepharitis
- UV keratitis
- Conjunctival foreign body
- Dry eye
- Subconjunctival hemorrhage
- Episcleritis
- Contact lens overwear syndrome

FIGURE 3-151 Algorithm showing diagnostic procedure for the acute red eye. *HSV,* Herpes simplex virus; *UV,* ultraviolet. (From Auerbach PS: *Wilderness medicine,* ed 5, St Louis, 2007, Mosby.)

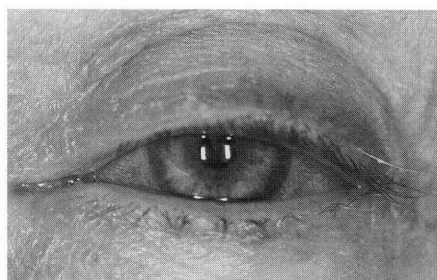

FIGURE 3-152 Contact lens acute red eye. This is often accompanied by pain and photophobia. (From Yanoff M, Duker JS: *Ophthalmology,* ed 2, St Louis, 2004, Mosby.)

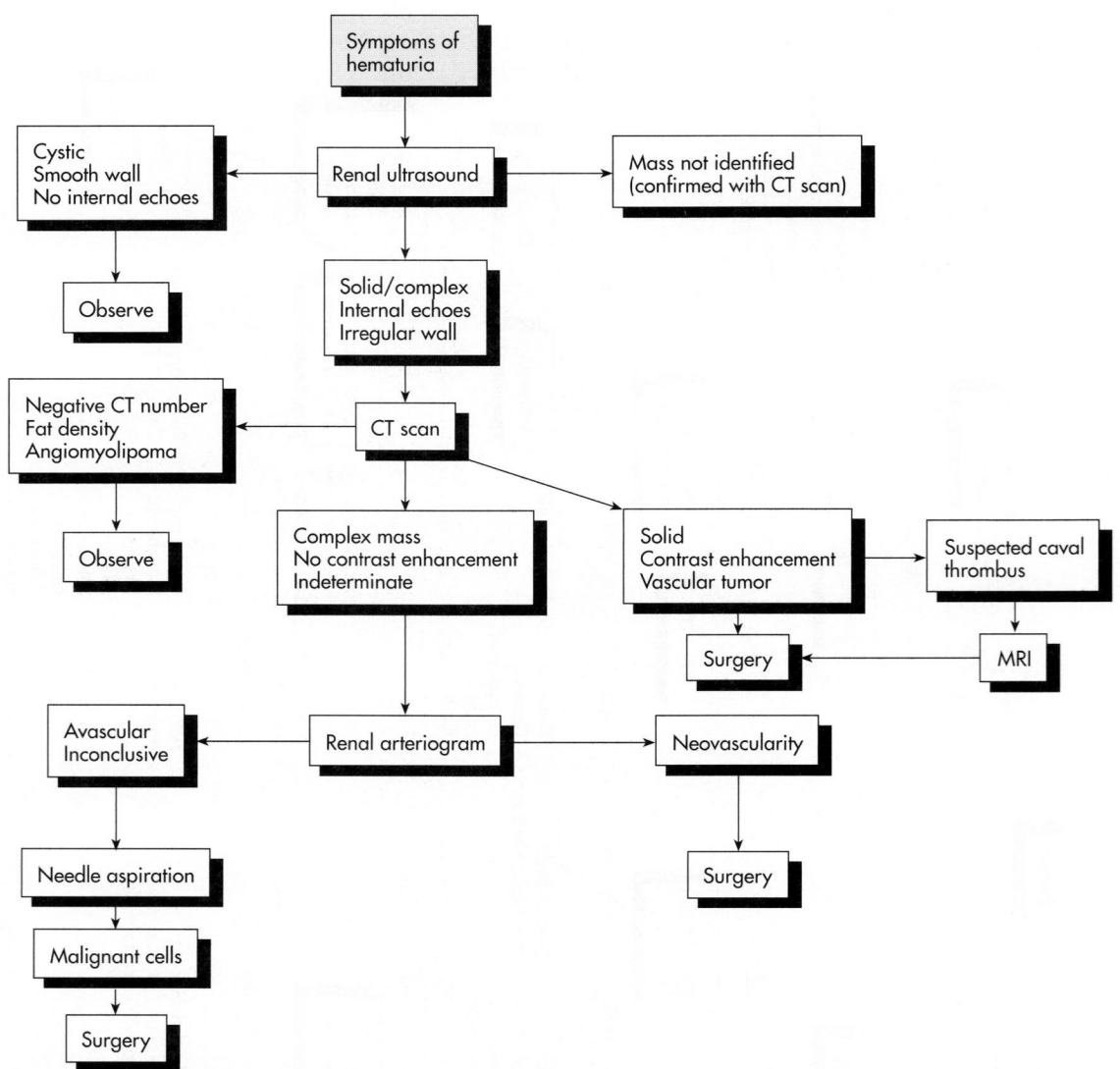

FIGURE 3-154 Evaluation of a patient with a renal mass. *CT,* Computed tomography; *MRI,* magnetic resonance imaging. (Modified from Williams RD: Tumors of the kidney, ureter, and bladder. In Goldman L, Ausiello D [eds]: *Cecil textbook of medicine,* ed 23, Philadelphia, 2008, Saunders.)

RESPIRATORY DISTRESS

ICD-9CM # 786.09 Respiratory distress NOS
518.82 Respiratory distress, acute

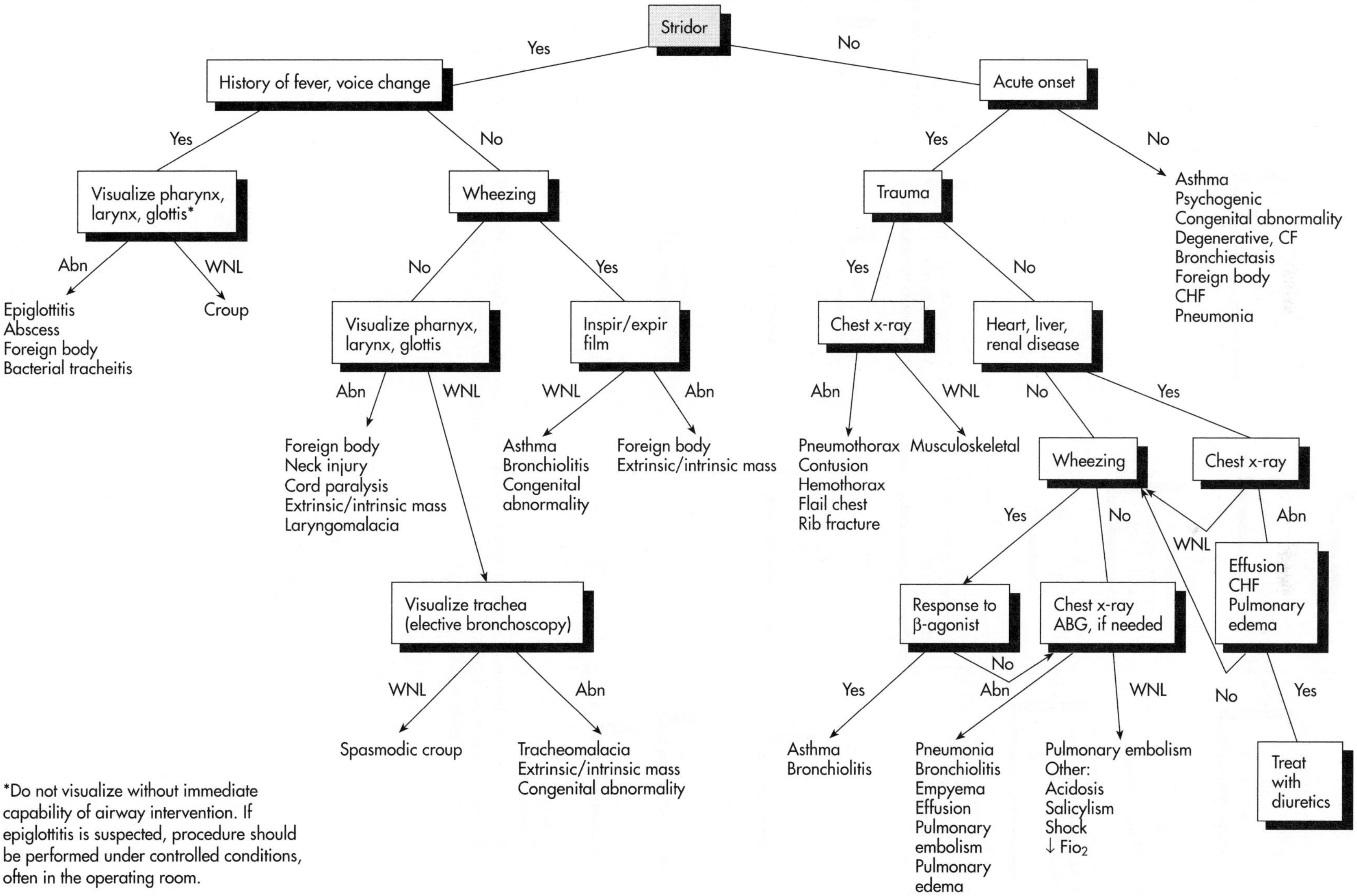

FIGURE 3-155 Respiratory distress in a pediatric patient. *ABG,* Arterial blood gas; *Abn,* abnormal; *CF,* cystic fibrosis; *CHF,* congestive heart failure; *WNL,* within normal limits. (From Barkin RM, Rosen P: *Emergency pediatrics,* St Louis, 1999, Mosby.)

*Do not visualize without immediate capability of airway intervention. If epiglottitis is suspected, procedure should be performed under controlled conditions, often in the operating room.

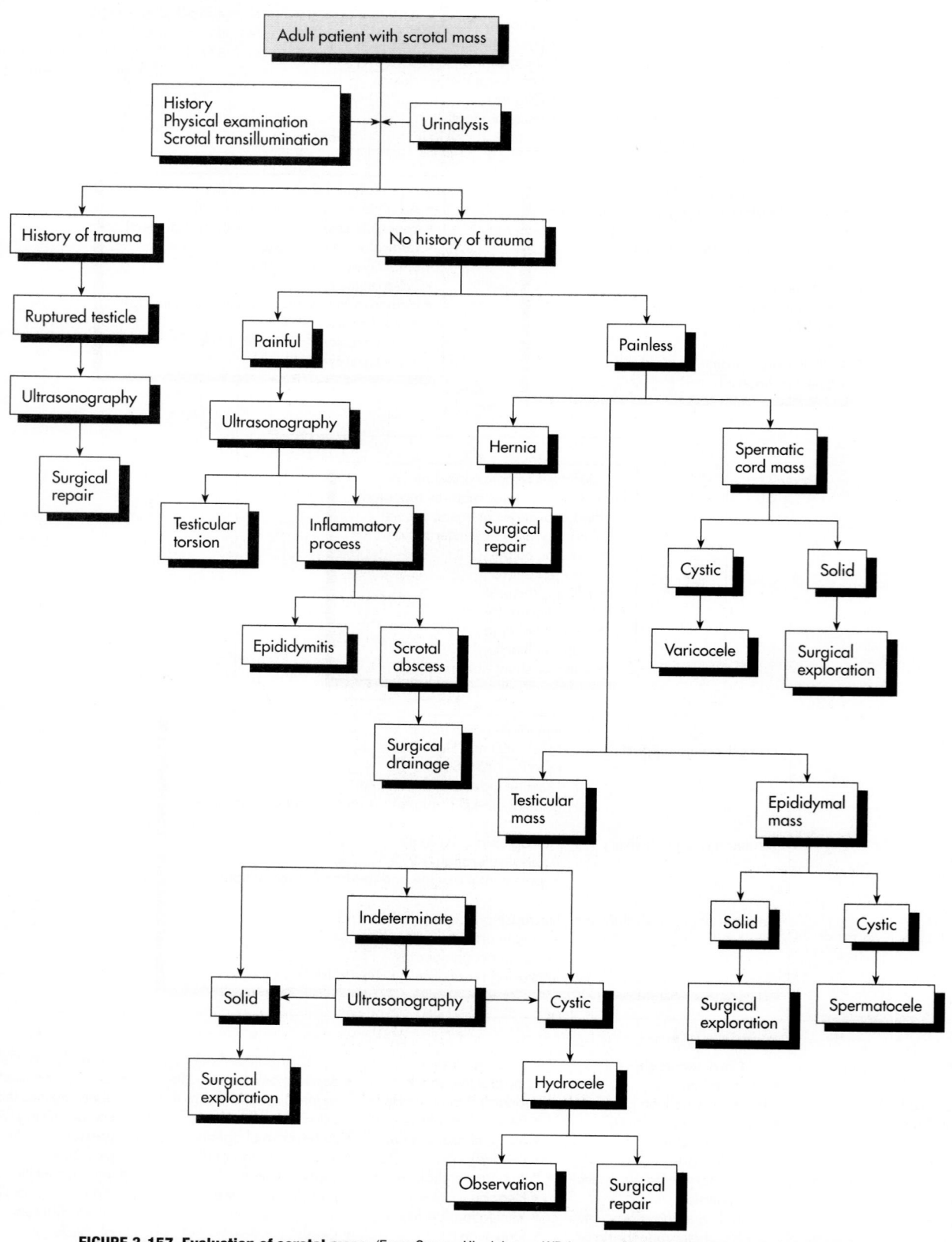

FIGURE 3-157 Evaluation of scrotal mass. (From Greene HL, Johnson WP, Lemcke DL [eds]: *Decision making in medicine,* ed 2, St Louis, 1998, Mosby.)

ICD-9CM # 785.50 Shock NOS
           995.0   Shock anaphylactic
           785.51 Shock cardiogenic
           785.59 Shock septic
           958.4   Shock traumatic
           977.9   Shock due to drug, medicine
                   incorrectly administered

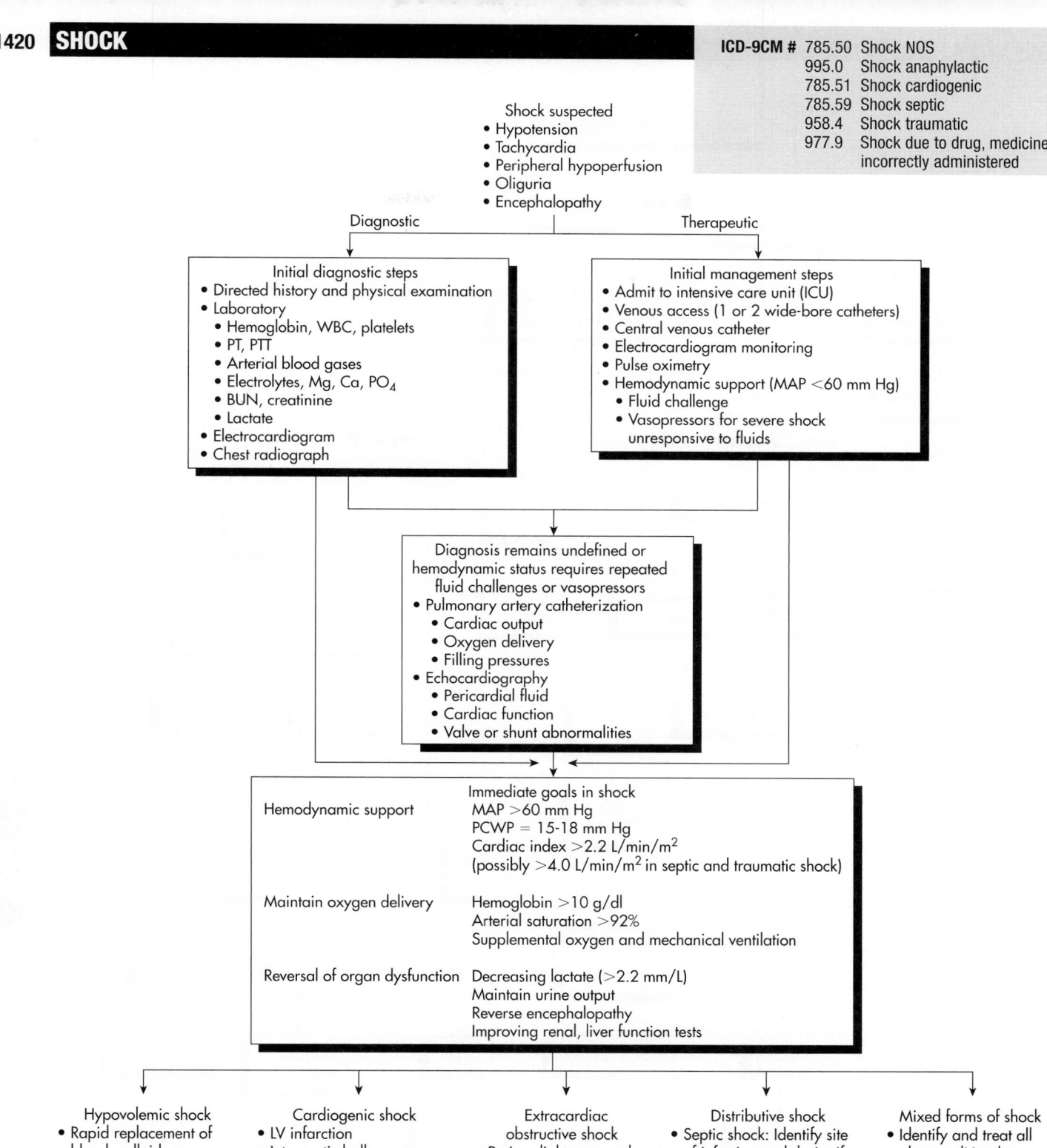

FIGURE 3-163 An approach to the diagnosis and treatment of shock. *BUN,* Blood urea nitrogen; *CT,* computed tomography; *LV,* left ventricular; *MAP,* mean arterial pressure; *MRI,* magnetic resonance imaging; *PA,* pulmonary arterial; *PCWP,* pulmonary capillary wedge pressure; *PT,* prothrombin time; *PTT,* partial thromboplastin time; *RV,* right ventricular; *WBC,* white blood cell count. (From Goldman L, Ausiello D [eds]: *Cecil textbook of medicine,* ed 24, Philadelphia, 2012, Saunders.)

SHOULDER PAIN

ICD-9CM # variable with specific disorder

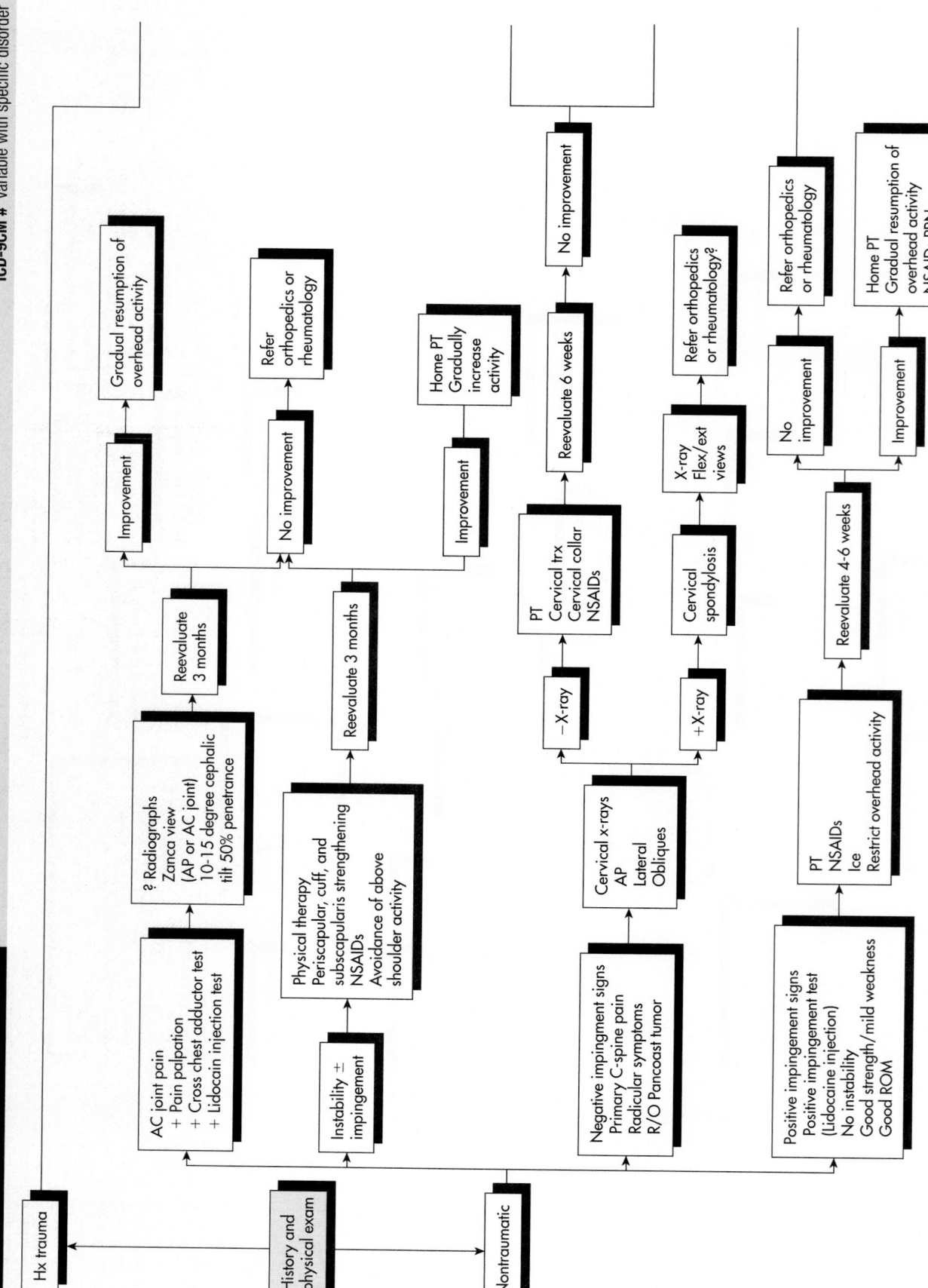

FIGURE 3-165 Algorithmic evaluation of shoulder pain. *AC,* Acromioclavicular; *AP,* anteroposterior; *GH,* glenohumeral; *Hx,* history; *MRI,* magnetic resonance imaging; *NSAIDs,* nonsteroidal anti-inflammatory drugs; *PRN,* as required; *PT,* physical therapy; *R/O,* rule out; *ROM,* range of motion; *Sx,* symptoms; *trx,* traction; *Tx,* therapy. (From Harris ED et al [eds]: *Kelley's textbook of rheumatology,* ed 7, Philadelphia, 2005, Saunders.)

(Continued on next page)

Clinical
Algorithms

III

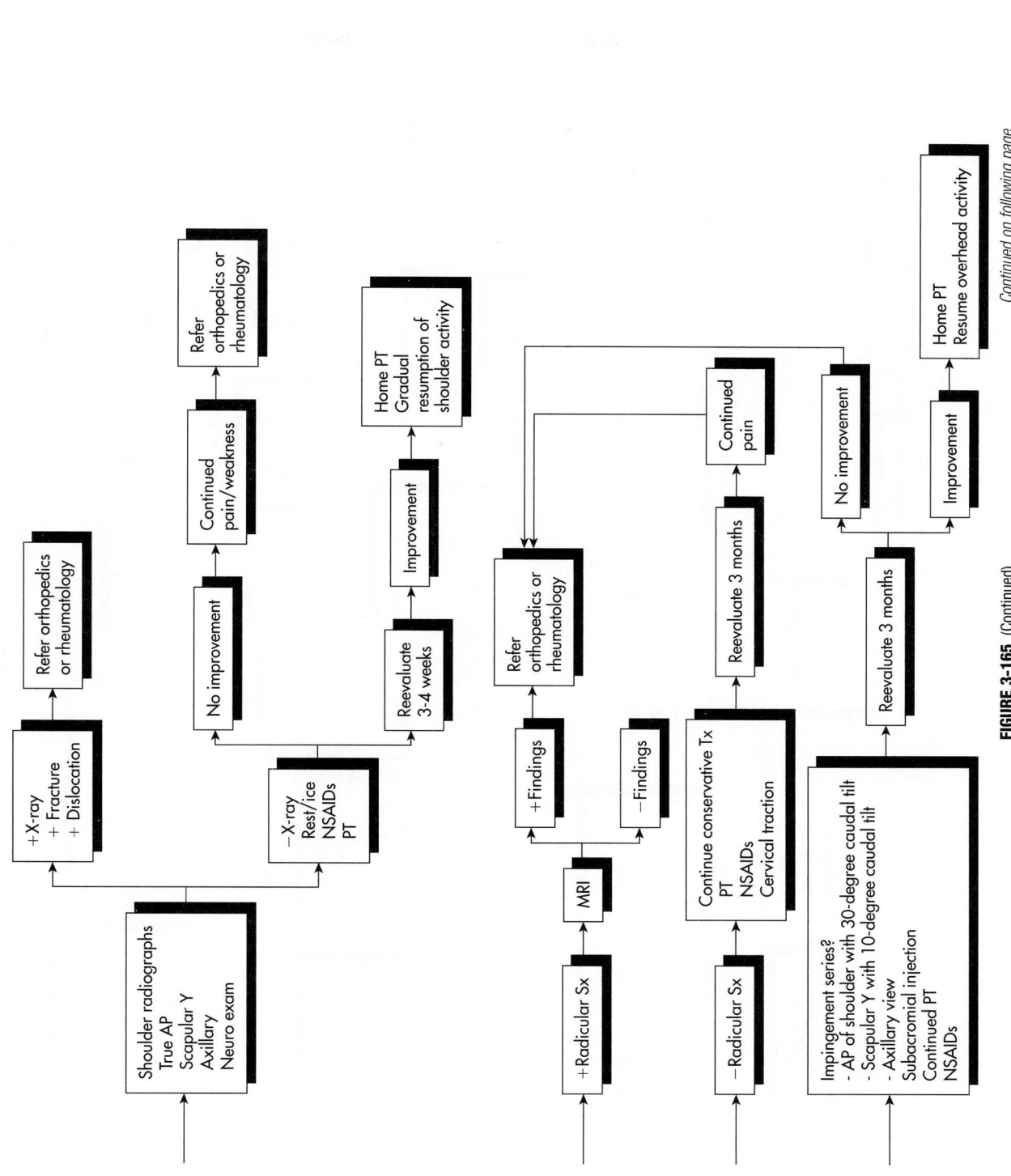

FIGURE 3-165 (Continued)

Continued on following page

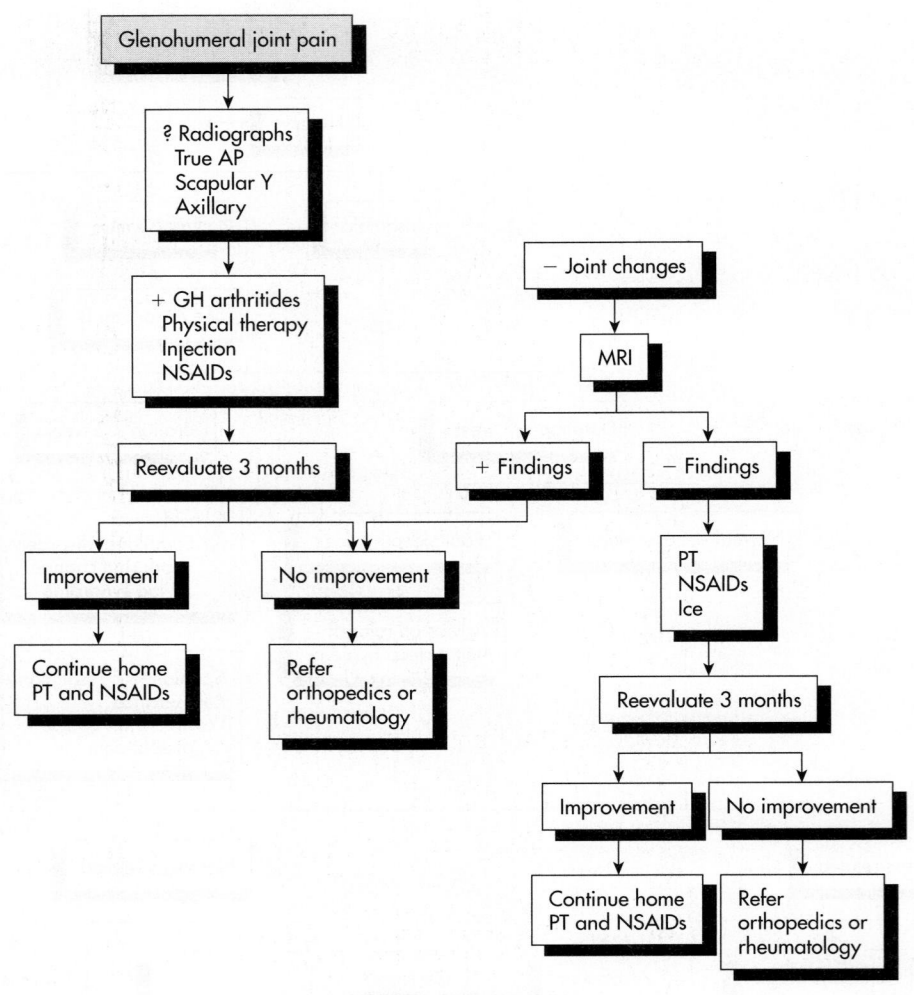

FIGURE 3-165 (Continued)

A

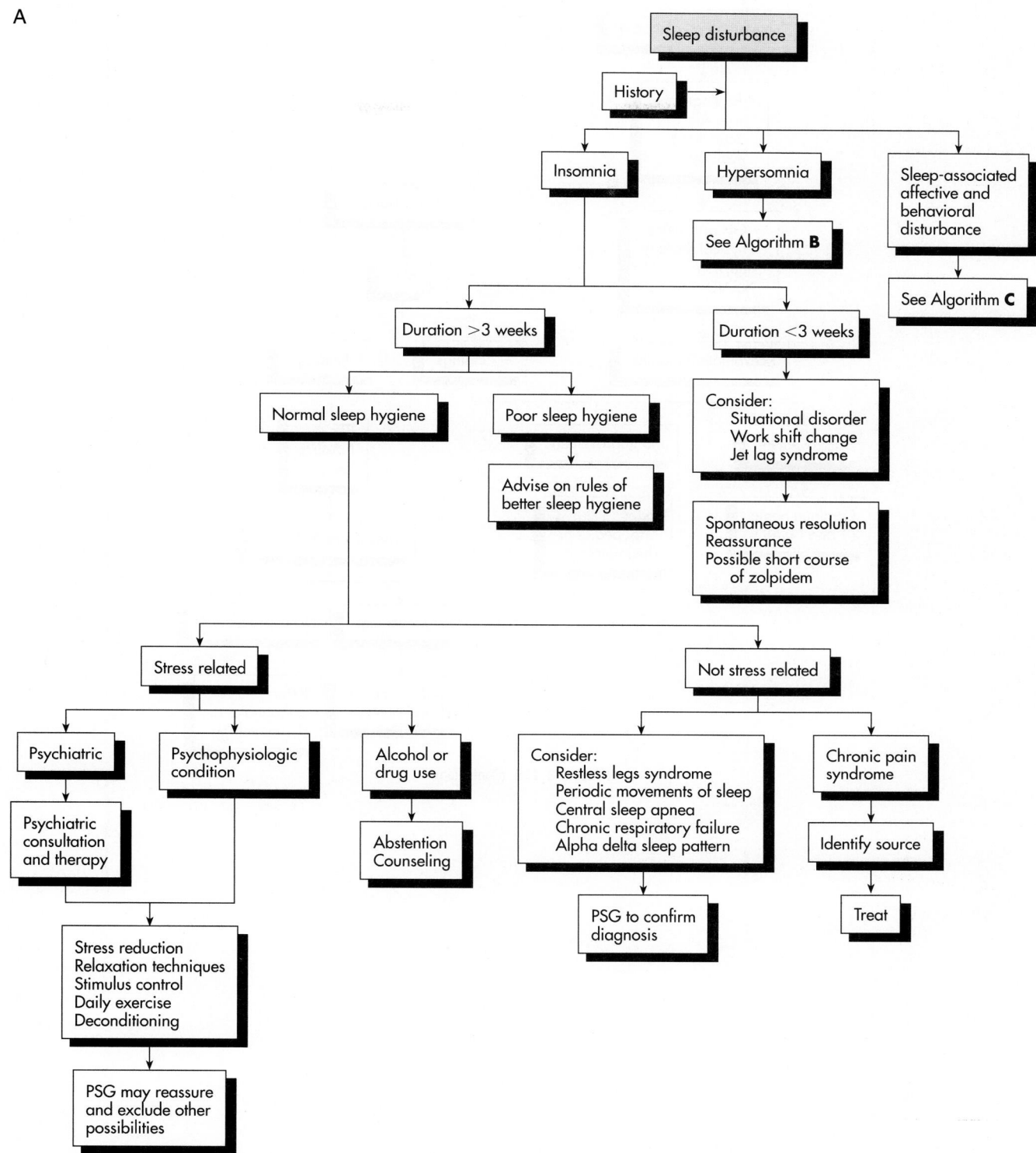

FIGURE 3-167 A, Patient with sleep disturbance. *PSG,* Polysomnography. (Modified from Greene HL, Johnson WP, Lemcke DL [eds]: *Decision making in medicine,* ed 2, St Louis, 1998, Mosby.)

B

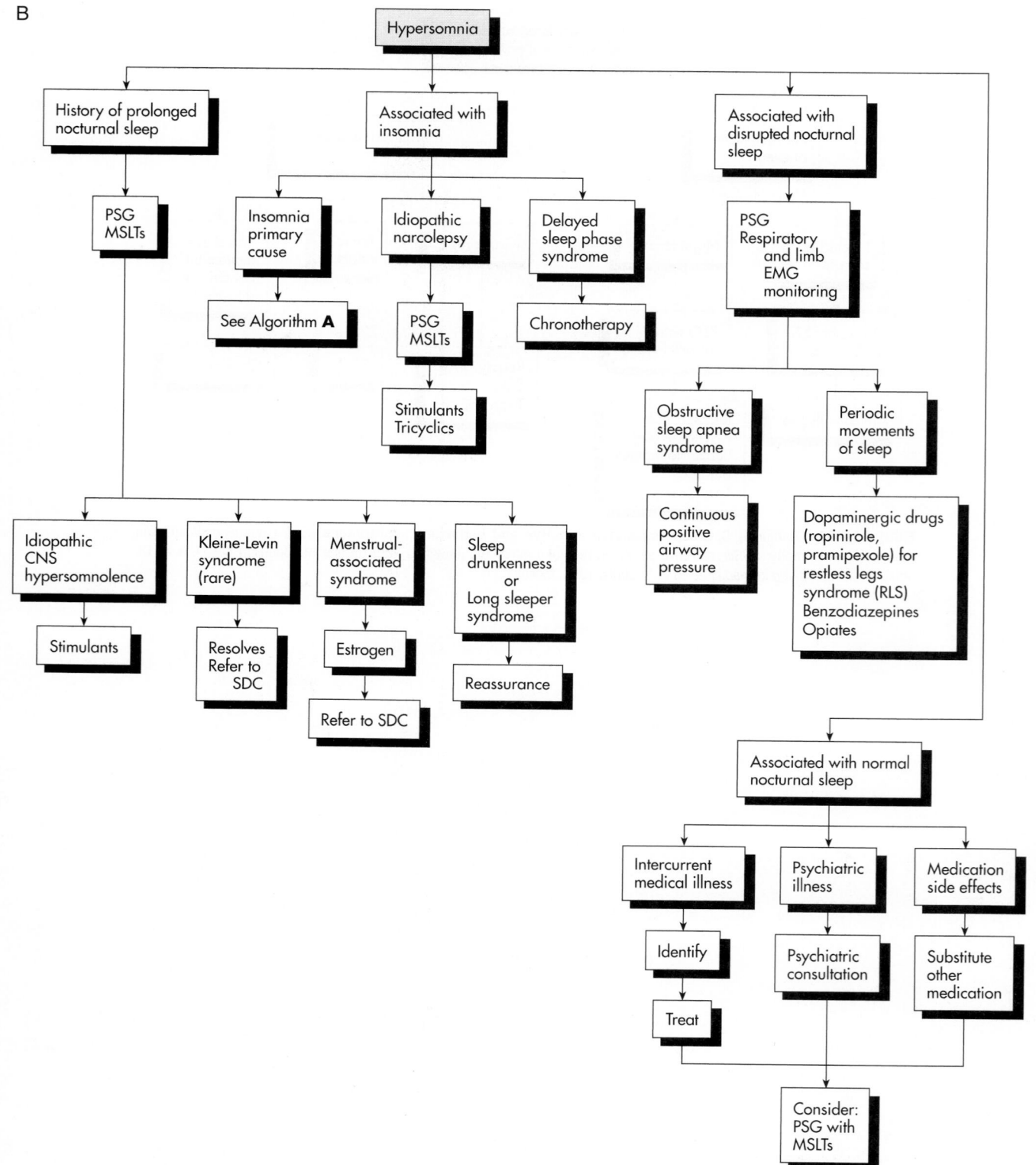

FIGURE 3-167 (Continued) **B, Hypersomnia.** *CNS,* Central nervous system; *EMG,* electromyelogram; *MSLTs,* multiple sleep latency tests; *PSG,* polysomnography; *SDC,* sleep disorders clinic. (Modified from Greene HL, Johnson WP, Lemcke DL [eds]: *Decision making in medicine,* ed 2, St Louis, 1998, Mosby.)

Continued on following page

C

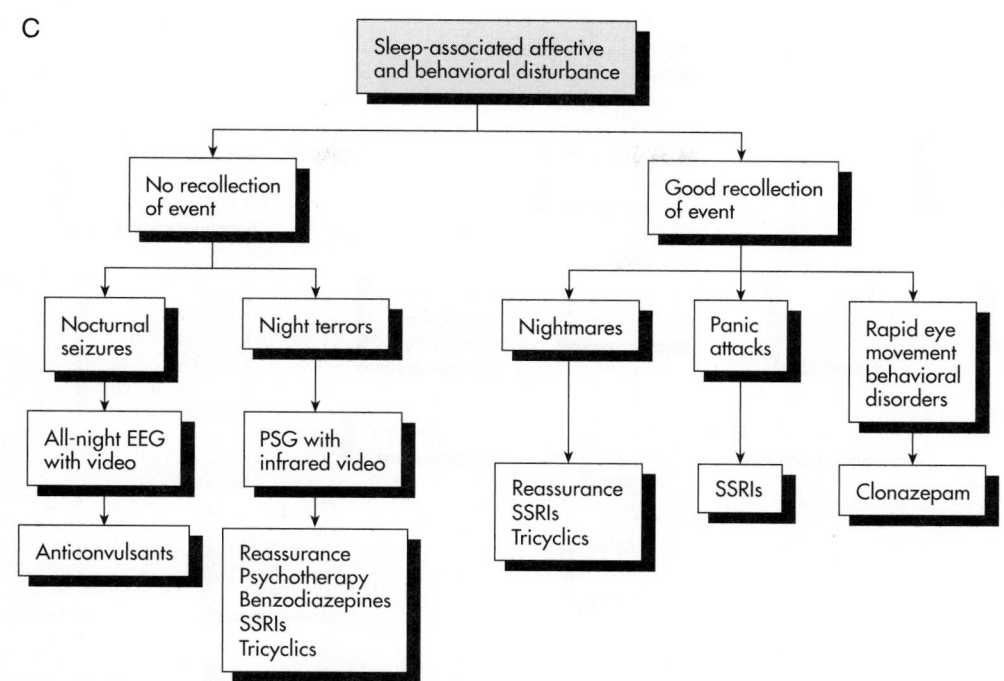

FIGURE 3-167 (Continued) **C, Sleep-associated affective and behavioral disturbance.** *EEG,* Electroencephalogram; *PSG,* polysomnography; *SSRIs,* selective serotonin reuptake inhibitors. (Modified from Greene HL, Johnson WP, Lemcke DL [eds]: *Decision making in medicine,* ed 2, St Louis, 1998, Mosby.)

SPLENOMEGALY

ICD-9CM # 789.2   Splenomegaly, unspecified
         289.51   Splenomegaly, chronic congestive
         759.0   Splenomegaly, congenital
         789.2   Splenomegaly, unknown etiology

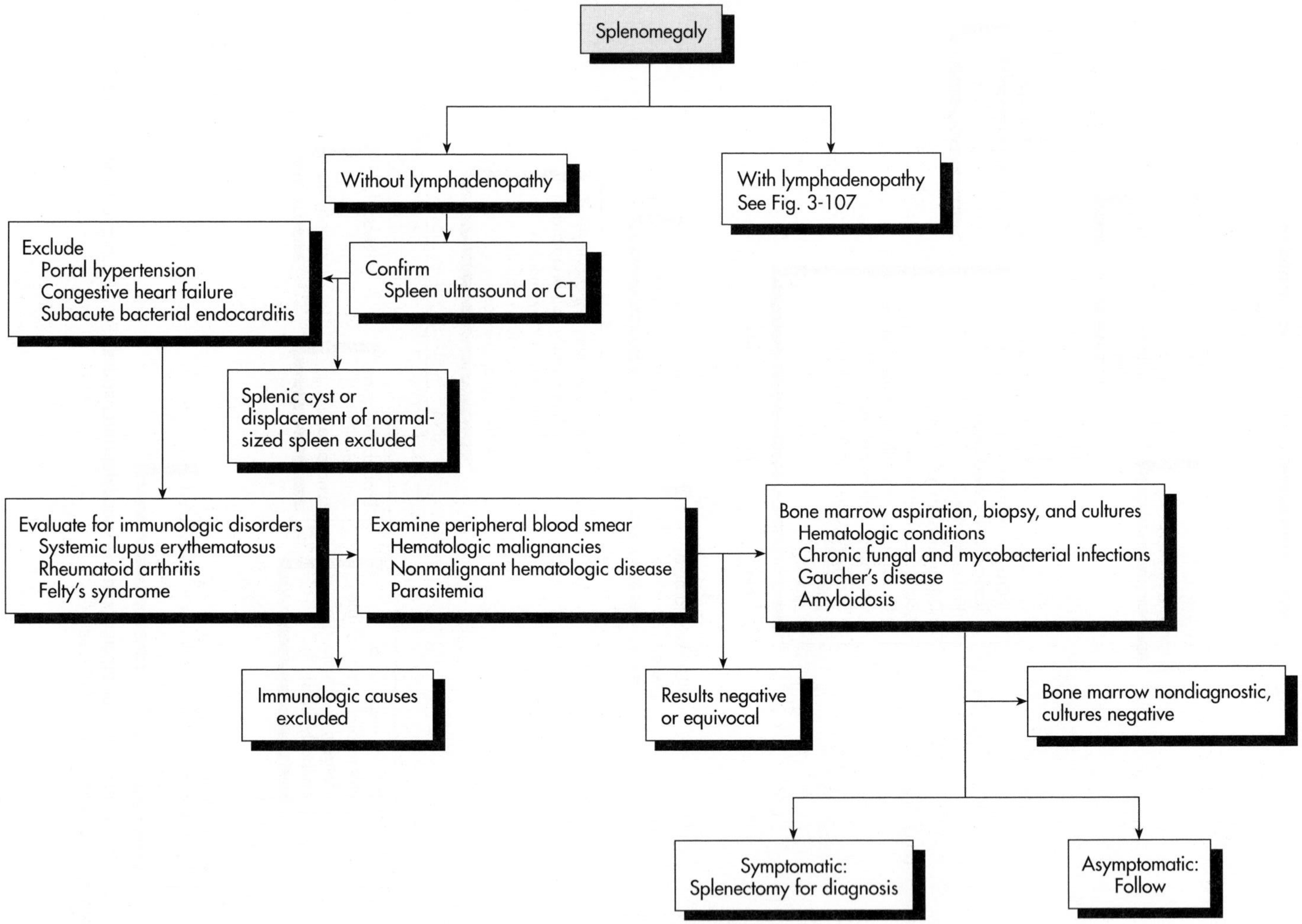

Splenomegaly

With lymphadenopathy
See Fig. 3-107

Without lymphadenopathy

Confirm
Spleen ultrasound or CT

Exclude
Portal hypertension
Congestive heart failure
Subacute bacterial endocarditis

Splenic cyst or
displacement of normal-
sized spleen excluded

Evaluate for immunologic disorders
Systemic lupus erythematosus
Rheumatoid arthritis
Felty's syndrome

Immunologic causes
excluded

Examine peripheral blood smear
Hematologic malignancies
Nonmalignant hematologic disease
Parasitemia

Results negative
or equivocal

Bone marrow aspiration, biopsy, and cultures
Hematologic conditions
Chronic fungal and mycobacterial infections
Gaucher's disease
Amyloidosis

Bone marrow nondiagnostic,
cultures negative

Asymptomatic:
Follow

Symptomatic:
Splenectomy for diagnosis

FIGURE 3-169 Clinical approach to patient with splenomegaly. *CT,* Computed tomography. (Modified from Stein JH [ed]: *Internal medicine,* ed 5, St Louis, 1998, Mosby.)

Clinical
Algorithms

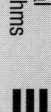

III

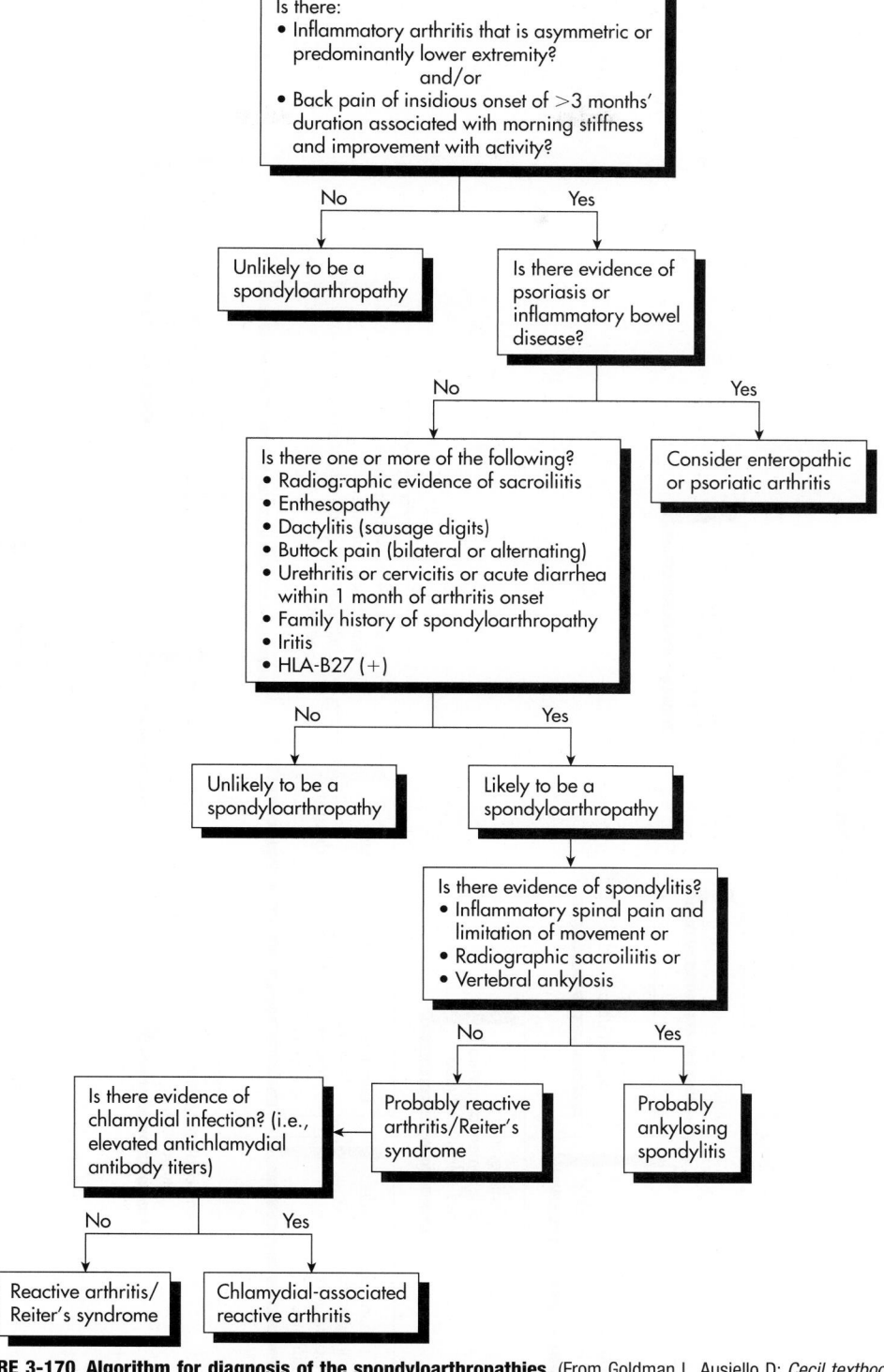

FIGURE 3-170 Algorithm for diagnosis of the spondyloarthropathies. (From Goldman L, Ausiello D: *Cecil textbook of medicine,* ed 24, Philadelphia, 2012, Saunders.)

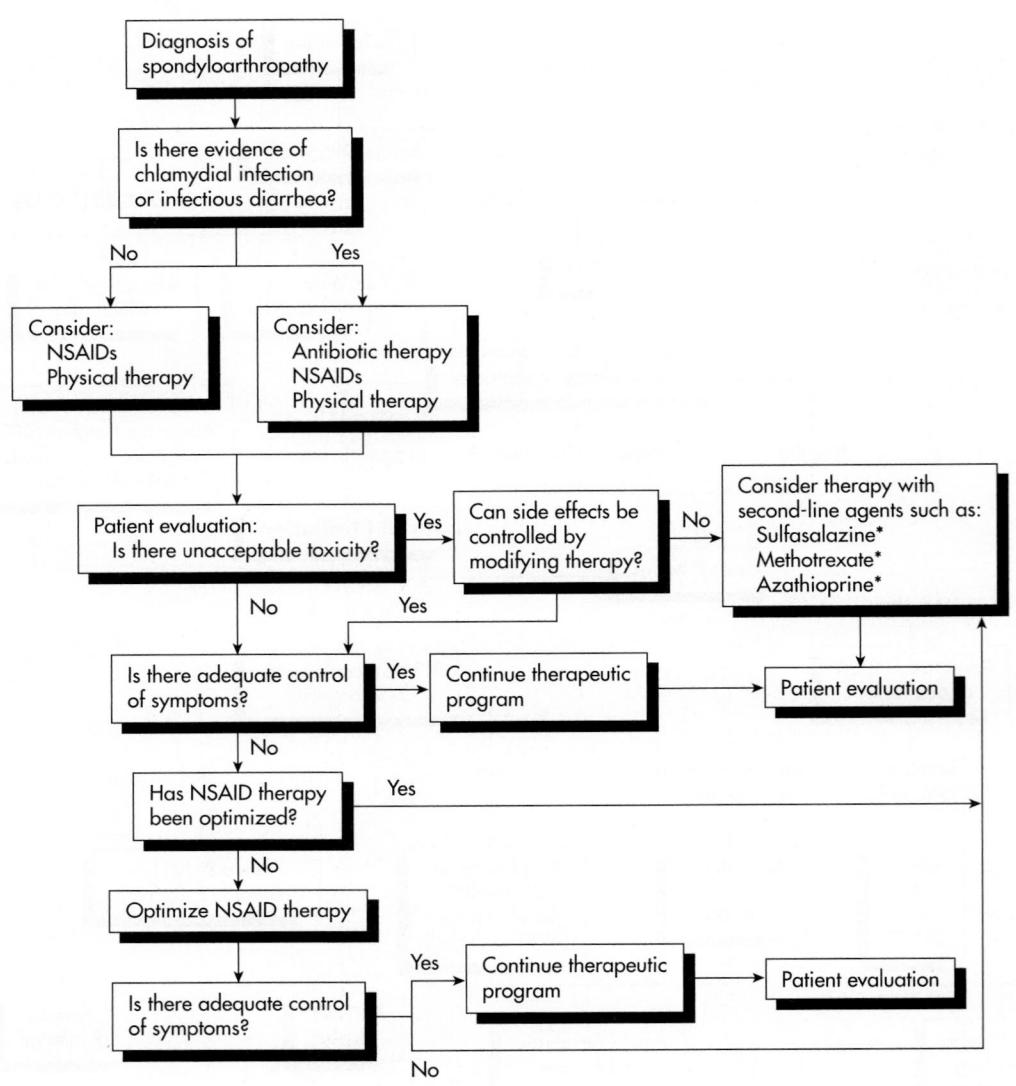

*Not approved by the FDA for treatment of spondyloarthropathies.

FIGURE 3-171 Treatment algorithm for patients with a spondyloarthropathy. *FDA,* Food and Drug Administration; *NSAID,* nonsteroidal anti-inflammatory drug. (From Goldman L, Ausiello D: *Cecil textbook of medicine,* ed 23, Philadelphia, 2008, Saunders.)

Clinical Algorithms

III

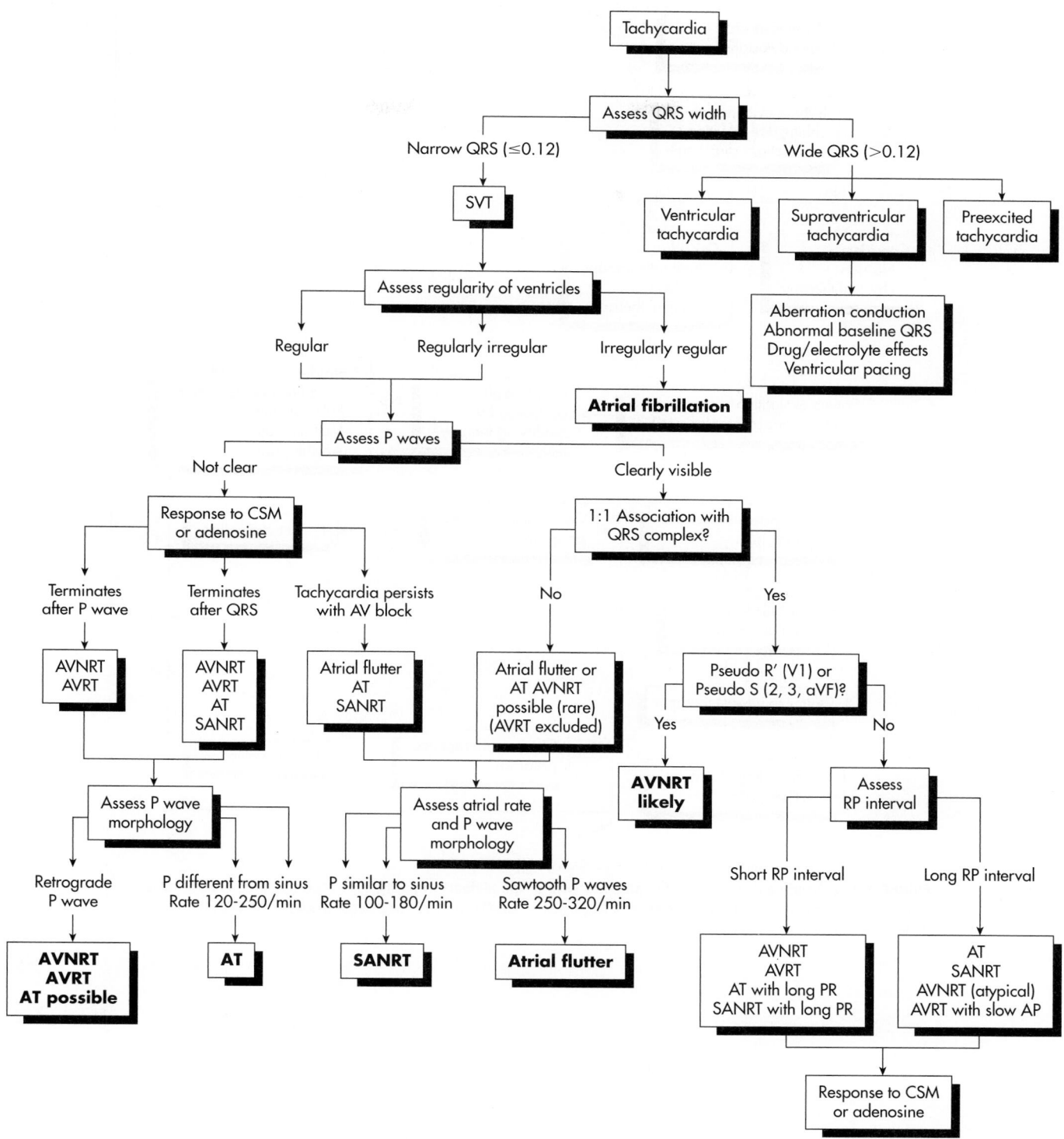

FIGURE 3-175 Stepwise approach to the diagnosis of type of tachycardia based on 12-lead electrocardiogram during the episode. The initial step is to determine whether the tachycardia has a wide or narrow QRS complex (see Fig. 3-176). For wide complex tachycardia, see Figure 3-178; the remainder of the algorithm is helpful in diagnosing the type of narrow-complex tachycardia. *AP,* Accessory pathway; *AT,* atrial tachycardia; *AV,* atrioventricular; *AVNRT,* AV nodal reentrant tachycardia; *AVRT,* AV reciprocating tachycardia; *CSM,* carotid sinus massage; *SANRT,* sinoatrial nodal reentry tachycardia; *SVT,* supraventricular tachycardia. (From Zipes DP, Libby P, Bonow RO, Braunwald E [eds]: *Braunwald's heart disease,* ed 7, Philadelphia, 2005, Saunders.)

ICD-9CM # 427.2   Paroxysmal tachycardia
427.0   Supraventricular paroxysmal tachycardia
427.42 Ventricular flutter
427.1   Ventricular paroxysmal tachycardia
427.89 Atrial tachycardia

1431

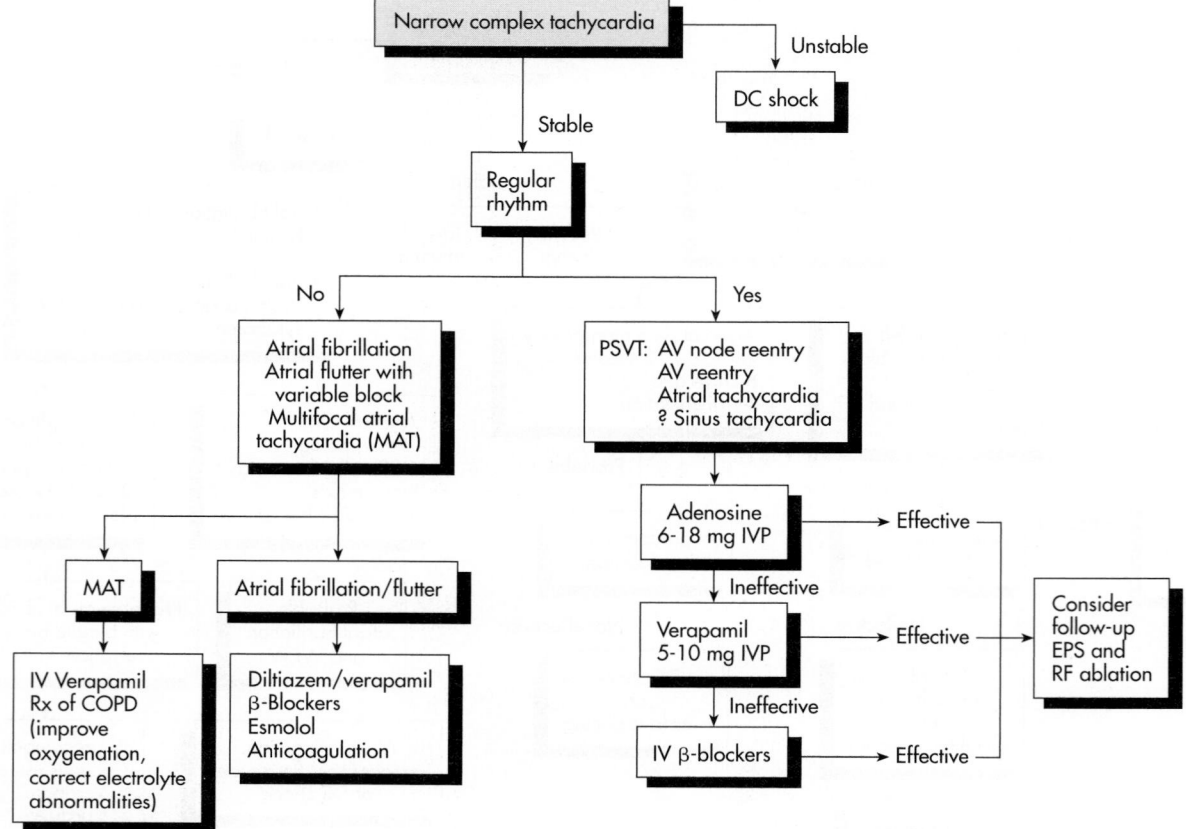

FIGURE 3-176 Evaluation and management of narrow complex tachycardia. *AV,* Atrioventricular; *COPD,* chronic obstructive pulmonary disease; *EPS,* electrophysiologic studies; *IV,* intravenous; *IVP,* intravenous push; *PSVT,* paroxysmal supraventricular tachycardia; *RF,* radiofrequency.

ICD-9CM # 427.2 Paroxysmal tachycardia
427.0 Supraventricular paroxysmal tachycardia
427.42 Ventricular flutter
427.1 Ventricular paroxysmal tachycardia
427.89 Atrial tachycardia

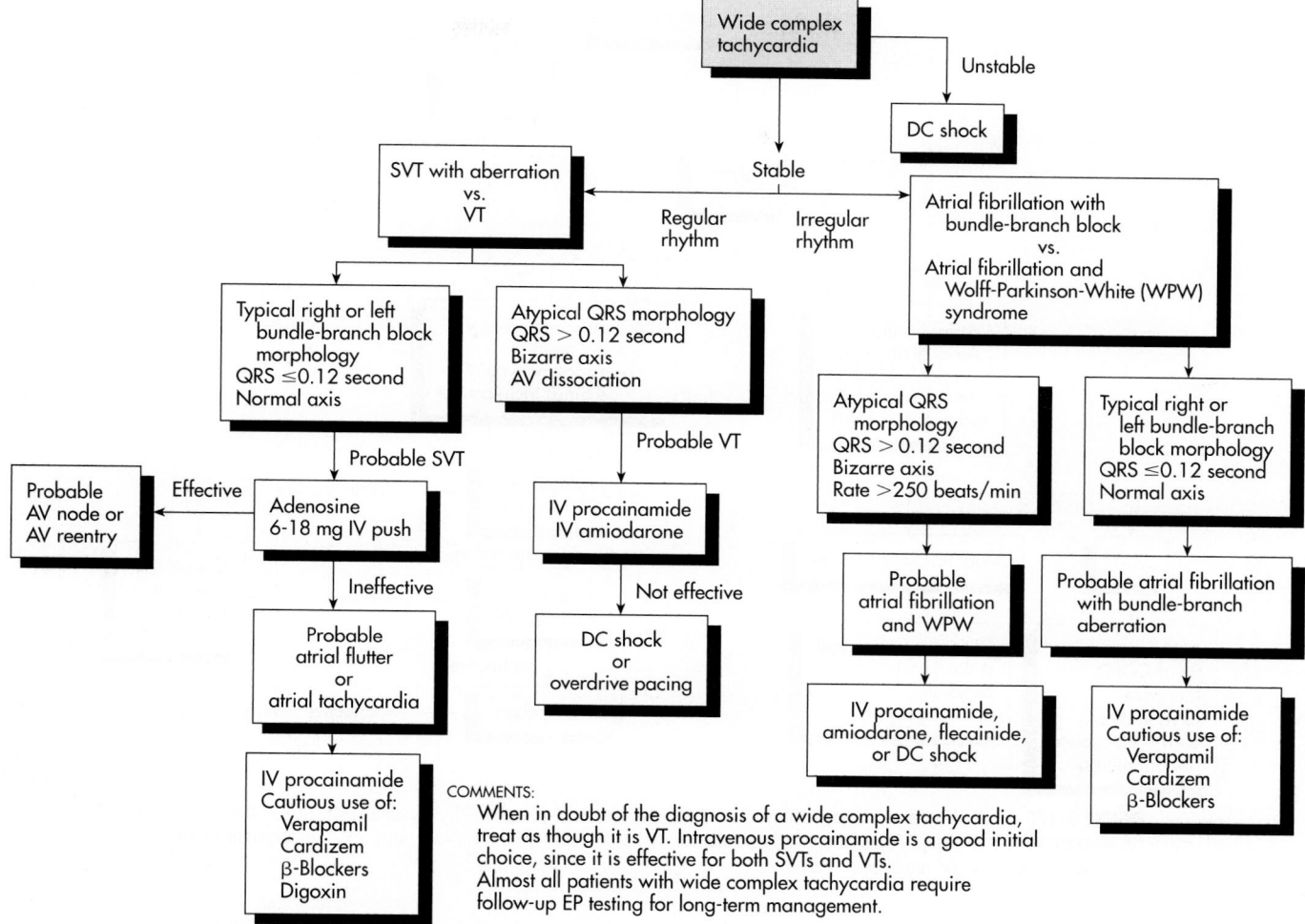

FIGURE 3-178 Evaluation and management of wide complex tachycardia. *AV,* Atrioventricular; *EP,* electrophysiologic; *IV,* intravenous; *SVT,* supraventricular tachycardia; *VT,* ventricular tachycardia. (From Driscoll CE et al: *The family practice desk reference,* ed 3, St Louis, 1996, Mosby.)

TABLE 3-27 Major Features in the Differential Diagnosis of Wide QRS Beats

Supports SVT	Supports VT
Slowing or termination by vagal tone	Fusion beats
Onset with premature P wave	Capture beats
RP interval ≤100 msec	AV dissociation
P and QRS rate and rhythm linked to suggest that ventricular activation depends on atrial discharge, e.g., 2:1 AV block rSR' V1	P and QRS rate and rhythm linked to suggest that atrial activation depends on ventricular discharge, e.g., 2:1 VA block
Long-short cycle sequence	"Compensatory" pause
	Left axis deviation; QRS duration >140 msec
	Specific QRS contours (see text)

From Zipes DP et al [eds]: *Braunwauld's heart disease,* ed 7, Philadelphia, 2005, Saunders.
SVT, Supraventricular tachycardia; *VT,* ventricular tachycardia.

ICD-9CM #   186.9   Testicular neoplasm
              M906/3   (seminoma)
              M9101/3 (embryonal carcinoma or teratoma)
              M9100/3 (choriocarcinoma)

1433

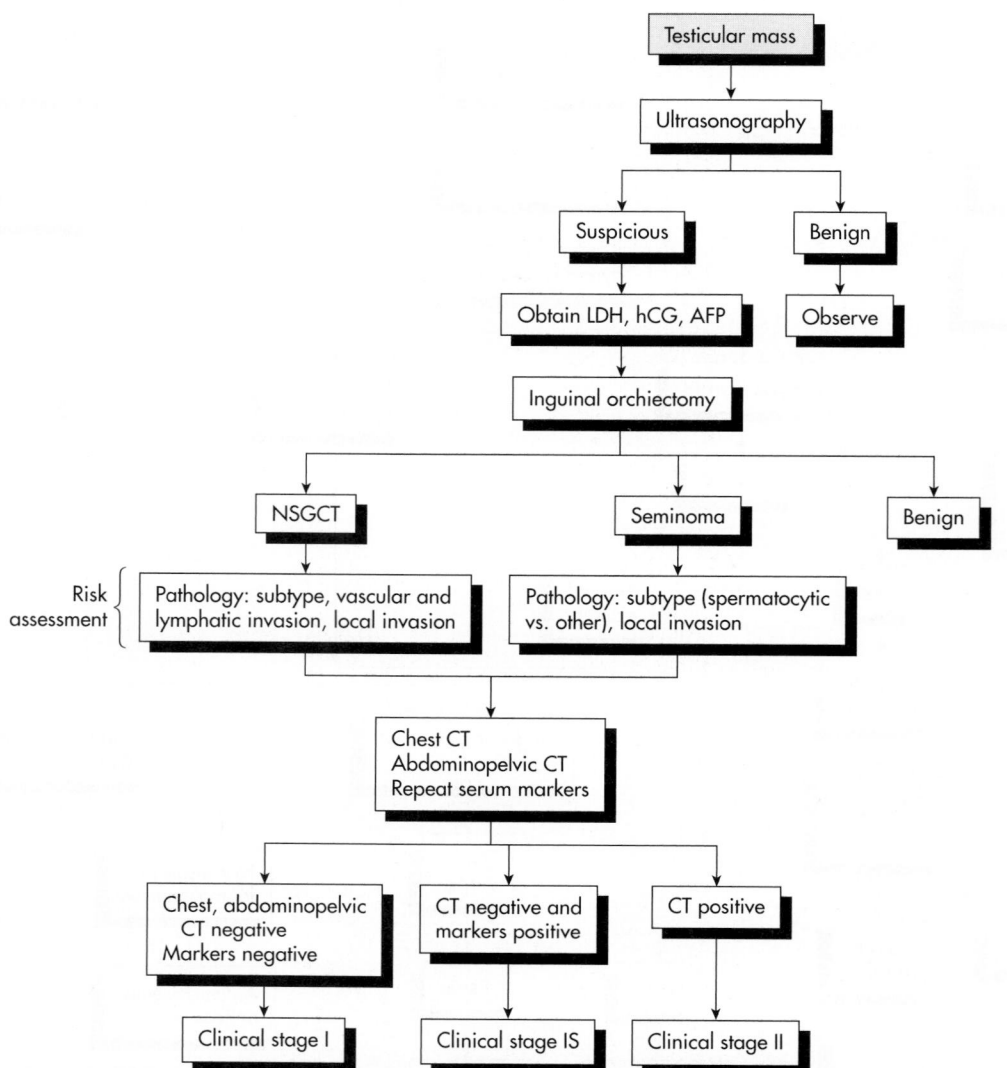

FIGURE 3-179 Diagnosis, staging, and risk assessment of patients with testicular germ cell tumor. *AFP,* α-fetoprotein; *CT,* computed tomography; *hCG,* human chorionic gonadotropin; *LDH,* lactic dehydrogenase; *NSGCT,* nonseminoma germ cell tumor. (From Abeloff MD: *Clinical oncology,* ed 4, New York, 2007, Churchill Livingstone.)

Clinical
Algorithms

III

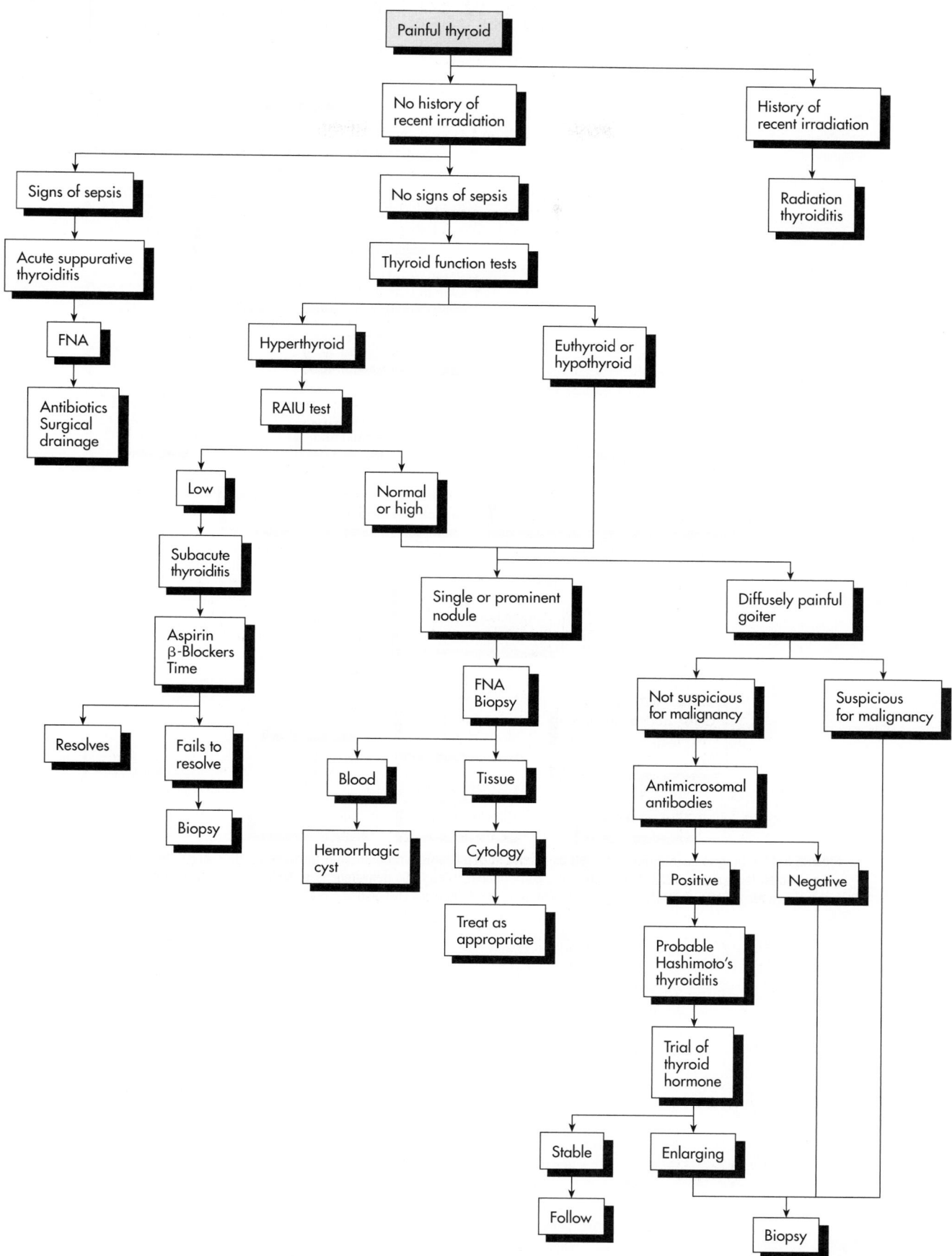

FIGURE 3-181 Painful thyroid. *FNA,* Fine-needle aspiration; *RAIU,* radioactive iodine uptake. (From Greene HL, Johnson WP, Lemcke DL [eds]: *Decision making in medicine,* ed 2, St Louis, 1998, Mosby.)

Investigation and Management of Suspected Urinary Tract Obstruction

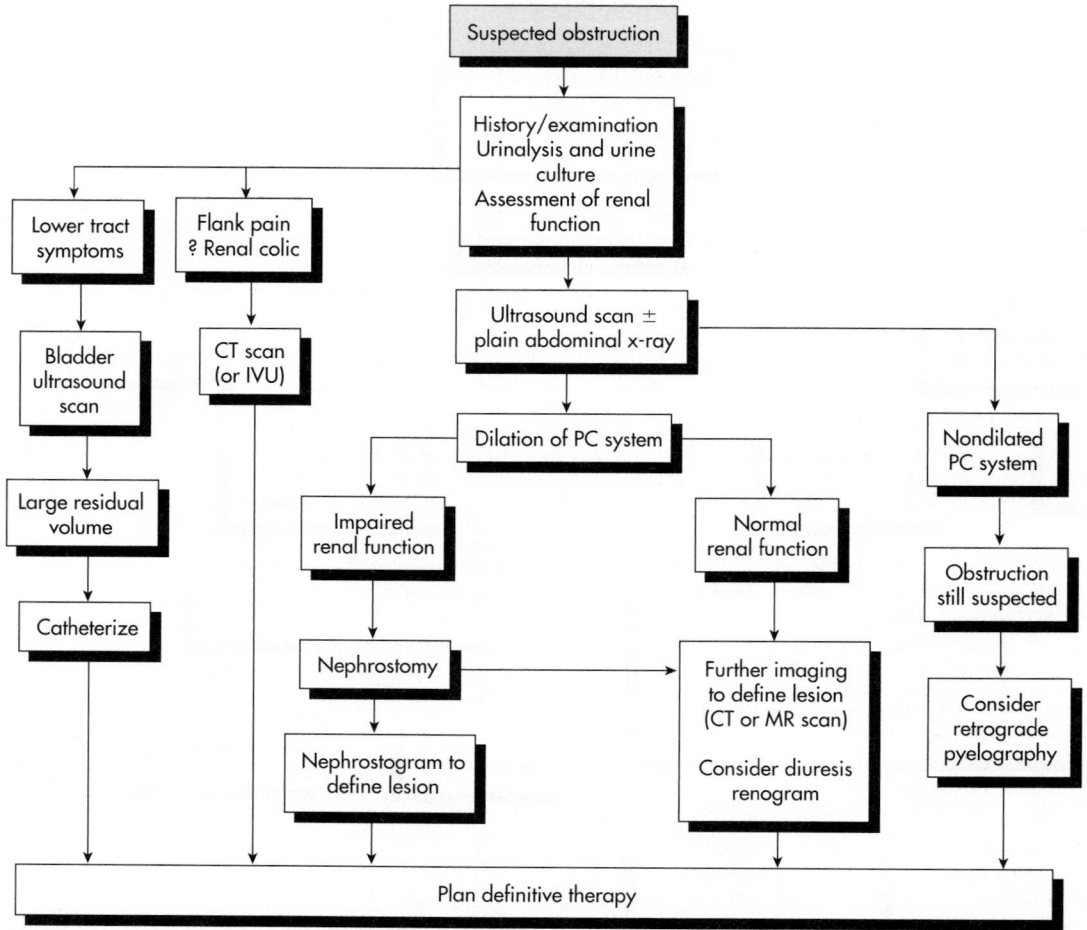

FIGURE 3-183 Investigation and management of suspected urinary tract obstruction. A full history and examination should be performed together with urinalysis, urine microscopy and culture, and measurement of renal function and serum electrolytes. Ultrasound is a useful first-line investigation for any patient with suspected urinary tract obstruction. Helical (spiral) computed tomography (CT) is now the preferred imaging technique when renal calculi are suspected. Either CT or magnetic resonance (MRI) urography can accurately diagnose both the site and the cause of obstruction in most cases. If there is renal impairment, insertion of a nephrostomy allows the effective relief of the obstruction and time for renal function to recover while definitive therapy is planned. *IVU,* Intravenous urography; *PC,* pelvicalyceal. (From Floege J et al: *Comprehensive clinical nephrology,* ed 4, Philadelphia, 2010, Saunders.)

BOX 3-6 Diagnostic Tests Used in Obstructive Uropathy

Upper Urinary Tract Obstruction
Sonography (ultrasound)
Plain films of the abdomen (KUB)
Excretory or intravenous pyelography
  (very rarely needed)
Retrograde pyelography
Isotopic renography
Computed tomography (helical CT)
Magnetic resonance imaging
Pressure flow studies (the Whitaker test)

Lower Urinary Tract Obstruction
Some of the tests listed at left
Cystoscopy
Voiding cystourethrogram
Retrograde urethrography
Urodynamic tests
Debimetry
Cystometrography
Electromyography
Urethral pressure profile

KUB, Kidneys, ureter, bladder.

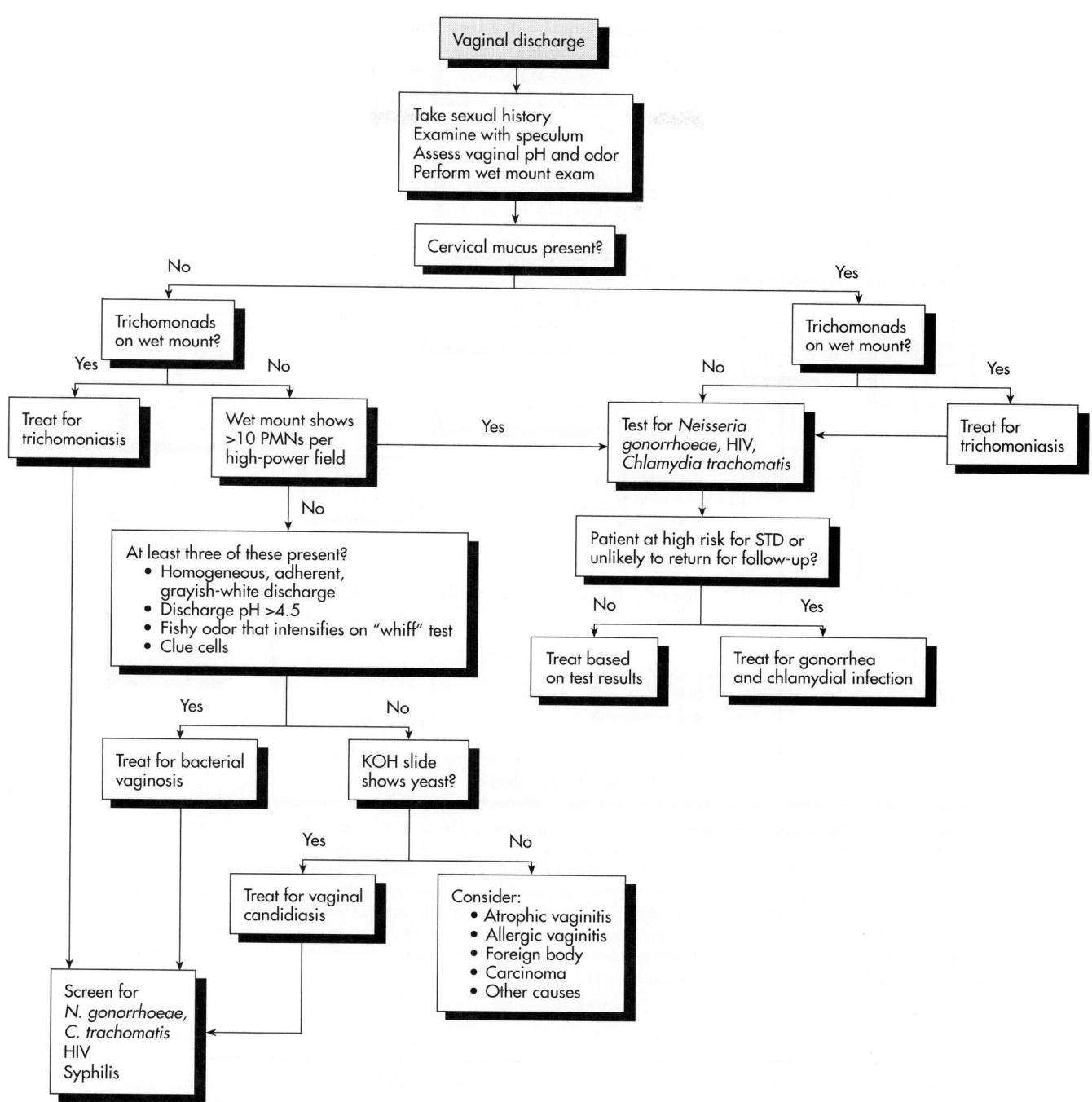

FIGURE 3-184 Evaluation of vaginal discharge. *HIV,* Human immunodeficiency virus; *KOH,* potassium hydroxide; *PMN,* polymorphonuclear leukocyte; *STD,* sexually transmitted disease.

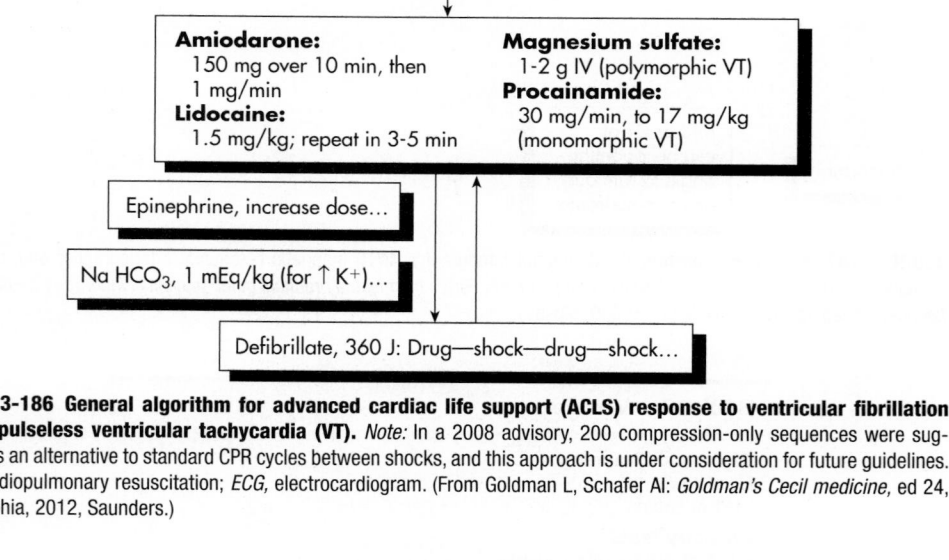

FIGURE 3-186 General algorithm for advanced cardiac life support (ACLS) response to ventricular fibrillation (VF) or pulseless ventricular tachycardia (VT). *Note:* In a 2008 advisory, 200 compression-only sequences were suggested as an alternative to standard CPR cycles between shocks, and this approach is under consideration for future guidelines. *CPR,* Cardiopulmonary resuscitation; *ECG,* electrocardiogram. (From Goldman L, Schafer AI: *Goldman's Cecil medicine,* ed 24, Philadelphia, 2012, Saunders.)

Clinical
Algorithms

III

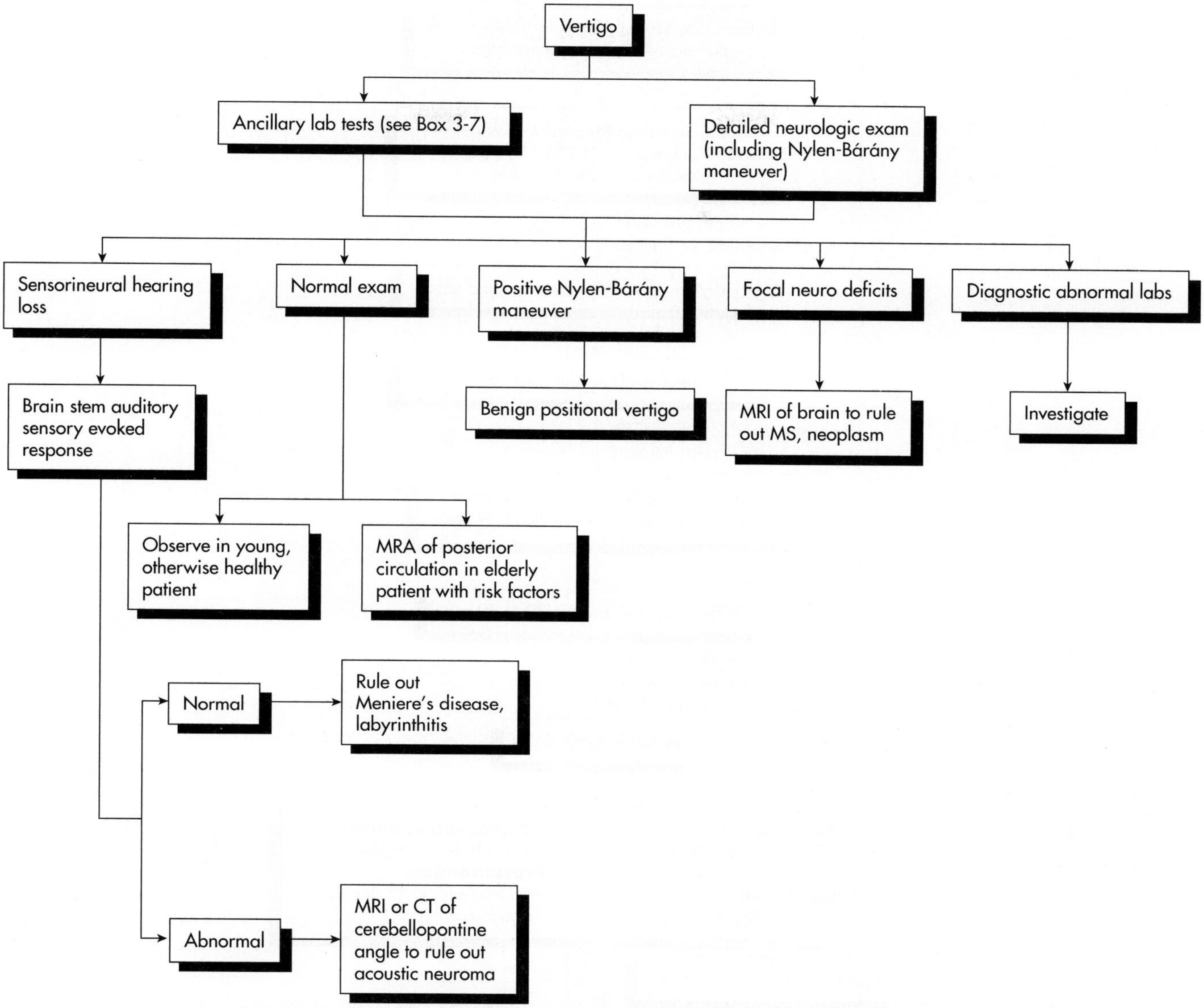

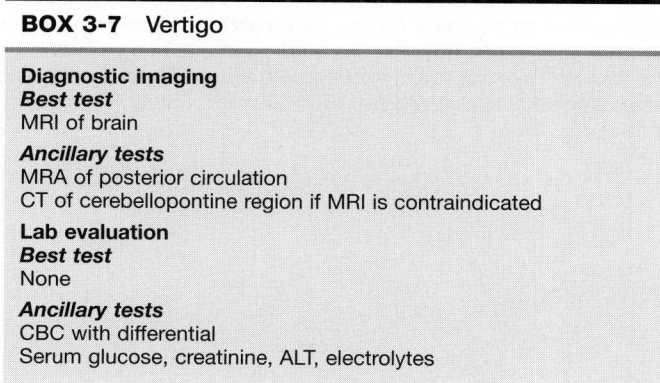

FIGURE 3-187 Vertigo evaluation. *CT,* Computed tomography; *MRA,* magnetic resonance arteriography; *MRI,* magnetic resonance imaging; *MS,* multiple sclerosis. (From Ferri FF: *Ferri's best test: a practical guide to clinical laboratory medicine and diagnostic imaging,* ed 2, Philadelphia, 2009, Mosby.)

BOX 3-7 Vertigo

Diagnostic imaging
Best test
MRI of brain

Ancillary tests
MRA of posterior circulation
CT of cerebellopontine region if MRI is contraindicated

Lab evaluation
Best test
None

Ancillary tests
CBC with differential
Serum glucose, creatinine, ALT, electrolytes

From Ferri FF: *Ferri's best test: a practical guide to clinical laboratory medicine and diagnostic imaging,* ed 2, Philadelphia, 2009, Elsevier Mosby.
ALT, Alanine aminotransferase; *CBC,* complete blood count; *CT,* computed tomography; *MRA,* magnetic resonance angiography; *MRI,* magnetic resonance imaging.

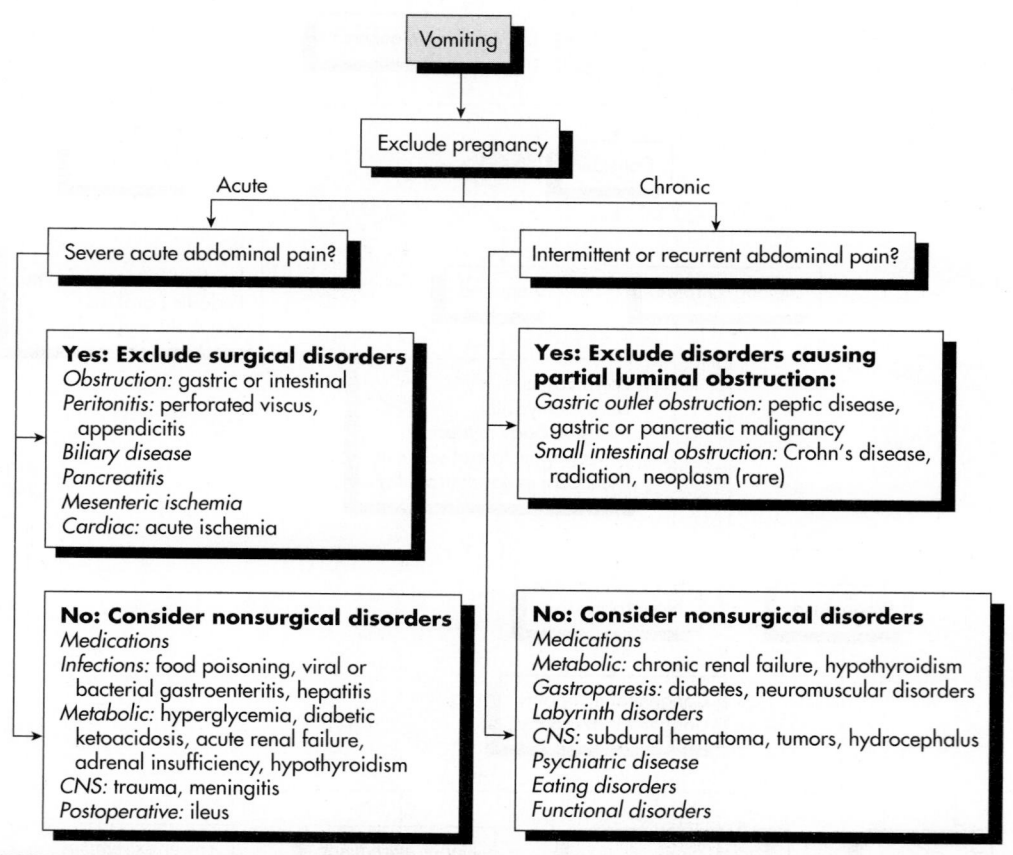

FIGURE 3-188 Approach to the patient with vomiting. *CNS*, Central nervous system. (From Goldman L, Schafer AI: *Goldman's Cecil medicine*, ed 24, Philadelphia, 2012, Saunders.)

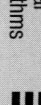

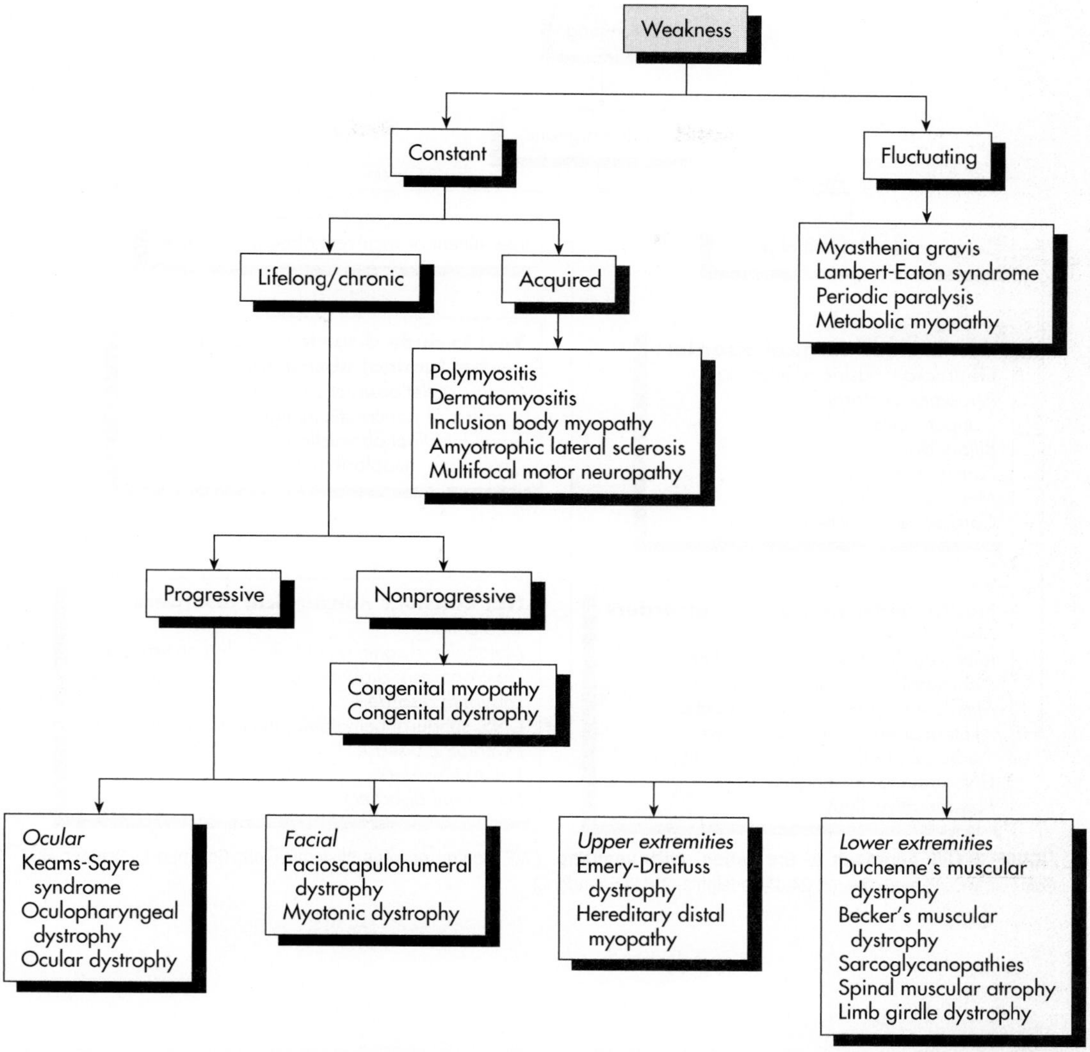

FIGURE 3-189 An algorithm for the approach to the patient with weakness. (From Bradley WG, Daroff RB, Fenichel GM, Jankovic J [eds]: *Neurology in clinical practice,* ed 4, Philadelphia, 2004, Butterworth Heinemann.)

ICD-9CM # 783.1 Abnormal weight gain
278.00 Obesity

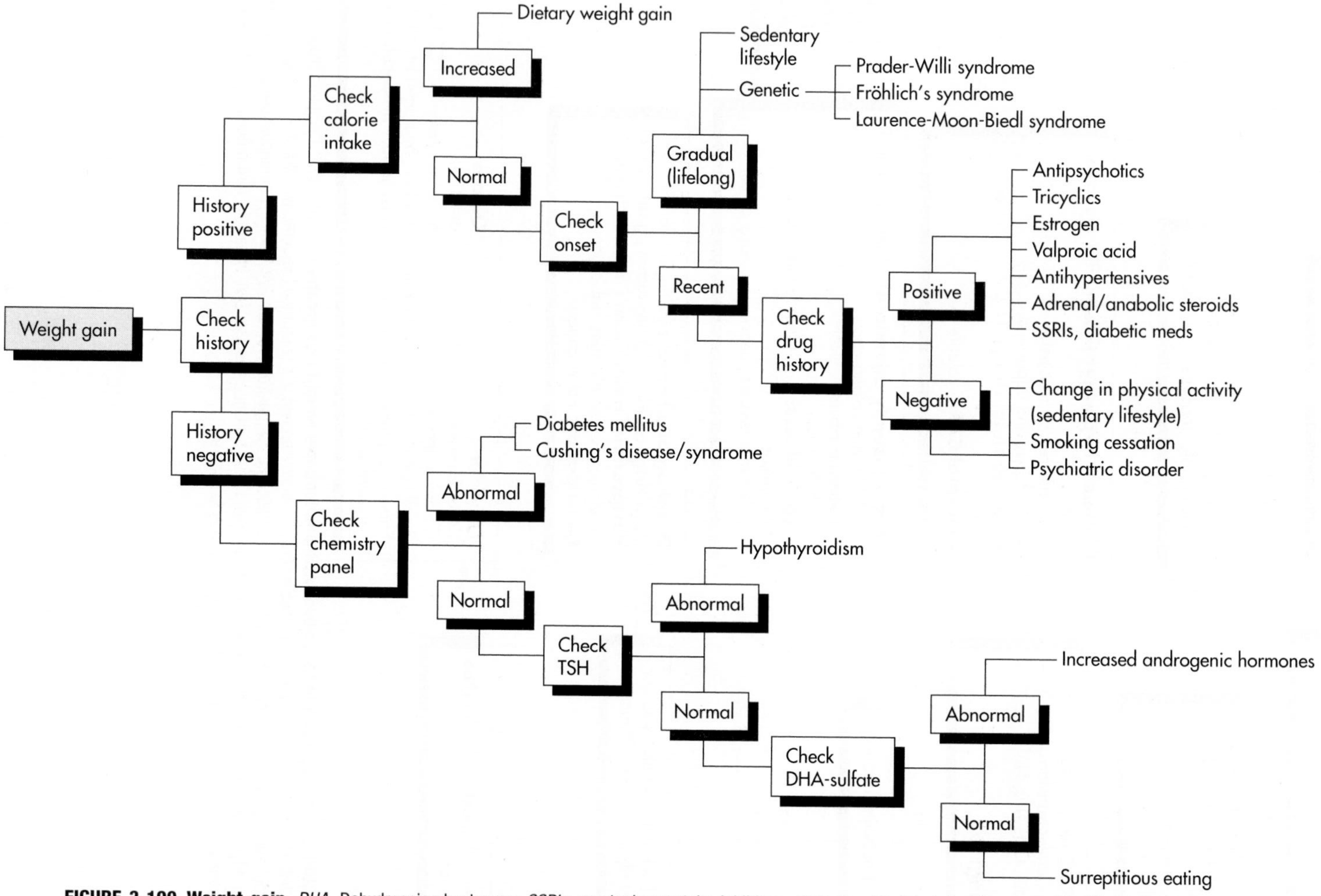

FIGURE 3-190 Weight gain. *DHA,* Dehydroepiandrosterone; *SSRIs,* serotonin reuptake inhibitors; *TSH,* thyroid-stimulating hormone. (Modified from Healey PM: *Common medical diagnosis: an algorithmic approach,* ed 3, Philadelphia, 2000, Saunders.)

Clinical
Algorithms

III

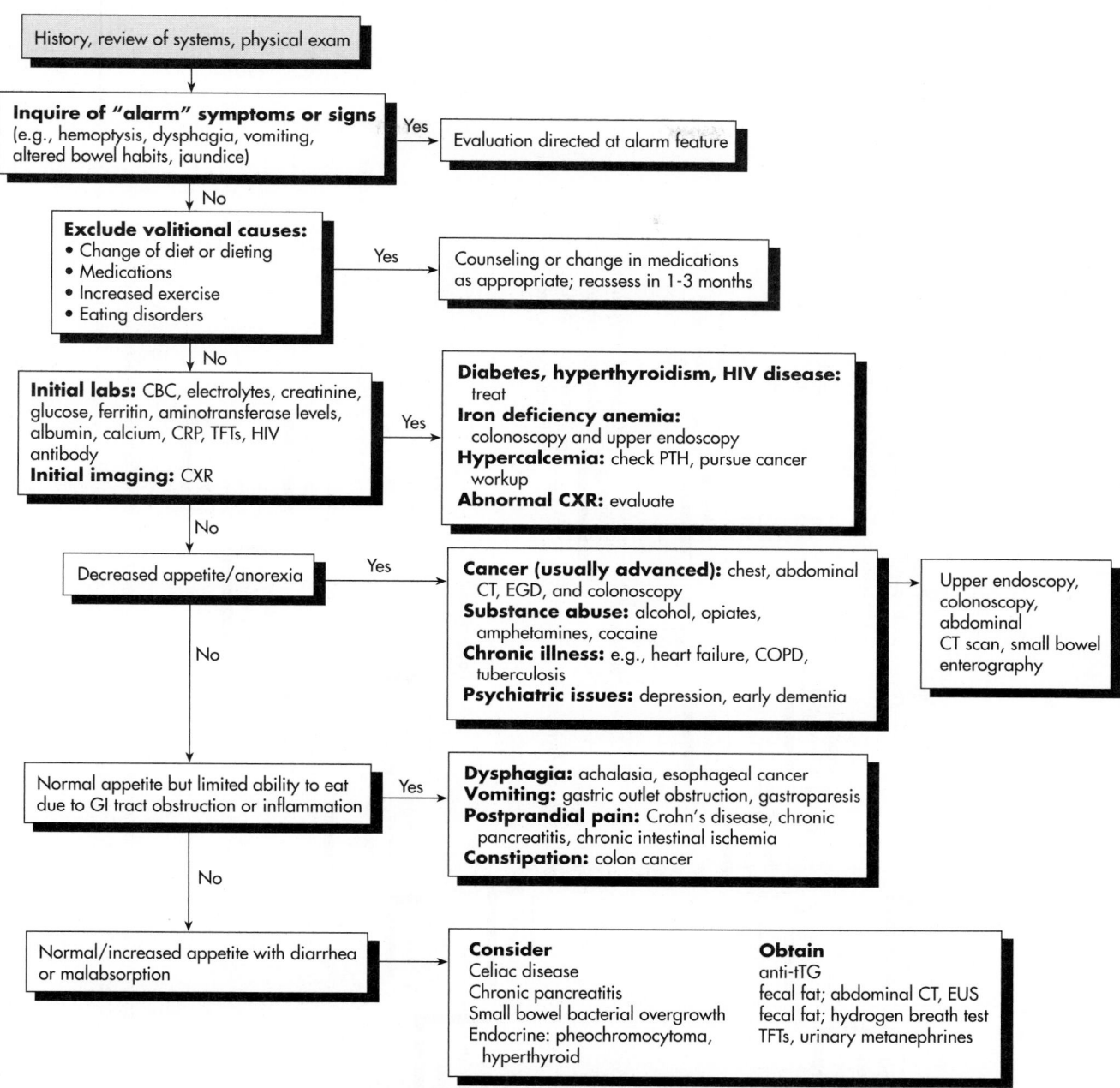

FIGURE 3-191 Approach to the patient with unintentional weight loss greater than 5%. *CBC*, Complete blood count; *COPD*, chronic obstructive pulmonary disease; *CRP*, C-reactive protein; *CT*, computed tomography; *CXR*, chest radiograph; *EGD*, esophagogastroduodenoscopy; *EUS*, endoscopic ultrasound; *GI*, gastrointestinal; *HIV*, human immunodeficiency virus; *PTH*, parathyroid hormone; *TFTs*, thyroid function tests; *tTG*, tissue transglutaminase; *U/A*, urinalysis. (From Goldman L, Schafer AI: *Goldman's Cecil Medicine*, ed 24, Philadelphia, 2012, Saunders.)

Laboratory Tests and Interpretation of Results

This section contains more than 300 commonly performed laboratory tests. In general, the tests are discussed in the following format:

1. Laboratory test.
2. Normal range in adult patients. Normal values are given using the present (traditional) reference interval, followed by the Système Internationale (SI) reference interval, the conversion factor (CF), and the suggested minimum increment (SMI).
3. Common abnormalities, such as positive test, increased or decreased value.
4. Causes of abnormal result.

The normal ranges may differ slightly, depending on the laboratory. The reader should be aware of the "normal range" of the particular laboratory performing the test. Every attempt has been made to present current laboratory test data, with emphasis on practical considerations.

ACE LEVEL

See ANGIOTENSIN-CONVERTING ENZYME

ACETONE (serum or plasma)

Normal: Negative
Elevated in: DKA, starvation, isopropanol ingestion

ACETYLCHOLINE RECEPTOR (AChR) ANTIBODY

Normal: <0.03 nmol/L
Elevated in: Myasthenia gravis. Changes in AChR concentration correlate with the clinical severity of myasthenia gravis following therapy and during therapy with prednisone and immunosuppressants. False-positive AChR antibody results may be found in patients with Eaton-Lambert syndrome.

ACID-BASE REFERENCE VALUES

See Tables 4-1 and 4-2.

ACID PHOSPHATASE (serum)

Normal range: 0-5.5 U/L (0-90 nkat/L [CF: 16.67; SMI: 2 nkat/L])
Elevated in: Carcinoma of prostate, other neoplasms (breast, bone), Paget's disease, osteogenesis imperfecta, malignant invasion of bone, Gaucher's disease, multiple myeloma, myeloproliferative disorders, benign prostatic hypertrophy, prostatic palpation or surgery, hyperparathyroidism, liver disease, chronic renal failure, idiopathic thrombocytopenic purpura, bronchitis

ACID SERUM TEST

See HAM TEST

ACTIVATED CLOTTING TIME (ACT)

Normal: This test is used to determine the dose of protamine sulfate to reverse the effect of heparin as an anticoagulant during angioplasty, cardiac surgery, and hemodialysis. The accepted goal during cardiopulmonary bypass surgery is usually 400-500 sec.

ACTIVATED PARTIAL THROMBOPLASTIN TIME (APTT, aPTT)

See PARTIAL THROMBOPLASTIN TIME

ADRENOCORTICOTROPIC HORMONE

Normal: 9-52 pg/ml
Elevated in: Addison's disease, ectopic ACTH-producing tumors, congenital adrenal hyperplasia, Nelson's syndrome, pituitary-dependent Cushing's disease
Decreased in: Secondary adrenocortical insufficiency, hypopituitarism, adrenal adenoma or adrenal carcinoma

ALANINE AMINOPEPTIDASE

Normal:
Male: 1.11-1.71 mcg/ml
Female: 0.96-1.52 mcg/ml
Elevated in: Liver or pancreatic disease, ethanol use, oral contraceptives use, malignancy, tobacco use, pregnancy
Decreased in: Abortion

ALANINE AMINOTRANSFERASE (ALT, SGPT)

See Fig. E4-1, an algorithm for evaluation of elevated ALT.
Normal range: 0-35 U/L (0.058 μkat/L [CF: 0.02 μkat/L])
Elevated in: Liver disease (hepatitis, cirrhosis, Reye's syndrome), hepatic congestion, infectious mononucleosis, myocardial infarction, myocarditis, severe muscle trauma, dermatomyositis/polymyositis, muscular dystrophy, drugs (antibiotics, narcotics, antihypertensive agents, heparin, labetalol,

TABLE 4-1 Commonly Used Acid-Base Reference Values for Arterial and Venous Plasma or Serum (Averaged from Various Sources)

	ARTERIAL		VENOUS	
	Conventional Units	SI Units*	Conventional Units	SI Units*
pH	7.40 (7.35-7.45)	7.40 (7.35-7.45)	7.37 (7.32-7.42)	7.37 (7.32-7.42)
Pco₂	40 mm Hg (35-45)	5.33 kPa (4.67-6.10)	45 mm Hg (45-50)	6.10 kPa (5.33-6.67)
Po₂	80-100 mm Hg	10.66-13.33 kPa	40 mm Hg (37-43)	5.33 kPa (4.93-5.73)
HCO₃ (CO₂ combining power)	24 mEq/L (20-28)	24 mmol/L (20-28)	26 mEq/L (22-30)	26 mmol/L (22-30)
CO₂ content	25 mEq/L (22-28)	25 mmol/L (22-28)	27 mEq/L (24-30)	27 mmol/L (24-30)

From Ravel R: *Clinical laboratory medicine,* ed 6, St Louis, 1995, Mosby.
*International system.

TABLE 4-2 Summary of Laboratory Findings in Primary Uncomplicated Respiratory and Metabolic Acid-Base Disorders*

Disorder	Pco₂	pH	Base Excess
Acute primary respiratory hypoactivity (respiratory acidosis)	Increase	Decrease	Normal/positive
Acute primary respiratory hyperactivity (respiratory alkalosis)	Decrease	Increase	Normal/negative
Uncompensated metabolic acidosis	Normal	Decrease	Negative
Uncompensated metabolic alkalosis	Normal	Increase	Positive
Partially compensated metabolic acidosis	Decrease	Decrease	Negative
Partially compensated metabolic alkalosis	Increase	Increase	Positive
Chronic primary respiratory hypoactivity (compensated respiratory acidosis)	Increase	Normal	Positive
Fully compensated metabolic alkalosis	Increase	Normal	Positive
Chronic primary respiratory hyperactivity (compensated respiratory alkalosis)	Decrease	Normal	Negative
Fully compensated metabolic acidosis	Decrease	Normal	Negative

From Ravel R: *Clinical laboratory medicine,* ed 6, St Louis, 1995, Mosby.
*Base excess results refer to negative (−) values more than 22 and positive (+) values more than 12.

statins, NSAIDs, amiodarone, chlorpromazine, phenytoin), malignancy, renal and pulmonary infarction, convulsions, eclampsia, shock liver

ALBUMIN (serum)
Normal range: 4-6 g/dl (40-60 g/L [CF: 10; SMI: 1 g/L])
Elevated in: Dehydration (relative increase)
Decreased in: Liver disease, nephrotic syndrome, poor nutritional status, rapid IV hydration, protein-losing enteropathies (e.g., inflammatory bowel disease), severe burns, neoplasia, chronic inflammatory diseases, pregnancy, oral contraceptives, prolonged immobilization, lymphomas, hypervitaminosis A, chronic glomerulonephritis

ALCOHOL DEHYDROGENASE
Normal: 0-7 U/L
Elevated in: Drug-induced hepatocellular damage, obstructive jaundice, malignancy, inflammation, infection

ALDOLASE (serum)
Normal range: 0-6 U/L (0-100 nkat/L [CF: 16.67; SMI: 20 nkat/L])
Elevated in: Muscular dystrophy, rhabdomyolysis, dermatomyositis/polymyositis, trichinosis, acute hepatitis and other liver diseases, myocardial infarction, prostatic carcinoma, hemorrhagic pancreatitis, gangrene, delirium tremens, burns
Decreased in: Loss of muscle mass, late stages of muscular dystrophy

ALDOSTERONE
Normal range:
Recumbent: 50-150 ng/L
Upright: 150-300 ng/L
(Highest levels in neonates, decreasing over time to adult levels)
Elevated in: Primary aldosteronism, secondary aldosteronism, pseudoprimary aldosteronism
Decreased in:
Patient with hypertension: diabetes mellitus, Turner's syndrome, acute alcohol intoxication, excess secretion of deoxycorticosterone, corticosterone, and 18-hydroxycorticosterone
Patient without hypertension: Addison's disease, hypoaldosteronism resulting from renin deficiency, isolated aldosterone deficiency

ALKALINE PHOSPHATASE (ALP) (serum)
See Fig. E4-2 for approach to elevated ALP.
Normal range: 30-120 U/L (0.5-2 μkat/L [CF: 0.01667; SMI: 0.1 μkat/L])
Elevated in:
LIVER AND BILIARY TRACT ORIGIN
Extrahepatic bile duct obstruction
Intrahepatic biliary obstruction
Liver cell acute injury
Liver passive congestion
Drug-induced liver cell dysfunction
Space-occupying lesions
Primary biliary cirrhosis
Sepsis
BONE ORIGIN (OSTEOBLAST HYPERACTIVITY)
Physiologic (rapid) bone growth (childhood and adolescence)
Metastatic tumor with osteoblastic reaction
Fracture healing
Paget's disease of bone
CAPILLARY ENDOTHELIAL ORIGIN
Granulation tissue formation (active)
PLACENTAL ORIGIN
Pregnancy
Some parenteral albumin preparations
OTHER
Thyrotoxicosis
Benign transient hyperphosphatasemia
Primary hyperparathyroidism
Decreased in: Hypothyroidism, pernicious anemia, hypophosphatemia, hypervitaminosis D, malnutrition

ALPHA-1-ANTITRYPSIN (serum)
Normal range: 110-140 mg/dl
Decreased in: Homozygous or heterozygous deficiency

ALPHA-1-FETOPROTEIN (serum)
See α-1 FETOPROTEIN

ALT
See ALANINE AMINOTRANSFERASE

ALUMINUM (serum)
Normal range: 0-6 ng/ml
Elevated in: Chronic renal failure on dialysis, parenteral nutrition, industrial exposure

AMEBIASIS SEROLOGIC TEST
Test description: Test is used to support diagnosis of amebiasis caused by *Entamoeba histolytica*. Serum acute and convalescent titers are drawn 1-3 weeks apart. A fourfold increase in titer is the most indicative result.

AMINOLEVULINIC ACID (δ-ALA) (24-hr urine collection)
Normal: 1.5-7.5 mg/day
Elevated in: Acute porphyrias, lead poisoning, DKA, pregnancy, anticonvulsant drugs, hereditary tyrosinemia
Decreased in: Alcoholic liver disease

AMMONIA (serum)
See Fig. E4-3 for approach to hyperammonemia in pediatric patients.
Normal range: 10-80 μg/dl (5-50 μmol/L [CF: 0.5872; SMI: 5 μmol/L])
Elevated in: Hepatic failure, hepatic encephalopathy, Reye's syndrome, portacaval shunt, drugs (diuretics, polymyxin B, methicillin)
Decreased in: Drugs (neomycin, lactulose, tetracycline), renal failure

AMYLASE (serum)
Normal range: 0-130 U/L (0-2.17 μkat/L [CF: 0.01667; SMI: 0.01 μkat/L])
Elevated in: Acute pancreatitis, pancreatic neoplasm, abscess, pseudocyst, ascites, macroamylasemia, perforated peptic ulcer, intestinal obstruction, intestinal infarction, acute cholecystitis, appendicitis, ruptured ectopic pregnancy, salivary gland inflammation, peritonitis, burns, diabetic ketoacidosis, renal insufficiency, drugs (morphine), carcinomatosis (of lung, esophagus, ovary), acute ethanol ingestion, mumps, prostate tumors, post–endoscopic retrograde cholangiopancreatography, bulimia, anorexia nervosa
Decreased in: Advanced chronic pancreatitis, hepatic necrosis, cystic fibrosis

AMYLASE, URINE
See URINE AMYLASE

AMYLOID A PROTEIN (serum)
Normal: <10 mcg/ml
Elevated in: Inflammatory disorders (acute phase–reacting protein), infections, acute coronary syndrome, malignancies

ANA
See ANTINUCLEAR ANTIBODY

ANCA
See ANTINEUTROPHIL CYTOPLASMIC ANTIBODY

ANDROSTENEDIONE (serum)
Normal:
Male: 75-205 ng/dl
Female: 85-275 ng/dl
Elevated in: Congenital adrenal hyperplasia, polycystic ovary syndrome, ectopic ACTH-producing tumor, Cushing's syndrome, hirsutism, hyperplasia of ovarian stroma, ovarian neoplasm
Decreased in: Ovarian failure, adrenal failure, sickle cell anemia

ANGIOTENSIN II

Normal: 10-60 pg/ml
Elevated in: Hypertension, CHF, cirrhosis, renin-secreting renal tumor, volume depletion
Decreased in: ACE inhibitor drugs, ARB drugs, primary aldosteronism, Cushing's syndrome

ANGIOTENSIN-CONVERTING ENZYME (ACE level)

Normal range: <40 nmol/ml/min (<670 nkat/L [CF: 16.67; SMI: 10 nkat/L])
Elevated in: Sarcoidosis, primary biliary cirrhosis, alcoholic liver disease, hyperthyroidism, hyperparathyroidism, diabetes mellitus, amyloidosis, multiple myeloma, lung disease (asbestosis, silicosis, berylliosis, allergic alveolitis, coccidioidomycosis), Gaucher's disease, leprosy

ANH

See ATRIAL NATRIURETIC HORMONE

ANION GAP

Normal range: 9-14 mEq/L
Elevated in: Lactic acidosis, ketoacidosis (diabetes, alcoholic starvation), uremia (chronic renal failure), ingestion of toxins (paraldehyde, methanol, salicylates, ethylene glycol), hyperosmolar nonketotic coma, antibiotics (carbenicillin)
Decreased in: Hypoalbuminemia, severe hypermagnesemia, IgG myeloma, lithium toxicity, laboratory error (falsely decreased sodium or overestimation of bicarbonate or chloride), hypercalcemia of parathyroid origin, antibiotics (e.g., polymyxin)

ANTICARDIOLIPIN ANTIBODY (ACA)

Normal range: Negative. Test includes detection of IgG, IgM, and IgA antibodies to phospholipid, cardiolipin
Present in: Antiphospholipid antibody syndrome, chronic hepatitis C

ANTICOAGULANT

See CIRCULATING ANTICOAGULANT

ANTIDIURETIC HORMONE

Normal range: mOsm/kg 295-300 4-12 pg/ml
Elevated in: SIADH, antipsychotic medications, ectopic ADH from systemic neoplasm, Guillain-Barré syndrome, CNS infections, brain tumors, nephrogenic diabetes insipidus
Decreased in: Central diabetes insipidus, nephritic syndrome, psychogenic polydipsias, demeclocycline, lithium, phenytoin, alcohol

ANTI-DNA

Normal range: Absent
Present in: Systemic lupus erythematosus, chronic active hepatitis, infectious mononucleosis, biliary cirrhosis

ANTI-ds DNA

Normal: <25 U
Elevated in: Systemic lupus erythematosus

ANTIGLOMERULAR BASEMENT ANTIBODY

See GLOMERULAR BASEMENT MEMBRANE ANTIBODY

ANTIHISTONE

Normal: <1 U
Elevated in: Drug-induced lupus erythematosus

ANTIMITOCHONDRIAL ANTIBODY

Normal range: <1:20 titer
Elevated in: Primary biliary cirrhosis (85%-95%), chronic active hepatitis (25%-30%), cryptogenic cirrhosis (25%-30%)

ANTINEUTROPHIL CYTOPLASMIC ANTIBODY (ANCA)

Positive test: Cytoplasmic pattern (cANCA): positive in Wegener's granulomatosis (see Fig. E4-4 and Table E4-3 for approach to patient with positive c-ANCA)

Perinuclear pattern (pANCA): positive in inflammatory bowel disease, primary biliary cirrhosis, primary sclerosing cholangitis, autoimmune chronic active hepatitis, crescentic glomerulonephritis (see Fig. E4-5 and Table E4-3 for approach to patient with positive P-ANCA)

ANTINUCLEAR ANTIBODY (ANA)

See Fig. E4-6 for approach to positive ANA pattern
Normal range: <1:20 titer
Positive test: Systemic lupus erythematosus (more significant if titer >1:160), drugs (phenytoin, ethosuximide, primidone, methyldopa, hydralazine, carbamazepine, penicillin, procainamide, chlorpromazine, griseofulvin, thiazides), chronic active hepatitis, age over 60 years (particularly age over 80 years), rheumatoid arthritis, scleroderma, mixed connective tissue disease, necrotizing vasculitis, Sjögren's syndrome, tuberculosis, pulmonary interstitial fibrosis. Table 4-4 describes diseases associated with ANA subtypes. Fig. 4-7 illustrates various fluorescent ANA test patterns.

ANTI-RNP ANTIBODY

See EXTRACTABLE NUCLEAR ANTIGEN

TABLE 4-4   Disease-Associated ANA Subtypes

Nuclear Location	Disease(s)
"Native" DNA (dsDNA, or dsDNA/ssDNA complex)	SLE (60%-70%; range, 35%-75%) Also PSS (5%-55%), MCTD (11%-25%), RA (5%-40%), DM (5%-25%), SS (5%)
sNP	SLE (50%) Also other collagen diseases
DNP (DNA-histone complex)	SLE (52%) Also MCTD (8%), RA (3%)
Histones	Drug-induced SLE (95%) Also SLE (30%), RA (15%-24%)
ENA Sm	SLE (30%-40%; range, 28%-40%) Also MCTD (0%-8%); RNP (U1-RNP) MCTD (in high titer without any other ANA subtype present: 95%-100%) Also SLE (26%-50%), PSS (11%-22%), RA (10%), SS (3%)
SS-A (Ro)*	SS without RA (60%-70%) Also SLE (26%-50%), neonatal SLE (over 95%), PSS (30%), MCTD (50%), SS with RA (9%), PBC (15%-19%)
SS-B (La)	SS without RA (40%-60%) Also SLE (5%-15%), SS with RA (5%)
Scl-70*	PSS (15%-43%)
Centromere*	CREST syndrome (70%-90%; range, 57%-96%) Also PSS (4%-20%), PBC (12%)
Nucleolar	PSS (scleroderma) (54%-90%) Also SLE (25%-26%), RA (9%)
RAP (RANA)	SS with RA (60%-76%) Also SS without RA (5%)
Jo-1	Polymyositis (30%)
PM-1	Polymyositis or PMS/PSS overlap syndrome (60%-90%) Also DM (17%)
ssDNA	SLE (60%-70%) Also CAH, infectious mononucleosis, RA, chronic GN, chronic infections, PBC

Cytoplasmic Location	Disease(s)
Mitochondrial	Primary biliary cirrhosis (90%-100%) Also CAH (7%-30%), cryptogenic cirrhosis (30%), acute hepatitis, viral hepatitis (3%), other liver diseases (0%-20%), SLE (5%), SS and PSS (8%)
Microsomal†	Chronic active hepatitis (60%-80%), Hashimoto's thyroiditis (97%)
Ribosomal	SLE (5%-12%)
Smooth muscle‡	Chronic active hepatitis (60%-91%) Also cryptogenic cirrhosis (28%), acute hepatitis, viral hepatitis (5%-87%), infectious mononucleosis (81%), MS (40%-50%), malignancy (67%), PBC (10%-50%)

From Ravel R: *Clinical laboratory medicine*, ed 6, St Louis, 1995, Mosby.
CAH, Chronic active hepatitis; *DM*, dermatomyositis; *GN*, glomerulonephritis; *MS*, multiple sclerosis; *PBC*, primary biliary cirrhosis; *SS*, Sjögren's syndrome.
*Not detected using rat or mouse liver or kidney tissue method.
†Not detected by cultured cell method.
‡Detected by cultured cells but better with rat or mouse tissue.

Laboratory Tests

IV

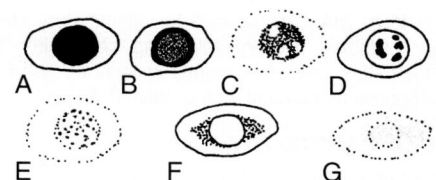

FIGURE 4-7 Fluorescent antinuclear antibody test patterns (HEP-2 cells).
A, Solid (homogeneous). **B,** Peripheral (rim). **C,** Speckled. **D,** Nucleolar. **E,** Anticentromere. **F,** Antimitochondrial. **G,** Normal (nonreactive). (From Ravel R [ed]: *Clinical laboratory medicine,* ed 6, St Louis, 1995, Mosby.)

ANTI-Scl-70
Normal: Absent
Elevated in: Scleroderma

ANTI-Sm (anti-Smith) ANTIBODY
See EXTRACTABLE NUCLEAR ANTIGEN

ANTI-SMOOTH MUSCLE ANTIBODY
See SMOOTH MUSCLE ANTIBODY

ANTISTREPTOLYSIN O TITER (Streptozyme, ASLO titer)
Normal range for adults: <160 Todd units
Elevated in: Streptococcal upper airway infection, acute rheumatic fever, acute glomerulonephritis, increased levels of β-lipoprotein
  NOTE: A fourfold increase in titer between acute and convalescent specimens is diagnostic of streptococcal upper airway infection regardless of the initial titer.

ANTITHROMBIN III
See Table 4-5.

TABLE 4-5 Assay Measurements in Heterozygous Antithrombin (ATIII) Deficiency for Diagnosis

Type	ACTIVITY		
	Antigen	Heparin Cofactor	Progressive ATIII
I	Low	Low	Low
II			
Active site defect	Normal	Low	Low
Heparin-binding site defect	Normal	Low	Normal

From Hoffman R et al: *Hematology: basic principles and practice,* ed 5, Philadelphia, 2009, Churchill Livingstone.

Normal range: 81%-120% of normal activity; 17-30 mg/dl
Decreased in: Hereditary deficiency of antithrombin III, disseminated intravascular coagulation, pulmonary embolism, cirrhosis, thrombolytic therapy, chronic liver failure, postsurgery, third trimester of pregnancy, oral contraceptives, nephrotic syndrome, IV heparin >3 days, sepsis, acute leukemia, carcinoma, thrombophlebitis
Elevated in: Warfarin drugs, post–myocardial infarction

APOLIPOPROTEIN A-1 (Apo A-1)
Normal: Recommended >120 mg/dl
Elevated in: Familial hyperalphalipoproteinemia, statins, niacin, estrogens, weight loss, familial cholesteryl ester transfer protein (CETP) deficiency
Decreased in: Familial hypoalphalipoproteinemia, Tangier disease, diuretics, androgens, cigarette smoking, hepatocellular disorders, chronic renal failure, nephritic syndrome, coronary heart disease, cholestasis

APOLIPOPROTEIN B (Apo B)
Normal: Desirable <100 mg/dl; high risk >120 mg/dl

Elevated in: High saturated fat diet, high-cholesterol diet, hyperapobetalipoproteinemia, familial combined hyperlipidemia, anabolic steroids, diuretics, beta-blockers, corticosteroids, progestins, diabetes, hypothyroidism, chronic renal failure, liver disease, Cushing's syndrome, coronary heart disease
Decreased in: Statins, niacin, low-cholesterol diet, malnutrition, abetalipoproteinemia, hypobetalipoproteinemia, hyperthyroidism

ARTERIAL BLOOD GASES
Normal range:
Po_2: 75-100 mm Hg
Pco_2: 35-45 mm Hg
HCO_3: 24-28 mEq/L
pH: 7.35-7.45
Abnormal values: Acid-base disturbances (see the following)
METABOLIC ACIDOSIS
Metabolic acidosis with increased AG (AG acidosis)
Lactic acidosis
Ketoacidosis (diabetes mellitus, alcoholic ketoacidosis)
Uremia (chronic renal failure)
Ingestion of toxins (paraldehyde, methanol, salicylate, ethylene glycol)
High-fat diet (mild acidosis)
Metabolic acidosis with normal AG (hyperchloremic acidosis)
Renal tubular acidosis (including acidosis of aldosterone deficiency)
Intestinal loss of HCO_3^- (diarrhea, pancreatic fistula)
Carbonic anhydrase inhibitors (e.g., acetazolamide)
Dilutional acidosis (as a result of rapid infusion of bicarbonate-free isotonic saline)
Ingestion of exogenous acids (ammonium chloride, methionine, cystine, calcium chloride)
Ileostomy
Ureterosigmoidostomy
Drugs: amiloride, triamterene, spironolactone, β-blockers
RESPIRATORY ACIDOSIS
Pulmonary disease (COPD, severe pneumonia, pulmonary edema, interstitial fibrosis)
Airway obstruction (foreign body, severe bronchospasm, laryngospasm)
Thoracic cage disorders (pneumothorax, flail chest, kyphoscoliosis)
Defects in muscles of respiration (myasthenia gravis, hypokalemia, muscular dystrophy)
Defects in peripheral nervous system (amyotrophic lateral sclerosis, poliomyelitis, Guillain-Barré syndrome, botulism, tetanus, organophosphate poisoning, spinal cord injury)
Depression of respiratory center (anesthesia, narcotics, sedatives, vertebral artery embolism or thrombosis, increased intracranial pressure)
Failure of mechanical ventilator
METABOLIC ALKALOSIS
Divided into chloride-responsive (urinary chloride <15 mEq/L) and chloride-resistant forms (urinary chloride level >15 mEq/L)
Chloride-responsive
Vomiting
Nasogastric (NG) suction
Diuretics
Posthypercapnic alkalosis
Stool losses (laxative abuse, cystic fibrosis, villous adenoma)
Massive blood transfusion
Exogenous alkali administration
Chloride-resistant
Hyperadrenocorticoid states (Cushing's syndrome, primary hyperaldosteronism, secondary mineralocorticoidism [licorice, chewing tobacco])
Hypomagnesemia
Hypokalemia
Bartter's syndrome
RESPIRATORY ALKALOSIS
Hypoxemia (pneumonia, pulmonary embolism, atelectasis, high-altitude living)
Drugs (salicylates, xanthines, progesterone, epinephrine, thyroxine, nicotine)
Central nervous system (CNS) disorders (tumor, cerebrovascular accident [CVA], trauma, infections)

Psychogenic hyperventilation (anxiety, hysteria)
Hepatic encephalopathy
Gram-negative sepsis
Hyponatremia
Sudden recovery from metabolic acidosis
Assisted ventilation

ARTHROCENTESIS FLUID
Interpretation of results:
1. **Color:** Normally it is clear or pale yellow; cloudiness indicates inflammatory process or presence of crystals, cell debris, fibrin, or triglycerides.
2. **Viscosity:** Normally it has a high viscosity because of hyaluronate; when fluid is placed on a slide, it can be stretched to a string >2 cm in length before separating (low viscosity indicates breakdown of hyaluronate [lysosomal enzymes from leukocytes] or the presence of edema fluid).
3. **Mucin clot:** Add 1 ml of fluid to 5 ml of a 5% acetic acid solution and allow 1 minute for the clot to form; a firm clot (does not fragment on shaking) is normal and indicates the presence of large molecules of hyaluronic acid (this test is nonspecific and infrequently done).
4. **Glucose:** Normally it approximately equals serum glucose level; a difference of more than 40 mg/dl is suggestive of infection.
5. **Protein:** Total protein concentration is <2.5 g/dl in the normal synovial fluid; it is elevated in inflammatory and septic arthritis.
6. **Microscopic examination for crystals**
   a. **Gout:** Monosodium urate crystals
   b. **Pseudogout:** Calcium pyrophosphate dihydrate crystals

ASLO TITER
See ANTISTREPTOLYSIN O TITER

ASPARTATE AMINOTRANSFERASE (AST, SGOT)
Normal range: 0-35 U/L (0-0.58 μkat/L [CF: 0.01667, SMI: 0.01μkat/L])
Elevated in:
HEART
Acute myocardial infarction
Pericarditis (active: some cases)
LIVER
Hepatitis virus, Epstein-Barr, or cytomegalovirus infection
Active cirrhosis
Liver passive congestion or hypoxia
Alcohol- or drug-induced liver dysfunction
Space-occupying lesions (active)
Fatty liver (severe)
Extrahepatic biliary obstruction (early)
Drug-induced
SKELETAL MUSCLE
Acute skeletal muscle injury
Muscle inflammation (infectious or noninfectious)
Muscular dystrophy (active)
Recent surgery
Delirium tremens
KIDNEY
Acute injury or damage
Renal infarct
OTHER
Intestinal infarction
Shock
Cholecystitis
Acute pancreatitis
Hypothyroidism
Heparin therapy (60%-80% of cases)
Fig. E4-1 describes an approach to the evaluation of AST elevation.

ATRIAL NATRIURETIC HORMONE (ANH)
Normal: 20-77 pg/ml
Elevated in: CHF, volume overload, cardiovascular disease with high filling pressure
Decreased with: Prazosin and other alpha-blockers

B-TYPE NATRIURETIC PEPTIDE (BNP)
Normal range: up to 100 mcg/L. Natriuretic peptides are secreted to regulate fluid volume, blood pressure, and electrolyte balance. They have activity in both the central and peripheral nervous systems. In humans the main source of circulatory BNP is the heart ventricles.
Elevated in: Heart failure. This test is useful in the emergency department setting to differentiate heart failure patients from those with chronic obstructive pulmonary disease presenting with dyspnea. Levels are also increased in asymptomatic left ventricular dysfunction, arterial and pulmonary hypertension, cardiac hypertrophy, valvular heart disease, arrhythmia, and acute coronary syndrome.

BASOPHIL COUNT
Normal range: 0.4%-1% of total WBC; 40-100/mm^3
Elevated in: Leukemia, inflammatory processes, polycythemia vera, Hodgkin's lymphoma, hemolytic anemia, after splenectomy, myeloid metaplasia, myxedema
Decreased in: Stress, hypersensitivity reaction, steroids, pregnancy, hyperthyroidism, postirradiation

BICARBONATE
Normal: Arterial: 21-28 mEq/L
Venous: 22-29 mEq/L
Elevated in: Metabolic alkalosis, compensated respiratory acidosis, diuretics, corticosteroids, laxative abuse
Decreased in: Metabolic acidosis, compensated respiratory alkalosis, acetazolamide, cyclosporine, cholestyramine, methanol or ethylene glycol poisoning

BILE ACID BREATH TEST (breath test, hydrogen breath test)
Normal: The test determines the radioactivity of $_{14}CO_2$ in breath samples at 2 and 4 hr.
  2 hr after dose: 0.11 ± 0.14
  4 hr after dose: 0.52 ± 0.09
Elevated in: GI bacterial overgrowth, disease or resection of terminal ileum and other H$_2$ blocker USF cimetidine

BILE, URINE
See URINE BILE

BILIRUBIN, DIRECT (conjugated bilirubin)
Normal range: 0-0.2 mg/dl (0-4 μmol/L [CF: 17.10; SMI: 2 μmol/L])
Elevated in: Hepatocellular disease, biliary obstruction, drug-induced cholestasis, hereditary disorders (Dubin-Johnson syndrome, Rotor's syndrome)

BILIRUBIN, INDIRECT (unconjugated bilirubin)
Normal range: 0-1.0 mg/dl (2-18 μmol/L [CF: 17.10; SMI: 2 μmol/L])
Elevated in:
A. Increased bilirubin production (if normal liver, serum unconjugated bilirubin is usually less than 4 mg/100 ml)
  1. Hemolytic anemia
    a. Acquired
    b. Congenital
  2. Resorption from extravascular sources
    a. Hematomas
    b. Pulmonary infarcts
  3. Excessive ineffective erythropoiesis
    a. Congenital (congenital dyserythropoietic anemias)
    b. Acquired (pernicious anemia, severe lead poisoning; if present, bilirubinemia is usually mild)
B. Defective hepatic unconjugated bilirubin clearance (defective uptake or conjugation)
  1. Severe liver disease
  2. Gilbert's syndrome
  3. Crigler-Najjar type I or II
  4. Drug-induced inhibition
  5. Portacaval shunt
  6. Congestive heart failure
  7. Hyperthyroidism (uncommon)

Laboratory Tests

IV

BILIRUBIN, TOTAL

See Fig. E4-8 and Table E4-6, for evaluation of hyperbilirubinemia and liver disease.

Normal range: 0-1.0 mg/dl (2-18 μmol/L [CF: 17.10, SMI: 2 μmol/L])

Elevated in: Liver disease (hepatitis, cirrhosis, cholangitis, neoplasm, biliary obstruction, infectious mononucleosis), hereditary disorders (Gilbert's disease, Dubin-Johnson syndrome), drugs (steroids, statins, niacin, acetaminophen, diphenylhydantoin, phenothiazines, penicillin, erythromycin, clindamycin, captopril, amphotericin B, sulfonamides, azathioprine, isoniazid, 5-aminosalicylic acid, allopurinol, methyldopa, indomethacin, halothane, oral contraceptives, procainamide, tolbutamide, labetalol), hemolysis, pulmonary embolism or infarct, hepatic congestion secondary to congestive heart failure

BILIRUBIN, URINE

See URINE BILE

BLADDER TUMOR ASSOCIATED ANTIGEN

Normal: ≤14 U/ml. Test is used to detect bladder cancer recurrence. Sensitivity 57%-83% and specificity 68%-72%.

Elevated in: Bladder cancer, renal stones, nephritis, UTI, hematuria, renal cancer, cystitis, recent bladder or urinary tract trauma

BLEEDING TIME (modified Ivy method)

See Fig. E4-9 for evaluation of patients with prolonged bleeding time.

Normal range: 2 to 9.5 min

Elevated in: Thrombocytopenia, capillary wall abnormalities, platelet abnormalities (Bernard-Soulier disease, Glanzmann's disease), drugs (aspirin, warfarin, anti-inflammatory medications, streptokinase, urokinase, dextran, β-lactam antibiotics, moxalactam), disseminated intravascular coagulation, cirrhosis, uremia, myeloproliferative disorders, von Willebrand's disease. Bleeding time tests are no longer performed at many hospitals and have been replaced by the platelet function analyzer (PFA-100) assay.

BLOOD VOLUME, TOTAL

Normal: 60-80 ml/kg

Elevated in: Polycythemia vera, pulmonary disease, CHF, renal insufficiency, pregnancy, acidosis, thyrotoxicosis

Decreased in: Anemia, hemorrhage, vomiting, diarrhea, dehydration, burns, starvation

BNP

See B-TYPE NATRIURETIC PEPTIDE

BORDETELLA PERTUSSIS SEROLOGY

Test description: PCR of nasopharyngeal aspirates or secretions is used to identify *Bordetella pertussis,* the organism responsible for whooping cough.

BRCA ANALYSIS
DESCRIPTION OF ANALYSIS
Comprehensive BRCA analysis:

BRCA1: Full sequence determination in both forward and reverse directions of approximately 5500 base pairs comprising 22 coding exons and one noncoding exon (exon 4) and approximately 800 adjacent base pairs in the noncoding intervening sequence (intron). Exon 1, which is noncoding, is not analyzed. The wild-type *BRCA1* gene encodes a protein comprising 1863 amino acids.

BRCA2: Full sequence determination in both forward and reverse directions of approximately 10,200 base pairs comprising 26 coding exons and approximately 900 adjacent base pairs in the noncoding intervening sequence (intron). Exon 1, which is noncoding, is not analyzed. The wild-type *BRCA2* gene encodes a protein comprising 3418 amino acids.

The noncoding intronic regions of *BRCA1* and *BRCA2* that are analyzed do not extend more than 20 base pairs proximal to the 5′ end and 10 base pairs distal to the 3′ end of each exon.

Single-site BRCA analysis: DNA sequence analysis for a specified mutation in *BRCA1* and/or *BRCA2.*

Multisite 3 BRCA analysis: DNA sequence analysis of specific portions of *BRCA1* exon 2, *BRCA1* exon 20, and *BRCA2* exon 11 designed to detect only mutations 187delAG and 5385insC in *BRCA1* and 6174delT in *BRCA2.*

Interpretive Criteria:

"Positive for a deleterious mutation": Includes all mutations (nonsense, insertions, deletions) that prematurely terminate ("truncate") the protein product of *BRCA1* at least 10 amino acids from the C-terminus, or the protein product of *BRCA2* at least 110 amino acids from the C-terminus (based on documentation of deleterious mutations in *BRCA1* and *BRCA2*).

In addition, specific missense mutations and noncoding intervening sequence (IVS) mutations are recognized as deleterious on the basis of data derived from linkage analysis of high-risk families, functional assays, biochemical evidence, and/or demonstration of abnormal mRNA transcript processing.

"Genetic variant, suspected deleterious": Includes genetic variants for which the available evidence indicates a likelihood, but not proof, that the mutation is deleterious. The specific evidence supporting such an interpretation will be summarized for individual variants on each such report.

"Genetic variant, favor polymorphism": Includes genetic variants for which available evidence indicates that the variant is highly unlikely to contribute substantially to cancer risk. The specific evidence supporting such an interpretation will be summarized for individual variants on each such report.

"Genetic variant of uncertain significance": Includes missense mutations and mutations that occur in analyzed intronic regions whose clinical significance has not yet been determined, as well as chain-terminating mutations that truncate *BRCA1* and *BRCA2* distal to amino acid positions 1853 and 3308, respectively.

"No deleterious mutation detected": Includes nontruncating genetic variants observed at an allele frequency of approximately 1% of a suitable control population (providing that no data suggest clinical significance), as well as all genetic variants for which published data demonstrate absence of substantial clinical significance. Also includes mutations in the protein-coding region that neither alter the amino acid sequence nor are predicted to significantly affect exon splicing, and base pair alterations in noncoding portions of the gene that have been demonstrated to have no deleterious effect on the length or stability of the mRNA transcript.

There may be uncommon genetic abnormalities in *BRCA1* and *BRCA2* that will not be detected by *BRCA* analysis. This analysis, however, is believed to rule out the majority of abnormalities in these genes, which are believed responsible for most hereditary susceptibility to breast and ovarian cancer.

"Specific variant/mutation not identified": Specific and designated deleterious mutations or variants of uncertain clinical significance are not present in the individual being tested. If one (or rarely two) specific deleterious mutations have been identified in a family member, a negative analysis for the specific mutation(s) indicates that the tested individual is at the general population risk of developing breast or ovarian cancer.

BREATH HYDROGEN TEST (hydrogen breath test)

Normal: This test is for bacterial overgrowth. H_2 excretion fasting: 4.6 ± 5.1, after lactulose, early increase <12. Lactulose usually results in a colonic response >30 min after ingestion.

Elevated in: A high fasting breath H_2 level and an increase of at least 12 ppm within 30 min after lactulose challenge are indicative of bacterial overgrowth in the small intestine. The increase must precede the colonic response.

False positives in: Accelerated gastric emptying, laxative use

False negatives in: Use of antibiotics and patients who are nonhydrogen producers

BUN

See UREA NITROGEN, BLOOD

C282Y AND H63D MUTATION ANALYSIS

Procedure: Detection of the C282Y and H63D mutations is accomplished by amplification of exons 2 and 4 of the *HFE* gene on chromosome 6 by polymerase chain reaction (PCR) followed by allele-specific hybridization and chemiluminescent detection of hybridized probes. H63D is viewed by some as a polymorphism rather than a mutation because of its prevalence

in the population, because 15% of the individuals affected with hereditary hemochromatosis (HH) are compound heterozygotes for C282Y and H63D and about 1% of patients are H63D homozygotes, which suggests that H63D may be causative in the development of the disorder at reduced penetrance.

Interpretation: Homozygosity for the C282Y mutation has been associated with an increased risk of being affected with HH compared with the general population. The genotype is observed in 60%-90% of individuals affected with HH and occurs in less than 1% of the general population. However, approximately 25% of asymptomatic individuals with this genotype do not develop the disorder.

C3

See COMPLEMENT

C4

See COMPLEMENT

CALCITONIN (serum)

Normal range: <100 pg/ml (<100 ng/L [CF: 1; SMI: 10 ng/L])
Elevated in: Medullary carcinoma of the thyroid (particularly if level >1500 pg/ml), carcinoma of the breast, apudomas, carcinoids, renal failure, thyroiditis

CALCIUM (serum)

See Fig. E4-10 for evaluation of hypercalcemia.
Normal range: 8.8-10.3 mg/dl (2.2-2.58 μmol/L [CF: 0.2495; SMI: 0.02 μmol/L])
ELEVATED
Relatively common:
Neoplasia
Bone primary
Myeloma
Acute leukemia
Nonbone solid tumors
Breast
Lung
Squamous nonpulmonary
Kidney
Neoplasm secretion of parathyroid hormone-related protein (PTHrP, "ectopic PTH")
Primary hyperparathyroidism

Thiazide diuretics
Tertiary (renal) hyperparathyroidism
Idiopathic
Spurious (artifactual) hypercalcemia
Dehydration
Serum protein elevation
Laboratory technical problem (lab error)
Relatively uncommon:
Sarcoidosis
Hyperthyroidism
Immobilization (mostly seen in children and adolescents)
Diuretic phase of acute renal tubular necrosis
Vitamin D intoxication
Milk-alkali syndrome
Addison's disease
Lithium therapy
Idiopathic hypercalcemia of infancy
Acromegaly
Theophylline toxicity

    Table 4-7 describes the laboratory differential diagnosis of hypercalcemia.

DECREASED
Artifactual
Hypoalbuminemia
Hemodilution
Primary hypoparathyroidism
Pseudohypoparathyroidism
Vitamin D–related
Vitamin D deficiency
Malabsorption
Renal failure
Magnesium deficiency
Sepsis
Chronic alcoholism
Tumor lysis syndrome
Rhabdomyolysis
Alkalosis (respiratory or metabolic)
Acute pancreatitis
Drug-induced hypocalcemia
Large doses of magnesium sulfate
Anticonvulsants
Mithramycin

TABLE 4-7 Laboratory Differential Diagnosis of Hypercalcemia

Diagnosis	PLASMA TESTS					URINE TESTS			Comments
	Ca	PO$_4$	PTH	25(OH)D	1,25(OH)$_2$D	cAMP	TmP/GFR	Ca	
Primary hyperparathyroidism	↑	N/↓	↑	N	N/↑	↑	↓	↑	Parathyroid adenoma most common
MEN I									Parathyroid hyperplasia; also includes pituitary and pancreatic neoplasms
MEN IIa									Parathyroid hyperplasia; also includes medullary thyroid carcinoma and pheochromocytoma
MEN IIb									Parathyroid disease uncommon, primarily medullary thyroid carcinoma and pheochromocytoma
FHH	↑	N	N/↑	N	N	N/↑	N/↓	↓↓	Autosomal dominant inheritance; hypercalcemia present within first decade; benign
Malignancy									
Solid tumor, humoral	↑	N/↓	↓	N	N	↑	↓	↑↑	Primarily epidermoid tumors; PTH-related protein(s) is mediator
Solid tumor, osteolytic	↑	N/↑	↓	N	N	↓	↑	↑↑	
Lymphoma	↑	N/↑	↓	N/↓	↑	↓	↑	↑↑	
Granulomatous disease	↑	N/↑	↓	N/↓	↑↑	↓	↑	↑↑	Sarcoid most common etiology
Vitamin D intoxication	↑	N/↑	↓	↑↑	N	↓	↑	↑↑	
Hyperthyroidism	↑	N	↓	N	N	N	N	↑↑	Plasma concentrations of T$_4$ and/or T$_3$ are elevated

From Moore WT, Eastman RC: *Diagnostic endocrinology*, ed 2, St Louis, 1996, Mosby.
Ca, Calcium; *cAMP*, cyclic adenosine monophosphate; *FHH*, familial hypocalciuric hypercalcemia; *GFR*, glomerular filtration rate; *MEN*, multiple endocrine neoplasia; *25(OH)D*, 25 hydroxyvitamin D; *PO$_4$*, phosphate; *PTH*, parathyroid hormone; *T$_3$*, triiodothyronine; *T$_4$*, thyroxine; *TmP*, renal threshold for phosphorus.

Laboratory Tests

IV

Gentamicin
Cimetidine
　Table 4-8 describes the laboratory differential diagnosis of hypocalcemia.

CALCIUM, URINE
See URINE CALCIUM

CANCER ANTIGEN 15-3 (CA 15-3)
Normal: <30 U/ml
Elevated in: Approximately 80% of women with metastatic breast cancer. Clinical sensitivity is 0.60, specificity 0.87, positive predictive value 0.91. This test is generally used to predict recurrence of breast cancer and evaluate response to therapy. May also be elevated in liver cancer, pancreatic cancer, ovarian cancer, colorectal cancer. Elevations can also occur with benign breast and liver disease.

CANCER ANTIGEN 27-29 (CA 27-29)
Normal: <38 U/ml
Elevated in: Approximately 75% of women with metastatic breast cancer. Clinical sensitivity is 0.57, specificity 0.97, positive predictive value 0.83, negative predictive value 0.92. This test is generally used to predict recurrence of breast cancer and evaluate response to therapy. May also be elevated in liver cancer, pancreatic cancer, ovarian cancer, colorectal cancer. Elevations can also occur with benign breast and liver disease.

CANCER ANTIGEN 72-4 (CA 72-4)
Normal: <4.0 ng/ml
Elevated in: Gastric cancer (elevated in >50% of patients). Often used in combination with CA 72-4, CA 19-9, and CEA to monitor gastric cancer after treatment.

CANCER ANTIGEN 125 (CA 125)
Normal range: <1.4%
This test uses an antibody against antigen from tissue culture of an ovarian tumor cell line. Various published evaluations report sensitivity of about 75%-80% in patients with ovarian carcinoma. There is also an appreciable incidence of elevated values in nonovarian malignancies and in certain benign conditions (see below). Test values may transiently increase during chemotherapy.
MALIGNANT
Epithelial ovarian carcinoma, 75%-80% (range, 25%-92%; better in serous than mucinous cystadenocarcinoma)
Endometrial carcinoma, 25%-48% (2%-90%)
Pancreatic carcinoma, 59%
Colorectal carcinoma, 20% (15%-56%)
Endocervical adenocarcinoma, 83%
Squamous cervical or vaginal carcinoma, 7%-14%
Lung carcinoma, 32%
Breast carcinoma, 12%-40%
Lymphoma, 35%
BENIGN
Cirrhosis, 40%-80%
Acute pancreatitis, 38%
Acute peritonitis, 75%
Endometriosis, 88%
Acute pelvic inflammatory disease, 33%
Pregnancy first trimester, 2%-24%
During menstruation (occasionally)
Renal failure (?frequency)
Normal persons, 0.6%-1.4%

CAPTOPRIL STIMULATION TEST
Normal: Test performed by giving 25 mg captopril orally after overnight fast. Patient should be seated during test. After captopril, aldosterone <15 ng/dl, renin >2 ng angiotensin I/ml/hr.
Interpretation: In patients with primary aldosteronism, plasma aldosterone remains high and plasma renin activity remains low after captopril.

CARBAMAZEPINE (Tegretol)
Normal therapeutic range: 4-12 mcg/ml

CARBOHYDRATE ANTIGEN 19-9
Normal: <37.0 U/ml
Elevated in: GI cancer, most frequently pancreatic cancer. Amount of elevation has no relation to tumor mass. Elevations can also occur with cirrhosis, cholangitis, and chronic or acute pancreatitis.

CARBON DIOXIDE, PARTIAL PRESSURE
Normal:
Male: 35-48 mm Hg
Female: 32-45 mm Hg
Elevated in: Respiratory acidosis
Decreased in: Respiratory alkalosis

CARBON MONOXIDE
See CARBOXYHEMOGLOBIN

TABLE 4-8　Laboratory Differential Diagnosis of Hypocalcemia

Diagnosis	PLASMA TESTS Ca	PO$_4$	PTH	25(OH)D	1,25(OH)$_2$D	URINE TESTS cAMP	cAMP after PTH	TmP/GFR	TmP/GFR after PTH	Ca	Comments
Hypoparathyroidism	↓	↑	N/↓	N	↓	↓	↑↑	↑	↓↓	N/↓	Deficiency of PTH
Pseudohypoparathyroidism											
Type I	↓	↑	↑↑	N	↓	↓	NC	↑	↑	N/↓	Resistance to PTH; patients may have Albright's hereditary osteodystrophy and resistance to multiple hormones
Type II	↓	N	↑↑	N	↓	↓	↑	↑	↑	N/↓	Renal resistance to cAMP
Vitamin D deficiency	↓	N/↓	↑↑	↓↓	N/↓	↑	↑	↓	↓	↓↓	Deficient supply (e.g., nutrition) or absorption (e.g., pancreatic insufficiency) of vitamin D
Vitamin D–dependent Rickets											
Type I	↓	N/↓	↑↑	N	↓	↑		↓		↓↓	Deficient activity of renal 25(OH) D-1α-hydroxylase
Type II	↓	N/↓	↑↑	N	↑↑	↑		↓		↓↓	Resistance to 1,25(OH)$_2$D

From Moore WT, Eastman RC: *Diagnostic endocrinology,* ed 2, St Louis, 1996, Mosby.
Ca, Calcium; *cAMP,* cyclic adenosine monophosphate; *FHH,* familial hypocalciuric hypercalcemia; *GFR,* glomerular filtration rate; *MEN,* multiple endocrine neoplasia; *NC,* no change or small increase; *(OH)D,* hydroxycalciferol D; *PO$_4$,* phosphate; *PTH,* parathyroid hormone; *T$_3$,* triiodothyronine; *T$_4$,* thyroxine; *TmP,* renal threshold for phosphorus.

CARBOXYHEMOGLOBIN

Normal range: Saturation of hemoglobin <2%; smokers <9%
Elevated in: Smoking, exposure to smoking, exposure to automobile exhaust fumes, malfunctioning gas-burning appliances

CARCINOEMBRYONIC ANTIGEN (CEA)

Normal range:
Nonsmokers: 0-2.5 ng/ml (0-2.5 μg/L [CF: 1; SMI: 0.1 μg/L])
Smokers: 0-5 ng/ml (0-5 μg/L [CF: 1; SMI: 0.1 μg/L])
Elevated in:
Colorectal carcinomas, pancreatic carcinomas, and metastatic disease (usually produce higher elevations: >20 ng/ml)
Carcinomas of the esophagus, stomach, small intestine, liver, breast, ovary, lung, and thyroid (usually produce lesser elevations)
Benign conditions (smoking, inflammatory bowel disease, hypothyroidism, cirrhosis, pancreatitis, infections) (usually produce levels <10 ng/ml)

CAROTENE (serum)

Normal range: 50-250 μg/dl (0.9-4.6 μmol/L [CF: 0.01863; SMI: 0.1 μmol/L])
Elevated in: Carotenemia, chronic nephritis, diabetes mellitus, hypothyroidism, nephrotic syndrome, hyperlipidemia
Decreased in: Fat malabsorption, steatorrhea, pancreatic insufficiency, lack of carotenoids in diet, high fever, liver disease

CATECHOLAMINES, URINE

See URINE CATECHOLAMINES

CBC

See COMPLETE BLOOD COUNT

CD40 LIGAND

Normal: <5 mcg/L. CD40 ligand is a soluble protein that is shed from activated leukocytes and platelets and used in risk stratification for acute coronary syndrome.
Elevated in: Acute coronary syndrome. Increased CD40 ligand is associated with higher incidence of death or nonfatal MI.

CD4+ T-LYMPHOCYTE COUNT (CD4+ T-cells)

Calculated as total WBC $\times$ % lymphocytes $\times$ % lymphocytes stained with CD4.

This test is used primarily to evaluate immune dysfunction in HIV infection. It is useful as a prognostic indicator and as a criterion for initiating prophylaxis for several opportunistic infections that are sequelae of HIV infection. Progressive depletion of CD4+ T-lymphocytes is associated with an increased likelihood of clinical complications (Table 4-9). Adolescents and adults with HIV are classified as having AIDS if their CD4+ lymphocyte count is under 200/μL and/or if their CD4+ T-lymphocyte percentage is less than 14%. HIV-infected patients whose CD4+ count is less than 200/μL and who acquire certain infectious diseases or malignancies are also classified as having AIDS. Corticosteroids decrease CD4+ T-cell percentage and absolute number.

CEA

See CARCINOEMBRYONIC ANTIGEN

CEREBROSPINAL FLUID (CSF)

Interpretation of results:
1. Appearance of the fluid
   a. Clear: normal.
   b. Yellow color (xanthochromia) in the supernatant of centrifuged CSF within 1 hour or less after collection is usually the result of previous bleeding (subarachnoid hemorrhage); it may also be caused by increased CSF protein, melanin from meningeal melanosarcomas, or carotenoids.
   c. Pinkish color is usually the result of a bloody tap; the color generally clears progressively from tubes 1 to 4 (the supernatant is usually crystal clear in traumatic taps).

TABLE 4-9 Relation of CD4 Lymphocyte Counts to the Onset of Certain HIV-Associated Infections and Neoplasms in North America

CD4 Count (Cells/mm^3)*	Opportunistic Infection or Neoplasm	Frequency (%)†
>500	Herpes zoster, polydermatomal	5-10
200-500	*Mycobacterium tuberculosis* infection, pulmonary and extrapulmonary	2-20
	Oral hairy leukoplakia	40-70
	Candida pharyngitis (thrush)	40-70
	Recurrent *Candida* vaginitis	15-30 (F)
	Kaposi's sarcoma, mucocutaneous	15-30 (M)
	Bacterial pneumonia, recurrent	15-20
	Cervical neoplasia	1-2 (F)
100-200	*Pneumocystis carinii* pneumonia	15-60
	Herpes simplex, chronic, ulcerative	5-10
	Histoplasma capsulatum infection, disseminated	0-20
	Kaposi's sarcoma, visceral	3-8 (M)
	Progressive multifocal leukoencephalopathy	2-3
	Lymphoma, non-Hodgkin's	2-5
<100	*Candida* esophagitis	15-20
	Mycobacterium avium-intracellulare, disseminated	25-40
	Toxoplasma gondii encephalitis	5-25
	Cryptosporidium enteritis	2-10
	CMV retinitis	20-35
	Cryptococcus neoformans encephalitis	2-5
	CMV esophagitis or colitis	6-12
	Lymphoma, central nervous system	4-8

From Andreoli TE (ed): *Cecil essentials of medicine*, ed 5, Philadelphia, 2000, Saunders.
CMV, Cytomegalovirus; *F*, exclusively in women; *HIV*, human immunodeficiency virus; *M*, almost exclusively in men.
*Table indicates CD4 count at which specific infections or neoplasms generally begin to appear. Each infection may recur or progress during the subsequent course of HIV disease.
†Even within the United States, great regional differences in the incidence of specific opportunistic infections are apparent. For example, disseminated histoplasmosis is common in the Mississippi River drainage area but very rare in individuals who have lived exclusively on the East or West Coast.

   d. Turbidity usually indicates the presence of leukocytes (bleeding introduces approximately 1 WBC/500 RBCs into the CSF).
2. CSF pressure: elevated pressure can be seen with meningitis, meningoencephalitis, pseudotumor cerebri, mass lesions, and intracerebral bleeding.
3. Cell count: in the adult the CSF is normally free of cells (although up to 5 mononuclear cells/mm^3 is considered normal); the presence of granulocytes is never normal.
   a. Neutrophils: seen in bacterial meningitis, early viral meningoencephalitis, and early tuberculosis (TB) meningitis.
   b. Increased lymphocytes: TB meningitis, viral meningoencephalitis, syphilitic meningoencephalitis, fungal meningitis.
4. Protein: serum proteins are generally too large to cross the normal blood–CSF barrier; however, increased CSF protein is seen with meningeal inflammation, traumatic tap, increased CNS synthesis, tissue degeneration, obstruction to CSF circulation, and Guillain-Barré syndrome.
5. Glucose
   a. Decreased glucose is seen with bacterial meningitis, TB meningitis, fungal meningitis, subarachnoid hemorrhage, and some cases of viral meningitis.
   b. A mild increase in CSF glucose can be seen in patients with very elevated serum glucose levels.
Table 4-10 describes CSF findings in central nervous system disorders.

CERULOPLASMIN (serum)

Normal range: 20-35 mg/dl (200-350 mg/L [CF: 10; SMI: 10 mg/L])
Elevated in: Pregnancy, estrogens, oral contraceptives, neoplastic diseases (leukemias, Hodgkin's lymphoma, carcinomas), inflammatory states, systemic lupus erythematosus, primary biliary cirrhosis, rheumatoid arthritis

Laboratory Tests

IV

TABLE 4-10   Cerebrospinal Fluid Findings in Central Nervous System Disorders

Condition	Pressure (mm H$_2$O)	Leukocytes (mm^3)	Protein (mg/dl)	Glucose (mg/dl)	Comments
Normal	50-80	<5, ≥75% lymphocytes	20-45	>50 (or 75% serum glucose)	
Common Forms of Meningitis					
Acute bacterial meningitis	Usually elevated (100-300)	100-10,000 or more; usually 300-2000; PMNs predominate	Usually 100-500	Decreased, usually <40 (or <66% serum glucose)	Organisms usually seen on Gram stain and recovered by culture; latex agglutination of CSF usually positive
Partially treated bacterial meningitis	Normal or elevated	5-10,000; PMNs usual but mononuclear cells may predominate if pretreated for extended period	Usually 100-500	Normal or decreased	Organisms may be seen on Gram stain; latex agglutination CSF may be positive; pretreatment may render CSF sterile
Viral meningitis or meningoencephalitis	Normal or slightly elevated (80-150)	Rarely >1000 cells; eastern equine encephalitis and lymphocytic choriomeningitis may have cell counts of several thousand; PMNs early but mononuclear cells predominate through most of the course	Usually 50-200	Generally normal; may be decreased to <40 in some viral diseases, particularly mumps (15%-20% of cases)	HSV encephalitis is suggested by focal seizures or by focal findings on CT or MRI scans or EEG. Enteroviruses and HSV infrequently recovered from CSF. HSV and enteroviruses may be detected by PCR of CSF.
Uncommon Forms of Meningitis					
Tuberculous meningitis	Usually elevated	10-500; PMNs early but lymphocytes predominate through most of the course	100-3000; may be higher in presence of block	<50 in most cases; decreases with time if treatment is not provided	Acid-fast organisms almost never seen on smear; organisms may be recovered in culture of large volumes of CSF; *Mycobacterium tuberculosis* may be detected by PCR of CSF
Fungal meningitis	Usually elevated	5-500; PMNs early but mononuclear cells predominate through most of the course; cryptococcal meningitis may have no cellular inflammatory response	25-500	<50; decreases with time if treatment is not provided	Budding yeast may be seen; organisms may be recovered in culture; cryptococcal antigen (CSF and serum) may be positive in cryptococcal infection
Syphilis (acute) and leptospirosis	Usually elevated	50-500; lymphocytes predominate	50-200	Usually normal	Positive CSF serology; spirochetes not demonstrable by usual techniques of smear or culture; dark-field examination may be positive
Amebic (*Naegleria*) meningoencephalitis	Elevated	1000-10,000 or more; PMNs predominate	50-500	Normal or slightly decreased	Mobile amebae may be seen by hanging-drop examination of CSF at room temperature
Brain and Parameningeal Abscesses					
Brain abscess	Usually elevated (100-300)	5-200; CSF rarely acellular; lymphocytes predominate; if abscess ruptures into ventricle, PMNs predominate and cell count may reach >100,000	75-500	Normal unless abscess ruptures into ventricular system	No organisms on smear or culture unless abscess ruptures into ventricular system
Subdural empyema	Usually elevated (100-300)	100-5000; PMNs predominate	100-500	Normal	No organisms on smear or culture of CSF unless meningitis also present; organisms found on tap of subdural fluid
Cerebral epidural abscess	Normal to slightly elevated	10-500; lymphocytes predominate	50-200	Normal	No organisms on smear or culture of CSF
Spinal epidural abscess	Usually low, with spinal block	10-100; lymphocytes predominate	50-400	Normal	No organisms on smear or culture of CSF
Chemical (drugs, dermoid cysts, myelography dye)	Usually elevated	100-1000 or more; PMNs predominate	50-100	Normal or slightly decreased	Epithelial cells may be seen within CSF by use of polarized light in some children with dermoids
Noninfectious Causes					
Sarcoidosis	Normal or elevated slightly	0-100; mononuclear	40-100	Normal	No specific findings
Systemic lupus erythematosus with CNS involvement	Slightly elevated	0-500; PMNs usually predominate; lymphocytes may be present	100	Normal or slightly decreased	No organisms on smear or culture; LE preparation may be positive; positive neuronal and ribosomal P protein antibodies in CSF
Tumor, leukemia	Slightly elevated to very high	0-100 or more; mononuclear or blast cells	50-1000	Normal to decreased (20-40)	Cytology may be positive

From Behrman RE: *Nelson textbook of pediatrics*, ed 17, Philadelphia, 2004, Saunders.

CNS, Central nervous system; *CSF,* cerebrospinal fluid; *CT,* computed tomography; *EEG,* electroencephalogram; *HSV,* herpes simplex virus; *MRI,* magnetic resonance imaging; *PCR,* polymerase chain reaction; *PMN,* polymorphonuclear neutrophils.

Decreased in: Wilson's disease (values often <10 mg/dl), nephrotic syndrome, advanced liver disease, malabsorption, total parenteral nutrition, Menkes' syndrome

CHLAMYDIA GROUP ANTIBODY SEROLOGIC TEST

Test description: Acute and convalescent sera is drawn 2-4 weeks apart. A fourfold increase in titer between acute and convalescent sera is necessary for confirmation. A single titer ≥1:64 is considered indicative of psittacosis or LGV.

CHLAMYDIA TRACHOMATIS PCR

Test description: Test is performed on endocervical swab, urine, and intraurethral swab
Normal: Negative

CHLORIDE (serum)

Normal range: 95-105 mEq/L (95-105 mmol/L [CF: 1; SMI: 1 mmol/L])
Elevated in: Dehydration, excessive infusion of normal saline solution, cystic fibrosis (sweat test), hyperparathyroidism, renal tubular disease, metabolic acidosis, prolonged diarrhea, drugs (ammonium chloride administration, acetazolamide, boric acid, triamterene)
Decreased in: Congestive heart failure, syndrome of inappropriate antidiuretic hormone secretion, Addison's disease, vomiting, gastric suction, salt-losing nephritis, continuous infusion of D_5W, thiazide diuretic administration, diaphoresis, diarrhea, burns, diabetic ketoacidosis

CHLORIDE (sweat)

Normal: 0-40 mmol/L
Borderline/indeterminate: 41-60 mmol/L
Consistent with cystic fibrosis: >60 mmol/L
False low results can occur with edema, excessive sweating, and hypoproteinemia.

CHLORIDE, URINE

See URINE CHLORIDE

CHOLECYSTOKININ-PANCREOZYMIN (CCK, CCK-PZ)

Normal: <80 pg/ml
Elevated in: Pancreatic disease, celiac disease, gastric ulcer, postgastrectomy, IBS, fatty food intolerance

CHOLESTEROL, HIGH-DENSITY LIPOPROTEIN

See HIGH-DENSITY LIPOPROTEIN CHOLESTEROL

CHOLESTEROL, LOW-DENSITY LIPOPROTEIN

See LOW-DENSITY LIPOPROTEIN CHOLESTEROL

CHOLESTEROL, TOTAL

Normal range: Varies with age
Generally <200 mg/dl (<5.20 mmol/L [CF: 0.02586; SMI: 0.05 mmol/L])
Elevated in: Primary hypercholesterolemia, biliary obstruction, diabetes mellitus, nephrotic syndrome, hypothyroidism, primary biliary cirrhosis, high-cholesterol diet, pregnancy third trimester, myocardial infarction, drugs (steroids, phenothiazines, oral contraceptives)
Decreased in: Medications (statins, niacin), starvation, malabsorption, sideroblastic anemia, thalassemia, abetalipoproteinemia, hyperthyroidism, Cushing's syndrome, hepatic failure, multiple myeloma, polycythemia vera, chronic myelocytic leukemia, myeloid metaplasia, Waldenström's macroglobulinemia, myelofibrosis

CHORIONIC GONADOTROPINS, HUMAN (serum)

Normal range, serum: Female, premenopausal: <0.8 IU/L; postmenopausal <3.3 IU/L
Male: <0.7 IU/L
Elevated in:
Pregnancy, choriocarcinoma, gestational trophoblastic neoplasia (including molar gestations), placental site trophoblastic tumors; human antimouse antibodies (HAMA) can produce false serum assay for hCG.

The principal use of this test is to diagnose pregnancy. The concentration of hCG increases significantly during the initial 6 weeks of pregnancy. Peak values approaching 100,000 IU/L occur 60-70 days following implantation.
hCG levels generally double every 1-3 days. In patients with concentration <2000 IU/L, an increase of serum hCG <66% after 2 days is suggestive of spontaneous abortion or ruptured ectopic gestation.

CHYMOTRYPSIN

Normal: <10 mcg/L
Elevated in: Acute pancreatitis, chronic renal failure, oral enzyme preparations, gastric cancer, pancreatic cancer
Decreased in: Chronic pancreatitis, late cystic fibrosis

CIRCULATING ANTICOAGULANT (lupus anticoagulant)

Normal: Negative
Detected in: Systemic lupus erythematosus, drug-induced lupus, long-term phenothiazine therapy, multiple myeloma, ulcerative colitis, rheumatoid arthritis, postpartum, hemophilia, neoplasms, chronic inflammatory states, AIDS, nephrotic syndrome
NOTE: The name is a misnomer because these patients are prone to hypercoagulability and thrombosis.

CK

See CREATINE KINASE

CLONIDINE SUPPRESSION TEST

Interpretation: Clonidine inhibits neurogenic catecholamine release and will cause a decrease in plasma norepinephrine into the reference interval in hypertensive subjects without pheochromocytoma. Test is performed by giving 4.3 mcg clonidine/kg orally after overnight fast. Norepinephrine is measured at 3 hr. Result should be within established reference range and decrease to <50% of baseline concentration. Lack of decrease in norepinephrine is suggestive of pheochromocytoma.

CLOSTRIDIUM DIFFICILE TOXIN ASSAY (stool)

Normal: Negative
Detected in: Antibiotic-associated diarrhea and pseudomembranous colitis

CO

See CARBOXYHEMOGLOBIN

COAGULATION FACTORS

See Table 4-11 for characteristics of coagulation factors.
Factor reference ranges:
V: >10%
VII: >10%
VIII: 50%-170%
IX: 60%-136%
X: >10%
XI: 50%-150%
XII: >30%
Table 4-12 describes screening laboratory results in coagulation factor deficiencies.

COLD AGGLUTININS TITER

Normal range: <1:32
Elevated in:
Primary atypical pneumonia (*Mycoplasma* pneumonia), infectious mononucleosis, CMV infection
Others: hepatic cirrhosis, acquired hemolytic anemia, frostbite, multiple myeloma, lymphoma, malaria

COMPLEMENT

Normal range:
C3: 70-160 mg/dl (0.7-1.6 g/L [CF: 0.01; SMI: 0.1 g/L])
C4: 20-40 mg/dl (0.2-0.4 g/L [CF: 0.01; SMI: 0.1 g/L])

TABLE 4-11   Characteristics of Coagulation Factors

Factor	Descriptive Name	Source	Approximate Half-Life (hr)	Function
I	Fibrinogen	Liver	120	Substrate for fibrin clot (CP)
II	Prothrombin	Liver (VKD)	60	Serine protease (CP)
V	Proaccelerin, labile factor	Liver	12-36	Cofactor (CP)
VII	Serum prothrombin conversion accelerator, proconvertin	Liver (VKD)	6	(?) Serine protease (EP)
VIII	Antihemophilic factor or globulin	Endothelial cells and (?) elsewhere	12	Cofactor (IP)
IX	Plasma thromboplastin component, Christmas factor	Liver (VKD)	24	Serine protease (IP)
X	Stuart-Prower factor	Liver (VKD)	36	Serine protease (CP)
XI	Plasma thromboplastin antecedent	(?) Liver	40-84	Serine protease (IP)
XII	Hageman factor	(?) Liver	50	Serine protease contact activation (IP)
XIII	Fibrin-stabilizing factor	(?) Liver	96-180	Transglutaminase (CP)
Prekallikrein	Fletcher factor	(?) Liver	?	Serine protease contact activation (IP)
High-molecular-weight kininogen	Fitzgerald factor, Flaujeac or Williams factor	(?) Liver	?	Cofactor, contact activation (IP)

From Noble J (ed): *Primary care medicine*, ed 3, St Louis, 2001, Mosby.
CP, Common pathway; *EP,* extrinsic pathway; *IP,* intrinsic pathway; *VKD,* vitamin K dependent.

TABLE 4-12   Screening Laboratory Results in Coagulation Factor Deficiencies

Deficient Factor	Frequency	PT	PTT	TT
I (fibrinogen)	Rare	↑	↑	↑
II (prothrombin)	Very rare	↑	↑	↑
V 1:1,000,000		↑	↑	NL
VII	1:500,000	↑	NL	NL
VIII	1:5000 (male)	NL	↑	NL
IX	1:30,000 (male)	NL	↑	NL
X 1:500,000		↑	↑	NL
XI	Rare*	NL	↑	NL
XII or HMWK or PK†	Rare	NL	↑	NL
XIII	Rare	NL	NL	NL

From Andreoli TE (ed): *Cecil essentials of medicine*, ed 5, Philadelphia, 2001, Saunders.
↑ Increased over normal range; *HMWK,* high-molecular-weight kininogen; *NL,* normal; *PK,* prekallikrein; *PT,* prothrombin time; *PTT,* partial thromboplastin time; *TT,* thrombin time.
*Except in those of Ashkenazi Jewish descent (approximately 4% are heterozygous for factor XI deficiency).
†Not associated with clinical bleeding.

Abnormal values:

Decreased C3: Active SLE, immune complex disease, acute glomerulonephritis, inborn C3 deficiency, membranoproliferative glomerulonephritis, infective endocarditis, serum sickness, autoimmune/chronic active hepatitis

Decreased C4: Immune complex disease, active SLE, infective endocarditis, inborn C4 deficiency, hereditary angioedema, hypergammaglobulinemic states, cryoglobulinemic vasculitis

COMPLEMENT DEFICIENCY

Table 4-13 describes complement deficiency states.

COMPLETE BLOOD COUNT (CBC)

See Fig. E4-11, which describes an algorithm for the evaluation of patients with neutropenia.
White blood cells 3200-9800/mm³ (3.2-9.8 × 10⁹/L [CF: 0.001; SMI: 0.1 × 10⁹/L])
Red blood cells
    Male: 4.3-5.9 × 10⁶/mm³ (4.3-5.9 × 10¹²/L [CF: 0.001; SMI: 0.1 × 10¹²/L])
    Female: 3.5-5 × 10⁶/mm³ (3.5-5 × 10¹²/L [CF: 0.001; SMI: 0.1 × 10¹²/L])
Hemoglobin
    Male: 13.6-17.7 g/dl (136-172 g/L [CF: 10; SMI: 1 g/L])
    Female: 12-15 g/dl (120-150 g/L [CF: 10; SMI: 1 g/L])

Hematocrit
    Male: 39%-49% (0.39-0.49 [CF: 0.01; SMI: 0.01])
    Female: 33%-43% (0.33-0.43 [CF: 0.01; SMI: 0.01])
Mean corpuscular volume (MCV): 76-100 μm³ (76-100 fL [CF: 1; SMI: 1 fL])
Mean corpuscular hemoglobin (MCH): 27-33 pg (27-33 pg [CF: 1; SMI: 1 pg])
Mean corpuscular hemoglobin concentration (MCHC): 33-37 g/dl (330-370 g/L [CF: 10; SMI: 10 g/L])
Red blood cell distribution width index (RDW): 11.5%-14.5%
Platelet count: 130-400 × 10³/mm³ (130-400 × 10⁹/L [CF: 1; SMI: 5 × 10⁹/L])
Differential:
    2-6 stabs (bands, early mature neutrophils)
    60-70 segs (mature neutrophils)
    1-4 eosinophils
    0-1 basophils
    2-8 monocytes
    25-40 lymphocytes

CONJUGATED BILIRUBIN

See BILIRUBIN, DIRECT

COOMBS, DIRECT

Normal: Negative
Positive: Autoimmune hemolytic anemia, erythroblastosis fetalis, transfusion reactions, drugs (α-methyldopa, penicillins, tetracycline, sulfonamides, levodopa, cephalosporins, quinidine, insulin)
False-positive: May be seen with cold agglutinins

COOMBS, INDIRECT

Normal: Negative
Positive: Acquired hemolytic anemia, incompatible cross-matched blood, anti-Rh antibodies, drugs (methyldopa, mefenamic acid, levodopa)

COPPER (serum)

Normal range: 70-140 μg/dl (11-22 μmol/L [CF: 0.1574, SMI: 0.2 μmol/L])
Decreased in: Wilson's disease, Menkes' syndrome, malabsorption, malnutrition, nephrosis, total parenteral nutrition, acute leukemia in remission
Elevated in: Aplastic anemia, biliary cirrhosis, systemic lupus erythematosus, hemochromatosis, hyperthyroidism, hypothyroidism, infection, iron deficiency anemia, leukemia, lymphoma, oral contraceptives, pernicious anemia, rheumatoid arthritis

COPPER, URINE

See URINE COPPER

TABLE 4-13 Complement Deficiency States

Component	No. of Reported Patients	Mode of Inheritance	Functional Defects	Disease Associations
Classic Pathway				
C1qrs	31	ACD	Impaired IC handling, delayed C' activation, impaired immune response	CVD, 48%; infection (encapsulated bacteria), 22%; both, 18%; healthy, 12%
C4	21	ACD	Impaired C' activation in absence of specific antibody	Infection (meningococcal), 74%; healthy, 26%
C2	109	ACD		
Alternative Pathway				
D	3	ACD	Impaired IC handling, opson/phag; granulocytosis, CTX, immune response and absent SBA	CVD, 79%; recurrent infection (encapsulated bacteria), 71%
P	70	XL		
Junction of Classic and Alternative Pathways				
C3	19	ACD	Impaired CTX; absent SBA	Infection (*Neisseria*, primarily meningococcal), 58%; CVD, 4%
Terminal Components				
C5	27	ACD	Absent SBA	Both, 1%
C6	77	ACD		Healthy, 25%
C7	73	ACD		
C8	73	ACD		
C9	165	ACD	Impaired SBA	Healthy, 91%; infection, 9%
Plasma Proteins Regulating C' Activation				
C1-INH	Many	AD	Uncontrolled generation of an inflammatory mediator on C' activation	Hereditary angioedema
H	13	Acq	Uncontrolled AP activation → low C3	CVD, 40%; CVD plus infection (encapsulated bacteria), 40%; healthy, 20%
I	14	ACD	Uncontrolled AP activation → low C3	Infection (encapsulated bacteria), 100%
Membrane proteins regulating C' activation	Many	Acq	Impaired regulation of C3b and C8 deposited on host RBCs; PMN, platelets → cell lysis	Paroxysmal nocturnal hemoglobinuria
Decay-accelerating factor				
Homologous restriction factor				
CD59	>20	ACD	Impaired PMN adhesive functions (i.e., margination), CTX, C3bi-mediated opson/phag	Infection (*Staphylococcus aureus, Pseudomonas* spp.), 100%
CR3 autoantibodies				
C3 nephritic factors	>59	Acq	Stabilize AP, convertase → low C3	MPGN, 41%; PLD, 25%; infection (encapsulated bacteria), 16%; MPGN plus PLD, 10%; PLD plus infection, 5%; MPGN plus PLD plus infection, 3%; MPGN plus infection, 2%
C4 nephritic factor		Acq	Stabilize CP, C3 convertase → low C3	Glomerulonephritis, 50%; CVD, 50%

From Mandell GL: *Mandell, Douglas, and Bennett's principles and practice of infectious diseases*, ed 6, New York, 2005, Churchill Livingstone.
ACD, Autosomal codominant; *Acq,* acquired; *AD,* autosomal dominant; *AP,* alternative pathway; *C',* complement; *CP,* classic pathway; *CTX,* chemotaxis; *CVD,* collagen-vascular disease; *IC,* immune complex, *MPGN,* membranoproliferative glomerulonephritis; *PLD,* partial lipodystrophy; *PMN,* polymorphonuclear neutrophil; *RBCs,* red blood cells; *SBA,* serum bactericidal activity; *XL,* X-linked.

CORTICOTROPIN RELEASING HORMONE (CRH) STIMULATION TEST

Normal: A dose of 0.5 mg of dexamethasone is given every 6 hours for 2 days; 2 hours after last dose 1 mcg/kg CRH is given IV. Samples are drawn after 15 min. Normally there is a twofold to fourfold increase in mean baseline concentration of ACTH or cortisol. Cortisol >1.4 mcg/L is virtually 100% specific and 100% diagnostic.

Interpretation:

Normal or exaggerated response: Pituitary Cushing's disease

No response: Ectopic ACTH-secreting tumor

A positive response to CRH or a suppressed response to high-dose dexamethasone has a 97% positive predictive value for Cushing's disease. However, a lack of response to either test excludes Cushing's disease in only 64%-78% of patients. When the tests are considered together, negative responses from both have a 100% predictive value for ectopic ACTH secretion.

CORTISOL, PLASMA

Normal range: Varies with time of collection (circadian variation):

8 AM: 4-19 μg/dl (110-520 nmol/L [CF: 27.59; SMI: 10 nmol/L])

4 PM: 2-15 μg/dl (50-410 nmol/L [CF: 27.59; SMI: 10 nmol/L])

Elevated in: Ectopic adrenocorticotropic hormone production (i.e., oat cell carcinoma of lung), loss of normal diurnal variation, pregnancy, chronic renal failure, iatrogenic, stress, adrenal or pituitary hyperplasia, or adenomas

Decreased in: Primary adrenocortical insufficiency, anterior pituitary hypofunction, secondary adrenocortical insufficiency, adrenogenital syndromes

C-PEPTIDE

Elevated in: Insulinoma, sulfonylurea administration

Decreased in: Insulin-dependent diabetes mellitus, factitious insulin administration

CPK

See CREATINE KINASE

C-REACTIVE PROTEIN

Normal range: 6.8-820 μg/dl (68-8200 μg/L [CF: 10; SMI: 10 μg/L])

Elevated in: Rheumatoid arthritis, rheumatic fever, inflammatory bowel disease, bacterial infections, myocardial infarction, oral contraceptives,

third trimester of pregnancy (acute phase reactant), inflammatory and neoplastic diseases

C-REACTIVE PROTEIN, HIGH SENSITIVITY (hs-CRP, cardio-CRP)

This is a cardiac risk marker. It is increased in patients with silent atherosclerosis years before a cardiovascular event and is independent of cholesterol level and other lipoproteins. It can be used to help stratify cardiac risk.

INTERPRETATION OF RESULTS:

Cardio-CRP result (mg/L)	Risk
0.6	Lowest risk
0.7-1.1	Low risk
1.2-1.9	Moderate risk
2.0-3.8	High risk
3.9-4.9	Highest risk
≥5.0	Results may be confounded by acute inflammatory disease. If clinically indicated, a repeat test should be performed in 2 or more weeks.

CREATINE KINASE (CK, CPK)

Fig. E4-12 describes a diagnostic approach to creatine kinase elevation.

Normal range: 0-130 U/L (0-2.16 μkat/L [CF: 0.01667; SMI: 0.01 μkat/L])

Elevated in: Myocardial infarction, myocarditis, rhabdomyolysis, myositis, crush injury/trauma, polymyositis, dermatomyositis, vigorous exercise, muscular dystrophy, myxedema, seizures, malignant hyperthermia syndrome, IM injections, cerebrovascular accident, pulmonary embolism and infarction, acute dissection of aorta

Decreased in: Steroids, decreased muscle mass, connective tissue disorders, alcoholic liver disease, metastatic neoplasms

CREATINE KINASE ISOENZYMES

CK-BB:

Elevated in: Cerebrovascular accident, subarachnoid hemorrhage, neoplasms (prostate, gastrointestinal tract, brain, ovary, breast, lung), severe shock, bowel infarction, hypothermia, meningitis

CK-MB:

Elevated in: Myocardial infarction (MI), myocarditis, pericarditis, muscular dystrophy, cardiac defibrillation, cardiac surgery, extensive rhabdomyolysis, strenuous exercise (marathon runners), mixed connective tissue disease, cardiomyopathy, hypothermia

NOTE: CK-MB exists in the blood in two subforms. MB_2 is released from cardiac cells and converted in the blood to MB_1. Rapid assay of CK-MB subforms can detect MI (CK-MB_2 ≥1.0 U/L, with a ratio of CK-MB_2/CK-MB_1 ≥1.5) within 6 hours of onset of symptoms.

Fig. 4-13 illustrates the time course of CK, AST, troponins, and LDH activity after acute MI.

CK-MM:

Elevated in: Crush injury, seizures, malignant hyperthermia syndrome, rhabdomyolysis, myositis, polymyositis, dermatomyositis, vigorous exercise, muscular dystrophy, IM injections, acute dissection of aorta

CREATININE (serum)

See Fig. 4-14.

Normal range: 0.6-1.2 mg/dl (50-110 μmol/L [CF: 88.4; SMI: 10 μmol/L])

Elevated in: Renal insufficiency (acute and chronic), decreased renal perfusion (hypotension, dehydration, congestive heart failure), urinary tract infection, rhabdomyolysis, ketonemia

Drugs (antibiotics [aminoglycosides, cephalosporins], hydantoin, diuretics, methyldopa)

Falsely elevated in: Diabetic ketoacidosis, administration of some cephalosporins (e.g., cefoxitin, cephalothin)

Decreased in: Decreased muscle mass (including amputees and older persons), pregnancy, prolonged debilitation

CREATININE CLEARANCE

Normal range: 75-124 ml/min (1.24-2.08 ml/sec [CF: 0.01667; SMI: 0.02 ml/sec])

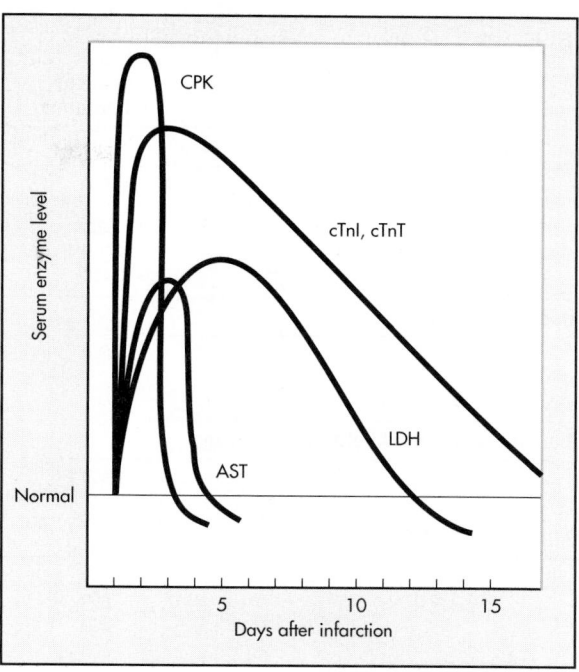

FIGURE 4-13 Evaluation of creatine kinase elevation. *CPK,* Creatine kinase; *cTnI,* cardiac troponin I; *cTnT,* cardiac troponin T; *AST,* aspartate aminotransferase; *LDH,* lactate dehydrogenase. (From Greene HL, Johnson WP, Lemcke D [eds]: *Decision making in medicine,* ed 2, St Louis, 1998, Mosby.)

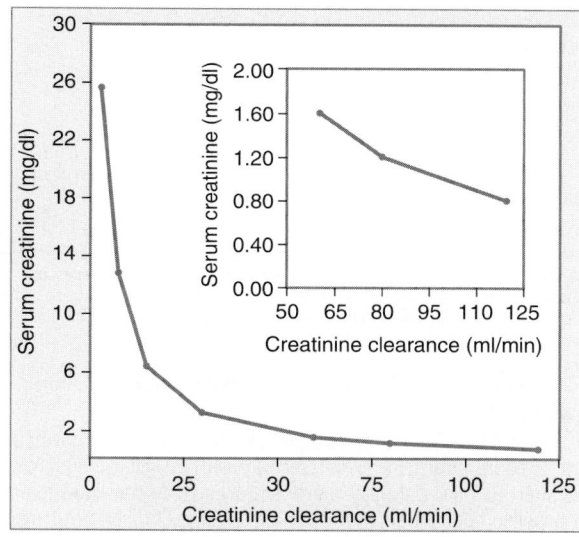

FIGURE 4-14 Relationship between creatinine clearance and serum creatinine. In steady state, serum creatinine should increase twofold for each 50% reduction in creatinine clearance. *Inset* represents enlarged view of changes in serum creatinine as creatinine clearance decreases from 120 to 60 ml/min. If serum creatinine is 0.8 mg/dl when creatinine clearance is 120 ml/min, creatinine clearance can decrease by 33% such that increased serum creatinine is still within normal range. (From Vincent JL et al: *Textbook of critical care,* ed 6, Philadelphia, 2011, Saunders.)

Box 4-1 describes a formula for calculation of creatinine clearance. The Cockcroft-Gault formula to calculate creatinine clearance is described in Box 4-2.

BOX 4-1   Calculation of the Creatinine Clearance

$C_{cr} = U_{cr} \times V/P_{cr}$
where C_{cr} = clearance of creatinine (ml/min)
   U_{cr} = urine creatinine (mg/dl)
   V = volume of urine (ml/min) (for 24-hr volume: divide by 1440)
   P_{cr} = plasma creatinine (mg/dl)
Normal range: 95 to 105 ml/min/1.75m^2

BOX 4-2   Cockcroft-Gault Formula to Calculate Creatinine Clearance (C_{cr})

$$C_{cr} = \frac{(140 - \text{age in year}) \times (\text{lean body weight in kg})}{S_{cr} \text{ in mg/dl} - 72}$$

Elevated in: Pregnancy, exercise
Decreased in: Renal insufficiency, drugs (cimetidine, procainamide, antibiotics, quinidine)

CREATININE, URINE
See URINE CREATININE

CRYOGLOBULINS (serum)
Normal range: Not detectable
Present in: Collagen vascular diseases, chronic lymphocytic leukemia, hemolytic anemias, multiple myeloma, Waldenström's macroglobulinemia, chronic active hepatitis, Hodgkin's disease

CRYPTOSPORIDIUM ANTIGEN BY EIA (stool)
Normal range: Not detected
Present in: Cryptosporidiosis

CSF
See CEREBROSPINAL FLUID

CYSTATIN C
Normal: Cystatin C is a cysteine protease inhibitor that is produced at a constant rate by all nucleated cells. It is freely filtered by the glomerulus and reabsorbed (but not secreted) by the renal tubules with no extrarenal excretion. Its concentration is not affected by diet, muscle mass, or acute inflammation. Normal range when measured by particle-enhanced nephelometric immunoassay (PENIA) is <0.28 mg/L.
Elevated in: Renal disorders. Good predictor of the severity of acute tubular necrosis. Cystatin C increases more rapidly than creatinine in the early stages of GFR impairment. The cystatin C concentration is an independent risk factor for heart failure in older adults and appears to provide a better measure of risk assessment than the serum creatinine concentration.

CYSTIC FIBROSIS PCR
Test description: Test can be performed on whole blood or tissue. Common mutations in the cystic fibrosis transmembrane regulator (CFTR) gene can be used to detect 75%-80% of mutant alleles.

CYTOMEGALOVIRUS BY PCR
Test description: Test can be performed on whole blood, plasma, or tissue. Qualitative PCR is highly sensitive but may not be able to differentiate between latent and active infection.

D-DIMER
Normal range: <0.5 mcg/ml
Elevated in:
DVT, pulmonary embolism, high levels of rheumatoid factor, activation of coagulation and fibrolytic system from any cause
D-dimer assay by ELISA assists in the diagnosis of DVT and pulmonary embolism. This test has significant limitations because it can be elevated whenever the coagulation and fibrinolytic systems are activated and can also be falsely elevated with high rheumatoid factor levels.

DEHYDROEPIANDROSTERONE SULFATE
Normal:
Males:
Ages 19-30:	125-619 mcg/dl
31-50:	59-452 mcg/dl
51-60:	20-413 mcg/dl
61-83:	10-285 mcg/dl

Females:
Ages 19-30:	29-781 mcg/dl
31-50:	12-379 mcg/dl
Postmenopausal:	30-260 mcg/dl

Elevated in: Hirsutism, congenital adrenal hyperplasia, adrenal carcinomas, adrenal adenomas, polycystic ovary syndrome, ectopic ACTH-producing tumors, Cushing's disease, spironolactone

DEHYDROTESTOSTERONE (serum, urine)
Normal:
Serum: Males: 30-85 ng/dl; females: 4-22 ng/dl
Urine, 24 h: Males: 20-50 mcg/day; females: <8 mcg/day
Elevated in: Hirsutism
Decreased in: 5-α-reductase deficiency, hypogonadism

DEOXYCORTICOSTERONE (11-deoxycorticosterone, DOC) (serum)
Normal: 2-19 ng/dl. Normal secretion depends on ACTH and is suppressible by dexamethasone.
Elevated in: Adrenogenital syndromes due to 17- and 11-hydroxylase deficiencies, pregnancy
Decreased in: Preeclampsia

DEXAMETHASONE SUPPRESSION TEST, OVERNIGHT
Normal: Test is performed by giving 1 mg dexamethasone orally at 11 PM and measuring serum cortisol at 8 AM the following morning. Normal response is cortisol suppression to <3 mcg/dl; If dose of 4 mg dexamethasone is given, cortisol suppression will be to <50% of baseline.
Interpretation: Cushing's syndrome (>10 mcg/dl), endogenous depression (half of patients suppress test values >5 mcg/dl). Most patients with pituitary Cushing's disease demonstrate suppression, whereas patients with adrenal adenoma, carcinoma, and ectopic ACTH-producing tumors do not.

DIGOXIN
Normal therapeutic range: 0.5-2 ng/ml
Elevated in: Impaired renal function, excessive dosing, concomitant use of quinidine, amiodarone, verapamil, fluoxetine, nifedipine. Toxicity may occur at a lower blood concentration in the presence of hypokalemia, hypomagnesemia, and hypercalcemia.

DILANTIN
See PHENYTOIN

DISACCHARIDE ABSORPTION TESTS
Normal: Test is used to diagnose malabsorption due to disaccharide deficiency. It is performed by giving disaccharide orally 1 g/kg body weight to a total of 25 g. Blood is drawn at 0, 30, 60, 90, and 120 min. Normal response is a change in glucose from fasting value >30 mg/dl, inconclusive when increase is 20-30 mg/dl, abnormal when increase is <20 mg/dl. Test can also be performed by measuring air at 0, 30, 60, 90, and 120 min. Normal is H$_2$ >20 ppm above baseline level before a colonic response.

Decreased in: Disaccharide deficiency (lactose, fructose, sorbitol), celiac disease, sprue, acute gastroenetetitis

DOC

See DEOXYCORTICOSTERONE

DONATH-LANDSTEINER (D-L) TEST FOR PAROXYSMAL COLD HEMOGLOBINURIA

Normal: No hemolysis
Interpretation: Hemolysis indicates presence of bithermic cold hemolysins or Donath-Landsteiner antibodies (D-L Ab)

DOPAMINE

Normal range: 175 pg/ml
Elevated in: Pheochromocytomas, neuroblastomas, stress, vigorous exercise, certain foods (bananas, chocolate, coffee, tea, vanilla)

D-XYLOSE ABSORPTION

Normal range: 21%-31% excreted in 5 hours
Decreased in: Malabsorption syndrome

D-XYLOSE ABSORPTION TEST

Normal range:
URINE: ≥4 g/5 hours (5-hour urine collection in adults >12 years [25-g dose])
SERUM: ≥25 mg/dl (adult, 1 hour, 25-g dose, normal renal function)
Normal results: In patients with malabsorption, normal results suggest pancreatic disease as an etiology of the malabsorption.
Abnormal results: Celiac disease, Crohn's disease, tropical sprue, surgical bowel resection, AIDS. False-positives can occur with decreased renal function, dehydration/hypovolemia, surgical blind loops, decreased gastric emptying, vomiting.

ELECTROPHORESIS, HEMOGLOBIN

See HEMOGLOBIN ELECTROPHORESIS

ELECTROPHORESIS, PROTEIN

See PROTEIN ELECTROPHORESIS

ENA COMPLEX

See EXTRACTABLE NUCLEAR ANTIGEN

ENDOMYSIAL ANTIBODIES

Normal: Not detected
Present in: Celiac disease, dermatitis herpetiformis

EOSINOPHIL COUNT

Normal range: 1%-4% eosinophils (0-440/mm^3)
Elevated in:
HELMINTHIC PARASITES
Ascaris lumbricoides (invasive larval stage)
Hookworms (invasive larval stage)
Strongyloides stercoralis (initial infection and autoinfection)
Trichinosis
Filariasis
Echinococcus granulosus and *E. multilocularis*
Toxocara species
Animal hookworms
Angiostrongylus cantonensis and *A. costaricensis*
Schistosomiasis
Liver flukes
Fasciolopsis buski
Anisakiasis
Capillaria philippinensis
Paragonimus westermani
"Tropical eosinophilia" (unidentified microfilariae)
OTHER INFECTIONS/INFESTATIONS
Pulmonary aspergillosis

Severe scabies
ALLERGIES
Asthma
Hay fever
Drug reactions
Atopic dermatitis
AUTOIMMUNE AND RELATED DISORDERS
Polyarteritis nodosa
Necrotizing vasculitis
Eosinophilic fasciitis
Pemphigus
NEOPLASTIC DISEASES
Hodgkin's disease
Mycosis fungoides
Chronic myelocytic leukemia
Eosinophilic leukemia
Polycythemia vera
Mucin-secreting adenocarcinomas
IMMUNODEFICIENCY STATES
Hyperimmunoglobulin E with recurrent infection
Wiskott-Aldrich syndrome
OTHER
Addison's disease
Inflammatory bowel disease
Dermatitis herpetiformis
Toxic/chemical syndrome
Eosinophilic myalgia syndrome, tryptophan, toxic oil syndrome
Hypereosinophilic syndrome (unknown etiology)

EPINEPHRINE, PLASMA

Normal range: 0-90 pg/ml
Elevated in: Pheochromocytomas, neuroblastomas, stress, vigorous exercise, certain foods (bananas, chocolate, coffee, tea, vanilla), hypoglycemia

EPSTEIN-BARR VIRUS SEROLOGY

Normal range: IgG anti-VCA <1:10 or negative
Abnormal:
IgG anti-VCA >1:10 or positive indicates either current or previous infection
IgM anti-VCA >1:10 or positive indicates current or recent infection
Anti-EBNA ≥1.5 or positive indicates previous infection
Table 4-14 and Fig. 4-15 describe test interpretation.

ERYTHROCYTE SEDIMENTATION RATE (ESR, sed rate, sedimentation rate)

Normal range:
Male: 0-15 mm/hr
Female: 0-20 mm/hr
Elevated in: Collagen vascular diseases, infections, myocardial infarction, neoplasms, inflammatory states (acute phase reactant), hyperthyroidism, hypothyroidism, rouleaux formation
Decreased in: Sickle cell disease, polycythemia, corticosteroids, spherocytosis, anisocytosis, hypofibrinogenemia, increased serum viscosity

ERYTHROPOIETIN (EP)

Normal: 3.7-16.0 IU/L by radioimmunoassay
Erythropoietin is a glycoprotein secreted by the kidneys that stimulates RBC production by acting on erythroid-committed stem cells.
Increased in:
Extremely high: Generally seen in patients with severe anemia (Hct <25, Hb, <7) such as in cases of aplastic anemia, severe hemolytic anemia, hematologic cancers
Very high: Patients with mild to moderate anemia (Hct, 25-35; Hb, 7-10)
High: Patients with mild anemia (e.g., AIDS, myelodysplasia)
Erythropoietin can be inappropriately elevated in patients with malignant neoplasms, renal cysts, postrenal transplant, meningioma, hemangioblastoma, and leiomyoma.
Decreased in: Renal failure, polycythemia vera, autonomic neuropathy

TABLE 4-14 Antibody Tests in Epstein-Barr Viral Infection

	Appearance	Peak	Disappears
Heterophil Ab	3-5 days after onset of Sx (range, 0-21 days)	During second wk after onset of Sx (1-4 wk)	2-3 mo after onset of Sx (still found at 1 yr in 20% of cases)
VCA-IgM	Beginning of Sx (1 wk before to 1 wk after Sx begin)	During first wk after onset of Sx (0-21 days)	2-3 mo after onset of Sx (1-6 mo)
VCA-IgG	3 days after onset of Sx (0-2 wk)	During second wk after onset of Sx (1-3 wk)	Decline to lower level, then persists for life
EBNA-IgG	3 wk after onset of Sx (1-4 wk)	8 mo after appearance (3-12 mo)	Lifelong
EA-D	5 days after onset of Sx (during first 1-2 wk after onset of Sx)	14-21 days after onset of Sx (1-4 wk)	9 wk after appearance (2-6 mo)
EBNA-IgM	Same as VCA-IgM	Same as VCA-IgM	Same as VCA-IgM

From Ravel R: *Clinical laboratory medicine,* ed 6, St Louis, 1995, Mosby.
Ab, Antibody; *EA,* early antigen; *EBNA,* Epstein-Barr virus nuclear antigen; *Sx,* symptoms; *VCA,* viral capsid antigen.

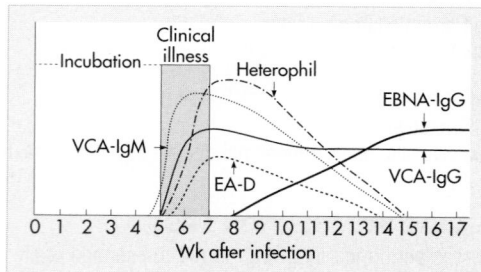

FIGURE 4-15 Tests in Epstein-Barr viral infection. See Table 4-14 for abbreviations. (From Ravel R [ed]: *Clinical laboratory medicine,* ed 6, St Louis, 1995, Mosby.)

ESTRADIOL (serum)

Normal range:
Female, premenopausal: 30-400 pg/ml, depending on phase of menstrual cycle
Female, postmenopausal: 0-30 pg/ml
Male, adult: 10-50 pg/ml
Decreased in: Ovarian failure
Elevated in: Tumors of ovary, testis, adrenal, or nonendocrine sites (rare)

ESTROGEN

Normal range (serum):
Males: 20-80 pg/ml
Females:
Follicular: 60-200 pg/ml
Luteal: 160-400 pg/ml
Postmenopausal: <130 pg/ml
Normal range (urine):
Males: 4-23 μg/g creatinine
Females:
Follicular: 7-65 μg/g creatinine
Midcycle: 32-104 μg/g creatinine
Luteal: 8-135 μg/g creatinine
Elevated in: Hyperplasia of adrenal cortex, ovarian tumors producing estrogen, granulosa and thecal cell tumors, testicular tumors
Decreased in: Menopause, hypopituitarism, primary ovarian malfunction, anorexia nervosa, hypofunction of adrenal cortex, ovarian agenesis, psychogenic stress, gonadotropin-releasing hormone deficiency

ETHANOL (blood)

Normal range:
Negative (values <10 mg/dl are considered negative)
Ethanol is metabolized at 10-25 mg/dl/hr. Levels ≥80 mg/dl are considered evidence of impairment for driving. Fatal blood concentration is considered to be >400 mg/dl.

EXTRACTABLE NUCLEAR ANTIGEN (ENA complex, anti-RNP antibody, anti-SM, anti-Smith)

Normal: Negative
Present in: Systemic lupus erythematosus, rheumatoid arthritis, Sjögren's syndrome, mixed connective tissue disease

FACTOR V LEIDEN

Test description: PCR test performed on whole blood or tissue. This single mutation, found in 2%-8% of the general Caucasian population, is the single most common cause of hereditary thrombophilia.

FASTING BLOOD SUGAR

See GLUCOSE, FASTING

FBS

See GLUCOSE, FASTING

FDP

See FIBRIN DEGRADATION PRODUCT

FECAL FAT, QUANTITATIVE (72-hr collection)

Normal range: 2-6 g/24 hr (7-21 mmol/dl [CF: 3.515; SMI: 1 mmol/dl])
Elevated in: Malabsorption syndrome

FECAL GLOBIN IMMUNOCHEMICAL TEST

Normal: Negative. This test is performed by immunochromatography on a cellulose strip that has been impregnated with various antibodies. The test uses a small amount of toilet water as the specimen and is placed onto absorbent pads of card similar to traditional OB card. There is no direct handling of stool. This test is specific for the globin portion of the hemoglobin molecule, which confers lower GI bleeding specificity. It specifically detects blood from the lower GI tract; guaic tests are not lower GI specific. It is more sensitive than typical Hemoccult test (detection limit 50 mcg Hb/g feces versus >500 mcg Hb/g feces for Hemoccult). It has no dietary restrictions and gives no false-positives due to plant peroxidases and red meats. It has no medication restrictions. Iron supplements and NSAIDs do not cause false-positives. Vitamin C does not cause false-negatives.
Positive in: Lower GI bleeding

FERRITIN (serum)

Normal range: 18-300 ng/ml (18-300 μg/L [CF: 1; SMI: 10 μg/L])
Elevated in: Hyperthyroidism, inflammatory states, liver disease (ferritin elevated from necrotic hepatocytes), neoplasms (neuroblastomas, lymphomas, leukemia, breast carcinoma), iron replacement therapy, hemochromatosis, hemosiderosis
Decreased in: Iron deficiency anemia

α-1 FETOPROTEIN

Normal range: 0-20 ng/ml (0-20 μg/L [CF: 1; SMI: 1 μg/L])
Elevated in: Hepatocellular carcinoma (usually values >1000 ng/ml), germinal neoplasms (testis, ovary, mediastinum, retroperitoneum), liver

disease (alcoholic cirrhosis, acute hepatitis, chronic active hepatitis), fetal anencephaly, spina bifida, basal cell carcinoma, breast carcinoma, pancreatic carcinoma, gastric carcinoma, retinoblastoma, esophageal atresia

FIBRIN DEGRADATION PRODUCT (FDP)

Normal range: <10 µg/ml
Elevated in: Disseminated intravascular coagulation, primary fibrinolysis, pulmonary embolism, severe liver disease
  NOTE: The presence of rheumatoid factor may cause falsely elevated FDP.

FIBRINOGEN

Normal range: 200-400 mg/dl (2-4 g/L [CF: 0.01; SMI: 0.1 g/L])
Elevated in: Tissue inflammation or damage (acute phase protein reactant), oral contraceptives, pregnancy, acute infection, myocardial infarction
Decreased in: Disseminated intravascular coagulation, hereditary afibrinogenemia, liver disease, primary or secondary fibrinolysis, cachexia

FOLATE (folic acid)

Normal range:
Plasma: 2-10 ng/ml (4-22 nmol/L [CF: 2.266; SMI: 2 nmol/L])
Red blood cells: 140-960 ng/ml (550-2200 nmol/L [CF: 2.266; SMI: 10 nmol/L])
Decreased in: Folic acid deficiency (inadequate intake, malabsorption), alcoholism, drugs (methotrexate, trimethoprim, phenytoin, oral contraceptives, Azulfidine), vitamin B_{12} deficiency (defective red cell folate absorption), hemolytic anemia
Elevated in: Folic acid therapy

FOLLICLE-STIMULATING HORMONE (FSH)

Normal range: 5-20 mIU/ml
Elevated in: Menopause, primary gonadal failure, alcoholism, castration, Klinefelter's syndrome, gonadotropin-secreting pituitary hormones
Decreased in: Pregnancy, polycystic ovary disease, anorexia nervosa, anterior pituitary hypofunction

FREE T_4

See T_4, FREE

FREE THYROXINE INDEX

Normal range: 1.1-4.3
INCREASED THYROXINE OR FREE THYROXINE VALUES
Laboratory error
Primary hyperthyroidism (T_4/T_3 type)
Severe thyroxine-binding globulin elevation
Excess therapy of hypothyroidism
Excessive dose of levothyroxine
Active thyroiditis (subacute, painless, early active Hashimoto's disease)
Familial dysalbuminemic hyperthyroxinemia (some FT_4 kits, especially analog types)
Peripheral resistance to T_4 syndrome
Amiodarone or propranolol
Postpartum transient toxicosis
Factitious hyperthyroidism
Jod-Basedow (iodine-induced) hyperthyroidism
Severe nonthyroid illness
Acute psychosis (especially paranoid schizophrenia)
T_4 sample drawn 2-4 hr after levothyroxine dose
Struma ovarii
Pituitary thyroid-stimulating hormone–secreting tumor
Certain x-ray contrast media (Telepaque and Oragrafin)
Acute porphyria
Heparin effect (some T_4 and FT_4 kits)
Amphetamine, heroin, methadone, and phencyclidine abuse
Perphenazine or 5-fluorouracil
Antithyroid or anti-IgG heterophil (HAMA) autoantibodies
"T_4" hyperthyroidism
Hyperemesis gravidarum; about 50% of patients
High altitudes

DECREASED THYROXINE OR FREE THYROXINE VALUES
Laboratory error
Primary hypothyroidism
Severe nonthyroid illness
Lithium therapy
Severe thyroxine-binding globulin decrease (congenital, disease, or drug-induced) or severe albumin decrease
Dilantin, Depakene, or high-dose salicylate drugs
Pituitary insufficiency
Large doses of inorganic iodide (e.g., saturated solution of potassium iodide)
Moderate or severe iodine deficiency
Cushing's syndrome
High-dose glucocorticoid drugs
Pregnancy, third trimester (low normal or small decrease)
Addison's disease; some patients (30%)
Heparin effect (a few FT_4 kits)
Desipramine or amiodarone drugs
Acute psychiatric illness

FTA-ABS (serum)

Normal: Nonreactive
Reactive in: Syphilis, other treponemal diseases (yaws, pinta, bejel), SLE, pregnancy

FUROSEMIDE STIMULATION TEST

Normal: Test is performed by giving 60 mg furosemide orally after overnight fast. Patient should be on a normal diet without medications the week before the test. Normal results: renin 1-6 ng angiotensin L/ml/hr.
Elevated in: Renovascular hypertension, Barrter's syndrome, high-renin essential hypertension, pheochromocytoma
No response in: Primary aldosteronism, low-renin essential hypertension, hyporeninemic hypoaldosteronism

GAMMA-GLUTAMYL TRANSFERASE (GGT)

See γ-GLUTAMYL TRANSFERASE

GASTRIN (serum)

Normal range: 0-180 pg/ml (0-180 ng/L [CF: 1; SMI: 10 ng/L])
Elevated in: Zollinger-Ellison syndrome (gastrinoma), pernicious anemia, hyperparathyroidism, retained gastric antrum, chronic renal failure, gastric ulcer, chronic atrophic gastritis, pyloric obstruction, malignant neoplasms of the stomach, H_2-blockers, omeprazole, calcium therapy, ulcerative colitis, rheumatoid arthritis

GASTRIN STIMULATION TEST

Normal: Gastrin stimulation test after calcium infusion is performed by giving a calcium infusion (15 mg Ca/kg in 500 ml normal saline over 4 hours). Serum is drawn in fasting state before infusion and at 1, 2, 3, and 4 hr. Normal response is little or no increase over baseline gastrin level.
Elevated in: Gastrinoma (gastrin >400 pg/ml), duodenal ulcer (gastrin level increase <400 ng/L)
Decreased in: Pernicious anemia, atrophic gastritis

GLIADIN ANTIBODIES, IgA AND IgG

Normal: <25 U, equivocal 20-25 U, positive >25 U. Test is useful to monitor compliance with gluten-free diet in patients with celiac disease.
Elevated in: Celiac disease with dietary noncompliance

GLOMERULAR BASEMENT MEMBRANE (gBm) ANTIBODY

Normal: Negative
Present in: Goodpasture's syndrome

GLOMERULAR FILTRATION RATE

See Box 4-3.

BOX 4-3   Common Equations for Estimating Glomerular Filtration Rate or Creatinine Clearance

Cockcoft-Gault ($C_{Cr} \cdot BSA/1.73 \ m^2$)
For men: $C_{Cr} = [(140 - age) \cdot weight \ (kg)]/S_{Cr} \cdot 72$
For women: $C_{Cr} = ([(140 - age) \cdot weight \ (kg)]/S_{Cr} \cdot 72) \cdot 0.85$

MDRD (1)
$GFR = 170 \cdot [S_{Cr}]^{-0.999} \cdot [age]^{-0.176} \cdot [0.762 \ if \ patient \ is \ female] \cdot [1.18 \ if \ patient \ is \ black] \cdot [BUN]^{-0170} \cdot [Alb]^{0.318}$

MDRD (2)
$GFR = 186 \cdot [S_{Cr}]^{-1.154} \cdot [age]^{-0.203} \cdot [0.742 \ if \ patient \ is \ female] \cdot [1.212 \ if \ patient \ is \ black]$

Jellife (1) ($C_{Cr} \cdot BSA/1.73 \ m^2$)
For men: $(98 - [0.8 \cdot (age - 20)])/S_{Cr}$
For women: $(98 - [0.8 \cdot (age - 20)])/S_{Cr} \cdot 0.90$

Jellife (2)
For men: $(100/S_{Cr}) - 12$
For women: $(80/S_{Cr}) - 7$

Mawer
For men: $weight \cdot [29.3 - (0.203 \cdot age)] \cdot [1 - (0.03 \cdot S_{Cr})]$
For women: $weight \cdot [25.3 - (0.175 \cdot age)] \cdot [1 - (0.03 \cdot S_{Cr})]$

Bjornsson
For men: $[27 - (0.173 \cdot age)] \cdot weight \cdot 0/S_{Cr}$
For women: $[25 - (0.175 \cdot age)] \cdot weight \cdot 0.07/S_{Cr}$

Gates
For men: $(89.4 \cdot S_{Cr}^{-1.2}) + (55 - age) \cdot (0.447 \cdot S_{Cr}^{-1.1})$
For women: $(89.4 \cdot S_{Cr}^{-1.2}) + (55 - age) \cdot (0.447 \cdot S_{Cr}^{-1.1})$

Salazar-Corcoran
For men: $[137 - age] \cdot [(0.285 \cdot weight) + (12.1 \cdot height^2)]/(51 \cdot S_{Cr})$
For women: $[146 - age] \cdot [(0.287 \cdot weight) + (9.74 \cdot height^2)]/(60 \cdot S_{Cr})$

From Vincent JL et al: *Textbook of critical care,* ed 6, Philadelphia, 2011, Saunders.

Normal:

Ages 20-29	116 ml/min/1.73 m²
Ages 30-39	107 ml/min/1.73 m²
Ages 40-49	99 ml/min/1.73 m²
Ages 50-59	93 ml/min/1.73 m²
Ages 60-69	85 ml/min/1.73 m²
Ages >75	75 ml/min/1.73 m²

Decreased in: Renal insufficiency, decreased renal blood flow

GLUCAGON

Normal: 20-100 pg/ml
Elevated in: Glucagonoma (900-7800 pg/ml), chronic renal failure, diabetes mellitus, glucocorticoids, insulin, nifedipine, danazol, sympathomimetic amines
Decreased in: Hyperlipoproteinemia (types III, IV), beta-blockers, secretin

GLUCOSE, FASTING (FBS, Fasting Blood Sugar)

Fig. E4-16 describes the approach to hypoglycemia. An algorithm for evaluation of hypoglycemia in children is described in Fig. E4-17.
Normal range: 60-99 mg/dl (3.8-6.0 mmol/L [CF: 0.05551; SMI: 0.1 mmol/L])
Elevated in: Diabetes mellitus, stress, infections, myocardial infarction, cerebrovascular accident, Cushing's syndrome, acromegaly, acute pancreatitis, glucagonoma, hemochromatosis, drugs (glucocorticoids, diuretics [thiazides, loop diuretics]), glucose intolerance, impaired fasting glucose
Decreased in: Sulfonylurea therapy, insulin therapy, reactive hypoglycemia (e.g., subtotal gastrectomy), starvation, insulinoma, glycogen storage disorders, severe liver disease or renal disease, ethanol-induced hypoglycemia, mesenchymal tumors that secrete insulin-like hormones

GLUCOSE, POSTPRANDIAL

Normal range: <140 mg/dl (<7.8 mmol/L [CF: 0.05551; SMI: 0.1 mmol/L])
Elevated in: Diabetes mellitus, glucose intolerance

Decreased in: Post–gastrointestinal resection, reactive hypoglycemia, hereditary fructose intolerance, galactosemia, leucine sensitivity

GLUCOSE TOLERANCE TEST

Normal values above fasting:
30 min: 30-60 mg/dl (1.65-3.3 mmol/L [CF: 0.05551; SMI: 0.1 mmol/L])
60 min: 20-50 mg/dl (1.1-2.75 mmol/L [CF: 0.05551; SMI: 0.1 mmol/L])
120 min: 5-15 mg/dl (0.28-0.83 mmol/L [CF: 0.05551; SMI: 0.1 mmol/L])
180 min: fasting level or below
Abnormal in: Glucose intolerance, diabetes mellitus, Cushing's syndrome, acromegaly, pheochromocytoma, gestational diabetes

GLUCOSE-6-PHOSPHATE DEHYDROGENASE (G6PD) SCREEN (blood)

Normal: G6PD enzyme activity detected
Abnormal: If a deficiency is detected, quantitation of G6PD is necessary; a G6PD screen may be falsely interpreted as "normal" after an episode of hemolysis because most G6PD-deficient cells have been destroyed.

γ-GLUTAMYL TRANSFERASE (GGT)

Normal range: 0-30 U/L (0.050 μkat/L [CF: 0.01667; SMI: 0.01 μkat/L])
Elevated in: Chronic alcoholic liver disease, neoplasms (hepatoma, metastatic disease to the liver, carcinoma of the pancreas), systemic lupus erythematosus, congestive heart failure, trauma, nephrotic syndrome, sepsis, cholestasis, drugs (phenytoin, barbiturates)

GLYCOHEMOGLOBIN (glycated [glycosylated] hemoglobin), (HbA$_{1c}$)

Normal range: 4.0%-5.9%
Elevated in: Uncontrolled diabetes mellitus (glycated hemoglobin levels reflect the level of glucose control over the preceding 120 days), lead toxicity, alcoholism, iron deficiency anemia, hypertriglyceridemia
Decreased in: Hemolytic anemias, decreased red blood cell survival, pregnancy, acute or chronic blood loss, chronic renal failure, insulinoma, congenital spherocytosis, hemoglobin S, C, and D diseases

GROWTH HORMONE

Normal: Male: 1-9 ng/ml; female: 1-16 ng/ml
Elevated in: Pituitary gigantism, acromegaly, ectopic GH secretion, cirrhosis, renal failure, anorexia nervosa, stress, exercise, prolonged fasting, amphetamines, beta-blockers, insulin, levodopa, metoclopramide, clonidine, vasopressin, human growth hormone (HGH) supplementation
Decreased in: Hypopituitarism, pituitary dwarfism, adrenocortical hyperfunction, bromocriptine, corticosteroids, glucose

GROWTH HORMONE RELEASING HORMONE (GHRH)

Normal: <50 pg/ml
Elevated in: Acromegaly caused by GHRH secretion by neoplasms

GROWTH HORMONE SUPPRESSION TEST (after glucose)

Normal: Test is done by giving 1.75 g glucose/kg orally after overnight fast. Blood is drawn at baseline, after 60 min, and after 120 min of glucose load. Normal response is growth hormone suppression to <2 ng/ml or undetectable levels.
Abnormal: There is no or incomplete suppression from the high basal level in gigantism or acromegaly.

HAM TEST (acid serum test)

Normal: Negative
Positive in: Paroxysmal nocturnal hemoglobinuria
False-positive in: Hereditary or acquired spherocytosis, recent transfusion with aged red blood cells, aplastic anemia, myeloproliferative syndromes, leukemia, hereditary dyserythropoietic anemia type II

HAPTOGLOBIN (serum)

Normal range: 50-220 mg/dl (0.50-2.2 g/L [CF: 0.01; SMI: 0.01 g/L])

Elevated in: Inflammation (acute phase reactant), collagen vascular diseases, infections (acute phase reactant), drugs (androgens), obstructive liver disease
Decreased in: Hemolysis (intravascular more than extravascular), megaloblastic anemia, severe liver disease, large tissue hematomas, infectious mononucleosis, drugs (oral contraceptives)

HBA₁c
See GLYCOHEMOGLOBIN

HDL
See HIGH-DENSITY LIPOPROTEIN CHOLESTEROL

HELICOBACTER PYLORI (serology, stool antigen)
Normal range: Not detected
Detected in: *H. pylori* infection. Positive serology can indicate current or past infection. Positive stool antigen test indicates acute infection (sensitivity and specificity >90%). Stool testing should be delayed at least 4 weeks after eradication therapy.

HEMATOCRIT
Normal range:
Male: 39%-49% (0.39-0.49 [CF: 0.01; SMI: 0.01])
Female: 33%-43% (0.33-0.43 [CF: 0.01; SMI: 0.01])
Elevated in: Polycythemia vera, smoking, chronic obstructive pulmonary disease, high altitudes, dehydration, hypovolemia
Decreased in: Blood loss (gastrointestinal, genitourinary) anemia

HEMOGLOBIN
Normal range:
Male: 13.6-17.7 g/dl (136-172 g/L [CF: 10; SMI: 1 g/L])
Female: 12.0-15.0 g/dl (120-150 g/L [CF: 10; SMI: 1 g/L])
Elevated in: Hemoconcentration, dehydration, polycythemia vera, chronic obstructive pulmonary disease, high altitudes, false elevations (hyperlipemic plasma, white blood cells >50,000/mm³), stress
Decreased in: Hemorrhagic (gastrointestinal, genitourinary) anemia

HEMOGLOBIN A₁c
See GLYCATED HEMOGLOBIN

HEMOGLOBIN ELECTROPHORESIS
Table 4-15 describes neonatal hemoglobin electrophoresis patterns, and Table 4-16 summarizes types of hemoglobin.
Normal range:HbA₁: 95%-98%
HbA₂: 1.5%-3.5%
HbF: <2%
HbC: absent
HbS: absent

HEMOGLOBIN, GLYCATED
See GLYCOHEMOGLOBIN

HEMOGLOBIN, GLYCOSYLATED
See GLYCOHEMOGLOBIN

HEMOGLOBIN H
See Table 4-16.
Normal: Negative
Present in: Hemoglobin H disease, alpha-thalassemia trait, unstable hemoglobin disorders

HEMOGLOBIN, URINE
See URINE HEMOGLOBIN, FREE

HEMOSIDERIN, URINE
See URINE HEMOGLOBIN, FREE

HEPARIN-INDUCED THROMBOCYTOPENIA ANTIBODIES
Normal: Antigen assay: Negative, <0.45; weak, 0.45-1.0; strong, >1.0
Elevated in: Heparin-induced thrombocytopenia

TABLE 4-15 Neonatal Hemoglobin (Hb) Electrophoresis Patterns*

FA	Fetal Hb and adult normal Hb; the normal newborn pattern.
FAV	Indicates the presence of both HbF and HbA. However, an anomalous band (V) is present, which does not appear to be any of the common Hb variants.
FAS	Indicates fetal Hb, adult normal HbA, and HbS, consistent with benign sickle cell trait.
FS	Fetal and sickle HbS without detectable adult normal HbA. Consistent with clinically significant homozygous sickle Hb genotype (S/S) or sickle β-thalassemia, with manifestations of sickle cell anemia during childhood.
FC†	Designates the presence of HbC without adult normal HbA. Consistent with clinically significant homozygous HbC genotype (C/C), resulting in a mild hematologic disorder presenting during childhood.
FSC	HbS and HbC present. This heterozygous condition could lead to the manifestations of sickle cell disease during childhood.
FAC	HbC and adult normal HbA present, consistent with benign HbC trait.
FSA	Heterozygous HbS/β-thalassemia, a clinically significant sickling disorder.
F†	Fetal HbF is present without adult normal HbA. Although this may indicate a delayed appearance of HbA, it is also consistent with homozygous β-thalassemia major, or homozygous hereditary persistence of fetal HbF.
FV†	Fetal HbF and an anomalous Hb variant (V) are present.
AF	May indicate prior blood transfusion. Submit another filter paper blood specimen when the infant is 4 mo of age, at which time the transfused blood cells should have been cleared.

From Tschudy MM, Arcara KM: *The Harriet Lane handbook,* ed 19, Philadelphia, 2012, Mosby.
NOTE: HbA: α2β2; HbF: α2γ2; HbA2: α2δ2.
*Hemoglobin variants are reported in order of decreasing abundance; for example, FA indicates more fetal than adult hemoglobin.
†Repeat blood specimen should be submitted to confirm the original interpretation.

TABLE 4-16 Types of Hemoglobin

	Hemoglobin	Structure	Comment
Normal	A	α₂β₂	97% of adult hemoglobin
	A₂	α₂δ₂	2% of adult Hb; elevated in β-thalassemia
	F	α₂γ₂	Normal Hb in fetus from 3rd to 9th month; increased in β-thalassemia
Abnormal chain production	H	β₄	Found in α-thalassemia, biologically useless
	Barts	γ₄	Found in α-thalassemia, biologically useless
Abnormal chain structure	S	α₂β₂	Substitution of valine for glutamic acid in position 6 of β chain
	C	α₂β₂	Substitution of lysine for glutamic acid in position 6 of β chain

From Ballinger A: *Kumar & Clark's essentials of clinical medicine,* ed 6, Edinburgh, 2012, Saunders.

HEPATITIS A ANTIBODY
Normal: Negative
Present in: Viral hepatitis A; can be IgM or IgG (if IgM, acute hepatitis A; if IgG, previous infection with hepatitis A)
See Fig. 4-18 for serologic tests in HAV infection.
HAV-IgM ANTIBODY
Appearance: About the same time as clinical symptoms (3-4 weeks after exposure; range, 14-60 days), or just before beginning of AST/ALT elevation (range, 10 days before to 7 days after)
Peak: About 3-4 weeks after onset of symptoms (1-6 weeks)
Becomes nondetectable: 3-4 months after onset of symptoms (1-6 months). In a few cases HAV-IgM antibody can persist as long as 12-14 months.
HAV TOTAL ANTIBODY
Appearance: About 3 weeks after IgM becomes detectable (therefore about the middle of clinical symptom period to early convalescence)
Peak: About 1-2 months after onset
Becomes nondetectable: Remains elevated for life but can somewhat slowly fall

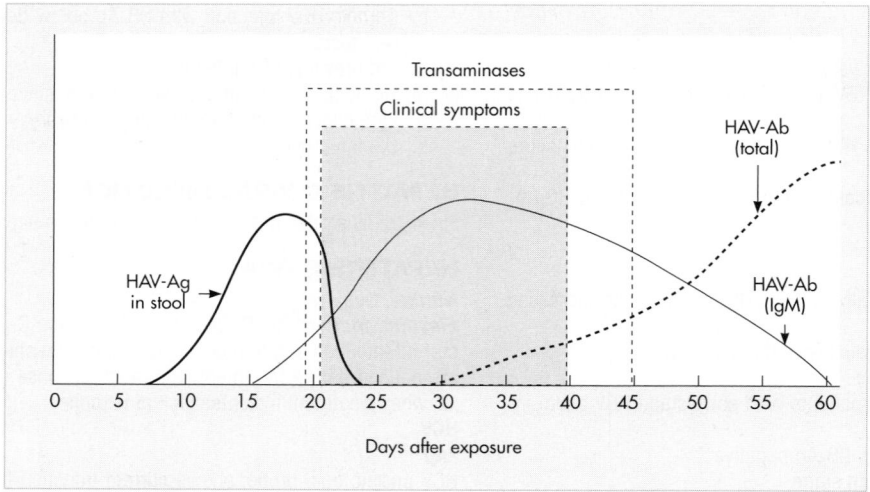

FIGURE 4-18 Serologic tests in HAV infection. (From Ravel R [ed]: *Clinical laboratory medicine,* ed 6, St Louis, 1995, Mosby.)

TABLE 4-17	Serologic Markers of Hepatitis B Infection			
	HBsAg	**anti-HBc**	**anti-HBs**	**IgM anti-HBc**
Susceptible to infection	Negative	Negative	Negative	Negative
Immune due to natural infection	Negative	Positive	Positive	Negative
Immune due to hepatitis B vaccination	Negative	Negative	Positive	Negative
Acutely infected	Positive	Positive	Negative	Positive
Chronically infected	Positive	Positive	Negative	Negative

From Ballinger A: *Kumar & Clark's essentials of clinical medicine,* ed 6, Edinburgh, 2012, Saunders.

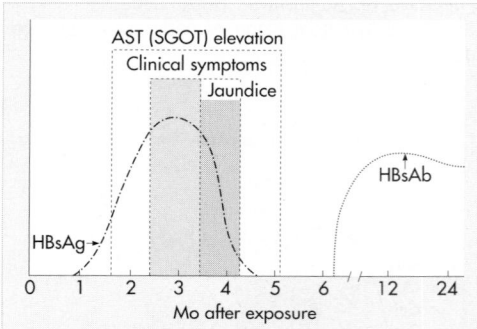

FIGURE 4-20 HBV surface antigen and antibody (HB$_S$Ag and HB$_S$Ab-total). (From Ravel R [ed]: *Clinical laboratory medicine,* ed 6, St Louis, 1995, Mosby.)

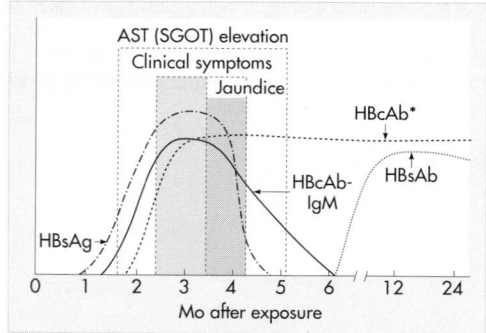

FIGURE 4-19 HBV surface antigen-antibody and core antibodies. Note "core window." *HB$_C$Ab = HB$_C$Ab-IgM + HBCAb-IgG (combined). (From Ravel R [ed]: *Clinical laboratory medicine,* ed 6, St Louis, 1995, Mosby.)

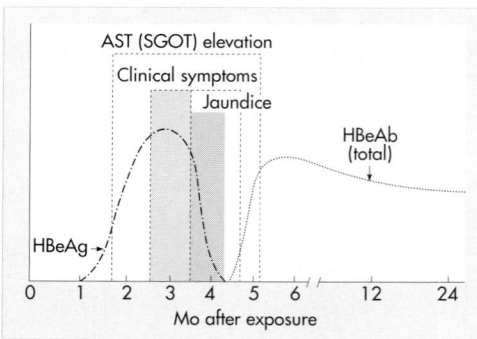

FIGURE 4-21 HBVe antigen and antibody. (From Ravel R [ed]: *Clinical laboratory medicine,* ed 6, St Louis, 1995, Mosby.)

HEPATITIS A VIRAL INFECTION

Best all-purpose test(s) to diagnose acute HAV infection = HAV-Ab (IgM)
Best all-purpose test(s) to demonstrate past HAV infection/immunity = HAV-Ab (total)

HEPATITIS B SURFACE ANTIGEN (HBsAg)

Normal: Not detected
Detected in: Acute viral hepatitis type B, chronic hepatitis B
Appearance: 2-6 weeks after exposure (range, 6 days to 6 months); 5%-15% of patients are negative at onset of jaundice
Peak: 1-2 weeks before to 1-2 weeks after onset of symptoms
Becomes nondetectable: 1-3 months after peak (range, 1 week to 5 months)

HEPATITIS B VIRAL INFECTION

See Table 4-17.
Figs. 4-19, 4-20, and 4-21 illustrate antigens and antibodies in hepatitis B infection.

HB$_S$

-Ag
HB$_S$Ag: shows current active HBV infection.
Persistence over 6 months indicates carrier/chronic HBV infection.
HBV nucleic acid probe: present before and longer than HB$_S$Ag.
More reliable marker for increased infectivity than HB$_S$Ag and/or HB$_e$Ag.

-Ab
HB$_S$Ab-total: shows previous healed HBV infection and evidence of immunity.

HB$_c$
-Ab

HB$_c$Ab-IgM: shows either acute or very recent infection by HBV.

In convalescent phase of acute HBV, may be elevated when HB$_S$Ag has disappeared (core window).

Negative HB$_c$Ab-IgM with positive HB$_S$Ag suggests either very early acute HBV or carrier/chronic HBV.

HB$_c$Ab-total: only useful to show past HBV infection if HB$_S$Ag and HB$_c$Ab-IgM are both negative.

HB$_e$
-Ag

HB$_e$-AbAg: when present, especially without HB$_e$Ab, suggests increased patient infectivity.

HB$_e$Ab-total: when present, suggests less patient infectivity.

I. HB$_S$Ag positive, HB$_c$Ab negative
   About 5% (range, 0%-17%) of patients with early-stage HBV acute infection (HB$_c$Ab rises later)
II. HB$_S$Ag positive, HB$_c$Ab positive, HB$_S$Ab negative
   a. Most of the clinical symptom stage
   b. Chronic HBV carriers without evidence of liver disease ("asymptomatic carriers")
   c. Chronic HBV hepatitis (chronic persistent type or chronic active type)
III. HB$_S$Ag negative, HB$_c$Ab positive,* HB$_S$Ab negative
   a. Late clinical symptom stage or early convalescence stage (core window)

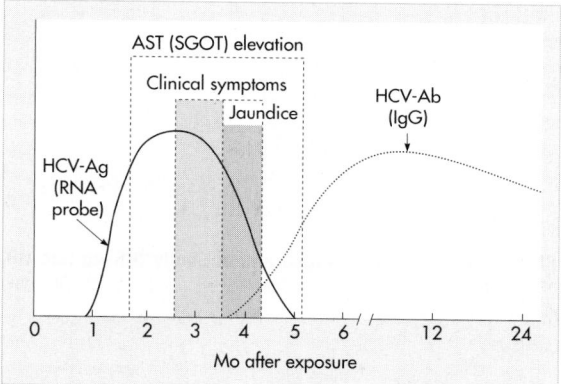

FIGURE 4-22 HCV antigen and antibody. (From Ravel R [ed]: *Clinical laboratory medicine,* ed 6, St Louis, 1995, Mosby.)

b. Chronic HBV infection with HB$_S$Ag below detection levels with current tests
c. Old previous HBV infection
IV. HB$_S$Ag negative, HB$_c$Ab positive, HB$_S$Ab positive
   a. Late convalescence to complete recovery
   b. Old infection

HEPATITIS C VIRAL INFECTION

Fig. 4-22 illustrates antigens and antibodies in hepatitis C infection.

HEPATITIS C RNA

Normal: Negative

Elevated in: Hepatitis C. Detection of hepatitis C-RNA is used to confirm current infection and to monitor treatment. Quantitative assays (viral load) are needed before treatment to assess response (<2 log decrease after 12-week treatment indicates lack of response).

HCV
-Ag

HCV nucleic acid probe: shows current infection by HCV (especially with PCR amplification).

-Ab

HCV-Ab (IgG): current, convalescent, or old HCV infection.

HAV
-Ag

HAV-Ag by EM: shows presence of virus in stool early in infection.

-Ab

HAV-Ab (IgM): current or recent HAV infection.
HAV-Ab (total): convalescent or old HAV infection.

HEPATITIS D VIRAL INFECTION

Fig. 4-23 illustrates antigens and antibodies in hepatitis D infection.
Best current all-purpose screening test = HDV-Ab (total)
Best test to differentiate acute from chronic infection = HDV-Ab (IgM)

DELTA HEPATITIS COINFECTION (acute HDV1 acute HBV) OR SUPERINFECTION (acute HDV1 chronic HBV)

HDV
-Ag

HDV-Ag: shows current infection (acute or chronic) by HDV.
HDV nucleic acid probe: detects antigen before and longer than HDV-Ag by EIA.

-Ab

HDV-Ab (IgM): high elevation in acute HDV; does not persist.
Low or moderate elevation in convalescent HDV; does not persist.

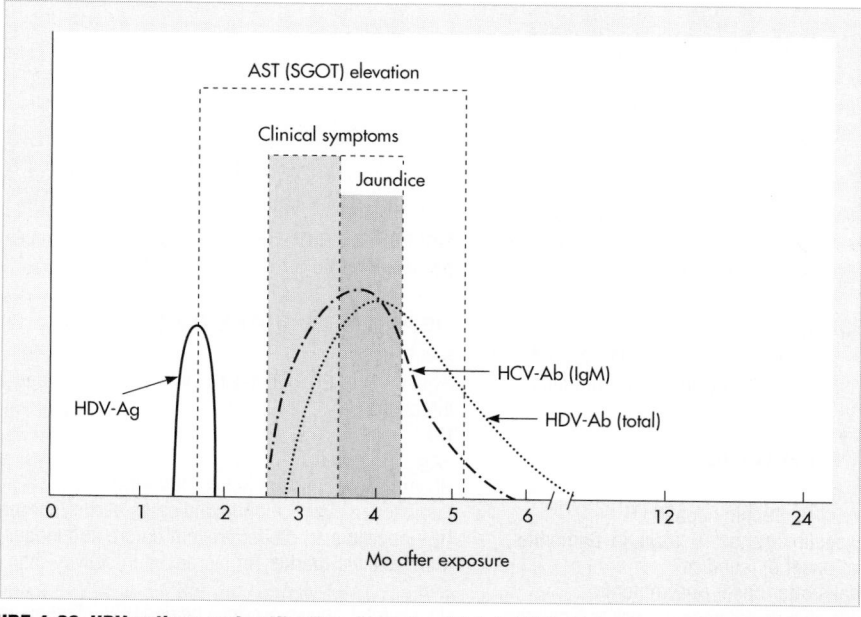

FIGURE 4-23 HDV antigen and antibodies. (From Ravel R [ed]: *Clinical laboratory medicine,* ed 6, St Louis, 1995, Mosby.)

Low to high persistent elevation in chronic HDV (depends on degree of cell injury and sensitivity of the assay).

HDV-Ab (total): high elevation in acute HDV; does not persist.

High persistent elevation in chronic HDV.

HDV-Ag

Detected by DNA probe, less often by immunoassay

Appearance: Prodromal stage (before symptoms); just at or after initial rise in ALT (about a week after appearance of HB_SAg and about the time HB_CAb-IgM level begins to rise)

Peak: 2-3 days after onset

Becomes nondetectable: 1-4 days (may persist until shortly after symptoms appear)

HDV-Ab (IgM)

Appearance: About 10 days after symptoms begin (range, 1-28 days)

Peak: About 2 weeks after first detection

Becomes nondetectable: About 35 days (range, 10-80 days) after first detection (most other IgM antibodies take 3-6 months to become nondetectable)

HDV-Ab (total)

Appearance: About 50 days after symptoms begin (range, 14-80 days); about 5 weeks after HDV-Ag (range, 3-11 weeks)

Peak: About 2 weeks after first detection

Becomes nondetectable: About 7 months after first detection (range, 4-14 months)

HER-2/NEU

Normal: Negative

Present in: 25%-30% of primary breast cancers. It can also be found in other epithelial tumors, including lung, hepatocellular, pancreatic, colon, stomach, ovarian, cervical, and bladder cancer. Trastuzumab (Herceptin) is a humanized monoclonal antibody against Her-2/*neu*. This test is useful to identify patients with metastatic; recurrent; and/or treatment refractory, unresectable, locally advanced breast cancer for trastuzumab treatment.

HERPES SIMPLEX VIRUS (HSV)

Test description: The PCR test can be performed on serum biopsy samples, CSF, vitreous humor.

HFE SCREEN FOR HEREDITARY HEMOCHROMATOSIS

Test description: PCR test can be performed on whole blood or tissue. One mutation (C282Y) and two polymorphisms (H63D, S65C) account for the majority of alleles associated with this disease.

HETEROPHIL ANTIBODY

Normal: Negative

Positive in: Infectious mononucleosis

HIGH-DENSITY LIPOPROTEIN (HDL) CHOLESTEROL

Normal range:

Male: 40-70 mg/dl (0.8-1.8 mmol/L [CF: 0.02586; SMI: 0.05 mmol/L])

Female: 50-90 mg/dl (1.1-2.35 mmol/L [CF: 0.02586; SMI: 0.05 mmol/L])

Increased in: Use of gemfibrozil, statins, fenofibrate, nicotinic acid, estrogens, regular aerobic exercise, small (1 oz) daily alcohol intake

Decreased in: Deficiency of apoproteins, liver disease, probucol ingestion, Tangier disease

NOTE: A cholesterol/HDL ratio >4.0 is associated with increased risk of coronary artery disease.

HLA ANTIGENS

Associated disorders: see Table 4-18.

HOMOCYSTEINE (plasma)

Normal range:

0-30 years: 4.6-8.1 mcmol/L

30-59 years: 6.3-11.2 mcmol/L (males), 4.5-7.9 mcmol/L (females)

>59 years: 5.8-11.9 mcmol/L

Increased: Thrombophilic states, B_6, B_{12}, folic acid, riboflavin deficiency, pregnancy, homocystinuria

NOTE: An increased homocysteine level is an independent risk factor for atherosclerosis.

HUMAN CHORIONIC GONADOTROPIN (hCG)

Normal range: Varies with gestational stage:

1 wk:	5-50 mU/ml
1-2 wk:	50-550 mU/ml
2-3 wk:	up to 5000 mU/ml
3-4 wk:	up to 10,000 mU/ml
4-5 wk:	up to 50,000 mU/ml
2-3 mo:	10,000-100,000 mU/ml

Elevated in: Normal pregnancy, hydatidiform mole, choriocarcinoma, germ cell tumors of testicle, some nontrophoblastic neoplasms (e.g., neoplasms of cervix, gastrointestinal tract, ovary, lung, breast)

HUMAN HERPES VIRUS 8 (HHV8)

Test description: PCR test can be performed on whole blood, tissue, bone marrow, and urine. HHV8 is found in all forms of Kaposi's sarcoma.

HUMAN IMMUNODEFICIENCY VIRUS ANTIBODY, TYPE 1 (HIV-1)

Normal range: Not detected

Abnormal result: HIV antibodies usually appear in the blood 1-4 months after infection.

Testing sequence:

1. ELISA is the recommended initial screening test. Sensitivity and specificity are >99%. False-positive ELISA may occur with autoimmune disorders, administration of immune globulin manufactured before 1985, within 6 weeks of testing, in the presence of rheumatoid factor, in the presence of DLA-DR antibodies in multigravida female, with administration of influenza vaccine within 3 months of testing, with hemodialysis, with positive plasma reagin test, and with certain medical disorders (hemophilia, hypergammaglobulinemia, alcoholic hepatitis).

2. A positive ELISA is confirmed with Western blot. False-positive Western blot may result from connective tissue disorders, human leukocyte antigen antibodies, polyclonal gammopathies, hyperbilirubinemia,

Laboratory Tests

IV

TABLE 4-18   HLA Antigens Associated with Specific Diseases

Antigen	Condition	Antigen	Condition
HLA-B27	Ankylosing spondylitis	HLA-B8, Dw3	Celiac disease
Reiter's syndrome	HLA-B8, Dw3	Dermatitis herpetiformis	
Psoriatic arthritis	HLA-B8	Myasthenia gravis	
HLA-A10, B18, Dw2	C2 deficiency	HLA-B8	Chronic active hepatitis in children
HLA-A2, B40, Cw3	C4 deficiency	HLA-Drw4	Active chronic hepatitis in adults
HLA-B7, Dw2	Multiple sclerosis	HLA-B13, Bw17	Psoriasis
HLA-A3	Hemochromatosis		

From Cerra FB: *Manual of critical care*, St Louis, 1987, Mosby.

HLA, Human leukocyte antigen.

presence of antibody to another human retrovirus, or cross-reaction with other non-virus-derived proteins in healthy persons. Undetermined Western blot may occur in AIDS patients with advanced immunodeficiency (caused by loss of antibodies) and in recent HIV infections.

3. PCR is used to confirm indeterminate Western blot results or negative results in persons with suspected HIV infection.

Fig. 4-24 describes tests in HIV infection; indications for plasma HIV RNA testing are described in Table 4-19.

HUMAN IMMUNODEFICIENCY VIRUS TYPE 1 (HIV-1) ANTIGEN (p24), QUALITATIVE (p24 antigen)

Normal range: Negative. This test detects uncomplexed HIV-1 p24 antigen. The core protein p24 is the first detectable protein encoded by the group-specific antigen *(gag)* gene. This protein is a marker for viremia. This test should not be used in place of HIV-1 antibody testing as a screen for HIV-1 infection. HIV-1 p24 may be detectable in the first month of acute HIV-1 infection and generally falls to undetectable levels during the asymptomatic stage of HIV-1 infection. A negative result does not exclude the possibility of infection or exposure to HIV-1. It is recommended that a negative result be followed with repeat testing at least 8 weeks after the original test. This test is used primarily for screening of donated blood and plasma and as an aid for the prognosis of HIV-1 infection.

HUMAN IMMUNODEFICIENCY VIRUS TYPE 1 (HIV-1) VIRAL LOAD

Normal range: HIV-1 RNA, quant. bDNA 3: less than 50 copies/ml or less than 1.7 log copies/ml

This test should be used only in individuals with documented HIV-1 infection for monitoring the progression of infection, response to antiretroviral therapy, and disease prognosis. It is not indicated for diagnosis of HIV infection.

HUMAN PAPILLOMA VIRUS (HPV)

Test description: PCR test can be performed on cervical smears, biopsies, scrapings, liquid cytology specimen, and anogenital tissues.

HUNTINGTON'S DISEASE PCR

Test description: PCR can be performed on whole blood. Huntington's disease is caused by the expansion of the trinucleotide repeat CAG within IT 15 (huntingtin). Pre- and post-test counseling should be performed when ordering this test.

HYDROGEN BREATH TEST

See BREATH HYDROGEN TEST

5-HYDROXYINDOLE-ACETIC ACID, URINE

See URINE 5-HYDROXYINDOLE-ACETIC ACID

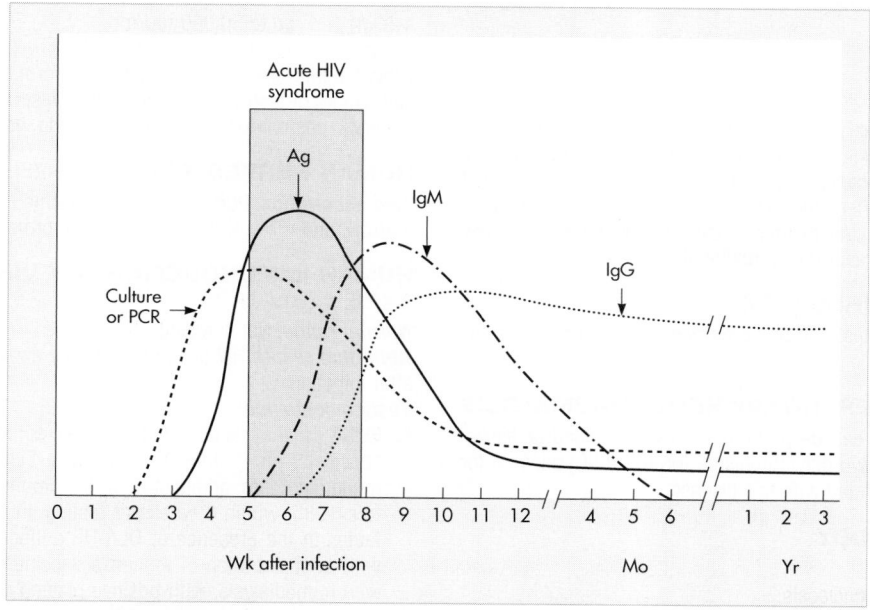

FIGURE 4-24 Tests in HIV-1 infection. (From Ravel R [ed]: *Clinical laboratory medicine,* ed 6, St Louis, 1995, Mosby.)

TABLE 4-19   Indications for Plasma HIV RNA Testing*

Clinical Indication	Information	Use
Syndrome consistent with acute HIV infection	Establishes diagnosis when HIV antibody test is negative or indeterminate	Diagnosis[†]
Initial evaluation of newly diagnosed HIV infection	Baseline viral load set point	Decision to start or defer therapy
Every 3-4 mo in patients not on therapy	Changes in viral load	Decision to start therapy
4-8 wk after initiation of antiretroviral therapy	Initial assessment of drug efficacy	Decision to continue or change therapy
3-4 mo after start of therapy	Maximal effect of therapy	Decision to continue or change therapy
Every 3-4 mo in patients on therapy	Durability of antiretroviral effect	Decision to continue or change therapy
Clinical event or significant decline in CD4+ T cells	Association with changing or stable	Decision to continue, initiate, or change

From Report of the NIH Panel to Define Principles of Therapy of HIV Infection, *MMWR Recomm Rep* 47(RR-5):1-41, 1998.

*Acute illness (e.g., bacterial pneumonia, tuberculosis, HSV, PCP) and immunizations can cause increase in plasma HIV RNA for 2-4 wk; viral load testing should not be performed during this time. Plasma HIV RNA results should usually be verified with a repeat determination before starting or making changes in therapy. HIV RNA should be measured using the same laboratory and the same assay.

[†]Diagnosis of HIV infection determined by HIV RNA testing should be confirmed by standard methods (e.g., Western blot serology) performed 2-4 mo after the initial indeterminate or negative test.

IMMUNE COMPLEX ASSAY

Normal: Negative
Detected in: Collagen vascular disorders, glomerulonephritis, neoplastic diseases, malaria, primary biliary cirrhosis, chronic acute hepatitis, bacterial endocarditis, vasculitis

IMMUNOGLOBULINS

Normal range:

IgA: 50-350 mg/dl (0.5-3.5 g/L [CF: 0.01; SMI: 0.01 g/L])
IgD: <6 mg/dl (<60 mg/L [CF: 0.01; SMI: 0.01 g/L])
IgE: <25 μg/dl (<0.00025 g/L [CF: 0.01; SMI: 0.01 g/L])
IgG: 800-1500 mg/dl (8-15 g/L [CF: 0.01; SMI: 0.01 g/L])
IgM: 45-150 mg/dl (0.45-1.5 g/L [CF: 0.01; SMI: 0.01 g/L])

Elevated in:

IgA: Lymphoproliferative disorders, Berger's nephropathy, chronic infections, autoimmune disorders, liver disease
IgE: Allergic disorders, parasitic infections, immunologic disorders, IgE myeloma
IgG: Chronic granulomatous infections, infectious diseases, inflammation, myeloma, liver disease
IgM: Primary biliary cirrhosis, infectious diseases (brucellosis, malaria), Waldenström's macroglobulinemia, liver disease

Decreased in:

IgA: Nephrotic syndrome, protein-losing enteropathy, congenital deficiency, lymphocytic leukemia, ataxia-telangiectasia, chronic sinopulmonary disease
IgE: Hypogammaglobulinemia, neoplasms (breast, bronchial, cervical), ataxia-telangiectasia
IgG: Congenital or acquired deficiency, lymphocytic leukemia, phenytoin, methylprednisolone, nephrotic syndrome, protein-losing enteropathy
IgM: Congenital deficiency, lymphocytic leukemia, nephrotic syndrome

INFLUENZA A AND B TESTS

Test description: PCR can be performed on nasopharyngeal swab, wash, or aspirate
Normal: Negative

INSULIN AUTOANTIBODIES

Normal: Negative
Present in: Exogenous insulin from insulin therapy. The presence of islet cell antibodies indicates ongoing beta cell destruction. This test is useful in the early diagnosis of type 1a diabetes mellitus and in the identification of patients at high risk for type 1a diabetes.

INSULIN, FREE

Normal: <17 mcU/ml
Elevated in: Insulin overdose, insulin resistance syndromes, endogenous hyperinsulinemia
Decreased in: Inadequately treated type 1 DM

INSULIN-LIKE GROWTH FACTOR-1 (IGF-1) (serum)

Normal range:

Ages 16-24: 182-780 ng/ml
Ages 25-39: 114-492 ng/ml
Ages 40-54: 90-360 ng/ml
Ages >55: 71-290 ng/ml

Elevated in: Adolescence, acromegaly, pregnancy, precocious puberty, obesity
Decreased in: Malnutrition, delayed puberty, diabetes mellitus, hypopituitarism, cirrhosis, old age

INSULIN-LIKE GROWTH FACTOR-II

Normal range: 288-736 ng/ml
Elevated in: Hypoglycemia associated with non–islet cell tumors, hepatoma, and Wilms' tumor
Decreased in: Growth hormone deficiency

INTERNATIONAL NORMALIZED RATIO (INR)

The INR is a comparative rating of prothrombin time (PT) ratios. The INR represents the observed PT ratio adjusted by the International Reference Thromboplastin. It provides a universal result indicative of what the patient's PT result would have been if measured using the primary World Health Organization International Reference reagent. For proper interpretation of INR values, the patient should be on stable anticoagulant therapy.

RECOMMENDED INR RANGES:

Proximal deep vein thrombosis:	2-3
Pulmonary embolism:	2-3
Transient ischemic attacks:	2-3
Atrial fibrillation:	2-3
Mechanical prosthetic valves:	2.5-3.5
Recurrent venous thromboembolic disease:	2.5-3.5

INTRINSIC FACTOR ANTIBODIES

Normal: Negative
Present in: Pernicious anemia (>50% of patients). Cyanocobalamin may give false-positive results.

IRON (serum)

Normal: Male: 65-175 mcg/dl; female: 50-1170 mcg/dl
Elevated in: Hemochromatosis, excessive iron therapy, repeated transfusions, lead poisoning, hemolytic anemia, aplastic anemia, pernicious anemia
Decreased in: Iron deficiency anemia, hypothyroidism, chronic infection

IRON-BINDING CAPACITY, TOTAL (TIBC)

Normal range: 250-460 μg/dl (45-82 μmol/L [CF: 0.1791; SMI: 1 μmol/L])
Elevated in: Iron deficiency anemia, pregnancy, polycythemia, hepatitis, weight loss
Decreased in: Anemia of chronic disease, hemochromatosis, chronic liver disease, hemolytic anemias, malnutrition (protein depletion)

Table 4-20 describes TIBC and serum iron abnormalities.

TABLE 4-20 Serum Iron and Total Iron-Binding Capacity Patterns

SI	TIBC	
SI↓	TIBC↓	Chronic diseases Uremia
SI↓	TIBC↑	Chronic iron deficiency anemia Pregnancy in third trimester
SI↑	TIBC↓	Hemachromatosis Iron therapy overload (TIBC may be normal) Hemolytic anemia; thalassemia; lead poisoning; megaloblastic anemia; aplastic, pyridoxine deficiency, or other sideroblastic anemias
SI↑	TIBC↑	Oral contraceptives Acute hepatitis (some report TIBC is low normal) Chronic hepatitis (some patients)
SI↑	TIBC NL	B₁₂ or folate deficiency
SI↓	TIBC NL	Chronic iron deficiency (some patients) Acute infection, surgery, tissue damage
SI NL	TIBC↑	B₁₂/folate deficiency plus iron deficiency

From Ravel R: *Clinical laboratory medicine,* ed 6, St Louis, 1995, Mosby.
NL, Normal; *SI,* serum iron; *TIBC,* total iron-binding capacity.

IRON SATURATION (% TRANSFERRIN SATURATION)

Normal:

Male: 20%-50%
Female: 15%-50%

Elevated in: Hemochromatosis, excessive iron intake, aplastic anemia, thalassemia, vitamin B₆ deficiency
Decreased in: hypochromic anemias, GI malignancy

Laboratory Tests

IV

LACTATE (blood)

Normal range: 0.5-2.0 mEq/L
Elevated in: Tissue hypoxia (shock, respiratory failure, severe CHF, severe anemia, carbon monoxide or cyanide poisoning), systemic disorders (liver or renal failure, seizures), abnormal intestinal flora (D-lactic acidosis), drugs or toxins (salicylates, ethanol, methanol, ethylene glycol), G6PD deficiency

LACTATE DEHYDROGENASE (LDH)

Normal range: 50-150 U/L (0.82-2.66 μkat/L [CF: 0.01667; SMI: 0.02 μkat/L])
Elevated in:
Infarction of myocardium, lung, kidney
Diseases of cardiopulmonary system, liver, collagen, central nervous system
Hemolytic anemias, megaloblastic anemias, transfusions, seizures, muscle trauma, muscular dystrophy, acute pancreatitis, hypotension, shock, infectious mononucleosis, inflammation, neoplasia, intestinal obstruction, hypothyroidism

LACTATE DEHYDROGENASE ISOENZYMES

Normal range:
LDH$_1$: 22%-36% (cardiac, red blood cell) (0.22-0.36 [CF: 0.01, SMI: 0.01])
LDH$_2$: 35%-46% (cardiac, red blood cell) (0.35-0.46)
LDH$_3$: 13%-26% (pulmonary) (0.15-0.26)
LDH$_4$: 3%-10% (striated muscle, liver) (0.03-0.1)
LDH$_5$: 2%-9% (striated muscle, liver) (0.02-0.09)
Normal ratios:
LDH$_1$<LDH$_2$
LDH$_5$<LDH$_4$
Abnormal values:
LDH$_1$>LDH$_2$: Myocardial infarction (can also be seen with hemolytic anemias, pernicious anemia, folate deficiency, renal infarct)
LDH$_5$>LDH$_4$: Liver disease (cirrhosis, hepatitis, hepatic congestion)

LACTOSE TOLERANCE TEST (serum)

Normal: Test is performed by giving 2 g/kg body weight lactose orally and drawing glucose level at 0, 30, 45, 60, and 90 min. Normal response is change in glucose from fasting value to >30 mg/dl. Inconclusive response is increase of 20-30 mg/dl, abnormal response is increase <20 mg/dl.
Abnormal in: Lactase deficiency

LAP SCORE

See LEUKOCYTE ALKALINE PHOSPHATASE

LEAD

Normal: Child, <10 mcg/dl; adult, <25 mcg/dl; acceptable for industrial exposure, <50 mcg/dl
Elevated in: Lead exposure, lead poisoning

LDH

See LACTATE DEHYDROGENASE

LDL

See LOW-DENSITY LIPOPROTEIN CHOLESTEROL

LEGIONELLA PNEUMOPHILA PCR

Test description: PCR can be performed on lung tissue, water sputum, bronchoalveolar lavage, and other respiratory fluids.

LEGIONELLA TITER

Normal: Negative
Positive in: Legionnaire's disease (presumptive: ≥1:256 titer; definitive: fourfold titer increase to ≥1:128)

LEUKOCYTE ALKALINE PHOSPHATASE (LAP)

Normal range: 13-100 (33-188 U)
Elevated in: Leukemoid reactions, neutrophilia secondary to infections (except in sickle cell crisis—no significant increase in LAP score), Hodgkin's disease, polycythemia vera, hairy cell leukemia, aplastic anemia, Down's syndrome, myelofibrosis
Decreased in: Acute and chronic granulocytic leukemia, thrombocytopenic purpura, paroxysmal nocturnal hemoglobinuria, hypophosphatemia, collagen disorders

LEUKOCYTE COUNT

See COMPLETE BLOOD COUNT

LIPASE

Normal range: 0-160 U/L (0-2.66 μkat/L [CF: 0.01667; SMI: 0.02 μkat/L])
Elevated in: Acute pancreatitis, perforated peptic ulcer, carcinoma of pancreas (early stage), pancreatic duct obstruction, bowel infarction, intestinal obstruction

LIPOPROTEIN(a)

Normal: Male: 1.35-19.6 mg/dl; female: 1.24-20.1 mg/dl
Elevated in: Coronary artery disease, uncontrolled diabetes, hypothyroidism, chronic renal failure, pregnancy, tobacco use, infections, nephritic syndrome
Decreased in: Niacin, omega-3 fatty acids, estrogens, tamoxifen, statins

LIPOPROTEIN CHOLESTEROL, HIGH-DENSITY

See HIGH-DENSITY LIPOPROTEIN CHOLESTEROL

LIPOPROTEIN CHOLESTEROL, LOW-DENSITY

See LOW-DENSITY LIPOPROTEIN CHOLESTEROL

LIVER KIDNEY MICROSOME TYPE 1 ANTIBODIES (LKM1)

Normal: <20 U
Elevated in: Autoimmune hepatitis type 2

LKM1

See LIVER KIDNEY MICROSOME TYPE 1 ANTIBODIES

LOW-DENSITY LIPOPROTEIN (LDL) CHOLESTEROL

Normal range: 50-130 mg/dl (1.30-1.68 mmol/L [CF: 0.02586; SMI: 0.05 mmol/L])

<70	Optimal in diabetics, prior MI, and patients with cardiac risk factors
100-129	Near or above optimal
130-159	Borderline high
160-189	High
≥190	Very high

LUPUS ANTICOAGULANT

See CIRCULATING ANTICOAGULANT

LUTEINIZING HORMONE

Normal range: 5-25 mIU/ml
Elevated in: Postmenopause, pituitary adenoma, primary gonadal dysfunction, polycystic ovary syndrome
Decreased in: Severe illness, anorexia nervosa, malnutrition, pituitary or hypothalamic impairment, severe stress

LYME DISEASE ANTIBODY TITER

Normal range: Negative
Positive result: Fig. 4-25 illustrates the usual serologic response in Lyme disease.
    A serologic test is not necessary or helpful for several days after a tick bite because it is only 40%-50% sensitive in this stage, and a negative test does not rule out the diagnosis.

LYMPHOCYTES

Normal range: 15%-40%
Total lymphocyte count = 800-2600/mm^3
Total T lymphocyte = 800-2200/mm^3
CD4 lymphocytes = ≥400/mm^3

CD8 lymphocytes = 200-800/mm³
    Normal CD4/CD8 ratio is 2.0.
Elevated in: Chronic infections, infectious mononucleosis and other viral infections, chronic lymphocytic leukemia, Hodgkin's disease, ulcerative colitis, hypoadrenalism, idiopathic thrombocytopenia
Decreased in:
AIDS, bone marrow suppression from chemotherapeutic agents or chemotherapy, aplastic anemia, neoplasms, steroids, adrenocortical hyperfunction, neurologic disorders (multiple sclerosis, myasthenia gravis, Guillain-Barré syndrome)
CD4 lymphocytes are calculated as total white blood cells × % lymphocytes × % lymphocytes stained with CD4. They are decreased in AIDS and other immune dysfunction.
    Table 4-21 describes various lymphocyte abnormalities in peripheral blood.

MAGNESIUM (serum)

See Fig. E4-26 for evaluation of hypermagnesemia and Fig. E4-27 for evaluation of hypomagnesemia.
Normal range: 1.8-3.0 mg/dl (0.80-1.20 mmol/L [CF: 0.4114; SMI: 0.02 mmol/L])
CAUSES OF HYPERMAGNESEMIA
I. Decreased renal excretion
    A. Renal failure—glomerular filtration rate less than 30 ml/min
    B. Hyperparathyroidism
    C. Hypothyroidism
    D. Addison's disease
    E. Lithium intoxication
    F. Familial hypocalciuric hypercalcemia
II. Other causes: usually in association with decrease in glomerular filtration rate
    A. Endogenous loads
        1. Diabetic ketoacidosis

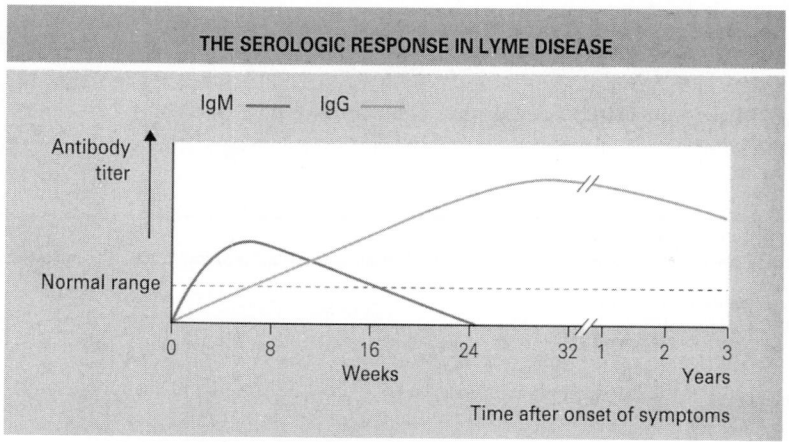

FIGURE 4-25 IgM and IgG responses in Lyme disease.

TABLE 4-21   Differential Diagnosis of Abnormal Lymphocytes in Peripheral Blood

Lymphocyte Type	Usual Disease Association	Cytologic Features	Laboratory Features	Clinical Features
Small lymphocyte	Chronic lymphocytic leukemia	B-cell surface markers with low concentration of surface immunoglobulin, CD5 antigen	Hypogammaglobulinemia in 50%; positive direct Coombs test in 15%; on node biopsy, diffuse, well-differentiated lymphocytic infiltrate	Elderly adults; presentation runs gamut from asymptomatic with lymphocytosis only to bulky disease with adenopathy, splenomegaly, and "packed" bone marrow
Atypical lymphocyte	Infectious mononucleosis, other viral illnesses	Suppressor T-cell markers	Heterophil agglutinin; positive serology for Epstein-Barr virus, cytomegalovirus, Toxoplasma, HBsAg	Pharyngitis, fever, adenopathy, rash, splenomegaly, palatal petechiae, jaundice
Plasmacytoid lymphocyte	Waldenström's macroglobulin anemia	Cytoplasmic IgM, periodic acid-Schiff positivity	IgM paraprotein, rouleaux, cryoglobulins	Adenopathy, splenomegaly, absence of bone lesions, hyperviscosity syndrome, cryopathic phenomena
Lymphoblast	ALL	Terminal transferase positivity, common ALL antigen, B- or T-precursor markers	Anemia, granulocytopenia, thrombocytopenia, hyperuricemia, diffuse bone marrow infiltration	Peak incidence in childhood, acute onset, bone pain frequent
Lymphosarcoma cell	Lymphocytic lymphoma	B-cell surface markers with high concentration of monoclonal surface immunoglobulin	Nodular or diffuse, poorly differentiated lymphocytic lymphoma on node biopsy, patchy, peritrabecular bone marrow involvement	Middle-aged to older adults, generalized adenopathy, constitutional symptoms
Sézary cell	Cutaneous lymphomas	T-lymphocyte surface markers	Skin biopsy is diagnostic	Exfoliative erythroderma, cutaneous plaques or tumors
Hairy cell	Hairy cell leukemia	B-lymphocyte markers, cytoplasmic projections, tartrate-resistant acid phosphatase, interleukin-2 receptors, CD11 antigen	Pancytopenia	Middle-aged males, moderate to marked splenomegaly without adenopathy
Prolymphocyte	Prolymphocytic leukemia	B-cell surface markers with high concentration of surface immunoglobulin, CD5 negative	Marked lymphocytosis (frequently >100 × 10⁹/L)	Elderly adults, massive splenomegaly, minimum adenopathy, poor response to therapy

From Stein JH (ed): *Internal medicine,* ed 5, St Louis, 1998, Mosby.
ALL, Acute lymphoblastic leukemia.

Laboratory Tests

IV

TABLE 4-22 Some Causes of Increased Mean Corpuscular Volume (Macrocytosis)

Causes	% of all Macrocytosis Patients*	% of Macrocytosis in Each Disease†
Common		
Folate or B_{12} deficiency	20-30 (5-50)‡	80-90 (4-100)
Chronic liver disease	15-20 (6-28)	25-30 (8-65)
Chronic alcoholism	10-12 (3-15)	60 (26-90)
Cytotoxic chemotherapy	10-15 (2-20)	30-40 (13-82)
Cardiorespiratory abnormality	8 (7-9.5)	?
Reticulocytosis	6-7 (0-15)	Depends on severity
Myelodysplastic syndromes	Frequent over age 40 yr	>60 in RAEB and RARS
Unexplained	25 (22.5-27)	—
Normal newborn		
Less Common	<4%	
Noncytotoxic drugs		
Zidovudine		
Phenytoin		30 (14-50)
Azathioprine		
Hypothyroidism		20-30 (8-55)
Chronic leukemia/myelofibrosis		
Radiotherapy for malignancy		
Chronic renal disease (occasional patients)		
Distance-runner macrocytosis (some persons)		
Down syndrome		
Artifactual (e.g., cold agglutinins)		

From Ravel R: *Clinical laboratory medicine,* ed 6, St Louis, 1995, Mosby.
RAEB, Refractory anemia with excessive blasts; *RARS,* refractory anemia with ring sideroblasts (formerly called "IASA," or idiopathic acquired sideroblastic anemia).
*Percentage of all patients with macrocytosis.
†Percentage of patients with each condition listed who have macrocytosis.
‡Numbers in parentheses are literature range.

    2. Severe tissue injury—burns
  B. Exogenous loads
    1. Gastrointestinal
      a. Magnesium-containing laxatives and antacids
      b. High-dose vitamin D analogs
    2. Parenteral: management of toxemia of pregnancy

CAUSES OF HYPOMAGNESEMIA
Alcoholic abuse
Diuretic use
Renal losses
Acute and chronic renal failure
Postobstructive diuresis
Acute tubular necrosis
Chronic glomerulonephritis
Chronic pyelonephritis
Interstitial nephropathy
Renal transplantation
Gastrointestinal losses
Chronic diarrhea
Nasogastric suctioning
Short bowel syndrome
Protein-calorie malnutrition
Bowel fistula
Total parenteral nutrition
Acute pancreatitis
Endocrine
Diabetes mellitus
Hyperaldosteronism
Hyperthyroidism
Hyperparathyroidism
Acute intermittent porphyria
Pregnancy
Drugs
Aminoglycosides
Amphotericin
β-agonists
Cisplatin
Cyclosporine
Diuretics
Foscarnet
Pentamidine
Theophylline
Congenital disorders
Familial hypomagnesemia
Maternal diabetes
Maternal hypothyroidism
Maternal hyperparathyroidism

MEAN CORPUSCULAR VOLUME (MCV)
Normal range: 76-100 μm^3 (76-100 fL) (76-100 fL [CF: 1; SMI: 1 fL])
  See Tables 4-22 and 4-23 for descriptions of MCV abnormalities.

TABLE 4-23 Some Causes of Decreased Mean Corpuscular Volume (Microcytosis)

Common	Less Common
Chronic iron deficiency	Some cases of polycythemia
α- or β-thalassemia (minor)	Some cases of lead poisoning
Anemia of chronic disease	Some cases of congenital spherocytosis
	Some cases of sideroblastic anemia
	Certain abnormal hemoglobins (HbE, Hb Lepore)

From Ravel R: *Clinical laboratory medicine,* ed 6, St Louis, 1995, Mosby.

METANEPHRINES, URINE
See URINE METANEPHRINES

METHYLMALONIC ACID (serum)
Normal: <0.2 mcmol/L
Elevated in: Vitamin B_{12} deficiency, pregnancy, methylmalonic acidemia

MITOCHONDRIAL ANTIBODY (AMA)
Normal: Negative
Present in: Primary biliary cirrhosis (>90% of patients)

MONOCYTE COUNT
Normal range: 2%-8%
Elevated in: Viral diseases, parasites, infections, neoplasms, inflammatory bowel disease, monocytic leukemia, lymphomas, myeloma, sarcoidosis
Decreased in: Aplastic anemia, lymphocytic leukemia, glucocorticoid administration

MYCOPLASMA PNEUMONIAE PCR
Test description: PCR can be performed on sputum, bronchoalveolar lavage, nasopharyngeal and throat swabs, other respiratory fluids, and lung tissue

MYELIN BASIC PROTEIN, CEREBROSPINAL FLUID
Normal: <2.5 ng/ml
Elevated in: Multiple sclerosis, CNS trauma, stroke, encephalitis

MYOGLOBIN, URINE
See URINE MYOGLOBIN

NEISSERIA GONORRHOEAE PCR
Test description: Test can be performed on endocervical swab, urine, and intraurethral swab
Normal: Negative

NEUTROPHIL COUNT
Normal range: 50%-70%
Subsets:
Stabs (bands, early mature neutrophils): 2%-6%
Segs (mature neutrophils): 60%-70%
Elevated in: Acute bacterial infections, acute myocardial infarction, stress, neoplasms, myelocytic leukemia
Decreased in: Viral infections, aplastic anemias, immunosuppressive drugs, radiation therapy to bone marrow, agranulocytosis, drugs (antibiotics, antithyroidals, clopidogrel), lymphocytic and monocytic leukemias
Box 4-4 describes various drugs that can cause neutropenia.

BOX 4-4   Drugs That Cause Neutropenia

Antiarrhythmics: tocainide, procainamide, propranolol, quinidine
Antibiotics: chloramphenicol, penicillins, sulfonamides, *p*-aminosalicylic acid (PAS), rifampin, vancomycin, isoniazid, nitrofurantoin
Antimalarials: dapsone, quinine, pyrimethamine
Anticonvulsants: phenytoin, mephenytoin, trimethadione, ethosuximide, carbamazepine
Hypoglycemic agents: tolbutamide, chlorpropamide
Antihistamines: cimetidine, brompheniramine, tripelennamine
Antihypertensives: methyldopa, captopril
Anti-inflammatory agents: aminopyrine, phenylbutazone, gold salts, ibuprofen, indomethacin
Antithyroid agents: propylthiouracil, methimazole, thiouracil
Diuretics: acetazolamide, hydrochlorothiazide, chlorthalidone
Phenothiazines: chlorpromazine, promazine, prochlorperazine
Immunosuppressive agents: antimetabolites
Cytotoxic agents: alkylating agents, antimetabolites, anthracyclines, *Vinca* alkaloids, cisplatin, hydroxyurea, dactinomycin
Other agents: recombinant interferons, allopurinol, ethanol, levamisole, penicillamine, zidovudine, streptokinase, carbamazepine, clopidogrel, ticlopidine

Modified from Goldman L, Ausiello D (eds): *Cecil textbook of medicine*, ed 22, Philadelphia, 2004, Saunders.

NOREPINEPHRINE
Normal range: 0-600 pg/ml
Elevated in: Pheochromocytomas, neuroblastomas, stress, vigorous exercise, certain foods (bananas, chocolate, coffee, tea, vanilla)

5'-NUCLEOTIDASE
Normal range: 2-16 IU/L (3-27 × 10^8 kat/L [CF: 1.67 × 10^8; SMI: 1 × 10^8 kat/L])
Elevated in: Biliary obstruction, metastatic neoplasms to liver, primary biliary cirrhosis, renal failure, pancreatic carcinoma, chronic active hepatitis

OSMOLALITY (serum)
Normal range: 280-300 mOsm/kg (280-300 mmol/kg [CF: 1; SMI: 1 mmol/kg])
It can also be estimated by the following formula:

$$2([Na] + [K]) + glucose/18 + BUN/2.8$$

Elevated in: Dehydration, hypernatremia, diabetes insipidus, uremia, hyperglycemia, mannitol therapy, ingestion of toxins (ethylene glycol, methanol, ethanol), hypercalcemia, diuretics
Decreased in: Syndrome of inappropriate diuretic hormone secretion, hyponatremia, overhydration, Addison's disease, hypothyroidism

OSMOLALITY, URINE
See URINE OSMOLALITY

OSMOTIC FRAGILITY TEST
Normal: Hemolysis begins at 0.50, w/v [5.0 g/L] and is complete at 0.30, w/v [3.0 g/L] NaCl.
Elevated in: Hereditary spherocytosis, hereditary stomatocytosis, spherocytosis associated with acquired immune hemolytic anemia
Decreased in: Iron deficiency anemia, thalassemias, liver disease, leptocytosis associated with asplenia

PARACENTESIS FLUID
Testing and evaluation of results:
1. Process the fluid as follows:
   a. Tube 1: LDH, glucose, albumin
   b. Tube 2: protein, specific gravity
   c. Tube 3: cell count and differential
   d. Tube 4: save until further notice
2. Draw serum LDH, protein, albumin.
3. Gram stain, AFB stain, bacterial and fungal cultures, amylase, and triglycerides should be ordered only when clearly indicated; bedside inoculation of blood-culture bottles with ascitic fluid improves sensitivity in detecting bacterial growth.
4. If malignant ascites is suspected, consider a carcinoembryonic antigen level on the paracentesis fluid and cytologic evaluation.
5. In suspected spontaneous bacterial peritonitis (SBP) the incidence of positive cultures can be increased by injecting 10 to 20 ml of ascitic fluid into blood culture bottles.
6. Peritoneal effusion can be subdivided as exudative or transudative based on its characteristics (see Section II).
7. The serum-ascites albumin gradient (serum albumin level–ascitic fluid albumin level [SAAG]) correlates directly with portal pressure and can also be used to classify ascites. Patients with gradients ≥1.1 g/dl have portal hypertension, and those with gradients ≤1.1 g/dl do not; the accuracy of this method is >95%.
8. For the differential diagnosis of ascites, refer to Section II.
9. An ascitic fluid polymorphonuclear leukocyte count >500/μl is suggestive of SBP.
10. A blood-ascitic fluid albumin gradient.

Laboratory Tests

IV

PARATHYROID HORMONE (PTH)
Normal:
Serum, intact molecule 10-65 pg/ml
Plasma 1.0-5.0 pmol/L
Elevated in: Hyperparathyroidism (primary or secondary), pseudohypoparathyroidism, anticonvulsants, corticosteroids, lithium, INH, rifampin, phosphates, Zollinger-Ellison syndrome, hereditary vitamin D deficiency
Decreased in: Hypoparathyroidism, sarcoidosis, cimetidine, beta-blockers, hyperthyroidism, hypomagnesemia

PARIETAL CELL ANTIBODIES
Normal: Negative
Present in: Pernicious anemia (>90%), atrophic gastritis (up to 50%), thyroiditis (30%), Addison's disease, myasthenia gravis, Sjögren's syndrome, type 1 DM

PARTIAL THROMBOPLASTIN TIME (PTT), ACTIVATED PARTIAL THROMBOPLASTIN TIME (APTT)
See Table 4-24.
Normal range: 25-41 sec
Elevated in: Heparin therapy, coagulation factor deficiency (I, II, V, VIII, IX, X, XI, XII), liver disease, vitamin K deficiency, disseminated intravascular coagulation, circulating anticoagulant, warfarin therapy, specific factor inhibition (PCN reaction, rheumatoid arthritis), thrombolytic therapy, nephrotic syndrome
NOTE: Useful to evaluate the intrinsic coagulation system.

TABLE 4-24 Clinical Peculiarities of Coagulation Protein Screening Tests

Long aPTT, normal or long PT, *no bleeding*	Normal aPTT, PT, *with bleeding*
Long APTT Only	
Factor XII deficiency	Factor XIII deficiency or inhibitor
Prekallikrein deficiency	α_2-Antiplasmin deficiency or defect
High-molecular-weight kininogen	Plasminogen activator inhibitor defiency or defect
Lupus anticoagulant	α_1-Antitrypsin Pittsburgh defect
Long APTT and PT	
Dysfibrinogenemia with fibrinopeptide B release	
Lupus anticoagulant	

From Hoffman R et al: *Hematology: basic principles and practice,* ed 5, Philadelphia, 2009, Churchill Livingstone.

PEPSINOGEN I
Normal: 124-142 ng/ml
Elevated in: ZE syndrome, duodenal ulcer, acute gastritis
Decreased in: Atrophic gastritis, gastric carcinoma, myxedema, pernicious anemia, Addison's disease

pH, BLOOD
Normal values:
Arterial: 7.35-7.45
Venous: 7.32-7.42
For abnormal values, refer to ARTERIAL BLOOD GASES.

pH, URINE
See URINE pH

PHENOBARBITAL
Normal therapeutic range: 15-30 mcg/ml for epilepsy control

PHENYTOIN (Dilantin)
Normal therapeutic range: 10-20 mcg/ml

PHOSPHATASE, ACID
See ACID PHOSPHATASE

PHOSPHATASE, ALKALINE
See ALKALINE PHOSPHATASE

PHOSPHATE (serum)
See Fig. E4-28 for approach to hyperphosphatemia and Fig. E4-29 for diagnostic evaluation of hypophosphatemia.
Normal range: 2.5-5 mg/dl (0.8-1.6 mmol/L [CF: 0.3229; SMI: 0.05 mmol/L])
DECREASED
Parenteral hyperalimentation
Diabetic acidosis
Alcohol withdrawal
Severe metabolic or respiratory alkalosis
Antacids that bind phosphorus
Malnutrition with refeeding using low-phosphorus nutrients
Renal tubule failure to reabsorb phosphate (Fanconi's syndrome; congenital disorder; vitamin D deficiency)
Glucose administration
Nasogastric suction
Malabsorption
Gram-negative sepsis
Primary hyperthyroidism
Chlorothiazide diuretics
Therapy of acute severe asthma
Acute respiratory failure with mechanical ventilation
INCREASED
Renal failure
Severe muscle injury
Phosphate-containing antacids
Hypoparathyroidism
Tumor lysis syndrome

PLASMINOGEN
Normal: Immunoassay (antigen): <20 mg/dl
Elevated in: Infection, trauma, neoplasm, myocardial infarction (acute phase reactant), pregnancy, bilirubinemia
Decreased in: DIC, severe liver disease, thrombolytic therapy with streptokinase or urokinase, alteplase

PLATELET AGGREGATION
Normal: Full aggregation (generally >60%) in response to epinephrine, thrombin, ristocetin, ADP, collagen
Elevated in: Heparin, hemolysis, lipemia, nicotine, hereditary and acquired disorders of platelet adhesion, activation, and aggregation
Decreased in: Aspirin, some penicillins, chloroquine, chlorpromazine, clofibrate, captopril, Glanzmann's thrombasthenia, Bernard-Soulier syndrome, Wiskott-Aldrich syndrome, cyclooxygenase deficiency. In von Willebrand's disease there is normal aggregation with ADP, collagen, and epinephrine but abnormal agglutination with ristocetin.

PLATELET ANTIBODIES
Normal: Absent
Present in: ITP (>90% of patients with chronic ITP). Patients with nonimmune thrombocytopenias may have false-positive results.

PLATELET COUNT
See Fig. E4-30 for evaluation of thrombocytosis. Box E4-5 describes testing for thrombocytopenia.
Normal range: 130-400 $\times 10^3$/mm^3 (130-400 $\times 10^9$/L [CF: 1; SMI: 5 $\times 10^9$/L])

Elevated in:
REACTIVE THROMBOCYTOSIS
Infections or inflammatory states—vasculitis, allergic reactions, etc.
Surgery and tissue damage—myocardial infarction, pancreatitis, etc.
Postsplenectomy state
Malignancy—solid tumors, lymphoma
Iron deficiency anemia, hemolytic anemia, acute blood loss
Uncertain etiology
Rebound effect after chemotherapy or immune thrombocytopenia
Renal disorders—renal failure, nephrotic syndrome
MYELOPROLIFERATIVE DISORDERS
Chronic myeloid leukemia
Primary thrombocythemia
Polycythemia vera
Idiopathic myelofibrosis
Decreased:
A. Increased destruction
　1. Immunologic
　　a. Drugs: quinine, quinidine, digitalis, procainamide, thiazide diuretics, sulfonamides, phenytoin, aspirin, penicillin, heparin, gold, meprobamate, sulfa drugs, phenylbutazone, NSAIDs, methyldopa, cimetidine, furosemide, INH, cephalosporins, chlorpropamide, organic arsenicals, chloroquine
　　b. Idiopathic thrombocytopenic purpura
　　c. Transfusion reaction: transfusion of platelets with platelet antigen HPA-1a (PL^{A1}) in recipients without PL^{A1}
　　d. Fetal/maternal incompatibility
　　e. Vasculitis (e.g., systemic lupus erythematosus)
　　f. Autoimmune hemolytic anemia
　　g. Lymphoreticular disorders (e.g., chronic lymphocytic leukemia)
　2. Nonimmunologic
　　a. Prosthetic heart valves
　　b. Thrombotic thrombocytopenic purpura
　　c. Sepsis
　　d. Disseminated intravascular coagulation
　　e. Hemolytic-uremic syndrome
　　f. Giant cavernous hemangioma
B. Decreased production
　1. Abnormal marrow
　　a. Marrow infiltration (e.g., leukemia, lymphoma, fibrosis)
　　b. Marrow suppression (e.g., chemotherapy, alcohol, radiation)
　2. Hereditary disorders
　　a. Wiskott-Aldrich syndrome: X-linked disorder characterized by thrombocytopenia, eczema, and repeated infections
　　b. May-Hegglin anomaly: increased megakaryocytes but ineffective thrombopoiesis
　3. Vitamin deficiencies (e.g., vitamin B$_{12}$, folic acid)
C. Splenic sequestration, hypersplenism
D. Dilutional, secondary to massive transfusion

PLATELET FUNCTION ANALYSIS 100 ASSAY (PFA)

Normal: This test is a two-component assay where blood is aspirated through two capillary tubes, one of which is coated with collagen and ADP (COL/ADP) and the other with collagen and epinephrine (COL/EPI). The test measures the ability of platelets to occlude an aperture in a biologically active membrane treated with COL/ADP and COL/EPI. During the test, the platelets adhere to the surface of the tube and cause blood flow to cease. The closing time refers to the cessation of blood flow and is reported in conjunction with the hematocrit and platelet count. Hematocrit count must be >25% and platelet count >50 K/microliter for the test to be performed
　COL/ADP: 70-120 sec
　COL/EPI: 75-120 sec
Elevated in: Acquired platelet dysfunction, von Willebrand's disease, anemia, thrombocytopenia, use of aspirin and NSAIDs

POTASSIUM (serum)

Normal range: 3.5-5 mEq/L (3.5-5 mmol/L [CF: 1; SMI: 0.1 mmol/L])
CAUSES OF HYPERKALEMIA (see Fig. E4-31 for diagnostic approach to hyperkalemia, Fig. E4-32 for evaluation and treatment of hyperkalemia, and Fig. E4-33 for electrocardiographic changes in hyperkalemia.)

I. Pseudohyperkalemia
　A. Hemolysis of sample
　B. Thrombocytosis
　C. Leukocytosis
　D. Laboratory error
II. Increased potassium intake and absorption
　A. Potassium supplements (oral and parenteral)
　B. Dietary—salt substitutes
　C. Stored blood
　D. Potassium-containing medications
III. Impaired renal excretion
　A. Acute renal failure
　B. Chronic renal failure
　C. Tubular defect in potassium secretion
　　1. Renal allograft
　　2. Analgesic nephropathy
　　3. Sickle cell disease
　　4. Obstructive uropathy
　　5. Interstitial nephritis
　　6. Chronic pyelonephritis
　　7. Potassium-sparing diuretics
　　8. Miscellaneous (lead, systemic lupus erythematosus, pseudohypoaldosteronism)
　D. Hypoaldosteronism
　　1. Primary (Addison's disease)
　　2. Secondary
　　　a. Hyporeninemic hypoaldosteronism (type IV RTA)
　　　b. Congenital adrenal hyperplasia
　　　c. Drug-induced
　　　　(1) NSAIDs
　　　　(2) ACE inhibitors
　　　　(3) Heparin
　　　　(4) Cyclosporine
IV. Transcellular shifts
　A. Acidosis
　B. Hypertonicity
　C. Insulin deficiency
　D. Drugs
　　1. β-blockers
　　2. Digitalis toxicity
　　3. Succinylcholine
　E. Exercise
　F. Hyperkalemic periodic paralysis
V. Cellular injury
　A. Rhabdomyolysis
　B. Severe intravascular hemolysis
　C. Acute tumor lysis syndrome
　D. Burns and crush injuries
CAUSES OF HYPOKALEMIA
See Fig. E4-34 for diagnostic evaluation of hypokalemia.
I. Decreased intake
　A. Decreased dietary potassium
　B. Impaired absorption of potassium
　C. Clay ingestion
　D. Kayexalate
II. Increased loss
　A. Renal
　　1. Hyperaldosteronism
　　　a. Primary
　　　　(1) Conn's syndrome
　　　　(2) Adrenal hyperplasia
　　　b. Secondary
　　　　(1) Congestive heart failure
　　　　(2) Cirrhosis
　　　　(3) Nephrotic syndrome
　　　　(4) Dehydration
　　　c. Bartter's syndrome
　　2. Glycyrrhizic acid (licorice, chewing tobacco)
　　3. Excessive adrenal corticosteroids
　　　a. Cushing's syndrome

    b. Steroid therapy
    c. Adrenogenital syndrome
  4. Renal tubular defects
    a. Renal tubular acidosis
    b. Obstructive uropathy
    c. Salt-wasting nephropathy
  5. Drugs
    a. Diuretics
    b. Aminoglycosides
    c. Mannitol
    d. Amphotericin
    e. Cisplatin
    f. Carbenicillin
 B. Gastrointestinal
  1. Vomiting
  2. Nasogastric suction
  3. Diarrhea
  4. Malabsorption
  5. Ileostomy
  6. Villous adenoma
  7. Laxative abuse
 C. Increased losses from the skin
  1. Excessive sweating
  2. Burns
III. Transcellular shifts
 A. Alkalosis
  1. Vomiting
  2. Diuretics
  3. Hyperventilation
  4. Bicarbonate therapy
 B. Insulin
  1. Exogenous
  2. Endogenous response to glucose
 C. β_2-Agonists (albuterol, terbutaline, epinephrine)
 D. Hypokalemia periodic paralysis
  1. Familial
  2. Thyrotoxic
IV. Miscellaneous
 A. Anabolic state
 B. Intravenous hyperalimentation
 C. Treatment of megaloblastic anemia
 D. Acute mountain sickness

POTASSIUM, URINE
See URINE POTASSIUM

PROCAINAMIDE
Normal therapeutic range: 4-10 mcg/ml

PROGESTERONE (serum)
Normal:
Female: Follicular phase: 15-70 ng/dl
Luteal phase: 200-2500 ng/dl
Male: 15-70 ng/dl
Elevated in: Congenital adrenal hyperplasia, clomiphene, corticosterone, 11-deoxycortisol, dihydroprogesterone, molar pregnancy, lipoid ovarian tumor
Decreased in: Primary or secondary hypogonadism, oral contraceptives, ampicillin, threatened abortion

PROLACTIN
See Fig. E4-35 for the evaluation of hyperprolactinemia.
Normal range: <20 ng/ml (<20 μg/L [CF: 1; SMI: 1 μg/L])
Elevated in: Prolactinomas (level >200 highly suggestive), drugs (phenothiazines, cimetidine, tricyclic antidepressants, metoclopramide, estrogens, antihypertensives [methyldopa], verapamil, haloperidol), postpartum, stress, hypoglycemia, hypothyroidism

PROSTATE-SPECIFIC ANTIGEN (PSA)
Normal range: 0-4 ng/ml
Table 4-25 describes age-specific reference ranges for PSA.
Elevated in: Benign prostatic hypertrophy, carcinoma of prostate, prostatitis, postrectal examination, prostate trauma.
Factors affecting serum PSA are described in Table 4-26.
NOTE: Measurement of free PSA is useful to assess the probability of prostate cancer in patients with normal digital rectal examination and total PSA between 4 and 10 ng/ml. In these patients, the global risk of prostate cancer is 25%; however, if the free PSA is >25%, the risk of prostate cancer decreases to 8%, whereas if the free PSA is <10%, the risk of cancer increases to 56%. Free PSA is also useful to evaluate the aggressiveness of prostate cancer. A low free PSA percentage generally indicates a high-grade cancer, whereas a high free PSA percentage is generally associated with a slower growing tumor.
Decreased in: 5-Alpha reductase inhibitors (finasteride, dutasteride), saw palmetto use, antiandrogens

TABLE 4-25 Age-Specific Reference Ranges for PSA

Age (yr)	Serum PSA (ng/ml)		
	Whites	Japanese	African Americans
40-49	0-2.5	0-2.0	0-2.0
50-59	0-3.5	0-3.0	0-4.0
60-69	0-4.5	0-4.0	0-4.5
70-79	0-6.5	0-5.0	0-5.5

From Nseyo UO (ed): *Urology for primary care physicians*, Philadelphia, 1999, Saunders. *PSA*, Prostate-specific antigen.

TABLE 4-26 Factors Affecting Serum PSA

Factors Affecting Serum PSA	Duration of Effect
Prostate cell number	NA
Prostate size	NA
Recent ejaculation	6-48 hours
Prostate manipulation	
Vigorous massage	1 week
Cystoscopy	1 week
Prostate biopsy	4-6 weeks
Prostatitis	
Acute	3-6 months
Chronic	Unknown
Prostate cancer	NA
Drugs: finasteride*	3-6 months

From Nseyo UO (ed): *Urology for primary care physicians*, Philadelphia, 1999, Saunders. *NA*, Not applicable; *PSA*, prostate-specific antigen. *Lowers PSA for as long as patient is on the medication.

PROSTATIC ACID PHOSPHATASE
Normal: 0-0.8 U/L
Elevated in: Prostate cancer (especially in metastatic prostate cancer), BPH, prostatitis, post–prostate surgery or manipulation, hemolysis, androgens, clofibrate
Decreased in: Ketoconazole

PROTEIN (serum)
Normal range: 6-8 g/dl (60-80 g/L [CF: 10; SMI: 1 g/L])
Elevated in: Dehydration, multiple myeloma, Waldenström's macroglobulinemia, sarcoidosis, collagen vascular diseases
Decreased in: Malnutrition, low-protein diet, overhydration, malabsorption, pregnancy, severe burns, neoplasms, chronic diseases, cirrhosis, nephrosis

PROTEIN C ASSAY

See Table 4-27.
Normal: 70%-140%
Elevated in: Oral contraceptives, stanozol
Decreased in: Congenital protein C deficiency, warfarin therapy, Vitamin K deficiency, renal insufficiency, consumptive coagulopathies

TABLE 4-27   Assay Measurement in Heterozygote Protein C Deficiency

	ACTIVITY		
Type	Antigen	Amidolytic	Coagulant
I	Low	Low	Low
II	Normal	Low	Low
	Normal	Normal	Low

From Hoffman R et al: *Hematology: basic principles and practice,* ed 5, Philadelphia, 2009, Churchill Livingstone.

PROTEIN ELECTROPHORESIS (serum)

Normal range:
Albumin: 60%-75% (0.6-0.75 [CF: 0.01; SMI: 0.01])
   α-1: 1.7%-5% (0.02-0.05)
   α-2: 6.7%-12.5% (0.07-0.13)
   β: 8.3%-16.3% (0.08-0.16)
   γ: 10.7%-20% (0.11-0.2)
Albumin: 3.6-5.2 g/dl (36-52 g/L [CF: 0.01; SMI: 1 g/L])
   α-1: 0.1-0.4 g/dl (1-4 g/L)
   α-2: 0.4-1 g/dl (4-10 g/L)
   β: 0.5-1.2 g/dl (5-12 g/L)
   γ: 0.6-1.6 g/dl (6-16 g/L)
Elevated in:
Albumin: dehydration
α-1: neoplastic diseases, inflammation
α-2: neoplasms, inflammation, infection, nephrotic syndrome
β: hypothyroidism, biliary cirrhosis, diabetes mellitus
γ: See IMMUNOGLOBULINS
Decreased in:
Albumin: malnutrition, chronic liver disease, malabsorption, nephrotic syndrome, burns, systemic lupus erythematosus
α-1: emphysema (α-1 antitrypsin deficiency), nephrosis
α-2: hemolytic anemias (decreased haptoglobin), severe hepatocellular damage
β: hypocholesterolemia, nephrosis
γ: See IMMUNOGLOBULINS
   Fig. 4-36 describes serum protein electrophoretic patterns.

PROTEIN S ASSAY

See Table 4-28.

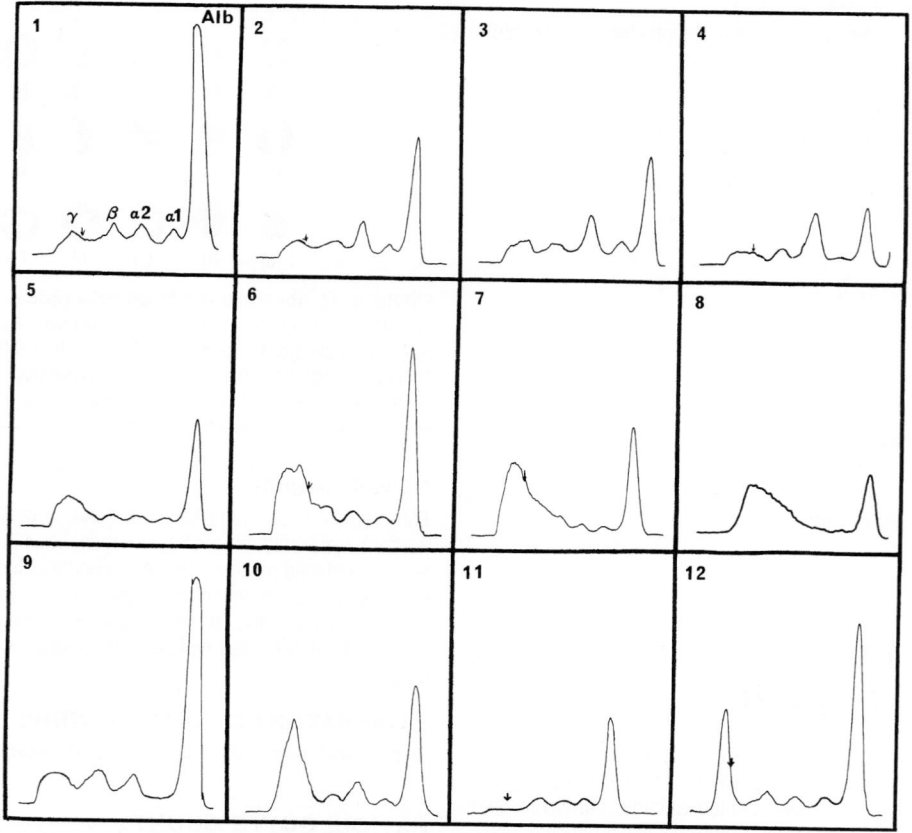

FIGURE 4-36 Typical serum protein electrophoretic patterns. *1,* Normal (*arrow* near γ region indicates serum application point). *2,* Acute reaction pattern. *3,* Acute reaction or nephrotic syndrome. *4,* Nephrotic syndrome. *5,* Chronic inflammation, cirrhosis, granulomatous diseases, rheumatoid-collagen group. *6,* Same as 5, but γ elevation is more pronounced. There is also partial (but not complete) β-γ fusion. *7,* Suggestive of cirrhosis but could be found in the granulomatous diseases or the rheumatoid-collagen group. *8,* Characteristic pattern of cirrhosis. *9,* α-1 Antitrypsin deficiency with mild γ elevation suggesting concurrent chronic disease. *10,* Same as 5, but the γ elevation is marked. The configuration of the γ peak superficially mimics that of myeloma, but is more broad-based. There are superimposed acute reaction changes. *11,* Hypogammaglobulinemia or light-chain myeloma. *12,* Myeloma, Waldenström's macroglobulinemia, idiopathic or secondary monoclonal gammopathy. (From Ravel R [ed]: *Clinical laboratory medicine,* ed 6, St Louis, 1995, Mosby.)

TABLE 4-28   Assay Measurements in Heterozygote Protein S Deficiency

	ACTIVITY		
Type	Protein S Total Antigen	Protein S Free Antigen	Protein S Activity
I (classic)	Low	Low	Low
II	Normal	Normal	Low
III	Normal	Low	Low

From Hoffman R et al: *Hematology: basic principles and practice*, ed 5, Philadelphia, 2009, Churchill Livingstone.

Normal: 65%-140%
Elevated in: Presence of lupus anticoagulant
Decreased in: Hereditary deficiency, acute thrombotic events, DIC, surgery, oral contraceptives, pregnancy, hormone replacement therapy, L-asparaginase treatment

PROTHROMBIN TIME (PT)

Normal range: 10-12 sec
Elevated in: Liver disease, oral anticoagulants (warfarin), heparin, factor deficiency (I, II, V, VII, X), disseminated intravascular coagulation, vitamin K deficiency, afibrinogenemia, dysfibrinogenemia, drugs (salicylate, chloral hydrate, diphenylhydantoin, estrogens, antacids, phenylbutazone, quinidine, antibiotics, allopurinol, anabolic steroids)
Decreased in: Vitamin K supplementation, thrombophlebitis, drugs (glutethimide, estrogens, griseofulvin, diphenhydramine)

PROTOPORPHYRIN (free erythrocyte)

Normal range: 16-36 μg/dl of red blood cells (0.28-0.64 μmol/L [CF: 0.0177; SMI: 0.02 μmol/L])
Elevated in: Iron deficiency, lead poisoning, sideroblastic anemias, anemia of chronic disease, hemolytic anemias, erythropoietic protoporphyria

PSA

See PROSTATE-SPECIFIC ANTIGEN

PT

See PROTHROMBIN TIME

PTH

See PARATHYROID HORMONE

PTT

See PARTIAL THROMBOPLASTIN TIME

RDW

See RED BLOOD CELL DISTRIBUTION WIDTH

RED BLOOD CELL (RBC) COUNT

Normal range:
Male: 4.3-5.9 $\times$ 10^6/mm^3 (4.3-5.9 $\times$ 10^{12}/L [CF: 1; SMI: 0.1 $\times$ 10^{12}/L])
Female: 3.5-5 $\times$ 10^6/mm^3 (3.5-5 $\times$ 10^{12}/L [CF: 1; SMI: 0.1 $\times$ 10^{12}/L])
Elevated in: Polycythemia vera, smokers, high altitude, cardiovascular disease, renal cell carcinoma and other erythropoietin-producing neoplasms, stress, hemoconcentration/dehydration
Decreased in: Anemias, hemolysis, chronic renal failure, hemorrhage, failure of marrow production

RED BLOOD CELL DISTRIBUTION WIDTH (RDW)

Measures variability of red cell size (anisocytosis)
Normal range: 11.5-14.5
Normal RDW and elevated mean corpuscular volume (MCV): Aplastic anemia, preleukemia

Normal MCV: Normal, anemia of chronic disease, acute blood loss or hemolysis, chronic lymphocytic leukemia (CLL), chronic myelocytic leukemia, nonanemic enzymopathy or hemoglobinopathy
Decreased MCV: Anemia of chronic disease, heterozygous thalassemia
Elevated RDW and elevated MCV: Vitamin B$_{12}$ deficiency, folate deficiency, immune hemolytic anemia, cold agglutinins, CLL with high count, liver disease
Normal MCV: Early iron deficiency, early vitamin B$_{12}$ deficiency, early folate deficiency, anemic globinopathy
Decreased MCV: Iron deficiency, red blood cell fragmentation, HbH disease, thalassemia intermedia

RED BLOOD CELL FOLATE

See FOLATE

RED BLOOD CELL MASS (volume)

Normal range:
Male: 20-36 ml/kg body weight (1.15-1.21 L/m^2 body surface area)
Female: 19-31 ml/kg body weight (0.95-1.00 L/m^2 body surface area)
Elevated in: Polycythemia vera, hypoxia (smokers, high altitude, cardiovascular disease), hemoglobinopathies with high oxygen affinity, erythropoietin-producing tumors (renal cell carcinoma)
Decreased in: Hemorrhage, chronic disease, failure of marrow production, anemias, hemolysis

RED BLOOD CELL MORPHOLOGY

See Fig. 4-37.

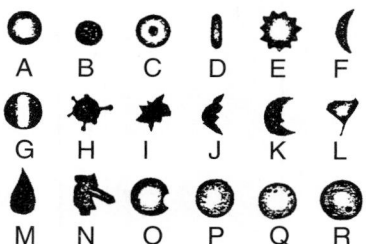

FIGURE 4-37 Abnormal red blood cells (RBCs). A, Normal RBC. **B,** Spherocyte. **C,** Target cell. **D,** Elliptocyte. **E,** Echinocyte. **F,** Sickle cell. **G,** Stomatocyte. **H,** Acanthocyte. **I to L,** Schistocytes. **M,** Teardrop RBC. **N,** Distorted RBC with Hb C crystal protruding. **O,** Degmacyte. **P,** Basophilic stippling. **Q,** Pappenheimer bodies. **R,** Howell-Jolly body. (From Ravel R [ed]: *Clinical laboratory medicine*, ed 6, St Louis, 1995, Mosby.)

RENIN (serum)

Elevated in: Drugs (thiazides, estrogen, minoxidil), chronic renal failure, Bartter's syndrome, pregnancy (normal), pheochromocytoma, renal hypertension, reduced plasma volume, secondary aldosteronism
Decreased in: Adrenocortical hypertension, increased plasma volume, primary aldosteronism, drugs (propranolol, reserpine, clonidine)
   Table 4-29 describes typical renin-aldosterone patterns in various conditions.

RESPIRATORY SYNCYTIAL VIRUS (RSV) SCREEN

Test description: PCR test can be performed on nasopharyngeal swab, wash, or aspirate

RETICULOCYTE COUNT

See Fig. E4-38 and Table 4-30.
Normal range: 0.5%-1.5%
Elevated in: Hemolytic anemia (sickle cell crisis, thalassemia major, autoimmune hemolysis), hemorrhage, postanemia therapy (folic acid, ferrous sulfate, vitamin B$_{12}$), chronic renal failure
Decreased in: Aplastic anemia, marrow suppression (sepsis, chemotherapeutic agents, radiation), hepatic cirrhosis, blood transfusion, anemias of disordered maturation (iron deficiency anemia, megaloblastic anemia, sideroblastic anemia, anemia of chronic disease)

TABLE 4-29   Typical Renin-Aldosterone Patterns in Various Conditions

	Plasma Renin	Aldosterone
Primary aldosteronism	Low	High
"Low-renin" essential hypertension	Low	Normal
Cushing's syndrome	Low	Low-normal
Licorice ingestion syndrome	Low	Low
High-salt diet	Low	Low
Oral contraceptives	High	Normal
Cirrhosis	High	High
Malignant hypertension	High	High
Unilateral renal disease	High	High
"High-renin" essential hypertension	High	High
Pregnancy	High	High
Diuretic overuse	High	High
Juxtaglomerular tumor (Bartter's syndrome)	High	High
Low-salt diet	High	High
Addison's disease	High	Low
Hypokalemia	High	Low

From Ravel R: *Clinical laboratory medicine*, ed 6, St Louis, 1995, Mosby.

TABLE 4-30   Combining the Reticulocyte Count and Red Blood Cell Parameters for Diagnosis

MCV, RDW	Reticulocyte Count <75,000/µL	Reticulocyte Count >100,000/µL
Low, Normal	Anemia of chronic disease	
Normal, Normal	Anemia of chronic disease	
High, Normal	Chemotherapy/antivirals/ alcohol	Chronic liver disease
	Aplastic anemia	
Low, High	Iron deficiency anemia	Sickle cell-β-thalassemia
Normal, High	Early iron, folate, vitamin B12 deficiency	Sickle cell anemia, sickle cell disease
	Myelodysplasia	
High, High	Folate or vitamin B12 deficiency	Immune hemolytic anemia
	Myelodysplasia	Chronic liver disease

From Hoffman R et al: *Hematology: basic principles and practice*, ed 5, Philadelphia, 2009, Churchill Livingstone.
MCV, Mean corpuscular volume; *RDW*, red blood cell distribution width.

RHEUMATOID FACTOR

Normal: Negative. Present in titer >1:20
RHEUMATIC DISEASES
Rheumatoid arthritis
Sjögren's syndrome
Systemic lupus erythematosus
Polymyositis/dermatomyositis
Mixed connective tissue disease
Scleroderma
INFECTIOUS DISEASES
Subacute bacterial endocarditis
Tuberculosis
Infectious mononucleosis
Hepatitis
Syphilis
Leprosy
Influenza
MALIGNANCIES
Lymphoma
Multiple myeloma
Waldenström's macroglobulinemia
Postradiation or postchemotherapy
MISCELLANEOUS
Normal adults, especially the elderly

Sarcoidosis
Chronic pulmonary disease (interstitial fibrosis)
Chronic liver disease (chronic active hepatitis, cirrhosis)
Mixed essential cryoglobulinemia
Hypergammaglobulinemic purpura

RNP
See EXTRACTABLE NUCLEAR ANTIGEN

ROTAVIRUS SEROLOGY
Test description: PCR test is performed on stool specimen
Normal: Negative

SED RATE
See ERYTHROCYTE SEDIMENTATION RATE

SEDIMENTATION RATE
See ERYTHROCYTE SEDIMENTATION RATE

SEMEN ANALYSIS
Table 4-31 describes semen analysis reference ranges.

TABLE 4-31   Semen Analysis Reference Ranges

Color	Grayish white
pH	7.3-7.8 (literature range, 7.0-7.8)
Volume	2.0-5.0 ml (literature range, 1.5-6.0 ml)
Sperm count	20-250 million/ml (literature range for upper limit varies from 100-250 million/ml)
Motility	>60% motile <3 hours after specimen is obtained (literature range, >40% to >70%)
% Normal sperm	>60% (literature range, >60% to >70%)
Viscosity	Can be poured from a pipet in droplets rather than a thick strand

From Ravel R (ed): *Clinical laboratory medicine*, ed 6, St Louis, 1995, Mosby.

SGOT
See ASPARTATE AMINOTRANSFERASE

SGPT
See ALANINE AMINOTRANSFERASE

SICKLE CELL TEST
Normal: Negative
Positive in: Sickle cell anemia, sickle cell trait, combination of *Hb S* gene with other disorders such as alpha-thalassemia, beta-thalassemia.

SMOOTH MUSCLE ANTIBODY
Normal: Negative
Present in: Chronic acute hepatitis (≥1:80), primary biliary cirrhosis (≤1:80), infectious mononucleosis

SODIUM (serum)
Normal range: 135-147 mEq/L (135-147 mmol/L [CF: 1; SMI: 1 mmol/L])
HYPONATREMIA
See Fig. E4-40 for the evaluation and treatment of hyponatremia. Table E4-32 describes drugs associated with hyponatremia.
A. Sodium and water depletion (deficit hyponatremia)
  1. Loss of gastrointestinal secretions with replacement of fluid but not electrolytes
    a. Vomiting
    b. Diarrhea
    c. Tube drainage
  2. Loss from skin with replacement of fluids but not electrolytes
    a. Excessive sweating
    b. Extensive burns
  3. Loss from kidney
    a. Diuretics
    b. Chronic renal insufficiency (uremia) with acidosis

4. Metabolic loss
   a. Starvation with acidosis
   b. Diabetic acidosis
5. Endocrine loss
   a. Addison's disease
   b. Sudden withdrawal of long-term steroid therapy
6. Iatrogenic loss from serous cavities
   a. Paracentesis or thoracentesis
B. Excessive water (dilution hyponatremia)
   1. Excessive water administration
   2. Congestive heart failure
   3. Cirrhosis
   4. Nephrotic syndrome
   5. Hypoalbuminemia (severe)
   6. Acute renal failure with oliguria
C. Inappropriate antidiuretic hormone (IADH) syndrome
D. Intracellular loss (reset osmostat syndrome)
E. False hyponatremia (actually a dilutional effect)
   1. Marked hypertriglyceridemia
   2. Marked hyperproteinemia
   3. Severe hyperglycemia

HYPERNATREMIA

See Fig. E4-39 for evaluation and treatment of hypernatremia. Dehydration is the most frequent overall clinical finding in hypernatremia.
1. Deficient water intake (either orally or intravenously)
2. Excess kidney water output (diabetes insipidus, osmotic diuresis)
3. Excess skin water output (excess sweating, loss from burns)
4. Excess gastrointestinal tract output (severe protracted vomiting or diarrhea without fluid therapy)
5. Accidental sodium overdose
6. High-protein tube feedings

STREPTOZYME

See ANTISTREPTOLYSIN O TITER

SUCROSE HEMOLYSIS TEST (sugar water test)

Normal: Absence of hemolysis
Positive in:
Paroxysmal nocturnal hemoglobinuria
False-positive: autoimmune hemolytic anemia, megaloblastic anemias
False-negative: may occur with use of heparin or EDTA

SUDAN III STAIN (qualitative screening for fecal fat)

Normal: Negative. Test should be preceded by diet containing 100-150 g of dietary fat/day for 1 week, avoidance of high-fiber diet, and avoidance of suppositories or oily material before specimen collection.
Positive in: Steatorrhea, use of castor oil or mineral oil droplets

SYNOVIAL FLUID ANALYSIS

Table 4-33 describes the classification and interpretation of synovial fluid analysis.

T_3 (triiodothyronine)

See Table 4-34 for T_3 abnormalities.
Normal range: 75-220 ng/dl (1.2-3.4 nmol/L [CF: 0.01536; SMI: 0.1 nmol/L])
Abnormal values:
A. Elevated in hyperthyroidism (usually earlier and to a greater extent than serum T_4).
B. Useful in diagnosing:
   1. T_3 hyperthyroidism (thyrotoxicosis): increased T_3, normal FTI.
   2. Toxic nodular goiter: increased T_3, normal or increased T_4.

TABLE 4-33 Classification and Interpretation of Synovial Fluid Analysis

Group	Diseases	Appearance	Viscosity	Mucin Clot	WBC/mm³	% PMN	Glucose (mg/dl) (Blood-Synovial Fluid)	Protein (g/dl)
Normal	—	Clear	↑	Firm	<200	<25	<10	<2.5
I (noninflammatory)	Osteoarthritis, aseptic necrosis, traumatic arthritis, erythema nodosum, osteochondritis dissecans	Clear, yellow (may be xanthochromic if traumatic arthritis)	↑	Firm	↑ Up to 10,000	<25	<10	<2.5
II (inflammatory)	Crystal-induced arthritis, rheumatoid arthritis, Reiter's syndrome, collagen vascular disease, psoriatic arthritis, serum sickness, rheumatic fever	Clear, yellow, turbid	↓	Friable	↑↑ Up to 100,000	40-90	<40	>2.5
III (septic)	Bacterial (staphylococcal, gonococcal, tuberculosis)	Turbid	↓/↑	Friable	↑↑↑ Up to 5 million	40-100	20-100	>2.5

↑, Elevated; ↑↑, markedly high; ↓, decreased; *PMN*, polymorphonuclear leukocytes. Note that there is considerable overlap in the numbers listed above.

TABLE 4-34 Findings in Thyroid Function Tests in Various Clinical Conditions

Condition	T_4	FT_4I	T_3	FT_3I	TSH	TSI	TRH Stimulation
Hyperthyroidism							
Graves' disease	↑	↑	↑	↑	↓	+	↓
Toxic nodular goiter	↑	↑	↑	↑	↓	−	↓
Pituitary TSH-secreting tumors	↑	↑	↑	↑	↑	−	↓
T_3 thyrotoxicosis	N	N	↑	↑	↓	+, −	↓
T_4 thyrotoxicosis	↑	↑	N	N	↓	+, −	↓
Hypothyroidism							
Primary	↓	↓	↓	↓	↑	+, −	↑
Secondary	↓	↓	↓	↓	↓ N	−	↓
Tertiary	↓	↓	↓	↓	↓, N	−	N
Peripheral unresponsiveness	↑, N	↑, N	↑, N	↑	↑, N	−	N, ↑

From Tilton RC, Barrows A: *Clinical laboratory medicine,* St Louis, 1992, Mosby.
↑, Increased; ↓, decreased; +, − variable; *N*, normal.

3. Iodine deficiency: normal T_3, possibly decreased T_4.
4. Thyroid replacement therapy with liothyronine (Cytomel): normal T_4, increased T_3 if patient is symptomatically hyperthyroid.

Not ordered routinely and indicated when hyperthyroidism is suspected and serum-free T_4 or FTI inconclusive.

T_3 RESIN UPTAKE (T_3RU)

Normal range: 25%-35%
Abnormal values: Increased in hyperthyroidism. T_3 resin uptake (T_3RU or RT_3U) measures the percentage of free T_4 (not bound to protein); it does not measure serum T_3 concentration; T_3RU and other tests that reflect thyroid hormone binding to plasma protein are also known as *thyroid hormone-binding ratios* (THBR).

T_4, FREE (free thyroxine)

Normal range: 0.8-2.8 ng/dl
Elevated in:

Graves' disease, toxic multinodular goiter, toxic adenoma, iatrogenic and factitious causes, transient hyperthyroidism

Serum-free T_4 directly measures unbound thyroxine. Free T_4 can be measured by equilibrium dialysis (gold standard of free T_4 assays) or by immunometric techniques (influenced by serum levels of lipids, proteins, and certain drugs). The free thyroxine index (FTI) can also be easily calculated by multiplying T_4 times T_3RU and dividing the result by 100; the FTI corrects for any abnormal T_4 values secondary to protein binding: $FTI = T_4 \times T_3RU/100$.
Normal values equal 1.1 to 4.3.

T_4, SERUM T_4

Normal range: 0.8-2.8 ng/dl (10-36 pmol/L [CF: 12.87; SMI: 1 pmol/L])
Abnormal values: Serum thyroxine (T_4)
Elevated in:

1. Graves' disease
2. Toxic multinodular goiter
3. Toxic adenoma
4. Iatrogenic and factitious
5. Transient hyperthyroidism
   a. Subacute thyroiditis
   b. Hashimoto's thyroiditis
   c. Silent thyroiditis
6. Rare causes: hypersecretion of TSH (e.g., pituitary neoplasms), struma ovarii, ingestion of large amounts of iodine in a patient with preexisting thyroid hyperplasia or adenoma (Jod-Basedow phenomenon), hydatidiform mole, carcinoma of thyroid, amiodarone therapy of arrhythmias.

Serum thyroxine test measures both circulating thyroxine bound to protein (represents >99% of circulating T_4) and unbound (free) thyroxine. Values vary with protein binding; changes in the concentration of T_4 secondary to changes in thyroxine-binding globulin (TBG) can be caused by the following:

Increased TBG ($\uparrow T_4$)	Decreased TBG ($\downarrow T_4$)
Pregnancy	Androgens, glucocorticoids
Estrogens	Nephrotic syndrome, cirrhosis
Acute infectious	Acromegaly
hepatitis	Hypoproteinemia
Oral contraceptives	Familial
Familial	Phenytoin, ASA and other NSAIDs, heroin,
Fluorouracil, clofibrate	methadone, high-dose penicillin,
	asparaginase
	Chronic debilitating illness

To eliminate the suspected influence of protein binding on thyroxine values, two additional tests are available: T_3 resin uptake and serum free thyroxine.

TEGRETOL

See CARBAMAZEPINE.

TESTOSTERONE (total testosterone)

Normal range: Variable with age and sex (see Fig. E4-41).
Serum/plasma

Males: 280-1100 ng/dl   Females: 15-70 ng/dl
Urine
Males: 50-135 μg/day   Females: 2-12 μg/day
Elevated in: Testicular tumors, ovarian masculinizing tumors, testosterone replacement therapy
Decreased in: Hypogonadism, sleep apnea

THEOPHYLLINE

Normal therapeutic range: 10-20 mcg/ml

THORACENTESIS FLUID

Testing and evaluation of results:
1. Pleural effusion fluid should be differentiated in exudate or transudate. The initial laboratory studies should be aimed only at distinguishing an exudate from a transudate.
   a. Tube 1: protein, LDH, albumin.
   b. Tubes 2, 3, 4: save the fluid until further notice. In selected patients with suspected empyema, a pH level may be useful (generally ≤7.0). See following for proper procedure to obtain a pH level from pleural fluid.
   NOTE: Do not order further tests until the presence of an exudate is confirmed on the basis of protein and LDH determinations; however, if the results of protein and LDH determinations cannot be obtained within a reasonable time (resulting in unnecessary delay), additional laboratory tests should be ordered at the time of thoracentesis.
2. A serum/effusion albumin gradient of ≤1.2 g/dl is indicative of exudative effusions, especially in patients with congestive heart failure (CHF) treated with diuretics.
3. Note the appearance of the fluid:
   a. A grossly hemorrhagic effusion can be a result of a traumatic tap, neoplasm, or an embolus with infarction.
   b. A milky appearance indicates either of the following:
      (1) Chylous effusion: caused by trauma or tumor invasion of the thoracic duct; lipoprotein electrophoresis of the effusion reveals chylomicrons and triglyceride levels >115 mg/dl.
      (2) Pseudochylous effusion: often seen with chronic inflammation of the pleural space (e.g., TB, connective tissue diseases).
4. If transudate, consider CHF, cirrhosis, chronic renal failure, and other hypoproteinemic states and perform subsequent workup accordingly.
5. If exudate, consider ordering these tests on the pleural fluid:
   a. Cytologic examination for malignant cells (for suspected neoplasm).
   b. Gram stain, cultures (aerobic and anaerobic), and sensitivities (for suspected infectious process).
   c. AFB stain and cultures (for suspected TB).
   d. pH: a value <7.0 suggests parapneumonic effusion or empyema; a pleural fluid pH must be drawn anaerobically and iced immediately; the syringe should be prerinsed with 0.2 ml of 1:1000 heparin.
   e. Glucose: a low glucose level suggests parapneumonic effusions and rheumatoid arthritis.
   f. Amylase: a high amylase level suggests pancreatitis or ruptured esophagus.
   g. Perplexing pleural effusions are often a result of malignancy (e.g., lymphoma, malignant mesothelioma, ovarian carcinoma), TB, subdiaphragmatic processes, prior asbestos exposure, and postcardiac injury syndrome.

THROMBIN TIME (TT)

Normal range: 11.3-18.5 sec
Elevated in: Thrombolytic and heparin therapy, disseminated intravascular coagulation, hypofibrinogenemia, dysfibrinogenemia

THYROGLOBULIN

Normal: 3-40 ng/ml. Thyroglobulin is a tumor marker for monitoring the status of patients with papillary or follicular thyroid cancer following resection.
Elevated in: Papillary or follicular thyroid cancer, Hashimoto's thyroiditis, Graves' disease, subacute thyroiditis

Laboratory Tests

IV

THYROID MICROSOMAL ANTIBODIES

Normal: Undetectable. Low titers may be present in 5%-10% of normal individuals
Elevated in: Hashimoto's disease, thyroid carcinoma, early hypothyroidism, pernicious anemia

THYROID-STIMULATING HORMONE (TSH)

See Fig. E4-42 for an algorithmic approach to thyroid testing.
Normal range: 2-11 μU/ml (2-11 mU/L [CF: 1; SMI: 1 mU/L])
CONDITIONS THAT INCREASE SERUM THYROID-STIMULATING HORMONE VALUES
Laboratory error
Primary hypothyroidism
Synthroid therapy with insufficient dose
Lithium or amiodarone; some patients
Hashimoto's thyroiditis in later stage
Large doses of inorganic iodide (e.g., SSKI)
Severe nonthyroid illness in recovery phase
Iodine deficiency (moderate or severe)
Addison's disease
TSH specimen drawn in evening (peak of diurnal variation)
Pituitary TSH-secreting tumor
Therapy of hypothyroidism (3-6 wk after beginning therapy [range, 1-8 wk]; sometimes longer when pretherapy TSH is over 100 μU/ml)
Acute psychiatric illness
Peripheral resistance to T_4 syndrome
Antibodies (e.g., HAMA) interfering with monoclonal sandwich method of TSH assay
Telepaque (iopanoic acid) and Oragrafin (ipodate) x-ray contrast media
Amphetamines
High altitudes
CONDITIONS THAT DECREASE SERUM THYROID-STIMULATING HORMONE VALUES
Laboratory error
T_4/T_3 toxicosis (diffuse or nodular etiology)
Excessive therapy for hypothyroidism
Active thyroiditis (subacute, painless, or early active Hashimoto's disease)
Multinodular goiter containing areas of autonomy
Severe nonthyroid illness (especially acute trauma, dopamine, or glucocorticoid)
T_3 toxicosis
Pituitary insufficiency
Cushing's syndrome (and some patients on high-dose glucocorticoid)
Jod-Basedow (iodine-induced) hyperthyroidism
Thyroid-stimulating hormone drawn 2-4 hr after levothyroxine dose
Postpartum transient toxicosis
Factitious hyperthyroidism
Struma ovarii
Radioimmunoassay, surgery, or antithyroid drug therapy for hyperthyroidism 4-6 weeks (range, 2 wk to 2 yr) after the treatment
Interleukin-2 drugs (3%-6% of cases) or α-interferon therapy (1% of cases)
Hyperemesis gravidarum
Amiodarone therapy

THYROTROPIN (TSH) RECEPTOR ANTIBODIES

Normal: <130% of basal activity
Elevated in: Values between 1.3 and 2.0 are found in 10% of patients with thyroid disease other than Graves' disease. Values >2.8 have been found only in patients with Graves' disease.

THYROTROPIN RELEASING HORMONE (TRH) STIMULATION TEST

Normal: Baseline TSH < 11 microU/ml; Stimulated TSH: more than double the baseline.
In primary hypothyroidism the TSH increase is 2× to 3× the normal result. In secondary hypothyroidism no TSH response occurs. In tertiary hypothyroidism (hypothalamic failure) there is a delayed rise in the TSH level.

THYROXINE (T_4)

Normal range: 4-11 μg/dl (51-142 nmol/L [CF: 12.87; SMI: 1 nmol/L])

TIBC

See IRON-BINDING CAPACITY, TOTAL

TISSUE TRANSGLUTAMINASE ANTIBODY

Normal: Negative
Present in: Celiac disease (specificity; 94%-97%, sensitivity, 90%-98%), dermatitis herpetiformis

TRANSFERRIN

Normal range: 170-370 mg/dl (1.7-3.7 g/L [CF: 0.01; SMI: 0.01 g/L])
Elevated in: Iron deficiency anemia, oral contraceptive administration, viral hepatitis, late pregnancy
Decreased in: Nephrotic syndrome, liver disease, hereditary deficiency, protein malnutrition, neoplasms, chronic inflammatory states, chronic illness, thalassemia, hemochromatosis, hemolytic anemia

TRIGLYCERIDES

Normal range: <150 mg/dl (<1.80 mmol/L [CF: 0.01129; SMI: 0.02 mmol/L])
Elevated in: Hyperlipoproteinemias (types I, IIb, III, IV, V), hypothyroidism, pregnancy, estrogens, acute myocardial infarction, pancreatitis, alcohol intake, nephrotic syndrome, diabetes mellitus, glycogen storage disease
Decreased in: Malnutrition, congenital abetalipoproteinemias, drugs (e.g., gemfibrozil, fenofibrate, nicotinic acid, clofibrate)

TRIIODOTHYRONINE

See T_3

TROPONINS (serum)

See Box 4-6 for causes of troponin elevations.

BOX 4-6 Causes of Serum Troponin T and I Elevations, Including Both Acute Coronary Syndromes, Noncoronary Cardiac Events, and Noncardiac Ailments

---

Acute coronary syndrome/acute myocardial infarction
Shock of any form (cardiogenic, obstructive, distributive)
Myocarditis and myopericarditis
Cardiomyopathies
Acute congestive heart failure (pulmonary edema)
Sepsis
Pulmonary embolism
Renal failure
Sympathomimetic ingestions
Polytrauma
Burns
Acute CNS event
Rhabdomyolysis
Cardiac neoplasm, inflammatory syndromes, and infiltrative diseases
Congenital coronary anomalies
Extreme physical exertion

From Vincent JL et al: *Textbook of critical care,* ed 6, Philadelphia, 2011, Saunders.

Normal range: 0-0.4 ng/ml (negative). If there is clinical suspicion of evolving acute MI or ischemic episode, repeat testing in 5-6 hours is recommended.
Indeterminate: 0.05-0.49 ng/ml. Suggest further tests. In a patient with unstable angina and this troponin I level, there is an increased risk of a cardiac event in the near future.
Strong probability of acute MI:
≥0.05 ng/ml
Cardiac troponin T (cTnT) is a highly sensitive marker for myocardial injury for the first 48 hours after MI and for up to 5-7 days (see Fig. 4-13, under "Creatine Kinase Isoenzymes"). It may also be elevated in renal failure, chronic muscle disease, and trauma.

Cardiac troponin I (cTnI) is highly sensitive and specific for myocardial injury (≥CK-MB) in the initial 8 hours, peaks within 24 hours and lasts up to 7 days. With progressively higher levels of cTnI, the risk of mortality increases because the amount of necrosis increases.

TSH
See THYROID-STIMULATING HORMONE

TT
See THROMBIN TIME

TUBERCULIN TEST (PPD)
Abnormal results: see Box 4-7.

BOX 4-7 PPD Reaction Size Considered "Positive" (Intracutaneous 5 TU Mantoux Test at 48 hr)

5 mm or More
- HIV infection or risk factors for HIV
- Close recent contact with active TB case
- Persons with chest x-ray consistent with healed TB

10 mm or More
- Foreign-born persons from countries with high TB prevalence in Asia, Africa, and Latin America
- IV drug users
- Medically underserved low-income population groups (including Native Americans, Hispanics, and blacks)
- Residents of long-term care facilities (nursing homes, mental institutions)
- Medical conditions that increase risk for TB (silicosis, gastrectomy, undernourishment, diabetes mellitus, high-dose corticosteroids or immunosuppression Rx, leukemia or lymphoma, other malignancies)
- Employees of long-term care facilities, schools, child-care facilities, health care facilities

15 mm or More
- All others not already listed

TB, Tuberculosis; *TU,* tuberculin units.

BOX 4-8 Factors Associated with False-Negative Tuberculin Tests

Technical Errors
- Improper administration
- Inaccurate reading
- Loss of potency of antigen

Patient-Related Factors (Anergy)
- Age (elderly)
- Nutritional status
- Medications: corticosteroids, immunosuppressive agents
- Severe tuberculosis
- Coexisting diseases
  - HIV infection
  - Viral illness or vaccination
  - Lymphoreticular malignancies
  - Sarcoidosis
  - Solid tumors
  - Lepromatous leprosy
  - Sjögren's syndrome
  - Ataxia telangiectasia
  - Uremia
  - Primary biliary cirrhosis
  - Systemic lupus erythematosus
- Severe systemic disease of any etiology

From Stein JH (ed): *Internal medicine,* ed 4, St Louis, 1994, Mosby.

UNCONJUGATED BILIRUBIN
See BILIRUBIN, DIRECT

UREA NITROGEN, BLOOD (BUN)
Normal range: 8-18 mg/dl (3-6.5 mmol/L [CF: 0.357; SMI: 0.5 mmol/L])

Box 4-9 describes factors affecting BUN level independent of renal function.

BOX 4-9 Factors Affecting Blood Urea Nitrogen Level Independent of Renal Function

Disproportionate Increase in Blood Urea Nitrogen
- Volume depletion ("prerenal azotemia")
- Gastrointestinal hemorrhage
- Corticosteroid or cytotoxic agents
- High-protein diet
- Obstructive uropathy
- Sepsis
- Catabolic states, tissue breakdown

Disproportionate Decrease in Blood Urea Nitrogen
- Low-protein diet
- Liver disease

From Andreoli TE (ed): *Cecil essentials of medicine,* ed 5, Philadelphia, 2001, Saunders.

Elevated in: Drugs (aminoglycosides and other antibiotics, diuretics, lithium, corticosteroids), dehydration, gastrointestinal bleeding, decreased renal blood flow (shock, congestive heart failure, myocardial infarction), renal disease (glomerulonephritis, pyelonephritis, diabetic nephropathy), urinary tract obstruction (prostatic hypertrophy)

Decreased in: Liver disease, malnutrition, third trimester of pregnancy, overhydration, acromegaly, celiac disease

URIC ACID (serum)
Normal range: 2-7 mg/dl

Elevated in: Renal failure, gout, excessive cell lysis (chemotherapeutic agents, radiation therapy, leukemia, lymphoma, hemolytic anemia), hereditary enzyme deficiency (hypoxanthine-guanine-phosphoribosyl transferase), acidosis, myeloproliferative disorders, diet high in purines or protein, drugs (diuretics, low doses of ASA, ethambutol, nicotinic acid), lead poisoning, hypothyroidism, Addison's disease, nephrogenic diabetes insipidus, active psoriasis, polycystic kidneys

Decreased in: Drugs (allopurinol, febuxostat, high doses of ASA, probenecid, warfarin, corticosteroid), deficiency of xanthine oxidase, syndrome of inappropriate antidiuretic hormone secretion, renal tubular deficits (Fanconi's syndrome), alcoholism, liver disease, diet deficient in protein or purines, Wilson's disease, hemochromatosis

URINALYSIS
Normal range:
Color: light straw
Appearance: clear
Ketones: absent
pH: 4.5-8 (average, 6)
Protein: absent
Glucose: absent
Specific gravity: 1.005-1.030
Occult blood absent
Microscopic examination:
    Red blood cells: 0-5 (high-power field)
    White blood cells: 0-5 (high-power field)
    Bacteria (spun specimen): absent
    Casts: 0-4 hyaline (low-power field)

Abnormalities in the microscopic examination of urine are described in Table 4-35.

TABLE 4-35   Microscopic Examination of the Urine

Finding	Associations
Casts	
Red blood cell	Glomerulonephritis, vasculitis
White blood cell	Interstitial nephritis, pyelonephritis
Epithelial cell	Acute tubular necrosis, interstitial nephritis, glomerulonephritis
Granular	Renal parenchymal disease (nonspecific)
Waxy, broad	Advanced renal failure
Hyaline	Normal finding in concentrated urine
Fatty	Heavy proteinuria
Cells	
Red blood cell	Urinary tract infection, urinary tract inflammation
White blood cell	Urinary tract infection, urinary tract inflammation
Eosinophil	Acute interstitial nephritis
(Squamous) epithelial cell	Contaminants
Crystals	
Uric acid	Acid urine, acute uric acid nephropathy, hyperuricosuria
Calcium phosphate	Alkaline urine
Calcium oxalate	Acid urine, hyperoxaluria, ethylene glycol poisoning
Cystine	Cystinuria
Sulfur	Sulfa-containing antibiotics

From Andreoli TE (ed): *Cecil essentials of medicine*, ed 5, Philadelphia, 2001, Saunders.

URINE AMYLASE

Normal range: 35-260 U Somogyi/hr (6.5-48.1 U/hr [CF: 0.185; SMI: 1 U/hr])
Elevated in: Pancreatitis, carcinoma of the pancreas

URINE BILE

Normal: Absent
Abnormal:
Urine bilirubin: hepatitis (viral, toxic, drug-induced), biliary obstruction
Urine urobilinogen: hepatitis (viral, toxic, drug-induced), hemolytic jaundice, liver cell dysfunction (cirrhosis, infection, metastases)

URINE CALCIUM

Normal range: <250 mg/24 hr (<6.2 mmol/dl [CF: 0.02495; SMI: 0.1 mmol/dl])
Elevated in: Primary hyperparathyroidism, hypervitaminosis D, bone metastases, multiple myeloma, increased calcium intake, steroids, prolonged immobilization, sarcoidosis, Paget's disease, idiopathic hypercalciuria, renal tubular acidosis
Decreased in: Hypoparathyroidism, pseudohypoparathyroidism, vitamin D deficiency, vitamin D–resistant rickets, diet low in calcium, drugs (thiazide diuretics, oral contraceptives), familial hypocalciuric hypercalcemia, renal osteodystrophy, potassium citrate therapy

URINE cAMP

Elevated in: Hypercalciuria, familial hypocalciuric hypercalcemia, primary hyperparathyroidism, pseudohypoparathyroidism, rickets
Decreased in: Vitamin D intoxication, sarcoidosis

URINE CATECHOLAMINES

Normal range:
Norepinephrine: <100 μg/24 hr (<590 nmol/day [CF: 5.911; SMI: 10 nmol/day])
Epinephrine: <10 μg/24 hr (55 nmol/day [CF: 5.458; SMI: 5 nmol/day])
Elevated in: Pheochromocytoma, neuroblastoma, severe stress

URINE CHLORIDE

Normal range: 110-250 mEq/day (110-250 mmol/day [CF: 1; SMI: 1 mmol/day])
Elevated in: Corticosteroids, Bartter's syndrome, diuretics, metabolic acidosis, severe hypokalemia
Decreased in: Chloride depletion (vomiting), colonic villous adenoma, chronic renal failure, renal tubular acidosis

URINE COPPER

Normal range: <40 μg/24 hr (<0.6 μmol/day [CF: 0.01574; SMI: 0.2 μmol/day])

URINE CORTISOL, FREE

Normal range: 10-110 μg/24 hr (30-300 nmol/day [CF: 2.759; SMI: 10 nmol/day])
Elevated: See CORTISOL, PLASMA

URINE CREATININE (24 hr)

Normal range:
Male: 0.8-1.8 g/day (7-16 mmol/day [CF: 8.840; SMI: 0.1 mmol/day])
Female: 0.6-1.6 g/day (5.3-14 mmol/day)
   NOTE: Useful test as an indicator of completeness of 24-hr urine collection.

URINE CRYSTALS

Uric acid: acid urine, hyperuricosuria, uric acid nephropathy
Sulfur: antibiotics containing sulfa
Calcium oxalate: ethylene glycol poisoning, acid urine, hyperoxaluria
Calcium phosphate: alkaline urine
Cystine: cystinuria

URINE EOSINOPHILS

Normal: Absent
Present in: Interstitial nephritis, acute tubular necrosis, urinary tract infection, kidney transplant rejection, hepatorenal syndrome

URINE GLUCOSE (qualitative)

Normal: Absent
Present in: Diabetes mellitus, renal glycosuria (decreased renal threshold for glucose), glucose intolerance

URINE HEMOGLOBIN, FREE

Normal: Absent
Present in: Hemolysis (with saturation of serum haptoglobin binding capacity and renal threshold for tubular absorption of hemoglobin)

URINE HEMOSIDERIN

Normal: Absent
Present in: Paroxysmal nocturnal hemoglobinuria, chronic hemolytic anemia, hemochromatosis, blood transfusion, thalassemias

URINE 5-HYDROXYINDOLE-ACETIC ACID
(URINE 5-HIAA)

Normal range: 2-8 mg/24 hr (10-40 μmol/day [CF: 5.23; SMI: 5 μmol/day])
Elevated in: Carcinoid tumors, after ingestion of certain foods (bananas, plums, tomatoes, avocados, pineapples, eggplant, walnuts), drugs (monoamine oxidase inhibitors, phenacetin, methyldopa, glycerol guaiacolate, acetaminophen, salicylates, phenothiazines, imipramine, methocarbamol, reserpine, methamphetamine)

URINE INDICAN

Normal: Absent
Present in: Malabsorption secondary to intestinal bacterial overgrowth

URINE KETONES (semiquantitative)

Normal: Absent
Present in: Diabetic ketoacidosis, alcoholic ketoacidosis, starvation, isopropanol ingestion

URINE METANEPHRINES

Normal range: 0-2.0 mg/24 hr (0-11.0 μmol/day [CF: 5.458; SMI: 0.5 μmol/day])

Elevated in: Pheochromocytoma, neuroblastoma, drugs (caffeine, pheno-thiazines, monoamine oxidase inhibitors), stress

URINE MYOGLOBIN

Normal: Absent
Present in: Severe trauma, hyperthermia, polymyositis/dermatomyositis, carbon monoxide poisoning, drugs (narcotic and amphetamine toxicity), hypothyroidism, muscle ischemia

URINE NITRITE

Normal: Absent
Present in: Urinary tract infections

URINE OCCULT BLOOD

Normal: Negative
Positive in: Trauma to urinary tract, renal disease (glomerulonephritis, pyelonephritis), renal or ureteral calculi, bladder lesions (carcinoma, cystitis), prostatitis, prostatic carcinoma, menstrual contamination, hematopoietic disorders (hemophilia, thrombocytopenia), anticoagulants, ASA

URINE OSMOLALITY

Normal range: 50-1200 mOsm/kg (50-1200 mmol/kg [CF: 1; SMI: 1 mmol/kg])
Elevated in: Syndrome of inappropriate antidiuretic hormone secretion, dehydration, glycosuria, adrenal insufficiency, high-protein diet
Decreased in: Diabetes insipidus, excessive water intake, IV hydration with D_5W, acute renal insufficiency, glomerulonephritis

URINE pH

Normal range: 4.6-8 (average, 6)
Elevated in: Bacteriuria, vegetarian diet, renal failure with inability to form ammonia, drugs (antibiotics, sodium bicarbonate, acetazolamide)
Decreased in: Acidosis (metabolic, respiratory), drugs (ammonium chloride, methenamine mandelate), diabetes mellitus, starvation, diarrhea

URINE PHOSPHATE

Normal range: 0.8-2.0 g/24 hr
Elevated in: Acute tubular necrosis (diuretic phase), chronic renal disease, uncontrolled diabetes mellitus, hyperparathyroidism, hypomagnesemia, metabolic acidosis, metabolic alkalosis, neurofibromatosis, adult-onset vitamin D–resistant hypophosphatemic osteomalacia
Decreased in: Acromegaly, acute renal failure, decreased dietary intake, hypoparathyroidism, respiratory acidosis

URINE POTASSIUM

Normal range: 25-100 mEq/24 hr (25-100 mmol/day [CF: 1; SMI: 1 mmol/day])
Elevated in: Aldosteronism (primary, secondary), glucocorticoids, alkalosis, renal tubular acidosis, excessive dietary potassium intake
Decreased in: Acute renal failure, potassium-sparing diuretics, diarrhea, hypokalemia

URINE PROTEIN (quantitative)

Normal range: <150 mg/24 hr (<0.15 g/day [CF: 0.001; SMI: 0.01 g/day])
Elevated in:
Nephrotic syndrome as a result of primary renal diseases
Malignant hypertension
Malignancies: multiple myeloma, leukemias, Hodgkin's disease
Congestive heart failure
Diabetes mellitus
Systemic lupus erythematosus, rheumatoid arthritis
Sickle cell disease
Goodpasture's syndrome
Malaria
Amyloidosis, sarcoidosis
Tubular lesions: cystinosis
Functional (after heavy exercise)
Pyelonephritis
Pregnancy

Constrictive pericarditis
Renal vein thrombosis
Toxic nephropathies: heavy metals, drugs
Radiation nephritis
Orthostatic (postural) proteinuria
Benign proteinuria: fever, heat or cold exposure

URINE SEDIMENT

See Fig. 4-43 for evaluation of common abnormalities.

URINE SODIUM (quantitative)

See Table 4-36 for use of urine electrolytes in the differential diagnosis of hypokalemia.
Normal range: 40-220 mEq/day (40-220 mmol/day [CF: 1; SMI: 1 mmol/day])
Elevated in: Diuretic administration, high sodium intake, salt-losing nephritis, acute tubular necrosis, vomiting, Addison's disease, syndrome of inappropriate antidiuretic hormone secretion, hypothyroidism, congestive heart failure, hepatic failure, chronic renal failure, Bartter's syndrome, glucocorticoid deficiency, interstitial nephritis caused by analgesic abuse, mannitol, dextran, or glycerol therapy, milk-alkali syndrome, decreased renin secretion, postobstructive diuresis
Decreased in: Increased aldosterone, glucocorticoid excess, hyponatremia, prerenal azotemia, decreased salt intake

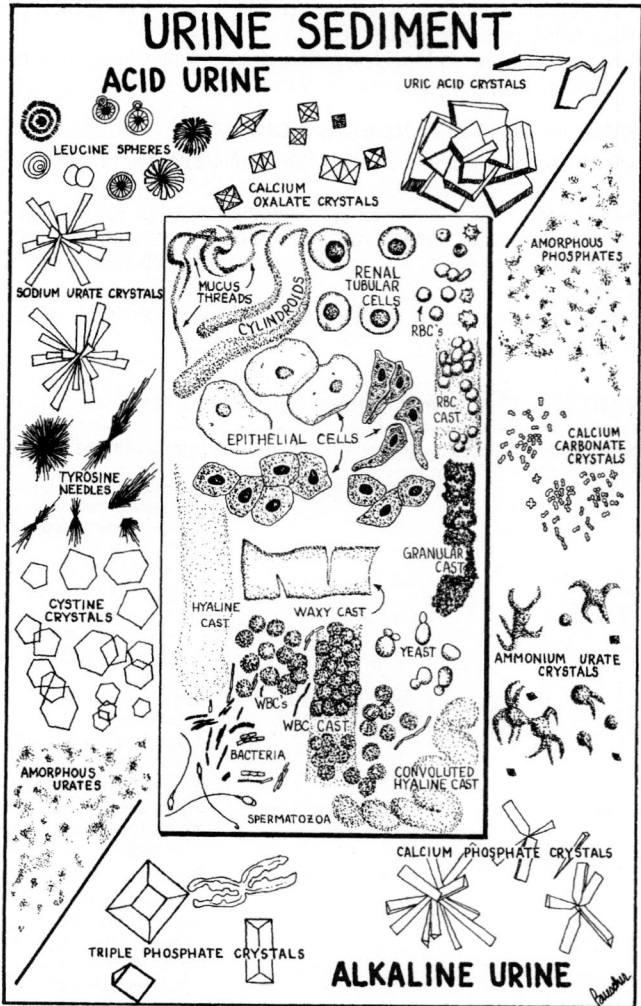

FIGURE 4-43 Microscopic examination of urinary sediment. (From Grigorian Greene M: *The Harriet Lane handbook: a manual for pediatric house officers,* ed 17, St Louis, 2007, Mosby.)

TABLE 4-36   Urine Electrolytes* in the Differential Diagnosis of Hypokalemia

Condition	Urine Electrolyte	
	Na$^+$	Cl$^-$
Vomiting		
Recent	High†	Low‡
Remote	Low	Low
Diuretics		
Recent	High	High
Remote	Low	Low
Diarrhea or Laxative Abuse	Low	High
Bartter's or Gitelman's Syndrome	High	High

From Vincent JL et al: *Textbook of Critical Care,* ed 6, Philadelphia, 2011, Saunders.
*Do not use the urine electrolytes in this fashion during polyuric states.
†High = urine concentration > 15 mmol/L.
‡Low = urine concentration < 15 mmol/L.

URINE SPECIFIC GRAVITY

Normal range: 1.005-1.030
Elevated in: Dehydration, excessive fluid losses (vomiting, diarrhea, fever), x-ray contrast media, diabetes mellitus, congestive heart failure, syndrome of inappropriate antidiuretic hormone secretion, adrenal insufficiency, decreased fluid intake
Decreased in: Diabetes insipidus, renal disease (glomerulonephritis, pyelonephritis), excessive fluid intake or IV hydration

URINE VANILLYLMANDELIC ACID (VMA)

Normal range: <6.8 mg/24 hr (<35 μmol/day [CF: 5.046; SMI: 1 μmol/day])
Elevated in: Pheochromocytoma, neuroblastoma, ganglioblastoma, drugs (isoproterenol, methocarbamol, levodopa, sulfonamides, chlorpromazine), severe stress, after ingestion of bananas, chocolate, vanilla, tea, coffee
Decreased in: Drugs (monoamine oxidase inhibitors, reserpine, guanethidine, methyldopa)

VARICELLA-ZOSTER VIRUS (VZV) SEROLOGY

Test description: Test can be performed on whole blood, tissue, skin lesions, and CSF

VASOACTIVE INTESTINAL PEPTIDE (VIP)

Normal: <50 pg/ml
Elevated in: Pancreatic VIP-omas, neuroblastoma, pancreatic islet call hyperplasia, liver disease, MEN I, ganglioneuroma, ganglioneuroblastoma

VDRL

Normal range: Negative
Positive test: Syphilis, other treponemal diseases (yaws, pinta, bejel)
   NOTE: A false-positive test may be seen in patients with systemic lupus erythematosus and other autoimmune diseases, infectious mononucleosis, HIV, atypical pneumonia, malaria, leprosy, typhus fever, rat-bite fever, relapsing fever.
   NOTE: See Table 4-37 for interpretation of serologic tests for syphilis.

VISCOSITY (serum)

Normal range: 1.4-1.8 relative to water (1.10-1.22 centipoise)
Elevated in: Monoclonal gammopathies (Waldenström's macroglobulinemia, multiple myeloma), hyperfibrinogenemia, systemic lupus erythematosus, rheumatoid arthritis, polycythemia, leukemia

VITAMIN B$_{12}$

See Fig. E4-44 for the Schilling test.
Normal:
190-900 ng/ml
Causes of vitamin B$_{12}$ deficiency:
1. Pernicious anemia (antibodies against intrinsic factor and gastric parietal cells)
2. Dietary (strict lacto-ovovegetarians, food faddists)
3. Malabsorption (achlorhydria, gastrectomy, ileal resection, pancreatic insufficiency, drugs [omeprazole, cholestyramine])
Falsely low levels occur in patients with severe folate deficiency, in patients using high doses of ascorbic acid, and when cobalamin levels are measured after nuclear medicine studies (radioactivity interferes with cobalamin radioimmunoassay).

TABLE 4-37   Interpretation of Serologic Tests for Syphilis*

Nontreponemal Tests	Treponemal Tests	Interpretation of Finding: Is Syphilis Present?*
Nonreactive	Nonreactive	Early primary syphilis is not ruled out by negative serologic tests. Early syphilis is present in 13%-30% of patients who have a negative microhemagglutination *Treponema pallidum* test; in about 30% of patients who present with chancre but have a nonreactive reagin test; and in about 10% of patients who have a negative FTA-ABS test. Late syphilis is present in a very small fraction of patients. Adequately treated syphilis in remote past may produce these results, but treponemal tests usually remain reactive.
	Reactive	Observed in about 10% of patients with chancre. The treponemal tests may turn positive shortly before the reagin tests. Reagin tests repeated after several days are generally positive. In adequately treated early syphilis, the reagin test may return to nonreactive within 1-2 yr, whereas the treponemal tests generally do not. Late syphilis is not ruled out by a negative reagin test. The sensitivity of the reagin tests is lower than that of treponemal tests in untreated late syphilis. In secondary syphilis, rarely, a highly reactive serum appears negative when tested undiluted with a reagin test because flocculation is inhibited by relative antibody excess. Not reported to occur with treponemal tests. Quantitative reagin tests are positive. False-positive treponemal tests occur in 40% of patients with Lyme disease.
Reactive	Nonreactive borderline (FTA-ABS)	Finding is not diagnostic of syphilis but constitutes a classic biologic false-positive reaction. Not diagnostic of syphilis; most patients (90%) with this pattern do not develop clinical or serologic evidence of syphilis. Repeat test is indicated. Chronic borderline results are associated with a variety of conditions other than syphilis.
	Beaded (FTA-ABS)	Not diagnostic of syphilis. Seen with collagen vascular disease.
	Reactive	Findings diagnostic of syphilis or other treponemal disease. In adequately treated syphilis, one would expect (1) a sustained fourfold drop in titer of reagin test, although reagin test may remain positive after adequate therapy; (2) treponemal tests remain positive after adequate therapy. Concurrent false-positive results on both nontreponemal and treponemal tests could occur in rare instances. It may be impossible to rule out syphilis in an individual with this test profile.

From Stein JH (ed): *Internal medicine,* ed 4, St Louis, 1994, Mosby.
FTA-ABS, Fluorescent treponemal antibody, absorbed.
*Serologic data must always be interpreted in the light of a total clinical evaluation. Diagnosis based on serologic criteria alone is fraught with error. Serologic tests apparently in conflict with clinical diagnosis should be confirmed by repetition or possibly referral to a reference laboratory.

Falsely high or normal levels in patients with cobalamin deficiency can occur in severe liver disease and chronic granulocytic leukemia.

The absence of anemia or macrocytosis does not exclude the diagnosis of cobalamin deficiency.

VITAMIN D, 1,25 DIHYDROXY CALCIFEROL

Normal: 16-65 pg/ml

Elevated in: Tumor calcinosis, primary hyperparathyroidism, sarcoidosis, tuberculosis, idiopathic hypercalciuria

Decreased in: Postmenopausal osteoporosis, chronic renal failure, hypoparathyroidism, tumor-induced osteomalacia, rickets, elevated blood lead levels

VITAMIN K

Normal: 0.10-2.20 ng/ml

Decreased in: Primary biliary cirrhosis, anticoagulants, antibiotics, cholestyramine, GI disease, pancreatic disease, cystic fibrosis, obstructive jaundice, hypoprothrombinemia, hemorrhagic disease of the newborn

VON WILLEBRAND FACTOR

Normal: Levels vary according to blood type; blood type O: 50-150 U/dl; blood type non-O: 90-200 U/dl

Decreased in: von Willebrand's disease (however, in type II von Willebrand's disease the antigen may be normal but the function is impaired)

WBC

See COMPLETE BLOOD COUNT

WESTERGREN

See ERYTHROCYTE SEDIMENTATION RATE

WHITE BLOOD COUNT

See COMPLETE BLOOD COUNT

Laboratory Tests

IV

Clinical Practice Guidelines

PART A
THE PERIODIC HEALTH EXAMINATION*

Age-Specific Charts, 1493

PART B
IMMUNIZATIONS AND CHEMOPROPHYLAXIS

Childhood and Adolescent Immunizations, 1503

General Recommendations on Immunization, 1508

*Data modified from U.S. Preventive Services Task Force: *Guide to clinical preventive services: report of the U.S. Preventive Services Task Force,* ed 2, Washington, DC, 1996 (revised 2001), U.S. Department of Health and Human Services. Text downloaded from http://text.nlm.nih.gov

Immunizations for Adults, 1520

PART A • THE PERIODIC HEALTH EXAMINATION

Age-Specific Charts

TABLE 5-1   Birth to 10 Years

Interventions considered and recommended for the Periodic Health Examination	Leading causes of death
	Conditions originating in perinatal period
	Congenital anomalies
	Sudden infant death syndrome
	Unintentional injuries (non–motor vehicle)
	Motor vehicle injuries

INTERVENTIONS FOR THE GENERAL POPULATION

Screening

Height and weight

Blood pressure

Vision screen (ages 3-4 yr)

Hemoglobinopathy screen (birth)[1]

Phenylalanine level (birth)[2]

Thyroxine and/or thyroid-stimulating hormone (birth)[3]

Lead level

Counseling

Injury prevention

Child safety car seats (age <5 yr)

Lap/shoulder belts (age ≥5 yr)

Bicycle helmet; avoid bicycling near traffic

Smoke detector, flame-retardant sleepwear

Hot water heater temperature <120°-130° F

Window/stair guards, pool fence

Safe storage of drugs, toxic substances, firearms, and matches

Syrup of ipecac, poison control phone number

CPR training for parents/caretakers

Diet and exercise

Breastfeeding, iron-enriched formula and foods (infants and toddlers)

Limit fat and cholesterol; maintain caloric balance; emphasize grains, fruits, vegetables (age ≥2 yr)

Regular physical activity*

Substance use

Effects of passive smoking*

Antitobacco message*

Dental health

Regular visits to dental care provider*

Floss, brush with fluoride toothpaste daily*

Advice about baby bottle tooth decay*

Immunizations

Diphtheria-tetanus-pertussis (DTaP)[4]

Inactivated poliovirus vaccine (IPV)[5]

Measles-mumps-rubella (MMR)[6]

Haemophilus influenzae type b (Hib) conjugate[7]

Hepatitis A vaccine (HR4)

Hepatitis B[8]

Varicella[9]

Pneumococcal vaccine[10]

Influenza[11]

Meningococcal conjugate vaccine (MCV)[12]

Rotavirus (RV)[13]

Human papillomavirus vaccine (HPV)[14]

Chemoprophylaxis

Ocular prophylaxis (birth)

INTERVENTIONS FOR HIGH-RISK POPULATIONS

Population	Potential Interventions (see detailed high-risk definitions)
Preterm or low birth weight	Hemoglobin/hematocrit (HR1)
Infants of mothers at risk for HIV	HIV testing (HR2)
Low income; immigrants	Hemoglobin/hematocrit (HR1); PPD (HR3)
TB contacts	PPD (HR3)
Native American/Alaska Native	Hemoglobin/hematocrit (HR1); PPD (HR3); pneumococcal vaccine (HR5)
Residents of long-term care facilities	PPD (HR3); hepatitis A vaccine (HR4); influenza vaccine (HR6)
Certain chronic medical conditions	PPD (HR3); pneumococcal vaccine (HR5); influenza vaccine (HR6)
Increased individual or community lead exposure	Blood lead level (HR7)
Inadequate water fluoridation	Daily fluoride supplement (HR8)
Family history of skin cancer; nevi; fair skin, eyes, hair	Avoid excess/midday sun, use protective clothing* (HR9)

CPR, Cardiopulmonary resuscitation; *HR*, high risk; *PPD*, purified protein derivative; *STDs*, sexually transmitted diseases; *TB*, tuberculosis.

[1]Whether screening should be universal or targeted to high-risk groups depends on the proportion of high-risk individuals in the screening area and other considerations. [2]If done during first 24 hr of life, repeat by age 2 wk. [3]Optimally between day 2 and 6, but in all cases before newborn nursery discharge. [4]2, 4, 6, and 12-18 mo; once between age 4-6 yr. [5]2, 4, 6-18 mo; once between age 4-6 yr. [6]12-15 mo and 4-6 yr. [7]2, 4, 6 and 12-15 mo; no dose needed at 6 mo if PRP-OMP vaccine is used for first 2 doses. [8]Birth, 1 mo, 6 mo; or, 0-2 mo, 1-2 mo later, and 6-18 mo. If not done in infancy: current visit, and 1 and 6 mo later. [9]12-18 mo; or any child without history of chickenpox or previous immunization. Include information on risk in adulthood, duration of immunity, and potential need for booster doses. Administer a second dose of varicella vaccine at age 4-6 yr. [10]Pneumococcal polysaccharide vaccine (PPSV) can be administered at the same time as the other childhood vaccines at a separate site. [11]Influenza vaccine is recommended in children 6 mo-18 yr of age. [12]Administer meningococcal conjugate vaccine (MCV) to children aged 2 through 10 yr with terminal complement component deficiency, anatomic or functional asplenia, and certain other high risk groups (see *MMWR* 54[RR-7], 2005). Persons who received MPSV 3 or more years previously and who remain at increased risk for meningococcal disease should be revaccinated with MCV. [13]Administer first dose at 2 mo. If Rotarix® is administered at ages 2 and 4 mo, a dose at 6 mo is not indicated. [14]HPV4 may be administered in a 3-dose series to males aged 9 through 26 yr and females aged 11 to 26 yr to reduce the likelihood of acquiring genital warts.

*The ability of clinician counseling to influence this behavior is unproven.

HR1: Infants aged 6-12 mo who are living in poverty, black, Native American or Alaska Native, immigrants from developing countries, preterm and low-birth-weight infants, infants whose principal dietary intake is unfortified cow's milk.

HR2: Infants born to high-risk mothers whose HIV status is unknown. Women at high risk include past or present injection drug users; persons who exchange sex for money or drugs and their sex partners; injection drug–using, bisexual, or HIV-positive sex partners currently or in past; persons seeking treatment for STDs; persons who received a blood transfusion between 1978 and 1985.

HR3: Persons infected with HIV, close contacts of persons with known or suspected TB, persons with medical risk factors associated with TB, immigrants from countries with high TB prevalence, medically underserved low-income populations (including homeless), residents of long-term care facilities.

HR4: Hepatitis A vaccine (Hep A) is recommended for all children at 1 yr of age (i.e., 12-23 mo). The two doses in the series should be administered at least 6 mo apart. Children who are not vaccinated by 2 yr of age can be vaccinated at subsequent visits.

HR5: Immunocompetent persons $\geq$2 yr with certain medical conditions, including chronic cardiac or pulmonary disease, diabetes mellitus, and anatomic asplenia, as well as cochlear implant candidates and recipients. Immunocompetent persons $\geq$2 yr living in high-risk environments or social settings (e.g., certain Native American and Alaska Native populations).

HR6: Annual vaccinations of children $\geq$6 mo who are residents of chronic care facilities or who have chronic cardiopulmonary disorders, metabolic diseases (including diabetes mellitus), hemoglobinopathies, immunosuppression, or renal dysfunction.

HR7: Children approximately age 12 mo who (1) live in communities in which the prevalence of lead levels requiring individual intervention, including residential lead hazard control or chelation, is high or undefined; (2) live in or frequently visit a home built before 1950 with dilapidated paint or with recent or ongoing renovation or remodeling; (3) have close contact with a person who has an elevated lead level; (4) live near lead industry or heavy traffic; (5) live with someone whose job or hobby involves lead exposure; (6) use lead-based pottery; or (7) take traditional ethnic remedies that contain lead.

HR8: Children living in areas with inadequate water fluoridation (<0.6 ppm).

HR9: Persons with a family history of skin cancer; a large number of moles; atypical moles; poor tanning ability; or light skin, hair, and eye color.

TABLE 5-2 Ages 11 to 24 Years

Interventions considered and recommended for the Periodic Health Examination	Leading causes of death
	Motor vehicle accidents/other unintentional injuries
	Homicide
	Suicide
	Malignant neoplasms
	Heart diseases

INTERVENTIONS FOR THE GENERAL POPULATION

Screening

Height and weight

Blood pressure[1]

Papanicolaou (Pap) test[2] (females)

Chlamydia screen[3] (females <25 yr)

HIV screening

Lipid panel (in high-risk young adults only)

Rubella serology or vaccination history[4] (females >12 yr)

Assess for problem drinking

Lead level

Counseling

Injury prevention

Lap/shoulder belts

Bicycle/motorcycle/ATV helmets*

Smoke detector*

Safe storage/removal of firearms*

Substance use

Avoid tobacco use

Avoid underage drinking and illicit drug use*

Avoid alcohol/drug use while driving, swimming, boating, etc.*

Sexual behavior

STD prevention: abstinence*; avoid high-risk behavior*; condoms/female barrier with spermicide*

Unintended pregnancy: contraception

Diet and exercise

Limit fat and cholesterol; maintain caloric balance; emphasize grains, fruits, vegetables

Adequate calcium intake (females)

Regular physical activity*

Dental health

Regular visits to dental care provider*

Floss, brush with fluoride toothpaste daily

Immunizations

Tetanus, diphtheria, pertussis[†]

Hepatitis B[5]

Measles-mumps-rubella (MMR) (11-12 yr)[6]

Varicella (11-12 yr)[7]

Rubella (females >12 yr)[4]

Meningococcal[8]

Human papilloma virus (females 11-26 yr, males 9-26 yr)[9]

Influenza[10]

Pneumococcal polysaccharide vaccine (PPSV)[11]

Chemoprophylaxis

Multivitamin with folic acid (females)

INTERVENTIONS FOR HIGH-RISK POPULATIONS

Population	Potential Interventions (see detailed high-risk definitions)
High-risk sexual behavior	RPR/VDRL (HR1); screen for gonorrhea (female) (HR2), HIV (HR3), chlamydia (female) (HR4); hepatitis A vaccine (HR5)
Injection or street drug use	RPR/VDRL (HR1); HIV screen (HR3); hepatitis A vaccine (HR5); PPD (HR6); advice to reduce infection risk (HR7)
TB contacts; immigrants; low income	PPD (HR6)
Native Americans/Alaska Natives	Hepatitis A vaccine (HR5); PPD (HR6); pneumococcal vaccine (HR8)
Travelers to developing countries	Hepatitis A vaccine (HR5)
Certain chronic medical conditions	PPD (HR6); pneumococcal vaccine (HR8); influenza vaccine (HR9)
Settings where adolescents and young adults congregate	Second MMR (HR10)
Susceptible to varicella, measles, mumps	Varicella vaccine (HR11); MMR (HR12)
Blood transfusion between 1975 and 1985	HIV screen (HR3)
Institutionalized persons; health care/lab workers	Hepatitis A vaccine (HR5); PPD (HR6); influenza vaccine (HR9)
Family history of skin cancer; nevi; fair skin, eyes, hair	Avoid excess/midday sun, use protective clothing* (HR13)
Prior pregnancy with neural tube defect	Folic acid 4.0 mg (HR14)
Inadequate water fluoridation	Daily fluoride supplement (HR15)
Pregnancy	HIV screen, Tdap vaccine (given in second or early third trimester of pregnancy)
Infants 6-11 mo of age travelling internationally	MMR

ATV, All-terrain vehicle; *HR,* high risk; *PPD,* purified protein derivative; *RPR,* rapid plasmin reagin; *STD,* sexually transmitted disease; *TB,* tuberculosis; *VDRL,* Venereal Disease Research Laboratory.
[1]Periodic blood pressure for persons aged ≥21 yr. [2]If sexually active at present or in the past: q ≤3 yr. If sexual history is unreliable, begin Pap tests at age 21 yr. [3]If sexually active. [4]Serologic testing, documented vaccination history, and routine vaccination against rubella (preferably with MMR) are equally acceptable alternatives. [5]If not previously immunized: current visit and 1 and 6 mo later. [6]If no previous second dose of MMR. [7]If susceptible to chickenpox. [8]Meningococcal conjugate vaccine (MCV) can be administered at 11-12 yr visit, at high school entry, or at beginning of college (especially indicated in students living in college dormitories). [9]Quadrivalent human papillomavirus (types 6, 11, 16, 18) recombinant vaccine (Gardasil) should be given to all females aged 11-26 yr who have not been previously vaccinated. The vaccine is indicated for the prevention of cervical cancer and genital warts caused by the human papilloma virus (HPV) 6, 11, 16, or 18. Gardasil is an intramuscular injection for administration to the thigh or upper arm. The schedule consists of three 0.5-ml doses, with the second dose given 2 mo after the first, and the final dose administered 6 mo after the initial dose. HPV4 may also be administered in a 3-dose series to males aged 9 through 26 years to reduce their likelihood of acquiring genital warts. A bivalent HPV vaccine is available for prevention of cervical dysplasia in females. [10]Influenza vaccine is recommended for children 6 mo to 18 yr of age. [11]Administer to children with certain underlying medical conditions (see *MMWR* 46[RR-8], 1997), including a cochlear implant. A single revaccination should be administered to children with functional or anatomic asplenia or other immunocompromising condition after 5 yr.
*The ability of clinician counseling to influence this behavior is unproven.
[†]Tdap vaccine is recommended for adolescents aged 11-12 yr who have completed the recommended childhood DTP/DTaP vaccination series and have not received a Td booster dose. Adolescents aged 13-18 yr who missed the 11-12-yr Td/Tdap booster dose should also receive a single dose of Tdap if they have completed the recommended childhood DTP/DTaP vaccination series. A 5-yr interval from the last Td dose is encouraged when Tdap is used as a booster drug; however, a shorter interval may be used if pertussis immunity is needed.

HR1: Persons who exchange sex for money or drugs and their sex partners, persons with other STDs (including HIV), and sexual contacts of persons with active syphilis. Clinicians should also consider local epidemiology.

HR2: Females who have had two or more sex partners in the last year or a sex partner with multiple sexual contacts; exchanged sex for money or drugs; or have a history of repeated episodes of gonorrhea. Clinicians should also consider local epidemiology.

HR3: Males who had sex with males after 1975; past or present injection drug users; persons who exchange sex for money or drugs and their sex partners; injection drug–using, bisexual, or HIV-positive sex partner currently or in the past; recipients of a blood transfusion between 1978 and 1985; persons seeking treatment for STDs. Clinicians should also consider local epidemiology and screening for HIV in general population.

HR4: Sexually active females with multiple risk factors, including history of prior STD, new or multiple sex partners, age <25 yr, nonuse or inconsistent use of barrier contraceptives, or cervical ectopy. Clinicians should consider local epidemiology of the disease in identifying other high-risk groups.

HR5: Persons living in, traveling to, or working in areas where the disease is endemic and where periodic outbreaks occur (e.g., countries with high or intermediate endemicity; certain Alaska Native, Pacific Island, Native American, and religious communities); men who have sex with men; injection or street drug users; persons with clotting factor disorders or chronic liver disease, diabetics. Vaccine may be considered for institutionalized persons and workers in these institutions; military personnel; and day-care, hospital, and laboratory workers. Clinicians should also consider local epidemiology.

HR6: HIV-positive, close contacts of persons with known or suspected TB, health care workers, persons with medical risk factors associated with TB, immigrants from countries with high TB prevalence, medically underserved low-income populations (including homeless), alcoholics, injection drug users, and residents of long-term care facilities.

HR7: Persons who continue to inject drugs.

HR8: Immunocompetent persons with certain medical conditions, including chronic cardiac, renal, or pulmonary disease; diabetes mellitus; cochlear implant candidates and recipients; and anatomic asplenia. Immunocompetent persons who live in high-risk environments or social settings (e.g., certain Native American and Alaska Native populations). Adults who smoke cigarettes, persons with asymptomatic or symptomatic HIV infection.

HR9: Annual vaccination of residents of chronic care facilities; persons with chronic cardiopulmonary disorders, metabolic diseases (including diabetes mellitus), hemoglobinopathies, immunosuppression, or renal dysfunction; and health care providers for high-risk patients.

HR10: Adolescents and young adults in settings where such individuals congregate (e.g., high schools and colleges) if they have not previously received a second dose.

HR11: Healthy persons aged ≥13 yr without a history of chickenpox or previous immunization. Consider serologic testing for presumed susceptible persons aged ≥13 yr.

HR12: Persons born after 1956 who lack evidence of immunity to measles or mumps (e.g., documented receipt of live vaccine on or after the first birthday, laboratory evidence of immunity, or a history of physician-diagnosed measles or mumps).

HR13: Persons with a family or personal history of skin cancer; a large number of moles; atypical moles; poor tanning ability; or light skin, hair, and eye color.

HR14: Women with prior pregnancy affected by neural tube defect who are planning pregnancy.

HR15: Persons aged <17 yr living in areas with inadequate water fluoridation (<0.6 ppm).

TABLE 5-3 Ages 25 to 64 Years

Interventions considered and recommended
  for the Periodic Health Examination

Leading causes of death
  Malignant neoplasms
  Heart diseases
  Motor vehicle and other unintentional injuries
  HIV infection
  Suicide and homicide

INTERVENTIONS FOR THE GENERAL POPULATION

Screening

Blood pressure

Height and weight

Lipid panel (men aged 35-64 yr, women aged 45-64 yr)

HIV screening

Papanicolaou (Pap) test (women)[1]

Fecal occult blood test[2] and/or colonoscopy (≥50 yr)

Mammogram ± clinical breast examination[3] (women 40-69 yr)

Bone density scan in postmenopausal women

Assess for problem drinking

Rubella serology or vaccination history[4] (women of childbearing age)

Counseling

Substance use

Tobacco cessation

Avoid alcohol/drug use while driving, swimming, boating, etc.*

Diet and exercise

Limit fat and cholesterol; maintain caloric balance; emphasize grains, fruits,
  vegetables

Adequate calcium intake (women)

Regular physical activity*

Injury prevention

Lap/shoulder belts

Motorcycle/bicycle/ATV helmets*

Smoke detector*

Safe storage/removal of firearms*

Sexual behavior

STD prevention: avoid high-risk behavior*; condoms/female barrier with spermicide*

Unintended pregnancy: contraception

Dental health

Regular visits to dental care provider*

Floss, brush with fluoride toothpaste daily*

Immunizations

Tetanus-diphtheria-pertussis (Tdap) booster

Rubella[4] (women of childbearing age)

Influenza vaccine[†]

Human papillomavirus[5]

Herpes zoster (≥60 yr)[6]

Chemoprophylaxis

Multivitamin with folic acid (women planning or capable of pregnancy)

INTERVENTIONS FOR HIGH-RISK POPULATIONS

Population	*Potential Interventions (see detailed high-risk definitions)*
High-risk sexual behavior	RPR/VDRL (HR1); screen for gonorrhea (female) (HR2), HIV (HR3), chlamydia (female) (HR4); hepatitis B vaccine (HR5); hepatitis A vaccine (HR6)
Injection or street drug use	RPR/VDRL (HR1); HIV screen (HR3); hepatitis B vaccine (HR5); hepatitis A vaccine (HR6); PPD (HR7); advice to reduce infection risk (HR8)
Low income; TB contacts; immigrants; alcoholics	PPD (HR7)
Native Americans/Alaska Natives	Hepatitis A vaccine (HR6); PPD (HR7); pneumococcal vaccine (HR9)
Travelers to developing countries	Hepatitis B vaccine (HR5); hepatitis A vaccine (HR6)
Certain chronic medical conditions	PPD (HR7); pneumococcal vaccine (HR9); influenza vaccine (HR10)
Blood product recipients	HIV screen (HR3); hepatitis B vaccine (HR5); hepatitis C screen
Susceptible to measles, mumps, or varicella	MMR (HR11); varicella vaccine (HR12)
Institutionalized persons	Hepatitis A vaccine (HR6); PPD (HR7); pneumococcal vaccine (HR9); influenza vaccine (HR10)
Health care/lab workers	Hepatitis B vaccine (HR5); hepatitis A vaccine (HR6); PPD (HR7); influenza vaccine (HR10)
Family history of skin cancer; fair skin, eyes, hair	Avoid excess/midday sun, use protective clothing* (HR13)
Previous pregnancy with neural tube defect	Folic acid 4.0 mg (HR14)
Cardiovascular risk factors	Lipid panel (HR 15)
Pregnancy	HIV screen, Tdap vaccine (in second or early third trimester of pregnancy)
Diabetes mellitus	Hepatitis B vaccine (HR5)

ATV, All-terrain vehicle; *HPV,* human papillomavirus; *HR,* high risk; *MMR,* measles-mumps-rubella; *PPD,* purified protein derivative; *RPR,* rapid plasma reagin; *STD,* sexually transmitted disease; *TB,* tuberculosis; *Tdap,* tetanus and diphtheria toxoids and acellular pertussis; *VDRL,* Venereal Disease Research Laboratory.

[1]Women who are or have been sexually active and who have a cervix: q ≤3 yr. Routine Pap smear screening is unnecessary for women who have undergone a complete hysterectomy for benign disease. The American College of Obstetricians and Gynecologists (ACOG) recommends that routine Pap smears should start at age 21. Women 30 and older should wait 3 yrs between paps once they have had three consecutive clear tests. [2]Annually. [3]Mammogram q1-2 yr, or mammogram q1-2 yr with annual clinical breast examination. [4]Serologic testing, documented vaccination history, and routine vaccination (preferably with MMR) are equally acceptable. [5]Quadrivalent human papillomavirus (types 6, 11, 16, 18) recombinant vaccine (Gardasil) should be given to all females aged 9-26 yr who have not been previously vaccinated. The vaccine is indicated for the prevention of cervical cancer and genital warts caused by the human papillomavirus (HPV) 6, 11, 16, or 18. Gardasil is an intramuscular injection for administration to the thigh or upper arm. The schedule consists of three 0.5-ml doses, with the second dose given 2 mo after the first, and the final dose administered 6 mo after the initial dose. Gardasil is also indicated in males aged 9 to 26 yr for prevention of genital warts. A bivalent HPV vaccine is available for prevention of cervical dysplasia in females. [6]Herpes zoster vaccine (Zostavax) is indicated for prevention of herpes zoster (shingles) in individuals 60 yr or older. Zostavax is administered as a single dose subcutaneously. It is a lyophilic preparation of the Oka/Merck strain of live, attenuated varicella-zoster virus (VZV). It should not be administered to individuals with a history of primary or acquired immunodeficiency states, persons on immunosuppressive therapy (including high-dose corticosteroids), those with active untreated tuberculosis, and those who may be pregnant.

*The ability of clinician counseling to influence this behavior is unproven.

[†]A live attenuated influenza vaccine (LAIV, Flumist) administered intranasally is available for healthy persons aged 2 to 49 yr.

HR1: Persons who exchange sex for money or drugs and their sex partners, persons with other STDs (including HIV), and sexual contacts of persons with active syphilis. Clinicians should also consider local epidemiology.

HR2: Women who exchange sex for money or drugs or who have had repeated episodes of gonorrhea. Clinicians should also consider local epidemiology.

HR3: Men who had sex with men after 1975; past or present injection drug users; persons who exchange sex for money or drugs and their sex partners; persons with current or past injection drug–using, bisexual, or HIV-positive sex partners; recipients of a blood transfusion between 1978 and 1985; persons seeking treatment for STDs. Clinicians should also consider local epidemiology and HIV screening in the general population.

HR4: Sexually active women with multiple risk factors, including history of STD, new or multiple sex partners, nonuse or inconsistent use of barrier contraceptives, or cervical ectopy. Clinicians should also consider local epidemiology.

HR5: Blood product recipients (including hemodialysis patients), persons with frequent occupational exposure to blood or blood products, men who have sex with men, injection drug users and their sex partners, persons with multiple recent sex partners, persons with other STDs (including HIV), travelers to countries with endemic hepatitis B, all diabetics age 19 to 59.

HR6: Persons living in, traveling to, or working in areas where the disease is endemic and where periodic outbreaks occur (e.g., countries with high or intermediate endemicity; certain Alaska Native, Pacific Island, Native American, and religious communities); men who have sex with men; injection or street drug users; patients with clotting factor disorders or chronic liver disease. Consider for institutionalized persons and workers in these institutions; military personnel; and day-care, hospital, and laboratory workers. Clinicians should also consider local epidemiology.

HR7: HIV-positive, close contacts of persons with known or suspected TB, health care workers, persons with medical risk factors associated with TB, immigrants from countries with high TB prevalence, medically underserved low-income populations (including homeless), alcoholics, injection drug users, and residents of long-term care facilities.

HR8: Persons who continue to inject drugs.

HR9: Immunocompetent institutionalized persons and immunocompetent persons with certain medical conditions, including chronic cardiac, renal, or pulmonary disease; anatomic asplenia; diabetes mellitus; or cochlear implant candidates and recipients. Immunocompetent persons who live in high-risk environments or social settings (e.g., certain Native American and Alaska Native populations), adults who smoke cigarettes, persons with asymptomatic or symptomatic HIV infection.

HR10: Annual vaccination of residents of long-term care facilities; persons with chronic cardiopulmonary disorders, metabolic diseases (including diabetes mellitus), hemoglobinopathies, immunosuppression, or renal dysfunction; and health care providers of high-risk patients.

HR11: Persons born after 1956 who lack evidence of immunity to measles or mumps (e.g., documented receipt of live vaccine on or after the first birthday, laboratory evidence of immunity, or a history of physician-diagnosed measles or mumps).

HR12: Healthy adults without a history of chickenpox or previous immunization. Consider serologic testing for presumed susceptible adults.

HR13: Persons with a family or personal history of skin cancer; a large number of moles; atypical moles; poor tanning ability; or light skin, hair, and eye color.

HR14: Women with previous pregnancy affected by neural tube disorder who are planning pregnancy.

HR15: Clinicians should consider a fasting serum lipid panel on a case-by-case basis.

TABLE 5-4 Ages 65 and Older

Interventions considered and recommended for the Periodic Health Examination	Leading causes of death
	Heart diseases
	Malignant neoplasms (lung, colorectal, breast)
	Cerebrovascular disease
	Chronic obstructive pulmonary disease
	Pneumonia and influenza

INTERVENTIONS FOR THE GENERAL POPULATION

Screening

Blood pressure

Height and weight

Fecal occult blood test[1] and/or colonoscopy

Mammogram $\pm$ clinical breast examination[2] (women ≤69 yr)

Papanicolaou (Pap) test (women)[3]

Bone density scan in postmenopausal patients

Vision screening

Assess for hearing impairment

Assess for problem drinking

Offer HIV screen

Counseling

Substance use

Tobacco cessation

Avoid alcohol/drug use while driving, swimming, boating, etc.*

Diet and exercise

Limit fat and cholesterol; maintain caloric balance; emphasize grains, fruits, vegetables

Adequate calcium intake (women)

Regular physical activity*

Injury prevention

Lap/shoulder belts

Motorcycle and bicycle helmets*

Fall prevention*

Safe storage/removal of firearms*

Smoke detector*

Set hot water heater to <120°-130° F

CPR training for household members

Dental health

Regular visits to dental care provider*

Floss, brush with fluoride toothpaste daily*

Sexual behavior

STD prevention: avoid high-risk sexual behavior*; use condoms

Immunizations

Pneumococcal vaccine

Influenza[1]

Tetanus-diphtheria (Td) boosters every 10 years, with 1 substitute Tdap dose

Herpes zoster[4]

INTERVENTIONS FOR HIGH-RISK POPULATIONS

Population	Potential Interventions (see detailed high-risk definitions)
Institutionalized persons	PPD (HR1); hepatitis A vaccine (HR2); amantadine/rimantadine (HR4)
Chronic medical conditions; TB contacts; low income; immigrants; alcoholics	PPD (HR1)
Persons ≥75 yr or ≥70 yr with risk factors for falls	Fall prevention intervention (HR5)
Cardiovascular disease risk factors	Consider lipid screening (HR6)
Family history of skin cancer; nevi; fair skin, eyes, hair	Avoid excess/midday sun, use protective clothing* (HR7)
Native Americans/Alaska Natives	PPD (HR1); hepatitis A vaccine (HR2)
Travelers to developing countries	Hepatitis A vaccine (HR2); hepatitis B vaccine (HR8)
Blood product recipients	HIV screen (HR3); hepatitis B vaccine (HR8)
High-risk sexual behavior	Hepatitis A vaccine (HR2); HIV screen (HR3); hepatitis B vaccine (HR8); RPR/VDRL (HR9)
Injection or street drug use	PPD (HR1); hepatitis A vaccine (HR2); HIV screen (HR3); hepatitis B vaccine (HR8); RPR/VDRL (HR9); advice to reduce infection risk (HR10)
Health care/lab workers	PPD (HR1); hepatitis A vaccine (HR2); amantadine/rimantadine (HR4); hepatitis B vaccine (HR8)
Persons susceptible to varicella	Varicella vaccine (HR11)
Men aged 65 to 75 who have ever smoked	Ultrasound of abdominal aorta (HR12)

HR, High risk; *PPD,* purified protein derivative; *RPR,* rapid plasma reagin; *STD,* sexually transmitted disease; *TB,* tuberculosis; *VDRL,* Venereal Disease Research Laboratory.

[1]Annually. [2]Mammogram q1-2 yr, or mammogram q1-2 yr with annual clinical breast exam. [3]The American Cancer Society (ACS) recommends that Pap testing can be discontinued at age 65 after three negative Pap tests or two negative HPV tests in past three years. ACOG (American College of Obstetricians and Gynecologists) recommends discontinuing Pap testing at age 65 to 70 after three negative tests in preceding 10 years. [4]Herpes zoster vaccine (Zostavax) is indicated for prevention of herpes zoster (shingles) in individuals age ≥60 yr. Zostavax is administered as a single dose subcutaneously. It is a lyophilic preparation of the Oka/Merck strain of live, attenuated varicella zoster virus (VZV). It should not be administered to individuals with a history of primary or acquired immunodeficiency states, persons on immunosuppressive therapy (including high-dose corticosteroids), those with active untreated tuberculosis, and those who may be pregnant.
*The ability of clinician counseling to influence this behavior is unproven.

HR1: HIV-positive, close contacts of persons with known or suspected TB, health care workers, persons with medical risk factors associated with TB, immigrants from countries with high TB prevalence, medically underserved low-income populations (including homeless), alcoholics, injection drug users, and residents of long-term care facilities.

HR2: Persons living in, traveling to, or working in areas where the disease is endemic and where periodic outbreaks occur (e.g., countries with high or intermediate endemicity; certain Alaska Native, Pacific Island, Native American, and religious communities); men who have sex with men; injection or street drug users; persons with clotting factor disorders or chronic liver disease. Consider for institutionalized persons and workers in these institutions and day-care, hospital, and laboratory workers. Clinicians should also consider local epidemiology and HIV screening in the general population.

HR3: Men who had sex with men after 1975; past or present injection drug users; persons who exchange sex for money or drugs and their sex partners; persons with current or past injection drug–using, bisexual, or HIV-positive sex partners; recipients of a blood transfusion between 1978 and 1985; persons seeking treatment for STDs. Clinicians should also consider local epidemiology.

HR4: Consider for persons who have not received influenza vaccine or are vaccinated late, when the vaccine may be ineffective because of major antigenic changes in the virus; for unvaccinated persons who provide home care for high-risk persons; as supplemental protection in persons who are expected to have a poor antibody response; and for high-risk persons in whom the vaccine is contraindicated.

HR5: Persons aged ≥75 yr or 70-74 yr with one or more additional risk factors, including use of certain psychoactive and cardiac medications (e.g., benzodiazepines, antihypertensives); use of four or more prescription medications; impaired cognition, strength, balance, or gait. Intensive individualized, home-based multifactorial fall prevention intervention is recommended in settings where adequate resources are available to deliver such services.

HR6: Clinicians should consider fasting lipid panel screening on a case-by-case basis for persons aged 65 to 75 yr, especially in those with additional risk factors (e.g., smoking, diabetes, or hypertension).

HR7: Persons with a family or personal history of skin cancer; a large number of moles; atypical moles; poor tanning ability; or light skin, hair, and eye color.

HR8: Blood product recipients (including hemodialysis patients), persons with frequent occupational exposure to blood or blood products, men who have sex with men, injection drug users and their sex partners, persons with multiple recent sex partners, persons with other STDs (including HIV), travelers to countries with endemic hepatitis B.

HR9: Persons who exchange sex for money or drugs and their sex partners, persons with other STDs (including HIV), and sexual contacts of persons with active syphilis. Clinicians should also consider local epidemiology.

HR10: Persons who continue to inject drugs.

HR11: Healthy adults without a history of chickenpox or previous immunization. Consider serologic testing for presumed susceptible adults.

HR12: Consider ultrasound of abdominal aorta to screen for abdominal aortic aneurysm in all men aged 65 to 75 yr who have ever smoked.

TABLE 5-5   Pregnant Women*

Interventions considered and recommended for the Periodic Health Examination

INTERVENTIONS FOR THE GENERAL POPULATION

Screening

First visit

Blood pressure

Hemoglobin/hematocrit

Hepatitis B surface antigen (HBsAg)

RPR/VDRL

Chlamydia screen (<25 yr)

Rubella serology or vaccination history

D(Rh) typing, antibody screen

Offer CVS (<13 wk)[1] or amniocentesis (15-18 wk)[1] (age ≥35 yr)

Offer hemoglobinopathy screening

Assess for problem or risk drinking

Offer HIV screening[2]

Follow-up visits

Blood pressure

Urine culture (12-16 wk)

Offer amniocentesis (15-18 wk)[1] (age ≥35 yr)

Offer multiple marker testing[1] (15-18 wk)

Offer serum α-fetoprotein[1] (16-18 wk)

Counseling

Tobacco cessation; effects of passive smoking

Alcohol/other drug use

Nutrition, including adequate calcium intake

Encourage breastfeeding

Lap/shoulder belts

Infant safety car seats

STD prevention: avoid high-risk sexual behavior[†]; use condoms[†]

Chemoprophylaxis

Multivitamin with folic acid[3]

INTERVENTIONS FOR HIGH-RISK POPULATIONS

Population	Potential Interventions (see detailed high-risk definitions)
High-risk sexual behavior	Screen for chlamydia (first visit) (HR1), gonorrhea (first visit) (HR2), HIV (first visit) (HR3); HBsAg (third trimester) (HR4); RPR/VDRL (third trimester) (HR5)
Blood transfusion between 1978 and 1985	HIV screen (first visit) (HR3)
Injection drug use	HIV screen (HR3); HBsAg (third trimester) (HR4); advice to reduce infection risk (HR6)
Unsensitized D-negative women	D(Rh) antibody testing (24-28 wk) (HR7)
Risk factors for Down syndrome	Offer CVS (first trimester), amniocentesis (15-18 wk)[1] (HR8)
Prior pregnancy with neural tube defect	Offer amniocentesis (15-18 wk),[1] folic acid 4.0 mg[3] (HR9)

CVS, Chorionic villus sampling; *HR,* high risk; *RPR,* rapid plasma reagin; *VDRL,* Venereal Disease Research Laboratory.

[1]Women with access to counseling and follow-up services, reliable standardized laboratories, skilled high-resolution ultrasound and, for those receiving serum marker testing, amniocentesis capabilities. [2]Universal screening is recommended. [3]Beginning at least 1 mo before conception and continuing through the first trimester.

*See Tables 5-2 and 5-3 for other preventive services recommended for women of this age group.

[†]The ability of clinician counseling to influence this behavior is unproven.

HR1: Women with history of STD or new or multiple sex partners. Clinicians should also consider local epidemiology. Chlamydia screen should be repeated in third trimester if at continued risk.

HR2: Women younger than 25 yr with two or more sex partners in the last year or whose sex partner has multiple sexual contacts, women who exchange sex for money or drugs, and women with a history of repeated episodes of gonorrhea. Clinicians should also consider local epidemiology. Gonorrhea screen should be repeated in the third trimester if at continued risk.

HR3: Universal screening for HIV infection is recommended for all pregnant women. It is especially important in women with the following individual risk factors: past or present injection drug use; history of exchanging sex for money or drugs; injection drug–using, bisexual, or HIV-positive sex partner currently or in the past; recipients of a blood transfusion between 1978 and 1985; persons seeking treatment for STDs.

HR4: Women who are initially HBsAg negative who are at high risk because of injection drug use, who have suspected exposure to hepatitis B during pregnancy, and who have had multiple sex partners.

HR5: Women who exchange sex for money or drugs, women with other STDs (including HIV), and sexual contacts of persons with active syphilis. Clinicians should also consider local epidemiology.

HR6: Women who continue to inject drugs.

HR7: Unsensitized D-negative women.

HR8: Prior pregnancy affected by Down syndrome, advanced maternal age (≥35 yr), known carriage of chromosome rearrangement.

HR9: Women with previous pregnancy affected by neural tube defect.

TABLE 5-6 Cervical Cancer Screening Guidelines

Group	ACOG 2009	USPSTF 2012	ACS 2012
Women age <21	No screening	No screening	No screening
Women age 21-29	Cytology every 2 years; HPV testing not recommended	Cytology every 3 years; HPV testing not recommended	Cytology every 3 years; HPV testing not recommended
Women age 30-65	Cytology every 3 years if three consecutive normal results; addition of HPV testing also appropriate	Cytology every 3 years or cytology plus HPV testing every 5 years	Cytology plus HPV every 5 years (preferred) or cytology alone every 3 years; both are regardless of screening history
Women age >65	Following three normal screening results and no abnormal results in the last 10 years, screening may be discontinued	If adequately screened in the past, screening should be discontinued	If adequately screened in the past, screening should be discontinued
Women with total hysterectomy and no prior history of high-grade CIN	No need to continue screening if hysterectomy was for benign indication	Screening should be discontinued	Screening should be discontinued

ACOG, American College of Obstetricians and Gynecologists; *ACS,* American Cancer Society; *CIN,* Cervical intraepithelial neoplasia; *HPV,* human papillomavirus; *USPSTF,* U.S. Preventive Services Task Force.

PART B • IMMUNIZATIONS AND CHEMOPROPHYLAXIS

Childhood and Adolescent Immunizations

TABLE 5-7 Recommended Immunization Schedule for Persons Aged 0 Through 18 Years: United States (For those who fall behind or start late, see the schedule below and the catch-up schedule [Table 5-8])

These recommendations must be read with the footnotes that follow. For those who fall behind or start late, provide catch-up vaccination at the earliest opportunity as indicated by the green bars. To determine minimum intervals between doses, see the catch-up schedule (Table 5-8). School entry and adolescent vaccine age groups are in bold.

Vaccines	Birth	1 mo	2 mos	4 mos	6 mos	9 mos	12 mos	15 mos	18 mos	19-23 mos	2-3 yrs	**4-6 yrs**	7-10 yrs	**11-12 yrs**	13-15 yrs	16-18 yrs
Hepatitis B[1] (HepB)	1st dose	2nd dose			← 3rd dose →											
Rotavirus[2] (RV) RV-1 (2-dose series); RV-5 (3-dose series)			1st dose	2nd dose	See footnote 2											
Diphtheria, tetanus, & acellular pertussis[3] (DTaP: <7 yrs)			1st dose	2nd dose	3rd dose		← 4th dose →					5th dose				
Tetanus, diphtheria, & acellular pertussis[4] (Tdap: ≥7 yrs)														(Tdap)		
Haemophilus influenzae type b[5] (Hib)			1st dose	2nd dose	See footnote 5		3rd or 4th dose see footnote 5									
Pneumococcal conjugate[6a,c] (PCV13)			1st dose	2nd dose	3rd dose		4th dose									
Pneumococcal polysaccharide[6b,c] (PPSV23)																
Inactivated poliovirus[7] (IPV) (<18years)			1st dose	2nd dose	← 3rd dose →							4th dose				
Influenza[8] (IIV; LAIV) 2 doses for some : see footnote 8					Annual vaccination (IIV only)						Annual vaccination (IIV or LAIV)					
Measles, mumps, rubella[9] (MMR)							1st dose					2nd dose				
Varicella[10] (VAR)							1st dose					2nd dose				
Hepatitis A[11] (HepA)							2 dose series see footnote 11									
Human papillomavirus[12] (HPV2: females only; HPV4: males and females)														(3 dose series)		
Meningococcal[13] (Hib-MenCY ≥ 6 wks; MCV4-D≥9 mos; MCV4-CRM ≥ 2 yrs.)					see footnote 13									1st dose		booster

Range of recommended ages for all children	Range of recommended ages for catch-up immunization	Range of recommended ages for certain high-risk groups	Range of recommended ages during which catch-up is encouraged and for certain high-risk groups	Not routinely recommended

This schedule includes recommendations in effect as of January 1, 2013. Any dose not administered at the recommended age should be administered at a subsequent visit, when indicated and feasible. The use of a combination vaccine generally is preferred over separate injections of its equivalent component vaccines. Vaccination providers should consult the relevant Advisory Committee on Immunization Practices (ACIP) statement for detailed recommendations, available online at http://www.cdc.gov/vaccines/pubs/acip-list.htm. Clinically significant adverse events that follow vaccination should be reported to the Vaccine Adverse Event Reporting System (VAERS) online (http://www.vaers.hhs.gov) or by telephone (800-822-7967). Suspected cases of vaccine-preventable diseases should be reported to the state or local health department. Additional information, including precautions and contraindications for vaccination, is available from CDC online (http://www.cdc.gov/vaccines) or by telephone (800-CDC-INFO [800-232-4636]).

This schedule is approved by the Advisory Committee on Immunization Practices (http://www.cdc.gov/vaccines/acip/index.html), the American Academy of Pediatrics (http://www.aap.org), the American Academy of Family Physicians (http://www.aafp.org), and the American College of Obstetricians and Gynecologists (http://www.acog.org).

NOTE: The above recommendations must be read along with the footnotes for Table 5-8.

TABLE 5-8 Catch-up Immunization Schedule for Persons Aged 4 Months Through 18 Years Who Start Late or Who Are More Than 1 Month Behind: United States

The table below provides catch-up schedules and minimum intervals between doses for children whose vaccinations have been delayed. A vaccine series does not need to be restarted, regardless of the time that has elapsed between doses. Use the section appropriate for the child's age. Always use this table in conjunction with Table 5-7 and the footnotes that follow.

		Persons aged 4 months through 6 years			
		Minimum Interval Between Doses			
Vaccine	Minimum Age for Dose 1	Dose 1 to dose 2	Dose 2 to dose 3	Dose 3 to dose 4	Dose 4 to dose 5
Hepatitis B[1]	Birth	4 weeks	8 weeks and at least 16 weeks after first dose; minimum age for the final dose is 24 weeks		
Rotavirus[2]	6 weeks	4 weeks	4 weeks[2]		
Diphtheria, tetanus, pertussis[3]	6 weeks	4 weeks	4 weeks	6 months	6 months[3]
Haemophilus influenzae type b[5]	6 weeks	4 weeks if first dose administered at younger than age 12 months 8 weeks (as final dose) if first dose administered at age 12–14 months No further doses needed if first dose administered at age 15 months or older	4 weeks[5] if current age is younger than 12 months 8 weeks (as final dose)[5] if current age is 12 months or older and first dose administered at younger than age 12 months and second dose administered at younger than 15 months No further doses needed if previous dose administered at age 15 months or older	8 weeks (as final dose) This dose only necessary for children aged 12 through 59 months who received 3 doses before age 12 months	
Pneumococcal[6]	6 weeks	4 weeks if first dose administered at younger than age 12 months 8 weeks (as final dose for healthy children) if first dose administered at age 12 months or older or current age 24 through 59 months No further doses needed for healthy children if first dose administered at age 24 months or older	4 weeks if current age is younger than 12 months 8 weeks (as final dose for healthy children) if current age is 12 months or older No further doses needed for healthy children if previous dose administered at age 24 months or older	8 weeks (as final dose) This dose only necessary for children aged 12 through 59 months who received 3 doses before age 12 months or for children at high risk who received 3 doses at any age	
Inactivated poliovirus[7]	6 weeks	4 weeks	4 weeks	6 months[7] minimum age 4 years for final dose	
Meningococcal[13]	6 weeks	8 weeks[13]	see footnote 13	see footnote 13	
Measles, mumps, rubella[9]	12 months	4 weeks			
Varicella[10]	12 months	3 months			
Hepatitis A[11]	12 months	6 months			
		Persons aged 7 through 18 years			
Tetanus, diphtheria; tetanus, diphtheria, pertussis[4]	7 years[4]	4 weeks	4 weeks if first dose administered at younger than age 12 months 6 months if first dose administered at 12 months or older	6 months if first dose administered at younger than age 12 months	
Human papillomavirus[12]	9 years	Routine dosing intervals are recommended[12]			
Hepatitis A[11]	12 months	6 months			
Hepatitis B[1]	Birth	4 weeks	8 weeks (and at least 16 weeks after first dose)		
Inactivated poliovirus[7]	6 weeks	4 weeks	4 weeks[7]	6 months[7]	
Meningococcal[13]	6 weeks	8 weeks[13]			
Measles, mumps, rubella[9]	12 months	4 weeks			
Varicella[10]	12 months	3 months if person is younger than age 13 years 4 weeks if person is aged 13 years or older			

NOTE: The above recommendations must be read along with the footnotes on the following pages.

Footnotes: Recommended Immunization Schedule for Persons Aged 0 Through 18 Years — United States, 2013

Additional guidance for use of the vaccines described in this publication is available at http://www.cdc.gov/vaccines/pubs/acip-list.htm

1. **Hepatitis B (HepB) vaccine. (Minimum age: birth)**
   Routine vaccination:
   At birth
   - Administer monovalent HepB vaccine to all newborns before hospital discharge.
   - For infants born to hepatitis B surface antigen (HBsAg)–positive mothers, administer HepB vaccine and 0.5 mL of hepatitis B immune globulin (HBIG) within 12 hours of birth. These infants should be tested for HBsAg and antibody to HBsAg (anti-HBs) 1 to 2 months after completion of the HepB series, at age 9 through 18 months (preferably at the next well-child visit).
   - If mother's HBsAg status is unknown, within 12 hours of birth administer HepB vaccine to all infants regardless of birth weight. For infants weighing <2,000 grams, administer HBIG in addition to HepB within 12 hours of birth. Determine mother's HBsAg status as soon as possible and, if she is HBsAg-positive, also administer HBIG for infants weighing ≥2,000 grams (no later than age 1 week).
   Doses following the birth dose
   - The second dose should be administered at age 1 or 2 months. Monovalent HepB vaccine should be used for doses administered before age 6 weeks.
   - Infants who did not receive a birth dose should receive 3 doses of a HepB-containing vaccine on a schedule of 0, 1 to 2 months, and 6 months starting as soon as feasible. See Table 5-8.
   - The minimum interval between dose 1 and dose 2 is 4 weeks and between dose 2 and 3 is 8 weeks. The final (third or fourth) dose in the HepB vaccine series should be administered no earlier than age 24 weeks, and at least 16 weeks after the first dose.
   - Administration of a total of 4 doses of HepB vaccine is recommended when a combination vaccine containing HepB is administered after the birth dose.
   Catch-up vaccination:
   - Unvaccinated persons should complete a 3-dose series.
   - A 2-dose series (doses separated by at least 4 months) of adult formulation Recombivax HB is licensed for use in children aged 11 through 15 years.
   - For other catch-up issues, see Table 5-8.

2. **Rotavirus (RV) vaccines. (Minimum age: 6 weeks for both RV-1 [Rotarix] and RV-5 [RotaTeq]).**
   Routine vaccination:
   - Administer a series of RV vaccine to all infants as follows:
     1. If RV-1 is used, administer a 2-dose series at 2 and 4 months of age.
     2. If RV-5 is used, administer a 3-dose series at ages 2, 4, and 6 months.
     3. If any dose in series was RV-5 or vaccine product is unknown for any dose in the series, a total of 3 doses of RV vaccine should be administered.
   Catch-up vaccination:
   - The maximum age for the first dose in the series is 14 weeks, 6 days.
   - Vaccination should not be initiated for infants aged 15 weeks 0 days or older.
   - The maximum age for the final dose in the series is 8 months, 0 days.
   - If RV-1(Rotarix) is administered for the first and second doses, a third dose is not indicated.
   - For other catch-up issues, see Table 5-8.

3. **Diphtheria and tetanus toxoids and acellular pertussis (DTaP) vaccine. (Minimum age: 6 weeks)**
   Routine vaccination:
   - Administer a 5-dose series of DTaP vaccine at ages 2, 4, 6, 15–18 months, and 4 through 6 years. The fourth dose may be administered as early as age 12 months, provided at least 6 months have elapsed since the third dose.
   Catch-up vaccination:
   - The fifth (booster) dose of DTaP vaccine is not necessary if the fourth dose was administered at age 4 years or older.
   - For other catch-up issues, see Table 5-8.

4. **Tetanus and diphtheria toxoids and acellular pertussis (Tdap) vaccine. (Minimum age: 10 years for Boostrix, 11 years for Adacel).**
   Routine vaccination:
   - Administer 1 dose of Tdap vaccine to all adolescents aged 11 through 12 years.
   - Tdap can be administered regardless of the interval since the last tetanus and diphtheria toxoid-containing vaccine.
   - Administer one dose of Tdap vaccine to pregnant adolescents during each pregnancy (preferred during 27 through 36 weeks gestation) regardless of number of years from prior Td or Tdap vaccination.

   Catch-up vaccination:
   - Persons aged 7 through 10 years who are not fully immunized with the childhood DTaP vaccine series, should receive Tdap vaccine as the first dose in the catch-up series; if additional doses are needed, use Td vaccine. For these children, an adolescent Tdap vaccine should not be given.
   - Persons aged 11 through 18 years who have not received Tdap vaccine should receive a dose followed by tetanus and diphtheria toxoids (Td) booster doses every 10 years thereafter.
   - An inadvertent dose of DTaP vaccine administered to children aged 7 through 10 years can count as part of the catch-up series. This dose can count as the adolescent Tdap dose, or the child can later receive a Tdap booster dose at age 11–12 years.
   - For other catch-up issues, see Table 5-8.

5. ***Haemophilus influenzae* type b (Hib) conjugate vaccine. (Minimum age: 6 weeks)**
   Routine vaccination:
   - Administer a Hib vaccine primary series and a booster dose to all infants. The primary series doses should be administered at 2, 4, and 6 months of age; however, if PRP-OMP (PedvaxHib or Comvax) is administered at 2 and 4 months of age, a dose at age 6 months is not indicated. One booster dose should be administered at age 12 through15 months.
   - Hiberix (PRP-T) should only be used for the booster (final) dose in children aged 12 months through 4 years, who have received at least 1 dose of Hib.
   Catch-up vaccination:
   - If dose 1 was administered at ages 12-14 months, administer booster (as final dose) at least 8 weeks after dose 1.
   - If the first 2 doses were PRP-OMP (PedvaxHIB or Comvax), and were administered at age 11 months or younger, the third (and final) dose should be administered at age 12 through 15 months and at least 8 weeks after the second dose.
   - If the first dose was administered at age 7 through 11 months, administer the second dose at least 4 weeks later and a final dose at age 12 through 15 months, regardless of Hib vaccine (PRP-T or PRP-OMP) used for first dose.
   - For unvaccinated children aged 15 months or older, administer only 1 dose.
   - For other catch-up issues, see Table 5-8.
   Vaccination of persons with high-risk conditions:
   - Hib vaccine is not routinely recommended for patients older than 5 years of age. However one dose of Hib vaccine should be administered to unvaccinated or partially vaccinated persons aged 5 years or older who have leukemia, malignant neoplasms, anatomic or functional asplenia (including sickle cell disease), human immunodeficiency virus (HIV) infection, or other immunocompromising conditions.

6a. **Pneumococcal conjugate vaccine (PCV). (Minimum age: 6 weeks)**
   Routine vaccination:
   - Administer a series of PCV13 vaccine at ages 2, 4, 6 months with a booster at age 12 through 15 months.
   - For children aged 14 through 59 months who have received an age-appropriate series of 7-valent PCV (PCV7), administer a single supplemental dose of 13-valent PCV (PCV13).
   Catch-up vaccination:
   - Administer 1 dose of PCV13 to all healthy children aged 24 through 59 months who are not completely vaccinated for their age.
   - For other catch-up issues, see Table 5-8.
   Vaccination of persons with high-risk conditions:
   - For children aged 24 through 71 months with certain underlying medical conditions (see footnote 6c), administer 1 dose of PCV13 if 3 doses of PCV were received previously, or administer 2 doses of PCV13 at least 8 weeks apart if fewer than 3 doses of PCV were received previously.
   - A single dose of PCV13 may be administered to previously unvaccinated children aged 6 through 18 years who have anatomic or functional asplenia (including sickle cell disease), HIV infection or an immunocompromising condition, cochlear implant or cerebrospinal fluid leak. See MMWR 2010;59 (No. RR-11), available at http://www.cdc.gov/mmwr/pdf/rr/rr5911.pdf.
   - Administer PPSV23 at least 8 weeks after the last dose of PCV to children aged 2 years or older with certain underlying medical conditions (see footnotes 6b and 6c).

6b. Pneumococcal polysaccharide vaccine (PPSV23). (Minimum age: 2 years)
Vaccination of persons with high-risk conditions:
- Administer PPSV23 at least 8 weeks after the last dose of PCV to children aged 2 years or older with certain underlying medical conditions (see footnote 6c). A single revaccination with PPSV should be administered after 5 years to children with anatomic or functional asplenia (including sickle cell disease) or an immunocompromising condition.

6c. Medical conditions for which PPSV23 is indicated in children aged 2 years and older and for which use of PCV13 is indicated in children aged 24 through 71 months:
- Immunocompetent children with chronic heart disease (particularly cyanotic congenital heart disease and cardiac failure); chronic lung disease (including asthma if treated with high-dose oral corticosteroid therapy), diabetes mellitus; cerebrospinal fluid leaks; or cochlear implant.
- Children with anatomic or functional asplenia (including sickle cell disease and other hemoglobinopathies, congenital or acquired asplenia, or splenic dysfunction);
- Children with immunocompromising conditions: HIV infection, chronic renal failure and nephrotic syndrome, diseases associated with treatment with immunosuppressive drugs or radiation therapy, including malignant neoplasms, leukemias, lymphomas and Hodgkin disease; or solid organ transplantation, congenital immunodeficiency.

7. Inactivated poliovirus vaccine (IPV). (Minimum age: 6 weeks)
Routine vaccination:
- Administer a series of IPV at ages 2, 4, 6–18 months, with a booster at age 4–6 years. The final dose in the series should be administered on or after the fourth birthday and at least 6 months after the previous dose.

Catch-up vaccination:
- In the first 6 months of life, minimum age and minimum intervals are only recommended if the person is at risk for imminent exposure to circulating poliovirus (i.e., travel to a polio-endemic region or during an outbreak).
- If 4 or more doses are administered before age 4 years, an additional dose should be administered at age 4 through 6 years.
- A fourth dose is not necessary if the third dose was administered at age 4 years or older and at least 6 months after the previous dose.
- If both OPV and IPV were administered as part of a series, a total of 4 doses should be administered, regardless of the child's current age.
- IPV is not routinely recommended for U.S. residents aged 18 years or older.
- For other catch-up issues, see Table 5-8.

8. Influenza vaccines. (Minimum age: 6 months for inactivated influenza vaccine [IIV]; 2 years for live, attenuated influenza vaccine [LAIV])
Routine vaccination:
- Administer influenza vaccine annually to all children beginning at age 6 months. For most healthy, nonpregnant persons aged 2 through 49 years, either LAIV or IIV may be used. However, LAIV should NOT be administered to some persons, including 1) those with asthma, 2) children 2 through 4 years who had wheezing in the past 12 months, or 3) those who have any other underlying medical conditions that predispose them to influenza complications. For all other contraindications to use of LAIV see MMWR 2010; 59 (No. RR-8), available at http://www.cdc.gov/mmwr/pdf/rr/rr5908.pdf.
- Administer 1 dose to persons aged 9 years and older.

For children aged 6 months through 8 years:
- For the 2012–13 season, administer 2 doses (separated by at least 4 weeks) to children who are receiving influenza vaccine for the first time. For additional guidance, follow dosing guidelines in the 2012 ACIP influenza vaccine recommendations, MMWR 2012; 61: 613–618, available at http://www.cdc.gov/mmwr/pdf/wk/mm6132.pdf.
- For the 2013–14 season, follow dosing guidelines in the 2013 ACIP influenza vaccine recommendations.

9. Measles, mumps, and rubella (MMR) vaccine. (Minimum age: 12 months for routine vaccination)
Routine vaccination:
- Administer the first dose of MMR vaccine at age 12 through 15 months, and the second dose at age 4 through 6 years. The second dose may be administered before age 4 years, provided at least 4 weeks have elapsed since the first dose.
- Administer 1 dose of MMR vaccine to infants aged 6 through 11 months before departure from the United States for international travel. These children should be revaccinated with 2 doses of MMR vaccine, the first at age 12 through 15 months (12 months if the child remains in an area where disease risk is high), and the second dose at least 4 weeks later.

- Administer 2 doses of MMR vaccine to children aged 12 months and older, before departure from the United States for international travel. The first dose should be administered on or after age 12 months and the second dose at least 4 weeks later.

Catch-up vaccination:
- Ensure that all school-aged children and adolescents have had 2 doses of MMR vaccine; the minimum interval between the 2 doses is 4 weeks.

10. Varicella (VAR) vaccine. (Minimum age: 12 months)
Routine vaccination:
- Administer the first dose of VAR vaccine at age 12 through 15 months, and the second dose at age 4 through 6 years. The second dose may be administered before age 4 years, provided at least 3 months have elapsed since the first dose. If the second dose was administered at least 4 weeks after the first dose, it can be accepted as valid.

Catch-up vaccination:
- Ensure that all persons aged 7 through 18 years without evidence of immunity (see MMWR 2007;56 [No. RR-4], available at http://www.cdc.gov/mmwr/pdf/rr/rr5604.pdf) have 2 doses of varicella vaccine. For children aged 7 through 12 years the recommended minimum interval between doses is 3 months (if the second dose was administered at least 4 weeks after the first dose, it can be accepted as valid); for persons aged 13 years and older, the minimum interval between doses is 4 weeks.

11. Hepatitis A vaccine (HepA). (Minimum age: 12 months)
Routine vaccination:
- Initiate the 2-dose HepA vaccine series for children aged 12 through 23 months; separate the 2 doses by 6 to 18 months.
- Children who have received 1 dose of HepA vaccine before age 24 months, should receive a second dose 6 to 18 months after the first dose.
- For any person aged 2 years and older who has not already received the HepA vaccine series, 2 doses of HepA vaccine separated by 6 to 18 months may be administered if immunity against hepatitis A virus infection is desired.

Catch-up vaccination:
- The minimum interval between the two doses is 6 months.

Special populations:
- Administer 2 doses of Hep A vaccine at least 6 months apart to previously unvaccinated persons who live in areas where vaccination programs target older children, or who are at increased risk for infection.

12. Human papillomavirus (HPV) vaccines. (HPV4 [Gardasil] and HPV2 [Cervarix]). (Minimum age: 9 years)
Routine vaccination:
- Administer a 3-dose series of HPV vaccine on a schedule of 0, 1-2, and 6 months to all adolescents aged 11-12 years. Either HPV4 or HPV2 may be used for females, and only HPV4 may be used for males.
- The vaccine series can be started beginning at age 9 years.
- Administer the second dose 1 to 2 months after the **first** dose and the third dose 6 months after the **first** dose (at least 24 weeks after the first dose).

Catch-up vaccination:
- Administer the vaccine series to females (either HPV2 or HPV4) and males (HPV4) at age 13 through 18 years if not previously vaccinated.
- Use recommended routine dosing intervals (see above) for vaccine series catch-up.

13. Meningococcal conjugate vaccines (MCV). (Minimum age: 6 weeks for Hib-MenCY, 9 months for Menactra [MCV4-D], 2 years for Menveo [MCV4-CRM]).
Routine vaccination:
- Administer MCV4 vaccine at age 11–12 years, with a booster dose at age 16 years.
- Adolescents aged 11 through 18 years with human immunodeficiency virus (HIV) infection should receive a 2-dose primary series of MCV4, with at least 8 weeks between doses. See MMWR 2011; 60:1018–1019 available at: http://www.cdc.gov/mmwr/pdf/wk/mm6030.pdf.
- For children aged 2 months through 10 years with high-risk conditions, see below.

Catch-up vaccination:
- Administer MCV4 vaccine at age 13 through 18 years if not previously vaccinated.
- If the first dose is administered at age 13 through 15 years, a booster dose should be administered at age 16 through 18 years with a minimum interval of at least 8 weeks between doses.
- If the first dose is administered at age 16 years or older, a booster dose is not needed.
- For other catch-up issues, see Table 5-8.

Vaccination of persons with high-risk conditions:

- For children younger than 19 months of age with anatomic or functional asplenia (including sickle cell disease), administer an infant series of Hib-MenCY at 2, 4, 6, and 12-15 months.
- For children aged 2 through 18 months with persistent complement component deficiency, administer either an infant series of Hib-MenCY at 2, 4, 6, and 12 through 15 months or a 2-dose primary series of MCV4-D starting at 9 months, with at least 8 weeks between doses. For children aged 19 through 23 months with persistent complement component deficiency who have not received a complete series of Hib-MenCY or MCV4-D, administer 2 primary doses of MCV4-D at least 8 weeks apart.
- For children aged 24 months and older with persistent complement component deficiency or anatomic or functional asplenia (including sickle cell disease), who have not received a complete series of Hib-MenCY or MCV4-D, administer 2 primary doses of either MCV4-D or MCV4-CRM. If MCV4-D (Menactra) is administered to a child with asplenia (including sickle cell disease), do not administer MCV4-D until 2 years of age and at least 4 weeks after the completion of all PCV13 doses. See MMWR 2011;60:1391–2, available at http://www.cdc.gov/mmwr/pdf/wk/mm6040.pdf.
- For children aged 9 months and older who are residents of or travelers to countries in the African meningitis belt or to the Hajj, administer an age appropriate formulation and series of MCV4 for protection against sero-groups A and W-135. Prior receipt of Hib-MenCY is not sufficient for children traveling to the meningitis belt or the Hajj. See MMWR 2011;60:1391–2, available at http://www.cdc.gov/mmwr/pdf/wk/mm6040.pdf.
- For children who are present during outbreaks caused by a vaccine sero-group, administer or complete an age and formulation-appropriate series of Hib-MenCY or MCV4.
- For booster doses among persons with high-risk conditions refer to http://www.cdc.gov/vaccines/pubs/acip-list.htm#mening.

Additional Vaccine Information

- For contraindications and precautions to use of a vaccine and for additional information regarding that vaccine, vaccination providers should consult the relevant ACIP statement available online at http://www.cdc.gov/vaccines/pubs/acip-list.htm.
- For the purposes of calculating intervals between doses, 4 weeks = 28 days. Intervals of 4 months or greater are determined by calendar months.
- Information on travel vaccine requirements and recommendations is available at http://wwwnc.cdc.gov/travel/page/vaccinations.htm.

- For vaccination of persons with primary and secondary immunodeficiencies, see Table 13, "Vaccination of persons with primary and secondary immunodeficiencies," in General Recommendations on Immunization (ACIP), available at http://www.cdc.gov/mmwr/preview/mmwrhtml/rr6002a1.htm; and American Academy of Pediatrics. Immunization in Special Clinical Circumstances. In: Pickering LK, Baker CJ, Kimberlin DW, Long SS eds. Red book: 2012 report of the Committee on Infectious Diseases. 29th ed. Elk Grove Village, IL: American Academy of Pediatrics.

General Recommendations on Immunization

TABLE 5-9 Recommended and Minimum Ages and Intervals between Vaccine Doses*†

Vaccine and Dose Number	Recommended Age for this Dose	Minimum Age for this Dose	Recommended Interval to Next Dose	Minimum Interval to Next Dose
HepB-1§	Birth	Birth	1-4 months	4 weeks
HepB-2	1-2 months	4 weeks	2-17 months	8 weeks
HepB-3¶	6-18 months	24 weeks	—	—
DTaP-1§	2 months	6 weeks	2 months	4 weeks
DTaP-2	4 months	10 weeks	2 months	4 weeks
DTaP-3	6 months	14 weeks	6-12 months	6 months**,††
DTaP-4	15-18 months	12 months	3 years	6 months**
DTaP-5	4-6 years	4 years	—	—
Hib-1§§§	2 months	6 weeks	2 months	4 weeks
Hib-2	4 months	10 weeks	2 months	4 weeks
Hib-3¶¶	6 months	14 weeks	6-9 months	8 weeks
Hib-4	12-15 months	12 months	—	—
IPV-1§	2 months	6 weeks	2 months	4 weeks
IPV-2	4 months	10 weeks	2-14 months	4 weeks
IPV-3	6-18 months	14 weeks	3-5 years	6 months
IPV-4***	4-6 years	4 years	—	—
PCV-1§§	2 months	6 weeks	8 weeks	4 weeks
PCV-2	4 months	10 weeks	8 weeks	4 weeks
PCV-3	6 months	14 weeks	6 months	8 weeks
PCV-4	12-15 months	12 months	—	—
MMR-1†††	12-15 months	12 months	3-5 years	4 weeks
MMR-2†††	4-6 years	13 months	—	—
Varicella-1†††	12-15 months	12 months	3-5 years	12 weeks§§§
Varicella-2†††	4-6 years	15 months	—	—
HepA-1	12-23 months	12 months	6-18 months**	6 months**
HepA-2	≥18 months	18 months	—	—
Influenza inactivated¶¶¶	≥6 months	6 months****	1 month	4 weeks
LAIV (intranasal)¶¶¶	2-49 years	2 years	1 month	4 weeks
MCV4-1††††	11-12 years	2 years	5 years	8 weeks
MCV4-2	16 years	11 years (+8 weeks)	—	—
MPSV4-1††††	—	2 years	5 years	5 years
MPSV4-2	—	7 years	—	—
Td	11-12 years	7 years	10 years	5 years
Tdap§§§§	≥11 years	7 years	—	—
PPSV-1	—	2 years	5 years	5 years
PPSV-2¶¶¶¶	—	7 years	—	—
HPV-1*****	11-12 years	9 years	2 months	4 weeks
HPV-2	11-12 years (+2 months)	9 years (+4 weeks)	4 months	12 weeks†††††
HPV-3†††††	11-12 years (+6 months)	9 years (+24 weeks)	—	—
Rotavirus-1§§§§§	2 months	6 weeks	2 months	4 weeks
Rotavirus-2	4 months	10 weeks	2 months	4 weeks
Rotavirus-3¶¶¶¶¶	6 months	14 weeks	—	—
Herpes zoster******	≥60 years	60 years	—	—

DTaP, Diphtheria and tetanus toxoids and acellular pertussis; *HepA*, hepatitis A; *HepB*, hepatitis B; *Hib*, *Haemophilus influenzae* type b; *HPV*, human papillomavirus; *IPV*, inactivated poliovirus; *LAIV*, live, attenuated influenza vaccine; *MCV4*, quadrivalent meningococcal conjugate vaccine; *MMR*, measles, mumps, and rubella; *MMRV*, measles, mumps, rubella, and varicella; *MPSV4*, quadrivalent meningococcal polysaccharide vaccine; *PCV*, pneumococcal conjugate vaccine; *PPSV*, pneumococcal polysaccharide vaccine; *PRP-OMB*, polyribosylribitol phosphate-meningococcal outer membrane protein conjugate; *Td*, tetanus and diphtheria toxoids; *Tdap*, tetanus toxoid, reduced diphtheria toxoid, and acellular pertussis.

*Combination vaccines are available. Use of licensed combination vaccines is generally preferred to separate injections of their equivalent component vaccines. When administering combination vaccines, the minimum age for administration is the oldest age for any of the individual components; the minimum interval between doses is equal to the greatest interval of any of the individual components.

†Information on travel vaccines, including typhoid, Japanese encephalitis, and yellow fever, is available at http://www.cdc.gov/travel. Information on other vaccines that are licensed in the United States but not distributed, including anthrax and smallpox, is available at http://www.bt.cdc.gov.

§Combination vaccines containing the hepatitis B component are available. These vaccines should not be administered to infants aged <6 weeks because of the other components (i.e., Hib, DTaP, HepA, and IPV).

¶HepB-3 should be administered at least 8 weeks after HepB-2 and at least 16 weeks after HepB-1 and should not be administered before age 24 weeks.

**Calendar months.

††The minimum recommended interval between DTaP-3 and DTaP-4 is 6 months. However, DTaP-4 need not be repeated if administered at least 4 months after DTaP-3.

§§For Hib and PCV, children receiving the first dose of vaccine at age ≥7 months require fewer doses to complete the series.

¶¶If PRP-QMP (Pedvax-Hib, Merck Vaccine Division) was administered at ages 2 and 4 months, a dose at age 6 months is not necessary.

***A fourth dose is not needed if the third dose was administered at ≥4 years and at least 6 months after the previous dose.

TABLE 5-9 Recommended and Minimum Ages and Intervals between Vaccine Doses—cont'd

†††Combination MMRV vaccine can be used for children aged 12 months to 12 years.

§§§The minimum interval from Varicella-1 to Varicella-2 for persons beginning the series at age ≥13 years is 4 weeks.

¶¶¶One dose of influenza vaccine per season is recommended for most persons. Children aged <9 years who are receiving influenza vaccine for the first time or who received only 1 dose the previous season (if it was their first vaccination season) should receive 2 doses this season.

****The minimum age for inactivated influenza vaccine varies by vaccine manufacturer. See package insert for vaccine-specific minimum ages.

††††Revaccination with meningococcal vaccine is recommended for previously vaccinated persons who remain at high risk for meningococcal disease. (Source: CDC. Updated recommendations from the Advisory Committee on Immunization Practices (ACIP) for revaccination of persons at prolonged increased risk for meningococcal disease. *MMWR* 2009;58:[1042-3]).

§§§§Only 1 dose of Tdap is recommended. Subsequent doses should be given as Td. For one brand of Tdap, the minimum age is 11 years. For management of a tetanus-prone wound in persons who have received a primary series of tetanus-toxoid–containing vaccine, the minimum interval after a previous dose of any tetanus-containing vaccine is 5 years.

¶¶¶¶A second dose of PPSV 5 years after the first dose is recommended for persons aged ≤65 years at highest risk for serious pneumococcal infection and those who are likely to have a rapid decline in pneumococcal antibody concentration. (Source: CDC. Prevention of pneumococcal disease: recommendations of the Advisory Committee on Immunization Practices [ACIP]. *MMWR* 1997;46[No. RR-8]).

*****Bivalent HPV vaccine is approved for females aged 10-25 years. Quadrivalent HPV vaccine is approved for males and females aged 9-26 years.

†††††The minimum age for HPV-3 is based on the baseline minimum age for the first dose (i.e., 108 months) and the minimum interval of 24 weeks between the first and third dose. Dose 3 need not be repeated if it is administered at least 16 weeks after the first dose.

§§§§§The first dose of rotavirus must be administered at age 6 weeks through 14 weeks and 6 days. The vaccine series should not be started for infants aged ≥15 weeks, 0 days. Rotavirus should not be administered to children older than 8 months, 0 days of age regardless of the number of doses received between 6 weeks and 8 months, 0 days of age.

¶¶¶¶¶If 2 doses of Rotarix (GlaxoSmithKline) are administered as age appropriate, a third dose is not necessary.

******Herpes zoster vaccine is recommended as a single dose for persons aged ≥60 years.

TABLE 5-10 Guidelines for Spacing of Live and Inactivated Antigens

Antigen Combination	Recommended Minimum Interval between Doses
Two or more inactivated*	May be administered simultaneously or at any interval between doses
Inactivated and live	May be administered simultaneously or at any interval between doses
Two or more live intranasal or injectable†	28 days minimum interval, if not administered simultaneously

From Centers for Disease Control and Prevention: General recommendations on immunization: recommendations of the Advisory Committee on Immunization Practices (ACIP), *MMWR* 60(2):38, 2011.

*Certain experts suggest a 28-day interval between tetanus toxoid, reduced diphtheria toxoid, and acellular pertussis (Tdap) vaccine and tetravalent meningococcal conjugate vaccine if they are not administered simultaneously.

†Live oral vaccines (e.g., Ty21a typhoid vaccine and rotavirus vaccine) may be administered simultaneously or at any interval before or after inactivated or live injectable vaccines.

TABLE 5-11 Guidelines for Administering Antibody-Containing Products* and Vaccines

Type of Administration	Products Administered		Recommended Minimum Interval Between Doses
Simultaneous (during the same office visit)	Antibody-containing products and inactivated antigen		Can be administered simultaneously at different anatomic sites or at any time interval between doses
	Antibody-containing products and live antigen		Should not be administered simultaneously.† If simultaneous administration of measles-containing vaccine or varicella vaccine is unavoidable, administer at different sites and revaccinate or test for seroconversion after the recommended interval
Nonsimultaneous	**Administered First**	**Administered Second**	
	Antibody-containing products	Inactivated antigen	No interval necessary
	Inactivated antigen	Antibody-containing products	No interval necessary
	Antibody-containing products	Live antigen	Dose related†,‡
	Live antigen	Antibody-containing products	2 weeks†

From Centers for Disease Control and Prevention: General recommendations on immunization: recommendations of the Advisory Committee on Immunization Practices (ACIP), *MMWR* 60:(RR-2), 2011.

*Blood products containing substantial amounts of immune globulin include intramuscular and intravenous immune globulin, specific hyperimmune globulin (e.g., hepatitis B immune globulin, tetanus immune globulin, varicella zoster immune globulin, and rabies immune globulin), whole blood, packed red blood cells, plasma, and platelet products.

†Yellow fever vaccine; rotavirus vaccine; oral Ty21a typhoid vaccine; live, attenuated influenza vaccine; and zoster vaccine are exceptions to these recommendations. These live, attenuated vaccines can be administered at any time before or after or simultaneously with an antibody-containing product.

‡The duration of interference of antibody-containing products with the immune response to the measles component of measles-containing vaccine, and possibly varicella vaccine, is dose related.

TABLE 5-12   Recommended Intervals between Administration of Antibody-Containing Products and Measles- or Varicella-Containing Vaccine, by Product and Indication for Vaccination

Product/Indication	Dose (mg IgG/kg) and Route*	Recommended Interval before Measles- or Varicella-Containing Vaccine[†] Administration (months)
Tetanus IG	250 units (10 mg IgG/kg) IM	3
Hepatitis A IG		
Contact prophylaxis	0.02 ml/kg (33 mg IgG/kg) IM	3
International travel	0.06 ml/kg (10 mg IgG/kg) IM	3
Hepatitis B IG	0.06 ml/kg (10 mg IgG/kg) IM	3
Rabies IG	20 IU/kg (22 mg IgG/kg) IM	4
Varicella IG	125 units/10 kg (60–200 mg IgG/kg) IM, maximum 625 units	5
Measles prophylaxis IG		
Standard (i.e., nonimmunocompromised) contact	0.25 ml/kg (40 mg IgG/kg) IM	5
Immunocompromised contact	0.50 ml/kg (80 mg IgG/kg) IM	6
Blood transfusion		
RBCs, washed	10 ml/kg negligible IgG/kg IV	None
RBCs, adenine-saline added	10 ml/kg (10 mg IgG/kg) IV	3
Packed RBCs (hematocrit 65%)[§]	10 ml/kg (60 mg IgG/kg) IV	6
Whole blood (hematocrit 35%-50%)[§]	10 ml/kg (80-100 mg IgG/kg) IV	6
Plasma/platelet products	10 ml/kg (160 mg IgG/kg) IV	7
Cytomegalovirus IGIV	150 mg/kg maximum	6
IGIV		
Replacement therapy for immune deficiencies[¶]	300-400 mg/kg IV[¶]	8
Immune thrombocytopenic purpura treatment	400 mg/kg IV	8
Postexposure varicella prophylaxis**	400 mg/kg IV	8
Immune thrombocytopenic purpura treatment	1000 mg/kg IV	10
Kawasaki disease	2 g/kg IV	11
Monoclonal antibody to respiratory syncytial virus F protein (Synagis [MedImmune])[††]	15 mg/kg IM	None

From Centers for Disease Control and Prevention: General recommendations on immunization: recommendations of the Advisory Committee on Immunization Practices (ACIP), *MMWR* 60:(RR-2), 2011.

HIV, human immunodeficiency virus; *IG,* immune globulin; *IgG,* immune globulin G; *IGIV,* intravenous immune globulin; *mg IgG/kg,* milligrams of immune globulin G per kilogram of body weight; *IM,* intramuscular; *IV,* intravenous; *RBCs,* red blood cells.

*This table is not intended for determining the correct indications and dosages for using antibody-containing products. Unvaccinated persons might not be protected fully against measles during the entire recommended interval, and additional doses of IG or measles vaccine might be indicated after measles exposure. Concentrations of measles antibody in an IG preparation can vary by manufacturer's lot. Rates of antibody clearance after receipt of an IG preparation also might vary. Recommended intervals are extrapolated from an estimated half-life of 30 days for passively acquired antibody and an observed interference with the immune response to measles vaccine for 5 months after a dose of 80 mg IgG/kg.

[†]Does not include zoster vaccine. Zoster vaccine may be given with antibody-containing blood products.

[§]Assumes a serum IgG concentration of 16 mg/mL.

[¶]Measles and varicella vaccinations are recommended for children with asymptomatic or mildly symptomatic HIV infection but are contraindicated for persons with severe immunosuppression from HIV or any other immunosuppressive disorder.

**The investigational VariZIG, similar to licensed varicella-zoster IG (VZIG), is a purified human IG preparation made from plasma containing high levels of antivaricella antibodies (IgG). The interval between VariZIG and varicella vaccine (Var or MMRV) is 5 months.

[††]Contains antibody only to respiratory syncytial virus.

TABLE 5-13 Contraindications and Precautions* to Commonly Used Vaccines

Vaccine	Contraindications	Precautions
DTaP	Severe allergic reaction (e.g., anaphylaxis) after a previous dose or to a vaccine component Encephalopathy (e.g., coma, decreased level of consciousness, or prolonged seizures), not attributable to another identifiable cause, within 7 days of administration of previous dose of DTP or DTaP	Progressive neurologic disorder, including infantile spasms, uncontrolled epilepsy, progressive encephalopathy; defer DTaP until neurologic status clarified and stabilized Temperature of ≥105°F (≥40°C) within 48 hours after vaccination with a previous dose of DTP or DTaP Collapse or shock-like state (i.e., hypotonic hyporesponsive episode) within 48 hours after receiving a previous dose of DTP/DTaP Seizure ≤3 days after receiving a previous dose of DTP/DTaP Persistent, inconsolable crying lasting ≥3 hours within 48 hours after receiving a previous dose of DTP/DTaP GBS <6 weeks after previous dose of tetanus toxoid-containing vaccine History of arthus-type hypersensitivity reactions after a previous dose of tetanus toxoid-containing vaccine; defer vaccination until at least 10 years have elapsed since the last tetanus-toxoid–containing vaccine Moderate or severe acute illness with or without fever
DT, Td	Severe allergic reaction (e.g., anaphylaxis) after a previous dose or to a vaccine component	GBS <6 weeks after previous dose of tetanus toxoid-containing vaccine History of Arthus-type hypersensitivity reactions after a previous dose of tetanus toxoid-containing vaccine; defer vaccination until at least 10 years have elapsed since the last tetanus-toxoid–containing vaccine Moderate or severe acute illness with or without fever
Tdap	Severe allergic reaction (e.g., anaphylaxis) after a previous dose or to a vaccine component Encephalopathy (e.g., coma, decreased level of consciousness, or prolonged seizures), not attributable to another identifiable cause, within 7 days of administration of previous dose of DTP, DTaP, or Tdap	GBS <6 weeks after a previous dose of tetanus toxoid-containing vaccine Progressive or unstable neurologic disorder, uncontrolled seizures, or progressive encephalopathy until a treatment regimen has been established and the condition has stabilized History of Arthus-type hypersensitivity reactions after a previous dose of tetanus toxoid-containing vaccine; defer vaccination until at least 10 years have elapsed since the last tetanus toxoid-containing vaccine Moderate or severe acute illness with or without fever
IPV	Severe allergic reaction (e.g., anaphylaxis) after a previous dose or to a vaccine component	Pregnancy Moderate or severe acute illness with or without fever
MMR[†,§]	Severe allergic reaction (e.g., anaphylaxis) after a previous dose or to a vaccine component Pregnancy Known severe immunodeficiency (e.g., from hematologic and solid tumors, receipt of chemotherapy, congenital immunodeficiency, or long-term immunosuppressive therapy[¶] or patients with HIV infection who are severely immunocompromised)[§]	Recent (≤11 months) receipt of antibody-containing blood product (specific interval depends on product) History of thrombocytopenia or thrombocytopenic purpura Need for tuberculin skin testing[††] Moderate or severe acute illness with or without fever
Hib	Severe allergic reaction (e.g., anaphylaxis) after a previous dose or to a vaccine component Age <6 weeks	Moderate or severe acute illness with or without fever
Hepatitis B	Severe allergic reaction (e.g., anaphylaxis) after a previous dose or to a vaccine component	Infant weight <2000 g[§§] Moderate or severe acute illness with or without fever
Hepatitis A	Severe allergic reaction (e.g., anaphylaxis) after a previous dose or to a vaccine component	Pregnancy Moderate or severe acute illness with or without fever
Varicella	Severe allergic reaction (e.g., anaphylaxis) after a previous dose or to a vaccine component Known severe immunodeficiency (e.g., from hematologic and solid tumors, receipt of chemotherapy, congenital immunodeficiency, or long-term immunosuppressive therapy[¶] or patients with HIV infection who are severely immunocompromised)[§] Pregnancy	Recent (≤11 months) receipt of antibody-containing blood product (specific interval depends on product)[¶¶] Moderate or severe acute illness with or without fever
PCV	Severe allergic reaction (e.g., anaphylaxis) after a previous dose (of PCV7, PCV13, or any diphtheria toxoid-containing vaccine) or to a component of a vaccine (PCV7, PCV13, or any diphtheria toxoid-containing vaccine)	Moderate or severe acute illness with or without fever
TIV	Severe allergic reaction (e.g., anaphylaxis) after a previous dose or to vaccine component, including egg protein	GBS <6 weeks after a previous dose of influenza vaccine Moderate or severe acute illness with or without fever
LAIV	Severe allergic reaction (e.g., anaphylaxis) after a previous dose or to vaccine component, including egg protein Pregnancy Immunosuppression Certain chronic medical conditions***	GBS <6 weeks after a previous dose of influenza vaccine Moderate or severe acute illness with or without fever
PPSV	Severe allergic reaction (e.g., anaphylaxis) after a previous dose or to a vaccine component	Moderate or severe acute illness with or without fever

TABLE 5-13   Contraindications and Precautions* to Commonly Used Vaccines—cont'd

Vaccine	Contraindications	Precautions
MCV4	Severe allergic reaction (e.g., anaphylaxis) after a previous dose or to a vaccine component	Moderate or severe acute illness with or without fever
MPSV4	Severe allergic reaction (e.g., anaphylaxis) after a previous dose or to a vaccine component	Moderate or severe acute illness with or without fever
HPV	Severe allergic reaction (e.g., anaphylaxis) after a previous dose or to a vaccine component	Pregnancy Moderate or severe acute illness with or without fever
Rotavirus	Severe allergic reaction (e.g., anaphylaxis) after a previous dose or to a vaccine component SCID	Altered immunocompetence other than SCID History of intussusception Chronic gastrointestinal disease††† Spina bifida or bladder exstrophy††† Moderate or severe acute illness with or without fever
Zoster	Severe allergic reaction (e.g., anaphylaxis) after a previous dose or to a vaccine component Substantial suppression of cellular immunity Pregnancy	Moderate or severe acute illness with or without fever

From Centers for Disease Control and Prevention: General recommendations on immunization: recommendations of the Advisory Committee on Immunization Practices (ACIP), *MMWR* 60:(RR-2), 2011.

DT, diphtheria and tetanus toxoids; *DTaP*, diphtheria and tetanus toxoids and acellular pertussis; *GBS*, Guillian-Barré syndrome; *HBsAg*, hepatitis B surface antigen; *Hib, Haemophilus influenzae* type b; *HIV*, human immunodeficiency virus; *HPV*, human papillomavirus; *IPV*, inactivated poliovirus; *LAIV*, live, attenuated influenza vaccine; *MCV4*, quadrivalent meningococcal conjugate vaccine; *MMRV* measles, mumps, rubella; *MPSV4*, quadrivalent meningococcal polysaccharide vaccine; *PCV*, pneumococcal conjugate vaccine; *PPSV*, pneumococcal polysaccharide vaccine; *SCID*, severe combined immunodeficiency; *Td*, tetanus and diphtheria toxoids; *Tdap*, tetanus toxoid, reduced diphtheria toxoid, and acellular pertussis; *TIV*, trivalent inactivated influenza vaccine.

*Events or conditions listed as precautions should be reviewed carefully. Benefits of and risks for administering a specific vaccine to a person under these circumstances should be considered. If the risk from the vaccine is believed to outweigh the benefit, the vaccine should not be administered. If the benefit of vaccination is believed to outweigh the risk, the vaccine should be administered. Whether and when to administer DTaP to children with proven or suspected underlying neurologic disorders should be decided on a case-by-case basis.

†HIV-infected children may receive varicella and measles vaccine if CD4+ T-lymphocyte count is >15%. (Source: Adapted from American Academy of Pediatrics. Passive immunization. In: Pickering LK, ed. Red book: 2009 report of the committee on infectious diseases. 28th ed. Elk Grove Village. IL: American Academy of Pediatrics: 2009.)

§MMR and varicella vaccines can be administered on the same day. If not administered on the same day, these vaccines should be separated by at least 28 days.

¶Substantially immunosuppressive steroid dose is considered to be ≥2 weeks of daily receipt of 20 mg or 2 mg/kg body weight of prednisone or equivalent.

††Measles vaccination might suppress tuberculin reactivity temporarily. Measles-containing vaccine can be administered on the same day as tuberculin skin testing. If testing cannot be performed until after the day of MMR vaccination, the test should be postponed for ≥4 weeks after the vaccination. If an urgent need exists to skin test, do so with the understanding that reactivity might be reduced by the vaccine.

§§Hepatitis B vaccination should be deferred for infants weighing <2000 g if the mother is documented to be HBsAg-negative at the time of the infant's birth. Vaccination can commence at chronological age 1 month or at hospital discharge. For infants born to HBsAg-positive women, hepatitis B immune globulin and hepatitis B vaccine should be administered within 12 hours after birth, regardless of weight.

¶¶Vaccine should be deferred for the appropriate interval if replacement immune globulin products are being administered.

***Source: CDC. Prevention and control of seasonal influenza with vaccines: recommendations of the Advisory Committee on Immunization Practices (ACIP), 2010. *MMWR* 2010;59(No. RR-8).

†††For details see CDC. Prevention of rotavirus gastroenteritis among infants and children: recommendations of the Advisory Committee on Immunization Practices. *MMWR* 2009;58(No. RR-2).

TABLE 5-14 Conditions Commonly Misperceived as Contraindications to Vaccination

Vaccine	Conditions Commonly Misperceived as Contraindications (i.e., Vaccination May be Administered under These Conditions)
General for all vaccines, including DTaP, pediatric DT, adult Td, adolescent-adult Tdap, IPV, MMR, Hib, hepatitis A, hepatitis B, varicella, rotavirus, PCV, TIV, LAIV, PPSV, MCV4, MPSV4, HPV, and herpes zoster	Mild acute illness with or without fever Mild-to-moderate local reaction (i.e., swelling, redness, soreness); low-grade or moderate fever after previous dose Lack of previous physical examination in well-appearing person Current antimicrobial therapy* Convalescent phase of illness Preterm birth (hepatitis B vaccine is an exception in certain circumstances)† Recent exposure to an infectious disease History of penicillin allergy, other nonvaccine allergies, relatives with allergies, or receiving allergen extract immunotherapy
DTaP	Fever of <105°F (<40°C), fussiness or mild drowsiness after a previous dose of DTP/DTaP Family history of seizures Family history of sudden infant death syndrome Family history of an adverse event after DTP or DTaP administration Stable neurologic conditions (e.g., cerebral palsy, well-controlled seizures, or developmental delay)
Tdap	Fever of ≥105°F (≥40°C) for <48 hours after vaccination with a previous dose of DTP or DTaP Collapse or shock-like state (i.e., hypotonic hyporesponsive episode) within 48 hours after receiving a previous dose of DTaP Seizure <3 days after receiving a previous dose of DTP/DTaP Persistent, inconsolable crying lasting >3 hours within 48 hours after receiving a previous dose of DTP/DTaP History of extensive limb swelling after DTP/DTaP/Td that is not an Arthus-type reaction Stable neurologic disorder History of brachial neuritis Latex allergy that is not anaphylactic Breastfeeding Immunosuppression
IPV	Previous receipt of ≥1 dose of oral polio vaccine
MMR§,¶	Positive tuberculin skin test Simultaneous tuberculin skin testing** Breastfeeding Pregnancy of recipient's mother or other close or household contact Recipient is female of childbearing age Immunodeficient family member or household contact Asymptomatic or mildly symptomatic HIV infection Allergy to eggs
Hepatitis B	Pregnancy Autoimmune disease (e.g., systemic lupus erythematosis or rheumatoid arthritis)
Varicella	Pregnancy of recipient's mother or other close or household contact Immunodeficient family member or household contact†† Asymptomatic or mildly symptomatic HIV infection Humoral immunodeficiency (e.g., agammaglobulinemia)
TIV	Nonsevere (e.g., contact) allergy to latex, thimerosal, or egg Concurrent administration of Coumadin or aminophylline
LAIV	Health care providers that see patients with chronic diseases or altered immunocompetence (an exception is providers for severely immunocompromised patients requiring care in a protected environment) Breastfeeding Contacts of persons with chronic disease or altered immunocompetence (an exception is contacts of severely immunocompromised patients requiring care in a protected environment)
PPSV	History of invasive pneumococcal disease or pneumonia
HPV	Immunosuppression Previous equivocal or abnormal Papanicolaou test Known HPV infection Breastfeeding History of genital warts
Rotavirus	Prematurity Immunosuppressed household contacts Pregnant household contacts
Zoster	Therapy with low-dose methotrexate (≤0.4 mg/kg/week), azathioprine (≤3.0 mg/kg/day), or 6-mercaptopurine (≤1.5 mg/kg/day) for treatment of rheumatoid arthritis, psoriasis, polymyositis, sarcoidosis, inflammatory bowel disease, or other conditions Health-care providers of patients with chronic diseases or altered immunocompetence Contacts of patients with chronic diseases or altered immunocompetence Unknown or uncertain history of varicella in a U.S.-born person

From Centers for Disease Control and Prevention: General recommendations on immunization: recommendations of the Advisory Committee on Immunization Practices (ACIP), *MMWR* 60:(RR-2), 2011.

DT, Diphtheria and tetanus toxoids; *DTP,* diphtheria toxoid, tetanus toxoid, and pertussis; *DTaP,* diphtheria and tetanus toxoids and acellular pertussis; *HBsAg,* hepatitis B surface antigen; *Hib, Haemophilus influenzae* type b; *HPV,* human papillomavirus; *IPV,* inactivated poliovirus; *LAIV,* live, attenuated influenza vaccine; *MCV4,* quadrivalent meningococcal conjugate vaccine; *MMR,* measles, mumps, and rubella; *MPSV4,* quadrivalent meningococcal polysaccharide vaccine; *PCV,* pneumococcal conjugate vaccine; *PPSV,* pneumococcal polysaccharide vaccine; *Td,* tetanus and diphtheria toxoids; *Tdap,* tetanus toxoid, reduced diphtheria toxoid, and acellular pertussis; *TIV,* trivalent inactivated influenza vaccine.
*Antibacterial drugs might interfere with Ty21a oral typhoid vaccine, and certain antiviral drugs might interfere with varicella-containing vaccines and LAIV.

TABLE 5-14 Conditions Commonly Misperceived as Contraindications to Vaccination—cont'd

†Hepatitis B vaccination should be deferred for infants weighing <2000 g if the mother is documented to be HBsAg-negative at the time of the infant's birth. Vaccination can commence at chronologic age 1 month or at hospital discharge. For infants born to HBsAg-positive women, hepatitis B immune globulin and hepatitis B vaccine should be administered within 12 hours after birth, regardless of weight.

§MMR and varicella vaccines can be administered on the same day. If not administered on the same day, these vaccines should be separated by at least 28 days.

¶HIV-infected children should receive immune globulin after exposure to measles. HIV-infected children can receive varicella and measles vaccine if CD4+ T-lymphocyte count is >15%. (Source: Adapted from American Academy of Pediatrics. Passive immunization. In: Pickering LK, ed. Red book: 2009 report of the Committee on Infectious Diseases, 28th ed. Elk Grove Village, IL: American Academy of Pediatrics; 2009.)

**Measles vaccination might suppress tuberculin reactivity temporarily. Measles-containing vaccine can be administered on the same day as tuberculin skin testing. If testing cannot be performed until after the day of MMR vaccination, the test should be postponed for at least 4 weeks after the vaccination. If an urgent need exists to skin test, do so with the understanding that reactivity might be reduced by the vaccine.

††If a vaccinee experiences a presumed vaccine-related rash 7–25 days after vaccination, the person should avoid direct contact with immunocompromised persons for the duration of the rash.

VACCINE ADMINISTRATION*

INFECTION CONTROL AND STERILE TECHNIQUE

Persons administering vaccines should follow appropriate precautions to minimize risk for spread of disease. Hands should be cleansed with an alcohol-based, waterless antiseptic hand rub or washed with soap and water between each patient contact. Occupational Safety and Health Administration (OSHA) regulations do not require that gloves be worn when administering vaccinations unless persons administering vaccinations are likely to come into contact with potentially infectious body fluids or have open lesions on their hands. Needles used for injections must be sterile and disposable to minimize the risk for contamination. A separate needle and syringe should be used for each injection. Changing needles between drawing vaccine from a vial and injecting it into a recipient is not necessary. Different vaccines should never be mixed in the same syringe unless specifically licensed for such use, and no attempt should be made to transfer between syringes.

For all intramuscular injections, the needle should be long enough to reach the muscle mass and prevent vaccine from seeping into subcutaneous tissue but not so long as to involve underlying nerves, blood vessels, or bone. Vaccinators should be familiar with the anatomy of the area where they are injecting vaccine. Intramuscular injections are administered at a 90-degree angle to the skin, preferably into the anterolateral aspect of the thigh or the deltoid muscle of the upper arm depending on the age of the patient.

Decision on needle size and site of injection must be made for each person on the basis of the size of the muscle, the thickness of adipose tissue at the injection site, the volume of the material to be administered, injection technique, and the depth below the muscle surface into which the material is to be injected (Fig. 5-1). Aspiration before injection of vaccines or toxoids (i.e., pulling back on the syringe plunger after needle insertion before injection) is not required because no large blood vessel exists at the recommended injection sites.

INFANTS (AGED <12 MONTHS)

For the majority of infants, the anterolateral aspect of the thigh is the recommended site for injection because it provides a large muscle mass (Fig. 5-2). The muscles of the buttock have not been used for administration of vaccines in infants and children because of concern about potential injury to the sciatic nerve, which is well documented after injection of antimicrobial agents into the buttock. If the gluteal muscle must be used, care

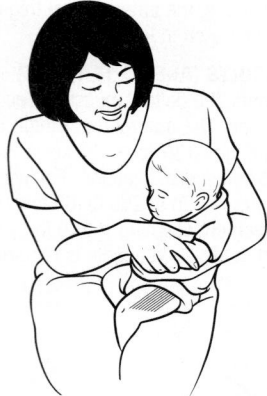

FIGURE 5-2 Intramuscular/subcutaneous site of administration: anterolateral thigh. (Adapted from Minnesota Department of Health. In Centers for Disease Control and Prevention: General recommendations on immunization: recommendations of the Advisory Committee on Immunization Practices [ACIP], *MMWR* 55[RR-15]:6, 2006.)

should be taken to define the anatomic landmarks.[†] Injection technique is the most important parameter to ensure efficient intramuscular vaccine delivery. If the subcutaneous and muscle tissue are bunched to minimize the chance of striking bone, a 1-inch needle is required to ensure intramuscular administration in infants. For the majority of infants, a 1-inch, 22- to 25-gauge needle is sufficient to penetrate muscle in an infant's thigh. For newborn (first 28 days of life) and premature infants, a ⅝-inch-long needle usually is adequate if the skin is stretched flat between thumb and forefinger and the needle inserted at a 90-degree angle to the skin.

TODDLERS AND OLDER CHILDREN (AGED 12 MONTHS TO 10 YEARS)

The deltoid muscle should be used if the muscle mass is adequate. The needle size for deltoid site injections can range from 22 to 25 gauge and from ⅝ to 1 inch on the basis of the size of the muscle and the thickness of adipose tissue at the injection site (Fig. 5-3). A ⅝-inch needle is adequate only for the deltoid muscle and only if the skin is stretched flat between the thumb and forefinger and the needle inserted at a 90-degree

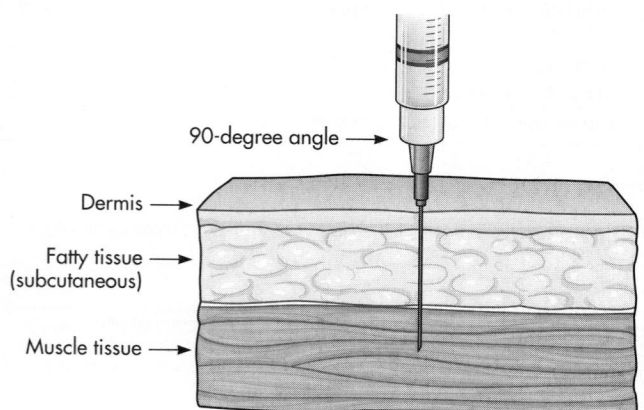

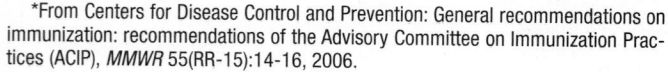

FIGURE 5-1 Intramuscular needle insertion. (Adapted from California Immunization Branch. In Centers for Disease Control and Prevention: General recommendations on immunization: recommendations of the Advisory Committee on Immunization Practices [ACIP], *MMWR* 55[RR-15]:16, 2006.)

Labels in Figure 5-1: 90-degree angle; Dermis; Fatty tissue (subcutaneous); Muscle tissue

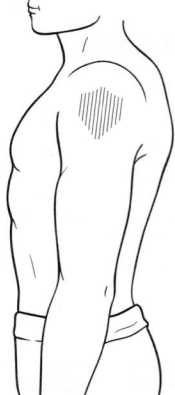

FIGURE 5-3 Intramuscular site of administration: deltoid. (Adapted from Minnesota Department of Health. In Centers for Disease Control and Prevention: General recommendations on immunization: recommendations of the Advisory Committee on Immunization Practices [ACIP], *MMWR* 55[RR-15]:17, 2006.)

---

*From Centers for Disease Control and Prevention: General recommendations on immunization: recommendations of the Advisory Committee on Immunization Practices (ACIP), *MMWR* 55(RR-15):14-16, 2006.

[†]If the gluteal muscle is chosen, injection should be administered lateral and superior to a line between the posterior superior iliac spine and the greater trochanter or in the ventrogluteal site, the center of a triangle bounded by the anterior superior iliac spine, the tubercle of the iliac crest, and the upper border of the greater trochanter.

angle to the skin. For toddlers, the anterolateral thigh can be used, but the needle should be at least 1 inch in length.

ADOLESCENTS AND ADULTS (AGED >11 YEARS)

For adults and adolescents, the deltoid muscle is recommended for routine intramuscular vaccinations. The anterolateral thigh also can be used. For men and women weighing <130 lb (<60 kg) a ⅝- to 1-inch needle is sufficient to ensure intramuscular injection. For women weighing 130 to 200 lb (60 to 90 kg) and men 130 to 260 lb (60 to 118 kg), a 1- to 1½-inch needle is needed. For women weighing >200 lb (>90 kg) or men weighing >260 lb (>118 kg), a 1½-inch needle is required.

SUBCUTANEOUS INJECTIONS

Subcutaneous injections are administered at a 45-degree angle, usually into the thigh for infants younger than 12 months and in the upper-outer triceps area of persons aged 12 months and older. Subcutaneous injections can be administered into the upper-outer triceps area of an infant if necessary. A ⅝-inch, 23- to 25-gauge needle should be inserted into the subcutaneous tissue (Figs. 5-4 and 5-5).

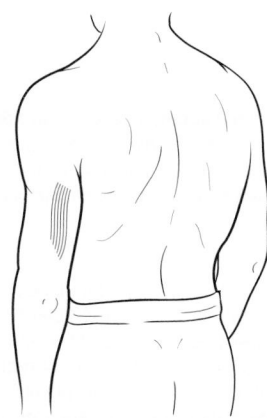

FIGURE 5-4 Subcutaneous site of administration: triceps. (Adapted from Minnesota Department of Health. In Centers for Disease Control and Prevention: General recommendations on immunization: recommendations of the Advisory Committee on Immunization Practices [ACIP], *MMWR* 55[RR-15]:17, 2006.)

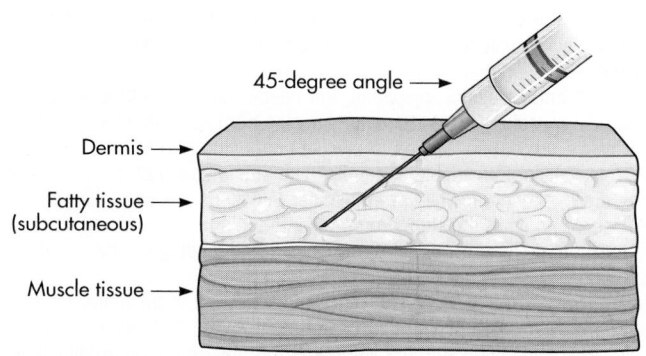

FIGURE 5-5 Subcutaneous needle insertion. (Adapted from California Administration Branch. In Centers for Disease Control and Prevention: General recommendations on immunization: recommendations of the Advisory Committee on Immunization Practices [ACIP], *MMWR* 55[RR-15]:17, 2006.)

TABLE 5-15 Treatment of Anaphylaxis in Children and Adults with Drugs Administered Intramuscularly or Orally

Drug	Dosage
Children	
Primary Regimen	
Epinephrine 1:1000 (aqueous) (1 mg/ml)*	0.01 mg/kg up to 0.5 mg (administer 0.01 ml/kg/dose up to 0.5 mL) IM repeated every 10–20 minutes up to 3 doses
Secondary Regimen	
Diphenhydramine	1–2 mg/kg oral, IM, or IV, every 4–6 hours (100 mg, maximum single dose)
Hydroxyzine	0.5–1 mg/kg oral, IM, every 4–6 hours (100 mg, maximum single dose)
Prednisone	1.5–2 mg/kg oral (60 mg, maximum single dose); use corticosteroids as long as needed
Adults	
Primary Regimen	
Epinephrine 1:1000 (aqueous)*	0.01 mg/kg up to 0.5 mg (administer 0.01 ml/kg/dose up to 0.5 ml) IM repeated every 10–20 minutes up to 3 doses
Secondary Regimen	
Diphenhydramine	1–2 mg/kg up to l00 mg IM or oral, every 4–6 hours

From Centers for Disease Control and Prevention: General recommendations on immunization: recommendations of the Advisory Committee on Immunization Practices (ACIP), *MMWR* 60:(RR-2), 2011. Adapted from American Academy of Pediatrics. Passive immunization. In: Pickering LK, Baker CJ, Kimberlin DW, Long SS, eds: *Red book: 2009 report of the Committee on Infectious Diseases*, 28th ed. Elk Grove Village, IL: American Academy of Pediatrics, 2009:66-7; Immunization Action Coalition. Medical management of vaccine reactions in adult patients (available at www.immunize.org/catg.d/p3082.pdf); and *Mosby's drug consult*, St Louis, 2005, Mosby.

IM, Intramuscular; *IV*, intravenous.

*If the agent causing the anaphylactic reaction was administered by injection, epinephrine may be injected into the same site to slow absorption.

TABLE 5-16 Vaccination of Persons with Primary and Secondary Immunodeficiencies

Primary	Specific Immunodeficiency	Contraindicated Vaccines*	Risk-Specific Recommended Vaccines*	Effectiveness and Comments
B-lymphocyte (humoral)	Severe antibody deficiencies (e.g., X-linked agammaglobulinemia and common variable immunodeficiency)	OPV[†] Smallpox LAIV BCG Ty21a (live typhoid) Yellow fever	Pneumococcal Consider measles and varicella vaccination	The effectiveness of any vaccine is uncertain if it depends only on the humoral response (e.g., PPSV or MPSV4). IGIV interferes with the immune response to measles vaccine and possibly varicella vaccine.
	Less severe antibody deficiencies (e.g., selective IgA deficiency and IgG subclass deficiency)	OPV[†] BCG Yellow fever Other live vaccines appear to be safe.	Pneumococcal	All vaccines likely effective; immune response might be attenuated.
T-lymphocyte (cell-mediated and humoral)	Complete deficits (e.g., severe combined immunodeficiency [SCID] disease, complete DiGeorge syndrome)	All live vaccines[§,¶,**]	Pneumococcal	Vaccines might be ineffective.
	Partial defects (e.g., most patients with DiGeorge syndrome, Wiskott-Aldrich syndrome, ataxia-telangiectasia)	All live vaccines[§,¶,**]	Pneumococcal Meningococcal Hib (if not administered in infancy)	Effectiveness of any vaccine depends on degree of immune suppression.
Complement	Persistent complement, properdin, or factor B deficiency	None	Pneumococcal Meningococcal	All routine vaccines likely effective.
Phagocytic function	Chronic granulomatous disease, leukocyte adhesion defect, and myeloperoxidase deficiency	Live bacterial vaccines[§]	Pneumococcal[††]	All inactivated vaccines safe and likely effective. Live viral vaccines likely safe and effective.
Secondary	HIV/AIDS	OPV[†] Smallpox BCG LAIV Withhold MMR and varicella in severely immunocompromised persons. Yellow fever vaccine might have a contraindication or a precaution depending on clinical parameters of immune function***	Pneumococcal Consider Hib (if not administered in infancy) and meningococcal vaccination.	MMR, varicella, rotavirus, and all inactivated vaccines, including inactivated influenza, might be effective.[§§]
	Malignant neoplasm, transplantation, immunosuppressive or radiation therapy	Live viral and bacterial, depending on immune status[§,¶]	Pneumococcal	Effectiveness of any vaccine depends on degree of immune suppression.
	Asplenia	None	Pneumococcal Meningococcal Hib (if not administered in infancy)	All routine vaccines likely effective.
	Chronic renal disease	LAIV	Pneumococcal Hepatitis B[¶¶]	All routine vaccines likely effective.

From Centers for Disease Control and Prevention: General recommendations on immunization: recommendations of the Advisory Committee on Immunization Practices (ACIP), *MMWR* 60:(RR-2), 2011. Adapted from American Academy of Pediatrics. Passive immunization. In: Pickering LK, Baker CJ, Kimberlin DW, Long SS, eds: *Red book: 2009 report of the Committee on Infectious Diseases*, 28th ed. Elk Grove Village, IL: American Academy of Pediatrics; 2009:74–5.

AIDS, acquired immunodeficiency syndrome; *BCG*, bacille Calmette-Guérin; *Hib*, *Haemophilus influenzae* type b; *HIV*, human immunodeficiency virus; *IG*, immunoglobulin; *IGIV*, immune globulin intravenous; *LAIV*, live, attenuated influenza vaccine; *MMR*, measles, mumps, and rubella; *MPSV4*, quadrivalent meningococcal polysaccharide vaccine; *OPV*, oral poliovirus polysaccharide vaccine; *PPSV*, pneumococcal polysaccharide vaccine.

*Other vaccines that are universally or routinely recommended should be given if not contraindicated.

[†]OPV is no longer available in the United States.

[§]Live bacterial vaccines: BCG and oral Ty21a *Salmonella typhi* vaccine.

[¶]Live viral vaccines: MMR, MMRV, OPV, LAIV, yellow fever, zoster, rotavirus, varicella, and vaccinia (smallpox). Smallpox vaccine is not recommended for children or the general public.

**Regarding T-lymphocyte immunodeficiency as a contraindication for rotavirus vaccine, data exist only for severe combined immunodeficiency.

[††]Pneumococcal vaccine is not indicated for children with chronic granulomatous disease beyond age-based universal recommendations for PCV. Children with chronic granulomatous disease are not at increased risk for pneumococcal disease.

[§§]HIV-infected children should receive IG after exposure to measles and may receive varicella and measles vaccine if CD4+ T-lymphocyte count is ≥15%.

[¶¶]Indicated based on the risk from dialysis-based bloodborne transmission.

***Symptomatic HIV infection or CD4+ T-lymphocyte count of <200/mm³ or <15% of total lymphocytes for children aged <6 years is a contraindication to yellow fever vaccine administration. Asymptomatic HIV infection with CD4+ T-lymphocyte count of 200–499/mm³ for persons aged ≥6 years or 15%–24% of total lymphocytes for children aged <6 years is a precaution for yellow fever vaccine administration. Details of yellow fever vaccine recommendations are available from CDC. (CDC. Yellow fever vaccine recommendations of the Advisory Committee on Immunization Practices [ACIP]. *MMWR* 2010;59[No. RR-7].)

TABLE 5-17	Immunizations for Pediatric Oncology Patients
Vaccine	**Indications and Comments**
DtaP	Indicated for incompletely immunized children <7 yr, even during active chemotherapy
Td	Indicated 1 yr after completion of therapy in children 7 yr
Hib	Indicated for incompletely immunized children if <7 yr
HBV	Indicated for incompletely immunized children
23PS	Indicated for asplenic patients
PCV13	Indicated for incompletely immunized children <5 yr
Meningococcus	Consider in asplenic patients
IPV	Indicated for incompletely immunized children; also recommended for all household contacts requiring immunization to reduce the risk of vaccine-associated polio
MMR	Contraindicated until child is in remission and finished with all chemotherapy for 3-6 mo; may need to reimmunize after chemotherapy if titers have fallen below protective levels
Influenza	Defer in active chemotherapy; may give as early as 3-4 wk after remission and off chemotherapy if during influenza season; peripheral granulocyte and lymphocyte counts should be >1000/μL; should also be given to household contact of children with cancer
Varicella	Consider immunizing children who have remained in remission and have finished chemotherapy for >1 yr; with absolute lymphocyte count of >700/μl and platelet count of >100,000/μL within 24 hr of immunization; check titers of previously immunized children to verify protective levels of antibodies

From *MMWR* 49(RR-10):1-147, 2000.
DtaP, Diphtheria, tetanus, and pertussis; *HBV,* hepatitis B virus; *Hib, Haemophilus influenzae* type b; *IPV,* inactivated polio vaccine; *MMR,* measles, mumps, rubella; *PCV13,* pneumococcal conjugate vaccine; *23PS,* 23-valent pneumococcal polysaccharide vaccine; *Td,* tetanus, diphtheria.

TABLE 5-18 Approaches to the Evaluation and Vaccination of Persons Vaccinated Outside the United States Who Have No (or Questionable) Vaccination Records

Vaccine	Recommended Approach	Alternative Approach*
MMR	Revaccination with MMR	Serologic testing for IgG antibodies to measles, mumps, and rubella
Hib	Age-appropriate revaccination	—
Hepatitis A	Age-appropriate revaccination	Serologic testing for IgG antibodies to hepatitis A
Hepatitis B	Age-appropriate revaccination and serologic testing for HBsAg†	—
Poliovirus	Revaccinate with inactivated poliovirus vaccine	Serologic testing for neutralizing antibody to poliovirus types 1, 2, and 3 (limited availability)
DTaP	Revaccination with DTaP, with serologic testing for specific IgG antibody to tetanus and diphtheria toxins in the event of a severe local reaction	Persons whose records indicate receipt of ≥3 doses: serologic testing for specific IgG antibody to diphtheria and tetanus toxins before administering additional doses, or administer a single booster dose of DTaP, followed by serologic testing after 1 month for specific IgG antibody to diphtheria and tetanus toxins with revaccination as appropriate
Tdap	Age-appropriate vaccination of persons who are candidates for Tdap vaccine on the basis of time since last diphtheria and tetanus-toxoid–containing vaccines.	—
Varicella	Age-appropriate vaccination of persons who lack evidence of varicella immunity	—
Pneumococcal conjugate	Age-appropriate vaccination	—
Rotavirus	Age-appropriate vaccination	—
HPV	Age-appropriate vaccination	—
Zoster	Age-appropriate vaccination	—

From Centers for Disease Control and Prevention: General recommendations on immunization: recommendations of the Advisory Committee on Immunization Practices (ACIP), *MMWR* 60:(RR-2), 2011.

DTaP, Diphtheria and tetanus toxoids and acellular pertussis; *HBsAg,* hepatitis B surface antigen; *Hib, Haemophilus influenzae* type b; *HPV,* human papillomavirus; *IgG,* immune globulin G; *MMR,* measles, mumps, and rubella; *Tdap,* tetanus toxoid, reduced diphtheria toxoid, and acellular pertussis.

*There is a recommended approach for all vaccines and an alternative approach for some vaccines.

†In rare instances, hepatitis B vaccine can give a false-positive HBsAg result up to 18 days after vaccination; therefore, blood should be drawn to test for HBsAg before vaccinating. (Source: CDC. A comprehensive immunization strategy to eliminate transmission of hepatitis B virus infection in the United States: recommendations of the Advisory Committee on Immunization Practices [ACIP]; Part I: Immunization in infants, children, and adolescents, *MMWR* 2005;54(No. RR-16.])

Immunizations for Adults

TABLE 5-19 Recommended Adult Immunization Schedule, by Vaccine and Age Group: United States[1]

These recommendations must be read with the footnotes that follow.

VACCINE ▼ AGE GROUP ▶	19-21 years	22-26 years	27-49 years	50-59 years	60-64 years	≥ 65 years
Influenza [2],*	1 dose annually					
Tetanus, diphtheria, pertussis (Td/Tdap) [3],*	Substitute 1-time dose of Tdap for Td booster; then boost with Td every 10 yrs					
Varicella [4],*	2 doses					
Human papillomavirus (HPV) Female [5],*	3 doses					
Human papillomavirus (HPV) Male [5],*	3 doses					
Zoster [6]					1 dose	
Measles, mumps, rubella (MMR) [7],*	1 or 2 doses					
Pneumococcal polysaccharide (PPSV23) [8,9]	1 or 2 doses					1 dose
Pneumococcal 13-valent conjugate (PCV13) [10]	1 dose					
Meningococcal [11],*	1 or more doses					
Hepatitis A [12],*	2 doses					
Hepatitis B [13],*	3 doses					

*Covered by the Vaccine Injury Compensation Program

☐ For all persons in this category who meet the age requirements and who lack documentation of vaccination or have no evidence of previous infection; zoster vaccine recommended regardless of prior episode of zoster

☐ Recommended if some other risk factor is present (e.g., on the basis of medical, occupational, lifestyle, or other indication)

☐ No recommendation

Report all clinically significant postvaccination reactions to the Vaccine Adverse Event Reporting System (VAERS). Reporting forms and instructions on filing a VAERS report are available at www.vaers.hhs.gov or by telephone, 800-822-7967.

Information on how to file a Vaccine Injury Compensation Program claim is available at www.hrsa.gov/vaccinecompensation or by telephone, 800-338-2382. To file a claim for vaccine injury, contact the U.S. Court of Federal Claims, 717 Madison Place, N.W., Washington, D.C. 20005; telephone, 202-357-6400.

Additional information about the vaccines in this schedule, extent of available data, and contraindications for vaccination is also available at www.cdc.gov/vaccines or from the CDC-INFO Contact Center at 800-CDC-INFO (800-232-4636) in English and Spanish, 8:00 a.m. - 8:00 p.m. Eastern Time, Monday - Friday, excluding holidays.

Use of trade names and commercial sources is for identification only and does not imply endorsement by the U.S. Department of Health and Human Services.

The recommendations in this schedule were approved by the Centers for Disease Control and Prevention's (CDC) Advisory Committee on Immunization Practices (ACIP), the American Academy of Family Physicians (AAFP), the American College of Physicians (ACP), American College of Obstetricians and Gynecologists and American College of Nurse-Midwives (ACNM).

TABLE 5-20A Vaccines That Might Be Indicated for Adults Based on Medical and Other Indications: United States[1]

Note: These recommendations *must* be read with the footnotes that follow containing number of doses, intervals between doses, and other important information.

VACCINE ▼ INDICATION ▶	Pregnancy	Immuno-compromising conditions (excluding human immunodeficiency virus [HIV])[4,6,7,10,15]	HIV infection CD4+ T lymphocyte count [4,6,7,10,14,15] < 200 cells/μL	HIV infection CD4+ T lymphocyte count ≥ 200 cells/μL	Men who have sex with men (MSM)	Heart disease, chronic lung disease, chronic alcoholism	Asplenia (including elective splenectomy and persistent complement component deficiencies) [10,14]	Chronic liver disease	Kidney failure, end-stage renal disease, receipt of hemodialysis	Diabetes	Healthcare personnel
Influenza [2,*]	1 dose IIV annually	1 dose IIV annually	1 dose IIV annually	1 dose IIV annually	1 dose IIV or LAIV annually	1 dose IIV annually	1 dose IIV annually	1 dose IIV annually	1 dose IIV annually	1 dose IIV annually	1 dose IIV or LAIV annually
Tetanus, diphtheria, pertussis (Td/Tdap) [3,*]	1 dose Tdap each pregnancy	Substitute 1-time dose of Tdap for Td booster; then boost with Td every 10 yrs									
Varicella [4,*]	Contraindicated	Contraindicated	Contraindicated	2 doses	2 doses	2 doses	2 doses	2 doses	2 doses	2 doses	2 doses
Human papillomavirus (HPV) Female [5,*]	3 doses through age 26 yrs	3 doses through age 26 yrs	3 doses through age 26 yrs	3 doses through age 26 yrs	3 doses through age 26 yrs	3 doses through age 26 yrs	3 doses through age 26 yrs	3 doses through age 26 yrs	3 doses through age 26 yrs	3 doses through age 26 yrs	3 doses through age 26 yrs
Human papillomavirus (HPV) Male [5,*]	3 doses through age 26 yrs	3 doses through age 26 yrs	3 doses through age 26 yrs	3 doses through age 21 yrs	3 doses through age 21 yrs	3 doses through age 21 yrs	3 doses through age 21 yrs	3 doses through age 21 yrs	3 doses through age 21 yrs	3 doses through age 21 yrs	3 doses through age 21 yrs
Zoster [6]	Contraindicated	Contraindicated	Contraindicated	1 dose	1 dose	1 dose	1 dose	1 dose	1 dose	1 dose	1 dose
Measles, mumps, rubella (MMR) [7,*]	Contraindicated	Contraindicated	Contraindicated	1 or 2 doses	1 or 2 doses	1 or 2 doses	1 or 2 doses	1 or 2 doses	1 or 2 doses	1 or 2 doses	1 or 2 doses
Pneumococcal polysaccharide (PPSV23) [8,9]	1 or 2 doses	1 or 2 doses	1 or 2 doses	1 or 2 doses	1 or 2 doses	1 or 2 doses	1 or 2 doses	1 or 2 doses	1 or 2 doses	1 or 2 doses	
Pneumococcal 13-valent conjugate (PCV13) [10]	1 dose	1 dose	1 dose	1 dose	1 dose	1 dose	1 dose	1 dose	1 dose	1 dose	
Meningococcal [11,*]	1 or more doses	1 or more doses	1 or more doses	1 or more doses	1 or more doses	1 or more doses	1 or more doses	1 or more doses	1 or more doses	1 or more doses	
Hepatitis A [12,*]	2 doses	2 doses	2 doses	2 doses	2 doses	2 doses	2 doses	2 doses	2 doses	2 doses	
Hepatitis B [13,*]	3 doses	3 doses	3 doses	3 doses	3 doses	3 doses	3 doses	3 doses	3 doses	3 doses	

*Covered by the Vaccine Injury Compensation Program

- For all persons in this category who meet the age requirements and who lack documentation of vaccination or have no evidence of previous infection; zoster vaccine recommended regardless of prior episode of zoster
- Recommended if some other risk factor is present (e.g., on the basis of medical, occupational, lifestyle, or other indications)
- No recommendation

These schedules indicate the recommended age groups and medical indications for which administration of currently licensed vaccines is commonly indicated for adults ages 19 years and older, as of January 1, 2013. For all vaccines being recommended on the Adult Immunization Schedule: a vaccine series does not need to be restarted, regardless of the time that has elapsed between doses. Licensed combination vaccines may be used whenever any components of the combination are indicated and when the vaccine's other components are not contraindicated. For detailed recommendations on all vaccines, including those used primarily for travelers or that are issued during the year, consult the manufacturers' package inserts and the complete statements from the Advisory Committee on Immunization Practices (www.cdc.gov/vaccines/pubs/acip-list.htm). Use of trade names and commercial sources is for identification only and does not imply endorsement by the U.S. Department of Health and Human Services.

Footnotes: Recommended Immunization Schedule for Adults Aged 19 Years and Older — United States, 2013

1. **Additional information**
   - Additional guidance for the use of the vaccines described in this supplement is available at http://www.cdc.gov/vaccines/pubs/acip-list.htm.
   - Information on vaccination recommendations when vaccination status is unknown and other general immunization information can be found in the General Recommendations on Immunization at http://www.cdc.gov/mmwr/preview/mmwrhtml/rr6002a1.htm.
   - Information on travel vaccine requirements and recommendations (e.g., for hepatitis A and B, meningococcal, and other vaccines) are available at http://wwwnc.cdc.gov/travel/page/vaccinations.htm.

2. **Influenza vaccination**
   - Annual vaccination against influenza is recommended for all persons aged 6 months and older.
   - Persons aged 6 months and older, including pregnant women, can receive the inactivated influenza vaccine (IIV).
   - Healthy, nonpregnant persons aged 2–49 years without high-risk medical conditions can receive either intranasally administered live, attenuated influenza vaccine (LAIV) (FluMist), or IIV. Health-care personnel who care for severely immunocompromised persons (i.e., those who require care in a protected environment) should receive IIV rather than LAIV.
   - The intramuscularly or intradermally administered IIV are options for adults aged 18–64 years.
   - Adults aged 65 years and older can receive the standard dose IIV or the high-dose IIV (Fluzone High-Dose).

3. **Tetanus, diphtheria, and acellular pertussis (Td/Tdap) vaccination**
   - Administer one dose of Tdap vaccine to pregnant women during each pregnancy (preferred during 27–36 weeks' gestation), regardless of number of years since prior Td or Tdap vaccination.
   - Administer Tdap to all other adults who have not previously received Tdap or for whom vaccine status is unknown. Tdap can be administered regardless of interval since the most recent tetanus or diphtheria-toxoid containing vaccine.
   - Adults with an unknown or incomplete history of completing a 3-dose primary vaccination series with Td-containing vaccines should begin or complete a primary vaccination series including a Tdap dose.

   - For unvaccinated adults, administer the first 2 doses at least 4 weeks apart and the third dose 6–12 months after the second.
   - For incompletely vaccinated (i.e., less than 3 doses) adults, administer remaining doses.
   - Refer to the Advisory Committee on Immunization Practices (ACIP) statement for recommendations for administering Td/Tdap as prophylaxis in wound management (see footnote #1).

4. **Varicella vaccination**
   - All adults without evidence of immunity to varicella (as defined below) should receive 2 doses of single-antigen varicella vaccine or a second dose if they have received only 1 dose.
   - Special consideration for vaccination should be given to those who have close contact with persons at high risk for severe disease (e.g., health-care personnel and family contacts of persons with immunocompromising conditions) or are at high risk for exposure or transmission (e.g., teachers; child care employees; residents and staff members of institutional settings, including correctional institutions; college students; military personnel; adolescents and adults living in households with children; nonpregnant women of childbearing age; and international travelers).
   - Pregnant women should be assessed for evidence of varicella immunity. Women who do not have evidence of immunity should receive the first dose of varicella vaccine upon completion or termination of pregnancy and before discharge from the health-care facility. The second dose should be administered 4–8 weeks after the first dose.
   - Evidence of immunity to varicella in adults includes any of the following:
     — documentation of 2 doses of varicella vaccine at least 4 weeks apart;
     — U.S.-born before 1980 except health-care personnel and pregnant women;
     — history of varicella based on diagnosis or verification of varicella disease by a health-care provider;
     — history of herpes zoster based on diagnosis or verification of herpes zoster disease by a health-care provider; or
     — laboratory evidence of immunity or laboratory confirmation of disease.

5. **Human papillomavirus (HPV) vaccination**
   - Two vaccines are licensed for use in females, bivalent HPV vaccine (HPV2) and quadrivalent HPV vaccine (HPV4), and one HPV vaccine for use in males (HPV4).
   - For females, either HPV4 or HPV2 is recommended in a 3-dose series for routine vaccination at age 11 or 12 years, and for those aged 13 through 26 years, if not previously vaccinated.
   - For males, HPV4 is recommended in a 3-dose series for routine vaccination at age 11 or 12 years, and for those aged 13 through 21 years, if not previously vaccinated. Males aged 22 through 26 years may be vaccinated.
   - HPV4 is recommended for men who have sex with men (MSM) through age 26 years for those who did not get any or all doses when they were younger.
   - Vaccination is recommended for immunocompromised persons (including those with HIV infection) through age 26 years for those who did not get any or all doses when they were younger.
   - A complete series for either HPV4 or HPV2 consists of 3 doses. The second dose should be administered 1–2 months after the first dose; the third dose should be administered 6 months after the first dose (at least 24 weeks after the first dose).
   - HPV vaccines are not recommended for use in pregnant women. However, pregnancy testing is not needed before vaccination. If a woman is found to be pregnant after initiating the vaccination series, no intervention is needed; the remainder of the 3-dose series should be delayed until completion of pregnancy.
   - Although HPV vaccination is not specifically recommended for health-care personnel (HCP) based on their occupation, HCP should receive the HPV vaccine as recommended (see above).

6. **Zoster vaccination**
   - A single dose of zoster vaccine is recommended for adults aged 60 years and older regardless of whether they report a prior episode of herpes zoster. Although the vaccine is licensed by the Food and Drug Administration (FDA) for use among and can be administered to persons aged 50 years and older, ACIP recommends that vaccination begins at age 60 years.
   - Persons aged 60 years and older with chronic medical conditions may be vaccinated unless their condition constitutes a contraindication, such as pregnancy or severe immunodeficiency.
   - Although zoster vaccination is not specifically recommended for HCP, they should receive the vaccine if they are in the recommended age group.

7. **Measles, mumps, rubella (MMR) vaccination**
   - Adults born before 1957 generally are considered immune to measles and mumps. All adults born in 1957 or later should have documentation of 1 or more doses of MMR vaccine unless they have a medical contraindication to the vaccine, or laboratory evidence of immunity to each of the three diseases. Documentation of provider-diagnosed disease is not considered acceptable evidence of immunity for measles, mumps, or rubella.

   Measles component:
   - A routine second dose of MMR vaccine, administered a minimum of 28 days after the first dose, is recommended for adults who
     —are students in postsecondary educational institutions;
     —work in a health-care facility; or
     —plan to travel internationally.
   - Persons who received inactivated (killed) measles vaccine or measles vaccine of unknown type during 1963–1967 should be revaccinated with 2 doses of MMR vaccine.

   Mumps component:
   - A routine second dose of MMR vaccine, administered a minimum of 28 days after the first dose, is recommended for adults who
     —are students in a postsecondary educational institution;
     —work in a health-care facility; or
     —plan to travel internationally.
   - Persons vaccinated before 1979 with either killed mumps vaccine or mumps vaccine of unknown type who are at high risk for mumps infection (e.g., persons who are working in a health-care facility) should be considered for revaccination with 2 doses of MMR vaccine.

   Rubella component:
   - For women of childbearing age, regardless of birth year, rubella immunity should be determined. If there is no evidence of immunity, women who are not pregnant should be vaccinated. Pregnant women who do not have evidence of immunity should receive MMR vaccine upon completion or termination of pregnancy and before discharge from the health-care facility.

   HCP born before 1957:
   - For unvaccinated health-care personnel born before 1957 who lack laboratory evidence of measles, mumps, and/or rubella immunity or laboratory confirmation of disease, health-care facilities should consider vaccinating personnel with 2 doses of MMR vaccine at the appropriate interval for measles and mumps or 1 dose of MMR vaccine for rubella.

8. **Pneumococcal polysaccharide (PPSV23) vaccination**
   - Vaccinate all persons with the following indications:
     —all adults aged 65 years and older;
     —adults younger than age 65 years with chronic lung disease (including chronic obstructive pulmonary disease, emphysema, and asthma); chronic cardiovascular diseases; diabetes mellitus; chronic renal failure; nephrotic syndrome; chronic liver disease (including cirrhosis); alcoholism; cochlear implants; cerebrospinal fluid leaks; immunocompromising conditions; and functional or anatomic asplenia (e.g., sickle cell disease and other hemoglobinopathies, congenital or acquired asplenia, splenic dysfunction, or splenectomy [if elective splenectomy is planned, vaccinate at least 2 weeks before surgery]);
     —residents of nursing homes or long-term care facilities; and
     —adults who smoke cigarettes.
   - Persons with immunocompromising conditions and other selected conditions are recommended to receive PCV13 and PPSV23 vaccines. See footnote #10 for information on timing of PCV13 and PPSV23 vaccinations.
   - Persons with asymptomatic or symptomatic HIV infection should be vaccinated as soon as possible after their diagnosis.
   - When cancer chemotherapy or other immunosuppressive therapy is being considered, the interval between vaccination and initiation of immunosuppressive therapy should be at least 2 weeks. Vaccination during chemotherapy or radiation therapy should be avoided.
   - Routine use of PPSV23 is not recommended for American Indians/Alaska Natives or other persons younger than age 65 years unless they have underlying medical conditions that are PPSV23 indications. However, public health authorities may consider recommending PPSV23 for American Indians/Alaska Natives who are living in areas where the risk for invasive pneumococcal disease is increased.
   - When indicated, PPSV23 should be administered to patients who are uncertain of their vaccination status and there is no record of previous vaccination. When PCV13 is also indicated, a dose of PCV13 should be given first (see footnote #10).

9. **Revaccination with PPSV23**
   - One-time revaccination 5 years after the first dose is recommended for persons aged 19 through 64 years with chronic renal failure or nephrotic syndrome; functional or anatomic asplenia (e.g., sickle cell disease or splenectomy); and for persons with immunocompromising conditions.
   - Persons who received 1 or 2 doses of PPSV23 before age 65 years for any indication should receive another dose of the vaccine at age 65 years or later if at least 5 years have passed since their previous dose.
   - No further doses are needed for persons vaccinated with PPSV23 at or after age 65 years.

10. **Pneumococcal conjugate 13-valent vaccination (PCV13)**
    - Adults aged 19 years or older with immunocompromising conditions (including chronic renal failure and nephrotic syndrome), functional or anatomic asplenia, CSF leaks or cochlear implants, and who have not previously received PCV13 or PPSV23 should receive a single dose of PCV13 followed by a dose of PPSV23 at least 8 weeks later.
    - Adults aged 19 years or older with the aforementioned conditions who have previously received one or more doses of PPSV23 should receive a dose of PCV13 one or more years after the last PPSV23 dose was received. For those that require additional doses of PPSV23, the first such dose should be given no sooner than 8 weeks after PCV13 and at least 5 years since the most recent dose of PPSV23.
    - When indicated, PCV13 should be administered to patients who are uncertain of their vaccination status history and there is no record of previous vaccination.
    - Although PCV13 is licensed by the Food and Drug Administration (FDA) for use among and can be administered to persons aged 50 years and older, ACIP recommends PCV13 for adults aged 19 years and older with the specific medical conditions noted above.

11. **Meningococcal vaccination**
    - Administer 2 doses of meningococcal conjugate vaccine quadrivalent (MCV4) at least 2 months apart to adults with functional asplenia or persistent complement component deficiencies.
    - HIV-infected persons who are vaccinated also should receive 2 doses.
    - Administer a single dose of meningococcal vaccine to microbiologists routinely exposed to isolates of *Neisseria meningitidis*, military recruits, and persons who travel to or live in countries in which meningococcal disease is hyperendemic or epidemic.
    - First-year college students up through age 21 years who are living in residence halls should be vaccinated if they have not received a dose on or after their 16th birthday.

- MCV4 is preferred for adults with any of the preceding indications who are aged 55 years and younger; meningococcal polysaccharide vaccine (MPSV4) is preferred for adults aged 56 years and older.
- Revaccination with MCV4 every 5 years is recommended for adults previously vaccinated with MCV4 or MPSV4 who remain at increased risk for infection (e.g., adults with anatomic or functional asplenia or persistent complement component deficiencies).

12. Hepatitis A vaccination

- Vaccinate any person seeking protection from hepatitis A virus (HAV) infection and persons with any of the following indications:
  — men who have sex with men and persons who use injection or non-injection illicit drugs;
  — persons working with HAV-infected primates or with HAV in a research laboratory setting;
  — persons with chronic liver disease and persons who receive clotting factor concentrates;
  — persons traveling to or working in countries that have high or intermediate endemicity of hepatitis A; and
  — unvaccinated persons who anticipate close personal contact (e.g., household or regular babysitting) with an international adoptee during the first 60 days after arrival in the United States from a country with high or intermediate endemicity. (See footnote #1 for more information on travel recommendations). The first dose of the 2-dose hepatitis A vaccine series should be administered as soon as adoption is planned, ideally 2 or more weeks before the arrival of the adoptee.
- Single-antigen vaccine formulations should be administered in a 2-dose schedule at either 0 and 6–12 months (Havrix), or 0 and 6–18 months (Vaqta). If the combined hepatitis A and hepatitis B vaccine (Twinrix) is used, administer 3 doses at 0, 1, and 6 months; alternatively, a 4-dose schedule may be used, administered on days 0, 7, and 21–30, followed by a booster dose at month 12.

13. Hepatitis B vaccination

- Vaccinate persons with any of the following indications and any person seeking protection from hepatitis B virus (HBV) infection:
  — sexually active persons who are not in a long-term, mutually monogamous relationship (e.g., persons with more than one sex partner during the previous 6 months); persons seeking evaluation or treatment for a sexually transmitted disease (STD); current or recent injection-drug users; and men who have sex with men;
  — health-care personnel and public-safety workers who are potentially exposed to blood or other infectious body fluids;
  — persons with diabetes younger than age 60 years as soon as feasible after diagnosis; persons with diabetes who are age 60 years or older

at the discretion of the treating clinician based on increased need for assisted blood glucose monitoring in long-term care facilities, likelihood of acquiring hepatitis B infection, its complications or chronic sequelae, and likelihood of immune response to vaccination;
  — persons with end-stage renal disease, including patients receiving hemodialysis; persons with HIV infection; and persons with chronic liver disease;
  — household contacts and sex partners of hepatitis B surface antigen-positive persons; clients and staff members of institutions for persons with developmental disabilities; and international travelers to countries with high or intermediate prevalence of chronic HBV infection; and
  — all adults in the following settings: STD treatment facilities; HIV testing and treatment facilities; facilities providing drug-abuse treatment and prevention services; health-care settings targeting services to injection-drug users or men who have sex with men; correctional facilities; end-stage renal disease programs and facilities for chronic hemodialysis patients; and institutions and nonresidential daycare facilities for persons with developmental disabilities.
- Administer missing doses to complete a 3-dose series of hepatitis B vaccine to those persons not vaccinated or not completely vaccinated. The second dose should be administered 1 month after the first dose; the third dose should be given at least 2 months after the second dose (and at least 4 months after the first dose). If the combined hepatitis A and hepatitis B vaccine (Twinrix) is used, give 3 doses at 0, 1, and 6 months; alternatively, a 4-dose Twinrix schedule, administered on days 0, 7, and 21–30 followed by a booster dose at month 12 may be used.
- Adult patients receiving hemodialysis or with other immunocompromising conditions should receive 1 dose of 40 µg/mL (Recombivax HB) administered on a 3-dose schedule at 0, 1, and 6 months or 2 doses of 20 µg/mL (Engerix-B) administered simultaneously on a 4-dose schedule at 0, 1, 2, and 6 months.

14. Selected conditions for which *Haemophilus influenzae* type b (Hib) vaccine may be used

- 1 dose of Hib vaccine should be considered for persons who have sickle cell disease, leukemia, or HIV infection, or who have anatomic or functional asplenia if they have not previously received Hib vaccine.

15. Immunocompromising conditions

- Inactivated vaccines generally are acceptable (e.g., pneumococcal, meningococcal, and influenza [inactivated influenza vaccine]), and live vaccines generally are avoided in persons with immune deficiencies or immunocompromising conditions. Information on specific conditions is available at http://www.cdc.gov/vaccines/pubs/acip-list.htm.

TABLE 5-20B Contraindications and Precautions to Commonly Used Vaccines in Adults[1]*[†]

Vaccine	Contraindications	Precautions
Influenza, inactivated vaccine (IIV)	Severe allergic reaction (e.g., anaphylaxis) after previous dose of any influenza vaccine or to a vaccine component, including egg protein.	Moderate or severe acute illness with or without fever. History of Guillain-Barré Syndrome (GBS) within 6 weeks of previous influenza vaccination. Persons who experience only hives with exposure to eggs should receive IIV with additional safety precautions.[2]
Influenza, live attenuated (LAIV)[3]	Severe allergic reaction (e.g., anaphylaxis) after previous dose of any influenza vaccine or to a vaccine component, including egg protein. Conditions for which the Advisory Committee on Immunization Practices (ACIP) recommends against use, but which are not contraindications in vaccine package insert: immune suppression, certain chronic medical conditions such as asthma, diabetes, heart or kidney disease. and pregnancy.[4]	Moderate or severe acute illness with or without fever. History of GBS within 6 weeks of previous influenza vaccination. Receipt of specific antivirals (i.e., amantadine, rimantadine, zanamivir, or oseltamivir) 48 hours before vaccination. Avoid use of these antiviral drugs for 14 days after vaccination.
Tetanus, diphtheria, pertussis (Tdap); tetanus, diphtheria (Td)	Severe allergic reaction (e.g., anaphylaxis) after a previous dose or to a vaccine component. For pertussis-containing vaccines: encephalopathy (e.g., coma, decreased level of consciousness, or prolonged seizures) not attributable to another identifiable cause within 7 days of administration of a previous dose of Tdap or diphtheria and tetanus toxoids and pertussis (DTP) or diphtheria and tetanus toxoids and acellular pertussis (DTaP) vaccine.	Moderate or severe acute illness with or without fever. GBS within 6 weeks after a previous dose of tetanus toxoid–containing vaccine. History of arthus-type hypersensitivity reactions after a previous dose of tetanus or diptheria toxoid–containing vaccine; defer vaccination until at least 10 years have elapsed since the last tetanus toxoid-containing vaccine. For pertussis-containing vaccines: progressive or unstable neurologic disorder, uncontrolled seizures, or progressive encephalopathy until a treatment regimen has been established and the condition has stabilized.
Varicella[2]	Severe allergic reaction (e.g., anaphylaxis) after a previous dose or to a vaccine component. Known severe immunodeficiency (e.g., from hematologic and solid tumors, receipt of chemotherapy, congenital immunodeficiency, or long-term immunosuppressive therapy[5] or patients with human immunodeficiency virus (HIV) infection who are severely immunocompromised). Pregnancy.	Recent (within 11 months) receipt of antibody-containing blood product (specific interval depends on product).[6,7] Moderate or severe acute illness with or without fever. Receipt of specific antivirals (i.e., acyclovir, famciclovir, or valacyclovir) 24 hours before vaccination; avoid use of these antiviral drugs for 14 days after vaccination.
Human papillomavirus (HPV)	Severe allergic reaction (e.g., anaphylaxis) after a previous dose or to a vaccine component.	Moderate or severe acute illness with or without fever. Pregnancy.
Zoster	Severe allergic reaction (e.g., anaphylaxis) to a vaccine component. Known severe immunodeficiency (e.g., from hematologic and solid tumors, receipt of chemotherapy, or long-term immunosuppressive therapy[5] or patients with HIV infection who are severely immunocompromised). Pregnancy.	Moderate or severe acute illness with or without fever. Receipt of specific antivirals (i.e., acyclovir, famciclovir, or valacyclovir) 24 hours before vaccination; avoid use of these antiviral drugs for 14 days after vaccination.
Measles, mumps, rubella (MMR)[3]	Severe allergic reaction (e.g., anaphylaxis) after a previous dose or to a vaccine component. Known severe immunodeficiency (e.g., from hematologic and solid tumors, receipt of chemotherapy, congenital immunodeficiency, or long-term immunosuppressive therapy[5] or patients with HIV infection who are severely immunocompromised). Pregnancy.	Moderate or severe acute illness with or without fever. Recent (within 11 months) receipt of antibody-containing blood product (specific interval depends on product).[6,7] History of thrombocytopenia or thrombocytopenic purpura. Need for tuberculin skin testing.[8]

TABLE 5-20B Contraindications and Precautions to Commonly Used Vaccines in Adults[1][*][†]—cont'd

Vaccine	Contraindications	Precautions
Pneumococcal polysaccharide (PPSV)	Severe allergic reaction (e.g., anaphylaxis) after a previous dose or to a vaccine component.	Moderate or severe acute illness with or without fever.
Pneumococcal conjugate (PCV13)	Severe allergic reaction (e.g., anaphylaxis) after a previous dose or to a vaccine component, including to any vaccine containing diphtheria toxoid.	Moderate or severe acute illness with or without fever.
Meningococcal, conjugate, (MCV4); meningococcal, polysaccharide (MPSV4)	Severe allergic reaction (e.g., anaphylaxis) after a previous dose or to a vaccine component.	Moderate or severe acute illness with or without fever.
Hepatitis A (HepA)	Severe allergic reaction (e.g., anaphylaxis) after a previous dose or to a vaccine component.	Moderate or severe acute illness with or without fever.
Hepatitis B (HepB)	Severe allergic reaction (e.g., anaphylaxis) after a previous dose or to a vaccine component.	Moderate or severe acute illness with or without fever.

1. Vaccine package inserts and the full ACIP recommendations for these vaccines should be consulted for additional information on vaccine-related contraindications and precautions and for more information on vaccine excipients. Events or conditions listed as precautions should be reviewed carefully. Benefits of and risks for administering a specific vaccine to a person under these circumstances should be considered. If the risk from the vaccine is believed to outweigh the benefit, the vaccine should not be administered. If the benefit of vaccination is believed to outweigh the risk, the vaccine should be administered. A contraindication is a condition in a recipient that increases the chance of a serious adverse reaction. Therefore, a vaccine should not be administered when a contraindication is present.
2. CDC. Prevention and control of influenza with vaccines: recommendations of the Advisory Committee on Immunization Practices (ACIP) — United States, 2012–13 influenza season. MMWR 2012;61:613-8.
3. LAIV, MMR, and varicella vaccines can be administered on the same day. If not administered on the same day, these live vaccines should be separated by at least 28 days.
4. For a complete list of conditions that CDC considers to be reasons to avoid getting LAIV, see CDC. Prevention and control of influenza with vaccines: recommendations of the Advisory Committee on Immunization Practices (ACIP), 2010. MMWR 2010;59(No. RR-8). Available at http://www.cdc.gov/vaccines/pubs/acip-list.htm.
5. Immunosuppressive steroid dose is considered to be 2 or more weeks of daily receipt of 20 mg prednisone or the equivalent. Vaccination should be deferred for at least 1 month after discontinuation of such therapy. Providers should consult ACIP recommendations for complete information on the use of specific live vaccines among persons on immune-suppressing medications or with immune suppression because of other reasons.
6. Vaccine should be deferred for the appropriate interval if replacement immune globulin products are being administered.
7. See CDC. General recommendations on immunization: recommendations of the Advisory Committee on Immunization Practices (ACIP). MMWR 2011;60(No. RR-2). Available at http://www.cdc.gov/vaccines/pubs/acip-list.htm.
8. Measles vaccination might suppress tuberculin reactivity temporarily. Measles-containing vaccine may be administered on the same day as tuberculin skin testing. If testing cannot be performed until after the day of MMR vaccination, the test should be postponed for at least 4 weeks after the vaccination. If an urgent need exists to skin test, do so with the understanding that reactivity might be reduced by the vaccine.

* Adapted from CDC. Table 6. Contraindications and precautions to commonly used vaccines. General recommendations on immunization: recommendations of the Advisory Committee on Immunization Practices. MMWR 2011;60(No. RR-2):40–41 and from Atkinson W, Wolfe S, Hamborsky J, eds. Appendix A. Epidemiology and prevention of vaccine preventable diseases. 12th ed. Washington, DC: Public Health Foundation, 2011. Available at http://www.cdc.gov/vaccines/pubs/pinkbook/index.html.
† Regarding latex allergy. Consult the package insert for any vaccine administered.

TABLE 5-21 Immunization and Pregnancy

Vaccine	Before Pregnancy	During Pregnancy	After Pregnancy	Type of Vaccine	Route
Hepatitis A	If at high risk for disease	If at high risk for disease	If at high risk for disease	Inactivated	IM
Hepatitis B	Yes, if at risk	Yes, if at risk	Yes, if at risk	Inactivated	IM
Human papillomavirus (HPV)	Yes, if 9 to 26 years of age	No, under study	Yes, if 9 to 26 years of age	Inactivated	IM
Influenza TIV	Yes	Yes	Yes	Inactivated	IM
Influenza LAIV	Yes, if <50 years and healthy; avoid conception for 4 weeks	No	Yes, if <50 years and healthy; avoid conception for 4 weeks	Live	Nasal spray
MMR	Yes, avoid conception for 4 weeks	No	Yes, give immediately postpartum if susceptible to rubella	Live	SC
Meningococcal:	If indicated	If indicated	If indicated		
• Polysaccharide				Inactivated	SC
• Conjugate				Inactivated	IM
Pneumococcal polysaccharide	If indicated	If indicated	If indicated	Inactivated	IM or SC
Tetanus/diphtheria Td	Yes, Tdap preferred	If indicated	Yes, Tdap preferred	Toxoid	IM
Tdap, one dose only	Yes, preferred	If high risk of pertussis; otherwise, Td preferred	Yes, preferred	Toxoid/inactivated	IM
Varicella	Yes, avoid conception for 4 weeks	No	Yes, give immediately postpartum if susceptible	Live	SC

IM, Intramuscular; *LAIV,* live, attenuated influenza vaccine; *SC,* subcutaneous; *Tdap,* tetanus and diphtheria toxoids and acellular pertussis; *TIV,* trivalent inactivated influenza vaccine.

TABLE 5-22 Immunizing Agents and Immunization Schedules for Health Care Workers (HCWs)*

Generic Name	Primary Schedule and Booster(s)	Indications	Major Precautions and Contraindications	Special Considerations
Immunizing Agents Strongly Recommended for Health Care Workers				
Hepatitis B (HB) recombinant vaccine	Two doses IM 4 wk apart; third dose 5 mo after second; booster doses not necessary	**Preexposure:** HCWs at risk for exposure to blood or body fluids	Based on limited data no risk of adverse effects to developing fetuses is apparent. Pregnancy should *not* be considered a contraindication to vaccination of women. Previous anaphylactic reaction to common baker's yeast is a contraindication to vaccination.	The vaccine produces neither therapeutic nor adverse effects on HB-infected persons. Prevaccination serologic screening is not indicated for persons being vaccinated because of occupational risk. HCWs who have contact with patients or blood should be tested 1-2 mo after vaccination to determine serologic response.
Hepatitis B immune globulin (HBIG)	0.06 ml/kg IM as soon as possible after exposure. A second dose of HBIG should be administered 1 mo later if the HB vaccine series has not been started.	**Postexposure prophylaxis:** For persons exposed to blood or body fluids containing HBsAg and who are not immune to HBV infection—0.06 ml/kg IM as soon as possible (but no later than 7 days after exposure)		
Influenza vaccine (inactivated whole-virus and split-virus vaccines)	Annual vaccination with current vaccine Administered IM	HCWs who have contact with patients at high risk for influenza or its complications; HCWs who work in long-term care facilities; HCWs with high-risk medical conditions or who are aged ≥65 yr	History of anaphylactic hypersensitivity to egg ingestion	No evidence exists of risk to mother or fetus when the vaccine is administered to a pregnant woman with an underlying high-risk condition. Influenza vaccination is recommended during second and third trimesters of pregnancy because of increased risk for hospitalization.
Measles live-virus vaccine	One dose SC; second dose at least 1 mo later	HCWs† born during or after 1957 who do not have documentation of having received two doses of live vaccine on or after the first birthday **or** a history of physician-diagnosed measles or serologic evidence of immunity. Vaccination should be considered for all HCWs who lack proof of immunity, including those born before 1957.	Pregnancy; immunocompromised persons,‡ including HIV-infected persons who have evidence of severe immunosuppression; anaphylaxis after gelatin ingestion or administration of neomycin; recent administration of immune globulin.	MMR is the vaccine of choice if recipients are likely to be susceptible to rubella and/or mumps as well as measles. Persons vaccinated between 1963 and 1967 with a killed measles vaccine alone, killed vaccine followed by live vaccine, or with a vaccine of unknown type should be revaccinated with two doses of live measles virus vaccine.
Mumps live-virus vaccine	One dose SC; second dose at least 1 mo later	HCWs† believed to be susceptible can be vaccinated. Adults born before 1957 can be considered immune.	Pregnancy; immunocompromised persons,‡ history of anaphylactic reaction after gelatin ingestion or administration of neomycin	MMR is the vaccine of choice if recipients are likely to be susceptible to measles and rubella, as well as mumps.
Hepatitis A virus (HAV) vaccine	Two doses of vaccine either 6-12 mo apart (HAVRIX), or 6 mo apart (VAQTA)	Not routinely indicated for HCWs in the United States. Persons who work with HAV-infected primates or with HAV in a research laboratory setting should be vaccinated.	History of anaphylactic hypersensitivity to alum or, for HAVRIX, the preservative 2-phenoxyethanol. The safety of the vaccine in pregnant women has not been determined; the risk associated with vaccination should be weighed against the risk for hepatitis A in women who may be at high risk for exposure to HAV.	
Meningococcal vaccine	One dose in volume and by route specified by manufacturer; single booster for adults 19 to 21 years of age if the first dose was given before age 16	Laboratory personnel and others with exposure risk.	The safety of the vaccine in pregnant women has not been evaluated; it should not be administered during pregnancy unless the risk for infection is high.	

TABLE 5-22   Immunizing Agents and Immunization Schedules for Health Care Workers (HCWs)—cont'd

Generic Name	Primary Schedule and Booster(s)	Indications	Major Precautions and Contraindications	Special Considerations
Typhoid vaccine, IM, SC, and oral	IM vaccine: One 0.5-ml/dose, booster 0.5 ml every 2 yr SC vaccine: Two 0.5-ml doses, ≥4 wk apart, booster 0.5 ml SC or 0.1 ID every 3 yr if exposure continues Oral vaccine: Four doses on alternate days. The manufacturer recommends revaccination with the entire 4-dose series every 5 yr	Workers in microbiology laboratories who frequently work with *Salmonella typhi*	Severe local or systemic reaction to a previous dose. Ty21a (oral) vaccine should not be administered to immunocompromised persons[†] or to persons receiving antimicrobial agents.	Vaccination should not be considered an alternative to the use of proper procedures when handling specimens and cultures in the laboratory.
Vaccinia vaccine (smallpox)	One dose administered with a bifurcated needle; boosters administered every 10 yr	Laboratory workers who directly handle cultures with vaccinia, recombinant vaccinia viruses, or orthopox viruses that infect human beings	The vaccine is contraindicated in pregnancy, in persons with eczema or a history of eczema, and in immunocompromised persons[†] and their household contacts.	Vaccination may be considered for HCWs who have direct contact with contaminated dressings or other infectious material from volunteers in clinical studies involving recombinant vaccinia virus.

Other Vaccine-Preventable Diseases

Generic Name	Primary Schedule and Booster(s)	Indications	Major Precautions and Contraindications	Special Considerations
Tetanus and diphtheria and pertussis (Tdap)	Two IM doses 4 wk apart or tetanus and diphtheria toxoid for adults with uncertain or incomplete primary vaccination; third dose 6-12 mo after second dose; booster every 10 yr. Substitute a one-time dose of Tdap for one of the doses of Td, either in the primary series or for the routine booster, whichever comes first.	All adults	Except in the first trimester, pregnancy is not a precaution. History of a neurologic reaction or immediate hypersensitivity reaction after a previous dose. History of severe local (Arthus-type) reaction after a previous dose. Such persons should not receive further routine or emergency doses of Td for 10 yr.	Tetanus prophylaxis in wound management[‡]
Pneumococcal polysaccharide vaccine (23 valent)	One dose, 0.5 ml, IM or SC; revaccination recommended for those at highest risk ≥5 yr after the first dose	Adults who are at increased risk of pneumococcal disease and its complications because of underlying health conditions; older adults, especially those age ≥65 who are healthy	The safety of vaccine in pregnant women has not been evaluated; it should not be administered during pregnancy unless the risk for infection is high. Previous recipients of any type of pneumococcal polysaccharide vaccine who are at highest risk for fatal infection or antibody loss may be revaccinated ≥5 yr after the first dose.	
Rubella live-virus vaccine	One dose SC; second dose at least 1 mo later	Indicated for HCWs,[†] both men and women, who do not have documentation of having received live vaccine on or after their first birthday **or** laboratory evidence of immunity. Adults born before 1957, **except women who can become pregnant,** can be considered immune.	Pregnancy; immunocompromised persons[†]; history of anaphylactic reaction after administration of neomycin	The risk for rubella vaccine–associated malformations in the offspring of women pregnant when vaccinated or who become pregnant within 3 mo after vaccination is negligible. Such women should be counseled regarding the theoretic basis of concern for the fetus. MMR is the vaccine of choice if recipients are likely to be susceptible to measles or mumps as well as rubella.
Varicella-zoster live-virus vaccine	Two 0.5-ml doses SC 4-8 wk apart if ≥13 yr	Indicated for HCWs[†] who do not have either a reliable history of varicella or serologic evidence of immunity	Pregnancy, immunocompromised persons,[‡] history of anaphylactic reaction after receipt of neomycin or gelatin. Avoid salicylate use for 6 wk after vaccination.	Vaccine is available from the manufacturer for certain patients with acute lymphocytic leukemia in remission. Because 71%-93% of persons without a history of varicella are immune, serologic testing before vaccination is likely to be cost effective.

TABLE 5-22 Immunizing Agents and Immunization Schedules for Health Care Workers (HCWs)—cont'd

Generic Name	Primary Schedule and Booster(s)	Indications	Major Precautions and Contraindications	Special Considerations
Varicella-zoster immune globulin (VZIG)	Persons <50 kg: 125 µg/10 kg IM; persons ≥50 kg: 625 µg§	Persons known or likely to be susceptible (particularly those at high risk for complications, e.g., pregnant women) who have close and prolonged exposure to a contact case or to an infectious hospital staff worker or patient		Serologic testing may help in assessing whether to administer VZIG. If use of VZIG prevents varicella disease, patient should be vaccinated subsequently.
BCG Vaccination				
Bacille Calmette-Guérin (BCG) vaccine (TB)	One percutaneous dose of 0.3 ml; no booster dose recommended	Should be considered only for HCWs in areas where multidrug TB is prevalent, a strong likelihood of infection exists, and where comprehensive infection control precautions have failed to prevent TB transmission to HCWs	Should not be administered to immunocompromised persons,‡ pregnant women	In the United States TB-control efforts are directed toward early identification, treatment of cases, and preventive therapy with isoniazid.
Other Immunobiologics That Are or May Be Indicated for HCWs				
Immune globulin (hepatitis A)	**Postexposure**—One IM dose of 0.02 ml/kg administered ≤2 wk after exposure	Indicated for HCWs exposed to feces of infectious patients	Contraindicated in persons with IgA deficiency; do not administer within 2 wk after MMR vaccine or 3 wk after varicella vaccine. Delay administration of MMR vaccine for ≥3 mo and varicella vaccine ≥5 mo after administration of immune globulin	Administer in large muscle mass (deltoid, gluteal).

Modified from *MMWR* 46(RR-18), 1998.

HBsAg, Hepatitis B surface antigen; *HBV,* hepatitis B virus; *HIV,* human immunodeficiency virus; *IM,* intramuscular; *MMR,* measles, mumps, rubella vaccine; *SC,* subcutaneous; *TB,* tuberculosis.

*Persons who provide health care to patients or work in institutions that provide patient care (e.g., physicians, nurses, emergency medical personnel, dental professionals and students, medical and nursing students, laboratory technicians, hospital volunteers, and administrative and support staff in health care institutions).

†All HCWs (i.e., medical or nonmedical, paid or volunteer, full time or part time, student or nonstudent, with or without patient-care responsibilities) who work in health care institutions (e.g., inpatient and outpatient, public and private) should be immune to measles, rubella, and varicella.

‡Persons immunocompromised because of immune deficiency diseases, HIV infection, leukemia, lymphoma or generalized malignancy, or immunosuppressed as a result of therapy with corticosteroids, alkylating drugs, antimetabolites, or radiation.

§Some experts recommend 125 µg/10 kg regardless of total body weight.

TABLE 5-23 Recommendations for Persons with Medical Conditions Requiring Special Vaccination Considerations

Condition	Tdap	MMR	Varicella	HBV	HAV	Pneumovax[a]	Influenza[b]	HbCV	Meningococcal	IPV	Other Live Vaccines[c]	Other Killed Vaccines[d]
HIV infection	Rou	Rou/Contr[e]	Contr[f]	Rou[g]	Rou	Rec	Rec	Cons	Rou	Rou	Contr	Rou
Severe immunocompromise[h]	Rou	Contr	Contr[f]	Rou[g]	Rou	Rec	Rec	Rou[i]	Rou	Rou	Contr	Rou
Renal failure	Rou	Rou	Rou	Rec[g]	Rou	Rec	Rec	Rou	Rou	Rou	Rou	Rou
Diabetes	Rou	Rou	Rou	Rou	Rou	Rec	Rec	Rou	Rou	Rou	Rou	Rou
Chronic liver disease	Rou	Rou	Rou	Rou	Rec	Rec	Rec	Rou	Rou	Rou	Rou	Rou
Cardiac disease	Rou	Rou	Rou	Rou	Rou	Rec	Rec	Rou	Rou	Rou	Rou	Rou
Pulmonary disease	Rou	Rou	Rou	Rou	Rou	Rec	Rec	Rou	Rou	Rou	Rou	Rou
Alcoholism	Rou	Rou	Rou	Rou	Rou	Rec	Rec	Rou	Rou	Rou	Rou	Rou
Functional/anatomic asplenia	Rou	Rou	Rou	Rou	Rou	Rec[i]	Rec	Rec[i]	Rec[i]	Rou	Rou	Rou
Terminal complement deficiency	Rou	Rou	Rou	Rou	Rou	Rou	Rou	Rou	Rec	Rou	Rou	
Clotting factor disorders	Rou	Rou	Rou	Rec	Rec	Rou	Rou	Rou	Rou	Rou	Rou	Rou

Modified and updated from *MMWR* 42(RR-4):16, 1993.

Cons, Consider vaccination; *Contr*, contraindicated; *HAV*, hepatitis A virus; *HbCV*, *Haemophilus influenzae* conjugate vaccine; *HBV*, hepatitis B virus; *IPV*, inactivated poliomyelitis vaccine; *MMR*, measles-mumps-rubella; *Rec*, recommended; *Rou*, routine as outlined for all adults; *Tdap*, tetanus and diphtheria toxoids and acellular pertussis.

[a]Pneumovax should be repeated in 5 yr for patients in whom vaccine is recommended. Asthma without chronic obstructive pulmonary disease is not an indication for the vaccine.

[b]Influenza vaccine should also be given to caregivers and household members.

[c]Includes bacille Calmette-Guérin, vaccinia, oral typhoid, yellow fever (if exposure cannot be avoided, persons with HIV can be given yellow fever vaccine; see text).

[d]Includes rabies (check postvaccination titers in HIV or severely immunocompromised persons), Lyme disease, inactivated typhoid, cholera, plague, and anthrax.

[e]For asymptomatic, nonseverely immunocompromised persons with HIV, MMR can be used; it is contraindicated in severely immunocompromised persons. MMR can be considered in symptomatic HIV patients without severe immunocompromise.

[f]Varicella can be given to household members and caregivers, but if varicella-like rash develops after vaccination, contact should be avoided.

[g]Recommended for persons with severe chronic renal failure approaching or already receiving dialysis, and higher doses should be given. Antibody titers should be measured after vaccination in these patients and in those with HIV or severe immunocompromise (who may require higher doses) to ensure adequate response. Yearly titers should be measured in dialysis patients.

[h]Severe immunocompromise can result from congenital immunodeficiency, leukemia, lymphoma, malignancy, organ transplant, chemotherapy, radiation therapy, or high-dose corticosteroids.

[i]Only for persons with Hodgkin's disease.

[j]Give at least 2 wk in advance of elective splenectomy.

TABLE 5-24 Vaccinations for International Travel

Disease*	Areas Affected†	Prophylaxis Recommended	Ideal Time between Last Vaccine Dose and Travel
Tetanus	All	All travelers; vaccine series/booster	Probably 30 days for series; anamnestic response to booster
Measles	All	If born after 1956; ensure immunity by antibody titer, diagnosed measles, or two doses of vaccine	As MMR, 7-14 days
Rubella	All	If born after 1956 and any female of childbearing age; rubella titer or one dose of vaccine	As MMR, 7-14 days
Mumps	All	If born after 1956; ensure immunity by antibody titer, diagnosed mumps, or one dose of vaccine	As MMR, 7-14 days
Varicella	All	All travelers; antibody titer, reported illness, or vaccine series	7-14 days
Hepatitis B	5%-20% of population are carriers in Africa, Middle East except Israel, all Southeast Asia, Amazon basin, Haiti, and Dominican Republic; 1%-5% of population are carriers in south-central and southwest Asia, Israel, Japan, Americas, Russia, and eastern and southern Europe	Travelers for more than 6 mo in close contact with population or for less time but with high-risk activities (close household contact, seeking dental or medical care, sex); vaccine series	Probably 30 days
Hepatitis A	Developing countries	Travelers to rural areas; eating and drinking in settings of poor sanitation; vaccine or pooled immune globulin	Vaccine, 30 days Pooled IG, 2 days
Influenza	Tropics throughout the year; southern hemisphere from April to September	Travelers for whom vaccine is otherwise indicated; give current vaccine and revaccinate in fall as usual	7-14 days
Meningococcus*	Sub-Saharan Africa "belt" (Senegal to Ethiopia) from December to June; required for pilgrims to Saudi Arabia during Hajj; epidemics reported in other African nations, India, Nepal, and Mongolia	All travelers; vaccine	7-10 days
Rabies	Endemic dog rabies exists in Mexico, El Salvador, Guatemala, Peru, Colombia, Ecuador, India, Nepal, Philippines, Sri Lanka, Thailand, and Vietnam	Travelers staying for more than 30 days or at high risk of exposure to domestic or wild animals; vaccine series/booster	7-14 days
Poliomyelitis	Developing countries not in western hemisphere; at risk all year in tropics; in temperate zones, incidence increases in summer and fall	All travelers; vaccine series/booster	Parenteral vaccine series, 28 day
Typhoid fever	Many countries in Asia, Africa, Central America, and South America	Travelers with prolonged stay in rural areas with poor sanitation; vaccine series/booster	Oral vaccine, 7 days Parenteral vaccine, probably 14 days
Yellow fever*	North and central South America, forest-savannah zones of Africa; some countries in Africa, Asia, and Middle East require travelers from endemic areas to be vaccinated	All travelers; vaccine/booster at approved yellow fever vaccination center.	10 days
Japanese encephalitis	Seasonally in most areas of Asia, Indian subcontinent, and western Pacific islands; in temperate zones, incidence increases in summer and early fall; in tropics, year-round incidence	Travelers staying for more than 30 days in high-risk rural areas; staying outdoors during transmission season; vaccine series	10 days
Cholera*	Certain undeveloped countries	If required by local authorities, one dose usually suffices; primary series only for those living in high-risk areas under poor sanitary conditions or those with compromised gastric defense mechanisms (achlorhydria, antacid therapy, previous ulcer surgery); booster every 6 mo	Probably 30 days
Plague	Africa, Asia, and Americas in rural mountainous or upland areas	Travelers whose research or field activities bring them in contact with rodents; vaccine series/booster; consider taking tetracycline (500 mg four times a day) for chemoprophylaxis (inferred from clinical experience in treating plague)	Probably 30 days

From Noble J: *Primary care medicine*, ed 3, St Louis, 2001, Mosby.
IG, Immune globulin; *MMR,* measles-mumps-rubella.
*Only yellow fever vaccine is required for entry by any country; cholera vaccine may be required by some local authorities. Meningococcus vaccine is required for pilgrims to Mecca, in Saudia Arabia, during Hajj. However, it is important to follow Centers for Disease Control and Prevention (CDC) recommendations for all vaccines to prevent disease. If a required vaccine is contraindicated or withheld for any reason, attempts should be made to obtain a waiver from the country's consulate or embassy.
†Because areas affected can change, and for more specific details, consult the CDC's traveler's hotline.

Recommendations and Implementation Strategies for Hepatitis B Vaccination of Adults

BOX 5-1 Adults Recommended to Receive Hepatitis B Vaccination

Persons at Risk for Infection by Sexual Exposure
- Sex partners of persons who are HBsAg positive
- Sexually active persons who are not in a long-term, mutually monogamous relationship (e.g., persons who have had more than one sex partner during the previous 6 months)
- Persons seeking evaluation or treatment for a sexually transmitted disease
- Men who have sex with men

Persons at Risk for Infection by Percutaneous or Mucosal Exposure to Blood
- Current or recent users of injection drugs
- Household contacts of persons who are HBsAg positive
- Residents and staff of facilities for developmentally disabled persons

- Health care and public safety workers with reasonably anticipated risk for exposure to blood or blood-contaminated body fluids
- Persons with end-stage renal disease, including predialysis, hemodialysis, peritoneal dialysis, and home dialysis patients

Others
- International travelers to regions with high or intermediate levels (HBsAg prevalence of ≥2%) of endemic HBV infection
- Persons with chronic liver disease
- Persons with HIV infection
- All other persons seeking protection from HBV infection

From CDC: A comprehensive immunization strategy to eliminate transmission of hepatitis B virus infection in the United States: recommendations of the Advisory Committee on Immunization Practices (ACIP), *MMWR* 55(RR-16):15, 2006.
  HbsAg, Hepatitis B surface antigen; *HBV,* hepatitis B virus.

BOX 5-2 Hepatitis B Vaccine Schedules for Adults (Aged ≥20 yr)*

0, 1, and 6 months
0, 1, and 4 months
0, 2, and 4 months
0, 1, 2, and 12 months[†]

From CDC: A comprehensive immunization strategy to eliminate transmission of hepatitis B virus infection in the United States: recommendations of the Advisory Committee on Immunization Practices (ACIP), *MMWR* 55(RR-16):15, 2006.
  *All schedules are applicable to single-antigen hepatitis B vaccines; Twinrix (combined hepatitis A and hepatitis B vaccine) may be administered at 0, 1, and 6 months.
  [†]A 4-dose schedule of Engerix-B is licensed for all age groups.

TABLE 5-25 Recommended Doses of Currently Licensed Formulations of Adult Hepatitis B Vaccine by Group and Vaccine Type

| | SINGLE-ANTIGEN VACCINE | | | | COMBINATION VACCINE | |
| | Recombivax HB[a] | | Engerix-B[b] | | Twinrix[b,c] | |
Group	Dose (μg)[d]	Vol. (ml)	Dose (μg)[d]	Vol. (ml)	Dose (μg)[d]	Vol. (ml)
Adults (aged ≥20 yr)	10	1.0	20	1.0	20	1.0
Hemodialysis patients and other immunocompromised persons aged ≥20 yr	40[e]	1.0	40[f]	2.0	—[g]	—

From Centers for Disease Control and Prevention: A comprehensive immunization strategy to eliminate transmission of hepatitis B virus infection in the United States: recommendations of the Advisory Committee on Immunization Practices (ACIP), *MMWR* 55(RR-16):10, 2006.
HB, Hepatitis B.
[a]Merck & Co., Inc., Whitehouse Station, New Jersey.
[b]GlaxoSmithKline Biologicals, Rixensart, Belgium.
[c]Combined hepatitis A and hepatitis B vaccine, recommended for persons aged >18 yr who are at increased risk for both hepatitis B virus and hepatitis A virus infections.
[d]Recombinant hepatitis B surface antigen protein dose.
[e]Dialysis formulation administered on a 3-dose schedule at 0, 1, and 6 mo.
[f]Two 1.0-ml doses administered in 1 or 2 injections on a 4-dose schedule at 0, 1, 2, and 6 mo.
[g]Not applicable.

TABLE 5-26 Recommended HIV/AIDS, Sexually Transmitted Disease (STD), and Viral Hepatitis Prevention Services by Risk Population

Risk Population[a]	Recommended Services
High-Risk Heterosexuals	
Persons seeking sexually transmitted disease evaluation or treatment	Hepatitis B vaccination Testing for HIV infection[b] Testing for syphilis, gonorrhea, and chlamydia, as clinically indicated[c]
Sexually active men not in a long-term, mutually monogamous relationship	Hepatitis B vaccination Annual testing for HIV infection[b,d]
Sexually active women not in a long-term, mutually monogamous relationship	Hepatitis B vaccination[e] Annual testing for HIV infection[b,d] Annual testing for chlamydia (NOTE: Also recommended for all sexually active females aged <25 yr)[c]
Men Who Have Sex with Men (MSM)	
All MSM	Hepatitis A vaccination Hepatitis B vaccination[e]
Sexually active MSM not in a long-term, mutually monogamous relationship	Hepatitis A vaccination Hepatitis B vaccination[e] Annual testing for HIV infection[b] Annual testing for syphilis, gonorrhea, and chlamydia[c]
Injection-Drug Users	
	Hepatitis A vaccination[f] Hepatitis B vaccination Testing for hepatitis C virus infection[g] Annual testing for HIV infection[b] Substance-abuse treatment[h]

From Centers for Disease Control and Prevention (CDC): A comprehensive immunization strategy to eliminate transmission of hepatitis B virus infection in the United States: recommendations of the Advisory Committee on Immunization Practices (ACIP), *MMWR* 55(RR-16):17, 2006.
[a]Testing for HIV infection, chlamydia, gonorrhea, syphilis, and hepatitis B surface antigen also is recommended for pregnant women. (CDC: Revised recommendations for HIV testing of adults, adolescents, and pregnant women in health care settings, *MMWR* 55[RR-14], 2006; CDC: Sexually transmitted diseases treatment guidelines, *MMWR* 55[RR-11], 2006; CDC: A comprehensive immunization strategy to eliminate transmission of hepatitis B virus infection in the United States: recommendations of the Advisory Committee on Immunization Practices [ACIP]. Part 1: immunization of infants, children, and adolescents, *MMWR* 54[RR-16], 2005.)
[b]CDC: Revised recommendations for HIV testing of adults, adolescents, and pregnant women in health care settings, *MMWR* 55(RR-14), 2006.
[c]CDC: Sexually transmitted diseases treatment guidelines 2006, *MMWR* 55(RR-11), 2006.
[d]HIV screening is recommended for all persons aged 13-64 yr. Repeat screening is recommended at least annually for persons likely to be at high risk for HIV infection, including MSM or heterosexuals who themselves or whose sex partners have had more than one partner since their most recent HIV test.
[e]Hepatitis B vaccination is recommended for persons who have had more than one sex partner during the previous 6 mo.
[f]CDC: Prevention of hepatitis A through active or passive immunization: recommendations of the Advisory Committee on Immunization Practices (ACIP), *MMWR* 55(RR-7), 2006.
[g]CDC: Recommendations for prevention and control of hepatitis C virus (HCV) infection and HCV-related chronic disease, *MMWR* 47(RR-19), 1998. Recommended frequency of testing for hepatitis C virus infection has not been determined.
[h]CDC: *Substance abuse treatment for injection drug users: a strategy with many benefits,* Atlanta, 2002, U.S. Department of Health and Human Services, CDC. Available at http://www.cdc.gov/idu/facts/treatment.htm.

Clinical Practice Guidelines

V

TABLE 5-27 Guidelines for Postexposure Prophylaxis* of Persons with Nonoccupational Exposures† to Blood or Body Fluids That Contain Blood by Exposure Type and Vaccination Status

	TREATMENT	
Exposure	Unvaccinated Person‡	Previously Vaccinated Person§
HBsAg-Positive Source		
Percutaneous (e.g., bite or needlestick) or mucosal exposure to HBsAg-positive blood or body fluids	Administer hepatitis B vaccine series and hepatitis B immune globulin (HBIG)	Administer hepatitis B vaccine booster dose
Sex or needle-sharing contact with a person who is HBsAg positive	Administer hepatitis B vaccine series and HBIG	Administer hepatitis B vaccine booster dose
Victim of sexual assault/abuse by a perpetrator who is HBsAg positive	Administer hepatitis B vaccine series and HBIG	Administer hepatitis B vaccine booster dose
Source with Unknown HBsAg Status		
Victim of sexual assault/abuse by a perpetrator with unknown HBsAg status	Administer hepatitis B vaccine series	No treatment
Percutaneous (e.g., bite or needlestick) or mucosal exposure to potentially infectious blood or body fluids from a source with unknown HBsAg status	Administer hepatitis B vaccine series	No treatment
Sexual or needle-sharing contact with person with unknown HBsAg status	Administer hepatitis B vaccine series	No treatment

From Centers for Disease Control and Prevention: A comprehensive immunization strategy to eliminate transmission of hepatitis B virus infection in the United States: recommendations of the Advisory Committee on Immunization Practices (ACIP), *MMWR* 55(RR-16):30, 2006.
HBsAg, Hepatitis B surface antigen.
*When indicated, immunoprophylaxis should be initiated as soon as possible, preferably within 24 hours. Studies are limited on the maximum interval after exposure during which postexposure prophylaxis is effective, but the interval is unlikely to exceed 7 days for percutaneous exposures or 14 days for sexual exposures. The hepatitis B vaccine series should be completed.
†These guidelines apply to nonoccupational exposures. Guidelines for management of occupational exposures have been published separately and also can be used for management of nonoccupational exposures if feasible.
‡A person who is in the process of being vaccinated but has not completed the vaccine series should complete the series and receive treatment as indicated.
§A person who has written documentation of a complete hepatitis B vaccine series and did not receive postvaccination testing.

TABLE 5-28 Typical Interpretation of Serologic Test Results for Hepatitis B Virus Infection

SEROLOGIC MARKER				
HBsAg	Total Anti-HBc	IgM Anti-HBc	Anti-HBs	Interpretation
−*	−	−	−	Never infected
+†‡	−	−	−	Early acute infection; transient (up to 18 days) after vaccination
+	+	+	−	Acute infection
−	+	+	+ or −	Acute resolving infection
−	+	−	+	Recovered from past infection and immune
+	+	−	−	Chronic infection
−	+	−	−	False-positive (i.e., susceptible), past infection, "low-level" chronic infection,§ or passive transfer of anti-HBc to infant born to mother who is HBsAg positive
−	−	−	+	Immune if concentration is >10 mIU/ml after vaccine series completion‖; passive transfer after hepatitis B immune globulin administration

From Centers for Disease Control and Prevention: A comprehensive immunization strategy to eliminate transmission of hepatitis B virus infection in the United States: recommendations of the Advisory Committee on Immunization Practices (ACIP), *MMWR* 55(RR-16):4, 2006.
HBc, Antibody to hepatitis B core antigen; *HBs*, antibody to HBsAg; *HBsAg*, hepatitis B surface antigen; *Ig*, immunoglobulin.
*Negative test result.
†Positive test result.
‡To ensure that an HBsAg-positive test result is not a false-positive, samples with reactive HBsAg results should be tested with a licensed neutralizing confirmatory test if recommended in the manufacturer's package insert.
§Persons positive only for anti-HBc are unlikely to be infectious except under unusual circumstances in which they are the source for direct percutaneous exposure of susceptible recipients to large quantities of virus (e.g., blood transfusion or organ transplant).
‖Milliinternational units per milliliter.

Hepatitis A Prophylaxis

TABLE 5-29 Recommended Dosages of Hepatitis A Immune Globulin

Setting	Duration of Coverage	Dose
Preexposure prophylaxis	Short term (<3 mo)	0.02 ml/kg
	Long term (3-5 mo)*	0.06 ml/kg
Postexposure prophylaxis	—	0.02 ml/kg

Modified from Centers for Disease Control and Prevention: Prevention of hepatitis A through active or passive immunization: recommendations of the Advisory Committee on Immunization Practices (ACIP), *MMWR* 55(RR-07):9, 2006.
NOTE: Immune globulin should be administered intramuscularly into the deltoid or gluteal muscle in children younger than 24 mo; it may be administered in the anterolateral thigh muscle.
*Repeat every 5 mo if continued exposure to hepatitis A virus occurs.

TABLE 5-30 Licensed Dosages of Hepatitis A Vaccines

Vaccine	Patient's Age	Dose	Volume (ml)	Number of Doses	Schedule (mo)*
Hepatitis A vaccine, inactivated (Havrix)	12 mo to 18 yr	720 EL.U.	0.5	2	0, 6-12
	≥19 yr	1440 EL.U.	1.0	2	0, 6-12
Hepatitis A vaccine, inactivated (Vaqta)	12 mo to 18 yr	25 U	0.5	2	0, 6-18
	≥19 yr	50 U	1.0	2	0, 6-18
Combined hepatitis A and hepatitis B vaccine (Twinrix)	≥18 yr	720 EL.U. of hepatitis A antigen and 20 mcg of hepatitis B surface antigen protein	1.0	3	0, 1, and 6

Modified from Centers for Disease Control and Prevention: Prevention of hepatitis A through active or passive immunization: recommendations of the Advisory Committee on Immunization Practices (ACIP), *MMWR* 55(RR-07):10, 2006.
*Zero represents the timing of the initial dose; subsequent numbers represent months after the initial dose.

Influenza Treatment and Prophylaxis

BOX 5-3 Summary of Seasonal Influenza Vaccination Recommendations

Children

All children aged 6 months-18 years should be vaccinated annually.

Children and adolescents at higher risk for influenza complications should continue to be a focus for vaccination efforts as providers and programs transition to routinely vaccinating all children and adolescents, including those who:
- are aged 6 months-4 years (59 months)
- have chronic pulmonary (including asthma), cardiovascular (except hypertension), renal, hepatic, cognitive, neurologic/neuromuscular, hematologic, or metabolic disorders (including diabetes mellitus)
- are immunosuppressed (including immunosuppression caused by medications or by human immunodeficiency virus)
- are receiving long-term aspirin therapy and therefore might be at risk for experiencing Reye's syndrome after influenza virus infection
- are residents of long-term care facilities
- will be pregnant during the influenza season

Note: Children aged <6 months cannot receive influenza vaccination. Household and other close contacts (e.g., day-care providers) of children aged <6 months, including older children and adolescents, should be vaccinated.

Adults

Annual vaccination against influenza is recommended for any adult who wants to reduce the risk of becoming ill with influenza or of transmitting it to others. Vaccination is recommended for all adults without contraindications in the following groups, because these persons either are at higher risk for influenza complications, or are close contacts of the persons at higher risk:
- persons aged ≥50 years
- women who will be pregnant during the influenza season
- persons who have chronic pulmonary (including asthma), cardiovascular (except hypertension), renal, hepatic, cognitive, neurologic/neuromuscular, hematologic, or metabolic disorders (including diabetes mellitus)
- persons who have immunosuppression (including immunosuppression caused by medications or by human immunodeficiency virus)
- residents of nursing homes and other long-term care facilities
- health-care personnel
- household contacts and caregivers of children aged <5 years and adults aged ≥50 years, with particular emphasis on vaccinating contacts of children aged <6 months
- household contacts and caregivers of persons with medical conditions that put them at higher risk for severe complications from influenza

Modified from *MMWR* 58:(RR-8), 2009.

RECOMMENDED VACCINES FOR DIFFERENT AGE GROUPS

When vaccinating children aged 6 to 35 months with TIV, health care providers should use TIV that has been licensed by the FDA for this age group (i.e., TIV manufactured by Sanofi Pasteur [FluZone]). TIV from Novartis (Fluvirin) is FDA approved in the United States for use among persons aged 4 years and older. TIV from GlaxoSmithKline (Fluarix and FluLaval) or CSL Biotherapies (Afluria) is labeled for use in persons aged 18 years and older because data to demonstrate efficacy among younger persons have not been provided to the FDA. LAIV from MedImmune (FluMist) is licensed for use by healthy, nonpregnant persons aged 2 to 49 years. A vaccine dose does not need to be repeated if inadvertently administered to a person who does not have an age indication for the vaccine formulation given. Expanded age and risk group indications for licensed vaccines are likely over the next several years, and vaccination providers should be alert to these changes. In addition, several new vaccine formulations are being evaluated in immunogenicity and efficacy trials; when licensed, these new products will increase the influenza vaccine supply and provide additional vaccine choices for practitioners and their patients.

INFLUENZA VACCINES AND USE OF INFLUENZA ANTIVIRAL MEDICATIONS

Administration of TIV and influenza antivirals during the same medical visit is acceptable. The effect on safety and effectiveness of LAIV coadministration with influenza antiviral medications has not been studied. However, because influenza antivirals reduce replication of influenza viruses, LAIV should not be administered until 48 hours after cessation of influenza antiviral therapy, and influenza antiviral medications should not be administered for 2 weeks after receipt of LAIV. Persons receiving antivirals within the period 2 days before to 14 days after vaccination with LAIV should be revaccinated at a later date.

PERSONS WHO SHOULD NOT BE VACCINATED WITH TIV

TIV should not be administered to persons known to have anaphylactic hypersensitivity to eggs or other components of the influenza vaccine. Prophylactic use of antiviral agents is an option for preventing influenza among such persons. Information about vaccine components is located in package inserts from each manufacturer. Persons with moderate to severe acute febrile illness usually should not be vaccinated until their symptoms have abated. However, minor illnesses with or without fever do not contraindicate use of influenza vaccine. Guillain-Barré syndrome within 6 weeks after a previous dose of TIV is considered a precaution for use of TIV.

CONSIDERATIONS WHEN USING LAIV

LAIV is an option for vaccination of healthy, nonpregnant persons aged 2 to 49 years, including health care providers and other close contacts of high-risk persons (except severely immunocompromised persons who require care in a protected environment). No preference is indicated for LAIV or TIV when considering vaccination of healthy, nonpregnant persons aged 2 to 49 years. Use of the term *healthy* in this recommendation refers to persons who do not have any of the underlying medical conditions that confer high risk for severe complications (see "Persons Who Should Not Be Vaccinated with LAIV"). However, during periods when inactivated vaccine is in short supply, use of LAIV is encouraged when feasible for eligible persons (including health care providers) because use of LAIV by these persons might increase availability of TIV for persons in groups targeted for vaccination but who cannot receive LAIV. Possible advantages of LAIV include its potential to induce a broad mucosal and systemic immune response in children, its ease of administration, and possibly increased acceptability of an intranasal rather than intramuscular route of administration.

If the vaccine recipient sneezes after administration, the dose should not be repeated. However, if nasal congestion is present that might impede delivery of the vaccine to the nasopharyngeal mucosa, deferral of administration should be considered until resolution of the illness, or TIV should be administered instead. No data exist about concomitant use of nasal corticosteroids or other intranasal medications.

Although FDA licensure of LAIV excludes children aged 2 to 4 years with a history of asthma or recurrent wheezing, the precise risk, if any, of wheezing caused by LAIV among these children is unknown because experience with LAIV among these young children is limited. Young children might not have a history of recurrent wheezing if their exposure to respiratory viruses has been limited because of their age. Certain children might have a history of wheezing with respiratory illnesses but have not had asthma diagnosed. The following screening recommendations should be used to assist persons who administer influenza vaccines in providing the appropriate vaccine for children aged 2 to 4 years.

Clinicians and vaccination programs should screen for possible reactive airways diseases when considering use of LAIV for children aged 2 to 4 years and should avoid use of this vaccine in children with asthma or a recent wheezing episode. Health care providers should consult the medical record, when available, to identify children aged 2 to 4 years with asthma or recurrent wheezing that might indicate asthma. In addition, to identify children who might be at greater risk for asthma and possibly at increased risk for wheezing after receiving LAIV, parents or caregivers of children aged 2 to 4 years should be asked, "In the past 12 months, has a health care provider ever told you that your child had wheezing or asthma?" Children whose parents or caregivers answer "yes" to this question and children who have asthma or who had a wheezing episode noted in the medical record during the preceding 12 months should not receive LAIV. TIV is available for use in children with asthma or possible reactive airways diseases.

LAIV can be administered to persons with minor acute illnesses (e.g., diarrhea or mild upper respiratory tract infection with or without fever). However, if nasal congestion is present that might impede delivery of the vaccine to the nasopharyngeal mucosa, deferral of administration should be considered until resolution of the illness.

PERSONS WHO SHOULD NOT BE VACCINATED WITH LAIV

The effectiveness or safety of LAIV is not known for the following groups, who should not be vaccinated with LAIV:

- Persons with a history of hypersensitivity, including anaphylaxis, to any of the components of LAIV or eggs
- Persons younger than 2 years or aged 50 years or older
- Persons with any of the underlying medical conditions that serve as an indication for routine influenza vaccination, including asthma, reactive airways disease, or other chronic disorders of the pulmonary or cardiovascular systems; other underlying medical conditions, including metabolic diseases such as diabetes, renal dysfunction, and hemoglobinopathies; or known or suspected immunodeficiency diseases or immunosuppressed states
- Children aged 2 to 4 years whose parents or caregivers report that a health care provider has told them during the preceding 12 months that their child had wheezing or asthma, or whose medical record indicates a wheezing episode has occurred during the preceding 12 months
- Children or adolescents receiving aspirin or other salicylates (because of the association of Reye syndrome with wild-type influenza virus infection)
- Persons with a history of Guillain-Barré syndrome after influenza vaccination
- Pregnant women

CONCURRENT ADMINISTRATION OF INFLUENZA VACCINE WITH OTHER VACCINES

Use of LAIV concurrently with measles, mumps, rubella (MMR) alone, and MMR and varicella vaccine among children aged 12 to 15 months has been studied, and no interference with immunogenicity to antigens in any of the vaccines was observed. Among adults aged 50 years or older, the safety and immunogenicity of zoster vaccine and TIV were similar whether administered simultaneously or spaced 4 weeks apart. In the absence of specific data indicating interference, following ACIP's general recommendations for vaccination is prudent. Inactivated vaccines do not interfere with the immune response to other inactivated vaccines or to live vaccines. Inactivated or live vaccines can be administered simultaneously with LAIV. However, after administration of a live vaccine, at least 4 weeks should pass before another live vaccine is administered.

TABLE 5-31 Live, Attenuated Influenza Vaccine (LAIV) Compared with Inactivated Influenza Vaccine (TIV) for Seasonal Influenza, United States Formulations

Factor	LAIV	TIV
Route of administration	Intranasal spray	Intramuscular injection
Type of vaccine	Live virus	Noninfectious virus (i.e.,inactivated)
Number of included virus strains	3 (2 influenza A, 1 influenza B)	3 (2 influenza A, 1 influenza B)
Vaccine virus strains updated	Annually	Annually
Frequency of administration	Annually*	Annually*
Approved age	Persons aged 2-49 yr	Persons aged ≥6 mo
Interval between 2 doses recommended for children aged ≥6 mo to 8 yr who are receiving influenza vaccine for the first time	4 wk	4 wk
Can be administered to persons with medical risk factors for influenza-related complications[†]	No	Yes
Can be administered to children with asthma or children aged 2-4 yr with wheezing during the preceding year[§]	No	Yes
Can be administered to family members or close contacts of immunosuppressed persons not requiring a protected environment	Yes	Yes
Can be administered to family members or close contacts of immunosuppressed persons requiring a protected environment (e.g., hematopoietic stem cell transplant recipient)	No	Yes
Can be administered to family members or close contacts of persons at high risk but not severely immunosuppressed	Yes	Yes
Can be simultaneously administered with other vaccines	Yes[¶]	Yes**
If not simultaneously administered, can be administered within 4 wk of another live vaccine	Prudent to space 4 wk apart	Yes
If not simultaneously administered, can be administered within 4 wk of an inactivated vaccine	Yes	Yes

Modified from *MMWR* 56(RR-6), 2007.

*Children aged 6 months-8 years who have never received influenza vaccine before should receive 2 doses. Those who only receive 1 dose in their first year of vaccination should receive 2 doses in the following year, spaced 4 weeks apart.

[†]Persons at higher risk for complications of influenza infection because of underlying medical conditions should not receive LAIV. Persons at higher risk for complications of influenza infection because of underlying medical conditions include adults and children with chronic disorders of the pulmonary or cardiovascular systems; adults and children with chronic metabolic diseases (including diabetes mellitus), renal dysfunction, hemoglobinopathies, or immunosuppression; children and adolescents receiving long-term aspirin therapy (at risk for developing Reye's syndrome after wild-type influenza infection); persons who have any condition (e.g., cognitive dysfunction, spinal cord injuries, seizure disorders, or other neuromuscular disorders) that can compromise respiratory function or the handling of respiratory secretions or that can increase the risk for aspiration; pregnant women; and residents of nursing homes and other chronic-care facilities that house persons with chronic medical conditions.

[§]Clinicians and immunization programs should screen for possible reactive airways diseases when considering use of LAIV for children aged 2-4 years and should avoid use of this vaccine in children with asthma or a recent wheezing episode. Health care providers should consult the medical record, when available, to identify children aged 2-4 years with asthma or recurrent wheezing that might indicate asthma. In addition, to identify children who might be at greater risk for asthma and possibly at increased risk for wheezing after receiving LAIV, parents or caregivers of children aged 2-4 years should be asked: "In the past 12 months, has a health care provider ever told you that your child had wheezing or asthma?" Children whose parents or caregivers answer "yes" to this question and children who have asthma or who had a wheezing episode noted in the medical record during the preceding 12 months should not receive LAIV.

[¶]LAIV coadministration has been evaluated systematically only among children aged 12–15 months who received measles, mumps, and rubella vaccine or varicella vaccine.

**TIV coadministration has been evaluated systematically only among adults who received pneumococcal polysaccharide or zoster vaccine.

INDICATIONS FOR USE OF ANTIVIRALS

PERSONS FOR WHOM ANTIVIRAL TREATMENT SHOULD BE CONSIDERED

If possible, antiviral treatment should be started within 48 hours of influenza illness onset. The effectiveness of initiating antiviral treatment more than 48 hours after illness onset has not been established. Persons for whom antiviral treatment should be considered include:

- Persons hospitalized with laboratory-confirmed influenza (limited data suggest benefit even for persons whose antiviral treatment is initiated more than 48 hours after illness onset)
- Persons with laboratory-confirmed influenza pneumonia
- Persons with laboratory-confirmed influenza and bacterial coinfection
- Persons with laboratory-confirmed influenza infection who are at higher risk for influenza complications
- Persons presenting to medical care with laboratory-confirmed influenza within 48 hours of influenza illness onset who want to decrease the duration or severity of their symptoms and transmission of influenza to others at higher risk for complications

PERSONS FOR WHOM ANTIVIRAL CHEMOPROPHYLAXIS SHOULD BE CONSIDERED DURING PERIODS OF INCREASED INFLUENZA ACTIVITY IN THE COMMUNITY

- Persons at high risk during the 2 weeks after influenza vaccination (after the second dose for children younger than 9 years who have not previously been vaccinated) if influenza viruses are circulating in the community

- Persons at high risk for whom influenza vaccine is contraindicated
- Family members or health care providers who are unvaccinated and are likely to have ongoing, close exposure to persons at high risk or unvaccinated persons or infants younger than 6 months
- Persons and their family members and close contacts and health care workers when circulating strains of influenza virus in the community are not matched with vaccine strains
- Persons with immune deficiencies or those who might not respond to vaccination (e.g., persons infected with HIV or other immunosuppressed conditions or who are receiving immunosuppressive medications)
- Unvaccinated staff and persons during response to an outbreak in a closed institutional setting with residents at high risk (e.g., extended-care facilities)

Modified from *MMWR* 57(RR-7), 2008.
Note: Recommended antiviral medications (neuraminidase inhibitors) are not licensed for chemoprophylaxis of children younger than 1 year (oseltamivir) or younger than 5 years (zanamivir). Updates or supplements to these recommendations (e.g., expanded age or risk group indications for licensed vaccines) might be required. Health care providers should be alert to announcements of recommendation updates and should check the CDC influenza website periodically for additional information (http://www.cdc.gov/flu).

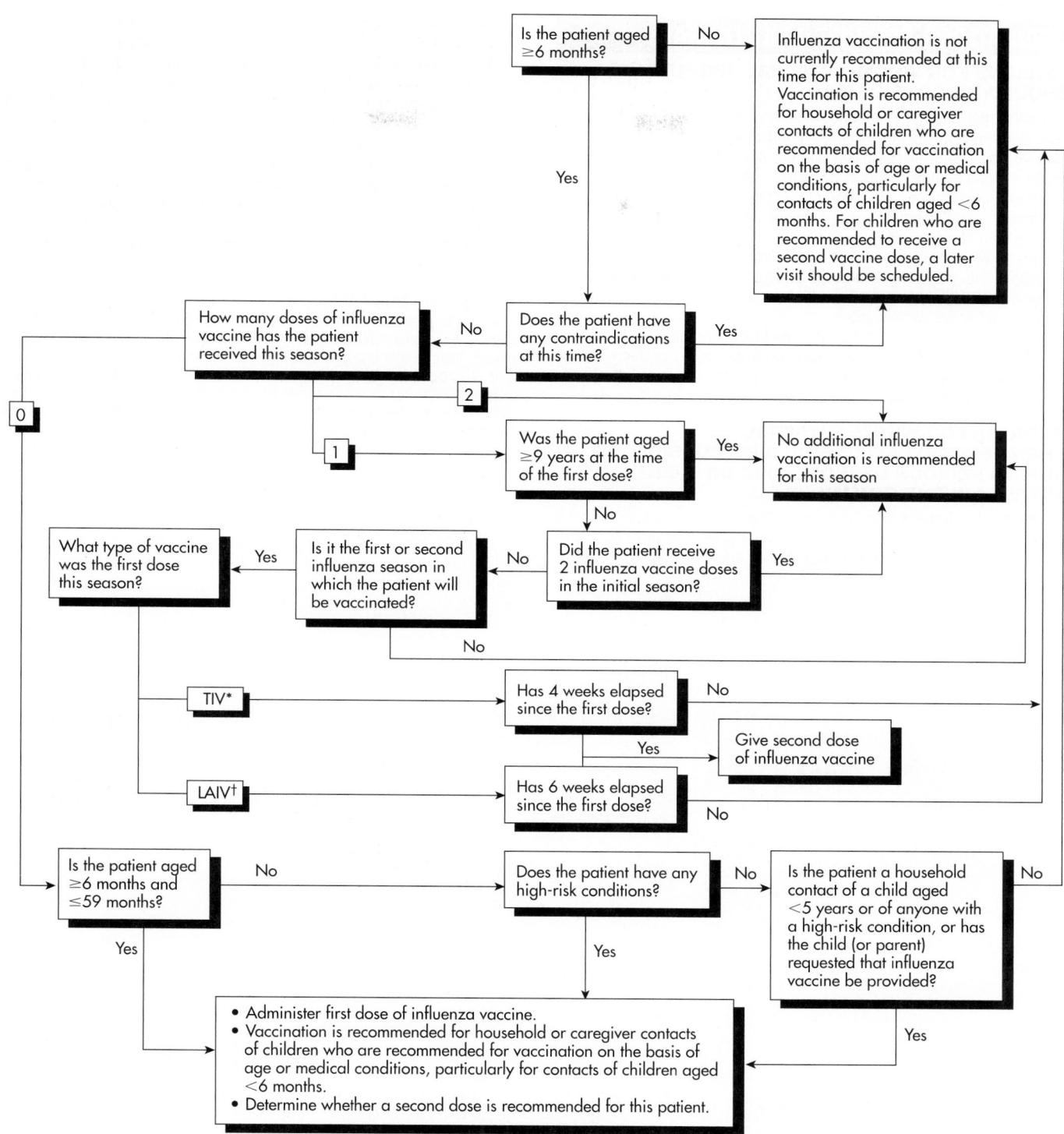

FIGURE 5-6 Algorithm for determining recommended influenza immunization actions for children. (Modified with permission from the American Academy of Pediatrics' Committee on Infectious Diseases: Prevention of influenza: recommendations for influenza immunization of children, 2006-2007, *Pediatrics* 119:846-51.315, 2007.)

*Trivalent inactivated influenza vaccine.
†Live, attenuated influenza vaccine.

HIV Testing and Postexposure Prophylaxis

RECOMMENDATIONS FOR HIV TESTING OF ADULTS, ADOLESCENTS, AND PREGNANT WOMEN

RECOMMENDATIONS FOR ADULTS AND ADOLESCENTS*

The CDC recommends that diagnostic human immunodeficiency virus (HIV) testing and opt-out HIV screening be a part of routine clinical care in all health care settings while also preserving the patient's option to decline HIV testing and ensuring a provider-patient relationship conducive to optimal clinical and preventive care. The recommendations are intended for providers in all health care settings, including hospital emergency departments, urgent-care clinics, inpatient services, sexually transmitted disease (STD) clinics or other venues offering clinical STD services, tuberculosis (TB) clinics, substance abuse treatment clinics, other public health clinics, community clinics, correctional health care facilities, and primary care settings. The guidelines address HIV testing in health care settings only; they do not modify existing guidelines concerning HIV counseling, testing, and referral for persons at high risk for HIV who seek or receive HIV testing in nonclinical settings (e.g., community-based organizations, outreach settings, or mobile vans).

SCREENING FOR HIV INFECTION

- In all health care settings, screening for HIV infection should be performed routinely for all patients aged 13 to 64 years. Health care providers should initiate screening unless prevalence of undiagnosed HIV infection in their patients has been documented to be less than 0.1%. In the absence of existing data for HIV prevalence, health care providers should initiate voluntary HIV screening until they establish that the diagnostic yield is less than 1 per 1000 patients screened, at which point such screening is no longer warranted.
- All patients initiating treatment for TB should be screened routinely for HIV infection.
- All patients seeking treatment for STDs, including all patients visiting STD clinics, should be screened routinely for HIV during each visit for a new complaint, regardless of whether the patient is known or suspected to have specific behavior risks for HIV infection.

REPEAT SCREENING

- Health care providers should subsequently test all persons likely to be at high risk for HIV at least annually. Persons likely to be at high risk include users of injection drugs and their sex partners, persons who exchange sex for money or drugs, sex partners of persons who are HIV infected, and men who have sex with men (MSM) or heterosexual persons who themselves or whose sex partners have had more than one sex partner since their most recent HIV test.
- Health care providers should encourage patients and their prospective sex partners to be tested before initiating a new sexual relationship.
- Repeat screening of persons not likely to be at high risk for HIV should be performed on the basis of clinical judgment.
- Unless recent HIV test results are immediately available, any person whose blood or body fluid is the source of an occupational exposure for a health care provider should be informed of the incident and tested for HIV infection at the time the exposure occurs.

CONSENT AND PRETEST INFORMATION

- Screening should be voluntary and undertaken only with the patient's knowledge and understanding that HIV testing is planned.
- Patients should be informed orally or in writing that HIV testing will be performed unless they decline (opt-out screening). Oral or written information should include an explanation of HIV infection and the meanings of positive and negative test results, and the patient should be offered an opportunity to ask questions and decline testing. With such notification, consent for HIV screening should be incorporated into the patient's

*Data from *MMWR* 57(RR-10), 2008.

general informed consent for medical care on the same basis as are other screening or diagnostic tests; a separate consent form for HIV testing is not recommended.
- Easily understood informational materials should be made available in the languages of the commonly encountered populations within the service area. The competence of interpreters and bilingual staff to provide language assistance to patients with limited English proficiency must be ensured.
- If a patient declines an HIV test, this decision should be documented in the medical record.

DIAGNOSTIC TESTING FOR HIV INFECTION

- All patients with signs or symptoms consistent with HIV infection or an opportunistic illness characteristic of acquired immunodeficiency syndrome (AIDS) should be tested for HIV.
- Clinicians should maintain a high level of suspicion for acute HIV infection in all patients who have a compatible clinical syndrome and who report recent high-risk behavior. When acute retroviral syndrome is a possibility, a plasma RNA test should be used in conjunction with an HIV antibody test to diagnose acute HIV infection.
- Patients or persons responsible for the patient's care should be notified orally that testing is planned, advised of the indication for testing and the implications of positive and negative test results, and offered an opportunity to ask questions and decline testing. With such notification, the patient's general consent for medical care is considered sufficient for diagnostic HIV testing.

HIV SCREENING FOR PREGNANT WOMEN AND THEIR INFANTS*

UNIVERSAL OPT-OUT SCREENING

- All pregnant women in the United States should be screened for HIV infection.
- Screening should occur after a woman is notified that HIV screening is recommended for all pregnant patients and that she will receive an HIV test as part of the routine panel of prenatal tests unless she declines (opt-out screening).
- HIV testing must be voluntary and free from coercion. No woman should be tested without her knowledge.
- Pregnant women should receive oral or written information that includes an explanation of HIV infection, a description of interventions that can reduce HIV transmission from mother to infant, and the meanings of positive and negative test results. They should be offered an opportunity to ask questions and decline testing.
- No additional process or written documentation of informed consent beyond what is required for other routine prenatal tests should be required for HIV testing.
- If a patient declines an HIV test, this decision should be documented in the medical record.

ADDRESSING REASONS FOR DECLINING TESTING

- Providers should discuss and address reasons for declining an HIV test (e.g., lack of perceived risk, fear of the disease, and concerns regarding partner violence or potential stigma or discrimination).
- Women who decline an HIV test because they have had a previous negative test result should be informed of the importance of retesting during each pregnancy.
- Logistical reasons for not testing (e.g., scheduling) should be resolved.
- Certain women who initially decline an HIV test might accept at a later date, especially if their concerns are discussed. Certain women will continue to decline testing, and their decisions should be respected and documented in the medical record.

TIMING OF HIV TESTING

- To promote informed and timely therapeutic decisions, health care providers should test women for HIV as early as possible during each pregnancy. Women who decline the test early in prenatal care should be encouraged to be tested at a subsequent visit.

- A second HIV test during the third trimester, preferably less than 36 weeks of gestation, is cost effective even in areas of low HIV prevalence and may be considered for all pregnant women. A second HIV test during the third trimester is recommended for women who meet one or more of the following criteria:
  - Women who receive health care in jurisdictions with elevated incidence of HIV or AIDS among women aged 15 to 45 years. In 2004, these jurisdictions included Alabama, Connecticut, Delaware, the District of Columbia, Florida, Georgia, Illinois, Louisiana, Maryland, Massachusetts, Mississippi, Nevada, New Jersey, New York, North Carolina, Pennsylvania, Puerto Rico, Rhode Island, South Carolina, Tennessee, Texas, and Virginia.[†]
  - Women who receive health care in facilities in which prenatal screening identifies at least one pregnant woman who is infected with HIV per 1000 women screened.
  - Women who are known to be at high risk for acquiring HIV (e.g., users of injection drugs and their sex partners, women who exchange sex for money or drugs, women who are sex partners of persons who are infected with HIV, and women who have had a new or more than one sex partner during this pregnancy).
  - Women who have signs or symptoms consistent with acute HIV infection. When acute retroviral syndrome is a possibility, a plasma RNA test should be used in conjunction with an HIV antibody test to diagnose acute HIV infection.

[†]A second HIV test in the third trimester is as cost effective as other common health interventions when HIV incidence among women of childbearing age is ≥17 HIV cases per 100,000 person-years. In 2004, in jurisdictions with available data on HIV case rates, a rate of 17 new HIV diagnoses per year per 100,000 women aged 15 to 45 years was associated with an AIDS case rate of at least nine AIDS diagnoses per year per 100,000 women aged 15 to 45 years (CDC, unpublished data, 2005). As of 2004, the jurisdictions listed above exceeded these thresholds. The list of specific jurisdictions where a second test in the third trimester is recommended will be updated periodically based on surveillance data.

RAPID TESTING DURING LABOR

- Any woman with undocumented HIV status at the time of labor should be screened with a rapid HIV test unless she declines (opt-out screening).
- Reasons for declining a rapid test should be explored (see "Addressing Reasons for Declining Testing").
- Immediate initiation of appropriate antiretroviral prophylaxis should be recommended to women on the basis of a reactive rapid test result without waiting for the result of a confirmatory test.

POSTPARTUM/NEWBORN TESTING

- When a woman's HIV status is still unknown at the time of delivery, she should be screened immediately postpartum with a rapid HIV test unless she declines (opt-out screening).
- When the mother's HIV status is unknown postpartum, rapid testing of the newborn as soon as possible after birth is recommended so that antiretroviral prophylaxis can be offered to infants exposed to HIV. Women should be informed that identifying HIV antibodies in the newborn indicates that the mother is infected.
- For infants whose HIV exposure status is unknown and who are in foster care, the person legally authorized to provide consent should be informed that rapid HIV testing is recommended for infants whose biologic mothers have not been tested.
- The benefits of neonatal antiretroviral prophylaxis are best realized when it is initiated within 12 hours after birth.

CONFIRMATORY TESTING

- Whenever possible, uncertainties regarding laboratory test results indicating HIV infection status should be resolved before final decisions are made regarding reproductive options, antiretroviral therapy, cesarean delivery, or other interventions.
- If the confirmatory test result is not available before delivery, immediate initiation of appropriate antiretroviral prophylaxis should be recommended to any pregnant patient whose HIV screening test result is reactive to reduce the risk for perinatal transmission.

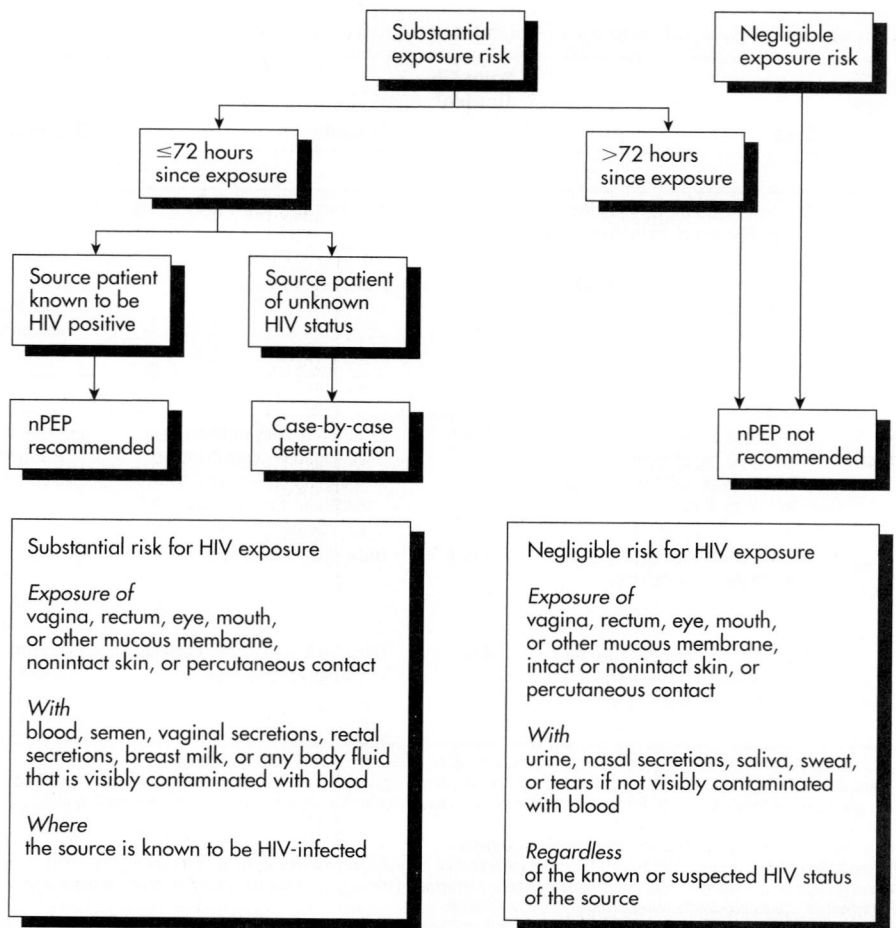

FIGURE 5-7 Algorithm for evaluation and treatment of possible nonoccupational HIV exposure. *nPEP,* Nonoccupational postexposure prophylaxis. (Modified from *MMWR* 54[RR-2], 2005.)

TABLE 5-32 HIV Exposure, Estimated Per-Act Risk

Exposure Route	Risk per 10,000 Exposures to an Infected Source
Blood transfusion	9000
Needle-sharing injection drug use	67
Receptive anal intercourse	50
Percutaneous needle stick	30
Receptive penile-vaginal intercourse	10
Insertive anal intercourse	6.5
Insertive penile-vaginal intercourse	5
Receptive oral intercourse	1
Insertive oral intercourse	0.5

Modified from *MMWR* 54(RR-2), 2005.
Estimates of risk for transmission from sexual exposures assume no condom use.
Source refers to oral intercourse performed on a man.

TABLE 5-33 Regimens for 28-Day Postexposure Prophylaxis for HIV Infection*

Regimen	Dose	Daily Pill Burden[†] no.	Advantages	Disadvantages
Two-Drug Regimens				
Tenofovir–emtricitabine (Truvada)[‡]	One tablet (300 mg of tenofovir with 200 mg of emtricitabine) once daily	1	Well-tolerated; once-daily dosing	Potential nephrotoxicity
Zidovudine–lamivudine (Combivir)[§]	One tablet (300 mg of zidovudine with 150 mg of lamivudine) twice daily	2	Preferred in pregnancy	Twice-daily dosing; less well-tolerated than tenofovir–emtricitabine (nausea, asthenia, neutropenia, anemia, abnormal liver-enzyme levels)
Three-Drug Regimens[¶]				
Ritonavir–lopinavir (Kaletra) (plus either tenofovir–emtricitabine or zidovudine–lamivudine)	Two tablets (50 mg of ritonavir with 200 mg of lopinavir per tablet) twice daily, or four tablets once daily	5 or 6	Either once-daily or twice-daily dosing; one copayment; no refrigeration required; most experience in pregnancy; high genetic barrier to resistance	Gastrointestinal side effects such as diarrhea; may cause elevated liver-enzyme levels or hepatitis
Ritonavir plus atazanavir (plus either tenofovir–emtricitabine or zidovudine–lamivudine)	100 mg of ritonavir plus 300 mg of atazanavir once daily	3 or 4	Once-daily dosing; well tolerated	Ritonavir must be refrigerated; potential for asymptomatic jaundice, renal stones; may cause elevated liver-enzyme levels or hepatitis
Ritonavir plus darunavir (plus either tenofovir–emtricitabine or zidovudine–lamivudine)	100 mg of ritonavir plus two tablets, each containing 400 mg of darunavir, once daily	4 or 5	Once-daily dosing; high genetic barrier to resistance	Ritonavir must be refrigerated; gastrointestinal side effects; may cause elevated liver-enzyme levels or hepatitis

From Landovitz RJ, Currier JS: Postexposure prophylaxis for HIV infection, *N Engl J Med* 361:1768-75, 2009.

*Tenofovir, emtricitabine, and lamivudine all have activity against hepatitis B. Patients with chronic active hepatitis B (i.e., patients who are positive for hepatitis B surface antigen) may have flares of hepatitis on withdrawal of these agents at the completion of postexposure prophylaxis treatment. Referral to a hepatitis specialist or serial monthly monitoring of liver-enzyme levels for up to 6 months after treatment should be considered.

[†]The daily pill burden in the three-drug regimens depends on which two-drug regimen is chosen.

[‡]The dose of tenofovir–emtricitabine should be reduced to one tablet every 48 hours in patients with a creatinine clearance of 30 to 49 ml per minute. Tenofovir–emtricitabine is not recommended in patients with a creatinine clearance of less than 30 ml per minute or in patients who are undergoing hemodialysis; see the guidelines from the Department of Health and Human Services for considerations regarding doses of individual agents in patients with advanced renal dysfunction.

[§]Zidovudine–lamivudine is not recommended in patients with a creatinine clearance of less than 50 ml per minute; see the guidelines from the Department of Health and Human Services for considerations regarding doses of individual agents in patients with renal dysfunction.

[¶]The boosting agent ritonavir is not considered to be an active drug in tabulating the number of agents in the three-drug regimen.

TABLE 5-34 Antiretroviral Therapy Medications, Adult Dosage, and Side Effects

Medication	Adult Dosage*	Side Effects and Toxicities
Combination Tablets		
Lopinavir/ritonavir (Kaletra)‡	3 tablets twice daily 400 mg lopinavir/100 mg ritonavir	Diarrhea, nausea, vomiting; asthenia; elevated transaminases; hyperglycemia; fat redistribution; lipid abnormalities; possible increased bleeding in persons with hemophilia; pancreatitis
Zidovudine/lamivudine (Combivir)	1 tablet twice daily 300 mg zidovudine/150 mg lamivudine	See following individual medications
Zidovudine/lamivudine/abacavir (Trizivir)	1 tablet twice daily 300 mg zidovudine/150 mg lamivudine/ 300 mg abacavir	See following individual medications
Lamivudine/abacavir (Epzicom)	1 tablet once daily 300 mg lamivudine/600 mg abacavir	See following individual medications
Emtricitabine/tenofovir (Truvada)	1 tablet once daily 200 mg emtricitabine/300 mg tenofovir	See following individual medications
Single Agents		
Nucleoside and nucleotide reverse transcriptase inhibitors (side effects as a class: lactic acidosis, severe hepatomegaly with steatosis, including some fatal cases)		
Abacavir (Ziagen, ABC)‡	300 mg twice daily or 600 mg once daily	Severe hypersensitivity reaction (can be fatal); nausea; vomiting
Didanosine (Videx, ddI)‡	>60 kg (132 lb) body weight: 200 mg twice daily or 400 mg daily; if with tenofovir, 250 mg/daily <60 kg (132 lb): 125 mg twice daily or 250 mg daily; if with tenofovir, dose not established Do not use with stavudine (d4T, Zerit) during pregnancy; avoid ddI/d4T combination in general because of increased risk for adverse events (e.g., neuropathy, pancreatitis, and hyperlactatemia)	Pancreatitis; nausea, diarrhea; peripheral neuropathy
Emtricitabine (Emtriva, FTC)	200 mg once daily	Minimal toxicity; lactic acidosis and hepatic steatosis a rare but possibly life-threatening event
Lamivudine (Epivir, 3TC)‡	150 mg twice daily or 300 mg once daily	Minimal toxicity; lactic acidosis and hepatic steatosis a rare but possibly life-threatening event
Stavudine (Zerit, d4T)‡	>60 kg (132 lb) body weight: 40 mg twice daily <60 kg (132 lb) body weight: 30 mg twice daily Do not use with didanosine (ddI, Videx) during pregnancy; avoid ddI/d4T combination in general because of increased risk of adverse events (e.g., neuropathy, pancreatitis, and hyperlactatemia)	Pancreatitis; peripheral neuropathy; rapidly progressive ascending neuromuscular weakness (rare)
Tenofovir (Viread)	300 mg daily	Nausea, vomiting, diarrhea; headache; asthenia; flatulence; renal impairment
Zidovudine (Retrovir, AZT)‡	200 mg three times daily or 300 mg twice daily	Bone marrow suppression (anemia, neutropenia); gastrointestinal intolerance; headache; insomnia; asthenia; and myopathy
Nonnucleoside reverse transcriptase inhibitors (side effects as a class: Stevens-Johnson syndrome)		
Efavirenz (Sustiva)	600 mg daily at bedtime	Rash; central nervous system symptoms (e.g., dizziness, impaired concentration, insomnia, and abnormal dreams); transaminase elevation; false-positive cannabinoid test
Protease inhibitors (side effects as a class: gastrointestinal intolerance, hyperlipidemia, hyperglycemia, diabetes, fat redistribution, and possible increased bleeding in hemophiliacs; do not use during known or possible pregnancy)		
Atazanavir (Reyataz)	400 mg once daily; if administered with tenofovir plus ritonavir, 300 mg once daily	Indirect hyperbilirubinemia; prolonged PR interval (use caution in patients with underlying cardiac conduction defects or on concomitant medications that can cause PR prolongation)
Fosamprenavir (Lexiva)‡	1400 mg twice daily	Gastrointestinal intolerance, nausea, vomiting, diarrhea; rash; elevated transaminases; headache
Indinavir (Crixivan)	800 mg q8h With ritonavir (might increase risk for renal adverse events): 800 mg indinavir and 100 mg ritonavir q12h or 800 mg indinavir and 200 mg ritonavir every q12h	Gastrointestinal intolerance, nausea; nephrolithiasis; headache; asthenia; blurred vision; metallic taste; thrombocytopenia; hemolytic anemia; indirect hyperbilirubinemia (inconsequential)
Nelfinavir (Viracept)‡	750 mg three times daily or one 250 mg twice daily	Diarrhea; elevated transaminases
Ritonavir (Norvir)‡	See doses used in combination with other specific protease inhibitors	Gastrointestinal intolerance; nausea, vomiting, diarrhea; paresthesias; hepatitis; pancreatitis; asthenia; taste perversion; many drug interactions
Saquinavir (hard-gel capsule) (Invirase)	With ritonavir: 400 mg saquinavir and 400 mg ritonavir twice daily or 1000 mg saquinavir and 100 mg ritonavir twice daily	Gastrointestinal intolerance; nausea, diarrhea; headache; elevated transaminases
Saquinavir (soft-gel capsule) (Fortavase)	With ritonavir: 400 mg saquinavir and 400 mg ritonavir twice daily or 1000 mg saquinavir and 100 mg ritonavir twice daily	Gastrointestinal intolerance; nausea, diarrhea; abdominal pain; dyspepsia; headache; elevated transaminases

*For pediatric dosing information, see *Guidelines for use of antiretroviral agents in pediatric HIV infection.* Available at http://www.aidsinfo.nih.gov/guidelines/default_db2.asp?id=51.
‡Pediatric formulation available.
Sources: Modified from U.S. Department of Health and Human Services and the Henry J. Kaiser Family Foundation: *Guidelines for the use of antiretroviral agents in HIV-infected adults and adolescents.* Available at http://www.aidsinfo.nih.gov/guidelines/default_db2.asp?id=50 (refer to website for updated versions); Bartlett JG, Finkbeiner AK: HIV drugs: the guide to living with HIV infection, 2001. Available at http://www.thebody.com/jh/bartlett/drugs.html.

TABLE 5-35 Laboratory Tests Generally Recommended for Persons after Exposure to HIV*

Test	RECOMMENDED DURING TREATMENT		RECOMMENDED AT FOLLOW-UP		
	Baseline	Symptom-Directed†	4-6 wk	12 wk	24 wk
ELISA for HIV antibodies	Yes	Yes	Yes	Yes	Yes
Creatinine, liver function, and complete blood count with differential count	Yes	Yes	No	No	No
HIV viral load	No	Yes	No	No	No
Anti-HBs antibodies	Yes‡	No	No	No	No
HBsAg	Yes‡§	No	No	No	No
HCV antibodies	Yes	No	Yes	Yes	Yes
HCV RNA¶	No	Yes	Yes	Yes	Yes
Screening, including rapid plasma reagin test, for other sexually transmitted infections‖	Yes	Yes	No	Yes	No

From Landovitz RJ, Currier JS: Postexposure prophylaxis for HIV infection, *N Engl J Med* 361:1768-1775, 2009.
Anti-HBs antibodies, Hepatitis B virus surface antibodies; *ELISA,* enzyme-linked immunosorbent assay; *HBsAg,* hepatitis B surface antigen; *HCV,* hepatitis C virus.
*Patients who receive zidovudine plus lamivudine–based regimens should have a complete blood count and measurement of liver-enzyme levels at 2 weeks of treatment, irrespective of the presence or absence of clinical symptoms. Tenofovir plus emtricitabine–based regimens generally involve few side effects, and symptom-directed assessment of serum creatinine or liver-enzyme levels should be considered. The addition of a ritonavir-boosted protease inhibitor should be followed by symptom-directed assessment of liver-enzyme levels, serum glucose levels, or both.
†Symptom-directed tests are for signs or symptoms of toxic effects (rash, nausea, vomiting, or abdominal pain) or HIV seroconversion (fever, fatigue, lymphadenopathy, rash, or oral or genital ulcers).
‡If tests for anti-HBs antibodies and HBsAg are both negative, a vaccination series against HBV infection should be initiated and completed.
§If the patient is HBsAg-positive, he or she should have monthly follow-up of liver function tests after discontinuation of postexposure prophylactic regimens containing tenofovir, lamivudine, or emtricitabine; referral to a specialist in viral hepatitis should be considered.
¶HCV RNA testing may identify early HCV seroconversion; early detection and treatment during acute HCV infection may avert or ameliorate chronic disease. Data are from Dienstag and McHutchison.
‖Rapid plasma reagin testing and testing of urethral-swab and rectal-swab specimens for gonorrhea and chlamydia and of pharyngeal-swab specimens for gonorrhea should be performed as appropriate, according to the patient's sexual risk-taking behaviors and the type of exposure to HIV.

BOX 5-4 Situations for Which Expert Consultation for HIV Postexposure Prophylaxis Is Advised*

- Delayed (i.e., later than 24-36 hours) exposure report
  - The interval after which there is no benefit from postexposure prophylaxis (PEP) is undefined
- Unknown source (e.g., needle in sharps disposal container or laundry)
  - Decide use of PEP on a case-by-case basis
  - Consider the severity of the exposure and the epidemiologic likelihood of HIV exposure
  - Do not test needles or other sharp instruments for HIV
- Known or suspected pregnancy in the exposed person
  - Does not preclude the use of optimal PEP regimens
  - Do not deny PEP solely on the basis of pregnancy
- Resistance of the source virus to antiretroviral agents
  - Influence of drug resistance on transmission risk is unknown
  - Selection of drugs to which the source person's virus is unlikely to be resistant is recommended if the source person's virus is known or suspected to be resistant to one or more of the drugs considered for the PEP regimen
  - Resistance testing of the source person's virus at the time of the exposure is not recommended
- Toxicity of the initial PEP regimen
  - Adverse symptoms such as nausea and diarrhea are common with PEP
  - Symptoms often can be managed without changing the PEP regimen by prescribing antimotility and/or antiemetic agents
  - Modification of dose intervals (i.e., administering a lower dose of drug more frequently throughout the day, as recommended by the manufacturer) in other situations might help alleviate symptoms

*Local experts and/or the National Clinicians' Postexposure Prophylaxis Hotline (PEPline [888-448-4911]).

BOX 5-5   Occupational Exposure Management Resources

National Clinicians' Postexposure Prophylaxis Hotline (PEPline)
Run by University of California–San Francisco/San Francisco General Hospital staff; supported by the Health Resources and Services Administration, Ryan White CARE Act, HIV/AIDS Bureau, AIDS Education and Training Centers, and CDC

Phone: 888-448-4911
Internet: http://www.ucsf.edu/hivcntr

Needlestick!
A website to help clinicians manage and document occupational blood and body fluid exposures. Developed and maintained by the University of California, Los Angeles (UCLA), Emergency Medicine Center, UCLA School of Medicine, and funded in part by CDC and the Agency for Healthcare Research and Quality

Internet: http://www.needlestick.mednet.ucla.edu

Hepatitis Hotline

Phone: 888-443-7232
Internet: http://www.cdc.gov/ncidod/diseases/hepatitis/index.htm

Reporting to CDC: Occupationally acquired HIV infections and failures of PEP

Phone: 800-893-0485

HIV Antiretroviral Pregnancy Registry

Phone: 800-258-4263
Fax: 800-800-1052
Address: 1410 Commonwealth Dr., Suite 215, Wilmington, NC 28405
Internet: http://www.glaxowellcome.com/preg_reg/antiretroviral

Food and Drug Administration
Report unusual or severe toxicity to antiretroviral agents

Phone: 800-332-1088
Address: MedWatch, HF-2, FDA, 5600 Fishers Lane, Rockville, MD 20857
Internet: http://www.fda.gov/medwatch

HIV/AIDS Treatment Information Service

Internet: http://www.hivatis.org

BOX 5-6   Management of Occupational Blood Exposures

Provide Immediate Care to the Exposure Site
- Wash wounds and skin with soap and water
- Flush mucous membranes with water

Determine Risk Associated with Exposure
- Type of fluid (e.g., blood, visibly bloody fluid, other potentially infectious fluid or tissue, and concentrated virus)
- Type of exposure (e.g., percutaneous injury, mucous membrane or nonintact skin exposure, and bites resulting in blood exposure)

Evaluate Exposure Source
- Assess the risk of infection using available information
- Test known sources for HBsAg, anti-HCV, and HIV antibodies (consider using rapid testing)
- For unknown sources, assess risk of exposure to HBV, HCV, or HIV infection
- Do not test discarded needles or syringes for virus contamination

Evaluate the Exposed Person
- Assess immune status for HBV infection (i.e., by history of hepatitis B vaccination and vaccine response)

Give PEP for Exposures Posing Risk of Infection Transmission
- HBV: See Table 5-27
- HCV: PEP not recommended
- HIV: See Tables 5-33, 5-34, and 5-35 and Figure 5-7
  - Initiate PEP as soon as possible, preferably within hours of exposure
  - Offer pregnancy testing to all women of childbearing age not known to be pregnant
  - Seek expert consultation if viral resistance is suspected
  - Administer PEP for 4 weeks if tolerated

Perform Follow-up Testing and Provide Counseling
- Advise exposed persons to seek medical evaluation for any acute illness occurring during follow-up

HBV Exposures
- Perform follow-up anti-HBs testing in persons who receive hepatitis B vaccine
  - Test for anti-HBs 1 to 2 months after last dose of vaccine
  - Anti-HBs response to vaccine cannot be ascertained if HBIG was received in the previous 3 to 4 months

HCV Exposures
- Perform baseline and follow-up testing for anti-HCV and alanine aminotransferase 4 to 6 months after exposures
- Perform HCV RNA at 4 to 6 weeks if earlier diagnosis of HCV infection desired
- Confirm repeatedly reactive anti-HCV enzyme immunoassays with supplemental tests

HIV Exposures
- Perform HIV-antibody testing for at least 6 months after exposure (e.g., at baseline, 6 weeks, 3 months, and 6 months)
- Perform HIV-antibody testing if illness compatible with an acute retroviral syndrome occurs
- Advise exposed persons to use precautions to prevent secondary transmission during the follow-up period
- Evaluate exposed persons taking PEP within 72 hr after exposure and monitor for drug toxicity for at least 2 weeks

HBIG, Hepatitis B immune globulin; *HBsAg,* hepatitis B surface antigen; *HBV,* hepatitis B virus; *HCV,* hepatitis C virus; *HIV,* human immunodeficiency virus; *PEP,* post-exposure prophylaxis; *RNA,* ribonucleic acid.

Endocarditis Prophylaxis*

TABLE 5-36 Cardiac Conditions Associated with the Highest Risk of Adverse Outcome from Endocarditis for Which Prophylaxis with Dental Procedures Is Recommended

Prosthetic cardiac valve
Previous infective endocarditis
CHD*
Unrepaired cyanotic CHD, including palliative shunts and conduits
Completely repaired congenital heart defect with prosthetic material or device, whether placed by surgery or by catheter intervention, during the first 6 mo after the procedure†
Repaired CHD with residual defects at the site or adjacent to the site of a prosthetic patch or prosthetic device (that inhibit endothelialization)
Cardiac transplant recipients who develop cardiac valvulopathy

CHD, Congenital heart disease.
*Except for the conditions listed above, antibiotic prophylaxis is no longer recommended for any other form of CHD.
†Prophylaxis is recommended because endothelialization of prosthetic material occurs within 6 mo after the procedure.

TABLE 5-37 Dental Procedures for Which Endocarditis Prophylaxis Is Recommended for Patients in Table 5-36

All dental procedures that involve manipulation of gingival tissue or the periapical region of teeth or perforation of the oral mucosa*

*The following procedures and events do not need prophylaxis: routine anesthetic injections through noninfected tissue, taking dental radiographs, placement of removable prosthodontic or orthodontic appliances, adjustment of orthodontic appliances, placement of orthodontic brackets, shedding of deciduous teeth, and bleeding from trauma to the lips or oral mucosa.

TABLE 5-38 Regimens for a Dental Procedure

| Situation | REGIMEN: SINGLE DOSE 30-60 MIN BEFORE PROCEDURE | | |
	Agent	Adults	Children
Oral	Amoxicillin	2 g	50 mg/kg
Unable to take oral medication	Ampicillin OR	2 g IM or IV	50 mg/kg IM or IV
	Cefazolin or ceftriaxone*	1 g IM or IV	50 mg/kg IM or IV
Allergic to penicillins or ampicillin, oral	Cephalexin*† OR	2 g	50 mg/kg
	Clindamycin OR	600 mg	20 mg/kg
	Azithromycin or clarithromycin	500 mg	15 mg/kg
Allergic to penicillins or ampicillin and unable to take oral medicine	Cefazolin or ceftriaxone† OR	1 g IM or IV	50 mg/kg IM or IV
	Clindamycin	600 mg IM or IV	20 mg/kg IM or IV

IM, Intramuscular; *IV*, intravenous.
*Or other first-generation or second-generation oral cephalosporin in equivalent adult or pediatric dosage.
†Cephalosporins should not be used in an individual with a history of anaphylaxis, angioedema, or urticaria with penicillins or ampicillin.

*From Prevention of infective endocarditis. A guideline from the American Heart Association Rheumatic Fever, Endocarditis, and Kawasaki Disease Committee, Council on Cardiovascular Disease in the Young, and the Council on Clinical Cardiology, Council on Cardiovascular Surgery and Anesthesia, and the Quality of Care and Outcomes Research Interdisciplinary Working Group. *Circulation* published online Apr 19, 2007, DOI: 10.1161/CIRCULATIONAHA.106.183095. Copyright © 2007 American Heart Association. All rights reserved. Print ISSN: 0009-7322. Online ISSN: 1524-4539.

TABLE 5-39 Summary of Major Changes in Updated Recommendations

We concluded that bacteremia resulting from daily activities is much more likely to cause IE than bacteremia associated with a dental procedure.

We concluded that only an extremely small number of cases of IE might be prevented by antibiotic prophylaxis even if prophylaxis is 100% effective.

Antibiotic prophylaxis is not recommended based solely on an increased lifetime risk of acquisition of IE.

Limit recommendations for IE prophylaxis only to those conditions listed in Table 5-36.

Antibiotic prophylaxis is no longer recommended for any other form of CHD, except for the conditions listed in Table 5-36.

Antibiotic prophylaxis is recommended for all dental procedures that involve manipulation of gingival tissues or periapical region of teeth or perforation of oral mucosa only for patients with underlying cardiac conditions associated with the highest risk of adverse outcome from IE (see Table 5-36).

Antibiotic prophylaxis is recommended for procedures on respiratory tract or infected skin, skin structures, or musculoskeletal tissue only for patients with underlying cardiac conditions associated with the highest risk of adverse outcome from IE (see Table 5-36).

Antibiotic prophylaxis solely to prevent IE is not recommended for GU or GI tract procedures.

The writing group reaffirms the procedures noted in the 1997 prophylaxis guidelines for which endocarditis prophylaxis is not recommended and extends this to other common procedures, including ear and body piercing, tattooing, and vaginal delivery and hysterectomy.

A guide to the clinical preventive services described is available online at http://www.ahrq.gov/clinic/pocketgd07/.

CHD, Congenital heart disease; *GI,* gastrointestinal; *GU,* genitourinary; *IE,* infective endocarditis.

I. Complementary and Alternative Medicine

II. Nutrition

III. Acute Poisoning

IV. Primary Care Procedures (available online)

V. Patient Teaching Guides (available online)

APPENDIX

I. Complementary and Alternative Medicine

II. Nutrition

III. Acute Poisoning

IV. Primary Care Procedures (available online)

V. Patient Teaching Guides (available online)

Definitions of Complementary and Alternative Medicine Terms

Acupuncture Thin needles are inserted superficially on the skin at locations throughout the body. These points are located along "channels" of energy. Heat can be applied by burning (moxibustion), electric current (electroacupuncture), or pressure (acupressure). Healing is proposed by the restoration of a balance of energy flow called *Qi.* Another explanation suggests that, possibly, the stimulation activates endorphin receptors.

Alexander Technique A bodywork technique in which rebalancing of "postural sets" (i.e., physical alignment) is taught by mentally focusing on the way correct alignments should look and feel and through verbal and tactile guidance by the practitioner.

Applied Kinesiology A form of treatment that uses nutrition, physical manipulation, vitamins, diets, and exercise to restore and energize the body. Weak muscles are proposed as a source of dysfunctional health.

Aromatherapy A form of herbal medicine that uses various oils from plants. Route of administration can be through absorption in the skin or inhalation. The aromatic biochemical structures of certain herbs are thought to act in areas of the brain related to past experiences and emotions (e.g., limbic system).

Ayurveda A major health system that originated in India and incorporates the body, mind, and spirit to prevent and treat disease. Includes special types of diets, herbs, and minerals.

Biofeedback A mind-body therapy procedure in which sensors are placed on the body to measure muscle tension, heart rate, and sweat responses or neural activity. Information is provided by visual, auditory, or body-muscle cell activation so as to teach either to increase or decrease physiologic activity, which, when reconstituted, is proposed to improve health problems (e.g., pain, anxiety, or high blood pressure). In some cases, relaxation exercises complement this procedure.

Chelation Therapy Involves the removal—through intravenous infusion of a chelating agent (synthetic amino acid ethylenediamine tetraacetic acid [EDTA])—of heavy metals, including lead, nickel, and cadmium, as a way to treat certain diseases. Ancillary treatments include the use of vitamins, changes in diet, and exercise.

Cognitive Therapy Psychological therapy in which the major focus is altering and changing irrational beliefs through a type of Socratic dialogue and self-evaluation of certain illogical thoughts. Conditioning and learning are important components of this therapy.

Craniosacral Therapy A form of gentle manual manipulation used for diagnosis and for making corrections in a system made up of cerebrospinal fluid, cranial and dural membranes, cranial bones, and sacrum. This system is proposed to be dynamic, with its own physiologic frequency. Through touch and pressure, tension is proposed to be reduced and cranial rhythms normalized, leading to improvement in health and disease.

Diathermy The use of high-frequency electrical currents as a form of physical therapy and in surgical procedures. The term *diathermy,* derived from the Greek words *dia* and *therma,* literally means "heating through." The three forms of diathermy used by physical therapists are short wave, ultrasound, and microwave.

Eye Movement Desensitization and Reprocessing (EMDR) A technique that proposes to remove painful memories by behavioral techniques. Rhythmic, multisaccadic eye movements are produced by allowing the patient to track and follow a moving object while imagining a stressful memory or event. By using deconditioning, including verbal interaction with the therapist, the painful memory is extinguished and health improved.

Feldenkrais Method A bodywork technique that integrates physics, judo, and yoga. The practitioner directs sequences of movement using verbal or hands-on techniques or teaches a system of self-directed exercise to treat physical impairments through the learning of new movement patterns.

Hatha Yoga The branch of yoga practice that involves physical exercise, breathing practices, and movement. These exercises are designed to have a salutary effect on posture, flexibility, and strength and are intended ultimately to prepare the body to remain still for long periods of meditation.

Hellerwork A bodywork technique that treats and improves proper body alignment through the development of a more complete awareness of the physical body. The goal is to realign fascia for improvement of standing, sitting, and breathing using "body energy," verbal feedback, and changing emotions and attitudes.

Homeopathy A form of treatment in which substances (minerals, plant extracts, chemicals, or disease-producing germs), which in sufficient doses would produce a set of illness symptoms in healthy individuals, are given in microdoses to produce a "cure" of those same symptoms. The *symptom* is not thought to be part of the illness but part of a curative process.

Hyperbaric Oxygen A therapy in which 100% oxygen is given at or above atmospheric pressure. An increase in oxygen in the tissue is proposed to increase blood circulation and improve healing and health and influence the course of disease.

Jin Shin Jyutsu An ancient bodywork technique to harmonize body, mind, and spirit by gentle touch that uses specific "healing points" at the body surface. The points are proposed to overlie flowing energy (Qi). The therapist's fingers are used to "redirect, balance, and provide a more efficient energy flow" to and throughout the body.

Light Therapy Natural light or light of specified wavelengths is used to treat disease. This may include ultraviolet light, colored light, or low-intensity laser light. Generally, the eye is the initial entry point for the light because of its direct connection to the brain.

Magnetic Therapy Magnets are placed directly on the skin, theoretically stimulating living cells and increasing blood flow by ionic currents that are created from polarities on the magnets.

Modified from Spencer JW: *Complementary/alternative medicine: an evidence-based approach,* St Louis, 1999, Mosby.

Mediterranean Diet   A diet that is thought to provide optimal distribution of daily caloric intake of different nutrients and includes 50% to 60% carbohydrates, 30% fats, and 10% proteins. The diet is derived from the eating habits of people in the Mediterranean area, who were shown to have reduced rates of cardiovascular disease.

Mind-Body Therapies   A group of therapies that emphasize using the mind or brain in conjunction with the body to assist healing. Mind-body therapies can involve varying degrees of levels of consciousness, including *hypnosis,* in which selective attention is used to induce a specific altered state (trance) for memory retrieval, relaxation, or suggestion; *visual imagery,* in which the focus is on a target visual stimulus; *yoga,* which involves integration of posture and controlled breathing, relaxation, and/or meditation; *relaxation,* which includes lighter levels of altered states of consciousness through indirect or direct focus; and *meditation,* in which there is an intentional use of posture, concentration, contemplation, and visualization.

Muscle Energy Technique   A manual therapy in osteopathic medicine that includes both passive mobilization and muscle reeducation. Diagnosis of somatic dysfunction is performed by the practitioner, after which the patient is guided to provide corrective muscle contraction.

Music Therapy   The use of music in an either active or passive mode. Used mainly to reduce stress, anxiety, and pain.

Naturopathy   A major health system that includes practices that emphasize diet, nutrition, homeopathy, acupuncture, herbal medicine, manipulation, and various mind-body therapies. Focal points include self-healing and treatment through changes in lifestyle and emphasis on health prevention.

Ornish Diet   A life-choice program based on eating a vegetarian diet containing less than 10% fat. The diet is high in complex carbohydrates and fiber. Meat and fish are generally avoided.

Oslo Diet   An eating plan that emphasizes increased intake of fish and reduced total fat intake. Diet is combined with regular endurance exercise.

Pilates   An educational and exercise approach using the proper body mechanics, movements, truncal and pelvic stabilization, coordinated breathing, and muscle contractions to promote strengthening. Attention is paid to the entire musculoskeletal system.

Prayer   The use of prayer(s) that are offered to "some higher being" or authority to heal and/or arrest disease. May be practiced by the individual patient, by groups, or by other(s) with or without the patient's knowledge (e.g., intercessory).

Pritikin Diet   A weight management plan that is based on a vegetarian framework. Meals are low in fat, high in fiber, and high in complex carbohydrates.

Qi Gong   A form of Chinese exercise-stimulation therapy that proposes to improve health by redirecting mental focus, breathing, coordination, and relaxation. The goal is to "rebalance" the body's own healing capacities by activating proposed electrical or energetic currents that flow along meridians located throughout the body. These meridians, however, do not follow conventional nerve or muscle pathways. In Chinese medical training and practice this therapy includes "external Qi," which is energy transmitted from one person to another so as to heal.

Raja Yoga   Yoga practice that includes all of the other forms of yoga. The practitioner is instructed to follow moral directives, physical exercises, breathing exercises, meditation, devotion, and service to others to facilitate religious awakening.

Reflexology   A bodywork technique that uses reflex points on the hands and feet. Pressure is applied at points that correspond to various body parts, to eliminate blockages thought to produce pain or disease.

Reiki   Comes from the Japanese word meaning "universal life force energy." The practitioner serves as a conduit for healing energy directed into the body or energy field of the recipient without physical contact with the body.

Rolfing   A bodywork technique that involves the myofascia. The body is realigned by using the hands to apply deep pressure and friction that allow more sufficient posture, movement, and the "release" of emotions from the body.

Shiatsu   A Japanese bodywork technique involving finger pressure at specific points on the body mainly to balance "energy" in the body. The major focus is on prevention by keeping the body healthy. The therapy uses more than 600 points on the skin that are proposed to be connected to pathways through which energy flows.

T'ai Chi   A technique that uses slow, purposeful motor-physical movements of the body to control and achieve a more balanced physiologic and psychological state.

Therapeutic Touch   A body energy field technique in which hands are passed over the body without actually touching to recreate and change proposed "energy imbalances" for restoring innate healing forces. Verbal interaction between patient and therapist helps maximize effects.

Traditional Chinese Medicine   An ancient form of medicine that focuses on prevention and secondarily treats disease with an emphasis on maintaining balance through the body by stimulating a constant, smooth-flowing Qi energy. Herbs, acupuncture, massage, diet, and exercise are also used.

Trager Psychophysical Integration   A bodywork technique in which the practitioner enters a meditative state and guides the client through gentle, light, rhythmic, nonintrusive movements. "Mentastics" exercises using self-healing movements are taught to the clients.

AUTHOR: **ANNE L. HUME, PHARM.D.**

Relaxation Techniques

Relaxation Techniques

Relaxation Technique	Summary	Further Resources
Breathing exercise	This is the foundation of most relaxation techniques. Have patients place one hand on the chest and the other on the abdomen. Instruct them to take a slow, deep breath, as if they were sucking in all the air in the room. While doing this, the hand on the abdomen should rise higher than the hand on the chest. This promotes diaphragmatic breathing that increases alveolar expansion in the bases of the lungs. Have them hold the breath for a count of 7 and then exhale. Exhalation should take twice as long as inhalation. Repeat this for a total of five breaths, and encourage patients to do this three times a day.	*Conscious Breathing* by Gay Hendricks is one of many good resources on using breathing for relaxation and health.
Meditation		
Transcendental/The relaxation response	To prevent distracting thoughts, the subject repeats a mantra (a word or sound) over and over again while sitting in a comfortable position. If a distracting thought comes to mind, it is accepted and let go, with the mind focusing again on the mantra.	www.mindbody.harvard.edu or *The Relaxation Response* by Herbert Benson; www.tm.org for information on transcendental meditation.
Mindful meditation	This represents the philosophy of living in the present or in the moment. The *body scan* is one technique where the subject uses breathing to obtain a relaxed state while lying or sitting. The mind progressively focuses on different parts of the body, where it feels any and all sensations intentionally but nonjudgmentally before moving on to another part of the body. A patient with back pain may focus on the quality and characteristics of the pain as if to better understand it and bring it under control.	*Full Catastrophe Living* by Jon Kabat-Zinn describes this technique in full and the program for stress reduction at the University of Massachusetts Medical Center.
Centering prayer	This is a form similar to transcendental meditation that has a more religious foundation. The subject repeats a "sacred word" similar to a mantra. As thoughts come to mind, they are accepted and let go, clearing the mind to become more centered on the spirit within, as if the mind's preoccupied thoughts are the layers of an onion that are peeled away, allowing better understanding of the spirit at the core.	www.Centeringprayer.com; look under "method of centering prayer" for a nondenominational discussion.
Progressive muscle relaxation (PMR)	A form of relaxation in which the subject is attuned to the difference in feeling when the muscles are tensed and then relaxed. In a comfortable position, start by tensing the whole body from head to toe. While doing this, notice the feelings of tightness. Take a deep breath in and as you let it out, let the tension release and the muscles relax. This is then followed by progressive tension and relaxation throughout the body. One may start by clenching the fists and then tensing the arms, shoulders, chest, abdomen, hips, legs, and so on, with each step followed by relaxation.	www.uaex.edu/publications/pub/fshei28.htm is a good review of PMR as well as other relaxation exercises. It is sponsored by the University of Arkansas. *You Must Relax* is a book by the founder of this technique, Edmund Jacobson.
Visualization/Self-hypnosis	The subject uses visualization to recruit images that create a relaxed state. For example, if a person is anxious, visualizing images of a place and a time that were peaceful and comforting would help induce relaxation. This is best used in conjunction with a breathing exercise.	There are many CDs, MP3s, and DVDs that can guide people through a visualization "script" that can result in relaxation. Emmett Miller is one well-known author.
Autogenic training	This induces a physiologic response by using simple phrases. For example, "My legs are heavy and warm" is meant to increase the blood flow to this area, resulting in relaxation. This is done progressively from head to toe with the use of deep breathing and repetition of the phrase. After completing this, focus attention on any body part that may still be tense, and then focus the breath and phrase to that area until the whole body is relaxed.	The British Autogenic Society at www.autogenictherapy.org.uk is a good resource for more information.

From Rakel RE (ed): *Principles of family practice,* ed 6, Philadelphia, 2002, Saunders.

Continued on following page

Relaxation Techniques—cont'd

Relaxation Technique	Summary	Further Resources
Exercise/Movement		
Aerobic	While performing an aerobic exercise, focus attention on a phrase, sound, word, or prayer and passively disregard other thoughts that may enter the mind. Some may focus on their breathing, saying to themselves, "In" with inhalation and "Out" with exhalation, or repeating "one-two, one-two" with each step they take with jogging. Doing this will help the mind focus, preventing other thoughts that may cause tension.	*Beyond the Relaxation Response* by Herbert Benson includes discussion of his research on inducing the relaxation response while exercising.
Yoga	This has been practiced for thousands of years in India. In America, it has been divided into three aspects: breathing (pranayama yoga), bodily postures or asanas (hatha yoga), and meditation to maintain balance and health. Regular practice induces relaxation.	For the following therapies, it is best to encourage patients to take a class at a local community center or gym and to pick up an introductory book at a library or bookstore.
T'ai chi	An ancient Chinese martial art that uses slow, graceful movements combined with inner mindfulness and breathing techniques to help bring balance between the mind and body.	See above.
Qi gong	A traditional Chinese practice that uses movement, meditation, and controlled breathing to balance the body's vital energy force, Qi.	See above.

Overview of Selected Natural Products

This table includes a few of the common uses and side effects of selected natural products. The evidence supporting the uses and side effects of these products varies considerably and may be based on anecdotal information or theoretical concerns with the natural products.

Natural Products	Common Use(s)	Adverse Effects/Potential Concerns
African plum (Pygeum)	Benign prostatic hyperplasia	Nausea and abdominal pain have been reported, but pygeum is generally well tolerated. Pygeum does not decrease prostate size or influence PSA concentrations.
Andrographis	Prevention and treatment of viral respiratory infections	Headache, fatigue, rash, diarrhea, and vomiting. Products are standardized to 4%-6% andrographolide; this botanical is commonly used in combination products.
Black cohosh	Menopausal symptoms (hot flashes), induction of labor in pregnant women, premenstrual syndrome	Dyspepsia, rash, weight gain, headache, and cramping have been reported. Concern exists that black cohosh causes liver toxicity. The potential development of mild estrogen-like adverse effects, especially endometrial hyperplasia, is of concern.
Butterbur	Prevention of migraine headaches; allergic rhinitis; urinary tract spasms; pain	Diarrhea, stomach upset, fatigue, belching, headache, and drowsiness may occur. Due to concern about hepatotoxicity, butterbur products should be free of pyrrolizidine alkaloids. Products should be standardized to 15% petasin and isopetasin.
Chamomile (German)	Motion sickness, anxiety, insomnia; gastrointestinal spasms; mucositis	Allergic reactions occur on rare occasion. Patients with a ragweed allergy should use chamomile with caution.
Chasteberry	Premenstrual dysphoric disorder, premenstrual syndrome, menopausal symptoms, female infertility, mastalgia	Gastrointestinal upset, headache, rash, acne, weight gain, and menstrual bleeding have been reported.
Chitosan	Weight loss, Crohn's disease, hypercholesterolemia, anemia	Gastrointestinal upset, nausea, flatulence, and constipation have been reported. Patients with a shellfish allergy should avoid the use of chitosan.
Chondroitin sulfate	Osteoarthritis, osteoporosis, hyperlipidemia	Gastrointestinal upset, nausea, diarrhea, constipation, and alopecia. Concern exists that chondroitin may have anticoagulant activity due to its structural similarity to part of heparin.
Cinnamon	Type 2 diabetes mellitus, flatulence, gastrointestinal spasms, anorexia, menopausal symptoms, impotence	Cassia cinnamon is one of three types of cinnamon in commercial food products; this is the only type that may have minor effects to improve blood glucose concentrations.
Coenzyme Q10	Congestive heart failure, angina, dilated cardiomyopathy, statin-induced myopathy, Parkinson's disease, chronic fatigue syndrome, HIV/AIDS	Nausea, vomiting, diarrhea, anorexia, heartburn, and rash have been reported. Coenzyme Q10 is structurally similar to vitamin K; concern exists about potential interaction with warfarin.
Cranberry	Prevention and treatment of urinary tract infections; type 2 diabetes mellitus; chronic fatigue syndrome; pleurisy	Gastrointestinal upset and diarrhea have been reported with large doses of cranberry. Uric acid kidney stone formation is also possible with large doses of cranberry over prolonged periods of time.
Dehydroepiandrosterone (DHEA)	Slow or reverse aging, weight loss, metabolic syndrome, erectile dysfunction, immune stimulant, osteoporosis, systemic lupus erythematosus, multiple sclerosis, depression, schizophrenia	Acne and other androgenic effects commonly occur in women. Alopecia, insulin resistance, hepatic dysfunction, and hypertension have been reported. Ingested wild yam and soy cannot be converted into DHEA by humans.
Devil's claw	Osteoarthritis, atherosclerosis, gout, myalgias, fever, migraines	Diarrhea, nausea, and vomiting, as well as allergic reactions, have been reported.

AIDS, Acquired immune deficiency syndrome; *HIV,* human immunodeficiency virus.

Continued on following page **1557**

Natural Products	Common Use(s)	Adverse Effects/Potential Concerns
Echinacea	Prevention and treatment of viral respiratory infections; urinary tract infections; chronic fatigue syndrome; attention deficit hyperactivity disorder	Nausea, vomiting, diarrhea, heartburn, headaches, dizziness, arthralgias, and allergic reactions have been reported with echinacea. Patients with a ragweed allergy should use echinacea with caution because the risk of allergic reactions may be increased.
Eleuthero (Siberian ginseng)	Maintenance of a normal blood pressure; atherosclerosis; Alzheimer's disease; chronic fatigue syndrome; diabetes; herpes simplex infections	Drowsiness, anxiety, and irritability have been reported.
Evening primrose oil (EPO)	Premenstrual syndrome, mastalgia, osteoporosis, asthma, menopausal symptoms, eczema, chronic fatigue syndrome	EPO is well tolerated.
Fenugreek	Type 2 diabetes mellitus, anorexia, atherosclerosis; also used as galactogogue	Gastrointestinal upset, flatulence, and hypoglycemia are possible side effects. Patients with a peanut allergy (and an allergy to related plants) should use fenugreek with caution. Nursing mothers who use fenugreek may notice a "maple syrup" smell in their sweat and in the urine of their infants. This may be mistaken to be maple syrup urine disease in the infant.
Feverfew	Prevention of migraines; fever; menstrual-related problems; arthritis; infertility; asthma	Gastrointestinal side effects are the most common with feverfew. A "post-feverfew syndrome" has been reported in individuals who have taken feverfew for prolonged periods of time and then have abruptly stopped the herbal.
Fish oil	Hypertriglyceridemia, coronary heart disease, hypertension, asthma, depression, rheumatoid arthritis, osteoporosis, psoriasis	Heartburn, nausea, rash, and a "fishy" aftertaste can occur. Contamination with pesticides (as well as with mercury and other heavy metals) is a potential concern, although this is unlikely.
Garlic	Hyperlipidemia, hypertension, peripheral arterial disease, type 2 diabetes mellitus	Nausea, vomiting, heartburn, and body odor are most common. "Deodorized" garlic products may lack the active ingredient, allicin.
Ginger	Nausea and vomiting secondary to pregnancy, chemotherapy, motion sickness, surgery	Heartburn, belching, and dermatitis have been reported. In overdoses, ginger has been associated with central nervous system depression and arrhythmias. Efficacy for hyperemesis gravidarum is unknown, and use is not recommended.
Ginkgo	Alzheimer's disease, vascular dementias, tinnitus, acute mountain sickness, intermittent claudication	Gastrointestinal side effects, headaches, dizziness, and allergic skin reactions. Seizures have been reported in several case reports. Products should contain 24% ginkgo flavone glycosides and 6% terpenoids.
Ginseng (Panax)	Increased resistance to stress and improved well-being; increased physical stamina; depression; diabetes; erectile dysfunction	Insomnia has been reported with ginseng. Vaginal bleeding, mastalgia, and amenorrhea have also been reported.
Glucosamine sulfate	Osteoarthritis	Nausea, heartburn, skin reactions, and headache have been reported. Increased glucose concentrations have been a concern but have not been well documented. Patients with a shellfish allergy should use glucosamine with caution.
Green tea	Improve cognitive performance; prevention of breast, prostate, and colon cancer; hyperlipidemia; Parkinson's disease; obesity; diabetes; cardiovascular disease	Nausea, vomiting, dyspepsia, dizziness, insomnia, and nervousness have been reported. Side effects may be a result of the large amount of caffeine in green tea products. Hepatotoxicity has been a potential concern with green tea.
Hawthorn	Mild heart failure, angina, arrhythmias, hypertension	Mild gastrointestinal effects, dizziness, rash, palpitations, and nervousness have been reported.
Hoodia	Obesity	Side effects have not been reported. Many products lack the actual ingredient.
Horse chestnut	Chronic venous insufficiency, including varicose veins; benign prostate hyperplasia; diarrhea	Mild nausea, vomiting, dizziness, headache, and itching. Products are standardized to 16%-20% aescin.
Huperzine	Alzheimer's disease, increased alertness and energy, myasthenia gravis, memory enhancement	Nausea, vomiting, diarrhea, sweating, and blurred vision as a result of the cholinergic effects of huperzine have been reported.
Kava	Anxiety, insomnia, restlessness, seizure disorders, depression, chronic fatigue syndrome	Gastrointestinal upset, headache, dizziness, "kava" dermopathy, and allergic skin reactions. Hepatotoxicity is the primary concern with kava; some countries have banned the use of kava.
Melatonin	Jet lag, insomnia, migraine, chronic fatigue syndrome, breast cancer, osteoporosis; also used for insomnia in children with ADHD	Daytime drowsiness, headache, and dizziness have been reported. Vaginal bleeding has occurred in perimenopausal women. Melatonin from animal sources should be avoided.
Melissa	Cold sores (topically), anxiety, insomnia, Alzheimer's disease, hypertension, dyspepsia	Nausea, vomiting, dizziness, and wheezing have occurred with oral melissa.
Methylsulfonylmethane (MSM)	Chronic pain, arthritis, diabetes, osteoporosis, allergies, obesity, premenstrual syndrome	Nausea, bloating, diarrhea, fatigue, and insomnia have been associated with MSM. This substance is used frequently in combination with glucosamine and chondroitin.
Milk thistle	Protective agent against liver damage due to alcohol, acetaminophen, and carbon tetrachloride; hepatitis C	Nausea, abdominal fullness, diarrhea, and allergic reactions. Patients with a ragweed allergy should use milk thistle with caution.
Peppermint	Irritable bowel syndrome, sinusitis, morning sickness, dysmenorrhea	Heartburn has been reported, as well as laryngeal and bronchial spasm in infants and children.

Natural Products	Common Use(s)	Adverse Effects/Potential Concerns
Policosanol	Hyperlipidemia, intermittent claudication, atherosclerosis	Migraines, insomnia, dizziness, skin rash, and bleeding have been reported with policosanol. The product has antiplatelet effects.
Probiotics	Treatment and prevention of diarrhea including antibiotic-associated diarrhea; irritable bowel syndrome; atopic dermatitis; Crohn's disease	Theoretically, probiotic products may increase risk of infections in immunocompromised individuals.
Red clover phytoestrogens	Menopausal symptoms, premenstrual syndrome, asthma	Rash, myalgias, headaches, and vaginal bleeding have been reported. Theoretically, endometrial hyperplasia is an adverse effect from the use of these compounds.
Red yeast rice	Hyperlipidemia, indigestion, diarrhea, circulatory conditions, HIV/AIDS	Gastrointestinal upset and dizziness may occur. Red yeast rice may contain lovastatin-like compounds and potentially cause rhabdomyolysis.
S-adenosylmethionine (SAM-e)	Depression, anxiety, dementia, osteoarthritis, heart disease	Nausea, vomiting, diarrhea, headache, and nervousness have been reported. Concern exists that SAM-e raises homocysteine levels.
St. John's wort	Depression, anxiety, chronic fatigue syndrome, HIV/AIDS	Anxiety, gastrointestinal upset, vaginal bleeding, neuropathy, and rash can occur. Hypomania has been induced by St. John's wort.
Tea tree oil	Topical use for acne, fungal infections, lice, scabies	Local inflammation and contact dermatitis may occur.
Valerian	Insomnia, depression, chronic fatigue syndrome, menstrual cramps	Headaches, gastrointestinal upset, and drowsiness can occur. Hepatotoxicity is a potential concern with valerian.

AUTHOR: **ANNE L. HUME, PHARM.D.**

Natural Products and Drug Interactions

This table lists interactions between selected natural products and prescription and nonprescription drugs. Although many of the listed interactions are theoretical in nature and have not been documented to occur in humans, those involving St. John's wort are potentially life threatening in nature, depending on the individual drug. Other interactions are based on small studies of healthy volunteers and use pharmaceutical-quality natural products that may or may not be commercially available.

Natural Products	Drugs	Interactions
Andrographis	Immune suppressants	Andrographis may stimulate immune function, potentially decreasing the effectiveness of drugs such as cyclosporine, tacrolimus, and prednisone.
	Antihypertensive agents	Andrographis may lower blood pressure, potentiating the hypotensive effects of antihypertensive agents.
	Antiplatelet and anticoagulant agents	Andrographis may have antiplatelet activity, potentially increasing the risk of bleeding.
Black cohosh	Hepatotoxic drugs	Concern exists that the risk of hepatotoxicity with black cohosh is increased in the presence of hepatotoxic drugs such as acetaminophen.
	Cisplatin	Animal studies suggest that the efficacy of cisplatin against breast cancer cells may be decreased by black cohosh.
	CYP2D6 substrates	Black cohosh may modestly inhibit CYP2D6 enzyme activity to result in higher drug concentrations.
Butterbur	CYP3A4 inducers (rifampin, carbamazepine, etc.)	Drugs that induce the activity of CYP3A4 increase the risk of the formation of hepatotoxic metabolites from pyrrolizidine alkaloids from some butterbur products.
Chamomile	CNS depressants (benzodiazepines, opiates, barbiturates, etc.)	Chamomile may have additive CNS depressant effects.
	CYP1A2 substrates	Chamomile may inhibit CYP1A2 enzyme activity to result in higher drug concentrations.
	CYP3A4 substrates	Chamomile may inhibit CYP3A4 enzyme activity to result in higher drug concentrations.
	Estrogens	Chamomile may compete for estrogen receptors.
	Tamoxifen	Chamomile may interfere with the effects of tamoxifen because of its estrogenic effects.
Chaste tree berry	Antipsychotic agents	Chaste tree berry may antagonize the effects of antipsychotic agents through its dopaminergic activity.
	Metoclopramide	Chaste tree berry may antagonize the effects of metoclopramide through its dopaminergic activity.
	Dopamine agonists	Chaste tree berry may possess additive effects to drugs such as levodopa and ropinirole through its dopaminergic activity.
	Oral contraceptives/estrogens	Chaste tree berry may possess additive hormonal effects.
Chondroitin	Warfarin	High-dose chondroitin has structural similarity to a heparinoid and may possess weak anticoagulant effects.
Cinnamon	Hypoglycemic agents	Cinnamon may possess additive effects on blood glucose to those of hypoglycemic agents.
Coenzyme Q10	Antihypertensive agents	Coenzyme Q10 may possess additive effects on blood pressure to those of antihypertensive agents.
	Warfarin	Coenzyme Q10 may lessen the anticoagulant effects of warfarin because of its structural similarity to vitamin K.
	Chemotherapy	The antioxidant effects of coenzyme Q10 may blunt the efficacy of certain chemotherapeutic agents that depend on the formation of free radicals.
Cranberry	CYP2C9 substrates (warfarin)	Cranberry may inhibit CYP2C9 enzyme activity to result in higher drug concentrations; evidence with warfarin is contradictory.
Dehydroepiandrosterone (DHEA)	Tamoxifen and aromatase inhibitors such as anastrozole and exemestane	DHEA may interfere with the antiestrogenic effects of these drugs.
	CYP3A4 substrates	DHEA may slightly inhibit CYP3A4 enzyme activity to result in higher drug concentrations.

AChE, Acetylcholinesterase; *CCBs,* calcium channel blockers; *CNS,* central nervous system; *MAOIs,* monoamine oxidase inhibitor; *PPIs,* proton pump inhibitors; *SSRIs,* selective serotonin reuptake inhibitors.

Continued on following page

Natural Products	Drugs	Interactions
Devil's claw	Antihypertensive agents	Devil's claw may possess additive effects on blood pressure to those of antihypertensive agents.
	Hypoglycemic agents	Devil's claw may possess additive effects on blood glucose to those of hypoglycemic agents.
	H_2 antagonists and PPIs	Devil's claw may raise gastric pH and blunt the efficacy of H_2 antagonists and PPIs.
	CYP3A4 substrates	Devil's claw may inhibit CYP3A4 enzyme activity to result in higher drug concentrations.
	CYP2C9 substrates	Devil's claw may inhibit CYP2C9 enzyme activity to result in higher drug concentrations.
	CYP2C19 substrates	Devil's claw may inhibit CYP2C19 enzyme activity to result in higher drug concentrations.
	Warfarin	Devil's claw may inhibit CYP2C9 enzyme activity to result in higher concentrations of warfarin; purpura has been reported.
Echinacea	Immune suppressants	Echinacea may stimulate immune function, potentially decreasing the effectiveness of drugs such as cyclosporine, tacrolimus, and prednisone.
	CYP3A4 substrates	Echinacea may modestly induce hepatic CYP3A4 enzyme activity to result in lower drug concentrations.
	CYP1A2 substrates	Echinacea may inhibit CYP1A2 enzyme activity to result in higher drug concentrations.
Eleuthero (Siberian ginseng)	CNS depressants (benzodiazepines, opiates, barbiturates, etc.)	Eleuthero may have additive CNS depressant effects.
	Antiplatelet and anticoagulant agents	Eleuthero may have antiplatelet activity, potentially increasing the risk of bleeding.
	CYP3A4 substrates	Eleuthero may inhibit CYP3A4 enzyme activity to result in higher drug concentrations.
	CYP1A2 substrates	Eleuthero may modestly inhibit CYP1A2 enzyme activity to result in higher drug concentrations.
	CYP2C9 substrates	Eleuthero may modestly inhibit CYP2C9 enzyme activity to result in higher drug concentrations.
	CYP2D6 substrates	Eleuthero may inhibit CYP2D6 enzyme activity to result in higher drug concentrations.
	Digoxin	Concentration of digoxin has been reported to increase but without evidence of toxicity.
Evening primrose oil (EPO)	Antiplatelet and anticoagulant agents	EPO may have anticoagulant activity, potentially increasing the risk of bleeding.
Fenugreek	Antiplatelet and anticoagulant agents	Fenugreek may have antiplatelet activity, potentially increasing the risk of bleeding.
	Hypoglycemic agents	Fenugreek may potentially lower blood glucose concentrations and have additive effects with hypoglycemic agents.
Feverfew	Antiplatelet and anticoagulant agents	Feverfew may have antiplatelet activity, potentially increasing the risk of bleeding.
	CYP3A4 substrates	Feverfew may inhibit CYP3A4 enzyme activity to result in higher drug concentrations.
	CYP1A2 substrates	Feverfew may inhibit CYP1A2 enzyme activity to result in higher drug concentrations.
	CYP2C9 substrates	Feverfew may inhibit CYP2C9 enzyme activity to result in higher drug concentrations.
	CYP2C19 substrates	Feverfew may inhibit CYP2C19 enzyme activity to result in higher drug concentrations.
Fish oils (omega-3 fatty acids)	Antiplatelet and anticoagulant agents	Fish oils may have antiplatelet activity, potentially increasing the risk of bleeding, although this has not been documented in humans.
	Antihypertensive agents	Fish oils may possess additive effects on blood pressure to those of antihypertensive agents.
	Oral contraceptives	Oral contraceptives may potentially interfere with the triglyceride-lowering effects of fish oil.
Garlic	Antiplatelet and anticoagulant agents	Garlic may have antiplatelet activity, potentially increasing the risk of bleeding.
	CYP3A4 substrates	Garlic may potentially induce CYP3A4 enzyme activity to result in lower drug concentrations; evidence is contradictory.
	CYP2E1 substrates	Garlic may modestly inhibit CYP2E1 enzyme activity to result in higher drug concentrations.
Ginger	Antiplatelet and anticoagulant agents	Ginger may have antiplatelet activity, potentially increasing the risk of bleeding.
	Hypoglycemic agents	Ginger may potentially lower blood glucose concentrations and have additive effects with hypoglycemic agents.
Ginkgo	Antiplatelet and anticoagulant agents	Ginkgo may have antiplatelet activity, potentially increasing the risk of bleeding.
	CYP2C19 substrates	Ginkgo may induce CYP2C19 enzyme activity to result in lower drug concentrations.
	CYP1A2 substrates	Ginkgo may modestly inhibit CYP1A2 enzyme activity to result in higher drug levels.
	CYP2C9 substrates	Ginkgo may modestly inhibit CYP2C9 enzyme activity to result in higher drug concentrations.
	CYP2D6 substrates	Ginkgo may inhibit CYP2D6 enzyme activity to result in higher drug concentrations.
Ginseng (Panax)	Antiplatelet and anticoagulant agents	Panax ginseng may have antiplatelet properties; American ginseng may decrease the effectiveness (international normalized ration [INR]) of warfarin.
	CYP2D6 substrates	Panax ginseng may modestly inhibit CYP2D6 enzyme activity to result in higher drug concentrations.
	Immune suppressants	Panax ginseng may stimulate immune function, potentially decreasing the effectiveness of drugs such as cyclosporine, tacrolimus, and prednisone.
	Hypoglycemic agents	Panax ginseng may potentially lower blood glucose levels and have additive effects with hypoglycemic agents.
Glucosamine	Warfarin	High-dose glucosamine (along with high-dose chondroitin) may have additive effects to those of warfarin because of structural similarity to heparin.

AChE, Acetylcholinesterase; *CCBs,* calcium channel blockers; *CNS,* central nervous system; *MAOIs,* monoamine oxidase inhibitor; *PPIs,* proton pump inhibitors; *SSRIs,* selective serotonin reuptake inhibitors.

Natural Products and Drug Interactions 1563

Natural Products	Drugs	Interactions
Green tea extract	Antiplatelet agents	Green tea possesses compounds that may have antiplatelet activity, potentially increasing the risk of bleeding.
	Amphetamines	Caffeine in green tea may increase the risk of CNS toxicity.
	Cocaine	Caffeine in green tea may increase the risk of CNS toxicity.
	Oral contraceptives	Oral contraceptives may decrease the clearance of caffeine in green tea.
	Warfarin	Small amounts of vitamin K have been reported to be present in green tea, potentially decreasing the effectiveness of warfarin.
	Theophylline	Caffeine potentially decreases theophylline clearance.
	Verapamil	Verapamil decreases caffeine clearance, resulting in increased concentrations.
	Quinolone antibiotics	Some quinolone antibiotics decrease the clearance of caffeine.
	Hepatotoxic drugs	Concern exists that the risk of hepatotoxicity with green tea is increased in the presence of hepatotoxic drugs such as acetaminophen.
Hawthorn	β-Blockers	Hawthorn and β-blockers may have additive effects on blood pressure and heart rate.
	CCBs, nitrates	Hawthorn and CCBs (or nitrates) may have additive effects due to coronary vasodilation.
	Digoxin	Hawthorn may have additive effects to those of digoxin.
	Phosphodiesterase inhibitors	Hawthorn may have additive vasodilatory and hypotensive effects with sildenafil, tadalafil, and vardenafil.
Horse chestnut seed extract (HCSE)	Antiplatelet and anticoagulant agents	HCSE may have antiplatelet activity, potentially increasing the risk of bleeding.
	Hypoglycemic agents	HCSE may potentially lower blood glucose concentrations and have additive effects with hypoglycemic agents.
Huperzine	AChE inhibitors (donepezil, etc.)	Huperzine may have additive effects when combined with AChE inhibitors.
	Anticholinergic drugs	The effectiveness of huperzine and/or the anticholinergic drug may be decreased by their concomitant administration.
	Cholinergic drugs (bethanechol, neostigmine, etc.)	Huperzine may have additive effects when combined with cholinergic drugs.
Kava	CYP3A4 substrates	Kava may inhibit CYP3A4 enzyme activity to result in higher drug concentrations.
	CYP1A2 substrates	Kava may inhibit CYP1A2 enzyme activity to result in higher drug concentrations.
	CYP2C9 substrates, CYP2C19 substrates	Kava may inhibit CYP2C9 and CYP2C19 enzyme activity to result in higher drug concentrations.
	CYP2D6 substrates	Kava may inhibit CYP2D6 enzyme activity to result in higher drug concentrations.
	P-glycoprotein substrates (digoxin; etoposide, paclitaxel, vinblastine, vincristine; itraconazole; diltiazem, verapamil; and many other drugs)	Kava may inhibit P-glycoprotein transporter systems.
	Hepatotoxic drugs	Concern exists that the risk of hepatotoxicity from kava is increased in the presence of hepatotoxic drugs such as acetaminophen.
Melatonin	Antiplatelet and anticoagulant agents	Melatonin may potentiate the effects of antiplatelets and anticoagulants, although the mechanism is unknown.
	CNS depressants	Melatonin may have additive CNS depressant effects.
	Fluvoxamine	Fluvoxamine may increase levels of melatonin.
	Immune suppressants	Melatonin may stimulate immune function, potentially decreasing the effectiveness of drugs such as cyclosporine, tacrolimus, and prednisone.
	Hypoglycemic agents	Melatonin may impair glucose utilization and may decrease the efficacy of hypoglycemic agents.
Milk thistle	Estrogens (and other drugs that undergo glucuronidation)	Silymarin may increase the clearance of estrogens.
	CYP2C9 substrates	Milk thistle may modestly inhibit CYP2C9 enzyme activity to result in higher drug concentrations.
Peppermint oil	H_2 antagonists and proton pump inhibitors	Peppermint oil may raise gastric pH and blunt efficacy of H_2 antagonists and PPIs.
	CYP3A4 substrates	Peppermint oil may modestly inhibit CYP3A4 enzyme activity to result in higher drug concentrations.
	CYP1A2 substrates	Peppermint oil may modestly inhibit CYP1A2 enzyme activity to result in higher drug concentrations.
	CYP2C9 substrates, CYP2C19 substrates	Peppermint oil may modestly inhibit CYP2C9 and CYP2C19 enzyme activity to result in higher drug concentrations.
Policosanol	Antiplatelet and anticoagulant agents	Policosanol may have antiplatelet activity, potentially increasing the risk of bleeding.
Probiotics	Antibiotics	Antibiotics may kill the live organisms in different probiotic preparations.
	Immune suppressants	Theoretically, probiotics may cause bacterial or fungal infections in patients who are taking immune suppressants chronically.

Continued on following page

Natural Products	Drugs	Interactions
Red clover phytoestrogens	Antiplatelet and anticoagulant agents	Theoretically, red clover may possess coumarins, which increase the risk of bleeding with antiplatelet and anticoagulants.
	CYP3A4 substrates	Red clover may inhibit CYP3A4 enzyme activity to result in higher drug concentrations.
	CYP2C9 substrates, CYP2C19 substrates	Red clover may inhibit CYP2C9 and CYP2C19 enzyme activity to result in higher drug concentrations.
	CYP1A2 substrates	Red clover may inhibit CYP1A2 enzyme activity to result in higher drug concentrations.
Red yeast rice	CYP3A4 inhibitors	Drugs that inhibit CYP3A4 may decrease the metabolism of lovastatin in red yeast rice.
	Statins	Red yeast rice contains lovastatin and increases the risk of myopathy (and hepatotoxicity).
	Fibrates and niacin	Fibrates and niacin may increase concentrations of lovastatin in red yeast rice.
S-adenosylmethionine (SAM-e)	Antidepressants (including MAOIs)	Additive effects are possible, and there is potential for toxicity.
	Serotonergic drugs (triptans, SSRIs, tramadol, meperidine, dextromethorphan, etc.)	SAM-e may increase the risk of development of serotonin syndrome when used concomitantly.
Soy phytoestrogens	Antibiotics	Antibiotics may decrease the efficacy of soy because intestinal bacteria convert isoflavones into more active forms.
	Estrogens	Soy potentially may inhibit the effects of estrogen.
	Tamoxifen/aromatase inhibitors	Soy's estrogenic effects may antagonize the antitumor effects of tamoxifen/aromatase inhibitors.
	MAOIs	Fermented soy products may contain tyramine.
St. John's wort	CYP3A4 substrates	St. John's wort strongly induces CYP3A4 enzyme activity to result in lower drug concentrations.
	CYP1A2 substrates	St. John's wort modestly induces CYP1A2 enzyme activity to result in lower drug levels.
	CYP2C9 substrates	St. John's wort induces CYP2C9 enzyme activity to result in lower drug concentrations.
	P-glycoprotein substrates (digoxin; etoposide, paclitaxel, vinblastine, vincristine; itraconazole; diltiazem, verapamil; and other drugs)	St. John's wort induces P-glycoprotein transporter systems.
	Serotonergic drugs (triptans, SSRIs, tramadol, meperidine, dextromethorphan, etc.)	St. John's wort may increase the risk of development of serotonin syndrome when used concomitantly.
Valerian	CNS depressants (benzodiazepines, opiates, barbiturates, alcohol, etc.)	Valerian may increase the sedative effects of CNS depressants.
	CYP3A4 substrates	Valerian may modestly inhibit the CYP3A4 enzyme activity.

AChE, Acetylcholinesterase; *CCBs,* calcium channel blockers; *CNS,* central nervous system; *MAOIs,* monoamine oxidase inhibitors; *PPIs,* proton pump inhibitors; *SSRIs,* selective serotonin reuptake inhibitors.

EXAMPLES OF DRUGS METABOLIZED BY CYP ENZYMES

The following are examples of drugs that are metabolized through the different cytochrome P450 isoenzymes:

CYP1A2 substrates: theophylline, imipramine, clozapine, naproxen

CYP2C9 substrates: warfarin, tamoxifen, irbesartan, ibuprofen, glipizide

CYP2C19 substrates: omeprazole and other proton pump inhibitors, phenytoin, phenobarbital, cyclophosphamide

CYP2D6 substrates: S-metoprolol, propafenone, paroxetine, risperidone, tramadol

CYP2E1 substrates: acetaminophen, alcohol

CYP3A4 substrates: most statins, indinavir, amlodipine, verapamil, alprazolam, buspirone

(For a complete list of drugs and their respective metabolic pathways through the cytochrome P450 isoenzyme systems go to http://medicine.iupui.edu/flockhart.)

AUTHOR: **ANNE L. HUME, PHARM.D.**

Commonly Ingested Plants with Significant Toxic Potential

Plant	Symptoms	Management
Autumn crocus (*Colchicum autumnale*)	Vomiting Diarrhea Initial leukocytosis followed by bone marrow failure Multisystem organ failure	Activated charcoal decontamination Aggressive fluid resuscitation and supportive care
Belladonna alkaloids: jimson weed (*Datura stramonium*) Belladonna ("deadly nightshade"; *Atropa belladonna*)	Anticholinergic toxidrome Seizures	Supportive care, benzodiazepines Consider physostigmine if patient is a threat to self or others; only use if no conduction delays on ECG
Cardiac glycoside–containing plants (foxglove, lily of the valley, oleander, yellow oleander, etc.)	Nausea Vomiting Bradycardia Dysrhythmias (AV block, ventricular ectopy) Hyperkalemia	Digoxin-specific Fab fragments
Jequirity bean and other abrin-containing species (e.g., rosary pea, precatory bean)	Oral pain Vomiting Diarrhea Shock Hemolysis Renal failure	Supportive care, including aggressive volume resuscitation and correction of electrolyte abnormalities
Monkshood (*Aconitum* species)	Numbness and tingling of lips/tongue Vomiting Bradycardia	Atropine for bradycardia Supportive care
Oxalate-containing plants: *Philodendron, Diffenbachia, Colocasia* ("elephant ear")	Local tissue injury Oral pain Vomiting	Supportive care, pain control
Poison hemlock (*Conium maculatum*)	Vomiting Agitation followed by CNS depression Paralysis Respiratory failure	Supportive care
Pokeweed	Hemorrhagic gastroenteritis Burning of mouth and throat	Supportive care
Rhododendron	Vomiting Diarrhea Bradycardia	Atropine for symptomatic bradycardia Supportive care
Tobacco	Vomiting Agitation Diaphoresis Fasciculations Seizures	Supportive care
Water hemlock (*Cicuta* species)	Abdominal pain Vomiting Delirium Seizures	Supportive care, including benzodiazepines for seizures
Yew (*Taxus* species)	GI symptoms QRS widening Hypotension CV collapse	Supportive care Atropine for bradycardia Sodium bicarbonate does not appear to be effective

AV, Atrioventricular; *CNS,* central nervous system; *CV,* cardiovascular; *ECG,* electrocardiogram; *Fab,* fragment, antigen binding; *GI,* gastrointestinal.
From Kliegman RM et al: *Nelson textbook of pediatrics,* ed 19, Philadelphia, 2011, Saunders.

Herbs Associated with Toxicity

Herbal Product	Toxic Chemicals	Toxic Effects
Aconite (*Aconitum* spp.)	Aconitine alkaloids	Nausea, vomiting, paresthesias, weakness, hypotension, asystole, arrhythmias, bradycardia
Chamomile (*Matricaria chamomilla, Anthemis nobilis*)	Allergens	Anaphylaxis, contact dermatitis
Chapparal (*Larrea divaricate, Larrea tridentate*)	Nordihydroguaiaretic acid	Nausea, vomiting, lethargy, hepatitis
Cinnamon oil (*Cinnamomum* spp.)	Cinnamaldehyde	Dermatitis, abuse syndrome
Coltsfoot (*Tussilago farfara*)	Pyrrolizidines	HVOD
Comfrey (*Symphytum officinale*)	Pyrrolizidines	HVOD
Crotalaria spp.	Pyrrolizidines	HVOD
Echinacea (*Echinacea angustifolia*, Compositae spp.)	Polysaccharides	Asthma, atopy, angioedema, anaphylaxis, urticaria
Eucalyptus (*Eucalyptus globulus*)	1,8-cineole	Drowsiness, ataxia, nausea, vomiting, seizures, coma, respiratory failure
Garlic (*Allium sativum*)	Allicin	Dermatitis, chemical burns, oxidizing agent
Germander (*Teucrium chamaedrys*)		Hepatotoxicity
Ginseng (*Panax ginseng*)	Ginsenoside	Ginseng abuse, diarrhea, anxiety, insomnia, hypertension
Glycerated asafetida	Oxidants	Methemoglobinemia
Groundsel (*Senecio longilobus*)	Pyrrolizidines	HVOD
Heliotrope, turnsole (*Crotalaria fulva, Heliotropium, Cynoglossum officinale*)	Pyrrolizidines	HVOD
Jin bu huan (*Stephania* spp., *Corydalis* spp.)	L-Tetrahydropalmitine	Hepatitis, lethargy, coma
Kava-kava (*Piper methysticum*)	Kawain, methysticin	Hepatic failure, "kavaism," neurotoxicity
Kelp	Iodine	Thyroid dysfunction
Laetrile	Cyanide	Coma, seizures, death
Licorice (*Glycyrrhiza glabra*)	Glycyrrhetic acid	Hypertension, cardiac arrhythmias, hypokalemia
Ma huang (*Ephedra sinica*)	Ephedrine	Cardiac arrhythmias, seizures, stroke, hypertension
Monkshood (*Aconitum napellus, A. columbianum*)	Aconite	Cardiac arrhythmias, weakness, coma, shock, paresthesias, vomiting, seizures
Nutmeg (*Myristica fragrans*)	Myristicin, eugenol	Hallucinations, emesis, headache
Nux vomica	Strychnine	Seizures, abdominal pain, respiratory arrest
Pennyroyal (*Mentha pulegium* or *Hedeoma* spp.)	Pulegone	Centrilobular liver necrosis, fetotoxicity, seizures, shock
Ragwort (golden) (*Senecio aureus, Echium*)	Pyrrolizidines	HVOD
Wormwood (*Artemisia* spp.)	Thujone	Seizures, dementia, tremors, headache

HVOD, Hepatic veno-occlusive disease.
From Fuhrman BP et al: *Pediatric critical care*, ed 4, Philadelphia, 2011, Saunders.

Websites Providing Data on Herbal Therapy Hazards

Web Address	Website
http://www.fda.gov or http://www.vmcfsan.fda.gov/~dms/aems/html	On the U.S. Food and Drug Administration website under the title "Medwatch," some herb warnings can be found ("special adverse event monitoring system" link)
http://www.faseb.org/aspet/H&MIG3.htm#top	ASPET Herbal and Medicinal Plant Interest Group: a site for an herb discussion group with pharmacologists
http://www.nnlm.nlm.nih.gov/pnr/uwmhg/	University of Washington Medicinal Herb Garden
http://www.nim.nih.gov/medlineplus/herbalmedicine.html	Provides an update on ongoing clinical studies involving herbal products, news, and many links
http://www.update-software.com/abstracts/mainindex.html	The Cochrane Collaboration maintains an updated international database of clinical trials involving complementary and alternative medicine
http://www.amfoundation.org/	Providing consumers and professionals with responsible evidence-based information on the integration of alternative and conventional medicine
http://www.herbmed.org/	An interactive electronic herbal database provides hyperlinked access to scientific data underlying the use of herbs for health; an evidence-based information resource for professionals, researchers, and general public
http://nccam.nih.gov/	The National Center for Complementary and Alternative Medicine is 1 of 27 institutes and centers that make up the U.S. National Institutes of Health; their mission is to support rigorous research on complementary and alternative medicine, train researchers, and disseminate information to the public and professionals
http://toxnet.nlm.nih.gov/	A cluster of databases on toxicology, hazardous chemicals, and related areas

From Floege J et al: *Comprehensive clinical nephrology,* ed 4, Philadelphia, 2010, Saunders.

Dietary Supplements: What Every Primary Care Provider Should Know

Primary care providers must be knowledgeable regarding the safety, efficacy, and drug interactions associated with common dietary supplements because of the following:

- An estimated 38% of adults ages 18 years and older reported the use of at least one form of complementary and alternative medicine (CAM) according to the National Health Interview Survey in 2007.
- Almost 17.8% of adults specifically reported the use of dietary supplements, with fish oil, glucosamine, echinacea, flaxseed, and ginseng most frequently used.
- Although the use of dietary supplements has plateaued as a result of consumer concerns about effectiveness and potential adverse effects, usage remains common and potentially dangerous.

COMMON TERMINOLOGY

- A *dietary supplement* is defined as an oral product containing vitamins, minerals, herbs, or other botanicals; amino acids; dietary substances used to supplement the diet by increasing the total dietary intake; or a concentrate, metabolite, constituent, extract, or combination.
- *CAM* refers to the broad domain of healing practices that include diverse health systems, modalities, and practices and their accompanying theories and beliefs (see glossary of terms in Appendix Ia).
- *Complementary therapies* are those that are used *in addition to* conventional therapies, whereas *alternative therapies* are those that are used *instead of* conventional therapies. Most consumers in the United States use dietary supplements as a complementary therapy.
- *Standardization* refers to the practice of producing dietary supplements with a specific amount of a given compound that may or may not include the actual active ingredient. For example, feverfew has been standardized to its parthenolide content.

LEGISLATION

The U.S. Food and Drug Administration (FDA) is frequently criticized for not closely regulating dietary supplements and monitoring their safety. However, although the agency regulates prescription drugs and over-the-counter (OTC) products, the FDA has limited regulatory authority over dietary supplements. This is because the Dietary Supplement and Health Education Act (DSHEA) of 1994 and its resulting regulations limit the FDA's authority. As a result of DSHEA, the FDA is able to act only when a dietary supplement has been documented to contain a prescription drug, as was the case with glyburide in a natural treatment for diabetes and diazepam in an osteoarthritis preparation. In addition, the FDA can act when safety issues related to a product have been clearly documented, although these cases are frequently challenged in the courts.

HEALTH CLAIMS

Dietary supplements generally are marketed under three types of health claims. The first category is the "nutrient content" claim, in which the product is identified as an excellent source of, typically, a mineral such as calcium, based on recommended daily values. The second type is the "significant scientific agreement" claim; these claims are used when some evidence of the product's efficacy exists (e.g., fish oil supplements). The third and most common type of health claim is called a "structure/function" claim; these claims state that the product has some effect on health—for example, "helps to maintain a healthy heart." However, dietary supplements are not permitted to carry claims stating that they are effective in preventing, treating, or curing diseases.

INFORMATION RESOURCES

Appendix Ic provides a brief overview of common dietary supplements. Until recently, few evidence-based resources on dietary supplements were available. Clinical studies and systematic reviews on dietary supplements are now widely available through PubMed, EMBASE, and the Cochrane Database of Systematic Reviews. Although more information is available, references on specific products vary in their interpretation of the available evidence and may exhibit an unintentional bias, either pro or con, regarding the safety and efficacy of dietary supplements.

"Gold standard" evidence-based databases on dietary supplements (subscription required) include the following:

- Natural Medicines Comprehensive Database (http://www.naturaldatabase.com): This database includes listings for many dietary supplements and is organized in a clinician-friendly manner. Monographs include the different common and scientific names; uses and likely effectiveness for different uses; chemical constituents; interactions with drugs, diseases, foods, and laboratory tests; adverse effects; and cautions. The information is extensively referenced and is updated on a daily basis. The primary limitation is that the evaluation of data on clinical effectiveness could be more rigorous.
- Natural Standard (http://www.naturalstandard.com): This database includes listings for dietary supplements and other forms of complementary and alternative medicine. The evidence supporting the assessments in this database is critically evaluated and rigorous in nature. The primary limitation is that many fewer dietary supplements are included in this database.

Evidence-based free websites on dietary supplements include the following:

- National Center for Complementary and Alternative Medicine (NCCAM) (http://nccam.nih.gov)
- Office of Dietary Supplements International Bibliographic Information on Dietary Supplements (http://dietary-supplements.info.nih.gov/Health_Information/IBIDS.aspx)
- Memorial Sloan-Kettering Cancer Center (http://www.mskcc.org/mskcc/html/11570.cfm)

DRUG INTERACTIONS

Clinically significant interactions have been documented between dietary supplements and prescription or OTC drugs. The challenge for primary care providers is to identify real, clinically relevant interactions versus potential or theoretical interactions. Data on interactions with dietary supplements are usually based on isolated case reports or on studies enrolling healthy volunteers. As with drug-drug interactions, the likelihood of an interaction and its severity are influenced especially by concomitant medical conditions, such as heart failure and presence or absence of impaired kidney and liver function.

Appendix Id lists interactions between selected natural products and prescription and nonprescription drugs. The following two broad interactions are particularly important in primary care practice:

- St. John's wort, commonly used for depression, is a potent inducer of cytochrome P450 3A4 isoenzymes and has been documented to increase the clearance of many drugs that are metabolized through this (and other) pathways. (For a list of common drugs cleared in this manner, readers should consult http://medicine.iupui.edu/flockhart/clinlist.htm.) In addition, St. John's wort may induce P-glycoprotein transporter systems that are important for digoxin and some chemotherapeutic agents. St. John's wort has also been associated with the development of serotonin syndrome when used with drugs that have significant serotonergic activity.
- Dietary supplements such as garlic, ginkgo, and feverfew, as well as many others, have been purported to either have antiplatelet activity or have effects on the clotting cascade. This may be important for adults also taking aspirin (and other platelet-active agents) or warfarin.

COUNSELING POINTS

The single most important counseling point related to dietary supplements is always to ask patients about their use of these products and to do so in an open, nonjudgmental manner. The approach should emphasize that many consumers have been interested in vitamins, minerals, herbs, teas, and so on, to maintain their health or to treat illness. If the clinician is unaware of the safety, efficacy, and interactions of a specific product, several websites are available to quickly scan for information. Also, access to drug information centers at colleges of pharmacy is almost always available, and some hospitals now offer programs in integrative medicine.

Patients should be asked about their goals in using the product, as well as how long they have taken it and in what dosage. Allergies to plants should be documented because cross-allergies are common. Clinicians should appreciate that individuals who use dietary supplements may be interested in making lifestyle changes and potentially decreasing their use of prescription drugs. In addition, if an individual is also consulting an alternative medicine practitioner, clinicians should recognize that some alternative health systems discourage the use of established therapies such as vaccines.

Although problems with safety and efficacy have been identified, many dietary supplements are benign except for their cost. Some patients are at higher risk for adverse outcomes from the use of dietary supplements (e.g., those with chronic kidney and liver disease). Patients should be counseled specifically to avoid purchasing dietary supplements over the Internet.

RESEARCH ISSUES

Many clinical and observational studies of dietary supplements have been published. In the past, clinicians frequently stated either that published studies of dietary supplements did not exist or that only a few were available. The reason for this finding was that until recently the National Library of Medicine did not abstract from the peer-reviewed alternative medicine literature. Fortunately, much more research is now readily available. As with all research, the more rigorous the study methodology, the less likely the dietary supplement is to demonstrate clinical benefit.

In evaluating published studies of dietary supplements, the following should be considered:

- Has the correct plant and part of the plant (root, stem, leaf) been used? This critical information may not be known to many clinicians. Consulting a resource such as the National Medicines Comprehensive Database can usually provide the needed information to judge this component of the study.
- Has the content of active ingredients been verified throughout the study? In a recent review of 81 major randomized controlled trials of herbal products, only 12 (15%) reported performing tests to quantify actual contents, and 3 (4%) provided adequate data to compare actual with expected content values of at least one chemical constituent.
- Is the severity of the disease appropriate for study? Negative studies with dietary supplements sometimes inappropriately enroll participants who have moderate-to-severe disease (e.g., those with depression or benign prostatic hyperplasia) when only mild disease would be appropriate.
- Is the duration of the study appropriate? Early studies comparing glucosamine and nonsteroidal anti-inflammatory agents (NSAIAs) demonstrated greater efficacy with the NSAIAs because of an inadequate study duration for glucosamine to show any benefit.
- Is a placebo group included? Recent studies with dietary supplements for menopausal symptoms and osteoarthritis have demonstrated placebo responses over 40% to 50%.
- Was the blinding maintained throughout the study? Some dietary supplements, such as saw palmetto, have distinctive odors and tastes that are not easily masked.
- Is the preparation commercially available? Most important, when a study with dietary supplements does show benefit, it frequently is difficult to use the product in practice because the specific formulation studied is not commercially available.

AUTHOR: **ANNE L. HUME, PHARM.D.**

Vitamins and Their Functions

	Biochemistry and Physiology	Deficiency [RDA*]	Toxicity [TUL†]	Assessment of Status
Fat-Soluble Vitamins				
Vitamin A	A family of the retinoid compounds, each member having biologic activity qualitatively similar to retinol. Carotenoids are structurally related to retinoids. Some carotenoids, most notably β-carotene, are metabolized into compounds with vitamin A activity and are therefore considered to be provitamin A compounds. Vitamin A is an integral component of rhodopsin and iodopsins, light-sensitive proteins in rod and cone cells in the retina. *Additional functions:* induction and maintenance of cellular differentiation in certain tissues; signal for appropriate morphogenesis in the developing embryo; maintenance of cell-mediated immunity. One microgram of retinol = 3.33 IU of vitamin A.	Follicular hyperkeratosis and night blindness are early indicators. Conjunctival xerosis, degeneration of the cornea (keratomalacia), and de-differentiation of rapidly proliferating epithelia are later indications of deficiency. *Bitot spots* (focal areas of the conjunctiva or cornea with foamy appearance) are an indication of xerosis. Blindness, due to corneal destruction and retinal dysfunction, ensues if left uncorrected. Increased susceptibility to infection is also a consequence. [F: 700 µg; M: 900 µg]	In adults, >150,000 µg may cause acute toxicity: fatal intracranial hypertension, skin exfoliation, and hepatocellular necrosis. *Chronic* toxicity may occur with habitual daily intake of >10,000 µg: alopecia, ataxia, bone and muscle pain, dermatitis, cheilitis, conjunctivitis, pseudotumor cerebri, hepatocellular necrosis, hyperlipidemia, and hyperostosis are common. Single, large doses of vitamin A (30,000 µg), or habitual intake of >4500 µg/day in early pregnancy can be teratogenic. Excessive intake of carotenoids causes a benign condition characterized by yellowish discoloration of the skin. Habitually large doses of canthaxanthin, a carotenoid, have the additional capability of inducing a retinopathy. [3000 µg]	Retinol concentration in the plasma and vitamin A concentrations in the milk and tears are reasonably accurate measures of adequate status. Toxicity is best assessed by elevated levels of retinyl esters in plasma. A quantitative measure of dark adaptation for night vision or an electroretinogram are useful functional tests.
Vitamin D	A group of sterol compounds whose parent structure is cholecalciferol (vitamin D₃). Cholecalciferol is formed in the skin from 7-dehydrocholesterol (provitamin D₃) by exposure to UVB radiation. A plant sterol, ergocalciferol (provitamin D₂) can be similarly converted into vitamin D₂ and has similar vitamin D activity. The vitamin undergoes sequential hydroxylations in the liver and kidney at the 25 and 1 positions, respectively, producing the most bioactive form of the vitamin, 1,25-dihydroxy vitamin D. Maintains intracellular and extracellular concentrations of calcium and phosphate by enhancing intestinal absorption of the two ions and, in conjunction with PTH, promoting their mobilization from bone mineral. Retards proliferation and promotes differentiation in certain epithelia. One microgram = 40 IU.	Deficiency results in disordered bone modeling called *rickets* in childhood and *osteomalacia* in adults. Expansion of the epiphyseal growth plates and replacement of normal bone with unmineralized bone matrix are the cardinal features of rickets; the latter feature also characterizes osteomalacia. Deformity of bone and pathologic fractures occur. Decreased serum concentrations of calcium and phosphate may occur. [15 µg, ages 19-70 yr; 20 µg, age >70 yr]	Excess amounts result in abnormally high concentrations of calcium and phosphate in the serum: metastatic calcifications, renal damage, and altered mentation may occur. [50 µg]	The serum concentration of the major circulating metabolite, 25-hydroxyvitamin D, is an excellent indicator of systemic status except in chronic renal failure, in which the impairment of renal L-hydroxylation results in disassociation of the mono- and dihydroxyvitamin concentrations. Measuring the serum concentration of 1,25-dihydroxyvitamin D is then necessary.

Continued on following page

	Biochemistry and Physiology	Deficiency [RDA*]	Toxicity [TUL†]	Assessment of Status
Vitamin E	A group of at least 8 naturally occurring compounds, some of which are tocopherols and some of which are tocotrienols. At present, the only dietary form that is thought to be biologically active in humans is α-tocopherol. Acts as an antioxidant and free radical scavenger in lipophilic environments, most notably in cell membranes. Acts in conjunction with other antioxidants such as selenium.	Deficiency due to dietary inadequacy rare. Usually seen in (1) premature infants, (2) individuals with fat malabsorption, and (3) individuals with abetalipoproteinemia. Red blood cell fragility occurs and can produce a hemolytic anemia. Neuronal degeneration produces peripheral neuropathies, ophthalmoplegia, and destruction of posterior columns of spinal cord. Neurologic disease is frequently irreversible if deficiency is not corrected early enough. May contribute to the hemolytic anemia and retrolental fibroplasia seen in premature infants. Reported to suppress cell-mediated immunity. [15 mg]	Depressed levels of vitamin K-dependent procoagulants and potentiation of oral anticoagulants have been reported, as has impaired WBC function. Doses of 800 mg/day have been reported to increase slightly the incidence of hemorrhagic stroke. [1000 mg]	Plasma or serum concentration of α-tocopherol is most commonly used. Additional accuracy is obtained by expressing this value per mg of total plasma lipid. RBC peroxide hemolysis test is not entirely specific but is a useful functional measure of the antioxidant potential of cell membranes.
Vitamin K	A family of naphthoquinone compounds with similar biologic activity. Phylloquinone (vitamin K_1) is derived from plants; a variety of menaquinones (vitamin K_2) is derived from bacterial sources. Serves as an essential cofactor in the post-translational γ-carboxylation of glutamic acid residues in many proteins. These proteins include several circulating procoagulants and anticoagulants as well as proteins in a variety of tissues.	Deficiency syndrome, uncommon except in (1) breast-fed newborns, in whom it may cause "hemorrhagic disease of the newborn," (2) adults with fat malabsorption or who are taking drugs that interfere with vitamin K metabolism (e.g., coumarin, phenytoin, broad-spectrum antibiotics), and (3) individuals taking large doses of vitamin E and anticoagulant drugs. Excessive hemorrhage is the usual manifestation. [F: 90 µg; M: 120 µg]	Rapid intravenous infusion of K_1 has been associated with dyspnea, flushing, and cardiovascular collapse; this is likely related to the dispersing agents in the solution. Supplementation may interfere with coumarin-based anticoagulation. Pregnant women taking large amounts of the provitamin menadione may deliver infants with hemolytic anemia, hyperbilirubinemia, and kernicterus. [no TUL established]	Prothrombin time is typically used as a measure of functional K status; it is neither sensitive nor specific for vitamin K deficiency. Determination of undercarboxylated prothrombin in the plasma is more accurate but less widely available.

Water-Soluble Vitamins

	Biochemistry and Physiology	Deficiency [RDA*]	Toxicity [TUL†]	Assessment of Status
Thiamine (vitamin B_1)	A water-soluble compound containing substituted pyrimidine and thiazole rings and a hydroxyethyl side chain. The coenzyme form is thiamine pyrophosphate (TPP). Serves as a coenzyme in many α-ketoacid decarboxylation and transketolation reactions. Inadequate thiamine availability leads to impairments of above reactions, resulting in inadequate adenosine triphosphate synthesis and abnormal carbohydrate metabolism, respectively. May have an additional role in neuronal conduction independent of aforementioned actions.	Classic deficiency syndrome ("beriberi") described in Asian populations consuming polished rice diet. Alcoholism and chronic renal dialysis are also common precipitants. High carbohydrate intake increases need for B_1. *Mild deficiency:* irritability, fatigue, and headaches. *More severe deficiency:* combinations of peripheral neuropathy, cardiovascular dysfunction, and cerebral dysfunction. Cardiovascular involvement ("wet beriberi"): congestive heart failure and low peripheral vascular resistance. Cerebral disease: nystagmus, ophthalmoplegia, and ataxia (Wernicke's encephalopathy); hallucinations, impaired short-term memory, and confabulation ("Korsakoff's psychosis"). Deficiency syndrome responds within 24 hr to parenteral thiamine but is partially or wholly irreversible after a certain stage. [F: 1.1 mg; M: 1.2 mg]	Excess intake is largely excreted in the urine, although parenteral doses of > 400 mg/day are reported to cause lethargy, ataxia, and reduced tone of the gastrointestinal tract. [TUL not established]	The most effective measure of B_1 status is the erythrocyte transketolase activity coefficient, which measures enzyme activity before and after addition of exogenous TPP: RBCs from a deficient individual express a substantial increase in enzyme activity with addition of TPP. Thiamine concentrations in blood or urine are also used.
Riboflavin (vitamin B_2)	Consists of a substituted isoalloxazine ring with a ribitol side chain. Serves as a coenzyme for a diverse array of biochemical reactions. The primary coenzymatic forms are flavin mononucleotide (FMN) and flavin adenine dinucleotide (FAD). Riboflavin holoenzymes participate in oxidation-reduction reactions in a myriad of metabolic pathways.	Deficiency is usually seen in conjunction with deficiencies of other B vitamins. Isolated deficiency of riboflavin produces hyperemia and edema of nasopharyngeal mucosa, cheilosis, angular stomatitis, glossitis, seborrheic dermatitis, and a normochromic, normocytic anemia. [F: 1.1; M: 1.3]	Toxicity not reported in humans. [TUL not established]	The most common method of assessment is determining the activity coefficient of glutathione reductase in RBCs (the test is invalid for individuals with glucose-6-phosphate dehydrogenase [G6PD] deficiency). Measurements of blood and urine concentrations are less desirable methods.

	Biochemistry and Physiology	Deficiency [RDA*]	Toxicity [TUL†]	Assessment of Status
Niacin (vitamin B$_3$)	Refers to nicotinic acid and the corresponding amide, nicotinamide. The active coenzymatic forms are composed of nicotinamide affixed to adenine dinucleotide, forming NAD or NADP. More than 200 apoenzymes use these compounds as electron acceptors or hydrogen donors, either as a coenzyme or as a co-substrate. The essential amino acid tryptophan is a precursor of niacin; 60 mg of dietary tryptophan yields approximately 1 mg of niacin. Dietary requirements thus depend partly on tryptophan intake. Requirement is often determined on basis of caloric intake (i.e., niacin equivalents/1000 kcal). Large doses of nicotinic acid (1.5-3 g/day) effectively lower low-density lipoprotein cholesterol and elevate high-density lipoprotein cholesterol.	Pellagra is the classic deficiency syndrome and is often seen in populations in which corn is the major source of energy. Still endemic in parts of China, Africa, and India. Diarrhea, dementia (or associated symptoms of anxiety or insomnia), and a pigmented dermatitis that develops in sun-exposed areas are typical features. Glossitis, stomatitis, vaginitis, vertigo, and burning dysesthesias are early signs. Reported to occasionally occur in carcinoid syndrome because tryptophan is diverted to other synthetic pathways. [F: 14 mg; M: 16 mg]	Human toxicity known largely through studies examining hypolipidemic effects. Includes vasomotor phenomenon (flushing), hyperglycemia, parenchymal liver damage, and hyperuricemia. [35 mg]	Assessment of status is problematic: blood levels of vitamin not reliable. Measurement of urinary excretion of the niacin metabolites, N-methylnicotinamide and 2-pyridone, is thought to be the most effective means of assessment at present.
Vitamin B$_6$	Refers to several derivatives of pyridine, including pyridoxine (PN), pyridoxal (PL), and pyridoxamine (PM), which are interconvertible in the body. The coenzymatic forms are pyridoxal-5-phosphate (PLP) and pyridoxamine-5-phosphate (PMP). As a coenzyme, B$_6$ is involved in many transamination reactions (and thereby in gluconeogenesis), in the synthesis of niacin from tryptophan, in the synthesis of several neurotransmitters, and in the synthesis of δ-aminolevulinic acid (and therefore in heme synthesis). It also has functions unrelated to coenzymatic activity: PL and PLP bind to hemoglobin and alter O$_2$ affinity; PLP also binds to steroid receptors, inhibiting receptor affinity to DNA and thereby modulating steroid activity.	Deficiency usually seen in conjunction with other water-soluble vitamin deficiencies. Stomatitis, angular cheilosis, glossitis, irritability, depression, and confusion occur in moderate to severe depletion; normochromic, normocytic anemia has been reported in severe deficiency. Abnormal electroencephalograms and, in infants, convulsions have also been observed. Some sideroblastic anemias respond to B$_6$ administration. Isoniazid, cycloserine, penicillamine, ethanol, and theophylline can inhibit B$_6$ metabolism. [Ages 19-50 yr: 1.3 mg; >50 yr: 1.5 mg for women, 1.7 mg for men]	Long-term use with doses exceeding 200 mg/day (in adults) may cause peripheral neuropathies and photosensitivity. [100 mg]	Many useful laboratory methods of assessment exist. The plasma or erythrocyte PLP levels are most common. Urinary excretion of xanthurenic acid after an oral tryptophan load or activity indices of RBC alanine or aspartic acid transaminases (ALT and AST, respectively) are all functional measures of B$_6$-dependent enzyme activity.
Folate	A group of related pterin compounds. More than 35 forms of the vitamin are found naturally. The fully oxidized form, folic acid, is not found in nature but is the pharmacologic form of the vitamin. All folate functions relate to its ability to transfer one-carbon groups. It is essential in the de novo synthesis of nucleotides and in the metabolism of several amino acids, and is an integral component for the regeneration of the "universal" methyl donor, S-adenosylmethionine. Inhibition of bacterial and cancer cell folate metabolism is the basis for the sulfonamide antibiotics and chemotherapeutic agents such as methotrexate and 5-fluorouracil, respectively.	Women of childbearing age are most likely to be deficient. *Classic deficiency syndrome:* megaloblastic anemia, diarrhea. The hematopoietic cells in bone marrow become enlarged and have immature nuclei, reflecting ineffective DNA synthesis. The peripheral blood smear demonstrates macro-ovalocytes and polymorphonuclear leukocytes with an average of more than 3.5 nuclear lobes. Megaloblastic changes also occur in other epithelia that proliferate rapidly (e.g., oral mucosa, gastrointestinal tract), producing glossitis and diarrhea, respectively. Sulfasalazine and diphenytoin inhibit absorption and predispose to deficiency. [400 µg of dietary folate equivalents (DFE); 1 DFE = 1 µg food folate = 0.6 µg folic acid]	Doses >1000 µg/day may partially correct the anemia of B$_{12}$ deficiency and may therefore mask (and perhaps exacerbate) the associated neuropathy. Large doses also reported to lower seizure threshold in individuals prone to seizures. Parenteral administration is rarely reported to cause allergic phenomena, which is probably due to dispersion agents. [1000 µg]	Serum folate measures short-term folate balance, whereas RBC folate is a better reflection of tissue status. Serum homocysteine rises early in deficiency but is nonspecific because B$_{12}$ or B$_6$ deficiency, renal insufficiency, and older age may also cause elevations.

Continued on following page

	Biochemistry and Physiology	Deficiency [RDA*]	Toxicity [TUL†]	Assessment of Status
Vitamin C (ascorbic and dehydro-ascorbic acid)	Ascorbic acid readily oxidizes to dehydroascorbic acid in aqueous solution. The latter can be reduced in vivo, so it possesses vitamin C activity. Total vitamin C is therefore the sum of ascorbic and dehydroascorbic acid content. It serves primarily as a biologic antioxidant in aqueous environments. Biosyntheses of collagen, carnitine, bile acids, and norepinephrine, as well as proper functioning of the hepatic mixed-function oxygenase system, depend on this property. Vitamin C in foodstuffs increases the intestinal absorption of nonheme iron.	Overt deficiency is uncommon in developed countries. The classic deficiency syndrome is scurvy: fatigue, depression, and widespread abnormalities in connective tissues, such as inflamed gingivae, petechiae, perifollicular hemorrhages, impaired wound healing, coiled hairs, hyperkeratosis, bleeding into body cavities. In infants, defects in ossification and bone growth may occur. Tobacco smoking lowers plasma and leukocyte vitamin C levels. [F: 75 mg; M: 90 mg; increase requirement for cigarette smokers by 35 mg/day]	$\geq$500 mg/day (in adults) may cause nausea and diarrhea. >1 g/day modestly increases risk for oxalate kidney stones. Supplementation may interfere with laboratory tests based on redox potential (e.g., fecal occult blood testing, serum cholesterol, and glucose). Withdrawal from chronic ingestion of high doses of vitamin C supplements should be done gradually because accommodation appears to occur, raising a concern of "rebound scurvy." [2 g]	Plasma ascorbic acid concentration reflects recent dietary intake, whereas WBC levels more closely reflect tissue stores. Women's plasma levels are approximately 20% higher than men's for any given dietary intake.
Vitamin B_{12}	A group of closely related cobalamin compounds composed of a corrin ring (with a cobalt atom in its center) connected to a ribonucleotide through an aminopropanol bridge. Microorganisms are the ultimate source of all naturally occurring B_{12}. The two active coenzyme forms are deoxyadenosylcobalamin and methylcobalamin. These coenzymes are needed for the synthesis of succinyl coenzyme A (CoA), which is essential in lipid and carbohydrate metabolism, and for the synthesis of methionine. The latter reaction is essential for amino acid metabolism, for purine and pyrimidine synthesis, for many methylation reactions, and for the intracellular retention of folates.	Dietary inadequacy is a rare cause of deficiency except in strict vegetarians. Most deficiencies arise from loss of intestinal absorption, which may occur with pernicious anemia, pancreatic insufficiency, atrophic gastritis, small bowel bacterial overgrowth, or ileal disease. Megaloblastic anemia and megaloblastic changes in other epithelia (see "Folate") are the result of sustained depletion. Demyelination of peripheral nerves, posterior and lateral columns of spinal cord, and nerves within the brain may occur. Altered mentation, depression, and psychoses occur. Hematologic and neurologic complications may occur independently. Folate supplementation, in doses of 1000 µg/day, may partly correct the anemia, thereby masking (or perhaps exacerbating) the neuropathic complication. [2.4 µg]	A few allergic reactions have been reported to crystalline B_{12} preparations and are probably due to impurities, not the vitamin. [TUL not established]	Serum, or plasma, concentrations are generally accurate. Subtle deficiency with neurologic complications, as described in the "Deficiency" column, can best be established by concurrently measuring the concentration of plasma B_{12} and serum methylmalonic acid because the latter is a sensitive indicator of cellular deficiency.
Biotin	A bi-cyclic compound consisting of a ureido ring fused to a substituted tetrahydrothiophene ring. Endogenous synthesis by intestinal flora may contribute significantly to biotin nurtiture. Most dietary biotin is linked to lysine, a compound called biotinyl lysine, or biocytin. The lysine must be hydrolyzed by an intestinal enzyme called biotinidase before intestinal absorption occurs. Acts primarily as a coenzyme for several carboxylases; each holoenzyme catalyzes an ATP-dependent CO_2 transfer. The carboxylases are critical enzymes in carbohydrate and lipid metabolism.	Isolated deficiency is rare. Deficiency in humans has been produced by prolonged total parenteral nutrition lacking the vitamin and by ingestion of large quantities of raw egg white, which contains avidin, a protein that binds biotin with such high affinity that it renders it biounavailable. Alterations in mental status, myalgias, hyperesthesias, and anorexia occur. Later, a seborrheic dermatitis and alopecia develop. Deficiency is usually accompanied by lactic acidosis and organic aciduria. [30 µg]	Toxicity has not been reported in humans with doses as high as 60 mg/day in children. [TUL not established]	Plasma and urine concentrations of biotin are diminished in the deficient state. Elevated urine concentrations of methyl citrate, 3-methylcrotonylglycine, and 3-hydroxyisovalerate are also observed in deficiency.

	Biochemistry and Physiology	Deficiency [RDA*]	Toxicity [TUL†]	Assessment of Status
Pantothenic acid	Consists of pantoic acid linked to β-alanine through an amide bond. An essential component of CoA and phosphopantetheine, which are essential for synthesis and β-oxidation of fatty acids, as well as synthesis of cholesterol, steroid hormones, vitamins A and D, and other isoprenoid derivatives. CoA is also involved in the synthesis of several amino acids and δ-aminolevulinic acid, a precursor for the corrin ring of vitamin B_{12}, the porphyrin ring of heme, and of cytochromes. CoA is also necessary for the acetylation and fatty acid acylation of a variety of proteins.	Deficiency rare: only reported as a result of feeding semisynthetic diets or an antagonist to the vitamin. Experimental, isolated deficiency in humans produces fatigue, abdominal pain, vomiting, insomnia, and paresthesias of the extremities. [5 mg]	In doses of 10 g/day, diarrhea is reported to occur. [TUL not established]	Whole blood and urine concentrations of pantothenate are indicators of status; serum levels are not thought to be accurate.

PTH, Parathyroid hormone; *UVB*, ultraviolet B.

*Recommended daily allowance (RDA) established for female (F) and male (M) adults by the U.S. Food and Nutrition Board, 1999-2001. In some instances, insufficient data exist to establish an RDA, in which case the adequate intake (AI) established by the board is listed.

†Tolerated upper intake (TUL) established for adults by the U.S. Food and Nutrition Board, 1999-2001.

From Goldman L, Schafer AI: *Goldman's Cecil medicine,* ed 24, Philadelphia, 2012, Saunders.

Nutritional Trace Elements and Their Clinical Implications

	Biochemistry and Physiology	Deficiency [RDA*]	Toxicity [TUL†]	Assessment of Status
Chromium	Dietary chromium consists of both inorganic and organic forms. Its primary function in humans is to potentiate insulin action. It accomplishes this function as a circulating complex called *glucose tolerance factor*, thereby affecting carbohydrate, fat, and protein metabolism.	Deficiency in humans only described in long-term total parenteral nutrition (TPN) patients receiving insufficient chromium. Hyperglycemia or impaired glucose tolerance occurs. Elevated plasma free fatty acid concentrations, neuropathy, encephalopathy, and abnormalities in nitrogen metabolism are also reported. Whether supplemental chromium may improve glucose tolerance in glucose-intolerant individuals remains controversial. [F: 25 µg; M: 35 µg]	Toxicity after oral ingestion is uncommon and seems confined to gastric irritation. Airborne exposure may cause contact dermatitis, eczema, skin ulcers, and bronchogenic carcinoma. [no TUL established]	Plasma or serum concentration of chromium is a crude indicator of chromium status; it appears to be meaningful when the value is markedly above or below the normal range.
Copper	Copper is absorbed by a specific intestinal transport mechanism. It is carried to the liver where it is bound to ceruloplasmin, which circulates systemically and delivers copper to target tissues in the body. Excretion of copper is largely through bile, and then into the feces. Absorptive and excretory processes vary with the levels of dietary copper, providing a means of copper homeostasis. Copper serves as a component of many enzymes, including amine oxidases, ferroxidases, cytochrome c oxidase, dopamine β-hydroxylase, superoxide dismutase, and tyrosinase.	Dietary deficiency is rare; it has been observed in premature and low-birth-weight infants fed exclusively a cow's milk diet and in individuals on long-term TPN without copper. Clinical manifestations include depigmentation of skin and hair, neurologic disturbances, leukopenia, hypochromic microcytic anemia, and skeletal abnormalities. Anemia arises from impaired utilization of iron and is therefore a conditioned form of iron deficiency anemia. The deficiency syndrome, except the anemia and leukopenia, is also observed in Menkes' disease, a rare inherited condition associated with impaired copper utilization. [900 µg]	Acute copper toxicity has been described after excessive oral intake and with absorption of copper salts applied to burned skin. Milder manifestations include nausea, vomiting, epigastric pain, and diarrhea; coma and hepatic necrosis may ensue in severe cases. Toxicity may be seen with doses as low as 70 µg/kg/day. Chronic toxicity is also described. Wilson's disease is a rare, inherited disease associated with abnormally low ceruloplasmin levels and accumulation of copper in the liver and brain, eventually leading to damage to these two organs. [10 mg]	Practical methods for detecting marginal deficiency are not available. Marked deficiency is reliably detected by diminished serum copper and ceruloplasmin concentrations as well as low red blood cell (RBC) superoxide dismutase activity.
Fluorine	Known more commonly by its ionic form, fluoride. It is incorporated into the crystalline structure of bone, thereby altering its physical characteristics.	Intake of <0.1 mg/day in infants and <0.5 mg/day in children is associated with an increased incidence of dental caries. Optimal intake in adults is between 1.5 and 4 mg/day. [F: 3 mg; M: 4 mg]	Acute ingestion of >30 mg/kg body weight is likely to cause death. Excessive chronic intake (0.1 mg/kg/day) leads to mottling of teeth (dental fluorosis), calcification of tendons and ligaments, and exostoses and may increase the brittleness of bones. [10 mg]	Estimates of intake or clinical assessment are used because no good laboratory test exists.
Iodine	Readily absorbed from the diet, concentrated in the thyroid, and integrated into the thyroid hormones, thyroxine (T$_4$) and triiodothyronine (T$_3$). These hormones circulate largely bound to thyroxine-binding globulin. They modulate resting energy expenditure and, in the developing human, growth and development.	In the absence of supplementation, populations relying primarily on food from soils with low iodine content have endemic iodine deficiency. Maternal iodine deficiency leads to fetal deficiency, which produces spontaneous abortions, stillbirths, hypothyroidism, cretinism, and dwarfism. Permanent cognitive deficits may result from iodine deficiency during first 2 years of life. In the adult, compensatory hypertrophy of the thyroid goiter occurs along with varying degrees of hypothyroidism. [150 µg]	Large doses (>2 mg/day in adults) may induce hypothyroidism by blocking thyroid hormone synthesis. Supplementation with >100 mg/day to an individual who was formerly deficient occasionally induces hyperthyroidism. [1.1 mg]	Iodine status of a population can be estimated by the prevalence of goiter. Urinary excretion of iodine is an effective laboratory means of assessment. Thyroid-stimulating hormone (TSH) blood level is an indirect, and therefore not entirely specific, means of assessment.

1579

Continued on following page

	Biochemistry and Physiology	Deficiency [RDA*]	Toxicity [TUL†]	Assessment of Status
Iron	Conveys the capacity to participate in redox reactions to a number of metalloproteins such as hemoglobin, myoglobin, cytochrome enzymes, and many oxidases and oxygenases. Primary storage form is ferritin and, to a lesser degree, hemosiderin. Intestinal absorption is 15%-20% for "heme" iron and 1%-8% for iron contained in vegetables. Absorption of the latter form is enhanced by the ascorbic acid in foodstuffs; by poultry, fish, or beef; and by an iron-deficient state. It is decreased by phytate and tannins.	The most common micronutrient deficiency in the world. Women of childbearing age are the highest-risk group because of menstrual blood losses, pregnancy, and lactation. The classic deficiency syndrome is hypochromic, microcytic anemia. Glossitis and koilonychia ("spoon" nails) are also observed. Easy fatigability often is an early symptom, before anemia appears. In children, mild deficiency of insufficient severity to cause anemia is associated with behavioral disturbances and poor school performance. [postmenopausal F and M: 8 mg; premenopausal F: 18 mg]	Iron overload typically occurs when habitual dietary intake is extremely high, intestinal absorption is excessive, repeated parenteral administration occurs, or a combination of these factors exists. Excessive iron stores usually accumulate in the reticuloendothelial tissues and cause little damage ("hemosiderosis"). If overload continues, iron eventually begins to accumulate in tissues such as the hepatic parenchyma, pancreas, heart, and synovium, causing hemochromatosis. Hereditary hemochromatosis results from homozygosity of a common recessive trait. Excessive intestinal absorption of iron is seen in homozygotes. [45 mg]	Negative iron balance initially leads to depletion of iron stores in the bone marrow: a bone marrow biopsy and the concentration of serum ferritin are accurate indicators of early depletion. As the severity of deficiency proceeds, serum iron (SI) decreases and total iron-binding capacity (TIBC) increases: an iron saturation (SI/TIBC) of <16% suggests iron deficiency. Microcytosis, hypochromia, and anemia ensue. Elevated levels of serum ferritin or an iron saturation of >60% suggest iron overload, although systemic inflammation elevates serum ferritin regardless of iron status.
Manganese	A component of several metalloenzymes. Most manganese is in mitochondria, where it is a component of manganese superoxide dismutase.	Manganese deficiency in the human has not been conclusively demonstrated. It is said to cause hypocholesterolemia, weight loss, hair and nail changes, dermatitis, and impaired synthesis of vitamin K–dependent proteins. [F: 1.8 mg; M: 2.3 mg]	Toxicity by oral ingestion is unknown in humans. Toxic inhalation causes hallucinations, other alterations in mentation, and extrapyramidal movement disorders. [11 mg]	Until the deficiency syndrome is better defined, an appropriate measure of status will be difficult to develop.
Molybdenum	A cofactor in several enzymes, most prominently xanthine oxidase and sulfite oxidase.	A probable case of human deficiency is described as being secondary to parenteral administration of sulfite and resulted in hyperoxypurinemia, hypouricemia, and low sulfate excretion. [45 μg]	Toxicity not well described in humans, although it may interfere with copper metabolism at high doses. [2 mg]	Laboratory means of assessment not meaningful until deficiency syndrome is better described.
Selenium	Most dietary selenium is in the form of an amino acid complex. Nearly complete absorption of such forms occurs. Homeostasis is largely performed by the kidney, which regulates urinary excretion as a function of selenium status. Selenium is a component of several enzymes, most notably glutathione peroxidase and superoxide dismutase. These enzymes protect against oxidative and free radical damage of various cell structures. The antioxidant protection conveyed by selenium apparently operates in conjunction with vitamin E because deficiency of one seems to potentiate damage induced by a deficiency of the other. Selenium also participates in the enzymatic conversion of thyroxine to its more active metabolite, triiodothyronine.	Deficiency is rare in North America but has been observed in individuals on long-term TPN lacking selenium. Such individuals have myalgias and/or cardiomyopathies. Populations in some regions of the world, most notably some parts of China, have marginal intake of selenium. In these regions Keshan's disease, a condition characterized by cardiomyopathy, is endemic; it can be prevented (but not treated) by selenium supplementation. [55 μg]	Toxicity is associated with nausea, diarrhea, alterations in mental status, peripheral neuropathy, loss of hair and nails: such symptoms were observed in adults who inadvertently consumed 27-2400 mg. [400 μg]	Erythrocyte glutathione peroxidase activity and plasma, or whole blood, selenium concentrations are the most commonly used methods of assessment. They are moderately accurate indicators of status.

	Biochemistry and Physiology	Deficiency [RDA*]	Toxicity [TUL†]	Assessment of Status
Zinc	Intestinal absorption occurs by a specific process that is enhanced by pregnancy and corticosteroids and diminished by coingestion of phytates, phosphates, iron, copper, lead, or calcium. Diminished intake of zinc leads to an increased efficiency of absorption and decreased fecal excretion, providing a means of zinc homeostasis. Zinc is a component of more than 100 enzymes, among which are DNA polymerase, RNA polymerase, and transfer RNA synthetase.	Zinc deficiency has its most profound effect on rapidly proliferating tissues. *Mild deficiency:* growth retardation in children. *More severe deficiency:* growth arrest, teratogenicity, hypogonadism and infertility, dysgeusia, poor wound healing, diarrhea, dermatitis on the extremities and around orifices, glossitis, alopecia, corneal clouding, loss of dark adaptation, and behavioral changes. Impaired cellular immunity is observed. Excessive loss of gastrointestinal secretions through chronic diarrhea and fistulas may precipitate deficiency. Acrodermatitis enteropathica is a rare, recessively inherited disease in which intestinal absorption of zinc is impaired. [F: 8 mg; M: 11 mg]	Acute zinc toxicity can usually be induced by ingestion of >200 mg of zinc in a single day (in adults). It is manifested as epigastric pain, nausea, vomiting, and diarrhea. Hyperpnea, diaphoresis, and weakness may follow inhalation of zinc fumes. Copper and zinc compete for intestinal absorption: long-term ingestion of >25 mg/day of zinc may lead to copper deficiency. Long-term ingestion of >150 mg/day has been reported to cause gastric erosions, low high-density lipoprotein cholesterol levels, and impaired cellular immunity. [40 mg]	No accurate indicators of zinc status exist for routine clinical use. Plasma, RBC, and hair zinc concentrations are often misleading. Acute illness, in particular, is known to diminish plasma zinc levels, in part by inducing a shift of zinc out of the plasma compartment and into the liver. Functional tests that determine dark adaptation, taste acuity, and rate of wound healing lack specificity.

*Recommended daily allowance (RDA) established for female (F) and male (M) adults by the U.S. Food and Nutrition Board, 1999-2001. In some instances, insufficient data exist to establish an RDA, in which case the adequate intake (AI) established by the board is listed.

†Tolerated upper limit (TUL) established for adults by the U.S. Food and Nutrition Board, 1999-2001.

From Goldman L, Schafer AI: *Goldman's Cecil medicine,* ed 24, Philadelphia, 2012, Saunders.

Summary of Vitamin and Mineral Deficiencies

Vitamin and Mineral Deficiencies	Neurologic Syndrome or Syndromes	Supporting Tests	Treatment	Causes (Other Than Malnutrition)
A (retinol)	Blindness from retinal or corneal damage	Visual fields, visual acuity Serum level <30-65 µg/dl	30,000 IU vitamin A daily × 1 wk	Hypothyroidism, diabetes, renal or liver failure
B_1 (thiamine)	Wernicke's encephalopathy: ataxia, nystagmus, ophthalmoparesis, confusion, delirium Korsakoff's syndrome: amnesia, confabulation Beriberi: axonal neuropathy	MRI: symmetric lesions of midbrain (periaqueductal area), pons, hypothalamus, thalamus, cerebellum MRI: necrosis of mamillary bodies, dorsomedial and anterior thalamus Nerve conduction tests: decreased amplitude Serum thiamine level <20 ng/dl Erythrocyte transketolase	Prevent by 100 mg PO daily before and 1 year after bariatric surgery, 100 mg IV before glucose administration or refeeding Treat Wernicke's encephalopathy with 5 days of thiamine, 100-500 mg IV or IM daily, then PO 100 mg daily Antioxidants (N-acetylcysteine)	Alcoholism, bariatric or other major GI surgery, prolonged vomiting, hemodialysis, diuretic treatment of heart failure, cachexia, 5-fluorouracil, other blockers of thiamine phosphate production
B_3 (niacin)	Pellagra: confusion, dementia, weakness, ataxia, spasticity, myoclonus, glossitis, dermatitis, photosensitivity	Erythrocyte NAD, plasma niacin, urinary N_1-methylnicotinamide	Nicotinic acid, 50 mg PO tid or 25 mg IV tid; nicotinamide, 50-100 mg IM or PO tid	Alcoholism, corn- or cereal-based diet, Hartnup's syndrome, carcinoid syndrome
B_5 (pantothenic acid)	Dysesthesias, foot paresthesias	Deficient coenzyme A	5 mg PO daily	Severe malnutrition
B_6 (pyridoxine)	Neuropathy, sensory ataxia, depression Infantile pyridoxine-deficient epilepsy	Plasma PLP <27 nmol/L; urinary 4-pyridoxic acid, <3 nmol ↑ Homocysteine after methionine loading challenge ↑ α-AASA in urine, plasma, CSF	50-100 mg PO daily for neuropathy (preventive use if taking B_6 antagonist) 100-200 mg daily for adult epilepsy	Diverticulosis, isoniazid, cycloserine, other antagonists Genetic defects in antiquitin (aldehyde dehydrogenase), pyridoxal synthesis
B_{12} (cobalamin)	Myelopathy with spastic paraparesis and sensory ataxia, peripheral neuropathy, optic neuropathy, memory loss, dementia; indirect contributor to stroke	Blood level <200 pg/ml ↑ Methylmalonic acid >145 nmol/L Intrinsic factor antibodies Schilling test, megaloblastic anemia Delayed somatosensory evoked potentials ↑ Homocysteine, total >12.5 µmol/L	IM B_{12}, 1000 µg daily for 1 week, then weekly for 1 month, then monthly or oral B_{12}, 1000 µg daily, or nasal B_{12}, 500 µg weekly for lifetime if abnormal absorption, 50-100 µg daily if normal absorption	Achlorhydria, gastric or ileal resection, blind loop syndrome, sprue, HIV infection, nitrous oxide anesthesia (especially abuse), fish tapeworm, vegan diet
D (calciferol)	Proximal myopathy, often painful; cognitive impairment Secondary compression of spinal cord, plexus, or peripheral nerves from rickets or osteomalacia	25-(OH) vitamin D_3 level <10 ng/ml in urine Serum calcium ↑ PTH >54 pg/ml Osteopenia/porosis on bone densitometry	Daily supplementation with 400 IU, >50,000 IU 3 times per wk if malabsorption; use blood level or urine calcium excretion to guide (should be >100 mg/day)	Lack of exposure to sunlight, including sunblock protection; chronic antiepileptic drug use
E (tocopherol)	Spinal and cerebellar ataxia, Babinski's sign, ophthalmoplegia, peripheral neuropathy, retinitis pigmentosa	Vitamin E level <2.5 mg/L (normal, 6-15 with normal lipid level) ↑ A-β-lipoprotein levels, antigliadin antibodies Genetic analysis to rule out other spinocerebellar ataxias such as Friedreich's ataxia	Supplement with 6-800 IU, 5-10 mg/kg twice daily, for ataxia of genetic causes, water-soluble 200 mg/kg/day or IM α-tocopherol for malabsorption	Biliary atresia, celiac sprue, Genetic: ↓ α-tocopherol transport protein (8q13), microsomal triglyceride transfer protein

Continued on following page

Vitamin and Mineral Deficiencies	Neurologic Syndrome or Syndromes	Supporting Tests	Treatment	Causes (Other Than Malnutrition)
Folate	Dementia, B_{12} deficiency, stroke	↑ Homocysteine, plasma level <2.5 µg/L	1 mg 3 times per day until normal level, then maintenance of 1 mg/day Pregnancy: additional 0.4 mg/day if taking a folate antagonist	Malabsorption or use of antagonist (methotrexate) or antiepileptic medication
K (phytonadione)	Intracranial hemorrhage	INR or PT elevation	IM phytonadione at birth, maternal vitamin K for last month of pregnancy	Medication use that increases metabolism, such as phenytoin
Copper	Myelopathy, neuropathy	Serum Cu <75 µg/dl, ↓ urinary Cu, ceruloplasmin <23 mg/dl MRI: ↑ T_2 signal in cervical cord, dorsal column Mutation in ATP7A gene (Menkes' disease)	Elemental Cu, 8 mg/day PO week 1, 6 mg/day week 2, 4 mg/day week 3, 2 mg/day ongoing malabsorption Menkes' disease: 250 mg SC bid	Wilson's disease, Menkes' disease, alcoholism, malabsorption, gastric bypass, zinc toxicity
Magnesium	Seizures, encephalopathy	Serum magnesium <1.5 mg/dl, correct for low albumin	Magnesium sulfate IV or PO Avoid magnesium-wasting drugs	Alcoholism, especially beer
Potassium	Muscle weakness, chronic, acute	Serum potassium <3.5 mEq/L, ECG	IV or PO KCl until normalized	Diuretic use, bulimia

AASA, Aminoadipic semialdehyde; *CSF,* cerebrospinal fluid; *ECG,* electrocardiography; *GI,* gastrointestinal; *HIV,* human immunodeficiency virus; *INR,* international normalized ratio; *MRI,* magnetic resonance imaging; *NAD,* nicotinamide adenine dinucleotide; *PLP,* pyridoxal-5-phosphate (active coenzyme of pyridoxine); *PT,* prothrombin time; *PTH,* parathyroid hormone.
From Goldman *L,* Schafer AI: *Goldman's Cecil medicine,* ed 24, Philadelphia, 2012, Saunders.

Historical and Physical Findings in Poisoning

Sign	Toxin
Odor	
Bitter almonds	Cyanide
Acetone	Isopropyl alcohol, methanol, paraldehyde, salicylates
Alcohol	Ethanol
Wintergreen	Methyl salicylate
Garlic	Arsenic, thallium, organophosphates, selenium
Ocular Signs	
Miosis	Opioids (except propoxyphene, meperidine, and pentazocine), organophosphates and other cholinergics, clonidine, phenothiazines, sedative-hypnotics, olanzapine
Mydriasis	Atropine, cocaine, amphetamines, antihistamines, TCAs, carbamazepine, serotonin syndrome, PCP, LSD, postanoxic encephalopathy
Nystagmus	Phenytoin, barbiturates, sedative-hypnotics, alcohols, carbamazepine, PCP, ketamine, dextromethorphan
Lacrimation	Organophosphates, irritant gas or vapors
Retinal hyperemia	Methanol
Cutaneous Signs	
Diaphoresis	Organophosphates, salicylates, cocaine and other sympathomimetics, serotonin syndrome, withdrawal syndromes
Alopecia	Thallium, arsenic
Erythema	Boric acid, elemental mercury, cyanide, carbon monoxide, disulfuram, scombroid, anticholinergics
Cyanosis (unresponsive to oxygen)	Methemoglobinemia (e.g., benzocaine, dapsone, nitrites, phenazopyridine), amiodarone, silver
Oral Signs	
Salivation	Organophosphates, salicylates, corrosives, ketamine, PCP, strychnine
Oral burns	Corrosives, oxalate-containing plants
Gum lines	Lead, mercury, arsenic, bismuth
Gastrointestinal Signs	
Diarrhea	Antimicrobials, arsenic, iron, boric acid, cholinergics, colchicine, withdrawal
Hematemesis	Arsenic, iron, caustics, NSAIDs, salicylates
Cardiac Signs	
Tachycardia	Sympathomimetics (e.g., amphetamines, cocaine), anticholinergics, antidepressants, theophylline, caffeine, antipsychotics, atropine, salicylates, cellular asphyxiants (cyanide, carbon monoxide, hydrogen sulfide), withdrawal
Bradycardia	β-Blockers, calcium channel blockers, digoxin, clonidine and other central α_2 agonists, organophosphates, opioids, sedative-hypnotics
Hypertension	Sympathomimetics (amphetamines, cocaine, LSD), anticholinergics, clonidine (early), monoamine oxidase inhibitors
Hypotension	β-Blockers, calcium channel blockers, cyclic antidepressants, iron, phenothiazines, barbiturates, clonidine, theophylline, opioids, arsenic, amatoxin mushrooms, cellular asphyxiants (cyanide, carbon monoxide, hydrogen sulfide), snake envenomation
Respiratory Signs	
Depressed respirations	Opioids, sedative-hypnotics, alcohol, clonidine, barbiturates
Tachypnea	Salicylates, amphetamines, caffeine, metabolic acidosis (ethylene glycol, methanol, cyanide), carbon monoxide, hydrocarbons

Continued on following page

Sign	Toxin
Central Nervous System Signs	
Ataxia	Alcohol, anticonvulsants, benzodiazepines, barbiturates, lithium, dextromethorphan, carbon monoxide, inhalants
Coma	Opioids, sedative-hypnotics, anticonvulsants, cyclic antidepressants, antipsychotics, ethanol, anticholinergics, clonidine, GHB, alcohols, salicylates, barbiturates
Seizures	Sympathomimetics, anticholinergics, antidepressants (especially TCAs, bupropion, venlafaxine), isoniazid, camphor, lindane, salicylates, lead, organophosphates, carbamazepine, tramadol, lithium, ginkgo seeds, water hemlock, withdrawal
Delirium/psychosis	Sympathomimetics, anticholinergics, LSD, PCP, hallucinogens, lithium, dextromethorphan, steroids, withdrawal
Peripheral neuropathy	Lead, arsenic, mercury, organophosphates

GHB, Gamma hydroxybutyrate; *LSD,* lysergic acid diethylamide; *NSAID,* nonsteroidal anti-inflammatory drug; *PCP,* phencyclidine; *TCA,* tricylic antidepressant.
From Goldman L, Schafer AI: *Goldman's Cecil medicine,* ed 24, Philadelphia, 2012, Saunders.

Recognizable Poison Syndromes

Poison Syndrome	SIGNS						Possible Toxins
	Vital	Mental Status	Pupils	Skin	Bowel Sounds	Other	
Sympathomimetic	Hypertension, tachycardia, hyperthermia	Agitated, psychosis, delirium	Dilated	Diaphoretic	Normal to increased		Amphetamines, cocaine, Ecstasy, pseudoephedrine, caffeine, theophylline
Anticholinergic	Hypertension, tachycardia, hyperthermia	Agitation, delirium, mumbling speech	Dilated	Dry	Decreased		Antihistamines, tricyclic antidepressants, atropine, jimson weed, phenothiazines
Cholinergic	Bradycardia (although may show tachycardia), BP and temp typically normal	Confusion, coma, fasciculations	Small	Diaphoretic	Hyperactive	Diarrhea, urination, bronchorrhea, bronchospasm, emesis, lacrimation, salivation	Organophosphates, nerve gases, Alzheimer medications
Opioids	Respiratory depression (hallmark of toxicity), bradycardia, hypotension, hypothermia	Depression, coma	Pinpoint	Normal	Normal to decreased		Methadone, suboxone, morphine, oxycodone, heroin, etc.
Sedative-hypnotics	Respiratory depression, HR normal to decreased, BP normal to decreased, temp normal to decreased	Somnolence, coma	Small	Normal	Normal		Barbiturates, benzodiazepines, ethanol
Serotonin syndrome	Hyperthermia, tachycardia, hypertension or hypotension (autonomic instability)	Agitation, confusion, coma	Dilated	Diaphoretic	Increased	Neuromuscular hyperexcitability: clonus, hyperreflexia (lower extremities > upper extremities)	SSRIs, lithium, MAOIs, linezolid, tramadol, meperidine, dextromethorphan
Salicylates	Tachypnea, hyperpnea, tachycardia, hyperthermia	Agitation, confusion, coma	Normal	Diaphoretic	Normal	Nausea, vomiting, tinnitus, ABG with primary respiratory alkalosis and primary metabolic acidosis	Aspirin, bismuth subsalicylate (Pepto-Bismol), methylsalicylates
Withdrawal	Tachycardia, tachypnea, hyperthermia	Lethargy, confusion, delirium	Dilated	Diaphoretic	Increased		Withdrawal from opioids, sedative-hypnotics, ethanol

ABG, Arterial blood gas; *BP,* blood pressure; *HR,* heart rate; *MAOI,* monoamine oxidase inhibitor; *SSRI,* selective serotonin reuptake inhibitor; *temp,* temperature.
From Kliegman RM et al: *Nelson textbook of pediatrics,* ed 19, Philadelphia, 2011, Saunders.

Antidotes and Indications for Use

Antidote	Indication for Use	Dose*	Treatment End Point	Comments
Antivenom (Fab)†	Crotalines	4-6 vials; repeat for persistent or worsening clinical condition; repeat doses of 2 vials at 6, 12, and 18 hr after initial antivenom dose(s) are recommended	Halt in progression of circumferential and proximal swelling Resolving systemic effects	Better safety profile than equine-derived antivenom Repetitive dosing indicated for recurrent soft tissue swelling
Antivenom, *Latrodectus* (equine)†	Black widow spider (*Latrodectus* sp.)	1 vial diluted in 100 ml NS, infused over 1 hr; can repeat	Resolution of symptoms, vital signs normal	Dilution and slow infusion rate are critical to avoid anaphylactoid reaction Indications include severe pain unresponsive to opioids and severe hypertension Serum sickness can occur IV calcium is ineffective
Atropine	Carbamates Nerve agents Organophosphorus compounds	2 mg IV; double the dose every 5 min to achieve atropinization and hemodynamic stability; then start continuous infusion of 10%-20% of total stabilizing dose per hr	Cessation of excessive oral and pulmonary secretions, >80 bpm, systolic blood pressure >80 mm Hg	Doubling of the dose every 5 min (e.g., 2 mg, 4 mg, 8 mg, 16 mg) estimated to achieve atropinization within 30 min Stop infusion if patient develops any signs or symptoms of anticholinergic toxidrome; restart infusion at lower rate when signs or symptoms abate
Calcium‡	Calcium-channel antagonists	Calcium chloride 10%, 20-50 mg (0.2-0.5 ml)/kg/hr	Reversal of hypotension; may not reverse bradycardia	All indications: Monitor ionized calcium levels IV extravasation causes tissue necrosis, especially with calcium chloride Can administer at faster than stated rates for immediate life-threatening conditions Taper infusions and monitor for relapse of toxicity when discontinuing therapy Calcium chloride contains three times more elemental calcium than calcium gluconate does Calcium-channel antagonists may be ineffective in severe toxicity
	Hydrofluoric acid	Systemic toxicity: calcium gluconate 10%, 1-3 g (10-30 ml) per dose IV over 10-min period; repeat as needed every 5-10 min	Reversal of life-threatening manifestations of hypocalcemia and hyperkalemia	Can dilute and give intraarterially or IV with a Bier block for extremity exposures and burns
	Hyperkalemia (except cardiac glycosides)	Calcium gluconate 10%, 1 g (10 ml) per dose IV over 10-min period; repeat as needed every 5-10 min	Reversal of myocardial depression and conduction delays	May precipitate ventricular arrhythmias
	Hypermagnesemia	Calcium gluconate 10%, 1-2 g (10-20 ml) per dose IV over 10-min period; repeat as needed every 5-10 min	Reversal of respiratory depression, hypotension, and cardiac conduction blocks	Simultaneous therapies to increase magnesium elimination should be instituted
	Hypocalcemia (e.g., ethylene glycol)	Calcium gluconate 10%, 0.5-1.0 g (5-10 ml) per dose over 10-min period; repeat as needed every 10 min	Reversal of tetany	Correct symptomatic hypocalcemia; avoid excessive administration that may increase production of calcium oxalate crystals in ethylene glycol poisoning

Continued on following page

Antidote	Indication for Use	Dose*	Treatment End Point	Comments
L-Carnitine	Valproate-induced hyperammonemia or hepatotoxicity	100 mg/kg (maximum 6 g) IV over 30 min, then 15 mg/kg IV over 30-min period q4h (max 6 g/day)	Treat until clinical improvement occurs	Levocarnitine is active form Adjust dose for end-stage renal disease
Cyanide antidote kit	Cyanide		Resolution of lactic acidosis and moderate to severe clinical signs and symptoms: seizures, coma, dyspnea, apnea, hypotension, bradycardia	
Amyl nitrate		Amyl nitrite: 0.3-ml pearls, crush and inhale over 30-sec period		Coordinate amyl nitrite with continued oxygenation and give only until sodium nitrite infusion is begun; nitrites may produce hypotension and excess methemoglobinemia
Sodium nitrite		Sodium nitrite 3%: 10 ml IV over 10-min period		Sodium nitrite dose must be adjusted if patient has hemoglobin <12 g/dl
Sodium thiosulfate		Sodium thiosulfate 25%: 50 ml (12.5 g) IV over 10-min period		Sodium thiosulfate dosing can be repeated
Deferoxamine	Iron	15 ml/kg/hr IV (max 8 g/day) Mild to moderate: administer for 6-12 hr Severe toxicity: administer 24 hr	Resolution of clinical signs and symptoms Do not use urine color, which is an unreliable marker for iron clearance	Indications: symptomatic patients with lethargy, severe abdominal pain, hypovolemia, acidosis, shock; any symptomatic patient with peak serum iron level >350 g/dl Prolonged therapy can cause pulmonary toxicity
Digoxin-specific antibody fragments (Fab)	Digoxin Digitalis Other cardiac glycosides (e.g., bufodienalides [*Bufo toads*], oleander)	Unknown digoxin dose or serum level or for plant or toad source: acute toxicity—10-20 vials; chronic toxicity—3-6 vials Digoxin dose known: number of vials = (mg ingested × 0.8) ÷ 0.5 Digoxin serum level known: number of vials = [serum level (ng/ml) × weight (kg)] ÷ 100	Resolution of hyperkalemia, symptomatic bradydysrhythmias, ventricular arrhythmias, Mobitz II or third-degree heart block	Each vial binds 0.5 mg of digoxin or digitoxin Monitor ECG and potassium levels Digoxin serum levels unreliable after antidote administered unless test is specific for free serum digoxin
Dimercaprol (BAL)	Arsenic Lead Mercury, elemental and inorganic salts	Arsenic: 3-5 mg/kg IM q4h Lead: 75 mg/m² (4 mg/kg) IM q4h for 5 days Inorganic mercury: 5 mg/kg IM, then 2.5 mg/kg IM q12h for 10 days or until patient clinically improved	Arsenic: 24-hr urinary arsenic <50 µg/L Lead: encephalopathy resolved, blood lead level <100 µg/dl, and succimer therapy can be started Mercury, elemental and inorganic: 24-hr urinary mercury <20 µg/L	Maximum adult dose is 3 g/day BAL started 4 hr before initiation of concomitant CaNa₂EDTA for lead encephalopathy Dosing not well established for arsenic and elemental or inorganic mercury toxicity; not used for organic mercury poisoning Adverse effects: painful injections, fever, diaphoresis, agitation, headache, salivation, nausea and vomiting, hemolysis in G6PD-deficient patients, chelation of essential metals Check essential metal levels if chelation is prolonged Succimer is replacing BAL for many indications except lead encephalopathy Treatment end points for arsenic and mercury include improving clinical condition
Edetate calcium disodium (CaNa₂EDTA)	Lead	1500 mg/m²/24 hr (max 3 g) by continuous infusion	Treat for 5 days, followed by 2-day hiatus; repeat until encephalopathy resolved, lead level <100 µg/dl, and succimer therapy can be started	Use in patients with lead encephalopathy or lead level >100 g/dl Administer BAL 4 hr before initiating CaNa₂EDTA Hydrate patient and establish good urinary output before starting therapy Avoid thrombophlebitis by diluting in NS or D₅W to a concentration ≤0.5% Substitution of Na₂EDTA can cause fatal hypocalcemia
Flumazenil	Benzodiazepines Venlafaxine	0.1 mg/min IV to a total dose of 1 mg	Reversal of respiratory depression	Limit use to reversal of inadequate respiration in benzodiazepine-toxic patients Increases intracranial pressure and risk for seizures in presence of underlying seizure disorder or ingestion of seizure-producing toxicants Monitor for resedation up to 2 hr after last dose

Antidote	Indication for Use	Dose*	Treatment End Point	Comments
Folinate (tetra-hydrofolic acid [leuco-vorin])	Methanol Methotrexate	Methanol: 50 mg IV q4h Methotrexate: 100 mg/m² IV q3-6h	Methanol: methanol undetect-able, metabolic acidosis cleared Methotrexate: serum level <1 × 10⁻⁸ mol/L	Essential therapy for both toxicants Methotrexate: large ingestions may require increased dose Glucarpidase administered 2-4 hr before or after folinate
Fomepizole	Ethylene glycol Methanol	Dose 1: 15 mg/kg IV Doses over next 48 hr: 10 mg/kg IV All subsequent doses: 15 mg/kg IV Administer q12h, except when HD per-formed: HD initiation: ½ next dose if >6 hr since last dose HD ongoing: q4h End of HD (based on time of last dose): <1 hr, no dose; 1-3 hr, ½ next dose; >3 hr, next dose	For both: serum level <20 mg/dl and metabolic acidosis resolved	Start immediately if toxic alcohol suspected, without waiting for confirmatory levels Dose amount is not affected by interval timing of doses
Glucagon	β-Adrenergic receptor antagonists Calcium-channel antagonists	Bolus of 3.5-5 mg IV; can repeat to achieve clinical effect, then infusion of 2-10 mg/hr	Reversal of hypotension and bradycardia; taper infusion	Can precipitate vomiting; be prepared to protect airway Mild hyperglycemia occurs Maximum dosing amounts unknown; bolus doses up to 30 mg reported Duration of effect is 15 min; thus infusion must be started immediately
Hydroxocobala-min	Cyanide	Initial: 5 g IV over 15-min period Second dose: 5 g IV over 15 min–2 hr; maximum total dose is 10 g Follow each hydroxocobalamin dose with sodium thiosulfate 25%: 50 ml (12.5 g) IV over 10-min period	Resolution of lactic acidosis and moderate to severe clinical signs and symp-toms: seizures, coma, dys-pnea, apnea, hypotension, bradycardia	Can be administered IV push if patient is in cardiac arrest Do not give hydroxocobalamin and sodium thiosulfate through the same IV line Adverse effects: red discoloration of plasma, urine, mucous membranes, skin; transient hypertension Interference with laboratory colorometric assays: Levels increased: bilirubin; creatinine; glucose; hemoglobin; magnesium; co-oximetry total Hb, COHb%, MetHb% Levels decreased: AST, ALT, creatinine, co-oximetry O₂Hb%
Hyperbaric oxy-gen (HBO)	Carbon monoxide Experimental: carbon tetrachloride, cya-nide, hydrogen sulfide	3.0 atm pressure for 60 min (25 min O₂, 5 min air, 25 min O₂, 5 min air), then 2.0 atm for 65 min (30 min O₂, 5 min air, 30 min O₂), then "surface" to 1.0 atm	One treatment Second treatment rarely ad-ministered (controversial)	Carbon monoxide: treatment protocols may vary HBO indicated for loss of consciousness; seizures; cerebellar dysfunction; impaired cognition; headache, nausea/vomiting persisting after 4 hr O₂ therapy regardless of carboxyhemoglobin level Experimental indications: treatment protocols not established
Insulin-glucose	Calcium-channel an-tagonists β-Adrenergic receptor antagonists	Regular insulin, 1 U/kg bolus, followed by 0.5-1 U/kg/hr Titrate 50% dextrose IV to avoid hypo-glycemia	Reversal of myocardial de-pression	Beneficial in case series and reports Initiate if glucagon and vasopressor or inotropic drugs fail to reverse myocardial depression; more effective if used before onset of cardiogenic shock Monitor glucose and potassium; hypoglyce-mia can occur during and after therapy Hyperglycemia results from toxicant-induced insulin resistance, and initial dextrose re-quirements may be less than anticipated. Recovery may be heralded by normalization of glucose levels, with increased dextrose required to avoid hypoglycemia
Intralipid	Cardiac toxicity from local anesthetics (e.g., bupivacaine, ropivacaine) Experimental: vera-pamil, diltiazem, tricyclic antidepres-sants, bupropion, propranolol	Use 20% formulation Initial bolus: 1.5 ml/kg IV over 1 min, followed immediately by infusion of 0.25 ml/kg/min for 30-60 min Can repeat bolus for asystole	Return of hemodynamic stability	Use based on animal experiments and human case reports; numerous dosing regimens have been used Use if advanced life support measures fail; continue CPR as needed during drug administration

Continued on following page

Antidote	Indication for Use	Dose*	Treatment End Point	Comments
Methylene blue	Methemoglobin-producing agents	1-2 mg/kg body weight (0.1-0.2 ml/kg) of 1% methylene blue is administered over 5-min period; repeat dose for persistent or recurrent symptoms or signs	Resolution of dyspnea and altered mental status	Use if patient is symptomatic (i.e., dyspneic, altered mental status) Maximum dose should not exceed 7 mg/kg (0.7 ml/kg) Contraindicated in G6PD-deficient patients; may cause hemolysis Some toxicants (e.g., dapsone) may require prolonged therapy
N-Acetylcysteine (NAC)	Acetaminophen Experimental: carbon tetrachloride, chloroform, pennyroyal oil	Oral: Load—140 mg/kg Maintenance (starting 4 hr after load)—70 mg/kg q4h IV: Load—150 mg/kg over 1-hr period Maintenance infusion—12.5 mg/kg over 4-hr period, then 6.25 mg/kg per hour as continuous infusion	Administer 24 hr of NAC and repeat AST and APAP levels: if AST normal and APAP not detected, stop NAC; if AST normal and APAP detected, continue NAC for 12 hr, then reassess AST and APAP levels; if AST elevated, continue NAC for total of 72 hr of therapy After 72 hr of therapy, if INR <2.0, stop NAC After patient has received 72 hr of therapy, if INR ≥2.0 or severe hepatotoxicity present, continue NAC until INR <2.0	Most effective if initiated within 8 hr after ingestion; may be started any time after ingestion and is beneficial in severe hepatotoxic states Use IV in patients unable to tolerate PO or with severe hepatotoxicity; the dose and timing differ from the oral regimen Dosage and administration of FDA-approved IV formulation assume early treatment of acute overdose without hepatotoxicity; longer duration of treatment required in patients with hepatotoxicity Treatment end points simplified for ease of use INR result not valid indicator if FFP recently administered
Naloxone	Opioids	Bolus: 0.4-2 mg via IV, sublingual injection, or endotracheal instillation; 0.4-0.8 mg SC Continuous infusion: establish bolus dose required to reverse respiratory depression Begin infusing two thirds of reversal dose every hour, and titrate to maintain adequate respirations Rebolus with half of reversal dose 15 min after reversing respiratory depression	Initial: reversal of respiratory depression with resolution of hypoxia and hypercapnia Final: resolution of CNS and respiratory depression	Preventilate patients with respiratory depression by bag-valve mask or intubation before administration Use smaller doses in opioid-dependent patients; some opioids (e.g., propoxyphene, pentazocine, fentanyls) may require larger doses of naloxone; use continuous infusion for recurrent symptoms and prolonged action of some formulations (e.g., sustained-release morphine, methadone) Resedation can occur Do not use nalmefene or naltrexone to reverse acute toxicity
Octreotide	Sulfonylureas	50 mg SC q6h	Resolution of hypoglycemia and dextrose not required	Maintain dextrose infusion as needed
Physostigmine	Anticholinergic agents (e.g., diphenhydramine, jimsonweed [*Datura* sp.], scopolamine)	1-2 mg IV over 5-min period; can repeat once after 10-15 min if no effect	Reversal of anticholinergic effects	Duration of effect is 60-90 min Benzodiazepine used for subsequent treatment of agitation and seizures; additional physostigmine used rarely (e.g., refractory seizures or agitation) Adverse effects include seizures, excessive oral secretions, bradyarrhythmias; contraindicated in cyclic antidepressant toxicity
Pralidoxime chloride	Organophosphorus compounds Nerve agents—sarin, VX	30 mg/kg IV bolus (max 2 g) over 30 min, followed by continuous infusion of 8-10 mg/kg/hr (max 650 mg/hr)	Resolution of signs and symptoms, atropine no longer required	Can give initial dose over 2-min period for life-threatening clinical effects Administer early when diagnosis known or strongly suspected Efficacy variable, depending on the organophosphate Fat-soluble organophosphates may require prolonged treatment
Pyridoxine	Ethylene glycol (theoretical efficacy)	100 mg IV	One dose	Efficacy theoretical Pyridoxine may stop seizures, but patient can remain comatose (isoniazid, mushrooms); use benzodiazepines and phenobarbital concomitantly to manage seizures Excessive dosing can cause neuropathy
	Isoniazid Monomethylhydrazine mushrooms	5 g IV, repeat for refractory seizures	Resolution of seizures	

Antidote	Indication for Use	Dose*	Treatment End Point	Comments
Sodium bicarbonate (NaHCO₃)	Reversal of myocardial sodium-channel blockers (e.g., cyclic antidepressants, cocaine, propoxyphene, sodium-channel-blocking antiarrhythmics with $\tau_{recovery}$ >1 sec, piperidine phenothiazines (thioridazine, mesoridazine)	1-2 mEq NaHCO₃/kg via intermittent bolus; repeat as needed	Narrowing of prolonged QRS, resolution of ventricular arrhythmias, reversal of hypotension	Monitor blood pH (optimal pH approximately 7.50); avoid pH > 7.55
	Altered tissue distribution or enhanced elimination of salicylates; may be used in chlorophenoxy herbicides, chlorpropamide, formic acid, methotrexate, phenobarbital	1-2 mEq NaHCO₃/kg, followed by 3 ampules (150 ml) NaHCO₃ (44 mEq per 50 ml) in 850 ml of D₅W, infused at 2-3 times normal maintenance fluid rate	Serum salicylate <30 mg/dl and patient clinically stable	Monitor urinary pH hourly; adjust infusion to maintain urine pH of 7.5-8.0 (avoid blood pH >7.55) Monitor ABGs Maintain normokalemia
Succimer (DMSA)	All forms: Arsenic Lead Mercury	10 mg/kg/dose q8h for 5 days, followed by q12h for 14 days Drug holiday for 2 wk; repeat if treatment end point not reached	Arsenic: 24-hr urinary arsenic <50 µg/L Lead: resolution of encephalopathy, gastrointestinal symptoms, neuropathy, nephropathy, arthralgias, myalgias, and blood lead level <70 µg/dl Mercury, elemental and inorganic: 24-hr urinary mercury <20 µg/L Mercury, organic: end point not well established	Oral chelator; adverse effects include rash, transient AST and alkaline phosphatase elevations, and gastrointestinal distress; minimal chelation of essential metals occurs Dosing for arsenic and mercury not well established Therapeutic end point for organic mercury not established; neurotoxicity not responsive to chelation therapy; suggest chelation until blood mercury level within normal value range for reference laboratory
Vitamin K	Anticoagulants (e.g., warfarin, long-acting anticoagulant rodenticides [LAARs])	Subcutaneous: AquaMEPHYTON (K₁), 10-25 mg, repeat every 6-12 hr until oral vitamin K₁ started Oral: 25-50 mg q6h; larger doses may be required	INR is normal 48-72 hr after stopping vitamin K₁ therapy Can also monitor factor VII activity	Anaphylactoid reaction can occur with IV administration Severe bleeding may also require FFP or factor concentrates Base decision to treat on finding of elevated INR; do not administer prophylactic vitamin K₁ Oral therapy has been required for months with LAAR poisoning because of lipophilicity of toxicant, with slow body clearance

ABG, Arterial blood gas; *ALT*, alanine aminotransferase; *APAP*, acetyl-para-aminophenol (acetaminophen); *AST*, aspartate aminotransferase; *BAL*, British antilewisite; bpm, beats per minute; *CNS*, central nervous system; *COHb%*, percent carboxyhemoglobin; *CPR*, cardiopulmonary resuscitation; *D₅W*, 5% dextrose in water; *DMSA*, 2,3-dimercaptosuccinic acid; *ECG*, electrocardiogram; *FDA*, Food and Drug Administration; *FFP*, fresh-frozen plasma; *G6PD*, glucose-6-phosphate dehydrogenase; *Hb*, hemoglobin; *HD*, hemodialysis; *IM*, intramuscular; *INR*, international normalized ratio; *IV*, intravenous; *MetHb%*, percent methemoglobinemia; *NS*, normal saline; *O₂Hb%*, percent oxyhemoglobin; *PO*, per os (by mouth); *SC*, subcutaneous; $\tau_{recovery}$, drug blockade recovery rate.

*Dose concentrations and infusion times are not given. Drug dosages may require adjustment in patients with renal or hepatic failure.

†Administer antivenom in a monitored setting; antivenom must be reconstituted and then diluted; initially infuse at a rate of 2 to 5 ml/hr, and double the infusion rate every 5 minutes as tolerated to administer antivenom over a 1-hour period.

‡Ten percent calcium chloride solution = 100 mg/ml (27.2 mg/ml elemental calcium); 10% calcium gluconate solution = 100 mg/ml (9 mg/ml elemental calcium).

From Goldman L, Schafer AI: *Goldman's Cecil medicine*, ed 24, Philadelphia, 2012, Saunders.

A

AA. *See* Secondary amyloidosis
AAA. *See* Abdominal aortic aneurysm
AADC. *See* Aromatic amino acid decarboxylase deficiency
AATD. *See* Alpha-1-antitrypsin deficiency
Abacavir (ABC)
  for AIDS, 33
  for HIV, 557
Abatacept
  for juvenile idiopathic arthritis, 632
  for RA, 977
ABCD. *See* Amphotericin B colloidal dispersion
Abciximab, for ACS, 41
Abdominal aortic aneurysm (AAA), **78–79, 79.e1**, 78f, 79f
  differential diagnosis for, 1322f
Abdominal calcification, non-visceral on x-ray, 1210–1211
Abdominal compartment syndrome (ACS), 284.e1b
Abdominal nodes, lymphadenopathy of, 1257
Abdominal pain
  adolescence, 1191
  arthritis and, 1201
  childhood, 1191
  chronic lower, 1191
  differential diagnosis of, 1191–1192
  diffuse, 1191
  epigastric, 1191, 1226
  fever and rash with, 1229
  infancy, 1191
  left lower quadrant, 1191
  left upper quadrant, 1191–1192
  by location, 1191–1192
  nonsurgical causes of, 1192
  poorly localized, 1192
  in pregnancy, 1192
  right lower quadrant, 1192
  right upper quadrant, 1192
  suprapubic, 1192
Abdominal pregnancy, **364–365, 365.e1**, 364f, 365.e1f
Abdominal wall masses, 1192–1193
Abetalipoproteinemia, 1340.e6f
ABI. *See* Ankle-brachial index
Abiraterone, for prostate cancer, 929
Ablation therapy
  for atrial fibrillation, 130, 131.e4f, 131.e3f
  for atrial flutter, 133
  for benign prostatic hyperplasia, 932
  for hyperparathyroidism, 577
ABLC. *See* Amphotericin B lipid complex
ABMT. *See* Allogenic bone marrow transplantation
Abortion
  recurrent, differential diagnosis of, 1193
  spontaneous, **1040**, 1040.e1f

Bolded page numbers indicate principal textual treatment.

Page numbers followed by f indicate figures; t, tables; b, boxes; e, online content.

ABPA. *See* Allergic bronchopulmonary aspergillosis
Abrasion, corneal, **297**, 297f
Abruptio placentae, **3–4**
Abscess
  anal, differential diagnosis of, 1197–1198
  brain, **4**, 4t, 5f, 5.e1b, 731, 1454t
  breast, **6, 6.e1**
  epidural, **7, 7.e1, 1035**, 1036f, 1036.e1f
  liver, **8–9, 9.e1**, 8t, 8b, 9f
  lung, **10–11, 11.e1**, 10t, 11f
  parameningeal, 1454t
  pelvic, **12, 12.e1**, 12.e1f
  perirectal, **13, 13.e1**, 13f
  peritonsillar, **14, 14.e1**, 14.e1f
  renal, **15, 15.e1**, 15f
  retropharyngeal, **16–17**, 16f, 17f
Absence seizures, **1001, 1001.e1**
ABSSSIs. *See* Acute bacterial skin and skin structure infections
Abuse
  alcohol, **21–23, 23.e1**, 21t, 22t, **51–53, 53.e1, 53.e2**, 52f, 53.e1t, 53.e2f, 53.e1b
  child, **18–20, 20.e1, 20.e2**, 18f, 19f, 19t, 20.e1b, 20.e2f
  drug, **21–23, 23.e1**, 21t, 22t, 23.e1b
  elder, **24, 24.e1, 24.e2**, 24.e1f
  narcotic, **793–794, 794.e1**
  opiate, **793–794, 794.e1**
Abusive head trauma, **1012**, 1012f
  child, **18–20, 20.e1, 20.e2**, 18f, 19f, 19t, 20.e1b, 20.e2f
ABVD. *See* Doxorubicin plus bleomycin plus vincristine plus dacarbazine
ACA. *See* Anticardiolipin antibody
Acamprosate, for alcohol abuse, 23, 53, 53.e1t
Acarbose
  for DM, 334, 335t
  for dumping syndrome, 348
Acceleration flexion-extension neck injury, **1182**, 1182t
Accutane. *See* Isotretinoin
ACD. *See* Anemia of chronic disease
ACE. *See* Angiotensin-converting enzyme
ACE inhibitors. *See also specific agents*
  for cardiorenal syndrome, 224
  for CKD, 257–258
  for dilated cardiomyopathy, 214–215
Acetadote. *See* N-acetylcysteine
Acetaminophen (APAP)
  jaundice due to, 629–630
  for osteoarthritis, 806
  for varicella, 1153
  for whiplash injury, 1182
Acetaminophen (APAP) poisoning, **25, 25.e1, 25.e2**, 25.e1b, 25.e2f
  pathophysiology, clinical effects, and management of, 1408–1411
Acetazolamide
  for high-altitude sickness, 537
  for idiopathic intracranial hypertension, 601
  for Meniere's disease, 697
Acetone, serum or plasma, 1445
Acetylcholine receptor (AChR) antibody, 1445

Achalasia, **26–27, 27.e1**, 26t, 27f, 27.e1b, 358.e1b
Aches and pains. *See also* Pain
  diffuse, differential diagnosis of, 1193
  muscle cramps and aches, 1390f
Achilles tendon rupture, **28, 28.e1**, 28f, 28.e1b
AChR. *See* Acetylcholine receptor
Acid phosphatase, serum, 1445
Acid serum test, 1463
Acid-base disorders, 1445t
Acid-base homeostasis, 1306f
Acid-base reference values, 1445t
Acidosis
  anion gap, differential diagnosis of, 1200
  differential diagnosis of, 1193–1194
  lactic, differential diagnosis of, 1193
  metabolic
    arterial blood gases, 1448
    assessment of, 1306f
    clinical algorithm for, 1307–1308
    differential diagnosis of, 1193
    hyperchloric, 1193
    laboratory findings in, 1445t
  renal tubular, **966**, 966.e1t, 966.e1f
  respiratory
    acute, clinical algorithm for, 1309f
    arterial blood gases, 1448
    assessment of, 1306f
    chronic, clinical algorithm for, 1310f
    differential diagnosis of, 1193–1194
    laboratory findings in, 1445t
Acitretin, for lichen planus, 658
Aclidinium, for COPD, 261
ACM. *See* Alcoholic cardiomyopathy
Acne, 30f, **29–30, 30.e1**, 29f, 30.e1b
Acne inversa, **534–535, 535.e1**, 534f
Acne rosacea, **981**, 981.e1b, 981.e1f
Acne vulgaris, 30f, **29–30, 30.e1**, 29f, 30.e1b
Acoustic neuroma, **31, 31.e1**, 31f
ACPE. *See* Acute cardiogenic pulmonary edema
ACPSs. *See* Acute chest pain syndromes
Acquired aplastic anemia, 1198
Acquired erythrocytosis, 1350f
Acquired idiopathic sideroblastic anemia (AISA), **77, 77.e1**, 77f, 77.e1f
Acquired immunodeficiency syndrome (AIDS), **32–33, 33.e1, 33.e2, 33.e3, 33.e4, 33.e5, 33.e6, 33.e7, 33.e8, 33.e9**, 33.e4f, 33.e3f, 33.e1f, 33.e6f, 33.e5f, 33.e2f, 33.e7f
  approach to acutely ill patient with, 33.e2f
  cardiac dysfunction in, 33.e7f
  CNS infection in, 33.e5f, 33.e6f
  diarrhea in, 33.e1f
  histoplasmoma with, 542, 543
  Kaposi's sarcoma in, 633, 633f, 633.e1f
  Pneumocystis jirovecii pneumonia in, 33, 33.e4f
  respiratory complaints in, 33.e3f
Acquired red blood cell aplasia, **951.e2**
  causes of, 951.e3t
  classification of, 951.e2f, 951.e2b
  diagnostic algorithm for, 951.e3f
  drugs and chemicals in, 951.e3f
  etiology of, 1282

1595

Craniopharyngioma	I
Cryptorchidism	I
Cystic fibrosis	I
Dehydration correction, pediatric patient	III
Developmental delay	III
Down syndrome	I
Ear pain	III
Encopresis	I
Enuresis	I
Epiglottitis	I
Failure to thrive	I
Fetal alcohol syndrome	I
Fever and neutropenia, pediatric patient	III
Fifth disease (parvovirus infection)	I
Food allergies	I
Friedreich's ataxia	I
Genitalia, ambiguous	III
Glomerulonephritis, acute	I
Hand-foot-mouth disease	I
Hematuria, pediatric patient	II, III
Hemophilia	I
Histiocytosis X	I
HIV: Recommended immunization schedule for HIV-infected children	V
Hypertension, in children	II
Hypogonadism, algorithm	III
Hypogonadism, differential diagnosis	II
Hypospadias	I
Immunizations, childhood, accelerated schedule	V
Immunizations, childhood and adolescent schedule	V
Immunizations, contraindications and precautions	V
Immunizations, immunocompromised infants and children	V
Impetigo	I
Infantile hypotonia	I
Intubation, pediatric patient	III
Jaundice, neonatal, algorithm	III
Juvenile rheumatoid arthritis	I
Kawasaki disease	I
Laryngotracheobronchitis	I
Marfan's syndrome	I
Measles (rubeola)	I
Meckel diverticulum	I
Mononucleosis	I
Mumps	I
Murmur, diastolic	III
Murmur, systolic	III
Muscular dystrophy	I
Nephroblastoma	I
Nephrotic syndrome	I
Neuroblastoma	I
Osgood-Schlatter disease	I
Otitis media	I
Papulosquamous disorders, pediatric patient	III
Pediatric medication errors	I
Pediculosis	I
Pertussis	I
Pharyngitis/tonsillitis	I
Pinworms	I
Poliomyelitis	I
Precocious puberty	I
Pseudohermaphroditism, female	II
Pseudohermaphroditism, male	II
Puberty, delayed, differential diagnosis	II
Puberty, precocious	II
Reactive erythema, pediatric patient	III
Reye's syndrome	I
Rh incompatibility	I
Rheumatic fever	I
Rickets	I
Roseola	I
Rubella (German measles)	I
Scabies	I
Scarlet fever	I
Seizures, absence	I
Seizures, febrile	I
Seizures, generalized onset	I
Seizures, partial onset	I
Sexual precocity, female breast development	III
Sexual precocity, female pubic hair development	III
Sexual precocity, male	III
Shaken baby syndrome	I
Short stature	III
Spina bifida	I
Splenomegaly, children	II
Status epilepticus	I
Stevens-Johnson syndrome	I
Strabismus	I
Sturge-Weber syndrome	I
Tetralogy of Fallot	I
Thrombocytopenia, inherited disorders	II
Torticollis	I
Tourette's syndrome	I
Tuberous sclerosis	I
Turner's syndrome	I

Urethral obstruction, children	II
Vaginitis, prepubescent	I
Varicella	I
Varicocele	I
Ventricular septal defect	I
Vision loss, children	II
Wilson's disease	I

PSYCHIATRY

Abuse, child	I
Abuse, drug	I
Abuse, elder	I
Alcoholism	I
Amnestic disorders	I
Anorexia nervosa	I
Anxiety (generalized anxiety disorder)	I
Autistic spectrum disorders	I
Bipolar disorder	I
Body dysmorphic disorder	I
Borderline personality disorder	I
Bruxism	I
Bulimia nervosa	I
Conduct disorder	I
Conversion disorder	I
Delirium	I
Delirium tremens	I
Delusions of parasitosis	I
Dementia	III
Dependent personality disorder	I
Depression, major	I
Dyspareunia	I
Ejaculation, premature	I
Encopresis	I
Enuresis	I
Erectile dysfunction	I
Fatigue, algorithm	III
Factitious disorder (including Munchausen's syndrome)	I
Gender dysphoria	I
Histrionic personality disorder	I
Hypochondriasis	I
Insomnia	I
Korsakoff's psychosis	I
Memory loss symptoms, elderly patients	II
Narcissistic personality disorder	I
Neuroleptic malignant syndrome	I
Obsessive-compulsive disorder (OCD)	I
Opioid dependence	I
Oppositional defiant disorder	I
Panic disorder, with or without agoraphobia	I
Paranoid personality disorder	I
Patient with ill-defined physical complaints, algorithm	III
Pedophilia	I
Phobias	I
Posttraumatic stress disorder	I
Premenstrual syndrome	I
Schizophrenia	I
Seasonal affective disorder	I
Serotonin syndrome	I
Sexual assault	I
Sexual dysfunction	III
Sexual dysfunction, female	II
Sleep disorders	III
Social anxiety disorder	I
Somatization disorder	I
Stuttering	I
Suicide	I
Tardive dyskinesia	I
Tourette's syndrome	I
Tricyclic antidepressant overdose	I

PULMONARY DISEASE

Abscess, lung	I
Acid-base homeostasis	III
Acidosis, respiratory, acute	III
Acidosis, respiratory, chronic	III
Acute bronchitis	I
Acute respiratory distress syndrome	I
Air-space opacification on x-ray	II
Alkalosis, respiratory, treatment	III
Alpha-1-antitrypsin deficiency	I
Asbestosis	I
Aspergillosis	I
Aspiration, gastric contents	III
Aspiration, oral contents	III
Asthma	I
Atelectasis	I
Bronchial obstruction	II
Bronchiectasis	I
Bronchopleural fistula	II
Chronic obstructive pulmonary disease	I
Churg-Strauss syndrome	I
Chylothorax	II
Cor pulmonale	I

Cough, chronic, algorithm	III
Cyanosis	II
Cyanosis, algorithm	III
Cystic fibrosis	I
Deep vein thrombosis	I
Diaphragm elevation, bilateral, symmetrical	II
Diaphragm elevation, unilateral	II
Dyspnea, diagnosis	III
Empyema	I
Eosinophilic lung disease	II
Eosinophilic pneumonias	I
Goodpasture's syndrome	I
Granulomatosis with polyangiitis (Wegener granulomatosis)	I
Hemoptysis	I
Hemoptysis, algorithm	III
Hepatopulmonary syndrome	I
High-altitude sickness	I
Hypersensitivity pneumonitis	I
Idiopathic pulmonary fibrosis	I
Interstitial lung disease	I
Lung cancer, occupational causes	II
Lung neoplasms, primary	I
Mesothelioma, malignant	I
Necrotizing pneumonias	II
Neurofibromatosis	I
Opacification of hemidiaphragm on x-ray	II
Pertussis	I
Pleural effusion, malignant	III
Pleural effusions, malignancy-associated	II
Pleural space fluid	III
Pleurisy	I
Pneumonia, aspiration	I
Pneumonia, bacterial	I
Pneumonia, *Mycoplasma*	I
Pneumonia, *Pneumocystis jiroveci (carinii)*	I
Pneumonia, viral	I
Psittacosis	I
Pulmonary cysts on x-ray	II
Pulmonary edema, non-cardiogenic	II
Pulmonary embolism	I
Pulmonary hemorrhagic syndromes, diffuse	II
Pulmonary hypertension	I
Pulmonary mass, solitary, causes	II
Pulmonary mass, solitary, mimics	II
Pulmonary nodule, algorithm	III
Pulmonary nodule, solitary, differential diagnosis	II
Sarcoidosis	I
Severe acute respiratory syndrome	I
Silicosis	I
Sleep apnea, obstructive	I
Tracheobronchial narrowing on x-ray	II
Tuberculosis, pulmonary	I
Ventilation-perfusion mismatch on lung scan	II

RHEUMATOLOGY

Ankylosing spondylitis	I
Antinuclear antibody (ANA)	IV
Antiphospholipid antibody syndrome	I
Arthralgia limited to one or few joints	III
Arthritis and abdominal pain	II
Arthritis and diarrhea	II
Aseptic necrosis	I
Back pain, algorithm	III
Back pain, low, acute	II
Baker's cyst	I
Biceps tendonitis	I
Bisphosphonate-related osteonecrosis of jaw	I
Bursitis	I
Carpal tunnel syndrome	I
Cerebral vasculitis	I
Cervical disk syndromes	I
Charcot's joint	I
Cogan's syndrome	I
Compartment syndrome	I
Complex regional pain syndrome	I
Costochondritis	I
Cryoglobulinemia	I
Cubital tunnel syndrome	I
De Quervain's tenosynovitis	I
Discoid lupus	I
Dupuytren's contracture	I
Ehlers-Danlos syndrome	I
Elbow pain	II
Epicondylitis	I
Erythema nodosum	I
Felty's syndrome	I
Fibromyalgia	I
Finger lesions, inflammatory	II
Foot and ankle pain, in different age groups	II
Frozen shoulder	I
Ganglia	I
Giant cell arteritis	I
Glenohumeral dislocation	I
Gout	I